Disease	Code
Laryngitis	464.0
Lead poisoning	984
Legionnaires' disease	482.83
Leishmaniasis	085, 089
Leprosy	030
Lichen planus	697.0
Low back pain	724.2
Lyme disease	088.81
Lymphogranuloma venereum	099.1
Malabsorption	579
Malaria	084.6
Measles (rubeola)	055.9
Meconium aspiration	770.1
Melanoma	172
Meniere's disease	386.0
Meningitis	320–322
Menopause	627.2
Migraine headache	346
Mitral valve prolapse	424.0
Monilial vulvovaginitis	112.1
Multiple myeloma	203.0
Multiple sclerosis	340
Mumps	072.9
Myasthenia gravis	358.0
Mycoplasmal pneumonia	483.0
Mycosis fungoides	202.1
Nausea and vomiting	787.01
Necrotizing skin and soft tissue infections	785.4
Neoplasms of the vulva	239.5
Neutropenia	288.0
Nevi	216, 448.1
Newborn physiologic jaundice	774.6
Nongonococcal urethritis	099.4
Non-Hodgkin's lymphomas	202
Nonimmune hemolytic anemia	283.1
Normal delivery	650
Obesity	278.0
Obsessive-compulsive disorders	300.3
Onychomycosis	110.1
Optic neuritis	377.3
Osteoarthritis	715
Osteomyelitis	730
Osteoporosis	733.0
Otitis externa	380.10
Paget's disease of bone	731.0
Panic disorder	300.01
Pap smear	V72.3
Parkinsonism	332.0
Paronychia	681.0
Partial epilepsy	345.4
Patent ductus arteriosus	747.0
Pediculosis	132
Pelvic inflammatory disease	614
Peptic ulcer disease	533
Pericarditis	423.9
Peripheral arterial disease	443.9
Peripheral neuropathies	356
Pernicious anemia and other megaloblastic anemias	281
Personality disorders	301
Pheochromocytoma	227.0
Phobia	300.2
Pigmentary disorders—vitiligo	709.01
Pinworms	127.4
Pityriasis rosea	696.3
Placenta previa	641.0
Plague	020
Platelet-mediated bleeding disorders	287.1
Pleural effusion	511.9
Polycythemia vera	238.4
Polymyalgia rheumatica	725
Porphyria	277.1
Postpartum hemorrhage	666.1
Post-traumatic stress disorder	309.81
Pregnancy	V22.2
Pregnancy-induced hypertension	642
Premature beats	427.6
Premenstrual syndrome (PMS)	625.4
Prescribing oral contraceptive	V25.01
Pressure ulcers	707.0
Preterm labor	644.2
Primary glomerular disease	581–583
Primary lung abscess	513.0
Primary lung cancer	162.9
Prostate cancer	185
Prostatitis	601
Pruritus	698.9
Pruritus ani	698.0
Pruritus vulvae	198.1
Psittacosis (ornithosis)	073
Psoriasis	696.1
Pulmonary embolism	415.1
Pyelonephritis	590
Q fever	083.0
Rabies	071
Rat-bite fever	026
Relapsing fever	087
Renal calculi	592
Reye's syndrome	331.81
Rheumatic fever	390
Rheumatoid arthritis	714.0
Rib fracture	807.0
Rocky Mountain spotted fever	082.0
Rosacea	695.3
Roseola	057.8
Rubella	056
Salmonellosis	003.0
Sarcoidosis	135
Scabies	133
Schizophrenia	295
Seborrheic dermatitis	690.1
Septicemia	038
Sézary's syndrome	202.2
Shoulder dislocation	831.0
Sickle cell anemia	282.6
Silicosis	502
Sinusitis	473
Skull fracture	800, 801, 803
Sleep apnea	780.57
Sleep disorders	780.5
Snakebite	989.5
Stasis ulcers	454.0
Status epilepticus	345.3
Stomach cancer	151
Streptococcal pharyngitis	034.0
Stroke	436
Strongyloides infection	127.2
Subdural or subarachnoid hemorrhage	852
Sunburn	692.71
Syphilis	090–097
Tachycardias	785.0
Tapeworm infections	123
Telogen effluvium	704.02
Temporomandibular joint syndrome	524.6
Tendinitis	726–727
Tetanus	037
Thalassemia	282.4
Therapeutic use of blood components	V59.0
Thrombotic thrombocytopenic purpura	446.6
Thyroid cancer	193
Thyroiditis	245
Tinea capitis	110.0
Tinnitus	388.3
Toe fracture	826.0
Toxic shock syndrome	040.89
Toxoplasmosis	130
Transient cerebral ischemia	435
Trauma to the genitourinary tract	958, 959
Trichinellosis	124
Trichomonal vaginitis	131.01
Trigeminal neuralgia	350.1
Tuberculosis	011
Tularemia	021
Typhoid fever	002.0
Typhus fevers	080, 081
Ulcerative colitis	556
Urethral stricture	598
Urinary incontinence	788.3
Urticaria	708
Uterine inertia	661.0
Uterine leiomyoma	218
Varicella (chickenpox)	052
Venous thrombosis	453.8
Viral pneumonia	480.0–480.9
Viral respiratory infections	465.0
Vitamin deficiency	264–269
Vitamin K deficiency	269.0
Warts (verruca)	078.10
Wegener's granulomatosis	446.4
Whooping cough (pertussis)	033
Wrist fracture	814.0

Adapted from Jones MK, Castillo LA, Hopkins CA, Aaron WS (eds): St. Anthony's ICD-9-CM Code Book for Physician Payment, Vols 1 and 2, 5th ed. Reston, VA, St. Anthony Publishing, 1996.

LATEST APPROVED METHODS OF TREATMENT
FOR THE PRACTICING PHYSICIAN

Edited by

ROBERT E. RAKEL, M.D.

Professor, Department of Family and Community Medicine
Baylor College of Medicine, Houston, Texas

W.B. SAUNDERS COMPANY
A Division of Harcourt Brace & Company
Philadelphia London Toronto Montreal Sydney Tokyo

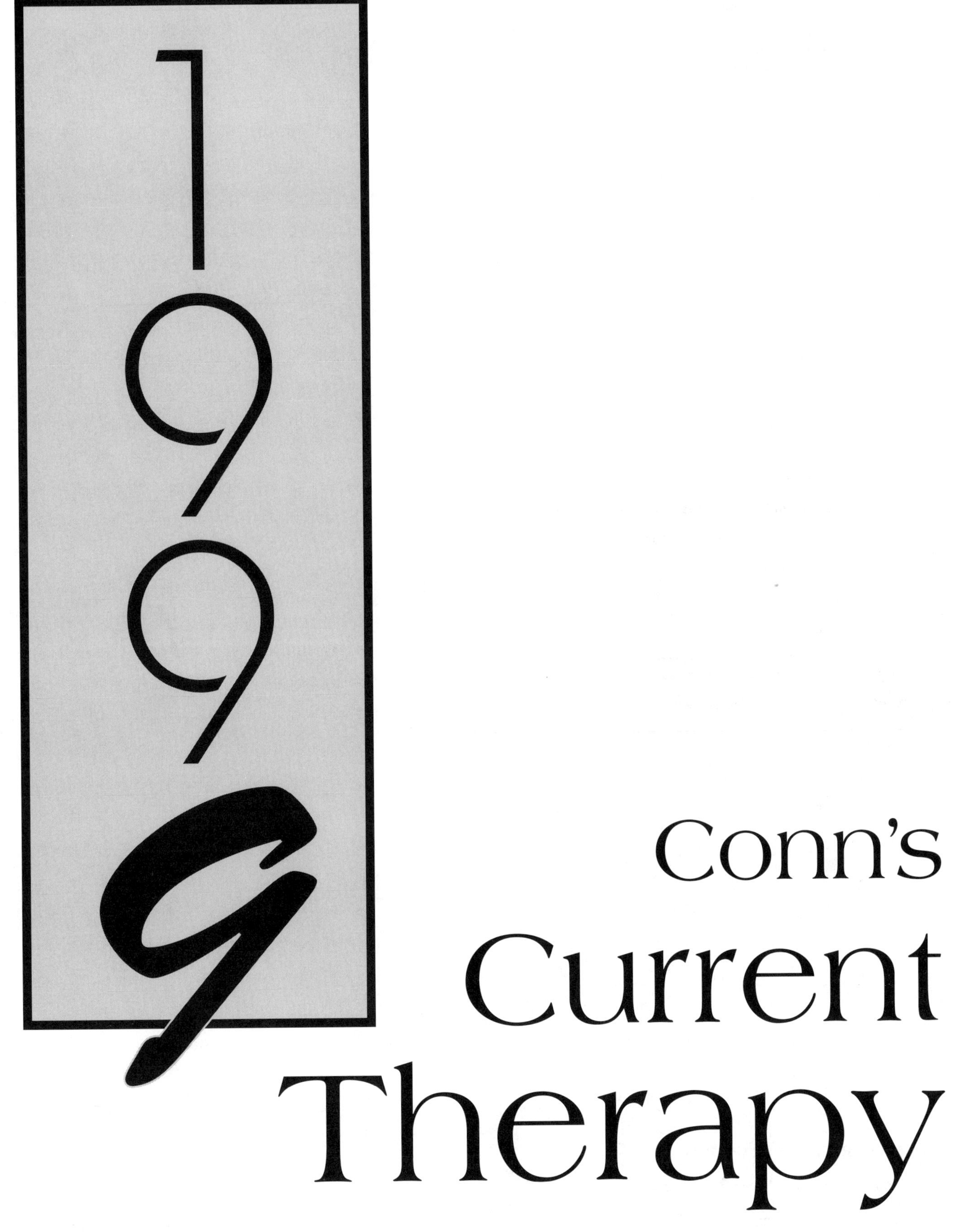

Conn's Current Therapy

W.B. SAUNDERS COMPANY
A Division of Harcourt Brace & Company

The Curtis Center
Independence Square West
Philadelphia, Pennsylvania 19106

Library of Congress Cataloging-in-Publication Data

Current therapy; latest approved methods of treatment for the practicing physician.

Editors: H. F. Conn and others

v. 28 cm. annual.

ISBN 0–7216–7224–8

1. Therapeutics. 2. Therapeutics, Surgical. 3. Medicine—Practice.
I. Conn, Howard Franklin, 1908–1982 ed.

RM101.C87 616.058 49–8328 rev*

CONN'S CURRENT THERAPY 1999 ISBN 0–7216–7224–8

Printed in the United States of America.

Last digit is the print number: 9 8 7 6 5 4 3 2 1

Contributors

WILLIAM ABRAMOVITS, M.D.
Assistant Clinical Professor, University of Texas Medical School at San Antonio, McAllen Branch, San Antonio; Baylor University Medical Center, Dallas, Texas
Papulosquamous Diseases

JAMES M. ADAMS, M.D.
Associate Professor of Pediatrics, Baylor College of Medicine; Medical Director, Special Care Nurseries, Texas Children's Hospital, Houston, Texas
Resuscitation and Stabilization of the Newborn

RAJEEV AGARWAL, M.B., B.S.
Fellow in Pediatric Nephrology, University of Florida, Gainesville, Florida; Fellow in Pediatric Nephrology, Children's Hospital, Ohio State University, Columbus, Ohio
Fluid and Electrolyte Abnormalities in Children

W. KEMPER ALSTON, M.D.
Assistant Professor, University of Vermont College of Medicine; Fletcher Allen Health Care, Burlington, Vermont
Rat-Bite Fever

NEIL M. AMPEL, M.D.
Associate Professor of Medicine, University of Arizona College of Medicine; Tucson Veterans Affairs Medical Center, Tucson, Arizona
Coccidioidomycosis

BRADLEY W. ANDERSON, M.D.
Chief Resident, Department of Urology, University of Oklahoma Health Sciences Center, Oklahoma City, Oklahoma
Benign Prostatic Hyperplasia

KENNETH C. ANDERSON, M.D.
Associate Professor of Medicine, Harvard Medical School; Department of Adult Oncology, Dana-Farber Cancer Institute, Boston, Massachusetts
Multiple Myeloma

GUNNAR B. J. ANDERSSON, M.D., PH.D.
Professor, Rush Medical College of Rush University; Chairman, Department of Orthopedic Surgery, Rush–Presbyterian–St. Luke's Medical Center, Chicago, Illinois
Low Back Pain

J. ANDRÉ, M.D.
Department of Dermatology, Saint-Pierre University Hospital, Brussels Free University, Brussels, Belgium
Diseases of the Nails

KENNETH ARNDT, M.D.
Professor of Dermatology, Harvard Medical School; Dermatologist-in-Chief, Beth Israel Deaconess Medical Center, Boston, Massachusetts
Erythema Multiforme

ASTA ASTRAUSKAS, M.D.
Pediatric Resident, Albany Medical College and Albany Medical Center, Albany, New York
Rubella and Congenital Rubella

PAUL S. AUERBACH, M.D., M.S.
Stanford University School of Medicine, Stanford; Chief Operating Officer, MedAmerica, Oakland, California
Hazardous Marine Animals

PHILIP L. BAILIN, M.D.
Professor of Medicine, Department of Dermatology, Ohio State University School of Medicine, Columbus; Chairman, Department of Dermatology, Cleveland Clinic Foundation, Cleveland, Ohio
Cancer of the Skin

CHANDRA P. BELANI, M.D.
Associate Professor of Medicine, University of Pittsburgh School of Medicine; Co-Director, Lung Cancer Program, University of Pittsburgh Cancer Institute, Pittsburgh, Pennsylvania
Primary Lung Cancer

WILLIAM R. BELL, M.D.
Professor of Medicine, Radiology and Nuclear Medicine; Clinical Director, Division of Hematology, Department of Medicine, Johns Hopkins University Hospital, Baltimore, Maryland
Disseminated Intravascular Coagulation

EDWARD J. BENZ, JR., M.D.
Physician-in-Chief, Johns Hopkins Hospital, Baltimore, Maryland
Thalassemia

ANDREW BERCHUCK, M.D.
Professor of Gynecologic Oncology, Department of Obstetrics and Gynecology, Duke University School of Medicine; Duke University Medical Center, Durham, North Carolina
Cancer of the Endometrium

PAMELA D. BERENS, M.D.
Assistant Professor, Department of Obstetrics, Gynecology, and Reproductive Services, University of Texas Health Science Center–Houston, Houston, Texas
Pelvic Inflammatory Disease

CHARLES S. BERENSON, M.D.
Associate Professor of Medicine, State University of New York at Buffalo School of Medicine and Biomedical Sciences; Veterans Affairs Medical Center–Western New York Healthcare System, Buffalo, New York
Tularemia

DANIEL N. BERGER, M.D.
Clinical Instructor, Division of Endocrinology, University of California, Los Angeles, UCLA School of Medicine, Los Angeles, California
Hypothyroidism

GREGORY KENT BERGEY, M.D.
Professor of Neurology and Physiology, University of Maryland School of Medicine; University of Maryland Medical System, Baltimore, Maryland
Tetanus

AGNETA BERGQVIST, M.D., PH.D.

Associate Professor and Senior Lecturer Karolinska Institute, Stockholm; Senior Consultant, Department of Obstetrics and Gynecology, Huddinge University Hospital, Huddinge, Sweden
Endometriosis

KARL R. BEUTNER, M.D., PH.D.

Associate Clinical Professor of Dermatology, University of California, San Francisco, School of Medicine, San Francisco, California
Warts

STEPHEN A. BEZRUCHKA, M.D., M.P.H.

Affiliate Assistant Professor, International Health Program, School of Public Health and Community Medicine, University of Washington, Seattle; Virginia Mason Medical Center, Seattle; Tacoma General Hospital, Tacoma, Washington
Altitude Illness

S. K. BHATTACHARYA, M.D.

Director, National Institute of Cholera and Enteric Diseases, Calcutta, India
Cholera

FRANK J. BIA, M.D., M.P.H.

Professor of Medicine and Laboratory Medicine, Yale University School of Medicine; Attending Physician, Infectious Disease Consult, Yale–New Haven Hospital, New Haven, Connecticut
Intestinal Parasites

HENRY R. BLACK, M.D.

Professor of Internal Medicine, Rush Medical College of Rush University; Charles J. and Margaret Roberts Professor and Chairman, Department of Preventive Medicine, Rush–Presbyterian–St. Luke's Medical Center, Chicago, Illinois
Hypertension

MICHAEL S. BLAISS, M.D.

Associate Professor of Pediatrics and Medicine, Division of Clinical Immunology, University of Tennessee, Memphis, College of Medicine; Chief of Allergy, LeBonheur Children's Medical Center, Memphis, Tennessee
Allergic Reactions to Drugs

JOEL A. BLOCK, M.D.

Associate Professor and Director, Section of Rheumatology, Rush Medical College of Rush University; Rush–Presbyterian–St. Luke's Medical Center, Chicago, Illinois
Osteoarthritis

JOHN F. BOHNSACK, M.D.

Associate Professor of Pediatrics, University of Utah School of Medicine; University of Utah Hospital and Clinics and Primary Children's Medical Center, Salt Lake City, Utah
Rheumatic Fever

GIANNI BONADONNA, M.D.

Director, Division of Medical Oncology, Istituto Nazionale per lo Studio e la Cura dei Tumori, Milan, Italy
Hodgkin's Disease: Chemotherapy

WILLIAM Z. BORER, M.D.

Professor of Pathology, Jefferson Medical College of Thomas Jefferson University; Thomas Jefferson University Hospital, Philadelphia, Pennsylvania
Reference Intervals for the Interpretation of Laboratory Tests

STEVEN BORZAK, M.D.

Assistant Professor of Medicine, Case Western Reserve University School of Medicine, Cleveland, Ohio; Director, Cardiac Intensive Care Unit, Henry Ford Heart and Vascular Institute, Detroit, Michigan
Acute Myocardial Infarction

HARISIOS BOUDOULAS, M.D., PH.D.

Professor of Medicine and Pharmacy, Division of Cardiology, Ohio State University College of Medicine; Director, Overstreet Teaching and Research Laboratory, Division of Cardiology, Ohio State University Medical Center, Columbus, Ohio
Mitral Valve Prolapse

MICHAEL C. BOYARS, M.D.

Associate Professor, Division of Pulmonary and Critical Care Medicine, University of Texas Medical Branch, Galveston, Texas
Acute Respiratory Failure

S. PHILIP BRALOW, M.D.

Clinical Professor of Medicine (retired), University of Pennsylvania School of Medicine, Philadelphia, Pennsylvania; Gastrointestinal Staff (emeritus), Sarasota Memorial Hospital, Sarasota, Florida
Diverticula of the Gastrointestinal Tract

GLENN D. BRAUNSTEIN, M.D.

Professor of Medicine, University of California, Los Angeles, UCLA School of Medicine; Chairman, Department of Medicine, Cedars-Sinai Medical Center, Los Angeles, California
Acromegaly

PETER E. BRAVERMAN, M.D.

Instructor, Department of Medicine, Johns Hopkins University School of Medicine; Johns Hopkins Hospital, Baltimore, Maryland
Disseminated Intravascular Coagulation

PAUL W. BRAZIS, M.D.

Associate Professor of Neurology, Mayo Medical School, Rochester, Minnesota; Consultant, Neurology, Mayo Clinic–Jacksonville, Jacksonville, Florida
Optic Neuritis

KENNETH H. BROOKLER, M.D.

Neurotologic Associates, P.C.; Attending Otolaryngologist, Lenox Hill Hospital; Associate Attending Surgeon, Manhattan Eye, Ear, and Throat Hospital, New York, New York
Tinnitus

RICHARD B. BROWN, M.D.

Professor of Medicine, Tufts University School of Medicine, Boston; Chief, Infectious Diseases Division, Baystate Medical Center, Springfield, Massachusetts
Streptococcal Pharyngitis

TIMOTHY P. BUKOWSKI, M.D.

Assistant Professor of Surgery and Pediatrics, University of North Carolina at Chapel Hill School of Medicine; Director of Pediatric Urology, University of North Carolina Hospital, Chapel Hill, North Carolina
Bacterial Infections of the Urinary Tract in Girls

JON M. BURCH, M.D.

Professor of Surgery, University of Colorado Health Sciences Center; Chief, General and Vascular Surgery, Denver Health and Hospitals, Denver, Colorado
Acute Pancreatitis

KIM J. BURCHIEL, M.D.

Chairman, Department of Neurological Surgery, Oregon Health Sciences University School of Medicine, Portland, Oregon
Trigeminal Neuralgia

JEFFREY BURGESS, D.D.S., M.S.D.

Clinical Assistant Professor, University of Washington, Seattle, Washington
Temporomandibular Disorders and Craniofacial Pain

FERNANDO CABANILLAS, M.D.
Ashbel Smith Professor of Medicine, Department of Hematology, University of Texas M. D. Anderson Cancer Center, Houston, Texas
Non-Hodgkin's Lymphoma

ANDRÉ CABIÉ, M.D.
Chef de Clinique, Université Paris VII, Service de Maladies Infectieuses et Tropicales, Hôpital Bichat Claude Bernard, Paris, France
Trichinellosis

MARLENE S. CALDERON, M.D.
Resident in Plastic Surgery, University of Michigan Medical Center, Ann Arbor, Michigan
Keloids

JEFFREY P. CALLEN, M.D.
Professor of Medicine and Chief, Division of Dermatology, University of Louisville School of Medicine, Louisville, Kentucky
Cutaneous Vasculitis

RICHARD P. CAMBRIA, M.D.
Associate Professor of Surgery, Harvard Medical School; Visiting Surgeon, Massachusetts General Hospital, Boston, Massachusetts
Acquired Diseases of the Aorta

DAVID B. CAMPBELL, M.D.
Professor of Surgery, Section of Cardiothoracic Surgery, Penn State–Geisinger Health System, Penn State–Milton S. Hershey Medical Center, Hershey, Pennsylvania
Atelectasis

ROBERT CANCRO, M.D., MED.D.SC.
Professor and Chairman, Department of Psychiatry, New York University School of Medicine; Director, Tisch Hospital, and Attending Physician, Bellevue Hospital Center, New York, New York
Schizophrenic Disorders

LOUIS R. CAPLAN, M.D.
Professor of Neurology, Harvard Medical School; Senior Neurologist, Beth Israel Deaconess Medical Center, Boston, Massachusetts
Intracerebral Hemorrhage

THOMAS R. CARACCIO, PHARM.D.
Assistant Professor of Emergency Medicine, State University of New York at Stony Brook Health Sciences Center School of Medicine, Stony Brook; Assistant Professor of Pharmacology/Toxicology, New York College of Osteopathic Medicine, Old Westbury; Assistant Professor of Clinical Pharmacy, St. John's University College of Pharmacy, Jamaica; Clinical Manager, Long Island Regional Poison Control Center, Winthrop University Hospital, Mineola, New York
Acute Poisonings

PAUL C. CARPENTER, M.D.
Assistant Professor, Mayo Medical School; Consulting Staff, St. Marys Hospital of Rochester and Rochester Methodist Hospital, Rochester, Minnesota
Adrenocortical Insufficiency

CULLEY C. CARSON III, M.D.
Professor and Chief of Urology, University of North Carolina at Chapel Hill School of Medicine, Chapel Hill, North Carolina
Erectile Dysfunction

MELISSA K. CAVAGHAN, M.D.
Instructor of Medicine, Section of Endocrinology, Department of Medicine, University of Chicago Pritzker School of Medicine, Chicago, Illinois
Hyperprolactinemia

JAMES J. CERDA, M.D.
Professor of Medicine and Chief, Nutrition Support, University of Florida College of Medicine; Attending Physician, Shands Hospital at the University of Florida, and Consultant, Veterans Affairs Medical Center, Gainesville, Florida
Giardiasis

MAURICE A. CERULLI, M.D.
Associate Professor of Clinical Medicine, New York University School of Medicine, New York; Chief, Division of Gastroenterology, Brooklyn Hospital Center–Downtown Campus, Brooklyn, New York
Gaseousness and Indigestion

JOSEPH C. CHAN, M.D.
Associate Professor of Medicine, Division of Infectious Diseases, University of Miami School of Medicine, Miami; Medical Director, Special Immunology Unit, Mt. Sinai Medical Center, Miami Beach; Attending Staff in Infectious Disease, Jackson Memorial Hospital, Miami, Florida
Primary Lung Abscess

ISRAEL CHANARIN, M.D.
Head, Section of Hematology (retired), Medical Research Council Clinical Research Centre, Northwick Park Hospital, Harrow, Middlesex, England
Pernicious Anemia and Other Megaloblastic Anemias

JOSEPH A. CHAZAN, M.D.
Clinical Professor of Medicine, Brown University School of Medicine; Director, Artificial Kidney Centers of Rhode Island, and Associate, Division of Renal Diseases, Rhode Island Hospital, Providence, Rhode Island
Chronic Renal Failure

LISA D. CHEW, M.D.
Acting Instructor, Department of Obstetrics and Gynecology, University of Washington School of Medicine; Attending Physician, Harborview Medical Center, Seattle, Washington
Bacterial Infections of the Urinary Tract in Women

LOLITA E. CHIU, M.D.
Fellow, Infectious Diseases, Brown University School of Medicine, Providence, Rhode Island
Bacteremia and Septicemia

INDER J. CHOPRA, M.D.
Professor of Medicine, University of California, Los Angeles, UCLA School of Medicine; Staff Physician, UCLA Center for Health Sciences, Los Angeles, California
Hypothyroidism

GEORGE P. CHROUSOS, M.D.
Chief, Section on Pediatric Endocrinology, National Institute for Child Health and Human Development, National Institute of Health, Bethesda, Maryland
Cushing's Syndrome

JONATHAN E. CLAIN, M.B., CH.B.
Associate Professor of Medicine and Consultant in Gastroenterology, Mayo Medical School, Mayo Graduate School, and Mayo Clinic; Consulting and Endoscopy, St. Mary's Hospital of Rochester and Rochester Methodist Hospital, Rochester, Minnesota
Chronic Pancreatitis

ARTHUR C. COFFEY, M.D.
Chief Resident, Thoracic and Cardiovascular Surgery, University of Virginia Health Science Center, Charlottesville, Virginia
Pleural Effusion and Empyema Thoracis

PETER F. COHN, M.D.

Professor of Medicine and Chief of Cardiology, State University of New York at Stony Brook Health Sciences Center School of Medicine, Stony Brook, New York
Angina Pectoris

JOHN CRAIG COLLINS, M.D.

Assistant Clinical Professor of Surgery, University of California, Irvine, College of Medicine, Irvine; Staff Surgeon, Kaiser Foundation Hospital, Los Angeles; Consultant Surgeon, Veterans Affairs Medical Center, Long Beach, California
Bleeding Esophageal Varices

BLAISE L. CONGENI, M.D.

Professor of Pediatrics, Professor of Microbiology/Immunology, Northeastern Ohio Universities College of Medicine, Rootstown; Director, Pediatric Infectious Diseases, Children's Hospital Medical Center of Akron, Akron, Ohio
Mumps

W. G. E. COOKSLEY, M.B., B.S., M.D.

Professor of Biochemistry, University of Queensland; Director, Clinical Research Centre, Royal Brisbane Hospital, Brisbane, Queensland, Australia
Acute and Chronic Viral Hepatitis

JOSE A. CORTES, M.D.

Resident, Department of Pediatrics, University of South Alabama, Mobile, Alabama
Pediatric Head Injury

RAYMOND A. COSTABILE, M.D.

Associate Professor of Surgery, Uniformed Services University of the Health Sciences, Bethesda, Maryland; Walter Reed Army Medical Center, Washington, D.C.
Malignant Tumors of the Urogenital Tract

SUSAN M. COX, M.D.

Associate Professor, Department of Maternal-Fetal Medicine, University of Texas Southwestern Medical Center at Dallas; Parkland Memorial Hospital, Dallas, Texas
Pyelonephritis

JOHN THORNE CRISSEY, M.D.

Clinical Professor of Medicine, Department of Dermatology, University of Southern California School of Medicine, Los Angeles; Attending Dermatologist, Los Angeles County–USC Medical Center, Los Angeles County, California
Fungal Diseases of the Skin

DANIEL J. CULKIN, M.D.

Professor and Chairman, Department of Urology, University of Oklahoma Health Sciences Center; Chief, Urology Section, The University Hospitals; Attending Physician, Presbyterian Hospital, Oklahoma City, Oklahoma
Benign Prostatic Hyperplasia

BURKE A. CUNHA, M.D.

Professor of Medicine, State University of New York at Stony Brook Health Sciences Center School of Medicine, Stony Brook; Chief, Infectious Disease Division, Winthrop University Hospital, Mineola, New York
Bacterial Pneumonias

GEORGE E. DAILEY III, M.D.

Clinical Professor of Medicine, University of California, San Diego, School of Medicine; Chairman, Department of Academic Affairs, and Head, Division of Diabetes and Endocrinology, Scripps Memorial Hospital–La Jolla, La Jolla, California
Diabetes Mellitus in Adults

MANISH N. DAMANI, M.D.

Chief Resident in Urology, University of North Carolina at Chapel Hill School of Medicine, Chapel Hill, North Carolina
Erectile Dysfunction

DENIS DANEMAN, M.B., B.CH.

Professor of Pediatrics, University of Toronto Faculty of Medicine; Chief, Division of Endocrinology, Hospital for Sick Children, Toronto, Ontario, Canada
Diabetes Mellitus in Childhood and Adolescence

DANIEL F. DANZL, M.D.

Professor and Chair, Department of Emergency Medicine, University of Louisville School of Medicine, Louisville, Kentucky
Disturbances Due to Cold

TONI DARVILLE, M.D.

Assistant Professor of Pediatrics, University of Arkansas College of Medicine; Arkansas Children's Hospital, Little Rock, Arkansas
Osteomyelitis

BRUCE L. DAVIDSON, M.D., M.P.H.

Clinical Associate Professor of Medicine, Division of Pulmonary and Critical Care Medicine, Allegheny University of the Health Sciences, MCP–Hahnemann School of Medicine; Attending Physician, Graduate Hospital and Hahnemann University Hospital, Philadelphia, Pennsylvania
Pulmonary Embolism

GEORGE S. DEEPE, JR., M.D.

Professor of Medicine, University of Cincinnati College of Medicine; Attending Physician, University Hospital, and Staff Physician, Veterans Affairs Medical Center, Cincinnati, Ohio
Histoplasmosis

PATRICIA DEMARAIS, M.D.

Associate Professor of Medicine, Rush Medical College of Rush University, Chicago; Oak Forest Hospital, Oak Forest; Cook County Hospital, Chicago, Illinois
Infectious Mononucleosis

PETER K. DEMPSEY, M.D.

Lahey Hitchcock Medical Center, Burlington, Massachusetts
Brain Tumors

MARGO A. DENKE, M.D.

Associate Professor of Medicine, University of Texas Southwestern Medical Center at Dallas; Director, Endocrine Clinic, Veterans Affairs North Texas Health Care System, Dallas, Texas
Hyperlipoproteinemias

SUSAN E. DENSON, M.D.

Professor of Pediatrics, Division of Neonatal-Perinatal Medicine, University of Texas Health Science Center at Houston; Medical Director, Neonatal Special Care Unit, Hermann Children's Hospital; Staff Physician, Lyndon Baines Johnson General Hospital, Houston, Texas
Care of the High-Risk Neonate

ROBERT L. DERESIEWICZ, M.D.

Assistant Professor of Medicine, Harvard Medical School; Associate Physician, Infectious Disease Division, Brigham and Women's Hospital, Boston, Massachusetts
Toxic Shock Syndrome

LUIS A. DIAZ, M.D.

Professor and Chairman, Department of Dermatology, Medical College of Wisconsin; Senior Attending Physician, Froedtert Memorial Lutheran Hospital, and Staff Physician, Veterans Affairs Medical Center, Milwaukee, Wisconsin
Bullous Diseases

EUGENE P. DIMAGNO, M.D.
Professor of Medicine, Mayo Medical School; Consultant, Division of Gastroenterology, Mayo Clinic, and Director, Gastroenterology Research Unit, Mayo Clinic and Mayo Foundation, Rochester, Minnesota
Chronic Pancreatitis

DGANIT DINOUR, M.D.
Attending Physician, Department of Nephrology, The Chaim Sheba Medical Center, Tel-Aviv University, Tel-Hashomer, Israel
Acute Renal Failure

ANANIAS C. DIOKNO, M.D.
Chief, Department of Urology, William Beaumont Hospital, Royal Oak, Michigan
Urinary Incontinence

GERALD R. DONOWITZ, M.D.
Associate Chair for Education, University of Virginia School of Medicine, Charlottesville, Virginia
Viral and Mycoplasmal Pneumonias

RACHELLE SMITH DOODY, M.D., PH.D.
Associate Professor of Neurology, Baylor College of Medicine; Methodist Hospital, Houston, Texas
Alzheimer's Disease

HAROLD O. DOUGLASS, JR., M.D.
Professor of Surgery, State University of New York at Buffalo; Vice Chair, Surgical Oncology, and Chief, Upper Gastrointestinal Oncology, Roswell Park Cancer Institute, Buffalo, New York
Tumors of the Stomach

ZOE DIANA DRAELOS, M.D.
Clinical Associate Professor, Department of Dermatology, Wake Forest University School of Medicine, Winston-Salem, North Carolina
Acne Vulgaris and Rosacea

NANCY E. DUNLAP, M.D., PH.D.
Professor of Medicine, Division of Pulmonary and Critical Care Medicine, University of Alabama at Birmingham School of Medicine; University of Alabama Hospital, Birmingham, Alabama
Tuberculosis and Other Mycobacterial Diseases

ERVIN Y. EAKER, JR., M.D.
Associate Professor, University of Kansas School of Medicine; Director of Gastrointestinal Motility, Kansas University Medical Center; Veterans Affairs Medical Center, Kansas City, Kansas
Irritable Bowel Syndrome

MARTIN J. EDELMAN, M.D.
Assistant Professor of Medicine, University of California, Davis, School of Medicine, Sacramento; Veterans Affairs Northern California Health Care System, Martinez, California
Nausea and Vomiting

ROBERT EDELMAN, M.D.
Professor of Medicine, Center for Vaccine Development, University of Maryland School of Medicine; University of Maryland Hospital and Baltimore Veterans Affairs Medical Center, Baltimore, Maryland
Typhoid Fever

LIBBY EDWARDS, M.D.
Associate Clinical Professor, Department of Dermatology, Bowman Gray School of Medicine of Wake Forest University, Winston-Salem; Chief of Dermatology, Carolinas Medical Center, Charlotte, North Carolina
Condylomata Acuminata

DAVID A. EHRMANN, M.D.
Associate Professor, Section of Endocrinology, University of Chicago Pritzker School of Medicine; University of Chicago Hospitals, Chicago, Illinois
Hyperprolactinemia

KENNETH A. ELLENBOGEN, M.D.
Professor of Medicine, Virginia Commonwealth University/Medical College of Virginia School of Medicine; Director, Clinical and Academic Cardiac Electrophysiology, Medical College of Virginia Hospitals and Hunter Holmes McGuire Veterans Affairs Medical Center, Richmond, Virginia
Atrial Fibrillation

DIRK M. ELSTON, M.D.
Chief, Department of Dermatology, Wilford Hall Air Force Medical Center, San Antonio, Texas
Hair Disorders

ADEL G. FAM, M.D.
Professor of Medicine and Head, Division of Rheumatology, University of Toronto Faculty of Medicine; Head, Division of Rheumatology, Sunnybrook Health Science Centre, Toronto, Ontario, Canada
Hyperuricemia and Gout

SEBASTIAN FARO, M.D., PH.D.
John M. Simpson Professor and Chairman, Department of Obstetrics and Gynecology, Rush Medical College of Rush University; Senior Attending Physician, Rush–Presbyterian–St. Luke's Medical Center, Chicago, Illinois
Chlamydia trachomatis *Infection; Vulvovaginitis*

R. WESLEY FARR, M.D.
Associate Professor of Medicine, Section of Infectious Diseases, West Virginia University School of Medicine; Director, International Health Program, Robert C. Byrd Health Sciences Center of West Virginia University, Morgantown, West Virginia
Relapsing Fever

PIERRE B. FAYAD, M.D.
Associate Professor of Neurology and Director, Yale Vascular Neurology Program, Yale University School of Medicine; Co-Director, Yale Cerebrovascular Center, Yale–New Haven Hospital, New Haven, Connecticut
Ischemic Cerebrovascular Disease

LEON A. FELDMAN, M.D.
Cardiology Fellow, Oregon Health Sciences University School of Medicine, Portland, Oregon
Infective Endocarditis

YEHUDI M. FELMAN, M.D.
Clinical Professor of Dermatology, State University of New York Health Sciences Center at Brooklyn College of Medicine; Attending Dermatologist, University Hospital of Brooklyn; Consultant Dermatologist, Maimonides Medical Center, Brooklyn, New York
Granuloma Inguinale (Donovanosis); Lymphogranuloma Venereum

TERRY D. FIFE, M.D.
Assistant Professor of Neurology, University of Arizona; Director, Balance Center, Barron Neurological Institute, Phoenix; St. Joseph's Hospital and Medical Center, Phoenix; University Medical Center, Tucson, Arizona
Episodic Vertigo

STEPHAN D. FIHN, M.D., M.P.H.
Professor of Medicine and of Health Service and Head, Division of General Internal Medicine, University of Washington School of Medicine, Seattle, Washington
Bacterial Infections of the Urinary Tract in Women

DOUGLAS P. FINE, M.D.

Professor and Chairman, Department of Medicine, University of Oklahoma Health Sciences Center; Staff Physician and Chairman of Medicine, University Hospital, Veterans Affairs Medical Center, Oklahoma City, Oklahoma
Rocky Mountain Spotted Fever

CATHERINE M. FLAITZ, D.D.S., M.S.

Associate Professor, Division of Oral and Maxillofacial Pathology, University of Texas Health Science Center at Houston, Dental Branch; Texas Children's Hospital, Houston, Texas
Diseases of the Mouth

JOHN A. FLEETHAM, M.D.

Professor of Medicine, University of British Columbia Faculty of Medicine; Head, Respiratory Division, Vancouver Hospital, Vancouver, British Columbia, Canada
Obstructive Sleep Apnea

SHARON A. FOLEY, M.D.

Assistant Professor, Medical College of Wisconsin; Fruedtert Hospital, Milwaukee, Wisconsin
Bullous Diseases

ROGER S. FOSTER, JR., M.D.

Wadley Glenn Professor of Surgery, Emory University School of Medicine; Chief of Surgical Services, Crawford Long Hospital of Emory University, Atlanta, Georgia
Diseases of the Breast

MITCHELL H. FRIEDLAENDER, M.D.

Adjunct Professor, Scripps Research Institute; Director, Cornea and Refractive Surgery, Scripps Clinic, La Jolla, California
Conjunctivitis

LAWRENCE S. FRIEDMAN, M.D.

Associate Professor of Medicine, Harvard Medical School; Physician, Gastrointestinal Unit, and Chief, Walter Bauer Firm, Massachusetts General Hospital, Boston, Massachusetts
Cirrhosis

RICK A. FRIEDMAN, M.D., PH.D.

Associate, House Ear Clinic, Inc.; St. Vincent Medical Center and Chapman Medical Center, Los Angeles, California
Otitis Media

J. C. GALLAGHER, M.D.

Professor of Medicine, Creighton University School of Medicine; St. Joseph's Hospital, Omaha, Nebraska
Osteoporosis

DAVID R. GANDARA, M.D.

Professor of Medicine, University of California, Davis, School of Medicine, Sacramento; Veterans Affairs Northern California Health Care System, Martinez, California
Nausea and Vomiting

WARREN L. GARNER, M.D.

Associate Professor of Surgery, University of Michigan Medical School, Ann Arbor, Michigan
Keloids

JOHN W. GEORGITIS, M.D.

Professor of Pediatrics, Section of Allergy, Immunology, and Respiratory Medicine, Bowman Gray School of Medicine of Wake Forest University; Wake Forest University Baptist Medical Center, Winston-Salem, North Carolina
Allergic Rhinitis Caused by Inhalant Factors

ARTHUR M. GERSHKOFF, M.D.

Associate Professor, Temple University School of Medicine; Clinical Director, Stroke and Neurological Diseases, MossRehab Hospital of Albert Einstein Health Care Network, Philadelphia, Pennsylvania
Rehabilitation of the Stroke Patient

DAVID M. GILLIGAN, M.D.

Assistant Professor of Medicine, Medical College of Virginia/Virginia Commonwealth University; Hunter Holmes McGuire Veterans Affairs Medical Center, Richmond, Virginia
Atrial Fibrillation

BARRY S. GOLD, M.D.

Assistant Professor of Medicine, Johns Hopkins University School of Medicine and University of Maryland School of Medicine; Johns Hopkins Hospital and Sinai Hospital of Baltimore, Baltimore, Maryland
Snake Venom Poisoning

LEONARD H. GOLDBERG, M.D.

Methodist Hospital and Ben Taub General Hospital, Houston, Texas
Premalignant Lesions

ADRIAN J. GOLDSZMIDT, M.D.

Director, Stroke Center, Sinai Hospital of Baltimore, Baltimore, Maryland
Intracerebral Hemorrhage

ANDREW E. GOOD, M.D.

Assistant Professor of Obstetrics and Gynecology, Mayo Medical School, Rochester, Minnesota
Dysfunctional Uterine Bleeding

JACK M. GORMAN, M.D.

Professor of Psychiatry, Columbia University College of Physicians and Surgeons; New York State Psychiatric Institute, New York, New York
Panic Disorder

LUIGI GRADONI, PH.D.

Senior Researcher and Director, Section of Protozoology, Parasitology Department, Istituto Superiore di Sanitá, Rome, Italy
Leishmaniasis

JENNIFER RUBIN GRANDIS, M.D.

Assistant Professor of Otolaryngology, University of Pittsburgh School of Medicine; Staff Surgeon, University of Pittsburgh Medical Center, Pittsburgh, Pennsylvania
Otitis Externa

MARK A. GRANNER, M.D.

Assistant Professor of Clinical Neurology, University of Iowa College of Medicine; Director, Epilepsy Monitoring Unit, University of Iowa Hospitals and Clinics, Iowa City, Iowa
Epilepsy in Adolescents and Adults

RICHARD N. GREENBERG, M.D.

Professor of Medicine, Division of Infectious Diseases, University of Kentucky School of Medicine; University of Kentucky Medical Center, Lexington, Kentucky
Food-Borne Illness

JOSEPH GREENSHER, M.D.

Professor of Pediatrics, State University of New York at Stony Brook, Health Sciences Center School of Medicine, Stony Brook; Medical Director, Associate Director, and Chairman, Department of Pediatrics, Winthrop University Hospital; Associate Director, Long Island Regional Poison Control Center, Winthrop University Hospital, Mineola, New York
Acute Poisonings

NICHOLAS J. GROSS, M.D., PH.D.
Professor, Departments of Medicine and Molecular Biochemistry, Loyola University of Chicago Stritch School of Medicine, Chicago; Edward Hines, Jr., Veterans Affairs Medical Center, Hines, Illinois
Chronic Obstructive Pulmonary Disease

EVA C. GUINAN, M.D.
Associate Professor of Pediatrics, Harvard Medical School; Attending Physician, Dana-Farber Cancer Institute and Children's Hospital, Boston, Massachusetts
Neutropenia

MADHAVI GUNDA, M.D.
Cardiology Fellow, Henry Ford Heart and Vascular Institute, Detroit, Michigan
Acute Myocardial Infarction

FADI F. HADDAD, M.D.
Clinical Research Fellow, H. Lee Moffitt Cancer Center, University of South Florida, Tampa, Florida
Malignant Melanoma

LISA A. HAGLUND, M.D.
Assistant Professor of Clinical Medicine, University of Cincinnati College of Medicine; University of Cincinnati Medical Center and Good Samaritan Hospital, Cincinnati, Ohio
Histoplasmosis

MOHAMED H. HAMDAN, M.D.
Assistant Professor of Medicine, Division of Cardiology, University of Texas Southwestern Medical Center at Dallas; Director, Electrophysiology Laboratory, VA Medical Center, Dallas, Texas
Premature Beats

SARAH E. HAMPL, M.D.
Assistant Professor of Pediatrics, University of Missouri–Kansas City School of Medicine; Pediatrician in General Pediatrics, Children's Mercy Hospital, Kansas City, Missouri
Pertussis

PHILIP HANNO, M.D.
Professor and Chairman, Department of Urology, Temple University Hospital, Philadelphia, Pennsylvania
Nongonococcal Urethritis

BRYAN D. HARRIS, M.D.
Senior Resident, Department of Dermatology, Cleveland Clinic Foundation, Cleveland, Ohio
Bacterial Diseases of the Skin

LAWRENCE E. HART, MB.B.CH., M.SC.
Associate Professor, Department of Medicine, McMaster University Faculty of Health Sciences; Chief of Rheumatology and Director, Rheumatic Disease Unit, Chedoke Site, Hamilton Health Sciences Corporation, Hamilton, Ontario, Canada
Disturbances Due to Heat

JOSEPH I. HARWELL, M.D.
Research Fellow in Medicine, Tufts University School of Medicine, Boston; Fellow in Infectious Diseases, Baystate Medical Center, Springfield, Massachusetts
Streptococcal Pharyngitis

RODRIGO HASBUN, M.D.
Postdoctoral Fellow in Infectious Diseases, Yale University School of Medicine, New Haven, Connecticut
Intestinal Parasites

IAN D. HAY, M.B., PH.D.
Professor of Medicine, Mayo Medical School; Consultant in Endocrinology and Internal Medicine, Mayo Clinic, Rochester, Minnesota
Thyroiditis

D. A. HEATH, M.B., CH.B.
Reader in Medicine, University of Birmingham; Honorary Consultant Physician, Selly Oak Hospital, Birmingham, England
Hyperparathyroidism and Hypoparathyroidism

VIVIEN HERMAN-BONERT, M.D.
Associate Professor of Medicine, University of California, Los Angeles, UCLA School of Medicine; Staff Endocrinologist, Cedars-Sinai Medical Center, Los Angeles, California
Acromegaly

DAVID N. HERNDON, M.D.
Jesse H. Jones Distinguished Chair in Burn Surgery and Professor of Surgery, University of Texas Medical Branch; Chief of Staff, Shriners Hospital for Crippled Children, Galveston Burn Unit, Galveston, Texas
Burns

HARRY R. HILL, M.D.
Professor of Pathology, Pediatrics, and Medicine, University of Utah School of Medicine; Attending Staff, University of Utah Hospital and Clinics, Primary Children's Medical Center, and Veterans Affairs Medical Center, Salt Lake City, Utah
Rheumatic Fever

CHRISTOPHER D. HILLYER, M.D.
Associate Professor, Department of Pathology and Laboratory Medicine, Emory University School of Medicine; Director, Transfusion Medicine Program, Emory University Hospital; Associate Professor and Deputy Director, Winship Cancer Center, Atlanta, Georgia
Therapeutic Use of Blood Components

JAY B. HOLLANDER, M.D.
Director of Urologic Education, William Beaumont Hospital, Royal Oak, Michigan
Urinary Incontinence

GREGORY L. HOLMES, M.D.
Professor of Neurology, Harvard Medical School; Children's Hospital, Boston, Massachusetts
Epilepsy in Infants and Children

G. RICHARD HOLT, M.D.
Head, Division of Facial and Reconstructive Surgery, Department of Otolaryngology–Head and Neck Surgery, Johns Hopkins Medical Institutions, Baltimore, Maryland
Hoarseness and Laryngitis

DOUGLAS B. HOOD, M.D.
Assistant Professor of Surgery, University of Southern California School of Medicine; USC University Hospital and Los Angeles County/USC Medical Center, Los Angeles, California
Peripheral Arterial Disease

W. KEITH HOOTS, M.D.
Pediatrician and Professor of Pediatrics, University of Texas Medical School at Houston; Professor of Pediatrics, University of Texas M. D. Anderson Cancer Center; Attending Physician, Hermann Children's Hospital, Houston, Texas
Hemophilia and Related Conditions

IRA R. HOROWITZ, M.D.
Assistant Professor and Director, Gynecologic Oncology, Emory University School of Medicine, Atlanta, Georgia
Neoplasms of the Vulva

DENISE L. HOWRIE, Pharm.D.
Associate Professor of Pharmacy and Pediatrics, Schools of Pharmacy and Medicine, University of Pittsburgh; Pharmacy Clinician, Department of Pharmacy, Children's Hospital of Pittsburgh, Pittsburgh, Pennsylvania
Viral Respiratory Infections

NANCY HURST, M.S.N., R.N.
Clinical Instructor, Baylor College of Medicine; Director, Lactation Program and Milk Bank, Texas Children's Hospital, Houston, Texas
Normal Infant Feeding

MARY ANNE JACKSON, M.D.
Professor of Pediatrics, University of Missouri–Kansas City School of Medicine; Pediatrician in Infectious Diseases, Children's Mercy Hospital, Kansas City, Missouri
Pertussis

DANNY O. JACOBS, M.D., M.P.H.
Associate Professor of Surgery, Harvard Medical School; Director, Metabolic Support Service, Department of Surgery, and Director, Laboratory for Surgical Metabolism and Nutrition, Brigham and Women's Hospital, Boston, Massachusetts
Parenteral Nutrition in Adults

RICHARD F. JACOBS, M.D.
Horace C. Cabe Professor of Pediatrics, University of Arkansas for Medical Sciences; Chief, Pediatric Infectious Diseases, Arkansas Children's Hospital, Little Rock, Arkansas
Osteomyelitis

THOMAS P. JACOBS, M.D.
Professor of Clinical Medicine, Columbia University College of Physicians and Surgeons; Attending Physician, Presbyterian Hospital, New York, New York
Hypopituitarism

LESLIE K. JACOBSEN, M.D.
Assistant Professor, Yale University School of Medicine, New Haven, Connecticut; Senior Staff Fellow, National Institute of Mental Health, Bethesda, Maryland
Drug Abuse

THOMAS W. JAMIESON, M.D.
Associate Professor of Clinical Medicine, Uniformed Services University of the Health Sciences; National Naval Medical Center, Bethesda, Maryland
Bursitis, Tendinitis, Myofascial Pain, and Fibromyalgia

JOSEPH JANKOVIC, M.D.
Professor of Neurology and Director, Parkinson's Disease Center and Movement Disorders Clinic, Baylor College of Medicine; Methodist Hospital, Houston, Texas
Gilles de la Tourette Syndrome

MICHAEL T. JELINEK, M.D.
McAllen Medical Center and Rio Grande Regional Hospital, McAllen, Texas
Rabies

GORDON L. JENSEN, M.D., Ph.D.
Associate Professor of Medicine, Vanderbilt University School of Medicine; Vanderbilt University Medical Center, Nashville, Tennessee
Obesity

BAOHONG JI, M.D.
Professor, Bactériologie et Hygiène, Faculté de Médecine Pitié-Salpêtrière, Paris, France
Leprosy (Hansen's Disease)

DAVID C. JIMERSON, M.D.
Associate Professor of Psychiatry, Harvard Medical School; Director of Research, Department of Psychiatry, Beth Israel Deaconess Medical Center, Boston, Massachusetts
Bulimia Nervosa

DARLENE S. JOHNSON, M.D.
Resident, Harvard Medical School; Massachusetts General Hospital and Beth Israel Deaconess Medical Center, Boston, Massachusetts
Erythema Multiforme

JAMES F. JONES, M.D.
Professor of Pediatrics, University of Colorado School of Medicine; National Jewish Medical and Research Center and Children's Hospital, Denver, Colorado
Chronic Fatigue Syndrome

CHRISTINE W. JORDAN, M.D.
Attending Physician, Lakeside Hospital and East Jefferson General Hospital, Metairie, Louisiana
Dysmenorrhea

STEPHEN M. JURD, M.B., B.S.
Clinical Senior Lecturer, University of Sydney, Sydney; Head, Department of Drug and Alcohol Services, Royal North Shore Hospital, St. Leonards, New South Wales, Australia
Alcoholism

MARILYN A. KACICA, M.D.
Associate Professor of Pediatrics, Albany Medical College; Attending Physician, Albany Medical Center Hospital, Albany, New York
Rubella and Congenital Rubella

MICHAEL A. KALINER, M.D.
Medical Director, Institute for Asthma and Allergy, Washington Hospital Center; Clinical Professor of Medicine, George Washington University Medical Center, Washington, D.C.
Anaphylaxis and Serum Sickness

JULIE P. KATKIN, M.D.
Assistant Professor of Pediatrics, Division of Pediatric Pulmonary Medicine, Baylor College of Medicine, Houston, Texas
Cystic Fibrosis

RALPH E. KAUFFMAN, M.D.
Professor of Pediatrics and Pharmacology and Marion Merrell Dow/Missouri Chair in Medical Research, University of Missouri–Kansas City School of Medicine; Director of Medical Research, Children's Mercy Hospital, Kansas City, Missouri
Fever

TARA L. KAUFMANN, B.S.
Medical Student, University Medical Center, Stony Brook, New York
Urticaria and Angioedema

ANDREW M. KAUNITZ, M.D.
Professor and Assistant Chairman, Department of Obstetrics and Gynecology, University of Florida Health Science Center/Jacksonville; Director, Division of Family Planning, University Medical Center, Jacksonville, Florida
Dysmenorrhea

DAVID W. KENNEDY, M.D.
Professor and Chairman, Department of Otorhinolaryngology, University of Pennsylvania School of Medicine; Hospital of the University of Pennsylvania, Philadelphia, Pennsylvania
Sinusitis

AMIR KHAN, M.D.

Fellow in Pediatrics, University of Texas Health Science Center at Houston; Hermann Hospital, Houston, Texas
Care of the High-Risk Neonate

MUHAMMAD ASIM KHAN, M.D.

Professor of Medicine, Case Western Reserve University School of Medicine; Department of Medicine, Division of Rheumatology, MetroHealth Medical Center, Cleveland, Ohio
Ankylosing Spondylitis

LOUISE S. KIESSLING, M.D.

Professor, Pediatrics and Family Medicine, Brown University School of Medicine, Providence; Memorial Hospital of Rhode Island, Pawtucket; Rhode Island Hospital, Providence, Rhode Island
Attention Deficit Hyperactivity Disorder (ADHD)

MICHAEL E. KIMERLING, M.D., M.P.H.

Assistant Professor of Medicine, University of Alabama at Birmingham School of Medicine and School of Public Health; Division of General Internal Medicine and Epidemiology, Cooper Green Hospital and University of Alabama Hospital, Birmingham, Alabama
Tuberculosis and Other Mycobacterial Diseases

MICHAEL B. KIMMEY, M.D.

Professor of Medicine, University of Washington School of Medicine; Director of Gastrointestinal Endoscopy and Section Chief of Gastroenterology, University of Washington Medical Center, Seattle, Washington
Gastritis and Peptic Ulcer Disease

LOUIS V. KIRCHHOFF, M.D., M.P.H.

Professor, Department of Internal Medicine, University of Iowa College of Medicine; University of Iowa Hospitals and Clinics and Veterans Affairs Medical Center, Iowa City, Iowa
American Trypanosomiasis (Chagas' Disease)

ROBERT S. KIRSNER, M.D.

Assistant Professor, University of Miami School of Medicine; Cedars Medical Center and Jackson Memorial Hospital, Miami, Florida
Venous Ulcers

ABBAS E. KITABCHI, PH.D., M.D.

Professor of Medicine and Biochemistry and Chief, Division of Endocrinology and Metabolism, University of Tennessee, Memphis, College of Medicine; Attending Physician, Bowld Hospital, and Consultant, Baptist Memorial Hospital, Memphis, Tennessee
Diabetic Ketoacidosis and Hyperglycemic Hyperosmolar Nonketotic State

AMY D. KLION, M.D.

Staff Physician, Laboratory of Parasitic Diseases, National Institutes of Allergy and Infectious Diseases, National Institutes of Health, Bethesda, Maryland
Parasitic Diseases of the Skin

WILLIAM J. KLISH, M.D.

Professor of Pediatrics, Baylor College of Medicine; Head, Pediatric Gastroenterology and Nutrition, Texas Children's Hospital, Houston, Texas
Normal Infant Feeding

ROBERT A. KLONER, M.D., PH.D.

Professor of Medicine, University of Southern California School of Medicine; Director of Research, Heart Institute, Good Samaritan Hospital, and Attending Cardiologist, Los Angeles County General Hospital, Los Angeles, California
Congestive Heart Failure

THOMAS R. KOSTEN, M.D.

Professor, Yale University School of Medicine; Chief of Psychiatry, Veterans Affairs Connecticut Healthcare System, New Haven, Connecticut
Drug Abuse

KEITH KRASINSKI, M.D.

Professor of Pediatrics and Environmental Medicine, New York University School of Medicine; Attending Physician, Tisch Hospital and Bellevue Hospital Center, New York, New York
Measles (Rubeola)

IRVING L. KRON, M.D.

Professor and Chief of Thoracic and Cardiovascular Surgery, University of Virginia School of Medicine and University of Virginia Health Sciences Center, Charlottesville, Virginia
Pleural Effusion and Empyema Thoracis

MARSHALL K. KUBOTA, M.D.

Associate Clinical Professor, Department of Family and Community Medicine, University of California, San Francisco, School of Medicine, San Francisco; Program Director, Family Practice Residency, Sutter Medical Center of Santa Rosa, Santa Rosa, California
Human Immunodeficiency Virus Infection and Its Complications

DANIEL H. LACHANCE, M.D.

Medical Associates Clinic, Mercy Hospital Center, Dubuque, Iowa
Brain Tumors

MARK D. LACY, M.D.

Fulbright Scholar, Faculty of Medicine, Infectious Diseases, Jordan University; Jordan University Hospital, Amman, Jordan
Relapsing Fever

BIMALIN LAHIRI, M.D.

Professor of Clinical Medicine, University of Connecticut School of Medicine, Farmington; Chief, Section of Pulmonary and Critical Care Medicine, St. Francis Hospital and Medical Center, Hartford, Connecticut
Cough

RICHARD A. LARSON, M.D.

Professor of Medicine, University of Chicago Pritzker School of Medicine; Director, Leukemia Program, University of Chicago Medical Center, Chicago, Illinois
Acute Leukemia in Adults

N. LATEUR, M.D.

Department of Dermatology, Chu Saint Pierre, Brussels Free University, Brussels, Belgium
Diseases of the Nails

YUNG R. LAU, M.D.

Assistant Professor of Pediatrics, University of Alabama at Birmingham School of Medicine, Birmingham, Alabama
Adult and Postoperative Congenital Heart Disease

SEAN F. LEAVEY, M.B., B.CHIR.

Lecturer, Internal Medicine, University of Michigan Medical School, Ann Arbor, Michigan
Primary Glomerular Diseases

LINE LEDUC, M.D.

Clinical Associate Professor, Department of Obstetrics and Gynecology, Université de Montréal Faculty of Medicine; Sainte-Justine Hospital, Montréal, Québec, Canada
Hypertensive Disorders of Pregnancy

ANDREW G. LEE, M.D.
Associate Professor of Ophthalmology, Neurology, and Neurosurgery, Baylor College of Medicine; Department of Neurosurgery, University of Texas M. D. Anderson Cancer Center, Houston, Texas
Optic Neuritis

LESLIE E. LEHMANN, M.D.
Instructor in Pediatrics, Harvard Medical School; Dana-Farber Cancer Institute and Children's Hospital, Boston, Massachusetts
Neutropenia

PHYLLIS A. LEVINE, M.D.
Clinical Assistant Professor, State University of New York Health Sciences Center at Brooklyn, Brooklyn; Lenox Hill Hospital, New York, New York
Carcinoma of the Uterine Cervix

SUE LEVKOFF, Sc.D.
Associate Professor, Department of Social Medicine and Division on Aging, Harvard Medical School, Boston, Massachusetts
Delirium

RICHARD F. LOCKEY, M.D.
Professor of Medicine, Pediatrics, and Public Health, Director, Division of Allergy and Immunology; and Joy McCann Culverhouse Professor in Allergy and Immunology, University of South Florida College of Medicine; James A. Haley Veterans Affairs Hospital and Tampa General Hospital, Tampa, Florida
Insect Sting Hypersensitivity

CHRISTY A. LORTON, M.D.
Clinical Preceptor, Medical College of Ohio, Toledo; Clinical Preceptor, W. W. Knight Residency Program; Consultant, Toledo Hospital and St. Luke's Hospital, Toledo, Ohio
Pigmentary Disorders

DEON LOUW, M.D.
Clinical Instructor, Oregon Health Sciences University School of Medicine, Portland, Oregon
Trigeminal Neuralgia

JERRY C. LUCK, M.D.
Professor of Medicine, Pennsylvania State University College of Medicine; Director, Clinical Electrophysiology, Penn State–Milton S. Hershey Medical Center, Hershey, Pennsylvania
Cardiac Arrest: Sudden Cardiac Death

CHARLES M. LUETJE, M.D.
Trinity Lutheran Hospital and St. Luke's Hospital of Kansas City, Kansas City, Missouri
Meniere's Disease

DONALD F. LUM, M.D.
Assistant Professor of Medicine, University of California, Davis, School of Medicine, Sacramento; Veterans Affairs Northern California Health Care System, Martinez, California
Nausea and Vomiting

RICHARD J. MACCHIA, M.D.
Professor and Chairman, Department of Urology, State University of New York Health Science Center at Brooklyn College of Medicine; Chief, Department of Urology, University Hospital of Brooklyn and Kings County Hospital Center, Brooklyn, New York
Trauma to the Genitourinary Tract

PAUL O. MADSEN, M.D., Ph.D.
Professor of Urology (emeritus), University of Wisconsin Medical School, Madison, Wisconsin
Prostatitis

MARK A. MALANGONI, M.D.
Professor and Vice Chairman, Department of Surgery, Case Western Reserve University School of Medicine; Chairperson, Department of Surgery, MetroHealth Medical Center, Cleveland, Ohio
Necrotizing Soft Tissue Infections

JULIE E. MANGINO, M.D.
Assistant Professor of Internal Medicine, Division of Infectious Diseases, Ohio State University Medical Center, Columbus, Ohio
Blastomycosis

MANUEL MAÑÓS-PUJOL, M.D., Ph.D.
Professor of Otorhinolaryngology, University of Barcelona; Head of Section, Department of Otorhinolaryngology, Civtat Sanitària Universitaria de Bellvitge, University of Barcelona, Barcelona, Spain
Acute Idiopathic Facial Palsy (Bell's Palsy)

ANDREW M. MARGILETH, M.D.
Clinical Professor of Pediatrics, Mercer University School of Medicine, Macon; Bachus Children's Hospital at Memorial Medical Center, Savannah, Georgia
Cat-Scratch Disease

MALCOLM L. MARGOLIN, M.D.
Clinical Professor of Obstetrics and Gynecology, University of Southern California School of Medicine; Clinical Chief of Obstetrics and Gynecology, Cedars-Sinai Medical Center, Los Angeles, California
Uterine Leiomyomata

ALI J. MARIAN, M.D.
Assistant Professor of Medicine, Baylor College of Medicine; Methodist Hospital and Ben Taub General Hospital, Houston, Texas
Hypertrophic Cardiomyopathy

DONALD W. MARION, M.D.
Professor of Neurological Surgery, Director, Brain Trauma Research Center, and Director, Center for Injury Research and Control, University of Pittsburgh School of Medicine; Attending Neurosurgeon, University of Pittsburgh Medical Center, Pittsburgh, Pennsylvania
Acute Head Injuries in Adults

PAULA MARLTON, M.B., B.S.
Senior Lecturer, Department of Pathology, University of Queensland; Assistant Director of Haematology, Princess Alexandra Hospital, Brisbane, Australia
Non-Hodgkin's Lymphoma

DAVID H. MARTIN, M.D.
Harry E. Dascomb, M.D., Professor of Medicine, Professor of Microbiology; and Chief, Section of Infectious Diseases, Louisiana State University School of Medicine in New Orleans, New Orleans, Louisiana
Chancroid

LUIGI MASTROIANNI, Jr., M.D.
William Goodell Professor of Obstetrics and Gynecology, University of Pennsylvania School of Medicine; Hospital of the University of Pennsylvania, Philadelphia, Pennsylvania
Contraception

ALEXANDER MAUSKOP, M.D.
Associate Professor of Clinical Neurology, State University of New York Health Science Center at Brooklyn, Brooklyn; Director, New York Headache Center, New York, New York
Headaches

HOWARD B. MAYER, M.D.
Clinical Instructor of Medicine, Yale University School of Medicine, New Haven; Attending Physician, Medical Service, Division of Infectious Diseases, Veterans Affairs Medical Center, West Haven, Connecticut
Acute Infectious Diarrhea

ERNEST L. MAZZAFERRI, M.D.
Professor and Chairman, Department of Internal Medicine, and Professor of Physiology, Ohio State University College of Medicine and Public Health; Ohio State University Medical Center, Columbus, Ohio
Thyroid Cancer

JOHN H. MCANULTY, M.D.
Professor and Head, Division of Cardiology, Oregon Health Sciences University School of Medicine, Portland, Oregon
Tachyarrhythmias

PHILIP L. MCCARTHY, JR., M.D.
Assistant Professor, State University of New York at Buffalo; Director, Clinical Blood and Marrow Transplantation, Roswell Park Cancer Institute, Buffalo, New York
Polycythemia Vera

S. TERI MCGILLIS, M.D.
Staff Physician, Department of Dermatology, Cleveland Clinic Foundation, Cleveland, Ohio
Cancer of the Skin

MARILYNNE MCKAY, M.D.
Professor of Dermatology and Executive Director, CME and Biomedical Media, Emory University School of Medicine; Emory University Hospital, Atlanta, Georgia
Pruritus Ani and Vulvae

PHILIP G. MCMANIS, M.D.
Senior Lecturer, University of Sydney; Staff Neurologist, Nepean Hospital, Sydney, Australia
Peripheral Neuropathies

KENNETH R. MCQUAID, M.D.
Associate Professor of Clinical Medicine, University of California, San Francisco, School of Medicine; Director of Endoscopy, Veterans Affairs Medical Center, San Francisco, California
Gastroesophageal Reflux Disease

ALAN MENTER, M.D.
Associate Clinical Professor of Dermatology, University of Texas Southwestern Medical School, Dallas; Chairman, Division of Dermatology, Baylor University Medical Center, Houston, Texas
Papulosquamous Diseases

PHILIP B. MINER, JR., M.D.
Clinical Professor of Medicine, University of Oklahoma School of Medicine, Oklahoma City, Oklahoma
Inflammatory Bowel Disease

HOWARD C. MOFENSON, M.D.
Professor of Pediatrics and Emergency Medicine, State University of New York at Stony Brook School of Medicine, Stony Brook; Professor of Pharmacology and Toxicology, New York School of Osteopathy, Westbury; St. John's University College of Pharmacy, Jamaica; Medical Director, Long Island Regional Poison Control Center, Winthrop University Hospital, Mineola, New York
Acute Poisonings

MARGARET MOLINE, PH.D.
Senior Research Associate, Cornell University Medical College, New York, New York
Premenstrual Dysphoric Disorder

GREGORY L. MONETA, M.D.
Professor of Surgery, Division of Vascular Surgery, Oregon Health Sciences University, Portland, Oregon
Venous Thrombosis

ANGELA YEN MOORE, M.D.
Assistant Professor in Dermatology and Assistant Professor in Pathology, University of Texas Medical Branch, University of Texas Medical School at Galveston, Galveston, Texas
Viral Diseases of the Skin

JOHN S. MORAN, M.D., M.P.H.
Division of STD Prevention, National Center for HIV, STD, and TB Prevention, Centers for Disease Control and Prevention, Atlanta, Georgia
Gonorrhea

WARWICK L. MORISON, M.D.
Professor of Dermatology, Johns Hopkins University School of Medicine; Johns Hopkins Medical Institutions and Greater Baltimore Medical Center, Baltimore, Maryland
Sunburn

JUDD W. MOUL, M.D.
Associate Professor, Department of Surgery, Uniformed Services University of the Health Sciences, Bethesda, Maryland; Attending Urologic-Oncologist, Walter Reed Army Medical Center, Washington, D.C.
Malignant Tumors of the Urogenital Tract

JOHN S. MUNGER, M.D.
Assistant Professor, New York University School of Medicine; Physician, Bellevue Hospital Center, New York, New York
Silicosis

EDWARD S. MURPHY, M.D.
Professor of Medicine, Division of Cardiology, Oregon Health Sciences University; Veterans Affairs Medical Center, Portland, Oregon
Infective Endocarditis

MARY BETH MURPHY, R.N., M.S., C.D.E., M.B.A.
Research Coordinator, University of Tennessee, Memphis, Memphis, Tennessee
Diabetic Ketoacidosis and Hyperglycemic Hyperosmolar Nonketotic State

PERTTI MUSTAJOKI, M.D.
Assistant Professor, Department of Medicine, University Central Hospital, Helsinki; Director, Department of Medicine, Peijas Hospital, Vantaa, Finland
The Porphyrias

SARAH A. MYERS, M.D.
Assistant Professor, Duke University Medical Center, Durham, North Carolina
Pruritus; Skin Diseases of Pregnancy

GERALD V. NACCARELLI, M.D.
Professor of Medicine; Head, Section of Cardiology; and Director, Cardiovascular Center; Pennsylvania State University College of Medicine; Head, Section of Cardiology, Penn State–Milton S. Hershey Medical Center, Penn State/Geisinger Health System, Hershey, Pennsylvania
Cardiac Arrest: Sudden Cardiac Death

LILA E. NACHTIGALL, M.D.
Professor of Obstetrics and Gynecology, New York University School of Medicine; Attending Physician, Tisch Hospital and Bellevue Hospital Center, New York, New York
Menopause

LISA B. NACHTIGALL, M.D.

Assistant Professor of Medicine, Tufts University School of Medicine; Director of Women's Endocrine Center, St. Elizabeth's Hospital, Boston, Massachusetts
Menopause

G. BALAKRISH NAIR, PH.D.

Deputy Director, Department of Microbiology, National Institute of Cholera and Enteric Diseases, Beliaghata, Calcutta, India
Cholera

HIDEKI NAKAKUMA, M.D., PH.D.

Associate Professor of Medicine, Kumamoto University School of Medicine; Division of Hematology Oncology, Department of Internal Medicine, Kumamoto University Hospital, Kumamoto, Japan
Nonimmune Hemolytic Anemia

GEETHA NARAYAN, M.D.

Assistant Professor of Medicine, Tufts University School of Medicine; Staff Nephrologist and Associate Director of Dialysis, St. Elizabeth's Medical Center of Boston, Boston, Massachusetts
Diabetes Insipidus

NAIEL N. NASSAR, M.D.

Assistant Professor of Medicine, University of Texas Southwestern Medical Center at Dallas, Southwestern Medical School; Director, HIV Program, Veterans Affairs Medical Center, Dallas, Texas
Bacterial Infections of the Urinary Tract in Men

NEENA NATT, M.B., B.CHIR.

Senior Clinical Fellow, Mayo Graduate School of Medicine; Senior Clinical Fellow, Division of Endocrinology, Mayo Clinic, Rochester, Minnesota
Thyroiditis

MARK R. NEHLER, M.D.

Assistant Professor of Surgery, Vascular Surgery Section, University of Colorado Health Sciences Center, Denver, Colorado
Venous Thrombosis

RICHARD E. NEIBERGER, M.D., PH.D.

Associate Professor of Pediatrics, University of Florida College of Medicine; Shands Hospital at the University of Florida, Gainesville, Florida
Fluid and Electrolyte Abnormalities in Children

ROBERT P. NELSON, JR., M.D.

Associate Professor of Medicine and Pediatrics, University of South Florida College of Medicine; All Children's Hospital, St. Petersburg, Florida
Insect Sting Hypersensitivity

VICTOR D. NEWCOMER, M.D.

Clinical Professor of Medicine/Dermatology, University of California, Los Angeles, UCLA School of Medicine; Senior Attending, Santa Monica–UCLA Medical Center, and Associate, St. John's, Santa Monica, California
Nevi

F. CARTER NEWTON, M.D.

Assistant Clinical Professor, University of California, Los Angeles, UCLA School of Medicine; Consulting Cardiologist, St. John's Hospital and UCLA Medical Center, Los Angeles, California
Care After Myocardial Infarction

RICHARD OHRBACH, D.D.S., PH.D.

Assistant Professor, School of Dental Medicine, State University of New York at Buffalo, Buffalo, New York
Temporomandibular Disorders and Craniofacial Pain

JAMES G. OLSON, PH.D.

Chief, Viral and Rickettsial Zoonoses Branch, Centers for Disease Control and Prevention, Atlanta, Georgia
Rickettsial and Ehrlichial Infections

STEVEN M. OPAL, M.D.

Professor of Medicine, Brown University School of Medicine, Providence; Infectious Disease Division, Memorial Hospital of Rhode Island, Pawtucket, Rhode Island
Bacteremia and Septicemia

RAUL C. ORDORICA, M.D.

Assistant Professor, University of South Florida College of Medicine; Chief, Urology Section, James A. Haley Veterans Affairs Hospital, Tampa, Florida
Urethral Strictures

BRUCE A. ORKIN, M.D.

Associate Professor; Director, Division of Colon and Rectal Surgery; and Director, Gastrointestinal Physiology Laboratory; George Washington University School of Medicine and Health Sciences; Attending Surgeon, George Washington University Hospital, and Consulting Surgeon, Children's National Medical Center, Washington, D.C.
Hemorrhoids, Anal Fissure, and Anorectal Abscess and Fistula

CHRISTOPHER D. PADDOCK, M.D., M.P.H.T.M.

Viral and Rickettsial Zoonoses Branch, Centers for Disease Control and Prevention, Atlanta, Georgia
Rickettsial and Ehrlichial Infections

DIMITRIS A. PAPANICOLAOU, M.D.

Chief, Adult Endocrine Ward and Clinics, Developmental Endocrinology Branch, National Institute of Child Health and Human Development, National Institutes of Health, Bethesda, Maryland
Cushing's Syndrome

LAWRENCE CHARLES PARISH, M.D.

Clinical Professor of Dermatology and Cutaneous Biology, Jefferson Medical College of Thomas Jefferson University; Director of the Jefferson Center for International Dermatology; Chief of Dermatology, Frankford Hospital, Philadelphia, and Consultant Dermatologist, Magee Rehabilitation Hospital, Philadelphia, Pennsylvania
Pressure Ulcers

CHARLES J. PARKER, M.D.

Professor of Medicine, University of Utah School of Medicine; Chief, Hematology/Oncology Division, Veterans Affairs Medical Center, Salt Lake City, Utah
Autoimmune Hemolytic Anemia

ROBERT M. PASCUZZI, M.D.

Professor and Vice Chairman, Department of Neurology, Indiana University School of Medicine; Chief, Department of Neurology, Wishard Health Services, Indianapolis, Indiana
Myasthenia Gravis

DAVID L. PATERSON, M.D.

Visiting Postdoctoral Scholar, University of Pittsburgh; Infectious Disease Section, Veterans Affairs Medical Center, Pittsburgh, Pennsylvania
Legionellosis (Legionnaires' Disease and Pontiac Fever)

ROY PATTERSON, M.D.

Professor of Medicine and Chief, Division of Allergy and Immunology, Department of Medicine, Northwestern University Medical School, Chicago, Illinois
Hypersensitivity Pneumonitis

TODD W. PERKINS, M.D.
Associate Professor, Department of Ophthalmology and Visual Sciences, University of Wisconsin Medical School; University of Wisconsin Hospital, Madison, Wisconsin
Glaucoma

KUSIEL PERLMAN, M.D.
Assistant Professor of Pediatrics, University of Toronto Faculty of Medicine; Staff Endocrinologist, Hospital for Sick Children, Toronto, Ontario, Canada
Diabetes Mellitus in Childhood and Adolescence

KENNETH M. PETERS, M.D.
Fellow, Department of Urology, William Beaumont Hospital, Royal Oak, Michigan
Urinary Incontinence

MARTIN D. PHILLIPS, M.D.
Director, Medical Affairs, Centeon, L.L.C., King of Prussia, Pennsylvania
Platelet-Mediated Bleeding Disorders

PAULA PIETRUCHA-DILANCHIAN, PHARM.D.
Clinical Manager, Owen Healthcare, Memorial Hospital–Pasadena, Pasadena, Texas
New Drugs for 1997

MARK H. POLLACK, M.D.
Associate Professor of Psychiatry, Harvard Medical School; Director, Anxiety Disorders Program, Massachusetts General Hospital, Boston, Massachusetts
Anxiety Disorders

DAVID G. POPLACK, M.D.
Elise C. Young Professor of Pediatric Oncology; and Head, Hematology-Oncology Section, Department of Pediatrics, Baylor College of Medicine; Director, Texas Children's Cancer Center, Texas Children's Hospital, Houston, Texas
Acute Leukemia in Childhood

J. GERALD QUIRK, M.D., PH.D.
Professor and Chairman, Department of Obstetrics and Gynecology, University of Arkansas for Medical Sciences, Little Rock, Arkansas
Antepartum Care

ELYSE S. RAFAL, M.D.
Assistant Professor of Clinical Dermatology, Director of Dermatopharmacology, and Assistant Director of Outpatient Clinical Dermatology, University Medical Center, Stony Brook, New York
Urticaria and Angioedema

DANIEL W. RAHN, M.D.
Professor of Medicine; Chief, Section of General Internal Medicine; and Vice Dean for Clinical Affairs, Medical College of Georgia Hospital and Clinics, Augusta, Georgia
Lyme Disease

RAMESH K. RAMANATHAN, M.D.
Assistant Professor of Medicine, University of Pittsburgh School of Medicine and University of Pittsburgh Cancer Institute, Pittsburgh, Pennsylvania
Primary Lung Cancer

FRANCISCO C. RAMIREZ, M.D.
Associate Chair of Medicine for Gastroenterology, Carl T. Hayden Veterans Affairs Medical Center, Phoenix; Assistant Professor of Clinical Medicine, University of Arizona College of Medicine, Tucson, Arizona
Hiccup

MARK X. RANSOM, M.D.
Clinical Assistant Professor, Mount Sinai School of Graduate Medical Education, New York, New York; Saint Joseph's Hospital and Medical Center, Paterson, New Jersey
Ectopic Pregnancy

SATISH S. C. RAO, M.D., PH.D.
Associate Professor of Medicine, University of Iowa College of Medicine; University of Iowa Hospitals and Clinics, Iowa City, Iowa
Constipation

DIDIER RAOULT, M.D., PH.D.
Professor, School of Medicine, Université de la Méditerranée; Chairman, Clinical Microbiology, Hôpital la Timone, Marseilles, France
Q Fever

JONATHAN I. RAVDIN, M.D.
Nesbitt Professor and Chair of Medicine, University of Minnesota Medical School–Minneapolis; Chief of Medicine, Fairview University Medical Center, Minneapolis, Minnesota
Amebiasis

ROBERT V. REGE, M.D.
Professor of Surgery, Northwestern University Medical School; Chief, Surgical Services, VA Chicago Health Care System, Lakeside Division Staff Surgeon, Northwestern Memorial Hospital, Chicago, Illinois
Cholelithiasis and Cholecystitis

MICHAEL F. REIN, M.D.
Professor of Medicine, Division of Infectious Diseases, University of Virginia School of Medicine; Attending Physician, University of Virginia Health Sciences Center, Charlottesville, Virginia
Syphilis

DOUGLAS S. REINTGEN, M.D.
Program Leader, Cutaneous Oncology, H. Lee Moffitt Cancer Center, University of South Florida; H. Lee Moffitt Cancer Center, Tampa, Florida
Malignant Melanoma

DOUGLAS S. RICHARDS, M.D.
Associate Professor of Obstetrics and Gynecology, University of Florida College of Medicine; Director of Obstetric and Gynecologic Ultrasound Section, University of Florida, Gainesville, Florida
Hemolytic Disease of the Fetus and Newborn

ELLIOTT RICHELSON, M.D.
Professor of Psychiatry and of Pharmacology, Mayo Medical School, Rochester, Minnesota; Consultant in Psychiatry and in Pharmacology, Mayo Clinic–Jacksonville; St. Luke's Hospital, Jacksonville, Florida
Mood Disorders

RICHARD S. RIVLIN, M.D.
Professor of Medicine, Cornell University Medical College; Program Director, Clinical Nutrition Research Unit, GI-Nutrition Service, Memorial Sloan-Kettering Cancer Center; Chief, Nutrition Division, Department of Medicine, New York Hospital–Cornell Medical Center, New York, New York
Vitamin Deficiency

JOHN D. ROBACK, M.D., PH.D.
Fellow, Transfusion Medicine Program, Department of Pathology and Laboratory Medicine, Emory University School of Medicine; Fellow, Transfusion Medicine Program, Emory University Hospital, Atlanta, Georgia
Therapeutic Use of Blood Components

DANIEL RODRIGUE, M.D.

Assistant Professor of Clinical Medicine, Division of Infectious Diseases, University of Southern California School of Medicine; Los Angeles County/USC Medical Center, Los Angeles, California
Salmonellosis

JAMES N. ROGERS, M.D.

Associate Professor of Anesthesiology, University of Texas Health Science Center at San Antonio; Chief, Audie L. Murphy Veterans Hospital Pain Clinic and University Health System Pain Management Center, San Antonio, Texas
Pain

WILLIAM N. ROM, M.D.

Professor of Medicine and Environmental Medicine, New York University School of Medicine; Director of Chest Service, Bellevue Hospital Center, New York, New York
Silicosis

KEVIN P. ROSENBACH, M.D.

Advanced Subspecialty Resident in Allergy and Immunology, University of South Florida College of Medicine; James A. Haley Veterans Affairs Hospital and Tampa General Hospital, Tampa, Florida
Insect Sting Hypersensitivity

PETER M. ROSENBERG, M.D.

Fellow in Medicine, Harvard Medical School; Clinical and Research Fellow, Gastrointestinal Unit, Massachusetts General Hospital, Boston, Massachusetts
Cirrhosis

RICHARD I. ROTHSTEIN, M.D.

Associate Professor of Medicine, Dartmouth Medical School, Hanover; Chief, Section of Gastroenterology, Dartmouth-Hitchcock Medical Center, Lebanon, New Hampshire
Dysphagia and Esophageal Obstruction

STEPHEN N. ROUS, M.D., M.S.

Professor of Surgery (Urology), Dartmouth Medical School, Hanover, New Hampshire; Staff Urologist, Dartmouth-Hitchcock Medical Center, Lebanon, New Hampshire; Chief of Urology, Veterans Affairs Medical Center, White River Junction, Vermont
Epididymitis

WILLIAM A. ROWE, M.D.

Assistant Professor, Section of Gastroenterology and Hepatology, Pennsylvania State University College of Medicine; Penn State–Milton S. Hershey Medical Center, Penn State/Geisinger Health System, Hershey, Pennsylvania
Malabsorption

FINDLAY E. RUSSELL, M.D., PH.D.

Professor, Pharmacology and Toxicology, University of Arizona College of Medicine, Tucson, Arizona; Adjunct Professor, University of Southern California School of Medicine, Los Angeles, California; University Medical Center, Tucson; Los Angeles County/USC Medical Center, Los Angeles, California
Spider Bites and Scorpion Stings

BIJAN SAFAI, M.D., D.SC.

Professor and Chairman, Department of Dermatology, New York Medical College; Director Dermatology, West Chester County Medical Center, Valhalla, New York
Cutaneous T Cell Lymphoma

ASH K. SAMANTA, M.D.

Clinical Teacher, Leicester University Medical School; Consultant Physician, Leicester Royal Infirmary, NHS Trust, Leicester, England
Brucellosis

I. JAMES SARFEH, M.D.

Professor of Surgery, University of California, Irvine, College of Medicine, Irvine; Chief of General Surgery, Veterans Affairs Medical Center, Long Beach; Staff Surgeon, University of California, Irvine, Medical Center, Orange, California
Bleeding Esophageal Varices

ARIF R. SARWARI, M.D., M.S.

Assistant Professor, Department of Medicine, Azia Khan University; Assistant Professor and Consultant, Infectious Diseases, Azia Khan University Hospital, Karachi, Pakistan
Typhoid Fever

KATHLEEN SAZAMA, M.D., J.D.

Professor of Pathology and Laboratory Medicine, Allegheny University of the Health Sciences; Hahnemann University Hospital and Medical College of Pennsylvania Hospital, Philadelphia, Pennsylvania
Adverse Effects of Blood Transfusion

THOMAS M. SCALEA, M.D.

Professor of Surgery and Director, Program of Trauma, University of Maryland School of Medicine; Physician in Chief, R. Adams Cowley Shock Trauma Center, Baltimore, Maryland
Trauma to the Genitourinary Tract

PHYLLIS L. SCHATZ, M.D.

Assistant Professor of Medicine, University of Connecticut School of Medicine, Farmington; Assistant Chief, Section of Pulmonary and Critical Care Medicine, and Associate Director, Medical Critical Care, St. Francis Hospital and Medical Center, Hartford, Connecticut
Cough

MELVIN SCHEINMAN, M.D.

Professor of Medicine, University of California, San Francisco, School of Medicine; Section of Cardiac Electrophysiology, Moffitt-Long Hospitals, San Francisco, California
Premature Beats

W. MICHAEL SCHELD, M.D.

Professor of Internal Medicine and Neurosurgery and Associate Chair for Residency Programs, University of Virginia School of Medicine; Attending Physician, University of Virginia Health System, Charlottesville, Virginia
Bacterial Meningitis

NOAH S. SCHENKMAN, M.D.

Clinical Instructor, Urology Department, University of California, San Francisco, School of Medicine; Urology Department, University of California–San Francisco Medical Center, San Francisco, California
Urinary Stone Disease

WILLIAM D. SCHLAFF, M.D.

Professor and Chief, Division of Reproductive Endocrinology, University of Colorado Health Sciences Center, Denver, Colorado
Amenorrhea

STANLEY B. SCHMIDT, M.D.

Professor of Medicine, West Virginia University School of Medicine; Director of Cardiac Electrophysiology, West Virginia University Hospitals, Morgantown, West Virginia
Heart Block

THOMAS J. SCHNITZER, M.D., PH.D.

Professor of Medicine, Northwestern University Medical School; Northwestern Memorial Hospital, Chicago, Illinois
Osteoarthritis

STEPHEN C. SCHOENBAUM, M.D., M.P.H.

Associate Professor of Medicine, Harvard Medical School, Boston, Massachusetts; Medical Director, Harvard Pilgrim Health Care of New England, Providence, Rhode Island
Influenza

PAMELA SCHUTZER, M.D.

Resident, Department of Dermatology, New York Medical College, Valhalla; Resident, Bayley Seton Hospital, Staten Island, New York
Cutaneous T Cell Lymphoma

STEPHEN M. SCOTT, M.D.

Assistant Professor, University of Colorado Health Sciences Center, Denver, Colorado
Amenorrhea

HEATHER SELMAN, M.D.

Resident, Department of Urology, Temple University Hospital, Philadelphia, Pennsylvania
Nongonococcal Urethritis

GIANPIETRO SEMENZATO, M.D.

Associate Professor of Medicine, Padua University School of Medicine; Chief, Clinical Immunology Branch, Department of Clinical and Experimental Medicine, Padua University, Padua, Italy
Sarcoidosis

LYLE L. SENSENBRENNER, M.D.

Professor of Medicine, Division of Hematology/Oncology, University of Maryland School of Medicine; University of Maryland Hospital, Baltimore, Maryland
Aplastic Anemia

GRAHAM R. SERJEANT, M.D.

Director, MRC Laboratories, University of the West Indies, Kingston, Jamaica, West Indies
Sickle Cell Disease

JESSICA L. SEVERSON, M.D.

Clinical Research Fellow, University of Texas Medical Branch at Galveston, Galveston, Texas
Viral Diseases of the Skin

MARTIN J. SHEARER, PH.D.

Principal Scientist, Head Vitamin K Diagnostic and Research Laboratories, Haemophilia Centre, St. Thomas's Hospital, London, England
Vitamin K Deficiency

JEANNE S. SHEFFIELD, M.D.

Fellow, Maternal Fetal Medicine, University of Texas Southwestern Medical Center at Dallas, Dallas, Texas
Pyelonephritis

DOUGLAS SHEMIN, M.D.

Clinical Assistant Professor of Medicine, Brown University Medical School; Director of Hemodialysis, Rhode Island Hospital, Providence, Rhode Island
Chronic Renal Failure

YORAM SHENKER, M.D.

Associate Professor of Medicine, University of Wisconsin Medical School; Head, Section of Endocrinology, Diabetes, and Metabolism, University of Wisconsin Hospital; Chief of Endocrinology, William S. Middleton Memorial Veterans Hospital, Madison, Wisconsin
Low-Renin Aldosteronism

JOSEPH B. SHUMWAY, M.D., M.P.H.

Assistant Professor of Obstetrics and Gynecology and Director of Ultrasound Program, St. Louis University School of Medicine; St. Mary's Health Center and DePaul Health Center, St. Louis, Missouri
Vaginal Bleeding Beyond the First Trimester of Pregnancy

RICHARD T. SILVER, M.D.

Clinical Professor of Medicine, Cornell University Medical College; Attending Physician, New York Hospital, New York, New York
Chronic Myeloid Leukemia

SUSAN L. SIMANDL, M.D.

Assistant Professor of Medicine and Director, Echocardiographic Laboratory, State University of New York at Stony Brook Health Sciences Center, Stony Brook, New York
Angina Pectoris

LEE S. SIMON, M.D.

Associate Professor of Medicine, Harvard Medical School; Director of Graduate Medical Education, Beth Israel Deaconess Medical Center, and Clinical Associate, Massachusetts General Hospital, Boston, Massachusetts
Rheumatoid Arthritis

NAOMI M. SIMON, M.D.

Instructor in Psychiatry, Harvard Medical School; Clinical Assistant in Psychiatry and Psychiatrist, Anxiety Disorders Program, Massachusetts General Hospital, Boston, Massachusetts
Anxiety Disorders

C. BLAKE SIMPSON, M.D.

Assistant Professor and Director of Residency Program, Department of Otolaryngology–Head and Neck Surgery, University of Texas Health Science Center at San Antonio, San Antonio, Texas
Hoarseness and Laryngitis

GARY L. SIMPSON, M.D., PH.D., M.P.H.

Research Professor, Department of Biology, University of New Mexico, Albuquerque; New Mexico Department of Health, Santa Fe, New Mexico
Plague

PETER A. SINGER, M.D.

Professor of Clinical Medicine and Chief, Clinical Endocrinology, University of Southern California School of Medicine, Los Angeles, California
Hyperthyroidism

SMIT S. SINHA, M.D.

Research Fellow, Department of Psychiatry, College of Physicians and Surgeons, Columbia University; New York State Psychiatric Institute, New York, New York
Panic Disorder

DAVID P. SKONER, M.D.

Associate Professor of Pediatrics and Otolaryngology, University of Pittsburgh School of Medicine; Chief, Allergy and Immunology, Children's Hospital of Pittsburgh, Pittsburgh, Pennsylvania
Viral Respiratory Infections

BRADLEY E. SMITH, M.D.

Professor of Anesthesiology, Vanderbilt University School of Medicine; Attending Physician, Vanderbilt University Hospital, Nashville, Tennessee
Obstetric Anesthesia

EDWIN A. SMITH, M.D.

Associate Professor of Medicine, Medical University of South Carolina, Charleston, South Carolina
Polymyalgia Rheumatica and Giant Cell Arteritis

JAMES W. SMITH, M.D.

Professor of Internal Medicine, University of Texas Southwestern Medical Center at Dallas, Southwestern Medical School; Staff Physician, Infectious Diseases Section, Veterans Affairs North Texas Health Care System, Dallas, Texas
Bacterial Infections of the Urinary Tract in Men

BRENT W. SNOW, M.D.

Professor of Surgery, University of Utah School of Medicine; Primary Children's Medical Center, Salt Lake City, Utah
Childhood Enuresis

WILLIAM B. SOLOMON, M.D.

Assistant Professor of Medicine and Microbiology/Immunology, State University of New York Health Science Center at Brooklyn; Attending Physician, University Hospital of Brooklyn and Kings County Hospital Center, Brooklyn, New York
Iron Deficiency Anemia

DENNIS P. SORRESSO, M.D.

Pulmonary Fellow, Foster G. McGaw Hospital, Loyola University Medical Center, Maywood, Illinois, and Edward Hines, Jr., Veterans Affairs Medical Center, Hines, Illinois
Chronic Obstructive Pulmonary Disease

MARK T. SPEAKMAN, M.D.

Senior Fellow in Cardiology, Division of Cardiology, University of Southern California School of Medicine, Los Angeles, California
Congestive Heart Failure

SHELDON L. SPECTOR, M.D.

Clinical Professor of Medicine, University of California, Los Angeles, UCLA School of Medicine; Director, Allergy Research Foundation; Attending Physician, UCLA Medical Center and Cedars-Sinai Medical Center, Los Angeles, California
Asthma in Adolescents and Adults

GWENDOLINE M. SPURLL, M.D.

Associate Professor, McGill University Faculty of Medicine; Associate Physician, Royal Victoria Hospital, Montreal, Québec, Canada
Thrombotic Thrombocytopenic Purpura

LYNN STAZZONE, R.N.

Nurse Practitioner, Multiple Sclerosis Program, Brigham and Women's Hospital, Boston, Massachusetts
Multiple Sclerosis

FERNANDO STEIN, M.D.

Associate Professor of Pediatrics, Baylor College of Medicine; Texas Children's Hospital and Ben Taub General Hospital, Houston, Texas
Pediatric Head Injury

C. PHILIP STEUBER, M.D.

Professor of Pediatrics, Section of Pediatric Hematology-Oncology, Baylor College of Medicine; Texas Children's Cancer Center and Hematology Service, Texas Children's Hospital, Houston, Texas
Acute Leukemia in Childhood

SETH R. STEVENS, M.D.

Assistant Professor of Dermatology, Case Western Reserve University; Director, Inpatient Services, Department of Dermatology, University Hospitals of Cleveland; Assistant Chief, Dermatology Service, Veterans Affairs Medical Center, Cleveland, Ohio
Atopic Dermatitis

CHRISTOPHER D. STILL, D.O., M.Sc.

Associate Physician, Department of Gastroenterology/Nutrition and General Internal Medicine; Section Head of Nutrition; and Director, High Risk Obesity Clinic, Penn State Geisinger Health Care System, Danville, Pennsylvania
Obesity

MARSHALL L. STOLLER, M.D.

Associate Professor of Urology, University of California, San Francisco, School of Medicine; University of California–San Francisco Medical Center, San Francisco, California
Urinary Stone Disease

JAMES A. STROM, M.D.

Associate Professor of Medicine, Tufts University School of Medicine; Chief of Nephrology, St. Elizabeth's Medical Center of Boston, Boston, Massachusetts
Diabetes Insipidus

RICARDO A. TAN, M.D.

Antelope Valley Allergy Medical Group, Palmdale, California
Asthma in Adolescents and Adults

ANTHONY S. TAVILL, M.D.

Professor of Medicine and Nutrition, Case Western Reserve University School of Medicine; Mathile and Morton J. Stone Professor of Digestive and Liver Disorders, Mt. Sinai Medical Center, Cleveland, Ohio
Hemochromatosis

RICHARD B. TENSER, M.D.

Professor of Neurology, Pennsylvania State University College of Medicine; Penn State–Milton S. Hershey Medical Center, Hershey, Pennsylvania
Viral Meningitis and Encephalitis (Meningoencephalitis)

ERICA R. THALER, M.D.

Assistant Professor, Department of Otorhinolaryngology, University of Pennsylvania School of Medicine; Hospital of the University of Pennsylvania, Children's Hospital of Philadelphia, Philadelphia, Pennsylvania
Sinusitis

RICHARD F. THOMPSON, M.D.

El Camino Hospital, Camino Medical Group, Sunnyvale, California
Immunization Practices

JAMES BRANTLEY THRASHER, M.D.

Associate Clinical Professor of Surgery, Uniformed Services University of the Health Sciences, Bethesda, Maryland; Associate Clinical Professor of Surgery, University of Washington, Seattle; Director, Urology Residency Program, Madigan Army Medical Center, Tacoma, Washington
Malignant Tumors of the Urogenital Tract

ROBERT D. TIEGS, M.D.

Associate Professor of Medicine, Mayo Medical School; Division of Endocrinology, Mayo Clinic, Rochester, Minnesota
Paget's Disease of Bone

KENNETH J. TOMECKI, M.D.

Department of Dermatology, Cleveland Clinic Foundation and Cleveland Clinic Hospital, Cleveland, Ohio
Bacterial Diseases of the Skin

ARIFA TOOR, M.D.

Instructor of Medicine, Dartmouth Medical School, Hanover; Gastroenterology Fellow, Dartmouth-Hitchcock Medical Center, Lebanon, New Hampshire
Dysphagia and Esophageal Obstruction

ELAINE B. TRUJILLO, M.S., R.D.

Clinical and Research Dietitian, Brigham and Women's Hospital, Boston, Massachusetts
Parenteral Nutrition in Adults

GUILLERMO E. UMPIERREZ, M.D.

Assistant Clinical Professor, Emory University School of Medicine; Director, Internal Medicine Residency Program, Georgia Baptist Medical Center, Atlanta, Georgia
Diabetic Ketoacidosis and Hyperglycemic Hyperosmolar Nonketotic State

STANLEY VAN DEN NOORT, M.D.

Professor and Chairman, Department of Neurology, University of California, Irvine, College of Medicine, Irvine; University of California, Irvine, Medical Center, Orange; Veterans Affairs Medical Center, Long Beach, California
Parkinson's Disease

L. GEORGE VEASY, M.D.

Professor of Pediatrics, University of Utah School of Medicine; Primary Children's Medical Center, Salt Lake City, Utah
Rheumatic Fever

JOAN VON FELDT, M.D.

Assistant Professor of Medicine, University of Pennsylvania School of Medicine; Hospital of the University of Pennsylvania, Philadelphia, Pennsylvania
Connective Tissue Disorders (Systemic Lupus Erythematosus, Dermatomyositis, and Scleroderma)

CHRISTINE A. WANKE, M.D.

Assistant Professor of Medicine, Harvard Medical School; Infectious Disease Division, Beth Israel Deaconess Medical Center, Boston, Massachusetts
Acute Infectious Diarrhea

ROBERT W. WARREN, M.D., PH.D., M.P.H.

Associate Professor and Head of the Section of Rheumatology, Department of Pediatrics, Baylor College of Medicine; Chief of Rheumatology Service, Texas Children's Hospital, Houston, Texas
Juvenile Rheumatoid Arthritis

BARBARA WATSON, M.B., CH.B.

Pediatrics/Infectious Diseases, Albert Einstein Medical Center; Immunization Specialist, Philadelphia Department of Public Health, Philadelphia, Pennsylvania
Varicella (Chickenpox, Herpes Zoster)

FRED A. WEAVER, M.D.

Associate Professor of Surgery, University of Southern California School of Medicine; Attending Staff, USC University Hospital, Los Angeles County/USC Medical Center, Los Angeles, California
Peripheral Arterial Disease

W. DOUGLAS WEAVER, M.D.

Division Head, Cardiovascular Medicine, and Co-Director, Henry Ford Heart and Vascular Institute, Detroit, Michigan
Acute Myocardial Infarction

IAIN J. WEBB, M.D.

Instructor in Medicine, Harvard Medical School; Medical Director, Cell Manipulation and Gene Transfer Laboratories, Dana-Farber Cancer Institute, Boston, Massachusetts
Multiple Myeloma

HOWARD L. WEINER, M.D.

Robert L. Kroc Professor of Neurology, Harvard Medical School; Co-Director, Center for Neurologic Diseases, and Director, Multiple Sclerosis Program, Brigham and Women's Hospital, Boston, Massachusetts
Multiple Sclerosis

LISA S. WEINSTOCK, M.D.

Instructor in Psychiatry, Cornell University Medical College, New York; Assistant Director, Anxiety and Depression Clinic, and Coordinator, Perinatal and Reproductive Psychiatry Service, New York Hospital–Cornell Medical Center–Westchester Division, White Plains, New York
Premenstrual Dysphonic Disorder

TONY WEN, M.D.

Assistant Professor, Division of Maternal Fetal Medicine, Department of Obstetrics and Gynecology, University of Texas Health Science Center at San Antonio, San Antonio, Texas
Postpartum Care

PAUL J. WENDEL, M.D.

Assistant Professor, Assistant Residency Director, and Director of Outpatient Obstetrical Services, University of Arkansas for Medical Sciences, Little Rock, Arkansas
Antepartum Care

VICTORIA P. WERTH, M.D.

Associate Professor of Dermatology and Medicine, University of Pennsylvania School of Medicine; Hospital of the University of Pennsylvania and Veterans Affairs Hospital, Philadelphia, Pennsylvania
Connective Tissue Disorders (Systemic Lupus Erythematosus, Dermatomyositis, and Scleroderma)

MARTHA V. WHITE, M.D.

Director of Research, Institute for Asthma and Allergy at Washington Hospital Center, Washington, D.C.
Asthma in Children

RUSSELL D. WHITE, M.D.

Clinical Associate Professor, University of South Florida College of Medicine, Tampa; Associate Director, Family Practice Residency, and Director, Sports Medicine Fellowship Program, Bayfront Medical Center, St. Petersburg, Florida
Common Sports Injuries

ROGER C. WIGGINS, M.B., B.CHIR.

Professor of Internal Medicine, University of Michigan Medical School; Professor of Internal Medicine and Chief, Nephrology Division, University of Michigan Health System, Ann Arbor, Michigan
Primary Glomerular Diseases

HAROLD A. WILLIAMSON, JR., M.D., M.S.P.H.

Professor of Family and Community Medicine, University of Missouri–Columbia School of Medicine; University of Missouri Health Sciences Center, Columbia, Missouri
Acute Bronchitis

SIDNEY J. WINAWER, M.D.

Professor of Medicine, Cornell University Medical College; Chairman, Cancer Prevention Control, Memorial Sloan-Kettering Cancer Center, New York, New York
Tumors of the Colon and Rectum

HUNG N. WINN, M.D.

Professor of Obstetrics and Gynecology, Director of Maternal-Fetal Medicine, and Chief of Obstetrics, St. Louis University School of Medicine; Chief of Obstetrics, St. Mary's Health Center, St. Louis, Missouri
Vaginal Bleeding Beyond the First Trimester of Pregnancy

PETER WINSTANLEY, M.D.

Reader in Clinical Pharmacology, Department of Pharmacology and Therapeutics, University of Liverpool; Consultant Physician, Royal Liverpool University Hospital, Liverpool, England
Malaria

J. H. WINTER, M.D.
Honorary Senior Lecturer, Department of Medicine, University of Dundee; Consultant Physician, Kings Cross Hospital, Dundee, Scotland
Psittacosis (Ornithosis)

JOSEPH A. WITKOWSKI, M.D.
Clinical Professor of Dermatology, University of Pennsylvania School of Medicine, and Professor of Dermatology, Pennsylvania College of Podiatric Medicine, Philadelphia, Pennsylvania
Pressure Ulcers

JOHN E. WOLF, JR., M.D.
Professor and Chairman, Department of Dermatology, Baylor College of Medicine; Chief of Dermatology Service, Methodist Hospital and Ben Taub General Hospital, Houston, Texas
Contact Dermatitis

STEVEN E. WOLF, M.D.
Assistant Professor of Surgery, University of Texas Medical Branch; Staff Surgeon, Shriners Hospital for Crippled Children, Galveston Burn Unit, Galveston, Texas
Burns

SIN-YEW WONG, M.B.B.S., M.MED.
Clinical Senior Lecturer, Department of Medicine, National University of Singapore; Clinical Director, Communicable Disease Centre; Head, Department of Infectious Diseases, Tan Tock Seng Hospital, Singapore
Toxoplasmosis

CHARLES F. WOOLEY, M.D.
Professor of Medicine, Division of Cardiology, Ohio State University College of Medicine; Ohio State University Medical Center, Columbus, Ohio
Mitral Valve Prolapse

VIRGIL D. WOOTEN, M.D.
Director, Sleep Disorders Center of Greater Cincinnati, Cincinnati, Ohio
Insomnia

JOACHIM YAHALOM, M.D.
Professor of Radiation Oncology, Cornell University Medical College; Member, Memorial Sloan-Kettering Cancer Center, New York, New York
Hodgkin's Disease: Radiation Therapy

LEMAN YEL, M.D.
Fellow, Division of Clinical Immunology, Department of Pediatrics, University of Tennessee, Memphis, College of Medicine, Memphis, Tennessee
Allergic Reactions to Drugs

JAMES B. YOUNG, M.D.
Medical Director, Kaufman Center for Heart Failure, and Head, Section of Heart Failure and Cardiac Transplant Medicine, Cleveland Clinic Foundation, Cleveland, Ohio
Pericarditis

WILLIAM F. YOUNG, JR., M.D.
Associate Professor of Medicine, Mayo Medical School; Consultant, Divisions of Hypertension, Endocrinology, and Internal Medicine, Mayo Clinic, Rochester, Minnesota
Pheochromocytoma

VICTOR L. YU, M.D.
Professor of Medicine, University of Pittsburgh School of Medicine; Chief, Infectious Disease Section, Veterans Affairs Medical Center, Pittsburgh, Pennsylvania
Legionellosis (Legionnaires' Disease and Pontiac Fever)

Preface

This is the 51st edition of *Current Therapy,* which was started by Howard Conn in 1949. I have been privileged to edit the last 16 editions, which have maintained Howard's original goal of providing physicians with up-to-date information on disease management in a format that makes material easy to find and assimilate. He also established the policy of inviting new authors each year so that the material remains as fresh and current as possible. This year is no exception, with 85% of the chapters written by new authors and the remaining 15% thoroughly updated.

Annual updating is essential if the practicing physician is to use this as a source for remaining current with the rapid advances in medicine. Take, for example, the recent changes in immunization requirements, management of patients with human immunodeficiency virus infection, chemotherapy of Hodgkin's disease, or treatments for Alzheimer's disease, impotence, and mood disorders.

Although most of the problems discussed in this book focus on diseases encountered in the United States, a significant number are primarily diseases of other countries that are of increasing importance to physicians in the United States because of international travel. Physicians in other countries may have more experience treating diseases such as malaria, cholera, leprosy, or trichinosis. Sometimes the world authority on a disease common in the United States is a citizen of another country, adding a fresh dimension to our usual method of treatment. This year 29 chapters are written by authorities in countries that include Belgium, France, India, Italy, Israel, Japan, Spain, and Sweden.

New topics added this year are cat-scratch disease, cystic fibrosis, and trypanosomiasis. Inflammatory bowel disease is also new, representing a combining of ulcerative colitis and Crohn's disease.

Because each year a new authority discusses his or her method of treating the problem, the reader is encouraged to compare the treatments presented in previous editions to see how different experts manage the same problem. The full institutional affiliation of each contributor is given if additional information or follow-up is needed.

The index has been painstakingly prepared to ensure completeness and to facilitate the rapid recovery of information. Many tables are used to give a maximum amount of information in the most concise manner.

My special thanks to Caroline Kosnik, my editorial assistant, who sees that all deadlines are met and that the book is published on time. It is also a pleasure to work with Ray Kersey and the excellent staff at W.B. Saunders, whose dedication to quality ensures that this book remains a valuable asset to physicians and their patients.

ROBERT E. RAKEL, M.D.

NOTICE

Medicine is an ever-changing field. Standard safety precautions must be followed, but as new research and clinical experience broaden our knowledge, changes in treatment and drug therapy become necessary or appropriate. Readers are advised to check the product information currently provided by the manufacturer of each drug to be administered to verify the recommended dose, the method and duration of administration, and the contraindications. It is the responsibility of the treating physician, relying on experience and knowledge of the patient, to determine dosages and the best treatment for the patient. Neither the publisher nor the editor assumes any responsibility for any injury and/or damage to persons or property.

THE PUBLISHER

Contents

SECTION 1. SYMPTOMATIC CARE PENDING DIAGNOSIS

SECTION 2. THE INFECTIOUS DISEASES

SECTION 3. THE RESPIRATORY SYSTEM

SECTION 4. THE CARDIOVASCULAR SYSTEM

SECTION 5. THE BLOOD AND SPLEEN

SECTION 6. THE DIGESTIVE SYSTEM

SECTION 7. METABOLIC DISORDERS

SECTION 8. THE ENDOCRINE SYSTEM

SECTION 9. THE UROGENITAL TRACT

SECTION 10. THE SEXUALLY TRANSMITTED DISEASES

SECTION 11. DISEASES OF ALLERGY

SECTION 12. DISEASES OF THE SKIN

SECTION 13. THE NERVOUS SYSTEM

SECTION 14. THE LOCOMOTOR SYSTEM

SECTION 15. OBSTETRICS AND GYNECOLOGY

SECTION 16. PSYCHIATRIC DISORDERS

SECTION 17. PHYSICAL AND CHEMICAL INJURIES

SECTION 18. APPENDICES AND INDEX

Section 1

Symptomatic Care Pending Diagnosis

PAIN

method of
JAMES N. ROGERS, M.D.
University of Texas Health Science Center at San Antonio
San Antonio, Texas

Pain is one of the biggest fears and a major source of morbidity for patients with cancer. Pain is common in cancer and becomes a significant factor in limiting the patient's function. Clinical experience suggests that patients with cancer pain are treated most effectively with a multidisciplinary approach, which may include appropriate analgesic drugs, multiple physical modalities, neurosurgical and anesthetic procedures, psychologic intervention, and supportive care. The goals of pain therapy for a cancer patient are significant relief of pain to maintain the functional status chosen by the patient, a reasonable quality of life, and, when applicable, a death relatively free of pain.

INCIDENCE

In the United States, approximately 1 million new cases of cancer will be diagnosed and approximately 510,000 deaths from cancer will occur yearly. Moderate-to-severe pain occurs in about 40 to 50% of patients with early or intermediate stage cancer and in 60 to 90% of patients with advanced cancer. It is estimated that cancer-related pain afflicts approximately 1.1 million Americans annually. Approximately 70 to 95% of terminal cancer patients have frequent or persistent pain before death. Pain varies by the stage, type, and site of the neoplasm. Pain is experienced by approximately 85% of patients with primary bone tumors, 70% of patients with cancer of the genitourinary tract, 50% of patients with breast cancer, 45% of patients with lung cancer, 20% of patients with lymphoma, and 5% of patients with leukemia. The prevalence of pain secondary to cancer is likely to continue to increase owing to multiple factors. These factors include longer survival times due to new cancer treatments that result in the increased likelihood of complex pain problems, increased prevalence of metastatic disease, and increased incidence of cancer secondary to an aging population.

PAIN ASSESSMENT

Failure to assess pain is a major reason for undertreatment. In fact, 76% of physicians have reported that poor pain assessment is the single most important barrier to adequate pain control. Lack of communication between those treating the cancer and those managing the pain contributes to inadequate treatment of pain. Effective communication is often a problem for patients, particularly elderly ones. Many patients see the pain associated with cancer as inevitable, and 70% have reported that cancer pain is a reason to stop life-prolonging treatment or a justifiable reason for committing suicide. More than 50% thought that cancer patients usually die a painful death. Many of these patients also have misconceptions about opioid analgesics. They feel that when opioid analgesics are prescribed, the active treatment of their disease is finished and they are near death. Because of these factors, cancer patients are often reluctant to discuss their pain with physicians and with their families. Reporting pain may also be viewed as a weakness or as drug-seeking behavior. Many patients may be afraid to report pain because of fear of the return of the cancer or of the treatments that may be necessary. Patients need to be taught that their pain can be treated effectively. They should be taught how to assess their pain and the efficacy of treatment and especially how to communicate with caregivers by using language, numeric scales, and visual scales. A standardized pain assessment protocol can improve communication among members of the health care team and patients (Figure 1).

EVALUATION

The initial evaluation of a cancer pain patient should include a detailed history and a thorough physical examination. Particular attention should be paid to the neurologic examination and the psychosocial evaluation. Determination of the source of the pain is important in developing the most effective treatment plan. Several different processes may cause pain in cancer patients. Pain secondary to direct tumor invasion is present in about 78% of cancer inpatients and about 62% of outpatients. Pain can result from infiltration of surrounding structures such as nerves, muscles, and visceral organs or from metastasis. Bony metastasis is responsible for pain in up to 50% of cancer patients. About one fourth of cancer pain is due to the treatment of the disease. Surgical procedures, radiotherapy, and chemotherapy can all induce pain syndromes. Postmastectomy syndrome, post-thoracotomy syndrome, and phantom pain syndrome can occur after surgery, even curative surgery. Radiation therapy can cause fibrosis, myelopathies, bony necrosis, and radiation-induced tumors. Chemotherapeutic agents can cause diffuse neuropathies, aseptic necrosis of joints, and postherpetic neuralgia. It is important to remember that not all the pain experienced by a patient with cancer results from the disease or its treatment. The presence of cancer does not make the patient immune to the other common causes of pain. Localized infections can cause pain and may be difficult to iden-

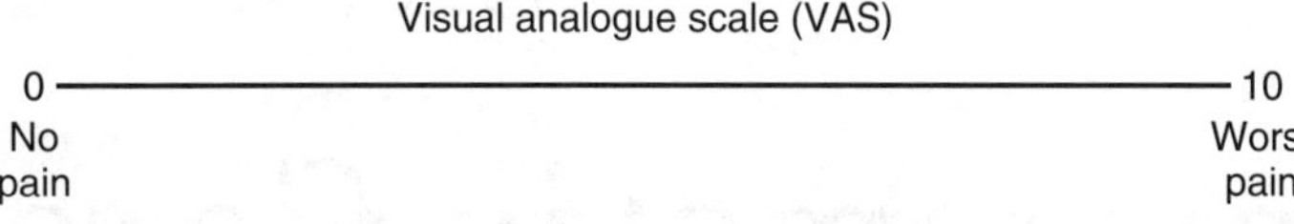

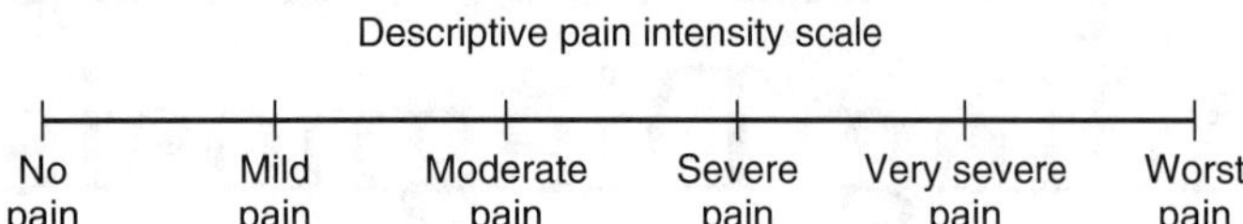

Figure 1. Pain assessment tools.

tify, particularly in patients with head and neck tumors. Fever and an increased white blood cell count may not be present because of the effects of the cancer or its treatment. Other causes of pain may include osteoporosis, degenerative joint disease, diabetic neuropathies, claudication, myofascial pain, and headaches. These pain syndromes should be treated aggressively as well.

PSYCHOSOCIAL EVALUATION

The various contributions of psychosocial factors, psychologic characteristics, and environmental factors to pain manifestations are poorly understood. No set of psychologic characteristics correlates with the development, exacerbation, and/or maintenance of cancer pain. This lack of consistency, however, does not preclude the role of psychologic factors in cancer pain. Anxiety and depression are often associated with an increase in pain intensity. The patient's social situation should be evaluated to ensure adequate support at home. Home hospice care should be considered when patients have less than 6 months of life expectancy. Hospice care can be especially helpful in providing terminally ill patients with pain relief and family support.

PHARMACOTHERAPY

Drug therapy is the cornerstone of the cancer pain management therapies. It is effective, inexpensive, and relatively low risk. It should be remembered that pain is an individual experience and that the treatment regimen should be individualized for each patient. Before one chooses drugs to treat the pain, it is important to identify the specific causes of the pain and then select the drugs accordingly. The three major classes of drugs used in managing cancer pain are nonsteroidal anti-inflammatory drugs (NSAIDs), opioids, and adjuvant analgesics. It is best to choose the simplest dosage schedule. In 1990 the World Health Organization (WHO) devised a simple, well-validated, and effective therapy rationale for the treatment of cancer pain. The WHO ladder has been shown to be effective in relieving pain in 90% of patients with cancer (Figure 2).

The essential features of this analgesic ladder are by mouth, by the clock, by the ladder, individualization, and attention to detail. It is important to remember that elderly patients are at increased risk for drug-drug and drug-disease interactions. Close attention to doses, concurrent medications, and side effects is required.

Nonsteroidal Anti-inflammatory Drugs

The first rung of the ladder is the use of NSAIDs for mild to moderate levels of pain. NSAIDs are effective and often are easily obtained. They do not produce tolerance or dependence (physical or psychologic) the way narcotics can. Pain relief occurs because of inhibition of the arachidonic acid cascade, reducing the levels of inflammatory mediators. Although there may be a central action of NSAIDs, they do not activate opioid receptors. NSAIDs therefore produce analgesia by a different mechanism. The concurrent use of NSAIDs or acetaminophen with opioids often produces a greater level of analgesia than does the use of either drug class alone. Acetaminophen is included in this group because even though it is not an anti-inflammatory drug, it has similar analgesic effects and pharmacologic characteristics.

Although effective, NSAIDs are more likely to cause gastric and renal toxicity in elderly patients. Platelet inhibition may pose a significant bleeding risk in elderly patients, who are already at greater

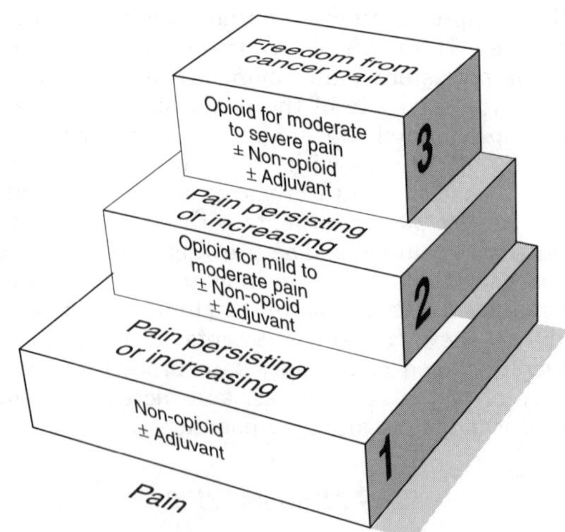

Figure 2. WHO analgesic ladder for cancer pain management. (Reproduced by permission of WHO from Cancer Pain Relief, 2nd ed. Geneva, World Health Organization, 1996.)

risk of sustaining falls. Aspirin causes an irreversible inhibition of platelet aggregation. Acetaminophen and the nonacetylated salicylates such as salsalate (Disalcid), sodium salicylate, and choline magnesium trisalicylate (Trilisate) do not affect platelet function and do not alter bleeding times. Other NSAIDs produce a reversible platelet inhibition. With the exception of acetaminophen and the nonacetylated salicylates, NSAIDs should be avoided in patients who are thrombocytopenic, have a bleeding disorder, or are at risk for falls or other injuries. Besides bleeding, the adverse effects of NSAIDs include renal failure, hepatic dysfunction, and gastric ulceration. The addition of a gastric protective agent such as misoprostol (Cytotec) may reduce the risk of gastric ulceration. No single NSAID has been shown to be superior to others in providing pain relief. It is also impossible to predict which NSAID will be best tolerated by an individual patient. When a specific agent has been selected, it should be titrated until pain relief is obtained. If the maximal dose has been reached or the side effects become intolerable, another NSAID should be selected. NSAIDs exhibit a ceiling effect to their efficacy, and exceeding the recommended maximal dose usually is not helpful. The choice of an NSAID should be based on efficacy, safety, and expense. In general, the least expensive NSAID should be chosen.

Narcotics

Opioids are the mainstay of management for moderate to severe cancer pain. They are very effective, are easily titratable, and have a favorable risk-benefit ratio. Commonly used opioids include morphine, hydromorphone (Dilaudid), codeine, oxycodone (Roxicodone), hydrocodone, methadone, levorphanol, and fentanyl. Opioid drugs are classified by their activity at opioid receptors. Full-agonist opioids do not have a ceiling to their analgesic efficacy. Partial agonists such as buprenorphine (Buprenex) have a lower intrinsic activity at opioid receptors and demonstrate a ceiling effect to analgesia. Mixed agonist-antagonists also exhibit a ceiling effect to analgesia. Patients who are receiving full-agonist opioids should not be given mixed agonist-antagonist drugs because this may precipitate withdrawal symptoms and increase pain.

Meperidine (Demerol) should not be used on a continuous basis for cancer pain management. Normeperidine, the metabolite of meperidine, accumulates when meperidine is used for more than several days and can cause central nervous system (CNS) stimulation that can result in seizures.

Opioid dosage titration requires the physician to take into account not only the analgesic effects but also the side effects that may occur. Besides cognitive impairment, opioid side effects that may be present include urinary retention, constipation, intestinal obstruction, respiratory depression, and exacerbation of Parkinson's disease. Opioid tolerance and physical dependence can be expected with long-term opioid pain management and should not be confused with psychologic dependence (addiction). Opioid tolerance may require an increased dose to achieve the same level of pain relief over time. Progressive disease is more likely to require a dose increase. Physical dependence may manifest as anxiety, irritability, chills, hot flashes, joint pain, lacrimation, rhinorrhea, diaphoresis, nausea, vomiting, abdominal cramps, and diarrhea if opioids are withdrawn. Mild withdrawal symptoms may resemble a viral flulike syndrome. The correct dose of an opioid should be one that controls pain with the fewest side effects. Medication should be scheduled to prevent pain rather than allowing pain to break through. Side effects should be treated aggressively. Constipation is a common problem and should be treated prophylactically. Increased fiber and mild laxatives should be administered on a regular schedule. A stimulating cathartic or hyperosmotic agent may be necessary to treat severe constipation. Antiemetics may be needed for opioid-induced nausea and vomiting but may increase sedation and other CNS side effects in the elderly.

Adjuvants

Adjuvant agents can be used to enhance the analgesic effects of opioids or to treat other symptoms of the disease or the side effects of the opioids. They can be used at any point on the WHO ladder. Tricyclic antidepressants* are helpful in treating pain of neuropathic origin, potentiating opioid analgesia, and elevating mood. Orthostatic hypotension, anticholinergic side effects (dry mouth, constipation, urinary retention), and sedation can be significant problems. The most extensive experience has been with amitriptyline. Treatment should be started at a low dose (10 to 25 mg orally) and increased slowly as tolerated. This approach minimizes the risk of falling from orthostatic hypotension.

Anticonvulsants are also useful in treating neuropathic pain, which is often described as lancinating, shooting, and burning pain. Anticonvulsants are thought to provide pain relief by suppressing spontaneous neuronal firing. Carbamazepine* (Tegretol) should be used with caution in patients receiving bone marrow–suppressive chemotherapeutic agents. Systemically administered local anesthetic-antiarrhythmic agents such as intravenous lidocaine, oral mexiletine* (Mexitil), and tocainide* (Tonocard) have also been used to treat neuropathic pain, although there is no current Food and Drug Administration (FDA)–approved indication for these drugs for pain. Psychostimulants such as dextroamphetamine* (Dexedrine) and methylphenidate* (Ritalin) can be used to improve opioid analgesia and treat excessive sedation from opioid medications. Antihistamines may reduce anxiety, insomnia, and nausea. Corticosteroids may elevate mood and provide anti-inflam-

*Not FDA approved for this indication.

matory, antiemetic, and appetite stimulation effects in cancer patients.

ROUTES OF ADMINISTRATION

The oral route of administration should be the preferred route for delivering analgesic medications. It is the most convenient and cost-effective method of administration. If the patient cannot take analgesic medications orally, other minimally invasive routes, such as rectal or transdermal, should be tried. Fentanyl, a synthetic opioid, is available in a transdermal delivery system that provides up to 3 days of constant, steady serum blood levels. NSAIDs, opioids, and many adjuvant agents are available in both oral and suppository preparations. If noninvasive routes are not tolerated or dose requirements make it impossible to meet the patient's analgesic needs, more invasive routes of administration may be used. These include the intravenous, subcutaneous, epidural, and intraspinal routes. These routes have been used primarily to deliver opioid medications, although adjuvant agents such as local anesthetics, clonidine, and baclofen have also been administered in this manner. Intramuscular administration should be avoided because it is painful and inconvenient and because absorption is unreliable. A major advantage of epidural and intrathecal narcotic management is the opportunity to perform a preimplantation trial. An epidural or intrathecal drug delivery system should not be considered without verification that it will alleviate the patient's pain. Preimplantation considerations should include a successful trial, no active infection, and no clotting disorders. Behavioral and psychologic abnormalities may interfere with the assessment of pain relief. Cost is a factor that should not be overlooked. Support systems, concurrent therapies, and life expectancy should be evaluated before one considers implantation. Standard percutaneous epidural catheters can be used to provide short-term pain relief. Subcutaneous tunneling of epidural and intrathecal catheters is useful in patients in whom several weeks to months of pain relief are necessary. Infection is a major concern, and careful attention to sterile technique is crucial. Prophylactic antibiotics should be considered during the placement of implanted systems. In patients with a life expectancy greater than 3 to 6 months, it is cost-effective to place a totally implantable infusion pump. With careful patient selection and screening, continuous intraspinal drug infusion of morphine has been especially helpful in managing lower body pain in up to 90% of patients.

INVASIVE THERAPIES

Noninvasive treatments should be exhausted before invasive approaches are attempted. Neurolytic peripheral neural blockade should be considered only after more conservative therapeutic modalities for treating the patient's pain have proved to be inadequate, poorly tolerated, or clinically inappropriate.

Nerve blocks with local anesthetics can be used to identify the source of the pain and provide prognostic information to predict the outcome of permanent neurolysis. Peripheral neurolysis can be accomplished by means of the injection of neurolytic agents such as alcohol and phenol or by means of thermocoagulation or cryoanalgesic techniques. Pancreatic cancer is particularly responsive to neurolytic celiac plexus blockage. Complications from neurolytic blockade may include hypotension, paresis, paralysis, and bowel or bladder dysfunction. If a patient becomes pain-free after neurolysis, narcotics should not be stopped abruptly, as this may precipitate narcotic withdrawal. Opioids should be tapered slowly to avoid withdrawal.

SUMMARY

Patients with cancer require comprehensive assessment and aggressive management of their pain. Issues that are important when treating cancer pain include the following.

Concurrent Medical Diseases and Noncancerous Pain. Patients often suffer from a wide variety of chronic diseases and may be on complex medication regimens that increase their risk of drug-drug and drug-disease interactions.

Physical and Cognitive Impairment. Pain assessment may be more difficult in patients with physical and cognitive impairment. It may be necessary to use behavior-based assessment tools to evaluate pain levels and the efficacy of pain management. Family members can also be taught how to assess pain.

Side Effects. Elderly patients are more likely to develop side effects from NSAIDs because of impaired metabolism and excretion related to age. Alternative NSAIDs with fewer gastrointestinal effects, such as choline magnesium trisalicylate, or the addition of misoprostol should be considered to reduce the risk of gastric toxicity. Increasing the dosage beyond the recommended dose is unlikely to improve pain relief and increases the risk of side effects. A different NSAID should be chosen if the first compound is poorly tolerated or if pain is not relieved.

Efficacy of Opioids. Opioids can provide significant pain relief in patients with cancer. Older patients may be more sensitive to opioids because the peak opioid effect is higher and the duration of pain relief is longer. The initial dosing requires caution and careful titration to achieve pain relief, and the patient should be monitored frequently for undesirable side effects.

Adjuvant Agents. Adjuvant agents are used to enhance analgesia and lessen side effects in pain patients. When these agents are combined with NSAIDs and opioids, cancer pain can often be relieved satisfactorily with a minimum of complications.

Route of Administration. The oral route is the preferred route of administration. In some patients, however, this route cannot be used. Alternatives include the rectal, subcutaneous, transdermal, intravenous, and intraspinal routes. Intramuscular injections should not be used to administer medication on a long-term basis.

Invasive Procedures. Invasive procedures such as peripheral and central neurolytic blockade and neuroablative surgical procedures should be considered only when other conservative methods have failed or the side effects cannot be tolerated. When appropriate, invasive procedures can alleviate pain and reduce opioid requirements. Informed consent is critical. The effects of permanent neurologic interruption may be more undesirable to the patient than is the pain itself.

Cancer pain can be treated adequately in most patients with careful use of medications, following the WHO analgesic ladder: NSAIDs for mild to moderate pain and increasingly potent opioids for more severe pain. Adjuvant agents can be used at any point on the ladder to enhance analgesia, treat side effects, and elevate mood. Each patient should have an individual pain management plan developed to allow for individual variations in the pain experience. Frequent reassessment of the pain management regimen is necessary to ensure continued adequate analgesia and monitoring for potentially devastating side effects. With care, most patients can receive significant relief of pain with minimal and tolerable side effects.

NAUSEA AND VOMITING

method of
MARTIN J. EDELMAN, M.D.,
DONALD F. LUM, M.D., and
DAVID R. GANDARA, M.D.
University of California, Davis
Sacramento, California
VA Northern California Health Care System
Martinez, California

Nausea and vomiting are common symptoms that occur throughout life. These symptoms may reflect benign, self-limiting illnesses or more serious, debilitating diseases. Nausea is a vague sensation of sickness or "queasiness" that refers to the urge to vomit. Vomiting refers to the expulsion of gastric contents up through and out of the mouth. This occurs by a forceful, sustained contraction of abdominal muscles and the diaphragm through a relaxed lower esophageal sphincter and contracted pylorus. Retching is the rhythmic movement of vomiting without expulsion of gastric contents (dry heaves). It consists of spasmodic respiratory and abdominal movements and often culminates in vomiting. Vomiting should be distinguished from regurgitation, which refers to the act by which gastric contents are brought back into the mouth without the motor and autonomic activity that characterizes vomiting. Regurgitation is a symptom of free gastroesophageal reflux or an obstructed esophagus, whether obstructed mechanically from a benign or malignant stricture or physiologically from an esophageal motility disorder.

Control of vomiting occurs in the vomiting center, which is felt to arise within the lateral reticular formation, adjacent to the medulla oblongata areas, that coordinates respiratory, salivary, and vasomotor centers and the vagus nervous innervation of the gastrointestinal tract. The vomiting center can be stimulated by four different sources of afferent input, which include the following:

1. The chemoreceptor trigger zone: located in the area postrema on the floor of the fourth ventricle. This area has chemoreceptors that are responsive to various drugs and chemotherapeutic agents, toxins, hypoxia, uremia, acidosis, and radiation therapy. Evidence suggests that type 3 serotonin, dopamine D2, and neurokinin-1 (NK-1) receptors as well as other neurotransmitters such as norepinephrine, glutamate, histamine, and endorphins play a role in mediating vomiting in the chemoreceptor trigger zone.
2. Higher central nervous system (CNS) centers: CNS disorders or certain smells, sights, or previously emotional experiences may result in nausea and vomiting.
3. The vestibular system: often stimulated by infections and motion. These fibers have high concentrations of muscarinic, cholinergic, and histamine H_1 receptors.
4. Afferent vagal fibers and splanchnic fibers from gastrointestinal viscera: often stimulated by gastrointestinal or biliary distention, peritoneal or mucosal irritation, or intra-abdominal infections.

Although nausea and vomiting may be evoked by disorders of the gastrointestinal tract, they may also reflect neurologic, psychogenic, endocrine, metabolic, toxic, or iatrogenic conditions and are common symptoms of pediatric illnesses (Table 1). Whereas nausea has few serious physical consequences, prolonged vomiting can lead to volume depletion, electrolyte depletion, acid-base disorders, malnutrition, pulmonary aspiration, esophageal rupture (Boerhaave's syndrome), and gastrointestinal hemorrhage secondary to mucosal tear at the gastroesophageal junction (Mallory-Weiss tear).

CLINICAL FINDINGS

Symptoms and Signs. A thorough medical history and physical examination are essential to determine the etiology of nausea and vomiting. Acute onset of symptoms without abdominal pain is typically associated with infectious causes (gastroenteritis, food poisoning) or medications. In these instances, a careful history should be taken, focusing on recent medications; food ingestions; related viral symptoms of fever, diarrhea, and malaise; and similar illnesses in family members or coworkers. The acute onset of pain suggests visceral involvement associated with peritoneal inflammation, pancreatobiliary illnesses, or intestinal obstruction. Special attention to the physical examination may reveal tympany, focal tenderness, rebound, and guarding.

Chronic nausea or vomiting may suggest gastric outlet obstruction, gastroparesis, intestinal dysmotility, psychogenic disorders, CNS diseases, pregnancy, or other systemic disorders. In these instances, the timing of the eme-

TABLE 1. **Causes of Nausea and Vomiting**

Acute Nausea and Vomiting

Pediatric

- Atresia
- Feeding disorder
- Foreign body
- Gastroesophageal reflux
- Hirschsprung's disease
- Intussusception
- Meconium-ileus
- Meningitis
- Necrotizing enterocolitis
- Peritonitis
- Pyloric stenosis
- Reye's syndrome
- Subdural hematoma
- Tracheoesophageal fistula
- Volvulus or malrotation of gut

Infections

- Viral gastroenteritis (Norwalk agent, rotavirus)
- Toxin-mediated (food poisoning)
  - *Staphylococcus aureus*
  - *Bacillus cereus*
  - *Clostridium perfringens*
- Acute systemic infections
- Infections in immunocompromised hosts

Central Nervous System

- Motion sickness
- Labyrinthitis (Meniere's)
- Migraine headaches
- Central nervous system (CNS) trauma
- CNS tumors or pseudotumors
- Meningitis, encephalitis, abscess
- Epilepsy

Gastrointestinal Mechanical Obstruction

- Acute gastric outlet obstruction
  - Pyloric channel ulcer (peptic ulcer disease)
- Constipation
  - Fecal impaction
  - Obstipation
- Extrinsic small bowel obstruction
- Incarcerated hernia
- Volvulus
- Adhesions
- Internal hernias
- Superior mesenteric artery syndrome
- Ileus
  - Postoperative
  - Medical illness
  - Gallstone

Visceral Pain

- Appendicitis
- Acute pancreatitis
- Acute cholecystitis
- Hepatitis
- Peritonitis from any cause
- Mesenteric ischemia

Systemic Conditions

- Pregnancy
- Myocardial infarction
- Renal failure
- Diabetic ketoacidosis
- Hypercalcemia
- Hyperparathyroidism
- Graft-versus-host disease

Iatrogenic

- Chemotherapeutic agents
- Radiation therapy
- Surgery
- Heavy ethanol ingestion
- Medications
  - Nonsteroidal anti-inflammatory drugs
  - Antibiotics
  - Digoxin
  - Theophylline
  - Narcotics
  - Niacin

Chronic Nausea and Vomiting

Gastrointestinal Mechanical Obstruction

- Chronic gastric outlet obstruction
  - Chronic peptic ulcer disease
  - Gastric malignancy
  - Crohn's disease with duodenal stricture
  - Pancreatic malignancy
- Small intestinal obstruction
- Peritoneal carcinomatosis

Motility Disorders

- Gastroparesis
  - Diabetes mellitus
  - Collagen vascular disorders (scleroderma)
  - Postgastric surgery
  - Idiopathic or iatrogenic
- Small intestine motility disorders
  - Chronic intestinal pseudo-obstruction
  - Paraneoplastic syndromes
  - Amyloidosis

Psychogenic

- Anorexia nervosa
- Bulimia
- Psychogenic, anxiety

Miscellaneous

- Increased intracranial pressure
- Pseudotumor
- Metabolic: hyperthyroidism, renal failure, Addison's disease
- Medications (cardiac glycosides, narcotics, theophylline)
- Pregnancy
- Idiopathic cyclic vomiting

sis in relation to meals and the nature of vomiting may provide clues to the specific etiology. Vomiting immediately after meals suggests bulimia or other psychogenic causes but may also occur in peptic ulcer disease with associated pyloric stenosis. Vomiting undigested food 1 hour or more after meals may be seen in esophageal dysmotility (achalasia), gastroparesis (diabetic, postvagotomy), or gastric outlet obstruction from malignancies (gastric or pancreatic) or peptic ulcer disease. Early morning vomiting may suggest pregnancy, alcoholism, or uremia. Vomiting associated with headache, neck stiffness, vertigo, paresthesias, or neuromuscular weakness may be related to CNS disorders and other causes of increased intracranial pressure. In these patients, a careful neurologic and funduscopic examination is essential.

Orthostatic vital signs, along with skin turgor and appearance of mucous membranes, should be checked to rule out volume depletion. Malnutrition and weight loss suggest more chronic conditions such as malignancy, inflammatory bowel disease, or scleroderma. Tympany and abdominal distention raise the suspicion of small intestinal obstruction. A succussion splash is usually present with gastric outlet obstruction or severe gastroparesis. A check of hernia orifices should be performed with careful attention to previous surgical scars.

Laboratory Findings. Depending on the clinical presentation, laboratory studies should include serum electrolytes, glucose, calcium, amylase, lipase, creatinine, liver panel, and β-human chorionic gonadotropin for females of child-bearing age. Protracted vomiting may result in various metabolic imbalances, including metabolic alkalosis, hypokalemia, hyponatremia, and prerenal azotemia.

Special Examinations. In addition to routine laboratory data, flat and upright plain films of the abdomen may be indicated to look for intestinal obstruction or free peritoneal air. In patients with suspected obstruction, a nasogastric tube may be inserted to relieve symptoms. Aspiration of more than 200 mL of gastric fluid in a patient who has been fasting suggests gastroparesis or gastric outlet obstruction. One can confirm this with a saline load test (greater than 400 mL residual 30 minutes after 750 mL instillation via nasogastric tube) or, better yet, with upper gastrointestinal endoscopy. Nuclear scintigraphy should be performed when upper endoscopy or barium upper gastrointestinal testing is unrevealing to confirm gastroparesis. Abdominal ultrasound or computed tomography (CT) scanning can be performed if laboratory data suggest hepatobiliary or pancreatic pathology. Head CT or magnetic resonance imaging (MRI) should be considered for suspected CNS disorders.

TREATMENT

General Measures. The treatment of nausea and vomiting should be directed at the underlying etiology as suggested by results of the history, physical examination, laboratory data, and other specific tests. The majority of acute causes are mild, self-limiting illnesses that often require no specific therapy. Patients should maintain hydration by ingesting clear liquids (broth, tea, carbonated beverages, sports beverages such as Gatorade) and small quantities of bland dry food. Hospitalization is required for more severe vomiting that leads to severe volume depletion and subsequent hypokalemia and metabolic alkalosis. Parenteral volume replacement using 0.45% saline with 20 mEq per liter potassium supplementation is often necessary. Placement of a nasogastic tube for suctioning promotes gastric decompression and enables a more accurate assessment of fluid losses.

Pharmacologic. If general measures fail to control the nausea and vomiting, pharmacologic therapy is given to prevent or control vomiting. Given the multitude of etiologies and various mechanisms involved in the control of nausea and vomiting, no single pharmacologic agent is effective in all patients. Table 2 lists many of the antiemetic agents available in the United States. Most of the agents listed are effective for nausea and vomiting due to a variety of etiologies. The type 3 serotonin antagonists are utilized primarily in the prevention and treatment of chemotherapy-, radiation-, and anesthesia-associated nausea and vomiting. They are relatively ineffective in the treatment of motion sickness. Conversely, transdermal scopolamine (Transderm Scōp) is primarily indicated for the treatment of motion sickness. Cisapride (Propulsid) and metoclopramide (Reglan), although effective in treating nausea and vomiting from a variety of causes, are particularly effective in treating gastroparesis-associated disease. Combination therapy with two or more agents from different drug classes is often required, and therapy should be individualized based on the etiology of vomiting. Most of the medications listed in Table 2 should be avoided in pregnancy; however, the use of the dopamine antagonist droperidol and the antihistamine trimethobenzamide (Tigan) are commonly utilized in pregnancy.

CHEMOTHERAPY-INDUCED EMESIS

Cancer chemotherapy is one of the most common causes of iatrogenic nausea and vomiting. Consequently, it is the best studied and serves as the model for other types of treatment-induced nausea and vomiting such as those that are induced by anesthesia or radiotherapy.

Significance of Chemotherapy-Induced Emesis. In addition to patient discomfort, chemotherapy-induced emesis may result in potentially life-threatening complications. Nausea and vomiting induced by chemotherapy may be so significant as to result in patient refusal to receive potentially curative chemotherapy. Before the introduction of the type 3 serotonin antagonist drugs, chemotherapy-induced nausea and vomiting was the most significant concern of cancer patients. In addition, the adverse effects on nutritional status, already frequently compromised as a result of malignancy, may be severely aggravated and may lead to diminished muscle mass, fatigue, and increased susceptibility to infection, with potentially fatal consequences.

Types of Chemotherapy-Induced Emesis. Three patterns of emetic response are associated with chemotherapy. Anticipatory vomiting occurs before therapy and usually, though not always, occurs after an initial adverse outcome (in terms of nausea and vomiting) in a prior cycle of treatment. Immediate vomiting occurs minutes to 24 hours after administration of chemotherapy and is the best understood. It is a result of release of serotonin from enterochromaffin cells in the gut mucosa. The surge in serotonin acts peripherally through the vagus nerve and centrally at the chemoreceptor trigger zone. Delayed vomiting occurs 24 to 120 hours after treatment and is poorly understood. It appears to be mediated at least partially by type 3 serotonin receptors, as some, but not all, studies indicate amelioration of this problem with continued administration of type 3 serotonin antagonists. An accumulating body of evidence implicates substance P, a tachykinin distributed throughout the peripheral and CNS that binds to NK-1 receptors, in this problem. Trials of substance P antagonists in humans are under way.

TABLE 2. **Antiemetic Drugs**

Agents	Dose/Schedule	Route	Cost (U.S.$)*
Phenothiazines			
Prochlorperazine (Compazine)	5–10 mg q 6–8 h	PO, IV, IM	.66/5-mg tab
	25 mg q 6–8 h	PR	
Thiethylperazine (Torecan)	10 mg q 8 h	PO, IV, IM, PR	.54/10-mg tab
Butyrophenones			
Droperidol (Inapsine)	5–15 mg × 1, 2–7.5 mg q 2 h	IV	3.16/5 mg IV
Cannabinoids			
Dronabinol (Marinol)	5–10 mg/m² q 3–4 h	PO	3.16/5-mg tab
Corticosteroids			
Dexamethasone	10–20 mg q 2–6 h	PO, IV	30.55/20 mg IV
Antihistamines			
Diphenhydramine (Benadryl)	50 mg q 4–6 h	IV, PO	1.52/50 mg IV
Substituted benzamides			
Metoclopramide (Reglan)	1–3 mg/kg† q 2 h × 2–5 doses	IV	24.52/150 mg IV
	0.5–3 mg/kg† q 2–6 h	PO	
Benzodiazepines			
Diazepam (Valium)	5 mg q 4 h	PO, IV	2.08/5 ml IV
	1.5–2.5 mg/m² q 4 h	IV, SL	
Lorazepam (Ativan)	1–4 mg q 4 h	PO	12.01/2 mg IV
Type 3 serotonin antagonists			
Ondansetron (Zofran)	32 mg/24 h	IV	206.41/32 mg IV
	8 mg/24 h‡	IV	
	8 mg bid	PO	19.62/8-mg tab
Granisetron (Kytril)	10 μg/kg/24 h	IV	173.95/1 mg IV
	2 mg/24 h	PO	41.28/1-mg tab
Dolasetron (Anzemet)	1.8 mg/kg/24 h	IV	149.88/100 mg IV
	100 mg/24 h	PO	66/100-mg tab
Tropisetron§ (Navoban)	5 mg/24 h	IV	
Prokinetic			
Cisapride (Propulsid)	10 mg 30 min ac and hs	PO	.75/10-mg tab
Anticholinergic			
Scopolamine	1 patch behind ear 30 min before travel	Transdermal	N/A

*Prices based on average wholesale price of brand name product in 1997 U.S. dollars.
†Exceeds dosage recommended by the manufacturer.
‡Recommended dose (see text).
§Not available in the United States.

Drugs Associated with Chemotherapy-Induced Emesis. There is enormous variation in the potential of various drugs to produce an emetic response. Many drugs have little or no emetic potential. In the case of glucocorticoids (e.g., dexamethasone, prednisone), which are integral parts of regimens in lymphoma and myeloma, they are antiemetic. Table 3 lists chemotherapy drugs with their degree of emetic potential. Recent research in antiemetics has focused on the problem of the emetic potential of combination chemotherapy regimens. As it is relatively rare for a patient to be treated with a single agent, it is important to assess the potential of a combination of drugs to produce emesis and prescribe an appropriate antiemetic regimen. A recently elucidated approach for determining the emetic potential of combination chemotherapy regimens is presented in Table 4.

Factors Contributing to Chemotherapy-Induced Emesis. It has long been recognized that patient variables significantly affect the occurrence and severity of chemotherapy-induced emesis. Factors predicting for emesis include female sex, age younger than 40 years, history of emesis associated with pregnancy, emesis associated with prior exposure to chemotherapy, and poor performance status. Factors conferring relative protection are male sex, age older than 65 years, and alcohol ingestion of more than 10 drinks per week.

Treatment. Many medications have demonstrated some degree of effectiveness in the prevention and treatment of chemotherapy-induced emesis. Table 2 lists currently available medications. The availability of type 3 serotonin receptor antagonist drugs, of which ondansetron (Zofran) is the prototype, has revolutionized the management of chemotherapy-induced emesis. As single agents, these drugs are 50 to 70% effective in the total protection from nausea and vomiting due to highly emetogenic chemotherapy exemplified by regimens containing more than 50 mg per m² of cisplatin. The addition of steroids, most typically dexamethasone at an intravenous dose of 10 to 20 mg, enhances the effectiveness of the type 3 serotonin antagonists, with some investigators reporting greater than 90% protection. These drugs are even more effective in the prevention of emesis due to moderately emetogenic chemotherapy such as cyclophosphamide. However, for mildly to moderately emetogenic chemotherapy regimens, a phenothiazine, butyrophenone, or steroid—alone or in combination—may provide equal antiemetic efficacy to 5-hydroxytryptamine$_3$ (5-HT$_3$) antagonists. The ad-

TABLE 3. **Emetogenic Potential of Single Chemotherapy Agents**

Level	Frequency of Emesis (%)	Agent
5	>90	Carmustine >250 mg/m²
		Cisplatin >50 mg/m²
		Cyclophosphamide >1500 mg/m²
		Dacarbazine
		Mechlorethamine
		Streptozocin
4	60–90	Carboplatin
		Carmustine <250 mg/m²
		Cisplatin <50 mg/m²
		Cyclophosphamide >750 mg/m² <1500 mg/m²
		Cytarabine >1 g/m²
		Doxorubicin >60 mg/m²
		Methotrexate >1000 mg/m²
		Procarbazine (oral)
3	30–60	Cyclophosphamide <750 mg/m²
		Cyclophosphamide (oral)
		Doxorubicin 20–60 mg/m²
		Epirubicin <90 mg/m²
		Hexamethylmelamine (oral)
		Idarubicin
		Ifosfamide
		Methotrexate 250–1000 mg/m²
		Mitoxantrone <15 mg/m²
2	10–30	Docetaxel
		Etoposide
		5-Fluorouracil <1000 mg/m²
		Gemcitabine
		Methotrexate >50 mg/m² <250 mg/m²
		Mitomycin
		Paclitaxel
1	<10	Bleomycin
		Busulfan
		Chlorambucil (oral)
		2-Chloro-2-deoxyadenosine
		Fludarabine
		Hydroxyurea
		Methotrexate <50 mg/m²
		L-phenylalanine mustard (oral)
		Thioguanine (oral)
		Vinblastine
		Vincristine
		Vinorelbine

Note: Proportion of patients who experience emesis in the absence of effective antiemetic prophylaxis.

From Hesketh PJ, Kris MG, Grunberg SM, et al: Proposal for classifying the acute emetogenicity of cancer chemotherapy. J Clin Oncol *15*:103–109, 1997.

dition of other antiemetic drugs such as prochlorperazine (C... pazine) may result in additional protec- tio...

...es in Antiemetic Research. Despite ... improvement in the prevention of ...ced emesis in the past 5 years, ...

...nd Schedule of Type 3 Sero- ...rkable variation in the ap- ...otonin antagonists exists ...d Europe. Ondansetron ...g per kg for 3 doses ...ours) in the United ...ed that a single ...ivided schedule

and is currently recommended. However, the approved ondansetron dose in Europe is 8 mg per 24 hours. Conversely, granisetron is approved at 10 μg per kg in the United States but at 3 mg (40 μg per kg) in Europe. These differences are a result of differences in pivotal studies employed by regulatory agencies. A consensus conference recommended that the lower doses of both drugs were appropriate for treating the effects of highly emetogenic chemotherapy. In addition, the divided dose schedule of the drugs appears to be unnecessary.

Route of Administration. All the serotonin antagonists were approved initially as intravenous formulations. Most now have an oral counterpart. Overwhelming evidence indicates that the oral version of these drugs in bioequivalent doses is equally efficacious for the prevention of nausea and vomiting due to moderately emetogenic chemotherapy. Emerging evidence supports the use of oral serotonin antagonists for treating the effects of highly emetogenic chemotherapy.

The Problem of Delayed Emesis. Delayed emesis from chemotherapy remains a problem despite the advent of the type 3 serotonin receptor antagonists. The mechanism is unclear but likely involves a distinct pathophysiology in comparison with immediate nausea and vomiting. Current management of a patient with delayed emesis is uncertain. The serotonin antagonists, metoclopramide, and steroids all appear to have some activity in the prevention and treatment of this complication.

Practical Approach. Antiemetic regimens for low, moderate, and highly emetogenic chemotherapy are given in Table 5. Other drugs may be substituted depending on individual patient features. For example, many younger patients who are on mild to moderately emetogenic regimens and who have experience inhaling marijuana may prefer the use of dronabinol (Marinol) to prochlorperazine (Compazine). Older patients frequently experience dysphoria with dronabinol, and its use is not recommended in that age group. Conversely, dystonic reactions are far more frequent in younger patients who use metoclopramide (Reglan) than in older patients. The use of type 3 serotonin antagonists should be reserved for

TABLE 4. **Algorithm for Defining the Emetogenicity of Combination Chemotherapy**

1. Identify the most emetogenic agent in the combination.
2. Assess the relative contribution of other agents to the emetogenicity of the combination. When considering other agents, the following rules apply:
   a. Level one agents do not contribute to the emetogenicity of a given regimen.
   b. Adding one or more level 2 agents increases the emetogenicity of the combination by one level greater than the most emetogenic agent in the combination.
   c. Adding level 3 or 4 agents increases the emetogenicity of the combination by one level per agent.

From Hesketh PJ, Kris MG, Grunberg SM, et al: Proposal for classifying the acute emetogenicity of cancer chemotherapy. J Clin Oncol *15*:103–109, 1997.

TABLE 5. **Prevention of Acute Nausea and Vomiting Due to Chemotherapy**

Emetogenic Potential	Regimen
Low (level 1 or 2)	No prophylaxis or single agent, e.g., dexamethasone (Decadron), 10–20 mg PO, or prochlorperazine (Compazine), 10 mg PO, or 15-mg spansule PO
Intermediate (level 3)	Dexamethasone (Decadron), 10–20 mg PO or IV, and/or prochlorperazine (Compazine), 10 mg PO or 15-mg spansule PO
Intermediate to high (level 4)	Type 3 serotonin antagonist PO or IV plus dexamethasone (Decadron), 10–20 mg PO or IV
High (level 5)	Type 3 serotonin antagonist PO or IV plus dexamethasone (Decadron), 20 mg IV ± prochlorperazine (Compazine), 10 mg PO or IV, or 15-mg spansule PO

For all levels—consider the addition of lorazepam (Ativan), 1–4 mg PO or IV, for anxious patients to prevent anticipatory vomiting. Additionally, for levels 2–5, all patients should have medication available for use at home, e.g., prochlorperazine (Compazine), 10 mg PO, 15-mg spansule PO, or pr q 6 h prn.

those on moderate to highly emetogenic regimens. Far less expensive alternatives usually suffice for regimens of lesser emetic potential. Should the patient experience nausea and vomiting despite appropriate prophylaxis, rescue medication in the form of phenothiazines and/or corticosteroids should be available. For patients with severe nausea and vomiting, intravenous hydration is indicated not only to replenish losses but also to relieve nausea by ameliorating orthostatic symptoms associated with dehydration. Furthermore, the patient with severe nausea and vomiting, particularly in the setting of advanced malignancy, should be evaluated for the possibility of non–chemotherapy-related etiologies. Specifically, electrolyte abnormalities (hyponatremia, hypercalcemia), gastrointestinal obstruction, and opiate intolerance should be considered.

GASEOUSNESS AND INDIGESTION

method of
MAURICE A. CERULLI, M.D.
Brooklyn Hospital Center–Downtown Campus
Brooklyn, New York

Indigestion or dyspepsia is a general term for upper abdominal discomfort. Patients may complain of eructation, gas, bloating, and heartburn in describing dyspepsia. Eliciting the relationship of the dyspepsia to eating or fasting, the timing of symptoms, and the choice of food can help in the diagnosis and management of this common complex of symptoms. This symptom complex gives the clinician an opportunity to assess the patient's diet and make important recommendations to reduce the risk of cardiovascular disease and colon cancer.

Studies of dyspepsia have shown, as with other symptoms of functional bowel disorders, that the patients who present with it tend to be more anxious and depressed than persons who do not come to see the physician even though they may have similar complaints.

Eructation involves the passing through the mouth of inspired air or gas from ingested carbonated beverages. No gases are produced in the stomach from digestive activity. The most common ways this may occur are when the patient eats rapidly, smokes cigarettes (inhaling smoke), chews gum, sighs frequently, or has developed a habit of aerophagia (especially seen in young males and anxious individuals). Anxiety can increase this symptom, with the patient often being able to produce symptoms for the examiner. This should be treated with reassurance and strategies to avoid aerophagia: no gum chewing, no smoking, eating slowly, and stress management. If the patient has vomiting, weight loss, or heartburn, then there may be such associated problems of gastric emptying as peptic ulcer disease, gastric cancer, or gastroparesis.

Another effect of inspired air is an increase in flatulence because nitrogen—80% of air—passes unaffected through the intestinal tract. Therefore, eructation and flatulence indicate inspired air is the cause of the symptoms. Flatulence without eructation also can be due to malassimilation (malabsorption and maldigestion) with a differential diagnosis of disaccharidase deficiency (most commonly from lactose), gas-forming vegetables (beans, broccoli, cauliflower), celiac sprue or gluten-sensitive enteropathy (common in western Ireland, associated with iron deficiency anemia, hypomagnesemia, or hypocalcemia), or pancreatic insufficiency (chronic pancreatitis can produce diabetes as well). Malassimilation syndromes are associated with weight loss.

Bloating or the sensation of fullness after eating can be due to delayed gastric emptying. Fat increases gastric emptying, as do commonly used medications (calcium channel blockers, tricyclic antidepressants, anticholinergic agents). Chronic constipation is commonly associated with bloating, but severe constipation may suggest a generalized motility problem such as colonic inertia. The bloating may be due to partial outlet obstruction as in a prepyloric, pyloric channel, or duodenal ulcer; a gastric cancer; a large pancreatic cancer; or gastroparesis. It can also be due to chronic cholelithiasis. Giardiasis can also produce bloating, often with diarrhea. Weight loss and vomiting associated with bloating are warning signs of serious illness requiring further work-up (gastric outlet ob[illegible] struction, progressive intestinal obstruction fr[illegible] colonic tumor, pancreatic cancer).

Recurrent abdominal pain or discom[illegible] about 25% of the populace; if freque[illegible] included, then the prevalence ap[illegible] the increase in knowledge of [illegible] infection is related to pe[illegible] proach to the dyspeptic patient has become more scientific but more problematic. *H. pylori* is the major etiologic factor in more than 90% of duodenal ulcers and 60% of gastric ulcers. It has been estimated that 40% of the world's population is infected in spite of the decreasing incidence of peptic ulcer disease. Therefore, if a patient has an acute duodenal ulcer or a past history of duodenal ulcer, the patient is very likely to be infected and to be at risk for recurrent ulcer if this pathogen is not eradicaded.

Of patients who present with ulcer-like symptoms, only about 20% will have an ulcer. Factors that increase the likelihood of finding an ulcer include (1) history of previous duodenal ulcer, (2) use of nonsteroidal anti-inflammatory drugs (NSAIDs) or aspirin (increased risk of gastric-duodenal ulcer), (3) nocturnal symptoms, and (4) symptoms relieved by antacids or food intake. It had been advocated that patients without warning signs be treated empirically for peptic ulcer disease. If they responded to initial therapy, then the therapy would be continued for 8 weeks; if not, then endoscopy would be performed to make an accurate diagnosis (ACP/ASGE consensus statement). In view of the recurrent nature of *H. pylori*–associated peptic ulcers, this approach can often lead to the patient re-presenting with the same symptoms after completing the course of ulcer therapy.

The two major figures in this debate are Talley and Fendrick. In Talley's decision tree analysis of the relative rates of nonulcer dyspepsia, gastroesophageal reflux, gastric and duodenal ulcer, and gastric cancer, the difference in cost of treating the patient empirically versus performing endoscopy for accurate diagnosis was less than 2%. However, Fendrick found that it was more advantageous to treat patients who were positive for *H. pylori* infection because of the cost of endoscopy. The National Institutes of Health (NIH) consensus conference in 1994 reviewed all the data available on *H. pylori* and concluded that only patients who tested positive for *H. pylori* infection and had ulcers should be treated. There is a burgeoning literature that has spilled over into a journal just for studies of *H. pylori*.

The main reasons *not* to treat unless the patient has a documented ulcer are as follows:

1. Studies of patients with nonulcer dyspepsia have not shown a clear benefit from treatment for *H. pylori* infection.
2. *H. pylori* eradication requires multidrug regimens, which are either complex (cheap) or require expensive proton pump inhibitors with expensive antibiotics.
3. *H. pylori* is difficult to eradicate and is becoming increasingly resistant to metronidazole.
4. Such treatment is not recommended by the NIH consensus conference on *H. pylori*.
5. Many patients are infected with *H. pylori* and do not have dyspepsia; in fact, 40% of office patients may test positive.
6. Pseudomembranous (*Clostridium difficile*) colitis may develop in regimens using amoxicillin.
7. It is difficult to agree that empirical *H. pylori* therapy is cost effective when most dyspeptic patients do not have ulcers.

There are possible reasons why some patients without ulcers may be treated:

1. Empirical therapy does not require endoscopy and may be cheaper, depending on the cost of endoscopy, although only a minority of patients will have documented ulcers.
2. The World Health Organization (WHO) has classified *H. pylori* as a co-carcinogen for gastric cancer (the number two cause of cancer deaths worldwide but decreasing in the United States).
3. The patient has tested positive for *H. pylori* and is concerned.
4. There is a history of gastric cancer in a first-degree relative.

The approach to this dilemma can be clarified by discussion with the patient about the use of empirical therapy or endoscopy, with a frank discussion of risks, benefits, and costs. Testing for *H. pylori* is not recommended unless treatment is contemplated for a positive result because of the expense of the test and the concern it may arouse in the patient. Testing for *H. pylori* will result in a number of positive results, which may force the clinician to treat the majority of patients. As the cost of upper endoscopy approaches the cost of treating patients with multiple drugs, this decision may become more straightforward. Complicating the picture is the fact that some recent evidence indicates that patients with *H. pylori* infection may be at an increased risk for the development of ulcers when treated with NSAIDs. Most patients requiring NSAID therapy are in the older age group, meaning that they would also be more likely to be *H. pylori* positive (incidence increases with age, perhaps because of poorer sanitary conditions in their childhood).

HICCUP

method of

FRANCISCO C. RAMIREZ, M.D.
Carl T. Hayden Veterans Affairs Medical Center
Phoenix, Arizona
University of Arizona College of Medicine
Tucson, Arizona

Hiccup, or singultus, is an abrupt, involuntary, repeated inspiratory muscle (diaphragmatic) contraction followed by closure of the glottis. It is usually unilateral, occurring more often on the left side, and it affects men more frequently than women. Hiccup may be detected as early as the second trimester. It increases in frequency during gestation and continues throughout the neonatal period. The specific physiologic role of this event is unknown, however. Hiccup is usually self-limited and temporary and may be considered a passing annoyance, but on occasion it may be chronic, persistent, and resistant to conventional forms of therapy, thus becoming intractable. The side effects or complications of temporary hiccup are minimal or nonexistent. Physiologic changes, such as a decrease in the systemic arterial pressure due to transient decrease in the intrathoracic pressure during the hiccup episodes, have been described, however. Transient esophageal manometric changes, including aperistalsis, poor clearance in the distal esophagus, and failure of the lower esophageal sphincter in response to swallowing—abnormalities similar to those observed in achalasia—have also been observed.

PATHOGENESIS

Although the exact pathogenesis of hiccup is unknown, experimental data in the animal model indicate that hiccups have been evoked by electrical stimulation of the medullary region, suggesting that the hiccup reflex center is located within the lower brain stem. Mechanical stimulation of the dorsal epipharynx has also been shown to evoke hiccup in the same animal model. The reported effects of intravenous lidocaine on the methohexitone-induced hiccup favor a decrease in the excitability of all nervous structures involved in the reflex by virtue of the membrane-stabilizing properties of lidocaine. Hiccup is regarded by some as an involuntary reflex mediated by sensory branches of the phrenic and vagus nerves as well as dorsal sympathetic afferents, with the main efferent limb mediated by motor fibers of the phrenic nerve. The center probably is located in the brain stem, with interactions among the respiratory center, phrenic nerve nucleus, medullary reticular formation, hypothalamus, and spinal connections. Because of studies that demonstrate an organic cause at the level of the brain stem and cervical spine, hiccup is considered by others as a myoclonus rather than an abnormal reflex. This myoclonus is proposed to have its genesis at the inspiratory solitary nucleus as a result of repetitive activity at that level due to release of higher nervous system inhibitory-regulatory control. Hiccup nevertheless is considered a neurogenic dysfunction of the "valve function" between the inspiratory complex and the glottis closure complex. Hiccup must be differentiated from a rare condition called diaphragmatic flutter, in which dyspnea, chest and abdominal wall pain, and epigastric pulsations are present due to involuntary contractions of the diaphragm.

ASSOCIATED CONDITIONS

Hiccup has been associated with many clinical conditions, both metabolic and organic, medical and surgical. They include sudden excitement; stress; cerebrovascular accident; brain tumor; tuberculoma of the brain stem; sarcoidosis of the central nervous system; recent intra-abdominal or open heart surgery; subdiaphragmatic irritation; gastric distention; hiatal hernia; gastroesophageal reflux; esophagitis; achalasia; diabetes mellitus; uremia; alcohol intoxication; pleurisy; and pharmacologic agents such as analeptics, short-acting barbiturates, antibiotics, and general anesthesia, to name a few (Table 1). None of these associated conditions or drugs has been consistently proved to be related in a causal manner to the development of hiccup, and any association has been mostly regarded as coincidental.

TABLE 1. **Conditions Associated with Hiccup**

Metabolic
Uremia
Diabetes mellitus
Alcohol intoxication
Addison's disease
Gout
Hyperventilation
Electrolyte abnormalities
Pharmacologic
Corticosteroids (i.e., high-dose intravenous methylprednisolone)
Benzodiazepines
Short-acting barbiturates
Analeptics
Antibiotics (sulfonamides, ceftriaxone, cefotetan, doxycycline, imipenem/cilastatin)
Methyldopa
Anesthetics (i.e., methohexital)
Central Nervous System
Cerebrovascular accidents
Tumors
Trauma (including surgical)
Infections (encephalitis, meningitis, tuberculoma)
Multiple sclerosis
Parkinson's disease
Sarcoidosis
Ventriculo-peritoneal shunt
Syringomyelia
Other
Gastroesophageal reflux
Esophagitis
Achalasia
Hiatal hernia
Gastric distention
Gastritis
Peptic ulcer disease
Hepatitis
Cholecystitis
Pancreatitis
Recent intra-abdominal, thoracic surgery
Subdiaphragmatic irritation (subphrenic abscess)
Peritonitis
Pericarditis
Myocardial infarction
Open-heart surgery
Pleurisy
Pneumonia
Tumors (ear, nose, and throat; cervical; pulmonary; mediastinal; abdominal)
Miscellaneous
Stress
Excitement
Anorexia nervosa
Idiopathic

MANAGEMENT

Treatment of the *occasional,* self-limited hiccup includes mostly home remedies that range from breath holding, drinking water without stopping to breathe, sudden fright, trying the Valsalva maneuver, swallowing granulated sugar, drinking water without turning the glass, coughing, gasping, and sneezing to hyperventilating, pulling hard on the tongue, instilling irritants such as ammonia or vinegar, and many others. Because *persistent* hiccup not only causes embarrassment and disruption of the patient's private and social life, but also may be associated with impairment of oral nutrition and consequent weight loss, disruption of the sleep pattern, potentially life-

TABLE 2. **Pharmacologic Therapy of Hiccup**

Amantadine hydrochloride: 100 mg PO/day
Amitriptyline hydrochloride (Elavil): 10 mg PO 3 times/day
Amphetamine sulfate (Adderall): 10–20 mg PO 2 times/day
Baclofen (Lioresal)*: 5–20 mg PO q 6–12 h
Carbamazepine (Tegretol): 200 mg PO 4 times/day
Chlorpromazine hydrochloride (Thorazine): 25–50 mg PO q 6 h. It may be tried intravenously at the same doses.
Ephedrine sulfate (Marax): 25 mg PO 3 times/day
Lidocaine hydrochloride (Xylocaine): 2–4 mg/min continuous IV infusion
Magnesium sulfate: 2 mL of a 50% solution IM
Methylphenidate hydrochloride (Ritalin): 6–20 mg IV bolus
Metoclopramide hydrochloride (Reglan): 10 mg PO q 6 h or 5–10 mg IM or IV q 8 h
Midazolam (Versed): 5–10 mg IV bolus followed by 40–120 mg/24 h as continuous subcutaneous infusion
Nifedipine (Adalat): 10 mg PO 2 times/day up to 20 mg PO 3 times/day
Ondansetron hydrochloride (Zofran): 8 mg PO 3 times/day or 4–32 mg IV bolus
Phenytoin (Dilantin): 200 mg IV bolus, followed by 100 mg PO 4 times/day
Quinidine sulfate: 200 mg PO 3 times/day
Valproic acid (Depakene): 15 mg/kg/day orally or rectally

*Only drug tested in a randomized, placebo-controlled manner.
Except for chlorpromazine, all drugs cited are not FDA approved for hiccup treatment.

threatening complications such as severe hyponatremic episodes resulting from water intoxication caused by psychogenic polydyspsia, or even severe respiratory alkalosis, multiple therapies have been proposed for its treatment without a clear understanding of its real mechanism. In the vast majority of cases, these therapies are the result of anecdotal experience rather than scientifically proven efficacy. Thus, treatment of intractable hiccup remains vastly empiric, nonreproducible, and often unsatisfactory when employed by persons other than the study's reporting authors. It is not surprising that the number of medical therapies, so varied in the case of hiccup, is in direct relation to their inability to provide sustained and consistent control (Table 2).

Therapies used for the management of intractable hiccup have included pharmacologic and surgical manipulations such as implantation of phrenic pacemakers, phrenic nerve transection or crushing, blockage with alcohol or local anesthesia, rectal massages, acupunture, and hypnosis, but again results have been inconsistent. Among the numerous pharmacologic agents reported to be effective in controlling hiccup, chlorpromazine (Thorazine) is the only approved drug for such purpose, a drug that may not work in all patients in a consistent and systematic manner. The most promising pharmacologic therapeutic modality described in the literature has been the γ-aminobutyric acid B (GABAB) agonist baclofen (Lioresal).* This drug is used primarily for the treatment of muscle spasms. It works at the cellular level by either inhibiting or releasing glutamate and aspartate (two excitatory amino acid neurotransmitters) or by increasing potassium flux in the neuronal cells, resulting in a blockade of mono- and polysynaptic reflexes. In addition to the multiple reports dealing with its efficacy for the treatment of intractable hiccup, baclofen is the only drug tested in a randomized, double-blind, placebo-controlled manner. In that study, contrary to the reported experience of decreasing the actual number of hiccup episodes and even the cessation of hiccup, baclofen was found not to affect the actual number of hiccups when compared with placebo. The subjective improvement noted by the patients, however, was greater with the active drug than with the placebo. It was postulated that this drug somehow decreases the perception of the severity of hiccup. There is some indirect evidence that baclofen induces central analgesia or antinociception, which supports this hypothesis. The reported inhibitory effect of baclofen on water intake, along with its effect on the perception of hiccup severity, may give it a role in treating patients with intractable hiccup and severe hyponatremic episodes due to psychogenic polydypsia, as has also been reported in the literature.

*Not FDA approved for this indication.

Given the lack of complete understanding of the pathophysiologic basis of hiccup and the consequent great variety of pharmacologic agents reported to be effective in treating this condition, it is imperative that these drugs must be tested in a more scientific manner to probe their real efficacy.

ACUTE INFECTIOUS DIARRHEA

method of
HOWARD B. MAYER, M.D.
Yale University School of Medicine
New Haven, Connecticut

and

CHRISTINE A. WANKE, M.D.
Beth Israel Deaconess Medical Center
and Harvard Medical School
Boston, Massachusetts

Diarrheal diseases represent the second most common cause of death worldwide and the leading cause of childhood death. Each year, as many as 6 million children die from diarrheal disease in Africa, Latin America, and Asia. Even in the United States, where diarrhea is more often than not a "nuisance disease" in the normally healthy individual, more than 10,000 deaths per year are attributed to this illness. In addition, morbidity rates in the United States are approximately 1.5 to 2 illnesses per person-year in adults, and 2 to 3 illnesses per child-year. It is imperative, therefore, that the general practitioner have the ability to diagnose and treat these illnesses.

Acute diarrheal disease is generally defined as three loose stools (or two loose stools with abdominal symptoms) or more than 250 grams of stool per day, for up to 7 days. Infectious or noninfectious causes may be responsible, and both may occur simultaneously. Noninfectious etiologies causing the acute onset of diarrhea include drugs (e.g., sorbitol, colchicine, theophylline, laxatives), food allergies, primary gastrointestinal diseases (e.g., sprue, inflammatory bowel disease, irritable bowel syndrome), and other disease states, such as thyroroxicosis and the carcinoid syndrome. Infectious etiologies include a wide variety of bacterial, viral, and protozoan pathogens.

Diarrheal syndromes due to infectious agents are generally grouped according to the epidemiologic setting in which the infection was acquired: diarrhea in the normal host, diarrhea in the immunocompromised host (e.g., the person with acquired immune deficiency syndrome [AIDS]), traveler's diarrhea, and diarrhea acquired in the hospital. In each of these settings, however, distinguishing between small bowel and large bowel diarrhea provides a more focused way of arriving at a diagnosis and may prevent the time, expense, and potential patient discomfort of a search for an unlikely pathogen (Table 1). By utilizing clues obtained from a careful history, physical examination, and evaluation of known laboratory data, a diagnosis can often be established.

DIAGNOSTIC EVALUATION

The small bowel functions as both a secretory and a nutrient-absorbing organ. Disease centered in the small bowel may have a distinctive presentation pertinent to dysregulation of these two processes. Small bowel diarrhea is generally watery and occurs in large volume (up to 10,000 mL per day). It may also be associated with abdominal cramping, bloating, gas, and weight loss. In a classic presentation fever is absent and stool examination results for occult blood and fecal leukocytes are negative. Cholera is the classic example of small bowel diarrhea. This is more commonly referred to as "noninflammatory diarrhea." In patients with AIDS this syndrome is classically caused by coccidian parasites, such as *Cryptosporidium* and *Microsporidium.* However, enterotoxigenic or enterohemorrhagic *Escherichia coli* (EHEC), *Clostridium perfringens,* Norwalk virus and related agents, and *Giardia lamblia* also cause this syndrome, both in immunocompetent and immunocompromised hosts.

TABLE 1. **Small Bowel and Large Bowel Pathogens**

	Small Bowel (Noninflammatory)	Colon (Inflammatory)
Bacteria	*Salmonella**	*Campylobacter**
	Escherichia coli†	*Shigella*
	Clostridium perfringens	*Clostridium difficile*
	Staphylococcus aureus	*Yersinia*
	Aeromonas hydrophila	*Vibrio parahaemolyticus*
	Bacillus cereus	Enteroinvasive *E. coli*
	Vibrio cholerae	*Plesiomonas shigelloides*
Viral	Rotavirus	Cytomegalovirus*
	Norwalk agent	Adenovirus
		Herpes simplex virus
Protozoa	*Cryptosporidium**	*Entamoeba histolytica*
	*Microsporidium**	
	Isospora	
	Cyclospora	
	Giardia lamblia	

*Can involve both the small and large bowel but are most likely to occur as listed.

†Enteropathogenic *E. coli,* enteroaggregative *E. coli,* enterohemorrhagic *E. coli,* and enterotoxic *E. coli* may all contribute. Routine laboratory tests and cultures will not differentiate these from *E. coli,* which are normal flora.

The large bowel functions more as a storage organ, and disease is therefore characterized by frequent, regular, small-volume, often painful bowel movements. Fever and bloody or mucoid stools are common, and stool study results for fecal leukocytes are positive. This syndrome, known as "dysentery" or "inflammatory diarrhea," is classically caused by *Shigella* but may also be the result of infection with a wide array of pathogens, such as enteroinvasive *E. coli, Clostridium difficile,* cytomegalovirus, and *Entamoeba histolytica.* This syndrome is often confused with ulcerative colitis in adults and with ischemic colitis in the elderly.

A third category of diarrheal disease is that which occurs in the setting of a systemic illness, such as with *Staphylococcus aureus* bacteremia. These diseases may also manifest as typhoidal illnesses with gastrointestinal complaints prominent among multiple other symptoms. As one example, *Salmonella* bacteremia has been associated with diarrhea but without stool isolation of the organism. Disseminated mycobacterial disease is another such example, most often described in patients with AIDS. Distinguishing among these three types of diarrheal syndromes, supplemented by data from a complete history and physical examination, can often lead to a more rational assessment of the necessary diagnostic studies and the need for empirical therapy.

In infectious diarrhea the single most important laboratory test is gross examination of the stool for blood, pus, and mucus. This should be followed by microscopic examination of the stool for leukocytes. At this point, if it seems appropriate from the patient's history (e.g., persistent diarrhea after travel, homosexual male), three separate stools for ova and parasites may be submitted. If these test results are negative but clinical suspicion is high, stool antigen for *Giardia* or sigmoidoscopy (with or without biopsy if amebiasis is suspected) may be performed. When leukocytes are present in the stool, *Shigella, Salmonella, Campylobacter, Yersinia,* and enteroinvasive *E. coli* or EHEC should be considered as potential pathogens and stool cultures should be obtained. Specific media or methods are generally required to isolate these organisms, and the laboratory must be notified of the concern for the particular pathogen. Certainly, in the hospitalized patient, *C. difficile* colitis should be suspected in this circumstance and toxin analysis should be performed on stool. Two sets of blood cultures should also be submitted if the patient is febrile. In patients infected with the human immunodeficiency virus (HIV), in whom the incidence of salmonellosis has been quite high, these tests may be of particular value. If no leukocytes are present in stool and symptoms persist, cultures may be submitted as indicated and sigmoidoscopy performed if these results are negative. A summary of this evaluation strategy may be found in Figure 1.

A thorough history and physical examination can be very instructive in patients with acute diarrhea. Duration of symptoms and frequency and characteristics of stools should be elicited. In addition, residence, occupational exposure, recent and remote travel, pets, hobbies (e.g., fishing, hunting, cooking), and water supply source may provide further diagnostic clues. History taking should include detailed questioning on recent dietary ingestions, which may facilitate a diagnosis and simplify the diagnostic tests ordered. Information on intake of potentially unpasteurized dairy products, raw or undercooked meat or fish, or organic vitamin preparations may be invaluable (Table 2). It is equally important to ask the patient about recent antibiotic use and other medications and to obtain a complete past medical history.

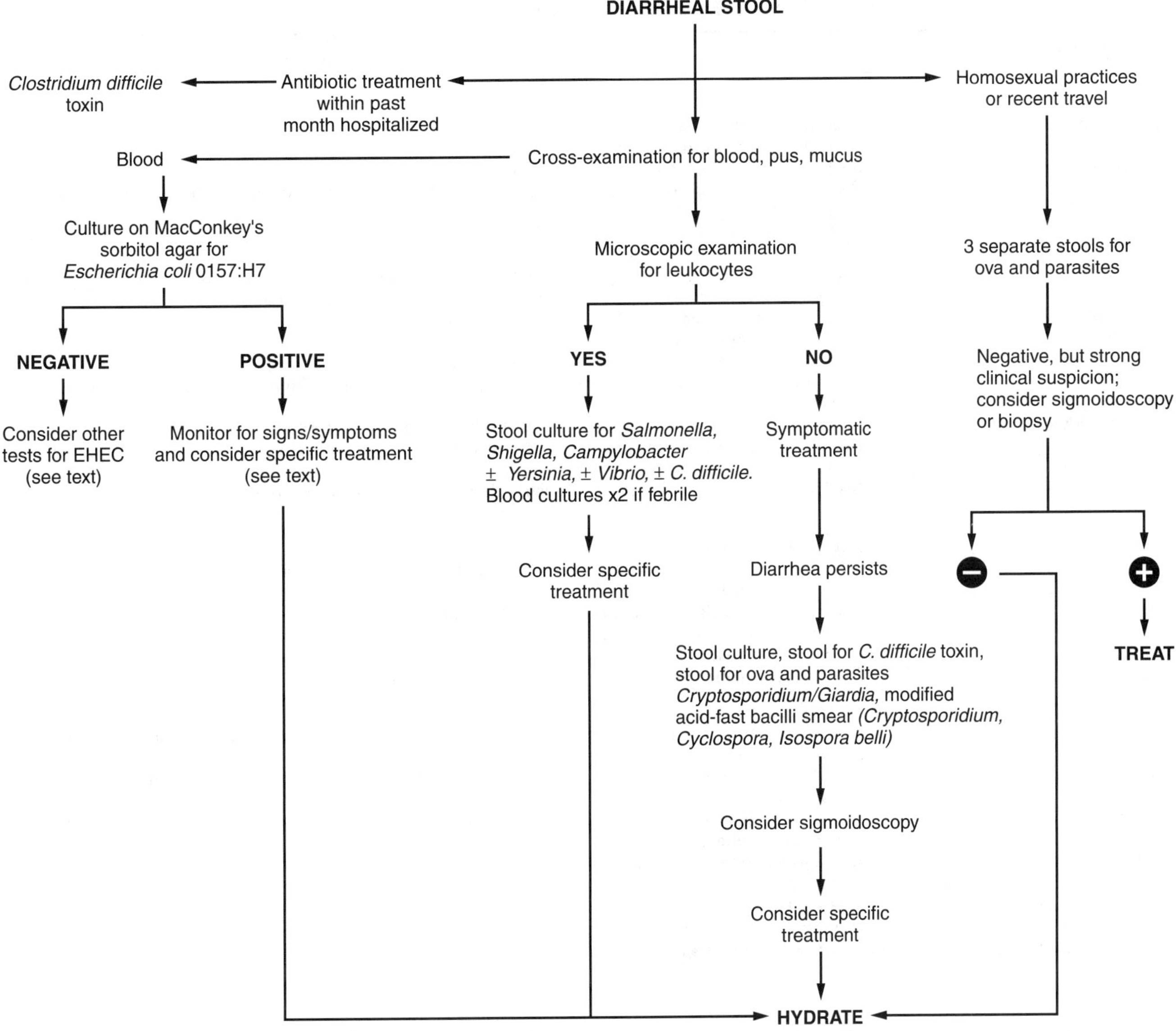

Figure 1. Clinical approach to the adult patient with acute infectious diarrhea.

Physical examination should include height and weight, temperature, and orthostatic blood pressure. Careful examination of the skin and mucous membranes may reveal petechiae, which may be seen in conjunction with cytotoxin-producing organisms, such as *Shigella* and *E. coli.* Endovascular infections caused by *Salmonella* or *Campylobacter* may give rise to a heart murmur or, alternatively, a palpable abdominal mass in the setting of an abdominal aortic aneurysm. An enlarged liver may be seen in the setting of acute infection with hepatitis A, and peritoneal signs are not infrequently seen in the setting of *C. difficile* colitis. Rarely, examination of the extremities may reveal a reactive polyarthritis, which may be seen with *Yersinia* infection or infection with the other invasive enteric pathogens. Finally, a detailed neurologic examination may reveal nuchal rigidity, which can be seen in the setting of *Listeria* infection, or early signs of Guillain-Barré syndrome, which are seen with acute *Campylobacter* infection. This is only a partial list of the clinical clues that may be obtained from a comprehensive evaluation.

SPECIFIC CLINICAL SYNDROMES

Diarrhea in the Normal Host

This category specifically refers to diarrhea in the nonimmunocompromised outpatient. These syndromes often occur in outbreaks because they may be food or water related (see Table 2). It is estimated that there are more than 10 million cases of food poisoning in the United States per year, perhaps costing billions of dollars annually. Food-borne diseases can be infectious or noninfectious in etiology. However, bacterial causes such as *Salmonella, Shigella, Campylobacter,* and EHEC account for the vast majority of cases in the United States.

Salmonella is the leading cause of food-borne disease in the United States and, like *Listeria* and *Campylobacter,* is associated with ingestion of poultry, eggs, and milk products. A 1995 outbreak in the midwestern United States due to the ingestion of contaminated ice cream highlights this point. Nontyphoidal *Salmonella* infection is most common during the summer and fall months, and risk factors

TABLE 2. **Epidemiologic Clues to Diagnosis**

Pathogen	Epidemiologic Clue(s) to Diagnosis
Bacteria	
Staphylococcus aureus	Beef, pork, poultry, eggs
Clostridium perfringens	Beef, pork, poultry, home-canned foods
Bacillus cereus	Beef, pork, fried rice (Chinese), vegetables
EHEC	Beef, pork, fast food restaurants (undercooked hamburger), apple cider, leaf lettuce, milk, cheese, extremes of age
EIEC	Milk, cheese
ETEC	Travelers to developing world
Salmonella	Beef, pork, poultry, eggs (e.g., Caesar salad), raw milk, ice cream, vegetables (e.g., alfalfa sprouts), unpasteurized orange juice, pet ducklings, lizards, rattlesnake meat
Campylobacter	Poultry (undercooked at barbecues), raw milk, and cheeses
Shigella	Day care centers, vegetables (e.g., green onions)
Yersinia	Pork (not common), beef, milk, cheeses, hemochromatosis
Vibrio cholerae	Inadequately cooked seafood from South America, coconut milk from Thailand, airline outbreaks, shellfish
Vibrio parahaemolyticus	Ingestion of raw seafood, particularly in East Asia, shellfish, cirrhosis
Clostridium difficile	Hospitalization, inpatient or outpatient antibiotic(s) or chemotherapy within the last several weeks, day care centers
Listeria	Beef, pork, poultry, milk, cheese, coleslaw, hot dogs, potato salad, pregnancy, neonates, "IC" patients
Viruses	
Rotavirus	Day care centers, nurseries, Australia
Norwalk-like viruses	Schools; nursing homes; cruise ships; camps; vegetables; water-borne, food-borne, and shellfish-associated outbreaks
Hepatitis A	Overcrowding, lack of clean water, patients and staff of institutions, day care centers, homosexual men, intravenous drug users, travelers, military barracks, shellfish (clams, oysters, mussels)
Adenovirus	Infantile diarrhea, ? AIDS
Cytomegalovirus	HIV-infected homosexual men with AIDS, organ transplantation
Protozoa	
Giardia lamblia	Day care centers, swimming pools, travel (e.g., Nepal, St. Petersburg, mountainous areas with ingestion of stream water), fruit salad
Entamoeba histolytica	Travelers to endemic areas (e.g., Mexico) for more than 1 month, sexually active male homosexuals, institutions
Cryptosporidium	Day care centers, swimming pools, AIDS, farm animal exposure, city water supply contamination (e.g., Milwaukee)
Cyclospora	Raspberries (from Guatemala, Nepal)
Isospora	Haiti, HIV infection
Microsporidium	AIDS (? travelers)

Abbreviations: EHEC = enterohemorrhagic *E. coli;* EIEC = enteroinvasive *E. coli;* ETEC = enterotoxic *E. coli;* IC = immunocompromised.

for infection include age younger than 5 years, altered intestinal flora due to antibiotics or surgery, inflammatory bowel disease, diseases associated with phagocytic overload or deficiency (e.g., schistosomiasis, malaria, sickle cell disease), lymphoproliferative diseases, and AIDS. Nontyphoidal *Salmonella* infection generally has an incubation period of from 6 hours to 2 days but is generally self-limited, lasting less than 1 week.

Shigella, the prototypical cause of bloody diarrhea, is the second most common documented cause of food-borne disease in the United States. As opposed to *Salmonella,* however, most cases of disease caused by *Shigella* are the result of person-to-person transmission. This is because only a small inoculum (10 organisms) is necessary to produce disease. Therefore, *Shigella* continues to be a major problem in day care centers for preschool children. The incubation period is similar to that of *Salmonella,* but symptoms can last as long as 1 month (average, 1 week). Like EHEC (see later discussion), *Shigella (dysenteriae)* produces a cytotoxin that may cause the hemolytic-uremic syndrome (HUS).

In developed countries, *Campylobacter* infection is generally acquired from undercooked infected poultry. The disease peaks in summer and early fall, during "barbecue" season. It is a worldwide commensal and is therefore also a cause of traveler's diarrhea. Unlike *Shigella,* person-to-person transmission of *Campylobacter* is rare. After a 2- to 4-day incubation period, there may be a 1-day prodrome of fever, headache, and malaise followed by up to 1 week of crampy abdominal pain and diarrhea, which can be watery or hemorrhagic. The disease is frequently misdiagnosed as inflammatory bowel disease in young adults; it may manifest as a pseudoappendicitis syndrome or toxic megacolon suggestive of ulcerative colitis. Increasingly, this pathogen has been linked with Guillain-Barré syndrome.

EHEC, most notably *E. coli* 0157:H7, is among the most common causes of infectious colitis. It has been estimated to cause more than 20,000 infections in the United States, although this is likely an underestimate because few laboratories test for its presence routinely. In addition, the diagnostic test that takes advantage of the inability of this pathogen to ferment sorbitol (MacConkey's sorbitol agar) does not routinely identify nonserogroup 0157 EHEC. There has been some recent work using the enzyme-linked immunosorbent assay (ELISA) method to test for Shiga-like toxin in stool samples, but these tests are not yet available commercially. The association of this pathogen with HUS and thrombotic thrombocytopenic purpura (TTP) has been well documented. As with *Salmonella* and *Campylobacter,* infections are more common during the warmer months. The most common mode of transmission is via ingestion of undercooked ground beef, and this has been responsible for numerous outbreaks. Other vehicles for transmission have also been documented, including unpasteurized apple cider. Secondary attack rates are high, suggesting that, as with *Shigella,* person-to-person transmission occurs frequently. It tends to affect patients at the extremes of age and therefore can mimic shigellosis in children and ischemic colitis in adults.

Other causes of diarrhea worth mentioning include those that are caused by preformed bacterial toxin, including *C. perfringens, Bacillus cereus,* and *S. aureus.* These illnesses cause noninflammatory diarrhea, which resolves with oral rehydration therapy alone. The category of watery diarrhea also includes viruses, which are among the leading causes of diarrhea in children (e.g., rotaviruses, Norwalk agent, enteric adenoviruses, astroviruses, and coronaviruses). *Yersinia enterocolitica* infection, also primarily a childhood malady, is more common in northern Europe than in the United States. Cholera is extremely uncommon in the United States, but noncholera vibrios, such as *Vibrio parahaemolyticus,* may cause diarrhea in coastal areas of the United States, where contaminated shellfish transmit the disease. Finally, *Aeromonas hydrophila* (watery nonbloody diarrhea) and *Plesiomonas shigelloides* (bloody diarrhea in up to one third of patients) have also been associated with outbreaks of diarrhea. Within the last year, *Cyclospora* has emerged as a diarrheal pathogen of note. Raspberries imported from Guatemala have been identified as the source of an outbreak that affected hundreds of individuals. The clinical course of *Cyclospora* diarrheal illness has been significant both for its duration and for the intense fatigue and malaise that accompany the diarrhea.

Diarrhea in the Immunocompromised Host

In the past decade this type of diarrhea has become synonymous with diarrhea in HIV-infected patients. Diarrhea has been reported in up to 60% of patients with AIDS from industrialized countries and in as many as 95% of patients with AIDS from the developing world. For many HIV-infected individuals, diarrhea is the presenting complaint and is often chronic. Patients with AIDS who have diarrhea tend to have lower CD4 counts and to have more extraintestinal opportunistic infections than AIDS patients without diarrhea.

The more usual enteric pathogens routinely cause enteric illnesses in HIV-infected individuals, and with the appropriate history, may lead one to suspect underlying HIV infection. For example, *Salmonella* is fairly common in previously asymptomatic HIV-infected individuals. However, septicemia with this bacterial enteric pathogen tends to occur more commonly in patients with a previous diagnosis of AIDS. *Campylobacter* enteritis also tends to occur more commonly in patients with AIDS and is distinctive in its ability to also cause a more prolonged diarrheal syndrome in these patients. Finally, bacteremia with *Shigella* may be more common in these patients, although infection with this pathogen does not appear to be more frequent than in homosexual men who are not HIV infected. In the homosexual patient with bloody or mucoid diarrhea, *Shigella* infection should be suspected along with *Campylobacter* and *Chlamydia* infection and amebiasis.

The coccidian parasites *Cryptosporidium* and *Microsporidium* are almost synonymous with chronic diarrhea in patients with AIDS. These pathogens may also cause extraintestinal disease, such as cholangitis and pneumonia in those with advanced HIV infection. In patients with CD4 counts higher than 150 cells per mm^3, however, infection with *Cryptosporidium* is generally self-limited, behaving as in the immunocompetent host (lasting only 1 to 2 weeks). This distinction was observed in the 1993 Milwaukee outbreak, in which only immunocompromised hosts had prolonged symptoms. In either setting these illnesses initially manifest acutely by definition and therefore may present a diagnostic challenge for the clinician. Cytomegalovirus, *Isospora belli,* and *Mycobacterium avium* are three other pathogens that cause diarrhea commonly and almost exclusively in patients with AIDS. In the current era of highly active antiretroviral therapy, the frequency of identification of *Cryptosporidium* and *Microsporidium* appears to be declining in some small surveys that looked at etiologies of diarrheal illness in HIV-infected patients. Diarrheal disease, however, remains a significant clinical problem in this patient population.

Diarrhea Acquired in the Hospital

Nosocomial diarrhea is most often defined as the new onset of diarrhea at least 72 hours after hospital admission with at least two to three loose stools per day for more than 2 to 3 days. Although comprehensive studies have been limited, nosocomial diarrhea has been shown to increase the length of stay in hospitalized adults by an average of more than 1 week and by more than 1 month in the elderly. Both the incidence and mortality rate are greatest in patients older than 70.

As in community-acquired diarrhea, causes of nosocomial diarrhea may be infectious or noninfectious. Although *C. difficile* has become almost synonymous with diarrhea acquired in the hospital, it arguably lags far behind the multiple noninfectious causes of this entity. These include medication intolerance, hyperalimentation, chronic underlying conditions, intestinal ischemia, procedures, and antibiotic-associated diarrhea that is not due to *C. difficile.* Pathogens identified as causing hospital-acquired diarrhea appear to vary with geographic location. In a study from Mexico, nosocomial diarrheal disease due to *Candida* and *E. histolytica* was reported more frequently than that due to *C. difficile.* In the United States, however, *C. difficile* may account for more than half of all cases when a pathogen is identified.

Pseudomembranous colitis is caused almost exclusively by *C. difficile,* which also accounts for up to 20% of antibiotic-associated diarrhea without colitis. These syndromes range from mild to moderate diarrhea to severe colitis. The latter may manifest with increased fecal leukocytes (which are found inconsistently in the majority of patients), peripheral blood leukocytosis, and peritonitis. Virtually all antibiotics have been associated with this infection, but broad-spectrum penicillins, cephalosporins, and clindamycin (Cleocin) are the most common culprits. Most patients develop symptoms while on antibiotics, but diarrhea may develop from 1 to 3 weeks after cessation of the drug. Diagnostic tests include the tissue culture assay, in which a positive result is based on cell rounding by *C. difficile* toxin B, which is neutralized by *Clostridium sordellii* antitoxin, and ELISAs for detection of toxin, which have the advantage of providing results rapidly. It is worth noting that these tests should not be utilized as a measure of "cure."

Diarrhea in Travelers

More than 300 million people travel abroad each year, and there are approximately 20 million travelers to the developing world per year. Traveler's diarrhea is generally defined as three or more unformed stools per day in a person living in an industrialized country who travels to the developing world. It is the most common medical problem encountered by travelers to high-risk areas, which include Latin America, Africa (except South Africa), the Middle East, and Asia (except Singapore). The incidence in these regions ranges from 20 to 50%. The chances of acquiring this infection may also be increased by the type and location of food consumed and by underlying host factors.

Travelers to high-risk areas should be advised to "cook it, boil it, peel it, or forget it." Salad bars, fruit bars, and steam tables should not be considered safe. More adventurous travelers who frequent street vendors have a greater risk of acquiring diarrheal disease. Other risks include using water from hot water taps (which are not hotter than 65°F) and alcohol or carbonated beverages to kill pathogens in ice. Finally, patients with underlying gastrointestinal disease (e.g., inflammatory bowel disease) may be at higher risk for developing traveler's diarrhea.

Bacterial enteric pathogens cause more than 75% of cases of traveler's diarrhea. Worldwide, ETEC is the most common causative agent (26 to 72%), but this varies according to location. For example, *V. parahaemolyticus* is a common cause of traveler's diarrhea in southeast Asia; *Aeromonas* infection appears to be common in Thailand. The parasites *Giardia* and *Cryptosporidium* are important causes of traveler's diarrhea in Russia, and *Giardia* and *Cyclospora* are common causes of traveler's diarrhea in Nepal. Seasonal variation exists as well. *Salmonella, Shigella,* and *E. coli* are common causes in the rainy summer season, whereas *Campylobacter* is a more common cause in the drier winter season.

TREATMENT

The most critical therapy in diarrheal illness is hydration, preferably with oral rehydration solution (ORS). This mode of therapy takes advantage of research done more than a quarter century ago that demonstrated that glucose-linked sodium absorption in the gut remains intact in secretory diarrhea. The advantage of ORS over intravenous hydration is that it is safer, less expensive, and easily available at home and that it stimulates the recovery of mucosal enzymes. World Health Organization (WHO) ORS was developed to replace stool losses of sodium, potassium, and bicarbonate by combining glucose with these electrolytes to achieve rapid absorption. The composition of this fluid is 90 mm sodium, 80 mm chloride, 111 mm glucose, and 10 mm citrate (or bicarbonate) per liter. Whereas antibiotic therapy is indicated only in a small number of instances, hydration remains the mainstay of diarrheal therapy.

In general, antimicrobial therapy is indicated in the following situations: treatment of infectious colitis due to *Shigella,* diarrhea due to *C. difficile,* cholera, traveler's diarrhea, amebiasis, and giardiasis. Gastroenteritis due to nontyphoidal *Salmonella* is usually self-limited (diarrhea lasting longer than 1 week should suggest an alternative diagnosis), and therefore antibiotic therapy is not indicated. It may, in fact, prolong carriage and lead to an increased rate of relapse in children. However, treatment should be strongly considered in newborns (to prevent meningitis); in patients older than 50 (especially those with atherosclerosis); in immunosuppressed patients (e.g., persons who have AIDS, organ transplant recipients); in patients with inflammatory bowel disease; and in patients with bone and joint prostheses, chronic arthritides, and hemoglobinopathies.

Antibiotic therapy may be withheld in most cases of diarrheal illness due to the other major bacterial enteric pathogens, as these are self-limited illnesses. Antibiotic therapy may be indicated in patients who present with high fever, bloody diarrhea, more than eight stools per day, dehydration, and symptoms for more than 1 week and in immunocompromised patients. Empirical antibiotics may be given to prevent the need for hospitalization in ill patients. A careful history should be taken before the institution of empirical antibiotics to ensure that there is no risk of *C. difficile* infection. The use of antibiotics for persons with hemorrhagic colitis due to *E. coli* 0157:H7 or related pathogens and for those at risk of developing HUS remains controversial. Although in vitro data suggest that exposure to antibiotics (e.g., trimethoprim-sulfamethoxazole, polymyxin B) enhances toxin production, the results of retrospective analyses have yielded mixed results. Many advocate the use of a quinolone agent in this setting, but no firm recommendations can be made at present. Treatment strategies for infection with these and other pathogens are summarized in Table 3. Whether patients are followed or treated, close contact to ensure resolution of symptoms is required.

Diarrhea due to *C. difficile* should be treated with oral metronidazole, 250 mg four times a day. Oral vancomycin, 125 mg four times a day, is equally effective but is much more expensive ($225 per day versus $18 per day) and should be avoided, as it is associated with the emergence of vancomycin-resistant enterococci. Patients who cannot tolerate oral medications (e.g., ileus, recent surgery) may be treated with intravenous metronidazole. In the severely ill patient, consideration can also be given to simultaneous therapy with vancomycin enemas. Intravenous vancomycin has not been shown to accumulate in the gut lumen and should therefore not be used. A second course of metronidazole therapy is recommended for the 10 to 20% of patients who relapse with diarrhea. Because most of these cases are not due to metronidazole-resistant *C. difficile,* oral vancomycin is unlikely to achieve superior results.

Prophylaxis of traveler's diarrhea has been a hotly contested issue for many years. Although several antibiotics have been shown to be of benefit in preventing this illness (e.g., doxycycline [Vibramycin], trimethoprim-sulfamethoxazole [Bactrim], norfloxacin* [Noroxin], ciprofloxacin [Cipro]), the routine use of these agents for prophylaxis is generally not recommended. Arguments against prophylaxis include the side effects of antimicrobial therapy (e.g., skin rashes including erythema multiforme, vaginal can-

*Not FDA approved for this indication.

TABLE 3. **Antimicrobial Therapy of Diarrheal Disease**

Pathogen	First Choice	Second Choice	Comments
Staphylococcus aureus, Bacillus cereus	Not required	Not required	Due to food poisoning and resolve with hydration only. TMP-SMX* can be used if susceptible; antibiotic therapy required only in severe cases (see text)
Salmonella	Usually not required (see text)	Oral quinolone† bid for 3–5 d	Same as above
Shigella	Oral quinolone bid for 5 d	TMP-SMX or ampicillin	Many strains now resistant to TMP-SMX, ampicillin
Campylobacter	Oral quinolone bid for 5 d	Macrolides‡ or doxycycline	Antibiotics only in severe cases (see text). Quinolone resistance has been reported
Yersinia	Oral quinolone bid for 7–10 d	TMP-SMX or doxycycline	Antibiotic therapy only in severe (systemic) cases
Clostridium difficile	Metronidazole (Flagyl), 250 mg PO qid	Vancomycin, 125 mg PO qid	Duration of therapy = 10 d; stop antibiotics, if possible; IV metronidazole if unable to tolerate PO therapy; IV metronidazole ± vancomycin fecal enemas for severe cases
Enterotoxic *Escherichia coli*	Oral quinolone bid for 1–3 d†	TMP-SMX, doxycycline, furazolidone	
Enteroinvasive *E. coli*	Same as for shigellosis		
Enterohemorrhagie *E. coli*	Not recommended at this time	? Oral quinolone†	
Vibrio cholerae	Doxycycline	TMP-SMX or ampicillin	
Amebiasis	Metronidazole, 750 mg PO tid for 10 d	Dehydroemetine 1–1.5 mg/kg/d IM for 5 d	Both plus a luminal amebicide for invasive intestinal infection and hepatic abscesses (iodoquinol [Yodoxin], 650 mg PO tid × 20 d; paromomycin, 500 mg PO tid × 7 d): cyst passers without symptoms require luminicidal agent only
Giardiasis	Metronidazole, 250 mg PO tid for 10 d	Tinidazole,§ quinacrine hydrochloride,§ furazolidone (Furoxone)	Relapses may occur
Cryptosporidium	Paromomycin (Humatin), 500 mg PO bid	Azithromycin, hyperimmune bovine colostrum, Nitazoxanide§	Benefit and duration of any therapy unclear; spontaneous resolution without specific therapy in immunocompetent hosts and in HIV-infected individuals with CD4 counts > 150 cells/mm^3
Microsporidium	Albendazole, 200–400 mg PO bid × 3 mo		Albendazole more effective for *Encephalitozoon intestinalis* than for *Enterocytozoon bieneusi;* available for compassionate use only
Isospora	TMP-SMX 1 DS PO qid × 10 d, then bid for 3 wk	Pyrimethamine + folinic acid	Maintenance therapy required in patients with AIDS
Cyclospora	TMP-SMX 1 DS PO bid × 3–5 d		

*Trimethoprim-sulfamethoxazole, 160/800 mg (DS tab) PO q 12h.
†Norfloxacin, 400 mg PO; ofloxacin, 400 mg PO; ciprofloxacin, 500 mg PO. Data regarding the use of the new once-a-day quinolones are not available.
‡Erythromycin, clarithromycin, azithromycin.
§Not available in the United States.
Abbreviations: TMP-SMX = trimethoprim-sulfamethoxazole.

didiasis, photosensitivity reactions, bone marrow toxicity, and anaphylaxis). In addition, altering gut flora may predispose to resistant pathogens. Many authorities, however, recommend antibiotic prophylaxis in the following situations: patients for whom dehydration would be problematic (e.g., patients who are receiving digoxin or diuretics or who have a history of stroke or coronary artery disease), patients with inflammatory bowel disease, and patients who are immunocompromised (e.g., HIV-infected persons or transplant recipients). A useful alternative is bismuth subsalicylate, which when taken in large enough quantities has been shown to decrease the incidence of diarrhea.

As in all patients with diarrheal disease, those with traveler's diarrhea should take fluids and electrolytes. Loperamide decreases intestinal motility and consequently reduces the severity of diarrheal illnesses and their duration. Although there are now some data regarding the safety of this agent in patients with dysenteric illnesses, its use should be limited to patients without fever or dysentery. Patients who use antimotility agents should be instructed to utilize adequate fluid replacement, as some of the intestinal fluid loss will continue and may be masked with the use of these agents. Empirical antibiotic therapy can be recommended after the third loose stool in a 24-hour period and in patients who have diarrhea associated with severe abdominal pain, fever, or dysentery. Fluoroquinolone antibiotics remain the drugs of choice for adults with traveler's diarrhea in all areas other than in inland Mexico, as widespread resistance of *E. coli* to usual agents such as trimethoprim-sulfamethoxazole is present elsewhere. In inland Mexico trimethoprim-sulfamethoxazole remains effective.

Diarrhea in the HIV-infected patient is complex, and a complete review is beyond the scope of this chapter. However, the treatment of patients with early HIV infection is essentially the same as that of nonimmunocompromised hosts. In general, more immunocompromised patients (absolute CD4 count less than 200 cells per mm^3) should be treated with antimicrobial therapy for the bacterial enteritides. The newer macrolide antibiotics clarithromycin and azithromycin have dramatically improved the therapy of diarrheal disease due to disseminated *M. avium* complex infection. Unfortunately, in the advanced stages of HIV infection, illnesses caused by the coccidian parasites become more frequent and far more difficult to treat. There are still no universally effective therapies for either *Cryptosporidium* or *Microsporidium* infection, which frequently leads to chronic debilitating diarrheal illnesses with wasting. The 1993 outbreak of *Cryptosporidium* in Milwaukee and of *Cyclospora* (due to contaminated raspberries) more recently has educated the medical community about these microbes and their ability to affect immunocompetent as well as immunocompromised hosts. These diseases, along with those mentioned elsewhere in this article, present a continued diagnostic and therapeutic challenge to the individual clinician and to the medical and scientific community at large.

CONSTIPATION

method of
SATISH S. C. RAO, M.D., PH.D.
*University of Iowa College of Medicine and University of Iowa Hospitals and Clinics
Iowa City, Iowa*

Constipation accounts for more than 2.5 million patient visits to physicians each year. In 1994, $840 million was spent on laxatives alone. Many patients self-treat their "constipation," either by using home remedies or by using laxatives, and often successfully. Hence, those who seek medical help merely constitute the tip of the "constipation iceberg." Most patients have a significant problem that requires a thoughtful appraisal.

DEFINITION

Constipation is a symptom, not a disease. It may be defined as the occurrence of two or more of the following symptoms for at least 12 months in a person who is not using laxatives: fewer than three bowel movements per week, excessive straining during at least 25% of bowel movements, a feeling of incomplete evacuation after at least 25% of bowel movements, and the passage of hard or pellet-like stools during at least 25% of bowel movements. Because patients may complain of one or more of the aforementioned symptoms, the physician must determine the exact nature of the problem.

ETIOLOGY

Constipation is often caused by a primary disturbance of colonic or anorectal neuromuscular function, but many other common conditions, including drugs, may lead to this problem (Table 1). Patients with depression, anorexia nervosa, and other psychiatric conditions also develop profound disturbances of gut motor function, including constipation.

PATHOPHYSIOLOGY

If secondary causes (see Table 1) can be excluded, most patients have idiopathic constipation, which is a functional and essentially a colorectal motility disorder. At least two subtypes have been recognized, although there is overlap. *Slow transit constipation* is characterized by prolonged delay of stool transit through the colon. This delay may

TABLE 1. **Common Secondary Causes of Constipation**

Anorectal and Colonic Disorders
Anal fissure
Hemorrhoids
Ulcerative colitis (proctitis)
Diverticulitis
Colorectal carcinoma
Inflammatory, postoperative, and radiation strictures
Drugs
Opioids and related agents
Anticholinergics and antispasmodics
Antidepressants
Antihypertensives, particularly calcium channel antagonists, methyldopa
Antiparkinsonian drugs
Anticonvulsants
Antihistamines
Diuretics
Metal ions such as antacids, iron supplements, and calcium supplements
Endocrine and Metabolic Disorders
Diabetes mellitus
Hypothyroidism
Hypokalemia
Hypercalcemia
Porphyria
Neuromuscular Disorders
Spinal cord lesions
Parkinson's disease
Multiple sclerosis
Stroke or cerebrovascular disease
Chagas' disease
Hirschsprung's disease

be due to primary dysfunction of colonic smooth muscle (myopathy) or nerve innervation (neuropathy), or it may be secondary to obstructive defecation. *Obstructive defecation,* also known as anismus or pelvic floor dyssynergia, is characterized by difficulty with expelling or inability to expell stools from the rectosigmoid region.

CLINICAL EVALUATION

History. A systematic and detailed history is extremely important. This should include an assessment of the duration, severity, onset, and precipitating event or events and an assessment of stool frequency, stool consistency (hard, formed, or soft), stool size (small, pellet-like or long column), degree of straining, a sensation of incomplete evacuation, and the need for digital disimpaction of stool. A history of repeatedly ignoring "a call to stool" and a history of travel or frequent changes in lifestyle, including shift work, are all important. Dietary history should include the amount of fiber and fluid intake, the number of meals per day, and the time of day when meals are consumed. In the elderly, stool impaction and overflow may manifest as fecal incontinence.

Physical Examination. A thorough examination, including a neurologic evaluation, should be performed to exclude systemic illnesses or abdominal masses that cause constipation. During digital rectal examination, it is important to ask the patient to bear down as if to defecate. Normally, one should perceive relaxation of the external anal sphincter together with perineal descent. If these are absent, one should suspect functional obstructive defecation.

DIAGNOSTIC PROCEDURES

General Measures. The first step is to exclude an underlying metabolic or pathologic disorder. A complete blood count, biochemical profile, serum calcium and glucose levels, and thyroid function tests are usually sufficient. Other investigations may include the following:

Flexible Sigmoidoscopy or Colonoscopy. This evaluation may help to detect mucosal lesions or abnormalities such as carcinoma, stricture, anal fissure, solitary rectal ulcer, diverticulosis, or proctitis.

Colon Transit Study. An assessment of colonic transit time enables the physician to understand better the rate of stool expulsion from the colon. This is particularly useful, because the patient's recall of stool habit is often inaccurate. The single capsule technique, which consists of administering one Sitzmarks capsule (Konsyl Pharmaceuticals, Fort Worth, TX) containing 24 radiopaque markers on day 1 and obtaining a plain radiograph of the abdomen on day 6 (i.e., 120 hours later), is usually adequate. The radiograph may reveal one of three patterns: *normal transit,* which consists of either no markers or fewer than 5 markers; *slow transit,* which consists of more than 5 markers that are scattered throughout the colon; or *obstructive defecation pattern,* which consists of more than 5 markers in the rectosigmoid region with a near normal transit through the rest of the colon.

Defecography. This procedure is performed by placing 150 mL of barium paste into the patient's rectum and by imaging the rectum with videofluoroscopy. When the patient tries to evacuate the barium, the morphologic and functional changes that occur in the anorectum are observed. This test provides useful information regarding abnormalities such as rectocele, intussusception, and rectal prolapse.

Anorectal Manometry. This test provides a comprehensive assessment of rectal sensation, rectoanal reflexes, rectal compliance, and anal sphincter pressures. Manometric abnormalities that are seen in patients with constipation include impaired rectal contraction, paradoxical anal contraction, absent rectoanal inhibitory reflex, and impaired rectal sensation.

When a balloon is distended in the rectum, there is reflex relaxation of the internal anal sphincter—rectoanal inhibitory reflex. This reflex is mediated by the myenteric plexus and is absent in patients with Hirschsprung's disease. Manometry may also detect abnormalities during maneuvers that simulate the act of defecation. Normally, when a subject bears down, there is a rise in intrarectal pressure associated with relaxation of the external anal sphincter. Inability to perform this coordinated movement represents the chief pathophysiologic abnormality in patients with functional obstructive defecation (anismus), a common cause of constipation.

TREATMENT

The first step is to elucidate an underlying cause or mechanism by performing appropriate tests as outlined earlier. An algorithmic approach to constipation is shown in Figure 1. It is worth reiterating that constipation is a common adverse effect of many *drugs,* a fact that is often overlooked. Some drugs have anticholinergic effects, others desiccate stool, and others affect rectal sensation and reduce awareness for stooling.

Education and General Advice. This should include instruction regarding normal bowel habits, diet, fluid intake, and exercise. Those who believe that bowels must move every day should be informed that a bowel movement every other day or sometimes every third day is not abnormal. Patients with poor eating habits, such as those who miss meals, should be encouraged to eat more regularly. Patients with inadequate fiber intake should be advised with the help of a dietitian to increase their intake of natural fiber with fruits and vegetables. It is useful to emphasize that 20 to 30 grams of fiber per day are essential to facilitate bowel movement. However, not every patient with constipation will benefit from a high-fiber diet. In one study, constipated patients who had either slow transit or pelvic floor dysfunction responded poorly to a diet containing 30 grams of fiber per day, whereas patients without an underlying motility disorder either improved or became symptom free. Thus, fiber intake may not be a panacea for all patients. Patients with sedentary habits should be encouraged to exercise or at least increase their physical activity. However, the benefit of exercise for patients with constipation is controversial.

Slow-Transit Constipation

Before labeling a patient as having slow-transit constipation, it is important to exclude pelvic floor dysfunction. Ideally, slow-transit constipation should be treated with a prokinetic agent that selectively stimulates colonic peristalsis. Unfortunately, such an

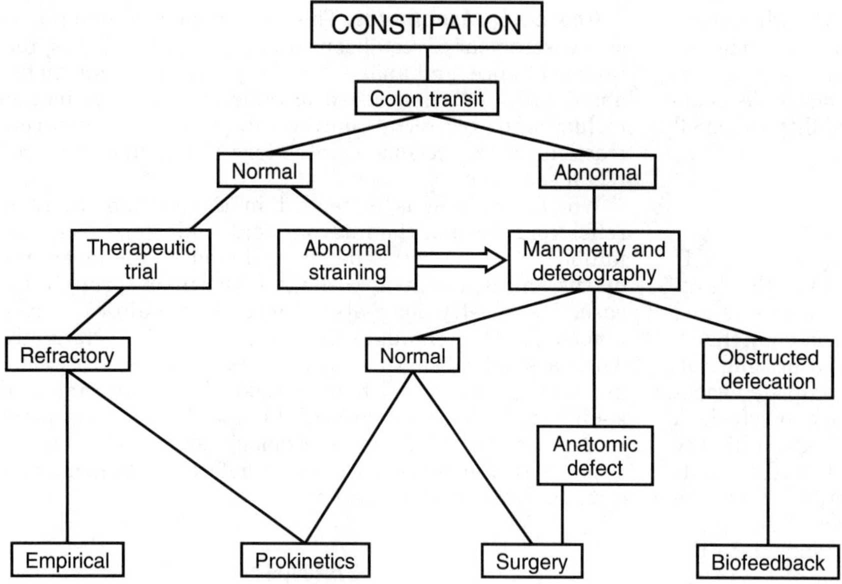

Figure 1. An algorithmic approach to the management of constipation. (From Rao SSC: Manometric evaluation of constipation—Part I. The Gastroenterologist 4:145–154, 1996.)

agent is not available. Prokinetic drugs such as cisapride* (Propulsid) and prostaglandin E analogues such as misoprostol* (Cytotec) have been tried with some success. Other agents that have been tried include a course of broad-spectrum antibiotics such as vancomycin (Vancocin),* anti-inflammatory drugs such as colchicine,* and synthetic bile acids such as ursodeoxycholic acid (Actigall),* although none of these drugs is approved by the U.S. Food and Drug Administration (FDA) for constipation. Laxatives remain the mainstay of treatment for slow-transit constipation. Based on their mode of action, laxatives can be classified into at least five groups. Frequently, over-the-counter laxatives contain more than one compound.

Bulk-Forming Laxatives. These laxatives consist of natural substances such as psyllium (Metamucil) or synthetic polysaccharides such as methylcellulose (Citrucel). These compounds resist digestion and retain water. Hence, they increase stool bulk and enhance colon transit. Because fermentation of psyllium can cause bloating and gas in some patients, nonfermentable products such as methylcellulose may be preferable. It is important to emphasize that fiber supplements should be accompanied by a generous intake of fluid. If not, the large bulky stool may become more difficult to expel. Because patients with chronic renal failure or heart failure are on fluid restriction, bulk laxatives are not advisable.

Emollients. These agents serve as anionic surfactants, that is, they can lower the surface tension of stool. This allows easy mixing of the fatty and aqueous contents of stool, and the softened stool permits easy defecation. The two most popular compounds are docusate sodium (Colace) or docusate calcium (Surfak).

Saline Laxatives. These include agents such as milk of magnesia, calcium citrate (Citracal), magnesium sulfate, sodium phosphate (Fleet Phospho-Soda), and those that contain a mixture of sodium and potassium salts or polyethylene glycol. These hyperosmolar salts exert an osmotic effect in the small bowel and the colon. This draws fluid into the lumen and increases intraluminal volume. Because up to 20% of magnesium can be absorbed, one should exert caution when treating patients with renal disease.

Osmotic Laxatives. This type of laxative includes lactulose (Cephulac, Chronulac), lactitol, sorbitol, mannitol, and polyethylene glycol solutions (Colyte, GoLYTELY, or NuLytely). Lactulose is a nonabsorbable disaccharide that passes unchanged through the stomach and small bowel and is fermented by anaerobic bacteria in the colon to produce fructose, galactose, short chain fatty acids, and gases. Similarly, sorbitol and mannitol are sugars that are poorly absorbed. In addition to diarrhea, all of these agents can cause bloating, distention, flatulence, and crampy discomfort.

Stimulant Laxatives. This group includes compounds such as anthraquinolones (cascara), senna (Senokot), bisacodyl (Dulcolax), castor oil, and phenolphthalein (Modane). If possible, one should avoid these agents. They act through a variety of mechanisms, but their net effect is to stimulate intestinal motility and secretion. They also reduce net absorption of fluid and electrolytes, which can lead to significant electrolyte disturbance. Some of these agents, particularly the anthraquinolones, have been reported to cause melanosis coli, a brownish pigmentation of the colonic mucosa.

Obstructive Defecation

This problem is best treated by neuromuscular conditioning and biofeedback techniques. The goal of biofeedback therapy is to restore a normal pattern of defecation. Patients with impaired rectal contraction

*Not FDA approved for this indication.

are taught diaphragmatic breathing exercises, which improve their intra-abdominal and rectal effort to defecate. Patients with paradoxical anal contraction are educated with the help of visual and audio feedback techniques to improve their rectoanal coordination. Because biofeedback therapy corrects the underlying pathophysiology, one can anticipate long-term benefits.

Stool Impaction

Patients with stool impaction or those with hard stools that are difficult to expel require digital disimpaction. This can be painful and may require sedation or anesthesia. Once the hard pellets have been removed, these patients require a bowel conditioning regimen of enemas, laxatives, and suppositories (glycerin or bisacodyl).

Refractory Constipation

In debilitated or neurologically impaired patients, a tap water, sodium phosphate (Fleet Enema) enema, or milk of molasses enema may be required to facilitate defecation. If the aforementioned measures fail, particularly in patients with slow transit constipation, surgery may be an option. However, before considering surgery, each patient must be carefully evaluated to exclude generalized neuromuscular dysfunction of the gut. Surgical options for refractory constipation include colectomy with ileostomy or an ileoanal pouch or a cecostomy. However, surgery should be regarded as a last resort for patients with constipation.

CONCLUSION

Constipation is a common clinical problem that is often misdiagnosed and inadequately managed. Today, technical advances, together with a better understanding of the underlying mechanisms, have led to real progress in the diagnosis and treatment of this condition.

FEVER

method of
RALPH E. KAUFFMAN, M.D.
Children's Mercy Hospital and University of Missouri—Kansas City School of Medicine
Kansas City, Missouri

Fever is one of the most common presenting complaints, particularly in pediatric patients, in whom it accounts for 10 to 15% of office and emergency department visits. Fever generates a great deal of anxiety on the part of patients and health care providers.

The febrile response involves complex physiologic and biochemical processes. A rational approach to the management of the febrile patient should be based on an understanding of these processes and their role in the host response to pyrogenic stimuli.

NORMAL THERMOREGULATION

Normal body temperature is regulated by complex interactions of thermosensitive neurons in the preoptic region of the anterior hypothalamus; these neurons communicate with modulating neurons in the posterior hypothalamus and other areas of the brain stem. When temperature adjustment is necessary, these thermosensitive neurons modulate the activity of thermostatic neurons located in the posterior hypothalamus to maintain the "set point" for body temperature. Under euthermic conditions, heat production and heat dissipation are balanced to maintain body temperature within a narrow physiologic range even though environmental temperatures may vary considerably. Normal body temperature averages 37°C, with inter-individual variation of 35.5 to 37.8°C. Diurnal variation about the individual mean is 0.5 to 1.0°C, with body temperature lowest in the morning and highest during the late afternoon. Normal temperature also varies seasonally and with ovulation in the female. Therefore, definition of fever must take into account the normal variation among individuals and normal diurnal fluctuation in body temperature.

Fever occurs when the hypothalamic set point is reset such that the mechanisms for thermoregulation are adjusted to maintain the body temperature at a new higher steady-state temperature. Readjustment of the set point initiates a number of physiologic processes, including peripheral vasoconstriction, central pooling of blood, increased heat conservation, shivering, a sensation of feeling cold, increased oxygen consumption, and rise in core temperature to a new steady-state level. Body temperature rarely, if ever, exceeds 41°C owing to set point regulated fever. Return of the set point to the euthermic range is accompanied by peripheral vasodilatation; perspiration; decreased oxygen consumption; heat loss by evaporation, convection, and conduction; and defervescence to normal body temperature.

THE BIOCHEMICAL MODULATION OF FEVER

Fever is an integral component of the "acute phase response," which is triggered by a wide variety of stimuli, including infection, burns, traumatic injury, autoimmune diseases, and certain neoplasms. Pyrogenic cytokines play a key role in mediation of the acute phase response. These peptides are produced in many different tissues by numerous cell types, including monocytes, macrophages, vascular endothelium, lymphocytes, mesangial cells, fibroblasts, and astrocytes. The principal pyrogenic cytokines are interleukin-1β (IL-1β), interleukin-6 (IL-6), and tumor necrosis factor (TNF). Pyrogenic cytokines initiate fever by acting at the hypothalamus. The exact mechanism is not fully understood. However, IL-1 is thought to act at the level of the organum vasculosum laminae terminalis, a circumventricular network of enlarged capillaries adjacent to the anterior hypothalamus, to stimulate local production of IL-1 and IL-6, which in turn induces increased local production of prostaglandin E_2 (PGE_2) A consequent increase in cyclic adenosine monophosphate (cAMP) mediates a rise in the hypothalamic set point to a new steady-state temperature. Local production of PGE_2 in the hypothalamus appears to be essential to the febrile response. Fever is a highly regulated physiologic response in which endogenous cryogens are thought to oppose the effect of endogenous pyrogens, thereby acting to modulate the elevated set point temperature within a range that is not harmful to the organism.

IL-1 also stimulates PGE_2 production peripherally. This has been shown to result in intralysosomal proteolysis of skeletal muscle and may explain the myalgia and negative nitrogen balance associated with fever.

FEVER AS A NORMAL HOST RESPONSE

Until the latter part of the 19th century, fever was viewed largely as a natural and beneficial adaptive host response. A change in perception of fever from that of an adaptive mechanism to that of a pathologic phenomenon occurred at the same time as the introduction of the thermometer and antipyretic drugs into medical practice. An extensive body of published information documents that fever is an adaptive mechanism that is extensively phylogenetically preserved over a wide range of animal species, from lower invertebrates to higher mammals. Animal studies of both warm- and cold-blooded species with experimental infections have shown improved survival associated with the febrile response and decreased survival when the febrile response is prevented. Similar evidence in humans is also available. Overuse of antipyretics for fever, particularly moderate fever of 39.5°C or lower, accompanying acute viral and bacterial infections may be more detrimental than beneficial. However, fever may be associated with considerable discomfort; increased caloric, oxygen, and fluid requirements; and increased risk of seizures in some children. The decision to use antipyretics should be governed more by the amount of discomfort, pain, and malaise than the degree of temperature elevation. There is little evidence that use of antipyretics following a febrile seizure reduces the risk of a subsequent seizure.

A PHYSIOLOGIC APPROACH TO FEVER REDUCTION

Treatment of fever should be directed toward the pathophysiologic mechanisms involved. This includes treating the underlying cause when possible, reducing the elevated hypothalamic set point, and, secondarily, enhancing physical removal of body heat.

Nonpharmacologic Methods

Nonpharmacologic management of fever includes management of increased fluid, oxygen, and caloric requirements along with measures to facilitate physical dissipation of body heat. Placing the patient in light clothing in a neutral ambient temperature may be adequate in many situations. Sponging with tepid water may be done to enhance heat loss by evaporation. Alcohol or cold water should never be used. Cold water induces vasoconstriction and shivering, which is counterproductive to heat loss. Measures to increase heat loss are counterproductive unless they are combined with antipyretic medication to lower the elevated hypothalamic set point temperature. Physical measures alone trigger reflex mechanisms that generate and conserve body heat to maintain the elevated temperature.

Antipyretic Drugs

All of the clinically useful antipyretics block production of PGE_2 in the hypothalamus, thereby inhibiting the febrile response. However, experimental evidence indicates that some antipyretic drugs also may lower body temperature by stimulating release of arginine vasopressin, which in turn induces release of α-melanocyte–stimulating hormone, which acts as a cryogen in the hypothalamus.

Acetaminophen

Acetaminophen (paracetamol—Tylenol, Panadol, Excedrin, and many combination products) is the most widely used antipyretic medication by individuals of all ages. It is a weak cyclooxygenase inhibitor peripherally but is metabolized in the central nervous system to a potent inhibitor of prostaglandin synthesis. Acetaminophen is rapidly and completely absorbed from the gastrointestinal tract when administered orally. When consumed in recommended doses, it is metabolized in the liver primarily to inactive water-soluble glucuronide and sulfate conjugates that are eliminated in the urine. Elimination half-life is 1 to 3 hours in individuals with normal hepatic and renal function.

Acute overdose leads to production of reactive metabolites, which, if not conjugated with glutathione, bind to cellular macromolecules and result in acute hepatotoxicity. Individuals who are taking drugs that induce cytochrome P450 activity, who smoke, or who are chronic alcohol users are particularly susceptible to acetaminophen toxicity. Children given excessive doses over a long term also may sustain severe hepatotoxicity. Acute acetaminophen overdose is treated successfully with *N*-acetyl-L-cysteine if treatment is started within 24 hours of acetaminophen ingestion. Acetaminophen does not cause gastric irritation, decrease platelet adhesion, or decrease renal blood flow as do the nonsteroidal anti-inflammatory drugs (NSAIDs). Notwithstanding the risk of hepatotoxicity with excessive doses, it remains the safest antipyretic currently available.

The recommended dose is 10 to 15 mg per kg every 4 to 6 hours in children and 325 to 650 mg every 3 to 4 hours in adults.

Multiple dosage formulations of acetaminophen are available, including infant drops, pediatric suspensions, chewable tablets, and tablets and caplets of various sizes. Adult formulations should never be used in children because this practice has resulted in tragic inadvertent overdoses. In addition, parents of infants and small children should be advised to always use the appropriate measuring device supplied in the product package to measure children's liquid preparations. The infant drops are three times as concentrated as the pediatric suspension and if administered in the volumes intended for the suspension may result in excessive and toxic doses.

Nonsteroidal Anti-inflammatory Drugs

Most of the NSAIDs are potent inhibitors of prostaglandin synthesis, both peripherally and in the central nervous system, and therefore are effective antipyretics. In addition, they may provide greater relief than acetaminophen from myalgia and malaise associated with systemic infections owing to their peripheral activity. Currently, only aspirin, ibuprofen, and naproxen are routinely used as antipyretics.

Ibuprofen (Advil, Motrin, Nuprin, and others) is the NSAID most commonly used for antipyresis. It is well absorbed after oral administration. Elimination is by hepatic oxidative metabolism and glucuronidation, with an elimination half-life of 1.5 to 2 hours in children and adults. Side effects are rare when ibuprofen is used in recommended doses for 1 to 3 days. In a double-blind randomized study of 84,000 children, the incidence of serious adverse events was no different between ibuprofen and acetaminophen. However, ibuprofen rarely may cause gastric irritation, occult gastrointestinal bleeding, reversible platelet dysfunction, abnormal liver function test results, exacerbation of asthma in aspirin-sensitive individuals, and decreased renal blood flow. Administration of ibuprofen in the presence of volume-contracted states such as dehydration may cause decreased renal blood flow, leading to acute renal failure. Acute overdose of ibuprofen less than 200 mg per kg rarely is associated with significant toxicity. Larger overdoses have been associated with acidosis, hepatotoxicity, and renal toxicity. The recommended ibuprofen dose is 8 to 10 mg per kg every 6 to 8 hours in children and 200 to 600 mg every 4 to 6 hours in adults. The antipyretic efficacy of acetaminophen and ibuprofen is approximately equivalent, although their respective dose-response curves differ. Eight mg per kg of ibuprofen provides approximately the same antipyretic effect as 15 mg per kg of acetaminophen. Ibuprofen is supplied in multiple dosage forms, including children's drops, children's suspension, tablets, caplets, and gelcaps.

Naproxen (Naprosyn, Aleve, Anaprox, and others) shares most of the antipyretic and side effect characteristics of ibuprofen. It differs from ibuprofen principally in its long elimination half-life, which ranges from 12 to 17 hours. Because of its long half-life, naproxen may be administered less frequently. The usual adult dose is 250 to 500 mg every 12 hours. Naproxen is not recommended for routine antipyretic use in young children. However, doses of 5 mg per kg every 8 to 12 hours have been shown to be well tolerated in children older than 2 years of age.

Aspirin is the original NSAID and remains a very effective antipyretic for adult use. The elimination half-life following antipyretic doses is 2 to 4 hours. However, metabolism of salicylate is saturable so that at higher doses the apparent half-life is longer and the concentration increases disproportionately to the dose. This increases the risk of significant toxicity. The propensity for gastrointestinal irritation, ulceration, and hemorrhage is greater than with acetaminophen, ibuprofen, or naproxen. Salicylate overdose causes uncoupling of oxidative metabolism, resulting in profound acidosis, fluid and electrolyte derangement, and metabolic abnormalities that may be lethal if not treated aggressively. Aspirin at low doses permanently acetylates platelets, resulting in noncompetitive inhibition of platelet function. The usual dose of aspirin is 325 to 650 mg every 4 hours in adults. Aspirin should not be used as a routine antipyretic in children and teenagers because of the associated increased risk of Reye's syndrome.

Combination Antipyretics

Use of two antipyretics with the same mechanism of action makes little sense pharmacologically or physiologically. Alternating doses of aspirin or ibuprofen with acetaminophen is no more effective than giving an equivalent dose of a single drug. In addition, this practice exposes the patient to potential toxicities of two drugs with little therapeutic advantage.

COUGH

method of
BIMALIN LAHIRI, M.D., and
PHYLLIS L. SCHATZ, M.D.
University of Connecticut School of Medicine and
St. Francis Hospital and Medical Center
Hartford, Connecticut

Cough is a defense mechanism for clearing secretions and inhaled and noxious substances from the tracheobronchial tree. Chronic cough, however, is a significant clinical problem and the most frequent chief complaint of patients presenting to primary care physicians. Cough is given as the reason for almost 4% of all office visits. Chronic cough is a complaint across all age groups and therefore is encountered by pediatricians, family physicians, and internists, as well as specialists in allergy and pulmonary medicine.

In approximately 50% of all presentations, the cough is chronic, which is commonly defined as longer than 3 weeks' duration. In the nonsmoking population, persistent cough is reported to occur in 14 to 23% of adults. Among smokers, chronic cough is reported in 25% of one-half-pack-per-day smokers and in more than 50% of those who smoke more than two packs per day. It is estimated that more than $600 million is spent annually in the United States for prescription and over-the-counter medications for the treatment of cough.

Constant coughing can become debilitating and can affect the patient's quality of life and work. Patients seek medical attention for various reasons, which include fear of having a serious disease such as cancer, acquired immune deficiency syndrome (AIDS), or tuberculosis; concern that something is wrong; change in lifestyle; embarrassment or distress; hoarseness; and symptomatic relief.

PATHOPHYSIOLOGY

Coughing may be voluntary but is more often the result of a complex involuntary reflex response to stimulation of cough receptors in the upper and lower airways. Each cough is generated in four steps that are coordinated by the cough center in the brain stem: (1) initial inspiratory gasp; (2) Valsalva maneuver with forceful contraction of the muscles of the chest wall, abdominal wall, and diaphragm against a closed glottis; (3) expiratory blast as the vocal cords abduct; and (4) post-tussive prolonged inspiration.

The removal of foreign material is accomplished during the expiratory phase, during which the expiratory flow rates can exceed 12 liters per second. This force can also result in characteristic sounds such as "whooping" cough or a brassy, barking quality. Cough effort can be diminished significantly owing to C6–7 spinal cord injury, resulting in loss of chest wall, intercostal, and abdominal muscles.

Pathologic cough in the absence of secretions or foreign material to be cleared results from stimulation of the cough reflex. Nerves that initiate cough are predominantly in the upper airway to protect the larynx from the entry of foreign material. The tracheobronchial tree contains several types of sensory nerves: (1) slowly adapting receptors known as stretch receptors, (2) rapidly adapting receptors ("irritant" receptors), (3) pulmonary C fiber or J-type receptors, and (4) bronchial C fiber receptors. Afferent impulses from stretch and irritant receptors are carried to the medulla via the vagus nerve as well as the glossopharyngeal and phrenic nerves. The vagus, phrenic, and other nerves carry efferent impulses as well to the diaphragm, glottis, and chest and abdominal wall muscles. Agents selective for C fibers, such as inhaled capsaicin and sulfur dioxide, also trigger cough and sneezing. Mechanical stimulation in the external auditory canal can trigger an afferent signal along the auricular branch of the vagus nerve. Cough receptors can also be found in the pericardium, tympanic membrane, and esophagus.

Complications from severe chronic cough are known. The Valsalva maneuver elevates intrathoracic pressure, causing decreased venous return and increased systemic blood pressure with reflex vasodilatation and bradycardia—this leading to post-tussive syncope. Pneumothorax and retinal vessel rupture can result from raised intrathoracic pressure. Tussive headache has been attributed to high venous pressure in cerebral vessels, causing increased intracranial pressure. Chest wall and abdominal muscle strain, as well as rib fracture, can result.

ACUTE COUGH

The most common cause of acute cough is a viral upper respiratory infection (URI), although bacterial infection, sinusitis, pharyngitis, bronchitis, or pneumonia can be involved. Acute inflammation with or without bronchospasm causes the cough, which is usually self-limited. Approximately 70 to 80% of cases of acute cough resolve spontaneously. Allergic rhinitis, asthma exacerbation, or exposure to irritants may also trigger cough. Treatment is ordered as appropriately directed toward specific infection or inflammation. On occasion, nonspecific symptomatic treatment is used while awaiting spontaneous resolution of the acute cough.

CHRONIC COUGH

The approach to the patient with chronic cough is based on knowledge of pre-existing pulmonary disease, other medical history, current medications, presence or absence of smoking or other exposures, and presence or absence of sputum and/or hemoptysis.

The most common causes of chronic cough include smoking and other environmental irritants, postnasal drip, asthma (including "cough-variant" asthma), gastroesophageal reflux (GER, GERD), chronic bronchitis, airway hyper-responsiveness (often following viral or atypical infection), and medications (especially angiotensin-converting enzyme [ACE] inhibitors and beta blockers). Less common causes include congestive heart failure, bronchogenic (or esophageal) carcinoma, interstitial lung disease, bronchiectasis, tuberculosis (and chronic fungal infection), cystic fibrosis, recurrent aspiration (after a cerebrovascular accident; frequent vomiting, bulimia, ethyl alcohol [ETOH] abuse), pressure from intrathoracic mass (e.g., thoracic aneurysm, thyromegaly, mediastinal lymphadenopathy), irritation of cough receptors in ear (e.g., impacted cerumen, hair), opportunistic infection, lymphangitic carcinomatosis, foreign body in the airway, chronic inhalation of bronchial irritants, and psychogenic factors.

HISTORY

A thorough history is important to help identify clues to specific causes of chronic cough.

1. *Smoking:* Quantify smoking history. Is the cough worse in the morning? Is the cough worse when the person is exposed to smoke?
2. *Postnasal drip:* Does the patient note mucous drainage from the nose? Is there a frequent need to "clear the throat" or swallow mucus? Is there a history of allergy, allergic rhinitis, or sinus infection or inflammation?
3. *Asthma:* Is coughing brought on by exercise or specific irritants (e.g., smoke, dust, pollen, fumes, chemicals, pets)? Is there a family history of allergies, asthma, or eczema? Is there associated wheezing, chest tightness, or dyspnea? Has there been a recent change in residence and/or working environment? Is there a seasonal component?
4. *Gastroesophageal reflux:* Does the patient complain of heartburn or a sour or an acid taste? Are symptoms worse when lying down? Is the cough improved by use of antacids or H_2 blockers?
5. *Chronic bronchitis:* Is the patient a smoker? Does the patient have a cough that has produced more than 30 mL of sputum daily for 3 months in 2 consecutive years?
6. *Medication related:* Review list; check especially for ACE inhibitors or beta blockers (including eye drops).
7. *Airway hyper-responsiveness following URI:* Did the cough begin during a URI? Is the cough usually nonproductive?
8. *Underlying malignancy or serious infection (e.g., tuberculosis):* Does the patient have fever, chills, night sweats, weight loss? Previous malignancy? Other risk factors? Has there been any hemoptysis? Take age, travel history, and country of origin into account.

PHYSICAL EXAMINATION

Increased accumulation of mucus and cobblestone appearance of the mucosa of the nasopharynx are typically seen in the postnasal drip syndrome. Patients with allergic rhinitis often exhibit nasal congestion with pale and boggy mucosa, a transverse crease over the bridge of the nose, and discoloration of the lower lids ("allergic shiners"). If tenderness is present over the maxillary or frontal sinuses, sinusitis is suggested as the cause of the postnasal drip.

Auscultation of the lungs can reveal prolonged expiratory phase and/or wheezing, which can also be induced by forced expiratory maneuver. End-inspiratory "squeaks, pops, and bubbles" are pathognomonic for postinfectious bronchiolitis. A careful examination for lymphadenopathy is important in the search for pulmonary tumor. Clubbing may be seen in lung carcinoma as well as in bronchiectasis. Fixed, late inspiratory ("Velcro") rales or crackles are commonly heard in interstitial lung disease. "Moist" rales and third heart sound are consistent with cardiac dysfunction.

For completeness, physical examination should include the ears to exclude the uncommon cause of a foreign body stimulating cough receptors.

GENERAL APPROACH TO EVALUATION OF CHRONIC COUGH

Initial screening must include a careful history and physical examination, with particular attention given to smoking history, occupational exposure or exposure to lung toxins or irritants, medication history, sputum production and/or hemoptysis, and pre-existing disease.

Cigarette smoke exposure must be eliminated as must other environmental toxins. Medications that could induce cough (ACE inhibitors, beta blockers) should be discontinued. If a preceding respiratory infection is apparent, post-URI hyper-reactivity and any residual bacterial or atypical infection should be treated. Postviral bronchiolitis is a relatively common but underdiagnosed clinical entity.

Patients with chronic bronchitis or bronchiectasis should be treated aggressively, as should patients with any subacute or suboptimally treated exacerbation of bronchial asthma. Similarly, acute or chronic sinus infection should be treated. A computed tomography (CT) scan may be beneficial as a diagnostic test.

When hyper-reactivity or infection is not apparent, the methacholine challenge test is an extremely important part of the patient's work-up.

If gastroesophageal reflux is obvious, aggressive antireflux therapy should be initiated. The diagnosis of GERD can be suggested by barium swallow or endoscopy or confirmed by more invasive esophageal pH monitoring. Reflux as the etiology of the patient's cough, however, is confirmed by response to therapy.

If specific therapy results in resolution of the cough in any of the above situations, further diagnostic studies are not uniformly required. Exceptions to this include patients with history of cigarette smoking and hemoptysis, in which case a chest radiograph must be obtained and consideration given to bronchoscopy. In patients who present with dyspnea and cough, pulmonary function tests should be obtained initially and repeated after therapy. Patients who have symptoms of weight loss and/or hemoptysis, fever, chills, or night sweats must have a chest radiograph and further diagnostic studies as indicated, especially purified protein derivative testing and sputum for acid-fast bacilli and cytology. Various factors such as the patient's age and country of origin and the findings on chest radiograph would then influence further investigations. If the chest radiograph result is equivocal, a CT scan of the thorax is advised. Pulmonary consultation with respect to bronchoscopy is recommended.

The algorithm presented in Figure 1 may be helpful in organizing the approach to the patient with chronic cough.

SPECIFIC THERAPY

As listed in Table 1, effective specific therapy for the common causes of chronic cough are outlined below:

Postnasal Drip. An antihistamine-decongestant combination such as brompheniramine and phenylpropanolamine (Dimetapp) or loratadine and pseudoephedrine (Claritin-D) or an antihistamine alone such as cetirizine (Zyrtec) is a common effective therapy. In patients with allergic rhinitis, or in whom the above is not sufficient, intranasal steroid (such as fluticasone [Flonase] or beclomethasone [Vancenase]) should be added. If vasomotor rhinitis is suspected, nasal ipratropium bromide (Atrovent 0.03%, 2 sprays two to four times daily) should be added. If symptoms persist, a CT scan of the sinuses and/or empirical treatment for sinusitis should be ordered (see "Sinusitis").

Sinusitis. Antibiotics should be chosen to treat the usual organisms (*Streptococcus pneumoniae, Haemophilus influenzae, Moraxella catarrhalis,* plus or minus anaerobes), such as amoxicillin-clavulanate (Augmentin), trimethoprim-sulfamethoxasole (Bactrim, Septra), or a second-generation cephalosporin (cefuroxime [Ceftin]), clarithromycin (Biaxin), or levofloxacin (Levaquin). A brief course (3 days) of intranasal decongestant spray (oxymetazoline [Afrin]) is sometimes helpful. In many cases of allergic or chronic sinusitis, intranasal corticosteroid will be beneficial.

Asthma and Cough-Variant Asthma. Beta agonists are effective bronchodilators and can improve cough. However, these agents do not reduce bronchial hyper-reactivity, which is recognized as being caused by chronic inflammation. Thus, a combination of a beta agonist metered-dose inhaler (e.g., albuterol [Proventil, Ventolin], 2 puffs four times daily as necessary) and an anti-inflammatory agent—either mast cell stabilizers such as cromolyn or nedocromil or inhaled steroid such as beclomethasone (Vanceril) or fluticasone (Flovent)—should be added. A long-acting theophylline preparation can be considered in nocturnal cough secondary to asthma.

If the patient is markedly symptomatic or dyspneic or has significantly abnormal pulmonary function test results, a course of oral corticosteroid (prednisone, 40 mg daily with tapering dose) should be utilized. Patients should avoid triggers of bronchospasm and hyper-reactivity. If the patient cannot be tapered off oral corticosteroid, an addition of the leukotriene receptor antagonist zafirlukast (Accolate) or 5-lipoxygenase inhibitor zileuton (Zyflo) can be considered.

Gastroesophageal Reflux. Antireflux measures in general include elevating the head approximately 20 to 30 degrees; avoiding eating 2 to 3 hours before going to sleep (or reclining); and avoiding aggravating factors such as coffee and alcohol and factors that decrease the lower esophageal sphincter pressure such as chocolate and theophylline. H_2 receptor antagonists such as ranitidine (Zantac) or famotidine (Pepcid) have been utilized, but the newer proton pump inhibitors such as omeprazole (Prilosec) appear to be more effective in blocking acid production in the stomach and relieving reflux symptoms. High protein and low fat meals may be considered as well. GER-induced cough appears to be secondary to stim-

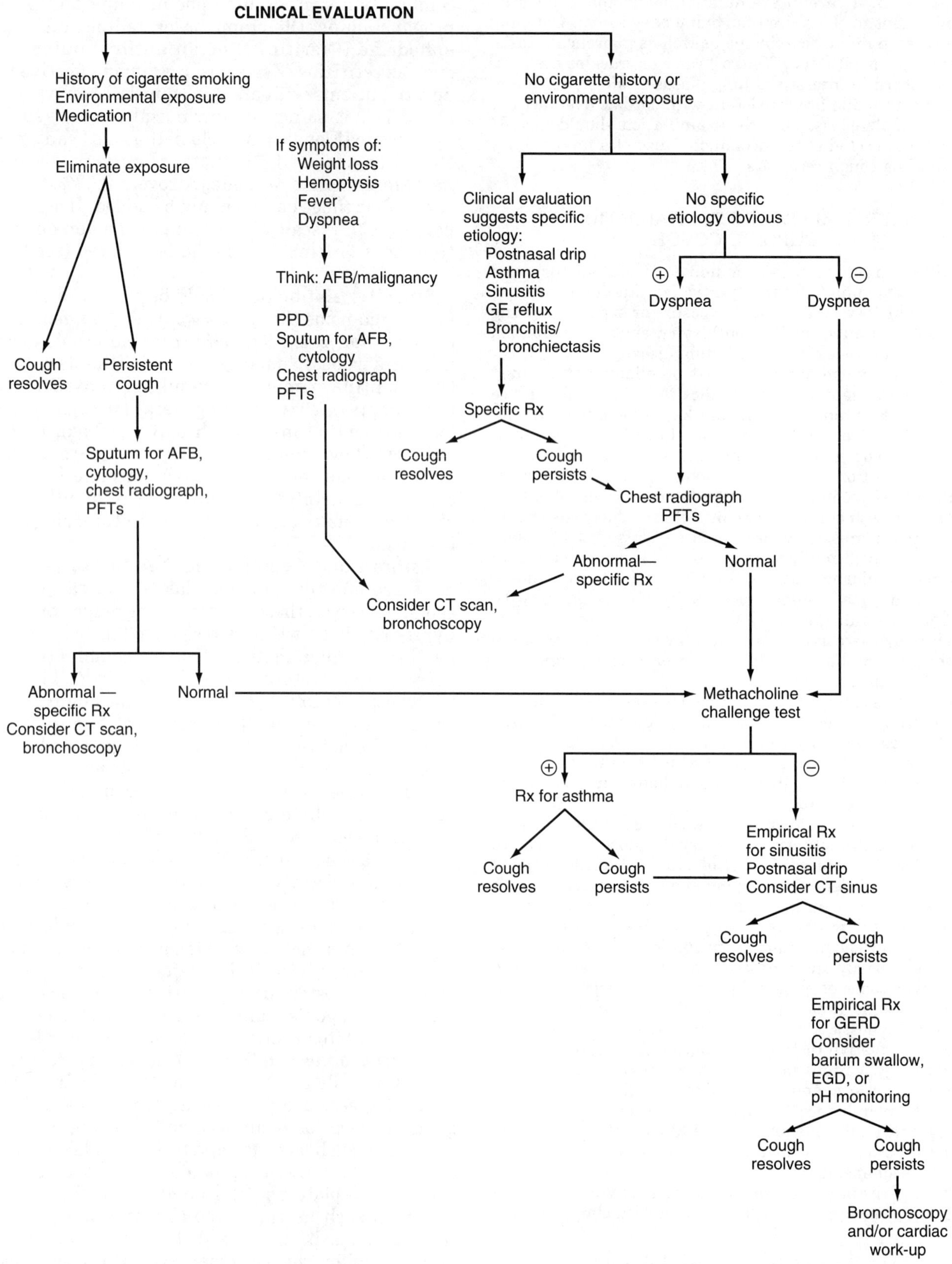

Figure 1. Approach to the patient with chronic cough. *Abbreviations:* AFB = acid-fast bacilli; PFT = pulmonary function test; Rx = treatment; CT = computed tomography; PPD = purified protein derivative; GERD = gastroesophageal reflux disease; EGD = esophagogastroduodenoscopy.

TABLE 1. **Specific Therapies by Etiology of Cough**

Cause	Generic Name	Brand Name	Dose
Postnasal drip	Brompheniramine plus phenylpropanolamine	Dimetapp	2 tsp q 4 hr
	Loratadine plus pseudoephedrine	Claritin-D	1 tablet PO bid
	Cetirizine	Zyrtec	10 mg PO qd
Sinusitis			
Antibiotic choices	Amoxicillin-clavulanate	Augmentin	250 mg PO tid
	Trimethoprim-sulfamethoxazole	Bactrim DS	1 tablet PO bid
	Cefuroxime	Ceftin	250 mg PO bid
	Clarithromycin	Biaxin	500 mg PO bid
	Levofloxacin	Levaquin	500 mg PO qd
Decongestant	Oxymetazolone	Afrin	2–3 sprays intranasally, each nostril bid (for 3 d)
	Loratadine plus pseudoephedrine	Claritin-D	1 tablet PO bid
Corticosteroid	Beclomethasone	Vancenase AQ	2 sprays each nostril bid
	Fluticasone	Flonase	1 spray each nostril qd
Asthma	Albuterol inhaler	Proventil/Ventolin	2 puffs qid prn
	Beclomethasone inhaler	Vanceril	2 puffs bid
	Fluticasone	Flovent	2 puffs bid
	Theophylline	Uniphyl	400 mg qd (PM)
	Corticosteroid	Prednisone	40 mg daily with taper
	Zafirlukast	Accolate	20 mg PO bid
	Zileuton	Zyflo	600 mg PO qid
Gastroesophageal reflux	Famotidine	Pepcid	20 mg PO bid
	Cisapride	Propulsid	10 mg PO qid (ac, hs)
	Omeprazole	Prilosec	20 mg PO qd
Bronchitis, bronchiectasis	Antibiotics as above		
	Albuterol/ipratropium	Ventolin and Atrovent (or Combivent)	2 puffs qid
Bronchiolitis	Corticosteroid	Prednisone	40 mg daily with prolonged taper over 6 wk

ulation of mucosal receptors in the distal esophagus and not necessarily due to aspiration. However, if the cough does not respond after 6 to 8 weeks of therapy, gastroenterology consultation for endoscopy and pulmonary consultation for bronchoscopy might be considered to detect aspiration.

Bronchitis, Bronchiectasis, and Postinfectious Bronchiolitis. Bronchodilator therapy—ipratropium (Atrovent) and albuterol (Proventil or Ventolin)—and appropriate antibiotic therapy are the mainstays of treatment. Effective clearance of secretions is often aided by chest percussion and postural drainage, especially in those with bronchiectasis. In patients with significant bronchospasm and hypersecretion of mucus, a course of oral corticosteroid is often beneficial (prednisone, 40 mg daily with taper). In patients with extremely tenacious secretions, a protussive agent such as iodinated glycerol or guaifenesin (Humibid) is beneficial. In patients with bronchiectasis, acetylcysteine (Mucomyst) via aerosol can be helpful but must be used with caution and in combination with a beta agonist bronchodilator because of its tendency to induce bronchospasm and mucosal irritation. In patients with postinfectious bronchiolitis, restrictive physiology and decreased diffusion capacity can be seen on pulmonary function test results. Prednisone, 40 mg a day orally, must be started, with a gradual decrease in dose over a 6-week period to prevent relapse.

Other Causes of Cough. Possible causes such as aspiration, interstitial lung disease, foreign body (in the airway or in the ear), and congestive heart failure should be suspected on the basis of history, physical examination, and/or chest radiograph. Further workup should be pursued as indicated. Psychogenic cough should be a diagnosis of exclusion. It is more common in children and adolescents and should be suspected when the cough disappears during sleep and seems to increase with attention from others.

NONSPECIFIC TREATMENT OF COUGH

In the small percentage of patients in whom it is not possible to ascertain or treat effectively the cause of the cough, or when the cough is not serving a useful function in clearing secretions and is disrupting sleep, it may be necessary to treat it in a nonspecific manner. An "annoying tickle" may be quieted by over-the-counter lozenges or honey or licorice or by using antitussive drugs (Table 2).

Effective nonspecific *antitussive therapy* can result from drugs that block various parts of the cough reflex.

1. Centrally acting drugs (that increase the threshold or latency of the cough center) such as narcotics (morphine, codeine) and non-narcotics (dextromethorphan, diphenhydramine).

TABLE 2. **Nonspecific Therapies for Cough**

	Generic Name	Trade Name	Dosage
Antihistamines	Loratadine	Claritin	10 mg qd
	Loratadine plus pseudoephedrine	Claritin-D	1 tablet bid
Non-narcotic antitussive	Guaifenesin	Robitussin	2–4 tsp q 4 h
	Guaifenesin plus dextromethorphan	Robitussin-DM	2 tsp q 4 h
Narcotic antitussive	Codeine		30–60 mg PO q 4 h
	Hydrocodone	Hycodan	1 tsp q 6–8 h
	Hydrocodone, chlorpheniramine	Tussionex	1 tsp q 8–12 h
Protussive	Acetylcysteine	Mucomyst	1–2 cc. of 10–20% via aerosol bid—qid
	Guaifenesin	Humibid L.A.	600 mg PO bid

2. Agents that block peripheral stretch receptors and mucociliary factors such as ipratropium bromide (Atrovent) and dexbrompheniramine maleate plus pseudoephedrine sulfate.

3. Drugs that may increase the threshold or latency of the efferent limb of the cough reflex such as ipratropium.

When the clearing of secretions is necessary but the cough is ineffective, *protussive therapy* may be beneficial. Drugs that provide such therapy include aerosolized amiloride (in cystic fibrosis), expectorants (such as guaifenesin, terpin hydrate), and iodinated glycerol. Mucolytics such as acetylcysteine liquefy thick mucus but must be used with caution, as mentioned previously, especially in the case of a patient with neuromuscular weakness or weak cough with inability to propel secretions centrally.

HOARSENESS AND LARYNGITIS

method of
C. BLAKE SIMPSON, M.D., and
G. RICHARD HOLT, M.D.
University of Texas Health Science Center at San Antonio
San Antonio, Texas

INITIAL EVALUATION OF VOCAL DISORDERS

Hoarseness and laryngitis are very common presenting symptoms to the primary care physician. Usually these symptoms are manifestations of benign and time-limited conditions; however, occasionally there is an underlying serious condition that must be diagnosed and treated expeditiously. The key is deciding which are not worrisome and which are indeed serious symptoms (Figure 1). In general, hoarseness that has an acute onset and is associated with systemic symptoms such as cough, malaise, and fever will be self-limited. Conversely, hoarseness that lasts more than 1 month, is generally painless, and is associated with smoking and drinking should be considered to be caused by a cancer until proven otherwise.

Obtaining a detailed medical history and review of symptoms is crucial to the diagnostic process. Information on respiratory and allergic symptoms, current drug therapy, vocal use or misuse, exposure to carcinogens and/or toxicants, and reflux symptoms is quite helpful in pointing to potential etiologies. Previous trauma, intubation, surgical procedures, and endoscopies may lead to the suspicion of laryngeal framework or nerve injuries. Hoarseness and laryngitis can even be symptoms of bulimia.

The physical examination of the head and neck as performed by a primary care physician should address neurologic, inflammatory, infectious, and traumatic abnormalities as a minimum. If possible, mirror examination of the larynx should be undertaken. A primary care physician who is proficient in flexible fiberoptic nasolaryngoscopy and comfortable with regard to the anatomy and appearance of the larynx and hypopharynx can perform this examination. One who is not should obtain an otolaryngologic consultation. A thorough neck examination, paying particular attention to the laryngeal anatomy, cervical lymph node areas, and thyroid gland, is critical.

Referral to an otolaryngologist or head and neck surgeon is appropriate when suspicious findings are present on the head and neck examination, when the patient is in a high-risk category, or when the hoarseness persists for more than 3 to 4 weeks (Table 1). Otherwise, the primary care physician may elect to treat the patient based on decisions derived from the history, examination, and likelihood of benign disease. Once the patient has been referred to the otolaryngologist, a more detailed head and neck examination will be performed, as well as fiberoptic laryngoscopy. Stroboscopic laryngoscopy (commonly referred to as a "videostrobe") may also be performed, particularly when a mucosal lesion or vocal use disorder is suspected. The specialist may decide to perform a computed tomography (CT) or magnetic resonance imaging (MRI) scan of the brain, neck, and/or chest, depending on the focus of the findings. Other tests available for providing additional information include 24-hour double pH probe with pharyngeal/esophageal monitoring, paranasal sinus radiographs, laryngeal electromyography, videofluoroscopic barium swallow, and thyroid function studies and scan. Endoscopy with biopsy of the lesion is usually the definitive diagnostic test if malignancy is suspected,

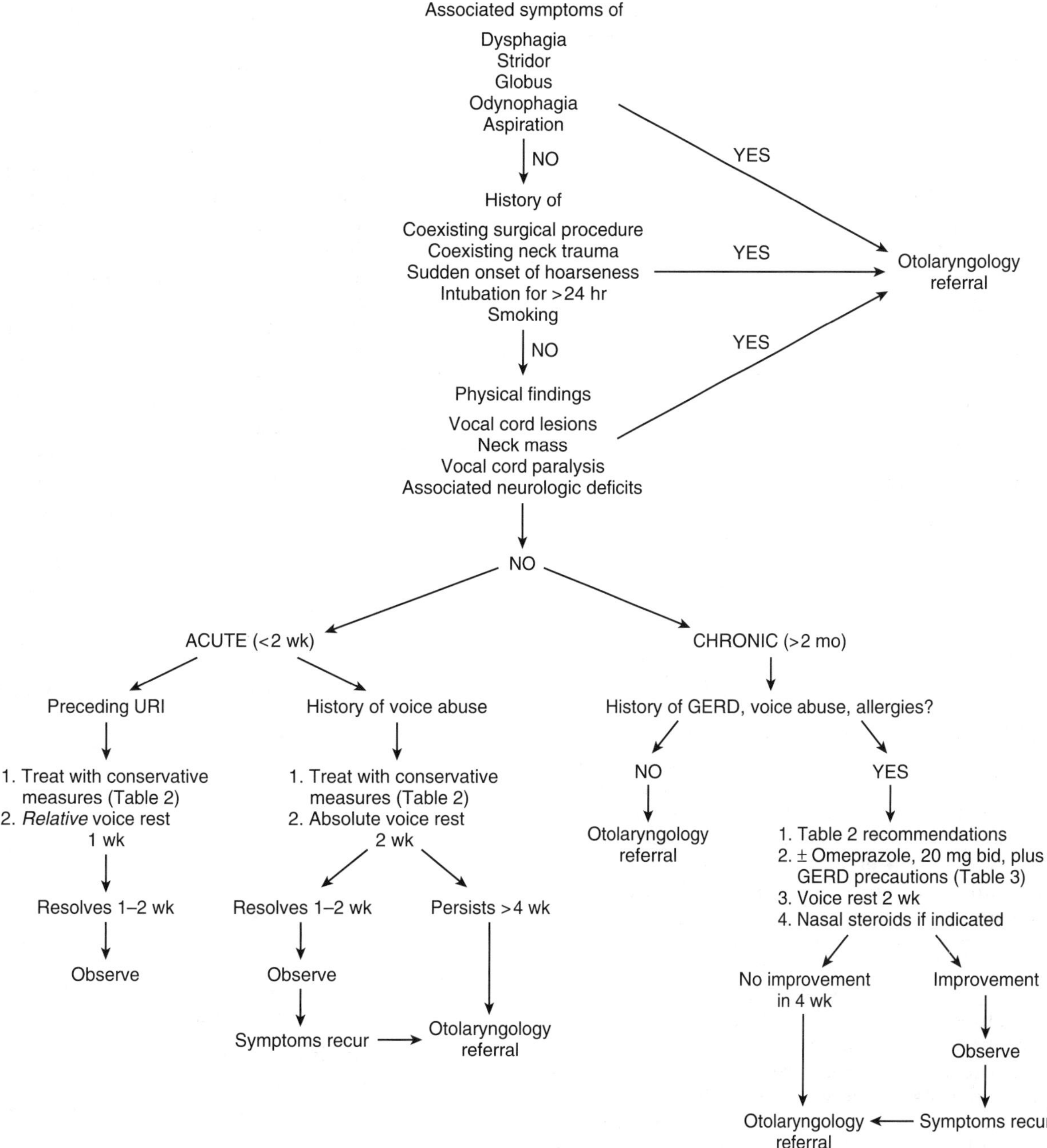

Figure 1. Hoarseness: evaluation and treatment. *Abbreviations*: URI = upper respiratory infection; GERD = gastroesophageal reflux disease.

whereas microsurgical excision is the gold standard for suspected benign pathology.

SPECIFIC CONDITIONS

Congenital/Pediatric

Vocal Cord Nodules. The most common cause of hoarseness in a child is vocal cord nodules, constituting almost 80% of cases. These lesions are most frequently seen in boys between the ages of 4 and 10 years old and are a direct result of vocal abuse. The common name, "screamer's nodules," indicates that there is almost always a history of excessive screaming and/or loud vocalization. The best objective method of diagnosis is careful examination of the larynx in the otolaryngologist's office, generally using a flexible nasolaryngoscope. Characteristically, the nodules are located at the junction of the anterior one third and the posterior two thirds of the vocal cords, which is the point of maximum impact on their vibratory surface. Treatment is conservative and consists of referral to a speech therapist who is knowledgeable in vocal misuse disorders and can attempt to reduce the child's vocal abuse behaviors. Surgical removal of vocal cord nodules is rarely recommended

TABLE 1. **Recommendations for Referral**

Hoarseness associated with any of the following symptoms
Dysphagia
Odynophagia (painful swallowing)
Aspiration
Stridor/partial airway obstruction
Globus (foreign body sensation)
Hoarseness associated with the following conditions
Following any surgical procedure, especially of the neck or chest
Sudden hoarseness after extreme vocal use or abuse
Neck trauma
Intubation, especially prolonged
Professional voice user with impending singing or speaking engagement
Hoarseness with the following physical findings
Neck mass
Vocal cord paralysis
Laryngeal lesion
Neurologic deficits
New-onset hoarseness in a smoker
Hoarseness that persists for longer than 4 weeks after initiating treatment

before puberty because of the high rate of recurrence. This is likely due to the tendency of the child to resume voice abuse behaviors after surgery.

Vocal Cord Paralysis. The second most common cause of hoarseness in children is unilateral vocal cord paralysis. This condition results in a hoarse, "breathy" voice or cry. Occasionally, there is a history of aspiration because of incomplete vocal cord closure and lack of airway protection during swallowing. Although vocal cord paralysis can be due to a congenital condition, there is often a history of trauma to the vagus or recurrent laryngeal nerves at some point along their course in the neck or upper chest. Common traumatic etiologies include prolonged intubation, traumatic (forceps, breech) delivery, neck surgery (tracheoesophageal fistula repair, thyroidectomy), thoracic surgery (e.g., repair of patent ductus arteriosus, double aortic arch, or pulmonary artery anomalies), or blunt trauma to the neck from a motor vehicle accident. A benign or malignant growth in the neck or chest can also cause vagus or recurrent laryngeal nerve compression, leading to vocal cord paralysis. All unexplained vocal cord paralysis should be evaluated with imaging studies mentioned later.

Diagnosis of this condition requires examination of the larynx by an otolarygologist, most often using a flexible nasolaryngoscope. In cases without an obvious etiology for the vocal cord paralysis, the otolaryngologist generally evaluates the entire course of the vagus and recurrent laryngeal nerve with an imaging study. Typically, a CT or MRI scan of the neck and upper chest is obtained to rule out a compressive or an infiltrative mass lesion.

Laryngeal Papillomatosis. The most common laryngeal tumor in children is papilloma. The condition is commonly contracted at birth, often from associated genital condylomas in the mother, although this has not been proven conclusively. The child is generally asymptomatic initially but will begin to have a progressively hoarse cry or voice in the first few months of life. The hoarseness may progress to airway obstruction eventually if no treatment is instituted. Diagnosis is generally suspected after fiberoptic nasolaryngoscopy reveals characteristic papillary lesions of the larynx. Surgery consists of direct laryngoscopy with biopsy and CO_2 laser excision. Surgical therapy is indicated to remove the papilloma, to establish a diagnosis, and to help alleviate symptoms of hoarseness/and or partial airway obstruction. Unfortunately, there is a strong tendency for recurrence of these lesions, requiring multiple surgeries. Systemic adjuvant therapy with interferon and other agents has been advocated for more advanced cases.

Other Disorders. Laryngomalacia typically appears with progressive inspiratory stridor in an infant in the first few weeks of life. Occasionally, however, the infant may have a watery or muffled cry. This condition is caused by neurologic immaturity of the larynx, resulting in a weakened, floppy larynx that tends to collapse with inspiration. Diagnosis is made by flexible nasolaryngoscopy. Typically, the child outgrows the condition by 1½ to 2 years of age. Very few children require tracheotomy or other surgical interventions.

Additional congenital causes of hoarseness include laryngeal web, vocal cord cysts, and saccular cysts of the larynx.

Traumatic

Paralyzed Vocal Cord. A paralyzed vocal cord does not necessarily suggest trauma to the vagus or recurrent laryngeal nerve; however this is often the case. The causes of a paralyzed cord are myriad, but the most common are the following:

- Surgical procedures of the neck
  - Thyroidectomy or parathyroidectomy
  - Anterior cervical spine procedures (diskectomy, fusion)
  - Carotid endarterectomy
  - Esophagectomy
- Surgical procedures of the chest
  - Repair of aortic aneurysm
  - Mediastinoscopy
  - Cardiac surgery
- Intubation, especially if prolonged
- External blow or trauma to the neck

The voice associated with a vocal cord paralysis is often very weak and breathy initially. The patient often complains of vocal fatigue, especially at the end of the day. Other prominent symptoms may include a weak cough and aspiration of liquids, characterized by choking and coughing with meals. Diagnosis is confirmed by visualization of an immobile, partially lateralized vocal cord on nasolaryngoscopy. Occasionally, electromyography (EMG) of the laryngeal muscles may be performed to assess the chances of recovery of vocal cord motion.

Treatment of the vocal cord paralysis by an otolaryngologist is extremely beneficial to the patient in most cases. This can be accomplished with injection of material into the larynx such as Gelfoam, fat, or collagen, which results in medialization of the paralyzed cord. These procedures can result in vast improvement in the voice and swallowing; however, the effects of injection laryngoplasty are often temporary and sometimes hard to predict. The current gold standard for management of chronic, long-standing vocal fold paralysis is medialization laryngoplasty with or without arytenoid adduction. Occasionally, medialization laryngoplasty alone can be performed in acute cases of paralysis in which recovery is possible. Again, significant improvement in the voice and elimination of aspiration can frequently be achieved with these procedures.

Dislocated Arytenoid. This is usually due to a traumatic intubation from either the force of the laryngoscope blade or the endotracheal tube itself. A red flag for this condition is hoarseness *and* odynophagia persisting longer than 2 days after extubation. Diagnosis is suspected by examination of the larynx with a flexible nasolaryngoscope, although direct laryngoscopy under anesthesia with palpation of the joint or laryngeal electromyography is often necessary to confirm the diagnosis. Relocation of the arytenoid is performed in the operating room as soon as possible. Referral for this condition, if suspected, must be quite prompt, as the cricoarytenoid joint may ankylose if left untreated for more than a few days or weeks.

Laryngeal Fracture. This is generally not a diagnostic problem for the otolaryngologist. Hoarseness following trauma to the neck should be referred as soon as possible to an otolaryngologist. Blunt trauma to the neck can be accompanied by fractures of the laryngeal skeleton with associated intralaryngeal hemorrhage and/or edema. The patient's symptoms can progress quickly from hoarseness to airway obstruction. A CT scan is helpful in establishing the site or sites of the injuries. Examination of the larynx with a flexible nasolaryngoscope is also necessary.

Vocal Process Granuloma. This lesion is sometimes referred to as an "intubation granuloma," although it can be caused by vocal abuse and chronic coughing. The common underlying factor is trauma to the posterior larynx, usually by an endotracheal tube, which causes an ulceration at the posterior aspect of the larynx. Gastroesophageal reflux into the larynx is thought to contribute to formation of granulation tissue at the site of the ulcer. Treatment is generally conservative, using high doses of proton pump inhibitors (omeprazole [Prilosec], 20 mg twice a day [bid]) and speech therapy. Surgical excision is used only for extremely large lesions, lack of response to therapy, or suspicion of malignancy. Botulinum toxin (Botox) injection into the laryngeal musculature has been shown to have promise in treating recalcitrant granulomas.

Infectious or Inflammatory

Benign Vocal Cord Lesions (Polyps, Nodules, Cysts, and Reinke's Edema). Technically, polyps and nodules are due to vocal abuse (phonotrauma), although many have an inflammatory component. Reinke's edema (polypoid corditis) is caused by a combination of inflammatory factors (smoking, gastroesophageal reflux disease [GERD]) as well as vocal abuse. All of these lesions have a fairly characteristic appearance and can be diagnosed with nasolaryngoscopy or videostroboscopy in the otolaryngologist's office.

Vocal fold polyps typically develop after a relatively short period of voice abuse, particularly when the patient has a coexisting upper respiratory tract infection (URI). Typical scenarios in which a polyp might develop would be screaming or yelling at a sporting event or amateur singing in a establishment in which there is a great deal of background noise, such as a karaoke bar. Polyps generally require direct laryngoscopy and excision with microsurgical techniques.

Vocal fold nodules, on the other hand, typically develop over a prolonged period of time and can occur in professionally trained singers as well as in untrained ones, although the latter are more prone to develop such lesions. Nodules are typically due to excessive voice use and chronic vocal abuse. Adult patients with nodules are almost always women between the ages of 20 and 40. Typical patients with nodules are semiprofessional singers, teachers, young mothers, and cheerleaders. Treatment is conservative, consisting of voice rest and speech therapy. Surgery is indicated only after failure of a prolonged trial of speech therapy, typically 3 to 6 months.

Reinke's edema is seen almost exclusively in elderly female smokers and is characterized by an unnaturally low-pitched, husky voice. The vocal cords are filled with a myxoid, edematous fluid just beneath the epithelium. The increased mass of the vocal cords results in the low pitch of the voice. This disorder requires microsurgical excision followed by smoking cessation. There is an extremely high rate of recurrence of this disease if the patient resumes smoking postoperatively. There is mounting evidence that gastroesophageal reflux is an important cofactor in this condition; therefore, most patients require aggressive treatment for their reflux, typically with omeprazole (Prilosec), 20 mg twice a day.

Vocal cord cysts are relatively rare and may arise from either mucous retention or ingrowth of vocal cord epithelium from the trauma associated with vocal abuse. These lesions are difficult to diagnose, even with nasolaryngoscopy. Often a videolaryngostroboscopy is necessary to detect the subtle loss of the vibratory "wave" that characterizes these lesions. Treatment of vocal cord cysts requires microsurgical excision.

Acute Laryngitis. The vast majority of cases of acute laryngitis are viral in origin, typically secondary to rhinoviruses or influenza viruses. Secondary bacterial laryngitis may develop, although this is quite rare. The most common pathogen in these cases is thought to be *Moraxella catarrhalis.* In the case of a typical acute viral laryngitis, the patient presents with signs and symptoms of a URI, such as sore throat, rhinorrhea, or cough, followed by increasing hoarseness, as an inflammatory edema of the vocal cords develops. When the patient does not have any pressing speaking engagements, the treatment of acute laryngitis is threefold: voice rest, hydration, and humidification.

Voice rest does not have to be absolute; instead it is recommended that the patient practice voice conservation, speaking in a normal voice only when absolutely necessary. It is important to emphasize that whispering is more traumatic than speaking in a normal voice. The period of voice rest recommended is typically about 1 week.

Hydration means taking in 6 to 8 8-ounce glasses of water per day. The goal for the patient is to drink enough water so that the urine is pale in color. Proper hydration results in a more thin, lubricating mucus on the surface of the vocal folds, resulting in more normal vibration. A useful adjunct to this recommendation is the use of a mucolytic to aid in further thinning of the thick laryngeal mucus associated with acute inflammatory conditions. We recommend guaifenesin (Humibid L.A.), 1200 mg bid. It is important to keep in mind that this medication is helpful only if accompanied by adequate hydration.

Humidification can be accomplished using a steam inhalation device or a room humidifier, if available; steam showers can be substituted if necessary.

If a dry, nonproductive cough is present, this can be an exacerbating factor for laryngeal edema. Repetitive coughing results in undue vocal cord trauma, as the vocal cords firmly contact with each tussive blast, worsening the laryngeal edema. Cough should be treated with an antitussive as outlined in Table 2.

Gastroesophageal Laryngitis (Laryngopharyngeal Reflux [LPR]). Reflux of gastric acid and pepsin into the laryngopharynx is almost certainly the most commonly missed cause of hoarseness. The reason that LPR is not commonly suspected in a hoarse patient is that a large percentage of the patients do not have heartburn or esophagitis. Reflux of only small amounts of acid and pepsin onto the larynx

TABLE 2. **Nonspecific Treatment of Hoarseness**

1. *Hydration*: Inflammatory conditions are often accompanied by a thick mucus, which impedes the normal vibratory mechanism of the vocal cords. Increasing the intake of water will cause the mucus glands to produce a thinner, lubricating mucus, resulting in an improved and a more consistent voice. Six to eight 8-oz glasses of water a day (48 to 64 oz per day) are recommended.
2. *Humidification*: A useful adjunct to systemic hydration is humidification of the air using a room air humidifier or inhaled steam. Frequent steam showers can also be beneficial.
3. *Mucolytics*: Thick mucus can also be treated with a mucolytic medication such as guaifenesin (Humibid L.A.), 1200 mg twice daily.
4. Treat associated conditions that could worsen the hoarseness:

   Cough: A chronic dry cough can promote further laryngeal edema because each tussive blast results in excessive trauma to the larynx. Over-the-counter preparations such as dextromethorphan can be used. Benzonatate (Tessalon Perles), 100 mg three times a day, is also frequently effective.

   Nasal congestion: The nasal cavity is normally the functional site for humidification of inspired air. When nasal congestion occurs, the job of humidification is shifted to the oral cavity, oropharynx, and larynx, resulting in dryness. Treatment of nasal congestion can be acute, using oxymetazoline spray (Afrin), 2 to 3 sprays twice a day for 3 days, or long term, using beclomethasone (Vancenase AQ), 2 sprays once a day. One should avoid the use of antihistamines and decongestants normally, as these dry the vocal cords.

   Sinusitis: Any associated sinusitis must be treated promptly, as nasal congestion and purulent drainage may worsen the hoarseness. Amoxicillin (Amoxil), 500 mg three times a day for 10 days, is usually adequate treatment for an acute infection. Three days of oxymetazoline spray (Afrin), as noted above, is also very useful. If resistant organisms are suspected, the following antibiotics are good choices: amoxicillin plus potassium clavulanate (Augmentin), 500 mg three times a day or 875 mg twice a day; cefuroxime (Ceftin), 250 mg twice daily; or azithromycin (Zithromax), 500 mg loading dose followed by 250 mg every day for 4 days.
5. Avoid medications that may worsen the hoarseness:

Medication	*Effect*
Antihistamines	Dries mucosa of respiratory tract
Decongestants	Dries mucosa of respiratory tract
Inhaled pulmonary steroids	Propellant causes laryngeal irritation
(e.g., triamcinolone [Azmacort])	Little appreciable effect on laryngeal edema

6. *Voice Rest*: Edema of the vocal cords is a common denominator in most causes of hoarseness, and voice rest results in a more rapid resolution of this edema. Absolute voice rest means not using the voice at all, whereas relative voice use indicates conservation of the voice, using it only when absolutely necessary. For specific recommendations regarding whether to use absolute or relative voice rest, please see the algorithm in Figure 1. Whispering must be avoided, as this results in more trauma than speaking in normal conversational tones. Typical recommendations for voice rest are between 1 and 2 weeks.
7. *Consider systemic corticosteroids in special circumstances*: When a professional voice user has an important upcoming performance that cannot be canceled or postponed, corticosteroids should be considered. Ideally in these instances, the vocal professional should be seen by an otolaryngologist, although this is not always possible. As would be true for a professional athlete, the vocal performer runs a risk of worsening the injury if he or she performs while using corticosteroids, especially if a lesion is present.

   Steroid medications can be given orally (prednisone, 1 mg per kg for 3 to 5 days followed by a rapid taper) or through an intramuscular route (dexamethasone acetate, 10 mg IM). It should be reiterated that steroid utilization to prepare for an important performance should be considered only when no other alternatives are available.

can result in inflammation and edema; generally these small amounts do not result in esophagitis and heartburn. In addition to hoarseness, patients with LPR commonly have "atypical" symptoms of reflux such as globus pharyngeus (sensation of a foreign body in the throat), chronic throat clearing, "postnasal drip," chronic cough, or sore throat. An empirical diagnosis of LPR can be made when the patient's symptoms are combined with the typical appearance of LPR changes of the larynx on nasolaryngoscopic examination: posterior commisure hypertrophy, erythema of the arytenoids, and laryngeal edema.

Suspected LPR is commonly treated aggressively with high-dose proton pump inhibitors such as omeprazole (Prilosec), 20 mg bid, and GERD precautions are initiated (Table 3). This aggressive therapy is warranted because near total acid suppression is needed for the inflammatory changes in the larynx to reverse. After weeks to months of this therapy, many patients can be tapered to an H_2 blocker and eventually weaned off therapy and maintained solely on GERD precautions.

In some cases, a *double probe* 24-hour pH study is needed to confirm that a patient has LPR, especially if he or she is not responding to empirical therapy or if the diagnosis is in question. This is the best method of confirming the diagnosis, although it is an expensive, somewhat cumbersome test that has a false-negative rate estimated between 10 and 20%.

Chronic Laryngitis. This is a wastebasket category that is often multifactorial in origin. Chronic laryngitis may have one or a combination of causes, including chronic voice abuse, inadequate hydration, gastroesophageal laryngitis, allergies or chronic sinusitis, muscular tension dysphonia, or exposure to environmental or occupational toxicants. Patients with chronic laryngitis are difficult to treat and often require a combination of medications, lifestyle modifications, and speech therapy.

Bacterial Supraglottitis or Epiglottitis. This condition has become quite rare in the pediatric population, since the implementation of the *Haemophilus influenzae* B vaccine. However, it is still present in the adult population, and can be life-threatening. The patient typically presents with a fever and a few hours to days of progressive sore throat, odynophagia, and sometimes a muffled or hoarse voice. As the disease advances, the patient may begin to drool and become stridorous. Examination of the oropharynx often produces completely normal results. Plain soft tissue films of the neck may reveal an enlarged soft tissue density above the vocal folds, sometimes referred to as a "thumb sign." Diagnosis is confirmed by examination of the larynx with a mirror or flexible nasolaryngoscope. The epiglottis and supraglottic structures are seen to be extremely edematous and to have a typical cherry-red color. Prompt consultation with an otolaryngologist is mandatory in cases of suspected supraglottitis, as airway management with a tracheostomy or controlled intubation in the operating room may be necessary.

Rheumatoid Arthritis. This is one of the few systemic diseases that may lead to development of hoarseness. The hoarseness is due to arthritis of the cricoarytenoid joint, which is responsible for vocal cord movement. Pain when speaking or swallowing may also be present. Diagnosis is suspected by examining the larynx with a fiberoptic nasolaryngoscope. Typical findings include limited mobility of the arytenoid and erythema over the arytenoid mucosa. Treatment is generally limited to anti-inflammatory medications, such as increasing the corticosteroid dosage over a 1- to 2-week period. If this is not successful, the patient can be taken to the operating room and corticosteroids can be injected directly into the cricoarytenoid joint. Progression of the patient's arthritis can lead to bilateral cricoarytenoid joint fixation with resultant airway obstruction, requiring a tracheostomy.

Other. Rare laryngeal infections that may result in hoarseness include *Candida* laryngitis (mucocutaneous), sometimes seen in patients with acquired immune deficiency syndrome and the immunosuppressed. Other infectious causes of laryngitis are diphtheria, tuberculous laryngitis, and rhinoscleroma.

TABLE 3. **Gastroesophageal Reflux Disease Precautions**

Dietary modifications

- Avoid caffeine (coffee, tea, many colas)
- Avoid chocolates and mints
- Avoid fatty, fried, and spicy foods
- Avoid alcohol, especially before bedtime
- Avoid large meals

Lifestyle modifications

- Stop smoking
- Avoid tight-fitting or binding clothing
- Lose weight
- Avoid eating 3 hours before bedtime
- Elevate head of bed 6 inches
- Exercise on an empty stomach

Neoplastic

Neoplastic causes of hoarseness can be broken down into two categories: (1) direct involvement of the vocal fold with tumor and (2) neoplasm of the neck or chest, resulting in compression of the 10th cranial nerve with vocal cord paralysis.

Direct neoplastic growth on the vocal folds almost always represents squamous cell carcinoma. This is most commonly seen in adults older than 40 years old who have a significant history of tobacco and alcohol abuse. Other common symptoms of squamous cell carcinoma of the larynx are dysphagia, odynophagia, and otalgia (referred ear pain from ulcerative tumor). The patient may also have a palpable neck mass, typically in the upper or mid levels of the anterior cervical chain. Neck disease may not be present until the tumor is very advanced. It is important to keep in mind that hoarseness may be the only symptom of early glottic carcinoma. For this reason, it is critical that a patient presenting with new-onset hoarseness and a significant history of tobacco and/or alcohol abuse be referred to an otolaryngologist as soon as possible. Delay in diagnosis can result in growth of tumor to the point that conservative, voice-sparing treatments are no longer possible.

Several tumors can cause compression of the 10th cranial nerve and its branches, with resulting vocal cord paralysis and hoarseness. The most common of these by far is a lung (endobronchial) tumor that has metastasized to the mediastinum, resulting in compression of the recurrent laryngeal nerve. This usually occurs on the left side, owing to the more inferior location of the nerve's course in the thorax. Typically the patient develops a weak, breathy, effortful voice. Other common symptoms include a weak cough and aspiration of liquids, manifested by choking and coughing with meals. This is due to loss of airway protection caused by the paralyzed vocal cord. In most cases, the compressing mass can be identified on a chest radiograph, although a CT scan of the chest may be needed to identify the mass. Diagnosis is confirmed by visualization of an immobile, partially lateralized vocal fold on nasolaryngoscopic examination. Treatment of the paralyzed vocal cord was previously covered in the "Traumatic" section of this chapter.

Other tumors that can lead to 10th cranial nerve compression are thyroid malignancies and neurogenic/paraganglioma tumors of the skull base. The former are generally associated with a palpable neck mass on examination, but the latter may be detectable only on CT or MRI scans, which reinforces the notion that all "unexplained" cases of vocal cord paralysis should be evaluated radiographically. Skull base malignancies may have coexisting cranial nerve palsies besides CN X, such as CN IX, XI, and XII.

In summary, all unexplained cases of vocal cord paralysis require radiographic evaluation with a CT or MRI scan of the neck and upper chest.

Neurologic

Cerebrovascular Accident (CVA). A CVA, or stroke, can cause hoarseness. Supranuclear damage from a stroke can lead to dysphonia that is associated with lack of voluntary speech, dysfunction of the oral phase of swallowing, hypoglossal weakness, and hemiplegia. Brain stem strokes that lead to hoarseness are most often due to occlusion of the posteroinferior cerebellar artery or vertebral artery producing a lateral medullary infarction (Wallenberg's syndrome). This can produce a vagal nerve paralysis that is associated with hoarseness, severe dysphagia, Horner's syndrome, vertigo, ataxia, and sensory deficits.

Spasmodic Dysphonia (SD). SD is becoming recognized as a more common cause of dysphonia. Although the cause of SD is thought to be neurologic, the exact pathophysiology has yet to be determined. The most common type of SD, adductor spasmodic dysphonia, is characterized by a "strained-strangled" sounding speech. The typical patient is a middle-aged or elderly female, with a relatively acute onset of hoarseness, sometimes following an emotionally traumatic event. Diagnosis is made subjectively by careful analysis of the patient's voice; however, observation of the larynx with a fiberoptic nasolaryngoscope may also be helpful. The current standard of therapy involves serial injections of botulinum toxin (Botox) into the thryoartenoid muscles of the larynx to weaken the adductor strength and reduce the spasmodic quality of the voice.

Other. Other neurologic causes of hoarseness include myasthenia gravis, Parkinson's disease, amyotrophic lateral sclerosis (ALS), and Guillain-Barré syndrome. Parkinson's disease can lead to a hypokinetic voice disorder, which manifests as a weak, breathy voice that is monotone in quality.

Other

Two other significant causes of dysphonia are muscular tension dysphonia (MTD) and age-related dysphonia (presbylaryngis).

Muscular Tension Dysphonia (MTD). This is a relatively common disorder that is caused by inappropriate use of the laryngeal musculature. Other names for this disorder include "laryngeal hyperfunction," "functional dysphonia," and "dysphonia plica ventricularis." The voice sounds very harsh and strained, somewhat similar to the voice of an SD patient. There is no organic pathology of the vocal folds; in fact, casual mirror examination of the vocal folds by an otolaryngologist may not reveal any abnormalities. More careful examination of the larynx with a flexible nasolaryngoscope commonly reveals hyperfunctional closure of the false vocal folds and/or anteroposterior "squeezing" of the supraglottis. Treatment consists of referral to a speech pathologist who is familiar with the treatment of vocal tension disorders. Therapy consists of relaxation of the laryngeal and cervical muscles, as well as using an efficient vocal mechanism with good breath support.

Presbylaryngis. Another important cause of hoarseness is presbylaryngis, or age-related changes in the voice. Interestingly, the effects in men and women are somewhat in opposition. In men there is a loss of muscle bulk and elasticity in the vocal cords with aging, which leads to a thin, reedy-sounding voice that is breathy and higher in pitch. This effect begins to occur after the patient reaches 60 years of age. In women, the relative increase in androgens that occurs with menopause leads to a slight masculinization of the voice characterized by a more harsh, lower pitch. Diagnosis of a male patient with presbylaryngis is made by videolaryngostroboscopy, which typically shows vocal fold "bowing." Common treatments for this condition include vocal cord fat injection or bilateral medialization laryngoplasty. As older men remain active, both socially and occupationally beyond the age of 70, more are electing to seek voice improvement through surgery. A successful treatment for age-related changes in the female voice has not yet been developed, although some have suggested that hormone replacement therapy may be of some benefit.

INSOMNIA

method of
VIRGIL D. WOOTEN, M.D.
Sleep Disorders Center of Greater Cincinnati
Cincinnati, Ohio

EPIDEMIOLOGY

Insomnia is the real or perceived inability to initiate and/or maintain sleep. Approximately 10% of the population has chronic and severe insomnia. At least half the population will experience significant insomnia at some point in their lives. Insomnia is more common with age and in women. Insomnia afflicts those in lower socioeconomic classes and those who are divorced, separated, or widowed more frequently. Insomnia is a major prodromal symptom of depression. About 40% of afflicted patients have major depression or anxiety disorders.

ETIOLOGIES

Insomnia is a complaint with numerous underlying causes. Most patients with insomnia have underlying psychologic or psychiatric issues; however, a number of patients also have a mix of problems contributing to their difficulty sleeping. Insomnia is relatively uncommon in childhood and is often related to poor bedtime habits and routines in this age group.

Societal, Behavioral, and Medication Factors

Young adults most often have sleep onset insomnia related to poor sleeping habits and psychologic issues. Acute stressors are the most common cause of sleep onset insomnia, and acute job stresses, marital problems, and life events can bring the patient in seeking relief. The use of caffeine, alcohol, tobacco products, and certain medications tends to aggravate insomnia. The most commonly offending medications are decongestants, diuretics, systemic corticosteroids, newer generation antidepressants, appetite suppressants, and any other medications with stimulating properties. Theophylline and other systemic bronchodilators can also aggravate insomnia. The medically ill elderly have insomnia more frequently than their healthy counterparts. Dementia, reduced sleep ability, security issues, lack of social activities, bereavement, and fear of nocturnal death of self or spouse are additional causes of insomnia in the elderly.

Some patients develop apprehension about their ability to sleep and develop a conditioned, or "performance," anxiety about going to bed. They often describe increasing tension as bedtime approaches, and they become increasingly frustrated when sleep does not occur. They often look at the clock, worrying about how long it is taking them to get to sleep, what time they awakened, and how they will feel the following day if they do not get enough sleep. Some patients, although not psychologically or psychiatrically abnormal, are somewhat hard driven, perfectionistic, or "type A" personalities. These patients often have difficulty letting go of their daily activities. They often use the bedroom to plan their future activities and obsess about things that they have done and that they are going to do.

Our 24-hour society also promotes difficulty sleeping. The variability in work and sleep schedules counters the normal biology, which is linked to the light and dark cycle inherent in our evolution. There is no way to perform optimally and to sleep optimally when engaging in shift work. Even with a fixed night shift schedule, normal sleep is not achieved during daytime sleeping hours. Daytime sleep interruptions, light exposure, and the tendency for shift workers to revert to a daytime schedule on their off days often prevent their accommodation to any fixed schedule at night. With rapidly rotating shifts, the internal timekeepers in the central nervous system become confused, and the ability to achieve sleep onset and maintain sleep are impaired. Shift work is less well tolerated with aging. Increased psychologic and health complaints are common in shift workers.

Psychiatric Factors

Major depression can result in rapid eye movement (REM) sleep architecture changes. The REM sleep onset latency may be less than 60 minutes. In severe depression, there may be prolonged REM sleep episodes in the first part of the night. An increase in rapid eye movements (increased REM density) may also be evident. Sleep is typically fragmented, and the amount of slow-wave sleep is reduced. Patients with major depression may also have terminal insomnia, awakening 1 to 2 hours before their normal waking time. Generalized anxiety results primarily in sleep onset insomnia. Panic attacks may occur either at sleep onset or in the middle of sleep. Sometimes, the patient confuses a panic attack with apnea. Although obstructive sleep apnea may cause patients to awaken with a feeling of dyspnea, the dyspnea is usually not prolonged and is not associated with prolonged palpitations or fearfulness as is often the case with panic attacks.

Patients with schizophrenia often complain of disturbed sleep, and they are more prone to have sleep state misperception. They may complain of not having slept at all for months and even years, yet they complain of little or no daytime impairment. In schizophrenic patients, hallucinations are often worse at night. Akathisia may also occur when antipsychotic medications are given at bedtime. In manic episodes, there is usually curtailed sleep. Patients engaging in drug and alcohol abuse often have very disturbed sleep. Alcohol may be used by the patient to assist sleep onset because of its central nervous system depressant and initial antianxiety properties; however, withdrawal effects appear within 2 to 3 hours and may cause difficulty with sleep maintenance. Sometimes patients who drink alcohol at bedtime will complain of awakening with anxiety. Drug withdrawal often aggravates sleeping difficulties, and the hallucinatory activity seen in drug and alcohol withdrawal cases may be related to REM sleep–related rebound phenomena.

TREATMENT OF NONORGANIC INSOMNIA

Treatment of insomnia due to psychophysiologic and psychiatric factors should include sleep hygiene techniques. These can include a regular bedtime with an appropriate number of bedtime hours; avoidance of clock watching; avoidance of excessive activity in bed or just before bedtime; and avoidance of substances such as tobacco, caffeine, alcohol, and other drugs or medications that can disturb sleep.

Patients should not spend long periods of time awake in bed. They should get up out of bed when they cannot achieve sleep onset after about 20 minutes. Something relaxing or boring should be done when out of bed before returning to sleep. Light snacks at night are sometimes helpful. Hot baths or exercise in the evening should be avoided, as these can stimulate instead of relax. A regular exercise program conducted in the morning or afternoon can be beneficial to sleep and can help in stress management. For patients able and willing to learn behavioral techniques, various methods can be taught. Behavioral techniques have been shown to be superior to sedative administration in the treatment of chronic insomnia. Progressive muscle relaxation is very useful and consists of progressively tensing and relaxing the muscles, usually beginning at the feet, and working up to the head over 30 minutes. Breathing exercises alone and other techniques can be employed. Visual imagery of relaxing or enjoyable activities sometimes distracts the person from worries and concerns. Thought-stopping techniques for obsessive individuals can also be useful. Biofeedback has limited effectiveness.

Restriction of time in bed to fewer hours than the person needs to sleep may initially deprive the person of sleep, causing him or her to go to sleep more quickly and maintain sleep better. The sleep hours can be increased gradually to the required sleep amount as the person achieves better habits and sleep.

Patients with acute insomnia due to acute psychologic stressors can be helped by short-acting and intermediate-acting sedatives. It is generally preferable to prescribe the sedatives for less than 1 month, but in certain circumstances, such as bereavement or a prolonged medical illness, it may be helpful for the patient to remain on the medication longer. If the patient remains on medication for more than 3 weeks, it is best to taper the medication rather than to discontinue it abruptly to avoid any withdrawal effects. During the same time of sedative application, behavioral techniques can be instituted.

Infants and toddlers sometimes have to be trained to sleep in bed on their own without the presence of the parent. Most commonly, they have become accustomed to falling asleep in the parent's bed or while being fed or rocked to sleep. When the child awakens in the night and is not in the parent's bed or is not being fed or rocked again, he or she may have difficulty returning to sleep. Simple weaning techniques (e.g., Ferber's) can be employed to improve the child's ability to sleep.

MEDICATION MANAGEMENT OF INSOMNIA

Benzodiazepine receptor agents (BRAs), which include benzodiazepines and newer nonbenzodiazepine drugs with ω_1-benzodiazepine receptor activity (e.g., zolpidem [Ambien]), are the preferred drugs in the treatment of insomnia. Their effectiveness, safety margin, and lower addictive potential make them better choices than other effective sedatives. These drugs also maintain their effectiveness longer than older sedatives. The antianxiety properties of the benzodiazepines lend themselves well to acute insomnia, especially in anxious patients. Short-acting BRAs (e.g., zolpidem, 5 to 10 mg; triazolam [Halcion], 0.125 to 0.25 mg) are useful for sleep onset insomnia, and intermediate BRAs (e.g., estazolam [Prosom], 1 to 2 mg; temazepam [Restoril], 15 to 30 mg) are useful for both sleep onset and sleep maintenance insomnia. Long-acting benzodiazepines such as flurazepam and quazepam are discouraged in the elderly because of cumulative cognitive and motor impairment. Lower initial doses of sedatives are recommended in the elderly.

Barbiturates, glutethimide, and methyprylon are discouraged because of their high toxicity and addictive potential. They also lose their effectiveness relatively rapidly. Antihistamines and chloral hydrate are weak sedatives and are generally not useful for most patients, especially if more than a brief interval of use is required. Antihistamines are especially prone to cause morning grogginess and anticholinergic side effects. Tricyclic antidepressants are generally not a good choice for sedation. Their side effect problems are the same as those encountered with antihistamines, and there is also added cardiovascular toxicity. Trazodone (Desyrel)* is sometimes useful in patients who cannot take BRAs owing to prior drug abuse or adverse cognitive effects (e.g., elderly patients). The starting dose can be as low as 25 mg, and it can be increased gradually as necessary to a maximum of 200 mg. It frequently causes nausea and dizziness; caution should be given about the side effects. There is also the rare side effect of priapism, which can cause permanent penile damage. In patients who are somewhat obsessive or who are type A personalities, selective serotonin reuptake inhibitors* are sometimes useful. Although these drugs sometimes fragment sleep, patients often have no perception of this effect and frequently report improved sleep. These drugs may also improve daytime relationships by reducing irritability and improving concentration and patience.

In patients with psychiatric disorders, the drug treatment needs to be tailored to the patient's particular problem. Antidepressants should be selected based on the patient's individual needs. Sedating antidepressants can be used in patients with major depression and insomnia, but the side effects of the sedating antidepressants can reduce patient compliance and delay the achievement of effective dose levels. The newer antidepressant agents, which are less sedating but sometimes stimulating, can be used with sometimes only temporary insomnia. Some BRAs can be combined with selective serotonin reup-

*Not FDA approved for this indication.

take inhibitors (SSRIs) to offset the insomnia, if necessary; however, the patient should be cautioned about the increased risk of adverse central nervous system complications. Patients with anxiety disorders may also respond to SSRIs.

Benzodiazepines and SSRIs may need to be used on a long-term basis for patients with chronic generalized anxiety or panic attacks unresponsive to other interventions. When benzodiazepines are used to control daytime anxiety, the same medication should be used as the sedative. Many of the benzodiazepines used for anxiety control have similar sedation, onset of action, and half-life as benzodiazepine sedatives; no benefit will be derived from administering two BRAs simultaneously. Behavioral techniques such as progressive muscle relaxation, cognitive interventions, and the like may be helpful for patients with anxiety disorders.

Patients with psychosis often present a challenge to the physician, and sometimes multiple psychotropic medications have to be employed to control the psychosis and to improve sleep. Akathisia at bedtime, which resembles restless legs syndrome, can be reduced by adding an antiparkinsonian drug. Excessive hallucinations at night in patients with schizophrenia may be helped by an increase in antipsychotic medication. Patients with bipolar disorder in the manic phase are particularly difficult to treat, and combination therapy with antimanic drugs as well as sedative medications may be necessary. Patients recovering from drug and alcohol abuse sometimes complain of continued insomnia. Trazodone is a useful nonaddictive sedative medication. SSRIs may be beneficial in drug-dependent patients who are somewhat obsessive or anxious.

RESTLESS LEGS SYNDROME AND PERIODIC LIMB MOVEMENTS OF SLEEP (NOCTURNAL MYOCLONUS)

Restless legs syndrome (RLS) is a common discomfort occurring in the lower extremities that is often difficult to describe by the patient. The lower extremities are usually affected, and sometimes the upper limbs may also become involved. There is usually no pain, burning, tingling, or cramping, although, as the illness progresses, leg aches and leg cramps can develop. The illness may have multiple etiologies. In some, it may be acquired through autosomal dominant transmission. The illness usually occurs after age 40, although in familial RLS, it may occur in childhood. The patient has an irresistible urge to move the legs to achieve comfort. Attempts to reduce the symptoms may include excessive walking, exercising, and taking hot baths. It is not uncommon for periodic limb movements of sleep (PLMS) to occur after sleep onset, further disrupting sleep. PLMS are leg movements that occur with a periodicity of about every 20 to 40 seconds. Most patients with periodic limb movements alone do not complain of significant sleep impairment or fatigue from this disorder, although in severe cases, insomnia, nocturnal leg cramps, daytime fatigue, and sleepiness may result. Patients with RLS, by contrast, may have severe distress, and suicide has occurred in afflicted patients. Underlying metabolic factors have been identified as aggravating causes. Patients with renal failure are very prone to develop RLS. Anemia and various vitamin deficiencies may play a role. Therefore, laboratory evaluations for anemia, electrolyte disturbances, uremia, and vitamin deficiencies are advised. Various medications can aggravate RLS, including diuretics, bronchodilators, antihistamines, decongestants, antipsychotics, and antidepressants. Caffeine and alcohol may also aggravate restless legs syndrome.

Treatment of Restless Legs Syndrome

The treatments of RLS and periodic limb movements are similar, as they both may have a common etiology. After excluding dietary, metabolic, and medicinal factors, various medications can be employed. Antiparkinsonian agents affecting the dopamine system appear to be very useful and are often used as first-line agents in treating RLS. Pergolide (Permax),* at 0.05 mg initially with sequential increases in dose over several days to control the symptoms, appears to have lasting effects. Levodopa (L-dopa)/carbidopa combinations* can also be used at a beginning dose of L-dopa, 100 mg, and carbidopa, 25 mg (Sinemet), at bedtime or in the evening. However, rebound RLS occurring in the middle of the night or the following day sometimes develops. Bromocriptine (Parlodel)* can also be used in the treatment of RLS. Patients on dopamine agents may need sequential increases to control the symptoms as tolerance ensues or as the illness progresses.

Clonazepam is also useful in the treatment of RLS, and the usual starting dose is 0.5 to 1.0 mg at bedtime. Narcotic analgesics are very effective, and propoxyphene (Darvon), oxycodone (Percocet), and hydrocodone (Vicodin) are the most often employed. A number of medications have been tried with variable success. Most of the reports are anecdotal, but supplemental vitamin E at 1000 units per day, calcium up to 1200 mg per day, and multivitamins may be beneficial. In very mild RLS, nonsteroidal anti-inflammatory agents or acetaminophen may be useful. A variety of medications such as quinine, clonidine* (Catapres), carbamazepine* (Tegretol), baclofen* (Lioresal), cyclobenzaprine* (Flexeril), SSRIs,* and tricyclic antidepressants* have been advocated. However, some of these drugs, particularly those related to tricyclic antidepressants, may aggravate RLS. In addition to the previously mentioned agents, trazodone has been used in the treatment of PLMS.

OTHER MEDICAL CAUSES OF INSOMNIA

A host of other medical factors play a role in insomnia, particularly in the elderly, and the treatment of

*Not FDA approved for this indication.

these is essential to the improvement of insomnia. Any medical problem causing pain or discomfort can cause insomnia. Pain should be addressed with analgesic medications. Treatment of discomfort due to respiratory insufficiency or other respiratory problems can improve sleep. Obstructive sleep apnea can be involved in insomnia by causing sleep disruption and nocturia, and its treatment can potentially eliminate insomnia. Nocturia due to prostatic hypertrophy can be addressed with terazosin (Hytrin) or finasteride (Proscar).

PRURITUS

method of
SARAH A. MYERS, M.D.
Duke University Medical Center
Durham, North Carolina

Pruritus, derived from the Latin word *prurire,* meaning "to itch," is the sensation in the skin that provokes one to scratch. Pruritus may be associated with a specific dermatologic condition and is the most common symptom in the dermatology setting (Table 1). In the absence of clinically evident primary skin disease, underlying systemic disease may be associated with generalized pruritus (Table 2). Skin lesions such as those created by rubbing, scratching, or infection are often present in this setting but are considered secondary to the underlying process and not a primary dermatologic condition. Treating pruritus can be frustrating to both the patient and the clinician, as scratching itchy skin is often inherently pleasurable and may lead to a vicious itch-scratch cycle that is very hard to break. Important aspects of management include accurate diagnosis, individualized treatment, and ongoing monitoring for new causes if the pruritus is persistent.

The precise neuroanatomy and neurophysiology of pruritus is not known. A specific end organ for the sensation of pruritus has not been found. The sensations of both itch and pain are transmitted via unmyelinated C fibers. Itch is generally felt to be a distinct sensory modality rather than a subthreshold pain; however, one patient's itch may be another patient's pain, as these sensations are closely related. Although histamine is the classic mediator of pruritus, there is evidence for other nonhistamine mediators and/or modulators as well. They include various proteases, peptides such as kinins and substance P, prostaglandins, serotonin, and physical stimuli. Opioid peptides appear to be important central modulators, as opioid antagonists may benefit some patients with pruritus.

TABLE 1. **Dermatologic Conditions Associated with Pruritus**

Inflammatory	Infestations
Atopic dermatitis	Insect bites
Bullous pemphigoid	Parasites
Contact dermatitis	Scabies
Dermatitis herpetiformis	**Neoplastic**
Dermatographism	Mycosis fungoides
Drug hypersensitivity	**Miscellaneous**
Folliculitis	Xerosis
Lichen planus	Sunburn
Miliaria	Anogenital pruritus
Psoriasis	Notalgia paresthetica
Urticaria	

TABLE 2. **Systemic Diseases Associated with Pruritus**

Hepatobiliary	Hematologic
Extrahepatic biliary obstruction	Iron deficiency anemia
Primary biliary cirrhosis	Polycythemia vera
Cholestasis of pregnancy	Paraproteinemia
Renal	**Malignancy**
Chronic renal failure	Hodgkin's and non-Hodgkin's lymphoma
Endocrine	Multiple myeloma
Hyperthyroidism	Visceral carcinoma
Hypothyroidism	Mycosis fungoides
Diabetes mellitus	Carcinoid syndrome
Infection	**Central Nervous System**
Human immunodeficiency virus	Multiple sclerosis
Autoimmune	Cerebrovascular accident
Sjögren's syndrome	Psychiatric disorders

DIAGNOSIS

Careful history taking, skin examination (often requiring repeated inspections), and selected laboratory tests are the most important aspects of evaluating patients with pruritus. Duration and characteristics of the itch as well as initiating, exacerbating, and relieving factors are helpful clues in the patient's history. Drugs and environmental factors (such as exposures to fiberglass, chemicals, irritating dusts, infested pets, other itching people) are important causes of generalized itching and should be evaluated thoroughly before undertaking a major systemic work-up. Characteristic skin lesions are usually associated with pruritic dermatologic conditions, but skin biopsy may be necessary to make a definitive diagnosis. Two dermatologic conditions that are often overlooked as a cause for pruritus include generalized xerosis (dry skin) and dermatographism. If no skin disease is evident to explain persistent pruritus (other than lesions produced by scratching), a work-up for underlying systemic disease should be performed. General history and review of systems and physical examination, with emphasis on adenopathy and organomegaly, are critical in this setting. Routine screening tests include complete blood count with differential, serum glucose, renal and liver panels, urinalysis, thyroid panel, sedimentation rate, serum protein electrophoresis, serum iron, stool for occult blood, and chest x-ray. A skin biopsy is rarely helpful if performed on normal skin. If laboratory test results are normal, conservative therapy can be initiated; however, the patient with persistent pruritus should be reassessed continually for the development of a primary dermatologic or systemic disease.

TOPICAL TREATMENT

Primary dermatologic conditions, when present, should be treated with therapy specific for the condition (e.g., permethrin [Elimite, Nix] for scabies infestation). Avoidance of causative or contributing factors involved in atopic, allergic, or other hypersensitivity dermatoses is important. Often, patients' behaviors such as taking long hot showers and self-treatments for pruritus (e.g., rubbing alcohol, witch hazel, or various over-the-counter products) may contribute to the problem even though they are temporarily soothing. Skin moisturization is critical, as dry skin frequently initiates pruritus or exacerbates other pruritic dermatoses such as atopic dermatitis and psoriasis. Mild, fragrance-free cleansing bars or liquids (Dove, Oil of Olay, Purpose, Basis, or Cetaphil) should replace harsh or deodorant soaps, and shorter, warm showers or baths should be stressed. Oatmeal baths (Aveeno) or baths with fragrance-free bath oils may also provide short-term symptomatic relief. Patting dry with a towel and immediately applying emollients such as Eucerin, Aquaphor, petroleum jelly, Theraplex clear lotion, Dermasil cream or lotion, or Cetaphil lotion should be undertaken after bathing. Emollients with camphor and menthol (e.g., Sarna Anti-Itch lotion), phenol, or pramoxine (e.g., PrameGel, Pramosone, or Aveeno Anti-Itch lotion) may provide safe relief from pruritus. Cool compresses and shake lotions (calamine) may also be highly efficacious. The use of the topical anesthetic benzocaine and the topical antihistamine diphenhydramine (Benadryl, Caladryl) is generally discouraged because of significant development of allergic contact sensitization.

Topical corticosteroids (even in the absence of skin eruption) may be useful adjunctive agents for pruritus control. For widespread pruritus, hydrocortisone (1 or 2.5%) or triamcinolone (0.025 or 0.1%) preparations are generally effective. Capsaicin cream (Zostrix) may be of some benefit in selected patients with a wide range of severe pruritic disorders. It is most practical for localized or particularly problematic pruritic areas. As it may produce burning or stinging sensations or superficial burns initially, careful patient instruction is required. In many cases, the burning sensation diminishes and relief from pruritus follows. Topical doxepin (Zonalon) is indicated for short-term relief of pruritus. It may be applied four times per day to affected skin for up to 8 days. Sedation can result if Zonalon is applied to extensive areas; therefore, it too is more useful in localized pruritus. A eutectic mixture of local anesthetics lidocaine and prilocaine (Emla cream) may be helpful in recalcitrant pruritic conditions.

SYSTEMIC THERAPY

Treatment of any underlying disorder, such as decreasing serum bile concentration in cholestatic liver disease, correcting secondary hyperparathyroidism in uremia, or treating a malignancy with chemotherapy, often leads to improvement or resolution of pruritus related to systemic disease. The use of systemic steroids, although often highly effective, is generally not recommended because of adverse sequelae associated with long-term use. As a result, symptomatic therapy with oral antihistamines is the mainstay of systemic therapy for pruritus. The H_1 histamine antagonists constitute the treatment of first choice. Hydroxyzine (Atarax) is frequently beneficial when dosed 10 to 25 mg every 6 hours daily, with upward titration based on response and toleration of side effects. Alternative H_1 blockers include diphenhydramine hydrochloride (Benadryl), 25 to 50 mg every 6 hours, or cyproheptadine (Periactin), 4 mg every 8 hours. The use of H_1 antihistamines needs to be accompanied with warnings of sedation, mental status changes, and urinary retention, especially in the elderly. Cetirizine (Zyrtec), 10 mg once daily, is less sedating than hydroxyzine and may be a useful alternative. In conditions other than urticaria, the nonsedating antihistamines, including terfenadine (Seldane, 60 mg every 12 hours), fexofenadine (Allegra, 60 mg every 12 hours), astemizole (hismanal, 10 mg once daily), and loratadine (Claritin, 10 mg once daily), may have only marginal therapeutic effect for pruritus. Because of potentially serious cardiac arrhythmias, the nonsedating antihistamines should not be used in patients also taking systemic agents, including azole antifungal agents and erythromycin. Another approach is to use tricyclic antidepressants, highly potent H_1 and H_2 antagonists. Doxepin (Sinequan),* 10 to 25 mg every 8 hours or in one nighttime dose (75 mg), can be highly effective in relieving pruritus.

A variety of other systemic agents have been used with some effect in specific disease states. Patients with cholestatic liver disease may experience relief from pruritus when serum bile concentration is lowered by oral cholestyramine (Questran), 4 grams twice daily, or colestipol hydrochloride (Colestid), which is less constipating. Activated charcoal can also be used as a potential binding agent to help reduce pruritus. Naloxone hydrochloride (Narcan),* an opiate antagonist, has demonstrated effectiveness in reducing pruritus and scratching activity in some patients with cholestasis. Erythropoietin therapy* (epoetin alfa [Epogen, Procrit]) (36 units per kg three times weekly) lowers histamine levels and relieves pruritus in patients with uremia.

Ultraviolet B phototherapy, and, less commonly, ultraviolet A and psoralen photochemotherapy (PUVA), can be successfully employed in a wide range of pruritic disorders, including atopic dermatitis, renal disease, and human immunodeficiency virus infection. Doses of ultraviolet therapy are usually administered three times per week and increased until mild erythema is attained. Therapy is then adjusted to accommodate the patient's level of photosensitivity. It may take 20 to 30 treatments to attain symptomatic relief, and patients often need encouragement to continue therapy. Ultraviolet therapy is best utilized with the input or supervision of a dermatologist.

*Not FDA approved for this indication.

TINNITUS

method of
KENNETH H. BROOKLER, M.D.
Neurotologic Associates, P.C.
New York, New York

Tinnitus is the perception of a sound or noise in the ears or head. It may be constant or intermittent. It has been described as up to 37 different sounds alone or in simultaneous combination. Tinnitus is a symptom, not a disease. Its successful treatment is based on understanding the causes of tinnitus and its effect on the person. It can have an insidious or a sudden onset. Sometimes it is noticed suddenly although it has been present for quite a while. As the perception of the tinnitus changes, its significance to the patient may become more prominent. The approach to tinnitus management discussed here will focus on the two areas of etiologic treatment and the use of therapeutic noise generators.

Tinnitus, as a symptom, should be considered at two different levels. One is the trigger, which is frequently believed to come from the inner ear or the cochlea. The other is the perception of the tinnitus, which is a brain response. This brain response may become habituated in some, making the tinnitus tolerable. In other patients there is a reflex limbic-hypothalamic stimulation in which the afflicted person lives in terror of the tinnitus.

DIAGNOSIS

The therapeutic response of a patient afflicted with tinnitus depends, in part, on the relationship with the physician. The beginning of the diagnosis and treatment of such a patient begins with the history. Part of the history taking is to allow the patient to vent concerns about the tinnitus and to find out how bothersome it is. The manner in which the history is elicited will give the patient some insight into the physician's experience in treating this symptom. If the patient senses that the physician is not familiar with this problem, a relationship beneficial to the tinnitus sufferer may not develop. Because part of the treatment attempts to change perception, the physician-patient relationship needs to be solid.

After the history is obtained, the physical examination usually demonstrates no obvious findings. The obvious findings include impacted cerumen, otitis media, and glomus tumor, to name a few. The next step is the performance of diagnostic tests to determine how well the hearing apparatus is functioning and to search for an etiologic explanation for the tinnitus. Tinnitus usually emanates from the cochlea, and tests of hearing function are necessary to examine and understand the tinnitus. Basic audiology tests, including speech testing and acoustic immittance (impedance) testing, are performed. This helps to define whether there is a coexistent alteration in the hearing mechanism. This is not to be confused with a loss of the ability to hear conversation, which is only a small portion of hearing function. Often there may be no difficulty in communication, but tests of hearing may show altered function. The portion of the acoustic immittance test called the stapedial reflex threshold frequently helps to determine whether there is a cochlear (inner ear) or neural (nerve) site for the tinnitus. Measurement of auditory brain stem–evoked potentials is a more expensive method of arriving at the same information.

When the tinnitus is unilateral, it may be a result of an acoustic tumor. At some point a decision needs to be made regarding magnetic resonance imaging (MRI) scanning. Millions of people have unilateral tinnitus but no acoustic tumor; thus, the decision whether to scan should be made on grounds of suspicion. However, more than 75% of patients with proven acoustic tumors have unilateral tinnitus as part of their symptom complex. Another reason to consider MRI scanning is to reduce the element of fear of a brain tumor in the patient. When the scan results are negative for either an acoustic neuroma or another intracranial pathologic condition, the fear level may be lowered, in turn reducing the anxiety associated with the tinnitus.

Small pixel size (0.007 mm) computed tomography (CT) of the temporal bones frequently provides two pieces of information regarding a possible etiology. First, the internal auditory canal may be larger on the side of a unilateral tinnitus, which would obligate one to obtain an MRI scan. If the internal auditory canals are symmetrical, there is less of a chance that an acoustic tumor is present. If other aspects of the examination suggest a retrocochlear or nerve site, an MRI scan with gadolinium enhancement is indicated. The other CT finding relates to the radiologic diagnosis of inner ear otosclerosis. Such a finding shows evidence of spongiotic or sclerotic plaque formation in the area of the oval window and the basal turns of the cochlea. There may also be evidence of pericochlear lucency, which is also a sign of otosclerosis.

A complete laboratory evaluation should be undertaken, including a thyroid-stimulating hormone test and a 5-hour glucose tolerance test. The laboratory evaluation may reveal anemia, various hyperlipidemias, and hypothyroidism. The glucose tolerance test may reveal a diabetic or extremely exaggerated response. In addition, there may be a flat blood sugar curve. Simultaneous insulin levels are requested. Some may reveal hyperinsulinemia, which frequently plays a role in the severity of the tinnitus.

TREATMENT

When an etiology other than an acoustic tumor is found, the treatment should be directed at the etiology. When otosclerosis is found, the physician needs to decide which of the now-available treatments is indicated. The oldest form of treatment is the use of sodium fluoride and calcium carbonate (Florical). The current similar product contains sodium monofluorophosphate and calcium carbonate (Monocal) and is taken two capsules or pills twice daily with food. It is important to take these preparations with food for two reasons. The first is to reduce any gastric irritation from the fluoride. The second is to mix the calcium with the food, which allows it to bind with any oxalate and therefore reduce the possibility of developing oxalate renal stones. The current use of bisphosphonates has revealed the efficacy of treating otosclerosis with a combination of agents compared with the use of fluoride alone. Therefore, etidronate* (Didronel), in the doses used for osteoporosis, or alendrolate* (Fosamax) may be helpful in reducing the cochlear trigger of the tinnitus. Otosclerosis is a demineralization of the capsule of the bone around the inner ear. The outcome of otic capsule bone demineralization is the deposit of enzyme by-products in the

*Not FDA approved for this indication.

inner ear fluids. These enzymes are toxic to the hair cells of the inner ear and may cause them to malfunction, producing the tinnitus or other inner ear symptoms. By slowing down this demineralization process with the use of fluoride or bisphosphonates, the amount of enzyme released into the inner ear fluids is reduced, thereby reducing the toxic effect on the hair cells.

When there is an exaggerated, flat, or diabetic response of the blood sugars to a standard glucose load for the tolerance test and/or when the insulin levels are higher than normal, a diet should be constructed to address these changes. The demands of the inner ear for blood sugar are three times greater than those for an equivalent volume of brain. Thus, when the inner ear is not working normally, it is very sensitive to even minor fluctuations in the blood sugar that may indicate neither diabetes nor hypoglycemia. These blood sugars may also be associated with abnormal elevations in the simultaneously measured insulin levels. When the diet is high in carbohydrates, the serum triglycerides may be elevated. Once the diet is under way, serial insulin levels or triglyceride levels help in monitoring dietary compliance. If the cholesterol is elevated, it must be addressed, as this may be an additional metabolic factor affecting inner ear function and may relate to the symptom of tinnitus. Any diet so constructed should also curtail the use of animal fats, such as those in meat and dairy products.

The effect of a treatment directed at an etiology takes about 6 to 12 weeks. If the hearing is in the normal range, special electrical high-frequency hearing tests may reveal findings that relate to the tinnitus and can be used for serial monitoring of auditory function. In addition, using these tests the tinnitus can be matched for the closest frequency and intensity. This matching technique can also help to interpret response to therapy. When the frequency match of the tinnitus is changing from visit to visit, it may be a sign that the treatment is affecting the mechanism of the tinnitus. In some instances, when the closest matched tinnitus frequency is dropping, the patient often observes that the tinnitus is becoming more tolerable. Once matched, attempts are made to suppress the tinnitus by increasing the volume. Success in suppressing the tinnitus gives more information about its character and can help to reduce patient anxiety about the tinnitus.

On the perceptual level, there are new concepts whose application may further benefit the patient afflicted with tinnitus of the severe disabling type. The first step is understanding the requirement of the brain for a minimum amount of sound stimulation or a set point of sound stimulation. This required sound stimulation need not be in the frequencies used for understanding words and not necessarily associated with a loss of hearing ability. Because most tinnitus is triggered by a disorder of the cochlea, this altered inner ear function results in reduced sound stimulation to the brain. The reduced stimulation below the set point leads to the brain's increasing its sensitivity to satisfy a requirement for minimum stimulation. This results in an amplification of the noise within the neuronal network from the inner ear to the brain and is perceived as tinnitus, or the emergence of tinnitus, when none existed before. In some instances, simultaneous hyperacusis (hypersensitivity to sound) occurs. Depending on the individual neuronal network, reflex stimulation of the limbic-hypothalamic areas may or may not occur, giving rise to the difference between tinnitus perceived as tolerable versus that which is perceived as severely disabling. From this concept evolved the use of "therapeutic noise generators," which are not to be confused with "tinnitus maskers." The goal is to habituate the tinnitus signal. Habituation is brought about by resetting or reprogramming neuronal networks involved in subcortical signal detection. Although maskers are hearing devices that mask the tinnitus while they are worn, noise generators are intended to reduce the brain's sensitivity by modifying the set point, resulting in a more tolerable degree of tinnitus. The idea behind the noise generators is to stimulate both ears with a low level of just-perceptible sound during 6 waking hours daily. This induces increased neuronal plasticity by the introduction of very low levels of wide band noise. This low level stimulation on a daily basis results in sound stimulation sufficient to begin reaching the brain's set point for stimulation. This results in reduced sensitivity, reduced limbic-hypothalamic stimulation, and a change in the perception of the tinnitus from severe and disabling to tolerable. These neuronal events are slow to occur and may require from 6 to 24 months before a change is perceived. This use of sound stimulation may be used in the absence of a treatment directed at the etiology of the inner ear disorder. However, by adding a treatment focused on the etiology of the inner ear disorder along with the therapeutic noise generators, the timetable for improvement of the tinnitus may be shortened.

LOW BACK PAIN

method of
GUNNAR B. J. ANDERSSON, M.D., PH.D.
Department of Orthopedic Surgery
Rush–Presbyterian–St. Luke's Medical Center
Chicago, Illinois

Back pain is so common that more than 85% of the population in the industrial world will experience it at some time in life. Although there are minor differences among countries in the prevalence and incidence of back pain, there are remarkable similarities. In the United States about 15% of all adults will have a back episode in a given year, and in about one third of these, the pain is severe and chronic. Back pain is the most frequent cause of activity limitation in people younger than 45 years, the second most common reason for patient visits, the fifth-ranking reason for hospitalization, and the third most common reason for surgical procedures. About 2% of the U.S.

workforce report compensable back injuries each year. Over the past few decades there has been a large increase in the number of surgical procedures back-related conditions. Thus, from 1979 to 1990 the frequency of back operations in the United States doubled, and between 1992 and 1996 the number of patients operated on for spinal conditions increased by 14% to 543,000.

Back pain remains, however, a generally benign condition. Some 60% of patients recover in a week and about 90% in 6 weeks. Advanced age, pain radiating into the leg, and psychosocial and occupational factors have all been identified as increasing the risk for long-term pain. Prevention strategies including education, lifestyle changes, and protective equipment have not proved to be significantly effective.

CAUSES OF BACK PAIN

Most patients with back pain never know the precise origin of their pain. Indeed, excluding degenerative changes, 85% of patients are given a symptom diagnosis only. Many textbooks classify back patients into more or less well-defined categories, as illustrated in Table 1. Although this is certainly helpful to make sure no disease entity is forgotten, it is often more useful to classify according to the patient's presenting symptoms. Using this method, you can early on focus on patients who require particular attention. Whenever a patient is evaluated for back pain, the history and physical examination should always consider the so-called red flags (Table 2). Usually, patients can be divided easily into six categories:

Back pain only
Back pain and leg pain, or leg pain mainly
Back pain, leg pain, and inability to void
Back and/or leg symptoms with walking
Severe, unremitting back pain (with or without leg pain)
Back pain in the morning improving over the day

TABLE 1. **Causes of Low Back Pain**

Developmental
Stenosis
Spondylolisthesis
Infectious
Diskitis
Vertebral osteomyelitis
Inflammatory
Seronegative spondyloarthropathies
Polymyalgia rheumatica
Traumatic
Fractures
Metabolic
Osteoporosis
Osteomalacia
Hyperparathyroidism
Iatrogenic (steroid use)
Neoplastic
Primary
Metastatic
Degenerative
Herniated disk
Degenerative disk disease
Facet arthropathy
Spinal stenosis
Spondylolisthesis
Referred
Vasculogenic
Aortic aneurysm, ischemia
Viscerogenic
Gastrointestinal, genitourinary, pancreatic
Hip osteoarthritis
Unknown
Musculoligamentous overuse
Psychosocial factors

TABLE 2. **The Red Flags of Low Back Pain**

Possible Condition	History	Physical
Fracture	Major trauma Minor trauma (older patient)	
Tumor	Age < 15 or > 50 years Known cancer Unexplained weight loss Night pain	
Infection	Recent fever or chills Recent bacterial infection (urinary tract) Intravenous drug use Immune suppression Unrelenting pain	Fever
Cauda Equina Syndrome	Saddle numbness Urinary retention, incontinence Severe (progressive) lower extremity neurologic deficit	Weak anal sphincter Perianal sensory loss Major motor weakness

Back pain only is the most frequent presentation. Often the patients associate the onset with a lift, a movement, or other physical activity, but not infrequently the pain developed for no obvious reason. The pain pattern is usually mechanical, increasing with activity, decreasing with rest. The source of the pain may be the muscles, ligaments, facet joints, disks, and even bone. Generally, the possibility of muscle and ligament being the source is higher in the young, whereas disk problems are more frequent in the 35- to 55-year age group; bone-related pain is more common in the elderly (osteoporosis). When leg pain is present, the probability of disk involvement increases, particularly when the pain is radicular. Inability to void or loss of bowel and bladder control suggests a cauda equina syndrome. Back and particularly leg symptoms, which occur when walking, suggest the possibility of spinal stenosis, particularly in the elderly. Stenosis patients often describe how their pain decreases when they bend forward (e.g., to push a grocery cart) or sit down, which enlarges the spinal canal and neuroforamina.

Severe, unremitting pain is one of the red flags (see Table 2). Patients with this type of pain have the greatest chance of having a life-threatening or disabling problem (tumor, infection, or fracture). Some patients may say that their pain is "present all the time." After further discussion, this can often be resolved. Morning pain and stiffness improving over the day suggest an inflammatory disease, of which ankylosing spondylitis is the most common. It is important to appreciate that degenerative changes do not equal pain and are the result of normal aging. Disks degenerate early, and by age 40 nuclear fissures and annular cracks are the rule, not the exception. Disk degeneration is almost a prerequisite for a disk herniation, which occurs first at the L4 and L5 disks and last at L1 and L2. The degenerative disk process shifts the loads in the facet joints, causing osteoarthritis. The combination of disk degeneration and facet osteoarthritis, in turn, causes spinal stenosis.

TREATMENT

Because back pain has such favorable natural history, treatment can often be simplified to pain relief, education, and activity alteration. Patients who present without red flags should be advised that they have no evidence of a severe underlying problem and that a rapid recovery can be expected. Many patients are concerned when experiencing back pain because they may have friends, relatives, or coworkers who have developed chronic or recurrent back problems. They need to know that this is the exception, not the rule. Patients with leg pain (particularly when dermatomal) have a slower recovery and a greater chance of future need for a specific treatment, yet the prognosis is excellent in these patients as well.

Pain relief is the primary concern and usually the reason for the visit to a physician. Activity alteration, analgesics and/or nonsteroidal anti-inflammatory drugs (NSAIDs), and various physical methods are available for symptomatic relief. Bed rest, long a cornerstone of back care, is rarely indicated and if so only for a day or two. Prolonged bed rest actually leads to deconditioning and is worse than a gradual return to normal activities, which is the advice of choice. Temporary activity limitations, including avoiding heavy lifts, bending and twisting of the back, and prolonged sitting, are indicated in patients with acute pain.

Analgesics, preferably acetaminophen, and NSAIDs are reasonably safe drugs and are helpful in accomplishing pain relief. NSAIDs have higher complication risks but are sometimes more effective. Muscle relaxants offer no particular advantage over NSAIDs and may cause drowsiness. Opioids are rarely indicated but occasionally are necessary to manage patients with very severe acute symptoms. They should be used sparingly and for short periods only. Steroids are not recommended for the treatment of acute lower back pain. In patients with radiculopathy, epidural injections or root blocks with steroids may be used as an attempt to avoid surgery. Antidepressants* may be useful in patients with chronic back pain but are not helpful in the acute stages of pain.

*Not FDA approved for this indication.

Physical agents and modalities are often used, including, ice, heat, diathermy, ultrasound, and massage. They have no documented effect on back pain, as such, but carry little risk of complications. Self-application of cold or heat often results in symptomatic but short-term relief. Physiologically, it makes more sense to use cold in the acute stages of back pain and heat in the later stages. Ultrasound and diathermy should not be used on pregnant women because of theoretical risks to the fetus. Transcutaneous electrical nerve stimulation (TENS) has no role in the treatment of acute back pain.

Corsets, braces, and back belts are widely used, but there is no evidence that they have any effect on acute back pain. In patients with chronic and recurrent problems, there is conflicting evidence, as is the case with the preventive use of back belts in industry. Continuous use of corsets can result in weakening of the trunk muscles and should be avoided. Traction has no documented effect on either back pain or sciatica.

Aerobic exercise programs (walking, biking, or swimming) should be started early in patients with acute back pain (after a week or two) and should continue indefinitely in patients with recurrent or chronic problems. Trunk muscle exercises and stretching are not particularly helpful during the first 2 weeks of acute pain but can be initiated later. It is often beneficial to have a physical therapist's advice on proper exercise routines. There is no specific advantage to one of many alternative philosophies used by therapists; the response is not universal. Although exercise programs cannot prevent recurrences, it appears that maintaining good physical fitness allows for a more rapid recovery.

Spinal manipulation (chiropractic, osteopathic, or other) can reduce pain and perhaps even speed recovery if applied during the first month of pain. Manipulations should not be used in patients with neurologic deficits and should not be continued if a few attempts are unsuccessful. The use of spinal manipulation in chronic back pain is controversial because study results remain inconclusive. Manipulation has no preventive value. Surgery is indicated primarily in patients with herniated disks, spinal stenosis, and spondylolisthesis. Even in those conditions, conservative treatment is often successful, and surgery should not be performed without attempts at such treatment. The cauda equina syndrome remains the exception and should be addressed surgically.

Section 2

The Infectious Diseases

HUMAN IMMUNODEFICIENCY VIRUS INFECTION AND ITS COMPLICATIONS

method of
MARSHALL K. KUBOTA, M.D.
*University of California, San Francisco, and Sutter Medical Center of Santa Rosa
Santa Rosa, California*

In 1981, clusters of *Pneumocystis carinii* pneumonia and Kaposi's sarcoma occurring among gay men living in large metropolitan areas defined the leading edge of the acquired immune deficiency syndrome (AIDS) epidemic in the United States. The syndrome encompassed immune dysfunction associated with a decrease in $CD4^+$ (T helper) lymphocytes, a markedly increased risk for non-Hodgkin's B-cell lymphomas and Kaposi's sarcoma, dementia and disorders of the peripheral nervous system, and metabolic disorders resulting in wasting. Discovery of the putative agent of AIDS, the human immunodeficiency virus type 1 (HIV-1), led to a fuller understanding of the epidemiology, pathogenesis, and treatment of this syndrome.

EPIDEMIOLOGY

From 1981 through 1996, the Centers for Disease Control and Prevention reported 573,800 adult and adolescent cases of HIV infection progressing to the stage of disease fulfilling the epidemiologic definition of AIDS. In 1996, for the first time in the epidemic, there was a decrease in the number of reported AIDS cases: 56,730 cases fitting the definition of AIDS were reported, representing a 6% decrease compared to 1995. Women (1992—14%; 1996—20% by gender) and black non-Hispanics (1992—33%; 1996—41% by ethnicity) have shown the largest proportional increases in reported AIDS cases. Deaths due to AIDS also decreased 23% in 1996 (38,780) compared with 1995. These reductions have been greater for men than women (−25% vs. −10%), white non-Hispanics vs. black non-Hispanics (−32% vs. −13%) and men having sex with men versus heterosexuals (−30% vs −8%). The overall improvements are due to the impact of prevention efforts of the mid-1980s resulting in reduced transmission and combination antiretroviral treatments resulting in reduced progression to AIDS and death. An estimated 40,000 to 60,000 Americans are infected by HIV-1 annually. There are currently about 235,470 Americans living with AIDS, representing an 11% increase from 1995 to 1996.

TRANSMISSION

The modes of transmission of HIV are sexual transmission, transmission through significant exposure to infected blood or blood products, and vertical transmission in utero, intrapartum, and by breast-feeding.

Blood, semen, and cervicovaginal secretions contain enough HIV-1 to be infectious. Uncontaminated saliva has not been implicated in transmission. Infection via the rectum, vagina, penile urethra, and direct vascular and tissue exposure is much more common than through the mouth or other mucous membranes. The volume of infected fluid, the exposure time, and the concentration of HIV in the fluid are also pertinent risk factors. Direct intravascular injection of infected blood into the veins carries a high risk for infection, as occurs with needle sharing by injection drug users or in occupational exposures (needlestick accidents). Infected males are more likely to transmit to females during vaginal intercourse than vice versa.

Vertical transmission from infected mother to her child occurs in utero, intrapartum, and in the postpartum period via breast-feeding. The overall risk for transmission in utero and intrapartum ranges from 13 to 40%. The risk of transmission to an uninfected newborn by breast-feeding from an infected mother is about 14%. Reduction of transmission in pregnancy can be achieved through antenatal HIV testing, treatment of the mother to reduce prenatal and intrapartum HIV-1 titers, reduction (as possible) of blood exposure to the infant during birth, and proscription of breast-feeding when safe alternatives exist.

HIV-1 KINETICS

Understanding the pathogenesis of HIV-1 infection and the kinetics of viral replication and mutation has aided the development of logical treatment strategies. The ability to precisely measure HIV-1 in the plasma coupled with the use of potent inhibitors of replication showed that HIV-1 infection is a dynamic process involving enormous levels of viral replication and immunologic destruction.

HIV-1 RNA in the plasma is measured by either a branched DNA (bDNA) assay or by quantitative polymerase chain reaction (PCR). Viral titers (loads) range from below the limits of detection (<25–100 copies of HIV-1 RNA per mL) to greater than 10^6 copies per mL. In an untreated state, higher titers are related to more rapid deterioration in the immune system as measured by $CD4^+$ counts and a poor prognosis. Daily virion production is in the range of 10^9 to 10^{10} particles daily.

Inherent in the replication of the virus is a high random mutation rate. Wild-type virus predominates but within the diverse population of HIV-1 in any individual exist viruses with mutations predetermined to be resistant to simple regimens of antiretroviral treatment.

Rapid destruction of the immune system is prevented only by robust $CD4^+$ cell replacement. The immune system is in a constant state of destruction with attempts at repair. The initial HIV infection set point of viral production along with intrinsic immune repair mechanisms determines the long-term progression of HIV infection (Figure 1).

Clinically, as long as immunologic replacement keeps pace with destruction there is a prolonged asymptomatic period. Throughout this clinically uneventful time, the vi-

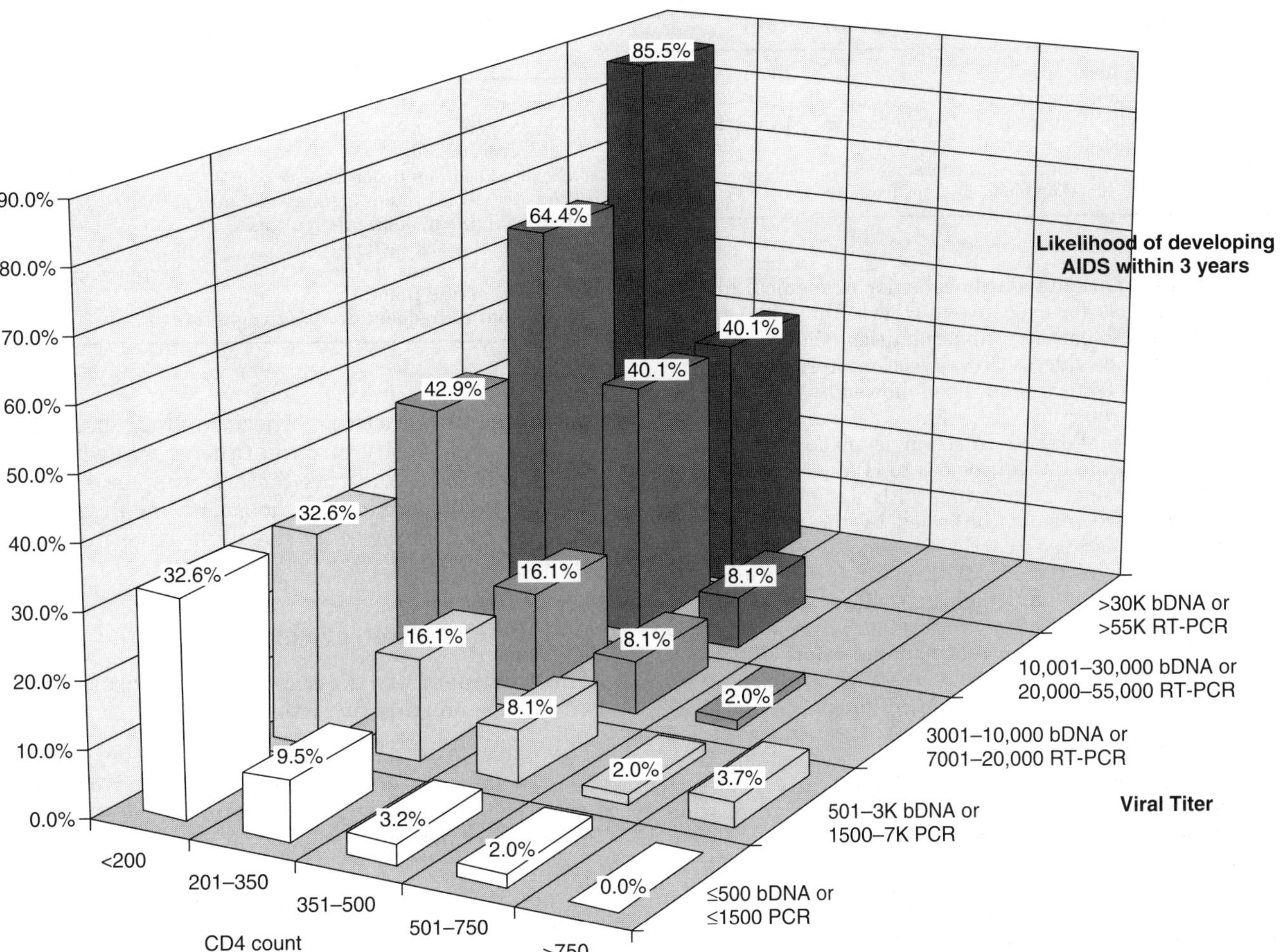

Figure 1. Progression of HIV-1. (Modified from Mellors JW, Kinsley LA, Rinaldo CR, et al: Quantitation of HIV-1 RNA in plasma predicts outcome after seroconversion. Ann Intern Med *122*:573–579, 1995.)

ral burden grows and immunologic deterioration ensues, characterized by falling CD4$^+$ cell counts. Eventually symptomatic HIV infection develops, leading to life-threatening opportunistic complications, neurologic dysfunction, and metabolic imbalances.

As the level of circulating CD4$^+$ cells declines, the immunologic protection afforded an individual passes down through succeeding layers of risk for specific opportunistic infections (OIs). Individuals with relatively normal levels of CD4$^+$ cells suffer from the same conditions as the immunocompetant population but with greater frequency or severity. If immunologic deterioration continues, OIs characteristic of AIDS become evident, and in an accumulation of risk, patients with very low CD4$^+$ cell counts are at risk for a large number of OIs.

The neurologic system is also the target of HIV-1 infection, either directly or indirectly. Minor cognitive/motor disorders, HIV-associated dementia, and peripheral neuropathies are the common sequelae of HIV infection. A prominent metabolic disorder is wasting syndrome.

ACUTE RETROVIRAL INFECTION

The response to initial HIV-1 infection has been described as a syndrome that varies from asymptomatic to the acute retroviral syndrome experienced by 50 to 90% of newly infected persons. The onset from exposure to symptoms is from 2 to 6 weeks. The acute illness lasts from 1 to 2 weeks and can vary from mild to a severity requiring hospitalization. A large burst of viral replication occurs prior to the immunologic response, resulting initially in high plasma titers of virus. Widespread dissemination into lymphatic tissues occurs, and individual viral titer set points are established as antibody responses are developed. Within 6 to 10 weeks, most individuals have developed specific HIV antibodies, although for conservative counseling a 3- to 6-month seronegative window period is used (Table 1).

DIAGNOSIS OF HIV INFECTION

Inquiries about risk behavior should be a routine part of history taking. HIV-1 testing and counseling should be

TABLE 1. **Signs and Symptoms of Acute Retroviral Syndrome**

Fever	Headache
Lymphadenopathy	Nausea/vomiting
Pharyngitis	Hepatosplenomegaly
Maculopapular rash	Thrush
Mucocutaneous ulcerations	Weight loss
Myalgias, arthralgias	Central and peripheral neurologic signs
Diarrhea	

TABLE 2. **Risk Factors for HIV Infection**

Illicit injection drug use
Male homosexual contact
Sexual contact with persons known to have HIV-1 infection or at high risk for infection
Multiple or anonymous sexual contacts
Transfusion of blood or blood product from 1977 to 1985

TABLE 3. **Clinically Common Conditions Associated with or Aggravated by HIV Infection**

Anemia
Lymphopenia
Thrombocytopenia
Elevated sedimentation rate
Elevated total protein (gamma globulin portion)
Bacterial pneumonia, tuberculosis
Shingles (herpes zoster)
Sexually transmitted diseases, including herpes simplex and hepatitis B and C
Persistent or frequent *Candida* vaginitis

considered for patients whose behavior or medical history puts them at risk for exposure to HIV-1 (Table 2). Clinical conditions and laboratory abnormalities, though nonspecific, that may be due to HIV infection or raise concerns about HIV risk factors should be followed by more specific tests for HIV-1 infection (Table 3).

The diagnosis of HIV-1 infection is made through the detection of specific IgG antibodies to HIV-1 viral proteins. These tests consist of screening with a sensitive ELISA test with positive results confirmed by the more specific Western blot. Testing is carried out on samples of blood, orally obtained oral mucosal transudate (OraSure), or urine (the Sentinel) and is highly specific and sensitive for HIV-1 antibodies once they are formed. A window period of 6 months may exist after infection and before the formation of detectable HIV-1 antibody. Tests for direct detection of the virus such as HIV-1 RNA, although specific, lack sensitivity. The reliability of the test, the window period between infection and the development of detectable HIV-1 antibody, and the medical benefits of early detection of HIV-1 infection including treatment and transmission prevention should be discussed. Home testing kits are commercially available and anonymous testing sites exist in many locales, providing patients with discreet testing with results and counseling given confidentially. Any patient presenting for treatment and claiming to have been diagnosed with HIV-1 infection through these sources should be retested in the office.

MEDICAL MANAGEMENT OF PATIENTS WITH HIV INFECTION

Management consists of baseline medical care, treatment of HIV infection with antiretroviral therapy, and prophylaxis and treatment of opportunistic infections, neoplasms, and metabolic disorders.

Baseline Medical Care

Initial data include a history or findings of current and past indicators of HIV-1 infection, how HIV-1 infection was acquired and ongoing risk behaviors (unsafe sexual practices, injection drug use), psychosocial and family circumstances (knowledge of current condition and risk factors, support systems, presence of depression), concurrent medical conditions and medications, and baseline laboratory data (Table 4).

Antiretroviral Therapy

The treatment of HIV infection comprises the following decisions and activities:

The decision to initiate antiretroviral therapy
Design of a durable and individualized combination antiretroviral treatment regimen
Monitoring for adequacy, maintenance, and failure of regimens
Secondary treatment in the event of failure of the primary regimen

The Decision to Begin Therapy

This requires a cooperative agreement and commitment between the patient and the physician and is based upon

The activity of viral replication as measured by plasma HIV-1 RNA titers
The degree of immunologic damage as determined by CD4+ cell count and patient symptoms
The patient's readiness and capability to adhere to demanding medication regimens

HIV-1 viral titer (viral load) is measured either by quantitative PCR or by branched DNA methods. As results vary depending upon the methodology used,

TABLE 4. **Medical Database**

Current and Past Symptom History	Baseline Laboratory Data	Baseline Therapy
Persistent dermatoses, herpes zoster	HIV-1 titer (PCR or bDNA)	Cervical cytology screening
Oral thrush, hairy leukoplakia, gingivitis	CD4+ cell count	Polyvalent pneumococcal vaccine
Chronic sinusitis	Complete blood count	Influenza vaccine
Diffuse, persistent adenopathy	Basic chemistry panel	Hepatitis vaccine as indicated
Persistent fevers	Syphilis serology	Contraception
Chronic diarrhea	Tuberculosis skin testing	
Weight loss	Chest radiography	
Distal symmetrical sensory neuropathy	Hepatitis B, C serology	
Memory disturbances	*Toxoplasma gondii* antibody	
Recurrent and/or severe herpes simplex labialis or genitalis		
Bacterial pneumonia by history		

TABLE 5. **1997 U.S. Public Health Service Treatment Guidelines**

Clinical	CD4+ Count	HIV-1 RNA Titer	Recommendation
Symptomatic	Any	Any	Treat
Asymptomatic	<500/mL or	>10,000 (bDNA) or >20,000 (PCR)	Treat
Asymptomatic	>500/mL and	<10,000 (bDNA) or <20,000 (PCR)	Treat or observe

it is advisable to utilize the same test with any one patient. As success in treatment is commonly measured in $\log_{10}$ reductions, familiarity with both forms of titer expression is useful. The same sample variance of HIV-1 titers can be as much as threefold. Both tests have active ranges from between 10^2 to 10^6 copies of viral RNA per mL. Ultrasensitive methodologies with active ranges from 25 to 80,000 copies ($\log_{10}$ 1.3 to 4.9) can be used in determining high-level viral suppression under treatment.

A viral titer greater than about 5000 copies per mL ($\log_{10}$ 3.7) is considered a level at which initiation of treatment is warranted. At titers less than 5000 copies per mL, treatment could be considered but should take into account the long-term trends established by the patient, the generally good prognosis at this level of viral activity, and the possible availability of improved treatments currently in development. However, some clinicians consider treatment at very low levels to have a greater chance of long-term success. As titers rise to greater than 10,000 copies per mL ($\log_{10}$ 4.0), the rationale to treat becomes strong. Because of intrinsic test variability, viral titers falling within values such that the decision to treat is still in question should be repeated. If the decision is made not to treat, viral titers should be monitored three to four times yearly.

$CD4^+$ cell counts should be monitored to determine the degree of immunologic damage. Counts greater than 500 $CD4^+$ cells per mm^3 are considered protective, whereas counts below 500 per mm^3 are generally indicative of immunologic damage, and treatment should be considered. Persistent constitutional symptoms attributed to HIV-1 infection (fever, weight loss, diarrhea, thrush, hairy leukoplakia) are reason enough to initiate antiretroviral treatment (Table 5).

Design of a Treatment Regimen

It is important to realize that the initial treatment regimen represents the best chance of success and must be carefully designed and critically examined (Table 6). The goal of antiretroviral treatment is to maximally reduce HIV-1 replication to levels that are below the detectable limits of HIV-1 plasma RNA tests. With such a reduction there is partial reconstitution of the immune system as evidenced by a rise in $CD4^+$ cells and clinical improvement. This also reduces the rate at which the virus acquires resistance to antiretroviral agents. Successful regimens greatly reduce the rate of viral replication and erect substantial genetic barriers to prevent the development of resistance. This combination of potency and genetic barrier endows a regimen with durability.

No single or two-drug therapies are durable. With the extensive inherent diversity of the virus, the mutations within target viral enzymes that result in high-level resistance to single drugs likely exist prior to the administration of the drugs.

Antiretroviral Drugs

Antiretroviral drugs work by inhibiting the action of two HIV-1–specific enzymes. Reverse transcriptase is the enzyme responsible for the transcription of intracellular viral RNA into a DNA analogue that is then integrated into the host CD4 cell chromosome. Drugs inhibiting this enzyme by a process of termination of DNA elongation are classified as nucleoside reverse transcriptase inhibitors (RTIs). Drugs targeting this enzyme through direct inhibition are referred to as non-nucleoside reverse transcriptase inhibitors (NNRTIs).

Protease inhibitors (PIs) target the viral protease enzyme that is responsible for the post-transcriptional modification of viral proteins during viral production. This class of antiretrovirals possesses the greatest potency and genetic barriers to the development of resistance. Durable regimens include one or two PIs.

Drug Combinations

In combining antiretroviral medications, the following steps should be followed:

1. Determine a regimen of adequate durability.
2. Evaluate the combination for pharmacologic and pharmacodynamic compatibility.

TABLE 6. **1997 International AIDS Society—U.S. Treatment Guidelines**

Clinical	CD4+ Count	HIV-1 RNA Titer	Recommendation
Symptomatic	Any	Any	Treat
Asymptomatic	<500/mL	Any	Treat
Asymptomatic	>500/mL	≥5,000/mL	Treat
Asymptomatic	>500/mL	<5,000/mL	Consider treatment

TABLE 7. **Antiretroviral Drugs with Substantial Resistance Profile Overlap**

DDC and DDI	RTV and IDV
NVP, DLV, and DMP	All PIs—partial overlap

Abbreviations: DDC = zalcitabine (Hivid); DDI = didanosine (Videx); NVP = nevirapine (Viramune); DLV = delavirdine (Rescriptor); DMP = efavirenz (Sustiva); RTV = ritonavir (Norvir); IDV = indinavir (Crixivan).

3. Evaluate the likelihood of patient adherence and tolerability.

4. Consider possible secondary regimens in case of failure.

Durable Regimens. Regimens of adequate durability contain two compatible inhibitors of reverse transcriptase (RTIs and NNRTIs) combined with one or two compatible PIs. 3TC (lamivudine [Epivir]), NVP (nevirapine [Viramune]), and DLV (delavirdine [Rescriptor]) are of specific concern in their contribution to a durable regimen because of a low genetic barrier to the development of resistance. These drugs should be used only in regimens expected to achieve undetectable levels of virus. Generally, any regimen that uses two of these drugs would be considered likely to have poor durability. Data that exist for regimens consisting of only combinations of RTIs (AZT [zidovudine, Retrovir] plus 3TC plus ABC [abacavir, Ziagen]*) or the regimen of two RTIs (AZT plus 3TC) in combination with the NNRTI DMP (efavirenz [Sustiva]*) demonstrate potent viral suppression but are limited to the duration of the current studies. These combinations have the advantages of reserving drug classes (NNRTIs and PIs in the former and PIs in the latter), avoidance of PI-associated side effects, low pill counts, and simple dosing schedules.

Pharmacologic and Pharmacodynamic Compatibility. Pharmacologic and pharmacodynamic compatibility takes into account interdrug antagonism, overlap in resistance profile, and drug interactions. Of particular importance is the high degree of cytochrome P4503A inhibition by ritonavir and to a lesser extent delavirdine (DLV). Careful examination of current and any future drugs (e.g., terfenadine, astemizole, cisapride) for interaction with these drugs is imperative. Hydroxyurea (Hydrea), 500 mg twice a day, potentiates DDI (didanosine [Videx]) by increasing its intracellular concentration. It is marrow suppressive, so decreases in viral titers may be seen without CD4$^+$ cell increases. Incompatibility exists between D4T (stavudine [Zerit]) and AZT, D4T and DDC (zalcitabine [Hivid]), DDC and 3TC, and possibly IDV (indinavir [Crixivan]) and SQV (saquinavir [Fortovase]), prohibiting their concomitant use. The resistance profiles of three sets of drugs (DDI/DDC, IDV/RTV, and NVP/DLV/DMP) overlap to the extent that, in regard to this characteristic they are considered interchangeable and when used together add little to the durability of a regimen. Similarly, virus resistant to one of the combinations will likely be resistant to the other(s). All PIs overlap with each other to some extent. RTV and IDV have the broadest genetic barrier to the development of resistance. If resistance develops to either RTV or IDV, subsequent use of NFV (nelfinavir [Viracept]) or SQV will give suboptimal results. Any PI not previously used may be used after SQV or NFV if changes are made as soon as treatment failure is suspected (Table 7). The use of drug interactions for therapeutic advantage is a complex but useful tool in which the effects of drugs on hepatic clearance via the cytochrome P450 system are examined for advantages and disadvantages for the regimen and patient. As a result, some drug combinations will be eliminated or dosages or dosing schedules will be increased or reduced. RTV and IDV can be paired to take advantage of pharmacokinetic interactions that reduce the dosing requirements of IDV (Table 8).

Compatible pairings of reverse transcriptase inhibitors with protease inhibitors are given in Table 9 and commonly utilized regimens are listed in Table 10.

Adherence to Regimens

A high degree of adherence to antiretroviral regimens is required to prevent continued replication and mutation, and eventual development of drug resistance. Regimens under consideration should be examined for factors that will either promote or re-

*Investigational drug in the United States.

TABLE 8. **Suggested Combination PI and NNRTI Doses**

	NVP	DLV	DMP	SQV	RTV	IDV
DLV	No use					
DMP	No use	No use				
SQV	Same	Same	Avoid			
RTV	Same	Same	No data	400/400 bid		
IDV	Same	IDV 600 q 8 h	IDV 1000 q 8 h	Avoid	400/400 bid	
NFV	Same	Avoid	Same	NFV same SQV 800 tid or 1250/1250 bid	NFV 750 bid RTV 400 bid	IDV 1000 NFV 1000–1250 bid

Abbreviations: DLV = delavirdine (Rescriptor); DMP = efavirenz (Sustiva); IDV = indinavir (Crixivan); NFV = nelfinavir (Viracept); NVP = nevirapine (Viramune); RTV = ritonavir (Norvir); SQV = saquinavir (Fortovase).

TABLE 9. **Compatible Combinations of Antiretroviral Medications**

RTI/NNRTI		PI
AZT + 3TC		RTV
AZT + DDI		IDV
AZT + DDC	in combination with	SQV
D4T + 3TC		NFV
D4T + DDI		RTV + SQV
ADF + 3TC*		NFV + SQV
ADF + AZT*		RTV + NFV
ADF + D4T*		RTV + IDV
ABC + RTI*		NFV + IDV
AZT + 3TC + ABC (with or without PIs)*		
AZT + 3TC + DMP (with or without PIs)*		
NNRTIs can be substituted for any RTI. Use of NVP or DLV in combinations containing 3TC raises durability concerns.		

*Limited data.
Abbreviations: AZT = zidovudine (Retrovir); 3TC = lamivudine (Epivir); RTV = ritonavir (Norvir); DDI = didanosine (Videx); IDV = indinavir (Crixivan); DDC = zalcitabine (Hivid); SQV = saquinavir (Fortovase); D4T = stavudine (Zerit); NFV = nelfinavir (Viracept).

duce adherence (Table 11). Missed doses will result in replication of HIV-1, which will in turn lead to the development of resistance to each drug and loss of durability of the combination. Factors that affect adherence can be inherent in the drug regimen, patient associated, or situation driven.

Failure of adherence increases as the frequency of daily doses rises. Single daily doses are most regularly taken; three-times-daily and every-8-hour dosing pose difficulties. Some medications must be taken with meals for adequate absorption (RTV, NFV, SQV), while others must be taken 1 hour before or 2 hours following meals (IDV, DDI). Further complicating this issue is the need to take IDV and DDI an hour apart. Combinations that mix these requirements are difficult to follow, leading to missed doses or poor absorption and the development of resistance. Some medications are being given in alternative dosing schedules with evidence that such changes are not harmful. Pharmacokinetic interactions, in particular the inhibition of cytochrome P450 3A by RTV and to a lesser extent NFV and DLV, can be used to advantageously alter drug dosing.

The number of pills in a given regimen can become a psychologic barrier for some patients. For example, SQV requires taking 18 capsules daily and DLV, 12 daily. Patients may poorly tolerate the taste and form of some of the drugs. The taste of chewable DDI or RTV solution is unacceptable to some patients. DDI and NFV are available in dissolvable powder, and AZT, 3TC, D4T, ABC, and RTV are available in liquid forms.

The potential for drug toxicity requires that clinical or laboratory parameters be closely monitored. The toxicities of some combinations may be additive (e.g., peripheral neuropathy) and these should be used with caution. DDI-related pancreatitis warrants special attention. Any persistent abdominal pain calls for an assessment of amylase and lipase levels to determine possible pancreatic injury. Patients should not be rechallenged. Neutropenia due to AZT is more frequent in advanced HIV infection. Levels down to 500 neutrophils per mL are protective. Filgrastim (Neupogen) can be used if AZT is continued. AZT anemia is macrocytic and if necessary can be treated with recombinant erythropoietin (Procrit) or discontinued. Prolonged AZT use (more than 9 months) can cause an aching myopathy with an elevated creatinine phosphokinase. It resolves on withholding AZT, after which there can be a rechallenge. The rash caused by NVP and to a lesser extent DLV can become severe. With NVP, gradual introduction lessens the risk of rash. Hypersensitivity to ABC, characterized by accumulation and escalation of fever, nausea, and malaise with or without rash, is a contraindication to further use or rechallenge. The use of ADF (adefovir [Preveon]) can result in Fanconi's syndrome (hypophosphatemia, proteinuria, glucosuria, low serum bicarbonate, or elevations in serum creatinine).

Patients should be advised to drink fluids to prevent IDV-associated kidney stones. Although painful, the stones, composed of crystallized IDV, usually pass unaided. All PIs (SQV, RTV, IDV, NFV) have been associated with the onset of glucose intolerance and non–insulin-dependent diabetes mellitus. The PIs have also been associated with elevations of cholesterol and triglycerides. Whether these abnormalities in lipids result in atherosclerotic disease or pancreatitis is not clear. An abnormal distribution of adipose tissue, with a loss of extremity and facial subcutaneous fat and deposition intra-abdominally, between the shoulders (buffalo hump) and in the breasts has been described in a significant number of patients on long-term PI-containing therapy. The risks of changing therapy (to other PIs or to non–PI-containing regimens) versus continued use recapitulates the principles of successful treatment of HIV-1 infection. At present, the benefit of direct treatment of these side effects (lipid-lowering agents, anabolic steroids) is unknown.

Specific drug side effects and their frequency and the tolerance for them vary among patients. Patients should be warned about these possible side effects. Drugs may have additive side effects. Side effects may either ameliorate with time or become tolerated by the patients.

The most important patient-associated factor in the ability to adhere to a medication regimen is patient acceptance and commitment to therapy. Patients unconvinced of the need to be treated may adhere poorly to treatment schedules. This commitment to treatment should be firm regardless of the immunologic situation. Psychiatric disorders, drug abuse, or homelessness can make compliance unlikely or impossible. Adherence to regimens will be aided by

A complete knowledge of medication names (generic, brand, alphanumeric) and dosing schedules

TABLE 10. **Commonly Utilized Regimens**

Regimen	Advantages	Disadvantages	Secondary Regimens
AZT 300 mg bid 3TC 150 mg bid IDV 800 mg q 8 h, empty stomach	Reserves DDI, D4T	q 8 h, empty stomach dosing AZT marrow suppression and nausea	(D4T + DDI) or (1 new RTI + NNRTI) plus (NFV + SQV)
AZT 300 mg bid 3TC 150 mg bid NFV 750 mg tid with meals	Can be taken with meals Reserves DDI, D4T Reserves IDV, RTV, SQV, RTV/SQV combination if failure not prolonged high titer	tid dosing AZT marrow suppression and nausea NFV-associated diarrhea	(D4T + DDI) or (1 new RTI + NNRTI) plus (SQV + RTV) or IDV alone or RTV alone
DDI 400 mg qd, empty stomach (separated from IDV by 1 h) D4T 40 mg bid IDV 800 mg q 8 h, empty stomach	Reserves AZT/3TC	DDI-associated diarrhea 4 dosing times daily Possible increased neuropathy Cannot be used with history of pancreatitis	(AZT + 3TC) or (AZT + NNRTI) plus SQV or NFV or (NFV + SQV)
DDI 400 mg q d, empty stomach D4T 40 mg bid NFV 750 mg tid with meals	Reserves AZT/3TC Reserves RTV, IDV, SQV, and RTV/SQV combination if failure not prolonged high titer	DDI and NFV associated diarrhea Cannot be used with history of pancreatitis Possible increased neuropathy 4 doses times daily	(AZT + 3TC) or (AZT + NNRTI) plus IDV alone or (RTV + SQV)
D4T 40 mg bid 3TC 150 mg bid + PI(s)	Low side effect RTIs After AZT resistance, AZT/3TC has effectiveness	Backup RTI combination of AZT/DDI may be poorly tolerated	(AZT + DDI) or (AZT + 3TC + DDI) or (new RTI + NNRTI) plus new PI
2 RTIs RTV 400 mg bid with meals SQV 400 mg bid with meals	Highly potent double protease inhibitor regimen (might be used in very high HIV titer patient) Interaction allows for reduced dosing of SQV and RTV to 400/mg/400/mg bid without regard to meals Fewer RTV side effect at lower dose	No good secondary therapy in case of failure May still have RTV-associated nausea RTV and SQV-associated diarrhea Possible hepatotoxicity due to high protease inhibitor levels—requires monitoring	No good secondary regimen because of high likelihood of broad PI resistance Possible use of 2 new RTIs or 1 new RTI + NNRTI plus NFV
2 RTIs SQV 1200 mg tid with meals NFV 750 mg tid with meals	Potent double protease inhibitor regimen, although likely less than RTV + SQV (might be used in very high HIV titer patient) Reserves IDV, RTV	SQV and NFV-associated diarrhea Large pill count, taken with meals (SQV—18/d, NFV—9/d)	2 new RTIs or 1 new RTI + NNRTI plus IDV or RTV
2 RTIs + NNRTI	Allow future use of all protease inhibitors Might be used in low HIV titer circumstances	May not be durable and therefore eliminates the accompanying RTIs from further use	2 new RITs or 1 new RTI + NNRTI plus 1 or 2 PIs

Abbreviations: AZT = zidovudine (Retrovir); 3TC = lamivudine (Epivir); RTV = ritonavir (Norvir); DDI = didanosine (Videx); IDV = indinavir (Crixivan); DDC = zalcitabine (Hivid); SQV = saquinavir (Fortovase); D4T = stavudine (Zerit); NFV = nelfinavir (Viracept).

TABLE 11. **Dosing and Prominent Side Effects of Antiretroviral Medications**

Drug	Unit Size	Dosing Options (mg per dose)			Prominent Side Effects																
		QD	*BID*	*TID or Q 8 hr*	*Nausea*	*Headache/ Insomnia*	*Dizziness*	*Diarrhea*	*Peripheral Neuropathy*	*Rash/ Hypersensitivity*	*Marrow Suppression*	*Pancreatitis*	*Aphthous Ulcers*	*Myositis*	*Oral Tingling*	*Kidney Stones*	*Increased Bilirubin*	*Renal*	*Glucose Intolerance/ Lipid Abnormalities*	*Decreased Carnitine*
Reverse Transcriptase Inhibitors																					
AZT (zidovudine, Retrovir)	100 mg, 300 mg, (300 mg + 150 mg 3TC)		300 mg	200 mg tid	X	X					X			X						
DDI (didanosine, Videx)	25 mg, 100 mg, 150 mg	400 mg (>60 kg) 240 mg (<60 kg) Empty stomach	200 mg (>60 kg) 120 mg (<60 kg) Empty stomach		X			X	X			X								
DDC (zalcitabine, Hivid)	0.375 mg, 0.75 mg			0.75 mg tid					X				X							
D4T (stavudine, Zerit)	20 mg, 30 mg, 40 mg		40 mg, 30 mg (<60 kg)						X											
3TC (lamivudine, Epivir)	150 mg, (150 mg + 300 mg AZT)		150 mg																	
AZT/3TC (Combivir)	AZT 300 mg + 3TC 150 mg		1 tablet		X	X					X			X						
Abacavir (Ziagen)*	300 mg		300 mg		X					X										
adefovir (Preveon)*	60 mg, 120 mg	120 mg + carnitine			X													XX		X
Non-nucleoside Reverse Transcriptase Inhibitors																					
NVP (nevirapine, Viramune)	200 mg		200 mg q d × 2 wk then 200 mg bid							XX										
DLV (delavirdine, Rescriptor)	100 mg			400 mg tid						X										
DMP (efavirenz, Sustiva)	200 mg	600 mg					X			X										
Protease Inhibitors																					
SQV (saquinavir, Fortovase)	200 mg			1200 mg tid with food				X											X	
RTV (ritonavir, Norvir)	100 mg refrigerated 80 mg/ml non-refrigerated		300 mg × 3 d, 400 mg × 4 d, 500 mg × 5 d, then 600 mg with food		XX			X							X				X	
IDV (indinavir, Crixivan)	400 mg			800 mg q 8 h Empty stomach, high fluid				X								X	X		X	
NFV (nelfinavir, Viracept)	250 mg			750 mg tid with food				XX											X	

*Investigational drug in the United States.

Reminders for dosing or association with routine daily events (brushing teeth, meals)

Medication sets, portable pill containers, emergency supplies

Planning for irregularities in the routine schedule—weekends, vacations, holidays

Special attention should be paid to mothers responsible for children (infected or not), midday doses for those working out of the home, shift workers, and changes brought upon by intercurrent illness.

Situational factors include financial status, transportation and living situations, and reliable medication refill systems.

Therapeutic Monitoring

Reductions in HIV-1 titers of greater than 1 $\log_{10}$ and a concomitant rise in $CD4^+$ counts determine effective therapy. First measurements are usually made 2 to 4 weeks after the initiation of treatment. Titers may continue to decline for a number of months before reaching maximal suppression. The long-term durability of a regimen is likely dependent upon reaching levels at least as low as 100 copies per mL ($\log_{10}$ 2) as measured by ultrasensitive quantitation. This should be achievable in about 80% of patients naive to prior therapy, more so in those with titers less than 20,000 copies per mL ($\log_{10}$ 4.3). If achieved, follow-up monitoring is done every 3 to 4 months. Any difficulties with adherence to a regimen should be ascertained and remedied.

Treatment Failure

Failure of a treatment regimen can be defined virologically as the existence of mutations or the stepwise acquisition of mutations resulting in HIV-1 drug resistance. This occurs when there is continued replication and evolution of the virus toward drug resistance under selective drug pressure. Viral titers will be inadequately suppressed and subsequently rise. Treatment failure can also be defined as the inability of a patient to adhere to a treatment regimen or intolerance of side effects or toxicities. Clinically this is seen as

Inadequate initial suppression of HIV-1

Confirmed trend of rising HIV-1 titers after initial suppression

Failure of $CD4^+$ cell response or loss of initial treatment gains

Clinical deterioration

Patient nonadherence or intolerable side effects or toxicities

Inability to achieve a $\log_{10}$ reduction in viral titers by 4 weeks or the inability to suppress viral titers to undetectable levels within 4 to 6 months signals failure of a regimen. Patients beginning with very high HIV-1 titers ($>10^5$ copies per mL), those with advanced disease, or those having had prior treatment and failure of antiretroviral therapy may be unable to achieve fully suppressed levels of HIV-1. The goal in this situation is to maximally suppress for as long as possible. A trend in HIV-1 titers rising from the nadir value under a treatment regimen signals the acquisition of drug resistance. This should take into account the variation in the precision of the HIV-1 viral titer testing, which can vary by threefold (0.5 $\log_{10}$). Repeated HIV-1 titer measurements may be required. Uncommonly, in spite of adequate suppression of HIV-1, a patient's $CD4^+$ gains may be lost or counts decline. Although controversial, an alternative regimen might be considered. Remediable causes for clinical deterioration (e.g., OIs) should be considered before an otherwise effective regimen is abandoned as failing.

Secondary Treatment

During treatment, any residual viral titer represents either the ongoing replication of resistant populations or production of virus from long-lived latently infected cells. If allowed to continue, replication results in a stepwise acquisition of the mutations within target viral enzymes and proteins until high-level resistance is achieved. Because of overlap in the mutations conferring viral drug resistance, prolonged administration of a failing antiretroviral regimen may result in viral resistance across a drug class. Remaining on a failing antiretroviral combination may threaten the durability of future regimens.

The addition or change of a single drug in a virologically failing combination regimen is tantamount to exposure of the residual HIV-1 to monotherapy. As with naive monotherapy, this will likely be of short-lived benefit to the patient, as resistance to the single new agent will arise quickly. When changes are necessary, residual HIV-1 should be treated with a regimen that contains at least two new antiretrovirals with a novel resistance profile. Preferably, the entire regimen is replaced. This proscribes the use of previously failed drugs and drugs of highly overlapping resistance profiles. The singular exception to this is the ability to reuse AZT if not previously combined with 3TC. The mutations associated with 3TC resistance re-establish sensitivity to AZT. In this setting, the combination of 3TC and AZT could be viewed as a "single" new RTI. If a patient is able to adequately suppress viral replication but cannot tolerate or fully adhere to a regimen, replacement of only the offending antiretroviral drugs is acceptable.

As a result of shared resistance profiles, PI-containing regimens following other failing PI-utilizing combinations perform poorly. This is accentuated if the failure continues for a prolonged period of time or leads to high viral titers. "All out" initial regimens, which might be used in advanced cases, leave little for secondary regimens. The use of regimens that are highly preferred by patients, which is important for adherence, may leave only poorly tolerated combinations as alternatives. Two novel reverse transcriptase inhibitors (RTI, NNRTI) should be reserved for the first protease inhibitor–containing regimen. The use of the RTI, the ABC, or the NNRTI, DMP in combination with the two RTIs (AZT plus 3TC) may hold promise as both potent and reserving of the PI class of antiretrovirals. Currently, these combinations have been shown to be effective in treatment of naïve patients from 16 to 24 weeks, respectively. Regimens designed beyond secondary levels are generally limited in capacity, for few novel antiretroviral drugs may remain. The current status of genotypic or phenotypic analysis for HIV-1 resistance to antiretrovirals is in evolution, and no firm recommendations have been developed.

Opportunistic Infections

With declining numbers of circulating $CD4^+$ cells, the immunologic protection of patients passes down through succeeding layers of risk for specific OIs. At relatively normal $CD4^+$ levels, the conditions seen are the same as those that affect the immunocompetent population but with greater frequency or severity. If immunologic deterioration continues, OIs characteristic of AIDS become evident, and in an accumulation of risk, patients with very low $CD4^+$ counts are at risk for a large number of OIs.

Although $CD4^+$ cell counts rise with treatment of HIV-1 and antiretroviral treatment has been shown to reduce the incidence of OIs, the immunologic competence achieved is not equivalent to the $CD4^+$ cell count attained. Because of this, the historic nadir $CD4^+$ cell count establishes the subsequent risk level for OIs. Prophylactic regimens are available for many OIs, with those for *P. carinii* pneumonia and *Mycobacterium avium* complex improving survival.

Although there is a large list of HIV-1–associated OIs, those of greatest clinical importance are *P. carinii* pneumonia, tuberculosis, cryptococcal meningitis, toxoplasmosis encephalitis, herpesvirus infections, mucosal candidiasis, and disseminated *Mycobacterium avium* complex. Other OIs are less common or will surrender to commonly utilized pathways of investigation and diagnosis.

Pneumocystis carinii *Pneumonia (PCP)*

The risk for PCP begins when $CD4^+$ cell counts fall to 200 cells per mL. Prophylactic antibiotics are indicated at this level. Patients with unexplained fevers of 100.2°F or with thrush should also receive prophylaxis. Trimethoprim-sulfamethoxazole (Septra, Bactrim), one double-strength tablet daily, is highly protective and provides prophylaxis against toxoplasmosis and bacterial infections. Adverse reactions to this prophylaxis can occur 7 to 14 days after institution with rash, nausea, and fevers. Severe reactions require discontinuing the drug—mild reactions may pass. A single-strength tablet daily may suffice with fewer side effects. Every effort, including desensitization, should be made to institute this medication. Alternative prophylactic regimens are dapsone*, 100 mg daily; dapsone, 50 mg daily, plus pyrimethamine* (Daraprim), 50 mg daily, plus leucovorin, 25 mg daily; aerosolized pentamidine (Pentam), 300 mg monthly administered via Respirgard II nebulizer; or atovaquone* (Mepron), 750 mg twice a day (bid) orally (PO). As a nonpyogenic interstitial pneumonia, PCP presents with fever, night sweats, and dyspnea on exertion progressing to shortness of breath at rest. Spasms of nonproductive cough are triggered by deep inspiration. On examination, respiration is restricted but is usually clear to auscultation. The chest film shows symmetrical interstitial infiltrates of varying amounts, depending on the degree of illness at presentation. Po_2 and oxygen saturation can be decreased or be shown to decrease with exercise. Without antecedent prophylaxis, induced sputum may show cyst forms. Direct fluorescent antibody staining is more sensitive. Prior prophylaxis alters the presentation and reduces the sensitivity of laboratory tests. Specimens obtained by bronchoalveolar lavage are 85 to 95% sensitive. Rarely, transbronchial biopsy may be required for definitive diagnosis. Treatment can be given empirically when the diagnosis is evident; however, in questionable cases definitive diagnosis is preferred. Treatment is curative and is followed by indefinite prophylaxis.

*Not FDA approved for this indication.

Treatment regimens for acute PCP (21-day regimens) include

Trimethoprim-sulfamethoxazole, 15 mg/kg per day divided every 8 hours IV until improvement then PO

Pentamidine, 3 to 4 mg per kg daily IV

Clindamycin (Cleocin), 600 mg IV or PO three times daily (tid) plus primaquine 30 mg as base PO daily

Dapsone, 50 mg bid, plus either trimethoprim, 15 mg per kg per day divided 3 to 4 times daily, or pyrimethamine, 50 to 75 mg daily PO

Trimetrexate (Neutrexin), 45 mg per m^2 plus dapsone, 50 mg bid, plus leucovorin, 24 days at 20 mg per m^2

Atovaquone suspension, 750 mg PO bid, plus pyrimethamine, 50 to 75 mg daily

Adjunctive corticosteroids added for Po_2 less than 70 mm Hg beginning at 40 mg prednisone or methylprednisolone (Solu-Medrol) and tapering over 2 weeks to reduce the risk of respiratory failure

Tuberculosis

Most active tuberculosis (TB) in patients with HIV-1 infection is a result of reactivation, although the risk of development of acute TB after exposure is high. The risk for reactivation of TB in persons with HIV-1 infection is 7% per year. PPD testing should be done at baseline and yearly. Anergy testing is not necessary. A 5-mm induration skin test or a history of untreated prior positive skin test or contact with a case of active TB are indications for prophylaxis regardless of age. Isoniazid, 300 mg daily, plus pyridoxine, 50 mg daily for 1 year, is the preferred prophylactic regimen. Isoniazid, 900 mg, plus pyridoxine, 50 mg, both twice weekly for 1 year is an alternative prophylactic regimen. Knowledge of local and population-based TB epidemiology in conjunc-

*Not FDA approved for this indication.

tion with HIV-1 infection is important in the consideration of the possibility of any pulmonary infiltrate being TB. Pulmonary TB presents with cough and fever but with greater immune suppression the presentation is atypical with constitutional symptoms predominating and extrapulmonary disease common. Chest films are variable with less cavitary and miliary disease. Mediastinal adenopathy, upper lobe disease, and pleural effusions as well as normal chest radiographs are seen. Extrapulmonary disease alone or with pulmonary infection occurs in 70% of cases with a bias toward advanced HIV disease. Blood, extrathoracic lymph nodes, and the genitourinary system are sites of infection and isolation of TB. Tuberculous meningitis presents with fever, headache and altered mental status and other signs of infection. In contrast to cryptococcal disease, cerebral spinal fluid (CSF) pleocytosis is common. Radiometric isolation (Bactec) with DNA probes allows for faster isolation and identification of TB. Drug sensitivities should be determined for all isolates. Unless local patterns of resistance dictate otherwise, initial treatment of active TB combines isoniazid, 300 mg daily PO, plus rifampin (Rifadin), 600 mg daily PO, plus pyrazinamide 15 to 30 mg daily PO (2 grams daily maximum), plus either ethambutol (Myambutol), 15 mg per kg daily PO, or streptomycin, 15 mg per kg intramuscularly (IM) daily (1 gram daily maximum) given for 2 months. This is followed by isoniazid plus rifampin alone for a minimum of 6 months beyond culture conversion and depending on sensitivities. Because of pharmcokinetic interactions between rifabutin and protease inhibitors, concomitant treatment of active TB and HIV-1 should be done with consultation. Strict adherence is necessary to avoid the development of resistant and multidrug-resistant disease.

Cryptococcal Meningitis

The risk for cryptococcal disease, which typically presents as meningitis, begins when the $CD4^+$ cell count fails to about 100 cells per mL. Prophylaxis with azole antifungals is effective, but the overall incidence of cryptococcal meningitis in the AIDS population is low, making this unnecessary. Baseline or screening serum cryptococcal antigen testing is not useful. Persistent headache with accompanying fever calls for a lumbar puncture. Meningeal signs are frequently absent. Combined CSF examination by India ink, cryptococcal antigen, and fungal cultures is highly sensitive. Cell counts and protein are commonly only slightly elevated. Elevated opening pressure, particularly if accompanied by altered mental status, is a poor prognostic sign and may require decompression by CSF removal. Serum cryptococcal antigen is also often positive, but this should not substitute for CSF sampling.

Preferred initial treatment is with intravenous amphotericin B (Fungizone), 0.3 to 1.25 mg per kg daily IV, or liposomal amphotericin B (Abelcet, AmBisome) which is further enhanced by the addition of flucytosine (Ancobon), 100 to 150 mg per kg per day in a divided dose. After 2 weeks of treatment, or after clear signs of clinical improvement, long-term suppressive treatment with fluconazole (Diflucan), 200 to 400 mg daily PO, is necessary to prevent relapse.

Toxoplasmosis Encephalitis

The risk for reactivation of *Toxoplasma gondii* infection, presenting as encephalitis, begins when the $CD4^+$ count is below 100 cells per mL. Those at greatest risk are positive for toxoplasmosis IgG antibodies. Trimethoprim-sulfamethoxazole provides prophylaxis for both PCP and toxoplasmosis. Alternatively, dapsone, 50 mg daily, plus pyrimethamine, 50 mg weekly, plus leucovorin, 25 mg weekly, will provide prophylaxis. Reactivation occurs as multiple focal brain lesions. Presentation is dependent upon location, with focal neurologic deficits, altered mental status, and fever. Diagnostic imaging can be done with CT or the more sensitive MRI. Characteristic multiple ring enhanced lesions are sufficient for a diagnostic/therapeutic trial of treatment. The primary differential diagnostic considerations include lymphoma and progressive multifocal leukoencephalopathy. Steroids hasten recovery by reducing brain edema but their use may lead to diagnostic confusion, as CNS lymphomas will also improve under their influence. Patients failing to show of signs of improvement after 7 to 9 days of treatment may require brain biopsy for definitive diagnosis. Initial treatment consists of the combination of pyrimethamine 200 mg loading followed by 100 mg daily, and sulfadiazine, 4 grams daily divided, plus leucovorin 10 to 20 mg daily. Alternatively, the same dose of pyrimethamine can be combined with clindamycin, 600 mg four times daily IV or PO. The dose of pyrimethamine is reduced to 25 to 50 mg daily for long-term suppression.

Herpesvirus Infection

Herpes Zoster. Herpes zoster is a common early manifestation of HIV-1–related immunologic damage. Education for early recognition by patients leads to prompt antiherpetic treatment and reduction in morbidity.

Herpes Simplex Virus Infection. Herpes simplex labialis or genitalis recurs with greater frequency, lasts longer, and is more severe than in immunologically competent persons. Untreated, large erosive ulcerations can occur and extension of genital herpes into the rectum can result in debilitating proctitis. Genital herpes may increase the sexual transmission of HIV-1. Episodic or suppressive therapy with acyclovir (Zovirax), 400 mg twice daily, is effective. With repeated exposure to acyclovir, there is a small risk for the development of resistant HSV requiring more intensive or alternative drug treatment.

Cytomegalovirus Infection. Cytomegalovirus (CMV) infections reactivate at $CD4^+$ cell counts below 100 cells per mL. Patients with CMV retinitis complain of fixed, progressive visual disturbances accompanied at times by floaters. An ophthalmoscopic examination may visualize the retinal-based "cottage cheese and ketchup" hemorrhages and infarctions; however, with peripheral lesions an ophthalmologic examination may be necessary. Prophylactic medication to prevent CMV opportunistic infection is available (ganciclovir [Cytovene]), but the toxicity, effectiveness, and limited ability to determine those at greatest risk for CMV infection makes prophylaxis of CMV of limited benefit. CMV ulcers in the gastrointestinal tract from the oropharynx to the colon cause localizable pain particularly in the esophagus, stomach, and fixed portions of the colon. CMV colitis of the cecum can be mistaken for appendicitis (or vice versa). CMV in body fluids turns all cultures positive, so a biopsy of involved gastrointestinal mucosa is necessary for histologic diagnosis.

Initial treatment consists of either ganciclovir or foscarnet (Foscavir) given intravenously. Ganciclovir can cause anemia and neutropenia. Absolute neutrophil counts (ANC) down to 500 cells per mL are protective. Filgrastim can be used to increase the ANC. Foscarnet can be nephrotoxic, and adjustment for serum creatinine or estimated glomerular filtration rate is necessary. For retinal disease, a ganciclovir ocular implant (Vitrasert) supplies high-concentration localized treatment but does not provide protection for other sites. After initial suppression of CMV activity, long-term suppressive treatment with oral ganciclovir, 1 gram three times daily, provides a less effective alternative to maintenance doses of ganciclovir or foscarnet. Oral ganciclovir is commonly used to provide systemic coverage in combination with intraocular ganciclovir implants. In cases of CMV resistant to single-drug therapy the combination of ganciclovir with foscarnet can be used. Cidofovir can be used for resistant CMV and other herpesvirus infections. Its high potential for nephrotoxicity requires the concomitant use of probenecid and hydration along with careful monitoring of renal function. Its infrequent dosing (every 2 weeks,) may obviate the need for permanent vascular access.

Mucosal Candidiasis

Candidal vaginitis is common at high $CD4^+$ cell counts. Oropharyngeal candidiasis (thrush) occurs with a $CD4^+$ cell count of about 400 cells per mL. Esophageal candidiasis develops at a $CD4^+$ count below 200 cells per mL. Because infection is generally uncomplicated and therapy straightforward, prophylaxis is optional. Recognizable mucosal white patches of vaginal and oropharyngeal candidiasis may make confirmatory testing by KOH preparation or culture unnecessary for diagnosis. Mild cases can be treated topically with nystatin, clotrimazole troches (Mycelex), oral amphotericin B concentrate (Fungizone), or itraconazole suspension (Sporanox); persistent or severe cases are treated with the systemic azole antifungals ketoconazole (Nizoral), fluconazole (Diflucan), or itraconazole. In the presence of oropharyngeal candidiasis and odynophagia at low $CD4^+$ cell counts, a diagnostic-therapeutic trial of systemic azole antifungals for the candidal esophagitis is warranted. Failure of clinical mucosal clearing or improvement may be due to infection with another yeast, and culture or esophagoscopy for further treatment guidance may be necessary. The need for suppressive therapy is made on a case-by-case basis.

Disseminated Mycobacterium avium *Complex (MAC)*

MAC is the most common cause of fever without source in a patient with a $CD4^+$ cell count of less than 50 cells per mL (others include subtle PCP, lymphoma, and drug fever). Night sweats, weight loss, anemia with an elevated band count, and elevation of liver-associated alkaline phosphatase diarrhea can accompany the fever. In the presence of protease inhibitor therapy, abdominal MAC adenitis occurs. Prophylaxis is recommended with a historic nadir $CD4^+$ count of 50 cells per mL or lower. Clarithromycin (Biaxin), 500 mg twice daily, or azithromycin (Zithromax), 1200 mg once weekly, has been shown to decrease the incidence of MAC. Rifabutin (Mycobutin), 300 mg daily PO, is effective but deleteriously interacts with protease inhibitors. IDV or NFV can be used with rifabutin at 150 mg daily. High blood levels of rifabutin are associated with uveitis. Active TB should be ruled out prior to the use of rifabutin. Diagnosis of MAC is most commonly made by isolation from the blood using specific media for acid-fast bacteria. MAC is detected faster with isotope-labeled media techniques (Bactec). Diagnosis can also be made by identification and culture from bone marrow, liver, lymph nodes, and intestinal mucosa. Life-prolonging treatment requires multiple antibiotics for an indefinite period. Azithromycin, 250 mg once or twice daily, or clarithromycin, 500 mg twice daily, is combined with ethambutol, 15 mg per kg daily. Ciprofloxacin (Cipro), 500 mg twice daily, may increase effectiveness. Amikacin, 10 mg per kg daily IV, is given in 2-week courses to reduce the initial burden of MAC or in cases of relapse. Dose-related nephrotoxicity and ototoxicity can occur.

HIV-1–Related Neoplasms

Of the numerous candidates for association with HIV-1 infection, the three most clinically relevant are Kaposi's sarcoma (KS), non-Hodgkin's B-cell lymphoma, and invasive cervical cancer. A rarely seen tumor prior to the HIV-1 epidemic, KS was one of the vanguard opportunistic processes bringing attention to the epidemic in 1981, constituting 50% of initial AIDS diagnoses. In subsequent years, the incidence has fallen dramatically. Because KS occurs primarily in gay men with HIV-1 infection, there is suspicion of a sexually transmitted cofactor. A likely candidate is human herpesvirus 8 (HHV-8), also referred to as Kaposi's Sarcoma–associated herpesvirus (KSHV). Controversy abounds about whether HHV-8 is necessary but not sufficient to cause KS or is in itself a transforming virus capable of causing KS.

KS presents as indurated, nonblanching pink to violaceous cutaneous nodules from 0.5 to 2 cm in diameter. Lesions are commonly distributed along

Langer's lines with a predilection for the inner aspects of the arms, thighs, and shins where they may coalesce into large plaques. The tip of the nose and penis and the palate are also commonly involved. Diagnosis is clinical to the experienced eye but biopsy will yield a definitive diagnosis and differentiate KS from the similar appearing bacillary angiomatosis caused by the opportunistic pathogen *Bartonella henselae*.

Untreated, the course is variable: the disease is indolent in some, but in others there is a rapid increase in the size and number of lesions. Large plaques, particularly of the lower extremities, cause distal edema. Confluent involvement of the feet can be debilitating and painful. Extensive facial involvement can result in social isolation for the patient. Visceral involvement is common but rarely causes symptoms. The exception is pulmonary KS, which can progress to the point of life-threatening respiratory failure. Pulmonary KS rarely occurs in isolation. Chest films shows variable patchy involvement and there may be pleural effusions, uncommon in PCP. Gallium scans are negative in pulmonary KS, and CT scans may show spread along bronchial pathways. Lesions can be seen at bronchoscopy but transbronchial biopsy rarely obtains diagnostic tissue.

Protease inhibitor–containing antiretroviral regimens have resulted in regression of KS. Apart from this, the decision to treat is based upon patient preference, rapidity of spread, pain, obstruction, peripheral edema, and cosmesis. Pulmonary KS should be treated to prevent respiratory complications. Therapy can be local, using cryotherapy, radiation, intralesional vinblastine [Velban], or systemic, employing regimens containing various combinations of vincristine [Oncovin], vinblastine [Velban], bleomycin [Blenoxane], doxorubicin [Adriamycin, Doxil], daunorubicin (DaunoXome), interferon alfa (Intron A, Roferon-A), etoposide (VePesid), or paclitaxel (Taxol).

Non-Hodgkin's B cell lymphomas (NHL) occur at a rate of about 1 to 2% per year in patients with advanced HIV-1 disease. The incidence may rise as survival is prolonged with antiretroviral treatment. Factors in the development of NHL are not fully elucidated, but Epstein-Barr virus is implicated as a potential causative agent. Non-CNS, peripheral NHL occurs at relatively high $CD4^+$ cell counts (~200 cells per mL), whereas CNS lymphoma is usually seen with $CD4^+$ cell counts below 50 cells per mL. Extranodal presentation of HIV-1–related NHL is common, with involvement of the marrow, and the CNS and the GI tract seen most often. NHL isolated to the CNS varies in presentation with its location. Confusion, lethargy, and personality changes along with focal neurologic signs or seizures can be presenting symptoms. Solitary contrast-enhanced lesions on brain imaging are more likely NHL than toxoplasmosis but solitary toxoplasmosis lesions are not rare. Conversely, CNS NHL is multiple in half the cases. In patients with positive toxoplasmosis serology, a diagnostic-therapeutic trial of toxoplasmosis treatment may be given, looking for improvement within a week. The use of steroids to reduce cerebral edema will result in improvement in either disease, a possible point of confusion. For definitive diagnosis, brain biopsy is necessary. Treatment response rates range from 21 to 64% and vary by morphologic cell type. Median survival times range from 4 to 7 months with predictors of poor survival being $CD4^+$ cell count below 100 cells per mL, Karnofsky score below 70, extranodal disease, and prior diagnosis of AIDS. Treatment regimens consist of variations of CHOP, m-BACOD, or the aggressive ACVB. The effect of current antiretroviral therapy on survival with NHL has not been determined.

The incidence of HPV infection and progressive cervical cytologic abnormalities is high in women with HIV-1 infection. Rates of invasive cervical cancer have not risen but this may be an artifact of aggressive screening and treatment, premature death due to other HIV-1–related causes, or cervical cancer cases not recognized as HIV-1 related. False-negative rates of Pap smears become more important in populations of women with high cervical cytologic abnormality rates. At a minimum there should be two initial normal Pap smears at 6 months, followed by annual examinations thereafter. Treatment of cervical disease is less successful than in HIV-1 negative women, and close follow-up is important.

Neurologic Disorders

Neurologic disorders due to HIV-1 itself, opportunistic processes, or medications occur in most cases of progressive HIV-1 infection. Cerebral opportunistic processes of highest concern are toxoplasmosis encephalitis, non-Hodgkin's lymphoma (NHL) (described elsewhere), and progressive multifocal leukoencephalopathy (PML). Central neurologic conditions due to HIV-1 itself are HIV-1–associated minor cognitive/motor disorder (MCMD) and HIV-associated dementia. PML is an OI caused by the human papovavirus. Pathologically, there is demyelination of subcortical white matter without surrounding mass effect. Patients present with focal neurologic deficits. CT or MRI is suggestive but brain biopsy may be necessary for definite diagnosis. The course is one of rapid deterioration. No successful treatments have been developed, although anecdotal regression has been seen with successful antiretroviral therapy.

HIV-1–associated minor cognitive/motor disorder occurs in up to 30% of patients and is more common in advanced HIV-1 infection. Neurologic deficits are minor in nature and reflect minimal neuronal dysfunction. Forgetfulness, inattentiveness, and decreased concentration not disruptive to daily activity or work characterize this disorder. Only some will progress to frank dementia, but prognostic factors are lacking. Treatment is aimed at HIV-1, with consideration given to the CSF penetration of the antiretrovirals used. However saquinavir, which poorly penetrates into the CSF, has been effective in reducing HIV-1 RNA in the CSF. HIV-associated dementia has an incidence of 15 to 20% and occurs in the setting of advanced HIV-1 infection. The most common complaint is of memory impairment, followed by gait impairment, mental slowing, and depressive symptoms. There can be also slowing of limb movement, hyperreflexia, hypertonia, and frontal release signs. These symptoms are more disabling than those seen in MCMD. On CSF examination, beta$_2$-microglobulin may be elevated. MRI shows cerebral atrophy and abnormal white matter signals. Other causes of these symptoms should be ruled out, including depression, drug use, and CNS OIs. AZT has reduced the incidence of this dementia in patients with advanced HIV-1 infection. The efficacy of current potent antiretroviral medications has yet to be evaluated, but their use is advisable.

Of the peripheral neuropathies seen in HIV-1 infection, distal symmetrical neuropathy is the most common. Pathologically a reduction in epidermal nerve fibers is seen. Although HIV-1 is directly implicated as the cause, medications (DDI, DDC, D4T, D4T plus DDC, INH, vincristine, dapsone) can also cause or worsen the condition. Patients complain of pain, tingling, or numbness in the ball of the foot, the toes, and the heel. Symptoms, which are worst in the morning and evening, move proximally, and in advanced cases can interfere with gait and balance and can involve the hands. Treatment is aimed at HIV-1 with care taken to avoid medications that can cause the disorder. Symptomatic treatment includes low-dose tricyclic antidepressants, phenytoin, analgesics, acupuncture, massage, and comfort measures.

AIDS-Related Weight Loss

Weight loss is common at all stages of HIV-1 infection. Low levels of albumin, cholesterol, and transferrin are correlated with decreased survival. Death occurs when a total weight loss of 66% or lean body mass loss of 54% is reached. Weight loss can be caused by inadequate nutrition, malabsorption, opportunistic processes, and HIV-1 infection itself. Nutrition can be affected by cognitive impairment, neurologic dysfunction, painful gastrointestinal conditions (aphthous or CMV ulcers, esophageal candidiasis), or nausea or anorexia caused by illness or medications. Malabsorption can be due to exocrine dysfunction, intestinal infection, or parasitosis (cryptosporidiosis, microsporidiosis) and HIV-1 enteropathy. Opportunistic infections induce both a hypermetabolic state and decreased caloric intake due to anorexia and cause rapid weight loss. HIV wasting, exclusive of the aforementioned causes of weight loss, occurs with altered metabolism and abnormal adaptive mechanisms due to cytokine dysfunction and results in a loss of lean body mass in excess of adipose tissue. Hypogonadism can be contributory. The treatment of weight loss is aimed at underlying causes. Diagnosis and treatment of OIs and neoplasms, intestinal causes of malabsorption, and manipulation of medications to reduce anorexia and nausea are therapeutic. Antinausea agents and appetite stimulants such as megestrol* (Megace) or dronabinol* (Marinol) are helpful. Lean body mass loss due to testosterone deficiency responds to anabolic replacement through injection (testosterone, nandrolone [Deca-Durabolin]), oral oxandrolone (Oxandrin), or cutaneous patch application (Testoderm, Androderm). Effective treatment of HIV-1 infection reverses HIV wasting. Protease inhibitors have been associated with lipid dysregulation and adipose deposits in the abdomen and across the shoulders. If treatment of HIV-1 infection is not adequate to reverse wasting, recombinant growth hormone (Somatropin [Serostim]) is effective at increasing lean body mass; however, the cost may be prohibitive. Anabolic steroids have been used for this indication.

*Not FDA approved for this indication.

AMEBIASIS

method of
JONATHAN I. RAVDIN, M.D.
University of Minnesota Medical School
Minneapolis, Minnesota

Amebiasis is a human disease due to the enteric protozoan *Entamoeba histolytica*. There are two morphologically identical *Entamoeba* species that infect humans, the noninvasive *Entamoeba dispar* and *E. histolytica*. Together they infect 10% of the world's population; approximately 1 in 10 of those infected harbors *E. histolytica*. *E. dispar* has never been associated with invasive colitis or liver abscess; intestinal infection clears spontaneously without treatment in 8 to 12 months. Apparently, all individuals with *E. histolytica* infection mount a serum antibody response, yet only 1 in 10 goes on to develop systemic invasive amebiasis. It is unknown whether clearance of *Entamoeba* infection, spontaneously or by chemotherapy, results in any degree of host immunity to prevent reinfection.

EPIDEMIOLOGY

It is important for clinicians to identify individuals at greater risk for infection and patients who are more likely to suffer severe invasive disease when they are infected. The infective dose can be as little as a single cyst, although a higher inoculum results in a shorter incubation period (1 to 3 days). High-risk groups for acquisition of infection include travelers to or immigrants from highly endemic areas (such as Mexico, India, Bangladesh, South Africa, and South America), sexually promiscuous individuals who engage in oral-anal or anal-genital-oral sex, chronically institutionalized populations (especially the mentally challenged), and Mexican Americans in the southwestern United States. Individuals who become at risk for fulminant amebiasis once they are infected include pregnant women, the malnourished, the very young (<1 year), and patients receiving corticosteroid therapy. Whether infection with human immunodeficiency virus results in increased frequency or severity of invasive amebiasis remains unclear.

CLINICAL SYNDROMES

The main clinical syndromes that result from *E. histolytica* infection include asymptomatic intestinal infection, acute amebic rectocolitis, chronic intestinal amebiasis, and amebic liver abscess. Infections of the peritoneum, lung, and pericardium are unusual manifestations resulting from extension of an amebic liver abscess or colonic perforation. Lung or brain abscesses are rare presentations resulting from hematogenous dissemination. In general, 60 to 90% of individuals with asymptomatic intestinal infection harbor *E. dispar*. Such patients are detected by routine or incidental stool examination. *E. dispar* infection does not elicit a serum antiamebic antibody response. Positive stool microscopy and serologic test results for antiamebic antibodies suggest infection with *E. histolytica*.

Acute amebic rectocolitis is characterized by bloody mucus in stools, tenesmus, and abdominal pain, with the onset of symptoms occurring in 7 to 10 days rather than more acutely. Only one third of patients are febrile; virtually all have stools positive for occult blood. Fulminant colitis is characterized by colonic dilatation, toxemia, and peritonitis (often with associated perforation). Chronic intestinal amebiasis is clinically identical to idiopathic inflammatory bowel disease. The disease can last for years, is intermittent in nature, and is characterized by abdominal pain with bloody diarrhea. The mistaken treatment of such patients with corticosteroids can result in fulminant disease. Ameboma, another form of chronic intestinal amebiasis, manifests as a focal colonic mass, usually in the right colon, and is often mistaken clinically for colonic carcinoma. Amebic liver abscess, which manifests acutely with right upper quadrant pain and fever, is indistinguishable from infection of the biliary tract. Patients with a more chronic infection have abdominal pain and weight loss. A minority are febrile, and many are initially misdiagnosed as having primary or metastatic liver cancer. Amebic liver abscess can be differentiated from pyogenic infection by its occurrence at any age, its association with specific epidemiologic risk factors, the finding of *E. histolytica* in the stool (20 to 60%), and the presence of serum antigen and antiamebic antibodies.

DIAGNOSIS

Diagnosis of intestinal infection still rests on expert microscopy of fecal samples. However, errors are frequent, and multiple stool samples are required. The finding of hematophagous (presence of ingested erythrocytes) trophozoites by microscopy is highly specific for amebic colitis. Antigen detection tests using enzyme-linked immunosorbent assays demonstrate *E. histolytica* antigen in serum and feces of patients with amebic liver abscess and colitis; a commercial assay for fecal testing is available from TechLab (Blacksburg, VA).

Serologic testing is extremely helpful in the diagnosis of invasive amebiasis or asymptomatic *E. histolytica* infection. Ninety percent of patients with invasive amebiasis are seropositive by the seventh day of illness. Asymptomatic patients harboring *E. histolytica* are also seropositive. In nonendemic areas, serologic testing is a cost-effective way to differentiate inflammatory bowel disease from chronic intestinal amebiasis. After the treatment of invasive amebiasis by most methods, patients remain seropositive for years, which is why up to 25% of noninfected control subjects in endemic areas have serum antiamebic antibodies. However, a negative test result does reduce the likelihood of invasive amebiasis.

Colonoscopy with scrapings or biopsy of the ulcer edge is the gold standard for diagnosis and is especially helpful in acute colitis or to rule out amebiasis before treatment of presumed inflammatory bowel disease with corticosteroids. A periodic acid–Schiff stain, which highlights trophozoites in tissues, should always be requested. Not only are barium studies not useful in diagnosis, but they also prevent any yield in stool examinations for ova and parasites for 1 to 2 weeks. Because it differentiates biliary tract disease from a primary liver process, abdominal ultrasonography is the most important study in evaluation of patients with right upper quadrant pain and fever. Amebic liver abscesses commonly appear as multiple nonhomogeneous defects by modern imaging techniques, especially in acute disease of less than 10 days' duration. Computed tomography (CT) and magnetic resonance imaging add little in evaluation at increased cost and radiation exposure. Amebic liver abscess cannot be differentiated from necrotic hepatoma or pyogenic abscess by imaging alone. The serologic results and the presence of epidemiologic risk factors are usually sufficient to establish the diagnosis. Well above 90% of patients will be seropositive after 7 days of symptomatic illness. If necessary, fine-needle aspiration under CT guidance can be used to rule out pyogenic disease, but this approach is rarely required for making an accurate diagnosis. Amebic liver abscesses contain proteinaceous fluid (not pus), and trophozoites are usually not found because they are in the tissues at the periphery of the lesion.

TREATMENT

Treatment of amebiasis is complicated by the need to use multiple agents and the lack of familiarity of physicians with an appropriate therapeutic response.

Pharmacology of Antiamebic Agents

The drugs recommended for use in treatment of amebiasis are listed in Table 1. Luminal agents include diloxanide furoate, paromomycin, and diiodo-

TABLE 1. **Drugs Recommended for Treatment of Amebiasis by Site of Action**

Drug	Advantages and Disadvantages
Luminal amebicides	
Diloxanide furoate (Furamide)	Low toxicity; high efficacy; available only from CDC
Paromomycin (Humatin)	Nonabsorbable; useful in pregnancy
Diiodohydroxyquin (Diiodoquin, Yodoxin)	20-d course required; potential optic toxicity
Useful in intestinal disease only	
Tetracyclines	Must combine with luminal agent against liver abscess
Erythromycin	
Active in all tissues	
Metronidazole (Flagyl)	Effective; in vitro resistance not described; frequent nausea and vomiting
Tinidazole (Simplotan)	Antabuse effect with ethanol
	Combine with luminal agent

Abbreviation: CDC = Centers for Disease Control and Prevention.

hydroxyquin. Diloxanide furoate* is highly efficacious (95% clearance of patients), relatively nontoxic, and clearly the drug of choice to eradicate *E. histolytica* from the intestinal lumen. However, it is not widely available except through the Drug Service at the Centers for Disease Control and Prevention in Atlanta, Georgia (telephone, 404–639–3670 during the daytime and 404–639–2888 in off-hours). Paromomycin, an oral aminoglycoside, is effective in clearing asymptomatic infection and is not absorbed in the setting of little or no inflammation. Therefore, this drug is especially helpful if one elects to treat asymptomatic infection in pregnant women. Paromomycin may cause mild gastrointestinal irritation or fungal overgrowth. Diiodohydroxyquin has been used extensively but requires high compliance to complete a 20-day course. Its accessibility is limited in the United States. This drug can cause optic atrophy, and I prefer to avoid its use for this reason. The tetracyclines and erythromycins have a long history of successful treatment of invasive intestinal disease; however, they are not nearly as active in vitro against trophozoites as metronidazole is and are ineffective in liver abscess. Therefore, these agents are usually used as second-line drugs in combination with a luminal agent to treat mild symptomatic amebic colitis. Given the risks of recurrent or chronic infection, I would reserve them for patients who experience neurotoxicity or otherwise cannot tolerate metronidazole. The nitroimidazoles are the mainstays of therapy for invasive amebiasis. They are directly amebicidal in vitro, penetrate well into all tissues, and have shown no parasite resistance to their amebicidal activity. However, gastrointestinal intolerance is common, and individuals must be cautioned to avoid ethanol due to a disulfiram (Antabuse) effect. These agents are metabolized in the liver, and high serum levels are associated with neurotoxicity, including seizures. However, most patients tolerate these drugs, and they have been used for years in the treatment of trichomoniasis. Carcinogenic risks suggested by in vitro mutagenesis studies have not been borne out by long-term follow-up (10 to 20 years); nevertheless, caution in the use of metronidazole should be exercised. Teratogenesis is a concern; however, uncontrolled studies suggested reasonable safety during the third trimester. Tinidazole* is better tolerated and highly efficacious but is not currently available in the United States.

Historically, emetines were used to treat invasive amebiasis. Although directly amebicidal, they are no longer recommended because of significant cardiovascular toxicity (hypotension, precordial chest pain, tachycardia). In addition, parenteral therapy with hospitalization is necessary, and neuromuscular toxicity is common. There are no studies that demonstrate that the addition of emetines to metronidazole improves the outcome in invasive amebiasis or is necessary in instances of initial treatment failure.

*Not available in the United States.

Asymptomatic Infection

This is an area of ongoing controversy. There is no evidence that infection with *E. dispar* represents a health risk to the index case or close contacts. However, long-term follow-up studies to assess symptoms and general health status have not been performed. The possibility of asymptomatic *E. histolytica* infection can be addressed by testing for serum antiamebic antibodies. A positive amebic serologic test result or detection of *E. histolytica*–specific antigen in feces is an indication for presumptive therapy, even in an endemic area. Treatment of asymptomatic infected patients who have negative results on Hemoccult and serologic testing should be individualized. In an endemic area, there are no indications for treating such individuals, but treatment is recommended when there is adequate sanitation and the risk for reinfection is low. This would prevent the spread of *E. dispar* infection and its subsequent confusion with *E. histolytica*. For seronegative individuals, treatment with a luminal agent (see Table 2 for regimens) is adequate. In asymptomatic seropositive individuals with no evidence of invasive disease, again a luminal agent is adequate. However, treatment of colitis is indicated if hematophagous trophozoites or occult blood is found in stool, even if the patient is asymptomatic. This may be the only circumstance in which the use of a tetracycline with a luminal agent seems a reasonable alternative to metronidazole.

Acute or Chronic Amebic Colitis

Metronidazole (see Table 2) is recommended for all invasive *E. histolytica* infections. Treatment with a luminal agent must follow, especially if shorter courses of metronidazole are used. It is unwise to use both agents simultaneously owing to gastrointestinal intolerance, but there is no direct contraindication if compliance is a major issue. Patients respond promptly to metronidazole therapy; there is no benefit from adding additional tissue amebicides. In patients with fulminant amebiasis, intestinal leakage and bacterial peritonitis may necessitate broader antibacterial therapy. Surgery is usually not indicated because it is difficult to handle colonic tissues and conservative management is more likely to be suc-

TABLE 2. **Therapeutic Regimens for Adults with Amebiasis**

Asymptomatic Infection
1. Diloxanide furoate, 500 mg PO tid for 10 d
2. Paromomycin, 10 mg/kg PO tid for 10 d
3. Diiodohydroxyquin, 650 mg PO tid for 20 d
Amebic Colitis
4. Metronidazole, 750 mg PO tid for 7 d followed by 1, 2, or 3
5. Doxycycline, 250 mg PO bid for 14 d followed by 1, 2, or 3
Invasive Liver Abscess
6. Metronidazole, 750 mg PO tid for 7–10 d, followed by 1, 2, or 3
7. Metronidazole, 2.4 gm PO once daily for 2 d, followed by 1, 2, or 3

cessful. The only (rare) exception is toxic megacolon, often a result of inadvertent corticosteroid therapy, which may require a total colectomy. Localized chronic amebiasis (ameboma) responds well to therapy with metronidazole.

It is imperative that successful clearance of infection be documented because relapses occur. At least two separate stool examinations or follow-up antigen detection tests should be performed after therapy to assess the patient's outcome. As mentioned, serum antiamebic antibody titers remain elevated for years and are not helpful in assessing the resolution of disease. In patients with persistent nonspecific abdominal complaints or underlying inflammatory bowel disease, post-treatment colonoscopy with biopsy is necessary to rule out relapse. In addition, occasional patients may experience the onset of an idiopathic colitis after treatment in which amebae cannot be demonstrated in biopsy samples of tissue. These patients do not respond to metronidazole, and standard therapy for inflammatory bowel disease is also usually not helpful. They are difficult to manage; however, their symptoms often resolve within a year after cure of the amebic infection. This syndrome is presumably an autoimmune phenomenon: circulating amebic antigen-antibody complexes have been identified during colonic amebiasis.

Amebic Liver Abscess

The overwhelming majority of patients with amebic liver abscess respond to therapy with metronidazole (see Table 2) with gradual defervescence, decreased pain, and improved appetite during a 3- to 5-day period. There is no need to add potentially toxic agents such as chloroquine or dehydroemetine. A lack of response to metronidazole indicates a need to reconsider the diagnosis and perform a fine-needle aspiration of the abscess under CT guidance. Patients with amebic liver abscess who respond promptly to aspiration should still receive a complete course of metronidazole therapy, and all patients should be treated with a luminal agent after completion of metronidazole therapy. Studies have suggested that intestinal colonization, leading to a recurrence of amebic liver abscess, is more frequent than previously recognized. Regardless of whether the stool examination was initially positive, a complete course of diloxanide furoate or paromomycin is essential.

Whether fine-needle aspiration of the liver abscess should be done immediately on presentation depends on the experience and skill of the physician and the resources of the local medical center. Although such aspiration is unnecessary in 90% of individuals, it is occasionally recommended. Examples include large abscesses with only a thin capsule of liver preventing rupture, a patient in extreme distress requiring rapid relief, and, last, a high likelihood that primary or secondary bacterial infection is present. Complications of amebic liver abscess such as peritonitis or lung involvement are best treated conservatively. However, an empyema or pericardial effusion must be drained. Amebic pericarditis is a fulminant disease that is often misdiagnosed; ultrasonography revealing a left lobe liver abscess suggests the diagnosis, and immediate action is necessary.

Once the patient responds, there is no need to monitor the hepatic lesion by expensive imaging studies. This creates undue anxiety and expense, because the lesion usually takes months to resolve. If the patient remains asymptomatic, there is no indication for therapy for a persistent defect, even 6 months after treatment. Only a recurrence of symptoms merits investigation.

GIARDIASIS

method of
JAMES J. CERDA, M.D.
University of Florida College of Medicine
Gainesville, Florida

As a challenge to diagnostic acumen and as a potential therapeutic triumph, the diagnosis and treatment of giardiasis is unexcelled in parasitology. *Giardia lamblia,* sometimes known as *Lamblia intestinalis*, is a flagellate, unicellular protozoan parasite inhabiting the upper small intestinal tract. *G. lamblia* is probably the most common cause of water-borne epidemic diarrheal disease in the United States. It is particularly common in day care centers; in travelers returning from Russia, Asia, and the Rocky Mountain states; and in any epidemic of gastroenteritis. Furthermore, *G. lamblia* infection is quite common in homosexual men who are both positive and negative for the human immunodeficiency virus, in whom it is presumed to be transmitted by anal receptive intercourse.

EPIDEMIOLOGY AND PATHOGENESIS

Giardia exists in two stages: trophozoite and cyst. The former inhabits the upper small intestine and appears to attach to the intestinal epithelium, where the parasites are shed every 48 to 72 hours in consonance with the intestinal cell cycle.

Although the exact mechanism of transmission is not clear, ingestion of surface water that has not been filtered effectively is a major mechanism. Interpersonal contact is also important in family and institutional transmission. Transmission by uncooked food and by vector is unlikely. Cross-transmission of giardial cysts among humans, dogs, and rabbits has been reported.

The pathogenesis of giardiasis is also not clear. Proposed mechanisms have included the parasite presenting a mechanical barrier to absorption, an inflammatory response to the mucosa, production of a toxin by the trophozoite, and an associated infection with either fungal or bacterial organisms resulting in malabsorption. Encystation usually occurs in the lower ileum. The cysts of *G. lamblia* are acid resistant and may survive for months in wet stools or in water. Trophozoites are seen with regularity only in stool specimens during episodes of severe diarrhea.

DIAGNOSIS

Infection with *G. lamblia* causes a diverse spectrum of symptoms and findings. Diarrhea is the usual common

TABLE 1. **Drugs for the Treatment of Giardiasis in the United States**

Drug	Adult Dosage	Pediatric Dosage	Side Effects
Metronidazole* (Flagyl)	250 mg 3 times/d for 10 d	5 mg/kg 3 times/d for 10 d	Nausea, headache, metallic aftertaste, abdominal pain after alcohol ingestion, brown discoloration of urine
Paromomycin (Humatin)	30 mg/kg/d in 3 divided doses for 7 d	Not recommended	Nausea, diarrhea, abdominal pain
Furazolidone (Furoxone)	100 mg 4 times/d for 7 d	1 mo to 1 y: ½–1 tsp 4 times/d for 10 d 1–4 y: 1–1½ tsp 4 times/d for 10 d 5 y and older: 1 tbsp 4 times/d for 10 d	Hemolysis, dermatitis, fever, nausea, vomiting, brown discoloration of urine

*Although used widely for giardiasis, metronidazole is not licensed by the FDA for this infection. May be mutagenic and carcinogenic (animal and bacterial studies only).

complaint. It can be either acute or chronic, continuous or intermittent. Not infrequently, patients with giardiasis present with alternating constipation and diarrhea, mimicking the irritable colon syndrome. Complaints of bloating and flatulence are frequent. Stools are usually watery and contain copious amounts of mucus. Blood is rarely noted in the stool. Less frequently, there can be generalized abdominal epigastric and crampy abdominal pain that resembles peptic ulcer disease. Other symptoms include headache, fatigue, weight loss, and depression. On occasion, patients may develop a syndrome resembling cholecystitis, commonly referred to as hepatobiliary giardiasis. It is for these reasons that giardiasis is usually included in virtually every differential diagnosis of abdominal pain.

The diagnosis of giardiasis is still based on obtaining adequate and fresh stool specimens. A mild purge with magnesium citrate is advised. Stools should be examined when they are fresh, and owing to the intermittent nature of the shedding of the parasite, several samples are suggested. A permanent record can be obtained by staining cysts with chlorazol black E. Other methods of diagnosis include duodenal aspiration, either with a Rehfuss tube or during endoscopy. A direct immunoflourescent-monoclonal antibody method may be the most sensitive method of detection of *G. lamblia.* If a small bowel biopsy has been obtained, an impression smear can be made at the time of biopsy. A modification of Masson's trichrome stain is recommended to recognize more easily the parasite usually seen adjacent to the epithelial cell.

TREATMENT

The time-honored drug of choice for symptomatic giardiasis in adults has been quinacrine hydochloride (Atabrine), but, unfortunately, it is no longer available.

Metronidazole (Flagyl) is effective in a dosage of 250 mg thrice daily for 10 days. Principal side effects include headache, nausea, and a metallic aftertaste. Ingestion of alcohol during metronidazole therapy may precipitate severe abdominal pain that mimics acute pancreatitis. Furazolidone (Furoxone) is less effective but is available as an oil suspension. It is popular with pediatricians for that reason. The recommended dosage for adults is 100 mg four times daily for 7 days. The pediatric dose should be adjusted according to the age of the child. Albendazole (Albenza) in a dosage of 400 mg per day for 5 days both for children and adults is available on compassionate clearance only from the manufacturer and is less effective than metronidazole. Paromomycin (Humatin) is seldom used in the United States but may be considered for treatment of infection during pregnancy.

Recommended dosages and significant side effects of these drugs are listed in Table 1. Asymptomatic cyst passers should be treated because of the potential for infecting others or for developing chronic symptoms themselves. During the course of treatment, patients may become lactose intolerant. Therefore, avoidance of milk, cheese, and ice cream during the treatment period and for 1 week thereafter is recommended.

The majority of patients will respond to monotherapy. Symptoms occurring 2 weeks after therapy suggest reinfection. A second course of therapy would seem reasonable and is recommended. Continued symptoms warrant a careful work-up, including a search for any of the immune deficiency syndromes.

PREVENTION

Because *G. lamblia* is the most common human parasitic infection in the United States and may cause a lengthy bout of diarrhea, prevention is of the utmost importance. The Environmental Protection Agency has regulated *Giardia* species in drinking water through the Safe Drinking Water Act. It is, therefore, of increasing importance that public health officials work with the water industry to ensure a pristine water supply. It goes without saying that good personal hygiene, particularly strict hand washing, and disposal of human and animal waste are important in the prevention of giardiasis. Proper education, particularly for hikers, travelers, and workers at day care centers, and explicit transmittal of information to patients with acquired immune deficiency syndrome regarding venereal transmission of this common parasite are strongly recommended.

BACTEREMIA AND SEPTICEMIA

method of
STEVEN M. OPAL, M.D.
Memorial Hospital of Rhode Island
Pawtucket, Rhode Island

and

LOLITA E. CHIU, M.D.
Brown University School of Medicine
Providence, Rhode Island

Bacteremia is the presence of viable bacteria in the bloodstream and can be transient, intermittent, or sustained. *Transient bacteremia,* which can occur after toothbrushing, chewing, bowel movements, and dental and certain medical procedures, is usually a common and benign process lasting no more than a few minutes. *Intermittent bacteremia* implies the presence of a localized extravascular infectious process, as can occur in the presence of abscess. *Sustained bacteremia* is the hallmark of endovascular infection and occurs in cases of endocarditis, suppurative thrombophlebitis, endarteritis, mycotic aneurysm, and infected arteriovenous fistula.

Bacteremia can also be *primary,* characterized by the absence of an identifiable source (often generated from vascular catheters), or *secondary,* complicating a focal infection such as a urinary tract infection, pneumonia, or cellulitis. Bacteremia may progress to sepsis, depending on its magnitude and duration, the infecting organism's intrinsic virulence, the patient's immune competence, and the presence of co-morbid underlying conditions.

DEFINITION OF TERMS

Infection is an inflammatory response to the presence of organisms or the invasion of a normally sterile site by organisms. *Systemic inflammatory response syndrome (SIRS)* is a clinical response arising from an insult, which could be infectious or noninfectious in origin. Examples of noninfectious causes of SIRS include trauma, burns, pancreatitis, ischemia, hemorrhagic shock, and immune-mediated organ injury. Two or more or these criteria must be present: (1) temperature higher than 38°C or lower than 36°C, (2) heart rate higher than 90 beats per minute, (3) respiratory rate higher than 20 breaths per minute or P_{CO_2} lower than 32 mm Hg, and (4) white blood cell count higher than 12×10^9/L, less than 4×10^9/L, or the presence of more than 10% immature neutrophils. *Sepsis* is the presence of SIRS caused by an infectious process; it is considered severe if either hypotension or systemic manifestations of hypoperfusion (lactic acidosis, oliguria, or change in mental status) are present. *Septic shock* is the presence of sepsis with hypotension in spite of adequate fluid resuscitation and is associated with hypoperfusion abnormalities.

These stages, usually starting with an infection and leading to sepsis with multiorgan dysfunction and shock, imply an increasing severity of the inflammatory response to infection rather than increasing severity of the infection itself.

PATHOGENESIS

In the presence of gram-negative infection, neutrophils attach to the endothelium, allowing them to migrate out of the vascular space to the site where bacteria are multiplying. Gram-negative organisms release endotoxin (also known as lipopolysaccharide [LPS]), which is found in their outer membranes. LPS then binds to the LPS-binding protein (LBP) found within the systemic circulation. LBP subsequently shuttles LPS to $CD14^+$-bearing myeloid effector cells (neutrophils, monocytes, macrophages). LPS triggers gene induction within these inflammatory cells for the production of cytokines, adhesive proteins, and enzymes with proinflammatory effects. Examples of substances released include tumor necrosis factor (TNF), interleukin-1 (IL-1), prostaglandins, leukotrienes, nitric oxide (NO), and platelet-activating factor. These mediators are capable of boosting host defense mechanisms, but they can also cause changes leading to septic shock and multiple organ dysfunction syndrome.

For gram-positive organisms, the cell wall components (teichoic acid, peptidoglycans) and/or their exotoxins act as the initiating event, causing the release of TNF and IL-1. Gram-positive bacterial superantigens (e.g., staphylococcal enterotoxins, toxic shock syndrome toxins) also increase endothelial membrane permeability and inhibit myocardial function, as seen in septic shock.

Furthermore, bacterial phagocytosis by polymorphonuclear neutrophils (PMNs) causes release of oxygen radicals, reactive nitrogen intermediates, and lysosomal enzymes. These neutrophil activation factors also contribute to additional microvascular injury.

CLINICAL MANIFESTATIONS

Accurate history taking and physical examination may offer certain clues regarding the possible focus of infection. Risk factors, such as intravenous drug use, presence of the human immunodeficiency virus (HIV) or acquired immune deficiency syndrome (AIDS), steroid use, recent administration of chemotherapy, other underlying illnesses, and previous use of antibiotics should be elicited. The severity

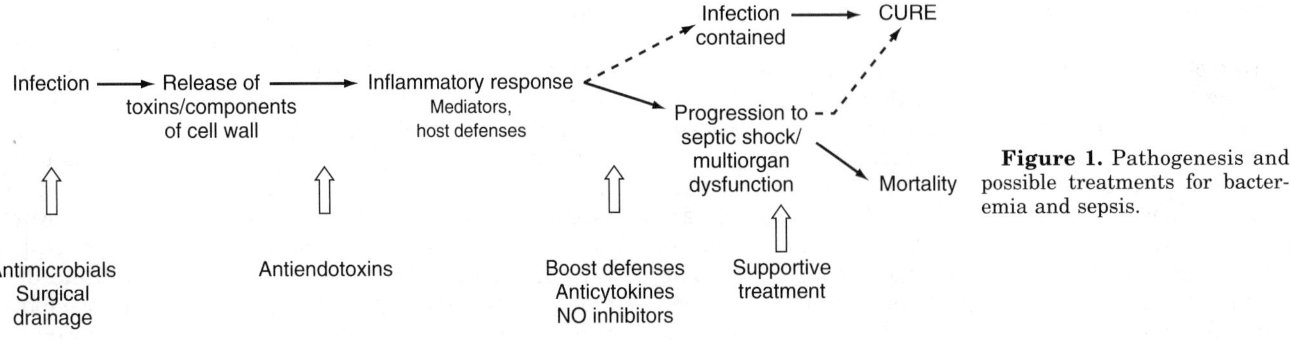

Figure 1. Pathogenesis and possible treatments for bacteremia and sepsis.

TABLE 1. **Empirical Therapy Based on Presumed Site of Infection**

Diseases	Common Organisms Involved	Recommended Antibiotics
Central Nervous System		
Adults, community acquired	*Streptococcus pneumoniae,* Neisseria meningitidis*	Ceftriaxone (Rocephin), cefotaxime (Claforan)†
Postneurosurgical	*Staphylococcus epidermidis, Staphylococcus aureus* Enterobacteriaceae, *Pseudomonas aeruginosa, S. pneumoniae*	Vancomycin (Vancocin) + ceftazidime (Fortaz)
Gastrointestinal Tract		
Gallbladder, biliary tree, peritonitis, abscess	Enterobacteriaceae, Enterococci, *Bacteroides, Clostridium*	Ampicillin + aminoglycosides + metronidazole (Flagyl) Ampicillin/sulbactam (Unasyn) or cefoxitin (Mefoxin) Clindamycin (Cleocin) + aminoglycosides
Kidney / Urinary Tract		
Community acquired	Enterobacteriaceae, Enterococci	TMP/SUL (Bactrim) or cephalosporins‡ Quinolones§
Nosocomial	Enterobacteriaceae, *P. aeruginosa*, Enterococci	Third-generation cephalosporins‖ or AP PCN¶ + aminoglycosides Quinolones§
Heart / Infective Endocarditis		
Native valve	*Streptococcus viridans, Streptococcus bovis,* other *Streptococcus* species	Penicillin** ± gentamicin Ceftriaxone (Rocephin) Vancomycin††
	Enterococci	Penicillin + gentamicin‡‡ Ampicillin + gentamicin‡‡ Vancomycin†† + gentamicin‡‡
	S. aureus	Nafcillin ± gentamicin Cefazolin (Ancef) ± gentamicin Vancomycin††
	HACEK organisms	Ceftriaxone (Rocephin) Ampicillin + gentamicin
Prosthetic valve	*S. aureus*, coagulase negative staphylococci	Nafcillin + gentamicin + rifampin Vancomycin†† + gentamicin + rifampin
Skin and Soft Tissue Infection	*S. aureus*, groups A, C, and G streptococci, Enterobacteriaceae	Nafcillin or cefazolin (Ancef) ± ciprofloxacin Ampicillin/sulbactam (Unasyn)
Pulmonary		
Pneumonia, community acquired	*S. pneumoniae, Haemophilus influenzae, Legionella*	Cephalosporins‡ + erythromycin if atypical organisms suspected
Hospital-acquired	*Enterobacter, Klebsiella, Pseudomonas, Legionella*, occasionally *S. aureus*	Third-generation cephalosporins‖ or AP PCN¶ ± erythromycin Imipenem-cilastatin (Primaxin)
Systemic Febrile Syndrome		
Nonimmunocompromise	Gram-positive cocci, aerobic bacilli, anaerobes	Third-generation cephalosporins‖ or AP PCN¶ + aminoglycosides + clindamycin or metronidazole (Flagyl)
Intravenous drug use	*S. aureus*	Nafcillin or cefazolin (Ancef) ± gentamicin Vancomycin†† ± gentamicin
Splenectomized	*S. pneumoniae, H. influenzae*, meningococci	Cefotaxime (Claforan) or ceftriaxone (Rocephin)
Neutropenia	Aerobic gram-negative bacilli (including *Pseudomonas*), others (e.g., *S. aureus*)	Ceftazidime (Fortaz) or cefepime (Maxipime) or imipenem-cilastin (Primaxin) or AP PCN¶ + aminoglycosides ± vancomycin
Vascular	*S. aureus, S. epidermidis*, group JK corynebacterium	Vancomycin ± gentamicin

*Add vancomycin if high rate of resistant *S. pneumoniae* is present.
†If *Listeria* is being considered (usually in elderly and in those with defective cell-mediated immunity), add ampicillin.
‡Cefuroxime (Ceftin), cefotaxime (Claforan), or ceftriaxone (Rocephin).
§Ciprofloxacin (Cipro), ofloxacin (Floxin), levofloxacin (Levaquin).
‖Ceftazidime (Fortaz); may use cefotaxime (Claforan) or ceftriaxone (Rocephin) if *Pseudomonas* is not strongly suspected.
¶Piperacillin, pip/tazobactam (Zosyn), ticarcillin, ticar/clavulanate (Timentin).
**For strep MIC ≤ 0.5.
††Use only if patient is allergic to PCN or organism resistant to initial options.
‡‡Organism needs to show sensitivity to both agents for synergy.
Abbreviations: HACEK = *Haemophilus aphrophilus, Haemophilus parainfluenzae, Actinobacillus, Cardiobacterium, Eikenella, Kingella; AP PCN = antipseudomonal penicillin.*

TABLE 2. **Drug Dosages**

Creatinine Clearance	>50	10–50	<10
Ampicillin	1–2 gm IV q 6 h	1–2 gm IV q 8–12 h	1–2 gm IV q 12–24 h
Ampicillin/sulbactam	3 gm IV q 6 h	3 gm IV q 8–12 h	3 gm IV q 12–24 h
Cefazolin	2 gm IV q 8 h	2 gm IV q 12 h	2 gm IV q 24–48 h
Cefepime	2 gm IV q 12 h	1–2 gm IV q 24 h	500 mg IV q 24 h
Cefotaxime	2 gm IV q 8 h	2 gm IV q 12–24 h	2 gm IV q 24 h
Cefoxitin	2 gm IV q 8 h	2 gm IV q 12 h	2 gm IV q 24–48 h
Ceftazidime	2 gm IV q 8 h	2 gm IV q 24–48 h	2 gm IV q 48 h
Ceftriaxone	1–2 gm IV q 24 h	Same	Same
Cefuroxime	1.5 gm IV q 8 h	1.5 gm IV q 12 h	1.5 gm IV q 24 h
Ciprofloxacin	400 mg IV q 12 h	400 mg IV q 24 h	400 mg IV q 24 h
Clindamycin	600–900 mg IV q 8 h	Same	Same
Erythromycin	1 gm IV q 6 h	Same	Same
Gentamicin	4–5 mg/kg/24 h	2–3 mg/kg/24 h	2 mg/kg/48 h
Imipenem	500 mg IV q 6 h	250 mg IV q 8–12 h	250 mg IV q 12 h
Levofloxacin	250–500 mg IV q 24 h	250 mg IV q 48 h	250 mg IV q 48 h
Metronidazole	500 mg IV q 6–8 h	Same	Same
Nafcillin	2 gm IV q 4 h	Same	Same
Ofloxacin	400 mg IV q 12 h	400 mg IV q 12 h	400 mg IV q 24 h
Piperacillin	4 gm IV q 4–6 h	4 gm IV q 8 h	4 gm IV q 12 h
Pip/tazobactam	3.375 IV q 6 h	2.25 IV q 6 h	2.25 IV q 8 h
Ticarcillin	3 gm IV q 4 h	2 gm IV q 6–8 h	2 gm IV q 12 h
Ticar/clavulanate	3.1 gm IV q 4 h	2 gm IV q 6–8 h	2 gm IV q 12 h
TMP-SUL	3–5 mg/kg q 6–12 h	3–5 mg/kg q 24 h	Avoid
Vancomycin	2 gm IV q 12 h	1 gm IV q 24 h	Monitor levels

of the illness can be determined by looking for signs of sepsis (temperature, heart and respiratory rates, white blood cell count, arterial blood gas) and organ system dysfunction. The presence of catheters and other foreign bodies should also be noted.

DIAGNOSIS

Blood cultures remain the cornerstone in the diagnosis of bacteremia. Certain factors can influence the diagnostic yield of blood cultures, however. The collection of an adequate number of specimens before antibiotic administration and the inoculation of a minimum of 10 ml of blood per set is required to increase diagnostic yield.

Aside from this, correct interpretation of the culture result is also needed. *Pseudobacteremia* is a phenomenon wherein bacteria isolated from blood cultures originated from outside the bloodstream. This occurs as a result of contamination at any stage of blood culturing—from drawing blood to processing in the laboratory. Coagulase-negative staphylococci, *Bacillus* species, and *Corynebacterium* species account for most of the cases. The number of positive blood culture sets, the intensity and rapidity of growth, the patient's clinical presentation, and the presence of risk factors (e.g., foreign bodies or catheters) may provide clues as to the "validity" of the result. Thus, it is important to distinguish a true-positive from a false-positive blood culture result to avoid the unnecessary risks and costs associated with inappropriate antimicrobial use for false-positive blood cultures.

TREATMENT

The management of bacteremia and sepsis involves three approaches: (1) antibiotic treatment with adequate surgical drainage as needed, aimed at the source of infection; (2) supportive treatment or intensive care unit care for sepsis-associated multiorgan dysfunction; and (3) inhibiting the formation and/or action of the mediators of sepsis (Figure 1).

Treatment Targeting the Source of Infection. The initial antibiotic choice depends on several components. First, the presumed site of infection needs to be identified. History, physical examination, and other laboratory studies (e.g., urinalysis, radiographs, Gram stain) may offer clues. Second, the most commonly reported microorganism causing infection at that site and its antimicrobial resistance patterns should be known. Based on this, an empirical choice of antibiotic or antibiotics can be made (Tables 1 and 2).

However, not all patients with sepsis present with an obvious focus of infection. In these clinical settings, a broad-spectrum antibiotic regimen may be chosen. Treatment should eventually be narrowed as the identification and susceptibilities of the organism become known.

Supportive Treatment. This includes intubation and mechanical ventilation in those with respiratory failure, hemodialysis in patients with renal failure, vasopressors and inotropic agents in persons with cardiovascular dysfunction, and use of blood and blood products in those with disseminated intravascular coagulation. Rapid recognition and initiation of measures to maintain perfusion to vital tissues is the key determinant of successful management of severe sepsis and septic shock.

Other Treatment Modalities

1. *Antiendotoxin monoclonal antibodies.* Half of the cases of sepsis are secondary to gram-negative bacteremia. As mentioned earlier, the presence of endotoxin initiates a cascade of events leading to the release of mediators—TNF, IL-1, and IL-6. Use of

antiendotoxin treatments attempts to block this release. Two types of methods had been used: (1) human monoclonal IgM antibody that binds specifically to the lipid A domain of the endotoxin (HA-IA) and (2) a murine monoclonal IgM antibody against gram-negative endotoxin (E5). Both had been considered safe; however uncertain benefits accrued from the use of these antibodies in clinical trials. Neither antibody is currently available for standard clinical use.

2. *Anticytokine therapy.* TNF and IL-1 are two of the proinflammatory cytokines noted to be increased in the presence of sepsis and septic shock. They, together with other mediators, are responsible for the myocardial depression, decreased systemic vascular resistance, and decreased consumption of oxygen by peripheral tissues seen in septic shock. Higher levels of these substances in the blood were noted to be associated with increased mortality. Thus, strategies to counteract their effects were developed. These include the use of recombinant human IL-1 receptor antagonist (RhIL-1RA), murine monoclonal anti-TNF, and recombinant human dimeric TNF receptor fused with the Fc component of IgG_1. Trials using these strategies have yet to show convincingly an improved outcome in the treatment of sepsis and septic shock. These agents may even be harmful in some cases. Part of the failure may be attributable to the fact that even though TNF and IL-1 can cause significant physiologic abnormalities, they also have protective effects. These include recruiting and activating PMNs, macrophages, and lymphocytes and promoting the release of acute phase reactant proteins, thus helping to contain the infection. The p55 TNF receptor: immunoglobulin fusion protein is currently in clinical trials in severe sepsis.

3. *Polymorphonuclear neutrophil inhibition or promotion.* Like the cytokines, PMNs also play a dual role. They can produce tissue injury and organ dysfunction through their by-products, but at the same time, they play a major role in host defenses. Because of the former, a monoclonal antibody directed against their adhesion site, CD 11/18, had been produced (thus decreasing the number of migrating PMNs to the site of infection). This strategy, however, proved harmful, as it impaired the clearance of bacteria and its toxins. However, augmentation of PMN numbers and function through the use of granulocyte colony–stimulating factor (G-CSF,* filgrastim [Neupogen]) may benefit some patients.

4. *NO inhibitors.* NO is a highly reactive gas produced by cells containing NO synthase (endothelial cells, neurons, and vascular smooth muscles) under normal conditions. It is responsible for regulation of vascular tone (producing vasodilatation) and has some antimicrobial properties. In the presence of other inflammatory mediators, increased production occurs. This can lead to hypotension, direct tissue injury, and organ dysfunction. NO synthase inhibitors were then developed to counteract this effect. So far, no proven benefits have been described in patients with septic shock. Clinical trials with NO synthase inhibitors are currently in progress.

The mechanisms surrounding the development of septic shock are interrelated, and some of these events are beneficial for the body's own defense mechanisms. Thus, a balance should be achieved. Also, individual patients respond differently to infection, so treatment measures should be tailored according to individual needs. Patients with intact immune systems may not benefit from anti-inflammatory measures because these may hinder their own defenses. By contrast, boosting host defenses can be the primary goal in those who are immunocompromised; anticytokine therapy can be given for those with extensive inflammatory mediator response. However, at present, despite reported failures of such treatment measures, investigators remain optimistic regarding the use of these substances.

*Not FDA approved for this indication.

BRUCELLOSIS

method of
ASH K. SAMANTA, M.D.
Leicester Royal Infirmary
Leicester, England

Brucellosis is transmitted to humans from infected animals. *Brucella* organisms are small, slow-growing, aerobic, gram-negative coccobacilli. Infection is due to *Brucella melitensis* (from sheep, goats, and camels), *Brucella abortus* (from cattle), *Brucella suis* (from swine), and *Brucella canis* (from dogs).

Approximately 500,000 cases are reported every year to the World Health Organization. Main endemic areas include the Mediterranean region, Latin America, and Asia. Infection occurs mainly in people such as farmers, shepherds, and veterinarians, who are occupationally exposed to animals. Also at risk are butchers and abattoir workers, as the organism can survive in animal carcasses for several weeks, and laboratory personnel who may come in direct contact with *Brucella.* Another high-risk group includes travelers from endemic areas.

Infection is acquired through lacerated or abraded skin, inhalation, or ingestion of infected milk or cheese (particularly goat cheese for *B. melitensis*). The organisms are initially phagocytosed by neutrophils and macrophages. Subsequently, they may spread to regional lymph nodes, and if host defenses are overwhelmed, then bacteremia occurs. The usual incubation period is 1 to 3 weeks and at times may be as long as several months.

Acute and subacute disease may occur with fever, malaise, chills and rigors, polyarthralgia, headache, fatigue, back pain, and myalgia. *Brucella* may localize in any organ but most commonly is found in bones, joints, heart, central nervous system, lungs, liver, and spleen. Endocarditis, osteomyelitis (particularly in the lumbosacral vertebrae), epididymo-orchitis, splenic abscess, and neurologic complications may occur. A chronic disease presentation, with insidious nonspecific symptoms for longer than 1 year, is also recognized.

As the manifestations of brucellosis are so protean, the

diagnosis depends on a high degree of suspicion, as well as a detailed history of occupational contact, travel to endemic areas, and exposure to high-risk foods. Other conditions such as typhoid, systemic lupus erythematosus, tuberculosis, infectious mononucleosis, toxoplasmosis, and hepatitis need to be considered in the differential diagnosis. Most routine laboratory tests are not helpful in making the diagnosis. Definitive evidence of *Brucella* infection is by positive blood cultures (which may be found in about 20% of acute cases). Culturing the organism may be dangerous for laboratory personnel, and suspected samples should be processed in laboratories with an appropriate biosafety level. Serologic confirmation is by the *Brucella* agglutination test. A titer of higher than 1:160 is considered positive. Recent exposure is indicated by a high titer of IgM antibodies or a fourfold rise in agglutination titer over 1 to 4 weeks. Enzyme immunoassay tests may be used for serologic diagnosis and are more sensitive than agglutination. Polymerase chain reaction methods using random or selected primers are potentially useful but require further evaluation. Radioisotope bone scans and magnetic resonance imaging scans may be useful in detecting vertebral and osteoarticular disease.

TREATMENT

As the *Brucella* organism is intracellular, the antibiotic chosen must have good tissue permeability. A synergistic combination of antimicrobials and prolonged therapy is recommended to reduce the chances of subsequent relapse.

Doxycycline (Vibramycin) has a long half-life (18 to 24 hours), excellent absorption, and good tissue permeability. Doxycycline 200 mg per day is recommended for a period of 6 weeks. Intramuscular streptomycin, 1 gram daily for the first 2 weeks, is recommended in combination with doxycycline. The dose of streptomycin may need to be decreased in older patients and in those with renal insufficiency, and renal function should be monitored. As an alternative to streptomycin, either netilmicin (Netromycin), 4 to 6 mg per kg once daily, or gentamicin (Garamycin), 2 to 5 mg per kg per day intramuscularly (IM) or intravenously (IV) in divided doses every 8 to 12 hours, may be used. Likewise, the dose of these agents may need careful adjustment depending on plasma levels and renal function.

Another very effective combination is doxycycline, 200 mg per day, and rifampin* (Rifadin), 600 to 900 mg per day, both given orally for 6 weeks. Hepatic function should be monitored with rifampin and the dose adjusted accordingly.

Other combinations include ofloxacin* (Floxin), 400 mg per day, with rifampin, 600 to 900 mg per day, or trimethoprim-sulfamethoxazole (Bactrim, Septra),* in a dose of 80/400 to 320/1600 mg per day given for 6 weeks. These are less effective but a reasonable substitute if the initially mentioned combinations cannot be used.

The combination of antibiotics used must be chosen according to each individual patient, bearing in mind adverse effects, hepatic and renal status of the patient, convenience of administration, and long-term compliance.

*Not FDA approved for this indication.

Children

Below the age of 8 years, rifampin, 10 mg per kg per day, with trimethoprim, 10 mg per kg per day, and sulfamethoxazole, 50 mg per kg per day, for 6 weeks is recommended. Older than 8 years, doxycycline, 3 mg per kg per day, with trimethoprim-sulfamethoxazole, 480 mg per day, for 6 weeks, or doxycycline, 3 mg per kg per day, with rifampin, 15 mg per kg per day, for 6 weeks may be used. Most physicians would avoid using aminoglycosides in children.

Pregnancy

Treatment is difficult due to the risk of harm to the fetus, and aminoglycosides and tetracyclines can be particularly toxic. A combination of rifampin, 600 to 900 mg per day, with trimethoprim-sulfamethoxazole, 480 mg per day, for 6 weeks is recommended.

Osteoarticular and Skeletal Disease

I prefer the combination of doxycycline, 200 mg per day, and an aminoglycoside (streptomycin, 1 gram per day for the initial 2 weeks) in this situation. I suggest that therapy be continued for a period of 12 weeks.

Cardiovascular and Neurologic Disease

These may be serious and life-threatening complications of brucellosis. Cardiovascular complications often occur in pre-existing damaged valves and may lead to acute cardiac failure. Early referral to a cardiac surgery unit is recommended, as valve replacement is frequently required.

Acute neurologic complications may include stroke and sudden intracranial bleeding from mycotic aneurysms. I use "triple therapy," with doxycycline, aminoglycoside, and rifampin, and believe that treatment should be continued for at least 12 weeks, and probably longer, if cardiac or intracranial surgery is performed.

Abscess

These should be drained, and appropriate antibiotic therapy should be continued for a longer period. Splenectomy has been recommended in relapse.

PREVENTION

The key lies in eradication of *Brucella* in animals, by a preventive program, and by immunization. There is no effective available vaccine for humans. Humans should avoid unpasteurized milk and milk products, and personnel at risk should be advised on appropriate protective clothing to protect the portals of entry of the organism.

ACKNOWLEDGMENTS

I am very grateful to Jo Beardsley for her help and support in preparing this article.

CONJUNCTIVITIS

method of
MITCHELL H. FRIEDLAENDER, M.D.
Scripps Clinic
La Jolla, California

The conjunctiva is the mucous membrane that covers the inner surface of the eyelids and the eyeball itself. It is divided into three anatomic areas: palpebral, forniceal (cul-de-sac), and bulbar. The conjunctiva is loosely attached to the eye and allows free movement. Like most mucous membranes, the conjunctiva has an epithelial layer and a deeper substantia propria.

Conjunctivitis is an inflammation of the conjunctiva that may have infectious or noninfectious etiologies (Table 1). Noninfectious entities include allergic-immunologic, toxic, and infectious agents, including bacteria, viruses, and *Chlamydia*.

ALLERGIC CONJUNCTIVITIS

Seasonal allergic conjunctivitis (SAC) is an acute process characterized by conjunctival edema, erythema, and itching. It is IgE mediated and triggered by airborne allergens such as pollen, dander, mold, and house dust, resulting in the degranulation of conjunctival mast cells and release of allergic mediators (such as histamines). Other more severe forms of allergic conjunctivitis include vernal keratoconjunctivitis (VKC), which affects mainly children, and atopic keratoconjunctivitis (AKC), which occurs in people with atopic dermatitis.

SAC is controlled by avoidance of the offending allergens, if possible. A topical antihistamine-decongestant can be used for treatment of the acute symptoms. The nonsteroidal anti-inflammatory agent ketorolac (Acular) is effective in relieving itching. Levocarbastine (Livostin) is a newer antihistamine that is very effective at eliminating symptoms. Cromolyn sodium 4% (Crolom) and lodoxamide (Alomide) are mast cell stabilizers and can be used before exposure to the offending allergen. Olopatadine (Patanol) is a mast cell stabilizer with antihistamine properties. Topical steroids can be very effective in controlling the symptoms of SAC; however, because of the side effects of cataract formation and secondary glaucoma they should be used with the supervision of an ophthalmologist. Patients with VKC and AKC should usually be referred to an ophthalmologist for management.

VIRAL CONJUNCTIVITIS

Many cases of conjunctivitis, or pink eye, are caused by adenovirus. Epidemic keratoconjunctivitis is a common form of conjunctivitis that is extremely infectious and caused by adenovirus, especially serotypes 8 and 19. Preauricular nodes are present in most cases, and the patient complains of redness, discharge, and eyelids sticking together in the morning. This follicular conjunctivitis runs a 1- to 2-week course and is often accompanied by subepithelial corneal infiltrates. The diagnosis is made by clinical signs and rarely by the use of cultures, Gram's stain, or immunofluorescent techniques. Other adenoviral infections are pharyngoconjunctival fever and hemorrhagic conjunctivitis. The treatment is supportive, but often artificial tears, topical decongestants, and even prophylactic topical antibiotics may be given. Topical steroids are controversial and should not be used without consultation with an ophthalmologist.

Primary herpetic conjunctivitis is follicular in nature and usually indistinguishable from an adenoviral infection unless the typical vesicular skin lesions

TABLE 1. **Differential Diagnosis of Conjunctivitis**

Etiology	Signs/Symptoms	Treatment
Bacterial	Discharge with lids sealed shut in AM, conjunctival injection	Polymyxin B/trimethoprim, quinolone, or aminoglycoside drops
Gonococcal	Hyperpurulent conjunctivitis Beefy-red conjunctival injection	Topical bacitracin, 500 U/gm 8 times daily *plus* Ceftriaxone, 1 gm intramuscularly every 24 hours for 5 days
Chlamydial	Chronic unilateral or bilateral mucopurulent conjunctivitis	Tetracyline, 500 mg, or erythromycin stearate, 500 mg, orally 4 times daily for 3 weeks
Viral	Serous discharge starting unilaterally, then spreading bilaterally, mild itching, moderate to severe conjunctival injection	Artificial tears, compresses, fomite precautions
Allergy	Bilateral itching, tearing, mild conjunctival injection, edema, associated systemic allergy	Topical antihistamine four times daily Consider prophylactic treatment with mast cell stabilizer or NSAID Cold compresses prn
Toxic	Unilateral/bilateral irritation with associated conjunctival injection	Artificial tears Removal of inciting agent

Modified from Frangie JP, Leibowitz HM: Conjunctivitis. *In* Rakel RE (ed): Conn's Current Therapy 1995. Philadelphia, WB Saunders Co, 1995, p 66.

are present in the periorbital region or a corneal dendrite is seen.

ACUTE BACTERIAL CONJUNCTIVITIS

This type of conjunctivitis is usually seen in children and is much less common in adults. It manifests with modest mucopurulent discharge and diffuse conjunctival hyperemia and a small or absent preauricular node. The most common causative organisms are *Staphylococcus aureus, Haemophilus influenzae,* and *Streptococcus pneumoniae.* Even though some cases may resolve spontaneously, topical treatment is recommended with a broad-spectrum topical antibiotic such as Polytrim (trimethoprim and polymyxin B), 1 drop four times a day for 10 days. Fluoroquinolones such as ofloxacin (Ocuflox) or ciprofloxacin (Ciloxan) are very potent broad-spectrum antibiotics widely used for the treatment of bacterial conjunctivitis. It is felt that topical therapy shortens the course and prevents complications such as corneal ulceration and permanent conjunctival changes.

HYPERACUTE BACTERIAL CONJUNCTIVITIS

This entity manifests with copious amounts of purulent discharge associated with marked lid swelling and conjunctival edema. The globe can be very tender, and a preauricular node is usually present. The causative organism is commonly *Neisseria gonorrhoeae*; however, other organisms such as *Neisseria meningitidis* have been reported. Gram's stain and cultures on Thayer-Martin and chocolate agar should be performed, followed by systemic and topical therapy.

CHRONIC BACTERIAL CONJUNCTIVITIS

S. aureus is the most common causative organism identified owing to its ability to colonize the eyelids. Lid hygiene using a washcloth and baby shampoo on the lashes and lid margins is indicated in most cases. This may be supplemented with topical or systemic antibiotics.

ADULT INCLUSION CONJUNCTIVITIS

This entity is caused by *Chlamydia trachomatis* and is characterized by a chronic follicular conjunctivitis associated with an enlarged preauricular lymph node. The diagnosis is made by a direct fluorescent antibody assay, an enzyme immunoassay, or a Giemsa stain of the conjunctiva. Treatment is with systemic tetracycline or erythromycin, and topical therapy is optional. Also, the patient's sexual contacts should be treated with systemic therapy.

OPHTHALMIA NEONATORUM

This particular entity requires special attention because it can have devastating effects on the eye and vision along with systemic manifestations (Table 2). It is defined as conjunctival inflammation occurring during the first 30 days of life.

The clinical signs and the age at presentation can be variable, making it imperative to use laboratory methods to assist in the differential diagnosis. An ophthalmologist should be consulted to participate in the management of these patients.

Chemical conjunctivitis has been reported in 10 to 100% of neonates treated with topical prophylactic agents at birth. Although it is 2.5 to 12 times more common when silver nitrate 1% is used, it has been reported with the use of topical erythromycin and tetracycline derivatives. Mild conjunctival erythema and lid edema manifest within the first 24 hours of life, and Gram's stain shows neutrophils with no organisms. This is a self-limited condition that resolves spontaneously in 48 hours in most cases.

Conjunctival cultures of vaginally delivered neonates reflect the flora of the vaginal canal, whereas the conjunctiva of neonates delivered by cesarean section within 3 hours of membrane rupture are culture negative. Therefore, the conjunctival flora of the neonate is correlated with the method of delivery. The most common organism isolated in bacterial ophthalmia neonatorum is *S. aureus,* followed in frequency by *Haemophilus* species, *S. pneumoniae,* enterococcus, *Pseudomonas aeruginosa,* and *N. gonorrhoeae.* Gram's stain and cultures are needed to make the diagnosis. With the exception of *N. gonorrhoeae* and *P. aeruginosa* infection, sight-threatening complications such as corneal ulcers, infiltrates, and endophthalmitis are rare, and topical therapy is adequate. Topical gentamicin (Genoptic) or tobramycin (Tobrex) drops are recommended for gram-negative organisms, and erythromycin ointment is recommended for gram-positive organisms.

P. aeruginosa is a very virulent organism that is rarely seen in healthy neonates but may be seen as a nosocomial pathogen in sick neonates. Corneal perforation and endophthalmitis can result from this organism, and an ophthalmologist should be consulted to participate in the management of patients with these conditions. These neonates should be hospitalized, isolated, and treated with fortified topical antibiotics; 1 drop every hour should be applied to the affected eye for the first 3 days. Systemic antibiotics are indicated only if other foci of infection are identified.

Gonococcal conjunctivitis in the neonate appears suddenly with eyelid edema and hyperpurulence. If left untreated, the gonococcal organism can perforate the intact cornea within 24 hours. This condition should be considered a medical emergency. Therapy must be started immediately based on a presumptive diagnosis made from the Gram stain that shows gram-negative intracellular diplococci. The neonate should be hospitalized in an isolation unit for systemic therapy (penicillin, kanamycin [Kantrex], cefotaxime [Claforan], or ceftriaxone [Rocephin], plus topical erythromycin ointment 0.5% applied four times a day) initiated with frequent saline irrigation

TABLE 2. **Differential Diagnosis and Treatment of Ophthalmia Neonatorum**

Etiology	Microscopic Features of Conjunctival Smears	Culture Media	Other Diagnostic Tests	Treatment
Chemical	Neutrophils, occasional lymphocytes (Gram)	None necessary		None necessary
Bacterial	Bacteria, neutrophils (Gram)	Reduced blood agar, thioglycolate broth, chocolate agar in CO_2, Thayer-Martin media	Drug sensitivity testing	Gram-positive organisms: erythromycin ointment Gram-negative organisms: gentamicin drops *Pseudomonas*-fortified topical antibiotics *Nesseria gonorrhoeae:* intravenous penicillin G Penicillin-resistant gonorrhea: intramuscular (Kantrex), cefotaxime (Claforan), or ceftriaxone (Rocephin) plus topical erythromycin or tetracycline
Chlamydial	Neutrophils, lymphocytes, plasma cells (Gram)	McCoy cell culture	ELISA, rapid fluorescent antibody test, in situ DNA hybridization	PO erythromycin estolate (Ilosone) or ethylsuccinate (EES) plus topical tetracycline, erythromycin, or sulfacetamide drops
Herpetic	Lymphocytes, plasma cells, multinucleate giant cells (Gram) Eosinophilic intranuclear inclusions in epithelial cells (Papanicolaou)	Viral cultures	Virus particle identification on electron microscopy, antigen detection tests	Intravenous acyclovir (Zovirax) plus topical trifluridine (Viroptic)

From O'Hara MA: Ophthalmia neonatorum. Pediatr Clin North Am *40:*715–725, 1993.

of the conjunctiva for several days until the purulence resolves. An ophthalmologist should be consulted to monitor the status of the eyes. The child's mother and her sexual contacts should be evaluated and treated.

C. trachomatis is a modified bacterium that is an obligate intracellular parasite; it can infect the genital tract, the respiratory tract, and the eye. The incidence of neonatal conjunctivitis due to *Chlamydia* in the United States is 8.2 per 1000 live births, or about 73,800 cases per year. It appears as mild to moderate erythema of the conjunctiva that is more apparent on the palpebral rather than the bulbar conjunctiva. No preauricular lymph nodes or follicles are present owing to the immaturity of the neonate's immune system. Treatment is with systemic erythromycin and topical erythromycin or tetracycline (erythromycin estolate [Ilosone], 10 mg per kg three times daily; or erythromycin ethylsuccinate [EES], 50 mg per kg per day in divided doses for 14 days; topical tetracycline or sulfacetamide [Sulamyd] drops or erythromycin ointment, four times daily for 2 to 3 weeks). The mother should be treated systemically; tetracycline should be avoided in mothers who are breast-feeding.

Viral conjunctivitis in the neonate is almost always herpetic and is seen in 40 to 60% of infants born to mothers with active genital infections. These infections are usually herpes type II; however, type I has been isolated. There is erythema of the conjunctiva and edema of the lids on presentation, with a mucopurulent discharge. This entity can be associated with central nervous system herpes or disseminated disease. The diagnosis is confirmed by the characteristic vesicular skin lesions or a corneal dendrite, if present; otherwise a maternal history of herpes is helpful in making the diagnosis. Conjunctival scrapings can be cultured and evaluated with the Papanicolaou technique, which shows eosinophilic intranuclear inclusion bodies. Antigen detection methods are also available. Treatment is with intravenous acyclovir (Zovirax), 10 mg per kg every 8 to 10 hours, and topical trifluridine (Viroptic), 1 drop five times per day. Overtreatment with topical antivirals should be avoided. Ophthalmic consultation is recommended.

IRRITATIVE CONJUNCTIVITIS

Many agents in the environment can cause irritation of the conjunctiva by direct contact. They include drugs, chemicals, foreign bodies, pollutants, and organic matter. The treatment usually involves removal of the toxic agent, if possible. Topical therapy can include artificial tears, topical antibiotics to prevent secondary infection, and topical steroids in a weak concentration. Consultation with an ophthalmologist is useful, especially if topical steroids are used. If the agent cannot be removed from the environment, measures must be taken to reduce the exposure, such as use of occlusive goggles.

VARICELLA

(Chickenpox, Herpes Zoster)

method of
BARBARA WATSON, M.B., CH.B.
Einstein Medical Center and Division of Disease Control
Philadelphia, Pennsylvania

Varicella-zoster virus (VZV) is a herpesvirus; only one strain is recognized. Humans are the only source of infection. Like other members of the herpesvirus family (cytomegalovirus, Epstein-Barr virus, herpes simplex virus), VZV establishes latency after primary infection; the clinical syndrome is described as chickenpox. Subclinical periodic reactivation of latent virus may occur; when clinical reactivation occurs, the clinical syndrome is described as herpes zoster (shingles).

PATHOPHYSIOLOGY OF VARICELLA-ZOSTER VIRUS

Humoral immunity is sometimes insufficient to provide protection. Severe varicella is due more to impairment of the cell-mediated immune response than to a defect in humoral immunity. Healthy children who develop cell-mediated immune response after the varicella exanthem have mild primary VZV infection, whereas immunodeficient children who fail to develop VZV-specific lymphocyte proliferation develop progressive disseminated varicella. Adults have impaired cell-mediated responses and are 35 times more likely to die of varicella than healthy children who contract chickenpox. Elderly adults and patients on immunosuppressive therapy have lower VZV-specific lymphocyte proliferation and are more likely to reactivate VZV, resulting in herpes zoster. A decrease in cell-mediated immunity is a necessary but insufficient setting for the development of zoster. Reactivation of the virus in the ganglia may occur sporadically without regard to immune function but may be more likely to be symptomatic if cell-mediated immunity is depressed.

EPIDEMIOLOGY

Person-to-person transmission occurs by direct contact between varicella or zoster and respiratory secretions. Varicella is most common during late winter and early spring in temperate climates and demonstrates cyclical peaks that correspond to the number of susceptible persons in the population. The most recent peak season was 1995. In tropical countries the disease is much less common in children, occurs more in urban than in rural areas, and therefore leaves many adults susceptible—a point that physicians who practice with a large immigrant population from tropical countries need to keep in mind. The introduction of an index case of varicella into a home results in transmission of the virus to susceptibles and secondary cases of disease in 98% of susceptibles. Secondary cases in this circumstance usually have more severe disease. Until recently, most reported cases occurred in children between the ages of 5 and 9 years. When both parents work and children are in day care, VZV infection has shifted to the 1- to 4-year-old age group and is associated with an increase in severity of complications. Immunity from natural disease is usually lifelong, but symptomatic reinfections do occur; more common are asymptomatic reinfections (with a fourfold boost in antibody level). Immunocompromised individuals with either primary varicella or zoster are at risk for severe disease. Disease is also more severe in infants (younger then 3 months), adolescents, adults, those on steroids or chronic aspirin, and those with pulmonary disorders.

The incubation period is 10 to 21 days after contact. Persons are most contagious 2 days before the rash appears and until 5 days after crops of lesions stop appearing (which takes longer in the immunocompromised).

The clinical diagnosis of VZV infection is made in accordance with time of year (for the United States and temperate countries, a typical rash that has multiple stages of macules, papules, vesicles, and pustules) and history of not previously having varicella. The macules evolve into papules and vesicles over a 24-hour period, with new lesions occurring at 3-day intervals. The vesicles become pustular if the person has a competent immune response; they proceed to rupture and crust over. In an immunocompetent host, this period takes 5 to 7 days. The most commonly associated symptom is high fever (higher than 40°C [104°F] in 30% of cases).

Other complications include secondary bacterial infection, particularly a notable increase in toxigenic group A streptococci and *Staphylococcus*. Varicella pneumonitis is more common in adults and infants. Gastrointestinal complications associated with viscous involvement, idiopathic thrombocytopenia (ITP) and bleeding diathesis, nephritis, transverse myelitis, and encephalitis can occur. Other complications include disseminated intravascular coagulation, which may occur at any time during the illness. These complications are associated with significant morbidity and may occur irrespective of the use of acyclovir (Zovirax).

Congenital varicella syndrome risk is about 2% and is greatest in the first trimester. The syndrome that occurs in the first or second trimester of pregnancy is characterized by limb atrophy and scarring of the extremities. Central nervous system and ocular manifestations also occur. A pregnant woman in the second or third trimester of pregnancy behaves like an immunocompromised host and has a higher incidence of the previously mentioned complications, with a mortality of 30% for the mother and the newborn who develops varicella.

LABORATORY AIDS TO DIAGNOSIS

VZV can be demonstrated in the vesicular lesions by immunoflourescence—this should be standard for most hospital viral laboratories. Also VZV may be cultured from skin lesions and nasopharyngeal or tracheal aspirates. The Tzanck preparation, a method of staining scrapings of the base of lesions with Giemsa or Wright's stain, demonstrates the multinucleated giant cells but does not differentiate between VZV and herpes simplex. Acute and convalescent sera are required for antibody testing. Various assays are used by different laboratories, including EIA, IFA, LA, FAMA. These tests can also be used to determine immunity; however, it is important to remember that immunity is also dependent on cell-mediated mechanisms. The absence of antibody by the previously mentioned commercially available serologic assays, which are not as sensitive as the glycoprotein ELISA assays that were performed to assess immune antibody response in the clinical trials of varicella vaccine, does not necessarily indicate susceptibility. The complement fixation test is not reliable for determining immunity in any setting.

DIFFERENTIAL DIAGNOSIS

The appearance of a typical rash that occurs in successive crops of macules, papules, and vesicles is distinctive.

However, with limited rash or mild rash, the differential diagnosis includes other causes of vesiculation, such as coxsackievirus infection with hand, foot, and mouth disease; rickettsialpox; infection with *Mycoplasma* or *Pseudomonas* (in immunocompromised individuals); eczema herpeticum or herpes zoster with dissemination; toxic epidermal necrolysis; scabies in infants; and various noninfectious vesicular conditions of the skin.

PROGNOSIS

Varicella-Zoster Virus

Fifty to 100 previously healthy children die each year from varicella and more than 9000 are hospitalized. Adults and immunocompromised persons die at a 35 times higher rate than healthy children. For most children, this childhood exanthem is a benign disease that lasts 6 to 8 days. With the advent of universal immunization, complications of varicella will become past history.

Herpes Zoster

In children herpes zoster occurs at an incidence of 77 per 100,000 of those who have had natural VZV infection and is usually a benign, self-limiting disease, rarely complicated by dissemination and postherpetic neuralgia. In adults the incidence of zoster rises to 131 per 100,000 of those who have had primary VZV infection and manifests with a typical rash, which occurs in successive crops of macules, papules, and vesicles involving one or more dermatomes unilaterally. The incidence of postherpetic neuralgia increases with age.

TREATMENT

Treatment of chickenpox in healthy children younger than 11 years is primarily symptomatic. Antihistamines (diphenhydramine [Benadryl] and hydroxyzine [Atarax]) are useful for pruritus. Colloidal oatmeal (Aveeno) baths or calamine lotion are topical agents that alleviate pruritus.

Acyclovir, vidarabine* (Vira-A), famciclovir* (Famvir),* foscarnet* (Foscavir), and a number of antivirals in clinical trials have been shown to be effective against VZV. At present acyclovir is the drug of choice, although a number of other antivirals have the advantage of increased half-life (reducing the timing of doses to three times a day).

Any child, adolescent, or adult who is ill enough to warrant hospitalization should be treated with acyclovir (IV dose of 1500 mg per m^2 divided into three doses every 8 hours). Oral acyclovir (adult dose is 800 mg four times daily for 5 days) should be prescribed for adolescents and adults, those with chronic cutaneous or pulmonary disorders, persons on short or intermittent corticosteroids or aerosolized corticosteroids, newborn infants, and selected immunocompromised persons at risk for severe varicella. Oral acyclovir (80 mg per kg per day divided in four doses every 6 hours) should be prescribed for children and adults who present with ophthalmic zoster, and these children should be referred to an ophthalmologist if ocular involvement beyond simple conjunctivitis is suspected. Consider oral acyclovir (80 mg per kg per day divided in four doses every 6 hours) for children older than 12 years of age.

Acyclovir and famciclovir, 500 mg three times a day for 7 days, and valacyclovir (Valtrex), 1 gram orally three times a day for 7 days, have been shown to reduce the incidence of postherpetic neuralgia, and thus I recommend the use of these antivirals in adults with herpes zoster. For immunocompromised adults with zoster, acyclovir administered intravenously initially (at the same dose described earlier for varicella) is preferred by most of our group practice; when patients demonstrate a prompt response to intravenous therapy, they can be switched to oral acyclovir.

Acyclovir is safe in pregnancy and should be given to pregnant women with varicella. Zoster in pregnancy has not been shown to be associated with increased complications for the mother or fetus, and thus use of antivirals is debatable.

Children with varicella should not receive salicylates because of the association with Reye's syndrome. Acetaminophen may be used to control the fever. Nonsteroidal anti-inflammatory drugs may increase the incidence of bacterial superinfection.

ISOLATION OF HOSPITALIZED PATIENTS WITH CHICKENPOX OR SHINGLES

Strict isolation for the duration of vesicular eruption (usually 5 days, longer in the immunocompromised) is recommended. Patients should be in negative pressure rooms if possible. Susceptible persons who have been exposed should be kept in strict isolation from 8 to 21 days after the onset of the rash in the index patient. Those who received varicella-zoster immune globulin (VZIG) should be kept in isolation for 28 days after exposure.

Immunocompromised patients who have zoster (localized or generalized) and normal patients with disseminated zoster should remain in strict isolation for the duration of the illness. For normal patients with localized zoster, drainage and secretion precautions are recommended until all lesions are crusted.

PREVENTION

All susceptible persons should undergo immunization; passive protection can be achieved with the use of VZIG.

Immunization

Extensive clinical trials have been conducted in Japan, Belgium, and the United States to evaluate the safety, immunogenicity, and transmissibility of vaccine virus, including comparative studies of various vaccine preparations, dose titration, efficacy (of which there is only one placebo-controlled study),

*Not FDA approved for this indication.

consistency, and persistence of the immune response and have resulted in licensure of the varicella vaccine. These guide recommendations for the proposed use of the vaccine in the following groups:

1. Healthy children: eventually if all children are immunized routinely against varicella, most children who become immunocompromised will have already been immunized (as is the case with measles-mumps rubella and *Haemophilus influenzae* type B).
2. Healthy adolescents and adults.
3. Immunocompromised individuals.
4. The elderly, to include adults older than 40 years of age, to prevent zoster by boosting the cell-mediated immune responses.
5. Possibly postexposure prophylaxis in preference to use of VZIG.
6. Vaccine is available by protocol for acute lymphatic leukemia in remission (telephone 215-283-0897).

For persons who cannot receive VZV vaccine on the basis of immunocompromised states, varicella-susceptible pregnant women (until the VZV vaccine registry has data to make alternate recommendations), and newborns, VZIG is still recommended. The Vaccine for Children Fund does cover VZV vaccine. It is unlikely that a booster dose of VZV vaccine will be necessary because 98% of individuals seroconvert with one dose and persistence of immunity during trials has been shown to be 10 years in the United States and 20 years in Japan. Also, surveillance procedures have been established to track the baseline incidence of varicella before licensure of the varicella vaccine and to follow the patterns of disease postlicensure. However, with licensure of an MMRV (measles-mumps-rubella-varicella vaccine)* that will have a two-dose schedule, the issue may be moot. Current immunization rates for 2-year-olds nationwide vary from 80% in some private pediatric offices to 18% in rural general practices. It is important that varicella immunization be as universal as measles to eliminate susceptibles who can then transmit the virus to members of the society who are at high risk for complications from VZV. In early studies in the elderly, use of VZV vaccine to boost cell-mediated immune responses has shown efficacy in preventing zoster. This may be a future use of the vaccine.

Passive Immunity

Treatment with VZIG is indicated for susceptible individuals at increased risk for severe disease, including pregnant women, newborns, and immunocompromised persons. The dose is 125 units (1 vial) per 10 kg body weight (minimum is 1 vial and maximum is 5 vials). This is available from the local Red Cross offices or blood banks.

Acyclovir has been used as postexposure prophylaxis and appears to give the most benefit in the second half of the incubation phase in immunocompetent individuals. Its use as a prophylaxis for individuals who are immunocompromised has not been established, and VZIG is recommended in those circumstances. With the advent of universal immunization, the need for postexposure prophylaxis should disappear.

*Not yet approved for use in the United States.

CHOLERA

method of
S. K. BHATTACHARYA, M.D., and
G. BALAKRISH NAIR, PH.D.
National Institute of Cholera and Enteric Diseases
Calcutta, India

Cholera, an ancient and dreadful disease, is characterized by uncontrolled purging of watery stools leading to life-threatening dehydration, hypovolemic shock, acidosis, and—if left untreated—death. Cholera is caused by *Vibrio cholerae,* a motile, gram-negative curved rod with a single polar flagellum. On the basis of the somatic O antigen, *V. cholerae* is classified into more than 155 serogroups, but only the O1 and O139 serogroups are capable of causing cholera. The O1 serogroup occurs as two biotypes—classic and ElTor—and each biotype has two serotypes, Ogawa and Inaba. From the beginning of the seventh pandemic of cholera between 1961 and 1992, the ElTor biotype was responsible for all cholera outbreaks, although cases caused by the classic biotype occurred till recently in southern Bangladesh. In September 1992, cholera workers and researchers noted an unprecedented event: the emergence of a new strain of *V. cholerae* non-O1 in southern India, which was responsible for explosive outbreaks of cholera. Within the span of a year, this new strain spread to all cholera endemic areas in India and neighboring countries; imported cases caused by this non-O1 strain were also reported from the United Kingdom, the United States, Germany, and Switzerland. The epidemic causing *V. cholerae* non-O1 strain was classified as *V. cholerae* O139 Bengal.

A feature that distinguishes both O1 and O139 from other serogroups of *V. cholerae* is their ability to produce cholera toxin (CT), a potent enterotoxin. Ingestion of as little as 5 μg of pure CT has caused between 1 and 6 liters of diarrheal stool in five of six human volunteers. The clinical state of cholera is, therefore, principally attributed to CT. The toxin is composed of one A (enzymatic) subunit and five identical B (binding) subunits. The molecular weights of the A and B subunits are 27 Kilodaltons and

TABLE 1. **Electrolyte Composition of Cholera Stool and Intravenous Solutions in Use**

	Mean Concentration (mmol/L)			
	Na^+	K^+	Cl^-	HCO_3
Cholera stool				
Adult	135	15	100	45
Children	105	25	90	30
Lactated Ringer's	131	4	109	28
Normal saline	154	0	154	0

11.7 Kilodaltons, respectively. Intact A subunit is not enzymatically active but must be nicked to produce fragments A1 (molecular weight 22 Kilodaltons) and A2 (molecular weight 5 Kilodaltons). The B subunit binds the toxin to the eukaryotic cell receptor, the G_{MI} ganglioside, which is ubiquitous in the body, whereas the A1 subunit functions intracellularly as an enzyme to activate adenylate cyclase, which results in increased levels of cyclic adenosine monophosphate, leading to hypersecretion of salt and water. The net effect of this is an outpouring of copious amount of fluids rich in electrolytes (Table 1), manifesting as watery stools. Other putative toxins produced by *V. cholerae* O1 or O139 such as the Zona occludens toxin and accessory cholera toxin are believed to exacerbate the fluid secretion process and thereby contribute to the disease but in ways not yet precisely discerned.

During the past 4 decades, intensive research has contributed substantially to our understanding of the epidemiology and clinical management of cholera. Now we know that in more than 90% of cases, cholera is mild and may therefore be difficult to distinguish from other causes of acute diarrhea, for example, diarrhea caused by enterotoxigenic *Escherichia coli.* In a minority of cases, however, the dramatic onset of severe watery diarrhea and vomiting results in the loss of large amounts of fluid and electrolytes from the body, so much so that an otherwise healthy adult quickly (within 2 to 3 hours) becomes thirsty, stops urinating, and becomes weak and dehydrated with imperceptible pulse. In fact, in a matter of few minutes the patient may collapse and die if not treated promptly and adequately. The response to proper treatment is so gratifying that within 3 to 4 hours the patient starts talking, may sit up, and even walk.

TREATMENT

The objective of treatment is essentially replacement of fluid and electrolyte losses. Use of an appropriate antibiotic in severe cases is only to reduce the purging rate. A typical patient with severe cholera is extremely floppy, lethargic, or even unconscious and has sunken and dry eyes. The mouth and tongue are very dry, the person drinks poorly or not at all, and the skin pinch goes back very slowly. The radial pulse is feeble or even imperceptible, and blood pressure is very low or at times unrecordable. Such patients often have cramps in the stomach, arms, and legs. The voice is hoarse. The cold and clammy extremities with wrinkled hands and feet are known as "washerwoman's hands." Oliguria and even anuria may ensue if dehydration is not corrected promptly by administration of intravenous (IV) fluids and electrolytes. The stools in a typical patient rapidly become clear without fecal matter, have a mild fishy odor, and contain only flecks of mucus (rice water stool). Children, particularly those who are malnourished, may develop profound hypoglycemia and have convulsions, or may be comatose.

REHYDRATION THERAPY

Rapid bedside clinical assessment is adequate for formulating a treatment plan for an individual patient; laboratory tests are not required in the majority of cases. Replacement of fluid and electrolytes (rehydration therapy) can be done by either oral or IV routes depending on the degree of dehydration with which the patient presents. The discovery of oral rehydration therapy (ORT) has revolutionized the treatment of cholera. Ninety percent of cases of cholera with mild to moderate dehydration are successfully rehydrated by oral rehydration solution (ORS) alone. The composition of ORS recommended by the World Health Organization (WHO) is shown in Table 2. This solution has a total osmolality of 331 or 311, depending on whether bicarbonate or citrate is used in preparing the ORS. Glucose in ORS facilitates the absorption of sodium (and water) from the intestine of cholera patients. As a general guide, the approximate amount of ORS required (in mL) can be calculated by multiplying the patient's weight (in kg) by 75. The calculated amount of ORS should be furnished to the care provider with the advice that if the patient is a child, the ORS should be given in small quantities at regular intervals during the first 4 to 6 hours, by which time the initial deficit should be corrected. If the child vomits, administration of ORS should be stopped for 5 to 10 minutes and restarted more slowly. Adults can drink as much as they desire. WHO ORS does not reduce the stool output and may be a cause for anxiety to the patient or the care provider. To overcome this drawback of WHO ORS, glucose in this formulation has been replaced by 50 grams of rice powder. Rice-based ORS may be available in packets containing precooked rice powder. Alternatively, uncooked rice powder may be added to water, boiled for 5 minutes, and allowed to cool before adding salts in the same concentration as that for standard WHO ORS. In cholera patients, rice ORS reduces stool output by about 35% compared with that in patients treated with standard WHO ORS. Use of reduced osmolarity of ORS solution may be of some clinical benefit in reducing stool output but requires further confirmation.

All cholera patients with severe dehydration should be rehydrated initially with IV fluid and electrolytes. The preferred solution is lactated Ringer's, which contains adequate amounts of sodium, potassium, and lactate (see Table 1); the lactate is converted in the liver to bicarbonate, which corrects the metabolic acidosis. If lactated Ringer's is not available, normal saline may be used with concurrent

TABLE 2. **World Health Organization–Recommended Oral Rehydration Salt Solution**

	Grams/L		Mmol/L
Sodium chloride	3.5	Sodium	90
Trisodium citrate, dihydrate	2.9	Chloride	80
or			
Sodium bicarbonate	2.5	Potassium	20
Potassium chloride	1.5	Citrate	10
		or	
Glucose (anhydrous)	20.0	Bicarbonate	30
		Glucose	111

administration of ORS. IV fluid should be given in a dose of 100 mL per kg; infants (younger than 12 months) should receive 30 mL per kg in the first hour and 70 mL per kg in the next 5 hours, whereas older children and adults should receive 30 mL per kg in the first 30 minutes and 70 mL per kg in the next 2½ hours. After starting the IV fluids, reassessment of the patient should be done every 1 to 2 hours. If dehydration does not improve, the fluid should be given more rapidly. After 6 hours (infants) or 3 hours (older patients), the patient's condition must be evaluated. If the radial pulse still remains very weak or undetectable, the same may be repeated once. Cholera patients started on IV therapy should be given ORS as soon as they can drink, even before the initial IV therapy has been completed. If possible, IV treatment should be done by admitting the patient to the hospital.

Once the initial deficit has been corrected, the state of hydration could be maintained by matching intake with output using ORS. Even in severe cholera after correction of initial deficit with IV fluid, maintenance may be done with ORS except in a few cases in which IV infusion may have to be given again due to continuing severe purging. As a guide, after each loose stool, children younger than 2 years of age should receive 50 to 100 mL of oral fluid, children aged 2 to 10 years 100 to 200 mL, and older children and adults should drink as much oral fluid as they want. Breast-feeding should be continued. Plain drinking water should be given as and when desired.

ROLE OF ANTIBIOTICS

Although virtually all cholera patients can be managed successfully with fluid therapy alone, a marked reduction of purging is achieved in severely dehydrated cholera patients by using appropriate antibiotic therapy as an adjunct to fluid replacement. Antibiotics also shorten the duration of excretion of vibrio in the stool and thereby reduce the period of hospitalization. Antibiotics should be started after the patient is rehydrated (usually 4 to 6 hours) and vomiting has stopped. The antibiotics of choice are oral tetracycline (50 mg per kg of body weight per day in four divided doses for 3 days), doxycycline (300 mg in a single dose for adults only), or furazolidone (Furoxone) (5 mg per kg per day in four divided doses for 3 days). Tetracycline may not be available for pediatric use in some countries owing to its ill effects of staining teeth and accumulation in the growing ends of the bone. Trimethoprim/sulfamethoxazole (Bactrim, Septra) is the antimicrobial of choice in children. However, *V. cholerae* O139 isolated in 1992 and the recent strains of *V. cholerae* O1 isolated in certain cholera endemic areas are resistant to trimethoprim/sulfamethoxazole. Erythromycin or chloramphenicol may be used when the antibiotics recommended earlier are not available or when *V. cholerae* O1 or O139 is resistant to them. In view of the reported emergence of resistant strains of *V. cholerae* O1 and O139 to some of these drugs in some areas, norfloxacin* (Noroxin) (400 mg twice daily for 3 days) and ciprofloxacin* (Cipro) (500 mg twice daily for 3 days) have been shown to be effective alternatives. Ciprofloxacin and norfloxacin have been incriminated as causing cartilage toxicity in experimental animals and hence are not currently recommended for use in children and pregnant women. Furazolidone is the antibiotic of choice for pregnant women. The choice of antibiotic should take into account local patterns of resistance to antibiotics. Antibiotic-resistant *V. cholerae* O1 or O139 should be suspected if diarrhea continues after 48 hours of antibiotic treatment.

Antidiarrheal agents and other drugs such as kaolin, pectin, activated charcoal, opium, diphenoxylate with atropine, loperamide, steroids, stimulants, and antiemetics are not indicated in the treatment of cholera patients. In fact, some of these drugs are very harmful, particularly in children, and their use should be discouraged. Antiemetics should not be used, as they produce sedation and interfere with ORT. They may also produce hypotension, which may interfere with renal filtration. Anticholinergic agents should not be used because they are useless and may produce paralytic ileus.

DIET

Maintenance of nutrition during an attack of cholera is also important. Uninterrupted breast-feeding along with easily digestible, energy-dense, high potassium–containing nonfibrous food should be given to children as soon as possible. Normal diet should be resumed in adults soon after initial rehydration.

COMPLICATIONS

Prompt and effective case management based on rehydration therapy will prevent most of the complications of cholera. Risk of pyrogen reaction, excessive hydration, or too-rapid correction of hypernatremia or hyponatremia or acidosis is minimized by optimal use of ORT, and early resumption of food will prevent the development of hypoglycemia. Renal failure may occur due to delay or insufficient fluid administration.

PREVENTION

With contaminated water being the most common source of infection, it is important to pay close attention to safe drinking water to prevent this illness. Raw vegetables or seafoods and other moist foods maintained at room temperature are also high-risk items, and therefore consumption of adequately heated or boiled food is important for prevention. Washing hands with soap and water, using clean water for drinking and washing utensils and other activities, and appropriate excreta disposal are useful preventive measures.

*Not FDA approved for this indication.

Vaccination against cholera is an attractive disease prevention strategy, because recovery from infection results in long-lived protective immunity. Parenteral inactivated whole cell cholera vaccines, which have been available for more than a century, offer only short-term protection and have been discontinued globally. Two new cholera vaccines—the inactivated oral whole cell recombinant B subunit vaccine and the live oral CVD-103HgR vaccine—are marketed in Sweden and Switzerland, respectively. A group of WHO experts observed that the killed whole cell B subunit oral vaccine (CHOLERIX)* could be considered for use in cholera prevention or control in emergencies. The recommendation for vaccination applies primarily to high-risk situations, such as refugee or displaced populations (either coming from or located in endemic areas) at risk or in natural disaster situations, when the crude death rates due to cholera are below 1 to 2 per 10,000 persons per day. WHO discourages vaccination as a means of personal protection for foreign travel.

*Not yet approved for use in the United States.

FOOD-BORNE ILLNESS

method of
RICHARD N. GREENBERG, M.D.
University of Kentucky School of Medicine
Lexington, Kentucky

The diagnosis of a food-borne illness mixes clinical and epidemiologic skills. The diagnosis includes a targeted history, physical examination, specific laboratory tests, and suspicion. Initially, treatment is directed at the symptoms. However, identification of the causative agent is important, not only for defining the treatment for a complicated illness but also for establishing a strategy to prevent additional cases and outbreaks.

The targeted history should include the timing of onset and duration of symptoms, a travel history, a detailed food history, and an inquiry about others with similar symptoms. Physical examination needs to establish the degree of dehydration as well as identification of other abnormalities. In severe disease, assessment of the circulatory, respiratory, and neurologic systems is essential.

Consultation with laboratory personnel may be necessary to establish the causative agent. In some instances, detection of the suspected agent may require special tests often not available in community hospitals. As most food-borne illnesses are self-limited, treatment is mostly symptomatic. Diarrheal illnesses not associated with inflammatory colitis are treated with antispasmodic agents such as loperamide (Imodium) or diphenoxylate (Lomotil). Vomiting is treated with antiemetics such as prochlorperazine (Compazine), promethazine (Phenergan), or trimethobenzamide (Tigan). Dehydration may be managed by oral rehydration if the patient is not septic, in shock, vomiting, obtunded, malabsorbing, or with an ileus. Oral rehydration fluid therapy should follow World Health Organization guidelines (i.e., per liter of water: 3.5 grams NaCl, 2.5 grams $NaHCO_3$, 1.5 grams KCl, and 20 grams glucose). A homemade recipe is ¾ tablespoon of table salt, 1 teaspoon of baking soda, 1 cup of orange juice, and 4 tablespoons of table sugar to 1.05 quarts of water. Commercial oral rehydration products are also available such as Pedialyte, Rehydralyte, Resol, and Infalyte. Less expensive oral rehydration therapy packets are available as "Oral Rehydration Salts" from Jianas Brothers Packaging Co., Kansas City, MO (816-421-2880), Travel Medicine, Northampton, MA (800-872-8633), and as "CeraLyte" from Cera Products, Inc., Columbia, MD (301-490-4941 or 888-237-2598).

Pursuing the causative agent requires developing a case definition based on symptoms and signs. If multiple individuals have been exposed, an excellent tool to establish the vehicle of transmission and clues to the cause of the outbreak is a food exposure questionnaire. The questionnaire should be administered to those who were potentially exposed, whether ill or not. A comparison of attack rates usually identifies the putative food item. A subsequent examination of how that item was prepared should expose the cause of the outbreak. Public health measures to curtail additional related outbreaks are then developed.

Food-borne disease may be caused by viruses, bacteria, protozoans, parasites, toxins, plants, and chemicals. Although most food-borne illnesses are caused by bacteria, other agents must be considered. Table 1 has been adapted from numerous sources. The table provides etiologic agents, associated food vehicles, and treatments and is organized according to incubation time. The case definition (signs and symptoms) and incubation time are key clinical clues. Differential diagnoses, laboratory tests, and treatments are based on these clues.

TRENDS IN FOOD-BORNE DISEASE

Current trends in food-borne illness are the emergence of newly recognized pathogens and the increase in prevalence of well-recognized pathogens. Food-borne disease is increasing in industrialized countries owing to changes in food processing, populations at risk, sabotage, "international" produce (i.e., produce shipped to another country), mass-distributed food products, and increases in the amount of food eaten away from home. More than 80% of reported outbreaks in the United States are due to food eaten outside the home.

Perhaps the most notorious newly identified agent is *Escherichia coli* O157:H7. Outbreaks and cases are often associated with consumption of undercooked ground beef (e.g., hamburgers), lettuce, raw milk, raw cider, untreated water, or foods cross-contaminated with beef. Person-to-person transmission occurs. In addition to causing bloody diarrhea, *E. coli* O157:H7 infection is the most common cause of the hemolytic uremic syndrome (HUS) and acute kidney failure in children in the United States. HUS is asso-

TABLE 1. **Agents Causing Food-Borne Illnesses**

Agent	Symptoms	Comments	Treatment
	Onset Within 6 Hours		
Staphylococcus aureus	Abrupt onset of nausea, vomiting, cramps, diarrhea, and prostration	Dairy products, custards, meats, due to ingestion of heat-stable enterotoxin	Self-limited, fluids
Bacillus cereus	Vomiting, nausea	Fried rice, due to heat-stable emetic toxin	Self-limited, fluids
Ciguatera fish poisoning	Nausea, vomiting, diarrhea, followed by pruritus, paresthesia, dry mouth, photophobia; severe poisoning: possible neuropathy, shock, and respiratory paralysis	Grouper, red snapper, barracuda, amberjack	Emesis induction, gastric lavage, atropine for brachycardia; intravenous mannitol may improve acute neurologic symptoms; tocainide may help with persistent dysesthesias
Scombroid poisoning	Histamine-like symptoms, flushing, pruritus, urticaria, headache, nausea, vomiting	Spoiled fish	Antihistamines, bronchodilator as needed
Puffer fish poisoning	Weakness, paresthesia, abdominal pain, general flaccid ascending paralysis; can be lethal	Puffer fish	Supportive treatment
Paralytic shellfish poisoning	Nausea, vomiting, diarrhea, facial paresthesias, paralysis including respiratory compromise	Mussels, clams, oysters; caused by neurotoxin (saxitoxin) associated with a red tide	Emetics and cathartics, fluids, supportive treatment
Neurotoxin shellfish poisoning	Nausea, vomiting, paresthesias	Shellfish from the Gulf Coast or Florida's Atlantic coast	Fluids
Amnesiac shellfish poisoning	Nausea, vomiting, diarrhea, confusion, cardiovascular compromise	Mussels contaminated with domoic acid	Fluids, supportive treatment
Mushroom poisoning	At least five syndromes occur within 2 hours		Cathartics, emetics, supportive treatment in addition to the following:
	(1) Delirium	*Amanita* spp.	Physostigmine may help
	(2) Parasympathetic hyperactivity	*Inocybe* spp. *Clitocybe* spp.	Atropine for bradycardia
	(3) Hallucinations	*Psilocybe* spp. *Panaeolus* spp.	
	(4) Disulfiram reaction	*Coprinus* spp.	Avoid alcohol
	(5) Gastroenteritis	Many	
	Two other syndromes have a longer incubation (6–24 h)	Illness is biphasic with self-limited gastroenteritis followed by organ failure	
	(6) Gastroenteritis, hepatorenal syndrome	*Gulerina* spp. *Amanita* spp.	Hemoperfusion, intravenous pyridoxine for neurologic symptoms, thioctic acid[1]
	(7) Gastroenteritis, hepatic failure	*Gyromitra* spp.	Hemoperfusion, intravenous pyridoxine for neurologic symptoms, thioctic acid[1]
Plant-derived foods	(1) Hemolytic crises	Fava beans	Blood transfusion may be necessary
	(2) Abdominal pain, diarrhea, confusion	Potato tubers (solanine poisoning)	Supportive treatment
	(3) Hyperventilation, headache, paralysis, seizures	Cyanide-containing plants (lima beans, unripe sorghum, bitter almonds, apricot almonds, apple seeds)	
Monosodium glutamate	Nausea, headache, flushing, burning sensation in skin	"Chinese restaurant syndrome"	Self-limited
Heavy metals	Nausea, vomiting, diarrhea, taste alterations, myalgias	Copper, zinc, tin, cadmium	Self-limited, fluids
	Onset Within 24 Hours		
Clostridium perfringens	Cramps, diarrhea, nausea, vomiting	Institutional settings, large quantities of food prepared, improper storage temperatures of large pieces of meat	Self-limited, fluids
Bacillus cereus	Cramps, diarrhea (rare hepatotoxicity)	Spices, meat, eggs, dairy products, soups, puddings, sauces; due to heat-labile enterotoxin	Fluids, self-limited

TABLE 1. **Agents Causing Food-Borne Illnesses** *Continued*

Agent	Symptoms	Comments	Treatment
Clostridium botulinum	Diplopia, drooping eyelids, slurred speech, difficulty swallowing, diarrhea, vomiting, paralysis	Onset as early as 6 h or as late as 10 d; home-canned foods (vegetables, fruits), chopped garlic in oil, chili peppers, tomatoes, fermented fish, improperly handled baked potatoes wrapped in aluminum foil	Antitoxin, supportive care; recovery can take months
Escherichia coli (not enterohemorrhagic or enteroinvasive)	Cramps, watery diarrhea, occasional fever	Travel (turista), tuna paste, contaminated water	Self-limited, fluids; may shorten illness with 3 days of either fluoroquinolone[2] or TMP-SMX[3]
Shigella spp. and enteroinvasive *E. coli*	Fever, tenesmus, dysentery	Eggs, vegetables, dairy products; *Shigella* spp. are easily spread owing to effectiveness of a low inoculum	Fluids, fluoroquinolone[2] or TMP-SMX[3] for 5 days
Yersinia enterocolitica	Fever, abdominal pain, diarrhea	Pork chitterlings, tofu, and contaminated milk; can cause persistent diarrhea	Fluids, antibiotics if disease becomes complicated and should be based on susceptibility pattern
Salmonella spp. (non-typhi)	Nausea, vomiting, cramps, diarrhea	Poultry, meat, eggs, fish, dairy products, pets, fresh produce, other raw foods	Fluids, antibiotics can shorten duration; if prosthetic material present or if immunocompromised, then a fluoroquinolone[2] is recommended until afebrile for 24 h
Salmonella typhi	Systemic disease, fever, splenomegaly	Human-to-human transmission (through contaminated food)	Fluoroquinolone[2], ceftriaxone (Rocephin),[4] TMP-SMX,[3] or chloramphenicol[5] for 2 wk
Vibrio parahaemolyticus	Fever, headache, cramps, nausea, diarrhea, dysentery	Fish, shellfish, can last 5 d	Fluids, self-limited
Vibrio cholerae	Watery diarrhea ("rice water" due to copious amounts of watery stool)	Seaweed, seafood	Fluids, antibiotic (tetracycline,[6] TMP-SMX[3] or furazolidone [Furoxone])[7] for 3–5 d
Norwalk-like viruses, SRSVs	Nausea, vomiting, watery diarrhea	Shellfish, salads	Self-limited, fluids
		Onset Within 3 Days	
E. coli (enterohemorrhagic)	Bloody (or nonbloody) diarrhea, in young (1–4 y) or elderly; can progress to hemolytic uremic syndrome or thrombotic thrombocytopenia	Undercooked ground beef, raw yogurt, lettuce, contaminated water, unpasteurized cider, apple juice, fermented meats (salami)	Supportive, avoid TMP-SMX; use of other antibiotics not fully established
Streptococcus pyogenes (group A)	Nausea, vomiting, fever, pharyngitis	Dairy products (milk, eggs), meats	Antibiotic for streptococcal pharyngitis (penicillin G or V, other β-lactams, macrolides)
Campylobacter jejuni	Nausea, fever, headache, cramps, vomiting, watery diarrhea, or dysentery can be persistent. Associated with sequelae of Guillain-Barré syndrome	Poultry, raw milk, contaminated water, pets	Erythromycin[8] or fluoroquinolone[2] for 7 d
		Onset After 3 Days	
Listeria monocytogenes	Flulike symptoms, bacteremia, meningitis, encephalitis, miscarriage	Onset up to 30 d after ingestion; unpasteurized milk, undercooked meat, poultry, or fish, ready-to-eat foods, soft cheese, deli, pâté	Ampicillin[9] ± gentamicin, SMX-TMP,[10] chloramphenicol,[5] or erythromycin[8] for 3–6 wk
Vibrio vulnificus	Hemorrhagic bullous skin lesions, septicemia; can rapidly progress to death	Onset up to 1 wk after eating raw shellfish; affects people with liver disease, diabetes, or disorders of the immune system	Tetracycline,[6] ceftazidime (Fortaz),[11] or ciprofloxacin (Cipro)[12] as soon as suspected
Hepatitis A	Anorexia, nausea, vomiting, fever, fatigue	Raw or partially cooked shellfish, food handled by an infected person, such as frozen strawberries, orange juice, and hamburgers; incubation period of 15–60 d	Immunoglobulin IM (0.2–0.6 mL/kg) within 2 wk of exposure
Brucella spp.	Systemic illness with fever, headache, back pains, splenomegaly	Raw milk, milk products (goat cheese), infected animal meat, blood or marrow	Doxycycline (Vibramycin, Doryx), 100 mg bid × 6 wk plus streptomycin, 1 gm IM/d × 3 wk

Table continued on following page

TABLE 1. **Agents Causing Food-Borne Illnesses** *Continued*

Agent	Symptoms	Comments	Treatment
Giardia lamblia	Persistent watery diarrhea, weight loss, flatulence, malaise, cramps, bloating, nausea, anorexia	Contaminated water associated with foreign travel or wilderness areas	Metronidazole (Flagyl), 250 mg tid × 5 d; alternatives: furazolidone[7] for 10 d or paramomycin (Humatin), 25–35 mg/kg/d as tid × 7 d
Entamoeba histolytica	Dysentery, fever, liver abscess; can be persistent	Foreign travel, raw or undercooked meats	Treat symptomatic patients; for intraluminal cysts—diloxanide furoate (Furamide [available through CDC]), 500 mg tid (pediatric: 20 mg/kg/d as tid) × 10 days, or paromomycin, 30 mg/kg/d as tid for 5–10 d; for invasive rectocolitis or hepatic abscess—metronidazole, 750 mg (pediatric: 35–50 mg/kg/d) as tid for 10 d
Trichinella spiralis	Fever, myalgia, malaise, edema, headache	Undercooked pork; also associated with bear, walrus, horse, and boar meat	Steroids for severe symptoms plus mebendazole* (Vermox), 200–400 mg tid × 3 d and then 400–500 mg tid × 10 d†; pediatric dosage unclear**
Toxoplasma gondii	Chorioretinitis, lymphadenitis	Food contaminated with feces from infected cats or undercooked meats (beef, venison, lamb, pork)	Pyrimethamine (Daraprim), 25 mg/d (pediatric: 2 mg/kg/d × 3 d, then 1 mg/kg/d up to 25 mg/d) × 4 wk and sulfadiazine, 1–1.5 g (pediatric: 100–200 mg/kg/d), as qid × 4 wk and leucovorin, 10 mg/d × 4 wk
Cryptosporidium parvum	Self-limited watery diarrhea in immunocompetent; nausea and vomiting in immunosuppressed; weight loss due to persistent watery diarrhea, anorexia, acalculous cholecystitis	Water reservoir contaminated by cats, dogs, horses, calves; secondary spread person to person is common	Fluids; no reliable curative treatment; some experts use paromomycin, 25–35 mg/kg/d in 3 or 4 divided doses
Cyclospora cayetanensis	Relapsing watery diarrhea that can last more than 20 d, fatigue, anorexia, abdominal pain	Incubation period is 2 to 11 (median 7) d; raspberries, undercooked meats	Fluids TMP-SMX[3] × 10 d
Cestode parasites (tapeworms)	Abdominal symptoms Seizures Vitamin B_{12} deficiency Mass effects	*Hymenolepis nana* *Taenia solium* (pork)[15] *Diphyllobothrium latum* (fish) *Echinococcus* spp. (canine contaminants)[16]	Niclosamide[13]‡—single dose Praziquantel (Biltricide)[14]—single dose

[1]Thioctic acid (α-lipoic acid) is an experimental drug that may be an effective antidote. The drug may be obtained from Burton Berkson, M.D., Ph.D., in Las Cruces, New Mexico (505-524-3720 or 505-521-1609; burt@zianet.com).
[2]Fluoroquinolone: ciprofloxacin, 500 mg PO as bid; norfloxacin, 400 mg PO as bid.*§
[3]TMP-SMX: trimethoprim-sulfamethoxazole-DS (double strength) (pediatric: 5 mg/kg TMP, 25 mg/kg SMX) bid.
[4]Ceftriaxone: 2 gm (pediatric: 50–100 mg/kg) daily IV.
[5]Chloramphenicol: 500 mg (pediatric: 50–100 mg/kg/d) PO as qid.
[6]Tetracycline: 500 mg PO as qid or 2 gm daily.§
[7]Furazolidone: 6 mg/kg/d qid (can be used in children and pregnant women).
[8]Erythromycin base: 250 mg (30–50 mg/kg/d) PO as qid.
[9]Ampicillin: 200 mg/kg/d as 6 doses/d.
[10]TMP-SMX: 20 mg TMP/kg/d as qid.
[11]Ceftazidime: 1–2 gm q (pediatric: 25–50 mg/kg) q 8 h IV.
[12]Ciprofloxacin: 750 mg PO bid or 400 mg q 12 h IV.
[13]Niclosamide: 500 mg tablet: adults—2 g (4 tablets); children >34 kg—1.5 g (3 tablets); children 11–34 kg—1 g (2 tablets).
[14]Praziquantel: 5–10 mg/kg dose except for *H. nana* (dose is 25 mg/kg).
[15]Neurocysticercosis: Prolonged administration of either praziquantel (50 mg/kg/d in 5 doses for 15–30 d) or albendazole (15 mg/kg/d in 2 doses for 8–30 d†). Also may require seizure control; hydrocephalus relief if symptomatic and concurrent use of dexamethasone; individualized therapy may be needed if responses are poor.
[16]Echinococcal disease: individualized therapy that may include surgery, CT-guided instillation of 95% ethanol, and albendazole.
*Not FDA approved for this indication.
†Exceeds dosage recommended by manufacturer.
‡Not available in the United States.
§Should not be given to children younger than 18 years of age.

ciated with long-term complications; 3 to 5% of patients with HUS die, and about 12% have sequelae, including end-stage renal disease, hypertension, and neurologic injury.

Campylobacter jejuni is now considered the leading cause of food-borne bacterial infection in the United States. Most sporadic infections are associated with mishandled poultry products. Outbreaks have been associated with consumption of raw milk or unchlorinated water. The Guillain-Barré syndrome, an acute paralytic illness that may leave chronic deficits, may follow *Campylobacter* infections.

Intestinal cryptosporidiosis caused by *Cryptosporidium parvum* has been associated with contaminated water supplies, children attending day care, and consumption of freshly pressed apple cider. Selected outbreaks of other food-borne illness in the United States from 1988 to 1997 include hepatitis A (frozen strawberries), *Cyclospora cayetanensis* (raspberries), *Salmonella enteritidis* (egg-containing foods, mass-distributed ice cream, sliced cantaloupe), Norwalk-like viruses (dining on cruise ships, eating oysters from the Gulf Coast), *Toxoplasma gondii* (uncooked pork), *Trichinella spiralis* (undercooked pork), *Vibrio cholerae* (seaweed, Thai coconut milk), *Vibrio vulnificus* (shellfish harvested from warm water areas), *Listeria monocytogenes* (ready-to-eat foods including coleslaw, milk inadequately pasteurized or contaminated after pasteurization, pâté, pork tongue in jelly, and soft cheese made with inadequately pasteurized milk), *Baylisacaris procyonis* (a raccoon roundworm that when ingested causes a neurologic disease), vancomycin-resistant enterococci, and *Yersinia entercolitica* (pork chitterlings).

The spread of the prion-associated cattle illness "mad cow disease" (bovine spongiform encephalopathy) has been suggested, but not proven, to be a food-borne disease due to changes in the rendering of animals used for bone meal. Although the mechanism for the spread of the agent for bovine spongiform encephalopathy is unknown, the concern of food-borne spread to humans exists.

RAPID ONSET FOOD-BORNE DISEASE

Timing is an important clue that often leads to the correct etiology. Nausea and vomiting, with or without diarrhea, within 6 hours of ingestion suggests preformed enterotoxin disease of *Staphylococcus aureus* or *Bacillus cereus,* heavy metal poisoning, ingestion of fish contaminated with ciguatoxin, scombroid fish poisoning, puffer fish poisoning, paralytic or neurotoxic shellfish poisoning, amnesic shellfish poisoning, mushroom poisoning, ingestion of toxic plant-derived foods such as fava beans or potato tubers, or ingestion of monosodium glutamate.

Ciguatoxin is a neurotoxin that originates from dinoflagellates and contaminates fish such as grouper, red snapper, and barracuda. Predicting contamination is difficult. Gastrointestinal symptoms may be followed by pruritus, paresthesias, dry mouth, photophobia, blurred vision, cranial nerve palsies, cardiovascular collapse, and respiratory paralysis. Scombrotoxicosis is a syndrome resembling a histamine overdose. Spoiled fish such as tuna, mackerel, skipjack, and mahi-mahi is associated with this food poisoning. Improperly prepared puffer fish may lead to tetrodotoxin poisoning. Tetrodotoxin causes a general flaccid paralysis with respiratory failure.

Paralytic shellfish poisoning is caused by eating shellfish contaminated with a potent alkaloid neurotoxin that interferes with sensory, cerebellar, and motor functions. The contamination of shellfish is associated with a "red tide" event. The neurotoxin (saxitoxin) causes gastrointestinal symptoms and facial paresthesias. Severe cases lead to paralysis and death. Shellfish obtained from waters with toxic algae blooms or red tide should not be consumed. Amnesic shellfish poisoning is associated with mussels contaminated with domoic acid and results in gastrointestinal symptoms followed by mental confusion and cardiovascular instability in severe cases. Owing to monitoring of shellfish beds, shellfish poisoning in the United States is very rare. From 1973 to 1987, only 19 outbreaks with an average of eight cases per outbreak were reported.

Mushroom poisoning is usually evident by the patient's history. The type of mushroom in question often requires an expert's evaluation. *Clitocybe* and *Inocybe* species cause an anticholinergic syndrome, whereas *Amanita phalloides* and other species produce toxins that can cause not only gastrointestinal symptoms but also more serious and life-threatening hemolysis and methemoglobinuria as well as hepatic and renal failure.

Fava beans are associated with acute hemolytic anemia in individuals with glucose-6-phosphate dehydrogenase deficiency. Potato tuber ingestion may lead to gastrointestinal symptoms and mental confusion. Monosodium glutamate may cause nausea, headache, flushing, and burning sensation in the skin that resolves within 4 hours. Heavy metal ingestion should be suspected when acidic fluid such as sodium carbonate or citric acid is allowed to contact metal tubing or structures. One such incident occurred when milk shake machines were used to mix carbonated drinks.

ONSET OF FOOD-BORNE ILLNESS WITHIN ONE DAY

Gastrointestinal disease within 1 day of ingestion (6 to 24 hours) suggests enterotoxigenic disease due to *B. cereus* or *Clostridium perfringens.*

Gastroenteritis occurring after a day or two of ingestion suggests Norwalk viruses and other small, round, structured viruses (SRSVs) and several bacterial pathogens including (1) enterotoxigenic *E. coli*; (2) inflammatory diarrhea-associated bacteria such as *Salmonella, Shigella, Campylobacter, Vibrio parahaemolyticus,* enteroinvasive *E. coli,* and *Y. enterocolitica*; (3) enterohemorrhagic *E. coli* (including O157:H7); and (4) neurologic disease associated with *Clostridium botulinum. C. botulinum* is suggested if ingestion of improperly canned foods or fish (contaminated with the botulinum toxin) is associated with a symmetrical descending paralysis. Early symptoms include blurred vision, photophobia, dry mouth, dysphagia, dysphonia, and signs of gastrointestinal disease.

E. coli have so many mechanisms to cause intestinal disease and are such a common cause of gastroenteritis that in outbreak situations they should always be considered a potential causative agent if no other agent has been identified.

FOOD-BORNE DISEASE WITH A DELAYED ONSET

Food-borne pathogens with an incubation period longer than 3 days include hepatitis A, *L. monocytogenes, V. vulnificus, Brucella* species, *T. gondii, Entamoeba histolytica, C. cayetanensis, Cryptosporidium parvum,* cestode parasites (tapeworms), and *T. spiralis.*

SAFETY AND PREVENTION

As there are more than 250 different diseases described that can be caused by contaminated food and drink, only those most common or of most concern at the moment are covered in this review. The great majority of food items that are associated with food-borne illness are undercooked, contaminated, or improperly stored foods of animal origin such as meat, milk, eggs, cheese, fish, or shellfish. Most cases are single cases never associated with any outbreak. Questions about the safety of a specific food can be answered by calling the Federal Drug Administration hotline: 1-301-443-1240. Questions about meat and poultry can be addressed to the United States Department of Agriculture Meat and Poultry Division hotline: 1-800-535-4555.

As always, the best advice for prevention of food-borne disease is "boil it, cook it, peel it, or forget it." Drinking water that is suspect, especially when traveling, should be avoided.

For travelers and for individuals in less than ideal situations, it is recommended to use bottled water or water boiled for 1 minute. Bottled carbonated water is safer than uncarbonated water. If unsure, it is best to avoid Popsicles or flavored ice and to prepare ice from bottled or boiled water. Washing vegetables thoroughly with safe water is difficult and not always effective. Raw vegetables and fruits that cannot be peeled should be avoided. It is best to peel the vegetables or fruits yourself. Lastly, avoid foods and beverages from street vendors.

NECROTIZING SOFT TISSUE INFECTIONS

method of
MARK A. MALANGONI, M.D.
*Case Western Reserve University School of Medicine and MetroHealth Medical Center
Cleveland, Ohio*

DEFINITION AND CLASSIFICATION

Necrotizing soft tissue infections comprise a spectrum of diseases characterized by extensive, rapidly progressive soft tissue necrosis that usually affects the muscular fascia and subcutaneous tissue but can also affect the skin and muscles. These infections can have either an indolent or a fulminant manifestation. Their clinical course is unpredictable, and mortality is usually high. These infections can appear on any part of the body; however, the lower extremities, groin, perineum, and abdominal wall are the most common sites of involvement. Necrotizing soft tissue infections can be classified as cellulitis, fasciitis, or myositis depending on the principal area involved with necrosis. Often there is involvement of multiple soft tissue layers, so classification systems based on anatomic location are not always accurate. This group of diseases also can be subdivided into clinical syndromes based on the causative organisms; however, this type of classification is usually retrospective and is not helpful to the clinician faced with an ill patient.

Necrotizing soft tissue infections can be either primary or secondary in origin. Primary or idiopathic infections are uncommon and occur in the absence of a portal of entry for bacteria. These infections result from hematogenous bacterial spread or from direct invasion through minuscule but unrecognized epidermal lesions. The halophilic marine *Vibrio* bacteria, most commonly *Vibrio vulnificus*, can cause primary necrotizing cellulitis that occurs in predisposed individuals following the ingestion of raw seafood. Secondary necrotizing soft tissue infections are much more common and occur in patients with some compromise of the skin, subcutaneous tissue, or muscle that increases their susceptibility to these infections.

MICROBIOLOGY

Necrotizing infections of the skin and soft tissues can be due to either a single bacterium or multiple organisms. Monomicrobic infections are caused principally by *Streptococcus pyogenes* or *Clostridium perfringens* and rarely by *Pseudomonas aeruginosa* or *V. vulnificus*. These infections tend to be fulminant early in their course, in contrast to the more insidious presentation of polymicrobic infections. The rapid onset and progression of monomicrobic infections is related to the production of bacterial exotoxins, which cause extensive local tissue damage and necrosis. Monomicrobic infections occur in approximately 20% of cases.

Polymicrobic infections are caused by the synergistic activity of facultative aerobes and anaerobes. The exact microbiology varies depending on the site of involvement but generally includes both gram-positive and gram-negative organisms (Table 1). Extensive necrosis is a common feature of this heterogeneous group of infections and can occur as a result of tissue ischemia, vascular thrombosis, bacterial exotoxin–induced injury, and pressure necrosis due to inflammatory edema within closed tissue spaces.

TABLE 1. **Causative Organisms for 45 Polymicrobic Necrotizing Soft Tissue Infections (n = 127)**

Aerobes (gram-positive)	51 (40%)
Enterococci	21
Streptococcal species	11
Coagulase-negative staphylococci	10
Staphylococcus aureus	6
Bacillus species	3
Aerobes (gram-negative)	54 (43%)
Escherichia coli	15
Pseudomonas aeruginosa	13
Enterobacter cloacae	5
Klebsiella species	5
Proteus species	4
Serratia species	4
Acinetobacter calcoaceticus	3
Other	4
Anaerobes	19 (15%)
Bacteroides species	12
Clostridium species	4
Others	5
Fungi	3 (2%)

From McHenry CR, Piotrowski JJ, Petrinic D, Malangoni MA: Determinants of mortality for necrotizing soft tissue infections. Ann Surg *221*(5):560, 1995.

Soft tissue gas results when the local environment allows facultative and anaerobic bacteria to produce insoluble gases such as hydrogen, nitrogen, and methane. The presence and amount of gas in the soft tissues are variable. Soft tissue gas is characteristically absent in monomicrobic infections caused by *S. pyogenes*.

PREDISPOSING FACTORS

Secondary necrotizing soft tissue infections generally occur after an operation or injury or as a complication of inadequately treated or unrecognized infections. Extensive blunt or penetrating injury to soft tissues; burns; skin closure after contaminated or dirty abdominal, pelvic, or perineal operations; use of unsterilized needles; and human, animal, and insect bites are accompanied by bacterial inoculation sufficient to result in necrotizing infections in susceptible patients. Diseases or conditions that predispose to the spread of these infections include diabetes mellitus, immunosuppressive states, chronic debilitating diseases, vascular insufficiency, and inadequate treatment of cutaneous infections, decubitus ulcers, iscemic ulcers of the leg, perirectal or Bartholin's cyst abscesses, and strangulated hernias.

DIAGNOSIS

The diagnosis of necrotizing soft tissue infections is primarily a clinical one and should be made based on the history and physical examination. Patients frequently complain of pain that is often disproportionately severe compared with the apparent physical findings. Skin necrosis usually underrepresents the amount of underlying necrotic soft tissue. Characteristic features on examination include edema, tenderness beyond the extent of cutaneous erythema, crepitus, skin vesicles, and bullae. As the infection progresses, cutaneous hypoesthesia and necrosis develop, along with signs of systemic sepsis including fever, tachycardia, changes in mental status, and hypotension. Other occasional manifestations of systemic toxicity include anemia, disseminated intravascular coagulation, and rhabdomyolysis.

Radiographs of the soft tissues should be obtained when the diagnosis is not clear from the examination results. These studies may demonstrate gas in the subcutaneous tissues even in patients without crepitus. Crepitus and radiographic demonstration of soft tissue gas are generally seen in patients with more advanced infection. Although computed tomography (CT) is not indicated in most patients with these disease states, CT may be performed to evaluate pain in patients without the obvious physical findings of necrotizing soft tissue infection and is a very sensitive test to demonstrate soft tissue gas. Asymmetric edema within tissue planes is another finding associated with but not diagnostic of necrotizing infections. An elevated serum creatine phosphokinase (CPK) level is a sensitive measure of the skeletal muscle destruction and may be useful to determine muscular involvement in these infections. A normal CPK level generally excludes muscle necrosis. Myoglobinuria can also occur in patients with muscular involvement. The white blood cell count is usually abnormal in patients with necrotizing skin and soft tissue infections, but this finding is variable and certainly not specific for this problem.

When unclear, the diagnosis may be made by fine needle aspiration cytology and Gram's stain or incisional biopsy with frozen section examination. In patients with atypical infections or equivocal history and physical findings, fine needle aspiration cytology can demonstrate the presence of organisms, necrosis, and various degrees of inflammatory cell infiltration. Definitive findings on frozen section examination include necrosis, vascular thrombosis, and the presence of microorganisms.

TREATMENT

The successful management of necrotizing soft tissue infections depends on early recognition and urgent operative treatment. Operative management always should be preceded by adequate fluid resuscitation and initiation of antibiotic therapy. Fluid resuscitation is best accomplished with a balanced isotonic electrolyte solution such as lactated Ringer's solution. Electrolyte abnormalities, particularly hypokalemia or hyperkalemia, should be corrected. Intravenous calcium gluconate is useful to correct the hypocalcemia that can result from calcium precipitation in the soft tissues when fat necrosis has been extensive. Red blood cell transfusions may be required to correct anemia related to intravascular hemolysis. Patients with traumatic wounds should receive tetanus toxoid or human tetanus immune globulin depending on their immunization status. The cumulative mortality of approximately 700 patients with necrotizing soft tissue infections is 34% and ranges from 6 to 76%. Delays in seeking or providing treatment are associated with an increased mortality.

The major objective of operation for necrotizing soft tissue infections is to débride all apparent necrotic and infected tissue. Underlying tissue necrosis typically extends beyond the obvious limits of cutaneous involvement, and therefore appropriate exposure and exploration are important. Débridement should be continued until viable tissue is reached. Any associated abscesses should be drained, and appropriate causative conditions should be treated appropriately.

Wound drainage, exudates, tissue specimens, and abscess contents should be submitted for Gram's stain as well as aerobic, anaerobic, and fungal cultures and antimicrobial sensitivity testing. Patients with extensive loss of the abdominal fascia may need prosthetic mesh placed to reconstruct the abdominal wall and prevent evisceration. Fasciotomies are necessary only in the unusual circumstance of a patient who develops a compartment syndrome. Primary amputation can be lifesaving in extensive necrotizing soft tissue infections of the extremities. A colostomy is helpful to prevent tissue contamination from defecation and to control wound sepsis in patients with necrotizing infections involving the perineal areas.

Routine re-exploration should be performed in the operating room within 24 hours in all but the most minor cases. Repeated débridement should continue in the operating room until the infection is controlled. Following débridements, the wound should be irrigated and packed lightly with gauze moistened with 0.9% normal saline. The use of various topical antiseptic and antibacterial solutions usually does little to inhibit bacterial growth.

Intravenous antimicrobial therapy is advocated in all patients with necrotizing soft tissue infections. The role of antibiotics is secondary to a prompt and adequate operative débridement. Because of the wide range of microorganisms that cause necrotizing soft tissue infections, initial empiric antibiotic therapy should be effective against a diverse group of potential pathogens. Current antibiotics with broad-spectrum coverage include imipenem/cilastatin (Primaxin) and extended-spectrum penicillins with a β-lactamase inhibitor such as piperacillin/tazobactam (Zosyn), ampicillin/sulbactam (Unasyn), or ticarcillin/clavulanate (Timentin). Trovafloxacin (Trovan) is a newer fluoroquinolone that can be used in these situations. Antibiotic combinations such as penicillin or ampicillin, an aminoglycoside, and either clindamycin (Cleocin) or metronidazole (Flagyl) also can be used.

Intravenous antimicrobial treatment should be continued until the signs of local wound sepsis and systemic toxicity have resolved. This includes eradication of fever and return of the white blood cell count to normal. Prolonged antibiotic therapy may be required in these circumstances. Occasionally, superinfection of the débrided site occurs 5 to 10 days following débridement. Additional systemic antibiotics and topical antibacterial or antiseptic agents may be needed in these circumstances.

Hyperbaric oxygen has been advocated by some as an adjunctive treatment for extensive necrotizing soft tissue infections, particularly those due to *Clostridium*. There are no data, however, demonstrating that the use of hyperbaric oxygen therapy leads to improved survival or earlier resolution of the infection. Because its role in treatment has been controversial, hyperbaric oxygen therapy should not delay operative débridement nor should it substitute for complete débridement of infected nonviable tissues.

Once wound sepsis is controlled, early soft tissue coverage by split thickness skin grafts or reconstructive flaps is recommended. Soft tissue coverage is necessary to preserve limb function and to protect exposed tendons, nerves, and bone. Premature closure of contaminated or persistently infected sites, however, will likely lead to recurrence of infection and increased mortality.

INFLUENZA

method of
STEPHEN C. SCHOENBAUM, M.D., M.P.H.
Harvard Pilgrim Health Care of New England
Providence, Rhode Island

THE ILLNESS

Humans, when infected by influenza viruses, may have different outcomes ranging from asymptomatic infection, which occurs about 30% of the time, to the more common and typical "influenza-like" illnesses, characterized by fever and cough, weakness, headache, myalgia, and anorexia not infrequently associated with nausea. The usual symptoms of influenza-like illness last 3 to 7 days and then begin to resolve, with most persons returning to their normal activities. On average, illnesses tend to cause 5 to 6 days of restricted activity, 3 to 4 days in bed, and 3 days lost from work or school. Furthermore, it is common for persons to have some residual symptoms—nonproductive cough and some degree of subjective weakness—often lasting for several weeks. Although influenza-like illness caused by influenza viruses is often considered mild, it is frequently associated with physician visits, laboratory tests or chest radiographs, and use of prescription and nonprescription drugs.

A small, but important, percentage of persons who are infected with influenza virus develop pneumonia as a complication. Early pneumonia is more likely to be due to primary viral infection; late pneumonia is more likely to be due to secondary bacterial infection. Both can lead to hospitalization, and both can be fatal. Most hospitalizations and fatalities associated with influenza virus infection are due to respiratory complications, such as pneumonia, and many of the fatalities occur among persons with underlying "high-risk" conditions, such as cardiovascular disease (particularly congestive heart failure), chronic pulmonary diseases, diabetes mellitus, chronic renal disease, and immune deficiency. Influenza infection in the later trimesters of pregnancy increases hospitalizations but usually is not associated with fatalities. The risk of complications from influenza does increase with both age (65 and older) and number of high-risk conditions a person has. In addition, the risk of complications from influenza increases with the severity of a high-risk condition, as evidenced by whether a person has needed recent medical care specifically for the condition or has been hospitalized in the recent past because of the condition. These characteristics of high-risk persons and conditions have influenced the development of policies and practices for the prevention and management of influenza.

EPIDEMICS AND THEIR SIGNIFICANCE

Although epidemics of influenza virus infection invariably include the occurrence of typical influenza-like illnesses, such illnesses are not specific to influenza virus infection—hence the term "influenza-like." These illnesses can occur as a result of infection by many different viruses. What makes influenza viruses important is their ability to spread rapidly through human populations, causing epidemics of 6 to 8 weeks' duration in which often 10 to 30% of persons in an affected geographic area become ill. Thus, influenza epidemics cause community disruption. They lead to absenteeism sufficient to close schools, interfere with the operation of assembly lines, and reduce the productivity of most types of workplace; they also lead to increases in doctors' office visits, emergency department visits, and hospitalizations, which strain, and potentially can exceed, the capacity of these services.

There are three types of influenza virus: A, B, and C. They are negatively stranded RNA viruses, classified in the orthomyxovirus family. Only types A and B cause epidemics. The occurrence of epidemics appears to be related to changes in the two surface antigens of the virus, the hemagglutinin and neuraminidase. Type A and B viruses both undergo point mutations in their viral genome, which lead to progressive changes in the surface antigens. This "antigenic drift" yields viral strains to which the population has partial immunity but not sufficient immunity to ward off epidemic transmission. In addition, influenza A viruses can undergo "antigenic shift" in which viruses carrying novel types of hemagglutinin and neuraminidase, believed to be derived from avian sources, possibly with an intermediate animal host such as pigs or horses, begin to circulate in the largely susceptible human population. When this happens, extremely extensive epidemics, called pandemics, can occur. The appearance of viruses in humans with novel types of hemagglutinin and neuraminidase is a necessary but not sufficient condition for a pandemic. This occurred in 1976 with the swine flu outbreak in Fort Dix, New Jersey, which did not lead to a pandemic; and it occurred again in 1997 with the H5N1 ("bird flu") outbreak in Hong Kong, at which time the likelihood of the new virus for causing a pandemic was unknown. There is no known genetic marker on the influenza virus signifying human virulence, so that each appearance of a new virus needs to be observed closely to determine its pandemic potential.

DIAGNOSIS

Most diagnoses of influenza are made clinically. These diagnoses are most likely to be accurate in the presence of an outbreak in the community; that is, the greater the number of influenza-like illnesses occurring at any time in the general population, the greater the likelihood that the cause is influenza. Clinical laboratories are not usually equipped to perform diagnostic testing by viral culture or serology but can generally process specimens for such testing. State and other governmental health authorities have set up surveillance networks consisting of clinicians in a variety of settings who send specimens from suspected cases of influenza to appropriate laboratories for diagnosis. There is now a surveillance network of laboratories throughout the world designed to look for novel strains of influenza.

PREVENTION

Vaccination is the principal preventive measure for influenza. Although the technology exists for making both live and inactivated influenza virus vaccines, in the United States all of the commercially available vaccine for many decades has been inactivated. There has been a progressive increase in the use of influenza vaccine in the United States, so that in each of the last few years approximately 50 to 60 million doses of vaccine have been distributed. Nevertheless, only about half of the population that would most benefit from annual vaccination has been receiving it.

The formulation of influenza vaccine is reconsidered annually, and the vaccine is administered annually for several reasons. First, vaccine-induced immunity is of relatively short duration, sometimes only a few months, particularly in the elderly whose antibody titers wane rapidly. Second, because of the continual changes in the virus' surface antigens, particularly the hemagglutinin, and because the protective effect of the vaccine is dependent on the antigenic relatedness of the vaccine virus with the viruses that subsequently circulate in the community, it is important to update the vaccine viruses frequently, with some change being made every year or two.

The effectiveness of influenza vaccine has been evaluated in numerous studies over a period of several decades. As previously noted, the effectiveness of influenza immunization varies with the relationship between the vaccine strain and the circulating strains; but it also varies with other factors such as age or the exact nature of a person's underlying clinical conditions or co-morbidities. Although one cannot give a single figure for the effectiveness of influenza vaccine, it can be considered to average in the range of 30 to 70% for preventing illness. Furthermore, the clinician needs to keep in mind that the overall effect of influenza vaccine is to shift the results of infection with influenza virus, should it occur at all, to less severe manifestations. Thus, even if an illness develops in someone who has been immunized, it is less likely, again by 30 to 70%, to lead to prostration, hospitalization, or death.

Influenza vaccine has been recommended consistently by the Centers for Disease Control and Prevention's Immunization Practices Advisory Committee for persons falling into two groups: persons at increased risk for influenza-related complications and persons who can transmit influenza to persons at high risk. Nevertheless, influenza vaccine can be given to children and the general adult population. Broader recommendations are usually made in years in which extensive disease is expected, assuming it is possible to make sufficient vaccine.

Persons at increased risk for influenza-related complications, who should receive annual vaccination, include all persons age 65 and older; residents of nursing homes and other long-term care facilities, regardless of age; adults and children with chronic pulmonary or cardiovascular disorders; adults and children who have been hospitalized or have required regular follow-up for chronic metabolic diseases, including diabetes mellitus, renal dysfunction, hemoglobinopathies, or immunosuppression; children 6 months to 18 years who are receiving chronic aspirin therapy and might be at risk for developing Reye's syndrome after influenza; and women who will be in the second or third trimester of pregnancy during the influenza season (winter-spring).

Persons who are more likely than average to transmit influenza to persons at high risk and thus should receive annual vaccination include health care personnel in hospital, nursing home, chronic care facility, and ambulatory settings; providers of home care to persons at high risk; and household members of persons at high risk.

The only persons for whom influenza vaccine is contraindicated are those who are known to have anaphylactic hypersensitivity to eggs (the vaccine virus, before inactivation, is grown in eggs), anaphylactic hypersensitivity to some other component of the vaccine (e.g., thiomersal), or a history of having developed Guillain-Barré syndrome within 6 weeks of a prior influenza immunization. There are some relatively mild adverse effects of the vaccine that are either local (e.g., erythema or pain) or systemic (e.g., fever, malaise, and myalgia). They usually begin within 6 to 12 hours and last 1 to 2 days. Inactivated influenza vaccines are highly purified, but the adverse reactions, when they occur, are presumably due to some residual toxic components. Because the vaccines are inactivated, they cannot cause influenza itself.

There are two types of inactivated vaccine: whole virus and split hemagglutinin. Owing to fewer side effects in children, only the split hemagglutinin vaccines should be used for children younger than age 13. Either vaccine may be used for persons 13 and older. When influenza vaccine is given to persons younger than 9 years for the first time, or when there is a new, potentially pandemic strain, two doses of vaccine, administered at a 4-week interval, are generally recommended. Otherwise, one dose is sufficient. The recommended route of injection is intramuscular. Although it is tempting to give smaller doses of vaccine intradermally when vaccine supplies are strained, the probability that the person will have a good antibody response is less, so this practice is not recommended.

Influenza vaccine can be administered simultaneously with pneumococcal vaccine (Pneumovax, Pnu-Imune). Because the groups at high risk for influenza and pneumococcal disease overlap, and because pneumococcal pneumonia is the most common cause of secondary bacterial pneumonia following acute influenza virus infection, it is important to take the time of administration of influenza vaccine as an opportunity to give pneumococcal vaccine to those for whom it is indicated.

The antiviral agents amantadine (Symmetrel) and rimantadine (Flumadine) may also be used to prevent influenza A but not influenza B. Even though various studies have shown these drugs to have been 70 to 90% effective at preventing influenza A, to be effective they must be taken daily throughout the period of potential exposure. For reasons of cost, adverse reactions, practicality, and the development of resistance, antiviral drugs should not be considered the primary approach to preventing influenza or a substitute for vaccination when it is available. There are, nonetheless, important niche uses for amantadine or rimantadine chemoprophylaxis, including for the following groups: (1) persons at high risk of complications of influenza who failed to be immunized in time and can be covered for a 2-week period following immunization when influenza A viruses are already circulating in the community; (2) persons at very high risk of complications of influenza due to very severe underlying conditions who might benefit from the combination of timely immunization and subsequent chemoprophylaxis when influenza A viruses are known to be present in the community; (3) previously unimmunized persons who provide care to high-risk persons, including both health care workers and household members, and can be covered for a 2-week period following immunization when influenza A viruses are present in the community; and (4) persons with immune deficiency conditions who might not have sufficient antibody response to immunization. Amantadine and rimantadine have also been used for control of outbreaks in populations of high-risk patients, such as nursing homes, irrespective of the immunization status of the members of the population. Finally, there may be times, such as the early stages of a pandemic, when a new strain of influenza A is circulating and there is no vaccine available yet, or an insufficient amount of vaccine available. At such times, amantadine or rimantadine could be used for persons for whom vaccine is normally indicated.

Although amantadine and rimantadine are generally similar, the former tends to be less expensive and the latter to have fewer side effects. Both drugs can cause central nervous system (e.g., insomnia, nervousness) and gastrointestinal (e.g., nausea) side effects. Overall, the side effects tend to be mild and the drugs well-tolerated. Nevertheless, some patients have developed congestive heart failure while receiving amantadine; also, amantadine has been associated with increased seizure activity in patients with prior epilepsy, whereas with rimantadine, seizure-like activity was seen in some persons with a history of prior seizures who were not on anticonvulsant drugs.

For both drugs, the usual dosage in children younger than age 10 is 2 to 5 mg per kg per day up to a total of 150 mg given in 2 divided doses. For persons aged 10 to 64, the usual dosage is 100 mg twice a day. A reduced dose of 100 mg per day or less is recommended for all persons aged 65 or older receiving amantadine and 100 mg per day for nursing home residents receiving rimantadine. Reduced dosages of both drugs are also recommended for persons with impaired renal function. Reduced dosage of rimantadine is recommended for persons with impaired hepatic function. For detailed adverse reaction and dosing information, please consult the package insert.

THERAPY

Both amantadine and rimantadine can shorten the duration and severity of symptoms and signs of influenza when administered within 48 hours of the onset of illness. Because the duration of therapy is short—the drugs should be discontinued after 3 to 5 days or within 1 to 2 days of disappearance of fever and major symptoms—the cost, risk of significant toxicity, and selection of antiviral resistant isolates are all relatively low. Recommended dosages are similar for treatment and prophylaxis; but rimantadine is not approved for treatment of influenza in children younger than age 10. Even though it has not been proved definitively that chemotherapy of influenza decreases the occurrence of complications among high-risk persons, it is likely that it does. Thus, antiviral drugs, although underused for treatment of influenza in high-risk persons for the past 30 years, can play an important role and should be considered an adjunct to vaccine as a means of decreasing the impact of influenza.

Most persons with influenza are treated symptomatically, with fluids and antipyretic analgesics. All persons with influenza should be observed for development of progressive respiratory symptoms, especially dyspnea, which could indicate development of primary viral pneumonia; and all persons with influenza should be cautioned about recurrence of fever or development of purulent sputum, usually in the second week of illness, which could indicate development of secondary bacterial pneumonia. Although the majority of cases of secondary bacterial pneumonia are due to pneumococci, those due to *Staphylococcus aureus* are disproportionately fatal. All patients with pneumonia should be evaluated and treated aggressively.

LEISHMANIASIS

method of
LUIGI GRADONI, Ph.D.
Istituto Superiore di Sanitá
Rome, Italy

Leishmaniasis is not a single disease but a variety of syndromes caused by infection with protozoan parasites of the genus *Leishmania.* The flagellated forms are transmitted by the bite of phlebotomine sandflies and multiply as aflagellated forms within cells of the mononuclear phagocyte system. Three main clinical syndromes, visceral leishmaniasis (VL), cutaneous leishmaniasis (CL), and mucocutaneous leishmaniasis (MCL) are widespread in tropical, subtropical, and temperate zones and often represent zoonotic infections. For some *Leishmania* species, humans are the principal or sole reservoir (anthroponotic leishmaniases). In the early 1990s the worldwide incidence of leishmaniases was estimated to be 400,000 cases. The current interest in leishmaniasis is probably due to the increasing importance of travel medicine, the medical problems encountered during the Persian Gulf War, and the inclusion of VL as a complication of acquired immune deficiency syndrome (AIDS).

The recent advances in biochemical taxonomy of *Leishmania* have made it possible to identify the parasite to the species and the strain levels and to define nosogeographic entities by which each of the 13 *Leishmania* species of medical interest is characterized by geographic distribution, clinical syndrome or syndromes provoked, vector, and host species. This information is of great medical importance, because different species that infect the same tissue may display different susceptibility to a drug, or the efficacy of a drug regimen against a viscerotropic *Leishmania* in one region does not ensure that such a regimen will be effective against dermotropic species in the same region.

CLINICAL LEISHMANIASIS

Visceral Disease

VL (kala-azar) results from multiplication of *Leishmania* in the phagocytes of the reticuloendothelial system. Anthroponotic VL is caused by *Leishmania donovani* in India and East Africa; zoonotic VL is caused by *Leishmania infantum* in Mediterranean regions and *Leishmania chagasi* in Latin America. These two species, however, are virtually identical by biochemical genotyping. In the endemic situation there are about 30 to 100 subclinical, self-healing infections for every case of acute VL. Healing is associated with the transient appearance of specific antibodies and a positive result on the leishmanin skin test (LST). In epidemic situations, as those caused by *L. donovani* in Sudan and India, subclinical cases are less common.

Classic VL manifests as fever, hepatosplenomegaly, pancytopenia, and hypergammaglobulinemia. The clinical incubation period ranges from 3 weeks to more than 2 years, but 2 to 4 months is average. Patients report a history of fever resistant to antibiotics, which is present at the time of medical consultation. On physical examination, the spleen is typically appreciated 5 to 15 cm below the left costal margin. Symptomatic VL is commonly fatal if left untreated. Post–kala-azar dermal leishmaniasis, a dermatologic complication characterized by macules, papules, or nodules, may develop months or years after treatment of Indian or African VL.

Other clinical presentations of VL have been described. Mild VL cases not progressing to symptomatic disease were reported among U.S. soldiers deployed to the Arabian peninsula during Operation Desert Storm. Fever and organomegaly were frequently absent, and all had normal hemoglobin concentrations. Instead, the patients complained of chronic fatigue, malaise, abdominal pain, and diarrhea. In southern Europe, the coexistence of the human immunodeficiency virus (HIV) and *L. infantum* leishmaniasis has resulted in a large number of dually infected individuals (by 1997 the total number of cases was approximately 1000). Although the clinical presentation of the disease in HIV-infected hosts is comparable to that in classic VL, the gastrointestinal tract is frequently involved and hepatosplenomegaly may be absent.

Cutaneous Disease

CL results from multiplication of *Leishmania* in the phagocytes of the skin. Anthroponotic CL is caused by *Leishmania tropica* in the Old World; zoonotic CL is caused by *Leishmania major, Leishmania aethiopica,* and dermotropic *L. infantum* in the Old World and by members of the

Leishmania mexicana complex (*L. mexicana, Leishmania amazonensis,* and *Leishmania venezuelensis*) and the *Leishmania braziliensis* complex (*L. braziliensis, Leishmania peruviana, Leishmania panamensis,* and *Leishmania guyanensis*) in the New World. In the classic course of this disease, lesions appear first as papules, progress to ulcers or nodules, then spontaneously heal with scarring over months to years. The incubation period ranges from 1 week to 8 months; lesions caused by some species (e.g., *L. major* and *L. mexicana*) tend to evolve and resolve quickly, whereas those caused by other species (e.g., *L. braziliensis, L. tropica,* and dermotropic *L. infantum*) have longer periods of incubation and spontaneous healing.

Mucocutaneous Disease

MCL results from parasitic metastasis in the nasal mucosa, which eventually extends to the oropharynx and larynx, which may develop from CL lesions caused by members of the *L. braziliensis* complex. Characteristically, MCL does not heal spontaneously and evolves slowly (mean time 3 years) before first being brought to medical attention.

IMMUNOLOGIC FEATURES

Leishmaniases have typical immunologic polarity: cure is associated with the presence of cellular immune responses, whereas chronic disease is associated with the absence of such responses and the presence of high levels of specific, nonprotective antibodies. Self-healing CL is characterized by positive LST results and high values for *Leishmania* antigen–induced lymphocyte transformation in vitro. Classic VL does not heal spontaneously, and LST results and in vitro lymphocyte transformation are negative in cases of acute disease but convert to positive after successful chemotherapy. In spite of this polarity, analysis of cytokine patterns reveals a less polar situation. Both the Th_1 and Th_2 cytokines are secreted in specimens of CL or MCL lesions and in bone marrow and lymph nodes of patients with acute VL. For only one Th_2 cytokine, interleukin-10 (IL-10), can a reasonable association between clinical course of VL and cytokine levels be made.

DIAGNOSTIC METHODS

The standard diagnosis of leishmaniasis is still made by classic microbiologic methods. Samples of infected tissue are obtained, and the organisms are either seen in Giemsa-stained impression smears or cultured from tissue. In general, both staining and culture should be performed to increase sensitivity. Cultured organisms can be identified by isoenzyme electrophoresis.

For VL, aspirates or biopsy specimens of spleen, bone marrow, liver, or enlarged lymph nodes are examined. Sensitivity is organ dependent; higher diagnostic yields of *Leishmania* are obtained with spleen aspirates (>98%), although bone marrow aspirates (80 to 98% of yield) are usually preferred. In Indian VL, as well as in Mediterranean HIV-VL, microscopy and culture of buffy coat from peripheral blood result in 64 to 75% of sensitivity.

For CL, material is obtained by scraping tissue juice from a nodular lesion or from the edge of an ulcer. By this method, *Leishmania* may be isolated from about 80% of sores during the first half of their natural course. After that, parasitologic diagnosis becomes more difficult. Biopsy specimens may also be used to make impression smears and cultures. Culture is more sensitive than microscopy for diagnosing MCL.

Immunologic tests are useful when the diagnosis of the disease proves difficult using standard methods, and these can be employed in deciding for or against treatment. In CL and MCL, LST results are positive in more than 90% of cases, whereas serologic results are often negative. In acute VL, LST results are negative, whereas antibodies are readily detectable by several techniques. Indirect immunofluorescence, standard enzyme-linked immunosorbent assay (ELISA), and direct agglutination test results are positive in 97 to 100% of patients (in HIV-VL, however, sensitivity of these tests may be as low as 40 to 60%). Specificity is also high (90 to 95%), although cross-reactions may occur with *Trypanosoma cruzi* infections in Latin America. A new recombinant antigen used for the ELISA, rK39, has the sensitivity to identify 98 to 100% of cases of acute VL and 75 to 80% of cases of HIV-VL but not to identify subclinical VL cases or nonleishmanial infections.

Attempts have been made to use polymerase chain reaction to eliminate the need for tissue samples. In one study of patients with VL from India, Kenya, and Brazil, assay of blood samples with use of this technique demonstrated high sensitivity (90%) and high specificity (100%).

TREATMENT

Pentavalent Antimonials

Organic salts of pentavalent antimony (Sb) are still the mainstay of therapy for all the leishmaniases. Two preparations are available, sodium stibogluconate (Pentostam), containing 100 mg of Sb per mL, and meglumine antimoniate (Glucantime), containing 85 mg of Sb per mL. The drugs are given intramuscularly or intravenously, and they are equal in efficacy and toxicity when used in equivalent Sb doses. As the leishmaniases became treated more extensively and studied more carefully, treatment failures with Sb became recognized. In the past few years alternatives to Sb have been found for some syndromes, and they are now used as first-line drugs in some countries.

The recommended dosage of Sb for all the leishmaniases is 20 mg per kg per day for 21 to 28 days and for 40 days in regions (e.g., in Bihar State, India) in which high rates of Sb-resistant VL have been documented. Uncomplicated CL may be treated at the same daily dose but for 10 days.

Clinical response to antimonials is rapid in CL cases, but complete reepithelialization of lesions is observed in only one third of patients by the end of a 3-week treatment course. In VL patients, fever recedes by day 4 to 5 of treatment, and well-being returns by the first week, whereas spleen size normalizes 1 to 2 months after the end of therapy. These observations indicate that Sb treatment should not be discontinued until all clinical parameters normalize. Relapses may occur after apparent clinical cure in both CL and VL, from 2 to 8 months after the Sb treatment is discontinued. In general, if the treatment schedule has been appropriate, relapses rarely occur, but in HIV-VL the frequency of relapses approaches 100%.

Systemic toxicity caused by the antimonials normally relates to total dose administered and includes anorexia, musculoskeletal pain, minor T wave and

ST segment changes on the electrocardiogram, and slow rise in hepatic enzymes. Moderate cytopenia may occur. Pancreatitis, revealed by elevation of serum levels of amylase or lipase, has been recognized as the commonest side effect of antimonial therapy, and pancreatic inflammation is probably the cause of the nausea and abdominal pain experienced by many patients. Doses in excess of 20 mg of Sb per kg per day require monitoring, especially for prolongation of QT interval, which may precede a dangerous arrythmia. Sudden death has been reported among Sb-treated adults, who tolerate antimonials poorly compared with children.

Amphotericin B and Lipid-Associated Amphotericin B

The antifungal amphotericin B has long been recognized as a powerful leishmanicidal drug. This drug activity results from the specific target of amphotericin B, which is ergosterol-like sterols, the major membrane sterols of *Leishmania* species as well as of fungi. However, amphotericin B was administered infrequently because of its infusion-related side effects (fever, chills, and bone pain) and delayed side effects (renal toxicity) when administered at the usual daily dose of 1 to 1.5 mg per kg. Owing to the increasing resistance of VL to antimonial therapy in different areas of the world and to the availability of less toxic formulations of the drug, amphotericin B has been increasingly used for VL and constitutes the major advance in antileishmanial chemotherapy during the last years.

Amphotericin B deoxycholate (Fungizone) administered at the low dosage of 0.5 mg per kg every other day for 14 days (total dose, 7 mg per kg) cured 98 to 100% of Indian VL patients who were either Sb resistant or had not been treated with drugs previously. In the same study area, primary Sb resistance was approximately 40%.

Liposomal amphotericin B (AmBisome) was shown effective and nontoxic at high daily doses of 2 to 4 mg per kg for VL treatment in immunocompetent individuals. A dose-finding study in Mediterranean VL showed that a total dose of around 20 mg per kg* of AmBisome requiring 5 to 6 days of hospitalization was optimal and cost-effective, especially for infantile cases. This regimen was found ineffective for HIV co-infected patients, who had VL relapses even when treated with a total dose of 40 mg per kg administered over 1 month. In a dose-finding study in Indian VL, a total dose of 6 mg of AmBisome per kg was shown to be 100% effective. A colloidal dispersion of amphotericin B, Amphocil, was found to be effective in Brazilian VL at the total dose of 10 mg per kg, but the drug showed serious side effects in patients younger than 6 years. A third lipid-associated amphotericin B (lipid complex, Abelcet) administered at the total dose of 15 mg per kg to Indian patients who had been unresponsive to Sb therapy resulted in full cure but also in significant adverse effects. Although showing some amphotericin B–associated toxicity, both Amphocil and Abelcet have more rapid efficacy compared with that of the conventional drug.

*Exceeds dosage recommended by the manufacturer.

Paromomycin (Humatin)

Paromomycin* is an aminoglycoside licensed in Europe for the parenteral treatment of bacterial diseases. Because the drug has revealed leishmanicidal activity in experimental leishmaniasis, injectable paromomycin has been used as monotherapy in patients with Sb-resistant VL in Kenya; the drug, given at the dosage of 14 to 16 mg per kg per day for a mean of 19 days, cured 79% of patients. The efficacy of paromomycin was augmented by administering it in combination with antimony for 20 days (82% of cure) in areas in which Sb treatment alone had to be given for twice as long (40 days) to obtain the same cure rate. In general, paromomycin monotherapy is probably not as effective as antimonial therapy in Sb-susceptible VL.

Other Parenteral Drugs

In Sb-resistant VL, pentamidine isethionate* (Pentam 300) may be used at the dosage of 4 mg per kg intramuscularly three times per week for 9 weeks. At this dosage, however, side effects such as myalgia, nausea, headache, and hypoglycemia are common. A lower dosage of pentamidine (2 mg per kg) for a shorter course (every other day for 7 days) was found to be effective and less toxic in the treatment of New World CL.

Cytokine therapy is limited to studies on human recombinant interferon-γ* (Actimmune). This cytokine was found only partially effective by itself in VL patients. When used at the intramuscular dosage of around 100 μg per m^2 per day in combination with 10 to 20 mg Sb per kg for 20 to 30 days, interferon-γ could speed the elimination of parasites in previously untreated Kenyan or Indian patients with VL and in patients with Sb-resistant New World CL or MCL. Side effects consisting of fever, chills, fatigue, myalgias, and headache occur in 30% of patients.

Pentamidine (2 mg per kg) and interferon-γ (175 μg)† have been used with some success in combination three times per week, 1 week per month, as maintenance therapy in HIV-infected patients with VL.

Oral and Local Agents

The ultimate goal for leishmaniasis treatment should be the replacement of long-term therapy using parenteral and moderately toxic drugs with shorter courses of nonparenteral, less toxic, and more effective agents.

Treatment with orally administered agents has

*Not FDA approved for this indication.
†Exceeds dosage recommended by the manufacturer.

been investigated for CL, which can be treated on an outpatient basis. The drugs used are inhibitors of ergosterol or purine biosynthesis, which have *Leishmania*-specific pathways. Ketoconazole* (Nizoral) was found to be effective at the dosage of 600 mg per day for 4 weeks against rapidly self-resolving disease due to *L. mexicana* or *L. major,* but not against "slow-evolving" species such as *L. braziliensis, L. tropica,* or dermotropic *L. infantum.* Itraconazole* (Sporanox), although more easily tolerated than ketoconazole, is probably less effective. Allopurinol* (Zyloprim) monotherapy at the dose of 20 mg per kg per day for 28 days was found to be ineffective against New World CL. Although this drug has been used extensively in combination with antimonials in VL patients, its role in the treatment of VL has to be definitively proven. Allopurinol and ketoconazole or itraconazole have been used together or in sequence for the treatment of complicated leishmaniasis cases or for maintenance therapy for HIV-VL.

Standard local treatment of CL consists of intralesional administration of antileishmanial agents, usually antimony, given intermittently over 20 to 30 days on an outpatient basis. The cure rate is around 75% in Old World CL. Use of this technique may cause problems when multiple lesions are present, when lesions are in face areas not suitable for injections, or when medical care centers are not readily accessible. Major emphasis has been placed on topical application of paromomycin (aminosidine)-containing formulations. *L. major* lesions treated with 15% paromomycin plus 12% methylbenzethonium chloride in soft white paraffin twice a day for 10 days cleared more rapidly than did untreated lesions on the same patients. Another paromomycin formulation in which the methylbenzethonium chloride has been replaced by 10% urea was found to be ineffective against CL caused by *L. major.* Topical miconazole* (Monistat) (2%) and topical clotrimazole* (Lotrimin) (1%) were administered twice a day for 30 days to patients with *L. major* CL, but the cure rate was unsatisfactory. Therapeutic failures using antileishmanial ointments may be due to the fact that CL is not a superficial problem as are infections due to the dermatophytes. *Leishmania*-infected macrophages reside deep in the dermis and also disseminate to the lymphatic system and mucosal membranes. Even when topical agents are effective in vitro they also must penetrate deeply to be effective against cutaneous lesions.

*Not FDA approved for this indication.

LEPROSY
(Hansen's Disease)

method of
BAOHONG JI, M.D.
Pitié-Salpêtrière, Paris, France

Leprosy is a chronic infectious disease caused by *Mycobacterium leprae.* Although the organism has not yet been cultivated in bacteriologic media or tissue cultures, it can be grown in the mouse footpad and in the armadillo. Although humans are considered the major host and reservoir of *M. leprae,* naturally acquired leprosy has been detected in armadillo, chimpanzee, and mangabey monkey, but the epidemiologic significance of the extra-human reservoirs is unknown and is likely to be very limited. The exact mode of transmission is not clear, but contacts of leprosy patients have a higher risk of contracting the disease. Millions of bacilli are released daily in the nasal discharges of untreated multibacillary leprosy patients, which then probably enter the body through the upper respiratory tract and possibly through broken skin. Over the last decade, tremendous progress has been made in controlling the disease worldwide. Compared with the global estimate of 10 to 12 million cases in the mid-1980s, it is estimated that, at the beginning of 1997, there were about 1.15 million leprosy cases in the world, out of whom 0.89 million were registered for treatment. Approximately 0.55 million new cases are diagnosed each year. To date, leprosy remains a public health problem in 55 countries or areas, but 16 top endemic countries contribute to 91% of the leprosy problem in the world. The leading six countries (number of registered cases at the beginning of 1997) are India (554,000), Brazil (106,000), Indonesia (34,000), Myanmar (19,000), Nigeria (14,000), and Bangladesh (13,000). Although 200 to 300 new leprosy cases are diagnosed each year in certain areas of the United States, mainly in southern Louisiana, Texas, southern California, and Hawaii, nearly 90% of these new cases are immigrants from endemic areas in Southeast Asia, Mexico, and the Philippines.

The manifestation of the disease varies from patient to patient in a continuous spectrum, which depends mainly on the immune response of the host. Based on clinical, bacteriologic, histologic, and immunologic findings, Ridley and Jopling proposed a classification dividing leprosy patients into five groups. At one end of the spectrum, tuberculoid leprosy (TT) patients develop a high level of cell-mediated immunity, which results in the killing and clearing of bacilli in the tissue; they present single or few skin lesions with sharply defined borders and localized but severe nerve involvement. At the other end, lepromatous leprosy (LL) patients exhibit a selective immunologic unresponsiveness to *M. leprae* antigens, so that the organisms inexorably multiply in the body and cause nerve damage as well as numerous bilaterally and symmetrically distributed skin lesions with diffused boundaries. The majority of patients are in the borderline categories between the two polar types and are further divided into three groups on an immunologic basis: borderline tuberculoid (BT, nearer the tuberculoid end), borderline lepromatous (BL, nearer the lepromatous end), and midborderline (BB), between BT and BL. Apart from the five groups, there is an indeterminate form (I) of leprosy, which is characterized by single or few macular lesions with alterations of color and impairment of sensation, and a primary neuritic (pure neural) form of leprosy. These two forms have been established as definite clinical entities, but their frequency, significance, and prognosis still remain unclear. Although the Ridley-Jopling classification is relatively precise, its application is mostly limited to research purposes; the majority of field workers are not able to apply the classification properly because of the limited facilities available under the field conditions. To simplify the classification, the World Health Organization (WHO) Study Group on Chemotherapy of Leprosy proposed in 1981 to classify the disease as multibacillary (MB) and paucibacillary (PB) leprosy according to the degree of skin-smear positivity. It was essentially an operational classification to serve as a basis for chemotherapy for the two different categories. The WHO Expert Committee on Leprosy at its sixth meeting (1987) endorsed the principles on which this classification was based, with the modification that all patients who are initially skin-smear positive should be classified as having MB leprosy and those who test negative be classified as having PB leprosy. The essential requirement for the new classification is the skin-smear services. It was gradually realized that the quality of skin smears and of microscopic examinations was probably the weakest link in most leprosy control programs, and it remains very poor even though tremendous efforts were made and resources were spent in trying to upgrade it. Because the skin-smear services are not always available in the field, the reliability of their results is often doubtful, and because more and more leprosy control programs classify leprosy cases based on clinical criteria, the WHO Expert Committee on Leprosy at its seventh meeting (1997) recommended new criteria for classification. They recommended that leprosy patients be classified into three groups based on the number of skin lesions: (1) PB single lesion leprosy (one skin lesion), (2) PB leprosy (two to five skin lesions), and (3) MB leprosy (more than five skin lesions). The PB single lesion leprosy is a newly defined clinical entity, which refers to patients who have a single hypopigmented or reddish skin lesion with definite loss of sensation but without nerve trunk involvement. Such patients represent an important proportion of newly diagnosed cases in certain countries such as India, have a strong tendency of self-healing, and can be cured by a significantly smaller amount of chemotherapy.

Because leprosy primarily affects the peripheral nerves and secondarily affects skin and certain other tissues, involvement and later destruction of peripheral nerves is a universal characteristic of the disease. Although leprosy mimics many dermatologic and neurologic disorders, the diagnosis can usually be made by careful clinical examination supported by skin smears. Occasionally, histologic examination may be helpful. The diagnosis is based on the presence of one or more of the following cardinal signs: (1) skin lesion(s) with definite loss of sensation, (2) thickening of peripheral nerve(s), and (3) presence of acid-fast bacilli in smears taken from the skin lesions. The first two signs are present in the vast majority of PB cases; in early MB cases, these two signs may not be evident, but acid-fast bacilli are always present and therefore support the diagnosis. It is important to remember that the diagnosis of leprosy is a very serious matter. If there is any doubt, an immediate diagnosis should be avoided. Physicians in the United States who are relatively unfamiliar with the disease may contact the U.S. Public Health Service, Gillis W. Long Hansen's Disease Center at Carville, Louisiana (phone: 1-800-642-2477), or a regional Hansen's disease center. Physicians from other countries may also be able to contact similar referral facilities in their own countries.

CHEMOTHERAPY OF LEPROSY

Effective chemotherapy of leprosy became possible for the first time with the introduction of dapsone. Since the late 1940s, dapsone monotherapy has been widely used for the treatment of all types of leprosy because it is an effective, cheap, and safe drug. However, the bacterial population in MB leprosy is very large. An untreated, advanced lepromatous patient may begin treatment with 10^{10} to 10^{11} viable organisms. Therefore, mutants that are resistant, separately, to dapsone and other drugs are present even before treatment. Although the majority of drug-susceptible organisms are killed during dapsone monotherapy, the dapsone-resistant mutants survive and multiply selectively, and finally they replace the susceptible organisms in the bacterial population, which results in secondary dapsone-resistant leprosy. In the course of time, primary dapsone-resistant leprosy, that is, the leprosy resistant to dapsone before treatment, also occurs as a result of infections with organisms from the secondary dapsone-resistant patients. Unlike secondary resistance, primary dapsone resistance probably occurs in at least as high a proportion of PB leprosy cases as of MB cases, although one cannot demonstrate resistance in PB patients through inoculation of mice, as they have too few bacilli in their skin biopsy specimens. Because of the widespread dapsone resistance by the end of the 1970s, a WHO Study Group recommended multidrug therapy (MDT) for both PB and MB leprosy. For the treatment of patients with PB leprosy, rifampin* should be administered along with dapsone, whereas at least two additional drugs should be combined with dapsone for patients with MB leprosy.

Currently Available Antileprosy Drugs

Unlike the usually lifelong monotherapy with dapsone, one of the basic concepts of MDT is that the treatment be administered for only a limited period and, by implication, that only bactericidal drugs be considered as components for MDT regimens. Currently, six drugs, which act by different bactericidal mechanisms against *M. leprae,* are available: dapsone, rifampin, clofazimine, ofloxacin, minocycline, and clarithromycin.

Dapsone. Dapsone (DDS) is available as 25-, 50-, and 100-mg tablets. The routine dosage is 100 mg daily for adults and 1 to 2 mg per kg body weight per day for children. It is rapidly and nearly completely absorbed when taken orally, well distributed throughout the body, and ultimately excreted for the most part in the urine. It acts as a synthetase inhibitor in the folate-synthesizing enzyme system of *M. leprae,* and a dose of 100 mg daily is weakly bactericidal. *M. leprae* is extremely susceptible to dapsone in the sense that the minimal inhibitory concentration (MIC) of dapsone is extremely low, being on the order of 3 ng per mL as studied through the mouse footpad experiments. Its half-life is relatively long, with an average of about 28 hours. Because of these characteristics, after ingestion of a single dose of 100 mg of dapsone, the peak blood level is 500 times the MIC and measurable amounts can be found in the blood even 10 days later.

Dapsone is relatively nontoxic in the routine dosage. A variety of side effects have been attributed to dapsone, including hemolytic anemia, skin rashes, gastrointestinal reactions, agranulocytosis, hepatitis,

*Not FDA approved for this indication.

psychosis, and peripheral neuropathies. Most of these effects are rare and mild. The so-called DDS syndrome, which is also rare, usually develops within the first 6 weeks after the start of therapy and consists of exfoliative dermatitis and/or other skin rashes, generalized lymphadenopathy, hepatosplenomegaly, and fever. When this syndrome does occur, dapsone should be discontinued immediately and corticosteroids should be given. The most common side effect with dapsone is anemia. However, this is usually very mild and well tolerated, unless the patient has a complete glucose-6-phosphate dehydrogenase (G6PD) deficiency. The safety of dapsone in pregnancy seems to be fairly well established, and no evidence of teratogenicity has been observed.

As mentioned earlier, dapsone resistance is a result of selective multiplication of resistant mutants during dapsone monotherapy, and it can be classified into three different levels of resistance: low-, intermediate-, or high-degree resistant, respectively, to a dose of up to 1 mg, 10 mg, or 100 mg of dapsone daily. Until now, the vast majority of secondary dapsone-resistant leprosy cases have high-degree resistance, whereas most of the primary dapsone-resistant leprosy cases have low or intermediate-degree resistance. The reason for this difference is still unclear. To date, dapsone is still one of the components of the MDT regimens for both PB and MB leprosy. Because the MDT regimens were designed on the principle that they would be effective against all the strains of *M. leprae* regardless of their susceptibility to dapsone, and because the testing for the drug susceptibility by the mouse footpad system is time-consuming and very expensive, whether the patient is resistant to dapsone or the global prevalence of dapsone resistance is increasing or declining is virtually irrelevant to the treatment of the individual patient or to the current strategy of eliminating leprosy. Hence, there is no need to test the dapsone susceptibility of the *M. leprae* strains as routine.

Rifampin. Rifampin (Rifadin, Rimactane), is available as 150- and 300-mg capsules. It acts by inhibiting the DNA-dependent RNA polymerase of the organisms, thereby interfering with bacterial RNA synthesis. Rifampin is absorbed rapidly from the gastrointestinal tract and distributed throughout the body. About two thirds of the absorbed drug is ultimately excreted via the gastrointestinal tract. It is by far the most powerful bactericidal drug against *M. leprae,* and its activity is greater than that of any single or combination of the other antileprosy drugs. It is, therefore, the key component of MDT regimens for both PB and MB leprosy and will continue to play a crucial role for the treatment of leprosy in the foreseeable future. Because of the evidence that no difference in the bactericidal activity, as measured by serial mouse footpad inoculations, has been detected between the daily and the monthly administration of rifampin, it is given at a dosage of 600 mg for an adult once monthly in the MDT regimens. The monthly rifampin administration not only reduces the costs greatly but also reduces the frequency and severity of side effects compared with those that are associated with the daily administration of the drug. During the treatment with MDT, one may assume that the elimination of drug-susceptible organisms is due almost entirely to the bactericidal effect of the initial doses of rifampin, because more than 99.999% (which is the limit of detectability by current technology) of viable *M. leprae* are killed by three monthly doses of rifampin administration.

The toxicity of rifampin is related to the dosage and the interval between doses. The standard dose of 600 mg monthly in MDT regimens has proved relatively nontoxic. Hepatotoxicity is extremely rare with monthly administration of rifampin. Although immunoallergic side effects, such as "flu" syndrome or syndrome consisting of shock, hemolytic anemia, and renal failure have been reported in the treatment of tuberculosis with once-weekly or twice-weekly rifampin administration, very few flu syndrome occurrences have been reported in leprosy patients with monthly administration of 600 mg of rifampin. Other side effects include skin rashes and mild gastrointestinal symptoms. Rifampin can be used safely during pregnancy.

Secondary rifampin-resistant leprosy has been detected after rifampin monotherapy in MB patients or after administration of rifampin plus dapsone in patients relapsed from previous dapsone monotherapy. A great majority of the latter cases end up with resistance to both dapsone and rifampin if there is further relapse. Rifampin should therefore always be combined with other antileprosy drugs, such as dapsone-clofazimine in the MDT regimen, which may ensure the elimination of rifampin-resistant mutants from the bacterial population. Among 9 million leprosy patients who have completed their treatment with MDT, the relapse rate is very low, and up to now no rifampin-resistant cases have been detected among patients relapsed after MDT.

Clofazimine. Clofazimine (Lamprene; B663) is an iminophenazine dye and is available as 50- and 100-mg capsules. It is weakly bactericidal against *M. leprae.* It also exhibits anti-inflammatory activity and, therefore, may be used for the treatment of erythema nodosum leprosum (ENL), but the mechanisms of action are unclear. It is absorbed to the extent of about 70% via the gastrointestinal tract and is deposited mostly in fatty tissues and cells of the reticuloendothelial system, including the skin. In humans, the half-life of clofazimine is extraordinarily long, at least 70 days. In the MDT regimen for the treatment of MB leprosy, it is given at 50 mg daily plus 300 mg monthly; for the treatment of ENL, higher doses, beginning with 200 to 300 mg once daily, or 100 mg two to three times daily* for reducing the gastrointestinal side effects, are required (see below).

The most common side effect is a reddish-black pigmentation of the skin, which normally develops within 4 to 8 weeks after the start of the therapy

*Exceeds dosage recommended by the manufacturer.

in patients with active skin lesions. The severity of pigmentation is dose dependent and is intensified in the areas of the lesions. The pigmentation diminishes gradually in 6 to 24 months after discontinuation of the drug. Pigmentation may also be seen in the mucous membrane. Sebum, sweat, faces, and urine also show a reddish coloration. Because of the pigmentation, some light-skinned patients refuse to take the drug. Gastrointestinal symptoms, such as nausea, vomiting, crampy abdominal pain, and diarrhea, are common but mild in patients treated with 50 mg daily. However, in patients receiving higher doses (usually more than 100 mg daily), these symptoms may appear more serious. Another common side effect is ichthyosis, resulting from the anticholinergic activity of the drug.

Although in the 1970s, clofazimine had been used as monotherapy for leprosy, or combined with dapsone after patients relapsed from previous dapsone monotherapy, secondary clofazimine-resistant leprosy is surprisingly very rare. The reason for this rarity remains unclear.

Ofloxacin* (Floxin). Although a large number of fluoroquinolones have been developed, some such as ciprofloxacin are inactive against *M. leprae.* Among those which are of most interest is ofloxacin. The most likely mechanism of action of ofloxacin against *M. leprae* is that it acts by inhibiting the DNA gyrase of the organisms. It is available as a 200-mg tablet. The results of clinical trials have indicated that its optimal dosage for the treatment of leprosy is 400 mg daily. Although a single dose of ofloxacin displayed a modest bactericidal effect against *M. leprae,* 22 daily doses killed 99.99% of the viable organisms in lepromatous patients. Because ofloxacin is still very expensive, it has not been used widely for the treatment of leprosy in routine programs, but it has begun to be used for the treatment of rifampin-resistant cases and as one of the components in the investigational short-course regimen (combined with rifampin daily for 4 weeks) or intermittent regimen (combined with rifampin and minocycline monthly). In vitro and in vivo experiments have demonstrated that, on a weight-to-weight basis, sparfloxacin* (Zagam) is more active against *M. leprae* than ofloxacin, but the recommended clinical dosage of sparfloxacin is 200 mg daily, only half of that of ofloxacin. The results of clinical trials have demonstrated that the therapeutic effect of sparfloxacin, 200 mg daily, for the treatment of leprosy did not differ significantly from that of ofloxacin, 400 mg daily, suggesting that the greater activity of sparfloxacin was offset by its lower daily dosage.

The most common side effects caused by ofloxacin are gastrointestinal reactions, such as nausea, vomiting, abdominal discomfort, and anorexia; a variety of central nervous system reactions, such as headache, dizziness, insomnia, anxiety, and hallucinations, have also been reported. Most of the side effects do not require discontinuing ofloxacin treatment, and serious problems are rare. Although photosensitivity reaction is one of the important side effects during fluoroquinolone treatment for various clinical conditions, up to now no such effect has been seen among leprosy patients treated with ofloxacin, probably because all the patients involved in the clinical trials are dark-skinned and may be less susceptible to the photosensitivity.

Minocycline* (Minocin). Due to its high lipophilicity, minocycline is the only member of the tetracycline group of antibiotics that has significant bactericidal activity against *M. leprae.* It binds to the 30S ribosomal subunits and, therefore, interferes with the protein synthesis of the microorganisms. It is available as a 100-mg tablet. After the administration of 100 mg of minocycline, the peak serum level exceeds the MIC of minocycline against *M. leprae* by a factor of 10 to 20. On weight-to-weight basis, its bactericidal activity is greater than that of clarithromycin; however, at the clinically tolerated dosages, that is, 100 mg daily for minocycline and 500 mg daily for clarithromycin* (Biaxin), the bactericidal effects were virtually the same between the two drugs, killing more than 99% of the viable *M. leprae* after 28 and 56 days of treatment.

Minocycline is commonly used for the long-term treatment of acne, indicating that in general it is well tolerated. Side effects of minocycline include central nervous system reactions (dizziness and unsteadiness), gastrointestinal reactions, and discoloration of teeth in infants and children. Normally the side effects are mild. However, a few serious side effects such as autoimmune hepatitis and systemic lupus erythematosus–like syndrome have been reported.

Clarithromycin.* Clarithromycin is the only macrolide that displays significant bactericidal effect against *M. leprae* in mice and in humans. As already mentioned, it showed very promising bactericidal effect in lepromatous patients.

Compared with other antileprosy drugs, clarithromycin is not well tolerated by patients. The most common side effects are the gastrointestinal reactions, including nausea, vomiting, abdominal pain, and diarrhea, which proved particularly common when the drug was given at a dosage of 1000 mg or beyond. Because of its cost and side effects, clarithromycin is reserved only for the treatment of rifampin-resistant leprosy patients.

Treatment Regimens

WHO Recommended Standard MDT Regimens

For adults, the standard MDT regimen for PB leprosy is as follows:

Rifampin, 600 mg once a month, supervised
Dapsone, 100 mg daily, self-administered
Duration: 6 months

*Not FDA approved for this indication.

For adults, the standard MDT regimen for MB leprosy is as follows:

Rifampin, 600 mg once a month, supervised
Dapsone, 100 mg daily, self-administered
Clofazimine, 300 mg once a month, supervised, and 50 mg daily, self-administered
Duration: 24 months

To improve the patients' compliance, to make sure that the patients always receive adequate quantities of different drugs, and to protect the drugs from various sources of damage, the monthly supply of all the drugs is currently packed in a calendar blister pack.

To ensure that the patients take the crucial monthly administered component of the MDT regimens, that is, rifampin for PB leprosy and rifampin plus a supplementary higher dosage of clofazimine for MB leprosy, these drugs should always be administered under supervision. In case it is impossible to organize the monthly supervision by health care workers, all efforts have to be made to identify a family or community member of the patient to supervise the monthly treatment. In addition, both the patients and family members should be educated about the importance of taking the daily, self-administered components regularly.

By June 1997, almost 9 million leprosy patients in the world have completed their treatment with MDT. The regimens have been well tolerated by the patients, and the side effects have been rare and mild. Both regimens are very effective, including for those patients who are resistant to dapsone. After completion of the treatment, the relapse rate has been very low, far below one per 1000 cases per year. Among the relapsed cases, none is resistant to rifampin or clofazimine, and they still respond favorably to retreatment with MDT.

Regimen for the Treatment of Rifampin-Resistant Leprosy

As already mentioned, the great majority of rifampin-resistant *M. leprae* are also resistant to dapsone, and, until recently, the treatment depended almost entirely on clofazimine. With the development of other antileprosy drugs, it is now possible to treat the rifampin-resistant patients with the following regimen:

Initial 6 months: daily administration of 50 mg clofazimine plus 400 mg ofloxacin *and* 100 mg of minocycline.

From the seventh to the 24th month: daily administration of 50 mg of clofazimine plus 400 mg ofloxacin *or* 100 mg of minocycline.

Regimens for Multibacillary Leprosy Patients Who Refuse to Take Clofazimine

Although the WHO Study Group (1994) recommended using daily ofloxacin, 400 mg, or minocycline, 100 mg, as an alternative to clofazimine, the WHO Expert Committee on Leprosy (1997) suggested treating such patients by monthly administration of a combination consisting of 600 mg of rifampin, 400 mg of ofloxacin, and 100 mg of minocycline for 24 months.

MANAGEMENT OF LEPROSY REACTION

During the long-term evolution of leprosy, immunologically mediated episodes of acute or subacute inflammation known as "reactions" may occur in any type of leprosy except the indeterminate. The mechanisms of such episodes are not entirely clear. Because peripheral nerve trunks are often involved, such episodes can result in permanent deformities unless reactions are promptly and adequately treated.

Most reactions belong to one of the two major types: reversal reaction (type 1 reaction) or erythema nodosum leprosum (ENL, or type 2 reaction).

Reversal Reaction and Its Treatment

Reversal reaction may occur throughout the whole spectrum of leprosy classification but is more frequent in patients with borderline leprosy. Usually it occurs soon after the onset of MDT, although it may also appear after the completion of MDT. During the reaction, some or all of the pre-existing skin lesions become raised, erythematous, and enlarged, and new lesions may appear. Nerve thickening may increase, and nerve pain and nerve tenderness may occur and be accompanied by deterioration of nerve function. In PB leprosy, especially if the episode occurs after the completion of MDT, it may be difficult to distinguish between reversal reaction and relapse. However, in general, in reversal reaction the onset is more acute, the skin lesions are considerably more raised and erythematous with severe edema, and the nerve involvement tends to be more serious. A 1-month course of corticosteroid therapy may help in the differential diagnosis, as reversal reaction normally responds rapidly to corticosteroids but relapse will not respond satisfactorily.

For mild reversal reactions (e.g., slight swelling and redness of skin lesions with or without appearance of new skin lesions, or mild nerve tenderness without pain or deterioration of nerve function) no specific treatment is required except analgesics, either aspirin or acetaminophen. However, the patients must be seen at least once every 2 weeks and asked to return immediately if the symptoms become more severe.

Reversal reactions are graded severe when there is marked fever and malaise; when there is edema of hands and feet; when the skin lesions ulcerate; when there is nerve pain and tenderness, with or without deterioration of nerve function; and when a mild reaction lasts more than 6 weeks. Because of the high risk of permanent damage to the peripheral nerve trunks, a severe reversal reaction should be considered as one of the very few emergency conditions in leprosy. Whenever possible, patients with severe reversal reaction should be hospitalized, and corticosteroids should be given immediately.

The treatment of choice is prednisone or prednisolone, the cheapest and most widely available corticosteroid. Its dosage should be sufficient to relieve both nerve pain and nerve tenderness as soon as possible and must be determined according to the severity of the reaction, the body weight of the patient, and the response to treatment. The usual course begins with 40 to 60 mg (not more than 1 mg per kg of body weight) daily of prednisone. As the acute symptoms of the reversal reaction are suppressed, generally within 2 to 3 days after starting treatment with prednisone, the dosage of prednisone can be reduced gradually at 5 to 10 mg for each reduction, weekly or biweekly. Most reversal reactions can be controlled successfully within 12 weeks of treatment. However, a maintenance dosage (e.g., prednisone 5 to 10 mg daily) lasting for several months may be necessary in some instances if there is a tendency for recurrence of reaction on complete stoppage of prednisone.

The potential risk of serious adverse effects caused by longer duration corticosteroid therapy must not be ignored, particularly under field conditions. The most common adverse effects include peptic ulcer, diabetes, reactivation of tuberculosis, menstrual irregularities, depression, and other emotional problems. If reversal reaction occurs during treatment with MDT, chemotherapy should not be discontinued.

Erythema Nodosum Leprosum and Its Management

Unlike reversal reaction, ENL occurs exclusively in patients with MB leprosy, especially lepromatous and BL lepromatous leprosy. In general, ENL reaction appears to be less of a problem among patients treated with MDT than among those treated with dapsone monotherapy, probably owing to the anti-inflammatory activity of clofazimine.

ENL is variable in severity, duration, and organ involvement. Mild ENL consists of crops of erythematous nodules with low-degree fever and malaise and can be treated with analgesics or antimonials.

ENL is graded severe when there is high fever along with severe general malaise; when a moderate fever lasts more than 4 weeks; when the erythematous nodules become pustular and progress to ulceration or coalesce to form hard, tender sheets in the skin; when the lymph nodes become enlarged and very tender; when the peripheral nerve trunks become painful or markedly tender or when there is any loss of nerve function; when there is iridocyclitis, orchitis, periostitis, or joint swelling; or when urine examinations reveal persistent albuminuria with red blood cells under the microscope. Such severe ENL patients should be hospitalized for treatment immediately.

The acute or subacute symptoms of ENL reactions can be suppressed rapidly by treatment with prednisone. However, certain seriously ill patients require continuous and often high dosages and may eventually become dependent on corticosteroids. The overall policy of using prednisone for the treatment of reversal reaction applies equally to the treatment of ENL.

Thalidomide, an investigational drug in the United States, is also highly effective for controlling ENL. Patients are given 200 mg twice daily, and with this dosage the symptoms of ENL reaction are usually alleviated within 2 to 3 days. The dosage can then be reduced gradually. It has fewer adverse effects than corticosteroids, but the consequences of its teratogenicity are very serious. Therefore, it may be used for the treatment of severe ENL only in male or postmenopausal female patients who have not responded to corticosteroids. In no case should thalidomide be given to females of childbearing age.

Clofazimine is also effective for ENL but is less potent than corticosteroids or thalidomide and often takes 4 to 6 weeks to develop its full effects, so it should never be started as the sole agent for the treatment of severe ENL. However, clofazimine may be extremely useful for reducing or withdrawing corticosteroids in corticosteroid-dependent patients. In that case, high dosages of clofazimine (e.g., 300 mg daily or 100 mg thrice daily to reduce the gastrointestinal side effects) are needed. Six to 8 weeks later, one may try to reduce the dosage of corticosteroids gradually. After the withdrawal of corticosteroids, the dosage of clofazimine can be gradually reduced. Ideally, the total duration of high-dosage clofazimine should not exceed 8 to 12 months.

The antileprosy chemotherapy should continue unchanged during leprosy reactions.

MALARIA

method of
PETER WINSTANLEY, M.D.
University of Liverpool
Liverpool, United Kingdom

As we approach the millennium, malaria, along with many infectious diseases, remains as prevalent and as grave a problem as ever; furthermore, we may yet see its prevalence and extent of geographic distribution increase as a result of global climate change. Most of the morbidity and mortality affect populations in the tropics, where malaria is mainly a disease of poverty and the cost of intervention is of enormous importance. Malaria also affects travelers, whose risk depends on the area visited and compliance with individual protective measures. The cost of intervention is considerably less important for this population.

There is no vaccine for malaria and little prospect of developing one that could be afforded by the vast majority of those at risk. Prevention currently hinges on avoidance of mosquito bites (relevant to both travelers and resident populations) and use of prophylactic antimalarial drugs (in practice, relevant only to travelers; most resident populations usually cannot afford them). Successful treatment, along with that of many other infectious diseases, depends on appropriate supportive care and use of appropriate antimicrobial drugs given at the correct dose by an appropriate route. Unfortunately, for sound economic reasons, the pharmaceutical industry has had little incentive to develop new antimalarial compounds, and resistance to the existing drugs is an ever-increasing problem.

THE HUMAN MALARIA PARASITES

Plasmodium falciparum

Four species of malaria parasite cause disease in humans, but it is *P. falciparum* with which we have the most problem, including its prevalence (about 120 million people worldwide have *P. falciparum* parasitemia at any one time, and there are about 12 million clinical cases of falciparum malaria annually), the severity of the clinical syndromes that it can cause (there are about 1.2 million deaths annually), and the development of drug resistance to it. The pathogenicity of this parasite results mainly from its rapid rate of asexual reproduction in the host and its ability to sequester in small blood vessels (especially in the brain). *P. falciparum* has no "dormant" liver stage, and cure depends on killing the asexual blood stages (in common with the other three species, the sexual forms of the parasite are nonpathogenic).

About 90% of the burden of falciparum malaria is carried by tropical Africa (which includes some of the poorest countries in the world), where most cases and deaths affect children younger than 5. The epidemiology of falciparum malaria, as a disease rather than as a parasitemic state, has been studied in depth only recently. Not surprisingly, there are enormous geographic variations in disease patterns. In most of tropical Africa everyone becomes infected with *P. falciparum* during childhood. The majority of children start to develop "partial immunity" to the strains they encounter, and this protects them, to a degree, from severe disease and death. A small proportion of those infected, but a numerically huge group, develops severe illness (mainly "cerebral malaria," anemia, and acidosis). The factors that determine the risk of severe disease are poorly understood, but, paradoxically, risk seems to be lowest among populations with high transmission rates and highest among those with low-to-moderate transmission rates, perhaps reflecting the need to develop "immunity" at a time when other protective mechanisms operate.

Falciparum malaria also affects generally richer areas such as South America, the Indian subcontinent, southeast Asia, and China. In these areas (which are vast so there is considerable variation in patterns), the disease tends to be less prevalent than in Africa, tends to be epidemic rather than endemic, and is (generally) managed by better-funded health services. Partial immunity does not develop as readily (because transmission is less intense and individuals are less frequently infected), and all age groups may be affected by severe disease.

P. falciparum has developed resistance to nearly all antimalarial drugs. Chloroquine resistance is encountered throughout the tropics, but multidrug resistance is mainly a problem in southeast Asia. Resistance to individual drugs is described in the appropriate sections of the article.

Plasmodium vivax, Plasmodium ovale, *and* Plasmodium malariae

P. vivax is encountered throughout the tropics but is relatively uncommon in tropical Africa. *P. ovale* is principally found in Africa, whereas *P. malariae* has a widespread, although patchy, distribution throughout the tropics and subtropics. None of these three species characteristically causes severe disease; they multiply more slowly in the host, achieving lower parasite "density" than *P. falciparum,* and do not sequester in small blood vessels. However, although acute mortality is low, all three species are important causes of morbidity, including anemia, low birth weight, splenomegaly (and occasional rupture, especially with *P. vivax*), and nephrosis (*P. malariae*). *P. vivax* and *P. ovale* have hepatic "hypnozoites," which, if uneradicated, may cause late relapse. The drugs used to achieve clinical cure do not eradicate hypnozoites, and a course of primaquine is needed after clinical recovery. *P. malariae* lacks hypnozoites but can persist in the blood for many years if inadequately treated. Blood forms of all three species are sensitive to chloroquine (although resistant isolates of *P. vivax* have been reported).

ANTIMALARIAL DRUGS

Some important points to remember.

1. It is not difficult to remember to exclude malaria in malaria-endemic countries; however, in countries in which malaria is uncommon it is easy to miss the diagnosis in travelers (often with fatal consequences), so inquiry about recent travel is an essential part of a medical history.
2. The gravity of detecting *P. falciparum* in the blood depends on the patient's level of immunity. In a nonimmune person a positive finding is a medical emergency, whereas in a semi-immune patient with uncomplicated clinical features outpatient management is usual in tropical Africa.
3. Usually uncomplicated malaria can be treated with oral medication (Table 1).
4. Severe falciparum malaria must be treated with parenteral antimalarials.
5. Expert advice should be sought on the optimal choice of drug when treating malaria imported into nonendemic countries. Attending physicians may be unfamiliar with patterns of drug resistance.

Chloroquine

Malaria Treatment. Chloroquine has been the mainstay of falciparum malaria chemotherapy for decades. It is cheap (the cost of an adult treatment course is around $0.12), safe, and practicable for outpatient use. Unfortunately, resistance, first noticed in South America and southeast Asia in the 1960s, has become ubiquitous throughout the tropics. In much of southeast Asia chloroquine cannot be relied on to produce clinical improvement or clearance of peripheral parasitemia. In contrast, chloroquine remains the most commonly used antimalarial drug in Africa, primarily because of its low cost. Efficacy figures vary geographically in Africa, but around 40% of patients treated with chloroquine now fail to achieve a clinical cure. As a result of the high risk of encountering resistant strains, chloroquine is generally used for only *uncomplicated* malaria in *semiimmune subjects.* However, when chloroquine is the only parenteral antimalarial drug available, it is still used in the treatment of severe disease. Dose calculations for parenteral use must be based on body

TABLE 1. **Use of Antimalarial Drugs**

Drug	Parasite	Clinical Severity	Dose		Route
Chloroquine (Aralen)	*P. vivax, P. ovale, P. malariae*		10 mg/kg* loading, then 5 mg/kg after 6, 24, and 48 h		PO
	P. falciparum	Uncomplicated†	Same		
	P. falciparum	Severe‡	10 mg/kg over 8 h, followed by 15 mg/kg over 24 h		IV§
			3.5 mg/kg every 6 h to total of 25 mg/kg		IM or SC
Quinine	*P. falciparum*	Uncomplicated	10 mg of the sulfate salt per kg every 8 h for 5 to 7 d		PO
	P. falciparum	Severe	*Adults*	Loading dose 20 mg of the dihydrochloride salt per kg, over 4 h;	IV§‖
				thereafter 10 mg of the salt per kg, over 2 h repeated 8 hourly until oral drugs possible	IV§
			Children	Loading dose 15 mg of the dihydrochloride salt per kg over 2 h;	IV§
				thereafter 10 mg of the salt per kg, over 2 h, repeated 12 hourly until oral drugs possible	IV§
Pyrimethamine-sulfadoxine‖	*P. falciparum*	Uncomplicated	*Adults*	Three tablets¶ once only	PO
			Children	<5 y 0.5 tablet; 5–8 yr 1 tablet; 9–14 y 2 tablets	PO
Artemether‖	*P. falciparum*	Severe	Loading dose 3.2 mg/kg, then 1.6 mg/kg daily for 5 d, or until patient can swallow oral drugs		IM
Artesunate‖	*P. falciparum*	Severe	Loading dose 2 mg/kg, then 1 mg/kg every 12 h for 5 d or until patient can swallow oral drugs		IV**
Mefloquine (Lariam)	*P. falciparum*	Uncomplicated	15 mg/kg as a single dose**		PO
Halofantrine (Halfan)	*P. falciparum*	Uncomplicated	*Adults*	500 mg at 6-h intervals to a total of 3 doses sometimes repeated after an interval of 1 wk**	PO
			Children	8 mg/kg at 6-h intervals to a total of 3 doses sometimes repeated after an interval of 1 wk	PO

* Chloroquine doses are calculated in terms of the free base.
† Not for use in nonimmune patients.
‡ See text. Resistance to chloroquine is common. Use chloroquine for severe disease only if other parenteral antimalarial drugs are not available, and be alert for drug failure.
§ Fixed-rate infusion.
‖ Not available in the United States.
¶ One tablet contains pyrimethamine, 25 mg, plus sulfadoxine, 500 mg.
** See text.

weight; the dose is routinely given in terms of the active base rather than the salt. Intravenous (IV) fixed-rate infusion is the preferred parenteral route; chloroquine must always be diluted and should never be given by rapid IV injection. If IV infusion is not possible, chloroquine may be given subcutaneously or intramuscularly. *P. ovale* and *P. malariae* retain sensitivity to chloroquine, as do all but a small minority of *P. vivax* isolates; treatment is with the oral drug.

Malaria Prevention. Weekly chloroquine, in combination with daily proguanil (see later), is still recommended by many countries for malaria chemoprophylaxis. Although chloroquine-resistant *P. falciparum* is prevalent throughout the tropics, this drug retains activity against all isolates of *P. ovale* and *P. malariae* and nearly all isolates of *P. vivax* and is a useful adjunct to proguanil, which has little innate activity against these three species. Proguanil-resistant *P. falciparum* is common throughout the tropics, but organisms resistant to both proguanil and chloroquine are less commonly encountered. The "protective efficacy" of the combination is about 70% in Africa (from whence come most of the data).

Adverse Effects. When used at the correct dose (and infused slowly if given intravenously), chloroquine is a very safe drug. Idiosyncratic adverse effects are remarkably uncommon, and chloroquine does not seem to be teratogenic. In self-poisoning, and if the drug is infused too quickly intravenously, shock and cardiac arrhythmias are the commonest problems. There is no specific antidote and dialysis is unhelpful, but adrenaline and diazepam (Valium) have been used in some series. Of its symptomatic adverse effects, pruritus is worthy of note: It is commoner in blacks than in whites, can be very unpleasant, and probably affects compliance. Cumulative chloroquine retinopathy is not encountered in malaria chemotherapy and is rare in chemoprophylaxis. Most cases occur during the treatment of rheumatoid disease, when large doses are used for prolonged periods. Even so, many ophthalmologists would advocate periodic screening of patients taking long-term chloroquine for chemoprophylaxis.

Quinine

Malaria Treatment. Quinine is a naturally occurring compound of relatively low potency and narrow therapeutic range. Because resistance to quinine is rare in Africa and uncommon elsewhere, quinine has become the first-choice drug for severe falciparum malaria (displacing chloroquine, which is more potent but with which resistant strains are much more commonly encountered). Like chloroquine, doses of parenteral quinine must be calculated from body weight; in contrast to chloroquine, parenteral doses of quinine are generally calculated in terms of the dihydrochloride salt rather than the active base. IV infusion is the preferred route, and, like chloroquine, it is essential that quinine be diluted and infused slowly. If IV infusion is not possible, quinine may be given by deep intramuscular (IM) injection. Doses should be diluted in water for injections, and the loading dose is best administered half into each thigh. The many disadvantages of quinine (it tastes very unpleasant, must be given at least twice daily for at least 5 days, and usually causes symptomatic toxicity) make it a difficult drug to use orally for uncomplicated malaria, although this is done in some countries. Furthermore, quinine is expensive ($2.28 for a 7-day oral course) and practicable only for the relatively small number with severe disease.

Malaria Prevention. Quinine is not used for chemoprophylaxis; there are more efficacious and safer alternatives.

Adverse Effects. Quinine is a relatively safe drug if dose recommendations are followed. Overdosage or rapid IV infusion can be serious and may result in retinal damage, QT prolongation, and arrhythmias. In the setting of overdose, stellate ganglion block is no longer considered useful to prevent or ameliorate retinal damage, but repeated doses of activated charcoal are used to increase quinine clearance. Idiosyncratic adverse reactions to quinine are not uncommon (but are seen mostly when the drug is used long-term in the prevention of night cramps) and include thrombocytopenia, pancytopenia, and coagulopathy.

Quinidine. In the United States quinine is often not available, and quinidine is used instead. Because of its plasma protein binding characteristics quinidine is more potent than quinine (both to the parasite and the host), and doses are slightly smaller. In severe falciparum malaria, a loading dose of 15 mg (of the base) per kg is given over 4 hours and is followed by 8 hourly maintenance doses of 7.5 mg (base) per kg each over 4 hours.

Pyrimethamine-Sulfadoxine (and Congeners)

Malaria Treatment. Pyrimethamine-sulfadoxine (PM/SD) (Fansidar) is cheap (cost for adult treatment around $0.20), practicable (only one dose is needed because both drugs are eliminated so slowly), and highly effective in much of Africa. In much of southeast Asia and parts of South America the combination is now useless. Even in areas where resistance is not a major problem, PM/SD is used only for uncomplicated cases of falciparum malaria. The parenteral formulation of PM/SD is used mainly for nonsevere falciparum malaria complicated by protracted vomiting. Theoretical concerns about the "speed" of onset of action and very practical worries about resistance make this an unwise choice for severe malaria. Plasmodia other than *P. falciparum* are innately less sensitive to PM/SD, and chloroquine is preferable.

Adverse Effects. PM/SD has a wide therapeutic range, and concentration-dependent toxicity is unusual except after overdose, when seizures and fatalities have been reported. Idiosyncratic toxicity to PM is unusual, but, like all sulfonamides, SD is prone to immune-mediated toxicity. Such reactions, usually dermatologic, have caused deaths but usually have been seen in the setting of prolonged exposure during chemoprophylaxis. Similarly, pyrimethamine-dapsone (PM/DDS), when used for chemoprophylaxis, was associated with a high risk of idiosyncratic agranulocytosis: this was thought to have been caused by the dapsone component. Neither PM/SD nor PM/DDS is now used for malaria prevention.

Proguanil

Daily proguanil* (Paludrine), combined with weekly chloroquine, is used for malaria chemoprophylaxis but is not used in the treatment of malaria. Proguanil has antimalarial activity but is not potent and can be regarded as a prodrug. It is metabolized to the potent antimalarial cycloguanil by hepatic mixed-function oxidases (specifically by CYP2C19 and CYP3A). Cycloguanil, like pyrimethamine, is an inhibitor of dihydrofolate reductase; also like pyrimethamine, cycloguanil is innately less active against *P. vivax, P. ovale,* and *P. malariae* than it is against *P. falciparum.* Proguanil has a reputation for safety, even after overdose. Self-limiting gastrointestinal adverse effects are common, but serious toxicity is rare.

Mefloquine

Malaria Treatment. Mefloquine (Lariam) is used only for uncomplicated falciparum malaria, because there is no parenteral formulation that might allow its use for severe disease. The drug is effective against all species of human malaria parasite. Mefloquine is mainly employed in richer countries in which multidrug resistance is a problem (e.g., Thailand); it is unaffordable for general use throughout tropical Africa ($2.40 for an adult treatment dose). Because of its extremely slow rate of elimination, mefloquine may be given as a single dose of 15 mg per kg; however, this dose is associated with much nausea, and many physicians would give the dose in two halves separated by several hours. In parts of

*Not available in the United States.

southeast Asia (especially the Thai-Burmese border), resistance to mefloquine is developing rapidly, and a higher dose (25 mg per kg in two halves, 6 hours apart) is employed.

Malaria Prevention. Once-weekly mefloquine (250 mg weekly for adults) is used extensively for chemoprophylaxis and currently gives the best degree of protection for visits to high-risk areas of Africa, with a protective efficacy of about 90%. Concerns about the risk/benefit ratio of prophylactic mefloquine have been expressed and are discussed briefly in what follows.

Adverse Effects. Like any drug, mefloquine can, rarely, cause serious idiosyncratic adverse reactions including exfoliative dermatitis, toxic epidermal necrolysis, cutaneous vasculitis, thyroid hormone perturbation, and aplastic anemia. Type A adverse effects are more common (particularly when high doses are given for malaria therapy), usually mild, and most frequently gastrointestinal. Mefloquine is not recommended in pregnancy, but this reflects caution rather than a reaction to known risk.

Much current interest centers on the "neuropsychiatric" adverse events associated with mefloquine prophylaxis. There is certainly a dose-related element to this group of adverse events, which are considerably more common during high-dose therapy with mefloquine for malaria treatment; however, whether all the events are straightforward type A reactions is unclear. "Serious" central nervous system (CNS) events, including seizures, are estimated to occur in about one in 10,000 prophylactic users, which is about the same rate as that for chloroquine. The estimated frequency of nonserious CNS events (including headache, dizziness, insomnia, and depression) varies between 1.8% and 7.6% and is generally higher in females than males; these proportions are similar to those for chloroquine but about five-fold higher than those reported by patients taking no prophylaxis. Direct comparisons have been made between mefloquine and chloroquine-proguanil in terms of the frequency, severity, and type of adverse reaction. In a retrospective questionnaire-based study, 1214 adults taking mefloquine and 1181 taking chloroquine plus proguanil were surveyed. Forty percent of both groups reported adverse events, but neuropsychiatric adverse events were significantly more common in travelers taking mefloquine (333/1214, compared with 189/1181 in the chloroquine-proguanil group). In contrast, a recent prospective randomized double-blind trial in soldiers found no difference in the prevalence of CNS toxicity between mefloquine users and those on chloroquine-proguanil; this latter study is in keeping with earlier findings in both military personnel and private travelers. In addition, a carefully conducted double-blind randomized placebo-controlled trial studied the prevalence of adverse effects to mefloquine in volunteers: mefloquine was associated with mild diarrhea, electrocardiographic QT-prolongation, and a mean drop in plasma glucose of 0.5 mmol per liter^{-1}, but there was no excess of CNS adverse events and "symbol digit modality" testing was unaffected by mefloquine.

Halofantrine*

Malaria Treatment. Like mefloquine, halofantrine (Halfan) is an expensive drug ($7.00 for an adult course) without a parenteral formulation. It is used frequently for uncomplicated malaria in richer countries in which multidrug resistance is a problem, but it is unaffordable for general use in poorer countries. Halofantrine is not an appropriate drug for chemoprophylaxis mainly for pharmacokinetic reasons but also because of concerns over cardiac toxicity. Halofantrine is poorly and unpredictably absorbed from the gut, the proportion of a dose absorbed declining with dose size; to reduce this problem the drug is taken in doses 6 hours apart (to a total of 24 mg per kg in children or 1.5 grams in adults). Resistance is already a problem, especially in parts of southeast Asia, where the same regimen is repeated 1 week after first treatment to reduce the risk of recrudescence.

Adverse Effects. Halofantrine is generally well tolerated, and idiosyncratic toxicity is rare, but it prolongs the electrocardiographic-corrected QT interval, especially in the high-dose regimen, and deaths from arrhythmias are recorded. It is possible that thiamine deficiency contributes to the cardiac effects of halofantrine.

Artemisinine Derivatives

Malaria Treatment. Artemisinine is a pharmacologically active molecule discovered in a herbal antimalarial remedy. It has been used successfully both by mouth and as a suppository, but several semisynthetic derivatives have been developed (two are described), with the advantages of greater antimalarial potency and stability but the disadvantage of higher cost. All compounds in the group are active antimalarials in their own right but are also metabolized to dihydroartemisinin, a pharmacologically active metabolite. The artemisinine group of drugs has two major advantages over other drugs for falciparum malaria: (1) resistance is not currently a problem, even in areas of multidrug resistance, and (2) the artemisinines have activity against circulating ring forms, which may confer clinical advantage in patients with severe malaria. Unfortunately, recrudescence rates are high if the course of treatment is shorter than 5 days. In the setting of severe malaria, clinical trials comparing the risks of death and sequelae in children treated with quinine and artemether have largely found that they are equivalent. However, there are concerns that, by chance, children randomized to artemether in such trials may have been worse than those randomized to quinine and that this may have caused bias. Meta-analysis stud-

*Not available in the United States.

ies are in hand, which may cast some light in this area.

Artemether. Artemether is available in ampules dissolved in arachis oil and is injected intramuscularly to treat severe falciparum malaria. There is a suspicion (based on one pharmacokinetic study) that the worst subgroup of children with cerebral malaria may absorb artemether poorly intramuscularly; this is currently being investigated further. Artemether is also available in an oral formulation for uncomplicated disease, but there is little reason to use this outside areas of multidrug resistance.

Artemether Plus Benflumitol.* Benflumitol is a long-acting, synthetic drug that is combined with artemether in tablet form for the treatment of uncomplicated malaria. It is hoped that recrudescence will be less of a problem than with the use of artemether alone.

Artesunate.* Artesunate is available as dry powder, which is first dissolved in 1 mL of 5% sodium bicarbonate and then further diluted in saline for either IV or IM injection. This formulation is intended for use in severe malaria. In addition, artesunate suppositories are being studied at the moment in the setting of children with nonsevere malaria who are unable to take drugs by mouth.

The cost of artemisinine derivatives (the critical determinant of their utility in Africa) is quite variable among countries, but they are expensive. In Thailand a standard 5-day course costs about $6.00 (parenteral therapy being about five-fold more expensive), but in Vietnam, where the drugs are manufactured locally, oral treatment courses cost about $1.00.

Malaria Prevention. Artemisinines are not recommended for chemoprophylaxis.

Adverse Effects. These are drugs with a wide therapeutic range and a very low risk of idiosyncratic toxicity. CNS toxicity can be produced in animal models when high doses are administered, but this is yet to be shown to be a problem in humans.

Doxycycline and Other Tetracyclines

Several groups of antibiotics, including the tetracyclines and the macrolides, have utility against *P. falciparum.* The commonest setting for their use is in southeast Asia, where tetracycline is often combined with quinine: The efficacy of the combination is greater than that of quinine alone in this region where quinine resistance is quickly emerging. Doxycycline (Vibramycin) is used for malaria prophylaxis. Experience with this drug is less extensive than that with other chemoprophylactic drugs, and its protective efficacy is less well established (some studies suggest good levels of protection). It tends to be given to travelers to high-risk areas who cannot take chloroquine-proguanil or mefloquine.

Primaquine

Pre-erythrocytic stages ("hypnozoites") of *P. vivax* and *P. ovale* (neither *P. falciparum* nor *P. malariae* has a hypnozoite form) are not eradicated by any of the drugs described thus far, which are capable of producing only a clinical cure, and may cause late relapse unless dealt with. The 8-aminoquinoline primaquine is the only drug available for this purpose at the moment. Primaquine is well absorbed after oral administration but has a short half-life and needs to be administered daily; the conventional adult regimen is 15 mg daily for 14 to 21 days. Mild gastrointestinal adverse effects are common. More serious toxicity includes reversible bone marrow depression and intravascular hemolysis; the latter may be a major problem in patients with glucose-6-phosphate dehydrogenase deficiency (which should be screened for before primaquine is prescribed to high-risk ethnic groups).

*Not available in the United States.

New Drugs

Atovaquone-Proguanil. Atovaquone (Mepron) is an antiprotozoan agent with activity against *P. falciparum, Pneumocystis carinii,* and *Toxoplasma gondii*; it probably works by blocking electron transport at the cytochrome-bc_1 complex of the respiratory chain, which results in inhibition of pyrimidine synthesis. Atovaquone synergises with proguanil against *P. falciparum* and has been shown (in an open trial) to be superior to amodiaquine in the treatment of uncomplicated falciparum malaria in Gabon. Most adverse effects are mild and usually gastrointestinal. Atovaquone-proguanil is likely to be relatively expensive and is of most value in areas of multidrug resistance, including southeast Asia. Its manufacturer has decided to provide the combination free to certain parts of Africa for the time being.

Pyronaridine. This synthetic Chinese drug is not yet available commercially. It is currently formulated as tablets, but because these have poor oral bioavailability, the drug is being reformulated by the World Health Organization. Pyronaridine is effective against multidrug-resistant *P. falciparum.* Unfortunately, resistance to pyronaridine develops readily, and the value of this compound in practice remains to be seen.

Chlorproguanil-Dapsone (Lapdap). This fixed-ratio combination of antifolate drugs is not yet available commercially. Lapdap is likely to have activity against PM/SD-resistant *P. falciparum* and has the promise of being low in cost. The combination is being developed with the treatment of uncomplicated malaria in Africa in mind. It remains to be seen how useful Lapdap will be.

WR 230609. This 8-aminoquinoline, which is not yet available commercially, promises to be less toxic than primaquine. Like primaquine, it will be used mainly for the "radical cure" of vivax and ovale malaria.

SUPPORTIVE THERAPY

In Africa, most patients with uncomplicated malaria are managed as outpatients; little supportive care is needed other than attention to the lowering of temperature, especially in young children who are at risk of febrile convulsions. Paracetamol (acetaminophen) is the first-choice antipyretic drug. Severe falciparum malaria, on the other hand, may require a full range of supportive care if the patient is to live long enough for the antiparasitic drugs described earlier to work. A detailed description of specific supportive measures is beyond the scope of this article and has been reviewed elsewhere.

AMERICAN TRYPANOSOMIASIS
(Chagas' Disease)

method of
LOUIS V. KIRCHHOFF, M.D., M.P.H.
University of Iowa College of Medicine
Iowa City, Iowa

American trypanosomiasis, or Chagas' disease, is a zoonosis caused by the protozoan parasite *Trypanosoma cruzi,* which is transmitted by triatomine insects. This organism is enzootic in Latin America and the southern and southwestern United States. Approximately 16 to 18 million people in Latin America are infected with *T. cruzi,* and 45,000 deaths per year are estimated to result from Chagas' disease. Only a handful of cases of insect-borne transmission of *T. cruzi* to humans in the United States have been reported. The number of *T. cruzi*–infected individuals living in the United States has increased markedly in recent decades, however, as several million persons have emigrated from endemic countries. These infected people will present diagnostic and therapeutic challenges to the physicians who provide their medical care. In addition, because most *T. cruzi*–infected persons harbor the parasite asymptomatically and are unaware of being infected, there is a risk of transmission of the parasite by blood transfusion; several such cases have been reported.

CLINICAL MANIFESTATIONS

Acute Chagas' disease is usually a mild illness and may include malaise, fever, edema of the face and lower extremities, hepatosplenomegaly, and generalized lymphadenopathy. Severe myocarditis develops in a small proportion of patients with acute infections, and meningoencephalitis is a rare complication. The death rate is less than 5%. In most patients, acute Chagas' disease resolves spontaneously over 4 to 8 weeks, after which they enter the indeterminate phase of *T. cruzi* infection. This asymptomatic phase is characterized by subpatent parasitemias and easily detectable anti–*T. cruzi* antibodies.

Years or decades after the resolution of acute *T. cruzi* infection, symptomatic chronic Chagas' disease develops in approximately 10 to 30% of infected persons. The heart is most commonly affected, leading to rhythm disturbances, congestive failure due to cardiomyopathy, and thromboembolic events. In some patients megaesophagus and/or megacolon develop and cause regurgitation, dysphagia, recurrent aspiration, and constipation. Immunosuppression of patients who harbor *T. cruzi* chronically can cause a recrudescence of acute Chagas' disease. This is particularly true in infected patients who undergo cardiac transplantation and in persons co-infected with *T. cruzi* and the human immunodeficiency virus.

DIAGNOSIS

The diagnosis of acute Chagas' disease is made by detecting parasites and should be considered in persons who have resided recently in an endemic area or in infants born to mothers at risk of harboring *T. cruzi.* In immunocompetent patients, examination of anticoagulated or Giemsa-stained blood is the cornerstone of diagnosing *T. cruzi* infection. In immunosuppressed persons suspected of having acute Chagas' disease, other specimens such as bone marrow, cerebrospinal fluid, pericardial fluid, and lymph nodes should be examined microscopically. Hemoculture and polymerase chain reaction–based assay are alternatives for cases in which the parasite cannot be seen, and both are available in my laboratory (telephone 319-335-6786).

Chronic Chagas' disease is diagnosed by detecting IgG antibodies to *T. cruzi,* and parasitologic studies are unnecessary. In the United States, enzyme-linked immunosorbent assay (ELISA)–based tests, manufactured by Abbott Laboratories (Abbott Park, IL), Gull Laboratories (Salt Lake City, UT), and Hemagen (Waltham, MA), have been cleared by the Food and Drug Administration for clinical use. A persistent problem with serologic tests for chronic *T. cruzi* infection, however, is the occurrence of false-positive results, which typically occur with sera from persons having other infectious or autoimmune diseases. A more specific radioimmune precipitation test is available in my laboratory for confirmatory testing.

TREATMENT

Antiparasitic Drugs

Current therapy for *T. cruzi* infection is unsatisfactory. Only two drugs have been shown to be useful. The first of these is nifurtimox (Lampit*), a nitrofuran derivative. Extensive clinical experience regarding its use has accumulated during the 3 decades that nifurtimox has been available. Its mechanism of action is not known. In patients with acute or congenital Chagas' disease, nifurtimox reduces the severity and duration of the illness and lessens mortality, but parasitologic cures are achieved in only 50% of these patients. Those not cured enter the indeterminate phase of *T. cruzi* infection and are at risk for symptomatic chronic Chagas' disease. Cure rates are also about 50% in patients with chronic *T. cruzi* infections. Nifurtimox can cause severe side effects, including gastrointestinal complaints such as nausea, vomiting, abdominal pain, anorexia, and weight loss. Some patients taking the drug also develop neurologic symptoms, such as restlessness, insomnia, twitching, paresthesias, polyneuritis, and seizures.

Nifurtimox can be obtained from the Centers for Disease Control and Prevention (CDC) Drug Service (telephone 770-639-3670 [working hours]; 770-639-2888 [off hours]). It is available in 30- and 120-mg tablets. For adults the recommended oral dosage is 8 to 10 mg per kg of body weight per day. For adoles-

*Investigational drug in the U.S.; available from CDC.

cents the dose is 12.5 to 15 mg per kg per day, and for children 1 to 10 years of age it is 15 to 20 mg per kg per day. The drug should be given each day in four divided doses, and treatment should be continued for 90 to 120 days.

The second drug useful for treating *T. cruzi* infections is benznidazole (Rachagan), which is also available from the CDC Drug Service. The effect of benznidazole on the clinical course of acute Chagas' disease is similar to that of nifurtimox, and cure rates are also roughly 50% in patients in either acute or chronic infections. Side effects can include granulocytopenia, rash, and peripheral neuropathy. The recommended oral dosage of benznidazole is 5 mg per kg of body weight per day for 60 days. The daily dose is given in two or three divided doses. I favor using benznidazole over nifurtimox because its side effects are less bothersome and its schedule of administration is simpler.

In terms of who should be treated, I feel that all patients infected with *T. cruzi* should be treated with either benznidazole or nifurtimox regardless of the stage of their infection. This view is based on the results of studies of *T. cruzi*–infected experimental animals and humans, which show that treatment with either of these drugs reduces the appearance and/or progression of cardiac lesions.

The usefulness of fluconazole (Diflucan), itraconazole (Sporanox), allopurinol (Zyloprim), and interferon-γ has been studied extensively in experimental animals and to a lesser extent in patients with acute Chagas' disease. None of these agents has shown a level of anti–*T. cruzi* activity warranting use in patients.

Treatment of Clinical Chagas' Disease

Beyond the use of nifurtimox and benznidazole, the treatment of both acute and chronic Chagas' disease is symptomatic. Patients with severe acute chagasic myocarditis should be supported as any patient with acute congestive cardiomyopathy. In patients with symptomatic chronic Chagas' heart disease, therapy is directed at ameliorating symptoms through the use of cardiotropic drugs and anticoagulants. Pacemakers have been shown to be useful in patients with ominous bradyarrhythmias or heart block.

Heart transplantation is an option for patients with end-stage chagasic cardiac disease. Several dozen *T. cruzi*–infected patients have undergone cardiac transplantation in Brazil and about a dozen have had the procedure in the United States. The degree of cardiac parasitization after transplantation and its impact on implant viability have not been defined. The experience with a handful of the U.S. patients suggests that intermittent prophylactic nifurtimox (three successive days of therapy each week) is useful in preventing recrudescence of acute Chagas' disease after transplant. It must be kept in mind, however, that the efficacy and adverse effects of long-term administration of nifurtimox or benznidazole are unknown. These uncertainties suggest that cardiac transplantation in patients with end-stage chagasic cardiac disease should be approached with caution, especially in view of the extremely limited availability of donor hearts. This view should not be applied to kidney transplantation, however, because postoperative immunosuppression is less intensive and the risk of reactivation is minimal.

Megaesophagus associated with Chagas' disease should be treated as idiopathic achalasia. Patients with megaesophagus who fail to respond to repeated balloon dilatation are treated surgically. The procedure most frequently used is wide esophagocardiomyectomy of the anterior gastroesophageal junction, combined with valvuloplasty to reduce reflux. Patients with severe distal esophageal dilatation are often treated with esophageal resection with reconstruction using an esophagogastroplasty. Laparoscopic myotomy is being used with increasing frequency in industrialized countries to treat patients with severe idiopathic achalasia, and this procedure may become the approach of choice for chagasic megaesophagus as well.

Patients with chronic Chagas' disease in the early stages of colonic dysfunction can be managed with a high-fiber diet and occasional laxatives and enemas. Fecal impaction requiring manual disempaction can occur, as can toxic megacolon or volvulus, both of which require surgery at some point. Endoscopic emptying can be done initially in patients with volvulus who have no clinical, endoscopic, or radiographic signs of ischemia in the affected area. Cases that are complicated should be treated with surgical decompression. In either case, however, surgical resection of the megacolon is ultimately necessary because of the frequent recurrence of volvulus. Several surgical procedures have been used to treat advanced chagasic megacolon, and all of them include resection of the sigmoid as well as removal of part of the rectum. The latter is performed to avoid subsequent recurrence of megacolon in the segment anastomosed to the rectum. The Haddad modification of the Duhamel procedure has been used with considerable success.

BACTERIAL MENINGITIS

method of
W. MICHAEL SCHELD, M.D.
University of Virginia School of Medicine
Charlottesville, Virginia

Despite the introduction of newer antimicrobial agents, the morbidity and mortality associated with bacterial meningitis remain unacceptably high. For example, approximately 60% of infants who survive gram-negative bacillary meningitis have developmental disabilities and/or neurologic sequelae. Similarly, in a review of 493 episodes of bacterial-meningitis in adults, the overall case-fatality rate was 25%. This brief discussion highlights epidemiologic trends of therapeutic importance, considers the potential

TABLE 1. **Bacterial Meningitis: Five States and Los Angeles County, 1986**

Organism	Total (%)	Case-Fatality Rate (%)
Haemophilus influenzae	45	3
Streptococcus pneumoniae	18	19
Neisseria meningitidis	14	13
Group B streptococci	5.7	12
Listeria monocytogenes	3.2	22
Other	15	28

Adapted from Wenger JD, Hightower AW, Facklam RR, et al: Bacterial meningitis in the United States, 1986: Report of a multistate surveillance study. J Infect Dis *162:*1316–1323, 1990. University of Chicago, publisher.

impact of new diagnostic tests, and focuses on the management of bacterial meningitis with antimicrobial agents, including the role of adjunctive therapy.

EPIDEMIOLOGIC TRENDS

In 1990, the Centers for Disease Control and Prevention published a multistate surveillance study of bacterial meningitis based on data collected in 1986 (Table 1). Although these data reflect a prospective laboratory-based study performed in five states and Los Angeles County, more recent trends have rendered the results out of date. In 1986, *Haemophilus influenzae* was the most common cause of bacterial meningitis, accounting for 45% of cases, with an overall fatality rate of 3%. *Streptococcus pneumoniae* (18%) and *Neisseria meningitidis* (14%) were isolated less commonly, with case-fatality rates in the 15 to 20% range. The incidence rates for specific pathogens were most influenced by age. In 1986, approximately 15,000 cases of bacterial meningitis occurred in the United States, and most cases were documented at the extremes of life (<1 month of age and >60 years of age).

The frequency of meningitis due to *H. influenzae* in children has declined dramatically because of widespread use of *H. influenzae* type b vaccines. For example, in the United States, as stated in one report, there was an 82% reduction in the incidence of *H. influenzae* meningitis in children 5 years of age and younger from 1985 through 1991. The changing epidemiology of meningitis from 1986 through 1995 is displayed in Table 2. These data were first presented at an international infectious diseases meeting in September 1996. The incidence per 100,000 population for *H. influenzae* disease has declined more than 95% in the past decade. This is the greatest achievement in the control of pediatric infectious diseases in this generation, and the scientists most responsible for this result received the Lasker Award in 1996. As can be seen, the overall incidence of pneumococcal and meningococcal meningitis has remained relatively stable in the United States during this interval. As shown in Table 3, the mortality for pneumococcal meningitis has remained approximately 20% during the past 10 years, but a dramatic decline in the mortality rate associated with meningococcal meningitis and meningitis due to group B streptococci (*Streptococcus agalactiae*) has been documented. Mortality associated with meningitis due to *Listeria monocytogenes* has remained relatively stable. Despite the overall reduction in *H. influenzae* disease, the overall rate of invasive disease due to *S. pneumoniae* and *S. agalactiae* has increased in the past 10 years (Table 4), whereas the incidence of invasive meningococcal disease has remained relatively stable. These epidemiologic trends have profound implications for the treatment of bacterial meningitis. *H. influenzae* meningitis has almost disappeared from the United States. Meningitis due to pneumococci and meningococci is now found more frequently in children.

Although penicillin resistance was first documented in *S. pneumoniae* in the late 1960s, the incidence of infection with *S. pneumoniae* resistant to penicillin, other β-lactam antibiotics, and other agents has increased worldwide in

TABLE 2. **Changing Epidemiology of Bacterial Meningitis: United States***

Organism	Incidence/100,000 Population	
	1986	*1995*
Haemophilus influenzae	2.9	0.2
Neisseria meningitidis	0.9	0.6
Streptococcus pneumoniae	1.1	1.1

*Data for 1995 represent race- and age-adjusted estimates and refer to surveillance for all pathogens listed from six counties in Maryland, eight in Georgia, five in Tennessee, and three in San Francisco. For San Francisco, surveillance occurred from October 1994 through September 1995.

Data from Schuchat A, Robinson KA, Wenger JD, et al: Bacterial meningitis in the United States in 1995. N Engl J Med *337:*970–976, 1997; and Wenger JD, Hightower AW, Facklam RR, et al: Bacterial meningitis in the United States, 1986: Report of a multistate surveillance study. J Infect Dis *162:*1316–1323, 1990.

TABLE 3. **Mortality for Bacterial Meningitis Caused by Selected Pathogens, 1986–1995**

Organism	Mortality (%)	
	1986	*1995*
Streptococcus pneumoniae	19	21
Neisseria meningitidis	13	3
Streptococcus agalactiae	12	7
Listeria monocytogenes	23	15

Data from Schuchat A, Robinson KA, Wenger JD, et al: Bacterial meningitis in the United States in 1995. N Engl J Med *337:*970–976, 1997; and Wenger JD, Hightower AW, Facklam RR, et al: Bacterial meningitis in the United States, 1986: Report of a multistate surveillance study. J Infect Dis *162:*1316–1323, 1990.

TABLE 4. **Invasive Disease Caused by Selected Pathogens, 1986–1995***

Organism	Incidence/100,000 Population	
	1986	*1995*
Streptococcus pneumoniae	15.0	26.1
Streptococcus agalactiae	3.7	8.1
Neisseria meningitidis	1.3	1.3
Listeria monocytogenes	0.7	0.5

*Data for 1995 represent race- and age-adjusted estimates and refer to surveillance for all pathogens listed from six counties in Maryland, eight in Georgia, five in Tennessee, and three in San Francisco. For San Francisco, surveillance occurred from October 1994 through September 1995.

Data from Schuchat A, Robinson KA, Wenger JD, et al: Bacterial meningitis in the United States in 1995. N Engl J Med *337:*970–976, 1997; and Wenger JD, Hightower AW, Facklam RR, et al: Bacterial meningitis in the United States, 1986: Report of a multistate surveillance study. J Infect Dis *162:*1316–1323, 1990.

TABLE 5. **Typical Cerebrospinal Fluid Findings in Patients with Bacterial Meningitis**

Cerebrospinal Fluid Parameter	Typical Findings
Opening pressure	>180 mm H_2O
Leukocyte count	1000–5000/mm^3 (range <100 to >10,000)
Percentage of neutrophils	≥80%
Protein concentration	100–500 mg/dL
Glucose concentration	≤40 mg/dL
Gram's stain	Positive in 60–90%
Culture	Positive in 70–85%

the last decade. This resistance is mediated not by β-lactamase production but by alterations in the penicillin binding proteins involved in bacterial cell wall synthesis. The global spread of penicillin-resistant pneumococci has important implications for the empirical treatment of meningitis (see later).

DIAGNOSTIC EVALUATION

The diagnosis of bacterial meningitis still rests on examination of the cerebrospinal fluid (CSF); the typical CSF abnormalities in patients with bacterial meningitis are shown in Table 5. In patients with typical CSF findings and a negative Gram stain, several other tests are available to assist in making an etiologic diagnosis, including counter-immunoelectrophoresis or latex agglutination tests for the detection of the antigens of common meningeal pathogens. The overall sensitivity of these tests ranges from 50 to 100%, but they are highly specific. Latex agglutination is currently favored. A positive test result establishes the diagnosis of bacterial meningitis caused by a specific pathogen, although a negative test result does not rule out this diagnosis. Examination of petechiae, if present, by scrapings with a touch preparation technique and proper staining will detect meningococci in approximately 70% of cases of meningococcemia. Similarly, in suspected meningococcemia, the organism may be apparent on the peripheral blood smear, especially a buffy coat preparation. The differential diagnosis of fever, altered sensorium, and petechial rash is shown in Table 6. This condition should be considered a medical emergency and promptly evaluated.

Several newer techniques have been proposed for the diagnosis of bacterial meningitis when the Gram stain of the CSF is negative. Elevation of the concentration of C-reactive protein in CSF is highly sensitive for the diagnosis of bacterial meningitis but is not specific. Nevertheless, a normal CSF C-reactive protein concentration excludes bacterial meningitis with nearly 99% certainty in the acute phase. CSF concentrations of tumor necrosis factor appear to be elevated in bacterial but not viral meningitis. The potential use of this technique in separating partially treated bacterial from viral meningitis remains uncertain but is promising. Similarly, the polymerase chain reaction (PCR) for the diagnosis of bacterial meningitis in the absence of a positive CSF Gram stain, latex agglutination test result, or culture may prove useful in the future. PCR for the diagnosis of tuberculous meningitis is particularly attractive because current diagnostic modalities are suboptimal.

TABLE 6. **Differential Diagnosis of Fever, Altered Sensorium, and Petechial Rash**

- Meningococcal disease
- Rickettsial infections (Rocky Mountain spotted fever, others)
- *Staphylococcus aureus* endocarditis
- *Streptococcus pneumoniae* or *Haemophilus influenzae* infection (especially with splenectomy)
- Septic shock
- Viral meningitis
- Viral hemorrhagic fevers
- "Noninfectious": thrombotic thrombocytopenic purpura, hemolytic-uremic syndrome, vasculitis, others

INITIAL APPROACH TO MANAGEMENT

A strategy, in algorithmic form, for the initial management of patients with suspected bacterial meningitis is shown in Figure 1. When a patient presents with clinical features suggestive of bacterial meningitis and displays an acute presentation (i.e., ≤24 hours from first symptom to presentation and/or stupor or coma), blood samples for two sets of cultures should be immediately obtained and the patient presumptively treated while lumbar puncture is performed. If the presentation is more subacute (i.e., >24 hours from the onset of symptoms to presentation, minimal alteration in mental status), a rapid neurologic examination should be performed. If focal findings are present (e.g., hemiparesis) or papilledema is documented, the patient should be evaluated first with computed tomography (CT). If bacterial meningitis is a strong consideration, blood samples should be drawn for cultures and the patient presumptively treated while undergoing CT. Appropriate treatment should be administered if a mass lesion is documented. If the CT result is normal or focal signs are absent on neurologic examination, the patient should immediately be subjected to lumbar puncture. On the basis of the results (CSF formula, Gram's stain, or antigen detection tests), empirical and/or specific treatment should be started. The interval from the onset of evaluation to the first dose of antimicrobial agent should not exceed 60 to 120

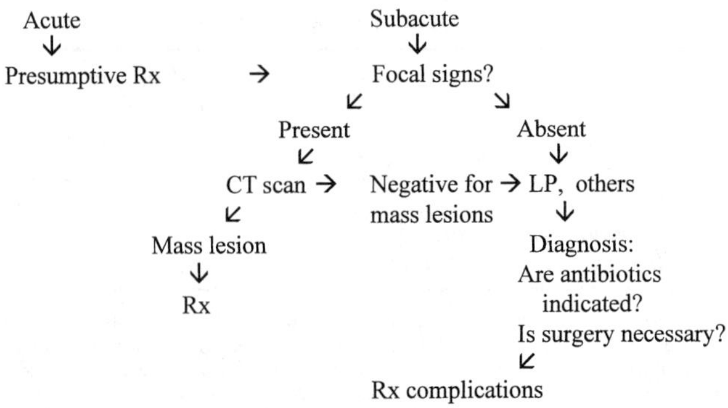

Figure 1. An algorithm for the initial strategy of management for patients with suspected bacterial meningitis.
Abbreviations: CT = computed tomography; LP = lumbar puncture; Rx = therapy.

minutes, although a delay in therapy has not been conclusively documented to adversely affect outcome in multiple studies in the medical literature. Nevertheless, in the absence of compelling clinical data and in the best interests of the patient, antimicrobial therapy should be initiated promptly in patients with suspected bacterial meningitis.

EMPIRICAL ANTIMICROBIAL THERAPY

When lumbar puncture is delayed or Gram's stain of the CSF is nondiagnostic, empirical therapy for presumed bacterial meningitis is essential and should be directed to the most likely pathogens based on the patient's age and the underlying host status (Table 7). In neonates, the major pathogens are group B streptococci, *Escherichia coli,* and *L. monocytogenes;* the empirical antimicrobial regimen of choice is ampicillin plus cefotaxime (Claforan), although some neonatologists still prefer ampicillin plus an aminoglycoside. Ceftriaxone is avoided in this age group because of concerns regarding protein binding and displacement of bilirubin. In older infants, the neonatal pathogens are joined by the three major meningeal pathogens, and ampicillin plus a third-generation cephalosporin is preferred. In children and young adults, a third-generation cephalosporin is often administered alone, although the addition of vancomycin must be considered, owing to the emergence of penicillin-resistant pneumococci (see later). Ampicillin plus chloramphenicol is probably inadequate. In older adults (i.e., >50 years), the pneumococcus is the most frequently isolated pathogen from CSF, but the organisms listed are more common in this age group than in younger adults; therefore, ampicillin plus a third-generation cephalosporin is the regimen of choice. These recommendations may require modification under special circumstances, most notably when penicillin-resistant pneumococci are prevalent in the community. In immunocompromised patients, such as those with a lymphoreticular malignant neoplasm or receiving cytotoxic or high-dose glucocorticoid therapy, *Listeria* is a major consideration and ampicillin should be added to any regimen. In penicillin-allergic patients, the drug of choice for potential *L. monocytogenes* meningitis is high-dose trimethoprim-sulfamethoxazole (Bactrim, Septra). For patients with recent head trauma or neurosurgery or those with indwelling CSF shunts, broad-spectrum antibiotics effective against both gram-positive and gram-negative organisms including staphylococci should be initiated (e.g., vancomycin [Vancocin] plus ceftazidime [Fortaz]). If identifiable bacteria are seen on Gram's stain of the CSF, antibiotic therapy remains empirical but should be directed toward the presumptive pathogen. These regimens are shown in Table 8 and are discussed in more detail in the following.

PATHOGEN-SPECIFIC THERAPY

Streptococcus pneumoniae

The recommendations for antimicrobial therapy for pneumococcal meningitis have been altered on the basis of changes in the pneumococcal susceptibility pattern to penicillin G. The susceptibility to penicillin G is based on the minimal inhibitory concentration (MIC) of this agent. Strains with an MIC of less than 0.1 μg per mL are considered susceptible. When the MIC is 0.1 to 1.0 μg per mL, the strains are termed relatively or intermediately resistant; strains with an MIC of 2 μg per mL or greater are considered highly resistant. Strains of pneumococci that are relatively or highly resistant to penicillin are at least as highly invasive as susceptible organisms. Recent data in the United States document penicillin resistance rates of approximately 25 to 35% overall among pneumococci (Table 9); higher rates have been reported from Spain, eastern Europe, South Africa, Japan, and other areas of the world. Factors that have been shown to predispose to the development of resistance include age younger than 10 or older than 50 years, immunosuppression, prolonged hospital stay, children in day care settings, infection by serotypes 14 and 23, and frequent or prophylactic use

TABLE 7. **Common Pathogens and Empirical Therapeutic Recommendations Based on Age in Patients with Bacterial Meningitis***

Age	Common Bacterial Pathogens	Empirical Antimicrobial Therapy
0–4 wk	*Streptococcus agalactiae, Escherichia coli, Listeria monocytogenes, Klebsiella pneumoniae*	Ampicillin plus cefotaxime, or ampicillin plus an aminoglycoside
4–12 wk	*S. agalactiae, E. coli, L. monocytogenes, Haemophilus influenzae, Streptococcus pneumoniae, Neisseria meningitidis*	Ampicillin plus a third-generation cephalosporin†
3 mo–18 y	*S. pneumoniae, N. meningitidis, H. influenzae*	Third-generation cephalosporin,† or ampicillin plus chloramphenicol
18–50 y	*S. pneumoniae, N. meningitidis*	Third-generation cephalosporin ± ampicillin‡
>50 y	*S. pneumoniae, N. meningitidis, L. monocytogenes,* aerobic gram-negative bacilli	Ampicillin plus a third-generation cephalosporin†

*Vancomycin should be added to empirical therapeutic regimens when pneumococcal meningitis is suspected with strains that are highly resistant to penicillin or cephalosporins.
†Cefotaxime or ceftriaxone.
‡Add ampicillin if meningitis caused by *L. monocytogenes* is suspected.

TABLE 8. **Specific Antimicrobial Therapy for Bacterial Meningitis**

Bacterial Pathogen	Standard Therapy	Alternative Therapy
Streptococcus pneumoniae		
Penicillin MIC ≤0.1 μg/mL	Penicillin G or ampicillin	Third-generation cephalosporin*; chloramphenicol; vancomycin
Penicillin MIC 0.1–1.0 μg/mL	Third-generation cephalosporin*	Vancomycin
Penicillin MIC ≥2.0 μg/mL	Vancomycin plus a third-generation cephalosporin*	Meropenem†
Neisseria meningitidis	Penicillin G or ampicillin	Third-generation cephalosporin*; chloramphenicol; fluoroquinolone
Haemophilus influenzae		
β-Lactamase–negative	Ampicillin	Third-generation cephalosporin*; chloramphenicol; aztreonam
β-Lactamase–positive	Third-generation cephalosporin*	Chloramphenicol; aztreonam; fluoroquinolone
Enterobacteriaceae	Third-generation cephalosporin*	Aztreonam; fluoroquinolone; trimethoprim-sulfamethoxazole; meropenem
Pseudomonas aeruginosa	Ceftazidime‡	Aztreonam; fluoroquinolone‡; meropenem
Listeria monocytogenes	Ampicillin or penicillin G‡	Trimethoprim-sulfamethoxazole
Streptococcus agalactiae	Ampicillin or penicillin G‡	Third-generation cephalosporin*; vancomycin
Staphylococcus aureus		
Methicillin sensitive	Nafcillin or oxacillin	Vancomycin
Methicillin resistant	Vancomycin	
Staphylococcus epidermidis	Vancomycin§	

*Cefotaxime or ceftriaxone.
†Currently under study in patients with pneumococcal meningitis.
‡Addition of an aminoglycoside should be considered.
§Addition of rifampin should be considered.
Abbreviation: MIC = minimal inhibitory concentration.

of antimicrobial therapy (e.g., for the prevention of otitis media).

Because of these considerations, penicillin, ampicillin, and related agents can no longer be recommended as empirical antimicrobial therapy when *S. pneumoniae* is considered a likely pathogen in patients with bacterial meningitis. Chloramphenicol, despite long-standing worldwide use, has proved disappointing in several areas, especially in South Africa where a poor outcome has been documented in approximately 80% of children with penicillin-resistant pneumococcal meningitis treated with this agent. The third-generation cephalosporins cefotaxime and ceftriaxone (Rocephin) have been effective in the therapy for meningitis caused by relatively penicillin-resistant pneumococci. Unfortunately, several reports of pneumococcal strains in patients with meningitis with relatively low MICs for the third-generation cephalosporins (approximately 0.5 to 1 μg per mL) have documented failures with conventional therapy with these agents. The current guidelines by the National Committee for Clinical Laboratory Standards state that CSF isolates of *S. pneumoniae* with MICs for cefotaxime or ceftriaxone of greater than 0.5 μg per mL be considered intermediately resistant to cephalosporins. Some regard this recommendation as too conservative. Nevertheless, third-generation cephalosporins are recommended for meningitis due to intermediately resistant strains (see Table 8). Pneumococcal isolates resistant to vancomycin have not been described, and this agent is commonly employed in the empirical regimens for adults and children when resistant pneumococci are of concern. CSF penetration of vancomycin in adults has been somewhat erratic and is reduced in the presence of dexamethasone therapy. Therefore, vancomycin should never be used alone in the empirical treatment of meningitis, especially when dexamethasone is administered as an adjunctive treatment. In experimental pneumococcal meningitis, the combination of vancomycin and ceftriaxone was synergistic when the disease was induced with ceftriaxone-resistant strains.

Several other agents have been investigated for the treatment of pneumococcal meningitis. Although imipenem has been used successfully, the proconvulsant activity of this drug precludes its use in patients with central nervous system infection. Meropenem (Merrem) appears to be less epileptogenic and has been evaluated with promising results, although only a few patients with resistant pneumococcal strains

TABLE 9. **Proportion of Pneumococcal Isolates Resistant to Selected Antimicrobial Agents: Atlanta, 1994**

Drug	% Resistant*
Penicillin	25 (7)
Cefotaxime	9 (4)
Erythromycin, clarithromycin	15
Trimethoprim-sulfamethoxazole	26
Tetracycline	8

*Numbers in parentheses indicate the percentage of strains with *high level* resistance.

Based on data in Hofmann J, Cetron MS, Farley MM, et al: The prevalence of drug-resistant *Streptococcus pneumoniae* in Atlanta. N Engl J Med *333*:481–486, 1995.

have been treated with this agent. Newer fluoroquinolones such as trovafloxacin (Trovan) appear to penetrate into the CSF in therapeutic concentrations and may be useful in the future. Trovafloxacin has also been used orally in therapy for meningococcal meningitis.

The empirical regimen for pneumococcal meningitis suspected to be caused by strains highly resistant to penicillin or cephalosporins remains controversial. The combination of vancomycin plus a third-generation cephalosporin (cefotaxime or ceftriaxone) is recommended at present. Some authorities have also suggested the addition of rifampin to this empirical regimen, but rifampin may be antagonistic when it is used in combination against some pneumococcal strains and is not preferred currently. Follow-up lumbar puncture to document clearance of the organism is essential in all cases of suspected penicillin-resistant pneumococcal meningitis. Again, once susceptibility studies are available, antimicrobial therapy can be modified (see Table 8).

Neisseria meningitidis

The antimicrobial agents of choice for the treatment of meningococcal meningitis remain penicillin G and ampicillin. Although meningococcal strains are now emerging that are relatively resistant to penicillin G (i.e., MIC range of 0.1 to 1 μg per mL), they remain unusual in the United States, and the clinical significance of these resistant isolates is unclear, because patients with meningitis caused by these strains have recovered with standard penicillin therapy. Third-generation cephalosporins are also acceptable as empirical therapy for meningococcal meningitis. Newer quinolones are not recommended as first-line agents pending further clinical experience.

Haemophilus influenzae

Approximately one third of *H. influenzae* type b strains in the United States produce β-lactamase and are therefore resistant to ampicillin and related agents. Resistance to chloramphenicol is unusual. The second-generation cephalosporin cefuroxime (Zinacef) was initially found to be as efficacious as the combination of ampicillin plus chloramphenicol in childhood bacterial meningitis caused predominantly by *H. influenzae* type b, but subsequent studies have questioned the efficacy of this agent, and ceftriaxone or cefotaxime is now considered the drug of choice. These agents sterilize the CSF more rapidly and are associated with a lower rate of hearing loss compared with older cephalosporins such as cefuroxime.

Enteric Gram-Negative Bacilli

Before the early 1980s, the outcome of therapy for bacterial meningitis caused by gram-negative aerobic bacilli was often poor. Chloramphenicol was ineffective because it was often bacteriostatic against these isolates, and aminoglycosides were not highly effective because of inadequate CSF concentrations. With the advent of the broad-spectrum cephalosporins, clinical outcomes were remarkably improved (85 to 90% success rates) owing to the high activity of these agents against gram-negative pathogens and their high CSF penetration. Ceftazidime (Fortaz) (and perhaps cefepime [Maxipime], pending further data) must be considered the drug of choice for *Pseudomonas aeruginosa* meningitis, often in combination with an aminoglycoside against this nosocomial pathogen.

Several other agents have been employed successfully in patients with enteric gram-negative bacillary meningitis; these include aztreonam (Azactam), imipenem (Primaxin) (to be avoided for the reasons cited before), meropenem, newer cephalosporins such as cefepime, and fluoroquinolones. In patients who fail to respond, intrathecal or intraventricular aminoglycosides or alternative systemic antimicrobial therapy may be necessary and should be based on susceptibility studies.

Listeria monocytogenes

Ampicillin or penicillin remains the agent of choice for a documented *L. monocytogenes* meningitis. However, neither agent is bactericidal against *Listeria,* and mortality rates remain as high as 30%. Therefore, gentamicin should be combined with ampicillin for this disease. In penicillin-allergic patients, trimethoprim-sulfamethoxazole is the agent of choice. Despite susceptibility data to the contrary, chloramphenicol and vancomycin have proved ineffective for patients with systemic *Listeria* infection. Meropenem is active in vitro and in experimental animal models of *Listeria* meningitis, but there are inadequate human data at present to recommend its use as a firstline agent.

Streptococcus agalactiae

For neonates with meningitis due to group B streptococci, the combination of ampicillin and gentamicin is the therapy of choice because of documented in vitro synergy and reports of penicillin-tolerant strains. For adults, the benefit of the combination therapy over penicillin or ampicillin alone is unproved, and mortality is chiefly influenced by the presence of underlying disease.

DURATION OF ANTIMICROBIAL THERAPY

The duration of antimicrobial therapy for patients with bacterial meningitis is based largely on tradition rather than rigorous scientific evidence. Nevertheless, the suggested duration of antimicrobial therapy for each of the major meningeal pathogens is shown in Table 10.

ADJUNCTIVE THERAPY

As stated before, the morbidity and mortality from bacterial meningitis remain unacceptably high. Mul-

TABLE 10. **Guidelines for Duration of Antibiotic Therapy**

Pathogen	Suggested Duration (d)
Haemophilus influenzae	7
Neisseria meningitidis	5–7
Streptococcus pneumoniae	10–14
Listeria monocytogenes	14–21
Group B streptococci	14–21
Gram-negative bacilli*	21

*Other than *H. influenzae.*

tiple studies in experimental animal models of infection conducted during the past 2 decades have elucidated many aspects of the pathogenesis and pathophysiology of bacterial meningitis. These studies have documented the inflammatory potential of the gram-positive cell wall and gram-negative lipopolysaccharide as mediated through host molecules, such as the proinflammatory cytokines interleukin-1, interleukin-6, and tumor necrosis factor. Similarly, adjunctive corticosteroid therapy has been shown to be effective in attenuating many of the pathophysiologic consequences during experimental meningitis, such as subarachnoid space inflammation, increased intracranial pressure, and cerebral edema.

On the basis of these experimental studies, multiple clinical trials have been undertaken to determine the effects of adjunctive dexamethasone or similar agents on outcome in patients with bacterial meningitis. Several major controversies remain, despite the accumulation of this clinical information. The majority of children enrolled in these trials were infected with *H. influenzae.* a pathogen that is disappearing from the United States as a cause of invasive infection. The benefits of dexamethasone in children infected with other pathogens, especially *S. pneumoniae,* are not as compelling, although trends suggest a reduction in audiologic and neurologic sequelae. Furthermore, the role of adjunctive glucocorticosteroid therapy for adults and neonates is less clear because these patient populations have not been studied in adequate detail. Adjunctive dexamethasone in a dose of 0.15 mg per kg every 6 hours for 2 to 4 days is recommended in children older than 2 months with suspected bacterial meningitis, particularly those suspected of being infected with *H. influenzae.* On the basis of a meta-analysis, dexamethasone should be initiated intravenously simultaneously with or slightly before the first dose of antimicrobial agent. When the delay in dexamethasone administration exceeds 3 to 4 hours beyond the first dose of antimicrobial agent, most beneficial effects are likely lost; therefore, the agent is not recommended in this setting. Data on the use of dexamethasone in the neonatal period are lacking. In adults, the benefits are less convincing, and dexamethasone reduces the penetration of several important agents such as vancomycin into the CSF. If dexamethasone is chosen as a component of the empirical regimen administered to adults with suspected bacterial meningitis, a combination regimen that covers penicillin-resistant pneumococci should be selected. Dexamethasone is appropriate when other indications for its use are present in patients with bacterial meningitis, such as a marked increase in intracranial pressure or the presence of cerebral edema at CT. When severe sepsis or septic shock is suspected or documented, corticosteroids should be avoided because the outcome is adversely affected. Plasmapheresis or plasma exchange has been used in small series of patients with meningococcemia and severe sepsis or septic shock (purpura fulminans). The initial results are extremely promising, but the use of these modalities in this desperately ill population of patients must be considered experimental at present.

INFECTIOUS MONONUCLEOSIS

method of
PATRICIA DEMARAIS, M.D.
Oak Forest Hospital
Oak Forest, Illinois
Cook County Hospital
Chicago, Illinois

THE CLINICAL SYNDROME

Infectious mononucleosis is the most common symptomatic manifestation of infection with Epstein-Barr virus (EBV). The classic syndrome consists of a triad of sore throat, fever, and lymphadenopathy. Other frequently described symptoms include headache, malaise, arthralgia, and anorexia. The signs noted on physical examination include fever, pharyngitis, lymphadenopathy, and hepatosplenomegaly. Rash is rarely seen unless the patient has inadvertently been treated with amoxicillin.

Infectious mononucleosis due to EBV usually occurs in late adolescence or early adulthood. Younger children tend to have a milder form of the illness. Most cases of infectious mononucleosis are self-limited, and symptoms resolve in 2 to 4 weeks. Uncommon complications of infectious mononucleosis due to EBV are numerous and involve many organ systems. Some of the more severe are autoimmune hemolytic anemia and thrombocytopenia, splenic rupture, upper airway obstruction, encephalitis and other central nervous system manifestations, Guillain-Barré syndrome, pericarditis, and renal failure. Fatal infections may occur in those with Duncan's X-linked recessive immunodeficiency.

Other infections such as cytomegalovirus; herpes simplex 1 and 2; hepatitis A, B, and C; toxoplasmosis; and human immunodeficiency virus can cause infectious mononucleosis syndrome. These should be considered when patients have known risk factors for any of these, have an atypical presentation, or have nondiagnostic EBV serology.

PATHOPHYSIOLOGY

The major route of transmission of EBV is through saliva (rarely through blood transfusion or bone marrow transplantation). The virus infects and replicates in mucous membrane cells, is released as infectious particles in secretions, and goes on to infect B lymphocytes. The viral replication induces a marked immune response. It is thought that the majority of symptoms and signs of infectious mononucleosis due to EBV are caused by this exuberant immune response.

DIAGNOSIS

The diagnosis is suggested by the clinical syndrome. About 70% of patients will have an atypical lymphocytosis, and 50% will have mild to moderate thrombocytopenia and elevated hepatocellular enzymes. The IgM heterophil antibody (monospot) test result is positive in 85 to 90% of adolescents and adults with infectious mononucleosis due to EBV. The test result is positive in only half of younger children with the disease. If the heterophil antibody test result is negative and EBV is considered to be a likely cause of the illness, EBV specific serology can be obtained. Patients with acute infectious mononucleosis due to EBV will have IgM and IgG antibodies to viral capsid antigen without antibody to EB nuclear antigen. The presence of antibody to early antigen is variable. The diagnosis can also be made through the detection of EBV DNA by a variety of methods.

TREATMENT

In the majority of cases, infectious mononucleosis due to EBV is a self-limited, uncomplicated disease. Symptomatic treatment with bed rest, saline gargles, and acetaminophen (650 to 1000 mg every 4 to 6 hours) or nonsteroidal anti-inflammatory agents (ibuprofen 200 to 600 mg every 6 hours). Aspirin should be avoided because of reported cases of Reye's syndrome. Antibiotics are not helpful, and, in fact, ampicillin causes a rash in most patients. Contact sports should be avoided in patients with splenomegaly to decrease the risk of splenic rupture.

Acyclovir* (Zovirax) has been used for the treatment of uncomplicated EBV-related infectious mononucleosis in several studies. It decreases EBV shedding during treatment but does not prevent shedding after treatment or significantly alter the clinical course of the disease. Therefore, acyclovir is not recommended for the treatment of uncomplicated infectious mononucleosis. The use of corticosteroids with or without acyclovir for the treatment of complicated infectious mononucleosis is controversial. Corticosteroids (methylprednisolone [Solu-Medrol], 60 mg intravenously every 6 hours, or prednisone, 60 to 80 mg daily, both tapered over 1 to 2 weeks) may be helpful in patients with obstructive tonsillar enlargement or severe autoimmune hemolytic anemia and thrombocytopenia. There is conflicting data regarding whether corticosteroids improve or exacerbate encephalitis, myocarditis, and pericarditis. Results of treatment of most of the other complications of infectious mononucleosis due to EBV are available only in case report form; the treatment usually involves both acyclovir and corticosteroids in varying doses, and the outcomes are variable.

Other drugs such as H_2 receptor antagonists (ranitidine [Zantac] and cimetidine [Tagamet])* employed as immune modulators have been used to treat infectious mononucleosis with varying results. A recent double-blind, placebo-controlled study with ranitidine did not show any alteration in the clinical course of the illness. There is some research being done to develop an EBV vaccine. Several prototypes have been developed and tested in small populations. The efficacy of these vaccines is not yet known. The target population and application of an EBV vaccine are still in question.

*Not FDA approved for this indication.

CHRONIC FATIGUE SYNDROME

method of
JAMES F. JONES, M.D.
University of Colorado School of Medicine and National Jewish Medical and Research Center
Denver, Colorado

Chronic fatigue syndrome (CFS) is the name applied to a chronic illness that at face value resembles unresolved infections, depression, endocrine and metabolic disorders, sleep disorders, and many other conditions that include fatigue in their diagnostic criteria. In the modern era, interest in this "illness" began with the question of a relationship with a chronic active Epstein-Barr virus infection. Subsequent studies did not support Epstein-Barr virus as the only cause of this syndrome, but several studies have found this agent to be one of the triggering infectious agents that are associated with the 25% of cases that follow an acute onset.

The lack of association with a specific infectious agent led to the generation in 1988 of a clinical definition based on the presence of incapacitating fatigue and varying combinations of signs and symptoms. Any pre-existing medical or psychiatric condition was exclusionary. The definition was subsequently altered so that pre-existing medical conditions that were treated satisfactorily were allowed as well as certain psychiatric diagnoses. Evaluation of this definition at a number of centers in the United States, Great Britain, and Australia led to the current definition published in 1994.

Changes in the definition included a decrease in the number of symptoms and removal of the signs. The signs had been shown to be somewhat arbitrary, and patients could be identified without their presence. The large number of symptoms did not allow identification of a specific illness, and they increased the possibility of mislabeling patients with primary psychiatric illnesses (e.g., somatiform disorders) with CFS. The 1994 definition still requires more than 6 months of fatigue, but it dropped the 50% level of activity because the requirement was impossible to apply evenly across all patients. Exclusion of other illnesses, as in the modifications listed in Table 1, remains a major requirement. The minor requirements that allow identification of patients include four of eight possible symptoms: sore throat, lymph node swelling or tenderness, myalgias, arthralgias, sleep problems, cognitive troubles, headaches, and an increase in the symptom complex 24 hours after increased level of physical or mental activity. This definition was designed as a research tool and included suggestions for unifying the measurement of fatigue and evaluation of the mental status of patients.

It is of interest to note that the number of patients

TABLE 1. **Exclusionary Illnesses**

Medical	Psychiatric
Untreated hypothyroidism	Psychotic depression
Sleep apnea	Schizophrenia
Chronic active hepatitis	Dementia
Severe obesity	Bipolar affective disorder
	Bulimia
	Anorexia nervosa
	Recent substance abuse

TABLE 2. **Screening Laboratory Tests**

Complete blood count
Erythrocyte sedimentation rate
Alanine aminotransferase
Total protein
Albumin
Globulin
Glucose
Electrolytes
Creatinine
Thyroid-stimulating hormone
Urinalysis
Alkaline phosphatase

that fulfilled the 1988 definition was approximately 13 per 100,000, whereas the 1994 definition identified approximately 300 per 100,000. Thus, the desire to ensure preclusion of one set of confounding illnesses may have allowed the inclusion of others. This possibility is illustrated by different patterns of the minor symptoms that allow fulfillment of the definition. For example, a patient with sore throat, lymph node swelling, arthralgia, and myalgia would be accepted, suggesting an infectious disease. A patient with headaches, sleep problems, cognitive problems, and increased symptoms following exercise would also fulfill the definition. It is therefore clear that patients fulfilling the definition might be heterogeneous in the origin of their illnesses. One demographic variable that has remained stable is the 3:1 ratio of women to men.

DIAGNOSIS

Diagnosis of CFS begins with suspicion of the syndrome after taking a history and performing a physical examination. Because the diagnosis of CFS continues to be based on clinical grounds alone, exclusion of other illness processes is paramount. It should not be assumed that a patient with fatigue as a presenting complaint has CFS. One commonly initiates evaluation of the patient by taking a history. This procedure allows an immediate determination of whether the illness began acutely or more gradually. It allows determination of pre-existing symptoms. It often allows insight into previously identified factors that influence patient perception of illness. Questioning about typical episodes provides information about cyclical events, possible triggers of symptoms, and possible exposures.

The interviewer gives the patients the opportunity to describe in their own words the history of their illness. The interviewer simply guides the patient and tries not to ask leading questions. This process not only gathers information, but also serves as an ice breaker between the interviewer and the patient. It allows interviewers to determine the mental status of the patients, their concentration and memory capabilities, and what may be on their agendas. It usually allows determination of the kind and scope of prior medical and alternative care evaluations the patients may have received.

One should question making a diagnosis of CFS on the first visit. Although not included in the working definition, attempts should be made to determine the duration, the mode of onset, the magnitude, and the consequences of each complaint. Only with such thorough questioning will an underlying process responsible for the illness be identified or suspected.

Routine laboratory evaluations are recommended (Table 2). It should be noted that routine testing does not include specific antibody testing; test of immune function per se, or single photon emission computed tomography (SPECT) and/or magnetic resonance imaging (MRI) scanning of the brain. Negative screening test results do not automatically exclude an alternative diagnosis. Specific testing, for example, for a sleep disorder or chronic sinusitis may be necessary. Performance of a mental status examination, either informally or by using a standard instrument when indicated, is equally important. A working diagnosis of CFS may then be made if the evaluation fails to identify an underlying problem. This approach is warranted because the patient's underlying disease may declare itself in the near or distant future. Continued adherence to a diagnosis of CFS in the face of an evolving or readily identifiable medical or psychiatric illness is the single most detrimental outcome of a premature or prolonged diagnosis of CFS.

Additional laboratory and/or other diagnostic testing is based on the individual patient's complaints. The interview techniques listed earlier assist in this process. An additional valuable tool that will lead the interviewer to specific illness identification and direct the therapy is simply to ask the patient to list the problems described in decreasing order of magnitude. Which problem causes the most difficulty? Or which problems interfere with the ability to carry out daily functions? Patients will often use this exercise to list the consequences of their illness. This latter information is valuable in formulating therapeutic goals, but it may not be germane to the diagnostic process.

THERAPY

Treatment regimens vary with the needs of the individual and how he or she perceives the illness (Table 3). The goals of treatment are dependent on the person within a framework of providing reentry into their premorbid condition. Complete return to "normal" may not be possible immediately, however.

TABLE 3. **Management of Patients**

Diagnosis

- Consideration of the diagnosis
- Accurate patient-initiated history
- Exclusion of other procedures
- Chronic fatigue syndrome (CFS) as a "working diagnosis"
- Identification of primary symptoms

Therapy

- Education regarding the advantages and disadvantages of CFS as a diagnosis
- Development of coping skills
- Initiation of a graded exercise program
- Symptomatic medication

In fact, the desire for total immediate recovery may hamper clinical improvement. Adaptation to their new, albeit temporary, state is frequently a more realistic short-term goal.

An important therapeutic component of the diagnostic process is the receipt of a name for the illness process. Many of the patients feel as if they are invalids. They perceive that they are literally "invalid" in the eyes of the medical profession and in some instances family members and employers. Acquisition of a name for their condition, even though descriptive, is enabling. It allows entry into diagnostic and therapeutic schema for patients who are floundering or entering unconventional or unaffordable treatment programs.

Therapeutic modalities include (1) education regarding the boundaries and limitations of the diagnosis, (2) development of coping skills, (3) institution of a graduated exercise program when possible, and (4) use of symptomatic medications. If the patient is being seen in a multidisciplinary setting, these approaches may be combined into a specific program. If CFS is an infrequent diagnosis, identification of the problems that cause loss of function becomes critical.

Education

Patients referred to clinics that deal with CFS frequently have a pre-existing diagnosis substantiated or are given this diagnosis and entered into a variety of treatment programs. Practitioners who see only an occasional patient often learn treatment from their patients. It is critical that all physicians who make the diagnosis provide information regarding the illness in general and the specific criteria that allowed recognition of the problem. Just as education regarding asthma and diabetes mellitus is a critical component of therapy for those diseases, education regarding the origin, specific components, and outcome of the syndrome is more critical in this situation. The literature supports CFS as a condition that is not life threatening or progressive. Lay representations, which are readily available, are often incorrect in painting a uniformly dismal outcome. Physicians should counsel their patients that all illness symptoms should not be attributed to CFS, and advice should be sought when new problems arise or old problems become more prominent. Patients should also be taught that persistent efforts to find a cure via experiences of their acquaintances or the newest information in magazines or on the Internet are not as productive as their participation in a specifically designed program as outlined here. Paramount in this process is their consideration of acceptance of their current, albeit temporary, status. Wanting their lives back and attempting to regain them with a pill are not effective approaches.

As mentioned earlier, a major part of the educational and treatment process is the interview process. Giving the patient the opportunity to describe the illness and its consequences in a nonjudgmental situation is critical to gaining patient confidence. A physician who makes the diagnosis of CFS literally establishes a contract for long-term care with the patient, and it must be based on mutual trust.

Development of Coping Skills

To recommend coping strategies, the provider must know the needs of the patient—another rationale for the patient-generated problem list. If the patient complains of problems with memory and concentration, simple advice regarding use of lists and audiotaping of activities or needs is logical. If they cannot perform on the job or their behavioral responses to these complaints aggravate the consequences, formal neuropsychologic testing and/or therapy is required. Assistance with understanding losses is also very important. Depending on the magnitude of the consequences of their illness, patients may lose self-respect and the appreciation of their families, employees, and coworkers. They need to learn that as individuals they are not responsible for these losses but that they are responsible, at least in part, for their recovery. They need to go through a grieving process and then learn how to adapt to their current state. They need to learn to accept and desire incremental levels of progress. Again, formal psychologic therapy may be required to achieve these goals.

The origin of the illness and the character of the fatigue dictate the approach in many cases. If the origin is with an apparent, usually unidentified, "flu-like" illness that does not resolve or the character of the fatigue simulates the malaise of such an illness, the patient needs to know that the magnitude and quality of the symptoms are normal responses. The duration and consequences in the eyes of society and the individual are the factors that differentiate a normal resolution of an illness from a prolonged or chronic condition. They also need to know that resumption of "normal" activity is not the correct approach. Most patients have symptoms on an everyday basis, but they also have days when the symptoms are more or less pronounced (bad and good days). A typical patient will perform on the good days as if there were no illness. This action is then followed in 1 or 2 days by an exacerbation of symptoms. Learning to compartmentalize activities and to never exceed their personal limits are critical steps in coping with CFS. On the other hand, total acceptance of such a program is not appropriate either. Usually acute onset patients will notice that they can be more active without exacerbation of symptoms regardless of their therapeutic program. This observation usually heralds resolution of the illness. In some instances, the illness is resolving, but the patient perceives the outcome of increased physical activity (e.g., muscle aches and tiredness) as illness symptoms rather than the simple, expected consequences of increased activity. The recurrence of the individual's whole syndrome following activity, however, suggests that resolution has not taken place.

Exercise

It seems contradictory to follow the previous discussion about listening to one's body and avoiding excessive activity with a section that recommends regular exercise. The studies on muscle function show that patients are tired after performing repetitive acts and that there appears to be no primary problem in muscle function. There does appear to be a problem in fitness or conditioning, however. Whether this result is a consequence of the illness or the inactivity that accompanies the syndrome is not known. Lessons from the rehabilitation of patients with cardiac and pulmonary diseases teach us that anaerobic exercise to regain strength should precede exercises to improve aerobic fitness and overall conditioning. A program that includes active stretching followed by range-of-motion contractions and extensions that eventually includes resistance is usually an effective start. Five minutes per day is a typical starting point for an individual who has been totally inactive. The end point of each session should be preset by the clock or number of repetitions and should be reached before the patient becomes tired. This end point is based on the fact that either tiredness is a trigger for the production of biologic changes that are a part of the host's attempt to limit activity or perception of tiredness triggers illness behavior. A reasonable long-term goal for the activity chosen by the patient (usually walking) is 30 minutes per day. As the patient is working toward that goal, the exercise time may be divided into three or more periods during the day. At this stage in the understanding of the illness, prevention of activation of either pathway and increasing overall fitness are appropriate goals. Graded exercise programs might be interpreted as increasing the magnitude of the effort during training. This connotation is appropriate once the patient is able to exercise without inducing an exacerbation of the illness. This section may be summarized by the adage that no exercise is bad, some is good, but too much needs to be avoided.

The previous sections on education, coping skills, and exercise provide the kinds of therapy that are offered in cognitive-behavioral therapy programs. These fixed-length programs have been helpful in some studies, but the duration of benefit may not be long term.

Symptomatic Therapy

One usually associates this form of therapy with medication. Some interventions require alterations in patient habits or changes in biologic processes that do not require medication per se. The primary example is treatment of sleep problems. A very large percentage of patients presenting for evaluation of fatigue, many of whom carry the diagnosis of CFS, have sleep disorders. Some have problems with sleep hygiene. They may read or watch television for prolonged periods (longer than 15 minutes) before trying to go to sleep. This habit may actually allow arousal of the brain within several hours following sleep onset, thus leading to interrupted sleep. Caffeine ingestion after 6 PM and exercise within 4 hours of bedtime may impede getting to sleep. Patients are frequently given medication for insomnia that is manifested by going to bed at 11 PM but not being able to get to sleep until 1 or 2 AM, with a waking time of 10 AM. A hypnotic is prescribed that allows induction of sleep at an earlier time, but the patient may still not experience restorative sleep. One explanation for this series of events is that the patient has a phase-delay syndrome and needs to alter the sleep cycle with AM light before improvement might be expected. Appropriate use of hypnotics may be important in allowing normalization of sleep cycling, but these are not sufficient as the sole mode of therapy.

Daytime sleepiness is another common problem. It can have a multitude of origins. Symptomatic therapy includes self-or physician-generated use of stimulants. These drugs include caffeine herbs that contain ephedrine and antidepressants that actually serve as stimulants (serotonin and norepinephrine reuptake inhibitors). These substances may allow improved functioning in the daytime, but they block identification of the underlying nighttime or daytime origin of the sleep problem.

It should be clear from these examples that premature treatment may prevent adequate diagnosis and treatment of readily remedial problems. However, symptomatic medications have a definite place in the therapy of CFS. It should be emphasized that many CFS patients do not tolerate standard doses of any of the medications listed below. For instance, the starting dose of the tricyclic antidepressants should be 10 mg or less. Their use should be based on symptoms that interfere with functioning for which an identifiable process has not been found. A symptom-based approach would be as follows:

1. Troubled sleep without a specific diagnosis: zolpidem (Ambien), 5 to 10 mg at bedtime (hs); triazolam (Halcion), 0.125 to 0.25 mg hs; temazepam (Restoril), 15 mg hs; and trazodone (Desyrel), 25 mg hs.
2. Troubled sleep with arthralgia: tricyclic antidepressants, for example, doxepin* (Sinequan), 10 to 50 mg hs (always begin with 10 mg; some patients require 2 to 5 mg as a starting dose), nortriptyline (Pamelor, Aventyl), and amitriptyline (Elavil). Doses for nortriptyline and amitriptyline are the same as for doxepin.
3. Troubled sleep with myalgias and general flu-like symptoms: clonazepam* (Klonopin), 0.125 to 0.5 mg hs; tricyclic antidepressants, bupropion (Wellbutrin), 75 mg hs; and cyclobenzaprine* (Flexeril), 10 to 30 mg hs.
4. Depressive symptoms (moodiness and lack of energy in the daytime): serotonin and serotonin-norepinephrine reuptake inhibitors: fluoxetine (Prozac), 10 to 20 mg every morning; paroxetine (Paxil), 10 to 20 mg every morning; venlafaxine (Effexor), 25 to 75

*Not FDA approved for this indication.

mg every morning; sertraline (Zoloft), 25 to 50 mg every morning; and nefazodone (Serzone), 50 to 100 mg every morning. The reader will notice that these are minimal doses.

5. Anxiety and panic attacks: short-term use of alprazolam (Xanax), 0.25 to 0.5 mg up to three times daily (tid); clonazepam (Klonopin), 0.25 to 0.5 mg twice daily (bid) and hs; trazodone (Desyrel), 25 mg up to tid; paroxetine (Paxil), 10 to 20 mg every morning; and buspirone (BuSpar), 2.5 to 5 mg tid.

6. Pain syndromes: fibromyalgia—tricyclic antidepressants, acetaminophen, tramadol (Ultram), 50–100 mg every 6 hours. Pain and fatigue without tender points—nonsteroidal anti-inflammatory agents, cyclobenzaprine (Flexeril), 10 mg tid.

7. Cognitive problems: clonazepam* (Klonopin), 0.25 to 0.5 mg hs; sertraline* (Zoloft), 25 to 50 mg every morning; paroxetine* (Paxil), 10 to 20 mg every morning; and pentoxifylline* (Trental), 400 mg one to three times daily.

8. Persistent flulike complex: benzodiazepine family members (particularly alprazolam and clonazepam), and tricyclic antidepressants have been shown to inhibit systemic flulike symptoms if given before interferon therapy and are sometimes useful in CFS if these symptoms are dominant. Dosages are the same as listed previously.

9. Allergy and sinusitis symptoms: normal saline nasal washes followed by short- or long-acting H_1 blockers and/or topical nasal anti-inflammatory agents—fluticasone (Flonase), beclomethasone dipropionate (Vancenase), triamcinolone (Nasacort), and cromolyn sodium (Nasalcrom). This latter group of agents is administered 1 to 2 times daily with two squirts in each nostril. IgE-mediated allergy may be important in symptom production in CFS. Up to 80% of patients in some studies have this type of allergy. Allergy shots or immunotherapy, although effective for allergic rhinitis and prevention of associated problems such as sinusitis, does not appear to positively influence CFS.

It is noteworthy that several of the medications are listed in multiple categories, particularly the tricyclic antidepressants. These agents have a variety of pharmacologic activities that appear to be beneficial in this setting. They are potent H_1 blockers and influence inflammation by prevention of production of mediators such as platelet-activating factor, a substance involved in the production of urticaria. Their usefulness in inducing sleep has been mentioned. Their apparent effect in altering norepinephrine metabolism, perhaps in boosting cardiovascular function, may be helpful in some patients with altered autonomic nervous system function. Whether they are effective in alleviating symptoms attributable to depression at the doses commonly used is unknown. Clonazepam (Klonopin) is another example. This drug is marketed as an antiseizure medication, but it influences muscle spasms, vertigo, paresthesias, restless leg syndrome, pain, flulike symptoms, delayed sleep onset, and anxiety. All of these problems are commonly seen in CFS patients, even though they all are not considered part of the syndrome.

*Not FDA approved for this indication.

Autonomic nervous system problems are present in some patients with CFS. It is not clear whether they play a role in the pathophysiology of the syndrome or whether they are consequences of prolonged inactivity. Therapy for neurally mediated hypotension is based on increased salt intake, along with fludrocortisone acetate* (Florinef) or midodrine* (ProAmatine). Postural orthostatic tachycardia syndrome is treated with beta blockers or calcium channel blockers. An unusual condition is postural hypertension, which is treated with clonidine* hydrochloride (Catapres) and angiotensin-converting enzyme (ACE) inhibitors.* All of these conditions can be identified only with tilt table testing. Therapy should not be instituted without a formal diagnosis. Occasionally patients will not generate the expected doubling of plasma norepinephrine that normally accompanies a 65-degree tilt. Tricyclic antidepressants are often effective in overcoming symptoms associated with this lack of response. If testing of autonomic cardiovascular responses is not available, increased salt intake and exercise may be the only therapeutic modalities that are required. Twice daily monitoring of supine and erect blood pressure and heart rate is required to evaluate efficacy of therapy for this group of problems. Clinical experience suggests that the mild cardiovascular problems discussed here respond well to treatment and are self-limited.

Many of the previously listed recommendations are successful in part because the patients have taught their health care providers these remedies. They also work because they involve the patient's participation. Because the previously mentioned medications are being used as adjuncts to the other modes of therapy, they are not always successful. They may need to be changed during the course of illness. Often patients come to the physician using a large number of medications. It may not be possible to determine by the history alone whether the patient's symptoms are not at least in part due to the medication regimen. Frequently the medications need to be tapered and stopped to sort out their influence on the presenting complaints.

Popular remedies for CFS are discussed primarily to familiarize the practitioner with them and to support previous warnings regarding lack of efficacy. The primary problem with their use is that proof is lacking that such intervention has been uniformly beneficial. This statement is particularly true in cases of parenteral (injectable) repetitious therapy with any substance. Three such substances are gamma globulin (either the intravenous or the intramuscular form), porcine liver extract* (Kutapressin), and mismatched double-stranded RNA* (Ampligen). These substances gained popularity when the syndrome

*Not FDA approved for this indication.

was thought primarily to be due to an ongoing virus infection or an immunologic abnormality. Likewise, the effectiveness of dietary, manipulations and ingestion of herbs, enzymes, amino acids, vitamins, minerals, or hormones, although usually safe, is equally unproven. Popular substances are coenzyme Q10 and carnitine to enhance muscle function. Herbs are particularly in vogue. Many of them have medicinal qualities and if taken in excessive amounts may be injurious. Because many of these substances are readily available, they will be utilized by patients who are anxious to get better. If the reader has such patients or is such a patient one must make sure that the remedy in question is safe and that its use is both affordable and does not hide illness parameters that require specific identification. If patients are intent on taking these types of remedies, they should be advised to at least seek the advice of a responsible care provider who is knowledgeable in their use and adverse consequences. Alternative care in many forms is also in vogue and may be helpful, again if provided in a responsible fashion. Some patients with myalgias and other pain complaints find particular benefit from acupuncture and therapeutic massage.

CONCLUSION

Therapy for CFS patients appears to be evolving at a faster rate than an understanding of this symptom complex. It is clear, however, that one approach or one medication is not satisfactory for all patients. Identifying the patient's most problematic symptoms and using a variety of modalities that address those problems in the treatment plan are the most effective ways of assisting the patient. Patients should be reminded not to expect total return to their premorbid state to occur immediately. Because the use of medications remains arbitrary, failure of one regimen may be followed by successful relief using another approach. In addition, one must always be careful that the treatment does not aggravate the illness.

MUMPS

method of
BLAISE L. CONGENI, M.D.
Children's Hospital Medical Center of Akron
Akron, Ohio

Since licensure of the mumps vaccine in the United States in 1967, cases of mumps have declined dramatically. Although only 3000 cases of mumps were reported annually in the United States between 1983 and 1985, a relative resurgence was seen between 1986 and 1987. Approximately 13,000 cases were reported in 1987. Since then the number of reported cases has continued to decline, and fewer than 2000 cases were reported in 1993.

Before the development of the vaccine, most cases occurred in children 5 to 9 years of age. In the late 1980s a shift toward older children was seen, with several outbreaks being reported on university campuses, in junior and senior high schools, and in the workplace. As a result of the improved immunization rates that have been achieved during the last 5 years and because of the initiation of the two-dose vaccination for mumps-measles-rubella (MMR), continued improvement from the already low levels reported in 1993 is anticipated.

CLINICAL FEATURES

Following an incubation period of 14 to 18 days with a range of 14 to 25 days, prodromal symptoms are seen. These are generally nonspecific and include myalgias and headache along with low-grade fever.

Parotitis is the most common clinical manifestation and occurs in approximately 30 to 40% of patients. The parotitis is more often bilateral but may be unilateral. This symptom occurs early, and its onset may be heralded by earache or jaw pain. With parotitis, obliteration of the angle of the jaw to palpation is most often noted. Symptoms tend to subside quickly and within 7 to 10 days are gone.

Thirty percent of cases are totally subclinical, and an additional 40 to 50% of patients experience nonspecific complaints. Even these cases confer durable immunity.

COMPLICATIONS

Mumps is generally considered to be a trivial illness in contrast to measles and rubella. Although complications are not uncommon, sequelae are rare.

Central nervous system involvement can occur frequently. Up to 50% of patients with mumps actually have aseptic meningitis based on cerebrospinal fluid findings. The majority of patients are relatively asymptomatic. Permanent sequelae with all central nervous system manifestations remain rare.

The most common complication seen in postpubertal males is orchitis (testicular inflammation). This is a complication that is most often feared and is usually seen following parotitis but may even precede it. The patient complains of the abrupt onset of acute testicular swelling and tenderness, and these symptoms may be associated with constitutional complaints including nausea, vomiting, and fever. Within a week, pain and swelling resolve. Although some patients may have testicular atrophy, sterility is rare. Oophoritis (ovarian inflammation) is much less common, occurring in less than 5% of postpubertal females. These patients present with pelvic pain, which may mimic appendicitis. As with orchitis, sterility is rare.

Nerve deafness is estimated to occur at 1 out of 20,000 cases and although rare is the most serious of the complications of mumps. Other infrequent complications that have been noted include mastitis, pancreatitis, nephritis, thyroiditis, myocarditis, arthritis, transverse myelitis, and thrombocytopenic purpura.

Only half of the patients with mumps might be sufficiently symptomatic that a visit to a physician would be necessary. Rarely dehydration will be seen, usually with pancreatitis or aseptic meningitis, necessitating a brief period of hospitalization for rehydration.

DIAGNOSIS

Diagnosis of mumps is usually made based on clinical grounds alone. Other possible causes of parotid gland swelling include other systemic viral infections (especially parainfluenza types I and III, coxsackievirus, and influenza A), acute suppurative parotitis, and obstruction in the parotid gland caused by either a stone or a tumor. In most cases when confirmation of the diagnosis is necessary, an elevated amylase confirms parotid gland inflammation as opposed to cervical adenitis. Mumps virus can be isolated from clinical specimens, especially saliva, urine, and cerebrospinal fluid.

Traditionally, physicians have relied on serology to confirm the diagnosis of mumps in difficult cases. The development of complement fixation (CF) antibody has been used traditionally, but both CF and hemagglutination inhibition antibody tests are too insensitive to be useful clinically. These tests have been replaced by neutralization assays as well as enzyme immunoassays (EIAs). The EIA is commercially available, and both IgM and IgG antibody can be measured. The development of IgM antibody, which becomes detectable a few days after the start of illness, or a fourfold rise in IgG antibody suggests mumps.

THERAPY

The treatment of mumps and its complications is generally supportive and symptomatic. Non-narcotic analgesics are generally all that is needed to relieve the discomfort associated with mumps. Rarely are narcotic analgesics needed for more severe discomfort associated with orchitis. Antiviral agents and intravenous gamma globulin* have not been shown to be of benefit therapeutically or following exposure.

PREVENTION

The live attenuated mumps vaccine is more than 95% effective in preventing disease following exposure. It is generally administered following the first birthday and the second dose is administered along with measles and rubella vaccine either on entry into school or before 12 years of age.

The mumps vaccine is well tolerated, and adverse reactions are extremely rare. A febrile illness associated with a mild upper respiratory infection is not a contraindication to administration. Recent administration of intravenous gamma globulin will necessitate a delay in administration of the vaccine. The length of the delay will depend on the dose of the intravenous gamma globulin employed. Although patients infected with the human immunodeficiency virus can be immunized safely, patients with altered immunity are best immunized once immunologic responsiveness has been restored. Patients receiving corticosteriods can generally be immunized safely 1 month following cessation of therapy. As with other live vaccines, pregnancy remains an absolute contraindication to immunization; nevertheless, children of pregnant women can safely receive the vaccine. During outbreaks, initiation of an immunization program has been shown to be effective in controlling the outbreak.

*Not FDA approved for this indication.

OTITIS EXTERNA

method of
JENNIFER RUBIN GRANDIS, M.D.
University of Pittsburgh School of Medicine
Pittsburgh, Pennsylvania

Otitis externa is a term used to describe a variety of infectious conditions involving the skin of the ear canal and pinna. The lateral third of the canal is composed of cartilage, with a thin layer of subcutaneous tissue between the cartilage and the skin. Cerumen is produced by glands in this portion of the canal. Medially, the canal is bony and is covered by a thin layer of skin with little subcutaneous tissue. The skin, cerumen, and resulting acidic environment generally protect the ear from infection. Any breakdown of this barrier may predispose to an infection. When complaints of otalgia are referable to disease in and around the external meatus, a careful history and physical examination should be performed to diagnose the specific malady. Treatment is then tailored to the individual etiology. The following discussion reviews the therapeutic options of the clinician when confronted with an inflammatory condition of the external ear.

ACUTE OTITIS EXTERNA

The diagnosis of an acute infection of the external auditory canal is generally uncomplicated. Inflammation of the external auditory canal is extremely common, with up to 10% of the population experiencing an episode of acute otitis externa. The disease occurs most commonly in warm, humid climates, especially during the summer months. A recent history of water exposure (e.g., swimming or diving), ear canal trauma (e.g., following ear cleaning with a cotton-tipped swab or long-term wearing of a hearing aid), or eczema is often present. The pain ranges from mild to severe, with the patient frequently requiring narcotic analgesics. Some degree of foul-smelling otorrhea may accompany the otalgia. On examination, the canal may appear erythematous and edematous, or, if the infection is severe, there can be complete obstruction secondary to the edema and the accumulation of desquamated debris. Redness of the preauricular region and pinna as well as adenopathy of the preauricular or postauricular cervical lymph node chain indicates extension beyond the ear canal.

Principles observed in the management of skin infections should apply to the treatment of acute external otitis. Initially, crusts, scales, and desquamated debris must be evacuated from the ear canal. Because the manipulation of an acutely infected canal can be painful, débridement should be performed gently. Once the canal has been cleaned, an ototopical agent may be applied directly into the meatus. Often, swelling of the canal may prohibit the topically applied medication from reaching the more medial aspects. In this case, a wick impregnated with an anti-inflammatory agent should be inserted carefully into the canal and left in place for several days or until the edema subsides and the wick falls out spontaneously. A wick can be made of a variety of materials, including 1/4-inch gauze or cotton or an expandable sponge. Once the wick is inserted, the patient (or family member) is instructed to saturate the material with drops several times a day. When the wick is removed (or falls out), the medication can be applied directly into the meatus until symptoms resolve (usually 7 to 10 days). The addition of a systemic antibiotic is generally unnecessary but may be indicated if the patient displays signs of regional or systemic illness (e.g., fever, cellulitis, cervical adenopathy). *Pseudomonas aeruginosa* and *Staphylococcus aureus* represent the most commonly cultured organisms. The ideal empirical agent would demonstrate antipseudomonal and antistaphylococcal activity (e.g., a quinolone such as levofloxacin [Levaquin]).

Several guidelines should be followed when selecting the appropriate ototopical agent. If the patient has a known or suspected tympanic membrane perforation, agents in the forms of solutions should be avoided in favor of suspensions because of the inflammatory properties of solutions when applied directly to the middle ear mucosa. Sometimes canal edema prevents this determination at the time of initial examination. The primary decision rests in whether to select a topical agent that contains an antibiotic. Antiseptics without an antimicrobial component have been shown in prospective clinical trials to be as effective as antibiotic-containing compounds in the treatment of acute external otitis. Although cultures generally reveal *Pseudomonas aeruginosa*, the favorable clinical response of patients to treatments that do not include antimicrobials highlights the undetermined pathogenic significance of these organisms. We prefer to institute empirical therapy with an agent such as 2% acetic acid plus 1% hydrocortisone in an acidic buffer (pH = 3.7; VōSol HC Otic), rather than the neomycin-containing drugs (e.g., polymyxin B, neomycin sulfate, hydrocortisone drops [Cortisporin Otic]; colistin sulfate, neomycin sulfate, thonzonium bromide [Coly-Mycin S Otic]) as a result of the frequent occurrence of neomycin-induced allergic contact dermatitis, which can result in an exacerbation of local symptoms. Topical aminoglycosides available as ophthalmic preparations may also be used (e.g., gentamicin [Genoptic] or tobramycin [TobraDex]). Many formulations of topical agents are effective, and the physician should be flexible about changing drugs if the initial empirical choice proves to be ineffective. Cultures of the aural discharge are generally reserved for patients who do not respond to treatment and should be obtained under direct visualization with a Venturi trap to avoid contact of the culture swab with the contaminated skin of the external canal. However, débriding the external canal (aural toilet) is more important than using topical or systemic antimicrobials.

After the resolution of the acute infection, preventive measures include maintenance of a dry ear canal. Water precautions include the use of ear plugs or petroleum jelly–coated cotton while swimming, showering, and shampooing. In addition, patients can be maintained on an acid-alcohol drop (5% boric acid saturated in a solution of 95% alcohol) to clean and dry the ear canal and prevent moisture damage. Hearing aids should be removed at night to allow the ear canal to dry.

CHRONIC OTITIS EXTERNA

Pruritus and decreased hearing due to external canal obstruction are characteristic of chronic infection of the external canal, in contrast to the pain and regional complications associated with acute inflammation. Although bacteria may be isolated from the ear canal, chronic otitis externa is primarily a dermatitis condition. Patients with this condition often have a history of contact dermatitis, eczema, or psoriasis. Chronic water exposure or use of cotton-tipped swabs may also contribute. As with acute infection, treatment includes débridement of the canal under direct visualization and avoidance of aural water exposure. The goal of therapy is to dry the ear. This may be accomplished by several methods, including the instillation of 70 to 95% alcohol at body temperature. Topical preparations that acidify the ear canal and are of appropriate viscosity to maintain contact with the affected skin for as long as possible are desired (e.g., 0.5 or 1% hydrocortisone cream or ointment). If a fingertip cannot apply the agent to the infected site, the medicine can be instilled under direct visualization using an angiocatheter-capped syringe.

OTOMYCOSIS

Fungi can be isolated in up to 40% of all cases of external otitis infection. These saprophytic fungi can become pathogenic under certain conditions such as immunosuppression or, more commonly, overuse of topical steroids or antibiotic-containing drops. Pruritus and otorrhea are more common than otalgia as a presenting complaint, and fungal mycelia are easily recognized on examination (the canal appears to be sprinkled with fine coal dust). *Aspergillus niger* is the most common cause of saprophytic fungal external otitis. As with bacterial infection, cleaning the canal is of utmost importance. Topical agents that can be used to treat this condition include cresyl acetate solution (Cresylate), 1% gentian violet, thimerosal (Merthiolate), topical amphotericin (Fungizone), or ketoconazole (Nizoral) cream. Drying the ear with boric acid may also reduce fungal growth. If the tympanic membrane is intact, an anhydrous solution of 4% boric acid and alcohol or 95% alcohol plus acetic acid may be used to keep the ear canal dry.

During the active phase of chronic otitis externa, surgery is not indicated. However, in patients with end-stage cutaneous changes of the ear canal that have resulted in canal stenosis, surgical correction is often beneficial. Excision of hypertrophied skin, enlargement of the bony meatus, and skin grafting generally lead to a functional ear canal. This procedure is not recommended until the underlying inflammatory condition has been stabilized.

NECROTIZING OTITIS EXTERNA

The most serious and potentially life-threatening form of otitis externa is necrotizing (or malignant) external otitis. This disease typically afflicts elderly patients with diabetes mellitus. Aural irrigation (e.g., for cerumen impaction) may be a predisposing factor. Immunosuppressed individuals, including patients with acquired immune deficiency syndrome, appear to have a higher incidence of this invasive external otitis. Exquisite otalgia accompanied by otorrhea are the typical presenting complaints. Examination characteristically shows granulation tissue at the bony cartilaginous junction, on which a biopsy should be performed to rule out carcinoma. The erythrocyte sedimentation rate is often elevated, and subtemporal extension of disease with bone erosion may be identified on imaging (computed tomography or magnetic resonance imaging). The most common pathogen is *Pseudomonas aeruginosa*, and therapy includes the prompt institution of a prolonged course (e.g., 4 to 6 weeks) of antispeudomonal antibiotics (e.g., ciprofloxacin [Cipro], 750 mg twice a day). In the absence of therapy, the infection progresses along the skull base and results in multiple cranial neuropathies.

PLAGUE

method of
GARY L. SIMPSON, M.D., PH.D., M.P.H.
New Mexico Department of Health
Santa Fe, New Mexico

Plague is an acute, febrile, and often fatal disease caused by the gram-negative bacillus *Yersinia pestis.* Human infection results primarily from the bites of infected rodent fleas. The incubation period is 2 to 8 days following the flea bite, and the clinical course can be rapidly fatal without prompt, appropriate antimicrobial chemotherapy. Although plague is endemic in many areas of the world, especially Asia and Africa, it is predominantly restricted in North America to the southwestern United States. From 1944 through 1994, approximately 90% of the nearly 400 cases of human plague in the United States were reported from four western states: Arizona, California, Colorado, and New Mexico. During each successive decade of this period, the number of states reporting cases has increased from three, between 1944 and 1953, to 13, between 1984 and 1993, indicating the spread of human plague infection eastward and northward to areas in which cases had not been reported previously. The ecology and the epidemiology of plague transmission are complex and differ for the epidemic urban form and the sporadic sylvatic form of disease transmission.

In the United States plague is a seasonal zoonotic infection concentrated in endemic foci throughout the southwest, with ground squirrels, prairie dogs, and wood rats being important natural reservoirs. Although human infection can result from direct contact with infected wild rodents or hares, approximately 85% of human infections are associated with bites of infected rodent fleas. Of note, 60% of plague cases occur in persons younger than 20 years of age, and attack rates are disproportionally high in Native Americans living in endemic areas. Other groups at higher risk of exposure include hikers, hunters, and campers, but domestic pets can provide exposure risks by returning infected rodents or infected fleas to their owners or by becoming infectious risks themselves (e.g., pneumonic plague in domestic cats).

CLINICAL FEATURES

Plague can manifest as any one or a combination of the following syndromes. Classic bubonic plague has a distinctive clinical presentation, described by sudden onset of fever, chills, and headache and followed shortly thereafter by the appearance of extremely painful, localized lymphadenitis (bubo). The majority of bubos are found in the groin (femoral and inguinal), but bubonic plague may appear in the axilla and cervical region. Gastrointestinal symptoms, including nausea, vomiting, abdominal pain, and diarrhea, are common. The liver and spleen may be tender and enlarged. Bubonic plague can progress from first onset of symptoms to rapid clinical deterioration and death in 2 to 4 days. In septicemic plague, bacilli disseminate rapidly from the initial focus of infection, resulting in the syndrome of septicemic plague. By definition, septicemic plague manifests with fever and hypotension but without bubo, in contrast to bubonic plague with septicemia. The importance of this distinction is highlighted by the observation that 25% of all cases of plague occurring over a 5-year period in New Mexico, a state with a high prevalence of plague, were, in fact, the septicemic form. The case-fatality rate was 33%, even in a region in which physicians are unusually sensitized to the possibility of human plague infections.

A remarkable feature of plague sepsis is high-density bacteremia, which premorbidly can reach concentrations of thousands of bacilli per milliliter of blood. Hematogenous dissemination of organisms to the lung with resultant, secondary pneumonia (pneumonic plague) is associated with mortality in excess of 75%. Plague transmitted by aerosols is highly contagious. Individuals exposed to the pneumonic form reportedly have become ill and died of primary inhalation plague pneumonia all in a single day. Unusual manifestations of plague infections include vesicular eruptions, eschar or ecthyma gangrenosum associated with a bubo, and a meningeal form usually seen as a late complication of inadequately treated bubonic plague. Risk of transmission of plague to close contacts (e.g., family, medical personnel) is related to exposure to respiratory aerosols from patients with pneumonia and to blood through needlesticks or aerosols in patients with high-density bacteremia.

From this discussion, it follows that the diagnosis of plague must be considered in certain clinical settings. If a patient has been in a plague-endemic region (New Mexico, Arizona, Utah, Colorado, or California) in the previous 10 to 14 days during the seasonal period of March to November and was exposed to rodents or mammals, plague must be included in the differential diagnosis of the following clinical presentations:

1. Sudden onset of fever and painful, localized unilateral lymphadenitis.
2. Clinical sepsis in an individual without obvious focus

of infection or without underlying conditions predisposing to sepsis.

3. Any community-acquired, gram-negative pneumonia.

DIAGNOSIS

A high index of suspicion in the context of the clinical settings outlined previously will lead to the timely diagnosis of plague. Routine laboratory evaluation typically reveals an elevated white blood cell count (in the range of 10,000 to 20,000 cells per mm^3) with neutrophil predominance, thrombocytopenia, and elevated serum aminotransferases.

The bacteriologic diagnosis is made by smear and routine culture of a bubo aspirate, blood, sputum, or cerebrospinal fluid. Because the bubo does not contain pus, it may be necessary to inject sterile saline into it. Much care, including mask and gloves for the clinician, is required in obtaining the specimens because of the highly contagious nature of *Y. pestis.* A sample of the aspirate should be placed on microscopic slides and air dried. A Gram's stain will reveal gram-negative coccobacilli, and Wayson stain will demonstrate light blue bacilli with dark blue bipolar staining. A specific, direct fluorescent antibody assay is available through public health reference laboratories. A passive hemagglutination, serologic test is also available.

TREATMENT

The successful treatment of plague is directly related to the timely institution of appropriate, empirical antimicrobial therapy. The mortality of untreated bubonic plague is estimated to be 50 to 60%, whereas early and effective antimicrobial therapy may decrease case-fatality rates to less than 10%. Streptomycin, 30 mg per kg of body weight per day, given in two divided daily doses intramuscularly (IM) is the therapy of choice. Other aminoglycosides (e.g., gentamicin) have demonstrated in vitro activity, but cumulative clinical experience is limited. For septic patients or those with meningitis, intravenous (IV) chloramphenicol is recommended at a loading dose of 25 mg per kg of body weight, followed by 60 mg per kg per day in four divided doses. Completion of a 10-day course of therapy is important to prevent relapse. Tetracycline is an effective oral agent and can be utilized to complete a 10-day course of therapy after initial response to parenteral treatment. The dosage is 30 to 40 mg per kg per day in four divided doses (to a maximum of 2 grams per day). All North American *Y. pestis* isolates have been shown to be uniformly susceptible to these antimicrobial agents. Notably, however, a recent report has described plasmid-mediated, multidrug resistance in a *Y. pestis* isolated from a patient in Madagascar.

PREVENTION

Hospitalized, suspect plague cases should be placed in strict respiratory isolation until the possibility of pneumonic involvement has been excluded. Active surveillance for febrile illness should be maintained for 8 days for family members and close contacts of an index case. Contacts of patients with pneumonic plague should receive prophylaxis with tetracycline or doxycycline for 7 days. Trimethoprim-sulfamethoxazole is an acceptable alternative chemoprophylaxis in children and pregnant women. A formalin-fixed vaccine is available for persons with high-risk occupational exposures, including laboratory personnel.

Of particular note, all suspect plague cases should be reported immediately to local and state public health authorities to facilitate diagnostic efforts and to manage chemoprophylaxis, when appropriate. Assistance can also be obtained from the Plague Branch Center for Disease Control and Prevention, Ft. Collins, Colorado.

PSITTACOSIS
(Ornithosis)

method of
J. H. WINTER, M.D.
Kings Cross Hospital
Dundee, Scotland

Psittacosis was recognized in humans more than 100 years ago when Ritter, a Swiss physician, described a severe outbreak of respiratory disease in a household exposed to recently imported sick parrots. The organism was originally classified as a virus when it was identified in 1930, but subsequently it was recognized to be a small bacterium that replicates intracellularly and is susceptible to certain antibiotics. Although initially identified in parrots, the organism has been found in many other birds, including parakeets, budgerigars, canaries, seagulls, pigeons, and domestic poultry. The carriage rate in parakeets has been estimated at 8%. Carriers may be asymptomatic, but when the bird becomes stressed, for example, by transportation, disease and shedding of the organism may occur. Transmission to humans is believed to be either from direct contact with an infected bird, its feathers, or its excreta or from inhalation of infected dried excreta. Although the majority of cases are believed to be contracted from birds, the minority of cases report bird contact on admission to hospital. Human-to-human transmission has been described but seems to be rare.

The number of cases of psittacosis reported in the United Kingdom is increasing. This may reflect a true increase in numbers or may relate to improved diagnosis and reporting. Studies of the etiology of community-acquired pneumonia have usually found that less than 5% of cases are attributable to psittacosis. A problem with a number of these studies is the use of complement fixation tests for making the diagnosis. These tests use a genus-specific antigen and do not differentiate between *Chlamydia psittaci, Chlamydia pneumoniae* and *Chlamydia trachomatis*; thus, it is probable that a number of cases of pneumonia attributed to *C. psittaci* may in fact have been related to infection with *C. pneumoniae.*

Psittacosis is a systemic infection with a predilection for the lungs that causes an atypical pneumonia. Many complications have been noted, including pancarditis, hepatitis, anemia, arthritis, skin lesions, meningoencephalitis, and, rarely, glomerular and tubular renal damage. The incubation period is usually 7 to 10 days but can extend to

TABLE 1. **Clinical Features of Psittacosis**

Usual: >50% of cases	Cough Fever Malaise Headache
Common: 10–50% of cases	Sputum Chest pain Vomiting Anorexia Myalgia Splenomegaly
Occasional: <20% of cases	Dyspnea Meningitis Confusion Arthralgia Lymphadenopathy Pharyngitis Horder's spots

up to a month. Clinical features are given in Table 1. The majority of these are nonspecific, and most diagnoses are made retrospectively when serologic results become available; nevertheless, an atypical pneumonia picture with subacute presentation, headache, and splenomegaly should raise the possibility of psittacosis and should lead to treatment with a tetracycline, with or without other agents, depending on the severity of the disease. The majority of patients have pulmonary infiltrates on their chest radiograph. Hilar lymphadenopathy has been described in up to two thirds of patients. A majority of cases have abnormal results on liver function tests, but this is frequently seen in pneumonia from other causes; rarely, significant hepatitis and jaundice occur.

DIAGNOSIS

The diagnosis is commonly made by serology; a fourfold rise in titer or a single high convalescent titer in an appropriate clinical context indicates recent infection. When a positive result on the complement fixation test for the chlamydial genus-specific antigen is obtained, further serologic studies can often indicate which chlamydial species is responsible. *Chlamydia* can be grown in cell culture, but *C. psittaci* is a category 3 pathogen, which requires specialized laboratory facilities. The use of enzyme immunoassay, direct fluorescent antibody staining, and polymerase chain reaction for the diagnosis of *C. psittaci* infection has been described, but these tests are largely experimental.

TREATMENT

The tetracyclines (e.g., tetracycline 250 to 500 mg every 6 hours) are the treatment of choice for psittacosis. If the disease is recognized, treatment should be prescribed for 2 to 3 weeks. Alternative antibiotics available for the treatment of psittacosis (e.g., in children or pregnant patients) include macrolides (e.g., clarithromycin [Biaxin], 500 mg every 12 hours), rifampin, 600 mg every 12 hours, and quinolones (e.g., ciprofloxacin [Cipro], 500 mg every 8 hours), all of which reach high intracellular concentrations appropriate for the treatment of intracellular infection.

Attempts should be made to identify an avian source for this infection. This is particularly important when outbreaks occur in, for example, the poultry industry. It may be possible to prevent further infection by exterminating the infected birds or by replacing the birds' feed with tetracycline-treated seed.

Q FEVER

method of
DIDIER RAOULT, M.D., PH.D.
Université de la Méditerranée
Marseille, France

Q fever is a widepread zoonosis caused by *Coxiella burnetii.* It is a strict intracellular gram-negative bacterium, small and coccoid. It lives within the phagolysosome of its eukariotic host cell at very low pH (4.5 to 4.8). It has been classified in the rickettsial family previously; however, recent phylogenic data based on the study of the 16S rRNA gene sequence have shown that it is distant from the other rickettsia, belonging to the gamma subgroup of proteobacteria. The more closely related bacteria are *Legionella* species and *Francisella tularensis*

The bacterium has a sporelike life cycle, which explains a marked resistance to physicochemical agents. It can also survive within free amoeba as *Legionella.* In cell cultures or embryonated eggs, *C. burnetii* exhibits a phase variation (from phase I to phase II) related to a lipopolysaccharide change equivalent to that observed in the smooth-rough variation in enterobacteria. The phase II organism is nonpathogenic but paradoxically generates high antibody levels in patients. A single phase I organism can cause a Q fever.

The reservoir of *C. burnetii* is wide, and nearly all tested mammals, many birds, and ticks could be infected. Outbreaks have been reported associated with birth products of mammals (including sheep, goats, cattle, humans, cats, and dogs), raw milk, abattoirs, and farm work. Laboratory outbreaks have also been reported. The disease is prevalent anywhere in the world, but as the clinical spectrum is wide and unspecific the observed incidence is directly connected to the physician interest in Q fever.

Q fever is not a reportable disease. In humans, infection is symptomatic in only 50% of patients. The majority of symptomatic patients experience a flulike syndrome lasting for 2 to 7 days with severe headaches and cough; 5 to 10% of infected patients may be sick enough to be investigated. They present with high fever and one or several of the following symptoms: pneumonia, hepatitis, meningoencephalitis, rash, myocarditis, and pericarditis. Routine laboratory values show frequently mildly elevated transaminases and mild thrombocytopenia. In special hosts *C. burnetii* can cause chronic infection in pregnant women; it can cause recurrent miscarriages, low birth weight of the fetus, and prematurity. In patients with valvular disease and in patients with arterial aneurysm or prosthesis it can cause chronic endocarditis or vascular infection, being spontaneously fatal in the majority of cases. The clinical presentation is that of a chronic blood culture–negative endocarditis; modified Duke criteria are of diagnostic value in such cases.

DIAGNOSIS

As Q fever is proteiform, diagnosis is based mainly on large prescribed serum testing in patients with unexplained infectious syndrome. Isolation of *C. burnetii* is no more difficult than that of cytomegalovirus by using the shell vial technique when the personnel are experienced; however, it is restricted to specialized laboratories. *C. burnetii* could be isolated from the blood of 17% of patients with acute Q fever and 53% of those with Q fever endocarditis when the sample is taken before antibiotic therapy is begun. Liver biopsy is of diagnostic value, as the typical doughnut granuloma is quasi-specific to Q fever. Valves obtained by surgery or autopsy can be used for culture, direct immunostaining, or polymerase chain reaction (PCR). Valves can be studied retrospectively, even when paraffin embedded, by immunostaining and PCR.

In fact, the vast majority of cases are diagnosed via the serology. Three techniques are used. Complement fixation lacks sensitivity, and one third of patients with acute Q fever will not exhibit complement-fixing antibodies within 1 month after the beginning of the disease. However, a fourfold increase to phase II antigen is indicative of acute Q fever, and antibody levels against phase I above 200 are indicative of chronic Q fever. Indirect immunofluorescence assay (IFA) is the reference method. A single titer of 200 for IgG antiphase II associated with a 50 titer for IgM is diagnostic of acute infection. IgG antibody levels against phase I above 800 and IgA above 50 are highly predictive of chronic infection. ELISA tests are currently evaluated and give promising results.

THERAPY

To be active against Q fever, an antibiotic compound has to enter the cell, enter the phagolysosome of the cell, be efficient at acidic pH, and have *C. burnetii* susceptible to it. No antibiotic is bactericidal in this condition. It was shown that acidic pH was critical, and rising phagolysosomal pH allows doxycycline (Vibramycin) to become bactericidal. This could be achieved by the addition of hydroxychloroquine. As for acute Q fever, the reference treatment is doxycycline, 100 mg orally twice daily (bid) for 2 to 3 weeks. Other compounds have been reported to be regularly efficient, such as co-trimoxazole* (Bactrim), rifampin* (Rifadin), 300 mg bid, and ofloxacin* (Floxin), 200 mg bid. In some cases of acute Q fever that resist the antibiotic treatment and exhibit auto antibodies (e.g., anti–smooth muscle antibodies, circulating anticoagulant), a rapid cure is obtained by using a short prescription of prednisone, 40 mg per day for 7 days.

Chronic endocarditis should be treated for years following antibody levels. IgG antiphase I should be inferior to 800 and IgA to 50 to stop the treatment. Two protocols have been evaluated: one associated doxycycline (200 mg daily) to ofloxacin (400 mg daily) prescribed 4 years to lifetime, and the other associated doxycyline and hydroxychloroquine* to obtain a 1 μg per mL of plasma concentration from 1.5 to 4 years. This last regimen is apparently more efficient in terms of relapses. However, a regular ophthalmologic surveillance is critical to detect retinal accumulation of chloroquine. Both regimens expose the patient to a major risk of photosensitization.

*Not FDA approved for this indication.

PREVENTION

Prevention depends on avoidance of exposure, specifically in pregnant women and in patients with a valvulopathy. No vaccine is currently available outside Australia.

RABIES

method of
MICHAEL T. JELINEK, M.D.
McAllen Medical Center
McAllen, Texas

Rabies is a much feared, widespread infection of certain animal species that is occasionally transmitted to humans and is virtually always fatal. It has been described in legal documents as far back as 2300 BC. Transmission of the infection from dog saliva was known to the Egyptians at the time of the pharaohs, and suggested methods of treatment were found in Chinese manuscripts from the fifth century BC. Democritus around 500 BC gives the first recorded description of canine rabies, and Aristotle in the fourth century BC described animal rabies. In the first century AD the Roman Celsius described the human condition with this disease, and the classic, clinical features of the disease were described by 16th-century Italian physician Fracastoro. John Hunter is credited with initiating the first scientific approach to rabies in 1793. Until Louis Pasteur's work in the 1880s, the treatment of choice remained cautery. Pasteur repeatedly passaged a virulent rabies virus in rabbits to an attenuated fixed laboratory strain and used this to make his first rabies vaccine. The virus has been grown in tissue cultures since the 1930s. There is still no effective cure for rabies. Treatment is only supportive, yet it is widely recognized that this disease is nearly completely preventable in humans.

THE VIRUS: MORPHOLOGY AND PATHOGENESIS

Rabies is a member of the family of Rhabdoviridae, which contains more than 200 definite members that infect vertebrates, invertebrates, or plants. The Rhabdoviridae that do infect animals and humans are divided into two genera: *Lyssavirus,* from the Greek *lyssa,* which means "frenzy," and *Vesiculovirus* from the Latin *vesicula,* meaning "little bladder." The lyssaviruses contain more than 80 members, of which six are clinically important in humans. Serotype I is classic rabies virus, which is the most common isolate from terrestrial mammals, including dogs, cats, and bats (both hematophagous and insectivorous) of North America. Other important lyssaviruses that are part of the rabies group include the Lagos bat virus, which comes from fruit-eating bats in Africa. Mokola virus is present in *Crocidura* shrews in Africa, humans, and dogs in Zimbabwe. Duvenhage virus has been recovered from humans in South Africa and insectivorous bats in South Africa and Zimbabwe. Two European bat lyssaviruses, serotype I and serotype II, have been isolated from European bats and from humans. The Mokola, Duvenhage, and

European bat lyssaviruses are known to cause human disease that is virtually indistinguishable from true rabies, yet these viruses are found only in the Old World.

There is considerable antigenic variation among rabies viruses; still it appears that there is adequate cross-protection from current vaccines made from relatively homogeneous laboratory-maintained or fixed laboratory strains that originated from street isolates of rabies several decades ago. The molecular structure of the virus itself reveals that it is a bullet-shaped virion that measures approximately 180 by 75 nm and contains a single strand of negative sense RNA, which is combined with nuclear protein and forms a helical coil. There are two other viral proteins, the phosphoprotein and RNA polymerase, which are associated with the coil. This whole structure is the ribonucleoprotein complex and is covered by matrix protein and then by a glycoprotein coat bearing club-shaped spikes that project outward through a host-derived lipid layer. The outer glycoprotein spikes are utilized by the virion in its attachment to the cell surface at nicotinic acetylcholine-binding sites.

The rabies virus is highly neurotropic without a viremic phase and is nearly completely restricted to the nervous tissue throughout the course of infection in animals and in humans. The virus may enter the peripheral nerves immediately, but most likely an incubation period follows inoculation. The length of the incubation period varies with the infecting strain and the size of the inoculant as well as the proximity of the bite to the central nervous system. While in the incubation phase, the virus is believed to be amplified until there is sufficient concentration to allow the infectious units, which are bare nucleocapsids, to cross the myoneural junction and enter the central nervous system through unmyelinated sensory and motor axon terminals. It is only during the incubation period that the disease can be prevented by immunization.

The virus travels to the central nervous system axonally through retrograde axoplasmic flow at a rate of approximately 12 to 24 mm a day until the virus reaches the spinal cord. It multiplies in the spinal ganglion, and the first symptoms of the disease may appear at that time such as pain or paresthesia at the wound site. Once in the spinal cord, the virus disseminates rapidly at a rate of 200 to 400 mm per day and symptoms of rapidly progressive encephalitis develop. There is a minimum of inflammatory response within the central nervous system both histopathologically and by gross visualization at this point. There follows a centrifugal spread of the virus through the peripheral nerves throughout the body and most notably to the salivary glands.

The virus has been isolated from human skeletal and cardiac muscle, skin, lung, kidney, adrenal, lacrimal, and, of course, salivary glands. In contrast to the pathogenesis in neurons, viral replication in the acinar cells of the salivary glands produces a large amount of extracellular virus. Rabies virus is shed in human lacrimal and respiratory secretions and has been demonstrated in the urine and possibly within milk. There is a striking difference in the behavior of street viruses and attenuated rabies strains, which has been linked to the presence of a particular amino acid component, which is arginine in position 333 of the glycoprotein molecule. Substitution of this marker apparently confers attenuation in virulence. There are other molecular sites that also influence virulence, but the mechanisms are unknown. Rabies virus escapes recognition by the immune system until the very late stages of the disease, yet there is a prompt and highly protective antibody response following vaccination with tissue culture–derived rabies vaccine.

Rabies virus is quickly inactivated by heat at 56°C. It takes less than a minute at 37°C. It is prolonged to several hours in moist conditions. The rabies virus is unstable at a pH of less than 3 or a pH of more than 11. The rabies virus can stay stable for many years when frozen at −70°C or freeze dried and held at 0 to −4°C. Agents that are effective at destroying the virus include 45% ethanol, iodine solutions that are 1 to 10,000 dilution, 1% benzalkonium chloride, and even simple 1% soap solution. It is also inactivated by drying, ultraviolet and x-radiation, and sunlight.

INCIDENCE OF RABIES

True occurrence of human rabies is unknown because of the inherent under-reporting in underdeveloped nations. In India, there are estimates of 25,000 to 50,000 cases of human rabies per year, in China between 1000 to 2000, and in Bangladesh about 2000 cases. Other countries with high incidence are Sri Lanka, Nepal, Ethiopia, Brazil, Mexico, Colombia, Ecuador, and El Salvador. Although there have been impressive reductions in the number of rabies cases in countries in which vector control campaigns have been undertaken (e.g., dog vaccination), the number of cases in tropical countries of the world has not declined for decades. Some areas of the world have eradicated rabies, such as Taiwan, Japan, and peninsular Malaysia, by means of vaccination and other vector control measures. There are very few cases of human rabies in temperate zones. In the United States, where rabies is endemic, there have been an average of 1.6 rabies deaths per year over the last 30 years, and 37% of these infections were acquired abroad.

Infected animals are almost always the source of human rabies, although there have been eight cases of human rabies transmitted via corneal transplant. In the United States animals most commonly infected with rabies are skunks, although bats are more widely distributed throughout 48 of the states and are a major source, as well as raccoons, foxes, and coyotes. All wild animal bites and the licking by wild animals of human mucosal tissue or open wounds are potential points for infection with rabies. Among domestic animals in the United States, the most common carriers are cattle, cats, and dogs. In Texas, U.S. Department of Agriculture inspectors were exposed to rabies in the process of autopsying several cattle who had died mysteriously and were subsequently found to have succumbed to rabies. In Europe, foxes are the most common carrier. Vampire bats, mongooses, jackals, and wolves are prominent sources of rabies elsewhere in the world. Rabies has very rarely been reported in rodents, and so far, no cases of human rabies have resulted from rodent bites.

Rabies is most often acquired by the bite of an infected animal, although mucous membrane contact is another means by which infection can occur. Inhalation of the virus, as in the case of spelunkers in bat-infested caves, and contamination of an open wound by licking have been reported as modes of transmission. In any situation in which a bat is present and the individual cannot strictly exclude the possibility of a bite or mucosal exposure, post-exposure prophylaxis should be given unless testing of the bat has excluded the presence of rabies virus.

CLINICAL MANIFESTATIONS

The interval between inoculation of the virus into the recipient and the onset of symptoms varies between 4 days and 19 years. However, in at least 60% of cases the onset of symptoms occurs within 20 to 90 days. The incubation period tends to be shorter in children and when bites are located on or near the head. There are three phases or stages of rabies. A prodromal stage that usually consists of apathy, malaise, anorexia, fatigue, chills, headache, fever, anxiety, irritability, and depression may occur. At this point at the bite wound site, there may be hyperesthesia, pruritus, or pain radiating proximally. Other symptoms include cough, sore throat, occasionally abdominal pain, vomiting, diarrhea, and dysuria. In some instances patients may be diagnosed as having gastroenteritis or an upper respiratory infection. The prodromal phase may last between 1 and 10 days. The second stage of rabies is the acute neurologic phase. Eighty percent of patients progress to furious rather than dumb or paralytic rabies. Furious rabies is so named because of the marked neurologic hyperactivity characterized by agitation, excitement, and increased motor activity followed by dysphagia and hydrophobia. Considered pathognomonic of rabies, hydrophobia is the result of the fear of pain and choking produced by laryngeal and pharyngeal muscle spasms in this stage of rabies when swallowing is attempted. There may be severe drooling from increased salivation and avoidance of swallowing. Hypersensitivity of the skin may also occur. There may be periods marked by thrashing about, disorientation, hallucinations, and even biting, which may last as long as 5 minutes and be followed by a period of full orientation and calmness. Seizures may also occur during this stage. There are also dysfunctions of the autonomic system characterized by supraventricular arrhythmias, tachypnea, and labile blood pressure. If during the acute neurologic stage death does not occur as a result of cardiopulmonary arrest, the final paralytic phase will follow. This invariably results in death 2 to 7 days after the onset of symptoms.

In approximately 20% of patients, paralytic rabies occurs. This appears to be more common in patients who have acquired rabies via vampire bats or have been given postexposure vaccination. Paralysis or paresis accompanied by constipation, urinary retention, respiratory failure and inability to swallow, and flaccid paralysis of the proximal muscles associated with loss of deep tendon reflexes occurs, but sensation remains normal. In paralytic rabies death follows on an average of 12 days after the onset of symptoms. Once any neurologic symptoms have started, survival is rare. Four individuals are claimed to have survived rabies encephalitis. Two patients had been given postexposure prophylaxis and then intensive care and recovered completely. Another patient had neurologic sequelae. The diagnoses were based on confirmatory rabies neutralizing antibody levels in the serum and cerebrospinal fluid (CSF) of the patients. The fourth patient was a microbiologist who apparently inhaled fixed rabies virus. He had previously been vaccinated, and he apparently has residual neurologic impairment.

The differential diagnosis antemortem can be very difficult if a clear history of exposure is not obtained. Tetanus, Guillain-Barré, other encephalitides, and toxic ingestions should also be considered in the differential. Recently, two patients were misdiagnosed as having Creutzfeldt-Jakob disease. Both patients were confirmed as having rabies by direct fluorescent antibody testing at the Centers for Disease Control and Prevention. No tests are available that can diagnose rabies before the onset of the disease. Diagnosis can be made by isolation of the virus by culture, by antigen detection, or by antibody detection. Isolation of rabies virus is most successful during the first week of illness from saliva, throat, tracheal, or eye swabs or brain biopsy samples, CSF, and occasionally from urine. The method is by inoculation of suckling mice, and the results are available in 1 to 3 weeks. This method is now being replaced by tissue culture techniques such as murine blastoma cells, which may still take as many as 4 days. Cell cultures are considered more sensitive to the toxic effects of contaminated inocula. There is a fluorescent antibody test available that detects antigen in skin biopsies usually taken from the nape of the neck. Frozen sections of these punch biopsies reveal rabies antigen in nerve twiglets throughout the base of hair follicles. This method is between 60 and 100% sensitive. No false-positive results have been reported.

In unvaccinated patients, rabies seroconversion occurs during the second week of illness and is diagnostic, but there may be a delay in antibody production of up to 24 days after the onset of symptoms. In vaccinated individuals very high levels of antibody in the serum and CSF are needed to make the diagnosis. Postmortem diagnosis is made by fluorescent antibody testing of brain tissue and by characteristic cytoplasmic inclusions (Negri bodies) that are present in 70 to 80% of cases. Negri bodies are sharply defined cytoplasmic inclusions that are round or oblong and vary in size from 2 to 10 μm. Negri bodies are eosinophilic and consist of viral nucleocapsid proteins.

TREATMENT

There are no specific chemotherapeutic regimens available for rabies encephalitis. Treatment consists of intensive supportive care concentrating on maintaining respiratory and cardiovascular support, together with sedation and pain control. Extreme care should be undertaken to protect hospital staff from the rabies virus, which is present in saliva, tears, urine, and other bodily fluids. Family members of the victim should be interrogated for any potential exposure. Standard (universal) precautions and respiratory precautions for suctioning are strongly recommended. Steroids should be avoided in the treatment of cerebral edema associated with rabies encephalitis. High-dose rabies immunoglobulin has been administered in several cases with no clear effect. The administration of vaccine after the onset of clinical illness is contraindicated.

PREVENTION

Because rabies has the highest case-fatality rate of any known human infection (essentially 100%), prevention is the key to control of this disease. The cornerstone of prevention is the control of rabies in animals, especially domestic animals, which very effectively decreases the exposure of humans to potentially infectious bites. Rabies vaccine is nearly always successfully protective against rabies when it is used in the appropriate fashion. Postexposure prophylaxis consists of local treatment of wounds and immunization, which includes the administration in most instances of both rabies immunoglobulin and vaccine. Local treatment of wounds cannot be overemphasized. Immediate and thorough cleansing of all wounds and scratches with soap and water is perhaps the most effective measure for preventing

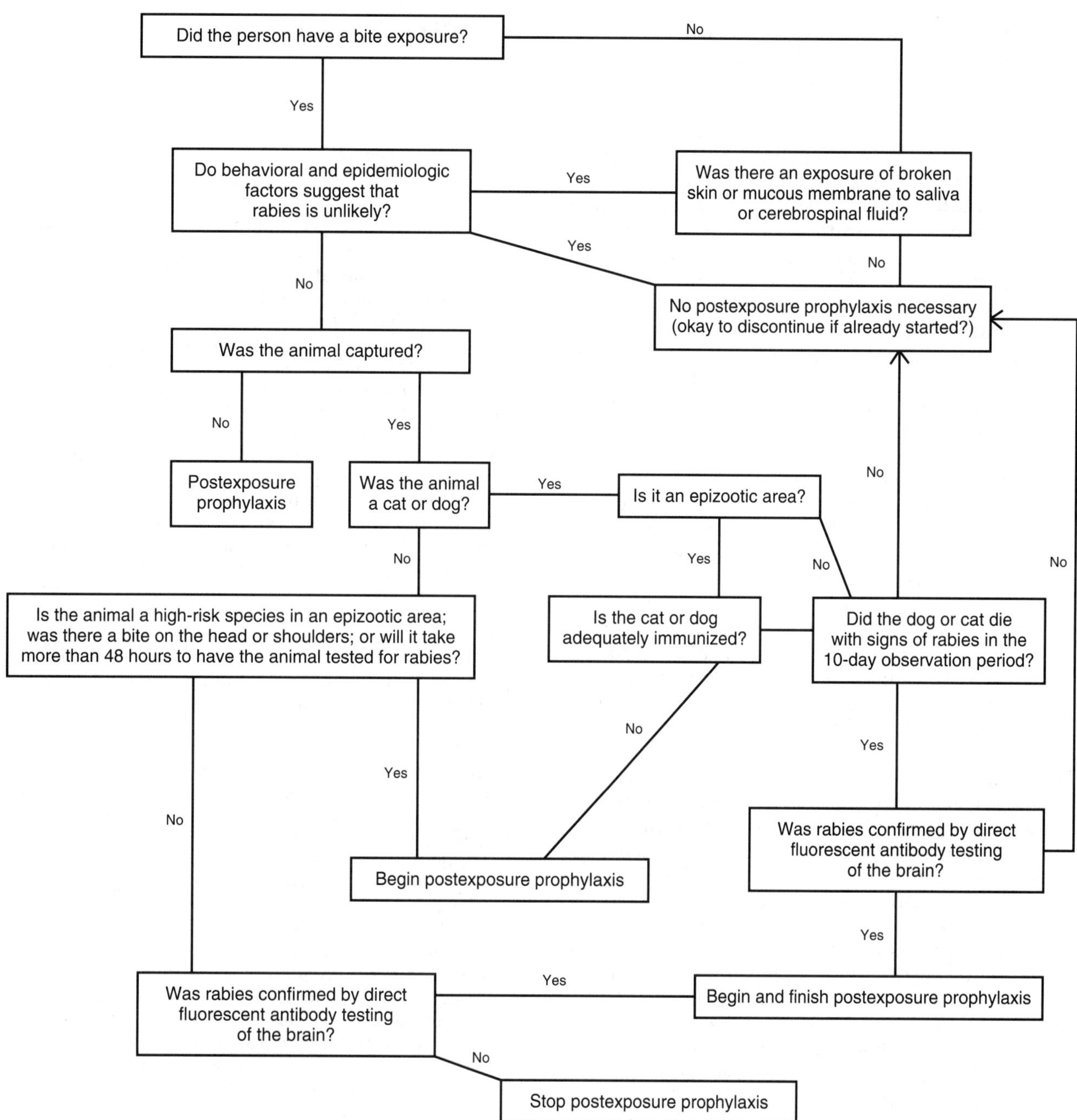

Figure 1. Rabies postexposure prophylaxis decision tree.

rabies. In experimental animals the simple local wound cleansing has been shown to markedly reduce the likelihood of rabies. Tetanus immunization and measures to control bacterial infections should be given as indicated.

The decision to treat or not treat must be based on information at hand about the patient (Figure 1). Postexposure antirabies immunization should always include administration of both human rabies immunoglobulin (HRIG) (Hyperab, Imogam) and the vaccine, either human diploid cell vaccine (HDCV) (Imovax) or rabies vaccine, adsorbed (RVA). RVA differs from HDCV in that a different virus strain, cell line, and concentration process are used in making the RVA vaccine. The only exception to giving rabies immunoglobulin along with vaccine is in patients who have previously received pre-exposure or postexposure regimens of HDCV or RVA or in those who have been immunized with other types of vaccine and have a history of documented adequate rabies antibody titer. In these cases alone HRIG would not be given, and only two doses of either vaccine would be given on day zero and on the third day after exposure.

It cannot be emphasized enough that the sooner treatment is begun after exposure, the better the chance of effectiveness of the vaccine. The vaccine is given in five 1-mL doses on days 0, 3, 7, 14, and 28.

The intramuscular injections for both vaccines should be given in the deltoid in adults and larger children. In infants and smaller children, the anterior lateral thigh should be used. HRIG is administered only once at the beginning of an antirabies prophylaxis to provide immediate antibody protection until the patient's immune system generates antibody to either HDCV or RVA. Rabies immunoglobulin can be given up to the eighth day after the first dose of vaccine was given. The dose of rabies immunoglobulin is 20 IU per kg or approximately 9 IU per pound of body weight. If it is anatomically feasible, half the dose of the human rabies immunoglobulin should be infiltrated in the area around the wound. The rest should be administered intramuscularly. The rabies immunoglobulin should be given in a separate anatomic site from that of the rabies vaccine.

Pre-exposure immunization is also very important. For pre-exposure immunization, HDCV is given in three 1-mL injections on days 0, 7, and 28, preferably in the deltoid area. Intradermal rabies vaccine (Imovax Rabies ID) has been used for pre-exposure immunization in a regimen of three 1-mL doses given intradermally in the lateral aspect of the arm over the deltoid area on the same administration schedule as that for HDCV. Caution must be taken in patients who are receiving either immunosuppressive drugs or chloroquine for malaria prophylaxis, as these agents may interfere with the antibody response to HDCV when this is given in the intradermal route. The intramuscular route of pre-exposure to prophylaxis appears to provide sufficient safety margin in this particular setting. Booster doses of vaccine are recommended for persons at high risk of rabies exposure; serologic testing should be done every 6 months to 2 years, depending on the severity of risk.

Adverse reactions to HDCV include local reactions such as pain, erythema, swelling, or itching at the injection site in about 25% of recipients and mild systemic reactions such as headache, nausea, abdominal pain, muscle aches, and dizziness in about 20%. About 6% of persons receiving booster doses of HDCV may experience immune complex reactions, which are characterized by the onset 2 to 21 days after the booster of generalized urticaria, arthralgias, arthritis, possible angioedema, nausea, vomiting, fever, and malaise. This phenomenon occurs very rarely with primary immunization with HDCV, and no life-threatening cases of immune complex–like illness have been reported. The source of the immune complex–like reactions appears to be sensitization to the β-propiolactone–treated human serum albumin present in HDCV. Reactions to rabies immunoglobulin consist basically of local pain and low-grade fever. There have been no specific reported adverse reactions to HRIG, although immunoglobulin itself has been associated with angioneurotic edema and nephrotic syndrome and anaphylaxis. These cases are so rare that a cause-effect relationship between immunoglobulin and these reactions is not clearly established.

RAT-BITE FEVER

method of
W. KEMPER ALSTON, M.D.
University of Vermont College of Medicine and Fletcher Allen Health Care
Burlington, Vermont

Rat-bite fever is a systemic infection caused by *Streptobacillus moniliformis* or *Spirillum minus* that occurs worldwide. It is considered to be rare in the United States and is not a reportable disease. Therefore, the true incidence of rat-bite fever in the United States is unknown. Cases of *S. moniliformis* (streptobacillary fever) predominate in North America, most commonly among laboratory workers who have contact with rodents. Several cases in children have also been reported in the literature following exposure to rats in the home, although the bite may occur at night and not be recalled. In Asia, rat-bite fever is caused by *S. minus* (spirillar fever, "Sodoku" in Japan).

These organisms are frequent commensals in the nasopharynx of wild and laboratory rats. *S. moniliformis* is a nonmotile, pleomorphic, gram-negative bacillus that grows in filamentous chains characterized by bulbous swellings. Culture usually requires microaerophilic conditions and medium enriched with serum. An ingredient of commercial blood culture systems, sodium polyanethol sulfonate (SPS), may inhibit growth. *S. minus* is a short, gram-negative, spiral rod that demonstrates motility under darkfield microscopy via terminal flagella. The organism is not culturable.

Rat-bite fever occurs following the bite of a rat, mouse, or other animal that has had contact with rodents. Cases may be sporadic or may occur in outbreaks. "Haverhill fever" refers to a form of *S. moniliformis* infection following the ingestion of raw milk or water contaminated by rats. An incubation period of less than 10 days characterizes *S. moniliformis* rat-bite fever. Headache, fever, chills, arthralgias, and myalgias predominate, followed by a maculopapular rash involving the palms, soles, and extremities. The initial wound, which served as the portal of entry, may have healed and may go unnoticed. Leukocytosis may be present. The infection is probably self-limited in most cases, but fever may persist and relapse. Polyarthritis, especially affecting the knees, as well as metastatic infection and infective endocarditis have been described.

S. minus infection typically has a longer incubation period of 1 to 4 weeks, which is followed by fever with pain and swelling at the site of the bite as well as prominent granulomatous regional lymphadenopathy. The wound eventually ulcerates, with eschar formation. As with *S. moniliformis,* infection is usually self-limited but may be complicated by wide dissemination and endocarditis. Fever may relapse over a period of weeks in untreated cases. Rat-bite fever should be suspected in an individual of any age who works with rodents or has been exposed to rats and presents with fever, centrifugal rash, and arthralgias. The differential diagnosis for both forms of the infection is broad and includes leptospirosis, Rocky Mountain spotted fever, secondary syphilis, neisserial infection, Lyme disease, enteroviral infection, and drug reaction.

DIAGNOSIS

The diagnosis of *S. moniliformis* rat-bite fever can be made by culture with enriched medium or direct smear of blood, synovial fluid, or pus with Giemsa stain. A serum agglutination titer may be useful in culture-negative cases. *S. minus* must be directly visualized because no serology or culture system is available.

TREATMENT

The treatment of choice for both forms of rat-bite fever remains penicillin. The paucity of reported cases in the literature, as well as the difficulties encountered with in vitro cultivation, limit the data available regarding treatment. The organisms do not produce β-lactamase and are sensitive in vitro to a wide range of antimicrobial agents. Severe cases complicated by endocarditis, septic arthritis, or other metastatic foci should be treated with intravenous penicillin G, 10 to 20 million units per day in divided doses. Milder infections can be treated with intramuscular procaine penicillin, 600,000 units every 12 hours, or oral penicillin V, 500 mg every 6 hours. Most infections have been treated for 10 to 14 days, although endocarditis is usually treated for 4 weeks. Some experts advocate adding an aminoglycoside, such as streptomycin, in severe cases, because penicillin-resistant "L-forms," which lack a cell wall, may exist. Patients allergic to penicillin have been treated successfully with tetracycline, 500 mg by mouth every 6 hours.

PREVENTION

Prevention of rat-bite fever is best accomplished by avoiding contact with rats. Laboratory workers should wear protective gloves and be vaccinated against tetanus. Any injuries should be cleansed promptly. The role of prophylactic oral penicillin following a rat bite remains unresolved but may be considered on an individual basis.

RELAPSING FEVER

method of
R. WESLEY FARR, M.D., and
MARK D. LACY, M.D.
West Virginia University School of Medicine
Morgantown, West Virginia

Relapsing fevers are arthropod-borne spirochetal infections characterized by recurrent febrile episodes followed by asymptomatic periods. The tick-borne variety is seen worldwide, including the western United States. The louse-borne variety is seen in the developing world but not in the United States unless imported.

ETIOLOGY, EPIDEMIOLOGY, AND PATHOPHYSIOLOGY

Various rodent ticks and the human body louse are the vectors by which humans acquire the spirochetal bacteria causing relapsing fever. These microbes are members of the *Borrelia* spirochete genus and are 8 to 30 μm long with a helix of three to 10 loose spirals. They cannot be cultivated in standard media, but, unlike other spirochetes causing human disease, they can be readily detected with Giemsa or Wright's stain.

Louse-borne disease is caused by *Borrelia recurrentis,* which is endemic in the highlands of Africa, South America, and foci in the Far East. It is not observed endemically in the United States. This form of relapsing fever usually occurs in the setting of overcrowding, in which the dissemination of body lice results in epidemics. Untreated, the mortality rate may reach 40% and is related to host factors such as malnutrition and concurrent illnesses.

More than 12 species of *Borrelia* produce the tick-borne variety of relapsing fever. The vectors are soft ticks of the genus *Ornithodoros.* The natural reservoirs are rodents and other small mammals residing in warm areas throughout the world at elevations of 1500 to 9600 feet. The ticks usually feed at night, have a painless bite, and feed for five to 20 minutes; hence, exposures to the vector may go unnoticed. Most cases in North America have occurred in the western forests; the number of reported cases there is growing because of increased intrusion of humans into the vectors' environment. Sixty-two visitors lodging in cabins at Grand Canyon National Park in Arizona in 1979 constituted the largest outbreak of the disease in the Western Hemisphere. The characteristic pattern of fevers interspersed with asymptomatic periods is related to the human immune response to the spirochete's ability to reconfigure its outer membrane antigens. A single borrelial spirochete may produce up to 40 different variants or serotype progeny by this multiphasic antigen variation during the same infection. Each surface antigen is encoded by a different gene that is activated to evade the host's serospecific antibody. Thus, after the first serotype wanes and the fever subsides because of an effective antibody response by the host, another antigen is expressed by a new bacterial variant. Several days later, as this new serotype multiplies, another febrile episode ensues, necessitating a new specific antibody response to clear the new variant. This cycle of genetic recombination and antigen expression followed by specific antibody response is repeated and is responsible for the periodicity distinctive in this disease.

SYMPTOMS, SIGNS, AND DIAGNOSIS

Tick-borne and louse-borne relapsing fevers have similar manifestations that develop after an incubation period of approximately 1 week. Symptoms begin suddenly with high fever, rigors, myalgia and arthralgia, weakness, and a severe headache. Nausea, abdominal pain, diarrhea, vomiting, or nonproductive cough is sometimes reported. During the febrile episodes, patients are acutely ill with lethargy, tachycardia, tachypnea, and occasionally confusion. Nonspecific maculopapular rashes may be seen; petechial rashes are less common. Hepatosplenomegaly is frequent in louse-borne disease but is unusual in the tick-borne variety. Lymphadenopathy usually affecting the cervical chains is not dramatic. Jaundice or mucosal bleeding is an infrequent sign of louse-borne relapsing fever and portends a worse prognosis. Myocarditis is a rare phenomenon. Central nervous system involvement, manifesting as meningitis or cranial nerve deficits, is occasionally seen, particularly in louse-borne disease. Laboratory parameters are nonspecific. Hemogram results are usually normal, although thrombocytopenia has been reported. Liver enzymes may be elevated, especially in severe cases of louse-borne relapsing fever. Positive serologic test results for

TABLE 1. **Preferred Therapy for Relapsing Fever**

	Drug	Adult Dosage	Duration
Louse-borne relapsing fever	Tetracycline*	500 mg PO	1 dose
	Doxycycline*	100 mg q 12 h PO	2 doses
Tick-borne relapsing fever	Doxycycline	100 mg q 12 h PO/IV	7–14 d
	Erythromycin	500 mg q 6 h PO/IV	7–14 d
Alternative drugs	Chloramphenicol	500 mg q 6 h PO/IV	
	Penicillin V	500 mg q 6 h PO	
	Penicillin G†	5 million units q 6 h IV	
	Ceftriaxone†	2 gm once daily IV	

* Substitute erythromycin, 500 mg PO, for pregnant women. In children younger than 8 years old, give 40 mg/kg/d in divided doses q 6–8 h.
† Use in patients with central nervous system manifestations.

Lyme disease and syphilis occur in less than 5% of patients.

The most useful laboratory study is a thick or thin smear of peripheral blood with a Wright's or Giemsa stain. Organisms may be detected only during febrile episodes. Repeated examinations may be necessary to demonstrate spirochetes. Darkfield and fluorescence microscopy may increase the sensitivity but require more laboratory expertise. Serologic tests are not widely available except in reference laboratories and often lack specificity.

The acute clinical syndrome lasts from 1 to 6 days and then terminates as abruptly as it began. Hypotension and shock have been observed in the primary episode. Subsequent relapses, occurring 7 to 10 days later, are usually less severe. In tick-borne disease, relapses may recur over several weeks; fewer relapses occur in louse-borne disease. The early stages of relapsing fever may simulate other disorders, so geographic and epidemiologic factors are important in the diagnosis. Tick-borne disease may be confused with Colorado tick fever or Rocky Mountain spotted fever. Early louse-borne relapsing fever may resemble malaria, dengue fever, typhoid fever, or leptospirosis.

TREATMENT

Tetracycline or doxycycline is the drug of choice and is usually given orally. Erythromycin is used in pregnant women and children. A single 500-mg dose of tetracycline or erythromycin is satisfactory for most episodes of louse-borne disease. A 500-mg oral dose of tetracycline or erythromycin four times daily for 7 to 10 days is given for the tick-borne variety owing to a higher rate of treatment failure and relapse. Penicillin or ceftriaxone (Rocephin) is recommended if central nervous system involvement is present. Chloramphenicol is another effective alternative therapy (Table 1).

Hospitalization may be necessary for very ill patients but also as a precaution in anticipation of a Jarisch-Herxheimer reaction (JHR). Frequently seen within 3 hours after treatment, the JHR elicits fever, increased rigors, and hypotension persisting for up to 24 hours. Management of JHR consists of supportive care. The JHR is associated with the systemic appearance of cytokines, such as tumor necrosis factor (TNF-α), interleukin-6, and interleukin-8. Corticosteroids, acetaminophen, and pentoxifylline* (Trental) fail to prevent or modify the JHR. Pretreatment with sheep polyclonal Fab antibody fragments against TNF-α (anti-TNF-α Fab, Therapeutic Antibodies, Inc., London) can suppress the JHR. Uncomplicated, adequately treated relapsing fever has a mortality rate of less than 5%.

*Not FDA approved for this indication.

PREVENTION

Louse-borne relapsing fever is best prevented by minimizing overcrowding and maintaining good hygiene. Malathion-type insecticides may be necessary to successfully delouse crowded housing facilities. Rodent-proofing of lodging facilities and the use of insect repellents may reduce the risk of tick-borne disease if vector habitats cannot be avoided. The Bacterial Zoonoses Branch, Division of Vector-Borne Infectious Diseases, Centers for Disease Control and Prevention, requests that serum samples from patients with documented infections be submitted for its International Borreliosis Reference Collection; telephone 1-970-221-6400. Cases should also be reported to state and local health departments.

RHEUMATIC FEVER

method of
JOHN F. BOHNSACK, M.D.,
L. GEORGE VEASY, M.D., and
HARRY R. HILL, M.D.
University of Utah School of Medicine
Salt Lake City, Utah

Acute rheumatic fever (ARF) is a nonsuppurative sequela of group A streptococcal pharyngitis that can affect the joints, heart, central nervous system, and skin. Although the incidence of rheumatic fever in developed countries has generally declined over the past 30 years, a resurgence of ARF occurred in several areas of the United States in the 1980s. In addition, ARF continues to be a significant problem in developing countries.

ARF occurs in early childhood through adult life but has its peak incidence in children between 5 and 15 years of age. Diagnosis of the initial attack of ARF is based on the revised Jones' criteria (Table 1). The presence of two major or one major and two minor manifestations indicates a

TABLE 1. **Updated Jones' Criteria for the Diagnosis of the Initial Attack of Acute Rheumatic Fever**

Major Manifestations	Minor Manifestations
Carditis	Fever
Polyarthritis	Arthralgia
Chorea	Elevated erythrocyte sedimentation rate or C-reactive protein
Erythema marginatum	Prolonged P-R interval
Subcutaneous nodules	*Doppler echocardiographic evidence of typical rheumatic valvular involvement**

The diagnosis of acute rheumatic fever is made when the patient has two major manifestations or one major and two minor manifestations,

plus

supporting evidence of preceding streptococcal infection: positive throat culture results for group A streptococcus or elevated or rising antistreptococcal antibody serum titer.

*The authors use echocardiographic evidence of mitral or aortic regurgitation typical of rheumatic fever as a minor manifestation (see text). The American Heart Association has not accepted this manifestation as minor criteria.

Adapted from the Special Writing Group of the Committee on Rheumatic Fever, Endocarditis, and Kawasaki Disease of the Council on Cardiovascular Disease in the Young of the American Heart Association: Guidelines for the diagnosis of rheumatic fever. Jones' criteria. 1992 Update. JAMA *268*:2069–2073, 1992. Copyright 1992, American Medical Association.

high probability of ARF, if supported by evidence of a recent streptococcal infection.

Arthritis is generally the first manifestation to occur during an episode of ARF. Arthritis occurs in as many as 70% of patients with ARF but is very nonspecific because many other disorders result in similar manifestations. In general, the arthritis in ARF is asymmetric, affects the large joints, and is fleeting or migratory in nature. The joints are painful and warm, but permanent damage does not occur. Septic arthritis or osteomyelitis should always be considered in patients with pronounced joint pain, particularly when a single joint is affected. Aspirin should not be administered before making a firm diagnosis of ARF because the arthritis of ARF is exquisitely sensitive to salicylate therapy.

Carditis, which occurs in approximately 50% of patients, is clearly the most important manifestation because it is the only life-threatening manifestation of ARF and because damage to the heart is the only significant cause of residual morbidity. In the past, emphasis has been placed on rheumatic carditis being a "pancarditis." Although myocarditis and pericarditis may occur, the specific lesions of rheumatic carditis are mitral and aortic regurgitation, and these lesions constitute "rheumatic heart disease," a term that is more specific than carditis.

Rheumatic heart disease in children is most often indicated by the murmur of mitral regurgitation, a high-frequency systolic murmur at the apex with transmission to the left axilla. In patients older than 30, the predominant manifestation of cardiac disease is mitral stenosis due to fusion and deformity of the mitral leaflets. Thus, a new murmur or a change in a previous murmur is required to make the diagnosis in an adult. Prolongation of the P-R interval (a minor criterion) is relatively nonspecific and is detected in only about 30 to 40% of young persons with ARF.

Doppler echocardiography can confirm regurgitant flow across the mitral valve that is suspected by physical examination and can differentiate the mitral regurgitation characteristic of ARF from benign or physiologic mitral regurgitation. Mitral regurgitation in patients with ARF is typically holosystolic, reflects posterolaterally at least 1 cm about the mitral annulus, is seen in two planes, and exhibits a mosaic pattern demonstrating high-turbulence, high-frequency flow. Strict adherence to these criteria will distinguish physiologic mitral regurgitation seen occasionally in individuals without heart disease from rheumatic mitral regurgitation. In addition, echocardiography can detect mitral regurgitation in patients with arthritis or chorea in whom a murmur is not audible. We believe that Doppler echocardiographic evidence of silent mitral regurgitation that is typical of rheumatic fever can be regarded as a minor manifestation of ARF and is particularly useful in diagnosing the patient with arthritis who does not have a murmur on physical examination (see Table 1). This approach increases the sensitivity of ARF diagnosis without leading to overdiagnosis and identifies patients needing more careful cardiac follow-up. This approach, however, has not been adopted by the American Heart Association in the current Jones' criteria.

Sydenham's chorea occurs in from 15 to 30% of ARF patients and follows the preceding streptococcal infection by 6 weeks to several months, making it difficult to establish a preceding streptococcal infection. Doppler echocardiography may be used to establish significant mitral regurgitation in patients with "pure" chorea as in patients with isolated arthritis.

The cutaneous manifestations of ARF, which include subcutaneous nodules and erythema marginatum, occur in 3% and 5% of patients, respectively. In the large series of cases seen by us in Utah, skin manifestations, although specific for the disease, were seldom valuable in establishing the diagnosis, because they most often occurred along with other major manifestations.

It is imperative to establish that there has been a recent streptococcal infection in all suspected cases of ARF. The pharynx should be cultured, although throat culture results are frequently negative at the time of presentation, and serum should be obtained for streptococcal antibody studies. The antistreptolysin O (ASO) and the antideoxyribonuclease B (anti-DNase B) tests should both be employed to increase sensitivity. The anti-DNase B titer remains elevated for 2 to 3 months, thereby increasing its value in patients with chorea.

TREATMENT

ARF varies in its presentation and severity. The following treatment recommendations are offered as guidelines to be adapted to the individual patient's particular manifestations. Every patient with ARF must be treated to eradicate residual streptococci and be given antibiotic prophylaxis to prevent recurrent attacks, because further cardiac damage results from recurrences of ARF.

Antibiotic Treatment to Eradicate Streptococci

Antibiotic therapy to eradicate group A streptococcus is instituted as soon as the diagnosis of ARF is established, even if the throat culture results are negative (Table 2). A single intramuscular injection of penicillin G benzathine is recommended. Oral penicillin V is an alternative to intramuscular penicillin.

TABLE 2. **Antibiotic Treatment of Streptococcal Pharyngitis**

Drug	Dosage, Route, and Duration
Penicillin G benzathine	<27 kg: 600,000 units single IM dose >27 kg: 1,200,000 units single IM dose
Penicillin V	Children: 250 mg PO tid × 10 d Adolescents and adults: 500 mg PO tid × 10 d
Erythromycin estolate	20–40 mg/kg/d bid to qid (maximum 1 g/d) × 10 d
Erythromycin ethylsuccinate	40 mg/kg/d bid to qid (maximum 1 g/d) × 10 d

Erythromycin may be substituted in patients who are allergic to penicillin if erythromycin-resistant group A streptococci are not prevalent in the area. Clindamycin (Cleocin) and first-generation cephalosporins may also be used to eradicate streptococci, but the broader spectrum cephalosporins have no clear-cut advantage over penicillin, particularly because as many as 15% of persons allergic to penicillin will also be allergic to cephalosporins. Tetracyclines and sulfa drugs should not be used to treat streptococcal pharyngitis. Prophylaxis of recurrent infection should begin immediately following the eradicating regimen (see later discussion).

Bed Rest

Although patients with ARF improve both symptomatically and objectively on bed rest, the value of prolonged bed rest in patients with ARF was probably overestimated in the past. Physicians should restrict activity and carefully observe patients with ARF during the first 2 weeks of illness because carditis usually appears during that time. Patients can return to full activity rapidly if they improve and there is no evidence of carditis. The patient with moderate to severe carditis should resume activity slowly and cautiously, with frequent and thorough clinical assessments. Return to full activity is permitted after symptoms and signs have resolved, and acute phase reactants have returned to normal.

Anti-inflammatory Agents

Therapy to suppress inflammation should not be instituted before the diagnosis of rheumatic fever is clearly established because the symptoms may dramatically improve or disappear in response to aspirin or corticosteroids.

Aspirin

Aspirin is extremely effective in the control of arthritis and is used to suppress carditis when there is no associated cardiomegaly and no evidence of congestive heart failure. Aspirin is generally started at a dose of 100 mg per kg per day given in 4 equally divided oral doses and can be decreased to 70 mg per kg per day after 2 to 3 days. The lower dose is usually adequate to maintain a therapeutic serum level of 20 to 25 mg per dL. It is advisable to measure a serum salicylate level 4 to 5 days after starting therapy and to adjust the dosage accordingly because absorption varies among individuals. It is also reasonable to measure a serum salicylate level if joint pain persists or if signs of salicylate toxicity occur. Parents and patients should be instructed about the signs of salicylate toxicity and about the risk and signs of Reye's syndrome. Aspirin should be discontinued immediately if the patient develops influenza or varicella or if a patient who is not immune to varicella is exposed to varicella. Aspirin should be given until the sedimentation rate returns to normal and then tapered over 4 weeks to prevent rebound.

Corticosteroids

Corticosteroids are recommended for moderate or severe carditis and often lead to dramatic symptomatic relief, although there is no documentation that steroids reduce residual cardiac disease. Oral prednisone is given at a dose of 2 mg per kg per day in 1 to 4 doses per day and continued until disease activity has disappeared and acute phase reactants have returned to normal. Prednisone should be tapered gradually over 2 to 3 weeks, and aspirin therapy instituted at 70 mg per kg per day at the start of the steroid taper and continued for 2 to 3 weeks after steroids are discontinued to prevent rebound. The doses of prednisone used are usually associated with significant side effects, including moon facies and hirsutism. The physician should also monitor the patient's blood pressure and be prepared to treat steroid-induced hypertension.

Congestive Heart Failure

Congestive heart failure is managed in a conventional manner with digoxin, diuretics, oxygen therapy, and rest to reduce cardiac demand. Rapid digitalization should be avoided because of possible sensitivity in the presence of myocarditis. Death from refractory congestive heart failure is rare during ARF. Surgical correction of valvular incompetence can be lifesaving when the patient fails to respond to vigorous medical management.

Sydenham's Chorea

Sydenham's chorea generally resolves after several months but may last for more than a year. Parents and patients should be informed of the self-limited nature of the disorder. Management of chorea varies with its severity. Patients with mild chorea can be managed by being placed in an environment that reduces stress. Some patients may also benefit from mild sedation. Patients with chorea so severe that they cannot feed or dress themselves or may injure themselves may require medication to control the chorea, and sometimes they need to be hospitalized. Haloperidol (Haldol), has been used to control chorea, but the patient needs to be monitored carefully for extrapyramidal side effects. Haloperidol is started as a single daily dose of 0.25 mg per day (0.5 mg in the adolescent) and increased by 0.25 mg per day (0.5 mg in the adolescent) every 7 days until symptoms are controlled. The drug is taken twice a day when the dosage is increased. Doses do not usually exceed 3 to 5 mg per day. The drug is administered until after the chorea is resolved for 1 to 2 weeks and then is tapered over several weeks. Both sodium valproate* and carbamazepine* (Tegretol) have also been reported to control chorea. Neurologists at our institution have also used short courses of prednisone to treat chorea with encouraging results. Prednisone is given for 2 weeks at 1 mg per kg per day and then tapered over 2 weeks.

PREVENTION OF PRIMARY AND RECURRENT RHEUMATIC FEVER

Prompt diagnosis and treatment of streptococcal pharyngitis with appropriate antibiotics reduce the risk of ARF and are therefore the primary means of preventing ARF. Recent outbreaks of rheumatic fever in the United States demonstrate that treatment of streptococcal pharyngitis is still warranted despite the overall decline in the incidence in rheumatic fever over the last 4 decades. (The management of streptococcal pharyngitis is discussed elsewhere in this text.)

Recurrent ARF occurs in from 5% to as high as 50% of cases, and the potential for cardiac damage resulting in rheumatic heart disease increases with each episode of ARF. All patients with ARF, including those without carditis, should receive antibiotic prophylaxis (Table 3). The best regimen is benzathine penicillin, 1.2 million units intramuscularly every 4 weeks, although some evidence from endemic areas suggests that the same dose given every 3 weeks is more efficacious at preventing recurrences of ARF. Oral penicillin V is an alternative, but compliance can be better ensured with intramuscular injections. The patient who is allergic to penicillin can be treated with sulfadiazine or sulfisoxazole. The rare patient who is allergic to both penicillin and sulfa drugs could be given erythromycin twice a day, but the physician should be aware that some group A streptococci are resistant to erythromycin.

Although the incidence of recurrent ARF decreases as the interval from the primary attack increases, it is prudent to administer lifelong antibiotic prophylaxis. Compliance with regimens requires considerable physician effort and education of the patient and parent. Special emphasis should be placed on ensuring antibiotic prophylaxis of high-risk patients: children and adolescents; those living in crowded conditions, such as military camps, prisons, or schools; teachers and others whose occupations bring them into contact with children; persons living in or visiting areas endemic for rheumatic fever or experiencing rheumatic fever outbreaks; and, most important, patients with residual rheumatic heart disease.

*Not FDA approved for this indication.

TABLE 3. **Antibiotic Prophylaxis of Recurrent Rheumatic Fever**

Drug	Dosage, Route, and Frequency
Benzathine penicillin	1.2 million units IM q 3–4 wk
Penicillin V	250 mg PO bid
Sulfadiazine or	<27 kg: 0.5 gm/d
sulfisoxazole	>27 kg: 1.0 gm/d
Erythromycin*	250 mg PO bid

*Use only in patients allergic to both penicillin and sulfa drugs.

The patient with ARF should be thoroughly educated about the seriousness of the disease and the need for close follow-up, continuing antibiotic prophylaxis, and periodic examination for evidence of valvular disease. Initially patients should be seen at least briefly every 3 to 4 weeks when they receive their intramuscular prophylaxis. A more thorough examination for residual cardiac abnormalities should also be carried out at least on a yearly basis.

Prophylaxis Against Bacterial Endocarditis

Patients with evidence of valvular involvement should be cautioned to maintain good dental and oral hygiene and to have prophylaxis for endocarditis when undergoing dental manipulations or gastrointestinal or genitourinary procedures. Recommendations for antibiotic prophylaxis to prevent bacterial endocarditis are discussed elsewhere in this book.

LYME DISEASE

method of
DANIEL W. RAHN, M.D.
Medical College of Georgia
Augusta, Georgia

Lyme disease is a complex, multisystem illness caused by *Borrelia burgdorferi*. Infection is transmitted to humans by hard-bodied tick vectors from the *Ixodes ricinus* complex. Although the geographic range of Lyme disease is broad, disease prevalence varies widely as a function of the prevalence of tick vectors and the rate of infection in the tick population. More than 95,000 cases have been reported to health authorities in the United States since the institution of systematic case reporting in 1982. In 1996 alone, 16,455 cases were reported, with 90% of cases occurring in endemic regions in the northeast, upper midwest, and northern California.

The principal vectors in the United States are *Ixodes scapularis* in the northeast and upper midwest and *Ixodes pacificus* in California. Although *I. scapularis* is widely distributed throughout the southeast, the rate of tick infection is very low, as is the incidence of Lyme disease.

Infection generally begins in spring or summer, the seasons when ticks are most active. Ixodid ticks have a three-stage life cycle (larva, nymph, and adult) that spans 2 years. The ticks take a single blood meal during each stage of development. Tick vectors themselves acquire infection from a reservoir host in their environment, most often from mice or other small mammals, and then become infectious to humans during subsequent feedings in later stages of development. Humans most often acquire infection from nymphs, so the time of greatest risk of acquiring infection is during the months that nymphs are active.

B. burgdorferi has been studied extensively in recent years. Three genospecies have been described. All human isolates in the United States have belonged to a single species, designated *Borrelia burgdorferi sensu stricto*. Isolates from Europe and Russia have been more diverse, belonging to three different species: *B. burgdorferi sensu stricto, Borrelia garinii*, and *Borrelia afzelii*. Differences in the clinical spectrum of Lyme disease in Europe and North America can be accounted for in part by differences in the pathogenicity of different species. *B. burgdorferi sensu stricto* has a propensity for early dissemination, often causing multiple secondary skin lesions and arthritis. *B. afzelii* has a greater tendency to persist in skin, causing the chronic skin lesion acrodermatitis chronicum atrophicans, which is seen almost exclusively in Europe. *B. garinii* may have a greater tendency to disseminate to the nervous system. Future treatment trials must take into account these differences in the natural history of infection caused by different species and must include efforts to isolate causative organisms.

The clinical spectrum of Lyme disease is broad, with manifestations varying among patients and over time in individual patients as the infection and immunologic response evolve. The wide geographic distribution, variable disease course, and differences among causative organisms all lead to the potential for diagnostic uncertainty. Almost regardless of clinical specialty, physicians practicing outside known endemic regions may be confronted with the question of whether a patient's symptoms could be due to Lyme disease. When diagnosis is based on serology in a patient with unusual complaints at unknown risk of exposure, the risk of misdiagnosis is considerable. Clinical experience, particularly in nonendemic areas, may be based on misdiagnoses (seropositivity in individuals with an alternative diagnosis), which underscores the need for precision in diagnosis.

Lyme disease typically begins with localized infection at the site of a bite by an infected tick (localized early Lyme disease). Infection spreads outward in the skin over a period of days, causing a slowly expanding skin lesion, erythema migrans. After a period of local spread, infection may disseminate hematogenously to secondary skin sites, heart, nervous system, and joints. During this stage of disseminated early Lyme disease, which generally occurs weeks after the onset of infection, a variety of symptoms may occur, including multiple erythematous skin lesions, fever, radiculoneuritis, meningitis, facial nerve palsy, cardiac conduction disturbance, and even arthritis. Symptoms of early Lyme disease generally remit even without antibiotic therapy. However, infection may persist in certain favored target organs, including nervous system and joints, in particular with the later emergence of more chronically persistent infection months to years after the onset of infection. This stage of illness, termed late Lyme disease, is the most difficult to diagnose and treat. Although all stages respond to appropriately chosen antibiotics, the illness is most responsive early in its course. Complete resolution of signs and symptoms after treatment is less certain in late disease.

Early detection and prompt institution of therapy is important in protecting against progression to later stages of illness. Signs and symptoms of Lyme disease result from both the direct tissue injury from infecting organisms and the immune response engendered by the organisms. As with many other infections, it is not necessary to treat until all evidence of inflammation has resolved; improvement commonly continues after completion of antibiotic therapy. In reported clinical series in the United States, the leading reason for patients' failure to respond to antibiotic therapy for Lyme disease has been incorrect diagnosis, often based on the results of serologic tests used indiscriminantly, which leads to low positive predictive value.

In this chapter, therapy is discussed according to the staging system in current use. Antibiotic recommendations are summarized in Table 1. Proper use of the laboratory is discussed by stage of illness.

EARLY LYME DISEASE

The characteristic clinical feature of early Lyme disease is erythema migrans. This largely asymptomatic skin lesion begins as an erythematous macule or papule at the site of a bite by a tick infected with *B. burgdorferi*. In general, ticks must be attached for more than 24 hours to transmit infection, but only a minority of patients recall being bitten. Lesions ex-

TABLE 1. **Antibiotic Recommendations for Treatment of Lyme Disease**

Early Lyme disease
Amoxicillin (Amoxil), 500 mg 3 times daily for 14–21 d
Doxycycline (Vibramycin), 100 mg twice daily for 14–21 d
Cefuroxime axetil (Ceftin), 500 mg twice daily for 14–21 d
Azithromycin (Zithromax), 500 mg daily for 7 days, is less effective than other regimens
Neurologic manifestations
Bell's palsy (no other neurologic abnormalities)
An oral regimen for 21–30 d
Meningitis (with or without radiculoneuropathy or encephalitis)*
Ceftriaxone (Rocephin), 2 g daily for 14–28 d
Penicillin G, 20 million units daily for 14–28 d
Doxycycline, 100 mg twice daily (oral or intravenous) for 14–28 d†
Chloramphenicol, 1 g 4 times daily for 14–28 d
Arthritis‡
Amoxicillin, 500 mg 3 times daily for 30 d§
Doxycycline, 100 mg twice daily for 30 d
Ceftriaxone, 2 g daily for 14–28 d
Penicillin G, 20 million units daily for 14–28 d
Carditis
Ceftriaxone, 2 g daily for 14 d
Penicillin G, 20 million units daily for 14 d
Doxycycline, 100 mg orally twice daily for 21 d‖
Amoxicillin, 500 mg 3 times daily for 21 d

*Optimal duration of therapy has not been established. Late manifestations are generally treated for 28 days. There are no controlled trials of therapy longer than 4 weeks for any manifestation of Lyme disease.

†No published experience in the United States.

‡An oral regimen should be selected if there is no neurologic involvement.

§Amoxicillin is generally administered 3 times daily, but the only trial of this agent for Lyme arthritis used a 4-times-daily regimen in conjunction with probenecid.

‖Oral regimens have been reserved for mild carditis without concomitant neurologic involvement.

pand in annular fashion at a rate of ½ to 1 centimeter per day, achieving a final diameter of 15 centimeters on average as spirochetes spread outward in skin. Lesions are erythematous, warm to touch, flat, sharply demarcated, and occasionally mildly tender. Ticks may attach to and infect any skin site, but the most common sites are skin folds (e.g., popliteal, fossa, groin, axillary folds). *B. burgdorferi* can be isolated by culture of skin biopsy samples in specialized media in 50 to 80% of cases, but culture is not routinely available because of the rigorous growth requirements of *B. burgdorferi* in culture. Diagnosis rests on recognition of this characteristic skin lesion.

Recently, erythema migrans–like lesions have been described in patients bitten by *Amblyomma americanum* (Lone Star) ticks in the southeastern United States. Efforts to isolate *B. burgdorferi* from these skin lesions have been unsuccessful so far, and serologic studies have not suggested a linkage to *B. burgdorferi* infection. Erythema migrans–like rashes in this region may be due to a related *Borrelia* or some other infectious agent. The importance of this observation is that it underscores that physician-diagnosed erythema migrans is not sufficient to establish a definite diagnosis of Lyme disease, especially in nonendemic regions.

If treatment is initiated promptly, there is often little in the way of systemic toxicity, and laboratory test results, including serologies, often remain negative. However, more than 50% of untreated patients develop disseminated early disease after a variable period of local infection in skin. Symptoms associated with disease dissemination include fever, chills, headache, arthralgias, myalgias, stiff neck, and often multiple secondary skin lesions. Cranial nerve palsies, especially Bell's palsy, are common, as is lymphocytic meningitis with or without radiculoneuropathy. Carditis characterized by atrioventricular conduction abnormalities also occurs during this stage of illness but less commonly. Frank arthritis may occur as well but usually later in the disease, as described subsequently. Spirochetes have been recovered from blood, secondary skin lesions, and cerebrospinal fluid during this stage of illness. In addition, spirochetes have been visualized in cardiac tissue by transvenous endomyocardial biopsy. All of these examples attest to direct spread of infection as the pathophysiologic mechanism driving symptoms at this stage of illness. Symptoms wax and wane and typically resolve completely after weeks to months, even without treatment, but without definitive antibiotic therapy, up to 80% of patients eventually progress to manifest signs and symptoms of late Lyme disease.

The diagnosis of early Lyme disease rests on clinical recognition with serologic testing used as an adjunct. Serologic tests are of limited value in the diagnosis of erythema migrans. Once infection has disseminated, however, most persons are seropositive. A two-stage procedure should be used. Initial serologic testing should be by enzyme-linked immunosorbent assay (ELISA). All positive ELISA results should be confirmed by Western blot. Both IgM and IgG blots should be performed. Standardized criteria for positive immunoblots have been adopted by a Centers for Disease Control and Prevention working group. Because of technical variability, it is not possible to make broad statements about specificity and sensitivity of serologic testing for Lyme disease. If all positive ELISA results are confirmed by Western blots and serologies are ordered only when clinical presentation truly suggests the diagnosis of Lyme disease, the predictive value of a positive or negative serology is as good as other commonly used serologic tests.

THERAPY

Imbedded ticks should be removed promptly and the site of the tick bite observed for the appearance of erythema migrans. Randomized controlled trials have shown that prophylactic antibiotic therapy is not necessary in ordinary circumstances following tick bites. Even in endemic regions, individuals with ixodid tick bites should simply remove the tick and watch the bite site expectantly; antibiotics should be reserved for individuals who develop erythema migrans.

A variety of antibiotic regimens have proved effective in the treatment of early Lyme disease. Amoxicillin (Amoxil), 500 mg three times daily, or doxycycline (Vibramycin), 100 mg twice daily, are preferred for most adults. Most experts currently recommend antibiotic courses of 2- to 3-weeks' duration because of the slow replication of *B. burgdorferi*. Skin lesions fade promptly, systemic symptoms subside, and later manifestations of disease are prevented. Individuals with disseminated early infection are at higher risk of failing antibiotic therapy than are those with disease limited to a single skin lesion and minor or no systemic symptoms. Macrolides (erythromycin, azithromycin [Zithromax], or clarithromycin [Biaxin]) are not recommended at present. A controlled trial comparing amoxicillin with azithromycin has shown azithromycin to be less effective than amoxicillin in preventing progression to later disease. Cefuroxime axetil (Ceftin), 500 mg twice daily, has been found equivalent to doxycycline and is an alternative for individuals who are allergic to amoxicillin. The pediatric dose of amoxicillin is 30 mg per kg per day in three divided doses, not to exceed the adult dose. Doxycycline and other tetracyclines should be avoided in children younger than 9 years of age because of the risk of staining the teeth. Doxycycline should be avoided in pregnancy. Cefuroxime axetil is classified in pregnancy category B and is excreted in breast milk, so it should be used in pregnancy only when clearly necessary, and consideration should be given to interrupting breast-feeding if this drug must be administered to women who are nursing.

Several studies have shown that individuals with disseminated early infection have a worse prognosis than those with localized early disease and have a higher rate of antibiotic failure and subsequent development of neurologic disease in particular. This clinical observation probably indicates that *B. burgdorferi* can spread to the nervous system early in the process of dissemination. Symptoms such as Bell's palsy, headache (even without meningismus), irritability, and paresthesias occurring in association with disseminated early Lyme disease may reflect central nervous system infection and should be evaluated by examination of cerebrospinal fluid before deciding on oral antibiotic therapy. If there is evidence of central nervous system inflammation, antibiotics should be administered intravenously as described later for late Lyme disease. Disseminated early Lyme disease complicated by Bell's palsy, without other neurologic abnormalities, has been treated successfully with oral antibiotics; most authorities recommend 3 to 4 weeks of treatment when Bell's palsy is present.

Carditis has been treated with both oral antibiotic therapy and intravenous therapy. Owing to its rarity, there have been no controlled clinical trials. In the absence of central nervous system involvement, my practice is to treat orally for 3 to 4 weeks. Observational studies have suggested that individuals with first-degree atrioventricular (AV) block and a PR interval longer than .3 seconds are at risk of progressing to high-degree AV block. Current practice is to hospitalize individuals with significant PR prolongation or second-degree or complete AV block until antibiotics have been initiated and the heart block has responded; temporary pacing may be necessary. Although carditis is usually self-limited, case reports have suggested that conduction disturbances may persist after antibiotic therapy.

Post-treatment sequelae, particularly a prolonged fatigue state and fibromyalgia, occur with some frequency after otherwise curative treatment of disseminated early Lyme disease. Although a subject of some controversy, current evidence suggests that these symptoms do not result from continued infection and do not respond to prolonged antibiotic therapy. For early Lyme disease without central nervous system involvement, no study has ever demonstrated the necessity of or benefit from therapy longer than 3 weeks.

LATE LYME DISEASE

The best information on the natural history of untreated Lyme disease in the United States comes from clinical observations of patients in Connecticut before the discovery of the spirochetal etiology of Lyme disease. In this cohort, 10% developed carditis, 15% neurologic abnormalities, and 60% arthritis. Arthritis and indolently progressive neurologic symptoms develop in some patients months after the onset of infection and may not first appear until years later. These late Lyme disease manifestations may be more resistant to antibiotic therapy and will be considered separately.

Lyme arthritis is typically asymmetrical and monoarticular, with 80% of cases involving one or both knees. Inflammation is most often characterized by intermittent attacks of pain and swelling lasting days to weeks, followed by spontaneous resolution. In a minority of patients, particularly individuals with HLA DR4 genotype, inflammation may become chronic. Studies utilizing the polymerase chain reaction (PCR) have shown that, at the onset of inflammation, spirochetal DNA is present in joint fluid and synovium, presumably indicating active infection. Patients with Lyme arthritis almost universally have strongly positive IgG serology and Western blot results.

Chronic neurologic Lyme disease (often termed neuroborreliosis) consists of a subtle encephalopathy and peripheral neuropathy. Cognitive impairment, primarily affecting short-term memory, can be demonstrated by psychometric testing. Paresthesias in a stocking or stocking/glove distribution also occur commonly; electromyogram results may be abnormal, but nerve conductions are typically normal. Cerebrospinal fluid may be normal or demonstrate elevated protein and a low-grade lymphocytic pleocytosis. Serologic test results are strongly positive in serum and usually positive on spinal fluid. These neurologic manifestations must be distinguished from chronic fatigue or fibromyalgia, which persists in some patients after treatment of Lyme disease but does not, in general, indicate persistent infection.

THERAPY

Late central nervous system Lyme disease must be treated with intravenous antibiotics. Optimal duration of treatment is unknown, but most experts recommend a 4-week course of a third-generation cephalosporin. The agent of choice has been ceftriaxone (Rocephin) in a dose of 2 grams daily by single intravenous injection, which can be given on an outpatient basis. Cefotaxime (Claforan) in a dose of 2 grams three times daily is equally effective. Neurologic signs and symptoms may resolve slowly, often continuing to resolve after completion of a 4-week course of antibiotics. If relapse or incomplete cure is suspected clinically, patients should be evaluated for evidence of persistent infection, and, if this is found, a repeat course of antibiotics may be indicated with carefully defined endpoints.

Lyme arthritis can be treated successfully with 4 weeks of oral therapy with amoxicillin or doxycycline. Joint inflammation may resolve gradually, particularly in individuals with chronic arthritis, often requiring up to 3 months for complete resolution. Patients who fail a 4-week course of oral therapy should be considered for a second 4-week course or 2 weeks of intravenous therapy with ceftriaxone or cefotaxime. Studies with PCR suggest that those who fail up to 8 weeks of oral therapy or 2 weeks of intravenous therapy may have immunologically mediated inflammation rather than persistent infection. Synovectomy has been curative in patients whose inflammation could not be controlled with anti-inflammatory therapy after completion of antibiotic therapy.

It is important to search for concomitant neurologic involvement in individuals with Lyme arthritis. Oral therapy that is effective for arthritis is ineffective for neurologic involvement.

There are no data at present to guide decision-making with regard to treatment of individuals who have rare manifestations of *B. burgdorferi* infection such as ocular involvement or myositis. Ocular infection should probably be treated intravenously to ensure adequate tissue penetration. Other manifestations can probably be treated orally.

LYME VACCINE

Two Lyme vaccines are under development at present. Both are based on an immunogenic outer surface protein of *B. burgdorferi*. Trials in mouse models and preliminary human trials have suggested efficacy and safety of these vaccines. No vaccine has been approved for human use at the time of this writing, but two are under Food and Drug Administration review. If approved, selection of proper candidates to receive vaccine will have to proceed deliberately to define who really needs protection.

ROCKY MOUNTAIN SPOTTED FEVER

method of
DOUGLAS P. FINE, M.D.
University of Oklahoma Health Sciences Center
Oklahoma City, Oklahoma

Rocky Mountain spotted fever, an acute systemic febrile illness with a prominent exanthem, is caused by infection with *Rickettsia rickettsii*. Despite the name, most cases now occur in the mid-Atlantic coastal states and the upper South, extending west to Oklahoma. Because of its rapid clinical evolution and potential lethality, this is a disease for which physicians should maintain a high index of suspicion and treat presumptively.

R. rickettsii is maintained in a tick reservoir: *Dermacentor andersoni* (the wood tick) in the western United States and *Dermacentor variabilis* (the dog tick) in the eastern United States. Most patients give a history of potential tick exposure (work or recreation in an outdoor setting or in close contact with dogs), and a sizable proportion recall a tick bite. Thus, questioning about tick exposure is useful, but the absence of such a history should not preclude the diagnosis. Rocky Mountain spotted fever tends to be a disease of spring and summer, when ticks are most active, but it may occur at other times of the year, particularly in warm climates.

CLINICAL MANIFESTATIONS

The clinical presentation of Rocky Mountain spotted fever reflects the diffuse vasculitic pathophysiology. A typical case begins with fairly abrupt onset of fever and headache, often severe. Rash follows in the majority of cases within a few days, usually beginning as erythematous maculopapular lesions on the wrists and ankles, spreading centripetally, and often becoming petechial or even purpuric. "Typical" involvement of palms and soles may not be obvious early. However, only about two thirds of patients have the triad of fever, headache, and rash, and presentation may be highly varied and subtle. Therefore, Rocky Mountain spotted fever must be considered in any febrile patient in an endemic area.

Neurologic symptoms in addition to headache are common and include depression or confusion, lethargy, dizziness, and irritability. Approximately one third of patients may have a stiff neck. Focal neurologic signs or coma can be seen in about 10% of hospitalized patients. Seizure disorders and focal paresis may be long-term sequelae. Gastrointestinal symptoms and signs are common but nonspecific: nausea, vomiting, abdominal pain or tenderness (at times manifesting as an acute abdomen), anorexia, diarrhea or constipation, and hepatomegaly. Myalgias and arthralgias are frequent. About 15% of patients report a nonproductive cough. The vasculitis may be severe enough to result in necrosis of skin, particularly on distal appendages, but fortunately this complication is rare.

When treated promptly, the mortality of Rocky Mountain spotted fever is thought to be less than 5 to 10%. This can be contrasted with a 25% or higher death rate before the introduction of effective chemotherapy.

DIAGNOSIS

In an endemic area, particularly if there is history of tick contact, presumptive diagnosis is based on the acute febrile presentation, especially if neurologic and cutaneous manifestations are present. Thrombocytopenia is a suggestive laboratory finding. Other hematologic changes are not specific or useful. Cerebrospinal fluid pleocytosis and elevated protein level are the rule; hypoglycorrhachia is rare.

If available, direct immunofluorescent antirickettsial antibody staining of organisms in tissue biopsy is useful for rapid diagnosis of Rocky Mountain spotted fever. Serologic tests are useful only for retrospective confirmation; therapy should not be delayed pending the results of these tests if Rocky Mountain spotted fever is suspected. Proteus OX-19 (Weil-Felix) agglutination and complement fixation tests are nonspecific and insensitive; microagglutination and indirect fluorescent antibody assays are more useful. Paired serum samples should be obtained approximately 2 weeks apart.

THERAPY

Tetracyclines are the primary therapeutic agents for Rocky Mountain spotted fever. Patients who are not severely ill and can tolerate oral medications can be treated with doxycycline (Vibramycin), 200 mg orally as a single loading dose, followed by 100 mg orally every 12 hours (2 to 2.5 mg per kg orally every 12 hours for children), or tetracycline (Achromycin), 500 mg orally every 6 hours (10 mg per kg orally every 6 hours for children older than 9 years). Tetracyclines should not be ingested at the same times as milk, milk products, antacids containing aluminum or magnesium, or iron because these agents interfere with absorption; however, tetracyclines can be administered with meals to minimize gastrointestinal toxicity.

Doxycycline and tetracycline can also be administered intravenously if needed for severe illness (nausea, vomiting, or excessive gastrointestinal toxicity precluding oral administration): doxycycline, 200 mg loading dose and 100 mg every 12 hours (4.4 mg per kg as a loading dose and 2.2 mg per kg every 12 hours in children), or tetracycline, 0.5 to 1.0 gram every 12 hours in adults.

The principal toxicity of tetracyclines is gastrointestinal, primarily nausea, vomiting, and cramping abdominal pain. Children younger than 9 years old may develop yellow staining of teeth from tetracyclines, usually only after receiving six or more courses of therapy. Tetracyclines may also cause severe hepatic disease in pregnant women and retard fetal bone growth. Photosensitization is an infrequent complication of tetracycline therapy and is unlikely to be a concern. Tetracycline should not be used in patients with renal failure, but doxycycline can be used, at a lower dosage (100 mg every 24 hours).

The alternative drug to tetracyclines is chloramphenicol (Chloromycetin), which is now available only in parenteral form. Usual dosage is 20 mg per kg intravenously every 6 hours (adults and children); the usual maximum is 4 grams daily. Chloramphenicol has heretofore been preferred for children younger than 9 years old, for pregnant women, and for patients unable to tolerate tetracyclines. However, for children who do not require parenteral therapy, doxycycline or tetracycline is considered an acceptable alternative. The principal toxicity of chloramphenicol is a rare but fatal idiosyncratic bone marrow aplasia. Young infants or children with underlying liver disease should have chloramphenicol blood levels monitored to ensure that these are within therapeutic and nontoxic ranges.

Antimicrobial therapy should be continued at least until the patient has been afebrile for 48 to 72 hours and probably for a minimum total of 7 to 10 days. Adjunctive therapy is symptomatic and depends on manifestations of the disease (e.g., fluids, pressor agents, oxygen, diuretics). No data suggest that anticoagulation or corticosteroid therapy is beneficial.

PREVENTION

Rickettsial vaccines are experimental at this time but have shown some promise. Prevention is primarily a matter of appropriate precautions to minimize chances of tick bites in an area of endemic disease; occlusive clothing and insect repellents such as permethrins are helpful. When ticks are removed from animals, care should be taken to avoid direct human contact with the tick, its secretions, or its blood. Each day after being in an outdoor environment or around tick-infested dogs, one should inspect all areas of the body for adherent ticks, particularly the legs and groin areas, external genitalia, and belt lines. Any ticks should be removed carefully to avoid further direct contact. Duration of tick attachment appears to be a factor in severity of disease. Postexposure antimicrobial prophylaxis cannot be recommended.

RUBELLA AND CONGENITAL RUBELLA

method of
ASTA ASTRAUSKAS, M.D., and
MARILYN A. KACICA, M.D.
Albany Medical College
Albany, New York

Rubella (German measles) is a systemic viral infection that is often subclinical. It is an RNA virus classified as a rubivirus in the Togaviridae family. When acquired in the first 12 weeks of pregnancy, it results in congenital infection associated with severe defects in about 80 to 90% of cases. Development of efficacious rubella vaccines has resulted in immeasurable benefit to human health throughout the world.

ETIOLOGY AND EPIDEMIOLOGY

Rubella as a disease was first recognized nearly 200 years ago. The peak incidence of disease occurs in late winter and early spring. Humans account for the only reservoir of rubella virus. Virus from an infected host is transmitted via nasopharyngeal secretions to a susceptible contact. Infrequently, transmission of the virus may occur in utero through the placenta at the time of primary maternal viremia. The majority of cases of rubella, before the widespread use of vaccine, occurred in children 5 to 9 years of age in 6- to 9-year cycles.

The incidence of rubella infection in the United States has declined by approximately 99% from the prevaccine era. Although the number of cases of infants born with the congenital rubella syndrome (CRS) decreased dramatically, recent serologio surveys have indicated that approximately 10% of young adults are susceptible to rubella virus. Worldwide, 78 countries reported a national policy of rubella vaccination.

CLINICAL PRESENTATIONS

Postnatal Rubella

The incubation period for postnatally acquired rubella ranges from 14 to 21 days, usually 16 to 18 days. A distinct prodromal period in children is rare. Adolescents and adults may experience prodromal symptoms such as low-grade fever, lymphadenopathy (most commonly suboccipital and postauricular), mild conjunctivitis, headache, malaise, anorexia, aches, chills, cough, and coryza up to 5 days before rash develops. The period of maximum communicability begins 1 to 2 days before the appearance of the rash and lasts about 7 days. The exanthem is a nonpruritic, erythematous-pinkish, fine maculopapular eruption that usually appears on the face and then spreads cephalocaudally within 24 hours over the entire body, including the extremities. The rash begins to fade in the same fashion during the second day of illness, clearing completely within 72 hours without pigmentation, peeling, or scaling. Most of the cases of rash are accompanied by transient polyarthralgia. Joint (large and small) involvement is rare in childhood but very common in adolescents and adults, especially in females (33 to 52%). Joint complaints usually begin 1 to 6 days after the onset of rash and can last up to several weeks. Chronicity is very rare. Forschheimer's spots, an enanthema consisting of reddish spots on the soft palate, can be seen in some patients at the onset of the rash and are helpful in diagnosis. Up to 25% of infected individuals may remain asymptomatic and yet be capable of transmitting virus.

Congenital Rubella

Congenital rubella infection is severe and damaging, resulting in spontaneous abortions, stillbirths, or severe congenital defects. The probability of fetal infection resulting in congenital abnormalities is almost 80 to 90% if passage of the virus across the placenta occurs within the first 12 weeks of pregnancy. When maternal infection occurs between 13 and 20 weeks, the risk of congenital defects declines to about 17%. Congenital rubella appears not to be fully established at birth but is a potentially progressive condition. CRS can manifest with transient sequelae that usually resolve over a period of weeks and include dermal erythropoiesis ("blueberry muffin" rash), abnormal radiographic test results, and meningoencephalitis. Permanent conditions of CRS include sensorineural deafness in up to 80% of patients, cardiovascular abnormalities (pulmonary artery and valvular stenosis, patent ductus arteriosus), ophthalmologic manifestations (cataracts, retinopathy, microphthalmia), and neurological impairment (mental retardation, motor weakness, microcephaly). Later sequelae include endocrinopathies (diabetes mellitus, growth hormone deficiency, thyroid disease). Clinical signs most frequently seen at birth are hypotonia and lethargy with a large and full anterior fontanel. In rare cases, CRS can be followed by progressive rubella panencephalitis, which is characterized pathologically by severe atrophy, periventricular dilatation, and diffuse neuronal loss.

COMPLICATIONS

Complications are very uncommon in childhood. The most common complication in postnatal rubella is arthritis. Thrombocytopenia and encephalitis are rare complications. Encephalitis occurs more often in children than in adults and has an incidence of one in 10,000 cases.

DIFFERENTIAL DIAGNOSIS

Rubella can be a difficult disease to diagnose because similar rashes and symptoms may occur with many other viral infections, such as adenovirus, parvovirus, Epstein-Barr virus, roseola infantum, enterovirus, and a mild case of scarlet fever. Drug rashes may manifest with rubelliform rash, and only characteristic lymphadenopathy may aid in the rubella diagnosis. Absence of occipital and postauricular lymphadenopathy distinguishes drug rashes from rubella infection.

DIAGNOSIS

Because clinical diagnosis of rubella infection is never definitive, confirmation of diagnosis requires laboratory testing. Virus isolation from nasopharyngeal secretions, blood, urine, and cerebrospinal fluid is a very slow and expensive procedure but highly sensitive. Serologic testing is useful in confirming acute infection when either a fourfold rise in antibody titer or a seroconversion is noted by testing sera from acute and convalescent patients. Serologic proof of congenital rubella can be demonstrated by detecting rubella-specific IgM in cord blood or by determining the presence of or an increase in the concentration of serum IgG throughout the first year of life. Occasionally, IgM assays may yield false-positive results with infectious mononucleosis and parvovirus group B19. Newer methods such as latex agglutination (LA), immunofluorescence assay (IFA), passive hemagglutination (PHA), hemolysis-in-gel, and enzyme-linked immunoassay have been replacing previous testing methods, being highly sensitive in the detection of rubella infection and immunity. Direct detection and semiquantitation of viral DNA in amniotic fluid samples by reverse transcription in polymerase chain reaction appears to be highly sensitive and specific for prenatal diagnosis of rubella virus infection.

TREATMENT

Management of acute rubella infections is only supportive. There is no specific treatment available for CRS. The administration of immune globulin to pregnant susceptible women after exposure may modify symptoms in the mother, but does not prevent infection in the fetus. Interferon has been used with questionable results.

IMMUNIZATIONS AND VACCINES

The objective of rubella immunization programs is to prevent fetal infection and subsequently CRS.

Passive Immunizations. Administration of intramuscular immune globulin to exposed susceptible persons in large doses (0.25 to 0.5 ml per kg) can prevent or modify clinical rubella. If a pregnant women has been exposed to rubella, antibody testing should be performed immediately. If protective antibody has not been found, passive immunization with 20 to 30 ml of intramuscular immune globulin should be administered immediately.

Active Immunizations. Since 1979 the RA 27/3 live rubella vaccine has been widely used and results in long-term immunity in more than 90% of vaccinees. It is administered by subcutaneous injection of 0.5 ml either alone or as combined vaccine (measles-mumps-rubella [MMR]) and can be given simultaneously with other vaccines. MMR vaccine is recommended for children 12 to 15 months of age as a first dose and at school entry at 4 to 6 years of age as a second dose. Otherwise, a second dose of MMR should be given at 11 to 12 years of age or before. Nonpregnant susceptible postpubertal females should all be immunized. Women should not become pregnant within 3 months after immunization. Women who are susceptible to rubella infection should receive vaccine immediately post partum. Breast-feeding is not a contraindication to immunization. All patients who have egg allergy can be immunized safely with MMR vaccine. Adverse reactions to vaccine include rash, lymphadenopathy, and low-grade fever; 5 to 15% of susceptible persons will develop these symptoms 5 to 12 days post vaccination. Twenty-five percent of women and 0.5% of children will develop transient arthritis or arthralgias post vaccination.

CONTRAINDICATIONS

Vaccine is contraindicated in pregnancy. Patients with immunodeficiency diseases and those receiving immunosuppressive chemotherapy, corticosteroids, or radiation should not receive the rubella vaccine. The exceptions are patients with asymptomatic human immunodeficiency virus infection who are not severely immunocompromised. Rubella vaccine should not be given 2 weeks before or 3 months after the administration of immune globulin or blood products.

MEASLES
(Rubeola)

method of
KEITH KRASINSKI, M.D.
New York University School of Medicine
New York, New York

Measles virus is a linear, single-stranded, negative sense, 15.9 kilodaltons, enveloped, human RNA *Morbillivirus* of the Paromyxoviridae family. A single serotype is recognized with a great deal of homogeneity among isolates of a given outbreak; however, genetic sequencing studies indicate relatively stable differences among strains in the viral nucleoprotein and hemagglutinin genes.

EPIDEMIOLOGY

Although measles is vaccine preventable, it and its complications continue to be important causes of morbidity and mortality worldwide, with an estimated 50 million cases resulting in more than 1 million deaths, principally in children. Infected individuals shed measles virus in respiratory secretions for approximately 2 days before the development of respiratory symptoms and 3 to 4 days before the development of rash; they continue to shed virus for approximately 4 days after the development of rash. The virus is spread by direct or indirect contact with virus-containing droplets, typically in crowded situations such as classrooms, day care centers, and residential care settings. Less commonly, measles virus is spread by the airborne route, with documented transmission in domed stadiums and in physicians' offices resulting from virus exposure hours after the index case has left. Measles is among the most contagious of diseases with more than 90% of closely-exposed and 25% of community-exposed susceptibles developing infection. Measles occurs worldwide. Among unimmunized populations, and in the prevaccine era in developed countries, measles was epidemic, with biennial cycles occurring in winter and spring in temperate climates; it tended to be a disease of infancy and childhood. The availability and use of a single-dose measles vaccine strategy has been associated with a 100-fold reduction in the incidence of measles and a change in the epidemiology to unimmunized preschool children and young adults. Improved efforts at immunization and use of a two-dose strategy has resulted in further reductions of measles. Passive maternal-to-infant transfer of immunoglobulins generally results in immunity in the first 4 to 5 months of life or longer; however, susceptible mothers deliver susceptible infants. One consequence of immunization is lower concentrations of measles-specific immunoglobulins, compared with concentrations that result from natural infection. Thus, less antibody is passed transplacentally, resulting in an earlier age of susceptibility of infants because of earlier waning of passive immunity. Although primary vaccine failure occurs in up to 5% of individuals immunized at or after 12 months of age and waning immunity contributes to the susceptible population, the overwhelming cause of continued transmission of measles is failure to immunize.

PATHOGENESIS

Measles virus attaches to the respiratory epithelium via its hemagglutinin. The virus replicates at the site of infection and in macrophages and regional lymph nodes, resulting in a primary viremia with extensive systemic spread to many organs and tissues. Subsequently, a secondary viremia develops coincident with clinical symptomatology. The human host responds with the development of a mononuclear cell response, the generation of specific T cell–mediated cytotoxic responses, and the production of specific IgM and IgG antibodies. Measles causes well-recognized suppression of cell-mediated immunity that may contribute to its complications. Immunologic abnormalities include depression of lymphoproliferative responses to mitogens, decreased natural killer cell activity, and altered production of cytokines, all at a time of intense immune activation. Measles binds to the CD46 receptor of monocyte/macrophages, interacting with the complement system at the binding site of C3b, causing cell aggregation and apoptosis.

Pathologically, large multinucleated giant cells develop in pharyngeal and bronchial mucosa as well as in the reticuloendothelial system, where they are known as Warthin-Finkeldey cells. The lungs develop peribronchiolar inflammation. The cutaneous and mucosal rashes also demonstrate focal syncytial epithelial giant cells with intranuclear aggregates of virus particles. When acute encephalomyelitis occurs, lymphocytic cellular infiltrates with perivascular hemorrhages occur and may be followed by demyelination.

CLINICAL FINDINGS

The incubation period to clinical illness ranges from 8 to 12 days and first manifests as fever, malaise, and mild respiratory involvement, followed, in approximately 24 hours, by progressive cough, coryza, and conjunctivitis accompanied by photophobia and occasionally by nausea and rising fever. Koplik spots develop 3 to 4 days after respiratory symptoms and are characterized as fine, irregular, bright red spots with a bluish-white center. Over the next 1 to 2 days, Koplik spots increase in number, coalesce, and then begin to slough. Concurrent with their regression, an erythematous macular rash appears at the hairline and over the next 3 days spreads cephalocaudad over the entire body, finally affecting the palms and soles. The rash may become hemorrhagic. It begins to fade by the third day in the order in which it appeared, leaving a brownish discoloration and then a fine desquamation at the sites of greatest involvement. In the absence of complications, fever also regresses. Vomiting and diarrhea may also occur and tend to be severe in malnourished children. Measles is usually accompanied by postauricular, cervical, and occipital lymphadenopathy and in more severe cases by generalized lymphadenopathy. Some manifestations of bronchitis, bronchiolitis, or pneumonia are typically present and may be severe, particularly in immunodeficient patients who may exhibit disease without the typical enanthem or exanthem. Severe laryngotracheobronchitis may also occur and sometimes requires intubation. Modified measles may occur following exposure in individuals with passively acquired humoral immunity, such as those who have used exogenous immunoglobulins and occasionally in infants with maternal antibody. Following an incubation period that can be prolonged to as much as 14 to 20 days, disease tends to be milder and of shorter duration. A syndrome of atypical measles occurs following measles exposure in individuals immunized with inactivated measles virus vaccine in use between 1963 and 1967. The inactivated vaccine failed to induce immunity to the fusion protein of the virus, and immunized persons are incapable of preventing the cell-to-cell spread of virus. Atypical measles manifests as fever; pneumonia, which may be associated with consolidation or pleural effusion; and unusual rash. Urticaria; maculopapular, petechial, or purpuric rashes; and occasionally vesicles, with a tendency to centrifugal distribution, have all been described. There may be associated edema, pain, and hyperesthesias of the extremities.

Confirmation of the clinical diagnosis of measles is usually established with the detection of IgG antibodies in samples collected 2 to 4 weeks after acute illness. Enzyme immunoassays are the most convenient and frequently used tests, although hemagglutination inhibition and neutralization assays are still performed. IgM antibodies may be detected as early as 72 hours after onset of rash; however, measles IgM assays may be less sensitive and less specific than IgG assays. Measles virus is recoverable in culture from respiratory secretions, urine, and blood, and a sensitive and specific reverse transcriptase-nested polymerase chain reaction test can be used for diagnosis, but, except in the presence of immunodeficiency or central nervous system disease, is rarely necessary for clinical purposes.

COMPLICATIONS

Otitis media is a common concomitant of measles. Viral pneumonia and supervening bacterial pneumonia with expected pathogens of children occur commonly and may be life-threatening. The well-known exacerbation of tuberculosis following measles is another recognized complication. Herpes simplex virus may also be reactivated.

Acute encephalomyelitis, apparently mediated by autoimmune mechanisms, is characterized by fever, headache, vomiting, changes in mental status, personality changes, seizures, and coma and occurs in approximately 0.1% of measles cases between the second and sixth days after onset of rash. The course is variable and carries a 15% mortality, with one third of survivors exhibiting evidence of brain damage. Cerebellar ataxia, retrobulbar neuritis, and hemiplegia may also occur. Subacute sclerosing panencephalitis (SSPE) is a rare (1 per 100,000 cases) complication of measles, with a long incubation period averaging 10.4 years. SSPE begins insidiously, first with subtle and then progressive mental deterioration, followed by motor dysfunction and seizures, coma, and death over a period of approximately 2 years. SSPE appears to result from persistence of measles virus that escapes immune surveillance because of defects in expression of viral matrix and/or hemagglutinin or fusion genes. Immunosuppressed patients exhibit another central nervous system syndrome characterized by generalized seizures and altered consciousness occurring weeks to 7 months after measles and progressing to death within 3 months in 85% of those affected. In this syndrome intact measles virus can be demonstrated.

Neutropenia and thrombocytopenia occur with measles. Keratoconjunctivitis is common, and corneal ulcerations may occur that can be aggravated by vitamin A deficiency that results in blindness. Appendicitis, often with rupture, also occurs. Infection during pregnancy is associated with excess fetal loss and prematurity; however, no congenital malformations have been identified. Putative associations of measles with Crohn's disease, Paget's disease of bone, autoimmune hepatitis, multiple sclerosis, and otosclerosis are controversial.

TREATMENT

Symptomatic therapy is indicated. Antipyretics are used for the management of high fever. Appropriate antibiotics are used for the management of bacterial complications but are not used routinely for the purposes of prophylaxis during acute measles because of problems with emergence of resistance. Because severe measles has been associated with low serum concentrations of vitamin A and outcome is improved with the administration of vitamin A, consideration should be given to the use of vitamin A in children 6 months to 2 years of age who have severe measles or its complications as well as in children older than 6 months who have immunodeficiency, ophthalmologic evidence of vitamin A deficiency, impaired intestinal absorption, or malnutrition, or who have immigrated from areas with high measles mortality. A single oral dose of 200,000 IU (100,000 IU for those younger than 1 year of age) is used but may be associated with vomiting and headache. For those with night blindness, Bitot's spots, or xerophthalmia the dose should be repeated in 24 hours and again in 4 weeks. Ribavirin* (Virazole) has activity in vitro against the virus and has been used in severe respiratory illness, central nervous system disease, and immunodeficiency but is not approved for these indications by the U.S. Food and Drug Administration.

PREVENTION

Measles vaccine is safe and effective in preventing measles and its complications, with 95% of vaccinees demonstrating serologic evidence of immunity. Susceptible individuals are those born after 1956 who have no documentation of measles vaccination or serologic evidence of immunity; they should be immunized using a two-dose regimen. Generally, the first dose is given at or after 12 months and the second at 5 years of age before school entry. If the second dose is not given at 5 years, it should be given as soon after as practical. Measles-mumps-rubella (MMR) vaccine is the preferred product, given in a dose of 0.5 mL subcutaneously. A monovalent product is also available and deserves consideration for immunization of children 6 to 12 months of age during an outbreak situation. Children vaccinated in this manner should be revaccinated with a two-dose MMR regimen as above.

Measles vaccination is generally contraindicated in individuals with significant immunocompromise;

*Not FDA approved for this indication.

however, asymptomatic and mildly symptomatic individuals infected with the human immunodeficiency virus without severe depression of CD4 count should be immunized, and the two-dose regimen should be accelerated to induce immunity before the progression of the underlying immunodeficiency. Measles vaccine may suppress delayed-type hypersensitivity but does not aggravate tuberculosis; therefore, tuberculin testing is not a precondition for immunization. To avoid false-negative purified protein derivative (PPD) responses, tuberculin testing is not performed in the 6 weeks following vaccination. Hypersensitivity to measles vaccine is rare. Children with egg allergies may be immunized safely. Children with a history of anaphylaxis to eggs have also been immunized safely. When anaphylaxis can be anticipated, prudence dictates vaccination in a setting in which it can be managed adequately. Anaphylaxis to measles vaccine or to neomycin are contraindications. Minor illnesses with or without fever are not contraindications to vaccination. Because exogenous antibody may interfere with the vaccine take, an immunization delay following the administration of antibodies, of 3 months for low-dose immunoglobulin-containing products and up to 11 months for very high doses, is recommended.

Vaccine administered within 72 hours after exposure may prevent measles. Immune globulin,* 0.25 mL/kg within 6 days after exposure, may also prevent measles. The dose of immune globulin is increased to 0.5 mL/kg in immunodeficient individuals who should receive prophylaxis despite prior active immunization. The maximum dose is 15 mL. In hospital settings, exposed susceptible individuals should be managed with infection control precautions from the fifth through the 21st day after contact or if they develop disease through the fifth day of rash. All suspected cases of measles should be reported promptly to the public health authorities.

*Not FDA approved for this indication.

TETANUS

method of
GREGORY KENT BERGEY, M.D.
University of Maryland School of Medicine
Baltimore, Maryland

PATHOPHYSIOLOGY

The clinical symptoms of tetanus result from the central nervous system (CNS) effects of tetanus toxin, an exquisitely toxic product of the spore-forming, gram-negative bacterium *Clostridium tetani.* The toxin is a protein of about 150,000 molecular weight, consists of a light and heavy chain, and is one of the most toxic biologic substances by weight (second only to botulinum toxin). The mechanism of transport and action of tetanus toxin is distinctive among biologic toxins; considerable recent research has finally elucidated the subcellular mechanism of action.

C. tetani bacteria are ubiquitous in most environments. When inoculated into a wound that permits anaerobic growth, the spores germinate, the bacteria multiply, and tetanus toxin is produced. If an individual has been immunized previously or has received recent passive immunization (see later discussion), the toxin is neutralized and no effects of the toxin are manifested. In the unprotected individual, the toxin is carried by blood throughout the body, where it then binds to presynaptic nerve terminals. Unlike botulinum toxin, which remains at the presynaptic site of the neuromuscular junction to block acetylcholine release and produce paralysis, tetanus toxin after binding is then transported by retrograde axonal transport to the spinal cord and the CNS. Also, unlike botulinum toxin, tetanus toxin is not toxic orally.

Once in the ventral horn of the spinal cord and other CNS sites, the toxin moves trans-synaptically across the synaptic cleft to the presynaptic terminals of other neurons and interneurons. At these loci the toxin produces its action: blockade of presynaptic neurotransmitter release. Although inhibitory neurotransmission (i.e., glycinergic and GABAergic) is preferentially affected, most neurotransmission can be affected by the actions of the toxin. In the ventral spinal cord, inhibitory inputs are preferentially located in the somatic and perisomatic region, so these anatomic considerations also serve to produce greater effects on inhibitory systems. Recent studies have determined that tetanus toxin is a zinc-dependent metalloprotease that cleaves synaptobrevin. This cleavage then blocks exocytosis of neurotransmitter. Both evoked and spontaneous synaptic vesicular release of neurotransmitter is blocked by tetanus toxin.

The difficulties in treating tetanus relate to its high potency and to the fact that once the toxin is bound to peripheral nerve endings or internalized, it is not accessible for neutralization by antibodies.

EPIDEMIOLOGY

Although active immunization has reduced dramatically the incidence of tetanus in the United States, about 50 cases per year are typically reported. The actual number of cases may be more than twice this number. As recently as 1965, 300 cases occurred in the United States. Tetanus most commonly occurs in more temperate climates and in unimmunized individuals and others who have not received recent booster immunizations. In the United States most cases of tetanus occur in adults older than 60 years of age, persons most likely to have inadequate antibody titers. Worldwide tetanus remains a major problem, with perhaps 1 million new cases per year. In some countries, due to inoculation of the umbilical stump at birth, neonatal tetanus constitutes more than half of all cases of tetanus and is a major cause of infant mortality. The difficulty of administering multistage immunizations requiring injections has made universal immunization difficult in developing countries.

CLINICAL PRESENTATION AND DIFFERENTIAL DIAGNOSIS

Injuries, particularly penetrating wounds, facilitate growth of the anaerobic bacteria. Historically, tetanus was common in wartime. Skin-popping drug abuse, ear piercing, and nonsterile surgery in unimmunized individuals may produce tetanus. In perhaps 20% of cases, however, there may be no history of a wound and in others the wound may be quite minor. Although in the United States tetanus is usually a disease of the elderly, who may no longer have protective antibody levels, in countries without effective immunization programs tetanus commonly affects infants, children, and young adults.

The diagnosis of tetanus today remains a clinical diagnosis. There are no laboratory tests that can confirm the diagnosis. Cultures of the wound are unreliable (and take time), and the serum titers of the toxin are too low for detection. A known history of adequate immunization with recent boosters (within 10 years) makes the diagnosis much less likely. Determination of a good protective titer of antitetanus antibody (requiring a bioassay that takes days) can provide strong evidence against the diagnosis of tetanus, but reports of clinical tetanus with detectable antibody titers indicate that the toxin load and other factors may also play a role. The history and examination remain the keystones to diagnosis.

The rapid onset of symptoms and the resultant mortality are directly related to the amount of toxin produced and transported to the CNS. In severe cases the onset of symptoms may occur several days after the wound inoculation; in mild cases, the first clinical symptoms may not appear until after 1 or even 2 weeks. Early tetanus begins with muscle aches and rigidity of a single limb, the wounded extremity (local tetanus). This local tetanus results from effects of the toxin on the local segmental motor system because toxin is transported to the spinal cord here first. This segmental dysinhibition may produce stiffness of a single limb, which may be confused with a stroke. Careful examination, however, will determine that weakness is not present; the stiffness and apparent weakness is produced by simultaneous contraction of agonist and antagonist muscles. Trismus, or "lockjaw," the classic symptom of tetanus, occurs relatively early because the trigeminal nerve is a short nerve and blood-borne toxin is transmitted to the trigeminal nucleus before toxin reaches other peripheral nerves. The clinical presentation may remain as local tetanus in some patients with some antibody present (to neutralize circulating toxin) or in other instances when only small amounts of toxin are produced.

Generalized tetanus occurs after the blood-borne toxin has been bound to remote nerve terminals and transported to the spinal cord and CNS. This produces central dysinhibition with severe and often painful rigidity produced by simultaneous contraction of all muscle groups instead of the normal pattern of contraction of agonist with relaxation of antagonist muscles. Physical stimuli or noise can produce painful spasms. The typical posture of flexed arms and extended legs reflects the relative strengths of the muscle groups. Sensory systems are not affected and cognitive function is preserved unless there is hypoxia.

A rare form of tetanus, cephalic tetanus, can be seen following facial wounds. It manifests with facial or ophthalmic weakness in addition to trismus and possible later generalized tetanus. The weakness in this form of tetanus may reflect the blockade of excitatory transmission in the facial and ophthalmic nuclei of the brain stem; peripheral neuromuscular blockade is typically not produced.

Neonatal tetanus is considered by some to be a separate type of tetanus, but in fact it represents generalized tetanus in the infant, often following inoculation of the umbilical cord. The child has generalized spasms (rarely diffuse weakness), including pharyngeal spasms and difficulty feeding. Mortality in neonatal tetanus is high.

The differential diagnosis of tetanus includes strychnine poisoning. Strychnine blocks postsynaptic inhibitory glycine responses and produces a clinical picture much like tetanus but of much more rapid onset and evolution. Dystonic reactions to dopamine blockade (e.g., phenothiazines) may be confused with tetanus. Other conditions at times confused with tetanus are listed in Table 1.

TABLE 1. **Differential Diagnosis of Tetanus**

Strychnine poisoning
Meningitis or encephalitis
Stiff-man syndrome
Dystonic reactions to dopamine blockade
Cerebrovascular accident
Alveolar abscess or other intraoral disease
Rabies
Acute abdomen
Hysteria

TREATMENT

Recognizing the signs of early and local tetanus can improve outcome. Human tetanus immune globulin (Hyper-Tet, 500 IU intramuscularly [IM]) should be administered to all patients with suspected tetanus, as well as those with high-risk wounds and unknown or incomplete immunization (Table 2). The preparations approved for intravenous administration may not provide consistent amounts of antitoxin and should not be used. The availability of human antitoxins has markedly reduced the risk of serum sickness, and therefore human antitoxin is preferred over previously used equine or bovine tetanus antiserum. Active immunization with tetanus toxoid should also begin because protective antibody levels take time to reach and will protect only against future events.

Prompt administration of antitoxin can neutralize unbound toxin. Once toxin is bound and internalized it is inaccessible to antitoxin. Intrathecal antitoxin or immunoglobulin fragments have been administered and reported by some (and not by others) to be beneficial (presumably by binding and neutralizing the toxin as it moves trans-synaptically), but this is not standardized treatment and the human antitoxin preparation available in the United States has a preservative that makes intrathecal administration undesirable. Débridement of the wound can reduce the toxin burden. Some authorities recommend waiting several hours after antitoxin administration be-

TABLE 2. **Treatment of Tetanus**

Specific
Human tetanus immune globulin (500 IU, IM)
Wound débridement
Antibiotics (metronidazole*)
Central inhibitory agents (benzodiazepines)
Supportive
Respiratory and cardiovascular support
Neuromuscular blockade if needed
Sedation
Analgesia
Minimization of patient stimulation and manipulation

*Not FDA approved for this indication.

fore wound débridement to allow for neutralization of circulating toxin; this seems to be a good solution. There appears to be no benefit to direct injection of antitoxin into the wound. Antibiotics effective against the *C. tetani* bacteria should be administered systemically. Penicillin (aqueous penicillin, 10 to 20 million units intravenously [IV] daily in divided doses every 4 to 6 hours) is commonly given, but one study showed that patients receiving metronidazole* (Flagyl), 500 mg orally every 6 hours, had shorter hospital courses than those treated with penicillin, and metronidazole is now preferred for a 7- to 14-day course. Another reason to prefer metronidazole is that high-dose penicillin can antagonize CNS GABAergic inhibition further.

The muscle spasms produced by tetanus are extremely painful and can produce rhabdomyolysis and vertebral compression fractures. The muscular spasms can be reduced by parenteral benzodiazepines, such as diazepam (Valium in repeated 5- to 10-mg doses IV) or lorazepam (Ativan in repeated 2-mg doses IV), which increase central GABAergic inhibition; these agents can also suppress respirations, particularly in the elderly. Intubation is often needed in severe generalized tetanus to provide airway protection and respiratory support and to allow administration of sufficient muscle relaxant because large doses of benzodiazepines are often needed. Once intubated, if benzodiazepines are insufficient to produce adequate muscle relaxation, full neuromuscular blockade (e.g., pancuronium bromide [Pavulon] or vecuronium bromide [Norcuron]) should be employed in conjunction with appropriate sedation and analgesia. It should be remembered that although these patients may appear to be having generalized convulsions, their consciousness is typically well preserved. Indeed, the spasms of tetanus are actually mediated by lower segmental centers without involvement of the cerebral cortex. Minimizing stimulation of the patient can also reduce the painful spasms.

Because recovery can take weeks, a tracheotomy should be performed early in patients who require intubation for management. Also because of the prolonged recovery period, parenteral feeding should be instituted in severe cases. Autonomic instability may be a feature of some severe cases and can be the most difficult management problem. Blood pressure can be quite labile, with broad swings between marked hypertension and overt symptomatic hypotension. The treatment of this autonomic instability can be difficult. Beta blockers have been reported by some to be beneficial; others report no benefits, and still other reports suggest adverse effects due to beta-adrengeric blockade. Others have recommended morphine (up to 0.5 mg IV per kg per hour) to assist management of autonomic instability; this also has the benefits of producing analgesia. Patients are at risk for all the complications of prolonged incapacity, including secondary infections (particularly pneumonia), thrombophlebitis, pulmonary emboli, and paralytic ileus.

*Not FDA approved for this indication.

Poor prognostic features in tetanus include rapid onset of symptoms, generalized tetanus, high frequency of spasms, occurrence in the neonate or elderly, and poor response to therapy. Modern intensive care has improved recovery, and most patients with mild or moderate tetanus can survive; however, mortality in severe generalized tetanus (including neonatal tetanus) is still higher than 50%. Without respiratory support, the mortality from severe tetanus is higher than 80%. Recovery results from toxin degradation. Whether neuronal sprouting plays a part in recovery (as it does in the periphery in botulism) has not been established.

PREVENTION AND PROPHYLAXIS

The key to reducing morbidity from tetanus is prevention. As mentioned earlier, the bacteria are ubiquitous; therefore, everyone must be protected. Infection with tetanus does not confer immunity because the amounts of toxin produced are not sufficient to produce an immune response. The standard immunization for tetanus (often combined with diphtheria or diphtheria and pertussis) is a series of three injections over a year. Immunity probably lasts for 10 years. Patients with clean or minor wounds should receive a booster if more than 10 years has elapsed since their last immunization, if their immunization history is unknown, or if fewer than three doses were administered. Clean, minor wounds do not require human tetanus immune globulin unless signs or symptoms of clinical tetanus appear.

Tetanus toxoid should be administered to patients who have not had a booster dose in the last 5 years and have received a tetanus-prone wound or severe injury. If the immunization history is incomplete or unknown, passive immunization with tetanus toxoid should be started, but active immunization with 500 IU of human tetanus immune globulin administered IM should also be given. These two types of immunotherapy do not interact.

PERTUSSIS

method of
MARY ANNE JACKSON, M.D., and
SARAH E. HAMPL, M.D.
Children's Mercy Hospital
Kansas City, Missouri

Pertussis is a respiratory illness caused primarily by the bacterium *Bordetella pertussis.* Recently, the incidence of pertussis has increased, despite the availability of immunization, and significant morbidity and mortality in infants continue to occur. Adolescents and adults with waning immunity represent the largest reservoir of susceptible individuals for this highly contagious disease. By focusing on improving vaccination levels for all infants and children, improving diagnostic tests for rapid detection of infection, utilizing prompt erythromycin therapy for those infected and their household contacts, and offering booster immunization for adolescents and adults, eradication of pertussis in the United States may finally be a reality in the next decade.

MICROBIOLOGY

B. pertussis, a small gram-negative coccobacillus, is the infectious agent implicated in the majority of cases of whooping cough. *Bordetella parapertussis* and *Bordetella bronchiseptica* account for as many as 10% and 5% of cases of whooping cough syndrome, generally producing a less severe clinical illness.

The pathogenesis of the disease begins with the transmission of respiratory droplets from an infected person to a susceptible person via cough. The role of the various toxins and adhesins elaborated by *B. pertussis* is a subject of ongoing investigation (Table 1). Pertussis toxin (PT) is a major virulence factor, and filamentous hemagglutinin (FHA) and pertactin, along with fimbriae, facilitate adhesion of *B. pertussis* to respiratory epithelium. *B. pertussis* also releases tracheal cytotoxin, which stimulates the production of interleukin-1α, which in turn catalyzes the synthesis of nitrous oxide (NO –). NO – not only is autotoxic to the cell that produced it but also mediates the destruction of surrounding ciliated respiratory epithelial cells. The eventual destruction of the host's mucociliary elevator allows *B. pertussis*–infected mucus to accumulate; hence the cough reflex is stimulated.

The regulation of the production of most *B. pertussis* toxins is controlled by the *BvgAS* (Bordetella virulence gene) system. *BvgS* acts on *BVgA,* a DNA-binding protein that activates the transcription of the virulence genes such as *fhaB,* which encodes FHA, and *ptxA,* which encodes the S1 subunit of PT. There is now evidence to support selective activation and suppression of the production of several *B. pertussis* toxins by the *BvgAS* system, perhaps in response to varying environmental conditions in the host.

EPIDEMIOLOGY

Pertussis, a highly communicable disease with epidemic cycles occurring every 2 to 5 years, is currently the most prevalent vaccine-preventable disease among U.S. children younger than 5 years of age. Significant mortality associated with pertussis is common, particularly in underimmunized populations, and globally more than 355,000 deaths are caused by pertussis annually. Humans are the only known host for *B. pertussis,* and virtually all susceptible persons in a household develop pertussis when exposed to a symptomatic individual.

Although most studies do not note a seasonal variation in pertussis infection rates, others have consistently observed a summer peak of disease. In our institution, from 1976 to 1996, 44% of pertussis cases occurred in summer, 14% in winter, 19% in spring, and 23% in the fall. All races appear to be affected equally, and a greater prevalence in girls has been noted.

In the prevaccine era, pertussis occurred with an annual incidence of 872 cases per 100,000 population. In the 30 years following widespread use of whole-cell pertussis vaccine, a 99% reduction in the annual incidence of disease was observed, correlating with an infection rate of 0.47 cases per 100,000 population.

Despite widespread immunization, a resurgence of disease in the United States had been noted since the mid-1980s. The growth of a susceptible adult population from 5 million in the 1970s to 70 million in the 1990s appears to be the key factor in accounting for this resurgence (Figure 1). Consequently, the incidence of disease appears to be increasing in older children and adults; 28% of recent pertussis cases reported to the Centers for Disease Control and Prevention (CDC) occurred in patients 10 years of age or older. In a prospective clinical study of health plan members aged 18 and older in California, the diagnosis of pertussis was confirmed in 12.4% of adults presenting with a persistent cough, a rate similar to that of peptic ulcer disease. Studies of household contacts of individuals with *B. pertussis* infection have shown that 53% of the primary or co-primary cases occurred in individuals older than 13 years of age. The large reservoir of susceptible adolescents and adults continues to represent the greatest stumbling block to eradication of pertussis globally.

The highest incidence and greatest morbidity of pertussis are still found in infants between 1 and 2 months of age. Pertussis-associated hospitalization and pneumonia have been noted in 82% and 20%, respectively, of infants younger than 2 months, and case fatality rates of 1% have been observed.

CLINICAL PRESENTATION

Clinical infection with pertussis may take many forms, depending on the age of the infected individual and prior

TABLE 1. **Pertussis Components, Function, and Contribution to Vaccine**

Name of Toxin	Toxin Function	Contribution to Vaccine
Pertussis toxin	Inactivates G proteins Causes lymphocytosis Possible adhesin	AV, CB, C-C, C-U, PM SKB-2, SKB-3, WLT
Filamentous hemagglutinin	Adhesin Possible synergy with fimbriae	CB, C-C, C-U, PM SKB-2, SKB-3, WLT
Pertactin	Adhesin, invasin	CB, C-C, SKB-3, WLT
Fimbriae	Adhesin	C-C, WLT
Adenylate cyclase	Intracellular hemolysin Causes elevated cAMP Causes phagocyte death	Future recombinant component?
Tracheal cytotoxin	Stimulates interleukin-1α Causes coughing paroxysms	Nonimmunogenic

Abbreviations: AV = Amvax; CB = Chiron-Biocine; C-C = Connaught-Canada; C-U = Connaught-US; PM = Pasteur-Mérieux; SKB 2 and 3 = SmithKline Beecham; WLT = Wyeth-Lederle/Lederle-Takeda; cAMP = cyclic adenosine monophosphate.

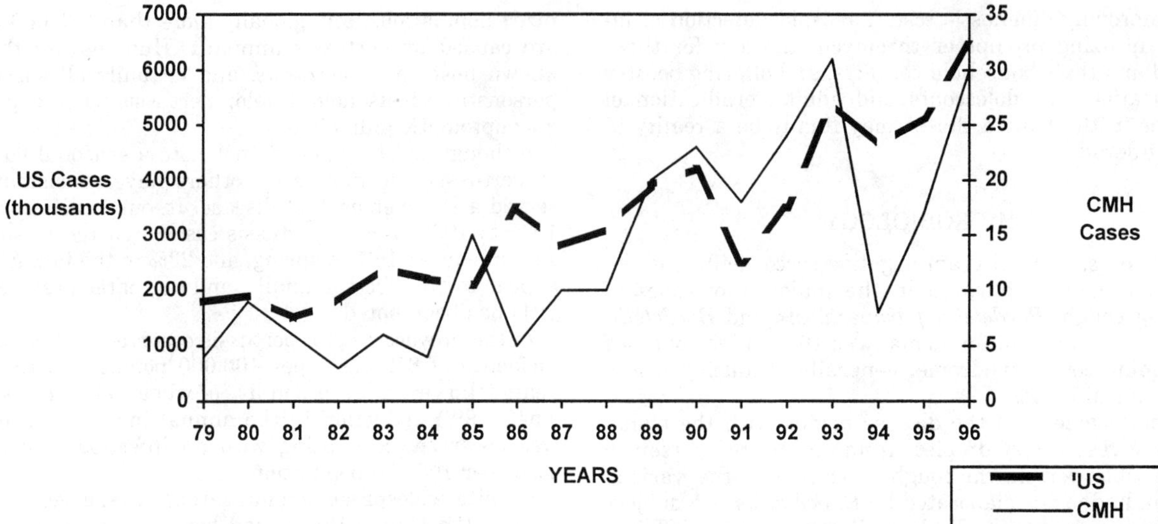

Figure 1. Reported cases of pertussis, 1979–1996, United States and Children's Mercy Hospital, Kansas City, MO.

infection, immunization, and treatment history. The incubation period ranges from 6 to 20 days, and the onset of most cases of pertussis occurs 7 to 10 days following exposure. The total duration of the illness is 6 to 10 weeks.

Classic pertussis infection has been divided into three stages. The catarrhal stage lasts 1 to 2 weeks and is characterized by upper respiratory tract infection symptoms, including mild cough, rhinorrhea, and occasional conjunctivitis with increased lacrimation. The nonspecific nature of these symptoms rarely leads to the suspicion of pertussis, although culture for pertussis is most likely to be positive at this stage. The cough increases in frequency and severity as the individual enters the paroxysmal stage, which typically lasts 2 to 4 weeks. Repetitive series of coughs are followed by a forceful inspiratory effort against a closed glottis, causing the familiar whoop. Cyanosis and increased lacrimation and salivation may accompany the paroxysmal cough, and post-tussive emesis may follow. Individuals may feel and appear well between paroxysms. If the classic paroxysmal cough is observed by a health care provider, the clinical diagnosis of pertussis is apparent, although culture may be negative as bacterial shedding decreases during the paroxysmal stage. The convalescent stage is the final stage of classic pertussis and lasts 1 to 2 weeks. The coughing paroxysms decrease and eventually disappear, although some individuals may experience reactivation of the cough with subsequent respiratory viral infections.

Complications encountered during the paroxysmal phase of pertussis include subconjunctival hemorrhage, rectal prolapse, malnutrition, dehydration, alkalosis, and otitis media. More serious complications usually occur in the younger patient and include pneumonia (22%), seizures (3%), and encephalopathy (0.9%).

The clinical course of pertussis in immunized children, adolescents, and adults is generally accepted to be less severe than in infants. However, prolonged cough remains a hallmark, with many reporting coughing paroxysms. Multiple health care provider visits, missed diagnosis, inappropriately prescribed medication, and days missed from work owing to illness make pertussis an economically burdensome disease as well.

DIAGNOSIS

The diagnosis of pertussis is rarely in question if the clinician witnesses a typical paroxysm of pertussis associated with a classic whoop. Unfortunately, a delay in diagnosis may occur if a careful history is not taken, as most patients appear completely well between paroxysms.

A clinical diagnosis of pertussis is suggested in the patient who presents with history of a cough that has been present longer than 2 weeks, particularly when associated with coughing in paroxysms, post-tussive emesis, or an inspiratory whoop (Table 2).

Although an absolute lymphocytosis of greater than 10,000 is a suggestive laboratory finding, it is not universally found, and culture remains the gold standard for diagnosis.

Nasopharyngeal mucus obtained by aspiration or with a Dacron or calcium alginate swab is inoculated onto Regan-Lowe or Bordet-Gengou medium. The medium must be prepared fresh, has a short shelf life, and is therefore not easily accessible to the practicing clinician. Recovery of the organism generally requires 10 to 14 days of incubation. Negative culture results are common, especially in those who have received prior antibiotics, children who have had one or more pertussis immunizations, and those beyond the fourth week of illness.

Direct immunofluorescent assay (DFA) of nasopharyngeal secretions, although offered by some laboratories, is generally considered unreliable because of low sensitivity and variable specificity.

Serologic studies including enzyme immunoassays for IgG antibody to pertussis toxin and IgA antibody to FHA are performed by many experienced research laboratories. Although these are reliable, they are not widely available to the clinician. Polymerase chain reaction assays of nasopharyngeal secretions, which are faster and more sensitive than culture, remain investigational.

TABLE 2. **Case Definition for Pertussis**

Cough for ≥ 14 days associated with one or more of the following:
Paroxysms of cough
Inspiratory whoop
Post-tussive emesis
Absolute lymphocyte count ≥ 10,000

TABLE 3. **Antimicrobial Treatment of Pertussis**

Drug	Dose (mg/kg/d)	Maximum Dose (gm)	Interval (h)	Duration (d)	Adult Dosage/Cost ($0.00)
Erythromycin	40–50	2	6	14	250 mg/0.19
Erythromycin estolate (Ilosone)	40–50	2	6	14	500 mg/0.28
Erythromycin ethylsuccinate (E.E.S.)	40–50	2	8	14	400 mg/0.22
Clarithromycin (Biaxin)	15	1	12	7	500 mg/3.45
Azithromycin (Zithromax)	12	0.5	24	5	250 mg/6.04

TREATMENT

Most infants with pertussis, including virtually all of those younger than 6 weeks of age, require hospitalization during the paroxysmal phase of pertussis. Supportive care should focus on management of paroxysms, especially those associated with apnea and cyanosis. Suctioning of secretions, oxygen, and hydration are usually necessary. Limited data suggest that inhaled albuterol may reduce the paroxysms of pertussis. Corticosteroids have been evaluated but in only a few placebe-controlled studies. One study suggested that a 7- to 10-day course of steroids reduced the frequency of whooping attacks and vomiting and shortened the duration of the disease; however, further controlled studies are necessary to recommend steroids as the standard of care for children hospitalized with pertussis.

Although antimicrobials may ameliorate disease if given during the catarrhal phase, most patients are not identified until paroxysmal cough is present and at that point, treatment has no effect on the clinical course. The primary reason to treat pertussis is to eradicate the organism and reduce the spread of the disease to others. Erythromycin, which is generally well tolerated in the young patient, is the drug of choice (Table 3). A dosage of 40 to 50 mg per kg per day orally in divided doses is recommended; some experts feel the estolate preparation is more effective. A recent study concluded that a 7-day course of erythromycin estolate is as effective as a 14-day course; however, many still believe that a 14-day course is necessary to prevent bacteriologic relapse. Newer macrolides such as clarithromycin* (Biaxin) and azithromycin* (Zithromax) have been shown to eradicate *B. pertussis* with an easier dosing schedule and less gastrointestinal upset; however, both of these drugs are relatively expensive. Nevertheless, because national surveillance data suggest that less than half of infected persons complete the 14-day course, the shorter course required for clarithromycin and azithromycin makes them attractive alternative drug choices in some cases.

*Not FDA approved for this indication.

Trimethroprim with sulfamethoxazole* (Bactrim, Septra) in a dose of 8 mg per kg per day of the trimethoprim component is considered a possible alternative in patients who are macrolide intolerant or in the rare patient in whom macrolide resistance is suspected.

Individuals with pertussis should be excluded from school and day care until erythromycin has been taken for 5 days. Treatment of household and day care center contacts is identical to that of the index case because as many as 90% of susceptible household contacts will develop infection. In addition, attention should be given to ensuring that pertussis immunization is current in young children who are likely to be exposed to pertussis. A heightened awareness is needed to identify individuals who develop symptoms for 14 days after contact with the index case; those who develop symptoms should be cultured promptly and treated for pertussis.

PREVENTION

Universal immunization against pertussis has effectively reduced the number of pertussis cases encountered in the United States. Whole-cell vaccine, in use since 1951, has resulted in a dramatic decline in cases from more than 250,000 per year in the prevaccine era to a nadir of 1000 annual cases in the mid 1970s. Although this vaccine has been the mainstay of pertussis prevention for more than 40 years, the success of whole-cell vaccine has always been overshadowed by a negative adverse event pro-

*Not FDA approved for this indication.

TABLE 4. **U.S. Food and Drug Administration–Licensed Acellular Pertussis Vaccines**

Trade Name	Manufacturer	Components			
		PT	*FHA*	*Pertactin*	*Fimbriae*
Tripedia	Connaught Laboratories, Inc.	+	+		
Infanrix	SmithKline Beecham	+	+	+	
Acel-Imune	Wyeth-Lederle Laboratories	+	+	+	+

TABLE 5. **Precautions Against and Contraindications to Use of DTaP Vaccine**

Event	Time from Vaccine
Precaution	
Seizure—febrile or afebrile	3 d
≥ 3 hours of inconsolable crying	48 h
Hypotonic/hyporesponsive episode	48 h
Fever ≥ 40.5°C	48 h
Contraindication	
Anaphylaxis	Immediate
Encephalopathy	7 d

file. More than 50% of recipients experienced fever and local reactions associated with the pertussis component of diphtheria, tetanus toxoids, and pertussis (DTP) vaccine. Less commonly observed but significant events related to whole-cell vaccine include anaphylaxis (2 cases per 100,000 injections), fever (≥40.5°C, 3 cases per 1000 injections), seizure (1 case per 1750 injections), hypotonic-hyporesponsive episodes (1 case per 1750 injections), and inconsolable crying for 3 hours or more (1 per 100 injections).

The development of acellular pertussis vaccines derived from *B. pertussis* immunogens that contain little or no endotoxin has provided the clinician with products that are immunogenic and efficacious as well as less likely to provoke an undesirable reaction than whole-cell vaccine. Acellular pertussis vaccines are available in combination with diphtheria and tetanus toxoids (DTaP) and are now the preferred vaccine in the United States (Table 4). All are given intramuscularly in a primary three-dose series at 2, 4, and 6 months in a dose of 0.5 ml; a reduced vaccine dose is not recommended for any group, including premature infants. Booster doses are recommended at 12 to 18 months and 4 to 6 years of age. Current immunization schemes do not include recommendations for use of acellular products in children 7 years or older; however, periodic booster immunization with adult tetanus/diphtheria toxoid in combination with an acellular pertussis vaccine component is anticipated for the adolescent in the near future.

Any licensed product is acceptable, and vaccines can be used interchangeably in the event that the type of DTaP vaccine received previously is not known or is unavailable. In the event of a pertussis outbreak, DTaP should be initiated at 6 weeks of age and subsequent doses given at 4-week intervals to complete the primary series.

Contraindications to future pertussis immunization include an immediate episode of anaphylaxis or encephalopathy. Precautions for which careful consideration should be given before further DTaP doses are noted in Table 5. Deferral of pertussis immunization is usually considered for infants who have underlying neurologic disorders such as infantile spasms or tuberous sclerosis or those who have an evolving neurologic disorder. In the event that vaccine is not given, diphtheria and tetanus (DT) vaccine should be substituted.

IMMUNIZATION PRACTICES

method of
RICHARD F. THOMPSON, M.D.
Camino Medical Group
Sunnyvale, California

During the past decade we have witnessed the introduction of very effective new vaccines, including *Haemophilus influenzae* type B (HIB), acellular pertussis, hepatitis A, and varicella. There is no longer any reason for major outbreaks of infectious pediatric diseases such as bacterial meningitis, pertussis, measles, mumps, or chickenpox. New immunizations, or combinations of immunizations, will continue to be introduced (e.g., hepatitis A, rotavirus, pneumococcal) into the "routine" immunization schedules. The issues concerning each new immunization will center on efficacy, duration of protection, severity of the disease, and economic impact of the disease on society.

Since 1995 the Advisory Committee on Immunization Practices (ACIP), the American Academy of Pediatrics (AAP), and the American Academy of Family Physicians (AAFP) have published an annual recommended childhood immunization schedule (Figure 1). The new "consensus" schedule allows increased flexibility and attempts to simplify the timing of immunization administration, recognizing the complexity of delivering as many as 20 immunizations to a single child before age 5 years. As the number of new and routine immunizations increases for the pediatric patient, combination immunizations will evolve.

In an attempt to improve the delivery of vaccination services in the United States, the ACIP recommends a routine vaccination assessment at age 11 to 12 and again at age 50 years. These assessments present an opportunity to initiate or update routine vaccines, that is, hepatitis B, measles-mumps-rubella (MMR), tetanus-diphtheria (Td) booster, and varicella vaccination. It is also an opportunity for the health care provider to administer other vaccines that may be recommended for certain persons, for example, influenza, pneumococcal, and hepatitis A vaccines (see Figure 1).

ROUTINE IMMUNIZATIONS

Diphtheria, Tetanus, and Pertussis Vaccine

Vaccines against diphtheria-tetanus-pertussis (DTP) during infancy and childhood have been administered routinely in the United States since the late 1940s. The introduction of these vaccines has been associated with a greater than 90% reduction in morbidity and mortality associated with infection by these organisms. In 1997 diphtheria-tetanus-acellular pertussis (DTaP) (Acel-Imune, Tripedia) became the preferred vaccine for all doses of the routine childhood immunization schedule (see Figure 1). DTaP is less likely to provoke adverse reactions because it contains purified antigenic components of *Bordetella pertussis.* In particular, infants and young children who have a history of previous seizures should be given DTaP because DTaP is less frequently associated with moderate to high fever.

Tetanus-diphtheria toxoid (Td) is recommended for

the routine immunization of persons 7 years of age and older. The recommended timing for the first Td booster is now age 11 to 12 years, maintaining an interval of at least 5 years since the last dose of diphtheria and tetanus (DT) toxoid, DTP, or DTaP. Thereafter, routinely boost every 10 years. Td is recommended over tetanus alone because adults in need of tetanus immunization are also considered susceptible to diphtheria.

Haemophilus influenzae Type B Vaccine

From December 1987—when HIB conjugate vaccines were introduced—through 1997, the incidence of invasive meningitis in children in the United States declined to such a low level that bacterial meningitis is now considered primarily a disease of adults. The success of this vaccine in eliminating bacterial meningitis and invasive bacterial disease in children younger than age 5 is extremely impressive and represents a major change in the epidemiology of HIB disease.

HIB vaccine is an inactivated bacterial vaccine that is available for reconstitution with DTP or DTaP. It is available in combination with DTP, DTaP, or hepatitis B vaccine. This conjugate vaccine is recommended for all healthy children from age 2 to 59 months (see Figure 1). Vaccination is also recommended for children 5 years of age or older who are at increased risk of invasive HIB disease, such as children with sickle cell disease, asplenia, human immunodeficiency virus (HIV) infection and certain immunodeficiency syndromes, and those receiving chemotherapy.

Hepatitis B Vaccine

Hepatitis B vaccine (Recombivax HB, Engerix-B) is a recombinant, inactivated viral vaccine that is recommended for all infants and children through adolescence as part of the routine immunization schedule (Table 1; see Figure 1). The dose and schedule of hepatitis B vaccine in infancy is dependent on the vaccine used, the age of the infant, and the hepatitis B surface antigen status of the mother. Timing and dosage of hepatitis B vaccine is extremely important for infants born to hepatitis B surface antigen–positive mothers or mothers with unknown hepatitis B antigen status.

Postvaccination testing for immunity (hepatitis B surface antibody [Hb_sAb]) is not routinely recommended, except when a suboptimal response is expected or patients are at risk for exposure and subsequent management depends on knowing their immune status. The ACIP recommends revaccination with one or more additional doses for persons who do not respond to an initial 3-dose regimen. Hb_sAb testing should then be repeated. The need for booster doses of hepatitis B vaccine has not yet been determined.

TABLE 1. **Indications for Hepatitis B Vaccination**

All infants born in the United States
Children aged 11 to 12 years who have not completed the 3-dose series
Adoptees from countries in which hepatitis B virus (HBV) infection is endemic
Health care workers (see "Immunization of Health Care Workers" in text)
Hemodialysis patients
Subpopulations with a known high incidence of hepatitis
Persons with clotting disorders (such as hemophilia) who receive blood products
Household contacts and sex partners of HBV carriers
Persons who test positive for hepatitis C virus
Staff and residents of institutions for the developmentally disabled
Injection drug users
Sexually active homosexual and bisexual men
Sexually active heterosexual men and women who have recently acquired a sexually transmitted disease, are prostitutes, or have a history of sexual activity with more than one partner in the past 6 months
Inmates of long-term correctional facilities who have histories of high-risk behavior
Some international travelers (see "Immunization of International Travelers" in text)
Component of the therapy used to prevent hepatitis B infection following HBV exposure

Influenza Vaccine

Influenza may be prevented in many cases by giving the appropriate influenza vaccine (Fluzone, Fluvirin, FluShield) at the proper time (ideally early October to mid-November) (Table 2). The composition of the influenza vaccine changes annually in anticipation of the expected flu strain for the upcoming winter. An intranasal influenza vaccine is expected as early as 1999.

Children aged 6 months to 8 years who have never received the vaccine require two injections, but children in the same age group who previously received the vaccine require only one injection. Children 9 years of age and older and all adults require only one injection. Only split-virus vaccines (labeled as "split," "subvirion," or "purified surface antigen") should be given to children younger than 13 years of age.

Measles-Mumps-Rubella Vaccine

The virtual elimination of these three infectious diseases since the introduction of MMR vaccine in

TABLE 2. **Indications for Influenza Vaccination**

All adults 65 years of age or older
All residents of long-term care facilities
Adults and children 6 months of age or older with chronic pulmonary, cardiac, or metabolic disease
Children and teenagers receiving long-term aspirin therapy
Pregnant women (see "Immunization of Pregnant Women" in text)
Health care workers
Persons who wish minimal disruption of their activities because of influenza

1971 has been a remarkable tribute to the effectiveness of modern vaccine technology combined with aggressive public health programs. There was a brief resurgence of measles from 1989 to 1991, but since then measles cases have been reported at record low levels. The second dose of MMR vaccine is now recommended at 4 to 6 years of age (see Figure 1) but may be administered during any visit, provided at least 1 month has elapsed since receipt of the first dose. All women of childbearing age should be immune to rubella.

Pneumococcal Vaccine

The 23-valent pneumococcal vaccine (Pneumovax 23, Pnu-Imune 23) is an inactivated bacteria vaccine that became available in the United States in 1977. Despite the efficacy, low cost, and minimal side effects of this vaccine, it remains underutilized in a large portion of the targeted population (Table 3). There is no recommendation for routine booster of healthy persons previously vaccinated with the current vaccine. However, for persons 65 years of age or older, a booster dose is recommended if the person received the vaccine more than 5 years previously and was younger than 65 years of age at the time of vaccination.

The current pneumococcal polysaccharide vaccine is poorly immunogenic and not effective in children younger than 2 years of age. Because of the rapidly

TABLE 3. **Indications for Pneumococcal Vaccine**

All adults 65 years of age and older
Adults and children 2 to 64 years of age with a chronic condition that increases the risk of pneumococcal disease
Persons 2 to 64 years of age who have functional or anatomic asplenia
Persons 2 to 64 years of age who are living in special environments or social settings (e.g., residents of nursing homes and other long-term care facilities and Alaskan Natives and certain American Indian populations)
Immunocompromised persons (2 years or older)

Vaccines are listed under the routinely recommended ages*

[shaded box] = Range of acceptable ages for vaccination; [open box] = "Catch-up" vaccination‡ ††; [oval] = Vaccines to be assessed and given if necessary

Vaccine	Age: Birth	1 mo	2 mo	4 mo	6 mo	12 mo	15 mo	18 mo	4–6 y	11–12 y	14–16 y	50 y	≥65 y
Hepatitis B†‡	Hep B-1 (Birth–2 mo)												
		Hep B-2 (1–4 mo)			Hep B-3 (6–18 mo)					Hep B‡			
Diphtheria, tetanus, pertussis§			DTaP or DTP	DTaP or DTP	DTaP or DTP		DTap or DTP‡ (15–18 mo)		DTP or DTaP	Td, booster every 10 y			
Haemophilus influenzae type b‖			HIB	HIB	HIB‖	HIB‖ (12–15 mo)							
Polio¶			Polio¶	Polio	Polio¶ (6–18 mo)				Polio				
Measles-mumps-rubella**						MMR (12–15 mo)			MMR**	MMR**			
Varicella zoster virus††						Var (12–18 mo)				Var††			
Influenza‡‡										Influ		Influ	Influ
Pneumococcal§§										Pneu		Pneu	Pneu
Hepatitis A§§										Hep A			

Figure 1. Recommended childhood and adult immunization schedule—United States, January–December 1998. (Adapted from Centers for Disease Control and Prevention: *Recommended Childhood Immunization Schedule—United States, 1998.* Approved by the Advisory Committee on Immunization Practices [ACIP], the American Academy of Pediatrics [AAP], and the American Academy of Family Physicians [AAFP].)

increasing number of pneumococcal strains resistant to penicillin, the development of an effective pneumococcal vaccine effective against *Streptococcus pneumoniae* infection in infancy and early childhood is an urgent national and worldwide public health concern.

Polio Vaccine

There has not been a case of wild-type polio in the Western Hemisphere since 1991, and polio is expected to be eliminated worldwide by 2002. Following the eradication of the disease, polio will most likely be eliminated from the routine pediatric vaccine schedule.

In 1997, the ACIP recommended that children in the United States receive 2 doses of injectable polio vaccine (IPV) followed by 2 doses of oral polio vaccine (OPV). This recommendation is expected to reduce the eight or nine cases of vaccine-associated paralytic poliomyelitis per year by 50 to 75%. The option to use the 4-dose OPV schedule or the 4-dose IPV schedule is still acceptable (see Figure 1).

An all-OPV schedule is recommended if the primary series is begun at age 6 months to 7 years. OPV is a live-virus vaccine and should not be administered to any person who is immunodeficient or living with someone who is immunodeficient. OPV may be given before, with, or after measles-containing vaccines, varicella vaccine, oral typhoid vaccine, or immune globulin. IPV is preferred for the primary immunization of persons older than 17 years of age.

Rotavirus Vaccine*

Rotavirus infection causes more than 3 million cases of gastroenteritis and diarrhea, 50,000 hospitalizations, and 40 deaths annually in the United States. The infection usually occurs annually between November and March and generally confers long-term immunity. In early 1998 the ACIP voted to recommend routine use of the rotavirus vaccine in infants at 2, 4, and 6 months of age. The new vaccine is an attenuated, oral, quadrivalent, live-virus vaccine that has demonstrated safety and efficacy in

*Not available in the United States.

---

*This schedule indicates the recommended age for routine administration of currently licensed childhood and adult vaccines. Catch-up immunization should be done during any visit when feasible. Some combination vaccines are available (HIB/DTP, HIB/DTaP and HIB/HBV). Providers should consult the manufacturers' package inserts for detailed recommendations.

†**Infants born to HBsAg-negative mothers** should receive 2.5 μg of Recombivax HB (Merck & Co., Inc.) or 10 μg of Engerix-B (SmithKline Beecham). The second dose should be administered ≥ 1 month after the first dose. The third dose should be given at least 2 months after the second dose but not before 6 months of age.

Infants born to HBsAg-positive mothers should receive 0.5 mL hepatitis B immune globulin (HBIG) within 12 hours of birth and either 5 μg of Recombivax HB or 10 μg of Engerix-B at a separate site. The second dose is recommended at 1–2 months of age and the third dose at 6 months of age.

Infants born to mothers whose HBsAg status is unknown should receive either 5 μg of Recombivax HB or 10 μg of Engerix-B within 12 hours of birth. The second dose of vaccine is recommended at age 1 month and the third dose at age 6 months. Blood should be drawn at the time of delivery to determine the mother's HBsAg status; if it is positive, the infant should receive HBIG as soon as possible (no later than 1 week of age). The dosage and timing of subsequent vaccine doses should be based on the mother's HBsAg status.

‡Children and adolescents who have not been vaccinated against hepatitis B in infancy may begin the series during any visit. Those who have not received 3 doses of hepatitis B vaccine previously should initiate or complete the series during the 11–12 year-old visit, and unvaccinated older adolescents should be vaccinated whenever possible. The second dose should be administered at least 1 month after the first dose, and the third dose should be administered at least 4 months after the first dose and at least 2 months after the second dose.

§DTaP (diphtheria and tetanus toxoids and acellular pertussis vaccine) is the preferred vaccine for all doses in the vaccination series, including completion of the series in children who have received ≥ 1 dose of whole-cell DTP vaccine. Whole-cell DTP is an acceptable alternative to DTaP. The fourth dose of DTaP or DTP may be administered as early as 12 months of age, provided 6 months have elapsed since the third dose, and if the child is considered unlikely to return at 15–18 months of age. Td (tetanus and diphtheria toxoids, adsorbed, for adult use) is recommended at age 11–12 years, if ≥ 5 years have elapsed since the last dose of DTP, DTaP, or DT (diphtheria and tetanus toxoids, adsorbed, for pediatric use). Subsequent routine boosters are recommended every 10 years.

‖Three *H. influenzae* type B (HIB) conjugate vaccines are licensed for infant use. If PRP-OMP (PedvaxHIB [Merck & Co., Inc.]) is administered at 2 and 4 months of age, a dose at 6 months of age is not required; however a booster is still required at 12–15 months and any HIB conjugate vaccine may be used.

¶Two poliovirus vaccines are currently licensed in the United States: inactivated poliovirus vaccine (IPV) and oral poliovirus vaccine (OPV). The following schedules are all acceptable by the ACIP, the AAP and the AAFP, and parents and providers may choose among them:

(1) 2 doses IPV followed by 2 doses OPV.
- The ACIP recommends IPV at 2 and 4 months of age followed by OPV at 12–18 months and 4–6 years of age.
- The AAP recommends IPV at 2 and 4 months of age followed by OPV at 6–18 months and 4–6 years of age.

(2) 4 doses IPV (2, 4, 6–18 months, and 4–6 years).
(3) 4 doses OPV (2, 4, 6–18 months, and 4–6 years).

IPV is the only poliovirus vaccine recommended for immunocompromised persons and their household contacts.

**The second dose of measles-mumps-rubella (MMR) vaccine is routinely recommended at age 4–6 years but may be administered during any visit, provided at least 1 month has elapsed since receipt of the first dose and that both doses are administered at or after 12 months of age. Those who have not *previously* received the second dose should complete the schedule no later than the routine 11–12 year visit.

††Susceptible children may receive varicella vaccine (Var) at any visit after the first birthday, and those who lack a reliable history of chickenpox should be immunized during the routine 11–12 year-old visit. Susceptible children ≥ 13 years of age should receive 2 doses, at least 1 month apart.

‡‡Administer any time after age 6 months if indicated by patient's health status or potential exposure.

§§Administer any time after age 2 years if indicated by patient's health status or potential exposure.

infants and young children. As soon as the U.S. Food and Drug Administration (FDA) licenses the vaccine, it will be placed on the recommended childhood immunization schedule. As with any new immunization, health care providers should carefully review the package insert as well as any published ACIP and AAP recommendations before giving this immunization.

Varicella Vaccine

Varicella vaccine (Varivax) became a part of the routine childhood vaccination schedule in 1996. It is an attenuated, live-viral vaccine that should be administered at 12 to 18 months of age (see Figure 1) but whose use is encouraged at any age older than that for individuals who have not been immunized previously and who lack a reliable history of the disease. It is particularly recommended for susceptible persons who will have close contact with those at high risk for serious complications, nonpregnant women of childbearing age, international travelers without evidence of immunity, and all susceptible health care workers (see "Immunization of Health Care Workers").

Children 12 months to 12 years receive a single injection. Adolescents (13 and older) and adults receive 2 doses 4 to 8 weeks apart. The vaccine must be stored frozen at −15°C (+5°F) and may be administered simultaneously with all other routine vaccines.

IMMUNIZATION OF INTERNATIONAL TRAVELERS

Twenty-five years ago it was thought that most of the common infectious diseases of international travelers would soon be eliminated. Since that time, despite an explosion of technologic advances in vaccine technology and increased understanding of virus and bacterial and parasitic biology, the eradication of most travel-related diseases is no longer considered attainable.

Hepatitis A vaccine (Havrix), was licensed in the United States in 1995 for use in susceptible persons, especially international travelers. It is approved for use as a 2-dose series in adults and children 2 years of age or older. The first dose should be administered at least 2 weeks before the expected exposure to hepatitis A virus. The duration of long-term protection is not known, but it could be as many as 20 years.

Even though hepatitis A vaccine is highly immunogenic with minimal side effects, it is not considered a "routine" vaccination at any age. It is indicated for some international travelers, children living in communities with high rates of hepatitis A, men who have sex with men, some users of illegal drugs, persons with chronic liver disease, persons with occupational exposure, and persons receiving clotting factor concentrates.

Hepatitis B remains a significant worldwide public health problem and is highly endemic in Asia, Africa, most Pacific islands, parts of the Middle East, the Amazon Basin, Haiti, and the Dominican Republic. Hepatitis B immunization is frequently recommended for international travelers, although the risk for infection is quite low for most short-term travelers (Table 4). There are two hepatitis B vaccines manufactured in the United States, and they may be used interchangeably.

Smallpox has disappeared, and the vaccination for this disease is no longer available. Parenteral cholera immunization is considered ineffective and obsolete and is no longer internationally regulated; hence it is rarely indicated. Polio may well be eradicated in the next few years, and there is very little reason to give this vaccine to most international travelers. Unfortunately, very little progress has been made in the development of immunizations for such common and destructive diseases as traveler's diarrhea, malaria, and dengue fever.

Per ACIP, unless contraindicated, either oral, live-attenuated typhoid Ty21a (Vivotif Berna) or injectable Vi capsular polysaccharide (Typhim Vi) is preferable to the older parenteral inactivated typhoid vaccine. The use of Japanese encephalitis, meningococcal, and rabies vaccines is always challenging because of the infrequency of their use, the dosing schedules, and the availability of multiple preparations (three typhoid and four rabies vaccine formulations). Their correct use depends on accurate, country-specific information and a thorough understanding of their administration schedules and dosing. Newer oral vaccines for cholera and typhoid appear imminent.

IMMUNIZATION OF PREGNANT WOMEN

In general, pregnant travelers should avoid live-antigen vaccines, such as MMR, OPV, varicella, yellow fever, and oral typhoid. There is an absolute contraindication to the administration of MMR during pregnancy. Women who receive MMR, measles-rubella, or single-antigen mumps or rubella vaccine should be counseled not to become pregnant for at least 3 months after immunization. Per ACIP, women should be counseled not to become pregnant for at

TABLE 4. **Indications for Hepatitis B Vaccination of International Travelers**

Working in health care fields for any duration of time in high or moderate areas endemic for hepatitis B (HBV) virus

Residing for 6 months or more in moderately or highly endemic areas, especially if the travelers will be living in rural areas, having daily physical contact with local populations (a particular risk for pediatric travelers), or receiving local medical or dental care

Traveling to areas with moderate to high levels of endemic HBV transmission and anticipating direct contact with blood or sexual contact with residents least 1 month after receiving the varicella immunization.

Td immunization is indicated for susceptible pregnant women to prevent neonatal tetanus. It should be given to pregnant women who have never received the primary series or who have not had a booster within 10 years, although use of the vaccine during the first trimester should be avoided, if possible. Influenza vaccine is indicated for pregnant women who will be beyond the first trimester of pregnancy (14 weeks' gestation) during the influenza season. In 1997, ACIP recommended that unimmunized women who need immediate protection against polio during pregnancy be given either OPV or IPV. Breast-feeding is not a contraindication to any immunization.

IMMUNIZATION OF IMMUNOCOMPROMISED PERSONS

Immunization of immunocompromised persons requires special attention and consideration. Individuals with weakened immune systems may face higher disease risks than the general citizenry. Further, many vaccines administered to this population may have a diminished antibody response. At times this may require that titers be checked or extra vaccine be given. All immunizations should be initiated as early as possible in the course of HIV infection.

In general, immunocompromised patients should not receive live-antigen vaccines—OPV, varicella, oral typhoid, yellow fever, or bacille Calmette-Guérin (BCG). MMR (a live-virus vaccine) is *not* recommended for HIV-infected persons who have evidence of severe immunosuppression. However, MMR is recommended for all asymptomatic HIV-infected persons who are not severely immunocompromised. Administration of MMR to HIV-infected persons who are symptomatic but do not have evidence of severe immunosuppression also should be considered.

Per the Centers for Disease Control and Prevention (CDC), persons using short-term (under 2 weeks), low- to moderate-dose systemic corticosteroid therapy; topical steroid therapy; long-term alternate-day treatment with low to moderate doses of short-acting systemic steroids; or intra-articular, bursal, or tendon injection with corticosteroids may receive live-virus immunizations. It is advisable, however, to wait at least 3 months before administering a live-virus vaccine to patients who have received high systemically absorbed doses of corticosteroids for 2 or more weeks (i.e., more than 2 mg per kg per day or more than 20 mg of prednisone per day).

IMMUNIZATION OF HEALTH CARE WORKERS

Health care workers (HCWs) at every level of employment may be exposed to infectious disease. They risk the morbidity and mortality of infectious disease; the secondary transmission of infectious disease to coworkers, family members, and other patients; and the possibility of significant loss of work because of illness. Screening and/or immunization for measles, mumps, rubella, varicella, influenza, and hepatitis B is strongly recommended for all HCWs. Hepatitis A immunization is not routinely recommended for HCWs.

HCWs are not at greater risk for diphtheria, tetanus, and pneumococcal disease than the general population, but, like all adults, they should be protected against these diseases by receiving routine immunizations per recommended schedules (see Figure 1). In unusual occupational environments, immunization for meningococcal disease, typhoid, polio, and vaccinia may be indicated.

CDC recommendations and Occupational Safety and Health Administration (OSHA) regulations govern most of the tuberculosis prevention and control efforts of health care institutions. Purified protein derivative screening of HCWs is determined by several factors, including the profile of tuberculosis in the community, the number of infectious patients with tuberculosis admitted to the facility, the estimated number of infectious tuberculosis patients to whom HCWs in an occupational group may be exposed, and the results of analyses of any skin test conversions among HCWs or review of any possible person-to-person transmission of *Mycobacterium tuberculosis.*

TOXOPLASMOSIS

method of
SIN-YEW WONG, M.B.B.S., M.Med.
Tan Tock Seng Hospital
Singapore

Toxoplasma gondii is a ubiquitous obligate intracellular protozoan parasite of humans and animals. Its definitive hosts are members of the cat family, in which *Toxoplasma* undergoes a sexual cycle in the intestine, resulting in the production of oocysts. All other animals including humans may be infected but are secondary hosts and have an extraintestinal asexual cycle with the production of tissue cysts. Infection in humans usually goes unnoticed or is a benign, self-limited disease in immunocompetent individuals. In contrast, congenital infection in the fetus or infection in the immunocompromised host may result in debilitating and life-threatening disease. Toxoplasmosis refers to the clinical and pathologic disease state caused by infection with *T. gondii.*

In humans, *Toxoplasma* infection is acquired primarily through ingestion of undercooked or raw meat containing tissue cysts or of food and water contaminated by oocysts. Following ingestion, the outer walls of the cysts or oocysts are disrupted by enzymatic degradation; the infective stages (bradyzoites and tachyzoites) are released. They rapidly invade and multiply within the surrounding nucleated cells, where they become tachyzoites. Intracellularly, the tachyzoites reside in a parasitophorous vacuole protected from the host cell–killing mechanisms. Further spread of the parasite follows its release from disrupted cells and dissemination via the blood and lymphatics. Because *T. gondii* may infect virtually all nucleated cells and tissues, the placenta of a pregnant woman may be infected during the parasitemic phase and result in congenital infection of the fetus. Development of immunity is associated with cessation of tachyzoite replication and invasion and formation of tissue cysts. These tissue cysts containing bradyzoites develop virtually in every organ, especially in brain, heart, and skeletal muscles, and persist for the life of the host. These persistent, slowly metabolizing forms of *T. gondii* are the most probable source of recrudescent infection in immunocompromised patients. Less common modes of acquiring the infection include blood and leukocyte transfusions, organ transplantation, and laboratory accident.

CLINICAL MANIFESTATIONS

Acute Acquired *Toxoplasma* Infection in the Immunocompetent Patient. Acute *Toxoplasma* infection is often asymptomatic and goes unrecognized in 80 to 90% of healthy immunocompetent adults and children. In the rest, symptomatic illness, usually painless lymphadenopathy or an "infectious mononucleosis–like" syndrome, develops. The enlarged nodes are usually discrete, of variable firmness, nontender, and nonsuppurative and may occur singly or in groups, or be diffusely enlarged in the cervical, suboccipital, supraclavicular, axillary, and inguinal areas. Rarely, an apparently immunocompetent patient may develop clinically overt illness with myocarditis, pneumonitis, or encephalitis with potentially fatal dissemination. Other than fatigue and lymphadenopathy, the signs and symptoms of acute *Toxoplasma* infection usually resolve within 1 to 3 weeks.

Toxoplasmosis in Pregnancy. Acute infection in the pregnant woman has similar manifestations as described earlier, with the majority being asymptomatic. More important, this infection may result in a tragic outcome in her offspring if it is left unrecognized. Transplacental transmission to the fetus has been limited almost solely to women who acquire the infection during gestation. The incidence of fetal infection relates to the stage of gestation at which a pregnant woman acquires the infection. Without treatment, the incidence is 10 to 15% in the first trimester, 30% in the second, and 60% in the third trimester. Approximately 85% of infants with congenital infection appear normal at birth, but this subclinical infection is associated with subsequent learning disabilities, psychomotor and mental retardation, and loss of vision from chorioretinitis. In the other 10 to 15%, the most severely damaged newborns are those born to mothers who acquired their infection in the first trimester, and these infants often have hydrocephalus, hepatosplenomegaly, growth retardation, or multiorgan dysfunction.

Rarely, reactivation of past infection in pregnant women may result in congenital infection. This has been reported in women who were severely immunocompromised by drugs, cancer, or human immunodeficiency virus (HIV) infection. In particular, women of childbearing age who are HIV-positive pose unique problems. They are at risk for acquiring acute toxoplasmosis during pregnancy if they are seronegative before onset of their pregnancy, and if they are seropositive for *Toxoplasma,* they may have reactivation of their latent infection. In either case, the fetus is at risk for congenital toxoplasmosis. In infants congenitally infected with HIV and *T. gondii, Toxoplasma* infection appears to have a more progressive course.

Ocular Toxoplasmosis. Up to one third of chorioretinitis in all age groups is thought to be caused by *T. gondii* infection. Toxoplasmic chorioretinitis usually reflects a late sequela of congenital infection. The patients usually complain of blurred vision, scotoma pain, photophobia, and epiphora. The characteristic lesion is a focal necrotizing retinitis that often appears as a yellowish-white cotton patch with indistinct margins ("headlights in the mist"). The lesions occur in small clusters, and panuveitis may occur. Relapses of chorioretinitis are observed in 13 to 30%, even with specific chemotherapy. Acute toxoplasmic chorioretinitis is being recognized with increasing frequency following postnatally acquired infection.

In patients with acquired immune deficiency syndrome (AIDS), ocular toxoplasmosis may develop but is far less frequent than retinitis caused by cytomegalovirus. The lesions, which are usually large and necrotic, progressively destroy retinal tissue. Definitive diagnosis requires either retinal biopsy and demonstration of the organisms in tissue specimens, isolation of *T. gondii,* or detection of *T. gondii* DNA by polymerase chain reaction from vitreous aspirate.

Acute Toxoplasmosis in the Immunocompromised Patient. This usually occurs because of reactivation of latent infection. The incidence of toxoplasmic encephalitis (TE) in AIDS patients is directly proportional to *Toxoplasma* seroprevalence in the population. In the United States, 10 to 40% of HIV-positive patients are latently infected with *Toxoplasma,* and of these, 30 to 50% develop TE, especially when their CD4 count falls below 100 per mm^3 and they are not on primary prophylaxis. In parts of western Europe and Africa, *Toxoplasma* seroprevalence among HIV-infected persons is much higher and hence is associated with a higher incidence of TE. In immunocompromised patients who are initially seronegative, acute disease may result from exogenous infection.

Focal necrotizing encephalitis is the most common manifestation of toxoplasmosis in patients with AIDS. The clinical presentation of TE is varied and may be difficult to differentiate from a number of other HIV-related conditions that affect the central nervous system (CNS). Magnetic resonance imaging (MRI) or computed tomography (CT) scans characteristically show multiple, bilateral cerebral lesions in patients with TE. The lesions on these scans are typically multiple and contrast enhancing, involving the basal ganglia and corticomedullary junction bilaterally. MRI is more sensitive than CT in the detection of multiple lesions. If a single lesion is seen using CT, then an MRI scan should be performed, if available.

The findings on MRI or CT scanning are not pathognomonic. However, a presumptive diagnosis of TE can be made based on the scan findings and positive toxoplasma serology in symptomatic AIDS patients, and treatment should be initiated promptly (Figure 1).

Other manifestations of toxoplasmosis in AIDS patients include pulmonary disease and chorioretinitis. Pulmonary toxoplasmosis is being increasingly recognized; it has a high mortality. The clinical picture may be indistinguishable from that of *Pneumocystis carinii* pneumonia.

Toxoplasmosis in immunocompromised patients who do not have AIDS, such as transplant recipients and patients with underlying malignancy (usually Hodgkin's disease and other lymphomas), is fatal if not recognized early and appropriate treatment given. In transplant recipients, toxoplasmosis may be newly acquired in seronegative patients from seropositive donor organs and less commonly via blood products. In addition, toxoplasmosis may result from reactivation of latent infection. Toxoplasmosis in transplant patients may affect the CNS (76%), myocardium (38%), or lung (23%) and may cause recurrent attacks

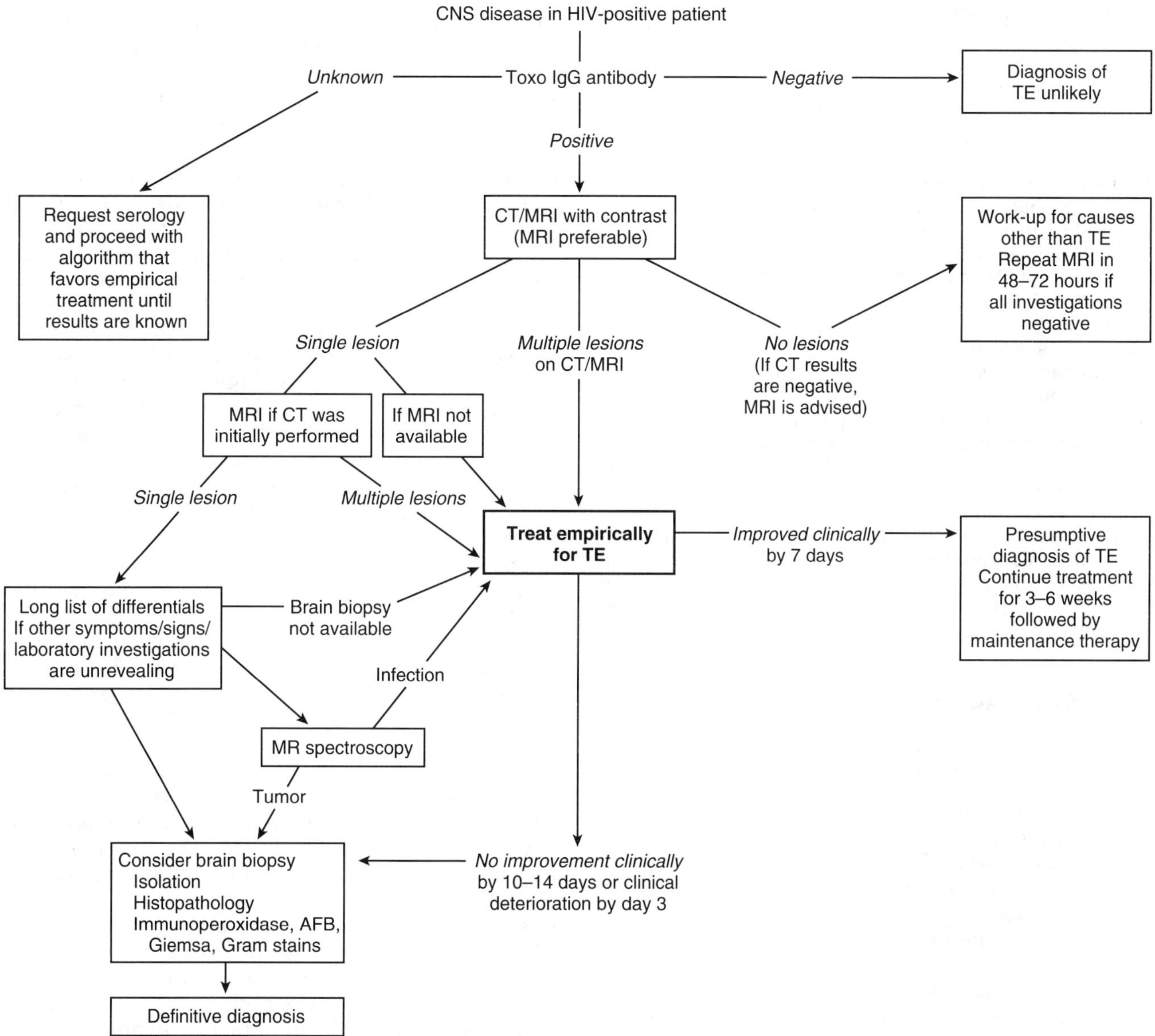

Figure 1. Clinical algorithm for HIV-infected patients suspected to have toxoplasmic encephalitis (TE).
(Modified from Wong SY, Remington JS: Toxoplasmosis in the setting of AIDS. *In* Broder S, Merigan TC Jr, Bolognesi D [eds]: Textbook of AIDS Medicine. Baltimore, Williams & Wilkins, 1994, pp 223–257.)
Abbreviations: CNS = central nervous system; HIV = human immunodeficiency virus; TE = toxoplasmic encephalitis; CT = computed tomography; MRI = magnetic resonance imaging; AFB = acid-fast bacilli.

of fever. In bone marrow transplant recipients, toxoplasmosis often results from reactivation of latent infection. In heart transplant recipients, toxoplasmosis frequently results when a seronegative recipient receives a heart from a seropositive donor.

DIAGNOSIS

Toxoplasma infection may result in protean clinical manifestations and must be carefully considered in the differential diagnosis of a variety of clinical presentations. The correct diagnostic test must be performed and interpreted appropriately in light of the patient's condition.

Serologic Test for Detection of Antibody. The use of serologic tests forms the primary method of diagnosis. A large number of tests have been reported to be useful, but only a few are widely available to clinicians. The most common are tests that detect IgG (Sabin-Feldman dye test, enzyme-linked immunosorbent assay [ELISA], indirect fluorescent antibody (IFA), and modified agglutination) and IgM (IFA, double sandwiched ELISA, and immunosorbent assay). Specific IgA and IgE antibodies may be detected in the sera of acutely infected individuals by ELISA and immunosorbent assay (ISAGA) methods and are particularly useful in the detection of congenitally infected infants. IgE antibodies have been discovered in approximately 40% of HIV-infected patients with TE; in contrast, IgA antibodies are rarely detected in the sera of such patients.

It is important to highlight the need for confirmatory testing for the diagnosis of recently acquired infection with *T. gondii* in pregnant women. A positive IgG titer in most tests is sufficient to establish that a patient is infected. However, because titers of IgM and IgA may remain detectable by any method for more than 1 year, a single positive result does not establish that the infection has been acquired recently. Physicians must be aware of this important issue, as a single set of positive IgG and IgM results may be interpreted as "acute and recent" infection and may lead to unnecessary abortion. A serologic diagnosis of acute infection in most instances requires the demonstration of a rise in antibody titer in serial serum samples, preferably obtained at least 3 weeks apart, that are tested in parallel. In such situations, the importance of testing by a reference laboratory cannot be overemphasized.

Isolation of *Toxoplasma*. Isolation of *T. gondii* establishes that infection is acute. Specimens are inoculated into the peritoneal cavity of mice or by tissue culture. The latter is less sensitive than mouse inoculation.

Histologic Diagnosis. Demonstration of tachyzoites in tissue sections or smear of body fluid establishes the diagnosis of acute *Toxoplasma* infection. Multiple cysts near an inflammatory necrotic lesion probably establish the diagnosis. Fluorescent antibody and immunoperoxidase staining techniques are more sensitive and specific for the detection of tachyzoites than is standard tissue staining.

Polymerase Chain Reaction (PCR). DNA amplification using PCR has been used successfully in body fluid and tissue to detect *T. gondii* DNA. It is now considered the method of choice for prenatal diagnosis of congenital infection.

DRUGS ACTIVE AGAINST *T. GONDII*

Drugs with anti-*Toxoplasma* activity can be broadly classified into the following categories:

1. Drugs interfering with folate metabolism
   a. Pyrimethamine
   b. Trimethoprim
   c. Sulfonamides, e.g., sulfadiazine
   d. Sulfones—dapsone
   e. Methotrexate analogues—trimetrexate,* piritrexim†
2. Drugs that inhibit protein synthesis
   a. Tetracyclines—chlortetracycline,† doxycycline, minocycline
   b. Macrolides—spiramycin, clarithromycin,* azithromycin,* roxithromycin†
   c. Lincosamides, e.g., clindamycin
   d. Ketolides
   e. Rifamycin derivatives—rifabutin,* rifapentine*
3. Drugs with an uncertain mechanism of action
   a. Hydroxynaphthoquinone—atovaquone*
4. Miscellaneous
   a. Diclazuril†
   b. Arprinocid
   c. Quinolones—trovafloxacin*

The first line of anti-infective therapy is a combination of drugs that inhibit folate metabolism. Pyrimethamine (a dihydrofolate reductase inhibitor) is combined with sulfadiazine (a dihydrofolate synthetase inhibitor) to block folate synthesis sequentially and produce synergistic activity against *T. gondii.* This combination is the most commonly used regimen. Folinic acid (leucovorin), which is preferentially utilized by mammalian cells and not by *T. gondii,* should be given to prevent pyrimethamine-induced hematologic toxicity. Folinic acid can be given orally, intravenously, or intramuscularly. The optimal dose of folinic acid is not known but should be individualized according to blood picture results. Although sulfadiazine is the most often used sulfonamide, sulfamethoxazole* and trisulfapyrimidines (no longer commercially available in the United States) can be used in conjunction with pyrimethamine. Other sulfonamides are less active against *T. gondii* and hence should not be used for the treatment of toxoplasmosis.

Dapsone is a sulfone with potent activity against *T. gondii.* It acts by inhibiting *T. gondii* dihydropteroate synthesis. Dapsone is well absorbed when given orally and has a long half-life and better toxicity profile than do sulfonamides, making it a good alternative to sulfadiazine for maintenance therapy. Trimethoprim* is markedly less active than pyrimethamine against the dihydrofolate reductase (DHFR) of *T. gondii.* Trimethoprim-sulfamethoxazole has been shown to have some activity against *T. gondii* in a number of animal models and has been used in a limited number of AIDS patients with TE. Low-dose trimethoprim-sulfamethoxazole given prophylactically for *P. carinii* infection was also found to prevent toxoplasmosis in AIDS patients.

In patients who are allergic to sulfonamides, a combination of pyrimethamine and clindamycin has shown efficacy equal to that of pyrimethamine/sulfonamide in patients with TE. The exact mode of action of clindamycin, especially in TE, is not known.

Other agents active against *T. gondii* have been less well studied in humans. Newer macrolides—roxithromycin, clarithromycin, and azithromycin—have been found to be highly active against *T. gondii* in animal models and have been used successfully in a limited number of patients in combination with pyrimethamine. These macrolide antibiotics have the advantage of greater bioavailability. Higher and more persistent serum and/or intracellular levels can be achieved with these agents. Additional studies are needed to determine the exact role of these drugs. Unlike pyrimethamine and sulfadiazine, which are active in animal models only against the tachyzoite form, azithromycin may have activity against both tachyzoites and the cyst forms (bradyzoites) of *T. gondii.*

The macrolides should not be used as single-agent therapy for toxoplasmosis, and this guideline is probably true for all the other agents as well. One exception is spiramycin, which is used to prevent placental infection in pregnant women during the first trimester when pyrimethamine is contraindicated. Although spiramycin alone is less effective than the standard regimen, it remains as a viable option for patients who cannot tolerate pyrimethamine, sulfonamide, and clindamycin. Spiramycin can be obtained in the

*Not available in the United States.
†Not FDA approved for this indication.

*Not FDA approved for this indication.

United States with permission of the U.S. Food and Drug Administration (FDA) (301-443-9550).

A newer class of macrolides, the ketolides (HMR 3647 and HMR 3004), has demonstrated remarkable in vitro and in vivo activity in animal models against *T. gondii* and may be useful in the treatment of toxoplasmosis in humans.

Atovaquone, a hydroxynaphthoquinone, has been shown in a small number of patients to produce a partial or complete clinical and radiologic response. Atovaquone acts by blocking electron transport in parasite mitochondria, which in turn inhibits pyrimidine synthesis in malarial parasites but does not appear to be the mechanism of action in *Toxoplasma.* Atovaquone has activity against both tachyzoites and tissue cysts of *T. gondii.* In vitro and animal studies have shown that atovaquone does not have synergistic effects when used with sulfadiazine, clarithromycin, or minocycline and in fact may even have an antagonistic effect with pyrimethamine. The exact clinical implications of these observations are not clear. Atovaquone is reasonably well tolerated. It is poorly absorbed from the gut, and the bioavailability is improved up to threefold when taken with a fatty meal. It has high protein-binding capacity and a long elimination half-life (50 to 70 hours). Relapse has occurred while on atovaquone maintenance therapy in several patients even after successful induction, thus limiting its use as a single agent in long-term treatment.

Trimetrexate, a lipid-soluble analogue of methotrexate and a potent inhibitor of *T. gondii* DHFR, has demonstrated activity against *T. gondii* in animal models. It is cleared both hepatically and renally, with up to 41% excreted unchanged in the urine. In a salvage trial of trimetrexate/leucovorin for TE in sulfonamide-intolerant AIDS patients, trimetrexate was given intravenously at a dose of 30 to 280 mg per m^2 per day with leucovorin. Although the drug was well tolerated and patients had dramatic but transient improvement, relapse was noted while the patients were still receiving the drug, thus limiting the role of trimetrexate as a single agent in the treatment of TE in AIDS patients.

Experimental and anecdotal clinical data suggest that tetracycline/doxycycline has anti-*Toxoplasma* activity. In a limited number of patients given doxycycline, relapses occurred while they were still on the drug, raising the possibility of the development of drug resistance.

Piritrexim, an analogue of methotrexate, is a lipid-soluble folate antagonist active against murine toxoplasmosis when combined with sulfadiazine. The nonclassic antifolates such as trimetrexate and piritrexim enter cells via passive diffusion, circumventing the need for the folate transport systems (which are absent in *T. gondii*) that are necessary for the uptake of classic antifolates, such as methotrexate. However, these nonclassic antifolates lack selectivity for parasite DHFR compared with mammalian DHFR, thus necessitating leucovorin rescue when used.

A variety of additional agents from different classes may have activity against *Toxoplasma,* including diclazuril, arprinocid,* and substituted pyridopyrimidine compounds. The clinical usefulness of these novel agents alone or in combination has not yet been established. Derivatives of rifamycin such as rifabutin and rifapentine have demonstrated in vitro and in vivo activity in the mouse model against *T. gondii* and may be useful agents in the treatment of toxoplasmosis in immunocompromised individuals. In the mouse model, the combination of rifabutin with atovaquone or clindamycin resulted in significant reduction in brain inflammation compared with the combination of rifabutin and pyrimethamine or sulfadiazine.

Of a group of quinolone agents tested against a murine model of toxoplasmosis, trovafloxacin† demonstrated remarkable in vitro and in vivo activity and may be useful in the treatment of toxoplasmosis in humans.

Because of their profound defect in cellular immunity, there is a possibility that biologic response modifiers may be useful as adjunctive therapy in treatment of AIDS-associated toxoplasmosis. Biologic response modifiers such as interferon gamma (IFN-γ),† interferon beta (IFN-β),† interleukin [IL]-2,† IL-7,* IL-12,* tumor necrosis factor (TNF),†‡ and granulocyte-macrophage colony-stimulating factor (GM-CSF)† have been studied and have demonstrated anti-*T. gondii* activity in experimental animal models. However, at this time, they have not yet been used therapeutically in AIDS-associated toxoplasmosis.

ISSUES IN THE MANAGEMENT OF TOXOPLASMOSIS

Acute Acquired Toxoplasmosis in Immunocompetent Persons

In the immunocompetent individual, acute toxoplasmosis may go unnoticed because of minimal symptoms. Isolation of *Toxoplasma* from blood and body fluid, demonstration of tachyzoites in tissue sections or smears of body fluids, detection of *T. gondii* DNA in blood and body fluid, or a typical histopathologic appearance of excised lymph nodes establishes the diagnosis of acute toxoplasmosis. A variety of serologic tests are also available, and a diagnosis of recently acquired infection is confirmed if there is seroconversion from a negative to a positive titer. A high IgM titer (measured either by IFA testing or by ELISA) and a positive Sabin-Feldman dye test result are probably diagnostic of recent acute infection, with or without symptoms. Traditionally, treatment is not given for acute acquired toxoplasmosis in immunocompetent patients unless there are severe and persistent symptoms or clinically overt disease with myocarditis, pneumonitis, or encephalitis, in which case, treatment is given for 2 or 4 weeks or longer, if warranted. Infection acquired by transfusion or laboratory accident should be treated promptly.

*Not available in the United States.
†Not FDA approved for this indication.
‡Investigational drug in the United States.

Acute Toxoplasmosis in Pregnancy and Congenital Toxoplasmosis

Treatment of women who acquire the infection during pregnancy can reduce the incidence and severity of fetal infection. The rationale for such treatment is the observation of a lag period between the onset of maternal infection and fetal infection. If treatment is to be given during the first trimester, spiramycin is the current drug of choice. In the United States, spiramycin may be obtained from the FDA, telephone number 301-443-4280. If the fetus is not infected, it is recommended that spiramycin be given without interruption until delivery. If spiramycin is not available, treatment with sulfadiazine alone (or with an equivalent sulfonamide) is recommended. Pyrimethamine is not used in the first trimester because of concerns of teratogenicity.

To determine whether fetal infection has occurred, prenatal diagnosis based on detection of the parasites or parasite DNA in amniotic fluid should be performed. PCR-based assays for the detection of *T. gondii* DNA are extremely promising and are considered by many authorities as the gold standard. Serologic tests that detect specific IgM and IgA in fetal serum may be performed, but they must be interpreted with caution because of the possibility of contamination with maternal blood. Fetal ultrasonography should be performed periodically to document evidence of fetal infection, including calcification, hydrocephalus, and the like.

In pregnancies with documented fetal infection, the combination of pyrimethamine/sulfadiazine is more effective than spiramycin in altering the severity of fetal infection. Spiramycin does not reliably cross the placenta, and this combination is superior to spiramycin alone when fetal infection has occurred. Pyrimethamine and sulfadiazine combined with leucovorin rescue should be given in the second and third trimesters. Folinic acid is included to reduce the pyrimethamine-induced myelosuppression.

Both symptomatic and asymptomatic infants with congenital toxoplasmosis can be treated with continuous sulfadiazine (50 mg per kg twice a day [bid]), pyrimethamine (2 mg per kg for 2 days, then 1 mg per kg per day for 2 to 6 months, followed by 1 mg per kg three times per week), and folinic acid (5 mg three times per week) for a total of 12 months. Serial follow-up to gauge the response of therapy should include serology, neuroradiology, and ophthalmologic and detailed neurologic examinations. Cerebrospinal fluid shunting should be performed as required.

HIV-infected pregnant women who are seropositive for toxoplasmosis pose therapeutic problems. Until further data are made available, these women should receive spiramycin during the first trimester of pregnancy if their CD4 lymphocyte counts are less than 200 per mm^3 and pyrimethamine/sulfadiazine or trimethoprim-sulfamethoxazole later in pregnancy to prevent vertical transmission.

Toxoplasmosis in Immunocompromised Patients

Toxoplasmosis is one of the most important opportunistic infections of the CNS in patients with AIDS, causing encephalitis or focal cerebral lesions. At present, treatment is usually initiated empirically in AIDS patients with multiple ring-enhancing lesions on CT scan or MRI of the brain and positive *Toxoplasma* serology (see Figure 1). The predictive value in such situations is approximately 80%. In empirically treated patients, clear clinical and radiologic response should be seen within 14 days (in one study of AIDS patients, 71% had complete or partial response, with 74% of the responders having clear evidence of improvement by day 7). If a single lesion is present on MRI, the probability of CNS lymphoma is at least equal or higher than the probability of TE. In such situations, proton magnetic resonance spectroscopy, if available, may be helpful in differentiating between tumor (lymphoma) and infection (possible TE or other brain "abscess" due to bacterial, mycobacterial, and fungal infection). Brain biopsy and attempts at definitive diagnosis should be made if empirically treated patients deteriorate clinically by 7 days or do not improve clinically by 10 days.

Extracerebral toxoplasmosis (ECT) with dissemination, although rare, is not uncommon in patients with advanced AIDS. Ocular toxoplasmosis is the most common manifestation of ECT and may be associated with cytomegalovirus (CMV) retinitis, making diagnosis difficult. Cerebral toxoplasmosis can occur before, during, or after ECT diagnosis. Involvement of other organ systems can occur during dissemination, or ECT may present as isolated, unexplained fevers. Demonstration of parasitemia establishes the diagnosis of ECT in AIDS patients with unexplained fevers. In patients with ECT, concomitant TE frequently occurs, and careful neurologic and neuroradiologic examinations are recommended.

Primary or induction therapy should be given for 3 to 6 weeks or more, depending on the severity of illness and response to therapy (Table 1). The combination of pyrimethamine and sulfadiazine with leucovorin rescue is the therapy of choice in TE. Unfortunately, some AIDS patients treated with this regimen had to discontinue therapy because of adverse reactions. The pyrimethamine and clindamycin combination is a reasonable alternative and appears to be comparable in efficacy to pyrimethamine/sulfadiazine, but it also has comparable side effects. Corticosteroids for reduction of cerebral edema and raised intracranial pressure have been used, but there are no controlled data for efficacy, and this treatment should best be limited to 2 weeks of therapy. Use of corticosteroids may complicate interpretation of response to empirical therapy for TE. Seizures occur in up to 35% of patients with TE, necessitating the use of anticonvulsants. However, anticonvulsants should be used only if seizures occur; they are not recommended for prophylactic use.

Sulfadiazine desensitization has been attempted under close in-hospital supervision in a limited number of AIDS patients who are allergic to sulfonamides and intolerant of clindamycin. One protocol is to administer gradually increasing amounts of sulfadiazine orally every 3 hours for 4 to 5 days, starting at 10 μg. Sulfadiazine suspensions can be prepared us-

TABLE 1. **Guidelines for Acute or Primary Treatment of AIDS Patients with Toxoplasmic Encephalitis**

Drug	Dosage
Recommended Regimens	
Pyrimethamine (Daraprim) *and* folinic acid	PO: 200 mg loading followed by 50–75 mg q 24 h PO, IV, or IM: 10–20 mg q 24 h
plus	
Sulfadiazine	PO: 1 g q 6 h
or	
Clindamycin* (Cleocin)	IV or PO: 600 mg q 6 h
Alternative Regimens	
Trimethoprim/ sulfamethoxazole* (Bactrim, Septra)	PO or IV: 5 mg (trimethoprim component)/kg q 6 h
Pyrimethamine and folinic acid *plus one of the following:*	As in recommended regimen
Clarithromycin* (Biaxin)	PO: 1 g q 12 h†
Atovaquone* (Mepron)	PO: 750 mg q 6 h†
Azithromycin* (Zithromax)	PO: 1200–1500 mg q 24 h†
Dapsone*	PO: 100 mg q 24 h

*Not FDA approved for this indication.
†Exceeds dosage recommended by the manufacturer.
Modified from Subauste CS, Wong SY, Remington JS: AIDS-associated toxoplasmosis. *In* Sande MA, Volberding P (eds): The Medical Management of AIDS, 5th ed. Philadelphia, WB Saunders Co, 1997, pp 343–362.

ing sulfadiazine and 2% methylcellulose mucilage. In patients who cannot tolerate the above-mentioned regimens, other agents have been used in a limited manner, including trimethoprim-sulfamethoxazole, pyrimethamine/atovaquone, pyrimethamine/azithromycin, pyrimethamine/clarithromycin, and pyrimethamine/dapsone.

Relapse of TE occurs, even after successful induction, in more than 50% of patients if they do not receive subsequent maintenance therapy. Pyrimethamine (25 to 50 mg per day) plus sulfadiazine (500 mg four times a day) is the recommended suppressive therapy (Table 2). If sulfonamides cannot be used, then pyrimethamine (25 to 50 mg per day) combined with clindamycin (600 mg four times a day*) should be given, although retrospective studies indicate a higher rate of relapse with this latter combination owing to poor tolerability. Alternative regimens include pyrimethamine plus atovaquone (750 mg every 6 hours), dapsone (100 mg per day), or azithromycin (1200 to 1500 mg per day*). Folinic acid should be given in conjunction with pyrimethamine.

TABLE 2. **Guidelines for Maintenance Treatment of AIDS Patients with Toxoplasmic Encephalitis**

	Oral Dose	Frequency
Recommended Regimens		
Pyrimethamine* *and*	25–50 mg	q 24 h
sulfadiazine	500 mg	q 6 h
Pyrimethamine *and* clindamycin	25–50 mg	q 24 h
	600 mg	q 6 h
Pyrimethamine/sulfadoxine (Fansidar)†	25 mg/500 mg (1 tablet)	TIW
Alternative Regimens		
Pyrimethamine *plus one of the following:*	25–50 mg	q 24 h
Dapsone†	100 mg	q 24 h
Atovaquone†	750 mg	q 6 h‡
Clarithromycin†	1000 mg	q 12 h‡
Azithromycin†	1200–1500 mg	q 24 h‡

*Folinic acid (leucovorin calcium), 10–20 mg q 24 h, is recommended for all patients receiving pyrimethamine to help reduce myelosuppressive effects associated with pyrimethamine. The dose of folinic acid is titrated against the patient's hematologic indices, and up to 50 mg of folinic acid has been used.
†Not FDA approved for this indication.
‡Exceeds dosage recommended by the manufacturer.
Modified from Subauste CS, Wong SY, Remington JS: AIDS-associated toxoplasmosis. *In* Sande MA, Volberding P (eds): The Medical Management of AIDS, 5th ed. Philadelphia, WB Saunders Co, 1997, pp 343–362.

Ocular Toxoplasmosis

Ocular toxoplasmosis usually occurs as a late sequela of congenital infection. Toxoplasmic chorioretinitis may also be a manifestation of extracerebral toxoplasmosis in AIDS patients. Specific treatment of patients with ocular toxoplasmosis has resulted in resolution of signs and symptoms. Clindamycin (300 mg every 6 hours for a minimum 3 weeks) or pyrimethamine with sulfadiazine (for 1 month) has been reported to be effective. Relapses occur and often necessitate repeated courses of treatment. When lesions affect the macula or optic nerve head or are threatening vision, systemic corticosteroids are usually given. Photocoagulation may be necessary both for the treatment of active lesions and for prophylaxis against spread of lesions.

PREVENTION

Education. Prevention of infection is extremely important for pregnant women and immunocompromised patients and is easily accomplished through physician education of patients. The goal is to avoid ingestion or contact with cysts and sporulated oocysts. Meats should be well cooked or frozen to −20°C or less to kill the cysts. Eggs should not be eaten raw, and unpasteurized milk should be avoided. Hands should be washed thoroughly after handling raw meat or vegetables. Fruits and vegetables may be contaminated with oocysts and hence must be thoroughly washed before eating. Direct contact with cat feces (clearing cat litter, working in the garden, or cleaning children's sandboxes) should be avoided.

Serologic Screening. May be used to prevent congenital infection and toxoplasmosis. For a successful screening program, appropriate tests must be used and interpreted correctly. The frequency of such screening is affected by epidemiology of the infection, cost of screening, and cost effectiveness of screening. The need for and the role of such a screening program in the United States remains controversial. Sporadic screening conducted in the absence of a systematic screening program may do more harm than good.

To prevent toxoplasmosis in HIV-infected patients, serologic testing for *Toxoplasma* antibodies will help

*This exceeds dose recommended by manufacturer.

TABLE 3. **Regimens Used for Primary Prophylaxis Against Toxoplasmosis in *Toxoplasma*-Seropositive HIV-Infected Individuals with CD4 Lymphocyte Count <200 mm³**

Drug	Dosage Schedule
Trimethoprim/sulfamethoxazole	PO: 1 DS† tab qd or 2 DS tab TIW
Pyrimethamine-dapsone*‡	PO: pyrimethamine, 50–75 mg once or twice a week, with dapsone, 50 mg qd, or 100 mg BIW or 200 mg once a week
Pyrimethamine/sulfadoxine (Fansidar)*‡§	PO: 3 tab every 2 wk or 1 tab BIW

*Not FDA approved for this indication.
†DS = double strength.
‡Folinic acid (Leucovorin), 25 mg qw, is recommended for all patients receiving pyrimethamine to help ameliorate the hematologic side effects associated with pyrimethamine. The dose of folinic acid is titrated against the patient's hematologic indices.
§Each tablet contains 25 mg of pyrimethamine and 500 mg of sulfadoxine.
Modified from Subauste CS, Wong SY, Remington JS: AIDS-associated toxoplasmosis. *In* Sande MA, Volberding P (eds): The Medical Management of AIDS, 5th ed. Philadelphia, WB Saunders Co, 1997, pp 343–362.

determine those at risk for reactivation from past infection and those at risk for acquisition of new infection. Those who are seronegative should be educated on how to prevent acquisition of new infection (described earlier). For those who are seropositive, the morbidity and mortality associated with toxoplasmosis in the patient population supports the use of prophylaxis in those whose CD4 lymphocyte counts fall below 200 per mm^3. A number of drugs appear to be useful in prophylaxis against TE, including trimethoprim-sulfamethoxazole, pyrimethamine/dapsone, or pyrimethamine/sulfadoxine (Table 3).

Prophylaxis with pyrimethamine (25 mg every day for 6 weeks) has been used with apparent success in seronegative recipients of hearts transplanted from seropositive donors.

TRICHINELLOSIS

method of
ANDRÉ CABIÉ, M.D.
Service des Maladies Infectieuses et Tropicales, Hôpital Bichat Claude Bernard
Paris, France

Trichinellosis is a parasitic infection due to *Trichinella* species that occurs worldwide. The adult worm infests the small intestine, and larvae live in the host's striated muscle cells. The pathology produced appears to be a combination of a vigorous host inflammatory response and direct damage caused by the larvae. Transmission to humans occurs through the ingestion of larva-infected undercooked meat. In the United States, the most common sources of infection are pork, bear, and walrus. In Europe since 1976, most cases of trichinellosis have been due to consumption of wild boar meat or horse meat, which has caused five epidemics in France since 1976 (21 to 642 cases by outbreak).

Most infections are asymptomatic. The presence of symptoms depends mainly on the number of ingested larvae. An initial intestinal phase, attributable to adult worms, is followed by a visceral phase, attributable to larvae dissemination. The intestinal phase may include diarrhea, abdominal discomfort, and/or vomiting. Symptoms associated with the visceral phase are common and appear during the second week after infection. Classic symptoms are fever; myositis with pain, swelling, and weakness; and periorbital edema, sometimes with subconjunctival hemorrhages and chemosis. Some patients may complain of headache, cough, dyspnea, hoarseness, and dysphagia. A macular or petechial rash can occur. These symptoms usually peak 2 to 3 weeks after infection and may persist for many weeks. Death can occur after myocarditis or encephalitis. The diagnosis is supported by the clinical triad of fever, myositis and periorbital edema, and eosinophilia. *Trichinella* antibodies that develop after 3 weeks are highly specific. Muscle biopsy is usually not necessary to confirm the diagnosis.

THERAPY

The goals of treatment of trichinellosis are to decrease the host's inflammatory response and to kill the different stages of the parasite. Nevertheless, this treatment has not yet been standardized. Available anthelmintic drugs are poorly active against *Trichinella* larvae, and to our knowledge, no controlled studies have proven the efficacy of antiparasitic treatment. Certain investigators recommend therapy with aspirin and bed rest for simple symptoms, reserving steroids for the more serious cases, whereas we and others prefer to use parasitic drugs routinely with the aim of limiting larval production by adult worms. Systemic steroid therapy has a remarkable impact on symptoms, which can be highly unpleasant, especially for the elderly. Thus, it is tempting to prescribe steroid therapy for all patients with clinical manifestations. Albendazole (Albenza), 800 mg (15 mg per kg) daily, should be prescribed for 10 days with prednisone, 0.75 mg per kg, for 10 days. Albendazole appears to be preferable to thiabendazole or mebendazole because of its markedly better tolerability.

Anthelmintic drugs can also be used as prophylactic drugs during the incubation phase in persons known to have ingested infected meat.

CAT-SCRATCH DISEASE

method of
ANDREW M. MARGILETH, M.D.
Mercer University School of Medicine
Macon, Georgia

Cat-scratch disease (CSD), a zoonotic bacterial infection, commonly manifests as a chronic (3 weeks or longer) lymphadenitis in the cervical or axillary areas that is usually benign and self-limited. About 24,000 cases occur annually in the United States, resulting in more than 2000

TABLE 1. **Clinical Features in 1722 Patients with Cat-Scratch Disease, April 1975 to December 31, 1997**

Symptoms and Signs	% of Patients*	Duration (Days)
Adenopathy	100.0†	14–730
Adenopathy only	50.0	14–730
Malaise/fatigue	29.5	1–21
Fever (38.3 to 41.2°C)	28.0	1–65
Headache	13.0	1–7
Anorexia, emesis	14.5	3–30
Splenomegaly	9.5	7–30
Sore throat	7.0	1–5
Exanthem	5.0	5–17
Conjunctivitis	3.3	1–20
Seizures/coma	2.7	1–5
Arthralgia	2.5‡	3–42‡
Blindness	2.0	30–200

*N = 1722.
†Three adults with systemic disease, neuroretinitis had no adenopathy.
‡Data from 1989 through 1997.

hospitalizations. Contact with a cat, especially a kitten, or cat fleas is a major risk factor for the disease. CSD is caused by a gram-negative pleomorphic bacillus *(Bartonella henselae)* that has been cultured from skin, blood, and lymph nodes. The adenopathy (10 mm or more) is commonly regional and is often tender initially. In one third of our patients multifocal adenitis occurred. Following cat contact (95%) or scratches (66%) but before the adenopathy, the patient or parent often notes a primary inoculation skin papule or eye lesion. Adenopathy invariably persists for several weeks to months and then gradually resolves spontaneously. However, 12% of patients have atypical manifestations, including the oculoglandular syndrome of Parinaud, encephalopathy, systemic disease, neuroretinitis, granulomatous hepatitis, thrombocytopenic purpura, osteomyelitis, thoracopulmonary disease, and, rarely, breast tumor. Clinical features in 1722 patients with CSD are noted (Table 1).

About 80% of patients are younger than 21 years of age. Systemic disease (severe malaise, weight loss, prolonged fevers, fatigue, encephalopathy) occurs in 2 to 3% of patients. Morbidity appears to be greater in adolescents and adults. Severe disseminated disease characterized by hepatic and/or splenic abscesses, neuroretinitis, pleuritis, and generalized lymphadenitis with epithelioid angiomatosis and granulomatous osteomyelitis has been reported in both immunocompetent and immunocompromised patients. Bacillary angiomatosis and bacillary peliosis (liver, spleen) are vascular proliferative manifestations of *Bartonella* infection *(B. henselae, Bartonella quintana)* that occur predominately in patients infected with the human immunodeficiency virus and affect skin, bone, brain, and lymph nodes.

Tuberculin tests should be performed routinely to rule out tuberculosis. Cat-scratch skin test antigens used since 1947, when available, provide a reliable and specific means of diagnosis. The diagnosis of CSD is based on clinical features and is confirmed with specific serologic studies. Performance of a *Bartonella* polymerase chain reaction (PCR) hybridization assay on lymph node and/or abscess aspirates or a biopsy specimen provide the highest diagnostic sensitivity. Serologic tests for diagnosis are available from several commercial laboratories. However, enzyme-linked immunoassay to detect IgM *B. henselae* antibodies are only 71% sensitive in patients who fulfilled two or more criteria for CSD. The Centers for Disease Control and Prevention perform the immunofluorescent antibody assay for *B. henselae* antibody, which has a 95% sensitivity. Serologic test results are usually negative during the first week of illness. Diagnostic criteria are noted in Table 2.

TABLE 2. **Diagnosis of Cat-Scratch Disease**

Lymphadenopathy (≥10 mm) present ≥3 weeks.*

1. Cat or flea contact: regional inoculation lesion (skin papule, eye granuloma, mucous membrane) and/or scratch mark.
2. Laboratory data negative for other infectious causes of adenopathy; sterile pus aspirated from node, polymerase chain reaction assay positive; *Bartonella henselae* or *Afipia felis,* highest sensitivity.
3. Positive enzyme-linked immunoassay or immunofluorescent antibody assay serology test >1:64 for *B. henselae* or *Bartonella clarridgeiae*. Fourfold rise in titer between acute and convalescent specimens is definitive.
4. Biopsy of node, skin, liver, bone, or eye granuloma showing granulomatous inflammation compatible with cat-scratch disease; positive Warthin-Starry silver stain.

*Three of four criteria confirm the diagnosis; in an atypical case all four criteria may be needed.

THERAPY

General

Management usually consists primarily of careful observation over several (2 to 6) months, during which time spontaneous involution of the lymphadenopathy should occur. Bed rest is rarely necessary; however, extreme fatigue may be lessened by frequent bed rest. Aspirin (65 mg per kg of body weight per day in 6 doses) or acetaminophen (60 mg per kg of body weight per day in 6 doses) is effective in treating the pain of tender adenitis. The local application of moist heat may provide relief and decrease swelling over several days. I have noted less pain, more rapid involution, and occasionally spontaneous drainage, especially from fluctuant lesions, with the application of warm, moist compresses to areas of lymph node swelling and to primary inoculation sites for 1 to 2 hours, four to six times daily.

If suppuration occurs (15% of patients), incision and drainage should be avoided because chronic sinus tract discharge may occur and persist for several months. Needle aspiration relieves painful adenopathy and provides material for cultures or PCR tests. After one or two aspirates, the patient usually becomes symptom-free within 24 to 48 hours. The technique for needle aspiration is as follows: after the area is washed with povidone-iodine cleanser, an 18- or 19-gauge needle is inserted through 1 to 2 cm of normal, unanesthetized skin at the base of the mass to avoid forming a chronic sinus tract in the event that a tuberculous lesion is present. Surgical excision of the nodes is usually not indicated unless one suspects a noninfectious etiology, such as a neoplasm.

Specific

A relatively healthy child, adolescent, or adult with typical CSD does not require antibiotic therapy. Re-

TABLE 3. **Antibiotic Therapy**

Antibiotic*	Route	Dosage	Frequency	Duration
Azithromycin (Zithromax)	PO	5–12 mg/kg (max 500 mg/d)	Once daily	7–10 d
Ciprofloxacin (Cipro)	PO	20–30 mg/kg	q 12 h	10–21 d or more
Gentamicin (Garamycin)	IM or IV	5 mg/kg	q 8 h	5–10 d
Rifampin (Rifadin)	PO	10–20 mg/kg (max 600 mg/d)	q 8–12 h	10–21 d
TMP-SMX (Bactrim, Septra)	PO	10–20 mg/kg TMP 50–100 mg/kg SMX	q 8–12 h	10–14 d or more

*A higher dose may be necessary if lymphadenopathy is over 5 cm or an abscess is present.
Abbreviation: TMP-SMX = trimethoprim-sulfamethoxazole.

cent literature reports that each of the following five drugs has been found efficacious in more than 60% of patients with systemic symptoms and/or severe lymphadenitis. Azithromycin (Zithromax), 5 to 12 mg per kg per day once daily for 7 to 10 days, is 90% effective (maximum daily dose is 500 mg). Trimethoprim-sulfamethoxazole (TMP-SMX [Bactrim, Septra]), 10 mg per kg of the trimethoprim component two or three times daily for 10 to 14 days, may effect prompt improvement. Rifampin (Rifadin), 10 to 20 mg per kg per day in 2 to 3 doses for 10 to 21 days, is 80% effective (maximum daily dose is 600 mg). In patients older than 12 years of age, ciprofloxacin (Cipro), 20 to 30 mg per kg per 24 hours in two divided doses for 10 to 14 or more days, may be very effective. In severely ill patients gentamicin sulfate, 5 mg per kg per 24 hours, given every 8 hours intramuscularly, was shown to be quite effective in selected patients (Table 3).

Other commonly used antibiotics are ineffective in patients with typical CSD. Paradoxically, CSD in patients with acquired immune deficiency syndrome (AIDS) has responded dramatically to erythromycin, doxycycline, or antimycobacterial antibiotics employed for several weeks to several months. Oral clarithromycin (Biaxin) 7.5 mg per kg in 2 doses, maximum daily dose, 1 gram, or azithromycin, 5 to 12 mg per kg once daily, maximum daily adult dose 600 mg, is also effective therapy for immunocompromised patients.

Oral glucocorticoids cannot be recommended in spite of anecdotal reports of several severely ill patients with systemic disease who responded to prednisone 2 mg per kg per 24 hours for 5 to 7 days.

PROGNOSIS

The prognosis for recovery is excellent. Lymphadenopathy usually regresses spontaneously in 2 to 6 months. One attack of CSD appears to confer lifelong immunity in children and adolescents. However, three adults have been reported with a recurrence of lymphadenopathy 6 to 13 months after their initial diagnosis. Fatal complications have not been documented. Most patients with encephalitis and neuroretinitis have recovered completely.

PREVENTION

The patient with CSD does not require isolation or quarantine; no evidence exists that the disease can spread directly from one person to another. Because the cats involved are invariably healthy, disposal is not recommended. The kitten appears to carry the bacillus for a few months. Control of flea infestation in pets is essential for immunocompromised persons. About 5% of other family members acquire the disease. Because 31% of U.S. households (about 60 million) own cats, and a larger number of households own cats worldwide, CSD is difficult to prevent. Preventive measures include declawing and regular nail clipping of young cats, keeping cats indoors, flea control, proper handling of the litter box, washing hands after close contact with a cat or especially a kitten, and washing bites and scratches with soap and water.

TULAREMIA

method of
CHARLES S. BERENSON, M.D.
State University of New York at Buffalo and Veterans Affairs Western New York Healthcare System
Buffalo, New York

Tularemia is an acute infectious zoonotic illness, caused by a small, gram-negative coccobacillus, *Francisella tularensis.* Although it was first isolated from wild rodents in Tulare County, California, and reported in 1912, worldwide outbreaks have been recorded. The onset of illness is relatively sudden and includes nonspecific findings of fever, chills, headache, myalgias, cough, pharyngitis, and fatigue. Unusual presenting features have included erythema multiforme and erythema nodosum. The latter was present, along with circulating immune complexes, in 13 of 98 victims in an outbreak in Turkey. Splenic nodules, presumed to be abscesses, may be seen on ultrasonography. The incubation period after exposure is 3 to 5 days (range 1 to 21 days). Classic syndromes of the disease are highly varied and often depend on the route of inoculation, the virulence of the strain, and the immune status of the victim. Division into clinical syndromes is somewhat arbitrary, and considerable overlap often occurs.

1. Ulceroglandular disease, the most common presentation (21 to 87%), is characterized by a painful ulcer at the site of inoculation and painful regional lymphadenopathy.
2. Glandular disease (3 to 20% in the United States) manifests with regional lymphadenopathy but without a skin ulcer. Both forms may resemble nodular lymphangitis,

which may also be caused by *Nocardia, Sporothrix*, and atypical mycobacteria, among others.

3. Typhoidal disease (5 to 30%) may be difficult to diagnose, as patients lack classic lymphadenopathy and skin ulcers and present with systemic symptoms only.

4. Tularemia pneumonia may appear with any form of the disease; it includes radiographic pleural effusions in 21 to 31% of patients. Effusions, which are classically exudative, with low glucose concentration and lymphocytic predominance, can be mistaken for tuberculosis.

5. Other syndromes include oculoglandular (<5%), oropharyngeal, and, less commonly, meningitis, osteomyelitis, and pericarditis.

Mortality with antibiotic treatment of uncomplicated disease is 1 to 3%, with higher mortality for typhoidal tularemia and tularemia complicated by secondary pneumonia. Severity of disease ranges from a mild, self-limited illness to fulminant septic shock or adult respiratory distress syndrome.

F. tularensis is primarily a pathogen of wild animals, but it also is found in domestic animals. Lagomorphs (rabbits and hares) and rodents, particularly squirrels, muskrats, and beavers, are the most important reservoirs. Transmission of disease from infected animals to humans may occur via several routes. Arthropod-borne transmission (ticks, deer flies, and mosquitoes) is particularly important in North America, where tick bites account for more than 50% of cases, particularly west of the Mississippi River. Major tick vectors in the United States include the lone star tick *(Amblyomma americanus)*, the wood tick *(Dermacentor andersoni)*, and the dog tick *(Dermacentor variabilis)*. Infection may also occur by direct contact with infected animal tissues, inhalation of aerosolized organisms, ingestion of infected meat or water, and bites from infected animals. Infections have been reported from domestic animal exposure, particularly cat bites. Disease may begin with the introduction of as few as 10 organisms intradermally or by aerosol.

In the United States tularemia has been reported in all 50 states but is most concentrated in Arkansas, Missouri, and Oklahoma. Increased seasonal incidence in spring and summer accompanies tick-borne disease. Approximately 150 to 300 cases are reported in the United States annually. Occupations that pose a risk for contracting tularemia include hunter, trapper, farmer, veterinarian, cook, meat handler, and laboratory worker.

Traditional teaching has supported a major role for T lymphocytes and macrophages in clearance of *F. tularensis* and survival of infection. Animal studies indicate a great overlap in specific subpopulations of T lymphocytes that are required for protective immunity. Cytokines, particularly interferon-γ, and tumor necrosis factor-α are involved in protective responses. Other studies support the importance of T lymphocyte–independent host defenses, including neutrophilic responses, in early phases of infection. Bacterial lipopolysaccharide and membrane lipoproteins may elicit protective host responses. Transfer of protective immunity to mice, with serum of vaccinated volunteers, also supports a protective role for B lymphocytes.

Although increased incidence is not documented in immunocompromised individuals, an unusual presentation of typhoidal tularemia in a child with acquired immune deficiency syndrome (AIDS) was described and included negative serologic test results for antibodies to *F. tularensis*. Tularemia pneumonia was also the presenting illness of underlying chronic granulomatous disease (CGD) in one report.

DIAGNOSIS

Because immediate laboratory diagnosis is often not possible, the diagnosis often rests on strong clinical suspicion when appropriate history and presentation are given. In these instances, empirical antibiotic therapy is given before the laboratory diagnosis is made. Definitive laboratory diagnosis may be made by isolation of *F. tularensis* from cultures of blood, lymph node aspirates, pleural fluid, sputum, or ulcers. In one instance, growth from only 10 to 20 μL of a lymph node aspirate grew *F. tularensis* 12 days after inoculation into a nonradiometric blood culture bottle. Media must include special supplements, including cysteine, to support growth. Because isolation of *F. tularensis* poses a danger to laboratory personnel, the clinical laboratory should be warned to implement precautions to prevent transmission. Serologic diagnosis, demonstrating a single positive agglutinating antibody titer of 1:160 or greater or a fourfold rise over the ensuing 2 to 6 weeks, has also been used. Agglutination tests may be positive by the end of the second week of illness and peak by 4 to 5 weeks. Antibodies may have low titer cross-reactivity with antigens of *Brucella, Proteus*, and *Yersinia* species. Reports of persistent immune responses years after exposure indicate that caution is warranted in interpretation of single, intermediate-titer serologic measurements.

Given the fastidious growth requirements of the organism, its potential danger to laboratory personnel, and delays in obtaining firm serologic diagnoses, alternative diagnostic methods have been investigated that may facilitate rapid diagnosis in the future. Direct immunofluorescence of organisms from infected tissues may be available from state public health laboratories. Successful identification from ulcers by polymerase chain reaction (PCR) was documented in 29 of 40 serologically confirmed cases of ulceroglandular disease in one report. Immunoelectron microscopy has been used with success on laboratory strains but has not yet been clinically utilized.

TREATMENT

The drug of first choice for all forms of tularemia, with the possible exception of meningitis, is streptomycin. One study indicated a 97% cure rate and no relapses among individuals treated with streptomycin. The effective dosage in adults is 7.5 to 10 mg per kg intramuscularly every 12 hours for 7 to 14 days. Shorter treatment regimens have been associated with more frequent relapses. Children account for a significant percentage of cases and should receive 20 to 40 mg per kg per day in two divided doses. Severely ill patients may be treated with higher doses (up to 30 mg per kg per day). Doses higher than 2 grams per day do not increase clinical efficacy and are associated with increased ototoxicity and nephrotoxicity. Dosages must be adjusted for patients with renal insufficiency to minimize toxicities. Rarely, initiation of streptomycin therapy may induce a Jarisch-Herxheimer reaction.

Tetracycline and chloramphenicol have also been used to treat tularemia. Both are bacteriostatic, possibly accounting for the higher relapse rates associated with their use. Cure rates of 88% and 77%, respectively, have been reported, with tetracycline having a 12% relapse rate. Tetracycline is given at 2 grams per day, and should not be used in children younger than 9 years of age and in pregnant or lactating women. Chloramphenicol (50 to 100 mg per kg per day intravenously) may be added to streptomycin for the treatment of meningitis.

Studies into the efficacy of alternative agents were in part prompted by lack of availability of streptomycin in the United States for a period before 1993. Gentamicin (Garamycin), 3 to 5 mg per kg per day intravenously in divided doses, is an effective alternative. Recent reports indicate an 86% cure rate and a 6% relapse rate. Retrospective review also supports gentamicin as a reasonable alternative in children. By contrast, the cure rate with tobramycin was reported as only 50%.

Third-generation cephalosporins have also been used as alternative agents. One report documented eight cases of treatment failure with outpatient ceftriaxone, despite prior acceptable in vitro susceptibilities. The latter point has prompted caution regarding the clinical usefulness of in vitro susceptibility data in selection of antibiotics to treat tularemia infections. Retrospective review also confirmed high failure rates for these agents in children.

Case reports have suggested a role for quinolone antibiotics in treatment of tularemia, possibly owing to efficacy against surviving intracellular *F. tularensis*. Animal studies have demonstrated improved outcome with liposomal ciprofloxacin,* administered intranasally and intravenously. Successes include oral treatment of an individual who relapsed after treatment with gentamicin. Isolated reports offer limited experience but provide encouragement for broader study of quinolones in treatment of tularemia.

Erythromycin has been used with variable success. In vitro susceptibilities have been highly variable. Therefore, use of macrolide antibiotics should not be relied on in seriously ill patients. Poor in vitro susceptibilities and clinical failures have also been documented with penicillins, ceftazidime (Fortaz), and carbapenems (imipenem-cilastatin [Primaxin] and meropenem [Merrem]). Nonetheless, one report noted successful treatment with imipenem.

PREVENTION

The best method of prevention is to minimize direct contact with infected animals. Individuals at risk may avoid exposure by wearing gloves, masks, and protective eye coverings while skinning or processing wild animals. Similarly, avoidance of contaminated wells is essential. Antibiotic prophylaxis for exposed individuals is not recommended. However, because streptomycin given in the incubation period after experimental inoculation is effective, accidental laboratory inoculations may be preventively treated with intramuscular streptomycin. Because person-to-person transmission does not occur, special isolation is not needed in hospitalized patients. Use of insect repellent and tight fitting clothing around wrists and ankles provides protection against arthropod-borne infection.

A live attenuated vaccine is available through the Centers for Disease Control and Prevention. It has provided partial protection in laboratory workers who work frequently with *F. tularensis*. Its use is not practical for protection against tick-borne tularemia. Murine model data indicate that immune response to the vaccine is relatively specific for *F. tularensis*. Previous infection generally results in lifelong immunity.

*Not FDA approved for this indication.

SALMONELLOSIS

method of
DANIEL RODRIGUE, M.D.
University of Southern California School of Medicine
Los Angeles, California

Salmonella infections increased over the past decade. The reasons are probably multifactorial, including changes in food production and delivery, increased numbers of immunocompromised hosts, and changes in the virulence of the organism. Salmonellae are named for the pathologist D. E. Salmon, who first isolated *Salmonella choleraesuis* from porcine intestines. Salmonellae are gram-negative, non–spore-forming, facultatively anaerobic bacilli that are motile (except for *Salmonella gallinarum-pullorum*), oxidase negative, and catalase positive; they do not ferment lactose and sucrose while producing acid, hydrogen sulfide, and gas (except *Salmonella typhi*). There are more than 2000 serotypes, and classification systems are confusing. Although the Kauffman-White classification scheme reports serovars based on different O (somatic), Vi (capsular), and H (flagellar) antigens, most laboratories perform simple agglutination reactions to the O antigens and place them into common serogroups, which include group A *(paratyphi)*, group B *(paratyphi, typhimurium)*, group C *(paratyphi, choleraesuis)*, group D *(enteritidis, typhi, dublin)*, and nontypable *(arizonae)*. Further epidemiologic differentiation of salmonellae can be obtained through antimicrobial resistance, plasmid profiles, phage typing, restriction fragment length polymorphisms, and pulsed-field gel electrophoresis. There are about 10 to 15 serotypes that cause the majority of human disease.

EPIDEMIOLOGY OF NONTYPHOIDAL SALMONELLOSIS

Salmonellae are animal and human-based commensals and pathogens. Most salmonellae have animal reservoirs (except *S. typhi, Salmonella sendai,* and *S. paratyphi A* and *B*—human). The most common serotypes associated with human disease are *S. typhimurium* and *S. enteriditis*. Fecal-oral transmission is the most important route. There are some specific epidemiologic associations with serotypes such as *S. arizonae* and ingestion of rattlesnakes (either through folk medicine "capsules" or as food), *Salmonella poona* (melons), *Salmonella chester* (cantaloupes), *Salmonella janiania* (tomatoes), *S. dublin* (unpasteurized milk and cow liver injections for malignancy), *Salmonella munchen* (contaminated marijuana), *Salmonella stanley* (alfalfa sprouts), and *S. enteritidis* (raw eggs plus others).

The most important reptile reservoir for *Salmonella* was pet turtles, but currently it is iguanas. The largest *Salmonella* outbreak occurred in Chicago in 1984 when approximately 200,000 persons acquired *S. typhimurium* through ingestion of contaminated milk. A breakdown in a pasteurization plant was thought to be responsible for the contaminated milk.

Antimicrobial resistance within *Salmonella* increased over the past decade and is continuing to increase. A multidrug-resistant strain of *S. typhimurium* known as DT104 (resistant to ampicillin, chloramphenicol, streptomycin, sulfonamides, and tetracycline) was reported in the United States in 1997. Ampicillin resistance may approach 50% in some areas.

HOST FACTORS AND SALMONELLOSIS

Salmonellae survive poorly at a pH of 1.5 or less but well at a pH of 4.0 or greater. Host risk factors that increase the risk of disease include a condition with reduced gastric acidity, such as induced or acquired achlorhydria, therapy with antacids or H_2 blockers, or gastric resection; decreased gastric motility with bacterial overgrowth; or alteration in the colonization resistance conferred by normal intestinal flora through the use of broad-spectrum antibiotics, purgatives, or bowel surgery. Volunteer studies have shown that nearly 10^6 to 10^7 organisms are needed in a normal host to cause disease, whereas as few as 10^2 to 10^3 organisms may cause disease in those with an identified host risk factor. Syndromes that are also associated with increased salmonellosis include acquired immune deficiency syndrome (AIDS) and syndromes with dysfunction of the reticuloendothelial system, including sickle cell anemia and other hemoglobinopathies, bartonellosis, malaria, and louse-borne relapsing fever.

PATHOGENESIS

Salmonellae are usually ingested through contaminated food or water, pass through the gastric acid barrier, and multiply in the small (Peyer's patches) and large intestines. Disease mechanisms are still not entirely understood and are probably the result of either production of enterotoxin or penetration of the epithelial cells, or both.

CLINICAL ILLNESS

Salmonella causes a number of clinical syndromes, which include enterocolitis (about 70% of cases), bacteremia, enteric fever, and the carrier state.

SYNDROMES AND THEIR TREATMENT

Enterocolitis

There are at least 2 to 4 million cases of *Salmonella* enterocolitis in the United States per year. Most cases are associated with ingestion of contaminated food or water.

Clinical

Salmonella enterocolitis is often clinically indistinguishable from that caused by common diarrheal pathogens such as *Campylobacter* species, *Escherichia coli, Clostridium difficile,* and *Yersinia enterocolitica.* It has an incubation period of about 48 hours (6 to 96 hours). A shorter incubation period may be associated with a larger inoculum. Onset is abrupt and includes nausea and crampy abdominal pain (>90%) with nonspecific headache, myalgias, and chills followed by loose, watery diarrhea. Most persons present with loose stool without blood or mucus, but a few contain one or both. Vomiting is not common. Fever (101 to 102°F) occurs in about 50 to 70% and usually resolves within 72 hours. The diarrhea in a normal host is self-limited and is less than 10 days. Positive blood cultures occur in less than 5% of immunocompetent patients. Persistent or high fever (104°F) may suggest bacteremia or metastatic infection. Immunocompromised patients are also predisposed to more severe disease. The mortality from enterocolitis is low (<0.5%) and more frequent in the elderly, immunocompromised, and diabetics. A reactive arthropathy may be seen in 7% of patients after infection is resolved, especially in those who have the HLA-B27 phenotype.

The diagnosis of infection is from stool or blood cultures and is usually available within 48 to 72 hours. Polymorphonuclear cells are often present in stool but may be absent. Serology is not a reliable diagnostic tool. The white blood cell count is usually normal or mildly elevated, with a left shift. Leukopenia with bands may indicate possible bacteremia. The mean duration of stool carriage after infection is 4 to 5 weeks, and less than 10% will carry it for 10 to 12 weeks.

Treatment

The most important aspect in the treatment of diarrhea of any cause (including salmonellosis) is fluid and electrolyte replacement. Patients should be assessed for the degree of dehydration and potential electrolyte deficits. Those who are severely dehydrated (>10% loss of body weight), in shock or coma, or showing signs of systemic toxicity or severe underlying diseases should be hospitalized for volume and electrolyte replacement. The majority of patients, however, can be treated successfully with oral rehydration therapy (ORT). Oral rehydration solutions are based on the concept that sodium and water absorption in the small intestine are facilitated by the active transport of glucose. The ORT solution recommended by the World Health Organization (WHO) includes sodium (90 mmol per liter), potassium (20 mmol per liter), chloride (80 mmol per liter), citrate (30 mmol per liter), and carbohydrate (20 grams per liter). It can be approximated by adding 1 teaspoon of table salt, ¼ teaspoon of baking soda, ⅛ teaspoon of salt substitute, and 8 teaspoons of sugar to 1 liter of water. The WHO solution should be supplemented with free water when used as a maintenance replacement because of its high sodium content. Other replacement fluids that are used frequently include Pedialyte and Infalyte. It should be noted that solutions such as Gatorade contain a reasonable concentration of sodium (about 23.5 mmol per liter) but less than 1 mmol per liter of potassium;

apple juice and orange juice are higher in potassium (25 to 50 mmol per liter) but low in sodium.

Antimotility agents such as loperamide (Imodium) or atropine-diphenoxylate (Lomotil) are not recommended because they are associated with increased severity of illness and bacteremia.

Antibiotics do not affect the clinical course for the immunocompetent and may prolong carriage and increase relapse rates. Antibiotic therapy, however, may be indicated for the immunocompromised patient to decrease bacteremia in such groups as newborns (<3 months, or 3 to 12 months who appear ill on re-evaluation, pending results of blood cultures); patients with AIDS; patients older than 50 years, especially those with anatomic cardiovascular abnormalities, sickle cell and hemoglobinopathies, joint prostheses, and inflammatory bowel disease; and organ transplant recipients. It may also be indicated if the patient appears "toxic," with a high fever (104°F) or other signs of possible bacteremia. Antimicrobial susceptibility should guide the choice of therapy. In patients in high-risk groups, for whom antibiotics are considered, ciprofloxacin (Cipro), 500 mg twice daily, ofloxacin (Floxin), 400 mg twice daily, or norfloxacin* (Noroxin), 400 mg twice daily, are effective. Quinolones are contraindicated in children and pregnant patients. Hospitalized patients may also be treated with intravenous third-generation cephalosporins such as cefotaxime (Claforan), 1 to 2 grams every 8 hours for adults or 100 to 200 mg per kg per day in three or four divided doses for children, or ceftriaxone (Rocephin), 1 gram every 12 hours for adults. If the organism is susceptible, trimethoprim-sulfamethoxazole (Bactrim, Septra), 5 to 8 mg of trimethoprim per kg every 12 hours for children, or 1 double-strength tablet (160 mg trimethoprim/800 mg sulfamethoxazole) every 12 hours for adults; or ampicillin, 50 mg per kg orally to 100 mg per kg per day intravenously, each in four divided doses for children, or 2 to 4 grams per day in four divided doses for adults, may be administered. The duration of therapy may range from 5 to 7 days depending on the clinical presentation. The presence of bacteremia or systemic infection would prolong the duration of antibiotics.

Bacteremia

Salmonella bacteremia occurs in about 5 to 10% of all cases of salmonellosis. It is most common in the young (<5 years) or older (>60 years) patient; in immunocompromised patients with such diseases as AIDS, hematologic malignancies or solid tumors, collagen-vascular diseases, sarcoidosis, or diabetes; in steroid users; and in transplantation patients. Certain serotypes are also associated with bacteremia such as *S. cholerasuis* (>50% cases) and *S. dublin.* Episodes of *Salmonella* bacteremia are associated with high mortality and septic complications, as well as relapse. The mortality rate from one recent study was 12%, and 16% of patients with bacteremia had at least one relapse. Relapse may be associated with AIDS, leukopenia, or concurrent infection with schistosomiasis. *Salmonella* has a propensity to metastasize, especially to sites of pre-existing abnormality. Common sites of metastatic infection include intravascular (such as atherosclerotic aorta aneurysms), skeletal (especially long bones, chondrosternal junction, and spine, and suppurative arthritis commonly in knees, shoulders, hips, and sacroiliac joints), and the meninges (principally in young children). An aortoduodenal fistula is a well-described complication. The risk of endovascular infection in a patient older than 50 years may be as high as 25% in those with bacteremia. Endocarditis, however, is rare and occurs in less than 5% of patients.

Clinical

Fever and gastrointestinal symptoms are present in more than 90% of patients without underlying disease. A clinically apparent enteritis, however, is often lacking (<20%) among immunosuppressed hosts (or the very elderly) who develop *Salmonella* bacteremia. In this subset of patients, a new infection or asymptomatic carriage may be a sufficient condition for the development of bacteremia. The high incidence of *Salmonella* bacteremias in hematologic malignancies may be partially explained by episodes of hemolysis often associated with this disease. Manifestations of *Salmonella* bacteremia are similar to those of other gram-negative bacteremias, namely, fever, chills, myalgias, and headache and occasional abdominal cramps. The differential diagnosis includes all acute infectious and noninfectious causes of fever, including those with bacteremias. The laboratory may reveal a relative leukopenia (with a left shift) and thrombocytopenia and mild elevations of liver transaminases. The diagnosis is confirmed by a positive blood culture result.

Treatment

Third-generation cephalosporins such as cefotaxime, 1 to 2 grams every 8 hours for adults or 100 to 200 mg per kg per day in three or four divided doses for children, or ceftriaxone, 1 gram every 12 hours for adults, or a fluoroquinolone such as ciprofloxacin or ofloxacin may be the best choices for treatment or to prevent relapses. Data do not indicate a clear choice. Duration of treatment is for 2 weeks in those without localization of organisms to metastatic sites. Surgical removal of foreign bodies is often needed to cure localized infection. Patients with endovascular lesions need surgical therapy in addition to medical therapy, especially those with aortic infection. Patients who resolve their bacteremic episodes with persistent leukopenia or corticosteroid treatment or who have recurrent episodes of bacteremia, especially in the setting of AIDS, should be considered for prophylactic therapy with a fluoroquinolone.

Enteric Fever

The term "enteric fever" was introduced in 1847 in an attempt to replace the term "typhoid fever" and

*Not FDA approved for this indication.

avoid the confusion with typhus. After ingestion, *S. paratyphi* (and *S. typhi*) bacilli reach the lamina propria of the small intestine. Despite being ingested by macrophages, they are not killed and remain in the reticuloendothelial system of the body, incubating about 10 to 14 days before the onset of clinical enteric fever. Clinical illness is accompanied by a fairly sustained "secondary" bacteremia. The *S. paratyphi* and *S. typhi* have strong predilections for the gallbladder, especially in females, the elderly, or those with previous gallbladder pathology. The gallbladder becomes chronically infected in approximately 2 to 5% (less with *S. paratyphi*).

Clinical

Nontyphoidal enteric fever is a severe systemic illness characterized by fever and abdominal symptoms. Although it is clinically indistinguishable from typhoid fever, which is discussed elsewhere in this publication, nontyphoidal enteric fever is a slightly milder illness. Higher morbidity and mortality are associated with delayed diagnosis and treatment and infection with the human immunodeficiency virus (HIV).

A number of infections can mimic enteric fever syndromes, including *Yersinia enterocolitica, Yersinia pseudotuberculosis, Campylobacter fetus, Francisella tularensis, Brucella* species, acute bartonellosis, rat-bite fever *(Streptobacillus moniliformis, Spirillum minus)*, leptospirosis, *Borrelia recurrentis,* rickettsial infections, *Babesia microti,* viral hepatitis, and Epstein-Barr virus infection. The differential diagnosis of a traveler with a fever, abdominal pain, and hepatosplenomegaly may also include malaria, amebic liver abscess, visceral leishmaniasis, and viral syndromes such as dengue fever. Although the above list is not complete, a thorough history for epidemiologic exposure and a physical examination may yield the diagnosis.

Treatment

The treatment of nontyphoidal enteric fever is similar to that of typhoid fever, and the reader is referred to the article on typhoid fever. Third-generation cephalosporins ceftriaxone and cefotaxime are effective agents for nontyphoidal enteric fever as are the fluoroquinolones ciprofloxacin or ofloxacin; however, treatment should be adjusted once the antimicrobial susceptibility results are known. Most studies administer the agents for 10 to 14 days, but smaller studies outside the United States have administered ceftriaxone or fluoroquinolones (ciprofloxacin or ofloxacin) for only 5 to 7 days, although not all studies have had adequate follow-up for relapse. Relapse usually occurs within 2 to 6 weeks of the end of therapy. Retreatment with the same antimicrobials (usually the organism remains sensitive) for a similar duration of time is appropriate. Clinically stable, compliant, healthy, young adult patients can finish treatment with an effective oral agent such as a quinolone after 1 to 5 days of intravenous therapy.

Adjunctive therapy with intravenous fluids and nutrition remain important in the care of the patient.

The Carrier State

The normal course after *Salmonella* enterocolitis is to resolve the infection. The mean duration of excretion of *Salmonella* in the stool, however, is 4 to 6 weeks after infection. Chronic carriers (>1 year) include less than 1% of those with nontyphoidal *Salmonella* enterocolitis (higher with *S. typhi* infections). The persistence of the organism is often associated with the biliary tract. Patients are usually asymptomatic. Clearance of the organism may be attempted with oral quinolones such as ciprofloxacin or ofloxacin or ampicillin (if sensitive) plus probenecid with a treatment course of 4 to 6 weeks. Cholecystectomy may be necessary in patients with recurrent salmonellosis, chronic carriage, and gallbladder disease with biliary calculi.

Other Sites of Disease

Salmonella osteomyelitis is commonly observed in patients with sickle cell disease. *Salmonella* infections of other sites include parotitis, urinary tract infections (including renal abscess, pyelonephritis, cystitis), neck abscess, hepatitis, thyroiditis, intra-abdominal abscess (such as splenic, pancreatic), pyomyositis, pulmonary abscess, mediastinitis, and mesenteric lymphadenitis.

PREVENTION

Salmonellosis can be prevented by proper food handling and education about the potential hazards of pets, such as reptiles. Immunocompromised patients such as those with AIDS should avoid raw eggs, unpasteurized milk and dairy products, and undercooked meat products.

TYPHOID FEVER

method of
ARIF R. SARWARI, M.D., M.S.
Aga Khan University Hospital
Karachi, Pakistan

and

ROBERT EDELMAN, M.D.
University of Maryland School of Medicine
Baltimore, Maryland

Typhoid fever remains a major global infectious disease with an estimated annual world incidence of 12 million cases with 500,000 deaths. In the United States, there are about 300 cases annually, and most of these occur in travelers who have recently returned from countries with high incidences of typhoid fever, such as Mexico, Peru, Pakistan, and India. The etiologic agents, *Salmonella typhi* and *Sal-*

monella paratyphi, have no reservoir other than the human carrier. Thus, typhoid or enteric fever remains largely a preventable food-borne disease whose transmission can be decreased greatly through improved sanitation and personal hygienic measures.

CLINICAL FEATURES

Transmission occurs through the ingestion of contaminated water or food. Persons at the extremes of age and those on antacids or with achlorhydria or gastric resection are at higher risk for developing infection. The organisms multiply in mononuclear phagocytes of Peyer's patches in the ileum and spread via the bloodstream to the liver, spleen, and bone marrow, where further intracellular multiplication occurs. After an incubation period of about 2 weeks, patients develop gradually worsening fever, chills, myalgia, headache, and fatigue. Most patients will complain of abdominal discomfort or distention, often with diarrhea or constipation. A few patients develop cough or rose spots early in the disease. Most patients have relative bradycardia, splenomegaly, hepatomegaly, and mild abdominal tenderness. After 2 to 3 weeks of untreated disease, mental confusion or delirium, rectal bleeding, or intestinal perforation may develop. Such patients are at greatest risk of dying.

DIAGNOSIS

The isolation of *S. typhi* from blood or feces confirms the clinical impression of typhoid fever. Blood cultures may be positive in only 50 to 70% of patients. Stool or rectal swab cultures will yield the organism in about 90% of patients if many attempts are made, but such cultures are positive in only 10 to 20% of patients early in their illness. Bone marrow culture, which is *S. typhi*–positive more often than blood, is advised for patients presenting after they have used antibiotics. A combination of cultures, including duodenal "string tests," provides the most sensitive diagnostic approach. Some laboratories employ the Widal anti-*Salmonella* agglutinins to detect antibodies against O or H antigens of *S. typhi.* Most patients with typhoid fever show elevated titers of these antibodies, but the results are not diagnostically specific, because many healthy persons who have lived in endemic areas have elevated titers.

TREATMENT

Antimicrobial Drugs

Local antimicrobial susceptibility patterns of *S. typhi* to the first-line drugs—ampicillin, chloramphenicol, and trimethoprim-sulfamethoxazole (Bactrim, Septra)—should be used to guide therapy while awaiting antibiotic sensitivity results. Chloramphenicol became the drug of choice in 1948 when it was shown to reduce the 15 to 20% mortality without antibiotics to 1% and to reduce the febrile course from 2 to 4 weeks to 3 to 5 days. This drug is inexpensive and remains the drug of choice in countries in which most *S. typhi* strains remain susceptible; these include Mexico, countries of Central and South America, and most countries of southern Europe and the Mediterranean region. In the United States and other industrialized countries, physicians are reluctant to employ chloramphenicol, because rarely it may induce idiosyncratic bone marrow aplasia. Accordingly, physicians in the United States have chosen alternative antimicrobial drugs (Table 1).

In 1989, strains of *S. typhi* showing multidrug resistance (MDR) to chloramphenicol, ampicillin, and trimethoprim-sulfamethoxazole emerged in China, India, and Pakistan. Over the ensuing years these MDR strains became prevalent in these and other Asian countries and some countries of Africa. Ciprofloxacin (Cipro), ofloxacin (Floxin),* and other fluoroquinolones were tested and found to be highly effective in adults. Fluoroquinolone use in children is problematic because it has the potential to damage developing cartilage. For children, the cephalosporins ceftriaxone (Rocephin),* cefotaxime (Claforan),* and cefoperazone (Cefobid)* have shown good results and are recommended. Other drugs that have shown satisfactory results in MDR typhoid fever are cefixime (Suprax),* ampicillin-sulbactam (Unasyn),* and furazolidone (Furoxone).

*Not FDA approved for this indication.

TABLE 1. **Antimicrobial Therapy for Typhoid Fever**

***Salmonella typhi* Characteristic**	**Drug of Choice**	**Alternative Drugs**
Chloramphenicol susceptible	Chloramphenicol 50–60 mg/kg/d PO or IV in 4 divided doses until defervescence, then 30–40 mg/kg/d to complete a 14-d course *or* *Adults*: ciprofloxacin (Cipro), 500 mg PO bid for 10–14 d	(1) Trimethoprim-sulfamethoxazole (Bactrim, Septra); *Adults*: one double-strength tablet bid for 14 d *Children*: 8–20 mg trimethoprim/kg/d IV *or* by oral suspension bid for 14 d (2) Amoxicillin: *Adults*: 1 gm PO q 8 h for 14 d. *Children*: 25 mg/kg/d PO q 8 h for 14 d
Multiple drug resistance to chloramphenicol, ampicillin, and trimethoprim-sulfamethoxazole	*Adults*: Ciprofloxacin, 500 mg PO bid for 10–14 d, or ofloxacin (Floxin), 400 mg PO bid for 10–14 d *Children*: Ceftriaxone, 50–75 mg/kg/d IV once daily for 10–14 d, or cefotaxime, 100–200 mg/kg/d IV bid for 10–14 d	*Adults:* Ceftriaxone (Rocephin), 2 gm IV once daily for 10–14 d, or cefotaxime (Claforan), 2–4 gm IV q 12 h for 10–14 d *Children*: Cefixime (Suprax), 20 mg/kg/d IV q 12 h for 10–14 d

The recommended duration of therapy for chloramphenicol was originally established at 14 days. Relapse, characterized by the return of fever and bacteremia within 6 weeks of stopping therapy, occurred in 10 to 25% of patients. For this reason, shorter courses of chloramphenicol have not been used. However, short parenteral courses (5 to 7 days) of ceftriaxone have been successful in small studies, with rates of relapse of less than 20%, although most investigators have administered the drug for 10 to 14 days. Many practitioners will switch to an oral antibiotic after control of initial symptoms with parenteral cephalosporins. Ciprofloxacin and ofloxacin have been successful in courses of 5 to 7 days, with relapse rates of less than 5%, although like ceftriaxone, most investigators have administered the drug for 10 to 14 days. For these reasons, and because they shorten the length of time of early *S. typhi* shedding and decrease the chronic carriage rate, fluoroquinolones are emerging as the first-line therapy for adults.

Following therapy, patients should be advised to return to their physician if fever recurs. Most relapses occur within 1 to 6 weeks of stopping therapy. A relapse should be treated the same as the first episode of illness.

Supportive Therapy

Patients with typhoid fever require attention to fluid and electrolyte balance. Patients with fever and anorexia for several days will be dehydrated. Some patients with vomiting or diarrhea will be salt depleted and develop acidosis or hypokalemia. Intravenous fluid support will be required for severely ill patients. Patients with severe anemia, sometimes caused by intestinal bleeding, will require blood transfusion.

Treatment of Complications

The most feared complication, intestinal perforation, develops in about 4% of hospitalized patients before or during antimicrobial therapy. Emergency surgical repair of the ileal or colonic perforation is mandatory. Another life-threatening complication, brisk intestinal hemorrhage from ileal ulcers, requires transfusions and, rarely, surgical resection of the ileum. Pulmonary complications that require treatment include pneumonia, which is usually a bacterial superinfection requiring additional antimicrobial therapy, and adult respiratory distress syndrome. The liver is frequently enlarged by the formation of typhoid nodules and "typhoid hepatitis," and in severe cases, patients are jaundiced. The liver dysfunction resolves during therapy and does not require special attention. Rare cases of acute typhoid cholecystitis requiring surgery have been described. In an Indonesian study, patients with severe disease, including delirium, coma, or shock, were shown to benefit from the addition of corticosteroid to the antibiotic regimen. Dexamethasone was given as 3 mg per kg initially, followed by 1 mg per kg every 6 hours for 48 hours.

The mortality rate of typhoid fever is considerably less than 1% in the United States and should approach zero in patients who receive appropriate antimicrobial therapy within a week of the onset of illness. In developing countries, the mortality rate is several times higher than 1% because of delayed presentation. Death may be caused by complications, such as intestinal perforation or hemorrhage, which are enhanced by nutritional deficiencies, especially in young children. Septic shock is a rare fatal complication.

Treatment of Chronic Fecal Carriers

About 3% of patients with typhoid fever treated successfully with antibiotics become chronic asymptomatic carriers. Chronic fecal shedders of *S. typhi* are more often women than children or men, because women are more likely to have gallstones or other diseases of the biliary tract, where the chronic *S. typhi* infection resides. These chronic carriers are an obvious threat to public health, because they represent a reservoir for spread to other persons in the home and in the community through food handling. For chloramphenicol-susceptible organisms, carriers should receive amoxicillin or ampicillin, 6 grams a day orally in three to four divided doses, for 6 weeks. For MDR *S. typhi* infection, ciprofloxacin, 500 mg orally twice daily for 4 weeks, is effective. Stool cultures need to be repeated at the end of therapy. Failure to eradicate infection is associated with the presence of gallstones. Cholecystectomy, if indicated for symptomatic biliary tract disease, will usually cure the infection.

PREVENTION

Infection can be prevented in many situations by ingesting potable water, freshly cooked foods, and fresh foods uncontaminated by human sewage. Travelers to the developing world should drink only bottled beverages or beverages made with recently boiled water without ice. They should avoid salads, dairy products, and cold dishes by choosing freshly cooked foods. Two newly improved vaccines offer additional protection for travelers to typhoid-endemic countries and to persons with intimate exposure to a typhoid carrier or to a microbiology laboratory. The live oral Ty21a vaccine (Vivotif Berna) is administered as 3 or 4 capsules, one every other day. For continuing exposure, travelers should repeat the oral vaccination every 5 years. The other vaccine, typhoid Vi capsular polysaccharide (Typhim Vi), is injected once, with reimmunization every 2 years. The protection provided by these two vaccines is equal to that of the parenteral whole-cell killed vaccine (typhoid vaccine, USP), but these two produce little or none of the fever and severe injection site reactions associated with the older whole-cell vaccine.

RICKETTSIAL AND EHRLICHIAL INFECTIONS

method of
CHRISTOPHER D. PADDOCK, M.D., and
JAMES G. OLSON, PH.D.
National Center for Infectious Diseases, Centers for Disease Control and Prevention
Atlanta, Georgia

Rickettsiae and ehrlichiae are small, gram-negative bacteria that produce a wide spectrum of human infections, from relatively mild flulike illnesses to overwhelming, fatal diseases. These pathogens account for some of the most ancient and some of the most contemporary human infections. Effective treatment exists for all the rickettsioses and ehrlichioses; however, these infections can be exceptionally difficult to diagnose in the early stages of disease, when antimicrobial therapy is most beneficial. Most antimicrobials used as empirical therapies for bacterial infections in febrile patients (e.g., β-lactams, macrolides, aminoglycosides, and sulfa-containing drugs) are characteristically ineffective in treating rickettsial and ehrlichial diseases; appropriate treatment is almost never given unless the diagnosis is suspected. Physician awareness of these diseases and early recognition of their salient epidemiologic and clinical features form the foundation of successful patient outcomes.

Table 1 describes selected features of the endemic and imported rickettsial and ehrlichial diseases most likely to be encountered by physicians in the United States. Q fever is distinct from the other rickettsioses in its clinical and epidemiologic characteristics and requires significantly different treatment strategies; these are considered in a separate chapter. Rocky Mountain spotted fever (also described in detail in a separate chapter), rickettsialpox, flea-borne (murine or endemic) typhus, cat flea typhus, recrudescent typhus (Brill-Zinsser disease), sylvatic (flying squirrel) typhus, human granulocytic ehrlichiosis (HGE), and *Ehrlichia chaffeensis* infection (human monocytic ehrlichiosis) represent diseases endemic to the United States. Flea-borne typhus, louse-borne (epidemic) typhus, African tick bite fever, Mediterranean spotted fever (MSF), and scrub typhus are occasionally imported infections recognized in travelers returning to the United States. Other diseases not described in Table 1 that reflect the cosmopolitan, albeit geographically distinct, distribution of specific rickettsial and ehrlichial diseases include Queensland tick typhus, Japanese spotted fever, Siberian tick typhus, Israeli spotted fever, Astrakan fever, and sennetsu fever. More than half of all known rickettsial and ehrlichial diseases have been characterized only in the last decade; additional pathogens undoubtedly will be discovered in the years to come.

CLINICAL MANIFESTATIONS

Patients with rickettsial and ehrlichial infections generally present to a physician in their first week of illness. Unfortunately, early clinical signs and symptoms of these diseases are remarkably nonspecific and may mimic various other infectious and noninfectious etiologies, including measles, infectious mononucleosis, rubella, enteroviral infections, typhoid fever, meningococcemia, secondary syphilis, disseminated gonococcal infection, leptospirosis, toxic shock syndrome, thrombotic thrombocytopenic purpura, idiopathic thrombocytopenic purpura, immune complex vasculitides, and drug reactions. Patients typically present with fever, headache, myalgias, and gastrointestinal symptoms. Rash is a well-recognized manifestation of the rickettsioses but is present in only a minority of infected persons when they present for care initially. Depending on the particular disease, a rash develops in 50 to 95% of patients, generally within 3 to 8 days after the onset of constitutional symptoms. The nature and distribution of the rashes vary among illnesses and in some patients may be evanescent over the course of the disease. Rash infrequently assists in the clinical diagnosis of ehrlichiosis in adults, but it is described in as many as 60 to 70% of pediatric patients with *E. chaffeensis* infection. Here again, the rash may be highly variable in appearance and distribution. Eschars are a prominent feature of several rickettsioses, including MSF, African tick bite fever, rickettsialpox, and scrub typhus; these lesions are frequently accompanied by regional adenopathy. Pulmonary manifestations of varying severity (e.g., from cough or dyspnea to adult respiratory distress syndrome) are noted in as many as 30 to 55% of patients with ehrlichial and rickettsial infections. Hematologic and blood chemistry abnormalities, particularly thrombocytopenia, anemia, elevated hepatic transaminases (especially aspartate aminotransferase), and hyponatremia, are often identified in rickettsioses and ehrlichioses. Leukopenia, particularly absolute lymphopenia, is a common manifestation of the ehrlichioses. Although certain rickettsioses (e.g., rickettsialpox) run a self-limited, relatively mild course in otherwise healthy patients, some of these diseases may progress to multiorgan system sequelae, including myocarditis, pulmonary hemorrhage, adult respiratory distress syndrome, disseminated intravascular coagulation, meningoencephalitis, acute renal failure, and gangrene. Case-fatality ratios for patients with untreated disease may exceed 25% with some of the rickettsioses (see Table 1).

DIAGNOSIS

At present, no routinely available laboratory test provides prompt confirmatory diagnosis for acute rickettsial and ehrlichial diseases. Successful patient outcomes are guided more by the perspicacity of the evaluating health care provider than the sensitivity or specificity of a retrospective confirmatory assay. Therapeutic decisions must be based on a presumptive diagnosis developed from clinical suspicion and the epidemiologic setting. Specific signs and symptoms early in course of infection may be sparse, so a careful history must be obtained. Points to be recognized and/or elicited by physicians in this process include the following.

Exposure. A history of arthropod (e.g., tick, mite, flea, or louse) bite or exposure may be elicited by questioning patients about leisure and/or occupational outdoor activities (e.g., hunting, fishing, hiking, gardening, forestry) in the weeks preceding the illness. Exposures to arthropods may also arise from contacts with certain animals, including rats, mice, flying squirrels, opossums, deer, or dogs; these vertebrates may serve as hosts for the arthropod and as reservoirs for various rickettsial and ehrlichial pathogens.

Geography. Awareness of disease endemicities is invaluable and may sensitize physicians to subtle clues observed in patients presenting with an otherwise unknown acute febrile illness. In addition, these infections may be acquired in travel-related activities in different states and on other continents. These diseases are not restricted to rural settings; in fact, some of the rickettsioses are more

TABLE 1. **Features of Selected Rickettsial and Ehrlichial Diseases**

Etiologic Agent	Disease	Case-Fatality Ratio Treated (Untreated)	Ecology of Exposure	Geographic Distribution
Rickettsia prowazekii	Louse-borne (epidemic typhus)	10% (up to 60%)	Crowded, squalid conditions created by war and natural disasters that lead to body louse infestations; exacerbated by cold weather or disruption of water supply for bathing	Endemic in highlands of Africa, Asia, and the Americas
R. prowazekii	Sylvatic (flying-squirrel) typhus*	No known fatalities	Houses (e.g., attics) or other areas where flying squirrels nest; most infections occur during the winter months	Eastern United States (especially Massachusetts, Virginia, North Carolina, and Georgia)
R. prowazekii	Brill-Zinsser disease (recrudescent typhus)*	No known fatalities	Debilitation caused by stress, malnutrition, or illness in chronically infected person leads to recrudescence	Worldwide; most common in areas in which louse-borne typhus occurs or has occurred in the past
Rickettsia typhi	Flea-borne (murine, endemic) typhus*	1–2% (6%)	Urban and suburban areas in which rats (*Rattus* spp.) and their fleas are common (in the United States most common from April to August)	Worldwide, particularly in coastal areas of tropics and subtropics
Rickettsia felis	Cat flea typhus*	No known fatalities	Contact with cat fleas and opossums in suburban areas	California, Texas, and Oklahoma
Rickettsia rickettsii	Rocky Mountain spotted fever*	4% (13–41%)	Grassy areas, forest edge, roadsides, hiking trails, stream banks, unmowed areas around homes (in United States, most common from May to September)	Throughout most of the United States (most common in the southeastern states), Central America, and South America
Rickettsia conorii	Mediterranean spotted fever	2–3% (unknown)	Peridomestic areas; contact with buildings in which dogs have been housed	Southern Europe, Africa, and Asia
Rickettsia africae	African tick-bite fever	Unknown	Camping, safaris, exposure in cattle farming areas	Eastern and sub-Saharan Africa, (South Africa Zimbabwe, and Ethiopia)
Rickettsia australis	Queensland tick typhus	<1% (1%)	Outdoor activities that involve contact with vegetation harboring questing ticks	Australia
Rickettsia akari	Rickettsialpox*	No known fatalities	Contact with urban dwellings infested by house mice and their mites (occurs year-round)	Worldwide; occasionally cases occur in large metropolitan centers in the United States, especially New York City. Also reported from Croatia, Ukraine, South Africa, and Korea
Ehrlichia chaffeensis	Human monocytic ehrlichiosis (HME)*	<4% (unknown)	Grassy areas, forest edges, roadsides, hiking trails, stream banks, unmowed areas around homes (most common from May to September)	Southeastern and southcentral United States (most common in Oklahoma, Missouri, Tennessee, Arkansas, Georgia); possibly Portugal, Mali, and Italy

Table continued on following page

TABLE 1. **Features of Selected Rickettsial and Ehrlichial Diseases** *Continued*

Etiologic Agent	Disease	Case-Fatality Ratio Treated (Untreated)	Ecology of Exposure	Geographic Distribution
The agent of human granulocytic ehrlichiosis (HGE) (closely related to or identical to *Ehrlichia equi*)	Human granulocytic ehrlichiosis (HGE)*	<5% (unknown)	Grassy areas, forest edges, roadsides, hiking trails, stream banks, unmowed areas around homes (most common from May to September)	Northeastern coastal and upper midwestern United States (most common in New York, Wisconsin, Minnesota, Connecticut, Massachusetts); Europe (Slovenia and possibly Germany, Sweden, Switzerland, and United Kingdom)
Orientia tsutsugamushi	Scrub typhus	<1% (<10–30%)	Areas in which regrowth of forest is occurring and contact with larval mites (chiggers) is common; plantations, clearings, building sites, river banks (most common during warmer temperatures in subtropics, and following onset of rains in tropics)	Asia (including southeastern Asia, Korea, China, far eastern Russia, Nepal, India, and Pakistan), Indonesia, northern Australia, and the Pacific islands (including Japan, Taiwan, Philippines, and Papua New Guinea)

*Diseases endemic in the United States.

frequently seen in urban or suburban habitats. Finally, distribution of these infections should be considered a dynamic process; expanding geographic boundaries of disease typically parallel changes in densities and distributions of vector and reservoir host populations.

Seasonality. The occurrence of these diseases is directly related to the life histories of their arthropod vectors; most rickettsioses and ehrlichioses encountered by health care providers in the United States occur between April and September, coincident with peak vector activity and abundance.

Serologic assays remain the primary confirmatory method for each of these infections. Depending on the patient and the particular disease, however, antibodies against these agents may not appear until 7 to 14 days after the onset of symptoms. Indirect immunofluorescence antibody assays are the most widely available tests for the rickettsioses and ehrlichioses and are offered through several commercial laboratories, state public health departments, and the Centers for Disease Control and Prevention. Availability of other techniques, including enzyme immunoassays of serum, polymerase chain reaction assays of acute phase whole blood or tissues, immunohistochemistry of biopsied tissues, and direct isolation, is generally restricted to public health reference laboratories or specialized research laboratories. The ehrlichioses are occasionally diagnosed by visualization of the distinctive intracytoplasmic aggregates of bacteria (known as morulae) in leukocytes in peripheral blood, bone marrow, or cerebrospinal fluid. However, this method lacks sensitivity, as morulae are identified in fewer than 10% and 25% of all patients with acute *E. chaffeensis* infection and HGE, respectively.

TREATMENT

Suggested treatment regimens are described in Table 2. In almost all clinical circumstances, tetracyclines are the drugs of choice. Tetracyclines are bacteriostatic against *Rickettsia* species and bactericidal against ehrlichiae. Doxycycline (e.g., Vibramycin, Doryx, Monodox) is generally preferred over other tetracyclines because of its reduced phototoxicity, safety in patients with renal insufficiency, reduced deposition in teeth and bones, and longer plasma half-life (18 hours). The most notorious side effect of the tetracyclines is their propensity to bind calcium,

TABLE 2. **Antimicrobial Therapy of Rickettsial and Ehrlichial Infections**

Drug	Dose	Route
Doxycycline*		
Adults and children >45 kg	200 mg/d, in 2 divided doses	PO or IV
Children <45 kg	3 mg/kg/d, in 2 divided doses	PO or IV
Tetracycline		
Adults and children >8 years	25–50 mg/kg/d, in 4 divided doses	PO
	10–20 mg/kg/d, in 4 divided doses	IV
Chloramphenicol†		
Adults	50 mg/kg/d, in 4 divided doses	PO or IV
Children	50 mg/kg/d, in 4 divided doses	PO
	50—75 mg/kg/d, in 4 divided doses	IV
Rifampin, ciprofloxacin‡		

*Doxycycline is the antimicrobial of choice for all ehrlichial and rickettsial infections in adults and children but is contraindicated in pregnancy.

†Efficacy of chloramphenicol in the treatment of ehrlichiosis is uncertain. Oral formulation is unavailable in the United States. Decreased dosages necessary in neonates.

‡Limited clinical data to suggest efficacy of these agents against specific diseases (i.e., rifampin as effective therapy in pregnant patients with ehrlichiosis, clinical success with ciprofloxacin in the treatment of Mediterranean spotted fever).

resulting in staining and hypoplasia of developing tooth enamel. For this reason, routine use of tetracyclines in children younger than 8 years of age has been discouraged. However, the benefit of tetracycline use in children with potentially life-threatening rickettsial and ehrlichial infections far exceeds the risks, and doxycycline remains the antimicrobial of choice in pediatric patients of any age. Indeed, as the degree of dental staining is dose- and duration-dependent (the threshold for cosmetically perceptible staining appears to be 6 or more multiple-day courses of therapy), the actual risk of discoloration appears minimal following a single short course of doxycycline. Doxycycline is effectively administered orally in most cases. Intravenous therapy is given to hospitalized patients with vomiting, severe multisystem disease, or obtundation. Tetracyclines are contraindicated in pregnant women because of the risk of severe maternal hepatotoxicity and pancreatitis and interference with normal development of teeth and long bones in the fetus.

Chloramphenicol (Chloromycetin) represents an alternate therapy for the rickettsioses and has been used with clinical success in pregnant patients who have severe rickettsial disease. Oral chloramphenicol is no longer manufactured in the United States. The only systemic formulation currently available is parenteral chloramphenicol sodium succinate. This drug provides broad-spectrum activity against agents of diseases that may mimic rickettsial infections (including *Neisseria meningitidis* and *Salmonella typhi*) and may be preferred in select critically ill patients when the etiology is uncertain and the differential diagnosis includes one or more of these pathogens. Chloramphenicol is neither bacteriostatic nor bactericidal against *Ehrlichia* species in vitro, and there are reports of treatment failures with this drug in some patients with ehrlichiosis. Idiosyncratic aplastic anemia, which occurs in one in 24,500 to 40,800 courses of treatment, is the most devastating adverse reaction caused by this antibiotic. There also appears to be a dose-response relationship between chloramphenicol use and some childhood leukemias (e.g., acute lymphocytic and nonlymphocytic leukemias). Chloramphenicol has a low therapeutic-to-toxic ratio, and a number of reversible, dose-related toxicities are associated with this drug, including bone marrow suppression (reticulocytopenia, granulocytopenia, and/or thrombocytopenia), cardiomyopathy, and gray baby syndrome in neonates. For this reason, serum concentrations should be monitored routinely, with the peak levels maintained between 10 and 20 μg per mL.

Rifampin (e.g., Rifadin, Rimactane) shows significant in vitro bactericidal activity against *E. chaffeensis* and the HGE agent, and anecdotal reports describe rapid clinical improvement in patients who have HGE and are treated with rifampin in the second and third trimesters of pregnancy. These data should be interpreted cautiously, however, and should not be applied uniformly to other rickettsial infections. Indeed, treatment failures have been documented in clinical trials evaluating rifampin for the treatment of MSF.

The efficacy of currently available quinolones against the ehrlichioses and rickettsioses other than MSF has not been evaluated in clinical trials. There are anecdotal reports of rapid clinical response with ciprofloxacin in the treatment of flea-borne and scrub typhus, and successful patient outcomes are well documented for MSF. Ciprofloxacin (Cipro), is not active against *Ehrlichia* species and should not be used to treat these infections. In vitro studies indicate that several newer generation quinolones possess bacteriostatic and/or bactericidal activities against spotted fever group rickettsiae (e.g., levofloxacin [Levaquin]) and ehrlichiae (e.g., trovafloxacin [Trovan]); however, these drugs have not been evaluated in patients with active disease.

Therapy with sulfa-containing antimicrobials is contraindicated, and there is evidence that these drugs may increase the severity of several rickettsial infections, including Rocky Mountain spotted fever, MSF, flea-borne typhus, and possibly ehrlichiosis.

Although no consensus exists regarding optimal duration of therapy, the best guide appears to be the clinical response: most clinicians advocate continuing antibiotic coverage for at least 2 to 3 days following defervescence, for a minimum total course of 5 days. In general, patients become afebrile within 24 to 48 hours after initiation of effective therapy, and the total duration of treatment is 5 to 10 days. Shortened (i.e., single-dose) regimens have been successfully implemented during outbreaks of louse-borne typhus, and effective single-day therapy for MSF has been reported. However, disease relapses within 2 to 8 days following termination of therapy have been described for several rickettsioses, including Rocky Mountain spotted fever, Israeli spotted fever, flea-borne typhus, and scrub typhus, particularly with abbreviated treatment regimens initiated very early in the course of infection. Relapses are more frequently associated with chloramphenicol use but have also been described with single-dose doxycycline. Longer courses of doxycycline (10 to 21 days) may be warranted in select patients with HGE if co-infection with *Borrelia burgdorferi* is suspected.

Severely ill patients may develop marked hypotension, oliguria, and shock from intravascular fluid losses. Close hemodynamic and electrolyte monitoring, coupled with careful fluid replacement and pharmacologic blood pressure support, may be warranted. Marked anemia and thrombocytopenia can develop in some patients, requiring close attention to blood counts. Standard criteria for transfusion of red blood cells and platelets should be followed. Use of high-dose corticosteroids late in the course of severe vasculotropic rickettsioses has been advocated by some clinicians, but there are no controlled trials to suggest that this therapy is efficacious.

Prophylactic therapy in non-ill patients who have had recent arthropod bites is not warranted. Administration of doxycycline before the onset of symptoms may only delay the onset of clinical disease with some rickettsial infections.

Section 3

The Respiratory System

ACUTE RESPIRATORY FAILURE

method of
MICHAEL C. BOYARS, M.D.
University of Texas Medical Branch
Galveston, Texas

Acute respiratory failure (ARF) is a sudden decompensation of the oxygenation and/or ventilation functions of the respiratory system. This leads to inadequate oxygen delivery and/or carbon dioxide removal, resulting in altered cellular function. Signs may include hypoxia, hypercapnia, and sometimes systemic acidosis. Dyspnea is the most common symptom of ARF but is too nonspecific to be helpful clinically. ARF is a clinical syndrome of acute respiratory decompensation, and as such its diagnosis is made from its clinical presentation more than from laboratory data such as arterial blood gas (ABG) analysis. The patient's chronic baseline pulmonary function, and hence pulmonary reserve, is most important in determining the course of ARF. Whereas an ABG determination on room air showing a Po_2 of 52 mm Hg, Pco_2 of 46 mm Hg, and pH of 7.35 may signify ARF in a 15-year-old asthmatic, it may represent a stable baseline for a 66-year-old patient with moderately advanced emphysema. Despite its limitation, ABG analysis plays an essential role in the diagnosis and follow-up of therapy for ARF. I find it useful clinically to divide causes of ARF into those in normal lungs and those in abnormal lungs (Table 1).

VENTILATORY SUPPORT

Adequate oxygenation and ventilation are the cornerstones of therapy for ARF. What defines adequate oxygenation is a more complex subject. Oxygenation is dependent on several factors, including (1) the partial pressure of arterial oxygen (Pao_2), because this determines oxygen saturation of hemoglobin; (2) the hemoglobin concentration; (3) the cardiac output (CO); (4) the blood pressure; and (5) the distribution of blood flow through the multiple vascular beds. Because tissue oxygenation is dependent on so many variables, it is difficult to determine when we are optimally oxygenating the patient. Calculation of total arterial transport seems to be the best single parameter to accurately assess adequacy of tissue oxygenation in a patient with ARF:

$$O_2 \text{ transport} = CO \times (\text{hemoglobin concentration} \times 1.34 \text{ mL } O_2 \times O_2 \text{ saturation } \%) + 0.003 \times Pao_2$$

Adequacy of alveolar ventilation is generally assessed by the level of $Paco_2$. With alveolar hyperventilation, there is relative hypocapnia; with alveolar hypoventilation, there is relative hypercapnia.

Treatment of ARF frequently requires intubation and mechanical ventilation. Regardless of the cause, when the patient's clinical parameters fall below those shown in Table 2, intubation and mechanical ventilation should be strongly considered. There are several modes of mechanical ventilation, as shown in Table 3. No one mode has been shown to be superior with respect to morbidity or mortality in clinical trials. Each mode has relative advantages and disadvantages that may make it more desirable in certain clinical situations. If you are inexperienced with a certain mode of ventilation, it is better to use one with which you are familiar rather than worry about which mode is best in a given clinical situation. Modes of ventilation can be divided into volume or pressure modes. With volume modes (assist/control [A/C] and synchronized intermittent mandatory ventilation [SIMV]), the patient is given a preset tidal volume (V_T) and the pressure rises to whatever is needed to deliver that volume. Pressure-mode ventilation (pressure-control ventilation [PCV] and pressure-support ventilation [PSV]) delivers a predetermined oxygen mixture until a specified peak airway pressure is reached, and the volume delivered varies directly with the stiffness or compliance of the lungs. Bilevel positive airway pressure (Bi-PAP) is a noninvasive mode of ventilation. General guidelines concerning each mode follow.

TABLE 1. **Causes of Acute Respiratory Failure**

In Normal Lungs	In Abnormal Lungs
Central nervous system causes	Obstructive airway disease
Sedative drug overdose	Asthma
Cerebrovascular disease	Chronic bronchitis
Infection	Emphysema
Tumor	Restrictive airway disease
Neuromuscular causes	Chronic pulmonary fibrosis
Guillain-Barré syndrome	Acute diffuse edema or inflammation
Myasthenia gravis	Space-occupying lesions
Amyotrophic lateral sclerosis	Pneumothorax
Drug induced	Pleural effusion
Aminoglycosides	Pneumonia—any cause
Organophosphates	Atelectasis
Muscular causes	Airway obstruction
Myositis	Pleural effusion
Hypophosphatemia	Pulmonary edema
Other causes	Hydrostatic (congestive heart failure)
Upper airway obstruction	Increased microvascular permeability (adult respiratory distress syndrome)
Sleep apnea syndrome	Pulmonary embolism
Enlarged tonsils (children)	

TABLE 2. **Guidelines for Initiation of Mechanical Ventilation**

Spontaneous respiratory rate	>30/min
Spontaneous tidal volume	<300 mL
Vital capacity	<20 mL/kg
Negative inspiratory pressure	<-30 cm H_2O
$Pa O_2$	<60 mm Hg on supplemental oxygen
$Pa CO_2$	>55 mm Hg or 10 mm Hg above baseline stable value
Poor clearance of secretions or ineffective cough	

Bi-PAP is a noninvasive mode of ventilation that may be used to support a patient with ARF and thus prevent the need for intubation and mechanical ventilation. Bi-PAP is delivered by a tight-fitting nasal mask. The patient's respiratory efforts are "sensed" by the Bi-PAP machine, which delivers a higher pressure during inspiration and a lower pressure during expiration. This provides for a measure of end-expiratory pressure that helps keep small airways open and improves gas exchange as well as drives a gas mixture into and out of the lungs. In this way, it works as a pressure respirator. This can decrease the patient's work of breathing and augment ventilation, and it has been reported to decrease the need for intubation and mechanical ventilation in some patients with ARF. The exact indication for this mode of therapy in ARF is not yet determined.

The goal of mechanical ventilation is to return the pH and $P CO_2$ to their previous stable values while maintaining adequate oxygenation. For volume-mode ventilation, initial settings are as follows. V_T should be set at 7 to 10 mL per kg of ideal body weight. Use lower volumes in patients with obstructive airway disease because the reduced lung compliance generates higher airway pressures, which results in a higher frequency of barotrauma. The initial rate should be 8 to 12 breaths per minute. The larger the V_T, the lower the rate. The initial fraction of inspired oxygen ($F IO_2$) is set at 0.50, and this should be adjusted to maintain a $Pa O_2$ in the range of 60 to 80 mm Hg. Blood samples for initial ABG analysis should be drawn in 30 to 45 minutes and adjustment made as necessary to keep $Pa O_2$ and pH values optimal. Marked respiratory alkalosis should be avoided because it can lead to seizures and cardiac arrhythmias and can be a negative stimulus to respiration.

TABLE 3. **Modes of Mechanical Ventilation**

Noninvasive
Bilevel positive airway pressure

Invasive
Volume cycled
- Assist/control
- Synchronized intermittent mandatory ventilation

Pressure cycled
- Pressure-control ventilation
  - Inverse ratio ventilation
- Pressure-support ventilation

A/C is the oldest mode of ventilation. The physician selects a V_T, a minimal respiratory rate, and an $F IO_2$. Each time an inspiratory effort is made, the patient gets a machine-delivered breath of predetermined V_T and $F IO_2$. If the patient's spontaneous rate falls below that set on the ventilator, the patient gets the preset rate. The greatest potential benefit of A/C is that unless the patient cannot make appropriate inspiratory efforts, the patient will not be "underventilated" and run the risk of worsening respiratory failure because of too low a preset rate. On the other hand, some believe that it is more difficult to wean patients from this mode because they tend to be "overventilated."

In the SIMV mode, the physician selects a V_T, a respiratory rate, and an $F IO_2$. Unlike in A/C ventilation, the rate cannot be increased by the patient's effort. The ventilator senses the patient's effort and delivers the preset V_T when an inspiratory effort is made. If an inspiratory effort is made in between the ventilator breath, the patient gets a V_T proportional to the inspiratory effort. The greater the effort, the greater the V_T. SIMV allows the patient to "actively participate" in respiration, and some think that this makes weaning easier. The most serious concern with SIMV is setting the spontaneous rate too low. If this is done, the patient will have increased work of breathing, which may eventually worsen the respiratory failure and prolong ventilator dependency.

PCV is similar to A/C, but rather than selecting a V_T, the physician chooses a peak inspiratory pressure. Each time the ventilator senses a patient's effort, the oxygen mixture is delivered to a preset peak airway pressure limit. The delivered V_T varies directly with the lung compliance. The more compliant the lungs, the greater the V_T; the stiffer the lungs, the less the V_T. This mode of ventilation guarantees that maximal peak airway pressure will not exceed the preset limit, thus minimizing the risk for barotrauma with resultant pneumothorax, subcutaneous emphysema, decreased venous return, and hemodynamic instability. Because of this, it is most useful in ventilating patients with obstructive airway disease. Initially, set the pressure at 30 cm H_2O, the respiratory rate at 8 to 10, and the $F IO_2$ at 0.50. Check the ABG values in 30 minutes, and make appropriate adjustments to keep the $Pa O_2$ in the 60 to 80 mm Hg range.

PSV delivers a preset pressure in the ventilator circuit when a patient's inspiratory effort is sensed by the ventilator. This is thought to decrease the patient's work of breathing. PSV can be used alone or combined with SIMV. When it is used in this way, combine a fixed rate volume-mode ventilator with a pressure-mode ventilator to assist the patient's spontaneous breaths. This mode of ventilation has its greatest utility in weaning. The amount of pressure to use initially is in the range of 15 to 25 cm H_2O. This can be increased or decreased on the basis of the patient's clinical status.

Permissive hypercapnia is an acceptable ventilatory strategy in which you ventilate with lower volumes and airway pressures and thus allow hypoventilation, and consequent $Pa{CO_2}$ elevation, to occur. This is done in an effort to lower the mean and peak airway pressures, which decreases the frequency of complications secondary to barotrauma. Critically ill patients can tolerate pH values in the range of 7.10 without significant consequences. Patients with significant heart disease do not tolerate a serum pH of less than 7.25, however. The level of pH, *not* the $Pa{CO_2}$, is the limiting factor.

Inverse ratio ventilation (IRV) is a ventilatory mode that is usually used with PCV. The normal inspiratory and expiratory time ratio (I/E ratio) is reversed, allowing a greater inspiratory than expiratory time. A normal I/E ratio is 1:2 to 1:3. The clinical indications for and exact place of IRV in supporting patients with ARF are controversial, and it should not be used unless one has extensive experience with it.

Intubation causes atelectasis and a fall in functional residual capacity (FRC) by unclear mechanisms. A small amount of positive end-expiratory pressure (PEEP) (2.5 to 5 cm H_2O) has been shown to prevent this and is routinely applied to most patients on ventilators. The use of PEEP may be harmful in some groups of patients. Patients with asthma or chronic obstructive pulmonary disease (COPD) usually have elevated baseline FRCs, and PEEP can worsen the hyperinflation and cause significant barotrauma. In patients with hypovolemia, relatively small increases in intrathoracic pressure may additionally reduce venous return significantly and cause hypotension.

Intubation and mechanical ventilation are uncomfortable and frightening for the patient. Because of this the patient should be sedated and have anxiety relieved. If the patient "fights" the ventilator, this will increase airway pressures, interfere with oxygenation and ventilation, and increase the rate of complications. Experience, personal preference, and the clinical situation dictate the agents used. It is best to use neuromuscular paralysis as a last choice because of the short- and long-term neuropathy and myopathy associated with these agents.

WEANING FROM MECHANICAL VENTILATION

Weaning is as much art as science. When the initial pathologic process that led to the ARF is treated or resolves, the patient is ready for weaning. If there is no objective improvement in this process, the patient will fail weaning attempts. Whereas no one or combination of clinical parameters can accurately predict the outcome of weaning attempts, I have found some to be clinically helpful (see Table 2). The patient has a greater chance at successful weaning if the spontaneous respiratory rate is 30 per minute or less, the spontaneous V_T is 300 mL or more, the vital capacity (VC) is 20 mL per kg or more, and the negative inspiratory pressure (NIP) is -30 cm H_2O or less. Patients who do not fulfill these criteria may be weaned; however, the better their "weaning parameters," the more likely weaning will be successful.

No one method of weaning has been shown to be uniformly superior in all clinical situations. If the patient is in the SIMV mode, one can simply reduce the SIMV rate progressively as the patient's clinical state allows until the patient is successfully weaned. This same strategy can be used with PSV. When the patient is ventilated with A/C or PCV, it is best to use a T tube trial. The patient is removed from the ventilator and given a T tube for a short time, 5 to 10 minutes initially, before being returned to ventilatory support. If this is tolerated, progressively longer periods of T tube support are used until the patient can breathe with the T tube without respiratory fatigue. The patient is then extubated and prescribed a Venturi or aerosol mask.

ACUTE RESPIRATORY FAILURE WITH NORMAL LUNGS

ARF with normal lungs usually results in a reduction in alveolar ventilation. The ventilatory function of the respiratory system serves to move gas into and out of the lungs during the respiratory cycle. Impulses originating in the "respiratory center" are transmitted down spinal tracts through peripheral nerves to the neuromuscular junction of the muscles of inspiration, causing them to contract. Expiration is a more passive process, effected largely by relaxation of the muscles of inspiration. Regardless of the cause, ventilatory failure leads to inadequate bellows function of the respiratory system, causing alveolar hypoventilation. This reduced ventilation causes inadequate removal of carbon dioxide from the alveoli, resulting in an increase in the alveolar $P{CO_2}$ ($P_A{CO_2}$). Because the total barometric pressure is unchanged, this increase in $P_A{CO_2}$ causes a decrease in alveolar $P{O_2}$ ($P_A{O_2}$), which results in a reduction in the $Pa{O_2}$. The difference or gradient between the alveolar and arterial $P{O_2}$ ($P_A{O_2} - Pa{O_2}$) remains normal in ARF caused by ventilatory failure with normal lungs, whereas it is always widened in ARF caused by ventilatory failure with abnormal lungs. The relationship between $P_A{O_2}$ and $Pa{CO_2}$ is described in the alveolar air equation (Table 4). Using it, we can calculate the $P_A{O_2}$ from the ABG values and then determine the alveolar-arterial $P{O_2}$ difference. When the alveolar-arterial $P{O_2}$ difference is widened (normal = 5 to 15 mm Hg), the ARF is secondary to ventilatory failure with abnormal lungs or oxygenation failure. When the alveolar-arterial $P{O_2}$ difference is normal, the ARF is secondary to ventilatory failure with normal lungs. Because the alveolar-arterial $P{O_2}$ difference widens with increasing concentrations of inspired oxygen, it is only clinically useful when the patient is breathing room air.

The rise in $Pa{CO_2}$ that occurs with ventilatory failure causes a respiratory acidosis. The more severe

TABLE 4. **Alveolar Air Equation**

P_{AO_2} = alveolar P_{O_2}	F_{IO_2} = fraction of O_2 in inspired air
Pa_{O_2} = arterial P_{O_2}	R = respiratory quotient
Pa_{CO_2} = arterial P_{CO_2}	$P_{AO_2} - Pa_{O_2}$ = alveolar-arterial P_{O_2} difference
P_{IO_2} = partial pressure of inspired O_2	

$$P_{AO_2} = P_{IO_2} - Pa_{CO_2}/R$$

$$P_{AO_2} = (\text{barometric pressure} - \text{water vapor pressure})(F_{IO_2}) - Pa_{CO_2}/R$$

At sea level on room air assuming R = 0.8

$$P_{AO_2} = (760 - 47)(0.21) - Pa_{CO_2}/0.8$$

$$P_{AO_2} = 150 - (Pa_{CO_2})(1.2)$$

Normal $P_{AO_2} - Pa_{O_2}$ = 5 to 15 mm Hg

the ventilatory failure, the greater the rise in Pa_{CO_2} and the more severe the respiratory acidosis. Acutely, every rise in Pa_{CO_2} of 10 mm Hg results in a decrease in pH of approximately 0.08. If the ventilatory insufficiency is more long-term (days, weeks, or longer), the kidneys partially compensate by retaining bicarbonate, and so the fall in pH is not as great. In this situation, for every rise of Pa_{CO_2} of 10 mm Hg, there is a fall in pH of approximately 0.03. Making this kind of calculation helps determine whether the ventilatory failure is acute or chronic.

Spirometry is the optimal way to monitor the day-to-day progression of ARF with normal lungs. VC, forced expiratory volume in 1 second (FEV_1), NIP, and maximal expiratory pressure can be easily and reliably measured at the bedside even in critically ill patients (see Table 2). In addition, they are relatively early indicators of change in the patient's clinical state. These parameters improve as the ventilatory failure resolves. If they worsen, intubation and mechanical ventilation may be necessary.

The treatment of ARF with normal lungs is mainly supportive. The etiologic process can be treated or addressed in some cases, but frequently one has to support respiration while the primary process resolves. If there is only mild respiratory depression with minimal hypoxemia and hypercapnia, supplemental oxygen by face mask or nasal cannula will suffice. With more profound degrees of respiratory depression, intubation and mechanical ventilation are required. The decision for intubation is predominantly a clinical one. Guidelines on when to intubate and mechanically ventilate a patient are given in Table 2. Measurement of FEV_1, VC, spontaneous respiratory rate and V_T, and NIP made at the bedside can be an invaluable aid. If these parameters deteriorate progressively during hours, this is a strong indication of progressive ventilatory failure and an urgent need for intubation and ventilation before complete respiratory collapse occurs. If the patient's bedside measurements are far outside the limits given in Table 2 and/or there is significant risk for aspiration, then intubation and mechanical ventilation should be considered immediately.

Sedative drug overdose is a frequent cause of ARF with normal lungs. The degree of respiratory depression generally correlates with the stage of coma. The greater the degree of coma and risk for vomiting and aspiration, the stronger the indication for intubation and mechanical ventilation. Naloxone (Narcan), 0.4 to 0.8 mg intravenously (IV), can be administered as a diagnostic test, because it will cause rapid improvement of narcotic sedation.

Central nervous system (CNS) infections are treated with appropriate antimicrobial agents coupled with ventilatory support. CNS tumors, cerebrovascular disease, and central apneas generally do not have a favorable response to specific therapy, and supportive care for the ARF is the mainstay of the treatment. Myasthenia gravis is treated with pyridostigmine (Mestinon), 60 mg three times daily initially. Plasmapheresis is effective in removing circulating antibody and has been found helpful in severely weak myasthenia patients in addition to supportive ventilatory care. Patients with the Guillain-Barré syndrome who develop severe weakness may be helped with plasmapheresis or intravenous immune globulin (0.4 gram per kg per day for 5 days).

Hypophosphatemia and hypokalemia are treated with the appropriate IV electrolyte solutions. Cholinergic crisis secondary to organophosphate poisoning should be managed with atropine, 2 to 5 mg IV. It is repeated every 15 minutes until atropinization occurs. To combat the muscle weakness, pralidoxime (Protopam), 1 gram IV given slowly, is used. It can be repeated three times in 8 to 12 hours if the muscle weakness is not relieved.

ACUTE RESPIRATORY FAILURE WITH ABNORMAL LUNGS

Asthma

Patients with ARF secondary to obstructive airway disease have special needs. The bronchial narrowing causes significant increases in airway resistance and hence work of breathing. Patients with asthma generally have more reversible obstruction than do those with COPD. They are generally younger in age and in better overall baseline health. Findings that indicate increased severity of an asthmatic attack are listed in Table 5.

Rapid IV hydration is always part of initial therapy in severe asthma. These patients are usually moderately dehydrated, which not only contracts their vascular volume but increases the viscosity of their secretions and exacerbates mucous plugging of the airways. In the first hour, 0.9% saline, 500 to 1000 mL, should be given unless it is contraindicated. This is followed by 100 to 200 mL per hour of 0.9% or 0.45% saline as indicated by the patient's cardiovascular and renal status.

Oxygen is administered to keep the minimum Pa_{O_2} in the 60 to 70 mm Hg range, which gives an oxygen saturation of greater than 90%. Unlike for patients with COPD, there is minimal risk for carbon dioxide narcosis with oxygen delivery to patients with asthma. Supplemental oxygen is most conveniently administered by nasal cannula at 1 to 2 liters per minute. The flow rate can be adjusted on the basis of the ABG results. Venturi or aerosol masks are also acceptable, although some asthmatic patients tolerate them poorly.

Initial drug therapy for ARF due to asthma is outlined in Table 6. Beta-adrenergic agents are first-line therapy and can be given by nebulizer or subcutaneously if the patient cannot tolerate use of a nebulizer. The nebulized route is preferred in older patients and those with known or suspected cardiac disease. IV theophylline therapy is usually started at the same time. In a patient who is already taking theophylline, a loading dose of 2 mg per kg can be given if there are no obvious signs of xanthine intoxication, such as nausea, vomiting, tremors, or seizures. This raises the serum level 5 to 8 mg per liter. Because of its narrow toxic/therapeutic ratio and variable rate of clearance, one must monitor serum theophylline levels and clinical effect closely.

Parenteral glucocorticoids should be used in all patients with asthma and ARF. Although there is no consensus on the precise dosage or which preparation is optimal, there is agreement that they should be given early, because a beneficial effect will not occur before 4 to 8 hours. Once stabilized, the patient should be switched to oral agents and then tapered slowly over 3 to 4 weeks to prevent rebound bronchospasm. There is little clinical evidence to support a beneficial effect of inhaled ipratropium bromide (Atrovent) solution in ARF due to asthma; however, because of its negligible side effects, it may be worth a therapeutic trial.

Factors that lead one to consider intubation and mechanical ventilation are marked with an asterisk in Table 5. Special care must be taken because of the high rate of complications due to elevated airway resistance and pressures in asthmatics. The goal of mechanical ventilation is to ventilate the patient at relatively low tidal volumes and respiratory rates. This prevents high airway pressures and excessive work of breathing. A good rule of thumb is to keep the respiratory rate less than 25 per minute and the airway plateau pressure less than 35 cm H_2O. The mode of ventilation used to achieve this is not important, because no one mode has proved to be superior to any other. ARF due to asthma is a relatively reversible process, and if you support the patient with ventilation while aggressively treating the bronchospasm, your patient is likely to have a favorable outcome.

TABLE 5. **Indications of a Severe Asthmatic Attack**

History
Previous recent severe attack
Prolonged attack (>24 h)
Previous steroid treatment within the last 6 mo
Previous hospitalization for asthma within the last 2 y

Physical Examination Findings
Pulsus paradoxus >15 mm Hg
Use of accessory muscles of respiration
Respiratory rate >30/min
Pulse >130/min
*Central cyanosis
*Disturbance of consciousness
*Subcutaneous emphysema
*Pneumothorax
*Silent chest in a tachypneic patient

Laboratory Data
*Pa_{CO_2} ≥40 mm Hg
*Pa_{O_2} <60 mm Hg on supplemental oxygen
*FEV_1 <30% predicted and no improvement with bronchodilators
*Vital capacity <1 L
*Electrocardiogram showing P pulmonale and right ventricular strain

*Strongly consider intubation and mechanical ventilation.

TABLE 6. **Initial Drug Therapy in Asthma**

IV hydration
Inhaled $beta_2$ agonists delivered by aerosol mist
  Albuterol (Ventolin), 0.5 mL of a 0.5% solution in 2.5 mL of 0.9% saline
  Metaproterenol (Alupent), 0.3 mL of a 5% solution in 2.5 mL of 0.9% saline
This can be administered q 20 min the first hour and q 2–4 h thereafter.
If the patient cannot use a nebulizer:
  Epinephrine in water 1:1000, 0.3–0.5 mL SC q 20 min for up to 3 doses
  or
  Terbutaline (Brethine), 0.25–0.50 mg SC as above
Intravenous theophylline (aminophylline)
  Loading dose 5–6 mg/kg in 0.9% saline in 20 min
  Initial maintenance dose 0.3–0.6 mg/kg/h
    Lower doses for older patients (>45 y) and those with active liver disease
    Higher doses in younger patients (<30 y); in cigarette smokers; and with certain drugs, e.g., cimetidine (Tagamet), barbiturates
  Obtain theophylline level at 12–24 h and maintain at 15–20 mg/L
Corticosteroids
  Initially 250–1000 mg of hydrocortisone or 50–200 mg of methylprednisolone IV
  Maintenance of 100–400 mg hydrocortisone IV q 4–6 h or 20–80 mg of methylprednisolone q 4–6 h
Inhaled parasympatholytic delivered by aerosol mist
  Ipratropium bromide (Atrovent), 2.5 mL of a 0.02% solution by nebulizer initially and q 2–4 h as indicated by clinical response

Chronic Obstructive Pulmonary Disease

ARF in patients with COPD usually results from an acute decompensation complicating their significant chronic underlying disease. Unlike asthmatics, these patients have little capacity to compensate for this insult. Therefore, a seemingly trivial event such as an upper respiratory tract infection may put them in ARF. In many patients, no obvious predisposing event can be found.

Patients with COPD may have chronic hypoxia, hypercapnia, and compensated respiratory acidosis. An ABG analysis at a time when the patient is clinically stable is invaluable. Indwelling arterial lines are useful to continuously monitor blood pressure and provide access for the frequent blood samples that must be drawn. Erythrocytosis (hematocrit greater than 50) is a clue to chronic hypoxia; a bicarbonate level of greater than 30 mEq per liter is a clue to chronic hypercapnia with renal compensation.

Carbon dioxide may not be the main respiratory stimulus in patients with COPD, as it is for patients with asthma, and one must be concerned about the development of carbon dioxide narcosis when administering oxygen. The lowest amount of oxygen needed to keep the $Paco_2$ around 60 mm Hg is used. This results in an oxygen saturation of more than 90%. Further increases in oxygen are not necessary because they will result only in increased risk for carbon dioxide narcosis with negligible increase in oxygen delivery.

Venturi and aerosol masks provide oxygen at a fixed concentration and so are the initial treatments of choice. Begin with 24% or 28% oxygen and adjust as indicated by ABG values and clinical response. Be more concerned by the level of pH than Pco_2, because it is the degree of acidosis that causes complications and not the level of Pco_2. Oxygen therapy frequently causes some carbon dioxide retention, which then reequilibrates at a higher level. If the Pco_2 continues to rise and the pH falls, you should reduce the oxygen concentration or consider mechanical ventilation.

Oxygen delivery by nasal cannula or prongs at a rate of 1 to 3 liters per minute is another option. This may be more comfortable for the patient, but the concentration of oxygen varies with the patient's minute ventilation. As the minute ventilation decreases, the oxygen concentration increases and so does the risk for carbon dioxide narcosis. Because of this, Venturi and aerosol masks are preferred.

Hypercapnia is tolerated well by patients with COPD. Hypoxia and acidosis are stronger indications for intubation and mechanical ventilation. Persistent severe acidosis, hypoxia, confusion, coma, decreased cough effectiveness, respiratory muscle fatigue, and use of accessory muscles of respiration are all indications for intubation and ventilation. The use of the largest possible endotracheal tube is recommended because this will allow more adequate suctioning, decrease resistive forces, and allow decreased work of breathing.

As in asthma, the choice of ventilator mode is not as important as keeping the respiratory rate below 25 per minute and the airway plateau pressure below 35 cm H_2O. The goal is to keep the Pao_2 around 60 mm Hg while avoiding marked respiratory acidosis or alkalosis. The use of bronchodilator therapy as outlined for ARF due to asthma is indicated but generally not as effective.

Adult Respiratory Distress Syndrome

The adult respiratory distress syndrome (ARDS) is the result of increased microvascular permeability secondary to another primary process that results in diffuse lung injury. The pulmonary capillaries are flooded with fluid, which causes impaired oxygenation and decreased lung compliance in the face of normal left-sided cardiac function. The primary process is frequently a systemic infection, but ARDS is the final common pathway of lung injury secondary to myriad conditions. The same principles described previously guide ventilator management in ARDS. In addition, because of the increased capillary microvascular permeability, one must be careful not to overhydrate these patients because the fluid will end up in the pulmonary capillaries, worsening the pulmonary edema.

Other Causes

For the other causes of ARF with abnormal lungs (see Table 1), the general principles of clinical management of the oxygenation and ventilation defects are the same as outlined earlier. In addition, the primary process needs to be addressed. For example, the patient with pneumonia needs appropriate antibiotics, the patient with significant pneumothorax or pleural effusion needs chest tube drainage, and the patient with pulmonary embolism needs heparin and/or fibrinolytic therapy. The indications for and management of ventilatory support are the same as previously outlined.

A Swan-Ganz catheter can be indispensable in distinguishing cardiogenic from noncardiogenic pulmonary edema as well as being a guide to respiratory and cardiovascular status. Hemodynamic parameters that should be obtained include CO, mixed venous Po_2, pulmonary capillary wedge pressure, central venous pressure, and pulmonary artery pressure. Systemic vascular resistance can be calculated by subtracting central venous pressure from the mean aortic pressure and dividing by the CO.

The treatment of the nonpulmonary factors is essential. Alimentation should be instituted from the onset. Enteral alimentation with a soft feeding tube is best if possible; if not, IV alimentation should be used. Low-dose heparin therapy should be instituted unless it is contraindicated. Last, the use of H_2 blockers to maintain the gastric pH above 4 for prophylaxis against stress ulceration is warranted.

ATELECTASIS

method of
DAVID B. CAMPBELL, M.D.
Penn State–Geisinger Health System
Hershey, Pennsylvania

DEFINITIONS

Fever, dyspnea, and imaging abnormalities are present in most forms of atelectasis ("airless lung"). *Obstructive* atelectasis is common and occurs secondary to intrabronchial mucous plugging (occurring with hypoventilation, poor cough, or copious and/or tenacious secretions), inflammation of the bronchi, or bronchogenic tumor blocking the clearance of normal mucus and other secretions. *Compressive* atelectasis occurs when tumor, a large space-occupying lesion, or effusion displaces and compresses lung tissue. *Adhesive* atelectasis refers to lung parenchymal collapse due to loss of surfactant (as in hyaline membrane disease); *cicatrization* atelectasis results from fibrosis and scarring within the lung (from chronic infections, irradiation, silicosis, or scleroderma).

RISK FACTORS

The quest for effective prevention and treatment schemes for atelectasis continues. Pulmonary complications are responsible for considerable patient morbidity and hospital cost; integration of effective prophylaxis against atelectasis is prudent. Many studies have documented the effectiveness of prophylactic routines in minimizing atelectasis and oxygen requirements for patients with normal lung function who are stressed with illness or surgery. The impact of these treatments on clinical outcome, length of hospital stay, and overall costs, however, has been minimal. In this group the appropriate strategy is to offer simple treatments that do not add significant cost.

Patients with identified risk factors for lung complications tend to develop such complications despite routine prophylactic measures, and the complications, once developed, tend to be refractory to treatment. Aggressive treatment options should be applied to these patients in hopes of minimizing morbidity and mortality. Risk factors for the development of pulmonary complications include poor baseline lung function (forced expiratory volume in 1 second [FEV_1] of less than 1000 mL, arterial partial pressures of oxygen and carbon dioxide [$Pa{O_2}$, $Pa{CO_2}$] that are abnormal ($Pa{O_2}<60$, $Pa{CO_2}>45$), neuromuscular disease, marked obesity, and advanced age in patients with coexistent cardiac disease. Trauma victims and institutionalized patients are also at increased risk. For surgical patients, the site of the incision and prolonged anesthesia time are additional factors. In evaluating a patient for lung resection, the high-risk indicators are similar, but a broad interpretation is appropriate.

TREATMENT: A THREE-TIERED APPROACH

For management of atelectasis, a three-tiered approach—comprising prophylaxis, intensive therapy, and the use of invasive techniques—is recommended. A positive response to treatment is indicated by normalization of temperature and breath sounds, the clinician's subjective impression of improvement in the patient's clinical status, decrease in sputum production, favorable changes in arterial blood gas values, and clearing of infiltrates on the chest x-ray film.

1. Routine Prophylaxis (low cost, appropriate for all patients; the type of treatment chosen is less important than the compulsiveness with which it is applied)

- Incentive breathing (includes preoperative teaching and practice)
- Vigilant, effective pain control (e.g., local and regional anesthesia, epidural analgesia, intravenous narcotics, splinting of wounds)
- Adequate hydration, humidification of inhaled gas, expectorants to thin secretions

2. Intensive Therapy (for high-risk patients and for those in whom routine preventive measures fail)

- Percussion and postural drainage: Known to be effective therapy for cystic fibrosis and bronchiectasis, percussion and postural drainage, particularly steep Trendelenburg positioning for 15 to 20 minutes, constitute an effective aid to lung segment re-expansion.
- Inhaled bronchodilator therapy: Anticholinergic (ipratropium bromide [Atrovent]) and sympathomimetic drugs (albuterol [Ventolin, Proventil]) augment secretion clearance. Given by metered dose inhalers, by supervised inhalation treatments, or in conjunction with intermittent positive-pressure breathing (IPPB), these drugs work in additive fashion.
- Mucolytic therapy: *N*-acetylcysteine (Mucomyst) reduces the viscosity of mucus and also incites cough. Aerosolized or nebulized sodium bicarbonate or hypertonic saline may also enhance mucociliary clearance.
- Positive-pressure interventions: Used to mobilize secretions and treat atelectasis, these measures include continuous positive airway pressure (CPAP), administered by oronasal mask, and positive end-expiratory pressure (PEEP) or expiratory positive airway pressure (EPAP), which employs a mouthpiece during expiration. Each creates a positive-pressure environment at a low pressure (5, 7.5, or 10 cm H_2O), which may recruit additional alveoli. Volume-delivered IPPB may be utilized selectively for patients who can receive a tidal volume of 10 to 15 mL per kg. An IPPB trial period of 24 hours (six treatments) will determine if any benefit is gained. Use of IPPB for up to 72 hours may be justified, but improvement should prompt substitution of incentive methods to maintain and augment the advantages gained.

3. Invasive Treatments (for incompetent patients with established alveolar collapse)

- Endobronchial suction, either blind nasotracheal suction or bronchoscopy with lavage, may be used for refractory cases in which the patient cannot clear secretions adequately.

- Selective endobronchial insufflation is performed by wedging the tip of a bronchoscope in a lobar or segmental bronchus and forcing small volumes of air and irrigant through the instrument's working channel. This invasive technique may be applied cautiously for refractory lobar collapse, but application in cases of less than 72-hours' duration is much more effective than in atelectasis of longer duration.
- Minitracheostomy for access and frequent suctioning may be appropriate for patients whose pulmonary problems are judged to be ongoing and complex in the setting of prolonged illness.
- Upcoming treatment strategies: Surfactant administration or use of drugs that promote surfactant synthesis shows promise in the prevention of postoperative bronchopulmonary complications. Intrabronchial proteolytic enzymes may be of value in patients with cystic fibrosis and for certain chronic infections, including tuberculosis.

CHRONIC OBSTRUCTIVE PULMONARY DISEASE

method of
DENNIS P. SORRESSO, M.D.
Loyola University Medical Center of Chicago and Edward Hines, Jr., Veterans Affairs Medical Center

and

NICHOLAS J. GROSS, M.D., PH.D.
Edward Hines, Jr., Veterans Affairs Medical Center Hines, Illinois

Chronic obstructive pulmonary disease (COPD) is a term used to describe airways obstruction associated with chronic bronchitis and/or emphysema. Obstruction is due to a lack of structural integrity of the lung needed to tether small airways during expiration in combination with airways remodeling. The disease may progress to bullous formation and emphysema.

Although the main risk factor for COPD is cigarette smoking, only 15% of smokers develop clinical disease. A minority of patients develop emphysema as a result of genetic alpha$_1$-antitrypsin deficiency. Other genetic risk factors are suspected but unknown.

The focus of this article on COPD is on the outpatient and inpatient management of the disease. The management of patients in the intensive care setting is not considered.

STAGES

COPD usually progresses through three stages (I, II, and III), which correlate with mild, moderate, and severe airways obstruction as measured by spirometry. In the normal individual, the forced expiratory volume in one second (FEV$_1$) declines by approximately 30 mL each year after the age of 35. An FEV$_1$ below 70% of the predicted value for age is indicative of airways obstruction. A response to bronchodilators is significant when the FEV$_1$ increases by 200 mL above the patient's prebronchodilator FEV$_1$ or there is a 12% change in FEV$_1$ following bronchodilator administration. Unfortunately, many patients show no response to bronchodilators spirometrically. However, many patients who do not have objective evidence of reversible airways disease still benefit clinically from bronchodilator therapy; this may be due to increased ciliary motility and the more efficient expectoration of secretions afforded by the beta$_2$ agonists. Furthermore, some individuals with COPD may have coexistent asthma or reactive airways syndrome. Patients who continue to smoke usually have airways that are prone to bronchospasm, inflammation, and hypersecretion of mucus.

Mild obstructive disease (stage I) typically involves an FEV$_1$ of 50% or more of predicted with intermittent symptoms relieved with bronchodilator therapy alone. Moderate disease (stage II) correlates with an FEV$_1$ between 35 and 49% of predicted with evidence of more chronic symptomatology and somewhat limited quality of life. Severe COPD (stage III) correlates with an FEV$_1$ less than 35% of predicted and severe restrictions of lifestyle. This is the stage in which the clinician may see end-stage sequelae of the disease process such as hypoxemia, evidence of both right and left heart failure, emphysema, erythrocytosis, cachexia, and depression, all resulting in more frequent exacerbations and hospitalizations. Despite the severity of the disease, mortality remains difficult to predict in this stage of COPD. Although an FEV$_1$ of 0.7 liters or less is associated with a very poor prognosis, these patients may live for another 5 years or more.

TREATMENT

Outpatient

A stepwise approach to managing COPD is displayed in Figure 1.

Smoking cessation is the cornerstone of therapy for all stages of COPD and is known to improve prognosis at any age. Unfortunately, this can be a formidable task for the primary caregiver. Quite a number of cessation programs are offered by both hospitals and voluntary agencies (e.g., American Lung Association's Freedom from Smoking clinics). However, despite a multidisciplinary approach involving physician, family, and outside agencies, highly dependent smokers may require pharmacologic intervention after multiple failed attempts at smoking cessation. In such case, nicotine replacement (e.g., nicotine transdermal patch [Habitrol, NicoDerm], 14 to 22 mg every day tapering after 6 weeks) may be helpful. Extended-release bupropion (Zyban) (150 mg orally twice daily for 6 weeks), previously used as an antidepressant, has been shown to reduce the severity of withdrawal symptoms.

For mild disease with intermittent symptoms, aerosol therapy via a metered dose inhaler (MDI) with a selective beta agonist, such as albuterol (Proventil, Ventolin), 1 to 2 puffs every 2 to 6 hours as needed, likely will suffice. However, an anticholinergic agent, such as ipratropium bromide (Atrovent), 2 to 6 puffs every 6 to 8 hours, should be prescribed first in all other presentations followed by a beta$_2$ agonist as needed. A combination MDI containing these two agents (albuterol and ipratropium bromide

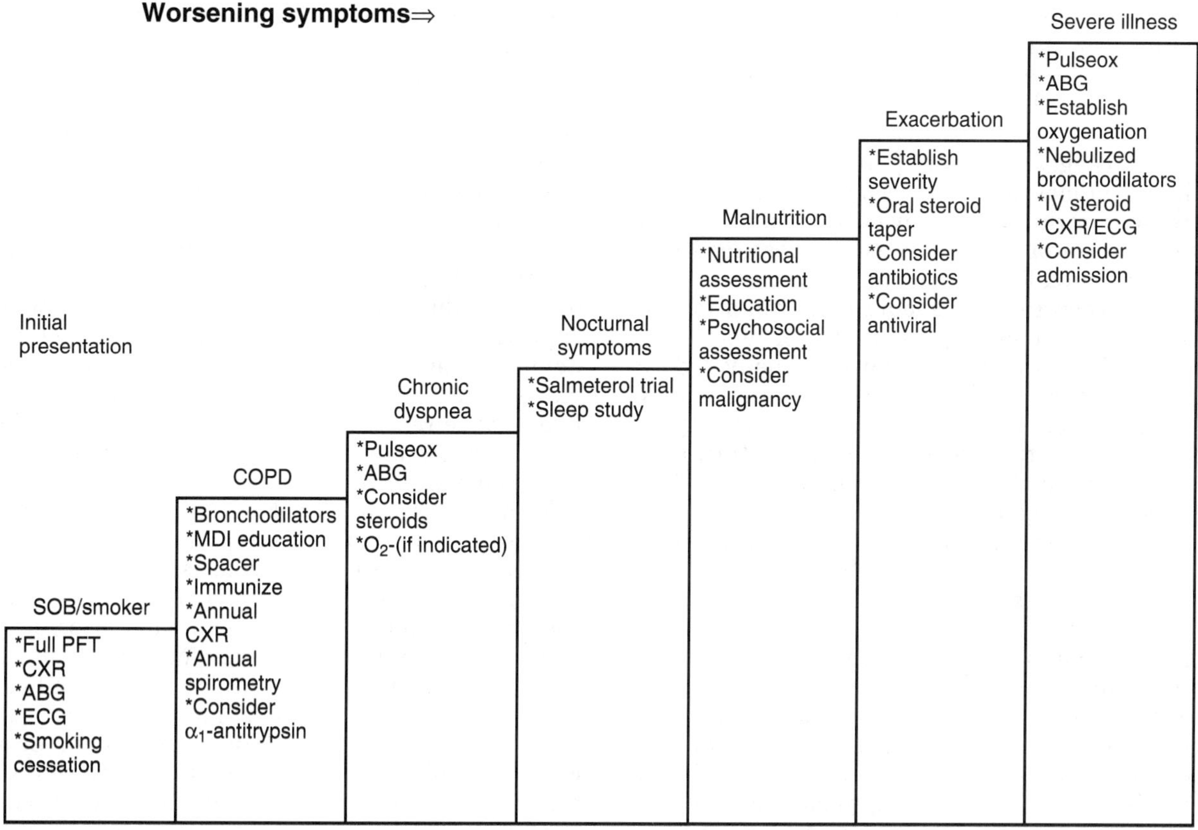

Figure 1. Stepwise summary of COPD management. Symptoms worsen with each step to the right.
Abbreviations: SOB = shortness of breath; PFT = pulmonary function tests; CXR = chest x-ray; ABG = arterial blood gases; ECG = electrocardiogram; COPD = chronic obstructive pulmonary disease; MDI = metered-dose inhaler.

[Combivent]) is now available; it may prove less expensive and more convenient for patients.

Chronic bronchitis with excessive sputum production is a common problem in COPD. Antibiotics should be instituted only when there is a change in the frequency, consistency, and/or color of sputum (i.e., clear or white [mucoid] to green, yellow, brown [purulent] secretions). Sputum cultures are not recommended and likely will not influence management.

Antibiotics should be chosen to ensure coverage of the most common pathogens (i.e., *Streptococcus pneumoniae, Haemophilus influenzae,* and *Moraxella catarrhalis*). Less expensive beta-lactam agents (e.g., amoxicillin [Amoxil], 250 to 500 mg orally three times a day), macrolides (e.g., erythromycin [E-mycin], 250 to 500 mg orally four times a day), or sulfa agents (e.g., trimethoprim/sulfamethoxazole [Bactrim], one double strength tablet twice a day) should be used for 7 to 10 days during mild to moderate exacerbations. Doxycycline (Vibramycin), 100 mg orally every 12 hours, is an acceptable alternative. These are considered adequate therapy when compared to the more expensive cephalosporins, macrolides, and newer quinolone agents.

All patients with COPD, regardless of age, should receive pneumococcal vaccination (Pneumovax, 0.5 mL intramuscularly) every 6 years and an influenza virus vaccine (0.5 mL intramuscularly) every fall unless contraindicated. Rimantadine [Flumadine] (100 mg orally twice daily for 2 to 7 days) should be used as an antiviral agent within the first 48 hours of a respiratory illness regardless of the patient's vaccine status. Caution must be taken in patients with renal or hepatic disease.

Intuitively, the use of expectorants and/or mucolytics (e.g., acetylcysteine, organic iodide) would seem practical. However, the available agents are either very expensive with little or no proven benefit or too toxic for the age group that would derive the most benefit. Adequate hydration in the absence of right and/or left heart failure coupled with guaifenesin (Robitussin) 5 to 20 mL orally every 4 hours, will likely be of the most benefit. Although Dornase alfa* (Pulmozyme), a DNAse, has proven efficacious in the treatment of tenacious secretions in cystic fibrosis patients, its benefit in COPD has yet to be proven.

Outpatient treatment of severe (stage III) COPD is challenging but feasible. COPD is known to be associated with hypoxemia leading to tissue hypoxia in more severe stages of the disease process. Long-term oxygen therapy (LTOT) is paramount during this stage, as it is the only therapy proven to *reduce mortality* and may dramatically improve the quality of life.

*Not FDA approved for this indication.

Current guidelines for the institution of LTOT rely heavily on $Pa{O_2}$ and $Sa{O_2}$ (i.e., $Pa{O_2}$ ≤55 mm Hg or $Sa{O_2}$ ≤88%). However, LTOT should still be instituted if a patient has a $Pa{O_2}$ between 55 and 59 (or $Sa{O_2}$ ≥89%) and erythrocytosis (hematocrit >55%), evidence of congestive heart failure, cor pulmonale, or a change in mental status. A patient who may not meet these criteria at rest may still qualify for LTOT during exercise or sleep. Moreover, resting LTOT should be titrated for exertion and sleep.

Ideally, oxygen therapy should maintain a $Pa{O_2}$ of 60 mm Hg or more or an $Sa{O_2}$ of 90% or more for at least 18 hours a day. Oxygen is usually delivered via a continuous-flow, dual-prong nasal cannula; however, many patients with severe hypoxemia may require a face mask to increase the inspired fraction of oxygen. Alternatively, reservoir cannulas are available to store oxygen during expiration, delivering oxygen at a higher concentration in early inspiration. Once LTOT is instituted, it should be continued indefinitely regardless of improvement in oxygenation when off therapy.

Anti-inflammatory therapy, such as corticosteroids, is still an unproven modality in the treatment of COPD. However, there is a subset of patients who benefit from long-term steroid use. For instance, a patient who responds dramatically to bronchodilator therapy during spirometry (i.e., attains a postbronchodilator FEV_1 of 200 mL above the prebronchodilator FEV_1 or a percent change in FEV_1 of ≥12%) likely has disease with an inflammatory or reactive airway component that would support the use of corticosteroids. For a patient who despite appropriate management for the degree of illness has persistent symptomatology, a trial of oral corticosteroids (prednisone 40 mg orally every day tapered to discontinue over 10 to 14 days) or inhaled steroids such as triamcinolone acetonide (Azmacort) (2 to 4 puffs two to three times a day), or more potent, longer acting flunisolide (AeroBid) or fluticasone (Flovent), 110 to 220 μg given in (2 to 4 puffs twice a day), would not be unreasonable.

Predicting which patients will respond to steroid therapy remains difficult. Follow-up spirometry after 2 weeks of an oral steroid trial is required to assess improvement in FEV_1. Oral steroids should be discontinued if symptoms have not clearly improved and spirometry results show no benefit. Otherwise, steroid dosage should be tapered to the lowest effective every-other-day dosage.

Unfortunately, *systemic* steroid therapy is not without serious side effects. Osteoporosis, diabetes mellitus, hypertension, weight gain, cataracts and mental status changes are some of the most worrisome sequelae. Monitoring for tuberculosis with a PPD skin test at the onset of therapy is recommended. Bone mineral density measurements via DEXA scanning (dual energy x-ray absorptiometry) should be obtained at baseline and 6 months after the initial institution of oral steroids. Values at least two standard deviations below normal are considered indicative of osteoporosis and warrant bisphosphonate therapy (e.g., alendronate [Fosamax], 10 mg orally once a day).

Education is one of the most important aspects in managing any of the three stages of COPD. First, the patient must be instructed in the proper use of an aerosol delivery system, preferably a metered-dose inhaler with a spacer device. Second, techniques such as diaphragmatic and pursed-lip breathing or the "huff cough" (open glottis coughing, which prevents increased intrathoracic pressures and dynamic airway collapse during cough) may prove useful during exacerbations of COPD. Lastly, new devices have been introduced that assist the patient in optimizing expiration and minimizing airway collapse. One such device is the PEP (positive expiratory pressure) valve, which allows the patient to exhale against a fixed-orifice resistor, thereby creating increased back pressures between 10 and 20 cm of H_2O to stent collapsible airways.

Many factors are involved in the chronic weight loss and respiratory muscle fatigue of end-stage COPD. Clearly, caloric intake is one of them. The depression, partly due to restrictions in daily living, that plagues many patients can cause loss of appetite. In addition to a full psychosocial evaluation and the possible institution of antidepressant medication, nutritional assessment during every outpatient visit is important. A 10% loss of ideal body weight or other clinical manifestations of weight loss are considered signs of malnutrition. Malnutrition can obviously have devastating effects on the overall health of the patient, causing respiratory failure secondary to atrophy of respiratory muscles as well as immunocompromise. Moreover, patients with COPD are considered relatively hypermetabolic due to the increased energy needs of the respiratory muscles. Consequently, patients with COPD should be educated about good nutritional habits, specifically frequent small meals and dietary supplements. In addition, appropriate electrolyte supplementation (i.e., phosphorus, calcium, and magnesium) is necessary to ensure adequate diaphragmatic function. Special diets to minimize CO_2 production or overfeeding beyond the caloric needs of the patient are not recommended and can be detrimental. Antioxidants may have a role in slowing progression of the disease, but at present vitamin supplementation in the form of one multivitamin tablet a day is considered adequate. If the patient is on long-term steroid therapy, calcium (500 mg orally twice daily) as well as vitamin D (400 IU once a day) supplementation should be started.

Rehabilitation has quickly come into vogue for the treatment of COPD, no doubt due to the beneficial effects demonstrated in potential lung volume reduction candidates. Before patients can even be considered for rehabilitation, they must undergo cardiopulmonary stress testing. Because most COPD patients are older and have a significant tobacco history, they may also have underlying cardiac disease. Pulmonary rehabilitation has reduced hospitalization in COPD patients. Specific guidelines for rehabilitation vary, but all stress aerobic activity. Brief (45 minute) sessions two to three times a week on calibrated cycle ergometers over a 6-week period are adequate. In addition, patients should be encouraged to walk for

1 hour a day and to maintain regular aerobic activity thereafter.

Nocturnal symptoms may often be associated with COPD. In the past, theophylline was commonly used to alleviate nocturnal dyspnea; however, salmeterol (Serevent), a longer acting $beta_2$ agonist (2 puffs twice a day or at bedtime) may be a better choice. In addition, one must always consider the possibility of oxygen desaturation during REM sleep or an overlap syndrome such as central or obstructive sleep apnea. Therefore, a sleep study is warranted in individuals who complain of nocturnal dyspnea regardless of daytime PaO_2 or SaO_2

Routine assessment of the COPD patient should include an annual chest roentgenogram. A smoking history is associated with malignancy. There is also some evidence to suggest that bullous disease, per se, is associated with lung cancer. In addition, assessment for adequate oxygenation (e.g., pulse oximetry or arterial blood gas testing) as well as decline in pulmonary function should be undertaken when a clinical change arises.

The primary caregiver should be aware of special cases concerning obstructive airways disease. For instance, if a patient presenting with emphysema is relatively young ($\leq$50 years old) or is a lifelong nonsmoker, one should consider the possibility of $alpha_1$-antitrypsin deficiency. This is a hereditary form of emphysema largely affecting whites. If $alpha_1$-antitrypsin levels are $\leq$11 μmol, $alpha_1$-proteinase inhibitor supplementation (Prolastin), 60 mg per kg body weight intravenously every week should be instituted. Of note, Prolastin is a human blood product that carries a relatively low risk of transmitting hepatitis B or C. Therefore, the patient should undergo hepatitis B vaccination several weeks prior to the initial dose.

Special cases arise with patients who are oxygen dependent, under the age of 65, and maximized on pharmacologic therapy but still have significant symptoms. In these situations, the primary caregiver must consider surgery as a therapeutic modality. Lung volume reduction surgery (LVRS) alone or as a bridge to lung transplant may be an option for patients who have not smoked for at least 6 months, have a PCO_2 of 45 or less, have relatively normal cardiac function, and have not had previous thoracic surgery. Studies have shown that the worst postoperative outcomes for LVRS occur in patients with a $PaCO_2$ of 45 or more and in patients unable to walk at least 200 feet in 6 minutes before or after pulmonary rehabilitation.

Inpatient

Patients with COPD are known to be prone to exacerbations, the cause of which is often not readily apparent. During the fall and winter months, a relatively innocuous viral upper respiratory infection can have devastating effects, leading to hospitalization and even intubation with mechanical ventilation. Other causes of decline may include gastroesophageal reflux disease, aspiration, bacterial infection, heart disease, environmental irritants, pulmonary embolus, spontaneous pneumothorax, and medication misuse or side effects. Good outpatient management, although helpful in reducing hospitalizations, will not prevent them.

In addition to the history and physical examination, evaluation of the patient with COPD in the emergency room includes a chest radiograph, electrocardiogram, arterial blood gas analysis, pulse oximetry, and theophylline level when indicated. Signs of respiratory muscle fatigue (e.g., accessory muscle use, paradoxical breathing, intercostal space retractions) will give the clinician an indication of the severity of illness.

Admission to the hospital for these patients should be geared toward the management of an acute deterioration, prevention of further decline, and transfer to an intensive care setting. Adequate oxygenation and reversal of tissue hypoxia are foremost in therapy. Supplemental oxygen should be given to ensure an SaO_2 of 90% or more or a PaO_2 of 60 or more. Oxygen supplementation to raise SaO_2 and PaO_2 above these values affords no benefit and is not recommended due to the added complication of CO_2 narcosis and hypercapnic respiratory failure.

Simultaneously, nebulized solutions of bronchodilators must be administered. A $beta_2$ agonist (albuterol, 2.5 mg nebulized every 1 to 2 hours) followed by or combined with an anticholinergic agent (ipratropium bromide 0.5 mg nebulized every 6 hours) is recommended. Some centers advocate the initial use of a metered-dose inhaler with spacer. Of note, high doses of a $beta_2$ agonist may cause tachycardia or other dysrhythmia.

Concomitant institution of parenteral corticosteroids such as methylprednisolone (Solu-Medrol), 50 to 80 mg intravenously every 6 hours for 24 to 72 hours, should begin immediately. Rapid taper with prednisone 40 mg orally every day tapered to discontinue over 10 to 14 days following parenteral steroid therapy is recommended. Although evidence to support the use of corticosteroids is unclear, they remain the mainstay of treatment for COPD exacerbation.

As mentioned earlier, selected antibiotics to cover common pathogens should be considered when sputum is purulent. When a viral illness is suspected, institution of antiviral therapy (e.g., rimantadine) within the first 48 hours is warranted regardless of immunization status. Sputum culture and Gram's stain are not recommended in the work-up as they are not likely to affect management.

In many instances, increased secretions seem to be a major problem. However, postural drainage with chest physiotherapy and mucolytics are of no proven benefit. Moreover, nebulized acetylcysteine has been known to cause bronchospasm.

Despite aggressive institution of the aforementioned modalities, many patients continue to deteriorate. Mechanical ventilation must be considered when the patient (1) has worsening respiratory acidosis, (2) has altered mental status or other signs of end-organ hypoxia, (3) has signs of severe respiratory distress or failure, (4) cannot be adequately oxygenated using conventional noninvasive means, or (5) has other comorbidities adding to the complexity of the clinical situation.

Patients who qualify for mechanical ventilation but remain lucid (e.g., hypercapnic respiratory failure without high oxygen requirements) may benefit from a trial of noninvasive positive-pressure ventilation (CPAP [continuous positive airway pressure] or BiPAP [bilevel positive airway pressure]). These modalities may provide enough assistance to reverse rapid shallow breathing and improve ventilation and oxygenation. Benzodiazepines and/or opiates to relieve anxiety and/or dyspnea are contraindicated due to their respiratory depressant effects unless the patient is being mechanically ventilated or is under terminal care.

Admission to the hospital should be taken as an opportunity to educate the patient and assess his or her psychosocial status, nutrition, and home environment. The average length of stay to allow maximum benefit and prevent readmission is 6 days. Discharge should be considered when the patient is off parenteral therapy, is able to ambulate and participate in activities of daily living, exhibits no indication of hypoxemia on minimal oxygen requirements, and needs bronchodilator therapy no more than every 4 hours. Both physician and family should feel sure that the patient can be managed successfully at home.

CYSTIC FIBROSIS

method of
JULIE P. KATKIN, M.D.
Baylor College of Medicine
Houston, Texas

Cystic fibrosis (CF) is the most common fatal autosomal recessive disease among Caucasian populations, with an incidence of one in 2000 to 3000 live births. CF is caused by mutations in the cystic fibrosis transmembrane conductance regulator (CFTR) protein, a complex chloride channel found in all exocrine tissues. Deranged chloride transport leads to thick, viscous secretions in the lungs, pancreas, liver, intestine, and reproductive tract, and to increased salt content in sweat gland secretions. The typical CF patient presents with multisystem disease involving several or all of these organs. However, many patients demonstrate mild or atypical symptoms, and clinicians should remain alert to the possibility of CF even when only a few of the usual features are present.

Diagnosis of CF is usually made in childhood, but patients with mild disease may not be identified until adolescence or adulthood. The classic presentation includes chronic obstructive lung disease, persistent lung infection (frequently with mucoid *Pseudomonas aeruginosa*), and steatorrhea with malnutrition or failure to thrive. Other associated findings include chronic sinusitis, nasal polyposis, and digital clubbing. Individuals with milder disease may present with a history of chronic bronchitis, atypical asthma, or infertility. In patients with a suggestive clinical history and physical findings, the diagnosis is confirmed by documentation of a sweat chloride level in excess of 60 mEq per liter or by the presence of pathologic CF mutations on both chromosomes. The sweat chloride test is technically difficult and should be obtained in a facility that performs it frequently to avoid inaccurate results.

Since cystic fibrosis was first recognized as a discrete clinical syndrome in the 1950s, average survival of patients has increased dramatically. The Cystic Fibrosis Foundation maintains a registry of more than 25,000 patients in the United States, and median survival in their cohort is currently approaching 31 years. Much of this improvement can be attributed to the development of centralized CF treatment centers, where patients have access to specialists with particular expertise in the treatment of CF. Data from the CF registry show that patients who are seen regularly in a CF center have less morbidity and slower progression of disease than patients who are seen infrequently or inconsistently.

PULMONARY MANIFESTATIONS

Although CF is a multisystem disease, respiratory symptoms remain the most common cause of morbidity and mortality in affected individuals. The disease process begins with thickened, hyperchloremic airway secretions. The increased viscosity limits ciliary motility and airway clearance, which permits bacterial colonization of the bronchi. Derangements in electrolyte balance lead to decreased function of airway defensins, proteins that normally provide local bactericidal activity. In this milieu, CF patients develop chronic infection with a variety of bacterial agents. *P. aeruginosa* and *Staphylococcus aureus* are particularly tenacious pathogens. *Pseudomonas* and some other gram-negative bacteria frequently assume a mucoid phenotype that is almost pathognomonic for CF-related disease.

Over time, CF patients develop chronic bronchitis with cough and regular sputum production. Typically, they experience episodic exacerbations of their disease associated with increased chest congestion, change in the amount or color of sputum, fatigue, weight loss, and generalized malaise. Although symptoms usually abate in response to antibiotics and chest physiotherapy, it is virtually impossible to eradicate *Pseudomonas* and other organisms from the airways once colonization occurs. Ultimately, the chronic infection causes irreversible airway damage and bronchiectasis, with cystic changes and abscess formation in the late stages of disease.

Monitoring Clinical Status

Regular pulmonary function testing is an essential component of routine care for all CF patients. Spirometry is noninvasive, is well studied, and can be performed by most children by 5 to 6 years of age. Because spirometric data represent the most reproducible, objective measurement of lung function available, routine pulmonary function tests should be obtained every 3 to 6 months in all patients. In childhood, spirometric measurements may remain stable for months or years at a time. Once pulmonary function begins to fall, patients usually experience a progressive decline, although there is wide variability in the rate of loss between individual patients. The earliest change is usually a drop in the forced expiratory flow from 25 to 75% of vital capacity ($FEF_{25\%-75\%}$), but wide variability precludes its use as a marker for disease progression. The forced vital capacity (FVC) and forced expiratory volume in 1 second (FEV_1) are most commonly used to follow lung function. Based on the Cystic Fibrosis Foundation's patient registry, the average yearly rate of decline in FEV_1 for children 6 to 18 years is 2%. Adults have an average decline of 1% per year. Patients with an FEV_1 less than 30% of predicted have a 2-year mortality rate of 50% and should be considered as candidates for lung transplantation.

Chest radiography is less quantitative than spirometry but continues to be a useful modality for monitoring the progression of CF lung disease. Hyperinflation is the earliest finding and may be the only apparent change in young children and adolescents. Increased interstitial markings and peribronchial thickening are a common early finding and may be more noticeable in the upper lobes. As the disease progresses, bronchiectasis and mucus plugging become increasingly obvious, often with a striking severity in the upper lobes. In late stages, cystic cavities may become prominent, and mucus plugs may be visible as nodular or tubular densities in the mid- to peripheral lung fields. High-resolution computed tomography (CT) provides a sensitive assay for the earliest airway changes and may be useful in confirming the diagnosis of bronchiectasis. Chest radiographs should be obtained every 2 to 4 years in patients with stable clinical status and at least yearly in those with deteriorating lung function.

Sputum cultures are essential to monitor the resident airway flora, particularly with regard to antibiotic sensitivity patterns. Cultures should be obtained at least yearly and at the time of pulmonary exacerbations to help guide antimicrobial therapy.

Maintenance Therapy

Routine pulmonary care in CF is designed to delay the onset and progression of pulmonary inflammation, infection, and bronchiectasis. Chest physiotherapy and intermittent antibiotic treatment have a time-honored role in CF treatment. More recent innovations include alternative airway clearance techniques, anti-inflammatory agents, inhaled recombinant DNase, and inhaled antibiotic therapy. CF patients should receive influenza vaccine on a yearly basis.

Routine chest physiotherapy (CPT) is the essential underpinning of pulmonary care in CF. Standard methods of manual percussion and postural drainage have been employed for years and are generally accepted as the "gold standard" against which other modalities are tested. Most practitioners prescribe 20- to 30-minute CPT sessions one to three times a day, depending on the severity of disease and the presence of intercurrent infection. Alternative methods of CPT may be more suitable for older CF patients who require greater autonomy. Available modalities include the positive expiratory pressure (PEP) mask, the Flutter device (Scandipharm, Birmingham, AL), and the ThAirapy Vest (American Biosystems, St. Paul, MN). The PEP mask contains a simple valve that increases resistance to expiratory airflow. The resulting positive end-expiratory pressure distends the large airways, facilitating the outward movement of mucus as the patient exhales. The Flutter consists of a metal ball encased in a plastic tube with a tapered diameter. The ball vibrates as the patient blows forcibly into the tube, creating a vibrating column of air under sustained pressure within the airways. The ThAirapy Vest is an inflatable jacket connected to a compressor that provides external, high-speed vibration of the chest wall. The ThAirapy Vest has efficacy similar to that of the Flutter and is preferred by many patients but is much more expensive. Finally, controlled breathing techniques such as autogenic drainage or active cycle of breathing may be useful modalities for some patients. These techniques must be taught by an experienced respiratory therapist, and patients' proficiency should be reviewed frequently if they are used as the primary modality of CPT.

Airway inflammation in CF may begin in very early childhood and has been shown to precede bacterial colonization in some children. For this reason, chronic use of anti-inflammatory agents is now accepted practice in some CF centers. Ibuprofen* has been studied in this regard and may reduce the rate of decline in lung function in patients with baseline FEV_1 between 40 and 70% of predicted when administered on a regular basis. A good starting dose is 20 mg per kg every 12 hours, but the quantity must be titrated to achieve a peak serum level of 50 to 100 μg per mL. This is accomplished by monitoring serum levels on an hourly basis over 4 hours following a test dose, and adjusting the level as needed. Several tests may be required to identify the proper dose for a given individual. Ibuprofen pharmacokinetics must be reassessed every 2 years or if there is a weight change of more than 25%; renal function should be monitored every 6 to 12 months. Because inadequate serum concentrations of ibuprofen can actually enhance neutrophil influx into the lungs of experimental animals, noncompliant patients should not be treated with this medication. Prednisone (1 to 2 mg per kg every other day) has also been shown to reduce the rate of decline of lung function, but may

*Not FDA approved for this indication.

be associated with multiple adverse effects including growth failure, abnormal glucose metabolism, hypertension, and cataracts. While oral steroids can be useful in selected settings, patients must be carefully monitored during treatment. Some practitioners use inhaled steroids to avoid systemic complications, but controlled trials of their utility have not yet been published.

Inhaled mucolytic agents have long been used by CF physicians to promote airway clearance. *N*-acetylcysteine (Mucomyst) has been used in this fashion for many years, by adding 1 to 2 mL of a 10 or 20% solution to routine inhalation treatments. There are no controlled clinical trials supporting its efficacy, however, and most patients find the taste and odor of the drug unpleasant. It has been largely supplanted by recombinant human DNase I, or dornase-α (Pulmozyme), a recently developed drug that has documented benefit in patients with 40 to 75% of normal lung function. Pulmozyme works by digesting the highly viscous DNA released by inflammatory cells within the airway. This helps to reduce the viscosity of the airway secretions, which then flow more easily along the airway surface. Pulmozyme is supplied in unit dose vials of 2.5 mg, which may be given once or twice daily depending on clinical severity. The drug must be delivered via a Hudson T-Updraft or a Marquest Acorn II nebulizer, either of which must not be used to deliver any other routine inhaled medications.

Chronic administration of oral antibiotics has been used to suppress infection with *S. aureus* and *P. aeruginosa* in some CF centers. Multiple studies have failed to show any long-term protective effects associated with this practice, however. In addition, increasing concern about the emergence of multiple-drug–resistant bacteria has caused many practicioners to be cautious in prescribing long-term systemic antibiotic therapy. Instead, inhaled antibiotics are being prescribed with increasing frequency for suppression of airway infection in CF patients. The FDA has recently approved the use of high-dose tobramycin for inhalation (TOBI) for this purpose. TOBI contains 300 mg of tobramycin in a more concentrated form than that in ordinary intravenous tobramycin solutions. Patients given TOBI twice daily on a 28-day cycle (28 days on the drug, 28 days off) showed improvement in FEV_1 and FVC when compared with placebo-treated controls. The TOBI aerosol must be generated by a PulmoAid or PulmoMate compressor and a Pari-LC Plus nebulizer to produce aerosol droplets of the proper size for airway deposition. Further clinical studies are currently underway to evaluate the long-term impact of this type of suppressive therapy. The potential for emergence of resistant strains of *Pseudomonas* remains an important concern, which will require careful evaluation.

Pulmonary Exacerbations

The phrase "pulmonary exacerbation" is used to describe a change in pulmonary symptoms from the patient's usual status that necessitates treatment with antibiotics and a supplemental airway clearance program. Exacerbations may be triggered by viral respiratory infections or episodes of asthma, but often no precipitating factor can be identified. No uniform criteria have been established to define the presence or severity of exacerbations, and symptoms can vary among individuals. In general, patients complain of increased chest congestion and cough with increased sputum production, sometimes associated with a change in the sputum color. New or increasing hemoptysis, decreased appetite, weight loss, fatigue, or generalized malaise are also common presenting symptoms. Physical examination may reveal increased respiratory rate, use of accessory muscles, new or increased crackles in the lung fields, tachycardia or fever, but some patients may have very few physical signs of increased disease. Spirometry frequently demonstrates a 10% or greater drop in FVC and/or FEV_1 when compared with the best value obtained in the previous 6 months. Other laboratory findings can include a new infiltrate on a chest radiograph, leukocytosis, and decreased oxygen saturation. Ultimately, the diagnosis and treatment of a pulmonary exacerbation is based on the clinician's judgment of the degree of change from the patient's usual baseline status.

Antibiotic therapy is almost always required for treatment of pulmonary exacerbations. The initial choice of antibiotics should be based on the identification and sensitivity patterns of flora grown from previous sputum cultures whenever possible. If previous cultures are not available, empiric therapy may be started with antimicrobial coverage directed against *S. aureus* and *P. aeruginosa*. Typically, initial therapy will consist of an aminoglycoside (gentamicin or tobramycin) and a semisynthetic penicillin with or without clavulanate (ticarcillin, piperacillin, or Timentin). Sputum cultures with antibiotic sensitivity panels should be obtained at the start of treatment for all patients, and the results should be used to adjust antibiotic therapy for patients who are not responding to treatment. Two antipseudomonal drugs should be administered to provide synergy, and to delay the emergence of resistant bacterial strains. CF patients are known to have an increased volume of distribution of medications, as well as increased rates of drug metabolism and clearance, and consequently, they typically require higher doses of many medications than other patients do. Table 1 shows usual starting doses of commonly used antibiotics for CF patients, along with optimum serum levels and potential toxicities where applicable.

Mild exacerbations may be treated with augmented airway clearance and a 10- to 14-day course of oral antibiotics effective against *Haemophilus influenzae* and *S. aureus*. Patients with documented *P. aeruginosa* colonization may require oral or inhaled antipseudomonal agents, which should be given for at least 14 days. Patients who have failed oral or inhaled antibiotic therapy, or who present with severe symptoms, will require intravenous antibiotics

TABLE 1. **Usual Antibiotic Doses for Cystic Fibrosis Patients**

Drug	Starting Dose	Levels	Comments
Aminoglycosides			
Tobramycin (Nebcin)	9 mg/kg/d IV unless renal impairment or known kinetics data Interval: divided q 8–12 h	Peak: 8–12 μg/mL Trough: ≤2 μg/mL	Monitor renal function Possible ototoxicity
Gentamicin (Garamycin)	9 mg/kg/d IV unless renal impairment or known kinetics data Interval: divided q 8–12 h	Peak: 8–12 μg/mL Trough: ≤2 μg/mL	Monitor renal function Possible ototoxicity
Amikacin (Amikin)	30 mg/kg/d IV unless renal impairment or known kinetics data Interval: divided q 8–12 h	Peak: 25–40 μg/mL Trough: ≤10 μg/mL	Monitor renal function Possible ototoxicity
Penicillins			
Piperacillin (Pipracil)	400–600 mg/kg/d IV unless renal impairment; maximum dose 24 gm/day Interval: divided q 4–6 h		
Ticarcillin (Ticar)	400–600 mg/kg/d IV; maximum 24 gm/day Interval: divided q 4–6 h		
Ticarcillin/clavulanic acid (Timentin)	400–600 mg/kg/d IV; maximum 24 gm/day Interval: divided q 4–6 h		Covers *S. aureus*
Nafcillin (Nafcil)	200 mg/kg/d IV; maximum 12 gm/day Interval: divided q 4–6 h		Covers *S. aureus*
Other			
Aztreonam (Azactam)	200 mg/kg/d IV unless renal impairment; maximum 8 gm/d Interval: divided q 6 h		Avoid use with imipenem, which can induce β-lactamase activity
Ceftazidime (Fortaz)	150 mg/kg/d IV unless renal impairment; maximum 6 gm/d Interval: divided q 8 h		
Imipenem (Primaxin)	60–75 mg/kg/day IV unless renal impairment; maximum 4 gm/d Interval: divided q 6 h		Nausea/vomiting common; may be reduced by longer infusion time or pretreating with antiemetics
Ciprofloxacin (Cipro)	10–15 mg/kg/dose IV; maximum 400 mg/dose Interval: q12 h Oral: <12 years: 500 mg/dose bid ≥12 years: 750 mg/dose bid		Monitor renal & hepatic function. Do not give with oral antacids. Do not give without 2nd antibiotic.
TMP-SMX (Bactrim, Septra)	10–20 mg/kg/d TMP orally; maximum 320 mg/d TMP Interval: divided q 8–12 h		

Abbreviation: TMP-SMX = trimethoprim-sulfamethoxazole.

for 10 to 14 days or longer. Asthma therapy should be initiated or intensified for all patients with symptoms of reactive airways disease.

Inhaled antibiotics may be prescribed for bacterial suppression, as previously described, or for treatment of acute exacerbations of disease. Gentamicin is prescribed in a dose of 80 mg three times a day (tid) for most patients, although adults may safely receive 160 mg tid. For an 80-mg dose, 2 mL of solution (40 mg per mL) are added to 1 mL of normal saline and administered via a standard home nebulizer unit with mask or mouthpiece. The 160 mg dose (4 mL of a 40 mg per mL solution) may be given without additional diluent. Inhaled tobramycin may be prescribed in doses of 80 to 160 mg tid for younger children and up to 400 to 600 mg tid for older children and adults with moderate to severe disease. The lower doses, supplied in a concentration of 40 mg per mL, may be delivered with a standard nebulizer in the same manner as gentamicin. High-dose tobramycin is supplied in a 1.2-mg vial, which is initially resuspended in 30 mL of 50% normal saline (40 mg per mL). The necessary drug is then removed and diluted in an equal volume of 50% normal saline, to a final concentration of 20 mg per mL, for aerosol delivery. The resulting large volume necessitates the use of an Ultraneb 99 ultrasonic nebulizer (Devilbiss), and the treatment may take from 30 to 45 minutes to complete. While this form of therapy is often very effective, it may become exhausting for sick patients who must also take asthma medications, perform airway clearance maneuvers, and consume 3000 to 5000 calories per day.

Most patients who require intravenous therapy should be hospitalized during the acute stage of their illness, because symptoms may worsen in the first few days of therapy as secretions are mobilized. Supplemental oxygen should be provided or increased based on the results of pulse oximetry or arterial blood gas analysis. Airway clearance therapy should be delivered three to four times daily based on the patient's usual regimen and the severity of the exacerbation. Aminoglycoside doses should be adjusted to provide optimum peak and trough serum levels, and renal function should be monitored at least weekly during therapy. Blood sugar levels should be monitored carefully in diabetic or prediabetic patients, as insulin requirements may be transiently increased during the acute stages of illness.

Patients who show clinical improvement may be eligible to complete their therapy at home if a capable caretaker is available to administer medications and assist in airway clearance. On occasion, an experienced patient may be able to receive a complete course of antibiotics at home, without an initial hospitalization. All candidates for home therapy, with or without an initial hospital stay, must have stable intravenous access, which can usually be managed by placement of a percutaneous central catheter for those who do not have surgically implanted central lines. Home nursing and infusion support services must be available and capable of obtaining blood tests and oximetry as needed. Patients who are prescribed antibiotics they have not previously used must receive at least the first dose in a monitored setting before completing the course of treatment at home. Patients who are not good candidates for home therapy include adult patients living alone (or who lack sufficient home support), patients with comorbidities that require close monitoring, patients with a history of poor compliance, and those who lack adequate utilities in the home to support high-tech care (e.g., telephone, electricity, refrigeration, plumbing).

The duration of treatment for a pulmonary exacerbation may range from 10 days to 3 to 4 weeks, depending on the severity of the symptoms and the degree of underlying disease. For most patients, treatment should continue until symptoms have resolved and pulmonary function tests have returned to baseline levels. On occasion, a patient will fail to have complete resolution of symptoms despite a prolonged course of antibiotic and airway clearance therapy. These patients may require further study to rule out pulmonary infection with atypical mycobacteria or fungi, previously undiagnosed reactive airway disease, gastroesophageal reflux, or overwhelming sinus infection, all of which can contribute to intractable symptoms. In some cases, patients will never return to their preillness state of health, and a new "baseline" of function will be established.

Hemoptysis

Hemoptysis occurs frequently in CF patients with moderate to severe lung disease. Bleeding originates in the bronchial arteries, which become enlarged and tortuous in bronchiectatic lung tissue. In older patients, collateral vessels connecting the bronchial circulation with major intrathoracic arteries increase the risk of serious blood loss. Minor hemoptysis, or "blood streaking" of the sputum, is fairly common and usually does not require specific therapy. Persistent streaking over several days may indicate the onset of a pulmonary exacerbation requiring appropriate therapy. Patients with recurrent streaking or frequent episodes of low-volume bleeding (1 to 2 tsp at a time) should have platelets, prothrombin time (PT), and partial thromboplastin time (PTT) checked and may need to discontinue use of aspirin or nonsteroidal anti-inflammatory drugs.

Major hemoptysis occurs in at least 1% of CF patients each year and is most common in those over 15 years of age. Major hemoptysis may present as a single episode of acute blood loss (usually defined as 240 mL within a 24-hour period) or as recurrent bleeding of a substantial volume (e.g., ≥100 mL per day) over several days. These episodes can produce airway obstruction, chemical pneumonitis, anemia, hypotension, or asphyxia, all of which are potentially life-threating for the CF patient. Hemoptysis must be differentiated from acute gastrointestinal bleeding, which can also occur in older CF patients. Sometimes patients can help to identify the site of bleeding by localizing sensations of "gurgling," warmth, discomfort, or fullness in the chest. A chest radiograph may also help by identifying infiltrates, cysts, or other new abnormalities. Useful laboratory studies include PT, PTT, liver function tests and sputum culture; patients should also have blood typed and cross-matched for possible transfusion.

Patients experiencing acute, severe hemoptysis should be reassured and calmed. Supplemental oxygen and mild sedation should be used as indicated. Coagulation defects should be corrected with vitamin K and/or fresh frozen plasma, and acute blood losses should be replaced with packed red cells as needed. Patients should be encouraged to cough frequently to keep the airways clear of blood. Life-threatening episodes may require emergent endotracheal intubation and ventilation to maintain airway patency. The most definitive therapy for major hemoptysis is bronchial artery embolization, which must be performed by a radiologist experienced in interventional angiography. Extreme cases may require resection of one or more lobes of the lung, so surgical support should also be readily available. For this reason, patients having major hemoptysis should be transferred to a medical treatment facility with experienced CF caretakers at the earliest opportunity.

Other Pulmonary Complications

Asthma occurs with greater frequency in CF patients than in the general population, and some studies have suggested that CF patients with asthma may have a more rapid deterioration of lung function than those without asthma. In affected patients, asthma exacerbations frequently coincide with episodes of worsening bacterial bronchitis, although it is not always clear which element flared first. Asthma therapy should follow the same principles used for other patients, with stepwise progression from intermittent bronchodilators to chronic inhaled anti-inflammatory medications as needed. In the setting of an acute exacerbation, both the asthma and the bronchitis may require aggressive therapy to achieve complete resolution of symptoms.

Pneumothorax occurs in approximately 1% of CF patients each year. The incidence increases with age and severity of disease; approximately 16 to 20% of adults with CF will experience a pneumothorax during their lifetime. Symptoms may be sudden and severe, including dyspnea, chest pain, tachypnea, and/or cyanosis. Other patients may be completely asymptomatic, presenting with an apparently incidental finding on chest radiograph. All patients with a newly diagnosed pneumothorax should be observed in the hospital for at least 24 hours, even if they are asymptomatic. Patients who remain stable and symptom-free with no increase in the amount of extrapulmonary air can be discharged home and followed closely as outpatients. Patients with pneumothoraces that occupy 20% or more of the hemithorax or that are increasing in size or patients who have increasing symptoms should be treated with tube thoracostomy. A pneumothorax associated with persistent air leak that fails to resolve after 5 days of negative pressure may require surgical intervention. This should be undertaken only by a clinician experienced in the care of CF patients, as invasive thoracic procedures can present a significant obstacle to later lung transplantation.

NUTRITIONAL MANAGEMENT AND PANCREATIC ENZYME SUPPLEMENTATION

Eighty percent of CF patients produce insufficient exocrine pancreatic enzymes to support digestion and absorption of ingested nutrients. In affected infants, failure to thrive is a common presenting symptom of CF. In older individuals, symptoms may include steatorrhea, abdominal distention and discomfort, fat-soluble vitamin deficiencies, and malnutrition despite high caloric intake. Pancreatic insufficiency is one of the few manifestations of CF that has a demonstrated relationship to genotype, and its presence or absence can sometimes be predicted on the basis of DNA analysis.

There is a clear association between malnutrition and deterioration of lung function in CF patients. For this reason, aggressive support with high caloric intake, vitamin supplementation, and pancreatic enzyme replacement is essential. Infants may be fed breast milk or normal cow's milk–based formula but sometimes require concentrated formula containing greater than the usual 20 kcal per ounce to maintain appropriate weight gain. Infants generally require supplementation with sodium chloride, especially during the summer. This can be conveniently accomplished by the addition of 1/8 to 1/4 tsp of salt to the day's intake. Older patients should eat a high-calorie diet with unrestricted fat, relying on enzyme supplementation to aid in digestion. School-aged children may require special dispensation to eat extra snacks during the day. Salt supplementation is usually not needed for older children and adults eating a regular diet but should be considered for patients engaged in strenuous work or play during the summer months.

Several commercial preparations of pancreatic enzymes are available. Some contain pancreatin and some pancrelipase but all are composed of porcine lipase, amylase, and trypsin. Most products come as capsules containing enteric-coated microencapsulated enzymes (e.g., Cotazym-S, Pancrease, Zymase, Creon, Ultrase). The enzyme dose is defined by the lipase content; most preparations are available in strengths ranging from 4000 to 20,000 units per capsule. Infants should be started with 1000 to 2000 lipase units per 120 mL of formula or breast-feeding, and which can be increased to a maximum of 4000 units per 120 mL feed as needed. Granular enzyme preparations that dissolve readily in formula are available (Cotazym, Viokase) but may cause excoriation of the oral and perianal mucosa. Most infants can be coaxed to swallow the microencapsulated form of enzyme beads if they are mixed in a small quantity of cereal or pureed fruit. The most convenient method for determining enzyme dosage is based on patient weight. First-time users should begin with 1000 lipase units per kg per meal in children under 4 years and 500 units per kg per meal in those over 4 years of age. One half of the usual mealtime dose can be given with snacks. The enzyme dosage can be slowly increased until signs and symptoms of malabsorption disappear, but changes should always be made in consultation with an experienced medical practitioner. Enzyme requirements vary among individuals but should not exceed 2500 units of lipase per kg per meal. Higher doses have been associated with the development of colonic strictures that may require surgical intervention. Persistent symptoms of malabsorption in the face of high doses of supplemental enzymes warrant further investigation.

GASTROINTESTINAL COMPLICATIONS

The earliest gastrointestinal complication of CF is meconium ileus, a condition that affects 10 to 20% of newborns with the disease. Thickened secretions during fetal development lead to intestinal obstruction, with abdominal distention and failure to pass meconium after birth. Surgical decompression is usually curative, and the presence of meconium ileus is not predictive of future gastrointestinal complications of CF. Meconium ileus is extremely rare in infants who do not have CF, and all affected babies should have sweat chloride testing at the earliest opportunity.

Older children and adults with CF may have intermittent episodes of partial intestinal obstruction known as distal intestinal obstruction syndrome (DIOS), caused by tenacious intestinal contents collecting in a thickened, edematous ileocecal bowel. Patients present with crampy abdominal pain, distention, flatulence, and anorexia. The symptoms may be acute or chronic and recurrent and can persist despite an apparently normal stool pattern. A right lower quadrant mass may be palpable in some patients, but the diagnosis is usually confirmed by evidence of obstruction and copious fecal matter on an abdominal radiograph. Care should be taken to rule out acute appendicitis or appendiceal abscess, which can present with a similar clinical picture. Complete bowel obstruction in DIOS mandates surgical consultation, but most episodes can be resolved by nonoperative means. Most patients respond to ingestion of a balanced polyethylene glycol–electrolyte solution (GoLYTELY, Colyte) given orally or by nasogastric tube. The dose is 20 to 40 mL per kg per hour, to a maximum volume of 1200 mL per hour. Associated nausea and bloating may be lessened by the concomitant use of prokinetic agents such as metoclopramide or cisapride. Resolution of symptoms is usually accomplished within 6 to 8 hours. Alternatively, the obstruction may be cleared by administration of a water-soluble contrast enema in the radiology suite. A large volume of contrast may be required to achieve reflux into the terminal ileum, and iso-osmolar agents should be used to avoid large fluid and electrolyte shifts. This method has the added advantage of immediate radiologic confirmation of the obstruction's removal.

Rectal prolapse may occur in up to 20% of patients with CF, and is commonly seen around the time of toilet training. Constipation, diarrhea, and malnutrition may all be contributing factors, as chronic cough may be in older patients. Rapid manual reduction of the prolapse will prevent bowel edema and usually forestalls the need for surgical intervention. Recurrent prolapse can usually be treated by improving nutritional status, and for many patients episodes decrease in frequency with age. Surgical treatment may be required for patients with frequent prolapse associated with pain and incontinence.

Gastroesophageal reflux (GER) is another common problem for CF patients, and occurs with increased frequency in patients who have relatively severe lung disease. Patients may present with the usual symptoms of epigastric or substernal pain, decreased appetite, regurgitation and dysphagia, but may also complain of worsening respiratory symptoms that are unresponsive to aggressive pulmonary therapy. Diagnostic evaluation and therapy should proceed as for other patients with GER. Prokinetic agents and H_2 blockers may be beneficial, particularly during episodes of acute respiratory exacerbations. GER in CF patients usually follows a relapsing course, and many patients will require repeated or chronic therapy to control their symptoms.

OTHER COMPLICATIONS

Diabetes Mellitus

Diabetes mellitus is a common complication associated with CF. The incidence increases with advancing age, probably as a result of progressive destruction of the pancreas. Recent evidence suggests that CF patients also have some degree of insulin receptor insensitivity, although the reason for this remains unclear. Ketoacidosis is unusual in CF patients, and the onset of diabetes is usually slow. Initial symptoms may occur only during periods of stress, such as during pulmonary exacerbations. The Cystic Fibrosis Foundation recommends screening with an oral glucose tolerance test (fasting and 2-hour postprandial glucose) every 2 years for patients 10 to 16 years of age and yearly for older individuals. Patients should also be monitored carefully during the first trimester of pregnancy and during pulmonary exacerbations. CF patients frequently require higher doses of insulin than do other diabetics to remain euglycemic. Systemic steroid medications, while useful for controlling some pulmonary symptoms, may cause serious derangements in blood glucose levels and should be used with caution in CF patients.

Chronic Sinusitis

Chronic sinusitis is an almost universal finding in CF patients. Viscous sinus secretions, reduced ciliary function, edema of the nasal mucosa, and nasal polyps may all contribute to the retention of mucus within the sinus cavities, where it is readily colonized with bacteria. *S. aureus, P. aeruginosa* (mucoid and nonmucoid), and *H. influenzae* are common pathogens in the sinuses of CF patients, as they are in the lungs. For some patients, sinus discomfort represents a major component of disease, while other patients are fairly asymptomatic despite persistent radiographic changes. Topical intranasal steroids may help promote sinus drainage by reducing mucosal edema, and intermittent courses of oral or intravenous antibiotics may be required to supress persistent infection. For some patients, sinus infections appear to trigger lower respiratory exacerbations of CF, and should therefore be treated aggressively. Large or copious nasal polyps or sinus discomfort unresponsive to antibiotic therapy is another indication for referral to an otolaryngologist experienced in the care of CF patients.

Hepatobiliary Disease

Hepatobiliary manifestations of CF occur in up to 20% of CF patients, with increasing incidence in adults. The pathognomic lesion in CF is focal biliary cirrhosis, which can remain completely asymptomatic or progress to multilobular biliary cirrhosis with portal hypertension and liver failure. Patients who have had meconium ileus or DIOS appear to have an increased incidence of hepatobiliary complications. Clinical findings in affected patients can include neonatal cholestasis, fatty liver and hepatomegaly, abdominal pain, cholecystitis, common bile duct obstruction, pancreatitis, or frank cirrhosis. Changes in liver enzymes may be present long before symptoms occur, so all patients should have annual evaluation of AST, ALT, alkaline phosphatase, GGT, and bilirubin levels. Gallstones in CF patients are usually low in cholesterol and unresponsive to lithotryptic agents, so that surgical intervention is often required to manage symptomatic cholecystitis. Liver transplants have been performed in some patients with end-stage hepatic disease.

Infertility

The vast majority of men with CF have azoospermia and infertility as a result of altered prostatic secretions and hypoplasia or absence of the vas deferens. In some cases, viable sperm can be recovered directly from the testis for in vitro fertilization procedures, but results vary widely among patients and medical practitioners. Women with CF frequently have reduced fertility, which is felt to be caused by increased viscosity of the cervical mucus. Despite this, many female CF patients conceive spontaneously and successfully carry pregnancies to full term. Intrauterine insemination can also be useful, as direct deposition of the sperm into the uterine cavity effectively bypasses the thickened mucus at the cervical os. All adults with CF desiring to have children should be carefully counseled about the certainty of passing a CF allele to their offspring. Partners of CF patients should have DNA testing to ensure that they do not carry a CF mutation, as the risk of an affected child for such a couple is 50%.

OBSTRUCTIVE SLEEP APNEA

method of
JOHN A. FLEETHAM, M.D.
Vancouver Hospital and Health Sciences Centre, University of British Columbia
Vancouver, British Columbia, Canada

Sleep-disordered breathing is characterized by recurrent obstruction of the upper airway, which results in episodic asphyxia and interruption of the normal sleep pattern. Although manifestations of sleep-disordered breathing have been described for many years, the condition has achieved wider recognition in the past decade. It comprises a continuum from asymptomatic snoring to obstructive sleep hypopnea to severe obstructive sleep apnea (OSA) associated with progressively increasing clinical consequences. Recent population-based studies have linked OSA with hypertension, motor vehicle accidents, increased medical care usage, and neuropsychologic impairment. OSA is a common condition, which is now thought to affect up to 4% of middle-aged men and 2% of middle-aged women. It is more common in patients who smoke or consume alcohol and increases with age and following menopause in women.

CLINICAL PRESENTATION

The clinical presentations of OSA are quite diverse (Table 1). It is essential to obtain a history from the patient's bed partner, as the patient may be unaware of any problem. Chronic loud snoring and excessive daytime sleepiness are the hallmark of OSA. Even though the results are completely normal in most patients with OSA, the physical examination is important because it may reveal signs related to the cause or effects of the disease. Many patients are overweight with short, thick necks and heavy jowls. Upper airway examination may reveal a specific abnormality, but more frequently any findings are subtle, including a narrow posterior oropharynx, long and redundant soft palate, or slight retrognathia. Systemic hypertension is common, and secondary polycythemia and right heart failure can occur in severe OSA.

TABLE 1. **Common Symptoms of Obstructive Sleep Apnea**

Loud snoring
Reported nocturnal apnea
Excessive daytime fatigue and sleepiness
Nocturnal choking or dyspnea
Recurrent nocturnal awakening
Unrefreshing sleep
Morning headache
Poor memory
Irritability
Depression
Reduced libido

CAUSES

OSA occurs because of recurrent upper airway obstruction. Upper airway patency during sleep is determined by upper airway size and neuromuscular activity. OSA is associated with a variety of conditions that reduce upper airway size (Table 2). Although the majority of patients do not have these conditions, the upper airways of patients with OSA are narrower and more compliant than in normal subjects. There is familial clustering of OSA and increasing evidence that this is due to similarities in upper airway structure. Upper airway muscle activity is reduced during sleep, resulting in increased airway resistance.

DIFFERENTIAL DIAGNOSIS

Conditions such as narcolepsy, periodic limb movement during sleep, central sleep apnea, and gastroesophageal reflux may present with symptoms suggestive of OSA. It is important to accurately diagnose OSA and determine the type and severity of sleep apnea before treatment. The majority of these patients demonstrate no abnormality while awake, so sleep studies are necessary. Case selection techniques such as overnight home oximetry may be useful in patients who are asymptomatic apart from snoring or reported nocturnal apnea (Figure 1). Definitive diagnosis in symptomatic patients usually requires a detailed overnight sleep study (polysomnogram). Guidelines have been developed for the indications and standards for polysomnography, which is usually performed in specialized referral centers. Split night studies (diagnostic and therapeutic) may be appropriate in selected patients. The role of portable diagnostic recordings is controversial. They should

TABLE 2. **Causes of Obstructive Sleep Apnea**

Obesity
Nasal obstruction (deviated septum, chronic rhinitis)
Enlarged tongue (Down syndrome, acromegaly, hypothyroidism)
Jaw malformations (rheumatoid arthritis, congenital craniofacial abnormalities)
Enlarged soft palate (cleft palate repair)
Upper airway tumor
Enlarged tonsils and adenoids
Paralyzed vocal cords
Drugs (alcohol, sedatives, androgens)

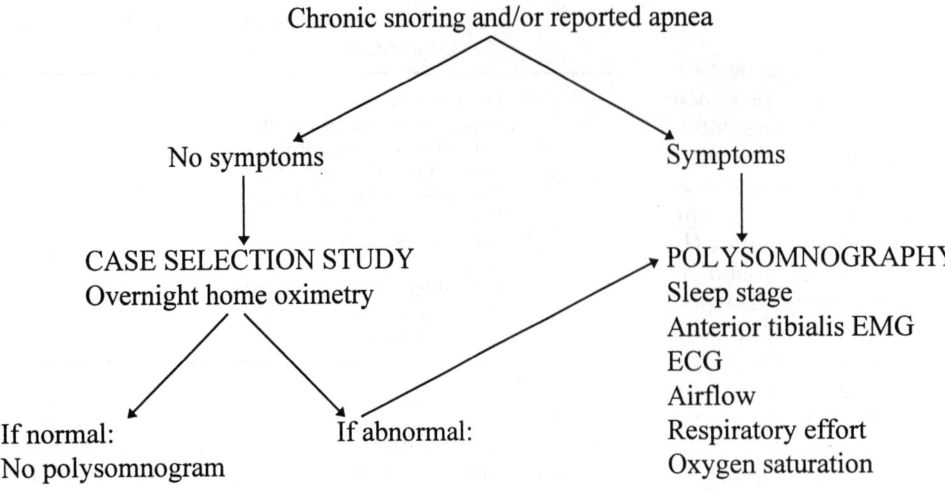

Figure 1. Investigation of suspected sleep apnea. *Abbreviations:* EMG = electromyogram; ECG = electrocardiogram.

probably be restricted to case-selection and follow-up studies until the accuracy and cost-effectiveness can be established.

TREATMENT

The treatment of OSA depends on the severity of symptoms, the magnitude of clinical complications, and the etiology of the airway obstruction. Simple measures such as weight reduction, smoking cessation, avoidance of alcohol, and relief of nasal obstruction should be addressed in every patient. Additional treatment is usually indicated following a failure of conservative treatment.

Nasal continuous positive airway pressure (CPAP) is both safe and effective and is generally established as the primary treatment for symptomatic OSA. Nasal CPAP acts as a "pneumatic splint," and its efficacy is dependent on the degree of positive pressure applied to the upper airway. Nasal CPAP reduces daytime sleepiness and improves both cognitive function and quality of life. Its long-term effects on systemic blood pressure and mortality are not yet established. Only 50 to 80% of patients continue to use this treatment on a long-term basis, and even in these patients, covert monitoring has shown that the average usage is less than 50% of night-time hours. Patient noncompliance is mainly due to the inherent cumbersomeness and inconvenience of nasal CPAP therapy.

The major side effects of nasal CPAP are rhinorrhea, nasal dryness, and eye and facial discomfort. A wide variety of nasal and oral masks are now available to help reduce the problems caused by a poor fitting mask. Claustrophobia can be reduced in some patients by use of a pressure "ramp," which slowly increases pressure at onset of sleep. "Intelligent" nasal CPAP has been developed that automatically varies the pressure to meet the changing needs of the patient. It is not yet clear whether this CPAP modality improves patient acceptance or compliance.

Oral appliances (OAs) are an effective alternative treatment in patients with mild to moderate OSA who are unwilling or unable to use nasal CPAP. There are major design differences in the OAs now available, which may have an impact on their success and compliance rates. The majority of OAs advance the mandible, utilizing traditional dental techniques to attach the appliance to one or both dental arches. Construction usually requires dental impressions, bite registration, and fabrication by a dental laboratory. However, at least one prefabricated appliance is available that can be molded to the patient's teeth in an office setting. Some appliances restrict mouth opening by means of clasps, whereas others allow relatively unhindered movement. OAs have been developed with an adjustable hinge that allows progressive advancement of the mandible after initial construction until an optimal mandibular position is achieved. Mandibular advancement OAs require at least 10 teeth in each of the maxillary and mandibular arches. In addition to advancing the mandible, they also produce downward rotation. The other type of OA available is a tongue retainer that keeps the tongue in an anterior position during sleep by means of negative pressure in a soft plastic bulb. This type of appliance is available in both a fabricated and prefabricated version and can be used in edentulous patients. The side effects of both types of OAs include excessive salivation, jaw discomfort, and sore teeth.

The role of upper airway surgery in the treatment of OSA is controversial. Tracheostomy is reserved for patients with severe OSA in whom all other treatments have been ineffective. Uvulopalatopharyngoplasty enlarges the upper airway by removing excessive distal palatal tissue while preserving the proximal palatal musculature. The success of this operation varies considerably, and it can compromise the ability to subsequently comply with nasal CPAP therapy. Laser-assisted uvulopalatoplasty (LAUP) is performed as an office procedure with less extensive resection of pharyngeal tissue. The long-term risks, benefits, and complications of LAUP in the treatment of OSA have not been established.

PRIMARY LUNG CANCER

method of
RAMESH K. RAMANATHAN, M.D., and
CHANDRA P. BELANI, M.D.
*University of Pittsburgh School of Medicine and University of Pittsburgh Cancer Institute
Pittsburgh, Pennsylvania*

Lung cancer is a major public health problem in the United States. It is one of the most common cancers worldwide, and the incidence is increasing by about 0.5% every year. In the United States, 171,500 new cases and 160,100 deaths were estimated for 1998. Lung cancer accounts for 29% of all cancer deaths and is the most common cause of cancer-related death in both sexes. In men, the incidence and death rate for lung cancer have declined; in women, recent data show that the incidence has started to decline, although death rates are still increasing. The 5-year survival for lung cancer has shown a small but significant improvement over the last 30 years, with current 5-year survival rates of about 14% for Caucasians and 11% for African-Americans.

ETIOLOGY

Cigarette smoking accounts for the vast majority of lung cancer cases and is related to the duration and number of cigarettes smoked in a lifetime. In heavy smokers (those who smoke more than 40 cigarettes per day), the risk of developing lung cancer is increased 18- to 24-fold compared with nonsmokers. Exposure to environmental tobacco smoke or second-hand smoke has been implicated as a risk factor in epidemiologic studies and may account for 2 to 3% of all lung cancer cases. Other risk factors for developing lung cancer include exposure to arsenic, some organic chemicals, asbestos, radon, chromium, nickel, and vinyl compounds.

CLINICAL MANIFESTATIONS

Early diagnosis of lung cancer is difficult, because most patients do not have symptoms until the cancer is advanced. Screening for lung cancer with sputum cytology or chest x-ray studies is imprecise and has not been shown to be cost-effective. The signs and symptoms of lung cancer vary, and patients can present with cough, hemoptysis, chest pain, weight loss, or recurrent lung infections. Generalized malaise and the anorexia-cachexia syndrome are common in advanced cancer. In metastatic cancer, different organ systems may be involved and give rise to various symptoms. A variety of paraneoplastic syndromes can be present and are more common in small cell lung cancer, except for hypercalcemia, which occurs more often with squamous cell carcinoma.

PATHOLOGY

The World Health Organization (WHO) lung cancer histologic classification is widely accepted. The histologic types are squamous cell carcinoma, adenocarcinoma, small cell cancer, and large cell carcinoma. Over the last several decades the incidence of adenocarcinoma has increased, and this entity has surpassed squamous cell carcinoma as the most common histologic type, at present accounting for about 31% of all cases. Well-differentiated squamous cell carcinoma usually presents as localized disease and is associated with the best outcome. Bronchoalveolar cell carcinoma, a variant of adenocarcinoma, appears to be increasing in incidence; the characteristic pathologic pattern is proliferating growth along the alveolar septa. Among tumors classified as non–small cell lung cancer (NSCLC), two distinct subtypes—well-differentiated squamous cell carcinoma and bronchoalveolar cell carcinoma—can be identified in this heterogeneous group. Small cell lung cancer (SCLC) accounts for about 20 to 25% of cases, and its differentiation from NSCLC is important for prognostication and treatment decisions. In some cases distinction between SCLC and NSCLC is difficult; disagreement among pathologists is seen in 5 to 7% of cases. Inadequate or crushed specimens may be the reason for diagnostic confusion, and rebiopsy may be needed.

DIAGNOSIS AND STAGING

In patients suspected of having lung cancer, a thorough history and physical examination are essential. Lung nodules are frequently first noted on the chest radiograph, and a computed tomography (CT) scan of the chest can confirm abnormalities and provide information for accurate staging. Pathologic confirmation of malignancy is mandatory. In centrally located tumors visualized through a flexible bronchoscope, the diagnosis can be established with an accuracy of more than 90%. In patients with peripheral lesions, percutaneous fine needle aspiration under fluoroscopic or CT guidance is useful to obtain tissue for pathologic analysis. Video-assisted minimally invasive thoracoscopy is increasingly being used in the diagnosis of lung cancer, because in addition to excision and biopsy of peripheral nodules, the mediastinum and pleura can also be examined by this procedure.

Once the diagnosis of lung cancer is made, the disease should be accurately staged. In the United States, most patients undergo CT scanning of the chest and upper abdomen, including the liver and adrenal gland. CT scans of the head and bone scans should be done if the history and findings on physical examination and biochemical tests suggest metastatic involvement. The International System for staging lung cancer, a classification for staging NSCLC, was first proposed in 1986 and is widely accepted throughout the world. Revisions to this staging system were made in 1997 (Table 1). The current guidelines differ from the previous version in that both stage I and stage II have been subdivided into A and B groupings. The group of patients who have T3N0M0 disease, previously included in stage IIIA, are now in stage IIA, as they have a better prognosis than other subgroups in stage IIIA. The new staging system also clarifies the role of the satellite nodules in the same lobe, now designated T4. The evaluation of mediastinal lymph nodes is of critical importance in determining prognosis and in formulating a treatment plan. In general, patients who have a small primary tumor and mediastinal lymph nodes less than 1 cm in diameter in greatest dimension on chest CT scans are unlikely to have mediastinal involvement. In this group of patients, mediastinal sampling may not be necessary. In all other patients with NSCLC, mediastinal lymph node sampling gives useful information and should be done either preoperatively or intraoperatively by the thoracic surgeon.

TREATMENT

Non–Small Cell Lung Cancer

Stage I/II Lung Cancer

Early-stage lung cancer is potentially curable by surgery, and every effort should be made to make

TABLE 1. **Tumor-Node-Metastasis (TNM) Staging in Non–Small Cell Lung Cancer**

Primary tumor (T)	
TX	Malignant cells in sputum or bronchial washings but not visualized by imaging or bronchoscopy
T0	No evidence of primary tumor
Tis	Carcinoma in situ
T1	Tumor ≤3 cm in greatest dimension, surrounded by lung or visceral pleura, without bronchoscopic evidence of invasion more proximal than the lobar bronchus
T2	Tumor with any of the following features of size or extent: • >3 cm in greatest dimension • Involves main bronchus, ≥2 cm distal to the carina • Invades the visceral pleura • Associated with atelectasis or obstructive pneumonitis that extends to the hilar region but does not involve the entire lung
T3	Tumor of any size that directly invades any of the following: chest wall, diaphragm, mediastinal pleura, parietal pericardium; or tumor in the main bronchus <2 cm distal to the carina, but without involvement of the carina; or associated atelectasis or obstructive pneumonitis of the entire lung
T4	Tumor of any size that invades any of the following: mediastinum, heart, great vessels, trachea, esophagus, vertebral body, carina; or tumor with a malignant pleural or pericardial effusion; or with satellite tumor nodule(s) within the ipsilateral primary tumor lobe of the lung
Regional lymph nodes (N)	
NX	Regional lymph nodes cannot be assessed
N0	No regional lymph node metastasis
N1	Metastasis to ipsilateral peribronchial and/or ipsilateral hilar lymph nodes, and intrapulmonary nodes involved by direct extension of the primary tumor
N2	Metastasis to ipsilateral mediastinal and/or subcarinal lymph node(s)
N3	Metastasis to contralateral mediastinal, contralateral hilar, ipsilateral or contralateral scalene, or supraclavicular lymph node(s)
Distant metastasis (M)	
MX	Presence of distant metastasis cannot be assessed
M0	No distant metastasis
M1	Distant metastasis present

Modified from Mountain CF: Revisions in the International System for staging lung cancer. Chest *111*:1710–1717, 1997.

affected patients eligible for the operation. Patients who have potentially resectable disease but are found to have isolated adrenal or liver metastasis on staging studies should have biopsy of these lesions to confirm metastatic disease. Patients with poor performance status or impaired pulmonary function who initially appear to be poor candidates for surgery may improve with intensive physical and pulmonary therapy. Smoking cessation is mandatory prior to surgery. In general, patients with a forced expiratory volume in 1 second (FEV_1) and diffusion capacity for carbon monoxide (DLCO) of more than 60% of predicted values have sufficient pulmonary reserve to tolerate surgery. In patients who have suboptimal FEV_1 and DLCO values, quantitative lung scans to predict postoperative lung function are needed. The operation of choice is a lobectomy or pneumonectomy, as limited resection has been shown to result in an increased incidence of local recurrence. The use of limited procedures such as segmental or wedge resection should be confined to patients with poor pulmonary reserve; these patients are also candidates for surgery by minimally invasive techniques such as video-assisted thoracoscopic surgery. The 5-year survival rate for resected stage I patients is 57 to 67% and for stage II patients is 39 to 55% (Table 2). Numerous studies reported in the literature have shown that chemotherapy or radiation therapy following surgical resection confers no benefit in overall survival. A recent randomized study from Japan utilizing UFT (uracil* and ftorafur*), an oral form of 5-fluorouracil, showed improvement in overall survival after surgical resection. Confirmatory studies need to be done, however, and at present postoperative thoracic radiotherapy or chemotherapy cannot be recommended as standard care.

Stage III NSCLC

Stage III disease can be divided into stage IIIA, which is potentially resectable, and stage IIIB, which is categorically unresectable. Patients diagnosed with stage III disease historically have had a poor prognosis, but with the advent of combined-modality therapy, the outlook appears to have improved for selected groups of patients.

Stage IIIA patients are a heterogeneous group with variable prognosis. Stage IIIA patients who have clinically evident N2 mediastinal nodal involvement treated with surgery alone have a 5-year survival rate of less than 10%, and many clinicians would consider these patients ineligible for surgery. Patients with T3N0 disease previously classified as stage IIIA have been reclassified as stage IIA in the new revised staging system, owing to a relatively favorable 5-year survival rate of 33% reported with surgery alone (Table 2).

*Not available in the United States.

TABLE 2. **Stage Grouping in Non–Small Cell Lung Cancer**

Stage	Tumor-Node-Metastasis (TNM) Subset	5-Year Survival Rate
IA	T1 N0 M0	67%
IB	T2 N0 M0	57%
IIA	T1 N1 M0	55%
IIB	T2 N1 M0	39%
	T3 N0 M0	
IIIA	T1–3 N2 M0	23%
	T3 N1 M0	
IIIB	T1–4 N3 M0	5%
IV	Any T, any N, M1	1%

Modified from Mountain CF: Revisions in the International System for staging lung cancer. Chest *111*:1710–1717, 1997.

Pancoast tumors are superior sulcus tumors in the apex of the lung that are associated with pain in the ipsilateral arm or shoulder, atrophy of the intrinsic muscles of the hand, and Horner's syndrome. This entity is most often due to NSCLC, although a few cases of SCLC have also been reported to present in this fashion. In the early stages of Pancoast tumors, symptoms such as cough, hemoptysis, and shortness of breath are not seen, and the tumor may not be evident on the chest film. For this reason the clinician should have a high index of suspicion for Pancoast tumor in a smoker who has pain in the arm or shoulder that is not otherwise explained. Pancoast tumors can be stage IIIA or stage IIIB, depending on the extent of local invasion. In patients with stage IIIA disease, the traditional treatment has been with preoperative radiation therapy followed by surgical resection, with 5-year survival rates of 40 to 50% in those who have complete resection of tumor. Current treatment strategies combine chemotherapy and radiation therapy in the preoperative setting for patients with superior sulcus tumors.

The traditional treatment for stage III patients who are not surgical candidates has been radiotherapy (RT). However, the impact of RT alone in unresectable locally advanced NSCLC has been minimal, and the use of this modality does not appear to prolong survival. This finding has led investigators to explore new modalities and to combine chemotherapy, aimed at controlling systemic disease, with radiation therapy or surgery for control of local disease. These studies of combined-modality therapy in stage III disease have yielded encouraging results, and these regimens are increasingly being used in community oncology practices.

In stage IIIA disease, systemic failure is common in patients who undergo surgery as the only modality of therapy. In stage IIIA patients with potentially resectable disease, induction or neoadjuvant therapy consisting of chemotherapy, RT, or both chemotherapy and RT has been used in an effort to "downstage" primary tumors and to increase the resectability rate. Early administration of chemotherapy may also eradicate systemic micrometastasis and hence improve overall survival. This concept was tested in phase II trials, with response to induction therapy seen in approximately 50 to 70% of patients, resectability rates of about 60 to 80%, and 2- to 3-year survival rates in the range of 30%. The therapy was well tolerated, and induction therapy did not appear to increase surgical complications.

Two recent randomized studies have evoked enthusiasm among the oncology community for use of a multidisciplinary approach to the management of lung cancer. The first study, published by the M. D. Anderson Cancer Center, randomized 60 patients with stage IIIA disease to surgery alone or to preoperative chemotherapy followed by surgery. The estimated median survival in the patients who underwent preoperative chemotherapy was 64 months, compared with 11 months in the surgery-only group. In the second study, reported from Spain, 60 patients were randomized either to chemotherapy followed by surgery or to surgery alone. All patients received postoperative RT to the mediastinum. The median survival was 24 months in the group of patients who underwent preoperative chemotherapy, compared with 8 months in the surgery-only group. The results in both studies were highly significant and led to early termination at interim analysis prior to completing planned accrual. Based on these two studies, it appears that chemotherapy given prior to surgical resection in patients with stage IIIA N2 disease improves overall survival and should be offered to patients with good performance status outside of a clinical trial. Further research is needed to improve on these results. New agents with activity in lung cancer, such as the taxanes, gemcitabine, and vinorelbine, need to be incorporated into induction regimens and tested in randomized studies.

In stage IIIB disease, which is categorically unresectable, combined-modality therapy with chemotherapy and RT appears to be of benefit in selected patients. As in stage IIIA disease, the exact sequence of chemotherapy and RT needs to be determined. Chemotherapy has been given sequentially followed by RT or given concurrently with RT. Chemotherapeutic agents with radiosensitizing properties are typically used in concurrent protocols to enhance the efficacy of RT. Most of the large randomized studies using concurrent or sequential chemoradiation therapy in inoperable NSCLC have shown a small survival benefit, although at the cost of increased toxicity. A meta-analysis of 52 randomized trials of radiotherapy with or without cisplatin-based chemotherapy revealed that the risk of death was reduced by 13% with the addition of chemotherapy. The absolute survival advantage at 2 years was modest (4%). Paclitaxel, a newer agent derived from the bark of the Pacific yew tree, *Taxus brevifolia,* has radiosensitizing properties. Preliminary studies with paclitaxel and RT in locally advanced NSCLC have shown encouraging activity with tolerable side effects, and these results need to be confirmed in large studies, which have been instituted.

Stage IV NSCLC

Stage IV NSCLC has a particularly poor prognosis and is incurable with currently available therapy. In the past, nihilistic attitudes prevailed among oncologists, with most electing not to offer chemotherapy to patients in view of the poor response rates and associated toxic effects. Early chemotherapy studies reported 1-year survival rates in the range of 12 to 15% for patients with metastatic NSCLC, and these results were similar to those in patients treated with supportive care alone. Progress appears to have been made, and in the last decade a number of new agents have been developed with promising activity in NSCLC. Use of the new generation of chemotherapeutic agents in combination with other established agents has yielded 1-year survival rates of 40 to 50% in recent trials.

Does chemotherapy improve survival in advanced

NSCLC? Meta-analysis of randomized trials has shown that median survival is prolonged by about 2 months with the administration of cisplatin-based chemotherapy. Quality of life also may be improved by chemotherapy, with diminution of symptoms and fewer days in the hospital necessitated by complications of cancer. A Canadian randomized study found that patients who received chemotherapy had improved quality of life indices and that use of chemotherapy resulted in cost savings in the long term compared with use of supportive therapy alone. At present the absolute survival advantage is modest with available chemotherapeutic regimens, and patients and physicians must weigh the potential benefits and risks of therapy on an individual basis.

Combination chemotherapy results in higher response rates and better median survival than those achievable with single-agent chemotherapy and should be used as first-line therapy. Cisplatin-based regimens have been the most commonly utilized regimens in NSCLC, and until recently, cisplatin (Platinol), in combination with etoposide (VePesid) or vinblastine (Velban), has been the reference regimen for randomized studies. Carboplatin (Paraplatin), an analogue of cisplatin, has the advantage of easy outpatient administration and has less ototoxicity and nephrotoxicity compared with cisplatin. The combination of carboplatin and etoposide appears to be as active as the cisplatin-etoposide combination in NSCLC and has gained popularity. In the last decade a number of new agents have been tested and have shown impressive activity in NSCLC. These agents include the taxanes (paclitaxel [Taxol]* and docetaxel [Taxotere]*), vinorelbine, gemcitabine (Gemzar),* and irinotecan (Camptosar).* These agents have shown consistent activity as single agents and are being tested in combination with cisplatin* and carboplatin.* The Eastern Cooperative Oncology Group (ECOG) tested the combination of cisplatin and paclitaxel at two dose levels against the standard regimen of cisplatin and etoposide in 560 patients with advanced NSCLC. The groups receiving the paclitaxel-containing regimens had the highest response rates (27 to 32%) and median survival times (9.6 to 10.0 months). In patients who received cisplatin and etoposide, the response rate was only 12% and median survival was 7.7 months. Patients who received cisplatin with the higher dose of paclitaxel had an increased incidence of neurotoxicity, and for future ECOG studies the reference regimen is cisplatin in combination with moderate-dose paclitaxel.

The combination of carboplatin and paclitaxel has shown impressive activity in early phase I and phase II studies and is being increasingly used in community practice. Vinorelbine in combination with cisplatin is another regimen recommended for patients with advanced and metastatic disease.

The optimum regimen for advanced NSCLC is not known at present. Results of an ongoing ECOG trial that randomizes patients to one of four regimens (cisplatin-paclitaxel, cisplatin-gemcitabine, cisplatin-vinorelbine, or carboplatin-paclitaxel) will help decipher some of these management issues for this difficult disease. Evidence-based medicine is developed systematically by review of the literature to assist patients and clinicians in selecting appropriate therapy and is increasingly being used in practice. The guidelines published by the American Society of Clinical Oncologists for management of patients with unresectable disease should help immensely with selecting appropriate therapy for this group of patients (Table 3). In the United States, only 2 to 3% of all patients receive treatment based on clinical protocols. Progress can be made only if new agents and therapies are tested in lung cancer, and patients should be encouraged to participate in clinical trials.

*Not FDA approved for this indication.

NSCLC: The Future

Although we have made advances in the overall management of NSCLC, we have not yet "hit a home run." The discovery of new and active chemotherapeutic agents must continue, and we must be cautious when incorporating these agents in combined-modality programs with radiation and/or surgery. Careful selection of doses and agents should be aimed at limiting the toxicity of therapy. Selective approaches such as insertion of adenovirus p53 (gene therapy) or introduction of antisense oligodeoxynucleotides are being explored and in the future will be combined with the known active chemotherapeutic agents. Most if not all patients with NSCLC will be offered chemotherapy in the years to come.

Small Cell Lung Cancer

SCLC accounts for about 25% of all lung cancer cases, and the vast majority of patients have had exposure to cigarette smoke. The incidence of SCLC appears to be increasing. This type of cancer is characterized by rapid growth, early systemic dissemination, and chemotherapy responsiveness. One third of patients diagnosed with SCLC have limited-stage disease, which is defined as tumor confined to one hemithorax and encompassable within a single RT portal, without evidence of pericardial or pleural involvement. The other two thirds of patients with SCLC have extensive-stage disease, which is disease extending outside of a hemithorax.

The aggressiveness and rapid growth of SCLC are evident in patients who do not receive treatment. The median survival with untreated limited-stage SCLC is about 12 weeks and with extensive-stage SCLC, little more than a month. SCLC is a systemic disease; in patients who undergo surgery or thoracic RT alone for limited-stage disease, the 2-year survival rate is less than 10%, with death due to systemic metastasis in most patients. However, there may be a role for surgery in patients who have a small lung nodule without any evidence of mediastinal involvement or metastatic disease. These pa-

TABLE 3. **Treatment Guidelines for Unresectable and Metastatic Non–Small Cell Lung Cancer (NSCLC)**

Modality	Comments
Chemotherapy	
Outcome	Chemotherapy in association with definitive thoracic irradiation is appropriate for selected patients with unresectable, locally advanced NSCLC. Chemotherapy is appropriate for selected patients with stage IV NSCLC.
Selection of drugs	Chemotherapy given to patients with NSCLC should be a platinum-based combination regimen.
Duration of therapy	In patients with unresectable stage III NSCLC who are candidates for combined chemotherapy and radiation therapy, and in patients with stage IV NSCLC, the duration of chemotherapy should be two to eight cycles.
Timing of treatment	In patients with unresectable stage III disease and stage IV disease, chemotherapy may best be started soon after the diagnosis of unresectable NSCLC has been made.
Second-line therapy	No current evidence either confirms or refutes that second-line chemotherapy improves survival in nonresponding or progressing patients with advanced NSCLC. Second-line treatment may be appropriate for good performance status patients for whom an investigational protocol is not available or desired, or for patients who respond to initial chemotherapy and then experience a long progression-free interval off treatment.
Role of investigational agents/options	Initial treatment with an investigational agent or regimen is appropriate for selected patients with stage IV NSCLC, provided that patients are crossed over to an active treatment regimen if they have not responded after two cycles of therapy.
Radiotherapy	
Radiation for locally advanced unresectable NSCLC	Radiation therapy should be included as part of treatment for selected patients with unresectable locally advanced NSCLC.
Patient selection	Candidates for definitive thoracic radiotherapy with curative intent should have good performance status, adequate pulmonary function, and disease confined to the thorax. Patients with malignant pleural effusion and those with distant metastatic disease are not candidates for definitive thoracic radiotherapy.
Dose and fractionation	The definitive radiation dose in thoracic radiotherapy should be no less than the biologic equivalent of 60 Gy, in 1.8- to 2-Gy fractions. Local symptoms from primary or metastatic NSCLC can be relieved by a variety of doses and fractionations of external-beam radiotherapy. In appropriately selected patients, hypofractionated palliative radiotherapy (using one to five fractions instead of 10) may provide symptomatic relief with acceptable toxicity in a more time-efficient and less costly manner.
Surgery	
Role of resection for distant metastases	In patients with controlled disease outside of the brain who have an isolated cerebral metastasis in a resectable area, resection followed by whole-brain radiotherapy is superior to whole-brain radiotherapy alone.

Modified from American Society of Clinical Oncologists: Clinical practice guidelines for the treatment of unresectable non–small cell lung cancer. J Clin Oncol *15*:2996–3018, 1997.

tients should receive postoperative chemotherapy and thoracic RT, as for other patients with limited-stage SCLC.

The role of chemotherapy in the treatment of SCLC has evolved over the last three decades. As it became evident that hematogenous metastases were present early in the course of the disease, investigators explored the role of single-agent and combination chemotherapy in the treatment of SCLC. A large number of phase II trials have been conducted in patients with SCLC, and a number of drugs with single-agent activity have been identified. Combination chemotherapy results in a superior response rate and survival compared with single-agent therapy. Although studies have been done using two to four agents in combination chemotherapy for SCLC, it is not clear if there is an advantage to using more than two or three drugs in the therapy of SCLC.

The most commonly used regimen for the treatment of SCLC in the United States is etoposide in combination with either cisplatin* or carboplatin.* The other regimens such as CAE (cyclophosphamide,* Adriamycin [doxorubicin], and etoposide), ICE (ifosfamide,* carboplatin, and etoposide) and CAV (cyclophosphamide, Adriamycin [doxorubicin], and vincristine*) are less commonly used as first-line therapy.

Limited-Stage SCLC

Although response rates as high as 70 to 80% and complete responses of up to 50% can be achieved with combination chemotherapy in limited-stage disease, most patients have recurrent disease, which ultimately causes death. The median survival time of patients who receive treatment ranges from 16 to 20 months. Several randomized studies have explored the use of concurrent thoracic RT to improve overall survival, but with conflicting results. Toxicity was

*Not FDA approved for this indication.

increased in patients who received combined chemoradiation therapy. However, a meta-analysis of randomized trials of chemotherapy with or without thoracic RT in patients with limited-stage SCLC revealed a 14% reduction in the mortality rate in the combined-modality groups. The survival difference is modest, with overall 3-year survival rate about 5.4% higher in patients who receive combined chemoradiation therapy.

Early thoracic RT appears to be superior to late thoracic RT. A randomized study showed that patients who received chemotherapy with thoracic RT during the second cycle of chemotherapy had a significantly improved median survival of 21.2 months, compared with 16 months in the group that received chemotherapy and thoracic RT starting with the last cycle of chemotherapy. The results of an ECOG randomized study lend further support to this observation. Based on these studies, most patients with limited-stage SCLC are given cisplatin or carboplatin in combination with etoposide and with the addition of early thoracic RT.

Although almost 50% of patients with limited-stage SCLC will exhibit a complete response to therapy, almost 70% of the complete responders will have recurrent disease within 2 years. The 5-year survival rate is only 15 to 20% for all patients with limited-stage SCLC.

Extensive-Stage SCLC

Systemic chemotherapy is the mainstay of treatment for patients with extensive disease. RT is useful for palliation of painful or symptomatic local disease. As in limited disease, combination chemotherapy employing etoposide with either cisplatin or carboplatin is commonly used as first-line therapy. These patients are also candidates for investigational protocols, as survival and overall prognosis do not seem to be affected by initial therapy with investigational agents if patients are crossed over to standard therapy at the first evidence of progression of disease. The response rate with use of combination chemotherapy is in the range of 60 to 80%, with a complete response seen in about 15 to 20% of patients. The median survival time for treated patients with extensive-stage SCLC is in the range of 7 to 9 months, and most patients will die of progressive or recurrent disease; 5-year survivors are rare.

Trials have been conducted with the addition of maintenance chemotherapy in patients who had a complete response to initial chemotherapy; however, use of maintenance did not yield a survival advantage but resulted in increased toxicity. Other studies have also shown that there is no advantage in administering more than 4 to 6 cycles of chemotherapy in patients with SCLC, despite the fact that the median duration of response is short. Patients who do not respond to chemotherapy have a poor prognosis. There is a small group of patients who may respond to the combination of PE (cisplatin [Platinol] and etoposide) if they initially are given the CAV regimen. However, if patients have received prior therapy with PE, there is no advantage to administering CAV. In patients who relapse 3 months or more after response to initial therapy, the cancer may still be chemoresponsive to a salvage regimen such as PE or oral etoposide. All patients with recurrent disease should be considered for participation in clinical protocol trials. The newer agents such as paclitaxel,* docetaxel,* topotecan,* CPT-11,* gemcitabine,* and vinorelbine have shown promising activity in SCLC. Two of these new agents, topotecan and paclitaxel, are worthy of mention in the treatment of SCLC, as they have shown substantial activity. These agents are currently being tested in combination regimens such as cisplatin-etoposide followed by topotecan, cisplatin-etoposide-paclitaxel, and topotecan-paclitaxel.

The role of alternating non–cross-resistant chemotherapy has been explored in SCLC, based on the Goldie-Coldman hypothesis that exposure to multiple non–cross-resistant drugs early in the course of the disease will reduce the development of drug-resistant clones. Some evidence suggests a survival benefit with alternating non–cross-resistant therapy, but controversy exists, and confirmatory studies are needed before this can be recommended as standard care.

Dose intensification of chemotherapeutic agents can be achieved by either increasing the doses of drugs or decreasing the interval between successive chemotherapy cycles. In order to achieve these goals and avoid toxicity, hematopoietic growth factor support may be necessary. This approach results in higher response rates, but overall survival appears similar to that achieved by conventional chemotherapy. Similarly, the use of high-dose chemotherapy with peripheral stem cell infusion or bone marrow transplantation can result in high response rates but without a clear survival advantage. In the absence of randomized trials comparing these dose-intensive approaches with standard chemotherapy, the role of dose-intensive approaches must remain investigational.

Prophylactic Cranial Irradiation

The role of prophylactic cranial irradiation (PCI) remains controversial. Brain metastasis is common in patients with SCLC; at diagnosis, 10 to 14% of patients have evidence of brain involvement, and at time of death, about a third of patients have clinically diagnosed brain involvement. Patients who present with brain metastasis after initial therapy have a very poor prognosis, as this finding is usually associated with systemic involvement. Although brain metastasis is associated with considerable morbidity, death is usually due to associated systemic disease. Randomized studies in SCLC patients have shown that PCI can reduce the incidence of brain metastasis by about 50% but without any improvement in overall survival. In addition, neurologic sequelae as a result of PCI, though rare, are known to occur in long-term survivors. At present, most oncologists

*Not FDA approved for this indication.

would offer PCI to patients with limited disease who achieve a complete response to therapy.

SCLC in the Elderly Patient

SCLC is a disease of the elderly, with median age at diagnosis ranging from 60 to 65 years. The relevance of age as a prognostic factor in patients with SCLC continues to be debated. Elderly patients vary in their ability to tolerate chemotherapy; those who are able to tolerate standard doses of therapy have survival rates similar to rates for younger patients. Elderly patients with a poor performance status and laboratory abnormalities in the white blood cell count or renal function appear to tolerate chemotherapy poorly and have inferior survival rates. In order to minimize toxicity, the role of single-agent chemotherapy has been explored in the elderly patient with SCLC. Oral etoposide has been extensively tested because it can be administered on an outpatient basis and is well tolerated. However, in a randomized study comparing oral etoposide with combination chemotherapy in elderly patients with SCLC, the use of etoposide alone was associated with inferior survival rates and yielded no advantage in palliation of symptoms. The elderly patient with SCLC should be offered combination chemotherapy with a regimen such as cisplatin and etoposide or carboplatin and etoposide, which is relatively well tolerated as initial therapy. In the patient with poor performance status or laboratory abnormalities, a reduced-dose combination regimen or single-agent therapy may be offered.

Future Directions

Vaccine strategies are also being explored in an attempt to decrease recurrence rates and increase overall survival of patients with SCLC. Other selective approaches such as use of monoclonal antibodies, inhibitors of angiogenesis, and gene therapy are being tested in ongoing studies. There will be continued efforts to refine present chemotherapeutic regimens and to develop new and active agents for treatment of this disease.

Chemoprevention

The rate of developing second malignancies in the lung and aerodigestive tract is about 10 times higher in persons with a history of smoking who have been treated for lung cancer than in other smokers. The risk of developing second malignancies is higher in SCLC patients (2 to 14% per patient per year) than in those with a history of NSCLC (1 to 2% per patient per year).

Smoking cessation is the most important factor in preventing second malignancies. Chemoprevention trials with 13-*cis*-retinoic acid (Accutane)* have shown promising activity in head and neck cancer in decreasing second malignancies, especially lung cancer, in these patients. A large randomized study evaluating the role of 13-*cis*-retinoic acid in resected stage I NSCLC patients in preventing second primary malignancies or recurrent lung cancer has completed data accrual and is awaiting final analysis. At present, apart from smoking cessation, other chemopreventive approaches remain investigational.

Palliative Care

Most patients who have locally advanced or metastatic disease will eventually die from progression of cancer. Pain is a frequent symptom, occurring in about 70% of patients with advanced cancer, and increases in severity with progression. Cancer pain has a substantial impact on the patient's physiologic, psychologic, and sociologic well-being and should be aggressively treated. Cancer pain is often underdiagnosed and undertreated by health care professionals. A multidisciplinary approach is essential, and patients should be questioned about symptoms of pain at every visit. In almost 90% of patients, cancer pain can be relieved with relatively simple measures such as oral, transdermal, or parenteral narcotics.

*Not FDA approved for this indication.

COCCIDIOIDOMYCOSIS

method of
NEIL M. AMPEL, M.D.
University of Arizona and
Tucson Veterans Affairs Medical Center
Tucson, Arizona

Coccidioidomycosis is an infection caused by the soil-dwelling fungus *Coccidioides immitis.* Infection is acquired when a susceptible host inhales a single-celled element of the fungus, called an arthroconidium. Once in the lung, the fungus undergoes a remarkable morphologic change, growing larger and rounder, to become a spherule containing smaller cellular forms, called endospores. Although the lungs are the most common site of initial infection, the fungus may spread beyond the confines of the thoracic cage and cause disseminated disease involving the skin and soft tissue, the bones and joints, and the meninges.

Coccidioidomycosis is geographically limited to certain regions of the Western Hemisphere that are characterized by aridity and lack of cold temperatures. In the United States, infection is endemic to the San Joaquin Valley in central California, whence the name "Valley Fever" is derived. In addition, coccidioidomycosis is extremely common in south-central Arizona, including the regions encompassing the cities of Phoenix and Tucson. Although infection may be acquired in New Mexico, western Texas, some areas of southern Nevada and Utah, and certain regions in southern California outside the San Joaquin Valley, infection is far less prevalent in these locales than in the San Joaquin Valley and Arizona.

CLINICAL MANIFESTATIONS AND NATURAL HISTORY

Coccidioidomycosis is completely asymptomatic in approximately two thirds of all people infected. In such individuals, the only manifestation of infection is a delayed-type hypersensitivity response to skin testing with a coccidioidal antigen such as coccidioidin (Spherulin). The other one third have a variety of symptoms during acute infection, most commonly the triad of fever, cough that is minimally productive of sputum, and pleuritic chest pain. Fatigue, at times profound, is a frequent manifestation of primary coccidioidal pulmonary infection. This characteristic distinguishes it from other common forms of pneumonia.

The vast majority of those infected with *C. immitis* experience complete resolution of their infection within 6 weeks and develop lifelong cellular immunity. In approximately 5 to 10% of individuals, however, infection is persistent. Such infection usually manifests itself in one of three ways. The first is a chronic pneumonia with symptoms lasting more than 6 weeks. Patients usually have persistent cough, fever, fatigue, and chest pain. Chest radiographs may show a variety of abnormalities, including focal consolidation, scarring, and cavities.

The second set of manifestations are pulmonary complications resulting from the coccidioidal infection but not necessarily indicative of active infection. Such complications include pyopneumothoraces due to rupture of subpleural granulomata, chronic hemoptysis because of a persistent coccidioidal cavity, and pulmonary nodules seen on chest radiograph that necessitate a diagnostic evaluation for malignancy.

The third presentation of chronic coccidioidomycosis is infection occurring beyond the thoracic cavity, known as disseminated extrathoracic infection. Such dissemination may occur in patients who were either symptomatic or asymptomatic during their initial coccidioidal infection. Common sites of extrathoracic disease include the skin and soft tissue, bones and joints, and the meninges. Extrathoracic infection rarely improves without prolonged antifungal therapy. One dire manifestation of dissemination is diffuse pulmonary involvement as a result of fungemia. This often occurs in highly immunosuppressed patients. The chest radiograph shows a reticulonodular infiltrate in both lungs, similar to that seen in miliary tuberculosis and *Pneumocystis carinii* pneumonia. More than half the patients with this form of coccidioidomycosis die within 1 month of diagnosis despite antifungal therapy.

Certain individuals are at markedly increased risk for developing either severe pulmonary disease or disseminated extrathoracic infection. Patients with insulin-dependent diabetes mellitus have an increased risk of chronic pulmonary infection. In addition, men in certain racial groups, particularly blacks and Filipinos, are at increased risk for extrathoracic dissemination.

Anyone with a deficit in cellular immunity is at particular risk for severe and disseminated coccidioidomycosis. This includes patients on chronic corticosteroid therapy, allogeneic transplant recipients, patients undergoing cancer chemotherapy, and individuals with human immunodeficiency virus infection. In addition, women who acquire coccidioidomycosis during the second or third month of pregnancy have a high risk of developing disseminated infection, particularly meningitis. This increased risk does not occur in women already infected with *C. immitis* who become pregnant.

Diagnosis

The diagnosis of coccidioidomycosis can be establish by serology, culture, or histology. For serologic diagnosis, the tube precipitin (TP) antibody test is usually positive in acute or reactivated infection. Testing for TP antibody is useful only on serum, and titers have no diagnostic importance. In addition to the standard TP assay, the immunodiffusion TP (IDTP) assay is also useful. The complement fixation (CF) antibody test is helpful not only in acute illness but also in tracking prognosis. Detection of antibody in serum and other body fluids, including cerebrospinal fluid (CSF), is generally considered diagnostic. Rising CF antibody titers suggest more active infection and possible dissemination. In addition to the true complement-fixing test, CF antibody can be detected by immunodiffusion (IDCF). A new enzyme immunoassay (EIA) test that measures IgM and IgG antibodies is commercially available. Although sensitive, it is not as specific as the TP and CF antibody tests, which should be used to confirm positive results obtained by EIA.

Unlike serologic tests, skin testing is not useful in establishing the diagnosis of active coccidioidomycosis. A positive skin test for coccidioidomycosis does not differentiate between prior and current infection, and a negative test does not preclude the diagnosis. However, skin testing may be useful in following the course of patients with active disease, since the development of a positive skin test appears to be associated with an improved outcome.

The diagnosis of coccidioidomycosis can also be established by culture of the organism. *C. immitis* will grow on a variety of culture media within 3 to 10 days. Samples appropriate for culture include expectorated sputum, bronchoalveolar lavage fluid and biopsies from clinical sites. The fungus rarely grows in a CSF sample. The diagnosis of meningitis is usually based on the finding of CF antibodies in the CSF with a lymphocytic pleocytosis.

Finally, identification of spherules in tissue sections or cytologic preparations is pathognomonic for coccidioidomycosis. The fungus is easily seen using the hematoxylin-eosin stain and is even more readily identified using the Gomori methenamine-silver stain.

TREATMENT

Because of the great variability in the individual response to therapy, even among patients with similar types of disease, making firm recommendations regarding the treatment of coccidioidomycosis is difficult. Moreover, no comparative trials of antifungal drugs for the treatment of coccidioidomycosis have been published. Despite this, some basic statements can be made regarding therapy (Table 1). In general, the oral triazole antifungals fluconazole (Diflucan) and itraconazole (Sporanox) are effective in most cases, particularly for patients not requiring hospitalization. Because of problems with absorption, drug interactions, and antifungal activity as compared with the newer agents, the older antifungal azole ketoconazole (Nizoral) can no longer be recommended for the treatment of coccidioidomycosis. Intravenous amphotericin B should be reserved for severe cases, especially for those with diffuse reticulonodular pulmonary disease and for those not responding to triazole therapy.

The most important therapeutic consideration is the type and extent of coccidioidal infection. In the patient without any underlying immunosuppressive condition, most cases of primary coccidioidal pneumonia will resolve spontaneously and therapy is not required. In patients with chronic pneumonia with symptoms persisting for more than 6 weeks, antifungal therapy is recommended. Treatment is required

TABLE 1. **Recommendations for Therapy of Different Forms of Coccidioidomycosis**

Manifestation	Primary Therapy	Secondary Therapy
Primary pulmonary	None	Fluconazole or itraconazole, 400 mg/d orally
Chronic pulmonary	Fluconazole or itraconazole, 400 mg/d orally	Amphotericin B, 1.0 mg/kg/d IV*
Diffuse reticulonodular pulmonary	Amphotericin B, 1.0 mg/kg/d IV	Fluconazole, 400 mg/d IV
Extrathoracic, nonmeningeal	Fluconazole or itraconazole, 400 mg/d orally	Amphotericin B, 1.0 mg/kg/d IV
Meningitis	Fluconazole or itraconazole, 800 mg/d orally†	Intrathecal amphotericin B‡

*Refers to deoxycholate form of amphotericin B (Fungizone).
†Fluconazole preferred over itraconazole for the treatment of meningitis.
‡Should be administered only by someone trained and experienced in this technique.

for all cases of extrathoracic disease, since the likelihood of improvement without therapy is small.

When treating with the triazole antifungals fluconazole,* and itraconazole,* the minimum starting dose in the adult is 400 mg per day. Higher doses should be used for severe disease. Triazole antifungals should be used with extreme caution or not at all in pregnant women. Congenital anomalies have been associated with the use of fluconazole.

Amphotericin B, formulated as a deoxycholate dispersion (Fungizone), has been available since the 1950s. Although effective for many forms of coccidioidomycosis, it has numerous dose-limiting toxicities. Newer formulations of amphotericin B (Abelcet, Amphotec, and AmBisome) are now available for use in the United States. While there are no data suggesting increased efficacy of these new preparations for the treatment of coccidioidomycosis, they all appear to be less toxic at higher doses than Fungizone and they should be considered when a patient has dose-limiting toxicity from that drug.

In all cases, antifungal treatment for coccidioidomycosis should be prolonged, on the order of months to years. Clinical endpoints, including changes in CF antibody titer of two or more dilutions, should be used to determine treatment efficacy. When amphotericin B is used as initial treatment, a switch to an oral triazole can be made once there is demonstrable clinical improvement. Once the patient is stable, the dose of the oral triazole can be reduced for cases of nonmeningeal disease. Because relapse is so frequent after triazole therapy is stopped, immediate discontinuation is discouraged. One approach is to halve the dose every 3 or 4 months, following the clinical course and CF titer.

Coccidioidal meningitis requires special consideration. Intravenous amphotericin B is not useful for this form of coccidioidomycosis. Both fluconazole and itraconazole, however, are effective in many cases. Because it has been more extensively studied and because it is well absorbed from the gastrointestinal tract, fluconazole is the preferred therapy for coccidioidal meningitis. A starting dose of 800 mg per day should be used. In patients who fail to respond, the dose should be increased. If there is still no response, intrathecal amphotericin B should be considered. The preferred approach is direct instillation into the cisterna magna, but this should be done only by an individual trained and experienced in this technique. Amphotericin B can also be instilled through either a ventricular or a lumbar reservoir. Because relapse of coccidioidal meningitis is extremely common if therapy is discontinued, life-long treatment is recommended.

*Not FDA approved for this indication.

HISTOPLASMOSIS

method of
LISA A. HAGLUND, M.D., and
GEORGE S. DEEPE, JR., M.D.
University of Cincinnati College of Medicine
Cincinnati, Ohio

Infection with the dimorphic fungus *Histoplasma capsulatum* is acquired by inhalation of mycelial fragments or microconidia, which are deposited within terminal bronchioles and alveoli. Within days, the mycelial-phase elements transform into yeast cells. These forms spread via the lymphohematogenous route within phagocytes to invade the reticuloendothelial system. Thus, most if not all cases of primary infection are disseminated. In tissues, yeast cells commonly evoke an inflammatory response that consists of formation of caseating or noncaseating granulomas. Virtually all the clinical manifestations of histoplasmosis are caused by yeast cells.

Cases of histoplasmosis have been reported from every continent except Antarctica. In the United States, this fungal infection is endemic to the mideastern and south central regions. Variations in the prevalence of infection in these areas are probably due to the presence of hyperendemic foci. Point sources for infection include caves, chicken houses, bird roosts, attics, and old buildings. Epidemics have been associated with mechanical disruption of infested areas by bulldozers, with exposure of accumulated bird or bat guano, or with renovation of old buildings.

Infection with *H. capsulatum* produces three distinct illnesses: acute pulmonary histoplasmosis, chronic pulmonary histoplasmosis, and progressive disseminated histoplasmosis. Acute pulmonary histoplasmosis (APH) often produces an influenza-like illness with cough, but it may be clinically inapparent. Severity of illness can be correlated directly with inoculum size. Each inhaled particle induces a small patch of bronchopneumonia. The primary lesions encapsulate, become necrotic in the center, and subsequently calcify.

Chronic pulmonary histoplasmosis (CPH) develops predominantly in older persons with structural lung damage such as obstructive lung disease. This form of histoplasmosis is characterized by weight loss, cough with abundant sputum production, and occasionally fever and hemoptysis.

It is believed that the yeast-phase organisms proliferate in bullae and slowly induce additional destruction of the lung parenchyma. *H. capsulatum* may rarely spread via the bronchi to the opposite lung.

In progressive disseminated histoplasmosis (PDH), there is widespread involvement of the mononuclear phagocyte system by yeast cells. Acute and chronic forms of PDH are seen. The acute form is associated with high fever, weight loss, hepatosplenomegaly, pancytopenia, and coagulation disturbances. The chronic form is characterized by low-grade fever, hepatosplenomegaly, and mucocutaneous ulcers affecting all areas of the gastrointestinal tract. Mucocutaneous ulcers of PDH may be mistaken for head and neck cancers, colonic polyps, colon cancers, or Crohn's disease and may cause small bowel obstruction and malabsorption. Findings on biopsy of bone marrow and other specimens may be misdiagnosed as acute leukemia, lymphoma, or lymphomatoid granulomatosis if silver stains for fungus and fungal cultures are not obtained. Patients with human immunodeficiency virus (HIV) infection may present with either form, manifestations of which can include skin lesions, pneumonia (seldom cavitary), and prostatic abscesses.

Serologic tests and fungal cultures both are useful in establishing the diagnosis of histoplasmosis. A complement fixation (CF) titer of 1:8 is considered a positive result, and a titer of 1:32 strongly suggests active disease. A fourfold rise in CF titers over 4 to 6 weeks is indicative of active histoplasmosis. The immunodiffusion test is less sensitive than the CF test. The presence of an H precipitin band indicates active disease, whereas an M band signifies past or recent infection. Both may be present in acute disease.

In immunosuppressed patients, serologic studies may be of limited value. Histopathologic examination of tissues, particularly bone marrow or liver, is a useful adjunct. Tissues should be silver-stained in order to visualize yeasts. Fungal culture of sputum and any tissue should be performed. The lysis-centrifugation blood culture system (Isolator) can detect *H. capsulatum* in patients with PDH in 1 to 2 weeks. Other blood culture systems (Septi-chek, BACTEC, and BacT/Alert) will not grow *H. capsulatum* unless the bottles are held 3 to 6 weeks (for example, when BACTEC TB media are used). There is a polysaccharide antigen detection system (most sensitive when performed on urine) available only in the laboratory of Dr. L. J. Wheat of the Indiana University School of Medicine (information accessible on the World Wide Web at www.iupui.edu/it/histodgn). It is especially helpful in identification of patients with PDH and can be used to follow the success of therapy.

TREATMENT

General Measures

Acute Pulmonary Histoplasmosis

Because APH is usually a self-limited illness, antifungal therapy is not required in most affected persons. Bed rest, antipyretics, and cough suppressants are effective for treatment of the influenza-like symptoms. Nevertheless, a few patients may experience a prolonged illness (2 to 4 weeks) that consists of fever, weight loss, chest pain, and cough. In these cases, antifungal therapy can hasten resolution of disease. In hospitalized patients, amphotericin B (Fungizone) should be given intravenously (IV) in a dose of 50 mg per day or every other day to a total dose of 500 mg to 1 gram, until the patient is well. Alternatively, this drug can be given until the patient is asymptomatic for 7 to 10 days. In children, 0.25 mg of amphotericin B per kg of body weight is given on the first day followed by 0.5 mg per kg on day 2 and 1 mg per kg thereafter. Itraconazole (Sporanox) may be used in less severely ill patients. A brief tapering course of corticosteroids will decrease acute high fever and chest pain dramatically but does not shorten the overall duration of fever.

Certain sequelae may be noted following acute histoplasmosis. Examples include pericariditis, fibrosing mediastinitis, lymphadenitis, and arthritis. Pericarditis may be manifested approximately 6 weeks after acute exposure to *H. capsulatum.* Yeast cells rarely are detected in pericardium or pericardial fluid. This illness is treated with anti-inflammatory agents such as salicylates or other nonsteroidal drugs. Uncommonly, the severity of illness may necessitate the use of corticosteroids. There is no role for antifungal treatment. If cardiac tamponade develops, pericardiocentesis is necessary. Pericardiectomy is indicated for constrictive pericarditis.

Fibrosing mediastinitis is a progressive illness that probably arises from an exuberant host response to the fungus. Proliferation of fibrous tissue leads to constriction of vital structures including bronchi, superior vena cava, and pulmonary arteries. Optimal therapy for this disorder has not been determined. Amphotericin B, surgery, corticosteroids, ketoconazole or itraconazole, or combinations thereof have been used, with inconsistent results. No controlled trials of any medical therapy or of the stenting of vascular obstructions have been done.

Chronic Pulmonary Histoplasmosis

Treatment of patients with cavitary lung disease or CPH should be instituted when there are thick-walled cavities, enlarging pneumonic lesions, progressive decline in pulmonary function, or persistent fever and weight loss. Itraconazole, 200 mg once daily, or ketoconazole (Nizoral), 400 mg once daily for at least 6 months, induces responses in 75 to 85% of patients. Fluconazole (Diflucan) is only moderately effective for CPH. If disease progresses despite oral therapy or if the patient is immunocompromised, amphotericin B should be substituted; a total of 30 to 35 mg per kg of body weight should be given over 6 to 8 weeks. Surgical resection of involved lung tissue should be considered in patients with massive hemoptysis or in those who fail to respond to medical therapy. Amphotericin B and the azoles are all less effective for CPH than for PDH, probably because of local factors in the cavitary pulmonary process that interfere with antifungal therapy.

Progressive Disseminated Histoplasmosis

If untreated, PDH is fatal in more than 80% of cases. Risk factors for the development of PDH are immunosuppressive drug treatment, lymphoreticular malignancy, HIV infection, and advanced age. Less frequently, persons without known pre-existing immune defects develop PDH. An interesting finding is that PDH may cause $CD4^+$ lymphocyte depletion in non–HIV-infected persons that is reversible with therapy. Reactivation is the most frequent cause of PDH; less commonly, overwhelming primary infection produces symptoms of PDH. Most HIV-infected patients have acquired immune deficiency syndrome (AIDS) with $CD4^+$ lymphocyte counts of less than 200 per mm^3 at the time of diagnosis of PDH. In endemic areas, 5% of AIDS patients are diagnosed with PDH, probably a result of reactivation. However, PDH has been reported in AIDS patients from nonendemic areas such as New York City or San Francisco.

Initial therapy of PDH depends on the severity of the presenting illness. Administration of amphotericin B remains the initial treatment of choice for more severe cases of PDH, as it acts more rapidly than the azole drugs. However, once the disease is controlled, drug therapy can be changed to administration of itraconazole, 200 mg once daily, or ketoconazole, 400 mg once daily, for at least 6 months. A total of 30 to 35 mg of amphotericin B per kg of body weight should be given if there is progression of disease during therapy with an azole drug. In patients with PDH with less severe illness (including HIV-infected patients), administration of itraconazole, 200 mg twice daily (following a loading dose of 200 mg three times daily for 3 days) for at least 12 weeks, is generally as efficacious as amphotericin B therapy. HIV-infected patients should receive 200 mg daily thereafter indefinitely as suppressive therapy. Ketoconazole and fluconazole both have unacceptably high failure rates when used for either initial therapy or chronic suppressive therapy given to HIV-infected patients with PDH. Amphotericin, 0.5 to 1.0 mg per kg IV weekly, has also been used. Whether it will be possible to safely discontinue long-term suppressive therapy in HIV-infected patients with PDH whose $CD4^+$ lymphocyte counts have been normalized through highly effective antiretroviral therapy is still unknown.

Antifungal Therapy

Antifungal agents effective in the treatment of histoplasmosis include amphotericin B and the azole drugs itraconazole, ketoconazole, and fluconazole. Significant drug interactions are possible; these are summarized in Table 1.

AMPHOTERICIN B

Amphotericin B (Fungizone) is a polyene antibiotic for which intravenous administration is required. This drug binds to membrane sterols, especially ergosterol, and increases permeability of fungal membranes, thus leading to loss of cell constituents and lysis of cells. The drug is insoluble in many solutions including saline and should be diluted in 5% dextrose in water at a concentration not to exceed 0.1 mg per mL. No loss of bioactivity occurs if amphotericin B is exposed to light. Although some clinicians begin with a test dose of 1 mg, we prefer to initiate therapy with 10 mg, which is infused over 2 to 4 hours. If this is tolerated, the dosage is increased by 10 to 15 mg per day until a maximal dose of 0.7 mg per kg is achieved. In adults, a dose of 50 mg given three times per week generally is a well-tolerated regimen. Electrolytes, renal function, and hemoglobin should be checked two to three times weekly during the first 3 weeks of therapy and then once weekly until completion.

Adverse side effects of amphotericin B include fever, chills, headache, hypotension or hypertension, anorexia, nausea, and vomiting. These signs and symptoms are observed frequently during the first few days of therapy and tend to subside thereafter. Fever, chills, and headache may be mitigated by premedication with acetaminophen (Tylenol), 650 mg orally (PO) in adults, and diphenhydramine hydrochloride (Benadryl), 25 to 50 mg PO or parenterally, one-half to one hour prior to amphotericin B administration. Slowing the rate of infusion may help, and premedication with ibuprofen (Motrin), 400 to 800 mg PO, or hydrocortisone (Solu-Cortef), 10 to 25 mg PO or parenterally, may be used if symptoms persist. Parenteral meperidine (Demerol), 25 mg, or dantrolene (Dantrium),* 25 to 50 mg, may abort symptoms, but these drugs should be reserved for difficult cases. In addition, amphotericin B often causes phlebitis, especially if it is infused through peripheral veins. Addition of 1000 to 2000 units of heparin* to the infusion is helpful in reducing phlebitis.

Renal dysfunction is the most serious toxic effect. The glomerular filtration rate is depressed in almost everyone who receives amphotericin B. Adequate prehydration and salt intake can minimize nephrotoxicity. Treatment should not be stopped until the serum creatinine or serum urea nitrogen exceeds 3.0 mg per dL or 50 mg per dL, respectively. When the creatinine falls to 2.5 mg per dL, the drug may be restarted. Moreover, because only a small fraction of amphotericin B is excreted by the kidneys, the dosage regimen does not need to be modified in renal failure. A high percentage of patients experience hypokalemia and hypomagnesemia owing to renal tubular damage, and thus potassium and magnesium supplementation are often necessary. This is especially true in patients receiving concomitant treatment with semisynthetic penicillins such as ticarcillin (Ticar) or carbenicillin (Geopen). Amphotericin B also adds to the nephrotoxicity of cyclosporine (Sandimmune). Anemia, presumed to result from direct marrow toxicity or inhibition of erythropoietin production or both, is also seen. Transfusion usually is not required, and hemoglobin returns to pretreatment levels after completion of therapy.

Recently, newer preparations of amphotericin B have become available: a lipid complex (Abelcet), a liposomal preparation (AmBisome), and a cholesteryl sulfate complex (Amphotec). Because these lipid-based drugs are associated with a lower incidence of nephrotoxicity, they are indicated when a patient has

*Not FDA approved for this indication.

TABLE 1. **Antifungal Azole Drug Interactions**

	Azole Drug		
Other Drug	*Ketoconazole (200-mg tablet PO)*	*Itraconazole (100-mg capsule PO)*	*Fluconazole (Various Doses; PO, IV)*
Phenytoin (Dilantin)	Increased phenytoin level, decreased ketoconazole level	Increased phenytoin level, decreased itraconazole level	Increased phenytoin level
Phenobarbital	—	Decreased itraconazole level	—
Carbamazepine (Tegretol)	—	Decreased itraconazole level	Increased carbamazepine level
Warfarin (Coumadin)	Increased anticoagulation effect	As for ketoconazole	As for ketoconazole
Oral hypoglycemics	Increased hypoglycemic effect	As for ketoconazole	As for ketoconazole
Cyclosporine (Sandimmune)	Increased cyclosporine level	As for ketoconazole	As for ketoconazole
Tacrolimus (Prograf)	Increased tacrolimus level	As for ketoconazole	As for ketoconazole
Digoxin	Increased digoxin level	As for ketoconazole	—
Terfenadine (Seldane),* astemizole (Hismanal)	Increased antihistamine level, possible fatal arrhythmia	Increased antihistamine level, possible fatal arrhythmia	Increased antihistamine level
Rifampin, isoniazid	Decreased ketoconazole level	Decreased itraconazole level	Decreased fluconazole level
Rifabutin (Mycobutin)	—	Increased rifabutin level, decreased itraconazole level	Increased rifabutin level
Midazolam (Versed), triazolam (Halcion), alprazolam (Xanax)	Increased sedative effect	As for ketoconazole	—
Felodipine (Plendil) (calcium channel blocker)	—	Increased felodipine level	—
Cisapride (Propulsid)	Increased cisapride level, possible fatal arrhythmia	As for ketoconazole	As for ketoconazole
Lovastatin (Mevacor), simvastatin (Zocor)	—	Possible rhabdomyolysis	—
Zidovudine (Retrovir)	—	—	Increased zidovudine level
Ritonavir (Norvir)	—	Increased ritonavir level	—
Indinavir (Crixivan)	—	Increased indinavir level	Increased indinavir level

*No longer marketed in the United States.

a marked increase in serum creatinine level with amphotericin B therapy (despite saline prehydration) or when pre-existing renal insufficiency is present (serum creatinine level of at least 2.5 mg per dL). Efficacy of the lipid-based preparations is no better than that of amphotericin, and is probably similar. The recommended dosage for histoplasmosis is 5 mg per kg per day, although the optimal dosage is not known.

ITRACONAZOLE

Itraconazole (Sporanox) is the newest of the azole antifungal compounds and, in capsular form, is FDA-approved for use in histoplasmosis, including chronic cavitary pulmonary disease and disseminated, non-meningeal histoplasmosis. Like amphotericin B, it is a highly lipophilic agent. It is entirely metabolized by the liver and is a potent inhibitor of the cytochrome P-450 3A enzyme system, resulting in multiple serious drug interactions, discussed later on. Itraconazole is available in 100-mg capsules for oral administration and in oral suspension; no intravenous form is available. Because 1 to 2 weeks may be required to reach steady-state concentration, a loading dose of itraconazole of 200 mg three times daily for the first 3 days is recommended. If more than 200 mg of itraconazole per day is given, divided doses are advised. A dose of 400 mg daily is recommended for initial therapy, and 200 mg daily for maintenance suppressive therapy, if needed.

Food increases absorption of itraconazole capsules; when the drug is taken on an empty stomach, serum levels are about one half of those achieved after the same dose is taken with a full meal. There is no experience yet with tube feedings, but it is not well absorbed when given through a nasogastric tube. Diarrhea has also been observed to interfere with absorption in some patients. Itraconazole oral suspension is best absorbed on an empty stomach; this formulation is not FDA-approved for the treatment of histoplasmosis.

The most common adverse reactions are nausea and vomiting with dosages of up to 400 mg per day. Rashes, elevation of serum transaminases, and edema, all reversible on discontinuation of itraconazole, have been described; rare cases of serious hepatotoxicity have occurred. Itraconazole-associated impotence and decreased libido have been reported; one case of reversible adrenal insufficiency has occurred with high doses (600 mg per day). No dosage adjustment is necessary in the presence of renal insufficiency, and it is not removed by either peritoneal or hemodialysis.

Drug interactions in this class of antifungal agents are summarized in Table 1, but two important itraconazole interactions are mentioned here. Co-administration of terfenadine (Seldane),* astemizole (Hismanal), or cisapride (Propulsid) with itraconazole is contraindicated because of possible fatal cardiac arrhythmias. Rhabdomyolysis has been reported in pa-

*No longer marketed in the United States.

tients taking lovastatin (Mevacor) and simvastatin (Zocor) along with itraconazole. It should also be noted that treatment failures in fungal diseases have resulted from co-administration of itraconazole with other drugs that lower itraconazole levels, either by increasing itraconazole clearance, such as rifampin, isoniazid, phenytoin (Dilantin), and carbamazepine (Tegretol), or by decreasing absorption by reducing gastric acidity, such as antacids, histamine H_2 blockers, and omeprazole (Prilosec).

There are no studies in pregnant women, and itraconazole should be used in pregnancy only if the potential benefit outweighs the risks, as teratogenicity has been observed in rats experimentally. Although the drug is not FDA-approved for pediatric use, 3 to 7 mg of itraconazole per kg per day has been given to children with PDH, with successful outcomes. Itraconazole should not be used in the critically ill patient, because absorption may be impaired owing both to the absence of food and to the frequent use of agents that reduce gastric acidity. Amphotericin B remains the drug of choice in patients extremely ill with histoplasmosis.

KETOCONAZOLE

Ketoconazole (Nizoral) is an imidazole that offers advantages because it is less toxic than amphotericin B and is administered orally. Recent studies have established, however, that ketoconazole should be used only as an alternative to itraconazole or amphotericin B for histoplasmosis. The combination of amphotericin B and ketoconazole does not offer any advantage over therapy with a single agent. Dosage is 400 mg PO once or twice daily. Twenty percent of patients receiving ketoconazole complain of nausea, vomiting, or anorexia. These symptoms can be reduced by giving the drug in two divided doses rather than in a single dose or by taking the drug with meals or at bedtime. The drug is well absorbed from the gastrointestinal tract, but absorption is diminished by achlorhydria or by drugs that lower gastric acidity. Ketoconazole blocks synthesis of testosterone, and high doses of the drug can produce oligospermia, gynecomastia, loss of libido, and loss of sexual potency. In addition, this agent inhibits cortisol secretion. To date, however, permanent hypoadrenalism has been reported in only one patient. Liver enzymes are elevated transiently in approximately 10% of patients, but there is symptomatic hepatic dysfunction in less than 0.1%. If jaundice or marked elevation of liver enzymes develops, ketoconazole must be discontinued; otherwise, fatal hepatic necrosis may result. Other drug interactions are discussed later on.

FLUCONAZOLE

Fluconazole (Diflucan),* a triazole antifungal agent, is a less effective treatment for histoplasmosis than is amphotericin B or itraconazole, even at high doses (800 mg per day). This is probably due both to reduced antifungal activity and to resistance arising during fluconazole therapy. Fortunately, cross-resistance between fluconazole and itraconazole has not been observed. It is available in 50-, 100-, and 200-mg tablets for oral administration and in 200- and 400-mg injections for intravenous administration. Adverse effects associated with fluconazole include gastrointestinal irritation (anorexia, nausea, and vomiting), hepatitis (usually clinically inapparent transaminase elevations, rarely hepatic necrosis), pruritic rashes, anaphylaxis, and Stevens-Johnson syndrome. Fluconazole is teratogenic in animals, and birth anomalies have been seen in infants exposed to the drug during pregnancy. Chapped lips and alopecia have been observed with prolonged courses. To date, the interference with human steroidogenesis seen with ketoconazole has not been reported with fluconazole.

*Not FDA approved for this indication.

DRUG INTERACTIONS WITH AZOLE ANTIFUNGAL AGENTS

The principal mechanism of action of the azole compounds is to preferentially inhibit cytochrome P-450 enzymes in fungal organisms. Because these enzymes are also present in mammalian cells, in which they play a key role in metabolic and detoxifying reactions, this class of drugs is well known to interfere with metabolism of other compounds (see Table 1).

Severe hypoglycemia has been reported in patients concomitantly receiving azole antifungal agents and oral hypoglycemic agents. Fluconazole, even at low doses (100 mg per day), markedly potentiates the anticoagulant activity of coumadin; itraconazole may have the same effect. Potentially fatal arrhythmias occurring with elevated levels of the newer antihistamines have been described with itraconazole. Drug interactions with the addition of itraconazole include decreased metabolism and therefore toxic levels of digoxin, dilantin, and cyclosporine. Ketoconazole also increases levels of cisapride. Plasma concentrations of azole antifungal agents are reduced when these drugs are given concurrently with isoniazid. Induction of hepatic microsomal enzymes by rifampin produces decreased serum concentrations of ketoconazole. Ketoconazole increases serum concentrations of cyclosporine. Although no studies have been conducted, case reports suggest that the dose of cyclosporine should be reduced by 50 percent when itraconazole is given. There is no information regarding cross-hypersensitivity among the azole antifungal agents.

BLASTOMYCOSIS

method of
JULIE E. MANGINO, M.D.
Ohio State University Medical Center
Columbus, Ohio

Blastomycosis, caused by *Blastomyces dermatitidis*, is one of the endemic mycoses, like histoplasmosis and coccidioidomycosis. All three illnesses are caused by dimorphic fungi, which exist in the yeast form in humans at body temperature and the hyphal or mycelial form in nature. Blastomycosis infections are confined geographically to the East Coast, Southeast, and Central United States as well as specific areas of South America, Western Europe, and Africa. In the United States, the natural reservoir for *B. dermatitidis* seems to be the riverbeds of wooded areas along the Mississippi, Ohio, and St. Lawrence rivers and the Great Lakes. Although blastomycosis is an uncommon infection, point source outbreaks have been described, yielding much information regarding the biology of this disease. It is not transmissible from person to person, and males are affected more often than females.

Infection is generally acquired via inhalation of spores, pneumonia being the most common manifestation of the disease. It may disseminate via the bloodstream, spreading characteristically to the skin, bones, and genitourinary tract (prostate, testes, and epididymis). Less commonly, infection spreads to the central nervous system (CNS) or to the liver, lymph nodes, and spleen.

The presentation is often subclinical or self-limited, with a mild influenza-like illness followed by eventual resolution of pulmonary infiltrates as *B. dermatitidis* disappears from the sputum. In rare cases, the patient presents with an acute community-acquired pneumonia and an alveolar or mass-like infiltrate, which does not respond to conventional antibiotics. Constitutional symptoms can include weight loss, fever, malaise, fatigue, and nonspecific complaints. In a subset of patients, the pulmonary infection can progress to chronic pneumonia with miliary or reticulonodular patterns on the chest film. These findings may persist for 2 to 6 months and are also associated with night sweats, fever, and pleuritic pain. Calcification, hilar adenopathy, and large pleural effusions are rare. In addition, some patients may have a solitary pulmonary nodule on the chest film and completely lack pulmonary symptoms. Surgical resection of such a nodule containing *B. dermatitidis* has led to resolution without further treatment. Spontaneous resolution of pneumonia has also been followed by reactivation at both pulmonary and extrapulmonary sites, even if the patient had received previous therapy. If therapy is not given, a prolonged follow-up period is recommended.

Immunosuppressed patients, such as those who chronically use steroids, have undergone organ transplantation, or have human immunodeficiency virus (HIV) infection, may have a fulminant pneumonic process with an adult respiratory distress syndrome (ARDS)–like picture ensuing. Blastomycosis, however, is a less common opportunistic infection than those due to other fungal pathogens, such as disseminated histoplasmosis or cryptococcosis.

The most common extrapulmonary manifestation of blastomycosis is skin disease. Lesions occur on exposed areas of the body, especially the face or the arms. Primary skin lesions due to direct inoculation may be associated with regional lymphadenopathy, while secondary skin lesions are not. The involved area begins as a subcutaneous papule or nodule that eventually ulcerates and develops into a raised, proliferative granulomatous lesion. As the lesions spread, central healing with scar formation occurs, while the outer margin can become verrucous with nodular plaques and a wartlike surface. They may resemble lesions due to atypical bacteria, mycobacteria, or syphilis, or they may be mistaken for skin cancer.

Inflammatory skin lesions are particularly common in patients with acquired immune deficiency syndrome (AIDS) and disseminated disease. They may be associated with fevers or pulmonary or neurologic symptoms. "Cold abscesses," or subcutaneous nodules, can be seen and are associated with a poorer clinical outcome. Blastomycosis has been documented in HIV-infected patients who have resided in endemic areas in the past; thus, the travel history can be an important clue to the diagnosis. Biopsy and culture of suspicious lesions should be performed early so that appropriate systemic therapy can be instituted.

Osteomyelitis due to *B. dermatitidis* is reported in up to 25% of extrapulmonary cases and may be the reason for seeking medical attention. The vertebrae, pelvis, sacrum, skull, ribs, and long bones are most commonly affected. The radiographic appearance is not specific. Débridement may be required for diagnosis or cure, although bone lesions usually resolve with antifungal therapy alone. CNS infection occurs in only 5 to 10% of patients with disseminated disease and more commonly presents as epidural or cranial abscess. Cerebrospinal fluid (CSF) appearance is not characteristic, and culture is often the only way to make a definitive diagnosis. In some cases of meningitis, yeast cells may be found within multinucleated giant cells in the CSF.

Presumptive diagnosis can be made via direct examination of a specimen such as sputum, bronchoscopic alveolar lavage (BAL) fluid, or pus after digestion with potassium hydroxide (KOH) to identify the yeast forms. *B. dermatitidis* has a very characteristic morphologic appearance. Identification of a broad-based budding yeast, often with a thick refractile wall and a single bud, attached by a wide septum is virtually diagnostic. Definitive diagnosis is made by concurrent culture on Sabouraud's agar, but the organisms may take 4 to 8 weeks to grow. Histologic examination of tissue to identify the organism can be made with periodic acid–Schiff (PAS) or Gomori methenamine silver (GMS) stains. Serologic tests such as complement fixation (CF) and immunodiffusion (ID) are of limited value. The blastomycin skin test antigen should not be used for diagnosis, as specificity and sensitivity are not well established. Colonization with *Blastomyces* species does not occur; therefore, detection of the fungus by direct or histologic examination or culture generally indicates true infection.

The specific therapy for blastomycosis is largely

dependent on the severity of illness, location of the disease, and the status of the host. Since resolution of infection without therapy has been seen in healthy patients exposed in an epidemic focus, observation without therapy may be considered. If the patient's condition deteriorates or progresses after 1 to 2 weeks, antifungal therapy should be started. As the diagnosis is often made when the culture grows the organism, therapy should be initiated if the patient is still symptomatic. Consequently, most cases of pulmonary disease and all cases of extrapulmonary disease should be treated.

Historically, amphotericin B (Fungizone) had been the cornerstone of therapy for blastomycosis. Over the last two decades, however, the azoles—ketoconazole (Nizoral), itraconazole (Sporanox), and most recently, fluconazole (Diflucan)—have been shown to be useful therapeutic options.

Cumulative doses of 1 to 2 grams of amphotericin B (Fungizone) have been shown to be effective in multiple series of patients, leading to clinical cure without relapse in 85 to 97% of cases. Unfortunately, amphotericin B is associated with a number of well-known adverse effects. These include anemia, nephrotoxicity, hypokalemia, and hypomagnesemia, along with the infusion-related effects of hypotension, nausea, vomiting, fever, rigors, and thrombophlebitis. Renal toxicity may be prevented by saline loading with 500 to 1000 mL of normal saline prior to the amphotericin B infusion, which is usually administered over 2 to 3 hours. Premedication with meperidine (Demerol), acetaminophen (Tylenol), and diphenhydramine (Benadryl) can abrogate the infusion-related events.

Amphotericin B should routinely be employed for life-threatening disease, such as disseminated pulmonary disease associated with hypoxia or noncardiogenic pulmonary edema and meningitis. It may be employed for "induction therapy" for treatment of chronic debilitating lesions, at least for the first few weeks to obtain control of the disease, followed by an azole for a minimum of 6 months. If amphotericin B alone is to be used for therapy, the infection should be treated for approximately 3 months with a total cumulative dose of at least 2.0 grams.

The Mycoses Study Group (MSG) established the efficacy of ketoconazole at doses of 400 to 800 mg per day for a minimum of 6 months in non–life-threatening disease in trials published in 1985. This agent may be less effective in bone disease, and because it does not penetrate the blood-brain barrier, it is not useful for treatment of CNS disease. As other azoles are generally better absorbed and tolerated, this drug has been less frequently recommended, but it should eradicate *B. dermatitidis* if the patient is compliant. It is notably the least expensive of the azoles currently available. Ketoconazole's mechanism of action is to disrupt the fungal cell membrane. It interacts with the cytochrome P-450 system; thus, drug-drug interactions are important to consider, especially with rifampin, cyclosporine, antiepileptic agents, and the protease inhibitors for HIV-related disease. Other adverse effects include elevated serum transaminases, hormonal abnormalities such as gynecomastia, dysfunctional uterine bleeding, and oligospermia. The absorption of ketoconazole requires an acidic gastric environment; therefore, antacids or histamine H_2-blocking agents are contraindicated while patients are on this agent.

Itraconazole, an orally administered triazole, is better absorbed and has substantially less endocrinopathy compared with ketoconazole. Drug-drug interactions include those enumerated for ketoconazole as well as those with antihistamines and oral anticoagulants. In a study published by the MSG in 1992, among 48 evaluable patients, 43 (89%) were successfully treated. Furthermore, if they received therapy for at least 2 months, 38 out of 40 (95%) were successfully treated. This efficacy is similar to that reported for amphotericin B and is somewhat better than that for ketoconazole. It is noteworthy that 4 of the 48 patients had had progression of disease while receiving ketoconazole and were cured with itraconazole. The mean duration of therapy in the study was 6.2 months. It is generally considered the drug of choice at a dose of 200 mg twice daily with food for those patients who have indolent nonmeningeal blastomycosis of mild to moderate severity. It too has poor CNS penetration. Therapy with itraconazole should be continued for a minimum of 6 months; ongoing evaluation of disease has required continuation for up to 12 months for both agents.

A pilot study of fluconazole* therapy in 23 patients with non–life-threatening blastomycosis, published in 1995, compared doses of 200 mg and 400 mg per day. Fluconazole was proved to be moderately effective, with an overall cure rate of 65%. The most recent MSG project, published in 1997, found fluconazole to be curative in doses of 400 and 800 mg for non–life-threatening blastomycosis in 89% and 85% of the patients, respectively. The mean duration of therapy for those successfully treated was 8.9 months. Fluconazole is a more hydrophilic agent that penetrates the CNS. It should be considered for maintenance therapy of CNS disease after initial response to amphotericin B, in cases of itraconazole intolerance, or in patients with contraindications to itraconazole because of potential drug-drug interactions.

In summary, the treatment of acute pulmonary blastomycosis in immunocompetent hosts is somewhat controversial, because some patients have spontaneous resolution of their disease without specific antifungal treatment. Without guidelines to distinguish those patients who will recover spontaneously from those in whom the disease will progress or disseminate, most authors recommend that every patient should receive treatment, especially since well-tolerated and effective oral agents are available. In addition, all patients with chronic and extrapulmonary disease should be treated with antifungal therapy. Itraconazole, 200 to 400 mg per day for at least

*Not FDA approved for this indication.

6 months, is the drug of choice, based on consistently favorable experience. At standard doses, fluconazole is less effective than itraconazole, but at higher doses (400 to 800 mg per day)* given for 8 to 9 months, it has efficacy nearly comparable to that of itraconazole. Fluconazole should be considered as a first-line alternative. Among those patients who are immunocompromised, amphotericin B may be necessary for initial treatment. Lifelong chronic suppressive therapy with an azole drug is ordinarily necessary to prevent relapse of disease.

*Exceeds dosage recommended by the manufacturer.

PLEURAL EFFUSION AND EMPYEMA THORACIS

method of
IRVING L. KRON, M.D., and
ARTHUR C. COFFEY, M.D.
University of Virginia Health Sciences Center
Charlottesville, Virginia

PLEURAL EFFUSION

A pleural effusion is a collection of fluid in the pleural space. Normally there are 3 to 10 mL of fluid in the pleural space, usually produced by the parietal pleura and reabsorbed by the visceral pleura. During a normal 24-hour period 5000 to 10,000 mL of fluid traverse the pleural space.

Pleural effusions develop when there is a change in the normal pleural physiology. Either an increase in production by the parietal pleura or a decrease in reabsorption by the visceral pleura can result in an accumulation of excessive pleural fluid. When present a pleural effusion can alter pulmonary physiology or be asymptomatic. Factors that determine whether an effusion will cause symptoms include size, nature of the effusion, whether it is unilateral or bilateral, and the status of the pulmonary parenchyma. Diagnosis of a pleural effusion is usually made by chest radiograph. At least 400 to 500 mL of fluid must be present before an effusion can be appreciated on a standard posterior-anterior upright radiograph. Other radiologic techniques are more sensitive in detecting pleural effusions; these include decubitus radiographs, computed tomography (CT) scans and transthoracic ultrasound.

Once radiographic confirmation of a pleural effusion is made, diagnostic as well as therapeutic procedures should be undertaken. Thoracentesis, either at the bedside or with radiologic guidance, will allow diagnosis and often treatment planning. Larger effusions may require placement of a chest tube with an underwater seal and suction apparatus. Pleural effusions have classically been divided into transudates and exudates. Transudates occur when the normal systemic physiologic state is disturbed but the mesothelial surfaces of the pleura are normal. For example, decreased serum oncotic pressure and increased pulmonary capillary pressure, as occur in nephrotic syndrome, can lead to transudation of fluid into the pleural space. Exudates result from disease processes of the pleura and its associated lymphatics. Common causes of exudates are neoplasm, infection, and inflammatory processes. A more complete list of common causes of pleural effusions is provided in Table 1.

TABLE 1. **Causes of Pleural Effusions**

Transudates	Exudates
Congestive heart failure	Neoplasm (pulmonary, mesothelial, metastatic)
Cirrhotic liver disease	Infection
Nephrotic syndrome	Pulmonary infarction
Glomerulonephritis	Subdiaphragmatic processes
Myxedema	Pancreatitis
Pulmonary emboli	Splenic or hepatic abscess
Peritoneal dialysis	Esophageal perforation
Pancreatitis	Inflammatory (rheumatic disease)
Hypoproteinemia	Chylothorax
Pericarditis	Hemothorax
Malignancy	Miscellaneous
Extravasated intravenous fluid	Postpericardiotomy syndrome
	Uremia
	Radiation

It is important to differentiate between transudates and exudates so the inciting disease process can be identified appropriately. This distinction can usually be made based on the protein and lactate dehydrogenase (LDH) concentrations of the pleural fluid. Table 2 lists the common laboratory values of transudates and exudates. An elevated amylase level in a sample of pleural fluid suggests pancreatitis as the etiology. Elevated triglycerides (>100 mg/dL) are associated with chylothorax. Bloody pleural effusions are associated with trauma or tumor. Leukocytosis in the pleural fluid or an odor is representative of empyema thoracis.

When thoracentesis and drainage cannot provide the correct diagnosis, more invasive procedures are needed. Percutaneous pleural biopsy can be helpful but often is not diagnostic. Thoracoscopically directed

TABLE 2. **Laboratory Values for Transudates and Exudates**

	Transudates	Exudates
Protein	<3 gm/dL	>3 gm/dL
Pleural fluid/serum protein ratio	<0.5	>0.5
pH		<7.2
Glucose	equal to serum	<60 mg/dL
Cytology	negative	positive in malignancy
Leukocyte count	<1000/mm^3	>1000/mm^3
Color	clear	cloudy
Specific gravity	<1.016	>1.106
Culture	negative	positive
Red blood cell count	<10,000/mm^3	>10,000/mm^3

biopsy of the parietal pleura, abnormal lung tissue, and lymph nodes will usually provide a correct diagnosis. Thoracoscopy can also allow instillation of sclerosing agents such as talc, tetracycline, or bleomycin that create a pleurodesis, thus preventing recurrence of the effusion.

EMPYEMA THORACIS

Empyema thoracis is a collection of pus between the parietal and visceral surfaces. Most often it results from the contamination of a parapneumonic effusion, but it can also occur secondary to a disease process in another body cavity or to iatrogenic causes. There are three characteristic phases through which an empyema evolves. Treatment is based on the particular phase a patient is in at the time of diagnosis. The evacuation of the empyema space and the restoration of the normal lung volume is essential in the treatment of all empyemas regardless of the phase at presentation.

The first phase is the exudative phase. Typically these patients present with a pleural effusion of 2 to 3 days' duration associated with a pneumonia. The fluid layers out on decubitus chest radiographs. Laboratory evaluation of the fluid shows negative Gram's stain, pH above 7.3, low to normal glucose, white blood cell (WBC) count of less than 15,000 per mm^3 and protein less than 2.5 mg per dL. Treatment of an empyema in the exudative phase consists of thoracentesis for complete removal of the exudative fluid and appropriate systemic antibiotics to cover the underlying infection. If the lung does not fully expand or there is residual fluid, tube thoracostomy should be performed.

An empyema left untreated will progress to the fibropurulent phase. As WBCs and bacteria move into the exudative fluid, there is loculation of the infected pleural fluid. Laboratory analysis of the fluid shows an increase in the protein concentration and WBC count and a decrease in the glucose concentration and pH.

Treatment of an empyema in the fibropurulent phase is somewhat controversial. Chest tube drainage with systemic antibiotics directed at the causative bacteria of a uniloculated fluid collection will result in resolution in approximately 75% of cases. If a multiloculated empyema is present by CT scan more invasive approaches may be indicated. Thoracoscopic decortication requires a general anesthetic with a double-lumen endotracheal tube. The loculations can be taken down through 1-cm incisions on the chest. The lung can then be freed circumferentially and chest tubes placed for drainage. If thoracoscopy is unavailable, a limited thoracotomy over the area of loculation followed by removal of a segment of rib and drainage of the pleural space with an empyema tube is effective. A nonsurgical alternative to the treatment of loculated empyemas is the use of fibrinolytic agents that are instilled directly into the pleural space. This modality is extremely expensive and not uniformly successful.

An empyema that has progressed for more than 7 days is said to be in the organization phase. In this phase, fibrosis of the parietal and visceral pleura results in a thick "peel" developing around the lung. This causes compression of the lung, a condition referred to as "trapped lung." A trapped lung is at risk for subsequent infection and does not fully expand during inspiration.

The only effective way to treat an organizing empyema is by surgical decortication. In this procedure, the fibrotic peel is removed from the parietal and visceral pleura and chest tubes are placed to keep the freed lung fully expanded. If a patient is unable to undergo a major surgical procedure such as a thoracotomy, an Eloesser flap (pleurocutaneous fistula) is an alternative.

PRIMARY LUNG ABSCESS

method of
JOSEPH C. CHAN, M.D.
Mount Sinai Medical Center
Miami Beach, Florida

Primary lung abscess is a suppurative and destructive pleuropulmonary infection often defined by the roentgenographic finding of a solitary or dominant lung cavity that measures more than 2 cm in diameter. On the other hand, small cavitary lesions within one or more segments of the lung are often referred to as necrotizing pneumonia. The basic pathologic process of the two entities is almost identical. The word "primary" implies that the illness develops in the community rather than in the hospital and that there is no obvious underlying medical condition to account for such a development. Therefore, lung abscess resulting from septic embolization to the lung from right-sided endocarditis would not be considered primary. Other conditions, such as the transdiaphragmatic spread of an amebic liver abscess or infection as a result of an obstructive bronchogenic carcinoma, should likewise not be included. Primary lung abscess develops because the lungs fail to defend themselves against a large inoculum of aspirated bacteria. Aspiration is a common daily event and it happens in about 50% of healthy persons during sleep. In individuals with impaired consciousness, the rate of aspiration can be as high as 70%. Gravitational flow dictates that the superior segments of the lower lobes and the posterior segments of the upper lobes are most often involved, because these segments are the most dependent in the recumbent position.

Patients who have primary lung abscess have a median duration of fever and productive cough of 2 weeks preceding hospitalization. It takes an average of 12 days after aspiration for a roentgenographically detectable lung cavity to develop. Weight loss, anemia, and putrid sputum are also commonly found in these patients. One third may have associated empyema, and pleuritic chest pain may be their presenting complaint.

Bacteria involved in lung abscesses are primarily endogenous in origin. Culture of these abscesses often yields three to five different species of bacteria with anaerobes predominating by a ratio of 3:1 to 5:1. Most of these bacteria belong to the normal flora of the oropharynx. Anaerobic gram-negative bacilli (AGNB) such as *Bacteroides, Prevotella, Porphyromonas,* and *Fusobacterium* species and anaerobic gram-positive cocci such as *Peptostreptococcus* species are important pathogens in this lung infection.

Nomenclature of anaerobic bacteria has been changing rapidly. Most of the pigmented *Bacteroides* species have been renamed *Prevotella* or *Porphyromonas. Prevotella* species are either pigmented (*P. melaninogenica, P. denticola, P. intermedia,* and *P. nigrescens*) or nonpigmented (*P. oris, P. buccae,* and *P. oralis*). *Porphyromonas* species are pigmented (*P. endodontalis* and *P. gingivalis*). Of the *Fusobacterium* species (*F. necrophorum, F. nucleatum, F. naviforme,* and *F. gonidiaformans*), *F. necrophorum* is the most virulent. It is the pathogen for the condition known as postanginal sepsis, or Lemierre's syndrome. In postanginal sepsis, lung abscesses occur as a consequence of septic embolizations from suppurative thrombophlebitis of the internal jugular vein.

Microaerophilic streptococci and *Eikenella corrodens* are the common aerobic counterparts in this mixed infection. *Pseudomonas aeruginosa, Staphylococcus aureus,* and other enterobacteriaceae are involved only in nosocomial cases of lung abscesses.

TREATMENT

A mixed infection is not just a simple microbiologic event; it also indicates that several organisms within this ecosystem are working together to contribute to the final pathogenic expression. Any successful treatment regimen must be capable of eradicating these organisms simultaneously. As a rule, the organisms of greatest importance are those that are most virulent and/or most resistant to antimicrobial agents generally employed in therapy. Therapy using antibiotics with selected activities against either aerobes or anaerobes often leads to disappointing results. The success of penicillin alone in the 1960s, despite known resistance among some of the so-called *Bacteroides fragilis* species, gave the impression that treating all the bacterial species in a complex polymicrobial infection might not be necessary to effect a cure. In 1983, when Levison and his associates demonstrated that penicillin G was inferior to clindamycin, the notion of benign neglect toward certain bacterial components could no longer be accepted.

Traditionally, the three antibiotics most commonly employed to treat primary lung abscesses were penicillin, clindamycin (Cleocin), and metronidazole (Flagyl). All three antibiotics could be given orally, and oral formulation was highly desirable because the patients often were required to take these drugs for 2 to 4 months. After Levison's publication, most authorities recommended clindamycin over penicillin. The addition of metronidazole to penicillin was considered a good alternative approach. For patients who might be colonized by gram-negative bacilli, as in certain nosocomial cases, an aminoglycoside such as gentamicin (Garamycin), should be included. Unfortunately, the development of resistance by AGNB to clindamycin and metronidazole suggested that newer agents with better anaerobic activities should probably be chosen instead.

There are three separate groups of antimicrobial agents available in the late 1990s that can be used alone to treat primary lung abscesses. They are the carbapenems (imipenem [Primaxin] and meropenem [Merrem]), the beta-lactam and beta-lactamase inhibitor combinations (ampicillin/sulbactam [Unasyn], ticarcillin/clavulanate [Timentin], and piperacillin/tazobactam [Zosyn]), and the third-generation fluoroquinolones (TGFs). There is very little difference between the two carbapenems, and they are probably the most active agents for this condition.

Piperacillin/tazobactam has better activity against *P. aeruginosa* than the other two inhibitors, a property that is useful occasionally. Unfortunately, both the carbapenems and the inhibitors require four intravenous administrations a day, which makes them less desirable agents for home therapy. Theoretically, ampicillin/sulbactam can be replaced by amoxicillin/clavulanate at the time of discharge, and home intravenous therapy may be avoided.

For outpatient therapy, only the TGFs (clinafloxacin, trovafloxacin, and grepafloxacin [Raxar]*) are available in oral formulations. At the time this chapter was submitted, clinical evaluations of these TGFs were incomplete, but the in vitro data appeared very promising. This author believes that these agents will make a significant impact in the treatment of anaerobic lung infections.

Most patients can drain the cavity spontaneously by coughing. Postural drainage with percussion is recommended but often unnecessary. Percutaneous needle drainage under computed tomographic guidance is rarely indicated, and this procedure can cause hemorrhage, pneumothorax, or bronchopleural fistula. Occasionally, it can allow the spread of infected material to other parts of the lung. The prognosis of most patients with primary lung abscess is very good. Mortality is low unless other causes of the lung abscesses were unrecognized.

*Not FDA approved for this indication.

OTITIS MEDIA

method of
RICK A. FRIEDMAN, M.D., Ph.D.
House Ear Clinic, Inc.
Los Angeles, California

Acute otitis media (AOM) is one of the most common diseases of infants and young children. Otitis media is by definition an inflammatory disorder of the mucoperiosteal lining of the middle ear. The mucosal inflammation of otitis media can extend from the eustachian tube to the mastoid cavity. Although there are a variety of classification schemes for effusions of the middle ear, most categorize the middle ear fluid as serous, mucinous, or purulent. The fluid in acute otitis media is largely purulent, and it is this type of effusion that will be the focus of this section.

EPIDEMIOLOGY

Acute otitis media affects children of all races and socioeconomic levels. The prevalence of the disease is directly related to age, with the vast majority of cases occurring in children 2 years of age or younger. More than 80% of children have at least one episode of AOM, and approximately 50% have multiple episodes.

There are several factors that correlate with an increased incidence of AOM. Certain ethnic groups such as Native Americans and Eskimos have a higher incidence, whereas blacks appear to have a lower incidence than whites. Environmental and seasonal factors influence disease prevalence. Children in day care are more prone to AOM. The incidence of disease peaks in the winter months and is lowest during the summer. Lastly, immunologic and genetic factors have been implicated as associated factors.

PATHOPHYSIOLOGY

The final common pathway in AOM is a suppurative infection of the mucosal lining of the tubotympanum, often resulting from eustachian tube dysfunction. The pediatric eustachian tube is inclined approximately 10° (45° in the adult), and the cartilaginous portion is far more pliable than in adults. Hence, when an upper respiratory tract infection causes congestion and edema of the tube, the middle ear can no longer aerate normally, resulting in stasis of secretions and local hypoxia and hypercarbia. All of these factors contribute to a breakdown in local immunity and proliferation of pathogens. It is likely that in many cases, AOM results from reflux of nasopharyngeal secretions into a patent tube. The net result is the same—purulent tubotympanitis.

CLINICAL COURSE

The clinical course can be separated into stages. The initial stage of hyperemia is characterized by otalgia and often fever. The vessels of the posterosuperior wall of the external canal and tympanic membrane become injected, and the tympanic membrane is dull, slightly bulging, and painful on pneumotoscopy. The exudative stage is associated with increasing fever, constitutional symptoms, and severe pain. The normal landmarks of the tympanic membrane, such as the short process of the malleus, may be lost. The suppurative stage is characterized by increasing temperature, pain, and constitutional symptoms. The tympanic membrane is often bulging, red, and immobile. It is not unusual for purulence to be noted in the external auditory canal after spontaneous rupture of the tympanic membrane. Complications are infrequent; however, the recurrence of pain 7 to 10 days after AOM may herald acute coalescent mastoiditis. Upon resolution, the pain, constitutional symptoms, and fever subside. Approximately 70% of children demonstrate a persistent serous effusion after AOM that is often associated with a conductive hearing loss. The vast majority of these effusions resolve spontaneously within 90 days.

MICROBIOLOGY

The most common organism cultured from middle ear aspirates of children with AOM is *Streptococcus pneumoniae. Haemophilus influenzae* is the second most common pathogen, and concomitant infection with these two organisms occurs in up to 3% of cases. A variety of other organisms have been implicated, including common respiratory viruses (Table 1). Neonatal AOM, although rare, warrants special mention. These children are often affected by gram-negative rods and in the course of a sepsis work-up may require tympanocentesis to direct therapy.

TABLE 1. **Specific Bacterial Isolates**

Specific Bacterial Isolates	Number of Occurrences* (%)
Streptococcus pneumoniae	770 (30.9)
Haemophilus influenzae	554 (22.2)
Moraxella catarrhalis	152 (6.1)
β-hemolytic streptococci, group A	44 (1.7)
Enteric bacteria	23 (0.9)
Staphylococcus aureus	18 (0.7)
Staphylococcus epidermidis	10 (0.4)
Pseudomonas aeruginosa	7 (0.25)
Others	63 (12.5)

*Total patients studied = 2251.
From Reichert TJ, Spector GJ: Acute Otitis Media. American Academy of Otolaryngology Self Instructional Package, 1979.

TREATMENT

Although antibiotic therapy is the standard treatment for AOM, in the preantibiotic era the vast majority of cases resolved spontaneously. The incidence of complications, such as coalescent mastoiditis, have been greatly reduced by antibiotics, however.

Appropriate treatment of AOM should be based upon the following: (1) knowledge of the age- and region-specific bacteriology; (2) sensitivities or patterns of resistance of causative organisms; and (3) antibiotic efficacy, complications, and cost. Antibiotic resistance rates are quite high for *H. influenzae* and *Moraxella catarrhalis,* and recent reports of *S. pneumoniae* resistance have appeared in the literature. These factors must be considered before therapy and in cases not responding to therapy. Table 2 lists the most commonly used antibiotics for AOM. Amoxicillin remains the mainstay of therapy for uncomplicated cases.

SEQUELAE

As alluded to earlier, with the advent of antibiotic therapy, complications of AOM have become exceedingly rare. However, virtually every case is associated with some degree of conductive hearing loss.

TABLE 2. **Antibiotic Therapy for Acute Otitis Media**

Initial Choice	Alternatives
Amoxicillin	Cefuroxime (Ceftin), cefprozil (Cefzil)
or	
Erythromycin plus sulfisoxazole (Pediazole)	Cefaclor (Ceclor), loracarbef (Lorabid) Cefpodoxime (Vantin), cefixime (Suprax)
or	
Amoxicillin/potassium clavulanate (Augmentin)	Trimethoprim/sulfamethoxazole (Bactrim)

The majority of children will display a persistent serous effusion that will spontaneously resolve over the ensuing several weeks. Intratemporal or intracranial complications such as mastoiditis, facial nerve paralysis, suppurative labyrinthitis, meningitis, and brain abscess are exceedingly rare, but suspected cases should be immediately referred to a specialist in otolaryngology and/or neurosurgery.

ACUTE BRONCHITIS

method of
HAROLD A. WILLIAMSON, Jr., M.D., M.S.P.H.
University of Missouri–Columbia School of Medicine
Columbia, Missouri

Acute bronchitis is a self-limited lower respiratory illness usually precipitated by a viral infection in which persistent and troubling cough is the predominant feature. It occurs in persons with structurally normal lungs and thus is distinct from acute exacerbations of chronic obstructive pulmonary disease.

Acute bronchitis is very common, resulting in more than 10 million annual physician visits. For family physicians, visits for acute bronchitis are 20 times more common than for pneumonia and 10 times more common than for asthma. Experienced physicians, therefore, develop an efficient approach that excludes other important diseases and deals with symptoms effectively and inexpensively.

Most cases of acute bronchitis are initiated by viral infections, and nearly any virus with a predilection for the respiratory tract may be involved. Influenza, rhinovirus, adenovirus, and coronaviruses are the most common causative organisms. Bacteria (*Pneumococcus* and *Haemophilus influenzae*) can occasionally be cultured from the sputum of such patients, but their causal role is uncertain. *Mycoplasma pneumoniae* and *Chlamydia* are important pathogens because of their potential treatability by antibiotics, but the frequency of these infections and the degree to which they respond to antibiotics remain unclear. Recently, *Bordetella pertussis* has been documented as an uncommon cause of prolonged cough.

Inflammation and ulceration of the trachea and bronchi accompany the clinical syndrome. Many viruses, especially influenza and respiratory syncytial viruses, cause an overproduction of histamine for approximately 5 weeks, roughly corresponding with the average cough duration. Patients diagnosed with acute bronchitis are much more likely than a control group to have a family history of atopy and a subsequent diagnosis of asthma. Pulmonary function tests demonstrate a reduced forced expiratory volume (FEV) in about half of patients with acute bronchitis. This information has caused speculation that acute bronchitis may best be considered as "temporary asthma," as opposed to a "chest infection."

TREATMENT

The typical patient is a young or middle-aged adult who may or may not be a cigarette smoker, and who reports that a "head cold has gone to my chest." A cough, intermittently productive, of 2 weeks' duration is usually the presenting complaint, but fatigue and loss of sleep may be more troublesome. Accompanying symptoms include scant sputum production, low-grade fever, chills but not rigor, and substernal pain with cough. The experienced clinician will quickly assess for other possibilities including asthma, chronic obstructive pulmonary disease, pulmonary embolism, and congestive heart failure.

Occasionally a white blood cell count or chest roentgenogram will help distinguish acute bronchitis from bacterial or viral pneumonia. The physical examination usually reveals evidence of upper respiratory infection only. Occasionally rhonchi or wheezes are noted. Rales, prominent wheezing, distended neck veins, cyanosis, and supraclavicular lymphadenopathy suggest other diagnoses.

Goals of treatment are alleviation of symptoms and improved functional capacity. Fluids and antipyretics are usually recommended. Cough suppression is best prescribed in a graded fashion. Dextromethorphan as an over-the-counter preparation may be used as an initial therapy, especially during the day time. Codeine, 10 to 30 mg every 4 hours, is helpful for more persistent cough; a bedtime dose may help with sleeplessness and minimizes side effects. If these are unsuccessful, benzonatate (Tessalon), 100 mg three times a day, may be tried.

Patients who have wheezing on examination or a strong personal or family history of atopic disease may benefit from use of an inhaled bronchodilator such as albuterol, 2 inhalations every 4 hours. Pulmonary function testing, while usually not indicated, may identify those patients who will benefit most from bronchodilators. Inhaled steroids have not yet been sufficiently tested in this disease to recommend them.

A majority of patients in the United States receive antibiotics for this disease, even though no compelling evidence supports their use. Indeed, six randomized control trials of antibiotics (doxycycline [Vibramycin], trimethoprim-sulfamethoxazole [Bactrim, Septra], and erythromycin) have not demonstrated a definite beneficial effect. Three studies comparing a bronchodilator to an antibiotic suggest that resolution of symptoms is the same with either treatment. Many clinicians use presence of fever, purulent sputum, and severe cough as indications for an antibiotic prescription, but there is no evidence that such subgroups respond better to antibiotics. If an antibiotic is used, it is sensible to choose a drug that has effectiveness against *Chlamydia* and *Mycoplasma,* is inexpensive, and has minimum side effects. For these reasons, erythromycin, 1 gram daily in divided doses, is probably the best choice, although 15 to 20% of patients may discontinue the drug because of side effects. Clarithromycin (Biaxin) and azithromycin (Zithromax) have fewer side effects but are more expensive.

During an epidemic, suspect influenza cases presenting with bronchitis may benefit from specific anti-influenza therapy.

Serious complications of acute bronchitis are uncommon. This disease only very rarely "goes into pneumonia," even though this is a common reason given for antibiotic use. Fatigue from sleeplessness is common, as is lateral chest pain from intercostal muscle tears. Occasionally, cough may be severe enough to fracture a rib, even in healthy patients. Severe coughs may also cause emesis (particularly in children), syncope, urinary incontinence, and elevated creatine phosphokinase (CPK).

Patient education is important because the benefits of therapy are not always striking, and return visits for unresolved symptoms are common. The natural history of the condition should be described as a viral infection that has caused airway inflammation. Patients may usually be told that improvement begins after 3 to 5 days but that another 2 or 3 weeks of cough are not uncommon. The average patient with acute bronchitis who seeks medical care coughs for nearly 4 weeks. Patients should be instructed to call or return if there is dyspnea, high fever, or failure to improve after a week.

Experienced clinicians avoid unnecessary antibiotic use by counseling patients about the lack of documented efficacy. Some physicians discuss the increasing incidence of antibiotic resistance, and some patients are familiar with these concerns from the lay press. An antibiotic prescription given with the advice to leave it unfilled for 72 hours while spontaneous improvement occurs sometimes avoids unnecessary antibiotic use.

In the future, rapid tests to identify *Mycoplasma* and *Chlamydia* may help direct antibiotic therapy. Randomized clinical trials of bronchodilators and perhaps steroids should help clarify their value.

BACTERIAL PNEUMONIAS

method of
BURKE A. CUNHA, M.D.
Winthrop University Hospital
Mineola, New York
State University of New York at Stony Brook School of Medicine
Stony Brook, New York

For the treatment of bacterial pneumonias to be effective, there must be an accurate presumptive diagnosis on which to base empirical therapy. Pneumonias can be classified by site of acquisition, by causative organism, or by severity. This clinical classification is useful because community-acquired pneumonias (CAPs) are caused by different organisms than nosocomial, or hospital-acquired, pneumonias. It is also useful to consider the infecting microorganism if known, because the clinical, radiologic, and laboratory features of each pathogen differ to varying degrees. The severity of a pneumonia clearly has therapeutic implications. Mild-to-moderate pneumonias may be treated in the ambulatory setting with oral antibiotics. Parenteral antibiotics are usually used for pneumonias requiring inpatient care, or if sufficiently severe, treatment in the critical care or intensive care setting. Pneumonias may also be classified as typical bacterial pneumonias, which are lower respiratory tract infections involving the lung parenchyma caused by typical respiratory pathogens, or as atypical pneumonias, which are systemic infectious diseases in which the lungs are only one of multiple organs involved. The clinician must be familiar with the differential diagnostic aspects of each of the varieties of pneumonia to formulate an effective therapeutic approach.

COMMUNITY-ACQUIRED PNEUMONIAS

CAPs are usually caused by *Streptococcus pneumoniae, Haemophilus influenzae,* or *Moraxella catarrhalis.* The clinical manifestations of these three infections overlap considerably, and they cannot be distinguished readily on clinical grounds. For this reason, antibiotics for typical bacterial pneumonias should cover all three of these key pathogens. It is equally important to recognize that other pathogens are uncommon and should be covered only under certain circumstances. *Staphylococcus aureus* pneumonia, for example, occurs almost exclusively in the postviral influenza setting. *Klebsiella pneumoniae* pneumonia occurs almost exclusively in chronic alcoholics, and *Pseudomonas aeruginosa* causes pneumonia in patients with bronchiectasis and cystic fibrosis but not in other individuals with CAPs. Therefore, *S. aureus, K. pneumoniae,* and *P. aeruginosa* need not be included in the spectrum of organisms covered in typical bacterial CAPs. Typical bacterial pneumonias are just that, and clinical findings are confined to the lungs.

Community-Acquired Aspiration Pneumonia

Aspiration pneumonia may be community acquired or nosocomial. Community-acquired pneumonia is caused by the aspiration of anaerobic oropharyngeal flora, (e.g., *Peptococcus, Veillonella, Fusobacterium, Peptostreptococcus, Bacteroides melaninogenicus, Prevotella,* and the oral pigmented *Bacteroides* species). Community-acquired aspiration pneumonia is caused by multiple organisms, in contrast to the typical bacterial pneumonias, in which only one organism is responsible for the pulmonary process. Therapeutically, the oral pigmented *Bacteroides* species and the other anaerobes of the oropharynx are susceptible to most antibiotics used to treat CAP. No additional antianaerobic coverage needs to be added for a patient with CAP when aspiration is suspected.

Community-Acquired Atypical Pneumonia

Atypical pneumonias are distinguished from the typical bacterial pneumonias by their extrapulmonary manifestations. The atypical pneumonias may be classified conveniently as zoonotic (e.g., psittacosis, tularemia, Q fever) or nonzoonotic (e.g., Legionnaires' disease, *Mycoplasma pneumoniae* pneumonia, *Chlamydia pneumoniae* pneumonia). Historical questioning regarding animal or bird contact will quickly rule in or rule out the zoonotic atypical pathogens. No single feature is diagnostic of any of the atypical pneumonias, but the pattern of organ involvement is characteristic and fairly specific. Whereas no patient has all of the symptoms associated with an atypical pneumonia due to a particular organism, all patients have several clinical and laboratory manifestations permitting an accurate presumptive clinical diagnosis.

Mycoplasma pneumonia and *Chlamydia* pneumonia occur in young adults or in adults who have had recent contact with young adults who are infected or are carrying the organisms. However, it is Legionnaires' disease that is most likely to be severe and sometimes life threatening. Therefore, the clinician's diagnostic approach should be focused on ruling in or ruling out *Legionella* from therapeutic consideration. This is important because β-lactams have traditionally been used to treat the typical CAPs but are ineffective against all of the atypical pathogens. Traditional coverage against the atypical pathogens has been with doxycycline or erythromycin. It should be noted that macrolides are relatively ineffective against *Chlamydia psittaci* and *C. pneumoniae,* and doxycycline should be used in preference to macrolides in treating chlamydial pneumonias in adults.

Legionnaires' disease can be treated with macrolides or doxycycline. However, quinolones are much more active against *Legionella* than the aforementioned drugs and should be used to treat severe cases of Legionnaires' disease or infection in compromised hosts. At the present time, quinolones provide the highest degree of anti-*Legionella* activity of the currently available antibiotics. Because it is rare for a typical and an atypical pathogen to coexist in the same patient, "double-drug" therapy to treat all CAPs is unnecessary and wasteful. The clinician should try to determine diagnostically whether the patient has a typical or an atypical pneumonia, then treat for either possibility but not both. If the clinician cannot clearly differentiate between typical and atypical pathogens, then monotherapy with an agent that covers both (e.g., levofloxacin [Levaquin]) is cost effective and the optimal therapeutic approach.

Severe Community-Acquired Pneumonia

It is a common misconception that patients presenting with severe CAP require a different therapeutic approach than patients with mild-to-moderate disease. Severe CAP is caused by the same pathogens that cause mild-to-moderate CAP, that is, the typical bacterial pathogens or Legionnella. Because the organisms causing severe CAP are the same as those causing mild-to-moderate disease, the antimicrobial therapy should be the same for both groups of patients.

The severity of pneumonia depends on the degree of immunocompromise as well as the underlying status of cardiopulmonary function. Obviously, patients with clinically significant cardiopulmonary disease are likely to have a severe CAP because they have little cardiopulmonary reserve and the pneumonia predictably will be serious regardless of the infecting pathogen. Even a mild pneumonia caused by a low-virulence pathogen (e.g., *M. catarrhalis*) can result in a severe CAP in a patient with underlying chronic bronchitis. Any CAP due to any pulmonary pathogen may be severe if superimposed on a pre-existing pulmonary disease, (e.g., cancer, connective tissue diseases, pulmonary drug reactions, pulmonary hemorrhage, pulmonary vasculitis, pulmonary fibrosis). Similarly, CAP in a patient with clinically significant coronary artery disease, valvular heart disease, or congestive heart failure often results in severe CAP.

Immunocompromised patients, especially those with impaired humoral immunity or B-lymphocyte function, are prone to severe pneumonia. Fulminant pneumococcal pneumonia with bacteremia and shock is a well-known infectious complication in asplenic individuals. The usual treatment for overwhelming pneumococcal sepsis is penicillin given at the same dose and dosing interval as for patients with intact immune systems and mild-to-moderate disease. The antibiotic approach is the same in mild-to-moderate and severe pneumonia because antibiotic therapy is directed against the pathogen and is not affected by host factors.

Indices of severity have been developed to classify patients with CAP. Such categorizations are useful prognostically since sicker patients are expected to have a stormier course and more complications. Importantly, however, the severity index has no bearing on the selection of initial empirical monotherapy for the treatment of a CAP. Therefore, initial antibiotic therapy is the same regardless of disease severity. Additional antibiotics are unnecessary and should not be given despite the presence of severe disease or co-morbid factors (Table 1).

Community-Acquired Pneumonia in a Compromised Host

Compromised hosts presenting with CAP are most often infected with the usual bacterial pathogens. However, viral pneumonias are also common in transplant and HIV-infected patients, and the clinical presentation is distinct from that of bacterial pneumonia. Viral pneumonia and *Pneumocystis carinii* pneumonia (PCP) are rarely if ever focal, segmental, or lobar in these patients; therefore, a discrete segmental infiltrate should be assumed to be bacterial until proved otherwise. Aerosolized PCP is an exception: bilateral apical infiltrates may occur in this patient subset.

If therapy with a respiratory quinolone such as levofloxacin does not result in prompt clinical improvement, the patient should undergo bronchoscopy for a definitive diagnosis (Table 2).

TABLE 1. **Differential Diagnosis of Severe CAP with Shock**

- CAP does not present with shock in normal hosts.
- If CAP presents with shock, look for impaired or absent splenic function.

Disorders associated with impaired splenic function:

Amyloidosis	Rheumatoid arthritis
Celiac disease	Sézary syndrome
Chronic active hepatitis	Sickle cell trait/disease
Chronic alcoholism	Splenectomy
Congenital asplenia	Splenic infarcts
Fanconi's syndrome	Splenic malignancies
Hyposplenism of old age	Steroid therapy
IgA deficiency	Systemic lupus erythematosus
Intestinal lymphangiectasia	Systemic mastocystosis
Intravenous gamma-globulin therapy	Systemic necrotizing vasculitis
Myeloproliferative disorders	Thyroiditis
Non-Hodgkin's lymphoma	Ulcerative coilitis
Regional enteritis	Waldenström's macroglobulinemia

- If CAP presents with shock in the absence of conditions associated with hyposplenism, look for "mimics of pneumonia" that present with pulmonary infiltrates on chest films, fever, leukocytosis, and hypotension, e.g., acute myocardial infarction (MI), acute pulmonary embolism (PE).
- If CAP presents with shock and there is no evidence of hyposplenia, acute MI, acute PE, etc., then consider an exacerbation of pre-existing advanced cardiopulmonary disease that presents with hypotension (e.g., coronary insufficiency, hypoxemia in emphysema) complicating CAP as the cause of shock.

Therapeutic Considerations

Intravenous to Oral Switch Therapy

It has been shown that in the treatment of typical bacterial CAP, 2 days of intravenous (IV) therapy followed by 12 days of oral (PO) therapy is therapeutically equivalent to a full 14-day course of intravenous antibiotics. This finding has important therapeutic and economic implications in the managed care era. Although patients in the critical care unit cannot take oral antibiotics after 48 hours, the majority of hospitalized patients can. Switching patients to an appropriate oral antibiotic after 48 hours has several clinical advantages: the length of stay is decreased, the costs of therapy are lower, and the incidence of IV line infections is greatly reduced.

The same considerations apply when selecting an antibiotic for an IV-to-PO transition program as in selecting an antibiotic for oral therapy. Oral antibiotics should have the same therapeutic spectrum as their IV counterparts, and bioavailability should be such that oral antibiotics achieve the same serum and tissue levels as their IV counterparts. Therefore, with the exception of those who cannot take oral medications, all patients with CAP should be placed on appropriate oral antibiotics after 48 hours, or in compromised hosts, as soon as there has been a clinical response and defervescence. As with oral antibiotics, the duration of therapy for typical bacterial CAPs is 14 days. This may be shortened in healthy normal individuals and may need to be extended in nonleukopenic compromised hosts and those with advanced cardiopulmonary disease (Tables 3 and 4).

Oral Antibiotic Treatment of Community-Acquired Pneumonia

Mild-to-moderate typical or atypical pneumonias may be treated solely with oral antibiotics. The choice of an oral antibiotic depends on the therapeutic spectrum, tissue penetration characteristics, resistance potential, safety profile, and cost. The ideal antibiotic for oral therapy has the same spectrum of activity as its IV counterpart and excellent bioavailability. Antibiotics with excellent bioavailability are equivalent to their intravenous counterparts attaining the same blood and tissue levels. Consequently, patients with moderately severe pneumonia who are able to take oral medications and do not require hospitalization may be treated entirely with carefully selected oral antibiotics.

Other important attributes of an orally administered antibiotic include a favorable safety profile and a convenient dosing regimen to assure compliance. Antibiotics that cause nausea and vomiting, gastrointestinal upset, or diarrhea should be used only if other alternatives cannot be found. Antibiotics that are taken once daily with few side effects have an advantage over antibiotics that must be taken more than once a day. The duration of oral antibiotic therapy to treat CAP is the same as that with intrave-

TABLE 2. **Empirical Antibiotic Therapy of CAP in Selected Compromised Hosts**

Immunodeficient State	Preferred Antibiotics*
Hyposplenism/Asplenia	
Streptococcus pneumoniae	Cefepime
Haemophilus influenzae	or
Neisseria meningitidis	Ceftriaxone
Klebsiella pneumoniae	or
	Levofloxacin
Febrile Leukopenia	
Pseudomonas aeruginosa	Cefepime
Serratia marcescens	plus
Klebsiella pneumoniae	Levofloxacin
	or
	Meropenem
Human Immunodeficiency Virus Infection (Excluding PCP)	
S. pneumoniae	Levofloxacin
H. influenzae	or
Salmonella	Trimethoprim/
Legionella	sulfamethoxazole
Nonleukopenic Compromised Hosts (SLE, DM, etc.)	
S. pneumoniae	Cefepime
H. influenzae	or
	Ceftriaxone

*Preferred in terms of spectrum, resistance potential, safety profile, and cost.
Abbreviations: PCP = *Pneumocystis carinii* pneumonia; SLE = systemic lupus erythematosus; DM = diabetes mellitus.

TABLE 3. **Therapeutic Approach to Community-Acquired Pneumonia (CAP)**

- Antibiotic coverage should be directed only against the most common community-acquired pathogens:
  - *Streptococcus pneumoniae*
  - *Haemophilus influenzae*
  - *Moraxella catarrhalis*
- Antibiotic coverage should be directed against unusual pathogens only under specific circumstances:
  - *Klebsiella pneumoniae* (only in chronic alcoholics)
  - *Staphylococcus aureus* (only in postviral influenza pneumonia)
  - *Pseudomonas aeruginosa* (only in cystic fibrosis/bronchiectasis)
- Compromised hosts (especially organ transplant recipients, febrile leukopenics, and patients with HIV infection) usually have the same bacterial pathogens as do normal hosts in CAP.
- Use monotherapy to treat CAP in compromised hosts. Do not use combination therapy just because the patient is a compromised host with CAP. Cover only the most likely pathogens, not the immune defect. Avoid "double-drug" therapy for presumed "double pathogens."
- CAP due to two or more organisms is extremely rare (except in aspiration pneumonia).
- Use appropriate monotherapy for severe CAP requiring CCU admission. Do not add antibiotics just because patient is critically ill. Severity is a function of:
  - Underlying cardiopulmonary disease or impaired splenic function

  Outcome with monotherapy is equal to that with double-drug therapy because the severity is not pathogen related.
- Clinically differentiate typical from atypical pneumonias and treat one group or the other group—but not both. CAP is caused by single and not multiple pathogens.
- If you cannot differentiate between typical and atypical pneumonias, treat with an antibiotic that optimally covers both groups, such as levofloxacin.
- Preferentially select antibiotics with a high degree of antipneumococcal activity that are unlikely to increase relative penicillin resistance of *S. pneumoniae* (e.g., doxycycline, levofloxacin).

nous preparations, that is, usually 14 days for typical pathogens and 4 weeks for Legionnaires' disease. Treatment may be shortened in healthy, immunocompetent hosts and extended in patients with impaired host defenses.

NOSOCOMIAL PNEUMONIAS

Nosocomial pneumonias may be acquired via inhalation or hematogenous dissemination to the lungs from a distant source. The former type usually demonstrates a segmental or lobar distribution on the chest film. In contrast, hematogenously acquired nosocomial pneumonia presents with bilateral symmetrical interstitial alveolar infiltrates resembling left ventricular failure, adult respiratory distress syndrome, or massive bilateral aspiration. The diagnosis of nosocomial pneumonia is difficult because there are many conditions with similar presentations. Many patients in the critical care unit or other hospital settings who have pulmonary infiltrates and fever with or without leukocytosis are treated empirically for hospital-acquired pneumonia but do not have a nosocomial pneumonia. The confirmation of the diagnosis of nosocomial pneumonia depends on isolating a known pulmonary pathogen in high concentration from a culture specimen of respiratory tract secretions obtained by protected bronchoscopic brushing. The mere recovery of respiratory pathogens from respiratory secretions in an intubated patient with fever, leukocytosis, and pulmonary infiltrates is not sufficient for the diagnosis.

There are many diseases that present with pulmonary findings that can be confused with hospital-acquired pneumonia (e.g., pulmonary embolism and collagen vascular diseases such as systemic lupus erythematosus). Clinicians should make every effort to rule out conditions that can mimic a nosocomial pneumonia before embarking on empirical therapy; treatment of pulmonary infiltrates accompanied by fever and leukocytosis that are not due to a nosocomial pneumonia results in needless and potentially harmful exposure to expensive antibiotics. If the common causes of pulmonary infiltrates with fever and leukocytosis in the intensive care unit can be eliminated, then the diagnosis of nosocomial pneumonia should be entertained. If the invasive methods required to make the diagnosis of nosocomial pneumonia cannot be done, then empirical therapy is a reasonable therapeutic approach.

A common therapeutic error in the treatment of nosocomial pneumonias is to assume that aerobic gram-negative pathogens isolated from respiratory secretions in intubated patients are responsible for the pulmonary infiltrates and fever. It is important to appreciate that certain organisms commonly seen in the critical care environment often colonize respiratory secretions but do not cause hospital-acquired pneumonias. These "common colonizers" include *Enterobacter* species, *Citrobacter* species, *Flavobacterium* species, *Xanthomonas maltophilia,* and *Pseudomonas cepacia.*

It is a general principle of infectious disease management that colonization should not be treated. Colonization with these organisms commonly recovered from the respiratory secretions of patients with pulmonary infiltrates, leukocytosis, and fever should never be considered as a pathogenic process or treated as a nosocomial pneumonia. It is vital to appreciate that known respiratory pathogens such as *P. aeruginosa, Serratia,* and *Klebsiella* are more often colonizers than pathogens in the critical care setting. Before these organisms are considered pathogenic, every attempt must be made to eliminate from diagnostic consideration the noninfectious causes of pulmonary infiltrates, leukocytosis, and fever and to arrive at a definitive diagnosis by semiquantitative cultures of respiratory tract secretions obtained by protected bronchoscopic brushings or lavage.

Nosocomial Aspiration Pneumonia

Community-acquired aspiration pneumonia is caused by aspirated oral anaerobic flora. If aspiration occurs after 7 days of hospitalization, then the pa-

TABLE 4. **Empirical Antibiotic Therapy of Community-Acquired Pneumonia (CAP)**

Typical Coverage	Atypical Coverage	Typical and Atypical Coverage
Mild/Moderate CAP (Oral Therapy)		
Typical Coverage	*Atypical Coverage*	*Typical and Atypical Coverage*
•Cefprozil Cefuroxime axetil Cefaclor	•Doxycycline Erythromycin Azithromycin	•Doxycycline Azithromycin Levofloxacin
Severe CAP (Initial IV Therapy)		
Typical Coverage	*Atypical Coverage*	*Typical and Atypical Coverage*
•Ceftriaxone Cefepime Levofloxacin	•Levofloxacin Ciprofloxacin	•Levofloxacin
IV/PO Switch Therapy for CAP		
Typical Coverage	*Atypical Coverage*	*Typical and Atypical Coverage*
•Cefprozil Cefuroxime axetil Cefaclor	•Levofloxacin Doxycycline Azithromycin	•Levofloxacin Doxycycline Azithromycin

• = Preferred antibiotic on the basis of cost, safety profile, and resistance potential.

tient has a hospital-acquired aspiration pneumonia. After a week or more of hospitalization, the predominant oropharyngeal flora are aerobic gram-negative bacilli acquired from the hospital environment.

Common nosocomial pathogens include *P. aeruginosa, Serratia marcescens,* and *K. pneumoniae* in addition to the oral anaerobic flora. Because most antibiotics including β-lactams are active against the oral aerobic flora, antibiotic therapy of nosocomial aspiration pneumonia should be directed against the hospital-acquired respiratory pathogens that cause nonaspiration nosocomial pneumonias. For these reasons, nosocomial aspiration pneumonia is treated in exactly the same way as hospital-acquired pneumonia. As with community-acquired aspiration pneumonia, there is no need to add separate antianerobic coverage. Nosocomial aspiration pneumonia is ordinarily treated for 2 weeks.

Nosocomial Atypical Pneumonia

Atypical pathogens (e.g., *Legionella, Mycoplasma, C. pneumoniae, Coxiella burnetii, Francisella tularensis, Chlamydia psittaci*) are often encountered in patients presenting with CAP but are uncommon causes of hospital-acquired pneumonia.

The only atypical pathogen likely to be acquired in the hospital setting is *Legionella.* Legionniares' disease can occur sporadically or in clusters during an outbreak, and any *Legionella* species can be involved in a sporadic case or an outbreak. The clinical presentation in nosocomial Legionnaires' disease is the same as in community-acquired cases; both have a characteristic pattern of extrapulmonary organ involvement. However, hospitalized patients usually have multiple underlying systemic disorders in addition to the disease responsible for hospital admission. The clinical manifestations of these conditions frequently involve different organ systems, making it more difficult to appreciate and recognize the extrapulmonary manifestations of Legionnaires' disease. If Legionnaires' disease is suspected, initial empirical treatment with a quinolone (e.g., levofloxacin) is recommended. Levofloxacin is more than twice as active against *Legionella* as ciprofloxacin (Cipro). Alternatively, doxycycline given in an initial loading dose of 200 mg (IV) every 12 hours for 72 hours followed by 100 mg (IV) every 12 hours can be used in less severe cases. Alternatively, doxycycline may be given as a single daily dose IV or PO every 24 hours. There is no reason to add rifampin to doxycycline for the treatment of Legionnaires' disease. Ordinarily, treatment is continued IV or PO for 4 weeks.

Therapeutic Considerations

Monotherapy Versus Combination Therapy

If bronchoscopy to obtain the diagnostic specimens is not possible, then empirical monotherapy should be instituted. Antimicrobial therapy should be directed primarily against *P. aeruginosa,* as this will cover all other common nosocomial pathogens, including *S. marcescens* and *K. pneumoniae.* Several therapeutic approaches have been utilized in the treatment of nosocomial pneumonias when *P. aeruginosa* is the most likely pathogen. Traditionally, two antibiotics with antipseudomonal activity have been given in a full 14-day course of therapy regardless of whether *P. aeruginosa* is proved to be the pathogen.

Two other more selective and cost-effective approaches are also commonly used. The first approach involves giving two antipseudomonal antibiotics for the first 72 hours while waiting for blood cultures and/or protected semiquantitative bronchial brushings to show whether *P. aeruginosa* is the primary pathogen. If *P. aeruginosa* is not cultured, then one of the antipseudomonal antibiotics is discontinued and the 14-day course of therapy is completed with the remaining antipseudomonal antibiotic.

The second, and better, approach is to use a single antipseudomonal agent with a high degree of activity against *P. aeruginosa* and a low resistance potential as initial therapy pending culture positivity for *P.*

aeruginosa. If *P. aeruginosa* is cultured from the blood or bronchoscopically obtained semiquantitative brushing specimens, then a second antipseudomonal antibiotic is added. This is the most cost-effective and logical approach because it minimizes needless double-drug therapy and does not compromise patient care while minimizing antibiotic cost. Therefore, monotherapy with an antibiotic with a high degree of anti–*P. aeruginosa* activity and minimal resistance potential is the preferred therapeutic approach.

For nosocomial pneumonias not due to *P. aeruginosa,* monotherapy has been shown to be at least as good as combination therapy. In the past, double-drug therapy has been advocated for nosocomial pneumonias based upon the assumption that *P. aeruginosa* is the causative organism in most cases. It is also based on the fact that organisms such as *Klebsiella* and *Serratia* required double-drug therapy in the past because the antibiotics available against these aerobic gram-negative bacilli were of modest efficacy. However, with the introduction of third- and fourth-generation cephalosporins, aztreonam (Azactam), quinolones, and carbapenems, all of which possess a high degree of activity when used alone, *P. aeruginosa* nosocomial pneumonias can be effectively treated with a single antibiotic (i.e., monotherapy) that has a high degree of activity against the common nosocomial pneumonia pathogens.

Antibiotic Resistance

The antibiotic selected for nosocomial pneumonia should possess a high degree of anti–*P. aeruginosa* activity and low resistance potential. Although antibiotics with a high resistance potential are equally efficacious in eliminating the organism in individual patients, the potential emergence of highly resistant strains is a concern for the critical care unit as well as the entire hospital. Antibiotics known to have a low resistance potential while possessing a high degree of anti–*P. aeruginosa* activity include cefepime (Maxipime), piperacillin (Pipracil), amikacin (Amikin), and meropenem (Merrem). Antipseudomonal antibotics with a high resistance potential include ceftazidime (Fortaz), ciprofloxacin (Cipro), and imipenem/cilastatin (Primaxin).

Antipseudomonal drugs with a high resistance potential should be used only when there are no other therapeutic alternatives. The problem of resistance is important because ciprofloxacin, imipenem, and ceftazidime have been associated not only with the emergence of resistant *P. aeruginosa,* but also with the emergence of methicillin-resistant *S. aureus,* especially in critical care units.

It is a misconception that the use of two antibiotics in combination will eliminate the resistance problems. The addition of an aminoglycoside to ciprofloxacin or ceftazidime does not prevent the emergence of ciprofloxacin- or ceftazidime-resistant *P. aeruginosa.* It is another common misconception that volume of use is related to the emergence of resistance. Antibiotics with a low resistance potential can be used without restriction in an unlimited volume without concern for the emergence of resistance. In contrast, antibiotics with a high resistance potential are associated with resistance problems even when used in low volume. Therefore, the best strategy to prevent the emergence of antibiotic resistance in the critical care unit is not to control volume of use per se but to restrict the use of antibiotics with a high resistance potential.

Cost Considerations

Cost considerations should be taken into account in selecting an antibiotic for nosocomial pneumonia. First, the antibiotic must have a spectrum that is appropriate (i.e., possesses a high degree of anti–*P. aeruginosa* activity, a low resistance potential, and a favorable side effect profile) before cost considerations can be entertained. Use of an "inexpensive" antibiotic that will result in therapeutic failure or resistance problems in the institution is not cost effective. It is important to take into account not only acquisition costs but also the cost of administration. To administer an antibiotic intravenously costs the institution approximately $10 per dose. Therefore, drugs with longer dosing intervals are less expensive, all other factors being equal. In addition to acquisition and administration charges, an assessment of the true cost of the antibiotic must take into account likely side effects as well as resistance potential. Thus, the total cost of an antibiotic to the institution may be vastly different than the acquisition cost to the pharmacy, and in the managed care era, it is the total cost to the institution that is important and not the acquisition cost.

As with CAPs, IV/PO switch therapy should be used for nosocomial pneumonia if at all possible. Of course, the switch will occur later than in patients with CAP, but even a few days of oral therapy and decreased length of stay are worth the effort. Only proven *P. aeruginosa* pneumonia should be treated intravenously for 14 days, because at present, oral antipseudomonal agents from different antibiotic classes are not available for use. For this reason, cefepime is preferred to ceftazidime, meropenem is preferable to imipenem, and levofloxacin is preferable to ciprofloxacin in the treatment of nosocomial pneumonias. If *P. aeruginosa* is the proven pathogen in hospital-acquired pneumonia, then the second antipseudomonal agent should also have a low resistance and a good side effect potential. The preferred agents to be added to cefepime, levofloxacin, or meropenem include piperacillin (Pipracil), aztreonam (Azactam), or an aminoglycoside (Tables 5 and 6).

Optimal Therapeutic Approach

Clinicians should make a concerted effort to be sure that the patient has a nosocomial pneumonia and not a condition that mimics a hospital-acquired pneumonia. Clinicians should avoid treating organisms recovered from respiratory secretions that are colonizers rather than pathogens, especially in patients with pulmonary infiltrates, fever, and leukocytosis who are on assisted ventilation. The clinician should attempt to arrive at a definitive diagnosis by demonstrating a nosocomial pathogen in the blood cultures or by semiquantitative culture of respiratory secretions obtained by protected bronchoscopic brushings. If bronchoscopy is not an option, then empirical treatment of nosocomial pneumonia is indicated. Whether the patient harbors *P. aeruginosa* or another common nosocomial pathogen, initial empirical monotherapy is the preferred approach. If *P. aeruginosa* is determined to be the cause of the nosocomial pneumonia, then a second antipseudomonal antibiotic can be added. Using this approach, if the patient does not have pseudomonal nosocomial pneumonia, the antipseudomonal antibiotic initially selected for monotherapy will still be highly effective against non–*P. aeruginosa* pathogens, such as *K. pneumoniae* and *S. marcescens*.

Therapy of nosocomial pneumonia is ordinarily continued for 14 days, but a longer course may be necessary in patients with impaired cardiopulmonary function or impaired B lymphocyte function. Patients with persistent or increasing pulmonary infiltrates in spite of appropriate antipseudomonal therapy should not be treated for longer than 14 days; the practice of treating persistent leukocytosis, low-grade fever, and unresolved pulmonary infiltrates beyond 14 days should be discouraged. If pulmonary infiltrates are still present after 2 weeks of effective antipseudomonal therapy the process is most likely noninfectious and not remediable by further antibiotic therapy. If diagnostic tests for pulmonary embolism, myocardial infarction, systemic lupus erythematosus, pulmonary drug reactions, left ventricular failure, ARDS, and related disorders are negative or equivocal, such patients should undergo bronchoscopy to allow definitive diagnosis of the cause of the pulmonary infiltrates.

TABLE 5. **Therapeutic Approach to Nosocomial Pneumonias**

- Coverage should be directed against only the most common nosocomial pathogens, focusing on *Pseudomonas aeruginosa*.
  - *Pseudomonas aeruginosa*
  - *Klebsiella pneumoniae*
  - *Serratia marcescens*
- Do not cover/treat nosocomial colonizers in respiratory secretions that do not cause nosocomial pneumonia.
  - *Enterobacter* spp.
  - *Citrobacter* spp.
  - *Enterococcus* spp.
  - *Flavobacterium meningosepticum*
  - *Pseudomonas cepacia*
  - *Xanthomonas maltophilia*
- Use monotherapy for nosocomial pneumonia, not double-drug therapy. Monotherapy is therapeutically equivalent to combination therapy in nosocomial pneumonia. Optimal monotherapy for nosocomial pneumonia is with cefepime or meropenem. If *P. aeruginosa* is cultured from blood or semiquantitative protected bronchial brushings (not respiratory secretions), add an additional anti-*P. aeruginosa* antibiotic, e.g., piperacillin, aztreonam, an aminoglycoside.
- Avoid using antibiotics with a high resistance potential for nosocomial pneumonia, i.e., ceftazidime, ciprofloxacin, or imipenem.
- Avoid covering/treating noninfectious conditions that "mimic" nosocomial pneumonia. Many patients are needlessly treated for unexplained or undiagnosed pulmonary infiltrates, fever, or leukocytosis with/without positive respiratory secretion cultures (including pathogens or colonizers).
- Give a full 14-day course and then discontinue antibiotics. Do not continue antibiotic therapy for persistent low-grade fever or pulmonary infiltrates (suggests a noninfectious disease etiology). Obtain an infectious disease consultation or perform a definitive diagnostic procedure.

TABLE 6. **Empirical Therapy of Nosocomial Pneumonia**

Hospital-Acquired Pneumonia	*Preferred Monotherapy*
Pseudomonas aeruginosa *Serratia marcescens* *Klebsiella pneumoniae* *Streptococcus pneumoniae*	Cefepime* or Meropenem
Nosocomial Atypical Pneumonia	
Legionella spp.	Levofloxacin
Nosocomial Aspiration Pneumonia	
Oral anaerobes *Pseudomonas aeruginosa* *Serratia marcescens* *Klebsiella pneumoniae* *Streptococcus pneumoniae*	Cefepime or Meropenem

*If *P. aeruginosa* is proved to be the pathogen by semiquantitative protected bronchial specimens, then an additional anti–*P. aeruginosa* antibiotic can be added to the initial antibiotic (i.e., levofloxacin, aztreonam, or an aminoglycoside).

VIRAL RESPIRATORY INFECTIONS

method of
DAVID P. SKONER, M.D., and
DENISE L. HOWRIE, PHARM.D.
University of Pittsburgh and
Children's Hospital of Pittsburgh
Pittsburgh, Pennsylvania

Viral respiratory infections are the most common human affliction and reason for physician office visits. Mild, self-limited upper respiratory symptoms—the common cold—are the usual presentation, but systemic symptoms and complications involving the sinuses, ears, or lower airways also occur. More than 100 serotypes of rhinoviruses cause over half of common colds, but coronaviruses and respiratory syncytial (RSV) viruses also contribute. Other viruses, including influenza, parainfluenza, and adenoviruses, can produce colds, but frequently cause lower respiratory or systemic symptoms as well. Colds develop year round but are less frequent during the summer months. Respiratory virus season starts with rhinovirus infections in August or September, followed by sequential outbreaks of different viral infections (e.g., RSV and influenza virus), and ends following a spring peak of rhinovirus infection in April or May. Identification of responsible viral pathogens is usually not necessary unless a complication develops or a community epidemic of influenza is suspected.

The average number of colds per year is 5 to 7 in most children (12 or more in 10% of children) and 2 to 3 in adults. In children, these numbers are influenced by a number of factors that increase exposure, including the presence of siblings and daycare attendance.

Cold symptoms characteristically begin 1 to 2 days after exposure, peak 2 to 4 days later, and usually resolve within 1 week. One quarter of colds last 2 weeks. Transient sore throat of 1 to 2 days' duration is typically the earliest symptom, followed by a more prolonged period of nasal congestion, rhinorrhea, and sneezing. Cough is present in about 30% of colds and peaks on day 4 to 5 when nasal symptoms are subsiding.

The most efficient mechanism of person-to-person transmission is direct contact for rhinoviruses and small particle aerosol dissemination for influenza virus. Therefore, maintaining a distance of at least 3 feet from an infected person may be helpful in preventing spread, although this is often impractical.

The absence of detectable histopathology during rhinovirus colds led to the hypothesis that host immune and inflammatory responses to the virus play a primary role in the production of symptoms, of which rhinorrhea and congestion are the most prominent. Implicated mechanisms involve increased vascular permeability and glandular secretions during the early and late stages of illness, respectively; humoral and cellular (neutrophils, lymphocytes) immune responses; and the release of inflammatory (some neurogenic) mediators and cytokines.

TREATMENT

Marketed specific antivirals include amantadine (Symmetrel) and rimantadine (Flumadine) for prophylaxis and treatment of influenza A virus infection. Drug resistance readily occurs with both compounds, but no reduction in efficacy has been demonstrated in epidemics. These drugs are about 50% effective in preventing infection in epidemics but are 70 to 90% effective in prevention or amelioration of clinical symptoms. Therapy following exposure should be initiated within 24 to 48 hours of first symptoms and given for 10 subsequent days; the duration of prophylaxis should be 4 to 8 weeks. Groups meriting special consideration for prophylactic treatment include high-risk populations (the elderly and those with chronic heart, respiratory, circulatory, or immunodeficiency diseases [whether immunized or not]) and special community groups (people in institutional settings, caretakers of high-risk individuals, physicians, nurses, and hospital employees).

Amantadine is extensively (90%) eliminated unchanged in the urine, while rimantadine is heavily (>80%) metabolized, indicating the need for caution and dose adjustment in the elderly and in patients with advanced renal or liver disease. Toxicity manifests principally as excitatory central nervous system and gastrointestinal effects, is dose related, and is particularly prominent in the elderly. Rimantadine, the preferred agent, does not cross the blood-brain barrier and is associated with significantly fewer adverse effects than is amantadine (5 to 10% versus 30%). The usual dose of amantadine in adults is 200 mg per day in a single dose or two divided doses, with adjustments necessary in children and lack of an indication in children under 1 year of age. Rimantadine is generally administered in adults in doses of 200 mg per day in two divided doses, with dose adjustment in children and the elderly.

Ribavirin (Virazole) is an expensive antiviral agent for RSV infection that is administered in doses of 6 grams per day via nebulization over 12 to 18 hours for 3 to 7 days. Initial enthusiasm for its use in infants with severe RSV bronchiolitis was tempered by more recent reports that ribavirin administration during mechanical ventilation in infants with RSV-precipitated respiratory failure was associated with excessive morbidity. Indications include severe RSV disease in infants with underlying conditions such as bronchopulmonary dysplasia, congenital heart diseases, and immunodeficiency states.

A high-titered RSV-neutralizing antibody preparation (RSV-IGIV, RespiGAM) may be administered intravenously in doses of 750 mg per kg per month for 4 to 6 months of RSV season (generally November through April) for prophylaxis for high-risk children under 2 years of age with bronchopulmonary dysplasia requiring oxygen therapy, prematurity (<32 weeks' gestation) with likely RSV exposure, or severe immunodeficiency states. No benefits of RSV-IGIV have been documented in the treatment of established RSV disease. The cost of such treatment with RespiGAM over one respiratory disease season is approximately $5000. Use of this product should be reduced when a monoclonal RSV vaccine currently undergoing clinical testing becomes available.

Antiviral treatments are under development for rhinovirus infection and are currently unavailable for parainfluenza virus infections. The influenza vaccine is recommended for those at risk for serious complications and death, especially the elderly, those with chronic disease, and health care workers. The large number of serotypes has precluded the development of a rhinovirus vaccine.

Symptomatic therapy is the mainstay of common cold treatment. The use of non-prescription remedies including antihistamines, decongestants, expectorants and/or antitussives has been the subject of considerable controversy, despite the billions of dollars spent each year on these products. Antihistamine-decongestant combinations relieve postnasal symptoms, cough, and nasal obstruction in adults; no benefit in children has been demonstrated although subjective rating scales have hampered efficacy measure. Of interest, parents who believe in the need for medicines were more likely to report benefit with placebo, demonstrating the patient/parent bias toward drug use. Although more conclusive testing needs to be performed in children, it seems reasonable to conclude that the effects observed in adults may also extend to older children.

First-generation sedating antihistamines such as

chlorpheniramine (Chlor-Trimeton) and clemastine fumarate (Tavist) have shown efficacy against rhinorrhea and sneezing, but not nasal congestion, in well-controlled cold trials. The mechanism(s), which may include anticholinergic effects on glandular secretion, is unclear, since attempts to demonstrate histamine release during colds produced conflicting results. Similar efficacy was not demonstrated for nonsedating antihistamines, thus preventing a similar recommendation regarding their use. Major side effects include sedation and drying of the eyes, mouth, and nose. These products should be used with caution in infants and young children, who may develop paradoxic excitability, and avoided in patients with attention-deficit hyperactivity disorder (ADHD), glaucoma, or prostatic hypertrophy.

Although topical and oral decongestants have not been compared, topical adrenergics such as phenylephrine (Neo-Synephrine; Nōstril) and oxymetazoline (Afrin) are superior for short-term use to avoid systemic side effects. Topical decongestant use is restricted to 3 to 5 days to prevent the development of rhinitis medicamentosa (rebound hyperemia upon discontinuation); these products should be avoided in children under 2 years of age. Oral agents such as pseudoephedrine (Sudafed, Novafed), phenylephrine (available only in combination products such as Triaminic Cold), and phenylpropanolamine (available in combination products such as Dimetapp Elixir, Naldecon, Hycomine) are also effective. However, these agents may produce central nervous system stimulation, hypertension, and palpitations and should be avoided in patients with diabetes mellitus, ADHD, hyperthyroidism, hypertension, or arrhythmias.

Nonsteroidal anti-inflammatory agents, such as naproxen (Aleve, Naprosyn) and ibuprofen (Motrin, Advil), may be beneficial for symptoms such as sore throat, headache, malaise, and myalgia. Over-the-counter cromolyn sodium (Nasalcrom) has shown modest efficacy in the common cold, but three- or four-times-daily dosing limits compliance. Rhinorrhea and sneezing, but not other nasal symptoms, can also be effectively treated with ipratropium bromide 0.06% nasal solution, 2 sprays four times a day (Atrovent). Dry mouth (25%), bad taste, nasal irritation, and bleeding are possible side effects.

Cough has several etiologies in colds, including postnasal drip and reactive lower airway disease. Cough in the former condition usually peaks in parallel with nasal symptoms and is antihistamine/decongestant responsive, while in the latter condition it can persist for days to weeks after acute illness and benefits from bronchodilator therapy. Persistent cough after resolution of cold symptoms can also indicate sinusitis, which may require antibiotic therapy.

Nonspecific cough suppression with diphenhydramine (Benylin Decongestant), dextromethorphan hydrobromide (Hold DM, Suppress, St. Joseph Cough Suppressant), a "sustained action" liquid dextromethorphan polistirex liquid (Delsym), or codeine has been tried, but efficacy in colds has not been demonstrated. Studies in children confirm a gradual decrease in cough severity with progressive days of illness and comparable symptom relief with placebo when compared to codeine or dextromethorphan. A modest effect of naproxen on cough during colds has been shown. Expectorants such as guaifenesin (Robitussin) have no conclusive antitussive efficacy; only mild subjective improvement in sputum thickness has been reported.

When begun on the first day of illness, zinc gluconate (13.3 mg zinc) every 2 hours while awake has significantly reduced many cold symptoms; contradictory studies may be the result of variable zinc product bioavailability. Frequent dosing and bitter taste limit compliance. Beneficial effects have not been conclusively demonstrated for other agents, including Echinacea, menthol, intranasal corticosteroids, steam or mist inhalation, and vitamins. Rest and increased fluid intake are generally recommended.

Osler's dictum still appears true: "There is just one way to treat a cold and that's with contempt."

VIRAL AND MYCOPLASMAL PNEUMONIAS

method of
GERALD R. DONOWITZ, M.D.
University of Virginia School of Medicine
Charlottesville, Virginia

MYCOPLASMAL PNEUMONIAS

The major etiologies of bacterial pneumonia had all been described by the 1930s. However, in 1938, a series of patients was reported with pneumonia that did not fit the usual clinical picture and was therefore considered "atypical." These episodes began as a mild respiratory illness followed by pneumonia in which constitutional symptoms rather than respiratory toxicity predominated. This atypical pneumonia syndrome is caused by a variety of respiratory viruses, *Chlamydia* species, and some bacteria, but is most commonly associated with *Mycoplasma pneumoniae*.

Infection with *M. pneumoniae* usually affects the older child, adolescent, or young adult; the majority of patients are younger than age 40. Although mycoplasmal infections occur throughout the year, an increased incidence is noted in late summer and fall. The course of disease is subacute, with up to 10 days of symptoms before presentation. Typically, mycoplasmal pneumonia begins with constitutional symptoms with progression from the upper to the lower respiratory tract. Sore throat is usually seen initially, followed by fever, malaise, myalgia, coryza, headache, and nonproductive cough. On physical examination, localized rales may be detected, but signs of consolidation are usually absent. Purulent sputum is absent in 50 to 60% of cases. Gram's stain and culture of sputum usually reveal oral flora or mixed respiratory pathogens. White blood cell counts are less than 10,000 in 80% of patients. Radiographic involvement is usually more extensive than the physical examination would suggest. Infiltrates are usually patchy, may be unilateral or bilateral, and usually occur in the lower lobes. The radiographic picture may progress despite an improving clinical course.

Mycoplasmal pneumonia is generally a benign disease. Constitutional symptoms usually resolve in 1 to 2 weeks, although cough may persist for several weeks. Occasionally, mycoplasmal infection presents as a severe community-acquired pneumonia that can require intensive care monitoring. Infection with mycoplasma may be associated with a variety of extrapulmonary manifestations involving the skin, central nervous system, blood, and kidney.

Serology has been the principal method used to diagnose mycoplasmal pneumonia infections; however, diagnostic antibody rises may take 2 to 3 weeks to manifest themselves. Cold agglutinins develop during the second week of illness but occur in only 50% of cases and are nonspecific. Although the organism can be cultured, special labor-intensive methods are required that have a sensitivity of approximately 26 to 64%. Polymerase chain reaction (PCR) has been utilized to detect mycoplasmal DNA within hours from respiratory secretions, throat swabs, nasopharyngeal aspirates, bronchovascular lavage fluid, and lung aspirates.

Standard therapy for mycoplasmal infections has traditionally been erythromycin or tetracycline, both drugs given at 500 mg orally (PO) four times a day, or doxycycline, 100 mg PO twice a day. Fourteen days of therapy is used as shorter durations have been associated with relapse. Newer azalide-macrolide compounds, such as azithromycin (Zithromax), 500 mg PO loading dose, then 250 mg PO daily for 4 more days, and clarithromycin (Biaxin), 250 to 500 mg PO twice daily, have been used successfully to treat mycoplasmal infections. The recently introduced quinolones sparfloxacin (Zagam), 400 mg loading dose followed by 200 mg PO daily, levofloxacin (Levaquin), 500 mg PO daily, and trovafloxacin (Trovan), 200 mg PO daily, have demonstrated excellent in vitro activity against *Mycoplasma* and have proven effective both in animal models and in small numbers of human cases (Table 1).

INFLUENZA

Influenza virus has been called the last great plague, having been responsible for at least 30 pandemics and numerous epidemics over the last 500 years. In the United States, influenza causes 10,000 to 20,000 deaths per year. While the most common manifestation of influenza is tracheobronchitis, pneumonia complicates up to 6% of cases.

Influenza is an RNA virus that changes its antigenic characteristics via alterations in the neuraminidase and hemagglutinin glycoproteins that project from its surface. Small changes, or "antigenic drift," cause partial loss of immunity in patients previously exposed to the virus; larger changes, or "antigenic shift," lead to complete loss of immunity and have been associated with large epidemics and pandemics. Three types of influenza virus have been recognized: influenza A has been responsible for pandemics and large epidemics; influenza B has been associated with both epidemics and smaller outbreaks; and influenza C, which may actually represent a separate genus, has been associated with sporadic cases of infection in children. In general, one cannot differentiate influenza A from influenza B clinically, although the latter usually causes less severe infection. Influenza epidemics usually occur from November through March in the Northern Hemisphere. The infection is associated with a constellation of well-recognized constitutional and upper respiratory symptoms, including fever, headache, myalgia, sore throat, malaise, anorexia, and photophobia. When it occurs, pneumonia may develop as a primary viral pneumonia or as a combined viral and bacterial infection. Chronic lung and heart disease are important risk factors for the development of pneumonia,

Primary viral pneumonia, which most often occurs in children, appears after several days of typical "flu" symptoms. Acute onset of dyspnea, tachypnea, and cyanosis is characteristic, and purulent or bloody sputum is frequently present. Physical examination reveals localized pulmonary findings, including rales and wheezing. Chest radiographs show diffuse, perihilar infiltrates or peribronchial infiltrates; more severe disease is associated with diffuse interstitial infiltrates. Combined viral and bacterial pneumonia occurs at least as commonly as primary viral pneumonia but is more frequent in adults. Marked respiratory toxicity with significant cyanosis associated with the production of bloody or purulent sputum are the major manifestations. Lobar, perihilar, and nodular infiltrates and, less commonly, pleural fluid or pneumatoceles have been described. The most common bacteria involved in co-infection are *Streptococcus pneumoniae, Haemophilus influenzae*, and *Staphylococcus aureus*.

In the past, laboratory diagnoses of influenza A and B depended on viral isolation in cell culture and diagnostic rises in antibody titer. Because only influenza A can be readily treated with currently available agents, more rapid identification of influenza virus has been sought. Immunofluorescence has been used to detect influenza A and B from respiratory epithelial cells. An enzyme-linked immunosorbent assay is also available that is sensitive and specific and does not require intact epithelial cells. Influenza A viral antigen detection is available commercially, is sensitive and specific, and can be performed in approximately 15 minutes.

At present, two oral agents are available for therapy of influenza A, amantadine (Symmetrel) and rimantadine (Flumadine) (see Table 1). Amantadine, 100 mg twice daily or 200 mg once a day, is associated with a variety of side effects, including insomnia, lightheadedness, and difficulty concentrating. A lower dose, 100 mg daily, is associated with fewer

TABLE 1. **Therapy for *Mycoplasma pneumoniae* and Viral Pneumonias**

Agent	Therapy	Comments
*Mycoplasma pneumoniae**	Erythromycin, 500 mg PO qid	May cause gastrointestinal toxicity
	Tetracycline, 500 mg PO qid	May be associated with phototoxicity and gastrointestinal toxicity
	Doxycycline, 100 mg PO bid	May be associated with phototoxicity
	Sparfloxacin (Zagam), 400 mg PO loading dose on day 1 followed by 200 mg PO daily	May be associated with phototoxicity
	Trovafloxacin (Trovan), 200 mg PO daily	
	Levofloxacin (Levaquin), 500 mg PO daily	
	Azithromycin (Zithromax), 500 mg PO loading dose on day 1 followed by 250 mg PO daily on days 2–5	Some data suggest that 500 mg daily × 3 days may be adequate therapy
	Clarithromycin, 250–500 mg PO bid	
Influenza A	Amantadine (Symmetrel), 100 mg PO bid or 200 mg PO qd	↑ Central nervous system side effects Dose should be halved for elderly Needs adjustment for renal insufficiency
	Rimantadine (Flumadine), 100 mg PO bid	Fewer side effects than amantadine Dose should be halved for elderly Needs adjustment for renal and hepatic failure
Respiratory syncytial virus	Ribavirin	Delivered as an aerosol via nebulizer, 20 mg/mL for 18–20 h/day
Herpes simplex virus Varicella-zoster virus	Acyclovir (Zovirax), 10 mg/kg IV q 8 h	Needs adjustment for renal failure
Cytomegalovirus	Ganciclovir (Cytovene), 5 mg/kg IV q 8 h† × 14–21 days then 5 mg/kg IV 3–5 times/wk as maintenance	Frequently associated with neutropenia Renal adjustment needed
	or	
	Foscarnet (Foscavir), 60 mg/kg q 8 h	Frequently associated with renal toxicity Renal adjustment needed
	plus	
	Immunoglobulin‡	

*Fourteen days for all agents is suggested with the exception of azithromycin, for which 3 to 5 days of therapy may be sufficient.
†Exceeds dosage recommended by the manufacturer.
‡Use of immunoglobulin may not be required for disease in non–bone marrow transplant patients.

side effects and is recommended for those older than 65 years of age. Because amantadine is excreted in the urine, the dose must be adjusted in the presence of renal disease. Rimantadine, 100 mg orally (PO) twice daily, has fewer side effects but needs adjustment for renal and hepatic insufficiency. A dose of 100 mg PO daily is suggested for the elderly. Neither agent is useful for treatment of influenza B infection. Ribavirin (Virazole),* (20 mg per mL, delivered continuously by aerosol at a rate of 12.5 liters per mm for 12 to 18 hours) is the only available agent with activity against influenza B, although it has been used in only a small number of cases. None of these agents is of proven usefulness in established influenza pneumonia.

RESPIRATORY SYNCYTIAL VIRUS

Respiratory syncytial virus (RSV) can cause pneumonia in normal and immunocompromised children and in immunocompromised adults, especially bone marrow transplant recipients. Both community-acquired and nosocomial acquisition have been well documented. Usually, pneumonia is preceded by signs of an upper respiratory tract infection, including sinusitis and bronchiolitis. Wheezing, rales, and hypoxia are the common manifestations of RSV pneumonia. Radiographs characteristically show interstitial infiltrates and hyperinflation. Mortality rates higher than 50% have been noted in immunocompromised patients. Ribavirin may be of benefit for treatment of RSV in infants and children. The drug is delivered as an aerosol, 20 mg per mL in a nebulizer, 18 to 20 hours per day for 5 days. Repeated courses of therapy may be necessary. Uncontrolled trials suggest that ribavirin may be beneficial for RSV infection in immunocompromised adults as well.

*Not FDA approved for this indication.

HERPES VIRUSES

Most members of the herpes family of viruses can cause pneumonia, especially in immunologically impaired hosts. Herpes simplex virus (HSV) can cause pneumonia in immunocompromised hosts, patients who are intubated, and those with damage to their respiratory epithelium. Localized disease is associated with herpetic tracheobronchitis, while diffuse disease is thought to occur as a result of viremia and is often associated with multiorgan involvement with herpes. Acyclovir (Zovirax), 10 mg per kg every 8 hours intravenously (IV), is the therapy of choice.

Varicella-zoster virus pneumonia can occur as a complication of chickenpox, especially in adults and in the compromised host. Pneumonia usually occurs 3 to 5 days after the onset of illness. Tachypnea, cough, and dyspnea are associated with diffuse nodular lesions or an interstitial infiltrate on chest radiographs. Acyclovir, 10 mg per kg IV every 8 hours, can be used as therapy though its efficacy in treating established varicella pneumonia remains unclear.

Cytomegalovirus (CMV) is an important cause of pneumonia in immunocompromised hosts, especially bone marrow and solid organ transplant recipients. Nonproductive cough, hypoxia, and fever in association with an interstitial pattern on chest radiographs are the common presenting findings for CMV pneumonia. Respiratory failure is not uncommon. Prognosis remains poor even with present management with a 30 to 50% mortality rate. Present strategies have been directed toward identifying patients at high risk for the development of CMV disease and treating them preemptively before they develop clinically active disease. Ganciclovir has been the agent most frequently utilized. In bone marrow transplant recipients who develop CMV pneumonia, therapy with ganciclovir (Cytovene), 5.0 mg per kg every 12 hours IV or 2.5 mg per kg every 8 hours* plus intravenous immunoglobulin† has been shown to reduce mortality. Fourteen to 21 days of therapy are usually indicated, and maintenance regimens are required. Foscarnet* (Foscavir), 60 mg per kg every 8 hours IV, is an alternative to ganciclovir. In solid organ transplant recipients, ganciclovir or foscarnet alone appears to effectively reduce mortality rates in patients with CMV pneumonia.

HANTAVIRUS

Hantavirus pulmonary syndrome (HPS) is an acute pneumonia caused by a hantavirus carried by rodents. Human infection was first described in the southwestern United States in 1993. Rapidly progressive respiratory failure, noncardiogenic pulmonary edema, and volume contraction with hemoconcentration are the hallmarks of disease. Signs of pulmonary edema develop early and progress rapidly to central alveolar infiltrates. Thrombocytopenia, a marked shift to the left of granulocytes, and immunoblastic lymphocytes are characteristic. Diagnosis can be made by detecting elevated antibodies or detecting viral RNA via PCR in mononuclear cells or other infected tissues. Aggressive supportive care with ventilation assistance and fluid resuscitation is a vital component of therapy. Ribavirin is presently being evaluated as antiviral therapy for HPS.

ADENOVIRUSES

Adenovirus infections are widespread in humans, although the majority of infections seem to be asymptomatic. Adenovirus pneumonia has been observed in children, military recruits, and immunocompromised adults. Signs of upper respiratory tract disease with fever, malaise, headache, and sore throat often accompany signs of lower respiratory tract infection (fever, cough, hypoxia). Gastrointestinal symptoms are frequent. In normal hosts, patchy basilar infiltrates are noted, while diffuse interstitial disease can be seen in the compromised host. Hemorrhagic pulmonary edema is noted in severe cases. There is no proven therapy at present.

PARAINFLUENZA VIRUS

Parainfluenza virus is a common cause of upper respiratory tract infection in children and adults. Although parainfluenza pneumonia is unusual in adults, it is the second most common type of severe pneumonia in infants. Diffuse interstitial infiltrates are noted, with fever, cough, and shortness of breath. Therapy of parainfluenza pneumonia involves supportive care only, although ribavirin has been used in a small number of cases.

*Exceeds dosage recommended by the manufacturer.
†Not FDA approved for this indication.

LEGIONELLOSIS
(Legionnaires' Disease and Pontiac Fever)

method of
DAVID L. PATERSON, M.D., and
VICTOR L. YU, M.D.
Veterans Affairs Medical Center
Pittsburgh, Pennsylvania

Legionellosis refers to infection caused by bacteria of the genus *Legionella*. Although *Legionella pneumophila* is the most common pathogenic species (accounting for up to 90% of human infections in some areas), 17 other species have been associated with human disease. Legionnaires' disease is the designation for pneumonia caused by any of the *Legionella* species, whereas Pontiac fever is an acute, self-limited, febrile illness without pneumonia, occurring in epidemics, which has been serologically linked to *Legionella* species. In addition, extrapulmonary legionellosis can occur, usually resulting from blood-borne dissemination from the lungs.

CLINICAL PRESENTATION

Legionnaires' disease is the most common syndrome produced by *Legionella* species. The infection can be community- or hospital-acquired, with the highest risk for those who are immunosuppressed (particularly solid organ transplant recipients). The incubation period is 2 to 10 days and is followed by cough (usually nonproductive), fever, malaise, and headache. Upper respiratory symptoms are rare. Virtually all patients have pulmonary infiltrates on chest radiography if it is performed at the time of clinical presentation. Rapid progression of disease with widespread pulmonary infiltrates and multisystem failure may occur. Clinical clues suggestive of Legionnaires' disease include diarrhea, high fever (>40°C), hyponatremia, and demonstration of numerous neutrophils but no organisms on Gram's staining of sputum.

DIAGNOSIS

Diagnosis can be made from culture of respiratory secretions using specialized media, which suppress the growth of competing bacteria. Rapid diagnosis can be made by way of detection of *Legionella* antigen in urine or by direct fluorescent antibody (DFA) staining of respiratory secretions. The urinary antigen test is available only for *L. pneumophila* serogroup 1, but in many areas this serogroup causes about 60% of all cases of Legionnaires' disease. Antibody testing of both acute and convalescent phase serum is available for many species, but since 4 to 12 weeks may be required to develop an antibody response, it may only provide a retrospective diagnosis. Polymerase chain reaction (PCR) for use on clinical specimens is being developed, but sensitivity is marginal at the present time.

THERAPY

In the 1976 American Legion outbreak in Philadelphia, patients treated with erythromycin or tetracycline appeared to have a better outcome than those treated with other antibiotics. Erythromycin was once regarded as the drug of choice for treatment of Legionnaires' disease, but other macrolides and quinolones have greater in vitro activity against *Legionella* and superior intracellular penetration. In addition, erythromycin is associated with venous irritation and gastrointestinal intolerance. It can cause prolongation of the QT interval and has been associated with symptomatic ototoxicity when given at a 4-gram daily dose.

In view of the demonstrated difficulties with erythromycin, newer macrolides or quinolones are now the preferred antibiotics in the treatment of Legionnaires' disease (Table 1). The new macrolides include azithromycin (Zithromax) and clarithromycin (Biaxin), as well as other drugs not available in the United States (roxithromycin and josamycin). Advantages of azithromycin include intravenous (IV) administration and once-daily dosing. A clinical response to IV therapy (for example, defervescence) usually occurs within 3 to 5 days, after which a switch to oral therapy can be made. Treatment duration is 10 to 14 days. Azithromycin, because of its longer half-life, should be given for only 7 to 10 days. A longer course (3 weeks) can be given to immunosuppressed patients who are severely ill. The newer macrolides also cover other common causes of community-acquired pneumonia, such as *Streptococcus pneumoniae, Haemophilus influenzae, Moraxella catarrhalis, Mycoplasma pneumoniae*, and *Chlamydia pneumoniae*. This makes them an ideal choice as empirical antibiotic therapy in immunocompetent hosts with community-acquired pneumonia.

The quinolones have greater in vitro activity against *Legionella* species than the macrolides. Although not evaluated in comparative studies, numerous patients with Legionnaires' disease have been successfully treated with ciprofloxacin (Cipro) and levofloxacin (Levaquin). Newer quinolones such as trovafloxacin (Trovan) and grepafloxacin (Raxar) would also be expected to have activity. The chosen quinolone should initially be given intravenously in patients with severe disease and, once a clinical response has occurred, switched to oral administration. Treatment should last for 10 to 14 days.

Comparative trials have not been performed to determine whether new macrolides or quinolones are superior. Quinolones are preferred in transplant recipients because macrolides can interact with the cytochrome P450 3A enzymes, leading to reduced metabolism of cyclosporine or tacrolimus.

A combination of rifampin* with a macrolide or quinolone should be considered for severely ill patients. Rifampin has excellent in vitro activity against *Legionella* but should never be used alone because of potential emergence of resistance.

Alternative agents include tetracycline, doxycycline (Vibramycin), minocycline (Minocin), and trimethoprim-sulfamethoxazole (Bactrim, Septra). Anecdotal successes with imipenem and clindamycin have been reported.

Pontiac fever requires symptomatic therapy, but not antimicrobial therapy, for clinical resolution.

*Not FDA approved for this indication.

TABLE 1. **Antibiotic Therapy for Legionnaires' Disease**

Antibiotic	Dose	Frequency	Route
Macrolides			
Azithromycin (Zithromax)	500 mg	q 24 h	IV, PO
Clarithromycin (Biaxin)	500 mg	q 12 h	PO
Erythromycin*	1 gm	q 6 h	IV
	500 mg	q 6 h	PO
Quinolones			
Ciprofloxacin (Cipro)	400 mg	q 8 h	IV
	750 mg	q 12 h	PO
Ofloxacin (Floxin)	400 mg	q 12 h	IV, PO
Levofloxacin (Levaquin)	500 mg	q 24 h	IV, PO
Rifampin†			
Rifampin‡	600 mg	q 12 h	IV, PO
Second-Line Agents§			
Doxycycline‖	100 mg	q 12 h	IV, PO
Trimethoprim-sulfamethoxazole¶	160/800 mg	q 8 h	IV
	160/800 mg	q 12 h	PO

*Trade names for erythromycin include Ilosone, E-Mycin, ERYC, Ery-Tab, PCE Dispertab.

†In combination with a macrolide or quinolone for severe disease.

‡Trade names for rifampin include Rifadin, Rifamate, Rifater, Rimactane.

§Should be used only if macrolides or quinolones cannot be given.

‖Trade names for doxycycline include Doryx, Vibramycin, Vibra-Tabs, Bio-Tab, Monodox.

¶Trade names for trimethoprim-sulfamethoxazole include Bactrim, Septra, and Cotrim.

PULMONARY EMBOLISM

method of
BRUCE L. DAVIDSON, M.D., M.P.H.
Allegheny University Hospitals—Graduate
Philadelphia, Pennsylvania

Few common diseases are as difficult to diagnose as pulmonary embolism (PE). Treatment is usually satisfactory, but optimal treatment is controversial. An estimated 300,000 Americans suffer from PE each year. It is the primary cause of death in 4% of patients in recent autopsy series, and in 70% of these patients it is completely unsuspected ante mortem. Among those in whom it is diagnosed, 2% die in the first day, but 10% suffer recurrent PE; the death rate among the latter is 45%. Thus, suspicion of PE and prevention are critically important, even while consensus on optimal treatment is not at hand.

DIAGNOSIS

PE occurs in the previously healthy and the sick, outpatients and inpatients. Because untreated symptomatic or asymptomatic PE may be fatal, a high index of suspicion and willingness to screen for PE are essential. That many patients will have negative results on evaluation studies reflects the lack of pathognomonic early findings, not lack of physician acuity. Table 1 presents a partial list of clinical findings and situations that should raise the possibility of PE. The presence or absence of any one or a combination of some features in Table 1 does not diagnose or exclude PE. Although venous thrombosis and PE are often spoken of as one disease and early literature suggested proximal deep vein thrombosis (DVT) always accompanies PE, recent series have shown that less than half of patients proved to have PE will have signs or symptoms in the legs, and many patients with proven PE will not have proximal DVT.

When a clinical assessment suggests PE may be present, diagnostic tests should promptly follow. The most valuable predictive tests are listed in Table 2, stratified by clinical suspicion. In apparently deterioriating patients it may be necessary to perform more than one test at a time: perfusion radionuclide lung scans (and sometimes ventilation scans), compression ultrasound studies of lower extremity proximal veins, and rapid D-dimer tests such as SimpliRed (American Diagnostica) can be performed nearly simultaneously in such patients, helping to make a rapid, minimally invasive diagnosis with minuscule risk. When experienced pulmonary angiographers are readily available and no contraindications are present, an indeterminate lung scan can lead directly to angiography. When spiral contrast computed tomography (CT) or contrast magnetic resonance imaging (MRI) scans are readily available from experienced radiologists with proven dye injection protocols, a positive scan for central vessel clot is convincing. However, these tests have both unacceptable rates of false-positive results and unsatisfactory sensitivity for subsegmental PE. Also, spiral CT scans poorly image clots in the (right) middle lobe and (left) lingular pulmonary arteries and their tributaries.

Echocardiography may assist in the diagnosis of PE, particularly in decision-making about treatment. When echocardiographic findings (tricuspid and/or pulmonic regurgitation, segmental wall motion abnormalities of the right ventricle) suggest pulmonary hypertension in patients with no other possible explanation and the right clinical setting (see Table 1), the diagnosis of PE is highly likely. Unfortunately, many patients with suspected PE have other reasons for pulmonary hypertension, including left ventricular failure, chronic (obstructive or restrictive) lung disease, sleep apnea syndrome, and hypoxia (acute or

TABLE 1. **Consider Pulmonary Embolism (PE) When These Clinical Features Present**

History

Recent surgery, including outpatient arthroscopic surgery
Recent or prolonged limb immobility
Prior PE or venous or arterial thrombosis
Drugs: estrogen, progesterone, warfarin, heparin, cancer chemotherapy
Family history of PE or venous or arterial thrombosis
Cancer
Laboratory coagulation abnormalities: presence of factor V Leiden, other activated protein C resistance, lupus anticoagulant, anticardiolipin antibody; deficiency of antithrombin III, protein C, or protein S

Physical Findings

Tachypnea
Fever (temperature of <102°F)
Obesity
Unilateral or bilateral leg swelling, erythema, tenderness
Right ventricular heave
Normal or low blood pressure

Atypical Clinical Settings

Failure of tachypnea to improve significantly after several days in patient with infiltrates on chest x-ray film who is being treated for pneumonia
Upper abdominal quadrant discomfort with pleural effusion and/or atelectasis and negative findings on abdominal work-up
Failure to wean from assisted ventilation or supplementary oxygen because of hypoxia unexplained by findings on chest x-ray film, e.g., in post–cardiac surgery patients

TABLE 2. **Using Tests and Clinical Suspicion for Managing Suspected Pulmonary Embolism (PE)**

	Clinical Suspicion	
Study/Result	*Moderate to High*	*Low (e.g., "Rule Out PE")*
Lung scan result		
High probability	Diagnosis confirmed; stop testing	Probably PE
Normal	Do not treat	Not PE
Indeterminate	Treat; test further	Treat ±; test further
After lung scan obtained:	*Moderate to High, Scan Indeterminate*	*Low, Scan Indeterminate or High Probability*
Compression ultrasound of proximal leg veins		
Abnormal	Probably PE; treat	Probably PE; treat
Normal	Test further	Test further
D-Dimer assay		
Elevated	Consistent with PE	Consistent with PE
Normal	Doubt PE; consider other diagnosis	Probably not PE
Spiral/electron beam contrast computed tomography or contrast magnetic resonance imaging		
Abnormal	Probably PE; treat	Probably; PE; treat
Normal	PE less likely	PE less likely
Pulmonary arteriogram		
Abnormal	Diagnosis confirmed; treat	Diagnosis confirmed; treat
Normal	Diagnosis probably excluded	Diagnosis excluded

chronic). The presence of akinesia of the mid–free wall of the right ventricle with normal motion of its apex has been reported to be relatively specific (94%) and predictive (71%) for PE compared with primary pulmonary hypertension, but among the group of patients with common secondary causes of pulmonary hypertension (e.g., those just described), the diagnostic accuracy of this finding is unknown.

Identifying thrombosis in the lower extremities can help diagnostically. Demonstration of venous clot by compression ultrasound studies (particularly in the popliteal vein or above, in which such tests are most accurate) in a patient with signs or symptoms in the leg warrants treatment irrespective of whether PE is ultimately proved. However, an abnormal result on proximal leg vein compression ultrasonography had a sensitivity of only 30% in patients with proven PE in one large series. Although a *normal* ultrasound examination missed 60% of the PE patients in this series, an *abnormal* compression ultrasound examination of the proximal veins correctly identified PE patients 90% of the time. Hence, an abnormal result on proximal ultrasound study should probably lead to treatment. If distal veins are also examined, the accuracy of ultrasonography in PE diagnosis is reduced. Other approaches to leg vein evaluation when PE is suspected include serial (repetitive) ultrasound studies or impedance plethysmography (up to five times in 2 weeks), MRI venous scanning from the pelvis to the foot, and contrast venography. Performing serial noninvasive tests in the legs is more appropriate for diagnosing DVT than for PE, because in PE treatment decisions (particularly for inpatients) usually must be made rapidly.

Upper extremity venous thrombosis, diagnosed by compression ultrasonography or venography, can also cause PE, particularly in patients with indwelling polyvinyl chloride or polyethylene catheters. Treatment is as described subsequently.

When PE is suspected in complicated cases (as in postoperative patients receiving assisted ventilation) or unfavorable practice situations (e.g., no pulmonary angiography available), clinicians must make their best estimates of the probability of PE and decide whether to treat. Because treatment is usually satisfactory and diagnosis is difficult, treatment without a secure diagnosis is not infrequent and is often appropriate.

TABLE 3. **Acute Treatment for Pulmonary Embolism (PE)**

Drug	Dose	Comments†
Standard heparin	5000 U bolus, then 1300 U/h IV* 80 U/kg bolus, then 18 U/kg/h IV	Check APTT q 4–6 h until in range and stable For heparin resistance, target anti-Xa level 0.35–0.7 U/mL
Low-molecular-weight heparin	100 anti-Xa U or 1 mg/kg q 12 h SC	Bolus not recommended Dosage may differ slightly by drug Divide total daily dose by 24 if hourly constant infusion is required If monitoring is required, target anti-Xa level 0.4–0.7 U/mL
Heparinoid		
Danaparoid (Orgaran)	2500 U bolus IV, then 400 U/h × 4 h, then 300 U/h × 4 h, then 200 U/h, all IV	Use for heparin-induced thrombocytopenia Target anti-Xa level 0.5–0.8 or even 1.0 U/mL
	20 U/kg q 12 h SC	Give by SC route after syndrome resolves unless constant infusion is required
Thrombolytics		Safest to withhold heparin until 3 h after thrombolytic infusion ends
Alteplase (Activase)	100 mg IV over 2 h*	2% incidence of cerebral bleeding
Streptokinase (Streptase)	250,000 U bolus, then 100,000 U/h for 24 h* 1,500,000 U over 1 h	Shorter infusion duration is probably safer
Urokinase (Abbokinase)	4400 U/kg bolus, then 4400 U/kg/h for 12 h*	

Abbreviation: APTT = activated partial thromboplastin time.
*This drug regimen has been approved by the Food and Drug Administration.
†See also text.

TREATMENT

The short-term prognosis in patients treated for PE is quite favorable. This outcome argues for considering empirical treatment in patients without substantial contraindications, both early and when a suspected diagnosis cannot be proved or refuted.

Aggressive supportive treatment is essential in many patients. Close monitoring, oxygen supplementation when oxygen saturation drops below 92%, and sometimes assisted ventilation are required. In patients with complicated medical problems and hypotension, a pulmonary artery catheter may be needed to help assure an adequate filling pressure.

Specific drug treatment options are presented in Table 3. Unfractionated standard heparin is safe and effective. It is customarily given by intravenous drip and must be monitored with a surrogate "heparin level"—the activated partial thromboplastin time (APTT)—to ensure that the dose is neither too high (bleeding risk is related to the intensity of anticoagulation) nor too low (published studies show that failure to reach the therapeutic level within 24 hours predisposes to recurrence). The desired APTT range (e.g., 60 to 85 seconds) depends on local reagents and equipment; it should correlate with a plasma heparin level of 0.2 to 0.4 units per mL by protamine titration or 0.35 to 0.7 anti-Xa units per mL. An intravenous bolus of 5000 USP units (or 80 units per kg of body weight) is given, and a drip (1300 units per hour or 18 units per kg per hour) is begun. Various nomograms have been published to assist in titrating unfractionated heparin therapy. Frequent monitoring (every 4 to 6 hours) of the APTT when heparin infusion rates are instituted and changed, until a reliable steady state is demonstrated by repetitive APTT values "in range," is essential.

Heparin resistance is said to occur when high dosages (e.g., more than 36,000 units of unfractionated heparin per 24 hours) are required to reach (or fail to reach) a therapeutic APTT. In this event, anticoagulant effect should be monitored instead by an anti-Xa assay, as indicated in Table 3, or a switch to low-molecular-weight (LMW) heparin should be made.

The use of subcutaneous LMW heparin,* administered twice daily in a dose based on patient weight and without monitoring anticoagulant effect, is an attractive and effective alternative. LMW heparin does not significantly prolong the APTT, probably because the APTT result reflects time to thrombin generation in vitro rather than overall inhibition of thrombin generation in vivo. Dosing is as described in Table 3, but each drug's package insert should be checked for exact recommendations. These drugs do not require routine monitoring because, as opposed to the case with use of unfractionated heparin, their nonspecific protein binding is minimal, and bioavailability after subcutaneous injection is over 90%. These characteristics considerably enhance predictability of heparin levels in most circumstances, so bleeding risk due to overly intense anticoagulation is minimized. Twice-daily therapy is probably safest, although the use of once-daily LMW heparin for PE has been studied and reported safe in highly selected patients. However, half-life of this preparation is 4 to 6 hours in the absence of substantial renal insufficiency; it dips to subtherapeutic levels at the end of a 24-hour period with once-daily dosing. Patients with PE face risk of clot extension from both the clot's thrombin generation and the suppression of their own protein C (the latter effect unavoidably accompanies warfarin use). With subtherapeutic heparin levels consequent to once-daily use, these actions are unopposed (to the patient's disadvantage) for several hours daily until the next injection.

Oral anticoagulant therapy (usually with warfarin) is begun concomitant with standard or LMW heparin and continued for a minimum of 3 months. In patients with venous thromboembolism that is recurrent, idiopathic, or associated with an unremitting risk factor (e.g., incurable cancer, limb paralysis, activated protein C resistance, chronic venous insufficiency), anticoagulation may need to be long-term.

Warfarin is begun at the estimated daily maintenance dose (5 to 7.5 mg daily), i.e., without a loading dose. Larger starting doses do not appear to substantially affect the rate of factor II (prothrombin) suppression but significantly reduce levels of the important endogenous anticoagulant protein C, possibly leading to thrombus extension unless heparin anticoagulation is at the proper level. Although the prothrombin time (PT) may be prolonged after one or two doses, this early prolongation reflects factor VII suppression. It is the suppression of longer lived prothrombin that is critical for prevention of thrombosis extension or recurrence. When the PT is therapeutically prolonged after 5 days of warfarin dosing, there is good confidence that the prothrombin level has been sufficiently suppressed without measuring it specifically. The PT has been relatively well standardized from laboratory to laboratory by use of the International Normalized Ratio (INR). For treating PE, the target INR range is 2.0 to 3.0. The INR is more accurate during chronic anticoagulation than during the first few weeks of anticoagulation therapy. The results of some PT assays (and their INRs) are affected by circulating heparin, so PT values during the heparin overlap period may be artifactually high or may be genuinely low when heparin is stopped. A minimum 4-day heparin-warfarin overlap with an in-range INR should be provided for 2 consecutive days. When warfarin dosage is adjusted early or late, the change should be 20% of the *weekly* dose; e.g., in a patient with an INR of 1.7 receiving 5 mg daily, an extra 1 mg daily should be given. Warfarin is often administered in the late afternoon, with PTs obtained in the morning—a protocol based on convenience but not science. If an increase in dosage is needed, it should be given immediately to save time.

If an INR is too high but less than 6 and the patient is not bleeding, warfarin can be withheld. In patients with INRs of more than 6 in whom oozing is noted and who are at risk for serious bleeding, rapid lowering to the therapeutic range is accomplished with a single dose of 2 mg vitamin K (Aqua-MEPHYTON), given subcutaneously. This low dose prevents rebound underanticoagulation as well as delays in re-establishing the proper anticoagulant state. For patients with elevated INRs consequent to warfarin use in need of urgent hemostasis, 10 mg of vitamin K given intramuscularly (or intravenously [IV] over 20 minutes) with fresh-frozen plasma infusion to correct the PT is effective. In such critically ill patients, infusion of unfractionated or LMW heparin can be restarted when some degree of anticoagulation is again deemed safe.

The following points apply to treatment with both unfractionated and LMW heparin and warfarin:

1. *Platelet counts*: A platelet count should be obtained at the start and after 4 days of treatment at a minimum. If longer heparin treatment is required, platelet counts are repeated every 2 to 3 days. LMW heparin is far less likely than standard heparin to provoke either antibody formation or a clinical thrombocytopenic syndrome.
2. *Heparin-induced thrombocytopenia (HIT)*: Both unfractionated and LMW heparin can induce immune thrombocytopenia, usually not before 5 days of treatment unless heparin has been recently given. HIT should be suspected when there is a significant drop (e.g., 50%) in platelet count even if it does not fall below 100,000 per mm^3. Heparin should be stopped because life-threatening or persistent HIT with thrombosis may develop without further warning. If a sufficient heparin-warfarin overlap has not

*Not FDA approved for this indication.

been accomplished (as described later), danaparoid* (as a heparin substitute) should be administered (see Table 3) and continued with warfarin. As the patient stabilizes, danaparoid may be given subcutaneously twice daily. When a thrombotic process and/or thrombocytopenia have resolved, warfarin alone should be continued. Giving warfarin without other anticoagulant therapy to a patient presenting with HIT is not recommended because it may aggravate thrombosis. Although danaparoid may cross-react in vitro to a small extent with antibodies in patients with HIT, it is highly effective clinically and more convenient for prolonged administration in HIT than are other drugs that must be given by intravenous drip, such as hirudin† and argatroban.†

3. *Reversing heparin effect*: Protamine sulfate should be used to reverse heparin in the case of serious bleeding. Protamine injections of up to 25 mg given over 5 minutes at 10-minute intervals are well tolerated. Protamine binds promptly to circulating heparin, but the complex may dissociate later, leaving residual but reduced heparin effect. Thus, if bleeding recurs or continues with a prolonged APTT, protamine should be readministered. For unfractionated heparin, the dosage is 1 mg given by slow intravenous push for every 100 units of heparin given IV in the past hour. If a large dose of subcutaneous unfractionated heparin was given, equal and proportional decay of the amount dosed over 12 hours should be assumed, and therapy aimed at reversing the heparin effect should take into consideration however much remains from the time of the injection to the end of the 12-hour period, plus 4 hours. For LMW heparin, the dosage is 1 mg protamine for every 1 mg or 100 anti-Xa units given. Protamine reverses the anti-IIa effect of LMW heparin but neutralizes its anti-Xa effect less well. It is probably an effective antidote nonetheless, although the prolonged half-life of LMW heparin compared with unfractionated heparin means that repeated protamine injections may be required.

4. *Apparent anticoagulation failure*: Up to 50% of patients presenting with leg vein thrombosis may have no PE symptoms but may have lung scan results highly suggestive of PE. These patients may subsequently develop chest symptoms, e.g., pleuritic-type pain, if pulmonary infarction evolves. Thus, apparent failure of anticoagulation therapy sometimes represents prior asymptomatic undiscovered disease. Prolonged treatment with heparin or LMW heparin can be more effective than and should be substituted for warfarin therapy in patients with a large clot burden and apparent PE recurrence.

5. *Heparin dosing in renal failure*: LMW heparin is eliminated by the kidneys and has a much-prolonged half-life in end-stage renal disease. Patients with renal failure should be monitored, after heparin loading, with plasma anti-Xa levels to determine the frequency of dosing.

*Not FDA approved for this indication.
†Not available in the United States.

Thrombolytic Therapy. Previously considered warranted for massive pulmonary embolism (unrelenting hypoxia with shock) in the absence of absolute contraindications, thrombolytic therapy is now also considered when there is echocardiographic evidence (as described previously) of right ventricular dysfunction without systemic hypotension. In a study reporting patient outcomes from a multicenter registry, the risk of cerebral hemorrhage with thrombolytic therapy was about 2% and of major hemorrhage, about 20%; the corresponding figures for heparin therapy were approximately 0.5% and 8%. Both 30-day mortality and recurrent PE rates were reduced by about 50% in the thrombolysis group. Although thrombolytic therapy for PE can apparently produce some benefit when given up to 14 days after the event, the 50% reductions were shown with early treatment (within 24 hours of diagnosis). The risk of major bleeding with thrombolysis is probably considerably reduced compared with its administration after prior invasive procedures. Contraindications to thrombolytic therapy are presented in Table 4.

Use of Vena Cava Filters. Conservative indications for the use of vena cava filters include proven new PE despite adequate anticoagulation, proven PE and venous thrombosis with hemodynamic compromise such that another PE may be lethal, and proven PE with an absolute contraindication to anticoagulation therapy. Free-floating clots, risk of PE, and central nervous system tumor are weak indications in my view. Complications of filter use include migration, thrombosis at the insertion site, caval thrombosis, and post-thrombotic syndrome. Patients with filters inserted for proven thrombosis should also receive therapeutic anticoagulation whenever possible.

Mechanical Clot Removal. Surgical embolectomy for massive PE unresponsive to other treatment and

TABLE 4. **Relative Contraindications to Thrombolytic Therapy in Pulmonary Embolism (PE)***

Relative Contraindications
Nearly Absolute Contraindications
Active aortic dissection
Active pericarditis
Active internal bleeding
Recent prior cerebral hemorrhage
Intracerebral vascular disease (arteriovenous malformation or aneurysm)
Cerebral or intraspinal neoplasm
Other Relative Contraindications
Major trauma or surgery within preceding 14 days
Hypertension (including diastolic blood pressure of >90 mm Hg)
Intracranial or intraspinal disease (including seizure disorder)
Recent internal bleeding
Hemorrhagic retinopathy
Significantly impaired hemostasis
Age >65 years
Significant anemia
Patient unacceptance of blood products
Pregnancy

*Some critically ill PE patients may derive overall benefit from thrombolytic therapy despite these relative contraindications.

intracardiac emboli has an 80% survival rate in experienced hands and is the treatment of choice. The prognosis is poorer but not hopeless in patients with prior cardiopulmonary arrest. If cardiopulmonary bypass and heart surgery are not immediately available, removal of emboli by directed suction catheter may be tried.

PREVENTION

Safe and effective PE prevention, if used routinely, would substantially reduce the risk of undiagnosed PE and death due to PE. It is difficult to justify the cost of preventive measures in general, and this is certainly true for PE prevention. Nonetheless, many specialty groups have reached consensus that sound medical practice includes PE prevention in patients at risk. These risk groups are discussed at length in the October 1998 supplement to the journal *Chest*. To summarize, all hospitalized patients should receive some form of proven effective pharmacologic or mechanical prophylaxis. The most effective pharmacologic prophylaxis, LMW heparin given twice daily subcutaneously without monitoring, should be used in the highest-risk groups, including knee replacement patients. Oral warfarin prophylaxis is somewhat less effective; unfractionated heparin given 2 or 3 times daily at 5000 units per dose is even less effective but acceptable in lower-risk patients. Knee-high pneumatic compression "boots" and other forms of mechanical prophylaxis, e.g., foot pumps, are effective only when actually worn and operating, but they may be preferred to the use of LMW heparin in patients at high risk for bleeding, such as those with very recent en bloc prostatic or other pelvic surgery. Some patients who undergo outpatient surgery, e.g., arthroscopic collateral ligament repair with use of a tourniquet during the procedure for over 60 minutes may also be at risk for PE and should be advised and monitored accordingly. An attractive alternative for asymptomatic patients at risk for thrombi despite prophylaxis, e.g., knee replacement patients receiving LMW heparin or less effective prophylaxis, is prolonged (1 to 2 months) outpatient prophylaxis with LMW heparin or warfarin. Adding once-daily aspirin may confer additional benefit against arterial thrombi.

SARCOIDOSIS

method of
GIANPIETRO SEMENZATO, M.D.
Padua University School of Medicine
Padua, Italy

Sarcoidosis is a multisystemic disease of unknown etiology characterized by an accumulation of immunocompetent cells at sites of disease activity, which include the lung, lymph nodes, eyes, skin, liver, and spleen. Owing to its diverse manifestations, affected patients may initially seek care from clinicians of different specialties.

CLINICAL FEATURES, NATURAL HISTORY, AND PROGNOSIS

The clinical picture, natural history, and prognosis in sarcoidosis are highly variable and depend on ethnicity, duration of the illness, and the site and extent of organ involvement. In Caucasians the disease is often asymptomatic; alternatively, sarcoidosis can have an acute onset, with erythema nodosum, fever, and polyarthritis. The triad of erythema nodosum, polyarthritis, and bilateral hilar lymphadenopathy is termed Löfgren's syndrome and usually portends a self-limited course and spontaneous resolution. Löfgren's syndrome is quite frequent in persons of Scandinavian origin but is rare in blacks. On the other hand, an insidious onset of the disease is associated with chronicity and tendency to progress to pulmonary fibrosis, lung function impairment, and multisystem involvement, and the condition is unlikely to resolve without therapy. In black persons, particularly women, it is associated with a higher rate of extrapulmonary involvement, chronic uveitis, lupus pernio, and cystic bone lesions, as well as a chronic progressive course, worse long-term prognosis, and a higher rate of relapse.

Sarcoidosis tends to resolve, either spontaneously or in response to therapy, with spontaneous remission occurring in nearly 50% of patients and progression in about 15% of the cases. Most patients improve or stabilize with treatment; in approximately 40% of the cases, relapse occurs as the therapy is tapered or discontinued. Five percent of patients with sarcoidosis present with severe extrapulmonary involvement (i.e., central nervous system, cardiac). Fatalities occur as a consequence of these latter complications or as a result of progressive respiratory failure in patients with end-stage lung disease.

ETIOLOGY AND PATHOGENESIS

Although the etiology of sarcoidosis is still unknown, cases in which sarcoidosis was transmitted by cardiac or bone marrow transplantation suggest that the causative agent may be infectious. The combination of the characteristic morphologic aspects and the immunohistologic patterns of the sarcoid granulomatous lesions suggests that they may be the result of an antigen-driven process. In particular, sarcoid granuloma is considered to be the consequence of an exaggerated immunologic response against an undefined antigen that has persisted at sites of disease involvement, perhaps because of its low solubility and degradability.

In terms of pathogenesis, the early sarcoid reaction is characterized by the accumulation of activated T cells and macrophages at different sites of ongoing inflammation, notably in the lung. Studies of sarcoid T lymphocytes in involved areas have shown that in most patients, cells bear the helper-related CD4 phenotype and spontaneously release interferon-γ (IFN-γ) and interleukin-2 (IL-2). On the other hand, sarcoid alveolar macrophages behave as versatile secretory cells that release a great variety of cytokines, including tumor necrosis factor-α (TNF-α), IL-12, IL-15, and other growth factors. All of these mediators trigger the two mechanisms that ultimately account for the increased number of cells in the tissues involved by the sarcoid inflammatory process: (1) a redistribution of immunocompetent cells from the peripheral blood to the areas of granuloma formation and

(2) an in situ cell proliferation. As far as the pathogenesis of the end-stage lung is concerned, a fibrotic process develops that is strictly correlated with the recruitment of fibroblasts and the increased production of matrix macromolecules.

DIAGNOSIS AND EVALUATION OF DISEASE ACTIVITY

The diagnosis is established when clinical and radiographic findings are supported by histologic demonstration of noncaseating granuloma and the exclusion of other diseases known to induce similar granulomatous lesions, in particular, those caused by infectious agents (negative special stains and cultures for acid-fast bacilli, fungi, bacteria, and protozoa). Biopsy specimens should be obtained from the most readily accessible organ with the least invasive method, usually the lung (transbronchial lung biopsy, video-assisted thoracoscopy, open lung biopsy), or from the lymph nodes (peripheral nodes, mediastinoscopy), conjunctival yellow nodules, skin, or liver. The Kveim-Siltzbach test is of help in formulating the diagnosis; however, homogenates of human sarcoid tissue are not widely available, nor have they been approved by the Food and Drug Administration (FDA). In patients with classic Löfgren's syndrome, the biopsy may not be required to make the diagnosis of sarcoidosis, provided that the acute episode resolves rapidly and spontaneously.

According to findings on the chest x-ray film, four stages can be identified: stage I disease—presence of hilar adenopathy without parenchymal infiltrates; stage II disease—hilar adenopathy with parenchymal infiltrates; stage III disease—infiltrates without hilar adenopathy; stage IV disease—pulmonary fibrosis.

The management of sarcoidosis depends upon whether the disease is acute or chronic, minimal (single organ involvement) or generalized, and mild or severe. The term "activity of the disease" is not yet precisely defined, and as noted at a recent American Thoracic Society, European Respiratory Society, and World Association of Sarcoidosis and Other Granulomatous Disorders Consensus Conference, there is no general agreement as to its meaning. The decisions thus are based mainly on the clinical picture (extent of disease, worsening respiratory symptoms), radiographic findings, and results of lung function tests (vital capacity, forced expiratory volume in 1 second [FEV_1], and diffusion capacity). These clinical features are integrated with findings on imaging and other studies as well as assays for biochemical-immunologic markers, which are referred to as markers of disease activity. These activity markers include morphologic and immunologic data from bronchoalveolar lavage (such as evidence of high-intensity alveolitis, in particular, increased numbers of $CD4^+$ lymphocytes), total-body gallium 67 scan (panda-plus-lambda sign), fluorescein angiography, biochemical markers (in particular, serum and bronchoalveolar lavage fluid levels of angiotensin-converting enzyme), and high-resolution computed tomography. This last study, providing excellent visualization of lung morphology, is likely to be the most promising technique to help guide therapy. None of these markers of activity, however, has a defined role in staging patients, and none can be used to establish the specific diagnosis of the disease. In specific cases they can help only in disease management, contributing to better define the degree of ongoing inflammation and the evolution of the granulomatous process.

TREATMENT

The wide spectrum of clinical manifestations of sarcoidosis is reflected in the heterogeneous nature of the treatment of the disease and in the difficulties inherent in its management. Patients should initially be observed without therapy, given the potential for spontaneous improvement observed in a significant number of cases (70% in stage I, 50% in stage II, less than 20% in stage III, none in stage IV). Therapeutic intervention should be considered in patients with severe, chronic, generalized, or progressive disease. The activity of the disease, as defined by the aforementioned parameters, may also be relevant in helping to formulate therapeutic decisions. Patients with pulmonary or extrapulmonary involvements are considered separately later in the discussion.

Pulmonary Involvement

Patients with *stage I disease* but without extrapulmonary involvement do not require treatment. In acute disease, such as Löfgren's syndrome, the administration of nonsteroidal anti-inflammatory drugs for several weeks is helpful in overcoming fever and joint pain. Rare patients presenting with airway obstruction should be closely monitored to detect early functional impairment and, on occasion, should be given corticosteroids to relieve symptoms.

Patients with *stage II disease* who are asymptomatic and have minimal impairment of lung function tests can be observed for several months. If a deterioration of lung function and/or other signs of disease activity are noted, treatment should be started. Symptomatic patients (with cough, dyspnea, chest pain, and so on) or patients who are asymptomatic but have severe impairment of lung function require treatment. Immunologic studies have shown that therapy in these cases should not be delayed, in order to prevent the inflammatory processes from progressing to a stage at which responsiveness to steroids may be reduced.

Patients with *stage III disease* usually suffer from progressive disease and require long-term steroid treatment and/or use of one of the alternative steroid-sparing drugs as described later.

In patients with *stage IV disease,* an initial course of steroid therapy is indicated. However, often these patients respond poorly to corticosteroids, and this type of treatment may increase the risk of infection in patients with bronchiectasis or cavitations. In these cases, other immunosuppressive drugs should be exploited before the possibility of lung transplantation is considered.

Extrapulmonary Involvement

Sarcoidosis can potentially affect any organ. In patients with extrapulmonary involvement, the indications for treatment are well defined, and specific tests are needed to define discrete tissue involvement. In particular, neurologic, ocular, cardiac, or skin involvement or malignant hypercalcemia necessitates steroid treatment with doses appropriate to the severity and extent of disease.

In patients whose disease is responsive to corticosteroids, after a period of treatment with high doses, the therapy must be tapered, and the lowest dose can be used on a long-term-therapy basis so long as no sign of relapse is present. In patients whose disease does not respond to corticosteroids, other immunosuppressive drugs are indicated. In particular, methotrexate* may be useful in neurologic involvement. Magnetic resonance imaging has proved useful in monitoring these manifestations of disease. Neurosarcoidosis sometimes responds to radiotherapy.

Cardiac involvement may remain clinically silent or may cause fatal arrhythmias with sudden death. Thallium-201 imaging is useful to confirm the suspicion of myocardial involvement. If the patient's disease is steroid-resistant (even at high doses), hydroxychloroquine (Plaquenil)* may be added to the steroid regimen. An implantable cardioverter-defibrillator should be applied after therapy is discontinued.

Skin involvement often requires the use of topical corticosteroids, whereas large or disfiguring dermatologic lesions necessitate systemic therapy; steroids must be tried, but the response is often disappointing. Methotrexate and/or hydroxychloroquine are currently given to patients with lupus pernio.

In ocular involvement, topical corticosteroids are used in patients with anterior uveitis. Administration of systemic steroids is indicated for treatment of retinal vasculitis, chorioretinitis and other manifestations of posterior segment inflammation, and granulomatous infiltration of lacrimal glands, orbit, and other structures. The use of cyclosporine in ocular involvement is still under evaluation.

Kidney involvement may present as hypercalcemic nephropathy, which usually requires steroid therapy. Calcium-chelating agents for hypercalciuria are recommended whenever steroid therapy must be discontinued. A diet low in calcium and avoidance of vitamin D supplements should be encouraged. Asymptomatic liver involvement requires no therapy, but regular follow-up evaluation must be planned.

Therapeutic Approaches: Drugs, Modalities of Administration, and Special Situations

DRUGS

When indicated, corticosteroids remain the mainstay of therapy for sarcoidosis even in the absence of well-controlled clinical trials showing the real efficacy of these drugs. However, corticosteroids have significantly influenced the natural history of sarcoidosis by preventing ocular fibrosis and blindness, pulmonary fibrosis, and pulmonary hypertension; overcoming the problem of nephrocalcinosis; and allowing most patients to follow a normal lifestyle. The mechanisms of action of steroids are still under study; these agents probably modulate the genes controlling the synthesis of cytokines and relevant cytokine receptors involved in the accumulation of immunocompetent cells at different sites of disease activity.

The standard dosage for prednisone is 40 to 50 mg daily given in a single dose. After a few months, the dose is gradually tapered to a maintenance level of 10 to 20 mg per day over an average period of 8 months. The duration of the treatment and the steroid dosage are determined by regular follow-up of clinical features and parameters of disease activity. Higher doses (1 to 1.5 mg per kg per day) are advocated to control severe disease (neurologic, ocular, cardiac, and skin involvement) or for relapses. Lower doses (15 to 20 mg per day) may be useful in special cases, such as in patients who do not respond to nonsteroidal anti-inflammatory drugs. A single daily dose of 40 mg of prednisone on an alternate-day regimen is helpful in reducing corticosteroid side effects and may be effective in treating the disease. Since long-term treatment is often required for sarcoidosis, the use of deflazacort,* a new bone-sparing corticosteroid, has been proposed to prevent osteoporosis. This approach, however, needs further confirmation.

Inhaled steroids can be used in cases with discrete pulmonary involvement and mild impairment of lung function; cough and signs of bronchial hyperreactivity can be suppressed. The use of inhaled steroids is otherwise not currently recommended. Oral corticosteroids may be reinforced under various circumstances by intravenous or intramuscular administration. Topical steroid therapy with creams, drops, and sprays is appropriate in the special circumstances described previously.

Although there is no good alternative to steroids, a variety of other pharmacologic approaches have been exploited in patients with disease refractory to corticosteroid treatment or as steroid-sparing adjuncts in patients requiring persistent steroid therapy and experiencing severe corticosteroid-induced side effects. Most reports supporting the use of methotrexate, hydroxychloroquine, azathioprine,† or cyclosporine† are in the form of uncontrolled studies or anecdotal reports. These drugs are not indicated in children and pregnancy.

Methotrexate, an antimetabolite, is an alternative drug for long-term therapy in severe disease (mostly neurosarcoidosis and dermatologic sarcoidosis, such as lupus pernio). The recommended dosage is 10 to 15 mg orally (PO) per week given in three divided doses at 12-hour intervals on a long-term basis (for 1 to 2 years or even longer). Monitoring of the white blood cell count and liver function is mandatory in patients undergoing this treatment.

Antimalarial agents, notably chloroquine (Aralen)†

*Not FDA approved for this indication.

*Not available in the United States.
†Not FDA approved for this indication.

and hydroxychloroquine, are given at doses of 200 to 400 mg in a daily or alternate-day regimen for several months. Eye examinations conducted on a regular basis are essential throughout the course of treatment. Hydroxychloroquine is the preferred agent because of the lower risk of ocular toxicity. Because hydroxychloroquine causes hepatic insulin degradation, suppresses gluconeogenesis, and increases peripheral tissue utilization of glucose, it is of benefit in diabetics with mild sarcoidosis.

When these drugs cannot be tolerated, or when contraindications to their use exist, a second-choice approach is administration of azathioprine (Imuran), 100 to 150 mg per day PO for a few months and cyclophosphamide (Cytoxan),* 50 to 100 mg per day PO for a few months. Various side effects, including the risk of therapy-induced cancer, must be taken into account. Despite its specific property of interfering with cytokine synthesis, cyclosporine, a fungus-derived drug, has been paradoxically ineffective in the treatment of sarcoidosis.

LUNG TRANSPLANTATION

In patients in whom other therapeutic approaches have failed and whose clinical status continues to deteriorate, mainly patients with stage III and stage IV sarcoidosis, single- or double-lung transplantation should be considered. Unfortunately, the recurrence of sarcoid lesions in lung allografts must be taken into account.

PREGNANCY

Sarcoidosis is one of the immunologic diseases that may regress during pregnancy; improvement is noted in approximately 65% of cases. If the pregnant patient is receiving oral steroids, the dose can be reduced and even discontinued. A flare-up of sarcoidosis may occur within the first 6 months after delivery; this may be controlled by a short course of corticosteroids. Nonetheless, in about 5% of patients the disease becomes worse during pregnancy. In these cases steroids are given cautiously. Methotrexate and other cytotoxic drugs as well as radiographic and isotopic monitoring should be avoided.

New therapeutic approaches to the management of sarcoidosis with pentoxifylline (Trental),* thalidomide,* or anti-cytokine molecules are still under evaluation.

*Not FDA approved for this indication.

SILICOSIS

method of
JOHN S. MUNGER, M.D., and
WILLIAM N. ROM, M.D.
New York University School of Medicine
New York, New York

Silicosis is an occupational lung disease caused by inhalation of crystalline silica particles. It is a disease of antiquity; descriptions date as far back as the ancient Greeks and Romans, and the disease may have occurred in prehistory. Although the causal relationship between silica and lung disease is known, and federal regulations on exposure are in effect that, if followed, would prevent virtually all cases, new cases of silicosis continue to occur.

Silica, also known as free silica, is silicon dioxide (SiO_2) and is abundant in the earth's crust. Silica can exist in an amorphous, relatively nontoxic form or as crystalline silica. Crystalline silica can take three forms: alpha quartz (the most common form), and cristobalite and tridymite, each of which can be formed from quartz at high temperatures. Silicates are a group of minerals composed of silicon dioxide combined with other elements (such as sodium, magnesium, aluminum, and fluorine). Silicates occur naturally and are used industrially in pure form (e.g., kaolin and talc) and as mixtures with silica. Exposure to silicate dusts alone can cause lung disease but not silicosis. The toxicity of silica appears to be reduced in occupational exposures that consist of mixtures of silica and nonquartz dusts.

EPIDEMIOLOGY

Silicosis can occur in occupations where small (less than 5 μm diameter) silica particles are formed and inhaled. Work that disrupts soil, sand, or rock, such as drilling, mining, excavating, quarrying, tunneling, and construction, can result in silicosis. Work in which silica is processed or used for its abrasive or insulative properties also poses a risk. These occupations include foundry work, sandblasting, ceramics manufacturing (e.g., pottery), production of silica flour, and stone cutting, grinding, and polishing. A small percentage of silicosis cases arise from other occupations or exposures, such as photocopier toner dust (siderosilicosis), souvenir statue casting, gemstone work, and dental technician work.

The current Occupational Safety and Health Administration (OSHA) permissible exposure limit is 100 μg of silica per cubic meter of air. If exposures are kept below this limit, virtually all cases of silicosis can be prevented. However, silicosis is still being diagnosed in the 1990s, largely due to occupational exposures occurring decades ago. Silicosis surveillance programs were established in the 1990s in Illinois, Michigan, New Jersey, North Carolina, Ohio, Texas, and Wisconsin. In 1993, 256 cases were documented in these seven states. Of ten workplaces in which airborne silica levels were measured, the OSHA limit was exceeded in six. Extrapolating these results to the national level, and recognizing that these studies underestimate cases, one would expect a few thousand new cases of silicosis annually. In Michigan, 577 silicosis cases were reported to state authorities between 1987 and 1995; of these, 3 patients began work with silica in the 1980s and 18 in the 1970s.

PATHOGENESIS AND CLASSIFICATION

The pathogenesis of silicosis involves the physicochemical properties of inhaled crystalline silica and resulting cellular responses. Large silica particles become impacted in the upper airway and are removed by the mucociliary escalator. These particles do not cause silicosis but may produce the bronchitis seen with dust exposure. Smaller particles (particularly under 1 μm diameter) are carried to the most distal airways and alveoli. There, they are internalized by alveolar macrophages and alveolar type I cells; penetrate to the interstitium, lymphatics, and regional lymph nodes; and provoke the cellular responses that lead to disease.

Free radicals are central to the disease process. The surface of silica particles, especially if freshly fractured, is catalytically reactive due to complexed iron. In the reduced state, iron forms highly damaging hydroxyl radicals from hydrogen peroxide in the Fenton reaction. Reactive oxygen species are also produced via the respiratory burst of phagocytes. A complex set of cellular responses ensues, prominently involving macrophages, lymphocytes, and fibroblasts and orchestrated by mediators such as interleukins-1 and -6, platelet-derived growth factor, transforming growth factor-beta, and tumor necrosis factor-alpha.

The initial response of the lung to silica exposure is a nonspecific injury pattern, but with time the pathognomonic lesion of silicosis, the silicotic nodule, develops. The fully developed nodule has a central zone of dense fibrous tissue, a second zone of concentric collagen fibers, and an outer zone of disorganized collagen fibers with macrophages and lymphoid cells. The nodules have a predilection for lymph nodes and, within the lung, subpleural and upper lobe locations. Nodules can encroach on and destroy pulmonary vessels, a process that may contribute to cor pulmonale in severe disease. Focal areas of air space enlargement can occur. The isolated finding of silicotic nodules in lymph nodes is evidence of exposure but is not classified as silicosis. Nodules can sometimes calcify centrally but rarely cavitate unless there is mycobacterial infection. Simple nodules are less than 1 cm in diameter. Nodules can enlarge after exposure ceases. In progressive massive fibrosis (PMF), nodules are larger and become confluent.

The silicotic nodule is the hallmark of both chronic and accelerated silicosis. These two categories of disease are defined by the duration of exposure leading to disease, as shown in Table 1. The accelerated form more frequently progresses to PMF, and interstitial fibrosis can be seen in addition to nodules in varying states of maturity. In contrast, acute silicosis occurs after as little as a few months of intense exposure, usually to very fine, highly reactive silica dust, and is characterized by an alveolar filling process like that of idiopathic alveolar proteinosis.

The radiograph in simple silicosis has rounded nodules smaller than 1 cm in diameter with an upper zone predominance. In complicated silicosis, nodules are greater than 1 cm and may become confluent. Cavitation and pleural disease are unusual without other causes (e.g., tuberculosis or heart failure). Hilar nodes may be enlarged and may have a peripheral "egg shell" pattern of calcification. In accelerated silicosis, there can be upper zone–predominant reticular changes in addition to nodules. Acute silicosis results in signs of air-space filling.

TABLE 1. **Classification of Disease**

Disease Category	Exposure	Typical Symptoms	Radiographic Findings
Chronic	>10 years		
Simple		None	<1 cm nodules, upper zones
Complicated		Dyspnea, cough	>1 cm confluent nodules, plus above
Accelerated	5–10 years		
Simple		None	As in chronic, simple
Complicated		Dyspnea, cough	As in chronic, complicated, plus interstitial changes
Acute	<5 years	Dyspnea, cough, fever, malaise	Diffuse alveolar filling

CLINICAL PRESENTATION AND DIAGNOSIS

Chronic, simple silicosis can occur without symptoms. The most common symptom in silicosis is dyspnea, initially with exertion and subsequently at rest. The degree of impairment and the rate of disease progression are greater in the accelerated and acute forms than in the chronic form; patients with chronic disease often die of other causes, whereas the more severe forms frequently cause death. Cough is a frequent manifestation and can be due to cigarette smoking, dust exposure, infection (bronchitis, tuberculosis), or involvement of large airways by enlarged hilar nodes. Acute silicosis presents with fever, malaise, weight loss, and dyspnea. Clubbing and chest pain are not expected with silicosis and should prompt evaluation for other causes.

In most cases, a history of silica exposure and a compatible chest radiograph are sufficient for the diagnosis. Most exposures occurred decades ago, so the clinician must conduct a detailed occupational history if silicosis is suspected. Bronchoscopic examination, biopsy, and lavage are not usually needed to confirm the diagnosis but may help exclude other diseases such as sarcoidosis, cancer, and mycobacterial infection. If the diagnosis is not certain and tissue is required, we favor open biopsy in most cases because bronchoscopic samples are often inadequate. Biopsy specimens should be analyzed for silica and other dusts. All biopsy slides and bronchoalveolar lavage cytospin slides should be examined under polarized light since silica is brightly birefringent. There are no characteristic findings on pulmonary function tests (PFTs); studies may be normal or may show various combinations of restrictive and obstructive ventilatory defects.

Silicosis patients are at increased risk of tuberculosis, presumably because of macrophage dysfunction stemming from the lung silica load. The earliest sign of infection may be a change in the radiograph (e.g., cavitation of a nodule) or clinical symptoms such as cough, hemoptysis, fever, weight loss, and night sweats. Patients should get purified protein derivative (PPD) tests at diagnosis and regularly thereafter regardless of symptoms; if active disease is suspected, sputum specimens should be obtained. If sputa are negative but concerns remain, bronchoscopy with lavage and biopsy is the next step in most cases.

Other complications of silicosis include infections (atypical mycobacteria, cryptococcosis, sporotrichosis), pneumothorax, central airway obstruction related to involved hilar nodes, and cor pulmonale. Associated conditions include connective tissue diseases (especially scleroderma), renal disease, and lung cancer. The International Agency for Research on Cancer has recently categorized respirable crystalline silica as a group 1 carcinogen.

TREATMENT AND PREVENTION

The management of silicosis patients is supportive (Table 2). Whole lung lavage, corticosteroids, inhaled aluminum citrate, tetrandrine, and poly-2[or 4]-vi-

TABLE 2. **Management Checklist**

Stop dust exposure
Notify occupational health authorities
Avoid cigarettes
PPD skin testing at diagnosis and annually thereafter
Influenza and pneumococcal vaccinations
TESTS
Sputum cultures for mycobacteria if PPD conversion, cavitation, or systemic symptoms occur
Chest radiograph for change in symptoms; consider annual radiography
PFTs, ABG (or oximetry) at baseline and as needed
MRI, CT, gallium scan, and bronchoscopy not routinely indicated
TREATMENTS
Airway obstruction: inhaled beta$_2$-agonists, anticholinergics; consider inhaled steroids, theophylline
Tuberculosis: INH, rifampin, ethambutol, pyrazinamide initially; at least two effective drugs for 1 year
Hypoxemia: supplemental O_2; check oxygenation with exercise and possibly at night
Cor pulmonale: supplemental O_2, diuretic
Pulmonary rehabilitation for moderate to severe impairment
Consider lung transplantation for severe disease; refer for early evaluation

Abbreviations: PPD = purified protein derivative; PFT = pulmonary function tests; ABG = arterial blood gases; MRI = magnetic resonance imaging; CT = computed tomography; INH = isoniazid.

nylpyridine-N-oxide (PVNO) have been used experimentally, but generally accepted treatments for the underlying disease do not exist. Further exposure to dusts should be eliminated. In one study, chronic silicosis patients treated for 6 months with prednisolone had improved lung function, but such treatment cannot be recommended without more information on outcome with more prolonged therapy. Patients with acute silicosis have been treated with whole lung lavage and steroids, but data are inadequate to assess effectiveness. Future therapies might involve specific anticytokine or antioxidant strategies. Lung transplantation should be considered in younger, otherwise healthy patients with severe disease.

Patients should get yearly influenza vaccinations and pneumococcal vaccination once every 10 years, and be instructed to report any possible symptoms of infection immediately. Episodes of bacterial bronchitis should be treated as discussed elsewhere in this book. All should be skin tested with intermediate-strength PPD intradermally at diagnosis and yearly. In most cases of new converters with silicosis we begin multiple drug therapy while awaiting culture data. If there is no evidence of active disease, isoniazid (INH) is given for 1 year to PPD converters. The physician must be alert to the possibility of reactivation tuberculosis occurring after a full course of INH. Treatment of active mycobacterial disease is discussed elsewhere and is the same in silicosis patients except that we treat for 12 months rather than 6 months because of a high risk of relapse.

Patients with airway obstruction should be treated with bronchodilators as discussed in the chapter on chronic obstructive pulmonary disease. Ideally, PFTs should be done before and after treatment is begun. If there is neither symptomatic nor objective improvement, treatment should be altered or stopped. This is particularly true if courses of oral steroids are tried. Progression of silicosis is monitored by chest radiographs, PFTs, arterial blood gas measurements, and oximetry measurements at rest and with exertion. Supplemental oxygen should be prescribed to keep Sa_{O_2} above 89% or Pa_{O_2} above 60 mm Hg. Some patients may benefit from a pulmonary rehabilitation program. Treatment of cor pulmonale requires supplemental oxygen, diuretics, and appropriate inotropes and vasodilators; an electrocardiogram and echocardiogram should be obtained in most cases. In selected patients sleep studies should be done to rule out nocturnal desaturation.

Although silicosis is not a reportable disease, the physician must make sure that appropriate authorities are aware of a newly diagnosed case of silicosis so that workplaces can be assessed if necessary. If the physician is not aware of the appropriate state authority to contact, we recommend consulting the National Institute for Occupational Safety and Health (NIOSH) (1-800-35NIOSH) for referral.

HYPERSENSITIVITY PNEUMONITIS

method of
ROY PATTERSON, M.D.
Northwestern University Medical School
Chicago, Illinois

Hypersensitivity pneumonitis (HP) is an immunologically mediated inflammatory disease of the lungs. It differs from IgE-mediated allergic asthma in symptoms, progression of disease, and the immunologic mechanisms responsible for the inflammation.

PATHOPHYSIOLOGY AND PATHOGENESIS

HP is the result of inhalation of foreign substances, which can include bacteria, fungal spores, foreign proteins, or reactive chemicals. The immunologic inflammation is the result of IgG antibodies reacting with inhaled antigens in pulmonary tissue, producing immune complexes that attract inflammatory cells that release biologic mediators and produce tissue damage. The IgG antibodies are the same antibodies that produce precipitin bands in immunoassays using double-diffusion gel reactions in laboratory tests. These precipitin reactions are useful diagnostic tools that demonstrate a significant immune response to the inhaled antigens.

CLINICAL PRESENTATION

The symptoms of HP can be acute, subacute, or chronic. These states relate to the amount of antigens inhaled, the degree of reactivity of the host, and the duration of exposure. Acute symptoms include cough, dyspnea, chills, fever, and malaise. In the subacute form, these symptoms are less severe, and anorexia and weight loss can occur. In the chronic form, all of these symptoms occur to a lesser degree but are more persistent.

DIAGNOSIS

Chest films show nodular infiltrates in the acute and subacute forms and fibrotic lesions in the chronic form. Pulmonary function tests show restriction in all three forms of HP to a variable degree, depending on the severity of disease.

Causative antigens are numerous. Unlike IgE-mediated asthma, which is seen in atopic individuals, anyone can develop HP. For example, bagassosis is caused by moldy sugar cane contaminated with organisms such as *Thermoactinomyces vulgaris*. The incidence of this disease decreased sharply once the pathogenesis was understood. Farmer's lung due to moldy hay can be caused by *Micropolyspora faeni* or other organisms. Ornithotic HP is due to avian proteins in bird droppings.

A more recent type of HP has been shown to be the result of chemicals reacting with human self proteins to form a chemical (hapten)–self protein complex that is antigenic to the host and produces inflammatory lung disease. Trimellitic anhydride is the prime model of this type of etiologic agent, and the chemical can also cause IgE-mediated diseases such as asthma and allergic rhinitis. Chemical sensitivities to phthalic anhydride and isocyanates can also produce HP. Lists of occupational exposures that cause HP are extensive and are available in textbooks of occupational and pulmonary medicine.

The diagnosis of HP is important because it can be a debilitating disease and lead to fibrotic end-stage lung disease if undiagnosed and untreated. HP is sufficiently uncommon that the diagnosis can be missed unless a correlation with exposure to organic dust or chemicals is sought, and even then the antigen may be obscure. The diagnosis is based on the previously described symptoms of HP and exclusion of infectious disease. An acute or chronic exposure to an antigen should be sought. Antibody assays such as precipitin reactions (e.g., against pigeon droppings) should be carried out in appropriate laboratories. The chest film and pulmonary function abnormalities should be compatible with the diagnosis of HP, and improvement should occur with avoidance of antigen exposure.

Problems with these diagnostic criteria are that idiopathic pulmonary fibrosis mimics chronic HP. A defined antigen may not be found, such as an antigen in the humidifier system, or may be obscure, such as an antigen contaminating water in a sauna. *Laboratories reporting serologic results may report false-negative precipitin reactions*. Subjects exposed to antigen such as pigeon droppings may have precipitating antibodies but no clinical disease. A patient with HP may not be able to avoid antigen exposure or may refuse to avoid exposure (e.g., bird handlers). Nevertheless, the astute clinician can arrive at a reasonable diagnosis, encourage the cessation of exposure, and initiate treatment.

TREATMENT

The treatment of HP focuses on avoidance of antigen exposure. Avoidance of moldy hay in Farmer's lung, bird droppings in pigeon breeder's disease, and chemical sensitizers in occupational HP is mandatory. The anti-inflammatory action of corticosteroids will accelerate resolution of acute and subacute cases of HP. Prednisone at 60 mg orally daily for 1 week followed by 60 mg on alternate days is appropriate, with gradual reduction and discontinuation in 4 to 6 weeks. The chest film should clear and pulmonary function tests should improve. It is not appropriate to treat patients with HP with prednisone when exposure to the antigen continues. In this situation, the patient will feel better or even become asymptomatic while damage to pulmonary tissue continues.

SINUSITIS

method of
ERICA R. THALER, M.D., and
DAVID W. KENNEDY, M.D.
University of Pennsylvania School of Medicine
Philadelphia, Pennsylvania

DEFINITION AND ETIOLOGY

Sinusitis is defined as an inflammatory condition involving the mucosa of the sinus cavities. Because involvement of the sinuses is usually accompanied by changes in the nasal mucosa, the American Academy of Otorhinolaryngology has recommended that the term sinusitis be replaced by rhinosinusitis. This new terminology also recognizes that when rhinitis is present, there is also typically some sinusitis present. A temporal distinction is also typically appended to the diagnosis: *acute*, lasting less than 4 weeks and of sudden onset, with complete resolution of symptoms; *subacute*, lasting between 1 and 3 months, again with resolution of symptoms; and *chronic*, lasting longer than 3 months, with no intervening symptom-free interval. Temporal distinctions are somewhat arbitrary, as there is no pathologic correlate that distinguishes the change from the inflammatory processes of acute sinusitis to those of the chronic condition.

A multitude of predisposing factors may make a person susceptible to the development of sinusitis. All such factors have the shared pathophysiology of impaired mucociliary clearance of secretions from the sinuses. Commonly, this involves blockage of the ostiomeatal complex (Figure 1),

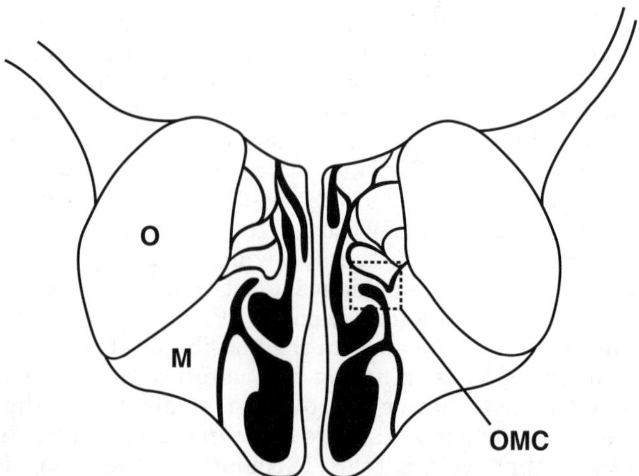

Figure 1. Coronal section of the paranasal sinuses at the level of the ostiomeatal complex (OMC).
Abbreviations: O = orbit; M = maxillary sinus.

which is the confluence of drainage of the frontal, anterior ethmoid, and maxillary sinuses, located under the middle turbinate. Pathologic narrowing of this anatomic complex is critical in the development of more pervasive sinus disease. Either anatomic narrowing or edematous mucosa impedes drainage from the sinuses. This allows trapped secretions to harbor bacteria, with subsequent overgrowth. Bacteria secrete toxins that impede ciliary motion, further limiting clearance of mucous.

The most common predisposing event for the development of sinusitis is a viral upper respiratory infection. Swollen mucosa blocks normal clearance of mucus, and bacterial superinfection may ensue. Other predisposing conditions include allergy, nasal polyposis, and exposure to mucosal irritants such as tobacco smoke and air pollution. Anatomic anomalies in the region of the ostiomeatal complex, such as a paradoxically curved middle turbinate or extreme septal deviation, may predispose patients to the development of sinusitis. Abnormalities in mucociliary clearance, abnormal mucus content, or mucosal edema from systemic medical conditions such as cystic fibrosis, Kartagener's syndrome, reactive airways disease, and immunodeficiency also predispose patients to the development of sinusitis.

The microbiology of sinusitis varies with the duration of infection. In chronic sinusitis, bacterial infection is often polymicrobial, with anaerobic organisms playing a role. Predominating aerobic organisms in acute bacterial sinusitis include *Streptococcus pneumoniae, Haemophilus influenzae*, and *Moraxella catarrhalis. Pseudomonas* species and *Staphylococcus aureus* are more prevalent in chronic sinus disease. Fungal organisms may be identified as colonies on inspissated secretions or may be present in allergic fungal sinusitis, a noninvasive form of fungal infection in immunocompetent hosts. *Aspergillus* species predominate, but in fulminant invasive fungal disease in an immunocompromised patient, organisms of the genus *Rhizopus* may be found.

DIAGNOSIS

The diagnosis of sinusitis is made by a careful history and confirmatory physical examination. Patients complain of facial pressure and pain, nasal congestion and obstruction, purulent nasal discharge, and hyposmia or anosmia. Patients with acute sinusitis may have associated fever. Less predominating but frequent complaints include fatigue, halitosis, dental pain, cough, and sensation of aural fullness. The location of pain and pressure may elucidate the involved sinus: maxillary sinusitis causes cheek and dental pain; ethmoid sinusitis causes periorbital and medial canthal pain; frontal sinusitis causes pain over the eyes and zygomatic arches; and sphenoid sinusitis causes deep retro-orbital and occipital pain.

Physical examination findings include hyperemic and edematous nasal mucosa, cheek and forehead tenderness, and purulent drainage visualized by nasal endoscopy. Although the diagnosis may be made accurately without nasal endoscopy, endoscopic visualization of the entire nasal anatomy, including the middle meatus and sphenoethmoid recess into which the sinuses drain, may secure the diagnosis. Endoscopy also allows for culture of purulent discharge, making antibiotic choice more appropriate.

The role of radiographic imaging in the diagnosis of sinusitis is restricted to complications of acute sinusitis and chronic sinusitis in which medical management is failing. Computed tomography (CT) imaging is the radiographic study of choice, using bone windows and 3-mm coronal cuts through the sinuses. Intravenous contrast is not necessary unless there is concern regarding potential spread of infection to the orbit or cranial vault. In the nonacute setting, CT scans should be obtained after the patient has been on maximal medical therapy for a minimum of 4 weeks. Residual mucosal thickening or obstructive anatomic anomalies may prompt surgical intervention. CT imaging is very important prior to surgical intervention. Evidence of persistent unilateral disease on CT is strongly suggestive of either fungal disease or neoplasia.

Plain films of the sinuses and ultrasound studies may be used to monitor the response of a sinus infection to medical therapy, but sensitivity and specificity are low with both imaging modalities. Magnetic resonance imaging is used rarely, because of its inferior ability to assess bone anatomy. It may be helpful in diagnosing fungal sinus disease and can distinguish secretions from soft tissue, which may be useful in differentiating a neoplastic process from chronic inflammation.

TREATMENT

Medical Therapy

Medical therapy differs for the acute and chronic forms of sinusitis. Acute sinusitis is treated with a broad-spectrum antibiotic for a minimum of 10 to 14 days. A 4-week course of antibiotics may be necessary in some cases. First-line agents include cefuroxime axetil (Ceftin), 250 mg twice daily (bid); amoxicillin-clavulanate (Augmentin), 875 mg bid; trimethoprim-sulfamethoxazole (Bactrim DS), one tablet bid; clarithromycin (Biaxin), 500 mg bid, and lorcarbef (Lorabid), 400 mg bid. Amoxicillin is no longer considered a first-line agent because of the prevalence of β-lactamase resistance. Topical and oral decongestants are important adjunctive agents in the treatment of acute sinusitis, assisting in reestablishing sinus drainage. Care should be used in administering systemic decongestants to patients with labile hypertension and prostate hypertrophy or prostatitis, as these conditions may be exacerbated. Topical nasal decongestants may be used for 3 to 5 days only, if the risk of rhinitis medicamentosus (rebound vasodilation of nasal mucosa) is to be avoided. Antihistamines have little role in the treatment of acute sinusitis, except when allergy has been the underlying cause of the acute infection. Mucolytic agents such as guaifenesin may help to enhance drainage by thinning secretions.

Chronic sinusitis may be treated with many of the same antibiotics that are used for acute disease. Quinolones may also be considered. The duration of therapy is longer, typically at least 4 to 6 weeks. Anaerobic coverage may be augmented with metronidazole. Culture-directed selection of antibiotics is of increasing importance, as resistant organisms may be present. Decongestants and antihistamines should be used sparingly, because these agents tend to dry secretions, which may impede drainage. Topical nasal steroids are important anti-inflammatory agents. In patients with nasal polyposis and reactive airways disease, oral steroids may also be required. They are also an important component of treatment for allergic fungal sinusitis.

Surgical Therapy

Surgery of the sinuses is reserved for cases in which medical management has been unsuccessful. Typically, the patient has had more than four episodes of acute disease per year or has chronic sinusitis with no symptom-free intervals. Endoscopic sinus surgery is currently considered first-line management and has largely replaced open procedures on the sinuses. Rigid nasal endoscopes are used to visualize the sinus anatomy, and compatible instruments are used to widen the natural drainage areas of the sinuses, most critically the ostiomeatal complex, while preserving as much native anatomy and mucosa as possible. This breaks the cycle of recurring infection and allows mucosa to heal. The extent of disease dictates the extent of surgery, but extensive endoscopic intervention may be required in diffuse sinonasal polyposis. Affected patients also require both long-term endoscopic follow-up and topical nasal steroids. Prolonged antibiotic therapy may also be necessary.

In occasional instances, open procedures on the sinuses are still necessary. For example, many surgeons continue to use an external ethmoidectomy approach to drain subperiosteal abscesses, a complication of acute sinusitis.

Complications

Complications of acute sinusitis may be divided by location: those that are extracranial and those that are intracranial. Extracranial complications of acute sinusitis involve the orbit and range from preseptal cellulitis (cellulitis of the lids with no significant visual compromise), to subperiosteal or orbital abscess (which typically leads to proptosis, impaired extraocular muscle mobility, and sometimes changes in visual acuity), to cavernous sinus thrombophlebitis (a life-threatening thrombosis of the cavernous sinus system). The use of broad-spectrum intravenous antibiotics to cover acute sinusitis pathogens is mandatory. If an abscess is present on CT scans or if orbital changes progress despite therapy, urgent surgical drainage is necessary.

Intracranial complications of acute sinusitis include meningitis and epidural or subdural abscess formation and are most likely to occur with frontal or sphenoid sinusitis. Adolescent males are at the highest risk. The use of intravenous antibiotics that penetrate the blood-brain barrier, as well as surgical drainage of abscess cavities, constitutes standard therapy.

The most common complication of chronic sinusitis is mucocele formation, in which encysted mucosa continues production of mucus, creating a slowly expanding cyst that erodes surrounding bone, frequently displacing the orbital globe. Treatment involves marsupialization of the mucocele cavity, with establishment of drainage into the surrounding sinonasal cavity.

STREPTOCOCCAL PHARYNGITIS

method of
RICHARD B. BROWN, M.D., and
JOSEPH I. HARWELL, M.D.
Baystate Medical Center
Springfield, Massachusetts
Tufts University School of Medicine
Boston, Massachusetts

Pharyngitis is one of the most common reasons why people seek medical care. However, it must be remembered that pharyngitis is merely a symptom, and the vast majority of sore throats are attributable to viruses. Even during the peak season for streptococcal pharyngitis (late fall through early spring), only 40% of children and 10% of adolescents and adults with clinical pharyngitis will be infected with this organism. With nearly two thirds of all office visits for upper respiratory infections, bronchitis, and colds resulting in the prescription of antibiotics, which in turn accounts for one fifth of all antibiotics prescribed in the United States, it is no wonder antibiotic resistance has become a major contributor to infectious morbidity and mortality. On the other hand, prompt initiation of antibiotic therapy can shorten the duration of symptoms and prevent the development of suppurative and nonsuppurative complications from pharyngitis caused by group A beta-hemolytic streptococci (GABHS). Appropriate diagnosis and treatment in this circumstance cannot be overemphasized.

Diagnosis and treatment of GABHS pharyngitis poses a number of dilemmas. Clinical findings are nonspecific, and laboratory data must be interpreted in context. As emphasized, there are risks both from over- and undertreatment. In addition, even with correct diagnosis and treatment, 10% of patients experience a relapse. This article reviews the epidemiology and microbiology of GABHS pharyngitis as well as current recommendations for diagnosis and treatment.

EPIDEMIOLOGY

Although household pets were at one time considered a possible reservoir for GABHS, this theory has not been substantiated and humans are considered the primary hosts. There is an approximately 15 to 20% asymptomatic carriage rate for the organism among school-aged children, who represent the group with the largest burden of acute disease. Pharyngitis is rare in children younger than 5 but an inflammatory nasal equivalent is seen in infants and toddlers, which has been referred to as "strep nose." The combination of improved hygiene and less school cohorting along with some immune maturation results in a lower incidence of active disease among adults.

Peak incidence occurs in the cold months with sporadic cases occurring throughout the year. Seasonal variability is probably related to social factors rather than microbiologic ones. During the winter months, carriers come into closer contact during school and other indoor activities. Most infections result from direct person-to-person contact with some infections probably caused by aerosolized respiratory droplets. Outbreaks among family members and schoolmates is common, and identification of index case contacts can help with diagnosis. Acutely ill patients should be considered infectious until completing 24 hours of antibiotic therapy. Carriers remain infectious longer, and reinfection from an asymptomatic family member is possible following otherwise adequate therapy.

MICROBIOLOGY

Streptococcus pyogenes is a gram-positive coccus that appears in chains on Gram's stain. When plated on blood agar it produces an area of clear (beta) hemolysis around each colony. A bacitracin disk produces a zone of inhibition helping to differentiate group A from other beta-hemolytic streptococci. Latex agglutination testing establishes Lancefield grouping of other streptococci.

Although associated with significant morbidity, GABHS is an uncommon cause of pharyngitis. Viral agents are responsible for the majority of cases of this illness. Table 1 presents a list of important organisms capable of producing acute pharyngitis. With the ongoing development of antiviral agents, it may become equally important to identify syndromes associated with these pathogens. As an example, acute retroviral syndrome may present with fever, adenopathy, and pharyngitis. Early recognition and treatment of human immunodeficiency virus (HIV) infection has a significant impact on long-term health. In the acute setting, HIV infection is associated with high levels of viremia with a negative antibody — the traditional diagnostic test for this infection. We would urge testing for HIV RNA in any patient with pharyngitis and risk factors. Other viral agents associated with significant morbidity include influenza virus, Epstein-Barr virus, cytomegalovirus, coxsackievirus, and herpes simplex virus.

Bacterial causes of pharyngitis have received more attention because of the availability of effective therapy for these organisms. Following GABHS, *Haemophilus influenzae* is a common cause of bacterial pharyngitis in all age groups, although the introduction of a type B vaccine has significantly reduced the number of cases among children as well as adults through herd immunity. *Moraxella catarrhalis* is emerging as an important upper respiratory pathogen, which along with *H. influenzae* and *Staphylococcus aureus*, can cause bacterial tracheitis presenting as a sore throat. These same organisms can cause sinusitis that presents with GABHS pharyngitis-like symptoms. *Neisseria gonorrhoeae* is an important cause of pharyngitis as a consequence of oral genital sex, again emphasizing the importance of a sexual history. This pathogen requires special culture collection and conditions. Other organisms to consider include *Mycoplasma* and *Chlamydia*, which are difficult to diagnose using standard laboratory techniques and require a high level of clinical suspicion. Different Lancefield group streptococci are responsible for sporadic cases of pharyngitis.

In the immunocompromised host opportunistic organisms may be implicated. Neutropenia itself can cause significant dysphagia in individuals who have received marrow-toxic drugs. Vasculitis syndromes such as Kawasaki disease and lupus erythematosus can usually be excluded through history and physical examination.

TABLE 1. **Differential Diagnosis of Streptococcal Pharyngitis (*S. pyogenes*)**

Common	Less Common
Epstein-Barr virus	*Corynebacterium hemolyticum*
Neisseria gonorrhoeae	*Yersinia enterocolitica*
Adenovirus, common cold viruses, coxsackievirus	*Corynebacterium diphtheriae*
Mycoplasma hominis	*Francisella tularensis*
Vincent's angina	Other "groupable" streptococci
Haemophilus influenzae	Acute retroviral syndrome

CLINICAL PRESENTATION

In a population with low prevalence, even experienced physicians overestimate the probability of positive throat cultures up to 80% of the time. The American Academy of Pediatrics recommends that additional microbiologic testing be done in patients suspected of having GABHS pharyngitis. The history and physical examination are sensitive for identifying patients unlikely to have GABHS pharyngitis, however. Clinical findings of rhinorrhea, conjunctivitis, cough, and diarrhea exclude the diagnosis of streptococcal pharyngitis, although they may be clues to other treatable infections. The urge to do further testing for GABHS in these individuals should be stifled so as to limit the identification and unnecessary treatment of incidental carriers.

Signs and symptoms most commonly associated with streptococcal pharyngitis include acute onset of high fever, tonsillar exudates, anterior cervical adenopathy, and headache. Children are also likely to have abdominal pain. Fairly specific for group A streptococcal infection in the setting of pharyngitis are the scarlet fever findings of palatal petechiae, strawberry tongue, sandpaper rash (with later desquamation), and reddened lines at skin folds (Pastia's lines).

DIAGNOSIS

Although clinical findings are not sufficient to make the diagnosis of GABHS pharyngitis, they are useful in deciding whether further testing is needed. There are a variety of rapid antigen detection systems with sufficiently high specificity to base treatment on a positive result in the right clinical setting. With most, however, the sensitivity is not reproducibly high enough to obviate backup culture with negative results. New optical immunoassays in some users' hands are approaching or exceeding the sensitivity of culture, sparking debate over the usefulness and cost effectiveness of the backup culture approach. Recent studies demonstrate this high sensitivity but also the interoperator variability of these tests. The time is approaching when greater experience with these tests will result in more standardized techniques and refined technology, such that routine backup culture may not be needed. Ever-increasing sensitivity of microbiologic testing, at times to a degree capable of detecting a single organism's nucleic acid, is not without drawbacks. Specimen contamination or detection of clinically insignificant organisms will make interpretation of these modern test results more difficult.

Our preference is to utilize the "low-tech" technique of Gram's stain and culture. An adequately collected swab of a tonsillar exudate demonstrating gram-positive cocci in chains and acute inflammatory cells is a quick, sensitive, and inexpensive way to diagnose streptococcal disease. Backup culture in this circumstance is recommended, but treatment can be delayed until the results are available. This approach avoids the possibility of missing pharyngitis caused by non–group A streptococci, which have been reported to cause nonsuppurative complications such as glomerulonephritis. Other potential causes for pharyngitis can similarly be detected on Gram's stain that would otherwise be missed by routine strep screens (*N. gonorrhoeae, H. influenzae, Corynebacterium diphtheriae*). In these days of increasing antibiotic resistance and virulent organism outbreaks, there is something to be said for having the organism on hand to do strain typing and sensitivities. Certainly in the case of treatment failures, cultures should be obtained and antibiotic sensitivities requested.

Antistreptolysin-O (ASO) serologic testing is quite specific and reasonably sensitive for past pharyngeal GABHS infections with no rise in titers following skin infections. The ASO tends to rise about a week after infection and peaks in 2 to 4 weeks. Prompt antibiotic therapy blunts this rise. If there are no complications or reinfections, the ASO titer falls to baseline in 6 to 12 months. Because of the late rise in titer, this test has little role in diagnosing acute infections and is used only to document a previous untreated GABHS infection. The goal of prompt antibiotic treatment is to prevent this rise in antibodies associated with the development of rheumatic fever. For these reasons, ASO titers are used for the diagnosis of rheumatic fever but not acute GABHS pharyngitis.

TREATMENT

Standard therapy for GABHS pharyngitis remains penicillin, which when taken reliably for the recommended length of time, will almost always eradicate the infection. Table 2 summarizes major treatment options. The most important criterion for successful therapy is adherence to dosing schedule: early discontinuation of medication is the leading cause of treatment failure. Longer dosing intervals improve compliance, and selected data support this approach. Some authors advocate the use of higher doses given twice daily. Single-dose benzathine penicillin eliminates the problem of compliance and is favored in outbreak situations and in penicillin-experienced patients for whom adherence to strict dosing is not practical or possible. This form of treatment may be more sensitizing and is associated with pain at the injection site. For children, amoxicillin is a reasonable alternative because it is available in a tasty suspension.

Cephalosporins are effective in eradicating GABHS but are generally more expensive and have an unnecessarily broad spectrum. Their use may occasionally be appropriate in the patient in whom treatment failure may be associated with β-lactamase–producing pathogens that inactivate penicillin. Some studies have shown efficacy with shorter courses (4 to 6 days) of long-acting second-generation cephalosporins. Although increased patient adherence to cephalosporin regimens may eventually outweigh financial considerations, the potential for generating resistance remains a very real concern.

For the penicillin-allergic patient, erythromycin has been the traditional alternative. There are more treatment failures with this drug, however, and side effects are considerable. Failure may be the result of poor adherence because of side effects, although macrolides tend to have lower blood and extracellular concentrations than β-lactams and thus may be prone to fail on a pharmacokinetic basis as well. Erythromycin is so poorly tolerated that it has been eliminated from the latest list of recommended alternatives for endocarditis prophylaxis in favor of newer macrolides and azalides. We favor a similar recommendation for the treatment of GABHS pharyngitis and suggest the use of the better tolerated azithromycin (Zithromax), or clarithromycin (Biaxin), requiring daily to twice-daily dosing, respectively. Although these drugs are considerably more expensive than erythromycin, the cost may be offset by a decrease in retreatment and complication costs resulting from drug failure.

Clindamycin (Cleocin), is another attractive penicillin alternative. The ribosomal target of clindamycin accounts for its bacteriostatic activity, which in scarlet fever has the added benefit of quickly shutting down toxin production. Clindamycin is comparable in cost to clarithromycin.

In all cases, the patient should be counseled to complete the full course of prescribed therapy to minimize relapses and complications. Incomplete therapy also facilitates antimicrobial resistance. Antibiotics to avoid include tetracyclines and trimethoprim-sulfamethoxazole because of unacceptably high failure rates. Nonpharmacologic treatment for symptom relief includes appropriate hydration and analgesia.

Special Considerations

Recurrences pose a major problem for treating physicians. The most common explanation for relapse

TABLE 2. **Antibiotic Therapy of GABHS Pharyngitis**

Drug	Dose Adult or Child (>40 kg)	Dose Child (<40 kg)	Duration*
Penicillin V (Pen-Vee K)	1000 mg bid	25–50 mg/kg/d bid	10 d
Amoxicillin (Amoxil)	500 mg tid	20–40 mg/kg/d tid	10 d
Benzathine penicillin (Bicillin)	1.2 mμ IM	25,000 μ/kg IM up to 1.2 mμ	Single dose (levels present for 2–4 wk)
Cephalexin (Keflex)	500 mg tid	25–50 mg/kg/d tid	10 d
Cefadroxil (Duricef)	1 gm qd	30 mg/kg/d qd	5–10 d*
Cefuroxime axetil (Ceftin)	250 mg bid	20 mg/kg/d bid	4–10 d*
Cefpodoxime proxetil (Vantin)	100 mg bid	10 mg/kg/d bid	5–10 d*
Azithromycin (Zithromax)	500 mg qd on d 1, 250 mg qd on d 2–5	12 mg/kg/d qd	5 d
Clarithromycin (Biaxin)	500 mg bid	15 mg/kg/d bid	10 d
Erythromycin estolate (Ilosone)	500 mg bid	40 mg/kg/d bid	10 d
Clindamycin (Cleocin)	150 mg tid	20 mg/kg/d tid	10 d

*With the exception of azithromycin, treatment for less than 10 days does not have FDA approval.

immediately following treatment is medical nonadherence. A significant number of patients report discontinuing therapy on resolution of symptoms, which can occur within the first 5 days of treatment. Standard oral regimens with penicillin do not effect microbiologic cure if taken for less than 10 days. Recent studies have also documented persistence of organisms on toothbrushes and dental appliances. If tonsils are significantly enlarged and exudative, organisms may remain in areas of poor penetration. β-lactamase production by coexisting organisms has also been proposed as an explanation for penicillin failures. Reinfection by family members who are asymptomatic carriers accounts for some relapses. Lastly, consideration should be given to the possibility that symptoms are the result of another infection (viral, gonococcal, *Haemophilus*) and the patient is an asymptomatic GABHS carrier. History and physical data can help in identifying these co-infections.

If compliance is the major issue, a single dose of intramuscular penicillin is usually the best course. Alternatively, a 4-day course of cefuroxime axetil (Ceftin), can improve compliance and prevent local β-lactamase production. Cephalexin is a cheap cephalosporin with similar β-lactamase resistance, but it must be taken three to four times daily for at least 10 days. Deeply sequestered organisms can require a prolonged course of treatment (2 to 3 weeks). In the outbreak situation, particularly with more virulent strains, culture of contacts and treatment of all carriers is an appropriate approach. Universal treatment is otherwise not indicated except in special circumstances. Cultures following completion of therapy are not recommended unless symptomatic relapse has occurred.

TUBERCULOSIS AND OTHER MYCOBACTERIAL DISEASES

method of
MICHAEL E. KIMERLING, M.D., M.P.H., and
NANCY E. DUNLAP, M.D., PH.D.
University of Alabama at Birmingham
Birmingham, Alabama

TUBERCULOSIS

Epidemiology

Tuberculosis (TB) is today the most common infectious cause of avoidable adult deaths in the world, accounting for 26% of such deaths in developing countries. In 1993, the World Health Organization (WHO) declared tuberculosis a "global emergency" and noted that one in three persons worldwide is infected with the *Mycobacterium tuberculosis* (MTB) organism. The WHO estimates that there are more than 10 million new cases annually, with 3 million deaths—more than those due to acquired immune deficiency syndrome (AIDS) and malaria combined. Globally, there has been a merging of the TB and human immunodeficiency virus (HIV) epidemics, complicated by rising rates of multidrug-resistant TB (MDR TB). In the United States, the impact of this epidemic is evident. In 1996, foreign-born persons, predominantly from high-prevalence countries, accounted for 37% of the 21,337 TB cases reported to the Centers for Disease Control and Prevention (CDC). While the TB upsurge over the past decade in the United States has gradually subsided, the basic challenges to control efforts continue to evolve. Primary among these is the maintenance of an adequate public health infrastructure in light of rising rates of poverty, homelessness and drug abuse, increasing globalization, and a rapidly changing health care delivery system. The observed epidemiologic shift toward hard-to-reach populations remains a key future challenge to ensuring the detection of cases as well as the initiation of and adherence to adequate antituberculosis therapy.

Diagnosis

The diagnosis of tuberculosis starts with its inclusion in the differential diagnosis based on the patient's complaints. It is made by sequential consideration of clinical symptoms, history of possible exposure (remote or recent), presence of certain risk factors, and results of purified protein derivative (PPD) skin testing and radiographic evaluation. Ultimately, sputum, tissue, or fluid smears must be examined for the presence of acid-fast bacilli (AFB), followed by culture confirmation.

Symptoms of Disease and Exposure History

The most common symptoms of TB disease are nonspecific but important to elicit if present: chronic productive cough of 2 to 3 weeks' duration (unresponsive to routine antibiotics), fever (usually low-grade), night sweats, chest pain with or without a pleuritic component, hemoptysis, weight loss, and fatigue. Although uncommon, hoarseness is suggestive of laryngeal TB, which is considered the most infectious form of the disease. Exposure history may be either remote (the patient may have a parent, grandparent, or other relative with a history of disease in the distant past) or recent, occurring within 2 years. Among the recent exposure possibilities are many that overlap with certain risk factors: residence in a long-term care facility, homelessness with use of shelters, incarceration or imprisonment, and chronic alcohol and substance abuse. Foreign-born persons from high-prevalence countries, especially those who have recently immigrated (within 5 years) or others who have resided in such places, should also be considered. Short periods of exposure are less likely to result in infection or subsequent development of disease.

At-Risk Groups and Purified Protein Derivative Status

Patients should be evaluated for both inclusion in a high-risk group and PPD status. Considerations in risk evaluation include age and coexisting medical conditions, in addition to the exposure history noted previously. Age-specific risk groups include persons under 4 years or over 60. Important comorbid conditions include diabetes mellitus, end-stage renal disease, head and neck cancer, hematologic and reticuloendothelial diseases, intestinal bypass or gastrectomy, prolonged corticosteroid use, and immunosuppressive therapy. The highest known risks associated with TB disease progression are HIV disease and AIDS. Persons with these conditions have an annual risk of developing disease nearly equal to the lifetime risk of a non-immunocompromised person (approximately 10%). High-risk institutional settings include nursing homes, correctional facilities, homeless shelters, drug treatment centers, and other locations in which intravenous drug users and HIV-infected persons may congregate.

The Mantoux skin test is administered by intradermal injection of 0.1 mL of PPD (containing 5 tuberculin units of PPD). Induration is measured in millimeters at 48 to 72 hours after PPD injection, using the transverse diameter. Surrounding erythema should be ignored in this measurement. Determining whether a reaction is significant (positive) or not is determined by the risk group of the person tested (Table 1). It is important to realize that a negative reaction does not rule out infection or disease. Overwhelming severity of disease such as seen in miliary infection or with severe weight loss/malnutrition may cause a false-negative result. Concurrent immunosuppression, HIV disease, sarcoidosis, overwhelming viral infection, and live-virus vaccination are other sources of a negative result on PPD skin testing when true MTB infection is present. A result may also initially be negative if the test is performed before the 10 to 12 weeks usually required for the host immune system to generate an appropriate response once infection occurs. Among elderly, in whom immune function may be diminished, a previously infected person may initially have a negative result but upon retesting 2 to 3 weeks later have a positive result. This "boosting" phenomenon is the basis for the two-step testing used in nursing homes when a new client is admitted. This approach ensures that a future "positive" test is not mistakenly considered a "recent" conversion that necessitates preventive therapy. Neither the CDC nor the American Thoracic Society (ATS) currently advocates anergy testing. It is not considered a sensitive test of immune function and increases confusion regarding interpretation of the PPD test.

On the other hand, false-positive results on PPD testing may be seen in regions where environmental mycobacteria are common or among persons with a history of bacille Calmette-Guérin (BCG) vaccination (mostly foreign-born persons). These cross-reactions generally result in smaller areas of induration than those found with true MTB infection; however, such findings constitute yet another potential cause of confusion in standard PPD test interpretation. In general, evaluation of skin test results should not take the patient's BCG status into consideration.

Chest Radiography

Chest radiography alone is never diagnostic of TB; however, it is useful for ruling out pulmonary disease in persons with a positive PPD reaction. Although apical disease with or without cavitation is typical of reactivated TB, primary TB may present as adenopathy, infiltrate, cavitation, pleural effusion, a miliary pattern, or even a solitary pulmonary nodule. Immunosuppression from any cause may be associated with atypical chest radiographic patterns and findings. No person with a positive result on PPD skin testing should be placed on preventive therapy until

TABLE 1. **Definition of Positive Result on PPD Skin Testing by Risk Factors and Lesion Diameter**

Risk Factors/Groups Signifying Positive Result with Specific Lesion Diameter*		
≥5 mm Induration	*≥10 mm Induration*	*≥15 mm Induration*
• Recent contact with a TB case • HIV infection • Immunosuppression • Abnormal chest radiograph consistent with prior TB • IVDA if HIV status unknown	• Foreign-born persons from high-prevalence countries • IVDA if HIV-negative • Age >60 y or <4 y • Residents of correctional institutions or nursing homes • Low-income, high-prevalence groups (homeless, migrant workers) • Nursing home and hospital employees • Mycobacteriology laboratory workers • Predisposing medical conditions Diabetes Corticosteroid therapy Post gastrectomy Silicosis	• General population, age ≥4 y (no known risk factors)

*Definition is based on the presence of any single risk factor or group.
Abbreviations: HIV = human immunodeficiency virus; IVDA = intravenous drug abuse; TB = tuberculosis.

a chest radiograph has been performed and active disease appropriately ruled out.

Clinical Specimens for Mycobacterium tuberculosis *Culture*

Owing to the lack of a single diagnostic test or method and the frequent complexity of the clinical scenarios, a definitive diagnosis depends upon visualization and isolation of the TB-causing organism from clinical specimens. A minimum of three sputum specimens obtained on three separate days should be collected from patients with suspected pulmonary TB. All specimens must be sent for AFB staining and mycobacterial culture. Although AFB staining is not a very sensitive test (requiring approximately 10,000 organisms per mL of stained material), this test is helpful in gauging a patient's infectiousness. Early-morning sputum specimens are generally preferable, and in some instances, it may be useful to induce sputum with saline inhalation. Bronchoscopy or gastric lavage may be required in patients unable to produce a clinical specimen. For suspected extrapulmonary disease, specimens collected directly from the suspected site are necessary for diagnosis: lymph node biopsy, cerebrospinal fluid, pleural tissue, and so on. Care should be taken to avoid placing any tissue specimen into formalin, which precludes subsequent culture possibilities. Results of smear for AFB should be available within 24 hours; use of concentration methods will improve smear sensitivity. Culture isolation with definitive species identification can take up to 8 weeks using solid culture media and 2 to 6 weeks by radiometric or nonradiometric liquid culture methods. Certain rapid methods, which are based on detecting unique DNA or RNA sequences in MTB organisms, are more sensitive and specific than AFB smears and take only hours to perform. However, these tests require a high level of laboratory quality control to prevent cross-contamination of samples and are thus more difficult and expensive to perform. These amplification tests are currently approved only for AFB smear–positive respiratory samples from patients who have not been on antituberculosis therapy for more than 7 days and have not been treated for TB within the past year. The sensitivity, specificity, and predictive value of the amplification tests are much lower in AFB-negative specimens, which significantly limits their clinical usefulness. Use of the amplification methods does not eliminate the need to submit all specimens for culture of MTB.

Management

Once a patient with suspected tuberculosis is identified and clinical specimens are collected, appropriate multidrug therapy should be started. Bacteriologic results are not required before initiation of such treatment. It is important that the local health department be informed of all suspected cases as soon as possible. Health department personnel will then conduct a contact investigation around the suspected case in order to identify other cases and to perform PPD skin testing where required. The health department may also have prior records for the patient that can help guide current management.

Directly Observed Therapy

Administration of multiple drugs will rapidly decrease the body's bacterial burden of disease and thus render the patient noninfectious sooner than if he or she took any single drug. In this way, the cycle of transmission is broken and the possibility of further spread to others not yet infected is stopped. Administration of multiple drugs simultaneously will also prevent the emergence of drug resistance, which can occur with all known antituberculosis medications. To further prevent the emergence of MDR TB, with the recognition that patient nonadherence with long-term therapy is common, directly observed therapy (DOT) is the established standard of care for treating both TB cases and suspects. Normally, DOT is administered by health department personnel in cooperation with private or public health physicians. The DOT approach also allows for continued evaluation of the patient, with frequent assessment for side effects to medications, clinical response to therapy, and necessary bacteriologic and radiographic follow-up studies. When DOT is not possible, the use of fixed-dose combination tablets containing both isoniazid (INH) and rifampin (RIF), or INH, RIF, and pyrazinamide (PZA), should be considered.

Specific Antituberculosis Agents

Five first-line antituberculosis medications are used in standard treatment regimens (Table 2): INH, RIF, PZA, ethambutol (EMB), and streptomycin (SM). Each drug is associated with potentially important adverse effects for which the patient should be monitored accordingly (Table 3). Baseline laboratory tests should include measurement of hepatic enzymes and total bilirubin, complete blood count with platelets, and determination of serum uric acid and creatinine levels. Patients should be clinically monitored regularly for the presence of adverse drug reactions, at least monthly. Patients taking ethambutol need regular assessment of their visual acuity and red-green color perception, while patients receiving streptomycin require hearing testing. Any change in a patient's visual or hearing abilities requires the immediate discontinuation of the offending drug until more thorough testing can be completed.

The goal of TB treatment is to cure every patient. The population of MTB organisms causing disease is a mixed one. Some are continually active growers (extracellular organisms), some grow best in a low-pH environment (intracellular bacilli and those in necrotic tissue), and some have the ability to lie dormant with only periodic spurts of active growth. Recognition of this heterogeneity underscores the importance of standardized multidrug regimens of long duration in order to prevent treatment failure and disease relapse.

Isoniazid. INH is the most important antituberculosis

TABLE 2. **Dosage Recommendations for the Treatment of Tuberculosis in Children* and Adults**

Drug	Daily Dosage		Twice-Weekly Dosage	
	Children	*Adults*	*Children*	*Adults*
Isoniazid	10–20 mg/kg Max. 300 mg	5 mg/kg Max. 300 mg	20–40 mg/kg Max. 900 mg	15 mg/kg Max. 900 mg
Rifampin	10–20 mg/kg Max. 600 mg	10 mg/kg Max. 600 mg	10–20 mg/kg Max. 600 mg	10 mg/kg Max. 600 mg
Pyrazinamide	15–30 mg/kg Max. 2 gm	15–30 mg/kg Max. 2 gm	50–70 mg/kg Max. 4 gm	50–70 mg/kg Max. 4 gm
Ethambutol†	15–25 mg/kg	15–25 mg/kg	50 mg/kg	50 mg/kg
Streptomycin	20–40 mg/kg Max. 1 gm	15 mg/kg Max. 1 gm	25–30 mg/kg Max. 1.5 gm	25–30 mg/kg Max. 1.5 gm
Ofloxacin‡		800 mg qd		
Ciprofloxacin‡		750 mg bid		

*Age of 12 years or less.
†Ethambutol is not recommended for children who are too young to be monitored for changes in vision (less than 8 years old). However, ethambutol should be considered for all children who have tuberculosis that is resistant to other drugs but susceptible to ethambutol. Quinolones (ofloxacin and ciprofloxacin) are not recommended for children or during pregnancy. Also, twice-weekly dosages have not been defined.
‡Not FDA approved for this indication.
Abbreviation: Max. = maximum dose.
From American Thoracic Society: Treatment of tuberculosis and tuberculosis infection in adults and children. Am J Respir Crit Care Med 149:1368, 1994.

losis drug. It is highly bactericidal, inexpensive, and easy to administer, on either a daily or twice- or thrice-weekly schedule. Absorption from the gastrointestinal tract is nearly complete, with good penetration into all body fluids and cavities. It is metabolized in the liver. The most toxic reaction is hepatitis, which increases with both age and frequent alcohol consumption. Peripheral neuropathy, associated with interference in pyridoxine metabolism, is another potential problem, found most commonly in malnourished persons and during pregnancy. Although neuropathy is uncommon at a dose of 5 mg per kg, pyridoxine (10 mg orally per day) should be given to those at risk and to those with conditions that

TABLE 3. **Adverse Reactions and Recommended Monitoring for Antituberculosis Medications**

Drug	Common Adverse Reactions	Signs and Symptoms	Recommended Regular Monitoring
Isoniazid	Abnormal results for liver function testing; hepatitis; peripheral neuropathy and other neurologic effects; drug interactions; rash	Nausea, vomiting, abdominal pain, fatigue, dark urine, tingling sensations in hands and feet	Liver function tests if baseline results are abnormal or if symptoms of adverse reactions occur (see text)
Rifampin	Orange discoloration of the urine and other body fluids; drug interactions; hepatitis; bleeding problems due to thrombocytopenia	Nausea, vomiting, abdominal pain, fatigue, dark urine, flu-like symptoms, weakness	Liver function tests if baseline results are abnormal or if symptoms of adverse reactions occur
Pyrazinamide	Abnormal results on liver function testing; rash; gout	Stomach upset, joint aches	Liver function tests if baseline results are abnormal or if symptoms of adverse reactions occur; measurement of uric acid level if joint symptoms occur
Ethambutol	Damage to optic nerve; elevation of uric acid	Changes in vision and color vision, joint aches	Monthly vision testing
Streptomycin	Damage to nerves of ear; abnormal kidney function	Hearing loss, balance problems	Hearing tests and kidney function tests
Quinolones (e.g., ofloxacin, ciprofloxacin)	Gastrointestinal upset is most common; hypersensitivity and mild central nervous system reactions have been reported		
Rifabutin	Uveitis; gastrointestinal upset, neutropenia, thrombocytopenia; arthralgia		

predispose to neuropathic complications (e.g., diabetes, uremia, alcoholism). Allergic skin reactions with fever may be seen as well as mild central nervous system effects. Potential drug-drug interactions are important and require more careful monitoring of levels. INH will increase levels of phenytoin, benzodiazepines, and oral anticoagulants while decreasing levels of ketoconazole.

Rifampin. RIF is also bactericidal for MTB and a potent drug. It is easily administered orally but somewhat less well absorbed than INH. Food can interfere with absorption. Penetration into cerebrospinal fluid (CSF) is adequate when the meninges are inflamed. RIF is metabolized in the liver, where it induces the cytochrome P-450 system, thereby reducing the effectiveness of many agents. Specifically, it interferes with the metabolism of protease inhibitors (PIs) and significantly reduces their levels. It has a similar effect on oral contraceptives, warfarin sodium, corticosteroids, theophyllines, phenytoin, methadone, beta-adrenergic blockers, itraconazole, fluconazole, and cyclosporine. RIF colors body fluids orange and may permanently discolor soft contact lenses. The principal adverse reactions are gastrointestinal upset, rash, and hepatitis. Rarely, thrombocytopenia, hemolytic anemia, and acute renal failure may occur, especially with intermittent therapy using higher-than-recommended dosages. Intermittent therapy may also be associated with an influenza-like syndrome, which may disappear when dosing is changed to a daily schedule. Dosing requirements are the same regardless of dosing frequency: 10 mg per kg up to a maximum dose of 600 mg. Rifabutin, a rifamycin derivative, is a potential substitute for RIF in HIV-infected TB patients receiving certain PIs. Its half-life is considerably longer than that of RIF, and dosage requirements are less when it is administered with a PI, which will raise serum rifabutin levels. Important toxic effects include leukopenia and uveitis, the latter occurring when the drug is given with clarithromycin. Use of rifabutin and a PI requires careful consultation and coordination between TB and HIV care providers.

Pyrazinamide. PZA is bactericidal for MTB in an acid environment (inside macrophages) and is given orally. It is well absorbed and penetrates into most tissues, including the CSF. Although metabolized in the kidney, its most important toxic effect is hepatitis. Skin rash and gastrointestinal upset may also occur. Owing to the inhibition of renal secretion of uric acid, hyperuricemia is common, occasionally accompanied by arthralgia. Acute gout, however, is uncommon. If gout occurs, the drug should be stopped; otherwise, nonsteroidal anti-inflammatory agents may be used for symptomatic relief. PZA is most important early in therapy and allows for a decrease in the length of chemotherapy (in combination with INH and RIF).

Ethambutol. EMB in usual doses is considered bacteriostatic for MTB. At the higher twice-weekly dose, it may be bactericidal. The drug is administered orally, well absorbed, and generally well tolerated. Penetration into the CSF is suboptimal. EMB is excreted by the kidneys and accumulates in persons with severe renal insufficiency. Therefore, the dose must be decreased in renal failure (by 50% with a glomerular filtration rate of less than 10 mL per minute). The major toxic effect is dose-related optic neuritis, which is rare with a dose of 15 mg per kg. Early symptoms include blurred vision, central scotomata, and problems with red-green color discrimination. Visual symptoms commonly precede a measurable decrease in visual acuity. Therefore, use of this drug in young children depends upon the ability to monitor changes in vision.

Streptomycin. SM is bactericidal in an alkaline environment and must be given parenterally. It has good tissue penetration but enters the CSF only in the presence of meningeal inflammation. It is an aminoglycoside and metabolized in the kidneys. As with other aminoglycosides, renal toxicity and ototoxicity (vertigo, hearing loss) can occur and are related to both the cumulative dose and peak serum concentrations. The dose should be reduced in elderly patients (age older than 60 years) and those with renal failure. A total cumulative dose above 120 grams should be avoided if possible. SM can be given two or three times weekly.

Preventive Therapy

Preventive therapy for persons with MTB infection is used to prevent progression to active disease and is considered to be 54 to 88% effective. In persons with a positive result on PPD skin testing, it is essential to rule out active disease before commencing such therapy. Otherwise, a standard regimen of monotherapy will be used, greatly increasing the chance of development of subsequent acquired drug resistance.

Isoniazid is the drug of choice for preventive therapy. If INH resistance is suspected, then rifampin may be used. The best choice of drugs for exposure to MDR TB is dependent on the resistance pattern of the infecting organism in the source case and should be made only after consultation with a TB expert.

INH may be given daily or twice or three times weekly. Adults should be treated for 6 consecutive months, HIV-infected persons for 12 months, and children for at least 6 months. Persons with silicosis or large fibrotic lesions on the chest radiograph consistent with old, untreated TB can be given either (1) 4 months of INH plus RIF or (2) 12 months of INH. Directly observed preventive therapy (DOPT) may be used for at-risk adults and children in whom reliable self-administration is unlikely. Pregnancy is not a contraindication to preventive therapy with INH when risk factors for progression to disease are present. Otherwise, therapy may be delayed until after delivery. All persons receiving preventive therapy should be questioned at monthly intervals about symptoms of adverse reactions. For persons 35 years and older, baseline hepatic enzymes are recommended followed by monthly monitoring. Those with other risk factors for hepatitis should also be closely followed.

Treatment of Tuberculosis Disease

The basis for modern "short-course" chemotherapy is that TB disease must be initially treated with multiple drugs to which the organism is susceptible. Normally, four drugs are recommended: INH, RIF, PZA, and EMB or SM. When there is little possibility of drug resistance (i.e., the rate of primary INH resistance in the community is less than 4%, and the patient has no prior history of taking TB medications and is not likely to have been exposed to a drug-resistant case), a three-drug regimen can be used: INH, RIF, and PZA. Treatment regimens generally consist of a 2-month intensive phase followed by a 4-month consolidation phase in which the patient is often asymptomatic (6 months total treatment). Duration of treatment for TB in an HIV-infected person is the same as for a person not infected with HIV. In the setting of MDR TB (involving resistance to INH and RIF), however, treatment must be individualized according to results of drug susceptibility testing. A minimum of three drugs should be used to treat MDR TB, and often up to five or six drugs may be employed. Such treatment is difficult and of long duration owing to increased drug toxicities and the use of second-line agents. DOT should be considered for all cases of tuberculosis and is essential for MDR TB cases. Intermittent drug regimens are easier to supervise; one of the following regimens can be used:

1. INH plus RIF plus PZA (plus EMB or SM) given daily for 8 weeks followed by twice- or thrice-weekly doses of INH plus RIF for an additional 16 weeks
2. INH plus RIF plus PZA (plus EMB or SM) given daily for 2 weeks (14 days) followed by the same drugs in twice- or thrice-weekly doses for another 6 weeks; then INH plus RIF, twice or three times weekly, for an additional 16 weeks
3. INH plus RIF plus PZA (plus EMB or SM) given three times weekly throughout the entire 6-month period

For patients who are unable to tolerate PZA, a 9-month regimen with INH plus RIF is effective. EMB or SM should initially be added to this regimen until drug susceptibility results are known.

Treatment of extrapulmonary TB generally follows that for pulmonary disease. Important exceptions include miliary, meningeal, and bone and joint disease in children. Such cases require a minimum of 12 months of therapy. Neither SM nor PZA should be used during pregnancy; however, lactating mothers do not have to stop breast-feeding while receiving standard antituberculosis medications (INH, RIF). Normally, patients should have negative results on smear and culture after 12 weeks of adequate therapy. If smear and culture results remain positive or the patient is symptomatic, it is important to ensure that the patient is taking the prescribed medicines. Drug susceptibilities should be rechecked and a TB medical expert consulted. Serum drug levels may be useful. A single drug should never be added to a failing drug regimen.

NONTUBERCULOUS MYCOBACTERIAL INFECTIONS

Infections with the nontuberculous mycobacteria (NTM) have taken on greater significance recently and are closely associated with advanced HIV disease, immunosuppressive therapy, and chronic lung disease. Chronic pulmonary disease is the most common localized clinical manifestation of NTM infection. Most NTM organisms have been isolated from natural water and soil. Both *Mycobacterium avium* complex and *Mycobacterium kansasii* are present in tap water, the former most commonly found in the Southeast. Despite a geographic predilection for NTM infection in the United States as shown by skin test reactivity, none appears to exist for disseminated disease. Infection by human-to-human contact is considered rare.

Diagnosis of NTM infection is by culture. However, it is difficult to distinguish "colonization" from disease. A positive result on PPD skin testing (5 to 10 mm of induration) may occur owing to cross-reactivity between NTM and MTB organisms. Chest radiographs of patients with NTM disease can be similar to those of patients with MTB disease. Since NTM organisms are also acid-fast bacilli indistinguishable from MTB organisms on smear, symptomatic patients should receive antituberculosis medications until species identification is made. Rapid broth culture systems in addition to rapid methods for species identification, such as commercial DNA probes, have greatly enhanced recovery and identification rates of NTM organisms, with results obtained within 1 to 4 weeks.

Mycobacterium avium Complex Infection

M. avium complex (MAC) causes disease in the lung, skin, and soft tissues. In HIV-negative patients, MAC lung disease is unpredictable. In some cases a stable clinical and radiographic pattern is maintained for years, while other cases rapidly progress with development of apical fibrocavitary lung disease (often occurring in middle-aged men with a history of heavy cigarette and alcohol use). The other primary presentation (often in elderly nonsmoking women) is nodular bronchiectasis, best seen on high-resolution computed tomography, and follows an intermediate course. Disseminated MAC disease in patients without AIDS usually presents as fever of unknown origin. In AIDS patients, it is very rare with $CD4^+$ cell counts higher than 100 and should be strongly considered in any person with fewer than 50 $CD4^+$ cells who has a history of fever, weight loss, anemia, diarrhea, or elevated alkaline phosphatase. Diagnosis of disseminated disease is best confirmed by isolation of *M. avium* in blood. Bacteremia is ongoing, and a single culture has a sensitivity of 90%. Diagnosis can also be made from culture of the bone marrow or a skin biopsy in the setting of multiple skin lesions.

Treatment of MAC pulmonary disease in the immunocompetent host should include daily clarithromycin or azithromycin, rifampin or rifabutin, and ethambutol. Streptomycin, twice or three times weekly, can be given during the first 8 weeks as tolerated. Treatment should be continued until the patient has negative results on culture for 1 year. Treatment of disseminated disease should include daily clarithromycin (Biaxin) or azithromycin (Zithromax), plus ethambutol (Myambutol). The addition of rifabutin also needs strong consideration, but use of this agent must be managed carefully in the patient taking a PI. Therapy should be continued for life until more data are available. Prophylaxis against disseminated MAC should be given to adults with AIDS and $CD4^+$ counts of fewer than 50 cells. Regimens include rifabutin, 300 mg per day; clarithromycin, 500 mg twice daily; and azithromycin, 1200 mg once weekly, plus or minus rifabutin, 300 mg per day. Treatment of NTM cervical lymphadenitis is primarily by surgical excision alone, with a 95% cure rate. A clarithromycin-containing regimen should be considered for patients with extensive disease or an inadequate response to surgery.

Mycobacterium kansasii Infection

M. kansasii is second only to MAC among NTM organisms as a cause of disease. It occurs in geographic clusters and affects primarily adult white males. Pulmonary disease with cavitary infiltrates is the most frequent clinical presentation; lymphadenitis and disseminated disease also occur, the latter usually associated with pulmonary findings. Clinically, infection is more closely related to *M. tuberculosis* than to NTM organisms. Treatment of pulmonary disease should include daily INH, RIF, and EMB (25 mg per kg for 2 months, then 15 mg per kg) for 18 months with a minimum of 12 months' culture negativity in adults. Clarithromycin or rifabutin should be substituted for RIF in HIV-infected patients receiving PIs. Treatment of *M. kansasii* infection is usually successful, and relapse is rare.

Other NTM Infections

M. fortuitum, M. abscessus, and *M. chelonae* are mycobacteria of rapidly increasing importance. Although resulting cutaneous disease is relatively common in the southeastern United States, these pathogens are also associated with wound infections, particularly following cardiac surgery or involving foreign bodies such as breast implants and percutaneous catheters, and pulmonary disease. Treatment is variable and depends on the clinical symptoms. Therapy for nonpulmonary disease should include drugs such as amikacin and clarithromycin, selected on the basis of in vitro susceptibility tests.

Section 4

The Cardiovascular System

ACQUIRED DISEASES OF THE AORTA

method of
RICHARD P. CAMBRIA, M.D.
Harvard Medical School and Massachusetts General Hospital
Boston, Massachusetts

Acquired diseases of the aorta generally are related to the sequelae of degenerative atherosclerosis; lesions related to trauma, aortic infection, and primary inflammatory diseases of the aorta are uncommon. Clinical problems referable to atherosclerosis include both occlusive disease, almost always centered on the aortic bifurcation and its primary iliac artery branches, and aneurysm formation with its potential for aneurysm rupture and death. Although there is considerable circumstantial evidence that at least in some patients, aneurysmal disease may have important genetic causative factors, most clinicians consider aortic aneurysm to be a sequelae of atherosclerosis. Because atherosclerosis accounts for the majority of acquired aortic pathology, patients presenting for treatment are typically older and frequently afflicted with other co-morbid conditions, especially coronary artery disease. Accordingly, the potential for complications during the course of treatment of aortic pathology, and the limitations on longevity imposed by concomitant coronary disease, are a constant in managing patients with aortic disease.

AORTOILIAC OCCLUSIVE DISEASE

Obstruction of the aorta related to atherosclerosis usually occurs in the context of combined aortic and iliac artery occlusive disease with its principal clinical manifestation being arterial insufficiency of the lower extremities. Association with atherosclerotic occlusive disease in other vascular territories is commonplace, and the risk factors for development of aortoiliac occlusive disease are those typically associated with vascular disease but with cigarette smoking being a nearly universal correlate. Certain patients with prominent risk factors, such as heavy cigarette smoking (particularly females) and familial hyperlipidemias, can develop clinically significant aortoiliac occlusive disease in the third and fourth decades of life, but the peak incidence occurs in older patients. Both the anatomic obstruction and its clinical manifestations tend to be gradually progressive, but acute thrombosis on pre-existent atherosclerotic disease can be one etiology of acute aortic occlusion.

Clinical syndromes related to aortoiliac occlusive disease include intermittent claudication, sexual dysfunction in males, and limb-threatening ischemia. The latter usually requires significant infrainguinal atherosclerosis to be present in conjunction with aortoiliac occlusive disease, whereas claudication alone can result from isolated aortoiliac occlusive disease. Whereas intermittent claudication can occasionally be confused with spinal pathology, the patient's history and a pulse examination combined with exercise-augmented lower extremity arterial noninvasive testing suffice to establish the diagnosis. Claudication alone is always a relative indication for intervention, and most patients tend to have long periods (years) of clinical stability. Furthermore, most patients will respond to a conservative regimen of risk factor control, particularly cessation of cigarette smoking, weight reduction, and a supervised exercise training program. A single pharmacologic agent, pentoxifylline (Trental) is approved for intermittent claudication. This hemorheologic agent is felt to improve microcirculatory flow, and several randomized placebo-controlled studies have shown increases in maximal walking distance for treated patients. However, this medication is relatively expensive, has significant gastrointestinal side effects, and in several studies has been demonstrated to improve symptoms in fewer than 25% of patients.

When intermittent claudication becomes truly disabling, interferes with work activities, or occurs in patients who are suitable candidates for intervention, effective symptom relief can be achieved by mechanical correction of the aortoiliac obstruction. There are two principal modes of intervention. Endovascular therapies include percutaneous balloon angioplasty, frequently augmented by endovascular stenting. Conventional surgical therapy, usually bypass grafting, remains the gold standard for the correction of aortoiliac occlusive disease but is, of course, a relatively invasive treatment. The choice among these various modes of intervention is anatomy driven, but co-morbidity frequently factors into the decision. More recently, these two therapeutic strategies have been joined in a single procedure in which open surgical access at the level of the femoral artery is combined with retrograde passage of stent-supported bypass grafts. With increasing experience with endovascular therapies, a wide variety of treatment options is now available for many patients with aortoiliac occlusive disease. The delineation of arterial anatomy with contrast arteriography while not necessary for diagnostic purposes, is mandatory in selecting a particular mode of therapy.

As a general rule, endovascular therapies produce results equivalent to those of surgical bypass when the disease is focal as opposed to diffuse and stenotic as opposed to totally occlusive. The more severe and extensive the occlusive process, the more likely that surgical reconstruction will be required. Surgical bypass from the unaffected aorta to both femoral arteries is a successful and durable form of therapy with 5-year primary patency rates in the 90% range. Historically, extra-anatomic bypass procedures (e.g., axillobifemoral bypass), which have the advantage of an extracavitary approach, have been plagued by significantly lower long-term success rates.

ACUTE AORTIC OCCLUSION

Acute aortic occlusion is a life-threatening surgical emergency because of the metabolic consequences of the large bulk of ischemic muscle, which in turn cause rapid cardiovascular and renal failure. There are four etiologies: aortic saddle embolism, acute thrombosis of a pre-existent abdominal aortic aneurysm (AAA), acute thrombosis superimposed on antecedent aortoiliac occlusive disease, and acute aortic dissection. The clinical presentation often involves collapse, weakness, and/or paralysis of the lower extremities, and diagnostic confusion with neurologic and central cardiovascular conditions is frequent. The key to the diagnosis is the absence of femoral pulses. Overall mortality is high and is related to delay in diagnosis and institution of appropriate therapy. Aortic saddle embolism is invariably cardiac in origin, and a typical history involves a recent transmural myocardial infarction with formation of cardiac mural thrombus and subsequent embolization. Retrograde catheter thrombectomy by a bilateral transfemoral route is simple and effective therapy. In the circumstance of thrombosed abdominal aneurysm or acute thrombosis on antecedent aortoiliac occlusive disease, rapid restoration of lower extremity and pelvic perfusion may be established by means of an extra-anatomic axillobifemoral bypass graft. Definitive therapy of an associated AAA is necessary at some point, as thrombosis of the iliac outflow of an abdominal aneurysm does not guarantee against rupture per se. Proximal propagation of thrombus so as to compromise renal and visceral vessels rarely occurs. Careful metabolic management in the operating room is mandatory to prevent the sequelae of reperfusion of a large bulk of muscle mass. Hyperkalemia, cardiac arrhythmias, and myoglobinuric renal failure are frequent causes of death, and appropriate methods to both anticipate and treat these sequelae are necessary for successful management.

AORTIC ANEURYSM

Although acute or remote trauma, infection, aortitis, and chronic dissection can all be potential etiologies of aortic aneurysm, the overwhelming majority are the sequelae of degenerative atherosclerosis. In some individuals, particularly when there is familial clustering of aneurysms, genetic factors are likely to be the principal etiology and atherosclerosis occurs as a secondary phenomenon. Aneurysms that occur as the sequelae of blunt or penetrating trauma are typically false aneurysms (i.e., not composed of all layers of the arterial wall). Once aneurysmal dilatation of the aorta begins, the expected natural history is that of progressive enlargement and eventual rupture if left untreated, although there is wide variability in the rate of aneurysm expansion. Data generated in the era before successful surgical management indicate a clear survival benefit for elective graft replacement of AAA as opposed to leaving the disease untreated. Virtually all natural history studies indicate that AAA size is the single most important correlate of risk of rupture, although other factors, including the presence of significant chronic obstructive pulmonary disease and uncontrolled diastolic hypertension, are known to increase the risk. The potential for rupture constitutes the rationale for treatment in the majority of aneurysm patients, although uncommon manifestations such as peripheral embolization can occur. In the circumstance of aneurysm of the ascending aorta, disruption of the aortic valvular apparatus may constitute a legitimate indication for intervention.

ABDOMINAL AORTIC ANEURYSM

The overwhelming majority of aortic aneurysms occur in the infrarenal aorta, and accordingly, AAA is the most frequently treated acquired pathology of the aorta. There are some 50,000 elective AAA operations carried out annually in the United States, representing a considerable expenditure of health care resources. In addition, some 15,000 operations for ruptured AAAs are also performed annually in the United States, at a far greater cost per patient and with significantly inferior results compared to surgery of intact AAA. The majority of AAAs cause no symptoms and are detected either on physical examination or as incidental findings on radiographic studies. AAA size is the most important variable in deciding whether surgical resection is indicated; in an otherwise fit patient, most clinicians use 5 cm as the size threshold for intervention. Whereas the survival benefit of elective aneurysm repair is not disputed, there is debate about how aggressive the posture should be with respect to small (4.5 to 5.5 cm) AAAs. Contemporary natural history studies have demonstrated that rupture of an AAA less than 5 cm in diameter is a rare clinical event; however, more than 50% of patients followed with small AAAs will eventually come to surgical correction within a few years because of expansion to 5 cm or more during sequential observation. The threshold for intervention in such patients is always a matter of clinical judgment, with patient age, presence of comorbid conditions, and predicted surgical results in terms of operative morbidity and mortality being the important variables.

Current surgical results for elective AAA correction are such that the majority of patients with 5-cm aneurysms should be advised to undergo elective correction unless there are clinically evident limitations on life expectancy or prohibitive surgical risk based on associated co-morbid conditions. Coronary artery disease is the most frequently encountered co-morbidity and is most often the focus for further evaluation prior to considering surgical intervention. Cardiac complications related to ischemic heart disease account for more than 50% of perioperative deaths after AAA repair, and associated coronary disease is the principal limitation on longevity in patients who undergo successful operation. Attention to preoperative cardiac risk stratification and greater awareness of the importance of the perioperative management of the frequently associated coronary disease have substantially reduced cardiac complications of AAA surgery over the past decade. In addition to coronary artery disease, significant azotemia and advanced COPD are important markers for potential perioperative morbidity. The best correlate of significant pulmonary or renal complications postoperatively is the presence of baseline abnormalities in these organ systems. When significant complications occur, operative mortality increases dramatically.

Abdominal ultrasound is the screening or initial diagnostic study most likely to be obtained before specialty referral. This study is cheap, rapidly performed, and virtually risk free, although it is somewhat operator dependent. It is a convenient way to sequentially follow small aneurysms. Abdominal computed tomography (CT) is the most accurate test for determining AAA size, and refinements in scan imaging provide the surgeon with clear-cut information with respect to aneurysm size and extent and consequently the extent of graft replacement. A majority of vascular surgeons will not order further imaging studies, and in contemporary practice, catheter-based contrast arteriography is usually reserved for selective indications such as aneurysm extent near or above the origin of the renal arteries, clinical indications to investigate potential renal artery or mesenteric artery stenosis, and associated aortoiliac occlusive disease. Magnetic resonance angiography can be substituted when there is a desire to avoid either contrast administration or excessive intra-arterial catheter manipulations.

Standard surgical therapy involves prosthetic graft replacement of the aneurysm via a transabdominal or retroperitoneal approach. Graft replacement is usually curative, although 5 to 8% of patients will ultimately undergo a second aneurysm operation. Operative mortality for elective AAA repair has steadily declined, and multiple clinical series from university-based medical centers for operations performed after 1980 indicate a perioperative mortality in the 3% range. Perhaps a more realistic view of the risk of operative mortality across a spectrum of hospital systems can be ascertained from geographically based studies that report for example, statewide mortality statistics for aneurysm repair. Such studies indicate that perioperative mortality can be as high as 5% even in contemporary practice. The risk of operative mortality is related to the clinical presentation and the presence or absence of co-morbid conditions. When operation is conducted under urgent circumstances, mortality even for intact aneurysms can approach 10% and operation for truly ruptured AAAs continues to be attended by a 50% mortality, a figure that has not changed substantially over the past decade. Late graft-related complications such as infection, enteric erosion, or fistula and anastomotic aneurysm are uncommon. Late survival after successful AAA replacement does not equate with that of an age- and sex-matched population unless patients with hypertension and coronary artery disease are subtracted out. Although the current risks of conventional surgery are low and the long-term results excellent, high-risk patients are often denied aneurysm repair, and considerable resource expenditure is necessary to bring these patients through successful conventional surgical repair. Clinical trials of minimally invasive surgical methods known as endovascular repair of AAA are under way to verify the anticipated decrease in overall morbidity associated with intervention. Endovascular repair involves transfemoral direct access to the arterial tree with retrograde passage of an aortic graft that is deployed from within the aneurysm under fluoroscopic control. The collapsible graft is affixed to the arterial tree above and below the aneurysm by one of several different types of attachment devices. Currently available delivery systems are inserted through open surgical access into the femoral artery. Despite the fact that there is little long-term durability data available on these endovascular stent/graft constructs, there is little doubt that they will soon become an important component in the vascular surgeon's armamentarium. At present, patient selection for treatment by the endovascular method is dictated strictly by arterial anatomy. With currently available devices, some 25% of AAA patients are potentially treatable by the endovascular method, and this figure is certain to increase in the future. Early technical results with this method have been satisfactory, with decreased morbidity in high-risk patients.

THORACIC AND THORACOABDOMINAL AORTIC ANEURYSMS

The descending thoracic aorta is the second most common location for degenerative aneurysms. Simultaneous involvement of the thoracic and abdominal aorta and/or that segment of the aorta from whence the visceral vessels arise (i.e., thoracoabdominal aneurysms) is rare, constituting less than 5% of patients afflicted with degenerative aortic aneurysm. Because of the extent of the aorta involved, the complexity of surgical repair, and the special risk of spinal cord ischemic injury, surgical repair of these extensive lesions with acceptable clinical results has been achieved only for the past decade. While size criteria for recommending intervention and predicting the risk of rupture are not as readily available for thoracoabdominal aneurysms because of their infrequent occurrence, it is clear that the potential for aneurysm rupture and the contribution to longevity from elective repair are similar to that for the more commonly encountered AAA.

Patients with complex aneurysm disease often have undergone multiple aortic resections, and associated COPD, smoking, and renovascular disease with severe hypertension are commonplace. Surgical repair of these extensive aneurysms can be accomplished in contemporary practice with a 5 to 10% risk of major morbidity-mortality, but the scope of the surgical undertaking is extensive. Resection of aneurysm limited to the descending thoracic aorta is usually performed with partial cardiopulmonary bypass and is considerably less complex than when the thoracoabdominal segment is involved. Focal aneurysms of the descending thoracic aorta have been treated with the endovascular stent graft repair approach outlined previously, but this approach is not possible when the aneurysm involves the visceral aortic segment.

AORTIC INFECTION

Primary infection of the aorta is usually manifest clinically as a mycotic aneurysm, a term originally coined by Osler to define the lesion caused by embolization of an infected cardiac vegetation. Although the term "infected aneurysm" is more appropriate in current parlance, "mycotic aneurysm" continues to be used for aneurysms that harbor active infection. Two etiologies are possible: the first is hematogenous seeding of a pre-existent degenerative aneurysm and the second involves blood-borne infection and seeding of aortic plaque with subsequent focal aortitis, aortic wall disruption, and formation of a false aneurysm, which is a contained aortic rupture. The latter is by far the more common pathogenesis, and the patients so afflicted are frequently immunocompromised. The clinical history often entails weeks to even months of malaise, weight loss, fever, and back pain. Since intravascular infection is present, positive blood cultures are usually noted. Diagnosis is usually confirmed with a CT scan.

Although an expanding false aneurysm is typically present for days to even weeks, ultimately rupture occurs irrespective of appropriate antibiotic therapy. When the process is confined to the infrarenal aorta, aortic resection and extra-anatomic revascularization with an axillobifemoral bypass graft is the preferred treatment. If the visceral or thoracoabdominal aortic segments are involved, treatment involves resection of the infected aorta and in situ graft replacement, generally with a PTFE prosthesis in addition to radical débridement of the infected aneurysm cavity and wrapping of the prosthesis with mobilized greater omentum. Permanent antibiotic suppression is an important adjunct when a prosthetic graft is placed in an infected field.

AORTITIS

Takayasu's aortitis and nonspecific giant cell arteritis of the aorta are autoimmune processes of unknown etiology. The patient typically afflicted with Takayasu's disease is a young woman with primary involvement of the aortic arch branches whose clinical manifestations may be related to occlusive lesions of the branch vessels. However, aortic aneurysm formation as the sequela of the aortic wall inflammatory process can and does occur. Nonspecific symptoms of malaise and fatigue, usually accompanied by an elevated sedimentation rate, are the clinical hallmarks of the disease. Smaller vessel arteritis of intracranial and/or mesenteric vessels, such as might occur in systemic lupus erythematosus and polyarteritis nodosum, can be noted with aortic involvement, but more often, giant cell aortitis is confined to the aorta and its principal branch vessels. Aortic aneurysm formation can follow either the acute or the inactive phase of the disease, and involvement of the abdominal aorta is frequently accompanied by stenotic lesions of the mesenteric and renal vessels with renovascular hypertension being a frequent finding. Steroid therapy is the principal management modality in the acute phase, and regression of stenotic lesions can be observed on this therapy. Surgery is generally reserved for correction of established aneurysm (preferably in the inactive phase of the disease), narrowing of the visceral abdominal aortic segment, or symptomatic aortic branch occlusion.

AORTIC DISSECTION

Acute aortic dissection is the most common catastrophic event affecting the aorta, with an incidence exceeding that of ruptured AAA. The diagnostic hallmark of dissection, both radiographically and pathologically, is an aortic intimal tear with propagating blood surging between the aortic layers and often re-entering the aortic lumen at some distal point. Although dissection frequently happens in a dilated aorta, it can also occur in an aorta with normal diameter and in young, otherwise healthy individuals. Patients with Marfan's syndrome are particularly prone to acute dissection and late chronic aneurysm formation. There may be confusion with other thoracic aortic pathology, such as penetrating aortic ulcer, intramural hematoma, or symptomatic or ruptured degenerative aortic aneurysms.

Dissections are classified according to the location of the intimal tear and the extent of the dissecting process in the aorta. The existence of two widely used classification systems can create confusion, and it is convenient to consider Stanford type A and Debakey types I and 2 as *proximal dissections* wherein the intimal tear is located in the ascending aorta. Distal dissections (Debakey types 3a and 3b and Stanford type B) are characterized by an intimal entry tear typically located just distal to the left subclavian artery. It is important to establish the location of the aortic intimal tear (i.e., whether the dissection is classified as proximal or distal), because this has direct implications for early management. Proximal aortic dissections are attended by a substantial risk of rupture of the ascending aorta and therefore constitute a surgical emergency, with emergency graft replacement of the ascending aorta being the preferred treatment. Alternatively, distal dissections typically do not rupture unless the aorta is extremely dilated at the site of the intimal tear. Accordingly, medical therapy as detailed later is the preferred treatment in patients with acute distal dissections.

An appropriate index of suspicion is the key to rapid diagnosis. Severe chest or back pain leading to presentation for treatment within hours of onset is reported by more than 90% of patients. Pulse deficits can be a helpful physical finding. Diagnostic confusion with acute coronary syndromes is usually eliminated with appropriate electrocardiography. Findings on plain chest films are generally not helpful. Although contrast arteriography was previously the diagnostic procedure of choice, rapid diagnosis in the emergency room can readily be made with transesophageal echocardiography or rapid-sequence dynamic computed tomography. Even after the diagnosis is confirmed by either of these two imaging modalities, aortography may be desirable to (1) assess the degree of aortic valvular insufficiency, (2) assess the distal extent of the dissection, and (3) elucidate the presence and mechanism of aortic branch compromise.

With rare exceptions, acute proximal dissection is a surgical emergency because of the threat of aortic rupture, acute aortic valvular insufficiency, and/or occlusion of the coronary artery ostia. Graft replacement for acute proximal dissection is accomplished with complete cardiopulmonary bypass. The aortic intimal tear is resected and graft replacement of the ascending aorta with or without concomitant aortic valve replacement is carried out with reapproximation of the aortic layers at the distal suture line, typically located in the proximal aortic arch. However, some 25 to 40% of patients will have persistent false lumen flow either from intimal fractures near the suture line or from distal spontaneous fenestration. In patients with Marfan's syndrome, a chronic "double barrel" aorta is to be anticipated as is late aneurysmal dilatation of the outer wall of the false lumen. Repetitive late operations for aneurysm formation are the rule in patients with this syndrome.

First described by Wheat and associates in 1965, urgent antihypertensive therapy has become the prime treatment modality for acute distal dissection. Emergency department management of all patients with acute dissection involves such therapy. The goals are to rapidly control mean arterial pressure, generally with sodium nitroprusside, and to decrease the $\Delta P/\Delta T$ of ventricular ejection with beta blockade. Such therapy must be monitored with arterial lines in an intensive care unit setting until the pain resolves and blood pressure control with an oral regimen is achieved. In addition to proximal aortic rupture, aortic branch compromise when the dissecting process proceeds into the abdomen can create life-threatening complications related to lower extremity ischemia from aortic obstruction and mesenteric or renal artery compromise. In such cases, the so-called complication specific approach, wherein peripheral vascular intervention is directed toward specific life-threatening complications, may involve surgical or endovascular treatment of aortic branch compromise. In fact, one third of patients with acute aortic dissection have evidence of some major aortic branch compromise, and the presence of such complications greatly increases the overall risk of mortality. Even with prompt surgical repair of the ascending aorta, mortality from proximal aortic dissection remains in the 25% range. With respect to distal dissections, the mortality is related to the extent of the dissecting process and the presence of significant aortic branch compromise.

AORTIC TRAUMA

Trauma to the aorta can be either blunt or penetrating and can present the threat of rupture and hemorrhage. In unusual cases, blunt trauma to the abdominal aorta can precipitate intimal fracture and abdominal aortic obstruction. Penetrating aortic injury is usually fatal. Blunt chest trauma, such as might occur with deceleration injury, can cause tears of the thoracic aorta typically in two locations. The first is at the aortic root; these are usually fatal in the field. The other site is just distal to the left subclavian artery beyond the point where the aorta is tethered to the central cardiac structures by the ligamentum arteriosum. Such tears are often contained temporarily by the aortic adventitia but have a high risk of rupture in the hours and days after injury. An appropriate level of clinical suspicion based on the mechanism of injury, and certain suggestive findings on plain chest films should lead to liberal use of contrast arteriography to confirm the diagnosis. Prompt surgical repair with a short Dacron graft is usually successful if associated injuries, primarily neurologic, are not severe.

ANGINA PECTORIS

method of
SUSAN L. SIMANDL, M.D., and
PETER F. COHN, M.D.
State University of New York Health Sciences Center
Stony Brook, New York

Angina pectoris was first described by the English physician Heberden in 1772 as a strangling sensation in the breast. Heberden related it to physical exertion, and his description has become synonymous with that of typical (or classic) angina pectoris. When angina pectoris is due to organic heart disease, most commonly coronary atherosclerosis, myocardial ischemia is the underlying pathophysiologic mechanism.

PATHOPHYSIOLOGY

Myocardial ischemia occurs when the coronary blood supply cannot meet myocardial demands. This discrepancy is termed a supply-demand mismatch. Coronary blood supply is determined by the oxygen-carrying capacity of the blood and the coronary blood flow, the latter being regulated by numerous interacting factors. Myocardial demands are affected by changes in heart rate, contractility, and systolic wall tension; increasing heart rate is believed to be the single most important determinant of increased myocardial oxygen consumption.

In the normal heart, the coronary blood supply increases to match increasing myocardial demands. In the patient with significant coronary atherosclerotic disease, however, myocardial oxygen consumption may exceed the coronary blood supply, resulting in myocardial ischemia. Because it is at the end of the arterial blood supply, the subendocardium is most vulnerable to ischemia.

The angina threshold is the level of metabolic activity (physical or emotional) at which myocardial ischemia ensues. If this threshold is fixed, as it is in some patients, the same amount of exertion, often expressed in metabolic equivalents or as a rate-pressure product (heart rate multiplied by systolic blood pressure), provokes the patient's angina. In other patients, the threshold varies throughout the day. These patients sometimes have angina while they are at rest or with minimal exertion; at other times, they are able to exercise more vigorously. Many patients have both fixed- and variable-threshold angina, which is described as mixed angina pectoris.

The clinical history may give clues to the mechanism of a patient's angina (increasing myocardial demands in exertional angina and decreasing coronary blood supply in patients with angina without obvious precipitants). This information may help to guide the physician in choosing a medication.

CLINICAL FEATURES

The clinical presentation of myocardial ischemia resulting from coronary artery disease ranges from asymptomatic disease (silent ischemia) to atypical chest pain syndromes to classic angina pectoris. The latter can be further classified as stable or unstable (see later discussion). Heberden's classic angina is defined as transient precordial discomfort provoked by exertion and relieved by rest or nitroglycerin. The discomfort can be heaviness, pressure, or tightness in the chest. It also can radiate to the arm, neck, jaw, or back and may be provoked by exercise; cold, hot, or humid weather; heavy meals; or emotional stress. The discomfort begins gradually and reaches maximal intensity over several minutes before resolving. Classic angina eases after rest or 2 to 3 minutes after sublingual nitroglycerin is taken. Most important, angina is *not* described as a brief, sharp, pleuritic, stabbing, localized, or migratory discomfort.

Atypical angina is a syndrome that has some symptoms that are similar to those of the classic one but lacks one or more of the criteria for classic angina. Angina equivalents are symptoms of myocardial ischemia other than angina, such as exertional dyspnea. Others use the term to describe pain in a referred location, such as isolated exertional arm or neck discomfort not accompanied by discomfort in the chest. Angina occurring only at rest and associated with transient ST-segment elevation (rather than depression) on electrocardiography is termed variant (Prinzmetal's) angina and has a different pathophysiologic mechanism: severe vasospasm.

DIFFERENTIATION BETWEEN UNSTABLE AND STABLE ANGINA

The predisposing pathologic alteration in *stable angina* is atherosclerosis with or without intimal fibrous proliferation. Coronary angiographic studies in patients with stable angina frequently reveal smooth, regular plaques with a low incidence of ulceration or thrombi (Table 1). Resting blood flow is little affected until stenosis reaches 85% of coronary luminal diameter. Another factor contributing to ischemia is the extent of collateral blood flow bypassing the stenotic segment. A third is the role played by the mediators of vasoconstriction, such as the sympathetic tone, histamine, serotonin, and the like. A fourth is the normal preferential distribution of blood flow to the endocardium at rest, resulting in diminished endocardial coronary flow reserve in response to stress.

Coronary angiography in patients with *unstable angina* reveals lesions that are often eccentric, with an irregular or scalloped margin, and a high incidence of thrombus. Plaque rupture and fissuring in the atherosclerotic coronary artery, platelet aggregation, and thrombus formation play critical roles in changing a stable lesion into an unstable one. As the plaque ruptures, it exposes several elements that are potent thrombogenic stimuli. Endothelial cell dysfunction over and near the plaque may result in vasoconstriction of the affected coronary segment, thus worsening the coronary luminal diameter. Vasoconstriction is accentuated by many factors produced by platelets, such as serotonin, platelet-derived growth factor, and other substances that possess vasoconstrictive properties. Another potential contributing factor in some patients is a low level of nitric oxide. Nitric oxide is generated by endothelial cells and produces vasodilatation and platelet inhibition. Dysfunctional endothelium may lack the ability to produce nitric oxide.

Depending on the thrombogenic stimulus and the balance between thrombogenic and vasoconstrictive factors on one hand and antithrombogenic and vasodilatory factors on the other, along with shear rate forces and the severity of the underlying stenosis, plaque rupture may result in thrombus formation that is either transient or permanent.

TABLE 1. **Differentiation Between Stable and Unstable Angina**

	Stable Angina	Unstable Angina
Pathoanatomy	Smooth, regular plaques with low evidence of thrombus formation	Eccentric lesions with irregular borders and high incidence of thrombus formation
Pathophysiology	Episodes have circadian pattern with most related to increased myocardial oxygen demand	Episodes have circadian pattern with most related to increased role of vasoconstriction, platelet adhesion, and/or plaque rupture
Clinical features	Most episodes usually related to physical exertion	Episodes can occur at rest as part of accelerated stable angina pattern, postinfarction angina, or new-onset angina

Progression can result from recurrent subclinical cycles of plaque rupture, hemorrhage, and organization.

Both unstable and stable angina have a circadian pattern of ischemic events. Many ischemic events, including angina, myocardial infarction, and ischemic stroke, occur in the morning hours between 6 AM and noon. This phenomenon is heterogeneous in origin and involves heart rate, blood pressure, and platelet and coagulation cascade activation, as well as variations in coronary artery tone variation.

DIAGNOSIS

The diagnosis of angina pectoris cannot be made on physical examination; however, some finding may increase clinical suspicion of coronary artery disease. One such example is systemic hypertension. Skin xanthomas are found in patients with familial hypercholesterolemia who have an increased incidence of premature coronary artery disease. The presence of carotid or femoral bruits, which are suggestive of peripheral vascular disease, increases the likelihood that the patient also has atherosclerotic heart disease. Cardiac examination may give clues to underlying organic heart disease (e.g., if pathologic murmurs or gallop sounds are noted), but it is by no means sensitive or specific for the diagnosis of coronary artery disease.

Noninvasive tests include the exercise ECG, ambulatory ECG monitoring, nuclear imaging, and echocardiography. The exercise stress test is best used in patients with chest pain syndrome who have normal findings on the resting ECG. The patient exercises, commonly with either a treadmill or a stationary bicycle, and the patient's exercise duration, symptoms, blood pressure, heart rate, heart rhythm, physical examination findings, and ECG findings are analyzed. In the context of the clinical history, these parameters are evaluated to formulate a diagnostic impression.

Exercise radionuclide ventriculography, thallium-201 stress testing, and stress echocardiography have increased the sensitivity for detecting coronary artery disease. These specialized tests are commonly used in patients with abnormal baseline ECG results that make the exercise ECG findings difficult to interpret. Radionuclide and echocardiographic studies are also commonly used in patients with poor exercise capacity and those who are unable to exercise. In these circumstances, pharmacologic stress agents such as dipyridamole, dobutamine, or adenosine have been employed. The sensitivity and specificity of dipyridamole-thallium stress testing are nearly comparable to those of exercise thallium stress testing. Because of their increased cost and time of performance as well as the marginal benefit for improved detection in some patients, however, nuclear and echocardiographic stress tests are not recommended as routine screening procedures.

In patients with chronic stable angina, the stress test has been said to provide little diagnostic information after clinical parameters are taken into account. However, the stress test can be used to monitor disease progression and the patient's response to medication. It can also assess the functional significance of a lesion detected angiographically, assess the benefits of revascularization via surgery or angioplasty, and, perhaps most important, provide a prognostic assessment (aid in risk stratification). The exercise test is not considered a standard procedure in unstable angina patients because of risk of complications.

PROGNOSIS

The prognosis in patients with angina pectoris can be determined by the patient history, physical examination, noninvasive data, and coronary angiographic results. With information obtained from the clinical examination, the clinician decides whether the patient is in a low-risk or high-risk group. In high-risk patients (those with unstable angina, or stable angina with frequent episodes of angina and evidence of left ventricular dysfunction on clinical examination), coronary angiography with an eye toward revascularization should be performed. In low-risk patients or those in a poorly defined risk category on clinical examination, stress test data have helped to delineate high-risk and low-risk groups. The specific criteria vary from report to report, but the conclusion remains the same: patients with poor exercise capacity and those with severe ischemia by ST response at a low workload compose a high-risk cohort.

Radionuclide stress tests (either with ventriculography demonstrating poor resting left ventricular function or failure of the left ventricular ejection fraction to increase with exercise, or with perfusion imaging showing severe ischemia as evidenced by multiple reversible thallium defects, thallium uptake in the lungs, and transient postexercise left ventricular dilatation) identify patients at high risk for cardiac events. Although left ventricular function is probably the strongest predictor of prognosis, the severity of the coronary artery disease has significant implications as well. Both the number of diseased vessels and the severity of the stenosis correlate with survival. Left ventricular function and severity of the coronary artery disease act synergistically to determine survival, and patients with left main coronary artery disease have been shown to have the worst prognosis, followed by those with severe three-vessel coronary artery disease.

THERAPY

The goals of therapy in managing angina patients are to prolong survival, reduce the incidence of disease progression, alleviate symptoms, and improve exercise capacity. Despite the increasing popularity of interventional procedures, noninvasive treatment continues to be the mainstay of anti-ischemic management. Many cardiologists regard combined administration of conventional antianginal medications (including nitrates, beta blockers and calcium channel blockers) rather than single-agent therapy as a more rational approach to the management of patients with angina. The rationale for this therapeutic strategy is based primarily on our knowledge of the pathophysiology of myocardial ischemia discussed previously and the mechanism of action of the various anti-ischemic drugs.

Nitrates. Of the various nitrate compounds, nitroglycerin is the most widely investigated (Table 2). The main effect of the drug is decreasing preload by dilating venous capacitance vessels. Dilating coronary arterial vessels, mainly the stenotic segment, is a secondary effect. In the acute setting, nitrates are delivered sublingually, by spray, or intravenously when available. When given intravenously in intensive care settings, as in unstable angina, close monitoring of blood pressure is mandatory. In stable angina, oral or transdermal preparations of nitrates may be used. A nitrate-free period is necessary to avoid tolerance. Typically, relatively long-acting and orally administered nitrates, such as isosorbide

TABLE 2. **Commonly Used Nitrates**

	Recommended Daily Dose (mg)	Duration of Action
Sublingual NTG	0.3–0.8	10–30 min
Oral NTG spray	0.4	10–30 min
Isosorbide mononitrate	40	7–12 h
Isosorbide dinitrate	10–160	2–6 h
NTG ointment (2%)	0.5–2 inches	3–8 h
Transdermal NTG disks	10–50	24 h

Abbreviation: NTG = nitroglycerin.
From Hanna GP, Smalling RW: Angina pectoris. *In* Rakel RE (ed): Conn's Current Therapy 1997. Philadelphia, WB Saunders Co, 1997, p 250.

mononitrate (Ismo) or dinitrate (Isordil), are given at 8- to 12-hour intervals during the day, and a nitroglycerin patch or paste is applied at night and removed the following morning after the patient arises. The mechanism of nitrate tolerance is not well understood, but there is evidence to suggest depletion of sulfhydryl groups. The nitrate's site of interaction with vascular smooth muscle may play an important role. Side effects of nitrates include hypotension, headache, flushing, and reflex tachycardia.

Beta Blockers. These are perhaps the most effective drugs for managing ischemic heart disease (Table 3). Beta blockers blunt sympathetic effects, thus reducing arrhythmias and ischemia and protecting the myocardium after infarction. Beta blockers with intrinsic sympathomimetic effects, however, are not as useful. Shorter-acting beta blockers are useful for titration of doses in the inpatient setting, whereas longer-acting preparations are desirable for outpatients to improve compliance. Potential side effects include bradycardia, hypotension, bronchospasm, inhibition of insulin release and blunting of metabolic response to hypoglycemia, lethargy, depression, and impotence. Fifteen such drugs are presently approved by the Food and Drug Administration (FDA). In addition to the agents listed in Table 3, the newly approved carvedilol will assume increasing importance because of its usefulness in heart failure patients.

TABLE 4. **Commonly Used Calcium Channel Blockers**

Name (Formulation)	Recommended Daily Dose	Duration of Action (h)
Diltiazem		
Cardizem	120–360 mg	6–8
Cardizem CD	120–360 mg	24
Cardizem SR	120–360 mg	12
Dilacor XR	60–120 mg	24
Injection	0.25 mg/kg bolus; 10 mg/h infusion	3
Nifedipine		
Adalat, Procardia	30–90 mg	4–8
Procardia XL	30–90 mg	16–24
Verapamil		
Calan, Isoptin	120–360 mg	8
Calan SR, Isoptin SR	120–240 mg	24
Injection	5–10 mg (may repeat in 30 min)	1–6
Nicardipine		
Cardene	60–120 mg	6–8
Cardene SR	60–120 mg	12
Amlodipine (Norvasc)	5–10 mg	24

From Hanna GP, Smalling RW: Angina pectoris. *In* Rakel RE (ed): Conn's Current Therapy 1997. Philadelphia, WB Saunders Co, 1997, p 251.

Calcium Channel Blockers. The three major groups of calcium channel blockers are the phenylalkylamines (e.g., verapamil), the benzodiazepines (e.g., diltiazem) and the dihydropyridines (e.g., nifedipine) (Table 4). Their mechanism of action is based mainly on blocking the calcium inward current, which plays an important role in the various physio-

TABLE 3. **Commonly Used Beta Blockers**

Name (Formulation)	Recommended Daily Dose	Duration of Action (h)
Cardioselective Preparations		
Acebutolol (Sectral)*	400–1800 mg†	24
Atenolol (Tenormin)	50–200 mg	24
Esmolol (Brevibloc) injection	Loading dose, 0.5 mg/kg Infusion, 50–300 μ/kg/min	10–20 min
Metoprolol		
Lopressor	15–240 mg	6–8
Lopressor SR, Toprol XL	50–400 mg	24
Injection	5 mg (may repeat q 5 min × 2–3)	5–8
Noncardioselective Preparations		
Nadolol (Corgard)*	80–240 mg	40
Propranolol		
Inderal	30–60 mg	3–6
Inderal LA	60–160 mg	24
Injection	1 mg (0.1 mg/kg) (may repeat q 4 h)	3–4
Pindolol (Visken)*	10–20 mg	8
Sotalol (Betapace)	240–480 mg	24
Timolol (Blocadren)	15–45 mg	6–12

* Significant intrinsic sympathomimetic activity.
† Exceeds dosage recommended by the manufacturer.
From Hanna GP, Smalling RW: Angina pectoris. *In* Rakel RE (ed): Conn's Current Therapy 1997. Philadelphia, WB Saunders Co, 1997, p 251.

logic processes of the myocardium and vascular smooth muscle. Therefore, calcium blockers dilate coronary and peripheral arteries. They can also cause negative inotropic effects. Nifedipine induces potent peripheral vasodilatation, resulting in reflex tachycardia. Eleven drugs are currently approved by the FDA. The newer dihydropyridines amlodipine (Norvasc), felodipine* (Plendil), and nimodipine* (Nimotop) have the benefit of inducing coronary vasodilatation with little negative inotropy; hence they possess potential benefit in ameliorating angina in patients with mildly depressed left ventricular function when other calcium blockers may be detrimental. However, it is important to keep in mind that all calcium antagonists, to varying degrees, may worsen congestive heart failure in patients with severely depressed left ventricular function. Diltiazem is intermediate with respect to the aforementioned effects. As with verapamil, side effects may include edema, headache, flushing, bradycardia, hypotension, and, as mentioned earlier, worsening ventricular function.

All three classes of antianginal drugs decrease the incidence of ischemia and improve exercise performance and are best used as combination therapies. However, these agents can be used as the sole therapy for patients stratified by noninvasive methods to a low-risk group for cardiac events. They are also often used as adjuncts to revascularization. In addition, because of its proven benefit in postmyocardial infarction, unstable angina, and postcoronary bypass patients, daily aspirin use is often recommended. Finally, risk modification with diet counseling, antilipemic therapy, smoking cessation, and exercise programs is also strongly advised. All of these measures can be initiated by the generalist; when revascularization is indicated by refractory symptoms or markedly abnormal stress test results, referral to a specialist is appropriate.

Coronary Artery Bypass Graft Surgery. This surgery is performed to improve quality of life and prolong survival. Coronary artery bypass grafting has been shown to relieve angina more effectively than medical therapy and is effective when angina is refractory to medical therapy. The poorer the prognosis (i.e., severe ischemia combined with poor left ventricular function), the greater the benefits of revascularization (albeit possibly at a higher operative risk).

Coronary Angioplasty. The role of coronary angioplasty in the treatment of chronic stable angina is evolving. A randomized trial comparing angioplasty with medical therapy in patients with single-vessel coronary artery disease reported a statistically significant improvement in exercise tolerance and anginal symptoms among the angioplasty group. The angioplasty patients had a greater number of hospital days, however, as well as a higher incidence of repeated angioplasty (with its associated risks) and a higher cost than the medically treated patients. Another randomized study, which compared angioplasty with coronary artery bypass surgery, showed no difference in the rate of death or nonfatal myocardial infarction between the two groups 2.5 years after enrollment. However, the angioplasty group had a statistically significant increase in subsequent revascularization procedures (repeated angioplasty, bypass surgery, or both) and need for repeated coronary arteriography. Surgical patients had less angina and required less antianginal therapy in this study. Diabetic patients are especially likely to benefit from surgery rather than angioplasty.

*Not FDA approved for this indication.

SILENT MYOCARDIAL ISCHEMIA

Although often considered a "separate" syndrome, silent ischemia is part of the ischemic spectrum. It is defined as objective evidence of transient myocardial ischemia without symptoms of chest pain or angina equivalent. We have classified it into three types:

1. Patients with asymptomatic coronary artery disease with silent ischemia detected by screening exercise testing.
2. Patients with silent ischemia postinfarction.
3. Patients with angina who also have episodes of silent ischemia. This is the most common type. It encompasses patients with stable, unstable, and variant (Prinzmetal's) angina.

In these groups, total ischemic time has been shown to correlate with poor clinical outcome, increased incidence of infarction, interventions, sudden cardiac death, and hospitalization. It has also been shown to correlate with the severity of coronary artery disease. Moreover, silent ischemia is associated with a high incidence of perioperative complications. Therefore, silent ischemia requires early detection by identifying high-risk patients so that pharmacologic therapy may be provided. The same agents described previously for treatment of angina are good for management of silent ischemia. However, persistent ischemia on objective stress testing despite maximal medical therapy may require early revascularization. In the Asymptomatic Cardiac Ischemia Pilot Study, silent ischemia and angina were relieved in more patients undergoing revascularization procedures (percutaneous transluminal coronary angioplasty and coronary artery bypass graft surgery) than patients receiving medical therapy alone.

CONCLUSIONS

It is important to emphasize that anti-ischemic medications eliminate or reduce angina by decreasing myocardial oxygen demand, increasing myocardial oxygen supply, or both. They do not correct the underlying cause of ischemia, although regression of atherosclerosis has been reported with aggressive lipid-lowering regimens in studies such as the Cholesterol Lowering Atherosclerosis Study (CLAS), the Monitored Atherosclerosis Regression study (MARS), and the Familial Atherosclerosis Treatment Study (FATS). Mechanical approaches to the treatment of myocardial ischemia do not alter myocardial oxygen demand but do improve myocardial oxygen supply by relieving or circumventing the atherosclerotic obstruction responsible for anginal symptoms. Initially successful revascularization procedures, however, may be followed by the recurrence of angina due to graft occlusion, restenosis after angioplasty, or the progression of coronary artery disease. There is no evidence to indicate that surgical treatment is superior to medical treatment in increasing longevity in patients with mild anginal symptoms and those with one or two diseased coronary arteries. For this reason such patients are best treated medically. Surgery has been shown to be more effective than medical therapy in increasing longevity in symptomatic and asymptomatic patients with significant stenosis of the left main coronary artery. Surgical management may also be preferable to medical therapy in patients with triple-vessel disease, regardless of symptoms, especially in those with continuing ischemia and impaired left ventricular function. Surgery is also recommended for patients with angina that fails to respond to medical therapy. Comparison of coronary angioplasty with bypass surgery has shown no clear-cut advantage in terms of morbidity and mortality. For patients in whom standard medical therapy and/or revascularization procedures have not proved to be successful in reducing angina and restoring an adequate quality of life, several new procedures have been introduced. These include spinal cord stimulation, transmyocardial laser revascularization, and enhanced external counterpulsation. The popularity of these procedures can be expected to grow as the patient base increases.

CARDIAC ARREST: SUDDEN CARDIAC DEATH

method of
JERRY C. LUCK, M.D., and
GERALD V. NACCARELLI, M.D.
Pennsylvania State University College of Medicine
Hershey, Pennsylvania

Although the actual number of persons experiencing out-of-hospital cardiac arrest has declined in the past two decades, nearly 300,000 people experience a cardiac arrest each year in the United States. Only 20% of these persons are resuscitated successfully and survive to be discharged from the hospital. Sudden death as viewed by the clinician involves unexpected collapse with cessation of circulation and breathing. Collapse is abrupt and not secondary to worsening angina or pulmonary congestion. Although sudden death can occur in the absence of heart disease, the clinician's definition implies that there is underlying heart disease. To the epidemiologist, sudden death means abrupt collapse with loss of consciousness within 1 hour of the onset of acute symptoms. This definition does not imply the presence of underlying heart disease, but the focus is directed more at the timing rather than the mode of death.

The reduction in sudden death cases parallels the reduction in total cardiovascular deaths. The introduction of medicines such as beta blockers has been shown to reduce the incidence of sudden death after acute myocardial infarction (MI). Coronary bypass surgery performed in patients without a history of infarction reduces the size of subsequent infarctions. Thrombolytic therapy in patients experiencing acute infarction reduces infarct size. Theoretically, the incidence should decrease further if use of an implantable cardioverter-defibrillator is shown to be beneficial in other patient groups at high risk for sudden death.

ETIOLOGY

About 80% of patients who die suddenly have underlying heart disease. Coronary artery disease is present in nearly 75% of these cases. Of those associated with coronary artery disease, less than 20% occur in the setting of acute MI. Seventy-five percent of patients with coronary artery disease who experience cardiac arrest have clinical evidence of a healed myocardial infarct. Cardiomyopathy occurs in 15%, valvular disease in 5%, and a primary conduction disorder in 5%, while less than 1% of cases are secondary to a vascular catastrophe (Table 1). As a rule, in the vast majority of cases of sudden death, evidence of structural cardiac disease is found at autopsy. Clearly, it is unusual for persons without a mechanical cardiac defect to suffer sudden death. The small number of sudden death cases that occur without evidence of a structural heart problem tend to have a primary conduction problem such as the long QT syndrome.

PATHOPHYSIOLOGY

The clinical syndrome of sudden death is best viewed by analyzing the cardiac rhythm at the time of the cardiac

TABLE 1. **Disorders Associated with Sudden Death**

Coronary artery disease
Acute myocardial infarction
Post myocardial infarction
Coronary artery spasm
Dilated cardiomyopathy
Idiopathic
Ischemic
Hypertrophic cardiomyopathy
Drug effects
Antiarrhythmic agent–related proarrhythmia
Recreational (e.g., cocaine)
Conduction abnormalities
Long QT syndrome
Atrioventricular block
Wolff-Parkinson-White syndrome
Primary electrical system disease
Arrhythmogenic right ventricular dysplasia
Congenital heart disease
Tetralogy of Fallot
Coronary anomalies
Double-outlet right ventricle
Transposition of the great vessels
Electrolyte abnormalities
Hypokalemia
Hypomagnesemia
Valvular heart disease
Aortic stenosis
Infiltrative
Myocarditis, amyloidosis, sarcoidosis
Cardiac tumors, Chagas' disease

arrest. Cardiac arrest in the hospital coronary care unit occurs generally as a result of either ventricular fibrillation or ventricular tachycardia (VT). Out-of-hospital cardiac arrest follows a similar pattern. About 70 to 80% of cases are secondary to ventricular fibrillation or sustained VT, while only 20 to 30% are thought to be caused by profound bradycardia or asystole. Ambulatory recordings of patients who suffer sudden death frequently show either monomorphic or polymorphic VT that degenerates into ventricular fibrillation. These Holter recordings produce clues as to why there is sudden collapse. Some recordings show an increase in heart rate before the actual collapse, reflecting changes in sympathetic tone. Occasionally, ischemic ST segment changes are documented prior to the actual event.

Ventricular fibrillation and VT are associated with structural cardiac problems. Classically, the mechanisms thought to cause most pathologic tachycardias are reentry, automaticity, and triggered activity. Reentry is the mechanism that underlies most cases of sustained monomorphic VT. In reentry, anatomic defects allow for areas of slow conduction and unidirectional block. Sustained monomorphic VT is seen post myocardial infarction, when scar and frequently a left ventricular aneurysm may be present. VT confined to reentry within the bundle branches is not uncommon in patients with dilated cardiomyopathy. Polymorphic VT with a changing QRS morphology is associated with acute ischemic heart disease or drug proarrhythmia. Torsades de pointes is a special VT (the term means "turning on its axis") that is associated with the prolonged QT syndrome. The mechanism underlying this polymorphic VT is triggered activity. Ventricular fibrillation is commonly seen with an acute myocardial infarction (Table 2).

Predisposing conditions for ventricular fibrillation and VT are myocardial infarction, cardiomyopathy, hypertrophy, and primary conduction system disorders. The healing phase of MI is characterized by fibrosis and scarring. In the human heart, islands of scarring form at the border of the infarct and normal myocardium. This predisposes to formation of areas of electrical inhomogeneity. Thus, areas of slow conduction and sites of unidirectional block permit reentry at the border zone of the healing infarct. Sustained monomorphic VT is recognized to occur in 6 to 8% of patients surviving MI. Those with larger areas of scar and aneurysm formation have a higher likelihood of developing VT or ventricular fibrillation. The loss of viable myocardium leads to reduced systolic function and the potential for congestive heart failure. Patients with a nonischemic dilated myocardium also have myocardial scarring and reduced myocardial function. Normally functioning myocytes are replaced by hypertrophied cells, and scar tissue interdigitates with myocardial tissue, producing islands of scarring, with an increased propensity for sudden death. Hypertrophic cardiomyopathy does not usually lead to congestive heart failure but is associated with the presence of thickened areas of cardiac muscle characterized by disorganized architecture. This promotes electrical instability as a result of anisotropic tissue structure. Reentry is thought to explain VT in this setting.

The actual triggers were originally thought to be premature ventricular complexes (PVCs). The "PVC theory" simply says that VT and ventricular fibrillation are initiated by PVCs. The more frequent and complex the PVCs, the higher the likelihood of initiating VT or ventricular fibrillation. Eliminating the PVCs should lower the incidence of sudden death. However, the Cardiac Arrhythmia Suppression Trial (CAST) disproved this hypothesis, because suppressing PVCs with several class IC antiarrhythmic agents (flecainide, encainide, moricizine) failed to decrease the incidence of sudden death. When the placebo group was compared with the treated group, patients who received antiarrhythmic therapy had a threefold higher incidence of death post MI.

The acute risk factors thought to trigger cardiac arrest include acute ischemia and possibly acute reperfusion; hemodynamic decompensation; acidosis and hypoxemia; electrolyte imbalance, particularly hypokalemia; autonomic nervous system fluctuations; and toxic effects of substances on the heart (e.g., class I antiarrhythmics) (Table 3). In the setting of an old MI, acute ischemia produces an increased propensity for VT and ventricular fibrillation. Left ventricular hypertrophy, old infarction, and subtotal coronary stenosis that produces ischemia can cause torsades de pointes and other types of polymorphic VT. Reperfusion, particularly with underlying hypertrophy, may produce VT by either reentry or triggered activity. The Framingham Study introduced the relationship between hypertrophy and sudden death. With left ventricular hypertrophy, the cell's action potential is prolonged as a result of altered calcium regulation. Thus, an increased inward current produces afterdepolarizations that may cause polymorphic VT. Worsening heart failure may lead to several events that

TABLE 2. **Possible Causes of Ventricular Tachycardia (VT)**

Sustained monomorphic VT (≥30s) with uniform and stable QRS morphology

Post myocardial infarction
Dilated cardiomyopathy (bundle branch reentrant VT)
Arrhythmogenic right ventricular dysplasia
Right ventriculotomy scar VT
Idiopathic—right ventricular outflow tract—repetitive VT

Nonsustained monomorphic VT (<30 s)

Coronary disease (post myocardial infarction)
Hypertrophic cardiomyopathy
Valvular heart disease
Acute myocarditis
Infiltrative diseases (sarcoidosis, amyloidosis)

Polymorphic VT with changing QRS morphology

Torsades: long QT syndromes
Bidirectional: digitalis intoxication
Multiformed: antiarrhythmics (class IA, III); tricyclics

TABLE 3. **Factors Predisposing to Sudden Death**

Anatomic Abnormalities

Ischemic heart disease with significant left ventricular dysfunction
Left ventricular hypertrophy
Cardiomyopathy
Primary conduction system disease

Triggering Factors

Acute ischemia and acute reperfusion
Hemodynamic decompensation
Metabolic disorders: acidosis and hypoxemia
Electrolyte disorders: hypokalemia, hypomagnesemia
Autonomic nervous system fluctuations: increased sympathetic tone
Toxic effects of cardiac medications: negative inotropes, proarrhythmia

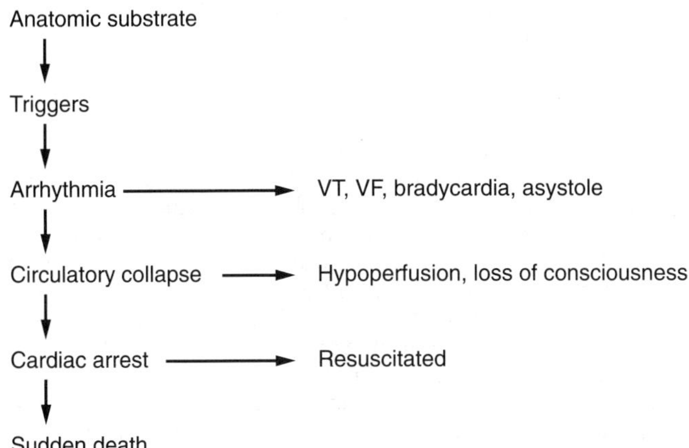

Figure 1. Mechanisms for ventricular fibrillation (VF). *Abbreviation*: VT = ventricular tachycardia.

could promote an episode of cardiac arrest. In addition to the problems of electrolyte imbalance, most notably hypokalemia and hypomagnesemia, these patients have altered mechanisms for metabolism of their prescribed antiarrhythmic drugs, which can on occasion become proarrhythmic. Acute cardiac decompensation can promote hypoxia, acidosis, and markedly elevated catecholamine levels. Sudden increases in catecholamines can rapidly shift electrolytes from the extracellular to the intracellular compartment and can precipitate ventricular fibrillation. Abnormalities in autonomic nervous system function have been linked to cardiac arrest. Sympathetic stimulation in the long QT syndrome has been linked to cardiac arrest. The mechanisms for sudden death are outlined in Figure 1.

RISK STRATIFICATION

The Seattle experience in the resuscitation of out-of-hospital cardiac arrest individuals has shown that success is mainly dependent on the time to arrival of trained paramedics and bystander-initiated cardiopulmonary resuscitation (CPR). Persons with cardiac arrest who receive a direct-current shock within 6 minutes of prompt CPR have a 70% survival rate. Persons receiving late (after 3 minutes) CPR have only a 39% survival rate. The in-field resuscitation rate is close to 60% for persons found in VT or ventricular fibrillation. Approximately 10% of patients are discharged neurologically intact after resuscitation. The Seattle data have been postulated to represent the best possible outcome that can be achieved realistically. Further expansion of the emergency response system nationally to the level of Seattle's may not be reasonable. It seems more efficacious to try to prevent sudden cardiac death.

Evidence of structural heart disease is found in the vast majority (nearly 80%) of out-of-hospital cardiac arrest survivors. Underlying ischemia or dilated cardiomyopathy is the cause of cardiac arrest in most cases (nearly 90%) of structural heart disease. To reduce the overall incidence of sudden death, the approach must include risk stratification in these two populations with the introduction of an effective intervention.

In patients with a recent MI, the factors associated with an increased risk for sudden death include a history of a complicated clinical course during acute infarction (e.g., congestive heart failure), a reduced left ventricular ejection fraction to below 0.40, complex ventricular ectopy (particularly nonsustained VT), abnormalities on a signal-averaged electrocardiogram (late potentials), inducible sustained VT using programmed ventricular extrastimuli, reduced heart rate variability, and depressed baroreceptor sensitivity. An ejection fraction of less than 0.40 is a sensitive predictor of sudden death. The incidence of nonsustained VT approaches 10 to 12% at 6 weeks post infarction. Patients with a reduced ejection fraction and nonsustained VT have a 3-year mortality rate of 17 to 21%. If systolic function is preserved and nonsustained VT is absent, then the incidence of sudden death drops to 2 to 3%. When ejection fraction is more than 0.50, the 5-year mortality rate is only 5%, but the 3-year mortality rate exceeds 50% when ejection fraction is less than 0.20.

The signal averaged electrocardiogram (SAECG) attempts to identify post-MI patients at high risk for sustained VT and presumably sudden death. Late potentials are high-frequency, low-amplitude signals continuous with the end of the QRS. They are present in 32 to 52% of patients at 1 week but disappear in a third of affected persons by 1 year after infarction. The SAECG study has a sensitivity of 80%, but its positive predictive value is less than 30%. However, the negative predictive value is high at more than 90%. If late potentials are absent, then there is a low incidence of sudden death at 1 to 3%.

Programmed ventricular extrastimulation (electrophysiologic testing) in post-MI patients with nonsustained VT induces sustained monomorphic VT in nearly 40% of individuals. A combination of reduced ejection fraction to less than 0.40, nonsustained VT, and inducible sustained monomorphic VT is associated with a 43% incidence of cardiac arrest at 2 years. Antiarrhythmic therapy guided by programmed electrical stimulation does little to reduce the risk of sudden death when left ventricular function is reduced to below 30%. Heart rate variability can predict ischemic ventricular fibrillation. Variability between successive QRS complexes tends to drop initially post MI, and lower values suggest increased sympathetic tone and reduced vagal tone. Post acute infarction, the relative risk of sudden death increases by three- to sevenfold if heart rate variability is markedly reduced. Similarly, baroreflex sensitivity drops as a result of increased sympathetic tone. Increases in sympathetic tone promote cardiac arrhythmias.

Data now exist for determining the risk of sudden death with dilated cardiomyopathy. Survival depends on the severity of left ventricular dysfunction. For patients with idiopathic dilated cardiomyopathy, the 1-year mortality rate averages 15%. Predictors of survival include left ventricular ejection fraction (less than 0.25: 1-year survival rate of about 50%), New York Heart Association functional class III, S_3 gallop, peak oxygen consumption (Vo_2 of 14 mL or less per kg per minute), low serum sodium (less than 133 mmol per liter), intraventricular conduction delay (0.12 second or less), pulmonary capillary wedge pressure, atrial fibrillation, and symptomatic sustained VT. The only etiologic risk factor that carries any significance is ischemic cardiomyopathy. Left ventricular dimension, findings on SAECG, and the presence of nonsustained VT are nonpredictors of sudden death in this patient population. In some studies of congestive heart failure, syncope is predictive of sudden death. It is reported to occur in about 12% of patients with dilated cardiomyopathy. About 35% of the cases of syncope are thought to be secondary to VT. Syncope does correlate with mortality. When syncope is present, the 1-year mortality rate is 45%, and when it is absent, the rate is only 12%.

Nonsustained VT correlates with overall mortality but

not consistently with the rate of sudden death in patients with dilated nonischemic cardiomyopathy. Neither do frequency and complexity of ventricular ectopy consistently correlate with the severity of ventricular dysfunction. The use of programmed ventricular extrastimuli in patients with dilated cardiomyopathy and nonsustained VT has not been shown to predict those at higher risk for sudden death. At present, electrophysiologic testing in this population is not routinely performed because it is rarely predictive of outcome.

The patient with hypertrophic cardiomyopathy is thought to be at increased risk for sudden death. It is the most common cause of sudden death in otherwise young and healthy persons. The prevalence of hypertrophic cardiomyopathy in the population is about 0.2%. Familial hypertrophic cardiomyopathy is inherited in an autosomal dominant pattern. The high-risk profile has been constructed and includes (1) a positive family history for sudden death that occurs prematurely (age of less than 55 years) and has affected two or more first-degree relatives, (2) nonsustained VT during ambulatory monitoring, and (3) syncope. However, none of these variables has been shown to reliably identify the patient who will have a cardiac arrest. It was initially thought that programmed ventricular extrastimuli might be more accurate at predicting patients at risk for sudden death. The data show that if among patients presenting with hypertrophic cardiomyopathy and cardiac arrest, 77% will have inducible VT on electrophysiologic testing. Patients with nonsustained VT clinically have a 20% induction rate. Thus, electrophysiologic testing appears to identify patients who have hypertrophic cardiomyopathy and have already progressed to a cardiac arrest.

Clearly, risk stratification can identify a group of patients with coronary artery disease who will experience sudden death. The profile for patients with congestive heart failure is also well defined. The hypertrophic cardiomyopathy high-risk group still needs better characterization. Methods of assessing the risk for sudden death post infarction—Holter monitoring, SAECG, heart rate variability, and electrophysiologic testing—have not been shown to alter management or survival. Thus, the routine use of specialized electrocardiographic testing cannot be vigorously recommended at present because of the lack of an intervention proven to be beneficial.

CLINICAL TRIALS AIMED AT PREVENTION OF SUDDEN DEATH

Prevention probably represents the best approach to reducing the incidence of cardiac arrest. Beta blockers remain the only group of agents that reduce total mortality and the incidence of sudden death post infarction. Multiple trials have demonstrated that beta blockers improve survival by 25 to 40%. Vasodilator therapy, particularly with angiotensin-converting enzyme (ACE) inhibitors, has been shown to improve survival in patients with congestive heart failure.

Several post-MI trials have helped to define the best approach to management of the high-risk patient with coronary artery disease. The Cardiac Arrhythmia Suppression Trials, CAST I and CAST II, demonstrated that suppression of frequent and complex PVCs will not reduce the incidence of cardiac arrest post infarction. The class I antiarrhythmics encainide, flecainide, and moricizine adversely affected patient survival despite significantly reducing PVC frequency and complexity. Meta-analysis of other class I antiarrhythmics has shown these agents to adversely affect survival post infarction. Few data exist to support the use of any class I antiarrhythmic agent to reduce the incidence of sudden death post acute infarction. Likewise, *d*-sotalol, a pure class III antiarrhythmic without beta-blocker activity, was shown in the Survival with Oral *dl*-sotalol (SWORD) trial to increase the incidence of sudden death compared to placebo. Post infarction, *dl*-sotalol, a combined beta blocker and class III agent, has been shown to have a neutral effect on survival. The Multicenter Automatic Defibrillator Implantation Trial (MADIT) also showed that use of the implantable cardioverter-defibrillator (ICD) produced a better survival than that obtained with conventional antiarrhythmic agents as predicted by electrophysiologic study. This was a primary prevention trial in a high-risk post-MI population. As the only trial of its kind, MADIT may well dictate future therapy for high-risk post-infarction patients.

Amiodarone (Cordarone) reduced arrhythmic mortality in two empirical post-infarction trials: the Basel Antiarrhythmic Study of Infarct Survival (BASIS) and the Polish Amiodarone Trial (PAT). Amiodarone reduced total mortality in BASIS and the PAT investigations. Two larger randomized placebo-controlled studies, the European Myocardial Infarct Amiodarone Trial (EMIAT) and the Canadian Amiodarone Myocardial Infarction Arrhythmia Trial (CAMIAT), confirmed that arrhythmic death is significantly reduced with use of this agent, but all-cause mortality was not significantly lowered. Patients taking beta blockers and amiodarone had a lower mortality. These trials demonstrate a consistent paucity of proarrhythmia. Should an antiarrhythmic agent be necessary post infarction and the patient is at high risk, amiodarone appears to be a safe alternative (Table 4).

In patients with congestive heart failure, therapies that are proved to prolong life include the use of ACE inhibitors, angiotensin A-II receptor blockers, the beta blocker carvedilol (Coreg), and the combination of nitrates and hydralazine. In mostly uncontrolled studies, the class I antiarrhythmics tend to be less effective and more detrimental owing to the risk of proarrhythmia in patients with poor systolic function (ejection fraction of less than 0.25). Several small pilot studies suggest that amiodarone may be useful in preventing sudden death in patients with congestive heart failure. The objective of the Grupo de Estudio de la Sobrevida en la Insuficiencia Cardiac en Argentina (GESICA) trial was to study the effect of amiodarone on asymptomatic ventricular arrhythmias in severe chronic heart failure. Amiodarone significantly reduced total mortality but did not reduce the incidence of sudden death. Another amiodarone congestive heart failure–asymptomatic VT trial was the Congestive Heart Failure–Survival Trial of Antiarrhythmic Therapy (CHF-STAT). Although amiodarone had little effect on overall mortality, it did tend to reduce mortality in patients with a nonischemic dilated myopathy. Those on amiodarone had an increase in ejection fraction. In both trials, amiodarone significantly benefited patients with a dilated nonischemic cardiomyopathy but had a neutral effect in those with an ischemic cardiomyopathy.

Prospective randomized trials have examined antiarrhythmic agents for secondary prevention of sudden death and sustained VT. Two of these trials, the Calgary trial and the Electrophysiologic Study Versus Electrocardiographic Monitoring (ESVEM) study, had divergent conclusions. Both were designed to compare electrophysiologic testing and ambulatory Holter monitoring in patients with VT or cardiac arrest and with both frequent ventricular premature contractions (VPCs) and inducible VT. The Calgary study concluded that the invasive method was superior to

TABLE 4. **Summary of Clinical Arrhythmia Trials**

Study	Results/Comments
Trials of Antiarrhythmics for VT	
Individualized antiarrhythmic therapy	EPS versus Holter: best guide; inconclusive.
Calgary Trial (1996)	EPS may be a better guide in drug-naive patients.
ESVEM Trial (1993)	Holter not very predictive in drug-naive patients.
	Neither EPS nor Holter effective in drug-resistant patients.
Empiric beta-blocker therapy	As primary therapy for VT/VF: data are not supportive.
	Important as concomitant therapy.
Empiric amiodarone therapy	Amiodarone is more effective than class I agents.
	Efficacy data are not overwhelming but are generally accepted as appropriate.
Post–Myocardial Infarction Trials	
Yusuf et al. (1988)	
Teo et al. (1993)	
Kendall et al. (1995)	
Beta-blocker trials	Reduce post-MI mortality by 25–40%.
	Decrease sudden death by 32–50%.
CAST I (1991) and CAST II (1992)	Disprove the PVC hypothesis.
	Class I antiarrhythmics tend to enhance mortality post MI.
Amiodarone post myocardial infarction	Amiodarone reduced arrhythmic but not total mortality.
EMIAT—Julian et al. (1997)	A beta blocker plus amiodarone improves survival.
CAMIAT—Cairns et al. (1997)	In high-risk patients, amiodarone is a safe alternative.
ACE inhibitors	ACE inhibitors should be started early post MI.
Latini et al. (1995)	
Ball et al. (1995)	Patients with heart failure benefit most.
Trials of Amiodarone in Congestive Heart Failure	
GESICA—Doval et al. (1994)	Beta blockers benefit CHF patients.
CHF-STAT—Singh et al. (1995)	Carvedilol improves survival.
	Nonsustained VT a marker for total mortality.
	Amiodarone no benefit.

Abbreviations: ACE = angiotensin-converting enzyme; CHF = congestive heart failure; EPS = electrophysiologic study; MI = myocardial infarction; PVC = premature ventricular complex; VF = ventricular fibrillation; VT = ventricular tachycardia.

Holter, while the ESVEM study concluded that there was no difference. The patient populations were distinctly different. In ESVEM, the beta blocker/class III agent *dl*-sotalol proved more effective than any class I antiarrhythmic.

In an out-of-hospital ventricular fibrillation population, the Cardiac Arrest Study in Seattle: Conventional versus Amiodarone Drug Evaluation (CASCADE) trial demonstrated that patients receiving empirical amiodarone therapy had better survival and less recurrence of VT than those receiving treatment with class I agents dictated by results of electrophysiologic study. In the Antiarrhythmics Versus Implantable Defibrillator (AVID) study, the ICD was more effective than amiodarone or sotalol in preventing recurrence of cardiac arrest. It appears that use of the ICD may prove the best approach to preventing recurrence of VT or cardiac arrest (Table 5).

DIAGNOSTIC EVALUATION

Patients who have had a cardiac arrest and are successfully resuscitated and stable from a neurologic standpoint have a 30% incidence of recurrence within 2 years. Table 6 summarizes the components of evaluation. A thorough history with a complete description of the acute event and a complete physical examination are required. Valuable clues are frequently obtained from persons witnessing the arrest and the emergency medical personnel attending the patient. Simple documentation of the initial rhythm may lead to an early diagnosis. Ruling out an acute MI with an ECG and assays for cardiac markers for myocardial cell damage including serum myoglobin, creatine kinase (CK)–MB fraction, and troponin should be routine. The initial chest radiograph may help with diagnosis and management of congestive heart failure. An echocardiogram will help to characterize ventricular function or detect the presence of regional wall motion abnormalities suggesting prior or acute infarction, valvular disease, ventricular hypertrophy, or pericardial effusion. Since the majority (80%) of sudden cardiac deaths are related to coronary disease, cardiac catheterization with attention to coronary arteriography is mandatory. Further assessment of global and

TABLE 5. **Summary of Trials of Implantable Cardioverter-Defibrillators**

Study	Results
Secondary Prevention Trials	
Cardiac Arrest Study Hamburg (CASH):	Interim report: Class I agents are not as effective as an ICD.
Efficacy of ICD versus antiarrhythmics in survivors of sudden death	ICD reduces sudden death mortality but not total mortality when compared with metoprolol or amiodarone.
Antiarrhythmics Versus Implantable Defibrillator (AVID):	
Efficacy of ICD versus empirical amiodarone or guided sotalol therapy in patients with VT or VF	ICD is superior to amiodarone and sotalol.
	Survival benefit persisted for 2–3 years.
Primary Prevention Trials	
Coronary Artery Bypass Graft (CABG) Patch:	
Prophylactic ICD in CABG patients with reduced ejection fraction	Prophylactic ICD did not improve survival over CABG alone.
Multicenter Automatic Defibrillator Implantation Trial (MADIT):	ICD does improve survival in a high-risk post-MI population.
Efficacy of ICD in high-risk patients/post–MI patients (EF <0.35)	

Abbreviations: EF = ejection fraction; ICD = implantable cardioverter-defibrillator; VF = ventricular fibrillation; VT = ventricular tachycardia.

TABLE 6. **Diagnostic Evaluation of Patients Surviving Cardiac Arrest**

Clinical Assessment

History and physical examination
Rhythm strips recorded at time of cardiac arrest
12-lead electrocardiogram
Chest radiography
Cardiac markers: myoglobin, creatine kinase-MB fraction, troponin
Echocardiography
Cardiac catheterization, coronary arteriography
Radionuclide ventriculography
Exercise testing

Electrical System Assessment

Ambulatory (Holter) monitoring
Electrophysiologic testing
Signal-averaged electrocardiography*
Heart rate variability, baroreceptor sensitivity*

*For post–myocardial infarction risk stratification.

regional ventricular function is best obtained with radionuclide ventriculography. On occasion, an exercise treadmill test with or without perfusion imaging will help to define the presence of active ischemia. These steps help to characterize the anatomic abnormalities predisposing to sudden cardiac death.

The conduction system is initially assessed by close analysis of the 12-lead ECG. Ambulatory (Holter) monitoring helps to quantitate baseline frequency and complexity of ventricular arrhythmia. Programmed ventricular stimulation at the time of electrophysiologic testing remains the best guide for characterization of the conduction system after cardiac arrest. It may replicate the sustained VT that precipitated the arrest. It also may help guide antiarrhythmic drug therapy as well as determine the usefulness of antitachycardia pacing modalities for termination of VT in selected cases. Electrophysiologic testing may provide information for choosing other nonpharmacologic approaches such as catheter ablation and surgical excision of a VT focus. As indicated previously, programmed ventricular stimulation and recording of high-frequency, low-amplitude late potentials on an SAECG are indicated in the post-MI patient for risk stratification. Characterization of the autonomic nervous system in patients at risk for sudden cardiac death may be obtained by measurement of T wave alternans, baroreceptor sensitivity, and assessment of heart rate variability. At present these tests of autonomic function are used to define prognosis and have not been shown to be useful in guiding treatment.

DIFFERENTIAL DIAGNOSIS AND EVALUATION OF CARDIAC SYNCOPE

Syncope in the absence of organic heart disease tends to have a benign outcome. Syncope due to a cardiac cause is secondary to either a mechanical defect or an arrhythmia. Arrhythmias account for 20% of all cases of syncope. Only a few arrhythmias cause syncope. The bradycardias frequently implicated are sinus node dysfunction and atrioventricular block. The tachycardias are nearly always ventricular and only rarely supraventricular. About 45% of all cardiac causes of syncope are secondary to VT. Patients with arrhythmia-induced syncope tend to be older and usually have little (less than 5 seconds) to no warning. Recurrent episodes of arrhythmia-induced syncope tend to be rare (fewer than two episodes) before the occurrence of a catastrophic event such as a cardiac arrest. Frequently, seizure activity is witnessed, and the patient is labeled as having epilepsy. The best indicators of a true seizure are disorientation surrounding the event, a young age, facial cyanosis, and tongue biting. Transient confusion may occur with cardiac syncope, but it rarely lasts more than 30 seconds.

Exercise-induced syncope is a significant problem, particularly in the young adult. The clinician must typically be concerned about dynamic left ventricular outflow tract obstruction caused by hypertrophic cardiomyopathy or an exercise-induced VT. Affected persons may have no history of heart disease. There is frequently a family history of sudden death at a young age in a close relative. In the absence of overt cardiac disease, an ECG may demonstrate a long QT interval, a short PR interval and delta wave consistent with Wolff-Parkinson-White syndrome, evidence of conduction system disease, or the rare right bundle branch block with persistent ST segment elevation syndrome. All can cause cardiac arrest. The long QT syndromes may be congenital or acquired. The congenital syndromes are characterized as "adrenergic-dependent" because the polymorphic VT is frequently triggered by adrenergic stimulation. The acquired forms of prolonged QT syndrome are characterized as "pause-dependent" because VT is frequently initiated by a sudden slowing in heart rate (Table 7).

The evaluation of syncope requires a detailed history (Figure 2). An ECG is mandatory in all cases of syncope. The type of organic heart disease can be characterized by an echocardiogram. An exercise treadmill-test may reproduce VT in persons with a history of exercise-induced syncope. Those with unexplained syncope and organic heart disease frequently require electrophysiologic study.

TREATMENT

Three groups of patients can be recommended for therapy. Patients with syncope and structural heart

TABLE 7. **Causes of Long QT Syndromes**

Congential	Jervell and Lange-Nielsen syndrome Romano-Ward syndrome
Drugs	Antiarrhythmics: IA—quinidine, procainamide; III—sotalol, ibutilide Tricyclic antidepressants: amitriptyline, imipramine, doxepin Phenothiazines: thioridazine, chlorpromazine Antibiotics: erythromycin, trimethoprim-sulfamethoxazole, ketoconazole, macrolide Antihistamines: terfenadine, astemizole Serotonin antagonists: ketanserin,* zimeldine*
Electrolytes	Hypokalemia, hypomagnesemia
Bradycardia	Sinus node dysfunction, atrioventricular block
Diet	Anorexia nervosa, starvation
Cerebrovascular diseases	Endocrine disturbance Hypothyroidism

*Not available in the United States.

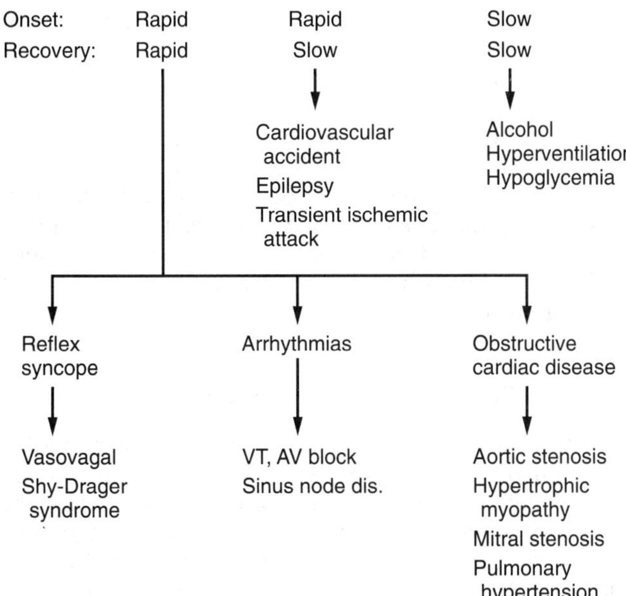

Figure 2. Classification of syncope based on presentation. *Abbreviations*: VT = ventricular tachycardia; AV = atrioventricular.

disease are best managed by removal or correction of the underlying cardiac abnormality. Patients with an electrical cause for syncope without overt structural disease need therapy directed at the underlying cause. Patients with symptomatic bradycardia from either sinus node dysfunction or type II second- or third-degree atrioventricular block should receive a permanent pacemaker. High-risk patients with congenital long QT syndrome must be identified so that the risk of sudden death can be eliminated by beta-blocker therapy in combination with atrial pacing and/or left cervical stellectomy. In contrast, persons with acquired long QT syndrome do well after removal of the offending agent causing QT interval prolongation. Occasionally, permanent pacing is warranted to prevent recurrent periods of bradycardia that predispose to torsades de pointes. Some patients with prolonged QT syndrome who are resuscitated from cardiac arrest require an implantable defibrillator.

The second group of patients requiring therapy comprises those with an increased risk for sudden death related to acute MI or to the presence of either hypertrophic or dilated cardiomyopathy. The degree of left ventricular dysfunction is the single factor that correlates with mortality in patients with coronary artery disease and in those with congestive heart failure. Prevention of cardiac arrest requires better risk stratification of patients with these two pathologic conditions. Effective treatment must be instituted to prevent or reverse ventricular fibrillation. Routine electrophysiologic testing in these patients has not proved effective in guiding antiarrhythmic drug therapy. It appears from studies such as MADIT that use of the implantable cardioverter-defibrillator may be the best therapy for preventing sudden death from VT or ventricular fibrillation. If trials such as the Multicenter Unsustained Tachycardia Trial (MUSTT) and Canadian Implantable Defibrillator Study confirm the superiority of the ICD to antiarrhythmic therapy, as recently concluded by the AVID study, then placement of an ICD may become an empirical standard of care for well-defined high-risk patients.

Patients resuscitated from out-of-hospital cardiac arrest constitute the third group. Documenting the initial arrhythmia at the time of collapse may help to establish a cause. About 80% of cases are related to the ventricular arrhythmias, VT, and ventricular fibrillation. At present, electrophysiologic testing is indicated in nearly all patients recovering from cardiac arrest. As concluded by the AVID trial, the ICD is superior to the antiarrhythmics amiodarone and sotalol in patients resuscitated from VT and ventricular fibrillation. Until future ICD trials confirm the hypothesis that these devices reduce the incidence of sudden death and total mortality, standard care will incorporate the use of electrophysiologic testing to guide either antiarrhythmic drug therapy, surgical or catheter ablation therapy, or device-based ICD therapy.

ATRIAL FIBRILLATION

method of
DAVID M. GILLIGAN, M.D., and
KENNETH A. ELLENBOGEN, M.D.
Medical College of Virginia, Virginia Commonwealth University, and the Hunter Holmes McGuire Veterans Affairs Medical Center
Richmond, Virginia

Atrial fibrillation is the most common arrhythmia encountered in clinical practice. It affects an estimated 1 million people in the United States. The management of atrial fibrillation has evolved significantly in recent years. Randomized trials have shown that anticoagulation markedly reduces the risk of stroke in patients with atrial fibrillation, and a number of new antiarrhythmic agents have become available. Procedures such as radiofrequency ablation of the atrioventricular (AV) node combined with permanent pacing are playing increasing roles in the management of patients with atrial fibrillation. Much of the following discussion is equally applicable to atrial flutter, which often occurs concomitantly in the same patient.

DIAGNOSIS

The diagnosis of atrial fibrillation can usually be made easily on clinical examination and 12-lead electrocardiography. The ventricular rate is typically "irregularly irregular," except in patients who have concomitant complete heart block or digoxin toxicity. Absent P waves and a variable degree of baseline fibrillatory activity on the electrocardiogram (ECG) confirm the diagnosis of atrial fibrillation. Atrial flutter is recognized as regular rapid flutter waves, with either a typical negative "saw-tooth" pattern

TABLE 1. **Principles of Management of Atrial Fibrillation**

- Identify any underlying cause(s) and/or precipitating factor(s).
- Control the ventricular rate, if necessary, in the short and long term.
- Decide whether restoration of sinus rhythm is to be undertaken, and if so, minimize thromboembolic risk.
- Decide how best to maintain sinus rhythm, should sinus rhythm be restored.
- Initiate long-term anticoagulation with warfarin or antiplatelet therapy with aspirin.

in the inferior leads or other atypical but regular patterns, and a regular ventricular response.

MANAGEMENT

The management of atrial fibrillation should be considered in five principal aspects. These are summarized in Table 1.

Identification of the Underlying Cause

In every patient presenting with atrial fibrillation, it is important to consider the possible underlying cause(s) and/or precipitating factors (Table 2). All patients presenting with new atrial fibrillation should have a complete evaluation including a detailed history, physical examination, 12-lead electrocardiography, chest radiography, laboratory tests including thyroid hormone levels, and transthoracic echocardiography. Echocardiography provides a measure of left ventricular function, which will influence further management such as the choice of antiarrhythmic agents and antithrombotic therapy, and may uncover structural heart disease, such as dilated cardiomyopathy or hypertensive heart disease, not suspected on the basis of the history and physical findings. A wide variety of cardiac or systemic conditions may cause atrial fibrillation, and a consideration of each possible cause is beyond the scope of this discussion. It is important to emphasize that treatment of the underlying cause or reversal of a precipitating factor may sometimes be the single most important factor in treating atrial fibrillation. However, regardless of the nature of the associated condition(s), the remaining four management issues will need to be addressed to a greater or lesser extent in each patient.

TABLE 2. **Causes and/or Precipitating Factors of Atrial Fibrillation**

Structural Heart Disease

Hypertensive heart disease
Coronary artery disease: chronic ventricular dysfunction, acute myocardial infarction
Valvular heart disease, especially mitral valve disease (rheumatic)
Cardiomyopathies: dilated, hypertrophic, restrictive
Prior cardiac surgery
Pericarditis
Congenital heart disease, e.g., atrial septal defect
Pulmonary hypertension

Systemic Conditions

Ethanol intoxication and withdrawal
Noncardiac surgery
Major infection(s), e.g., pneumonia
Hyperthyroidism/hypothyroidism
Electrolyte disturbance (severe)
Malignancy, especially lung and mediastinal, primary or metastatic
Systemic illnesses: sarcoidosis, pheochromocytoma, amyloidosis

Control of the Ventricular Rate

It is important to decide (1) whether ventricular rate control is necessary and, if so, (2) how quickly control needs to be achieved, and (3) which drugs are to be used and by which route. Initial management should follow the guidelines for Advanced Cardiac Life Support of the American Heart Association. Patients who are hemodynamically unstable owing to a rapid ventricular response require urgent synchronized, direct-current (DC) cardioversion.

Intravenous Drug Therapy

The initial rate control strategy in patients with stable hemodynamics will be determined by the rapidity of the ventricular rate and the presence of associated symptoms. A summary of available drugs is given in Table 3. Intravenous therapy is indicated for control of rapid ventricular rates (more than 150 beats per minute) that are accompanied by clinical manifestations. Intravenous diltiazem (Cardizem) has become the drug of choice. The slowing of AV node conduction with intravenous diltiazem occurs rapidly and can be maintained by titrating a continuous infusion. Intravenous beta blockers may also be used to control the ventricular rate, especially in situations of high sympathetic drive, e.g., postoperatively. Intravenous digoxin (Lanoxin) does not provide immediate heart rate control—onset of effect occurs in from 1 to 6 hours—and digoxin is typically ineffective in settings of high sympathetic tone. Preliminary reports show that intravenous amiodarone (Cordarone) may be effective in slowing the ventricular response in patients who are critically ill or have severe left ventricular dysfunction. Intravenous amiodarone, at a dose identical to that used for patients with ventricular tachyarrhythmias, is capable of causing a 20% or greater decrease in heart rate within 1 to 3 hours in critically ill patients with atrial fibrillation, including patients on intravenous vasopressors. Finally, in the Wolff-Parkinson-White syndrome, antegrade conduction of atrial fibrillation over an accessory bypass tract will produce wide-complex tachycardia, and very rapid conduction is associated with a risk of ventricular fibrillation. Drugs that block AV node conduction should not be used. DC cardioversion or intravenous procainamide should be used to terminate atrial fibrillation in the setting of Wolf-Parkinson-White syndrome.

TABLE 3. **Pharmacologic Control of Ventricular Rate in Atrial Fibrillation**

Clinical Setting	Drug	Dosing	Efficacy	Comments
	Intravenous Drugs			
Rapid ventricular rate (>150 bpm) Associated symptoms	Diltiazem (Cardizem)	20-mg bolus IV over 2 min; at 15 min, 25 mg over 2 min; infusion 5–15 mg/h	Rapid rate control	Well tolerated
	Verapamil (Isoptin)	5–10 mg IV, repeat after 10 min		Hypotension may occur
	Metoprolol (Lopressor)	5 mg IV q 5 min, total 15 mg	Rapid rate control	Useful in postoperative setting
	Esmolol (Brevibloc)	0.5 mg/kg over 1 min; 0.05 mg/kg/min infusion	Short-acting	Hypotension may occur
	Digoxin (Lanoxin)	0.25–0.5 mg IV, total 1 mg/24 h	Moderate to low efficacy	Delayed onset of AV slowing
	Amiodarone (Cordarone)*	200 mg IV, then 1 mg/min for 6 h, then 0.5 mg/min for 18 h	Acts within 1–2 h	Tolerated by patients with moderate to severe LV dysfunction
	Oral Drugs			
Ventricular rate mildly or moderately increased at rest and/or with exercise	Verapamil (Calan, Isoptin, Verelan)	120–480 mg PO qd	Reduces rest and exercise rate	
	Diltiazem (Cardizem, Dilacor)	90–360 mg PO qd	Reduces rest and exercise rate	
	Atenolol (Tenormin)	25–100 mg PO qd	Reduces exercise rate most effectively	Any beta blocker may be used
	Digoxin (Lanoxin)	0.1–0.75 mg PO qd	Reduces resting rate	Exercise tachycardia persists

*Not FDA approved for this indication.
Abbreviations: AV = atrioventricular; bpm = beats per minute; LV = left ventricular.

Oral Drug Therapy

In less acute situations, when the ventricular rate is not very rapid and there are mild or minimal symptoms, oral therapy is appropriate. In chronic sustained or paroxysmal atrial fibrillation, ventricular rate control is important to minimize symptoms and reduce the risk of tachycardia-induced ventricular dysfunction. In the past, digoxin therapy has been the mainstay of treatment. However, because digoxin's effect is primarily to increase vagal tone in the AV node, it may have little effect on exercise heart rate. Monotherapy with digoxin may be appropriate in sedentary patients or in those requiring its inotropic support. Other agents, used either alone or in combination with digoxin, provide better control of the ventricular response in chronic atrial fibrillation. The calcium channel blockers diltiazem (Cardizem, Dilacor) and verapamil (Calan, Isoptin, Verelan), best given in slow-release, once-daily preparations reduce both rest and exercise heart rate. Beta blockers are also effective in controlling the ventricular response, especially during exercise. Whichever drugs are used, it is important to assess whether control of the ventricular rate is adequate. This can be achieved by Holter monitoring, formal exercise testing, or measuring the apical heart rate after a hall walk at the physician's office.

Nonpharmacologic Therapy

Some patients with chronic atrial fibrillation have persistently rapid ventricular rates despite drug therapy with AV node–blocking drugs and continue to be symptomatic or have left ventricular dysfunction that may be secondary to or exacerbated by the high rates. In addition, the use of AV-slowing drugs may be limited in patients with left ventricular dysfunction because of the negative inotropic effects of beta blockers and calcium channel blockers. These patients should be referred to a cardiac electrophysiologist for consideration of radio frequency ablation of the AV node coupled with implantation of a ventricular rate–responsive permanent pacemaker.

Patients with intrinsic conduction system disease may present with a slow ventricular response to atrial fibrillation, generally less than 70 beats per minute, or demonstrate prolonged pauses. AV node–blocking drugs should initially be avoided in such patients, but the heart rate response to exercise should be assessed, as some patients may have concomitant exercise tachycardia. Patients with a symptomatic slow ventricular rate in atrial fibrillation, either due to intrinsic conduction system disease or secondary to AV node–blocking drugs that are required to control the exercise heart rate, should receive a permanent pacemaker.

Restoration of Sinus Rhythm

DC cardioversion should be performed urgently in patients with atrial fibrillation and a rapid ventricular response who are hemodynamically unstable. Elective restoration of sinus rhythm should be considered in all other patients. It should be remembered that approximately 50% of patients with recent-onset atrial fibrillation will revert spontaneously to sinus rhythm within 48 hours. The AV node–blocking agents (digoxin, beta blockers, calcium channel blockers) probably do not have any specific effect in restoring sinus rhythm. Elective cardioversion is probably indicated for all patients with a first episode of atrial fibrillation unless relative contraindications exist (Table 4). The advantages of restoring sinus rhythm include relief of symptoms, improvement in hemodynamics, and possible avoidance of long-term anticoagulation. The advantages of allowing atrial fibrillation to persist are the avoidance of further procedures and antiarrhythmic drugs with their concomitant side effects. Therefore, the decision to attempt restoration of sinus rhythm must be individualized for each patient. If the decision is made to restore sinus rhythm, this can be achieved by one of two methods: synchronized DC cardioversion or antiarrhythmic drug therapy. Before either procedure, the thromboembolic risk of restoring sinus rhythm must be minimized.

Anticoagulation Strategies Before Cardioversion

A common approach is to assume that patients with atrial fibrillation of less than 48 hours' duration may undergo conversion to sinus rhythm with a low risk of thromboembolism, but recent studies suggest that in some of these patients, clot may be present in the left atrial appendage. Thus, patients with atrial fibrillation occurring in hospital or with a clear symptomatic onset within a 48-hour window may undergo chemical or elective cardioversion. However, it has been our practice in these cases to administer heparin therapy in hospital and warfarin (Coumadin) after cardioversion (as described later).

In patients with atrial fibrillation of more than 48 hours' duration, or when time of onset of the arrhythmia is unclear, anticoagulation should be initiated with intravenous heparin and oral warfarin. A therapeutic International Normalized Ratio (INR) is achieved (2.0 to 3.0) and should be maintained for at least 4 weeks prior to cardioversion. The rationale for this period of anticoagulation prior to cardioversion is to allow any pre-existing atrial thrombus to dissolve or endothelialize and to prevent the formation of new thrombi. Following conversion, the patient should remain anticoagulated for at least 4 weeks, as left atrial mechanical function does not recover immediately and stasis may persist for days to weeks following conversion. Continuing anticoagulation for up to 4 weeks also protects the patient during the period when arrhythmia recurrence is highest.

Another strategy, especially when conversion to sinus rhythm must proceed because of marked symptoms, is to perform transesophageal echocardiography to exclude thrombus in the left atrium (transthoracic echocardiography is inadequate for this purpose). If thrombus is excluded, studies show that cardioversion can proceed with minimal risk of thromboembolism. In these studies, the patients were anticoagulated with heparin around the time of echocardiography and for 3 to 4 weeks after conversion.

TABLE 4. **Relative Contraindications to Attempting Restoration of Sinus Rhythm in Atrial Fibrillation**

Acutely Unsafe
No anticoagulation therapy given
High anesthetic risk, e.g., in severe respiratory disease
Digoxin toxicity
Electrolyte imbalance
Unlikely to Succeed
Long-standing atrial fibrillation (>3 years' duration)
Very enlarged left atrium (>6 cm)
Prior failed cardioversion attempts
Unlikely to Benefit
Spontaneously self-terminating or intermittent atrial fibrillation
Poor prognosis, e.g., with advanced malignancy
Other severe functional limitation
Well-controlled ventricular rate with minimal or no symptoms

Pharmacologic Cardioversion

Class IA, class IC, and class III antiarrhythmic agents are all modestly effective in restoring and maintaining sinus rhythm. The important features and dosing of these drugs are summarized in Table 5 and also discussed later on in the section on maintaining sinus rhythm. Several drugs are available, and it is best to become familiar with the use and side effects of one or two drugs. For all agents, the likelihood of conversion is related to the duration of atrial fibrillation: sinus rhythm may be restored in up to 80% of patients with recent-onset atrial fibrillation (of less than 48 hours' duration), while conversion of long-standing atrial fibrillation is unlikely. All antiarrhythmic agents have a risk of proarrhythmia; therefore, we recommend that these drugs be initiated in hospital with continuous electrocardiographic monitoring.

Of the oral agents, quinidine (Quinaglute, Quinidex) has traditionally been used for pharmacologic cardioversion to sinus rhythm, formerly in high doses (until conversion or side effects occurred) but now in regular dosing schedules. Procainamide (Procan SR) is another commonly used class IA agent for pharmacologic cardioversion. Other oral agents, probably of similar efficacy, for atrial fibrillation conversion are the class IC drugs flecainide acetate (Tambocor) and propafenone (Rythmol) and the class III drugs sotalol (Betapace) and amiodarone.

To use intravenous therapy for pharmacologic con-

TABLE 5. **Antiarrhythmic Drug Therapy in Atrial Fibrillation**

	Oral Drug Dose	Useful in	Avoid in
Class IA			
Quinidine gluconate (Quinaglute)	324–648 mg q 8–12 h	Chronic renal failure	CHF Liver failure
Procainamide (Procan SR)	0.5–1.5 gm q 6 h	Men, short-term therapy	Renal failure CHF Joint disease
Disopyramide (Norpace CR)	200–400 mg q 12 h	Women	Older men at risk of urinary retention Glaucoma Renal failure, CHF
Class IC			
Flecainide acetate (Tambocor)	50–150 mg q 12 h	Failure of class IA agents Structurally normal heart	Any LV dysfunction, CAD
Propafenone (Rythmol)	150–300 mg q 8 h	Failure of class IA agents Structurally normal heart	Any LV dysfunction
Class III			
Sotalol (Betapace)	80–240 mg q 12 h	Failure of IA, IC agents May be used with mild to moderate LV dysfunction	Cases in which beta blockers are contraindicated
Amiodarone (Cordarone)	1200 mg qd × 5 d followed by 400 mg qd × 1 mo; then 200–400 mg qd Many alternative dosing regimens	Severe LV dysfunction Failure of other drugs CHF Renal failure	Young patients Pulmonary disease Multiple systemic effects; close monitoring for lung, thyroid, neurologic, ophthalmologic effects needed

Abbreviations: CAD = coronary artery disease; CHF = congestive heart failure; LV = left ventricular.

version, procainamide may be given in a bolus of 10 to 15 mg per kg at a rate of 50 mg per minute followed by an infusion of 1 to 4 mg per minute. Hypotension is the major side effect. Ibutilide (Corvert) was approved for the acute termination of atrial fibrillation in 1996. It is a class III agent that has a rapid onset of action, leading to arrhythmia termination in up to 50% of patients with atrial fibrillation or flutter within 30 minutes. The drug is administered as a 1-mg infusion over 10 minutes, which may be repeated once. Ibutilide does not cause hypotension but does prolong the QT intervals and polymorphic ventricular tachycardia occurs in 2 to 3% of patients. Patients receiving ibutilide must have electrocardiographic monitoring for up to 4 hours following infusion because of the risk of proarrhythmia. Equipment for DC cardioversion should be available nearby. Ibutilide may be useful in the emergency room in patients with atrial fibrillation of acute or recent onset, as well as in the postoperative setting or in patients in whom the need for chronic antiarrhythmic drug therapy is not anticipated. Intravenous amiodarone appears to have a low efficacy in conversion of atrial fibrillation, but its AV conduction–slowing properties may be helpful as described previously.

Direct-Current Cardioversion

If the chosen drug has not achieved conversion in 24 hours, DC cardioversion is usually performed, or DC cardioversion may often be the first-line therapeutic modality to restore sinus rhythm. Patients on antiarrhythmic drug therapy should be monitored for proarrhythmia for up to 24 hours following restoration of sinus rhythm. DC cardioversion should be performed in an environment in which full resuscitation equipment is available. The patient should fast for a minimum of 6 hours. The procedure should be carried out with the assistance of either an anesthesiologist or a cardiologist experienced in airway management and ventilation during sedation and anesthesia. Usually, deep sedation is achieved with a rapid, short-acting intravenous agent, such as methohexital (Brevital), and a short-acting benzodiazepine. We use adhesive chest patches placed in the anteroposterior position and give a synchronized shock, initially at 200 joules; if this is unsuccessful, two additional shocks of 360 joules each are delivered, usually with slightly different patch positions. DC cardioversion of atrial fibrillation is successful in over 90% of cases. In patients refractory to external cardioversion, we and others have had experience that suggests that successful cardioversion may still be possible with use of an internal technique. Internal cardioversion is performed by placing two multipolar catheters in the heart, one in the lateral right atrium and one in the coronary sinus. A shock is delivered between the two catheters from an external defibrillator. Internal cardioversion may be particularly effective in patients in whom delivery of external energy to the atrial myocardium is inefficient (e.g., obese patients).

Maintenance of Sinus Rhythm

When atrial fibrillation converts spontaneously or is converted to sinus rhythm, the question of maintaining sinus rhythm must be addressed. If there is a clear underlying cause or precipitating factor that can be reversed, it should be corrected. Infrequent episodes of atrial fibrillation can be managed with repeated pharmacologic or electrical cardioversion to sinus rhythm if it is acceptable to the patient and the physician. When occurrences are more frequent, consideration must be given to long-term antiarrhythmic drug therapy.

Chronic Antiarrhythmic Drug Therapy

Antiarrhythmic agents have only modest efficacy in maintaining sinus rhythm and are expensive; all have side effects, and proarrhythmia is a major concern. A meta-analysis of six trials of quinidine for maintaining sinus rhythm in atrial fibrillation found an increased mortality in patients taking quinidine, suggesting that quinidine may worsen survival, especially in patients with congestive heart failure. Despite these concerns, the careful use of antiarrhythmic drugs has an important role in the management of atrial fibrillation. Any one of the several agents described for pharmacologic conversion would be modestly effective in maintaining sinus rhythm (see Table 5). Again, it is best to become familiar with the use of one or two drugs. If long-term antiarrhythmic drug therapy is used to maintain sinus rhythm, patients should be seen regularly and monitored for proarrhythmia. Standard 12-lead ECGs are helpful to follow the PR, QRS, and QT intervals.

The class IA agents have modest efficacy, with approximately 50% of patients in sinus rhythm at 1 year. Long-term quinidine use is limited by its systemic side effects, particularly gastrointestinal intolerance. Long-term use of procainamide is also limited by side effects including gastrointestinal disturbances and arthralgias. Disopyramide (Norpace) is another class IA agent that has some effectiveness in prevention of atrial fibrillation; in extended-release form, it can be given either two or three times a day. However, it has prominent anticholinergic side effects. The class IC drugs flecainide acetate and propafenone have at least equivalent efficacy to that of class IA drugs and are usually better tolerated. With class IA and class IC drugs, the risk of proarrhythmia depends to some degree on the presence of left ventricular dysfunction and coexistent structural heart disease. Class IC agents should be avoided in patients with structural heart disease, in particular coronary artery disease. Class IA agents and class III agents prolong the QT interval and may give rise to torsades de pointes. With class IA agents, this type of proarrhythmia usually occurs within 48 hours of initiation of drug therapy. Sotalol, a beta blocker with class III antiarrhythmic properties, is at least as effective as quinidine in maintaining sinus rhythm. It does cause progressive prolongation of the QT interval that is directly correlated with the risk of torsades. It is wise to avoid a greater than 25 to 30% increase in the QT or a corrected QT interval of more than 500 milliseconds. Amiodarone is considered to be the most effective antiarrhythmic agent with the lowest incidence of proarrhythmia. However, amiodarone has other potentially serious side effects that involve the lungs, thyroid, skin, and nervous system. These toxic effects may be more likely to occur with long-term and higher-dose therapy.

Class IA agents do not slow AV nodal conduction and can at times accelerate it. Therefore, these drugs should be combined with an AV node–blocking drug. In contrast, class III agents have independent AV node conduction–slowing properties, and when these drugs are used, it is often necessary to reduce the dosage or even discontinue other drugs that block AV node conduction. Patients who continue to have symptomatic episodes of atrial fibrillation despite antiarrhythmic drug therapy should be referred to a cardiac electrophysiologist for radiofrequency ablation of the AV node coupled with implantation of a dual-chamber permanent pacemaker with mode-switching capabilities. Although this will not necessarily reduce the occurrence of atrial fibrillation, several observational studies and one controlled trial have shown marked reduction in symptoms following this procedure.

Nonpharmacologic Methods

Other methods of maintaining sinus rhythm are currently being explored. The most aggressive of these requires open heart surgery and is called the "maze procedure." This procedure involves breaking up potential macro-reentrant circuits in the right and left atria by making a series of incisions in each atrium. The operation is associated with a 95% cure rate for atrial fibrillation but has 1 to 5% morbidity and mortality rates, and patients often require permanent pacemakers following this procedure. Similar atrial compartmentalization procedures using catheter-based techniques with radiofrequency energy have been reported. A catheter-based "maze procedure" may become a clinical reality in the coming years. In patients who require permanent cardiac pacing for sick sinus syndrome or conduction disease, multiple retrospective studies and one prospective randomized clinical trial have shown that atrium-based pacing (or dual-chamber pacing) is associated with a decrease in the subsequent occurrence of atrial fibrillation compared with ventricle-based pacing. New forms of multisite or biatrial pacing are being actively investigated to determine whether they offer an advantage over standard pacing from the right atrial appendage in terms of decreasing the incidence of paroxysmal atrial fibrillation. Finally, an implantable atrial defibrillator has been developed and is undergoing clinical trials. This device is implanted like a pacemaker. Leads placed in the right atrium and coronary sinus can internally cardiovert atrial fibrillation with energies of 1 to 4 joules. Synchronization and back-up ventricular pacing are provided by a lead in the right ventricle. Early results suggest that the device is effective and safe, but issues of cost and patient tolerance of shocks remain.

Chronic Anticoagulation and Antiplatelet Therapy

The final but most important consideration in long-term management of patients with atrial fibrillation is the need for anticoagulation. The most serious complication of atrial fibrillation is thromboembolism. About 90% of embolic events occurring in patients with atrial fibrillation are strokes. These strokes tend to be large, with 50 to 60% of patients experiencing death or major long-term sequelae.

Five large, multicenter randomized trials have demonstrated the ability of warfarin to reduce the risk of thromboembolism in patients with atrial fibrillation. The average risk of embolic stroke in these studies was 4 to 6% per year in patients taking placebo drug and, on the average, 70% less, or approximately 1 to 1.5% per year, in patients taking warfarin. Two of these studies incorporated the use of aspirin, and although aspirin also reduced the risk of stroke, its effects were more modest (a reduction rate of approximately 20%). These studies also identified risk factors for systemic embolism in patients with atrial fibrillation (Table 6).

The decision to use anticoagulation in a patient with atrial fibrillation must be individualized, and the associated bleeding risk must always be considered. For patients less than 75 years of age who have structural heart disease or systemic risk factors for stroke, anticoagulation with warfarin is recommended to achieve an INR of 2.0 to 3.0. Higher INRs increase the risk of bleeding significantly. Lower INRs are associated with a decreased efficacy in preventing strokes. In patients less than 65 years of age with no structural heart disease or risk factors for stroke, the risk of thromboembolism is low, and aspirin alone (in a dose of 81–325 mg per day) appears adequate in these patients. In patients more than 75 years of age, warfarin is indicated, but there appears to be an increased risk of bleeding complications with anticoagulation. Thus, anticoagulation should be undertaken with great care. Evidence documenting the risk-benefit ratio with anticoagulation in patients with paroxysmal atrial fibrillation is much less firm. In our opinion, patients with frequent or prolonged episodes of atrial fibrillation or those who are asymptomatic during atrial fibrillation should receive anticoagulation. Those with rare, brief, and highly symptomatic spells of atrial fibrillation should have the benefits and risks of anticoagulation carefully weighed and individualized to their risk factors.

TABLE 6. **Risk Factors for Thromboembolism in Atrial Fibrillation**

Cardiac Factors

Valvular heart disease, especially rheumatic mitral valve disease
Coronary artery disease: history of prior myocardial infarction, angina
History of congestive heart failure
Depressed left ventricular systolic function
Left atrial enlargement

Systemic Factors

Age >75 years (possibly >65)
Prior thromboembolic event
Hypertension
Diabetes mellitus

ATRIAL FLUTTER

The management of atrial flutter follows the approach described for atrial fibrillation except in a number of aspects. First, ventricular rate control is often more difficult to achieve in atrial flutter, and conversion to sinus rhythm is usually a better long-term option. Second, the risk of thromboembolism has traditionally been considered low in atrial flutter, but this may not always be the case, especially if there is significant structural heart disease or coexistent atrial fibrillation. In these situations, the decision to use anticoagulation should follow the guidelines for atrial fibrillation. Finally, for patients with recurrent typical atrial flutter, radiofrequency ablation of a predictable macro-reentrant circuit in the low right atrium has shown considerable promise for preventing recurrences. Immediate success rates of 80 to 95% have been reported, with long-term success rates somewhat lower and recurrence rates for atrial flutter of 10 to 20%. After successful ablation of atrial flutter, some patients may continue to experience atrial fibrillation. On the basis of the high success rates noted after ablation of atrial flutter, some investigators have advocated ablation as first-line therapy, while the majority of investigators recommend ablation for patients with recurrences of arrhythmia on drug therapy or patients intolerant of or unwilling to take drug therapy.

PREMATURE BEATS

method of
MOHAMED H. HAMDAN, M.D.
University of Texas Southwest Medical Center and Dallas Medical Center
Dallas, Texas

and

MELVIN SCHEINMAN, M.D.
University of California, San Francisco
San Francisco, California

Atrial depolarization is driven by the sinus node, which is located in the high right atrium along the crista terminalis. This waveform propagates down the atrioventricular (AV) node and His-Purkinje system, resulting in synchronized activation of both ventricles. An early depolarization occurring before the anticipated normal sinus beat will result in a premature beat. The site of origin defines the beat as an atrial, junctional, or ventricular premature beat. This premature activation of the cardiac chambers can occasionally impair hemodynamic function and/or trigger other sustained arrhythmias. The clinical presentation can be palpitations, fatigue and shortness of breath resulting from poor perfusion, or no symptoms at all. In addition to producing clinical symptoms, premature beats may indicate an increased risk for sudden death. Therefore, the management of patients with premature beats not only should address the presence or absence of symptoms but must also evaluate their prognostic significance.

PATHOGENETIC MECHANISMS

The common electrophysiologic mechanisms responsible for the genesis of premature beats are similar to those involved in the pathogenesis of sustained tachyarrhythmias, namely, reentry, abnormal automaticity, and triggered activity.

Reentry

Reentry is the most common mechanism of arrhythmogenesis. During reentry, a depolarization propagates in one direction while being blocked in adjacent tissue, returns to depolarize the area not initially excited, and, if successful, will travel around repeating its course. Therefore, three criteria are needed for reentry to be present: unidirectional block in one of two available pathways, conduction in the other, and return excitation. Based on these general concepts, three types of reentry have been described: anatomic, functional (leading circle or anisotropic reentry), and reentry by reflection. Detailed description of the types of reentry is beyond the scope of this discussion; however, it should be emphasized that the presence of a discrete anatomic obstacle (such as a scar) is not always needed for reentry, because conduction delay and block can be caused by many factors including differences in refractoriness, ischemia, fibrosis, electrolyte abnormalities, and drug toxicity.

Abnormal Automaticity

Abnormal automaticity refers to spontaneous (phase 4) depolarization resulting in impulse formation in cardiac tissues that normally lack intrinsic automaticity. Atrial and ventricular myocytes normally exhibit a fast-response type of action potential that lacks phase 4 depolarization. Under certain conditions, these cells may show spontaneous automaticity, resulting in premature depolarizations, which, if repetitive, can lead to tachycardia. On the other hand, increased automaticity in tissue that is "automatic" under physiologic conditions can also result in similar findings. Because the tissue has intrinsic automaticity at baseline, such a change is called enhanced automaticity. A classic example of such a tissue is the His-Purkinje system. Ischemia, digoxin and methylxanthine toxicity, electrolyte abnormalities, and high-catecholamine states are well-known causes of abnormal and enhanced automaticity.

Triggered Activity

Triggered activity means impulse initiation caused by afterdepolarizations. Afterdepolarizations are oscillations in membrane potentials that occur after the upstroke of the action potential. Afterdepolarizations during repolarization are called "early afterdepolarizations," and those that occur after full repolarization are called "delayed afterdepolarizations." If the amplitude is large enough for the potential to reach threshold, afterdepolarizations will result in propagated responses. By definition, afterdepolarizations must be preceded by at least one action potential—hence the term "triggered activity." Early afterdepolarizations are usually the result of drugs; they may be catecholamine-driven or provoked by a critical heart rate. On the other hand, delayed afterdepolarizations are usually caused by ischemia, catecholamines, and digitalis.

TYPES OF PREMATURE BEATS

Atrial Premature Depolarizations

An atrial premature depolarization (APD) is defined as a premature activation of the atria arising from a site other than the sinus node. APDs appear on the surface electrocardiogram (ECG) as P waves with morphologic characteristics different from those of the sinus P wave occurring before the anticipated sinus beat. They occur in both normal and abnormal hearts. The cellular mechanism responsible for APDs is not clear. Intra-atrial reentry, abnormal automaticity, and triggered activity all are considered likely mechanisms.

Electrocardiographic Manifestation

An APD may conduct with a short, normal, or prolonged PR interval, or it may not conduct at all. The PR interval is determined by the site of origin and the degree of prematurity. A site of origin close to the AV node is likely to result in a short PR interval. On the other hand, the more premature APD will produce a longer PR interval. If conducted, an APD may be associated with either a normal or a wide QRS complex. An early APD is likely to impinge upon the refractory period of the His-Purkinje conduction system, resulting in various degrees of aberration. Because the right bundle branch has a longer refractory period than the left bundle branch, right bundle branch block aberrancy is more common. If nonconducted, an APD may give the false appearance of a sinus pause (Figure 1). This is the result of the APD impulse's penetrating and resetting the sinus node. Careful analysis of all 12 leads is crucial for the recognition of nonconducted APDs, as they may manifest only as small deformities on the T wave.

Clinical Presentation

Twenty-four-hour Holter studies have shown that APD frequency increases with age. APDs occur in patients with normal hearts but appear to be more frequent in patients with structural heart disease and in the setting of other medical conditions such as chronic renal failure and chronic pulmonary disease. APDs have been shown to increase in the early stages of a myocardial infarction (MI), with a subsequent decrease in frequency after 10 days. This may be related to atrial ischemia, increased filling pressures, or the increased-catecholamine state often

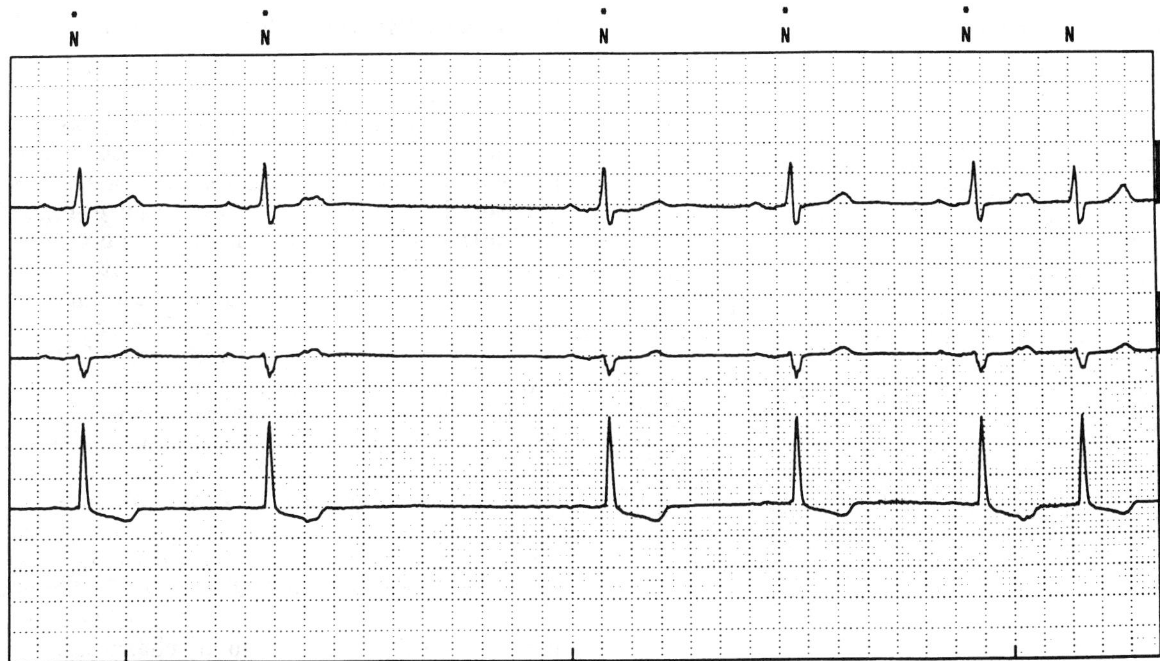

Figure 1. Tracing during normal sinus rhythm showing two atrial premature depolarizations (APDs). The first one is noted on the T wave of the second QRS complex and is not conducted, resulting in a pause. This pause is due to resetting of the sinus node by the APD. The second APD is seen on the T wave of the fifth QRS complex and is conducted with a long PR interval. Beware of nonconducted APDs, as they may give the appearance of sinus pauses.

seen during MI. APDs also appear to be frequent in the setting of pericarditis, suggesting that inflammation and/or increased atrial pressure in the atria may be causing these depolarizations. Patients with APDs may have palpitations or the sensation of skipped beats. If atrial bigeminy with nonconducted APDs is present, the effective heart rate can be as low as 30 beats per minute, resulting in decreased cardiac output symptoms.

Management

In the asymptomatic patient with APDs, no treatment is needed. In the presence of symptoms, treatment of the underlying cardiac disease and elimination of provoking factors such as alcohol and coffee intake are usually enough. Every effort should be made to reassure the patient, as APDs alone are without any significance. If drug therapy is needed, the physician should start with beta blockers and use drugs with little adverse effects. Other antiarrhythmic agents such as class IA or IC and class III drugs should not be used unless the benefit far outweighs the risk of proarrhythmia associated with these agents.

Junctional Premature Depolarizations

The AV junction includes the approaches to the AV node, the compact node, and the His bundle. Any of these areas except for the central area of the compact zone may demonstrate automaticity. Junctional premature depolarizations (JPDs) occur in both normal and abnormal hearts. They are more common in the setting of digitalis toxicity, hypokalemia, and high-cathecholamine states. They also occur in the setting of acute MI. The pathogenetic mechanism in JPDs is believed to be abnormal automaticity, although triggered activity may also be a potential mechanism.

Electrocardiographic Manifestation

The electrocardiographic manifestation of a JPD depends on its site of origin and the relative antegrade and retrograde conduction velocities. As a rule, JPDs originating from the perinodal area result in a retrograde P wave preceding or buried in the QRS complex with a PR interval less than 90 milliseconds. On the other hand, JPDs originating from the His bundle result in P waves that follow the QRS. As with APDs, the degree of prematurity will determine whether the QRS is normal or aberrant. If it is aberrant, APDs may be hard to distinguish from ventricular premature depolarizations (VPDs). The presence of a full compensatory pause suggests lack of sinus node resetting, thus favoring a ventricular rather than a junctional site of origin. JPDs may not conduct in the antegrade direction, so that only retrograde atrial depolarizations occur, thus mimicking APDs. Finally, JPDs may not conduct in either direction. Such APDs, though nonconducted (concealed), may affect the conduction of subsequent impulses, resulting in all types of AV block. The diagnosis of concealed JPDs as a cause of AV block can be impossible from the surface ECG alone. A helpful finding is the presence of manifest JPDs in a patient with a normal QRS complex and evidence of intermittent AV block.

Clinical Presentation

Most patients with JPDs have no symptoms. When symptoms are present, skipped beats or palpitations are common complaints. In the case of concealed JPDs resulting in 2:1 or third-degree AV block, lightheadedness and dizziness may occur.

Management

As with all premature depolarizations, correction of the underlying problem should be the first step in the management of patients with JPDs. In patients with no precipitating factors, treatment should be initiated only in the presence of symptoms. Because abnormal automaticity is the most common mechanism, beta blockers may be successful in suppressing JPDs. Class IC and class III agents may be used only after careful consideration of their adverse effects. In the case of concealed JPDs resulting in heart block, the focus should be suppression of JPDs rather than pacemaker implantation.

Ventricular Premature Beats

VPDs are very common, occurring in normal and abnormal hearts. Their importance relates not only to the associated symptoms but also to their prognostic value. High-density VPDs or nonsustained ventricular tachycardia in patients with structural heart disease may signal an increased risk of death, whereas their presence in persons with normal hearts has little significance. The pathogenetic mechanism for VPDs may be reentry, abnormal automaticity, or triggered activity.

Electrocardiographic Manifestation

VPDs are manifested on the ECG as a wide QRS complex (longer than 120 milliseconds) with a T wave vector opposite the main QRS vector. Quite often, the ventricular impulse does not conduct to the atria, and when it does, it fails to reset the sinus node, resulting in a fully compensatory pause (Figure 2). If the VPD resets the sinus node, a noncompensatory pause will be inscribed. An interpolated VPD is an early ventricular depolarization that fails to affect the sinus node and AV node. With an interpolated VPD, the RR interval surrounding the VPD is equal to the sinus RR interval.

A wide QRS complex may also represent a supraventricular premature beat with aberration. Criteria that favor aberration include (1) antecedent premature P wave, (2) typical right or left bundle branch block, and (3) the presence of a noncompensatory pause. Criteria in favor of a ventricular origin include (1) AV dissociation, (2) marked left axis deviation, (3) a QRS interval longer than 160 milliseconds, and (4) certain configurational characteristics such as Rsr′ in lead V1, QS or rS in lead V6, and concordance (upright or downward QRSs in all precordial leads).

Clinical Presentation

VPDs may result in palpitations or the sensation of skipped beats. Patients usually complain of the forceful contraction that follows the VPD. Others feel that the heart has stopped with every post-VPD pause. If VPDs occur in bigeminy, the effective heart rate may be too slow, resulting in symptoms of poor cardiac output such as dizziness and fatigue.

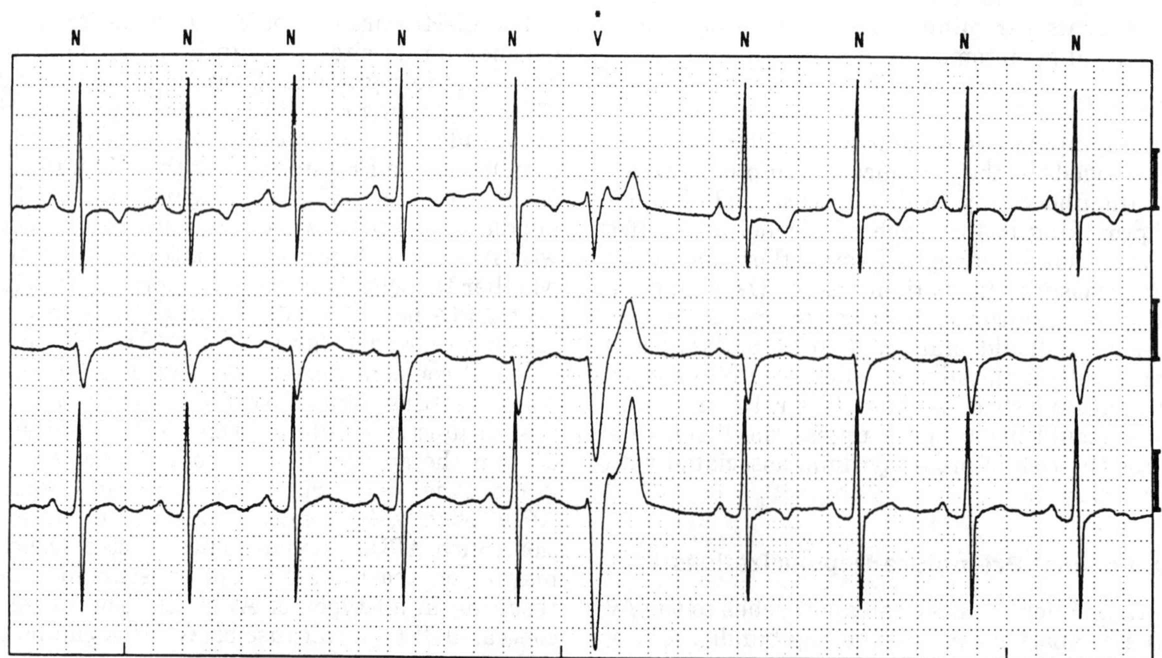

Figure 2. Normal sinus rhythm with evidence of a wide complex premature depolarization. The pause following this beat is a full compensatory pause (R-R interval surrounding the premature beat = 2 x sinus cycle length). This suggests lack of sinus node resetting and thus a ventricular origin. Furthermore, close analysis reveals a sinus P wave at the terminal portion of the QRS, giving the appearance of an R′.

Management

The prognosis in patients with ventricular ectopy (i.e., VPDs) and no structural heart disease is very good, with a long-term survival similar to that in patients without ventricular ectopy. Therefore, these patients should be reassured and require no medical therapy. On the other hand, the presence of ventricular ectopy in patients with a previous MI is a well-recognized risk factor for death. The presence of frequent ventricular premature beats (more than 10 per hour) during ambulatory electrocardiographic monitoring is an independent risk factor for sudden death. The curve relating mortality rate to ventricular premature depolarization frequency in postinfarct patients rises steeply between 1 and 10 VPDs per hour, with annual mortality rates of approximately 20%.

For this reason, several studies were initiated with the hypothesis that reducing ventricular ectopy would reduce the risk of sudden death. The Cardiac Arrhythmia Suppression Trial (CAST) was designed to test this hypothesis. Recruitment for the trial began in June 1987. Suppression was evaluated using encainide (Enkaid), flecainide (Tambocor), or moricizine (Ethmozine) in an open-label titration period before randomization. Arrhythmia suppression was defined as 80% suppression of VPDs and at least 90% suppression of runs of ventricular tachycardia. Patients in whom arrhythmias were suppressed were then randomized to receive either the actual drug or placebo. In April 1989, encainide and flecainide were discontinued from the study because they were shown to be probably causing harm, but a favorable trend was noted with moricizine. The study was then continued as CAST II with moricizine. However, CAST II was also stopped early because it appeared unlikely that long-term use of moricizine would show benefit over placebo.

Beta blockers have been shown to improve survival in patients with a history of previous MI but were never used to test the suppression hypothesis. On the other hand, calcium channel blockers have been shown to have a negative effect on survival in post-MI patients, especially those with left ventricular dysfunction.

Sotalol (Betapace) was tested in patients with a history of MI. Patients received, in a double-blind randomized fashion, sotalol, 320 mg per day, or placebo on post-MI days 5 to 14. and were followed for 1 year. The difference in mortality rates was not statistically significant in the two groups (7.3% in the sotalol group versus 8.9% in the placebo group); however, this 18% reduction in mortality rate was very consistent with the known beneficial effect of beta blockers in this patient population. Therefore, another trial was designed to assess the effect of the *d*-stereoisomer of sotalol* (which lacks the beta-blocking effect) on mortality in post-MI patients with left ventricular dysfunction. After enrolling more than 3000 patients, the trial was stopped because of increased mortality in the treatment group. The investigators concluded that the use of *d*-sotalol in post-MI patients with left ventricular dysfunction may be associated with an increased mortality.

Amiodarone has been used in many trials in post-MI patients. The early experience is best summarized by the results of the Basel Antiarrhythmic Study of Infarct Survival (BASIS), the Polish Trial, and the Canadian Pilot Study. In all these trials, arrhythmic events and total mortality were reduced with amiodarone therapy. On the basis of these promising results, the benefit of amiodarone was tested in two large trials: the Canadian Amiodarone Myocardial Infarction Arrhythmia Trial (CAMIAT) and the European Myocardial Infarction Amiodarone Trial (EMIAT). The CAMIAT trial was designed to test the effect of amiodarone on the risk of arrhythmic death or resuscitated ventricular fibrillation among survivors of MI with frequent or repetitive premature ventricular contractions, i.e., the occurrence of 10 or more per hour or one episode of nonsustained ventricular tachycardia. After a mean follow-up period of 1.79 years, the event rate was reduced by 48.5% with amiodarone therapy ($P < .01$). All-cause mortality, although not a primary end point, was also reduced in the amiodarone group by 21.2% (not significant). A major limitation of this study was the lack of assessment of left ventricular dysfunction, which is known to be an independent predictor of arrhythmic events and mortality in post-MI patients. The EMIAT study assessed the effect of amiodarone on all-cause mortality in post-MI patients with left ventricular dysfunction. After a median follow-up period of 21 months, there was a 35% reduction in risk of sudden death in the amiodarone treatment group but no difference in total mortality. The investigators did not recommend the routine use of amiodarone in post-MI patients because of its lack of effect on total mortality. However, all trials have found that amiodarone is not associated with excess risk of death.

Summary and Recommendations

In patients without structural heart disease, the presence of ventricular ectopy has no effect on prognosis. Therefore, in the absence of symptoms, no treatment is required. In the symptomatic patient, reassurance and elimination of known precipitating factors such as alcohol consumption, coffee intake, and smoking should be the first line of therapy. If this approach fails, the use of beta blockers may be helpful. The use of other antiarrhythmic agents such as class I and class III agents should be avoided and should be considered only as a last resort for very symptomatic patients.

In patients with structural heart disease, the presence of ectopy carries a poor prognosis. Whether suppression of ectopy has any effect on prognosis is unknown. In the asymptomatic patient, no treatment is indicated. In the symptomatic patient, beta blockers may be used, especially when there is a history of myocardial infarction, in which a clear beneficial effect on mortality has been demonstrated. If ventricu-

*Not available in the United States.

lar ectopy persists or the patient cannot tolerate beta blockers, amiodarone may be used with caution. Class IA agents should not be used because of their proarrhythmic effect, especially in the setting of left ventricular hypertrophy. Class IC agents are contraindicated in the setting of coronary artery disease because of the proven increased mortality in these patients.

HEART BLOCK

method of
STANLEY B. SCHMIDT, M.D.
West Virginia University School of Medicine
Morgantown, West Virginia

In a broad sense "heart block" refers to any impairment in conduction of the cardiac electrical impulse as it travels from the sinus node to the ventricular myocardium. The term is often applied specifically to slowing or failure of conduction ("block") at the level of the atrioventricular (AV) junction, which includes the AV node. It also encompasses blocks between the sinus node and atrial tissue (sinoatrial exit block), within the atria, and within the His-Purkinje system, including the left and right bundle branches. Blocks may be caused by physiologic stimuli, drugs, and a number of pathologic conditions. Treatment may be influenced by the location of the block and its cause, hemodynamic impact, and anticipated duration and progression.

SINOATRIAL BLOCK AND SINUS NODE DYSFUNCTION

Electrical impulses arising in the sinus node may occasionally fail to conduct to the surrounding atrial tissue, a condition called sinoatrial (SA) exit block. In one typical pattern (SA Wenckebach), there is a progressive delay in conduction of each successive sinus beat until conduction to the atria fails, causing the rhythm to pause until the cycle repeats itself. This is diagnosed by recognizing grouped beating on the surface electrocardiogram, in which brief pauses are preceded by progressive shortening in the intervals between successive P waves. Higher grades of SA exit block may cause sinus bradycardia or sinus arrest. SA Wenckebach is a common benign finding in young people and rarely needs any treatment. In older populations it is usually associated with abnormal impulse formation in the sinus node as part of the sick sinus syndrome. Manifestations of the latter may also include intermittent or persistent sinus bradycardia, sinus pauses, inadequate heart rate acceleration during exercise or other stress (chronotropic incompetence), and increased propensity to atrial tachyarrhythmias (including fibrillation) and thromboembolic events.

In adults, the cause of sinus node dysfunction is usually undetermined. In the young it may occur with untreated or particularly with surgically treated congenital heart disease. A variety of drugs may cause or contribute to sinus node dysfunction, including beta blockers, calcium channel blockers, digoxin, amiodarone, and other antiarrhythmics.

If the patient with sinus node dysfunction experiences symptomatic slow heart rates that cannot be reversed by removal or treatment of correctable factors, permanent pacing is indicated. It is often necessary to use permanent pacing therapy in conjunction with rate-slowing drugs in patients who suffer from both symptomatic brady- and tachyarrhythmias (bradycardia-tachycardia syndrome).

Establishing a correlation between intermittent symptoms and bradyarrhythmias is often difficult. Holter monitoring and in-hospital telemetry may provide relatively short-term data. Longer periods of observation, extending over weeks or months, are available by employing various event recorders. Electrophysiologic testing can provide additional data about sinus node function but is generally much less useful than these noninvasive modalities in determining the need for permanent pacing.

INTERATRIAL BLOCK

Delayed conduction from the right to the left atrium, manifested by a broad notched P wave, is usually not of much clinical significance. In some patients, though, it may promote atrial tachyarrhythmias such as fibrillation. In others with impaired left ventricular filling, delayed left atrial contraction may be disadvantageous from a hemodynamic viewpoint. Novel approaches to cardiac pacing are being evaluated in some of these patient groups.

ATRIOVENTRICULAR BLOCK

AV block is subdivided into several categories, depending on the relationship between atrial and ventricular electrical activity. AV block may occur coincidentally with various atrial arrhythmias, but the simplest case to consider is that with underlying sinus rhythm. In first-degree AV block, all P waves conduct to the ventricles, but they do so more slowly than normal, prolonging the surface PR interval above the normal upper limit of 0.20 second. In second-degree AV block, some, but not all, P waves fail to conduct to the ventricles, and in third-degree, or complete, AV block, no P waves conduct to the ventricles.

Second-degree AV block is further divided into Mobitz type I, or Wenckebach, block, in which the first PR interval after the blocked P wave is shorter than the last PR interval before the blocked P wave; Mobitz type II, in which the PR interval is fixed before and after the blocked P wave; and "advanced" second-degree AV block. The latter includes 2:1 AV block, in which alternate P waves are blocked, and higher conduction ratios, in which two or more consecutive P waves fail to conduct. Second-degree AV block must not be confused with premature atrial beats that block because of normal refractoriness in the AV junctional tissues ("blocked PACs"). Diagnosis of second-degree AV block requires that the nonconducted P wave be "on time" rather than premature. Third-degree AV block must be distinguished from the broader category of AV dissociation, which indicates relative independence of atrial and ventricular beating. The latter may exist when the ventricular rate exceeds the atrial rate, as during most ventricular tachycardias, without any true impairment in AV conduction.

When AV block occurs at the level of the AV node it is said to be proximal. Distal AV block is located in the His-Purkinje system. Distal AV block is often associated with other evidence of disease in the Purkinje system, including nonspecific intraventricular conduction delays or bundle branch block, with resulting widening of the QRS complex. Distal block is generally less favorable prognostically, because of the reduced rate and reliability of the associated escape rhythms. Although type II second-degree AV block is distal, the terms are not synonymous. Some type I second-degree AV block occurs distally as well, although a proximal location is more typical. Intracardiac electrophysiologic recordings can define the level of AV block but are usually not required for patient management. Some of the more frequent causes of AV block are listed in Table 1.

First-degree AV block is usually asymptomatic and rarely requires specific treatment by permanent pacing. AV block of any degree that is symptomatic and not due to an acute reversible cause requires treatment with permanent pacing. Heart block associated with Lyme disease generally resolves with antibiotic therapy and therefore does not usually require permanent pacing, although temporary pacing is often needed.

Generally, persistent second-degree AV block should be treated with permanent pacing. Data are limited, but one prospective study in older patients suggests a high mortality without pacing for all subtypes of chronic second-degree AV block, even without associated symptoms or bundle branch block.

Transient isolated asymptomatic type I second-degree AV block is often seen in the young or well conditioned and is not an indication for permanent pacing. Type II second-degree AV block, even when transient, is usually treated with permanent pacing. Transient advanced second-degree AV block is not rare and is often due to an acute reversible cause such as high vagal tone or profound hypoxemia. Most of these patients do not require cardiac pacing. However, if no reversible factors are identified, or if distal conduction disease is present, pacing is usually recommended. Transient advanced second-degree AV block has been observed during exercise testing. In the few cases studied and reported, electrophysiologic testing showed distal conduction disease, and pacing was performed. The natural history of these patients is unknown.

TABLE 1. **Causes of Atrioventricular Block**

Drugs—digoxin, beta blockers, verapamil, diltiazem, others	Lyme disease
Fibrodegenerative	Congenital
High vagal tone	Acute rheumatic fever
Myocardial infarction or ischemia	Hypoxia
Cardiac surgery	Amyloidosis
Valve ring abscess	Sarcoidosis
Muscular dystrophies—myotonic, others	Connective tissue diseases
Myocarditis	Radiation
	Malignancy
	Catheter ablation

Asymptomatic third-degree AV block is not rare. In young patients it is usually congenital and is located at the level of the AV node. Patients with this type of block typically have stable junctional (narrow QRS) escape rhythms. Traditionally, they have been felt to have a favorable prognosis as adults, but a recent prospective study points to a significant risk of sudden death and improved survival with pacing. Acquired third-degree AV block is prognostically unfavorable and is usually an indication for permanent pacing. Such block is usually distal, and distal third-degree AV block requires pacing, even if asymptomatic.

In the setting of acute myocardial infarction, type I second-degree AV block often responds to atropine. Type II and advanced second-degree AV block, along with third-degree AV block, are generally treated with temporary pacing. There is little sentiment in favor of prophylactic permanent pacing for those whose AV block resolves.

BUNDLE BRANCH AND FASCICULAR BLOCKS

Blocks in the distal conduction system are relatively common electrocardiographic findings. In older populations they usually reflect fibrodegenerative changes in the conduction system and by themselves do not generally require specific work-up or therapy. In younger populations they may be a presenting finding of myocarditis or other significant pathology. Alternating bundle branch block, in which both left and right bundle branch blocks are seen either on alternate beats or at different times, is reported to carry a high risk for complete heart block and should be treated by permanent pacing.

So-called bifascicular block has been used to describe right bundle branch block associated with left anterior or posterior fascicular block. "Trifascicular" block has been used to refer to the combination of bifascicular block with first-degree AV block, or the association of right bundle branch block with alternating left anterior and posterior fascicular blocks. These two terms are imprecise and are less favored than specific description of combinations of blocks.

In myotonic muscular dystrophy, distal conduction system disease can progress rapidly and unpredictably (independent of baseline HV [His-to-ventricular conduction time] measurement). When identified, early consideration should be given to permanent pacing.

In patients with distal conduction system disease, symptoms such as syncope should not necessarily be attributed to transient complete heart block. Significant underlying myocardial disease may be present, along with potentially malignant ventricular tachyarrhythmias. These patients merit thorough evaluation, usually including intracardiac electrophysiologic testing.

TACHYARRHYTHMIAS

method of
JOHN H. MCANULTY, M.D.
*Oregon Health Sciences University
Portland, Oregon*

APPROACH TO THE ARRHYTHMIA PATIENTS (Table 1)

Immediate Concerns

Some arrhythmias have immediate, potentially severe consequences. Hemodynamic stability has to be the first concern. In trying to think of some way to remind myself of what to do, I start with the question Is there time to think? The irony, of course, is that if there is *no* time to think, immediate action must be taken. A patient in severe hemodynamic distress requires emergency resuscitation measures. If stability of the patient allows, the next approach is to document the rhythm. A rhythm strip should be recorded, and if at all possible, more than one lead (preferably 12 leads) should be recorded. The rules for diagnosis of the tachycardias follow, but as shown in Figure 1, there are some important first questions. First, even with the electrocardiogram (ECG) in hand, it is worth determining whether there is, or is not, an arrhythmia. Many patients have been treated for arrhythmias when none occurred; artifact was misinterpreted as an arrhythmia. If it is convincing that an arrhythmia did occur, it is next appropriate to classify it as slow or fast and then to attempt to classify it as to the specific type of arrhythmia (Figure 1).

Chronic Concerns

Once an arrhythmia is terminated, or if the patient is stabilized, the "chronic" phase of management ensues and two additional questions are appropriate.

TABLE 1. **Arrhythmia Management**

Immediate	Chronic
Ask One Question:	*Ask Two Questions:*
Is there time to think?	1. What is the rhythm trying to tell us? That is, what is the cause?
No Take immediate lifesaving action (cardioversion, CPR)	*Outside the body causes* Drugs, drugs, drugs *Inside the body causes* Metabolic abnormalities Endocrine abnormalities *Cardiac causes*
Yes Record and interpret rhythm Apply specific therapy	2. Is treatment needed? For symptoms? For safety?

Abbreviation: CPR = cardiopulmonary resuscitation.

Arrhythmia
Yes — No
Yes: Bradycardia / Tachycardia
Tachycardia: *Irregular* / *Regular*

Irregular: *Atrial Fibrillation*; *Multifocal Atrial Tachycardia*

Regular: *The Important 4:* *Sinus Tachycardia*; *Paroxysmal Supraventricular Tachycardia (PSVT)*; *Atrial Flutter*; *Ventricular Tachycardia*

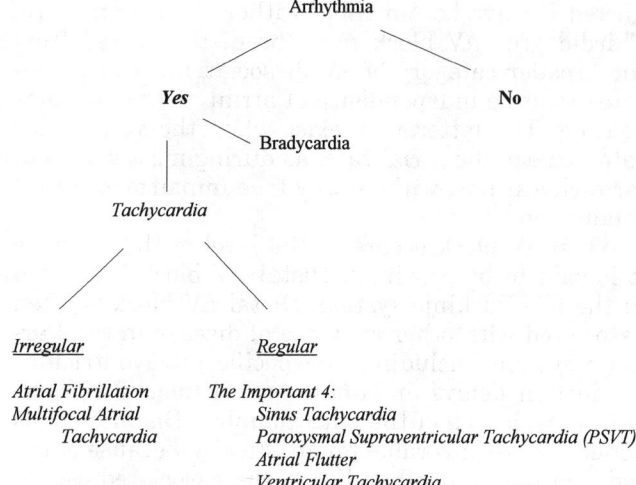

Figure 1. Analysis of arrhythmia on the electrocardiogram (ECG).

1. What is the rhythm trying to tell us? That is, what is the cause? Whereas the rhythm itself may be important, it may simply be a marker for something else that should be addressed. This is a concern whether the rhythm is or was atrial premature beats or ventricular fibrillation. In an approach that seems too simple-minded to put into an article like this (but does happen to be that used by me), causes can originate from *outside* the body, from *inside* the body, and finally as the result of a *cardiac* abnormality. The point of this approach is that to treat rhythms when they are only secondary to other problems may not be appropriate. In considering outside the body causes, drugs are the overwhelming explanation, and when drugs do not explain the problems, drugs should be considered again. Arrhythmias are commonly caused by prescription drugs, over-the-counter drugs, caffeine, tobacco, or illicit or recreational drugs. Causes inside the body that are potentially correctable include metabolic and endocrine abnormalities, particularly thyroid problems. And finally, an arrhythmia may be a marker for a cardiac abnormality that requires treatment. Although not totally satisfying, if a cause cannot be found, a patient can at times be comforted by knowing there is no dangerous underlying explanation.

2. Is treatment required? Many arrhythmias do not require treatment. Treatment should be considered if the rhythm causes intolerable symptoms or increases the risk of sudden death.

DIAGNOSIS OF TACHYCARDIAS

Treatment is usually safer and more effective when the rhythm is defined. Start with assessment of the regularity of the tachycardia. Is the rhythm regular or irregular? Sometimes determination of this is difficult because even regular rhythms have minor rate variation, but if there is less than a 10% variability of R-R intervals, for the most part, a rhythm can be classified within the regular category. Next, assess the QRS duration. A "narrow" QRS complex (≤0.10 second) defines the rhythm as being supraventricular in origin; a "wide" QRS complex may occur with a ventricular or a supraventricular rhythm. Identification of P waves and their relationship to the QRS complex is important but often difficult; on occasion, an esophageal or atrial lead can help. The response to a vagal maneuver (5 to 10 seconds of firm, brisk massage of a carotid vessel without a bruit) will help in diagnosis and sometimes in treatment of the regular tachyarrhythmias. A drug challenge can also safely achieve diagnosis and treatment (Table 2). Short-acting drugs are preferable when feasible ("if you're wrong, you're not wrong for long"). Adenosine (Adenocard 12 mg by rapid intravenous [IV] bolus) is almost always the most appropriate. Esmolol (Brevibloc 0.5 mg per kg bolus followed by drip of 0.05 to 0.2 mg per kg per minute) is a short-acting alternative. Although not short acting, verapamil (Isoptin or Calan 2.5- to 5-mg bolus, repeat with 5 to 10 mg at 10 minutes) can be used for *narrow* QRS complex rhythms.

Irregular Tachycardias

Chaotically irregular rhythms are usually atrial fibrillation. The R-R interval patterns are unpredictable, and there are no recognizable consistent P waves. Atrial flutter with extremely variable ventricular conduction can occasionally appear to be atrial fibrillation (the diagnosis is made by looking for a regular P wave pattern). Multifocal atrial tachycardia can also present as a chaotically irregular rhythm. It is not atrial fibrillation because P waves are distinct (usually three or more P wave morphologies). For the most part, however, whether the QRS is narrow or wide, if the ventricular response rate is chaotically irregular, assuming the rhythm to be atrial fibrillation is appropriate.

Regular Tachycardias

These are the most difficult to define, are common, and are the most interesting! Although they are intimidating, there is good news. For all practical purposes, it is necessary to remember the rules for only four—they compose 95% of the regular clinical tachycardias (Table 3).

Sinus Tachycardia. In the nonexercising patient, sinus tachycardia is usually 150 beats per minute or less. In the young, or in those receiving large amounts of sympathomimetic agents, it may be as fast as 160 or 170 beats per minute, but for every increment greater than 150 beats per minute, the diagnosis of sinus tachycardia becomes less secure. When identified, the P waves (upright or "positive" in leads I and II) have a 1:1 relationship to the QRS. On occasion, a vagal maneuver or adenosine will result in transient, gradual slowing of the sinus node (and thus the P and QRS complexes). On rare occasions, the adenosine may cause transient atrioventricular (AV) block defining the P wave and its rate.

Paroxysmal Supraventricular Tachycardia (PSVT). This rhythm, also known as paroxysmal atrial tachycardia (PAT), is due almost exclusively to the mechanisms of reentry within the AV node ("AV node reentry" based on "dual" AV node pathways) or reentry using an accessory pathway ("AV reentry" using an accessory pathway connecting the atrium to the ventricle; this accessory pathway, also called a Kent bundle, occasionally results in pre-excitation on the sinus rhythm ECG, leading to the diagnosis of the Wolff-Parkinson-White syndrome). In either case, the rules for paroxysmal supraventricular tachycardia are about the same. There is a 1:1 P to QRS relationship (again when P waves can be seen), and the rate of each ranges from 150 to 250 beats per minute (occasionally 130 to 260 beats per minute). When the P waves are seen, they immediately follow the QRS (generally by less than 150 milliseconds; thus, these are "short RP" tachycardias). The QRS may be narrow or wide. An excellent vagal maneuver may not affect the rhythm, but the expected response is an abrupt termination of the rhythm with return to sinus rhythm. Adenosine defines and stops PSVT almost 95% of the time. There can be clues in the QRS and the ST-T segments to suggest the rhythm mechanism (AV node reentry versus AV reentry), but management approaches are not greatly affected by this differentiation.

Atrial Flutter. A red-light rule: a QRS or pulse of 150 beats per minute is atrial flutter until proved otherwise. This rule is applicable because atrial flutter is common, the atrial rate often approximates 300 beats per minute (it is "allowed" to be between 250 and 350 beats per minute), and the AV node generally allows 2:1 conduction; thus, the ventricular response rate of around 150 beats per minute. When the rule is ignored, a search for two P waves may not occur, and the diagnosis is often missed (the reason for the rule). The QRS complex may be narrow or wide. A vagal maneuver or adenosine may have no effect, but a transient slowing of the ventricular response with no effect of the P (or flutter) waves is diagnostic. There are different types of atrial flutter, but a common ("typical") form results in the "sawtooth" pattern of the baseline (the flutter waves) best seen in the inferior leads.

Ventricular Tachycardia. The QRS complex is always wide (exceptions are quite rare). The ventricular rate can be as slow as 100 beats per minute and as fast as 300 beats per minute. (Some call a rate faster than 250 beats per minute ventricular flutter.) If P waves can be seen and they are clearly slower than the ventricular rate, the diagnosis is reasonably secure. P waves, however, are often difficult to recognize; even if they are found, there can be a 1:1 P to QRS relationship owing to the retrograde ventricular to atrial conduction observed in 10 to 30% of ventricular tachycardias. Ventricular tachycardia usually (95% of the time) does not respond to a vagal maneuver or adenosine.

Unexplained Wide QRS Complex Tachycardia. Although there are only four important common clinical regular tachycardias, it is this rhythm that is the most difficult to explain and treat because it can be any of the others. The ECG rules (see Table 3) may make the diagnosis obvious. When this rhythm is encountered, it is most important to consider the clinical status. If the patient has known coronary artery disease, and especially if the patient has had a previous myocardial infarction, the rhythm should be diagnosed and treated as ventricular tachycardia. There are many rules for determining whether a wide QRS complex tachycardia is supraventricular or ventricular in origin. A ventricular origin is more likely if the QRS width is greater than 0.14 second (recognizing that it is often difficult to assess a QRS width during a tachycardia), if there is a left axis deviation in the limb leads, or if there is a concordance of appearance of the QRS morphologies (either all positive or all negative) in the precordial leads. Other rules are both difficult to remember and apply infrequently enough that they are less useful. Diagnostic procedures can again include transesophageal or atrial recordings of the atrial complex. A drug challenge with adenosine (12 mg IV) can be helpful but—a warning—verapamil should *not* routinely be used as a diagnostic maneuver because of potential hypotension and negative inotropic effects from the drug.

MANAGEMENT OF TACHYARRHYTHMIAS

(See Table 2 for drug doses)

Sinus Tachycardia

Do not treat it. Look for and correct the cause (see Figure 1). If a patient is having angina, the first

TABLE 2. **Drugs Used to Treat Tachyarrhythmias**

Drug	Dose	Comment
AV-Node–Blocking Drugs		
INTRAVENOUS		
Adenosine (Adenocard)	12 mg rapid "push"	The rapid push (followed immediately by rapid flush if a peripheral vein is used) improves the chance of response. If no response to 12 mg in a large person (arbitrarily >75 kg), 18 mg can be given.
Calcium channel blockers		
Verapamil (Calan, Isoptin)	5-mg bolus; repeat with 5 or 10 mg if no response	Avoid in undiagnosed regular wide QRS tachycardia.
Diltiazem (Cardizem)	10- to 20-mg bolus followed by infusion of 10–15 mg/h	
Beta blockers		
Metoprolol (Lopressor)	5 mg IV q 5 min × 3	Avoid when reactive airway disease is a concern. CHF is not an absolute contraindication but should be monitored and treated. If there is concern about either (airway disease or CHF), esmolol is the appropriate choice because of its 10-min half-life.
Propranolol (Inderal)	0.15 mg/kg bolus	
Esmolol (Brevibloc)	0.5 mg/kg bolus followed by infusion of 0.05–0.2 mg/kg/min	
ORAL		
Beta blockers		If there is concern about toxicity, start with short-acting agents and, if tolerated, switch to once-daily preparations.
Atenolol (Tenormin)*	50–100 mg once daily	
Metoprolol (Lopressor)	25–50 mg tid of the short-acting preparation or 50–200 mg of the once-daily preparations	There are 14 beta-blocking preparations; I use these almost exclusively because on the basis of efficacy, side effect profile, and expense, there are no advantages to the others. If intrinsic sympathomimetic activity is desired, acebutalol (200–400 mg qd) is effective.
Calcium blockers		
Verapamil, sustained-release (Calan SR)*	180–360 mg qd	Verapamil is generally more effective.
Diltiazem, sustained-release (Cardizem SR)*		
Digoxin	0.25 mg qd	Load with 1–1.5 mg in first 24 h. Daily dose lower with renal failure.
Antiarrhythmia Drugs		
INTRAVENOUS		
Lidocaine (Xylocaine)	1.5 mg/kg bolus, repeat ½ in 15 min and infuse at 0.05 mg/kg/min	Whereas mg/kg dosing is optimal, an initial dose of 50 mg (small person), 75 mg (medium-sized person), or 100 mg (large person) is more practical with administration of one half to two thirds of that dose at 15 min.
Procainamide (Pronestyl)	15 mg/kg IV in 30 min and then infuse at 0.08 mg/kg/min	May contribute to hypertension.
Bretylium (Bretylol)	5 mg/kg bolus followed by infusion of 1–2 mg/min	
Amiodarone (Cordarone)	150-mg IV bolus followed by infusion of 1 mg/min for 6 h, then 0.75 mg/min	
Ibutilide fumarate (Corvert)	If >60 kg, infuse 1 mg over 10 min; repeat if no conversion by 10 min If <60 kg, infuse 0.01 mg/kg over 10 min; repeat if no conversion by 10 min	A 1–3% incidence of ventricular arrhythmias within the first 12 hr is a reason to use guardedly in outpatients
ORAL		
Flecainide (Tambocor)	100–150 mg bid	
Mexiletine (Mexitil)	250 mg tid	Important to take with meals to prevent gastric instability.
Sotalol (Betapace)	80 mg bid × 3 d; increase to 160 mg bid if needed for desired effect	The beta-blocker effect is approximately two thirds of that of propranolol.
Amiodarone (Cordarone)	400 mg tid × 2 wk, then 400 mg bid × 2 wk, then 400 mg qd (for VT or VF) or 200–400 mg qd for supraventricular rhythm	

*Not FDA approved for this indication.
Abbreviations: CHF = congestive heart failure; VT = ventricular tachycardia; VF = ventricular fibrillation.

TABLE 3. **The "Important" Four Regular Tachycardias**

Tachycardia	Onset and Termination	Rate (bpm)*		QRS Width	Response to Vagal Maneuver or to Adenosine
		P Wave	*QRS Complex*		
Sinus tachycardia	Gradual	100–150	100–150	Narrow or wide	None or transient gradual slowing
Paroxysmal supraventricular tachycardia (PSVT)	Abrupt	150–250	150–250	Narrow or wide	None or abrupt termination
Atrial flutter	Abrupt	250–350	<P wave rate: often one half the P wave rate	Narrow or wide	None or transient ventricular slowing
Ventricular tachycardia	Abrupt	≤ QRS rate	100–300	Wide	None

*These values apply about 95% of the time. Sinus tachycardia will occasionally be greater than 150, but the farther it strays above this value, the stronger other rhythms should be considered. Likewise, PSVT may be less than 150, but the same thought process applies. Wide QRS ≥0.12 s.

recommendation can be ignored and beta-blocker therapy is appropriate. Rare patients have chronic symptomatic sinus tachycardia unexplained despite an exhaustive search for a cause. Again, beta-blocker therapy may decrease associated symptoms. If not, or if the drug is poorly tolerated or ineffective, catheter ablation techniques can be applied to stop the rhythm or to cause AV block (a pacemaker is required if AV block is created).

Paroxysmal Supraventricular Tachycardia

Patients, of course, learn that they can often stop PSVT with their own vagal maneuver (in particular, a Valsalva maneuver). If a patient presents for medical care with this arrhythmia, a Valsalva maneuver or carotid massage (5 to 10 seconds of firm, almost painful massage) may provide the diagnosis and treatment. IV adenosine or verapamil is effective more than 90% (almost 95%) of the time. IV beta blockers (esmolol, metoprolol,* propranolol) may also convert the rhythm. Digoxin is less effective and takes 2 to 3 hours to have any effect. A refractory rhythm with deteriorating hemodynamics should be treated with synchronized, direct-current (DC) cardioversion (100 joules, after deep sedation using anterior-posterior paddles).

After an episode of PSVT, a decision about chronic management is required. Daily antiarrhythmic therapy is not appropriate for a first or rare episode. If an individual tolerated the rhythm well, an argument can be made for giving no therapy other than instruction about a vagal maneuver. An alternative is to provide an individual with medication on an as-needed basis—a beta blocker (propranolol 160 mg or metoprolol 100 mg). The patient should be advised to try a vagal maneuver if the rhythm occurs. If the rhythm does not stop, the patient should take the medication and then relax for 1.5 hours. Vagal maneuvers should be tried again. The combination of the drug, the time, the relaxation, and the maneuvers may be enough to convert the rhythm back to normal and avoid a hospital visit. Individuals bothered by recurrent episodes should be treated with a daily AV-node–blocking agent (beta blockers or verapamil). If an accessory AV pathway is potentially a part of the rhythm mechanism, it is optimal to avoid digoxin or verapamil because they can speed conduction through this pathway—a problem if the individual should develop atrial fibrillation.

Radiofrequency catheter ablation is an increasingly used alternative for chronic management. When the mechanism of the rhythm is accessory pathway or dual AV nodal conduction, success again hovers around 95%. Currently, indications for its use include drug failure for control of the rhythms, drug side effects, or an unwillingness to take long-term medications. It is also indicated in the person who is limiting his or her life because of constant concern that an arrhythmia will occur. Although expensive (often $10,000 to $12,000 per procedure), this approach is low risk (rare valve damage, extremely rare death, and rare need for permanent pacemaker); may decrease expense in the long term; and has freed many patients from rhythms, limitations, and apprehension.

Atrial Fibrillation

Although treatment of the rhythm for hemodynamic stability is often a pressing concern, it still seems important to first emphasize the need for *stroke prevention* with this rhythm. This issue should be addressed each time a patient with atrial fibrillation is seen. A concept: *Once an atrial fibrillation patient, always an atrial fibrillation patient.* In considering stroke prevention, this concept is particularly important because there is no evidence that the 3 to 8% per year chance of a stroke is any less when a patient is in sinus rhythm. Fortunately, antithrombotic therapy can reduce the risk of this complication by 70% with reasonable bleeding complication rates (1 to 2% per year).

A large amount of recently accumulated information influences treatment recommendations. I use the following approaches as general rules. In patients with chronic atrial fibrillation, whether persistent or

*Not FDA approved for this indication.

intermittent (paroxysmal), antithrombotic therapy is addressed with each interaction. If an atrial fibrillation patient has one of the risk factors that increase the risk of thromboemboli (has left ventricular dysfunction, uncontrolled systolic hypertension [blood pressure above 160 mm Hg], or a previous thromboembolic episode, or is a woman older than 75 years) and is a reasonable warfarin (Coumadin) candidate, use of that drug maintaining an International Normalized Ratio of 2 to 3 is recommended. A previous thromboembolism is the factor of greatest concern and the most important reason to attempt to use warfarin. If an atrial fibrillation patient does not have one of these risk factors, aspirin 325 mg per day offers stroke prevention. If an individual has one of the risk factors but is a poor warfarin candidate, again, aspirin 325 mg per day is appropriate treatment. A patient with "lone" atrial fibrillation (atrial fibrillation occurring in individuals younger than 60 years with no recognizable heart disease) is at such low risk of an embolus that an argument can be made for no treatment. Still, it is recommended that the patient be treated with aspirin 325 mg per day. If a patient goes for some prolonged time with no recognized atrial fibrillation (for example, longer than 6 months to a year), it could again be argued that antithrombotic therapy could be stopped, but until more is known (some large prospective studies are addressing this issue), antithrombotic therapy is recommended for life.

There is less information available on which to base the decision about antithrombotic therapy requirements at the time of a cardioversion. If it can be certain that the atrial fibrillation has existed for a short time (somewhat arbitrarily chosen as less than 48 hours), cardioversion can be performed without initiating antithrombotic therapy (although the therapy should be initiated for the long term). If the duration of atrial fibrillation is uncertain or known to be greater than 48 hours, when possible, rate control should be achieved, warfarin therapy started, and the patient returned in 4 to 6 weeks for an elective cardioversion. If the logistics of this delay are difficult, transesophageal echocardiography can be performed, and if there is no intra-atrial thrombus, the cardioversion can be performed without anticoagulation. This approach is expensive and, in most situations, not required.

Acute Atrial Fibrillation

Most individuals presenting with this rhythm have a ventricular response rate between 100 and 200 beats per minute with some associated symptoms. If there is severe hemodynamic compromise, urgent cardioversion is required (synchronized 200 joules, DC energy using anterior-posterior paddles in a sedated patient). Rate control is preferable in most patients with verapamil (5 mg IV followed in 10 minutes by 5 to 10 mg IV) or diltiazem (10 to 20 mg IV followed by an IV drip at 1 to 2 mg per minute). If an individual is hypotensive, vasodilator drugs must be used with caution, but in almost all cases, the hypotension is related to the rate, and the pressure will improve as the rate is controlled. At this point, the patient is either in sinus rhythm or in atrial fibrillation with a controlled ventricular response (depending on the approach used). In either case, this is still an atrial fibrillation patient.

If the patient remains in atrial fibrillation, cardioversion can be considered if the rhythm is thought to have been present less than 48 hours. If the rhythm duration is longer or uncertain, the rate should be controlled with an oral regimen (verapamil, beta blocker, or digoxin; see Table 2), and warfarin therapy should be started. If an individual is asymptomatic while in atrial fibrillation, an argument can be made for simply maintaining rate control and continuing treatment for prevention of stroke. There are also arguments for cardioversion (currently large ongoing prospective studies are evaluating which approach is optimal). Until the answers are known, at least one attempt to achieve normal sinus rhythm seems appropriate. After 4 to 6 weeks of warfarin therapy, cardioversion can be performed (generally requiring only a few hours under hospital observation). If sinus rhythm is achieved, warfarin should be continued for 2 weeks (to allow time for recovery of atrial contractile function), and then the appropriate long-term antithrombotic program should be initiated (see earlier). If sinus rhythm is maintained for 3 months, the rate control medication can be stopped (unless the patient tolerated the initial atrial fibrillation with a fast response poorly, in which case long-term continuation of medication is appropriate). If the patient is not successfully cardioverted and remains asymptomatic, atrial fibrillation can be accepted with reasonable rate control and attention to stroke prevention. If a patient is symptomatic despite rate control, initiation of an oral antiarrhythmic drug is appropriate. Because all antiarrhythmic drugs have the potential 1 to 2% risk of creating ventricular arrhythmias, the issue of hospitalization for initiation of the drug should be considered. This is not practical in most cases, and hospitalization should be reserved for the individual who has associated severe heart failure or perhaps a recent severe ischemia when the chance of the proarrhythmic effect of the drug may be enhanced.

Flecainide (Tambocor) is usually an appropriate first drug. It has the advantage of being effective with a twice-daily regimen and with a low side effect profile. It should be avoided in those with *severe* heart failure (it has a negative inotropic effect) and in those with recent significant ischemia. When evaluated in recently ischemic patients in the Cardiac Arrhythmia Suppression Trial, it was shown to be proarrhythmic. Other available drugs were not assessed in that trial, so it is not clear that they are any safer for use. Once flecainide is started, the patient can be brought back in a few days for an attempt at repeated cardioversion. If sinus rhythm is achieved, long-term antiarrhythmic drug therapy is warranted. If flecainide fails, sotalol or amiodarone is a reasonable next choice. The list of complications associated with amiodarone is long, and some are severe (potentially severe lung disease, liver disease, or possibly optic neuritis). The risks of using either drug would have to be balanced against the hope for benefit of making an individual feel better.

Many patients have reasonable freedom from symptoms with rate control alone. If drugs are not effective, AV node ablation has a high success rate, although it does obligate the patient to a permanent pacemaker; rate modification with AV node ablation techniques is of uncertain benefit. In a rare individual unwilling to accept atrial fibrillation, a surgical atrial dissection procedure (the maze procedure) has been applied with success in eliminating this rhythm.

Atrial Flutter

Atrial flutter is atrial fibrillation. Of course that is not true, but the statement is made because management should be nearly identical. The differences are worth discussion. First, there is less known about the thromboembolic risk with this rhythm. Because emboli have occurred when the rhythm is chronic and at the time of cardioversion, and because many people with atrial flutter frequently have episodes of atrial fibrillation, the antithrombotic regimen just presented for atrial fibrillation is also recommended for patients with atrial flutter. A second difference with atrial flutter is that it is often more difficult to control the ventricular response rate with the AV-node–blocking drugs—a reason to consider cardioversion earlier. A third difference is that some atrial flutters, particularly those with the typical form with the appearance of negative flutter waves in the inferior leads (sawtooth pattern), with the atrial rate being approximately 300 beats per minute, lend themselves to the possibility of elimination with atrial catheter ablation techniques. The ablation can eliminate the rhythm mechanism but allow maintenance of AV conduction. If that does not work, as with atrial fibrillation, an AV node ablation can be performed, although this results in the need for permanent ventricular pacing.

Ventricular Tachycardia

When ventricular tachycardia is associated with significant hemodynamic embarrassment, immediate sedation followed by cardioversion (synchronized DC 100 to 200 joules) is the treatment of choice. In the patient with sufficiently stable hemodynamics, drug therapy using IV lidocaine (Xylocaine), procainamide (Pronestyl), or amiodarone (Cordarone), in that order, is appropriate. In the refractory patient or in a patient with recurrent rhythms, IV beta blockers can also be helpful.

Long-Term Therapy

Ventricular tachycardia resulting from coronary artery disease or cardiomyopathies has a 20 to 40% chance of recurrence in the first year. Treatment can reduce the mortality to 5 to 15% in that year. Therapeutic options include drug therapy—amiodarone or sotalol (Betapace)—or an implantable cardioverter defibrillator (ICD). The just completed AVID trial (antiarrhythmics vs. implantable defibrillator trial) demonstrated improved survival with the device, compared with drug therapy. A similar Canadian trial, Canadian Implantable Defibrillator Study (CIDS), showed the same trend. Quality of life and financial impact are still being assessed, but, on the basis of these studies, an ICD is the preferred treatment in suitable candidates.

An individual will occasionally present with exercise-induced ventricular tachycardia. Particularly when it has an appearance of coming from the right ventricular outflow track (usually a left bundle branch block morphology with an inferiorly directed axis), beta-blocker therapy can be highly effective. If these rhythms are recurrent, they can often be eliminated with radiofrequency catheter ablation.

Another somewhat unusual tachycardia is that arising from the inferior aspect of the left side of the ventricular septum (generally a right bundle branch block morphology with a superior axis). These rhythms respond to treatment with verapamil and can also be treated with catheter ablation.

Ventricular Fibrillation

Complete life support and emergency treatment are of course required. Early defibrillation offers the best chance of survival. Cardiopulmonary resuscitative measures should be undertaken until conversion of the rhythm to normal can be achieved. A sudden death rate of 20 to 40% in the next year can be reduced to 5 to 15% with drug therapy—again sotalol or amiodarone—or with insertion of the ICD. The previously mentioned AVID and CIDS trials also demonstrated improved survival when the ICD was used to treat survivors of ventricular fibrillation.

Nonsustained Ventricular Tachycardia

The role and optimal treatment of this rhythm are not yet fully understood. In the patient with recurrent unacceptable symptoms, drug therapy may be beneficial, and sotalol or amiodarone is most likely to be effective. Alternatives (quinidine, procainamide, mexiletine, or propranolol) are less likely to be effective and have their own set of potential side effects. In the patient with this rhythm with associated coronary artery disease and a reduced ejection fraction (below 0.35), electrophysiologic testing may determine those whose life would be better protected with an implantable defibrillator (i.e., those in whom sustained ventricular tachycardia can be induced and not suppressed by procainamide in the rhythm laboratory).

THE OTHER FIVE PERCENT

These uncommon rhythms still occur often enough that a comment in regard to each seems appropriate. They are often dangerous and even more difficult to treat than the more common rhythms and thus fortunately *are* rare.

The Rapid Irregular Wide QRS Tachycardia (Often with a Rate Above 250 Beats per Minute)

Irregularity makes ventricular tachycardia an unlikely diagnosis, so atrial fibrillation, as noted before, should be considered. The rapid rate suggests that conduction may be not through the AV node but rather through an accessory pathway. AV-node–blocking drugs will not work and may actually exacerbate the rhythms by increasing accessory pathway conduction or by decreasing blood pressure and ventricular function. The treatment of choice for this rhythm is DC cardioversion. IV procainamide or lidocaine can block accessory pathway conduction in some patients.

Torsades de Pointes

This is perhaps the most confusing of all rhythms; different causes of this rhythm require opposite treatments. The rhythm is recognized by a rapid wide QRS complex tachycardia with a gradually changing morphology. It usually recurs as repetitive nonsustained episodes, so cardioversion should be avoided (and frequently is ineffective). It is difficult to differentiate from a "polymorphic" ventricular tachycardia; the presence of a prolonged QT interval on the sinus rhythm electrocardiogram (a Qt_e >500 milliseconds) is the major reason to consider the rhythm as torsades de pointes. This prolonged QT interval syndrome can be "acquired" and due to drugs (quinidine, class IA antiarrhythmic agents, tricyclic antidepressants, phenothiazine drugs, and the antihistamines astemizole [Hismanal] and terfenadine [Seldane], particularly when used in combination with a macrolide antibiotic) or to metabolic abnormalities (hypokalemia, hypomagnesemia). Treatment consists of identification of and stopping the offending agent, use of magnesium sulfate (2 to 4 grams IV), and potassium repletion. Until the effect of the drug dissipates, the torsades de pointes may be suppressed by initiation of isoproterenol or atrial pacing (to a heart rate of 120 beats per minute).

Torsades de pointes can also occur as the result of a congenital abnormal prolonged QT interval. This should be suspected if these rhythms are documented in the young, in those with a history of recurrent unexplained syncope, and in those with a family history of syncope or early sudden death. In patients with a congenital prolonged QT syndrome, the rhythm is often induced by sudden increase in adrenergic tone, e.g., when an affected person is startled by an alarm. IV beta-blocking agents will suppress the rhythm acutely. Chronic beta-blocker therapy should be initiated. In patients with the chronic syndrome and recurrent rhythms, if beta-blocker therapy does not work, an implantable defibrillator is an occasional consideration.

Abnormal Sinus Node and Atrial Rhythms

Sinus tachycardia, PSVT, atrial flutter, and atrial fibrillation have been discussed. There are other supraventricular rhythms. Sinoatrial reentry tachycardia can appear to be sinus tachycardia but is distinguished by its abrupt onset and termination. Beta-blocking agents or an antiarrhythmia agent can on occasion correct the rhythm. Atrial tachycardia may appear to be PSVT, but it behaves more like atrial flutter. The P waves may be more apparent than they are with PSVT and often are midway between QRS complexes (a "long RP" tachycardia). AV-node–blocking agents do not stop the rhythm (as they may with PSVT) but rather cause an increase in AV block. These rhythms can occur as the result of drug toxicity (e.g., digitalis). In general, treatment should consist of AV nodal blockade (with verapamil or beta blockers) and antiarrhythmia drugs; catheter ablation techniques can eliminate some of these rhythms.

ADULT AND POSTOPERATIVE CONGENITAL HEART DISEASE

method of
YUNG R. LAU, M.D.
University of Alabama at Birmingham
Birmingham, Alabama

The number of teenagers and adults with congenital heart disease, especially those who have had a surgical procedure, is increasing. About 90% of children born with congenital heart disease will reach adulthood, predominantly owing to improving surgical techniques. However, even successful surgical palliation or "repair" often does not eliminate sequelae and residua. The management of these problems is ever changing as new problem patterns are discovered and more tools for dealing with newly discovered and well-delineated problems become available. With the use of balloons, stents, and coils, interventionalists are often able to relieve stenosis and close unwanted vessels, and with the advances in catheter ablation, electrophysiologists have another tool for managing arrhythmias. This article highlights the unique problems in the more common congenital heart conditions. It begins with a discussion of the adult with congenital heart disease, then looks at the hemodynamic and electrophysiologic aspects of common lesions, and ends with a few comments about reproductive issues, bacterial endocarditis, and other miscellaneous issues.

CYANOTIC CONGENITAL HEART DISEASE

Patients can reach adulthood with persistent cyanotic heart disease for a number of reasons. In some, the defect will go undiscovered until irreversible pulmonary hypertension has occurred; others will have a cyanotic cardiac anomaly that was or is irreparable. Thankfully, owing to improvement in surgical skill, the increased awareness of primary care physicians, and greater availability and utility of diagnostic techniques, these patients are becoming fewer. Unfortunately, there have been no recent advances in the medical treatment of these patients, but surgical intervention with heart-lung transplantation or with single- or double-lung transplantation with concomitant intracardiac repair offers hope for increased longevity. Nontransplanted patients are a management challenge; in particular, attention must be paid to hematologic status, renal function, and urate metabolism.

The two hematologic complications of concern in adults with cyanotic heart disease are erythrocytosis and homeostatic abnormalities. Erythrocytosis can be compensated or decompensated. Despite hematocrit levels of 70% or more, patients with compensated erythrocytosis in the setting of appropriate iron levels do not experience symptoms attributed to hyperviscosity, such as headaches, dizziness, visual disturbances, fatigue, myalgias, or paresthesias. On the other hand, patients with decompensated erythrocytosis experience rising hematocrit levels and symptoms of hyperviscosity. The precise mechanisms of decompensated erythrocytosis are complex but are probably related to tissue hypoxia, iron deficiency, and hyperviscosity. Of these factors, iron deficiency is probably the most important for a couple of reasons. Iron supplementation should be used in patients with symptomatic iron deficiency. The dose should be small (65 mg per day of elemental iron in adults) and the response monitored for a rise in the hematocrit level. Once a rise is detected, supplementation should be stopped.

The risk of cerebrovascular accidents appears to be highest in the younger patient. Dehydration, inappropriate phlebotomies, or injudicious use of anticoagulants raise the risk. These patients are also at risk for paradoxical emboli and brain abscesses. Any patient with cyanotic congenital heart disease who presents with a new-onset focal seizure should undergo cranial computed tomography.

Phlebotomy is not recommended in the asymptomatic or mildly symptomatic patient with compensated erythrocytosis even with high hematocrit levels. In the patient with significant symptoms, phlebotomy is often helpful once dehydration has been ruled out. Generally, removal of 500 mL of blood with concurrent volume replacement with isotonic saline will provide relief of symptoms within 24 hours.

The bleeding diathesis seen in these patients seems to correlate with the degree of erythrocytosis and the level of hypoxemia. This is distinct from congenital hematologic abnormalities that are sometimes associated with congenital heart disease and that should be treated as is appropriate for the specific disorder. All three mechanisms of coagulation (platelet, intrinsic, and extrinsic) appear to be affected. The platelet counts are generally in the low range of normal or may be quite depressed. These abnormalities will be exacerbated by aspirin and other nonsteroidal anti-inflammatory agents, and therefore these drugs should not be used in the cyanotic patient.

These patients confront a significant risk of bleeding during surgery. Phlebotomy has been used to improve hemostasis with the goal of gradually reducing the hematocrit to just below 65% and normalizing the partial thromboplastin time. In addition, fresh frozen plasma should be available perioperatively.

High plasma urate levels can occasionally lead to urate nephropathy and urolithiasis. While arthralgias are quite common in this patient population, acute gouty arthritis is not. Nonsteroidal anti-inflammatory agents should be used with great caution because of their antihemostatic effects on platelets. Medications such as salsalate (Disalcid) that do not interfere with platelet function can be helpful for arthralgias. Colchicine is useful in the treatment of acute gout, and probenecid or sulfinpyrazone (Anturane) can be used for patients with hyperuricemia and gouty arthritis. Allopurinol (Zyloprim) should be considered for symptomatic hyperuricemia that is refractory to other medications.

ATRIAL SEPTAL DEFECT

There are three types of atrial septal defects: ostium secundum, sinus venosus, and ostium primum. Atrial septal defects (ASDs) are probably the most common congenital cardiac defects that physicians manage. Because of the absence of recognized symptoms and subtle physical signs, an ASD can go undiagnosed for decades. Traditionally, repair of these lesions has been surgical, but transcatheter devices are being developed and show promise. The typical patient with a significant uncorrected ASD will survive into adulthood, but survival after 40 to 50 years is less than 50%. Those who do survive will have worsening of symptoms owing to increasing left-to-right shunting, atrial arrhythmias, and mild to moderate pulmonary hypertension. In addition, the risk of pulmonary artery thrombosis is thought to be increased. Infrequently, patients may have paradoxical emboli.

On the other hand, those patients whose ASD was repaired early in life before significant pulmonary hypertension developed have a survival equal to that of the normal healthy population. Those with significant preoperative pulmonary hypertension (systolic pressure >40 mm Hg) have a late survival rate only one half that of healthy controls. If the preoperative pulmonary resistance is less than 14 Wood's units per m^2, symptoms of dyspnea and fatigue will regress after repair; if it is greater than 15 Wood's units per m², symptoms will progress. No additional significant hemodynamic issues for the ostium secundum or sinus venosus defects exist. The patient with an ostium primum defect, however, may have important postoperative hemodynamic residua. The mitral valve is invariably malformed; almost all patients will have at least mild mitral valve incompetence in the immediate postoperative period, and 10% will have late progressive mitral regurgitation requiring valvuloplasty or valve replacement.

Electrophysiologic residua are uncommon, but some patients with all three types of ASDs experience atrial flutter, atrial fibrillation, or sinus node dysfunction. The efficacious treatment of atrial fibrillation is elusive, but new catheter ablation techniques are being developed that show some promise in controlling and sometimes curing this arrhythmia. Catheter ablation has already been found to be highly successful in the treatment of atrial flutter in this population. New activity-sensing pacemakers are coming closer to mimicking normal sinus node function for those with sinus node dysfunction syndrome.

COMPLETE ATRIOVENTRICULAR SEPTAL DEFECT

Most of these patients have Down syndrome, which remains an important residuum. The postoperative course is similar to that in patients with a primum ASD, and the prognosis is excellent. Concerns about the mitral valve and its competency make long-term follow-up necessary. In addition, a small segment of patients with Down syndrome will have early pulmonary vascular disease that persists and progresses postoperatively.

Electrocardiography (ECG) in these patients shows a distinctive left axis deviation. Postoperatively, there is often a right bundle branch block as well. Late development of atrial flutter after repair occurs in approximately 5% of patients. Catheter ablation is highly successful in curing this arrhythmia. With improved understanding of the anatomy of the conduction system, complete atrioventricular block is rarely seen, but when it occurs pacing is usually needed.

VENTRICULAR SEPTAL DEFECTS

Ventricular septal defects (VSDs) come in a variety of sizes and locations. VSDs in the perimembranous and muscular sites have a tendency to decrease in size, whereas those in the inlet and infundibular septum (doubly committed) locations do not. Unrepaired VSDs in adults are either small ($Q_p/Q_s < 1.5$) and have not damaged the pulmonary vascular bed or at least moderate in size and may pose risk of Eisenmenger's syndrome. (The treatment of Eisenmenger's syndrome is delineated in the section on cyanotic heart disease.) Patients with a small muscular defect need minimal follow-up for their cardiac lesions, although antibiotic prophylaxis should be emphasized, as there is a cumulative risk of infective endocarditis. For patients with infundibular and perimembranous defects, even if the shunt is small, close follow-up to ascertain continued integrity of the aortic valve is necessary. With the available echocardiographic technology, even trivial regurgitation can be seen and necessitates closure of the VSD. Once this has been done, the aortic regurgitation is arrested and often improves.

The long-term prognosis for patients with surgically closed VSDs is excellent. Hemodynamically, no sequelae have been reported. Electrophysiologically, most patients will have a right bundle branch block pattern on their ECG postoperatively. Fewer patients are experiencing even transient complete heart block. Atrial and ventricular arrhythmias are rare but have been reported. Catheter ablation is quite successful in these patients.

TETRALOGY OF FALLOT

Patients who have undergone repair of tetralogy of Fallot have an excellent prognosis with survival rates from 80 to 94% at 20 years after the operation. Most are free from significant symptoms and are able to lead normal lives. Although all patients with repaired tetralogy of Fallot are at risk for hemodynamic and electrophysiologic complications, those undergoing late correction appear to be at greater risk. Hemodynamic residua include right ventricular failure (relatively common), right ventricular aneurysms (rare), and left ventricular dysfunction (rare). Electrophysiologic complications include heart block, ventricular arrhythmias, and atrial arrhythmias.

Right ventricular failure is often the cause of significant hemodynamic sequelae. This failure usually occurs because of chronically high pressures due to outflow and pulmonary arterial obstruction and/or volume overload due to the free pulmonary insufficiency. Even patients with right ventricular hypertension (systolic >40 mm Hg) and significant volume overload are asymptomatic during the first decade of life, and it is not until the third or fourth decade that symptoms of right ventricular failure are experienced. In those with symptomatic right ventricular failure, severe tricuspid regurgitation, or progressive right ventricular dilatation, placement of a valve in the pulmonary position should be considered. Obstruction in the outflow or pulmonary arteries can often be improved with catheter techniques and should be attempted before reoperation.

Heart block has become less common postoperatively as surgeons have developed techniques to avoid the AV node. However, those who experience transient postoperative complete heart block and those who have bifascicular block appear to be at higher risk for late heart block. These patients should be followed closely with ECGs and ambulatory monitors. Atrial arrhythmias, usually atrial flutter, are relatively uncommon and can be cured with catheter ablation.

Sudden death (0.5 to 5.5%) after repair of tetralogy

of Fallot has been presumed to be due to ventricular arrhythmias. Risk stratification for these patients has been a source of controversy among pediatric electrophysiologists. Some earlier studies reported that ventricular ectopic rhythms and elevated right ventricular pressures identify patients at risk for life-threatening ventricular arrhythmias, but others have disputed this. More recent studies have looked at the QRS duration and QRS dispersion on the ECG. For patients who have had documented ventricular tachycardias, therapy depends on hemodynamic stability while in tachycardia. If the patient is stable, catheter ablation has been found to be successful in eliminating the tachycardia. If the patient is not stable during the tachycardia, then placement of an internal cardioverter/defibrillator can be lifesaving.

TRANSPOSITION OF THE GREAT ARTERIES

The surgical treatment of complete transposition of the great arteries underwent a dramatic shift 5 to 10 years ago. The atrial switch operations pioneered by Drs. Senning and Mustard had a very high immediate postoperative survival but the 30-year survival is approximately 50%. The declining long-term survival of these patients as well as improved survival after the arterial switch operation has made it the procedure of choice. However, there are large numbers of patients who underwent the atrial switch operation, and it is in these patients that the hemodynamic and electrophysiologic problems are seen.

Two areas are of hemodynamic concern. The long-term performance of the morphologic right ventricle as the systemic pump declines with time, although the timeline is highly variable. The diagnosis of right ventricular failure is based primarily on the patient history as commonly available imaging techniques seem to correlate only loosely. Traditional medical therapy often relieves mild to moderate symptoms of heart failure, but some of these patients will eventually have to undergo heart transplantation.

Other hemodynamic residua include intra-atrial baffle obstruction and leaks. Baffle obstructions are less common in the inferior than in the superior vena cava. Both types can cause protein-losing enteropathy many years after the operation. Balloon dilatation with stent placement has been effective in relieving baffle obstructions. Late obstruction of the pulmonary venous baffle is uncommon. Relief of obstruction in the pulmonary venous baffles using catheter techniques is technically challenging but has been reported. Large leaks in the baffles are uncommon and require reoperation. Trivial or small leaks occur in 15% of patients and are bidirectional. They are usually of no hemodynamic significance but do increase the risk of paradoxical emboli and are a concern if a pacing device is needed.

Atrial tachycardias, bradyarrhythmias, and ventricular tachycardias have all been reported after the atrial switch operation. These arrhythmias are of significance, as 2 to 8% of these patients die suddenly, a fatal arrhythmia being the presumed cause. Some studies have found that the risk of sudden death is increased after a documented episode of atrial flutter, although the mechanism underlying this relationship is unclear. Symptomatic sinus node dysfunction requires a pacemaker, although placement of an endocardial system is predicated on the lack of baffle leaks or obstruction and requisite center expertise.

The diagnosis of atrial tachycardia is sometimes based on quite subtle findings. The atrial flutter (or intra-atrial reentry tachycardia) can be slower than typical atrial flutter and the P waves on the surface ECG are small. Any postoperative atrial switch patient with a heart rate of greater than 100 beats per minute should be suspected of being in atrial flutter. Yearly monitoring with 24-hour ambulatory systems is probably warranted.

Because of the association between sudden death and atrial flutter, treatment has been aggressively pursued. Initial cardioversion can be done using DC current, transesophageal or intracardiac overdrive pacing, or pharmacologic cardioversion with an intravenous class I or class III antiarrhythmic. Long-term treatment has included antitachycardia pacing as well as antiarrhythmic medications with varying success. Generally, long-term therapy for atrial flutter begins with digoxin and/or a beta blocker with careful monitoring of bradyarrhythmias. Beyond that, the next step is controversial. Some institutions would attempt catheter ablation, although the application of this technique for atrial flutter in the postoperative atrial switch patient is still being defined. Other centers recommend an implanted antitachycardia pacing system. Still others begin antiarrhythmia medications and implant a pacing system because these medications exacerbate bradyarrhythmias. Given the anatomic complications, procedures such as catheter ablation and pacemaker placement should be done in a center experienced in congenital heart disease.

It is becoming evident that ventricular arrhythmias also play a role in these patients. Management after a syncopal episode is especially difficult. When the history is consistent with a life-threatening arrhythmia or a ventricular tachycardia can be induced with electrophysiologic testing, implantable cardioverter defibrillators should be used.

Hemodynamic residua after the arterial switch operation are uncommon. Improvement in surgical skill has made coronary artery kinking rare. Supravalvular stenosis at both the ascending aorta and the main pulmonary anastomosis is unusual. Some patients will also have long-segment stenosis of the branch pulmonary arteries as they straddle the aorta, and 14% will have mild aortic regurgitation, the natural history of which is unclear. Unlike in the atrial switch operation, no significant postoperative arrhythmias have been found in arterial switch patients.

POSTOPERATIVE FONTAN DEFECTS

The Fontan operation and its modifications have been used in situations in which there is an underdeveloped ventricle. The older Fontan operations closed any communication between the right atrium and the rest of the heart and connected the roof of the atrium or the appendage directly to the pulmonary arteries. Currently the most common technique requires two surgical stages. The first stage, done during infancy, is a modified Glenn-type operation in which the superior vena cava is connected directly to the right pulmonary artery. The second stage, done between 1 and 3 years of age, involves directing the inferior vena cava flow to the pulmonary arteries by using a straight "tube." Operative results have been variable. Although the quality of life improves, the survival rate is only 87% at 5 years and 60 to 73% at 15 years.

The hemodynamic sequelae depend on a number of factors but largely depend on the long-term ventricular function. Morphologic left ventricles (e.g., tricuspid atresia) perform better than morphologic right ventricles (e.g., hypoplastic left heart). Some patients have remained in the New York Heart Association functional class I or II as long as 15 years after the operation. However, in some there is late progressive deterioration of ventricular function and transplantation becomes the only option. Obstruction within the Fontan circulation is serious. If any obstruction exists (even low gradients of less than 5 mm Hg), either catheter balloon dilatation with or without stent placement or reoperation should be considered. Any patient with new-onset atrial arrhythmias, decreasing functional capacity, fluid retention, or protein-losing enteropathy should be investigated for obstruction. It is hoped that the newer surgical techniques will improve the flow dynamics of the Fontan system and thus reduce the degree of postoperative fluid retention and lessen the incidence of protein-losing enteropathy. Another anticipated benefit of the newer operations is a lower incidence of atrial thrombi. In the dilated right atrium, flow is sluggish and thrombi can form. The risk of thrombi is increased in patients with atrial arrhythmias. All patients having the Fontan procedure should be placed on long-term anticoagulation.

The arrhythmias seen after the Fontan procedure are similar to those seen after an atrial switch operation but have more of a hemodynamic impact, as atrial tachyarrhythmias can adversely affect left ventricular function and thus cause a rise in end-diastolic pressure, which will be reflected in a rise in right atrial pressure transferred through the pulmonary circulation. In addition to atrial tachyarrhythmias, sinus bradycardia that predisposes patients to these tachyarrhythmias becomes common as time passes. As with the atrial switch, vigilance is needed in the diagnosis as the ECG findings can be subtle.

The approach for the treatment of atrial arrhythmias is similar to that for postoperative atrial switch patients (described in the preceding section), except for these notable differences. Before DC cardioversion, intracardiac thrombi should be ruled out with echocardiography. If thrombi are present, alternative methods of cardioversion should be used, such as transesophageal or intracardiac overdrive pacing or pharmacologic cardioversion with an intravenous class I or III antiarrhythmic. In patients who had the older type of operation that connected the right atrium directly to the pulmonary arteries, access to the entire right atrium for catheter ablation is easier, and if no right atrial–to–left atrial leaks exist, transvenous atrial pacing devices can be placed. With the newer type of operations in which a "tube" is used to direct inferior vena caval flow to the pulmonary arteries, access to the right atrium for catheter ablation or pacing lead placement is eliminated. Although the hemodynamics in these patients are presumably better, atrial tachyarrhythmias still occur. Medical therapy is the main treatment modality.

In addition to atrial arrhythmias, ventricular arrhythmias are a cause of late death. The incidence is probably related to the degree of systemic ventricular dysfunction. Treatment consists of antiarrythmics (e.g., amiodarone) and/or implantation of an epicardial implantable cardioverter defibrillator.

CORRECTED TRANSPOSITION OF THE GREAT ARTERIES

Even when there are no coexisting cardiac malformations, these patients have a shortened life span; survival into the sixth decade is uncommon. This is primarily because of the right ventricle's inability to maintain its function as the systemic ventricle instead of its usual role as the pulmonary ventricle. The left-sided atrioventricular valve is often malformed, and incompetence can develop later in life.

Electrophysiologically, the risk of developing complete heart block is constant at a rate of 2% per year. Ambulatory 24-hour ECG should be done at least annually as surveillance for heart block. If there is evidence of second-degree heart block or transient complete heart block occurs, a pacing system should probably be placed.

COARCTATION OF THE AORTA

Coarctation of the aorta can appear at two times; in the first few weeks of life or, more typically, in adolescence or adulthood. The presenting sign in the older patient is often hypertension. Less commonly, undiagnosed patients present with an aneurysm of the circle of Willis or a dissecting aneurysm of the aorta.

Even after repair, significant residua and sequelae can occur, including hypertension, recoarctation, aortic aneurysm, premature coronary artery disease, cerebrovascular accident, congenital mitral valve disease, and degenerative disease of the hip. Postoperative systemic hypertension is most common. The older the patient is at the time of repair, the more likely residual systemic hypertension will occur, even when there is no residual obstruction. This underscores the importance of early diagnosis, usually during careful well child examinations. In fact, even patients who are normotensive in the immediate postoperative period may have inappropriate blood pressure responses during exercise and can develop hypertension in later years. Antihypertensive medications, primarily angiotension-converting enzyme inhibitors, are used to control hypertension.

Newer techniques have minimized the incidence of recoarctation. Recoarctation or residual coarctations are diagnosed when the arm-to-leg systolic pressure difference is greater than 20 mm Hg. In these patients, balloon angioplasty has been effective in relieving the stenosis. True and false aneurysms at the site of repair occur mainly in those who had patch aortoplasty, and vigilant follow-up is needed. Chest films are often a good screen for aneurysms, but further work-up with echocardiography or magnetic resonance imaging is warranted if the patient complains of chest or back pain. Premature coronary artery disease primarily seen late in the postoperative course. Cerebrovascular accidents are usually caused by rupture of a concurrent aneurysm in the circle of Willis and can even occur when the patient is normotensive. These strokes usually occur in the second or third decade of life. Concomitant congenital mitral valve dysmorphology is seen in 20% of the patients and involves a wide pathologic spectrum, ranging from clinically insignificant disease to gross incompetence and/or stenosis. One report indicates that up to 20% of postoperative patients followed for more than 26 years will develop degenerative disease of the hip; the mechanism is unclear.

PULMONARY VALVE STENOSIS

Pulmonary valve stenosis is usually diagnosed early in life as the murmur is obvious. Those with mild stenosis (renal vein to pulmonary artery gradient of <50 mm Hg) are generally asymptomatic. Those with significant pulmonary valve stenosis are usually treated efficaciously with balloon valvuloplasty. Their long-term survival is excellent and similar to that of age- and sex-matched controls. The exception is the patient with a dysplastic stenotic valve with or without supravalvar pulmonary stenosis, who occasionally requires surgical excision of a leaflet and sometimes a transannular patch and then is left with significant valve regurgitation, which can cause right ventricular volume overload and eventually right ventricular failure. As in the patient with repaired tetralogy of Fallot, placement of a valve in the pulmonary position often relieves the symptoms.

AORTIC STENOSIS

Bicuspid aortic valves are the most common cause of aortic valve disease. These patients often are functionally normal in childhood or have only mild stenosis or regurgitation. The natural history is highly variable. Some cases remain mild and do not cause any trouble throughout life, while others will worsen, slowly or quickly, and require surgical intervention. Valve replacement is usually needed by the fourth to sixth decade of life.

When significant aortic valve stenosis (>50 mm Hg) occurs early in life, balloon valvuloplasty or valvotomy can often provide temporary relief of the stenosis. However, this valve still has a tendency to thicken, calcify, and become stenotic with time, and close follow-up is needed. Several options are available when valve replacement is needed. These include replacement with a mechanical valve, a cryopreserved homograft, or an autograft procedure. For younger patients, particularly females at or below child-bearing age, an autograft (Ross) procedure should be considered.

Discrete subaortic stenosis is important not only because of the hemodynamic effects on the left ventricular myocardium but also because of the damage it often inflicts on the aortic valve. The resulting aortic regurgitation can be significant. Previously, discovery of this lesion required prompt resection of the offending membrane, but with the advance in color-flow Doppler, even the most trivial regurgitation can be detected, allowing close follow-up with careful attention to regurgitation and progression to significant stenosis.

PATENT DUCTUS ARTERIOSUS

Adults diagnosed with patent ductus arteriosus (PDA) either have a PDA large enough to cause chronic volume overload or a very small one. In patients with a large PDA, closure should be done if the increased pulmonary vascular resistance is reversible. A small PDA with an audible murmur carries a cumulative lifetime risk for bacterial endocarditis, and closure is recommended in most centers. A more recent phenomenon is silent PDA detected by echocardiography. In these patients, the risk is unknown and generally endocarditis prophylaxis is recommended instead of closure.

Until recently, surgical ligation was the only operative option, but in many centers, closure of the PDA with catheter techniques (use of a coil) is now the treatment of choice. Initial studies have shown a high rate of success.

REPRODUCTIVE ISSUES

Pregnant patients with congenital heart disease may face a substantial risk or no significant increased risk or may need to be managed on a case-by-case basis. A markedly increased risk of morbidity and mortality exists with pulmonary hypertension (mortality of up to 30% per pregnancy), uncorrected or recurrent coarctation of the aorta, and Marfan's syndrome with aortic involvement (aortic root >4 cm). Defects with no significant increased risk include repaired ASD; repaired, closed, or small VSD; and closed PDA. Postoperative Fontan defects, postoperative atrial switch defects, single ventricle defects, and tetralogy of Fallot should be managed on a case-by-case basis. In general, patients in New York Heart Association functional class III or IV should avoid pregnancy.

Patients with a right-to-left shunt are at greater risk for paradoxical emboli. The management of bacterial endocarditis during delivery is controversial. For those with repaired ASDs or VSDs or closed PDAs, prophylaxis is not required. Antibiotic prophylaxis should probably be administered for most other lesions.

The incidence of congenital heart lesions in the offspring of affected parents is 5 to 16% depending on the defect. Genetic counseling for patients with congenital heart disease interested in having children is advisable. Fetal echocardiography is feasible after 15 weeks' gestational age and is recommended to assess cardiac anatomy.

Contraception counseling should be done, as unplanned pregnancies can be devastating. Contraceptive methods should be chosen carefully with consideration given to the cardiac lesion. In those at high risk, tubal ligation may be appropriate. In general, estrogen-progesterone products should not be used by those with pulmonary hypertension or venous stasis (i.e., postoperative Fontan defects). Intrauterine devices are contraindicated in patients at risk for endocarditis.

MISCELLANEOUS ISSUES

Bacterial endocarditis prophylaxis is recommended in all patients with congenital heart disease with the exception of secundum ASDs and mitral valve prolapse without regurgitation. It need not be continued beyond 6 months following repair of secundum ASD, VSD (without residual) and PDA (without residual).*

Athletic participation by patients with congenital heart disease is dependent on the lesion. The overall goal is to maximize such activity.†

*Specific recommendations have been recently revised: Dajani AS, Taubert KA, Wilson W, et al.: Prevention of bacterial endocarditis. JAMA *277*:1794–1801, 1997; and Dajani AS, Taubert KA, Wilson W, et al.: Prevention of bacterial endocarditis. Circulation *96*:358–366, 1997. Alternatively, they can be found on the World Wide Web at http://www.americanheart.org/pubs/scipub/statements/.

†Specific guidelines were published in 26th Bethesda Conference: Recommendations for determining eligibility for competition in athletes with cardiovascular abnormalities. JACC *24*:845–899, 1994.

HYPERTROPHIC CARDIOMYOPATHY

method of
ALI J. MARIAN, M.D.
Baylor College of Medicine
Houston, Texas

Hypertrophic cardiomyopathy (HCM) was first reported by two French pathologists in the 19th century; however, modern interest in various features of HCM began approximately 30 years ago and paralleled the development of modern diagnostic tools. During the 1960s, HCM was recognized as a clinical and hemodynamic entity. During this period, reports emphasized the significance of subaortic stenosis, and the term "idiopathic hypertrophic subaortic stenosis" was commonly used. Advances in echocardiography in the 1970s led to characterization of hypertrophy, and the term "asymmetrical septal hypertrophy" was coined to emphasize its asymmetrical nature with predominant involvement of the interventricular septum. In the 1980s, routine use of Doppler echocardiography led to a better understanding of the dynamics of outflow tract obstruction, intracavitary gradient, and diastolic dysfunction. In the 1990s, advances in molecular genetic techniques elucidated the molecular basis of HCM and led to identification of a number of responsible genes. Despite such major advances, many questions remain unanswered, and the study of HCM is likely to expand into the new millennium.

Hypertrophic cardiomyopathy is an autosomal dominant disease that primarily involves the myocardium and is caused by mutations in sarcomeric proteins. It is characterized by the presence of left ventricular hypertrophy (LVH) in the absence of an increased external load, myofibrillar disarray, and a hyperdynamic left ventricle with a small cavity. Although LVH is a common cardiac response to a variety of injuries, disarray is the pathologic hallmark of HCM.

PREVALENCE

The true prevalence of HCM is not known, but echocardiographic studies of individuals 25 to 35 years old indicates a prevalence of 1 to 2 cases per 1000 population. Given the age-dependent penetrance of the disease, it may be more common in older populations.

GENETICS

Hypertrophic cardiomyopathy is a genetically heterogeneous disease. Over 70 mutations in seven different genes have been identified (Table 1), βMyHC being the first. Beta-MyHC is the predominant form of myosin in the human heart and constitutes more than 95% of the total myosin in the human ventricles. It is the motor unit of the myocardium, and its interaction with thin filaments during cardiac cycle generates the force of contraction. Most of the mutations in the βMyHC gene are missense mutations and are located within the globular head of the myosin molecule. The two apparent hot spots for mutations in the βMyHC gene are codons 403 and 719. Mutations in the βMyHC gene are responsible for about 30% of all HCM cases.

Another major gene for HCM is the cardiac troponin T gene, which is located on chromosome 1q3. Troponin T is an important component of the thin filaments and consti-

TABLE 1. **Gene Loci and Frequency in Hypertrophic Cardiomyopathy**

Gene	Locus	Frequency (%)
βMyHC	14q1	25–30
cTnT	1q3	15–20
α-tropomyosin	15q2	<5
MyBP-C	11q11	10–15
?	7q3	?
vMLC-1	3p	<1
vMLC-2	12q	<1
cTnI	19p13.2	3–5

tutes approximately 5% of the total myofibrillar protein. It positions the troponin complex on tropomyosin, and along with troponins C and I, plays a major role in the Ca^{2+} regulation of cardiac contraction and relaxation. A number of mutations in troponin T, mostly missense, have been identified, and codon 92 is considered a hot spot for mutations. Mutations in cTnT account for approximately 15 to 20% of HCM cases. An interesting feature of cTnT mutations is the high incidence of sudden cardiac death (SCD) in affected families, despite a mild degree of LVH.

The third most common gene for HCM is the MyBP-C gene on chromosome 11q1. This gene codes for another sarcomeric protein that binds to MyHC and titin, which helps to stabilize the sarcomere. Phosphorylation of MyBP-C domains modulates cardiac contractility. A number of mutations, mostly deletion mutations, in MyBP-C have been identified that commonly affect the binding sites for MyHC or titin. It is estimated that mutations in MyBP-C account for approximately 10 to 15% of HCM cases.

Other known genes for HCM are α-tropomyosin, cardiac troponin I, and myosin light chains 1 (essential) and 2 (regulatory), all of which code for the components of sarcomeres. Mutations in these genes are uncommon, and altogether they account for less than 10% of HCM cases.

MOLECULAR PATHOGENESIS

It is generally believed that hypertrophy is a compensatory process due to an impetus provided by the mutant sarcomeric proteins. Experimental data suggest that mutant sarcomeric proteins are assembled into the myofibrils, but the assembled myofibrils exhibit impaired mechanical performance, providing the impetus for a compensatory hypertrophy. The molecular mechanism of impaired myofibrillar function is poorly understood. The majority of mutant sarcomeric proteins probably function as "poison peptides" and act through a dominant-negative effect (i.e., impairing function at a low level of expression). Deletion mutations can function as null alleles (haplo-insufficiency) and alter the stoichiometry of the sarcomeric proteins, leading to impaired structure or function.

PATHOLOGY

Cardiac hypertrophy is the common morphologic feature of HCM. The left ventricle is the common site of hypertrophy, and the interventricular septum is predominantly involved, leading to asymmetrical hypertrophy. Hypertrophy rarely involves the right ventricle. Occasionally it is restricted to the apex (apical HCM); this is most common in Japan. The development of hypertrophy is age dependent and frequently accelerates during adolescence and puberty. The extent of hypertrophy is variable and is, in part, determined by the underlying mutations, genetic background, and possibly environmental factors. Other morphologic features of HCM include small ventricular cavities, dilated and hypertrophied atria, elongated and enlarged mitral leaflets, anomalous insertion of papillary muscles, and thickening of media of the intramural small coronary arteries.

The pathologic hallmark of HCM is myofibrillar and cardiac myocyte disarray. Cardiac myocytes are hypertrophied, have large nuclei, and are distributed in an unorganized manner. Disarray predominantly involves the interventricular septum. Myocardial interstitial collagen content is also increased and fibrosis is common.

CLINICAL MANIFESTATIONS

Hypertrophic cardiomyopathy varies in severity from a benign asymptomatic condition to severe heart failure and SCD, but the majority of patients are asymptomatic or mildly symptomatic. The disease often presents in middle age. The main symptoms are dyspnea and chest pain, predominantly due to left ventricular diastolic dysfunction. Diastolic dysfunction leads to increased left ventricular end-diastolic pressure and pulmonary venous congestion. It also results in diminished coronary perfusion pressure, which in the presence of hypertrophied myocardium leads to relative myocardial ischemia and thus chest pain. Other common symptoms include fatigue, palpitations, lightheadedness, and syncope.

DIAGNOSIS

Physical Examination

Physical findings are reflective of LVH and outflow tract obstruction. Therefore, in those without outflow tract obstruction or significant hypertrophy, the physical examination results may be completely normal. The typical arterial pulse has two components: percussion waves and tidal waves. The percussion wave is due to abrupt and brisk ejection of blood from the left ventricle in early systole. However, in those with outflow tract obstruction, a midsystolic decline and then a secondary rise (tidal wave) follow it. The jugular vein may show a prominent a wave reflective of poor right ventricular compliance. The apical impulse is strong and commonly bifid. The first component is due to forceful contraction of the atrium against a poorly compliant left ventricle. The second component is due to early systolic contraction of the left ventricle. A third component due to late systolic bulge of the left ventricle is present in some patients. The most common finding on physical examination is a midsystolic murmur in the left sternal border that is a harsh crescendo-decrescendo type that terminates with aortic closure. It rarely radiates to the carotid arteries. It is accentuated by maneuvers that diminish left ventricular volume (e.g., amyl nitrate inhalation) or increase left ventricular contractility. Postextrasystolic potentiation of the left ventricular outflow tract gradient increases the intensity of the murmur and is accompanied by a diminished arterial pulse (Brockenbrough's phenomenon). Maneuvers that increase left ventricular volume (e.g., squatting) diminish the intensity of the murmur. A significant number of patients with outflow tract obstruction also have mitral regurgitation and thus a pansystolic blowing murmur that radiates to the axillae. A loud S4 and/or S3 heart sound and a diastolic rumble may also be noted.

Laboratory Studies

The electrocardiogram (ECG) is usually abnormal in patients with significant disease. The predominant ECG findings are those of LVH with repolarization abnormalities, prominent Q waves in inferior and anterolateral leads, left anterior fascicular block, and left atrial enlargement. A small fraction of patients may also exhibit a short PR interval and evidence of preexcitation. There is no specific ECG finding that is pathognomonic for HCM, except for the giant negative T waves often seen in patients with apical HCM. Atrial fibrillation is present in 10 to 15% of cases.

Arrhythmias are common and usually poorly tolerated. Atrial fibrillation is particularly troublesome, as it is commonly associated with worsening of symptoms and increased risk of thromboembolism. Ventricular arrhythmias are found in the majority of patients on Holter monitoring, and the presence of repetitive nonsustained ventricular tachycardia is considered a risk factor for SCD. Routine electrophysiologic testing is not indicated. Induction of sustained ventricular tachycardia on electrophysiologic testing carries a low positive predictive value for SCD. However, noninducibility of sustained ventricular tachycardia identifies patients who are at low risk for SCD.

Echocardiography is the main diagnostic technique. The clinical diagnosis of HCM is based on the presence of LVH with a wall thickness of 13 mm or greater in the absence of a secondary cause for hypertrophy. Typical echocardiographic findings include a small left ventricular cavity with an increased ejection fraction, asymmetrical septal hypertrophy (ASH), septal hypokinesis, systolic anterior motion (SAM) of the mitral leaflet, and an intracavitary gradient. The latter is a characteristic feature of HCM; however, it may be labile (requires provocation) or absent in the majority of cases. A significant portion of patients also have mild to moderate mitral regurgitation. Echocardiography is also extremely useful in assessing left ventricular diastolic function. Isovolumic relaxation time is prolonged and early diastolic filling (E) is reduced, while the contribution of atrial contraction (A) is significantly increased.

Cardiac catheterization can be used to document the presence of an outflow tract gradient, mitral regurgitation, and concomitant diseases; to delineate coronary anatomy; or for ethanol ablation of septal hypertrophy. Left ventriculography shows a hypertrophic and hypercontractile left ventricle with cavity obliteration, SAM of mitral leaflets, and a spade-shaped configuration in apical HCM.

NATURAL COURSE

The annual mortality from HCM in adults is approximately 1%, with SCD accounting for approximately half of the deaths. Overall, the incidence of SCD is higher in younger patients. Hypertrophic cardiomyopathy is the most common cause of SCD in young athletes and accounts for 35% of SCDs in competitive athletes.

A number of clinical variables are considered risk factors for SCD in patients with HCM (Table 2). Genetic factors are also predictors of SCD. The majority of mutations in cardiac troponin T and certain mutations in βMyHC such as $Arg^{403}Gln$, $Arg^{453}Cys$, and $Arg^{719}Trp$ are associated with a high incidence of SCD, particularly in young adult males. Approximately 50% of the affected individuals with these mutations die prematurely, half from SCD. In contrast, other βMyHC mutations such as $Gly^{256}Glu$, and $Leu^{908}Val$, mutations in the MyBP-C, and α-tropomyosin are associated with a mild form of the disease and a low incidence of SCD. Genetic factors other than the underlying mutations also influence the phenotypic expression of HCM.

TABLE 2. **Risk Factors for Sudden Cardiac Death in Hypertrophic Cardiomyopathy Patients**

Family history of sudden cardiac death ("malignant hypertrophic cardiomyopathy")
Mutations in cTnT, βMyHC ($Arg^{403}Gln$, $Arg^{453}Cys$, $Arg^{719}Trp$) and genetic background
Early onset of clinical manifestations
History of syncope
Sustained and repetitive nonsustained ventricular tachycardia
Abnormal blood pressure response to exercise
Myocardial ischemia
Severity of hypertrophy

TREATMENT

Medical Management

The majority of patients with HCM are asymptomatic or mildly symptomatic. Routine prophylactic treatment is not indicated in asymptomatic patients, unless they are considered at high risk for SCD. The majority of symptomatic patients respond well to pharmacologic therapy with either beta blockers or verapamil (Calan SR) or a combination of both. Beta blockers are preferred in patients with an outflow tract gradient at rest, as verapamil can induce hypotension and worsen the gradient. Palpitations, dizziness, and syncope should be investigated before empirical therapy. Patients with atrial fibrillation should receive anticoagulation and electrical cardioversion should be attempted in those with new-onset atrial fibrillation. Patients with chronic or paroxysmal atrial fibrillation should be treated with beta blockers, verapamil, or amiodarone (Cordarone). Patients with repetitive bursts of nonsustained ventricular tachycardia on Holter monitoring and those with sustained ventricular tachycardia are candidates for amiodarone or cardioverter-defibrillator implantation.

Surgical Myomectomy-Myectomy

A small fraction of patients who are refractory to pharmacologic therapy and have significant outflow tract obstruction (>50 mm Hg at rest) are candidates for surgical resection of a small portion of the interventricular septum (Morrow's procedure). The merits of myomectomy in reducing or abolishing outflow tract gradients and improving symptoms has been well documented. However, its impact on overall survival and the risk of SCD remains to be established. Surgical mortality is approximately 1% and is higher in elderly patients, in those with concomitant diseases, and in inexperienced hands. Mitral valve replacement has been advocated in selected patients with severe mitral regurgitation or anomalous insertion of papillary muscles.

Dual-Chamber Pacing

Dual-chamber pacing has been proposed as a treatment modality in symptomatic patients who are refractory to pharmacologic therapy and have outflow tract obstruction. The principle of dual-chamber pacing is based on modification of the left ventricular excitation pattern, which leads to relief of outflow tract obstruction. Optimal timing of the atrioventricular (AV) interval is an important aspect of the pacing strategy: initial observational studies showed a significant improvement in symptoms along with a major reduction in outflow tract obstruction. However, preliminary results of randomized multicenter studies show a placebo effect of pacing as well as a true reduction in outflow tract obstruction without improvement in exercise tolerance.

Ethanol Ablation of Septal Hypertrophy

Injection of alcohol into a major septal branch results in septal infarct and reduction of outflow tract gradient. Initial observational studies show improvement in symptoms and a reduction in the outflow tract gradient. However, a significant number of these patients also develop complete AV block and require pacemaker implantation. Further refinement of this technique is needed before it is a viable therapeutic option.

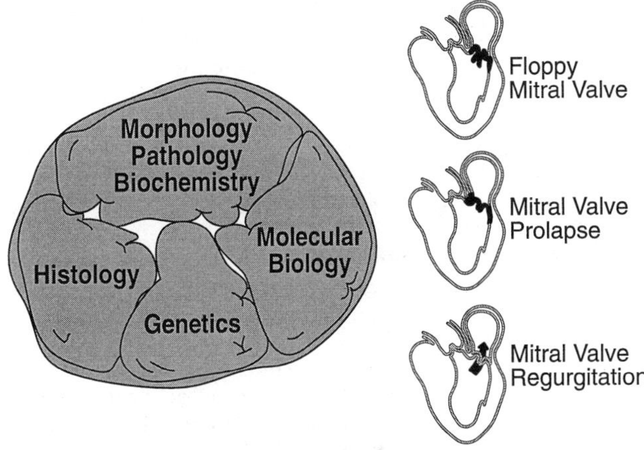

Figure 1. Floppy mitral valve–mitral valve prolapse–mitral valve regurgitation triad. Emphasis on the central role of the floppy mitral valve with tissue characteristics that reflect basic morphology, pathology, and biochemistry regulated by molecular biologic and genetic factors.

MITRAL VALVE PROLAPSE

method of
CHARLES F. WOOLEY, M.D., and
HARISIOS BOUDOULAS, M.D., PH.D.
Ohio State University College of Medicine
Columbus, Ohio

Each cardiac valvular lesion has its own lineage. Murmur identification correlated with anatomic pathology in the 19th century resulted in diagnostic profiles for patients with valvular heart disease. Although this reliance on autopsy confirmation was effective in patients with inflammatory valvular lesions of rheumatic or syphilitic origin who died at relatively young ages, the floppy mitral valve (FMV) was the exception to the rule, because identifying and separating the FMV as a discrete pathologic entity distinct from rheumatic mitral valvular disease were gradual processes. In addition, the long natural history of the FMV was not apparent when the life span of patient and physician was short. Although the hypothesis that certain forms of mitral regurgitation resulted from prolapse of the mitral valve into the left atrium was advanced in the 19th century, the proof awaited 20th-century surgical observations and imaging techniques. Early 20th-century clinical use of the radiograph, the electrocardiogram, and the phonocardiogram was followed at midcentury by clinical use of cardiac catheterization, angiography, and cardiac surgery, a process that accelerated with the introduction of increasingly sophisticated imaging techniques during the latter part of the century.

FLOPPY MITRAL VALVE

Three major themes in our understanding of mitral valvular disease during the last 50 years include (1) recognition of the FMV as a discrete pathologic entity producing mitral valve dysfunction; (2) mitral valve dysfunction associated with the FMV resulted in prolapse of the mitral valve into the left atrium mitral valve prolapse [MVP]; and (3) the FMV with MVP resulted in a specific form of mitral valvular regurgitation (MVR) (Figure 1).

FMV description and definition began at autopsy when the pathologists and morphologists pointed out the discrete nature of floppy mitral valves in the 1940s, emphasized that these valves were not the result of rheumatic fever, and recognized certain of the clinical correlates. These correlates were the long natural history of the disorder, FMV susceptibility to infectious endocarditis, the occurrence of ruptured chordae tendinae, and the late onset of rapidly progressive congestive heart failure associated with progressive MVR. Although FMV morphology and the clinical implications were well described in the 1940s, the clinicians' preoccupation with rheumatic fever as the predominant cause of valvular heart disease obscured the FMV etiologic and pathodynamic significance for another 2 decades.

The early cardiovascular surgeons visualized the mitral valve in the beating heart, using the term "floppy valve syndrome" in 1965 to describe patients with significant mitral and aortic valvular regurgitation due to myxomatous transformation of the mitral and aortic valves and the mechanism for valvular regurgitation as "valve prolapse." Visualization of the redundant FMV prolapsing into the left atrium resulted in the introduction of descriptive terminology including "floppy valve," as a term for myxomatous changes in mitral valve tissue, and mitral valve "prolapse", as the mechanism for MVR. Emphasis shifted to the etiologic significance of the connective tissue changes in the FMV rather than the traditional rheumatic or inflammatory etiology.

Physical Diagnosis

The clinicians approached the FMV from different directions. Apical systolic sounds, described during the 19th century, were called systolic clicks or systolic gallop sounds; however, their significance was uncertain, and the sounds were usually considered to be extracardiac in origin. Although the loud, apical holosystolic murmur of advanced MVR transmitted to the axilla and the back was well recognized by 19th-century auscultors, the fact that apical mid or late systolic murmurs were not transmitted puzzled auscultors for 150 years. As a result, apical systolic clicks and nontransmitted apical midsystolic and late systolic murmurs were long considered to be extracardiac, innocent, or functional. During the 1960s, systematic study of patients with apical midsystolic or late systolic clicks, and apical midsystolic and late systolic murmurs showed that these auscultatory phenomena were of intracardiac origin associated with the FMV prolapsing into the left atrium (MVP). These auscultatory tenets were established using phonocardiographic recordings correlated with left ventricular angiography (i.e., the diagnoses were based on coherence among auscultation, phonocardiography, and angiography, important distinctions in diagnostic sensitivity and specificity).

The systolic clicks correlated with the abrupt termination of the motion of the FMV apparatus into the left atrium, whereas the midsystolic or late systolic murmurs were due to mitral regurgitation occurring during midsystole or late systole. The timing and intensity of the systolic click or clicks, and the duration and intensity of the apical midsystolic or late systolic murmurs change with body posture (Figure 2). These changes are often dramatic, reflecting changes in the timing of the MVP and in the timing and extent of the MVR. In general, these auscultatory and hemodynamic changes parallel the expected changes in left ventricular volume and left ventricular dynamics with changes in body posture. Thus, dynamic cardiac auscultation expands the role of cardiac physical diagnosis in patients with MVP, providing clinicians with important physical diagnostic criteria for the clinical approach to patients with FMV producing MVP with or without MVR.

Cardiac Imaging

Prolapse of the FMV into the left atrium, first visualized under direct observation at surgery, was confirmed with left ventricular cineangiography during the 1960s. Angiographic criteria for normal mitral valve morphology and function were established and a reasonable degree of consensus was reached about FMV-MVP correlates. Thus, FMV-MVP diagnostic criteria were initially based on auscultatory, phonocardiographic, and angiographic correlates. The advent of ultrasonography provided new imaging modalities for definition of mitral valve function and dysfunction. Major problems in diagnosis, specificity, and sensitivity were introduced with the early M-mode imaging modalities when the imaging studies were dissociated from the established pathologic criteria for the FMV and from auscultatory-phonocardiographic-angiographic criteria. A period of diagnostic confusion followed during which the prevalence of MVP using M-mode criteria was grossly exaggerated.

Echo-Doppler studies using the transthoracic or transesophageal approach correlating FMV pathologic criteria with strict FMV-MVP criteria, and color-flow imaging with analysis of MVR jet phenomena provide contemporary diagnostic precision. Three-dimensional echo imaging of the mitral valve adds an additional approach to definition of individual mitral valve leaflet scallops. FMV patients without MVR in the recumbent position or at rest may develop MVR with posture change or exercise, extending the scope of such diagnostic testing. The net effect of informed imaging studies has been a refocusing of attention of the central role of the FMV in the pathogenesis of MVP, enhancing the diagnosis of the FMV-MVP-MVR triad.

Understanding these inter-relationships within the FMV-MVP-MVR triad are important because diagnostic criteria have been changing as technology advances. Clinicians should use rigid criteria for the clinical, auscultatory, phonocardiographic, angiographic, or echo-Doppler definition of patients with FMV producing MVP with or without MVR, enhancing diagnostic sensitivity and specificity. The result is a dimunition of the controversy surrounding the FMV-MVP-MVR triad.

Floppy Mitral Valve Characteristics: Clinical Implications

The characteristics of the FMV that form the bases for mitral valve dysfunction, specifically MVP and MVR, are inherent in the FMV pathology. Myxomatous degeneration, collagen disruption and dissolution, and proteoglycan accumulation, with changes in the extracellular matrix, alter intrinsic mitral valve structure and organization, resulting in a spectrum of pathologic change involving the entire mitral valve complex (see Figure 1). As a result, the FMV surface area is greater than normal, and the FMV is thicker than the normal mitral valve. Abnormal stress-strain relationships of the mitral valve leaflets and support structures provide the setting for valve stretching or redundancy, chordal elongation, and chordal rupture. Redundancy of the enlarged anterior, posterior, or both mitral leaflets, or one or more of the posterior leaflet scallops, or the presence of elongated mitral chordae results in MVP. FMV enlargement and redundancy may occur with or without mitral annular enlargement. Valve surface changes that occur as the result of the intrinsic valve pathology alter valve surface endothelium and provide the environment for the complications of infectious endocarditis and thromboemboli.

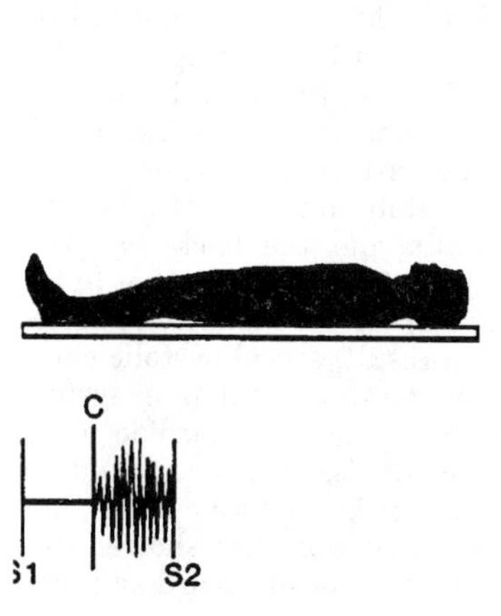

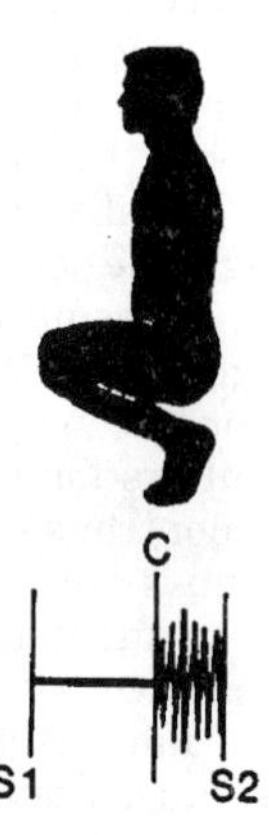

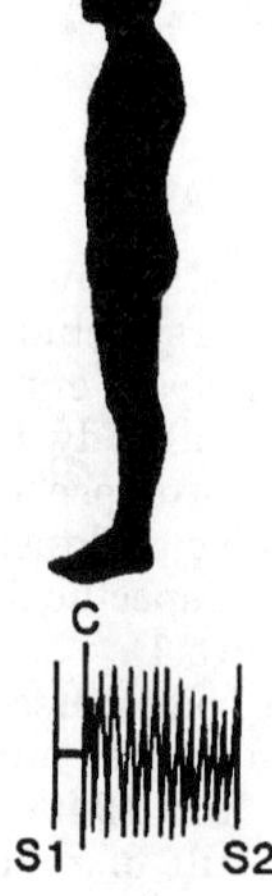

Figure 2. Floppy mitral valve–mitral valve prolapse: a postural auscultatory complex.

The Clinical Setting

The FMV may occur as an isolated phenomenon: as a familial disorder associated with congenital cardiac abnormalities, as the cardiac manifestation of a well-defined heritable disorder of connective tissue such as the Marfan syndrome, as the cardiac manifestation of incompletely defined connective tissue disorders, or in association with autonomic nervous system disorders and vasomotor instability. These clinical settings become apparent if the clinician performs a careful history, pedigree analysis, and a comprehensive physical examination.

The occurrence of the FMV-MVP in families, frequently as an autosomal dominant trait, is well recognized and has important diagnostic implications. FMV genetic diagnostic testing has not entered clinical practice, but such approaches open up diagnostic pathways for 21st-century clinicians. Separating the click-murmur auscultatory findings of the FMV-MVP-MVR triad from the so-called innocent murmurs in young children and adolescents continues to be a diagnostic challenge and a source of incorrect or missed diagnoses. This becomes apparent in long-term studies when adults with the triad recall being told of an innocent murmur in childhood and adolescence.

FLOPPY MITRAL VALVE–MITRAL VALVE PROLAPSE–MITRAL VALVULAR REGURGITATION: NATURAL HISTORY

Although the FMV-MVP may be genetically determined, clinical manifestations do not usually become evident before childhood. Although children and adolescents with FMV-MVP may have the same symptoms as adults, the frequency of symptoms appears to be less in children. The FMV-MVP association may lead to progressive mitral valvular dysfunction and progressive MVR over time; however, 7 or 8 decades may elapse before the individual patient's natural history is defined. The FMV has been documented as one of the leading causes of MVR requiring mitral valve surgery in the United States. Surface phenomena, including infectious endocarditis, thrombi, and thromboemboli phenomena, occur as complications in patients with the FMV. The FMV is particularly vulnerable to infection and is a universal etiologic factor for infectious endocarditis. Progressive MVR, left atrial and left ventricular failure, atrial and ventricular arrhythmias, and FMV chordal rupture occur as late complications in certain patients with FMV. Identification of FMV-MVP-MVR patients at high risk for these complications is obviously a high priority in their care and management.

High-Risk Patients

Individuals with FMV-MVP and thick, redundant mitral valve leaflets are at high risk for developing complications; those older than 50 years of age are at particularly high risk. A mitral systolic murmur has also been shown to be a risk factor for complications. Left ventricular enlargement in patients with FMV-MVP-MVR is a good predictor for the subsequent need for mitral valve surgery. When two or more of these abnormalities coexist, the possibility of complications increases. In contrast, the absence of all three of these features identifies patients with MVP of very low risk (Figure 3).

Classification

The classification of cardiovascular diseases is constantly evolving, which is not always reflected in the literature. At present, we classify patients with the FMV-MVP-MVR triad in two general categories. The first includes patients whose symptoms, physical findings, laboratory abnormalities, and clinical course are directly related to the mitral valve dysfunction and complications associated with the FMV-MVP-MVR triad (Table 1). The second category includes patients with FMV-MVP whose symptoms cannot be explained on the basis of valvular abnormality alone but result from the occurrence, or coexistence, of various forms of neuroendocrine or autonomic nervous system dys-

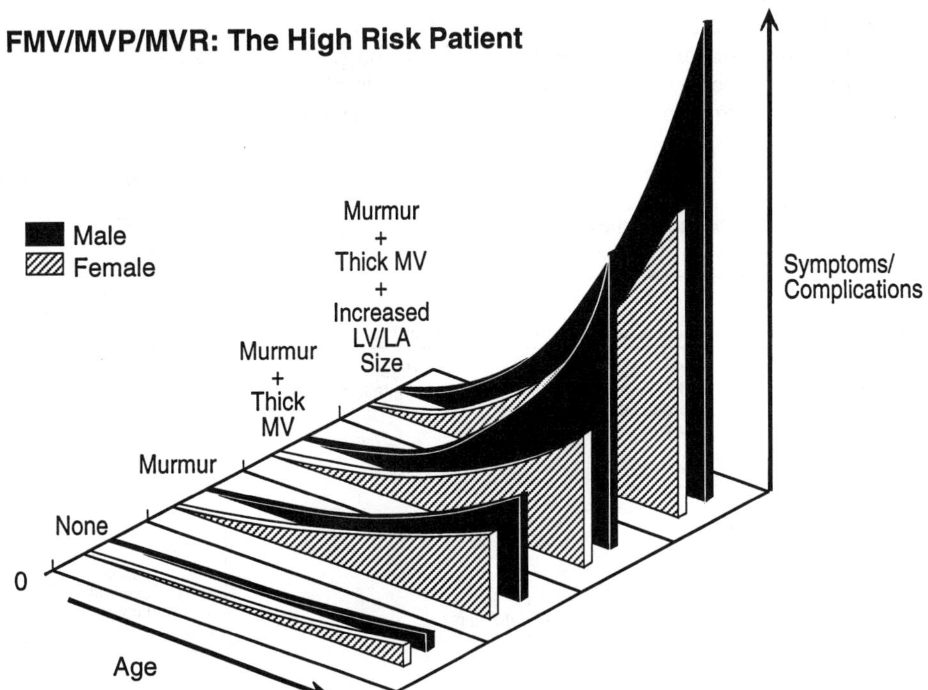

Figure 3. FMV-MVP-MVR: the high-risk patient. Symptoms and complications plotted against age. Details in text.

TABLE 1. **Classification of Floppy Mitral Valve–Mitral Valve Prolapse–Mitral Valvular Regurgitation (FMV-MVP-MVR)**

FMV/MVP/MVR	FMV/MVP/MVR Syndrome
• Common mitral valve abnormality with a spectrum of structural and functional changes, mild to severe *The basis for* • Systolic click; mid-late systolic murmur • Mild or progressive mitral valve dysfunction • Progressive mitral regurgitation, atrial fibrillation, congestive heart failure • Infectious endocarditis • Embolic phenomena • Characterized by long natural history • May be heritable, or associated with heritable disorders of connective tissue • Conduction system involvement possibly leading to arrhythmias and conduction defects	• Patients with mitral valve prolapse • Symptom complex: chest pain, palpitations, arrhythmias, fatigue, exercise intolerance, dyspnea, postural phenomena, syncope-presyncope, neuropsychiatric symptoms • Neuroendocrine or autonomic dysfunction (high catecholamines, catecholamine regulation abnormality, hyperresponse to adrenergic stimulation, parasympathetic abnormality, baroreflex modulation abnormality, renin-aldosterone regulation abnormality, decreased intravascular volume, decreased ventricular diastolic volume in the upright posture, atrial natriuretic factor secretion abnormality) may provide explanation for symptoms • Mitral valve prolapse—a possible marker for autonomic dysfunction

function. This classification scheme is clinically useful with important therapeutic implications because it separates patients with MVP and symptoms related to mitral valve dysfunction from those whose symptoms may be secondary to autonomic dysfunction.

The demonstration of MVP with imaging studies without any clinical correlates and without FMV characteristics may occur in individuals with decreased intravascular volumes, small left ventricular chamber size, or hyperdynamic circulatory states. We do not consider these circumstances to fall within the FMV-MVP-MVR triad.

THERAPEUTIC IMPLICATIONS

For all of the reasons just described, the FMV may be dangerous to one's health. To understand the long-term significance of the FMV, both the patient and physician must live a long time. Thus, the need for long-term, periodic follow-up will frequently clarify matters that are unclear in an initial evaluation.

The primary concern is the certainty of the diagnosis (Figure 4). Does this individual have an FMV? Does the FMV prolapse into the left atrium? Does the mitral valve leak because of FMV dysfunction? If so, how severe is the leak? Is the individual symptomatic? Are the symptoms related to valvular dysfunction, or are the symptoms more likely related to autonomic dysfunction or neuroendocrine abnormalities? Answering these questions may require assessment of left atrial and left ventricular function. Each question and each answer call forth a different therapeutic response.

From the clinical viewpoint, if the individual has a mitral systolic click or clicks with a mid or late apical systolic murmur, further evaluation is indicated including postural auscultation and a contemporary imaging study. If the ausculatory findings are not clear, the individual should either be re-examined or referred to someone with more experience in this area.

If the individual is shown to have an FMV, with ausculatory-imaging coherence, the primary emphasis is on explanation and prevention (Figure 5). The

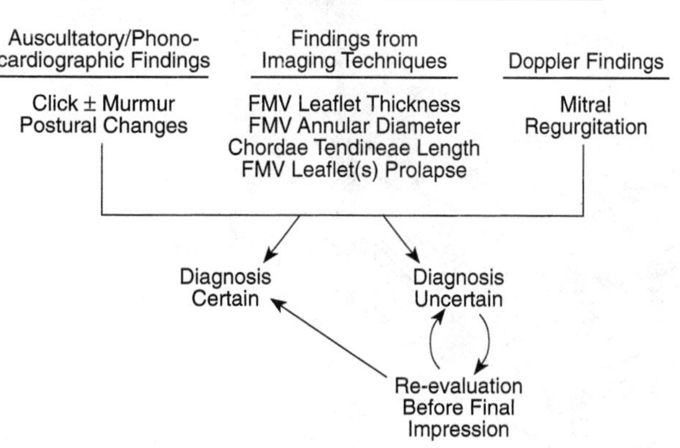

Figure 4.

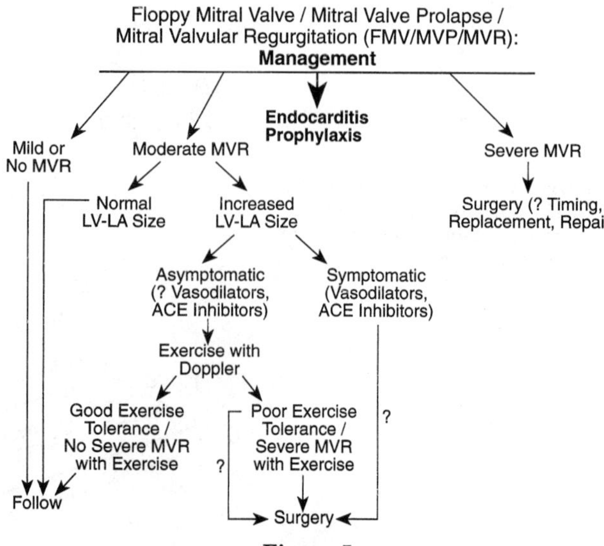

Figure 5.

individual should receive appropriate infectious endocarditis phrophylaxis according to the most recent antibiotic usage format established by The American Heart Association. If the FMV results in MVP with MVR, the explanation and prevention approach is supplemented by management. Infectious endocarditis prophylaxis is indicated, along with documentation of the extent of the valvular dysfunction. These individuals, whether symptomatic or not, may require more sophisticated imaging studies, exercise testing, or hemodynamic and angiographic assessment. Individuals with a history of atrial or ventricular arrhythmias should be evaluated with contemporary electrophysiologic monitoring or testing. Patients who have a history of syncope, light-headedness, or unexplained collapse or who are post-resuscitation require further diagnostic testing.

Careful explanation of the clinical findings and the nature of MVP will help reassure the anxious patient with the MVP syndrome. Patients with MVP syndrome are sensitive to volume depletion and increased adrenergic activity. Thus, prophylaxis for volume depletion before, during, or immediately after physical exercise may be particularly beneficial to patients with low intravascular volume. Removing catecholamine and cyclic AMP stimulation by abstaining from caffeine, tobacco, alcohol, and prescription or over-the-counter drugs containing epinephrine or ephedrine may help. Low doses of beta-blocking drugs administered for a short time during stressful periods or in a single dose may be beneficial. A gradual exercise program is frequently beneficial in patients with the MVP syndrome.

As is always the case, individual patient evaluation and diagnostic certainty precede rational therapy.

CONGESTIVE HEART FAILURE

method of
MARK T. SPEAKMAN, M.D., and
ROBERT A. KLONER, M.D., PH.D.
Good Samaritan Hospital and University of Southern California
Los Angeles, California

Congestive heart failure (CHF) is a common clinical problem in the United States, estimated to affect 1 to 2 million individuals. There are 400,000 new cases per year, and 60 to 70% of these patients will have repeated recurrences within 6 years. Approximately $8 billion per year is being spent on total care.

Heart failure has been defined variously. The syndrome may be described as inability of the heart to maintain adequate vital organ perfusion, resulting in impairment of exercise capacity. It is associated with a constellation of predictable neurohumoral, autocrine, and paracrine features that are initially generally compensatory but later become maladaptive. CHF is the syndrome of heart failure and its associated congestive symptoms: pulmonary and peripheral edema, hepatic congestion, and ascites. We will use the terms CHF and heart failure interchangeably. Heart failure also has been categorized as backward versus forward, right versus left, acute versus chronic, and systolic versus diastolic; the latter three distinctions are the most clinically useful.

CAUSES AND PATHOPHYSIOLOGY

Hypertension alone or in combination with coronary artery disease accounts for approximately 70% of cases of heart failure in the United States. Ischemic heart disease (IHD) alone accounts for 10 to 20% of cases, and the remaining cases are due to cardiomyopathies and valvular and congenital heart disease. Table 1 outlines the major causes of heart failure. A number of illnesses may exacerbate or precipitate bouts of heart failure. These include anemia, infection, hyperthyroidism, arrhythmias, uncontrolled hypertension, pulmonary embolism, and lack of compliance with diet or drugs.

Heart failure is characterized by increased vascular tone mediated by elevated levels of plasma norepinephrine, angiotensin II, and endothelin. Retention of sodium and water is effected by elevations of aldosterone and arginine vasopressin. Elevation of atrial natriuretic peptide (ANP) is an early phenomenon in CHF that is responsible for natriuresis, diuresis, and vasodilatation.

CLINICAL EVALUATION

Dyspnea on exertion, orthopnea, paroxysmal nocturnal dyspnea, and cough are the principal symptoms of left-sided heart failure and relate to elevated filling pressures. Fatigue is a common feature and is due to hypoperfusion of skeletal muscle. Right-sided heart failure is typified by peripheral edema and in the later stages by right upper quadrant discomfort from hepatic congestion and dyspnea due to reduced right ventricular output and the effect of ascites on lung mechanics. The New York Heart Association classification is useful for prognosis and tailoring therapy. It can be summarized as follows:

Class I. No limitation of ordinary physical activity.
Class II. Slight limitation with fatigue, dyspnea, palpitations, or angina resulting from ordinary physical activity.
Class III. Marked limitation; symptomatic with less than ordinary activity.
Class IV. Symptoms present while at rest.

A careful clinical examination is often diagnostic. Common physical findings include tachycardia, S_3 gallop, murmurs, rales, jugular venous distention, hepatic distention and tenderness, peripheral edema, and ascites. The presence of hepatojugular reflux is a sign we find particularly helpful. Evidence of the precipitant should be sought, and a basic work-up should include serum electrolytes, renal function, liver function, blood count, urinalysis, electrocardiogram, and chest radiograph. Echocardiography is of particular value in confirming valvular disease, systolic and

TABLE 1. **Causes of Heart Failure**

Hypertension	Hypertrophic cardiomyopathy
Ischemic heart disease	Restrictive cardiomyopathy
Dilated cardiomyopathy	Arrhythmias
Valvular disease	Drugs
Congenital heart disease	High-output states
Pericardial disease	

diastolic dysfunction, and hypertrophy and chamber enlargement and in assessing both global function as well as regional wall motion. Doppler evaluation allows measurement of hemodynamics, including pressure gradients and cardiac output.

THERAPY

Acute Left Ventricular Failure

Patients with pulmonary edema secondary to acute left ventricular failure require emergent attention focused on correcting hypoxemia, reducing filling pressures, and, if low, increasing cardiac output. Oxygen is administered via a face mask, and oxygenation is assessed by pulse oximetry and arterial blood gas analysis. Continuous positive airway pressure ventilation is of value in more acutely ill patients who do not warrant mechanical ventilation. Morphine, 2 to 4 mg intravenously (IV) over 5 minutes, is used to reduce afterload and anxiety. Diuretics are given, but bear in mind that intravascular volume may not be elevated in all patients. Furosemide (Lasix), 10 to 40 mg IV, is given over 2 minutes, and this can be increased to 80 mg IV over 2 minutes after 1 hour if diuresis is insufficient. Alternatively, bumetanide (Bumex), 0.5 to 1 mg IV over 2 minutes is given as the initial dose. A pulmonary arterial catheter is used to monitor hemodynamically unstable patients with hypotension or shock. Nitroglycerin (Nitro-Bid) is the intravenous agent we use most commonly in acute exacerbations and is of particular value in IHD. Sublingual nitroglycerin is used to lower filling pressure until an intravenous preparation is started; 0.3 to 0.6 mg is given every 5 to 10 minutes (up to 4 doses). Intravenous nitroglycerin is started at 5 μg per minute and titrated upward according to hemodynamic response. Nitrate tolerance necessitates keeping infusion periods short (<72 hours) and using escalating doses.

Nitroprusside (Nipride) is a powerful vasodilator and is ideal in heart failure associated with uncontrolled hypertension and aortic and mitral regurgitation. It is employed for short-term use at a dose of 0.1 to 0.3 μg per kg per minute IV and titrated according to filling pressures and blood pressure. The most common side effects are hypotension and a coronary steal phenomenon in IHD. Thiocyanate and cyanide toxicities are rare outside of renal dysfunction or prolonged (>72 hours) use.

Dobutamine, a $beta_1$ agonist, increases cardiac contractility and via its $beta_2$ and $alpha_1$ stimulation has a mild vasodilatory effect. It is used in decompensated heart failure and as support before transplantation. There is general agreement regarding its short-term use at a starting dose of 2.5 μg per kg per minute, increasing up to 15 μg per kg per minute or until hemodynamic goals are achieved. Higher infusion rates (up to 40 μg per kg per minute) are rarely required. Its use on a long-term intermittent basis is controversial owing to negative reports of sudden death and increased mortality. Dopamine is used for inotropic support in patients with cardiogenic shock and low systemic vascular resistance. A starting dose of 2 μg per kg per minute IV infusion is titrated upward based on hemodynamics. Adverse effects include tachycardia and arrhythmias.

Milrinone (Primacor), a phosphodiesterase inhibitor that increases contractility and decreases vascular resistance, is available for short-term use in decompensated patients. A loading dose of 50 μg per kg is given over 10 minutes followed by an infusion up to a maximum of 0.75 μg per kg per minute. In our opinion, given the cost differential of dobutamine and milrinone and their equal efficacy, there is little to be gained from milrinone as a first-line agent; the vasodilatory effect of milrinone can be equalled by adding nitroprusside or nitroglycerin to dobutamine.

CHRONIC HEART FAILURE

A suggested general approach to the management of chronic CHF is outlined in Table 2. The specifics are outlined below.

Angiotensin-Converting Enzyme Inhibitors

Angiotensin-converting enzyme inhibitors (ACEIs) are first-line vasodilators that are considered the cornerstone of therapy. They decrease mortality in patients with class II, III, and IV heart failure and delay progression to overt heart failure in those with asymptomatic left ventricular dysfunction. There are very few patients with heart failure who should not receive ACEIs. Concerns regarding baseline renal function or modest decreases with therapy are outweighed by the benefit in terms of survival. Patients at greatest risk for renal deterioration are those with severe heart failure, underlying renal dysfunction, and volume depletion (usually secondary to diuretics). The risk of ACEI-related renal insufficiency can be reduced by cautious dose titration or temporary drug discontinuation, avoidance of nonsteroidal anti-inflammatory drugs, liberalizing salt intake, and adjusting the diuretic dosage. Renal function and serum potassium are assessed 2 to 3 days after initia-

TABLE 2. **Treatment Guidelines for Chronic Congestive Heart Failure**

Class I: ACEI + ? beta blockers
Class II: ACEI, low-dose loop or thiazide diuretic, digoxin + ? beta blockers
Class III: ACEI, loop diuretic, digoxin ± nitrates and hydralazine + ? beta blockers
Class IV: ACEI, loop diuretic, digoxin, ± nitrates and hydralazine
Acute exacerbations: consider
Intravenous diuresis
Dobutamine
Dopamine
Milrinone
Nitroglycerin
Nitroprusside
Treatment of underlying cause

Abbreviation: ACEI = angiotensin-converting enzyme inhibitors.

tion of ACEIs in those at higher risk and at 1 week in lower risk patients. Except for fosinopril, which has both renal and hepatic routes of elimination, baseline serum creatinine is important in determining the initial dose to avoid drug accumulation.

Other significant adverse effects of ACEIs include hypotension, hyperkalemia, cough, and angioneurotic edema. Hypotension per se should not mandate discontinuing the drug unless the patient experiences dizziness or syncope. Hyperkalemia can be avoided or minimized by ensuring that potassium supplements are stopped; concomitant diuretic use will offset the potassium retention provided they are not potassium sparing (e.g., spironolactone). Pregnant patients should not receive ACEIs because of their teratogenic effects.

Several ACEIs are approved for use in CHF in the United States, including captopril (Capoten), enalapril (Vasotec), ramipril (Altace), lisinopril (Prinivil), quinapril (Accupril), and fosinopril (Monopril). In patients at higher risk, as defined earlier, we start with captopril (6.25 mg orally [PO] three times daily [tid]) because it has its peak effect within 1 to 2 hours and is more easily monitored than other ACEIs. It is titrated upward as tolerated to 50 mg tid, usually over 1 to 2 weeks. Once patients have stabilized, a longer-acting agent (enalapril or lisinopril) can be substituted. In low-risk patients, enalapril is started at 2.5 mg PO twice a day (bid) with a target dose of 10 to 20 mg bid achieved over 1 to 2 weeks. Lisinopril is started at 5 mg PO every day (qd) and titrated to a maximum of 20 mg qd.

Although not yet approved by the Food and Drug Administration (FDA) for treating CHF, the angiotensin II receptor blockers have shown promise in clinical trials. In one study the angiotensin II receptor blocker losartan (Cozaar)* was associated with better survival than captopril. These new agents have the advantage of not causing cough.

Nitrates and Hydralazine

Isosorbide dinitrate (Isordil), hydralazine (Apresoline), and the combination have been studied in large trials. The drugs are used either singly or in combination in patients on ACEIs, diuretics, and digoxin who remain symptomatic. Nitrates, as venodilators, improve symptoms related to pulmonary congestion and improve exercise tolerance. In patients with IHD and CHF with predominantly pulmonary symptoms, isosorbide dinitrate is started at 20 mg PO tid, aiming for a maximum of 40 mg PO tid, with a dose-free interval of at least 14 hours at night to avoid tolerance. Alternatively, the extended-release preparation of isosorbide mononitrate (Imdur) is started at 30 mg PO qd and increased to a maximum of 240 mg PO qd. The combination of hydralazine (200 to 300 mg per day) and isosorbide dinitrate (120 to 160 mg per day) improves survival in heart failure, albeit less so than enalapril. The target dose of hydralazine was 300 mg per day in the large trials. The starting dose is 10 mg PO qid, increasing after 3 days to 25 mg PO qid for 1 week and then sequentially increasing each week to the target dose. Hydralazine is avoided in IHD because it can cause reflex tachycardia and hence worsen ischemia. Hypotension, gastrointestinal upset, and a lupus-like syndrome are other adverse effects.

*Not FDA approved for this indication.

Calcium Channel Blockers

Although some calcium channel blockers such as verapamil, diltiazem, and nifedipine may worsen heart failure in some patients, newer agents such as amlodipine (Norvasc), felodipine (Plendil), and nisoldipine (Sular) do not appear to do so. In the Prospective Randomized Amlodipine Survival Evaluation (PRAISE) study, mortality was reduced by amlodipine in class III/IV patients with nonischemic dilated cardiomyopathy, whereas ischemic cardiomyopathy patients had a mortality rate similar to those on placebo. Other studies have shown amlodipine's beneficial effect on exercise time and hemodynamics. In patients on ACEIs, diuretics, and digoxin, it is an appropriate drug for control of angina or hypertension. It is started at 5 mg PO qd and increased to 10 mg PO qd as tolerated after 2 weeks. Broader indications for its use depend on the results of the ongoing PRAISE-2 trial. A large veterans affairs trial suggested that felodipine (Plendil) may be safe to use in CHF, but it does not carry a survival benefit.

Diuretics

CHF is associated with an increase in total body water, and diuretics are used to control related symptoms: peripheral edema, pulmonary congestion, and ascites. There are no data to show a survival benefit from the use of diuretics. Patients with asymptomatic left ventricular dysfunction can be managed with dietary sodium restriction (<2500 mg per day) and ACE inhibition alone. Loop diuretics (furosemide, bumetanide, ethacrynic acid, and torsemide) are the most widely used class of diuretic because of their potency and because they, unlike the thiazides, remain effective at lower glomerular filtration rates (< 30 mL per minute).

In symptomatic patients, furosemide (Lasix), 20 to 80 mg PO, is given as a single daily dose. Alternatively, it can be given twice daily (e.g., at 8 AM and 2 PM). As renal function declines, the dose should be increased; the risk of ototoxicity is low with large oral doses of furosemide in severe heart failure as the rate of absorption is slower and peak serum levels are therefore lower. It is rarely necessary to exceed more than 300 mg per day. Bumetanide (Bumex) is usually given as a single oral dose of 0.5 to 2 mg per day. Thiazides and related drugs including hydrochlorothiazide (HydroDIURIL), chlorthalidone (Thalitone), and indapamide (Lozol) can be used alone in mild CHF. Hydrochlorothiazide is started at 25 mg PO qd and increased to a ceiling of 100 mg.

Diuretic therapy should be individualized; administration schedules using alternate days or 3 to 4 consecutive days per week often achieve superior results.

Diuretic resistance is said to occur when patients require escalating doses of diuretic to manage their symptoms. Declining renal function, decreased oral bioavailability, use of nonsteroidal anti-inflammatory drugs, and hypertrophy of the ascending loop of Henle are among the causes. In this situation a thiazide-like diuretic, for example, metolazone (Zaroxolyn), 5 to 10 mg PO, can be given 30 to 60 minutes before the daily Lasix dose; metolazone may take several days to achieve its maximal effect. Careful monitoring of serum potassium is essential, and we generally use this diuretic on a short-term basis only. Continuous infusions may benefit refractory hospitalized patients. One such regimen is an intravenous bolus of 40 to 60 mg furosemide followed by an infusion of furosemide, 10 to 20 mg per hour for 6 to 10 hours with electrolyte monitoring. Spironolactone (Aldactone), is occasionally used in combination with a loop diuretic in the patient prone to hypokalemia. Hypokalemia is seen particularly with loop and thiazide agents and is often offset by concomitant use of an ACEI or by potassium supplementation (e.g., KCl 20 to 40 mEq per day).

Inotropes

The use of dobutamine, dopamine, and milrinone in decompensated chronic heart failure is referred to earlier in the section on acute left ventricular failure. Digoxin (Lanoxin) is of hemodynamic benefit to patients in CHF due to systolic dysfunction. It increases forward output and reduces pulmonary capillary wedge pressure. Its benefit in asymptomatic left ventricular dysfunction is unclear. It does not affect mortality, but its withdrawal from patients with CHF increases hospitalizations for CHF. The benefit is greater in patients with more advanced heart failure. An oral dose of 0.125 to 0.25 mg PO qd is usually sufficient to maintain levels of 1 to 2 ng per mL; loading is only used in the setting of an acute supraventricular arrhythmia. Clinicians should be mindful of electrolyte disturbances (especially potassium but also magnesium, calcium, and sodium), alterations in renal clearance by drugs such as amiodarone and verapamil, advanced age, thyroid disease, and renal insufficiency. We do not routinely monitor digoxin levels except in patients with altered clearance rates. The role of other oral inotropes including pimobendan, levosimendan, and vesnarinone remains to be clarified. A randomized trial of oral milrinone was stopped early because of increased mortality.

Beta Blockers

Selective and nonselective beta blockers improve left ventricular function and exercise capacity, and decrease hospitalizations for CHF. The precise mechanism for this benefit is unclear but may relate to blockade of the "cardiotoxic" effects of catecholamines, heart rate reduction, and prolongation of diastole. The drugs should be administered in a controlled environment by experienced clinicians starting at very low doses because of the potential for worsening CHF. Carvedilol (Coreg) reduces the combined risk of mortality and cardiovascular morbidity in patients with mild to moderate heart failure and is started at 3.125 mg PO bid for 2 weeks. If tolerated, it can be increased to 6.25 mg bid and the dose doubled every 2 weeks to a maximum of 25 to 50 mg bid depending on body weight. Although not FDA approved for use in CHF, metoprolol (Lopressor) is started at 5 mg PO bid and is increased as tolerated to 50 mg tid over 6 weeks; pharmacies can be helpful in customizing such small starting doses. At this time, the use of beta blockers in class IV patients or in unstable heart failure is not recommended.

Diastolic Dysfunction

Our approach to treating diastolic dysfunction includes aggressive control of hypertension, careful reduction of preload, treating ischemia and tachycardia, and considering invasive options such as revascularization and valve surgery. Nitrates improve coronary flow and reduce preload. Diuretics are used to reduce preload, but care should be emphasized as patients with diastolic dysfunction rely on adequate preload to maintain cardiac output. Calcium channel and beta blockers are appropriate for patients with ischemia and hypertension-related diastolic dysfunction and for reducing heart rate (beta blockers, diltiazem, and verapamil). Nisoldipine has been shown to improve diastolic function in post–myocardial infarction patients with mild left ventricular dysfunction. Verapamil is of particular value in hypertrophic cardiomyopathy. Digoxin has no role outside of controlling atrial fibrillation or treating concomitant systolic dysfunction. ACEIs may improve diastolic dysfunction and may inhibit fibrosis related to hypertrophy. Currently there are no drugs specifically approved by the FDA for heart failure due to diastolic dysfunction.

Anticoagulation

Although not uncommon, thromboembolic events are less frequent than some early trials suggested. There are insufficient data to support the use of antiplatelet agents or anticoagulants in patients with CHF who are in sinus rhythm. There are also data that suggest a negative impact on survival from the combination of aspirin and ACEIs. Patients with CHF and atrial fibrillation or a prior embolic event are given anticoagulants such as warfarin (Coumadin), aiming for an international normalized ratio (INR) of 2 to 3. Aspirin is avoided in CHF in view of the potential interaction with ACEIs. In patients with left ventricular mural thrombus, acute infarction, and ventricular dysfunction, anticoagulation is continued with Coumadin for 3 to 6 months.

Although likely, there is no proven benefit from anticoagulation for ventricular thrombi in nonischemic cardiomyopathy; in this situation, risk and benefit are assessed in each individual case.

Ventricular Arrhythmias in Congestive Heart Failure

Complex ventricular arrhythmias and sudden cardiac death are common in CHF. Ventricular function is the strongest predictor of sudden death in patients with CHF. Reversible causes such as electrolyte disturbances, ischemia, and drug effects should be considered. Data from the Multicenter Automatic Defibrillator Implantation Trial (MADIT) strongly support the use of implantable cardiac defibrillators (ICDs) as first-line therapy for patients with a prior myocardial infarction, ejection fraction of less than 35%, and asymptomatic nonsustained ventricular tachycardia that is inducible at electrophysiologic study but not suppressed by intravenous procainamide. The antiarrhythmic versus implantable defibrillator trial showed that ICD therapy reduced overall mortality, compared with antiarrhythmic drugs, in patients with ventricular fibrillation, sustained ventricular tachycardia with syncope, or sustained ventricular tachycardia with an ejection fraction of 40% or less with symptoms suggesting hemodynamic compromise. The results of trials designed more specifically to evaluate the efficacy of prophylactic ICD use compared with that of antiarrhythmic drugs and placebo in patients with CHF are awaited. Amiodarone (Cordarone) is currently the antiarrhythmic drug of choice for ventricular arrhythmias in class III or IV CHF, particularly those of nonischemic origin.

Transplantation and Ventricular Assistance

The number of patients listed for transplantation continues to increase relative to the availability of donors. Ninety percent of those listed have ischemic or nonischemic dilated cardiomyopathy. Patients must undergo tailored therapy with invasive hemodynamic monitoring before they are considered for transplantation; class IV patients can often undergo dramatic improvement with aggressive tailored therapy. The indications for transplantation take into account the extent of refractory ischemia and arrhythmias, maximal oxygen consumption, and lability of fluid balance and electrolytes despite adherence to a diet and drug regimen. Contraindications have been loosened in recent years and include, among others, the presence of a second disease that would limit life expectancy, age greater than 70, diabetes with end-organ damage, severe pulmonary hypertension, and psychosocial factors.

The intra-aortic balloon pump is placed in the descending aorta, usually via the femoral artery, and it decreases afterload and increases cardiac output and coronary perfusion. It is indicated in patients with cardiogenic shock following myocardial infarction or its mechanical complications (ventricular septal defect or papillary muscle rupture with mitral regurgitation), refractory ventricular arrhythmias, and unstable angina and in decompensated patients awaiting transplantation. Contraindications include aortic regurgitation and dissection.

Ventricular assist devices include those assisting the left or right ventricle, or both. Outcome figures are best for the left ventricular device. Generally, the role of these devices is one of support before transplantation. However, devices (e.g., the HeartMate system) are now being implanted permanently, and their performance is under assessment. Complications include bleeding and coagulopathy, infection, renal failure, and thromboembolism. The Batista procedure is an experimental procedure whereby a wedge of myocardium is resected to decrease ventricular volume. Some centers have reported promising early results; long-term results are pending.

INFECTIVE ENDOCARDITIS

method of
LEON A. FELDMAN, M.D.
Oregon Health Sciences University

and

EDWARD S. MURPHY, M.D.
Oregon Health Sciences University and Portland Veterans Affairs Medical Center
Portland, Oregon

Acute and subacute bacterial endocarditis are classic clinical syndromes of infected heart valves, and these distinctions are useful when making empirical management decisions. However, most authorities use the broader term "infective endocarditis" (IE). IE often presents with protean symptoms and signs that may result in a missed or delayed diagnosis. Before the antibiotic era, IE was a uniformly fatal disease. This outcome suggests that host defense mechanisms play a relatively minor role in the eradication of this infectious process and highlights the importance of effective antimicrobial therapy and/or timely surgical intervention. Despite meaningful advances, the overall mortality rate remains significant at approximately 10 to 20%. Basic principles of management are important in all forms of IE. They include recognition of the clinical syndrome, isolation of the organisms, appropriate antimicrobial therapy, prompt recognition and treatment of complications, prophylaxis for individuals at risk, and identification of the significant percentage of patients who will need eventual valve surgery despite bacterial cure.

PATHOGENESIS

Animal models have been used to study the mechanisms leading to the formation of bacterial vegetations, the pathologic hallmark of IE. This infectious process is thought to begin with endothelial damage resulting from immune complex deposition or hemodynamic alterations such as regurgitant blood flow, high pressure gradients, or turbulent flow through narrow orifices. This leads to the accumulation of platelets, red blood cells, and fibrin strands, termed "nonbacterial thrombotic endocarditis," which adhere to the endothelial surface of the valve. These microthrombi appear to be a prerequisite for IE and form the nidus for bacterial growth as a result of seeding during transient bacteremia. Bacterial adherence is an important component of this process; elaboration of dextran by the organisms and binding to fibronectin are likely pathogenic mechanisms. Further platelet, fibrin, and bacterial deposition occur, creating a series of layers that ultimately forms a vegetation. This allows both rapid unrestricted growth of bacterial colonies within the vegetation and protection from normal host defense mechanisms. Depending on host factors and the virulence of the microorganism, the presentation may be acute, subacute, or chronic.

EPIDEMIOLOGY

Based on data from tertiary care hospitals, the estimated incidence of IE is approximately 1 per 1000 hospital admissions, or 3 to 4 cases per 100,000 person-years. Although the incidence has remained relatively unchanged, several clinical and microbiologic features have evolved. As in other illnesses, the mean age of affected individuals has increased.

Previously, chronic rheumatic valvular heart disease was the most common predisposing cardiac lesion. This has been supplanted by mitral valve disease and hypertrophic cardiomyopathy. There is also an increasing proportion of patients over the age of 65 with IE who have minimal or no identifiable underlying structural heart disease. A relatively new group of affected individuals are intravenous drug users. Additionally, there is a growing population with prosthetic valves, which are prone to endocarditis. Among children, congenital heart disease is the most common predisposing cause, especially in those with cyanotic heart disease associated with shunts and stenotic valves. These children remain at risk, as the advances in surgery have allowed an increasing number to become adults with congenital heart disease.

The microbiologic spectrum has been altered by the aging population, the increase in the number of intravenous drug users, and the aggressive use of medical interventions (e.g., intravascular prostheses and monitoring equipment). Further apparent microbiologic diversity is due to improved culture techniques that have demonstrated an increased prevalence of nutritionally variant streptococci, *Chlamydia*, *Legionella*, *Coxiella burnetii* (Q fever), and other fastidious organisms.

ETIOLOGY

Streptococci and staphylococci continue to be the most prevalent isolates, affecting at least 75% of patients who are not intravenous drug users (Table 1). Intravenous drug use (IVDU)–associated IE is most often caused by *Staphylococcus aureus*, *Staphylococcus epidermidis*, gram-negative bacilli, or *Candida*. Prosthetic valve endocarditis (PVE) can be divided into early onset, less than 60 days postoperatively, or late onset, greater than 60 days postoperatively. Early PVE is most commonly due to *S. epidermidis* and *S. aureus*. Other organisms include aerobic gram-negative bacilli and fungi (usually *Candida* or *Aspergillus*). In contrast, the organisms responsible for late PVE are similar to those that cause native valve endocarditis.

Culture-negative endocarditis occurs in less than 5% of cases of IE and is usually the result of prior antibiotic therapy. Other causes include failure to grow fastidious organisms, such as the HACEK group (*Haemophilus* species, *Actinobacillus actinomycetemcomitans*, *Cardiobacterium hominis*, *Eikenella* species, and *Kingella kingae*), nutritionally variant streptococci, *Corynebacterium*, *Legionella*, and fungi, such as *Aspergillus*. These organisms may require specialized culture techniques for isolation. Rare causes of sterile blood cultures include IE with *C. burnetii* (Q fever) and *Chlamydia*. Systemic illnesses such as systemic lupus erythematosus and malignancies may also give rise to syndromes of noninfective endocarditis, termed "Libman-Sacks" and "marantic" endocarditis, respectively.

Polymicrobial IE is a relatively recent problem that has predominantly affected intravenous drug users and patients with indwelling central venous catheters. These patients have an overall mortality of 30%, and prognosis is worse with infections involving *Candida*, *Pseudomonas*, and enterococci.

A thorough history and physical examination should alert the physician to the potential "portal of entry" for the infection such as cutaneous lesions or poor dentition. Furthermore, positive isolates of *Streptococcus bovis* should raise the suspicion for a gastrointestinal malignancy.

TABLE 1. **Etiologic Agents of Infective Endocarditis**

Organism	Approximate Percentage	
	Native Valve	*Prosthetic Valve*
Streptococci		
Alpha-hemolytic	60	10–30
Enterococci	10	5–10
Pneumococci	1–2	<1
Beta-hemolytic	<1	<1
Others	<1	<1
Staphylococci		
Staphylococcus aureus	25	15–20
Coagulase-negative	<1	25–30
Gram-Negative Organisms		
Enterics	<5	<5
Pseudomonas spp	<5	<5
HACEK	<5	<1
Neisseria spp	<1	<1
Fungi		
Candida spp	<1	5–10
Others	<1	<1

Abbreviation: HACEK = *Haemophilus* spp, *Actinobacillus actinomycetemcomitans*, *Cardiobacterium hominis*, *Eikenella* spp, and *Kingella kingae*.

From Dajani AS: Infective endocarditis. *In* Rakel RE (ed): Conn's Current Therapy 1994. Philadelphia, WB Saunders, 1994.

CLINICAL FEATURES

The presentation of IE is quite variable. The virulence of the organism and the host response in large part determine the presentation of the illness. Previously used diagnostic criteria lacked sensitivity, and therefore IE was uniformly underdiagnosed. A more recent classification scheme developed by the Duke University Endocarditis Service incorporates diagnostic criteria that more closely reflect the changing epidemiology of IE and also consider advances in echocardiographic diagnosis. These are modeled after the Jones criteria for rheumatic fever (Tables 2 and 3). Several different investigators have demonstrated the validity of these criteria when compared with the gold

TABLE 2. **Duke Criteria for Diagnosis of Infective Endocarditis**

Definite Infective Endocarditis

Pathologic Criteria

Microorganisms: Demonstrated by culture or histologic appearance in a vegetation, *or* in a vegetation that has embolized, *or* in an intracardiac abscess, *or*

Pathologic Lesions: Vegetation or intracardiac abscess present, confirmed by histologic examination showing active endocarditis

Clinical Criteria Using Specific Definitions Listed in Table 3

2 major criteria, *or*

1 major and 3 minor criteria, *or*

5 minor criteria

Possible Infective Endocarditis

Findings consistent with infective endocarditis that fall short of "definite," but not "rejected"

Rejected

Firm alternative diagnosis for manifestations of endocarditis, *or*

Resolution of manifestations of endocarditis, with antibiotic therapy for ≤ 4 days, *or*

No pathologic evidence of infective endocarditis at surgery or autopsy, after antibiotic therapy for ≥4 days

Reprinted from Durack DT, Lukes AS, Bright DK: New criteria for diagnosis of infective endocarditis: Utilization of specific echocardiographic findings. Am J Med *96*:200–209, 1994. Copyright 1994 with permission from Excerpta Medica Inc.

standard of IE diagnosis, namely, pathologic confirmation of valvular vegetations at surgery or autopsy. Sensitivity and, in particular, specificity have been improved with a negative predictive value greater than 90%. However, further evaluation of these criteria is required, especially in situations such as PVE and IE in children.

Clinical features of IE are a reflection of systemic toxicity, localized intracardiac infection, embolic phenomena (bland or septic), and immune complex disease. Systemic features usually include fever, and in subacute forms there may be complaints of malaise, weight loss, myalgias, and arthralgias.

Intracardiac infection primarily affects the valvular apparatus and usually results in a regurgitant murmur. The sensitivity of this finding for detection of endocarditis increases significantly if the murmur is new onset or has changed in character. Rupture of chordae tendineae or papillary muscle and perforation of a valve leaflet commonly result in significant regurgitation and the abrupt onset of congestive heart failure (CHF), which confer a poor prognosis.

Acute onset of aortic insufficiency (AI) can produce a short diastolic murmur that may actually decrease in intensity as regurgitation progresses. There may be rapid elevation of left ventricular (LV) end-diastolic pressure and pronounced pulmonary congestion without prominent LV dilatation. More chronic progression of AI often produces greater LV enlargement and the eventual development of CHF.

Acute mitral insufficiency may result from destruction of the chordae, the papillary muscle, or the valve leaflet itself. Examination reveals a hyperdynamic precordium with evidence of pulmonary congestion and a systolic murmur of variable quality.

Tricuspid valve endocarditis with regurgitation is most often associated with IVDU, although rare causes such as an intracardiac lead (pacemaker or defibrillator) or alcoholic cirrhosis have been reported. Quite often there is no discernible murmur. However, the peripheral manifestations of tricuspid regurgitation are usually obvious. These include a large V wave in the jugular venous pulse, an enlarged pulsatile liver, and peripheral edema in the absence of pulmonary congestion.

Prosthetic valve dysfunction may manifest with a new regurgitant murmur and/or loss of appropriate opening and closing sounds.

Occasionally intramyocardial abscesses may form and rupture, resulting in a variety of intracardiac shunts or purulent pericarditis. Rarely, valvular stenosis may result from an obstructing vegetation or thrombus.

Clinically evident emboli occur in approximately 25% of patients. The classic embolic findings consist of Osler's nodes (painful nodules on the pads of the fingers and toes), Janeway's lesions (nontender hemorrhagic lesions on the palms and soles), Roth's spots (white-centered hemorrhages in the fundus), splinter hemorrhages (linear red streaks in the nail beds), and petechiae (conjunctiva,

TABLE 3. **Definitions of Terminology Used in the Proposed New Criteria**

Major Criteria

1. *Positive blood culture for infective endocarditis*
   Typical microorganism for infective endocarditis from two separate blood cultures
   Viridans streptococci,* *Streptococcus bovis,* HACEK group, *or*
   Community-acquired *Staphylococcus aureus* or enterococci, in absence of primary focus, *or*
   Persistently positive blood culture, defined as recovery of microorganism consistent with infective endocarditis, from
   (a) Blood cultures drawn more than 12 h apart, *or*
   (b) All of three sets, or majority of four or more separate sets of blood cultures, with first and last drawn at least 1 h apart
2. *Evidence of endocardial involvement*
   Positive echocardiogram for infective endocarditis
   (a) Oscillating intracardiac mass, on valve or supporting structures, *or* in path of regurgitant jets, *or* on implanted material, in absence of alternative anatomic explanation, *or*
   (b) Abscess, *or*
   (c) New partial dehiscence of prosthetic valve, *or*
   (c) New valvular regurgitation (increase or change in preexisting murmur not sufficient)

Minor Criteria

1. *Predisposition:* Predisposing heart condition *or* intravenous drug use
2. *Fever:* ≥38.0°C (100.4°F)
3. *Vascular phenomena:* Major arterial emboli, septic pulmonary infarcts, mycotic aneurysm, intracranial hemorrhage, conjunctival hemorrhages, Janeway's lesions
4. *Immunologic phenomena:* Glomerulonephritis, Osler's nodes, Roth's spots, rheumatoid factor
5. *Microbiologic evidence:* Positive blood culture but not meeting major criteria as noted previously† *or* serologic evidence of active infection with organism consistent with infective endocarditis
6. *Echocardiogram:* Consistent with infective endocarditis but not meeting major criteria as noted previously

*Including nutritional variant strains.

†Excluding single positive cultures for coagulase-negative staphylococci and organisms that do not cause endocarditis.

Reprinted from Durack DT, Lukes AS, Bright DK: New criteria for diagnosis of infective endocarditis: Utilization of specific echocardiographic findings. Am J Med *96*:200–209, 1994. Copyright 1994 with permission from Excerpta Medica Inc.

palate, buccal mucosa, and skin above the clavicle). These classic findings are more often seen in the subacute form of IE. It should be noted that although these are considered classic embolic phenomena, they might instead be related to immune complex formation. In addition, emboli may travel to the cerebral circulation resulting in stroke or mycotic aneurysm formation. Mycotic aneurysms may occur in any part of the arterial tree and are due to bacterial seeding of the endothelial surface with structural damage to the arterial wall and subsequent aneurysmal dilatation and possible rupture. Other organs such as the spleen and rarely the kidney may be sites for systemic emboli. A common feature among IVDU-associated IE is septic pulmonary emboli that appear as nodules, infiltrates, and cavitary lesions on chest films.

The immune system is broadly activated in IE. The formation of circulating immune complexes may be responsible for Osler's nodes and also for the glomerulonephritis that sometimes accompanies IE. Splenomegaly is present in approximately 30% of affected individuals and may also be related to immune system activation, although it can also reflect splenic infarcts. Clubbing is a chronic manifestation of IE and is typically seen in illnesses lasting longer than 6 weeks.

LABORATORY EVALUATION

The presence of continuous bacteremia with an organism known to cause endocarditis in the appropriate clinical setting confirms the diagnosis of IE. Therefore, the most important diagnostic test is properly obtained blood cultures.

Because the number of colony-forming units per milliliter of blood is relatively low, it has been shown that at least 10 mL of blood is necessary per culture. To demonstrate continuous bacteremia, three sets should be collected at 1-hour intervals or longer. At least two of the three sets should be positive. If antibiotics have been used previously, it may be more beneficial to wait 48 hours before drawing blood to improve the chances of isolating the infecting organism. However, if the clinical course is fulminant, three blood samples for culture should be obtained at 30-minute intervals and empirical antibiotic therapy initiated.

It is extremely important to alert the microbiology laboratory that the diagnosis of IE is being considered. This enables the laboratory to hold cultures for longer periods and also to initiate any specialized techniques that may be necessary to isolate fastidious organisms.

Other laboratory parameters may be abnormal but are not diagnostic. Normochromic, normocytic anemia is usually present, and the white blood cell count may be normal or elevated depending on the acuity of the illness. Thrombocytopenia may occur, and the erythrocyte sedimentation rate is usually elevated. Up to 50% of patients with IE develop a positive rheumatoid factor. The urinalysis may be abnormal, with the presence of microscopic hematuria and/or proteinuria. This may indicate immune complex–mediated glomerulonephritis or renal emboli. A reduction in serum complement levels usually parallels abnormal renal function.

An electrocardiogram (ECG) is an important tool in the assessment of conduction system disease that may result from extension of the infection into the septum, particularly from the aortic valve. Abnormalities in conduction typically manifest as atrioventricular (AV) block, hemiblock, or bundle branch block. Conduction system disease may be transient or permanent, reflecting either edema or invasion of the conduction system. Higher degrees of AV block and bundle branch block are more specific for the detection of septal extension of the infective process. The sensitivity of ECG abnormalities for this condition, however, remains low and should not be relied on to rule out intramyocardial infection.

The chest roentgenogram is valuable in the assessment of the hemodynamic status and complements the physical examination findings of left heart failure. In tricuspid valve endocarditis, the x-ray film is an important tool to demonstrate infiltrates and cavitary lesions indicative of septic pulmonary emboli.

ECHOCARDIOGRAPHY

The advances in echocardiographic technology along with its relative ease and noninvasiveness have made it a frequently used test in the evaluation of patients with suspected IE. The Duke University criteria for IE incorporate echocardiographic abnormalities in the diagnostic schema; however, the definitive diagnosis of IE must be made in conjunction with clinical and microbiologic findings. The existing echocardiographic technology includes two-dimensional color-flow and Doppler evaluation. Imaging can be performed using either transthoracic echocardiography (TTE) or transesophageal echocardiography (TEE).

The issue of vegetation size and its prognostic significance have been the subject of much debate. The overall consensus suggests that larger vegetations (>10 mm) are associated with a higher embolic rate. However, whether this embolic potential predicts progression to heart failure, the development of perivalvular extension of infection, the need for valve surgery, or death remains controversial. What is clear is that the decision to proceed with valve surgery should not be based exclusively on vegetation size. Furthermore, follow-up studies to document the resolution of vegetations have not provided any greater prognostic information than can be obtained clinically.

In cases of CHF, echocardiography is useful to evaluate the degree of valvular abnormality, define underlying structural heart disease, and assess left ventricular function. With the addition of color mapping and Doppler flow techniques, it is possible to define in a semiquantitative fashion the degree and nature of the valvular regurgitation. In addition, these modalities can be helpful in the diagnosis of fistulous tracts and intracardiac shunts, which can develop as complications of IE. An absolute indication for either TEE or TTE would be persistent bacteremia despite adequate antibiotic therapy, suggesting perivalvular extension of infection.

Some debate still exists in the choice of TTE versus TEE. In general, TTE and TEE are complementary in the assessment of LV function. Furthermore, the relative ease of performing a TTE tends to favor this technique as the initial approach followed by the TEE if there is inadequate visualization or further information is required, as is often the case in patients with prosthetic valves.

Screening for IE by echocardiography is a complex issue, and several factors need to be considered. Because a missed diagnosis and delayed therapy can be fatal, echocardiography by itself, even by the transesophageal approach, cannot entirely rule out the diagnosis of IE. This is true for several reasons, including the inability to resolve structures less than 2 mm and impaired visualization in the presence of heavily calcified leaflets or prosthetic valves. On one hand, in the specific case of nosocomial *S. aureus* bacteremia, screening for IE is not cost-effective unless there is a new regurgitant murmur, underlying structural heart disease, or persistent bacteremia. On the other hand, community-acquired *S. aureus* bacteremias with no clinical stigmata of IE are associated with a 20% likelihood of having occult vegetations or predisposing structural heart disease. Finally, not all cases of endocarditis are associated with vegetations, particularly early in the course of the disease. For all these reasons, echocardiography should be used thoughtfully, and, more important, the findings must be integrated with the existing clinical and microbiologic information.

CARDIAC CATHETERIZATION

The primary role of cardiac catheterization is the preoperative evaluation of patients who require surgery for complications related to IE. Preoperative catheterization is a useful step to assess hemodynamics and LV function, define aortic root anatomy, and detect significant coronary artery disease, especially when there are uncertainties regarding the echocardiographic assessment. Prosthetic valves can also be evaluated visually under fluoroscopy, especially for a characteristic rocking motion suggestive of valve dehiscence.

TREATMENT

The cornerstones of the management of IE are organism identification, appropriate antimicrobial therapy (Table 4), recognition of complications, and prompt surgical intervention when indicated. The principles of antimicrobial therapy are to ensure adequate serum levels of bactericidal agents, utilize synergistic combinations when possible, and maintain therapy for an appropriate duration. In general, all forms of IE should be treated for no less than 4 weeks. The two notable exceptions are IE caused by penicillin-susceptible *Streptococcus viridans* and selected cases of right-sided endocarditis resulting from *S. aureus*.

Acute IE is usually fulminant and is accompanied by some degree of sepsis syndrome; therefore therapy should not be delayed. In the subacute form, therapy may be initiated after identification of the organism. In the case of previous antibiotic therapy, organism recovery is extremely low for approximately 2 weeks; therefore, the risk of delayed therapy must be weighed against the benefit of organism isolation. Despite these uncertainties in diagnosis, fairly reliable empirical judgments can be made based on the acuity of the clinical presentation and also the site and type of valvular involvement. The major categories of IE are native valve endocarditis (NVE), PVE, and right-sided endocarditis, which is usually associated with IVDU.

The vast majority of NVE cases are caused by viridans streptococci, enterococci, and staphylococci. A combination of penicillin G, gentamicin (Garamycin), and nafcillin (Unipen) is a reasonable choice if one cannot wait for the results of microbiologic cultures. In the setting of early PVE, there is a greater concern for *S. epidermidis* infections; therefore vancomycin should be used in place of nafcillin. Late-onset PVE has organisms similar to those of NVE; therefore a similar empirical regimen may be used. Infective endocarditis related to IVDU is predominantly *S. aureus* infection, and a combination of nafcillin and gentamicin would be a reasonable choice. It should be emphasized that these are short-term empirical regimens that should be modified as soon as culture and susceptibility testing are available.

Susceptible viridans streptococci are defined by the minimal inhibitory concentration (MIC) of antibiotics, which is the minimal concentration of antibiotic that inhibits the growth of the organism in a test tube. Organisms with MICs of 0.1 μg per mL or less can be effectively treated with a 2-week course of penicillin G and gentamicin. The concentrations of gentamicin required to act synergistically with penicillin G are quite low (peak of 3μg per mL or less; trough of 1μg per mL or less) and minimize the risk of nephrotoxicity and eighth cranial nerve damage. Recent studies have demonstrated efficacy with a 4-week regime of ceftriaxone (Rocephin), 2 grams per day intravenously or intramuscularly. This antibiotic course offers the possibility of outpatient therapy that could reduce health care costs and at the same time be safe, effective, and convenient. However, only patients with uncomplicated IE who are hemodynamically stable and have documented clearance of bacteremia would qualify for this treatment option. For relatively resistant strains of viridans streptococci (MIC 0.1 to 0.5 μg per mL), for example, nutritionally variant streptococci, *S. bovis*, a 4-week course of penicillin G along with gentamicin in the first 2 weeks is recommended. Resistant viridans streptococci (MIC of 0.5 μg per mL or more) are treated with a 4- to 6-week course of penicillin G and gentamicin.

Enterococci *(Streptococcus faecalis, Streptococcus faecium, Streptococcus durans)* are the third most common cause of NVE and occur more commonly in elderly men. Such NVE is best treated with a 4-week course of both penicillin G and gentamicin, or ampicillin and gentamicin. The likelihood of cure using antibiotics alone improves if the infection has been less than 3 months in duration. Highly gentamicin-resistant strains may require surgical removal of the infected valve for a complete cure. Enterococci causing PVE should be treated with the same regimen as described previously for 6 weeks. In the last several years, the emergence of vancomycin-resistant enterococci (VRE) has complicated therapy. No reliably effective regimen for VRE has been established, and therapy should be guided by antibiotic sensitivity testing. The combination of quinupristin and dalfopristin (Synercid) has been suggested. Consultation with an infectious disease specialist and early surgical intervention should be considered.

Staphylococcal IE is treated on the basis of methicillin susceptibility or resistance, left- versus right-sided valvular involvement, and the presence or absence of prosthetic material. Methicillin-susceptible staphylococcal left-sided NVE or PVE (right- or left-sided) can be treated with 6 weeks of nafcillin alone or it can be combined with low-dose gentamicin for 3

TABLE 4. **Antimicrobial Therapy for Endocarditis***

Microorganism	Regimen	Duration (Weeks)
Penicillin-Susceptible Streptococci (Viridans streptococci)		
Native valve (Relatively resistant viridans streptococci and *Streptococcus bovis* should be treated with 4 weeks of penicillin G and 2 weeks of gentamicin.)	Aqueous penicillin G 10–20 × 10^6 U IV q 24 h + Gentamicin 1 mg/kg IM or IV q 8 h	2 2
	or Aqueous penicillin G 10–20 × 10^6 U IV q 24 h	4
	or Ceftriaxone (Rocephin) 2 gm IV or IM single daily dose	4
	or Vancomycin 15 mg/kg IV q 12 h	4
Prosthetic valve	Aqueous penicillin G *or* vancomycin in same dose as above	4–6
	+ Gentamicin 1 mg/kg IM or IV q 8 h	2
Enterococci (Streptococcus faecalis, Streptococcus faecium, Streptococcus durans) *and resistant viridans streptococci*† Native valve and infections of <3 months' duration (For prosthetic valves and infections of >3 months' duration, 6 weeks of therapy is recommended.)	Aqueous penicillin 20–30 × 10^6 U IV q 24 h + Gentamicin 1 mg/kg IV q 8 h	4 4
	or Vancomycin 15 mg/kg IV q 12 h + Gentamicin 1 mg/kg IV or IM q 8 h	4 4
Coagulase-Positive Staphylococci		
Native valve		
Staphylococcus aureus, methicillin-susceptible	Nafcillin (Unipen) *or* oxacillin (Bactocill) 2 gm IV q 4 h	6
	or Cefazolin (Ancef) 2 gm IV q 8 h	6
	or Vancomycin 15 mg/kg IV q 12 h	6
S. aureus, right-sided, methicillin-susceptible (If extrapulmonary infection exists, nafcillin should be continued for 4–6 weeks.)	Nafcillin *or* oxacillin 2 gm IV q 4 h	2
	+ Tobramycin (Nebcin) *or* gentamicin 1 mg/kg IV q 12 h	2
S. aureus, methicillin-resistant	Vancomycin 15 mg/kg IV q 12 h	6
Prosthetic valve		
S. aureus, methicillin-susceptible (The use of rifampin in this setting is controversial.)	Vancomycin 15 mg/kg IV q 12 h	≥6
	+ Rifampin (Rifadin) 300 mg PO q 8 h	≥6
	+ Gentamicin 1 mg/kg IV or IM q 8 h	2
Coagulase-Negative Staphylococci (*Staphylococcus epidermidis,* methicillin-resistant)‡		
Native valve	Vancomycin 15 mg/kg IV q 12 h	6
Prosthetic valve	Vancomycin 15 mg/kg IV q 12 h	≥6
	+ Rifampin 300 mg PO q 8 h	≥6
	+ Gentamicin 1 mg/kg IV or IM q 8 h	2
Diphtheroids	Vancomycin 15 mg/kg IV q 12 h	6
HACEK organisms	Ceftriaxone 2 gm IV *or* IM q 24 h single dose	4
	or Ampicillin 2 gm IV q 4 h + Gentamicin 1.0 mg/kg IV q 8 h	4 3
Gram-Negative Organisms (Should be treated according to antibiotic susceptibility; suggested regimens are listed.)		
Pseudomonas aeruginosa	Piperacillin (Pipracil) 3 gm IV q 4 h *or* ceftazidime (Fortaz, Tazicef) 2 gm IV q 8 h *or* Aztreonam (Azactam) 2 gm IV q 6 h *or* imipenem 0.5–1 gm IV q 6 h	6
	+ Tobramycin 1.7 mg/kg IV q 6 h	6
Enterobacteriaceae	Cefotaxime 2 gm IV q 6 h *or* imipenem 0.5–1 gm q 6 h *or* aztreonam 2 gm IV q 6 h	4–6
	+ Tobramycin 1.7 mg/kg IV q 8 h	6
Q-Fever Bacteria and Chlamydia	Doxycycline 100 mg PO q 12 h *or* Tetracycline 500 mg PO q 6 h + Co-trimoxazole (160 mg trimethoprim and 800 mg sulfamethoxazole) PO q 8 h	1–2 y or longer
Fungi	Amphotericin B (Fungizone) IV 1 mg/kg/24 h	6–8
	+ Flucytosine (Ancobon) 37.5 mg/kg PO q 6 h	6
Culture-Negative (empirical therapy)	Vancomycin 15 mg/kg IV q 12 h	
	+ Gentamicin 1 mg/kg IV or IM q 8 h	6

*Dosages recommended are for patients with normal renal and hepatic function.
†Standard antimicrobial regimen for vanomycin-resistant enterorocci not established (see text).
‡Antimicrobial therapy for methicillin-susceptible strains is identical to that for methicillin-susceptible *S. aureus*.
From Wilson WR, Thandroyen FT: Infective endocarditis. *In* Willerson JT, Cohn JN (eds): Cardiovascular Medicine. New York, Churchill Livingstone, 1995.

TABLE 5. **Complications of Infective Endocarditis**

Local valvular destruction, which often accounts for
- Congestive heart failure
- Aortic insufficiency
- Mitral regurgitation
- Tricuspid regurgitation (right-sided heart failure, particularly in the presence of pulmonary hypertension)

Perivalvular extension of infection, may be associated with
- Persistent, uncontrolled infection
- Valvular insufficiency
- Cardiac conduction defects
- Left-to-right shunts
- Arrhythmias

Embolic phenomena
- Systemic: cerebrovascular accidents, splenic or renal infarcts, myocardial infarction, mesenteric/limb ischemia, or metastatic abscesses
- Pulmonary: cavitary lesions or pneumonia

Other
- Systemic sepsis (usually secondary to staphylococcal or gram-negative infections)
- Mycotic aneurysms
- Valve obstruction by vegetation (rare, but may occur with exuberant growth of large, bulky vegetations, particularly on prosthetic valves)

From Larsen G, Greenberg B: Infective endocarditis. *In* Rakel RE (ed): Conn's Current Therapy 1988. Philadelphia, WB Saunders, 1988.

to 5 days. The addition of gentamicin decreases the duration of bacteremia but does not improve survival or reduce complications. Methicillin-susceptible right-sided staphylococcal NVE (typically IVDU-related) not associated with an extrapulmonary focus of infection can be treated successfully with a 2-week course of nafcillin and tobramycin, or nafcillin and gentamicin. Those with extrapulmonary involvement should receive a 4- to 6-week course of nafcillin, combined in the initial 2 weeks with tobramycin or gentamicin. *S. aureus* (methicillin-resistant) NVE should be treated with vancomycin for 6 weeks. Methicillin-resistant strains of *S. epidermidis* are typically associated with early-onset PVE and are best treated with a combination of vancomycin and rifampin for 6 weeks, with gentamicin added in the first 2 weeks.

Endocarditis associated with the HACEK group of organisms accounts for approximately 9% of non–IVDU-associated cases. These can be effectively treated with 3 weeks of ampicillin. In penicillinase-producing strains, ceftriaxone may be substituted.

Gram-negative infections with other than the HACEK group account for 5% of NVE-, 13% of PVE-, and 30% of IVDU-associated IE. According to their in vitro susceptibility, these infections should be treated for 4 to 6 weeks with cefotaxime, imipenem, or aztreonam in combination with high-dose gentamicin. There is some evidence to suggest that intravenous ciprofloxacin* may now be the preferred therapy in Enterobacteriaceae and *Pseudomonas aeruginosa* infections. A combination of an extended-spectrum penicillin (piperacillin or azlocillin) combined with high-dose tobramycin also appears to be an effective regimen for *P. aeruginosa* IE. This combi-

*Not FDA approved for this indication.

TABLE 6. **Indications for Surgery in Infective Endocarditis**

Generally Accepted Indications
- Congestive heart failure refractory to routine management
- Uncontrolled infection despite appropriate antimicrobial therapy
- Fungal endocarditis
- Suppurative pericarditis
- Unstable prosthetic valve
- Recurrent disabling systemic emboli after 1–2 weeks of adequate antimicrobial therapy
- Mycotic aneurysms

Relative Indications
- Infection with gram-negative organism
- *Staphylococcus aureus* infection of left-sided valve (particularly aortic)
- Recurrent relapse after apparent cure
- Evidence of perivalvular extension of infection
- Rupture of sinus of Valsalva or of ventricular septum
- Early prosthetic valve endocarditis
- New periprosthetic leak
- Metastatic abscesses not responding to antimicrobial therapy

From Larsen G, Greenberg B: Infective endocarditis. *In* Rakel RE (ed): Conn's Current Therapy 1988. Philadelphia, WB Saunders, 1988.

TABLE 7. **Cardiac Conditions Associated with Endocarditis**

Endocarditis prophylaxis recommended

High-risk category
- Prosthetic cardiac valves, including bioprosthetic and homograft valves
- Previous bacterial endocarditis
- Complex cyanotic congenital heart disease (e.g., single ventricle states, transposition of the great arteries, tetralogy of Fallot)
- Surgically constructed systemic pulmonary shunts or conduits

Moderate-risk category
- Most other congenital cardiac malformations (other than above and below)
- Acquired valvar dysfunction (e.g., rheumatic heart disease)
- Hypertrophic cardiomyopathy
- Mitral valve prolapse with valvar regurgitation and/or thickened leaflets

Endocarditis prophylaxis not recommended

Negligible-risk category (no greater risk than the general population)
- Isolated secundum atrial septal defect
- Surgical repair of atrial septal defect, ventricular septal defect, or patent ductus arteriosus (without residual beyond 6 mo)
- Previous coronary artery bypass graft surgery
- Mitral valve prolapse without valvar regurgitation
- Physiologic, functional, or innocent heart murmurs
- Previous Kawasaki disease without valvar dysfunction
- Previous rheumatic fever without valvar dysfunction
- Cardiac pacemakers (intravascular and epicardial) and implanted defibrillators

From Dajani AS, et al: Prevention of bacterial endocarditis. Circulation *96*(1):359, 1997.

TABLE 8. **Dental Procedures and Endocarditis Prophylaxis**

Endocarditis prophylaxis recommended*

- Dental extractions
- Periodontal procedures including surgery, scaling and root planing, probing, and recall maintenance
- Dental implant placement and reimplantation of avulsed teeth
- Endodontic (root canal) instrumentation or surgery only beyond the apex
- Subgingival placement of antibiotic fibers or strips
- Initial placement of orthodontic bands but not brackets
- Intraligamentary local anesthetic injections
- Prophylactic cleaning of teeth or implants where bleeding is anticipated

Endocarditis prophylaxis not recommended

- Restorative dentistry† (operative and prosthodontic) with or without retraction cord‡
- Local anesthetic injections (nonintraligamentary)
- Intracanal endodontic treatment; postplacement and buildup
- Placement of rubber dams
- Postoperative suture removal
- Placement of removable prosthodontic or orthodontic appliances
- Taking of oral impressions
- Fluoride treatments
- Taking of oral radiographs
- Orthodontic appliance adjustment
- Shedding of primary teeth

*Prophylaxis is recommended for patients with high- and moderate-risk cardiac conditions.

†This includes restoration of decayed teeth (filling cavities) and replacement of missing teeth.

‡Clinical judgment may indicate antibiotic use in selected circumstances that may create significant bleeding.

From Dajani AS, et al: Prevention of bacterial endocarditis. Circulation *96*(1):361, 1997.

nation therapy may be effective in right-sided NVE; however, the cure rate for left-sided infections is quite dismal, and early valve replacement is recommended.

COMPLICATIONS

The vast majority of deaths related to IE result from CHF. The major complications can be broadly divided into (1) local valvular destruction, (2) perivalvular extension of infection, (3) embolic complications, (4) systemic sepsis, and (5) intractable infection (Table 5).

Local valvular destruction caused by bacterial vegetations constitutes the most common cause of valvular regurgitation; however, infection of the chordal apparatus or perivalvular abscess formation may also give rise to insufficiency of the affected valve. In the case of acute aortic insufficiency or mitral regurgitation, rapid evaluation of the hemodynamic status and prompt intervention form the basis for effective therapy. Right heart catheterization can be helpful in making this important assessment. If the patient is poorly responsive to medical therapy or initial catheterization reveals severe elevation in the pulmonary capillary wedge pressure, urgent surgical evaluation should be obtained with concomitant aggressive treatment of CHF. Failure to proceed with surgical therapy within 24 to 48 hours after the diagnosis of severe progressive heart failure usually results in cardiogenic shock and death. Even mild acute CHF requires surgical intervention in the setting of a regurgitant aortic valve. The clinician also must be alert to the development of CHF several weeks or months after the acute infection is believed to be cured. Despite successful bacterial eradication, the hemodynamic effects of valvular dysfunction may take time to manifest.

Right-sided endocarditis differs in that the effects of tricuspid valvular regurgitation with right ventricular volume overload can often be controlled with diuretic therapy. However, if right-sided heart failure becomes intractable, a number of surgical procedures may be considered. These include replacement with

TABLE 9. **Other Procedures and Endocarditis Prophylaxis**

Endocarditis prophylaxis recommended

- Respiratory tract
  - Tonsillectomy and/or adenoidectomy
  - Surgical operations that involve respiratory mucosa
  - Bronchoscopy with a rigid bronchoscope
- Gastrointestinal tract*
  - Sclerotherapy for esophageal varices
  - Esophageal stricture dilatation
  - Endoscopic retrograde cholangiography with biliary obstruction
  - Biliary tract surgery
  - Surgical operations that involve intestinal mucosa
- Genitourinary tract
  - Prostatic surgery
  - Cystoscopy
  - Urethral dilatation

Endocarditis prophylaxis not recommended

- Respiratory tract
  - Endotracheal intubation
  - Bronchoscopy with a flexible bronchoscope, with or without biopsy†
  - Tympanostomy tube insertion
- Gastrointestinal tract
  - Transesophageal echocardiography†
  - Endoscopy with or without gastrointestinal biopsy†
- Genitourinary tract
  - Vaginal hysterectomy†
  - Vaginal delivery†
  - Cesarean section
  - In uninfected tissue:
    - Urethral catheterization
    - Uterine dilatation and curettage
    - Therapeutic abortion
    - Sterilization procedures
    - Insertion or removal of intrauterine devices
- Other
  - Cardiac catheterization, including balloon angioplasty
  - Implanted cardiac pacemakers, implanted defibrillators, and coronary stents
  - Incision or biopsy of surgically scrubbed skin
  - Circumcision

*Prophylaxis is recommended for high-risk patients; it is optional for medium-risk patients.

†Prophylaxis is optional for high-risk patients.

From Dajani AS, et al: Prevention of bacterial endocarditis. Circulation *96*(1):362, 1997.

TABLE 10. **Prophylactic Regimens for Dental, Oral, Respiratory Tract, or Esophageal Procedures**

Situation	Agents	Regimen*
Standard general prophylaxis	Amoxicillin	Adults: 2.0 gm; children: 50 mg/kg orally 1 h before procedure
Unable to take oral medications	Ampicillin	Adults: 2.0 gm IM or IV; children: 50 mg/kg IM or IV within 30 min before procedure
Allergic to penicillin	Clindamycin	Adults: 600 mg; children: 20 mg/kg orally 1 h before procedure
	or cephalexin† or cefadroxil†	Adults: 2.0 gm; children: 50 mg/kg orally 1 h before procedure
	or azithromycin or clarithromycin	Adults: 500 mg; children: 15 mg/kg orally 1 h before procedure
Allergic to penicillin and unable to take oral medications	Clindamycin	Adults: 600 mg; children: 20 mg/kg IV within 30 min before procedure
	or cefazolin†	Adults: 1.0 gm; children: 25 mg/kg IM or IV within 30 min before procedure

*Total children's dose should not exceed adult dose.
†Cephalosporins should not be used in individuals with immediate-type hypersensitivity reaction (urticaria, angioedema, or anaphylaxis) to penicillins.
From Dajani AS, et al: Prevention of bacterial endocarditis. Circulation *96*(1):363, 1997.

a prosthetic valve and valvuloplasty. Because most cases of right-sided IE are found in intravenous drug users, there are significant implications when considering the placement of prosthetic valves in these patients. Unfortunately, a large percentage of these individuals continue to use intravenous drugs and therefore put themselves at significant risk for PVE, which carries a higher mortality and almost always requires surgical intervention. This has led several groups to consider valvuloplasty as a possible alternative. Initial reports have been encouraging; however, these were at fairly specialized centers, and therefore their wider application must await larger clinical experience.

The incidence of perivalvular extension of infection (PVEI) varies considerably, depending on the series that is studied. The incidence among NVE patients is approximately 10%, and the incidence among PVE patients is approximately 50 to 60%. Aortic valve infections are the most common source of PVEI. Typically, PVEI comes to the attention of the clinician as persistent bacteremia despite adequate antibiotic therapy, or as worsening CHF. In both these situations, TTE and TEE become invaluable for appro-

TABLE 11. **Prophylactic Regimens for Genitourinary/Gastrointestinal (Excluding Esophageal) Procedures**

Situation	Agents	Regimen*†
High-risk patients	Ampicillin plus gentamicin	Adults: ampicillin 2.0 gm IM or IV plus gentamicin 1.5 mg/kg (not to exceed 120 mg) within 30 min of starting procedure; 6 h later, ampicillin 1 gm IM/IV or amoxicillin 1 gm orally Children: ampicillin 50 mg/kg IM or IV (not to exceed 2.0 gm) plus gentamicin 1.5 mg/kg within 30 min of starting procedure; 6 h later, ampicillin 25 mg/kg IM/IV or amoxicillin 25 mg/kg orally
High-risk patients allergic to ampicillin/amoxicillin	Vancomycin plus gentamicin	Adults: vancomycin 1.0 gm IV over 1–2 h plus gentamicin 1.5 mg/kg IV/IM (not to exceed 120 mg); complete injection/infusion within 30 min of starting procedure Children: vancomycin 20 mg/kg IV over 1–2 h plus gentamicin 1.5 mg/kg IV/IM; complete injection/infusion within 30 min of starting procedure
Moderate-risk patients	Amoxicillin or ampicillin	Adults: amoxicillin 2.0 gm orally 1 h before procedure, or ampicillin 2.0 gm IM/IV within 30 min of starting procedure Children: amoxicillin 50 mg/kg orally 1 h before procedure, or ampicillin 50 mg/kg IM/IV within 30 min of starting procedure
Moderate-risk patients allergic to ampicillin/amoxicillin	Vancomycin	Adults: vancomycin 1.0 gm IV over 1–2 h; complete infusion within 30 min of starting procedure Children: vancomycin 20 mg/kg IV over 1–2 h; complete infusion within 30 min of starting procedure

*Total children's dose should not exceed adult dose.
†No second dose of vancomycin or gentamicin is recommended.
From Dajani AS, et al: Prevention of bacterial endocarditis. Circulation *96*(1):364, 1997.

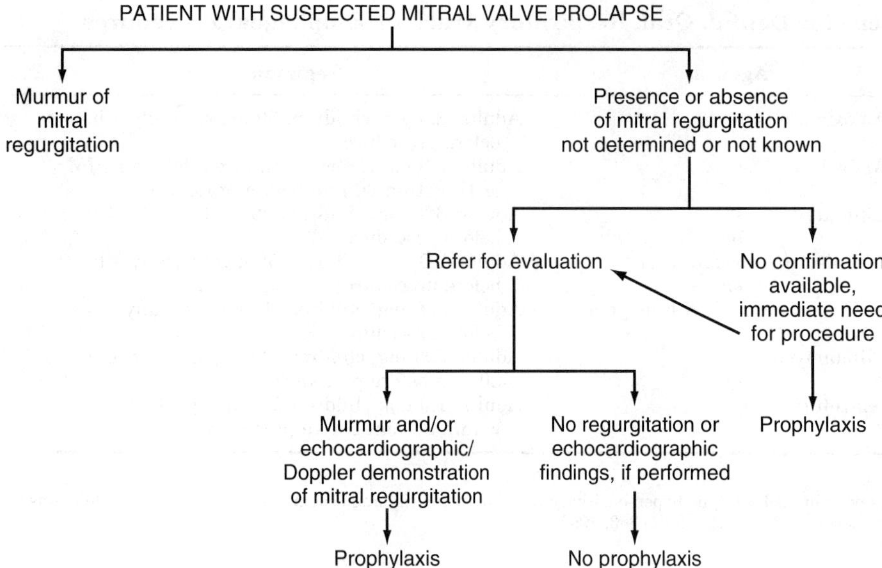

Figure 1. American Heart Association algorithm for infective endocarditis prophylaxis in mitral valve prolapse. (From Dajani AS, et al: Prevention of bacterial endocarditis. Circulation *96*: 359–364, 1997.)

priate management. The manifestations of PVEI may reflect both its extent and its location. PVEI secondary to prosthetic valve endocarditis may result in paravalvular regurgitation, as well as valve dehiscence. From 5 to 10% of patients may develop arrhythmias and heart block as a result of PVEI; therefore the ECG remains a valuable, although somewhat insensitive, tool for diagnosis. Occasionally, infection may spread to the pericardium, resulting in purulent pericarditis that requires prompt surgical drainage. Infection may also involve the papillary muscles, causing disruption of the subvalvular apparatus and resulting in mitral regurgitation. Destruction of the intracardiac septum may result in shunt formation with consequent volume overload. All these conditions may be associated with myocardial abscess formation, and surgery is usually indicated.

Clinically evident embolic phenomena occur in 22 to 43% of patients with IE. There are also likely to be a large number of clinically silent events, particularly affecting the spleen or kidney. They may also present dramatically with an acute arterial occlusion in the limb or mesentery. Rarely, vegetations may embolize to the coronary arteries producing a myocardial infarction. However, cerebral emboli remain the most profound embolic complication because of their potential for causing death and long-term disability. The embolic risks appear to be related to the size of the vegetation, the duration of antimicrobial therapy, and the type of organism. Despite the advances in echocardiographic technique, valvular surgery cannot be recommended strictly on the basis of vegetation size. However, if there are recurrent embolic events despite adequate antimicrobial therapy, especially in the presence of organisms such as group B streptococci, nutritionally variant streptococci, HACEK organisms, or fungi, a stronger consideration could be given for surgical intervention. Currently the most effective treatment for reduction of embolic risk is prompt antimicrobial therapy, which results in a significant reduction in embolic rates in the second and third week of treatment.

Septic embolization can result in metastatic abscesses and mycotic aneurysms. Metastatic abscesses are most often caused by *S. aureus* and in general require surgical drainage. However, certain clinical situations may resolve with antibiotic therapy alone such as with septic emboli to the lung from right-sided IE. Cerebral mycotic aneurysms typically present with unremitting headache and homonymous hemianopsia, and this symptom complex should alert the physician to the possibility of a serious intracranial complication. In general, if mycotic aneurysms are detected, the therapy of choice is surgical excision.

Systemic complications include systemic inflammatory response syndrome (SIRS), particularly with *S. aureus* and aerobic gram-negative infections. These complications may not reverse immediately with prompt antibiotic therapy and therefore require supportive treatment in an intensive care setting. In addition, meningitis and encephalopathy may result secondary to the bacteremia and sepsis.

Intractable infection may occur in the setting of fungal, gram-negative bacterial, or staphylococcal infection of prosthetic valves. Consequently these infections are associated with a greater incidence of complications including valve dysfunction and PVEI. In addition native valve infections resulting from aminoglycoside- (or vancomycin-) resistant enterococcus and *P. aeruginosa* have a poor response to antimicrobial therapy; therefore early valve replacement may be the only viable option.

In general most IE relapses occur between 4 and 8 weeks after stopping antimicrobial therapy and tend to be rare, less than 5%. Although there are no clear guidelines, most authorities agree that IE relapse caused by antibiotic-sensitive viridans streptococci and enterococci can be treated successfully with a repeat course of antibiotics. In cases of multiple relapses and in first-time infections involving Q fever or other resistant organisms, cardiac valve replacement is the appropriate approach.

The decision to proceed to surgical intervention and valve replacement must be made carefully after assessing all the available clinical, laboratory, echocardiographic, and hemodynamic information (Table 6). Long-term cardiologic follow-up is prudent, as studies have suggested that nearly 50% of patients that are medically cured of IE will eventually need valve surgery. Patients with aortic valve involvement are at particular risk.

PREVENTION

The data from controlled trials are insufficient to support the strong association between medical and surgical instrumentation and IE in individuals with underlying structural heart disease. Nevertheless, antibiotic prophylaxis has assumed a widespread role in the prevention of IE in such individuals. The American Heart Association (AHA) in 1997 revised these guidelines (Tables 7 through 11). They represent a consensus approach to endocarditis prophylaxis, incorporating the extent to which a cardiac abnormality predisposes to IE, the risk of bacteremia with a particular procedure, the potential for antibiotic adverse effects, and a cost-benefit analysis.

These newer guidelines stratify cardiac conditions into high, moderate, and negligible risk categories and clearly outline procedures that may cause bacteremia and for which prophylaxis is recommended. The AHA algorithm for IE prophylaxis in mitral valve prolapse is presented in Figure 1. New recommendations no longer suggest a postoperative antibiotic dose for oral/dental procedures, and regimens have been simplified for gastrointestinal/genitourinary procedures. In addition, general measures that include the maintenance of excellent oral hygiene and the use of chlorhexidine (Peridex) mouthwash before dental procedures can significantly decrease the amount of subsequent bacteremia. As a corollary to these preventive measures, there is a need to improve awareness among physicians, dentists, and patients with regard to antibiotic prophylaxis and the maintenance of good oral health.

HYPERTENSION

method of
HENRY R. BLACK, M.D.
Rush Medical College of Rush University
Chicago, Illinois

Hypertension is the most common disease-specific reason for which Americans visit a physician. The third National Health and Nutrition Survey (NHANES III), conducted in 1988–1991, estimated that 50 million Americans are hypertensive, compared with 58 million in the 1976–1980 survey. Of those 50 million, 43 million persons either were hypertensive when evaluated or were receiving antihypertensive drug therapy. The other 7 million persons had been told they had an elevated blood pressure but were not receiving antihypertensive therapy, nor were they found to have an elevated blood pressure at the time of screening by the NHANES III field staff. In this group, the apparent reduction in blood pressure might have been due to lifestyle modification, or these persons were erroneously diagnosed as being hypertensive initially.

Because hypertension is so common, all physicians and health care providers will encounter hypertensive patients on an almost daily basis. The provider treating the hypertension must know how to estimate the patient's cardiovascular risk and how that patient's hypertension should be classified and treated. This is especially pertinent now that the Sixth Joint National Committee on the Prevention, Detection, Evaluation, and Treatment of High Blood Pressure (JNC VI) has recommended different treatment approaches based on the level of blood pressure and risk assessment (Tables 1, 2, and 3).

The change in classification is a result of greater understanding and appreciation of the importance of *absolute* or *attributable risk* and resultant *absolute benefit* of treatment. In earlier classification systems, only *relative risk* (RR) was considered. The RR associated with hypertension is the measure of risk of events and/or mortality when an individual or a population with a particular level of high or high-normal blood pressure is compared with another individual or population whose blood pressure is at an optimal or lower level. RR progressively increases as both systolic and diastolic blood pressures rise. Absolute risk reflects the risk associated with the elevated reading in an individual patient (or group of patients) and takes into account other conditions that increase risk. Although hypertension is the risk factor that contributes most to overall cardiovascular disease and especially to stroke, there are many other important antecedents of cardiovascular disease, i.e., risk factors (see Table 3). Elevated lipid levels, age, the presence of diabetes or glucose intolerance, obesity, family history, sedentary lifestyle, and smoking are but a few of the well-established risk factors for cardiovascular disease. The Framingham Heart Study (FHS) and many other observational studies have clearly demonstrated that risk factors have an additive, if not multiplicative, impact on risk.

TABLE 1. **Classification of Blood Pressure Levels in Adults ≥18 Years of Age***

Category	Blood Pressure (mm Hg)		
	Systolic		*Diastolic*
Optimal†	<120	and	<80
Normal	<130	and	<85
High-normal	130–139	or	85–89
Hypertension‡			
Stage 1	140–159	or	90–99
Stage 2	160–179	or	100–109
Stage 3	≥180	or	≥110

*Not taking antihypertensive drugs and not acutely ill.
†Optimal blood pressure with respect to cardiovascular risk: below 120/80 mm Hg. However, unusually low readings should be evaluated for clinical significance.
‡Based on the average of two or more readings taken at each of two or more visits after an initial screening.
Adapted from the Sixth Report of the Joint National Committee on Prevention, Detection, Evaluation, and Treatment of High Blood Pressure. Arch Intern Med *157*:2413–2446, 1997. Copyright 1997, American Medical Association.

TABLE 2. **Risk Stratification and Treatment for Blood Pressure Risk Groups**

Blood Pressure Stage (diastolic/systolic, mm Hg)	**Treatment Recommendation** *Risk Group A (no risk factors; no TOD/CCD)*	*Risk Group B (at least 1 risk factor, not including diabetes; no TOD/CCD)*	*Risk Group C (TOD/CCD and/or diabetes, ± other risk factors)*
High-normal (130–139/85–89)	Lifestyle modification	Lifestyle modification	Drug therapy Lifestyle modification
Stage I (140–159/90–99)	Lifestyle modification (up to 12 mo)	Lifestyle modification (up to 6 mo)	Drug therapy Lifestyle modification
Stages II and III (≥160/≥100)	Drug therapy Lifestyle modification	Drug therapy Lifestyle modification	Drug therapy Lifestyle modification

For example, a patient with diabetes and a blood pressure of 142/94 mm Hg plus left ventricular hypertrophy should be classified as having stage I hypertension with TOD (i.e., left ventricular hypertrophy) and with another major risk factor (diabetes). This patient would be categorized as stage I, Risk Group C.

Abbreviation: TOD/CCD = target organ disease/clinical cardiovascular disease (see Table 3).
Adapted from the Sixth Report of the Joint National Committee on Prevention, Detection, Evaluation, and Treatment of High Blood Pressure. Arch Intern Med *157*:2413–2446, 1997. Copyright 1997, American Medical Association.

The presence of demonstrable target organ damage or clinical disease such as left ventricular hypertrophy, heart failure, angina, retinopathy, or prior stroke and/or myocardial infarction has a similar if not even more powerful effect on prognosis (see Table 3). A patient with only a minimal (if any) elevation in blood pressure is much more likely to experience a cardiovascular or other event if he or she also has other risk factors or target organ damage than is a patient with a significantly higher blood pressure who is free of other comorbid conditions or risk factors.

Similar analyses have shown that the absolute benefit of treatment (the overall number of lives saved or events prevented) is considerably greater in high-risk cohorts (those groups in which absolute risk is high) than that demonstrated in low-risk groups. *The goal in treatment of hypertension is to reduce the excess morbidity and mortality related to having an elevated blood pressure and not simply to lower blood pressure.* Thus, it appears that concentrating our efforts on the treatment of hypertension in high-risk patients, as determined by absolute risk, sooner and more aggressively will have a much more dramatic and beneficial impact on individual and public health than that achieved by focusing simply on the level of blood pressure, as determined by relative risk, as we have in the past.

TABLE 3. **Components of Cardiovascular Risk Stratification in Patients with Hypertension**

Major risk factors
Smoking
Dyslipidemia
Diabetes mellitus
Age older than 60 years
Gender: men and postmenopausal women
Family history of cardiovascular disease, in women under age 65 or in men under age 55

Target organ damage/clinical cardiovascular disease
Heart disease

- Left ventricular hypertrophy
- Angina/prior myocardial infarction
- Prior coronary revascularization
- Heart failure

Stroke or transient ischemic attack
Nephropathy
Peripheral arterial disease
Retinopathy

Adapted from the Sixth Report of the Joint National Committee on Prevention, Detection, Evaluation, and Treatment of High Blood Pressure. Arch Intern Med *157*:2413–2446, 1997. Copyright 1997, American Medical Association.

CLASSIFICATION AND STRATIFICATION OF HYPERTENSIVE PATIENTS

JNC VI modified the classification system first proposed in 1993 by the Fifth Joint National Committee on the Detection, Evaluation, and Treatment of Hypertension (JNC V) (see Table 1). The new system continues to include both systolic and diastolic blood pressures and uses the same levels for optimal, high-normal, and stage I and stage II hypertension. Stage IV hypertension (a separate category for patients with a systolic blood pressure of 210 mm Hg or higher and/or a diastolic blood pressure of 120 mm Hg or higher in JNC V) has been eliminated. Any hypertensive patient with a systolic blood pressure of 180 mm Hg or higher or a diastolic blood pressure of 110 mm Hg or higher is now classified as stage III. This change was adopted because a very small number of Americans were in stage IV.

As in JNC V, the stage assigned reflects the higher of the two categories into which the patient falls. Thus, a patient whose blood pressure is 182/88 mm Hg is classified as stage III, as determined by the systolic level, and not high-normal, which is the level of the diastolic blood pressure.

This system has, as did JNC V, continued to acknowledge the importance of systolic blood pressure as a predictor of risk but perhaps did not emphasize it enough. In 1993, the FHS highlighted the risk for persons with stage I isolated systolic hypertension (systolic blood pressure of 140 to 159 mm Hg with a diastolic blood pressure of less than 90 mm Hg). After 34 years of follow-up, the likelihood of cardiovascular disease, including myocardial infarction, stroke, and heart failure, was 50 to 85% higher in FHS volunteers with stage I systolic hypertension at the initial screening, than in those with normal blood pressures (less than 140 mm Hg systolic and less than 90 mm Hg diastolic). The risk of all-cause mortality was also elevated by more than 20%. All of these differences were statistically significant. These patients with stage I systolic hypertension are often ignored and usually are not offered treatment, and they represent a very large group at risk of probably preventable events and premature death. The Physicians Health Study has recently confirmed the increased risk for cardiovascular disease and death for persons with stage I systolic hypertension. The physicians in the study with that level of blood pressure at entry had an intermediate risk between that of physicians with normal blood pressure and that of physicians with stage II or III hypertension. To date, however, no clinical trials have clearly established the benefit of treatment in these hypertensive patients.

Earlier surveys emphasized the impact of systolic blood pressure in older persons with systolic blood pressure readings of 160 mm Hg or higher. More recent epidemiologic studies, however, have clearly extended these findings to younger people and have shown that risk increases dramatically with lesser increases in systolic blood pressure than had been previously appreciated. The Physicians Health Study and the Multiple Risk Factor Intervention Trial, for example, have now demonstrated that risk for cardiovascular events and end-stage renal disease increases significantly as systolic blood pressure rises from 120 mm Hg to 139 mm Hg. These data suggest that the currently accepted boundary between hypertension and high-normal blood pressure may still be set too high and that future classification systems should continue the trend to recommend diagnosing hypertension at lower levels than has been customary.

The JNC VI classification has also ignored the potential importance of pulse pressure, the difference between systolic and diastolic blood pressures. All population-based surveys have shown that while the average systolic blood pressure rises with age, average diastolic blood pressure rises until approximately age 55 years and then falls, resulting in the wider pulse pressure characteristic of older persons. In well-characterized populations, this increase in pulse pressure with age can also be seen in the segment of the population with the lowest level of blood pressure. The pathophysiologic correlate of the widening of the pulse pressure is progression of the atherosclerotic process. Increasing systolic pressure results from a loss of vascular compliance in large conduit arteries. This stiffening of the large arteries is due to increasing collagen formation, possibly resulting from barotrauma due to excessively forceful systolic contraction of the heart. When arteries stiffen, they become less compliant, store less blood, and encounter longer and slower run-off during diastole, resulting in a lower diastolic blood pressure.

Data now available from case-control studies, clinical trials, and observational studies in populations and cohorts have convincingly demonstrated that persons or groups of persons with wide pulse pressures, generally 60 mm Hg or more, have a higher rate of cardiovascular, cerebrovascular, and renal complications. The effect of pulse pressure is independent of the level of systolic or diastolic blood pressure and has often been a more robust predictor of those events than either systolic or diastolic blood pressure.

The fall in diastolic blood pressure seen in persons with wide pulse pressures due to worsening arterial disease is characteristic of aging and may be the explanation for the "J-curve" hypothesis. In 1979, an English practitioner first described the phenomenon. He noted that coronary mortality was higher in patients in his practice whose diastolic blood pressure was lowered *with treatment* to below 90 mm Hg (phase IV Korotkoff sound) than in patients with more modest reductions in blood pressure. Numerous further analyses in clinical trials confirmed this observation and suggested that excessive reduction in diastolic blood pressure (the observation was not seen with systolic blood pressure) could lead to increased coronary artery disease morbidity and mortality. A diastolic blood pressure of 83 mm Hg with treatment appeared to be optimal and has been suggested as a reason not to treat hypertensive patients with coronary artery disease too aggressively. Yet other studies showed that this relationship between diastolic blood pressure and coronary disease outcomes was also noted in untreated populations and in the placebo groups in clinical trials. Furtheremore, in two large trials in elderly patients with stage II or III isolated systolic hypertension (pretreatment diastolic blood pressure of 77 mm Hg), the group receiving active treatment had a clear reduction in coronary events even though diastolic blood pressure was lowered to below 70 mm Hg.

It is certainly plausible that the lower diastolic pressure that results from arterial stiffening could explain the seeming increase in cardiovascular and other events in persons with lower diastolic blood pressure. If anything, our efforts to treat hypertension should not be timid but rather should be even more aggressive if patients are to get the most from therapy. When the results of the Hypertension Optimal Treatment (HOT) study are available, we will have a clear understanding about whether we may do harm by reducing diastolic blood pressure too aggressively.

EVALUATION

The evaluation of the hypertensive patient is directed at answering the following questions:

1. What is the appropriate classification and stratification for that patient?
2. Are other risk factors present?
3. Is target organ damage present?
4. Is there an identifiable cause for that patient's hypertension?
5. Are there any features in this patient's history, physical examination, or routine laboratory evaluation that will influence the choice of therapy?

In most cases these questions can be answered during one or two office visits and without resorting to expensive or risky laboratory testing or prolonged periods of observation.

The need to measure blood pressure accurately cannot be overemphasized. A properly trained person using a well-functioning and calibrated sphygmomanometer should measure blood pressure. Regular calibration of the instruments used is especially crucial now that concerns about the environmental effects of mercury have severely limited the use of mercury sphygmomanometers, and most measurements are done with aneroid devices. Automated electronic devices may be accurate but should not replace blood pressure measured by a health care professional.

The measurement should be done when the patient is relaxed and after at least 5 minutes of rest. At the first visit, especially in older persons, it is useful to measure the blood pressure with the patient both supine and standing to ascertain whether postural hypotension (a drop in systolic blood pressure of 20 mm Hg or greater upon standing) is present. Sitting blood pressure with the back supported should also be measured and used as a baseline for all subsequent readings unless substantial postural hypotension was noted, or unless the patient complains of symptoms, particularly dizziness, suggesting that standing blood pressure is too low for adequate cerebral perfusion. The arm should be bared, and the cuff chosen for use must be of adequate size. The bladder of the cuff should encircle at least 80% of the arm. If a cuff is too small, the blood pressure reading may be artifactually high and the patient inappropriately diagnosed and treated as hypertensive. At least two and probably three readings should be taken. The second two should be averaged and used as the blood pressure for that visit. The diagnosis of hypertension should not be made until elevated readings are found on three visits separated by at least a week. Patients whose blood pressure readings classify them as having stage II or III hypertension, especially if typical hypertension-related target organ damage is present, should probably be diagnosed as hypertensive sooner so that appropriate action can be taken.

Those patients whose readings fluctuate greatly, especially if some readings are below 140/90 mm Hg, may need additional observation and further measurements before the diagnosis of hypertension can be firmly established. Some of these patients with so-called labile hypertension, as well as persons who are hypertensive in the office but normotensive elsewhere (such patients are said to have "white coat hypertension") may be candidates for home blood pressure or ambulatory blood pressure monitoring. Should patients wish to follow their blood pressures with home monitoring, it is important to have them take blood pressure measurements at pre-specified times of day to avoid the bias associated with measuring blood pressure only when they are feeling well or poorly. It is very important to ensure that the instrument used is accurate. Although many devices are marketed, only a few have been rated as acceptable by independent testing organizations.

A complete history should be taken and a thorough physical examination should be done, directed at looking for evidence of target organ damage, other risk factors, comorbid conditions, and features suggesting secondary hypertension. Every hypertensive patient should be weighed on the first and each subsequent visit, and the eye grounds should be carefully examined to look for hypertensive retinopathy. Because the presence of bruits in the carotid arteries, abdomen, or lower extremities is important evidence of vascular disease, these should be looked for carefully in every hypertensive patient.

The laboratory evaluation is performed for the same purposes—assessing risk, discovering identifiable causes for secondary hypertension, and planning therapy—and must be done in a cost-effective manner. Only a few simple and inexpensive laboratory tests should be ordered in every hypertensive patient (Table 4). These tests are recommended because they are useful in assessing risk (serum creatinine, fasting blood glucose, total and high-density lipoprotein cholesterol, 12-lead electrocardiogram), diagnosing identifiable secondary causes of hypertension (urinalysis, serum potassium, serum creatinine), and/or guiding therapy (serum creatinine, serum potassium, fasting blood glucose). Other laboratory tests are useful should the history and findings on physical examination and routine laboratory studies suggest that further evaluation is necessary to assess risk or to find an identifiable secondary cause for the patient's hypertension (Table 5). Certain highly specialized tests can also be valuable. For example, in an elderly smoker with refractory hypertension and carotid bruits (a typical history and physical findings in a hypertensive patient with renal artery stenosis), a captopril renogram would be appropriate. A hypertensive patient with headaches, diaphoresis, and palpitations may need urinary studies to exclude a pheochromocytoma. The use of a combination of clinical skills and judgment to identify a probable secondary cause of hypertension, together with the judicious use of the laboratory, is the optimal way to evaluate hypertensive patients and patients in general. In this manner the clinician can avoid errors of omission, which could lead to inadequate or inappropriate treatment, as well as to the excessive use of expensive and risky laboratory evaluations.

TABLE 4. **Routine Laboratory Tests for Diagnosis of Hypertension**

Test
Urinalysis
Complete blood cell count
Blood chemistry
Potassium
Sodium
Creatinine
Fasting glucose
Total cholesterol
High-density lipoprotein (HDL) cholesterol
12-lead electrocardiography

Adapted from the Sixth Report of the Joint National Committee on Prevention, Detection, Evaluation, and Treatment of High Blood Pressure. Arch Intern Med *157*:2413–2446, 1997. Copyright 1997, American Medical Association.

TABLE 5. **Optional Tests for Diagnosis of Hypertension**

Test
24-hour urinary protein
Blood calcium
Uric acid
Fasting triglycerides
Low-density lipoprotein (LDL) cholesterol
Glycosylated hemoglobin
Thyroid-stimulating hormone
Limited echocardiography
Captopril renogram (when renovascular hypertension suspected)
Duplex renal ultrasonography (when renovascular hypertension suspected)
Urinary or plasma catecholamines and/or metabolites (when pheochromocytoma suspected)
Abdominal computed tomography scan (when pheochromocytoma or hyperaldosteronism suspected)
Renin/aldosterone ratio (when hyperaldosteronism suspected)
24-hour aldosterone excretion (when hyperaldosteronism suspected)

Adapted from the Sixth Report of the Joint National Committee on Prevention, Detection, Evaluation, and Treatment of High Blood Pressure. Arch Intern Med *157*:2413–2446, 1997. Copyright 1997, American Medical Association.

TREATMENT

Lifestyle Modification

The approach to treatment of patients with hypertension has undergone subtle but important changes in the recommendation of JNC VI compared with earlier guidelines. Although JNC VI still recognizes the value of lifestyle modification for all patients, it does not suggest that this measure alone should constitute initial therapy for all persons with hypertension—an approach favored in earlier reports for all patients but those with the highest levels of blood pressure. In JNC VI the recommendations are that patients with systolic blood pressures of 160 mm Hg or greater or diastolic blood pressures of 100 mm Hg or greater (stage II or III) and all hypertensive patients in Risk Group C should receive pharmacologic therapy once the diagnosis is confirmed. Furthermore, the time period for the use of lifestyle modification alone before the initiation of drug therapy has been clarified in JNC VI and is based on risk, not just on the level of blood pressure (see Table 2). Patients with stage I hypertension (systolic blood pressure of 140 to 159 mm Hg and/or diastolic blood pressure of 90 to 99 mm Hg) who have no other risk factors or end-organ damage (Risk Group A) can be managed with lifestyle modification for up to 1 year if goal blood pressure is not reached (discussed later), before pharmacologic therapy is considered to be required. Patients with stage I hypertension in Risk Group B (with other risk factors present) should receive drug therapy after only a 6-month trial of lifestyle modification.

A number of approaches to lowering blood pressure and treating hypertension with lifestyle modifications have been suggested and evaluated (Table 6). Of these, weight loss has generally been the most successful when compared with other strategies in appropriately done clinical trials. In the first phase of the Trials of Hypertension Prevention (TOHP I), more than 2000 volunteers were randomized to one of five groups: a weight loss program; a diet to reduce sodium intake; supplementation of potassium, calcium, magnesium, or fish oil; stress management; and usual care in the control group. This 18-month controlled trial confirmed the value of weight loss and sodium reduction, because only these two approaches were successful in lowering blood pressure. The other lifestyle modification modalities failed to reduce blood pressure or prevent the development of hypertension when compared with control. TOHP I demonstrated that modest weight loss of approximately 10 pounds was adequate to bring diastolic/systolic blood pressure down by 2.9/2.1 mm Hg, while a decrease in sodium level of 50 mmol per day was only slightly less effective (a fall of 2.1/1.2 mm Hg). The second phase of TOHP was completed in 1997.

TABLE 6. **Lifestyle Modifications**

- Nutritional changes
  - Weight loss
  - Sodium (as chloride) reduction
  - Potassium supplementation
  - Calcium supplementation
  - Magnesium supplementation
  - Fish oil supplementation
  - Fiber supplementation
  - Saturated fat and dietary cholesterol reduction
  - Alcohol reduction
- Isotonic exercise
- Stress reduction
  - Relaxation
  - Biofeedback—generalized and specific

In this trial, the effects of weight loss were compared with those of sodium reduction, and the combined results with these approaches were compared with those with usual care. At 3 years, the results were disappointing. Patients in the group receiving the combination reduced their blood pressure by 1.2/0.6 mm Hg from levels seen with usual care, while weight loss alone (a reduction of 1.3/0.9 mm Hg) and sodium restriction alone (a reduction of 1.2/0.7 mm Hg) did equally well. The results at 6 months were much more impressive, but as in so many trials of weight loss, subjects tended to gain back weight after 6 to 18 months and had half the weight loss at 36 months that they had achieved at 6 months. More hypertension was prevented in the active-care groups than in the usual-care group, emphasizing the value of lifestyle modification to *prevent* hypertension but also highlighting the lack of efficacy of a nondrug approach to *treat* established hypertension.

Although other lifestyle modification modalities may not be particularly effective at lowering blood pressure, these approaches play a role in overall cardiovascular and general health. Stopping cigarette smoking is recommended strongly and unambiguously in all smokers, not just hypertensive persons. Moderation of alcohol intake can prevent alcohol-related conditions such as cirrhosis, although consumption of up to two or even more drinks per day does seem to offer protection against cardiovascular disease. Calcium supplementation may increase bone density and prevent osteoporotic fractures and possibly colon cancer. Physical activity has benefit for overall cardiovascular health. Maintaining potassium and magnesium intake at high levels (90 mmol per day or more for potassium) has been associated with some lowering of blood pressure and prevention of hypertension, and reducing dietary intake of saturated fat and cholesterol intake can be effective at lowering serum cholesterol. Stress reduction can improve the patient's sense of well-being, even if blood pressure is not reduced by this approach.

The most interesting new clinical trial of a nonpharmacologic approach to reducing blood pressure is the Dietary Approaches to Stop Hypertension (DASH) study, also completed in 1997. This trial compared the hypotensive effects of three diets: a 2000-calorie diet with 3 grams of sodium and 25th-percentile intake of calcium, magnesium, and fiber (the usual or control diet); a diet containing the same sodium and calories but with increased magnesium, potassium, and fiber intake (the fruit and vegetable diet); and a diet that was similar to the fruit and vegetable diet but also was low in saturated fat and cholesterol (the combination diet). At the end of 8 weeks, both the fruit and vegetable and the combination diets were more effective at lowering blood pressure than the usual diet. The combination diet was superior and, for the hypertensive patients in DASH, as good as many pharmacologic agents given for a similar time period. It is now clear that hypertensive patients will benefit from a diet low in saturated fat

TABLE 7. **Oral Antihypertensive Drugs**

Drug	Trade Name	Usual Dose Range: total mg/d* (frequency/d)	Selected Side Effects and Comments*
Diuretics (partial list)			Short-term: increases cholesterol and glucose levels; biochemical abnormalities: decreases potassium, sodium, and magnesium levels, increases uric acid and calcium levels
Chlorthalidone (G)	Hygroton	12.5–50 (1)	
Hydrochlorothiazide (G)	HydroDIURIL, Microzide, Esidrix	12.5–50 (1)	
Indapamide	Lozol	1.25–5 (1)	(Milder or no hypercholesterolemia)
Metolazone	Mykrox	0.5–1.0 (1)	
	Zaroxolyn	2.5–10 (1)	
Loop diuretics			
Bumetanide (G)	Bumex	0.5–4 (2–3)	(Short duration of action, no hypercalcemia)
Ethacrynic acid	Edecrin	25–100 (2–3)	(The only non-sulfonamide diuretic; ototoxicity)
Furosemide (G)	Lasix	40–240 (2–3)	(Short duration of action, no hypercalcemia)
Torsemide	Demadex	5–100 (1–2)	
Potassium-sparing agents			Hyperkalemia
Amiloride hydrochloride (G)	Midamor	5–10 (1)	
Spironolactone (G)	Aldactone	25–100 (1)	(Gynecomastia)
Triamterene (G)	Dyrenium	25–100 (1)	
Adrenergic inhibitors			
Peripheral agents			
Guanadrel	Hylorel	10–75 (2)	(Postural hypotension, diarrhea)
Guanethidine monosulfate	Ismelin	10–150 (1)	(Postural hypotension, diarrhea)
Reserpine (G)	Serpasil	0.05–0.25 (1)	(Also acts centrally; nasal congestion, sedation, depression, activation of peptic ulcer)
Central alpha agonists			Sedation, dry mouth, bradycardia, withdrawal hypertension
Clonidine hydrochloride (G)	Catapres	0.2–1.2 (2–3)	(More withdrawal)
Guanabenz acetate (G)	Wytensin	8–32 (2)	
Guanfacine hydrochloride (G)	Tenex	1–3 (1)	(Less withdrawal)
Methyldopa (G)	Aldomet	500–3000 (2)	(Hepatic and "autoimmune" disorders)
Alpha blockers			Postural hypotension
Doxazosin mesylate	Cardura	1–16 (1)	
Prazosin hydrochloride (G)	Minipress	2–30 (2–3)	
Terazosin hydrochloride	Hytrin	1–20 (1)	
Adrenoreceptors			
Acebutolol†‡	Sectral	200–800 (1)	Bronchospasm, bradycardia, heart failure; may mask insulin-induced hypoglycemia; impaired peripheral circulation, insomnia, fatigue, decreased exercise tolerance, hypertriglyceridemia (except agents with intrinsic sympathomimetic activity)
Atenolol (G)‡	Tenormin	25–100 (1–2)	
Betaxolol‡	Kerlone	5–20 (1)	
Bisoprolol fumarate‡	Zebeta	2.5–10 (1)	
Carteolol hydrochloride†	Cartrol	2.5–10 (1)	
Metoprolol tartrate (G)‡	Lopressor	50–300 (2)	
Metoprolol succinate (G)‡	Toprol XL	50–300 (1)	
Nadolol (G)	Corgard	40–320 (1)	
Penbutolol sulfate†	Levatol	10–20 (1)	
Pindolol (G)†	Visken	10–60 (2)	
Propranolol hydrochloride (G)	Inderal	40–480 (1)	
	Inderal LA	40–480 (2)	
Timolol maleate (G)	Blocadren	20–60 (2)	
Combined alpha- and beta-adrenoreceptor blockers			
Carvedilol	Coreg	12.5–50 (2)	Postural hypotension, bronchospasm
Labetalol hydrochloride (G)	Normodyne, Trandate	200–1200 (2)	
Direct vasodilators			Headaches, fluid retention, tachycardia
Hydralazine hydrochloride (G)	Apresoline	50–300 (2)	(Lupus syndrome)
Minoxidil (G)	Loniten	5–100 (1)	(Hirsutism)

TABLE 7. **Oral Antihypertensive Drugs** *Continued*

Drug	Trade Name	Usual Dose Range: total mg/d* (frequency/d)	Selected Side Effects and Comments*
Calcium antagonists			
Non-dihydropyridines			Conduction defects, systolic dysfunction, gingival hyperplasia
Diltiazem hydrochloride	Cardizem SR	120–360 (2)	(Nausea, headache)
	Cardizem CD, Dilacor XR, Tiazac	120–360 (1)	
Verapamil hydrochloride	Isoptin SR, Calan SR	90–480 (2)	(Constipation)
	Verelan, Covera-HS	120–480 (1)	
Dihydropyridines			Edema, flushing, headache, gingival hyperplasia
Amlodipine besylate	Norvasc	2.5–10 (1)	
Felodipine	Plendil	2.5–20 (1)§	
Isradipine	DynaCirc	5–20 (2)	
	DynaCirc CR	5–20 (1)	
Nicardipine	Cardene SR	60–90 (2)	
Nifedipine	Procardia XL, Adalat CC	30–120 (1)	
Nisoldipine	Sular	20–60 (1)	
ACE inhibitors			Common: cough; rare: angioedema, hyperkalemia, rash, loss of taste, leukopenia
Benazepril hydrochloride	Lotensin	5–40 (1–2)	
Captopril (G)	Capoten	25–150 (2–3)	
Enalapril maleate	Vasotec	5–40 (1–2)	
Fosinopril sodium	Monopril	10–40 (1–2)	
Lisinopril	Prinivil, Zestril	5–40 (1)	
Moexipril	Univasc	7.5–15 (2)	
Quinapril hydrochloride	Accupril	5–80 (1–2)	
Ramipril	Altace	1.25–20 (1–2)	
Trandolapril	Mavik	1–4 (1)	
Angiotensin II receptor blockers			Hyperkalemia
Losartan potassium	Cozaar	25–100 (1–2)	
Valsartan	Diovan	80–320 (1)	
Irbesartan	Avapro	150–300 (1)	

*These dosages may vary from those listed in the *Physicians' Desk Reference* (51st edition), which may be consulted for additional information. The listing of side effects is not all-inclusive, and side effects are for the class of drugs except where noted for individual drugs (in parentheses); clinicians are urged to refer to the package insert for a more detailed listing.

†Has intrinsic sympathomimetic activity.

‡Cardioselective.

§Exceeds dosage recommended by the manufacturer.

Abbreviation: G = generic available.

Adapted from the Sixth Report of the Joint National Committee on Prevention, Detection, Evaluation, and Treatment of High Blood Pressure. Arch Intern Med *157*:2413–2446, 1997. Copyright 1997, American Medical Association.

and cholesterol, for the effects on not only lipid levels but also blood pressure.

Pharmacologic Therapy

The proper selection of an antihypertensive regimen is one of the more frequent and challenging decisions that physicians regularly have to make. Fortunately more than 80 effective antihypertensive drugs are available from which to choose. All of these agents lower blood pressure and reduce the incidence and severity of many of its consequences.

A variety of ways exist to classify antihypertensive agents. In general, these drugs can be classified as those that are effective parenterally and are indicated only for a hypertensive crisis and those that work orally. These agents can be further subclassified by pharmacologic class and alleged primary mechanism of action. A partial list of currently available antihypertensive drugs and combination preparations, with the usual starting and maximum doses for adults under 60 years of age, is shown in Tables 7 and 8, respectively. In hypertensive patients over the age of 60, I recommend starting therapy with half the dose used in younger patients. Such precautions may not be necessary with angiotensin-converting enzyme (ACE) inhibitors and angiotensin receptor blockers (ARBs), whose adverse reactions are not dose-dependent. For young children in whom a secondary cause of hypertension has been excluded, drug therapy has not been well studied, and lifestyle modification should be given a thorough trial before pharmacologic therapy is started. Most agents that are safe and effective in adults will also work in children with appropriate adjustment in dose.

The choice of the drug with which to begin therapy

TABLE 8. **Combination Drugs for Hypertension**

Combination	Trade Name
Beta-adrenergic blocker/diuretic	
Atenolol, 50 or 100 mg/chlorthalidone, 25 mg	Tenoretic
Bisoprolol fumarate, 2.5, 5, or 10 mg/hydrochlorothiazide, 6.25 mg	Ziac*
Metoprolol tartrate, 50 or 100 mg/hydrochlorothiazide, 25 or 50 mg	Lopressor HCT
Nadolol, 40 or 80 mg/bendroflumethiazide, 5 mg	Corzide
Propranolol hydrochloride, 40 or 80 mg/hydrochlorothiazide, 25 mg	Inderide
Propranolol hydrochloride (extended-release), 80, 120, or 160 mg/hydrochlorothiazide, 50 mg	Inderide LA
Timolol maleate, 10 mg/hydrochlorothiazide, 25 mg	Timolide
ACE inhibitor/diuretic	
Benazepril hydrochloride, 5, 10, or 20 mg/hydrochlorothiazide, 6.25, 12.5, or 25 mg	Lotensin HCT
Captopril, 25 or 50 mg/hydrochlorothiazide, 15 or 25 mg	Capozide*
Enalapril maleate, 5 or 10 mg/hydrochlorothiazide, 12.5 or 25 mg	Vaseretic
Lisinopril, 10 or 20 mg/hydrochlorothiazide, 12.5 or 25 mg	Prinzide, Zestoretic
Angiotensin A-II receptor antagonist/diuretic	
Losartan potassium, 50 mg/hydrochlorothiazide, 12.5 mg	Hyzaar
Calcium antagonist/ACE inhibitor	
Amlodipine besylate, 2.5 or 5 mg/benazepril hydrochloride, 10 or 20 mg	Lotrel
Diltiazem hydrochloride, 180 mg/enalapril maleate, 5 mg	Teczem
Verapamil hydrochloride (extended-release), 180 or 240 mg/trandolapril, 1, 2, or 4 mg	Tarka
Felodipine, 5 mg/enalapril maleate, 5 mg	Lexxel
Other combinations	
Triamterene, 37.5, 50, or 75 mg/hydrochlorothiazide, 25 or 50 mg	Dyazide, Maxide
Spironolactone, 25 or 50 mg/hydrochlorothiazide, 25 or 50 mg	Aldactazide
Amiloride hydrochloride, 5 mg/hydrochlorothiazide, 50 mg	Moduretic
Guanethidine monosulfate, 10 mg/hydrochlorothiazide, 25 mg	Esimil
Hydralazine hydrochloride, 25, 50, or 100 mg/hydrochlorothiazide, 25 or 50 mg	Apresazide
Methyldopa, 250 or 500 mg/hydrochlorothiazide, 15, 25, 30, or 50 mg	Aldoril
Reserpine, 0.125 mg/hydrochlorothiazide, 25 or 50 mg	Hydropres
Reserpine, 0.10 mg/hydralazine hydrochloride, 25 mg/hydrochlorothiazide, 15 mg	Ser-Ap-Es
Clonidine hydrochloride, 0.1, 0.2, or 0.3 mg/chlorthalidone, 15 mg	Combipres
Methyldopa, 250 mg/chlorothiazide, 150 or 250 mg	Aldochlor
Reserpine, 0.125 or 0.25 mg/chlorthalidone, 25 or 50 mg	Demi-Regroton
Reserpine, 0.125 or 0.25 mg/chlorothiazide, 250 or 500 mg	Diupres
Prazosin hydrochloride, 1, 2, or 5 mg/polythiazide, 0.5 mg	Minizide

*Approved for initial therapy by the FDA.
Abbreviation: ACE = angiotensin-converting enzyme.
Adapted from the Sixth Report of the Joint National Committee on Prevention, Detection, Evaluation, and Treatment of High Blood Pressure. Arch Intern Med *157*:2413–2446, 1997. Copyright 1997, American Medical Association.

is probably the most important decision for the clinician to make. Approximately half of the patients will respond to and tolerate most rationally chosen options. If the clinician chooses wisely, the first-choice drug will be successful in getting blood pressure to goal, and that will be the drug the patient remains on for the usually indefinite period of therapy. The clinician must select a regimen that is affordable and compatible with the patient's lifestyle and job requirements. In view of all of the effective options available, the clinician must pay very close attention to the patient's specific needs and plan the regimen accordingly. Whatever drug is chosen, the aim of treatment is to reduce systolic blood pressure to a goal of below 140 mm Hg *and* to reduce diastolic blood pressure to below 90 mm Hg. In diabetics, a goal of below 130 mm Hg for systolic blood pressure and below 85 mm Hg for diastolic blood pressure has been recommended by JNC VI. In patients with renal disease and marked proteinuria (a urinary excretion rate of 1 gram or more per day), the goal is even lower (below 125/75 mm Hg). Although the benefits of this level of aggressive therapy have not yet been proved, results of clinical trials suggest that use of these treatment goals will prevent substantially more cardiovascular or other untoward events than

TABLE 9. **Factors in the Choice of Agents for Antihypertensive Therapy**

- Efficacy
  - Clinical end points
  - Surrogate end points
- Safety
  - Clinical side effects
  - Biochemical side effects
- Co-morbidity and other risk factors
- Special populations
- Dosage schedule
- Drug interactions
- Cost
- Mechanism of action of the drug
- Pathophysiology of the patient's hypertension

would otherwise occur, with little if any harm to the patient.

The clinician should consider several factors when selecting a drug for initial antihypertensive therapy, as summarized in Table 9. In practice, more than half of the patients will not achieve target blood pressure levels with monotherapy; therefore, these recommendations are also appropriate for selecting additional agents required to bring blood pressure to goal.

Efficacy

JNC VI has properly distinguished between clinical end points and surrogate end points in selecting its treatment recommendations (Table 10). *Clinical end points* are the cardiovascular and other events for which hypertension is treated, while *surrogate* (or intermediate) *end points* are factors that may contribute to clinical end points and can be favorably or unfavorably affected by treatment. To date, thiazide diuretics, beta-adrenoreceptor blockers, and dihydropyridine calcium antagonists have been shown to reduce the frequency of clinical end points when these agents are used for initial therapy in appropriately designed and implemented clinical trials. Other agents such as ACE inhibitors (enalapril), peripheral sympatholytics (reserpine and guanethidine), and centrally acting $alpha_2$ agonists (methyldopa) and vasodilators (hydralazine) have also been used in clinical trials as the second, third, or even fourth agents to be added to bring blood pressure under control. Of these, only ACE inhibitors represent an option for initial therapy. Reliable data from long-term, properly performed clinical trials that focused on cardiovascular or other untoward events formed the basis for the JNC VI recommendations. JNC VI has also recognized two other critical factors that enter into the process of making the most efficacious choice for treatment in an individual hypertensive patient:

- Considerable data are derived from trials conducted in hypertensive patients who were enrolled because of other conditions (type 1 diabetes mellitus or heart failure, for example).
- Individual patients may have certain co-morbid conditions for which a specific agent might be appropriate, but no trial is yet completed in which that agent has been compared with drugs for which clinical trial data are available (Table 11).

TABLE 10. **End Points for Initiation of Antihypertensive Therapy**

Clinical End Points
Mortality from all causes
Cardiovascular mortality
Coronary artery disease
Cerebrovascular disease
Heart failure
Progressive renal insufficiency and end-stage renal disease
Peripheral vascular disease
Aortic dissection
Progression to stage III hypertension
Hypertensive crises
Surrogate End Points
Cardiac
Left ventricular hypertrophy
Systolic dysfunction
Diastolic dysfunction
Renal
Proteinuria
Decline in glomerular filtration rate
Vascular
Atherosclerosis
Blood pressure
Metabolic
Potassium—decreased
Magnesium—decreased
Uric acid—increased
Total cholesterol—increased
LDL cholesterol—increased
HDL cholesterol—decreased
Triglycerides—increased
Insulin resistance—increased
Fibrinogen—increased

Abbreviations: LDL = low-density lipoprotein; HDL = high-density lipoprotein.

Adverse Reactions and Side Effects

Two primary types of adverse reactions or side effects may occur with antihypertensive therapy: clinical and biochemical (Table 12). Clinical side effects are directly evident to the patient and are perceived to be related to the medication. These adverse reactions or side effects require that the drug be stopped or the dose reduced, or that the patient be willing to remain on therapy until he or she becomes tolerant of the reaction or it disappears. All antihypertensive agents, with the exception of ACE inhibitors and ARBs, have dose-dependent side effects, and a drug should not necessarily be abandoned if a lower dose is tolerable. Biochemical side effects may lead to clinical side effects (e.g., hypokalemia from thiazide diuretics causing muscle weakness, palpitations, nocturia, or polyuria), but usually the biochemical side effects that occur with antihypertensives are more troublesome to the provider than to the patient. The drugs recommended for initial therapy generally cause few clinical side effects at the doses that lower blood pressure. Drugs not recommended for initial or monotherapy are either ineffective alone or substantially less well tolerated than those chosen as appropriate for starting treatment. A series of fixed-dose combinations have been introduced that have fewer clinical side effects than some of the component drugs have when used for monotherapy (see Table 8). The best example is the combination of dihydropyridine calcium antagonists with ACE inhibitors. Data for all of these fixed-dose combinations have shown a significantly lower incidence of edema formation when the two agents are given together than that experienced with dihydropyridine calcium antagonists given alone. The most likely explanation for this observation relates to the mechanism of action of the two classes of agents: ACE inhibitors dilate both arterioles and venules, providing balanced reduction of pressure at the capillary level. Dihydropyridine calcium antagonists dilate the arteriolar bed but do

TABLE 11. **Considerations in Individualizing Antihypertensive Drug Therapy**

Indication	Therapeutic Agent(s)
Compelling Indications Unless Contraindicated	
Diabetes mellitus (type 1) with proteinuria	ACE I
Heart failure	ACE I, diuretics
Isolated systolic hypertension (older patients)	Diuretics (preferred), CA (long-acting DHP)
Myocardial infarction	Beta-adrenoreceptor blockers (non-ISA), ACE I (with systolic dysfunction)
May Have Favorable Effects on Co-morbid Conditions*	
Angina	Beta-adrenoreceptor blockers, CA
Atrial tachycardia and fibrillation	Beta-adrenoreceptor blockers, CA (non-DHP)
Cyclosporine-induced hypertension (caution with the dose of cyclosporine)	CA
Diabetes mellitus (types 1 and 2) with proteinuria	ACE I (preferred)
Diabetes mellitus (type 2)	Low-dose diuretics
Dyslipidemia	Peripheral alpha$_1$-adrenoreceptor blockers
Essential tremor	Beta-adrenoreceptor blockers (non-CS)
Heart failure	Carvedilol, losartan potassium
Hyperthyroidism	Beta-adrenoreceptor blockers
Migraine	Beta-adrenoreceptor blockers (non-CS), CA (non-DHP)
Myocardial infarction	Diltiazem hydrochloride, verapamil hydrochloride
Osteoporosis	Thiazide diuretics
Preoperative hypertension	Beta-adrenoreceptor blockers
Prostatism (BHP)	Peripheral alpha$_1$-adrenoreceptor blockers
Renal insufficiency (caution in renovascular hypertension and serum creatinine ≥3 mg/dL)	ACE I, angiotensin receptor blockers
May Have Unfavorable Effects on Co-morbid Conditions*†	
Bronchospastic disease	Beta-adrenoreceptor blockers‡
Depression	Beta-adrenoreceptor blockers, central alpha agonists, reserpine‡
Diabetes mellitus (types 1 and 2)	Beta-adrenoreceptor blockers, high-dose diuretics
Dyslipidemia	Beta-adrenoreceptor blockers (non-ISA), diuretics (high-dose)
Gout	Diuretics
Second- or third-degree heart block	Beta-adrenoreceptor blockers,‡ CA (non-DHP)‡
Heart failure	Beta-adrenoreceptor blockers (except carvedilol) CA (except amlodipine besylate, felodipine)
Liver disease	Labetalol hydrochloride, methyldopa‡
Peripheral vascular disease	Beta-adrenoreceptor blockers
Pregnancy	ACE I,‡ angiotensin receptor blockers‡
Renal insufficiency	Potassium-sparing agents
Renovascular disease	ACE I, angiotensin receptor blockers

*Conditions and (nonpreferred) drugs are listed in alphabetical order.
†These drugs may be used with special monitoring unless contraindicated.
‡Contraindicated.
Abbreviations: ACE I = angiotensin-converting enzyme inhibitors; BPH = benign prostatic hyperplasia; CA = calcium antagonist; DHP = dihydropyridine; ISA = intrinsic sympathomimetic activity; MI = myocardial infarction; CS = cardioselective.
Adapted from the Sixth Report of the Joint National Committee on Prevention, Detection, Evaluation, and Treatment of High Blood Pressure. Arch Intern Med *157*:2413–2446, 1997. Copyright 1997, American Medical Association.

little to the venous side of the microcirculation, which may lead to leakage of fluid from capillaries. The additional venular dilation from the ACE inhibitor prevents much of this fluid loss, so there is much less clinical edema.

The importance of biochemical side effects lies in the danger that these permutations of lipids, glucose, and insulin may aggravate other risk factors and accelerate the clinical impact of dyslipidemias and/or glucose intolerance and insulin resistance. Whether the minor and often short-term effects on total serum cholesterol, high-density lipoprotein cholesterol (HDL-C), or triglycerides (TGs) resulting from therapy with thiazides or beta-adrenoreceptor blockers are responsible for an increase in coronary artery disease remains to be proved. When these agents are given in the doses recommended, these changes and the accompanying electrolyte disturbances are modest, although it is still possible that at high doses, thiazides could reduce serum potassium sufficiently to increase the rate of sudden cardiac death. Whether the increase in insulin resistance seen with thiazide diuretics and beta-adrenoreceptor blockers or the hypokalemia from thiazide diuretics has precipitated diabetes mellitus sooner, or in patients who would not otherwise have become diabetic, remains to be proved. Although it is not certain that these metabolic adverse reactions are clinically relevant, I often treat patients with diabetes mellitus or dyslipidemias with another antihypertensive, so long as blood

TABLE 12. **Selected Important Adverse Reactions to Antihypertensive Agents**

Drug	Adverse Effects — *Clinical*	Adverse Effects — *Biochemical*
Diuretics		
Thiazides	Weakness Sexual dysfunction Diabetes mellitus Gout	Hypokalemia Hyponatremia Hypomagnesemia Hyperglycemia Hypertriglyceridemia Hypercholesterolemia Hyperuricemia Hypercalcemia Reduction in HDL cholesterol
Loop-active agents	Volume depletion	Same as thiazides except for hypercalcemia
Potassium-sparing agents	Gynecomastia and breast tenderness Sexual dysfunction Menstrual irregularities (spironolactone only)	Hyperkalemia (all)
Sympatholytics		
Beta-adrenoreceptor blockers	Fatigue Bronchospasm Intermittent claudication Bradycardia and heart block Systolic dysfunction Sleep disturbances Diabetes mellitus	Hypertriglyceridemia Reduction in HDL cholesterol Hyperglycemia
Peripheral $alpha_1$-adrenoreceptor	Syncope Orthostatic hypotension Headache	
Alpha/beta-adrenoreceptor blockers	Syncope Orthostatic hypotension Headache	
Central $alpha_2$ agonists	Sedation Dry mouth Orthostatic hypotension Fatigue Rebound hypertension Liver toxicity (methyldopa) Hemolytic anemia (methyldopa) Rash (clonidine patch)	
Peripherally acting sympatholytics	Orthostatic hypotension Retrograde ejaculation (guanethidine) Lethargy Depression (reserpine) Dizziness (reserpine) Dyspepsia	
Angiotensin-converting enzyme inhibitors	Cough Angioedema Renal failure	Hyperkalemia
Angiotensin receptor blockers	Renal failure	Hyperkalemia
Calcium entry blockers		
Non-dihydropyridines	Bradycardia Heart block Constipation (verapamil) Headache (diltiazem)	
Dihydropyridines	Headache Dizziness Edema Palpitations	
Direct vasodilators	Palpitations Edema Headache Hirsutism (minoxidil)	

Abbreviation: HDL = high-density lipoprotein.

pressure is successfully controlled. Fixed-dose combinations may also ameliorate biochemical adverse reactions. ACE inhibitors (and ARBs) and thiazides, when given together, produce few if any of the metabolic abnormalities associated with thiazides and are also available as fixed-dose combinations.

With the exception of ACE inhibitors and ARBs, the incidence of clinical side effects tends to increase with increasing doses. In patients who develop an adverse reaction to a drug given in a high dose or in a dose previously well tolerated, discontinuation of the drug is not necessarily the solution. Instead, the dose can be lowered and another antihypertensive added to reduce blood pressure to goal. The primary problems with ACE inhibitors are cough and angioedema. Both of these adverse reactions tend to be idiosyncratic, occur with all representatives of that class of agents, and are not dose-related. Thus, reducing the dose or changing to a different ACE inhibitor is rarely helpful. Because other clinical side effects are unusual, ACE inhibitors can and should be increased to the maximum recommended dose before therapy is abandoned or another agent is added. ARBs as a class appear to be the best tolerated of all currently available antihypertensives and can be used for initial therapy in cases in which ACE inhibitors appear to be a good option.

Co-morbidity and Other Risk Factors

The presence of other risk factors and active clinical problems may exert a profound influence on the initial and subsequent choices for antihypertensive therapy. The appreciation that the drugs prescribed to reduce blood pressure can either improve or adversely affect other conditions that may exist in the patient provides a strong rationale for obtaining a thorough history, performing a complete physical examination, and determining certain laboratory parameters before the initiation of treatment. This fact is the basis for the JNC VI recommendations that diuretics and beta-adrenoreceptor blockers be used when a patient has "uncomplicated" hypertension but that these co-morbid conditions may and should alter the choice, even though a randomized clinical trial is not yet available to support the decision (see Table 11). The regimen selected must be tailored to the one that best suits the needs of the patient.

DYSLIPIDEMIAS

Hypertensive patients with lipid abnormalities probably should not receive therapy with drugs that worsen their particular dyslipidemia. This is an important issue, because perhaps as many as half of the patients presenting with hypertension also have an abnormal lipid profile. Although it has not as yet been possible to prove that the minimal changes in serum lipids caused by certain classes of antihypertensives are harmful, it is certainly prudent to choose an equally effective drug that is "lipid-neutral," or to select one that may even improve the lipid profile. Peripheral alpha$_1$-adrenoreceptor blockers, for example, reduce total cholesterol and low-density lipoprotein cholesterol (LDL-C) by approximately 8 to 10% and reduce serum TG by 15% and HDL-C by 10 to 15%. Although these alterations are modest, the overall cardiovascular risk of a hypertensive patient whose lipid levels are changed in this fashion is clearly improved. ACE inhibitors do not affect serum lipids, and in some studies benefits similar to those seen with use of peripheral alpha$_1$-adrenoreceptor blockers have been observed. ARBs and calcium antagonists are lipid-neutral.

In large doses (more than 25 mg per day), thiazide diuretics and related compounds such as chlorthalidone at least transiently raise total cholesterol and LDL-C (by 5 to 10%) and may lower HDL-C (by 2 to 4%). Triglycerides are increased by 15 to 30%. With the doses currently recommended, few if any changes in these parameters are seen. The clinical relevance of these adverse reactions is unclear. Beta-adrenoreceptor blockers without intrinsic sympathomimetic activity (ISA) lower HDL-C even more (10%) and also raise TG (approximately 20%) without affecting total cholesterol or LDL-C. Those agents with ISA and combined alpha- and beta-adrenoreceptor blockers are lipid-neutral. Other sympatholytics do not affect the lipid profile, and direct vasodilators (e.g., hydralazine) raise HDL-C and lower total cholesterol and LDL-C and TG levels even when used in combination with thiazide diuretics.

GLUCOSE AND INSULIN

Antihypertensive drugs also affect glucose metabolism and may worsen or improve insulin sensitivity. The results with use of various agents reflect the changes that occur in the lipid profile. Peripheral alpha$_1$-adrenoreceptor blockers and ACE inhibitors improve insulin sensitivity, although this property may be limited to captopril, enalapril, and perindopril. Both thiazides and beta-adrenoreceptor blockers worsen insulin sensitivity and may occasionally precipitate glucose intolerance and clinical diabetes mellitus. Very few data exist for other classes of antihypertensives, although some preliminary studies with ARBs (candasartan* and irbesartan) are promising. JNC VI recommends that hypertensive patients with type 1 diabetes mellitus be given ACE inhibitors, based on data from a randomized clinical trial. To date, no studies yet completed prove the value of these drugs in patients with type 2 diabetes, although many experts believe that the benefit shown with type 1 diabetes will also be shown with non–insulin-dependent diabetes mellitus. Some still preliminary analyses have raised concerns about the safety of dihydropyridine calcium antagonists in patients with type 2 diabetes, suggesting that these agents may increase cardiovascular events and proteinuria. Non-dihydropyridine calcium antagonists alone and in combination with ACE inhibitors may lower urinary protein and may be particularly useful in diabetic patients with nephropathy. Even though thiazide diuretics may adversely affect insulin sensi-

*Not available in the United States.

tivity, data from the Systolic Hypertension in the Elderly Program (SHEP) showed that clinical events were statistically significantly reduced by low-dose chlorthalidone (plus atenolol in some volunteers); therefore, the use of these agents is considered appropriate in older hypertensive patients with non–insulin-dependent diabetes mellitus. At this time, it appears that no drugs are contraindicated in hypertensive patients with diabetes mellitus. What is most important is getting blood pressure to goal, which is less than 130/85 mm Hg in this subgroup of hypertensive patients.

LEFT VENTRICULAR HYPERTROPHY

Left ventricular hypertrophy is a common consequence of hypertension and an important independent risk factor for cardiovascular disease and premature mortality. It is especially common in the elderly, especially women, and is often associated with diastolic dysfunction. It appears that all drugs that reduce blood pressure (with the possible exception of direct vasodilators) will reduce left ventricular mass. Data from meta-analyses suggest that agents that block the renin-angiotensin-aldosterone (RAA) system reduce left ventricular mass better than do other antihypertensives. However, neither the Treatment of Mild Hypertension Study (TOMHS) nor the most recent Veterans Administration Trial of Monotherapy supports this contention. In those studies, all classes of commonly used antihypertensives were successful at reducing left ventricular mass. Thiazide diuretics were the most successful. Salt restriction and weight loss also are effective.

SYSTOLIC AND DIASTOLIC DYSFUNCTION AND HEART FAILURE

In patients with heart failure caused by systolic dysfunction, ACE inhibitors, diuretics, and possibly ARBs should be included in the antihypertensive regimen. Dihydropyridine calcium antagonists (amlodipine and felodipine, in particular) and carvedilol, a combined alpha- and beta-adrenoreceptor blocker, may also be useful in these patients. The role of beta-adrenoreceptor blockers when systolic dysfunction is present still needs to be elucidated. For patients with diastolic dysfunction, non-dihydropyridine calcium antagonists, particularly verapamil, and beta-adrenoreceptor blockers may provide a distinct advantage over other antihypertensives.

OTHER CONDITIONS

The presence of certain other co-morbid conditions also influences the choice of an antihypertensive agent. Hypertensive patients with bronchospasm should not, for example, be treated with beta-adrenoreceptor blockers, and patients with gout should not receive thiazide diuretics. Patients with renal insufficiency usually need loop-active diuretics to achieve the reduction in plasma volume necessary to reduce their blood pressure. Although the efficacy of ACE inhibitors has been proved only for patients with type 1 diabetes and proteinuria, patients with renal insufficiency and proteinuria from type 2 diabetes may also benefit from ACE inhibitors and possibly ARBs; therefore, these agents should be part of the antihypertensive regimen for this group as well.

Some studies in humans have suggested that the combination of ACE inhibitors and non-dihydropyridine calcium antagonists may slow the decline of glomerular filtration rate in patients with renal insufficiency and may therefore be the agents of choice in such patients. Before an ACE inhibitor or ARB is used, the presence of bilateral renal artery stenosis or renal artery stenosis to a single kidney must be ruled out if the clinical profile of the patient suggests the possibility of either condition. Serum potassium must be carefully monitored, although the likelihood of clinically significant hyperkalemia is small.

Hypertensive patients with angina pectoris should be given a beta-adrenoreceptor blocker or calcium antagonist, and those who have had a myocardial infarction should receive a beta-adrenoreceptor blocker without ISA if they do not have systolic dysfunction. Those with low ejection fractions will almost surely benefit from treatment with an ACE inhibitor and possibly an ARB. Cigarette smokers may not respond to non-cardioselective beta-adrenoreceptor blockers without ISA, and obese patients may do better with thiazide diuretics, because volume is often expanded in obesity-related hypertension.

Patients who wish to perform at maximum activity levels may not do well with beta-adrenoreceptor blockers, and those with peripheral vascular disease or cardiac conduction defects may also be harmed by these drugs; those with anxiety may be helped. Non-dihydropyridine calcium antagonists should also be avoided in patients with cardiac conduction defects, and patients with esophageal strictures or reduced esophageal motility may have problems with some sustained-release preparations. Hypertensive patients with osteoporosis may do especially well with thiazide diuretics, which increase bone mass and prevent osteoporotic fractures. In elderly men with prostatism, blood pressure will improve and symptoms will be ameliorated by treatment with peripheral alpha$_1$-adrenoreceptor blockers.

Special Populations and Special Situations

The choice of antihypertensive therapy is often influenced by whether the patient is a member of a particular demographic group or by the severity or lack of responsiveness of the hypertension. Different therapies are indicated for pregnant hypertensive women and for hypertensive patients undergoing surgery.

DEMOGRAPHIC CONSIDERATIONS

African-Americans and Other Ethnic Minority Groups. Some classes of antihypertensive agents reduce blood pressure more or less effectively in certain ethnic groups. Thiazide diuretics, for example, are more effective in African-Americans than in whites, while ACE inhibitors, ARBs, and beta-adrenoreceptor blockers are more effective at lower doses in whites. Many African-Americans will respond to agents that block the RAA system (ACE inhibitors, ARBs, and beta-adrenoreceptor blockers) but often need higher doses than do whites or Asians. If an African-American patient with hypertension will benefit from the adjunctive pharmacologic effects of a drug on type 1 diabetes or heart failure, for example, the drug should definitely be used even if additional agents will be needed to reduce blood pressure to goal. Peripheral alpha$_1$-adrenoreceptor blockers, combined alpha- and beta-adrenoreceptor blockers, and calcium antagonists are equally effective in all hypertensive patients in all ethnic groups. In general, the response rates to antihypertensives in persons of Hispanic heritage is usually intermediate between those seen in whites and in African-Americans, while East Asians, although not necessarily South Asians (patients from the Indian subcontinent), often need smaller doses than do whites.

Age. All classes of antihypertensives lower blood pressure effectively in older persons, although often the doses needed to reach goal are lower than those necessary in young and middle-aged hypertensive patients. Certain drugs and certain classes of drugs, however, should be avoided or used with caution in older patients. Agents such as peripheral alpha$_1$-adrenoreceptor blockers and some sympatholytics can exacerbate the postural fall in blood pressure seen more frequently in older persons who have baroreceptor dysfunction and can lead to symptomatic postural hypotension. Non-dihydropyridine calcium antagonists and beta-adrenoreceptor blockers may aggravate subtle or subclinical conduction defects or precipitate systolic dysfunction and heart failure. Verapamil may not be well tolerated in some older persons who are bothered by constipation, while giving alpha$_1$-adrenoreceptor blockers to men with prostatism may be especially beneficial. Cough from ACE inhibitors may be more common in older women. In elderly patients with isolated systolic hypertension, diuretics may be particularly effective at lowering blood pressure, and both diuretics and dihydropyridine calcium antagonists have been shown to reduce morbidity and mortality in older persons with stage II and stage III isolated systolic hypertension.

The approach to the management of hypertension in adolescents is similar to that used for adults, with only some minor variations. For the most part, adolescent patients have essential hypertension, and very little evaluation for secondary causes of hypertension is appropriate, unless a feature of the patient's clinical or laboratory presentation of hypertension suggests an identifiable cause. It is appropriate to implement lifestyle modification if it can be achieved and to delay starting pharmacologic therapy unless the patient has stage III hypertension or end-organ damage. ACE inhibitors and ARBs should not be given to female adolescents or adults who are likely to become pregnant because of the high likelihood of fetal wastage and congenital abnormalities. Less is known about the safety and efficacy of newer agents in young children; therefore, the therapeutic approach tends to rely on drugs that have been available longer.

Gender. There is no evidence of any difference in response to antihypertensives between men and women. The results of clinical trials in which higher risk women have been included show almost identical benefits in both genders. Concerns that women would not have the same good results with treatment as those seen in men have turned out to be groundless.

PREGNANCY

In women with pregnancy-induced hypertension, methyldopa and hydralazine have been the therapeutic agents of choice for decades and remain so. There has been some favorable experience with beta-adrenoreceptor blockers, particularly atenolol, and calcium antagonists, especially nifedipine, but little is known about the efficacy of other drugs. Diuretics can be used if the patient had used them before pregnancy, but these agents should be used with caution in the second and third trimesters or if preeclampsia is suspected. Pregnant women can generally stay on the regimen that was successful before pregnancy, with the exception of ACE inhibitors and ARBs.

HYPERTENSIVE CRISES

The proper management of hypertensive crises requires rapid and accurate diagnosis and careful selection of therapeutic agents. Hypertensive emergencies are those conditions that require blood pressure to be reduced within minutes. For hypertensive crises classified as urgent, the reduction can proceed over hours. For both types of crises, the clinician must assiduously avoid an overzealous approach to blood pressure reduction and should try only to prevent acute target organ damage. Hypotension and decreased organ perfusion from overaggressive therapy usually pose a bigger threat to the patient than does the elevated blood pressure at clinical presentation. The ideal drug with which to treat a hypertensive emergency is one that is effective parenterally, virtually always works, has an almost instant onset of action, and has a very short duration of action so that therapy can be stopped or the dose reduced if blood pressure is lowered too far. The drug should be easy to titrate and not cause cerebral or cardiac dysfunction.

The ideal drug for use in urgencies is one that is orally active and almost always effective, but the onset and the duration of action can be longer than those for drugs used for emergencies. Drugs useful for the urgent treatment of hypertension should also not cause dysfunction of vital organs and ideally should be an appropriate choice for long-term therapy. In bona fide urgencies, the patient should be started on an oral regimen that is acceptable for long-term treatment, and the treating clinician must be certain that the patient is seen within 24 to 48 hours. Table 13 lists selected examples of hyperten-

TABLE 13. **Parenteral Drugs for Treatment of Hypertensive Emergencies***

Drug	Dose	Onset of Action	Duration of Action	Adverse Effects†	Special Indications
Vasodilators					
Sodium nitroprusside (Nitropress)	0.25–10 μg/kg/min IV as infusion‡ (maximal dose for 10 min only)	Immediate	1–2 min	Nausea, vomiting, muscle twitching, sweating, thiocyanate and cyanide intoxication	Most hypertensive emergencies; caution with high intracranial pressure or azotemia
Nicardipine hydrochloride (Cardene I.V.)	5–15 mg/h IV	5–10 min	1–4 h	Tachycardia, headache, flushing, local phlebitis	Most hypertensive emergencies except acute heart failure; caution with coronary ischemia
Fenoldopam (Corlopam)	0.1–0.3 μg/kg/min IV as infusion	<5 min	30 min	Tachycardia, headache, nausea, flushing	Most hypertensive emergencies; caution with glaucoma
Nitroglycerin	5–100 μg/min IV as infusion‡	2–5 min	3–5 min	Headache, vomiting, methemoglobinemia, tolerance with prolonged use	Coronary ischemia
Enalaprilat (Vasotec I.V.)	1.25–5 mg q 6 h IV	15–30 min	6 h	Precipitous fall in pressure in high-renin states; response variable	Acute left ventricular failure; avoid in acute myocardial infarction
Hydralazine hydrochloride (Apresoline)	10–20 mg IV 10–50 mg IM	10–20 min 20–30 min	3–8 h	Tachycardia, flushing, headache, vomiting, aggravation of angina	Eclampsia
Diazoxide (Hyperstat)	50–100 mg IV, bolus repeated, or 15–30 mg/min as infusion	2–4 min	6–12 h	Nausea, flushing, tachycardia, chest pain	Now obsolete when no intensive monitoring available
Adrenergic inhibitors					
Labetalol hydrochloride (Normodyne, Trandate)	20–80 mg IV as bolus every 10 min; 0.5–2.0 mg/min IV as infusion	5–10 min	3–6 h	Vomiting, scalp tingling, burning in throat, dizziness, nausea, heart block, orthostatic hypotension	Most hypertensive emergencies except acute heart failure
Esmolol hydrochloride (Brevibloc)	250–500 μg/kg/min for 1 min, then 50–100 μg/kg/min for 4 min; may repeat sequence	1–2 min	10–20 min	Hypotension, nausea	Aortic dissection, perioperative
Phentolamine (Regitine)	5–15 mg IV	1–2 min	3–10 min	Tachycardia, flushing, headache	Catecholamine excess

*These doses may differ from those in the *Physicians' Desk Reference* (51st edition).
†Hypotension may occur with all agents.
‡Requires special delivery system.
Adapted from the Sixth Report of the Joint National Committee on Prevention, Detection, Evaluation, and Treatment of High Blood Pressure. Arch Intern Med *157*:2413–2446, 1997. Copyright 1997, American Medical Association.

sive crises and gives recommendations as to what to use and what to avoid.

REFRACTORY HYPERTENSION

Hypertension can be considered to be refractory or resistant to treatment if the patient's blood pressure remains elevated (at 140 mm Hg systolic or 90 mm Hg diastolic, or higher) on the maximum dose of two or more appropriately chosen antihypertensive agents. The common reasons why some cases are refractory to treatment are usually related to clinician and/or patient behavior. The clinician, for example, may not be prescribing the right drugs or may not be giving them in the right dose or time schedule, or may not recognize that the patient has an identifiable secondary cause for hypertension, which often may not respond well to conventional therapy. For example, hypertensive patients with renal disease need loop-active agents, whereas those with normal renal function respond better to a thiazide. A different clinician may have prescribed another drug, such as a nonsteroidal anti-inflammatory drug (NSAID), which may interfere with the antihypertensive effect of the agent chosen to reduce blood pressure. Patient-related behavior can also result in apparent unresponsiveness to therapy. In fact, in most analyses of refractory hypertension, failure properly to adhere to the medical regimen is the most common reason for resistance to treatment. Nonadherence should be considered in all patients whose blood pressure is not at goal. No reliable clinical or biochemical clues to nonadherence exist, although patients who fail to keep appointments and those who do not appear to be filling their prescriptions as often as they should are more likely to be not taking their medication properly. Obese patients may not respond as well to treatment as do hypertensive patients of normal weight. Also, patients may be ingesting excessive alcohol or using over-the-counter preparations such as sympathomimetic amines (e.g., nasal decongestants or NSAIDs). In addition, a number of patients with seemingly refractory hypertension that is actually adequately controlled out of the office may still have elevated measurements when the clinician or other staff do the readings. These persons have "office resistance," which should be distinguished from "white coat hypertension"—a term that should be reserved to describe the presence of elevated readings obtained in the office, but not in other settings, in patients who are not receiving antihypertensive therapy.

Dosage Schedule

Two elements of dosage scheduling need to be considered in prescribing antihypertensive therapy. One is the ability of patients to comply with the regimen and the other is the need to treat hypertension for all 24 hours of the day and night. Patients are much more likely to take their medications as prescribed if the agent is effective when taken once or, at most, twice a day (see Table 7). Adherence to any therapy falls dramatically when more than three pills per day of any kind are needed; therefore, all unnecessary elements of a regimen should be stopped. Fixed-dose combinations that provide the right amounts of the desired agents can be used to reduce the number of pills taken daily and could improve adherence to the antihypertensive regimen.

It has become apparent that a greater-than-expected percentage of myocardial infarctions, strokes, and episodes of sudden death occur between 6 AM and noon or within 1 hour of awakening. One possible explanation for this phenomenon relates to the circadian pattern of blood pressure during the day and night in both normal and hypertensive persons. Blood pressure tends to be at its lowest level from midnight to 4 AM, at which time it rises and peaks at approximately noon. It gradually falls until 2 to 4 AM, when, coincident with secretion of cortisol and catecholamines, blood pressure begins to rise again. An increasing number of investigators believe that this rise in blood pressure predisposes to the rupture of vulnerable plaque and results in the greater frequency of cardiovascular events in the morning hours. Appreciation of the importance of the circadian variation in blood pressure and cardiovascular events has two therapeutic ramifications. The first is the appreciation that for drugs to be classified as once-a-day agents, their blood pressure–lowering effect at trough should be at least 50% of their effect at peak. Some drugs once classified as once-a-day antihypertensives, such as atenolol and enalapril, may not meet these criteria and may be better used twice a day. The second ramification is the development of a "chronobiologic" approach to antihypertensive therapy, which uses a drug delivery system that releases active drug for 18 hours beginning about 2 to 4 AM, leaving the patient with no active drug from about 10 PM to 2 AM. The rationale for this approach is to avoid excessive blood pressure lowering during the middle of the night, when blood pressure falls coincident with the usual circadian rhythm. This sustained-release preparation provides adequate active drug when the blood pressure rises prior to awakening and during the peak time of cardiovascular events, that period between 6 AM and noon.

Drug Interactions

The selection of an agent for initial therapy of hypertension must be done with the understanding that perhaps as many as 40 to 50% of persons receiving monotherapy may not reach goal blood pressure on that agent alone. Certain combinations of antihypertensives are particularly effective, such as thiazide diuretics with beta-adrenoreceptor blockers or with ACE inhibitors and ARBs. Four new fixed-dose combinations of ACE inhibitors with calcium antagonists (dihydropyridine and non-dihydropyridines) have been released, reflecting how effective these agents are when used together. Thiazide diuretics are also effective with central and peripheral sympatholytics and peripheral alpha$_1$-adrenoreceptor blockers. Although there was some doubt about whether calcium antagonists and thiazides provide additive blood pressure reduction, recent studies have clearly shown that this combination is effective.

Cost

Cost considerations are playing an increasingly important role in the pharmacologic management of hypertension. No regimen, no matter how carefully and appropriately selected, will work if the patient cannot afford to buy it or if the agents do not appear on the formulary of the dispensing agency from which the patient gets medication. Thiazide diuretics and beta-adrenoreceptor blockers, for which generic preparations are available, tend to be the least expensive agents for initial therapy, although generics are available for every class of antihypertensives except for ARBs. In general, branded calcium antagonists are the most expensive agents. ARBs and ACE inhibitors are the next most expensive drugs, with others following. Some of the more recently marketed ACE inhibitors and calcium antagonists are less expensive than older ones and cost the same for each dose level. For many of the fixed-dose combinations, the cost is actually less than what would be paid for the individual components. It is customary with those fixed-dose combinations that include a thiazide for there to be no additional cost for the diuretic.

The true cost of antihypertensive therapy, however, involves more than just the price of the drug. Pharmacy fees to fill the prescription are the same regardless of the cost of the drug. Office visits are necessary to evaluate the response to therapy, and blood tests must be conducted to look for adverse biochemical reactions. In addition, a vast potential for cost to society or individuals exists if one choice of antihypertensive agent is not as effective as others in preventing the complications of hypertension. Unfortunately, it is still not known whether newer and more expensive agents that have theoretical advantages over older and cheaper drugs would actually save money and suffering overall, even though they would be more costly at the point of service. If these drugs actually added "value" by reducing the frequency of strokes, heart failure, myocardial infarctions, and renal disease more effectively than less expensive agents, they would be well worth the incremental cost.

Mechanism of Action of the Drug and Pathophysiology of the Patient's Hypertension

If we really understood exactly how the drugs we use worked and precisely why an individual patient was hypertensive, and if we could easily, safely, and reliably obtain that information, treating hypertension would be relatively simple. Attempts to profile patients, either biochemically using plasma renin activity (PRA), for example, or hemodynamically, are intellectually appealing but are too expensive to do in all cases and would not always provide the necessarily definitive information needed to predict the response to therapy in a particular patient. Although it is true that African-Americans and the elderly tend to have low or suppressed PRA, many do not. Many who do will respond to drugs, such as ACE-inhibitors or ARBs, that are less effective, on the average, in hypertensive persons with low PRA. Although it is true that hypertensive older persons tend to have a modestly decreased plasma volume compared with younger hypertensive patients, thiazide diuretics are not only effective but also very well tolerated in the elderly. Although it is true that ACE inhibitors usually suppress the endocrine RAA system, the antihypertensive effect is still evident even when plasma angiotensin levels return to pretreatment levels. This is compelling evidence that either there is a tissue site of action for these drugs or that other mechanisms, perhaps the stimulation of bradykinin or nitric oxide formation, participate in how they lower blood pressure. This persistence of the antihypertensive effect also explains why some patients with low PRA (the PRA value being a measure of endocrine RAA system function) respond well to ACE inhibitors or to ARBs, which suppress the RAA system at angiotensin A-I receptors throughout the body. All effective antihypertensives, not only calcium antagonists, reduce intracellular calcium, an excess of which may be the primary abnormality in essential hypertension. Perhaps the major flaw in the reasoning that drugs can be used to "probe" the pathophysiologic abnormality causing a patient's hypertension is the concept that there is one overriding abnormality responsible for the elevation in blood pressure. In all likelihood, more than one, if not many, of the systems that control blood pressure are dysfunctional simultaneously, and pharmacologic agents that reduce blood pressure alone or in combination do so by correcting more than one abnormality.

Despite the facts that the mechanism or mechanisms of action of antihypertensive drugs have not yet been precisely determined, and that we cannot precisely elucidate why a particular patient is hypertensive, the use of an empirical and aggressive approach to treating hypertension has dramatically reduced the rates of stroke and coronary heart disease. This approach, though far from perfect, has paid great dividends.

Summary and Recommendations

Although there are numerous options and many sources for error, the successful pharmacologic treatment of hypertension need not be too complicated, nor should it be oversimplified. Once the diagnosis has been established and the routine evaluation and any more complex testing believed to be necessary are completed, lifestyle modification should be begun. Adequate encouragement and time to work should be given, unless the patient falls in a group for which drug therapy (together with lifestyle modification) is indicated at the initiation of treatment. Drug therapy is indicated in all hypertensive patients if goal blood pressure is not reached with lifestyle modification.

The following steps are recommended in choosing a regimen and altering it until goal blood pressure is reached:

1. Deal first with cost. If the patient is unable to afford any but the least expensive drugs or cannot pay for the agent selected, price becomes the primary issue.
2. Ascertain whether or not other risk factors or co-morbid conditions are present. Avoid drugs that may worsen those factors or conditions and choose ones that might tend to improve them.
3. Find out what clinical adverse reactions the patient would find the most troublesome, and avoid agents that are more likely to cause these problems. Some patients are not at all concerned by side effects that would be very troublesome for others.
4. Consider demographic issues, and make the

selection with a higher probability of success should options be available.

5. Start with the lowest effective dose and plan to see the patient within 2 to 4 weeks unless the severity of the patient's hypertension or another problem warrants a visit sooner. Do appropriate biochemical monitoring when necessary. In some patients, start with a fixed-dose combination when it appears appropriate.

6. Increase the dose if goal blood pressure has not been reached, or if there has been only a minimal response. Do not increase the first dose or any dose prematurely. Give each dose adequate time to be fully effective. If intolerable side effects occur and are likely to be drug-related, or if there has been no response, then switch to another appropriate agent for monotherapy.

7. Continue the process of dose titration and monitoring until the maximum recommended dose has been reached. Stopping before full dose has been reached can lead to a situation in which the patient is receiving multiple agents at subtherapeutic doses when the use of only one or two drugs is necessary.

8. Should the first-choice agent fail to reduce blood pressure to goal, add a second agent with a different mechanism of action and that is known to have additive antihypertensive effects to those of the first-choice agent. A fixed-dose combination that combines two drugs in the doses desired could also be used at this time.

9. Titrate the second drug to full dose, as was done for the first, and continue appropriate monitoring.

10. Should the two-drug combination fail, consider a specific cause for the patient's refractory hypertension.

11. Should none be evident, add a third drug, after ensuring that a diuretic is part of the regimen, and/or consider a referral to a hypertension specialist.

12. Plan to see the patient who is at goal at least every 3 months to ensure that blood pressure control is sustained.

13. If control is achieved for 18 to 24 months, consider slowly reducing the doses of one or more components of the regimen, especially if the patient has made substantial adjustments in lifestyle.

14. Plan to do a re-evaluation similar to the initial evaluation annually and even more frequently for certain parameters.

15. Reinforce the need for adherence to the regimen and always question the patient carefully about adverse reactions.

16. Encourage the patient to communicate any problems with the therapeutic regimen.

Although some patients will not reach goal with this approach, even with the many effective treatment options available, most will come under or close to control. Those who do can anticipate substantial long-term benefit with an extended life expectancy and a much reduced risk of stroke, coronary artery disease, heart failure, and probably renal failure and dementia.

Although treating high blood pressure can be costly and at times seemingly unrewarding, the benefits to individual patients and to society make the effort worthwhile. Clinicians must be careful not to become apathetic about hypertension. The problem is not solved and will not be until all persons with hypertension are able to avail themselves of what has been among the most successful examples of preventive medicine.

ACUTE MYOCARDIAL INFARCTION

method of
MADHAVI GUNDA, M.D.,
W. DOUGLAS WEAVER, M.D., and
STEVEN BORZAK, M.D.
Henry Ford Heart and Vascular Institute
Detroit, Michigan

Acute myocardial infarction (MI) remains the leading cause of death worldwide. Annually about 1,500,000 patients suffer from MI in the United States. Despite advances in both coronary artery disease prevention and acute myocardial infarction treatment over the last 3 decades, significant morbidity and mortality remain as evidenced by the fact that as many as one half of people with acute MI die before they even reach the hospital.

PATHOGENESIS

Coronary atherosclerosis is responsible for almost all myocardial infarctions. Superficial "fatty" streaks appear to be the initial lesions and can be identified as early as childhood. These lesions progress to fibrous plaques, especially in the presence of risk factors known to cause endothelial injury such as hypertension, elevated low-density lipoprotein (LDL) cholesterol, diabetes mellitus, smoking, and perhaps local infection and inflammation. These complex plaques can rupture, leading to platelet aggregation, vasoconstriction, and thrombus formation, which is the precipitating cause of acute coronary syndromes. The degree and duration of coronary obstruction along with the extent of collateral blood supply to the affected area determine the extent of myocardial injury.

Precipitating factors include sudden strenuous exertion, emotional stress, direct trauma, and other types of physiologic stress (e.g., anemia, circadian rhythms, noncardiac surgery). An identifiable precipitant can be identified in as many as 50% of patients with an acute MI.

CLINICAL PRESENTATION AND DIAGNOSIS

The history still has tremendous diagnostic value in the evaluation of a patient with acute angina. Approximately 50% of patients suffer from prodromal angina. MI pain is usually similar in quality, but more intense and persistent and can occur at rest or with less activity than usual. There is great variability in clinical presentations, and a classic presentation is often not found, especially in the elderly, women, and African-Americans. Therefore, one cannot rely on the history alone to make a diagnosis of MI. When a patient presents with acute onset of severe chest discomfort, important differential diagnostic considera-

TABLE 1. **Differential Diagnosis of Acute Chest Pain**

Diagnosis	Symptoms	Physical Findings
Pericarditis	"Sharp" pleuritic chest pain	Pericardial rub
Aortic dissection	"Ripping or tearing" pain in chest radiating to the back or abdominal quadrants; pain worst at onset	Blood pressure discrepancy between upper and lower extremities, aortic insufficiency, stroke, loss of peripheral pulses
Pulmonary embolism	Acute-onset shortness of breath Pleuritic chest pain	Tachypnea
Musculoskeletal pain	Pain with movement	Tenderness to palpation of affected muscles or joints
Costochondritis	Pleuritic chest pain	Reproducible tenderness to palpation of the costochondral junction
Gastroesophageal reflux	"Heartburn" related to food, supine position, dysphagia	Usually normal
Peptic ulcer disease	Aggravated or relieved by food Epigastric pain	Epigastric or upper abdominal tenderness to palpation Guaiac (+) stools

tions need to be kept in mind and systematically excluded (Table 1).

A carefully obtained history and physical examination will strongly suggest the diagnosis of MI in the majority of patients. Additional essential information includes an electrocardiogram (ECG) and serum analysis of cardiac proteins or enzyme markers of necrosis. Because of the considerable variability in the clinical presentation of an MI with respect to the classic history, ECG changes, and the rise and fall pattern of serum markers, the World Health Organization criteria for the diagnosis of MI require that at least two of these three elements be present.

The diagnosis of MI by ECG criteria includes ST segment elevation of at least 0.1 mV in at least two contiguous leads of MI location. Reciprocal ST segment depression, although not always present, is a helpful associated finding that makes the possibility of diagnostic confusion with acute pericarditis less likely. ST segment elevation is felt to represent acute myocardial injury, whereas Q wave formation is reflective of infarction. Q waves in the setting of ST elevation are best labeled as acute infarction, whereas in the absence of ST elevation, Q waves are indicative of an MI of indeterminate age.

In various series, 40 to 60% of patients with MI have ST elevation at initial presentation. The only patients who have been shown to benefit from thrombolytic therapy are those with ST elevation or left bundle branch block with MI serum markers. Patients who present with ST depression are at high risk for death or major complications but have not yet been shown to benefit from thrombolysis. MI patients can thus be classified by the presence or absence of ST elevation initially, which determines immediate therapy. The subsequent classification of Q wave or non–Q wave infarction has less prognostic meaning and should guide therapy to a lesser degree than clinical markers of risk, such as heart failure, recurrent chest pain, late (>48 hours) ventricular arrhythmias, and persistent ST-segment depression.

TREATMENT

All patients with acute MI warrant hospitalization and telemetry monitoring, often in the intensive care unit. Since time is of the essence in preserving myocardium, the initial triage and assessment of these patients in the emergency room should be a coordinated effort among physicians, nurses, and other support staff in order to implement effective therapy as quickly as possible. Initial therapy should feature those medications that have been proven effective in reducing mortality.

Pharmacologic Therapy (Table 2)

Aspirin

Aspirin inhibits cyclooxygenase activity and therefore thromboxane A_2 formation, which is a potent mediator of platelet aggregation. Because low doses can take several days to achieve their full antiplatelet effect, non–enteric coated aspirin should be given promptly at a dose of at least 160 to 325 mg and chewed initially to ensure rapid absorption. The Second International Study of Infarct Survival (ISIS-2) clearly demonstrated the efficacy of aspirin with a 35-day mortality reduction of 23%; when aspirin was combined with streptokinase, the mortality benefit was additive and reached 42%. In addition, aspirin has been shown to reduce the incidence of coronary reocclusion, recurrent ischemia, and stroke. With the exception of patients with known hypersensitivity to aspirin, every patient suspected of having an MI should be given aspirin.

Beta Blockers

Beta blockers appear to limit infarct size, relieve the pain associated with an MI, and reduce short- and long-term cardiac morbidity and mortality. Once contraindications to beta-blocker therapy have been excluded, such as cardiogenic shock, second- and third-degree heart block, severe bradycardia (heart rate <60 beats per minute), moderate or severe heart failure, hypotension (systolic blood pressure <90 mm Hg), and obstructive airway disease, patients should be considered for intravenous administration of beta blockers followed by oral therapy early in the course of an MI.

In the prethrombolytic era, intravenous atenolol (Tenormin) produced a 14% reduction in mortality, with the greatest benefit occurring during the first 2 days after an MI. In the postthrombolytic era, there is much less data; however, the Thrombolysis in Myocardial Infarction (TIMI-2B) trial tested the possibil-

TABLE 2. **Pharmacologic Therapy in the Presence or Absence of Thrombolysis**

Drug	Dose and Titration	Patient Selection	Contraindications
Aspirin	160–325 mg PO immediately and daily	All patients	Aspirin allergy
Ticlopidine*	250 mg PO twice daily	Aspirin allergy	None
Heparin	5000 U bolus at initiation of thrombolytics, 800–1000 U/h with a PTT-defined dose adjustment	With alteplase or reteplase or in absence of thrombolysis	Streptokinase, high bleeding risk
Beta blockers	IV followed by PO†‡	All patients	Heart block, hypotension, obstructive lung disease with wheezing, moderate and severe heart failure
ACE inhibitors	Oral considered within first 24 h§	All patients	ACE inhibitor allergy, hypotension, renal failure
Cholesterol-lowering agents	HMG Co A reductase inhibitor PO prior to discharge	LDL cholesterol >100 mg/dL	Severe liver dysfunction

* Not FDA approved for this indication.
† Metoprolol, 5 mg IV at 5-min intervals × three doses, then 50 mg PO qid × 48 h, then 100 mg PO bid.
‡ Atenolol, 5 mg IV over 5 min, repeat 10 min later, then 50 mg PO 10 min later, then 50–100 mg daily.
§ Captopril, 50 mg PO tid or its equivalent.
Abbreviations: ACE = angiotensin-converting enzyme; PTT = partial thromboplastin time; LDL = low-density lipoprotein.

ity of a complementary role for beta blockade and thrombolytic therapy and reported a reduction in early, nonfatal reinfarction rates, but the patient population was too small to determine any survival advantage.

Many large studies from the 1980s examined the long-term effects of beta-blocker therapy after hospital discharge and showed a 25% reduction in mortality. Recent studies have indicated that many eligible patients remain untreated with beta blockers, representing an important opportunity to reduce further death and disability following MI.

Thrombolytics

Thrombolytic therapy for MI significantly reduces mortality, but this benefit declines steadily with the passage of time after the onset of symptoms. The survival benefit is greatest in patients with anterior infarction, prior MI, younger age, and diabetes mellitus. Thrombolytics have not demonstrated a proven benefit in patients with ST segment depression, nonspecific T-waves, or other nonspecific changes on ECG.

Streptokinase is a protein formed by beta-hemolytic streptococci that complexes to fibrin-bound and free plasminogen, resulting in plasmin formation and producing a hypocoagulable state that may protect against reocclusion after thrombolysis. In fact, the use of heparin following streptokinase has not been shown to improve survival and in fact is associated with an increased risk of intracranial hemorrhage and is therefore contraindicated. Streptokinase can cause transient hypotension, which is felt to be bradykinin mediated but is usually responsive to volume infusion. Anisoylated plasminogen-streptokinase activator complex (Eminase), is more active than streptokinase and has a longer half-life; however, its clinical effect appears to be similar to that of streptokinase in comparative trials with the disadvantage of being more expensive.

Recombinant tissue plasminogen activator, (t-PA) (alteplase [Activase]) becomes a very potent plasminogen activator once bound to fibrin (and is therefore referred to as "clot specific"), resulting in less fibrinogen depletion. Following thrombolysis, however, there is no anticoagulant effect, and in fact, there may be a prothrombotic state, suggesting a theoretical need for heparin to prevent reocclusion.

Streptokinase was compared with alteplase in two major European trials and no difference was found with respect to mortality. More recently, the first Global Utilization of Streptokinase and Tissue Plasminogen Activator for Occluded Coronary Arteries (GUSTO) study did show a modest reduction in mortality of 9 lives saved per 1000 patients treated with front-loaded t-PA and aggressive intravenous heparin regimens compared with streptokinase, especially in patients younger than age 75 and those with an anterior infarction. Whether to give timely thrombolytic therapy is a more important decision than which thrombolytic agent to use. However, alteplase with intravenous heparin is recommended over streptokinase for younger patients with anterior and/or larger inferior MIs, prior streptokinase use, and presentations within 4 to 6 hours from the onset of pain.

Molecular biology and genetic engineering have been used to modify the plasminogen activators. Reteplase (r-PA) (Retavase), a mutant of wild-type alteplase has a longer half-life and is intermediate in fibrin specificity between streptokinase and t-PA and thus can be given as a bolus. Recently the Global Use of Strategies to Open Occluded Coronary Arteries Investigators (GUSTO III) concluded that although reteplase was easier to administer, it did not provide any additional survival benefit or reduction in major bleeding compared to front-loaded alteplase.

Contraindications to thrombolytic therapy must be assessed when contemplating their use in MI patients and include the following: (1) history of intracranial hemorrhage or surgery, (2) history of nonhemorrhagic stroke within 6 months, (3) active peptic ulcer disease within 3 months, (4) surgery within

2 weeks, (5) pericarditis, (6) aortic dissection, (7) traumatic resuscitation or prolonged cardiopulmonary resuscitation, (8) active bleeding or a bleeding diathesis, excluding menstruation, (9) pregnancy, (10) uncontrolled hypertension with persistent systolic blood pressure of more than 200 mm Hg or diastolic blood pressure above 110 mm Hg.

Heparin

Limited data support the use of heparin plus aspirin in patients ineligible for or not receiving thrombolysis. In thrombolytic-treated patients, heparin increases bleeding risk above that of aspirin plus thrombolysis alone. Heparin combined with streptokinase and aspirin has no clinical benefit but increases serious bleeding. Heparin plus aspirin and fibrin-specific agents has not been evaluated in large trials but is a rational approach for reasons described previously. To minimize bleeding risk, the activated partial thromboplastin time (APTT) should be monitored beginning at 6 hours, and the dose of heparin should be adjusted to maintain APTT between 50 and 85 seconds. Heparin is appropriate for 24 to 48 hours, unless atrial fibrillation is present or left ventricular thrombus is visualized or clinically suspected. In these cases, warfarin should be started and heparin continued until the International Normalized Ratio approaches the target range of 2 to 3.

Angiotensin-Converting Enzyme Inhibitors

Angiotensin-converting enzyme (ACE) inhibitors are effective afterload-reducing agents and appear to influence the remodeling of myocardium following an MI. Several trials demonstrated a reduction in death and heart failure in patients with a large MI and left ventricular dysfunction (ejection fraction <40%) when ACE inhibitors were started during the first week following an MI. More recent trials have also unequivocally shown that mortality is further reduced when an ACE is started within 24 hours of an acute MI in patients without hypotension.

ACE inhibitors should be considered on the first day, provided there is no history of an anaphylactic allergic reaction or bilateral renal artery stenosis and the blood pressure is adequate. The importance of initiating, as well as maintaining, ACE inhibitors beyond 6 weeks is much greater in the presence of clinically evident heart failure or asymptomatic left ventricular dysfunction.

Lipid-Lowering Agents

The National Cholesterol Education Panel II has recommended that a complete blood lipid profile be done in all patients with established coronary heart disease. In MI patients, this should ideally be done within the first 24 hours after onset to ensure accurate readings. During this time, all patients should be treated with a low-cholesterol, low–saturated fat diet. Drug therapy with HMG-CoA reductase inhibitors (statins) should be started with the goal of achieving an LDL level of less than 100 mg per dL. Recently, the Scandinavian Simvastatin Survival Study (4S) reported that coronary heart disease mortality was reduced by 42% and total mortality by 30% among men and women with coronary heart disease and hypercholesterolemia treated with simvastatin (Zocor) compared with placebo.

A low high-density lipoprotein (HDL) cholesterol level (<35 mg per dL) is also recognized as an independent risk factor, and therefore patients should be advised to exercise in the context of a structured cardiac rehabilitation program in order to raise it. In the setting of an elevated LDL level, statins raise the HDL level modestly. There is no evidence as yet that raising HDL levels alone improves survival.

Nitrates

Nitroglycerin has been used for many years in the treatment of MI and is frequently first-line therapy for chest pain in the emergency department. No reduction in mortality, however, has been shown in two very large trials in the postthrombolytic era. The pharmacologic effects of nitrates include redistribution of coronary blood flow to the subendocardium, reduction in preload and afterload by dilatation of venous capacitance vessels and systemic arteries, and dilatation of coronary vessels. Clinically, this may result in relief of ischemic pain, control of hypertension and a reduction in symptoms of pulmonary vascular congestion acutely, although hypotension is a risk, especially in the setting of volume depletion or right ventricular infarction. There does not appear to be any long-term benefit with oral nitrates unless there is persistent angina or ventricular failure.

Calcium Channel Blockers

Most randomized trials that have studied calcium channel blocker therapy during MI have found no beneficial effect on mortality, infarct size, or left ventricular function. The Multicenter Diltiazem Postinfarction Trial followed patients for 2 years and observed no reduction in cardiac events, death, or MI with diltiazem, but in fact an increased risk of mortality in patients with poor left ventricular function. A more recent study of amlodipine (Norvasc) in patients with chronic heart failure has shown no hazard of treatment but also no significant improvement in outcomes, including survival.

A review of all randomized trials using calcium antagonists for MI by Yusuf and colleagues noted a trend toward higher mortality and reinfarction among patients treated with short-acting nifedipine. In contrast, trials using diltiazem and verapamil showed no difference in mortality and less reinfarction. This difference between nifedipine and the other agents may be secondary to the reflex tachycardia or platelet aggregation that results from nifedipine. Calcium channel blockers are not presently recommended for routine treatment or secondary prevention of MI and should be discontinued in favor of beta blockers or ACE inhibitors when hypertension requires treatment after MI.

Analgesia

Control of pain is an important aspect of management of MI patients. Ongoing chest discomfort causes increased sympathetic output, leading to a rise in heart rate, blood pressure, and ultimately myocardial oxygen demand. Pharmacologic measures to control pain include oxygen, nitrates, morphine, and beta blockers, all of which aim to improve the myocardial oxygen supply and demand relationship and thereby reduce ongoing ischemia.

Interventional Therapy (Table 3)

Primary Percutaneous Transluminal Coronary Angioplasty

Among the many limitations of thrombolytic therapy are (1) 90-minute infarct-related vessel patency rates of only 35 to 75% compared to 85 to 95% with primary percutaneous transluminal coronary angioplasty (PTCA), (2) serious bleeding complications, (3) higher rates of coronary reocclusion and recurrent ischemia, and (4) limited patient eligibility due to contraindications.

Several investigations have evaluated the efficacy of PTCA as an initial treatment strategy for MI. It appears that in the hands of experienced interventional cardiologists, primary PTCA is at least as clinically effective as, and may be superior to, thrombolytic therapy by achieving more complete reperfusion of the infarct-related vessel with a resultant lower rate of reocclusion. The long-term comparative effectiveness of the two strategies is less clear. One study showed a 30-day advantage of primary PTCA using a composite end point of death, MI, or nonfatal disabling stroke, but the advantage was attenuated and not statistically significant at 6 months. Thrombolysis has been studied in trials consisting of more than 100,000 patients; an exact role for PTCA will be better defined when it has been evaluated in more than the few thousand patients so far reported.

Secondary Percutaneous Transluminal Coronary Angioplasty

Early and mandatory use of PTCA following thrombolytic therapy in uncomplicated or stable patients has no proven benefit over thrombolysis alone, and in fact, has been associated with a trend toward increased mortality, higher rates of abrupt reocclusion, and reinfarction necessitating emergent coronary artery bypass grafting. It is therefore not recommended.

Rescue angioplasty, (i.e., PTCA in patients who failed to initially achieve reperfusion with thrombolytic therapy) may be considered in hemodynamically unstable patients or those with heart failure or large infarctions. Limited data are available to evaluate this strategy.

After 24 hours, routine coronary angiography in uncomplicated patients has not been shown to be beneficial unless the patient develops postinfarction angina, heart failure, other complications, or a positive low-level stress test before discharge.

In patients who present with cardiogenic shock or who develop it during their hospital stay, nonrandomized observational data suggest that urgent revascularization is associated with reduced mortality compared with 80% or more in medically treated patients.

Intra-aortic Balloon Pump

Intra-aortic counterpulsation is achieved by advancing a balloon in the descending aorta through the femoral artery, which inflates with diastole and deflates with systole. The net effect is a reduction in afterload during systole and an increase in the coronary artery perfusion pressure during diastole.

Although balloon pumping has not been shown to improve survival, it may be useful in hemodynamically stabilizing patients in shock and, therefore, used as a bridge to other procedures such as PTCA, coronary artery bypass graft, mitral valve replace-

TABLE 3. **Revascularization and Other Interventions**

Intervention	Patient Selection	Status
Primary PTCA	Thrombolytic therapy ineligible	Established
	Cardiogenic shock	Recommended based on nonrandomized observational data
Rescue PTCA after thrombolytics	Failed thrombolysis Large MI	Theoretically appropriate but limited data
Intra-aortic balloon counterpulsation	Cardiogenic shock Persistent ischemic pain refractory to medical therapy	Theoretically appropriate based on retrospective observational studies
Elective catheterization ± revascularization	Postinfarction angina	Established
	Positive predischarge stress test	Established
	Serious arrhythmias (beyond 24 hr)	Rational
	Heart failure	Rational
Emergency catheterization	Mechanical complication of MI (ventricular septal rupture, severe mitral regurgitation)	Rational
	Cardiogenic shock	Rational; under investigation
Echocardiography	LV function unknown	Established
	Suspected mechanical complications	Established

Abbreviations: PTCA = percutaneous transluminal coronary angioplasty; MI = myocardial infarction; LV = left ventricular.

ment, and ventricular septal repair. Recently, randomized trials have shown that the routine prophylactic use of intra-aortic balloon pumping following primary PTCA had no clinical benefit.

CONCLUSIONS

MI management has undergone major evolution over the last decade. Five drugs have unequivocally reduced mortality: aspirin, thrombolytics, beta blockers, ACE inhibitors, and HMG-CoA reductase inhibitors. Primary PTCA is at least as good if not superior to thrombolysis when done in experienced centers without extremely long delays. Multidisciplinary institutional efforts to rapidly assess patients and promptly and efficiently deploy effective strategies offer the opportunity to simultaneously reduce mortality and the cost of hospitalization.

CARE AFTER MYOCARDIAL INFARCTION

method of
F. CARTER NEWTON, M.D.
University of California, Los Angeles, UCLA School of Medicine
Los Angeles, California
Pacific Heart Institute
Santa Monica, California

Following an actual or aborted myocardial infarction the clinical phase of coronary atherosclerosis begins. This condition has both a short- and a long-term outcome, and the healing process is both mental and physical. In the United States, 40% of patients with acute myocardial infarction never make it to the hospital alive; for the 60% who survive, recognize the illness, and come to the hospital, clinical pathways have been refined that limit infarct size and thereby change the natural history of atherosclerosis. Beyond the acute phase of the illness, the outcome pathways are strongly influenced by cardiac rehabilitation, an individualized and shared activity involving the patient, the treating consultant, the nursing staff, the dietary staff, and the counseling and vocational resources of the hospital. The primary physician has the medicolegal responsibility for clinical decisions and must therefore be the final decision-maker about the active and passive strategies involved in recovery. Active strategies are interventions such as drug therapy that are intended to limit the risk of infarct expansion. Passive strategies steer the patient away from risky activities, unnecessary medications, or even surgical therapy that is not of proven benefit for a given situation.

Heart disease amenable to rehabilitation has three phases:

1. *The Acute Illness.* This could be an acute myocardial infarction for which thrombolytic therapy has been given or a case of severe angina pectoris for which a coronary artery bypass graft operation has just been performed.
2. *The Stabilization Phase.* Examples include paroxysmal intervals of sustained ventricular tachycardia following successful reperfusion of an occluded coronary artery or an interval of hypotension during recovery from a late-arriving myocardial infarction as antiremodeling medication such as angiotensin-converting enzyme (ACE) inhibitors are titrated.
3. *The Recovery Phase.* This, in very large measure, represents the simple spontaneous miracle of healing (e.g., endothelialization of a coronary artery stent surface). But there can be a contribution from the directed pathways of the treating medical rehabilitation team. The pathways to in-hospital recovery may be circuitous and involve arrhythmia management and treatment for congestive heart failure, or they may be as simple as early and progressive mobilization to minimize the risks of inactivity. In stable patients, outpatient cardiac rehabilitation is a continuing effort at guidance to return to normal activities, minimize symptoms, and maximize the length and quality of life.

This article discusses the goals of cardiac rehabilitation, the structure of an inpatient and an outpatient program, the value of secondary prevention in coronary atherosclerosis, and the special requirements for exercise programs for patients with the collateral problems of diabetes mellitus and/or congestive heart failure.

PHASE I: INPATIENT REHABILITATION

Cardiac rehabilitation in the hospital begins as soon as the patient is hemodynamically stable and abnormal heart rhythms have quieted. At our facility, patients are seen by a cardiac rehabilitation nurse specialist on arrival at the step-down telemetry unit. With the increasing pressure to minimize patient length of stay, rehabilitation emphasis is on physical rather than psychologic recovery; consequently, patients now leave the hospital when it is "safe" rather than when they are "ready."

The goals in the phase are the following:

1. To minimize the deleterious effects of inactivity, e.g., skeletal muscle weakness, rapid deconditioning, development of a catabolic state, contraction of the circulating blood volume, loss of orthostatic reflexes, and a high likelihood of venous thromboembolism.
2. To initiate and titrate appropriate medications that will minimize subsequent ventricular remodeling (ACE inhibitors), limit subsequent ischemia (beta blockers), and reduce the likelihood of recurrent arterial thrombus formation (antiplatelet agents).
3. To provide risk stratification based on the predischarge symptoms and the results of an exercise test.
4. To identify appropriate patients (i.e., high-risk patients) for revascularization therapy.

5. To gather information to allow physical, psychologic, vocational, and medical profiling for creation of an individualized outpatient treatment plan. This includes the details of the acute illness, such as angiographic and echocardiographic information, as well as personal data, such as risk factor problems, concurrent illnesses, and psychosocial status.

6. To improve the patient's psychologic state, thereby limiting disability, potentially shortening the hospital stay, and prompting a more rapid return to work.

While still in the intensive care unit, the patient sits on the edge of the bed and then in a chair for up to a half hour. The extremities are put through range of motion exercises, initially passive, then active, and then the patient can stand at the bedside and use a bedside commode.

Transfer to a step-down unit follows with ongoing telemetry until discharge. Activity progresses from longer periods of time out of bed in a chair to strolling in the halls and finally climbing a flight of stairs under supervision. During this time, the patient is weaned from narcotic analgesics, eating and bowel and bladder activity are observed, and medications are titrated up to discharge levels and tolerance assessed (beta blockers, ACE inhibitors, aspirin, anticoagulants, etc., as appropriate). Concurrently with these activities, the cardiac rehabilitation nurse, dietitian, and patient meet. The pathologic process is explained, and basic dietary instruction is begun and a low-fat diet prescribed. The patient should not leave the hospital until he or she is physiologically stable and understands the medication regimen.

Before discharge, the patient's risk for future adverse events must be assessed so that more aggressive therapy can be given in appropriate cases. Obviously the nature of the illness dictates not only the duration of the hospital stay but also the level of risk that exists at the time of discharge. For example, a patient undergoing a simple angioplasty for unstable angina can usually leave the hospital the following day. In contrast, someone having coronary artery bypass graft surgery for three-vessel coronary disease with depression of left ventricular function may remain in the hospital 7 to 9 days or more. A low-level walking exercise test to a heart rate of 120 beats per minute or a symptom limit of moderate fatigue is most helpful before discharge. Patients can then be stratified to a low-, medium-, or high-risk cohort for subsequent adverse events.

- *Low-risk patients* retain good left ventricular function; signs and symptoms of myocardial ischemia at rest or with effort are absent; the hospital procedure was successful and uncomplicated; and complex ventricular arrhythmias have not been observed.
- *Moderate-risk patients* have some, but not severe, impairment of left ventricular function (e.g., echo ejection fraction ≥35%). Low-level exercise testing with or without nuclear imaging suggests that a residual reversible ischemic burden remains, but signs of severity are not present. Personality profiling suggests that long-term risk factor modification such as cigarette smoking cessation is not likely to occur or medication compliance is likely to be poor.
- In addition to the aforementioned adverse lifestyle factors, *high-risk patients* have severe impairment of left ventricular function (echo ejection fraction <30%). Complex ventricular arrhythmias may have been present in the latter phase of hospitalization and a low-level exercise test suggests the possibility of moderate to severe residual myocardial ischemia.

Higher levels of risk do not preclude an exercise/cardiac rehabilitation program, but they do identify those needing continuous electrocardiographic monitoring, more cautious observation, and lower intensity and briefer intervals of exercise. Coordination between the primary physician and the rehabilitation team becomes essential for these patients as their clinical course can change abruptly and their medication regimen may be more complex.

Regardless of these factors, at the time of discharge patients should have an activity level beyond that anticipated at home. The discharge plan should include a visit to the outpatient rehabilitation facility within 2 weeks as well as immediate follow-up with the treating physician.

PHASE II: OUTPATIENT CARDIAC REHABILITATION

Patients begin outpatient rehabilitation as soon as they become outpatients. They are encouraged to be independent at home, to dress in street clothes, to avoid prolonged time in bed in favor of a chair, and to stroll out of doors at a casual as-tolerated pace twice a day. As a general rule, patients should not have sex or lift more than 25 pounds before visiting the outpatient facility or undergoing an exercise test. If tolerated, patients may enjoy casual social activity and do light housework. Perhaps the ultimate goal for this period is confidence building.

Two to 4 weeks postevent, regular attendance at the rehabilitation facility should begin. At this point a symptom-limited ramped exercise test should be performed by a protocol that allows observation of at least 9 minutes of incremental work, either on a treadmill or on a supine bicycle. The results of this test, performed with patients on their usual medication regimen, are used to plan the exercise program and to define a target heart rate and heart rate range for training. At our facility, this range is calculated to be 60 to 80% of the maximal heart rate achieved at the time of the stress test. If a patient's heart rate response is limited by his or her own constitution or by the effects of beta blockers, then a level of perceived exertion that is moderate but permits a comfortable target heart rate is considered the training effort range.

A priority at our inpatient rehabilitation facility

is creating a happy atmosphere where a spirit of camaraderie and team effort is fostered. The atmosphere is relaxed and supportive but always medically professional. The rehabilitation team is made up of nurses skilled in cardiac patient assessment, ECG telemetry interpretation, and counseling. Exercise physiologists organize and lead the stretching exercises and workouts with exercise machines and free weights. A nutritionist gives classes on food preparation and food composition. The team provides for patient and family counseling and organizes group encounters to talk about psychologic issues. Additionally, classes are presented on different aspects of heart disease, sources of problems, symptom recognition and management, and cardiopulmonary resuscitation. It is a place where medications and new procedures on the horizon are discussed. Support groups for smoking cessation and weight control meet regularly.

The cardiac rehabilitation team is responsible for maintaining the patient chart, documenting each session's progress, and observing symptomatic or telemetry problems. Weight, pre- and postexercise heart rate, and blood pressure are recorded, a sample rhythm strip is saved, and symptoms of medication intolerance or new disease activity are noted and communicated to the primary physician. Updates are mailed to the treating physician on a monthly basis if the patient is stable or urgently if the patient is not or if it is felt that formal psychologic counseling is indicated.

Patients in this phase initiate what are intended to be lifelong changes in exercise and lifestyle habits. The goals of exercise should be clear: Training will restore and increase functional capacity and effort-related symptoms will improve. Each exercise session should last roughly 1 hour. As a warm-up, 10 to 15 minutes are spent stretching and strolling. Then initially 20 and eventually 40 to 50 minutes are spent doing sustained aerobic exercise such as treadmill walking, stationary cycling, or arm ergometry within the target heart range. Ten to 15 minutes are spent in cool-down, strolling, and more stretching. An additional 10 to 15 minutes of resistive exercises can take place after the cool-down period. Continuous telemetry should be done during the initial 8 to 12 visits. If complex atrial or ventricular arrhythmias have not occurred, a periodic check with the "quick look" defibrillator paddles at peak work intensity will suffice to document the maximum pulse rate and record any perceived arrhythmia.

Exercise sessions should take place three to five times weekly at first, then as fitness increases, the intensity and duration of each session can be increased. At 3 months, a follow-up lipid profile and symptom-maximum stress test are repeated. The adequacy of the antilipidemic interventions can then be assessed and appropriately modified. Similarly, functional capacity improvement can be measured by comparing pre- and postrehabilitation stress test performance. A training effect can be documented if at a given level of protocol work the heart rate and blood pressure have declined from baseline levels. With exercise, ischemic symptoms may abate and the range of activities the patient is capable of can expand.

PHASE III: LONG-TERM MAINTENANCE REHABILITATION

The goals of long-term rehabilitation (beyond 4 to 6 months following a myocardial infarction) are to continue the momentum of secondary disease prevention established in phase II. By this time patients have returned to work, resumed normal sexual activity, and hopefully achieved optimal functional capacity and are maintaining a salutary lifestyle by avoiding cigarettes and optimizing their weight. The rehabilitation team continues to encourage lifestyle changes, reinforce antilipidemic medication compliance, and promote exercise in a group environment for psychosocial support. Stress reduction and a positive attitude contribute to the maintenance of all the secondary prevention elements. Regular exercise sessions of up to five times per week at a perceived exertion level of moderate severity continue indefinitely.

EXERCISE SAFETY

It has been shown that early ambulation following acute myocardial infarction does not lead to an increase in in- or out-of-hospital follow-up complications (e.g., worsening of angina or the development of congestive heart failure). Furthermore, predischarge stress testing is safe and useful in identifying the cohort of high-risk patients who should have further invasive studies and may benefit from predischarge revascularization.

The Thrombolysis and Myocardial Infarction II Trial reported an incidence of exercise-associated myocardial infarction as high as 20%. Although this figure perhaps overestimates the actual incidence, this fact, as well as the association of myocardial infarction with stress, raises important safety questions. It is reassuring however, that in the Determinance of Myocardial Infarction Onset Study a nearly 50-fold risk reduction for exercise-triggered myocardial infarction was observed in habitual exercisers versus the inactive patient controls.

In addition, cardiovascular complications in coronary artery disease are in fact extremely low, as evidenced by a 1978 study of 30 supervised U.S. rehabilitation centers. The rate of nonfatal myocardial infarction was one per 326,000 patient exercise hours, and the rate of fatal myocardial infarction was one per 800,000 patient exercise hours.

EXPECTATIONS AND GOALS OF EXERCISE TRAINING

Cardiovascular fitness is defined by maximal oxygen uptake, or $\dot{V}O_2max$. This can increase up to 30% or more with training in the elderly as well as the young. The product of heart rate × systolic blood pressure (double product) is a rough approximation of cardiac work for a given amount of exercise. With training, a smaller percentage of $\dot{V}O_2max$ is utilized and this in large part is the basis of symptom improvement. However, studies have shown that objective evidence of myocardial ischemia at a given double-rate product can actually be reduced with training. This implies improved coronary circulation perhaps via enhanced collateral blood flow in addition to peripheral vascular training. An analysis of pooled data of 4554 post–myocardial infarction patients followed for 3 years showed a 20% reduction in total mortality in cardiac rehabilitation–trained patients versus nontrained controls. Clearly, exercise training following myocardial infarction is not only safe but can also improve survival.

IMPORTANCE OF RISK FACTOR MODIFICATION

A good rehabilitation program will share the accumulating evidence about the value of lowering cholesterol in changing the natural history of atherosclerosis. Controlled trials have amply demonstrated the value of lowering cholesterol, particularly low-density lipoprotein (LDL) cholesterol, in both primary and secondary disease prevention strategies. Lowering risk, stabilizing ulcerative plaques, and indeed potentially reversing the actual atherosclerotic burden are clearly possible in a significant percentage of patients. Similarly, a rehabilitation program will provide smoking intervention programs and antismoking education. Smokers experience a rapid relative risk decline after cessation that approaches 1.0 after 3 years in some studies. Randomized interventional trials of smoking cessation have repeatedly shown a reduced incidence of myocardial infarction.

EXERCISE WITH IMPAIRED LEFT VENTRICULAR FUNCTION OR CHRONIC HEART FAILURE

It is well known that patients with chronic heart failure are at a higher risk for all causes of mortality. These patients reach their anaerobic threshold sooner and cannot increase their cardiac output by normal preload responsiveness or endogenous catecholamine stimulation. Exercising skeletal muscles are underperfused, leading to early fatigue, and sustained exercise raises the left ventricular filling pressures, resulting in early dyspnea.

Despite this, exercise programs have been shown to safely increase work capacity, reduce resting heart rate, increase peak cardiac output, and enhance a sense of well-being even in patients with severe depression of left ventricular function. Importantly, a training program does not increase the risk or the severity of post–myocardial infarction ventricular remodeling and infarct expansion. Patients in this category should train at approximately one half of their functional capacity and exercise for shorter intervals (5 to 15 minutes), at least initially. Supervision should be closer, including telemetry at each session. There should be a heightened awareness of signs of worsening heart failure and the risk of serious ventricular arrhythmias (heightened by digitalis toxicity, hypomagnesemia, and hypokalemia).

EXERCISE AND DIABETES

Both type I (insulin-dependent) and type II (non–insulin-dependent, insulin-resistant) diabetics can safely train for the same goals as nondiabetics. Their disease should ideally be controlled and the hypoglycemic effect of training exercise anticipated. This is due both to the enhanced mobilization of depot exogenous insulin and the insulin-like effect of aerobic exercise. Blood sugar should be monitored closely before and after the training session. Daily training is ideal so that the necessary adjustments (decreased insulin requirements and increased caloric intake 1 to 2 hours before each session) can be empirically determined and maintained. For exercise lasting more than 30 minutes, supplemental carbohydrates should be ingested during the activity. Perhaps most importantly, the usual symptoms of myocardial ischemia are often absent in these patients and therefore noninvasive surveillance for objective changes in the size of ischemic burden (i.e., routine symptom–maximal stress testing) should be performed more often (i.e., at 6-month intervals).

CONCLUSION

With each passing year it becomes more evident that the natural history of coronary atherosclerosis can be modified with an expanding therapeutic arsenal. A cardiac rehabilitation program, be it in an institutional outpatient setting or self-directed at home, helps patients to regain lost fitness, reduce symptoms, and lower the risk of subsequent cardiac events and need for rehospitalization. The safety and value of exercise in coronary patients is well established, and it is this activity that forms the backbone of secondary prevention programs. More will become known about the role of endothelial function, infection, and inflammation in acute myocardial infarction. Techniques of transcatheter interventions and minimally invasive surgery will improve. The cardiac rehabilitation centers will be an additional source of patient information and education about these and other new therapies. To quote Jay Leno, "Patients will be living so long we won't know what to do with them all."

PERICARDITIS

method of
JAMES B. YOUNG, M.D.
Cleveland Clinic Foundation
Cleveland, Ohio

Pericarditis, though not a rare condition, is not necessarily common. It challenges the diagnostic acumen of physicians because it mimics many other conditions, some of which are extraordinarily important not to misdiagnose, such as acute myocardial infarction. Pericarditis is caused by inflammation of the mesothelial lining of the pericardium. The most common symptom is chest pain, and because patients with chest pain frequently present initially to their primary care physician, the nuances of pericarditis must be understood so that a correct diagnosis can be made and appropriate therapies begun. Also important is the fact that inflammatory conditions of the pericardium are frequently accompanied by an effusive process that can be life-threatening, depending on the volume and rapidity of fluid build-up within the pericardium. Fortunately, inflammatory pericarditis usually responds to rather simple therapeutic maneuvers generally based on prescription of nonsteroidal anti-inflammatory medications. Occasionally, steroids are required, as is specific antimicrobial therapy for bacterial, fungal, tuberculous, and other specific infective processes amenable to such treatment. Malignant processes must be correctly identified and diagnosed so that antineoplastic therapies can be instituted.

PATHOPHYSIOLOGY

The pericardial sac is a fibrous structure with a mesothelial cell lining that suspends the heart within the mediastinum. Under normal circumstances, about 50 mL of serous fluid is present in the pericardial space. The fluid is rich in phospholipids that reduce friction between the heart and mediastinal contents during heart beat and body motion. The major function of the pericardium appears to be limiting excessive cardiac motion with body movement and the creation of a barrier between the heart and other mediastinal organs and the lungs. This protective effect is particularly important when infection or malignancy exists in structures contiguous to the heart, such as the lung or esophagus. This also explains why some conditions, such as carcinoma of the lung or pneumococcal pneumonia, often cause pericarditis. Although individuals with congenital absence of the pericardium do not have dramatic abnormalities of circulatory function, the pericardium does play a role in optimizing cardiac filling and emptying dynamics. Specifically, excessive acute cardiac dilation is prevented by the fibrous pericardium, and diastolic coupling of right and left ventricular filling and emptying is effected.

ETIOLOGY

Table 1 summarizes many, but certainly not all, of the etiologies of pericarditis. It is a good reference point to start from when pericardial disease is suspected. As can be seen from this list, causes of pericarditis range from common maladies, such as adenovirus infection, mumps, and pneumococcal pneumonia, to more obscure difficulties, such as autoimmune diseases and tuberculosis. Because pericarditis rarely represents a process affecting the pericardium alone, it is important to diagnosis underlying diseases promptly and accurately, because therapy of the primary problem is mandatory if pericarditis is to be cured and, in particular, significant pericardial effusions are to be prevented. Whenever a chest pain syndrome accompanies any of the situations listed in Table 1, pericarditis should be considered, and whenever pericarditis is considered, the presence of a pericardial effusion must also be suspected. Sometimes patients, particularly younger patients, present with a history of chest pain suggesting pericarditis and have physical findings of a pericardial friction rub with diagnostic electrocardiographic patterns but no obvious primary disease process that can be blamed for the inflammatory pericardial states. This is generally labeled "idiopathic pericarditis," but a careful review of the history or serial viral titers often implicate a prior viral infection.

TABLE 1. **Etiology of Pericarditis/Pericardial Effusion**

- Viral infections (Coxsackie, adenovirus, echovirus, mumps, mononucleosis, varicella, hepatitis, AIDS)
- Acute bacterial infection (*Pneumococcus, Staphylococcus, Streptococcus, Neisseria gonorrhoeae, Neisseria meningitidis, Legionella*)
- Fungal infections (histoplasmosis, coccidioidomycosis, candidiasis, blastomycosis)
- Tuberculosis
- Unusual infections (*Nocardia,* Lyme disease, toxoplasmosis, mycoplasma, amebiasis, actinomycosis, echinococcosis)
- Uremia (de novo, dialysis-associated)
- Neoplastic diseases (lung cancer, breast cancer, melanoma, leukemia, lymphoma, Hodgkin's disease)
- Myocardial infarction (acute evolving infarction, Dressler's syndrome)
- Inflammatory disease states (systemic lupus erythematosus, rheumatoid arthritis, rheumatic fever, scleroderma, polyarteritis nodosa, sarcoidosis, amyloidosis, inflammatory bowel disease, cardiac allograft rejection)
- Radiation injury
- Drug reactions (hydralazine, procainamide, phenytoin, isoniazid, phenylbutazone, dantrolene, doxorubicin, methysergide, cyclophosphamide)
- Myxedema
- Dissecting aortic aneurysm
- Chylopericardium
- Trauma (blunt, penetrating, cardiac catheterization complications)
- Idiopathic

DIAGNOSIS

Chest pain is the most frequent symptom of acute pericarditis, and because angina pectoris caused by obstructive coronary artery disease also produces a chest pain syndrome, it is important to differentiate these two conditions (Table 2). Acute pericarditis generally manifests with the insidious onset of sharp or stabbing precordial chest discomfort that often has a pleuritic component and is posi-

TABLE 2. **Differentiating Ischemic from Pericardial Pain**

Pain/ECG Characteristics	Angina/Infarct	Pericarditis
Location	Precordial	Precordial
Radiation	Shoulder, arms	Scapular region
Description	Pressure, burning, oppression	Sharp, stabbing dull ache
Pleurisy	No	Yes
Fever	Unusual	Common
Posture related	No	Yes (worse supine)
Effort related	Yes	No
Time course	Minutes–hours	Hours–days
Concomitant disease related	Not usually	Frequently
Q waves	Present	Absent
ST elevation	Localized	Diffuse
PR depression	Absent	Diffuse

tional, being particularly worse when patients are supine. The pain sometimes is described as dull and aching and a hallmark is its persistence over many hours and days. Exertion generally does not make the discomfort worse. Radiation to the back, especially the scapular region, is common, and this pain distribution may be particularly noted with deep inspiration. Low-grade fever is frequently reported, as is malaise, myalgias, and arthralgias; these symptoms likely represent the underlying inflammatory cytokine perturbation.

As mentioned, pericarditis is often caused by other concomitant diseases. Symptoms specific to conditions noted in Table 1 should be seriously considered and pursued. For example, arthralgias and claudication might suggest systemic lupus erythematosus or polyarteritis nodosa. Patients with cough, concomitant pleurisy, hard shaking chills, and high fever might have pneumonia, and therefore an infectious process, particularly a bacterial pneumonia, needs to be excluded. Patients sometimes complain of palpitations or arrhythmias, and atrial fibrillation is a common hallmark of pericarditis. Pericardial disease should always be considered when atrial arrhythmias are detected. Ventricular arrhythmias are less commonly caused by pericarditis; nevertheless, pericarditis should be considered. Obviously, in all of these situations, angina pectoris with ischemic heart disease is a possible cause, and appropriate diagnostic tests should be done. Because post–myocardial infarction pericarditis usually appears 7 days after the index event, recurrent chest pain in this setting is not always ischemic in origin, and careful evaluation of the patient is required to differentiate pericarditis from ischemia causing postinfarction angina pectoris. Drugs are an often overlooked cause of pericarditis: hydralazine, procainamide, phenytoins, and chemotherapeutic agents such as doxorubicin and cyclophosphamide have all been implicated.

Physical findings in patients with pericarditis are generally due to either the pericardial inflammation or the effusion resulting in hemodynamic disturbances. A pericardial friction rub is often present, although it may be transient and difficult to hear. Significant pericardial effusion can cause the disappearance of a previously easily heard rub, elevated venous pressure, paradoxical inspiratory fall in systemic blood pressure (greater than 10 mm Hg during quiet respiration), and tachycardia. Cardiogenic shock can become apparent suddenly when effusions grow to such a size that cardiac filling (and thus emptying) becomes significantly impaired. It is critically important to determine the presence of pericardial effusion early so that progression to cardiac tamponade can be prevented. One should strongly consider echocardiographic evaluation in all patients presenting with suspected pericarditis. Two-dimensional echocardiography can give valuable insight into the presence of clinically silent but hemodynamically significant pericardial effusion.

An electrocardiogram should also be obtained in all patients suspected of having pericarditis and scrutinized carefully for findings diagnostic of this difficulty, in particular QRS complex and ST segment patterns that might make one more suspicious of ischemic heart disease. Diffuse ST segment elevation with PR segment depression should suggest pericarditis; focal Q waves with ST segment elevation and T wave inversion point toward myocardial infarction. Atrial and sometimes ventricular arrhythmias may be seen. When particularly large pericardial effusions are present, low QRS voltage can be apparent with the characteristic pattern of beat-to-beat QRS voltage change (electrical alternans) that is produced by rotational alteration in the QRS axis as the heart swings to and fro in the large fluid-filled cavity. When this finding or rhythmic inspiratory progressive diminution of QRS voltage is noted, the clinician should be concerned about the possibility of cardiac tamponade. A chest film may not be helpful when looking for small pericardial effusions (which can be hemodynamically significant), but large ones can cause cardiomegaly. Chest roentgenography is important, however, because it can give insight into concomitant pathology such as pneumonia or pulmonary malignancy. As mentioned, echocardiography is the most practical way to detect and size pericardial effusions. Computed tomographic scans of the chest and magnetic resonance imaging of the heart are alternative methods of assessing pericardial pathology, particularly pericardial thickening.

When other concomitant diseases are suspected or known to be present, disease-specific tests and evaluations must be ordered. This is particularly important when an infectious cause is possible or when pericardial disease is likely produced by systemic illnesses such as those causing collagen vascular disorders.

TREATMENT

Pericarditis should be treated with disease-specific therapies and anti-inflammatory agents to prevent development or enlargement of pericardial effusion. Pericarditis and pericardial effusions are responsible for many difficulties, such as acute and chronic pain syndromes, cardiac tamponade, and chronic constrictive hemodynamic syndromes when inflammation causes excessive pericardial fibrosis. Pain syndromes, purulent effusions with sepsis, cardiac tamponade, and pericardial constriction of ventricular filling are the most frequent problems that require therapeutic attention. The pain of acute pericarditis generally responds well to nonsteroidal anti-inflammatory medications. Aspirin, 650 mg every 3 to 4 hours, or indomethacin, 25 to 50 mg four times daily, are very effective remedies. Indomethacin can be reserved for more severe pain syndromes because of the frequency of gastrointestinal difficulties encountered with this drug. Alternatively, other nonsteroidal anti-inflammatory agents, such as ibuprofen, can be used. Steroids should be reserved for patients with pain syndromes persisting after 48 to 72 hours of treatment despite adequate doses of nonsteroidal anti-inflammatory drugs. Chronic pain syndromes, or recurrent relapsing pericarditis, tend to respond better to a course of steroids. One must remember, however, that steroids can adversely affect the situation when purulent pericardial effusions are present. When using steroids, one approach is to give prednisone (approximately 1 mg per kg) daily for 1 week with a slow subsequent dose taper (decreasing by 5 mg per day) when symptoms have abated. Rarely, the combination of prednisone and a nonsteroidal agent is necessary, but combining these two drugs may simply increase the risk of significant gastrointestinal toxicity. Chronic pain syndromes may require pericardiectomy to achieve symptom relief; however, selecting patients for this operation is extraordinarily difficult, and all other causes of chest pain must be excluded with a reasonable degree of certainty before subjecting the patient to this type of operation. Unfortunately, it is very difficult to resect the entire pericardium, and pain syndromes can persist even when only small pieces of the pericardium remain.

Treatment must also focus on concomitant disease processes if associated pericarditis is to be resolved. This is particularly important when purulent pericarditis is present. Care must be taken to prescribe the proper antimicrobial agent while draining the effusion and avoiding steroid administration (which might make the infectious process worse). Anticoagulants should be discontinued when pericarditis is diagnosed because of the risk of increasing effusion size from hemorrhage into the pericardial cavity, which could precipitate cardiac tamponade and cardiogenic shock. Patient management is particularly problematic in individuals with prosthetic heart valves or early post–myocardial infarction when thrombolytics have been used. If anticoagulation must be given, continuous intravenous heparin infusion seems preferable, so that clotting times can be frequently and precisely monitored.

Atrial arrhythmias are common in patients with pericarditis. Premature atrial contractions, atrial flutter, and atrial fibrillation often respond to anti-inflammatory therapy and antiarrhythmic drug administration. It is best to control the ventricular response rate in patients with atrial fibrillation with beta blockers, calcium channel blockers, and digoxin while attention is being directed toward resolution of the inflammatory state. Frequently, the rhythm will spontaneously revert back to a normal sinus rhythm without cardiac-specific drugs before all problems are definitively addressed. One should not wait to intervene because patients in atrial fibrillation for longer than 48 or 72 hours are at risk for intracardiac thrombi formation with stroke or other peripheral embolic events. Indeed, when atrial fibrillation occurs in the setting of pericarditis, prompt consideration of cardioversion is appropriate to avoid the need for longer term anticoagulant therapy.

Management of Pericardial Effusions

It should be re-emphasized that all patients with suspected pericarditis should undergo echocardiography to determine whether or not a pericardial effusion is present and, if so, its size. Echocardiographic evidence of cardiac tamponade (inspiratory atrial or right ventricular chamber collapse) must be excluded if conservative medical management of the effusion is to be pursued. Large effusions, effusions with evidence of tamponade, and those that may be purulent must be tapped expeditiously. Also, when the cause of an effusion is in doubt, pericardiocentesis should be performed. This is particularly the case if a malignant pericardial effusion is suspected. One should remember that asymptomatic pericardial effusion is most frequently secondary to concomitant ailments. When a large effusion is encountered, an indwelling drainage catheter can be left in place and frequently, with treatment of the underlying difficulty, the rate of fluid production will slow dramatically. Pericardial tube placement generally prevents tamponade, allows estimation of speed of fluid build-up, and, if necessary, provides access for installation of sclerosing, antineoplastic, or antimicrobial agents.

If a patient with pericarditis and known effusion becomes tachycardiac, hypotensive, or tachypneic, cardiac tamponade may be occurring. Volume expansion with isotonic fluid or nitroprusside infusion coupled with volume expansion may initially stabilize the situation while preparations for urgent pericardiocentesis are made. Whenever cardiac tamponade is suspected, echocardiography should be expeditiously performed so that appropriate therapy can be planned. Isoproterenol (Isuprel) or dopamine (Intropin) is also sometimes helpful by increasing cardiac filling pressures while augmenting contractility and countering the effects of external compression of the heart by the pericardial fluid. Volume expansion and inotropic or vasodilator infusion are temporizing measures, and more definitive pericardial drainage procedures must be planned. In chronic effusions that cannot be controlled with ordinary medical therapy or therapy directed at the underlying problem (such as a malignancy), surgical resection of a portion of the pericardium and creation of a "window" that allows fluid to drain into the pericardial sac or peritoneum can prevent recurrent tamponade.

Chronic pericarditis can cause a concomitant effusive process. Sometimes occult constrictive hemodynamics are unmasked during cardiac catheterization and hemodynamic evaluation with rapid volume expansion. In any event, one must be absolutely certain that a patient's symptoms and functional limitations are, for the most part, related to constrictive, or effusive constrictive, pericarditis. Certain intrinsic myocardial diseases such as hemochromatoses and cardiac amyloidoses can produce restrictive hemodynamic physiology with symptoms and findings similar to those of chronic constrictive pericarditis. Patient should not, therefore, be referred for pericardiectomy for constrictive pericardial disease without exclusion of infiltrative myocardial processes by endomyocardial biopsy. Careful hemodynamic study is required to document significant hemodynamic perturbations from constrictive pericardial disease.

PERIPHERAL ARTERIAL DISEASE

method of
DOUGLAS B. HOOD, M.D., and
FRED A. WEAVER, M.D.
University of Southern California School of Medicine
Los Angeles, California

"Peripheral arterial disease" is a term used to describe a number of different pathologic processes that affect the peripheral arterial tree, including occlusive disease arising from atherosclerotic and nonatherosclerotic causes and aneurysmal disease. Atherosclerotic occlusive disease of the lower extremity circulation is the most common of these entities and is the focus of the following discussion.

RISK FACTORS

Atherosclerosis is a generalized process affecting all vascular beds (i.e., coronary, carotid, visceral, and extremity circulations). A patient with manifestations of atherosclerosis at one site can be assumed to have atherosclerosis of various degrees at other sites as well, although the process may be clinically silent. Several well-defined risk factors for atherosclerosis have been identified. Factors that cannot be modified include age, male gender, and diabetes mellitus. The prevalence of symptomatic lower extremity atherosclerosis increases after the age of 50 years in both men and women. The onset of symptoms tends to be several years later in women, but gender prevalence rates tend to become equal by the age of 70. The association of atherosclerosis and diabetes is well established. Although there is evidence that strict control of hyperglycemia in patients with diabetes can delay the clinical onset and progression of atherosclerosis, strict control still does not completely negate diabetes as a risk factor. Risk factors for atherosclerosis that can be modified include smoking, hypertension, hyperlipidemia, and obesity. Not only do smokers have an increased incidence of symptomatic lower extremity atherosclerosis, but the onset of symptoms in this group is also about 10 years earlier than in nonsmokers. Good control of hypertension and hyperlipidemia may reduce the incidence and the rate of progression of atherosclerotic occlusive disease.

CLINICAL PRESENTATION

Mild lower extremity arterial occlusive disease frequently remains asymptomatic and is discovered only by detection of a pulse deficit or bruit on routine physical examination. More severe occlusive disease is clinically manifested as one of several well-defined patterns of symptoms. *Intermittent claudication* is usually described as a cramping or aching pain that occurs in the large muscle groups of the lower extremities. Symptoms occur with physical exertion or exercise and are relieved by a few minutes of rest; symptoms do not occur in the absence of physical exertion. In patients with claudication, arterial perfusion at rest is sufficient to supply the metabolic demands of the tissues. The normal response to exercise is arterial dilatation, which increases blood flow several-fold to the now more metabolically active tissues. However, in arterial segments with fixed proximal atherosclerotic obstruction, exercise-induced vasodilatation results in a decrease in the arterial pressure and relative ischemia distal to the atherosclerotic obstruction.

Claudication symptoms occur in the calves, thighs, or buttocks, depending on the level of occlusive disease. Those patients with significant aortoiliac obstruction experience symptoms in the buttocks, thighs, or calves, while those patients with primarily femoropopliteal disease complain of symptoms isolated to the calves. *Leriche syndrome* describes a clinical triad of findings that are a consequence of severe proximal aortoiliac occlusive disease, including thigh or buttock claudication, impotence, and diminished or absent femoral pulses. Claudication is usually quantitated in terms of the distance that can be walked before symptoms occur. The usual measure of distance is city blocks, although this is a highly variable distance and poorly reproducible. A better, more reproducible measure is the distance or time that can be walked on a treadmill at a standardized speed and degree of incline.

Longitudinal studies of patients with claudication have shown that the risk of progression to more severe, disabling claudication or to severe ischemia and threatened limb loss is approximately 15 to 20% at 5 years. In the majority of patients, symptoms remain stable and do not necessitate major changes in lifestyle to accommodate the disease. Because of this low risk of progression compared with the risks and benefits of revascularization, mild to moderate claudication is not usually an indication for intervention other than risk factor modification. Most physicians would agree that claudication symptoms must be truly disabling before therapeutic intervention is considered.

Patients with more severe degrees of ischemia present with tissue loss (nonhealing ulcers or gangrene) or impending tissue loss (ischemic rest pain). In such cases the condition is known as limb-threatening ischemia because of the high risk of amputation (roughly 50% at 2 years) if intervention is not performed to improve the blood supply to the affected limb. *Rest pain* is an aching, boring pain that occurs in the forefoot. Ischemic rest pain does not occur more proximally in the ankle or calf. The pain results from severe ischemia of distal nerve endings in the foot. Rest pain commonly occurs when the foot is elevated in bed at night and is frequently relieved by placing the affected foot in a dependent position, resulting in a small but sufficient augmentation of blood flow to the foot by the force of gravity.

Nonhealing (ischemic) ulcers may occur anywhere on the foot but typically occur on the toes. These lesions arise from minor trauma such as that associated with tight-fitting shoes or nail clipping. The ulcers are usually painful, except in diabetic patients with peripheral neuropathy, and have a poorly granulating wound bed. Ischemic ulcers should be differentiated from the neuropathic ulcers that occur over pressure points, such as the plantar surface of the foot beneath the metatarsal heads, in patients with peripheral neuropathy. Neuropathic ulcers are nonpainful and typically have a red, granulating wound bed. Ischemic ulcers should also be distinguished from ulcers that arise from chronic venous insufficiency and commonly occur near the medial and lateral malleoli. Ischemia may occasionally contribute to nonhealing of both neuropathic and venous ulcers, which necessitates assessment of the arterial circulation in all patients presenting with lower extremity ulcerations. However, the majority of patients with these latter conditions have a normal pulse on examination and adequate arterial perfusion to support wound healing, and the pathophysiology of delayed healing of these ulcers is quite distinct from that of true ischemic ulceration.

Gangrene of the toes and forefoot may arise spontaneously in patients with especially severe ischemia or may be the result of seemingly minor trauma. In addition, gangrene may be the result of microvascular thrombosis associated with infection. Wet (infected) gangrene is heralded by foul-smelling, purulent drainage and surrounding cellulitis; wet gangrene is a surgical emergency, and débridement of infected tissues should be performed as soon as possible to prevent spread of infection along tendon sheaths into the deeper spaces of the foot. Débridement and drainage of infected tissues should not be delayed for the purposes of evaluating the patient for possible associated ischemia. Although important, the evaluation can be postponed until after the infection is controlled. In contrast, peripheral vascular evaluation for noninfected, dry gangrene should be performed prior to surgical débridement. Revascularization, if needed, should be performed before or at the time of amputation for dry gangrene to maximize chances for primary wound healing.

The physical examination is of paramount importance in the evaluation of peripheral arterial occlusive disease. Chronically diminished blood flow to the distal extremities results in trophic changes of the skin and its epithelial appendages, including loss of hair, thinning of the skin, and thickening of the nails. Patients with severe ischemia may have pallor of the foot on elevation of the affected extremity, with rubor on dependency that results from maximal cutaneous vasodilatation. The affected extremity may be cool to the touch. Coolness is not a reliable finding in the presence of the sympathetic dysfunction with loss of vasomotor tone that occurs in some diabetic patients. The presence and location of ulcerations and gangrene of the lower extremities should be noted. In examining the feet, it is important to look in the web spaces between the toes, because ulcerations and sinus tracts in these spaces may be easily overlooked.

The pulses of both extremities should be assessed and compared, including the femoral pulses at the groins, the popliteal pulses behind the knees, and the dorsalis pedis and posterior tibial pulses at the ankles. The amplitude of the pulse at each of these locations can be graded as normal, diminished, or absent. The pulse distal to hemodynamically significant lesions in the more proximal arteries will be diminished or absent. For example, patients with significant aortoiliac disease have diminished femoral pulses at the groin, whereas patients with isolated femoropopliteal disease may have normal femoral pulses but decreased popliteal pulses behind the knee. Bruits, which signify turbulent blood flow, may be auscultated at or just distal to significant occlusive lesions and are commonly heard in the inguinal crease or in the distal thigh where the superficial femoral artery traverses the adductor hiatus.

ADJUNCTIVE DIAGNOSTIC TESTING

Peripheral arterial occlusive disease can usually be diagnosed on the basis of the history and physical examination alone. In patients presenting with the aforementioned complaints and physical findings, no further studies are necessary to ascertain the diagnosis. However, noninvasive evaluation in the vascular laboratory is helpful to provide objective data that confirm the diagnosis, document and quantify the hemodynamic severity of the occlusive process, and provide a baseline with which later findings can be compared. The simplest and most useful noninvasive test is determination of the ankle-brachial index (ABI), which may be performed in the clinic or at the bedside. The ABI is determined by dividing the Doppler-derived blood pressure at the ankle by the Doppler-derived pressure of the brachial artery. A blood pressure cuff is inflated just above the malleoli at the ankle. The systolic opening pressure in the dorsalis pedis and posterior tibial arteries is determined by listening for the return of a Doppler signal in the artery while the cuff is slowly deflated. Similarly, the brachial pressure is determined by insonating with the Doppler device at the antecubital fossa after a blood pressure cuff has been placed around the upper arm. To correct for occlusive disease, which is occasionally present in one of the upper extremity arteries, the pressure should be determined in both arms, and the higher value used for calculation of the ABI. A normal ABI value is 0.92 or greater. In patients with claudication, the ABI is generally in the range of 0.50 to 0.92; patients with limb-threatening ischemia generally have ABIs of less than 0.50. Caution must be exercised in evaluating ABIs in diabetic patients, who frequently have calcification of the ankle arteries, leading to noncompressibility of these vessels. The blood pressure cuff in such patients can be inflated to pressures of greater than 200 to 300 mm Hg without diminution of the Doppler signal in the more distal arteries. Vessel noncompressibility results in falsely elevated pressure readings and a falsely elevated ABI. The digital arteries to the toes are usually spared the calcification process. Toe pressures obtained with small cuffs on the toes and photoplethysmographic (PPG) tracings may be more reliable than ankle pressures and ABIs in the diabetic population. A normal toe-brachial index is 0.7 or greater; an absolute toe pressure of 50 mm Hg or greater usually signifies adequate perfusion to the forefoot to support wound healing.

Another physiologic test that we have found increasingly useful for the evaluation of healing potential is measurement of transcutaneous oxygen tension (Tco_2). By means of sensors applied to the external surface of the skin, the partial pressure of oxygen in the interstitial space at this region can be determined. The equipment is small, lightweight, and highly portable and can easily be taken to the bedside. The normal Tco_2 value is 40 mm Hg or above. A value of 30 mm Hg or above signifies good (more than 80%) wound healing potential, while a value of 20 mm Hg or below signifies poor (less than 5%) chance of wound healing. This information is very useful for determining if revascularization will be necessary for a given ulcer to heal or if observation is warranted. It is also useful for selecting the level of amputation at which wound healing will occur without preliminary revascularization. Tco_2 measurement is inaccurate in the presence of edema or cellulitis.

The use of noninvasive color-flow duplex ultrasonography has been a major advance in the diagnosis and treatment of peripheral vascular disease. It can be used to evaluate both occlusive and aneurysmal lesions and to provide information regarding the physiologic significance of these lesions. Color-flow scanning is increasingly used in lieu of arteriography to evaluate candidates for potential therapeutic intervention. Compared with arteriography, color-flow scanning is noninvasive, nonpainful, and less expensive and has a complication rate of virtually zero. The indications for color-flow duplex examination in the evaluation of peripheral arterial occlusive disease are still evolving. At present, it seems that the most useful application is to determine whether symptomatic lesions are amenable to endovascular versus open operative methods of treatment. Localization and evaluation of these lesions prior to the patient's arrival in the angiographic suite may then direct the appropriate placement of arterial access sheaths, helping to limit the amount of radiographic contrast necessary to complete the examination.

Color-flow scanning may also sometimes be useful to evaluate the hemodynamic significance of questionable anatomic lesions seen with arteriography. At present, patients who are to undergo operative revascularization are better evaluated with arteriography than with duplex alone, although suitable distal tibial or pedal targets for bypass that cannot be demonstrated arteriographically occasionally are confirmed to be patent with duplex scanning.

TREATMENT

Lower extremity occlusive disease is only one manifestation of the generalized process of atherosclerosis. Affected patients have a significantly increased risk of stroke, myocardial infarction, and cardiovascular death. In fact, a diminished ABI has been shown to be an independent predictor of cardiovascular and all-cause mortality, even in patients with asymptomatic peripheral arterial occlusive disease. Of patients with lower extremity arterial disease, 75% will die of a coronary or cerebrovascular event. For this reason, all patients with peripheral atherosclerosis, regardless of symptom status, should receive treatment for systemic atherosclerosis. Risk factor modification is the cornerstone of such therapy. Smoking cessation should be strongly encouraged. Reduction of low-density lipoprotein (LDL) cholesterol levels in hypercholesterolemic persons has been shown to reduce the incidence of coronary events. Although there is no current evidence indicating a beneficial effect on the course of peripheral atherosclerotic disease, the incidence of cardiovascular events in such patients may be reduced. Maintenance of euglycemia in diabetics and control of hypertension may also delay the progression of the atherosclerotic process.

To date, results with pharmacologic management of peripheral vascular disease have been disappointing. Pentoxifylline (Trental), a rheologic agent that has Food and Drug Administration (FDA) approval for the treatment of intermittent claudication, has shown mixed efficacy in randomized, placebo-controlled trials. Clinical benefit may be achieved in about one third of patients receiving this drug, but the expense of therapy probably does not justify its widespread use. Aspirin, although beneficial in reducing coronary and cerebrovascular events, has not been demonstrated to relieve symptoms of claudication or retard the progression of atherosclerosis. However, aspirin has been shown to improve long-term patency of peripheral and coronary bypass grafts that were performed for atherosclerotic occlusive disease. There is no role for warfarin (Coumadin) in the treatment of peripheral occlusive disease.

Perhaps the most important measure in the nonoperative treatment of lower extremity claudication is a regular program of exercise. Patients should be encouraged to walk to the point of tolerance on a daily basis, with expected doubling or more of walking distance after 3 to 6 months. Although it was previously thought that the mechanism of improved exercise tolerance was recruitment of collateral blood supply, this is probably not the case. Other possibilities include improved metabolic efficiency of the muscles and changes in the perception and tolerance of pain symptoms.

The indications for therapeutic intervention by endovascular or open operative methods in peripheral arterial occlusive disease are limb-threatening findings of rest pain, nonhealing ulcers, and gangrene and claudication that produces true disability and limitation of lifestyle. It is necessary to consider the systemic nature of atherosclerosis and the incidence of periprocedural complications in evaluating the risks and benefits of revascularization for each patient.

Arteriography is virtually always recommended prior to elective revascularization by endovascular or open procedures. Arteriography provides definitive assessment of the extent of the occlusive process, including the status of the inflow and outflow components of circulation above and below the site of most severe disease. Because of the attendant risks and expense of the procedure, arteriography should not be performed unless assessment of the history, physical findings, results of noninvasive testing, and comorbid conditions indicates that the patient is indeed a candidate for revascularization. Arteriography is not a diagnostic procedure; it should be used only as a tool to plan operative strategy.

Most patients with severe ischemia requiring intervention are found to have multilevel occlusive disease on arteriography. Patients may have aortoiliac and femoropopliteal disease, femoropopliteal and infrapopliteal disease, or a combination of all three. For patients with aortoiliac and infrainguinal disease, correction of the inflow (aortoiliac) disease should be performed first. If the aortoiliac disease is severe, up to 80% of patients will improve sufficiently with an inflow procedure alone and not require correction of the infrainguinal disease. The necessity for concurrent correction of inflow and infrainguinal occlusive disease relies on clinical judgment and experience; there is presently not a good objective test to determine which patients will improve sufficiently with an inflow procedure alone. It is usually best to correct all levels of disease in patients with isolated infrainguinal lesions.

The selection of an endovascular or a traditional, open operative procedure to correct significant atherosclerotic occlusive disease should be based on reported intermediate- and long-term results with each method. Endovascular methods of treatment, including percutaneous transluminal angioplasty (PTA) with or without stent placement, are most appropriate for focal lesions of short length in the large, proximal, high-flow vessels. Results are better in patients with claudication than in those with limb-threatening ischemia, because the patients with claudication tend to have less extensive disease with better run-off. Patency rates are approximately 70% at 2 years in the iliac arteries, 50% at 2 years in the femoropopliteal segment, and less than 50% at 2 years in the infrapopliteal vessels. The role of intravascular stenting as an adjunct to PTA is still evolving. Stenting is definitely indicated for the treatment of PTA-related dissection and restenosis. There is also evidence that stenting improves the long-term primary patency rates with common iliac artery PTA from approximately 60% to 70% or more at 5 years, although definitive confirmation of this awaits the results of ongoing prospective trials. There appears to be no benefit to routine stenting in combination with infrainguinal PTA.

More diffuse disease in the aortoiliac segment and nearly all cases of disease in the smaller infrainguinal arteries are best treated with traditional bypass procedures. Aortofemoral bypass procedures using prosthetic conduit have excellent patency rates of 85% or more at 5 years and 70% or more at 10 years. Autogenous conduit (usually the greater saphenous vein, if it is available) is nearly always preferable to prosthetic graft materials for infrainguinal bypass procedures, with the possible exception of grafts to the above-knee popliteal artery. Some reports indicate equivalent patency rates for autogenous and prosthetic grafts that do not cross the knee. The 5-year patency rate with above-knee grafts is approximately 70%. With grafts to the tibial arteries below the knee, 5-year patency rates in the range of 50 to 80% are reported. A program of routine surveillance duplex scanning of autogenous grafts to detect any abnormalities before failure and thrombosis of the grafts occur has had an extremely beneficial effect on patency rates. Up to one third of grafts will have abnormalities, usually intimal hyperplasia developing either at venous valve sites or at the anastomoses, that require minor revision.

VENOUS THROMBOSIS

method of
MARK R. NEHLER, M.D.
University of Colorado Health Sciences Center
Denver, Colorado

and

GREGORY L. MONETA, M.D.
Oregon Health Sciences University
Portland, Oregon

Multiple advances in understanding and management of deep venous thrombosis (DVT) have occurred in the last decade. Increased knowledge of hypercoagulation disorders, both congenital and acquired, has made the diagnosis of truly idiopathic DVT unusual. Understanding of the prevention, management, and natural history of catheter-related axillary or subclavian DVT has been refined. Serial duplex examinations have documented the natural history of recanalization and valvular incompetence in thrombosed venous segments. Improved methods of catheter-directed thrombolysis and potential benefits for subsequent valvular function with early recanalization have fueled an interest in early regional thrombolytic therapy for proximal lower extremity DVT. The availability of accurate methods of tibial venous duplex scanning using color-flow technology has led to re-examination of the controversy regarding the potential danger of isolated calf DVT.

Prophylaxis of DVT has also changed. The use of plantar venous plexus compression devices is applicable in a greater number of orthopedic and trauma patients. Multiple-decade follow-up results are now available to document safety of the Greenfield vena cava filter, and large series of prophylactic percutaneous placement of vena cava filters in high-risk patients have been reported. Perhaps the most important development has been the proven efficacy of low-molecular-weight (LMW) heparins in both prophylaxis and therapy for DVT. These drugs can be given subcutaneously without need for activated partial thromboplastin time (APTT) monitoring. The potential exists to transform DVT from an inpatient to an outpatient disease.

ETIOLOGY

DVT is best understood as a continuous, progressive, frequently multifocal disease process rather than a single localized event with a low likelihood of recurrence. Predisposing events (trauma, surgery, intravenous catheters) are often implicated in the final formation of DVT, but evidence supporting the importance of underlying systemic factors is increasing. Not surprisingly, the list of potential risk factors (Table 1) has grown substantially in the past decade, making truly idiopathic DVT an increasingly rare entity. Significant new developments have evolved in understanding the genesis of DVT with respect to systemic factors (congenital and acquired hypercoagulable states) and local factors (intravenous catheters, operative manipulation).

An important advance in the etiology of DVT has been the discovery of an inherited factor V resistant to activated protein C (factor V Leiden, resulting from an autosomal dominant single-point amino acid substitution of glutamine to arginine). The protein C system is critical in limiting thrombosis. Binding of thrombin to thrombomodulin on the endothelial surface activates the protein C complex. Activated protein C keeps thrombosis in check by degrading factors V and VIII_a. Factor V Leiden, due to the amino acid substitution, is resistant to this degradation, promoting an imbalance in favor of thrombosis. The prevalence of this mutation in the normal population is 2 to 4%, making it the most common genetic factor predisposing to thrombosis. Several clinical studies of DVT in a variety of patient populations document a 10 to 30% incidence of factor V Leiden. This genetic defect is also associated with DVT recurrence. At the present time, it is unclear whether patients with DVT who have factor V Leiden should undergo lifetime anticoagulation or limited anticoagulation of higher intensity and/or longer duration.

Another recently described genetic coagulation abnormality is a point mutation in the 3′ untranslated region of the prothrombin gene. This defect results in elevated plasma prothrombin levels and a three- to fivefold increased risk of DVT. Heterozygosity for this gene has been demonstrated in 5 to 18% of patients with DVT and in 1.2% of normal persons.

Other hereditary hypercoagulation disorders include protein C deficiency, protein S deficiency, antithrombin III deficiency, the presence of lupus anticoagulant, and plasminogen activator deficiency. These defects are very rare, and routine screening for them in all cases of DVT is probably not cost-effective. Conversely, high levels of factor VIII are found in 11% of the population and reportedly increase the DVT risk sixfold. Traditionally, treatment for symptomatic patients with hypercoagulation disorders is

TABLE 1. **Risk Factors for Deep Venous Thrombosis**

Surgery	Antithrombin III deficiency
Trauma	Homocystinemia
Paralysis	Lupus anticoagulant
Malignancy	Plasminogen activator deficiency
Pregnancy	Increased factor VIII levels
Factor V Leiden	Intravenous lines
Protein C deficiency	Prothrombin gene mutation
Protein S deficiency	

lifetime anticoagulation. Asymptomatic patients appear to be at increased risk for DVT (2.5 to 3.5% cases of DVT per year) and should receive prophylactic anticoagulation at periods of high risk (pregnancy, surgery, trauma).

Homocystinemia is another newly recognized risk factor for DVT. Homocystinuria is a rare inherited disorder of methionine metabolism (most frequently due to a homozygous defect in cystathionine β-synthase activity) that results in accumulation of homocystine in the plasma, with untreated afflicted patients dying of multiple arterial and venous thromboses in the second or third decade. Several clinical studies of idiopathic DVT have demonstrated homocystinemia in 10 to 20% of patients. The mechanism promoting thrombosis in homocystinemia is not completely understood, but may involve the potential production of toxic by-products by the thiol side group of the homocystine molecule with resultant endothelial damage. Abundant information indicates elevated plasma homocystine can be predictably normalized with oral folate in most patients.

Oral contraceptive regimens have historically been considered a risk factor for DVT. Newer preparations with diminished estrogen content have been designed to lower this risk. Despite this, a recent study from the World Health Organization determined that the use of oral contraceptives increased the risk of DVT by more than fourfold. Risk correlated significantly with increased body mass index. The increased risk was apparent within 4 months of starting the oral contraceptives and resolved within 3 months of discontinuing them. Surprisingly, the new third-generation progestins (with the lowest dose of estrogen) are associated with the greatest risk.

The association of DVT and malignancy is well known. Potential mechanisms include increased platelet aggregation, thrombocytosis, hypercalcemia, activation of factor X by tumor-produced serine proteases, and acquired antithrombin III deficiency. Several recent studies have demonstrated a 5 to 25% chance of coexistent or subsequent occult malignancy in patients with apparently idiopathic DVT. Therefore, a careful screening examination for occult malignancies (physical examination including rectal examination, testicular examination, prostate examination, and prostate-specific antigen assay in male patients; pelvic examination, breast examination, and mammography in female patients; and chorioembryonic antigen assay and chest radiography in all patients) should be performed in older patients with DVT and no clear-cut underlying cause.

The influence of local mechanical factors on DVT formation has also been examined. Studies of these factors provide insight for improved prevention strategies, particularly regarding intravenous dialysis catheters. A review of outcomes in more than 1700 patients undergoing percutaneous hemodialysis access demonstrated a 0.3% incidence of DVT/stenosis from internal jugular catheters compared with 8.2% from subclavian catheters. Another review cites an incidence of subsequent subclavian/superior vena cava (SVC) stenosis from subclavian hemodialysis catheters of 20 to 50%, presumably due to repetitive endothelial trauma at multiple sites secondary to the angulated route from the subclavian vein to the SVC. At present the less tortuous internal jugular route for SVC access is preferred because of the probability of decreased endothelial trauma. Research is ongoing to develop new catheter systems that will further minimize endothelial trauma.

The femoral vein as a site for central venous access has undergone re-evaluation. A small prospective randomized trial comparing internal jugular/subclavian lines with femoral lines demonstrated DVT in 25% of the femoral line group of 24 patients and in none of the 21 patients in the upper access group. A prospective ultrasound study of 56 femoral catheters placed in 54 pediatric patients demonstrated inferior vena cava occlusion in 10.7% (correlated with catheter duration). A prospective evaluation of femoral catheters in trauma patients monitored with venous duplex scanning demonstrated DVT in 9 of the 76 patients (12%). Clearly, femoral vein catheterization should be avoided if possible.

Operative manipulation may predispose to the development of DVT. A venographic survey of 745 consecutive patients undergoing total hip replacement with use of heparin or LMW heparin for anticoagulation demonstrated DVT in 81 (10.8%) patients (half of the thrombi involved the femoral vein). The investigators then performed necropsy studies in 10 cadaver limbs using either anterior or posterior approaches for total hip replacement. Using standard operative manipulations (medial rotation of up to 110 degrees in combination with varying degrees of adduction and/or flexion), they demonstrated significant folding of the femoral vein at the level of the lesser trochanter. These authors concluded that the combination of adduction and flexion should be minimized to avoid femoral venous trauma when using either the anterior or posterior approach for total hip replacement.

Intra-abdominal venous compression from insufflation for laparoscopic procedures has the potential to compromise venous flow. Eight patients undergoing laparoscopic cholecystectomy had left common femoral venous duplex scanning performed before and after abdominal insufflation. Abdominal insufflation caused significant venous stasis and elevated venous pressures. Some version of DVT prophylaxis may be prudent in patients undergoing laparoscopy.

Operative positioning may also increase DVT risk. Popliteal venous duplex scanning was performed in 100 normal persons with the lower limbs in full knee extension and demonstrated total compression in 17 and more than 50% compression in another 10. These findings suggest that full knee extension in supine patients on the operating table is undesirable, and that some effort to provide partial knee flexion should be attempted if possible.

NATURAL HISTORY

Recent clinical trials emphasize the dynamic and recurrent natural history of DVT. A European trial of 6-week versus 6-month oral anticoagulation therapy for DVT examined recurrence rates. Of 897 patients, 123 had clinically evident episodes of recurrent DVT (18.9% in the 6-week group and 9.5% in the 6-month group). The difference in the groups represented recurrences at between 2 and 6 months. After this point, the recurrence rate in both groups was 5 to 6%.

Another study randomized 90 patients with DVT to anticoagulation or to phenylbutazone and early ambulation. Serial venography documented thrombus progression in almost 50% of limbs, with no significant difference between the two treatment groups. The same authors, using ventilation-perfusion (V/Q) scans at the time of DVT diagnosis, demonstrated clinically silent pulmonary embolus in almost 50% of patients, a finding confirmed by others.

Serial venous duplex scanning has greatly expanded understanding of the natural history of DVT. A prospective study of 177 patients with DVT in 204 extremities that used serial duplex examinations at 1 day, 1 week, 1 month, every 3 months for 1 year, and then annually has provided important data on the dynamic nature of DVT. Thrombi propagated to new segments in 30% of initially involved extremities, and rethrombosis occurred in 31%. Thirteen percent of venous segments had both rethrombosis and propagation. Valvular reflux occurred most often in initially uninvolved venous segments that were subsequently involved with thrombus propagation. Known clinical risk factors were not helpful in predicting propagation or rethrombosis. A smaller study demonstrated a 16% incidence of progression/rethrombosis in 19 patients followed sequentially with venous duplex scanning. In addition, plasma markers of systemic fibrinolysis were measured. Thrombus regression was evident by 1 to 2 weeks, and by 24 to 36 weeks only 26% of residual thrombus remained. Complete resolution of thrombus occurred in 56% of patients. Tissue plasminogen activator (TPA) activity increased within 2 weeks, remained elevated through week 8, and then dropped to baseline levels by 24 to 36 weeks. Elevated TPA activity correlated with the time course of maximal venous segment recanalization. Patients with thrombus progression/rethrombosis appeared to have slightly less systemic TPA activity. Other serial venous duplex studies have confirmed that lysis appears to continue through at least 6 months, 75% of thrombosed segments will undergo recanalization, and up to 50% of limbs with DVT will undergo complete thrombus resolution by 6 months. Conversely, DVT propagation occurs in 20 to 40% of limbs despite apparently adequate anticoagulant therapy. Of interest, patients with lower extremity motor paralysis have been shown to have a significantly longer DVT recanalization period.

The development of valvular reflux continues long after the initial onset of DVT. In 123 limbs studied for a mean of 1 year, reflux was present at DVT diagnosis in 14%, occurred in another 17% within 1 week, and by 1 year affected almost two thirds of all extremities. The popliteal and femoral venous segments were most commonly affected. Reflux developed predominantly in segments initially thrombosed but was not entirely limited to those areas. This finding has potential implications regarding thrombolytic therapy for DVT.

The controversy regarding the natural history and optimal management of isolated calf DVT continues. Historically, this entity has been considered relatively benign, with a low risk of pulmonary embolism. Primary management consisted of serial noninvasive examinations of the limb to detect thrombus progression into the popliteal vein (incidence of less than 20%), which would then mandate anticoagulation. Recent data challenge this. Serial duplex examinations in 288 patients with isolated calf vein DVT demonstrated propagation in 28% (none in patients receiving heparin therapy). Patients with symptomatic calf DVT treated for 1 week were found to have a significantly greater recurrence rate than those who received treatment for 3 months. Nine pulmonary emboli (two fatal) diagnosed with high-probability V/Q scan or pulmonary angiogram in 26 patients with isolated calf DVT and pulmonary symptoms have been reported. One fourth of 58 patients with isolated calf DVT monitored with serial duplex examinations had persistent symptoms and valvular reflux in these segments at 1 year. Eleven percent of these patients had pulmonary emboli diagnosed at DVT presentation.

Catheter-related subclavian/axillary DVT also has undergone re-evaluation. Eighty-five consecutive patients with subclavian/axillary DVT associated with use of intravenous catheters were managed aggressively with intravenous heparin and catheter removal and evaluated prospectively. A V/Q scan was performed within 24 hours. Thirteen patients (15%) had pulmonary embolism, which was fatal in two cases. A larger retrospective review of 170 patients with axillary/subclavian DVT (only half of whom received anticoagulation) demonstrated pulmonary embolism in 7% but a 3-month mortality rate of 34%. It appears that patients with axillary/subclavian DVT have approximately a 10% incidence of pulmonary emboli, which are occasionally fatal, and a high short-term mortality related to systemic diseases (such as malignancy).

Free-floating deep vein thrombi are occasionally visualized in the iliofemoral system by venography or, more commonly, duplex scanning. Two recent studies have demonstrated a relatively moderate incidence of pulmonary embolism (10%) in patients with free-floating thrombi. The majority of the pulmonary emboli occurred by the time the free-floating thrombi were discovered. Over time, the majority of these thrombi become adherent to the venous wall.

DIAGNOSIS

Color-flow duplex scanning has been accepted as the diagnostic method of choice for detecting infrainguinal DVT both above and below the knee. A recent prospective evaluation in 75 patients with suspected DVT demonstrated 100% sensitivity and 98% specificity for DVT above the knee, and 94% sensitivity and 75% specificity for DVT below the knee. The investigators also surveyed 190 limbs in 99 patients considered at high risk for postoperative DVT and demonstrated DVT in 23% (more than 90% were isolated thrombi below the knee). The sensitivity of duplex scanning in these asymptomatic patients was only 55%. Therefore, although color-flow duplex examination is highly accurate in evaluating symptomatic patients, this may not be true for surveillance of asymptomatic high-risk groups. Color-flow duplex scanning has proved to be the initial diagnostic procedure of choice for axillary/subclavian DVT, with a sensitivity of nearly 90% and a specificity approaching 100%.

Several large DVT series in which the DVT was diagnosed by duplex scanning have detailed the incidence and anatomic distribution of thrombus. These studies indicate that the incidence of DVT in symptomatic patients referred to a vascular laboratory for evaluation of the presence of DVT is between 12 to 25%. Ninety-five percent of these thrombi are located in the popliteal or proximal veins. In addition, patients with superficial phlebitis harbored occult DVT in 23% when examined with venous duplex scanning. Forty percent of these DVT lesions were in or proximal to the popliteal vein. Based on these data, venous duplex imaging is probably indicated for patients with any leg symptoms potentially consistent with DVT or with evident superficial phlebitis.

Several reports have questioned the need to perform bilateral venous duplex studies in patients with unilateral symptoms. Strothman and colleagues retrospectively reviewed a 2-year experience with venous duplex imaging performed to rule out DVT. In 248 patients with DVT, every patient with DVT in the asymptomatic limb had DVT in the symptomatic limb. The authors concluded that treatment would be unchanged, so that contralateral examination is unnecessary. Another group prospectively examined 50 patients with bilateral symptoms consistent with DVT and found no DVT. They concluded that venous duplex examination was not indicated in patients with bilateral symptoms. However, a review of 2511 bilateral venous duplex studies demonstrated DVT in 43% (30% with unilateral symptoms and 13% with bilateral symptoms). Thirty-six percent of unilateral DVTs were in limbs contralateral to the symptomatic ones. Therefore, bilateral venous imaging in patients suspected of DVT seems prudent. A major limitation of venous duplex imaging for DVT has been the inability to consistently differentiate new from old thrombus in patients suspected of having recurrent DVT. Experimentally produced red blood cell–fibrin mesh acute thrombus demonstrates an initial higher decibel signal intensity that diminishes over time. This work has recently been duplicated in human patients with DVT undergoing serial examinations.

Another major limitation of venous duplex imaging is the inability to consistently visualize the pelvic veins. Magnetic resonance imaging (MRI) with spin echo imaging has been used to detect DVT in the pelvis and abdomen with some success. A review of abdominal MRI scans in 72 patients with suspected intra-abdominal DVT using both spin echo and gradient echo imaging demonstrated a sensitivity of 88%. Spin echo images are viewed in transverse sections and can demonstrate inflammatory changes in the venous wall that may help differentiate acute and chronic thrombus. Also, visualization of soft tissue changes may delineate the underlying cause of DVT. The major limitation has been false-positive readings due to sluggish flow rather than to thrombus.

Magnetic resonance venography (MRV), using flow-sensitive techniques, has been developed to avoid this problem. Eighty-five patients with suspected DVT underwent both MRV and contrast venography ranging from the vena cava to the popliteal veins. Of the 101 venous systems studied, 27 had DVT. All were correctly identified with MRV, but MRV also had false-positive results in three cases, due to extrinsic venous compression, for a sensitivity of 100% and specificity of 96%. A similar evaluation in 61 patients demonstrated almost identical values for MRV in detecting pelvic DVT. Considerable research has also focused on the role of noninvasive tests in the diagnosis of pulmonary embolism. The most important study was the Prospective Investigation of Pulmonary Embolism Diagnosis (PIOPED) trial. This multicenter study has provided the best data on sensitivity and specificity of V/Q scanning in the diagnosis of pulmonary embolism. A random sample of 933 patients was obtained from a total of 1493 patients undergoing evaluation for pulmonary embolism. All except 2 patients (931) underwent V/Q scans, and 755 also underwent pulmonary angiography. The remaining 176 patients did not undergo pulmonary angiography owing to normal V/Q scans or patient refusal. Each study was independently evaluated by two examiners. Agreement for V/Q scans and pulmonary angiography was more than 90% for both very low- and high-probability studies, but only 70 to 75% for intermediate- and low-probability V/Q scans. Seventy-three percent of V/Q scans were intermediate- or low-probability scans. Thirteen percent were high-probability scans. Of the 755 pulmonary angiograms, 251 demonstrated emboli. Twenty-four (3%) were considered inconclusive. A high-probability V/Q scan had a sensitivity of 41% but a specificity of 97% (this was reduced in patients with a prior history of pulmonary embolism). High-probability or intermediate-probability V/Q scans had a sensitivity of 82% but a specificity of only 52%. These data settle some controversy regarding V/Q scanning with the following conclusions. A high-probability V/Q scan indicates pulmonary embolism (unless recurrent), but only a minority of patients with pulmonary emboli have a high-probability V/Q scan. A normal or near-normal V/Q scan essentially eliminates pulmonary embolism as the diagnosis. A low-probability scan with a low index of clinical suspicion makes the diagnosis of pulmonary embolism unlikely. An intermediate-probability V/Q scan is not helpful in the diagnosis of pulmonary embolism.

Owing to the lack of sensitivity of the majority of V/Q scans obtained to investigate pulmonary embolism, some interest has also focused on venous duplex examination of the lower extremities to document DVT in patients with possible pulmonary emboli. However, although it has been assumed that more than 90% of pulmonary emboli arise from the lower extremities, negative results on duplex scanning are observed in more than 50% of cases of pulmonary embolism documented by pulmonary angiography. Thus, a negative result on duplex examination of the lower extremity veins cannot be used to rule out a diagnosis of pulmonary embolism in a patient with clinical signs or symptoms suggestive of pulmonary embolism. A positive result on duplex scanning for DVT certainly provides grounds for anticoagulation therapy but does not confirm pulmonary embolism. Because the length and intensity of anticoagulation may be influenced by the presence of pulmonary embolism, a confirmatory study documenting pulmonary embolism is advisable in most cases.

Testing for plasma D-dimer in patients suspected of having pulmonary embolus is evolving as a means of excluding the diagnosis of pulmonary embolism. Plasma D-dimer is a plasmin degradation product of cross-linked fibrin clot, and its level is elevated in a number of thrombotic states. An elevated level does not confirm a diagnosis of pulmonary embolism; a normal level, however, virtually excludes the diagnosis (false-negative results were noted in 3 of a total of 148 patients in several studies).

PROPHYLAXIS

Intermittent pneumatic compression devices have become a standard method of DVT prophylaxis. Comparative studies of surgical patients at high risk have demonstrated a reduction in the frequency of DVT from 20 to 40% to 5 to 15% when these devices are used (Table 2). However, a moderate number of patients are unable to be fitted with these devices because of the location of injury or operative sites. These devices are uncomfortable for many patients and difficult to place properly on the limb. Peroneal neuropathy complicating their use has been reported. Improper application by hospital personnel was reported in up to 50% of surveillance examinations in either routine nursing units or intensive care units despite nursing education.

The plantar venous plexus is recognized as an important peripheral venous pump, and compression during ambulation is partially responsible for venous return. A number of new devices designed to compress the plantar venous plexus alone have undergone evaluation. These devices cover only the foot and offer the advantages of increased patient applicability, comfort, and ease of placement and appear to provide augmentation of blood flow in the deep veins of the leg equal to or better than that achieved with standard full-size leg compression devices. A single randomized clinical trial of 75 patients undergoing total hip surgery demonstrated use of the plantar compression device to be more effective prophylaxis for DVT than administration of aspirin and subcutaneous heparin.

TABLE 2. **Comparative Studies Using Intermittent External Pneumatic Compression (EPC) for Postoperative Deep Vein Thrombosis (DVT) Prophylaxis**

Author	Year	No. of Patients	Type of Surgery	Incidence of DVT (%)	
				Control	*EPC*
Hull	1990	310	Orthopedic	49	24
Turpie	1977	128	Neurosurgery	19	2
Clarke-Pearson	1984	107	Gynecology	35	13
Hartman	1982	104	Orthopedic	19	2
Hills	1972	100	General surgery	30	12
Skillman	1978	95	Neurosurgery	25	9
Borow	1981	168	Mixed	36	11
Hull	1979	61	Orthopedic	66	6
Coe	1978	53	Urology	25	7
Black	1986	146	Neurosurgery	18	6

Titanium Greenfield vena cava filters can be placed percutaneously. Use of this new device, similar to the older stainless steel Greenfield filter, which required transvenous placement, appears to be associated with a minimal rate of long-term adverse events (pulmonary embolism in less than 5%, cava occlusion in less than 5%). It has not, however, been evaluated for the same length of time as has the older vena cava filter. Several clinical series of high-risk trauma patients who underwent prophylactic placement of Greenfield filters have been reported. Patients selected for study had high injury severity scores, and despite the prophylactic goal of preventing DVT, the mean time from admission to filter placement in these trials ranged from 4 to 9 days. Only 1 patient of the combined 171 patients in these series developed a pulmonary embolism. There were two procedure-related complications (one misplaced filter requiring thoracotomy and one internal jugular DVT). The vena cava patency rate was 96% at one year (reported in only one study). Problems include the lack of a randomized control group for these evaluations and the minimal follow-up time in these predominantly young patients with indwelling devices.

Prophylactic vena cava filters have also been used in cancer patients, and a recent Medicare analysis demonstrated an increase in their use in older patients despite the stable incidence of DVT in this population. Similar concerns regarding justification for increased use of prophylactic vena cava filters have been reported by others. Postprocedure femoral vein thrombosis at the access site has been reported in 35%; 10% of these thrombi were occlusive. Harris and coworkers reported phlegmasia cerulea dolens in 4 of 17 patients (with one fatal case) who underwent filter placement without anticoagulation. They caution against the use of prophylactic vena cava filters and recommend continuing anticoagulation in patients in whom filters have been placed.

The use of LMW heparin has had a profound impact on DVT prophylaxis and treatment. These compounds inhibit factor X_a activity and factor II_a activity. Compared with unfractionated heparin, LMW heparin preparations have a longer half-life, improved bioavailability, and less variability in anticoagulant response to a fixed dose. They can be administered subcutaneously once or twice daily with no need for laboratory monitoring. They are currently approved in the United States for prophylaxis in general surgery and orthopedic patients.

A meta-analysis of the use of LMW heparin for DVT prophylaxis in general and orthopedic surgery summarizes the available data for prophylaxis. Studies comparing LMW heparin with placebo have demonstrated considerable efficacy for LMW heparin. Seventeen trials of LMW heparin versus twice-daily, low-dose unfractionated heparin demonstrated increased effectiveness of LMW heparin in some but not all studies (Table 3). LMW heparin was more effective than thrice-daily, low-dose unfractionated heparin. These studies suffer from nonuniform designs and the use of differing preparations of LMW heparin. Subsequent to this analysis, a large randomized trial of trauma patients demonstrated that LMW heparin reduces proximal DVT by 50% compared with unfractionated heparin (5000 units subcutaneously twice daily).

The duration of risk for DVT at the time of elective surgery is not clear. Traditionally, patients receive prophylaxis until the time of hospital discharge. A prospective study of 42 patients discharged free of DVT (as determined by venography or duplex scanning) demonstrated proximal DVT in 4 patients within 2 months of discharge during follow-up surveillance. The incidence of symptomatic pulmonary embolism has been demonstrated to increase by 30% if carefully sought for after hospital discharge. In response to these concerns, a recent randomized trial included 262 patients who all received LMW heparin for prophylaxis during their hospitalization for total hip arthroplasty. They were then randomized at discharge to receive either LMW heparin or placebo for outpatient therapy until the total time of prophylaxis reached 1 month. Serial venography was used to detect DVT. At 1-month follow-up, patients who received LMW heparin had no pulmonary emboli and 21 DVTs, compared with 2 pulmonary emboli and 43

TABLE 3. **Low-Molecular-Weight Heparin versus Low-Dose Heparin for Prevention of Deep Venous Thrombosis (DVT) in General Surgery and Orthopedic Patients**

		Low-Molecular-Weight Heparin		**Low-Dose Heparin**		
Author	**Year**	*Cases of DVT*	*Total No. of Patients*	*Cases of DVT*	*Total No. of Patients*	*No. of Daily Doses*
Schmitz-Huebner	1984	3	81	0	80	2
Kakkar	1986	5	196	15	134	2
Sashara	1986	14	126	14	134	2
Onarheim	1986	1	24	0	27	2
Bergqvist	1986	13	215	9	217	2
Koller	1986	2	70	2	68	2
Bergqvist	1988	28	505	41	497	2
Briel	1988	1	95	1	98	2
Borstad	1988	0	105	0	110	2
Caen	1988	6	195	7	190	2
Kakkar	1989	8	88	10	91	2
PLSG	1989	34	861	26	868	2
Baumgartner	1989	6	87	7	89	2
Verardi	1989	1	44	3	44	2
Speziale	1989	3	46	4	49	2
FSG	1988	27	960	42	936	3
Samama	1988	13	406	20	406	3
Flicker	1988	2	40	0	40	3
Dahan	1989	0	50	0	50	3
Kruck	1989	2	150	8	150	3
Adolf	1989	16	202	14	202	3
Planes	1988	15	120	27	108	3
Eriksson	1989	13	70	18	70	3
Chiapuzzo	1988	5	70	7	70	3
Dechavanne	1989	5	77	8	76	3
Koringer	1989	3	35	7	33	2
Monreal	1989	14	32	6	30	3
Lassen	1989	14	53	23	54	2
Breyer	1986	5	70	7	70	2
Total		258	5073	316	5061	

DVTs in those receiving heparin only during hospitalization and placebo thereafter.

THERAPY

The importance of early therapeutic anticoagulation is illustrated by a European randomized trial of DVT therapy either with heparin followed by acenocoumarol or with acenocoumarol alone. The trial was terminated early owing to 40% DVT extension in the acenocoumarol-only group. Traditional therapy for DVT with unfractionated intravenous heparin suffers from difficulties in establishing expedient therapeutic anticoagulation. Patients are frequently underanticoagulated early in the course of therapy. There is also an apparent diurnal variation in anticoagulant response to heparin, with the maximal response occurring between 4 and 6 AM and the minimal response occurring near noon. The greatest interpatient changes occur between 6 and 8 AM, frequently the time at which morning blood specimens are drawn. It has been suggested that daily APTT be assessed at standard times (10 AM and/or 10 PM) to minimize this variability. There is also a difference in responsiveness of various activated APTT reagents to heparin. Use of a protamine titration method to determine the therapeutic range of heparin may be more reliable.

A nomogram method of administration of heparin, as bolus of 5000 units followed by either 40,000 units per 24 hours or 30,000 units per 24 hours, with or without simultaneous warfarin therapy, was prospectively evaluated in 199 consecutive patients with proximal DVT to attempt to eliminate problems with undertreatment when heparin is given intuitively. Accordingly, subtherapeutic APTTs (less than 55 seconds) were seen in less than 2% of patients in the first 24 hours of therapy. However, supratherapeutic APPTs (greater than 85 seconds) were seen in 69% of the combined-therapy group and in 24% of the heparin group, with bleeding occurring in 9 and 12%, respectively. Recurrent DVT was documented in 7% of patients in both groups. The authors concluded that supratherapeutic APTTs with an aggressive heparin dosage nomogram are associated with a decreased thrombotic risk without increased risk of bleeding. A further study confirms the safety of initiating early (within 48 hours of diagnosis), simultaneous warfarin therapy with initial heparin therapy for DVT.

A meta-analysis summarizes the available published randomized trials of LMW heparin in the treatment of DVT. Importantly, in the 10 randomized trials reviewed, the incidence of recurrent DVT or pulmonary embolism was reduced by 50% with LMW heparin compared with unfractionated heparin. The incidence of major bleeding episodes was reduced by almost 70% and mortality was reduced by almost 50% with LMW heparin compared with unfractionated heparin. A recent prospective trial of 10-day therapy with LMW heparin for DVT demonstrated that twice-daily therapy was more effective than once-a-day dosing. Patients were kept ambulatory with leg compression bandages from the time of diagnosis, with warfarin anticoagulation initiated during hospitalization. Several patients with symptomatic pulmonary embolism on presentation were included in this trial.

The logical extension of results of the foregoing research is outpatient therapy for DVT with LMW heparin. A prospective randomized trial from Canada and England examined treatment for proximal DVT with at least 5 days of either inpatient intravenous unfractionated heparin (in 253 patients) or outpatient twice-daily subcutaneous LMW heparin (in 247 patients). Warfarin was begun on day 2, with the goal of an International Normalized Ratio (INR) of 2 to 3. Serial examinations (duplex scanning, impedence plethysmography, or venography) were performed to evaluate for recurrent DVT. There was no difference in the rate of recurrent DVT between the two groups (5.3% versus 6.7%). A similar trial with duplicate findings was conducted in Europe. At present, however, LMW heparin is not approved for DVT treatment in the United States, although approval is expected.

Recombinant hirudin is a pure, specific antithrombin agent that effectively inactivates clot-bound thrombin in vitro. It has an extremely short half-life and requires a constant infusion when given intravenously. A pilot study of twice-daily hirudin therapy given subcutaneously for 5 days followed by acenocoumarol in 10 patients with DVT demonstrated stable APTT levels paralleling the plasma hirudin level. One patient had recurrent DVT. Hirudin has also been used successfully to treat DVT in a patient who suffered heparin-associated thrombocytopenia, as has the rapidly acting defibrinogenating drug ancrod. The development of additional drugs for use in patients with heparin antibodies is important. LMW heparin is not a useful agent for this condition because of cross-reactivity.

The use of systemic thrombolytic therapy for DVT compared with standard anticoagulation has been reported in multiple prospective trials. A recent review summarizes the data. This approach is expensive. Only 10 to 20% of patients with DVT are potential candidates for systemic thrombolytic therapy. Only 50% of patients treated will have successful lysis of thrombus (however, a majority of patients in these trials had extensive DVT in the iliofemoral system, perhaps predisposing them to an inability to respond to systemic administration of the agents). Thrombus of more than 1 week's duration is unlikely to undergo lysis (at present there is no accepted method to accurately determine the age of DVT lesions). Patients who demonstrate no clinical response venographically at 24 hours are unlikely to respond, and treatment should be stopped. However, a long-term follow-up study demonstrated popliteal valvular reflux in only 9% of patients with successful initial lysis, but reflux occurred in 75% of patients without successful initial lysis. This finding, combined with some of the duplex study–derived natural history data, has continued to fuel an interest in thrombolytic therapy for acute DVT, particularly extensive iliofemoral DVT. According to other studies, only a fraction of all patients with DVT in tertiary care hospitals are potential candidates for systemic thrombolytic therapy.

Owing to the relative lack of success with systemic thrombolysis for DVT, catheter-directed regional thrombolysis has been tried in selected patients with iliofemoral DVT. This regional approach to thrombolytic therapy has several advantages. The dose of lyric agent is usually half that required to achieve success when delivered systemically, thus decreasing the bleeding risk and increasing the number of patients for whom this approach may be suitable. Older thrombus can be effectively treated with regional therapy (if the lesion can be crossed with a guidewire, it can usually be lysed). The presence of catheters in the area of DVT allows potential interventions for residual lesions (angioplasty and/or stent placement) that may theoretically improve long-term success. A potential problem is pulmonary embolism. The placement of a temporary or permanent vena cava filter was therefore used initially by several groups. The presence of the filter often made treating the lesion more cumbersome. In addition, dislodgement of the filter with catheter manipulations was also a possibility. Most investigators have therefore abandoned routine filter placement in patients undergoing catheter-directed thrombolysis.

Dake reported on the use of regional thrombolysis via the transjugular approach in 27 consecutive limbs in 21 patients with iliofemoral DVT. Catheters crossed the lesion in 93% of cases, with an initial success rate of 85%. Average duration of therapy was 30 hours. Complete lysis was achieved in 72% and partial lysis in 20%. Eighteen limbs had residual stenosis with more than 50% occlusion, and 16 limbs underwent further interventions (angioplasty alone in 2 and angioplasty followed by stent placement in 14). However, only 52% of the 23 successfully treated limbs underwent follow-up evaluation (by duplex scanning for confirmation of patency at 3 months). Comerota reported regional thrombolysis via the contralateral groin or transjugular in 7 patients with iliofemoral DVT in a combined report with surgical thrombectomy with or without bypass. Complete clot lysis was achieved in the five patients with successful catheter positioning. None of these patients experienced reocclusion at a mean of 38 months.

Hirsch and colleagues have reported the largest prospective series of regional thrombolysis for iliofemoral DVT to date. Eighty-seven limbs in 77 patients have been treated since 1990. The majority were approached by the transjugular route. The average duration of therapy was 75 hours, and 79% of lesions were successfully lysed. Eighty-six endoluminal stents were placed in 38 limbs for residual stenoses (defined as lesions with pressure gradients of 3 mm Hg or greater or with collateral flow visualized). In 15 limbs, arteriovenous fistulas were placed for low velocities as determined on postprocedural duplex scanning. Three patients in whom thrombolysis failed to achieve lysis underwent venous bypass, and adjunctive mechanical thrombectomy was performed in 17 limbs. Five patients had major bleeding, and one patient had pulmonary embolism. All patients received at least 6 months of warfarin therapy. Postprocedural duplex examinations were performed at 1 month, 3 months, 6 months, and then annually. The life table 2-year primary and secondary iliac vein segment patency rates were 60% and 78%, respectively. However, the 2-year primary and secondary patency rates for the femoral vein segments were only 37% and 51%, respectively. An ongoing multicenter venous registry of patients undergoing regional thrombolysis for both suprainguinal and infrainguinal DVT has enrolled more than 160 patients with at least 6 months' follow-up.

Recent experience with surgical thrombectomy for iliofemoral DVT has primarily been in Europe. This technique has not been popular in the United States owing to widely reported operative mortality rates of approximately 10% and high early and late rethrombosis rates of more than 50%. Proponents claim that with use of modern anesthesia techniques and intraoperative positive end-expiratory pressure during thrombus manipulation to minimize pulmonary embolism, and creation of adjunctive arteriovenous fistulas (with later percutaneous closure) to improve perioperative venous flow during the endothelial healing phase, results have substantially improved. Juhan reported on 77 iliofemoral venous thrombectomies performed in 75 patients. Operations were performed at a mean of 6 days from onset of symptoms. The surgical approach was a common femoral venotomy using balloon catheters and suction maneuvers to remove the iliac vein thrombus. External compression was used to extrude distal thrombus in the femoral and popliteal veins. When inferior vena cava control was required, a right subcostal transperitoneal incision was used. An arteriovenous fistula was constructed from the common femoral vein and ligated at 6 to 8 weeks postoperatively. There were no perioperative deaths. The mean follow-up period was 8.5 years. Patency was assessed with either ascending venography or venous duplex scanning. Life table results demonstrate that after early failure with iliofemoral rethrombosis in 12 limbs by 1 year, the remaining iliofemoral segments continued patent, with 5- and 10-year combined patency rates of 84%. Valvular competence was less durable. Although 80% of femoropopliteal venous segments were competent at 5 years, only 56% were competent at 10 years (however, the small number of segments evaluable at this time interval precluded accurate statistical analysis). Only 10% of patients developed moderate or severe symptoms of chronic venous insufficiency. Unfortunately, a high proportion of the patients (35% of the total and 41% of those with early rethrombosis) was lost to follow-up. Neglen reported 48 consecutive patients with iliofemoral DVT treated with thrombectomy and construction of an arteriovenous fistula. At 2 years, 88% of the iliac segments were patent, but only 56% of the femoropopliteal segments were competent. Nineteen percent of patients had symptoms requiring use of compression stockings.

Several small comparative trials of thrombectomy versus anticoagulation or thrombolysis for iliofemoral DVT have been performed in Europe. The results have been mixed. Eklof, in a randomized trial of thrombectomy versus standard anticoagulation, reported significantly more asymptomatic patients in the surgical management group at 5 years but could not correlate clinical findings with convincing hemodynamic differences. Hold, in a nonrandomized comparison of anticoagulation, systemic thrombolysis, and thrombectomy, also could not correlate subjective improvements with objective findings. Ganger, in a randomized trial of thrombectomy versus anticoagulation, found that the significant benefits of thrombectomy (increased venous recovery times, diminished edema) were maintained only in patients operated on within 3 days of onset of symptoms. At present, iliofemoral venous thrombectomy is performed in multiple centers in Europe but only occasionally in the United States.

Thrombolysis and embolectomy have also been studied in patients with acute symptomatic pulmonary embolism. The majority of patients in these trials have been hemodynamically unstable, and the diagnosis has frequently been made by bedside echocardiography demonstrating acute right heart failure. A multicenter registry of patients with symptomatic pulmonary embolism documented the results of systemic thrombolysis in 478 patients with pulmonary embolism. Mortality rates ranged from 8.1% of hemodynamically stable patients to 65% of patients needing cardiopulmonary resuscitation. Despite the presence of contraindications to thrombolysis in 40% of the treated patients, major bleeding occurred in only 9.2%. The registry data also demonstrated reduced mortality rates (4.7% versus 11.1%), reduced recurrence rates (7.7% versus 18.7%), but an increased incidence of bleeding episodes (21.9% versus 7.8%) in all patients receiving thrombolytic therapy compared with anticoagulation. The investigators speculated that thrombolytic therapy may be superior to anticoagulation regardless of hemodynamic presentation. As with DVT, the success of thrombolytic therapy is inversely correlated with duration of symptoms. In one additional study, 46 patients with symptomatic pulmonary embolism were randomized to receive thrombolytic therapy or heparin therapy. Echocardiography demonstrated improvement in right ventricular wall motion in 39% of the thrombolytic therapy group but in only 17% of the heparin therapy group. No clinical recurrent pulmonary emboli were observed in the thrombolytic therapy group, but there were five recurrences, two of which were fatal, in the heparin therapy group.

Pulmonary embolectomy is for patients with acute pulmonary embolism and hemodynamic instability. Most patients have either failure of or contraindications to systemic thrombolytic therapy. Cardiopulmonary bypass is routinely used. Mortality rates in small series range from 20 to 40%. Up to half of the mortality is due to right heart failure or recurrent pulmonary emboli, prompting most authors to advocate use of vena cava filters in these patients postoperatively.

Section 5

The Blood and Spleen

APLASTIC ANEMIA

method of
LYLE L. SENSENBRENNER, M.D.
University of Maryland School of Medicine
Baltimore, Maryland

Aplastic anemia is a clinical syndrome characterized by pancytopenia of varying degree and a demonstrated hypoplastic marrow with no evidence of infiltrating disease. What hematopoietic cells remain must show no evidence of dysplasia. Macrocytosis may be seen in the erythroid lines, but no dyserythropoiesis or dysplastic changes of the granulocytic or megakaryocytic lines should be present. Chromosomal analysis of those hematopoietic cells present in the marrow must show no clonal abnormalities (e.g., deletions, translocations).

Aplastic anemia is classified in several ways (Table 1). The two most commonly used classifications are by severity of the pancytopenia (severe, super severe, and not severe or moderate) and etiologic, that is, whether there is an inherited condition predisposing to the disorder or the disease is acquired in the absence of a recognized underlying predisposition (inherited versus acquired aplastic anemia).

The end result of the pathogenic process is the failure of the marrow to produce an adequate number of precursors and mature cells. Toxins and other marrow-damaging agents act either by directly destroying the earliest stem cells in the marrow or by causing nonlethal damage to progenitor cells, exposing antigens that induce an autoimmune destruction of early marrow cells. Whatever the pathogenesis or etiology, replacement of stem cells from a normal donor appears able to correct the defect, because allogeneic marrow transplantation has been reported to be successful in restoring normal hematopoiesis in all forms of aplastic anemia.

TABLE 1. **Classification of Aplastic Anemia**

Severity	
Super severe	Neutrophils <200/mm^3 Platelets <20,000/mm^3 Reticulocytes <40,000/mm^3
Severe (2 of 3)	Neutrophils <500/mm^3 Platelets <20,000/mm^3 Reticulocytes <40,000/mm^3
Moderate	Pancytopenia less than severe
Etiologic Classification	
Acquired aplastic anemia	
Idiopathic	
Secondary to a recognized etiologic agent	
Toxins and chemicals—benzene, trinitrotoluene, chlorophenol pesticides	
Drugs—chloramphenicol, hydantoins, gold, carbamazepine, phenylbutazone, sulfonamides, penicillamine, cancer chemotherapeutics	
Viruses—Epstein-Barr virus, hepatitis (not hepatitis A, B, C, or G)	
Autoimmune disorders	
Radiation	
Pregnancy	
Inherited aplastic anemia	
Fanconi's anemia	
Dyskeratosis congenita	
Shwachman-Diamond syndrome	
Amegakaryocytic thrombocytopenia	
Familial aplastic anemia	

CLINICAL PRESENTATION

A complication of one of the cytopenias usually results in the symptoms that compel the patient to seek medical attention. The most common presenting feature is bleeding secondary to thrombocytopenia. This is first manifested by either petechiae, especially of the dependent portions of the body, or minor bleeding from other sources, such as the gums during tooth-brushing. The petechiae frequently progress to ecchymoses, and the patient has no history of trauma to explain their presence.

The second most common presenting symptom is frequent or severe infections with no clear explanation. These infections are commonly at the sites of minor trauma, such as a small cut or a skin or mucosal abrasion. They frequently occur in the mouth, throat, nasal passages, and sinuses.

Anemia, along with its symptoms of fatigue, shortness of breath on exertion, and weakness, is occasionally the factor initiating the patient's visit to the physician's office.

DIAGNOSIS

The diagnosis of aplastic anemia is made by a complete blood count to determine the severity of pancytopenia. In addition, a careful inspection of the peripheral blood smear and marrow aspirate is essential to rule out any dysplastic changes. A bone marrow biopsy is essential to accurately assess cellularity and to detect the presence of any infiltrating diseases, such as metastatic cancer, leukemia, or lymphoma. Chromosomal analysis of the marrow aspirate cells should also be done to rule out clonal dysplastic disorders. Careful attention should be paid to the physical examination to rule out Fanconi's anemia. If the patient is younger than 30 years or there is any suspicion that Fanconi's anemia might be the underlying cause (short stature, history of or presence of extra or missing digits on the hands, numerous café au lait spots, or congenital renal abnormalities), a clastogen-induced chromosomal breakage study of peripheral blood lymphocytes should be done to exclude the disorder. A careful history, elucidating an underlying etiology or familial incidence, is of value for determining the type of aplastic anemia, because the approach to therapy in some cases varies with the etiology of the disorder.

THERAPY

Supportive Care

Blood Product Support (Table 2)

Because pancytopenia is the major manifestation of aplastic anemia, supportive measures are directed primarily at correcting bleeding, infections, and anemia. Thrombocytopenic bleeding can be a serious and even lethal complication of aplastic anemia, and it is corrected primarily by the use of platelet transfusions. Major bleeding almost never occurs in patients with aplastic anemia in whom the platelet count is higher than 20,000 per mm^3. Significant bleeding usually occurs only when the platelet count has fallen to 5000 per mm^3 or less.

Platelet transfusions can and often do lead to severe alloimmunization, resulting in refractoriness to further platelet infusions. The fewer transfusions given the patient, the less likely that alloimmunization will result. Therefore, my colleagues and I give platelet transfusions only if one of the following conditions is present: (1) the platelet count is 5000 per mm^3 or less, (2) the patient is bleeding, (3) the patient is febrile with a platelet count of 10,000 per mm^3 or less, (4) the patient has demonstrated bleeding at a platelet count greater than 5000 per mm^3 and the count is now that low, or (5) the patient is to undergo a procedure that could cause bleeding, such as surgery, a diagnostic "scoping" procedure, or tooth extraction.

To prevent alloimmunization, the use of leukocyte-depleted platelet products should be standard practice for any transfusion for aplastic anemia patients. If platelet support is required, 10-minute post-transfusion platelet counts are obtained to determine whether an adequate incremental rise in platelet count is obtained with each transfusion. If a poor response to the transfused platelets is detected, studies of lymphocytotoxic antibody should be carried out. If evidence of severe alloimmunization is detected, the use of either crossmatched platelets or of platelets matched for the class 1 HLA antigens may be required to obtain an adequate increment in the platelet count with transfusion.

TABLE 2. **Therapeutic Approaches to Aplastic Anemia**

Immunosuppressive Regimens	
ATG, 40 mg/kg/d IV × 4 d, plus cyclosporine, 2–5 mg/kg/d IV, or 2.5–7.5 mg/kg q 12 h PO for 3–4 mo	
or	
Cyclophosphamide, 45–50 mg/kg/d × 4 d IV over 1–2 h	
Supportive Care	
Transfusions	Use leukocyte-depleted products. For potential transplant patients, use only CMV-negative products unless patient and/or donor is CMV-positive.
Platelets	Only if patient is bleeding or count <5000/mm^3, or if count <10,000/mm^3 and patient is febrile, or if count <50,000/mm^3 and patient is to undergo a surgical procedure.
Red blood cells	When hemoglobin <7.0 gm/dL or patient is symptomatic from anemia (9.0 gm/dL if patient is having bleeding problems).
Neutropenic fever	Imipenem, 500–1000 mg q 6 h IV *or* Ceftazidime, 1–2 gm q 8 h IV If fever persists, add vancomycin, 1 gm q 12 h IV If fever persists, add amphotericin, 0.75 mg/kg/d IV

Abbreviations: ATG = antithymocyte globulin; CMV = cytomegalovirus.

Alloimmunization becomes a severe problem for patients who might be candidates for allogeneic bone marrow transplantation. Many of the antigens that are important for rejection of transfused platelets are also responsible for the rejection of an allogeneic marrow graft. Thus, it has been shown that the fewer the number of platelet transfusions a patient with aplastic anemia has received, the more likely that patient is to accept an allograft. It is important that patients who might be candidates for a transplant receive as few platelet transfusions as possible and that all such transfusions be leukocyte depleted.

As the disease progresses, red blood cell transfusions are required. Most patients can tolerate a slowly developing anemia as long as the hemoglobin level remains above 7 grams per dL. If the patient is symptomatic from the anemia at a level greater than 7 grams per dL and is unable to carry out normal activities of daily living, transfusions of red blood cells are indicated. In patients in whom bleeding is a problem, or who are to undergo a procedure that could result in bleeding, the hemoglobin level should be kept at least 2 grams per dL higher, that is, above 9 grams per dL or 2 grams per dL above the symptomatic level if that level is higher than 7 grams per dL.

All red blood cell products should be leukocyte depleted to prevent alloimmunization. Each unit of red blood cells contains about 250 mg of iron, an element the body has no mechanism for removing. If iron stores develop to a high level, damage to pancreas, liver, and heart can result, with lethal consequences. To prevent such complications, chelation therapy should be instituted early in the course of the disease. At present, the only chelating agent available is deferoxamine (Desferal), which must be administered either quite slowly intravenously or by subcutaneous infusion. The usual dose of deferoxamine is 1.5 to 2.5 grams per day given subcutaneously and using a portable pump to administer the drug. Chelation therapy should begin after 20 to 50 units of red blood cells have been administered or when the serum ferritin level is greater than 600 ng per mL.

For the severely neutropenic patient, meticulous care should be taken to prevent infections, including careful cleansing and prevention of breaks in the skin if at all possible. Finger or earlobe sticks to obtain blood should be avoided. Careful hand washing is essential, as are good oral hygiene and dental care to prevent infectious sites from developing. The use of prophylactic antibiotics is to be avoided except for coverage during an invasive procedure such as tooth extraction or colonoscopy. The use of antifungal prophylaxis with an agent such as fluconazole (Diflucan) can and often does lead to overgrowth of resistant fungi. Infections that do occur in neutropenic patients must be treated promptly with empirically chosen broad-spectrum antibiotics while awaiting the results of cultures of blood, urine, throat, sputum, and any potentially infected site. Imipenem (Primaxin), 500 to 1000 mg intravenously every 6 hours, or ceftazidime (Fortaz, Tazicef, or Tazidime), 1.0 to 2.0 grams every 8 hours intravenously, is an effective empirical antibiotic regimen that can be used while awaiting culture results. If after 48 to 72 hours the patient remains febrile with little in the way of signs of improvement, vancomycin (Vancocin, Vancoled), 1 gram every 12 hours intravenously, is added to cover possible gram-positive organisms. If fever continues more than 72 hours longer with the double-antibiotic regimen and a source and organism have not been determined, or if the patient's condition appears to be deteriorating, antifungal coverage with amphotericin B (Fungizone), 0.25 to 0.75 mg per kg per day intravenously, should be added. If the patient demonstrates a serious infection with an organism shown to be resistant to antibiotics, granulocyte transfusions may be considered, but they are associated with severe reactions in addition to alloimmunization. In patients with no defined period of neutropenia, granulocytes are frequently ineffective in the long run.

Blood products can jeopardize a later marrow transplant by transmitting cytomegalovirus (CMV) as well as other viruses with the transfusions. Marrow recipients who are serologically negative for CMV and who have a donor who is negative have the best chance of not having problems with the virus during the transplantation. Therefore, all blood products given to a patient with aplastic anemia should be from a CMV-negative donor until the CMV serologic status of the patient has been established. If the patient is CMV-negative or of indeterminate status, all blood products should be CMV-negative. If CMV-negative products are not available and transfusion is necessary, a filter to remove any white blood cells should be used in the administration of the product. If the patient or the donor is serologically CMV-positive, the status of the blood product is not important. Because family members could share minor antigens with the donor, antigens that the patient may not have, family members should not be used as blood product donors for potential transplant candidates.

Hematopoietic Growth Factors

If the granulocyte count is less than 500 per mm^3, granulocyte colony-stimulating factor (Neupogen) or granulocyte-macrophage colony-stimulating factor (Leukine) may be used to temporally raise the granulocyte counts. The usual dosage is 250 μg per m^2 per day given subcutaneously. However, this dosage rarely causes a rise in the hemoglobin level or the platelet count, and the granulocyte count drops back to the pretreatment level shortly after the drug is stopped.

Specific Therapy (Table 3)

Bone Marrow Transplantation

For patients younger than 50 years who have severe acquired aplastic anemia and for whom an HLA-identical donor is available, the therapy of choice is marrow transplantation. A sibling donor is preferred. If none is available, one can occasionally find a perfectly matched donor in the unrelated donor registry. Because the earlier in the course of the disease one attempts transplantation, the more successful the procedure is, one should refer all potential transplant recipients to a transplant center immediately after making the diagnosis of severe aplastic anemia. With allogeneic marrow transplantation utilizing an HLA-matched sibling donor, one expects a long-term disease-free survival of greater than 75%. If radiation is not utilized in the regimen to prepare the patient for transplantation, the rate of post-transplantation neoplastic complications is low (<5%).

Patients with inherited forms of aplastic anemia are also candidates for marrow transplantation if a suitable donor can be found. However, it is essential to determine the underlying disease process, such as Fanconi's anemia, because patients with such processes are exceedingly sensitive to agents such as

TABLE 3. **Approach for Treating Patients with Aplastic Anemia**

I. Severe aplastic anemia.
   A. If patient is younger than 55 years, perform HLA typing of siblings and other potential family member matches.
      1. If a match, proceed to marrow (stem cell) transplantation.
      2. If no match in family, proceed to immunosuppressive therapy and begin searching the unrelated donor registries for a marrow donor.
         a. If anemia responds to immunosuppressive therapy, follow patient with no further therapy.
         b. If anemia fails to respond to immunosuppressive therapy, give supportive therapy while pursuing an unrelated marrow donor. Consider androgens, cytokines, or experimental therapies.
   B. If patient is 55 years or older, give immunosuppressive therapy along with supportive care.
      1. If anemia responds to immunosuppressive therapy, follow patient with no further therapy.
      2. If anemia fails to respond to immunosuppressive therapy, give supportive therapy and consider androgens, cytokines, or experimental therapies.

II. Moderate aplastic anemia.
   A. Transfusion independent: observe patient.
   B. Transfusion dependent: immunosuppressive therapy.
      1. If anemia responds, observe patient.
      2. If no response and the transfusion requirements are more frequent than once a month, consider androgens, cytokines, or experimental therapies. If patient is younger than 55 years, consider for transplantation.

cyclophosphamide and radiation, and they must be prepared for transplantation with a much milder regimen.

Immunosuppressive Therapy

If the patient with acquired severe aplastic anemia is older than 50 years, or no donor for a younger patient can be readily identified, immunosuppressive therapy should first be attempted. The most commonly used regimen for immunosuppression is antithymocyte globulin (ATG) (Atgam), 40 mg per kg per day intravenously for 4 consecutive days, followed by 3 to 4 months of cyclosporine (Sandimmune),* starting at 5 mg per kg per day as a continuous infusion, and after 5 days gradually tapering the dose to maintain a blood level of between 150 and 450 ng per mL of whole blood. If the patient can tolerate the drug orally, it may be given in doses of 5 to 10 mg per kg every 12 hours. Careful attention to blood levels of cyclosporine and creatinine is necessary, with adjustments in the cyclosporine dose if toxicity occurs. Serum sickness, manifested as arthralgias, arthritis, fever, proteinuria, and rash, is a common complication of ATG therapy and is treated with a steroid such as prednisone or methylprednisolone (Solu-Medrol) at a dose of 0.5 to 1.0 mg per kg per day. This dose should be tapered and the steroid discontinued as soon as the process subsides.

If a patient has not shown response to the therapy by 4 months after starting the cyclosporine, it should be stopped. If, however, the patient has shown a response, the cyclosporine is tapered slowly, being reduced by no more than 5% a week, while the blood counts are carefully monitored and higher doses are instituted if the counts begin to fall. Another immunosuppressive regimen reported to be quite effective in a small series of patients with severe acquired aplastic anemia is the use of cyclophosphamide (Cytoxan),* 45 to 50 mg per kg per day for 4 days given as an intravenous infusion over 1 to 2 hours. The patients in the small series who showed a response to cyclophosphamide had no episodes of relapse of disease and no late clonal disorders.

Immunosuppressive therapy has been tried in patients with aplastic anemia secondary to Fanconi's anemia, with little success.

Androgens

Androgens, either alone or in combination with immunosuppressive therapy, have had some degree of efficacy, but the results have been extremely variable. Reported results vary from no response to more than 30% of patients showing response. The most commonly used agents are oxymethalone (Anadrol-50), at a dose of 3 to 5 mg per kg per day orally. At present, however, this compound is no longer available in the United States. Nandrolone deconate (Deca-Durabolin), a compound that is as effective as oxymethalone, is available and possibly has less hepatotoxicity. It is given intramuscularly (deep in the buttocks), a potential problem in patients with pancytopenia. The dosage is 3 to 5 mg per kg weekly for up to 12 weeks. We have also used danazol (Danocrine),* 400 to 800 mg per day orally, with some success.

Androgens have been shown to be effective in Fanconi's anemia as well and have resulted in remissions of the pancytopenia for months to even years in some patients.

*Not yet approved for this use in the United States.

IRON DEFICIENCY ANEMIA

method of
WILLIAM B. SOLOMON, M.D.
State University of New York Health Science Center at Brooklyn
Brooklyn, New York

Iron, the fourth most abundant element in the earth's crust and the most abundant transition metal in living organisms, is required for oxygen transport, electron transfer reactions, and deoxynucleotide synthesis; ironically, molecular iron is poorly absorbed in the gastrointestinal tract, making iron deficiency the most common cause of anemia in the world. In the United States, 4 to 5% of women of childbearing age (an estimated 3.3 million) have iron deficiency anemia, and an additional 7% (an estimated 4.3 million) have depleted iron stores; 1 to 2% of men above age 50 have iron deficiency anemia; of infants 1 to 2 years of age, 3% (an estimated 240,000) have iron deficiency anemia, and 6% (an estimated 460,000) have depleted iron stores.

MECHANISMS OF IRON DEFICIENCY

Depletion of iron stores is usually defined as a serum ferritin of less than 15 ng per mL; when this is accompanied by a hemoglobin of less than 10.5 grams per dL in children or women of childbearing age, or less than 13.5 grams per dL in adult males, the criteria for the diagnosis of iron deficiency anemia are met (Table 1). When iron depletion is sufficient to cause anemia, erythrocytes are hypochromic, as evidenced by a decreased mean cell hemoglobin (MCH); microcytic, with a decreased mean cell volume (MCV) to less than 80 fL; and anisocytotic, with an

TABLE 1. **Diagnostic Criteria for Iron Deficiency Anemia**

Hemoglobin
Children or women: <10.5 gm/dL
Men: <13.5 gm/dL
AND
Mean cell volume <80 fL
AND
Serum ferritin <15 ng/mL
OR
Serum soluble transferrin receptor >28 nM
OR
Absent stainable iron stores in macrophages obtained from bone marrow aspirate

increased range distribution of width (RDW) to more than 16%.

In infants and toddlers, iron depletion, even in the absence of anemia, may lead to psychomotor retardation. When deficiency of iron leads to a hemoglobin of less than 9 grams per dL, during activity there is accelerated production of blood lactate and tachycardia, leading to a decrease in exercise capacity and work performance. The impairment in performance and anemia can be reversed by repletion of iron stores.

In infants, iron depletion and iron deficiency anemia are usually caused by poor intake of dietary iron. Multiparous women, vegetarians, athletes, frequent blood donors, persons experiencing gastrointestinal blood loss, patients who have undergone gastric surgery, users of antacid medications or nonsteroidal anti-inflammatory drugs (NSAIDs), and recent immigrants from hookworm-endemic regions have an increased risk of iron deficiency anemia (Table 2). In adults older than 50 years of age, iron deficiency anemia is almost always secondary to blood loss in the lower or upper gastrointestinal tract, necessitating investigation to locate a bleeding site or sites.

BODY IRON STORES, DAILY UTILIZATION, AND DIETARY REQUIREMENTS

Iron most commonly exists in either of two valency states, Fe^{3+} (ferric) or Fe^{2+} (ferrous), permitting it to participate in many oxidation-reduction reactions. Since free ferric iron is difficult to absorb and also highly destructive to cellular enzymes and DNA, the body has developed homeostatic mechanisms to absorb, transport, and retain iron.

The total quantity of tissue iron in the average adult is 3800 mg. About two thirds (2500 mg) is found in the red cell mass as the iron atoms that carry oxygen within the heme moieties of hemoglobin. The muscle masses contain myoglobin, the resident oxygen transport molecule, which in total contains about 500 mg of iron. The mitochondrial heme-containing enzymes account for about 50 mg, and other iron-containing enzymes, about 200 mg. The major iron storage protein ferritin, which is synthesized in all cells, and its lysosomal breakdown product hemosiderin contain approximately 750 mg of iron in adult males and 250 mg in adult females. Each ng per mL of serum ferritin is equivalent to body stores of approximately 8 mg of elemental iron. About 15 mg of iron is found on transferrin, which is the only circulating iron transport molecule.

Because iron is always tightly bound to proteins and is otherwise highly insoluble, there is no mechanism for excretion of iron save for the normal loss of about 1 mg per day occurring with the exfoliation of cells from the gastrointestinal (GI) mucosae and skin. Blood loss is the other source of iron loss; in females of childbearing age, an additional 1.5 mg per day (on average) is lost, because the average monthly loss in menstrual blood is 40 ± 20 mL (about 0.5 mg of iron is lost with every mL of blood loss). Each full-term pregnancy results in a net utilization of about 800 to 1000 mg of iron.

The daily utilization of iron is about 35 mg. Almost all of this requirement is supplied from endogenous sources. About 25 mg is obtained by recycling the iron removed from the heme moieties when hemoglobin is released from senescent red cells removed from the circulation. An additional 5 to 7 mg of iron is obtained after its release from ferritin storage. Therefore, there is a requirement for absorption of 1 to 2 mg of dietary iron each day. Because an adequate delivery of iron to the tissues is maintained across a wide variety of iron intakes, the rate-limiting step in iron delivery to the cells appears to be its absorption.

When food iron is obtained from animal sources such as meat, chicken, and fish, it is in the more readily soluble heme molecule (iron protoporphyrin IX). When it is obtained from vegetable sources, it is in the insoluble ferric (Fe^{3+}) state. The action of the acidic gastric contents reduces ferric iron to soluble ferrous iron. Persons who have undergone gastrectomy and those who take medicines that block gastric acid secretion, so that gastric acid produced is insufficient to reduce ferric to ferrous iron, are at increased risk for iron deficiency.

In the duodenum, soluble ferrous iron is absorbed across a polarized cell by the iron (divalent metal atom) transporter termed natural resistance-associated macrophage protein-2 (Nramp-2). Heme iron is absorbed more readily than ferrous iron by a separate transport process. Heme iron and other animal proteins also help to promote the absorption of non-heme iron in the proximal small bowel. Malabsorption of iron in the proximal small bowel occurs in persons following ulcer surgery and can also occur in celiac (nontropical sprue) disease of the duodenum.

The mechanism for pumping iron out of the intestinal mucosal cell into the blood onto circulating transferrin is not well understood. Transferrin, bearing two atoms of ferric iron, binds to the dimeric transferrin receptor that is synthesized by all cells. The transferrin receptors on dividing erythroid precursor cells of the bone marrow account for about 80% of all transferrin receptors. The transferrin receptor is subject to proteolytic cleavage, resulting in the soluble transferrin receptor that circulates in the blood. Within the bone marrow, iron-laden macrophages give up their iron by a poorly understood process to erythroid precursor cells. Indeed, it is the absence of stainable

TABLE 2. **Risk Factors for the Development of Iron Deficiency Anemia**

Demographic Factors

Age
- Infants, especially premature
- Adolescents
- Elderly

Females
- Menorrhagia
- Multiparity

Recent immigrants from hookworm-endemic regions (hookworm infestation is the most common cause of iron deficiency worldwide)

Diet

Vegetarian diet
Excess tannins (tea/coffee)
Excess phytates (brans and cereals)
Alcohol abuse

Gastrointestinal Diseases

Blood loss
Celiac disease
Atrophic gastritis

Drug History

Aspirin
Nonsteroidal anti-inflammatory drugs

Iron deficiency anemia is most often found in persons with at least two risk factors.

iron within bone marrow macrophages obtained by needle aspiration that is considered to be the definitive criterion for a diagnosis of iron deficiency anemia.

The amounts of all of the known proteins involved in iron absorption, transport, and storage are regulated by the level of cellular iron. Increased amounts of the iron absorber Nramp-2, the transporter transferrin, and transferrin receptor are required during times when cellular iron is lean; when the cells are redolent with iron an increased amount of the storage protein ferritin is required. Regulation of the amount of all of these proteins appears to be mainly at the post-transcriptional level in human cells and is controlled by the activity of the iron response element–binding protein (IRE-BP) found in the cytosol that binds to specific iron-responsive elements (IREs) formed by sequences within mRNA for the aforementioned proteins (except for transferrin). The IRE-BP is related to the iron:sulfur ring containing the enzyme mitochondrial aconitase, whose function is to convert citrate to isocitrate. The enzymatic activity of cytosolic aconitase is increased when the cells are iron-replete, and the number of iron atoms per aconitase molecule increases to four. When cells are iron-deficient, the number of iron atoms per cytosolic aconitase decreases to three, which alters its molecular conformation, permitting it to bind to the IREs. The IRE for the transferrin receptor or Nramp-2 mRNA is located at its 3′ untranslated end; when bound by the IRE-BP, the mRNA is inhibited from being degraded, leading to an increase in transferrin receptor protein and Nramp-2 protein when cellular iron is in short supply. The IREs of the ferritin mRNA are located in the 5′ untranslated end of the mRNA; when bound by IRE-BP, the translation of ferritin is suppressed, leading to decreased amounts of ferritin when cells are depleted of iron. Therefore, the levels of soluble transferrin receptor and ferritin directly reflect the level of intracellular iron and can be used as diagnostic tests for iron depletion and iron deficiency anemia. A caveat remains: Ferritin is an acute phase reactant protein, and its level may be elevated during inflammatory states even with iron deficiency. The serum level of soluble transferrin receptor is not increased in inflammatory states.

DIAGNOSIS OF DEPLETED IRON STORES OR IRON DEFICIENCY ANEMIA

There are three levels of iron deficiency: The first, depletion of iron stores, is detected by a decreased serum ferritin level to below 15 ng per mL. Persons with decreased iron stores, although they may not be anemic, will very probably benefit from increased iron intake. As the level of iron stores continues to drop, the amount of transferrin increases, so that the total iron-binding capacity (TIBC) increases and the amount of saturated transferrin decreases. Finally, the last manifestation of iron deficiency is the development of a hypochromic, microcytic anemia. A complete blood count (CBC) demonstrates a decreased MCH and a decreased MCV to less than 80 fL. With iron deficiency, hemoglobinization of each erythrocyte is quite variable, resulting in anisocytosis, which on a CBC is demonstrated by an elevated RDW to more than 16%.

The difficulty in establishing a diagnosis of iron deficiency anemia is due to the fact that not all cases of anemia that is hypochromic and microcytic are secondary to iron deficiency. There are two other common causes of hypochromic and microcytic anemias that must be distinguished from iron deficiency anemia, and that on occasion can coexist with iron deficiency anemia. The *thalassemias* are a group of anemias characterized by a deficiency of globin chain synthesis, either alpha or beta, which leads to cells that have decreased hemoglobinization. The consequence is a decrease in both MCH and MCV. However, the defect appears to affect every red cell equally, leading to a normal RDW. Furthermore, the absorption of iron may be increased in these disorders, often leading to a serum ferritin above 50 ng per mL. Perhaps the most important laboratory finding that distinguishes the thalassemias from iron deficiency anemia is that the red blood cell count is normal or elevated. It is therefore said that microcytosis in the presence of a red blood cell count greater than 4.5×10^6 per μL is diagnostic for thalassemia and essentially rules out iron deficiency anemia. A diagnosis of β-thalassemia can be confirmed by hemoglobin electrophoresis demonstrating an elevation of hemoglobin A_2 (and also by column chromatography for hemoglobin A_2). The diagnosis of α-thalassemia, which is common in African-Americans and Asian-Americans, can be confirmed, when warranted, by Southern blot analysis of the alpha globin gene domain, which most often will detect deletions of one or both of the two alpha globin genes located on one or both chromosome 16's.

Also difficult to distinguish from iron deficiency anemia is *anemia of chronic disease* (ACD), which can coexist with iron deficiency anemia. This form of anemia is thought to be secondary to the secretion of inflammatory cytokines that inhibit erythropoiesis, such as interferon-γ, interleukin-1, and tumor necrosis factor. Most often, ACD is a normochromic, normocytic anemia, although on occasion the erythrocytes can be frankly hypochromic and microcytic. Furthermore, individuals with chronic inflammatory diseases such as rheumatoid arthritis often take aspirin or other NSAIDs, which can lead to GI blood loss, so that ACD can coexist with iron deficiency anemia.

Certain findings are useful to distinguish iron deficiency anemia from ACD from a combination of iron deficiency anemia and ACD. In healthy individuals, a serum ferritin of 15 ng per mL or less is considered to be evidence of iron depletion likely to require supplemental oral iron for repletion of seriously diminished iron stores. Since serum ferritin is an acute phase reactant, in patients with a chronic disease such as a collagen-vascular disorder, cancer, or rheumatoid arthritis, a serum ferritin of less than 40 ng per mL should be considered evidence of iron depletion; these patients may receive a trial of iron supplementation to determine whether they can benefit from iron treatment.

Some patients with ACD coexistent with iron deficiency anemia will have a serum ferritin greater than 40 ng per mL. To help confirm that these persons indeed have iron deficiency anemia, a soluble transferrin receptor assay can be performed. The transferrin receptor is found on all cells; by far the great mass of soluble transferrin receptor is produced by the erythroid component of the bone marrow. About 80% of all iron-containing tissue and of all transferrin receptors is found in this compartment. Therefore, any disorder that increases the amount of erythroid precursor cells in the bone marrow, such as a hemolytic anemia or thalassemia, will increase the amount of serum soluble transferrin receptor. If there is no increase in the number of erythroid bone marrow cells, then the other mechanism of increasing the amount of serum soluble transferrin receptor is via iron deficiency: In iron-deficient individuals there is an increase in the activity of the iron-binding protein, leading to increased translation of the mRNA encoding for the transferrin receptor, with a consequent increase in the amount of serum soluble transferrin receptor protein produced by each erythroid bone marrow cell.

There is no increase in the soluble transferrin receptor in individuals with ACD (i.e., no increase in erythroid compartment mass and no change in the activity of the iron-binding protein). However, there is an increase in the binding activity of the iron-binding protein in iron deficiency anemia or in those persons with ACD combined with iron deficiency anemia, leading to increased amounts of serum soluble transferrin receptor, to more than 28 nM.

Another feature distinguishing iron deficiency anemia from ACD is that in most cases, ACD responds to erythropoietin. A series of erythropoietin (Epogen) injections can be used to raise red cell mass in persons with ACD in whom the hematocrit is low, particularly those who have cardiopulmonary diseases. In contrast, iron deficiency anemia does not respond to erythropoietin.

To further complicate matters, the entity deemed "iron-deficient erythropoiesis" seen in iron-replete patients is frequently found in patients with the anemia of renal failure who receive erythropoietin injections. Individuals in whom hematocrit fails to increase after erythropoietin injections may benefit from the addition of supplemental iron, often given parenterally, resulting in an hematocrit increase.

ETIOLOGY

Deficiency of iron in children and adolescents of both sexes is almost always secondary to inadequate intake. In adults, iron deficiency is both an illness and a sign of blood loss. In menstruating women, especially those who have had full-term pregnancies, iron deficiency is common and is almost always secondary to menstrual blood loss or the requirements of the fetus for iron. In adult males, iron deficiency is considered to be a herald sign of blood loss, and in the absence of an easily identifiable source of blood loss such as hemorrhoids, it is a mandate for a GI blood loss work-up. In men, and in women older than 50 years, iron deficiency anemia requires a full work-up even in the face of an obvious site of GI blood loss because of the increased incidence of colorectal adenocarcinoma.

TREATMENT

Once the diagnosis of iron deficiency anemia is established, treatment is initiated with oral iron supplements. The standard oral preparation for iron replacement therapy is ferrous sulfate 325 mg (5 grains) tablets. Each ferrous sulfate tablet contains 65 mg of elemental iron (some pharmacies carry 300 mg ferrous sulfate tablets equivalent to 60 mg of elemental iron or Feosol, which contains 200 mg of dried ferrous sulfate equivalent to 325 mg of ferrous sulfate). At best, an individual with iron deficiency anemia will absorb (on average) no more than 20 mg of elemental iron per day. Thus, treatment can begin with just one ferrous sulfate 325-mg tablet per day. Because oral ferrous sulfate can cause gastrointestinal discomfort, each tablet should be taken with food. Ideally, the tablet should be taken with a meal containing foods rich in animal proteins and vitamin C, which promote iron absorption. The tablet should not be taken with meals rich in cereals or calcium, or with tea or coffee, all of which inhibit iron absorption. If one tablet a day is well tolerated, the dose of iron supplementation can be increased during the second week of treatment to two a day and then to three a day in the subsequent weeks of treatment. If ferrous sulfate tablets cannot be tolerated, an alternative oral treatment is a polysaccharide-iron complex capsule that contains elemental iron. Preparations are marketed under a number of names, including Niferex-150 and Nu-Iron 150; each capsule contains 150 mg of elemental iron and is taken once daily.

The response to treatment with oral iron can be ascertained by following the patient's reticulocyte count. Within 7 to 10 days after commencement of supplemental iron by mouth there is an increase in the reticulocyte count. A two- to fourfold increase above the baseline reticulocyte count is considered evidence of a response. To further confirm this reticulocyte response, the hemoglobin and hematocrit are monitored and should be increased by at least 2 grams per dL at 1 month following commencement of therapy. To confirm that iron stores are increased there should be an increase in serum ferritin and a decrease in serum TIBC (transferrin levels).

Treatment with oral iron preparations should be continued for 4 to 6 months after return of the hematocrit to normal levels so that iron stores are replenished. To confirm that iron stores are adequate a serum ferritin level can be obtained; this should be greater than 20 ng per mL.

What if there is no response to oral iron supplementation after 1 month of compliance with therapy? With ongoing GI blood loss, an acute inflammatory process such as a urinary tract infection, or renal insufficiency, or if excess calcium, phytates, or tannins are taken with the iron, then the response to iron can be inhibited. If after remediation of any of these factors there is still no response to iron, then the data leading to the diagnosis of iron deficiency anemia should be reviewed.

It is the rare patient with iron deficiency anemia who does not respond to oral iron supplementation. Lack of response to oral iron usually indicates persistent blood loss or true oral iron malabsorption secondary to nontropical sprue or other abnormalities of the proximal small bowel. For this rare patient, intravenous or intramuscular iron can be given.

Two parenteral iron preparations have been used extensively outside of the United States—ferric gluconate (Ferrlecit) and ferric saccharate; each of these preparations should be approved for use in the United States soon. The advantage of either of these preparations over iron dextran, which is the standard parenteral iron preparation used in the United States, is the absence of anaphylactic responses. The only approved parenteral iron preparation in the United States is iron dextran injection (InFeD). A formula to calculate the amount of iron dextran needed is

$$\text{Iron needed (mg)} = [15 - \text{hemoglobin (gm/dL)}] \times [\text{body weight (lb)}] + 1000$$

Since each mL of iron dextran contains 50 mg of iron,

the total number of milliliters required is obtained by dividing the mg of iron needed by 50.

Parenteral iron is toxic, and deaths due to anaphylactic reaction to intramuscular or intravenous iron dextran have been reported. In most cases up to 1000 mg of parenteral iron dextran replacement can be given intravenously in each monitored sitting. The dose of iron dextran is diluted into 1 liter of 5% dextrose in water or normal saline and is infused over 6 to 8 hours. The patient should be monitored every 15 minutes during the first hour of infusion and every 30 minutes after the first hour. Parenteral steroids and epinephrine should be readily available in case the patient develops signs of anaphylaxis such as hives, bronchospasm, hypotension, or stridor. Parenteral iron can also be given as a series of intramuscular injections; however, no more than 2 mL of intramuscular iron can be given at any one time. Most patients will require at least 15 to 20 intramuscular injections to replenish their iron stores.

It is the rare case in which it is necessary to use toxic parenteral iron preparations; before embarking on this course of treatment the patient should be seen by a hematologist.

AUTOIMMUNE HEMOLYTIC ANEMIA

method of
CHARLES J. PARKER, M.D.
University of Utah School of Medicine and the Veterans Affairs Medical Center
Salt Lake City, Utah

There are three general categories of autoimmune hemolytic anemia (AIHA), with each group having idiopathic and secondary forms (Table 1). In this article, drug-induced immune hemolytic anemia is treated as a subcategory of warm antibody AIHA.

TABLE 1. **Classification of Autoimmune Hemolytic Anemias**

Warm Antibody Autoimmune Hemolytic Anemia (approximately 80% of cases)
- Idiopathic
- Secondary (associated with chronic lymphocytic leukemia, Hodgkin's and non-Hodgkin's lymphoma, connective tissue diseases [primarily SLE], ulcerative colitis, ovarian cysts, immunodeficiency syndromes [including AIDS], antiphospholipid syndrome)
- Drug-induced

Cold Agglutinin Syndrome (approximately 18% of cases)
- Idiopathic
- Secondary (associated with *Mycoplasma pneumoniae* infection, infectious mononucleosis, lymphoreticular malignancy, viral infections)

Paroxysmal Cold Hemoglobinuria (approximately 2% of cases)
- Idiopathic (associated with chronic autoimmune disease in adults)
- Secondary (associated with viral illnesses, typically in children; also associated with syphilis)

Modified from Parker CJ: Acute hemolytic disorders. *In* Carlson RW, Geheb MH (eds): Principles and Practice of Medical Intensive Care. Philadelphia, WB Saunders Co, 1993, p 1376.

TABLE 2. **Laboratory Values That Suggest Hemolysis**

1. Reticulocytosis >125,000/μL of blood*
2. Indirect bilirubin between 1 and 5 mg/dL†
3. Haptoglobin <50 mg/dL‡
4. Elevated lactic dehydrogenase§

*If automated determination of reticulocyte concentration is unavailable, the value can be derived by multiplying the reticulocyte count (reported in percent) by the red cell concentration (RBC/μL) and dividing the total by 100. For example, if the reticulocyte count is 1 and the RBC concentration is 5,000,000/μL, the number of reticulocytes/μL of blood is 50,000.

†Patients with Gilbert's disease have increased indirect bilirubin in the absence of hemolysis. Unless there is underlying liver disease, the direct bilirubin is rarely elevated in association with hemolysis.

‡Haptoglobin is an acute phase reactant. When hemolysis occurs in association with inflammatory processes or with steroid administration, haptoglobin levels may be within the normal range.

§The normal range for LDH depends on the assay and the units of measurement and therefore varies among laboratories. LDH is mildly to moderately elevated in cases of extravascular hemolysis. Values are much higher in cases of intravascular hemolysis.

Modified from Parker CJ: Acute hemolytic disorders. *In* Carlson RW, Geheb MH (eds): Principles and Practice of Medical Intensive Care. Philadelphia, WB Saunders Co, 1993, p 1370.

WARM ANTIBODY AUTOIMMUNE HEMOLYTIC ANEMIA

Immune hemolytic anemia should be included in the differential diagnosis of patients who have laboratory evidence of hemolysis (Table 2). The diagnostic criteria for warm antibody AIHA are shown in Table 3. In addition to the general laboratory signs of hemolysis (Table 2), patients with warm antibody AIHA

TABLE 3. **Diagnostic Criteria for Warm Antibody Autoimmune Hemolytic Anemia and Cold Agglutinin Syndrome**

Criteria for Diagnosis of Warm Antibody AIHA
- Patient has not been transfused during previous four months*
- Laboratory evidence of hemolysis†
- A positive direct Coombs' test for IgG, complement C3, or both
- Absence of a cold agglutinin of high thermal amplitude‡
- Patient has a warm antibody with broad reactivity in the serum or eluted from the red cell§

Criteria for Diagnosis of Cold Agglutinin Syndrome
- Clinical evidence of acquired hemolytic anemia†
- A positive Coombs' test result for complement C3
- A negative Coombs' test result for IgG‖
- The presence of a cold agglutinin with reactivity up to at least 30°C¶

*Patient may still have AIHA, but delayed transfusion reaction should be excluded.

†See Table 2. In addition, the peripheral blood film shows microspherocytes.

‡Reactivity up to 30°C.

§If the antibody is not present in the plasma (indirect Coombs' test is negative), it can be eluted from the red cell membrane and its reactivity subsequently characterized.

‖Cold agglutinins are almost invariably IgM antibodies that activate complement.

¶The antibody causes agglutination at temperatures up to 30°C.

Modified with permission from Parker CJ: Acute hemolytic disorders. *In* Carlson RW, Geheb MH (eds): Principles and Practice of Medical Intensive Care. Philadelphia, WB Saunders Co, 1993, p 1376.

present with two other important laboratory features. First, the peripheral blood film shows microspherocytes; and second, the direct antiglobulin (Coombs') test result is positive. In approximately 67% of patients, the Coombs' test result is positive for both IgG and complement, in 20% the test is positive for IgG but not complement, and in the remaining 13%, it is positive for complement but not IgG. The indirect Coombs' test result is positive in approximately 60% of cases. "Coombs'-negative" warm antibody AIHA is uncommon but not rare (~5% of cases). These patients have laboratory evidence of hemolysis and the peripheral blood film shows microspherocytes, but the standard Coombs' test result is negative. The presence of IgG and/or complement, however, can often be demonstrated using more sensitive assays available in reference laboratories (e.g., radioimmunobinding assays using monoclonal antibodies or enzyme-linked antiglobulin tests). The clinical diagnosis of Coombs' negative AIHA is also supported by observing a response to an empirical trial of corticosteroids (see further on).

The anti-RBC antibodies of warm antibody AIHA are almost invariably classified as panagglutinins because they cause agglutination of all of the erythrocytes (RBCs) that are part of the standard test panel used by the blood bank to characterize the reactivity of anti-RBC antibodies. More detailed analysis often shows that the antibodies are directed against antigenic determinants within the Rh system (although many other specificities have been reported).

Idiopathic Warm Antibody Antoimmune Hemolytic Anemia

An approach to treatment of warm antibody AIHA is shown in Table 4. All patients should receive folate supplementation to compensate for the increased utilization that is due to the compensatory enhancement of erythropoiesis. Approximately 80% of patients with warm antibody AIHA will respond to steroids, and the response is usually rapid (within a few days). Unfortunately, permanent remissions are observed in less than 20% of cases. The decision to recommend splenectomy should be based on clinical criteria (see Table 4) because splenic sequestration studies using radiolabeled erythrocytes have not proved to be predictive of a response to splenectomy. In patients who relapse after splenectomy, low doses of prednisone (5 mg per day orally or less) may be effective in controlling the hemolytic process. Immunosuppressive therapy (see Table 4) is often beneficial in patients who have failed splenectomy. Plasmapheresis with plasma exchange is unconventional therapy but offers the possibility of rapidly ameliorating the hemolysis in emergency situations. In contrast to its value in the management of immune thrombocytopenia, intravenous immunoglobulin therapy appears to be significantly less efficacious in AIHA. Approximately 30% of patients will respond to intravenous immunoglobulin G (IVIgG), but responses are not durable, and maintenance therapy given every 3 to 4 weeks is usually required. Occasionally, patients respond to the synthetic androgen danazol* (Danocrine), and anecdotal reports suggest that some patients with AIHA may respond to immunoadsorbent therapy using immobilized protein A from *Staphylococcus aureus*.

TABLE 4. **Treatment of Warm Antibody Hemolytic Anemia**

Prednisone (1.0–1.5 mg/kg/d)*
Splenectomy†
Immunosuppressive therapy‡
Other§

*Patients who fail to respond after 3 weeks are considered to be treatment failures. If patients respond, steroids should be tapered gradually (over 3–4 mo).

†Indications: (1) failure to respond to steroids; (2) steroid dose required to maintain remission unacceptably high (>10 mg/d or 15 mg/qod).

‡Indications: (1) failure to respond to splenectomy (or a combination of splenectomy and low-dose prednisone); (2) patients who cannot tolerate splenectomy. Cyclophosphamide (Cytoxan) (1.5–2.0 mg/kg/d) or azathioprine (Imuran) (2.0–2.5 mg/kg/d) is recommended. Treatment should continue for at least 3 months.

§Plasmapheresis with plasma exchange may be beneficial in emergency situations. IVIgG produces a transient response in ~30% of patients. Responses to danazol (Danocrine) and immunoadsorption columns have been reported. All patients should be supplemented with 1 mg/d of folate.

Modified from Parker CJ: Acute hemolytic disorders. *In* Carlson RW, Geheb MH (eds): Principles and Practice of Medical Intensive Care. Philadelphia, WB Saunders Co, 1993, p 1377.

Secondary Warm Antibody Autoimmune Hemolytic Anemia

The approach to management of patients with secondary AIHA is similar to that described for idiopathic AIHA. In the case of patients with chronic lymphocytic leukemia (CLL), it is particularly important to emphasize that treating the underlying disease is unlikely to ameliorate immune-mediated processes (e.g., AIHA or immune thrombocytopenic purpura [ITP]). In fact, treatment of CLL with purine nucleoside analogues, particularly fludarabine (Fludara), has been associated with the development of AIHA and ITP. Patients who develop AIHA or ITP following fludarabine should never receive additional fludarabine or other purine nucleoside analogues, as recent reports suggest that such treatment can exacerbate AIHA or ITP, causing these processes to become intractable, with alarmingly high morbidity and mortality rates.

In general, for patients with secondary warm antibody AIHA, the decision to treat the primary disease should be made separately from the decision to treat the hemolytic anemia. For example, a patient with Rai stage 0 CLL who has AIHA but no other symptoms should receive treatment for AIHA but not CLL. In some instances, however, secondary AIHA may respond to treatment of the primary disease (e.g., treatment of lymphoma with combination chemotherapy). In other cases, treatment of the primary disease

*Not FDA approved for this indication.

overlaps with treatment for AIHA (e.g., steroid therapy for systemic lupus erythematosus).

Response to Therapy

It is not necessary that the hematocrit be normal for the patient to be classified as a treatment success. The goal of therapy is to restore the hematocrit to a level that provides adequate oxygenating capacity (usually >30% unless there are attendant problems). Further, although the titer of the direct antiglobulin (Coombs') test may fall in response to therapy, it is unusual for test results to become negative. Thus, normalization of the Coombs' test should not be a therapeutic goal.

It is important to keep in mind that idiopathic warm AIHA is a chronic disease and that relapses are common. Steroids should be tapered very slowly (over several months); however, disease exacerbations during the taper are frequent and are frustrating for both patient and physician. Patients requiring more than 10 mg per day or more than 15 mg every other day of prednisone for more than a few months are candidates for splenectomy. Patients undergoing splenectomy should receive preoperative vaccinations against pneumococcal and meningococal disease and against *Haemophilus influenzae* type B. Management of chronic AIHA is challenging, and it is not unusual for patients to require a combination of steroids, splenectomy, and immunosuppressive therapy. Patients should be informed that the disease is usually chronic and that relapses are common. Physicians should be prepared to monitor the patient frequently so that relapses can be treated promptly and therapy-related problems avoided. Prolonged use of steroids at unacceptably high levels is the most frequent cause of iatrogenic problems associated with treatment of chronic warm antibody AIHA. After splenectomy, if the dose of prednisone required to maintain an appropriate hematocrit is unacceptably high, immunosuppressive therapy should be initiated. In patients younger than 70 years, azathioprine* (Imuran) is preferred over cyclophosphamide* (Cytoxan) because the former is less leukemogenic than the latter. During the course of treatment, the hematocrit, reticulocyte count, and lactate dehydrogenase (LDH) should be monitored regularly. A rising hematocrit in association with a falling reticulocyte count and LDH is consistent with a response to therapy. On the other hand, a falling hematocrit in association with a falling reticulocyte count suggests a superimposed bone marrow problem (e.g., parvovirus infection or megaloblastic crisis associated with folate deficiency) that requires further evaluation.

Transfusion

Transfusion of patients with warm antibody AHIA should be undertaken with caution. It is important to remember that response to steroid therapy is usually rapid (within a few days). Thus, in most instances, transfusion can be avoided by reducing oxygen demand by placing the patient at rest. Nonetheless, in cases of fulminant hemolysis, or when a patient at rest becomes symptomatic while awaiting a response to therapy, transfusion can be lifesaving. Careful consideration should be given to the volume of blood to be infused since overtransfusion can be dangerous for two reasons. First, patients may experience volume overload, causing further cardiopulmonary embarrassment. Second, the rate of hemolysis of donor red cells is exponentially related to the amount of blood infused. Consequently, problems associated with acute hemolysis are more likely to occur in patients who have received relatively large amounts of blood. Accordingly, the amount of blood transfused should be the minimum required to control the patient's symptoms (e.g., 100 mL of packed cells twice a day may be sufficient to prevent high-output heart failure).

Inasmuch as the autoantibody is almost always a panagglutinin, it is virtually impossible to find donor cells that are not recognized by the patient's antibody. Therefore, the goal of the blood bank staff is not to find donor cells that are unreactive in the crossmatching studies, but rather to insure that the patient's ABO and Rh phenotypes are properly determined and that the patient does not have an alloantibody in addition to an autoantibody. A detailed history of previous pregnancies and transfusions is important as patients with warm antibody AIHA who have never been pregnant or transfused are unlikely to have become alloimmunized. A number of assays are available to identify a concurrent alloantibody, but these types of studies are usually not performed routinely. Accordingly, it is important that the blood bank have a level of sophistication and experience that insures competence in the performance and interpretation of these critical studies.

Some immunohematologists advocate that studies be undertaken to determine the relative specificity of the autoantibody so that donor cells that lack the antigen can be transfused. For example, the antibody may react more strongly with cells that have the "little e" antigen than with those that have the "big E" antigen (E and e are part of the Rh antigen system). In this case, the antibody is said to have relative specificity for "little e". However, data from limited studies suggesting that a clinical benefit results from transfusing cells that lack the antigen of relative specificity are not compelling. Nonetheless, it seems prudent to determine the relative specificity of the antibody and to avoid transfusing cells that express the antigen, especially if in vitro studies indicate a strong degree of specificity (e.g., if the antibody induces hemolysis of antigen-positive but not antigen-negative cells).

Patients with AIHA who are being transfused should be monitored closely both during and after the infusion. Laboratory studies to document the extent of hemolysis (e.g., LDH, haptoglobin, plasma free hemoglobin, and hemoglobinuria) and the development of renal compromise should be obtained.

*Not FDA approved for this indication.

Drug-Induced Immune Hemolytic Anemia

In reviews of drug-induced hemolytic anemia from 20 years ago, methyldopa (Aldomet) was reported to be the responsible agent in the majority of cases. Because the use of methyldopa as an antihypertensive has markedly declined over the last 20 years, the incidence of drug-induced hemolytic anemia has probably fallen. Nonetheless, drug-induced hemolytic anemia continues to account for a significant proportion of all cases of acquired immune hemolytic anemia. Accordingly, when evaluating patients with evidence of immune hemolysis, a detailed drug history is essential. In addition, a temporal relationship between drug administration and the development of hemolysis should be sought. Unfortunately, such relationships are often ambiguous because patients are taking multiple drugs. While some drugs induce immune hemolytic anemia more frequently than others, any drug must be considered potentially culpable in a given patient.

There are three mechanisms by which drugs can induce immune hemolytic anemia (Table 5). Prototypical drugs are included for each mechanism, but it is important to keep in mind that these drugs are only the best characterized examples and that other drugs can induce hemolysis by the same mechanisms. For example, levodopa (Larodopa) and procainamide (Procan) have been reported to induce immune hemolytic anemia in a manner analogous to that of methyldopa. A detailed review of all of the drugs that have been implicated in the production of AIHA is beyond the purview of this chapter.

Recent reports strongly suggest that quinine can induce the hemolytic uremic syndrome (HUS). Patients present with chills, sweats, nausea and vomiting, abdominal pain, oliguria, and petechiae following exposure to quinine in medications or beverages.

TABLE 5. **Characteristics of Drug-Induced Hemolytic Anemias**

Quinidine/quinine prototype
- Proposed mechanism: The drug acts as a hapten after binding to a cell membrane protein. Consequently, antibodies against constituents of the drug-membrane protein complex arise.
- Clinical characteristics
  - Small doses of drug induce the process.
  - Intravascular hemolysis is common; hemolysis may be severe and life-threatening. Can produce hemolytic uremic syndrome (HUS).
- Laboratory findings
  - Direct Coombs' test result positive for complement but not IgG.
  - Antibody may be IgG or IgM.
  - Positivity of the indirect Coombs' test depends on having the drug present in the reaction mixture, thus demonstrating the drug-dependent nature of the antibody.
- Therapy
  - Discontinue drug.
  - Supportive care (maintain renal blood flow, transfuse as needed).
  - In patients with severe hemolysis, an empirical trial of steroids is warranted.
  - Patients with HUS appear to benefit from plasma exchange. Dialysis is often required.

Penicillin prototype
- Proposed mechanism: Drug binds tightly to red cell. Antidrug antibody binds to drug on red cell surface.
- Clinical characteristics
  - Large doses of drug required (10 million units or more/d)
  - Hemolysis is usually subacute, developing over 1–2 wk.
  - Patients may have positive Coombs' test results without clinical evidence of hemolysis.
  - In rare instances, the process may be life-threatening.
- Laboratory findings
  - Direct Coombs' test positive for IgG, rarely positive for complement.
  - Patient's serum will react in indirect Coombs' test with red blood cells coated with drug.
- Therapy
  - Discontinue drug in cases of overt hemolysis.
  - If hemolysis is clinically insignificant, the drug can be continued while monitoring the patient closely.

Methyldopa (Aldomet) prototype
- Proposed mechanism: Speculative, but may alter the immune system resulting in a pathophysiologic process similar to that observed in idiopathic autoimmune hemolytic anemia.
- Clinical characteristics
  - Dose and time dependent (patient will have taken drug for at least 3 mo).
  - Hemolysis is usually mild, and resolves gradually over several weeks after cessation of the drug.
  - Patients may have positive Coombs' test results without clinical evidence of hemolysis.
- Laboratory findings
  - Direct Coombs' test result positive for IgG, rarely for complement. When hemolysis is present, indirect Coombs' test is invariably positive.
  - Positivity of Coombs' test is not dependent on having the drug in the reaction mixture.
  - Coombs' test result may be positive for months after cessation of drug.
- Therapy
  - Discontinue drug in cases of overt hemolysis.
  - If hemolysis is clinically insignificant, the drug can be continued while monitoring the patient closely. However, the availability of other effective agents makes it prudent to switch to a structurally unrelated alternative antihypertensive agent.

Modified with permission from Parker CJ: Acute hemolytic disorders. *In* Carlson RW, Geheb MH (eds): Principles and Practice of Medical Intensive Care. Philadelphia, WB Saunders Co, 1993, p 1379.

Laboratory studies show anemia, severe thrombocytopenia, markedly elevated serum LDH, and azotemia. Drug-dependent antibodies reactive with platelets, erythrocytes, and granulocytes have been identified. These patients have a favorable outcome when treated with plasmapheresis with plasma exchange and dialysis as indicated. Prompt recognition and appropriate treatment of this clinical entity are imperative.

In a given patient, almost any drug can produce an idiosyncratic reaction resulting in immune hemolytic anemia. Therefore, for patients with newly diagnosed acquired immune hemolytic anemia, all drugs that are not absolutely essential should be discontinued. Further, if temporal events implicate a drug (particularly one that has been previously reported to induce immune hemolysis), that drug should be stopped and alternative therapy using a structurally unrelated compound should be initiated. A causal role for a particular drug can be established by using an in vitro assay based on a modified indirect Coombs' test to determine if antibody binding to the red cell is drug dependent. The technical aspects of the test (particularly the concentration of drug to use) can be obtained from published reports if studies have been done on a particular drug. If a drug that has not been previously shown to induce immune hemolysis is suspected, experiments to establish the optimal conditions for testing are required. Unfortunately drug-related antibodies cannot be conclusively demonstrated in many cases in which clinical suspicion is strong. Further adding to the problem is the fact that antibodies may be directed against metabolites rather than the whole drug. In these cases, ex vivo antigens (present in the serum or urine of the patient) may be required to demonstrate the drug-dependent nature of the antibody.

COLD AGGLUTININ SYNDROME

Although the presence of cold agglutinins in the plasma is relatively common, cold agglutinins that produce clinically significant hemolysis are relatively uncommon. A cold agglutinin titer of less than 1:64 is normal. Patients with cold agglutinin syndrome may complain of Raynaud's phenomenon or acrocyanosis of the ears, nose tip, fingers, and toes that occurs at cold temperatures and vanishes upon warming. These symptoms arise because as the blood flows through skin capillaries, the intravascular temperature drops to levels at which the cold agglutinin is functional. As a consequence of the agglutination, blood flow through the small vessels is restricted. Hemoglobinuria following exposure to cold may be part of the history, but in general, this symptom is unusual. Hepatosplenomegaly is not usually prominent, and lymphadenopathy is uncommon. Agglutination of the red blood cells at room temperature is an obvious consequence of the disease.

The criteria for diagnosis of cold agglutinin syndrome are shown in Table 3. It should be emphasized that mere observance of cold agglutination is not diagnostic of cold agglutinin disease. The antibodies involved in cold agglutinin disease are almost invariably IgM, and in the vast majority of cases, they are directed against determinants of the I antigen system. Although in most instances, the cold agglutinin titer in cold agglutinin syndrome is above 1:1000, the titer at 4°C does not correlate well with the hemolytic potential of the antibody. A more useful characterization is determination of the thermal amplitude of the antibody (defined as the highest temperature at which it causes agglutination). The majority of cold agglutinins that produce clinically significant hemolysis have a thermal amplitude of at least 30°C; if the thermal amplitude is less, the antibody will not fully activate the complement system.

Treatment

Treatment of cold agglutinin syndrome is mainly supportive because patients tend to have a low grade, compensated anemia, and currently available therapeutic modalities (i.e., corticosteroids, splenectomy, and alkylating agents) are relatively ineffective. A small minority of patients appear to benefit from chlorambucil* (Leukeran) (0.1 to 0.2 mg per kg per day) or cyclophosphamide* (Cytoxan) (1.5 to 2.0 mg per kg per day), and these agents should be prescribed if the disease is complicated by severe anemia. In situations in which the cold agglutinin syndrome is associated with underlying neoplasia, the hemolytic process often ameliorates in response to treatment of the underlying disease. Patients should avoid cold conditions, and in some instances it may be necessary for the patient to move to a warm climate. Inasmuch as the antibody is IgM, plasmapheresis can lower the antibody concentrations in emergency situations.

Transfusion. Because the I antigen is present on all adult red blood cells, it is not possible to transfuse unreactive donor cells. Difficulties in establishing ABO and Rh phenotypes and in identifying alloantibodies are usually not encountered, however, because tests can be performed at a temperature above that at which the cold agglutinin is active. The clinical benefit of using in-line blood warmers during transfusion of patients with cold agglutinin disease (or paroxysmal cold hemoglobinuria, see further on) has not been clearly established. In general, properly crossmatched blood can be transfused safely if it is warmed to room temperature and infused slowly. In cases of particularly severe cold agglutinin syndrome or paroxysmal cold hemoglobinuria, however, it seems prudent to use an in-line warmer.

Secondary Cold Agglutinin Syndrome

Whereas the finding of cold agglutinins in association with infectious processes is relatively common (particularly for *Mycoplasma pneumoniae* and infectious mononucleosis), clinically significant hemolysis in this setting is unusual. The association of cold

*Not FDA approved for this indication.

agglutinin disease with lymphoproliferative neoplasias is also uncommon. Some of the features of secondary cold agglutinin disease are shown in Table 6.

PAROXYSMAL COLD HEMOGLOBINURIA

Paroxysmal cold hemoglobinuria (PCH) is an uncommon disease that can have a dramatic presentation. Patients with PCH (usually children) experience acute attacks of shaking chills, fever, malaise, and aching pains involving the abdomen, back, and legs. Hemoglobin is usually present in the first urine passed after the attack. A history of exposure to cold is usually elicited, although the extent of the exposure may be modest. In rare instances, cold exposure is not part of the presenting history. Often there is a history of a flulike prodromal illness. The anemia is usually moderate to severe at the time of presentation and may be progressive despite the fact that the patient is kept warm.

The diagnosis of PCH is made by finding the Donath-Landsteiner antibody in the patient's plasma. This IgG antibody is directed against the P blood group antigen and is identified by using a bithermal assay. First, the patient's serum is incubated with erythrocytes at 4°C, and the cold-reacting antibody binds to the red cells. Subsequently, the reaction mixture is warmed to 37°C, and the cells hemolyze as a result of complement activation initiated by the Donath-Landsteiner antibody.

Management

Most patients with PCH require only supportive care as the process is usually transient. The patient should be kept warm at all times. Guidelines for transfusion are the same as those for patients with cold agglutinin syndrome (see previous discussion). In severe cases, an empirical trial of corticosteroids is warranted. Although the association is now rare, patients with PCH should be evaluated for syphilis. PCH has also been reported as part of a chronic autoimmune process in adults.

TABLE 6. **Secondary Chronic Cold Agglutinin Disease**

Mycoplasma pneumoniae Infections
- Approximately 50% of patients have elevated cold agglutinin titers, but overt hemolysis is rare.
- When it does occur, the hemolytic process begins in the second or third week of the infection and the onset is rapid. Fatalities have been reported.
- Characteristically, the cold reacting antibody is an IgM that recognizes I antigens. The antibody may cross-react with mycoplasma antigens.
- The hemolysis is self-limited and steroids are ineffective.

Infectious Mononucleosis
- Clinically significant hemolysis occurs infrequently.
- Hemolysis occurs 1–2 wk after onset of the infection.
- The antibody may be IgM anti-i, IgM anti-I, or IgG anti-i.*
- Hemolysis is usually self-limited, but steroids may be of benefit.

Association with reticuloendothelial neoplasia is unusual.

*The I antigen is found predominantly on adult red blood cells, while the i antigen is found primarily on fetal red cells. In primary cold agglutinin disease, the antibody is almost invariably IgM anti-I. The cold agglutinins associated with infectious mononucleosis are unusual in that they may have specificity for the i antigen and they may be IgG.

Modified from Parker CJ: Acute hemolytic disorders. *In* Carlson RW, Geheb MH (eds): Principles and Practice of Medical Intensive Care. Philadelphia, WB Saunders Co, 1993, p 1378.

NONIMMUNE HEMOLYTIC ANEMIA

method of
HIDEKI NAKAKUMA, M.D., PH.D.
Kumamoto University School of Medicine
Kumamoto, Japan

Normal red blood cells (RBCs) survive for approximately 90 to 120 days in the circulation. Senescent RBCs are cleared from the circulation by reticuloendothelial cells in such organs as the spleen and liver. The progression from normal erythropoiesis to extravascular destruction of senescent RBCs is physiologically regulated. Reference ranges for the RBC count and RBC degradation products, such as serum bilirubin are based on the kinetics of this process.

Premature destruction of RBCs is termed "hemolysis." Brisk hemolysis leads to an increase in serum bilirubin, resulting in jaundice. When compensatory erythopoiesis is inadequate, hemolytic anemia results. Low-level hemolysis causes neither anemia nor jaundice. Hemolytic anemia thus represents a clinically advanced hemolytic disorder. In general, hemolysis associated with ineffective hematopoiesis in impaired bone marrow is not grouped with other hemolytic disorders. Hemolytic disorders can be classified chronologically (congenital or acquired), pathogenetically (intrinsic or extrinsic), or by destruction in reticuloendothelial organs (extravascular hemolysis) or in the circulation (intravascular hemolysis). Despite this heterogeneity, there are common symptoms and signs. For accurate diagnosis and therapeutic decision-making, characteristic findings of some special disorders need to be appreciated, and careful history taking is essential.

CLASSIFICATION

Table 1 shows the classification of relatively common nonimmune hemolytic disorders. Inherited defects that cause hemolysis are often found in the RBC membrane, hemoglobin, and enzymes. In acquired hemolytic disorders, intrinsic membrane defects are rare (an exception is paroxysmal nocturnal hemoglobinuria [PNH]). Extrinsic causes are frequently implicated in mechanical hemolysis, hypersplenism, infection, and hemolysis caused by physical and chemical agents.

SIGNS AND SYMPTOMS

The hemolytic disorders share common symptoms and signs, including easy fatigability, palpitations, shortness of breath, faintness, appetite loss, pallor, slight fever, heart murmur, and tachycardia. Table 2 shows relatively common physical and laboratory findings indicative of hemolytic anemia. A decrease in the RBC count and reticulocytosis reflecting erythroid hyperplasia in bone marrow is observed. Destruction of RBCs releases lactate dehydrogenase (LDH) and hemoglobin into the circulation. Serum

TABLE 1. **Relatively Common Nonimmune Hemolytic Anemia**

Classification	Diagnostic Information
Congenital	Family history, DNA analysis
Membrane defect	Osmotic fragility
Hereditary spherocytosis	Spherocytes, autosomal dominant
Hereditary elliptocytosis	Elliptocytes, autosomal dominant
Hereditary acanthocytosis	Acanthocytes, abetalipoproteinemia
LCAT deficiency	Target cells, cholesterol, corneal lesions
Hemoglobinopathy	Hemoglobin analysis, target cells
Thalassemia	Microcytic hypochromic anemia
Sickle cell anemia	Sickled cells, vaso-occlusive episode
Unstable hemoglobins	Heat instability, Heinz bodies, isopropanol precipitation test
Enzyme defect	Enzyme activity
G6PD deficiency	Drug-evoked hemolysis, sex-linked heredity, Heinz bodies, fluorescent spot test
Pyruvate kinase deficiency	
Pyrimidine 5′-nucleotidase deficiency	Basophilic stippling of erythrocytes
Erythropoietic porphyria	Cutaneous photosensitivity
Acquired	
Paroxysmal nocturnal hemoglobinuria	Ham's test, sugar-water test, GPI-anchored protein defect
Mechanical hemolysis	Schistocytes, plasma hemoglobin
March hemoglobinuria	History
Traumatic cardiac hemolysis	
Microangiopathic hemolysis (DIC, HUS, TTP)	
Hypersplenism	Splenomegaly
Chemical and physical agents	Oxidants, venoms, thermal injury
Infectious agents	Malaria, cholera, Oroya fever
Spur cell anemia	Spur cells in severe liver disease
Hypophosphatemia	
Vitamin E deficiency	Newborns

Abbreviations: LCAT = lecithin-cholesterol acyltransferase; DIC = disseminated intravascular coagulation; HUS = hemolytic uremic syndrome; TTP = thrombotic thrombocytopenic purpura.

haptoglobin is rapidly consumed as a consequence of binding of liberated hemoglobin. Uncomplexed hemoglobin circulates and is excreted into the urine. Iron from hemoglobin is partly absorbed and stored in tubular cells and is finally excreted together with the renal tubular cells into the urine (hemosiderinuria). Degradation of liberated hemoglobin causes an increase in bilirubin, resulting in jaundice, and in cases of chronic hemolysis, cholelithiasis. Splenomegaly is an indicator of activation of the reticuloendothelial system, which traps affected RBCs. Hemolysis is often precipitated by infections with various pathogens. These are rarely life-threatening, except in PNH patients with a high population of complement-sensitive cells. Selective infection of erythroid progenitor cells with parvovirus B19 in patients with severe hemolytic anemia may cause an anemic crisis, which may be prolonged in patients with coexisting immunodeficiency. Surgery and pregnancy infrequently accelerate hemolysis; the mechanism is unclear.

DIAGNOSIS

General Approach

Hemolytic anemia is diagnosed on the basis of clinical and laboratory evidence of hemolysis and resultant anemia. Anemia-associated symptoms were described previously. Important clinical findings of hemolysis are jaundice, splenomegaly, and cholelithiasis. Laboratory findings are shown in Table 2. Despite manifestation of anemia and jaundice, megaloblastic anemia, erythroleukemia, congenital dyserythropoietic anemia, liver diseases, and myelodysplastic syndromes including refractory anemia and sideroblastic anemia are generally easily distinguishable from hemolytic disorders. Usually, hemolytic anemia includes a normocytic, normochromic anemia. Because of the increased reticulocytosis, a mild increase in macrocytic indices may be observed. Hemolysis in PNH causes urinary loss of iron, sometimes resulting in microcytic, hypochromic anemia. Subclinical hemolytic disorders may become manifest by transient hemolytic exacerbation induced by various causes.

Specific Plan

Table 1 lists the characteristic findings useful for diagnosis of nonimmune hemolytic disorders. For example, family history and DNA analysis are essential for the diagnosis of congenital disorders. Osmotic fragility may be useful as an indicator of a defect of the erythrocyte membrane. Membrane defects induce morphologic changes in RBCs (e.g., spherocytes, elliptocytes or rod cells, and acanthocytes). Hemoglobinopathy is diagnosed by biochemical analysis of hemoglobin and molecular analysis of its gene. Microcytic, hypochromic anemia is observed in thalassemia. Sickle cells and vaso-occlusive episodes are helpful for diagnosis of sickle cell anemia. Enzyme analysis is needed to confirm enzyme defects. Glucose-6-phosphate dehydrogenase (G6PD) deficiency shows sex-linked heredity and is exacerbated by drugs such as antimalarials that increase the oxidative stress placed on erythrocytes. Abundant basophilic stippling of RBCs is a distinct characteristic of pyrimidine 5′-nucleotidase deficiency. Lead inhibits this enzyme, and consequently lead intoxication shows similar stippling. Some acquired hemolytic disorders have unique characteristic markers for diagnosis. PNH shows Coombs'-negative intravascular hemolysis of complement sensitive RBCs, which are detected by conventional hemolysis tests such as Ham's acidified serum test and the sugar-water test. PNH cells are also detectable by flow cytometry with antibodies to glycosylphosphatidylinositol (GPI)-anchored membrane proteins including decay-accelerating factor (DAF) and CD59, which are complement

TABLE 2. **Clinical Manifestations of Hemolytic Anemia**

Physical findings	Anemia, jaundice, splenomegaly, hemoglobinuria, cholelithiasis
Laboratory findings	
Blood cell count	Erythrocytopenia reticulocytosis
Bone marrow	Erythroid hyperplasia
Serum	Increased lactate dehydrogenase and unconjugated bilirubin, decreased haptoglobin
Plasma	Increased free hemoglobin
Urine	Hemoglobin, hemosiderin
Life span	Shortened life span of erythrocytes
Exacerbation	
Infection	Virus, bacteria, protozoa
Chemicals	Antimalaria drugs, vitamin C
Aplastic crisis	Parvovirus B19
Pregnancy	
Surgery	

regulatory membrane proteins. Because PNH cells are unable to generate the GPI anchor, they are negative for GPI-anchored membrane proteins. At present, flow cytometry is the best method of diagnosing PNH. Affected cells are also detected by molecular analysis of *PIG-A,* the gene that is responsible for the synthetic defect of GPI anchor. For the diagnosis of mechanical hemolysis, which is also called red cell fragmentation syndrome, presence of schistocytes and an increase of plasma free hemoglobin level due to intravascular hemolysis are helpful.

TREATMENT

In general, treatment of hemolytic disorders requires the control of chronic mild hemolysis, hemolytic precipitation, and various complications. Specific therapy depends on the etiology. Hemolysis caused by extrinsic factors can be prevented and is discussed elsewhere. The focus here is mainly on hemolysis associated with intrinsic abnormalities.

Patient Education

To maintain a good quality of life, education of both patients and their families is essential. Patients should be informed about the nature of their disorder, including the pathophysiology, symptoms and signs, factors that trigger critical exacerbation of hemolysis, complications, therapy and its side effects, and prognosis. For example, to prevent hemolytic precipitation, patients with G6PD deficiency are advised to avoid antimalarial drugs (primaquine, pamaquine, pentaquine), sulfa drugs (sulfamethoxazole [Gantanol], sulfanilamide), some antibiotics such as nalidixic acid (NegGram) and nitrofurantoin (Macrodantin, Furadantin), analgesics (acetanilid), water-soluble vitamin K, doxorubicin, methylene blue, furazolidone (Furoxone), niridazole, phenazopyridine (Pyridium), diaphenylsulfone (DDS, dapsone), naphthalene, and fava beans. Some patients with unstable hemoglobin show exacerbation of hemolysis with the same drugs that intensify hemolysis in G6PD deficiency. A large dose of ascorbic acid (vitamin C) rarely worsens the hemolysis in patients with G6PD deficiency and PNH.

Of the other notorious causes of hemolytic attacks, infection is particularly troublesome. Even a clinically mild common cold accelerates hemolysis markedly in PNH. To minimize respiratory infections, the oral cavity and hands should be kept clean. Immunization against common pathogens, including hepatitis viruses and influenza should be considered.

Patients with PNH should be aware of potential serious complications such as venous thrombosis and marrow failure. Abdominal pains and headache are warning signs for thrombosis. Frequent episodes of infection, anemic symptoms, and bleeding tendency are indicative of pancytopenia due to marrow failure. Patients with sickle cell anemia need be advised to avoid infection, fever, dehydration, and exposure to cold, which trigger vaso-occlusive attacks. Further, genetic counseling for hereditary diseases is indispensable. Birth control for sexually active women should be discussed with the patient.

Pregnancy often exacerbates anemia partly due to hypersplenism and folic acid deficiency. Folic acid supplementation is necessary for pregnant women with thalassemia and other hemoglobinopathies. It may be helpful to prepare blood bank files that include information regarding blood genotypes.

Transfusions

Transfusion of healthy RBCs rapidly improves anemia and subsequently suppresses the production of affected RBCs. Transfusion also alleviates the infection-associated precipitation of hemolysis in patients with PNH. This therapy may be life-saving in episodes of hemolytic and aplastic crises. Clinically stable chronic anemia does not usually require transfusion, except in seriously anemic patients with thalassemia and G6PD deficiency. For those patients, the goal is to keep the hemoglobin level above 7 grams per dL. Maintenance of the hemoglobin concentration above 10 grams per dL permits normal growth and development in children and minimizes the risk of life-threatening aplastic crises. When the hemoglobin level exceeds 9 grams per dL, erythropoiesis of affected cells is effectively suppressed in patients with PNH.

The clinical importance of hypertransfusion to keep the hemoglobin level above 12 grams per dL is not fully established in hemolytic disorders. In contrast, transfusion therapy is of limited benefit in patients with spur cell anemia, because transfused healthy RBCs undergo spur formation. Transfusion with RBCs and platelets is required in severe pancytopenia due to marrow failure in patients with PNH. Because of the risk of thrombosis, platelet transfusion should not be given to patients with red cell fragmentation syndromes. Exchange transfusion may be of value in sickle cell anemia with abnormal viscosity and microangiopathic red cell fragmentation syndromes, such as hemolytic uremic syndrome (HUS) and thrombotic thrombocytopenic purpura (TTP).

Untoward consequences of transfusion include blood product–mediated infection with such pathogens as hepatitis viruses and human immunodeficiency virus (HIV), immunologic reaction against exogenous antigens on donor blood cells, graft-versus-host reaction (GVHR) of donor lymphocytes against organs of the recipient, and iron overload. The benefit/toxicity ratio should always be considered in deciding whether to transfuse. In practice, transfusion with washed and leukocyte-depleted RBCs may be useful in reducing donor serum–associated hemolysis of recipient RBCs and donor leukocyte-associated immunoreaction to recipient organs, respectively. Membrane filtration (membrane filter: Sepacell, Pall RC) and irradiation (15 to 50 Gy) of blood products are used to deplete and inactivate donor leukocytes, respectively.

Drug Therapy

It is important to treat infection-induced hemolytic attacks that manifest with rapidly progressive anemia, hypotension, and serious damage to critical organs, such as the kidney. It is prudent to try to prevent infection or to begin therapy promptly with pathogen-sensitive drugs at an early stage of infection. Intravenous infusion of both haptoglobin (4000 units every 24 hours for at least 3 consecutive days) and saline is of benefit to facilitate the clearance of liberated hemoglobin, preserve intravascular volume, and protect the kidney. Diuretics are useful to maintain adequate urine output (100 mL per hour). Acidosis, if present, needs to be corrected. For pregnant women with hemoglobinopathy, folic acid (0.2 to 1.0 mg per day) is recommended. Patients with TTP should receive glucocorticoids and undergo plasmapheresis with plasma exchange. For patients whose hemolysis is insensitive to plasmapheresis, immunosuppressants (vincristine,* cyclophosphamide*) have been used. For PNH with severe anemia due to marrow failure, immunosuppressive therapy with antithymocyte globulin* (Atgam) or cyclosporine* should be considered. Rarely, hematopoietic cytokines such as erythropoietin* (Epogen) and granulocyte-colony stimulating factor* (G-CSF) are also useful. Although glucocorticoids are often used for therapy of PNH hemolysis, responses are not always observed. Frequent episodes of abdominal pain indicative of thrombosis subside after intravenous heparin (10,000 units per day for several days) and subsequent warfarin. Warfarin action is modified by various drugs: suppressed by barbiturates, carbamazepine (Tegretol), and vitamin K; and enhanced by aspirin, antibiotics, and allopurinol (Zyloprim). The appropriate dose of warfarin is determined by using the international normalized ratio converted from the prothrombin time. In fact, prophylactic use of 2 mg per day of warfarin may be effective for abdominal thrombosis in PNH. On the other hand, persistent intravascular hemolysis in patients with PNH leads to urinary excretion of iron in the form of hemoglobin and hemosiderin, resulting in iron deficiency anemia. This type of anemia needs to be corrected by oral administration of iron.

In contrast, iron is contraindicated in patients with thalassemia, unstable hemoglobinopathy, and hereditary spherocytosis (HS). Iron accumulates steadily as a consequence of iron administration and frequent transfusion in these patients, who do not show pathologic loss of iron. To prevent iron overload that can result in hemosiderosis and hemochromatosis in such critical organs as heart, liver, and pancreas, therapy with deferoxamine (Desferal) for iron chelation is useful when the serum ferritin level is above 2000 μg per mL. Vitamin C (50 to 100 mg per day) may facilitate the iron chelation. Attention should be paid to deferoxamine-induced damage of the optic and auditory nerves. Twice-yearly audiometry and ophthalmologic examination is recommended.

*Not FDA approved for this indication.

Splenectomy

Splenectomy reliably corrects the anemia due to spleen-mediated destruction of RBCs (e.g., erythrocyte membrane defects such as HS and hereditary elliptocytosis), although the defect and abnormal morphology persist after the operation. Patients with pyruvate kinase deficiency may benefit from splenectomy if they show splenomegaly, no signs of infection, and transfusion-dependent anemia. Patients with mild to moderate unstable hemoglobinopathy improve after splenectomy, whereas patients with the severe type do not. In patients with thalassemia, the clinical benefit of splenectomy is variable; however, surgery may be performed in cases of extreme anemia and splenomegaly. Splenectomy is of limited benefit in patients with intravascular hemolysis due to PNH. When gallstones cause symptoms, splenectomy should be performed first, followed by cholecystectomy, or intrahepatic cholelithiasis may develop. To minimize the risk of severe infections, it is recommended that splenectomy be postponed until children have reached school age (at least 5 to 10 years of age). Immunization against pneumococci, meningococcis, and *Haemophilus influenzae* should be given preoperatively for all patients. When splenectomy does not alleviate the hemolytic manifestation, the presence of an accessory spleen or misdiagnosis should be considered.

Bone Marrow Transplantation

Therapy with splenectomy, drugs, and transfusion does not eliminate affected cells. When hemolytic disorders due to intrinsic RBC abnormalities are uncontrollable by these measures, bone marrow transplantation (BMT) using bone marrow or peripheral blood stem cells from an HLA-identical donor should be considered. BMT is the treatment of choice for severe thalassemia in patients younger than 5 years. Overall event-free survival for thalassemia patients younger than 16 years of age is 75% after BMT, and 3-year event-free survival exceeds 90%. Older patients with transfusion-dependent thalassemia show advanced iron overload, leading to liver failure, and liver function is a critical factor in the success of BMT. Patients with severe sickle cell anemia or pyruvate kinase deficiency are also candidates for BMT.

Because most hemolytic disorders due to intrinsic RBC abnormalities are hereditary, the same abnormality may be observed in siblings; thus, the probability of finding an HLA-identical healthy sibling is comparatively lower. For children without HLA-compatible siblings, cord blood stem cell transplantation may be an option, because the transplantation appears to permit one locus mismatch of HLA between donor and recipient. On the other hand, PNH is an acquired stem cell disorder that shows an intrinsic erythrocyte membrane defect leading to hemolysis. PNH has a much better prognosis than other acquired stem cell disorders (e.g., leukemia). Therefore,

BMT is recommended in PNH only for cases of serious marrow failure or life-threatening thrombotic episodes. PNH patients need myeloablation before BMT, or affected clones soon emerge.

Gene Therapy

Gene therapy holds promise for the prevention and treatment of hemolytic diseases caused by genetic defects. Patients with congenital abnormalities such as hemoblobinopathies, enzyme defects, and membrane defects are good candidates for this therapy. Paroxysmal nocturnal hemoglobinuria may also be an indication for this type of therapy, because the *PIG-A* gene responsible for the membrane defect leading to hemolysis has been cloned. However, it is not yet clear whether the *PIG-A* mutation explains such clinical manifestations as thrombosis, marrow failure, and leukemic conversion observed in patients with PNH. Unlike congenital diseases, each of which has a single pathogenic gene, the possibility of involvement of multiple genes in the pathogenesis is not excluded in PNH. At present, introduction of gene therapy for PNH awaits the elucidation of the whole complex pathophysiology. On the other hand, insertion of cloned healthy genes into the fertilized egg is not clinically applicable. Instead, insertion and expression of the cloned genes in hematopoietic progenitors might permit repopulation with cells that are genetically repaired using retroviral vectors. Elaborate efforts have been made to improve vectors for stem cell gene transfer in regard to effective introduction, specific expression of the cloned genes in the target cells, and clinical safety.

PERNICIOUS ANEMIA AND OTHER MEGALOBLASTIC ANEMIAS

method of
ISRAEL CHANARIN, M.D.
Medical Research Council Clinical Research Centre, Northwick Park Hospital
Harrow, Middlesex, England

Most patients with megaloblastic anemia (MA) have a deficiency of cobalamin (vitamin B_{12}, Cbl), usually due to pernicious anemia (PA); a smaller number have a deficiency of folate (folic acid, pteroylglutamic acid). Of 1.8 million persons enrolled in Medicare in the United States, 1% made claims related to Cbl deficiency in 1991; thus, about 1% of the population older than age 65 is receiving treatment for Cbl deficiency. Under some circumstances Cbl or folate is given prophylactically. Cbl is widely used as a tonic, but as the recipients are not Cbl deficient, they are not likely to derive material benefit.

Appropriate treatment requires correct diagnosis. Deficiencies of Cbl or folate are almost invariably accompanied by hematologic changes, and in the case of Cbl deficiency, not infrequently by neuropathy. Cbl neuropathy is a diagnosis that must not be missed, as early treatment will reverse the process; the serum Cbl level must be measured in patients with appropriate neurologic changes irrespective of the blood findings.

Folate is present in multivitamin preparations taken regularly by about 40% of American adults; in addition, folate is added to wheat products in the United States to increase dietary folate intake to prevent neural tube defects. A significantly increased folate intake can suppress the blood changes due to Cbl deficiency while allowing the neuropathy to progress. Awareness of the signs and symptoms of Cbl neuropathy is all important.

Causes of Cbl and folate deficiency are presented in Table 1.

CLINICAL AND LABORATORY FINDINGS

Clinical and hematologic presentation is usually similar in both Cbl and folate deficiencies. Cbl neuropathy in the absence of blood changes is rare.

About 90% of patients with MA are tired and lack energy,

TABLE 1. **Causes of Cobalamin and Folate Deficiency**

Causes of Cobalamin Deficiency

- Dietary (Cbl) deficiency
  - Strict vegetarian diet
  - Neonates born to mothers with Cbl deficiency
- Gastric causes
  - Pernicious anemia
  - Gastrectomy
  - Infant with absent or abnormal intrinsic factor
- Intestinal causes
  - Anatomic abnormalities of the small gut (blind loops, strictures, fistulae, ileal resection, small gut diverticulitis, poorly functioning gastroenterostomy)
  - Pelvic (ileal) irradiation
  - Abnormal gut bacterial flora
  - Chronic tropical sprue
  - Hypogammaglobulinemia with associated pernicious anemia
  - *Diphyllobothrium latum* (fish tapeworm) infestation
  - Congenital Cbl malabsorption (Imerslund-Gräsbeck syndrome)
- Transport defects
  - Transcobalamin II deficiency
- Metabolic defects
  - Impaired cellular metabolism of Cbl (including methylmalonylacidurias)
  - Chronic nitrous oxide addiction

Causes of Folate Deficiency

- Dietary folate deficiency
  - May be associated with pregnancy, alcohol abuse, scurvy, prematurity, goat's milk anemia
- Intestinal causes
  - Celiac disease
  - Tropical sprue
  - Congenital folate malabsorption in infants
- Increased folate requirement
  - Pregnancy
  - Chronic hemolytic anemia
  - Hemoglobinopathy
  - Malaria
  - Exfoliative skin disorders
  - Agnogenic myeloid metaplasia
- Drugs
  - Methotrexate
  - Pyrimethamine (Daraprim)
  - Trimethoprim (Trimpex)
  - Triamterene (Dyrenium)
  - Sulfasalazine
  - Anticonvulsants (diphenylhydantoin, phenobarbital, primidone)

about half are short of breath, and about one in five has a sore mouth and tongue. One third of patients with Cbl deficiency have a tingling sensation in the hands and/or feet, which is almost always symmetrical. There may be micturition problems such as hesitancy and poor urinary flow. The patient may be irritable with fluctuations of mood. Gait changes may be seen.

DIAGNOSIS

Patients may show evidence of an underlying disorder causing the MA. Patients with MA due to folate deficiency in celiac disease may have bulky stools, short stature, and other signs of malnutrition. Mild jaundice may occur in MA but may be more marked if folate deficiency has developed as a result of a hemolytic anemia. Alcohol excess is strongly associated with MA. Those with neuropathy may have impaired vibration sense, inability to detect passive movement, reflex abnormalities, and related signs.

Hematologic Diagnosis

The commonest change in the blood is macrocytosis, which is usually assessed by the red blood cell (RBC) mean corpuscular volume (MCV). The normal range is 80 to 94 femtoliters (fl), although the stated upper limit varies in different laboratories. Concurrent thalassemia trait or iron deficiency may prevent the emergence of macrocytosis.

As the hemoglobin level falls, there is a decrease in the white cell and platelet counts. The blood film now shows not only macrocytes, but also variation in size of red cells (anisocytosis) and red cell fragments as well as pear-shaped red cells (poikilocytes). Some hypersegmented neutrophils may be present.

A blood film showing target cells, Howell-Jolly bodies, normoblasts or even megaloblasts, and red cell fragments suggests loss of splenic function and hence celiac disease as a diagnosis unless the patient has previously undergone a splenectomy.

If there is any doubt, a bone marrow aspiration should be done to establish megaloblastic hematopoiesis, especially if the clinical situation is not straightforward. Macrocytosis can be due to many causes other than MA.

Diagnosis of MA depends entirely on the changes present in the blood and bone marrow. Because these disappear post-therapy, treatment before a firm diagnosis is made should be avoided.

NATURE OF THE DEFICIENCY

It is necessary to determine whether the MA is due to Cbl or folate deficiency. Most are due to Cbl deficiency. When the MA accompanies pregnancy, hemolytic anemia, celiac disease, or chronic myelofibrosis it is probably due to folate deficiency.

The standard diagnostic tests are serum Cbl level and red cell folate level. A low serum folate level may signify a negative folate balance, but this finding is too common to be helpful in diagnosis. Similarly, an elevated serum methylmalonic acid is usually present in Cbl deficiency; however, current assay techniques produce many false-positive results with sera from subjects with normal serum Cbl levels, and consequently it is of little help in diagnosis.

SERUM COBALAMIN LEVEL

A low serum Cbl level (below 170 pg per mL) is present in virtually all patients with Cbl deficiency. The rare exception occurs in patients with myeloproliferative disorders who have high levels of Cbl-binding proteins. Low serum Cbl levels can occur in situations other than MA. A low level is significant only in the presence of blood or marrow changes or an appropriate neuropathy. MA with a normal serum Cbl level indicates folate deficiency as the etiology.

RED CELL FOLATE LEVEL

The normal range is about 140 to 450 ng per mL packed red cells. Levels below 140 indicate folate deficiency even in the absence of MA.

COBALAMIN ABSORPTION TESTS

These are needed in the evaluation of Cbl deficiency. With the exception of nutritional Cbl deficiency, all patients with MA due to Cbl deficiency have impaired Cbl absorption. Whole-body counting has much to commend it for measuring Cbl absorption. If facilities are not available, the urinary excretion (Schilling) test is used. A low urinary excretion of isotope-labeled Cbl (less than 10% of a 1.0 μg oral dose) indicates Cbl malabsorption provided that the 24-hour urine collection is complete. Because it is often incomplete, a plasma sample should be taken 8 to 10 hours after the start of the test and the plasma radioactivity is counted. The normal range is 0.6 to 2.2% of the oral Cbl dose per liter of plasma. Normal plasma radioactivity with a low urine count means normal Cbl absorption with incomplete urine collection and is found in a quarter of all tests.

Normal Cbl absorption, other than in nutritional Cbl deficiency, excludes Cbl deficiency and means that the MA is due to folate deficiency. Impaired Cbl absorption corrected by repeating the test with the addition of intrinsic factor to the oral dose of isotope-labelled Cbl indicates the presence of severe gastric atrophy as in PA or gastrectomy. Failure to improve Cbl absorption with intrinsic factor suggests intestinal malabsorption but can be due to PA with potent intrinsic-factor antibodies.

Finally, Cbl absorption tests involving an injection of Cbl should be done only after all samples needed for diagnosis have been collected and assessed, as the injection is complete initial treatment for Cbl deficiency.

SERUM ANTIBODIES

Parietal cell antibodies, usually present in sera in PA, are not helpful in diagnosis, but intrinsic factor antibodies, present in about 57% of PA sera, are rare in the absence of PA; a positive result strongly supports a diagnosis of PA.

SOME USEFUL ADDITIONAL TESTS

There are many causes of macrocytosis other than MA; it is useful to arrange further tests when requesting Cbl and folate assays. These tests should be for thyroid-stimulating hormone (TSH), liver function, reticulocyte count, and as part of a blood count, proper scrutiny of a stained blood film. Hypothyroidism, alcoholism, chronic hemolytic states such as may accompany G6PD deficiency and blood disorders such as leukemia, myeloma, sideroblastic anemia, and hypoplastic anemias as well as a number of therapeutic drugs are some of the other causes of macrocytosis.

RESPONSE TO TREATMENT

Unless one has good reason to suspect folate deficiency, treatment is started with Cbl alone. An optimal response to Cbl is confirmation of Cbl deficiency. All patients, including those with Cbl deficiency, show response to folate; folate-deficient patients, however, do not respond in any significant way to Cbl.

FINAL EVALUATION

Occasionally, final assessment of the situation can be made only when all the features of the case are brought together. Table 1 lists the disorders producing MA, and appropriate steps should be taken to elucidate the underlying diagnosis. Failure to make a firm diagnosis is usually due to inadequate hematology or premature treatment, as discussed previously.

TREATMENT OF COBALAMIN DEFICIENCY

Two forms of supplemental Cbl are available: cyanocobalamin (cyanoCbl) and hydroxocobalamin (hydroxoCbl); both are equally efficacious. They are given by injection as most patients with Cbl deficiency have malabsorption of Cbl. As hydroxoCbl is better retained after injection than cyanoCbl, it is often preferred for treatment. However, cyanoCbl should be used as the flushing dose in the Schilling test as there is little experience with the use of hydroxoCbl for this purpose.

The usual starting dose of Cbl is 1000 μg, and in an attempt to replenish stores of Cbl, another six to eight injections are given over the next few weeks. This is less important than ensuring that maintenance therapy is given as 1000 μg Cbl every 2 months. The injection, given deep subcutaneously (SC) or intramuscularly (IM), usually causes a localized ache of short duration.

Adverse reactions to Cbl are rare. There have been two reports of anaphylactic reactions with shivering, bronchospasm, dyspnea, and urticaria. One fatal reaction has been reported. Among 168 patients receiving Cbl, 3 noted skin reactions, including a morbilliform rash in one, urticaria in a second, and pruritus in a third. Equally rare is sensitivity to cobalt in Cbl and to preservatives, such as benzyl alcohol, that may be present in the Cbl preparation.

Assessment of Response

Most patients with Cbl deficiency show a rapid response to Cbl. Within 1 to 2 days, there is return of alertness, appetite, and general well being. Mouth soreness improves rapidly as do disorders of taste and smell and psychiatric manifestations. The rise in reticulocytes reaches a peak 5 to 7 days after the Cbl injection and a steady rise in hemoglobin. If this does not happen in an anemic patient, either the diagnosis is wrong or there is an intercurrent disorder interfering with the response, such as infection, renal failure, or undetected thyroid disease. Neuropathy responds more slowly but manifestations of less than 6 months' duration should disappear; however, all patients benefit considerably. Loss of vibration sense and extensor plantar response is not correctable.

Blood Transfusion

A difficult decision is whether to transfuse elderly, anemic patients with incipient cardiac failure as overloading the circulation can be fatal. After collection of samples needed for diagnosis, 1000 μg Cbl and 5 mg folate can be given SC or IM. If there is no response within 36 hours, packed red cells from a single unit of blood can be given slowly over 6 hours. This is combined with a diuretic (which is monitored to ensure diuresis). The patient is propped up in bed and kept warm. A rise in venous pressure, restlessness, dry cough, and an increase in moist sounds in the chest suggest circulatory overload. Removal of 100 mL of blood from the other arm and an intravenous (IV) diuretic may be needed. Such patients should be given an oral potassium supplement over the first week.

Other Routes of Administration

Those with nutritional Cbl deficiency can be treated with oral Cbl given daily (5 μg or more), as they have normal Cbl absorption. Patients unable to tolerate injections can be treated with large doses of oral Cbl, as about 1% is absorbed by passive diffusion; thus 10 μg is absorbed from a 1000 μg oral dose and is taken several times a week. The daily requirement is 1 to 2 μg, and oral intake must be scheduled to ensure this. Adequacy of intake can be monitored by the serum Cbl level, which should be above 170 pg per mL.

Pernicious Anemia

This type of MA is due to Cbl deficiency. There is gastric atrophy with loss of intrinsic factor secretion and hence Cbl malabsorption. More than half the patients have serum intrinsic factor antibodies. After a few months of Cbl treatment, many patients run out of iron. This is shown by a fall in the MCV below 80 fl and confirmed by the usual tests for iron deficiency. These patients should be given oral iron. Patients with PA do not have iron deficiency on initial presentation. Megaloblastic anemia with iron deficiency de novo is seen after gastrectomy and in celiac disease.

In addition to gastric atrophy, there is an increased incidence of gastric carcinoma, polyps, and small carcinoid tumors. Endoscopy is therefore necessary.

There is a strong association with other autoimmune disorders. Hypothyroidism is present in 10% of patients and thyrotoxicosis in 2.4%; adrenal failure, hypoparathyroidism, premature ovarian failure, and pure red cell aplasia are other less common associations. Appropriate tests for these should be done.

Small Intestinal Disease

Because Cbl is absorbed in the distal ileum, ileal disease and an abnormal intestinal bacterial flora can cause Cbl deficiency. Ileal disease can involve surgical resection, bypass, or ileal irradiation as a result of treatment of carcinoma of the cervix, bladder, ovary, uterus, or prostate. Abnormal bacterial flora is associated with intestinal stasis; small intestinal diverticulosis is a well-known cause of Cbl neuropathy. In some patients, surgery may correct a gut defect. Otherwise long-term Cbl therapy is given, and when indicated, measures to control the steatorrhea are used.

Although one third of patients with untreated celiac disease, which affects the upper gut, have low serum Cbl levels and malabsorb Cbl, they have a complete hematologic response with folate (and a gluten-free diet) alone and do not require Cbl therapy.

Megaloblastic anemia due to the fish tapeworm has become rare as pollution of fresh-water lakes has killed off the fish that carried the tapeworm larvae. If infection does occur, expulsion of the worm and short-term Cbl therapy are required.

Tropical sprue is associated with folate deficiency in its earlier stages but with Cbl deficiency in its more chronic form.

Nutritional Cobalamin Deficiency

Cbl is present only in animal-derived foods; it is totally absent from plants. Vegetarians who do not consume any food of animal origin do not have any Cbl in their diet other than that derived from bacterial contamination of food or water. This is the case with many millions of Hindu Indians, and to a lesser extent, with other strict vegetarians. Occasional consumption of eggs, milk, or cheese will not supply enough Cbl. The affected age group ranges from 13 to over 80 years and half the population may have low serum Cbl levels without MA. As iron is poorly available from a vegetarian diet, iron deficiency is common, as is bone pain from osteomalacia due to low intake of calcium and vitamin D. PA is the alternative diagnosis; thus proper investigation is required. These patients respond slowly to 5 μg Cbl by mouth daily, and the return to normality establishes the diagnosis. Diagnosis is also made by response to injected Cbl with normal Cbl absorption. Pernicious anemia does not respond to small doses of oral Cbl. Advice on broadening the diet to include food of animal origin and on the need for oral supplements of Cbl and calcium/vitamin D should be given.

Megaloblastic Anemia in the Young

Women who are deficient in Cbl, either PA or because of a vegetarian diet, are usually infertile. Occasionally they do become pregnant and have an uncomplicated pregnancy. As their Cbl stores are very low, they do not supply enough Cbl to the fetus in utero and to the neonate during lactation. The infant develops normally for the first 4 months of life but thereafter becomes lethargic and hyperirritable. Such infants are weak and cannot support their heads or turn over. They stop smiling and become inactive and withdrawn. They may show hypotonia, exaggerated reflexes, extensor plantars, and even diffuse brain atrophy and coma. They are usually underweight and some have increased pigmentation on the back of the hands and feet. They can be severely anemic with all the features of a megaloblastic anemia. Once diagnosed and treated with Cbl, they respond dramatically with return to normality. The mothers must be investigated and treated as well.

There are other uncommon inherited defects of Cbl absorption and metabolism that manifest as either megaloblastic anemia or methylmalonicaciduria in very early life. These include abnormal intrinsic factor production, failure to produce the normal Cbl transport protein, transcobalamin II, and failure to absorb the intrinsic factor–Cbl complex (Imerslund-Gräsbeck syndrome), which is associated with proteinuria. Transcobalamin II deficiency is treated with 1000 μg Cbl two to three times a week. The frequency of Cbl injections in Cbl-responsive methylmalonicaciduria has to be assessed in each patient. Failure of functional intrinsic factor production and Imerslund-Gräsbeck syndrome are treated as for PA.

Prophylactic Use of Cobalamin

After total gastrectomy, 1000 μg Cbl is given every second month as in PA. Strict vegetarians should take oral Cbl to ensure an intake of more than 2 μg daily. Those who have had resection of more than 6 feet of distal small gut and have malabsorption of Cbl should receive Cbl injections.

TREATMENT OF FOLATE DEFICIENCY

Some 80% of an oral dose of pteroylglutamic acid is absorbed; after the first one or two doses, most of the absorbed folate is excreted largely in the urine and probably less than 0.5 mg is retained. The total body content of folate in an adult is about 15 to 20 mg, and the normal daily adult requirement is 0.2 mg daily. Tablets of folic acid containing 0.4, 0.8, 1.0 and 5.0 mg are available. Preparations for injection contain 5 and 15 mg per mL as the sodium salt.

Folinic acid (D/L-5-formyltetrahydrofolate) is available as a solution of the sodium salt containing 15 mg per mL; only the L form (half the folate in the mixture) is biologically active. It is given to reverse toxic effects of folate antagonists such as methotrexate. In treatment of MA, 5-mg tablets are given once or twice daily for 4 to 6 weeks, and any underlying disorders are addressed.

Adverse effects are few. Rarely an individual can be sensitized by the initial dose, and a second exposure produces a generalized pruritic, erythematous rash, malaise, and bronchospasm. Long-term folate therapy has been found by some to increase seizure frequency in epileptics; this is managed by adjustment of antiepileptic therapy. A single dose of folate has precipitated status epilepticus. In long-term folate administration in untreated PA, the initial hematologic response is followed by neurologic relapse, anemia, and glossitis.

Nutritional Folate Deficiency

This is common in poor countries but uncommon in industrialized societies in the absence of excess alcohol intake, pregnancy, hemolysis, anticonvulsants, and other risk factors. Folate is present in all foods; natural folates are labile and destroyed by oxidation, sunlight, and heat. Folates are protected by reducing agents such as ascorbate. Assessment of the diet and exclusion of other causes of MA are necessary for the diagnosis of nutritional folate deficiency. Treatment is with oral folate.

Pregnancy

There is an increased demand for folate during pregnancy, which has to be met from the diet and from folate stores. If dietary folate intake has been inadequate, folate deficiency will develop.

Anemia in pregnancy is usually due to iron deficiency, and recognition of the added complication of folate deficiency can be difficult. Failure of the anemia to respond to iron suggests folate deficiency. Hematologic findings are those of iron deficiency with occasional macrocytes and some hypersegmented neutrophils; the findings in treated iron deficiency can be very similar. The red cell folate level may be low, but this occurs in a quarter of healthy pregnant women at the same stage of pregnancy; in others, insufficient time has elapsed to allow the development of a low red cell folate level as the red cell has a mean lifespan of about 110 days. A firm diagnosis requires a bone marrow aspiration; this will demonstrate both iron deficiency and megaloblastic hematopoiesis. Sometimes the blood studies show a frank, macrocytic blood picture.

The anemia is usually diagnosed in the last few weeks of pregnancy or in the puerperium; the incidence of MA in twin pregnancies is ten times that in singleton pregnancies. Bone marrow aspiration in the last few weeks of pregnancy has shown megaloblastic hematopoiesis in one quarter of all women in Western countries including the United States, Canada, and England, and there are much higher frequencies in developing countries. In most of these women, the megaloblastic process does not come to clinical notice and, with delivery, remits spontaneously.

The minimum dose for folate supplementation in pregnancy is 200 μg daily. This is often combined with oral iron in a single daily supplement, a strategy that has been so successful in preventing anemia in pregnancy that a generation of obstetricians and midwives are unfamiliar with the condition and do not advocate hematinics until anemia appears. This is to be deplored. Overt MA anemia in pregnancy should be treated with iron and 5 mg folate once or twice daily for up to 6 weeks postpartum.

Apart from the effect on the blood, folate deficiency is associated with prematurity, low birth weight, and a small placenta. Controlled trials around the world have established that these complications can be prevented by maternal folate supplements during pregnancy.

Prevention of Neural Tube Defects

Normally, the neural tube closes at about 2 weeks after conception, but failure to close occurs in about 4 per 1000 pregnancies. In most cases, these anomalies are detected and the pregnancy terminated. However, in about 0.3 per 1000 births the neural tube defect (NTD) is not detected antenatally.

About 70% of NTDs can be prevented by administering folate supplementation exceeding 0.4 mg daily from conception through the fourth week of pregnancy. Unfortunately, most women are not even certain that they are pregnant during this early period. When there is a history of NTDs the woman can start taking oral folate supplements before conception, but there is no certain way to reach other women who might benefit. To overcome this, folate has been added to wheat flour in the United States. Despite the increased folate in the diet, it is probably advisable for those who plan to become pregnant to take about 1 mg additional folate for the first 4 weeks of an anticipated pregnancy and thereafter to take a combined iron-folate tablet daily throughout pregnancy.

Prematurity

Premature infants fail to build up adequate stores of iron and folate in utero. The fall in red cell folate is more rapid than in full term infants, being evident at 7 weeks in premature infants as compared with 11 weeks in full-term infants. Storage and warming of milk is accompanied by loss of up to 80% of folate. Anemia not responding to oral iron suggests folate deficiency. A folate supplement of about 30 μg daily is recommended for the first 12 weeks of life; anemia should be treated with iron and 50 μg folate daily.

Goat's Milk Anemia

Children thought to be sensitive to cow's milk, are often given goat's milk instead. Goat's milk has a very low content of both Cbl and folate, and after a few months on such a diet, severe folate deficiency and MA develop, which respond completely to folic acid supplements. If goat's milk needs to be given, a folate supplement of 50 μg folate daily has to be added. Although goat's milk anemia was described more than 80 years ago, new cases continue to be reported.

Anticonvulsant Drugs

Megaloblastic anemia is associated with a number of anticonvulsants, including phenobarbital and other barbiturates, primidone (Mysoline), phenytoin (Dilantin), carbamazepine (Tegretol), and valproic acid (Depakene). The way these drugs produce MA is not clear, but most likely multiple factors are involved, including a poor diet, interference with DNA synthesis, and enzyme induction with increased folate catabolism.

Treatment is with folate, and the anticonvulsant drugs are continued with dose adjustment, if necessary, to ensure proper seizure control.

Chronic Myelofibrosis (Agnogenic Myeloid Metaplasia)

This disorder is associated with an increased folate requirement and, not uncommonly, with MA that, unfortunately, is usually not diagnosed clinically. The MA may manifest as a new transfusion requirement that disappears when folate is given or as isolated thrombocytopenia sometimes accompanied by neutropenia and anemia. Because marrow cannot be aspirated readily it is more difficult to demonstrate megaloblasts, but these may be seen in the peripheral blood using blood films made from the buffy coat on centrifugation of the blood and even from a speck of fluid in the marrow needle after a so-called dry tap. Of 49 patients seen over a 10-year period, 17 had frank MA, 16 had mild changes, and 16 were normoblastic. Recognition of MA was sometimes lifesaving. Megaloblastic anemia is treated in the usual way, and all patients should receive 5 mg of folate twice weekly for life.

Chronic Hemolytic Anemia

An increased folate requirement occurs in sickle cell disease and sickle cell–hemoglobin C disease, as well as in S-thalassemia, hereditary spherocytosis, autoimmune hemolytic anemia, including that complicating chronic lymphocytic leukemia, and less severe hemolytic states such as some forms of G6PD deficiency. Usually a poor diet or pregnancy precipitates the folate deficiency and MA; in pregnancy accompanying hemolytic anemia the MA may appear as early as the twentieth week of pregnancy.

In adolescents there may be delayed puberty and failure to menstruate, both of which are dramatically reversed by folate. The blood shows the changes of MA with far lower reticulocyte levels than expected for the hemolytic state; anemia may be very severe. Where the diet is poor, folic acid, 5 mg twice weekly, should be given long term; when MA has developed, 5 mg of folate daily is given.

Alcohol and Folate

Alcohol has a direct toxic action on marrow cells, producing megaloblastic changes, vacuolation of blood cell precursors, and iron accumulation in erythroblasts forming a ring of iron granules around the cell nucleus, termed a ringed sideroblast. All these disappear within 10 days of cessation of alcohol intake. The effect on the blood is macrocytosis; there is no effect on folate metabolism. These changes are present in most severe alcoholics who drink spirits or wine; changes are seen in a smaller proportion of less severe alcoholics, particularly if they drink beer, which has significant amounts of folate.

About a third of alcoholics have a poor diet; they substitute alcohol for food and do not take a proper meal during the day. They develop MA due to the accompanying folate deficiency; these patients have low red cell folate values but usually relatively high serum Cbl levels due to liver damage. They require folate supplementation as well as interventions for alcoholism. Excess alcohol intake is often the explanation for puzzling MA in otherwise apparently well patients when tests fail to establish PA or another obvious cause. Indeed, when there is macrocytosis with a normal hemoglobin level, excess alcohol intake should be the first diagnostic consideration.

THALASSEMIA

method of
EDWARD J. BENZ, JR., M.D.
Johns Hopkins University School of Medicine
Baltimore, Maryland

PATHOPHYSIOLOGY: BASIC MECHANISMS OF HEMOGLOBIN SYNTHESIS

The sequential expression of the different globin genes is responsible for the production of specific types of hemoglobins at different stages of development. At about 12 weeks of gestation, there is a transition from embryonic to fetal hemoglobin, followed at 38 weeks by the switch to adult hemoglobin. Hemoglobin production occurs in bone marrow erythroblasts. The stable accumulation exclusively of fully formed hemoglobin tetramers (e.g., hemoglobin A $= \alpha_2\beta_2$) requires that the production of alpha-like globins equal that of beta-like globins by the globin gene clusters (alpha-like genes on chromosome 16; beta-like genes on chromosome 11) at all times.

Thalassemia syndromes result from deficiencies in the production of either alpha-globin (α-thalassemia) or beta-globin (β-thalassemia) chains. The disease becomes apparent when production of the affected globin is first required during development. α-Thalassemia is thus symptomatic during gestation. Because beta globin is not required before birth, β-thalassemia is asymptomatic until 6 to 12 months after birth.

An obvious consequence of the biosynthetic defect in thalassemia is the microcytosis and hypochromia owing to reduced amounts of hemoglobin tetramer in each red blood cell. However, the major pathologic process in the thalassemias is caused by the imbalance of alpha and non-alpha chain accumulation. Aggregation of the *unaffected chains* produced in normal amount occurs because the surplus chains are unable to find a heterologous counterpart to which to bind; these precipitate during erythropoiesis because free globin is far less soluble than intact tetramers. In β-thalassemia, the precipitated alpha globin forms inclusion bodies that damage the red blood cell membrane and cause cell death (ineffective intramedullary erythropoiesis); decreased red blood cell survival also occurs because of uptake in the splenic reticuloendothelial system (splenomegaly). A dramatic expansion of the bone marrow compartment then results from erythropoietin stimulation of further ineffective erythropoiesis. The marrow overgrowth leads to cortical thinning, pathologic fractures, and deformities of bones. Hypersplenism worsens the anemia by causing increased trapping of the formed elements of the blood. An increase in plasma volume, a consequence of the marrow and splenic expansion, also lowers the effective level of hemoglobin.

In α-thalassemic fetuses, excessive gamma globin forms tetramers (γ_4 = hemoglobin Bart's) during the fetal and neonatal period; excess beta globin (β_4 = hemoglobin H) accumulates after birth. Hemoglobin Bart's and hemoglobin H are somewhat more soluble and result in a milder ineffective erythropoiesis than is seen in β-thalassemia. These tetramers, however, exhibit abnormal oxygen binding and sensitivity to oxidant stress (see later).

The alpha-globin gene is duplicated. There is a good correlation between the number of abnormal alpha-globin loci inherited and the clinical presentation. Loss of all four globin genes results in a lethal intrauterine condition, hydrops fetalis. Only hemoglobin Bart's can form; this hemoglobin has a massively left-shifted oxygen dissociation curve that supports almost no oxygen delivery to tissues. Deletion of three alpha loci produces a chronic hemolytic anemia, hemoglobin H disease. Hemoglobin A production is sufficient for survival, but hemoglobin H is moderately unstable and oxidant sensitive, causing hemolysis. Deletion of only one (α-thalassemia-2) or two (α-thalassemia-1) loci is asymptomatic, although the latter condition produces hypochromia and microcytosis.

Severe forms of α-thalassemia are common in Asians and in Mediterranean populations. In black (African) populations, severe disease is almost never seen, even though the α-thalassemia-2 deletion is extremely common (5 to 15% gene frequency). The virtual absence of mutations that inactivate both loci on the same chromosome in black persons explains this discrepancy.

In β-thalassemia, clinically significant disease is seen only when both beta-globin alleles are impaired by mutation. Direct globin gene analysis in affected patients and their families indicates whether the expression of each of the two affected genes is completely absent (β^0-thalassemia) or partially reduced (β^+-thalassemia). A large number of different molecular lesions of the gene, mostly point mutations, cause these defects.

Thalassemia syndromes are commonly graded according to the severity of the anemia. Severe anemia presenting in the first 6 to 9 months after birth (thalassemia major) is usually caused by the inheritance of two seriously impaired beta-globin alleles. The heterozygous state (inheritance of a single defective allele) is characterized by a mild hypochromic and microcytic anemia (thalassemia minor). Under certain circumstances, the "homozygous" state has a milder than usual presentation, for example, when there is a relatively mild reduction in globin synthesis attributable to one or both thalassemic alleles, when there is a higher than usual compensatory increase in gamma chain production, or when the co-inheritance of α-thalassemia decreases the net imbalance and alpha- and beta-globin synthesis. This condition, termed "thalassemia intermedia," exhibits stigmas of anemia, hemolysis, and marrow expansion but no requirement for chronic transfusions for survival.

DIAGNOSIS

The diagnosis of severe thalassemia is usually straightforward. The family history, especially in ethnic groups at high risk (Italian, Greek, black, Asian, North African), is often a solid lead. Thalassemia major or thalassemia intermedia is marked by microcytic anemia associated with jaundice, bone deformities, and splenomegaly appearing during gestation (α-thalassemia) or in the first 2 years of life. Hydrops fetalis typically presents as polyhydramnios and fetal distress during the second trimester.

Peripheral blood films show characteristic features that distinguish thalassemia from iron deficiency. For the same level of anemia, thalassemic smears exhibit more pronounced microcytosis with anisocytosis and *relative* hypochromia, punctate basophilic stippling, and a high percentage of target cells (up to 30%). The last two phenomena are less dramatically expressed in iron deficiency. The reticulocyte count is deceptively low for the degree of anemia (2 to 8%) because of the ineffective erythropoiesis. In hemoglobin H disease, the diagnosis can be suspected by in vitro precipitation of hemoglobin H with brilliant cresyl blue.

β-Thalassemia trait (β-thalassemia minor) is recognized by mild anemia (hematocrit of >30) with dramatically low mean corpuscular volume (<75 fL) and erythrocytosis (red blood cell count of $>5 \times 10^6$ per mm^3), near-normal "red blood cell distribution width" and mean corpuscular hemoglobin concentration values, a normal serum iron concentration and total iron-binding capacity, and normal ferritin level. A microcytic blood picture is also seen in cases of congenital sideroblastic anemia, but the classic dimorphic picture and the higher degree of transferrin saturation in this disorder usually permit discrimination.

Hemoglobin electrophoresis, including a quantitative search for the elevation of hemoglobin A and F levels characteristic of β-thalassemia or for hemoglobin H or Bart's, is a useful adjunct, but normal results do not rule out the diagnosis of heterozygous thalassemia. In most heterozygotes, elevations of hemoglobin A_2 and/or hemoglobin F confirm the diagnosis of β-thalassemia. Rare forms of β-thalassemia (e.g., δ β-thalassemia) do not cause elevated hemoglobin A_2 levels. α-Thalassemia trait can be completely silent or similar to β-thalassemia trait, except for an absence of changes in hemoglobin A_2 or F levels. Iron deficiency can mask β-thalassemia trait by decreasing the hemoglobin A_2 level. Coexisting thalassemia trait may thus be overlooked in an iron-deficient individual. If microcytic anemia does not respond completely to iron therapy, hemoglobin electrophoresis should be reconsidered.

The prenatal diagnosis of thalassemia can now be accomplished with a high degree of safety and reliability by direct polymerase chain reaction analysis of fetal DNA obtained by amniocentesis or chorionic villus biopsy. Fetal cell DNA is obtained by amniocentesis after 14 weeks of gestation or by chorionic villus biopsy any time in the first trimester. Direct isolation of fetal cells from maternal blood for DNA analysis by ultrasensitive polymerase chain reaction methods has been shown to be technically feasible but remains clinically unproven as a noninvasive method of antenatal diagnosis.

The large variety of DNA sequence defects that can cause thalassemia require that these analyses be done by experts. Many mutations must be screened to achieve useful predictability. One major improvement has been the tailoring of these searches within each ethnic group on the basis of molecular epidemiologic surveys. These have shown that a few mutations account for the majority of serious cases within virtually every ethnic group. This greatly simplifies the analyses. The small size of the globin genes also permits rapid and direct DNA sequencing of the inherited alleles in cases in which clear diagnosis is not apparent from the standardized assays. Widespread application of molecular epidemiology, genetic counseling, and antenatal diagnosis has virtually eliminated the appearance of new cases of thalassemias in some areas of the Mediterranean basin.

THERAPY

β-Thalassemia

In heterozygous α- or β-thalassemias, close monitoring of the hematocrit is necessary during pregnancy to avoid a harmful drop, but patients are otherwise asymptomatic. Genetic counseling is mandatory.

Transfusion Therapy

In β-thalassemia major, red blood cell transfusion is the mainstay of supportive therapy. Transfusions should be administered in sufficient quantity and frequency to achieve a hemoglobin level of *at least* 9.3 grams per dL; this level partly suppresses the erythropoietic drive. A regimen that maintains the mean hemoglobin level above 10.5 to 11 grams per dL reduces marrow expansion, leading to a reduction in plasma volume and thus in the amount of blood required to achieve the same level of hemoglobin, especially in splenectomized patients. Bone changes are arrested or even regress, splenomegaly is retarded or recedes, growth improves, and improved physical activity can be expected. The increased transfusional iron load is partially compensated for by decreased gastrointestinal iron absorption. *Most* experts maintain patients in the range of 9.5 to 11 grams per dL.

With regard to initiation of chronic transfusions, one can safely follow the recommendations of the guide of the Cooley's Anemia Foundation: transfusion should be started for a persistent and otherwise unexplained fall in hemoglobin below 7 grams per dL. Patients with higher hemoglobin levels may require chronic transfusions to address significant growth impairment, serious bone changes, or progressive splenomegaly. A maintenance hemoglobin level above 10.5 to 11 grams per dL in nonhypersplenic patients is recommended. Frequent (one or two per week) infusions of small quantities of red blood cells provide the most "physiologic" support, but the psychologic burden, especially for children, and logistic issues render this strategy impractical. In general, transfusion of about 15 mL of red blood cells per kg at 3- to 5-week intervals is feasible for most patients and families. Transfusion records should be kept to measure the annual mean hemoglobin level and the annual blood consumption.

A complete genotype of the patient's red blood cells should be established before any transfusion treatment occurs; this information simplifies later identification of the involved antigens should isoimmunization occur. Only fresh ABO- and Rh_0D-compatible crossmatched blood should be given. I advocate continuous monitoring for isoantibodies to critical red blood cell antigens, using indirect antiglobulin testing. When patients develop febrile reactions during transfusions, filters retaining the leukocytes should be installed or red blood cells frozen in glycerol used instead. If this is unsuccessful, washing the red blood cells is the next option. Aspirin taken before the transfusion often reduces the reaction. Increased transfusion requirements should alert the physician to possible hypersplenism, alloimmunization, or the presence of an accessory spleen. In addition to the rigorous screening of donor blood for hepatitis antigens, patients should be immunized early for hepatitis B. When titers drop to low levels, booster immunizations are suggested. The danger of human immunodeficiency virus (HIV) infection acquired from blood transfusion depends on the incidence of the disease in the donor pool but is favorably influenced by the intensity of the donor blood screening program, which has considerably diminished the risk for HIV infection in the United States. The possible use of irradiated and cytomegalovirus-free preparations is relevant in potential bone marrow transplant candidates and should be approached in that fashion, in consultation with transfusion medicine experts who are conversant with this rapidly evolving area.

Splenectomy

Massive splenomegaly is usually avoided or delayed by a proper hypertransfusion regimen. However, splenic sequestration of donor cells can eventually cause an excessive transfusion requirement. A 50% or greater increase in the transfusion requirements during a 1-year period is the major indication for surgical removal of the spleen. A transfusion requirement of more than 200 mL per kg per year of packed red blood cells is also an indication for splenectomy if there is no serologic evidence of isoimmunization. Significant leukopenia and thrombocytopenia by splenic trapping are other indications, but these rarely occur without the aforementioned increase in the red blood cell requirement.

Splenectomy significantly increases the risk of overwhelming sepsis, especially in young children. Encapsulated pneumococci are responsible in two thirds of the cases. The other two most frequent pathogens are *Haemophilus influenzae* and *Neisseria meningitidis* (meningococcus). *Yersinia enterocolitica* or *Yersinia pseudotuberculosis* is also found, especially in patients undergoing deferoxamine mesylate (Desferal) treatment (these organisms use the iron bound to the chelator). Because the risk of infections is greatest if patients undergo splenectomy during infancy, one should attempt to defer the operation until the age of 6 years.

Polyvalent pneumococcal vaccine should be administered 1 month before splenectomy. Many experts advocate the administration of oral penicillin V (250 mg per day) as prophylaxis after the procedure for at least 2 years in children younger than 10 years. Trimethoprim-sulfamethoxazole is an alternative in case of allergy. Parents should be instructed to seek immediate medical attention when significant fever develops (>101°F). Such patients are at risk for a fulminant course leading to death within 6 hours. Broad-spectrum antibiotics should be given immediately, even before the results of any laboratory investigations are obtained. Splenectomized patients undergoing invasive procedures (e.g., dental work, endoscopy) should be given prophylactic penicillin (or alternative drugs in allergic patients, as stated earlier) for 24 hours before and after the procedure.

Treatment of Iron Overload

Each unit of blood contains approximately 250 mg of iron. A typical hypertransfusion regimen encumbers each patient *each year* with an average of four times the normal total body iron burden. There is no compensatory mechanism of sufficient magnitude to eliminate this iron; the decrease in intestinal absorption typical of the iron overloaded state is inadequate. Indeed, many transfused thalassemic patients continue to absorb dietary iron at high rates, probably because of signals from the expanded erythropoietic drive. By the time most of these patients reach adolescence, their iron stores have risen to toxic levels (transfusional hemosiderosis).

Before effective iron chelation therapy was developed, the dramatic multiorgan toxicity of iron was the major determinant in the fatal progression of the disease. The complications have a more subtle presentation in patients maintained with chelation therapy. Hemosiderosis causes the most striking clinical dysfunction in the endocrine organs, liver, and heart.

One common endocrinologic complication is glucose intolerance. Insulin-dependent diabetes mellitus occurs in a smaller group. Laboratory evidence of primary hypothyroidism, hypoparathyroidism, and other endocrinopathies can often be detected in the absence of symptoms; digoxin refractoriness in such patients should lead one to suspect hypocalcemia on this basis. One should be alert to diminished adrenal reserves during periods of metabolic stress in these patients. Delayed puberty is common and is probably the result of iron deposition in the hypothalamus. Retarded growth in the hypertransfused patients is less striking in the early years but becomes pronounced at puberty. The exact mechanism is unclear.

Hepatic toxicity can lead to cirrhosis, but progression to symptomatic liver disease before the era of sustained chelation therapy was unusual because of the superseding onset of lethal cardiac complications. Subclinical cardiac dysfunction usually begins in the early teens; it is detectable by the reduced ejection fractions in exercising patients or by wall motion anomalies. Onset of clinical symptoms usually begins with arrhythmias or pericarditis, followed by congestive failure in the late teens and death at about the age of 20 years.

The iron chelator deferoxamine mesylate is an effective agent when it is administered as a continuous subcutaneous or intravenous infusion. This maneuver markedly improves urinary iron excretion in comparison with intramuscular injections. When given as a continuous infusion in high enough doses in *most* patients, the drug maintains a negative iron balance despite continuing blood transfusions. When started before 5 to 8 years of age, these regimens are proving to be effective in delaying cardiac disease in some patients, potentially prolonging survival.

In the presence of a significant iron burden before the onset of therapy, complete reversibility of the lesions by deferoxamine cannot be reliably predicted. If therapy is started after 10 years of age, progressive cardiac dysfunction may not be completely prevented. Early initiation of therapy is thus advocated.

Iron overload should be documented first in candidates for iron chelation by a deferoxamine test. The 24-hour urinary excretion after injection of 500 mg of deferoxamine should exceed 1 mg to consider chelation therapy (or the serum ferritin level should be above 1000 ng per mL). Another option, gaining increasing favor and preferred by me, is to start the deferoxamine therapy at the same time as the transfusions.

A small infusion pump is used to administer a dose of about 40 mg per kg per day during a period of 10 hours into the abdominal subcutaneous fat, with rotation of the sites. Hypertonicity of the solution can be prevented by increasing the volume of water for the delivery of a given dose. Local allergic reactions (pruritus, hyperemia) can be suppressed by adding hydrocortisone (up to 2 mg per mL) to the solution or by using topical diphenhydramine. A number of cases of severe arrhythmias and severe congestive heart failure have been temporarily reversed with high-dose (15 mg per kg per hour for 10 hours) deferoxamine through a central venous catheter.

The drug is generally well tolerated. Anaphylactic reactions are rare and can be treated with desensitization. A number of patients treated with high-dose intravenous deferoxamine developed optic and acoustic neuritis, with only partial reversibility. Periodic vision and hearing tests are advocated. If the abnormalities disappear after discontinuation of the drug, the treatment can be cautiously reinitiated, beginning with lower doses.

Iron overload causes depletion of vitamin C. This deficiency inhibits iron release from the reticuloendothelial cells. Sudden availability of vitamin C can lead to a massive, abrupt release of iron, a situation that can cause serious cardiotoxicity. It is therefore advisable to start exogenous vitamin C administration only *after* the first cycle of treatment with deferoxamine. The dose should be about 5 mg per kg, should not exceed 100 mg per day when deferoxamine is given, and should be given only while the deferoxamine infusion is actually in progress. Ascorbate can be replaced by oranges (75 mg per orange) or orange juice (50 mg per 100 mL).

The major problem with deferoxamine therapy is noncompliance because of the inconvenience of using the pump. Regular monitoring and psychologic support are important for the success of the treatment. In addition to specialized assistance from social workers and child psychologists, patients' advocacy associations can help the patient cope with the emotional burden of the disease. There is reason to hope that the inconvenience of the present chelation therapy will disappear in the near future. Clinical trials with a promising oral chelator (L1) suggest possible clinical efficacy, although further testing for long-term effectiveness and safety is still in progress.

Thalassemia Intermedia

A number of patients with symptomatic β-thalassemia do not develop a debilitating anemia. These patients should not be committed to a lifelong transfusion regimen. In general, when the hemoglobin level remains above 8 grams per dL, patients lead a relatively normal life. However, regardless of the steady-state hemoglobin level, the patient should be watched closely for signs of bone marrow expansion, increasing spleen size, or growth retardation. These are all indications to initiate transfusion, usually the same regimen used to treat thalassemia major. If the fall of the mean hemoglobin level to unsuitable values parallels an increase in spleen size, splenectomy should be considered. Hypertransfusion can be delayed or avoided by splenectomy in some cases.

The hyperplastic marrow in thalassemia intermedia stimulates intestinal iron absorption, resulting in iron overload. Deferoxamine therapy should probably be started when the ferritin level rises above normal; one or two subcutaneous infusions a week generally suffice. Deferoxamine therapy is stopped during pregnancy, and a regular transfusion regimen during this period should be considered. The avoidance of iron-rich meats (liver and spleen), the ingestion of cereals, and the regular drinking of a cup of tea are advocated by some as dietary measures.

Other complications of chronic hemolysis are relative folate deficiency, gallstones, leg ulcers, and, rarely, compression syndromes. Vitamin deficiency can be avoided by a daily supplement of 1 mg of folic acid. Patients should be evaluated promptly for symptoms suggestive of cholecystitis. In addition to local treatment of leg ulcers, leg elevation and peroral zinc sulfate are useful; ulcers in a nontransfused patient may require at least temporary hypertransfusion. Radiotherapy may be needed to treat spinal cord compression from marrow expansion in vertebrae.

α-Thalassemia

Often no treatment is indicated with this disorder. The homozygous form is usually lethal in utero. Cases have been described of neonates who were kept alive with exchange transfusions. Patients with hemoglobin H disease usually present with moderate anemia. They should be monitored for worsening of the anemia during infections. If it is persistent and is associated with increasing splenomegaly, splenectomy should be considered; as in other forms of unstable hemoglobin disease, a substantial increase in red blood cell survival and in hemoglobin level often follows removal of the spleen. Another characteristic in common with unstable hemoglobin variants is the sensitivity of hemoglobin H to oxidant stress; drugs such as sulfonamides exacerbate the effect of the infection in worsening the anemia. Oxidant drugs should thus be avoided in this disease. Folic acid supplements are indicated, as in other cases of chronic hemolysis. Iron overload is a real issue in these patients, by analogy to patients with β-thalassemia intermedia, and becomes a major issue in late adolescence and adult life; iron status should thus be monitored even in the absence of transfusions.

EXPERIMENTAL THERAPY

Bone Marrow Transplantation

Allogeneic bone marrow transplantation can be curative by replacing stem cells harboring defective globin genes with normal cells. Transplantation is associated with significant mortality and morbidity resulting from the toxicity of the conditioning regimen and from the pancytopenia and acute and chronic graft-versus-host disease after the procedure. Because of the immediate risks, only a few centers have systematically used this therapeutic option in the last decade. Data emerging from these centers suggest short-term mortality rates of 10 to 15%, with good long-term results in survivors; risk of dying is greatest in patients with the greatest degree of iron overload at the time of transplantation. Organ hemosiderosis is considered the age-related risk factor. Relapse occurred in 13% of the younger patients and 5% of the older ones. Moderate to severe graft-versus-host disease was present in 5% of patients younger than 7 years and in 13% of the older group.

I believe that if a patient has an HLA-matched sibling, marrow transplantation should be considered in the earlier years. The risks of this curative therapeutic modality must be weighed against the lifelong burden of hypertransfusion regimens and iron-chelating therapy. This balance may be shifted in the near future by the introduction of oral chelating agents and by improvement in the transplantation regimens.

Activation of Fetal Globin Synthesis

In a limited number of patients studied for a short period of observation, gamma-globin chain expression was stimulated by the use of the chemotherapeutic agent 5-azacitidine. The increased gamma chain synthesis resulted in a significant decrease in the transfusion requirement that lasted for several days after discontinuation of the drug. Initially, the effect of the drug was thought to be mediated by the DNA hypomethylating activity of this agent, because gamma-globin gene expression was inversely correlated with the methylation status of gamma-globin gene DNA. (DNA *hypermethylation* often correlates with inactivation of a gene.) Other cytotoxic agents (hydroxyurea and cytosine arabinoside) with no direct demethylating activity have subsequently been shown to be efficacious, suggesting strongly that the clinical effect arises from cell selection and reprogramming of globin gene regulation by mechanisms not dependent on demethylating activity. The uncertainty about the carcinogenic side effects resulting from long-term use of these drugs has, until recently, limited this therapy to adult patients with advanced disease in the controlled setting of experimental trials in a few centers. Although significant favorable clinical experiences have been reported with the use of hydroxyurea in sickle cell anemia, suggesting that this drug might be useful for wider application to thalassemic patients, results in this group have been disappointing. Until more information about long-term toxicity and efficacy is available from these studies, this therapy should still be considered experimental and used in major centers in the context of longitudinal studies. Butyric acid derivatives also appear to promote gamma-globin synthesis; they are also under active investigation.

Gene Transfer

Many are investigating the biologic mechanisms necessary to achieve the long-term goal of correcting the defective genes in the stem cells of a thalassemic patient. At present, the most efficient system for transferring globin genes in hematopoietic stem cells is the retroviral vector, but many alternative systems are being studied because of disappointing results with this vector. Recent research has defined the major DNA control elements ("locus control region" sequences) that must be introduced with the structural globin sequences in retroviral vectors for controlled, abundant expression in erythroid progenitors. Several important problems must be solved before gene transfer systems can be applied in a curative mode to human thalassemic, hematopoietic stem cells. No definite time frame for the introduction of gene therapy in thalassemia can be anticipated at this moment.

SICKLE CELL DISEASE

method of
GRAHAM R. SERJEANT, M.D.
MRC Laboratories (Jamaica), University of the West Indies
Kingston, Jamaica, West Indies

The experience presented here draws heavily, but not entirely, on Jamaican practice evolved from the management of more than 5000 patients with sickle cell disease. These groups of patients include the Jamaican Cohort Study (approximately 550 children with sickle cell disease followed up from birth) and a large group of patients acquired predominantly by symptomatic referral. With the limited resources available for care, this treatment approach has had to be confined to methods for which there is good scientific and experimental evidence. Costly and often arbitrary therapies such as blood transfusion have been used only if there was clear evidence of a benefit. It is suggested that the rigorous discipline imposed by limited resources has rarely compromised the quality of medical care. This, then, is a Jamaican perspective of the therapy for sickle cell disease.

PATHOPHYSIOLOGY

The single nucleotide mutation determining the insertion of valine for glutamic acid at the sixth position from the amino terminus of the beta chain significantly changes the behavior of the hemoglobin (Hb) molecule. When deoxygenated, molecules of sickle hemoglobin (HbS) polymerize, raising the internal cellular viscosity, reducing membrane pliability, and distorting the red blood cell (RBC). Such cells have difficulty negotiating capillary beds, resulting in the two independent but closely interrelated pathophysiologic features of the disease, hemolysis and vaso-occlusion.

Hemolysis reduces RBC survival from a normal mean of 120 days to an average of 10 to 18 days, resulting in anemia (average Hb value, 6 to 9 grams per dL in homozygous sickle cell [SS] disease), jaundice, increased prevalence of pigment gallstones, and expansion of the bone marrow spaces. The expanded bone marrow can change the configuration of some bones, and its metabolic and nutritional demands may compromise growth and development. Generally, the hemolytic features are well tolerated and, with the exception of a superimposed aplastic crisis, rarely lead to mortality. The tendency to compromise blood flow damages the tissue supplied, the features depending on the site of nonperfusion. This ischemia most commonly affects the bone marrow (dactylitis, painful crisis, avascular necrosis of the femoral head), skin (leg ulceration), spleen (acute and chronic sequestration, impaired function), brain (stroke), and lungs (acute chest syndrome).

GENOTYPES OF SICKLE CELL DISEASE

Among communities in which sickle cell disease is predominantly of African origin, there are four principal genotypes (Table 1). SS disease and sickle cell–β^0-thalassemia manifest greater anemia and generally more severe clinical courses, although both show extreme variability in clinical features. Patients with sickle cell–hemoglobin C (SC) disease and sickle cell–β^+-thalassemia are less anemic, with he-

TABLE 1. **Major Genotypes of Sickle Cell Disease and Their Frequency in Jamaica**

Genotype	Abbreviated Form	Frequency
Homozygous sickle cell disease	SS disease	1 in 300 births
Sickle cell–hemoglobin C disease	SC disease	1 in 500 births
Sickle cell–β^+-thalassemia	Sβ^+-thalassemia	1 in 3000 births
Sickle cell–β^0-thalassemia	Sβ^0-thalassemia	1 in 7000 births

moglobin levels reaching into the normal range, and generally have mild manifestations. Most complications of sickle cell disease occur in all genotypes, although the frequency and severity are greater in the severe forms. The following discussion relates primarily to SS disease, and the complications believed to be related to hemolytic rate are discussed first.

ANEMIA

Steady State

Most patients with SS disease have steady-state hemoglobin levels of 6 to 9 grams per dL. At steady-state levels, symptoms of anemia are unusual, and oxygen carriage appears to be close to normal. This is because HbS within the RBC manifests a low oxygen affinity, becoming almost fully saturated in the lungs but releasing more oxygen per gram of hemoglobin in the periphery compared with normal hemoglobin A (HbA). Furthermore, the severity of anemia correlates with the extent of shift in the oxygen dissociation curve, patients with the largest shifts (lowest affinity) manifesting the lowest hemoglobin levels. These observations imply that erythropoiesis is switched off at submaximal levels (average reticulocyte counts 10 to 12%), not because the bone marrow cannot sustain greater erythropoietic activity, but because higher levels are not necessary to maintain adequate oxygen carriage. Transfusion of patients with hemoglobin at their steady-state levels is therefore not justified on the basis of improving oxygen carriage.

Lowered Hemoglobin Levels

A variety of complications are associated with acute and chronic lowering of hemoglobin below steady-state values. In each case, the physician should seek and treat the cause rather than resorting to the blanket therapy of transfusion. Reticulocyte counts, as indicators of bone marrow activity, are essential to diagnosis, and mean cell volume (MCV) is helpful in distinguishing iron deficiency or megaloblastic change from folate deficiency (Table 2). Megaloblastic change should be treated with folic acid. Regular folate supplementation is not practiced in Jamaica, because dietary folate levels appear adequate, but folate supplementation may be given at times of additional requirements, such as rapid growth periods or pregnancy. Unnecessary supplementation should be avoided, and patients encouraged to eat fresh fruit and vegetables.

Iron deficiency may occur without obvious cause and is presumed to be dietary in origin, although causes of iron loss may need investigating. There is usually a rapid response to oral iron therapy. Occasionally, combined iron and folic acid deficiencies may cause diagnostic confusion, because there may be no change in RBC characteristics, but both serum folate and iron levels are low. Supplementation with folate reveals iron-limited erythropoiesis, and the MCV falls; supplementation with iron reveals folate-limited erythropoiesis, and the MCV rises. Aplastic crisis and acute splenic sequestration generally require urgent transfusion and are discussed later. A variety of hypoplastic situations manifest low hemoglobin levels, and low levels but not absence of reticulocytes and can occur with infections and chronic renal failure.

APLASTIC CRISIS

Aplastic crisis affected 30% of patients with SS disease in the Jamaican Cohort Study by the age of 15 years. Defined clinically by marked lowering of hemoglobin level and absence of reticulocytes from the peripheral blood, aplastic crises are most common before 15 years of age, occur in epidemics, and cluster in families. The cause is human parvovirus infection. Bone marrow aplasia lasts 7 to 10 days, and the bone marrow always recovers provided that oxygen carriage is maintained by transfusion. A single unit of blood (1 pint for age 15 years and older; 10 mL per kg for younger than this age) achieves this goal, and the clinical course is so predictable and benign that the transfusion is usually performed as an outpatient procedure; the patient is seen after 3 to 4 days to ensure that the reticulocytosis of spontaneous marrow recovery has occurred. The strong

TABLE 2. **Features Associated with Lowered Hemoglobin Levels in SS Disease**

Complication	Hb Range (gm/dL)	Reticulocytes (%)	MCV (fL)	Other Features
Normal average	6–9	10–12	75–95	
Acute lowering				
Acute splenic sequestration	1–4	20–30	Unchanged	Splenomegaly, 3–5 cm
Aplastic crisis	2–5	0	Unchanged	
Chronic lowering				
Iron deficiency	4–6	1–8	67–75	Iron stores low
Folate deficiency	3–4	1–10	100–120*	
Chronic hypersplenism	3–5	20–40	Unchanged	Splenomegaly, 5–15 cm
Infection	4–6	1–8	Unchanged	
Chronic renal failure	3–5	1–8	Unchanged	Renal impairment

*Degree of change in MCV is important; some patients with genetically determined microcytosis, such as those with SS and α-thalassemia, with a steady-state MCV of 65 fL may manifest megaloblastic change with a rise in MCV to 85 fL (i.e., increase of 20 fL).

Abbreviations: SS = homozygous sickle cell; Hb = hemoglobin; MCV = mean cell volume.

family history (50% chance of susceptible siblings being affected within 3 weeks) implies that the patient's siblings with SS should be closely monitored. A human parvovirus vaccine has been developed and is currently undergoing early trials. Recurrence of human parvovirus-induced aplastic crisis has never been described, and immunity appears to be lifelong.

ACUTE SPLENIC SEQUESTRATION

Acute enlargement of the spleen with pooling of a significant proportion of the RBC mass may lead to a life-threatening anemia in young children. In the Jamaican Cohort Study, this complication had affected 25% of children by 2 years and 30% by 5 years of age. If the patient survives the first episode, there is a 50% chance of recurrence, with repeated episodes occurring at shorter intervals. Transfusion of a single unit of blood is the treatment of the acute attack, and splenectomy is recommended after two attacks. Parental education in the detection and significance of acute splenic sequestration (ASS) has reduced mortality from this complication by 90%.

CHRONIC HYPERSPLENISM

Chronic splenic sequestration or hypersplenism differs from ASS in its gradual development, greater degree of splenomegaly, and markedly expanded bone marrow activity, which allows a new hematologic equilibrium but at a greatly increased hemolytic rate (mean RBC life, 1 to 3 days). The metabolic demands of the expanded bone marrow compete with those of growth, which frequently slows or ceases, and rapid increase in growth follows splenectomy. The very low hemoglobin level (3 to 5 grams per dL) is associated with high cardiac output and increased cardiac work. Death may occur from superimposed acute sequestration, incidental aplastic crisis, or hemorrhage consequent to the low platelet counts. Hypersplenism may resolve spontaneously, so the condition is usually monitored for 4 to 6 months to assess any resolution before splenectomy is recommended. Patients may be managed by regular transfusion for a limited period, but splenectomy after a period of monitoring is the preferred option.

CHRONIC RENAL FAILURE

Renal tubular damage is common in SS disease, resulting in an inability to concentrate urine and in other functional tubular abnormalities, but the progressive loss of glomeruli results in chronic renal failure. The most likely mechanism is glomerular hyperfiltration leading to glomerulosclerosis and a progressive fall in glomerular filtration rate with eventual elevation of serum creatinine level. Reduced erythropoietin production by the kidney leads to an increased anemia. This is initially well tolerated; indeed, many patients experience a "honeymoon period" free of painful crises. As hemoglobin falls to a level compromising cardiac function, simple "top-up" transfusion may alleviate symptoms. Patients are often the best judges of when transfusion is required, and 1 to 2 units may be given to raise the hemoglobin to 5 to 6 grams per dL. Higher levels are not necessary, and sudden changes in hematocrit may actually further compromise renal function. The anemia of renal failure has been treated with recombinant human erythropoietin, most effectively given by subcutaneous injection at least twice weekly. The most appropriate dose is not known, experience with this expensive drug in sickle cell disease is limited, and poor response is common. Correction of anemia by this method rather than by transfusion increases circulating HbS. Sudden increases in hemoglobin level may induce iatrogenic painful crises, and careful follow-up by clinicians experienced in the use of this agent is recommended. Where renal replacement therapy is an option, early referral to a renal physician is recommended. The severity of renal impairment in SS disease may be underestimated from serum creatinine levels, which are usually lower than those in normal people. Impaired cardiac or respiratory function may necessitate early entry of an SS patient into a dialysis program. Renal transplantation has been successful in SS disease, although sickle-induced damage may occur in the transplanted kidney.

INFECTIONS

Patients with SS disease are more prone to several bacterial infections. Early loss of the splenic filtering capacity for removing blood-borne antigens results in a tendency to overwhelming septicemia, most commonly with *Streptococcus pneumoniae* and *Haemophilus influenzae* type b (Hib).

Prevention

Pneumococcal septicemia may be prevented in a child with SS disease by regular penicillin, given in Jamaica by monthly intramuscular depot preparations, from 4 months to 4 years of age (penicillin G benzathine, 300,000 units from 4 months to 3 years; 600,000 units from 3 to 4 years), and then administering the 23-valent pneumococcal vaccine (Pneumovax 23) before stopping the penicillin. It is vital that penicillin prophylaxis is not stopped before the vaccine is given, because the child has little naturally acquired immunity and is therefore especially susceptible to infection. The capsular polysaccharide vaccines appear to be poorly antigenic in children younger than 4 years, and there is no convincing evidence that booster vaccines provoke a better response than the age-related increase in maturity of the immune system. Two factors may cause this policy to be modified in the near future: the increasing frequency of penicillin-resistant pneumococci and the advent of a conjugated pneumococcal vaccine that may be effective when given at 2, 4, and 6 months and that is currently undergoing trial in SS disease.

Hib infection is also increased in SS disease and

becomes more apparent with the prevention of pneumococcal disease. Prevention is based on a conjugated Hib vaccine (HibTITER), which appears to induce good antibody levels and the clinical efficacy of which is being assessed. This may be given with other immunizations at 2, 4, and 6 months.

Areas of avascular necrosis of bone have long been known to be susceptible to infection by *Salmonella* species, causing salmonella osteomyelitis (see later). Salmonella septicemia may also occur in the absence of bone involvement, and the low index of suspicion for this organism in a "septicemic" patient may result in high mortality.

Treatment

Septic patients with high fever must be assumed to have infections with *S. pneumoniae*, Hib, or *Salmonella* and should be given suitable antibiotics pending the results of blood culture. Most effective, if available, is ceftriaxone (Rocephin), 100 mg per kg per day twice daily intravenously for at least 7 days. Less expensive alternatives are crystalline penicillin, 200,000 units per kg per day, and chloramphenicol, 75 to 100 mg per kg per day, both intravenously every 6 hours for at least 7 days.

Although infections are commonly associated with reduced bone marrow activity and an increasing anemia, primary therapy must be directed against the cause of the infection and only secondarily against the anemia, which may require transfusion.

JAUNDICE, BILIRUBIN EXCRETION, AND GALLSTONES

The increased bilirubin production consequent to hemolysis is associated with both clinical jaundice and pigment gallstones. The severity of clinical jaundice varies among patients and also in the same patient, becoming more obvious during fever, dehydration, or painful crises. This feature causes concern, but patients may be reassured that such jaundice is a harmless side effect of hemolysis and does not have the serious significance of jaundice in otherwise normal people (e.g., indicative of hepatitis). Occasionally, marked increases in bilirubin level may occur consequent to acute cholestasis or obstruction of the common bile duct by a gallstone. The distinction by ultrasonography is vital, because acute cholestasis generally resolves with conservative therapy, whereas an obstructed common bile duct may need removal at surgery or endoscopy.

Gallstones have been observed in children as young as 3 to 4 years and reached an incidence of 40% by age 20 years in the Jamaican Cohort Study. Most gallstones are asymptomatic, and there is no evidence justifying surgical removal of asymptomatic stones. Cholecystectomy should be performed for specific symptoms, including acute and chronic cholecystitis, empyema, and obstruction of the cystic duct or of the common bile duct. Nonspecific abdominal pain should not be considered an indication for cholecystectomy, because it frequently coincides with gallstones, but studies have shown that both factors reflect an underlying clinical severity and that they are not causally related. Nonspecific abdominal pain may continue after cholecystectomy for gallstones.

BONE PROBLEMS

Dactylitis

A common early manifestation of SS disease, dactylitis affects 50% of Jamaican Cohort Study children by the age of 2 years. Because it may start in children as young as 3 to 4 months and is almost synonymous with sickle cell disease, it is a common cause of the initial diagnosis of sickle cell disease. Painful swelling of the small bones of the hands and feet affects single or multiple bones and results from bone marrow necrosis. Dactylitis frequently recurs, but attacks become rare after age 5 to 6 years. Generally, clinical and radiologic resolution is complete, although sometimes, probably as a result of superimposed infection, there may be premature fusion of the epiphysis and a permanent shortening and deformity of small bones. Treatment consists of pain relief and reassurance that the complication is not serious.

Painful Crisis

With increasing age, erythropoietic activity ceases in the bone marrow of the small bones of the hands and feet, and greatest activity occurs in the juxta-articular areas of the long bones, the spine, and the flat bones of the sternum, ribs, and pelvis. Avascular necrosis of bone marrow at these sites causes the typical painful crisis that may thus be viewed as the adult counterpart of dactylitis in childhood. It is believed that the necrosis is probably painless but that the inflammatory response associated with the repair and healing of dead bone marrow increases intramedullary pressure and may cause extreme pain. There are well-recognized precipitating factors that, in Jamaica, include skin cooling, dehydration, infection, pregnancy, and the immediate postpartum period. Cold is most common, and many painful crises may be prevented by avoiding getting caught in the rain, not taking cold baths, and keeping warm in winter and at night. Risk factors include a high hemoglobin level, most common in adolescent male patients. The natural history is for pains to become less frequent and less severe after age 30 years, and, in most patients, they cease entirely after age 40 years. Patients who seem to be exceptions to this pattern should be carefully assessed for social, psychologic, and other possible factors.

Pain relief is a clinical challenge in the painful crisis. Human response to pain and the ability to cope with pain are notably influenced by many social and cultural factors. Examination of the clinical course in some patients manifesting frequent painful crises in Jamaica shows amelioration of symptoms during periods of social stability and recurrence of pains when support systems disappear. Patients in painful crisis often do not understand the cause or mechanism of the pains, and they experience panic and a sense of impending doom. Patients in painful crisis have stated that they have only to reach the doors of the Sickle Cell Clinic in Jamaica and they start to feel better. It is clear that reassurance can do much to alleviate anxiety and increase the ability to cope with pain.

The objectives of management should therefore be reassurance, treatment or alleviation of any underlying cause if identified, hydration (by intravenous fluid if the patient is vomiting or unable to take fluids orally), and pain relief sufficient to allow the patient to rest and sleep. Most patients keep acetaminophen (Tylenol) at home and have used it before reaching the clinic, but if not, this would be the first line of treatment for all but severe bone pain. Codeine, 30 mg orally, may be helpful in children. Patients with severe bone pains may be given pentazocine (Talwin), 1 mg per kg intramuscularly, or meperidine (Demerol), 1.5 mg per kg intramuscularly, with further assessment and additional doses after 2 to 3 hours. Anti-inflammatory agents such as diclofenac (Voltaren), 1.5 mg per kg intramuscularly, may relieve pain and reduce narcotic requirements. Most patients are treated in a day care center, where, after being monitored for 6 to 7 hours, they are offered the option of admission to hospital or discharge home with the same analgesics in oral form. More than 90% of patients with pain of sufficient severity to require narcotic analgesia in the morning elect to go home in the evening with the assurance that they can return to the day care center on the following day.

Avascular Necrosis of the Femoral Head

Avascular necrosis of bone marrow may also occur in the femoral head and, with continued weight bearing, may result in permanent deformity. Treatment depends on early diagnosis and avoidance of weight bearing for approximately 6 months to allow the femoral head to heal without deformity. Traction may be necessary, but many cases, especially in children and adolescents, may be managed with plaster casts and crutches, alternating a hip spica cast for 6 weeks with a bent-knee cast for 6 weeks, preventing weight bearing on the affected hip, and allowing the patient to continue attending school. In the belief that a high pressure within the femoral head may exacerbate further necrosis, core decompression of the femoral head has been proposed but is untested in controlled trials. Permanent deformity of the femoral head with persistent pain and limitation of movement may be alleviated by a limited remodeling of the head or an osteotomy, but extensive damage and severe symptoms often require total hip replacement (THR). There has been reluctance to perform THR in younger patients because of concern about life of the prosthesis or the need to revise the operation when such patients are older. Experience suggests that many patients have 10 to 15 years of good function with THR before revision and that the operation should be performed on the basis of severity of symptoms rather than concern about future needs for revision.

Avascular Necrosis of Bone

Avascular necrosis forms part of the spectrum of syndromes resulting from bone marrow necrosis, but rather than the commonly symmetrical distribution of sites seen in the painful crisis, the term "avascular necrosis of bone" is usually reserved to describe involvement of one or two sites that is associated with marked, persistent pain and swelling. Commonly affected sites are the humerus, radius and ulna, clavicle, and tibia. Repeated blood cultures are sterile. Treatment consists of pain relief, restriction of movement, rest of the affected area, and, usually, antibiotics to decrease the risk of secondary infection of dead bone marrow. Differentiating this complication from osteomyelitis may be difficult.

Osteomyelitis

Osteomyelitis, usually caused by *Salmonella* organisms, although occasionally by Hib, *Staphylococcus*, or *Escherichia coli*, is a well-recognized complication. It is believed to be secondary to sterile avascular necrosis. The distribution reflects that of underlying avascular necrosis, most commonly affecting the femur, tibia and fibula, humerus, radius and ulna, small bones of the hands and feet secondary to dactylitis, and, occasionally, femoral head, causing a rapid bone destruction. The diagnosis may be obvious, with gross pain and swelling, high fever, marked radiologic change, suppuration, and positive blood cultures, but some cases are difficult to distinguish from sterile avascular necrosis of bone. There is no acceptable standard for diagnosis in this situation. Treatment requires antibiotics for at least 4 to 6 weeks. Choice of antibiotic is usually based (pending the results of culture) on the typical sensitivity of *Salmonella* (i.e., with chloramphenicol or ampicillin). Surgical drainage and removal of a sequestrum, if formed, are also done. Gentamicin-impregnated beads inserted into the site of osteomyelitis release high concentrations of antibiotic locally, but there is no evidence of their efficacy from controlled trials.

ACUTE CHEST SYNDROME

The acute chest syndrome covers a spectrum of lung disease characterized by fever, cough, pleuritic pain, clinical signs, and radiologic evidence of new pulmonary infiltrates. It is one of the major manifestations of SS disease and a principal cause of death at all ages after 2 years. The pathogenesis includes elements of infection, infarction, fat embolism, and pulmonary sequestration. A patient's condition may deteriorate rapidly, especially with acute pulmonary sequestration, and should be monitored by pulse oximetry. Respiratory distress with a rapid fall in oxygen saturation is an emergency requiring immediate exchange transfusion (performed in Jamaica manually, with 1 unit of blood removed and 2 units of HbA blood given), which may be repeated after 4 to 6 hours. In successful cases, respiratory distress and a pulmonary "whiteout" may be reversed within 24 hours, indicating an acutely reversible vascular phenomenon. Although evidence of infection is uncommon, all cases of acute chest syndrome should be treated with broad-spectrum antibiotics and physiotherapy. Oxygen is usually given on basic principles, but there is no proof of its benefit. Rib and sternal infarction may also cause pleuritic pain, and voluntary splinting of the chest wall may give rise to secondary atelectasis and the acute chest syndrome. In such cases, incentive spirometry significantly reduces the risks of secondary acute chest syndrome.

BRAIN AND EYES

Stroke

Stroke occurred in 8% of patients in the Jamaican Cohort Study by 14 years and at a median age of 8 years. The risk factors for initial stroke are largely unknown, so prevention is not possible. The risk of recurrence is 50 to 70% within 3 years, and treatment at other centers is currently based on preventing recurrent events through long-term transfusion programs aimed at maintaining HbS levels below 30%. There are many problems with such programs, including the development of alloimmunization, iron overload, maintenance of venous access, transfusion-acquired infections, duration of necessary transfusion, and determining the most appropriate methods of monitoring.

Stroke recurrence has been seen with "successful" programs that maintain HbS levels below 25%. Transfusion reactions continue to be a problem despite the use of leukocyte- and platelet-depleted blood, and some patients develop so many antibodies that they can not undergo transfusion. Prevention of iron overload requires subcutaneous chelation with desferrioxamine and the use of syringe driving pumps for at least 5 nights each week. This treatment is expensive and commonly fails because of lack of compliance in adolescence. Many patients lose peripheral veins and require permanent ports such as Port-A-Caths or Hickman's catheters, both of which are subject to infection and thrombosis.

Transfusion-acquired infections have been reduced by screening of transfused blood, but there remains a period during which infection with human immunodeficiency virus may be undetectable. Cessation of transfusion programs after periods up to 10 to 12 years suggests that the recurrence rate for strokes is higher than if transfusion had never been commenced, resulting in a policy of transfusion for life. The enormous cost and logistic difficulties with such treatment place it beyond the resources in Jamaica, so long-term transfusion programs are not offered. Exchange transfusion is recommended for the acute event, and a limited transfusion program (approximately 1 unit per month) is offered for 1 year only because of the risks of iron accumulation. A final disadvantage of current therapy is that it cannot be commenced until the child develops the initial stroke.

There is a need to understand the risk factors for initial stroke to institute prevention. This is currently being addressed by two initiatives, a trial of transcranial Doppler ultrasonography to detect cerebral vessel stenoses predictive of stroke and an assessment of the predictive role of upper airway obstruction and episodic hypoxemia in stroke. The transcranial Doppler study has shown that transfusion therapy in patients with evidence of stenosis significantly reduces the incidence of stroke. In the meantime, management of stroke represents a major problem and may justify the risks of bone marrow transplantation (see later).

Eyes

Retinal vaso-occlusion, affecting predominantly the peripheral retina, results in the development of fragile new vessel systems in the periphery supplied by feeding arterioles. These proliferative sickle retinopathy (PSR) lesions may bleed, causing vitreous hemorrhage with transient blurring of vision, and large lesions with associated fibrosis may cause retinal detachment and permanent visual loss. Efforts to prevent these symptoms have led to attempts to render PSR lesions avascular by coagulating the feeding arterioles with a xenon arc or argon laser and also by ablating the ischemic retina with an argon laser. Three trials involving much effort, expense, and potential complications confirmed a significant decrease in the risk of vitreous hemorrhage, but it was clear that although PSR was common (occurring in approximately 70% of adult patients with SC disease), visual loss was relatively rare. It is now recognized that spontaneous nonperfusion (autoinfarction) of these lesions is common, and there is a moratorium on such treatment in Jamaica until the risk factors for autoinfarction are better understood. It is hoped that treatment may be focused on patients in whom spontaneous autoinfarction of PSR lesions is unlikely and in whom the risks of visual loss justify the potential complications of treatment.

LEG ULCERS

Chronic leg ulcers around the ankles are particularly common in Jamaica, affecting 75% of adults with SS disease at some time. They are believed to be multifactorial, with components from trauma, skin infarction, and high venous pressure. Prevention depends on avoiding skin trauma and treating early lesions seriously and intensively. All ulcer swabs yield a variety of bacteria, but these are generally colonizers, and antibiotics do not promote healing unless there is evidence of invasion, such as cellulitis.

Standard treatment consists of regular dressing at

home twice daily with mild antiseptic agents such as half-strength Eusol* or 0.01% potassium permanganate. Débridement is achieved when necessary by the use of crushed papaya, which has a proteolytic enzyme. Oral zinc sulfate, 200 mg three times daily, significantly improved healing in a controlled trial. Skin grafting (only pinch grafts, and not split-skin or full-thickness grafts) may be used in clean vascular ulcers, but ambulation before complete healing commonly leads to failure of the pinch grafts. This feature requires complete bed rest in hospital for 2 to 4 months, and the recurrence rate after complete healing is 80 to 90% within 2 years. Complete bed rest always improves ulcer healing, and there is no evidence for a beneficial effect of transfusion or hyperbaric oxygen. In Jamaica, ulceration usually commences in patients between 15 and 20 years of age, at a critical time for education, and there is a direct relationship between age at ulceration and educational attainment. In the absence of the ability to reliably heal ulcers quickly, this secondary educational deprivation may be avoided by persuading teachers and parents to allow children to continue attending school and to dress their ulcers at home at the beginning and end of each day.

PRIAPISM

Involuntary painful erection of the penis unassociated with sexual desire affects approximately 30 to 40% of postpubertal Jamaican male patients with SS disease. It is commonly not reported because of embarrassment or lack of realization that it is related to sickle cell disease. There are two clinical patterns: stuttering priapism, which is generally nocturnal, lasts 3 to 4 hours, is relieved by simple physical measures such as exercise, and is associated with normal intervening sexual function; and major attacks lasting longer than 24 hours, with extreme pain, often penile edema, and usually followed by irreversible damage to the vascular erectile system and impotence. Stuttering attacks are commonly a prodrome for a major attack, although some major attacks occur de novo.

The physician should always inquire directly about stuttering priapism and should reassure patients that these attacks are a common complication of sickle cell disease. If they occur more than 2 nights per week, they may be stopped by stilbestrol.† After the attacks have been stopped, the dose should be rapidly decreased to the minimal amount required to prevent stuttering priapism but to allow normal erections and avoid gynecomastia. The usual regimen is 5 mg daily for 3 days to stop the attacks, then 5 mg twice weekly for 2 weeks, 2.5 mg twice weekly for 2 weeks, 2.5 mg weekly for 2 weeks, and then 2.5 mg on alternate weeks for 2 weeks. At that point, the drug is stopped to see whether the attacks return. Cases of priapism vary in the dosage required; some are controlled by almost homeopathic doses of 1 mg every 3 weeks but attacks recur if this dose is stopped or replaced by a placebo. An alternative but more expensive approach is the use of injections of luteinizing hormone–releasing hormone, but these have not been tested in controlled trials. Lack of understanding of the association of stuttering priapism with sickle cell disease and the anxiety involved may result in frequent painful crises, otherwise uncharacteristic of the patient, which resolve with the successful prevention of priapism with stilbestrol.

Major attacks do not respond to stilbestrol and require surgical relief, which should be minimal. Aspiration and irrigation of the corpora by wide-bore needles allow detumescence, and a spongiosocavernosal shunt is a simple procedure giving more permanent relief. In the past, surgical drainage was avoided in the belief that it induced impotence, but this complication is now recognized to result from the permanent damage to the erectile vascular system. Vascular function may recover in patients sustaining major attacks before the age of 15 years, and occasionally, other patients recover some erectile function in 1 to 2 years after a major attack; usually, however, impotence results. Ejaculation is normal, and the mechanical problems of impotence may be treated with penile prostheses. The dense fibrosis of the corpora renders insertion of even simple rigid prostheses, such as the Small-Carrion prosthesis, difficult, and there is no place for the more sophisticated pneumatic penile prostheses.

PREGNANCY AND CONTRACEPTION

Pregnancy

Sexual development is retarded in patients with sickle cell disease, with a mean delay in menarche of 2.5 years. The interval between first unprotected sexual exposure and pregnancy is similar in SS disease and normal control subjects, contrary to the concept of relative infertility in this condition. Pregnancy is associated with a higher risk of painful crises and acute chest syndrome, especially in the third trimester and the immediate postpartum period. The risk of fetal loss is increased at every stage of pregnancy, and the infant is usually of low birth weight. Delivery should be by the normal vaginal route unless there are obstetric contraindications. All mothers should receive regular antenatal care with daily supplementation with iron and folic acid and should be booked for delivery in a hospital. There is no evidence that prophylactic transfusion improves fetal outcome, and this measure is not performed in Jamaican management of pregnancy in sickle cell disease. Many pregnant women with SS disease continue in good health throughout pregnancy and have normal deliveries, but some are seriously ill, and the maternal mortality in Jamaica is 1%.

Contraception

Patients requesting contraception should be given the best methods available. The frequent assumption

*Not available in the United States.
†Not FDA approved for this indication.

that there are serious risks to contraception in SS disease is unjustified, and the risks of pregnancy, although small, far outweigh the theoretical risks of contraception. The injectable contraceptive medroxyprogesterone (Depo-Provera), which is not only an effective contraceptive agent but also increases RBC survival and decreases bone pain in SS disease, is the method of choice. Many Jamaican patients prefer to have regular menstruation and choose the low-estrogen pill. Those requiring longer lasting methods are offered the intrauterine device, or tubal ligation if a permanent method is requested.

SURGERY AND ANESTHESIA

Surgery is performed as infrequently as possible in patients with SS disease, conservative management being preferred for asymptomatic gallstones and nonspecific abdominal pain. Common causes of surgery are splenectomy, orthopedic procedures, and operations unassociated with sickle cell disease, such as tonsillectomy and adenoidectomy. Elective surgery should be performed only with the patient clinically well and at a steady-state hemoglobin level. Preoperative transfusion is not performed, but blood is crossmatched to replace that lost at surgery. Most patients are preoxygenated before induction, and close monitoring is essential in the immediate postoperative period, when anesthesia-induced respiratory depression is common. Continued oxygenation and physiotherapy are important after upper abdominal surgery to prevent postoperative acute chest syndrome. The randomized study of transfusion in the Cooperative Study of Sickle Cell Disease in the United States found no difference between preoperative simple transfusion and exchange transfusion but did not assess a group without transfusion. Jamaican experience without transfusion shows a morbidity similar to that observed in transfused groups elsewhere, casting doubt on the value of routine preoperative transfusion.

DIAGNOSIS AND COUNSELING

The many ways in which early morbidity and mortality may be ameliorated in SS disease imply that early diagnosis is essential to implement educational and preventive programs. Diagnosis at birth is a simple cost-effective exercise and should be the objective in all communities. Only then can penicillin prophylaxis, parental education about ASS, complete immunization, better management of the aplastic crisis, and general education about disease management have their full potential impact on improving survival of the patient with SS disease.

Counseling services should explain the basic genetics of the disease and the chances that another child of parents with an SS child will be affected. Prenatal diagnosis should be available for couples who wish to make informed decisions about whether to complete an affected pregnancy. Social and general support services can help patients and their families find solutions to the social and other problems that are so often manifest in symptoms of the disease.

NEW APPROACHES TO TREATMENT

There have been many attempts to find effective antisickling agents, on the assumption that inhibition of sickling may ameliorate manifestations of the disease. Inducing higher levels of fetal hemoglobin has been achieved by hydroxyurea, with significant reductions in the prevalence of painful crises and transfusion requirements in a selected group of severely affected adults. Long-term transfusion programs have been grossly overutilized and, although leading to some short-term benefits, have often induced serious iatrogenic pathology. In Jamaica, no patients receive regular transfusion with the exception of a small group with chronic renal failure, and no patients are receiving hydroxyurea for prevention of painful crises. There seem to be other, more appropriate ways of preventing and managing painful crises, and because a high hemoglobin level is a clearly documented risk factor, venesection is currently being assessed by controlled trial. Currently, our knowledge of the natural history of sickle cell disease is not sufficiently detailed to be able to predict the most appropriate forms of intervention. Bone marrow transplantation may represent a treatment option in the prevention of stroke recurrence. However, the cost, the short-term mortality of 10%, the limited availability of suitable compatible donors, and the long-term risks of sterility mandate a cautious approach.

OPTIMAL CARE

Care is best provided in specialized centers with extensive experience with the disease and familiar, competent staff in whom the patient has confidence. Patients should be regularly reviewed every 3 to 6 months when clinically well and should be encouraged to visit the center at any time if ill. Steady-state hematologic assessments are performed in Jamaica every 2 years, or more frequently if clinically indicated, and allow earlier detection of problems such as chronic renal failure. Counseling and other support services should be available within the center. A day care approach to pain management for the painful crisis may provide a more acceptable alternative to frequent emergency room attendance or hospital admission. The average survival of patients with SS disease is currently approximately 50 years and will continue to improve with better medical and social care.

NEUTROPENIA

method of
LESLIE E. LEHMANN, M.D., and
EVA C. GUINAN, M.D.
Dana-Farber Cancer Institute and Children's Hospital
Boston, Massachusetts

Neutropenia is defined by a lower-than-expected number of neutrophils circulating in the peripheral blood. Neutrophil numbers are expressed using the absolute neutrophil count (ANC), which is calculated by multiplying the total white blood cell count by the percentage of neutrophils (including both mature and immature or band forms) on the differential. Normal values vary with age and race, but an ANC of less than 1500 μL is generally considered to be abnormal in persons beyond infancy. An ANC of less than 500 μL conventionally defines severe neutropenia and is associated with a markedly increased risk of life-threatening infections. Consequently, patients with this degree of neutropenia require prompt medical evaluation if a fever develops, and intravenous antibiotic therapy is initiated in most circumstances.

ETIOLOGY

There are many causes of neutropenia, and effective therapy is closely linked to the underlying disorder. Spurious neutropenia can be seen with excessive white blood cell clumping in the setting of abnormal proteins in the blood or can occur if blood counts are performed long after the blood sample has been drawn. In considering the causes of true neutropenia, it is useful to group them into two categories: decreased production and increased destruction of neutrophils. The most common problem is decreased production: Either an insufficient number of neutrophil precursors are generated, or the precursors are unable to develop into functional mature forms. These conditions can be congenital or acquired.

Decreased Production of Neutrophils

Congenital neutropenia, presenting as an isolated hematologic finding, often reflects a problem with hematopoietic precursors. For example, cyclic neutropenia, a dominantly inherited disorder due to a presumed defect in stem cell regulation, results in predictable, intermittent episodes of neutropenia and associated infections, mild or severe, that recur every 15 to 35 days. Alternatively, Kostmann's syndrome (infantile agranulocytosis), an autosomal recessive disorder in which progenitor cells are arrested at an immature stage of development, results in persistent neutropenia. Affected patients maintain an ANC of less than 200 μL and are often plagued by serious bacterial infections. In contrast, patients with chronic benign or idiopathic neutropenia, a poorly understood syndrome that appears to represent a late-stage arrest of neutrophil maturation, may have an equivalent degree of neutropenia but generally have a relatively low risk of serious infection and are otherwise completely well. Their neutrophil count remains stable over time, and the condition may spontaneously remit in early childhood.

Congenital neutropenia can also be part of other well-described syndromes with protean associated manifestations. Examples include Shwachman-Diamond syndrome (neutropenia and exocrine pancreatic insufficiency), cartilage-hair syndrome (an autosomal recessive disorder characterized by dwarfism and fine hair), dyskeratosis congenita (an X-linked recessive disorder characterized by nail dystrophy, leukoplakia, and hyperpigmentation of the skin), and Chédiak-Higashi syndrome (oculocutaneous albinism, progressive neurologic impairment, and giant granules in granulocytes). Many immunologic disorders also have associated neutropenia, including hypo- and hypergammaglobulinemia, T-cell defects, and autoimmune syndromes. Many patients have a family history of neutropenia and recurrent infections. Neutropenia can also be the presenting sign of inherited bone marrow failure states such as Fanconi's anemia.

Isolated acquired neutropenia can be induced by exposure to a wide variety of drugs. Any of various cytotoxic drugs or irradiation of the bone marrow predictably causes a fall in the ANC, and patients are at greatly increased risk of bacterial infection during the time of neutropenia. Neutropenia may also appear as an idiosyncratic drug reaction, either from a direct toxic effect or due to maturational arrest. Commonly cited offenders include antimicrobial agents, especially the penicillins and sulfonamides, anticonvulsants, anti-inflammatory agents, antithyroid drugs, diuretics, and phenothiazines. The neutropenia usually begins 7 to 14 days after the first exposure to the drug or immediately following re-exposure. In almost all instances this is a reversible phenomenon and the leukocyte count will begin to recover within 1 week of drug cessation. Rare instances of irreversible drug-induced neutropenia have been described in association with chloramphenicol or phenylbutazone.

Infection is another cause of neutropenia. Viral infections often result in an isolated decrease in the ANC, especially in children. Hepatitis A and B, influenza, rubella, varicella, Ebstein-Barr virus or respiratory syncytial virus infection, and measles all have been reported to cause a transient neutropenia that develops during the first days of infection and persists for 1 to 2 weeks. Neutropenia is seen in the majority of patients with acquired immune deficiency syndrome (AIDS), usually as a result of late myeloid arrest. Although bacterial infections traditionally cause an increase in neutrophil number, infections such as typhoid, paratyphoid, tuberculosis, brucellosis, tularemia, and rickettsioses can result in neutropenia.

Acquired neutropenia due to ineffective granulopoiesis may be seen in the setting of folate, vitamin B_{12}, or copper deficiency and is accompanied by associated megaloblastic changes in the bone marrow. Infiltrative processes in the bone marrow may lead to loss of normal hematopoietic cells, with resultant neutropenia or pancytopenia. This may be observed in hematologic malignancies such as leukemia, lymphoma or myeloma, myeloproliferative syndromes and myelofibrosis and in solid tumors with a propensity for marrow metastasis, including breast cancer and neuroblastoma. It occurs as well as in nonmalignant conditions such as glycogen storage diseases and mucopolysaccharidoses.

Increased Destruction of Neutrophils

Neutrophil destruction is commonly immune-mediated and can occur as either an isoimmune or an autoimmune process. Neonatal isoimmune neutropenia is the result of maternal sensitization to fetal neutrophil antigens during gestation and occurs in approximately 3% of live births. Affected infants will normalize their neutrophil count by a median age of 7 weeks, reflective of the half-life of maternal IgG. Autoimmune neutropenia with circulating antineutrophil-specific antibodies is analogous to autoimmune hemolytic anemia. Patients usually have moderate to severe neutropenia with associated monocytosis. As an isolated condition it most often presents in infants under 2 years of age but has been reported in all age groups. Autoimmune neutropenia also occurs in association with collagen-vascular or other autoimmune diseases, such as systemic lupus erythematosus or Felty's syndrome (rheumatoid arthritis, splenomegaly, and leukopenia).

Splenic enlargement alone can lead to neutropenia from reticuloendothelial sequestration. This may be seen in the setting of portal hypertension, intrinsic splenic disease, or splenic hyperplasia. Neutropenia is usually modest in degree and is often accompanied by anemia and thrombocytopenia. Last, overwhelming sepsis with endotoxinemia causes excessive destruction of neutrophils from phagocyte ingestion or activation of the complement system.

PRESENTATION AND EVALUATION

Some patients are asymptomatic, and neutropenia is diagnosed in the context of a routine medical examination. Owing to the increased incidence of infection, other patients present with fever; this is more likely in those with severe neutropenia. There may be no localizing signs to point to the origin of the infection, especially because patients with few neutrophils form abscesses slowly, if at all. Common sites of infection are the skin (cellulitis, furunculitis), lymph nodes (adenitis), lung, and gastrointestinal tract. Stomatitis, gingivitis, or perirectal inflammation may be nidi of infection that can be easily overlooked. Patients may have bacteremia with or without an identified origin.

A complete medical history is essential for the evaluation of a patient with neutropenia. The clinician should attempt to determine the duration of neutropenia and whether there are associated medical conditions or a family history suggestive of similarly affected relatives. A dietary history and a thorough drug history, including use of nonprescription drugs such as ibuprofen, should be elicited. Physical examination may reveal evidence of splenomegaly, an associated congenital syndrome or autoimmune disease, or evidence of an active infection. Vitamin and trace mineral levels can be obtained to detect specific deficiencies. Serial weekly or semiweekly neutrophil counts over a period of 2 months are required to diagnose cyclic neutropenia. The presence of antineutrophil antibodies can be evaluated by sending serum to an appropriate referral laboratory, but interpretation of borderline results is difficult. Examination of a bone marrow aspirate and biopsy specimen will rule out neoplastic or infiltrative processes, assess cellularity, and determine if there is an arrest in myeloid maturation or other evidence of dysmyelopoiesis. In addition, the presence of granulocyte hyperplasia and normal maturation of neutrophils may suggest the occurrence of peripheral destruction.

TREATMENT

The most important facet of treatment with neutropenia of any cause is the prevention and control of infection. Patients with chronic neutropenia should be instructed in good oral hygiene and meticulous skin care to prevent recurrent infections in these areas. They should also receive regular dental care, because chronic gingivitis can be problematic. In most patients with an ANC of less than 500 μL, a body temperature of greater than 38.5°C, or greater than 38.3°C on two occasions, requires immediate evaluation and institution of antibiotic therapy after blood samples for culture have been obtained. This may not be necessary in cases of autoimmune or chronic benign neutropenia. Except in the rare instances in which a specific organism can be identified, the initial choice of antibiotics will be empirical. Most documented infections in the neutropenic host are due to endogenous organisms such as *Staphylococcus aureus* and enteric gram-negative rods. The literature regarding the most efficacious empirical therapy in these circumstances derives mostly from patients receiving chemotherapy. In this setting, a combination of broad-spectrum antibiotics such as an aminoglycoside, in addition to either a semisynthetic penicillin or a third-generation cephalosporin, or use of an extended-spectrum single agent is recommended. If the patient becomes afebrile and results of blood cultures are negative, antibiotics should be continued until the ANC is rising (in the case of chemotherapy-induced neutropenia) or until 3 days beyond the last fever (in patients with chronic neutropenia). If fever persists beyond 2 days without identification of a source, addition of antifungal therapy such as amphotericin B (Fungizone) should be strongly considered.

Interventions designed to increase the neutrophil count depend to a large extent on the underlying causative disorder. Corticosteroids or other methods of immunosuppression can increase the ANC in patients with autoimmune neutropenia. Likewise, high-dose intravenous gamma globulin (1 to 2 grams per kg as a single dose or divided daily over 3 to 4 days) may be helpful. Unfortunately, most of the responses seen with either therapy are transient. In addition, the use of steroids further impairs the host defense system and increases the risk of fungal infection.

The use of recombinant human colony-stimulating factors constitutes a recent advance in the treatment of some forms of neutropenia. Granulocyte colony–stimulating factor, or G-CSF (filgrastim [Neupogen]), acts by stimulating production of granulocytes; granulocyte-macrophage colony–stimulating factor, or GM-CSF (sargramostim [Leukine]), stimulates production of granulocytes and monocytes. In addition, these agents enhance the functional activity of mature myeloid cells. Side effects are usually mild and include low-grade fevers, myalgia, headache, and faint macular rash. Significant bone pain or splenomegaly may also result.

Colony-stimulating factors have been used most often in patients recovering from myelosuppressive chemotherapy, in whom they have been well documented to shorten the duration of neutropenia in specific settings. They may also decrease infectious complications and shorten hospital stay, but these findings have not been as consistently demonstrated. Both G-CSF and GM-CSF (at doses of 5 to 10 μg per kg per day) have been successfully used to accelerate neutrophil recovery after stem cell transplantation and may contribute to a shorter period of hospitalization.

The use of G-CSF in patients with cyclic neutropenia or chronic benign neutropenia can increase the ANC and ameliorate stomatitis, unexplained fevers, and documented infections. Patients with Kostmann's syndrome can also benefit from treatment. Sensitivity to G-CSF varies, so dosages must be individually titrated. The usual range is between 1 and 20 μg per kg per day. The toxicities associated with long-term use of G-CSF are unknown, however, and there is concern that chronic marrow stimulation may initiate or accelerate conversion to myelodysplasia or leukemia, especially in patients with Kostmann's syndrome. Malignant transformation has been most often accompanied by acquired chromosome 7 abnormalities. Therefore, bone marrow cytogenetic studies must be performed prior to G-CSF initiation in these patients and at periodic intervals during chronic administration. Because the true risk for malignant transformation is not yet known, growth factor administration should be reserved for frequently symptomatic or severely affected patients.

HEMOLYTIC DISEASE OF THE FETUS AND NEWBORN

method of
DOUGLAS S. RICHARDS, M.D.
University of Florida College of Medicine
Gainesville, Florida

Since the 1960s, there has been a marked reduction in the number of fetuses and neonates dying from isoimmune hemolytic anemia. This is primarily because the administration of Rh immune globulin (RhoGAM) to Rh-negative pregnant women has been very effective in preventing sensitization. This article emphasizes measures that ensure adequate prophylaxis but also discusses the intensive management that is required for the few women who become sensitized.

THE Rh ANTIGEN

In the 1940s, the Rh antigen was discovered in Rhesus monkeys, and it was determined that antibodies against this antigen were responsible for most cases of hemolytic disease of the human newborn. Of two widely used systems for describing the Rh status of an individual, the Fisher-Race system is the most commonly used in obstetrics. It assumes three very closely linked genetic loci, termed C, D, and E, each of which has two possible alleles. The most common genotype is CDe/cde. If the D allele is present on either chromosome, the individual is said to be Rh positive.

The D^u antigen is a weakly expressed D antigen. Clinically, D^u-positive individuals should be managed the same as Rh-positive individuals. A D^u-positive mother is not at risk for the development of Rh antibodies if her fetus is Rh positive. Conversely, an Rh-negative mother should receive Rh immune globulin if she delivers a D^u-positive baby since the D^u variant is capable of stimulating the production of anti-D antibodies.

MINOR ANTIGENS

Historically, less than 2% of cases of hemolytic disease of the newborn were caused by antigens other than the Rh antigen. With the successful elimination of most cases of Rh sensitization in recent years, the so-called minor antigens have assumed a relatively greater importance. Multiparous women and individuals who have received blood transfusions are at a higher risk of sensitization to these antigens. Several of the minor antigens are capable of causing clinically significant hemolytic disease (Table 1). Sensitization against the Lewis antigen does not cause hemolytic disease in the fetus, since anti-Lewis antibodies are of the IgM type and do not cross the placenta.

ISOIMMUNIZATION

Isoimmunization can occur when fetal cells bearing an antigen foreign to the mother enter the maternal circulation. As little as 0.1 mL of Rh-positive blood is sufficient to cause sensitization in an Rh-negative woman. The risk of fetomaternal hemorrhage is low in the first and second trimesters but increases in the third trimester, and at delivery up to 50% of women have sufficient fetomaternal hemorrhage to be at risk for sensitization. Pathologic processes such as abortion and ectopic pregnancy and invasive procedures such as amniocentesis and chorionic villus sampling are associated with an increased risk of fetomaternal hemorrhage and maternal sensitization.

CHANCE OF Rh INCOMPATIBILITY AND ISOIMMUNIZATION

For isoimmunization to occur, the mother must be negative and the fetus must be positive for a particular antigen. An Rh-negative woman has an 85% chance of mating with an Rh-positive man. Because 60% of Rh-positive individuals are heterozygous, there is a 70% chance that the fetus of an Rh-negative woman and an Rh-positive man will be Rh positive. In whites, if the father's blood type is unknown, there is a 60% chance that the child of an Rh-negative woman will be Rh positive. The chance of Rh incompatibility is lower in African-Americans and Asians, because the incidence of Rh negativity is only 8% and 2% in these populations, respectively.

Without the administration of Rh immune globulin, the chance of sensitization is highly influenced by ABO incompatibility between the fetus and mother. Because fetal cells are more rapidly cleared from the maternal circulation in ABO incompatible pregnancies, the incidence of Rh sensitization in untreated pregnancies is only 5%, compared to 16% in pregnancies in which ABO incompatibility does not exist.

TABLE 1. **Partial List of Antigens Capable of Causing Hemolytic Disease of the Newborn**

Antigen System	Antigen Name
Duffy	Fy^a, Fy^b
Lutheran	Lu^a, Lu^b
Kell	K, k, Kp^a, Kp^b, Js^a
Kidd	Jk^a, Jk^b, Jk3
MNS	M, S, s, U
Rh	D, C, c, E, e

SUPPRESSION OF IMMUNIZATION

The principle of antibody-mediated immune suppression was first applied to the Rh problem in the 1960s. In initial trials, Rh immune globulin was administered to Rh-negative male volunteers who were exposed to small amounts of Rh-positive blood. Success in these experiments led to trials of postpartum Rh immune globulin administration in Rh-negative pregnant women. In these trials, only 1.3% of women became sensitized, a 10-fold reduction compared to untreated controls. Subsequent larger studies demonstrated similar reductions in sensitization rates, and the administration of Rh immune globulin to Rh-negative women after the delivery of Rh-positive infants quickly became the standard of care.

Studies have subsequently been performed evaluating the use of Rh immune globulin to prevent third-trimester sensitization. The benefits are not so clear-cut as with peripartum Rh immune globulin administration, but it is now generally accepted that it is cost-effective to give Rh immune globulin to Rh-negative women at 28 weeks' gestation. Although sensitization can rarely occur before 28 weeks, Rh immune globulin is indicated only when there are complications or when invasive procedures are performed (Table 2).

MANAGEMENT OF PREGNANT WOMEN NOT KNOWN TO BE SENSITIZED

A blood type and antibody screen should be performed at the first prenatal visit on all pregnant women. Because of the possibility of laboratory and clerical errors, repeat typing is indicated even if the woman has previously been typed. The antibody screen is performed on all women, even those who are Rh positive, to allow detection of antibodies against the minor antigens.

Antepartum Rh Immune Globulin

Rh-negative women with an initial negative antibody screen should have the screen repeated at 28 weeks' gestation. If the antibody screen is still negative, Rh immune globulin, 300 μg, should be given. If anti-Rh antibodies are detected at the time of the repeat screen, the patient is already sensitized, and Rh immune globulin will be of no benefit. Rh immune globulin administration is not harmful in this setting, so it is permissible to administer it before the results of the antibody screen are available.

Because more than 85% of partners of Rh-negative women are Rh positive, and because paternity is not always certain, it is usually best to assume the possibility of an Rh-positive fetus. If a woman declines to receive antepartum Rh immune globulin because she believes her husband has Rh-negative blood, I have her sign the following statement in her chart. "I understand that if the father of my baby has Rh-positive blood I should receive Rh immune globulin. Knowing this, I decline to receive Rh immune globulin."

TABLE 2. **Indications for Rh Immune Globulin**

Induced abortion	Chorionic villus sampling
Spontaneous abortion	Amniocentesis
Vaginal bleeding in pregnancy	Abdominal trauma in pregnancy
Ectopic pregnancy	

When Rh immune globulin is indicated before 12 weeks' gestation for the conditions listed in Table 2, a 50 μg dose is adequate to cover any potential fetomaternal bleed. At the University of Florida clinics, however, it has been our practice to administer the full 300 μg dose to all women requiring antepartum RhoGAM. The higher dose is not associated with any adverse maternal effects, and it is more convenient for the clinic to stock only one dosage form. When there is an ongoing risk of fetomaternal hemorrhage in pregnancy, such as in the patient with repetitive spotting, Rh immune globulin should be repeated at least every 12 weeks.

Based on the initial studies with male volunteers, it is recommended that Rh immune globulin be administered within 72 hours of the time of suspected fetomaternal hemorrhage. However, it has never been shown that Rh immune globulin is ineffective if the interval is longer. Therefore, even if there is a delay of greater than 72 hours, Rh immune globulin should be given.

Postpartum Rh Immune Globulin

Delivery represents the time of greatest risk for fetomaternal hemorrhage. At birth, the antibody screen should be repeated, and the neonatal blood type should be determined. If the baby is Rh positive or D^u positive, Rh immune globulin should be given. If the mother received antepartum Rh immune globulin at 28 weeks, it is not uncommon for there to be low levels of residual passive antibodies. This does not represent sensitization, and Rh immune globulin should be given. If the last dose of antepartum Rh immune globulin was given within 3 weeks of delivery, and there was no large fetomaternal hemorrhage, Rh immune globulin does not need to be repeated.

A standard 300 μg vial of Rh immune globulin is sufficient to cover a fetomaternal bleed of 15 mL of red blood cells (30 mL of whole blood). To avoid sensitization in the 1% of women in whom there is a larger bleed, a screening test for the presence of Rh-positive cells in the maternal circulation is recommended. In a commercially available "rosette" test (Fetalscreen), anti-D antibodies, then Rh-positive indicator cells are added to a maternal blood sample. If there are a significant number of Rh-positive cells in the maternal blood sample, the indicator cells form rosettes, that is, clumps of Rh-positive indicator cells surrounding Rh-positive fetal cells.

If rosettes are seen, the Kleihauer-Betke test is performed to quantify the fetomaternal hemorrhage. One 300 μg vial of Rh immune globulin should be given to the mother for every 15 mL of fetal red blood cells that have entered the maternal circulation. Because the calculated fetomaternal hemorrhage from the Kleihauer-Betke test is not precise, it is best to be liberal in calculating the Rh immune globulin dose.

MANAGEMENT OF SENSITIZED WOMEN

Antibody Titers

An initial positive antibody screen with a titer of 1:4 or greater indicates that the patient is sensitized. Titers of 1:2 are sometimes due to laboratory error, so they should be repeated. The prognosis for the Rh-sensitized pregnancy depends in part on the antibody titer, and in part on the prior obstetric history. Fetal and neonatal outcomes tend to get worse with subsequent pregnancies, so a history of a prior fetal death or hydrops from hemolytic disease carries a poor prognosis.

Because of the intensive work-up that is required in sensitized women, it is appropriate to test the father's blood for the antigen against which the mother is sensitized. If the father is negative, the fetus is not at risk. If the father is Rh positive but there is a chance that he is heterozygous, the fetal Rh antigen status can be tested by polymerase chain reaction (PCR) methods from an amniotic fluid sample if amniocentesis is eventually required.

If the initial titer is less than 1:16 and there is no history of a previously affected infant, titers should be repeated monthly after 20 weeks. Antibody titers of 1:16 or greater are considered to be above the critical threshold. Once titers are above this threshold, the fetus should be considered to be at risk for significant hemolytic disease, and subsequent titers are not helpful.

Amniocentesis

Amniocentesis with spectrophotometric analysis of the amniotic fluid is the standard method of determining the degree of hemolysis in an at-risk fetus. Amniocentesis is performed with ultrasound guidance, with care to avoid the placenta. The amniotic fluid sample is transported to the laboratory in a light-resistant container to prevent degradation of bilirubin. Optical density readings are made and plotted on a graph that has the wavelength of light on the horizontal axis and the optical density on the logarithmic vertical axis. The deviation from the plotted line at 450 nm (the ΔOD 450 reading) is reflective of the amount of bilirubin in the amniotic fluid, and is directly related to the severity of hemolysis.

The ΔOD 450 value is plotted on a semilogarithmic graph that has weeks gestation on the horizontal axis and the ΔOD 450 on the logarithmic vertical axis. Based on Liley's pioneering work in the 1960s, the graph is divided into three zones that describe the degree of fetal risk. Zone I, the lowest zone, indicates mild or no hemolytic disease, while Zone III, the upper zone, indicates severe hemolytic disease. Without treatment, there is a high probability of fetal hydrops and death for fetuses in this zone. Outcomes of fetuses with initial values in zone II are highly variable. In these cases, the trend of subsequent values is important for determining the fetal status.

Initial ΔOD values obtained before 28 weeks' gestation must be interpreted with caution, because relatively high levels of amniotic fluid bilirubin are present early in normal pregnancies. With mildly affected and unaffected fetuses, subsequent values show a clear downward trend, whereas the trend is upward when severe erythroblastosis is present. In normal pregnancy, borders between zones slope downward, reflecting the normal fall in amniotic fluid bilirubin levels as pregnancy advances.

The timing of the first amniocentesis depends on the likelihood that severe hemolysis exists and the possibility of transfusing the fetus if severe hemolysis is discovered. Because fetal transfusion is now possible at 20 to 22 weeks' gestation, amniocentesis should be performed at this gestational age if there is a history of a previous severely affected pregnancy. With no such history, the first amniocentesis can be delayed until 26 weeks. The timing of repeat amniocentesis depends on the results of prior tests and trends of ΔOD values. Values that are in the low zone and falling can be repeated in 2 to 3 weeks. Midzone results should lead to repeat amniocentesis in 10 to 14 days. If the initial value is in the high zone, fetal blood sampling should be performed without delay.

Fetal Blood Sampling and Intravascular Transfusions

In recent years there has been a trend toward more liberal use of fetal blood sampling to determine directly and precisely the degree of fetal anemia. Risks of umbilical cord blood sampling include fetal bradycardia, fetal hemorrhage from the puncture site, and umbilical cord hematoma. Fortunately, serious complications occur in only 1 to 2% of sampling procedures.

Intrauterine fetal blood transfusions are begun when the hematocrit falls to a value less than 25 to 30%. Historically, fetal blood transfusions were given into the peritoneal cavity, from which about 50% of the transfused red cells are absorbed. Most practitioners now give the transfusion directly into the umbilical vein. Advantages of this approach include a more rapid correction of fetal anemia, and because the starting hematocrit is known, a more rational calculation of the amount and timing of blood transfusions is possible.

Intravascular transfusion can be performed as early as 22 weeks' gestation. If the procedure is done at a time when the fetus is potentially viable, intramuscular betamethasone (Celestone, 12 mg intramuscularly) is given to the mother 48 and 24 hours before the transfusion in case a transfusion-related complication leads to delivery. An ultrasound estimate of the fetal weight is obtained to aid in the calculation of the required transfusion volume. The blood bank is asked to prepare irradiated, leukocyte poor, cytomegalovirus-negative, type O–negative blood with a hematocrit of 80 to 85%, crossmatched against the mother. We perform the procedure in an operating room, observing full OR sterile technique. Before we begin, we give an intravenous dose of cefazolin (Kefzol, 1 g IV) for antimicrobial prophylaxis. The mother is administered agents to obtain light conscious sedation.

Under ultrasound guidance, a 20- or 22-gauge needle is advanced into the umbilical vein at the point that the cord inserts into the placenta. A transplacental approach is often easier with an anterior placenta, but this is avoided because of a greater chance of a fetomaternal hemorrhage, which could augment the mother's immune response.

Once intravascular access is obtained, an aliquot of fetal blood is aspirated for initial hematocrit determination. The amount of blood to be transfused is calculated, based on the initial fetal hematocrit, the estimated fetal blood volume, the desired final hematocrit, and the hematocrit of the transfused blood. Because fetal movement can dislodge the needle from the vessel, vecuronium bromide (Norcuron), 0.3 mg per kg, is injected directly into the umbilical vein to paralyze the fetus. The transfusion is then begun, pushing the very viscous blood with steady continuous pressure. It is important to visualize the blood streaming into the umbilical vein, with flow away from the placenta. If streaming is not seen, it is possible that the needle has become dislodged into the vessel wall, which can rapidly cause a life-threatening hematoma.

Previously, attempts were made to perform exchange transfusions to avoid overloading the fetal circulation. It has since been recognized that the placenta acts as a good reservoir, and that concerns about overloading the fetal circulation by too rapid or large a transfusion are unwarranted. Once the desired volume is transfused, a fetal blood sample is drawn to check the final hematocrit, the needle is withdrawn, and the cord is observed for bleeding, which usually stops within 1 minute. The mother is kept under close observation in the labor and delivery suite for at least 4 hours, with continuous electronic monitoring to look for signs of fetal distress or premature labor.

Timing of Subsequent Transfusions

The fetal hematocrit falls rapidly after the first transfusion, because ongoing hemolysis of the remaining Rh-positive cells occurs and because fetal hematopoiesis slows dramatically. For this reason, the second transfusion is scheduled about 10 days after the first. After the second transfusion, the majority of cells in the fetal circulation are Rh negative, so the rate of fall of the hematocrit is governed by the natural senescence of the donor cells. A good rule of thumb is to expect a 1 point drop in the hematocrit per day. Subsequent transfusions are given when the calculated hematocrit falls below 25%. Intervals of 2 to 4 weeks are often possible.

Controversy exists about whether to transfuse a fetus who is due for a final transfusion between 32 and 34 weeks' gestation. Because the chance of extrauterine survival is excellent at this age, one could argue that the risks of transfusion outweigh any benefit of additional maturity gained by performing another intrauterine transfusion. I make this determination based on the lecithin/sphingomyelin (L/S) ratio, the expected difficulty of performing the transfusion, and the desires of the patient.

Intraperitoneal Transfusions

Intraperitoneal transfusions are still sometimes performed when severe hemolytic disease occurs at a gestational age at which an intravascular access is not yet possible. After a successful intravascular transfusion, an intraperitoneal transfusion can be performed to increase the interval between scheduled transfusions. Intraperitoneal transfusions are done via a 20-gauge needle placed through the anterior fetal abdominal wall into the region of small bowel. The quantity of blood that can be transfused is limited by the amount the peritoneal cavity can hold without an increase in pressure.

Timing of Delivery

For fetuses in sensitized pregnancies who do not require a transfusion, early delivery is sometimes desirable. If the ΔOD 450 values remain in zone II, delivery is performed as soon after 35 weeks' gestation as a mature L/S can be obtained. An Rh-positive fetus with a ΔOD in zone I is delivered when the cervix becomes favorable after 37 weeks.

Fetal Monitoring

The health of fetuses who are receiving transfusions and those whose ΔOD values are in zone II should be monitored with daily fetal movement counts. Weekly nonstress tests and weekly ultrasound examinations are performed on fetuses receiving transfusions. When the ΔOD is in zone II, ultrasound is performed with each amniocentesis, and fetal well-being is assessed with weekly nonstress tests starting at 34 weeks' gestation. Ultrasound is also useful for the weekly evaluation of fetuses at 22 to 26 weeks' gestation who are not thought, based on history, to be at high enough risk to warrant invasive testing. If there is an ultrasound finding suggestive of severe fetal anemia (hepatomegaly, placentomegaly, polyhydramnios, fetal skin edema, pericardial or pleural effusion, ascites, or cardiomegaly), then fetal blood sampling should be performed without delay to confirm the suspected anemia.

Neonatal Care

The three greatest problems facing the neonate from an isoimmunized pregnancy are prematurity, hyperbilirubinemia, and anemia. When the management scheme outlined previously is followed, serious problems from prematurity are uncommon, because almost all fetuses can be successfully transfused in utero until near term. When there have been two or more intrauterine transfusions, neonatal hyperbilirubinemia is not a serious problem. Most of the circulating red cells are Rh-negative donor cells, and significant hemolysis has long since ceased. Hyperbilirubinemia can usually be managed with phototherapy, and it is uncommon for exchange transfusions to be required.

Hematopoiesis is severely depressed in neonates who have been transfused in utero. It is expected that the postnatal hematocrit will gradually fall, and it often reaches a nadir of 15 to 20%. In order not to further depress hematopoiesis, blood transfusions are given only to symptomatic neonates. In recent years, administration of erythropoietin (Epogen) has proven useful in stimulating neonatal reticulocytosis.

ABO Incompatibility

There is the potential for ABO incompatibility in 20 to 25% of pregnancies. This occurs when a fetus carries an A and/or B antigen that the mother lacks. ABO incompatibility is a common cause of neonatal hyperbilirubinemia, but it rarely results in the need for neonatal exchange transfusion, and it is not a cause of fetal hydrops.

HEMOPHILIA AND RELATED CONDITIONS

method of
W. KEITH HOOTS, M.D.
Gulf States Hemophilia Center
Houston, Texas

Hemophilia A (factor VIII deficiency) and hemophilia B (factor IX deficiency) are X-linked hereditary bleeding disorders. By contrast, von Willebrand's disease (vWD) is autosomally inherited, so that males and females are affected equally. Hemophilia A and hemophilia B present as clinically identical conditions, with joint bleeding (hemarthrosis) and joint destructions constituting the primary morbid manifestations. The reason that the clinical findings are indistinguishable is that factor VIIIc (hemophilia A) and factor IX (hemophilia B) are essential cofactors for activating factor Xa in the intrinsic clotting pathway. Each of these factors is primarily produced in the liver. Factor IX is a serine protease and factor VIII is a large glycoprotein essential for configuring the clotting enzymes on the platelet surface so that enzyme-substrate reactions occur at optimal maximal kinetics.

Both hemophilia A and B exhibit a range of clinical severities that correlate fairly well with assayed factor levels. Specifically, severe disease is defined as less than 1% assayed clotting factor in plasma; approximately 1 to 5% and more than 5% of normal are defined as moderate and mild disease, respectively. Males within a family almost always have the same degree of impairment because they share the same defect in the DNA coding for the clotting protein.

Both hemophilia A and B are coded for by DNA on the long arm (q) of the X chromosome. The factor VIII gene, coding as it does for a glycoprotein that is substantially larger than the factor IX protein (approximately 340,000 daltons versus approximately 70,000 daltons), has been demonstrated to be highly susceptible to mutation events, including deletions, insertions, and missense and nonsense mutations. In addition, an inversion sequence of intron 22 of the gene encoding factor VIII is now known to account for more than 34% of mutations giving rise to hemophilia A. This inversion involves a crossover between the intragenic and extragenic copies of factor VIII on the X chromosome (the so-called flip-tip inversion).

Although significantly smaller than the gene encoding factor VIII, the gene encoding factor IX also has been shown to be prone to new mutation events, particularly of the missense and nonsense type. In practical terms, this results in approximately 25 to 30% of newly diagnosed cases of either hemophilia A or B representing a *new* mutation event within a family previously unaffected by hemophilia. This also accounts for the exceptional consistency of prevalence and incidence of both hemophilia A and B across all racial and ethnic groups.

The incidence of hemophilia A and B together is between 1 in 5000 and 1 in 10,000 live male births. Approximately 80 to 85% of these affected neonates have hemophilia A. Approximately two thirds of those with hemophilia A have severe or moderately severe ($\leq$1% factor VIII) disease. By contrast, almost half of hemophilia B individuals have factor IX levels of more than 1%. Patients with hemophilia A and B of comparable severities bleed with similar frequency.

vWD results when there is a defect in the gene for von Willebrand factor (vWF), which is located on chromosome 12. The disease is among the most prevalent of genetic diseases. As high of 1% of certain cohort studies using molecular biologic analyses for gene mutation have shown abnormalities. The glycoprotein coded for by the vWF gene is a large subunit of approximately 226,000 daltons that multimerizes into large cell-adhesive molecules that are essential both for platelet aggregation by cross-linking of glycoprotein Ib receptors between platelets and for platelet adhesion at the site of blood vessel endothelial cell injury. In addition, these vWF multimers, which are secreted from both endothelial cells and platelets, are essential for stabilizing factor VIIIc from proteolysis in the circulating plasma. This explains the low level of factor VIIIc seen in several types of vWD (see later) despite the fact that both the factor VIIIc gene and its coded protein are entirely normal.

Unlike hemophilia A and B, the clinical bleeding pattern for vWD is primarily localized to mucous membrane surface. Hence, epistaxis, menorrhagia, postdental surgical bleeding, and gastrointestinal bleeding are common manifestations for individuals with vWD. Postsurgical bleeding or hemorrhage secondary to significant trauma occurs to varying degrees, depending on the qualitative or quantitative defect or deficiency in the circulating vWF molecule.

Despite the heterogeneity of the molecular defects of vWF, the categorization of clinical vWD is based on the amount and the functional capacity of the vWF protein in the plasma. Abnormalities have been divided into three major types on the basis of the specific laboratory tests that assess both quantity and function of vWF in the plasma of an affected individual.

Type 1 vWD (formally type I) is a heterozygous state in which the genetic defect inherited from one parent (or representing a new mutation) is partially compensated for by normal vWF production directed by the normal gene from the other parent. This type or classic vWD is the clinical state most commonly diagnosed. Laboratory studies that measure *quantitative* vWF protein immunologically (factor VIII–related antigen) are abnormal. *Functional* studies that measure qualitative function of vWF (factor VIII von Willebrand factor:ristocetin cofactor activity [VIII vWF:RCoF]) are proportionally reduced in the plasma. Further, as noted before, the factor VIIIc level in the plasma is frequently abnormal as well because the diminished VIII vWF:RCoF results in a decreased plasma half-life for the factor VIIIc molecules produced by the hepatocyte.

Type 2 vWD consists of multiple genetic defects sharing one common defining characteristic: there is normal production of vWF protein, which is measured by protein antigen assays in the plasma; however, these vWF molecules are defective to varying degrees in their function. A comprehensive discussion of all the type 2 variants of vWD is beyond the scope of this article. Nonetheless, several distinct categories of these that create the heterogeneity can be listed; examples include abnormalities in the multimerization of the vWF subunits, a defective factor VIIIc binding site, and a defective secretion of vWF from platelets despite normal plasma vWF structure and function. Any and all may produce clinical bleeding syndromes. Further, as with vWD in general, there is often substantial clinical heterogeneity between individuals of the same type 2 variant.

Persons with type 3 vWD have a defect in the vWF genes of both chromosomes 12. In many cases, neither parent will have a clinically significant bleeding history because subclinical disease among type 1 heterozygotes is common. By contrast, the individual with type 3 homozygous vWD will have severe clinical bleeding because he or she has little if any vWF protein or circulating factor VIIIc. The latter is deficient because a paucity of vWF in plasma results in rapid proteolysis of the factor VIIIc even though its production is normal. Hence, individuals with type 3 vWD may experience both the mucous membrane hemorrhage pattern seen with vWD as well as the bleeding into deep tissue or organs (e.g., hemarthroses) seen more commonly in hemophilic persons. Further, chronic morbidity is much more commonly observed in these individuals.

Inherited bleeding diatheses secondary to other plasma proteins, platelets, or blood vessels are much less common than either hemophilia or vWD. Genetic defects in factors XI, prekallikrein, and high-molecular-weight kininogen will result in prolongation of the activated partial thromboplastin time (APTT) and may cause clinical bleeding syndromes, although usually less severe than hemophilia A or B. By contrast, inherited factor XII deficiency, although prolonging the APTT, produces no clinical bleeding.

Autosomally inherited factors VII, V, and X and prothrombin deficiencies are rare. When diagnosed, they may produce a significant hemorrhagic state the severity of which correlates inversely with the circulating plasma concentration of the deficient protease (factors II, VII, and X) or glycoprotein (factor V).

Factor VII deficiency is suggested when the prothrombin time (PT) is prolonged but the APTT is normal. Homozygous factor VII deficiency is exceedingly rare and may suggest consanguinity. However, the clinical course is often quite severe, and infants are at significant risk for intracranial hemorrhage. Homozygous autosomal afibrinogenemia, the clinical incidence of which is approximately 1 in 1 million live births, may present in the neonatal period with life-threatening hemorrhage necessitating emergent and aggressive replacement therapy with cryoprecipitate. Abnormalities of factors II, V, and X and fibrinogen prolong both the PT and the APTT.

Two inherited protein deficiencies are notable for their likelihood for producing hemorrhagic syndromes despite normal PT and APTT screening test results. The first, factor XIII deficiency, frequently presents with an indicative clinical history: delayed bleeding after initial adequate hemostasis. This occurs because factor XIII is required for clot stabilization. The second is homozygous deficiency of the inhibitor α_2-antiplasmin, which also produces a bleeding diathesis. Deficiency of this natural inhibitor for the fibrinolytic protein plasmin permits exaggerated clot lysis, thus producing clinical bleeding after tissue injury. Inherited disorders of platelet and endothelial cell function do, in a number of circumstances, cause clinical bleeding. These are discussed elsewhere.

TREATMENT

Hemostatic Abnormalities

Replacement Therapy

For the majority of inherited coagulation disorders, primary therapy consists of infusing a protein product that repletes the deficient clotting component. The source for these replacement clotting proteins has historically been human plasma. The majority of these clotting proteins have their hemostatic activity defined as unit of clotting activity per milliliter of pooled normal human plasma. Hence, the blood banking and pharmaceutical strategy for improving the replacement capacity for the specific deficient factor has been to concentrate the specific protein. In some cases, similar proteins co-purify in the concentration process from the source plasma. An example is cryoprecipitate, which results from the slow thawing of fresh-frozen plasma (FFP) and results in a severalfold concentration of the following clotting proteins: factor VIIIc, factor VIII vWF, fibrinogen, factor XIII, and fibronectin.

Commercial fractionation of cryoprecipitate yielded the first generation of lyophilized factor VIII concentrates, which resulted in an approximate 100-fold increase per mL of infusate in the concentration of factor VIII. This commercial scale-up resulted when source plasma from 5000 to 25,000 donors was converted into lyophilized vials of factor VIII. These vials range in potency from 200 to 1500 units (20 to 35 units per mg of protein) per vial. For the first time, convenient home infusion treatment of hemophilia-associated hemorrhage was feasible. Unfortunately, because of the number of donors contributing to the commercial plasma pool, transfusion-transmitted viral disease (particularly transfusion-associated hepatitis and human immunodeficiency virus [HIV] infection) became a common complication in the hemophilia A population. Purification strategies to alleviate or ultimately eliminate this viral risk required advances in technology. A discussion of this evaluation in purity follows.

Similar viral transmission risk existed for the fractionated therapeutic clotting factor produced for hemophilia B. Because cryoprecipitation does not enrich factor IX, the initial step in fractionation of factor IX clotting factor products has traditionally been barium or aluminum sulfate absorption followed by further column fractionation. For therapies used in the 1970s and 1980s, this resulted in co-purification of all the molecularly similar vitamin K–dependent factors (II, VII, IX, and X), yielding a final product called prothrombin complex concentrates (PCCs). Like factor VIII products, production of PCCs yielded a final concentration of 200 to 1500 units (20 to 40 units per mg of protein) per vial. Like the factor VIII products, these commercially produced factor concentrates, in the years before more effective viral attenuation techniques, almost invariably had viral contamination, notably several species of hepatitis and HIV (after 1979).

The co-purification of factors II, VII, and X in the preparation of factor IX concentrates sometimes resulted in selective conversion of one or more of these zymogen proteases to its active enzyme (e.g., factor VII is converted in trace amounts to factor VIIa). This trace contamination with active proteases creates a thrombogenic potential for PCCs. Indeed, PCCs given therapeutically in high and recurrent dosing schedules have produced significant and sometimes fatal clotting events in patients with hemophilia B, particularly among individuals receiving the PCCs to provide hemostasis in association with orthopedic surgery. Other clinical situations in which thrombogenesis may be associated with the infusion of PCCs include (1) sustained crush injuries, (2) large intramuscular bleeds (e.g., psoas or thigh), (3) treatment of neonates with hemophilia B who have immature natural anticoagulation, and (4) hemostatic therapy given to individuals with severe chronic hepatitis (because this may adversely affect their ability to make antithrombin III and the vitamin K–dependent inhibitors protein C and protein S in their hepatocytes). In its most severe manifestations, dosing with PCCs has produced acute myocardial infarction and disseminated intravascular coagulation. The risk for disseminated intravascular coagulation may be mitigated by not infusing more than 50 to 75 units per kg per 24 hours when recurrent dosing is required (e.g., after surgery or to treat life-threatening hemorrhage) and by adding small amounts of heparin to each infusate. Fortunately, as discussed subsequently, more advanced purification technologies have resulted in the production of single-component factor IX products that are free of any significant trace-activated proteases. These now provide the mainstay of therapy for hemophilia B patients and are obligatory when high-dose, recurrent infusion therapy is required.

Later Generation Clotting Factor Concentrates

THERAPEUTIC OPTIONS FOR TREATMENT OF HEMOPHILIA A AND B IN THE LATE-1990s

Factor VIII Products. Because of the high frequency and profound clinical impact of transfusion-associated transmission of the hepatitis virus and HIV in the hemophilia population during the 1970s and 1980s, there were exigent and profound advances in the attenuation (and even elimination) of these and other viral contaminants. The first step in this evolution was heat treatment of factor VIII products first licensed for use in 1983. Subsequent advances included the following: pasteurization, solvent detergent treatment to eliminate lipid envelope viruses, advanced Sepharose chromatography, affinity chromatography with monoclonal antibodies directed against the factor VIIIc–factor VIII vWF complex or against factor IX, and most recently the commercial production of a recombinant factor VIIIc product in transfected mammalian cell systems. Each non-recombinant clotting factor concentrate presently produced in the United States is made from a donor pool screened for HIV, hepatitis B virus, and hepatitis C virus. In addition, each of the currently marketed products undergoes either heating to high temperatures and of long duration or solvent detergent treatment. Both processes appear sufficient to remove the risk for HIV transmission. Hepatitis risk is further reduced when concomitant donor screening is used.

This degree of confidence of safety from HIV infection does not exist for cryoprecipitate and FFP, which typically undergo no viral attenuation other than donor screening (an exception is the investigational pasteurized FFP product made by the New York Blood Center). Efficient donor screening has reduced the relative risk from either of these single-donor products to between 1 in 40,000 and 1 in 100,000 per donor unit for HIV infection and to 0.03% or less per donor unit for hepatitis C. Even though the risk for hepatitis B from single-donor cryoprecipitate or FFP is similarly low, anyone likely to be treated with *any* plasma-derived product (whether single-donor or pooled, attenuated product) *should* receive a full three-inoculation course of the hepatitis B vaccine.

Each one of the factor VIII concentrates available at this time is considered safe from HIV and similar retroviral transmission. However, not all are free of hepatitis C virus transmission risk. Fortunately, the relative risk that any single lot of any of the products will transmit hepatitis C appears low. Nonetheless, transmissions of hepatitis C virus, hepatitis A virus, and human parvovirus B19 from some existing factor VIII products have been documented. A product-by-product comparison of the relative risk for transmission of these viruses is beyond the scope of this discussion and would quickly become outdated as technology advances. However, a basic stratification of relative product purity is discussed by the following product groupings after a definition of each is provided: (1) intermediate-purity products, (2) high-purity products, (3) ultra–high-purity products.

The intermediate-purity factor concentrates are so designated because even though they undergo aggressive viral inactivation with heat (even pasteurization) and/or solvent detergent, the final concentration of factor VIII in the end product represents a small percentage of the total heterogeneous plasma proteins present (6 to 10 units of factor VIIIc per mg of total protein, excluding albumin).

High-purity products are factor concentrates that have at least 50 units (range, 50 to 150) of factor VIIIc per mg of protein (excluding albumin for stabilization). In the majority of cases, specialized column chromatographic techniques (e.g., heparin Sepharose) result in the significantly higher purity, although there still is trace contamination with immunoglobulins or other plasma proteins. The chromatographic technique provides some viral attenuation, but enhanced viral safety is dependent on postchromatographic pasteurization or solvent detergent treatment. These products are considered safe from HIV in the end product and relatively but not absolutely safe for hepatitis C.

Ultra–high-purity products are the monoclonal antibody affinity-purified plasma-derived factor concentrates and the recombinant factor VIII products. For the former, the affinity chromatography step not only is efficient at removing all non–factor VIIIc protein but also is an efficient viral attenuation process. Nonetheless, effective elimination of hepatitis C from the monoclonal products has required subsequent treatment with either pasteurization or solvent detergent. The specific activity of the monoclonal preparations (before the addition of human serum albumin) is 3000 units of factor VIIIc per mg of protein. This is essentially identical to the effective purity of the licensed recombinant products, which also require comparable dilution with albumin to maintain stability after lyophilization.

There is a notable distinction with regard to theoretical viral safety to be made between the monoclonal and the recombinant products. Because the recombinant factor VIII products are affinity purified from the cell culture of transfected hamster-derived cell lines, there is no requirement for any further viral attenuation. The addition of human serum albumin constitutes the sole theoretical source for human viral contamination. There remains a theoretical risk for other nonhuman, mammalian viruses or other infective species.

Frequent infusions of ultrapure products (specifically the monoclonal products) have been shown in scientific studies to produce a stabilization of the $CD4^+$ cell count in HIV-infected hemophiliacs compared with chronic infusion of similar amounts of intermediate clotting factor concentrates. It is suspected that this results from the absence of other protein contamination in these ultrapure products rather than from greater purity from viral contamination. Nonetheless, most physicians treating hemophilia have opted to use one of these products to treat their HIV-infected patients. Many have also chosen to treat their previously untreated hemophilia A patients (particularly the young children) with these products because of a perceived theoretical viral safety. This safety margin is inferred from (1) studies showing enhanced capacity to remove surrogate viruses during the monoclonal processing and (2) the bypassing of a human plasma source (with the exception of the added human serum albumin) from the recombinant products.

Clinical trials are ongoing at this time of a recombinant factor VIIIc preparation from which the B domain of the gene has been removed before transfection of the hamster cell lines. The protein portion of factor VIII coded for by the B domain of the gene is not required for efficient clotting function; further, its deletion confers greater stability on the resultant smaller factor VIIIc molecule. Hence, there is no requirement for human serum albumin to stabilize the final lyophilized product. This may provide a higher level of confidence against any future microbiologic contamination. It is not yet apparent when this product will be available for clinical use.

Factor IX Products. The clotting factor products available for treating hemophilia B must be assessed for two potential complications: (1) theoretical viral safety and viral purity (activity per mg protein) and (2) thrombogenicity. The factor IX products determined to be free of thrombogenic potential are those preparations that have effectively purified the factor IX protein from the other prothrombin complex proteins (factors II, VII, and X). Two technical strategies have been used to purify factor IX from the other vitamin K factors and thereby to remove the thrombogenic risk: (1) chromatographic partitioning followed by solvent detergent treatment and (2) monoclonal affinity purification of factor IX. The product produced by the former process contains some residual nonclotting plasma proteins. By contrast, the monoclonal product is free of other plasma proteins. Viral attenuation to remove HIV appears effective for both processes. The hepatitis virus risk is significantly reduced by both processes. However, studies using surrogate viruses imply greater safety from hepatitis C or similar viruses with the monoclonal factor IX concentrate.

The other plasma-derived clotting factor concentrates available for treating hemophilia B patients are PCCs. They can, therefore, produce thrombotic complications when given in high dose or after repeated sequential dosing. Viral attenuation strategies for PCCs are either solvent detergent treatment or heating to 80°C for more than 10 hours. PCCs using the heat process may provide a greater viral attenuation for some viruses, although this has not been proved scientifically. As discussed later, either of these PCCs may prove efficacious for treating moderate bleeding (e.g., hemarthrosis) in individuals with high responsive factor VIII inhibitors for whom factor VIIIc concentrates are nonhemostatic because of the factor VIII antibody.

Recombinant factor IX clotting factor concentrate has recently been licensed. Unlike the presently licensed recombinant factor VIII preparations, recombinant factor IX has no human albumin in the viral product. The theoretical advantages of this are discussed earlier with the B domain–deleted recombinant factor VIII. The in vivo half-life of recombinant factor IX concentrate is identical to that of plasma-derived monoclonal factor IX concentrate. Because of a slightly different volume of distribution, recombinant factor IX recovery may vary a small amount from monoclonal factor IX.

Anti-inhibitor Clotting Preparations. Because PCCs are thrombogenic owing to their trace contamination with the active proteases (e.g., factor VIIa or factor Xa), they have been used for nearly 2 decades to treat bleeding in factor VIII-deficient patients with high responsive (i.e., anamnestic) factor VIII antibodies. Later manufacturers of PCCs increased the trace amounts of these active proteases to produce activated prothrombin complex concentrates (APCCs). There is no in vitro assay for either of the two licensed APCC products that correlates with in vivo hemostatic efficacy. Hence, it is often difficult to predict the hemostatic efficacy of APCCs. Both individual response and therapeutic efficacy for specific hemorrhagic episodes vary widely. Stated another way, it is difficult, if not impossible, to predict a priori whether a given dose (units per kilogram of body weight) will provide the necessary hemostasis after a single infusion in a patient with no prior use of APCC. This is true even though the factor VIIIc "bypassing" activity of APCCs is supplied according to units of hemostatic activity per vial and is dosed accordingly. (Typical dosing for hemarthroses is 75 to 100 units per kg per dose.) To further complicate the issue, there are two APCC preparations. One may be ineffective in an individual, whereas the other may provide effective hemostasis for an acute bleeding episode. Because of this capriciousness of the use of APCC in individuals with inhibitors, an individualized therapeutic plan needs to be established empirically. However, certain principles generally apply: (1) Effective dosing of APCCs is minimally 75 to 100 units per kg; (2) dosing frequency more often than every 6 hours predisposes to significant thrombogenicity, particularly after the third to fourth consecutive dose (hence, monitoring for markers of disseminated intravascular coagulation is warranted when sequential dosing for several days is required); and (3) because the activated proteases that account for the procoagulant activity of APCCs are short-lived, initial hemostasis may be followed by breakthrough bleeding between doses that may create difficulty for maintenance hemostatic therapy. Therapy with APCCs is expensive, is less than reliable, and carries risk for significant complications. Experience and expertise in their use help to mitigate these risks and to differentiate the appropriate use of APCCs from the other alternatives for inhibitor therapy cited in the following.

One alternative therapy for treating patients with inhibitors is porcine factor VIII. This product is produced from porcine plasma by use of a polyelectrolyte resin separation technology. The residual nonhuman protein is relatively low, although this does not completely eliminate the anaphylactoid potential of this product. Another characteristic of porcine factor VIII will often limit its efficacy in many individuals with inhibitors. In many cases, the specific anamnestic antibody directed against the human factor VIIIc glycoprotein cross-reacts with shared epitopes on the porcine molecule. Therefore, before the therapeutic efficacy of the product of porcine factor VIII can be assessed in an individual, it is necessary to quantitate the neutralizing capacity of the antibody against both the porcine and the human factor VIII product by use of the Bethesda assay. In those instances in which the antiporcine Bethesda unit titer is significantly lower (<10 Bethesda units) than the corresponding antihuman Bethesda titer, therapy with porcine factor VIII may be the therapy of choice. Before the first dose of porcine factor VIII is infused at a starting dose of approximately 100 units per kg, there is need to infuse a test dose of approximately 100 units to ensure that there is no immediate hypersensitivity reaction. If none occurs, a slow infusion during 20 to 30 minutes with careful monitoring for allergic symptoms can proceed. Further, because the porcine Bethesda unit inhibitor assay provides only an in vitro estimate of the neutralizing capacity of the anti–factor VIII antibody against porcine factor VIII, it is essential to monitor factor VIII levels in these patients. As with most therapies for hemophilia A patients with inhibitors, therapy with porcine factor VIII is costly.

The indications for use of other more esoteric and experimental therapies for factor VIII inhibitors (e.g., factor VIIa, immune tolerance induction, or antibody depletion using a staphylococcal protein A Sepharose chromatographic column) are beyond the scope of this discussion. Comprehensive hemophilia treatment centers provide expertise for these specialized therapeutic procedures. Further, because optimal methodologies are still to be determined by collaborative research protocols, discussion with physician-scientists at these centers offers the best prospect for providing clinicians with up-to-date information about therapeutic options for treating complex inhibitor patients.

Therapies for von Willebrand's Disease

Patients with type 1 and most with type 2 vWD may often be treated with desmopressin acetate (DDAVP), a synthetic analogue of the antidiuretic hormone 8-arginine vasopressin. Similarly, because of its efficacy in inducing release of vWF multimers from endothelial cells, it results in a concomitant rise in factor VIIIc (because vWF spares the latter molecule from rapid proteolysis in plasma). Desmopressin at a dose of 0.3 μg per kg (maximal dose is 25 μg per dose) by slow intravenous infusion will increase circulating vWF by approximately 250% in the average individual and factor VIIIc approximately 300%. Therefore, it becomes a treatment of choice for mild to moderate bleeding in most individuals with both mild hemophilia A (e.g., >5% factor VIII activity) and types 1 and 2 vWD. (Note: In type 2B vWD in which the largest vWF multimers are missing from plasma but are released in excess after desmopressin use, there is a theoretical risk for thrombocytopenia from excessive platelet aggregation. Hence, its use in this subgroup must be evaluated on an individual case basis.) Because a 2.5- to threefold increase in both factor VIIIc and factor VIII vWF is often sufficient to raise both to normal ranges in vWD patients, many such individuals may never require any other type of therapy for either acute hemorrhage or prophylaxis for surgical or dental procedures. Tachyphylaxis after repeated dosing with desmopressin can occur because of depletion of the vWF stores in the endothelial cells. Therefore, monitoring of levels in those individuals requiring frequent dosing (e.g., daily or more often) is indicated.

A highly concentrated (150 μg per spray = 1.5 mg per mL) intranasal form of desmopressin is also available for use in vWD and mild hemophilia A. Two inhalations in a single nostril acutely in adults and one in children will typically achieve approximately two thirds of the intravenous dosing. As with the intravenous preparation, facial flushing, mild to moderate blood pressure elevation, and antidiuretic side effects are expected.

For individuals with type 3 vWD, for those with types 1 and 2 who either fail to respond to desmopressin or respond to a degree inadequate to achieve complete and predictable hemostasis, and for those vWF patients who experience tachyphylaxis precluding required repeated therapy, other therapeutic options are needed. Cryoprecipitate administered in a dose calculated to elevate factor VIIIc or factor VIII vWF or both to the normal range has traditionally been the most effective means for achieving hemostasis in such patients. However, as noted previously, single-donor cryoprecipitate has a small but finite risk for hepatitis and even HIV infection, and for this reason caution must be exercised before cryoprecipitate is administered. Accordingly, most coagulationists have chosen one of three intermediate- or high-purity factor VIII concentrates that have been demonstrated to have most sizes of vWF multimers present after reconstitution to treat vWD patients when desmopressin is deemed inadequate for hemostasis. Unlike cryoprecipitate, these concentrates may not have the ideal ratio of vWF multimers compared with that in the physiologic state. Nonetheless, the theoretical viral safety conferred by the attenuation they undergo in preparation more than compensates for this theoretical hemostatic deficit. Several studies have shown clinical efficacy to be good even when individuals with severe disease (type 3) have experienced potential or actual life-threatening hemorrhage.

Antifibrinolytic Agents

Tranexamic acid and ϵ-aminocaproic acid (EACA) act by inhibiting plasminogen activation, thereby enhancing clot stability. These two agents are useful therapeutic adjuncts to stabilize clots that have formed after therapy in individuals with underlying hemostatic defects. For patients with inherited clotting disorders, they have proved particularly efficacious for bleeding in the oral cavity (e.g., after dental or oral surgical procedures or trauma to the mouth) and for epistaxis. Dosing for tranexamic acid is 25 mg per kg per dose every 6 to 8 hours; for EACA, it is 75 to 100 mg per kg per dose every 6 hours (maximal dose, 3 to 4 grams every 6 hours). For patients with hemophilia and vWD, treatment may be required for 7 to 14 days, depending on the amount of tissue injury. In hemophilia B, it is prudent to use a purified factor IX preparation rather than PCC when concomitant antifibrinolytic therapy is contemplated because of the added thrombotic risks of the PCC and antifibrinolytic agents together.

PREVENTIVE CARE

Male infants born to known or suspected hemophilic carrier mothers should not be circumcised until hemophilia in the infant has been excluded by laboratory testing. Blood for assay for APTT and factor VIII or factor IX assay (or both if family history is uncertain) should be obtained from cord blood. When a cord blood sample is not available, venipuncture should be performed from a superficial limb vein to lessen the likelihood of producing a hematoma that might then require replacement therapy. Femoral and jugular sites must be avoided.

Routine immunizations requiring injection, such as diphtheria-pertussis-tetanus or measles-mumps-rubella vaccines, may be given in the deep subcutaneous tissue (rather than by deep intramuscular injection as is the usual practice), using the smallest gauge needle that is feasible. Hepatitis B vaccine should be given as soon after birth as possible to all infants with confirmed diagnosis of hemophilia. The live attenuated oral poliovirus vaccine should not be given to an infant whose hemophilic older brother (or grandfather in the household) is known to be HIV immune suppressed; Salk vaccine may be substituted. Hepatitis A vaccine should also be administered to those individuals with hemophilia who have no hepatitis A virus antibody in their serum.

Early dental examination of the infant is recommended to teach proper tooth-brushing and to ensure adequate household water fluoridation. In addition to education about hemophilia, both genetic counseling and psychosocial counseling are important for the mother of a newborn with hemophilia. This is particularly true for the approximately 30% for whom hemophilia represents a new mutation and for whom there is no previous family experience with the disease. Reluctance to clean the teeth routinely should be dispelled early, and anticipated problem areas for causing bleeding should be discussed.

Both parents should be encouraged to participate intensively in every part of the infant's care. Further, normal socialization opportunities must not be limited because of the hemophilia. Experienced personnel should discuss specifically what minimal limitations are reasonable versus what constitutes overprotection that may jeopardize the child's normal development.

An appropriate exercise regimen that excludes "contact" sports (e.g., tackle football) should be encouraged as a daily routine. Further, the role of such a program for the child and adult after episodes of hemarthrosis is best discussed before the child has a joint bleed.

SPECIAL CONSIDERATION FOR HEMOPHILIC BLEEDING

Early treatment improves the quality of life. It is not only necessary but will in many cases diminish the ultimate duration of therapy. For example, infusion for an acute hemarthrosis with an appropriate dose of factor concentrate (generally 15 to 25 units per kg of body weight) immediately on recognition of pain may often obviate the need for a second infusion by forestalling the inflammatory response in the joint. This may curtail the predisposition for rebleeding in the same joint. Appropriate dosage is chosen to ensure some circulating factor level for at least 48 hours. The strategy for maintaining such a minimal level always is known as prophylaxis and has been demonstrated to be efficacious in preventing essentially all joint bleeding in patients with both hemophilia A and B. A decision to undertake primary prophylaxis requires extensive prospective evaluation and is best done in close consultation between the parent of the hemophilic child and professionals in the comprehensive hemophilia treatment center.

For life-threatening bleeding in a hemophiliac, the exigency for immediate infusion is superseded only by resuscitative requirements. Every effort should be made to keep the factor level in the normal range (e.g., >50%) until this bleeding emergency has passed. Further, an acutely hemorrhaging hemophiliac should be transported, if at all possible, to an emergency center that stocks appropriate clotting factor products. All head injuries must be considered nontrivial unless proved otherwise by observation and computed tomography or magnetic resonance imaging. Late bleeding after head trauma can occur as long as 3 to 4 weeks after the injury. Hence, patients with head and neck injuries should be infused immediately unless one is totally convinced that the injury is insignificant. In addition, if the patient is not hospitalized, the patient and his or her family should be instructed in the neurologic signs and symptoms of central nervous system bleeding so that the patient will return for reinfusion, clinical and radiologic reassessment, and hospitalization at the earliest manifestation of bleeding.

Bleeding from the floor of the mouth or the pharynx or epiglottic region frequently results in partial or complete airway obstruction. Therefore, such bleeding should be treated with an aggressive infusion program with extended clinical follow-up to ensure resolution. Such bleeding may be precipitated by coughing, tonsillitis, oral or otolaryngologic surgery (e.g., extraction of wisdom teeth, tonsillectomy, adenoidectomy), or regional block anesthesia. For surgery and anesthesia, prophylaxis with appropriate infusion therapy before the procedure usually obviates the need for further treatment.

Patients with hemophilia who have gastrointestinal lesions, such as ulcers, varices, or hemorrhoids, must be managed with an appropriate continuous infusion regimen that maintains nearly normal circulating levels for factor VIIIc or factor IX until some healing has been achieved. Concomitant transfusion with packed red blood cells may also be required.

Selected types of hemarthroses may be a particular problem. Hip joint or acetabular hemorrhages can be dangerous because increased intra-articular pressure from bleeding and the associated inflammation may lead to aseptic necrosis of the femoral head. Twice-daily infusion therapy designed to sustain a factor level above 10 units per dL for at least 3 days should be given, along with enforced bed rest that includes Buck's traction for immobilization.

A hemarthrosis of the hip joint may, at first appearance, be difficult to differentiate from a bleed in the iliopsoas muscle. The iliopsoas bleed limits primary hip extension, whereas a bleed in the joint makes any motion of the hip excruciatingly painful. Further, an iliopsoas bleed may decrease sensation over the ipsilateral thigh because of compression of the sacral plexus root of the femoral nerve. Ultrasonography may demonstrate a hematoma in the iliopsoas region. Treatment of the two is similar, although rehabilitation from the hip bleed is more protracted. Both conditions will benefit from a physical therapy regimen that strengthens the supporting musculature while slowly mobilizing the affected area. Closed compartment muscle and soft tissue hemorrhages are dangerous because they frequently impinge on the neurovascular bundle. These can occur in the upper arm, forearm, wrist, and volar aspect of the hand as well as in the anterior or posterior filial compartments. Swelling and pain precede tingling, numbness, and loss of distal arterial pulses. Infusion must maintain an adequate hemostatic level of factor VIIIc or factor IX. Other possible therapeutic maneuvers include elevation to enhance venous return and, as a last resort, surgical decompression if medical therapy fails to forestall progression.

COMPREHENSIVE CARE

Special treatment centers have been established in the United States and many other countries to provide multidisciplinary care of hemophilia and related disorders. Many patients infused with plasma-derived factor concentrates before 1985 were infected with HIV and/or one of the hepatitis viruses. The comprehensive hemophilia centers provide voluntary testing for these viruses, counseling of patients found seropositive for previous infection, and access to appropriate care and therapy. Risk reduction counseling and education are essential elements of comprehensive treatment centers, as is repeated testing for evidence of hepatitis infection.

Comprehensive hemophilia treatment centers are also the mainstay for ongoing education of patients and families about the management of their bleeding disorder. The centers coordinate home therapy and preventive services and work closely with hemophilia consumer organizations to advocate advances in therapy and care.

Further information about hemophilia care, hemophilia centers, and HIV infection risk reduction and counseling is available through the National Hemophilia Foundation, The Soho Building, 110 Green Street, Suite 303, New York, NY 10012 (telephone, 212-219-8180) or from its local chapter.

PLATELET-MEDIATED BLEEDING DISORDERS

method of
MARTIN D. PHILLIPS, M.D.
Centeon, L.L.C.
King of Prussia, Pennsylvania

Thrombocytopenia may present as spontaneous hemorrhage, as bleeding out of proportion to what is expected, or as an incidental finding on a routine blood count. Petechial hemorrhage and epistaxis are particularly common physical findings. A careful history and physical examination, an assessment of the hemorrhagic risk, and a diagnosis of the underlying disorder are essential elements for successful therapy. Table 1 lists some factors indicating that prompt assessment and therapy are needed.

THROMBOCYTOPENIA

Spurious Thrombocytopenia

In evaluating causes of thrombocytopenia, it is important to exclude a relatively common and benign cause of a low platelet count. The platelets of a few people have the characteristic of aggregating in vitro when exposed to the anticoagulant ethylenediaminetetraaceticacid (EDTA). An unexpected finding of low or widely fluctuating platelet counts may indicate spurious thrombocytopenia. In all thrombocytopenic patients the blood smear should be examined. Clumps of platelets may indicate spurious thrombocytopenia, or abnormalities indicative of other causes could be seen. The definitive test is to repeat a platelet count using blood anticoagulated with sodium citrate or to perform a manual platelet count.

TABLE 1. **Factors Requiring Urgent Assessment in Thrombocytopenia**

Significant, active hemorrhage
Platelet count less than 20,000/μL
Neurologic dysfunction
Evidence of microangiopathic hemolytic anemia
Concomitant unexplained renal dysfunction
Concomitant heparin use
Pregnancy
Recent or impending invasive procedure or thrombolytic therapy
Risk of significant hemorrhage

True Thrombocytopenia

Once spurious thrombocytopenia has been ruled out, management is directed at (1) assessment of the risk of bleeding due to thrombocytopenia, (2) determination of the cause of the thrombocytopenia, and (3) selection of the type of therapy, if any, that is required.

Risk Assessment

The likelihood of hemorrhage due to thrombocytopenia is affected by the degree of thrombocytopenia, the necessity of invasive procedures, a recent history of trauma, concurrent coagulopathy, and medication use. Table 1 lists factors that require urgent evaluation.

In the absence of invasive procedures or trauma, it has long been held that the risk of severe hemorrhage is low if the platelet count is greater than 20,000 per μL. Recently this estimate has been revised downward. Many hematologists now regard 10,000 per μL as a relatively safe level. However, the need for invasive procedures or a recent history of surgery or trauma requires a higher platelet count. Any elective procedure should be postponed until the cause of thrombocytopenia can be determined and treated. The risk associated with any planned procedure or any adverse effect of delaying the procedure should be considered. Minimally invasive procedures require a minimum platelet count of 50,000 per μL, and major procedures require 100,000 per μL. There is no need to delay bone marrow aspiration and biopsy owing to thrombocytopenia; in fact, a low platelet count is often an *indication* for a bone marrow examination. There is likely to be bruising, but significant hemorrhage is extremely rare.

The risk of hemorrhage is increased by concomitant abnormality of the coagulation system, either congenital or acquired, or by the use of drugs that inhibit platelet function, such as aspirin or other nonsteroidal anti-inflammatory drugs (NSAIDs), abciximab (ReoPro), or ticlopidine (Ticlid). Thrombolytic therapy carries additional risk.

Some thrombocytopenic disorders require urgent attention. These include the thrombotic microangiopathies: thrombotic thrombocytopenic purpura (TTP), hemolytic-uremic syndrome (HUS), and the HELLP syndrome of pregnancy (*h*emolysis, *e*levated *l*iver enzymes, and *l*ow *p*latelets). Signs of these disorders may include evidence of microangiopathic hemolytic anemia (fragmented erythrocytes, anemia, high reticulocyte count, elevated lactic dehydrogenase levels), unexplained renal dysfunction, or neurologic dysfunction. Any neurologic dysfunction in the setting of thrombocytopenia may also signify intracranial hemorrhage and should be evaluated promptly.

Heparin use in thrombocytopenic patients is potentially problematic for two reasons. First, the anticoagulant effect of heparin may increase the risk of bleeding due to thrombocytopenia. Second, heparin causes a specific type of immune thrombocytopenia, discussed later on. Unlike other drug-induced thrombocytopenias, the heparin-induced variety can activate platelets and be a source of life- and limb-threatening arterial or venous thrombosis. The paradoxical finding of thrombosis in a thrombocytopenic patient should raise this diagnostic possibility. Heparin should be considered as the cause in any thrombocytopenic patient receiving any amount or form of heparin.

The occurrence of thrombocytopenia during pregnancy deserves a careful evaluation. In addition to all of the causes of thrombocytopenia discussed subsequently, three entities need to be considered: the HELLP syndrome, benign gestational thrombocytopenia, and a rare subtype of von Willebrand's disease (type 2b). The concerns are for the safety of both fetus and mother during gestation and in the peripartum and postpartum periods. The choice of methods for anesthesia and delivery must include consideration of the risks of thrombocytopenia.

Determining Cause

Evaluation to identify the cause of thrombocytopenia is important to determine prognosis and therapy. The two major mechanisms of thrombocytopenia are (1) an increased rate of platelet destruction and (2) decreased platelet production. In cases of increased destruction, especially immune-mediated destruction, it may be fruitless to attempt to increase the platelet count by transfusion.

DESTRUCTIVE CAUSES

Idiopathic Thrombocytopenic Purpura

Idiopathic thrombocytopenic purpura (ITP) is a frequent cause of thrombocytopenia. Although persons of any age or either gender may be affected, it is most common in young women. ITP is a clinical "diagnosis of exclusion," made by ruling out other causes. There are no specific diagnostic tests that are helpful. ITP may be associated with viral infections, especially in children, and in those cases is transient. Adults usually have a chronic waxing and waning course and require treatment intermittently. ITP may be a presenting sign of HIV infection. The American Society of Hematology reported in 1996 the consensus of experts on treating ITP. If the platelet count is over 50,000 per μL and the course is otherwise uncomplicated, observation is sufficient. If the platelet count is less than 50,000 per μL and the course is uncomplicated, administration of oral prednisone in a dose of 1 mg per kg per day is adequate therapy. Prophylactic platelet transfusions are not indicated. After the platelet count has reached greater than 100,000 per μL, the dose should be decreased to 0.6 mg per kg per day for 10 days and then to 0.3 mg per kg per day for 10 days and then tapered to zero over 4 weeks. The platelet count should be monitored weekly, and bleeding symptoms reported immediately. If the platelet count falls below 50,000 per μL, the original dose of prednisone should be restarted.

If there is evidence of significant bleeding, immune globulin intravenous (IGIV) should be given at 1 gram per kg per day for 2 days, in addition to prednisone and platelet transfusion (1 pheresis unit or 6 random donor units). The effect of IGIV lasts about 3 weeks. Hospitalization is necessary only for severe mucous membrane bleeding or other hemorrhage.

If the platelet count does not increase sufficiently with use of steroids and/or IGIV or falls too low when steroids are tapered, or if the patient has frequent relapses of ITP after discontinuation of medication, then splenectomy should be considered. Splenectomy is curative in more than three fourths of the cases. Pneumococcal, *Haemophilus influenzae*, and meningococcal vaccines should be given if splenectomy is being considered.

Danazol (Danocrine),* in a dose of 600 mg per day to start, tapered to the lowest effective dose, may replace prednisone for chronic use in some cases. It may take 8 weeks to have its full effect. Danazol is an attenuated androgen and can cause reversible hirsutism and irreversible lowering of the voice in women. Liver function tests should be monitored monthly.

There has been increasing use of Rh_0(D) immune globulin (WinRho SD) as a substitute for IGIV. Additional studies are ongoing to determine its place in the therapeutic armamentarium.

Medications and Drugs

Many medicines, prescription and nonprescription, cause thrombocytopenia. Antibiotics (particularly sulfa derivatives), antiepileptic medications, and histamine H_2 receptor-blocking drugs are frequently implicated in mild or moderate thrombocytopenia. Quinine and quinidine are notorious for causing a profound thrombocytopenia, with a propensity for hemorrhage. Recreational drugs, particularly those used intravenously (IV), may cause thrombocytopenia.

The course is dependent upon the rate of metabolism of the parent drug and its metabolites. Some metabolites have antiplatelet activity and may have a very long half-life.

All nonessential medicines should be stopped. If an offending agent can be identified, it should be avoided, with substitution of an alternative agent of a different chemical class whenever possible. Steroids are not necessary when a particular drug can be implicated. Prophylactic platelet transfusions are usually futile, as the mechanism of platelet clearance is at least partly immunologic.

Sepsis/Bacteremia

Bacteremia causes thrombocytopenia in the majority of cases; one third of patients will have platelet counts of less than 50,000 per μL. Pathogenetic mechanisms include the opsonization of platelets with immune complexes and the elaboration of in-

*Not FDA approved for this indication.

flammatory cytokines that suppress megakaryocytes. There is no specific therapy other than correction of the underlying infection. Platelets usually have such a short life span that prophylactic platelet transfusions are useless. However, these patients frequently are quite ill and require invasive diagnostic and therapeutic procedures, for which platelet transfusions are indicated to bring the platelet count to a safe level (50,000 per μL for minor procedures).

Disseminated Intravascular Coagulation

Disseminated intravascular coagulation (DIC) is a systemic condition characterized by inappropriate activation of thrombin and consumption of fibrinogen and platelets, usually caused by the exposure of blood to tissue factor. Acute DIC may be secondary to bacteremia or sepsis, obstetric complications, trauma (especially head trauma), and snakebite. A chronic, compensated form of DIC may be a complication of cancer. While the patient is in a compensated state, thrombocytopenia is minimal; however, the compensation is fragile and can deteriorate to acute DIC with minimal provocation.

Findings in acute DIC are a decrease in platelet count and fibrinogen, a prolonged prothrombin time (PT) and activated partial thromboplastin time (APTT), and an increase in fibrin(ogen) split products. The thrombocytopenia may be moderate or marked; counts as low as 20,000 per μL are not uncommon. The bleeding propensity is worsened by the consumption of clotting factors. Therapy of the thrombocytopenia and the DIC must be directed at the underlying cause. Replacement of platelets and clotting factors is often futile and generally should be reserved for clinically significant bleeding. The role of heparin is often controversial. Heparin should be reserved for cases in which the thrombotic manifestations outweigh the hemorrhagic manifestations.

Thrombotic Microangiopathies

Thrombotic microangiopathies are disorders that result in the agglutination of platelets in small vessels, with resultant organ ischemia and dysfunction. Three syndromes are recognized: TTP, HUS, and HELLP. The major features are as described previously. Early recognition and treatment are essential to a successful outcome. The treatment of each condition is somewhat different. TTP definitely should be treated with daily plasma exchanges of 40 mL per kg using fresh-frozen plasma or "cryoprecipitate-poor" plasma ("cryosupernatant"), not colloid, crystalloid, or IGIV. Prednisone, 1 mg per kg, appears to be a useful adjunct. The therapy of HUS is similar, but the benefit of plasma exchange is less well documented. HELLP, which usually occurs in the last weeks of pregnancy, often resolves with delivery of the fetus. The only role of platelet transfusion in any of these disorders is to stop active hemorrhage due to thrombocytopenia or to raise the platelet count temporarily for necessary procedures.

Heparin-Induced Thrombocytopenia

Heparin-induced thrombocytopenia (HIT) is a special case of drug-induced thrombocytopenia, caused by the formation of a complex of heparin and a platelet surface molecule, platelet factor 4 (PF4). Unlike in other drug-induced thrombocytopenias, which are due simply to immune-mediated platelet clearance, heparin causes activation and aggregation of the platelets, resulting in arterial and/or venous occlusion. The clinical finding of thrombocytopenia and arterial or venous thrombosis in a patient receiving heparin should raise this diagnostic possibility. Heparin in any amount and by any route of administration can cause the syndrome, including intravenous therapeutic doses, "flush" doses, subcutaneous prophylaxis, or trace amounts in intravenous solutions or in renal dialysis solutions. Until the diagnosis can be ascertained, all forms of heparin should be stopped. This is particularly problematic in patients receiving therapeutic heparin. Other parenteral anticoagulants such as argatroban are in clinical trials, but at present none of these is FDA licensed. The syndrome occurs less frequently with low-molecular-weight heparin (LMWH). However, these antibodies may cross-react, and LMWH should not be substituted for standard heparin in the setting of HIT. Although the data are still evolving, heparinoids such as danaparoid (Orgaran) may be useful in this setting.

Hypersplenism

Excessive macrophage activity of the spleen is a frequent cause of moderate thrombocytopenia. Often, there is hepatic cirrhosis associated with portal hypertension and splenomegaly. An incidental finding of thrombocytopenia may be the first recognized sign of splenomegaly. The diagnosis rests on ruling out other causes of thrombocytopenia and ascertaining the cause for the splenomegaly. A bone marrow examination may be helpful. As the thrombocytopenia is usually of moderate degree, no therapy may be required. In any case, platelet transfusions are futile, except for management of thrombocytopenic hemorrhage.

Post-transfusion Purpura

Post-transfusion purpura (PTP) is an infrequent cause of severe thrombocytopenia occurring 5 to 10 days after the transfusion of any cellular blood product, caused by alloimmunization to a polymorphic form of platelet glycoprotein, GP IIb/IIIa, also known as the Pla antigen system. Patients who possess the normal allele can develop an antibody response to the transfusion of a rare mutant allele. The resultant antibodies can cross-react with the patient's own platelets, causing profound thrombocytopenia. Platelet transfusions should be reserved for symptomatic bleeding. IGIV and steroids are not documented to be useful.

Alcohol Use

Overuse of alcohol causes thrombocytopenia by several mechanisms, including direct bone marrow toxicity. The thrombocytopenia is usually mild and reversible with abstinence. After years of chronic overuse, cirrhosis, portal hypertension, and splenomegaly can cause moderate thrombocytopenia. At this stage, there is no effective therapy. Abstinence will decrease further damage.

PRODUCTION DEFECTS

Aplastic Anemia

Aplastic anemia is a rare but serious cause of thrombocytopenia. Platelets, leukocytes, and erythrocytes all may be severely decreased in number. A bone marrow examination is necessary for diagnosis. Thrombocytopenia in aplastic anemia should be treated conservatively. Platelet transfusions should be minimized, and single-donor platelets utilized to prevent alloimmunization. Platelets from unrelated donors are preferable to those from family members to facilitate potential bone marrow transplantation. The underlying aplastic anemia should be treated with immunosuppression and bone marrow transplantation should be considered.

Myelodysplasia, Myelophthisis

Myelodysplasia is a state of disordered production of blood cells by the bone marrow, leading to a decrease in any or all blood cell lines. The incidence increases with age. Myelodysplasia may degenerate into leukemia. Myelophthisis is the replacement of the bone marrow by fibrotic tissue or abnormal cells, such as metastatic tumor cells. Diagnosis is made by bone marrow examination. Again, it is difficult to provide adequate support with chronic platelet transfusions, owing to frequent alloimmunization and the 3- to 5-day lifespan of transfused platelets. The risk of bleeding should be weighed against the risks of transfusion.

Nutrient Deficiencies: Folate and Vitamin B_{12}

Vitamin B_{12} or folate deficiency may lead to pancytopenia. Diagnosis is made by measuring blood levels of the vitamins. Replacement therapy usually results in a rapid normalization of blood counts. After blood specimens have been sent to the laboratory, both vitamin B_{12}, 1000 μg intramuscularly (IM) daily for 1 week and then weekly for 1 month, and folate, 1 mg orally per day, should be given until the results of the blood tests are known. Performance of Schilling's test should be delayed for 3 months to allow regrowth of the intestinal epithelium. The maintenance dose of B_{12} is 1000 μg IM once a month for life.

Chemotherapy

Chemotherapy for cancer or immune suppression also suppresses the bone marrow. Usually the clinical situation is sufficiently clear-cut to make the diagnosis. If the risk of bleeding is high, platelet transfusions are indicated to temporarily maintain the platelet count.

FUNCTIONAL PLATELET DEFECTS

Bleeding in the setting of a normal platelet count and a normal coagulation system raises the possibility of von Willebrand's disease or a functional platelet defect.

Von Willebrand's Disease

Von Willebrand's disease (vWD) is the partial or complete absence of von Willebrand factor (vWF), which functions in both primary and secondary hemostasis. Common symptoms are mucosal hemorrhage, menorrhagia, and easy bruising. The diagnosis is made by blood tests of vWF quantity (antigen) and function (ristocetin cofactor activity). The therapy varies with the subtype of vWD. Type 1 vWD may be managed with intranasal or intravenous desmopressin acetate (DDAVP), once it has been demonstrated that the patient responds appropriately. The intravenous dose is 0.3 to 0.4 μg per kg, given over 30 minutes. Intranasal therapy must be with the high-concentration formulation, Stimate, 150 to 300 μg per dose. In the absence of a satisfactory response to desmopressin acetate, or in type 2 or type 3 vWD, the only FDA-licensed agent is cryoprecipitate. However, two factor VIII concentrates (Humate-P and Alphanate) contain a significant amount of vWF and are in frequent use.

Congenital Platelet Defects

Congenital defects of platelet function include deficiencies of specific surface receptors (deficiency of GP Ib receptors in Bernard-Soulier syndrome and of GP IIb/IIIa receptors in Glanzmanns's thrombasthenia) or a variety of defects in the contents of the platelet granules. The diagnosis is made by specialized platelet function tests. The therapy is platelet transfusion for specific bleeding episodes or prophylaxis. Complete deficiency of a surface glycoprotein may lead to alloimmunization against normal platelets, for which there is no effective therapy.

Acquired Platelet Defects

Several medications induce platelet function defects, including aspirin, ticlopidine, anagrelide, NSAIDs, and abciximab. The half-life and degree of platelet inhibition are different for each agent. For bleeding episodes, the drug should be stopped and platelet transfusions may be needed.

Uremia also causes platelet dysfunction that is reversed by about 2 weeks of adequate dialysis. Although cryoprecipitate has been used in the past for uremia-induced hemorrhage, platelet transfusions are more effective. Patients may be prepared for necessary surgical procedures with desmopressin acetate and/or conjugated estrogens.

DETERMINING THERAPY

There are three essential questions about the use of platelet transfusions in thrombocytopenia: Is any treatment necessary? Will it be possible to raise the platelet count with transfusions? What are the risks of platelet transfusions?

As previously noted, in most cases a numeric "trigger" for platelet transfusion is not warranted. The necessity of transfusion depends on the clinical situation and the likelihood of bleeding due to a low platelet count. The necessity of achieving a higher platelet count should also be considered. If the additional platelets will correct or prevent bleeding, the benefit is obvious. If the outcome is merely a higher count in a patient at low risk of bleeding, then the benefit is insignificant.

As noted, in most cases of destructive thrombocytopenia, it is not possible to raise and maintain a platelet count by transfusion of blood bank platelets, because transfused platelets are destroyed at the same rate as that of the patient's own platelets, or at an even higher rate. In cases of decreased production of platelets, transfused platelets will have a transient effect. However, if the cause of the decreased production is chronic, such as in myelodysplasia, it is very difficult for the patient to be maintained on platelet transfusions.

One of the risks of frequent platelet transfusion is alloimmunization, which probably occurs in response to human leukocyte antigens (HLAs) on the platelet surface. The result of alloimmunization is a very short life span of the transfused platelets and resultant inability of transfused platelets to increase the platelet count. There is no way to predict nor prevent this complication. Leukocyte filters are minimally effective. HLA typing of donors is logistically difficult and very expensive. The use of platelets from related donors may be helpful, as well as the use of single-donor platelets collected by platelet pheresis.

Each unit of platelets exposes the recipient to one blood donor. There is a small but finite risk of transmission of human immunodeficiency virus (HIV) infection or hepatitis. Therefore, platelet transfusion should be used only when clearly indicated.

Finally, intramuscular injections and platelet-inhibitory drugs should be avoided in thrombocytopenic patients.

DISSEMINATED INTRAVASCULAR COAGULATION

method of
PETER E. BRAVERMAN, M.D., and
WILLIAM R. BELL, M.D.
Johns Hopkins University School of Medicine
Baltimore, Maryland

Disseminated intravascular coagulation (DIC) is an acquired coagulopathy that is best understood as an epiphenomenon of a broad variety of disease states. The effects of this clinicopathologic entity encompass a spectrum ranging from asymptomatic laboratory abnormalities, to "chronic compensated" coagulopathies, to acute and fulminant catastrophic bleeding and thrombosis. The diagnosis and especially the management of this disorder remain controversial topics, but progress has been made in the appreciation that DIC represents a group of disorders of variable etiology and expression, and that treatment may differ greatly depending upon the clinical setting.

The first experimental demonstration of this entity was described in 1834, when injection of emulsified brain tissue into animals induced lethal clotting. If the infusion was given more slowly, thrombi did not develop, but the blood became incoagulable. Since then, many triggering factors have been identified that disrupt the complex balance between activation and inhibition of the coagulation and fibrinolytic systems. Tissue factor, or thromboplastin, probably plays a major role in the initiation of this process and may be derived directly from tissue injury (brain trauma), fetal-uterine tissue, invading bacteria, or inflammatory cells (monocytes), or from neoplastic cells.

Supported in part by NIH research grant HL 36260 from the NHL BI of the National Institutes of Health, Bethesda, Maryland.

DIAGNOSIS

The DIC syndrome will be obvious when unusual bleeding and thrombosis occur in the appropriate clinical settings, such as those listed in Table 1. Abnormally prolonged prothrombin time (PT) and activated partial thromboplastin time (APTT) and thrombocytopenia are the immediately obvious supporting laboratory features but are not always present. Plasma levels of fibrinogen, an acute phase reactant, are often elevated early on in these settings and will usually but not always decline as the DIC process progressively develops. The most reliable and specific laboratory indicators of the DIC syndrome are elevated fibrinogen/fibrin degradation (or split) products (FDPs), elevated levels of soluble fibrin monomers, and reduced antithrombin III (AT-III) levels. Some authors have developed DIC scoring systems that quantify the severity of the coagulopathy, adding points for lower platelet counts, lower fibrinogen levels, higher FDP titers, and so on.

TREATMENT

There are three general elements in the management of DIC: (1) treatment of the underlying cause or trigger, (2) replacement of depleted platelets and/or coagulation factors, and (3) the use of inhibitors of coagulation and/or fibrinolysis. By far the most

TABLE 1. **Conditions Associated with Disseminated Intravascular Coagulation**

Any cause of extensive tissue damage and necrosis (resulting in massive release of tissue factor):
Shock, burns, trauma, brain injury, heat stroke, acidosis, rhabdomyolysis
Infections, especially:
Sepsis (gram-negative and gram-positive)
Rickettsial (Rocky Mountain spotted fever)
Post-splenectomy bacteremia
Viral "hemorrhagic" fevers
Malignancy, especially:
Leukemia (promyelocytic and others)
Mucin-producing adenocarcinomas and others
Obstetric complications, especially:
Abruptio placentae
Retained dead fetus
Amniotic fluid embolism
Toxemia of pregnancy
Vascular diseases, especially:
Giant hemangiomas
Aortic aneurysm
Miscellaneous:
Hemolytic transfusion reactions
Hyperacute allograft rejection
Venomous snake bites
Peritoneovenous shunts (liver disease)

important of these remains the prompt identification, reversal, and eradication (or at least control) of the condition that caused the coagulopathy. If this cannot be accomplished, all other treatment modalities are only temporizing and are doomed to failure. In some situations, control or reversal of the underlying trigger alone will be sufficient, such as evacuation of the fetus in abruptio placentae, but in other disease entities, replacement and inhibitor therapy may significantly reduce morbidity and mortality. Management must be individualized to the particular setting and circumstances in which the coagulopathy is occurring, but the following general guidelines are appropriate.

Along with prompt treatment of the underlying trigger, general supportive care is crucial, especially with regard to limiting further tissue damage, infarction, or any complication that may release more tissue factor and contribute further to the coagulopathy. This includes maintenance of circulatory volume and of sufficient blood pressure for organ perfusion, correction of hypoxemia, and prevention of venous stasis. Whenever possible, and especially when peripheral ischemia and thrombosis are in evidence (e.g., with purpura fulminans), aggressive volume support should be given in preference to administration of adrenergic vasopressors, to limit vasoconstriction in the acral distribution.

There is little evidence to support the long-held notion that factor replacement in DIC "fuels the fire" and worsens outcome. In general, if platelet counts or fibrinogen levels are dangerously low or hemorrhage is occurring, replacement attempts should be made along with a vigorous attack on the underlying disorder. Post-infusion incremental increases must be demonstrated (5000 to 10,000 platelets per mL for each unit given, and 10 mg of fibrinogen per dL for each unit of cryoprecipitate given), and if improvement is not observed, additional replacements should not be given. When such immediate "consumption" is evident, repeat infusions after the start of low-dose (500 to 800 units per hour) heparin may, in some circumstances, produce more sustained increments. When bleeding is a problem, the approximate goal for platelets is a count of at least 50,000 per mL, and for fibrinogen, a level of at least 100 mg per dL. When there is no bleeding, we attempt to give replacement therapy "prophylactically" for platelet levels below 10,000 to 20,000 per mL, and for fibrinogen levels less than 50 mg per dL. Effective replacement therapy is more important when insufficient production is a feature of the disease state (e.g., with platelets in leukemic patients or with coagulation factors in cirrhotic patients).

Although bleeding is often the most salient and dramatic feature of the DIC syndrome, in our experience it is thrombosis that produces most of the end-organ damage and morbidity, including renal and respiratory failure, stroke, and gangrene. Although the use of heparin in conditions involving factor consumption and bleeding remains extremely controversial, its use is clearly indicated in any setting of DIC complicated by large-vessel thromboembolism or by the dermal necrosis of purpura fulminans. In these situations, if there is no active bleeding, full-dose heparin therapy (1000 to 1600 units per hour) should be given. If the APTT is already prolonged by the DIC, we either estimate appropriate infusion rates from published weight tables or mix the patient's plasma 1:1 with normal plasma and then adjust for a target of 1.5 to 2.0 times the APTT control. These recommendations constitute guidelines only, and it is more informative to consider the efficacy of different treatment modalities for DIC in each clinical setting.

When DIC accompanies septic shock, survival is probably more directly related to the severity of the infection and hypotension than it is to the complications of DIC. Nevertheless, the issue of the value of coagulation inhibitors in this situation remains a subject of heated controversy in this disease and has historically been dominated more by anecdote and dogma than by data. Even now, despite accumulating publications on the possible efficacy of heparin and AT-III in these patients, there is still no prospective controlled trial with the power to demonstrate a survival advantage. Recent work with AT-III is promising but typically demonstrates far greater improvements in laboratory abnormalities than in clinical outcomes. A French study of AT-III administration in sepsis showed a trend toward improved survival but did not have the numbers to show statistical significance. Nevertheless, some experts in the field now tout AT-III therapy as the treatment of choice for fulminant DIC in septic shock, given in an intravenous dose of approximately 100 IU per kg per day. Our experience with this agent is limited.

For the subset of septic patients with features of classic purpura fulminans, we almost always advocate the use of heparin. Studies clearly support its efficacy in pediatric patients, but we also see this catastrophe in adult asplenic patients and support its use here as well. Unfortunately we are usually consulted only after the patient has progressed to advanced gangrene of the digits. It must be emphasized that heparin should be started at the very first sign of dermal or acral ischemia, such as livedo reticularis, and so long as there are no contraindications such as excessive or central nervous system bleeding, heparin should be given at full dose (1000 to 1600 units per hour).

Other Conditions That Affect Treatment

Certain malignancy states deserve special mention. When DIC complicates acute promyelocytic leukemia (APL), it is usually manifested by more hemorrhage than thrombosis, perhaps as a consequence of more fibrinolytic activity. Many practitioners still use heparin "prophylactically" prior to chemotherapy in this disease, but without the support of good data. A few studies have documented a reduction in hemorrhagic events with the use of inhibitors of fibrinolysis, such as tranexamic acid used alone in a dose of 2 grams every 8 hours intravenously, or ε-aminocaproic acid (EACA) combined with heparin, but our experience with these agents is limited. It should be noted that DIC has been less of a problem in APL with the introduction of all-*trans*-retinoic acid (tretinoin) induction therapy.

In the special circumstance of malignancy-associated chronic compensated DIC, heparin therapy is absolutely essential. Heralded by migrating superficial thrombophlebitis and complicated by both venous and arterial large-vessel thromboembolism, this syndrome will respond only to heparin therapy. Indeed, any hypercoagulable state that does not respond to warfarin treatment should immediately suggest Trousseau's syndrome, and the search for an occult malignancy should begin. Heparin should be given in full dose, either intravenously, to achieve an APTT of 1.5 to 2.0 times control, or in an equivalent low-molecular-weight subcutaneous form, such as enoxaparin (Lovenox),* 30 mg every 12 hours, or dalteparin (Fragmin),* 200 units per kg per day.

Obstetric problems complicated by DIC also need to be addressed individually. In the case of abruptio placentae, heparin therapy has no role. In this situation, bleeding predominates over thrombosis. Cryoprecipitate should be given to maintain a fibrinogen level above 150 mg per dL if hemorrhage commences, but nothing should delay evacuation of the uterus, as this is the only assured way to arrest the coagulopathy. In the case of a retained dead fetus, a low-grade chronic hemorrhagic diathesis may ensue, and heparin is often effective in raising fibrinogen levels and improving hemostasis in preparation for evacuation. If delivery is already under way and hypofibrinogenemia is present, however, cryoprecipitate—not heparin—should be given. With intrauterine death of a twin, in most cases, subcutaneous heparin can control the consumption of fibrinogen while the living twin matures. In amniotic fluid embolism, survivors of sudden death develop excessive bleeding related to uncontrolled fibrinolysis, and EACA may be useful in this circumstance.

Entities causing localized vascular coagulation also require separate consideration. In Kasabach-Merritt syndrome, characterized by giant cavernous hemangiomas and a bleeding tendency secondary to local platelet and fibrinogen consumption, the use of EACA has proved successful, inducing local thrombosis and normalizing counts. In some cases of aortic aneurysm, a compensated form of DIC with low fibrinogen levels and thrombocytopenia may occur. In preparation for surgery, if vessel leaking is ruled out, low-dose heparin will often stop the consumptive process and return these clotting factors to normal levels, allowing surgical repair to safely proceed.

Newer agents that remain under investigation have shown promise in initial experimental studies. Infusions of other natural anticoagulants such as protein C and soluble thrombomodulin, direct inhibitors of the tissue factor–factor VIIa complex and factor Xa, and agents that act on both thrombin and plasmin, such as the protease inhibitor gabexate and the combination of hirudin and tissue plasminogen activator have produced impressive results in animal studies of DIC and are soon to make their debut in human trials.

*Not FDA approved for this indication.

THROMBOTIC THROMBOCYTOPENIC PURPURA

method of
GWENDOLINE M. SPURLL, M.D.
McGill University and Royal Victoria Hospital
Montreal, Quebec, Canada

Thrombotic thrombocytopenic purpura (TTP) and hemolytic-uremic syndrome (HUS) are related clinical syndromes characterized by thrombocytopenia and microangiopathic hemolytic anemia, variably accompanied by renal failure, altered mental function, and fever. In HUS the main end-organ affected is the kidney, and in children it is usually preceded by a diarrheal illness. In adults the underlying causes of HUS are more heterogeneous. TTP occurs more typically in adults and may result in damage to any organ, though renal and central nervous system signs are most prominent. A viral syndrome or diarrhea may precede TTP/HUS. The patient typically presents with confusion, fluctuating focal neurologic defects, fever, or renal failure.

Prompt diagnosis and treatment of patients with TTP/HUS are critical, because without treatment the fatality rate is 90%, whereas with optimal treatment 70 to 90% of the patients survive.

PATHOPHYSIOLOGY

The clinical syndrome of TTP/HUS represents the final common pathway of a number of disorders characterized by endothelial damage and/or platelet activation, with deposition of platelet/fibrin clots (hyaline clots) in arteries, arterioles, and capillaries. Scission of red cells by fibrin strands or abnormal adhesion of erythrocytes to the endothelium causes red cell fragmentation. This is detected as the presence of schistocytes on the blood smear (microangiopathic change). Interruption of blood supply to end-organs impairs organ function, resulting in renal failure, fluctuating mental change, and other evidence of end-organ failure. In diarrhea-associated TTP/HUS any organ may be affected, whereas in sporadic TTP the lung and liver are usually spared.

Etiology

Normally, platelets circulate singly, each in the form of a disk. They do not bind to unstimulated endothelium. Platelets remain in this state until they are stimulated by soluble platelet-aggregating agents or by adhesion to damaged endothelium. Production of prostacyclin by endothelial cells aids in maintaining the quiescent state of the platelet.

Damage to the endothelium causes platelet adhesion and aggregation by exposure of underlying collagen and release of high-molecular-weight von Willebrand factor (vWF) from endothelial cells. Binding to collagen and platelet aggrega-

TABLE 1. **Differential Diagnosis for Thrombocytopenia and Microangiopathy**

Disease	Platelets	Smear	PT	APTT	Fbg	ALT	LDH
TTP	↓	Schistocytes, polychromasia	↑ ↓	↑ ↓	↑ ↓	↑ ↓	↑ ↑
DIC	↓	Schistocytes	↑	↑	↓ or ↑ ↓	↑ ↓	↑ or ↑ ↓
ITP	↓	Normal RBCs	↑ ↓	↑ ↓	↑ ↓	↑ ↓	↑ ↓
Evans' syndrome	↓	Spherocytes, polychromasia	↑ ↓	↑ ↓	↑ ↓	↑ ↓	↑ ↓ or ↑
HELLP	↓	Schistocytes	↑ ↓	↑ ↓	↑ ↓	↑ ↑	↑
AFLP	↓ or ↑ ↓	Normal RBCs or schistocytes	↑ or ↑ ↓	↑ or ↑ ↓	↓ or ↑ ↓	↑ ↑	↑

Abbreviations: ALT = alanine aminotransferase; APTT = activated partial thromboplastin time; Fbg = fibrinogen; LDH = lactate dehydrogenase; PT = prothrombin time; RBC = red blood cell.

tion are both mediated by vWF, and the higher the molecular weight of the vWF, the more active it is in mediating adhesion.

The precise pathophysiology is still not clear, but a number of abnormalities have been noted in patients with TTP/HUS that might cause abnormal platelet aggregation and endothelial damage. Abnormal circulating platelet-aggregating agents, an increase in platelet microparticles with calpain (a calcium-activated protease that cleaves von Willebrand multimers to low-molecular-weight fragments), and a relative decrease in prostacyclin levels have been demonstrated in patients with TTP. Patients with relapsing TTP often have unusually high-molecular-weight circulating vWF. Some patients with sporadic or human immunodeficiency virus (HIV)-associated TTP have a serum factor that causes apoptotic death of endothelial cells. Patients with chemotherapy-associated TTP/HUS have increased circulating immune complexes and decreased complement levels. Clearance of these complexes after treatment is associated with resolution of the illness. It is unclear which if any of these processes represents the primary event and which are secondary.

EPIDEMIOLOGY

TTP is a rare disorder, with an incidence of 1 case per million population per year and a female predominance. Most adult cases are sporadic, but associated disorders include diarrhea due to verocytotoxin-producing organisms (e.g., *Escherichia coli* O157:H7), HIV infection, autoimmune disorders such as systemic lupus erythematosus (SLE), cancer chemotherapy (particularly with 5-fluorouracil [Adrucil] and mitomycin [Mutamycin], and combination bleomycin [Blenoxane] and cisplatin [Platinol-AQ]), post–bone marrow or organ transplant state, immunosuppressive medication (cyclosporine [Sandimmune], tacrolimus [Prograf], or monoclonal antibodies), pregnancy, and hormonal contraceptive use.

DIAGNOSTIC WORK-UP

The diagnosis of TTP/HUS should be suspected in any patient presenting with thrombocytopenia and renal failure or mental changes. A review of the peripheral blood smear reveals schistocytes. The presence of hemolysis is confirmed by the finding of an increased serum lactate dehydrogenase (LDH), usually in the presence of normal serum alanine aminotransferase (ALT), aspartate aminotransferase (AST), and alkaline phosphatase.

Other causes of thrombocytopenia and microangiopathy, such as disseminated intravascular coagulation (DIC), idiopathic thrombocytopenic purpura (ITP), Evans' syndrome, and the obstetric syndromes of hemolysis, elevated liver enzymes, and low platelets (HELLP) and acute fatty liver of pregnancy (AFLP), must be ruled out (Table 1). In DIC there is an increase in prothrombin time (PT) and activated partial thromboplastin time (APTT) and a decrease in fibrinogen, as well as an increase in fibrin degradation products. In ITP there are no schistocytes and serum LDH is normal, and renal and mental changes are absent unless there is intracranial hemorrhage. In Evans' syndrome there is autoimmune thrombocytopenia and autoimmune hemolytic anemia, with spherocytes and positive results on direct Coombs' test, rather than microangiopathic hemolysis. In pregnancy with thrombocytopenia elevated levels of liver enzymes suggest the HELLP syndrome or AFLP, which may be associated with DIC, rather than TTP. Thrombocytopenia associated with eclampsia may be difficult to differentiate from TTP, and careful monitoring of the clinical state and the peripheral smear is essential.

TREATMENT AND PROGNOSIS

The key to a successful outcome in TTP is prompt initiation of treatment (Table 2). The shorter the interval to beginning treatment, the better the outcome.

Plasma exchange is the cornerstone of treatment in TTP and should be begun as soon as the diagnosis is suspected. This process, in which the patient's plasma is removed and replaced with normal plasma, has been shown to be superior to plasma infusion alone. It is unclear whether this is because pathogenetic mediators are being removed by the process of plasma removal or whether the removal of the patient's plasma simply allows the infusion of larger

TABLE 2. **Treatment of TTP/HUS**

Clearly Indicated

Plasma exchange with plasma replacement

Probably Indicated

Acetylsalicylic acid (aspirin)
Dipyridamole (Persantine)
High-dose corticosteroids

Useful in Refractory or Relapsing Disease

Splenectomy
Vincristine (Oncovin)* or vinblastine (Velban)*
Repeated plasma infusion
Staphylococcal A immunoabsorbent column (IMRE column)
Intravenous immune globulin*

* Not FDA approved for this indication.

amounts of normal plasma. The usual protocol is daily exchange, with an exchange volume in the first three plasma exchanges of 1.5 times the patient's plasma volume. In subsequent exchanges an exchange volume equal to the patient's plasma volume is used. Plasma exchanges are continued daily, usually for at least 7 to 9 days, until a normalization of the serum LDH and the platelet count is seen. The platelet count, peripheral smear, LDH, and liver and renal function should be monitored daily.

If plasmapheresis cannot be initiated immediately, temporizing treatment with plasma infusion should be begun.

The studies showing the effectiveness of plasma exchange used fresh frozen plasma as replacement. However, cryodepleted plasma (plasma relatively depleted of factor VIII, vWF, fibrinogen, and fibronectin) may be more effective than fresh frozen plasma. This is currently under study by the Canadian Apheresis Study Group.

In the studies demonstrating the effectiveness of plasma exchange in TTP/HUS, the antiplatelet agents acetylsalicylic acid (aspirin) and dipyridamole (Persantine) were used to block platelet aggregation. Although these agents are relatively ineffective *alone* in the treatment of TTP, they may aid in inducing and maintaining a remission. In addition, many treatment centers regularly use corticosteroids at high dose.

Some patients have deteriorated rapidly and dramatically after platelet transfusion, with fatal outcome. For this reason, platelet transfusion is considered relatively contraindicated in TTP, and platelets are not transfused unless there is major active bleeding.

Patients with chemotherapy-related TTP/HUS have a particularly poor outcome but may respond to passage of plasma over a staphylococcal A immunoabsorption column (IMRĒ). High-dose intravenous immune globulin* may be effective in some refractory patients.

Sixty to 90% of patients will go into remission with resolution of the thrombocytopenia and microangiopathy. However, 20 to 46% of patients will eventually relapse. Some patients have repeated relapses, and in these patients splenectomy may be of benefit. Pregnancy-related TTP may recur in a subsequent pregnancy, though in most cases it does not. Renal failure usually resolves in pediatric HUS but may persist in adults. Fetal and maternal mortality rates in pregnancy-associated cases are high. Neurologic defects may persist although the patient is in remission. The overall prognosis depends on the underlying disease, because many patients with cancer and HIV infection–related TTP die of the underlying disease.

*Not FDA approved for this indication.

HEMOCHROMATOSIS

method of
ANTHONY S. TAVILL, M.D.
Mt. Sinai Medical Center and Case Western Reserve University School of Medicine
Cleveland, Ohio

Hemochromatosis is a diagnosis that signifies a group of disorders with a common feature of pathologic deposition of iron in the parenchymal cells of many organs, leading to cell damage and functional insufficiency. Because the liver is the primary site of iron storage, the earliest accumulation is evident within the hepatocytes, and the evidence for toxicity is related to the quantitative degree of iron overload. Other organs and structures such as the pancreas, heart, and joints are variably affected, either as a result of the overloaded capacity of the liver to accommodate storage iron or as a consequence of a particular vulnerability to iron toxicity of the functional cell in that structure (e.g., the cardiomyocyte, the pancreatic islet cell).

When the condition of iron overload is genetically determined, the condition is termed genetic or hereditary hemochromatosis (HH), previously called primary or idiopathic hemochromatosis. The candidate gene for HH, now termed the *HFE* gene, was identified in 1996 by means of a positional cloning technique and has been implicated in the pathogenesis of the disease in the vast majority of phenotypically diagnosed patients. These persons stand in contrast to those with a disorder of secondary hemochromatosis, in which iron overload occurs secondary to an underlying condition, leading to increased intestinal iron absorption, decreased iron utilization, and/or increased parenteral iron availability such as occurs in conditions requiring red blood cell transfusion. Chronic anemias associated with ineffective erythropoiesis, chronic liver disease (particularly of alcoholic etiology), and African hemochromatosis fall into the category of secondary hemochromatosis.

GENETIC BASIS OF HEREDITARY HEMOCHROMATOSIS

Studies available since 1977, based on pedigree analysis and histocompatibility (i.e., HLA) typing of families of probands with HH, showed that the gene was located on the short arm of chromosome 6 in proximity to the *HLA A3* locus. It became apparent that the disease was inherited in an autosomal recessive fashion, with phenotypic expression occurring only in homozygotes possessing abnormal alleles on the chromosome 6 pair. It was also evident that the candidate gene was confined to Caucasians of northern European origin, with the likelihood that the ancestral gene originated in a Celtic population. Homozygotes occur with a frequency of 1:250 to 1:300 in such Caucasian populations, making HH the most common single-gene hereditary disorder. Heterozygotes constitute 10 to 12% of such populations, and although occasionally showing some phenotypic diagnostic features (e.g., increased transferrin iron saturation), these persons, possessing only one gene on a pair of chromosomes, do not go on to develop the full phenotypic expression of the disorder with its signs of cellular and organ toxicity.

In 1996 the candidate gene, now termed *HFE* under International System for Human Gene Nomenclature (ISGN) terminology, was first described by a group of workers in the United States. Its nucleotide sequence indicated the transcriptional coding for a major histocompatibility complex (MHC) class 1–like molecule with four domains, one of which binds beta$_2$-microglobulin, a ligand necessary for presentation of the molecule on the plasma membrane of the cell. By means of histochemical techniques specific for the normal gene product, workers have shown that the predominant site of expression of the gene is the crypt cell of the upper small intestine, the precursor of the absorptive cell of the villus.

In patients with HH, two missense mutations of the *HFE* gene have been identified. One is a substitution of tyrosine for cysteine at position 282 (C282Y); the other is a substitution of aspartic acid for histidine at position 63 (H63D). The former mutation has been described in approximately 84% of the patients in several series from varied geographic regions in North America, Europe, and Australia, with a lower prevalence in Italy (64%) and the highest in Australia (100% in one series). The H63D mutation occurs in 15 to 20% of the population (of Caucasian origin) but does not appear in isolation to be associated with HH. It does, however, occur in a compound heterozygous state (C282Y, H63D) in about 5% of patients with phenotypically characteristic HH. Because the pathogenetic role of the gene product (or products) is not yet identified, the possible synergy between the two genes has not been elucidated. It is important to emphasize that at present, a significant minority of patients with typical HH do not demonstrate the C282Y mutation. In certain populations (e.g., African, African-American), there may be alternative gene-linked disorders of iron overload—a situation that may also account for the emerging group of Caucasian persons with familial iron overload who also do not possess the C282Y gene.

DIAGNOSIS

The diagnosis of hemochromatosis is traditionally predicated on the confirmation of iron overload. However, because the accumulation of excessive storage iron is a lifelong process, determined by the translational product of the inherited gene, it is now possible to detect the disorder of HH before disease has occurred by means of sensitive early phenotypic markers and, more recently, by the identification of the homozygous genotype. It is a salutary observation that 30 to 40 years ago the diagnosis of HH was almost invariably made in clinically detected probands over the age of 45 years with established cirrhosis and diabetes. With current access to suspected family members, recognized as homozygous for HH by HLA typing or, more recently, by identification of the C282Y mutation, the majority of cases in recent series have been made up of asymptomatic persons without organ damage who are detected before they have accumulated large iron stores (usually less than 5 grams based on amounts removed by phlebotomy).

As indicated previously, the diagnosis of HH may be made in three groups of individuals: (1) patients with symptoms and signs suggestive of clinical HH; (2) asymptomatic relatives of such patients; and (3) asymptomatic persons suspected of having HH on the basis of a chance finding of an abnormal blood test.

Routine assays of transferrin iron saturation and serum ferritin concentration have been suggested in persons over the age of 20 years as useful screening tools during periodic health examinations. Preliminary cost-effectiveness studies have provided feasibility data for such an approach, particularly if the tests can be targeted to susceptible populations.

Recent data have been used to examine the value of a fasting transferrin iron saturation in defining populations of persons homozygous for HH, heterozygous for HH, and without evidence for HH. A level of saturation greater than 45% detected 98% of patients with HH and included no normal persons. Such a value did, however, capture 22% of nonaffected persons with heterozygous HH, necessitating further evaluation to eliminate the presence of significant iron overload. Some of these unnecessary evaluations could have been avoided by conducting follow-up evaluation only in persons with both an elevated serum ferritin *and* elevated transferrin iron saturation. In another study of 128 persons with HH, 54 were discovered by family evaluations. These persons were all homozygous for the C282Y mutation; 86% had elevated transferrin saturation, and 90% had elevated serum ferritin. It is apparent, therefore, that some affected persons, homozygous for HH, particularly young people, may have normal indirect iron studies. Similarly, the sensitivity and specificity of iron studies may be limited by other inflammatory disorders, particularly those involving the liver (e.g., viral hepatitis, steatohepatitis, alcoholic liver disease).

In such circumstances liver biopsy provides the means to document both excessive storage iron and the pathologic effects of excessive iron, in particular fibrosis and cirrhosis. The semiquantitative grading system based on Perls' Prussian blue staining requires confirmation by quantitative biochemical iron measurement. The latter may be performed on formalin-fixed or frozen tissue, subsequently taken to dryness in the laboratory. Normal values of up to 1800 μg per gram of dry weight are most often quoted. Patients with symptomatic HH usually have hepatic iron concentration (HIC) levels of greater than 10,000 μg per gram, whereas asymptomatic younger homozygotes will show variably elevated levels depending on age, gender, and dietary and other factors (e.g., service as a blood donor). Based on the concept that patients with HH progressively accumulate iron throughout life, the hepatic iron index, or HII (HIC in micromoles per gram divided by age in years), was devised as a means to exclude heterozygotes and others with liver disease associated with moderate iron overload. At least seven studies from around the world have confirmed a very high predictive accuracy for an HII in excess of 1.9. It should be emphasized that patients with some forms of secondary hemochromatosis, particularly those associated with dyserythropoiesis and blood transfusion requirements, will also have a greatly elevated HII. Furthermore, a recent study of a large number of explanted livers removed prior to liver transplantation showed an HII of greater than 1.9 in 8.5% of cases that could not be ascribed to HH.

In 1998, we are now in a position to validate the aforementioned phenotypic diagnostic features with genotypic determination. The prevalence of the C282Y-homozygous genotype ranges from 93 to 100% in well-defined pedigrees, and from 64 to 83% in nonfamilial studies; accordingly, the presence of the homozygous genotype provides very strong supportive evidence for the diagnosis of HH. While virtually 100% of patients homozygous for C282Y will have elevated transferrin saturation (greater than 45%), and serum ferritin, a significant minority (up to 15%) may have an HII of less than 1.9, even though their HIC is above the upper limit of normal.

It is therefore suggested that the finding of a transferrin saturation greater than 45%, particularly when supported by an elevated serum ferritin level, should be followed by genetic testing (request for hemochromatosis genotyping for both C282Y and H63D mutations). In persons homozygous for C282Y or compound heterozygotes (C282Y, H63D) with abnormal results on liver function testing or over the age of 30 years, a liver biopsy for pathologic evaluation and quantitative determination of liver iron should be carried out. In younger C282Y-homozygous patients with normal liver test results, it is reasonable to proceed to prophylactic therapeutic phlebotomy without the need for liver biopsy, because fibrosis and cirrhosis are very rare below the age of 30 years. Genotyping has supplanted HLA typing in the assessment of both probands and first-degree relatives.

TREATMENT

Hereditary Hemochromatosis

The mainstay of treatment for hemochromatosis remains phlebotomy (Table 1). Adequate phlebotomy aggressively instituted before the onset of cirrhosis or diabetes prevents the development of these complications and promotes normal life expectancy. With once-weekly or biweekly removal of one unit of blood (equivalent to about 250 mg of iron), patients with a heavy (greater than 30 grams) iron burden may take 2 to 3 years to complete primary therapy. Furthermore, because the diagnosis can now be made in presymptomatic homozygotes by the methods previously outlined, as soon as evidence of iron overload has been established, these patients should also be treated prophylactically. Criteria for completion of iron removal are a fall in transferrin saturation to normal levels, a reduction in serum ferritin to below 50 ng per mL, and a hematocrit that fails to return to within 5 to 10% below its baseline value. In practice it is not necessary to determine transferrin saturation or serum ferritin levels more than once every 3 to 4 months.

At the point at which the preceding criteria indicating incipient iron deficiency occur, frequent phlebotomy can be stopped and a maintenance schedule started. The frequency of maintenance phlebotomies is extremely variable. Some persons (both male and female) require up to 6 to 8 phlebotomies per year, whereas others, who presumptively reaccumulate iron at a slower rate, require fewer procedures. There is no need for repeated liver biopsy for documentation of iron removal. Rather, reliance on the indirect iron markers is sufficient for assurance of adequate "deironing." The only circumstance in which repeated liver biopsy may be indicated is when the initial biopsy suggested early fibrosis; in such cases it may be reassuring to ascertain that phlebotomy has achieved reversal or prevention of progression to cirrhosis. It is noteworthy that the complication of primary hepatocellular cancer has been confined almost invariably to patients with already-established cirrhosis. My experience has been that phlebotomy can be completed over a period of 12 to 24 months, with most persons able to replenish their hematocrit levels prior to each blood donation. Currently, in the United States, blood acquired by therapeutic phlebotomy in these circumstances may not be used for blood donation.

TABLE 1. **Treatment of Hemochromatosis**

Genetic (Hereditary) Hemochromatosis

- One phlebotomy (with removal of 500 mL of blood) weekly or biweekly
- Check hemoglobin and hematocrit prior to each phlebotomy; proceed if within 10% of baseline value
- Check transferrin saturation and serum ferritin levels every 3 months
- Stop frequent phlebotomy when serum ferritin falls below 50 ng/mL
- Continue phlebotomy with removal of one unit of blood at 2- to 3-month intervals or less to keep serum ferritin at or about 50 ng/mL

Secondary Hemochromatosis Associated with Dyserythropoiesis

- Deferoxamine (Desferal) at dose of 20 to 40 mg/kg per day administered SC over 24 hours (by mini-pump) or over 8 to 12 hours during the night by infusion
- Use serum ferritin in similar fashion to judge adequacy of iron removal

Several studies have established the benefits of iron depletion by phlebotomy. Subjective symptoms are relieved, a sense of well-being is restored, and survival is improved. Although a few scattered reports of regression of fibrosis and cirrhosis have been published, for the most part cirrhosis is irreversible, even though survival in such patients is improved by iron removal. Because cardiac dysrhythmia and cardiomyopathy are the most common causes of sudden death in iron overload states, there is a need for accelerated iron removal in the face of warning signs of cardiac complications. This can be achieved by a combination of phlebotomy and chelation therapy with deferoxamine (see later on).

Secondary Hemochromatosis

Phlebotomy has been used in certain forms of secondary hemochromatosis with improved survival (African hemochromatosis and porphyria cutanea tarda, for example). In secondary hemochromatosis associated with ineffective erythropoiesis, deferoxamine therapy has been shown to prevent hepatic fibrosis and cirrhosis and to increase life expectancy.

Deferoxamine mesylate (Desferal) in a dose of 20 to 40 mg per kg of body weight is administered subcutaneously, using an implanted mini-pump, by continuous infusion over a 24-hour cycle. Usually, no more than a total of 2 grams per 24 hours is needed to achieve maximum excretion. Alternatively, deferoxamine may be administered by subcutaneous infusion during the 8- to 12-hour overnight period. Such prophylactic treatment should be started early in life in patients with thalassemia major, who are dependent on blood transfusions. The value of deferoxamine therapy is limited by cost, the need for parenteral administration and the associated discomfort, and neurotoxicity. In addition, a variety of opportunistic infections have been described after prolonged chelation therapy.

In patients with end-stage liver disease, hepatic

decompensation is now manageable by orthotopic liver transplantation (OLT). Recent studies in the United States suggest that survival after OLT for this indication is not as favorable as for other causes of end-stage liver disease. Most of the deaths occurred in the perioperative period from cardiac or infection-related complications. Nevertheless, OLT offers an alternative when all other therapeutic approaches have been exhausted. In patients who have undergone successful transplantation for management of HH, there has been no evidence for recurrence of disease. This finding is supportive of the notion that the abnormal gene product exerts its effects on the absorptive intestinal cell rather than on the liver.

HODGKIN'S DISEASE: CHEMOTHERAPY

method of
GIANNI BONADONNA, M.D.
Istituto Nazionale per lo Studio e la Cura dei Tumori
Milan, Italy

At the end of this century the prognostic outlook for Hodgkin's disease is definitely more favorable than in previous decades. An extraordinary amount of important information is now available on the natural history of this lymphoma, its excellent response to various forms of treatment, and the types and frequencies of delayed morbidities, such as organ damage (e.g., heart, lung) and second malignancies produced by the therapeutic strategies applied.

Certain procedures and indications that were routine in the past 2 decades (e.g., staging laparotomy, primary radiotherapy for almost all patient subsets with nodal disease, a single polydrug regimen such as MOPP [nitrogen mustard, vincristine, procarbazine, and prednisone]) should now enjoy more flexible applications in the light of modern diagnostic tools and newly identified prognostic factors as well as a variety of treatment options. The complexity of the clinical evaluation and modern sophisticated treatment approaches demands considerable technical resources and qualified personnel. Despite the high cure rate now achieved in Hodgkin's disease, practicing physicians should carefully and honestly evaluate whether their own experience and the facilities available to them are adequate. If not, referral of patients to specialized centers remains a wise practice. Appropriate management of Hodgkin's disease still relies on complex programs and is not yet ready to be relegated to the care of a single physician in a private office or local hospital.

DIAGNOSIS AND STAGING

The vast majority of patients present with supradiaphragmatic disease, primarily cervical (approximately 70%), mediastinal, and axillary adenopathy. Inguinal involvement alone occurs in less than 10% of patients. The ideal method of establishing or confirming a pathologic diagnosis of Hodgkin's disease is excision biopsy of one or more enlarged lymph nodes. This procedure also provides sufficient material for immunophenotyping and cytogenetic studies as well as long-term storage. Aspiration cytology and drill biopsies have generally been thought to be unrewarding and unreliable because the amount of tissue obtained is small and there may be significant cellular trauma and architectural distortion. Although in experienced hands the diagnostic accuracy of fine-needle aspiration can be as high as 90%, subtype classification can be done in only about 60% of cases.

During the past 25 years, efforts have been made to improve the staging of malignant lymphomas. The goal of systematic documentation of the extent of disease is to make appropriate treatment decisions, delineate prognosis, and continue research. Over the years, lymphography, needle marrow biopsy, laparotomy, and laparoscopy have become important steps in the accurate staging of both adults and children. In recent years, computed tomography (CT) and magnetic resonance imaging (MRI) have made staging procedures simpler and less invasive. In deciding what examination to perform, a general guideline is that if localization of the lymphoma to a specific anatomic site would have a great impact on the treatment approach, the test is warranted. Conversely, a test of limited accuracy probably should not be performed.

The latest international staging classification was proposed and adopted in 1989 during a meeting held in Cotswold, England. The Cotswold classification (Table 1) maintained the framework of the Ann Arbor staging system in use at that time, implementing a few new elements derived from the experience gained in the preceding years. In par-

TABLE 1. **The Cotswold Staging Classification**

Stage I
Involvement of a single lymph node region or lymphoid structure (e.g., spleen, thymus, Waldeyer's ring) or involvement of a single extralymphatic site (I_E)

Stage II
Involvement of two or more lymph node regions on the same side of the diaphragm (hilar nodes, when involved on both sides, constitute stage II disease); localized contiguous involvement of only one extranodal organ or site and lymph node region(s) on the same side of the diaphragm (II_E)
The number of anatomic regions involved should be indicated by a subscript (e.g. II_3)

Stage III
Involvement of lymph node regions on both sides of the diaphragm (III), which may also be accompanied by involvement of the spleen (III_S) or by localized contiguous involvement of only one extranodal organ site (III_E) or both (III_{SE})
III_1 With or without involvement of splenic, hilar, celiac, or portal nodes
III_2 With involvement of paraortic, iliac, and mesenteric nodes

Stage IV
Diffuse or disseminated involvement of one or more extranodal organs or tissues, with or without associated lymph node involvement

Designations applicable to any disease stage

A	No symptoms
B	Fever (temperature >38°C), drenching night sweats, unexplained loss of >10% of body weight within the preceding 6 months
X	Bulky disease (a widening of the mediastinum by more than one third or the presence of a nodal mass with a maximal dimension >10 cm)
E	Involvement of a single extranodal site that is contiguous or proximal to the known nodal site
CS	Clinical stage
PS	Pathologic stage

ticular, it was recommended that CT be used to evaluate intrathoracic and infradiaphragmatic lymph nodes, that the criteria for clinical involvement of the spleen and liver be modified to include evidence of focal defects with two imaging techniques, and that abnormalities of liver function be ignored.

Certain selected patients with localized extranodal disease (e.g., Waldeyer's ring, muscle, bone, skin) contiguous to involved nodes are classified in the appropriate lymph node system stage followed by the subscript "E." The E patients have a more favorable prognosis than those showing clearly disseminated involvement (stage IV) with the exception of patients having Hodgkin's disease with direct extension into pulmonary parenchyma from a bulky mediastinal mass. The E designation thus excludes multiple extranodal deposits or bilateral lung extension, which constitutes stage IV disease.

Staging procedures for pediatric Hodgkin's disease are practically identical to those utilized in adults. Children usually show a comparatively lower incidence of liver infiltration and a high incidence of splenic involvement. Laparotomy and splenectomy in children were once considered important for accurate staging but carried a significant risk of infection. Splenectomy is definitely contraindicated in a child younger than 5 years because of the increased risk of fulminant septicemia. For these reasons as well as because of growth retardation following mantle field irradiation (shoulders and clavicles) and extended field irradiation (decreased sitting height), staging laparotomy has been progressively abandoned by all centers, and current treatment for children with Hodgkin's disease consists of chemotherapy with low-dose involved-field irradiation.

Staging classification applies only to the patient at the time of disease presentation and before the first treatment. Although it is usually both feasible and desirable to complete the diagnostic work-up before starting treatment, there are situations that call for a modified approach. For example, in the presence of massive mediastinal and/or hilar adenopathy compromising a major airway, it is recommended that 15 to 20 Gy be delivered in more than 2 weeks to shrink the lymph node masses before performing staging work-up.

Table 2 outlines the procedures deemed necessary to carry out correct staging. As previously mentioned, an adequate surgical biopsy, possibly of more than one intact lymph node, should be undertaken for pathologic examination. Inguinal nodes should not be biopsied if equally suspicious peripheral nodes are present elsewhere.

A variety of imaging techniques are available to assist in the initial staging of patients with histologically documented, previously untreated Hodgkin's disease. The usefulness of a specific imaging test can be defined in terms of sensitivity, specificity, and overall accuracy. The following guidelines are suggested:

1. The radiographic studies should include chest films and thoracic CT scan or MRI to evaluate the mediastinal adenopathy and any extension of it into the surrounding viscera. In addition, it is important to assess the bulk of disease, which is one of the most important prognostic factors.

2. Abdominal involvement must be evaluated using bipedal lymphography and abdominal CT scan. Lymphography remains the most accurate diagnostic tool for the assessment of low para-aortic and para-aortic and paracaval nodal disease.

3. Routine screening is of little value in sites infrequently involved with disease, but suggestive symptoms and signs at specific sites should prompt performance of pertinent imaging examinations. Gallium-67 scanning can be useful in determining the extent of nodal involvement, particularly in the chest. The technique may also be advantageous in the reassessment of residual nodal abnormality at the end of therapy. Gallium scanning is of limited value in assessing infradiaphragmatic disease, with false-positive findings due to normal gallium accumulation in the liver, spleen, and feces.

TABLE 2. **Recommended Procedures for Proper Staging**

Mandatory Procedures
Adequate surgical biopsy reviewed by an experienced hemopathologist. In primary extranodal lymphomas, biopsy should also include a lymph node when palpable.
Detailed history with special attention to the presence or absence of systemic symptoms
Careful physical examination, emphasizing node chains, size of liver and spleen, Waldeyer's ring inspection, and bony tenderness
Routine laboratory tests, including complete blood count, erythrosedimentation rate, liver function tests, serum uric acid, serum copper
Chest films (posteroanterior and lateral) with measurement of mass/thoracic ratio, chest and abdominal CT scan or MRI
Bipedal lymphography
Core needle biopsy of bone marrow from posterior iliac crest. Biopsy should be bilateral, especially in the presence of clinical stage III disease and in patients with systemic symptoms
Procedures Done Under Certain Circumstances
Needle or surgical biopsy of any suspicious extranodal (e.g., hepatic, splenic, osseous, pulmonary, cutaneous) lesion(s)
Cytologic examination of any effusion
Radioisotopic evaluation with gallium-67 when the results of other conventional diagnostic procedures are not conclusive
Staging laparotomy with splenectomy, needle and wedge biopsy of liver, and biopsies of para-aortic, mesenteric, portal, and splenic hilar lymph nodes indicated after negative bone marrow biopsy in initial stages (clinical stage I to II) only if therapeutic decisions will depend on the identification of occult abdominal involvement

Bilateral bone marrow biopsy (not aspiration) is required in all patients. Biopsy of specific sites to determine involvement is helpful only if a positive result would alter the treatment approach. A guided bone biopsy using CT or a percutaneous or even open lung biopsy may be necessary when evidence of involvement is otherwise equivocal.

Although the laboratory investigations listed in Table 2 may not necessarily contribute directly to staging, they may influence treatment modification and guide further investigations to other possible sites of disease. Most of these studies should be repeated after the initial treatment to assess remission status or to restage in the presence of a single recurrence. Once a patient has been determined to be free of Hodgkin's disease, follow-up examinations are recommended every 2 to 3 months for the first year, with physical examinations, chest radiographs, and abdominal radiographs for patients who had a prior positive lymphangiogram. In addition to routine laboratory tests, determination of sequential erythrocyte sedimentation rate and serum lactate dehydrogenase levels is helpful in following patients with Hodgkin's disease. A serial increase in either of these two laboratory tests from previously normal values is predictive of recurrent lymphoma. From time to time, patients in continuous complete remission should be carefully evaluated to rule out delayed iatrogenic morbidity (e.g., sterility, cardiac and pulmonary damage, second malignancies).

PROGNOSTIC INDICATORS

The major unfavorable prognostic factor is tumor mass (e.g., bulky mediastinal lymphoma, multiple extranodal involvement, five or more splenic nodules). The biologic implications of large tumor volume have been extensively studied: the greater the tumor cell population, the more likely it is to contain significant numbers of various classes of drug-resistant cells. Disease progression while on chemotherapy or short-term complete remission despite intensive multiple drug regimens indicates poor prognosis because of primary cell resistance. In general, prognosis is inversely related to age, because children and young adults fare better than older people. In particular, patients older than 60 years often present with advanced disease and other medical problems that cause difficulties in the proper staging and treatment of their lymphoma. Recent observations have confirmed that lymphocyte-depleted Hodgkin's disease is a rare but very aggressive form of lymphoma whose prognosis is unfavorable because of widespread nodal and extranodal involvement. In general, the presence of systemic (B) symptoms and male gender carry unfavorable prognostic significance, especially in patients with advanced disease.

PRINCIPLES OF MANAGEMENT

As a consequence of multiple trials, there are a variety of treatment options for almost every disease stage. Physicians should not forget these points: (1) Total tumor cell burden and optimal drug dose intensity remain the most critical treatment variables. (2) Primary tumor cell resistance is the major stumbling block for all chemotherapy regimens. (3) Mainly because of the known limitations of radiotherapy alone in stages II and III and the risk that splenectomy might contribute to the incidence of fulminant infections and second malignancies, staging laparotomy has been almost completely abandoned. (4) Lymphography is likewise falling into disuse, and consequently the decrease in intensity and accuracy of staging procedures makes combined-modality treatment a necessity to ensure optimal results in terms of cure rate with the first treatment approach. However, careful patient selection remains important to identify patients who will benefit from combined modality therapy.

Among the several polydrug regimens available for the treatment of Hodgkin's disease (Table 3), doxorubicin (Adriamycin), bleomycin, vinblastine, dacarbazine (ABVD) has been confirmed in recent years to

TABLE 3. **Commonly Used Drug Regimens in the Treatment of Hodgkin's Disease**

Drug Regimen	Conventional Dose (mg/m²)	Route	Cycle Days*
ABVD			
Doxorubicin (Adriamycin)	25	IV	1 and 15
Bleomycin (Blenoxane)	10	IV	1 and 15
Vinblastine (Velban)	6	IV	1 and 15
Dacarbazine (DTIC-Dome)	375	IV	1 and 15
MOPP			
Nitrogen mustard (Mustargen)	6	IV	1 and 8
Vincristine (Oncovin)	1.4	IV	1 and 8
Procarbazine (Matulane)	100	PO	1 to 14
Prednisone†	40	PO	1 to 14
ChlVPP			
Chlorambucil (Leukeran)	6	PO	1 to 14
Vinblastine	6	IV	1 and 8
Procarbazine	100	PO	1 to 14
Prednisone	40	PO	1 to 14
LOPP			
Chlorambucil	6	PO	1 to 14
Vincristine	1.4	IV	1 and 8
Procarbazine	100	PO	1 to 14
Prednisone	40	PO	1 to 14
VBM			
Vinblastine	6	IV	1 and 8
Bleomycin	10	IV	1 and 8
Methotrexate	30	IV	1 and 8
MOPP-ABVD in alternating monthly cycles—Same as for MOPP and ABVD			
MOPP-ABV hybrid			
Nitrogen mustard	6	IV	1
Vincristine	1.4 (maximum 2)	IV	1
Procarbazine	100	PO	1 to 7
Prednisone	40	PO	1 to 14
Doxorubicin	35	IV	8
Bleomycin	10	IV	8
Vinblastine	6	IV	8

* Each cycle lasts 28 days.
† During cycles 1 and 4.
Abbreviations: IV = intravenously; PO = orally.

be superior, alone or with irradiation, to the classic MOPP. In fact, ABVD is able to achieve a comparatively high incidence and duration of complete remission with less severe myelosuppression, allowing a more intensive dose administration of doxorubicin and vinblastine than nitrogen mustard and procarbazine, and a virtual absence of alkylating-induced sterility and acute leukemia. VBM combined with radiation has been shown in a long-term experience at Stanford University to be practically devoid of sterility and leukemogenesis.

TREATMENT GUIDELINES

Stage I and II with No Bulky Adenopathy

Many physicians still prefer to use staging laparotomy. After this surgical procedure, patients with supradiaphragmatic disease and no bulky mediastinal or extranodal involvement are treated with subtotal nodal irradiation delivered with high-energy equipment at conventional tumoricidal doses (involved areas, 40 to 44 Gy; uninvolved areas, 35 Gy). In rare patients (4 to 5%) with subdiaphragmatic nonbulky Hodgkin's disease, radiotherapy is administered through an inverted Y field including the splenic pedicle in stage I and through total nodal irradiation (including the mediastinum) in stage II, respectively. With this strategy, if radiotherapy is impeccably delivered, the 10-year relapse-free survival (RFS) is about 80% in patients with stage I disease or those without systemic symptoms. In contrast, in stage IIB patients presenting with all three systemic symptoms, prognosis following extensive radiotherapy alone is extremely poor, because the 5-year freedom from relapse is only about 40%. In this subset of patients, however, laparotomy is no longer performed, and combined-modality therapy is recommended. Late relapses, (i.e., 3 years or more after completion of radiotherapy) are 10 to 20% and are often related to technique; also, they occur more often in patients with stage I disease and a nodular sclerosis histology.

Treatment guidelines for patients not subjected to staging laparotomy are less well defined. A full course of MOPP chemotherapy was reported by the National Cancer Institute to yield relapse-free survival of 86% and a total survival of 92% at 10 years. Most clinicians now prefer to use a combined-modality approach with three to four cycles of combination chemotherapy followed by radiotherapy limited to the involved nodal regions. The chemotherapy regimen of choice should exclude alkylating agents (see Table 3) to reduce the risk of second malignancies and drug-related sterility.

Stage I and II with Bulky Adenopathy and/or Limited Extranodal Extension

The large majority of oncologists agree that this stage group should be managed with combined-modality therapy. In general, patients present with multiple supradiaphragmatic adenopathies and may have extension of tumor into the lung, pericardium, or chest wall. Because effective combination chemotherapy is able to induce prompt tumor shrinkage and amelioration of compressive symptoms from mediastinal-hilar adenopathy, medical treatment should precede radiotherapy, which can be delivered as mantle or subtotal nodal irradiation including spleen once four to six cycles of the selected combination are completed (i.e., ABVD or MOPP alternated with ABVD). With this treatment approach, the vast majority of patients begin the radiation program in complete or almost complete clinical remission, and cardiac and pulmonary sequelae following high-dose primary irradiation of huge mediastinal-hilar adenopathy can be reduced, if not avoided. With a combined modality approach, the 5-year remission-free survival (RFS) is approximately 85 to 90%.

Stage IIIA

There is still debate as how to treat this group of patients, which includes various prognostic subsets depending on the extent and the bulkiness of disease. If after careful surgical staging, patients with clinical stage I or II show histologic involvement limited to the lymphatic structures in the upper abdomen that accompany the celiac-axis group of arteries (substage III_1), subtotal or total nodal irradiation may still be the treatment of choice in the absence of bulky adenopathy and extensive splenic involvement.

The controversy arises when there is involvement of low para-aortic nodes and iliac nodes (substage III_2). The results of numerous trials of systemic drug therapy when the lymphographic patterns appear typical for retroperitoneal node involvement have prompted clinicians to avoid staging laparotomy and to use combination chemotherapy with or without radiotherapy. A once-common approach was total nodal irradiation followed by chemotherapy, usually six cycles of MOPP, but this form of treatment carried a high risk of acute leukemia. More recently, in the experience of the Milan Cancer Institute, three cycles of ABVD delivered before and after radiotherapy yielded superior 10-year results (RFS 97%, survival 80%) to those of MOPP plus radiotherapy (RFS 64%, survival 63%) and was devoid of leukemogenesis, irreversible gonadal dysfunction, and clinical or laboratory signs of doxorubicin-related myocardial damage.

In light of contemporary concepts about drug-resistant tumor cells, it appears highly questionable whether further chemotherapy with the same drug regimen after completion of the irradiation program will influence the duration of complete remission. A more recent approach consists first in the delivery of four to six cycles of ABVD chemotherapy to be followed by total nodal irradiation with 30 to 36 Gy if the patient achieves complete or almost complete remission after drug therapy. This approach is particularly useful in patients with extensive Hodgkin's disease and in the presence of bulky mediastinal or para-aortic nodes. To make combined treatment more tolerable, one can limit the radiation program to involved fields or even to the bulky sites of lymphoma. Also, the radiotherapy dose to the mediastinum should not exceed 36 Gy in complete responders to avoid or limit delayed cardiac complications.

Stage IIIB

The treatment options are similar to those for stage $IIIA_2$. Modern chemotherapy regimens often involve ABVD, MOPP alternated with ABVD, or MOPP-ABV (see Table 3). Six cycles are sufficient to achieve complete remission in about 90% of cases. Most clinicians prefer to supplement drug therapy with radiation to previously involved nodal sites in order to maximize tumor cell eradication. Irradiation is deemed necessary in critical areas if adenopathies were bulky at the start of treatment.

Stage IVA and IVB

This group is best managed with intensive full-dose combination chemotherapy. However, it is possible that irradiation limited to the site(s) of initial bulky disease can further improve the long-term RFS. During the past decade, MOPP alternated with ABVD was shown by the Milan Cancer Institute to be superior to MOPP alone in terms of complete remission (89 versus 74%), 10-year freedom from progression (61 versus 37%) and total survival (69 versus 58%). In particular, the superiority of alternating chemotherapy was evident in the subsets known to be prognostically unfavorable or less affected by MOPP chemotherapy. Comparable results were achieved by investigators of the American Intergroup using the MOPP-ABV hybrid regimen and the Cancer and Acute Leukemia Group B using ABVD alone.

It is important to administer chemotherapy through six to eight cycles with the appropriate dose intensity unless peripheral leukocytes are below 3500 per mm^3 and/or platelets are below 100,000 per mm^3, respectively, on the planned day of drug administration. In this case, physicians can decide whether to delay therapy for a few days or continue chemotherapy, reducing temporarily by 50% the dose of myelosuppressive drugs such as nitrogen mustard, procarbazine, doxorubicin, and vinblastine.

Treatment in Children and Adolescents

The biology, natural history, and staging of Hodgkin's disease are no different in children and adolescents than in adults. For many years the treatment of children paralleled that of adults, using large-field radiotherapy and combination chemotherapy. It became clear that a number of sequelae of radiotherapy and chemotherapy were more severe in children than in adults, with an inverse relationship to age. The most widely recognized complication was the impairment of soft tissue and bone growth that accompanied high-dose radiotherapy. More recently, it has become evident that mediastinal radiation of 40 to 44 Gy affects the pericardium, myocardium, endocardium, valves, conduction system, coronary arteries, and other vessels. As far as chemotherapy is concerned, gonadal toxicity in boys and girls remains a major problem when the drug regimen includes alkylating agents. Because most children effectively treated are expected to be long-term survivors, the most serious of all iatrogenic sequelae is a second malignant neoplasm.

With the aim of decreasing undesirable side effects of therapy, a new treatment strategy for children and adolescents actively growing and developing at the time of diagnosis was devised in the late 1960s at Stanford University. The strategy consisted of low-dose radiotherapy (20 to 25 Gy) and combination chemotherapy. Because of its enormous success regardless of stage, this combined modality approach has become the standard treatment for children who have not yet attained full growth. With time, staging laparotomy was omitted and ABVD or MOPP-ABVD replaced MOPP and its variants. Furthermore, 6 monthly cycles of chemotherapy preceded radiotherapy. In experienced hands, long-term survival rates range from 84 to 95%. The incidence of severe late sequelae has dramatically decreased, although some late effects of therapy (e.g., solid tumors, coronary artery disease) beyond the fifteenth year from the time of diagnosis will require longer follow-up investigation.

Salvage Chemotherapy

Relapse from Primary Radiotherapy. After proper restaging, further irradiation can be delivered, if technically feasible, when the relapse occurs in a single lymph node chain after 5 years from completion of the primary irradiation program. In all other instances, combination chemotherapy should be preferred. Recent results indicate that doxorubicin-containing regimens (ABVD, MOPP-ABVD) can yield superior results to those of MOPP. Chemotherapy should be administered for a minimum of six cycles or to complete tumor remission plus two consolidation cycles.

Relapse After a Year. If the first complete remission lasts longer than 12 months, retreatment with the original drug regimen or a program that does not involve cross-resistance remains the standard approach; it can yield a second complete remission in about 80% of patients, and in about half of the cases remission is durable.

Relapse in Resistant Patients. Most patients who do not attain complete remission following adequately delivered chemotherapy and those with complete remission lasting less than 12 months are considered resistant to conventional drug programs. Although treatment with non–cross-resistant drugs can be tried, objective tumor response occurs in only 40% of patients, complete durable remissions are rare, and the 5-year survival rate is about 20%. Thus, in these resistant tumors, a program of high-dose chemotherapy with autologous stem cell or bone marrow transplantation is indicated.

Bone Marrow Transplantation. In recent years intensive (myeloablative) chemotherapy followed by the reinfusion of autologous bone marrow and/or circulating progenitor cells has been applied to patients with advanced Hodgkin's disease in relapse or refractory to first- or second-line chemotherapy. Several drug regimens are being tested with the support of hematopoietic growth factors. At present, this promising form of salvage therapy remains experimental, and patients should be referred to specialized centers for proper evaluation and treatment. The experience of the Milan Cancer Institute in resistant Hodgkin's disease has been favorable without treatment-induced mortality. Following high-dose sequential chemotherapy, patients relapsing within 12 months from a complete remission achieved after MOPP, ABVD or MOPP-ABVD, experienced a 6-year RFS of 78%. More recently, high-dose chemotherapy strategies have become more manageable and safer, and it is quite possible that in the future the indications to use this new intensive approach will be further expanded to other patient subsets.

Treatment-Related Morbidity

The most serious consequence of curative therapy for Hodgkin's disease is second malignancies, most commonly acute nonlymphocytic leukemia, myelodysplastic syndromes including preleukemia, and diffuse aggressive non-Hodgkin's lymphomas. In patients treated with alkylating agents, procarbazine, or nitrosourea derivatives (BCNU, CCNU), the risk of leukemia within 10 years is 3 to 4%, while after ABVD the figure is around 1%. This risk seems to be increased when patients are subjected to splenectomy or are older than 40 years at the time of systemic treatment and when combined treatment modality is used, especially if salvage MOPP is given after radiation failure (over 15%). The overall risk of non-Hodgkin's lymphomas is about 2%. The risk of developing a secondary solid tumor is continuing to increase beyond 10 years (a finding not seen with leukemia), and the risk is highest in older patients; so far, approximately two thirds of the tumors have occurred in the radiotherapy field.

Gonadal dysfunction is another important iatrogenic toxicity that has a considerable effect on the quality of life of patients with Hodgkin's disease. A few cycles of MOPP or MOPP-like combinations induce azoospermia in 90 to 100% of patients, and this finding is associated with germinal hyperplasia and increased follicle-stimulating hormone levels, with normal levels of luteinizing hormone and testosterone. In addition, only 10 to 20% of patients eventually show recovery of spermatogenesis after as much as 10 years. ABVD chemotherapy produces only a limited and transient germ cell toxicity; following MOPP alternated with ABVD, the incidence of permanent azoospermia is about 50%. Young men undergoing MOPP or MOPP-ABVD can store their sperm prior to chemotherapy; however, both physicians and patients should be aware that about one third of male patients with Hodgkin's disease have low sperm count or sperm motility before starting cytotoxic treatment. About half of women become amenorrheic, and premature ovarian failure appears to depend on age (over 30 years, 75 to 85%; under 30 years, about 20%). This is most probably related to the total dose of drugs and is a progressive rather than an all-or-none phenomenon.

Pericarditis, both acute and chronic, is the most common symptomatic cardiovascular complication of mediastinal irradiation. The incidence of pericarditis is related to the dose, dose rate, and volume irradiated. Clinically evident pericarditis occurs in about 15% of patients following anteroposterior fields from a linear accelerator to a mean mediastinal dose of 44 Gy. Pericardial effusions develop in 25 to 30% of patients within 2 years of radiation. Surgical stripping of the pericardium remains the only definitive therapy for chronic constrictive pericarditis. Radiation-induced myocardial fibrosis at the subclinical level occurs in more than 50% of irradiated patients. Those who receive mediastinal irradiation of 40 to 44 Gy, particularly children and adolescents, run an increased risk of death from coronary artery and other cardiac diseases. Chronic cardiomyopathy may occur after anthracycline administration if the cumulative dose of doxorubicin exceeds 400 to 450 mg per m^2. Careful cardiac screening of treated patients is now highly recommended, for high-dose mediastinal irradiation can predispose to premature coronary artery disease, and this risk may be further increased by the administration of anthracyclines.

Acute radiation pneumonitis and chronic restrictive fibrosis are the most important pulmonary complications of mantle irradiation. Both are related to the total dose, dose rate, and volume of lung tissue irradiated. The overall incidence is about 20%. Patients with relapsed Hodgkin's disease who receive total body irradiation in preparation for bone marrow transplantation are also at risk for pneumonitis. The drugs with greatest potential for pulmonary toxicity are bleomycin and BCNU. In patients treated with ABVD followed by radiotherapy, overt bleomycin-related lung toxicity is uncommon, and no pulmonary damage was seen in patients given MOPP alternated with ABVD.

HODGKIN'S DISEASE: RADIATION THERAPY

method of
JOACHIM YAHALOM, M.D.
Memorial Sloan-Kettering Cancer Center
New York, New York

Radiation therapy (RT) plays an important role in the management of all stages of Hodgkin's disease (HD). The overall cure rate for HD is 75%, and since HD is sensitive to radiation and to many chemotherapeutic drugs, more than one effective treatment option often exists. Although RT alone maintains an excellent track record as a primary treatment for early-stage HD, a combined-modality approach (chemotherapy followed by radiotherapy) has become in recent years a popular and effective alternative to RT alone in most centers. Combined-modality therapy requires less stringent staging methods compared with those used for RT alone and allows a reduction in field size and radiation dose in many patients. The decrease in extent of RT may theoretically reduce future long-term complications attributed to irradiation. As the most potent single treatment modality, RT also plays an important role in the management of advanced-stage HD and in salvage programs that include high-dose chemoradiotherapy with stem cell transplantation.

Effective treatment of HD is complex and requires the skills of a multidisciplinary team during staging of the disease and subsequent treatment. In addition, the use of a modern, high-quality radiotherapy facility staffed with an experienced team has been shown to significantly affect the treatment results.

STAGING

Precise delineation of the extent of nodal and extranodal involvement with HD according to a standard staging classification system is critical for selection of the proper treatment strategy. Detailed documentation of the extent of disease will also provide the baseline for evaluating the response to therapy and for monitoring for potential relapse. Accurate determination of disease sites is mandatory for the design of RT fields. The use of a standard staging system also allows comparison of the results of therapeutic interventions in different clinical trials.

The Ann Arbor staging classification has been the basis for treatment decisions for patients with HD since 1971. It was originally designed to distinguish between patients who would benefit from extended-field radiotherapy from those who would require systemic chemotherapy. Thus, the staging system is an anatomic one that describes the sites of tumor in relation to the diaphragm. The Ann Arbor staging classification was revised at a meeting in Cotswold, England. The most important contribution of the Cotswold classification is the recognition of the importance of tumor bulk, with addition of a definition of bulky disease. The updated staging classification is detailed in Table 1.

The assignment of stage is based upon the number of sites of involvement, whether lymph nodes are involved on both sides of the diaphragm, whether this involvement is bulky (particularly in the mediastinum), whether there is contiguous extranodal involvement (E sites) or disseminated extranodal disease, and in addition, whether typical systemic symptoms (B symptoms) are present. In defining the stage of disease, it is important to note how the information was obtained, because this reflects on remaining uncertainties in the extent of disease evaluation. The clinical stage (CS) refers to information that has been obtained by initial biopsy, history and physical examination, and radiographic studies only. The pathologic stage (PS) is determined by more extensive surgical assessment of potentially involved sites, e.g., by surgical staging laparotomy and splenectomy.

The presence of B symptoms also affects the prognosis with HD. In obtaining the history, attention should be paid to the presence or absence of unexplained fever, drenching night sweats, or significant weight loss—the B symptoms. In our experience, the presence of generalized pruritus is also a serious adverse prognostic symptom.

In addition to a careful physical examination, the following laboratory studies are important. Blood studies include a complete blood count, erythrocyte sedimentation rate (ESR), and liver function tests. Abnormalities should lead to careful evaluation for the presence of disease in bone marrow, liver, or bone. The ESR has some prognostic importance and is useful as an indicator of potential relapse. In all patients, a bone marrow biopsy is obtained for pathologic examination.

TABLE 1. **Cotswold Staging Classification for Hodgkin's Disease**

Stage I	Involvement of a single lymph node region or a lymphoid structure (e.g., spleen, thymus, Waldeyer's ring)
Stage II	Involvement of two or more lymph node regions on the same side of the diaphragm (i.e., the mediastinum is a single site, hilar lymph nodes are lateralized); the number of anatomic sites should be indicated by a subscript (e.g., II_2)
Stage III	Involvement of lymph node regions or structures on both sides of the diaphragm III_1: With or without involvement of splenic, hilar, celiac, or portal nodes III_2: With involvement of para-aortic, iliac, or mesenteric nodes
Stage IV	Involvement of extranodal site(s) beyond that designated E
Designations applicable to any stage	
A:	No symptoms
B:	Fever, drenching sweats, weight loss
X:	Bulky disease More than one third the width of the mediastinum Maximal dimension of nodal mass of more than 10 cm
E:	Involvement of a single extranodal site contiguous or proximal to a known involved nodal site
CS:	Clinical stage
PS:	Pathologic stage

From Portlock CS, Yahalom J: Hodgkin's disease. *In* Bennett JC, Plum F (eds): Cecil Textbook of Medicine, 20th ed. Philadelphia, WB Saunders Co, 1996, p 949.

Evaluation of the Chest

The standard chest film provides basic information regarding the extent of disease in the chest. We also perform routine thoracic computed tomography (CT) scanning in all patients. The incremental data on thoracic involvement obtained with CT scans of the chest are important for the design of the radiation field and for assessment of response. Since the thoracic CT scan can remain abnormal for a long period after completion of therapy, evaluation of pretreatment involvement and of response to a therapy is assisted by a gallium scan, a sensitive indicator of disease above the diaphragm, particularly when a dose of 10 millicuries and single photon emission computed tomography (SPECT) are employed. Negative results on a follow-up gallium scan support the supposition that there is no active disease after completion of treatment even in the presence of residual abnormality on the CT scan.

Evaluation of the Abdomen and Pelvis

CT scanning and bipedal lymphography are essential complementary imaging studies for the evaluation of the abdomen and pelvis. Lymphography accurately evaluates the opacified retroperitoneal and pelvic lymph nodes and is helpful in the design of radiation fields and in assessing the response to therapy. The celiac, splenic hilar, porta hepatis, and mesenteric nodes are not opacified during lymphography and are best evaluated with a CT scan. Unfortunately, even modern imaging studies fail to detect abdominal disease (mostly splenic involvement) in approximately 20 to 30% of patients with CS I or II HD. Hence, surgical staging by laparotomy is appropriate if the findings will influence the subsequent treatment plan. Negative findings at staging laparotomy may allow treatment of early-stage supradiaphragmatic HD with a mantle radiation field alone, eliminating the need to irradiate the para-aortic nodes and the spleen. In recent years, most of our patients have been staged clinically (without a staging laparotomy) and received combined-modality therapy or RT alone, the selection being based on clinical prognostic factors and patient preference.

During the staging process and prior to possible splenectomy or splenic RT, patients should receive a pneumococcal vaccine (Pneumovax), and the option of sperm banking should be presented to male patients.

RADIATION THERAPY

Proper irradiation technique requires the use of linear accelerators that produce 6- to 10-MV photons and have a source-to-skin distance of 120 to 150 cm to permit the delivery of a relatively homogeneous dose to large fields. Careful treatment planning is based on the imaging information obtained during the staging process and transfer of the disease volumes into the simulation films manually or, preferably, using CT-simulation equipment and software such as Aqusim. Simulation is performed on a simulator that duplicates the features of the treatment unit and should be done with the patient in the treatment position with appropriate immobilization devices. Port film verification is obtained on a weekly basis and the clinical set-up is checked regularly.

Radiation Fields

Successful therapy with radiation alone requires treatment of all clinically involved lymph nodes and all nodal and extranodal regions at risk for subclinical involvement. The HD radiation fields were designed to conform to the philosophy of extending treatment beyond the immediately involved area, while accounting for normal tissue tolerance and the technical constraints of field size. To avoid excessive toxicity, the radiation fields are treated sequentially, the total dose is fractionated, and the irradiated volumes are carefully tailored with the use of individualized cerrobend blocks. When patients require separate treatment of adjacent regions, the calculation of field separation is exceedingly important to avoid overlap at the spinal cord.

The Involved Field

The involved field of irradiation refers to the site or sites of clinical involvement but may be extended to adjacent clinically uninvolved lymph node sites (usually immediately above and below the involved site). Involved-field irradiation is commonly used when RT is given as an adjunct to chemotherapy.

The Mantle Field

The radiation field that covers most lymph node areas above the diaphragm is called the "mantle." Extending from the base of the mandible to the diaphragm, the mantle field covers the submandibular, cervical, supraclavicular, infraclavicular, axillary, mediastinal, and hilar nodal areas. Individually contoured cerrobend blocks shield the lungs and the cardiac apex. In addition, depending on anatomy and disease location, supplementary blocks are placed over the humeral heads, occiput, and mouth posteriorly and anteriorly. We also insert half-value-layer blocks to shield the larynx anteriorly and the cervical cord posteriorly throughout the treatment course. If high cervical lymph nodes (above the thyroid notch) are involved, the preauricular nodes are treated prophylactically with a dose of 30 to 36 Gy.

The Subdiaphragmatic Fields

The classic subdiaphragmatic radiation field for HD is the inverted Y, which includes the major lymph node regions from the diaphragm to the femoral areas. Sequential treatment to the mantle and inverted Y fields is termed "total lymphoid irradiation" (TLI). When TLI is indicated, we often divide the inverted Y field into two fields that are irradiated sequentially, with a 2-week break in between to allow bone marrow recovery. The upper field, called the "para-aortic field," includes all the para-aortic lymph nodes between the aortic bifurcation and the bottom of the mantle field. The para-aortic field is normally positioned to encompass the lateral transverse processes of the lumbar vertebrae unless imaging data or surgical findings indicate more extensive disease. This field also includes the spleen and the splenic hilar nodes. If the spleen has been removed, only the splenic pedicle is included. Attention should be paid to the location of the kidneys, as they may be partially included in the field and proper shielding can decrease the irradiated renal volume. The inferior border of the para-aortic field is placed at the bottom of the L4 vertebral body.

The pelvic field encompasses the iliac, inguinal, and femoral nodes. The superior border is at the level of L5, matched with an appropriate gap to the bottom of the para-aortic field. A customized cerrobend block shields the midline structures that are not at risk. The large central block covers the bladder, rectum, and centrally transposed ovaries in women and the testes in male patients. We use a double-thickness midline block and, in males, a scrotal shield to decrease the dose to the testes or centrally placed ovaries to 3 to 8% of the fractionated total dose. Iliac wing blocks are placed to spare bone marrow.

Often, it is not necessary to treat the pelvic lymph nodes, and only the mantle and the para-aortic fields are irradiated in sequence. The treatment is then termed "subtotal lymphoid irradiation" (STLI).

Dose Considerations

When radiation alone is used for the treatment of HD, the standard total dose to each field is 36 Gy delivered in daily fractions of 1.8 Gy over a period of 4 weeks. In patients who receive RT as their only treatment, irradiation is intensified in clinically involved areas by the addition of an individually tailored boost of 5.4 Gy to 9 Gy in three to five fractions to bring the total dose to these areas to 41.4 to 45 Gy. Patients who receive RT for consolidation after chemotherapy receive a total dose of 30 to 36 Gy in fractions of 1.5 to 1.8 Gy.

We use opposed anterior and posterior fields that are evenly weighted, and both fields are treated daily. Special clinical situations may require treatment of the entire cardiac silhouette to a dose of 15 Gy. When irradiation of the whole lung is considered, treatment with partial (37%) transmission blocks allows concomitant low-dose irradiation of the lungs during full-dose mantle irradiation. When whole-liver irradiation is considered, the use of a partial (50%) transmission liver block during irradiation of the para-aortic field will keep the dose below the radiation tolerance of the liver.

Treatment Recommendation by Stage

Stages I and II

For patients with stage IA or IIA disease and no unfavorable features (such as the presence of bulky disease or more than 3 involved sites), RT alone is an excellent treatment option. Treatment includes mantle irradiation to a dose of 36 Gy, followed by a boost of 5.4 to 9 Gy to clinically involved areas. This is followed by prophylactic para-aortic and splenic-field irradiation to a total dose of 36 Gy. Patients in whom a staging laparotomy showed no disease below the diaphragm can be given mantle irradiation alone. Patients with lymphocyte-predominance histology rarely have involvement of the mediastinum and can be given "mini-mantle" irradiation (with the mediastinum fully shielded) or involved-field irradiation.

With subtotal lymphoid irradiation, approximately 70 to 80% of CS/PS I and II patients will achieve a complete response (CR) and never have a relapse. The remaining 20 to 30% generally enter CR but later relapse. Most of these relapsing patients, however, are subsequently cured with combination chemotherapy, so that the overall cure rate (10-year actuarial survival) for CS/PS I and II patients is about 90%.

An alternative treatment approach for patients with stage I or II disease (including those with unfavorable features such as B symptoms, bulky disease, and more than three sites) is four to six cycles of ABVD (doxorubicin [Adriamycin], bleomycin, vinblastine, dacarbazine) chemotherapy followed by mantle or involved-field RT to a dose of 30 to 36 Gy. The cure rate for the group with early-stage disease but unfavorable features is approximately 80%. There are insufficient data to recommend treatment with chemotherapy alone for patients with early-stage HD.

Stage IIIA

For most patients with stage IIIA HD, the recommended treatment is chemotherapy followed by irradiation of the initially involved sites. We achieved encouraging results by combining ABVD chemotherapy with subsequent mantle and para-aortic/splenic-field irradiation to a dose of 30 to 36 Gy in patients with CS IIIA disease. We add a pelvic field only when this area is clinically involved. The 5-year relapse-free survival rate with this program is 80 to 90%.

Stages IIIB, IVA, and IVB

In stages IIIB and IV, the primary treatment modality is clearly combination chemotherapy. However, subsequent to effective chemotherapy, adjunctive RT has an important role in decreasing the relapse rate in patients with advanced-stage disease who have attained a complete response with chemotherapy. In our experience, most of the relapses in patients with advanced-stage disease occur in unirradiated nodal sites that were originally documented to be involved with HD.

This predictable pattern of relapse is not limited to bulky sites alone but extends to all sites of clinically detectable disease. Studies at Memorial Sloan-Kettering Cancer Center (MSKCC) and other institutions have demonstrated a significant improvement in disease-free survival and in overall survival for patients who received adjuvant radiation therapy to all sites of initial involvement, compared with patients who received chemotherapy alone or received post-chemotherapy irradiation to only selected sites. We advocate detailed delineation of all sites of disease prior to the initiation of chemotherapy in patients with stage III or IV disease to assist in defining the irradiated volumes. Following induction of response with effective chemotherapy regimens such as ABVD, MOPP/ABVD (mechlorethamine, vincristine [Oncovin], procarbazine, and prednisone with the ABVD agents), or Stanford V (mechlorethamine, doxorubicin, vinblastine, vincristine, bleomycin, etoposide, and prednisone), the patients undergo rigorous restaging to confirm CR. Those in CR receive irradiation to all originally involved sites. In general, the design of treatment fields follows the same outline described for primary irradiation fields. The fields are irradiated sequentially to a total dose of 30 to 36 Gy.

Salvage Therapy in Refractory or Relapsed Disease

The majority of HD patients who relapse after RT alone are managed successfully with combination chemotherapy. ABVD is our regimen of choice, and RT to previously unirradiated areas of relapse is added. On the other hand, patients with advanced-stage HD whose disease remains refractory to chemotherapy or who relapse within the first year after completion of chemotherapy have a poor prognosis with standard-dose chemotherapy salvage regimens. At MSKCC we developed a salvage program for patients who had not previously received radiotherapy and who failed to respond to multiple chemotherapy regimens. This treatment program incorporates reinduction with ifosfamide, carboplatin, and etoposide (ICE) and involved-field RT, followed by accelerated hyperfractionated TLI with high-dose chemotherapy and autologous peripheral blood stem cell transplantation (PBSCT). Patients who received prior RT receive ICE, pre-transplant involved-field RT, and high-dose chemotherapy followed by PBSCT. High-dose chemoradiation salvage programs at MSKCC have yielded a 5-year event-free survival rate of 50%.

Special Considerations in the Treatment of Children

The cure rate for children with stage I and stage II HD is excellent. However, prepubertal children who have not completed their growth may develop intraclavicular narrowing and a decreased crown-to-rump length following mantle and para-aortic irradiation. In prepubertal children, treatment with chemotherapy and low-dose (21 to 24 Gy) involved-field or extended-field irradiation is the preferred approach. The cure rate is approximately 90%, and with low-dose irradiation the effect on growing bones and muscles is minimal.

Side Effects and Complications

Acute Side Effects

Expected transient side effects during mantle irradiation can include localized hair loss in irradiated areas, mild pharyngitis, mouth dryness, change in taste, dry cough, mild dysphagia, nausea and loss of appetite, mild skin reaction, and fatigue and loss of energy. Generally, these side effects can be managed symptomatically and subside gradually after the completion of RT.

The main side effects of subdiaphragmatic irradiation are loss of appetite, nausea and vomiting, mild diarrhea, and urinary frequency. These reactions are usually mild, can be minimized with standard appropriate medications, and disappear shortly after the completion of treatment.

Subacute Side Effects

Fatigue and loss of energy are common symptoms during and after radiotherapy. Although most patients are able to continue their routine activities during treatment, it often takes 6 months after completion of RT for restoration of full baseline energy levels.

Patients with HD have a propensity to develop herpes zoster infection within 2 years after treatment. Usually the infection is confined to a single dermatome and is self-limited. If the cutaneous eruption is identified promptly, systemic acyclovir (Zovirax) will limit the duration and intensity of the infection.

L'hermitte's sign develops in approximately 15% of patients receiving mantle irradiation. The syndrome is characterized by an electric shock sensation radiating down the backs of both legs when the head is flexed. Onset is generally at 6 weeks to 3 months after completion of mantle RT, and the problem resolves spontaneously after a few months. It may be secondary to transient demyelinization of the spinal cord and is not associated with late or permanent damage to the cord.

Radiation pneumonitis occurs in fewer than 5% of patients; those who had extensive mediastinal disease are affected more often. Symptomatic management may be adequate, but some patients require corticosteroids. Acute pericarditis occurs in 2 to 5% of patients; this complication has become rare with modern radiotherapy techniques. It can be managed with nonsteroidal anti-inflammatory drugs, and symptoms usually subside within a few weeks.

Late Complications

Late complications include hypothyroidism, sterility, pulmonary fibrosis, cardiac damage, transverse myelitis, growth abnormalities in children, and secondary malignancies.

Subclinical hypothyroidism develops in about one third of patients after mantle irradiation. This is detected by elevation of the sensitive thyroid-stimulating hormone (TSH). Thyroid replacement with L-thyroxine is recommended, even for asymptomatic patients, to prevent overt hypothyroidism and to decrease the risk for development of benign thyroid nodules.

Irradiation of the pelvis may have deleterious effects on fertility and gonadal function. Irradiation of the mantle and para-aortic fields alone does not increase the risk of sterility. However, chemotherapy, particularly the MOPP regimen, has detrimental effects on the fertility of almost all men and most women.

With modern radiotherapy techniques, constrictive pericarditis and symptomatic pulmonary fibrosis are very rare complications of mantle irradiation. Mediastinal irradiation is associated with an increased risk of coronary heart disease. Long-term observations of morbidity patterns in survivors of HD indicate that mediastinal irradiation carries an increased risk of coronary heart disease. To minimize this complication, patients should be monitored and advised about the control of other established risk factors for coronary heart disease such as smoking, hyperlipidemia, hypertension, and poor dietary and exercise habits.

Development of a second cancer is a well-recognized hazard for patients cured of HD. Secondary acute nonlymphocytic leukemia (ANLL) is clearly evoked by certain chemotherapy regimens (e.g., MOPP or MOPP-like combinations) with or without radiotherapy. Secondary solid tumors were observed after RT alone, chemotherapy alone, and combined-modality therapy. The most frequent solid tumors reported after HD are lung cancer, breast cancer, stomach cancer, and melanoma. Patients cured of HD are also at high risk for late (10 to 15 years) development of non-Hodgkin's lymphoma. Cigarette smoking should be strongly discouraged because the increase in lung cancer after mantle irradiation has been detected mostly in smokers. The increase in breast cancer is inversely related to the age at HD treatment: in women irradiated after the age of 30 years, no increase in the risk of breast cancer has been found. Breast cancer is curable in its early stages, and early detection has a significant impact on survival. Breast examination should be part of the routine follow-up program for women cured of HD, and routine mammography should begin about 8 years after treatment of HD.

ACUTE LEUKEMIA IN ADULTS

method of
RICHARD A. LARSON, M.D.
University of Chicago Pritzker School of Medicine
Chicago, Illinois

After two decades of incremental improvements in therapy, acute myeloid leukemia (AML) and acute lymphoblastic leukemia (ALL) are now curable in approximately 50% of adults with good risk features. An improved understanding of prognostic factors has allowed risk stratification, and more appropriate management strategies have led to better outcomes for patients with acute leukemia. Recent trials have tested the concepts of dose intensification and the use of multiple non–cross-resistant agents. New drug development has had relatively little clinical impact, except for the introduction of all-*trans*-retinoic acid (tretinoin [Vesanoid]; ATRA) for acute promyelocytic leukemia (APL). The appropriate role of bone marrow transplantation (BMT) remains to be defined, but progress has been made in elucidating the graft-versus-leukemia effect of donor lymphocytes. Improved antifungal and antiviral therapies have contributed to better supportive care. The ancillary role of hematopoietic growth factors in antileukemia treatment strategies and in supportive care remains investigational.

Management of acute leukemia remains complex, requiring a multidisciplinary and dedicated team approach for optimal results. Therapy remains hazardous, unpleasant, and costly. Most adult patients with acute leukemia still die from the disease. Progress in understanding the molecular biology of leukemia has not yet translated into improved management and survival. Little progress has been made in improving the survival of poor-prognosis groups, especially the elderly, those who develop leukemia after a myelodysplastic syndrome (MDS) or prior cytotoxic exposure (therapy-related leukemia [t-AML]), and those with complex or unfavorable cytogenetic features. Nevertheless, considerable progress has been made. Initial response rates are high, and most patients achieve a remission and recover normal hematopoiesis, at least transiently. The current challenge has shifted from achieving remission to the ultimate eradication of the disease to prevent relapse.

DIAGNOSIS, CLASSIFICATION, AND PROGNOSTIC FACTORS

Acute leukemia is a malignant neoplasm of hematopoietic tissue characterized by the clonal accumulation of immature blood cells in the bone marrow. These abnormal cells are generally arrested in the blast stage of the normal maturation pathway. Aberrations in differentiation and function of blood cells are common. Normal hematopoiesis is suppressed.

Acute leukemia usually manifests with the clinical features of bone marrow failure. Patients may have infection, anemia, or bleeding. Rare presentations include granulocytic sarcoma and skin or central nervous system (CNS) manifestations. The blood usually shows a leukocytosis with normocytic anemia and thrombocytopenia. Circulating blast cells are often present. Sometimes the leukocyte count is low, which is a common feature in APL, for example. In rare cases, patients may present with thrombocytosis.

The most precise diagnosis is made by examining the morphology, cytochemistry, immunophenotype, and chromosomal abnormalities of bone marrow and peripheral blood cells. Bone marrow aspiration and biopsy are the standard diagnostic procedures. Aspiration may be difficult or impossible, (i.e., a "dry tap") in patients with very high marrow cellularity ("packed marrow"). In the most widely used morphologic classification scheme, published by the French-American-British (FAB) Cooperative Group, subgroups of AML are distinguished according to features of lineage differentiation (Table 1). Flow cytometric analysis of cell surface markers is widely available and can accurately distinguish myeloid from lymphoid (and B-cell from T-cell) lineage in most cases. Clear distinction between AML and ALL is not always possible. Rarely, null, biphenotypic, or bilineal acute leukemias occur.

Cytogenetic analysis of an individual patient's leukemia cells has become an increasingly important component of diagnosis before treatment in both AML and ALL. An adequate (>2 mL) sample of bone marrow aspirate from a fresh puncture site should be submitted for cytogenetic

TABLE 1. **French-American-British (FAB) Classification of Acute Leukemia**

FAB Subtype	Morphologic Description	Frequency (%)
M0	Minimally differentiated acute myeloid leukemia (AML)	2–3
M1	Acute myeloblastic leukemia without differentiation	20
M2	Acute myeloblastic leukemia with maturation	25–30
M3	Acute promyelocytic leukemia (APL)	8–15
M4	Acute myelomonocytic leukemia (AMMoL)	20–25
M4Eo	Acute myelomonocytic leukemia with abnormal eosinophils	5
M5	Acute monoblastic leukemia (AMoL) A: poorly differentiated B: well-differentiated	10
M6	Acute erythroblastic leukemia (AEL)	5
M7	Acute megakaryoblastic leukemia (AMegaL)	1–2
	Acute lymphoblastic leukemia (ALL)	
L1	Small, homogeneous lymphoblasts	30–40
L2	Large, heterogeneous lymphoblasts	50–60
L3	Burkitt-type ALL	5

analysis in all patients suspected of having leukemia. Specific and well-characterized recurring chromosomal abnormalities facilitate diagnosis, confirm subtype classification, and have major prognostic value for treatment planning (Table 2).

Age is the most important independent patient variable in determining outcome. Treatment results are best in young adults and are considerably poorer in patients older than 60 years. In addition, young or middle-aged adults may benefit from the availability of BMT for postrelapse rescue. Elderly patients have a lower response rate to remission induction chemotherapy and increased treatment toxicity, in part due to their high incidence of comorbid disorders. The poor survival of elderly patients, however, is not fully explained by their lower tolerance for intensive treatment; the disease itself appears to have a different natural history in this group. Elderly patients with AML are more likely to have had an MDS and are also more likely to have unfavorable cytogenetic features.

Antecedent hematologic disorders such as MDS are a major adverse prognostic factor. Acute leukemia following treatment with alkylating agents or topoisomerase II inhibitors or radiotherapy for a prior cancer has been well described and has a similarly poor outcome with conventional chemotherapy programs.

TREATMENT

General Principles

The goal of remission induction chemotherapy is the rapid restoration of normal bone marrow function. The term "complete remission" (CR) is reserved for patients who have full recovery of normal peripheral blood counts and bone marrow cellularity with less than 5% residual blast cells. Induction therapy aims to reduce the total body leukemia cell population from approximately 10^{12} to below the cytologically detectable level of about 10^9 cells. This is followed by postinduction or remission consolidation therapy, usually comprising one or more courses of chemotherapy designed to eradicate residual leukemia, allowing the possibility of cure. Multiple chemotherapy drugs in high doses are typically used to prevent the emergence of resistant subclones and to limit cumulative and overlapping toxicities. The adjunctive use of lower doses of prolonged remission maintenance therapy lasting 1 to 2 years is commonly used in ALL but has minimal value in AML.

Bone marrow transplantation using an HLA-identical sibling donor is an established treatment modality in acute leukemia and is indicated for suitable high-risk patients in first remission or for any young or middle-aged patient in first relapse or second remission. Allogeneic BMT (alloBMT) has two therapeutic components. Intensive myeloablative therapy is used to eradicate all tumor cells, if possible. In addition, T cells in the donor marrow can produce a graft-versus-leukemia (GvL) immune response that can destroy remaining leukemia cells; this effect has been correlated with improved disease-free survival. Unfortunately, this beneficial immune response is closely associated with acute and chronic graft-versus-host disease (GvHD), a major cause of morbidity and mortality following alloBMT. GvHD can be reduced by T-cell depletion from the donor marrow, but only at the cost of increased rates of graft failure and leukemia relapse. Because the risk of treatment-related mortality increases with age, most centers restrict BMT to patients younger than 60 years old. The use of alloBMT is also limited in part by donor availability: a patient has only a 25 to 30% chance that a sibling will be HLA identical.

Autologous BMT allows the use of myeloablative therapy in patients who lack an allogeneic marrow donor as well as in older patients. The appropriate role for this treatment modality is controversial. Treatment-related morbidity and mortality (<5%) are relatively low, but relapse rates are high, and overall outcomes are not clearly better than in patients who receive intensive but nonablative therapy. The relative contribution to relapse of tumor cell contamination in the reinfused cryopreserved marrow versus the failure of the high-dose therapy to

TABLE 2. **Cytogenetic Subsets in Acute Myeloid Leukemia and Acute Lymphoblastic Leukemia**

Karyotype	Complete Remission Rate	Remission Duration	Treatment Approach
t(8;21)	High	Long	Standard induction with an anthracycline and intensive consolidation with high-dose cytarabine
inv(16)(p13q22) or t(16;16)	High	Intermediate to long	Standard induction with an anthracycline. Intensive consolidation chemotherapy with high-dose cytarabine
t(15;17)	High	Intermediate to long	All-*trans* retinoic acid (ATRA) together with chemotherapy
t(9;11)	High	Intermediate	Standard induction with an anthracycline. Intensive consolidation chemotherapy with high-dose cytarabine
del(5q), +13, +8, −7, inv(3), del(12p), t(9;22), or complex abnormalities	Low	Short	New induction regimens, including use of growth factors during chemotherapy or modulators of drug resistance. BMT in first CR.
t(9;22); t(4;11)	High	Low	Standard ALL remission induction followed by allogeneic BMT in first CR.
t(8;14) or t(2;8) or t(8;22)	High	Intermediate to long	Short duration, high intensity chemotherapy with CNS prophylaxis.

Abbreviations: BMT = bone marrow transplantation; CR = complete remission; CNS = central nervous system.

eradicate all disease in vivo has not been determined. Hematopoietic cells capable of reconstituting bone marrow function can be harvested for autologous transplantation by direct bone marrow aspiration or by apheresis of progenitor cells from peripheral blood. The use of peripheral blood stem cells has not been proven to decrease the risk of relapse, but it does accelerate the rate of hematopoietic reconstitution.

Remission Induction Therapy for Acute Myeloid Leukemia

The most common remission induction regimen used for patients with AML is cytarabine (Cytosar-U) given by continuous intravenous (IV) infusion daily for 7 days plus daunorubicin (Cerubidine) given daily for 3 days (7+3 regimen). Depending on age and patient selection, 60 to 80% of patients achieve a CR. The outcome in general has not been improved by the substitution of other anthracyclines, increasing the dose of cytarabine, or adding a third or fourth drug (Table 3).

Cytarabine in conventional doses of 100 to 200 mg per m^2 per day is generally given by continuous IV infusion for 7 to 10 days. High-dose cytarabine (HDAC) regimens typically use 1000 to 3000 mg per m^2 given intravenously over 1 to 3 hours every 12 hours for 8 to 12 doses. HDAC increases the CR rate to 75 to 90% but at the cost of increased toxicity. Treatment mortality, the rate of early relapse, and overall survival are not clearly improved. In a recent trial, high-dose cytarabine was given for 3 days immediately following a standard 7+3 regimen. The CR rate was 89% among patients less than 65 years old with no prior myelodysplasia.

Attempts have been made to improve the CR rate of induction therapy by adding potentially non–cross-resistant drugs. Etoposide has activity as a single agent in approximately 25% of patients with previously treated AML. In a randomized trial among newly diagnosed patients, the addition of etoposide (VePesid), at 75 mg per m^2 per day for 7 days to cytarabine and daunorubicin (7+3 regimen) produced increased toxicity but also prolonged remission duration in the etoposide arm. There was no survival benefit. A randomized comparison between cytarabine at standard doses versus high doses, both in combination with daunorubicin and etoposide, showed no improvement in the CR rate or overall survival in the HDAC arm, although disease-free survival was significantly prolonged.

Postremission Therapy of Acute Myeloid Leukemia

Additional chemotherapy after a successful remission induction is mandatory to cure AML. The median disease-free survival for patients who receive no additional therapy is 4 to 8 months. When several courses of consolidation chemotherapy are given, survival at 2 to 3 years is 35 to 50% for young and middle-aged adults.

The same induction therapy may be repeated for one or more cycles, with or without dose intensification, or non–cross-resistant drugs can be used for consolidation. There is increasing evidence that high-dose cytarabine (HDAC) provides the best survival for good- and intermediate-prognosis patients. HDAC

TABLE 3. **Acute Myeloid Leukemia Remission Induction Chemotherapy Regimens**

Drugs	Dose	Comment
Cytarabine + Daunorubicin	100 mg/m^2 daily as a continuous infusion for 7 days; 45 mg/m^2 IV push on each of the first 3 days of treatment	"Standard" induction regimen resulting in approximately 60 to 80% remission rate and acceptable toxicity in patients <60 years old.
Cytarabine + Daunorubicin	3 g/m^2 twice daily for a total of 12 doses; 45 mg/m^2 IV push for 3 days following cytarabine	Yields a 90% remission rate, but substantial toxicity precludes postremission therapy in a high proportion of patients.
Cytarabine + Idarubicin	100 mg/m^2 daily as a continuous infusion for 7 days; 13 mg/m^2 IV push on each of first 3 days of treatment	Has produced a greater CR rate (88 vs. 70%) compared to cytarabine/daunorubicin in younger patients. Appears superior to daunorubicin in patients with hyperleukocytosis. Overall survival not clearly superior to "standard" regimen.
Cytarabine + Daunorubicin + Etoposide	100 mg/m^2 daily as a continuous infusion for 7 days; 50 mg/m^2 IV push on each of first 3 days of treatment; 75 mg/m^2 daily for 7 days	Remission rates similar to "standard" induction regimen. Remission duration significantly improved but overall survival comparable to "standard" regimen. May prolong survival in patients <55 years old but at expense of increased toxicity.
Cytarabine + Daunorubicin + Cytarabine (high-dose)	100 mg/m^2 daily as a continuous infusion for 7 days; 45 mg/m^2 IV push on each of the first 3 days of treatment; 2 g/m^2 twice daily on days 8, 9, and 10	High rate of CR after first course in patients <65 years old.

Abbreviations: CR = complete remission.

may be effective in eliminating resistant cell populations that survive induction therapy. The Cancer and Leukemia Group B (CALGB) conducted a randomized trial of consolidation therapy using four courses of cytarabine at low (100 mg per m^2 per day) or intermediate doses (400 mg per m^2 per day) as continuous IV infusions for 5 days or at high doses (3 g per m^2 every 12 hours on days 1, 3, and 5). For patients less than 60 years old with a good or intermediate prognosis, disease-free survival in the HDAC arm was 46% at 3 years compared with 35% for the intermediate-dose and 31% for the low-dose group ($P = 0.003$). There were relatively few relapses in the HDAC group more than 2 years after attaining CR. The best results from consolidation therapy in patients older than 60 years are likely to be achieved with two cycles of daunorubicin (30 to 45 mg per m^2 for 2 days) and cytarabine (100 mg per m^2 per day for 5 days). Alternating courses of other two-drug combinations (e.g., etoposide/cyclophosphamide, mitoxantrone/etoposide, mitoxantrone/cytarabine, or mitoxantrone/diaziquone) appear to provide equivalent disease-free survival.

Most studies reporting on allogeneic or autologous BMT for AML patients in first CR are nonrandomized, and many are retrospective. Considerable selection bias is generated by the delay between remission induction and transplantation and by the entry requirements for good performance status for most trials. Prospective randomized studies comparing intensive consolidation therapy and BMT for patients in first CR have failed to show a clear survival advantage.

Acute Promyelocytic Leukemia

Acute promyelocytic leukemia (FAB M3) is a biologically distinct disease with characteristic clinical, morphologic, and cytogenetic features. Disseminated intravascular coagulation at presentation or soon after the initiation of cytotoxic chemotherapy can cause severe hemorrhage in up to 40% of patients and a high mortality rate. The cytoplasmic granules in the leukemic blasts contain factors with procoagulant as well as fibrinolytic activity.

ATRA (tretinoin) has proved to be a highly effective remission induction agent. ATRA accelerates the terminal differentiation of malignant promyelocytes to mature neutrophils, leading to apoptosis and CR without bone marrow hypoplasia. This effect is a unique consequence of the rearranged PML-RARα gene resulting from the t(15;17), which defines APL. ATRA induction therapy produces CR rates of 80 to 95% in both previously untreated and relapsed patients. Most treatment failure is due to early mortality. Primary resistance is rare. ATRA is neither immunosuppressive nor myelosuppressive. The coagulopathy of APL typically improves rapidly with initiation of treatment. The median times to CR range from 38 to 44 days but may take as long as 90 days. As yet, the drug is available only as an oral preparation. The recommended daily dose is 45 mg per m^2, and ATRA may work best in combination with daunorubicin for remission induction.

One serious and specific complication may occur with ATRA treatment of APL. In 25 to 40% of patients, the retinoic acid syndrome develops within 2 to 21 days after initiation of treatment and is characterized by fever, peripheral edema, pulmonary infiltrates and respiratory distress, hypertension, renal and hepatic dysfunction, and serositis resulting in pleural and pericardial effusions. The syndrome is possibly due to tissue infiltration by maturing malignant promyelocytes and the systemic effects of cytokine release. Many cases are associated with hyperleukocytosis, but the retinoic acid syndrome occurs with normal leukocyte counts in a third of cases. Early recognition and aggressive management with high-dose dexamethasone therapy (10 mg IV every 12 hours for 6 doses) has been effective. Cessation of ATRA therapy alone does not reverse the syndrome. However, once the complication resolves, ATRA can be restarted in most cases.

Management of the coagulopathy associated with APL may be difficult and should be expectant. Coagulation parameters, including fibrinogen, D-dimer, and platelet levels, should be monitored closely. Platelet transfusions and cryoprecipitate or fresh frozen plasma are used to maintain the fibrinogen level above 100 mg per dL and the platelet count above 20,000 per μL. The role of heparin is controversial. Continuous infusions of 5 to 10 units per kg per hour are widely used and appear effective at stopping the consumption of clotting factors. Inhibitors of fibrinolysis should be considered only for life-threatening hemorrhage.

Acute Lymphoblastic Leukemia

Treatment regimens for ALL have evolved empirically into complex schemes that use numerous agents in various doses, combinations, and schedules. Few of the individual components have been tested rigorously in randomized trials; thus, it is difficult to analyze critically the absolute contribution of each drug or dose schedule to the ultimate outcome. Steady improvements in the cure rate for adults have been achieved through more accurate diagnoses, the use of intensive multiagent chemotherapy, attention to potential sanctuary sites such as the CNS, and the appropriate use of allogeneic bone marrow transplantation. Further progress will require large numbers of uniformly evaluated patients to be entered into randomized clinical trials, testing various components of the total therapy that have heretofore been added empirically.

In two sequential trials by the CALGB involving 379 adults, a five-drug induction regimen produced a CR rate of 85% and median duration of remission of 28 months. Cyclophosphamide (1200 mg per m^2) was given on day 1 with daunorubicin (45 mg per m^2) on days 1, 2, and 3. Vincristine (2 mg) was given on days 1, 8, 15, and 22 together with 21 days of prednisone (60 mg per m^2). L-Asparaginase (6000 units per m^2) was given subcutaneously twice per week starting on day 5. The median duration of remission was 34 months for the 237 patients who rapidly achieved CR within 30 days compared with 20 months for the 88 patients who required more than 30 days to enter remission.

Consolidation and Maintenance

Eradication of subclinical or "minimal" residual disease during hematologic remission is the primary aim of the consolidation or intensification phases. Once normal hematopoiesis has been restored, patients are good candidates for aggressive attempts at cure. However, it remains controversial as to how intensive this phase of treatment should be and whether, in fact, relative drug resistance can be overcome by myelosuppressive combinations including bone marrow transplantation. Several nonrandomized studies strongly suggest a benefit from intensive multiagent postremission therapy.

Remission maintenance therapy is still a standard component of the management of ALL, although its benefit has not been established in adults. Standard outpatient maintenance therapy typically utilizes oral 6-mercaptopurine (60 mg per m^2 per day) and methotrexate (20 mg per m^2 per week) with monthly pulses of vincristine and prednisone for 1 to 3 years. The optimal duration for maintenance treatment is unknown.

Central Nervous System Prophylaxis

Central nervous system prophylaxis is an integral step in ALL treatment. The CNS is a common sanctuary for ALL cells as indicated by its frequent involvement at the time of relapse. CNS leukemia is more easily prevented than treated. Less than 10% of adults with ALL have CNS leukemia at diagnosis. Examination of spinal fluid at diagnosis is not necessary in asymptomatic patients. However, without specific attention to CNS prophylaxis, CNS relapse rates range from 21 to 50%. Cranial neuropathies are common sequelae. Symptoms resulting from increased intracranial pressure include headaches, nausea, vomiting, lethargy and papilledema, as well as irritability and nuchal rigidity.

Several methods are currently used for prevention of meningeal leukemia. These include intrathecal (IT) injection of methotrexate and/or cytarabine together with hydrocortisone, intravenous administration of the same chemotherapy agents in high doses with the goal of achieving therapeutic levels in the cerebrospinal fluid (CSF), and cranial irradiation (2400 cGy). Irradiation of the entire spinal cord is quite myelosuppressive and is rarely done.

Hematopoietic Growth Factors

Myelosuppression and the infections that result are common and sometimes fatal complications of intensive chemotherapy. Prolonged myelosuppression can also necessitate long hospital stays and lead to unacceptable delays between scheduled courses of treatment. Such delays compromise dose intensity. With the use of hematopoietic growth factors, neutrophil recovery has been accelerated following chemotherapy for solid tumors as well as after myeloablative therapy and bone marrow transplantation. Several clinical trials now suggest that hematopoietic growth factors may provide important ancillary benefits for adults undergoing treatment for ALL. The major benefit is in older patients.

As yet, growth factors have not had a marked impact on survival or remission duration for patients with AML. Data from several large controlled trials have recently been reported, but the issue remains unsettled. Differences in dose and schedule, and the specific growth factor and chemotherapy agents used, as well as the age group studied, prevent firm conclusions. Even though a more rapid recovery of neutrophils has been observed in some trials, the nadir has not been affected, and thus the incidence of severe infection remains high. At the same time, stimulation of leukemia regrowth by myeloid growth factors appears to be uncommon in vivo. A recent clinical trial suggested that granulocyte colony-stimulating factor (G-CSF) was beneficial when used after consolidation chemotherapy for AML.

ACUTE LEUKEMIA IN CHILDHOOD

method of
C. PHILIP STEUBER, M.D., and
DAVID G. POPLACK, M.D.
Baylor College of Medicine and Texas Children's Cancer Center
Houston, Texas

The acute leukemias constitute approximately 28% of malignancies occurring in children younger than 15 years of age. In contradistinction to adult acute leukemias, in children, acute leukemias of lymphoid origin comprise approximately 80 to 85% of cases, and the remainder are nonlymphoid or myeloid in origin. Using current methodologies, there are very few cases that are not classifiable into one of these two subsets. These infrequent cases may demonstrate features of neither and are considered truly undifferentiated. Although the causes and mechanisms of leukemogenesis remain elusive, associations are recognized with both congenital and acquired predisposing factors such as Down syndrome, familial myeloproliferative disorders, exposure to ionizing radiation, chemical exposures, and immune deficiency states. These circumstances account for only a small portion of all acute leukemia cases in children. The complexity of diagnostic tools and the intensity of modern therapies dictate that children and adolescents with acute leukemia be evaluated and treated in established pediatric treatment facilities.

PRESENTATION AND DIAGNOSIS

Children with acute leukemia generally present with complaints resulting from sequelae of marrow involvement or replacement such as bleeding from thrombocytopenia, pallor due to anemia, infection with neutropenia, and bone or joint pain. Commonly, the child and family members relate a history of nonspecific symptoms that have evolved insidiously, and it is not unusual for the history of the illness to span several weeks before recognition. There may also be objective or subjective findings secondary to extramedullary tissue infiltration with leukemic cells (i.e., hepatosplenomegaly and associated abdominal pain, lymphadenopathy, chloromas, or respiratory distress due to mediastinal masses). In addition to the carefully done history and physical examination, the initial diagnostic evaluation should include a complete blood count, urinalysis, blood chemistries, coagulation studies, and chest radiograph.

Although there may be significant numbers of circulating malignant cells in the peripheral blood at the time of presentation, the diagnosis of acute leukemia is definitively established by evaluation of a bone marrow aspirate. Because the initial diagnosis is the major determinant of therapy, it is of paramount importance that the diagnostic specimen be accurately and thoroughly characterized. It is well recognized that the acute leukemias are a heterogeneous group of disorders exhibiting a variety of clinical and laboratory features at presentation. Consequently, the leukemic cells should undergo meticulous examination including appropriate immunophenotyping and cytogenetic analysis as well as morphologic characterization and cytochemical staining. Errors, omissions, or inadequacies in the evaluation of the diagnostic bone marrow or peripheral blood specimen usually cannot be rectified at a later date.

Acute leukemia is commonly classified or diagnosed using the combination of morphologic features and cytochemical staining patterns defined by the FAB (French-American-British) Cooperative Working Group. Immunologic identification of specific lineage-associated antigens on the surface of the malignant cell is of diagnostic and also prognostic importance. The common, cell differentiation–directed monoclonal antibodies frequently used to diagnose and classify acute leukemia are listed in Table 1.

In addition to providing insights into the biology of acute leukemia, cytogenetic studies are performed to determine structural as well as numeric abnormalities, because both the presence of specific translocations and/or changes in ploidy can have significant diagnostic and prognostic implications. It is commonly a composite of the morphologic, immunologic, and cytogenetic features of the malignant cell population that substantiates the final diagnosis and influences the selection of therapy.

INITIAL MANAGEMENT

At the time of presentation, transfusion support is frequently required to correct the potential or actual complications of anemia and thrombocytopenia. If fever is present, a careful evaluation for infection is necessary, and, particularly if the fever is associated with neutropenia, the empirical use of broad-spectrum antibiotics is indicated. Patients with significant tumor burden, as manifested by extreme leukocytosis, visceromegaly, or metabolic derangements, and who have actual or impending hyperuricemia, with or without renal dysfunction, require careful fluid management accompanied by treatment with urate oxidase or a xanthine oxidase inhibitor. Rarely, such patients may require leukapheresis to reduce the circulating white blood cell (WBC) numbers or dialysis to manage renal failure secondary to disease- or therapy-induced nephropathy.

TABLE 1. **Antibodies Commonly Used to Designate Immunophenotype in Acute Leukemia**

Reactive Cell Type	Cluster of Differentiation (CD) Designation
T cell lineage	2, 3, 5, 7, 8
B cell lineage	10, 19, 20, 21, 24
Myeloid cell lineage	11, 13, 14, 15, 33

ACUTE LYMPHOID LEUKEMIA

Evaluation

The most common childhood malignancy, acute lymphoid leukemia (ALL) has an annual frequency in the United States of approximately 2000 cases. The peak incidence occurs at approximately 2 to 4 years of age. For reasons unknown, there is a slight male and Caucasian predominance. Fever, bleeding, and pain are the most common presenting manifestations. Lymphadenopathy, hepatomegaly, and splenomegaly are the most common findings on physical examination at the time of diagnosis.

The initial evaluation, in addition to comprehensive history and physical examination and laboratory studies, should include a lumbar puncture for cerebrospinal fluid examination. In the majority of cases, the complete blood count shows some degree of anemia and thrombocytopenia. The WBC count is less than 10,000 per μL in a little over half of the cases, and the differential count usually demonstrates circulating blast forms.

As noted previously, the diagnosis is established by precise evaluation of the leukemic cell population. The sample is usually obtained by bone marrow aspiration. The majority (84%) of ALL cases are recognized as FAB-L1, 15% are FAB-L2, and 1% are FAB-L3. Immunophenotyping is done using a panel of monoclonal antibodies specific for various stages of B cell, T cell, and myeloid cell differentiation (see Table 1). Approximately 15% of ALL cases have predominantly T cell markers, another 1 to 2% exhibit mature B cell characteristics (almost all of these are FAB-L3), and in the remaining cases, the leukemic cells are of early B lineage and the disease is termed B-precursor ALL.

Prognostic Factors and Risk Group Assignment

The last three decades have witnessed a dramatic improvement in the outcome for children with ALL. This success is attributed not only to new drug development and the subsequent expanded use of drug combinations but also to the recognition of therapeutic principles and strategies for management of childhood ALL such as the use of preventive central nervous system (CNS) therapy and the use of risk-based individualized systemic therapy regimens. The significance of prognostic factors such as age, WBC count, immunophenotype, and chromosomal patterns has been first established by retrospective analysis of clinical trial outcomes and then subsequently confirmed by prospective studies. As therapy has progressed, emphasis is shifting from the use of clinically determined risk factors to the use of more laboratory-derived ones in selecting treatments. A number of clinical and laboratory characteristics determined at diagnosis are known to be predictive of outcome and are used to select therapies. Patients with ALL are placed into risk groups based on criteria using combinations of these variables that predict clinical outcomes.

Although a multitude of potential prognostic variables have been recognized and incorporated into treatment-assignment algorithms, the relative importance of the presence of any one feature may vary from therapy to therapy. Age at presentation and WBC count are universally accepted as key among these prognostic features. A recent workshop sponsored by the Cancer Treatment Evaluation Program (CTEP) resulted in uniform recommendations for risk assignment using age and WBC count, shown in Table 2. Standardization of these parameters will allow for ease of comparison of outcomes among the various treatment approaches. All B-precursor ALL patients with WBC counts of more than 50,000 per μL are assigned to higher risk groups, as are all patients under age 1 year or over age 10 years. These patients should receive more aggressive treatment regimens. Approximately two thirds of patients are in the standard-risk group, and the rest are in the high-risk group. Using these risk group parameters, the 4-year event-free survival rate for the standard-risk group is 80% and for the high-risk group is 64%.

Among immunophenotypic characteristics, leukemic cell populations that have T cell, mature B cell, or mixed-lineage features (demonstrating both lymphoid and myeloid antigens) have been associated with unfavorable outcome and the need for specific aggressive therapies. As mentioned previously, the majority of ALL cases are recognized as being of early B lineage. However, the independent prognostic significance of the immunophenotypic characteristics of leukemia cells is the subject of some controversy, and although the potential high-risk nature of these findings has been suggested, their eventual role in the evolution of therapeutic strategies and treatment assignment remains to be established.

TABLE 2. **Uniform Age and White Blood Cell (WBC) Count Criteria for Risk Assignment in B-Precursor Acute Lymphocytic Leukemia**

	WBC Count (cell/μL)	
Age	*<50,000*	*≥50,000*
1.00–9.99 y	Standard risk	High risk
<1 y, >10 y	High risk	High risk

Selected cytogenetic aberrations have prognostic connotation. Patients with more than 50 chromosomes per leukemia cell—hyperdiploidy—have demonstrated favorable response patterns to appropriate standard-risk therapies and constitute about 27% of all B-precursor ALL cases. This chromosomal number correlates with a DNA Index (DI) of greater than 1.16. In approximately 42% of cases, the leukemia cell is pseudodiploid, and in 8% of cases it is diploid. Translocations are the most common structural abnormality and occur most frequently in the pseudodiploid and hypodiploid groups. With the exception of the recently described t(12;21), the presence of any translocation in the malignant lymphoid cells at diagnosis has been associated with higher risk of treatment failure. Three specific translocations found in B-precursor ALL — t(4;11), t(1;19), and t(9;22)— are associated with particularly poor outcomes and occur respectively in 5%, 6%, and 4% of newly diagnosed cases.

As therapy has evolved, the relative importance of various risk factors has shifted or vanished, emphasizing the role of the therapy itself as a prognostic determinant. Most children with ALL in the United States are managed using risk-based protocols developed by the two major cooperative groups, the Children's Cancer Group (CCG) and the Pediatric Oncology Group (POG).

Therapy

Modern ALL treatment regimens divide therapy into four main elements: remission induction therapy, consolidation or intensification therapy, CNS preventive therapy, and continuation or maintenance therapy.

Remission Induction

Achievement of completion remission is the first step in the successful therapy of ALL. This is most commonly accomplished by the administration of a 4-week course of weekly vincristine (Oncovin) and a corticosteroid (usually prednisone), accompanied by a third and often a fourth agent such as L-asparaginase (Elspar) and/or an anthracycline such as doxorubicin (Adriamycin) or daunorubicin (Cerubidine). Using three- or four-drug therapy, remission induction rates are commonly reported to be 90 to 95%. It is common practice to use a less toxic three-drug regimen for standard- or low-risk patients and to reserve the more intense regimens of four or more drugs for the higher risk patients. It has been suggested but not firmly established that the use of more intensive induction regimens, although increasing the toxicity of the early treatment, will result in improved long-term outcome. Rate of response during this first month of therapy has been shown to correlate directly with risk of recurrence, and patients whose disease responds rapidly are more likely to have a favorable outcome. During the induction phase it is common practice to initiate some early CNS preventive therapy using intrathecal chemotherapy.

Consolidation or Intensification Therapy

Once complete remission is achieved, a significant amount of additional therapy is required to prevent recurrence. A subsequent period of intensified therapy is recommended and is most often administered immediately following completion of the induction period. This consolidation phase usually lasts approximately 6 months. Consolidation therapy frequently includes the use of multiple agents with differing modes of action given consecutively in different combinations and is intended to eliminate the development of drug resistance. These regimens often use repeated doses of cytarabine, epipodophyllotoxins, anthracyclines, and intermediate- or high-dose methotrexate (Mexate) as well as those drugs given during the successful induction regimen. Another strategy is the use of delayed-intensification "pulses" whereby an intensive multiple-drug regimen is given once or more than once during the first 6 to 12 months of remission, with some form of less intense therapy in the intervening times. No one regimen has recognized superiority, and a wide variety of intensification approaches is currently in use. As with induction therapy, the intensity (and toxicity) of such consolidation programs varies directly with the perceived risk of treatment failure. For patients with mature B-cell ALL, no therapy is recommended after completion of the intensive phase, which lasts approximately 6 months.

Central Nervous System Preventive Therapy

The principle of directed CNS preventive therapy in the management of ALL was one of the major therapeutic advances responsible for the current favorable event-free survival rates. It was long recognized that the development of overt CNS leukemia, which occurred with a high incidence, was a manifestation of treatment failure. It was established that prevention of that occurrence improves overall outcome. In current therapies for lower risk patients, CNS preventive therapy is accomplished by the use of single- or multiple-agent intrathecal therapy. Methotrexate is the most effective single agent in current usage and may be combined with cytarabine and/or hydrocortisone. A series of lumbar punctures—usually totaling 16 to 18 in number—are performed at varying intervals over the duration of the treatment program in order to administer intrathecal medications. The majority of these instillations are given during the early phases of therapy. Patients with high-risk features or those who demonstrate evidence of CNS leukemia at diagnosis require intrathecal chemotherapy and a course of cranial or craniospinal irradiation for optimal management. With modern approaches to treatment, the overall incidence of CNS involvement has been reduced to 5% or less. The optimal timing of cranial or craniospinal radiation therapy for ALL is not established, but when indicated, it is usually administered during the first 3 to 6 months of treatment once remission is well established.

Continuation or Maintenance Therapy

Continuing therapy for 2 to 3 years after remission induction has been established as the standard of care for most forms of B-precursor ALL. For the majority of patients, such maintenance regimens are less intensive than induction and consolidation regimens. They are based on the use of the antimetabolites methotrexate, given intermittently, and 6-mercaptopurine (Purinethol), given daily. Occasional pulses of additional agents such as vincristine and prednisone may be given as adjunctive therapy.

Maintenance therapy may be initiated after the completion of consolidation therapy or administered between intensification pulses and then continued. For select high-risk patients such as older children with T cell ALL, there may be little de-escalation of the intensity of therapy during the later phase of therapy, and continued intensive treatment during maintenance may be recommended. Efforts are currently under way to re-examine the required duration of therapy in the context of modern regimens, with the hope that in some patients it may be possible to shorten maintenance therapy.

Relapse

Even with optimal modern therapy, one fourth of patients with ALL will experience relapse, usually in the bone marrow. Most will respond favorably to reinduction therapy. Those in whom relapse occurs while they are still receiving initial therapy respond less well to subsequent management, particularly if the relapse occurs during the first 18 months after the original diagnosis. Bone marrow transplantation should be considered as an alternative therapy for patients with ALL in whom relapse occurs during administration of initial treatment regimens. Patients in whom relapse occurs later than 6 months after completion of their initial treatment program may have an excellent response to another chemotherapy-based regimen, especially if the initial therapy regimen employed only a few drugs, usually antimetabolites. However, transplantation is an important treatment option. Patients experiencing initial relapse in an isolated extramedullary site such as the CNS or testis may be given salvage therapy using intensified systemic chemotherapy accompanied by local irradiation; transplantation is reserved for those who then experience subsequent marrow relapse.

ACUTE MYELOID LEUKEMIA

Evaluation

Acute myeloid leukemia (AML) in children occurs with an annual frequency of approximately 500 cases and accounts for 15 to 20% of cases of acute leukemia in the pediatric age group. Presenting symptoms and physical findings are generally not distinguishable from those of ALL. In childhood AML there is an increase in gingival involvement and retroorbital tumors known as chloromas or granulocytic sarcomas. The FAB classification system recognizes seven subgroups of AML, as listed in Table 3. The relative incidence of the seven types is also shown.

With the exception of a presenting WBC count of more than 100,000 per μL and the presence of certain cytogenetic abnormalities as noted later on, consistent favorable or unfavorable prognostic factors have not been identified in childhood cases of AML. Persons who develop AML following myeloproliferative disorders (MDs) and those with secondary AML are well recognized to have relatively refractory disease that responds poorly to any form of therapy. Immunophenotyping has proved to be of diagnostic value, but surface antigen characteristics have no independent prognostic value. Most if not all patients have chromosomal abnormalities. The t(8;21), t(9;11), and inv(16) rearrangements are associated with a better outcome, and monosomy 7 is associated with poorer outcome.

Treatment

Induction Therapy

Standard induction therapy for AML includes the combination of three daily doses of an anthracycline, usually daunorubicin, and cytarabine given over 7 to 10 days according to a variety of dosage schedules. Often other drugs such as 6-thioguanine and/or an epipodophyllotoxin are added. With the use of modern therapies, induction response rates range from 80 to 85%. It is not clear, however, whether rate of response is predictive of remission duration. Frequently, the anthracycline-cytarabine combination is followed by a regimen using high-dose (1 to 3 grams per m^2 per dose) cytarabine (Cytosar-U). The majority of patients who go on to receive postremission chemotherapy regimens will experience relapse, and event-free survival rates are usually 35 to 40%. An exception is the group of patients (8%) with acute promyelocytic leukemia (FAB-M3), who receive a combination of all-*trans*-retinoic acid (ATRA) plus standard induction chemotherapy. These children have a favorable outcome, with observed long-term survival rates of 80 to 90%. Another exception is children with Down syndrome who develop AML. These patients have also been noted to respond well to moderately aggressive chemotherapy regimens and should not be considered bone marrow transplantation candidates in first remission.

TABLE 3. **FAB Subgroups of Acute Myeloid Leukemia (AML)**

AML Subgroup	Approximate Incidence (%)
M0: acute undifferentiated nonlymphoid leukemia	2
M1: acute myeloid leukemia without maturation	14
M2: acute myeloid leukemia with differentiation	28
M3: acute promyelocytic leukemia	8
M4: acute monomyelogenous leukemia	21
M5: acute monocytic leukemia	19
M6: erythroblastic leukemia	2
M7: megakaryocytic leukemia	6

Abbreviation: FAB = French-American-British classification.

Central Nervous System Management

Among children with AML, CNS involvement at diagnosis is noted in 10 to 15%, and an equal number of cases may be recognized during therapy. Most treatment regimens employ intrathecal chemotherapy for early management and prophylaxis of CNS leukemia. The role of CNS irradiation in preventive therapy for children with AML is not established, although this strategy is routinely recommended in some therapy regimens. Irradiation is commonly used to treat overt CNS disease in patients with AML.

Postremission Management

For the majority of AML patients achieving remission, postinduction therapy may take a variety of forms. Although data may be conflicting, bone marrow transplantation using an HLA-matched sibling, if there is one, as donor is considered by many to be the treatment of choice for most AML patients in remission and should be performed early. Post-transplant disease-free survival rates are reported at from 55 to 70% in selected patients receiving bone marrow transplants in first remission. As noted previously, superior outcomes may be noted in certain subsets of AML patients receiving chemotherapy regimens, and these patients are not candidates for transplantation in first remission. For patients not eligible for bone marrow transplantation for whatever reason who receive postremission chemotherapy, optimal management recommendations remain uncertain. In the immediate postinduction period, a course of intensive-dose cytarabine is commonly given. Thereafter, some treatment strategies have recommended a shortened (2 to 6 months) course of intensive, high-dose combination chemotherapy. Other, less intense treatment regimens have been given but over a longer period of time (1 to 2 years). In either circumstance, the majority of patients relapse, usually within 12 months of diagnosis. Postinduction intensification with marrow-ablative chemotherapy and autologous marrow rescue yields survival rates equivalent to those with intensive chemotherapy. Alternative intensive therapies using rescue with harvested autologous peripheral stem cells or marrow or using marrow grafts from matched unrelated donors or mismatched related donors are being investigated but do not have a clearly established role in the management of AML in children.

CHRONIC MYELOID LEUKEMIA

method of
RICHARD T. SILVER, M.D.
New York Hospital–Cornell Medical Center
New York, New York

Chronic myeloid leukemia (CML) is a chronic myeloproliferative disorder of a pluripotent stem cell with a specific cytogenetic abnormality—the Philadelphia (Ph) chromosome—that involves myeloid, erythroid, megakaryocyte, and occasionally B lymphoid cells. Recent advances in cell biology and molecular genetics have yielded much new data regarding this disease. Advances in bone marrow transplantation (BMT) and the effects of recombinant interferon-alpha have been significant, and have played a major role in the overall treatment of the illness.

The clinical, cytogenetic, and molecular abnormalities in CML must be appreciated in order to understand both the diagnosis and treatment of CML, which is characterized by two phases. The "benign," or "chronic," phase, which usually lasts about 3 years, terminates in a second more acute or abrupt illness, called the "accelerated," "terminal," or "blast" phase.

In the chronic phase, symptoms and signs usually develop insidiously and can include fatigue, anemia, progressive splenomegaly, and leukocytosis. The white blood cell (WBC) count approximates 200,000 per μL. The myeloid cells in the peripheral blood show all stages of differentiation, but the myelocyte predominates. Basophils and eosinophils are prominent. More than half the patients have platelet counts above one million per μL. A slight degree of anemia is common.

Terminal CML can develop at any time but usually occurs after a median interval of 36 to 48 months. A number of criteria can be used to define this relatively abrupt change in disease status, the most reliable being the presence in the peripheral blood and/or bone marrow of myeloblasts and promyelocytes exceeding 30% of the differential distribution. This occurs in about 70% of cases. In the absence of frank blast crisis, other criteria for defining terminal-phase CML include fever of undetermined origin, increasing splenomegaly, a rising WBC count, an increased degree of basophilia or anemia and thrombocytopenia, and refractoriness to previously effective therapy such as busulfan and hydroxyurea. The median survival in this phase is approximately 3 months.

The blast crises are divided into two general types, myeloid and lymphoid. A lymphoid blast crisis occurs in 20 to 30% of patients. The cells often resemble those seen in acute lymphocytic leukemia and contain terminal deoxynucleotidyl transferase (Tdt). This transferase is found mainly in normal and malignant lymphoid cells of T cell and B cell origin and is lost as these lymphocytes differentiate and mature.

The basic mechanism by which chronic-phase disease transforms into blast-phase disease is not understood. Although additional cytogenetic abnormalities are seen as patients enter the blast phase, they may not necessarily be causally related to the transformation.

CYTOGENETIC AND MOLECULAR ABNORMALITIES

The Ph chromosome, the hallmark of CML, appears following reciprocal translocation of cytogenetic material from chromosomes 9 and 22. This chromosome is found in approximately 85% of all patients diagnosed with CML. In another 5%, the Ph chromosome results from complex chromosome translocations always involving chromosomes 9 and 22 and usually three or more chromosomes. In the remaining 10% of cases, a Ph chromosome cannot be detected by conventional cytogenetics. In this group, about half the patients have a characteristic molecular abnormality, the BCR/ABL oncogene, which can be found by sophisticated but widely available molecular tests obtained at centers specializing in this disease or through commercial sources that demonstrate the typical BCR/ABL rearrangement. The clinical course and response to treatment of patients who have masked Ph chromosomes or who are Ph-negative/BCR positive are like those with the classic translocation. In less than 5% of patients with the *clinical* diagnosis of CML, neither the Ph chromosome nor the molecular abnormality of the BCR/ABL gene can be demonstrated. For the purpose of this chapter, it is assumed that the patients have either the cytogenetic or molecular abnormality. The treatment of patients with some manifestations of CML but who are Ph negative and BCR/ABL negative is not addressed in this chapter.

TREATMENT

Chronic Phase

The cardinal therapeutic principle in CML is that initially the great majority of patients respond to many drugs and also to radiation therapy. Although the quality of life in CML may be improved by such treatment, no evidence exists that survival is prolonged by conventional agents because neither the Ph chromosome nor the BCR/ABL gene is affected.

Recent studies have indicated that hydroxyurea (Hydrea) is superior to busulfan (Myleran) with respect to survival. Therefore, the use of busulfan is not discussed.

Hydroxyurea

Hydroxyurea is an S-phase–specific inhibitor of ribonucleotidase. The starting dose ranges from 15 to 30 mg per kg per day orally depending upon the WBC and platelet counts, then tapered as these counts fall. Caution must be exercised with respect to the serum uric acid levels, since as the count falls, serum uric acid values may increase. Therefore, allopurinol (Zyloprim), at a dose of 300 mg daily, should be given as soon the diagnosis is made and continued thereafter. In general, if the platelet count is sufficiently elevated, the target should be 600,000 per μL or less. It is not necessary to reduce the WBC count to a given absolute number although in general, a target number of 15,000 to 20,000 per μL is adequate. This is because CML leukocytes retain virtually all normal function so that it is not necessary to insist upon a normal WBC count in the 5000 to 10,000 per μL range. In general, the dose of hydroxyurea must be continued since its discontinuation leads to prompt rise in the white cell and platelet counts. Occasional attacks of gout that may occur should be treated in the usual fashion with colchicine or a nonsteroidal agent.

Side effects of hydroxyurea include stomatitis, nausea, vomiting and a maculopapular rash. Generally, no transfusions are necessary because as the WBC falls, the hematocrit, if initially low, rises.

Blast Phase

No substantial progress has been made in the treatment of terminal or blast phase disease. We and others have tested a large series of drugs and drug regimens, including those used for the acute leukemias, without success. In view of this, I prefer to use a combination of agents that can be given on an outpatient basis. A combination of hydroxyurea, 6-mercaptopurine (Purinethol), and prednisone in patients (especially for patients who may not have received prior therapy with hydroxyurea) yields a response rate of approximately 30%. This modest improvement in response is characterized by a remission duration of about 7 months, compared with 2 or 3 months for patients with no response. Hospitalized patients with myeloid blast crisis can be given an anthracycline and intravenous cytosine arabinoside in the same dosage as used in de novo acute myeloid leukemia. Although vincristine/prednisone with or without other drugs is useful in lymphoid blast crises, in my experience survival is not significantly increased over myeloid blast crisis even with such "tailored" chemotherapy. These results suggest that therapeutic responsiveness in blast crisis depends on the inherent sensitivity of the blast cells rather than on the effectiveness of any therapeutic regimen.

Elevated Platelet Counts

Within recent years, we have observed a significant number of patients with CML who developed refractory thrombocytosis resistant to hydroxyurea (or interferon) that was associated with significant thrombotic and hemorrhagic complications. A new agent, anagrelide, (Agrylin)* is highly effective in reducing the platelet count in this situation. (It is also effective against the thrombocythemia associated with other myeloproliferative diseases.) Using a dose of approximately 0.5 mg four times a day, a significant fall in the platelet count can occur within 4 to 6 weeks. Dose adjustment may be required depending on response.

Interferons

The interferons have a wide variety of biologic activities including antiproliferative and oncogene regulatory effects. Sufficient evidence has accrued that interferon can prolong the lives of a small but significant number of patients with CML. Furthermore, randomized trials indicate interferon alpha (rIFN-alpha)–based therapy is superior to conventional treatment. Overall, cytogenetic remissions can be achieved with interferon alpha-2a (Roferon-A) or alpha-2b (Intron A) in approximately 40 to 50% of patients, particularly those defined as "good risk" and a major or complete cytogenetic response can be obtained in 20 to 25%. The recommended dose is 5 million units per m^2 per day subcutaneously for either interferon alpha 2a or 2b. The median time to complete cytogenetic remission ranges between 12 and 17 months, but complete cytogenetic remission may occur 36 months after the start of interferon therapy and even later. In some patients, rIFN-alpha results in 100% Ph-negative marrows but the more sensitive molecular abnormality (BCR/ABL rearrangement) persists. Data suggest that these patients have a significantly improved survival time, for the majority of these remissions are relatively stable and long-lasting (up to 6 years and longer).

Although, as mentioned, cytogenetic response has been correlated with improved survival, recent studies from England and Italy have indicated a survival advantage for interferon-alpha even in patients who did *not* have a cytogenetic response. Thus, if the patient tolerates the drug and is in clinical remission, rIFN should be continued.

The side effects of rIFN-alpha are not trivial, and not all patients can tolerate it indefinitely. Nonhematologic effects include fever, chills, malaise, headache, impotence, anorexia, joint pain, changes in mood and concentration, and abnormalities of liver enzymes. Nevertheless, dose intensity with rIFN-alpha is important because it is necessary to produce leukopenia of approximately 2000 to 3000 per μL in order to obtain a cytogenetic response. Therefore, it is wise to warn patients of the side effects of interferon in advance. Over time, these effects become less severe. The constitutional symptoms often respond to acetaminophen. Impotence can be helped by the use of androgens, although the usual caveat with respect to prostate cancer must be made. Mood changes and depression can be dealt with by employing the usual psychotropic drugs. Hypothyroidism, autoimmune disease, and neuritis and other neurologic complications can be seen with long-term administration.

The use of interferon with chemotherapy has been evaluated recently. If the full dose cannot be resumed, hydroxyurea can be added with the aim of keeping the leukocyte count between 2000 and 4000 per μL. The recent publication of a randomized multicenter French trial comparing interferon-alpha alone versus interferon-alpha plus low-dose cytarabine (ara-C) is provocative. The rate of major and complete cytogenetic responses was significantly greater in those patients who received cytarabine. The initial dose of interferon-alpha was 5 million units per m^2 per day with a reduction in the dose when the WBC count fell below 1500 per μL and/or the platelet count below 100,000 per μL. Interferon was discontinued when the granulocyte count fell below 1000 per μL and/or the platelet count below

*Distributed by Roberts Pharmaceutical Company, Eatontown, N.J.

50,000 per μL. Each month, cytarabine was used in a single dose of 20 mg per m^2 per day for 10 days. Cytarabine was discontinued if the granulocyte count fell below 1000 per μL or the platelet count dropped below 50,000 per μL. It was also discontinued if chromosome analysis on two consecutive occasions revealed a complete cytogenetic response. Interferon was continued unless there were reasons for stopping it. Although interferon plus cytarabine has been employed in other doses in the United States, the correct method remains to be determined.

Allogeneic Stem Cell Transplantation

There is little doubt that in selected patients with CML, allogeneic bone marrow transplantation (BMT) can cure the disease. The limiting factor in BMT in CML relates to the often overlooked fact that only 10 to 15% of patients are eligible for this procedure. Age and histocompatibility requirements eliminate most CML patients. Major questions remain, including selection criteria for eligible patients, choice of the appropriate donor, timing of the transplant in the chronic phase, technical features of the actual transplant, preoperative regimens, and most aspects of matched unrelated donor transplantation. These issues are beyond the scope of this chapter. Although there is general agreement that the risk of transplant mortality increases with the age of the patient, there is no general agreement regarding the maximum age for transplantation using a genetically HLA-identical sibling. This is even more true for matched *unrelated* donors. Although most transplantation centers reluctantly offer allogeneic donor transplantations to patients older than 50, some specialty centers do use higher age limits. Their successful results, however, may be due to a high degree of selectivity. It is clearly established that the risk of relapse and transplant-related mortality is substantially higher if the transplant is performed in advanced-phase rather than chronic-phase disease. Although the recommendation has been made that patients should undergo BMT within the first 12 months of their illness, this is true of patients treated with busulfan or hydroxyurea and may not apply to those treated with interferon only. Nevertheless, since the onset of transformation cannot be predicted with assurance, it probably is wise to proceed with a BMT as soon as possible in any eligible individual.

With the caveat that there may be major disagreement among different experts treating patients with CML, what is a reasonable algorithm for the practicing hematologist? General agreement suggests that a patient younger than 20 should receive a BMT initially using a matched-unrelated donor if necessary. For patients younger than 45 years without a match, I prefer a trial of rINF-alpha for 12 months while a search for an unrelated donor is made. For patients 70 years or older, conventional chemotherapy with hydroxyurea may be appropriate, although the option of interferon therapy should be offered. In general, adults between the ages of 45 to 70 in any risk category should receive a trial of interferon, although high-risk patients may be considered for BMT if there is no response after 12 months.

NON-HODGKIN'S LYMPHOMA

method of
PAULA MARLTON, M.B., B.S.
Princess Alexandra Hospital
Brisbane, Australia

and

FERNANDO CABANILLAS, M.D.
M. D. Anderson Cancer Center
Houston, Texas

The non-Hodgkin's lymphomas (NHLs) constitute a clinically and biologically diverse group of malignant disorders involving lymph nodes and extranodal lymphoid tissue. The incidence of lymphoma in Western societies has been steadily increasing for more than two decades, with a more rapid rise noted in recent years. Acquired immune deficiency syndrome (AIDS)-related lymphomas and an aging population are both contributing to this rise, but other etiologic factors remain poorly understood. The introduction of chemotherapy dramatically improved outcomes for many subsets of patients with these previously untreatable disorders; however, despite the progressive introduction of new treatment strategies, the majority of lymphoma patients are not cured. Herein lies the challenge to hematologists and oncologists for the new millennium.

CLASSIFICATION

Although all NHLs are clonal disorders of cells derived from the lymphoid lineage, they encompass a great diversity of diseases. Initial histologic classification is an essential first step in clarifying the diagnosis of NHL. This almost always requires an excisional lymph node biopsy, although in some institutions with extensive experience, computed tomography (CT)–guided needle core biopsy or fine-needle aspiration is a useful alternative to major surgery, particularly in very ill patients. Classification of the lymphoma provides useful clinical information about the likely natural history and prognosis of the disease. The interpretation of nodal histology is a challenging field, with several classification systems in use. The most recent of these is the Revised European and American Lymphoma (REAL) classification (Table 1), which is gradually replacing both the Working Formulation (WF), entrenched in U.S. practice since 1982, and the Kiel classification, popular in Europe. Entities defined in the REAL classification are described in terms of several features in addition to the fundamental histology, including immunohistochemistry, flow cytometric characteristics, clinical features, and, where applicable, cytogenetic and molecular findings. It includes several categories that have been recognized as distinct entities since the advent of the WF system, providing greater accuracy in subset definition. Since its publication in late 1994, the REAL classification has been validated clinically in several retrospective analyses. The next major landmark in classification will be the completion of

TABLE 1. **REAL Classification: Non-Hodgkin's Lymphoid Neoplasms Recognized by the International Lymphoma Study Group**

B Cell Neoplasms
Precursor B cell neoplasm: Precursor B-lymphoblastic leukemia/lymphoma
Peripheral B cell neoplasms
- B cell chronic lymphocytic leukemia/prolymphocytic leukemia/small cell lymphocytic lymphoma
- Lymphoplasmacytoid lymphoma/immunocytoma
- Mantle cell lymphoma
- Follicle center lymphoma, follicular
  - Provisional cytologic grades: I (small cell), II (mixed small and large cell), III (large cell)
  - Provisional subtype: Diffuse, predominantly small cell type
- Marginal zone B cell lymphoma
  - Extranodal (MALT-type ± monocytoid B cells)
  - Provisional subtype: Nodal (± monocytoid B cells)
- Provisional entity: Splenic marginal zone lymphoma (± villous lymphocytes)
- Hairy cell leukemia
- Plasmacytoma/plasma cell myeloma
- Diffuse large B cell lymphoma
  - Subtype: Primary mediastinal (thymic) B cell lymphoma
- Burkitt's lymphoma
- Provisional entity: High-grade B cell lymphoma, Burkitt's-like

T Cell and Putative Natural Killer (NK) Cell Neoplasms
Precursor T cell neoplasm: Precursor T-lymphoblastic lymphoma/leukemia
Peripheral T cell and NK cell neoplasms
- T cell chronic lymphocytic leukemia/prolymphocytic leukemia
- Large granular lymphocyte leukemia (LGL)
  - T cell type
  - NK cell type
- Mycosis fungoides/Sézary syndrome
- Peripheral T cell lymphomas, unspecified
  - Provisional cytologic categories: Medium-sized cell, mixed medium and large cell, large cell, lymphoepithelioid cell
  - Provisional subtype: Hepatosplenic $\gamma\delta$ T cell lymphoma
  - Provisional subtype: Subcutaneous panniculitic T cell lymphoma
- Angioimmunoblastic T cell lymphoma (AILD)
- Angiocentric lymphoma
- Intestinal T cell lymphoma (± enteropathy-associated)
- Adult T cell lymphoma/leukemia (ATL/L)
- Anaplastic large cell lymphoma (ALCL), $CD30^+$, T cell and null cell types
- Provisional entity: Anaplastic large cell lymphoma, Hodgkin's-like

Modified from Harris NL, Jaffe ES, Stein H, et al: Perspective: A revised European-American classification of lymphoid neoplasm: A proposal from the International Lymphoma Study Group. Blood *84*:1361–1392, 1994.

the WHO classification, described by many as a refined version of the REAL.

STAGING AND PROGNOSTIC FACTOR ASSESSMENT

After histopathologic classification, the next important assessment in lymphoma management is to determine the extent or stage of disease. Staging procedures define the anatomic sites of disease; the findings are then systematized into a shorthand notation. The almost universally used staging classification is the Ann Arbor system (Table 2) originally devised for use in Hodgkin's disease, which is imperfect in its application to NHL. However, it remains central to determining prognosis and appropriate treatment.

TABLE 2. **Ann Arbor Staging System**

Stage I	One lymph node (LN) region or one extranodal organ or site (IE)
Stage II	Two or more LN regions on the same side of the diaphragm, or one localized extranodal organ or site (IIE) and one or more LN regions on the same side of the diaphragm
Stage III	LN regions on both sides of the diaphragm
Stage IIIE	Stage III plus localized involvement of one extranodal organ or site or spleen (IIIS) or both (IIISE)
Stage IV	One or more extranodal organs with or without associated LN involvement (diffuse or disseminated)

Augmenting our ability to predict prognosis has been the identification of a range of other pretreatment variables besides stage that have been shown to correlate with outcome. An extensive analysis of more than 2000 patients with aggressive lymphomas performed by the International Non-Hodgkin's Prognostic Factor Project culminated in the "International Index," presented in Table 3. This index defines four distinct risk categories based on five pretreatment characteristics. At M. D. Anderson Cancer Center a similar analysis led to development of a "Tumor Score System" that defines low-risk and high-risk aggressive lymphomas based on five parameters (see Table 3). Other variables known to correlate with outcome include

TABLE 3. **Alternative Prognosticating Systems for Non-Hodgkin's Lymphoma**

International Index

Parameter	Criteria	Score
Age	<60 y	0
	>60 y	1
Ann Arbor stage	I–II	0
	III–IV	1
Serum LDH level	Normal	0
	Higher than normal	1
Performance status	0–1	0
	>1	1
Extranodal sites	0–1	0
	>1	1

Score	Risk
0, 1	Low
2	Low intermediate
3	High intermediate
4, 5	High risk

Tumor Score System

Parameter	Adverse Feature
Ann Arbor stage	III–IV
Symptoms	Presence of B symptoms
Tumor bulk	Mass >7 cm, or detectable mediastinal mass on chest x-ray film
β-2M fraction	>3.0 mg/L
Serum LDH level	≥685 IU/L

Each adverse feature scores one point. Totals of 3 or greater define poor-risk status.

Abbreviations: β-2M = β_2-microglobulin; LDH = lactate dehydrogenase; B symptoms = weight loss > 10 lb, fever, night sweats.

certain cytokine levels (interleukins IL-6 and IL-14), S-phase fraction, and specific cytogenetic and molecular variables. With these aggressive lymphomas, the risk of central nervous system (CNS) disease must also be evaluated to define appropriate therapy. With indolent lymphomas, risk factor identification analysis has shown that the serum β_2-microglobulin (beta-2M) fraction is highly predictive of outcome. Several groups of investigators have shown that the International Index can also be applied successfully in patients with indolent lymphomas.

A guide to appropriate evaluation of stage and prognosis is outlined in Table 4. Restaging or response evaluation is always undertaken at defined intervals during and after therapy and consists of repeating tests that had positive results at the time of diagnosis. Other patient evaluations are included to predict tolerance to treatment and to assess toxicity when indicated.

MANAGEMENT

In the following discussion, approaches to management of NHL are considered for the broad categories of indolent, aggressive, and highly aggressive lymphomas.

Indolent B Cell Lymphomas

Representing 40 to 50% of all NHLs, indolent B cell lymphoma is the most common subtype in Western countries. The vast majority of these tumors are follicular lymphomas (follicle center lymphoma or follicular lymphoma grade I or II in the REAL classification or follicular small cleaved cell and mixed small cleaved and large cell in the WF). Other entities encompassed in this category include small lymphocytic lymphoma and its subtypes and marginal zone lymphomas, including mucosa-associated lymphoid tissue (MALT) lymphomas. Characterizing the common indolent lymphomas (follicular lymphomas) are the following features: advanced stage at presentation, long median survival of 7 to 9 years; high response rates to initial chemotherapy; gradual development of chemoresistance with subsequent courses of therapy; propensity to transform to more aggressive histology subtypes over time; and low curability with stage IV presentation. Despite these generalizations, the prognosis for patients with indolent lymphoma is variable, and prognostic factor assessment may identify subgroups with better or worse outcomes.

Management of Localized Disease

For the small group of patients (15 to 20%) with localized indolent lymphoma, cure is a realistic treatment goal. In stage I and nonbulky stage II disease, involved field (IF) radiation therapy with small doses of 30 to 40 Gy will achieve long-term disease-free survival in at least 50% of cases. This has been most convincingly demonstrated in laparotomy staged patients. Relapse within the radiation field occurs in less than 10% of cases, with the majority of recurrences therefore occurring outside the original sites of known disease. Thus, the use of systemic chemotherapy in combination with IF radiation therapy has been evaluated; although this approach is not definitively superior in terms of overall survival, relapse-free survival is improved. Our preferred approach is therefore chemotherapy based on the combination of cyclophosphamide (Cytoxan), doxorubicin (Adriamycin), vincristine (Oncovin), and prednisone—CHOP (Table 5)—followed by IF radiotherapy.

Management of Disseminated Disease

Advanced-stage disease has been approached from widely disparate treatment philosophies. On the one hand, advocates of a conservative approach have quoted the long median survival and incurability as justification for minimally toxic therapy (using a sin-

TABLE 4. **Staging Work-up**

- History of B symptoms: fever, sweats, weight loss
- Detailed physical examination
- Adequate node biopsy
- Blood work: complete blood count, biochemical profile including serum LDH and β-2M, serum protein electrophoresis, ESR, HIV serology
- Bone marrow aspirate and biopsy (bilateral in indolent lymphoma)
- Chest x-ray film
- CT scans of chest, abdomen, and pelvis
- Lymphangiogram
- Gallium scan
- ± Bone scan, GI work-up, CSF examination

Abbreviations: CBC = complete blood count; LDH = lactate dehydrogenase; β-2M = β_2-microglobulin; ESR = erythrocyte sedimentation rate; HIV = human immunodeficiency virus; CT = computed tomography; GI = gastrointestinal; CSF = cerebrospinal fluid.

TABLE 5. **Chemotherapy for Indolent Lymphomas**

Regimen	Dose
Single-Agent	
Chlorambucil (Leukeran)	14–16 mg/m² daily × 5 d PO q 21–28 d, or 0.1–0.2 mg/kg daily for 4–6 wk
Cyclophosphamide (Cytoxan)	500–1000 mg/m² IV q 21–28 d, or 60–100 mg/m² PO q d
Combination	
CVP (21-day cycle)	
Cyclophosphamide	400 mg/m² daily PO d 1–5
Vincristine (Oncovin)	1.4 mg/m² IV d 1
Prednisone	100 mg/m² daily PO d 1–5
CHOP (21-day cycle)	
Cyclophosphamide	750 mg/m² IV d 1
Doxorubicin* (Adriamycin)	50 mg/m² IV d 1 or infused over 72 h
Vincristine	1.4 mg/m² IV d 1
Prednisone	100 mg/m² daily PO d 1–5
Purine Analogues	
Fludarabine (Fludara) (4-week cycle)	25 mg/m² daily IV d 1–5
Cladribine† (Leustatin)	0.14 mg/kg daily IV d 1–5

*Formerly hydroxydaunomycin.
†Cladribine is 2-chlorodeoxyadenosine (2-CDA).

gle-agent regimen) or no therapy until a symptomatic indication occurs (watchful waiting). On the other hand, investigators seeking curative treatment have considered the chemosensitivity of the disease and the poor long-term outlook as justification for investigational strategies.

Watchful waiting has not been shown to compromise overall survival in the limited studies available; however, disease-free survival rates are clearly much higher in patients who receive treatment, so that consequent quality of life may be improved. Minimally toxic therapy, once considered the standard approach, consists of administration of a single alkylating agent (chlorambucil [Leukeran] or cyclophosphamide) in varying schedules (see Table 5). Such conservative strategies are still useful in specific clinical situations, particularly in elderly patients. More aggressive approaches to therapy began with simple combinations of chemotherapy. The cyclophosphamide-vincristine-prednisone (CVP) regimen (see Table 5) has not been convincingly demonstrated to be superior to single agents. However, the additional use of doxorubicin as in the CHOP or CHOP plus bleomycin (CHOP-Bleo) regimen (Table 6) is associated with more rapid responses, but whether it leads to superior survival remains controversial. Relapse rates remain very high, however, and treatment intensification has been tested in an attempt to improve the continuous remission rate. We have used alternating regimens of aggressive non–cross-resistant chemotherapy and observed a very high remission rate; in many cases, this was confirmed even at the molecular level. The durability of the remissions appears better, but results of longer follow-up studies are awaited.

High-dose chemotherapy (HDCT) with autologous bone marrow or peripheral blood stem cell (PBSC) rescue is increasingly utilized as a therapeutic option in the treatment of indolent lymphomas. Data supporting this approach are gradually accumulating. The optimal timing for a potentially toxic therapy is a difficult issue in disorders with a long natural history. The inevitability of relapse and emergence of chemoresistance have encouraged its use earlier in the course of the disease. HDCT in first relapse or even in first remission in young patients or those with poor prognostic features is being studied extensively. Several high-dose regimens are in common use such as BEAM, which employs carmustine (BCNU [bis-chloroethyl-nitroso-urea]), etoposide (VePesid), cytarabine (Cytosar-U), and melphalan (Alkeran). One of the factors complicating the use of autologous PBSC rescue in the indolent lymphomas is the high frequency of bone marrow involvement with disease. Attempts to purge contaminating lymphoma cells from the stem cell harvest using monoclonal antibodies to remove B cells or to positively select stem cells have been successful in some studies.

Alpha interferon has also found a role in the treatment of indolent lymphomas. Several studies since the early work at M. D. Anderson Cancer Center have confirmed the efficacy of interferon in prolonging remission duration when used in the minimal residual disease setting after initial chemotherapy. Interferon has also been shown to improve remission duration when used concurrently with initial chemotherapy and may have a favorable effect on overall survival in this setting.

Alternative chemotherapy agents have been studied. The most successful among these are the purine analogues fludarabine* (Fludara) and 2-chlorodeoxyadenosine (cladribine* [Leustatin]) (Table 5). At the M. D. Anderson Cancer Center, after demonstrating initial single-agent activity we studied fludarabine in combination with mitoxantrone (Novantrone)* and dexamethasone (Decadron), with excellent response rates in patients with recurrent disease. Other new approaches being investigated follow exciting developments in the immunotherapy field. Humanized monoclonal antibodies to CD20, which target B cells, have been used alone and in combination with CHOP chemotherapy. Early results indicate that the antibodies have activity in approximately 50% of patients with recurrent indolent lymphoma, with responses lasting a median of 12 months. Additional studies using murine monoclonal antibodies conjugated to toxins or radionuclides are ongoing and show early promising results. Finally, the explosive developments in dendritic cell immunotherapy in many areas of cancer medicine are also being applied to the treatment of indolent lymphomas.

Salvage therapies for relapsed indolent lymphoma include several options already discussed, including HDCT with autologous PBSC rescue, allogeneic bone marrow transplant in young patients with a matched sibling donor, monoclonal anti-CD20 antibodies, purine analogue–based therapy, or other active chemotherapy regimens including cytarabine and cisplatin* (Platinol) combinations.

Aggressive Lymphomas

The aggressive lymphomas include the following entities identified in the REAL classification: diffuse large B cell lymphoma (diffuse large cell lymphoma and immunoblastic lymphoma in the WF), primary mediastinal large B cell lymphoma, anaplastic large B cell lymphoma, anaplastic large cell lymphoma of T cell and null cell types, and peripheral T cell lymphoma. The cornerstone of treatment for essentially all patients with aggressive NHL is initial combination chemotherapy. Several principles have been established. First, chemotherapy is administered with curative intent in all cases, and the regimen must therefore achieve a high rate of complete response (CR). Second, dose intensity is very important for the attainment of durable CRs; thus, drugs must be delivered in full therapeutic doses without treatment delays, particularly in patients up to 60 years of age. Third, toxicities must be predicted and precautions taken to reduce these wherever possible.

---

*Not FDA approved for this indication.

TABLE 6. **Chemotherapy for Aggressive Lymphomas**

Regimen	Dose
First-Generation	
CHOP	
Cyclophosphamide (Cytoxan)	750 mg/m² IV d 1
Doxorubicin (Adriamycin)	50 mg/m² IV d 1 or infused over 72 h
Vincristine (Oncovin)	1.4 mg/m² IV d 1
Prednisone	100 mg/m² daily PO d 1–5
CHOP-Bleo (CHOP plus bleomycin)	
Bleomycin (Blenoxane)	10 U/m² IV d 1
Second-Generation	
M-BACOD (21-day cycle)	
Bleomycin	4 U/m² IV d 1
Doxorubicin	45 mg/m² IV d 1
Cyclophosphamide	600 mg/m² IV d 1
Vincristine	1 mg/m² d 1
Dexamethasone (Decadron)	6 mg/m² daily PO d 1–5
Methotrexate	3 gm/m² IV d 14
Leucovorin (rescue agent)	10 mg/m² IV 24 h after methotrexate infusion, then 10 mg/m² PO q 6 h for 72 h
Third-Generation	
MACOP-B	
Methotrexate	400 mg/m² IV wk 2, 6, and 10
Leucovorin	15 mg PO q 6 h × 6 doses commencing 24 h after start of methotrexate
Doxorubicin	50 mg/m² IV wk 1, 3, 5, 7, 9, 11
Cyclophosphamide	350 mg/m² IV wk 1, 3, 5, 7, 9, 11
Vincristine	1.4 mg/m² IV wk 2, 4, 6, 8, 10, 12
Prednisone	75 mg/m² daily PO, taper wk 11 and 12
Bleomycin	10 U/m² IV wk 4, 8, 12
Alternating Triple Therapy (ATT)	
ASHAP (IdSHAP)*	
Doxorubicin	50 mg/m² over 48 h
Methylprednisolone (Solu-Medrol)	500 mg daily IV d 1–5
Cytarabine [ara-C†] (Cytosar-U)	1.5 gm/m² over 2 h after cisplatin d 5
Cisplatin (Platinol)	100 mg/m² over 96 h (25 mg/m² daily)
M-BACOS (M-BIdCOS)*	
Methotrexate	1 gm/m² IV d 2
Leucovorin (rescue agent)	15 mg PO q 6 h × 8 doses starting 24 h after start of methotrexate
Bleomycin	10 U/m² d 1
Doxorubicin	50 mg/m² over 48 h
Cyclophosphamide	750 mg/m² IV d 1
Vincristine	1.4 mg/m² IV d 1
Methylprednisolone	500 mg daily IV d 1–3
MINE	
Mesna (Mesnex)	500 mg/m² daily PO d 1–3 plus 1.5 gm/m² daily IV d 1–3
Ifosfamide (Ifex)	1.5 gm/m² daily d 1–3
Mitoxantrone (Novantrone)	10 mg/m² IV d 1
Etoposide (VePesid)	80 mg/m² daily IV d 1–3
Salvage Regimen	
ESHAP	
Etoposide	40 mg/m² daily IV d 1–3
Solu-Medrol	500 mg daily IV d 1–5
Cytarabine	2.0 gm/m² IV d 5
Cisplatin	100 mg/m² IV over 96 h (25 mg/m² daily)

*Idarubicin (Idamycin) is substituted for doxorubicin in the alternatives IdSHAP and M-BIdCOS.
†Ara-C is cytosine arabinoside (cytarabine).

Management of Localized Disease

Early-stage disease is less uncommon than in indolent lymphoma accounting for approximately 40% of patients. Previous recommendations for radiation therapy alone in this group have gradually been abandoned. The best long-term disease-free survival rates of 70% or more with radiation therapy alone were originally attained in patients who had laparotomy-proven stage I disease. The unacceptably low survival rate of 30% or less for stage II patients treated with radiation therapy alone indicated their need for systemic chemotherapy. The morbidity associated with laparotomy staging can no longer be justified for this group of patients, however, and thus systemic chemotherapy has been used for all stage I and stage II patients. An update on the British experience has rekindled some interest in the use of radiotherapy alone for highly selected patients: An 80% 10-year survival rate was reported in younger patients with favorable prognostic features such as low bulk, early stage disease.

Chemotherapy has been combined with radiotherapy in a variety of ways, with excellent survival rates of greater than 80% in most series. Short-course combination chemotherapy (e.g., three courses of CHOP) followed by IF radiotherapy is currently the most widely used approach. This strategy proved superior in terms of overall survival to a full course of chemotherapy alone (eight courses of CHOP) in a recent randomized study. It is important to recognize, however, that patients with limited-stage disease but unfavorable associated prognostic features, such as raised serum lactate dehydrogenase levels or β_2-microglobulin fraction or large tumor bulk, will not share the same favorable outlook and must be considered for more aggressive therapy.

Management of Disseminated Disease

Front line therapy for all advanced-stage patients consists of multiagent chemotherapy. Regimens in common use are outlined in Table 6. Still considered standard among these is the original CHOP regimen introduced more than 20 years ago. The subsequent second- and third-generation regimens were the fruit of attempts to improve on CHOP by incorporating additional active agents and intensifying dosing schedules. Early single-institution data yielded greatly improved CR rates (70 to 80%) and survival rates (50 to 60%) over those (58% and 30%, respectively) CHOP had been shown to achieve. Disappointment was great, therefore, when more definitive randomized studies directly comparing CHOP with other regimens failed to detect any advantages in terms of CR rates or overall survival. Small differences have been reported with longer follow-up in specific patient subsets in a small number of studies; however, the great hopes for the more toxic regimens have not been realized.

Current investigation is focused less on new regimen design and more on dose intensification principles and patient stratification according to prognosis prediction. Our current studies utilize the Tumor Score System to select patients with poor-risk disease for intensive alternating triple therapy (ATT) with non–cross-resistant regimens. As outlined in Table 6, ATT consists of a course of doxorubicin, methylprednisolone (Solu-Medrol), cytarabine, and cisplatin, or ASHAP; followed by a course of methotrexate with leucovorin rescue, bleomycin (Blenoxane), doxorubicin, cyclophosphamide, vincristine, and methylprednisolone, or M-BACOS; followed by consolidation with mesna (Mesnex), ifosfamide (Ifox), mitoxantrone (Novantrone), and etoposide, or MINE. In alternatives to the ASHAP and M-BACOS regimens, IdSHAP and M-BIdCOS, respectively, idarubicin* (Idamycin) is substituted for doxorubicin. An integral part of this approach is thorough restaging to identify patients with residual active disease after four courses, who are then directed to investigational approaches incorporating HDCT and autologous PBSC rescue. The ATT regimen based on doxorubicin appears better than other regimens tested in patients younger than 61 years who have poor prognostic features, i.e., a tumor score of 3 or higher. On the other hand, the idarubicin-based ATT regimen has less toxicity than its doxorubicin-based counterpart, and for that reason the survival was better with regimens incorporating idarubicin when used in patients older than 60 years of age with poor prognostic features.

The role of high-dose therapy with stem cell rescue has been clearly established in recurrent aggressive NHL, where it is the treatment of choice in chemotherapy-sensitive relapse. Its position earlier in therapy remains less well defined. Two studies investigating its usefulness as a consolidative procedure in patients with high-risk disease have yielded conflicting results. In two further studies it has failed to show a convincing impact on outcome when compared with further conventional chemotherapy in patients who have not achieved complete remission after initial response evaluation during standard front line treatment. Thus, HDCT and autologous PBSC rescue should still be considered investigational in the front line setting.

Salvage chemotherapy regimens for relapsed patients utilize additional active agents that have not been used in the front line combination. Cytarabine-based and cisplatin-based combinations (e.g., ESHAP; see Table 6) are effective in patients who have received initial CHOP therapy. In those with responsive disease who are eligible, HDCT with autologous PBSC rescue improves survival over that achieved with standard chemotherapy alone. Paclitaxel* (Taxol) is a newer agent with modest activity in relapsed aggressive NHL.

Mantle cell lymphoma is now recognized as a distinct entity with very poor prognosis. Categorized histologically in the WF most often with the low-grade lymphomas, it has a vastly different median survival of 36 months or less, with only 8% of pa-

*Not FDA approved for this indication.

tients alive at 10 years. Standard therapies have not demonstrated any significant cure fraction among this group of patients, and thus investigation of more aggressive therapy is under way. HDCT with PBSC rescue is being explored in some centers. At M. D. Anderson Cancer Center, an intensive protocol incorporating cyclophosphamide, mesna, vincristine, doxorubicin, dexamethasone (Decadron), methotrexate, cytarabine, and granulocyte colony–stimulating factor (G-CSF—filgrastim [Neupogen]), termed HyperCVAD (Table 7), is being tested, with very encouraging early results.

Highly Aggressive Lymphomas

Highly aggressive lymphomas include Burkitt's lymphoma, Burkitt's-like lymphoma, and lymphoblastic lymphoma. Burkitt's lymphoma occurs in endemic (African—Epstein-Barr virus–associated) and sporadic forms. It is more common in children and AIDS patients and is characterized molecularly by a unique translocation between chromosomes 8 and 14. Burkitt's lymphoma is among the most rapidly growing of all neoplasms, with very high S-phase fractions, rendering it exquisitely sensitive to chemotherapy. Consequently, tumor lysis syndrome not infrequently complicates initial management. Hydration, urinary alkalinization, allopurinol (Zyloprim) therapy, and careful monitoring are all integral to managing highly aggressive lymphomas.

TABLE 7. **Chemotherapy for Highly Aggressive Lymphomas**

Regimen	Dose
HyperCVAD	
Cyclophosphamide (Cytoxan)	300 mg/m² IV q 12 h d 1–3 (6 doses)
Mesna (Mesnex)	450 mg/m² IV at 1 h pre-cyclophosphamide d 1–3 and d 4
Vincristine (Oncovin)	2 mg IV d 4 and d 11
Doxorubicin (Adriamycin)	50 mg/m² IV d 4
Dexamethasone (Decadron)	40 mg IV or PO d 1–4 and d 11–14
Methotrexate	12 mg intrathecally d 2
Cytarabine (Cytosar-U)	100 mg intrathecally d 7
G-CSF (filgrastim [Neupogen])	5 μg/kg SC d 5 until white cell recovery
Alternates with HiDAC/MTX	
Methotrexate	200 mg/m² IV over 2 h d 1, then 800 mg/m² IV over 22 h d 1
Leucovorin (rescue agent)	60 mg IV or PO 12 h after methotrexate infusion completed, then 15 mg q 6 h × 8 doses
Cytarabine	3 gm/m² IV q 12 h × 4 doses d 2–3
G-CSF	5 μg/kg SC d 4 until white cell recovery
Intrathecal therapy as for HyperCVAD in high-risk cases	

Abbreviations: ara-C = cytosine arabinoside; G-CSF = granulocyte colony–stimulating factor; HiDAC = high-dose ara-C; MTX = methotrexate.

Diagnosis and staging may need to be curtailed if a medical emergency supervenes demanding urgent definitive therapy. The highly aggressive lymphomas are also associated with a high propensity for CNS involvement. Cerebrospinal fluid (CSF) must be examined prior to therapy, and CNS prophylaxis incorporated into the treatment protocol. Staging systems in use for Burkitt's lymphoma differ from the Ann Arbor system. The Ziegler and St. Jude's systems are commonly used. These emphasize the importance of abdominal disease and bone marrow involvement as poor prognostic features.

Intensive multiagent chemotherapy is the only curative approach to nonendemic Burkitt's lymphoma. Much progress has been made in recent years with regard to outcome for patients with this disease. The pediatric experience has led the way, with cures in more than 80% of patients now reported in this previously fatal disorder. Therapeutic principles for Burkitt's lymphoma have largely been borrowed from acute lymphoblastic leukemia (ALL) treatments, with current emphasis on brief but very intense chemotherapy supported by administration of growth factors. Therapy is tailored according to individual risk assessment, with the use of alternating non–cross-resistant regimens in the highest risk groups. The most encouraging results to date have come from the National Cancer Institute studies of the CODOX-M protocol, which utilizes cyclophosphamide, vincristine, doxorubicin, and methotrexate, alternating with non–cross-resistant drugs (ifosphamide,* etoposide,* and high-dose cytarabine*), in high-risk patients. The 2-year event-free survival rate has been reported at 92%. At M. D. Anderson we have used the HyperCVAD protocol (Table 7), originally developed for the treatment of ALL, which utilizes the principle of hyperfractionated delivery of cyclophosphamide to overcome the very rapid cycling of tumor cells. Results are very favorable to date.

Lymphoblastic lymphoma is another rare subtype, accounting for only 5% of adult cases of lymphoma. This is usually a T cell disorder, and patients frequently present with a large mediastinal mass. It is generally considered indistinguishable from T cell ALL, and treatment principles are the same. Thus, identical or similar regimens to those used in Burkitt's lymphoma are employed (HyperCVAD at M. D. Anderson Cancer Center). Cure rates are variable, with approximately 50% of adult patients cured overall. As with the other diseases in this category, the highest risk patients fare less well, and adults invariably have inferior outcomes compared with children.

There is no well-established role for HDCT with autologous bone marrow or PBSC rescue as part of initial therapy. The superior cure rates observed with the newer treatment regimens have not been improved upon by this approach, although it is still being investigated in the highest risk patient groups.

*Not FDA approved for this indication.

AIDS-Related Lymphoma

AIDS-related lymphoma (ARL) is worthy of separate discussion, because NHL occurring in the setting of human immunodeficiency virus (HIV) infection manifests differences in both natural history and therapeutic outcome. The probability of the development of NHL in AIDS patients is clearly higher than in the general population. The distribution of histologic subtypes differs from that in the non-AIDS population and appears to vary with stage of HIV-related disease. Almost 75% of tumors are aggressive or highly aggressive tumors of diffuse large B cell or Burkitt's types. Widely disseminated extranodal disease is present in the majority of patients at presentation.

Chemotherapy for patients with ARL is often compromised by poor bone marrow reserve exacerbated by antiretroviral therapy, and by the development of intercurrent opportunistic infections. Consequently, the high CR rates as expected in the nonimmunocompromised population are diminished significantly. The $CD4^+$ count, pre-existing opportunistic infections, and performance status all are important prognostic indicators. Overall median survival has been reported at less than 6 months. Attempts to improve therapeutic outcomes have used lower doses of standard regimens and hematopoietic growth factors. Reduced-dose M-BACOD (see Table 6) was tried with no reduction in median survival but less toxicity. This approach has been validated in a randomized study comparing full-dose and reduced-dose therapies, with improved outcome in the reduced-dose cohort. Growth factors to reduce the incidence of febrile neutropenic episodes, prophylaxis against *Pneumocystis* pneumonia, and concurrent antiretroviral therapy all are important aspects of treatment.

At M.D. Anderson Cancer Center, our own approach has been to utilize a novel, minimally myelosuppressive regimen for patients with $CD4^+$ counts of less than 200 mm^3. This incorporates continuous-infusion 5-fluorouracil (5-FU), leucovorin, and cisplatin with provision for use of G-CSF. For patients whose $CD4^+$ counts are higher than 200 mm^3 and who have no prior history of opportunistic infections, standard-intensity regimens are used. Patients with localized nonbulky disease and histologic subtype other than Burkitt's lymphoma are given abbreviated chemotherapy (three courses of CHOP-Bleo) and local radiotherapy.

Primary CNS lymphoma accounts for 17 to 42% of cases of lymphoma in AIDS patients but only 1 to 2% in nonimmunocompromised patients. The majority of patients have low $CD4^+$ counts and prior AIDS-defining opportunistic infections. The diagnosis should be confirmed by brain biopsy, particularly important in distinguishing lymphoma from toxoplasmosis, which may have an identical appearance on CT scan. The lesions are usually multifocal and often disseminate to the CSF, and the prognosis is poor. Standard therapy has been with whole-brain irradiation and steroids. This has improved median survival from 42 days in untreated cases to 136 days in one series. Chemotherapy has proved extremely difficult to deliver effectively to this group of patients, and no consistently good results have been achieved. Chemotherapy may benefit those patients in the better prognostic categories with greater tolerance to toxicity. Non–HIV-positive patients with primary CNS lymphoma have been given cytarabine-* and methotrexate-based chemotherapy in combination with brain irradiation, with a better although still poor median survival of approximately 18 months.

Gastrointestinal Lymphoma

As many as 25% of NHLs are extranodal in origin. The most common site for extranodal lymphoma is the gastrointestinal (GI) tract, accounting for 30 to 40%, and the majority of these are gastric (in the Western world). The histologic subtype varies, ranging from indolent MALT lymphomas to the more common aggressive lymphomas, most of which are diffuse large B cell in type. Diagnostic material is usually obtained at endoscopic biopsy, and the remaining staging work-up should proceed along standard lines.

Optimal management of aggressive GI lymphoma remains an equivocal issue with an absence of randomized trial evidence. In gastric lymphoma, the relative roles of surgery and chemotherapy have altered over time. Historically, surgery was the mainstay of treatment; however, its role more recently has been re-evaluated. In locally advanced or disseminated disease, where surgical resection is not possible or very difficult, combination chemotherapy is the treatment of choice. Response rates in patients with advanced gastric lymphoma are comparable to those in patients with advanced nodal disease, with a survival rate of approximately 40%. The regimens used are the same as for nodal aggressive lymphoma. In localized gastric lymphoma, curability with surgery alone has been well established; however, even partial gastrectomy remains a procedure with considerable attendant morbidity, and alternative nonsurgical management has therefore been advocated. This approach has been validated by the observation that the majority of recurrences after surgery are at distant sites, suggesting that local treatment may not be sufficient. Extensive experience with stomach conservation and front line chemotherapy has now accrued at M. D. Anderson Cancer Center and elsewhere, with very favorable outcomes, and this is our recommended approach. Few patients require subsequent surgical intervention, and perforation has been an uncommon complication. Survival rates upwards of 70% can be expected in stage I patients. Radiotherapy was traditionally used as an adjuvant to surgery in patients with early-stage disease. It has not been proved definitively to improve outcome in patients who have received chemotherapy but is a useful modality in patients unable to tolerate chemotherapy or

*Not FDA approved for this indication.

as an adjunct in bulky disease. It can also be used to complement a brief chemotherapy protocol (three courses of CHOP) in very limited and localized disease.

The indolent MALT lymphomas are characterized by a long natural history and prolonged confinement to the site of origin. Local surgical treatment has been used with excellent results; however, there is increasing evidence that surgery may not be necessary. A strong association between the presence of *Helicobacter pylori* and the development of gastric MALT lymphoma has been shown. Eradication of the organism with appropriate antibiotic therapy has been associated with regression of MALT lymphomas, both histologically and on molecular studies, in more than half the patients. In view of the long natural history and feasibility of close endoscopic monitoring, this is now considered appropriate initial treatment. In the majority of patients, this approach will avert the need for surgical intervention. Current studies are exploring the combination of *H. pylori* eradication and chlorambucil therapy in an attempt to improve regression rates.

MULTIPLE MYELOMA

method of
IAIN J. WEBB, M.D., and
KENNETH C. ANDERSON, M.D.
Dana-Farber Cancer Institute and Harvard Medical School
Boston, Massachusetts

MULTIPLE MYELOMA

Multiple myeloma is a malignant proliferation of plasma cells and plasmacytoid cells nearly always characterized by the presence of a monoclonal immunoglobulin (Ig) or Ig fragment in the serum and/or urine. Both major and minor criteria for the diagnosis of myeloma have been defined. These include the presence of excess monotypic marrow plasma cells, monoclonal Ig in serum and/or urine, decreased normal serum Ig levels, and lytic bone disease. Myeloma must be distinguished from other disorders characterized by monoclonal gammopathies, both malignant and otherwise. These include monoclonal gammopathy of unclear significance (MGUS), macroglobulinemia, non-Hodgkin's lymphoma, primary amyloidosis, idiopathic cold agglutinin disease, essential cryoglobulinemia, and heavy chain disease.

Treatment

Patients undergoing therapy for myeloma should have clinical and laboratory assessment to ensure both safety and efficacy of treatment. Before each course of treatment, a complete blood count, including differential and platelets, should be done. Serum chemistries should be measured at least every 3 months or more often if clinically indicated. Concomitantly, monoclonal protein in the serum and/or urine should be measured by immunoelectrophoresis, or preferably by more sensitive immunofixation techniques. A skeletal survey should be done annually, with bone marrow examination reserved for diagnosis or when there have been changes in clinical status, in monoclonal Ig, or in the hemogram. It is important to remember that when reduction of serum or urine M component is regarded as objective evidence of tumor response, the decrease could reflect increased protein catabolism, decreased protein production, or both. Moreover, non–M protein-secreting myeloma clones can emerge during treatment, so that even a marked reduction in monoclonal Ig may not correlate with a decrease in the tumor burden.

Two major definitions of response in myeloma have been widely utilized: that of the Chronic Leukemia-Myeloma Task Force and that of the Southwest Oncology Group (SWOG). The former requires a decrease of 50% or more in monoclonal serum or urine protein and in cross sectional areas of plasmacytoma as well as some recalcification of bone lesions (without new lesions), whereas the latter requires a 75% reduction in production of myeloma protein. However, the frequency of responses by either definition is similar in previously untreated patients receiving melphalan and prednisone: 32 to 53% response rates were noted by SWOG criteria and 33 to 56% responses by the Task Force criteria. The need for, and the response to, treatment may be a more important determinant of survival than initial tumor stage. For example, a low labeling index may define patients who may not need therapy irrespective of stage: such patients may have a long course before the need for therapy, a gradual response to treatment, and prolonged survival.

High-Dose Therapies

High-dose therapy with hematopoietic stem cell support has been utilized to treat patients with relapsed myeloma and as up-front therapy. Complete clinical remissions are seen after the administration of alkylating agents (melphalan [Alkeran], cyclophosphamide [Cytoxan], busulfan [Myleran]) in a higher-than-conventional dose with or without total body irradiation, followed by transplantation of syngeneic, allogeneic, or autologous marrow or of autologous peripheral blood stem cells. Reduction in tumor mass in some cases has been dramatic, with complete response rates ranging up to 50 to 60%. Moreover, there are reports of relapse-free survival for as long as 15 years, 7 years, and 5 years after syngeneic, allogeneic, and autologous marrow grafting, respectively. Nonetheless, the median response duration in most studies is only 16 to 24 months.

A recent randomized study has demonstrated statistically significant improvements in disease-free and overall survival with high-dose therapy and autologous bone marrow transplantation in previously untreated patients. In contrast, despite high response rates, only a minority of patients achieve prolonged disease-free survival after high-dose therapy for relapsed or refractory disease. Preliminary studies suggest that interferon (IFN) may prolong these responses when high-dose therapy and stem cell grafting are used as up-front therapy. The need for purging of tumor cells within the graft remains unproven but continues to be evaluated.

Autologous Stem Cell Transplantation. High-dose chemoradiotherapy followed by transplantation of either autologous bone marrow (BM) or peripheral blood progenitor cell (PBPCs) has achieved high (40%) complete response (CR) rates, but the median duration of these responses has unfortunately been only 24 to 36 months at best. Patients who have sensitive disease and who are less heavily pretreated have the most favorable outcomes. Most importantly, a recently completed national French trial of 200 patients with myeloma who received either conventional or high-dose chemotherapy followed by autologous bone marrow transplantation (BMT) has demonstrated significantly higher rates for therapeutic response, event-free survival (EFS), and overall survival (OS) for patients treated with high-dose versus conventional therapy.

Allogeneic Stem Cell Transplantation. A most encouraging lead for new treatment approaches for myeloma also stems from reports of CRs after the administration of alkylating agents in higher-than-conventional doses with or without total body irradiation (TBI), followed by syngeneic or allogeneic BMT. Reduction in tumor mass in some cases has been dramatic, with CR rates commonly in the 40% range and a similar number of partial responses (PRs). Of major concern, however, is the 40 to 44% transplant-related mortality. Improving the outcome of allogeneic transplantation for myeloma therefore requires addressing two major concerns. The first is avoiding transplant-related toxicity, especially graft-versus-host disease (GVHD) and the second is preventing relapse.

Recent data have shown that infusions of lymphocytes collected from the marrow donor (donor lymphocyte infusion [DLI]) can achieve marked responses when administered to treat relapsed myeloma after allografting, providing for the first time direct evidence of a graft-versus-myeloma effect. Studies at our institute have shown that CD8-depleted DLI resulted in responses in the majority of cases, in some patients in the absence of GVHD. Given the high rate of relapse after allografting noted in all series to date, we are currently using CD8-depleted DLI at 6 months postallografting, when donor hematopoiesis is achieved, in an attempt to prevent relapse in patients who have achieved CR and to treat residual disease in patients with PRs after allografting.

Conventional Therapy

Oral administration of melphalan and prednisone (MP) is a standard form of therapy that produces objective responses in up to 50 to 60% of patients. Due to the potential damage to normal hematopoietic progenitors from alkylating agents, MP and other regimens containing alkylating agents should not be administered to patients being considered for high-dose therapy. Combination therapy with vincristine (Oncovin), doxorubicin (Adriamycin), and dexamethasone (VAD) or single-agent dexamethasone is preferred for these patients. Melphalan is given at 0.15 mg per kg per day for 7 days with prednisone, 20 mg orally (PO) three times daily for 7 days. Due to the variability of absorption, the dosage of melphalan should be modified if necessary so that some reduction in leukocytes and platelets occurs 3 to 4 weeks after the beginning of each cycle. Melphalan should be given every 6 weeks but should be discontinued if the monoclonal Ig levels in the serum and/or urine have been stable for at least 6 months (plateau state) and if the patient has no other evidence of active disease. Chemotherapy should not be discontinued during the first year unless there is definite evidence of progression of disease, because some patients with a low plasma cell proliferative index do not obtain an objective response until the second year. Patients who remain stable should not be switched to other therapy, as they appear to do as well as responders.

Although some studies have demonstrated that combination chemotherapy (CCT) is superior to MP, 10 prospective randomized trials of MP versus a drug combination failed to clearly show that drug combinations were better than MP in the treatment of multiple myeloma. Improved response rates may not translate into prolonged survival. Patients who progress with initial therapy have a 40% response to high-dose or pulsed corticosteroid therapy. Patients who relapse during therapy or within 6 months of stopping initial treatment have a 75% response rate to VAD therapy. Patients receive both vincristine, 0.4 mg per day, and doxorubicin, 10 mg per m^2 per day via an intravenous (IV) continuous infusion for 4 days, along with dexamethasone (Decadron), 40 mg PO daily for 12 days, as follows: days 1 to 4, 9 to 12, and 17 to 20. Patients who relapse more than 6 months after stopping therapy have a 60 to 70% response rate when initial therapy is reinstituted; if no response is achieved, then VAD or alternate regimens can be used. VAD or single-agent dexamethasone, given according to the same schedule as in the VAD regimen, is the treatment of choice for patients being considered for high-dose therapy approaches.

Alpha-2b Interferon* (Intron A). Recombinant interferon (IFN), a biologic response modifier, can be effective in initial therapy when used in conjunction with alkylating agents and in delaying relapse after induction chemotherapy. Patients can develop flulike symptoms and anorexia as well as myelosuppression related to IFN therapy, but only a fraction of patients, primarily the elderly, require either dose reduction or discontinuation of IFN. At present IFN treatment appears to benefit patients who have a low tumor burden. However, additional studies are

---

*Not FDA approved for this indication.

needed to define subgroups of myeloma patients who benefit from IFN treatment.

Radiation Therapy. Radiation therapy is used for treatment of localized disease, including plasmacytoma or spinal cord compression syndrome, and is frequently given for palliation. Hemibody radiation therapy has been utilized either as consolidation therapy following induction combination chemotherapy or as salvage therapy for chemotherapy-resistant disease. As discussed previously, total body irradiation can also be a component of ablative therapy before hematopoietic stem cell transplantation.

OTHER PLASMA CELL DYSCRASIAS

Plasmacytomas

Plasmacytomas are collections of monoclonal plasma cells originating either in bone (solitary osseous plasmacytoma, SOP) or in soft tissue (extramedullary plasmacytoma, EMP). They comprise less than 10% of plasma cell dyscrasias. Myeloma must be excluded before the diagnosis of SOP or EMP can be made. Magnetic resonance imaging can show additional marrow abnormalities consistent with myeloma. Primary treatment for SOP and EMP is local therapy, primarily radiotherapy, with surgery as needed for structural anatomic support. The benefit of chemotherapy, either alone or in combination with radiotherapy and surgery, as primary therapy for SOP or EMP has not been proven. Moreover, the benefit of adjuvant chemotherapy, given to prevent recurrent disease and/or progression to myeloma, is also undefined. One report suggests that the disappearance of protein after involved-field radiotherapy predicts for long-term disease-free survival and possible cure. Conversely, nonsecretory disease and persistent monoclonal protein after treatment are adverse prognostic factors for which adjuvant therapy with IFN should be considered.

IgM Monoclonal Gammopathy

Excess monoclonal IgM in the serum can occur in a variety of diseases, including monoclonal gammopathy of uncertain significance, Waldenström's macroglobulinemia, lymphoma, chronic lymphocytic leukemia, primary amyloidosis, and other malignant lymphoproliferative diseases.

The diagnosis of Waldenström's macroglobulinemia requires an IgM serum level of at least 3.0 grams per dL in association with an increase in lymphocytes or plasmacytoid lymphocytes in the bone marrow. Fatigue and bleeding are the most common symptoms. Lymphadenopathy, splenomegaly, and/or hepatomegaly are present in 30 to 40% of cases, and at least 20 to 25% lymphoplasmacytoid cells are usually present in the marrow. Visceral involvement of the kidney, lung, small bowel, and peripheral nerves can also cause the clinical sequelae of infiltration (e.g., malabsorption in the setting of gastrointestinal involvement or neuropathy). Hemorrhagic complications are common, attributable to abnormal bleeding times, decreased platelet adhesion, or direct interference by the IgM protein with the release of platelet factor 3 or coagulation factors. Primary systemic amyloidosis occurs rarely. Hyperviscosity syndrome, a rare complication of myeloma, is seen more commonly in the setting of excess IgM and is characterized by mucosal bleeding and neurologic, ocular, and cardiovascular abnormalities. Plasmapheresis is more useful to remove excess IgM than it is in the setting of excess IgG monoclonal proteins and related hyperviscosity in myeloma.

Plasmapheresis can be considered only as adjunctive therapy. Treatment regimens are similar to those for low-grade lymphomas and myeloma (e.g., chlorambucil, cyclophosphamide, melphalan, and corticosteroids), either as single agents or in combination. In contrast to persons with myeloma, however, many individuals with Waldenström's macroglobulinemia have indolent disease requiring no therapy for long periods of time, with survival in excess of 20 years. Pretreatment parameters including older age, male sex, constitutional symptoms, and cytopenias define a high-risk population that could perhaps benefit from newer therapeutic approaches. Acute leukemia has developed in patients with Waldenström's macroglobulinemia, emphasizing a potential complication of premature and prolonged low-dose therapy with alkylating agents. Recently 2-chlorodeoxyadenosine (Leustatin),* which has achieved high response rates and durable responses in hairy cell leukemia, has also been shown to be effective in newly diagnosed as well as refractory Waldenström's macroglobulinemia.

Heavy Chain Diseases

These diseases are characterized by the presence of a portion of the Ig heavy chain in the serum or urine or both. The most common presenting symptoms are weakness, fatigue, and fever associated with lymphadenopathy and hepatosplenomegaly. In addition to Ig heavy chains in serum or urine, a lymphoplasmacytic marrow infiltrate is noted in most cases. The clinical course can be fulminant and rapidly progressive; alternatively, the monoclonal γ heavy chain can persist for years in otherwise asymptomatic patients. Treatment options for progressive disease are similar to those for lymphoma or myeloma, whereas patients with the more indolent form should be followed expectantly without therapy.

Amyloidosis

Amyloidosis is relatively rare as a clinically significant disease. It has been classified as follows: (1) primary, with or without plasma cell and lymphoid neoplasms; (2) secondary, associated with chronic infections or autoimmune disease; (3) heredofamilial, associated with familial Mediterranean fever, Portu-

*Not FDA approved for this indication.

guese lower limb neuropathy, and others; (4) amyloidosis associated with aging; and (5) amyloidosis of endocrine glands, with medullary thyroid carcinoma and multiple endocrine neoplasia type 2. The amyloid found in most cases of amyloidosis is classified according to whether the fibrils consist mainly of the variable region of Ig light chains (AL, primary amyloidosis) or protein A (AA, secondary amyloidosis).

Treatment for AL has been unsatisfactory, although alkylating agent–based chemotherapy may be beneficial for a subset of patients and result in prolonged survival. In an exciting development, dose-intensive melphalan with blood stem cell support has been noted to achieve complete remissions, with improvement in performance status and clinical remission of organ-specific disease.

COMPLICATIONS

Complications of myeloma include bone disease and hypercalcemia, hyperviscosity, recurrent infections, renal failure, and cardiac failure.

Bone Disease and Hypercalcemia

As noted earlier, 80% of patients with myeloma present with bone pain. Bone lesions can manifest as isolated, discrete lytic lesions or diffuse osteopenia. Bone scans and serum alkaline phosphatase are usually not abnormal. Radiographic evaluation is standard. Although patients with normal renal function can increase urine calcium excretion, those with renal failure develop hypercalcemia. Therefore hypercalcemia is more likely to occur in the setting of Bence Jones proteinuria, myeloma kidney, chronic infection, or uric acid nephropathy. Overall, hypercalcemia occurs in 20 to 40% of patients with myeloma.

Treatment

Pamidronate (Aredia), an inhibitor of bone resorption, has been shown in a randomized trial to reduce skeletal complications, including pathologic fractures, need for radiation to bone, and spinal cord compression in patients with Durie-Salmon stage III myeloma and one or more lytic bone lesions. Interestingly, patients in this study who failed first-line chemotherapy had improved survival, suggesting that bisphosphonates may also have antimyeloma activity. More potent bisphosphonates (e.g., zoledronate) are currently undergoing clinical evaluation.

Hypercalcemia is managed by inhibition of osteoclastic bone resorption with corticosteroids, calcitonin, mithramycin, and/or bisphosphonates, as well as the primary treatment for the myeloma.

Hyperviscosity

Hyperviscosity is characterized clinically by spontaneous bleeding with neurologic and ocular disorders. It can result from elevated serum viscosity, increased numbers of cells (polycythemia or leukemia), or increased resistance of cells to deformation (sickle cell anemia or spherocytosis). In myeloma with hyperglobulinemia, coagulopathy has also been attributed to adsorption of minor clotting proteins onto the abnormal globulin. The severity of the syndrome is not directly related to the serum viscosity. Clinical findings improve with vigorous plasmapheresis, however, which reduces both myeloma protein concentration and serum viscosity.

Recurrent Infections

As noted previously, infection is a common cause of both morbidity and mortality. *Streptococcus pneumoniae* and *Haemophilus* infections usually occur early, during the response to chemotherapy. Gram-negative infections occur in refractory, advancing disease and are associated with previous antibiotic therapy, instrumentation, immobilization, colonization with hospital flora, and azotemia. Fatal infections may be hospital acquired, emphasizing the need to minimize indwelling devices in patients with myeloma. There is lack of correlation between bacteremia (either gram-negative or gram-positive) and chemotherapy-induced neutropenia. Fungal, herpes, mycobacterial, and *Pneumocystis* infections are only rarely described in myeloma patients.

Infection Prophylaxis

Due to its low cost and possible benefit to some patients, pneumococcal vaccination has been recommended. Repeated immunizations, not usually recommended due to local and systemic reactions, have not been studied in myeloma but may be useful. In a double-blind randomized trial of gammaglobulin prophylaxis in 48 patients with myeloma, no benefit was noted. At present gammaglobulin is reserved only for those with recurrent or life-threatening infections. The role of prophylactic antibiotics remains controversial.

Renal Failure

Renal failure in myeloma can predict poor outcome. The causes of renal failure in myeloma may be multifactorial and include hypercalcemia; myeloma kidney, with distal and proximal tubules obstructed by large laminated casts containing albumin, IgG, κ and λ light chains, surrounded by giant cells; hyperuricemia; intravenous urography; dehydration; plasma cell infiltration; pyelonephritis; and amyloidosis. The most important predisposing factor is dehydration; aggressive hydration is therefore crucial to avoid irreversible renal dysfunction. Otherwise treatment is for the underlying myeloma along with avoidance of intravenous urography. Combination chemotherapy is preferred due to the more rapid response than that obtained with melphalan and prednisone. The type and quantity of proteinuria can distinguish myeloma kidney, with larger amounts of light chains and less albuminuria; light chain deposition disease, characterized by low levels of both light chains and albumin in urine; and amyloidosis, in which there are large amounts of albuminuria and less light chain proteinuria.

Cardiac Failure

The mean and median age of patients with myeloma is approximately 60 years, and affected patients are also frequently at risk for cardiovascular disease. However, patients can be uniquely susceptible to cardiac ischemia and/or congestive heart failure (CHF) due to myocardial infiltration with amyloid causing dilated or restricted cardiomyopathy, hyperviscosity syndrome, and/or anemia. Myeloma patients are also susceptible to high-output CHF of unclear etiology.

Anemia

Anemia in myeloma can be due to a number of factors, including tumor infiltration of the bone marrow, renal impairment, myelosuppressive effects of chemotherapy, and deficient production of erythropoietin (EPO) compared with the degree of anemia. Pilot studies demonstrated efficacy of exogenous EPO in myeloma; 10,000 units per day subcutaneously three times weekly was the optimal starting dose.

POLYCYTHEMIA VERA

method of
PHILIP L. McCARTHY, Jr., M.D.
Roswell Park Cancer Institute
Buffalo, New York

Polycythemia vera (PV) is a clonal myeloproliferative disease resulting in dysregulated production of hematopoietic cells. An elevated red blood cell mass is a primary feature of this disorder. Other features of PV include an increased platelet and neutrophil count, confirming the pan-myeloid nature of this disease. PV has been considered part of a family of myeloproliferative disorders including essential thrombocytosis (ET), agnogenic myeloid metaplasia, and chronic myeloid leukemia. PV is an unusual disease, with an incidence of 0.5 to 1.5 cases per 100,000 population per year. The median age at presentation is 60 years. A literary reference to an elevated red blood cell mass can be found in Shakespeare's *Macbeth*. Following the murder of Lord Duncan, Lady Macbeth suffers nightmares. She complains of bloodstains that do not wash out: "Out damned spot! out I say! . . . Yet who would have thought the old man to have had so much blood in him?" Did the murdered king have PV?

Presenting symptoms and signs of PV are related to microcirculatory and macrocirculatory disturbances associated primarily with an elevated red cell mass and increased viscosity that may be accompanied by thrombocytosis and platelet dysfunction. Symptoms include headache, dizziness, visual changes, fatigue, and pruritus, which can be severe following warm water exposure. Signs of PV may include erythema, erythromelalgia (swelling), and ecchymoses, along with chronic eczematous skin changes. Hemorrhage and thrombosis are severe complications of PV. Hemorrhagic manifestations may include intracranial and gastrointestinal bleeding. Thrombotic events include Budd-Chiari syndrome and portal, splenic, and mesenteric vein thrombosis. Atypical cerebral ischemic attacks and cerebrovascular accidents also may result from uncontrolled PV. Despite these complications, the survival of PV patients is similar to that of age-matched controls if the disease is managed with appropriate care.

DIAGNOSIS

Patients with an increased hemoglobin, hematocrit, and red blood cell count may be evaluated for PV. The diagnosis of PV is based on the original criteria of the Polycythemia Vera Study Group in 1971 (Table 1). An elevated red blood cell mass is a requirement for diagnosis. Splenomegaly and a normal O_2 saturation are the other major criteria that determine the diagnosis of PV. An elevated red cell mass and normal O_2 saturation plus any two minor criteria (the B criteria in Table 1) also are diagnostic. Evidence of clonal hematopoiesis, autonomous bone marrow erythroid growth, and a decreased serum erythropoietin (EPO) level have also been proposed as diagnostic criteria. A bone marrow test will demonstrate a hypercellular marrow and an increase in number and size of megakaryocytic and erythroid precursors. Bone marrow morphologic abnormalities may include multilobulated megakaryocytes and increased reticulin staining. Clonal cytogenetic abnormalities may be seen in up to 50% of cases at presentation. Bone marrow culture by methylcellulose assay will demonstrate erythroid colony growth independent of EPO. Other peripheral blood laboratory abnormalities may include basophilia, eosinophilia, elevated uric acid, platelet aggregation abnormalities, and an increase in bleeding time. Artifactual hyperkalemia and hypoglycemia may result from

TABLE 1. **Polycythemia Vera: PVSG Major and Minor Diagnostic Criteria**

Major Criteria	Minor Criteria
A1: Increased red cell mass >32 mL/kg for females >36 mL/kg for males	B1: Platelet count $>400 \times 10^9$/L
A2: Normal arterial O_2 saturation (in the absence of a cause of secondary polycythemia)	B2: Neutrophil count $>10 \times 10^9$/L (in the absence of infection)
A3: Splenomegaly	B3: Elevated leukocyte alkaline phosphatase (in the absence of infection)
	B4: Elevated serum vitamin B_{12} level or unbound vitamin B_{12}-binding protein
	*Marker of clonal hematopoiesis
	*Autonomous erythroid colony growth
	*Decreased serum erythropoietin level

Abbreviation: PVSG = Polycythemia Vera Study Group.
The following combinations establish the diagnosis: A1 plus A2 plus A3, or A1 plus A2 plus any two minor (B) criteria. Proposed new criteria are labeled with an asterisk.

TABLE 2. **Causes of Secondary Polycythemia**

Cardiopulmonary disease
Altitude elevation
Abnormal hemoglobin with altered O_2 affinity
Methemoglobinemia
Drug-induced
Exogenous erythropoietin (EPO)
Androgens
Carcinomas
Hepatoma
Renal carcinoma
Other tumors
EPO receptor mutation
Abnormal EPO production

cellular release and metabolic turnover in vitro before blood sample analysis. Correction for this phenomenon can be achieved by plasma sampling and rapid analysis.

Considerations in the differential diagnosis for PV are the causes of secondary polycythemia (Table 2). The most common cause of secondary polycythemia is cardiopulmonary disease. Persons who live at high altitudes develop polycythemia owing to relative hypoxia. Unusual causes of polycythemia are hemoglobin mutations that result in abnormal O_2 binding. This abnormality can be detected by hemoglobin O_2-binding determination. Other unusual causes of secondary polycythemia include methemoglobinemia, drugs, carcinomas, mutations of the EPO receptor, and abnormal EPO production.

THERAPY

The therapy of PV has not changed significantly over the past three decades. Major therapeutic options are outlined in Table 3, and guidelines for treatment, in Table 4. Phlebotomy (with removal of 250 to 500 mL of whole blood) should be performed at 1- to 2-day intervals to decrease the hematocrit to less than 45%. Maintenance phlebotomy should occur at 2- to 8-week intervals to maintain the hematocrit at less than 45%. All patients will develop iron deficiency that may necessitate reducing the frequency of phlebotomy. Iron deficiency in PV patients does not result in nonhematologic complications. Iron replacement can exacerbate PV, causing a rapid rise in hematocrit and is not recommended.

In younger patients the platelet count may be maintained between 400 and 1000 × 10^9 per liter in the absence of thrombotic complications. Patients older than 50 years and especially those older than 70, as well as those patients with platelet-associated thromboses, should have platelet counts maintained at less than 400 × 10^9 per liter owing to the risk of hemorrhage and thrombosis. PV platelets may have a qualitative functional defect that results in bleeding despite normal or high platelet counts. Some clinicians recommend the use of low-dose aspirin at 40 mg per day for patients with a history of thrombosis or with high and difficult-to-control platelet counts, although this is an area of some controversy.

TABLE 3. **Options for Treatment of Polycythemia Vera**

Phlebotomy
Hydroxyurea (Hydrea)
Interferon alfa-2a (Roferon-A) and interferon alfa-2b (Intron A)
Anagrelide (Agrelin)
Radioactive phosphorus (^{32}P)
Aspirin (low dose for elevated platelet count?)

TABLE 4. **Age-Related Guidelines for Treatment of Polycythemia Vera**

Age <50 y	Age >50 y
Maintain hematocrit at <45%	Maintain hematocrit at <45%
Maintain platelet count <400 to 1000 × 10^9/L	Maintain platelet count <400 × 10^9/L

Antimetabolites and other agents have been used to control the elevated platelet count and hematocrit associated with PV. Hydroxyurea (HU) (Hydrea),* at doses usually ranging from 10 to 30 mg per kg per day (500 to 2000 mg), may be used to lower the platelet count and assist in control of the red cell count. HU has a low or minimal risk for the development of leukemia and is widely used for control of blood counts, unlike chlorambucil, which is leukemogenic and is not recommended. Interferon alfa has been used to control the platelet count and hematocrit at doses of 6 to 27 × 10^6 units given three times weekly. In addition, interferon alfa may control the symptoms of pruritus and erythromelalgia. Pipobroman,† an unusual alkylating agent, has been used for the control of PV with initial dosing of 1 to 3 mg per kg per day, up to 30 days, and maintenance therapy at 0.1 to 0.2 mg per kg per day. There is a suggestion that patients receiving pipobroman may be less likely than those on HU therapy to develop myelofibrosis and acute leukemia. Anagrelide (Agrelin), at doses of 0.5 to 2 mg per day in divided doses, with adjustment to a lower maintenance dose, has been approved for ET and the thrombocytosis associated with PV. Radioactive phosphorus (^{32}P) may be used for the control of excessive platelet and red blood cell counts in elderly (older than 70 years) patients refractory to other therapy and/or not tolerant of phlebotomy. The dose is 2.3 mCi per m^2 (maximum dose 5 mCi) intravenously (IV) at 12-week intervals, with a maximum yearly dose of 15 mCi. There is a 10% risk of leukemogenesis over a 10-year period, and this therapy should not be used in a younger patient. Blood counts may need to be monitored weekly during early therapy and monthly when the counts are stable. The neutrophil count with any treatment should not fall below 1500 per μL, and a falling white blood cell count despite therapeutic modification may signal a change of the disease to a myelofibrotic phase or transition to acute leukemia.

Symptoms of pruritus may be severe even with

*Not FDA approved for this indication.
†Not available in the United States.

control of the hematocrit. Hydroxyzine (Vistaril), 50 to 100 mg given four times daily; or cimetidine (Tagamet),* 300 mg, four times daily; or cyproheptadine (Periactin), 4 to 8 mg, four times daily, may be necessary for control of these symptoms. Hyperuricemia may predispose to gout and is treated with allopurinol (Zyloprim) at doses of 100 to 300 mg per day depending on renal function.

LONG-TERM HEMATOLOGIC SEQUELAE OF POLYCYTHEMIA VERA

Less than 10% of PV patients may develop acute myeloid leukemia (AML) as a consequence of their disease and unrelated to the use of leukemogenic therapeutic agents. Another unusual consequence of PV is post–polycythemic myeloid metaplasia, which may occur several years into the course of PV. This disease is similar to agnogenic myeloid metaplasia, with the development of bone marrow myelofibrosis. It is accompanied by splenomegaly and cytopenias including anemia and thrombocytopenia. The development of post–polycythemic myeloid metaplasia may herald the onset of AML. Results of treatment of AML arising from PV are similar to those with other secondary acute leukemias arising from myeloproliferative disorders. Aggressive therapy such as allogeneic hematopoietic stem cell transplantation may be considered for young PV patients who develop AML or an aggressive form of myeloid metaplasia.

ACKNOWLEDGMENTS

I thank Dr. S. Jack Mitus for the quotation from *Macbeth* and for encouraging my interest in hematology, and Dr. David S. Rosenthal, who is the consummate clinician and teacher.

THE PORPHYRIAS

method of
PERTTI MUSTAJOKI, M.D.
University Central Hospital of Helsinki
Helsinki, Finland

Porphyrias are a group of diseases caused by defective functions of the enzymes of heme biosynthesis. Seven different porphyrias are known, each corresponding to an abnormality of a specific enzyme of the pathway (Table 1). The genes coding for the enzymes are known in all porphyrias, and several mutations have been identified in porphyric patients.

Two major types of clinical manifestations occur in porphyrias. Acute porphyric attack, which is characterized by abdominal pain and neurologic manifestations, is a feature in acute intermittent porphyria, variegate porphyria, and hereditary coproporphyria. In all three conditions the porphyrin precursors porphobilinogen and 5-aminolevulinic acid are accumulated during attacks. In other porphyrias cutaneous symptoms are the principal manifestations.

In symptomatic patients the specific porphyria can easily be diagnosed by specific laboratory tests (Table 2). Most porphyrias are inherited in autosomal dominant fashion, but the penetrance of the disease varies greatly. In many porphyrias, the majority of patients remain asymptomatic throughout their lives. Biochemical tests are often inaccurate in the diagnosis of latent cases of porphyria. When the underlying mutation in an affected family is known, the DNA diagnosis is accurate, but the genetic heterogeneity of individual porphyrias restricts usefulness of this method.

ACUTE PORPHYRIAS

The acute porphyrias—acute intermittent porphyria, porphyria variegata, and hereditary coproporphyria— are characterized by episodic acute attacks. During an acute attack, symptoms include severe abdominal pain, vomiting, constipation, often pain in the extremities and in the back, and psychologic symptoms that range from anxiety to delirium. Urine may be dark or red in color because of increased amounts of porphobilin and porphyrins. Sometimes the disease progresses to peripheral motor neuropathy with the onset of seizures or cranial nerve palsies. Common clinical findings are hypertension and sinus tachycardia, and routine laboratory findings may include low serum sodium values.

All symptoms during acute attacks are nonspecific, and the diagnosis must be confirmed by appropriate laboratory tests. Laboratory diagnosis is easy, because during attacks all patients, irrespective of the type of porphyria, excrete great amounts of the porphyrin precursors porphobilinogen and 5-aminolevulinic acid. A rapid and relatively reliable qualitative test for porphobilinogen is available. A clearly positive qualitative test is a strong indicator of acute porphyria and allows beginning of therapy. However, the diagnosis must always be confirmed by quantitative tests for porphobilinogen and 5-aminolevulinic acid. During acute attacks the values are usually more than 10 times higher than reference values.

Treatment of the Acute Attack

Treatment of acute porphyric attacks includes three different approaches: elimination of precipitating factors, specific therapy, and symptomatic treatment. Summary of treatment is outlined in Table 3.

Elimination of Precipitating Factors

Acute porphyric attacks are often precipitated by factors such as certain drugs, excessive alcohol consumption, and fasting. Lists of precipitating drugs and safe drugs are available in textbooks and on the

*Not FDA approved for this indication.

TABLE 1. **Characteristics of Individual Porphyrias**

Porphyria	Inheritance	Enzyme Defect	Main Clinical Symptoms	Main Biochemical Tests
Acute intermittent porphyria	Autosomal dominant	Porphobilinogen deaminase	Acute attacks	Urinary porphobilinogen and 5-aminolevulinic acid, erythrocyte porphobilinogen deaminase
Variegate porphyria (porphyria variegata)	Autosomal dominant	Protoporphyrinogen oxidase	Acute attacks and skin fragility	Fecal protoporphyrin, plasma fluorescence
Hereditary coproporphyria	Autosomal dominant	Coproporphyrinogen oxidase	Acute attacks and skin fragility	Fecal and urinary coproporphyrin
Porphyria cutanea tarda	Acquired or autosomal dominant	Uroporphyrinogen decarboxylase	Skin fragility and liver disease	Urinary uroporphyrin, plasma fluorescence
Erythropoietic protoporphyria	Autosomal dominant, sometimes recessive	Ferrochelatase	Photosensitivity, liver damage	Erythrocyte protoporphyrin, plasma fluorescence
Congenital erythropoietic porphyria	Autosomal recessive	Uroporphyrinogen III synthase	Severe skin symptoms, hemolysis	Urinary and erythrocyte uroporphyrin I

Internet.* All drugs listed as unsafe must be avoided in patients with acute symptoms. Because fasting or a hypocaloric state may precipitate attacks, nutrition allowing enough calories as carbohydrates is important. If nausea prevents eating, feeding via nasogastric tube or parenteral nutrition is necessary.

Specific Therapy

Heme therapy and carbohydrate loading are specific therapies for acute porphyric attacks because these agents are able to reduce the overproduction of excess amounts of porphyrin precursors. Heme is much more effective in this regard than glucose.

Specific treatment is justified only when a patient has symptoms and signs compatible with an acute attack and increased excretion of porphobilinogen in the urine. The presence of symptoms without raised levels of porphobilinogen, or the finding of raised levels of porphobilinogen, 5-aminolevulinic acid, or porphyrins without symptoms, is not an indication for specific treatment.

Mild attacks are sometimes treated with glucose loading (by the oral or intravenous route, 400 to 500 grams daily) rather than heme. Severe attacks or symptoms that on the basis of clinical findings seem likely to progress should be treated with heme. When indicated, heme therapy should be started without delay because the effect of any treatment may be poor later in an attack after onset of neuropathy. Patients who have received heme may still require administration of some intravenous glucose and other nutrients for nutritional support.

The usual dose of heme is 3 mg per kg daily given intravenously for 4 consecutive days. The course may be shorter if the patient responds quickly or longer if the attack persists more than 4 days. There are two commercial heme preparations: hemin (Panhematin) and heme arginate (Normosang). Heme arginate is

*Home page of the American Porphyria Foundation (PO Box 22712, Houston, TX 77227, telephone number 713-266-9617): http://www.enterprise.net/apf/drugs.html.

TABLE 2. **Problem-Based Approach to Diagnosis of Porphyrias**

Symptoms Suggesting Porphyria	Diagnostic Tests	Interpretation
Classic features of an acute porphyric attack (e.g., abdominal pain, vomiting, extremity pain, psychologic symptoms)	Qualitative urinary porphobilinogen Quantitative urinary porphobilinogen and 5-aminolevulinic acid	• Qualitative test clearly positive, quantitative tests give clearly increased values → **acute porphyric attack**
Increased fragility of sun-exposed skin	Urinary total porphyrins or uroporphyrin Fecal protoporphyrin Plasma fluorescence spectrum	• Urinary uroporphyrin markedly increased and a characteristic fluorescence spectrum → **porphyria cutanea tarda** • Fecal protoporphyrin content clearly increased and a characteristic plasma fluorescence spectrum → **variegate porphyria** • Fecal coproporphyrin content increased and a characteristic plasma fluorescence spectrum → **hereditary coproporphyria**
Acute photosensitivity	Erythrocyte protoporphyrin Urinary porphyrins Plasma fluorescence spectrum	• Erythrocyte protoporphyrin concentration increased more than 5 to 10 times normal, characteristic plasma fluorescence spectrum → **erythropoietic protoporphyria** • Urinary porphyrins (uroporphyrin I) massively increased → **congenital erythropoietic porphyria**

TABLE 3. **Treatment of Symptoms of Acute Porphyria**

Elimination of precipitating factors
- Eliminate all unsafe drugs
- Attend to adequate calories and nutrition

Specific therapy
- Heme, 3 mg/kg for 4 days
- Mild attacks may be treated with glucose 400 to 500 gm/day

Symptomatic and supportive therapy
- Severe pain: opiates in appropriate doses
- Hypertension: propranolol or other beta-adrenergic blocking agents
- Hyponatremia: saline infusion, fluid restriction if signs of inappropriate antidiuretic hormone secretion develop
- Psychologic symptoms: chlorpromazine
- Epileptic seizures: diazepam or clonazepam (no barbiturates or phenytoin!); correction of hyponatremia
- Motor neuropathy: physiotherapy

the preferred preparation for intravenous use because it has been studied intensively and seems to have fewer side effects than hemin. Heme arginate has been registered in many European and other countries. In the United States, heme arginate has been under investigation but will be available soon. Hemin has been long available in the United States.

Symptomatic Therapy

Patients with acute attacks usually have symptoms that may necessitate medication or other therapies, summarized in Table 3. Pain is typically severe, often requiring opiate analgesics for control; morphine, meperidine, or other opiates in normal doses may be used. For insomnia, chloral hydrate or benzodiazepines can be used. Chlorpromazine (Thorazine), up to 25 mg three or four times a day, can be given for major psychologic symptoms.

Seizures, which may occur during acute attacks, should not be treated with phenytoin or barbiturates because they are porphyric attack–precipitating drugs. Diazepam (Valium) and clonazepam (Klonopin) are probably safe and can be used in appropriate doses. Peripheral motor neuropathy tends to resolve slowly, with improvement to normal over weeks or months. Thus, it should be treated with effective physiotherapy and, if respiratory muscles are involved, with mechanical ventilation.

Prevention of Acute Attacks

After an acute attack the patient must be informed about precipitating factors to prevent future episodes. A list of unsafe drugs should be provided, and avoidance of alcohol consumption should be emphasized. Some authors recommend more strict regulation of dietary intake, e.g., a carbohydrate intake of 55 to 60% of total energy intake, but there is no evidence that this regimen improves the outcome. Our policy is to instruct the patient to avoid fasting or vigorous weight reduction but otherwise not to regulate food intake.

A few female patients with acute porphyria may have frequent symptoms associated with menstrual cycles. The symptoms usually develop during the premenstrual phase. Various hormonal manipulations have been tried for prevention of symptoms. Exogenous estrogens and progestins, e.g., oral contraceptive pills, have been reported to prevent attacks in some patients. These agents must be administered with caution, because female sex hormones are also regarded as precipitating drugs. In some patients, symptoms can be prevented by using gonadotropin-releasing hormone analogues. If there is a good response to one of these agents for several months, low doses of estradiol can be added to control the adverse effects of inadequate endogenous estrogens. Hormonal treatment for cyclical attacks is seldom needed for more than 1 to 3 years, which suggests that such attacks do not occur throughout the reproductive period of life. If hormonal manipulation does not control cyclical attacks, prophylactic heme administration can be used. The dose of heme in the prophylactic use is not established, but most treatment centers administer one infusion of 3 mg per kg weekly or, in milder cases, biweekly. An alternative approach is to administer heme only during the luteal phase of the cycle if the symptoms occur regularly premenstrually.

Management of acute attacks does not require identification of the exact type of acute porphyria, because the treatment and prevention are the same in all three types of acute porphyria. Prevention of attacks also includes evaluation of family members to find asymptomatic individuals with porphyria. In the asymptomatic phase, each of the acute porphyrias (acute intermittent porphyria, variegate porphyria, and hereditary coproporphyria) has characteristic biochemical findings (see Table 1). Thus, choosing appropriate laboratory tests for screening family members calls for precise identification of the type of porphyria. Biochemical tests identify most asymptomatic individuals with porphyria, but normal results do not exclude porphyria. The genes coding for the enzymes of heme biosynthesis are known, and various mutations have been described in patients with all three types of acute porphyria. Because of genetic heterogeneity, no universal DNA tests are available for acute porphyrias, but whenever the mutation is known a DNA analysis is the method of choice to diagnose or exclude porphyria among family members.

Also, asymptomatic family members should be informed about precipitating factors. Susceptibility to precipitating agents varies greatly, and many persons with latent porphyria tolerate them without harm. For that reason, in porphyric individuals who previously have been asymptomatic, strict avoiding of all drugs listed as unsafe is not necessary. Thus, for example, moderate alcohol intake is not necessarily prohibited, and contraceptive pills or postmenopausal hormone preparations can be allowed when appropriate.

PORPHYRIA CUTANEA TARDA

Porphyria cutanea porphyria is the most common type of porphyria in the United States and Europe.

Onset is usually during the fourth or fifth decade of life, and the disorder is manifested mainly as cutaneous symptoms and hepatopathy. Characteristic skin lesions are blistering and erosions on sun-exposed areas, mainly on the backs of the hands. Porphyria cutanea tarda is usually associated with chronic liver disease. Many patients consume excessive amounts of alcohol, and there is a high prevalence of hepatitis C infection among patients with porphyria cutanea tarda. In susceptible persons, hepatic siderosis is a common histopathologic finding, and accumulation of iron plays a pathogenetic role, probably by inhibiting uroporphyrinogen decarboxylase. In many countries, patients with porphyria cutanea tarda have an increased prevalence of genetic hemochromatosis, some 35 to 45% being heterozygous and 10 to 15% homozygous for major hemochromatosis mutations.

The main biochemical feature in porphyria cutanea tarda is massive overproduction of uroporphyrin. Urinary excretion of uroporphyrin in symptomatic patients is usually more than 2000 nmol per 24 hours (the normal value is less than 100 nmol). Other diagnostic characteristics are increased urinary 7-COOH porphyrin excretion, increased fecal isocoproporphyrin content, and a typical pattern in the plasma fluorescence spectrum.

Treatment

Predisposing factors such as alcohol, iron supplements, and estrogen preparations should be eliminated. In some cases this may result in clinical and biochemical remission.

Two specific and effective treatments for porphyria cutanea tarda are known, namely, iron removal by phlebotomy and low-dose chloroquine therapy.* There is no general agreement on which is preferable; the use of chloroquine is more frequent in many European countries than in the United States, where chloroquine is recommended only if phlebotomy is contraindicated. In patients with significant iron overload, phlebotomy is the preferred therapy; in other cases, either treatment may be efficacious. Combination therapy with chloroquine and phlebotomy has also been reported to be useful.

In phlebotomy, 400 to 500 mL of blood is removed at weekly or biweekly intervals until the blood hemoglobin concentration falls to 100 to 110 grams per liter. Usually, 4 to 10 liters of blood must be removed before therapeutic effects are seen. Measurement of urinary excretion of uroporphyrin or total porphyrins is useful for monitoring the therapeutic effect, and phlebotomies can be discontinued when uroporphyrin excretion falls below 500 nmol per 24 hours. Clinical remission occurs usually within 6 months and biochemical remission within 12 months.

In low-dose chloroquine therapy, chloroquine (Aralen) or hydroxychloroquine (Plaquenil) is administered orally 125 mg twice a week. The time needed for clinical and biochemical remission is usually the same as with phlebotomies.

After remission induced by phlebotomy or chloroquine, a relapse usually occurs within 1 to 2 years. Clinical relapse can be predicted by monitoring urinary excretion of porphyrins at intervals of 3 to 6 months. Treatment can be started if porphyrin levels are increasing (e.g., with uroporphyrin levels of 500 to 1000 nmol per 24 hours), which will prevent the occurrence of clinical manifestations.

ERYTHROPOIETIC PROTOPORPHYRIA

Erythropoietic protoporphyria is manifested as acute photoreactivity of the skin in childhood. Typical symptoms are stinging pain or itching with subsequent swelling and erythema of the exposed skin within minutes to hours after sun exposure. Hepatobiliary complications may be associated with protoporphyria: early-onset cholelithiasis is found in 10% and signs of parenchymal liver disease are seen in 5 to 20% of patients.

The main biochemical finding is massively increased concentrations of free erythrocyte protoporphyrin: the values in symptomatic patients are usually more than 10 μmol per liter (the normal value is less than 1.0 μmol). Other biochemical findings are increased fecal protoporphyrin content in most patients and a characteristic plasma fluorescence spectrum.

Treatment

There is no specific treatment for erythropoietic protoporphyria. In most patients, beta carotene* increases tolerance to sunlight, but it has no influence on the erythrocyte or plasma porphyrin concentrations. The dosage of beta carotene must be adjusted to the level that clearly reduces photosensitivity. The daily effective dose varies, being 30 to 120 mg for children and 120 to 300 mg for adults. For therapeutic effects, the serum beta carotene concentration should be at least 600 to 800 μg per dL. The clinical effect is achieved concomitantly with carotenodermia, which develops over 3 to 6 weeks. In addition to beta carotene, topical sunscreens with high protection factor against long-wave ultraviolet radiation may be useful.

At present there is no effective treatment for prevention of liver complications. Many drugs such as cholestyramine,* chenodeoxycholic acid,* and heme have been used but without significant clinical effect. A liver transplantation is at present the only therapy for terminal liver failure associated with erythropoietic protoporphyria, although it poses specific problems. During surgery, phototoxic damage of abdominal wall and intestine, caused by standard lamps used in the operating room, has been reported. Thus, careful protection of the skin and modification of operating room lighting are needed. A long-term problem may be that protoporphyrin-induced damage may develop in the transplanted liver as well.

*Not FDA approved for this indication.

CONGENITAL ERYTHROPOIETIC PORPHYRIA

Congenital erythropoietic protoporphyria (Gunther's disease) is a rare autosomal recessive disease that is manifested as severe photosensitivity. This leads to bullae, scarring, and, ultimately, mutilation of the hands, nose, ears, and so on. Hemolysis is often present, but its mechanism is poorly understood. Congenital erythropoietic porphyria is an incapacitating disease with considerable mortality. The patients excrete massive amounts of porphyrins (mainly uroporphyrin I). Many organs, including the teeth, accumulate porphyrins, which can be detected by red fluorescence under ultraviolet light.

There is no effective therapy. Protection of the skin from sunlight is important to prevent skin reactions, skin infections, and mutilation. Topical sunscreens that give protection against radiation in the 400-nm region may be used, but their value has not been proved. Transfusion of packed red cells effectively suppresses the overproduction of porphyrins, but weekly transfusions are impracticable and lead to iron accumulation. Charcoal (60 grams three times daily) has been reported to lead to clinical improvement and to long-term reduction in the levels of porphyrins. It is not known whether charcoal is effective in every patient.

The site of overproduction of porphyrins in congenital erytropoietic porphyria is erythropoietic tissue. Bone marrow or stem cell transplantation replaces abnormally functioning cells with normal erythropoietic tissue. Some recent case reports suggest that these therapies can effect dramatic reversals of the clinical and biochemical abnormalities. At present, bone marrow or stem cell transplantation is the only curative treatment for patients with congenital erythropietic porphyrias. Although long-term results are lacking, this approach is the treatment of choice in severely disabled patients.

RARE TYPES OF PORPHYRIAS

5-Aminolevulinic acid (ALA) dehydratase defect porphyria is a very rare type of porphyria that is caused by severe deficiency of 5-aminolevulinic acid dehydratase, the second enzyme of the heme biosynthetic pathway. It is inherited in autosomal recessive fashion, and fewer than 10 cases have been reported. The disease manifests itself in childhood and is usually associated with severe neurologic abnormalities suggestive of acute porphyric attacks. No effective therapy is known. Heme therapy or liver transplantation has had little effect on clinical course.

Porphyrias that are inherited in autosomal dominant fashion and thus are manifested in the heterozygous state may rarely occur in homozygous forms. Homozygous cases of variegate porphyria and hereditary coproporphyria have been described. Onset is in childhood, with presenting manifestations of severe photosensitivity and nonspecific neurologic symptoms. No specific treatments have been reported.

Hepatoerythropoietic porphyria is a homozygous form of porphyria cutanea tarda. The disease manifests itself in early childhood with severe skin problems that may lead to scarring and mutilation as in congenital erythropoietic porphyria. No effective treatment has been reported. According to one report, phlebotomy had no effect on porphyrin excretion or skin lesions.

THERAPEUTIC USE OF BLOOD COMPONENTS

method of
JOHN D. ROBACK, M.D., PH.D., and
CHRISTOPHER D. HILLYER, M.D.
Emory University Hospital
Atlanta, Georgia

Before the 1960s, the primary blood product available for transfusion was whole blood. Today, however, donated whole blood is processed into a number of components including red blood cells (RBCs), platelets (PLTs), fresh frozen plasma (FFP), and cryoprecipitated antihemophilic factor (cryoprecipitate, or CRYO). In addition, plasma can also be fractionated into derivatives including albumin, immune globulin intravenous (IGIV), and clotting factor concentrates (factor VIII, factor IX, antithrombin III [ATIII], and others). Each of these components or derivatives has substantial therapeutic value in specific clinical settings. However, each also has the potential to cause adverse effects that may be associated with significant morbidity and mortality. Thus, these products must be used judiciously, which requires careful consideration of the patient's clinical condition, laboratory results, and alternatives to blood component transfusion.

DONOR SCREENING AND THE RISKS OF TRANSFUSION

Blood donors must answer confidential questions regarding their medical health, sexual practices, travel history, and any other factors that increase their likelihood of harboring transmissible infectious diseases. The donated blood then undergoes specific testing for human immunodeficiency virus-1 and -2 (HIV), hepatitis B virus (HBV), hepatitis C virus (HCV), human T-lymphotropic virus-I and -II (HTLV), and syphilis. Alanine aminotransferase (ALT) levels may also be determined. Blood units with repeat reactive infectious disease markers are destroyed, and if the test result is confirmed, the donor is prohibited from future donation in order to safeguard the blood supply.

Because of these screening procedures, the blood supply is safer today than at any time in recent history. Table 1 lists recent estimates of the risk of infectious disease transmission from blood transfu-

TABLE 1. **Transfusion-Associated Infection**

Infectious Agent	Estimated Transmission Incidence (per Number of Units)
Viruses	
HIV-1 and 2	1 in 493,000 (1 in 676,000)*
HAV	1 in 1,000,000
HBV	1 in 63,000
HCV	1 in 103,000
Non-ABC hepatitis	1 in 5900
HTLV-I and II	1 in 641,000
Bacteria/spirochetes	
Yersinia enterocolitica	1 in 500,000
Borrelia burgdorferi (Lyme disease)	NE
Rickettsia spp. (spotted fever)	NE
Parasites	
Trypanosoma cruzi (Chagas disease)	1 in 42,000
Trypanosoma gambiense, T. rhodesiense (African trypanosomiasis)	NE
Plasmodium sp. (malaria)	NE
Babesia microcoti (babesiosis)	NE
Toxoplasma gondii (toxoplasmosis)	NE
Leishmania tropica (leishmaniasis)	NE
Other	
Prions (Creutzfeldt-Jakob disease)	NE

*The lower incidence of 1:676,000 is estimated based on the inclusion of an HIV p24 antigen determination in the screening protocol; some authorities consider these estimates to be high and suggest that the actual incidence of HIV transmission by transfusion may be less than 1 in 1,000,000.
Abbreviations: HAV = hepatitis A virus; HBV = hepatitis B virus; HCV = hepatitis C virus; NE = not estimated.

sion; many authorities consider these estimates to be conservative. In general, these risks are small, especially when it has been estimated that up to 50% of patients who require RBC transfusion may die without transfusion.

In addition to infectious disease transmission, there are other adverse transfusion effects that are categorized as immune- or non–immune-mediated; these are listed in Table 2. Adverse reactions to blood transfusions are described in more detail in the following article, "Adverse Effects of Blood Transfusion."

TABLE 2. **Immune- and Nonimmune-Mediated Transfusion Reactions**

Immunologic	Nonimmunologic
Hemolysis (ABO incompatibility)	Infectious disease transmission
Anaphylaxis (IgA deficiency)	Volume overload
Hypotension	Hemolysis (physical)
TRALI	Hypothermia
Febrile nonhemolytic reaction	Hyperkalemia
Allergic (urticarial) reaction	Hypocalcemia
TA-GVHD	Iron overload
Posttransfusion purpura	
Alloimmunization	
Immunomodulation	

Abbreviations: TRALI = transfusion-related acute lung injury; TA-GVHD = transfusion-associated graft-versus-host disease.

BLOOD COMPONENT PREPARATION

Whole blood, donated into a preservative/anticoagulant solution, is separated into components by differential centrifugation. Initially, packed erythrocytes (RBCs, stored at 1 to 6°C for up to 42 days) are sedimented by low-speed centrifugation, leaving a platelet-rich plasma supernatant. This supernatant is subsequently centrifuged at a higher speed to make a platelet concentrate (PLT, stored at 20 to 24°C with continuous agitation up to 5 days) and supernatant plasma, which if frozen at −18°C or less within 8 hours of collection is termed FFP. If FFP is thawed at 1 to 6°C, a precipitate forms (CRYO), which can then be separated from the thawed plasma unit and refrozen for later use. Both FFP and CRYO can be stored at −18°C for up to 1 year.

INDIVIDUAL BLOOD COMPONENTS

Red Blood Cells

Constituents. Each RBC unit in Adsol-1 preservative/anticoagulant solution contains about 3×10^{12} erythrocytes at a hematocrit of about 60%. In addition, 3×10^9 leukocytes and a small residual amount of platelet-containing plasma are also present.

Indications. RBC transfusions are indicated to increase peripheral oxygen delivery in patients with signs and/or symptoms of anemia. Hemoglobin quantitation can be used to broadly categorize patients into those who are likely or unlikely to benefit from RBC transfusion (Table 3). However, the final transfusion decision must be based on a careful clinical evaluation. Signs and symptoms of decreased oxygen delivery include dyspnea (with and without exertion), tachycardia, and angina. The rapidity with which anemia develops, the likelihood of ongoing blood loss, and the coexistence of conditions such as coronary artery disease must also be considered (see Table 3).

Dosage. The current standard of care is evolving and varies among institutions. Usually, an initial transfusion of 2 RBC units is given, followed by repeat hemoglobin quantitation and clinical evaluation to determine whether or not additional transfusions are needed. Each RBC unit should increase the he-

TABLE 3. **Indications for Red Blood Cell Transfusion**

Hemoglobin (g/dL)	Transfusion Priority	Clinical Factors that Increase Transfusion Priority	
<7	Usually transfuse	Dyspnea	Acute anemia
7–10	May transfuse	Tachypnea	Continued bleeding
>10	Rarely transfuse	Angina	Coronary artery disease

moglobin concentration of an average-sized adult by approximately 1 gram per dL.

Contraindications and Alternative Therapies. Transfusion of RBCs is usually not appropriate in patients without symptomatic anemia regardless of hemoglobin concentration. In patients with volume depletion and adequate oxygen-carrying capacity, crystalloid or colloid infusion is indicated. In chronically anemic patients with inadequate nutrition, hematinic therapy (iron, vitamin B_{12}, and folate) should be administered based on the specific deficiency. Preoperative autologous RBC donations and intraoperative RBC salvage methodologies are alternatives to the use of allogeneic RBC units during surgery. Concomitant use of epoetin alfa (Procrit) allows preoperative autologous blood donations by some patients who would otherwise be deterred from donating, or in those patients who are unable to donate autologous blood and have a hemoglobin of 10 to 13 grams per dL, prior to elective surgery to raise the hematocrit. Erythropoietin is also beneficial in patients whose anemia is due to chronic renal disease, AZT therapy (in patients infected with HIV), or cancer therapy. Leukoreduced units (LR-RBCs) can be used to decrease the incidence of recurrent febrile transfusion reactions, cytomegalovirus (CMV) transmission, and HLA alloimmunization (see further on). CMV-seronegative units are also available. Washed units (W-RBCs) and gamma-irradiated units (I-RBCs) should be used to prevent repetitive allergic transfusion reactions, and transfusion-associated graft-versus-host disease (TA-GVHD), respectively. Washing and gamma irradiation may require 1 to 2 hours extra preparation time (see discussion of special processing).

Platelets

Constituents. PLT units should contain a minimum of 5.5×10^{10} platelets (and an average of 7 to 8×10^{10} platelets) in plasma and preservative/anticoagulant solution with a final volume of about 50 mL. Pools of six platelet concentrates are usually considered to be an adequate dose (see further on) and contain about 10^8 leukocytes. Single donor platelet pheresis units (SD-PLT) should contain a minimum of 3×10^{11} platelets (and an average of 4 to 5×10^{11} platelets) in a volume of approximately 200 mL. In addition, about 10^6 leukocytes are present. SD-PLT units are often considered to be a superior product as they expose the recipient to only one donor's infectious disease risk, can be efficiently crossmatched or HLA-matched, and are significantly leukoreduced (about 100-fold compared to PLT concentrates) without filtration. The coagulation factors II, VII, IX, X and fibrinogen present in the plasma are stable during storage, while the others are more labile.

Indications. PLT transfusions are indicated in patients with active generalized bleeding (petechiae, bleeding from mucosal surfaces including the gastrointestinal and urinary tracts) *and* a decreased peripheral blood platelet count. Rarely, these patients may have a platelet function defect, which should be diagnosed in consultation with a coagulation specialist. There are also indications for prophylactic platelet transfusions in nonbleeding patients, including patients with platelet counts less than 10,000 to 20,000 per μL, patients undergoing minor surgery with counts less than 50,000 per μL, and those with platelet counts less than 100,000 per μL before major surgery. The bleeding time test is generally not considered reliable for determining the need for PLT transfusions, and should not be used for this purpose.

Dosage. Platelet concentrates are usually given in pools of 6 to 8 units, or 1 unit per 10 kg of patient weight. A pool of six PLT concentrates can increase the platelet count of a 75-kg patient by 30 to 60,000 per μL at 10 to 60 minutes posttransfusion. SD-PLT units are usually given individually and can produce an increase in platelet count of the same magnitude.

Contraindications and Alternative Therapies. PLT transfusions should not be used for control of localized bleeding, which frequently requires local intervention including suturing. PLT transfusions are also contraindicated in thrombotic thrombocytopenic purpura (TTP) and heparin-induced thrombocytopenia, where they may exacerbate the thrombotic complications; TTP should be treated with plasma exchange using FFP as the replacement fluid (see following section). PLT transfusions are usually unsuccessful in patients with idiopathic thrombocytopenic purpura (ITP) where there is immunologic destruction of autologous and transfused platelets; corticosteroids, IGIV, and splenectomy are preferred treatments. In uremic patients with bleeding, DDAVP is the treatment of choice; however, platelet transfusion in conjunction with dialysis may provide clinical benefit. Uremic platelet dysfunction is reversible with correction of the underlying cause.

Specialized platelet products are often helpful in patients requiring chronic platelet support. Some patients become unresponsive to PLT transfusions; that is, bleeding does not stop after transfusion and the patient fails to obtain a corrected count increment (CCI) of at least 7 to 10,000 per μL. The CCI is calculated as follows:

$$\begin{aligned} \text{CCI} = {} & (\text{1 hour posttransfusion PLT count} \\ & - \text{pretransfusion PLT count}) \\ & \times (\text{body surface area in m}^2) \\ & \div (\text{number of PLT concentrates transfused}) \\ & \times (0.7) \end{aligned}$$

where the surface area of an average-sized adult is 1.7 m^2, and the constant 0.7 in the denominator is based on PLT units with an average of 7×10^{10} (or 0.7×10^{11}) platelets per μL. Unresponsiveness to PLT transfusions may be due to immune-mediated refractoriness or to clinical factors, including fever and/or sepsis, splenomegaly, continued bleeding and/or disseminated intravascular coagulation (DIC), and amphotericin B treatment. If these clinical factors are not present, immune refractoriness is presumed, and the patient should be given trials of ABO-matched, crossmatched, or HLA-matched platelet units in order to find a specialized component that produces an adequate platelet response. Leukoreduced, washed, and irradiated PLT units are used for the same indications as similarly processed RBC units.

Fresh Frozen Plasma

Constituents. FFP contains all the proteins normally present in the plasma from whole blood, including coagulation factors, immunoglobulins, and albumin. On average, FFP contains 0.7 to 1 units per mL of each coagulation factor and 2 to 3 mg per mL of fibrinogen. Volume averages 250 mL.

Indications. There are relatively few accepted indications for FFP, most of which are specific to its coagulation factor content. FFP is indicated for congenital deficiencies of coagulation factors for which no factor concentrates are currently available (e.g., factor V, factor VII, factor XI, protein C, and protein S) and for C1-esterase inhibitor deficiency. FFP is also indicated in liver disease and transplantation where there are multiple factor deficiencies and bleeding, in DIC, and for rapid reversal of a warfarin (Coumadin) overdose. In patients undergoing cardiopulmonary bypass or massive transfusion (replacement of one blood volume [about 5 liters] within 24 hours), FFP is indicated for symptomatic bleeding but not for bleeding prophylaxis. FFP is also indicated for therapeutic plasma exchange in patients with TTP and Refsum's disease.

Dosage. Typically, an order of FFP consists of 2 to 4 units. However, the appropriate dose may best be calculated from the plasma volume, the desired increment of factor activity, and the expected half-life of the factor being replaced. Alternatively, FFP dosage may be estimated as 8 to 10 mL per kg, and can be ordered as the number of milliliters to be infused. The frequency of administration depends on the clinical response to the infusion and improvement in laboratory values, although complete correction of laboratory abnormalities may not occur and should not be used to define the endpoint for FFP transfusion.

Contraindications and Alternative Therapies. FFP is not indicated for volume expansion, nutritional supplementation, or reconstitution of RBCs into whole blood. FFP is not appropriate for prophylaxis in nonbleeding patients with liver disease or those undergoing cardiopulmonary bypass or massive transfusion. In patients with hypoalbuminemia or protein deficiency, FFP is not indicated; in patients with immunoglobulin deficiencies, IGIV should be used (see further on). In nonbleeding patients with deficiencies in vitamin K–dependent coagulation factors, vitamin K administration is first-line therapy but requires about 8 hours for an observable effect. FFP is not indicated for deficiencies of specific factors (such as factor VIII, factor IX, and ATIII) for which concentrates are available. For patients with von Willebrand's disease, hypofibrinogenemia, or dysfibrinogenemia, CRYO is preferred to FFP because a smaller volume can be administered. Mild type I von Willebrand's disease may also respond to DDAVP therapy. FFP is strongly contraindicated for heparin neutralization, since the ATIII content of FFP may be sufficient, when bound to heparin, to inactivate thrombin and factor Xa and thus actually exacerbate the bleeding tendency.

As an alternative to FFP, solvent/detergent-treated plasma (SD-plasma), is prepared from pools of FFP by combined solvent and detergent treatments to inactivate enveloped viruses. SD-plasma has recently received FDA approval and may become preferred to FFP because of a decreased risk of infectious disease transmission.

Cryoprecipitate

Constituents. CRYO is a concentrate of factor VIII (minimum 80 IU; average of 100 to 120 IU), fibrinogen (100 to 350 mg), and factor VIII:von Willebrand's factor (factor VIII:vWF). CRYO also contains fibronectin (50 to 60 mg) and factor XIII. The volume of a single unit is 5 to 15 mL, depending on the method of preparation.

Indications. CRYO is indicated for bleeding related to a deficiency of one of its component factors, such as occurs in hemophilia A (*only* when factor VIII concentrate is unavailable), von Willebrand's disease, factor XIII deficiency, and hypofibrinogenemia and dysfibrinogenemia seen in severe liver disease and DIC. CRYO is also used to prepare fibrin sealant in surgical procedures.

Dosage. Initially, 1 to 2 CRYO units should be transfused per 10 kg of patient weight. Subsequent transfusions should be based on the resulting factor levels.

Contraindications and Alternative Therapies. CRYO is contraindicated in patients with hemophilia A if purified factor VIII concentrates are available. CRYO should not be used routinely to manage uremic bleeding.

PLASMA DERIVATIVES

Albumin

Constituents. Albumin is available in three preparations for clinical use: 5% solution in saline, 25% solution in distilled water, and a purified protein fraction that contains globulins in addition to albumin. Albumin has been treated and rendered free of the risk of viral transmission.

Indications. There is extensive debate concerning the acceptable uses of albumin. The indications are strongest for nephrotic syndrome resistant to diuretics, fluid replacement in plasmapheresis, following large-volume paracentesis, adult respiratory distress syndrome, priming of cardiopulmonary bypass pumps, fluid resuscitation in shock or sepsis, neonatal kernicterus, ovarian hyperstimulation syndrome,* and enteral feeding intolerance.*

Dosage. The dosage depends on the clinical indication. If infusion volume is an important consideration, 25% albumin in distilled water is preferred.

Contraindications and Alternative Therapies. Albumin replacement is contraindicated in patients with mild edema secondary to mild hypoalbuminemia, nutritional deficiencies, or pre-eclampsia; it also should not be used to promote wound healing. Many situations requiring volume expansion can be treated initially with crystalloid solutions.

Immune Globulin Intravenous (IGIV)

Constituents. Immunoglobulins are prepared from large pools of donor plasma by fractionation. Like albumin, IGIV has been treated and poses no risk of viral transmission.

Indications. IGIV is indicated for primary immunodeficiency syndromes, including X-linked agammaglobulinemia, severe combined immunodeficiency, Wiskott-Aldrich syndrome, IgG subclass deficiency, common variable immunodeficiency, and ataxia-telangiectasia. IGIV has also been shown to be beneficial in patients with childhood ITP, ITP refractory to corticosteroid therapy, CMV interstitial pneumonitis after bone marrow transplantation, chronic lymphocytic leukemia, pediatric HIV infection, and mucocutaneous lymph node syndrome. IGIV may also be useful in warm-type autoimmune hemolytic anemia unresponsive to prednisone therapy, Guillain-Barré syndrome,* refractory myasthenia gravis,* burn patients,* chronic fatigue syndrome,* and multiple sclerosis.*

Dosage. Most patients require 100 to 200 mg per kg every 3 to 4 weeks. In patients with ITP, the usual administration schedules are 400 mg per kg per day for 5 days or 1000 mg per kg per day for 2 days.

Contraindications and Alternative Therapies. Given that many uses of IGIV are still experimental, there are few well-documented contraindications; however, prior to the use of IGIV for these investigational indications, serious consideration should be given to the cost:benefit ratio.

SPECIAL PROCESSING OF BLOOD COMPONENTS

There are occasions when RBCs and PLT units require special processing prior to transfusion, including leukoreduction, washing, and gamma irradiation. Special processing techniques sometimes require significant time to perform and can alter the expiration date of the component.

Leukoreduction. Leukoreduction, most commonly achieved by filtration, is indicated to reduce the incidence of febrile nonhemolytic transfusion reactions, CMV transmission, and HLA alloimmunization. It has been stated that for febrile nonhemolytic transfusion reactions, leukocytes should be reduced to less than 5×10^8 per unit and to less than 5×10^6 to reduce CMV transmission and alloimmunization; however, these numbers have not been determined in randomized trials. Filtration can be performed either at the time of blood product preparation (prestorage leukoreduction or blood bank leukoreduction) or at the time of transfusion (bedside leukoreduction). Prestorage leukoreduction offers the advantages of decreasing cytokine contamination from white blood cells (responsible for febrile reactions), closely monitored quality control, and the ability to ensure the desired reduction prior to transfusion.

Washing. Washing of RBCs and PLT units with 1 to 2 liters of saline produces a significant reduction in the plasma components that can cause repeated allergic transfusion reactions in the recipient. If the units are washed more extensively, they may also reduce the incidence of anaphylactic reactions, such as those seen in patients who are IgA deficient; however, components made from IgA-deficient donors constitute first-line therapy.

Gamma Irradiation. TA-GVHD occurs when immunocompetent donor leukocytes transfused with the blood product engraft, recognize the transfusion recipient's cells as foreign, and initiate an antirecipient immune response. In immunocompetent recipients, the donor leukocytes are rapidly eliminated before TA-GVHD can develop. However, patients with immature immune systems (fetuses and neonates), congenital immunodeficiencies, or hematologic malignancies such as Hodgkin's disease or those receiving chemotherapy or immunosuppressive agents cannot mount a sufficient immune response to the donor leukocytes. In addition, patients receiving directed donations from first-degree relatives or HLA-matched PLT units may also have difficulty eliminating the donor leukocytes and should receive irradiated products.

TRANSFUSION LOGISTICS

Informed Consent. After the clinical and laboratory indications for transfusion have been determined to outweigh the potential risks, the patient should give informed consent for the transfusion. The physician and patient should discuss the indications, potential benefits, possible risks, and alternatives to transfusion. This discussion must be documented.

Type and Screen, Type and Crossmatch. Blood banks choose ABO-appropriate units to transfuse based on the presence of naturally occurring anti-A and anti-B antibodies in the recipient. In addition, the presence of RBC alloantibodies (such as Rh, Kell, Kidd, and Duffy), which are generated in an unpredictable fashion after exposure to foreign RBCs during previous pregnancy or transfusion, is used to select RBC units for transfusion. Table 4 displays a compatibility matrix for component transfusion. In patients without unexpected antibodies, the process of providing compatible blood to patients is simple and straightforward. In contrast, it can occasionally

*Not FDA approved for these indications.

TABLE 4. **Compatibility Matrix for Component Transfusions**

Patient's Blood Type	Compatible Red Blood Cells	Compatible Plasma Components (Suggested, Not Required)
A	A, O	A, AB
B	B, O	B, AB
AB	A, B, AB, O	AB
O	O	A, B, AB, O
Rh-positive	Rh-positive, Rh-negative	NA
Rh-negative	Rh-negative	NA

take 24 hours or more to provide compatible blood for patients expressing a spectrum of alloantibodies. Thus, in addition to making an assessment of the likelihood and urgency of transfusion, the clinician must also determine how difficult it may be to provide blood for the patient. The order sent to the blood bank should reflect this assessment.

The *type and screen order* is appropriate if the anticipated likelihood of transfusion is low or if there is not an urgent need for transfusion. If no alloantibodies are identified on the screen, crossmatch-compatible units can be provided within 1 hour of the order to transfuse. If alloantibodies are identified, the blood bank then has sufficient time to identify compatible units (either from inventory or from outside sources) and to reserve the units for the patient.

The *type and crossmatch* should be ordered when transfusion is required in 2 to 4 hours or prior to surgery based on the hospital surgical blood-ordering schedule. When a type and crossmatch is unnecessarily ordered for every patient, regardless of the likelihood of transfusion, valuable resources are wasted, including RBC units that may be reserved for the patient and are thus unavailable for transfusion to other patients. In contrast, failing to order a type and screen on a patient whose clinical history suggests the possibility of RBC alloantibodies may make it extremely difficult to provide RBCs when they are needed. In both cases, patient care is unnecessarily compromised.

Patient and Component Identification. Clinical staff must exercise great care to avoid patient or component misidentification during all stages of the transfusion process. Initially, they must confirm that the blood sample sent to the blood bank is labeled with the patient's name and hospital identification number and exactly matches that on the patient's hospital ID bracelet. After a crossmatch-compatible unit has been identified in the blood bank, it must again pass appropriate clerical checks prior to transfusion. Hospital protocol must be rigorously followed in order to confirm the identity of the patient via the attached ID bracelet and the proper identification of the unit before transfusion. Clerical errors leading to misidentification of either the recipient or the product are the primary cause of fatal hemolytic transfusion reactions.

Component Transfusion. RBC units must have a clot filter interposed between the unit and the patient during infusion to trap clots that may develop during product storage. PLT and RBC units may also have leukoreduction filters placed in the circuit to remove leukocytes from the product as it is being infused. No filters are necessary for FFP or CRYO. Under no circumstances can medications be added to the product. Except for normal saline, no other solutions should be added to or infused through the same tubing as the component unless (1) they have been approved by the FDA for this use, or there is documentation of their safety and efficacy for this use, and (2) there is physician approval for their use. In particular, lactated Ringer's or other electrolyte solutions containing calcium can never be used as they can cause clotting of the component during infusion.

The initial transfusion should proceed at a rate of 5 mL per minute or less for the first 15 minutes. The transfusion should be completed within 4 hours of starting and prior to the component expiration date. During the initial infusion period, the patient should be carefully observed by medical personnel for signs and symptoms of a transfusion reaction: fever (greater than 1°C rise in temperature), chills, pain (chest, back, or infusion site), hypotension, flushing, nausea, dyspnea, wheezing, urticaria, or rash. Less frequently observed are shock, generalized bleeding, oliguria, and hemoglobinuria. Should any of the adverse effects occur, the transfusion should be stopped immediately and the IV should be kept open with normal saline. The reaction should be reported to the blood bank immediately in order to initiate a transfusion reaction investigation.

ADVERSE EFFECTS OF BLOOD TRANSFUSION

method of
KATHLEEN SAZAMA, M.D., J.D.
Allegheny University of the Health Sciences
Philadelphia, Pennsylvania

Adverse effects occur in less than 0.2% of all transfusions (the rate is higher in chronically transfused patients) and frequently cause only mild and transient morbidity. However, certain adverse effects may lead to significant morbidity or even death. Because transfusion of blood cannot be made entirely risk-free, patients should provide informed consent based on their understanding of the risks, benefits, and alternatives, prior to undergoing transfusion. Systems to rapidly identify and manage life-threatening adverse effects for every component type used, including autologous collections and reinfusions, should be implemented both within and outside of hospitals, wherever transfusions occur. New federal regulations mandate reporting of such events, annually and periodically, as often as every 45 days, as errors or accidents.

Transmission of infectious diseases, some of which can be fatal, is not further discussed here except as noted:

1. The risk of transfusion that is most feared by patients, namely, infection with the human immunodeficiency virus (HIV), is one of the least likely adverse effects of transfusion, with current estimated rates of 1 case per 800,000 units. Risks of transmission of the hepatitis viruses, hepatitis B virus (HBV) (1 case per 50,000 to 250,000 units) and hepatitis C virus (HCV) (1 case per 10,000 to 100,000 units) are far higher. Virally inactivated plasma for transfusion has been submitted for FDA approval and will soon be available for use, probably in selected patients for massive or chronic plasma therapy.

2. Bacterial contamination of platelets, which is detected by concurrent methods in as many as 1 per 900 to 2000 units but leads to symptoms far less frequently, is the subject of a current national study by the Centers for Disease Control and Prevention (CDC). Methods to prospectively identify bacteria in platelets prior to issuance for transfusion are under active investigation.

3. Transmission of other pathogens such as the causative agents of syphilis, malaria, babesiosis, and Chagas' disease and parvovirus B-19 is the subject of occasional case reports but not commonly seen.

Most transfusion reactions can be categorized by time to onset of symptoms and the underlying mechanisms, whether immunologic or nonimmunologic (Table 1). These reactions occur with use of both allogeneic and autologous units, the latter generally being due to errors in patient identification, but even with correct autologous blood use, adverse effects, including fatalities, may occur.

TABLE 1. **Adverse Effects of Transfusion***

Acute	Delayed
Immunologic	
Fever without hemolysis (FNHTR)	Alloimmunization
Urticaria	Delayed hemolysis
Acute lung injury (TRALI)	Platelet refractoriness†
Acute hemolysis	Immune modulation/ suppression
Anaphylaxis	Graft-versus-host disease†
Fatal acute hemolysis	Post-transfusion purpura
Nonimmunologic	
Bacterial contamination, platelets	Hepatitis C
Hypervolemia†	Hepatitis B
Chemical effects, hypothermia, coagulopathy†	HTLV-I
Nonimmune hemolysis	HIV-1
Sepsis, RBCs	Hemosiderosis (RBCs only)

* Listed by frequency of occurrence.
† In selected patients or clinical circumstances.
Abbreviations: FNHTR = febrile, nonhemolytic transfusion reaction; HIV-1 = human immunodeficiency virus type 1; HTLV-I = human T-lymphotropic virus type 1; RBCs = red blood cells; TRALI = transfusion-related acute lung injury.

TABLE 2. **Immediate Management of Acute Adverse Effects of Transfusion**

Step 1:	**STOP THE TRANSFUSION**
Step 2:	Manage the patient • Keep intravenous line open with normal saline or equivalent • Consult with treating physician for treatment/ intervention • Administer treatment*
Step 3:	Notify the transfusion service (TS) staff and physician • Obtain and begin to complete TRANSFUSION REACTION REPORT form • Perform and DOCUMENT clerical recheck of patient wristband (or other identification) with information ATTACHED TO the component bag • Disconnect the component bag and administration set from the patient; dispose of as advised by TS staff or according to institution policy • Obtain blood samples from patient; some institutions also request a urine sample • Send samples, test orders, and transfusion reaction report form (and bag/tubing, if requested) to TS

* If the only manifestation is urticaria, the transfusion may be resumed once it has resolved. In some institutions, transfusions are resumed after antipyretics are administered for febrile reactions, but this practice is not recommended.

ACUTE ADVERSE EFFECTS

Immunologic

Febrile Nonhemolytic Transfusion Reaction (FNHTR). FNHTR is a diagnosis of exclusion. Fever, the most commonly observed adverse effect with transfusions of all types of components (occurring in 0.1 to 1% of cases), can be a mild symptom, easily treated by antipyretic medication, or it can signal the onset of serious consequences, including death, due to sepsis or hemolysis. Consequently, when fever occurs during transfusion of any blood component, it must be considered an ominous sign. Transfusions must be stopped while investigation for possible hemolytic or septic reactions is undertaken (Table 2). Although some institutions permit resumption of transfusion after hemolysis and sepsis have been excluded and symptomatic febrile relief has occurred, most still recommend discarding the implicated component.

The mechanism of fever with transfusion is now thought to be usually related to infused cytokines (interleukin-6 and tumor necrosis factor) that accumulate in stored components owing to leukocyte metabolism, but the interaction of recipient antibodies (HLA or granulocyte) with infused leukocytes may also play a role. The widespread practice of premedicating all patients to prevent FNHTR should probably be abandoned now that a more effective intervention can be selectively applied. Because only about 15% of recipients ever experience a second FNHTR, use of any additional preventive measures is not recommended until a repeat febrile event occurs. When recurrent febrile reactions have been documented, use of leukoreduction, either pre-storage or by bedside filtration, depending on the local cost of such options, is recommended. The definition of fever varies between institutions and may contribute to the differences in reported rates. Use of a definition of temperature elevation above baseline (pre-transfusion) levels of more than 1.5 to 2°C (more than 2.7 to 3.8°F) may permit proper patient management and more efficient use of blood. When fever is the only symptom, use of antipyretics is appropriate. When chills, especially shaking chills, also occur, meperidine (Demerol) may be required for symptomatic relief.

Urticaria with No Other Signs or Symptoms. The appearance of an itchy rash during component transfusion, frequently seen with transfusion of platelets or plasma, is a common occurrence. The mechanism is histamine release after degranulation of basophils or mast cells due to immunoglobulin E (IgE) antibody interaction with transfused plasma proteins. Because local or generalized rash with itching can be relieved quickly by administration of antihistamine, typically 50 mg of diphenhydramine (Benadryl), this adverse effect should be managed symptomatically. Once rash and/or itchiness has subsided, the transfusion can be safely continued to completion. This is the *only* acute adverse effect for which resumption of transfusion is considered to be safe, once symptoms have resolved. Because these reactions are idiosyncratic, premedication is not recommended. Only rarely does a patient have a recurrence, generally when a component from the same donor is used.

Transfusion-Related Acute Lung Injury. The abrupt onset, usually within 2 to 4 hours of a transfusion, of acute respiratory distress, hypotension, and fever with documented hypoxemia and bilateral pulmonary edema may signal the potentially life-threatening complication termed transfusion-related acute lung injury (TRALI). These symptoms define adult respiratory distress syndrome (ARDS), which may occur in numerous other clinical settings. When transfusion-related, ARDS carries a much more favorable prognosis than when associated with other causes, with a fatality rate limited to 10% if the disorder is properly diagnosed and managed. Prompt administration of respiratory support with mechanical ventilation and oxygen supplementation is essential. The mechanism of this reaction is not well understood. Donor HLA and/or granulocyte antibodies that react with recipient cells within the pulmonary vasculature are thought to activate complement and cause granulocyte aggregation with consequent damage to the pulmonary parenchyma.

Acute Hemolysis. Acute hemolysis of transfused red blood cells (RBCs) generally occurs owing to an error in patient identification, most often at the time of phlebotomy for laboratory testing or at the moment of blood administration. In the overwhelming majority of cases, the error is ABO mismatch, although occasionally other antigens are implicated (Kell, Kidd, and Rh antibodies have been reported). The usual clinical scenario is transfusion of Group A blood in a Group O patient, but other combinations have been reported. These errors occur with a frequency of 1 in 20,000 transfusions, with the likelihood of fatality of about 1 in 12 to 30 cases once the error has occurred. All such errors now must be reported to the U.S. Food and Drug Administration (FDA), whether or not a fatality has occurred.

Hemolysis may be clinically silent, with only an unexplained hyperbilirubinemia or anemia, particularly if no clinical signs alert the caregivers to its presence. However, it can also be severe and life-threatening when it is due to disseminated intravascular coagulation (DIC), shock, hypotension, or acute renal failure. Published cases describe a classic picture of abrupt onset of acute flank pain, bright red urine, fever, and often a patient's complaint that "something is wrong." Fever (body temperature elevation of greater than 1°C above normal) and chills are commonly seen. In anesthetized or comatose patients, the onset of unexplained oozing from venipuncture sites and the appearance of hemoglobinuria may be the only signs. In some patients, for reasons not fully understood, a very small volume (less than 25 mL) of incompatible RBCs can trigger a violent and fatal outcome, while others tolerate multiunit transfusions with no apparent clinical harm.

If signs and symptoms occur, the steps outlined in Table 2 constitute the basic approach to management. Each institution should have a formal transfusion reaction protocol that provides guidance to the transfusion technician, the treating physician, the transfusion service technical staff, the transfusion service physician, and hospital administration (or equivalent oversight group for out-of-hospital transfusions). Prompt and vigorous hydration and the use of vasoactive drugs such as dopamine may be helpful. Because the vast majority of these adverse events are due to failure to properly identify the patient, systems to improve patient identification, including policies that enforce use of objective patient identifiers, are strongly recommended.

Anaphylaxis. Anaphylaxis is a life-threatening adverse event, typically occurring within minutes of beginning a transfusion, that is characterized by abrupt respiratory distress, shock, hypotension, and angioedema, sometimes with gastrointestinal symptoms. Prompt administration of epinephrine (0.3 mL of 1:1000 epinephrine given intramuscularly) and airway support are essential. The most common mechanism underlying this reaction is administration of IgA-containing plasma to a recipient who is IgA-deficient and has developed anti-IgA antibodies. IgA deficiency is relatively common, affecting 1 in 200 to 500 persons in the United States, but few develop anti-IgA antibodies. Because this is a rare situation, most cases are diagnosed only when the reaction occurs. Subsequent treatment alternatives include use of plasma-reduced or IgA-deficient components.

Nonimmunologic

With the exception of the problem of bacterial contamination of platelets, the other effects occur rarely.

They should be considered in the appropriate clinical setting as described subsequently.

Bacterial Contamination of Platelets. A national investigation of this adverse effect is under way and should provide additional guidance for identifying and avoiding this problem.

Hypervolemia. This problem arises generally in two clinical situations: during massive replacement until bleeding can be controlled and in very young or elderly patients. The clinical signs are dyspnea, tachycardia, and hypertension from pulmonary edema due to congestive heart failure, with onset during or within 6 hours after transfusion. Affected patients should be managed with diuretics and supplemental oxygen; occasionally, therapeutic phlebotomy may be needed.

Chemical Effects

CITRATE TOXICITY. Citrate toxicity is a rare adverse event. Citrate is the anticoagulant used in whole blood and component collection because it chelates calcium and prevents clotting. In massive transfusion settings in which components are being replaced at rates of 1 unit per 5 to 10 minutes, it is possible to cause hypocalcemia in the recipient, who may exhibit cardiac arrhythmias, muscle spasms, and tetany. Such patients can be managed by careful cardiac monitoring and, occasionally, slow infusions of calcium bicarbonate.

HYPERKALEMIA AND HYPOKALEMIA. Hyperkalemia is of concern only in very small infants who are undergoing exchange transfusions using RBCs that are near the end of their usable life. In massive transfusions, hypokalemia may also be seen; it can be managed by administering potassium. The mechanism for development of hypokalemia in massive transfusions is the metabolism of citrate to bicarbonate, which drives potassium into cells.

HYPOTHERMIA AND COAGULOPATHY. In a rapidly bleeding patient with massive blood component replacement, generally defined as total blood volume replaced within 24 hours, a dilutional coagulopathy can be anticipated. In practice, it is infrequently seen, probably because extravascular reservoirs of essential coagulation factors, e.g., platelets and plasma coagulation factors such as von Willebrand factor, factor V, factor VIII, and fibrinogen, exist to maintain levels of at least 20 to 25% of normal. If readily available, laboratory testing should be done to assess the need for replacement of coagulation factors. However, in the presence of shock and severe blood loss with hypothermia, some institutions continue to use a standardized replacement protocol to avoid microvascular coagulopathies in affected patients.

Nonimmune Hemolysis. Patients may have red urine with or without fever because the transfused RBCs have been lysed by external processes during or prior to entering the patient's circulation. RBCs that are subjected to chemical (e.g., osmotic) or thermal extremes will lyse. For this reason, RBCs should be transfused using only 0.9% normal saline or any FDA-approved iso-osmotic fluid. For example, use of D5W is contraindicated because if it is mixed with RBCs, the rapid uptake of glucose will cause intracellular hyperosmolality with a rapid uptake of water, causing lysis. Similarly, if RBCs are frozen without use of appropriate concentrations of cryoprotectant agents or warmed beyond recommended temperatures, they will lyse. Strict regulatory temperature requirements exist for maintaining RBCs; these are met only through use of carefully monitored refrigerators and validated transport containers.

Sepsis, RBCs. Although morbidity and even fatality from bacterially contaminated RBCs continue to be reported, the incidence of such events is estimated to be less than 1 in 1,000,000 cases. However, this is a known risk for autologous units that should be weighed when re-transfusion of such units is commonly practiced.

DELAYED ADVERSE EFFECTS

Immunologic

Alloimmunization. The most common adverse effect that occurs days to months after transfusion is the detection of alloantibody(ies) to antigens that were present on the transfused cells or platelets and were foreign to the recipient. Because we routinely crossmatch only RBCs (not platelets) and only for the most common and strongest-reacting antigens, namely, A, B, and D, the other antigens (more than 50) present on such cells have the potential for eliciting an immune response. In fact, it is common practice in many busy trauma centers to routinely administer D-positive RBCs to D-negative (or D-unknown) male patients and to D-negative female patients who are beyond their child-bearing years. This practice is necessitated by the chronic national shortage of D-negative RBC units (which are reserved for use in D-negative females younger than 45 to 50 years of age to prevent possible hemolytic disease of the newborn). Alloimmunization may also occur in women owing to pregnancy.

The mere presence of an alloantibody is not usually harmful to the recipient (as with the presence of immune-stimulated antibodies to various childhood diseases), but such antibodies can be problematic in two clinical situations. In the first setting, if the alloantibody was present but undetected prior to a current transfusion and the RBCs transfused contain the corresponding antigen, then such RBCs will be destroyed, and a delayed hemolytic transfusion reaction (discussed subsequently) may result. The second clinical situation involves detection of the alloantibody prior to a subsequent transfusion, which leads to a delay in location of a suitable antigen-negative unit. This most often occurs for patients with hemoglobinopathies (e.g., sickle cell disease or thalassemia) who are frequently transfused.

It is common for transfusion services to provide treating physicians and/or patients with information about the occurrence of alloantibodies so that appropriate adjustments in treatment planning can be made. In most cases of alloimmunization, the transfusion is easily managed without delay, but in some instances, only very rare donor units will provide therapeutic benefit to the alloimmunized patient. Careful planning and cooperation may be necessary.

Delayed Hemolysis. When a patient experiences unexplained hyperbilirubinemia, anemia, or lack of increase in hemoglobin level within 5 to 10 days after appropriate RBC transfusion, delayed hemolysis should be suspected. If an alloantibody was not detected prior to transfusion of RBCs containing the corresponding antigen, it will react with the antigen on the RBC surface. This RBC antigen-antibody complex, which generally does not fix complement, is removed by extravascular means. (Rarely, a brisk intravascular hemolysis occurs.)

A positive result on a direct antiglobulin test (DAT) or the presence of alloantibodies, now sufficiently immune-stimulated to be detectable, is often detected by transfusion service technicians when a new sample is sent for evaluation. The implicated antibodies are frequently directed against antigens in the Kidd (Jk^a), Duffy (Fy^a), or Rh (E, c, C) system.

Generally, no treatment is needed for the delayed hemolysis reaction, but all future RBC transfusions should be with RBCs that lack the implicated antigen(s).

Platelet Refractoriness. In selected disease conditions, generally those associated with hematologic or oncologic diagnoses, patients may be chronically supported with platelet transfusions. Generally, no platelet crossmatching or pre-selection of antigen-negative donors is done until the patient shows evidence of platelet refractoriness. Patients whose platelet count does not increase after transfusion of an appropriate platelet dose may be refractory to platelet transfusions owing to nonimmune or immune mechanisms. If sources of platelet loss, destruction, or consumption (e.g., bleeding, sepsis, DIC, fever) have been eliminated, then immune destruction due to antiplatelet (most often, anti-HPA-1a) or anti-HLA antibodies may be occurring. Supportive therapy for the underlying disease states and use of random- or single-donor platelets should be continued for the patient with nonimmune platelet destruction. If continued platelet transfusion support is indicated in the patient with documented immune destruction, consultation is appropriate because special arrangements or testing to obtain suitable platelets for transfusion is probably necessary.

Immune Modulation/Suppression. A growing body of literature, disputed by some investigators, suggests that transfusions may alter immune status in selected surgical patients as evidenced by earlier recurrence of malignancy after resection and/or increased rates of infections in the postoperative period. Currently, the only intervention is to treat the malignancy or infection according to standard approaches. The use of "leukoreduced" RBCs and platelets is being debated.

Graft-Versus-Host Disease. Certain patients may experience the onset of a rash, fever, nausea or vomiting, and unexplained peripheral cytopenias within 3 to 15 days after transfusion; these are manifestations of graft-versus-host disease (GVHD). GVHD, which is nearly always fatal in the transfusion setting, can occur when the recipient is immunocompromised (e.g., in congenital immunodeficiency states) or when the recipient receives a blood component containing an HLA antigen identical to that in one of the recipient's own HLA haplotypes. If the blood component is HLA haplotype–homozygous (i.e., contains two copies of exactly the same HLA antigens) and the recipient is HLA haplotype–heterozygous (has two different HLA antigens), then GVHD can occur. The only effective measure to address GVHD is to prevent it by gamma irradiation of cellular blood components at a sufficiently high dose (2500 cGy) to inhibit mitosis of any donor lymphocytes. Because the particular HLA setting is more likely to exist among biologic relatives than between strangers, all directed blood donations are routinely irradiated to prevent this catastrophic disease. There is no effective treatment once transfusion-associated GVHD occurs.

Post-Transfusion Purpura. Women who have been pregnant or have received transfusions have the highest risk for development of post-transfusion purpura (PTP) (the male-female ratio of affected patients is 1:26). Patients with PTP have a profound thrombocytopenia (with counts of usually less than 10,000 per mL) occurring within 5 to 10 days after transfusion of either RBCs or platelets. This thrombocytopenia can last days to weeks and is treated with therapeutic plasma exchange, intravenous immune globulin, and/or high-dose steroids. Generally, an anti-HPA-1a (antiplatelet) antibody is thought to cause the immune destruction of both transfused and autologous HPA-1a–negative platelets (the latter by an unknown mechanism). If transfusion is required, use of HPA-1a–negative platelets is recommended, even though they will probably undergo accelerated destruction.

Nonimmunologic

Hemosiderosis. Iron accumulation (hemosiderosis) occurs in patients who have received RBC transfusions over long periods of time. The hemosiderosis is sometimes manifested as cardiomyopathies, cirrhosis, and "bronze diabetes." The 250 mg of iron in each transfused RBC unit accumulates in the reticuloendothelial system until the tissues are saturated; then the iron begins to be deposited in various other sites such as heart, skin, and pancreas and other endocrine organs. Some benefit may derive from use of an iron-chelating agent, deferoxamine.

Section 6

The Digestive System

CHOLELITHIASIS AND CHOLECYSTITIS

method of
ROBERT V. REGE, M.D.
Northwestern University Medical School and Veterans Affairs Chicago Health Care System, Lakeside Division
Chicago, Illinois

Gallstones are very common, occurring in 11 to 15% of women and 3 to 11% of men younger than age 50. They are even more common in individuals with obesity, diabetes mellitus, ileal disease, or a family history of gallstones; in certain ethnic groups (e.g., Native Americans); and in patients on parenteral nutrition or undergoing rapid weight loss. Gallstones can cause severe abdominal pain and lead to serious complications, such as acute cholecystitis, obstructive jaundice, pancreatitis, gallstone ileus, and ascending cholangitis. Gallstones account for more than 500,000 operations and several billion dollars in health care expenditures in the United States each year.

Although the general principles of gallstone management have not changed appreciably, methods of treatment have. Laparoscopic cholecystectomy, lithotripsy, gallstone dissolution, endoscopic retrograde management of bile duct stones, and percutaneous approaches to the biliary tract now play a role in the treatment of gallstones, and a comprehensive approach to biliary tract disease requires a team of well-trained surgeons, interventional gastroenterologists, and interventional radiologists. Moreover, the evolution of laparoscopic cholecystectomy has necessitated the reeducation and retraining of surgeons. Nonetheless, cholecystectomy remains the treatment of choice for gallstones, and gallstone disease remains the purview of the surgeon.

TYPES OF GALLSTONES

Gallstones are classified as cholesterol, mixed, and pigment gallstones by gross and compositional analysis. Selected patients with single, nearly pure cholesterol (but not pigment) gallstones may be treated with gallstone dissolution and/or extracorporeal lithotripsy. Cholesterol and mixed gallstones are both composed primarily of cholesterol. Together, they account for 80% of gallstones in the West. Two types of pigment gallstones, black pigment and calcium bilirubinate, account for 10 to 27% of all gallstones. Black pigment gallstones, composed mainly of an amorphous bilirubin polymer and calcium salts, develop when there is excessive bilirubin in bile. Most patients with pigment gallstones do not have predisposing factors, but black pigment gallstones are more common in the elderly and in patients with hemolytic anemia or cirrhosis. Calcium bilirubinate stones usually form behind biliary strictures or in bile containing bacteria or parasites. They are mainly composed of calcium bilirubinate, free fatty acids, and up to 10% cholesterol.

Asymptomatic Gallstones

Most gallstones remain asymptomatic for many years; symptoms and complications develop in only 1 to 2% of patients per year. Observation of patients with asymptomatic gallstones is currently recommended since the risk of observation is less than the risk of prophylactic surgery. However, certain patients with gallstones, including children, patients with congenital hemolytic anemia, and those with large (>2.5 cm) gallstones or nonfunctioning gallbladders, may benefit from prophylactic cholecystectomy. In addition, symptoms develop in more than 36% of morbidly obese patients who have undergone barosurgery, and 20% of colectomy patients with gallstones develop symptoms within 5 years. Prophylactic cholecystectomy adds no significant morbidity or mortality to either of these operations, and it should be considered for these patients during their primary operation. Incidental cholecystectomy during other abdominal operations may not be prudent in some situations (e.g., when prosthetic material is required) and must be left to the discretion of the surgeon. In the past, it was taught that diabetic patients were more likely to develop gallstones, complications of gallstones, and complications after emergent/urgent biliary tract surgery. However, recent studies have demonstrated similar outcomes in diabetic and nondiabetic patients, and prophylactic operation for diabetic patients is no longer recommended.

Symptomatic Gallstones

Right upper quadrant and epigastric pain 15 to 60 minutes after meals is quite specific for gallstone disease. The pain often occurs after ingesting fatty foods, onions, cabbage, spicy foods, or dairy products. It lasts from 20 minutes to several hours; pain lasting longer suggests acute cholecystitis or acute pancreatitis. Severe episodes of pain associated with nausea and vomiting have been called "biliary colic," although the pain is constant, not colicky. Patients with symptomatic gallstones are said to have chronic cholecystitis. They can expect continued episodes of pain, which often increase in frequency and severity. Complications develop more frequently in symptomatic than in asymptomatic patients, and as many as 40 to 50% require operative treatment within 2 to 5 years. The risks incurred by merely following symptomatic patients is higher than the risk of operation, and cholecystectomy is clearly indicated.

Patients who present with vague, mild pain, indigestion, flatulence, and nausea without vomiting are now classified as being mildly symptomatic, although these symptoms are not specific for gallstones, as they can be caused by many other disorders of the gastrointestinal tract. Mildly symptomatic disease is much like asymptomatic disease; only 1 to 2% of patients per year require cholecystectomy. Operation should be recommended with care if only mild symptoms are present. Cholecystectomy may, however, give relief in 50 to 70% of patients with persistent symptoms, especially if they significantly interfere with lifestyle. Patients must be warned that cholecystectomy may not relieve their symptoms as they may be due to other disorders.

CHRONIC CHOLECYSTITIS

Diagnosis and treatment of chronic cholecystitis are frequently straightforward. Biliary colic combined with the presence of gallstones on an imaging study is sufficient for the diagnosis. Ultrasonography is the study of choice, successfully demonstrating gallstones in 90 to 95% of patients. Plain films of the abdomen and computed tomography (CT) scan are not very sensitive, demonstrating gallstones in only 20% of patients. However, positive findings on these studies are very reliable. In some individuals, gallstone disease mimics another abdominal disease, or other gastrointestinal disorders mimic gallstone disease, making diagnosis challenging. Extensive testing may be required to exclude gastroesophageal reflux, peptic ulcer disease, hepatitis, pancreatitis, intestinal pathology, and malignant tumors of the stomach, bile duct, duodenum, or pancreas. Chronic acalculous cholecystitis and cholesterolosis of the gallbladder may cause symptoms identical to those of gallstones, but specific tests do not exist for these disorders. An oral cholecystogram may reveal no, or only faint, visualization of the gallbladder, demonstrating impaired gallbladder function. Impaired gallbladder emptying measured with ultrasound or gallbladder scintigraphy (HIDA scan) after administration of cholecystokinin may also suggest gallbladder disease in some of these patients.

Cholecystectomy is the treatment of choice for patients with symptomatic cholelithiasis. This operation carries a mortality rate of less than 0.3% and relieves symptoms in 95% of patients. When performed by experienced surgeons, laparoscopic cholecystectomy can be successful in more than 95% of patients, and the rate of complications, including bile duct injury, is comparable to that with open cholecystectomy. The laparoscopic approach is not safe or prudent in 5 to 10% of patients, and the surgeon should convert to open operation. Conversion of the operation to open cholecystectomy should not be considered a failure.

Common bile ducts stones are present in as many as 10 to 20% of patients undergoing cholecystectomy. Only about 4% of patients without any preoperative risk factors will have "silent" common bile duct stones. Intraoperative cholangiography can be performed either routinely or selectively with the laparoscope, but it should always be used in patients at high risk for choledocholithiasis (Table 1) and whenever biliary anatomy is not well-defined by operative dissection. In contrast, dissolution therapy and extracorporeal shock wave lithotripsy eliminate gallstones in less than 50% of selected patients, and at least half of these patients experience recurrence. If used at all, these methods of treatment should be limited to patients with single, "nearly pure" cholesterol gallstones less than 2 cm in diameter.

ACUTE CHOLECYSTITIS

Acute cholecystitis is the most common complication of gallstones, occurring in about 10% of patients. It is caused by cystic duct obstruction by a gallstone, tumor, or swelling. Bacteria grow in bile, and infection develops in the gallbladder wall. If unchecked, acute cholecystitis can lead to gallbladder perforation, pericholecystic abscess, or peritonitis. Patients present with unremitting right upper quadrant pain, fever, elevated white blood cell count, nausea and vomiting, and gallstones. Ultrasonography is the most common confirming test in demonstrating the presence of gallstones. It may also show a thickened gallbladder wall, a gallbladder "rim" sign, or an ultrasonographic Murphy's sign (pain when the gallbladder is compressed with the ultrasound probe). Gallbladder scintigraphy (HIDA scan) is helpful in patients with less typical signs and symptoms. HIDA scans are very sensitive and specific for acute cholecystitis as the gallbladder cannot be visualized in 98% of patients due to cystic duct obstruction. Gallbladder visualization occurs in a few patients with acute acalculous cholecystitis (false negative), and the test is not reliable in critically ill patients and patients on parenteral nutrition who have not emptied their gallbladders. Percutaneous aspiration of

TABLE 1. **Factors That Increase the Risk of Choledocholithiasis**

History of acute jaundice
History of pancreatitis
Dilated biliary tree
  Ultrasound—Dilated intrahepatic ducts
    Common bile duct >7 mm
  CT scan—Dilated intra- and extrahepatic ducts
Elevated serum bilirubin, liver enzymes, or amylase
Episode of acute cholangitis

the gallbladder with Gram's stain examination and cultures may be helpful in these patients.

Patients with acute cholecystitis should be admitted to the hospital, given nothing by mouth, and treated with broad-spectrum parenteral antibiotics. A second-generation cephalosporin or a combination of ampicillin/sulbactam (Unasyn) and an aminoglycoside will suffice and should be continued postoperatively. A nasogastric tube is placed if there is persistent vomiting. Operation is performed in the next 24 to 72 hours. The complication rate and chance of successfully performing the procedure are not improved by delaying cholecystectomy for 6 weeks. Perforation of the gallbladder occurs in some patients despite clinical improvement, and 20 to 30% of patients develop recurrent symptoms while waiting for operation. Delayed treatment is indicated in patients with medical conditions precluding operation, especially if improvement is expected during the waiting period. Critically ill patients who do not respond to medical therapy and who are not candidates for operation are treated with percutaneous cholecystostomy.

Acute cholecystitis is not a contraindication to laparoscopic cholecystectomy. The procedure can be performed safely, although conversion to open operation is necessary in 10 to 30% of patients. It is prudent to convert to an open operation if dissection does not progress or if biliary tract anatomy cannot be defined by intraoperative cholangiography. Laparoscopic cholecystectomy is more likely to be successful when performed within 3 days of the onset of symptoms. Conversion rates are higher later when edema is replaced by inflammatory tissue and fibrosis or when gangrene is present.

About 5% of patients with acute cholecystitis do not have gallstones. Often these patients are critically ill. The diagnosis is frequently delayed because signs and symptoms of cholecystitis cannot be elicited due to the patient's medical condition, ultrasound may be unremarkable, and the HIDA scan is not reliable in patients who have not eaten and emptied their gallbladder. Urgent cholecystectomy or percutaneous cholecystostomy is warranted in patients with acalculous cholecystitis as this disease may rapidly progress to gangrene and perforation.

OTHER COMPLICATIONS OF GALLSTONES

Gangrenous cholecystitis, gallbladder empyema, emphysematous cholecystitis, and gallbladder perforation represent advanced presentations of acute cholecystitis. Patients with these complications often present with higher than expected white blood cell counts, severe abdominal pain often associated with abdominal guarding or rebound tenderness, high fever, and failure to respond to medical therapy. Abdominal radiography or CT scan shows air in the gallbladder wall or lumen with emphysematous cholecystitis. Ultrasound or CT scan demonstrates pericholecystic fluid, subhepatic fluid, or abscess with gallbladder perforation. Urgent abdominal exploration is indicated as these complications are associated with significant mortality and morbidity.

Acute gallstone pancreatitis results when a gallstone passes into and through the common bile duct. Attacks range from very mild and transient to life-threatening. Patients present with severe epigastric pain, left upper quadrant pain, elevated serum amylase or lipase levels, gallstones, and no other obvious causes for pancreatitis. If the attack resolves quickly, only 20 to 30% of patients will have a retained gallstone in their common bile duct. Cholecystectomy with intraoperative cholangiography in these patients is reasonable from both a medical and a cost perspective. The patients with retained stones may have them removed at surgery or postoperatively using endoscopic retrograde cholangiopancreatography (ERCP). Common bile duct stones are present in 50 to 80% of patients with persistent symptoms, elevated liver tests, and jaundice, and this group of patients should undergo ERCP and stone removal before cholecystectomy.

Choledocholithiasis also causes obstructive jaundice. Gallstones are more likely to cause both jaundice and pain; bile duct stricture and malignancies are more likely to cause "silent" jaundice. Ultrasonography is used to document stones in the gallbladder and dilated intra- and extrahepatic ducts. It will occasionally demonstrate the stone in the common bile duct. The CT scan also demonstrates dilated intra- and extrahepatic bile ducts and excludes mass lesions in the pancreas. The cause of jaundice is best ascertained by directly imaging the biliary tract. ERCP is the procedure of choice because it is successful in 90 to 95% of patients and has low complication rates. Percutaneous transhepatic cholangiography is reserved for patients in whom ERCP cannot visualize the proximal biliary tract. It is successful and safe in more than 90% of patients with dilated intrahepatic ducts but is more likely to result in complications, such as bile leakage and hemorrhage.

Choledocholithiasis is most often treated endoscopically before operation. Endoscopic approaches are successful in more than 95% of patients when performed by an experienced interventional gastroenterologist. Gallstones that cannot be removed because they are too large or because of anatomic considerations are removed operatively. Common duct exploration currently can be performed using laparoscopic as well as open techniques.

Gallstone ileus refers to intestinal obstruction caused by a gallstone that has eroded from the gallbladder into the intestinal tract. The gallstone usually causes obstruction at the ileocecal valve or in the sigmoid colon. By necessity, a fistula is present between the gallbladder and the stomach, duodenum, or colon. Besides dilated loops of bowel, abdominal films demonstrate air in the biliary tract. Occasionally, the gallstone can be seen if it is calcified. Treatment should relieve the bowel obstruction by removing the gallstone. The fistula is treated later, although this is often not necessary if the patient is asymptomatic.

CIRRHOSIS

method of
PETER M. ROSENBERG, M.D., and
LAWRENCE S. FRIEDMAN, M.D.
Massachusetts General Hospital
Boston, Massachusetts

Cirrhosis is the final common pathway in the course of a variety of chronic, progressive liver diseases. Strictly defined, cirrhosis is a histologic diagnosis, based on the presence of hepatocellular necrosis, fibrosis, and regenerative nodules. From a clinical point of view, however, cirrhosis represents a constellation of symptoms, signs, and laboratory abnormalities reflecting underlying hepatocellular dysfunction, portal hypertension, and portosystemic shunting. Typically, cirrhosis follows a slow, insidious course and often culminates in dramatic and fatal complications. The cornerstone of management is the prevention and treatment of these complications.

The prognosis for patients with cirrhosis varies according to clinical stage and etiology. It is clearly best for patients with well-compensated disease. For example, in patients with well-compensated cirrhosis due to chronic hepatitis C, the 10-year survival rate has been estimated to be approximately 80%. Regardless of etiology, prognosis correlates with the Child-Pugh classification (Table 1). Mean survival periods for patients with class A, class B, and class C cirrhosis are 40, 32, and 8 months, respectively. Whereas patients with class A cirrhosis may benefit from treatment of the underlying chronic liver disease, patients with class B or C cirrhosis should generally be evaluated for liver transplantation.

DIAGNOSIS

In clinical practice, the diagnosis of cirrhosis is usually based on the presence of suggestive symptoms, signs, and laboratory abnormalities. Possible symptoms and signs include fatigue, nausea, vomiting, diarrhea, amenorrhea, easy bruising, jaundice, increased abdominal girth, leg swelling, evidence of upper gastrointestinal bleeding, and confusion. Other physical signs include jaundice, spider angiomata, palmar erythema, ascites, peripheral edema, a firm and nodular liver edge, splenomegaly, caput medusae, gynecomastia, testicular atrophy, and gastric or esophageal varices (on endoscopic examination). Characteristic laboratory abnormalities include an elevated serum bilirubin level, decreased serum albumin level, elevated serum globulin levels, an elevated prothrombin time (PT), and thrombocytopenia.

If at least several of these features are present in a patient, the diagnosis of cirrhosis is usually secure. Their absence, however, does not exclude a diagnosis of cirrhosis, especially in patients with compensated disease. In such cases, the disease is subclinical, and liver biopsy may be necessary for definitive diagnosis. Ultrasonography with Doppler flow studies may show abnormalities in liver size, surface patterns, and homogeneity and may detect splenomegaly, portal vein enlargement, caudate lobe enlargement, and the presence of collateral circulation, all of which are suggestive of cirrhosis. However, ultrasonography is not as sensitive as liver biopsy and fails to provide information on the underlying cause of cirrhosis. Various serum markers of fibrosis have been reported to aid in the noninvasive diagnosis of cirrhosis, and recently, an elevated serum hyaluronate level has been suggested to be a sensitive and specific marker. However, this test is not widely available and has not been validated in a large population.

It should be noted that overt clinical signs of portal hypertension, portosystemic shunting, and hepatic synthetic dysfunction may also be seen with acute alcoholic hepatitis and, less commonly, with flares of chronic hepatitis B, in the absence of cirrhosis. Without a liver biopsy, distinguishing decompensation due to one of these acute processes (or both) from cirrhosis may be impossible. When percutaneous liver biopsy is precluded by marked coagulopathy (PT prolonged by at least 3 seconds or a platelet count of 75,000 per mm^3 or less), a transjugular approach may be used for biopsy.

TABLE 1. **Child-Pugh Classification of Cirrhosis**

	Score		
Feature	*1*	*2*	*3*
Encephalopathy (stage)	0	1–2	3–4
Ascites	Absent	Slight	Poorly controlled
Bilirubin (mg/dL)	<2.0	2.0–3.0	>3.0
Albumin (gm/dL)	>3.5	2.8–3.5	<2.8
Prothrombin time (seconds prolonged)	1.0–4.0	4.0–6.0	>6.0

Each feature is assigned 1, 2, or 3 points.

Class A: 5–6 points **Class B:** 7–9 points **Class C:** 10–15 points

CAUSES OF CIRRHOSIS: EVALUATION AND SPECIFIC THERAPY

The causes of cirrhosis are numerous (Table 2). In the United States, the majority of cases can be attributed to alcohol or hepatitis C virus infection, or both. Despite the discovery of hepatitis C virus in 1989, many cases of cirrhosis are still considered cryptogenic. It has recently been suggested that nonalcoholic steatohepatitis (NASH) may account for many of these cases, because cryptogenic cirrhosis is found in a substantial number of obese diabetic patients with hypertriglyceridemia.

Often, the cause of cirrhosis can be determined by the history and noninvasive testing alone. Standard work-up should include serologic tests for viral hepatitis, including assays for hepatitis B surface antigen and antibody to hepatitis C; determination of serum iron, total iron-binding capacity (TIBC), ferritin, ceruloplasmin, and alpha$_1$-antitrypsin levels; assays for antinuclear, anti–smooth muscle, and antimitochondrial antibodies; and, as noted previously, an abdominal ultrasound scan with Doppler flow studies. If the presence and cause of cirrhosis in a given patient can

TABLE 2. **Causes of Cirrhosis in Adults in the United States**

Chronic viral hepatitis	Drugs
Hepatitis C	Methotrexate
Hepatitis B (with or without delta co-infection)	Isoniazid
Alcohol	Methyldopa
Cryptogenic cirrhosis	Amiodarone
Nonalcoholic steatohepatitis	Halogenated hydrocarbons
Autoimmune diseases	Hypervitaminosis A
Primary biliary cirrhosis	Nonviral infections
Autoimmune hepatitis	Schistosomiasis
Primary sclerosing cholangitis	Brucellosis
Metabolic diseases	Syphilis
Hemochromatosis	Nonautoimmune biliary disease
Wilson's disease	Chronic biliary obstruction
Alpha$_1$-antitrypsin deficiency	Biliary atresia
Galactosemia	Cystic fibrosis
Hereditary fructose intolerance	Chronic graft-versus-host disease
Tyrosinemia	Vascular disorders
Glycogen storage disease (types III and IV)	Chronic Budd-Chiari syndrome
Abetalipoproteinemia	Veno-occlusive disease
	Chronic heart failure
	Sarcoidosis
	Jejunoileal bypass

be inferred from results of this noninvasive work-up a liver biopsy may not be needed. If, however, the results are negative or ambiguous, liver biopsy should be performed. In suspected primary sclerosing cholangitis, endoscopic retrograde cholangiopancreatography should be performed; anti-neutrophil cytoplasmic antibody (p-ANCA) may be detected in 70% of affected persons.

Knowledge of the exact cause of cirrhosis in a patient may allow treatment of the underlying disorder. Although cirrhosis is generally thought to be irreversible, treatment of the underlying disease may slow the progression of cirrhosis, ameliorate the clinical course, reduce the risk of hepatocellular carcinoma, and, in rare cases, lead to regression of cirrhosis. In general, such treatment is most effective and best tolerated when initiated in the precirrhotic or Child class A phase. Regardless of the cause of cirrhosis, treatment with colchicine to inhibit hepatic fibrogenesis may be considered. In a long-term study, 5- and 10-year survival rates for patients with early-stage cirrhosis were found to be significantly higher for those who received oral colchicine, in a dose of 1 mg daily, than for those who received placebo. In the future, more specific antifibrotic agents will probably become available.

Alcoholic Cirrhosis

Alcoholic cirrhosis typically results from repeated bouts of alcoholic hepatitis, either overt or subclinical. Acute alcoholic hepatitis is generally self-limited, and abstinence can clearly prevent progression to cirrhosis. Treatment with corticosteroids may be beneficial for selected patients with severe alcoholic hepatitis. Even once cirrhosis develops, abstinence from alcohol improves the prognosis. In patients with decompensated alcoholic cirrhosis who continue to drink, the 5-year survival rate is less than 50%, but in those who remain abstinent, survival is improved and the incidence of liver-related complications decreased. Both ascites and esophageal varices have been observed to regress and portal pressure to decrease with abstinence. Therefore, every effort should be made to enter patients with alcoholic cirrhosis into organized alcohol counseling programs.

Nutrition also plays a role in therapy for the alcoholic patient with cirrhosis. Adequate caloric intake should be ensured, and vitamin and electrolyte deficiencies should be corrected. It is generally advisable to maintain patients on a multivitamin, folic acid 1 mg, and thiamine 100 mg daily. Hypomagnesemia and hypophosphatemia are common and should be corrected, initially with intravenous therapy.

Cirrhosis Due to Chronic Viral Hepatitis

Worldwide, chronic hepatitis B is probably the most common cause of cirrhosis and liver-related death. The active, or replicative, phase of chronic hepatitis B is characterized by the presence in serum of the hepatitis B e antigen (HBeAg) and hepatitis B virus (HBV) DNA. Standard treatment for patients with chronic hepatitis B is administration of interferon alfa-2b (Intron-A), 5 million units subcutaneously (SC) daily or 10 million units SC three times per week, for 4 months (see the article "Acute and Chronic Viral Hepatitis" for more detail on treatment). Response to interferon in hepatitis B is typically accompanied by a mild flare of hepatitis. In HBeAg-positive patients with compensated cirrhosis, response to interferon treatment has been shown to be associated with improved survival and decreased incidence of hepatic decompensation. However, interferon should not be used in patients with decompensated liver disease, because the treatment-induced flare of hepatitis may precipitate liver failure. More promising for patients with advanced liver disease caused by chronic hepatitis B are nucleoside analogues such as lamivudine, although these drugs are not yet approved for treatment of hepatitis B. These drugs may also prove effective in diminishing the risk of recurrent hepatitis B after liver transplantation.

Interferon therapy, alone or with ribavirin, has not been shown to improve the prognosis of hepatitis C–related cirrhosis. In fact, the presence of cirrhosis predicts a poor response to interferon, although therapy may be considered in patients with well-compensated cirrhosis and active inflammation on liver biopsy. There is some evidence that such therapy reduces the risk of hepatocellular carcinoma. Unfortunately, there are as yet no therapeutic alternatives to interferon for treatment of hepatitis C. Therefore, the only treatment for advanced hepatitis C–related cirrhosis is liver transplantation, if indicated.

Primary Biliary Cirrhosis

Primary biliary cirrhosis (PBC) is a chronic cholestatic disease caused by immunologic reactivity against the epithelium of the intrahepatic bile ductules. The disorder typically affects middle-aged women and follows a slow but progressive course, characterized eventually by pruritus, jaundice, steatorrhea, fat-soluble vitamin deficiencies, and ultimately end-stage liver disease. Laboratory hallmarks of PBC are an elevated serum alkaline phosphatase level, the presence of antimitochondrial antibody, and hypercholesterolemia. Prognosis is closely related to the serum bilirubin level as well as to the patient's age, presence of edema, prolongation of PT, and variceal bleeding.

At present, the mainstay of treatment for PBC is administration of ursodeoxycholic acid, or ursodiol (Actigall),* given orally (PO) in a daily dose of 10 to 15 mg/kg,† generally in divided doses. Ursodeoxycholic acid is a hydrophilic bile acid that is absorbed from the gastrointestinal tract after oral ingestion and displaces more toxic bile acids from the enterohepatic circulation and thus from the bile pool. It also improves bile flow and appears to modulate the humoral immune response. Treatment with ursodeoxycholic acid has been shown to reduce pruritus, improve biochemical parameters (especially serum bilirubin levels), delay progression to cirrhosis, and improve survival, as measured by time to liver transplantation. However, the drug has not been shown to induce histologic improvement in patients with PBC. The survival benefit has been shown even in patients with stage IV disease (i.e., cirrhosis). Therefore, ursodeoxycholic acid is clearly indicated in the treatment of cirrhosis due to PBC.

Other pharmacologic agents for treatment of PBC that have been studied include colchicine,* prednisone, D-penicillamine,* azathioprine,* cyclosporine,* chlorambucil,* and methotrexate.* Colchicine,* 0.6 mg twice daily (bid), may slow the rate of progression to cirrhosis but has not been shown to improve survival. Dramatic results have been reported with long-term methotrexate therapy (in weekly "pulses" of 15 mg) in a small series of patients, and complete histologic remission was observed in several patients. Further trials are needed to define the subgroup likely to benefit from methotrexate therapy, and the drug should still be considered investigational. Trials of the other agents have been disappointing, and the toxic effects of these drugs appear to outweigh their benefits.

Several unique complications of PBC may require specific treatment. Pruritus may be treated with cholestyramine (Questran) in doses of 4 grams PO in water or juice, bid or three times daily (tid); colestipol, 5 grams bid or tid; or oral antihistamines such as hydroxyzine (Atarax), in a dose of 25 mg four times a day as needed. Additional treatments for refractory pruritus include rifampin (Rifadin),* 300 mg PO bid; phenobarbital,* 2 to 4 mg per kg per day, with a target serum level of 10 μm per mL; and phototherapy. The oral opiate antagonist naltrexone (ReVia) has shown particular promise in the treatment of pruritus associated with cholestasis. Patients with PBC also require supplementation to compensate for malabsorption of fat-soluble vitamins. In general, calcium, 1000–1500 mg daily, and vitamin D, 50,000 units PO per week, should be prescribed. Vitamin K, 10 mg SC daily for 2 to 3 days and then 10 mg SC per month should be given to patients with a prolonged PT, and vitamin A, 25,000 units PO per day, to those with night blindness. The value of bisphosphonates and estrogen in the prevention and treatment of osteoporosis associated with PBC is uncertain.

*Not FDA approved for this indication.
†Exceeds dosage recommended by the manufacturer.

Hemochromatosis

Hereditary hemochromatosis is an autosomal recessive disorder characterized by excessive intestinal absorption of iron, with resulting iron deposition in the liver, heart, pituitary, and pancreas and eventual cirrhosis, dilated cardiomyopathy, panhypopituitarism, and diabetes mellitus. Initial testing for suspected hemochromatosis should include determination of serum iron level, TIBC, and ferritin level; a fasting transferrin saturation (defined as the serum iron level divided by the TIBC) of greater than 50% is suggestive of hemochromatosis. However, the transferrin saturation and serum ferritin level are also elevated in up to half of patients with chronic viral hepatitis, alcoholic liver disease, and NASH. Definitive diagnosis of hemochromatosis has traditionally been made by liver biopsy with quantitative hepatic iron determination, which should be performed in all patients with an elevated transferrin saturation or serum ferritin level. The recent identification of a single mutation *(HFE)* in a human leukocyte antigen (HLA)–like gene *(HLA-H)* has made it possible to perform genetic testing for hemochromatosis. Two copies of the *HFE* gene mutation are present in more than 90% of patients with biochemical and histologic evidence of hemochromatosis.

Identifying hemochromatosis as the underlying cause of cirrhosis in a given patient is of great importance, because treatment with iron depletion therapy ameliorates the liver dysfunction and other systemic manifestations of hemochromatosis, even in patients who already have cirrhosis. In rare cases, phlebotomy therapy has been reported to reverse cirrhosis. Phlebotomy with removal of 500 mL of whole blood should be performed weekly until the transferrin saturation falls below 50% and the ferritin level below 50 ng per mL, or until the hemoglobin level falls to 10 mg per dL. Preoperative iron depletion is particularly important in optimizing outcome after liver transplantation. For patients with cirrhosis who are too ill or anemic to tolerate phlebotomy, iron chelation

*Not FDA approved for this indication.

therapy with deferoxamine (Desferal) may be considered but is less effective than phlebotomy. Finally, first-degree relatives of patients with hemochromatosis should undergo screening with serum iron studies and, if the proband has the *HFE* gene, genetic testing.

Wilson's Disease

Wilson's disease is an uncommon disease, inherited as an autosomal recessive trait, resulting in copper accumulation in the liver, central nervous system (CNS), and kidneys. The disorder tends to manifest in childhood or early adulthood. The diagnosis is made on the basis of detection of Kayser-Fleischer rings in the cornea, a serum ceruloplasmin level of less than 20 mg per dL, an elevated urinary copper level, and an elevated hepatic copper concentration on liver biopsy. However, Kayser-Fleischer rings may be absent, particularly in patients without neuropsychiatric features of Wilson's disease. Medical therapy with D-penicillamine (Cuprimine), 1–2 grams daily in four divided doses, is effective in preventing copper accumulation but has not been shown to induce regression of established cirrhosis. Side effects of D-penicillamine include rash, fever, bone marrow suppression, and glomerulonephritis and may necessitate a reduction in dosage or use of an alternative agent such as trientine hydrochloride (Syprine), 750 to 2000 mg per day in two to four divided doses. Zinc may be used for maintenance therapy after copper depletion has been achieved or in pregnant and presymptomatic patients. End-stage liver disease due to Wilson's disease carries an especially poor prognosis, and liver transplantation should be strongly considered in such cases; copper levels return to normal after transplantation.

Autoimmune Hepatitis

Classic (type 1) autoimmune hepatitis typically affects women in the third to fifth decades of life and is often associated with high globulin levels and the presence of antinuclear and anti–smooth muscle antibodies in serum. The disease is generally very sensitive to therapy with corticosteroids, which is indicated in patients with symptoms, serum aminotransferase elevations at least 10 times the upper limit of normal (or 5 times the upper limit of normal and a serum globulin level at least twice the upper limit of normal), or histologic evidence of severe chronic hepatitis. Prednisone should be initiated at a dose of 40 to 60 mg daily for 1 to 2 weeks and then tapered over several weeks to a maintenance dose of 10 to 15 mg. Azathioprine (Imuran),* in a dose of 50 to 100 mg daily, is useful in allowing a lower dose of prednisone in these patients. Maintenance therapy should be continued until biochemical and histologic remission occurs, which may take more than 18 months. Thereafter, therapy may be discontinued, but relapse is common. In patients who experience repeated relapses long-term suppressive therapy should be used; in some cases, long-term therapy with azathioprine alone in a dose of 2 mg per kg per day, may maintain remission. Treatment of autoimmune hepatitis should be initiated even if cirrhosis has already supervened, and complete regression of established cirrhosis has been reported. Liver transplantation should be considered for patients with progressive liver dysfunction that does not respond to immunosuppressive therapy; clinical recurrence of autoimmune hepatitis is uncommon after transplantation.

*Not FDA approved for this indication.

PREVENTION AND TREATMENT OF COMPLICATIONS

Variceal Bleeding

Bleeding from ruptured esophageal or gastric varices is one of the most common and potentially catastrophic complications of cirrhosis. Prevention and treatment of variceal bleeding are addressed in the article "Bleeding Esophageal Varices."

Ascites

Ascites is the most common and often the earliest major complication of cirrhosis and occurs in 50% of patients within 10 years of the diagnosis of compensated cirrhosis. Pathogenetic factors include (1) increased hydrostatic pressure in the portal circulation due to distortion of the hepatic vasculature, (2) decreased plasma oncotic pressure due to impaired albumin synthesis, (3) transudation of lymph from the liver surface due to hepatic sinusoidal obstruction, and (4) renal fluid retention mediated by activation of the renin-angiotensin-aldosterone system. Ascites signals a poor prognosis in chronic liver disease and is associated with a 2-year survival rate of approximately 50%. Morbidity may result directly from tense abdominal distention; thus, findings may include abdominal discomfort, anorexia, early satiety, respiratory compromise, and renal insufficiency. Massive ascites may also lead to the formation of inguinal or umbilical hernias. When the hernias become large and the overlying skin becomes excoriated, life-threatening rupture of the hernia may occur, necessitating urgent surgical repair. Superinfection of ascites may result in spontaneous bacterial peritonitis (see later on), and translocation of ascitic fluid across the diaphragm may lead to hepatic hydrothorax (see later on).

Diagnostic paracentesis should be performed in any patient with new or worsening ascites, as well as in any patient with established ascites in whom abdominal pain, fever, or encephalopathy develops. When performed with a 21-gauge needle, paracentesis is safe even in patients with significant coagulopathy. The fluid obtained should be sent for cell and differential counts; total protein, albumin, amylase, and triglyceride levels; and cytologic studies and culture (by direct inoculation into blood culture bottles at the bedside). A serum albumin level should be obtained on the same day. Ascitic fluid glucose and lactate dehydrogenase (LDH) concentrations and a Gram's stain are useful only when secondary bacterial peritonitis is a diagnostic consideration. When tuberculous ascites is a possibility, an acid-fast stain should be obtained and a specimen submitted for mycobacterial cultures. Cirrhotic ascites is typified by a low total protein concentration, less than 2.5 grams per dL and often less than 1 gram per dL, and a high serum-ascites albumin gradient. The serum-ascites albumin gradient correlates directly with portal pressure, and gradients of 1.1 grams per dL or greater signify the presence of portal hypertension.

Therapy of cirrhotic ascites begins with dietary modification. Initial restriction of sodium chloride intake to 2 grams per day results in resolution of ascites in some patients and is crucial to the effectiveness of diuretics in the remainder. Patients with new ascites and normal renal function may respond to salt restriction alone. Counseling by a dietitian on how to implement such a diet leads to improved compliance. Fluid restriction is unnecessary unless significant hyponatremia (serum sodium concentration of less than 120 mEq per liter) develops.

The majority of patients with cirrhotic ascites require diuretic therapy in addition to dietary salt restriction. Such therapy requires vigilant monitoring to avoid electrolyte disturbances and volume depletion. Before initiation of diuretic therapy, the patient's baseline body weight, serum electrolyte values, and urinary sodium and potassium concentrations should be measured and tests of renal function conducted. In patients with hyperkalemia, such as those with type IV renal tubular acidosis related to diabetes mellitus, cautious treatment, if indicated at all, with potassium-sparing diuretics is in order. Patients with abnormal renal function at baseline must be monitored carefully in order to avoid precipitating prerenal azotemia or hepatorenal syndrome. In most patients with cirrhosis, the urinary potassium concentration exceeds that of sodium owing to hypersecretion of aldosterone. In these patients, the goal of diuretic therapy is to induce natriuresis and reduce kaliuresis, so that the ratio of urinary sodium to potassium concentration is greater than 1.

The first diuretic prescribed for most patients should be spironolactone (Aldactone), a direct aldosterone receptor antagonist and potassium-sparing agent. The starting dose is 100 mg per day which may be given initially in divided doses and after several days as a single dose. The dose may be increased to a maximum of 400 to 600 mg per day, but dose changes should be made no more often than every 4 days, owing to the long half-life of the drug. The dosage should be considered optimal once urine sodium concentration exceeds urine potassium concentration. The most common complication of spironolactone therapy is hyperkalemia, which is usually avoidable if serum electrolytes are monitored. Spironolactone may cause painful gynecomastia because it is an androgen receptor antagonist. If this occurs, triamterene (Dyrenium) may be substituted in a dose of 50 mg bid, with increases to 150 mg bid.

Optimal diuresis should result in weight loss of approximately 0.5 kg per day; weight loss of up to 1.0 kg per day is well tolerated in patients with concomitant peripheral edema. Although spironolactone antagonizes the sodium-retaining effect of aldosterone, additional stimuli to sodium retention remain, and effective diuresis often requires addition of another agent, usually a loop diuretic such as furosemide (Lasix). In patients with large-volume ascites, it is reasonable to begin administration of furosemide simultaneously with spironolactone. Otherwise, furosemide can be withheld until it has been established that the dosage of spironolactone has been optimized without adequate diuresis. The usual starting dose of furosemide is 40 mg once daily, and the dose may be doubled every several days to a maximum of 160 mg per day if necessary. When given intravenously (IV), furosemide diminishes renal perfusion significantly in patients with cirrhosis; therefore, this route of administration should be avoided. Occasionally, the addition of a third diuretic, such as hydrochlorothiazide, may be considered.

Failure to respond to medical therapy defines refractory ascites; failure of ascites to resolve despite maximal doses of diuretics (400 mg of spironolactone and 160 mg of furosemide daily) defines "diuretic-resistant" ascites, whereas failure due to intolerance of maximal doses of diuretics defines "diuretic-intractable" ascites. Surreptitious salt ingestion should be ruled out in patients who fail to lose weight despite adequate natriuresis. In patients with diuretic-resistant or diuretic-intractable ascites, the next therapeutic option is generally large-volume paracentesis, which should be initial therapy in any patient with respiratory compromise from tense ascites. In this procedure, 5 or more liters of fluid is removed using an 18-gauge needle connected by phlebotomy or peritoneal dialysis tubing to vacuum bottles. This procedure has been shown to be safe and effective in relieving tense ascites. Complete paracentesis, in which the entire volume of ascites is drained, has also been shown to be safe and effective. Although our approach is controversial, we prefer to administer approximately 10 grams of salt-poor albumin IV per liter of ascites removed in order to minimize the risk of renal insufficiency and hyponatremia. Large-volume paracentesis may be repeated regularly, with careful monitoring of hemodynamics, electrolytes, and renal function. For hospitalized patients with tenuous renal function, tense ascites, and significant hypoalbuminemia, infusion of salt-poor albumin without paracentesis probably enhances diuresis over the short term without a detrimental hemodynamic effect. In such patients, infusions of 25 to 50 grams per day should be continued until a target serum albumin of 3.0 grams per dL is reached. However, excessive albumin administration may increase the risk of variceal bleeding by increasing intravascular volume.

Other therapies for refractory ascites include insertion of a peritoneovenous (Le Veen) shunt and placement of a transjugular intrahepatic portosystemic shunt (TIPS). A LeVeen shunt connects the peritoneal cavity directly to the internal jugular vein, allowing decompression of ascites by drainage into the vascular system. However, the use of such shunts is associated with a high incidence of serious complications, most notably disseminated intravascular coagulation (DIC) and sepsis, and such devices have fallen out of favor. Placement of a TIPS is performed by an interventional radiologist and may lead to dramatic resolution of ascites in as many as 75% of patients in whom the condition is refractory to diuretics. Natriuresis may be delayed up to 4 weeks after a TIPS insertion. Unfortunately, shunt thrombosis is a common early complication, and stent occlusion due to pseudointimal hyperplasia is nearly universal in the first 1 to 2 years after placement of a TIPS. Therefore, frequent shunt revisions are usually necessary. In addition, the use of a TIPS poses an increased risk of portosystemic encephalopathy and has not been shown to reduce overall mortality. In selected patients, refractory ascites is an indication for liver transplantation (see later on).

Spontaneous Bacterial Peritonitis

An ominous complication in patients with cirrhotic ascites is spontaneous bacterial peritonitis (SBP), which is associated with a short-term mortality rate of approximately 50%, and a 1-year mortality rate of 62% even after recovery from a first episode. SBP results from hematogenous superinfection of ascites stemming from prolonged bacteremia due to decreased reticuloendothelial (RE) function, portosystemic shunting, and deficiency of complement and immunoglobulins in ascitic fluid. Because the ascitic fluid total protein concentration correlates directly with the opsonic activity of ascitic fluid, patients with an ascitic fluid total protein concentration of less than 1 gram per dL are at highest risk of developing SBP. The most common pathogens in SBP are gram-negative enteric bacteria, especially *Escherichia coli* and *Klebsiella pneumoniae,* but streptococci, including pneumococci, and also enterococci account for a significant minority of cases. In contrast, anaerobic bacteria rarely cause SBP.

The manifestations of SBP may be protean. Abdominal pain and fever are typical but often absent. Abdominal tenderness, sometimes with peritoneal signs, is present in approximately half the patients. In many cases, the only clue to the presence of the infection is worsening encephalopathy, renal function, or ascites. In fact, up to one third of affected patients may be completely asymptomatic. Therefore, a high index of suspicion for SBP is necessary, and the clinician should have a low threshold for performing diagnostic paracentesis. Paracentesis should be performed in any patient with ascites and fever, new abdominal pain, or new encephalopathy.

The diagnosis of SBP is based on an ascitic fluid polymorphonuclear neutrophil (PMN) count of 500 per mm^3 or higher (or 250 per mm^3 or higher if the patient has any symptoms of SBP) and absence of an underlying intra-abdominal focus of infection, whether or not the ascitic fluid culture is positive. At least 10 mL of fluid should be inoculated directly into blood culture bottles at the bedside to maximize the sensitivity of the culture. Culture-negative neutrocytic ascites, defined as ascites with a fluid PMN count of 500 cells per mm^3 or higher in the absence of a positive fluid culture and recent antibiotic therapy, should be treated as for SBP. On the other hand, monomicrobial non-neutrocytic "bacterascites," defined as ascites with positive results on fluid culture but an ascitic fluid PMN count of less than 250 per mm^3, is generally transient and often does not require treatment.

The antibiotic of choice for treatment of SBP is the third-generation cephalosporin cefotaxime (Claforan) in a dose of 2 grams IV every 8 hours. Alternatives include ceftriaxone (Rocephin), ampicillin-sulbactam (Unasyn), ticarcillin–clavulanic acid (Timentin), and piperacillin-tazobactam (Zosyn). Recently, oral ofloxacin (Floxin) has been shown to be highly effective for treatment of SBP, but additional studies are needed before oral antibiotic therapy alone can be recommended. Use of aminoglycosides should be avoided, because patients with cirrhosis are particularly prone to aminoglycoside-induced nephrotoxicity. Antibiotic therapy should be started immediately after paracentesis, pending culture results. If SBP is confirmed, antibiotics should be continued for at least 5 days. So long as the patient improves clinically, another paracentesis procedure is not necessary. If the patient does not improve by 48 hours, paracentesis should be repeated; if the ascitic PMN count has not fallen by 50%, antibiotic coverage should be broadened and other causes of peritonitis should be considered. Secondary bacterial peritonitis should also be considered when the initial ascitic fluid PMN count is greater than 10,000 per mm^3, the ascitic fluid glucose level is less than 50 mg per dL, or the culture is positive for more than one organism.

Prophylactic administration of oral nonabsorbable antibiotics has proved effective in preventing SBP in high-risk patients. The goal of prophylaxis is selective elimination of gram-negative bacteria from the intestinal flora. The most effective antibiotic studied has been norfloxacin (Noroxin),* in a dose of 400 mg daily. High-risk patients who may warrant prophylactic therapy include those with a previous episode of SBP, with a recent episode of gastrointestinal hemorrhage, or awaiting liver transplantation, and possibly those with an extremely low ascitic fluid total protein concentration (less than 1 gram per dL). Because candidal overgrowth is a possible side effect of prophylactic antibiotic therapy, liver transplant candidates on long-term antibiotic prophylaxis should also receive either clotrimazole (Mycelex),

*Not FDA approved for this indication.

1 troche tid, or nystatin (Mycostatin), swish and swallow 10 mL, tid.

Hepatorenal Syndrome

Progressive renal failure often heralds the cirrhotic patient's demise and may be the primary cause of death. Although the pathogenesis is not completely understood, hepatorenal syndrome (HRS) results from renal cortical hypoperfusion related to the complex hemodynamic alterations induced by cirrhosis. Portal hypertension results in decreased systemic vascular resistance and relative hypovolemia as well as increased renal vascular resistance due to increased sympathetic nervous system output and elevated levels of various renal arteriolar vasoconstrictors, including angiotensin, vasopressin, endothelin, and leukotrienes. The effect of these renal vasoconstrictors may be offset by secretion of prostaglandins and kallikreins, but the compensatory mechanisms may eventually be overwhelmed, resulting in HRS. Nevertheless, kidneys from patients with HRS remain structurally normal and can even be used as donor organs for transplantation.

Major criteria for the diagnosis of HRS include advanced hepatic failure and portal hypertension; a low glomerular filtration rate, as indicated by a serum creatinine level of greater than 1.5 mg per dL or a 24-hour creatinine clearance of less than 40 mL per minute; absence of shock, sepsis, drug-induced nephrotoxicity, and gastrointestinal or diuretic-induced fluid losses; lack of improvement in renal function following diuretic withdrawal and expansion of plasma volume with 1.5 liters of normal saline; and absence of significant proteinuria or ultrasonographic evidence of obstructive or parenchymal renal disease. Additional criteria that support the diagnosis of HRS, but which may not be present in all cases, include oliguria (urine volume of less than 500 mL per day), low urine sodium concentration (less than 10 mEq per liter), and urine osmolality greater than plasma osmolality. Fractional excretion of sodium is characteristically less than 1%.

The only effective treatment of HRS is liver transplantation. Short of transplantation, intravascular volume should be optimized using blood products or albumin, diuretics should be withheld, and any other potentially aggravating drugs (such as nonsteroidal anti-inflammatory drugs and aminoglycosides) should be avoided. Intravenous infusion of "renal-dose" dopamine (1 to 3 μg per kg per minute) may help to maintain urine output. Intravenous infusion of ornipressin (6 International Units per hour), a vasoconstrictor that does not increase renal vascular resistance, has been reported to be useful in stabilizing renal function in patients with HRS awaiting liver transplantation. The use of TIPS may also be beneficial but has not been studied systematically in patients with HRS. Dialysis may be necessary to maintain intravascular volume, electrolyte levels, and acid-base homeostasis, but survival is poor once this stage is reached.

Hepatic Hydrothorax

A pleural effusion due to portal hypertension, also known as hepatic hydrothorax, affects 5 to 10% of patients with cirrhosis. Most cases occur in patients with poorly controlled ascites, but a pleural effusion may occur in the absence of ascites. The effusion is typically right-sided and may be massive. Diagnosis requires exclusion of other causes of pleural effusion, including cardiac or pulmonary disease. Diagnostic thoracentesis should be performed on any new pleural effusion in a cirrhotic patient; low ascitic fluid values of LDH and total protein as well as negative results of microbiologic studies are consistent with hepatic hydrothorax. In addition, analogous to SBP, "spontaneous bacterial empyema" may occur owing to superinfection of chronic hepatic hydrothorax. Therefore, diagnostic thoracentesis should be considered in any cirrhotic patient with a pleural effusion and encephalopathy or fever of unknown source.

The pathogenesis of hepatic hydrothorax appears to be related to small diaphragmatic defects that allow passage of ascitic fluid into the thorax. Therefore, treatment is generally the same as that for ascites—namely, salt restriction, diuretics, and large-volume paracentesis when appropriate. Serial therapeutic thoracenteses may be performed, but rapid reaccumulation of fluid usually follows. Chemical pleurodesis has been attempted, but results are poor owing to reaccumulation of fluid before the desired effect can be achieved. In refractory cases, the use of TIPS is often successful and has been proposed as the treatment of choice. In selected cases, thoracoscopic closure of diaphragmatic defects has been used with excellent results, but this approach is unlikely to be necessary with the advent of TIPS.

Hepatic Encephalopathy

Cirrhosis may result in disturbance of CNS function by several mechanisms. The diagnostic and pathophysiologic hallmark of hepatic encephalopathy is hyperammonemia, which results from reduced hepatic clearance of gut-derived ammonia from portal venous blood because of both portosystemic shunting and hepatocellular dysfunction. Effects of ammonia on the CNS include alterations in membrane transport, decreases in oxidation-reduction potential and energy stores, and depletion of the excitatory neurotransmitter glutamate in neurons. When the serum ammonia concentration increases acutely, accumulation of glutamine in astrocytes can result in lethal cerebral edema. Other factors that may contribute to hepatic encephalopathy include gut-derived mercaptans, elevated serum levels of aromatic amino acids, increased sensitivity to γ-aminobutyric acid (GABA) and endogenous benzodiazepine-like compounds, zinc deficiency, and deposition of manganese in the basal ganglia.

Clinical manifestations of hepatic encephalopathy vary considerably depending in part on the severity of hepatic dysfunction and portosystemic shunting

TABLE 3. **Clinical Stages of Hepatic Encephalopathy**

	Findings			
Grade	*Level of Consciousness*	*Personality and Intellect*	*Neurologic Abnormalities*	*EEG Abnormalities*
0	Normal	No abnormality	None	None
1	Reversed sleep pattern, restless	Forgetful, agitated, irritable, mildly confused	Tremor, apraxia, incoordination, poor handwriting	Slowing 5-cps triphasic waves
2	Lethargic	Disoriented to time, amnesia, disinhibited, poor judgment	Asterixis, dysarthria, ataxia, hyporeflexia	Slowing 5-cps triphasic waves
3	Somnolent	Disoriented to place, aggressive	Asterixis, rigidity, hyperreflexia	Slowing 5-cps triphasic waves
4	Comatose	None	Decerebrate	Slow 2- to 3-cps delta activity

Abbreviations: EEG = electroencephalogram; cps = counts per second.

(Table 3). Patients with mild encephalopathy may present clinically with reversal of the sleep-wake cycle. Mild personality changes may also be noted, but asterixis is often absent. Patients with moderately severe encephalopathy experience either drowsiness or agitation, and asterixis is usually present. Severe acute encephalopathy is marked by somnolence, deep confusion, asterixis, and hyper-reflexia. At this stage, airway protection is compromised, and endotracheal intubation should be considered to prevent aspiration pneumonia. Coma may ultimately supervene, with decerebrate posturing followed by death. Patients with chronic encephalopathy often display personality changes, dementia, memory loss, and occasionally movement disorders.

Most episodes of acute hepatic encephalopathy are precipitated by a potentially reversible factor. Precipitants include dehydration, constipation, excessive dietary protein intake, hypokalemia, metabolic alkalosis, sepsis (especially SBP), gastrointestinal bleeding, renal failure, and use of benzodiazepines or other sedatives. Identification and removal of the relevant precipitant(s) are the first steps in the treatment of acute encephalopathy. Other causes of mental status changes, such as subdural hematoma, alcohol withdrawal, Wernicke's encephalopathy, hypoglycemia, and drug or alcohol intoxication, should be ruled out.

Further treatment of acute encephalopathy centers on facilitating net ammonia excretion. Dietary protein should be restricted, initially to as little as 20 grams per day. Lactulose syrup should be administered in doses of 30 mL PO every hour until diarrhea occurs and then every 4 to 6 hours as needed to achieve two to four loose bowel movements per day. Lactulose is a nonabsorbable disaccharide that passes unchanged into the colon, where it is fermented by colonic flora. It reduces ammonia absorption by producing diarrhea and by acidifying the colonic lumen, thereby trapping ammonia as nondiffusible ammonium ion. In patients with severely depressed levels of consciousness, a nasogastric tube may be required for the administration of lactulose. If ileus is present, lactulose may be administered as a retention enema, using 300 mL of lactulose suspended in 700 mL of water. In patients who fail to respond to lactulose alone, oral neomycin,* 6 grams per day initially and then 1 gram bid, or metronidazole (Flagyl),* 250 mg tid, may be added. However, neomycin is absorbed by the intestine to some extent in patients with cirrhosis and may thus cause nephrotoxicity and ototoxicity.

Other treatments may be beneficial in selected cases. Administration of the short-acting benzodiazepine antagonist flumazenil (Romazicon)* leads to improvement in up to 40% of patients unresponsive to lactulose, but the response is transient, the drug must be administered parenterally, and the medication is expensive. Oral sodium benzoate or phenylacetate may facilitate renal excretion of ammonia, and ornithine aspartate, which enhances ureagenesis, may also lower the serum ammonia level, but these agents are not widely used for treatment of hepatic encephalopathy due to cirrhosis. Zinc deficiency, if present, should be corrected, because several enzymes in the urea cycle are zinc-dependent. Finally, *Helicobacter pylori,* a urea-splitting bacterium that commonly colonizes the stomach, may add in small measure to the generation of ammonia in the gastrointestinal tract, and anecdotal reports suggest that encephalopathy may lessen following eradication of *H. pylori.*

Prevention of recurrent encephalopathy requires extensive counseling and close monitoring of the patient. Dietary protein should be restricted, but usually to no less than 60 to 80 grams per day, so that protein malnutrition does not worsen. Formal consultation with a dietitian is essential to achieving this goal. Lactulose should be continued at a dose of 15 to 30 mL bid or tid as needed to achieve two or three loose stools per day. Excessive diuresis and use of sedative medications should be avoided.

Hepatopulmonary Syndrome

Hepatopulmonary syndrome (HPS) is defined as the presence of an increased alveolar-arterial oxygen gradient and intrapulmonary vascular dilatations in a patient with chronic liver disease. Affected persons

*Not FDA approved for this indication.

may become markedly debilitated owing to severe hypoxemia (partial pressure of oxygen [Pao_2] of less than 50 mm Hg) and may require continuous oxygen supplementation. Typically, oxygenation worsens as the patient moves from the supine to the standing position (orthodeoxia). The pathophysiology of the syndrome relates to intrapulmonary right-to-left shunting through vascular dilatations of varying size. Type I HPS is characterized by diffuse small precapillary dilatations scattered throughout the lung parenchyma, whereas type II HPS is characterized by discrete, large pulmonary arteriovenous malformations (AVMs). The diagnosis of HPS may be made by contrast echocardiography, radiolabeled albumin scanning, or pulmonary angiography, but only angiography differentiates type I from type II HPS. Angiography is potentially therapeutic in the case of type II HPS; large AVMs can sometimes be ablated by spring-coil embolization. Unfortunately, for most patients with HPS there is no effective therapy. However, recent experience indicates that HPS is reversible after liver transplantation so long as pulmonary hypertension has not developed. Therefore, patients with debilitating hypoxemia from HPS should be considered candidates for liver transplantation.

Coagulopathy

The liver synthesizes fibrinogen and coagulation factors II, V, VII, IX, and X; factors II, VII, IX, and X require vitamin K for their activity. Deficiency of one or more of these clotting factors in cirrhosis typically results in prolongation of the prothrombin time (PT); with severe synthetic dysfunction, the activated partial thromboplastin time (aPTT) may also be prolonged. Caution must be used in differentiating the coagulopathy of liver disease from DIC; in both conditions, PT and aPTT are elevated, the platelet count is decreased, fibrinogen levels are decreased, and fibrin split products are elevated. The most useful laboratory parameter for differentiating the two processes is the factor VIII level; because factor VIII is not synthesized by the liver, levels are preserved in cirrhosis but markedly decreased in DIC.

Additional hematologic consequences of chronic liver disease include anemia, leukopenia, and thrombocytopenia. Hypersplenism due to portal hypertension is the most common mechanism underlying these abnormalities, although leukopenia and thrombocytopenia do not resolve consistently after placement of a TIPS. Iron deficiency due to chronic or recurrent gastrointestinal bleeding may also contribute to anemia. Folic acid deficiency, which is common in alcoholic patients, may also contribute to both anemia and thrombocytopenia. Polycythemia should alert the clinician to the possibility of an occult hepatocellular carcinoma.

Coagulopathy should be corrected, if possible, in any cirrhotic patient with bleeding or before an invasive procedure. In general, invasive procedures, including percutaneous liver biopsy, should not be performed if the PT is prolonged by more than 3 seconds or if the platelet count is less than 75,000 per mm^3. Administration of vitamin K, 10 mg SC daily for 1 to 3 days, can lower the PT in patients with vitamin K deficiency, including those with predominantly cholestatic disease such as PBC or primary sclerosing cholangitis, those who are malnourished (especially alcoholic patients), and those receiving chronic antibiotic therapy. However, vitamin K does not reverse coagulopathy due to impaired hepatocellular function. Moreover, because the effect of vitamin K depends on synthesis of new clotting factors, the onset of action is slow. In most patients, therefore, fresh-frozen plasma (FFP) is needed to reverse significant coagulopathy, and FFP should be administered in doses of 1 to 2 units per hour IV until bleeding stops or the PT is corrected. If coagulopathy fails to respond to large quantities of FFP and if the fibrinogen level falls below 100 mg per dL, cryoprecipitate should be administered. Platelet infusions are also indicated in patients with active bleeding or before invasive procedures when the platelet count is less than 75,000 per mm^3. Desmopressin (DDAVP), in a dose of 0.3 μg per kg diluted in 50 mL of normal saline and infused over 30 minutes, may also be used to improve the bleeding time and aPTT; the drug, an analogue of vasopressin, increases factor VIII and von Willebrand factor activities.

Blood products carry a risk, albeit small, of viral transmission or transfusion reactions, as well as overexpansion of the intravascular space and precipitation of variceal bleeding. Therefore, they should not be administered to nonbleeding patients with cirrhosis and laboratory evidence of coagulopathy.

Susceptibility to Infection

Cirrhosis induces a relatively immunocompromised state owing to impaired RE function. Malnutrition, when present, further impairs both humoral and cell-mediated immunity. Therefore, several steps should be taken to protect cirrhotic patients from infection. Polyvalent pneumococcal vaccine (Pneumovax) should be administered to all patients with cirrhosis. Hemophilus b conjugate vaccine is also recommended by some authorities, although *Haemophilus influenzae* serotype b is an uncommon cause of respiratory infections in adults. Influenza vaccine should be administered yearly. Finally, vaccination against hepatitis A (Havrix or Vaqta) and hepatitis B (Engerix-B or Recombivax HB) should be offered to seronegative patients, because acute viral hepatitis is more likely to lead to hepatic failure in a patient with already compromised hepatic function.

Hepatocellular Carcinoma

Patients with cirrhosis of any cause are at increased risk of hepatocellular carcinoma (HCC). The risk varies with the cause of cirrhosis; patients with chronic viral hepatitis and hemochromatosis are at especially high risk, while those with primary biliary cirrhosis and Wilson's disease are at lowest risk. A diagnosis of HCC should be considered in any patient with cirrhosis in whom clinical decompensation is observed. Specifically, HCC may underlie variceal bleeding, worsening ascites, encephalopathy, or cachexia in a previously well-compensated patient. We screen all patients with cirrhosis for HCC using ultrasonography and serum alpha-fetoprotein testing every 6 months, although the cost-effectiveness of this strategy is uncertain. To evaluate focal hepatic lesions detected by ultrasound studies, magnetic resonance imaging and computed tomography (CT) with arterial-phase imaging after the administration of IV contrast are useful. Definitive diagnosis may be obtained by ultrasound- or CT-guided needle biopsy. In patients with cirrhosis, resection of the tumor may be precluded by limited hepatic reserve. Therefore, liver transplantation should be considered in any patient with cirrhosis and HCC, provided that the tumor is smaller than 5 cm in diameter and confined to the liver or, if several lesions are present, the largest is no more than 3 cm in diameter and there is no invasion of the portal vein. In patients who are not candidates for surgery or transplantation, percutaneous ethanol injection to ablate small tumors may be considered. For large, unresectable tumors, chemoembolization via the hepatic artery may provide palliation.

ORTHOTOPIC LIVER TRANSPLANTATION

For cirrhosis of most causes, orthotopic liver transplantation is the only curative therapy. Proper timing of transplantation is crucial; patients with far-advanced cirrhosis and several serious complications have a higher mortality rate than do patients with relatively compensated cirrhosis who undergo liver transplantation, whereas patients with fully compensated cirrhosis do not require transplantation. In general, patients with cirrhosis should be referred to a transplant center at the first sign of decompensation or when death due to liver disease is expected within several years.

In preparation for liver transplantation, the following tests should be performed: identification of ABO blood type, determination of human immunodeficiency virus (HIV) status, measurement of cytomegalovirus (CMV) and varicella-zoster virus titers, tuberculin skin test, abdominal ultrasound scan with Doppler flow studies, pulmonary function tests, and measurement of serum alpha-fetoprotein level. If HCC is present, CT scanning of the chest and abdomen is necessary to rule out extrahepatic spread. In addition, formal psychiatric evaluation should be obtained. In patients who are CMV-seronegative, filtered or CMV-safe blood products should be used to avoid transfusion-borne infection, because CMV infection has been shown to increase mortality after liver transplantation.

Absolute contraindications to liver transplantation include sepsis, extrahepatic malignancy, advanced cardiac or pulmonary disease, acquired immunodeficiency syndrome (AIDS), and inability to understand the procedure and post-transplant regimen. Relative contraindications include age greater than 70 years, active alcohol or drug use, HCC, mesenteric vein thrombosis, hepatobiliary sepsis, HIV infection, pulmonary hypertension, advanced chronic renal insufficiency, and severe malnutrition.

Five-year survival rates after liver transplantation are approximately 70%, and most post-transplant deaths occur in the first 6 months and are due to perioperative complications, acute graft rejection, or sepsis. After transplantation, patients are maintained on lifelong immunosuppression. The standard regimen consists of cyclosporine or tacrolimus (FK 506, Prograf), azathioprine, and prednisone. Patients must be willing and able to comply with a complicated medical regimen and intensive follow-up. The original liver disease may recur in the transplanted organ. In particular, the risk of recurrent hepatitis B after liver transplantation is high, but can be reduced with hepatitis B immune globulin (HBIG) or treatment with the oral nucleoside analogue lamivudine. Hepatitis C almost invariably recurs after transplantation but follows a relatively benign course in many patients.

BLEEDING ESOPHAGEAL VARICES

method of
JOHN CRAIG COLLINS, M.D., and
I. JAMES SARFEH, M.D.
University of California, Irvine, College of Medicine
Irvine, California

Advances in several areas—portacaval shunt surgery, endoscopic therapy, pharmaceuticals, and transjugular intrahepatic portosystemic shunts (TIPS)—have made clinical management of bleeding esophageal varices even more complex. Notwithstanding the accelerating progress of the last 25 years, variceal hemorrhage remains a highly lethal condition that will occur in approximately one third of patients with portal hypertension. There is no reliable means to predict a priori the subset of patients at greatest risk. Once a given patient has bled from varices, the probability of rebleeding is 50 to 80% unless the underlying portal hypertension is corrected. About 30% of acute episodes are fatal.

Of all upper gastrointestinal hemorrhages among patients with portal hypertension, approximately half are due to rupture of esophageal varices. Peptic ulcer disease and portal hypertensive gastropathy are other common causes of bleeding. Less frequent causes include Mallory-Weiss tears and sclerotherapy-induced esophageal ulcers. Rapid and accurate diagnosis should guide therapy.

Peptic ulcer disease in this population follows a natural history similar to that in normal patients, except that the underlying liver disease reduces tolerance of physiologic stress and worsens coagulopathy in response to blood loss. Portal hypertensive gastropathy (PHG) is a process in which microvessels in the gastric mucosa become ectatic and congested. Mucosal blood loss usually is chronic. Proton pump inhibitors and treatment of *Helicobacter pylori* have little effect on PHG; definitive treatment requires reduction of the portacaval pressure gradient. Mallory-Weiss tears usually are self-limited but may require endoscopic or operative treatment. Sclerotherapy-induced ulcers can be a cause of catastrophic arterial bleeding that is rapidly fatal unless corrected by emergency operation.

Prompt video endoscopy of the esophagus, stomach, and duodenum is the mainstay of diagnosis and can provide an avenue for emergency treatment. The characteristics of any varices should be recorded carefully, as the size and appearance of varices may provide an index of the risk of rebleeding. Larger varices bleed twice as frequently as smaller ones. Red wale markings, cherry-red spots, and "varices on varices" are further predictors of rebleeding risk.

Once varices are implicated as the cause of bleeding, attempts should be made to define their etiology. In North America, alcoholic cirrhosis is the most common cause of portal hypertension. Chronic infectious hepatitis and "cryptogenic" cirrhosis account for smaller shares. In addition to the intrahepatic causes just mentioned, there are less common prehepatic (portal or splenic vein thromboses) and posthepatic causes (Budd-Chiari syndrome). Portal hypertension caused by schistosomiasis is the prevalent etiology of variceal hemorrhage in developing nations. Unusual causes of portal hypertension may influence definitive treatment.

TREATMENT

Prophylaxis

Beta-adrenergic blockade with propranolol (Inderal) and related drugs is currently the only proven means to prevent the first episode of variceal bleeding. Investigation of other agents for pharmacologic prophylaxis of portal hypertension is proceeding, although compliance becomes a problem with any lifelong intervention that lacks visible benefit.

Studies of portacaval shunts and endoscopic sclerotherapy for prophylaxis have demonstrated that neither approach is warranted for this indication. Surgical shunts, because of the limitations of the "total" portacaval shunt procedures then available, resulted in encephalopathy and accelerated liver failure. Sclerotherapy is costly, has its own risks and, because it does not correct the underlying portal hypertension, does not reliably prevent initial episodes of variceal bleeding.

Better means of predicting precisely which 30% of cirrhotic patients are destined to bleed from varices must be devised. Proper risk stratification should guide the rational application of preventive measures in the future.

ELECTIVE THERAPY

Pharmacologic

Despite a number of studies using beta blockers for prevention of variceal rebleeding, no consensus has been reached regarding long-term effectiveness in this setting. Drugs that reduce portal pressure may find their ultimate role in combination with other modalities, such as endoscopic treatment.

Endotherapy

Sclerotherapy (using paravariceal or intravariceal injections of sclerosant agents) is gradually giving way to the newer method of endoscopic rubber band ligation as a primary means of endoscopic treatment for varices. Ligation requires fewer sessions for complete eradication of visible varices and had a lower rate of complications than sclerotherapy in a prospective, randomized trial. The combination of sclerosis and ligation has also been advocated.

The larger question is the overall place of endoscopic therapy in the therapeutic algorithm. Randomized trials of endotherapy versus TIPS were beginning to appear in 1997; as in earlier studies comparing sclerotherapy with portacaval shunts, endoscopic treatment (ligation and/or sclerosis) generally resulted in a lesser incidence of encephalopathy and similar survival but a higher risk of rebleeding. Advantages of endotherapy include the following:

1. Avoidance of a major operation
2. Wide availability
3. Very low risk of postprocedural encephalopathy
4. Comparable survival to other forms of therapy

Disadvantages are these:

1. The potential for complications, including arterial bleeding and esophageal stricture or perforation
2. The requirement for multiple treatment sessions to achieve complete eradication of esophageal varices
3. Exacerbation of portal hypertensive gastropathy and the appearance of extraesophageal varices (e.g., gastric, duodenal) as a consequence of uncorrected portal hypertension
4. Much higher rates of rebleeding compared with procedures that reduce portal pressure

Proper end points for endoscopic therapy remain controversial. Most authorities define failure of *elective* treatment as any rebleeding that occurs after complete eradication of varices, or two episodes of bleeding during the course of treatment. Some proponents of endoscopic therapy have been criticized for persisting in the face of severe recurrent bleeding, a situation in which TIPS or portacaval shunt operations become more appropriate. It is important for the endotherapist to work closely with the surgeon and interventional radiologist so that decisions of this sort can be made with a full understanding of local expertise and capabilities.

Transjugular Intrahepatic Portosystemic Shunts

An ingenious percutaneous method of inserting an expandable stent to connect the portal and systemic circulations within the liver substance has been accepted rapidly since its clinical debut in 1989. TIPS was initially touted as a quantum advance that would render all other forms of therapy for portal hypertension obsolete. As the strengths and limitations of the technique have come to light, it becomes clear that TIPS is not yet a mature technology. Existing nonrandomized series suggest that a patent TIPS stent is as effective as a surgical portacaval shunt in preventing recurrent variceal hemorrhage.

Unfortunately, TIPS has been plagued by progressive stenoses and occlusions, limiting its long-term usefulness in elective cases. The most optimistic current reports place the median "assisted" patency at 12 to 24 months. A recent prospective, randomized trial compared TIPS with the partial portacaval shunt for mostly elective indications. TIPS had higher rates of death and rebleeding, as well as a doubled incidence of treatment failure.

Although the eventual prospects for elective TIPS are promising, current evidence suggests that its major role should be that of a temporizing measure or a bridge to transplantation for patients with advanced (Child C) cirrhosis.

Surgical Procedures

Operative approaches include nonshunt procedures and three main types of shunts: total, selective, and partial.

Nonshunt Procedures

The goal of such operations is to interrupt flow to varices by ablation of collaterals. The limitation of these operations is that uncorrected portal hypertension persists and rebleeding, therefore, is likely (up to 50% at 2 years). The most popular variant is a combination of splenectomy, gastric devascularization, and transection-reanastomosis of the esophagus using a circular stapling device. Devascularization procedures are accepted in Europe but are used less frequently in the United States. The main indication has been acute hemorrhage that fails endoscopic therapy, although TIPS is probably a better choice in this circumstance.

Total Shunts

Operations that divert all portal venous blood flow into the systemic circulation are classified as total shunts. This category includes end-to-side and side-to-side portacaval shunts, as well as mesocaval interposition and proximal splenorenal shunts. They are extremely effective in controlling variceal hemorrhage but deprive the liver of a large share of its nutrient blood flow. As shown in multiple randomized trials, total shunts are associated with high rates of hepatic encephalopathy and accelerated mortality due to liver failure. Despite their disadvantages, these operations are widely performed because of their familiarity and reliability. Because they completely decompress the liver and portal vein, the side-to-side varieties are therapeutic for ascites.

Selective Shunts

The main example of a selective shunt is the distal splenorenal shunt, devised by Warren and Zeppa to maintain portal flow to the liver. The splenic vein is divided at its confluence with the superior mesenteric vein and anastomosed to the side of the left renal vein. The coronary and gastroepiploic veins, as well as other spontaneous collateral vessels feeding the azygous system, are ligated. The aim is to maintain right-sided portal hypertension and forward flow in the portal vein while decompressing gastroesophageal varices through the left-sided shunt. This complex operation is challenging and rarely used in emergencies; ascites is a relative contraindication. Evidence suggests that the benefits of the procedure eventually are diminished in alcoholic patients, who tend to develop new collaterals connecting the portal-mesenteric system to the shunt with resultant loss of prograde portal flow. In nonalcoholic patients, studies have demonstrated prolonged maintenance of portal flow and low rates of encephalopathy.

Partial Shunts

This procedure was developed in the 1980s by Sarfeh and Rypins and is based on the observation that variceal bleeding occurs above a critical pressure gradient of 12 mm Hg as measured between the portal vein and vena cava. Partial shunting is accomplished by a small-diameter portacaval H graft combined with collateral ablation. This reduces portal pressure sufficiently to prevent rupture of varices, yet preserves prograde flow to the liver. The goal of the operation is to replace abnormal collateral vessels with a prosthetic conduit of fixed size and resistance carrying a similar volume of blood. In this concept of *collateral substitution*, portal hemodynamics are minimally altered except that the risk of variceal bleeding is markedly reduced. Compared with total shunts in a randomized trial, partial shunts were associated with significantly less postoperative encephalopathy and equivalent (100%) control of variceal rebleeding. Longitudinal follow-up has demonstrated durable patency and effectiveness. The operation is technically less demanding than the Warren shunt and has few contraindications. Its principal indication is the long-term prevention of variceal rebleeding in Child A and B alcoholics.

Hepatic Transplantation

Orthotopic liver transplantation is the only option for patients with irreversible liver disease, but its availability has been limited by expense and the chronic shortage of donor organs. Transplantation reverses portal hypertension and thus abolishes variceal bleeding and ascites. Although indications have been liberalized at many transplant centers, active substance abuse remains an absolute contraindication.

For patients who are not immediate candidates for transplantation, a sustained reduction in portal hypertension can be achieved with any of the surgical shunt procedures. A similar but shorter lived result is available through TIPS.

EMERGENCY TREATMENT

Beginning with the initial evaluation of any major episode of upper gastrointestinal hemorrhage, it is critical to establish adequate intravenous access, proceed with appropriate pharmacotherapy and fluid resuscitation, transfuse liberally, maintain normothermia, and prevent coagulopathy. Regardless of the etiology of bleeding, a hypovolemic, anemic, cold, coagulopathic patient is unlikely to survive.

During this phase of initial resuscitation, endoscopy should be performed and, if the diagnosis of variceal bleeding is confirmed, emergency endotherapy (sclerotherapy or ligation) can be done. Endoscopic treatment, performed simultaneously with fluid resuscitation and pharmacotherapy, is effective about 90% of the time. Balloon tamponade with the Sengstaken-Blakemore or Linton tube is a temporizing maneuver when bleeding cannot be stopped by endotherapy. Emergency TIPS, operative devascularization, or portacaval shunt are additional options for refractory bleeding. Many approaches to this problem have been described. This is our recommended treatment:

1. Establish access with at least two 14- to 16-gauge peripheral intravenous catheters. Maintain normovolemia and keep the hematocrit above 30%.
2. Infuse octreotide (Sandostatin), (somatostatin analogue) or a combination of vasopressin (Pitressin) and nitroglycerin, or terlipressin (Glypressin).*
3. If bleeding continues, add balloon tamponade (after endotracheal intubation). Institute sclerotherapy or ligation.
4. After 12 hours, deflate the balloon. If bleeding recurs, give a second course of endotherapy and then reinflate the balloon.
5. Deflate the balloon after another 12 hours and wean the pharmacotherapeutic agent(s). Rebleeding at this point constitutes failure of initial treatment; the patient should promptly undergo emergency TIPS, devascularization, or shunt.
6. If bleeding stops, treat electively with partial or selective shunt (Child A and B) or TIPS with consideration of liver transplantation (Child C). Many centers would substitute sclerotherapy or endoscopic ligation as "definitive" elective treatment, although the risk of rebleeding remains high.

Mortality for prolonged acute bleeding episodes is dismal, the more so for patients with advanced liver disease and poor hepatic functional reserve. TIPS is a major advance in the emergency treatment of variceal hemorrhage and can be expected to lead to improved survival compared with emergency portacaval shunt in high-risk patients. Rapid diagnosis and resuscitation leading to prompt definitive treatment ensure the best attainable outcomes.

*Orphan drug.

DYSPHAGIA AND ESOPHAGEAL OBSTRUCTION

method of
RICHARD I. ROTHSTEIN, M.D., and
ARIFA TOOR, M.D.
Dartmouth-Hitchcock Medical Center and Dartmouth Medical School
Lebanon, New Hampshire

Dysphagia is defined as difficulty in swallowing and literally comes from the Greek words *dys* (hard) and *phagein* (to eat). Dysphagia is a symptom that affects up to 15 million people in the United States and is usually experienced as a sensation of food or other ingested substance "sticking" at some point between mouth and stomach. The sensation that follows a difficult swallow is described as "choking," "hanging up," "catching," "slow passage," and "trouble swallowing." With esophageal dysphagia, there may be some associated chest pain, but painful swallowing alone is called odynophagia and should evoke a distinct differential diagnosis and etiology. Pyrosis (heartburn), weight loss, or respiratory symptoms may be part of the clinical presentation. Careful attention to the history of the dysphagia and its associated symptoms will direct the clinician toward identification of the underlying cause and the appropriate evaluation and treatment.

NORMAL SWALLOWING

Normal swallowing, which occurs about 600 times a day in most healthy individuals, is accomplished with a series of finely coordinated neural and muscular events. Swallows begin voluntarily with an oral phase in which food is prepared by the muscles of the jaw, face, and tongue into a bolus of appropriate size and consistency. Food needing to be chewed is mixed with saliva and compacted. The tip of the tongue then presses against the palate, and contractions of the tongue squeeze the bolus toward the pharynx, initiating the pharyngeal phase of swallowing. A rapid series of involuntary events then take place in the pharynx: (1) elevation and retraction of the soft palate with complete closure of the nasopharynx to prevent swallowed material from entering the nasal cavity, (2) elevation of the larynx with epiglottal closure over the airway, briefly interrupting respiration to prevent aspiration, (3) relaxation and opening of the upper esophageal sphincter (UES), and (4) initiation of pharyngeal peristalsis that provides a driving force to propel the bolus into the esophagus. This entire sequence takes approximately 1 second. The neural mediation of the swallowing reflex involves sensory input to the medullary swallowing center by way of cranial nerves V, X, and XI and motor activity transmitted through cranial nerves V, VII, IX, X, and XII.

The primary peristaltic wave initiated in the pharynx continues into the upper portion of the cervical esophagus, beginning the esophageal phase of swallowing. As the bolus enters the body of the esophagus, it descends by gravity and is propelled by peristalsis, taking about 6 to 9 seconds to reach the distal portion. Peristalsis is controlled primarily by intrinsic neural networks located between the longitudinal and circular muscle layers (Auerbach's plexus) and in the submucosa (Meissner's plexus) and is modulated by central mechanisms in the swallowing center. Relaxation of the lower esophageal sphincter (LES), initiated when the ingested bolus reaches the midesophagus, allows passage of the food bolus into the stomach. This relaxation lasts about 5 seconds and continues until the bolus is propelled into the stomach. The phenomenon of "chug-a-lug," whereby large volumes of liquid beverages are swallowed rapidly, can occur owing to prolonged relaxation of the LES when multiple swallows occur in sequence within 1 to 2 seconds of each other. This permits unobstructed passage of liquids through the esophagus into the stomach by gravity. After the last clearing swallow of a rapid series, the LES contracts, as after a single swallow, and resumes its resting tone.

ABNORMAL SWALLOWING

Multiple pathologic processes can disrupt the normal physiology of swallowing, producing the symptom of dysphagia. Clinically, dysphagia can be divided into two syndromes. Oropharyngeal (transfer) dysphagia involves the inability to move food or other material from the mouth to the upper esophagus. It is caused by abnormalities affecting the neuromuscular mechanisms of the mouth, pharynx, or UES. Patients describe difficulty initiating a swallow and often attempt to swallow repeatedly. They may report food sticking in the throat, nasal regurgitation, or coughing during swallowing. Esophageal (transport) dysphagia involves difficulty with the movement of ingested food, liquid, or other material down the esophagus. Aboral movement of the bolus may be inhibited by intraluminal obstruction from anatomic (e.g., ring, stricture, cancer, extrinsic compression) or functional (e.g., spasm, motor failure) mechanisms. Patients usually complain of food sticking somewhere in the throat or chest after it is swallowed. These two types of dysphagia are generally readily distinguished by a careful history.

When obtaining a history from a patient, it is important to distinguish true dysphagia from globus. Globus is the sensation of a lump, fullness, or constant "tickle" in the throat. It does not interfere with swallowing, and the sensation is often relieved by swallowing food. True dysphagia occurs only during swallow attempts, and can usually be easily distinguished from globus by the clinical history. Globus is a functional disorder that can be worsened by stress and anxiety, and may result in part from spasm of the cricopharyngeus or pharyngeal muscles. The diagnosis of globus is appropriate only after organic esophageal and pharyngeal pathology has been excluded by direct visualization and radiologic evaluation.

OROPHARYNGEAL DYSPHAGIA

Oropharyngeal dysphagia is caused by a wide variety of local, neurologic, and muscular diseases (Table 1). The symptoms suggesting transfer dysphagia usu-

TABLE 1. **Disorders Associated with Oropharyngeal Dysphagia**

Neuromuscular Disorders

Neurologic Disorders
- Cerebrovascular accidents
- Transient ischemic attacks
- Cranial nerve palsies
- Brain stem stroke
- Amyotrophic lateral sclerosis
- Multiple sclerosis
- Parkinson's disease
- Huntington's chorea
- Wilson's disease
- Spinocerebral degeneration
- Poliomyelitis
- Tabes dorsalis
- Neurosyphilis
- Botulism
- Tetanus
- Diphtheria

Skeletal Muscle Disorders
- Polymyositis
- Dermatomyositis
- Myasthenia gravis
- Myotonic dystrophy
- Oculopharyngeal dystrophy
- Metabolic myopathy (steroid myopathy, thyrotoxicosis, myxedema)
- Amyloidosis

Structural Abnormalities
- Oropharyngeal malignancy
- Inflammation (pharyngitis, tonsillar abscess, syphilis, tuberculosis)
- Postresective surgery for head/neck tumor
- Postradiation therapy to the neck
- Extrinsic compression (cervical spur, thyromegaly, lymphadenopathy)
- Zenker's diverticulum
- Cricopharyngeal bar
- Cricopharyngeal web
- Xerostomia (Sjögren's, sicca syndrome, anticholinergic drugs, dehydration)

Motility Disorders of the Upper Esophageal Sphincter (UES)
- Hypertensive UES
- Hypotensive UES
- Abnormal UES relaxation (cricopharyngeal "achalasia")

ally begin within 1 second of swallowing. Patients often describe coughing during a meal, suggesting tracheobronchial aspiration from inadequate laryngeal protection. Weakness or impaired control of the musculature of the soft palate may result in nasal speech or dysarthria. Swallowing associated with a gurgling noise, cough, and neck fullness can indicate the presence of a Zenker's diverticulum. In severe cases, patients cannot swallow their saliva and may drool.

Because oropharyngeal dysphagia is often associated with a known systemic illness such as a stroke or a neuromuscular disorder, the underlying cause of the dysphagia is frequently identifiable and does not pose a diagnostic problem. Regardless of the underlying disease, dysphagia must be fully evaluated to direct therapy. Appropriate diagnostic testing may include cineradiography, direct laryngoscopy, and esophagoscopy. Cineradiography is the most useful initial study; it involves recording, on videotape, the movements of the mouth, pharynx, and upper esophagus during a barium swallow. Frame-by-frame analysis (30 to 100 frames/second) of individual swallows is needed to delineate the complex and rapid sequence of events occurring in this region and provides much more information than a routine barium swallow. This study can identify oral or pharyngeal muscular weakness or discoordination, inadequate laryngeal closure, incomplete or premature cricopharyngeal relaxation often described as a "bar," or a Zenker's diverticulum.

Direct laryngoscopy may be helpful to evaluate the oral, pharyngeal, and laryngeal mucosa for inflammatory or neoplastic processes. Esophagoscopy plays a minor role in the diagnosis of diseases of the oropharynx and upper esophagus; however, it is useful in evaluating the esophageal body, which may be the source of proximally referred symptoms. Traditional esophageal manometry has been less helpful in patients with oropharyngeal dysphagia than in those with disorders of the esophageal body. Newer techniques incorporating circumferential pressure transducers now permit elegant manometric recordings of oropharyngeal swallowing, but at present they are available only in specialized motility laboratories.

Laryngopharyngeal (LP) sensory testing has been shown to improve the prognostication of outcome for dysphagic stroke patients when performed with a modified barium swallow. LP sensory assessment involves discrete pulsing of air endoscopically directed onto the mucosa innervated by the superior laryngeal nerve and directly observing reflex vocal fold closure. Although the modified barium swallow is useful for demonstrating aspiration, it specifically visualizes the motor component of swallowing and can underpredict the development of aspiration in stroke patients. LP sensory discrimination testing can identify patients at risk for aspiration who have bilateral laryngopharyngeal sensory deficits.

Management of oropharyngeal dysphagia first involves recognition and treatment of potentially reversible causes including hypothyroidism or hyperthyroidism, myasthenia gravis, Parkinson's disease, and polymyositis/dermatomyositis. In addition to disease-specific therapy, the overall approach to management should be aimed at developing safe techniques for swallowing without aspiration and providing adequate nutrition. Stroke patients with dysphagia often need temporary feeding by a nasoenteric feeding tube or percutaneous endoscopic gastrostomy (PEG) tube, with the expectation of symptom improvement over time. Unfortunately, many of the other neuromuscular disorders are progressive or untreatable (e.g., stroke, head and neck tumors, postglossectomy or other tumor resection, brain tumor, severe neurologic disease). Patients with these disorders require video esophagrams to assess whether they can swallow safely without tracheal aspiration and to plan therapy. Some individuals can be trained by a speech pathologist to use compensatory measures to improve their swallowing function. Examples of these include reducing the bolus size, thickening the consistency of the bolus, and using head posture to control the bolus in the oral cavity during initiation of a swallow. Patients who aspirate when swallowing can be taught the supraglottic swallow, in which the breath is held after a deep inspiration and released as a forceful cough to clear the airway.

Maintaining adequate nutritional status is essential, and enteral feedings via a nasoenteric or gastrostomy tube may become necessary if a patient is unable to maintain weight with oral intake using compensatory measures. Patients who have difficulty with liquids, but not solids, can have liquids thickened to facilitate swallowing or obtain liquids through tube feedings while continuing to eat solids. Patients with swallowing difficulties to all consistencies of food will likely need long-term support with a PEG feeding tube. Patients with gastroesophageal reflux who are concerned that it contributes to aspiration can have the PEG tube converted to a PEJ (jejunostomy) tube, so that the enteral formula enters somewhat more distal in the small intestine to diminish the reflux potential, although the benefit of this modification is not certain. Patients who aspirate their salivary secretions with unprotected airways and recurrent pneumonia can be best served with a surgical laryngeal closure and tracheostomy.

Patients with oropharyngeal dysphagia may benefit from a surgical cricopharyngeal myotomy. This procedure is designed to weaken or abolish the high pressure zone of the UES by sectioning the cricopharyngeal muscle and the proximal 3 to 4 cm of the striated muscle of the cervical esophagus. Clinical improvement from this procedure is variable, depending on the degree of pharyngeal dysfunction or cricopharyngeal obstruction. Patients with a Zenker's diverticulum usually benefit from diverticulectomy and cricopharyngeal myotomy. Patients with oculopharyngeal syndrome (who are often of French-Canadian descent), in which there is cricopharyngeal dysfunction and bilateral eyelid ptosis, in our experience benefit from myotomy to improve the passage of food through the UES.

The best evaluative and treatment approach for patients with oropharyngeal dysphagia is involvement of a multidisciplinary team composed of speech pathologists, otolaryngologists, gastroenterologists, neurologists, radiologists, and dietitians. Specific diseases can thus be identified and treated, and appropriate attention can be given to nutritional management.

ESOPHAGEAL DYSPHAGIA

Esophageal dysphagia means difficulty in transporting food down the esophagus after it has been successfully transferred from the mouth and pharynx. The patient will often describe a sensation of food sticking somewhere in the chest. The level where the patient locates the hang-up is often not the actual level of the obstruction, and the sticking sensation is often referred to an area above the actual level of blockage. For example, in a distal esophageal obstruction, the sensation of dysphagia may be referred to the neck, but without the associated symptoms of aspiration, nasopharyngeal regurgitation, or drooling that are seen in disturbances affecting oropharyngeal swallowing. Several important questions need to be asked to narrow the differential diagnosis in a patient with esophageal dysphagia:

1. What kind of foods (solids, liquids, or both) elicit the symptom?
2. If both solids and liquids induce the problem, was it initially solids that then progressed to include liquids, or was it dysphagia to both liquids and solids at the onset?
3. Are the symptoms intermittent, constant, or progressive?
4. Has there been associated weight loss?

When a patient reports that dysphagia occurs with both solids and liquids from the onset of symptoms, and that even water sometimes seems to stop, the cause is most likely an esophageal motility disorder. In contrast, if the dysphagia occurs only after swallowing a large piece of meat or other solid and never with liquids, it suggests a mechanical obstruction. Intermittent dysphagia to large solids in a patient who is otherwise asymptomatic generally suggests a lower esophageal B (Schatzki) ring. Patients with carcinoma of the esophagus usually have progressive dysphagia for solids, with marked weight loss that may be disproportionate to the swallowing difficulty. Patients with mainly solids dysphagia secondary to a peptic stricture may also have progressive symptoms, but generally do not have marked weight loss, and will usually admit to a long history of heartburn and/or antacid use. Thus, a careful history will often strongly suggest the diagnosis before further diagnostic testing is begun.

The evaluation of a patient with esophageal dysphagia should begin with a barium swallow. It is important to ask the radiologist to give a solid bolus, such as a barium pill or barium-soaked piece of bagel or marshmallow, during the study. This will help to identify subtle abnormalities such as rings or webs, thus demonstrating the level of hang-up, and is especially important when the patient's complaint is dysphagia only for solids. If the radiographic findings are normal or suggest a motility disorder, esophageal manometry should be performed. Demonstration by the barium study of an obstructing lesion should result in endoscopy. In the following section, the clinical presentation, assessment, and treatment of the more common disorders causing esophageal dysphagia are described. Table 2 contains a more complete list of disorders.

Esophageal Webs and Rings

Webs are concentric or eccentric membranous narrowings covered entirely by squamous mucosa. They can occur anywhere above the gastroesophageal junc-

TABLE 2. **Conditions Causing Esophageal Dysphagia**

Structural Lesions
Esophageal rings
Mucosal (Schatzki "B" ring)
Muscular ("A" ring)
Esophageal webs
Esophageal diverticula
Esophagitis: reflux, pill, radiation, infection, caustic injury
Benign esophageal strictures
Peptic stricture
Postcaustic injury
Postradiation esophagitis
Postpill-induced esophagitis
Malignant tumors
Squamous cell carcinoma of the esophagus
Adenocarcinoma of the esophagus or gastroesophageal junction
Lymphoma
Melanoma
Kaposi's sarcoma
Benign tumors
Leiomyoma
Lipoma
Angioma
Epithelial papilloma
Inflammatory fibroid polyp
Extrinsic Compression
Vascular compression
Aberrant right subclavian artery (dysphagia lusoria)
Right-sided aorta
Left atrial enlargement
Aortic aneurysm (dysphagia aortica)
Mediastinal mass
Motility Disorders of the Esophagus
Achalasia
Scleroderma/CREST
Diabetes mellitus
Hypothyroidism
Chagas' disease
Presbyesophagus
Spastic motility disorders
Diffuse esophageal spasm
Nutcracker esophagus
Hypertensive lower esophageal sphincter
Vigorous achalasia
Nonspecific esophageal dysmotility

tion, but more commonly are found in the cervical and midesophagus. Their etiology is unknown, although likely congenital, and there is an association of upper esophageal webs with iron deficiency anemia and dysphagia (Plummer-Vinson, Paterson–Brown Kelly syndromes). Many asymptomatic webs are identified as incidental radiographic findings. Symptomatic patients usually report intermittent dysphagia to solids. Diagnosis is best made radiographically with careful attention to the postcricoid area. Webs are often missed endoscopically but, when seen, appear as a thin, intraluminal constriction of tissue with normal overlying mucosa. Thin mucosal webs of the midesophagus can obstruct the passage of a food bolus resulting in intermittent dysphagia. Symptomatic webs can be successfully treated with bougienage or avulsion during endoscopy.

Lower esophageal rings (also known as Schatzki or B rings) are one of the most common causes of dysphagia seen by primary care clinicians. They are sharply defined, thin, circumferential mucosal narrowings at the gastroesophageal junction just above a hiatal hernia. Microscopically, the mucosa on the upper surface of the ring is esophageal tissue while the underside is gastric tissue. The origin of Schatzki rings is unknown, but many consider them to be a congenital structural variant, whereas others believe that they arise from chronic gastroesophageal reflux. Symptoms generally do not occur unless the luminal diameter is less than 12 mm. Characteristically, the dysphagia is episodic and not progressive. The classic presentation is that of sudden, severe dysphagia occurring while the patient is eating rapidly, often after swallowing steak or bread. The patient usually will attempt to dislodge the bolus by drinking liquids to wash it through, but sometimes may need to regurgitate to relieve the obstruction. Subsequently he or she can complete the meal by chewing more carefully and slowly. The diagnosis can be made by history and barium studies. Adequate esophageal distention during the barium swallow is essential in making the diagnosis radiologically. Giving a 13-mm barium tablet or barium-soaked bread, or marshmallow will identify the area of obstruction. Management consists of reassurance for the infrequently symptomatic patient, who can eat slower and chew food more thoroughly before swallowing. More symptomatic rings can usually be treated in a single session by passage of a no. 50 or 60 French mercury-weighted bougie. Endoscopic pneumatic balloon dilatation has also been a successful intervention. Endoscopic disruption of persistent esophageal rings using a cutting papillotome has been beneficial to relieve obstructive symptoms for some patients, and surgery for symptomatic rings not responding to dilatation is rarely needed.

Another ring in the lower esophagus is the muscular or "A" ring. These are less common than mucosal rings and are rarely symptomatic. If symptoms do occur, they are identical to those of "B" rings. On barium esophagrams, these muscular rings appear as broad constrictions a few centimeters above the gastroesophageal junction and may change in size and shape from one examination to another. When symptomatic, these rings may also be treated with dilatation.

Benign Esophageal Strictures

Severe mucosal injury to the esophagus can lead to stricture formation. Stenoses secondary to chronic severe acid reflux are known as peptic strictures and are the most common type of benign esophageal stricture. These represent an end stage of chronic reflux, mucosal damage, and fibrosis. Use of nonsteroidal anti-inflammatory agents may be a risk factor for peptic stricture. Patients typically present with slowly progressive dysphagia for solids and eventually liquids with minimal associated weight loss. Long-standing antecedent heartburn is present in the majority of patients.

Certain drugs can cause esophageal injury by being retained in the esophagus (pill esophagitis), which sometimes leads to stricture formation. The more common agents include doxycycline, potassium supplements, and quinidine preparations. Patients receiving radiation treatment for lung, mediastinal, or esophageal cancer can develop radiation esophagitis, which results in severe odynophagia. This is sometimes complicated by the development of an esophageal stricture several months later. Similarly, patients who incur severe corrosive injury to the esophagus from ingestion of a caustic substance can develop a stricture weeks to months later.

Barium radiographic studies demonstrate benign esophageal stenoses as smooth tapered strictures, variable in length, and usually in the lower third of the esophagus. Associated ulcerations or mucosal irregularities can also be seen, and peptic strictures may be identified in the proximal esophagus at the upper margin of a segment of Barrett's esophagus in some patients with gastroesophageal reflux disease. Evaluation must include endoscopy with biopsy to exclude malignancy. Treatment consists of dilatation with mercury-filled bougies, guide wire–directed polyvinyl dilators, or polyethylene balloons to achieve a stricture diameter of greater than 12 mm, if possible. Unlike the forceful rupture of the pliable lower esophageal ring accomplished with the passage of one large dilator, treatment of fibrotic, stiff peptic strictures usually requires passing sequential dilators or inflating balloons of increasing diameter. For most benign strictures, and especially for peptic ones, aggressive antireflux therapy with a proton pump inhibitor is essential to prevent recurrence of the stenosis and decreases the need for repeated stricture dilatations.

Esophageal Cancer

Patients with early esophageal cancer are usually asymptomatic or have only mild, nonspecific symptoms for which they often fail to seek medical attention. These symptoms may be minor complaints related to eating such as retrosternal discomfort, intermittent dysphagia, a foreign body sensation, or odynophagia. As the tumor grows, solid food dysphagia occurs and can rapidly progress to a point where liquids or even saliva cannot be swallowed. The majority of patients are older and present with progressive dysphagia, anorexia, and weight loss. The barium esophagram strongly suggests the diagnosis, with advanced carcinomas appearing ulcerated and circumferential, and early tumors appearing as irregular plaques or polyps. Unfortunately, most esophageal carcinomas are far advanced at the time of diagnosis, resulting in a poor prognosis. Endoscopy with biopsy is necessary to confirm the diagnosis. In North America, patients with squamous cell carcinoma usually have a history of alcohol and/or tobacco use. Most esophageal adenocarcinomas develop as a complication of Barrett's esophagus. Adenocarcinomas of the gastric cardia may arise in short segments of Barrett's metaplasia. Although once considered rare, the incidence of Barrett's-associated adenocarcinomas has risen sharply over the last 2 decades, and the annual incidence of esophageal squamous cell carcinoma equals esophageal adenocarcinoma in the United States (about 6000 cases each). Adenocarcinomas tend to occur in the distal esophagus, whereas squamous cell carcinomas occur in the mid- or more proximal esophagus.

Once the diagnosis of either type of esophageal cancer is made, one must determine the stage of disease on which appropriate therapy depends. Computed tomography (CT) scanning and endoscopic ultrasound are useful in determining depth of invasion, lymph node involvement, and tumor resectability. Endoscopic ultrasound has been shown to be more accurate than CT scanning, especially for early tumors. Small tumors without local extension should be referred for surgical resection. Larger and locally advanced tumors are candidates for radiation and chemotherapy with possible resection if there is a significant response. In patients with advanced disease at the time of presentation, palliative therapy to relieve dysphagia and maintain adequate oral intake is the main goal of therapy. Palliative modalities include surgical resection, chemotherapy, radiotherapy, endoscopic laser ablation, endoscopic bipolar electrocoagulation, electrocautery tumor probe therapy, and esophageal endoprosthesis placement. The choice of treatment depends on the patient's desires, tumor characteristics, and the experience and capabilities of local endoscopists. Placement of a feeding gastrostomy tube may be necessary for nutritional support.

Foreign Body Ingestion

The esophagus is the most common site of foreign body obstruction in the gastrointestinal tract. Symptoms associated with impactions include chest or neck discomfort, odynophagia, increased salivation, and a persistent feeling of esophageal obstruction when swallowing. Children who cannot communicate their symptoms may present with excessive salivation, recurrent emesis, or failure to eat. Coins are the objects most commonly ingested by children. Acute esophageal obstruction in adults is usually a result of food bolus impaction at the site of a structural lesion such as a ring, stricture, or web. There is often a history of previous intermittent solid food dysphagia. Poorly fitting dentures may be a contributing factor. Prisoners and psychiatric patients have been known to swallow foreign objects that can become lodged in the esophagus. Typically these items tend to lodge in areas of normal anatomic narrowing: the cervical esophagus, the level of the aortic arch, and the esophagogastric junction. Inadvertent ingestion of bones, fruit pits, and dentures behaves similarly.

All patients who present with intentional or inadvertent foreign body ingestion should have anteroposterior and lateral radiographs of the neck and chest to evaluate the size, shape, and location of the object. All sharp and pointed foreign bodies should be removed before they pass into the stomach to prevent intestinal perforation. Alkaline batteries can cause severe corrosive injury if not removed. Retrieval is best accomplished by flexible endoscopy with the use of an overtube to protect the airway from aspiration of the object. Some objects impacted in the cervical esophagus may require rigid esophagoscopy and general anesthesia for safe removal.

Food impaction represents a special case of foreign body impaction. Steak is the most common food causing this type of obstruction. It generally occurs in the setting of rapid eating, often combined with imbibing of alcohol. Food usually impacts in the distal esophagus and is almost always associated with underlying esophageal disease. Sublingual nitroglycerin* may produce smooth muscle relaxation and occasionally allows the food to pass. Glucagon decreases the lower esophageal sphincter pressure, and its administration in 0.5-mg boluses up to 2 mg may relieve esophageal food impaction. Most patients who present to the emergency department with esophageal food impaction have had the symptoms for several hours before reporting. By that time the food impaction has produced localized edema, making the bolus even harder to pass; therefore these pharmacologic measures will often be ineffective. Flexible upper endoscopy is usually successful in removing the impaction. The bolus can be pushed into the stomach with gentle pressure, or it can be removed through the mouth using an overtube for airway protection. The patient should then be placed on acid blockers and a soft diet for several days while the inflammation and edema from the obstruction resolve. Such patients should undergo upper endoscopy several weeks after the episode, as there is usually an underlying esophageal lesion such as a web, ring, or stricture that requires dilatation.

---

*Not FDA approved for this indication.

Achalasia

Idiopathic achalasia is an esophageal motility disorder characterized by slowly progressive dysphagia to solids and liquids and often regurgitation of undigested foods. The two major defects in achalasia are obstruction of the esophagogastric junction owing to incomplete relaxation of the LES, which may be hypertensive, and aperistalsis or motor failure in the esophageal body. The pathophysiology involves loss of ganglion cells within the myenteric (Auerbach's) plexus, as well as reduction of nerve fibers within the wall of the esophagus. A specific etiology has not been identified. The majority of patients present between the ages of 20 and 40 years, but it can occur in children and in elderly patients. The most common initial complaint is progressive dysphagia for liquids and solids. Patients may report the use of specific maneuvers to improve esophageal emptying such as throwing the shoulders back, lifting the neck, and performing rapid Valsalva maneuvers. Frequent regurgitation of undigested food is common, often causing pulmonary symptoms of wheezing, coughing, and choking that awaken the patient at night.

The diagnosis can sometimes be suggested on a routine chest radiograph. Findings include absence of a gastric air bubble, mediastinal widening from a dilated esophagus, and evidence of aspiration pneumonia. A barium esophagram is the most appropriate first study in patients suspected of having achalasia. Characteristic features are esophageal dilatation with a smoothly tapered narrowing at the distal end ("bird's beak"). An air-fluid level in the upper esophagus may also be seen owing to retention of esophageal secretions and ingested food.

Esophageal manometry should be performed to confirm the diagnosis of achalasia. Four manometric features are characteristic: (1) absence of peristalsis in the body of the esophagus, (2) absent or incomplete relaxation of the LES, (3) elevated LES pressure, and (4) elevated intraesophageal pressure relative to intragastric pressure.

Endoscopic examination is always required to exclude malignancy at the esophagogastric junction and to evaluate the esophageal mucosa before therapeutic manipulations. Adenocarcinoma of the gastroesophageal junction can mimic achalasia; and less commonly lymphomas and pancreatic, lung, and esophageal squamous cell carcinomas can invade the region of the LES and mimic achalasia (so-called "secondary" achalasia). In true achalasia, the LES has a puckered appearance that does not open with air insufflation; however the instrument should pass with gentle pressure. Inability or excessive difficulty in passing the endoscope raises the suspicion of malignancy or benign stricture.

Treatment of achalasia is aimed at reducing the esophageal obstruction to relieve the symptoms of dysphagia and regurgitation and to prevent aspiration pneumonia and weight loss. In otherwise healthy patients, the initial treatment of choice is either pneumatic balloon dilatation of the LES or surgical myotomy. There have been few comparative studies of the two procedures.

Pneumatic dilatation with at least a 90 French (30-mm) diameter rigid balloon is performed over a guide wire placed during esophagogastroduodenoscopy. Measurement from incisors to gastroesophageal junction permits the balloon catheter to be marked so that the midpoint of the balloon straddles the LES zone. The balloon is inflated for 2 minutes, during which fluoroscopic monitoring is done to observe the elimination of the "waist" of the balloon, correlating to effective dilatation. Pneumatic dilatation is generally successful in relieving symptoms in more than 60% of cases, with a risk of esophageal perforation ranging from 2 to 5%, most of which can be treated conservatively. Subsequent dilatations in patients with recurrent symptoms can be done using larger diameter balloons, but they tend to be less successful if symptoms recur soon after the first dilatation.

Surgical myotomy reduces LES pressure more dependably than does pneumatic dilatation, resulting in slightly greater efficacy in reducing symptoms. Myotomy divides the muscle layer of the most proximal 1 cm of stomach and several centimeters of distal esophagus. The most significant complication of surgical myotomy is gastroesophageal reflux. Gastroesophageal reflux is more damaging in patients with achalasia, as esophageal clearance is affected by the aperistalsis. For this reason, surgical myotomy procedures are often combined with fundoplication. Recent experience with thoracoscopic and laparoscopic esophagomyotomy has made the surgical approach more attractive by decreasing postoperative pain, morbidity, and recovery time.

Another option for the treatment of achalasia in elderly patients and in patients with medical problems prohibiting surgery or pneumatic dilatation is botulinum toxin, a potent inhibitor of the release of acetylcholine from nerve terminals. With the use of a sclerotherapy needle, endoscopic circumferential injection of 80 or 100 units of this toxin into the area of the LES safely and rapidly relieves the symptom of dysphagia. The effect persists from 3 months to more than 1 year after initial injection therapy and may be repeated. At present, the long-term results of botulinum injections and the outcomes of repeated injections are under study.

Other Esophageal Dysmotility Syndromes

Dysphagia and chest pain are the presenting complaints in patients with one of several spastic motility conditions of the esophageal smooth muscle. These disorders have been defined by their manometric patterns and are characterized by normal peristalsis that is intermittently interrupted by simultaneous (nonpropagating) contractions, high amplitude or long duration contractions, or dysfunction of the LES. Dysphagia is for liquids and solids and is intermittent in nature. There is considerable clinical overlap in the different dysmotility syndromes, and they are mainly differentiated from each other by defined manometric criteria.

Diffuse Esophageal Spasm

The major manometric characteristics include high-amplitude, simultaneous, nonperistaltic contractions occurring with intermittent normal peristalsis. Other features include repetitive contractions, high amplitude contractions, contractions of prolonged duration, and abnormalities of the LES.

Nutcracker Esophagus

This is a descriptive term for the manometric findings characterized by very high distal esophageal contraction pressures, which are all peristaltic. The pressures should be greater than two standard deviations above the normal range, and are frequently more than 300 mm Hg. This condition may be an epiphenomenon in chest–pain-prone patients, and there may be no causation of chest pain by the dysmotility.

Hypertensive Lower Esophageal Sphincter

This is characterized by higher than normal resting esophageal sphincter pressure. It may be associated with mildly abnormal sphincter relaxation. Peristalsis of the esophageal body is normal, but many have high amplitude contractions as seen in nutcracker esophagus.

Nonspecific Esophageal Dysmotility

Many patients who undergo esophageal manometry for dysphagia have abnormal findings that do not clearly fit into the preceding syndromes. These miscellaneous abnormalities have been classified as "nonspecific esophageal dysmotility." The findings include frequent nontransmitted contractions, retrograde contractions, low-amplitude contractions, prolonged duration peristaltic waves, and isolated incomplete relaxation. The clinical significance of these findings is unclear.

Test Results and Therapy for Esophageal Dysmotility

The radiographic findings in patients with these esophageal dysmotilities are variable. The syndrome most likely to show abnormalities on barium esophagram is diffuse esophageal spasm. Classically, simultaneous, nonperistaltic contractions result in segmentation of the barium column in the lower half of the esophagus. The distorted radiographic appearance has been descriptively termed "corkscrew esophagus" or "rosary bead esophagus." Endoscopic inspection of the esophagus in a patient with esophageal dysmotility is generally normal. Provocative testing with edrophonium injection or balloon distention may elicit pain and reproduce the patient's symptoms.

Medical therapy for these disorders has not been uniformly successful. An empirical trial of antireflux therapy may be worthwhile because reflux may provoke dysmotility. Drugs that relax the esophageal smooth muscle have been tried with variable success in controlling chest pain or dysphagia. These include nitroglycerin, 0.4 mg SL,* isosorbide dinitrate (Isordil), 10–20 mg four times daily,* dicyclomine (Bentyl),* 10–20 mg four times daily, hydralazine* (Apresoline), 25 to 50 mg four times daily, and calcium channel blockers* (nifedipine [Procardia], 10 to 30 mg four times daily and diltiazem [Cardizem], 30 to 90 mg four times daily). A trial of anxiolytics or antidepressants may be effective in the right setting. Behavioral modification and biofeedback can be helpful for treating symptoms associated with dysmotility.

Scleroderma/Systemic Disease

Numerous systemic diseases affect esophageal motility (see Table 2); of these, scleroderma has been best characterized. The esophagus is involved in 75 to 85% of scleroderma patients by radiographic and manometric studies. The lower two thirds (the smooth muscle portion) of the esophagus, including the LES, is affected. The pathologic process is atrophy of the smooth muscle with subsequent replacement and fibrosis of the submucosa and muscularis, resulting in absent peristalsis in the lower esophagus and an incompetent LES. In those patients with symptoms, heartburn and dysphagia predominate. The gastroesophageal reflux can be quite severe because of an incompetent LES and poor clearance of noxious refluxate. Erosive esophagitis therefore is common, and patients are at increased risk for developing Barrett's esophagus and peptic strictures as complications of the reflux.

Characteristic barium esophagrams show a dilated esophagus with aperistalsis involving the distal portion. Esophageal emptying occurs normally if the patient is upright, but if the patient lies down, the barium remains in the esophagus. Free-flowing gastroesophageal reflux is usually apparent. Esophageal manometry typically reveals low to absent LES pressure, weak or absent distal esophageal peristalsis, and preserved normal upper esophageal peristalsis in the striated segment.

There is no effective treatment for esophageal dysfunction in the patient with scleroderma. Gastroesophageal reflux needs to be recognized and treated aggressively with acid suppression to prevent stricture formation. Peptic strictures that do form often need frequent dilatation. In severe cases, antireflux surgery may be required.

Systemic diseases including diabetes mellitus, amyloidosis, thyroid disease, and other metabolic disorders may affect esophageal motility, as may aging (presbyesophagus). Extraesophageal causes of dysphagia, usually identified by barium swallow, include extrinsic compression owing to aortic aneurysm or a rigid atherosclerotic aorta (dysphagia aortica), vascular anomalies (dysphagia lusoria), hypertrophic cer-

*Not FDA approved for this indication.

vical vertebral spurs, or mediastinal adenopathy (bronchial carcinoma, lymphoma, sarcoidosis).

DIVERTICULA OF THE GASTROINTESTINAL TRACT

method of
S. PHILIP BRALOW, M.D.
Sarasota Memorial Hospital
Sarasota, Florida

The term "diverticulum" is derived from the Latin root for "by-road" and is used to describe an outpouching of the gastrointestinal tract. Diverticula can be classified according to their etiology (congenital or acquired); completeness of the herniated wall (true or false); pathophysiology (pulsion or traction); and location (Table 1). Most diverticula are acquired, false, and of the pulsion type. Diverticula were attributed to functional motility disorders by Sir Charles Bell in 1816. The site of the herniation was felt to be an area of structural weakness of the muscle coat of the gut.

Most diverticula are asymptomatic and are found incidentally on radiographic studies for other disease states. Symptoms such as dysphagia, obstruction, bleeding, or malabsorption should not be attributed to diverticula until other more likely causes are ruled out. Attempts should be made to directly visualize the offending diverticulum before resorting to surgery unless the diverticulum is clearly the source of significant symptoms that are not responsive to conservative medical management.

TABLE 1. **Classification of Diverticula of the Intestinal Tract**

Types
True—congenital, all layers of wall intact
False—no muscle coat, acquired
Pulsion—most common, increased intraluminal pressure
Traction—rare; due to adhesions, neoplasms, lymph nodes
Presentation
Diverticulum—single, located anywhere in GI tract
Diverticulosis—multiple, esophagus, small bowel, colon
Diverticulitis—single or multiple, sigmoid
Esophageal diverticula
Hypopharyngeal—Zenker's—hypertrophic, cricopharyngeal muscle
Midesophageal—single—pulsion
Diffuse intramural pseudodiverticulosis—motor abnormality
Epiphrenic—distal esophagus, single, hypertensive LES
Gastric diverticula
Congenital—cardia, single
Pulsion—single, antrum
Pseudodiverticulosis—single or multiple, pyloric, healed ulcer or chronic perforation
Small intestinal diverticula
Duodenal—bulb, postulcer deformity
Periampullary—single, biliary stones
Mesenteric—multiple, pulsion, occasionally intraluminal
Meckel's—single, ileal
Colonic diverticula
Diverticulosis—multiple, mostly sigmoid
Diverticulitis—mostly left colon, obstruction, perforation, acute

Abbreviations: GI = gastrointestinal; LES = lower esophageal sphincter.

ESOPHAGEAL DIVERTICULA

Diverticula of the esophagus have aroused much surgical attention, although only the rare lesion will require surgical intervention. Many different procedures have been advocated but have been discarded because of poor results. These failures have been due to lack of understanding of the underlying motor abnormalities and the resultant increase in intraluminal pressures. Currently, diverticula of the esophagus are classified according to their location: hypopharyngeal (Zenker's), midesophageal, epiphrenic, and intramural pseudodiverticulosis.

Zenker's Diverticula

A Zenker's diverticulum is an acquired pulsion type that has herniated through the cricopharyngeal portion of the inferior constrictor muscle posteriorly. The inferior constrictor muscle courses downward to blend with the circular bundles of the esophageal wall forming a slinglike muscle called the cricopharyngeal muscle. This slinglike arrangement produces the upper esophageal sphincter and is usually at the level of C5 and C6. Between the cricopharyngeal muscle and the thyropharyngeal muscle is an area of muscle weakness (Killian's triangle) that is the most common site for a Zenker's diverticulum. This anatomic predilection was first described by Ludlow in 1769.

The current explanation for this type of pulsion herniation at the site of muscle weakness is that an area of localized spasm, stricture, or hypertrophy of the cricopharyngeal muscle increases the intraluminal pressure. Incoordination of pharyngeal relaxation during swallowing may be the underlying mechanism. These functional abnormalities may be absent when the patient is asymptomatic or is not swallowing. Zenker's diverticula are more common in male adults during the sixth and seventh decades. Congenital diverticula are occasionally seen in young children. The diverticula are found incidentally in about 2% of upper gastrointestinal radiographic studies but may be noted as an air-filled sac or cystic shadow on the left side of the neck on routine chest films or on palpation.

Dysphagia is the most common symptom but probably relates to the functional abnormality rather than the anatomic change. Frequent regurgitation of recently digested food, halitosis, globus sensation, odontophagia, and neck pain have all been described. Chronic food aspiration at night may occur if the herniated sac is moderately or massively enlarged, retaining large volumes of food or secretions. Endoscopic evaluation is usually not necessary and may be risky. If the sac appears irregular or seems to have fixed filling defects, malignancy must be ruled out. Computed tomography scans and ultrasound studies of these lesions do not appear to be additive or necessary unless a malignancy is being considered.

Treatment is usually observational but the patient should be instructed to carefully chew food and to increase fluid intake at meal time. Patients should be warned not to lie down after eating and to avoid nocturnal snacks for 2 to 3 hours before bedtime. When symptoms are severe, with nocturnal coughing or weight loss, surgical intervention is usually necessary. Cricopharyngeal myotomy is the simplest procedure and can be done under local anesthesia on an outpatient basis or with a one night hospital stay. It is most effective for smaller lesions (up to 5 cm). More extensive procedures need to be done on the larger pouches or those with local inflammation. Diverticulopexy is the next most frequently done procedure, in which the pouch is inverted back into the lumen with or without a concomitant myotomy. Patients who have had previous surgery or fistualization may require a diverticulectomy in one or two stages. Endoscopic diverticulotomy was described by Mosher in 1906, using the old rigid esophagoscope and dividing the wall between the pharynx and the diverticulum, creating an internal myotomy with free drainage. Dohlman recently revised the procedure, using diathermy with a CO_2 laser. This procedure is best suited for elderly patients at increased operative risk. Although it requires less operative time and hospitalization, it does have a higher recurrence rate.

Midesophageal Diverticula

Both Mondierl (1833) and Rokitansky (1840) attributed the single diverticulum occasionally seen projecting from the middle of the esophagus to traction from fibrinous adhesions or chronic lymphadenopathy. Current thought is that these sacs are the result of abnormal motility and can be demonstrated on manometry. These diverticula should be classified as acquired, pulsion type. They are generally asymptomatic and do not retain food or secretions. Symptoms of dysphagia or chest pain are best explained by the motor abnormalities. Isolated cases of perforation, fistulization, vomiting, and even bleeding have been reported. Usually no treatment is necessary except for these complications.

Epiphrenic Diverticula

These diverticula usually project from the right posterior wall between 8 and 10 cm above the cardioesophageal junction. They may be single or multiple. At least 60% are associated with dysmotility and high lower esophageal sphincter pressure–associated achalasia or diffuse spasm. Reflux esophagitis may lead to multiple diverticula, which have been reported to disappear after adequate treatment of the esophagitis. Isolated cases of congenital diverticula with an intact muscle coat have been reported in this area.

Dysphagia, chest pain, and aspiration due to regurgitated undigested food occur in about 20% of cases. Surgical intervention is usually not necessary and medical treatment of the achalasia or stricture with endoscopic dilatation or botulinum toxin may be all that is necessary. Complications such as abscess, phlegmonous esophagitis, or malignancy require appropriate surgical therapy. If a diverticulectomy is performed, a myotomy should also be done.

Diffuse Intramural Pseudodiverticulosis

This is a rare condition characterized by multiple tiny flask-shaped outpouchings of the submucosal glands. These lesions are most commonly associated with infections (e.g., candidiasis) and areas of narrowing or stasis. They are usually seen in clusters in the upper third of the esophagus and less often in the most distal portion. These outpouchings are usually asymptomatic, but dysphagia may result from the infection. Treatment is directed at the areas of narrowing and stasis as seen radiographically or during endoscopic study. Endoscopic-controlled dilatation and treatment of the infection are usually adequate.

GASTRIC DIVERTICULA

Congenital diverticula of the cardia are rare, being reported in only 0.04% of upper gastrointestinal radiographic studies. These lesions were first reported by Moebius in 1661 and were fully described by Baille in 1793. The pouches are almost always single and arise high on the posterior wall about 2 cm below the esophagogastric junction and toward the lesser curvature. Congenital diverticula can enlarge up to 10 cm and cause postprandial fullness, lower chest pain, nausea, vomiting, heartburn, and dysphagia. These symptoms may be relieved by postural drainage after meals. Since symptoms occur so rarely, other causes should be ruled out before surgical intervention is contemplated.

The diagnosis is not difficult because the radiographic appearance is characteristic. Mucosal folds radiating through the neck of the diverticula differentiate them from ulcers of walled-off perforations (Hudek diverticula). Endoscopy may be slightly risky and should be performed with caution if the pouch appears irregular or has filling defects and malignancy is a possibility. Isolated instances of complications have been reported, including hemorrhage, perforation, and tumor formation. Surgery is rarely necessary and invagination of the diverticulum may be performed surgically or endoscopically with laser ablation. Diverticulectomy is necessary only in the face of complications or recurrences.

Between 10 and 15% of gastric diverticula occur in the antrum or prepyloric areas. These are occasionally congenital or embryonic with aberrant pancreatic tissue. The most common diverticula in this area are acquired and are caused by inflammation or ulceration. Endoscopy is an important diagnostic procedure to rule out malignancy. Usually these lesions are asymptomatic and require no specific treatment.

SMALL INTESTINAL DIVERTICULA

Duodenal diverticula are usually asymptomatic and are an incidental finding in 1% of routine upper gastrointestinal radiographic studies. Autopsy data suggest an incidence of between 3 and 22%. With endoscopic retrograde cholangiopancreatography (ERCP), an incidence of 29% has been reported. Postbulbar diverticula were first reported by Morgagni in 1770. These pouches are usually single and occur in the medial portion of the second to fourth portion of the duodenal sweep. They range in size from 1 to 5 cm. Commonly these diverticula are extraluminal, but in about 20% they appear to be intraluminal, and tumors must be ruled out, preferably by endoscopic biopsy. Most are thought to be congenital with no clinical significance, and no treatment is necessary. Occasional cases of complications have been reported: massive hemorrhage has been controlled by endoscopic coagulation, and perforation and obstruction have required diverticulectomy.

Periampullary diverticula are frequently seen on both radiographic studies and ERCP. Choledocholithiasis is frequently found with these lesions, but the relationship to pancreatitis has not been universally accepted.

Diverticula of the jejunum and ileum are rare, usually multiple, and can enlarge to 10 cm or more. These acquired lesions are a complication of motility disorders such as scleroderma, visceral neuropathies, and myopathies. Bacterial overgrowth can occur with resultant malabsorption. Cultures are difficult to obtain but breath tests with 14C-d xylose are usually diagnostic. Surgical intervention should be considered only if the symptoms of malabsorption are not controlled with adequate aerobic and anerobic antibiotics. Massive hemorrhage linked to aspirin intake or an obstruction due to an enlarged pouch may require resection.

Meckel's Diverticulum

Meckel's diverticula are the most frequent congenital lesions of the gastrointestinal tract, occurring in about 20% of the general population. Characteristically, they are single blind sacs arising from the distal ileum within 100 cm of the ileocecal valve. They are the residua of the vitelline duct, which was not completely obliterated during development. The diverticula average 5 cm in length and up to 2 cm in diameter. They are true diverticula—all the layers of the ileal wall are intact. Gastric mucosa is found in the sac in about 45% of the cases, while heterotopic mucosa make up the rest. Ulcerations, bleeding, intussusception, and volvulus have been documented. *Helicobacter pylori* has been isolated from the gastric mucosa. There is a tendency for the mucosa to bleed after aspirin ingestion. Technetium-99m scans can identify the aberrant gastric mucosa. An inverted diverticulum may be difficult to differentiate from a neoplasm. Filling defects in the pouch may represent enteroliths or a malignancy and require further study. Adenocarcinoma can arise from the aberrant gastric mucosa and remain undiagnosed until it is far advanced.

Diverticulitis occurs in about 12% of cases and is difficult to differentiate from acute appendicitis. Only 6% of cases are diagnosed before surgery or autopsy. A high index of suspicion can be confirmed by sonography, radionuclide scanning, or angiography. Fortunately the vast majority of these diverticula are asymptomatic, and less than 20% require surgery. An asymptomatic Meckel's diverticulum found incidentally at surgery does not require resection unless it contains gastric mucosa or has a narrow neck.

COLONIC DIVERTICULA

Diverticula of the colon were first identified by Cruveilhier in 1849, but were not commonly reported before the 20th century. These pouches occur mostly in Westernized and industrialized populations and are still rare in Africa and the developing countries. This difference in incidence is probably related to dietary fiber intake. The increasing age of the population is also significant: diverticula of the colon are found in more than 50% of individuals older than 70 years.

These diverticula are of the false pulsion type, and up to 90% herniate through the wall of the sigmoid flexure. They are usually multiple, but occasionally a single congenital diverticulum is found in the right colon. The distinction between diverticulitis, and diverticulosis should be explained to the patient.

Diverticulosis

Asymptomatic diverticula of the colon are so common that they may be considered a normal consequence of aging rather than a distinct disease. These pouches are frequently found incidentally during a barium study or by colonoscopy. The true incidence is unknown. The etiology appears to be a motility disorder with an exaggerated intracolonic pressure and areas of segmentation, physiologic factors that allow increased water absorption. The protective effect of a high-fiber diet is due to the formation of bulkier stools that expand the lumen, thereby lowering the intracolonic pressure.

The great majority of patients with uncomplicated diverticulosis remain asymptomatic. Occasionally, a patient will complain of left lower quadrant colic that is relieved by a bowel movement. The stool may be mucoid and accompanied by gas. These symptoms are usually due to a concomitant irritable bowel syndrome, which should be managed with the judicious use of antispasmodics and an increase in dietary fiber.

Diverticolosis is the most common cause of massive lower gastrointestinal bleeding, which rarely occurs with diverticulitis. The bleeding which may be brisk and may derive from a single diverticulum, can present as hematochezia rather than melena. The bleeding usually subsides spontaneously within 24 to 48 hours, but recurrences are frequent. Precise identification of the bleeding site may be difficult; red cell nuclear scanning and mesenteric angiography may be helpful if the bleeding is active and brisk. If the offending vessel can be identified, the bleeding can be controlled by embolization or injection of vasoconstrictors via a mesenteric catheter. Surgical colectomy should be considered for exsanguinating hemorrhage that cannot be controlled by less invasive techniques or for recurrent episodes. Blind colectomy of the right colon should be reserved for dire situations when the site of bleeding remains unknown. Colonoscopy may be helpful in therapeutic decision-making if the colon can be adequately cleared. Mild bleeding can be controlled with injections of absolute alcohol or epinephrine.

Diverticulitis

Inflammation of a diverticulum is usually acute and results from blockage of the neck of the pouch leading to microperforation. The clinical course depends on the size of the perforation and the degree of involvement of the pericolic tissue. A large perforation can result in a frank abscess or fistulization into an adjacent viscera. A small perforation is usually immediately walled off, presents with only mild symptoms, and is self limited. Intestinal stricture or obstruction can result from recurrent infections. Tenderness associated with diverticulitis is usually well localized, and occasionally a mass can be palpated with signs of peritonitis. Hematochezia and iron deficiency are seldom the result of acute diverticulitis, and neoplasm should be considered in these circumstances.

During the acute phase of the illness, the patient may be toxic and febrile, and interventional diagnostic procedures such as barium enemas and colonoscopy should be avoided. The inflammation usually subsides in 7 to 10 days, after which further studies can be performed. Early intervention can convert a microperforation into a major perforation with abscess formation and should be avoided. Computed tomography can further define the process by demonstrating pericolic inflammation, abscess, or a walled-off perforation. Tomographically guided drainage of the abscess can resolve the inflammation and limit the complications.

The inflammatory process can lead to stricture formation with radiographic narrowing of the lumen, a finding that may be difficult to differentiate from malignancy. It may be difficult or impossible to pass the colonoscope through the narrowed area safely. Biopsies can be helpful if available. Radiographic evidence of intraluminal and extramural extravasation of the contrast material and thickening of the mucosa and colonic wall is helpful in ruling out malignancy.

Mild diverticulitis (no significant fever, leukocytosis but with normal peristalsis) can usually be managed at home. Bed rest, a liquid diet, and oral antibiotics should bring a resolution in 5 to 7 days. If the patient develops signs of toxicity, hospitalization with intravenous fluids and antibiotics is necessary. Watchful waiting over the next 48 to 72 hours is the best conservative approach.

If the patient remains toxic, surgical intervention may be necessary. The type of surgery will depend upon the type of complication. Either a one-stage resection or a two-stage procedure with a transverse colostomy can be performed. Elective surgery with a primary resection is indicated for fistulization, abscess formation, or two or more recurrences. Surgery may be necessary if malignancy cannot be completely ruled out.

Diverticular Disease Associated with Chronic Colitis

A syndrome of chronic colitis located in the sigmoid flexure and diverticulosis has recently been reported. It is characterized by a patchy area of inflammation, granularity, and friability. Mucosal biopsy reveals an idiopathic inflammation with plasma cells and eosinophilic expansion of the lamina propria. Neutrophilic cryptitis and crypt abscesses are frequent as is Paneth cell metaplasia. Granulomas are frequently seen. The coexistence of these two lesions has been infrequently reported and the syndrome must be differentiated from Crohn's disease or ulcerative colitis sparing the rectum.

These patients respond to oral sulfasalazine (Azulfidine) and topical steroids. A high fiber diet and antibiotics have also been successful. The clinical response does not correlate with changes in the histology. Surgical intervention may be necessary to control bleeding or recurrences.

INFLAMMATORY BOWEL DISEASE

method of
PHILIP B. MINER, Jr., M.D.
University of Oklahoma School of Medicine and Oklahoma Foundation for Digestive Research
Oklahoma City, Oklahoma

Inflammatory bowel disease (IBD) is a complex disorder principally involving the small bowel and colon of young patients. Numerous systemic symptoms can become bothersome and require management; however, the principal symptoms are abdominal pain, diarrhea, incontinence, and blood in the stool. There is a genetic influence, most obviously in Crohn's disease. It appears that an environmental influence is necessary to activate the aggressive inflammation that causes colonic injury. Many important advances have been made in our understanding of the pathogenesis of the disordered immune regulation both from a genetic and environmental point of view.

IDENTIFICATION OF THE DISEASE

The definition of IBD distinguishes between broad groups of patients. The principal distinction is between transmural, discontinuous disease—Crohn's disease—and continuous, mucosal disease—ulcerative colitis. Identifying Crohn's disease or ulcerative colitis may not ensure a diagnosis that clarifies the pathophysiology of the patient's problems. These disease labels are applied once the extent of disease is understood by imaging studies (radiography or endoscopy with biopsy) and other problems such as infectious colitis, ischemic colitis, or radiation injury to the bowel are excluded. Exclusion of treatable causes of colitis is the goal of initial diagnostic evaluation in patients with IBD. Table 1 lists many of the identifiable causes of intestinal inflammation.

Classic features help distinguish ulcerative colitis from Crohn's disease. Crohn's disease is characterized by discontinuous disease, small bowel involvement, fistulas or abscesses, and severe perineal disease. Ulcerative colitis is limited to the colon. A few exceptions to these basic principles have been recognized and are important to our understanding of ulcerative colitis.

During phase II and III protocols evaluating mesalamine compounds for approval by the Food and Drug Administration for the treatment of ulcerative colitis, total colonoscopy was part of the initial evaluation of patients with suspected left-sided disease. Many of these patients had an area of cecal inflammation. This observation initiated considerable debate over whether these patients had subclinical Crohn's disease, universal ulcerative colitis with an area of uneven improvement in the colonic mucosa, or left-sided disease with a large skip area. Experts ultimately agreed that a cecal patch can be present in patients who have left-sided ulcerative colitis. Their disease should not be classified as pancolitis when the visible disease is clearly demarcated in the left colon.

The second issue concerning disease distribution is rectal sparing, which has classically defined Crohn's disease. As early as the 1960s, it was noted that occasional patients with ulcerative colitis had near-normal rectal mucosa or at least rectal mucosa that was less inflamed than the rest of the colon. This was attributed to topical rectal therapy with steroids. Experience with numerous oral agents for the management of inflammatory bowel disease demonstrates less involvement in the rectum than the sigmoid colon in patients with ulcerative colitis. These two endoscopic findings should not influence the diagnosis in a patient with strong clinical evidence of ulcerative colitis.

Other confusing issues are related to perineal disease in which it may be difficult to differentiate a patient with ulcerative colitis and a perirectal abscess from one with Crohn's disease. Hemorrhoidal disease may appear to be present in ulcerative colitis or Crohn's disease. Large, fleshy tags (elephant ears), which are often present in Crohn's disease, should be considered a diagnostic feature and not confused with severe hemorrhoidal disease. Microscopic ileal inflammation may be present in biopsies obtained at colonoscopy or surgical resection in patients with ulcerative colitis. The most common useful features distinguishing Crohn's disease from ulcerative colitis are the visible areas of inflammation identified at the time of endoscopy or after x-ray studies. Microscopic inflammation may be confusing, as it is commonly present in areas with no apparent disease. This important observation helps explain some of the changes that occur in ulcerative colitis and that appear to influence small bowel function.

TABLE 1. **Infectious Causes of Intestinal Inflammation**

Bacterial	Viral
Campylobacter jejuni	Cytomegalovirus
Shigella	Herpes simplex
Salmonella	**Parasitic**
Aeromonas hydrophila	*Entamoeba histolytica*
Yersinia enterocolitica	
Clostridium difficile	
Escherichia coli O157:H7	
Tuberculosis	
Neisseria gonorrhoeae	
Chlamydia trachomatis	
Treponema pallidum	

DIAGNOSTIC TESTS

The goals of diagnostic tests are to identify treatable causes of colonic inflammation and to distinguish ulcerative colitis from Crohn's disease. All patients presenting with chronic diarrhea, bloody or nonbloody, should be evaluated by (1) stool cultures, (2) a microscopic search for ova and parasites, and (3) *Clostridium difficile* toxin. These diagnostic tests identify treatable infectious diseases that mimic IBD; many of these infections can last for weeks to months. In the acute initial phase of IBD and with relapses, fecal leukocytes, eosinophils, and Charcot-Leyden crystals are also important stool studies. Blood tests including a complete blood count, chemistries, and indices of inflammation (e.g., erythrocyte sedimentation rate, C-reactive protein) can be useful in identifying disease severity.

Urinalysis identifies dehydration from the severity of diarrhea, the presence of oxalate crystals as a cause for nephrolithiasis, and multiorganism urinary tract infection due to fistulous tracts into the bladder. Pneumaturia is the passage of air during the process of micturition and nearly always indicates multiorganism bladder infection and enterovesical fistulous tract seen in Crohn's disease.

Endoscopy has advanced our understanding of Crohn's disease and ulcerative colitis. Endoscopic procedures include colonoscopy, esophagogastroduodenoscopy, endoscopic retrograde cholangiopancreatography (ERCP), and ultrasound. Colonoscopy perhaps is the single-most valuable test in management of IBD, as it allows visualization of the mucosa to distinguish the smooth, granular, friable mucosa of ulcerative colitis from the edematous irregular appearance of Crohn's disease. Colonoscopy allows biopsies of the ileum and colon to define the extent of disease. In ulcerative colitis, not only the severity of inflammation but also the extent of colonic involvement influences therapy and symptomatic management. Upper gastrointestinal endoscopy may identify inflammation of the mucosa typical of Crohn's disease, but it is more important in identifying histologic changes of focal gastritis not associated with *Helicobacter pylori* in the mucosa of the antrum. Antral biopsies are useful in children to identify Crohn's disease in the early stages. ERCP plays an important role in patients who have abnormal liver function tests because of sclerosing cholangitis, an important complication of IBD. Sclerosing cholangitis may lead to hepatic transplantation and also carries the risk of cholangiocarcinoma. Endoscopic ultrasonography is emerging as an important diagnostic test for numerous disorders. It can identify the thickness of the layers of the mucosa and may be able to distinguish colonic ulcerative colitis from Crohn's disease. This emerging technology has not been validated in IBD.

Histologic evaluation of biopsies obtained by endoscopy is important in distinguishing ulcerative colitis from Crohn's disease and in identifying other causes of inflammation. Rectal Crohn's disease must be distinguished from solitary rectal ulcer syndrome (SRUS). SRUS often manifests as edematous ulcerative mucosa from the distal rectum. Biopsies have a classic appearance of disturbed muscle fibers extending into the lamina propria. This lesion is thought to be due to ischemia from intussusception of the rectal mucosa down into the anal canal. *C. difficile* causes acute, aggressive colitis in patients with IBD. Typical histology is a volcanic-appearing eruption of inflammatory cells from the mucosa. Because *C. difficile* can often appear with colitis, its histologic distinguishing characteristics are useful for identifying patients who should be treated with metronidazole or vancomycin.

Identification of ischemia is also important in the management of patients with IBD, particularly in elderly patients who present with acute colitis. In the past, we believed that ischemia always had a progressive, destructive, and deadly course. However, it often is chronic, with an indolent course presenting with changes of mucosal function without transmural injury, infarction, or perforation. A classic histologic finding indicative of inflammatory disease is crypt distortion. In acute self-limiting colitis, which is likely an infectious illness with prolonged course, there is no crypt distortion. The straight linear crypts seen in acute self-limiting colitis predict resolution of the disease and identify patients who do not need long-term maintenance therapy.

Granulomas are not as useful as we would like them to be in separating Crohn's disease from ulcerative colitis because they are often absent in Crohn's disease, and pseudogranulomas may present a confusing picture in ulcerative colitis. True granulomas found in gastric biopsies are helpful, especially when associated with focal *H. pylori*–negative gastritis. Since the early 1960s, dense eosinophil infiltration has been recognized as a prominent feature of the histologic changes of serious IBD. Eosinophil migration and eosinophil crypt abscesses are important in distinguishing the cause of disease relapse. The pathologist should be aware that migration of the eosinophils between mucosal cells or into the crypts is useful diagnostic information. Another important histologic feature is dysplasia, which should be managed by colectomy to avoid complications of cancer.

Computed tomography and magnetic resonance imaging identify perineal disease and abscess formation. Newer techniques (e.g., virtual endoscopy) are being developed to demonstrate luminal changes to distinguish ulcerative colitis from Crohn's disease.

Breath tests detect (1) bacterial overgrowth in the small bowel associated with small bowel strictures or (2) carbohydrate malabsorption as a contributing cause of diarrhea in Crohn's disease. These standard, simple, noninvasive tests can provide useful diagnostic information.

Nuclear medicine scans with labeled white blood cell scan localize areas of inflammation of the colon. This information is helpful when contemplating surgical intervention while noninvasively assessing disease state and response to therapy. These nuclear medicine tests are currently limited to research applications but soon should be available to help with diagnosis and management.

An important emerging aspect of treating patients with IBD is focusing on the patient's principal complaint. This is especially valuable in Crohn's disease, as the principal complaint may indicate the type of therapy. The World Health Organization toxicity scale is a useful assessment tool for identifying and following severe symptomatic complaints.

Emerging blood tests may distinguish between patients with ulcerative colitis and those with Crohn's disease and stratify them into important subgroups. Currently, these diagnostic tests have limited clinical applicability but are important for long-term longitudinal and family research studies. In the next 5 to 10 years, these tests may be valuable for initial diagnosis in management of patients. Within the next decade, the genetics of IBD will define family patterns and may influence management decisions of active and subclinical disease.

INTRODUCTION TO MANAGEMENT

Management of IBD involves treating patient symptoms and inflammation of the mucosa. Symptomatic management is related to the patient's principal complaint and includes managing diarrhea, bleeding, tenesmus, fecal incontinence, nutritional failure, fatigue, fever, perineal pain, abdominal pain, and joint symptoms. All of these symptoms affect the patient's quality of life. Focusing attention on symptomatic management is as important as decreasing the inflammation in the mucosa. Managing mucosa inflammation is the physician's principal goal. During the diagnostic phase, attention is directed toward identifying the location and severity of inflammation. After controlling active disease, the focus shifts to early, aggressive management of relapses of disease. Serious complications of IBD must be avoided or managed carefully. These include risk of cancer, short-bowel syndrome, and sclerosing cholangitis.

MANAGING SYMPTOMS

Diarrhea is one of the prominent features of IBD. Small mucoid stools are usually due to rectal inflammation, whereas large volume watery stools indicate small bowel dysfunction. Symptomatic treatment includes (1) driving water absorption by using sodium and glucose in the small bowel, (2) eliminating osmoles entering the colon by managing diet, (3) binding bile acids in patients with ileal failure due to surgery or disease or in whom small bowel bacterial overgrowth causes deconjugation of bile acids, (4) eliminating bacterial overgrowth in patients who have partial strictures or obstructions in Crohn's disease or who have a period of small bowel contamination because of partial resection, (5) treating rectal inflammation to try to decrease rectal sensitivity, and (6) decreasing rectal contractility by using antihistamines or by slowing motility with the use of motility agents.

Tenesmus reflects active inflammation of the rectum. Decreasing rectal inflammation improves tenesmus. Topical rectal therapy with mesalamine or glucocorticoids improves rectal inflammation. Antihistamines are useful adjunctive therapy, because they decrease rectal contractility and inhibit the rapid and deep relaxation of the internal anal sphincter, which is associated with tenesmus.

Bleeding is best managed by treating active inflammation. The changes that occur in anorectal and colonic physiology with active inflammation of the colon make topical rectal therapy better than oral therapy.

Fecal incontinence occurs for several reasons. Pelvic floor dysfunction associated with fecal incontinence occurs when active inflammation of the colon changes rectal sensitivity in conjunction with enhanced rectal contraction. The internal anal sphincter relaxes in concert with rectal contractility, increasing the risk of incontinence. Although decreasing the inflammation in the rectum modifies these changes, patients with visibly normal mucosa may have persistent changes. In these patients, the symptoms, as well as the rectal contractility and internal sphincter relaxation, can be modified with antihistamines. An often overlooked reason for fecal incontinence in patients with Crohn's disease is bile acid malabsorption, which responds to bile acid–binding agents. A related issue is deconjugation of bile acids by bacterial overgrowth. This also can be managed by primary treatment of bacterial overgrowth or by binding bile acids with bile acid–binding resins.

Nutritional failure occurs because of mucosal failure and the metabolic stress of inflammation and anorexia or systemic illness. Dietary supplements, parenteral alimentation, and vitamin therapy can improve nutrition. Bacterial overgrowth is the commonly overlooked reason for poor nutrition in Crohn's disease, but active inflammation in the small bowel is the principal cause for nutritional failure.

Perineal pain generally occurs because of abscesses or perineal disease. Decreasing inflammation in the perineum with antibiotics or surgical drainage provides important long-term relief. Decreasing diarrhea in patients who have fistulous disease improves symptoms as increasing stool viscosity limits passage through the fistula and decreases contamination of the perineum. Managing some of the perineal pain in patients who do not have fistulous disease includes topical therapy to the skin, which has been injured by liquid diarrhea. Balneol therapy is useful in many patients for relieving the symptoms of perineal pain.

Abdominal pain is complex and often associated with activity of disease. Identifying the source of abdominal pain is critical for its management. For example, a stricture and abscess produce abdominal pain that can be modified by surgical intervention. Abdominal pain occurs for several reasons. Substance P, serotonin, and histamine are mediators of abdominal pain; interfering with these pathways is often useful. The antihistamine cyproheptadine (Periactin), is extremely valuable because it blocks both serotonin and histamine but often causes severe fatigue. The role of capsaicin-sensitive pain pathways is being investigated and may provide new management strategies.

Joint symptoms are common, and management is difficult. Nonsteroidal anti-inflammatory drugs (NSAIDs) activate IBD and should be avoided. I approach these problems by first eliminating the possibility of enteric enteropathy associated with enteric infection by a therapeutic trial of metronidazole* (Flagyl). The next step is to try to manage patients with pain medication that does not carry the risk of activating intestinal inflammation. These medications include acetaminophen (Tylenol), propoxyphene (Darvon), or tramadol (Ultram). Blocking the leukotriene pathway may be useful for management of joint symptoms. This strategy includes shifting the leukotrienes from the four series to the five series by supplementing the diet with eicosapentaenoic acid, which changes the substrate for leukotrienes. If patients improve with the use of eicosapentaenoic acid, then blocking 5-lipoxygenase using zileuton* (Zyflo) may enhance the benefit.

MANAGING INFLAMMATION

The severity of ulcerative colitis is determined by the extent of mucosal involvement and the degree of inflammation. Management of Crohn's disease is influenced by the location of intestinal inflammation and complications of the disease.

Aminosalicylates

Development of sulfasalazine (Azulfidine) was an early attempt to design a drug to manage arthritis by targeting joints with a salicylate and then applying an antibiotic to decrease the infectious component of arthritis. Not only did the enteric arthropathy improve, but so did IBD. From the early 1940s until mid-1950s, this observation had clinical importance but was not verified by controlled clinical trials. Early controlled trials proved that sulfasalazine was important in management of acute IBD. By the mid-1960s, sulfasalazine became accepted as maintenance therapy in patients with ulcerative colitis. It was not until 1977 that the emergence of the aminosalicylate component of sulfasalazine was shown to be an important factor in decreasing colonic inflammation. Azad-Kahn's classic experiment using enemas of sulfasalazine, 5-aminosalicylic acid (5-ASA), and sulfapyridine demonstrated efficacy with sulfasalazine and 5-ASA. Sulfapyridine is responsible for most of the adverse reactions in patients taking sulfasalazine. Sulfasalazine continues to be a useful medication in management of IBD and is the first of the 5-ASA drugs. All aminosalicylate therapy is topical. Sulfasalazine arrives in the colon intact where it is separated into 5-ASA and sulfapyridine by bacterial azoreductase.

Because all aminosalicylate therapy is topical, colonic and anorectal physiology influences the effectiveness of the drugs by affecting distribution in the inflamed and noninflamed portions of the small bowel and colon. These effects occur whether these

*Not FDA approved for this indication.

topical drugs are given orally or rectally. When a liquid enters the rectum and pelvic floor, contractility activates either expulsion of the fluid from the rectum or movement of the fluid into the proximal colon. When it is not possible to empty the contents of the rectum back into the sigmoid colon, the constant urge to defecate is present. The patient will either have a voluntary bowel movement or suffer incontinence. In IBD, the process is complicated by greater sensitivity in the left colon and impaired motility in the right colon. The exposure of the left colon to orally administered drugs is limited because of stasis in the right colon and rapid transit through the inflamed portion of the colon. Combined topical rectal and oral therapy results in a speedy remission of the disease because of the improved mucosal coating from rectal therapy and the ability of oral therapy to work on the proximal extent of the disease. Topical rectal mesalamine therapy consists of suppositories and enemas. The suppositories (Rowasa) cover 15 to 20 cm from the anal canal with tenacious adherence to the mucosa. Enemas are more fluid and spread to the splenic flexure, thereby improving the inflammation in the rectosigmoid area and markedly decreasing symptoms. It is impressive how rapidly patients can be brought into symptomatic remission by using topical rectal therapy. Initial studies of 5-ASA enemas found that visible bleeding stopped in approximately 50% of the patients with left-sided ulcerative colitis within 3 days of enema therapy. Oral approaches to 5-ASA therapy include the use of bacterial azoreductase–dependent compounds (sulfasalazine, olsalazine,* and balsalazide*), all of which require bacteria to separate the 5-ASA from a second compound. Eudragit-coated mesalamine (Asacol) requires a pH change in the cecum to dissolve the coating and release the mesalamine compound, whereas ethylcellulose beads (Pentasa) slowly release 5-ASA into the colon. Table 2 lists the options for aminosalicylate therapy and the unique characteristics of each compound.

*Not available in the United States.

The value of aminosalicylates for managing ulcerative colitis is undisputed. They have emerged as the first-line therapy for all but severely ill hospitalized patients with ulcerative colitis and have long-term value in maintaining remission. In Crohn's disease the issue is less clear. The response to the aminosalicylates is not as dramatic as with ulcerative colitis; however, most experienced clinicians use 5-ASA compounds for managing Crohn's disease of mild-to-moderate severity. The value of the aminosalicylates in maintaining remission in Crohn's patients is debatable; however, studies suggest the use of mesalamine decreases the number of patients who experience relapse after surgical intervention.

Glucocorticoids

Glucocorticoids have been used for decades for management of IBD based on the supposition that decreasing the active inflammation in the colon will improve the inflamed mucosa and prognosis. Topical rectal steroids were used in the 1960s and 1970s with obvious benefit. During the early development of these drugs, it was believed that the inflamed mucosa actively absorbed glucocorticoids with decreased absorption following improvement in the disease. Now it is known that rectal glucocorticoids are well absorbed by the healed mucosa. Oral strategies are emerging to try to take advantage of some of the unique aspects of a glucocorticoid intervention.

The use of every-other-day steroids in IBD has not been studied adequately, but many gastroenterologists use this strategy in patients in whom they are trying to decrease toxicity. In instances of active disease associated with eosinophil proliferation, high-dose, short-term steroids, such as methylprednisolone (Medrol Dosepak) can be useful.

The debate surrounding intravenous steroids in hospitalized patients is over intermittent versus continuous dosing. Newer steroids are being developed that have active mucosal metabolism and a resultant decrease in systemic toxicity. As these compounds emerge, it will be important to focus attention on

TABLE 2. **Mesalamine Preparations**

Type of Formulation	Name of Medication	Comment
Bacterial azoreductase	Sulfasalazine (Azulfidine)	First of the compounds requiring bacterial azoreductase to separate the 5-aminosalicylate (ASA) from sulfapyridine
	Balsalazide (Colazide)	5-ASA bonded with an inert carrier to decrease the toxicity associated with sulfapyridine
	Olsalazine (Dipentum)	Two 5-ASA molecules combined to give the theoretical advantage of the bacterial azoreductase without the toxicity of the carrier; the dimer may cause diarrhea
Topical rectal therapy	Rowasa suppositories (500 mg)	Covers about 20 cm of distal colon; safe and effective with negligible toxicity
	Rowasa enemas (4 gm)	Extends topical rectal therapy into the descending colon; safe and effective
Delayed release oral	Pentasa	Microencapsulated sustained release; has the theoretical advantage of delivery to the small intestine and colon
	Asacol	Eudragit coating dissolves in the pH of the distal ileum and cecum, allowing safe passage through the small intestine and delivery to the colon

whether a systemic effect is necessary. In studies of patients with Crohn's disease, budesonide improves symptoms; however, management is most effective when systemic effects of these steroids can be demonstrated by sensitive tests of adrenal function. As new glucocorticoids evolve and safety issues become less of a problem, we may be able to change our opinion regarding the use of steroids. With the currently available steroids, there is no role for long-term maintenance glucocorticoid therapy. In summary, current glucocorticoid therapy has shifted from primary therapy to rescue therapy.

6-Mercaptopurine* and Azathioprine*

In the mid-1970s, evaluation of 6-mercaptopurine (Purinethol), and azathioprine (Imuran), in Crohn's disease began. Initially used for perineal disease, these drugs gradually have become acceptable for all patients with refractory or steroid-dependent IBD. Toxicity includes leukopenia, aplastic anemia, hepatitis, and pancreatitis. Possible complications should be evaluated prospectively during therapy using doses of between 50 and 100 mg of 6-mercaptopurine and 50 and 150 mg of azathioprine.

Methotrexate*

Methotrexate is a fascinating drug because of its implications with regard to the pathophysiology of IBD more than because of its practical use. Studies have shown good early response to methotrexate, 15 to 25 mg intramuscularly per week, but early relapses are common. Methotrexate acts as an interleukin (IL)-1 receptor antagonist modifying the immune response.

Antibiotics

Antibiotic therapy has been used for years with variable success. This approach began because of the supposition that IBD must be an infectious problem. The combination of metronidazole (1 gm per day) and ciprofloxacin* (Cipro), (1 gm per day) has been shown to be as effective as prednisone in management of acute Crohn's disease. These drugs may decrease the luminal antigen load, but in addition to their antibacterial action, they affect the immune system. Nonantibiotic quinolones are being designed to explore the immunosupressive effects of this class of drugs. Clarithromycin* (Biaxin) has also been useful in patients with IBD but is not widely used because the response is only moderate in these patients.

Biologics

There is tremendous interest in cytokine therapies using anti-tumor necrosis factor (TNF), IL-11, IL-10, IL-2, and a host of other active inflammatory cytokines. These are valuable in modulating the immune system; however, none are currently available, and there is no documentation of their long-term value.

Cyclosporine* (Sandimmune), transformed transplant medicine by decreasing transplant organ rejection by modulating T-cell function. The drug is remarkable in management of IBD. Dramatic improvement can be seen in as little as 7 days after initiating IV cyclosporine, 4 mg per kg per day. My personal experience with cyclosporine supports enthusiasm early in the course of the disease, but I am disappointed with long-term management. I have been unable to move patients from a regimen of cyclosporine to other immunosupressive agents. Although this may represent referral bias, I am currently using cyclosporine only as a bridge to surgical intervention by improving patient's symptoms and nutritional status.

Modulating the Neuroimmune System

The most exciting area of gastrointestinal research is the discovery that the enteric nervous system influences the immune system. Studies with lidocaine,* clonidine,* and nicotine* show that modulating the neuroimmune system can induce remission of IBD. In folk medicine, capsaicin* has been used for improvement of IBD. The scientific explanation for the success of this drug is the modulation of neuroimmune function. None of the studies investigating lidocaine, clonidine, and nicotine report sufficient therapeutic benefit to advocate common usage; however, they do open modulating neuroimmune function as an emerging area of possible management.

Leukotrienes

Leukotriene modulation may influence IBD. It is known that Leukotriene-B4 is 100- to 1000-fold higher in rectal dialysis fluid of patients with IBD than in fluid of normal subjects. This observation led to a trial of a 5-lipoxygenase inhibitor (Zileuton) in patients with IBD. Control trials failed to show any therapeutic benefit; however, eicosapentaenoic acid, which shifts the leukotrienes from the four series to the five series, may decrease the intensity of some complications of IBD (e.g., joint problems) and has been reported to prolong remission after surgical resection in patients with Crohn's disease.

Antioxidants

One of the proposed mechanisms of action of mesalamine is the scavaging of oxygen-derived free radicals. Anecdotal reports support the use of allopurinol* (Zyloprim) and vitamin E derivatives in treatment of IBD by focusing on scavenging oxygen-derived free radicals. This area is important because it represents development of a new domain in control of intestinal inflammation—a reduction in the toxic

*Not FDA approved for this indication.

*Not available in the United States.

tissue effects of substances released after the induction of inflammation.

Nutritional Therapy

Short-chain fatty acids are one of the substrates for oxidative metabolism for the mucosa of the left side of the colon. Rectal therapy with short-chain fatty acids has been beneficial in improving refractory left-sided colitis. Glutamine acts in the same capacity in the small intestine and right colon, opening a new area of mucosal nutrition provided by the luminal contents. Elemental diet decreases the exposure of the gastrointestinal tract to potential antigens. Effective improvement in nutrition and symptoms in children with IBD may be due to the immune down-regulation caused by a decrease in luminal antigens. Parenteral nutrition has also been used for supplementing nutrition in patients who have short-bowel syndrome due to small intestinal Crohn's disease or surgery. Parenteral nutrition is useful in improving growth in children, although long-term complications of parenteral nutrition must be considered before initiating this treatment regimen.

SPECIAL CONSIDERATIONS IN IBD

Toxic megacolon is a complicated and difficult problem that often requires urgent colectomy. It has become rare in today's medical environment and has been replaced by subfulminant colitis as the most frequent reason for nonelective colectomy. Pregnancy and fertility are also important, as the majority of patients with IBD are young. Unlike Azulfidine, 5-ASA compounds do not decrease sperm motility and viability. Replacing Azulfidine with one of the newer mesalamine derivatives often reverses male infertility. I approach management of pregnancy by focusing on maternal health and nutrition. I use whatever medications are necessary to keep IBD in remission. Fortunately, the natural immunosupression of pregnancy that allows women to maintain their fetuses helps suppress intestinal inflammation, making the task of disease control easier after the first trimester.

Managing perineal disease can be challenging, particularly painful perineal disease resulting from abscesses or fistulas. Metronidazole and 6-mercaptopurine improve fistula closure, but better drugs are needed. Decreasing the liquid content of the stools helps decrease perineal contamination and improves the chemical dermatitis associated with fistula leakage. New drugs such as anti-TNF may help provide management strategies that will be useful for decreasing perineal disease and fistula formation. Therapeutic trials of Balneol (Solvay Pharmaceuticals), charcoal, or bile-acid binding agents may improve the chemical dermatitis associated with perineal discomfort.

Stenotic disease presenting with pain, obstruction, or fistulae is an important indication for surgery in Crohn's disease. Fistula tracts should be explored by a fistulogram to identify distal luminal stenosis and the need for surgical intervention. Many patients with Crohn's disease have partial short-term obstruction due to food, which can be managed conservatively by short-term hospital stays with hydration and subsequent avoidance of obstructing foods. Common foods associated with transient obstruction are popcorn, nuts, shredded coconut, and other fibrous food components.

Anemia

Chronic anemia occurs because of nutritional factors related to intolerance to iron and failure to absorb vitamin B_{12} and folate. Once these have been replaced, anemia may persist as a consequence of impaired hematopoiesis secondary to chronic disease. Erythropoietin* (Epogen) is useful in improving the status of anemia in these patients. Bacterial overgrowth occurs as a natural consequence of partially obstructive intestinal disease, but also occurs after surgery by contamination of the small bowel via the open small bowel to colon anastomosis. Bacterial overgrowth is often overlooked as a cause of diarrhea and nutritional failure. It should be sought by breath test or empirically treated with antibiotics. The hallmark of bile acid–induced enteropathy is fecal incontinence. In the single study assessing fecal incontinence in patients with Crohn's disease, all of them had ileal disease. Incontinence improved following the use of bile acid–binding agents. Fecal incontinence also may occur because of an over-reactive rectum and anal canal. Because histamine causes relaxation of the internal anal sphincter and rectal contractility, modulation with antihistamines is often helpful.

Dysplasia and Cancer

Dysplasia and cancer are feared complications of ulcerative colitis. Recently we have become aware of an increased incidence of cancer in patients with Crohn's disease. Patients should undergo periodic endoscopy for dysplasia to identify those at risk for cancer so that colectomy can be done. Dysplasia needs to be confirmed by expert pathologists. Sclerosing cholangitis should not be overlooked as a complication of IBD. Patients with cholestasis should be assessed by ERCP. Abdominal ultrasonography may be useful in identifying sclerotic bile ducts. The clinician should be alert for the development of cancer in patients with sclerosing cholangitis. Liver transplantation should be considered when sclerosing cholangitis becomes advanced. Total colectomy has little value in decreasing the inexorable course of sclerosing cholangitis. Liver transplant recipients who are managed with high-dose immunosuppression also may have active colonic disease requiring treatment.

*Not FDA approved for this indication.

Surgical Intervention

Surgical intervention should not be ignored as an appropriate therapeutic mode, as surgery is the best option in numerous clinical situations. Surgical intervention for patients with strictures from Crohn's disease and total colectomy with the new surgical anastomotic techniques for patients with ulcerative colitis should be considered.

MAINTENANCE THERAPY

Maintenance therapy for ulcerative colitis has been recognized as an important part of disease management since the early 1960s. Options for maintenance therapy include topical rectal therapy, which can occur every day, every other day, every third day, or 7 consecutive days each month. Guidelines for oral therapy generally begin with approximately one-half the oral dose required for remission; however, some patients will require the full oral dose that placed the patient in remission for long-term management. 6-Mercaptopurine and azathioprine decrease the dependency on glucocorticoids and thus are important for maintenance therapy. Long-term management of patients with these drugs is one of the important improvements in treatment of IBD because of the decreased risk of glucocorticoid toxicity. Methotrexate may also be used in some patients; however, it is not particularly of value because of the recognized relapses. Glucocorticoids should rarely be used for maintenance therapy because of the toxicity associated with them; however, strategy using every-other-day therapy may be necessary in some patients. Only during the last few years has maintenance therapy for Crohn's disease been considered. The use of 5-ASA, metronidazole, or 6-mercaptopurine may delay recurrence of the disease after surgery.

WHY DO PATIENTS EXPERIENCE RELAPSE?

Patients with IBD experience relapse for specific reasons. The first is a change in smoking status. Cessation of smoking is associated with the onset of active ulcerative colitis or an increase in disease activity. Although I do not advocate treating patients by having them smoke, the use of nicotine patches may be useful. Crohn's disease appears to be made worse by smoking, and all patients with Crohn's disease should be counseled not to smoke.

Mesalamine toxicity is also recognized as a cause of active inflammation. It has occurred with all of the mesalamine derivatives and is a chemical sensitivity probably due to the mesalamine, although other chemical constituents of the preparations may play a role in activating chemical colitis. Withdrawal of the mesalamine drugs is an important diagnostic test. It is also important to try to rechallenge patients to be certain that mesalamine is the cause of their active IBD.

The third reason for relapse is seasonal variation, which may cause an allergic reaction. An allergic reaction can activate IBD by two processes: up-regulation of the immune system through nonspecific stimulation of eosinophilic function and direct intestinal induction by swallowed inhaled antigens brought into the posterior pharynx through pulmonary secretions. The diagnosis is supported by eosinophils or their toxic products and Charcot-Leyden crystals in the stools. The presence of Charcot-Leyden crystals is evidence of sufficient eosinophil concentration in the intestinal mucosa to cause tissue injury. Treatment with methylprednisolone is often effective in decreasing the number of eosinophils and improving the colitis without commitment to long-term steroids.

The fourth reason for relapse is infection. As the allergic pathway, infection up-regulates the immune system in nonspecific and specific ways. Enteric infections expose the gastrointestinal immune system to pathogens, which activate the inflammatory process. Systemic infections also have repercussions in the gastrointestinal tract. There are numerous examples in which systemic infection can activate IBD 5 to 7 days after the onset of the infection.

The fifth cause for activation of IBD is the use of NSAIDs. Activation can occur through several pathways: (1) inducing intestinal inflammation by the drug itself, (2) impairing oxidative phosphorylation, (3) decreasing the synthesis of protective prostaglandins, and (4) producing a change in intestinal permeability. Studies are in progress to identify the reason for flares in the disease.

IRRITABLE BOWEL SYNDROME

method of
ERVIN Y. EAKER, Jr., M.D.
Kansas University Medical Center
Kansas City, Kansas

Irritable bowel syndrome is a complex, symptom-based disorder characterized by abdominal discomfort and altered bowel habits. In fact, it is defined by the presence of recurrent or continuous abdominal discomfort relieved with bowel movement and/or associated with altered bowel habits in the absence of "organic" disease. The inability of objective tests such as barium enema, colonoscopy, ultrasound, and computed tomography (CT) of the abdomen to demonstrate any structural abnormalities has placed this syndrome in the "functional" bowel disorder group. Because of the elusive nature of this syndrome, diagnosis is more difficult and less tenable to both the physician and patient. A consensus opinion by experts in gastroenterology has provided us with a standard by which the diagnosis can be considered more efficiently. As shown in Table 1, the Rome criteria for irritable bowel syndrome allow both clinicians and investigators to better select patients who fit these criteria. This has led to more awareness and a minimization of the repetitive testing that is precipitated by such chronic abdominal complaints. Even more exciting

TABLE 1. **Rome Criteria for Diagnosis of Irritable Bowel Syndrome**

At least 3 months of continuous or recurrent symptoms must be present:

1. Abdominal pain relieved by defecation and/or associated with a change in frequency or consistency of stool

   AND

2. Two or more of the following (at least 25% of the time):
   - Altered frequency of bowel movements
   - Altered consistency of stool (hard or loose and watery)
   - Altered stool passage (straining, urgency, incomplete evacuation)
   - Passage of mucus
   - Bloating or abdominal distention

are recent advances in our abilities to recognize that both motor and sensory abnormalities may be present in the gut of individuals with irritable bowel syndrome. Thus, it is possible that more specific objective testing will allow us to define the individuals who have this syndrome and to identify more specific and appropriate treatments.

PREVALENCE

Although the true prevalence of irritable bowel syndrome in the United States is not known, estimates based on a variety of surveys suggest the prevalence may be in the range of 15 to 25% of all adults. Irritable bowel symptoms seem to be present predominantly in young women, with an incidence six times more frequent than in men. Some have suggested this may, in part, reflect a greater likelihood to seek medical care. Up to 40% of individuals who present to an outpatient gastrointestinal practice have symptoms consistent with irritable bowel syndrome.

The costs associated with irritable bowel syndrome are enormous. In fact, a recent study has suggested that the cost in health care dollars in the United States may be as high as $8 billion a year, with nearly $800 more in yearly medical costs per patient with irritable bowel syndrome compared with a matched control population. Much of this comes from multiple visits to the physician, who at times is ill prepared to deal with this elusive set of symptoms. As we better define this symptom complex and improve our understanding of the pathophysiology, we may be able to become more efficient in diagnosis and reduce the costs of managing this syndrome.

PATHOPHYSIOLOGY

The use of a number of different terms such as spastic colon, irritable gut, and irritable bowel syndrome is a reflection of our limited understanding of the true pathophysiology of this complex disorder. This is an idiopathic syndrome, but our attention has been focused on neuromuscular control of "spastic" problems of the colon. Investigators have now incorporated the possibility of microscopic inflammation and humeral, hormonal, and sensory influences on this vast syndrome. Early descriptions of an excess number of colonic contractions in some patients with irritable bowel were followed by the realization that hormonal influences such as the change in menstrual cycling or stressful influences may precipitate or worsen symptoms. We now appreciate that thresholds for pain from the viscera of the gut in individuals with irritable bowel syndrome may be quite distinct from asymptomatic control subjects. In fact, ongoing research suggests that irritable bowel syndrome is, in fact, a brain/gut disorder incorporating disturbances of gut wall muscular activity and abnormal sensory perceptions. At the root of these abnormalities, however, are a variety of etiologies including microscopic colitis (including mast cell disorders), hormonal influences, and stress. Epidemiologic evidence suggests that many patients with irritable bowel syndrome have a history of either psychologic or sexual abuse. These factors may be strong contributors to underlying pathophysiology including effects on sensory perceptions. Some studies suggest that patients with irritable bowel syndrome who do not seek significant medical attention have a different psychologic profile than those with irritable bowel syndrome who repetitively seek medical care. The importance of those observations is not yet clearly understood. In the past, irritable bowel syndrome has been a diagnosis of exclusion. It has required exclusion of organic disease that might be obtained from colonoscopy, barium enema, ultrasound, or CT scans. With the Rome criteria, we are able to focus attention on criteria for diagnosis rather than placing everyone with abdominal symptoms but negative evaluations into the classification of irritable bowel syndrome. As our understanding of the pathophysiology of this disorder expands, particularly in the area of sensory threshold abnormalities, further tests such as balloon distention of the rectum with assessment of altered threshold to pain may provide a more clear diagnosis.

TREATMENT

In a disease that is idiopathic and as poorly understood as irritable bowel syndrome, multiple treatment regimens have been proposed. Most important, clarity of the diagnosis based on rational criteria such as the Rome criteria is essential. In fact, one of the most important treatments for this disorder is patient education as to the reality of this syndrome. Support and reduction in test seeking from the patient are also essential. Once a strong physician-patient relationship is established, it is much more likely that therapy will be effective.

We have paid a great deal of attention to dietary therapies for this disorder, and none has proved effective in prospective blinded trials. However, logic dictates that treatment be tailored to the individual's history and symptoms as they relate to exacerbation of complaints. This is particularly true in relationship to changes in diet. We have appreciated that in some individuals certain foods and components of foods such as lactose-containing dairy products, fructose and sorbitol, caffeine, carbonated beverages, and high fat can result in the exacerbation of symptoms. Also implicated in some individuals are tyramine-containing foods such as aged cheese, beer, liquor, chocolate, and red meat. A well-balanced, low-fat diet is probably the most appropriate initial suggestion. Certain foods that historically have caused problems in specific patients should be avoided if at all possible, but general dietary restrictions in every patient should not be advised.

A lack of dietary fiber has been strongly linked epidemiologically with disorders of the colon such as diverticulosis and irritable bowel. However, prospective studies of supplemental dietary fiber have had mixed results. With the classic alteration in bowel habits seen in patients with irritable bowel syndrome (i.e., constipation, diarrhea, or an alternation of the two), attention to regulation of the bowels makes sense. A high-fiber diet with addition of fiber supplementation (in higher doses than are used in mild constipation) (Table 2) has been the mainstay therapy for irritable bowel syndrome. If attention is paid to what the fiber supplement is trying to accomplish and the patient is educated to that goal, it is more likely that the therapy will be continued and that positive effects will be achieved. Regulation of the patient's bowels should afford overall improvement in well-being, even if some of the symptoms are not ameliorated.

Other therapies to control either constipation or diarrhea should be considered on a patient-by-patient basis. The patient should be informed that these agents will be prescribed to correct a specific bowel problem without expressing the expectation that such therapy will ameliorate all irritable bowel symptoms. Agents such as diphenoxylate HCl with atropine sulfate (Lomotil) or loperamide HCl (Imodium) have been useful in the intermittent treatment of diarrhea-prone irritable bowel syndrome. At the other extreme, constipation-prone irritable bowel can be approached with agents such as milk of magnesia or lactulose in low dose (Chronulac).

TABLE 2. **Medications**

Type	Dosing
Fiber Supplements	
Psyllium (Konsyl, Metamucil, Perdiem)	1–2 tbsp qd-bid
Polycarbophil* (FiberCon)	1–3 tablets bid
Methylcellulose (Citrucel)	1–2 tbsp qd-bid
Antispasmodic Agents	
Belladonna and phenobarbital (Donnatal)	1–2 po tid-qid
Dicyclomine HCl* (Bentyl)	10–20 mg po tid-qid
Clidinium and chlordiazepoxide HCl (Librax)	1 cap po tid to qid
Hyoscyamine sulfate	
(Levbid, Levsin)	0.375 mg po qd-bid
(Levsin SL)*	0.125 mg sublingual prn
Bowel Regulation	
ANTIDIARRHEAL	
Diphenoxylate HCl with atropine sulfate (Lomotil)	2.5 mg po q 4 h prn
Difenoxin HCl with atropine sulfate (Motofen)	1 mg po q 4 h prn
Loperamide HCl* (Imodium)	2 mg po q 4 h prn
LAXATIVE	
Milk of magnesia*	2–4 tbsp po q hs-bid
Lactulose (Chronulac)	2–4 tbsp po bid-tid
Tricyclic Antidepressants (Pain Management)	
Amitriptyline HCl* (Elavil)	25–50 mg q hs
Nortriptyline HCl (Pamelor)	25–50 mg q hs
Trazodone (Desyrel)	50 mg q hs or bid
Other Agents	
Anxiolytics† (Ativan, Librium, Valium, Xanax)	Varying doses, up to qid
Selective serotonin re-uptake inhibitors† (Paxil, Prozac, Zoloft)	qd

*Author's first choice.
†Not FDA approved for this indication.

As would belie the term *spastic colon*, some physicians have suggested the use of antispasmodic agents in the treatment of irritable bowel syndrome. In individuals with a history of crampy abdominal pain, particularly in association with their bowel movements, agents such as hyoscyamine sulfate (Levsin/SL), dicyclomine HCl (Bentyl), belladonna alkaloids (Donnatal), or clidinium and chlordiazepoxide HCl (Librax) have been recommended and may provide some symptomatic improvement. (See Table 2 for the recommended dosing for these agents.)

In regard to the altered pain threshold and the interaction of the brain and gut, other agents have been used. In particular, tricyclic antidepressants such as amitriptyline HCl* (Elavil), trazodone HCl* (Desyrel), or nortriptyline HCl* (Pamelor) have been used. These agents have been used for the treatment of depression but also have been shown to modulate pain responses in individuals with chronic pain, including visceral pain. Because of the high association of psychological problems in functional bowel, including anxiety, anxiolytics such as lorazepam (Ativan) or alprazolam (Xanax) have also been used. The newer selective serotonin re-uptake inhibitors have been tried, but prospective analysis of their effects has not been undertaken.

Besides medical therapy and the establishment of a strong patient/physician relationship, some individuals require additional therapy including a referral to a psychiatrist or psychologist. This strategy can be quite beneficial in individuals who have a significant number of psychological problems associated with their irritable bowel syndrome, and lack of attention to these important details will significantly reduce the ability of other treatments to improve overall patient well-being.

Some investigational agents for individuals with irritable bowel syndrome are on the horizon. As we draw closer to a better understanding of the pathophysiology, our ability to specifically treat or even prevent irritable bowel syndrome will improve. Agents directed at better control of symptoms have been proposed and are in the investigational arm. These include fedotozine, a kappa-opioid agonist with potential effects on visceral pain thresholds and 5HT3 receptor antagonists such as alosetron. Gonadotropin-releasing hormone agonists such as leuprolide acetate* (Lupron) have shown some efficacy in patients with severe functional bowel complaints. Treatment with antihistamines and mast cell stablizers such as cromolyn sodium* (Gastrocrom) have produced limited results. Prospective studies of these therapies are limited, and the experience of many who treat individuals with irritable bowel syndrome has not produced the enthusiasm necessary to make

*Not FDA approved for this indication.

any of these investigational approaches generally recommended. However, each of these agents focuses on poorly understood potential mechanisms for individuals with irritable bowel syndrome and deserve continued investigation as to their role in the pathophysiology or improved treatment.

HEMORRHOIDS, ANAL FISSURE, AND ANORECTAL ABSCESS AND FISTULA

method of
BRUCE A. ORKIN, M.D.
George Washington University
Washington, D.C.

Anorectal disorders are extremely common; more than 50% of the population will experience one at some time during their lives. It is important for the clinician to be familiar with these problems as many are easily treated without referral to a colorectal surgeon. On the other hand, it is critical that patients who do not respond to initial conservative therapy or who have an acute problem be referred promptly. Many patients with anorectal complaints attribute it to "hemorrhoids" ("Doc, my hemorrhoids are killing me!" or "My hemorrhoids are bleeding again"). Although hemorrhoids may be the cause of these patients' complaints, more than half have another problem, such as a fissure, abscess, fistula, hypertrophied anal papilla, or pruritus ani (anal irritation).

ANATOMY

An appreciation of the anatomy of the anorectal region is necessary to understand the pathophysiology of these disorders. The rectum is the distal compartment of the gastrointestinal tract and is fixed posteriorly to the sacrum. As it descends into the pelvis, it becomes completely retroperitoneal. The lower end of the rectum is the anorectal ring, which marks the transition between the rectum and anal canal. At this point, the lumen, which has been turning anteriorly around the sacral curve, angles down and posteriorly as it penetrates the pelvic floor, or levator ani, muscles. This forms the anorectal angle, which is accentuated by contraction of the puborectalis muscle, the innermost of the pelvic floor muscles. This U-shaped muscle arises from the pubic bone and swings posteriorly around the anorectal junction to return to the pubis. The surgical anal canal starts at the anorectal junction and ends at the anal verge. When the buttocks are separated during an examination the anal verge is the highest portion of the skin generally visible. The anal canal is closed at rest.

The rectum expands as it fills, staying at a relatively low pressure until its threshold for emptying is reached. This is termed the rectal compliance. The anal canal is surrounded by two cylindrical sphincter muscles, one inside the other (*not* above and below), the internal anal sphincter and the external anal sphincter. The internal anal sphincter consists of smooth muscle, and as such, is an involuntary muscle. It is a continuation of the circular fibers of the rectal wall. The internal sphincter muscle contributes 80 to 90% of the resting tone of the anal canal. The external anal sphincter muscle, composed of striated, voluntary muscle, contributes about 10 to 20% of the resting tone of the anal canal and is one of the few striated muscles in the body that is active at rest. The upper end of the external sphincter is contiguous with the puborectalis muscle and the pelvic floor. All of the squeezing pressure of the anal canal comes from these striated muscles. The anal canal is closed at rest and may be further tightened to protect against leakage. During evacuation, these muscles must relax to allow the bolus to pass.

The anal canal is 2 to 4 cm long. The dentate line is found about halfway up the canal; this is where the anal skin (anoderm) stops and the mucosal lining (transitional zone) starts. The dentate line curves up and down like a sine wave: the upper points are called the papillae and the lower curves are the crypts. Many crypts lead into ducts and anal glands, which can become plugged, resulting in abscesses. Superior to the dentate line and deep to the mucosa lie the internal hemorrhoidal vessels, composed of both arteries and veins. The external hemorrhoidal vessels lie inferior to the dentate line and beneath the skin. These vessels are the normal blood supply to this area. When they become dilated and symptomatic they are termed internal or external hemorrhoids.

The perirectal and perianal region is divided into spaces, and these are the locations of most abscesses. The four major spaces are the *perianal space* below the dentate line and the skin and superficial to the muscles, the *ischiorectal space* between the external sphincter and the pelvic walls below the pelvic floor muscles, the *intersphincteric space* between the internal and external sphincters, and the *supralevator space* above the pelvic floor muscles.

HISTORY

Most anorectal disorders can be diagnosed by the history alone and then confirmed on physical examination. Again, many patients complaining of "hemorrhoids" do not have symptomatic hemorrhoids, and the physician should concentrate on the actual symptoms and not the patient's self-diagnosis. Patients typically present with one or more of the following four complaints: pain, bleeding, a change in bowel habits (constipation or diarrhea), or a mass. The history should include inquiries about all of these even if not brought up by the patient. Pain may be sharp or dull, mild or severe, stabbing, burning, or aching. Its duration, frequency, and relationship to bowel movements should be established. Bleeding is a very common problem that is often ignored when mild. The extent, character, and timing of bleeding should be ascertained. There may be pink staining on the toilet tissue or bright red blood dripping into the bowel or squirting from a vessel. Blood can be seen on the tissue alone or it can coat the stool or be mixed with it. It may be difficult to determine quantity accurately as a few drops of blood will turn the toilet water red and cause great alarm. The bleeding can accompany bowel movements and stop promptly, can last many minutes, or can occur between movements. Altered or difficult bowel movements are a very common finding with anorectal disorders. Constipation with infrequent movements, laxative use, or straining is often causative. Diarrhea or incontinence may also contribute. A recent change in bowel habits may be a sign of colorectal cancer or other problems.

In addition, sexual habits and orientation are important factors in many situations. Anoreceptive intercourse or manipulation and sexually transmitted diseases often give rise to anorectal complaints. Other medical conditions associated with anorectal conditions include rectal carcinoma and polyps, inflammatory bowel disease (particularly Crohn's disease), immune system compromise such as human immunodeficiency virus (HIV) infection or transplant suppression, and neuromuscular disorders.

Most anorectal disorders are easily identified by a careful history and examination. Table 1 lists the most common disorders along with their typical symptoms and signs.

PHYSICAL EXAMINATION

Physician visits for anorectal problems can be anxiety provoking and embarrassing for patients and they often postpone the visit rather than submit to questioning or examination. The examiner should be comfortable with the topic and should reassure the patient, explaining each step of the examination. This will go a long way toward alleviating their concerns. The examiner should be organized and gentle. A general and abdominal examination are performed as indicated. The patient is then placed in the jackknife (preferred) knee-chest position or on the side with the legs pulled up. First, the perineum is visually inspected. Then the examiner digitally palpates the skin, anal canal, and lower rectum and, as indicated, vagina. In men, the prostate should be carefully palpated. In women, anterior weakness of the rectovaginal septum is felt as a rectocele. Anoscopy is performed with a short, angled or side-viewing instrument, followed by rigid proctoscopy or flexible sigmoidoscopy. Flexible instruments do not allow visualization of the anal canal and should not be substituted for careful anoscopy. Visual inspection will identify pruritus ani with erythema and excoriation of the skin, skin tags, thrombosed external hemorrhoids, low anal cancers, and scars. Careful separation of the anal verge and inspection between the folds is the only way to adequately identify anal fissures, which are often missed. The patient is asked to squeeze and bear down, during both the inspection and the digital examination. Prolapsing internal hemorrhoids, polyps, hypertrophied anal papillae, full-thickness rectal prolapse, and even cancers may be seen. If prolapse is suspected but not demonstrated, the patient should be asked to sit on the commode in the bathroom and strain. The examiner can then observe the perineum while the patient leans forward. Digital examination will identify anorectal masses (hard, soft, or fluctuant), tenderness, rectoceles, and prostate lesions and allow a gross assessment of internal and external sphincter tone. Anoscopy is the only appropriate way to examine the internal hemorrhoidal vessels and the anal canal; inflammation, hypertrophied anal papillae, and other conditions may be seen. Endoscopic evaluation of the rectum and sigmoid is essential in all patients to rule out contributing disorders and to screen for neoplasia.

On occasion, a portion of the proctologic examination may be deferred to a later time. This is appropriate when a patient has an acutely painful fissure or an abscess that requires drainage. Further evaluation of the gastrointestinal tract may be in order at times to rule out other problems such as Crohn's disease, polyps, or cancer.

BOWEL MANAGEMENT PROGRAM

Regular bowel habits are important in preventing diverticular disease, hemorrhoids, and fissures. They can also reduce the risk of colorectal neoplasia and abscesses and fistulas. Normal bowel habits are defined as the evacu-

TABLE 1. **Differential Diagnosis of Common Anorectal Disorders**

Disorder	Duration	Symptoms	Signs
Skin tags	Chronic	Soft mass Irritation	Soft Floppy tag
Pruritus ani	Acute or chronic Often intermittent	Itching Irritation Staining or bleeding	Erythema Excoriations Ulceration
Hypertrophied anal papilla	Chronic	None Mass Prolapse "Polyp"	Firm mass on digital examination May prolapse Skin covered extension of the dentate line
Internal hemorrhoids	Chronic	Bleeding Prolapse	Dilated vessels, loose mucosa above dentate line May prolapse
External hemorrhoids	Acute	Pain Mass	Bluish, tender, rubbery mass Not fluctuant
Anal fissure—acute	Acute	Severe pain with bowel movement Bleeding	Fissure or cut in anal canal skin
Anal fissure—chronic	Chronic	Pain Tag Bleeding	Fissure Tag Hypertrophied anal papilla
Anorectal abscess	Acute	Pain Swelling/mass Fever Chills	Marked tenderness Swelling, induration Erythema Fluctuance
Anorectal fistula	Chronic	Discharge Pruritus Intermittent swelling and pain ± History of abscess	External opening Palpable cord
Anal carcinoma	Gradual	Mass Bleeding Constipation	Hard mass Nontender Skin breakdown/replacement

ation of formed, soft stools that pass easily and without trauma to the anal canal between three times a day and two to three times a week. All patients with any suggestion of abnormal bowel habits should be placed on a bowel management program (Table 2).

A high-fiber diet is recommended on a routine basis. A wide variety of foods contain soluble and insoluble fiber, including fruits, vegetable, and grains. The best source of fiber is wheat bran, although oats, rye, and other cereals are also good sources. Bran cereal, whole-wheat breads, and miller's bran are other good sources. A bowl of bran cereal that has 5 to 7 grams of dietary fiber per serving along with a glass of milk and/or juice is a good way to start the day. Each box of cereal lists the amount of dietary fiber and the number of calories per serving. Alternatives to cereal include a bran muffin or 2 or 3 tablespoons of miller's bran mixed into hot cereal. About 25 to 30 grams of fiber per day is reasonable.

Since the major function of fiber is to hold fluid in the stool, it is important to drink enough water and other liquids during the day. At least 6 to 8 glasses of water and other liquids should be taken during each day. Like a sponge, fiber becomes hard and stiff if it does not contain enough water.

In addition to the high-fiber diet, some patients require a fiber supplement and/or stool softeners. Fiber supplements or bulking agents function in the same way as dietary fiber and bran. They are taken by mouth once or twice a day and are not absorbed. As fiber travels down the bowel, it absorbs water and keeps the stool in a semisolid state. The stools remain moist and soft, instead of becoming dried out as they pass through the colon. Most of these products contain psyllium, which is a seed product. Many pharmacies and grocery stores have their own generic brands, which are often much less expensive than the name brands. One tablespoon of the powder or one premeasured package is mixed in a glass of water or juice and taken once or twice each day. Alternately, four to six fiber tablets can be taken with one or two large glasses of liquid once or twice each day. Stool softeners lubricate the stools and allow them to pass more easily; they are not laxatives. The most commonly used agents contain either docusate sodium (Colace) or docusate calcium (Surfak). Generic docusate is available at low cost. One or two capsules are taken in the morning and evening. Laxatives and enemas are rarely needed, and prolonged use of laxatives can be harmful. Patients should be told to respond promptly to the urge for evacuation and to avoid straining and prolonged periods on the toilet. With this simple approach, most people will develop regular bowel habits. A small percentage of individuals will have persistent problems and may require further evaluation.

TABLE 2. **Bowel Management Program**

High-fiber diet	25–30 grams of fiber per day Bran cereal or muffin, 5–7 grams of fiber per serving Whole-wheat breads, other grains Fruits, vegetables
Fluids	6–8 glasses per day
Fiber supplement	Psyllium (Konsyl, Metamucil, Citrucel, or generic), 1 tbsp powder mixed in a glass of fluid once or twice each day
Stool softener	Generic docusate sodium (Colace) or docusate calcium (Surfak), 1 tablet once or twice each day
Bowel habits	Do not defer movements Avoid excessive straining Do not read or spend long periods on the commode Carefully cleanse perianal area with moistened towelettes or baby wipes, pat dry

HEMORRHOIDS

Hemorrhoids are a very common complaint but are often misdiagnosed and inappropriately treated. There are really two types of hemorrhoids, and they behave entirely differently and are treated differently.

Internal Hemorrhoids

Internal hemorrhoids arise from the normal internal hemorrhoidal vessels that lie beneath the mucosa proximal to the dentate line. These vessels can dilate and become thin walled and easily damaged. As they dilate, the overlying mucosa becomes detached from the muscle wall and the tissue bulges. Internal hemorrhoids are typically associated with a history of constipation, straining, and prolonged sitting on the toilet. They are commonly a problem after labor and delivery. Symptoms include painless bleeding with bowel movements and prolapsing tissue. Pain is rarely a primary symptom of internal hemorrhoids, contrary to product advertising. Bleeding is bright red in nature and blood may be seen on the toilet tissue, coating the stools, or squirting from a vessel in a prolapsed hemorrhoidal mass. Minor bleeding is found in many other conditions including carcinomas, and these must be ruled out before attributing bleeding to minor internal hemorrhoids. Usually, the bleeding is limited, and it is extremely rare to find anemia due to hemorrhoids. Prolapse is common, and mucus and particles of stool may be deposited on the perianal skin, causing secondary pruritus ani.

Treatment of internal hemorrhoids depends on the symptoms and degree of prolapse (Table 3). All patients are placed on a bowel management program. There is no role for topical agents or suppositories. There are three levels of treatment:

1. Bowel management as outlined previously. This may be all that is necessary for minimally symptomatic disease and is a component of all other treatment regimens.
2. Office treatment. This is appropriate for bleeding first-degree internal hemorrhoids and for second- and some third-degree prolapsing hemorrhoids. Methods such as rubber band ligation, infrared coagulation, and sclerotherapy are commonly employed. Laser treatment is no more effective and tends to be more expensive and more of a marketing gimmick. Ninety percent of patients with symptomatic hemorrhoids are adequately treated without surgery.
3. Formal operative hemorrhoidectomy. This is necessary in a small number of patients with fourth-degree chronically prolapsed and extensive third-degree bleeding and prolapsing internal hemorrhoids.

TABLE 3. **Degree of Prolapse and Treatment Options for Internal Hemorrhoids**

	Characteristics	Treatment
First degree	Do not prolapse, may bleed, often asymptomatic	Bowel management, IRC, ST
Second degree	Prolapse with BM and reduce spontaneously	Bowel management, IRC, RBL
Third degree	Prolapse with BM or spontaneously and are manually reducible	Bowel management, RBL, occasionally hemorrhoidectomy
Fourth degree	Chronically prolapsed, either are not reducible or do not stay reduced	Operative hemorrhoidectomy

Abbreviations: BM = bowel movement; IRC = infrared coagulation; ST = sclerotherapy; RBL = rubber band ligation.

Most hemorrhoidectomies are now performed in an ambulatory setting. Pain is significant for 1 to 2 weeks after hemorrhoidectomy but results are impressive, with recurrence rates of only 2 to 5%. Rarely, internal hemorrhoids may prolapse and become incarcerated and extensively thrombosed. These patients present with severe pain and require emergent surgery.

External Hemorrhoids

External hemorrhoids are generally asymptomatic unless acutely thrombosed. Most lesions labeled external hemorrhoids are, in reality, just skin tags. Skin tags may be the residual stretched skin found after resolution of a thrombosed external hemorrhoid or the lower end of a prolapsing internal hemorrhoid and may be found distal to a chronic fissure or arise de novo. Patients with a thrombosed external hemorrhoid present with the sudden onset of acute perianal pain associated with a tender lump. This may come on after a difficult bowel movement and straining or after prolonged sitting or travel. They are very common after labor and delivery. External hemorrhoids always develop beneath the skin at the anal verge and do not extend into the anal canal significantly. On examination, they are found at the anal verge as a bluish, tender, rubbery lump. Bleeding is not a major symptom of external hemorrhoids except in the occasional patient in whom the skin has ulcerated and some of the clot extrudes.

Treatment depends on symptoms. During the first 2 to 3 days, the pain is fairly severe and local excision of the vessel and clot along with a small wedge of overlying skin is warranted. Unless the hemorrhoids are extensive, this is usually done in the office using local anesthesia. This procedure gives prompt relief. The skin is left open and heals over in 2 to 3 weeks. Incision with clot evacuation is not recommended, as the thrombosis will recur and there may be persistent bleeding. If the symptoms are waning, symptomatic relief with tub baths and oral analgesics is all that is necessary. All patients are placed on a bowel management program. There is no role for topical agents or suppositories.

ANAL FISSURE

An anal fissure starts as a simple cut or split in the skin of the lower anal canal, usually due to altered bowel habits, primarily constipation and hard stools. Diarrhea can also be causative. Excessive tension within the anal canal due to a tight internal sphincter muscle is the culprit in a minority of patients. Fissures may be single or multiple and acute or chronic. Acute fissures are quite painful and may be associated with bleeding. Pain is sharp and stabbing with bowel movements and can last from minutes to hours afterwards. It may be annoying or incapacitating. Bleeding is bright red in color and may be seen on the toilet tissue or streaking the stools. The vast majority of fissures are located posteriorly in the anoderm, although occasionally they are found anteriorly. Laterally positioned fissures are uncommon and raise the issue of an associated disorder such as Crohn's disease, HIV infection, anal sepsis, or trauma. Occasionally, a fissure may develop into a fistula, more commonly when one of the above disorders is present. Chronic fissures may be intermittently or persistently symptomatic; the typical triad of findings on examination is composed of the fissure itself, a skin tag below at the anal verge, and a hypertrophied papilla above at the dentate line. Examination must be performed very gently because the patient is often anxious and in pain. The perineum is inspected and the anal verge is slightly separated to see into the low canal. All fissures arise in this region and most are not visible until the anal verge is separated. Once visualization is achieved, the examination can be stopped if the patient is in too much pain and completed at a later date after the acute process is resolved.

Acute fissures are treated conservatively with a rigorous bowel management program, warm tub baths several times a day for pain relief and sphincter relaxation, and oral and occasionally topical analgesics. There is no role for topical agents containing steroids or suppositories of any kind. The vast majority of fissures (90 to 95%) heal completely within 6 to 8 weeks with symptomatic improvement in days to weeks. Patients with a fissure that fails to heal are candidates for lateral internal sphincterotomy to reduce the resting pressure of the internal sphincter. Anorectal manometry to document high resting pressures is useful. Sphincterotomy is successful in 95% of patients with persistent fissures but carries a small risk of some degree of incontinence. Topical 0.2% Nitropaste placed in the anal canal may reduce spasms and has recently been used with some success, although it is not yet felt to be standard therapy. Some patients experience severe headaches with this drug.

ANORECTAL ABSCESS

Anorectal abscesses are the acute manifestation of perirectal sepsis, while fistulas are the chronic result. Most perirectal abscesses start with occlusion of one of the anal gland ducts in the dentate line crypts by feces, inflammation, or trauma. The bacteria that normally live in the ducts and glands then multiply, causing the infection (the cryptoglandular theory of perirectal sepsis). As the infection expands, it extends along the path of least resistance. The cavity may be primarily located in one of the four spaces previously described: perianal, ischiorectal, intersphincteric, or supralevator. The perianal and ischiorectal types of abscesses are by far the most common. (Abscesses and fistulas are always described by their relationship to the sphincter muscles because of the implications for treatment.) The differential diagnosis of a perirectal abscess includes hidradenitis suppurativa and pilonidal disease. Patients present with complaints of increasing, persistent, and often severe pain usually lasting 1 to 4 days. They notice an enlarging mass, which is very tender, and they may have fever, chills, sweating, and malaise if the infection is extensive. Occasionally, the abscess will have spontaneously drained and the patient will have a malodorous discharge and some relief. There may be a history of prior abscesses with spontaneous or surgical drainage. On examination, there is an erythematous, indurated mass that is extremely tender, and fluctuance may be palpated. If the abscess is high in the ischiorectal fossa or dissecting up to the supralevator space, there may be nothing visible externally, but there will be fullness and marked tenderness in one quadrant on digital examination.

Initially, treatment is the same as for any abscess—incision and drainage. Antibiotics are not necessary unless there is extensive cellulitis or the patient is diabetic or markedly immunocompromised. Antibiotics alone are never indicated, and if there is suspicion of an abscess, the patient should never be sent home with instructions to return when the abscess has "come to a head" or "matured." Referral to a surgeon is preferable. Incision and drainage are usually performed in the office or emergency department, but occasionally patients with extensive processes or possible necrotizing fasciitis may be taken to the operating room. Successful drainage requires an adequate opening or unroofing of the cavity to promote prolonged drainage and avoid premature closure. A local anesthetic is used, and an opening 1 to 2 cm in diameter is created over the area of maximal fluctuance but tending toward the anal verge and avoiding the sphincter muscle. The cavity does not need to be explored or packed. Occasionally, higher cavities may be drained with a mushroom or Pezzer catheter placed to promote drainage. Patients are placed on a bowel management program and given a prescription for an oral analgesic. Dressings are changed two to four times each day in conjunction with a warm tub bath.

FISTULA IN ANO

A fistula is a communicating tract between two epithelially lined surfaces. An anorectal fistula starts in the anal canal or rectum and ends in the perianal skin. Most fistulas arise from the dentate line and are felt to be the consequence of cryptoglandular infection. Anorectal abscesses recur or develop into a fistula roughly 50% of the time, and this is due to a persistent internal opening. Patients presenting with a fistula often have a history of an acute abscess. They note persistent perianal discharge or soreness. Often intermittent discharge alternates with periods of quiescence or gradual swelling followed by rupture with drainage and relief. Examination reveals an external fistula opening on the perianal skin, which may be surrounded by sclerosis or heaped-up skin resembling a nodule. Probing will demonstrate the fistula opening. The tract toward the anal canal may be palpable as a cord of fibrotic tissue. Anoscopy and probing either internally at the dentate line or externally through the opening may identify the course of the fistula, but this may be too uncomfortable to do in the office.

Virtually all fistulas require surgical treatment, the particular procedure depending on the relationship of the fistula tract to the anal sphincter muscles. Low fistulas that traverse only the internal sphincter or a small portion of the external sphincter can be laid open as a primary fistulotomy with the expectation of secondary healing in 1 to 2 months and good function. Midlevel fistulas with more than 40 to 50% of the sphincter below the tract are treated with a staged fistulotomy. At the first procedure the skin and fat are cut, leaving the sphincter intact. The tract and any associated cavity are curetted and a circular drain, or seton, is placed to keep the transsphincteric portion of the tract open and draining while the remaining wound heals. A second-stage fistulotomy is performed 1 to 3 months later to divide the remaining tissues. This reduces the risk of incontinence and improves results dramatically. High fistulas, which account for only a small percentage of fistulas, are repaired with an advancement flap after interval drainage with a seton.

GASTRITIS AND PEPTIC ULCER DISEASE

method of
MICHAEL B. KIMMEY, M.D.
University of Washington Medical Center
Seattle, Washington

Medical practitioners consider the diagnoses of gastritis and peptic ulcer disease together in several clinical situations. Whereas there is overlap between these two diagnoses, they are different pathologically. In many cases, pathologic and diagnostic tests are not available, so a diagnosis is given on the basis of symptoms alone. The astute clinician should distinguish symptoms from a specific diagnosis and tailor therapy for the individual patient on the basis of a current knowledge of the pathophysiologic mechanisms of these diverse conditions.

In this article, the treatment of several upper gastrointestinal problems is divided into categories based on what information is known to the treating clinician. In some instances, this is only symptoms; in other situations, specific diagnostic information is available. An effort to separate these different situations is made because the best prescribing will be done by the clinician who can separate symptoms from diagnosis.

DYSPEPSIA

Dyspepsia is a term used to describe a range of symptoms that originate in the upper gastrointestinal tract. Epigastric pain or discomfort, usually of mild to moderate severity, is the predominant component of dyspepsia. Nausea, vomiting, a sense of indigestion, and anorexia may also be present. The relationship of the symptoms to eating is variable but should be sought. The pain may be relieved, exacerbated, or unaffected by all or only certain types of food.

There are numerous causes of dyspepsia. It is a common symptom of patients with peptic ulcer disease (see later); however, only about 20% of patients with dyspepsia have an ulcer. On evaluation with endoscopy or radiographic contrast-enhanced studies, those without an ulcer are often said to have "nonulcer dyspepsia." This term is also not a specific diagnosis and refers to patients with the symptom of dyspepsia in whom no organic cause can be found. It is usually not possible to distinguish patients with nonulcer dyspepsia from those with an ulcer by symptoms alone. Histologically confirmed gastritis and *Helicobacter pylori* infection (see later) are infrequent causes of dyspepsia.

Several other gastrointestinal conditions may present with dyspepsia as the predominant symptom. Gastroesophageal reflux disease is probably the most common cause when one is identifiable (see the article on gastroesophageal reflux disease). These patients often describe a burning retrosternal discomfort and regurgitation of stomach contents into their mouths or throats. Motility disturbances of the stomach or upper intestine may also cause dyspepsia. Nausea, bloating, and early satiety are other frequent complaints of patients with motility disorders. These patients may also have other intestinal complaints such as diarrhea and/or constipation and are probably afflicted with a variant of the irritable bowel syndrome (see the article on irritable bowel syndrome). Lactose intolerance may also cause dyspepsia along with more typical symptoms of bloating and diarrhea.

Dyspepsia may also be a side effect of several medications, including some antibiotics, medications for osteoporosis, and nonsteroidal anti-inflammatory drugs (NSAIDs). Drugs in this class more commonly cause dyspepsia than ulcers, and most patients with NSAID-associated dyspepsia do not have ulcers.

Cholelithiasis and chronic pancreatitis can sometimes manifest with dyspepsia, although other features usually suggest these diagnoses. When symptomatic, cholelithiasis generally results in severe epigastric pain with radiation to the back or right scapula that lasts for several hours after being precipitated by eating. Pain from chronic pancreatitis may also be precipitated by meals and radiates to the back but is more of a dull, boring pain and is often accompanied by nausea or vomiting.

Evaluation of the Dyspeptic Patient

A complete history and physical examination should be performed to recognize possible causes of dyspepsia and also to identify patients with findings that cause concern for the presence of a more serious problem. Simple laboratory tests such as a blood count, liver enzyme activities, and a serum amylase determination can also be helpful in this regard. Abdominal ultrasonography is an effective screening test when considering gallstones or pancreatitis as a cause of the symptoms. An aggressive diagnostic evaluation is recommended for patients with fever, weight loss, dysphagia, new onset of dyspepsia in individuals older than 45 years, anemia, melena, and hematemesis. Other patients may be candidates for empirical treatment, with further evaluation reserved for those patients whose symptoms are refractory to empirical therapy.

Treatment

Symptoms of dyspepsia usually resolve with effective treatment of its underlying cause (see later). When the cause of dyspepsia is not known, empirical treatment may be attempted if there are no findings to suggest the presence of a serious underlying disease. Reassurance and alleviation of anxiety are sometimes the only interventions required. Some patients may also benefit from treatment with medications.

Drugs that reduce gastric acid are used most commonly for this purpose. In fact, patients often have treated themselves with antacids or over-the-counter (OTC) histamine H_2-receptor blockers before they see a physician. The response to antacids may be of limited duration or associated with side effects of diarrhea when these agents are taken in sufficient quantity. If the response to the OTC H_2 blockers is partial, then prescribing prescription doses of the same medication (two times greater than the OTC dose) will often be effective. A 6-week course of therapy is usually prescribed if there is a beneficial response to allow time for healing of undiagnosed ulcers.

When the patient's dyspepsia is associated with

significant heartburn and regurgitation, use of a proton pump inhibitor may be necessary to control symptoms. Cisapride (Propulsid) may also be useful if the reflux occurs primarily at night or after late evening meals. Cisapride may also be useful for the dyspeptic patient with an underlying motility disorder.

Empirical treatment of dyspepsia with antibiotics is discouraged. Serologic diagnosis of *H. pylori* infection is inexpensive, sensitive, and specific and should be pursued before antibiotics are prescribed (see later). Other medications that have been used with variable success in the treatment of dyspepsia include sucralfate (Carafate) and anticholinergic drugs with or without a sedative or benzodiazepine (Levsin, Donnatal, Librium, others). When nausea is a prominent symptom, use of cisapride, metoclopramide (Reglan), or phenothiazine-type antiemetics (prochlorperazine [Compazine], others) can be helpful.

The empirical treatment of dyspepsia without a firm diagnosis has its drawbacks. The duration of therapy, what to do with relapses on discontinuation of therapy, and how closely to observe the patient all become potential problems for the clinician. Many of these patients ultimately undergo further diagnostic testing including upper endoscopy such that the cost savings from avoiding endoscopy in the short term may not be realized in the long term.

GASTRITIS

The correct definition of gastritis is "inflammation of the stomach." This can be detected reliably only with histologic evaluation of the gastric mucosa. Symptoms of dyspepsia should not be called gastritis. Endoscopic and radiographic appearances are also unreliable and should not be used to make the diagnosis of gastritis.

The main cause of true gastritis is *H. pylori* infection. This common infection causes gastric inflammation but is asymptomatic in the overwhelming majority of those who have it. NSAIDs and bile reflux, especially after gastric surgery, also cause gastritis. Other less frequent causes of gastritis include autoimmune disease associated with vitamin B_{12} deficiency, Crohn's disease of the stomach, sarcoidosis, and rarely syphilis and other infections. Other manifestations of these diseases are usually present that direct the alert physician to the correct diagnosis.

Treatment

Effective treatment of *H. pylori* infection causes resolution of gastric inflammation. The presence of gastritis alone, however, is not an indication for antibiotic treatment. Specific treatment of other causes of gastritis (e.g., avoidance of NSAIDs, prednisone for Crohn's or eosinophilic gastritis, antibiotics for syphilitic gastritis) usually leads to resolution of gastric inflammation.

PEPTIC ULCER DISEASE

Ulcers are breaks or defects in the gastrointestinal mucosal lining that extend into deeper parts of the gastrointestinal wall. They may occur in the esophagus, usually caused by gastroesophageal reflux disease, or in the stomach or duodenum. The latter ulcers have traditionally been called peptic ulcers, although this term implies nothing about etiology. The majority of these ulcers are benign and heal with medical treatment. Duodenal ulcers are rarely malignant; however, between 2 and 4% of otherwise benign-appearing gastric ulcers are really ulcerated adenocarcinomas. This risk for malignant change mandates that all gastric ulcers either be examined by biopsy at the time of diagnosis or have healing confirmed with follow-up imaging studies.

There are other less dramatic differences between gastric and duodenal ulcers. Duodenal ulcers are associated with *H. pylori* infection 80 to 90% of the time, whereas only 70% of patients with gastric ulcers have this infection. The remainder of gastric ulcers are caused predominantly by NSAIDs, medications that have a greater effect on the stomach than on the duodenum. Gastric ulcers are also more difficult to treat than duodenal ulcers, often requiring longer courses of more potent medications.

Cigarette smoking is another factor that contributes to ulcer disease. Smokers have a twofold greater risk for developing an ulcer than do nonsmokers. Smokers are also more likely to have an ulcer complication and have delayed ulcer healing with standard medications. The problem of delayed healing is less pronounced if concomitant *H. pylori* infection is treated. Stress and diet do not contribute significantly to ulcer development. Other rare causes of ulcers include gastric acid hypersecretion (e.g., gastrinoma) and Crohn's disease.

The typical symptoms of a duodenal ulcer are a burning epigastric pain without radiation that is most apparent a few hours after eating or at night. The pain is usually relieved by eating or taking antacids. Gastric ulcers may cause similar symptoms or may be associated with pain that is increased by eating and may be located in the left upper quadrant. Nausea or vomiting may accompany the pain. Ulcers associated with NSAID use are often painless.

Ulcers can also cause life-threatening problems. Bleeding is the most common ulcer complication and may present with anemia, melena, or hematemesis. Prompt gastrointestinal endoscopy is desirable to accurately diagnose and often treat the cause of bleeding. Endoscopic findings also assist in the decision on whether to hospitalize the patient. Perforated ulcers can cause peritonitis and require emergency surgery. Chronic recurrent ulcers can also lead to strictures of the pylorus or duodenum, resulting in gastric outlet obstruction.

The diagnosis of an ulcer is usually made with an upper gastrointestinal x-ray study or with endoscopy. Endoscopy is more sensitive than radiography and allows biopsy of gastric ulcers to exclude malignant disease. However, endoscopy is more expensive than radiography. Upper gastrointestinal x-ray studies are less useful in detecting ulcer recurrences and ulcers after gastric surgery because of scarring and other anatomic alterations.

Treatment

The goals of treating the patient with peptic ulcer disease are the alleviation of symptoms, the avoidance of complications, and the prevention of ulcer recurrence. Pain usually responds within 1 week of beginning medications that inhibit acid secretion (Table 1). Breakthrough pain can be managed with antacids as needed; liquid antacids may be more effective than tablets. Avoiding ulcer complications requires ulcer healing. This is also usually achievable with the same antisecretory medications given for 4 to 12 weeks. Proton pump inhibitors heal most ulcers an average of 2 weeks (for duodenal ulcers) to 4 weeks (for gastric ulcers) faster than H_2 blockers.

Other treatments that promote ulcer healing are also available. Sucralfate is an organic complex of aluminum that binds to ulcers and promotes healing through several potential mechanisms. The prostaglandin analogue misoprostol (Cytotec)* also promotes ulcer healing, but medication-related side effects limit compliance with this drug. Stopping NSAIDs and treating *H. pylori* infection also have beneficial effects on ulcer healing that are independent of the prevention of recurrence. Diet and reduction in activity have no role in the treatment of peptic ulcer disease.

Surgery for uncomplicated ulcer disease is fortunately only of historical interest. Vagotomy with or without antrectomy cured ulcers but at the expense of numerous side effects, such as dumping syndrome and bile reflux gastritis. Surgery is now reserved for ulcer complications: bleeding ulcers that cannot be stopped with endoscopy, perforated ulcers, and gastric outlet obstruction that is not adequately treated with endoscopic balloon dilatation.

Approximately two thirds of ulcers recur within 1 year of ulcer healing, and about half of these recurrences are symptomatic. Successful treatment of *H. pylori* infection reduces annual ulcer recurrences to less than 10%. *H. pylori* infection should be sought and treated if it is present in all patients with ulcers. Even if the patient has another potential reason for ulcers, such as NSAID use, the *H. pylori* infection should still be treated.

The majority of ulcer patients without *H. pylori* infection are taking NSAIDs. These drugs should be avoided if possible and less ulcerogenic medications substituted (Table 2). When NSAIDs are required for inflammatory-type pain, co-therapy with misoprostol has been shown to reduce the frequency of recurrent ulcers and ulcer complications. When misoprostol is not tolerated owing to side effects of diarrhea and abdominal cramping, use of a proton pump inhibitor also reduces the frequency of ulcer recurrence. Avoidance of NSAIDs is the best strategy because none of the prophylactic regimens completely eliminates the risk for recurrent ulcers and ulcer complications.

Patients who do not have *H. pylori* infection and who are not taking NSAIDs require special consideration. Serum gastrin levels should be checked to detect the rare patient with gastrinoma. In this condition, ulcers are typically multiple and may be associated with diarrhea caused by the high levels of acid secretion. Long-term treatment of ulcer patients who do not have an underlying cause identified has not been well defined. Those without ulcer complications can be followed up after ulcer healing. If they have recurrent ulcers or if an ulcer complication is present, maintenance therapy should be considered. Full doses of H_2 blockers, twice-daily sucralfate, or single doses of a proton pump inhibitor are all reasonable options for these infrequent patients.

TABLE 1. **Drugs Used for Ulcer Healing**

Agent	Dose	Duration (wk)	
		Duodenal Ulcer	*Gastric Ulcer*
Antacids			
Magnesium-aluminum hydroxides (Mylanta, Maalox, Riopan, others)	30 mL qid	6	Not advised
Aluminum hydroxides (Amphojel, ALternaGEL)	30 mL qid	6	Not advised
Calcium carbonates (Tums, others)	1000 mg qid	6	Not advised
H_2-Receptor Antagonists			
Cimetidine (Tagamet)	400 mg bid	6	8–12*
Ranitidine (Zantac)	150 mg bid	6	8–12*
Nizatidine (Axid)	150 mg bid	6	8–12*
Famotidine (Pepcid)	20 mg bid *or* 40 mg hs	6	8–12*
Proton Pump Inhibitors			
Omeprazole (Prilosec)	20 mg qd	4	—
	20 mg bid	—	4–8*
Lansoprazole (Prevacid)	30 mg qd	4	—
	30 mg bid	—	4–8*
Others			
Sucralfate (Carafate)	1 gm qid	8	8–12*

*Longer durations are recommended for large (>2 cm) ulcers.

HELICOBACTER PYLORI INFECTION

H. pylori selectively colonizes gastric-type epithelium, leading to a local inflammatory reaction (gastri-

*Not FDA approved for this indication.

TABLE 2. **Ulcer Risk of Analgesic and Anti-inflammatory Drugs**

No risk
Acetaminophen (Tylenol)
Tramadol (Ultram)
Narcotics (numerous agents)
Low risk
Nonacetylated salicylates
Salsalate (Disalcid)
Choline-magnesium trisalicylate (Trilisate)
Moderate risk
Low-dose aspirin (<325 mg/d)
Etodolac (Lodine)
Nabumetone (Relafen)
Higher risk
Aspirin (in higher doses)
Diclofenac (Voltaren, Cataflam)
Diflunisal (Dolobid)
Fenoprofen (Nalfon)
Ibuprofen (Motrin, Advil,* Nuprin*)
Indomethacin (Indocin)
Ketoprofen (Orudis, Oruvail, Actron*)
Ketorolac (Toradol)
Mefenamic acid (Ponstel)
Meclofenamate
Naproxen (Naprosyn, Aleve*)
Oxaprozin (Daypro)
Piroxicam (Feldene)
Tolmetin (Tolectin)
Highest risk for ulcer bleeding
NSAIDs plus steroids or oral anticoagulants

*Available without a prescription in the United States.
Abbreviation: NSAIDs = nonsteroidal anti-inflammatory drugs.

tis) and a systemic immune response. This is probably the most common bacterial infection of humans. Most evidence suggests that it is transmitted between humans by the fecal-oral or oral-oral routes. It is more common in developing than in developed countries and is more prevalent in lower socioeconomic groups. In developed countries, infection is much more common in those born before World War II than in those born later.

Acute infection with *H. pylori* causes abdominal pain and a temporary reduction in acid secretion by the stomach. Chronic infection with its resultant gastritis is usually asymptomatic, however. As discussed before, *H. pylori* is associated with most cases of ulcers, probably through a variety of mechanisms. These include increased levels of acid secretion and reduced mucosal defenses caused by the infection. *H. pylori* infection is also associated with gastric cancer and gastric lymphoma, although other factors are likely to play a role in the pathogenesis of these malignant neoplasms.

There are several ways to diagnose *H. pylori* infection. All of the available tests have sensitivities and specificities above 90% for detecting *H. pylori* infection. The choice of test depends primarily on the specific clinical situation. Detection of antibodies to *H. pylori* in either serum or whole blood is the least invasive and least expensive. Serology should be used for diagnosis of infection when endoscopy is not required. Serology is less useful for documenting treatment response because antibodies persist for years after successful treatment. When endoscopy is being done for other reasons, three biopsy specimens should be taken from the gastric antrum. One of the biopsy specimens can be placed into one of several available rapid urease tests, which may give a positive result within 1 hour. If the rapid urease test result is negative, the other two biopsy specimens can be sent for histologic evaluation of the presence of gastritis and for special stains that demonstrate *H. pylori*. Confirmation of effective *H. pylori* treatment, when needed (see later), is best achieved by a carbon-labeled urea breath test administered at least 1 month after antibiotics have been stopped.

Treatment

The primary indication for treating *H. pylori* is current or past ulcer disease. Other less common indications include the rare patient who has gastric mucosa-associated lymphoid tissue (MALT) lymphoma and possibly the patient who has a first-degree relative with gastric cancer. Less accepted indications are patients with nonulcer dyspepsia. Most double-blind, placebo-controlled studies in *H. pylori*–positive dyspeptic subjects have not shown a significant advantage to *H. pylori* eradication.

Numerous antibiotic regimens have been proposed for the treatment of *H. pylori* infection (Table 3). Combinations of two or three antibiotics are required to eradicate this organism. Adding an agent that reduces gastric acid secretion (e.g., omeprazole [Prilosec], lansoprazole [Prevacid], or ranitidine [Zantac]) improves eradication rates and reduces the upper gastrointestinal side effects that are associated with the antibiotics. When an ulcer is present, these drugs also reduce ulcer pain and speed ulcer healing. Compliance with these often complicated multidrug regimens is also important. All of the regimens listed in Table 3 should achieve eradication of *H. pylori* in more than 80% of patients if they are compliant with taking the medications.

Several factors should be considered in selecting an *H. pylori* treatment regimen for the individual patient. Up to one half of isolates of *H. pylori* are resistant to metronidazole (Flagyl), so this antibiotic should not be used if the patient has had metronidazole use in the past. Resistance to clarithromycin (Biaxin) is less common (less than 10%), and resistance to amoxicillin (Amoxil) is nonexistent currently. Reliability and compliance of the patient, cost of treatment regimen, and whether a coexisting ulcer is present are other factors that affect treatment choice. For most patients, the 10-day, twice-daily regimen of a proton pump inhibitor (omeprazole or lansoprazole) with two antibiotics (clarithromycin and either amoxicillin or metronidazole) is the treatment of choice because it is simple and effective in more than 90% of patients.

Recurrence of infection after successful treatment is uncommon. Recurrence rates of about 2% in the first year and less than 1% annually in subsequent years have been reported. Routine surveillance for

TABLE 3. **Treatment Regimens for *Helicobacter pylori***

Agent	Dose	Duration (d)
Bismuth-Based Therapy		
Triple therapy*		14
Bismuth subsalicylate (Pepto-Bismol)	525 mg qid	
Tetracycline†	500 mg qid	
Metronidazole (Flagyl)	250 mg qid	
Triple therapy + proton pump inhibitor	(see above)	
Omeprazole (Prilosec)	20 mg bid	7
or		
Lansoprazole (Prevacid)	30 mg bid	7
Ranitidine bismuth citrate (Tritec)	400 mg bid	14‡
plus		
Clarithromycin (Biaxin)	500 mg tid	14
Dual Therapy		
Omeprazole (Prilosec)	20 mg bid	14
or		
Lansoprazole (Prevacid)	30 mg bid	14
plus		
Clarithromycin (Biaxin)§	500 mg tid	14
Proton Pump Inhibitor with Two Antibiotics		
Omeprazole (Prilosec)	20 mg bid	10
or		
Lansoprazole (Prevacid)	30 mg bid	10
plus		
Clarithromycin (Biaxin)	500 mg bid	10
plus		
Amoxicillin (Amoxil)‖	1000 mg bid	10

*Also available in a prepackaged multidose form (Helidac).
†Amoxicillin (500 mg qid) can be substituted for tetracycline, but efficacy is reduced by about 20%.
‡Can be continued for an additional 2 wk to achieve duodenal ulcer healing.
§Use of amoxicillin instead of clarithromycin has unacceptably low success rates and should not be a first-line regimen.
‖Metronidazole (500 mg bid) can be substituted for amoxicillin if there is a history of penicillin allergy.

recurrent infection and even for the effectiveness of eradication is not advised for most patients. The main exception is patients who have had ulcer complications and those with MALT lymphoma. Eradication should be confirmed in these patients by repeated endoscopy and biopsy or the urea breath test before antisecretory therapy is discontinued.

SUMMARY

A knowledge of the differences and overlaps between dyspepsia, gastritis, and peptic ulcer disease will lead to more effective prescribing practices. These conditions are common, so diagnostic testing is used selectively. However, widespread treatment of *H. pylori* infection is not advocated because of limited information about the effectiveness and consequences of this treatment except in patients with ulcer disease. In these patients, *H. pylori* eradication can produce a dramatic reduction in health care costs and improvement in the quality of the patient's life.

ACUTE AND CHRONIC VIRAL HEPATITIS

method of
W. G. E. COOKSLEY, M.B., B.S., M.D.
Royal Brisbane Hospital
Brisbane, Queensland, Australia

The terms "acute" and "chronic hepatitis" refer to a group of hepatotrophic viral diseases with the nomenclature A to E (and possibly G). Hepatitis B is a DNA virus, while the others are RNA viruses. Hepatitis A and E are spread by the gastrointestinal route and hepatitis B, C, and D by the parenteral route. Hepatitis A and E produce acute hepatitis only, whereas the others can all progress to chronic liver disease. In most cases the liver damage is due to immune elimination of infected liver cells. Other viruses such as yellow fever virus, Epstein-Barr virus, rubella and cytomegalovirus can also cause hepatitis. Furthermore, nonviral liver diseases such as alcoholic liver disease, Wilson's disease, and autoimmune hepatitis can also simulate viral hepatitis.

HEPATITIS A

Hepatitis A virus is transmitted via contaminated food or water. Following a short incubation period of 3 to 6 weeks, there may be a mild, often subclinical infection in children, most of whom are anicteric, whereas the majority of adults are icteric. The disease is characterized by elevation of alanine aminotransferase (ALT) and IgM anti-HAV followed by clinical and biochemical resolution. About 20% of patients will have a biochemical or clinical relapse, but chronicity does not occur. Mortality is low overall but may be substantial in middle-aged or elderly patients. The pattern of infection varies throughout the world. In industrialized countries, most people have not been exposed to the virus unless they are middle-aged or older. In developing countries hepatitis A is uncommon in urban environments but is still a major problem in rural areas where sanitation is poor. In some parts of the world, infection is still hyperendemic, with most people being infected in childhood. As a result, the presence of antibodies and therefore immunity follows a sigmoid-shaped curve with age, with different proportions of the population at risk. Outside developing countries, the major risk is now to travelers visiting underdeveloped or developing countries. Other at-risk groups include institutionalized people, the military, and staff, children, and parents at preschool centers. The virus is transmitted by the fecal/oral route prior to the development of symptoms, and since children are usually anicteric, infection spreads from them to their parents, leading to miniepidemics. Intravenous drug users may also be at risk due to poor personal hygiene. Finally, it is recommended that restaurant workers be immunized to protect their patrons.

All of these high-risk groups should be vaccinated against hepatitis A. Immune globulin (ISG)* is still available and should be offered to close contacts of patients with acute hepatitis A at a dosage of 0.02 to 0.06 mL per kg, provided it can be administered within 10 days of exposure. These individuals, of course, will not be protected against future exposure. Hepatitis A remains the most prevalent serious infection for which travelers are at risk, and vaccine (Havrix) should be offered to anyone planning to visit an endemic area. Since travelers requiring vaccination often seek advice too late to receive two injections of vaccine of 720 IU at monthly intervals, a single injection of 1440 units is recommended. A third injection 6 months later will offer maximum long-term protection.

There are no antiviral agents for hepatitis A, and treatment is essentially symptomatic, with recommendations for rest, a low-fat, high-carbohydrate diet, adequate fluids, and avoidance of alcohol. Hospitalization is usually unnecessary unless there is prolongation of the prothrombin time, edema, or clouding of consciousness. Such patients should be referred to a liver center, as transplantation may be necessary for fulminant hepatitis.

HEPATITIS B

Despite effective vaccines and treatments for hepatitis B, this disease still remains a major cause of chronic liver disease and hepatocellular carcinoma. In Asia and sub-Saharan Africa, the most common route of transmission is from mother to baby in the perinatal period. In contrast, in countries with a low frequency of hepatitis B such as in Europe and North America, infection usually occurs in adults as a result of sexual spread. Virtually 100% of patients infected in the neonatal period become chronic carriers, whereas those infected as adults usually recover, with only a few percent becoming chronic carriers. Childhood infection carries an intermediate risk of becoming a carrier.

The World Health Organization targeted 1997 as the year for all countries to introduce universal immunization to eradicate hepatitis B. The first injection of vaccine is administered as close to birth as possible (particularly within 24 hours), and subsequent injections as part of the expanded program for immunization. Some countries have also introduced catch-up programs for preschool children and for preadolescents to provide immunity before sexual maturity. A number of vaccines are available, including both recombinant and plasma-derived types. These contain the surface antigen and may have preS antigen in addition. Hyperimmune globulin (HBIG) is also available but is expensive and in limited supply. It is usually administered within a few hours of birth, in addition to vaccine, to those babies whose mothers are carriers of hepatitis B surface antigen.

Other modes of infection include transfusion of blood or blood products, needlestick injuries in health care workers and intravenous drug users, and tattoos and other skin piercing. Childhood acquisition can occur, usually within the first few years of life, often from a family member or from children at a preschool center. Infection during the school years is less common but can occur when children have skin lesions, sores, cuts, or wounds. Participation in contact sports appears to be another means of transmission. Although the vaccines available are highly effective, experience in high-incidence countries has shown that the carrier rate is reduced from about 10% to about 1% of the population, and it will probably be many decades before this disease is eradicated. Nonresponse to the vaccine can occur, particularly in middle-aged people who are overweight, who smoke, or who are immunosuppressed. Further injections may be necessary, but even then some people will fail to respond to the vaccine. If they are health care workers, exposure to hepatitis B should be treated with HBIG.

In assessing hepatitis B infection, HBsAg indicates the presence of infection. Antibodies to HBs indicate recovery from infection. In a person who is HBsAg positive, replication is indicated by serum HBeAg and HBV DNA. Loss of replication is marked by anti-HBe and undetectable HBV DNA.

Following perinatal transmission of hepatitis B, the child is asymptomatic with normal ALT but very high levels of virus. This is referred to as the immunotolerant phase of infection and usually remains until adolescence, but with wide variation. Loss of tolerance to the virus then occurs, resulting in elevation of ALT. HBeAg and HBV DNA are still detectable, although the levels are lower than in the immunotolerant phase. This phase is referred to as the immunoeliminative phase and may be successful with loss of HBeAg and HBV DNA and normalization of ALT (the latent phase). Unsuccessful attempts at eradication of infection lead to liver damage. Ongoing chronic hepatitis may eventually lead to cirrhosis and hepatocellular cancer.

In adult infection, about one third of patients will have a clinical illness with anorexia, lethargy, and sometimes jaundice, while others will simply have a biochemical and virologic hepatitis. The hallmark of an acute viral infection is the presence of IgM anti-HBc. Since there is no tolerance to the virus, the ALT level will rise immediately, and in more than 95% of individuals loss of HBeAg and HBsAg will occur, with normalization of ALT over the next few weeks or months. Failure to eliminate the virus, however, leads to the chronic carrier stage (i.e., HBsAg-positive status for more than 6 months). While patients remain HBeAg positive, they continue to have ongoing liver damage, often with lethargy, which may progress to cirrhosis within a few years. These patients lose HBeAg with normalization of ALT at the rate of about 5% per annum. Transplantation may be necessary in those progressing to end-stage liver disease.

In patients with cirrhosis, particularly those who

*Not available in the United States.

have had perinatal infection, hepatocellular carcinoma (HCC) can develop, but it can also occur in the absence of cirrhosis. In cirrhotic patients over the age of 40, a surveillance program should be set up with ultrasound examination and measurement of alpha fetoprotein measurements every 4 to 6 months. Treatment of HCC is complex but includes surgical excision and percutaneous ethanol injection.

Treatment of hepatitis B is restricted to those patients who have viral replication (positive HBeAg and detectable HBV DNA) and liver damage (elevated ALT). In such patients, the optimal treatment is 9 mIU subcutaneously of interferon alfa-2a (Roferon-A) or 10 mIU of interferon alfa-2b (Intron A), three times a week for 4 to 6 months. After several months, a seroconversion flare is noted with an increase in ALT followed by loss of HBeAg and normalization of ALT. This seroconversion occurs in about 30 to 40% of patients and is more likely in those whose HBV DNA is low (less than 100 pg per mL by the liquid hybridization assay or less than 1000 pg per mL by the RNA hybrid capture assay) and who have moderately active disease (ALT more than three times the reference range). Patients who fail to respond should be reassessed in 6 to 12 months. A further course of treatment possibly with a higher dose or with pretreatment pulse steroids may be considered. The same interferon treatment program should be offered to those who acquired the infection perinatally once they are in the immunoeliminative phase with elevated ALT and reduced HBV DNA. Treatment during the immunotolerant phase has been shown to be ineffective. Some studies suggest that the treatment in patients with perinatal acquisition is probably less successful than in those who acquired the infection as an adult. Although loss of HBeAg alone is sufficient to lead to normalization of ALT, about a third of those patients undergoing loss of HBeAg will also lose surface antigen.

Treatment of children with elevated ALT, patients co-infected with human immunodeficiency virus (HIV) or hepatitis C virus (HCV), patients who are immunosuppressed (e.g., renal disease or liver transplantation), and patients with precore mutants is more complex and should be undertaken in specialist units. Although patients with well-compensated cirrhosis can be treated with interferon, patients with decompensated cirrhosis should not be so treated due to high morbidity and mortality.

Because less than half the patients respond to interferon, newer antiviral agents are undergoing trials, including famciclovir* (Famvir) and lamivudine* (Epiver, Zeflex). The latter agent has been shown to be particularly effective in post-transplantation situations but has also been effective in patients with chronic hepatitis B. The two major problems are the development of lamivudine-resistant mutants and the need for long-term therapy (more than 1 year) to prevent relapse on cessation of the antiviral agents.

*Not available in the United States.

Other novel therapies include therapeutic vaccines. Patients with long-standing chronic hepatitis B are more likely to develop cirrhosis, mutations, and disease that may fluctuate with spontaneous hepatitis flares and remissions. Treatment of these patients is difficult, and response to interferon is often disappointing.

Liver disease in a chronic carrier is not always the result of hepatitis B. In patients who lack HBeAg, active disease may be due to other diseases such as concurrent hepatitis C or D or alcoholic or other liver disease. It may also be due to the development of a precore mutant or to replicating virus whose HBV DNA level is insufficient to be detected by standard assays.

In HBeAg-negative patients, polymerase chain reaction (PCR) is usually positive, and the loss of virus detectable by PCR may indicate that the subject may subsequently lose surface antigen as well. Large studies indicate that spontaneous loss of surface antigen is a relatively rare event, occurring at a rate of about 1% per annum.

HEPATITIS C

Since the development of assays for hepatitis C, this virus has been found to be responsible for the vast majority of cases of what was previously referred to as non-A, non-B hepatitis. The diagnostic test is an enzyme-linked immunosorbent assay (ELISA) test for the presence of antibodies to the virus. The third-generation ELISAs currently in use are directed against a number of viral epitopes, and false-positive and false-negative results are very rare. Confirmation can be carried out using a recombinant immunoblot assay (RIBA) in those patients with a borderline or unconfirmed ELISA. In addition, both qualitative and quantitative PCR tests are available to detect the presence of virus itself. These may occasionally be negative, usually in patients with low levels of virus.

The natural history of this disease is of an often asymptomatic illness following infection with the virus, which resolves in only 10 to 20% of patients and progresses to chronicity in the vast majority. The ELISA usually becomes positive within a month or two after infection. Although hepatitis C–induced end-stage liver disease is now the major indicator for liver transplantation in most developed countries, the majority of infected patients have much milder disease, with about 80% remaining noncirrhotic. The disease is characterized by slow progression histologically, with about 20% of patients developing cirrhosis after 20 years. Follow-up studies in post-transfusional hepatitis 20 years after infection indicate a small increase in liver-related mortality only. Studies from Italy in elderly patients suggest the majority of patients will remain infected for most of their lives and be ELISA and PCR positive, although many will have normal ALT. Therefore, in management of hepatitis C, liver biopsy is performed on those with elevated ALT. Indications for therapy include symptoms, medium or severe hepatitis histologically, or the presence of fibrosis on biopsy.

Risk factors for hepatitis C include transfusion of blood or blood products prior to screening with ELISA; a history of IV drug use, even on only one or two occasions; and other forms of body piercing such as tattoos. Health care workers may be at higher risk, with data indicating that about 5% of needlestick injuries result in hepatitis C. Sexual spread is uncommon (0 to 5%). Perinatal acquisition is also uncommon, with 1 to 5% of HCV-positive mothers infecting their babies (provided the mother is HIV negative). Infection seems to be dependent on the level of virus titer. In various Mediterranean and Asian countries, there is a higher risk of sporadic infection, particularly in older people; this may be due to medical procedures undergone in the pre-disposables era (e.g., vaccination). Nosocomial infections have been recognized in dialysis units and hematology units and can be spread by surgeons. Household spread probably occurs rarely, but sharing of personal items like toothbrushes and razors should be avoided.

Following infection, the majority of patients are asymptomatic and seek testing because of the risk of exposure. Most symptomatic patients present because of lethargy; few have clinical evidence of liver disease. Liver function tests usually indicate a mild elevation in ALT and AST, but synthetic function usually remains intact. Excess alcohol probably has an additive effect, causing a more rapid progression to cirrhosis. Viral genotypes, viral load, age, gender, iron intake, quasispecies, and nonalcoholic steatohepatitis may all promote progression. The clinical course fluctuates in some patients, and symptoms do not correlate with the severity of the disease. Patients are usually referred to as having chronic hepatitis with inflammation in the portal tracts in the periportal region and within the lobules. The terms "chronic persistent" and "chronic active hepatitis" are no longer used. The duration of infection is the major determinant of the extent of fibrosis. Cirrhosis is often present histologically in the absence of clinical findings. Hepatocellular carcinoma is a complication of cirrhosis, occurring at a rate of about 2% per annum.

The goals of treatment are to eradicate the infection before the development of cirrhosis and, if cirrhosis has occurred, to prevent progression to liver failure or transplant. Patients with cirrhosis may need to undergo a surveillance program with alphafetoprotein measurements and ultrasound every 6 months. The basis for treatment is interferon-alfa, which occurs in several forms: interferon alfa-2a (Roferon-A),* alfa-2b (Intron A), lymphoblastoid (natural) interferon† (Wellferon), and consensus interferon (Interferon con1).* Many studies around the world have shown that treatment with interferon alfa, 3 mIU three times a week subcutaneously for 6 months, will normalize ALT in about half the patients. However by the end of therapy about half will have experienced relapse, so that a response sustained for more than 6 months occurs in only about a quarter of patients. Long-term follow-up studies indicate that most patients who relapse will do so within the first 6 to 12 months.

*Not available in the United States.
†Orphan drug in the United States.

Fever, myalgias and arthralgias, headache, particularly within the first 2 weeks, and change in mood with irritability and mild depression are the most common of a large number of reported side effects. About 10% of patients will withdraw from the program because of side effects. In view of the relatively low proportion of successful outcomes and the frequency of side effects, the decision to treat is made on the basis of symptoms and presence of fibrosis or active hepatitis histologically in patients without a significant psychiatric history. Patients with cirrhosis can be treated, but the results are fairly disappointing unless high doses and/or longer duration are offered. Patients with Child's stage B or C cirrhosis should not be treated due to potential complications but instead referred for liver transplant.

Negative predictors of response include age older than 60 and cirrhosis. Genotype and pretreatment virus level also appear to be important.

Nonresponders rarely respond to a second course of therapy, and only about 10% of relapsers will respond to a second course. In the last few years, new protocols have undergone clinical trials, and current data indicate that ribavirin† (Virazole) (a nucleoside analogue) in combination with interferon is likely to be effective in about 50% of relapsers. Studies have also indicated that patients are less likely to relapse following 12 months rather than 6 months of therapy. Higher doses initially (induction therapy) cause a more rapid decrease in HCV RNA levels. To maximize these and to minimize side effects, it has been suggested that optimal therapy may be interferon, 6 mIU three times a week for 4 months, followed by 3 mIU three times a week for 8 months. Even higher induction doses may be advocated in future in relapsers and nonresponders, and studies are in progress.

It has been suggested that if the ALT is still abnormal at 3 or 4 months, interferon therapy should be stopped. Patients who are negative for HCV-RNA by PCR at 1 month are more likely to be sustained responders. Long-term follow-up studies indicate that of patients who have normal ALT at the end of the study and remain that way for 6 more months, about half will still be PCR positive, albeit at very low levels. Those at higher levels are more likely to relapse. Clearly, with the large number of new protocols, modified interferons, and antiviral agents undergoing evaluation at present, optimal treatment

*Not available in the United States.
†Not FDA approved for this indication.

for this disease is likely to change over the next few years.

There have also been suggestions that interferon can prevent the development of hepatocellular carcinoma in patients with cirrhosis. This remains a controversial area.

HEPATITIS D

The causative agent of hepatitis D is a defective RNA viroid that expresses hepatitis D antigen surrounded by a core of HBsAg. Hepatitis D, therefore, occurs only in patients who are also carriers for hepatitis B. Its geographic distribution is similar to that of hepatitis B, except that the disease is relatively uncommon in Asia. Infection produces serious liver disease in some individuals and relatively mild illness in others. In Western countries, hepatitis D infection is usually seen in people with a past history of IV drug sharing, and these patients will usually be positive for hepatitis B, C, and D as a result. The disease cannot be differentiated from hepatitis B and C clinically and the diagnosis is serologic. Patients with hepatitis D may be co-infected with hepatitis B or the hepatitis D may be superimposed in a hepatitis B carrier. Usually patients with hepatitis D will have more severe liver disease and often will have progressed to cirrhosis at the time of the initial diagnosis. The frequency of hepatitis D is decreasing in many countries.

Treatment is rather disappointing, as standard doses of interferon are usually ineffective. A higher dose of interferon, perhaps 9 mIU daily* for a longer period of time, may be helpful, but many patients cannot tolerate the side effects. Patients with end-stage liver disease due to hepatitis D who require transplantation may not experience re-infection of their new liver. Prevention of hepatitis D largely depends on prevention of hepatitis B by immunization, but this does not offer protection to people who are already hepatitis B carriers.

HEPATITIS E

Hepatitis E virus is an enterically transmitted virus that causes extensive epidemics in a broad belt across the tropical and subtropical areas of the world, particularly central America, India, Asia, and Africa. The incubation period of approximately 6 weeks is followed by acute, self-limited hepatitis with no chronicity. A high mortality rate has been noted in epidemics, particularly among pregnant women. A specific assay is available, and it should be performed in travelers returning with hepatitis.

HEPATITIS F

The putative identification of a new virus, hepatitis F, in samples from a patient with hepatitis has been retracted.

*Exceeds dosage recommended by the manufacturer.

HEPATITIS G VIRUS (GBV-C AGENT)

It is still uncertain whether this agent is hepatotropic or gives rise to clinical liver disease. Following its discovery several years ago, measurement of the virus by PCR has shown it to be common in blood donors, with up to 4% being positive for RNA and a similar percentage having antibodies. It is also frequent in patients who have had parenteral exposure, such as IV drug users, patients with chronic hepatitis C, and patients who have had multiple blood transfusions such as hemophiliacs. Well-controlled trials including longitudinal studies have failed to show evidence of hepatic damage. For example, the frequency of infection is identical in blood donors with normal ALT and those with elevated ALT. There still are claims that this virus can give rise to acute, and indeed fulminant, hepatitis, but other studies dispute this. It does not appear to be the cause of non–A to E hepatitis.

MALABSORPTION

method of
WILLIAM A. ROWE, M.D.
Pennsylvania State University College of Medicine
Hershey, Pennsylvania

The primary function of the gastrointestinal tract is the absorption of fluid and nutrients. Failure of this absorptive process is generally referred to as malabsorption. Malabsorption is most commonly caused by dysfunction in the upper gastrointestinal tract. It can be generalized and affect all nutrients, or it can be specific, involving a single substance.

Evaluation of malabsorption relies heavily on an understanding of normal physiology. In this article, most attention is given to fat malabsorption, or steatorrhea. This is because the methods of detecting increased fecal fat are relatively simple, and colonic bacteria metabolize only a very small fraction of unabsorbed fat during its transit through the colon. Although malabsorption of carbohydrate and protein can occur in the adult patient, with the exception of lactose intolerance, these disorders are much more likely to present in childhood.

PROTEIN MALABSORPTION

After ingestion, proteins are emulsified in the mouth and in the stomach and digested by gastric and pancreatic proteases and peptidases. The products of digestion that are delivered to the small bowel for absorption are free amino acids and small peptides. Because of the ability of the intestinal mucosa to absorb incompletely digested peptides, it is very unusual to observe protein malabsorption in the absence of fat and/or carbohydrate malabsorption. The peptides are absorbed and further broken down in the enterocyte into free amino acids and together with the absorbed amino acids are delivered into the portal vein.

Enzymatic deficiencies in protein digestion can occur in

pancreatic insufficiency, but, as noted, this is almost always accompanied by steatorrhea. Mucosal uptake abnormalities (not diagnosed in infancy) occur with substantial loss of intestinal mucosa and are often associated not just with protein malabsorption but often with a protein-losing enteropathy (such as inflammatory bowel disease).

CARBOHYDRATE MALABSORPTION

Carbohydrates are ingested primarily as disaccharides and polysaccharides. Digestion begins with salivary amylase, and intestinal carbohydrases break down more complex polysaccharides into mono- and disaccharides. Associated with the intestinal mucosa are multiple disaccharidases (sucrase, lactase, isomaltase, maltase), which break down the disaccharides into monosaccharides. The monosaccharides are then absorbed by a large variety of monosaccharide transport proteins and passed without alteration into the portal vein.

Because of the abundance of disaccharides in the diet, malabsorption of carbohydrate is generally caused by a deficiency of one of the mucosal disaccharidases. Although deficiencies in one of the other disaccharidases are occasionally seen in the neonatal and pediatric population, lactase deficiency is by far the most common in both pediatric and adult populations. Lactase deficiency can be either congenital or acquired; acquired lactase deficiency can occur after a viral gastroenteritis as well as with normal aging if lactose (milk sugar) is only rarely consumed. Deficiency of lactase causes lactose to pass unabsorbed into the colon, where the osmotic load of the lactose and its breakdown products cause an osmotic diarrhea.

FAT MALABSORPTION

Triglycerides, the major chemical constituent of animal fat and vegetable oil, are an important caloric source, accounting for 36% of calories in the typical American diet. Fat contains 9 calories per gram and as such it is a concentrated caloric source.

The evaluation of fat malabsorption is based on knowledge of the normal physiology of fat absorption and upon evaluation of potential defects in one of the steps involved in normal fat absorption. The treatment of malabsorption is then generally aimed at correction of the underlying defect.

Mechanism of Fat Absorption

FAT EMULSIFICATION

The initial step in fat absorption is the emulsification of dietary fat (Figure 1). This initially occurs by mastication, followed by gastric mixing. The gastric contractions move material toward an initially closed pylorus, with a resultant retrograde current of gastric contents. This movement creates a shearing action, which helps emulsify the fat, with the emulsified fat generally being stabilized by other dietary constituents. Within the small intestine, peristalsis continues to assist in fat emulsification, although in the small intestine, bile is the usual stabilizing agent. The end result of this emulsification is an increase in the surface area of the fatty constituents of the diet that can be exposed to luminal contents, and thus there is an increase in the amount of lipolysis that can take place. Lipolysis is also initiated in the stomach to a small but significant degree by gastric lipase.

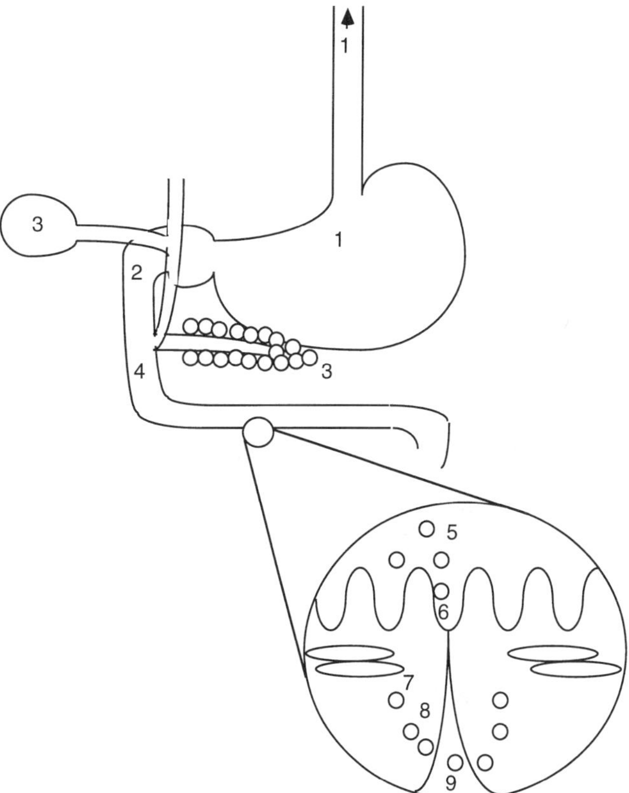

Figure 1. Normal physiology of fat absorption. (1) Emulsification; (2) stimulation of cholecystokinin release; (3) stimulation of bile and pancreatic enzyme release; (4) pancreatic lipolysis; (5) micellar solubilization by bile acids; (6) mucosal uptake of mixed micelles; (7) triglyceride resynthesis; (8) chylomicron formation; (9) lymphatic transport.

CHOLECYSTOKININ RELEASE

The next step in fat absorption occurs when fatty acids (as well as amino acids and peptides) enter the duodenum. As fat enters the duodenum, cholecystokinin is released.

STIMULATION OF BILE AND PANCREATIC ENZYME RELEASE

Cholecystokinin in turn stimulates gallbladder contraction and pancreatic secretion. It also causes relaxation of the sphincter of Oddi. As a result, bile is discharged into the duodenum. Cholecystokinin also induces the discharge of zymogen granules into the pancreatic acini. These pancreatic enzymes and proenzymes then enter the duodenum, where the proenzymes are activated by enzyme enterokinase (located on the surface of intestinal enterocytes). The active enzymes then hydrolyze dietary fat, releasing more fatty acids, which in turn provide positive feedback as the increasing concentration of fatty acids in the intestinal lumen stimulates the release of more cholecystokinin.

PANCREATIC LIPOLYSIS

Breakdown of triglycerides into fatty acids is essential for micelle formation and fat absorption. Although a small amount of lipolysis occurs in the stomach, pancreatic lipase is responsible for the vast majority of hydrolysis of dietary triglyceride. Pancreatic lipase is secreted by the pancreas in its active form and has both hydrophilic and hydrophobic portions. It binds to the lipid-water interface, where it hydrolyzes triglycerides. The enzyme does have positional specificity and attacks only the alpha ester bonds, generating two fatty acids and one monoglyceride from each triglyceride molecule. The enzyme works rapidly, and in the presence of bile acids has a pH optima of between 6 and 7, which is the pH found in the duodenum and jejunum during fat digestion. Pancreatic lipase in the healthy subject is excreted at approximately 10 times the amount required for breakdown of dietary triglycerides; thus, a 90% reduction in the lipase concentration must occur before steatorrhea is observed. Additional enzymes involved in digestion are present in the pancreatic juice; these include esterases and a phospholipase.

MICELLAR SOLUBILIZATION BY BILE ACIDS

The products of lipolysis, free fatty acids and monoglycerides, are insoluble in water. This problem is overcome by the formation of bile acid micelles, which requires a bile acid concentration of greater than 2 mM, the critical micellar concentration. Micellar dispersion increases the concentration of lipolytic products in the aqueous phase approximately 1000-fold.

Bile acids are synthesized by the liver from cholesterol and conjugated with glycine or taurine and stored in the gallbladder. Upon release, they form solubilized lipolytic products for efficient absorption in the jejunum. As they continue to pass down the small intestine, they are actively absorbed in the ileum and returned to the liver via the portal vein; they are then taken up and re-excreted into the bile. This cycle, referred to as enterohepatic circulation of bile acids, represents an extremely efficient reuse of bile acids, as more than 95% are absorbed in the intestine.

MUCOSAL UPTAKE

After micellar dispersion of lipolytic products by bile salts, diffusion to the cell membrane occurs. A fatty acid–binding protein then assists in the passive diffusion of the micellar lipid into the enterocyte.

TRIGLYCERIDE RESYNTHESIS

Triglycerides are then resynthesized within the cell by the joining of a monoglyceride with two fatty acid-CoA molecules.

CHYLOMICRON FORMATION

Chylomicrons are formed to carry the resynthesized triglycerides in an aqueous-soluble form. A lipoprotein coat is formed around the lipid droplets, and they are extruded through the basolateral membrane of the enterocyte.

LYMPHATIC TRANSPORT

Chylomicrons are carried by the lymphatics to the thoracic duct and then into the systemic circulation.

Defects in Fat Absorption

A defect in any of the steps required for proper fat absorption can result in steatorrhea. Loss of emulsification, as with surgical gastrectomy, can be a contributory factor. In addition, a duodenal bypass is part of many gastric ulcer surgeries (e.g., Bilroth II gastrojejunostomy or a Roux-en-Y gastrojejunostomy), resulting in decreased pancreatic and biliary secretion of bile acids and lipase. This reduced secretion can play a role in postgastrectomy malabsorption.

Any form of exocrine pancreatic insufficiency can cause steatorrhea if pancreatic lipase concentration falls to a low enough level. In addition to decreased production, diminished lipase function can occur at a low duodenal pH, as can occur in gastric acid hypersecretory states.

Liver and biliary diseases that cause decreased bile acid secretion can interfere with micellar solubilization of lipids. If the intestinal lumen has a low pH, bile salts can precipitate and micellar solubilization will not occur. Bile acids can also be deconjugated by bacterial overgrowth in the small intestine, and any disruption in the enterohepatic circulation (such as by ileectomy or problems with bile excretion) can result in a deficiency of bile acids being delivered to the intestine. Although the liver can compensate for interference in the enterohepatic circulation to a certain extent, that capacity is limited.

Mucosal uptake of solubilized lipid is impaired in a variety of diseases in which the intestinal mucosa is damaged. Although there is no known defect in the resynthesis of triglycerides after absorption, failure of packaging and lymphatic transport does occur. Failure to synthesize the protein coat of chylomicrons occurs in abetalipoproteinemia, and any disruption of lymphatic transport, whether congenital or acquired, will interfere with transport of lipid from the intestine and likewise result in steatorrhea.

Clinical Evaluation of Fat Malabsorption

The clinical manifestations of fat malabsorption are associated with steatorrhea (Figure 2). Typically, the stool is malodorous and large in quantity. There may be an oily sheen on the surface of the water in the toilet. The stool may tend to float (although this commonly occurs with air in the stool as well) and is typically difficult to flush, tending to stick to the porcelain surface of the toilet. Weight loss and abdominal cramping are also frequent complaints.

Physical findings suggestive of fat malabsorption tend to be nonspecific. Weight loss may be clinically apparent but is frequently absent. As fat malabsorption often causes deficiencies in vitamins A, D, E, or K, ecchymoses may be present because of an elevated prothrombin time. The patient may have night blindness secondary to vitamin A deficiency or may present with osteoporosis from calcium malabsorption (vitamin D deficiency). There may be peripheral edema from hypoalbuminemia.

CONFIRMATORY TEST

Without evidence pointing toward one single cause of steatorrhea, a relatively simple algorithm can be followed (see Figure 2). The first step in any evaluation of fat malabsorption is to confirm that steatorrhea is indeed present. A quick screening test is a Sudan stain of a single stool specimen (generally ordered as a "spot" or "qualitative" fecal fat study); the presence of large globules of fat is strongly suggestive. This can be confirmed by obtaining a 48- or 72-hour fecal fat study. For this, the patient is placed on a high-fat diet (100 grams fat per day), and stool is collected in a 1-gallon paint can (supplied by the laboratory) for 48 or (preferably) 72 hours. A "typical" American diet contains approximately 100 grams of fat per day; patients in whom dietary intake is substantially decreased can take a high-fat supplement such as Pulmocare to ensure an adequate fat intake for this study. More than 7 grams of fat in the stool per 24-hour period is considered abnormal. This study has the advantage of quantifying both the degree of fat malabsorption and total stool output. The degree of fat malabsorption may be a useful indicator of the cause of the malabsorption; pancreatic insufficiency tends to have a higher degree of malabsorption then does an intestinal mucosal defect. If the 72-hour fecal fat study does not reveal steatorrhea, then the quantification of total stool output is useful for the evaluation of other nonmalabsorptive causes of diarrhea.

Once steatorrhea has been confirmed, a review of the patient's medical and surgical history is useful. Has the patient undergone gastric or intestinal surgery that may

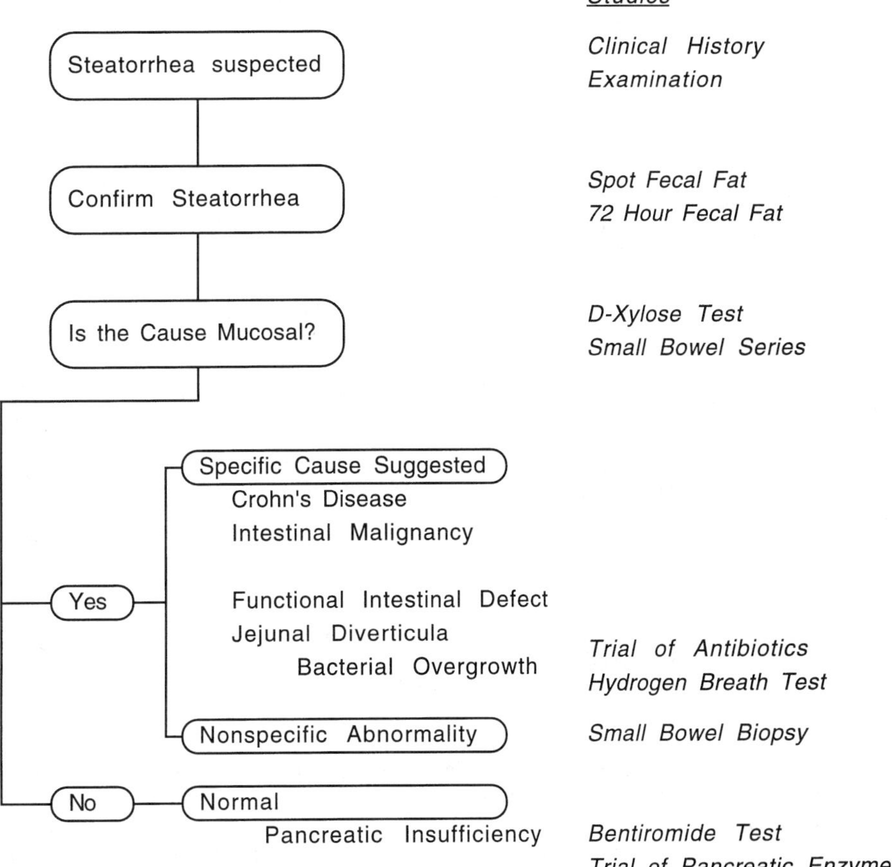

Figure 2. Suggested algorithm for the evaluation of fat malabsorption. The algorithm is primarily intended for situations in which the cause of the fat malabsorption is not immediately clinically apparent.

alter emulsification or enterohepatic circulation? Has the patient had any recent major abdominal or thoracic trauma that may disrupt lymphatic drainage? Does the patient have any underlying disease that might suggest a particular etiology (e.g., chronic pancreatitis)?

TESTS FOR MUCOSAL ABNORMALITIES

Unless the history suggests a likely cause of malabsorption, the first step is to determine whether the malabsorption is due to a problem in digesting the lipid (i.e., an intraluminal disorder) or to a defect in mucosal uptake and removal. This usually involves evaluation of mucosal function and/or integrity. This is easily accomplished with a small bowel series, which can provide clues as to the diagnosis of a mucosal dysfunction (such as Crohn's disease) or to a predisposition for other causes of the steatorrhea (such as the presence of large jejunal diverticula, which may predispose to bacterial overgrowth, or pancreatic calcifications, which are associated with chronic pancreatitis).

The D-xylose test is a simple and rapid method of assessing mucosal integrity. Twenty-five grams of D-xylose are ingested, and under normal conditions, approximately 50% is absorbed in the small intestine. Of the 50% absorbed, approximately half is metabolized by the liver, with the remaining amount being excreted unchanged by the kidney. Urine is collected for 5 hours after the oral ingestion of the D-xylose and the amount excreted quantified. If 5 grams or more of the D-xylose appears in the urine, mucosal absorption is most likely intact.

The D-xylose test is limited in its specificity for mucosal disease. A decrease in the glomerular filtration rate of the kidney can decrease the amount of D-xylose in urine, as can significant third-space fluid (as in ascites or anasarca), bacterial overgrowth in the small intestine, unusually rapid transit through the small intestine, or incomplete collection of urine by the patient. Hepatic decompensation can result in a falsely elevated level of D-xylose in the urine.

TESTS FOR PANCREATIC INSUFFICIENCY

If the small bowel series and D-xylose study are both unremarkable, the most likely cause of steatorrhea is pancreatic insufficiency. A useful study for pancreatic insufficiency is the noninvasive bentiromide test in which an analog of para-amino benzoic acid (PABA), which is rapidly absorbed in the intestine, conjugated in the liver, and excreted in the urine, is photometrically measured in a 6-hour urine sample. PABA is provided bound to an *N*-benzoyl-L-tyrosyl group (bentiromide), in a 500-mg oral dose. The active pancreatic enzyme chymotrypsin is necessary to free the PABA, which is then rapidly absorbed and excreted. A low urinary level of PABA is strongly suggestive of pancreatic exocrine insufficiency (in the absence of liver disease).

The utility of this test has been severely hampered in recent years by the inconsistent availability of bentiromide. A reasonable alternative is a therapeutic trial of pancreatic enzyme replacements. The enzymes must be given in sufficient amount (a minimum of 20,000 to 40,000 units of lipase [one or two Pancrease MT-20 capsules]) before each meal, and the clinical response to enzyme replacement monitored. Although a symptomatic response can be utilized, re-evaluation of a 72-hour fecal fat provides a firmer basis for diagnosis.

TESTS FOR BACTERIAL OVERGROWTH

Bacterial overgrowth is suspected when there are suggestive radiographic findings (e.g., jejunal diverticula, a blind intestinal loop, or other functional intestinal defect), or when the D-xylose test is abnormal but the small bowel series and/or mucosal biopsies are normal. The best readily available diagnostic test for bacterial overgrowth of the small intestine is the breath hydrogen test. A 50- to 80-gram dose of glucose is consumed, and serial measurements of breath hydrogen are made (the patient exhales into a bag at fixed intervals). An early rise in exhaled hydrogen concentration suggests bacterial overgrowth. An alternative method is a therapeutic trial of antibiotics and observation for clinical response. Typically, metronidazole (Flagyl), tetracycline, or trimethoprim-sulfamethoxazole (TMP-SMX, Bactrim) is used in standard therapeutic doses. A clinical response should be observed within 1 week.

SMALL BOWEL BIOPSIES

Endoscopic small bowel biopsies are easily obtained and can provide valuable clues to the cause of steatorrhea in patients in whom the evaluation has suggested a disorder of mucosal function. The small bowel biopsy can occasionally be diagnostic but is more often suggestive. Nonspecific or normal biopsies make it likely that the studies suggesting mucosal disease were misleading and that the diagnosis is more likely pancreatic insufficiency, bile salt deficiency, or small intestinal bacterial overgrowth.

Diagnostic small bowel biopsies can be obtained in Whipple's disease. These tissue specimens have PAS-positive (and AFB-negative) macrophages in the lamina propria. In addition to steatorrhea, polyarticular arthritis, lymphadenopathy, and neurologic problems (from concurrent central nervous system infection) are usually present.

Other mucosal infections can also be diagnosed by biopsy. Steatorrhea is often the sole presenting sign in giardiasis. The beaver is the natural reservoir for *Giardia lamblia*, so a recent history of camping or consumption of water of unproven potability is common. Some outbreaks have been reported in municipal water systems as well; it can take a year or more for the water system to be purged of *Giardia*. In immunosuppressed patients, cryptosporidia, mycobacteria, and cytomegalovirus can be seen; these organisms are also occasionally found in patients without other clinical evidence of immunosuppression.

Diagnostic intestinal biopsies can also be obtained in noninfectious mucosal abnormalities. Abetalipoproteinemia is caused by a defect in the packaging of chylomicrons. Intestinal lymphangectasia occurs when the flow of chyle from the intestine is obstructed, and can be congenital, caused by trauma (disruption of the thoracic duct), or associated with medical illnesses (severe pancreatitis). Amyloidosis can also be diagnosed by intestinal biopsy, although rectal biopsies are more commonly performed if this diagnosis is suspected (e.g., in myeloma or connective tissue disorders).

The majority of mucosal biopsies, however, are more likely to be suggestive rather than diagnostic in and of themselves. In celiac disease (nontropical sprue, gluten-sensitive enteropathy) the small bowel biopsy reveals a flattened mucosal surface, villus blunting, elongated crypts, and an inflammatory infiltrate of the lamina propria with a predominance of lymphocytes and plasma cells. Gliadin, a component of the wheat protein gluten, appears to be the causative agent of celiac disease. The diagnosis of celiac disease is made after dietary modification (gluten-free diet) and demonstration of improvement of villus architecture by repeat endoscopic mucosal biopsies.

Mucosal biopsies can also suggest the diagnosis in tropical sprue (similar biopsy appearance to celiac sprue but with a history of travel to tropical areas). Eosinophilic gastroenteritis is suggested by the presence of eosinophils in unusual amounts in the mucosa. The presence of mucosal ulceration or noncaseating granulomata raises the suspicion of Crohn's disease. Granulomata can also be seen in intestinal sarcoid. Intestinal tuberculosis is unlikely to be present unless pulmonary tuberculosis is clinically apparent.

Exceptions to the Algorithm Approach

There are many clinical situations in which a full malabsorption evaluation may not be necessary, even in the presence of significant steatorrhea. A patient with known chronic pancreatitis, for example, who presents with foul-smelling, oily stools is very likely to have pancreatic insufficiency. In this situation, it would be reasonable to start pancreatic enzyme replacement without further evaluation and pursue evaluation only if there is no appropriate clinical response. Likewise, the clinical manifestations and laboratory or radiologic studies may suggest a cause of the malabsorption prior to the initiation of a full evaluation. In these situations, it is reasonable to evaluate the most likely cause of the malabsorption first, and if the presumptive diagnosis appears to be correct, treat appropriately and observe for a reduction in steatorrhea. If the expected reduction does not occur, then a more complete evaluation for steatorrhea is certainly warranted.

DISEASE STATES ASSOCIATED WITH MALABSORPTION AND THEIR TREATMENT

Protein Malabsorption

There is an essential requirement for exogenous protein in order to avoid protein deficiency in all parts of the body. During illness, nitrogen (and protein) loss is exacerbated and intake requirements tend to be higher. The normal adult requires approximately 1 gram of protein per kilogram body weight per day. If an adequate intestinal mucosa is present, it is generally possible to attain protein needs with an oral diet, but some patients may need high-protein supplements.

If protein malabsorption is due to pancreatic enzyme deficiency, these peptidases can be easily replaced with virtually any of the pancreatic enzyme supplements. An inadequately functioning mucosa is much more difficult to manage, however, as the uptake of amino acids and peptides is dependent on transport proteins that are an integral part of the mucosa. If significant mucosal inflammation is present, it can often be decreased with a variety of anti-inflammatory agents, such as aminosalicylates or steroids. In some situations, especially when there is inadequate functioning mucosa because of surgical removal (short bowel syndrome), it may be necessary to provide protein in the form of parenteral amino acids.

Carbohydrate Malabsorption

As most carbohydrate malabsorption syndromes occur because of a deficiency of an individual disaccharidase, the mainstay of treatment is to eliminate problematic disaccharide from the diet. By far the most common disaccharidase deficiency is of lactase. If dairy products and other rich sources of lactose (regular chewing gum, many presweetened cereals) are avoided, the patient tends to do quite well. As the disaccharidases work within the intestinal lumen, enzyme replacements can be provided orally. There are several commercially available lactase supplements (e.g., Lactaid), which, when taken before ingestion of lactose-containing foods, can ameliorate the malabsorption associated with the native enzyme deficiency.

It is not uncommon for a transient lactase deficiency to develop after an episode of viral gastroenteritis. This is treated by avoiding dairy products for a few weeks, after which they may slowly be reintroduced. As lactase is an inducible enzyme, once the brush border of the intestine is re-established, the enzyme will slowly return to its previously normal levels.

Fat Malabsorption

Treatment of fat malabsorption is primarily based on the underlying cause of the malabsorption, which is why determination of the defective step in fat absorption is of importance. A defect in any of the steps required for proper fat absorption can result in steatorrhea.

Defects in fat emulsification occur most commonly after surgical gastrectomy. In this situation, an inadequate amount of surface area of the lipid is exposed for lipolysis and micelle formation. The main treatment for this condition is to limit dietary fat intake or to alter the lipid ratio toward shorter-chain fatty acids; the assistance of a registered dietitian may be useful for dietary instruction.

Other surgical interventions in the upper gastrointestinal tract may also have adverse effects on the stimulation of bile and pancreatic enzyme release. As mentioned, most gastric ulcer surgeries (Bilroth II gastrojejunostomy or Roux-en-Y gastrojejunostomy) bypass the duodenum and thus decrease pancreatic and biliary secretion of bile acids and lipase. Although the flow of bile and pancreatic secretions is maintained, pancreatic enzyme supplementation may be necessary.

Any significant decrease in exocrine pancreatic function can lead to a defect in pancreatic lipolysis. The primary treatment for pancreatic insufficiency is oral pancreatic enzyme replacement. The degree of pancreatic insufficiency is highly variable, and dose titration for pancreatic enzymes is necessary. Most pancreatic enzyme preparations are labeled according to the lipase content, with the more recent formulations containing 5, 10, or 20 thousand international units of lipase (e.g., Creon 10 and Pancrease MT10 both contain 10,000 IU lipase). To avoid fat malabsorption after a typical meal, approximately 28,000 IU active lipase must be in the duodenum during the 4-hour postprandial period. The amount that the patient is supplying from the pancreas cannot be easily measured. In addition, given that substantial amounts of lipase can be degraded by acid pepsin in the stomach, it is clear that inadequate supplementation is a frequent problem. Pancreatic enzyme replacement should start at 10,000 to 20,000 IU lipase at a minimum, and increase from there. Occasionally, the requirement for pancreatic enzyme replacement is lower in borderline cases of steatorrhea. Although histamine-2 receptor antagonists (Tagamet, Zantac, Pepcid, Axid) are often given with pancreatic enzymes, there does not appear to be any advantage to further acid suppression with proton pump inhibitors (Prilosec, Prevacid). In gastric acid hypersecretory states, however, even high doses of lipase can be degraded, and more aggressive gastric acid suppression may be required.

Liver and biliary diseases that cause a decrease in bile acid secretion can interfere with micellar solubilization of lipids. Disruption of the enterohepatic circulation by significant (usually greater than 100 cm) ileectomy can result in a deficiency of bile acids being delivered to the intestine. Although the liver can compensate for interference in the hepatic circulation to a certain extent, that capacity is limited. The steatorrhea from disruption of enterohepatic circulation is controlled by limiting fat intake or by correcting the interruption. Biliary obstruction caused by malignancy of the pancreas or bile duct (cholangiocarcinoma) can often be alleviated by endoscopic stent placement. Use of the bile salt–binding agent cholestyramine can also cause a relative deficiency of bile salts, but this is reversible by lowering the dose of the cholestyramine or discontinuing it altogether.

Bile acids can also be deconjugated by bacterial overgrowth in the small intestine. Bacterial overgrowth is treated with metronidazole (Flagyl), tetracycline, or TMP-SMX in standard therapeutic doses. Clinical response is usually rapid. Given that there is often an anatomic defect that allows the bacterial overgrowth, retreatment is frequently required, often with rotation of the antibiotics used.

Mucosal uptake of solubilized lipid is impaired in a number of diseases in which the intestinal mucosa is damaged. The prototypical mucosal disorder is celiac disease (also called celiac sprue, gluten-sensitive enteropathy, and nontropical sprue). Strict adherence to a gluten-free diet is the most effective therapy for celiac disease, although the diet may be difficult to maintain because it requires avoidance of not only wheat, but also barley and rye cereals and flour. Rice, soybean, and corn flours do not induce celiac disease. This is a disease in which early referral to a registered dietitian is beneficial; unfortunately, insurance coverage for this is spotty. No patient with a biopsy suggestive for celiac disease should be labeled a diet failure without a thorough dietary review. There are some patients who are refractory to dietary treatment; oral prednisone (10 to 20 mg per day) may be required. If a patient with previously well-controlled celiac disease develops a recurrence of steatorrhea, the most likely explanation is dietary indiscretion; the most worrisome is intestinal lymphoma.

The diagnosis of tropical sprue is likewise suggested by biopsies that have villus blunting and inflammation very similar to that seen with nontropical (celiac) sprue. This disease occurs primarily (but not universally) in adults who have lived in tropical regions for a year or more, most commonly India, southeast Asia, and the Caribbean. Treatment involves pharmacologic replacement of vitamins and antibiotic treatment of the contaminating coliform bacteria that are thought to cause the disease. Specifically, folate, 5 mg orally (PO) every day with parenteral vitamin B_{12}, 1000 μg every week, along with tetracycline, 250 mg PO four times a day, is curative in patients who have returned to a temperate climate. Treatment should be given for at least 2 months and can be needed for as long as 6 months, until the intestinal abnormalities disappear. Recurrence has been reported only in those who have returned to the tropical region where the disease was acquired.

The etiology of eosinophilic gastroenteritis has not been determined. In young children, sensitivity to milk is not uncommon, but in other populations evidence for an immune (allergic) pathogenesis is inconclusive and response to dietary elimination is usually disappointing. A stool study for intestinal parasites is warranted, and diagnostic consideration should be given to Crohn's disease and intestinal lymphoma. Effective symptomatic treatment of eosinophilic gastroenteritis is usually obtained with prednisone, 20 to 40 mg PO every day for 7 to 10 days. Retreatment is frequently necessary, and prolonged treatment with steroids is sometimes required. The disease typically waxes and wanes in severity, but the overall prognosis is usually good. Parenteral nutrition is required rarely in patients with refractory disease.

The diagnosis of Crohn's disease, suggested by mucosal ulceration and/or noncaseating granulomata (present in less than half of biopsy tissue), is effectively treated with aminosalicylates, steroids (if more severe), and occasionally immune modifying agents such as azathioprine* (Imuran) or 6-mercaptopurine* (Purinethol). Because active drug is released more proximally in the time-release formulation of the aminosalicylate mesalamine (Pentasa), there are theoretical advantages to using this drug to treat proximal intestinal disease. However, no studies have demonstrated that Pentasa is any more effective for the treatment of proximal intestinal Crohn's than any of the other aminosalicylate preparations (sulfasalazine [Azulfidine], mesalamine [Asacol], olsalazine [Dipentum]).

Whipple's disease, although uncommon, is readily treatable. Identification of the organism is made by genetic analysis (polymerase chain reaction) of biopsy tissue; the organism is resistant to culture. Initial treatment should be with penicillin G (1.2 million units) and streptomycin (1 gram) daily for 10 to 14 days, followed by double-strength TMP-SMX, one tablet PO twice a day for 1 year. Relapses occur in as many as one third of patients but usually respond to repeated twice a day antibiotic therapy.

*Not FDA approved for this indication.

Infection with *Giardia lamblia* is treated with metronidazole, 500 mg three times a day for 1 to 2 weeks. Cryptosporidiosis, mycobacterial infection, and cytomegalovirus infection are not uncommon in immunocompromised patients. Cytomegalovirus infection of the intestinal tract is treated with ganciclovir* (Cytovene), 5 mg per kg every 12 hours intravenously or 1000 mg orally three times a day. The duration of treatment is dependent on the cause of immune suppression and whether it can be reversed. If possible, immunosuppression should be lessened (e.g., by decreasing doses of immunosuppressive agents).

Abnormalities in chylomicron formation occur in abetalipoproteinemia. The only effective treatment for this disorder is reduction in dietary lipid consumption. Additionally, pharmacologic replacement of vitamin E (100 mg per kg per day) and supplemental vitamin A and K are given. Likewise, the treatment for defects in lymphatic transport, such as lymphangiectasia, also revolves around dietary fat restriction. If the intestinal lymphangiectasia is secondary (i.e., caused by another disease process blocking the lymphatic drainage of the intestinal tract), then therapy should be aimed at the underlying disease process (e.g., tuberculosis, lymphoma, sarcoidosis, constrictive pericarditis). Malabsorption from congenital lymphangiectasia (Milroy's disease), as well as from secondary lymphangiectasia, is treated by reduction of long chain triglycerides in the diet and substitution with short and medium chain dietary triglycerides. Because of their higher water solubility, the shorter chain fatty acids are more readily absorbed through the portal venous system than through the lymphatics. By manipulating the dietary fatty acid mix to decrease the rate of chylomicron formation, the associated protein-losing enteropathy is generally also decreased.

Finally, steatorrhea can occur from consumption of a nonabsorbable fat product. Olestra (Olean) is a sucrose-lipid polymer that has many of the cooking properties of natural fat but is not absorbed in the human gastrointestinal tract. Olestra's current use is limited to snack foods such as potato chips (fat-free Pringles) or corn chips (Frito Lay MAX chips). Although normal serving sizes of snacks containing olestra are unlikely to cause overt steatorrhea, the likelihood of developing symptoms increases with greater consumption. Because the fat-soluble vitamins can be adsorbed by and excreted with the olestra, vitamins A, D, E, and K are added by federal regulation as a precautionary measure. Avoidance of olestra is curative if symptomatic steatorrhea occurs when consuming this product.

*Not FDA approved for this indication.

The evaluation and treatment of patients with malabsorption can be intellectually rewarding for the physician. Once the clinical suspicion of malabsorption arises, a careful history, examination, and selective diagnostic evaluation can quickly be performed based upon the knowledge of the normal physiology of absorption. This evaluation almost always leads to establishment of a cause of the malabsorption, which in turn allows initiation of appropriate treatment, and, in the majority of patients, an appreciable clinical response.

ACUTE PANCREATITIS

method of
JON M. BURCH, M.D.
Denver Health Medical Center and University of Colorado Health Sciences Center
Denver, Colorado

Eighty to 90% of all cases of acute pancreatitis are caused either by gallstones or by alcohol abuse. Other known factors include hyperparathyroidism, hyperlipemia, postoperative states, trauma, hereditary conditions, drugs, and infectious diseases. In about 10% of cases, the cause is not clear, and these cases are referred to as idiopathic. The frequency with which a particular etiologic factor is noted depends on the population of patients in question.

In the United States, gallstones are the most common cause of acute pancreatitis. Although the relationship between gallstones and the development of pancreatitis is clear, the mechanism is not well understood. At the turn of the century, Opie hypothesized that a stone could occlude the ductal ampulla distal to the junction of the common bile duct and pancreatic duct, thereby permitting bile to flow into the pancreatic duct and activate pancreatic enzymes. Subsequent experiments have shown that this is unlikely to occur. It has been demonstrated that patients with gallstone pancreatitis have a high rate of gallstones that can be recovered in the feces. These stones appear to either transiently obstruct the pancreatic duct or create a temporary path that permits duodenal contents to enter the pancreatic duct and induce the development of pancreatitis.

The mechanism by which alcohol causes acute pancreatitis is also unknown. Current theories have incriminated an alteration of the normal constituents of pancreatic secretions resulting in concretions in the pancreatic ducts. It is also possible that alcohol exerts a direct toxic effect on the pancreatic parenchyma as it does in the liver.

DIAGNOSIS

Patients usually give a history of progressive epigastric or right upper quadrant pain that radiates in a bandlike distribution or straight through to the back. The pain is sharp and stabbing or boring in nature, and nothing the patient can do will ameliorate the discomfort. Nausea and vomiting almost always accompany the pain.

On physical examination, the patient appears acutely ill and dehydrated. Fever is not uncommon but is usually of low grade; tachycardia and tachypnea may be present. Blood pressure is normal except in a few patients with severe disease who may be in shock. Bowel sounds can be absent because of ileus, and the abdomen may be distended. Palpation reveals epigastric tenderness with voluntary or involuntary guarding. True abdominal rigidity is rare. A mass may be palpable in the upper abdomen, suggesting a pseudocyst, an abscess, or a diffuse enlargement of the pancreas.

The laboratory hallmark of acute pancreatitis is elevation of the serum amylase level, in most cases to three or more times the upper limit of normal. Patients with gallstone pancreatitis tend to have higher peak amylase levels than those with alcohol pancreatitis. Regardless of etiology, the serum amylase value falls to nearly normal levels within 2 to 3 days in most patients. A persistently elevated amylase level suggests the development of pseudocyst.

Unfortunately, serum amylase alone is neither sensitive nor specific for acute pancreatitis. Indeed, some of the most critically ill patients with pancreatitis have a normal serum amylase level when they are first seen by a physician. Furthermore, many other abdominal and extra-abdominal diseases may be associated with hyperamylasemia. Alternative available enzyme analyses include measurement of urinary amylase and serum lipase. Urinary amylase concentration parallels serum amylase and does not enhance the accuracy of diagnosis. Serum lipase does improve specificity, although it may not be elevated in all cases.

Because of the difficulties with serum amylase interpretation, two modifications have been proposed. The ratio of amylase clearance to creatinine clearance yields a percentage that, if greater than 5, is said to be compatible with acute pancreatitis. Although the test is more precise than serum amylase alone, it is not uniquely specific for pancreatitis. Furthermore, the sensitivity of the test is diminished in patients with near-normal serum amylase levels. Preliminary evidence suggests that isoenzyme determinations of pancreatic amylase may improve specificity. Pancreatic isoamylase levels are not currently available for routine use in many hospitals.

An upright chest film and plain abdominal radiographs should be obtained in all patients suspected of having acute pancreatitis. Although such films may not aid in diagnosis of pancreatitis, they do help to avoid missing other diseases that can mimic pancreatitis, such as a perforated ulcer.

Ultrasonography is a valuable screening test because it is both sensitive and specific for identifying concomitant gallstones, and it is inexpensive. It can also detect the presence of associated fluid collections. The major disadvantage of ultrasonography is its inability to consistently image the pancreas, especially in obese individuals or when surrounding gas shadows prevent penetration of the beam.

Computed tomography (CT) can be used to identify gallstones, masses within the pancreas, fluid collection, and diffuse enlargement of the gland. The advantages of CT over ultrasonography are that the overlying gas shadows do not obscure the pancreas, and anatomic relationships can be precisely defined. The major disadvantage of CT is its cost. For this reason, CT is not recommended for early diagnostic use in uncomplicated cases. The primary role of CT is to clarify the diagnosis in questionable cases and to survey for septic intra-abdominal complications in patients with severe disease.

In making the diagnosis of acute pancreatitis, the clinician must always be on guard for the possibility that the diagnosis is in error. Several abdominal surgical emergencies can resemble acute pancreatitis, including perforated ulcer without free intraperitoneal air, bowel obstruction (especially closed loop obstructions), acute cholecystitis, and small bowel infarction. At times, patients with persistent severe symptoms may require diagnostic laparotomy with the knowledge that the cause could be acute pancreatitis. However, CT has reduced the need for exploratory laparotomy to a low level.

TERMINOLOGY

The most important development in the management of acute pancreatitis during the past decade has been the creation and acceptance of a consistent terminology (Table 1). Note that the term hemorrhagic pancreatitis is no longer used. Formerly, hemorrhagic pancreatitis and necrotizing pancreatitis were used interchangeably. Another important step has been the abandonment of the Marseille classification. The original system described the course of some patients with alcoholic pancreatitis but in no way described the course of patients with gallstone pancreatitis. Even the simplified revised version is largely ignored.

TREATMENT

Mild to Moderate Disease

All patients with a tentative diagnosis of acute pancreatitis should be hospitalized for observation and supportive care. Patients with mild to moderate disease can be cared for on a general ward provided that close observation is maintained. Because of the capricious nature of the disease, some patients who appear well when they are first seen may deteriorate rapidly; therefore, vigilant observation should be maintained for 24 to 48 hours.

Most patients demonstrate some degree of dehydration, and all should receive intravenous fluids. This can be accomplished with 2 liters of D5 half-normal saline with 30 mEq potassium chloride per liter each day. In addition, nasogastric losses should be replaced on a volume-per-volume basis with normal saline to prevent alkalosis. Patients who are seriously dehydrated require resuscitation with isotonic fluids such as lactated Ringer's. In this situation, serum electrolyte levels should be obtained and the hourly urine output monitored with a Foley catheter. When the urine output reaches 0.5 mL per kg per hour, routine fluid orders can be resumed.

The patient should take nothing by mouth, and a nasogastric tube should be inserted. Prospective studies in patients with mild to moderate pancreatitis have shown that the use of a nasogastric tube does not significantly alter the course of the disease. However, I continue to recommend this therapy because it effectively relieves nausea and vomiting.

Acute pancreatitis causes severe pain, and the use of parenteral narcotics is an important adjunct to general supportive care. The selection of a specific narcotic agent is not important. Patient-controlled analgesia pumps have become increasingly popular. Reasonable starting doses for an alert and competent adult receiving intravenous morphine sulfate are a basal rate of 1 mg per hour and a patient-controlled additional dose of 1 mg every 15 minutes. Dosage should be adjusted according to the patient's age, weight, general condition, and response to the medication.

The prophylactic use of antibiotics is controversial. Prospective studies have suggested that antibiotics do not help prevent the septic complications of acute pancreatitis in patients with mild or moderately severe disease.

Many other medications have been used in an attempt to alter the course of acute pancreatitis, but virtually all have been ineffective to date. Parasympatholytic drugs such as atropine have had little effect in improving the course of the disease and because of their unpleasant side effects are not recommended. H_2 blockers have been used to reduce the secretin-mediated stimulation of the pancreas by decreasing gastric acid secretion. Unfortunately, these drugs have not been effective. Either H_2 blockers or antacids should be used in critically ill patients with necrotizing pancreatitis to reduce the possibility of acute gastric mucosal hemorrhage. The enzyme inhibitor aprotinin (Trasylol)*† has been shown to improve the course of acute pancreatitis in laboratory animals if the drug is administered before the induction of pancreatitis. In humans, aprotinin has not been shown to be beneficial and is not recommended. Somatostatin† and gabexate mesylate (the latter being a protease inhibitor similar to aprotinin but much lower in molecular weight) can now be added to the long list of medications that have been shown in clinical trials to be ineffective in altering the course of acute pancreatitis.

When patients begin to recover from the acute attack as evidenced by the return of bowel function and disappearance of epigastric pain and tenderness,

TABLE 1. **Terminology in Acute Pancreatitis**

Term	Definition
Acute interstitial pancreatitis	Sterile inflammation and edema of the pancreas
Necrotizing pancreatitis	Same as above but with necrosis of peripancreatic fat (mostly transverse mesocolon) and/or pancreas
Infected pancreatic necrosis	Necrotizing pancreatitis that has become infected
Pancreatic abscess	A collection of peripancreatic pus surrounded by an inflammatory wall; includes "infected pseudocysts"
Pseudocyst	A collection of sterile peripancreatic fluid, high in amylase, which is surrounded by an inflammatory wall
Fat sequestra	A collection of sterile necrotic fat surrounded by an inflammatory wall

*Not available in the United States.
†Not FDA approved for this indication.

oral feedings should be resumed. The diet should be low in fat and other gastropancreatic secretagogues. Some patients will have a prolonged ileus, and parenteral hyperalimentation should be initiated if they are unable to eat by the fifth to seventh day after admission.

Severe Disease

Virtually all patients who become critically ill with pancreatitis have necrotizing pancreatitis, infected necrosis, or pancreatic abscess. All patients with potentially severe pancreatitis should be admitted to an intensive care unit for careful monitoring and prompt intervention if necessary. Life-threatening complications include shock, respiratory failure, renal failure, infection, and hemorrhage. Invasive monitoring with an arterial line, a Foley catheter, and a central venous catheter is essential in these patients.

Patients with severe pancreatitis may experience hypotension or shock soon after admission. The shock is primarily hypovolemic and is due to the sequestration of fluid in the abdominal cavity. Because several liters of crystalloid solution may be required for volume resuscitation, isotonic solutions such as lactated Ringer's or Plasma-Lyte should be used to avoid acute hyponatremia. The end point for resuscitation is a clear sensorium and normal urine output. For patients who fail to respond to the usual regimen of fluid resuscitation, a Swan-Ganz catheter should be inserted and intravenous fluids administered until the pulmonary artery wedge pressure reaches approximately 15 to 18 mm Hg. If oliguria or anuria persists, acute renal failure has almost certainly occurred and appropriate consultations should be sought. Some authorities advocate the addition of albumin to resuscitation solutions for patients with severe disease. I subscribe to this view although I acknowledge the lack of supporting data.

When fluid resuscitation is completed, some patients may remain hypotensive. Mild hypotension, systolic blood pressure of 90 to 100 mm Hg, does not necessarily require further blood pressure support if urine output is good and the patient's sensorium is clear. For patients with severe hypotension (systolic blood pressure less than 80 mm Hg) and oliguria, inotropes to enhance cardiac output and/or vasomotor tone are indicated. The preferred drug in this circumstance is dopamine, which should be started at 3 to 5 μg per kg per minute. Further adjustments should be made according to hemodynamic parameters and urine output.

Respiratory failure is common in patients with severe pancreatitis and is indistinguishable from adult respiratory distress syndrome of other causes. For this reason, at least one determination of arterial blood gases should be made for all patients admitted with acute pancreatitis. Those with persistent tachypnea require frequent blood gas measurements. A falling PO_2 is an ominous sign, and endotracheal intubation and mechanical ventilation may be required. Positive end-expiratory pressure is helpful in maintaining an adequate PO_2 in hypoxemic patients who require high fractional inspired oxygen concentrations (FIO_2 more than 50%).

Renal failure may occur and is usually related to hypovolemia and shock. Although azotemia is often prerenal in nature, acute tubular necrosis or cortical necrosis can occur if the early prerenal phase is not treated aggressively. This requires careful monitoring of urine output, suitable administration of crystalloid solutions, and avoidance of nephrotoxic medications.

Potentially severe metabolic complications include hypocalcemia and hyperglycemia. A falling serum calcium level is a sign of poor prognosis, and treatment may be required to prevent tetany. Calcium gluconate should be administered by careful intravenous infusion with electrocardiographic monitoring if the patient becomes symptomatic or if the serum calcium reaches levels inappropriately below 8 mg per dL. Hyperglycemia is also a serious sign in patients who are not already diabetic and suggests extensive damage to the pancreas. A sliding scale of regular insulin based on the patient's serum glucose level can be used to treat this problem. In a few patients, continuous insulin infusion (insulin drip) may be necessary.

Evidence is slowly accumulating that the broad-spectrum antibiotic imipenem-cilastatin (Primaxin) may reduce the rate of septic complications for patients with necrotizing pancreatitis and perhaps improve survival. This drug can penetrate both pancreatic and necrotic peripancreatic tissue while retaining activity against organisms usually found in infected necrosis. Doses in the literature are in the range of 0.5 gram intravenously every 8 hours. Administration of the drug is begun when the diagnosis is made. The appropriate duration of treatment is unknown; it varies in the literature from 3 to 14 days.

COMPLICATIONS REQUIRING SURGICAL TREATMENT

The most serious of all complications is the development of intra-abdominal infection. This may take the form of a pancreatic abscess or infection of necrotic peripancreatic tissue (infected necrosis). Patients with continued elevation of the white blood cell count or persistent unexplained fever should be suspected of having intra-abdominal infection. CT is the most reliable test for diagnosing this condition. It may reveal abnormal lucencies, suggesting gas accumulation within necrotic tissue or well-delineated fluid collections. If the patient appears septic, CT-directed percutaneous aspiration of suspicious fluid collections is an effective method for the surveillance of intra-abdominal infection. This procedure can be repeated as often as necessary. If pus is aspirated or if enteric bacteria are grown on culture, laparotomy is indicated.

Proper therapy for intra-abdominal infection includes laparotomy with débridement of necrotic tissue, adequate drainage, and culture-specific antibiotics. Attempts to treat infected necrosis or pancreatic abscesses with percutaneous drainage have been largely unsuccessful because of necrotic debris and multiple loculations that are often present.

The necrotizing nature of severe pancreatic inflammation renders patients susceptible to the development of enteric fistulas. These may involve the colon, stomach, or small intestine. Treatment consists of establishing adequate drainage and general supportive care until the fistula heals. Persistent fistulas may require operative intervention as the patient's condition permits.

Life-threatening hemorrhage is uncommon. If it occurs, it is usually related to bleeding into a pseudocyst or erosion of a necrotizing process into an adjacent blood vessel. A falling hematocrit, unexplained shock, or sudden bleeding from surgical drains may be the first signs of severe hemorrhage. Profuse bleeding is best controlled by immediate laparotomy and oversewing of the offending vessel. The use of arteriography with embolization of the bleeding site should be reserved for patients who cannot tolerate laparotomy.

Pancreatic pseudocyst is another complication of acute pancreatitis. The diagnosis should be considered in all patients with pancreatitis whose serum amylase levels remain elevated for more than a few days. Ultrasonography is the most cost-effective technique for the diagnosis and surveillance of a pseudocyst. If this study is obtained early in the course of acute pancreatitis, peripancreatic fluid collections are often visualized. These collections tend to come and go and are seen at different times in different areas juxtaposed to the pancreas. This phenomenon has led to a misunderstanding that pseudocysts frequently resolve without surgical treatment. True pseudocysts do not disappear and are consistently found in the same location. In general, a pseudocyst requires 4 to 6 weeks from the onset of symptoms of acute pancreatitis to develop. These rare and potentially lethal cysts require treatment once the diagnosis is made. The timing of invasive intervention is based on the natural history of the disease or evidence of maturation (a thickened capsule) on ultrasound or CT examination. Ideal management consists of internal drainage, usually into the stomach. Complications of pseudocyst include hemorrhage, infection, or rupture, all of which can be prevented by timely invasive intervention.

Endoscopists are now performing transgastric endoscopic drainage, and interventional radiologists are treating pseudocysts by percutaneous drainage. The role of these new procedures remains to be determined, but they are reasonable options in patients who are poor operative candidates.

ADDITIONAL INDICATIONS FOR SURGERY

It is clear that cholecystectomy in patients with gallstone pancreatitis will prevent further attacks. It has been demonstrated that the gallbladder can be safely removed during the initial hospitalization. This can be accomplished within a few days of admission when the patient shows signs of clinical improvement.

Emergency endoscopic sphincterotomy has been advocated as an alternative to cholecystectomy for definitive treatment of gallstone pancreatitis. At present, there is no evidence that this procedure alters the course of the disease. Because cholecystectomy will still be necessary, needless risk and expense are incurred by patients so treated. This technique may have a place in those patients who also have obstructive jaundice or cholangitis.

A few patients with necrotizing pancreatitis who are not infected experience progressive systemic failure in spite of intensive support and should be considered candidates for surgical exploration. Laparotomy under these conditions is hazardous, and expert judgment is essential. At the time of surgery, extensive necrosis of the pancreas and peripancreatic tissue may be found. Appropriate treatment includes resection of all necrotic tissue. Understandably, the mortality rate for these patients is high, but some may be saved.

PROGNOSIS

Overall, acute pancreatitis in my institution is associated with a mortality rate of less than 4%. Many factors influence prognosis, including etiology, history of previous attacks, age, and pre-existing comorbidity. It is generally recognized that most patients who die of acute pancreatitis do so with the first attack. The natural history of alcoholic pancreatitis is one of frequent recurrences. The mortality rate for each subsequent attack is less than for the previous one. Consideration should be given to performing endoscopic retrograde cholangiopancreatography for any patient who requires repeated admissions to the hospital for pancreatitis. In some of these individuals, surgically correctable lesions, such as pancreatic ductal strictures, may be identified.

The prognosis for gallstone pancreatitis during the first attack is similar to that for the first attack of

TABLE 2. **Ranson's Criteria for Prognosis in Acute Pancreatitis**

At Admission
Age > 55 y
White blood cell count > 16,000/mm^3
Blood glucose level > 200 mg/dL
Serum lactate dehydrogenase level > 350 U/L
Serum aspartate aminotransferase level > 250 U/dL
Within 48 Hours
Hematocrit value decrease > 10%
Blood urea nitrogen level rise > 5 mg/dL
Serum calcium level > 8 mg/dL
Arterial Po_2 <60 mm Hg
Base deficit > 4 mEq/L
Estimated fluid sequestration > 6 L

alcoholic pancreatitis. Recurrent attacks of pancreatitis or biliary tract disease can occur in as many as 50% of patients if the gallbladder is not removed. Once the gallbladder has been removed and the common duct is noted to be free of stones, recurrent pancreatitis is rare.

As noted earlier, the course of acute pancreatitis is difficult to predict when patients are first seen. To address this problem, early clinical and laboratory prognostic indicators of the severity of disease have been developed. The most popular of these is Ranson's criteria (Table 2). This system contains 11 elements, some of which are determined at the time of admission and others 48 hours later. Patients with fewer than three positive criteria almost always have mild disease. Those with three or more criteria may have severe disease with a significantly higher mortality rate; patients in this category deserve early admission to an intensive care unit and careful monitoring.

CHRONIC PANCREATITIS

method of
JONATHAN E. CLAIN, M.B., Ch.B., and
EUGENE P. DiMAGNO, M.D.
Mayo Clinic
Rochester, Minnesota

The first modern description of chronic pancreatitis was made in 1946 when the association between long-standing alcohol ingestion and the development of chronic relapsing pancreatitis was first documented. It was subsequently recognized that gallstone pancreatitis rarely, if ever, resulted in chronic pancreatitis.

Since those observations were made, knowledge of chronic pancreatitis has greatly increased because of continued clinical observations and the development of imaging techniques such as computed tomography (CT), ultrasound (US), and endoscopic retrograde cholangiopancreatography (ERCP), as well as both noninvasive and invasive pancreatic function tests.

CLASSIFICATION AND EPIDEMIOLOGY

The diagnosis of chronic pancreatitis assumes progressive and irreversible changes in the pancreatic parenchyma. The pathologic changes in chronic pancreatitis include inflammatory changes and necrosis, with fibrosis and loss of both exocrine and endocrine elements. Ductal changes, including dilatation and protein plug formations, which ultimately calcify, are seen in more advanced disease. The use of the term chronic calcific pancreatitis, although useful to characterize the advanced form of the disease, implies unity of etiology and of clinical manifestations, which is not necessarily true when considering the spectrum of chronic pancreatitis.

Because pathologic material cannot be obtained from the pancreas for examination except after surgery, the lack of a practical pathology-based classification continues to be a problem in terms of separating acute pancreatitis from chronic pancreatitis with acute attacks. Several attempts to address this have been made in the past. The Marseilles classifications of 1963 and 1984 rely heavily on pain for diagnosis, and the Cambridge classification of 1983 incorporates imaging tests to diagnose the grade and severity of disease. The Marseilles-Rome classification of 1988 divides pancreatitis into acute and chronic and includes clinical, morphologic, and etiologic factors, but this does not always resolve the problem of classification and staging in an individual patient.

The incidence of chronic pancreatitis, especially that related to alcohol use, has increased over the years and in a number of series from different countries is currently reported at 5 to 10 per 100,000 per year.

ETIOLOGY AND PATHOGENESIS

In contrast to the multiple etiologies that can result in episodes of acute pancreatitis, the causes of chronic pancreatitis are few. Alcohol is the most important cause, and in most series constitutes approximately 70% of patients. Idiopathic pancreatitis constitutes almost all of the remaining patients. Hereditary pancreatitis is a rare condition, in which a genetic defect in the trypsinogen gene has been recently identified. Patients with the disease produce trypsin with a mutation at the cleavage site that is resistant to proteolysis. It has been postulated that this mutation prevents inactivation of intrapancreatic trypsin and that persistent trypsin leads to episodes of pancreatitis. In other parts of the world, including the tropics, nonalcoholic disease may predominate; it is of unknown etiology, although both nutritional and toxic causes have been proposed. Other causes of pancreatitis are rare and are listed in Table 1. Pancreatic insufficiency may occur without evidence of pancreatitis due to primary causes or to secondary causes, which results in the failure of release, failure of activation, or poor mixing of released pancreatic enzymes and intestinal contents.

Table 1. **Etiology of Chronic Pancreatic Insufficiency**

Chronic Pancreatitis
Alcohol-induced
Idiopathic
Tropical (nutritional)
Hereditary
Trauma-induced
Hypercalcemia-induced

Pancreatic Insufficiency Without Pancreatitis

Primary Pancreatic Insufficiency
Cystic fibrosis
Pancreatic, papillary, and duodenal tumors
Shwachman-Diamond syndrome
Primary pancreatic atrophy of childhood
Adult pancreatic lipomatosis or atrophy
Kwashiorkor protein-calorie malnutrition
Isolated lipase deficiency
Pancreatic resection

Secondary Pancreatic Insufficiency
Mucosal small bowel disease—decreased CCK release
Gastrinoma—intraluminal destruction of enzymes
Billroth II anastomosis—"poor mixing" or "decreased hormonal release"
Enterokinase deficiency

The pathogenetic mechanisms responsible for the development of chronic pancreatitis are speculative. There are several theories as to how alcohol may cause pancreatitis, including the following (1) Disturbance of acinar and ductular function with diffusion of proteins into the ducts, formation of protein plugs, and obstruction of ducts with subsequent inflammation and fibrosis. (2) A toxic metabolic cause, whereby alcohol results in pancreatic lipid deposition and inflammatory and fibrotic changes. (3) Oxidation stress, whereby excess free radicals ultimately lead to mast cell degranulation, platelet activation, and an inflammatory response. Abnormally large intrapancreatic nerves in close contact with inflammatory cells have recently been demonstrated and support this concept. (4) The necrosis-fibrosis sequence presumes repeated insults resulting in focal necrosis, inflammation, and scarring and is similar to hypothesis 3. These hypotheses are not mutually exclusive, and pancreatitis could plausibly be caused by one or more mechanism.

CLINICAL PRESENTATION

Pain. Characteristic pain is the commonest presenting symptom followed by exocrine and endocrine insufficiency. In our series, pain was present in 77% of alcoholic and 96 and 54% of early-onset and late-onset idiopathic pancreatitis, respectively. Pain continued over time, but over 14 to 27 years the pain decreased or disappeared in 64 to 77% of patients and frequently coincided with the presence of exocrine or endocrine insufficiency. Others have also reported that amelioration or disappearance of pain is coincident with the appearance of calcification in exocrine insufficiency.

A frequent error is to assume that pain in the presence of chronic pancreatitis is pancreatic in origin. Peptic ulcer disease should always be excluded and a careful history taken to distinguish alcoholic pancreatitis from a history of alcoholic gastritis. Most patients with pancreatic pain will give an initial history of an episode of acute pancreatitis. In alcoholic patients, abstaining from alcohol after an initial attack usually prevents further symptoms. Most patients continue to drink, however, and the chief problem is intermittent pain related to acute flares of the disease. In patients whose initial presentation of alcoholic pancreatitis is an acute episode and who do not exhibit evidence of exocrine or endocrine insufficiency, pancreatic function test results are abnormal in about 70% when tested 6 weeks or more after the attack. This is in keeping with the known pathogenesis of the disease, namely, that morphologic changes in the pancreas occur over many years—usually 5 to 10—of excess alcohol ingestion and that the acute episode is simply the first expression of what is already a chronic disease.

MECHANISM OF PAIN. The origin of pain in chronic pancreatitis is not clearly understood, but two main mechanisms are proposed: (1) Disruption of the perineural sheath in nerves within and around the pancreas, thus exposing these nerves to bioactive materials from inflammatory cells or pancreatic enzymes, which in turn cause pain perception. (2) Ductal hypertension as a result of obstruction of the secondary pancreatic ducts and perhaps the main pancreatic duct, although the lack of obstructive changes on ERCP in some patients with pain indicates that main duct obstruction may not be the major problem. This theory is supported by demonstration of ductal hypertension and increased pancreatic tissue fluid pressure in some patients with chronic pancreatitis. It is also indirectly supported by the benefit obtained by decompressive surgery of the pancreas. How ductal hypertension causes pain is unknown, but ischemia of the gland may be an important factor. Furthermore, ductal hypertension is a popular theory because several studies have correlated the appearance of calcification and exocrine insufficiency with pain disappearance or improvement.

Malabsorption. Overt steatorrhea occurs in about 30% of patients with chronic pancreatitis. When mild, it may not be clinically apparent and may not result in weight loss. A normal-appearing stool does not exclude biochemical steatorrhea. When steatorrhea is overt, it may occasionally result in leakage of oil from the anus, and when present, this symptom is virtually pathognomonic of steatorrhea of pancreatic origin. The degree of steatorrhea in pancreatic insufficiency exceeds that from other causes of malabsorption.

The exocrine pancreas has a large reserve capacity, and steaorrhea and azotorrhea do not occur until there is at least 90% reduction in lipase and trypsin secretion.

Pancreatic Diabetes. Diabetes is common in chronic pancreatitis and occurs with increasing frequency with the advance of the disease; in our series, it occurred in approximately one third or more of patients irrespective of alcoholic or nonalcoholic etiology, but in the alcoholic form of the disease, the time to development of diabetes was shorter. Diabetes is usually mild, and ketoacidosis is very unusual. In patients presenting with diabetes and diarrhea, a careful history may reveal episodes of pain consistent with acute pancreatitis, or an abdominal radiograph may demonstrate pancreatic calcification. When the patient gives a history of steatorrhea with or without the previously mentioned symptoms, chronic pancreatitis should be suspected rather than the autonomic diarrhea associated with diabetes mellitus, and the appropriate tests for pancreatitis, including a stool fat estimation, should be requested. Although initial observations were that diabetic vascular complications were rare in chronic pancreatitis, subsequent reports have refuted this. Peripheral neuropathy, however, is common in alcoholic pancreatitis, because of the additive effects of alcohol and malnutrition.

DIAGNOSIS OF CHRONIC PANCREATITIS

The history of characteristic abdominal pain with or without exocrine and/or endocrine insufficiency, or occasionally in patients with "painless pancreatitis" the presence of insufficiency alone should raise the suspicion of pancreatitis, especially in the presence of a long history of excessive alcohol ingestion. The diagnosis of mild forms of the disease remains difficult, but in overt disease the presence of calcification on plain abdominal films should first be sought. Modern imaging tests, namely, CT and US, depend on enlargement or atrophy of the gland or changes in the morphology of the pancreatic duct (dilatation, stricture, or calcified stones) or compression of the distal bile duct with biliary dilatation. The presence of pancreatic calcification is seen far more readily on a CT scan than on a plain abdominal film.

In mild forms of chronic pancreatitis, results of these studies are frequently negative, and unfortunately, the search for a simple noninvasive test for chronic pancreatitis continues. ERCP is an imaging test of the pancreatic ducts that can be performed when the initial imaging study results are negative. The diagnosis of chronic pancreatitis is classified as minimal, moderate, or advanced, depending on the degree of abnormality. In mild cases, the secondary ducts are abnormal, and only in the more advanced stages of the disease does the main ductal system becomes abnormally beaded or dilated, until in the advanced stages of the disease it assumes a "chain of lakes" appearance due to consecutive dilatation and stenosis of the duct. Overall, the sensitivity and specificity of ERCP in the diagnosis of pancreatitis is about 90%.

The pancreas can be viewed from the stomach and duodenum by means of endoscopic ultrasonography (EUS). Technically, placement of the instrument, which has a high-resolution transducer incorporated in the tip of the endoscope, is no more difficult or hazardous than that in upper gastrointestinal endoscopy. Changes thought to indicate pancreatitis include hyperechoic foci, lobulation of the gland, irregular main duct margins, and visible side branches. These changes may correlate with mild or moderate changes seen at pancreatography. However, correlation of EUS findings with standard pancreatic function test results has not been done. Although EUS results are intriguing, they are not yet reliable or consistent enough for the diagnosis of early chronic pancreatitis.

PANCREATIC FUNCTION TESTS

Tests of pancreatic function can be divided into those that are noninvasive and those that are invasive.

Noninvasive Tests

Serum Tests. Total serum amylase is of little use to diagnose chronic pancreatitis because it is usually normal even in advanced disease. The total serum amylase consists of both salivary (S) and pancreatic (P) isoenzymes. P amylase can be measured and would be expected to be low in chronic pancreatitis, but it is only 60% sensitive in advanced disease and far less sensitive in mild or moderate disease. Serum lipase and serum trypsinogen measurements are subject to the same shortcomings.

Other Noninvasive Tests. The so-called tubeless tests depend on the ability of pancreatic enzymes to digest a nonabsorbable substrate, with subsequent absorption of its product. In chronic pancreatitis, with decreased pancreatic enzyme secretion, the urinary recovery of the product should be diminished. The NBT-PABA test is based on the hydrolysis of a synthetic tripeptide N-benzoyl-L-tyrosyl-p-aminobenzoic acid by chymotrypsin, the release of PABA, and its subsequent absorption in the intestine and recovery in the urine. However, it is nonspecific (it can be abnormal with previous gastric surgery, diseases of the intestinal mucosa, and renal insufficiency) and 37 to 100% sensitive in chronic pancreatitis. Thus, it is useful in advanced pancreatic insufficiency, when the diagnosis of chronic pancreatitis is more simply established by other means, and least reliable in patients with mild or moderate disease.

The same principles and problems apply to the other tubeless tests. In the pancreolauryl test, fluorescein dilaurate is hydrolyzed by pancreatic arylesterases to water-soluble fluorescein, which is then absorbed by the small intestine, conjugated in the liver, and excreted in the urine. This test has been reported to be more reliable than the PABA test, but it is also insensitive in mild forms of the disease. A dual-labeled Schilling test, which relies on the ability of pancreatic enzymes to displaced R protein from cobalamin and permit its subsequent binding to intrinsic factor, has not been widely tested, nor is it widely available.

We do not use any of the previously mentioned tests. They are insensitive, and test results do not add any clear diagnostic benefit in our practice when we have an invasive pancreatic function test (see later discussion) and imaging tests available. In other clinical settings, however, the NBT-PABA test may play a role in diagnosis but should not be relied on in isolation.

Breath Tests. Fat malabsorption can be detected by measuring $^{14}CO_2$ or hydrogen in the breath after ingesting radiolabeled fat or a starch load. None of these tests has come into general use because they are not sufficiently sensitive and specific. Any breath test based on measurement of breath $^{14}CO_2$ after intestinal hydrolysis of a substrate will be subject to false-positive test results in patients with diabetes mellitus, obesity, diseases or resection of the small bowel, and hepatic or pulmonary disease.

Invasive Tests

Oroduodenal intubation is required in these tests to collect samples for enzymes and/or bicarbonate. The pancreas is usually stimulated with intravenous administration of secretin or cholecystokinin octapeptide (CCK-OP). Gastric juice is aspirated during the test through a gastric tube. Measuring bicarbonate concentrations after secretin or measuring pancreatic enzyme output during a constant intravenous infusion of CCK-OP is 90% sensitive and specific. However, in about 5% of patients with advanced disease as evidenced by pancreatic calcification, normal test results can be obtained.

SUMMARY OF DIAGNOSTIC TESTS

An algorithm of diagnostic tests in chronic pancreatitis is presented in Figure 1. Note that in some patients who do not have clear clinical evidence of pancreatic disease and present with symptoms of malabsorption, the starting point of investigation may be a quantitative stool fat to confirm the diagnosis of steatorrhea. If malabsorption is present, confirmation of pancreatic disease should be obtained with a pancreatic function test. Because pancreatic function tests are not available in many centers, structural studies such as CT, US, and ERCP may be employed to establish the diagnosis. Alternatively, pancreatic enzymes can be administered, and the clinical response and/or quantitative stool fat estimation while the patient is on therapy can be determined.

TREATMENT OF CHRONIC PANCREATITIS

Pain

Control of pain is the most challenging and unsatisfactory aspect of the management of chronic pancreatitis (Figure 2). In patients with alcoholic pancreatitis, we initially advise total abstinence from alcohol. Reports indicate that up to 75% of patients obtain pain relief after stopping alcohol. This may be true in early chronic pancreatitis, but in patients with advanced disease, about 50% of patients with both painful or painless disease continue to drink. This is most likely explained by the fact that in early chronic pancreatitis in which pancreatic secretion is well preserved, alcohol acting as a secretogogue may

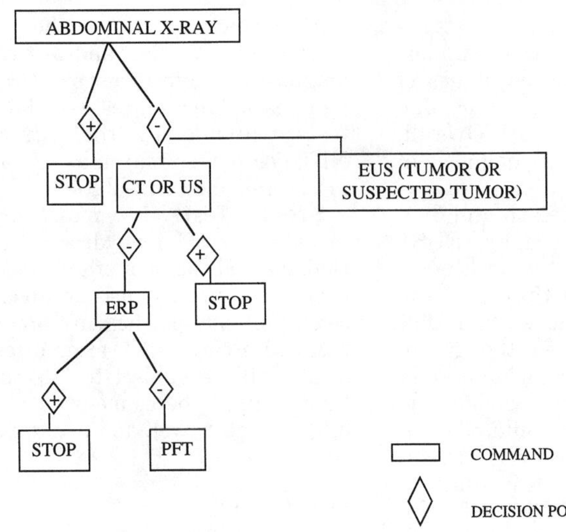

Figure 1. Algorithm for the diagnosis of suspected chronic pancreatitis.

induce pain, but in end-stage disease with malabsorption, alcohol no longer plays a role in the production of pain. Small meals and the use of simple analgesics may also be helpful and should be advised.

It has been proposed that pancreatic enzyme administration is helpful for the treatment of pain in chronic pancreatitis. In rats and other experimental animals, diversion of pancreatic proteases from the duodenum results in increased pancreatic secretion. In fasting rats, pancreatic proteases hydrolyze CCK-releasing factor (CCK-RF) secreted into the duodenum and thus prevent CCK release. This protease-dependent negative feedback system is difficult to demonstrate in humans. In theory, in chronic pancreatitis, the low levels of intraduodenal proteases cannot hydrolyze CCK-RF, which in turn leads to CCK release and chronic fasting stimulation of pancreatic secretion with resultant pain. The oral administration of pancreatic enzymes is hypothesized to restore the normal suppressive mechanism described earlier. Consequently, CCK is not released, fasting pancreatic secretion is not stimulated, and pain is therefore relieved.

In humans, studies testing the efficacy of pancreatic enzymes for pain relief have had mixed results. Proponents of the use of pancreatic enzymes claim it is effective only in patients with mild, usually idiopathic, disease who do not have malabsorption. They further point out that studies that produced negative results have employed enteric-coated preparations that are not likely to release their enzymes in the duodenum. This issue remains unresolved, but because oral administration of pancreatic enzymes is safe, most clinicians prescribe them. In clinical practice, we have not been impressed by their effects but agree that a trial is reasonable, provided that a nonenteric-coated preparation is used in the subset of patients described earlier.

Other suppressors of pancreatic secretion are CCK-receptor antagonists and the somatostatin analogue

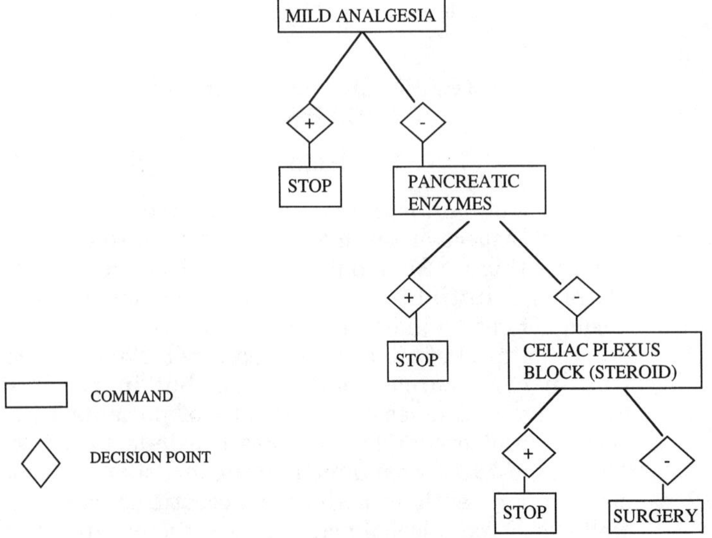

Figure 2. Algorithm for the treatment of pain in chronic pancreatitis.

octreotide (Sandostatin).* The former have not been evaluated clinically; in a pilot study of octreotide in a dose of 200 μg administered subcutaneously three times a day, pain was reduced in 65% of patients receiving the active drug compared with 35% of patients receiving placebo. No further studies have been performed; further data are required before this expensive parenterally administered agent can be recommended. Of interest, if octreotide is proved to be effective in reducing pain, it may not be via the mechanism of decreased pancreatic secretion but because it inhibits secretion of neurotransmitters.

Opiates, except for occasional use in controlling severe exacerbations of pain, cannot be recommended, although there are proponents who claim that in carefully planned and supervised situations, they can be useful without causing abuse. This may be true of a small number of patients with nonalcoholic chronic pancreatitis, but we would not recommend this strategy in alcoholic patients.

Celiac plexus blocks have been evaluated for the management of pain. In general, alcohol-based blocks have been useful in the treatment of pancreatic cancer but ineffective in the treatment of the pain of chronic pancreatitis. At the Mayo Clinic, short-term benefit has been obtained with steroid, but not alcohol, blocks. Not all patients benefit; in those who benefit, pain relief lasts a few months only, but the block can be repeated. In our view, this is sometimes a useful strategy to tide patients over episodes of pain.

Surgical and Endoscopic Management of Pain in Chronic Pancreatitis. Endoscopic therapy relies on the hypothesis that establishing better duct drainage will improve pain in chronic pancreatitis. This can be achieved by the placement of stents in the pancreatic duct endoscopically. Although reports were initially enthusiastic, and remain so in some quarters, it should be recognized that the data are uncontrolled and these are mostly short-term nonrandomized studies. There is little or no information regarding the precise nature of the pain in terms of its frequency, severity, and duration in these studies. Because 35% of patients with chronic pancreatitis may respond to placebo therapy, it is important to perform controlled trials before accepting the efficacy of a procedure. Studies that combine duct drainage with removal of duct stones by extracorporeal shock-wave lithotripsy or endoscopic removal confuse what may be the potentially useful modality. Stent placement over a long period of time has been reported to have significant complications, including acute pancreatitis, pancreatic abscess formation, and duct damage simulating findings in chronic pancreatitis, stressing the need for further data. Although the idea of being able to treat painful pancreatitis endoscopically is attractive, we believe it is experimental and should be done only under the conditions of a prospective, randomized, controlled trial.

*Not FDA approved for this indication.

The two surgical methods that are generally accepted as relieving pain are pancreatic duct drainage procedures or some form of pancreatic resection. The indication for surgery in chronic pancreatitis is almost always intractable pain, but in some patients the inability to exclude a pancreatic neoplasm based on localized changes in the pancreas on CT, US, or ERCP provides an additional reason. Pancreatic pseudocysts and biliary obstruction are also indications for surgery and should always be considered in attempting to explain an individual patient's pain.

Lateral pancreaticojejunostomy requires a dilated pancreatic duct, and therefore patients with small duct chronic pancreatitis are not candidates for this procedure. In technical terms, the duct is opened from the tail of the pancreas through to the head, and stone material is removed when present. Approximately 75 to 80% of patients are reported to obtain benefit from the procedure, but several reports indicate that over a number of years the pain recurs. Unfortunately, although the results in the surgical literature are impressive, they are diminished by subjective and nonuniform methods for evaluating the efficacy of surgery. The advantage of a lateral pancreaticojejunostomy is that it does not remove any portion of the pancreas and thus does not hasten (or obviously retard) the onset of exocrine or endocrine insufficiency.

Other surgical procedures such as sphincteroplasty and distal pancreatectomy with pancreaticojejunostomy have been virtually abandoned because they are ineffective.

Pancreatic Resection. The major drawback to pancreatic resection is the development of insulin-dependent diabetes and pancreatic exocrine insufficiency. Thus, although distal pancreatectomy ranging from 40 to 80% of the gland was once popular, this operation has now been discarded except for truly focal disease involving the tail. Most surgeons today agree that in patients with chronic pancreatitis the disease is usually dominant in the pancreatic head. A standard Whipple's procedure or pancreaticoduodenectomy produces late postoperative mortality and morbidity related to diabetes and malnutrition, and this has led to the adoption of the pylorus-preserving Whipple's procedure. Beger in Germany devised a procedure that preserves the stomach, duodenum, and bile duct while resecting the head of the gland, preserving only a juxtaduodenal rim. Seventy percent of patients in his series are reported to be totally pain free after follow-up of 3.6 years. The Frey procedure, popularized in the United States, is similar in concept and provides similar results.

At our tertiary referral center, about 30% of patients with chronic pancreatitis have surgery but only after careful evaluation and when all medical options have been exhausted. Patients with chronic pain and diffuse small duct disease remain a difficult problem, and there are no established surgical techniques that deal reliably with this form of the disease.

Malabsorption

Uncertainties remain as to the most effective manner in which to treat malabsorption. Although there is general agreement that currently available commercial preparations contain too little lipolytic activity, there is no unanimity of opinion with regard to the best type of enzyme preparation to use. Enzyme preparations fall under two main categories: (1) pancreatin, uncoated (Viokase) or enteric-coated, and (2) microencapsulated preparations (Creon, Pancrease) that consist of pancreatic enzyme coated with a pH-sensitive material that dissolves when the pH is 5 or above, are available as so-called high-potency preparations, and have the advantage that somewhat fewer capsules are required with each meal. Many studies of in vitro and in vivo efficacy of pancreatic enzyme preparations have been conducted and show that steatorrhea is improved but rarely completely corrected; with the addition of an H_2 blocker or proton pump inhibitor, complete correction can be achieved in 40% of patients. Although the in vitro and in vivo therapeutic effects of pancreatin are well established, the large number of tablets that need to be taken with meals to overcome both the low specific activity of the preparation and the gastric acidity that can irreversibly inactivate much of the lipolytic activity remain disadvantages. We recommend 8 Viokase tablets, 2 after a few bites of a meal, 4 during, and 2 at the end of the meal, and 4 tablets with snacks, in conjunction with an acid-reducing agent. In this way, the approximately 30,000 IU of lipase that are required in the duodenum during the 4-hour postprandial phase can be delivered. Fewer capsules of the high-potency microsphere preparations are required to deliver the same amount of lipolytic activity to the duodenum. Because microsphere coating dissolves at pH 5, acid conditions in the duodenum can potentially prevent the release of enzyme, and the use of acid-reducing agents may still be required. The high-potency microsphere preparations have been associated with colonic strictures in children with cystic fibrosis, leading to the recommendation that doses of no more than 10,000 USP units of lipase per kg per day should be used.

Much of the data with regard to Pancreatin was obtained by in vitro studies in which the enzyme activity of an individual preparation was measured and by detailed in vivo studies. The same detailed studies have not been performed with the newer preparations. Wide discrepancies between advertised enzyme activity in a preparation and that measured in individual investigators' laboratories have been recorded; there is a difference in activity not only from one preparation to another, but also within different batches of the same preparation. Lack of uniform methods and units (IU vs. USP units) to describe the lipase content of a preparation confuses an already difficult subject. Because therapy is lifelong for patients with steatorrhea, all of these issues should be considered carefully when patients do not respond appropriately to what appears to be adequate therapy.

In contrast to steatorrhea, treatment of azotorrhea is not a problem because ingested trypsin survives the passage through the stomach and the duodenum much better than does lipase.

Pancreatic Diabetes

Although principles of management are similar to those for diabetes mellitus, there is a tendency to hypoglycemia in patients with chronic pancreatitis who receive insulin, which can be explained on the basis of continued alcohol use with decreased calorie intake or impaired release of glucagon or hepatic glycogen. Under these circumstances, undertreatment of hyperglycemia may be necessary, especially in patients considered to be unreliable.

OTHER MANIFESTATIONS OF CHRONIC PANCREATITIS

Complications of chronic pancreatitis are listed in Table 2.

Pancreatic Pseudocysts

Pseudocysts have no epithelial lining and, therefore, are not true cysts. Pancreatic pseudocysts may occur in acute or chronic pancreatitis. In chronic pancreatitis, they can be asymptomatic and generally observed, or they can manifest insidiously and cause pain or jaundice owing to bile duct obstruction. Cyst drainage should be performed when pseudocysts are symptomatic. Historically, cyst drainage has been achieved by surgical cystgastrostomy or cystenterostomy. Percutaneous radiologic placement of a drainage catheter, which can be left in position for 6 weeks or longer, has been reported to be successful in treating pancreatic pseudocyst in about 85% of patients, but persistence of a pancreaticocutaneous fistula and infection are potential complications. Endoscopic drainage of pseudocysts into the stomach or the duodenum after confirmation of suitable anatomy and absence of large vessels by endoscopic ultrasound has assumed a definite role in management and has the advantage that there is no potential for an external fistula. Multiloculated cysts present a special challenge if drainage is attempted by radiologic or endoscopic techniques. Pseudocysts that become infected either primarily or after drainage procedures should be treated with antibiotics and may then require more effective drainage. Bleeding from pancreatic

TABLE 2. **Complications of Chronic Pancreatitis**

- Pancreatic pseudocyst
- Pancreatic ascites or pleural effusion
- Common bile duct stricture resulting in:
  - Jaundice
  - Secondary biliary cirrhosis
  - Cholangitis
- Splenic vein thrombosis
- Pancreatic cancer

pseudocysts is a serious but fortunately a rare complication and is managed by either arterial embolization or surgery.

Extrahepatic Biliary Obstruction

Fibrosis of the head of the pancreas may result in a long tapered stricture of the common bile duct. About 5 to 10% of patients with calcific pancreatitis have been reported to present initially with jaundice, but asymptomatic elevations in alkaline phosphatase are far more common. Biliary obstruction may lead to episodes of cholangitis or secondary biliary cirrhosis. Biliary strictures must always be distinguished from malignant strictures due to pancreatic cancer, and abnormalities in liver test results must be differentiated from those abnormalities found in alcoholic steatosis or cirrhosis. Surgery is indicated in the presence of increasing cholestasis and liver biopsy–proven secondary biliary cirrhosis. When treatment is required, biliary sphincterotomy is inadequate to relieve the long stricture. Placement of endoscopic metal stents is reported to relieve jaundice, but we do not endorse their use in benign disease and recommend surgery.

Pancreatic Ascites and Pancreatic Pleural Effusion

This relatively uncommon disorder results when a pancreatic cyst or duct ruptures into the lesser sac or peritoneal cavity, or tracks into the mediastinum or pleural space via the retroperitoneum. Diagnosis is made by demonstrating greatly elevated amylase levels in the peritoneal or ascitic fluid, at least twice as high and usually many times higher than the serum amylase. Malignant ascites and tuberculous peritonitis need to be considered in these patients, particularly because all of these conditions have a high protein content in the ascitic fluid. Treatment initially should always be conservative, by stopping oral intake and providing parenteral nutrition. Pancreatic secretion can be reduced by means of intravenous octreotide administration. In patients with persistent ascites, endoscopic retrograde pancreatography should be performed to determine the site of the leak from the cyst or duct rupture. An endoscopic stent placed in the pancreatic duct may seal the leak successfully. All efforts at conservative management should be undertaken because, owing to their poor physical status, there is a 15 to 20% mortality in patients who undergo surgery.

Gastrointestinal Bleeding

In the setting of chronic pancreatitis, the commonest cause of gastrointestinal bleeding is nonsteroidal anti-inflammatory drug–induced erosive gastritis or peptic ulcer disease. However, splenic vein thrombosis may occur and should always be considered when gastric varices are identified in the absence of esophageal varices; splenectomy is curative. On very rare occasions, bleeding into the pancreatic duct may occur after erosion into the gastroduodenal or splenic artery.

PROGNOSIS OF CHRONIC PANCREATITIS

Prognosis depends on the cause of pancreatitis. Survival in patients with alcoholic pancreatitis is less than that in patients with idiopathic pancreatitis and is less than that in the general population, 72 versus 80 years. In our series, death was related to pancreatitis in 15% of patients and complicating pancreatic cancer in 3%. The majority of patients do not die directly as a result of pancreatitis, and this is in keeping with other reported series.

GASTROESOPHAGEAL REFLUX DISEASE

method of
KENNETH R. McQUAID, M.D.
San Francisco Veterans Affairs Medical Center and University of California, San Francisco
San Francisco, California

Gastroesophageal reflux disease (GERD) is a broad term that refers to the symptoms and/or tissue damage caused by the reflux of gastric contents into the esophagus. The occurrence of minor gastroesophageal reflux in the postprandial period that does not cause symptoms or tissue injury is physiologically normal. Gastroesophageal reflux may be considered a "disease" when it leads to symptoms that prompt patients to self-medicate or to seek a medical opinion or when it results in complications.

MANIFESTATIONS

Typical Symptoms. The typical symptoms of GERD are heartburn (retrosternal burning caused by acid reflux), regurgitation (reflux of gastric contents into the mouth occurring without effort), and/or dysphagia (sensation of "sticking" of swallowed material). Heartburn commonly occurs 30 to 60 minutes after meals or upon reclining and may be relieved by antacids. Half of patients report nocturnal symptoms. Nearly 40% of adults experience heartburn monthly, 15% weekly, and 7% daily. Symptom prevalence rates are similar for men and women and for different age groups. The majority of patients with heartburn self-medicate with over-the-counter (OTC) medications; less than 20% seek medical attention. Dysphagia is present in one third of patients, in whom it may be due to abnormal peristalsis or peptic stricture. Up to half of patients have other associated postprandial symptoms, including belching, bloating, and early satiety.

Atypical Symptoms. Gastroesophageal reflux can cause or exacerbate a host of respiratory and otolaryngologic conditions. GERD symptoms are present in more than half of asthmatic patients; however, establishing a causal relationship with reflux is difficult. GERD-related asthma should be suspected when there is nocturnal cough or when asthmatic symptoms occur after meals or with recumbency. It should also be considered in asthmatic patients who present in adulthood and whose disease lacks an allergic component and is refractory to inhaled steroid therapy. GERD accounts for 25% of patients with non-cardiac chest pain, recurrent hoarseness, chronic cough, or chronic laryngitis. Significantly, many of these patients do not have typical GERD symptoms, arguing for increased awareness among practitioners for these atypical GERD manifestations.

Esophageal Tissue Damage

REFLUX ESOPHAGITIS. An endoscopically normal esophagus is present in the majority of GERD patients, indicating mild mucosal acid exposure. When there are repeated and/or prolonged episodes of acid reflux, damage to the esophageal epithelium is visible in the distal esophagus as erythema, friability of the squamocolumnar junction, or erosions. These changes, known as "reflux esophagitis," occur in a minority of the entire GERD population but are present in 50% of patients with frequent heartburn. Reflux esophagitis is graded as follows: grade I: erythema, friability; grade II: distal linear erosions; grade III: erosions encompassing 20 to 50% of distal mucosal surface; grade IV: circumferential erosions, ulcers, Barrett's esophagus–type changes, or peptic stricture. The severity or frequency of heartburn is not a reliable index of the severity of reflux esophagitis. Over 10% of patients with severe erosive GERD deny heartburn.

ESOPHAGEAL STRICTURE. Ten percent of patients with untreated reflux esophagitis develop circumferential strictures in the distal esophagus, resulting in slowly progressive dysphagia for solid foods, especially bread and meats. Paradoxically, as the stricture lumen narrows, reflux symptoms may diminish.

BARRETT'S ESOPHAGUS. In long-standing reflux esophagitis the normal squamous epithelium may undergo metaplasia to columnar epithelium, resulting in a premalignant condition known as Barrett's esophagus. This condition is more common in middle-aged or elderly white men, especially those with severe and/or chronic GERD symptoms. However, it appears that many patients with Barrett's esophagus have minimal or no GERD symptoms and do not seek medical attention unless a complication (e.g., dysphagia or adenocarcinoma) develops. The incidence of adenocarcinoma in patients with Barrett's esophagus is 0.8% per year (1 case per 125 patient-years of observation). Mucosal changes characteristic of Barrett's esophagus are present in 10% of patients with GERD who undergo endoscopy. The affected mucosa may appear as jagged "tongues" or a long tubular segment of orange gastric-type epithelium extending upward from the gastroesophageal junction, or there may be patches of orange mucosa surrounded by normal yellow distal esophageal mucosa. Histologically, three types of columnar epithelium occur: gastric cardia–type; gastric fundic–type (with parietal cells); and specialized columnar (also known as intestinal-type) epithelium, which contains goblet cells. Only the specialized columnar epithelium is associated with an increased risk of esophageal adenocarcinoma, warranting periodic endoscopic surveillance. Recent studies reveal specialized columnar epithelium in biopsies from the squamocolumnar junction in 18% of patients undergoing endoscopy who do not have visible Barrett's-type changes. The significance of this histologic observation at present is unclear.

DIAGNOSIS

Clinical Diagnosis. Dominant symptoms of heartburn and regurgitation suggest a diagnosis of GERD with a high degree of reliability. Many patients, however, have presentations that suggest other diagnoses, including peptic ulcer disease, nonulcer dyspepsia, and malignancy. Overall, the use of clinical findings to make a diagnosis of GERD has a sensitivity of 78% but a specificity of only 68% when pH monitoring is used as the gold standard to determine the presence of significant acid reflux. The possibility of GERD should be entertained in patients with refractory respiratory or ear-nose-throat (ENT) symptoms, including noncardiac chest pain, asthma, laryngitis, and hoarseness.

Diagnostic Tests. With a history suggestive of uncomplicated GERD, a presumptive diagnosis is made without initial diagnostic testing, and empirical therapy is initiated. The majority respond to such treatment, obviating the need for diagnostic work-up. Further evaluation is indicated for patients with symptoms that do not respond to empirical antireflux therapy, as well as patients with atypical symptoms (e.g., asthma, hoarseness, noncardiac chest pain) or signs suggestive of complications, e.g., dysphagia, weight loss, vomiting, occult blood–positive stool, or anemia.

UPPER ENDOSCOPY OR BARIUM SWALLOW. Upper endoscopy is the study of first choice in suspected GERD. Findings typical for reflux esophagitis establish the diagnosis. Half of GERD patients have a normal esophagus, however, which does not eliminate acid reflux as a cause of symptoms. Endoscopy is also useful to look for Barrett's esophagus and peptic stricture, which require biopsy. Barium swallow is less sensitive for detecting reflux esophagitis. Although barium swallow is useful in the evaluation of dysphagia to distinguish peristaltic dysfunction from a peptic stricture, patients with stricture must undergo subsequent endoscopic evaluation and biopsy.

AMBULATORY ESOPHAGEAL pH MONITORING. The most sensitive and specific diagnostic study is esophageal pH monitoring. For this study, a small pH probe is placed in the distal esophagus to measure the pattern, frequency, and duration of acid reflux. In normal persons, esophageal pH is lower than 4 for less than 5% of a 24-hour period. Normal results argue against significant acid reflux. A correlation can be sought between reflux episodes and symptoms, such as heartburn, chest pain, cough, or asthma. Thus, it is useful both in patients with typical GERD symptoms unresponsive to antireflux therapy and in patients with atypical symptoms.

TREATMENT

The efficacy of antireflux therapy is related to the presence and severity of underlying reflux esophagitis. The majority of patients have so-called nonerosive GERD, in which the esophagus appears normal. For these patients, therapy with antacids, H_2-receptor antagonists, or promotility agents is usually efficacious. Patients with erosive esophagitis, however, are better managed initially with use of potent acid-suppressive agents, i.e., proton pump inhibitors (PPIs).

In most patients with uncomplicated typical GERD symptoms, initial antireflux therapy is administered empirically, i.e., without benefit of an upper endoscopy to distinguish nonerosive from erosive GERD. Generally, a step-wise approach to treatment is undertaken, as outlined below (Figure 1).

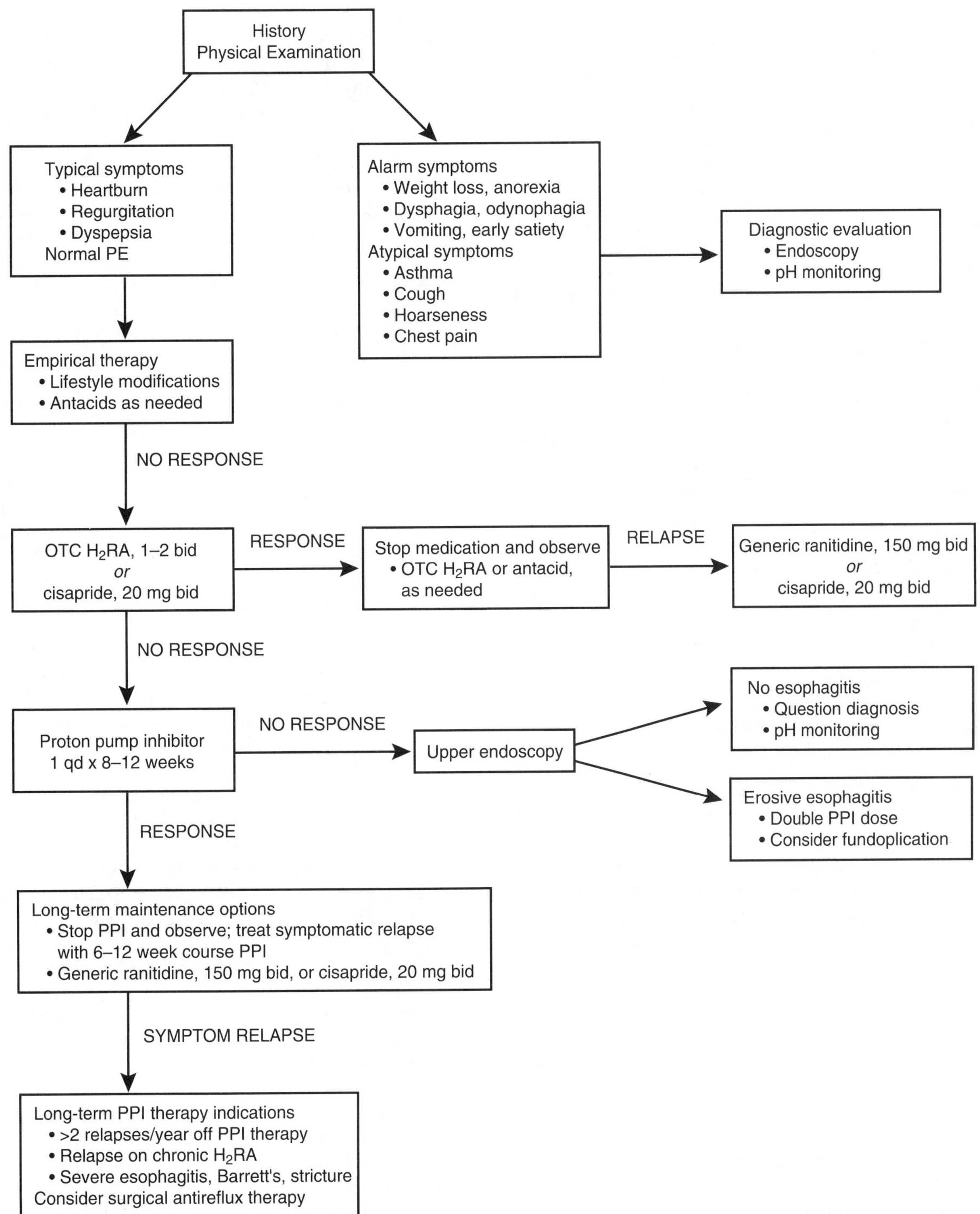

Figure 1. Algorithm for management of gastroesophageal reflux disease. *Abbreviations*: PE = physical examination; OTC = over-the-counter; H_2RA = H_2-receptor antagonist; PPI = proton pump inhibitor.

Lifestyle Modifications and Antacids

Changes in lifestyle are recommended to all patients. Modifications are aimed at reducing the number and duration of reflux episodes. Reflux is especially damaging during sleep, when swallowing and salivation decrease, leading to delays in acid clearance in the recumbent position. Therefore, the most important admonition is to elevate the head of the bed by 4 to 6 inches and to avoid meals within 3 hours of bedtime, when most reflux events occur. Other recommendations include elimination of smoking, moderation in alcohol use, reduction of meal size, and weight loss. Foods that relax the lower esophageal sphincter are prescribed, including fried or fatty foods, peppermint, chocolate, and coffee. Citrus, tomatoes, and spicy foods are direct mucosal irritants. Drugs with anticholinergic action, theophylline, and calcium channel blockers decrease lower esophageal sphincter pressure and/or delay gastric emptying. Nonsteroidal anti-inflammatory drugs (NSAIDs), alendronate (Fosamax), quinidine, potassium tablets, zidovudine (Retrovir), and some antibiotics can cause direct esophageal mucosal injury.

Antacids are the mainstay of therapy for occasional heartburn, providing relief within 15 minutes. Symptoms may recur within the hour. Commonly used formulations are Maalox and Mylanta, available either as a liquid (10–15 mL) or as tablets (2 to 4). Gaviscon is an alginate-antacid combination that decreases reflux in the upright position and is superior to antacids alone.

H_2-Receptor Antagonists or Promotility Agents

The advent of OTC histamine H_2-receptor antagonists (H_2RAs) has altered the initial management of mild GERD. These agents provide heartburn relief within 30 to 45 minutes lasting 5 to 9 hours. Patients with occasional symptoms should take them as needed or prophylactically before a meal likely to cause symptoms. Currently available are cimetidine (Tagamet) 200-mg tablets; ranitidine (Zantac 75) and nizatidine (Axid), 75-mg tablets; and famotidine (Pepcid AC), 10 mg; these OTC drugs are formulated at half the standard doses of their prescription counterparts. Patients experiencing frequent heartburn should try an OTC H_2RA, 1 or 2 tablets twice daily. For self-paying patients, these drugs are significantly less expensive than prescription H_2RAs. The cost of a 30-day supply (60 tablets) is less than $20 retail. Administered as 2 pills twice daily, for doses equivalent to those of prescription H_2RAs, OTC H_2RAs cost less than half the *wholesale* price of prescription H_2RAs, including generics. H_2RAs provide heartburn relief in 50 to 75% of patients. After symptoms remit, these medications should be discontinued; they can be resumed as needed for symptom relapses. Depending upon health insurance, patients purchasing regular OTC H_2RAs may fare better with a prescription H_2RA. Of the agents available, ranitidine and cimetidine are offered in the less expensive generic form. For most patients, there does not appear to be any advantage of one drug over another, and choice should be driven by cost. Standard prescription doses of these agents for GERD are as follows: famotidine, 20 mg twice daily (bid); nizatidine or ranitidine, 150 mg bid; and cimetidine, 400 to 800 mg bid. Although double doses of H_2RAs are more effective, this approach should not be used, because the cost exceeds that of a PPI.

The promotility agent cisapride (Propulsid) is a serotonin 5-HT_4 agonist that enhances acetylcholine release from the gut myenteric plexus, resulting in improvements in lower esophageal sphincter pressure, esophageal peristalsis, and gastric emptying. Cisapride, 10 mg qid or 20 mg bid, provides heartburn relief equivalent to that achieved with H_2RAs but is superior in treating belching and regurgitation. Thus, it is useful either alone or in combination with acid inhibitory agents to treat associated dyspeptic symptoms. It is more expensive than OTC or generic H_2RAs but less expensive than proprietary H_2RAs or PPIs.

Neither cisapride nor H_2RAs given in standard doses are very effective in healing erosive esophagitis; hence PPIs should be employed first for patients with proven reflux esophagitis at endoscopy.

Proton Pump Inhibitors

Patients with persistent symptoms despite H_2RA and/or cisapride therapy should be given a PPI. Some investigators argue that an upper endoscopy study should first be performed to document the presence or severity of esophagitis and to screen for Barrett's esophagus, but results seldom influence therapy, and such studies are not cost-effective and are unnecessary in uncomplicated cases. PPI administration is the best initial therapy for erosive reflux esophagitis, Barrett's esophagus, and peptic stricture.

PPIs permanently inactivate the parietal cell acid-secreting pump, blocking more than 90% of 24-hour acid secretion. Two agents (omeprazole [Prilosec], 20-mg capsules, and lansoprazole [Prevacid], 30-mg capsules), are available, and two others (rabeprazole and pantoprazole) are anticipated in 1998. There is no clinical advantage of one PPI over another. PPIs afford heartburn relief and healing of reflux esophagitis in more than 80% of patients when given once daily and in more than 95% when given twice daily for 6 to 8 weeks. Patient satisfaction with PPIs is high, side effects are uncommon, and long-term safety concerns have been dispelled. For these reasons, use of H_2RAs for GERD has fallen steadily, and PPIs account for more than 50% of GERD prescriptions. If drug costs were not a consideration, PPIs would be the agents of choice for almost all patients with regular GERD symptoms. It must be recognized, however, that the majority of GERD patients have mild to moderate symptoms and do not have reflux esophagitis, and their disease is well controlled on less expensive agents, i.e., H_2RA or cisapride.

Maintenance Therapy

For most patients, GERD is a chronic condition. After acute therapy, the likelihood of symptom recurrence is related to the presence of reflux esophagitis. Patients who have a rapid response to therapy with H_2RAs or cisapride should discontinue these agents after 6 to 8 weeks, resuming them as needed for symptom relapses. Frequent relapses dictate the need for chronic daily therapy.

After discontinuation of acute PPI therapy, over 70% of patients experience return of symptoms and esophagitis within 6 months. These symptoms can have a substantial impact upon quality of life and medical costs. The optimal, cost-effective management of these patients is hotly debated. Options include the following approaches: (1) Stop PPI therapy and administer an H_2RA or cisapride twice daily. With this approach, approximately 40% of patients remain in remission; the remainder may be managed with chronic PPI therapy at full dose (lansoprazole, 30 mg, or omeprazole, 20 mg) or half dose (lansoprazole, 15 mg). (2) Stop all medications and treat symptom recurrences as needed with a course of PPI therapy. Recent decision analyses suggest that for patients with fewer than 2 relapses per year, this is the most cost-effective option. Patients with more frequent relapses and those with known severe esophagitis (grade IV: Barrett's esophagus or peptic stricture) warrant chronic PPI therapy.

Given the expense of chronic therapy, an attempt should be made at least once to discontinue PPI therapy employing one of the strategies just described. Of patients who do require chronic PPI therapy, one third require doubling the PPI dose to maintain remission.

Laparoscopic Antireflux Surgery

Laparoscopic antireflux surgery represents a major advancement in the treatment of GERD and has supplanted traditional open procedures owing to the shorter hospital stays and lower complication rates associated with this technique. It provides excellent symptom relief, healing of esophagitis, and patient satisfaction in more than 90% of patients. Although the surgical approach is more costly initially, aggregate expenses may be less than those for medical treatment over a 10-year period for patients requiring chronic PPI therapy.

Currently, antireflux surgery should be considered for (1) younger patients with severe esophagitis who prefer surgery to the inconvenience and expense of chronic PPI therapy; (2) patients with respiratory or ENT symptoms thought to be secondary to GERD—although medical therapy may relieve these atypical symptoms, uncontrolled surgical studies suggest dramatic improvement in carefully selected patients; and (3) GERD refractory to medical therapy. With the advent of PPIs, however, medical failure now is uncommon.

MANAGEMENT OF COMPLICATIONS

Barrett's Esophagus. All patients with Barrett's esophagus should receive chronic PPI therapy, regardless of symptoms or esophagitis severity. They should also undergo endoscopy with biopsy every 24 months to look for dysplasia, unless contraindicated by comorbidity. With high-grade dysplasia, one in four patients will develop adenocarcinoma within 5 years, and esophagectomy is therefore recommended. For poor operative candidates or patients refusing surgery, biopsy every 6 months is recommended. Recently, ablation of Barrett's epithelium by laser, contact cautery, or photodynamic therapy, followed by high-dose PPI therapy to achieve compete acid suppression, has been shown to result in esophageal reepithelialization with squamous epithelium. Patients who are poor risks for esophagectomy may be referred to clinical trials for this therapy. Low-grade dysplasia should be followed with intensive endoscopic surveillance every 12 months.

Esophageal Stricture. Mechanical dilation to a luminal diameter of 14 mm or larger provides excellent symptomatic relief from dysphagia. For uncomplicated strictures, dilation may be achieved by blind or fluoroscopically guided passage of weighted flexible Maloney dilators. For tortuous or tight strictures, dilation is achieved with balloons or plastic dilators passed over a guide wire under fluoroscopic or endoscopic guidance. Mild strictures often require only one dilation procedure; severe strictures may require several. Chronic PPI therapy dramatically reduces the recurrence of strictures. The need for surgical treatment of refractory strictures now is uncommon.

TUMORS OF THE STOMACH

method of
HAROLD O. DOUGLASS, Jr., M.D.
State University of New York at Buffalo and Roswell Park Cancer Institute
Buffalo, New York

GASTRIC TUMORS

Benign Tumors

Benign gastric tumors constitute less than 5% of all neoplastic lesions of the stomach. Among the mesenchymal tumors are leiomyomas and neurofibromas. Epithelial tumors include inflammatory, hyperplastic, juvenile, hamartomatous, adenomatous, and villous polyps. Heterotopic pancreatic tissue consisting of acini and ducts, but rarely islets, usually appears as a submucosal lesion projecting into the lumen of the antrum or pylorus. Hypertrophic gastritis (Ménétrier's disease) can present as multiple gastric polypoid lesions in the gastric fundus and body but not in the antrum.

Leiomyomas and Leiomyoblastoma

Leiomyomas, the most common benign neoplasms of the stomach, arise from smooth muscle fibers of the muscularis mucosa, the muscularis propria, or the muscularis of vessel walls and may be multiple. They generally arise in the body or antrum but can arise from the gastroesophageal junction. Most are discovered incidentally at autopsy. Leiomyomas larger than 3 cm tend to develop a central ulceration that penetrates deeply into the tumor, causing significant bleeding. With central necrosis, they may cause pain but rarely obstruction. Leiomyomas are often diagnosed on an upper gastrointestinal series, in which the "target" appearance of central ulceration and smoothly elevated surrounding mucosa is a typical presentation. Histologically benign lesions may be distinguished from leiomyosarcomas as less cellular tumors with fewer bizarre nuclei and mitotic figures. Myxoid changes, hyalinization, and calcification also suggest benignity. Because the correlation between histologic appearance and clinical behavior is less than perfect, enucleation is inadequate treatment. Proper treatment requires complete excision with confirmation of normal tissue in all margins.

Neuroendocrine tumors may be similar in clinical presentation to leiomyomas or can present as submucosal masses. Leiomyoblastomas show a predominance of clear or epithelioid cells but can be difficult to distinguish from malignant spindle cell tumors. They also require complete surgical excision with normal tissue in all margins.

Polyps

The most common types of gastric polyps—hyperplastic, inflammatory, and hamartomatous—have no exact counterpart elsewhere in the bowel. Randomly distributed in the stomach, these tumors are often small and multiple and have a smooth or lobulated contour. They are sometimes found at gastroenteric stomas. Microscopically, they are composed of dilated or cystic glands, fibrous stroma, inflammatory cells, and occasional smooth muscle bundles from the muscularis mucosa. Atypia is rare, but carcinoma can be found in as many as 8 to 28% of these lesions.

Adenomatous polyps tend to be single and larger and are occasionally villous in appearance and often antral in location. Carcinoma may be found in half of these lesions. Patients with familial adenomatous polyposis may present with adenomatous or villous gastric polyps. Cancer or carcinoids may appear in familial polyps. With all adenomatous polyps, the risk of cancer is proportional to polyp size, being less than 5% in small (0–12 cm) polyps but as high as 80% in much larger polyps with irregular shapes.

Complete endoscopic polypectomy is the procedure of choice after identification of the site in the stomach from which the polyp is to be removed. If the polyps are benign, no further treatment other than follow-up is necessary. Villous polyps, polyps that cannot be completely excised endoscopically, and those with a focus of malignancy require complete surgical excision, with an appropriate extension of resection if cancer is present.

Malignant Tumors

Leiomyosarcoma

Although occasionally clinically silent until the advent of liver metastases, most gastric leiomyosarcomas are diagnosed after an episode of upper gastrointestinal bleeding. Although generally large in size (>4 cm to 10 cm or more), leiomyosarcomas rarely cause vomiting unless they are very large (>10 cm), invade adjacent organs, or metastasize, usually to the liver. Histologic discrimination between small low-grade sarcomas and benign leiomyomas can be difficult or impossible.

The surgical approach to leiomyosarcoma depends on its location within the stomach. There is no evidence that survival after extensive gastric resection is superior to that after regional resection, so long as the tumor is surrounded by a disease-free margin greater than 2 cm. Obviously, this requires partial gastrectomy in many locations, but along the greater curvature a local resection may be sufficient. There is no survival benefit for resection of regional lymph nodes (to which metastases are uncommon) or uninvolved adjacent structures such as the spleen. Overall 5-year survival rates range from 45% to 60%, being higher for small low-grade tumors but practically zero when adjacent organs are invaded, despite attempts at cure by extensive resection. Median survival is approximately 4 years for patients with localized disease and 3 years for those with contiguous organ invasion or peritoneal implants. Benefit for adjuvant radiation or chemotherapy has yet to be demonstrated.

Malignant leiomyoblastomas are handled in the same manner as for leiomyosarcomas. Histologic grade is the best determinant of survival. Although the overall 5-year survival rate is about 33%, few if any patients with high-grade leiomyoblastomas survive 3 years.

Neuroendocrine Tumors

The two most common neuroendocrine tumors of the stomach are carcinoids and gastrinomas, most of which arise in the distal stomach within the "gastrinoma triangle" (based on the duodenum and the origin of the superior mesenteric artery). These tumors may appear as submucosal nodules or present a "target" appearance on gastrointestinal series similar to that of leiomyomas. However, many gastric carcinoids are readily confused radiographically and endoscopically with gastric adenocarcinoma. Both metastasize to regional lymph nodes and to the liver. Surgical resection should include the primary tumor and adjacent stomach and at least N1 lymph nodes. Liver metastases from these usually slowly growing cancers can be treated by resection (multiple wedge resections), cryosurgery, infusion chemotherapy with dacarbazine (DTIC) and floxuridine (FUDR), or chemoembolization using doxorubicin (Adriamycin), 30 mg, and powdered oxidized cellulose (Gelfoam). Endocrine symptoms often respond to somatostatin analogue (Sandostatin), 100 to 600 μg/day in divided doses. Bone metastases respond to radiotherapy. A variety of combination chemotherapy regimens for systemic disease provide remissions of 3 to 12 months or longer; the agents used are doxorubicin (Adriamycin), 5-fluorouracil (5-FU), dacarbazine (DTIC), streptozotocin (Zanosar), and cyclophosphamide (Cytoxan).

Lymphomas

Approximately 5% of the malignant tumors of the stomach are lymphomas. Presenting signs and symptoms are nausea, vomiting, weight loss, gastrointestinal bleeding (generally occult, but occasionally with hematemesis), early satiety, and epigastric pain. Endoscopic biopsy usually provides sufficient tissue for diagnosis and histologic typing. Physical examination, chest x-ray study, computed tomography of the abdomen, and a bone marrow biopsy are necessary to ensure that the gastric tumor does not represent extension into the stomach of an advanced lymphoma. Endoscopy should be complemented by biopsy and rapid urease assay (CLO test) for urea-splitting *Helicobacter pylori*, which can be associated with the usually low- or intermediate-grade, often indolent MALT (mucosa-associated lymphoid tissue) B cell lymphomas. Lymphomas of the stomach can be localized or diffuse and are frequently quite large (>10 cm in diameter), often extending beyond the serosa.

In the 1950s and 1960s, gastric lymphomas were treated by surgical resection. If the tumor could be completely resected, 5-year survival rates ranged between 45% and 70%. The addition of radiation therapy and/or chemotherapy after complete resection did not improve survival but was of benefit if there was residual lymphoma after surgery. It was necessary to distinguish between a primary lymphoma of the stomach and non-Hodgkin's lymphoma (NHL) secondarily involving the stomach, for which surgery was of little if any benefit. The development of the CHOP chemotherapy regimen—cyclophosphamide (Cytoxan), 600 to 700 mg/m^2 of body surface, plus doxorubicin (formerly hydroxydaunorubicin; Adriamycin), 40 to 50 mg/m^2, plus vincristine (Oncovin), 1.4 mg/m^2, to a maximum dose of 2 mg, all on the first day, with prednisone, 60 mg/m^2 daily on days 1 to 5, by mouth, all repeated every 21 or 28 days—administered after resection was associated with increased 5-year survival rates of 75 to 95% in patients with localized disease but only 25% in patients with advanced stage IV lymphomas. Most patients had IWG (International Working Group) mid- or high-grade lymphomas. More rigorous chemotherapy regimens had little further impact on survival. Radiation therapy (25–35 Gy) was often added, but there was little evidence that it affected survival favorably.

Recent studies suggest that patients who receive chemotherapy, with or without radiation therapy, but without surgery, have 5- and 10-year survival rates equivalent to those in patients who undergo gastrectomy, without the 2 to 11% surgical mortality rates in most surgical series. Treatment-related complications of bleeding and perforation of the lymphoma are rare (<4%). Although patients with smaller tumors (<7 cm) are usually cured by chemotherapy, with or without surgery, there is some evidence that the clinical course of patients older than 60 years with larger lymphomas may be more favorable after gastric resection. The current standard of care for patients with stage IE (confined to the stomach) and IIE (involvement of contiguous lymph nodes) lymphomas of the stomach is complete surgical resection so long as no other organs are involved.

More than 75% of "pseudolymphomas"—the subject of numerous publications in the 1980s—have been reclassified as MALT lymphomas, usually IWF low-grade B cell gastric lymphomas associated with *H. pylori* infestation. These low-grade MALT lymphomas may spread to distant sites, and some may have a high-grade component. However, several investigators have demonstrated regression of 50 to 80% of true low-grade B cell MALT lymphomas confined to the stomach after eradication of *H. pylori* by bismuth and combination antibiotic regimens. Regression may take 1 year or more. About one third of these patients relapse, sometimes with transformation into a higher grade (e.g., large cell, IWF IIG) lymphoma.

Adenocarcinomas

Since the mid-1930s, when gastric cancer was the leading cause of cancer death in the United States, the incidence of typical gastric cancer has fallen precipitously. Recently, the incidence has stabilized, owing in part to an increase in the Asian American population and to immigration from Southeast Asia, and also to a rapidly increasing incidence in cancer at the gastroesophageal junction, frequently in a younger patient population.

With more than 15,000 deaths from gastric cancer occurring annually in the United States, of which 95% are adenocarcinomas, stomach cancer is the sixth most common cause of cancer-related mortality. The disease is slightly more common in men than women, and 60 to 70% of cases are associated with the presence of *H. pylori* in the gastric mucosa. Elsewhere in the world, particularly where salting and smoking are common means of food preservation, the incidence of gastric cancer is higher. Diets and water sources high in nitrates have similarly been associated with increased gastric cancer incidence.

Early (mucosal or submucosal, T1) gastric cancer causes a variety of dyspeptic symptoms, none of which is specific. With more advanced disease come pain, nausea, anorexia, weakness, early satiety, and regurgitation. Endoscopic examination of small cancers can suggest prognosis, although there is an inexact correlation between Boorman classification and depth of invasion: type 1 includes polypoid and fungating cancers, type 2 are ulcerated lesions with elevated borders, type 3 are ulcerated lesions infiltrating the gastric wall, and type 4 are diffusely infiltrating cancers, often without an obvious mucosal lesion. These infiltrating cancers (linitis plastica type) are associated with a thickened gastric wall covered with normal mucosa in an often nondistensible stomach and can be missed by the endoscopist unless random gastric brushings precede deep (submucosal) biopsies. Mucosal biopsies often fail to reveal the cancer.

Histologically, gastric cancer is divided by the Lauren classification into intestinal and diffuse. Intestinal cancers carry a better prognosis and are more common in endemic areas and are often associated with intestinal metaplasia and chronic gastritis. Diffuse cancers include linitis plastica and signet ring cell tumors, for which the prognosis can be grim. After three decades, the three major staging systems (American Joint Committee on Cancer, International Union Against Cancer, and Japanese Society for the Research of Gastric Cancer) are now virtually identical.

TREATMENT OF GASTRIC CANCER

Treatment of gastric cancer is stage-dependent: surgery plays a major role in stages I, II, and III, but radiation therapy and chemotherapy are the primary therapeutic modes used in stage IV (metastatic cancer), with surgery only rarely indicated. Numerous cooperative trials have failed to confirm a benefit for postoperative adjuvant therapy, a fact that has led to experimental neoadjuvant treatment programs. Overall 5-year survival rates for gastric cancer patients as reported by the American College of Surgeons in 1987 are 56.8% for stage I, 33.9% for stage II, 17.1% for stage III, and 5.6% for stage IV. Individual institutions usually report higher survival rates, but the extent of resection and surgical selection bias may affect their data.

Surgery

There is a continuing debate with regard to the extent of surgical resection, and particularly of the lymphadenectomy that should be performed on patients with gastric adenocarcinoma. Five-year survival data for patients with stages I through III cancers show little improvement since the 1970s. However, Japanese investigators report that overall survival approaches 60%, with survival rates for stages I, II, and III approaching 95%, 70%, and 35%, respectively. Overall survival reflects the results of screening for early disease. Nearly half of Japanese patients are diagnosed at stage I or II. However, stage for stage, improved survival may reflect the results of systematic, more aggressive surgery.

Results reported by individual institutions from Germany and the United States are similar to those reported from Japan. Generally, these institutions have used "Japanese-type" surgery, involving resection of the second-echelon (N2) lymph nodes—that is, D2 dissection. The main criticism of D2 resection is increased surgical morbidity compared with that with limited, D1 resection, but reports from institutions where this operation is performed routinely suggest that D2 lymphadenectomies can be performed without a significant increase in morbidity or mortality, particularly when lymph nodes are dissected without resection of adjacent organs (e.g., pancreas). The survival rate of patients with positive lymph nodes in the second echelon (N2), when these nodes are all methodically resected, can be 35% or higher. In contrast, when individual N2 nodes or groups are resected, the 5-year survival rate is less than 15%.

Two randomized trials are ongoing to compare limited D1 resection and the D2 procedure. Thus far, neither shows a survival advantage for D2 resection, and both revealed significant increases in morbidity when D2 resections are performed by surgeons who have traditionally performed D1 limited procedures.

Whether total gastrectomy is necessary is another unresolved question. Although total gastrectomy does not increase operative morbidity or mortality, long-term digestive complaints and difficulty in weight stabilization are quality-of-life issues that must be considered.

In general, patients with tumors of antrum and distal stomach can be treated by distal subtotal gastrectomy, while patients with cancers in the gastric cardia and fundus can be treated by proximal esophagogastrectomy. A 6-m margin between the gross tumor and the specimen margin is necessary, and very small gastric pouches are of almost no value. Cancers of the body of the stomach generally require total gastrectomy. As a rule, any cancer that impinges on an imaginary line running from the incisura on the lesser curvature to the "bare area" between the branches of the right gastroepiploic artery and the short gastric branches of the splenic artery will require a total gastrectomy for a curative resection.

Adjuvant Therapy

Twenty-five years of postoperative adjuvant therapy trials in the United States and throughout the world have left most investigators convinced that an active treatment program has yet to be identified. In Japan and Korea, a number of trials comparing postoperative chemotherapy and "chemoimmunotherapy" using streptococcal (PSK) or nocardial (OK432) cell wall antigens as the immunologic adjuvant strongly suggest benefit for immunologically enhanced treatment. Unfortunately, the original controlled chemotherapy studies, which are now 20 to 30 years old, showed advantages generally confined to subpopulations and could not always be duplicated.

This result has led to exploration of a variety of neoadjuvant and perioperative adjuvant phase II (uncontrolled) studies, some of which have introduced intraperitoneal or intra-arterial (via the celiac artery) drug infusions. Early promising results need to be retested in controlled trials.

Therapeutic Approaches with Advanced Disease

The role of radiation therapy in gastric cancer is largely limited to control of surgically and endoscopically uncontrollable bleeding (usually a continuous slow ooze from the tumor) and the relief of pain, particularly if bone metastases are present. Radiopotentiation with 5-FU, with or without cisplatin (DDP), is currently standard treatment. The future may see gemcitabine (Gemzar) as the radiopotentiating agent, if a safe radiopotentiating dose of gemcitabine in combinination with abdominal radiation can be identified. However, current regimens carry unacceptable risks of ulceration and bleeding from both normal and malignant gastrointestinal tissue.

Although numerous chemotherapy regimens have been proposed for treatment of patients with advanced metastatic gastric cancer, most add considerable drug toxicity with little evidence that they are more effective than single-agent 5-FU. Two regimens of European origin that appear to be useful are ELF (etoposide [VePesid], leucovorin [Wellcovorin], and 5-FU) and FAMTX (5-FU, doxorubicin, and high-dose methotrexate). ELF was designed for older patients with limited bone marrow reserve, but the hematologic toxicity (and mucous membrane toxicity) of FAMTX can be formidable. There is still considerable room for exploratory phase II trials, the more promising of which include taxines with carboplatin.

In general, gastric cancer spreads transperitoneally (to peritoneal surfaces including the surface of the liver and ovaries), via the lymphatics (to lungs and bone), via the (portal vein) bloodstream (to the liver), and by direct extension to the pancreas, mesocolon, liver, and spleen. Although liver metastases are considered the prominent feature in gastrointestinal metastasis, the peritoneum and lymphatics are the major routes of gastric cancer dissemination. Dissemination of gastric cancer to the liver is much less common in autopsy series. Thus, multimodality approaches of the future will have to include therapy with agents that will reach the peritoneal cavity and retroperitoneal lymphatics—areas reached by little if any drug in currently used systemic chemotherapy regimens.

TUMORS OF THE COLON AND RECTUM

method of
SIDNEY J. WINAWER, M.D.
Memorial Sloan-Kettering Cancer Center
New York, New York

Adenocarcinoma accounts for nearly 98% of the malignant tumors arising in the colon and rectum. The three most common nonadenocarcinoma cancers at these anatomic sites are carcinoids, lymphomas, and sarcomas. The colon and rectum can also be the site of metastatic cancer and a variety of benign tumors, the most common of which is the adenomatous polyp. This article focuses on adenocarcinoma of the colon and rectum, commonly called colorectal cancer. The most frequent cancers in patients in the United States and most Western countries are cancers of the breast, lung, colon, rectum, and prostate. The number of new colorectal cancer cases in the United States in 1998 will be 135,000, and the number of deaths 50,000, making colorectal cancer the second leading cause of cancer death in the United States after lung cancer. The incidence of and death rate from this cancer are the same for women as for men. The mortality has been gradually declining during the last few years, attributable to improved therapy and earlier diagnosis. The incidence has also shown a downward trend, the reason as yet being unclear but possibly the result of increasingly widespread use of colonoscopy and polypectomy with removal of the premalignant stage of this disease.

PATHOLOGY

Adenocarcinoma of the colon is almost always preceded by a precursor lesion, the benign adenomatous polyp. The concept of the adenoma as a precursor of adenocarcinoma of the colon is strongly supported by epidemiologic and pathologic studies. In addition, clinical studies have provided evidence that polypectomy dramatically reduces the risk of subsequent colorectal cancer. Approximately two thirds of polyps encountered in the clinical setting are adenomas. These are classified histologically as tubular, tubulovillous, and villous and according to whether high-grade dysplasia is present. The most prevalent histologic growth pattern is tubular. Adenomas with a villous pattern are more likely to show high-grade dysplasia and transform into invasive malignant tumors. Other colorectal polyps include hyperplastic polyps, mucosal tags, inflammatory polyps, juvenile polyps, hamartomas, and a variety of nonmucosal lesions. Adenomas represent a monoclonal proliferation of stem cell progeny. The acquired mutation that underlies sporadic adenoma formation is not known, but it is speculated that it may be related to the familial adenomatous polyposis (FAP) gene locus. Two thirds of the adenomatous polyps are distal to the splenic flexure in clinical studies. This parallels the distribution of adenocarcinoma of the colon.

Colorectal cancer can be tiny to massive. The size is not predictive of metastatic potential. The tumors can be exophytic and polypoid with variable extension into the lumen or endophytic with little luminal involvement. The exophytic tumors can be broad based and sessile or, less commonly, pedunculated. New tumors tend to grow circumferentially, especially in the distal colon, producing obstruction, and often have ulcerations with associated bleeding. Staging is based on the degree of penetration into the bowel wall, the presence or absence of lymph node metastases, and the presence or absence of distant metastases (Table 1). The tumor can spread by direct extension to involve not only lymph nodes and mesentery but adjacent organs, and it can spread through vascular and lymphatic routes to distant sites, the most common of which are the liver and lung. Direct extension to surrounding pelvic tissues is especially seen with rectal cancers. Synchronous lesions are seen in about 3 to 5% of patients. The majority of these tumors are moderately well-differentiated, gland-forming adenocarcinomas with typical characteristic histo-

TABLE 1. **Comparison of TNM and Dukes' Staging Systems for Colorectal Cancer**

Stage	TNM Designation			Dukes' Designation
0	Tis	N0	M0	—
I	T1	N0	M0	A
	T2	N0	M0	
II	T3	N0	M0	B
	T4	N0	M0	
III	Any T	N1	M0	C
	Any T	N2, N3	M0	
IV	Any T	Any N	M1	D

Abbreviations: Tis = tumor in situ; T1 = tumor invades submucosa; T2 = tumor invades muscularis propria; T3 = tumor invades through muscularis propria; T4 = tumor invades serosa ± adjacent organs; N0 = negative lymph nodes; N1 = one to three positive nodes; N2 = more than three positive nodes; N3 = positive nodes on vascular trunk; M0 = no distant metastases; M1 = distant metastases.

logic features. Tumors that have abundant mucin in the cytoplasm, especially when forming a "signet cell" appearance, are usually aggressive tumors with poor prognosis. Residual adenomatous tissue is often seen, especially when the cancers are small.

A number of genetic abnormalities have been demonstrated in adenomatous polyps and cancers as adenomas form, grow, and transform to cancer and the cancer advances. The most common genetic abnormalities are mutations and deletions in chromosomes 5 (*APC* [adenomatous polyposis coli] genes), 17 (*p53* genes), and 18 (*DCC* [deleted in colorectal cancer] genes) and mutations in the K-*ras* oncogene. In a small percentage of colorectal cancers, a "mutator" phenotype has been demonstrated that is characterized by genomic instability at simple repeated sequences in DNA, thought to be a consequence of a mutation in genes involved in DNA repair. This abnormal phenotype is commonly seen as a germline or inherited abnormality in hereditary nonpolyposis colorectal cancer (HNPCC or the Lynch syndrome). Growth factors, immunologic factors, and factors associated specifically with invasiveness and metastatic potential have also been described.

ETIOLOGY

Colorectal cancer is associated with age; more than 90% of cases occur in men and women older than 50 years (Table 2). Rectal cancer, in contrast to colon cancer, is more common in men than in women. Lifestyle factors have been shown to be important in the causation. A positive association has been demonstrated with a diet high in fat and low in fiber, fruits, and vegetables; sedentary lifestyle; lack of exercise; cigarette smoking; and excess alcohol consumption.

Individuals with a prior history of colorectal cancer or adenomatous polyps have a higher risk of subsequent colorectal cancer if their colon has not been cleared of polyps. Individuals with inflammatory bowel disease (IBD) are at increased risk, which is related to the length of time of their ulcerative or granulomatous colitis and the extent of the anatomic involvement. IBD accounts for 1% of the new cases of colon cancer in the United States each year, usually in those who have involvement of the entire bowel 8 years or longer or involvement of the distal bowel 15 years or longer. Women with a prior cancer of the endometrium, breast, or ovary may have an increased risk of colorectal cancer, the magnitude of which is unclear but may be related to the age at diagnosis and family history of cancer.

There is an increased susceptibility to colorectal cancer with a family history of colorectal cancer, especially when the diagnosis of colorectal cancer is made before the age of 55 years or adenomatous polyps are diagnosed before the age of 60 years. The overall increased risk for first-degree relatives (siblings, parents, children) of these patients is twofold. A greater increase in risk for colorectal cancer is present in individuals who are in families demonstrating a strong pattern of inheritance based on transmission of germline mutations. The two major inherited genetic syndromes are FAP and Gardner's syndrome, which is a full expression of FAP, and HNPCC. FAP accounts for approximately 1% and HNPCC for approximately 5% of the new cancers diagnosed each year (Figure 1). Both are inherited in an autosomal dominant pattern. In FAP, the colon is studded with thousands of adenomatous polyps throughout, beginning in adolescence, with cancers being seen in the twenties and thirties. In HNPCC, the polyps are fewer and are found mostly on the right side of the colon, with cancer occurring in the forties and fifties compared with the average age of 67 years at diagnosis of colorectal cancer in the general population. FAP is associated with inheritance in gene carriers of mutations on chromosome 5; HNPCC is associated with mutations on chromosomes 2, 3, and 7. FAP is associated with other cancers, including those of the stomach and duodenum, and with desmoid tumors. HNPCC is associated with a variety of tumors including stomach, pancreas, uterus, melanoma, and others.

SYMPTOMS, SIGNS, AND DIAGNOSIS

Symptoms occur after an adenoma has formed, grown, and transformed into cancer and the cancer has advanced. It has been estimated that this takes on the average 10 to 15 years. The earliest symptoms may be fatigue as a result of anemia, especially from right-sided lesions. Changes in bowel habits with constipation and irregularities may occur especially from left-sided lesions, which may also be associated with abdominal discomfort, mild distention, and

TABLE 2. **Risk Factors for Colorectal Cancer**

Average Risk

Age 50 y and older, asymptomatic

High Risk

Inflammatory bowel disease
- Chronic ulcerative colitis
- Chronic granulomatous colitis

Familial adenomatous polyposis
- Familial polyposis
- Gardner's syndrome

Turcot's syndrome

Oldfield's syndrome

Juvenile polyposis

Hereditary nonpolyposis colorectal cancer
- Family cancer syndrome
- Site-specific inherited colorectal cancer

Family history
- Colorectal adenomas
- Colorectal cancer

Past history
- Colorectal adenomas
- Colorectal cancer
- Breast, ovarian, and uterine cancer

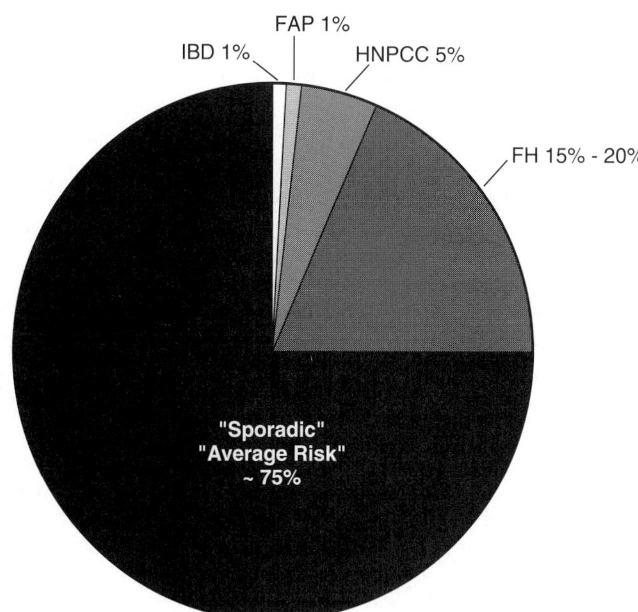

Figure 1. Factors associated with annual new cases of colorectal cancer.

Abbreviations: Sporadic = men and women age 50 years and older with no special risk factors; IBD = inflammatory bowel disease; FAP = familial adenomatous polyposis; HNPCC = hereditary nonpolyposis colorectal cancer; FH = positive family history.

(From Winawer SJ, Schottenfeld D, Flehinger BJ: Colorectal cancer screening. J Natl Cancer Inst *83*:243–253, 1991.)

cramps. Rectal lesions may be associated with tenesmus, rectal bleeding, and pelvic discomfort. Any of these symptoms requires a diagnostic work-up, which would include a digital rectal examination and either flexible sigmoidoscopy and double-contrast barium enema examination or colonoscopy. If a cancer is not found in the lower bowel by sigmoidoscopy, the remainder of the bowel needs to be evaluated. One should not be satisfied with a diagnosis of hemorrhoids in a patient with bright red rectal bleeding. The advantage of the endoscopic methods are biopsy for tissue diagnosis of observed abnormalities and the ability to remove polyps, which are found more commonly than cancer in symptomatic patients, especially those with rectal bleeding.

SCREENING

Although it is important to perform an aggressive work-up for individuals with symptoms suggestive of neoplasia, the diagnosis of cancer in asymptomatic patients as a result of screening more often results in an earlier diagnosis, with a much higher probability of survival, and will be associated with less morbidity and a much lower likelihood of additional treatment with radiation and chemotherapy. Screening approaches should be divided into those for average-risk men and women with no other risk factors and for high-risk individuals who have factors that increase their risk, including familial factors, IBD, or prior history of polyps or colorectal cancer.

There is strong evidence now that screening with fecal occult blood testing (FOBT) annually and flexible sigmoidoscopy every 5 years reduces the mortality from colorectal cancer. This should be offered to all men and women older than 50 years with no other risk factors. Other options for screening average-risk individuals include colonoscopy or double-contrast barium enema examination with flexible sigmoidoscopy. There are good reasons to consider these other options in individual people but insufficient evidence to recommend them as general guidelines.

Individuals who have one or two first relatives with colorectal cancer, particularly before the age of 55 years or adenomatous polyps before the age of 60 years, should be encouraged to have the same screening as the average-risk individuals but starting at age 40 years, because there is evidence that a family history is associated with younger age at onset of the cancer or adenomatous polyps. Many physicians and patients prefer either colonoscopy or double-contrast barium enema examination and flexible sigmoidoscopy rather than FOBT and flexible sigmoidoscopy in these families. I recommend colonoscopy every 5 years for these people. Individuals and families identified as having either FAP or HNPCC need to have individualized screening at a young age and should be referred to genetic counselors for full discussion of their risk, age at which they should start screening for colorectal cancer, and recommendations for other cancer screening. Genetic testing is of value only in these families at present. Obtaining a family history is a powerful clinical tool for identifying those at increased risk for these syndromes as well as those at increased risk because of one or two first relatives with colorectal cancer or adenomatous polyps. The latter accounts for 15 to 20% of individuals destined to develop colorectal cancer each year.

People with IBD need to be examined by colonoscopy every 1 to 2 years after disease for 8 years involving the entire colon or 15 years involving the distal colon. The search for early cancer and the premalignant dysplasia in the colon is the goal of these examinations. Prophylactic colectomy is an alternative approach that should be seriously considered, especially in young individuals.

People who have their colon cancer resected need to have periodic follow-up to search for additional adenomatous polyps. I prefer a complete colonoscopy before surgery, if it is possible to pass the endoscope beyond the cancer, a second complete examination or colonoscopy 1 year later, and less frequent colonoscopies thereafter. Individuals who have had adenomatous polyps removed from their colon can have their first follow-up colonoscopy 3 years later provided that their first colonoscopy completely removed all polyps from rectum to cecum, unless there were numerous polyps, malignant polyps, or a large sessile polyp, in which case an earlier examination is in order. At the 3-year follow-up, little in the way of significant disease is found. Subsequent follow-ups can be at 5 years.

MANAGEMENT

Surgical resection provides the best opportunity for cure. This can be done as the sole modality of treatment or in conjunction with radiation or chemotherapy. There is evidence that colon cancer involving lymph nodes is associated with better survival in patients who are treated with a course of postoperative chemotherapy with a combination of either 5-fluorouracil and levamisole (Ergamisol) or 5-fluorouracil and leucovorin (Wellcovorin). The survival of patients with rectal cancer that has penetrated through the bowel wall with or without lymph node involvement is improved with a combination of radiation therapy and chemotherapy postoperatively. This is considered to be adjuvant treatment of patients with no known residual disease. In some patients, radiation therapy given preoperatively may convert a potentially unresectable rectal cancer into one that is resectable. The approach to each patient is individualized and is based on physical examination, digital rectal examination, imaging with computed tomography (CT), and in the case of rectal cancer, endoscopic ultrasonography. The standard treatment of resectable colon cancer is a hemicolectomy and a regional lymphadenectomy based on the regional vascular supply. Rectal cancers can usually be resected by an abdominal approach (low anterior resection) even when they are within 3 to 4 cm of the anal verge. Permanent colostomies are necessary in few patients today. Laparoscopic colectomy is being evaluated within the framework of clinical studies as an alternative to open laparotomy.

There are special considerations for the surgical approach in some patients. Patients with IBD having prophylactic colectomy can now have the option of either an ileostomy or a pouch reconstruction. Individuals with FAP need a total colectomy, and patients with HNPCC who are having surgery for colorectal cancer, usually on the right side of the colon, should have a subtotal colectomy at that time if possible to reduce their future risk for additional cancers. Patients having had a polyp removed that histologically is found to have an invasive cancer will require follow-up surgical intervention only if the malignant tumor has encroached on the cautery line or involved vascular or lymphatic spaces. The location of the polyp and co-morbidity are other factors that need to be considered in this decision.

After curative resection, I usually follow-up patients with office visits, carcinoembryonic antigen (CEA) determination, and other blood tests every 3 months, and chest radiography and CT of the abdomen annually in patients who are at high risk for recurrence because of the stage of the disease at the time of surgery.

TREATMENT OF RECURRENT AND METASTATIC DISEASE

At the time of surgery, it will usually be clear whether the patient has gross residual disease after the resection. This will commonly be in the form of nodules on the liver or peritoneal surface that are too small to have been detected by preoperative imaging. A solitary implant or a small number of implants in the liver can be resected at that time or subsequently. A single pulmonary nodule is usually resected because it may be a new primary cancer of the lung rather than a metastatic focus from the colon. Residual disease after surgery may also be suspected if a preoperative CEA level has not fallen to normal in spite of the absence of gross residual disease observed at the time of surgery or on postoperative imaging.

Recurrent colon cancer is usually outside the bowel. Rarely, primary anastomotic recurrences are found after low anterior resections. Anastomotic recurrences are usually secondary to intra-abdominal recurrent tumor. Recurrent cancer that is nonresectable is usually treated with 5-fluorouracil, which is the most active agent, in combination with another agent, usually leucovorin. Other agents are used less successfully. Direct infusion into the liver of fluorodeoxyuridine (floxuridine, FUDR) has been shown to have significant response rates compared with systemic chemotherapy, but it is not clear whether it increases chances for survival. Radiation therapy is usually reserved for painful pelvic or bone disease and for the less common brain metastases. Patients who present initially with metastatic incurable disease may nevertheless have surgery offered, especially if the primary colon cancer is associated with bleeding or obstruction, provided that the patient has a reasonable performance status.

CONCLUDING COMMENTS

It is clear that colorectal cancer is a highly curable disease when it is detected at an early stage. This can be accomplished in a high percentage of people in the general population by use of FOBT and flexible sigmoidoscopy. More aggressive screening with colonoscopy has the potential for being highly effective in individuals at high risk for colorectal cancer, especially in those with a family history. In all of these patients, adenomatous polyps are often identified and removed with a dramatic reduction in the likelihood of developing colorectal cancer. This is a unique opportunity for cancer prevention. Thus, cancer deaths can be prevented not only by detecting the cancer at an earlier stage but by finding the precursor lesions, the adenomatous polyps, and removing them, thus avoiding the occurrence of cancer. In addition, we know much about lifestyle and its relationship to colorectal cancer, modification of which can dramatically reduce the probability of developing colorectal cancer and precursor adenomatous polyps. At present, we can identify genetic syndromes in only 5 or 6% of the people who are destined to get colorectal cancer. With future advances in molecular genetics, the percentage of individuals who will be identified as being susceptible to colorectal cancer may increase considerably. We will then be able to target a smaller subset of the general population for colonoscopy and polypectomy to reduce colon cancer incidence. There is also considerable interest in research into better methods for screening, including more sensitive FOBT and noninvasive means of examining the colon in the general population by "virtual colonoscopy." While we await results regarding these promising developments, we need to aggressively increase the participation of people in techniques now available that can dramatically reduce the incidence, morbidity, and mortality of this disease.

INTESTINAL PARASITES

method of
RODRIGO HASBUN, M.D., and
FRANK J. BIA, M.D., M.P.H.
Yale University School of Medicine
New Haven, Connecticut

INTESTINAL PROTOZOA

Giardia intestinalis is an enteric protozoan pathogen with a worldwide distribution that is not limited to the tropics. Giardiasis can manifest as an asymptomatic carrier state, acute diarrhea, or chronic diarrhea with clinical evidence of severe malabsorption. In North America, giardiasis is seen more frequently in children, travelers, or immunocompromised persons. It is estimated that approximately 10% of children attending some day care centers are asymptomatic carriers. Travelers in the developing world or domestic travelers, such as hikers who drink untreated ground water, are also at risk of acquiring giardiasis. *G. intestinalis* has been implicated in large water-borne outbreaks of disease both in the Rocky Mountains and Appalachian Mountains of western and eastern North America. Although immunodeficiency states, such as IgA deficiency, predispose patients to chronic giardiasis, symptomatic infection has not been a major clinical problem for human immunodeficiency virus (HIV)-infected individuals.

The different classes of drugs that are efficacious in treating giardiasis include the nitroimidazoles (metronidazole and tinidazole*), quinacrine,* furazolidone, and paromomycin. Both metronidazole (Flagyl), administered orally at 250 mg three times a day for 5 days, and tinidazole (Fasigyn), administered as a single 2-gm oral dose, have excellent cure rates and are considered the drugs of choice for adults with giardiasis. Tinidazole has side effects similar to those of metronidazole, but this agent is not available in the United States. Patients receiving metronidazole should be warned against drinking alcoholic beverages, because alcohol may cause a disulfiram-like reaction. The most common side effects of metronidazole include nausea, vomiting, metallic taste, rashes, and urticaria. Other less common adverse reactions include drowsiness, headache, dizziness, and ataxia. Nitroimidazoles such as metronidazole should be avoided early in pregnancy and during breast-feeding. Metronidazole is in Food and Drug Administration (FDA) pregnancy category B.

Furazolidone (Furoxone) is the least effective antigiardial agent (20% failure rate), but, because of its availability in suspension form, furazolidone is the most frequently used therapy for children with giardiasis. It is commonly associated with nausea and vomiting but less commonly causes headache, allergic reactions, or hypoglycemia. It can induce hemolysis in patients with glucose-6-phosphate dehydrogenase deficiency. Paromomycin (Humatin), a nonabsorbable aminoglycoside, used for giardiasis therapy during pregnancy, has only a 50% cure rate. Albendazole (Albenza), a recently approved benzimidazole agent given as 400 mg daily for 5 days, has been shown to be useful in treating giardiasis, but with variable efficacy. It is not recommended over metronidazole. Quinacrine is no longer available in the United States.

Entamoeba histolytica is an important cause of invasive colitis and liver abscesses in patients of lower socioeconomic status, among the institutionalized, and among immigrants from the developing world. Occult blood is found in nearly all patients with invasive colitis, but fecal leukocytes may be absent because they are lysed by these parasites. A newly described species, *Entamoeba dispar*, has been characterized. It is morphologically identical to *E. histolytica* but is not pathogenic. *E. dispar* is about 10 times more prevalent than *E. histolytica*, but causes an asymptomatic carrier state. The presence of serum antibodies directed against amebae and the observation of ingested erythrocytes within protozoa indicate *E. histolytica* infection. Asymptomatic carriers of *E. dispar* do not require therapy, but if serology is unavailable in nonendemic areas, therapy is advised to eliminate any potential pathogenic *E. histolytica* infection. All patients with *E. histolytica* infection should be treated.

Iodoquinol (Yodoxin) is the preferred agent for eradicating intraluminal infection. In addition to gastrointestinal side effects, it may interfere with thyroid function tests because of its high iodine content. It has rarely been associated with optic neuritis or optic atrophy if given in high doses, or over a prolonged time. Iodoquinol is equally effective as another alternative agent, diloxanide furoate, but iodoquinol must be administered for 20 days. Diloxanide furoate is relatively nontoxic, and a 10-day course has an 85% efficacy rate. Paromomycin is also effective and can be used in pregnancy because it is not well absorbed from the gastrointestinal tract.

Metronidazole is the drug of choice for patients with invasive intestinal disease and/or amebic liver abscess. It has a cure rate of 90%, and despite widespread use, metronidazole-resistant *E. histolytica* trophozoites have not been reported. The recommended duration of therapy for amebic colitis is 7 to 10 days, but recent studies indicate that 2.5 grams of oral metronidazole, given once daily for 3 days, are equally effective. Although metronidazole is not recommended for use during early pregnancy, therapy of severe, invasive amebiasis is warranted because of complication risks. Outside the United States, tinidazole is the preferred drug because it has fewer gastrointestinal side effects. The dose is 2 grams per day orally for 3 days. Therapy with either metronidazole or tinidazole should be followed with a lumen-active agent such as iodoquinol, paromomycin, or diloxanide furoate to effectively eliminate cyst carriage. When combined with another lumen-active agent, either tetracycline or erythromycin alone has

*Not available in the United States.

been used as an alternative for treating mild cases of amebic colitis in metronidazole-intolerant patients. However, neither agent will eradicate trophozoites from the liver.

Amebic liver abscess is usually managed with medical therapy alone. Metronidazole is the drug of choice, but it should be followed by a lumen-active agent. The recommended duration of therapy is 10 days, but single-dose therapy with 2.5 grams has also been effective. The recommended dose of tinidazole for liver abscess is 1200 to 2400 mg per day for 5 days, in divided doses (Table 1). Drainage of the abscess is indicated if there is no clinical improvement within 3 days on medical therapy; if the abscess has ruptured into the peritoneum or adjacent organs; if an abscess is located in the left hepatic lobe adjacent to the pericardium; or if the abscess is simply large, possesses a thin capsule, or is otherwise in danger of rupture.

Cryptosporidium parvum has been a well-known and well-characterized coccidian protozoan of animals for almost a century, but human infections were uncommonly recognized until the HIV pandemic brought them to the attention of clinicians. In immunocompetent patients, cryptosporidiosis causes a self-limited gastroenteritis, but in patients with acquired immune deficiency syndrome (AIDS) it causes a refractory, chronic diarrhea leading to a severe wasting syndrome. In the immunocompromised host, organisms can disseminate and cause respiratory disease, cholecystitis, and pancreatitis. Diagnosis is made by examination of stool specimens for either oocysts, using a modified acid-fast stain or for antigen, using an enzyme-linked immunosorbent assay (ELISA) test. Several forms of therapy have been evaluated in clinical studies with variable success rates. In adults, paromomycin, 500 mg four times a day, is effective in clearing *Cryptosporidium* oocysts and relieving clinical symptoms. Once a clinical response has been achieved in a patient with AIDS, a continuous maintenance dose of paromomycin, 1 to 2 grams per day, is recommended indefinitely for suppression. The somatostatin analogue octreotide* (Sandostatin), at doses of 300 to 500 μg subcutaneously three times a day, can be used to decrease fluid losses but is expensive and has variable efficacy. Another therapeutic approach for HIV-infected patients is to boost the immune system with highly active antiretroviral therapy (HAART). Since the introduction of protease inhibitors in France, investigators were unable to recruit enough AIDS patients with cryptosporidiosis for clinical studies because of a marked decrease in the incidence of this disease.

Isospora belli is also a coccidian protozoan, usually encountered in the tropics, where it causes a self-limited gastroenteritis in normal hosts. In patients with AIDS, it causes severe chronic diarrhea. The diagnosis is established by identifying oocysts in stool specimens with an acid-fast stain. The treatment of choice is oral trimethoprim-sulfamethoxazole (160 mg trimethoprim, 800 mg sulfamethoxazole [Bactrim DS, Septra DS]), four times per day for 10 days, then twice a day for 3 more weeks. HIV-infected patients may require a higher dosage and long-term maintenance therapy. In patients who are allergic to sulfa drugs, pyrimethamine, 50 to 75 mg daily, has been effective. Because approximately half of those patients with AIDS who are infected with *I. belli* will have relapses, maintenance therapy with oral trimethoprim-sulfamethoxazole three times a week or pyrimethamine (25 mg) and sulfadoxine (Fansidar) (500 mg) once each week can be used for suppression of infections.

Intestinal microsporidiosis, commonly caused by *Enterocytozoon bieneusi* or *Encephalitozoon [Septata] intestinalis*, has been implicated as a cause of chronic diarrhea and cholangiopathy in patients with advanced HIV infection. *E. intestinalis* may also disseminate systemically. The diagnosis is established by electron microscopy of biopsy specimens obtained from the small bowel or biliary mucosa. Antimotility agents should be the first line of therapy. Both metronidazole, 500 mg orally four times a day, and albendazole, 400 mg orally twice daily for 28 days, have been effective in improving symptoms. Albendazole is now considered the agent of choice for these infections. Long-term suppressive therapy is necessary because no pharmacologic agent has been able to eradicate the organisms from immunocompromised patients. Recent data suggest that patients receiving highly active antiretroviral therapy can clear their infections.

Cyclospora cayetanensis, also known as the "large cryptosporidium" and formerly as the cyanobacterium-like agent, is a recently described coccidian protozoan that causes gastroenteritis in normal hosts. It has been implicated as the etiologic agent of gastroenteritis outbreaks associated with fecally contaminated raspberries imported into the United States. In a placebo-controlled study of immunocompetent patients with cyclosporiasis in Nepal, trimethoprim-sulfamethoxazole given as one double-strength tablet twice daily for 7 days was effective in eradicating infection (see Table 1). In a large open-label study of HIV-infected patients with cyclospora infections in Haiti, treatment with trimethoprim-sulfamethoxazole, one double-strength tablet four times a day for 10 days, controlled the infection. This course of therapy was followed by secondary prophylaxis using one double-strength tablet three times a week. Currently, there are no known alternative effective therapies.

INTESTINAL HELMINTHS

The intestinal helminths are classified into nematodes (roundworms) or platyhelminths (flatworms); the latter are further subclassified into cestodes (tapeworms) and trematodes (flukes). The classification is helpful because members of each group are generally susceptible to similar pharmacologic agents.

*Not FDA approved for this indication.

TABLE 1. **Drugs for the Treatment of Protozoan Infections**

Infection	Drug	Adult Dosage	Pediatric Dosage
Amebiasis *(Entamoeba histolytica)*			
Asymptomatic			
Drug of choice:	Iodoquinol	650 mg tid × 20 d	30–40 mg/kg/d (max 2 gm) in 3 doses × 20 d
OR	Paromomycin	25–35 mg/kg/d in 3 doses × 7 d	25–35 mg/kg/d in 3 doses × 7 d
Alternative:	Diloxanide furoate	500 mg tid × 10 d	20 mg/kg/d in 3 doses × 10 d
Mild to Moderate Intestinal Disease			
Drug of choice[6]:	Metronidazole	500–750 mg tid × 10 d	35–50 mg/kg/d in 3 doses × 10 d
OR	Tinidazole[1]	2 gm/d × 3 d	50 mg/kg (max 2 gm) qd × 3 d
Severe Intestinal Disease, Hepatic Abscess			
Drug of choice[6]:	Metronidazole	750 mg tid × 10 d	35–50 mg/kg/d in 3 doses × 10 d
OR	Tinidazole[1]	600 mg bid or 800 mg tid × 5 d	50 mg/kg or 60 mg/kg (max 2 gm) qd × 5 d
Balantidiasis *(Balantidium coli)*			
Drug of choice:	Tetracycline[2,3]	500 mg qid × 10 d	40 mg/kg/d (max 2 gm) in 4 doses × 10 d
Alternatives:	Iodoquinol[2]	650 mg tid × 20 d	40 mg/kg/d in 3 doses × 20 d
	Metronidazole[2]	750 mg tid × 5 d	35–50 mg/kg/d in 3 doses × 5 d
Blastocystis hominis infection			
Drug of choice:	See footnote[4]		
Cryptosporidiosis *(Cryptosporidium)*			
Drug of choice:	Paromomycin[2]	25–35 mg/kg/d in 3 or 4 doses	
Cyclospora infection			
Drug of choice:	Trimethoprim-sulfamethoxazole[2,5]	TMP 160 mg, SMX 800 mg bid × 7 d	TMP 5 mg/kg, SMX 25 mg/kg bid × 7 d
Dientamoeba fragilis infection			
Drug of choice:	Iodoquinol	650 mg tid × 20 d	40 mg/kg/d (max 2 gm) in 3 doses × 20 d
OR	Paromomycin[2]	25–30 mg/kg/d in 3 doses × 7 d	25–30 mg/kg/d in 3 doses × 7 d
OR	Tetracycline[2,3]	500 mg qid × 10 d	40 mg/kg/d (max 2 gm) in 4 doses × 10 d
Entamoeba polecki infection			
Drug of choice:	Metronidazole[2]	750 mg tid × 10 d	35–50 mg/kg/d in 3 doses × 10 d
Giardiasis *(Giardia lamblia)*			
Drug of choice:	Metronidazole[2]	250 mg tid × 5 d	15 mg/kg/d in 3 doses × 5 d
Alternatives[8]:	Tinidazole[6]	2 gm once	50 mg/kg once (max 2 gm)
	Furazolidone	100 mg qid × 7–10 d	6 mg/kg/d in 4 doses × 7–10 d
	Paromomycin[2,7]	25–35 mg/kg/d in 3 doses × 7 d	
Isosporiasis *(Isospora belli)*			
Drug of choice:	Trimethoprim-sulfamethoxazole[2,9]	160 mg TMP, 800 mg SMX qid × 10 d, then bid × 3 wk	
Microsporidiosis			
Ocular (*Encephalitozoon hellem, Encephalitozoon cuniculi, Vittaforma corneae* [*Nosema corneum*])			
Drug of choice[10]:	Albendazole[2]	400 mg bid	
Intestinal (*Enterocytozoon bieneusi, Encephalitozoon* [*Septata*] *intestinalis*)			
Drug of choice[11]:	Albendazole[2]	400 mg bid	
Disseminated (*E. hellem, E. cuniculi, E. intestinalis, Pleistophora* sp.)			
Drug of choice[12]:	Albendazole[2]	400 mg bid	

[1]A nitroimidazole similar to metronidazole, but not marketed in the United States, tinidazole appears to be at least as effective as metronidazole and better tolerated. Ornidazole, a similar drug, is also used outside the United States. Higher dosage is for hepatic abscess.

[2]An approved drug, but considered investigational for this condition by the US FDA.

[3]Use of tetracyclines is contraindicated in pregnancy and in children younger than 8 years old.

[4]Clinical significance of these organisms is controversial, but metronidazole, 750 mg tid × 10 d or iodoquinol, 650 mg tid × 20 d, anecdotally has been reported to be effective (from Boreham PFL, Stenzel D: Adv Parasitol *32*:2, 1993; Keystone JS, Markell EK: Clin Infect Dis *21*:102, 104, 1995).

[5]HIV-infected patients may need higher dosage and long-term maintenance (from Pape JW et al: Ann Intern Med *121*:654, 1994).

[6]Treatment should be followed by a course of iodoquinol or paromomycin in the dosage used to treat asymptomatic amebiasis.

[7]Not absorbed; may be useful for treatment of giardiasis in pregnancy.

[8]Albendazole, 400 mg daily × 5 d, may be effective (from Hall A, Nahar Q: Trans R Soc Trop Med Hyg *87*:84, 1993.) Bacitracin zinc or bacitracin 120,000 U bid for 10 days may also be effective (from Andrews BJ, et al: Am J Trop Med Hyg *52*:318, 1995).

[9]In sulfonamide-sensitive patients, pyrimethamine, 50–75 mg daily, has been effective (from Ackers JP: Semin Gastrointest Dis *8*:33, 1997).

[10]Ocular lesions caused by *E. hellem* in HIV-infected patients have responded to fumagillin eyedrops prepared from Fumidil-B, a commercial product (Mid-Continent Agrimarketing, Inc., Olathe, Kansas, 1-800-547-1392) used to control a microsporidial disease of honey bees (from Diesenhouse MC: Am J Ophthalmol *115*:293, 1993). For lesions caused by *V. corneae,* topical therapy is generally not effective and keratoplasty may be required (from Davis RM et al: Ophthalmology *97*:953, 1990).

[11]Octreotide (*Sandostatin*) has provided symptomatic relief in some patients with large volume diarrhea. Oral fumagillin (see footnote 10) has been effective in treating *E. bieneusi* (from Molina J-M, et al: AIDS *11*:1603, 1997) but has been associated with thrombocytopenia.

[12] There is no established treatment for *Pleistophora* infection (from Molina J-M, et al: J Infect Dis *171*:245, 1995).

Modified with special permission of the publisher from Drugs for Parasitic Infections. Med Lett Drugs Ther *40*:1–12, 1998. The CDC Drug Service, Centers for Disease Control and Prevention in Atlanta, Georgia 30333 can be contacted at 404-639-3670 (evenings, weekends, or holidays at 404-639-2888).

Soil-transmitted nematodes, such as *Ascaris lumbricoides*, hookworm infections, and *Trichuris trichiura*, are quite common in developing countries. In the United States they are more frequently diagnosed among immigrants, returning expatriates, and travelers. Mebendazole (Vermox), a benzimidazole agent, given at a dose of 100 mg twice a day for 3 days, has been the standard therapy for these helminth infections. Mebendazole is contraindicated in pregnancy, particularly during the first trimester. Even though it is usually well tolerated, it can cause diarrhea, abdominal pain, migration and expulsion of *Ascaris* through the mouth and nose, hypersensitivity reactions, and, rarely, leukopenia, agranulocytosis, or hypospermia.

Albendazole, the most recently introduced benzimidazole agent, has also been shown to be effective against some nematodes. It has the advantage of being administered as a single dose, which has encouraged mass chemotherapy for school-aged children and improved both their growth rates and scholastic performances. Albendazole is usually well tolerated; its occasional side effects include diarrhea, abdominal pain, migration of *Ascaris*, reversible alopecia, elevated transaminases, and, rarely, leukopenia, rash, or renal toxicity. Pyrantel pamoate (Antiminth), a depolarizing neuromuscular blocking agent, given at 11 mg per kg body weight to a maximum single dosage of 1 gram, is effective against *A. lumbricoides* and hookworm but not against *T. trichiura*. Although pyrantel pamoate is usually well tolerated, it can cause headaches, dizziness, fever, rash, and gastrointestinal disturbances.

Ivermectin (Stromectol), is a potent broad-spectrum, antihelmintic drug that is effective against *A. lumbricoides* and *T. trichiura* but ineffective against hookworms. In the United States, ivermectin was recently released for treatment of other parasitic infections. It has been used to treat strongyloidiasis but has not yet been included as alternative therapy for other nematode infections in the most recent *Medical Letter* recommendations (Tables 1 and 2).

The pinworm *Enterobius vermicularis* has a worldwide distribution and primarily affects children within all socioeconomic classes in both temperate and tropical climates. The main symptoms are anal or vaginal pruritus caused by the irritation from worms and ova deposition. The diagnosis is made by identifying either ova or characteristic small adult worms in the perianal region, or by examining the stool for ova. Effective agents for therapy of *E. vermicularis* infections include mebendazole, albendazole, pyrantel pamoate, and, more recently, ivermectin. All agents can be given in a single oral dose with a recommendation for retreatment of the patient in 2 weeks to eradicate infections contracted at the time of initial therapy. Patients and/or parents should be instructed during therapy to carefully wash bed sheets and underwear, to cut and clean fingernails, and to thoroughly vacuum affected children's rooms. Between treatment courses, patients should wear pajamas and underwear to sleep and bathe in the morning to remove any ova deposited on the perianal area during the night.

Strongyloides stercoralis is a widely prevalent nematode infection in tropical regions, but it can also be found as an endemic infection in the southeastern United States. In North America patients at risk for strongyloidiasis include recent and not-so-recent immigrants, travelers returning from tropical regions, and veterans of World War II or the Vietnam War. An important feature in the life cycle of *S. stercoralis* is its ability to autoinfect the human host, permitting chronic, low-grade strongyloidiasis to persist for years after leaving an endemic area. Immunocompromised individuals (e.g., patients with malnutrition, immunosuppressed organ transplant recipients, lymphoma patients, and those receiving other forms of immunosuppressive chemotherapy) can develop extensive infections of the intestinal mucosa and lungs (hyperinfection) or dissemination of larvae to other anatomic sites, including the brain and meninges. *S. stercoralis* has not been an important opportunistic pathogen for HIV-infected individuals unless they are co-infected with human T cell lymphotropic virus type I (HTLV-I).

Oral thiabendazole has been a standard treatment of uncomplicated strongyloidiasis, but it is only 75% effective in eradicating infections. Alternative therapies have been sought. One or two doses of ivermectin (Stromectol), 200 μg per kg, is as effective as thiabendazole (Mintezol), 50 mg/kg/day given in two doses for 3 days, but with less adverse reactions and better compliance. Ivermectin is usually given as a one or two 12-mg doses (see Table 2), and the most common side effects include mild pruritus, rash, and dizziness. Occasionally headache, tender lumph nodes, and bone or joint pain are observed. A single dose of ivermectin is more effective than albendazole, given at a dose of 400 mg daily for 3 days (83% and 45% cure rates, respectively).

Several other unusual intestinal helminths occasionally present for medical therapy or possible surgical intervention. For patients who acquire anisakiasis by ingesting raw or inadequately prepared fish (sushi) infected with *Anisakis* species, there is presently no effective pharmacologic intervention. These larvae may cause painful inflammatory lesions of the stomach, small intestine, or colon. Treatment is surgical or endoscopic removal of the larvae.

Trichinella spiralis is the agent of both human and animal trichinosis. This organism may be acquired by ingestion of infected meat obtained from a variety of sources besides undercooked pork products. After an initial phase of intestinal infection, characterized by abdominal pain and diarrhea, larvae migrate to muscle and other organs, causing myalgias, periorbital edema, eosinophilia, and occasionally splinter hemorrhages. *Trichinella* larvae can invade the central nervous system, producing hemorrhagic infarcts by occlusion of cerebral small vessels. Therapy with mebendazole is outlined in Table 2, but albendazole or flubendazole (not available in the United States) also may be effective. Corticosteroids are used to control inflammation and the severe symptoms of trichinosis associated with larval invasion.

In the returning traveler, expatriate, or immigrant who appears chronically ill with severe diarrhea, malabsorption and wasting, these are serious symptoms of infection with *Capillaria philippinensis*, a possible etiology of the syndrome. Infection is acquired from contaminated or undercooked fish. The treatment of choice still includes a long, 20-day course of mebendazole, but albendazole is an alternative that can be used in a shorter 10-day course of therapy.

Rarely, patients from rural areas where cattle are raised can acquire a *Trichostrongylus* infection. Most human infections with *Trichostrongylus* species are acquired by fecal-oral transmission of this pathogen, which is found largely in cattle. Most human infections are either mild or asymptomatic, and the drug of choice for treatment is pyrantel pamoate. Mebendazole and albendazole are alternative therapies with known efficacy.

CESTODES (TAPEWORMS)

The treatment of human tapeworm infections involves the use of two agents, praziquantel (Biltricide), and albendazole, depending on the infecting species and the expected complications from infection. Praziquantel has a fairly broad spectrum of antiparasitic activity that includes tapeworms, schistosomes, and lung and liver flukes. However, its role in the treatment of neurocysticercosis is gradually being supplanted by albendazole.

Although praziquantel's precise mechanism of action is not known, it appears to increase cell permeability in susceptible helminths, which results in loss of intracellular calcium; rapid, massive muscle contractions; and cellular death. Adverse effects include malaise, headache, and dizziness, which have been reported frequently. Occasionally abdominal discomfort, sedation, sweating, fever, eosinophilia, and fatigue are noted. Rarely pruritus and rash have been seen. Praziquantel is in FDA pregnancy category B.

Humans are the definitive hosts for several gastrointestinal tapeworms. Rarely the dog tapeworm, *Dipylidium caninum*, infects children and requires therapy. The beef tapeworm is acquired by humans from infected beef and is notorious for the prodigious size it reaches within the human intestine without causing major symptoms. The pork tapeworm presents a different and more threatening clinical problem, as humans are potentially both the definitive and intermediate hosts for *Taenia solium*. When ova of this parasite are ingested by humans, there is the potential for evolution into cysticercosis, often with serious neurologic consequences requiring specific therapy for neurocysticercosis. The latter cannot be treated in the same manner as intestinal infection with *T. solium*. The adult intestinal stage of each of these three tapeworms can be treated with a single oral dose of praziquantel, 5 to 10 mg per kg. Praziquantel is an approved drug, but it is still considered investigational by the FDA. The treatment of yet another common cestode known as the dwarf tapeworm, *Hymenolepis nana*, requires a somewhat higher single dose of praziquantel, 25 mg per kg, to eradicate infection. Praziquantel is also useful as an alternative agent for the treatment of cysticercosis, at a dose of 50 mg per kg per day in three doses for 15 days; however, the drug of choice for this infection is now albendazole.

Albendazole has several interesting properties. It binds to colchicine-sensitive intracellular sites and inhibits the formation of parasitic microtubules. The organisms lose their ability to take up glucose and thus deplete their glycogen energy stores, resulting in their immobilization and death. Although albendazole is poorly absorbed from the gastrointestinal tract, absorption increases markedly if it is taken with a fatty meal. It is distributed into bile, cerebrospinal fluid, hydatid cyst fluid, and serum. Because of its teratogenic effects in animals, albendazole is not recommended for use in pregnant women. Contraceptive measures should be used for the duration of treatment and for 1 month after the cessation of treatment with albendazole. Therapy is occasionally associated with abdominal pain, increased serum liver transaminase levels, or reversible alopecia. *Ascaris* may migrate if not treated before using albendazole. Rarely leukopenia, rash, and nephrotoxicity have occurred.

Human infections with the larval stage of *Echinococcus granulosus* may produce hydatid cysts, which are treated with a 4-week course of oral albendazole, 400 mg twice daily. This regimen can be repeated as often as necessary, and some patients benefit from adjunctive surgical resection of cysts. If spillage from cysts occurs during surgery, praziquantel can be used to control the potential spread of infection. Hepatic cysts have also been managed with ultrasound-guided percutaneous drainage and oral albendazole therapy. In contrast, infections caused by *Echinococcus multilocularis* are not readily amenable to pharmacotherapy. These alveolar echinococcal infections generally require surgical excision, which is still considered the only reliable means of therapy.

For the treatment of cysticercosis, the drug of choice is albendazole, 400 mg twice daily for 8 to 30 days, and praziquantel is now considered an alternative therapy for this infection. Corticosteroids are generally given 2 to 3 days before and during treatment for neurocysticercosis. An ophthalmologic examination should be performed before treatment for cysticercosis because any cysticercocidal agent may cause ocular damage when ocular cysts are present. The same is true for spinal cysts.

Schistosomiasis (bilharziasis) results from chronic infection with adult *Schistosoma* species that live in either the vesical or mesenteric plexus of venules. These organisms are blood flukes, or trematodes, which infect several hundred million people worldwide. They infect by skin invasion in contrast to foodborne trematodes, which are acquired by eating raw

TABLE 2. **Drugs for the Treatment of Helminth Infections**

Infection	Drug	Adult Dosage	Pediatric Dosage
Ancylostoma caninum (Eosinophilic enterocolitis)			
Drug of choice:	Mebendazole	100 mg bid × 3 d	100 mg bid × 3 d
	OR Pyrantel pamoate[1]	11 mg/kg (max 1 gm) × 3 d	11 mg/kg (max 1 gm) × 3 d
	OR Albendazole[1]	400 mg once	400 mg once
Anisakiasis *(Anisakis)*			
Treatment of choice:	Surgical or endoscopic removal		
Angiostrongyliasis			
Angiostrongylus cantonensis			
Drug of choice[2]:	Mebendazole[1]	100 mg bid × 5 d	100 mg bid × 5 d
Angiostrongylus costaricensis			
Drug of choice:	Mebendazole	200–400 mg tid × 10 d	200–400 mg tid × 10 d
Alternative:	Thiabendazole[1]	75 mg/kg/d in 3 doses × 3 d (max 3 gm/d)[14]	75 mg/kg/d in 3 doses × 3 d (max 3 gm/d)[14]
Ascariasis *(Ascaris lumbricoides,* roundworm)			
Drug of choice:	Mebendazole	100 mg bid × 3 d or 500 mg once	100 mg bid × 3 d or 500 mg once
	OR Pyrantel pamoate[1]	11 mg/kg once (max 1 gm)	11 mg/kg once (max 1 gm)
	OR Albendazole[1]	400 mg once	400 mg once
Capillariasis *(Capillaria philippinensis)*			
Drug of choice:	Mebendazole[1]	200 mg bid × 20 d	200 mg bid × 20 d
Alternative:	Albendazole[1]	400 mg daily × 10 d	400 mg daily × 10 d
Enterobius vermicularis (pinworm) infection			
Drug of choice:	Pyrantel pamoate	11 mg/kg once (max 1 gm); repeat in 2 wk	11 mg/kg once (max 1 gm); repeat in 2 wk
	OR Mebendazole	100 mg once; repeat in 2 wk	100 mg once; repeat in 2 wk
	OR Albendazole[1]	400 mg once; repeat in 2 wk	400 mg once; repeat in 2 wk
Hookworm infection *(Ancylostoma duodenale, Necator americanus)*			
Drug of choice:	Mebendazole	100 mg bid × 3 d or 500 mg once	100 mg bid × 3 d or 500 mg once
	OR Pyrantel pamoate[1]	11 mg/kg (max 1 gm) × 3 d	11 mg/kg (max 1 gm) × 3 d
	OR Albendazole[1]	400 mg once	400 mg once
Fluke, hermaphroditic, infection			
Clonorchis sinensis (Chinese liver fluke)			
Drug of choice:	Praziquantel	75 mg/kg/d in 3 doses × 1 d	75 mg/kg/d in 3 doses × 1 d
	OR Albendazole	10 mg/kg × 7 d	
Fasciola hepatica (sheep liver fluke)			
Drug of choice[3]:	Bithionol	30–50 mg/kg on alternate days × 10–15 doses	30–50 mg/kg on alternate days × 10–15 doses
	OR Triclabendazole*	10 mg/kg once	
Fasciolopsis buski, Heterophyes heterophyes, Metagonimus yokogawai (intestinal flukes)			
Drug of choice:	Praziquantel[1]	75 mg/kg/d in 3 doses × 1 d	75 mg/kg/d in 3 doses × 1 d
Metorchis conjunctus (North American liver fluke)[4]			
Drug of choice:	Praziquantel[1]	75 mg/kg/d in 3 doses × 1 d	75 mg/kg/d in 3 doses × 1 d
Nanophyetus salmincola			
Drug of choice:	Praziquantel[1]	60 mg/kg/d in 3 doses × 1 d	60 mg/kg/d in 3 doses × 1 d
Opisthorchis viverrini (Southeast Asian liver fluke)			
Drug of choice:	Praziquantel	75 mg/kg/d in 3 doses × 1 d	75 mg/kg/d in 3 doses × 1 d
Paragonimus westermani (lung fluke)			
Drug of choice:	Praziquantel[1]	75 mg/kg/d in 3 doses × 2 d	75 mg/kg/d in 3 doses × 2 d
Alternative[5]:	Bithionol	30–50 mg/kg on alternate days × 10–15 doses	30–50 mg/kg on alternate days × 10–15 doses
Schistosomiasis (bilharziasis)			
S. haematobium			
Drug of choice:	Praziquantel	40 mg/kg/d in 2 doses × 1 d	40 mg/kg/d in 2 doses × 1 d
S. japonicum			
Drug of choice:	Praziquantel	60 mg/kg/d in 3 doses × 1 d	60 mg/kg/d in 3 doses × 1 d
S. mansoni			
Drug of choice:	Praziquantel	40 mg/kg/d in 2 doses × 1 d	40 mg/kg/d in 2 doses × 1 d
Alternative:	Oxamniquine[6]	15 mg/kg once[7]	20 mg/kg/d in 2 doses × 1 d[7]
S. mekongi			
Drug of choice:	Praziquantel	60 mg/kg/d in 3 doses × 1 d	60 mg/kg/d in 3 doses × 1 d

Table continued on opposite page

or undercooked plants and animals containing parasitic larvae. *Schistosoma hematobium* is endemic within Africa and the Middle East and its presence within the vesical plexus results in urinary tract pathology from deposition of ova. *Schistosoma mansoni, Schistosoma japonicum,* and *Schistosoma mekongi* are the important intestinal schistosomes. *S. mansoni* is found in Africa, the Middle East, South America, and the Caribbean region; and *S. japonicum* is endemic throughout the Far East. Their ova are released in venules and pass through the microvasculature, where they can either be retained in the

TABLE 2. **Drugs for the Treatment of Helminth Infections** *Continued*

Infection	Drug	Adult Dosage	Pediatric Dosage
Strongyloidiasis *(Strongyloides stercoralis)*			
Drug of choice[8,9]:	Ivermectin	200 μg/kg/d × 1–2 d	200 μg/kg/d × 1–2 d
Alternative:	Thiabendazole	50 mg/kg/d in 2 doses (max 3 gm/d) × 2 d[14]	50 mg/kg/d in 2 doses (max 3 gm/d) × 2 d[14]
Tapeworm infection—adult (intestinal stage)			
Diphyllobothrium latum (fish), *Taenia saginata* (beef), *Taenia solium* (pork), *Dipylidium caninum* (dog)			
Drug of choice:	Praziquantel[1]	5–10 mg/kg once	5–10 mg/kg once
Hymenolepis nana (dwarf tapeworm)			
Drug of choice:	Praziquantel[1]	25 mg/kg once	25 mg/kg once
—Larval (tissue stage)			
Echinococcus granulosus (hydatid cyst)			
Drug of choice[10,11]:	Albendazole	400 mg bid × 28 d, repeated as necessary	15 mg/kg/d × 28 d, repeated as necessary
Echinococcus multilocularis			
Treatment of choice:	See footnote[13]		
Cysticercus cellulosae (cysticercosis)			
Drug of choice[13]:	Albendazole	400 mg bid × 8–30 d, repeated as necessary	15 mg/kg/d (max 800 mg) in 2 doses × 8–30 d, repeated as necessary
OR	Praziquantel[1]	50 mg/kg/d in 3 doses × 15 d	50 mg/kg/d in 3 doss × 15 d
Alternative:	Surgery		
Trichinosis *(Trichinella spiralis)*			
Drugs of choice:	Steroids for severe symptoms plus Mebendazole[1,15]	200–400 mg tid × 3 d, then 400–500 mg tid × 10 d	
Trichostrongylus infection			
Drug of choice:	Pyrantel pamoate[1]	11 mg/kg once (max 1 gm)	11 mg/kg once (max 1 gm)
Alternative:	Mebendazole[1]	100 mg bid × 3 d	100 mg bid × 3 d
OR	Albendazole[1]	400 mg once	400 mg once
Trichuriasis *(Trichuris trichiura,* whipworm*)*			
Drug of choice:	Mebendazole	100 mg bid × 3 d or 500 mg once	100 mg bid × 3 d or 500 mg once
Alternative:	Albendazole[1]	400 mg once[16]	400 mg once[16]

*Not available in the United States.

[1]An approved drug, but considered investigational for this condition by the US FDA.

[2]Antiparasitic drugs can provoke neurologic symptoms, and most patients recover spontaneously without them. Analgesics, corticosteroids, and careful removal of cerebrospinal fluid at frequent intervals can relieve symptoms (from Koo J, et al: Rev Infect Dis *10:*1155, 1988). Albendazole, levamisole (Ergamisol), or ivermectin have been used successfully in animals.

[3]Unlike infections with other flukes, *Fasciola hepatica* infections may not respond to praziquantel. Triclabendazole (Fasinex–Novartis), a veterinary fasciolide, has been safe and effective (from Apt W, et al: Am J Trop Med Hyg *52:*532, 1995).

[4]From MacLean JD et al: Lancet *347:*154, 1996.

[5]Unpublished data indicate triclabendazole (Fasinex), a veterinary fasciolide, may be effective in a dosage of 5 mg/kg once daily for 3 days or 10 mg/kg twice in 1 day.

[6]Oxamniquine has been effective in some areas in which praziquantel is less effective (from Stelma FF, et al: J Infect Dis *176:*304, 1997). Oxamniquine is contraindicated in pregnancy.

[7]In East Africa, the dose should be increased to 30 mg/kg, and in Egypt and South Africa, 30 mg/kg/d × 2 d. Some experts recommend 40–60 mg/kg over 2–3 days in all of Africa (from Shekhar KC, Drugs *42:*379, 1991).

[8]In immunocompromised patients or disseminated disease, it may be necessary to prolong or repeat therapy or use other agents.

[9]Ivermectin is not FDA-approved for disseminated strongyloidiasis, and thiabendazole may be preferred.

[10]Some patients may benefit from or require surgical resection of cysts (from Tompkins RK: Mayo Clin Proc *66:*1281, 1991). Praziquantel may be useful preoperatively or in case of spill during surgery.

[11]Percutaneous drainage with ultrasound guidance plus albendazole therapy has been effective for management of hepatic hydatid cyst disease (from Khuroo MS, et al: N Engl J Med *337:*881, 1997).

[12]Surgical excision is the only reliable means of treatment. Some reports have suggested use of albendazole or mebendazole (from Hao W, et al: Trans R Soc Trop Med Hyg *88:*340, 1994; WHO Group: Bull WHO *74:*231, 1996).

[13]Corticosteroids should be given for 2 to 3 days before and during drug therapy for neurocysticercosis. Any cysticercocidal drug may cause irreparable damage when used to treat ocular or spinal cysts, even when corticosteroids are used (from White AC Jr: Clin Infect Dis *24:*101, 1997). An ophthalmic examination should be done before treatment.

[14]This dose is likely to be toxic and may have to be decreased.

[15]Albendazole or flubendazole (not available in the United States) may also be effective.

[16]In heavy infection, it may be necessary to extend therapy to 3 days.

Modified with special permission of the publisher from Drugs for Parasitic Infections. Med Lett Drugs Ther *40:*1–12, 1998. The CDC Drug Service, Centers for Disease Control and Prevention in Atlanta, Georgia 30333 can be contacted at 404-639-3670 (evenings, weekends, or holidays at 404-639-2888).

host bowel wall, pass into the bowel lumen, or be distributed hematogenously to the liver, lung, and other internal organs. The presence of ova in tissues and the immune response to them cause hypertrophy of tissues, inflammation, or ulcerative lesions. Chronic infection results in egg granuloma formation and tissue fibrosis.

The mainstay of therapy for the chronic forms of schistosomiasis is praziquantel and the doses are indicated in Table 2. In some cases, *S. mansoni* infections may not respond to praziquantel, and oxamniquine (Vansil) has been used successfully to treat such infections. However, oxamniquine cannot be used during pregnancy and is associated with other side effects such as headache, dizziness, nausea, diarrhea, rash, and orange-red discoloration of the urine. Acute schistosomiasis (Katayama fever) appears within 2 to 8 weeks of initial infection and is typically treated with both praziquantel and corticosteroids for life-threatening conditions such as deposition of ova in the spinal cord. Supportive data for such therapy are not as clear as for chronic disease. Cercarial dermatitis for other avian or mammalian schistosomes is treated symptomatically with antihistamines and antipruritic lotions.

There are more than 50 different species of intestinal flukes and many additional liver and lung flukes, all with complex life cycles involving one or more intermediate hosts. Sources of infection include freshwater plants, crayfish, snails, frogs, fish, or crabs; and clinical manifestations of infection include recurrent cholangitis (opisthorchiasis, clonorchiasis), biliary obstruction (fascioliasis), and pleuropulmonary disease (paragonimiasis). Table 2 summarizes the use of praziquantel for treatment of these fluke infections. The one exception is *Fasciola hepatica*, which may not respond to praziquantel and could be treated with bithionol (Bitin), obtainable from the Centers for Disease Control and Prevention (CDC) Drug Service. Bithionol frequently causes photosensitivity reactions, abdominal pain, vomiting, diarrhea, or urticaria. Triclabendazole (Fasinex) is an alternative veterinary agent, which is considered both safe and effective for fascioliasis, but it is not available in the United States. Refer to the tables included in this chapter for additional information, which has been adapted from the most recent 1998 recommendations published in *The Medical Letter.*

Section 7

Metabolic Disorders

DIABETES MELLITUS IN ADULTS

method of
GEORGE E. DAILEY III, M.D.
Scripps Clinic
La Jolla, California

Promising new approaches to the treatment of diabetes mellitus have evolved with important studies on plasma glucose control and with the development of alternative antidiabetic agents. Originally, only one class of oral medication—the sulfonylureas—was available for the treatment of type II diabetes. Three "new" classes of medications, introduced into the United States between 1995 and 1997, have now been added. However, two of these have been in use elsewhere in the world for a number of years. Furthermore, a new definition of diabetes has been adopted worldwide that reflects the importance of earlier diagnosis in treatment of diabetes.

MAGNITUDE OF THE PROBLEM

Data from the National Health and Nutrition Examination Survey II (NHANES) showed that about 3% of people in the United States were aware of having diabetes. However, a total of 15 million people (1 in every 17 Americans) are estimated to have diabetes, for an overall incidence of approximately 6%. Therefore, approximately half of all diabetic individuals did not know they had diabetes. Over 90% of affected persons in the United States have type II or non–insulin-dependent diabetes. The prevalence ranges from less than 2% of persons less than 45 years of age to 18% of persons between the ages of 65 and 74. Prevalence rates are lowest in Caucasians and highest among Native American individuals. Overall mortality among type II diabetics is two- to fourfold that of unaffected persons of similar age. Likewise, health care costs are also approximately two- to fourfold those of age-matched individuals. Diabetes accounts for 20% of all new cases of blindness among adults and is the leading cause of chronic renal insufficiency. However, approximately 75% of all individuals with diabetes die of cardiovascular disease. Their mortality risk is also two- to fourfold that of age-matched individuals. The presence of diabetes or impaired glucose tolerance magnifies all other risk factors. Furthermore, there is a clustering of risk factors probably operating through the common mechanism of the insulin resistance syndrome (IRS) or syndrome X, thought to be present in as many as 25% of Caucasians and in higher proportions in other ethnic groups. It may explain the extremely high prevalence of hypertension, hypertriglyceridemia, low HDL cholesterol, small dense LDL cholesterol, hyperuricemia, and obesity in diabetes. This association has implications for treatment, because at least two agents are capable of reducing endogenous insulin levels, thereby correcting, at least in part, the insulin resistance that may underlie much of the atherosclerotic risk.

A large-scale type II diabetes prevention study is under way (DPT II). In this study, individuals with impaired glucose tolerance but without frank diabetes are randomized to receive one of four treatment regimens: (1) diet and exercise, (2) placebo, (3) metformin, 850 mg twice daily, or (4) troglitazone, 400 mg per day. Modeling studies suggest that it may be possible to prevent as many as half of the cases of frank diabetes by early treatment. Also, earlier treatment may be able to preserve beta cell function and avoid the otherwise inexorable decline in beta cell insulin secretion, which ultimately requires insulin therapy, in a large number of individuals with type II diabetes. Thus, it is currently believed that the "clock starts ticking" long before the development of frank diabetes in terms of macrovascular complications. The microvascular complications of the disease, in contrast, appear to be clearly linked to duration and degree of hyperglycemia, as Diabetes Control and Complications Trial (DCCT).

The new definition of diabetes is a fasting plasma glucose value of 126 mg per dL (7 mmol) (Table 1). This definition is consistent with that previously adopted by the World Health Organization. Impaired glucose tolerance is present when the fasting blood sugar is between 110 and 125 mg per dL. Postprandial or casual glucose values defining diabetes remain those above 200 mg per dL. It is now apparent that a large number of individuals have relatively preserved fasting blood sugar levels correlating with hepatic glucose output but strikingly elevated postprandial values early in the course of diabetes. The term "mild diabetes" should be abandoned, as was recommended in the case of hypertension, because it suggests to patients and physicians that the condition is not too serious and need not be treated aggressively.

OVERVIEW OF TREATMENT

It is reasonable to classify the severity of type II diabetes on the basis of the fasting plasma glucose, because it is the most reproducible measurement (Table 2). In *early diabetes*, the fasting value is relatively normal—say, less than 130 mg per dL—and postprandial values are generally 180 to 240 mg per dL. Early in this stage, endogenous insulin is almost always elevated. As the fasting plasma glucose rises toward 200, endogenous insulin levels begin to fall. This is in part due to the effects of "glucotoxicity" on beta cell function. A period of relative normalization of glucose will help to restore beta cell function in these persons. Once the fasting plasma glucose rises above 200 to 250 mg per dL, endogenous insulin levels are almost always low. Treatment options will be governed by the amount of remaining endogenous insulin.

TABLE 1. **Plasma Glucose Levels for Diagnosis of Diabetes Mellitus**

Glycemic Status	Plasma Glucose Level (mg/dL)		
	Fasting	*Casual*	*Oral Glucose Tolerance Test (OGTT)*
Diabetes	≥126 (7 mmol)	≥200 (11.1 mmol) plus symptoms	2-h post-OGTT: ≥200
Impaired glucose tolerance (IGT)	110–125		2-h post-OGTT: 140–200
Normal	<110		2-h plasma glucose: <140

Adapted from Report of the Expert Committee on the Diagnosis and Classification of Diabetes Mellitus. Diabetes Care *21*(Suppl 1):S5–S19, 1998; and Lorber DL: Redefining diabetes (commentary). Practical Diabetology *16*(3):22, 1997. Reprinted with permission from R. A. Rapaport Publishing, Inc.

Approximately 15% of whites who appear to have typical type II diabetes presenting after age 40 can be found to have some autoimmune markers and actually have an indolent form of autoimmune or type I diabetes. This finding probably accounts for "primary failures" to oral medications such as sulfonylureas. At present, measurement of endogenous insulin reserve in the form of insulin or C peptide is not usual clinical practice, although it may become so in the future. One can generally predict these values from the clinical presentation and plasma glucose. Early diet therapy is certainly the cornerstone of diabetes treatment in any stage of the disease. Persons who are not particularly symptomatic may reasonably be given a trial of diet therapy, particularly if there is significant weight to lose. However, data from the United Kingdom Perspective Diabetes Study (UKPDS) suggest that less than 10% of individuals with a frankly elevated fasting plasma glucose will achieve normal glucose levels by means of diet alone. It is often prudent to begin an oral medication to achieve control and reduce glucose toxicity; the drug can always be withdrawn later if the patient achieves a good degree of control.

Stage II or *moderate diabetes* is present when the fasting plasma glucose is frankly elevated between 130 and 200 mg per dL. It is prudent to begin medication in affected persons while instructing them in diet. Here the treatment algorithm becomes more complex. At present, there is considerable experience with the use of sulfonylurea as well as metformin for initial monotherapy. The oral agents acarbose and troglitazone both have been studied in small numbers of subjects, and both seem reasonable choices for monotherapy. However, there is significantly less experience with their use. In this stage of diabetes, the UKPDS and other studies have shown that approximately 80% of individuals will respond initially to either agent when used for monotherapy. However, approximately 10% per year develop "secondary failure" at some point. Perhaps earlier treatment will reduce this number or at least the rapidity of progression. Happily, in any case, adding the other agent "rescues" control for a substantial period of time. It is quite clear, in contrast, that simply substituting another agent (e.g., metformin for sulfonylurea or troglitazone for sulfonylurea) will not control diabetes in a person who has developed secondary failure. Combination treatment is definitely required in such cases. Three- and even four-drug combination oral regimens are just now coming into use. Therefore, it is difficult to define the precise sequence of timing and selection. However, this sequence should be based on the known different mechanisms of action. The use of combination agents is very much analogous to the use of several classes of antihypertensive agents in more complicated cases of hypertension or, correspondingly, antimicrobial agents in complex cases of infection. There are good reasons, at least in theory, for avoiding insulin therapy as long as possible in type II diabetes and then for using it in the lowest possible and most physiologic dose and fashion.

Individuals with severe diabetes, i.e., who are substantially symptomatic, particularly when fasting plasma glucose is above 250 mg per dL, require rapid control. It is often prudent to begin insulin therapy immediately. If control is achieved rapidly, withdrawal of insulin is possible later. The presence of significant ketonuria should suggest a more severe degree of insulin deficiency.

Table 3 summarizes therapeutic approaches for the stages of diabetes.

TABLE 2. **Classification of Severity of Diabetes Mellitus**

Stage of Disease	Plasma Glucose Level (mg/dL)		Endogenous Insulin Level
	Fasting	*Postprandial*	
Stage I: Early diabetes	<130	180–240	Elevated
Stage II: Moderate diabetes	130–200	200–300	Beginning to fall
Stage III: Severe diabetes	>200–250	300–400	Low

TABLE 3. **Selection of Initial Therapy in Diabetes Mellitus**

Stage of Disease	Symptoms	Initial Therapy
Stage I: Early diabetes	Few or none	Trial of diet or oral agent
Stage II: Moderate diabetes	Mild to moderate	Oral agent (e.g., metformin, sulfonylurea)
Stage III: Severe diabetes	Usually significant	Consider insulin; follow closely

THE MAJOR ORAL AGENTS

(Table 4)

Sulfonylureas

Sulfonylureas have been in use since around 1950. The major agents available in the United States and their dosages are listed in Table 5. There are some pharmacologic differences, but it is not clear that any one is more effective than another. Therefore, changing from one sulfonylurea to another rarely improves the therapeutic response. Another underappreciated feature of this class of medications is that approximately 80 to 90% of the clinical effect is seen at so-called "half-maximal" doses (e.g., 10 mg of glyburide or glipizide, 4 mg of glimepiride). Going higher rarely achieves much additional therapeutic response in most patients. Starting doses are generally 2.5 to 5 mg for glyburide or glipizide and 1 mg for glimepiride. Older patients may be particularly prone to hypoglycemia, the most serious side effect with these agents. They act on a potassium channel, the so-called sulfonylurea receptor, in the beta cell to permit enhanced insulin secretion. Generally, a therapeutic response to a given dose can be seen within 1 to 2 weeks. Therefore, I suggest beginning with one tablet and increasing to three tablets over 3 to 4 weeks, particularly in symptomatic individuals.

Metformin

Metformin (Glucophage) has been used for more than 30 years in 90 countries but just reached the U.S. market in mid-1995. It is the first "insulin-sensitizing" agent available in that it reduces endogenous insulin levels as well as glucose. Its principal effect appears to be in reducing hepatic glucose output. It is also unique among antidiabetic agents in that it promotes weight loss despite improved blood glucose. This effect has to do in part with reduced appetite and intake, but there may also be some selective effects on adipose tissue as well. Triglycerides are generally significantly reduced. Because most individuals with type II diabetes are obese at the onset, this agent is an attractive initial choice for monotherapy. Another significant advantage is that it does not cause hypoglycemia when used for monotherapy even in overdoses.

The principal side effects are gastrointestinal and occur in as many as 25 to 30% of persons initially. Fortunately, most can acclimate to the drug over a 2- to 4-week period. Thus, it is advisable to begin with one 500-mg tablet given once or twice a day with meals and increase by one tablet per week up to 2000 mg, which appears to be the maximum effective dose in most individuals. The availability of an 850-mg tablet makes it convenient to take two or three per day when maximal doses are needed. Data from the UKPDS suggest that compliance with this drug is as

TABLE 5. **Sulfonylureas: Insulin Mutation**

Agent	Initial Dose	Probable Maximal Dose
First Generation		
Tolbutamide (Orinase)	500 mg	500 mg PO tid
Tolazamide (Tolinase)	250–500 mg qd	500 mg bid
Acetohexamide (Dymelor)	250–500 mg/dL	500 mg bid
Chlorpropramide (Diabinese)	125–250 mg qd	375 mg qd
Second Generation		
Glyburide (DiaBeta, Micronase)	2.5–5.0 mg qd	10 mg qd
Micronized glyburide (Glynase)	1.5–3.0 mg	6 mg qd
Glipizide (Glucotrol)	5 mg qd	10–20 mg qd
Glipizide GTS (Glucotrol XL)	5 mg	10–20 mg
Glimepiride (Amaryl)	0.5–1 mg	4–8 mg qd
Repaglinide (Prandin)	1 mg before meals (0.5 mg in elderly)	2 mg PO tid, before meals

TABLE 4. **Oral Agents for Initial Therapy of Diabetes Mellitus**

Agent	Principal Mechanism (of Action)	Ideal Patient Type	Principal Side Effect
Sulfonylurea	Insulin release stimulation	Insulinopenic	Hypoglycemia
Metformin (Glucophage)	Decrease in hepatic glucose output	Insulin-resistant obese	Gastrointestinal in 20–30% (bloating, diarrhea)
Acarbose (Precose)	Impairment of carbohydrate absorption	Postprandial hyperglycemic	Gastrointestinal (flatulence)
Troglitazone (Rezulin)	Increase in peripheral muscle glucose utilization	Insulin-resistant renal impaired	Hepatic (in <2%)

Adapted from Report of the Expert Committee on the Diagnosis and Classification of Diabetes Mellitus. Diabetes Care *21*(Suppl 1):S5–S19, 1998.

good as with sulfonylurea (i.e., approximately 90% at 5 years). However, approximately 5 to 10% of individuals are unable to tolerate the drug, owing principally to persistent gastrointestinal side effects, generally bloating and diarrhea.

The most feared side effect, lactic acidosis, is extremely rare, occurring in approximately 1 in 50,000 patient-years of treatment. This problem has occurred principally in individuals having impaired renal function who were given the drug inappropriately. The drug is highly dependent upon normal renal function for clearance. With a significant reduction in glomerular filtration rate, plasma levels will rise. Nevertheless, the risk of lactic acidosis appears to be less than 5% that associated with the related drug phenformin, which was removed from the market in the United States and most other countries in 1977. The product information for metformin contains a warning about concomitant use in individuals receiving iodinated contrast material, which has to do with the risk of contrast-induced renal dysfunction. This has created much confusion. A total of 14 cases of lactic acidosis associated with contrast-induced renal dysfunction have been reported. In virtually all instances, the individuals had pre-existing renal disease and the medication was not stopped prior to or at the time of the procedure. The plasma half-life of the drug is approximately 6 hours. The risk of contrast-induced renal dysfunction is 1 to 2% in diabetic individuals with normal renal function. However, this risk rises sharply when there is any degree of pre-existing renal dysfunction. Renal dysfunction rarely develops in less than 12 to 24 hours following contrast administration. It is generally safe to stop the drug 12 to 24 hours before an elective procedure. However, patients should not be denied a needed contrast procedure even if they have just taken the drug. With a half-life of 6 hours, as noted, the plasma level will generally drop quickly. It is, of course, important to confirm normal renal function following the contrast procedure before the drug is resumed.

Alpha-Glucosidase Inhibitors

Acarbose (Precose) is the prototype of alpha-glucosidase inhibitors, although several others are under development. All of these agents act by inhibiting small intestinal brush border glucosidase, which break down complex carbohydrates. This has the effect of reducing postprandial glucose, particularly in individuals on a higher carbohydrate diet. It has been in use in Germany since 1990, and more than 500,000 patients have been treated. Only 1 to 2% of the drug is absorbed. Therefore, side effects are almost exclusively confined to colon gas. This is due to the breakdown or fermentation of undigested carbohydrates in the colon by bacteria normally residing there. The key to the use of this agent is to begin with a low dose and increase it slowly. Tolerance develops, apparently through the induction of glucosidases, throughout the small bowel. Normally these are concentrated in the first third of the small intestine. Therefore, best success will generally be achieved by starting with one-half tablet (25 mg) at the beginning of a meal, e.g., the evening meal. If this is tolerated it may be increased slowly over a 4- to 8-week period up to the recommended dose of one tablet at the beginning of each meal. It is important that the tablet be ingested within the first 10 minutes of the meal to achieve a maximum effect as it has a very short duration of action. The effects on postprandial glucose may be a reduction of as much as 60 to 80 mg per dL. However, the effect on fasting blood glucose is minimal—generally only 10 to 15 mg per dL, as would be expected. This agent could be used for monotherapy in early diabetes; however, it is most commonly used for "add-on" therapy in individuals with persistently elevated postprandial glucose levels. Unfortunately, it is rarely feasible to use the drug only with larger meals, because regular use is necessary in order to achieve the tolerance described. This agent does not cause weight gain or hypoglycemia, because endogenous insulin levels are not directly affected.

Thiazolidenediones

The thiazolidenediones (troglitazone [Rezulin]) are the newest oral medications available for the treatment of diabetes and act by yet another unique principal mechanism. At doses of at least 400 mg and below for troglitazone, the principal effect appears to be enhancement of insulin sensitivity at peripheral muscle, the chief organ for glucose disposal. With a 600-mg dose, there is also an effect on the hepatic glucose output. Preliminary data with this agent suggest that secondary failures do not occur, at least after 2 to 3 years of therapy. However, the agent is considerably more expensive than others and is therefore less commonly used for initial or monotherapy. This may change when more data on cost-effectiveness become available.

Troglitazone therapy can be begun with 200 to 400 mg taken once daily with a meal. The drug is unique in that 2 to 4 weeks are required for an initial response and 2 to 3 months may be needed for the maximal response. Thus, if troglitazone is to be used for "add-on" therapy, the other drugs including insulin should be continued unchanged until it is clear that the glucose level is falling. Side effects are unusual. Slightly less than 2% of patients develop some elevation in liver function tests that requires monitoring every 1 to 2 months for the first year. However, rare cases of severe hepatocellular injury have been reported after both short- and long-term treatment.

INSULIN THERAPY: IMPORTANCE OF BEDTIME INSULIN

One of the more important advances in insulin therapy of diabetes has been the recognition of the value of bedtime intermediate-acting insulin (NPH or Lente). A relatively small amount of intermediate-acting insulin such as 0.1 unit per kg of body weight is often sufficient to normalize the fasting plasma glucose. Then oral medication can manage glucose control through the remainder of the day. In a feasibility trial conducted by the Veterans Administration, the principal benefit in sulfonylurea-failure type II diabetics was with the addition of bedtime NPH insulin. There is clearly much less risk of overnight hypoglycemia or weight gain with this strategy, and I generally try to employ it initially if possible.

However, some persons with type II diabetes will inevitably become sufficiently insulin-deficient that they require twice-daily insulin. This is usually most effectively given as a premixed 70/30 insulin. I rarely use once-a-day morning NPH except in patients receiving corticosteroids. Generally, a dose of 0.7 unit per kg given as two thirds in the morning and one third at night, or as one half each time, will suffice. However, very insulin-resistant individuals may require up to 1.3 units per kg.

The use of twice-daily insulin in most of these individuals seems at first a reasonable alternative. It is less expensive. However, studies have shown that this approach is accompanied by inevitable weight gain, often of substantial magnitude, even when individuals reduce their oral intake. In addition, control of glucose is achieved at the expense of substantial hyperinsulinemia, which at least in theory could exacerbate atherosclerotic risk. This does not mean, however, that the glucose should be left uncontrolled. We know the risks of hyperglycemia.

TARGETS AND TESTING

Recommended pre-meal target values for plasma glucose are generally 80 to 120 mg per dL (Table 6). Self-testing is essential for all persons with significant diabetes. The most important and underappreciated test is the *postprandial glucose*. Studies have shown that a 1- to 2-hour postprandial glucose value correlates better with glycohemoglobin levels and overall control than does a fasting plasma glucose or any other pre-meal measurement. It is extremely common to find that the patient has been testing only a fasting blood sugar, which often grossly underestimates the degree of glucose control. Drawing the patient's attention to the striking elevations in postprandial glucose values will provide strong reinforcement to respond much earlier and more effectively to worsening glucose control. This is important in early as well as insulin-treated diabetes.

TABLE 6. **Suggested Target Levels for Plasma Glucose**

Test	Level (mg/dL)		
	Ideal	*Acceptable*	*Suggested Modification*
Fasting plasma glucose (and pre-meal)	70–110	80–140	>140
1- to 2-hour postprandial glucose*	80–140	140–180	>180
HbA_{1C}†	<6%	<7%	>8%

*Most important test for monitoring.
†Normal range 4–6%.
Adapted from Report of the Expert Committee on the Diagnosis and Classification of Diabetes Mellitus. Diabetic Care *21*(Suppl 1):S5–S19, 1998.

Fortunately, the risk of serious hypoglycemia is only about 5% of that in intensively treated type I diabetics according to the UKPDS. Therefore, it should be possible to achieve near-normal glucose control in the majority of type II diabetics, particularly with earlier treatment. A number of studies have suggested that individuals treated by heretofore conventional means typically have blood sugars in the mid to high 200-mg per dL range. This clearly greatly accelerates the risk of microvascular complications and may contribute to macrovascular risk as well. According to the DCCT, each 1% reduction in glycohemoglobin (approximately 30 mg per dL of glucose) reduces the risk of retinopathy progression by 35 to 40%. Thus, any improvement in control will significantly reduce this risk.

PREVENTION OF COMPLICATIONS

Early surveillance for complications of diabetes should be part of the treatment protocol for all diabetic patients.

Cardiovascular Complications

As noted initially, diabetic individuals are at enormous risk for cardiovascular complications, and meticulous monitoring of other cardiovascular risk factors such as lipid levels and blood pressure is essential. Of the newer tests, measurement of urinary microalbumin is the most important. This can be done easily with a dip stick capable of detecting 20 μg per dL of albumin, versus 300 mg per dL for the traditional urine dip sticks. Microalbuminuria generally occurs 6 to 8 years prior to the development of macroproteinuria (more than 500 mg per 24 hours). Persons with microalbuminuria are at greatly increased risk not only for renal failure but also for microvascular and macrovascular complications. The reason for this increased risk is not entirely clear. However, albuminuria appears to be a "downstream marker" for serious microvascular and macrovascular dysfunction. Therefore, microalbuminuric individuals should have a target blood pressure of less than 130/80 mm Hg, as recommended by the American Diabetes Association.

Likewise, lowering the LDL cholesterol to 100 mg per dL or less is desirable. This will require the use of medication in about one half of diabetic individuals. Hypertriglyceridemia is the most common dyslipidemia. However, since currently we have fewer drugs for treatment of hypertriglyceridemia and much less information on its risks, it seems prudent to target the LDL cholesterol. More specific data should become available in the future from diabetic dyslipidemia intervention studies.

Retinopathy

The importance of annual ophthalmologic screening cannot be overemphasized. The Early Treatment of Diabetes Retinopathy Study (ETDRS) clearly established the value of early laser therapy in diabetic retinopathy, and this is an important surrogate measure of diabetes care according to the Health Plan Data and Information Set (HEDIS) and the National Committee for Quality Assurance (NCQA), among other agencies.

The opportunities for prevention of complications of diabetes such as renal failure, blindness, amputation, and heart disease have enormous public health implications. It seems highly likely that shifting some of the funds currently spent on end-stage complications into outpatient preventive measures will pay great dividends both for patients and for payers and providers in the future.

DIABETES MELLITUS IN CHILDHOOD AND ADOLESCENCE

method of
DENIS DANEMAN, M.B., B.CH., and
KUSIEL PERLMAN, M.D.
University of Toronto and The Hospital for Sick Children
Toronto, Ontario, Canada

Diabetes mellitus is one of the chronic disorders most frequently encountered in childhood and adolescence. It can be classified as follows.

Type I diabetes (formerly insulin-dependent diabetes mellitus, or IDDM) accounts for the vast majority of cases in this age group. The incidence of type I diabetes varies more than 20-fold around the world, being highest in Scandinavia, intermediate in North America, and lowest in places like Japan. In the United States and Canada, the incidence ranges from 9 to 25 new cases per 100,000 population per year, so that by 18 years of age about 1 in 400 to 500 individuals will have developed the disorder. In most cases, type I diabetes is the result of autoimmune destruction of the insulin-producing beta cells of the pancreas. However, more recently, a nonimmune variety of type I diabetes has been described, particularly in African-American youths.

Type II diabetes (formerly non–insulin-dependent diabetes mellitus, or NIDDM) accounts for a small but perhaps steadily increasing proportion of children and adolescents with diabetes. Those with type II diabetes in this age group are more likely to be from a high-risk group, such as Native Americans, African-Americans, or Hispanics. The steady increase in the prevalence of obesity in North America probably plays an important role in the expression of type II diabetes in younger individuals.

Other types of diabetes are relatively uncommon but should be considered when the presentation of diabetes is atypical or in the presence of other clinical features. In those with a strong family history suggestive of an autosomal dominant pattern of inheritance, *maturity-onset diabetes of the young* (MODY) may be present. At least three different genetic conditions have been found in people with MODY. Also, mutations in mitochondrial DNA have been found to be associated with diabetes, as well as with other specific findings such as deafness, ptosis, and short stature.

There are a number of other chronic diseases in which the primary disease itself or its management may be associated with the development of permanent or transient diabetes, including cystic fibrosis–related diabetes (CFRD); iron-overload diabetes, due to transfusion therapy for thalassemia major; and diabetes resulting from drug administration, such as corticosteroids alone or in combination with L-asparaginase or other chemotherapeutic agents. Rarely, secondary diabetes in childhood may be associated with conditions such as Cushing's disease, pheochromocytoma, or growth hormone excess. Glucose intolerance of variable severity may also be found in association with a variety of genetic conditions, including Friedreich's ataxia, Refsum's syndrome, Prader-Willi syndrome, and Turner syndrome.

Children with new-onset type I diabetes generally present with the classic symptoms of polyuria, polydipsia, polyphagia, and weight loss. The finding of glycosuria and ketonuria confirms the diagnosis. Increasing severity of insulin deficiency will lead to diabetic ketoacidosis (DKA), characterized by dehydration with nausea, vomiting, abdominal pain, and deep (Kussmaul's) respirations. Currently less than 20% of these children and adolescents in our center present with florid DKA. This article focuses only on type I diabetes and its management in childhood and adolescence.

ETIOLOGY OF TYPE I DIABETES

Current information suggests very strongly that in most cases, type I diabetes results from the autoimmune destruction of beta cells. Susceptibility to the disease has been localized to polymorphisms in an increasing number of genes. The most important genetic susceptibility is determined by the class II antigens (HLA-D haplotypes) residing on the short arm of chromosome 6. However, genetic susceptibility appears to be insufficient to allow expression of the disease, and data suggest that environmental "trigger(s)" are required to initiate beta cell destruction. The exact nature of the environmental factors remains unknown, but candidates include viruses, toxins, and food products.

Immune destruction appears to progress relatively slowly, starting with the appearance of immune markers (e.g., islet cell antibodies, antibodies to glutamic acid decarboxylase, insulin, and other islet peptides), followed by loss of first-phase insulin secretion to an intravenous glucose load, and then progression to clinical diabetes. The rate of destruction of the islets (and, by inference, the timing of diabetes presentation) will depend on the degree of genetic susceptibility plus the severity of the islet insult(s).

Although determination of susceptibility to type I diabetes is becoming increasingly sophisticated, there are still no interventions available that have proven safe and effective in preventing the progression to overt diabetes. A number of immune interventions (e.g., administration of insulin or nicotinamide) are currently under intensive research evaluation. Until the results of these studies are available, programs for prediction and prevention of type I diabetes will remain experimental.

PHILOSOPHY OF CARE

We believe that all children and adolescents with diabetes and their families should have access to the services of a multidisciplinary diabetes health care team, consisting of physicians, nurses, dietitians, and behavioral specialists (social worker, psychologist) experienced in their care. It is also important, when necessary, to expand the team to include community services beneficial to these children's care, e.g., contact with visiting nurses or school and sports personnel. Our approach to the care of these patients is a family-centered one, in which the child or adolescent and the family play a pivotal role in the decision-making processes. Furthermore, careful attention must be paid to the normal developmental processes of childhood and adolescence, with age and stage-appropriate goals set and supervision provided.

Over the past number of years, and particularly with the completion of the Diabetes Control and Complications Trial (DCCT) in 1993, there has been an increasing move toward tighter metabolic control in all persons with type I diabetes. This has been facilitated by a number of advances in diabetes care: availability of accurate and simple techniques for self-monitoring of blood glucose concentrations; assays for measurement of hemoglobin A_{1c} (HbA_{1c}), the best indicator of long-term metabolic control; new insulins and insulin delivery systems (intensive diabetes management); ever-improving techniques for detection and treatment of early diabetes-related complications (e.g., urine assays for microalbuminuria; angiotensin-converting enzyme inhibitors for early nephropathy; fundus photography for detection of early retinopathy; laser therapy for proliferative vascular retinal changes).

With regard to the changing philosophy of diabetes management in childhood and adolescence, three issues underline the need to define changing glucose targets as they pass through the different ages and stages of development. First, increasingly intensive diabetes management is associated with a two- to threefold increased risk of severe hypoglycemia. This has the greatest implication for infants and younger children, who may be susceptible to mild cognitive deficits if severe hypoglycemia complicates the early course of their diabetes. Second, the DCCT results included an adolescent but not a preadolescent cohort; it is uncertain whether the findings of this study can be extrapolated to the younger age group. Finally, there is ongoing controversy as to when the "clock starts ticking" on the development of microvascular complications. Some of the available data suggest that the prepubertal years of diabetes contribute less toward complication development.

A second change in health care delivery to children and adolescents with diabetes has been the decreasing emphasis on hospitalization, with a corresponding increase in the need to enhance ambulatory services. It is our philosophy that children with diabetes should be admitted to the hospital only if their medical condition (e.g., DKA) or social situation (e.g., travel from a far distance, language difficulties) demands it.

Finally, we recognize that parents of children and younger adolescents with diabetes need to play a close supervisory role in their care. The placing of undue pressure on these children and adolescents to take primary responsibility for many, if not most, aspects of their daily routines often results in poor metabolic control and increasing family tensions. Furthermore, health care professionals need to avoid placing unrealistic expectations on these children and their families in terms of their ability to achieve metabolic targets. The supportive role of the health care team is an essential component of diabetes management.

GOALS OF DIABETES MANAGEMENT IN CHILDREN AND ADOLESCENTS

The following objectives should be pursued in the treatment of children and adolescents with diabetes.

1. Set realistic goals for each child or adolescent with diabetes and the family. This includes the best possible metabolic control achievable in each individual, based on age, developmental stage, hypoglycemia history, and psychosocial and economic factors.
2. Control of symptoms of hyperglycemia and prevention of DKA.
3. Avoidance of severe hypoglycemia. Mild, occasional hypoglycemia that can be easily recognized and treated is an unavoidable part of routine diabetes care.
4. Maintenance of normal growth and physical development.
5. Availability of personnel to ensure an optimum understanding of diabetes and its implications by each child or adolescent and the family.
6. Provision of adequate psychosocial support.
7. Surveillance for diabetes-related complications.
8. Smooth transition from pediatric to adult diabetes care when appropriate.

INITIAL MANAGEMENT OF THE CHILD OR ADOLESCENT WITH NEW-ONSET DIABETES

The diagnosis of diabetes mellitus in a child or adolescent is an important event with significant emotional impact on the family. It has been widely believed that admitting the child to the hospital, even if the child is not gravely ill, facilitates the family's acquisition of "survival skills" by provision of a safe and supportive environment. More recently, published data support the possibility of ambulatory care for the child with newly diagnosed diabetes who is not in a state of acute metabolic decompensation. In our center, initial management and education of the child or adolescent follow a three-phase ambulatory program: first, the phase of diagnosis and stabilization; a second phase for the acquisition of "survival skills"; and the third phase, during which diabetes education is completed, and the family is "empowered" to provide day-to-day care for the child.

Phase 1. For the child or adolescent who is not acutely ill, insulin therapy is initiated in the emergency department. If the diagnosis is made in the middle of the day, the child is given 0.1 to 0.15 unit of rapid-acting insulin per kg of body weight subcutaneously. Before the evening meal, 0.25 to 0.5 unit of intermediate-acting insulin per year of age is prescribed, combined with rapid-acting insulin depending on the blood glucose concentration. The family is provided with limited factual information concerning the etiology of diabetes, and the parents are reassured, in this regard, that there is no known activity, food, or exposure that has been proved responsible for the child's developing diabetes. Using this approach, none of the children has experienced hypoglycemic symptoms with the initiation of insulin therapy; nevertheless, the family is informed of possible signs that may indicate an exaggerated response to the initial dose of insulin. Arrangements are then made for the child to return to the diabetes day care unit the following morning before breakfast.

Phase 2. This phase is a 2- to 3-day period in the day care unit during which the child and family receive instruction in the specific tasks that need to be accomplished to provide day-to-day management at home—i.e., insulin injections, blood glucose monitoring, and the essentials of meal planning. A core multidisciplinary team, consisting of a pediatric endocrinologist, a diabetes nurse, a dietitian, and a social worker, is assigned to each child and family. Each day the child receives his or her morning insulin dose in the unit and remains there until after the evening meal. The child then returns home to sleep. We have found that with the support of the diabetes team members, the families are very comfortable and relaxed with this approach. We have experienced extremely few situations in which children need to be admitted after initiating care on an ambulatory basis.

During Phase 2, information is provided concerning the pathophysiology of the symptoms of hyperglycemia and hypoglycemia. The family and the child, if old enough, are taught about the types of insulin, where and how to inject insulin, how to mix insulin, and how to rotate the injection sites. To appropriately monitor therapy, family members are taught how to measure the blood sugar level and how to test the urine for sugar and ketones. Other tasks that need to be accomplished during this phase include acquiring an understanding of the simplest guidelines for planning meals and snacks and an awareness of what to expect over the first few weeks if the blood glucose level is very high or too low. At this time, the child is encouraged to eat three meals and two or three snacks each day at around the same time, eating a balanced diet with a variety of foods from the four basic food groups. The family is instructed to avoid excessive amounts of foods high in simple carbohydrates. With this approach, the symptoms of diabetes rapidly disappear.

The child or adolescent returns to school as soon as he or she is discharged from the diabetes day care unit and the family is managing the diabetes at home. The school needs some basic information, and printed material should be provided by the diabetes team. Since not every family's schedule is similar, the diabetes nurse works with family members on an individual basis to fit the diabetes routines into the home schedule. The family is provided with the telephone numbers for its team members, and the schedule is arranged for the educational program to be completed over the subsequent 2 to 3 weeks.

Phase 3. This consists of four sessions with the diabetes nurse, two to three with the dietitian, and one to two with the social worker. Topics for these sessions include the pathophysiology of type I diabetes, insulin and its formulations, nutritional planning, blood glucose target levels, and frequency of blood and urine monitoring. The family is instructed in principles related to prevention, detection, and treatment of hypoglycemia, including the use of glucagon for severe reactions. Management of intercurrent illness is stressed, as is the role of activity and its impact on diabetes control. Preliminary information is also provided on long-term complications and appropriate surveillance. The meetings with the social worker provide the family members with an opportunity to specifically discuss their feelings, develop coping strategies, and access community resources as necessary.

Daily telephone contact for insulin dose adjustment, ongoing education, and advice are instituted at the start of this phase. The frequency of such contact is diminished as the family and diabetes team gain confidence in the child's home management. We suggest that daily blood glucose measurements be done before each meal and the bedtime snack, and once weekly at 2 to 4 AM.

Blood Glucose Targets. The target blood glucose levels vary depending on the age of the child. In infants and toddlers, we aim for pre-meal blood glucose concentrations of 6 to 12 mmoles per liter (110 to 220 mg per dL). In the school-age child, we lower the target to 4 to 10 mmoles per liter (72 to 180 mg per dL), and in adolescents to 4 to 8 mmoles per liter (72 to 144 mg per dL). Blood glucose values are recorded in a diary. Beyond the first few weeks, insulin dose is adjusted in 10% increments based on patterns of consistently elevated or low blood glucose levels. The total daily insulin requirement for most children beyond the "honeymoon period" is 0.5 to 1 unit per kg, increasing to as much as 1.5 units per kg during puberty.

Insulin Preparations. There are currently four major categories of insulin preparations available for the management of type I diabetes in children and adolescents. As shown in Table 1, these preparations differ primarily in their time to onset, period of peak action, and duration of activity. Most children are started on twice-daily injections of insulin, with a combination of rapid- and intermediate-acting insulins before breakfast and dinner until the completion of Phase 2. Many children are now started on the very-rapid-acting insulin analogue insulin lispro (Humalog) in place of regular insulin. The initial dose of insulin usually consists of about 0.3 to 0.6

TABLE 1. **Insulin Preparations**

Type	Action	Onset of Action (h)	Peak Action (h)	Duration of Action (h)
Regular	Rapid	0.5–1	2–4	6–8
Humalog	Very rapid	0.1–0.5	0.5–2.5	3–4
NPH (isophane)	Intermediate	1–3	6–12	18–24
Lente	Intermediate	1–3	6–12	18–24

Data are for human insulin preparations and are approximations based on controlled laboratory studies. The time course will often vary from subject to subject and will be affected by injection site, insulin dose, and ambient temperature.

unit per kg of body weight per day, with approximately two thirds given before breakfast and one third before dinner. The initial dose must be individualized depending on the clinical situation. The ratio of intermediate-acting insulin to short-acting insulin is similarly about 2 to 1. At the start of Phase 3, we split the evening injection for most older children and adolescents so that the rapid-acting insulin is given before dinner and the intermediate-acting insulin at bedtime.

Meal Planning. In order to achieve the blood glucose targets, attention must be paid to nutritional planning to ensure that substrate provision matches the availability of insulin. The diet, therefore, evolves from the low refined carbohydrate diet in the first stage of diabetes management to one of more regulated content and amount. A method commonly used to estimate the child's initial daily caloric requirement is 1000 kcal plus 100 kcal for each year of age. This amount must often be increased at the time of puberty or during the first couple of months of diabetes management when the child is regaining lost weight. In prescribing this diet, our nutritionists generally follow the principles of 50 to 60% of the total calories as carbohydrate, approximately 15 to 20% as protein, and less than 30 to 35% as fat, provided as three meals and three snacks. In older children the midmorning snack is often omitted.

Consistency in timing and content of meals and snacks is stressed, and an individualized nutritional plan formulated according to the child's food preferences and activity pattern. The exchange system is generally followed based on the seven food groups of milk, fruit, vegetables, starch, protein, fat, and sugars. For some older adolescents, and particularly those opting for more intensive diabetes management routines, carbohydrate counting may provide a more appropriate approach to nutritional planning.

Physical Activity. Since physical activity can significantly affect blood glucose control, it is essential that families understand the effects of exercise and know how to compensate for them. Except for acute bursts of very strenuous exercise, which may increase blood glucose levels by increasing counterregulatory hormones, exercise generally lowers the blood glucose concentration. Children and adolescents with diabetes are encouraged to exercise on a regular basis, performing those activities that they find enjoyable. Exercise should not become a punishment but should be encouraged to promote positive self-image and generalized well-being.

Although children and adolescents with diabetes tend to have very individualized responses to physical activity, it is prudent, at least initially, to provide extra calories during periods of extra physical activity. By monitoring blood glucose responses to such activities, the family can better gauge the need for the quantity of food required to prevent hypoglycemia associated with exercise. Avoidance of low blood sugar reactions with exercise can be achieved by providing a snack of one bread or fruit exchange for every 30 to 60 minutes of regular physical activity. If the increased physical activity can be anticipated, extra food may be avoided by decreasing the appropriate insulin dose by 10 to 20%. For those involved in physical activities late in the day, the problem of late post-exercise hypoglycemia needs to be considered.

ACUTE COMPLICATIONS

Avoidance of severe hypoglycemia and of DKA and minimization of the metabolic disturbances associated with intercurrent illness are important objectives of diabetes management in children and adolescence.

Hypoglycemia. The primary goal should be the prevention of hypoglycemia. This requires a clear understanding of the actions of the insulin preparations, the role of activity in blood glucose control, and the importance of consistency in dietary content and timing. The family must be taught how to anticipate low blood glucose levels and, in this way, avoid their occurrence. However, occasional mild episodes of hypoglycemia are an inevitable consequence of insulin therapy. The symptoms of hypoglycemia include those related to increased adrenergic output (i.e., shakiness, sweating, blurred vision, hunger, tiredness), as well as to neuroglycopenia (i.e., confusion, coma, convulsion) if more severe. Although the list of potential symptoms and signs of hypoglycemia is quite extensive, for each child the constellation of symptoms is usually fairly consistent. The family and the patient should be trained to recognize these findings and act accordingly. In the infant or toddler, in whom communication is more limited, the findings are usually of a behavioral nature and the family should be taught to check the blood glucose level to confirm the association between the child's altered mood and the ambient glucose level.

In a school-age child or adolescent, most episodes of hypoglycemia can be self-detected and self-treated with 10 to 15 grams of rapidly absorbed glucose. Suitable forms of rapidly absorbed carbohydrate for the treatment of hypoglycemia include glucose tablets (each containing about 5 grams of glucose), granulated table sugar (4 grams/teaspoon), and 150 mL of apple juice or 120 mL of orange juice. Overtreatment of mild hypoglycemic episodes should be avoided, because it may contribute to overall poor metabolic control.

Glucagon should be available at home for the treatment of severe hypoglycemia when the level of consciousness is decreased or if one is concerned about the safety of providing glucose orally. The glucagon emergency kit includes a syringe pre-filled with diluent and a vial of lyophilized hormone. The diluent is injected into the bottle and 0.5 mL is injected subcutaneously in the infant or toddler; the dose is 1 mL in the older child or adolescent. The blood glucose level generally rises within 5 to 15 minutes. Nausea and vomiting may follow glucagon administration. To avoid further hypoglycemia, oral glucose should be provided within 15 to 20 minutes of glucagon injection. Following the severe hypoglycemic reaction, some children continue to have symptoms for an extended period of time despite a blood glucose level that appears to be within the normal range. It is important to provide intravenous glucose at a sufficient rate to maintain the blood glucose above 8 to 10 mmoles per liter if these symptoms are to resolve.

Diabetic Ketoacidosis. DKA is a medical emergency and should be avoidable. At presentation, a child with DKA is usually moderately to severely dehydrated owing to the osmotic diuresis caused by the hyperglycemia. Despite a loss of potassium in the urine, the serum potassium concentration initially rises because of failure of this ion to enter the cells and to increase efflux from the cells in exchange for hydrogen ions. The sodium concentration, on the other hand, will usually be low because of the osmotic effect of glucose in the intravascular space. A high serum sodium concentration suggests extreme free water loss and severe dehydration. In treating DKA, care must be taken not to overhydrate the child, because this may predispose to the development of cerebral edema—a complication with a high mortality rate. The exact cause of cerebral edema remains unknown.

A key to successful management of DKA is careful monitoring of the child's clinical status as well as the fluid balance. All intravenous fluid administration must be carefully documented, with each urine sample measured for glucose, ketones, and volume. In addition to hourly assessments of the level of consciousness, blood pressure, pulse, and blood glucose should be measured every hour for the first 4 to 6 hours and every 2 hours thereafter. Acid-base and electrolyte status should be determined every 4 hours until correction has been obtained. Particular attention should be paid to the corrected sodium concentration, which is calculated as follows:

$$\text{Corrected Na} = \text{measured Na} + 1.5\left(\frac{\text{measured glucose} - 5}{5}\right)$$

In general, children should not be given anything by mouth, at least during the early stage of therapy, so long as the tachypnea persists. The use of nasogastric tubes or urinary catheters should be avoided unless the child is comatose. Specific guidelines for the management of DKA are described in Table 2. In addition to cerebral edema, the major complications of the treatment of DKA, which should be anticipated and avoided, are hypokalemia and hypoglycemia.

Once the acidosis has been corrected and it is the appropriate time for the usual subcutaneous (SC) injection, the intravenous (IV) insulin should be discontinued. Since the plasma half life of IV insulin is very short, the infusion should be maintained for at least half an hour if the SC injection includes regular insulin, and for about 2 hours if only intermediate-acting insulin is being administered.

Management of Sick Days. Intercurrent illnesses

TABLE 2. **Management of Diabetic Ketoacidosis**

Fluids	Initial management should consist of normal saline infused at 10 ml/kg of body weight for the first hour and then at approximately 5 ml/kg/h, depending upon the degree of dehydration. When the plasma glucose concentration falls below 15 mmol/L or if it falls at a rate greater than 5–10 mmol/h, the fluid should be changed to 5% dextrose in 0.45–0.9% saline. The sodium concentration of the infusate should be adjusted to avoid a drop in the corrected sodium of more than 1 mmol/L/h. In general one should aim to correct any fluid deficit over 24–36 h.
Insulin	Once rehydration with IV fluids has been initiated, IV regular insulin is started at a rate of 0.1 unit/kg/h, controlled by an infusion pump. When the plasma glucose concentration falls to less than 15 mmol/L, the insulin infusion can be decreased to 0.03–0.05 unit/kg/h to maintain a rate of insulin infusion above normal basal requirements. The objective is to maintain a glucose concentration in the 6–15 mmol/L range to avoid either hypo- or hyperglycemia. If intravenous infusion is not possible, insulin may also be administered by the IM or SC route at 0.25 unit/kg every 4 h.
Alkali	We administer bicarbonate only if the DKA is fairly severe, with a pH of <7.1 and a serum bicarbonate of <10 mmol/L. The amount of bicarbonate is calculated to increase the serum concentration to 12 mmol/L, with half the repletion given over the first 30 minutes and the remainder over the subsequent 2–4 h.
Potassium	After the child has voided, KCl should be added to the IV fluid at a concentration of 20–30 mmol/L if the potassium concentration is above 4.5 mmol/L, and 30–40 mmol/L if it is below this level. It is particularly important to start KCl infusion early when the serum potassium concentration is below 4.5 mmol/L.

are common in the childhood age group. The avoidance of both hypoglycemia and dehydration leading to DKA are the major objectives in managing intercurrent illness in a child with diabetes. If the child is not eating, sugar-containing fluids should be given on a regular basis between the usual mealtimes. During intercurrent illness, the blood glucose and urinary ketones should be checked every 4 hours. If the child vomits more than twice within a 12-hour period, a member of the diabetes team should be contacted, and the child seen at the emergency department to assess the need for intravenous fluids. In our center, the intermediate-acting insulin is not discontinued but extra regular insulin is administered according to Table 3. This aggressive approach to the management of intercurrent illness has significantly reduced the frequency of hospital admissions for DKA at our center.

ONGOING MANAGEMENT

The complex and ongoing requirements of diabetes management demand that these children and their families be seen by the health care team at regular intervals (three to four times per year) in order to evaluate their status. At these visits, focus should be placed on diabetes-related issues, such as insulin dose requirements, dietary satisfaction and compliance, results of self-monitoring of blood glucose, symptoms and frequency of hypoglycemia and hyperglycemia, sick days and their impact on diabetes control, and adequacy of growth and sexual maturation. Assessment should also focus on psychosocial adjustment to the diabetes, which includes evaluation of school attendance and performance, behavioral issues, and, in the teen, such issues as smoking, alcohol and drug use, sexuality, career planning, and when the time comes, transition to adult care. Physical examination should include height and weight measurement with plotting on appropriate growth curves, blood pressure determination, palpation of thyroid and liver size, fundus examination, and inspection of insulin injection sites.

The purpose of the routine clinic visits is also to provide the opportunity for improving the child's and the family's understanding of diabetes and its implications, to make appropriate adjustments in the treatment regimen to improve metabolic control and/or decrease the frequency of symptoms of hypoglycemia and hyperglycemia, and to intervene should any medical or psychosocial problems be detected. Availability in the clinic setting of all members of the health care team facilitates evaluation of insulin and blood monitoring techniques, and ongoing meal planning.

HbA_{1c} levels should be measured at each clinic visit and the families informed of the results. Furthermore, regular checks of serum thyroid hormone and lipid levels can be accomplished at clinic visits. It is our current practice to measure these levels about 6 months after diagnosis of diabetes. If the lipid (total cholesterol and triglyceride) levels are normal, we measure them again only during puberty. If the lipid levels are abnormal, steps are taken to reduce them, first with dietary interventions and attempts to optimize metabolic control and then, if these fail, with lipid-lowering medications. Serum thyroid-stimulating hormone values are measured annually.

Since the needs of children with diabetes change as they progress through different maturational stages, it is imperative that there be ample opportunity for them and their families to meet with the members of their diabetes team for refresher courses. These courses can often be conducted in the context of group meetings. However, some degree of individual counseling is advisable, because it helps to build the relationship between the team members and the maturing child or adolescent. Such sessions are most urgently needed in those experiencing difficulties in achieving blood glucose targets but should also be provided to those with excellent or good control as a means of anticipatory guidance.

Table 4 outlines the factors associated with poor metabolic control in children and adolescents with type I diabetes. It should be noted that the majority of these fall into the psychologic or psychosocial area, rather than being due to biologic problems.

INTENSIVE DIABETES MANAGEMENT PROTOCOL

The results of the DCCT and other intervention trials clearly demonstrate a close relationship be-

TABLE 3. **Guidelines for Insulin Adjustment During Intercurrent Illness**

	Sickness Profile				
	A	*B*	*C*	*D*	*E*
Blood glucose (mmol/L)	>4–6* and <13	>13 and <17	>17	>13	<4–6
Urine ketones	Negative or positive	Negative	Negative	Positive	Negative or positive
Action	Wait; continue to monitor carefully	Wait; if condition persists, increase insulin next day by 10–20%/day until aims achieved	Give extra regular insulin q 4 h, equal to 10–20% of total daily dose, until urine ketones clear and/or blood sugar <11 mmol/L; then proceed as for regimen in columns A and B		Decrease daily insulin by 20%/day until blood glucose is between 4 and 11 mmol/L

* Depends on the patient's age and target blood glucose concentrations.

TABLE 4. **Factors Associated with Poor Metabolic Control in Children and Adolescents with Diabetes Mellitus**

Biologic
Impaired insulin action during adolescence
Exaggerated counterregulatory hormone responses

Medical
Acute intercurrent illness
(e.g., viral or bacterial illness)
Chronic disease
Diabetes-related
(e.g., thyroid disease, celiac disease)
Unrelated to diabetes
(e.g., chronic infection, malignancy)

Psychologic
Lack of knowledge of diabetes and its management
Poor social support
Unrealistic expectations for self-care
in children and younger adolescents
Specific psychosocial issues
Psychiatric disease (e.g., depression)
Adolescent noncompliance
Family dysfunction
Eating disorders in adolescent females
Sexual or physical abuse

tween metabolic control and the onset and progression of diabetes-related microvascular complications in adolescents and adults with type I diabetes. To achieve the goals of intensive diabetes management, a multifaceted plan is required that includes all of the following components:

1. Patient motivation and more intensive education.
2. Frequent contact between the patient and members of the patient's team experienced in the provision of this type of care.
3. Four or more daily blood glucose measurements.
4. Careful attention to the balance among food intake, physical activity, and insulin dosage.
5. A multiple-dose daily insulin injection routine (e.g., rapid-acting insulin before each meal and intermediate-acting insulin at bedtime) or use of a continuous SC insulin infusion pump.
6. Adjustment of insulin dosage at each injection time according to an algorithm geared to meet specific blood glucose targets.

This treatment approach provides the opportunity to achieve tighter levels of metabolic control than can generally be achieved with more conventional therapeutic approaches. The side effects of intensive diabetes management include a two- to threefold increase in the risk of severe hypoglycemia, as well as the potential for excessive weight gain.

COMPLICATION SURVEILLANCE

Significant diabetes-related microvascular and macrovascular complications are exceptionally rare in prepubertal children and in those with diabetes of less than 10 years' duration. It is therefore distinctly unusual to encounter other than the early manifestations of these complications during the adolescent years. Nevertheless, early detection provides the potential for early intervention before the changes become permanent. Information regarding the complications of diabetes should start at the time of initial diabetes education, and reinforcement should be provided throughout the course of the disease. The message should be given that although the complications are serious and potentially life-threatening, good glycemic control plus surveillance will allow for either prevention of complication onset or early detection and intervention.

Retinopathy. We recommend that all adolescents with diabetes receive an annual eye examination by a practitioner experienced in the evaluation of diabetic retinopathy once they have reached 15 years of age and have had diabetes for more than 5 years. Earlier and/or more frequent evaluation is not thought to be required and may overburden already limited resources for diabetic retinopathy management.

Nephropathy. Regular checks of blood pressure should be a part of routine diabetes management. For patients with persistently elevated blood pressure, consideration should be given to the use of antihypertensive therapy.

All patients older than 15 years of age who have had diabetes for more than 3 years should be screened annually for microalbuminuria. We have performed two timed overnight urine collections for this purpose, with further attention to patients with albumin excretion rates above 15 μg per minute. More recent data suggest that the albumin-creatinine ratio in a spot urine specimen may be an acceptable way to screen for early nephropathy. Detection of microalbuminuria during adolescence is a fairly good predictor of those likely to show evidence of progressive nephropathy. Attention should be paid to the achievement of excellent metabolic control, as well as to the use of angiotensin-converting enzyme inhibitors, in these youngsters.

Macrovascular Complications. Surveillance for macrovascular disease implies regular blood pressure measurement, screening for hyperlipidemia, avoidance or cessation of smoking, and attention to weight management. For those adolescents with long-duration diabetes, regular foot examination and neurologic assessment are advisable.

SUMMARY AND CONCLUSIONS

Type I diabetes in childhood and adolescence is a common and complex metabolic disorder with important implications for both short-term and long-term health. A multidisciplinary approach is necessary to help these children and their families deal with the medical and psychosocial impact of the disease. Advances over the past 20 years have served only to increase further the complexity of diabetes management. It is hoped that ongoing research endeavors will allow prevention of diabetes in children at high risk for its development, as well as simplifying the management of those already affected.

DIABETIC KETOACIDOSIS AND HYPERGLYCEMIC HYPEROSMOLAR NONKETOTIC STATE

method of
ABBAS E. KITABCHI, PH.D., M.D.
*University of Tennessee, Memphis
Memphis, Tennessee*

GUILLERMO E. UMPIERREZ, M.D.
*Georgia Baptist Medical Center and Emory University School of Medicine
Atlanta, Georgia*

and

MARY BETH MURPHY, R.N., M.S., C.D.E., M.B.A.
*University of Tennessee, Memphis
Memphis, Tennessee*

Diabetic ketoacidosis (DKA) and hyperglycemic hyperosmolar nonketotic state (HHNS) are the two most serious metabolic complications of diabetes mellitus even if managed properly.

Although the mortality rate in patients with DKA has significantly decreased, to less than 5%, since the advent of low-dose insulin protocols, the mortality rate in patients with HHNS is still alarmingly high at approximately 30%. The prognosis is substantially worsened with increased age, presence of coma, and hypotension.

PATHOGENESIS

Although the pathogenesis of DKA is better understood than that of HHNS, the basic underlying mechanism for both disorders is a reduction in the net effective concentration of circulating insulin coupled with a concomitant elevation of counterregulatory hormones such as glucagon, catecholamines, cortisol, and growth hormone. These hormonal alterations in DKA and HHNS lead to increased hepatic glucose production and impaired glucose utilization in peripheral tissues, with resulting hyperglycemia. Furthermore, the combination of insulin deficiency and increased counterregulatory hormones in DKA also leads to an excessive release of free fatty acids into the circulation from adipose tissue (lipolysis), and to unrestrained oxidation of hepatic fatty acids to ketone bodies (β-hydroxybutyric and acetoacetic acids), with resulting ketonemia and metabolic acidosis.

HHNS may also be due to plasma insulin concentration insufficient to facilitate glucose utilization by insulin-sensitive tissues but adequate (as determined by residual C peptide) to prevent lipolysis (and subsequent ketogenesis). This, along with severe dehydration, results in the characteristic laboratory and clinical findings with HHNS. The characteristic laboratory findings in both DKA and HHNS including water and electrolyte deficits are summarized in Table 1. As can be seen, the two conditions differ in the magnitude of dehydration and degree of ketosis (and acidosis).

TABLE 1. **Diagnostic Laboratory Criteria and Typical Water/Electrolyte Deficits for DKA and HHNS**

	DKA	HHNS
Diagnostic Criteria		
Plasma glucose (mg/dL)	>250	>600
pH	<7.3	>7.3
Serum HCO_3^- (mEq/L)	<15	>15
Urine ketones*	≥3+	≤1+
Serum ketones*	Positive at 1:2 dilution	Negative at 1:2 dilution
Serum osmolality	Variable	≥330 mOsm/kg
Typical Deficits		
Water (L)	6	9
Water (mL/kg)	100	100–200
Na^+ (mEq/kg)	7–10	5–13
K^+ (mEq/kg)	3–5	5–15

*Nitroprusside reaction method.
Abbreviations: DKA = diabetic ketoacidosis; HHNS = hyperglycemic hyperosmolar nonketotic state.

The most frequent precipitating factors in DKA, in known diabetics, are infection and discontination of or inadequate insulin. In HHNS, infection is by far the most frequent precipitating event, followed by new-onset diabetes; affected persons are often elderly residents of nursing homes or persons who have not sought medical care early enough owing to delayed recognition of hyperglycemia.

The most common types of precipitating infection in either condition are urinary tract infection and pneumonia. Other acute conditions that may precipitate hyperglycemic crises include cerebrovascular accident, alcohol abuse, pancreatitis, myocardial infarction, and trauma. Drugs that affect carbohydrate metabolism such as corticosteroids, thiazides, and sympathomimetic agents (e.g., dobutamine, terbutaline) may also precipitate the development of hyperglycemia and DKA. In young female patients with type I diabetes, psychologic problems complicated by eating disorders may be a contributing factor in 20% of cases of recurrent ketoacidosis. Factors that may lead to insulin omission in younger patients include fear of gaining weight with good metabolic control, fear of hypoglycemia, rebellion against authority, and diabetes-related stress. Recently, noncompliance with insulin therapy has been reported to be a major cause for DKA in urban black and medically indigent patients.

DIAGNOSIS

History and Physical Examination

Whereas the clinical presentation of DKA usually develops rapidly, over a time span of less than 24 hours, HHNS symptoms may occur more insidiously, with gradual clouding of the sensorium progressing to mental obtundation and coma. Vomiting and abdominal pain are frequently the presenting symptoms. The importance of a good history and physical examination cannot be overemphasized. The physical examination reveals signs of dehydration, including loss of skin turgor, dry mucous membranes, tachycardia, and hypotension. Mental status can vary from full alertness to profound lethargy; however, less than 20% of patients with DKA present with loss of consciousness. Other findings include acetone on the breath and labored (Kussmaul's) respirations. In HHNS, mental obtundation and coma are more frequent because in the majority of cases, by definition, a state of hyperosmolarity exists. As mentioned earlier, although the most common precipitating event is infection, most patients are normothermic or even hypothermic at presentation.

Laboratory Findings

The initial laboratory evaluation of patients with DKA or HHNS should include arterial blood gases, complete blood count with differential, urinalysis, blood glucose, blood urea nitrogen (BUN), and serum ketones, electrolytes, and creatinine level (all obtained immediately). Table 1 presents the laboratory characteristics of most patients with severe DKA and HHNS. Although these data are empirical, they constitute the most accepted criteria for diagnosis. Accumulation of ketoacids in DKA usually results in an increased anion gap metabolic acidosis. The anion gap is calculated by subtracting the sum of chloride and bicarbonate from the sodium concentration: $Na-(Cl + HCO_3)$. The normal anion gap is 12 ± 2 mEq per liter. Patients with DKA generally present with an anion gap greater than 20 mEq per liter. In some cases, the diagnosis of DKA can be confounded by the coexistence of other acid-base disorders.

The majority of patients with hyperglycemic emergencies present with leukocytosis, but a white blood cell count greater than 25,000 per mm^3 is seldom seen in the absence of bacterial infection. In DKA the serum sodium at presentation is usually decreased because of the osmotic flux of water from the intracellular to the extracellular space in the presence of hyperglycemia. To assess the severity of sodium and water deficit, serum sodium may be corrected by adding 1.6 mg per dL of sodium for each 100 mg of glucose per dL above 100 mg per dL. The serum potassium concentration at presentation is usually elevated because of a shift of potassium from the intracellular to the extracellular space due to acidemia, insulin deficiency, and hypertonicity. On the other hand, in HHNS, serum sodium is usually normal or elevated, with elevated BUN and serum creatinine.

Differential Diagnosis

Not all patients who present with ketoacidosis have DKA. Patients with chronic ethanol abuse with a recent binge culminating in nausea, vomiting, and acute starvation may present with alcoholic ketoacidosis (AKA). In virtually all reported series of AKA, the elevation of total body ketone concentration (7 to 10 mM) is comparable to that reported in patients with DKA. However, because of the altered intracellular redox state caused by increased reduced nicotinamide adenine dinucleotide (NADH)/nicotinamide adenine dinucleotide (NAD) levels in AKA, the β-hydroxybutyrate–acetoacetate equilibrium reaction is shifted toward β-hydroxybutyrate production. Consequently, in AKA, levels of β-hydroxybutyrate are much higher than acetoacetate levels, and the average β-hydroxybutyrate/acetoacetate ratio observed in AKA may be as high as 7 to 10:1, as opposed to a 3:1 ratio observed in DKA. The variable that differentiates diabetic and alcohol-induced ketoacidosis is the concentration of blood glucose. Whereas DKA is characterized by severe hyperglycemia, the presence of ketoacidosis with normal or low glucose levels in an alcoholic patient is virtually diagnostic of AKA.

Some patients with decreased food intake (lower than 500 calories per day) for several days may present with starvation ketosis. However, in a healthy subject, the body is able to adapt to prolonged fasting by increasing the clearance of ketone bodies in peripheral tissues (brain and muscle), and by enhancing the kidney's ability to excrete ammonia to compensate for the increased ketoacid production. Thus, patients with starvation ketosis rarely present with serum bicarbonate concentrations less than 18 mEq per liter.

DKA must also be distinguished from other causes of high anion gap metabolic acidosis including lactic acidosis, chronic renal failure, and ingestion of drugs such as salicylate, methanol, ethylene glycol, and paraldehyde. Measuring blood lactate concentration easily establishes the diagnosis of lactic acidosis, with a value of greater than 5 mM considered diagnostic, because patients with DKA seldom demonstrate this level of serum lactate. Salicylate overdose is suspected in the presence of mixed acid-base disorder (primary respiratory alkalosis and high anion gap metabolic acidosis) in the absence of increased ketone levels. The diagnosis is confirmed by measuring a serum salicylate level in excess of 80 to 100 mg per dL. Methanol ingestion results in acidosis from the formation of formic acid and, to a lesser extent, lactic acid. Methanol intoxication develops within 24 hours after ingestion, and patients usually present with abdominal pain secondary to gastritis or pancreatitis and visual disturbances that range from blurred vision to blindness (optic neuritis). The diagnosis is confirmed by the presence of an elevated blood methanol level. Ethylene glycol (antifreeze) ingestion leads to excessive production of oxalic acid. The diagnosis of ethylene glycol intoxication is suggested by the presence of an increased osmolality and anion gap acidosis without ketonemia, as well as neurologic and cardiovascular abnormalities (seizures and cardiovascular collapse), and the presence of calcium oxalate and hippurate crystals in the urine. Paraldehyde ingestion is suspected by its characteristic strong odor on the breath.

In HHNS, patients are usually more hyperglycemic, with an increased serum osmolality (normal values are 290 ± 5 mOsm per kg H_2O). Serum osmolality may be calculated using the following formula:

$$\text{Serum osmolality} = 2[Na^+](\text{mEq/L}) + \text{glucose (mg/dL)}/18 + \text{BUN (mg/dL)}/2.8$$

In the laboratory diagnosis of DKA, two points need to be emphasized: (1) The use of nitroprusside for the assessment of ketone bodies does not measure the most abundant ketone, β-hydroxybutyrate, but reacts with acetoacetate and a nonketoacid compound, acetone. However, as the DKA begins to resolve, more β-hydroxybutyrate is converted to acetoacetate. Therefore, ketone levels as measured by the nitroprusside method during the course of therapy are misleadingly higher as the patient improves. Therefore, we do not recommend the measurement of ketones by the nitroprusside method for follow-up of patients in DKA. (2) Ketone bodies interfere with the standard laboratory test for creatinine (colorimetric method), leading to falsely elevated serum creatinine values (sometimes as high as 4 to 5 mg per dL) in the absence of any renal problems. This high value usually normalizes once ketosis is resolved and hydration is adequate.

TREATMENT

Successful treatment of DKA and HHNS requires frequent monitoring of patients, improvement of circulatory volume and tissue perfusion, correction of hyperglycemia and electrolyte imbalances, and identification of precipitating events.

Fluid Therapy

Patients with DKA and HHNS are invariably volume-depleted, with an estimated water deficit of approximately 100 mL per kg of body weight. The initial fluid therapy is directed toward expansion of the intravascular volume and restoration of renal perfusion. The initial fluid of choice is isotonic saline (0.9% NaCl), which is infused at a rate of 500 to 1000 mL per hour during the first 2 hours. After the intravascular volume depletion has been corrected, the rate of normal saline infusion should be reduced to 250 mL per hour, or the infusate should be changed to 0.45% saline (250–500 mL per hour) depending upon the serum sodium concentration and state of hydration. The water deficit can be estimated, based on a corrected serum sodium concentration, using the following equation:

$$\text{Water deficit} = (0.6)(\text{body weight [kg]}) \times (1 - [\text{corrected sodium}/140]).$$

The goal is to replace half the estimated water deficit over a period of 12 to 24 hours.

Dextrose should be added to replacement fluids when the plasma glucose concentration reaches 200 mg per dL for DKA and 300 mg per dL for HHNS. This allows continued insulin administration until acidosis and hyperosmolality, respectively, are controlled while avoiding hypoglycemia. An additional important aspect of fluid management in hyperglycemic states is to replace the volume of urinary losses. Failure to adjust fluid replacement for urinary losses may delay correction of the electrolyte and water deficits.

Insulin Therapy

The cornerstone of DKA and HHNS management after initial hydration is insulin therapy. Continuous intravenous (IV) infusion of regular insulin is the treatment of choice for severely dehydrated and mentally obtunded patients. In such patients, we recommend admission to an ICU, step-down unit, or similar facility in which adequate nursing care and quick turn-around of laboratory test results are available. Such patients should first receive a hydrating solution until the results of serum potassium determination are known. Once hypokalemia ($[K^+] < 3.3$ mEq per liter) is excluded, an IV bolus of regular insulin of 0.15 unit per kg of body weight, followed by a continuous infusion of regular insulin at a dose of 0.1 unit per kg per hour (5–7 units per hour), should be administered. This will result in a fairly predictable decrease in plasma glucose concentration at a rate of 65 to 125 mg per hour. When plasma glucose reaches 200 mg per dL in DKA or 300 mg per dL in HHNS, the insulin infusion rate should be decreased to 0.05 unit per kg per hour (3 to 5 units per hour), and dextrose (5 to 10% dextrose) should be added to intravenous fluids. Thereafter, the rate of insulin administration may need to be adjusted to maintain the foregoing glucose values until acidosis in DKA or mental obtundation and hyperosmolality in HHNS are resolved. During therapy, capillary blood glucose should be determined every 1 to 2 hours at the bedside using a glucose oxidase reagent strip; and blood should be drawn every 4 to 6 hours for determination of BUN and serum electrolytes, glucose, and creatinine, and for DKA, venous pH. During follow-up, we recommend pH determination by venous rather than repeated arterial punctures, because arterial blood gases are seldom needed. In patients who do not need frequent monitoring of blood gases, we prefer to obtain blood pH by the venous route, because venous pH values are usually 0.03 unit lower than arterial.

In a conscious patient admitted to a general hospital ward with mild DKA or HHNS (without coma or obtundation), the administration of regular insulin every 1 to 2 hours by the subcutaneous or intramuscular route has been shown to be as effective in lowering blood glucose and ketone levels as giving the entire insulin dose by intravenous infusion. Such patients should receive first the recommended hydrating solution, followed by an initial "priming" dose of regular insulin of 0.3 to 0.4 unit per kg of body weight, given half as intravenous bolus and half as a subcutaneous (SC) or intramuscular (IM) injection. Subsequently, all insulin injections are changed to SC injections of 10 units of regular insulin every 2 hours for DKA or HHNS. The effectiveness of IM and SC administration is essentially the same; however, SC injections are easier and less painful.

The criteria for resolution of DKA include a blood glucose lower than 200 mg per dL, a serum bicarbonate level equal to or greater than 18 mEq per liter, a venous pH greater than 7.3, and a calculated anion gap equal to or lower than 14 mEq per liter. After resolution of DKA in patients with newly diagnosed diabetes who are able to eat, they should be placed on an American Diabetes Association (ADA) diet and be given split-dose insulin therapy with both regular and intermediate-acting insulin, for an initial total insulin dose of 0.6 to 0.7 unit per kg per day. This is usually sufficient to achieve metabolic control, but final adjustment may require modification of the insulin schedule to multiple-dose insulin injections. However, as an initial approach, two thirds of this total daily dose can be given in the morning and one third in the evening as a split-mixed dose. It is extremely important to remember that blood glucose values should be monitored at least before meals and at bedtime. Complete diabetes education should be provided for these patients.

Potassium

Mild to moderate hyperkalemia is commonly found in patients in hyperglycemic crisis despite total body potassium depletion. The serum potassium deficit in both conditions is rather severe. During treatment, there is typically a rapid decline in plasma potassium concentration. Insulin therapy and correction of acidosis decrease serum potassium by increasing cellular potassium uptake in peripheral tissues. In addition, IV fluids exert a dilutional effect and increase urinary potassium excretion. Therefore, to prevent hypokalemia, we recommend that potassium replacement be initiated after serum levels fall below 5.5 mEq per liter in the presence of adequate urine output. Generally, potassium replacement at a rate of 20 to 30 mEq in each liter of infusion is appropriate, and the goal is to maintain a serum potassium concentration within the normal range of 4 to 5 mEq per liter. In some rare patients with DKA presenting with significant hypokalemia, insulin administration may precipitate profound hypokalemia, which can induce life-threatening arrhythmias and respiratory muscle weakness. In such patients, insulin therapy should not be started until potassium replacement has been initiated.

Bicarbonate

The use of bicarbonate administration in the therapy of DKA is highly controversial. Arguments that favor the use of alkali therapy are based on the assumption that severe metabolic acidosis can lead to organ dysfunction such as impaired myocardial contractility, coma, and gastrointestinal complications. Potential adverse effects of alkali therapy include hypokalemia, worsening of intracellular acidosis due to increased carbon dioxide production, delayed ketoanion metabolism, and development of paradoxical central nervous system acidosis.

Prospective randomized studies have failed to show any positive changes in morbidity or mortality with bicarbonate therapy in patients with DKA in whom blood pH is between 6.9 and 7.1. No prospective, randomized studies concerning the use of bicarbonate in DKA with pH values of less than 6.9 have been reported. Despite the absence of such studies, we empirically recommend that in patients with a blood PH of less than 6.9, 88 mEq of sodium bicarbonate be added to 250 mL of hypotonic saline and given over 30 minutes. Thereafter, venous pH should be assessed every 2 hours until the pH rises to 7.0. Furthermore, unless the bicarbonate is given in the presence of hyperkalemia (serum K^+ value of more than 5.5 mEq per liter), 15 mEq of KCl per liter should be given with each ampule of bicarbonate to prevent hypokalemia. We recommend no bicarbonate administration in patients with HHNS or in DKA patients with blood pH of greater than 7.0.

Phosphate

The phosphate deficit in DKA averages approximately 1.0 mmol per kg of body weight; however, as with potassium, serum levels of phosphate at presentation are often normal or increased, and levels rapidly decrease after initiation of insulin therapy. Prospective randomized studies on the use of phosphate therapy in DKA have failed to show any beneficial effect of phosphate replacement on clinical outcome. Furthermore, aggressive phosphate therapy may result in hypocalcemia. Because potential complications of hypophosphatemia include cardiac and skeletal muscle weakness and respiratory depression, careful phosphate replacement may be indicated in patients with cardiac dysfunction, anemia, or respiratory depression and in those with serum phosphate concentration lower than 1.0 to 1.5 mg per dL. When needed, 20 to 30 mEq of potassium phosphate per liter can be added to replacement fluids.

Figures 1 and 2 are detailed flow charts of our recommended protocols for treatment of DKA and HHNS, respectively.

COMPLICATIONS AND PROGNOSIS

Symptomatic and even fatal cerebral edema has been reported in pediatric patients with DKA, but fortunately this is a very rare complication. It usually occurs in newly diagnosed diabetic patients during their first episode of ketoacidosis. The clinical presentation of cerebral edema is characterized by headache and lethargy followed by seizures and the development of papilledema and other signs of increased intracranial pressure. Although the mechanism of cerebral edema is not known, it appears to result from osmotic disequilibrium with failure of the intracellular osmolality to adjust to rapid changes in extracellular osmolality. During treatment of DKA, the resolution of hyperglycemia leads to a progressive decrease in plasma osmolality, which favors the shift of water into the intracellular space. In addition, insulin therapy per se also promotes the membrane transport of sodium and water into the intracellular space. Although in most reported cases a specific cause could not be found, a rapid correction of hyperglycemia and plasma osmolality by excessive water replacement may contribute to the development of cerebral edema. Preventive measures that might decrease the onset of cerebral edema are a gradual replacement of sodium and water deficit and avoidance of an excessively rapid decline in blood glucose concentration. Similarly, fatal cases of HHNS have been reported, with the most likely cause being a rapid correction of hyperglycemia. For this reason, we and others recommend that a gradual, slower decrease of blood glucose in HHNS be accomplished with smaller doses of insulin, and most important, that dextrose be added to the hydrating solution once blood glucose reaches 300 mg per dL. A level of 250 to 300 mg per dL should be maintained until hyperosmolality and mental status improve and the patient becomes stable.

Hypoglycemia and hypokalemia result from overzealous treatment with high-dose insulin and inadequate monitoring of glucose and potassium concentrations during therapy. The frequency of these complications is significantly decreased by the use of low-dose insulin protocols, frequent monitoring of

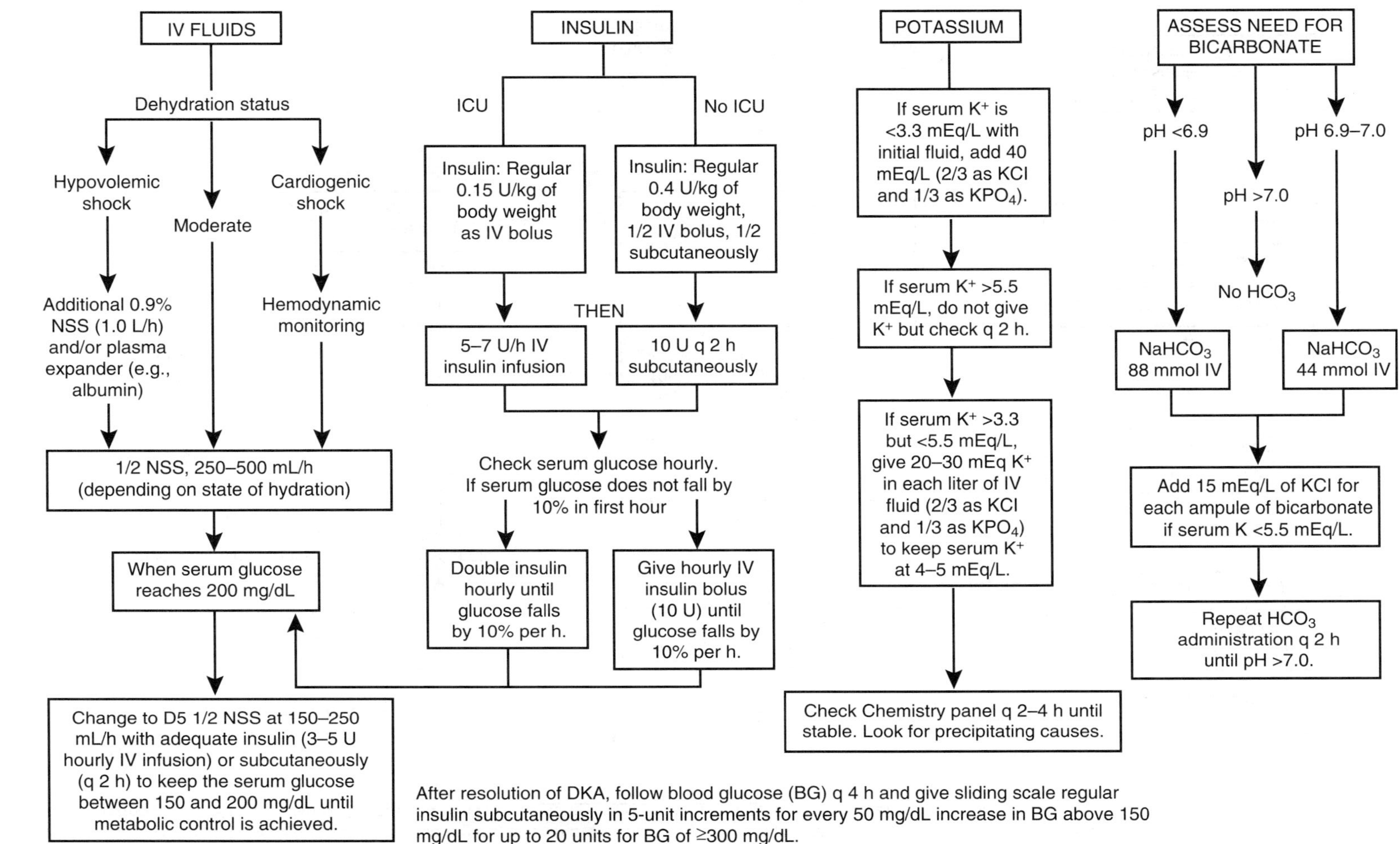

Figure 1. Protocol for management of diabetic ketoacidosis (DKA). *Abbreviation*: NSS = normal saline solution.

Initial evaluation: History and physical examination, arterial blood gases, complete blood counts with differentials, serum "ketones," Chemistry panel, and urinalysis, STAT. Start IV fluid, 1.0 L of 0.9% NSS/h initially, then reassess.

Diagnostic criteria: Blood glucose >600 mg/dL, arterial pH >7.3, HCO_3 >15 mEq/L, mild ketonemia (negative at 1:2 dil), osmolality ≥330 mOsm/kg [calculated as : $2(Na) + \frac{glucose\ (mg/dL)}{18} + \frac{BUN\ (mg/dL)}{2.8}$], and mental obtundation.

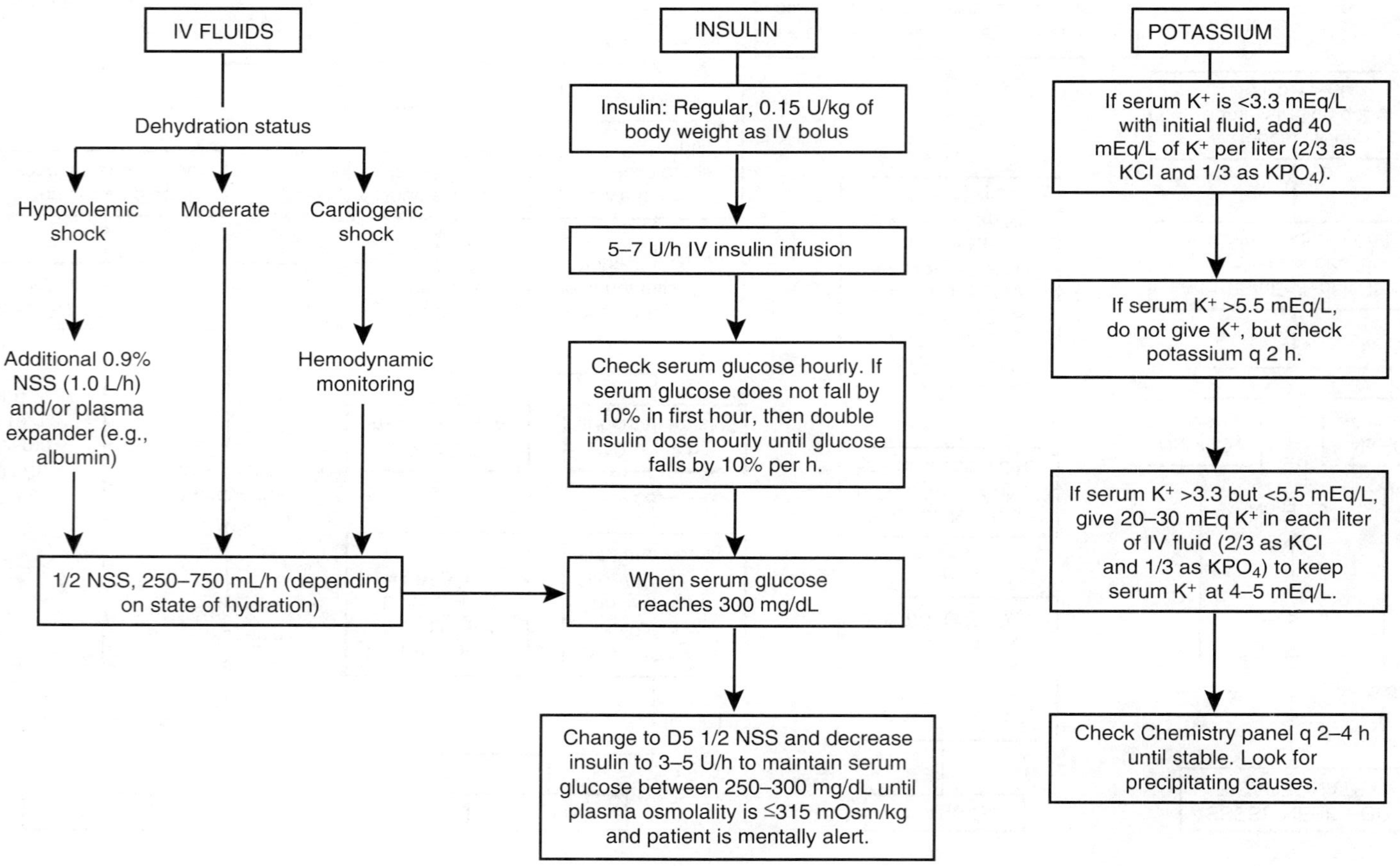

IV FLUIDS

Dehydration status

Hypovolemic shock → Additional 0.9% NSS (1.0 L/h) and/or plasma expander (e.g., albumin) → 1/2 NSS, 250–750 mL/h (depending on state of hydration)

Moderate → 1/2 NSS, 250–750 mL/h (depending on state of hydration)

Cardiogenic shock → Hemodynamic monitoring → 1/2 NSS, 250–750 mL/h (depending on state of hydration)

1/2 NSS, 250–750 mL/h (depending on state of hydration) → When serum glucose reaches 300 mg/dL

INSULIN

Insulin: Regular, 0.15 U/kg of body weight as IV bolus → 5–7 U/h IV insulin infusion → Check serum glucose hourly. If serum glucose does not fall by 10% in first hour, then double insulin dose hourly until glucose falls by 10% per h. → When serum glucose reaches 300 mg/dL → Change to D5 1/2 NSS and decrease insulin to 3–5 U/h to maintain serum glucose between 250–300 mg/dL until plasma osmolality is ≤315 mOsm/kg and patient is mentally alert.

POTASSIUM

If serum K^+ is <3.3 mEq/L with initial fluid, add 40 mEq/L of K^+ per liter (2/3 as KCl and 1/3 as KPO_4). → If serum K^+ >5.5 mEq/L, do not give K^+, but check potassium q 2 h. → If serum K^+ >3.3 but <5.5 mEq/L, give 20–30 mEq K^+ in each liter of IV fluid (2/3 as KCl and 1/3 as KPO_4) to keep serum K^+ at 4–5 mEq/L. → Check Chemistry panel q 2–4 h until stable. Look for precipitating causes.

After resolution of HHNS, follow blood glucose (BG) q 4 h and give sliding scale regular insulin subcutaneously in 5-unit increments for every 50 mg/dL increase in BG above 150 mg/dL for up to 20 units for BG ≥300 mg/dL.

Figure 2. Protocol for management of hyperglycemic hyperosmolar, nonketotic state (HHNS) in critical care units. *Abbreviation:* NSS = normal saline solution.

serum glucose and electrolytes charted on a flow sheet, and judicious use of glucose and potassium replacement.

The development of hypoxemia and, in rare instances, noncardiogenic pulmonary edema may complicate the treatment of DKA. Hypoxemia and increased alveolar-arterial oxygen gradient have been noted during treatment in approximately half of the patients with DKA. This is attributable to a reduction in colloid osmotic pressure, which results in increased lung water content and decreased lung compliance. In the majority of patients, these changes do not produce symptoms and are not clinically significant, and the chest x-ray appearance remains normal. A small number of patients receiving treatment for DKA progress to adult respiratory distress syndrome (ARDS). Patients with DKA who have a widened alveolar-arterial oxygen gradient or with pulmonary rales on physical examination appear to be at higher risk for the development of ARDS.

Patients recovering from DKA commonly develop hyperchloremia and a transient non–anion gap metabolic acidosis. Indeed, by 4 hours of therapy, 46% of patients develop a non–anion gap acidosis, and by 8 hours of therapy, 91% demonstrate a hyperchloremic non–anion gap metabolic acidosis. Although the pathogenesis of hyperchloremic acidosis during the recovery phase of DKA is not well understood, postulated mechanisms include the loss of large quantities of ketoanions occurring during the development of DKA. Because ketoanions are metabolized with regeneration of bicarbonate, the prior loss of ketoacid anions in the urine hinders regeneration of bicarbonate during treatment. Other mechanisms that contribute to the development of hyperchloremic acidosis during treatment of DKA include the administration of intravenous fluids containing chloride that exceed the plasma chloride concentration, resulting in intracellular shifts of sodium during correction of DKA.

IMMEDIATE POST–HYPERGLYCEMIC CRISIS FOLLOW-UP CARE

The use of low-dose insulin protocols provides an ambient serum insulin concentration of approximately 100 microunits per mL, but owing to the short half-life of insulin (a few minutes), any sudden interruption of insulin treatment will immediately lower this ambient insulin level, resulting in relapse into DKA or HHNS. We therefore recommend that in such patients, while they are still on IV infusion and not eating, blood glucose be checked every 4 hours, with sliding-scale regular insulin given if the blood glucose concentration is greater than 150 mg per dL (with 5-unit increments given for every 50 mg per dL increase in blood glucose above 150, for up to 20 units of regular insulin given for a blood glucose of 300 mg per dL or higher). Once DKA or HHNS is resolved and the patient can take food by mouth, blood glucose should be monitored before meals and at bedtime, with sliding-scale regular insulin given during this time in addition to an intermediate-acting preparation, as discussed under Insulin Therapy.

HYPERURICEMIA AND GOUT

method of
ADEL G. FAM, M.D.
University of Toronto
Toronto, Ontario, Canada

CLINICAL FEATURES

Gout is characterized by chronic hyperuricemia, recurrent attacks of acute arthritis provoked by release of monosodium urate crystals into joint cavities, and development in some patients of gross urate deposit (tophi). It chiefly affects middle-aged and elderly men, and the incidence in women increases after menopause. Gout occurs in three overlapping phases: a long phase of asymptomatic hyperuricemia, a period of recurrent acute gouty attacks separated by symptom-free intervals (interval gout), followed in about 10% of patients by the development of chronic tophaceous gouty arthritis.

In the majority of patients, gout is a primary disorder. Less commonly, hyperuricemia and gout are secondary to purine enzyme defects, myeloproliferative or lymphoproliferative disorders, renal failure, drugs, or other conditions (Table 1). Measurement of 24-hour urinary uric acid excretion in patients with primary gout can often indicate whether the hyperuricemia is the result of overproduction or underexcretion of urate. In most patients (80 to 90%), hyperuricemia is due to a renal tubular defect in the excretion of uric acid (gouty underexcretors). These patients excrete either normal or reduced amounts of uric acid (< 600 mg or 3.6 mmol per day on a purine-restricted diet),

TABLE 1. **Classification of Hyperuricemia and Gout**

Primary
Uric acid overproduction: 10 to 20%
Uric acid renal underexcretion: 80 to 90%
Secondary
Uric acid overproduction:
Purine enzyme defects:
HGPRT deficiency
PRPP synthetase overactivity
Glucose-6-phosphatase deficiency
Increase nucleotide turnover
Myelo- and lymphoproliferative disorders
Hemolytic anemia
Psoriasis
Cytotoxic drugs (tumor lysis syndrome)
Excessive dietary purines and ethanol abuse
Uric acid renal underexcretion:
Renal failure
Acidosis, lactic: ethanol ketoacidosis: diabetic, dieting
Drugs: low-dose ASA, diuretics, cyclosporin A, pyrazinamide, ethambutol
Chronic lead nephropathy (saturnine gout)
Uncertain mechanisms:
Hypothyroidism
Hyperparathyroidism
Eclampsia

Abbreviations: HGPRT = hypoxanthine guanine phosphoribosyltransferase; PRPP = phosphoribosyl pyrophosphate.

and their urate clearance is lower than that in normal individuals (< 6 mL per minute, compared with 6 to 11 mL per minute). They have a limited capacity to eliminate a urate (purine) load, and excretion of normal amounts of uric acid is accomplished only at inappropriately high serum urate levels. In a minority of patients with primary gout (10 to 20%), hyperuricemia is caused by overproduction of uric acid. These patients also excrete excessive quantities of uric acid (> 800 to 1000 mg or > 4.5 to 5.5 mmol per day while on a regular diet) (gouty overproducer overexcretors). Their urate clearance is often normal and studies using isotope-labeled urate invariably demonstrate an increased rate of de novo purine (and uric acid) biosynthesis.

Acute Gouty Arthritis

Gouty attacks commonly affect the joints of the lower extremity, particularly the metatarsophalangeal (MTP) joint of the great toe (acute podagra). The intertarsal, ankle, knee, elbow, and wrist joints and olecranon bursae are next in order of frequency. The onset, which typically occurs at night, is rapid; and the acute arthritis often peaks within 24 hours, producing a painful, warm, red, tender, swollen joint, as well as diffuse erythema of the surrounding soft tissues, resembling cellulitis. In the early stages of gout, the attacks are few and far between, with the affected joints returning to normal between attacks. Late in the disease, the acute episodes become more frequent, longer lasting, with a tendency toward incomplete resolution and polyarticular involvement.

Chronic Tophaceous Gouty Arthritis

Before the introduction of effective urate-lowering drugs, approximately 20 to 40% of untreated patients developed chronic tophaceous gouty arthritis. Recent data suggest a much lower incidence (about 10%). However, every so often, one encounters individuals in whom failure to properly diagnose or treat has permitted full expression of the disease. The average time from the initial gouty attack to the occurrence of tophi is 11 years. Tophi are typically located in periarticular sites about the feet, fingers, and knees; in and around bursae (olecranon, prepatellar, and bunion); and in the subcutaneous tissues over the Achilles tendon and ear pinnae. Chronic gouty arthritis is characterized by persistent aching, stiffness, swelling, punched out erosions with overhanging margins, and joint deformity. Superimposed episodes of acute gouty inflammation are common. Medical disorders frequently associated with gout include obesity, hyperlipidemia, hypertension, and vascular disease.

DIAGNOSIS

A firm diagnosis of gout can be secured by demonstration with compensated polarized light microscopy of intracellular or extracellular needle-shaped negatively bi-refringent monosodium urate crystals in joint fluids, bursal effusions, or in aspirates from tophi. However, this may not be possible in all patients for a number of reasons: absence of a detectable joint effusion or visible tophi, an inaccessible joint, inexperience with either joint aspiration or evaluation of synovial fluid for crystals, or presence of a few urate crystals or crystals too small (< 1 μm) to be seen by light microscopy. Under these circumstances, the diagnosis of gout can be made on the basis of a typical clinical history in association with documented hyperuricemia. The diagnosis can sometimes be confirmed in these individuals by demonstrating urate crystals in fluid aspirates from previously affected but asymptomatic knee or first MTP joint.

Hyperuricemia, elevated serum urate greater than 7.0 mg/dL (450 μmol per liter) in men and greater than 6.0 mg/dL (360 μmol/L) in women, is the biochemical hallmark of gout. However, it is improper to equate the finding of hyperuricemia with gout; many individuals who have lifelong hyperuricemia do not develop gouty arthritis (asymptomatic hyperuricemia). Serum urate levels may be normal in some patients with gout, particularly during the early phases of gout, following alcoholic excesses or withdrawal of diuretic therapy, and during initial therapy with allopurinol or uricosuric drugs.

TREATMENT

Gouty arthritis nearly always occurs in the setting of chronic hyperuricemia. Management of a patient with gout, therefore, requires that two objectives be considered independently: immediate control of the acute gouty episode, and treatment of chronic hyperuricemia to prevent subsequent attacks and long-term complications, such as chronic tophaceous gouty arthritis, uric acid urolithiasis, and urate nephropathy.

Acute Gouty Arthritis

Standard therapy for acute gouty arthritis includes nonsalicylate nonsteroidal anti-inflammatory drugs (NSAIDs), colchicine, and corticosteroids (Table 2).

Nonsteroidal Anti-inflammatory Drugs

NSAIDs are preferred by most clinicians as the drugs of first choice in the treatment of acute gout. They are generally better tolerated and more predictable in their therapeutic effects than is oral colchicine. There is no clear advantage of any one preparation, but a large dose of indomethacin (Indocin), naproxen (Naprosyn), or diclofenac sodium (Voltaren) on the first 1 to 3 days, with a reduction thereafter,

TABLE 2. **Drugs in the Treatment of Acute Gouty Arthritis**

Nonsteroidal Anti-inflammatory Drugs	
Indomethacin (Indocin)	50 mg qid for 3–5 d
Naproxen (Naprosyn)	500 mg bid or tid for 3–5 d
Diclofenac sodium (Voltaren)	50 mg tid for 3–5 d
Tolmetin sodium (Tolectin)	600 mg tid for 3–5 d
Colchicine	
0.6 mg q 1–2 h until relief occurs, gastrointestinal toxicity or a maximum dose of 4–6 mg/d has been reached.	
Corticosteroids	
Monarticular or oligoarticular gouty attacks:	
IA methylprednisolone acetate (Depo-Medrol) 5–40 mg	
Polyarticular gouty attacks:	
IM triamcinolone acetonide (Kenalog) 60 mg q 1–4 d	
IM methylprednisolone acetate (Depo-Medrol) 40 mg q 1–4 d or IM ACTH (corticotropin) 40–80 IU q 6–24 h	
Ambulatory treatment of gouty attacks:	
Oral prednisone 20–40 mg first day, then taper in 4–8 d	

is generally effective. Whatever drug is used, it should be started as early as possible after the onset of an acute episode. It is important, therefore, to supply the patient with the appropriate NSAID (preferably kept in a convenient pocket, for gout often strikes when the patient is far from home) and instructions on how to self-treat acute flares at the first "twinge" of an attack.

Although adverse reactions (e.g., nausea, dyspepsia, diarrhea, headache, confusion) can occur, the duration of NSAID therapy is usually short, and serious toxicity leading to drug withdrawal (e.g., gastrointestinal [GI] bleeding) is rare (<10% of patients).

NSAIDs are potentially hazardous and are not recommended for the treatment of acute gouty events in aged patients and in those with co-morbid medical conditions such as congestive heart failure, renal impairment, peptic ulcer disease, GI bleeding, and hepatic insufficiency. Parenteral NSAIDs, such as intramuscular (IM) ketorolac (Toradol), offer no safety advantage.

Colchicine

Although colchicine has traditionally been used in the treatment of acute gouty arthritis, its use has steadily declined. Its drawbacks include (1) slow onset of action, (2) narrow benefit/toxicity ratio, with about 80% of patients experiencing GI toxicity (nausea, diarrhea, and abdominal pain) after oral administration, and (3) reduced therapeutic efficacy when administered 24 hours or longer after the onset of acute gouty inflammation (a frequent occurrence). It is administered orally in a dose of 0.6 mg every 1 to 2 hours until acute joint pain is relieved, the patient develops GI toxicity, or a maximum of 4 to 6 mg per day has been administered. Colchicine is efficacious in about two thirds of patients. It is primarily useful for those without renal or hepatic disease who are intolerant or hypersensitive to NSAIDs.

The role of intravenous (IV) colchicine in the treatment of acute gout has come under close scrutiny in light of growing concerns about its safety. A major drawback is the drug's potential for serious toxicity (bone marrow suppression, oliguric renal failure, hepatic necrosis, diarrhea, seizures, and death), particularly in elderly patients with renal and/or hepatic impairment. This controversy has led to the publication of a set of guidelines for the IV administration of colchicine. However, inappropriate use of the drug is relatively common, and many clinicians have advocated restriction or an outright ban on the use of IV colchicine.

Corticosteroids Including Corticotropin (ACTH)

Intra-articular (IA) corticosteroid therapy and both systemic corticosteroids and ACTH are indicated for the treatment of acute gouty episodes in patients with coexisting medical illnesses, contraindicating the use of NSAIDs (Table 3). Such treatment is also efficacious in the management of acute gout occurring during the postoperative period, for those with NSAID hypersensitivity, and for severe gouty attacks refractory to both NSAIDs and colchicine.

TABLE 3. **Indications for Corticosteroid Drugs in the Treatment of Acute Gouty Arthritis**

Co-morbid medical conditions:
Cardiac failure, hypertension
Renal insufficiency
Peptic ulcer, gastrointestinal bleeding
Hepatic insufficiency
Chronic alcoholism
Bleeding diathesis, anticoagulants
Advanced age
Postoperative state
NSAID hypersensitivity
Severe attacks refractory to both NSAIDs and colchicine

Abbreviation: NSAID = nonsteroidal anti-inflammatory drug.

IA corticosteroid injections, such as methylprednisolone acetate (Depo-Medrol) 5 to 40 mg IA, are particularly useful for the treatment of acute monoarticular and oligoarticular gouty episodes in these patients. However, such therapy is not practical for those with polyarticular gouty attacks. Concern about coexistent joint infection, concomitant anticoagulant therapy, and fear of needle injection may also preclude IA corticosteroid administration. In these clinical situations, IM triamcinolone acetonide (Kenalog), 60 mg, or IM methylprednisolone acetate, 40 mg repeated every 1 to 4 days as required, can be used to provide rapid control of acute attacks, thereby circumventing delayed absorption after oral administration. IV methylprednisolone sodium succinate (Solu-Medrol), 40 to 160 mg repeated every 1 to 4 days as required, is indicated for those receiving anticoagulant therapy.

Oral prednisone, 20 to 40 mg on the first day, followed by gradual tapering over 4 to 8 days, is particularly useful for the ambulatory treatment of acute gouty flares in outpatients with co-morbid conditions contraindicating the use of NSAIDs.

Although the efficacy and safety of IM ACTH* (corticotropin [Acthar]), 40 to 80 IU repeated every 6 to 24 hours as required, in the treatment of acute gout have been demonstrated in a number of studies, there is no convincing evidence that such therapy is superior to corticosteroids. Drawbacks of ACTH include dependence of therapeutic effects on sensitivity of the adrenal cortex (drug may be ineffective in subjects previously treated with corticosteroids); increased release of adrenal androgens and mineralocorticoids, which can lead to fluid overload; and a relatively short duration of action, with a greater potential for rebound attacks and treatment failures compared to IM corticosteroids.

Chronic Gouty Arthritis

Corrective measures including weight reduction for obesity, elimination of drugs causing hyperuricemia

*Not FDA approved for this indication.

(e.g., aspirin [ASA], diuretics), and restriction of alcohol intake and purine-rich foods, constitute sufficient therapy for many patients with infrequent gouty attacks and mild hyperuricemia. The frequency of gouty attacks can be reduced by prophylactic administration of colchicine, 0.6 mg once or twice daily. However, such therapy does not correct the hyperuricemia, does not prevent silent progression of tophaceous lesions, and can lead to a number of toxic reactions including neuromyopathy, myelotoxicity, alopecia, and malabsorption syndrome.

The ultimate treatment of established gout requires long-term control of hyperuricemia. Two types of urate-lowering drugs are available: allopurinol, a xanthine oxidase inhibitor that decreases uric acid synthesis, and uricosuric agents, which act by competitive inhibition of postsecretory renal tubular reabsorption of urate, thus increasing urate excretion and lowering serum urate.

Not every patient with gout requires treatment with urate-lowering drugs (Table 4). The administration of a drug to normalize serum urate is usually a lifelong commitment to regular daily therapy. Frequent measurement of serum urate concentrations is important in monitoring the patient's compliance and the effectiveness of urate-lowering treatment. To prevent further gouty attacks and ensure resorption of tophaceous deposits, serum urate should be reduced and sustained to less than 4–6 mg per dL or less than 250 to 350 μmol per liter, well below the concentration at which urate saturates the extracellular fluid (approximately 6.8 mg per dL or 404 μmol per liter at 37°C).

Initiation or interruption of urate-lowering therapy during an acute attack of gout is not recommended; a major change in serum urate concentration, induced by starting or stopping allopurinol or a uricosuric drug, may prolong an attack already in progress.

TABLE 4. **Urate-Lowering Drugs**

Indications for Allopurinol Therapy
Dose: Allopurinol (Zyloprim) 100–600 mg/d (single dose)
Frequent gouty attacks despite corrective measures (>4 attacks/y)
Major overproduction of uric acid with hyperuricosuria including HGPRTase deficiency and PRPP synthetase overactivity
Chronic tophaceous gouty arthritis
Gout complicated by urate nephropathy, uric acid nephrolithiasis, or renal insufficiency
Hyperuricemia secondary to lymphoma, leukemia, and myeloproliferative disorders treated with cytotoxics or radiotherapy (to prevent tumor lysis syndrome)
Failure of uricosuric drugs
Recurrent calcium oxalate urinary calculi associated with hyperuricosuria
Indications for Uricosuric Drugs
Dose: probenecid (Benemid): 1–3 gm/d (divided doses) sulfinpyrazone (Anturane): 100–800 mg/d (divided doses)
Patients under 60 years of age with primary gout, frequent gouty attacks, normal renal function, and urinary uric acid excretion who have no history of urinary calculi
Allergy or intolerance to allopurinol
Combined allopurinol-uricosuric treatment for patients with massive tophaceous deposits

Abbreviations: HGPRTase = hypoxanthine guanine phosphoribosyltransferase; PRPP = phosphoribosyl pyrophosphate.

The sharp reduction in serum urate level that takes place early in the course of urate-lowering treatment may be associated with flares of gout. These flares may be mistaken for a poor response to treatment. Some physicians advocate prophylactic colchicine, 0.6 mg once or twice daily during the first 1 to 12 months of initiating antihyperuricemic therapy. However, this practice cannot be routinely recommended, given the potential toxicity of prolonged use of colchicine (neuromyopathy, myelotoxicity, alopecia, malabsorption syndrome) and the fact that only a minority (about 10 to 25%) of patients develop flares of gouty arthritis after initiation of allopurinol or uricosuric treatment. Instead, many clinicians advocate the temporary use of a supplemental NSAID to control these attacks. Colchicine prophylaxis is of special value, however, in those patients who continue to experience frequent gouty flares precipitated by urate-lowering therapy.

Allopurinol

Allopurinol (Zyloprim) is the urate-lowering drug of choice. As a xanthine oxidase inhibitor, it interferes with the conversion of hypoxanthine to xanthine and of xanthine to uric acid, leading to a reduction of serum and urinary urate concentrations, and a concomitant increase in serum and urinary hypoxanthine and xanthine concentrations. Allopurinol is rapidly oxidized in the body to its principal metabolite oxipurinol, which is also a potent xanthine oxidase inhibitor. The plasma half-life of allopurinol is 1 to 3 hours, whereas that of oxipurinol is 14 to 26 hours. Thus, allopurinol can be administered as a single daily dose. Because oxipurinol is excreted solely through the kidneys, reduction of allopurinol dose is indicated in elderly patients and in those with renal impairment. The starting dose of allopurinol is 50 to 300 mg per day (formulations: 100 mg, 200 mg, and 300 mg tablets), and the total daily dose ranges between 100 mg and 600 mg, with most patients requiring 300 mg per day. Reduction of serum urate concentration is noted within 2 days of starting therapy. The level usually falls to normal within 7 to 14 days, although it may take much longer in patients with extensive tophaceous deposits. Gouty attacks often cease within 3 to 6 months of continuous therapy, but dissolution of the tophi may take 6 to 24 months. Discontinuation of allopurinol is followed by a rapid rise of serum urate concentration to pretreatment levels, although recurrence of acute gouty attacks may not occur for long periods. Specific indications for the use of allopurinol are outlined in Table 4.

Allopurinol is well tolerated by the majority of patients, and adverse reactions are rare (about 3.5%). Precipitation of acute gouty arthritis and allergic dermatitis are the most frequent adverse reactions. Cautious reintroduction of allopurinol after cutaneous reactions may be possible using a schedule of gradually increasing doses. An initial oral dose of 50 μg allopurinol daily is progressively increased every 3 to 7 days to 100 μg, 200 μg, 500 μg, 1 mg, 5 mg, 10 mg, 25 mg and finally to a target dose of 50 to 100 mg daily. Further dose adjustments are based on the patient's serum urate and creatinine levels. This desensitization regimen is particularly useful in patients with impaired renal function that prohibit the use of uricosuric drugs.

Allopurinol hypersensitivity syndrome is a rare, life-threatening toxic reaction characterized by fever, severe dermatitis (usually toxic epidermal necrolysis), hepatitis, renal failure, eosinophilia, and leukocytosis. It occurs most frequently in elderly patients with renal impairment in whom the dose of allopurinol has not been reduced appropriately.

Uricosuric Drugs

Uricosuric drugs increase the renal excretion of urate and thereby reduce serum concentration. The intense initial uricosuria can result in the deposition of uric acid crystals in renal tubules and formation of urinary calculi, which in turn can cause renal colic or deterioration of renal function. To minimize this risk and to prevent the precipitation of acute gouty attacks associated with rapid decline in serum urate concentration, uricosuric drugs are started at low doses and gradually increased over 2 to 4 weeks. The risk of uric acid stones can be further reduced by maintenance of a high urine volume (> 2 liters per day) and/or alkalization of urine with sodium bicarbonate, 1 gram four times daily, particularly during the first 4 to 6 weeks of therapy when the uricosuria is greatest. After serum urate normalizes, the intense uricosuria subsides, and renal urate excretion approaches pretreatment levels.

Two uricosuric drugs are used to manage chronic gout. Probenecid (Benemid), 250 mg twice daily, is given for 1 to 2 weeks, followed by 500 mg twice daily, increasing the dose thereafter to 1000 mg two or three times daily if required. Sulfinpyrazone (Anturane), 50 to 100 mg, is administered twice daily for 1 to 2 weeks, followed by 100 to 200 mg twice daily, increasing to 400 mg twice daily if needed. Side effects of each drug include nausea, abdominal pain, and allergic rash.

In the absence of clear-cut indications for treatment with allopurinol (see Table 4), uricosuric drugs can be used in patients younger than 60 years old with primary gout, frequent gouty attacks, normal renal function and 24-hour urinary uric values, and no gross tophi or a history of urinary calculi. Other specific indications for uricosurics include patients who are allergic or intolerant to allopurinol, and those with massive tophaceous deposits who may require treatment with both allopurinol to block uric acid synthesis and a uricosuric to increase uric acid excretion (Table 4).

About 75% of patients respond to uricosuric drugs with normalization of serum urate, control of gouty attacks, and resorption of tophaceous deposits. Most failures, in the remaining 25% of patients, are due to intolerable side effects (particularly GI upset), concomitant intake of salicylates (which nullify the uricosuric action), or the presence of renal impairment; uricosurics are ineffective at a creatinine clearance of less than 50 to 60 mL per minute.

Patients with Massive Tophaceous Deposits

Patients with massive tophaceous deposits who do not respond to either allopurinol or a uricosuric drug alone may benefit from a combination of these drugs. Serum urate concentrations should be kept consistently below 5 mg per dL (300 μmol per liter) to ensure complete resolution of the tophaceous deposits. Surgical excision of bulky tophi may be required, and restriction of both purine-rich foods (e.g., meats, liver, kidney, peas, beans) and alcoholic beverages is helpful.

Patients with Gout and Renal Impairment

Uricosuric drugs are generally ineffective in patients with renal insufficiency. Allopurinol therapy in these individuals is associated with an increased incidence of both cutaneous and severe hypersensitivity reactions. To minimize this risk, the drug is introduced in reduced doses, starting at 50 mg on alternate days and gradually increasing to a maximal daily dose based on the patient's creatinine clearance: 200 mg daily for clearance of 60 mL per minute, 100 mg daily for clearance of 20 mL per minute, and 50 to 100 mg on alternate days for clearance of 10 mL per minute or less.

Gout in the Elderly

Co-morbid medical illnesses, including hypertension, cardiac failure, and renal impairment, are common in elderly patients with gout. NSAIDs are potentially hazardous and are not recommended for the control of acute gouty episodes in these patients. Oral colchicine is also poorly tolerated by the elderly and is best avoided. Oral, IM, IV, or IA corticosteroids are increasingly being used for treating acute gouty flares in aged patients with multiple medical conditions, contraindicating NSAID therapy.

Urate-lowering therapy should be approached with caution in the elderly. Because of concomitant renal impairment, uricosuric drugs are unlikely to be efficacious and are best avoided. Allopurinol therapy is associated with an increased incidence of both cutaneous and severe hypersensitivity reactions. To minimize this risk, the doses of allopurinol must be kept low. A starting dose of 50 to 100 mg on alternate days, to a maximum daily dose of 100 to 300 mg, is recommended.

Gout in the Transplant Recipient

Both hyperuricemia and severe tophaceous gouty arthritis occur with increased frequency in cyclosporine-treated kidney, heart, or lung/heart allograft transplant recipients. Cyclosporine induces hyperuricemia by both inhibiting renal tubular urate secretion and enhancing postsecretory tubular urate reabsorption. Concurrent diuretic therapy and coexistent renal insufficiency are important contributing factors.

Both NSAIDs and colchicine are hazardous and are not recommended for the treatment of acute gouty arthritis in these patients. Corticosteroids, administered intra-articularly or systematically, are the preferred drugs. Resistance to ACTH from adrenal suppression by corticosteroids is common.

Uricosuric drugs are generally ineffective in cyclosporine-treated transplant recipients with renal impairment. Allopurinol is the preferred urate-lowering drug. Its toxicity can be minimized by adjusting the initial dose according to the creatinine clearance.

Because azathioprine* (Imuran) is inactivated by xanthine oxidase, inhibition of this enzyme by allopurinol markedly enhances azathioprine toxicity. In transplant patients receiving both azathioprine and allopurinol, reduction of the initial doses of both drugs by about two thirds is recommended.

Asymptomatic Hyperuricemia

Most individuals with asymptomatic hyperuricemia do not develop clinical gout, and there is no evidence that hyperuricemia per se adversely affects renal function. For these reasons, and because of concerns about cost and potential hazards of unnecessary drug therapy, there seems to be no rationale for treating these individuals with allopurinol. Exceptions include acute urate overproduction owing to tumor lysis syndrome, and patients with severe hyperuricemia (> 12 mg per dL or 700 μmol per liter) and hyperuricosuria who are at an increased risk of developing both gout and nephrolithiasis. For most other patients, corrective measures including weight reduction, restriction of alcoholic beverages and purine-rich foods, and elimination of drugs such as aspirin and thiazides, constitute sufficient treatment.

*Not FDA approved for this indication.

HYPERLIPOPROTEINEMIAS

method of
MARGO A. DENKE, M.D.
University of Texas Southwestern Medical Center at Dallas
Dallas, Texas

Lipoproteins are spherical particles whose core of nonpolar fat is surrounded by a water-soluble protein/phospholipid coat. Lipoproteins can be characterized by size, density, type of lipid carried, and type of apoproteins on the coat. Using size and density, four major classes have been described: chylomicrons, very-low-density lipoprotein (VLDL), low-density lipoprotein (LDL), and high-density lipoprotein (HDL). All lipoprotein particles contain both triglycerides and cholesterol. Two classes of lipoproteins, chylomicrons and VLDL, mainly carry triglyceride; the other two, LDL and HDL, mainly carry cholesterol. The apoproteins on the surface of lipoproteins serve as ligands for receptors and as cofactors for many enzymes in lipid metabolism.

METABOLISM OF LIPOPROTEINS

Chylomicrons are synthesized in the intestine, from which they transport newly ingested dietary cholesterol and triglycerides to the liver and other sites. The half-life of a chylomicron is 20 to 30 minutes. Chylomicrons are recognized by an enzyme on the capillary wall, lipoprotein lipase, which permits release of triglycerides to peripheral tissues. Delivery of core triglycerides leads to the formation of a smaller remnant particle, which is cleared from circulation by specific hepatic receptors.

In the fasting state, peripheral tissues receive triglycerides from the other major triglyceride-carrying lipoprotein, VLDL. VLDLs are synthesized in the liver, have a half-life of 4 to 6 hours, and deliver triglycerides to peripheral tissue via the same mechanism as for chylomicrons. Both VLDLs and chylomicrons are thought to be atherogenic. Like chylomicrons, VLDLs participate in cholesterol transfer reactions and become more cholesterol-enriched the longer they stay in circulation. Unlike chylomicrons, VLDL remnants have two possible fates: they can be taken up directly by the liver via specific cellular receptors, or they can become further cholesterol-enriched and triglyceride-poor, forming LDLs.

LDL is the major cholesterol-carrying lipoprotein, and LDL cholesterol typically accounts for 65 to 70% of the total serum cholesterol. This lipoprotein has a half-life of 2 to 3 days. LDL delivers cholesterol to tissues by specific cellular receptors. There is conclusive evidence that LDL is atherogenic, and the means by which LDL serves as a source for the cholesterol found in arterial plaques is now clear: If LDL becomes oxidized, its apoprotein is no longer recognized by LDL receptors but instead is recognized by scavenger receptors found on macrophages. Arterial wall macrophages that ingest oxidized LDL become "foam cells," an early step in the atherogenic process. The use of antioxidants to prevent LDL modification and their subsequent deposition into arterial wall plaques is an active area of research.

HDL is a complex lipoprotein whose metabolism is less well understood. HDL is derived from the liver and intestine and has a half-life of 5 to 6 days. HDL cholesterol typically accounts for 20 to 25% of the total serum cholesterol. HDL cholesterol levels are inversely associated with coronary disease. Why HDL is protective has not been fully elucidated. HDL may serve as an antioxidant, may promote transfer of cholesterol from cells to the liver, and may have endothelial actions that promote antiatherogenesis.

DIAGNOSIS OF AND MANAGEMENT CONSIDERATIONS IN HYPERLIPOPROTEINEMIAS

Fredrickson and Lees first classified hyperlipidemias in the 1960s. Since lipoproteins were not easily assayed, their classification relied on interpretation of an agarose gel electrophoresis of the patient's serum. According to their size and electrical charge, lipoproteins migrate down the gel, forming one of five characteristic patterns. Types I and V were associated with pancreatitis, and types II, III, IV, and V were associated with coronary heart disease.

Some laboratories still offer a lipoprotein electrophoresis, but it is preferable to classify a patient's lipoprotein disorder by directly quantitating lipoproteins. Although a true measurement of lipoprotein cholesterol and triglyceride can be done only in research laboratories, commercial laboratories can reliably estimate lipoprotein cholesterol by measuring total cholesterol and total triglycerides and by precipitating out apoprotein B–containing lipoprotein (VLDL and LDL) and measuring the cholesterol remaining in solution (HDL). Measurements of the common apoproteins—apoprotein B, found in VLDL and LDL, and apoprotein A-I, found in HDL—add little information beyond that of lipoprotein cholesterol and should not be routinely performed.

Current treatment guidelines recommend measurement of total and HDL cholesterol levels in all adults at least once every 5 years. The long half-life of LDL and HDL, together with recognition of the small contribution of dietary cholesterol to total cholesterol level, makes fasting unnecessary for this determination. If either total or HDL cholesterol is abnormal, or if the patient is at high risk for disease, the next step is to order a fasting lipid profile, for which, in addition to total and HDL cholesterol levels, the laboratory will quantitate triglycerides.

Before measurement of a lipoprotein profile, the patient should be instructed to fast for 10 to 12 hours, with nothing to eat or drink except water, black coffee, or plain tea. In the majority of cases, fasting will allow all chylomicron particles to be cleared, so that the total triglyceride level becomes a surrogate for VLDL triglyceride. Taking advantage of the observation that normal VLDL carries a 1:5 ratio of cholesterol to triglyceride, the cholesterol content of VLDL can be estimated, and the cholesterol content of LDL can be calculated by subtracting this VLDL cholesterol estimate plus the HDL cholesterol measurement from the total cholesterol. A new technique has been developed to directly measure LDL cholesterol. The measurement appears accurate and does not necessitate fasting, but accurate categorization of the lipid disorder still requires determination of a fasting triglyceride level. Direct measurement of LDL cholesterol level can be useful in confirming the presence of type III hyperlipidemia.

Most commercial laboratories perform reliable determinations for total cholesterol, with less than a 3% assay variation. Greater assay variations can be seen with triglycerides and HDL, so that laboratory variation can complicate the evaluation of patients who have had determinations from several places. Furthermore, lipid levels can be falsely elevated from hemoconcentration if a patient stands more than 20 minutes before phlebotomy, if the tourniquet is kept in place for more than 2 minutes, and if vigorous exercise is performed just prior to phlebotomy. Disease states can also alter lipids: recent surgery, infection, and myocardial infarction are all associated with transient reductions in serum cholesterol levels and increases in triglyceride levels that may last several months. Pregnancy raises serum cholesterol levels. Several conditions can cause secondary hyperlipidemias, and the most common are listed in Table 1.

TABLE 1. **Secondary Causes of Dyslipidemias**

Condition	Lipoprotein Disorder	Treatment Nuances
Diet		
>3% calories from alcohol	↑ ↑ TG, ↑ ↑ HDL rarely ↑ Chol	Effect more pronounced in patients with triglyceride disorders
Disease		
Obesity	↑ TG, ↑ VLDL, ↓ HDL	30–50 lb of excess weight may lower HDL levels by 5–10 mg/dL
Diabetes mellitus	↑ ↑ ↑ TG, ↑ Chol ↑ ↑ VLDL ↓ HDL in type II	Improved glucose control will improve dyslipidemia; in type II diabetes, HDL may remain low secondary to obesity
Hypothyroidism	↑ Chol, ↑ LDL, ↑ HDL ± ↑ TG	Subclinical hypothyroidism can raise LDL by 5–20 mg/dL
Cholestasis	↑ ↑ Chol in the form of lipoprotein X, a disk-shaped phospholipid particle	Improves when cholestasis is relieved or when liver disease progresses; may respond to diet and bile acid resins
Nephrotic syndrome	↑ ↑ Chol, ↑ TG ± HDL	Steroid treatment of renal disease may exacerbate dyslipidemia; reductase inhibitors may improve lipids
Chronic renal failure	↑ ↑ TG, ↑ ↑ VLDL, ± ↓ HDL	Renal transplant may improve dyslipidemia; reductase inhibitors may be of benefit
Drug Therapy		
Beta blockers	↑ VLDL, ↓ HDL	Labetolol and those with intrinsic sympathomimetic activity have little lipid effect
Thiazide diuretics	↑ LDL, ↑ VLDL	Increases may be greater at higher doses
Oral contraceptives	May increase or decrease LDL and HDL depending on the progestogen used and dose of estrogen	Low-dose oral contraceptives have little effect
Hormone replacement therapy	↓ LDL ± ↑ HDL depending on the type and dose of estrogen/progestogen	May be an effective therapy for postmenopausal hypercholesterolemia
Corticosteroids, cyclosporine	↑ Chol, ↑ TG	Dose-dependent, but increases still detectable at small doses
Dilantin, griseofulvin	↑ HDL	Drugs increasing cytochrome P-450 raise HDL, but their toxicity prevents use as HDL-raising agents

Abbreviations: Chol = cholesterol; HDL = high-density lipoprotein; LDL = low-density lipoprotein; TG = triglyceride; VLDL = very-low-density lipoprotein.

TABLE 2. **Patterns of Dyslipidemia**

Dyslipidemia	Total Cholesterol	LDL	HDL	TG
Isolated hypercholesterolemia	>200 mg/dL	>160 mg/dL	Normal or low	<200 mg/dL
Isolated borderline to high hypertriglyceridemia	<200 mg/dL	Variable	Normal or low	200–400 mg/dL
Mixed dyslipidemia	200–400 mg/dL	Variable	Normal or low	200–400 mg/dL
Moderate or severe hypertriglyceridemia	Typically >240 mg/dL	Variable	Typically low	400–800 mg/dL = moderate >800 mg/dL = severe
Isolated low HDL	<200 mg/dL	Variable	<35 mg/dL	<200 mg/dL

Abbreviations: HDL = high-density lipoprotein; LDL = low-density lipoprotein; TG = triglyceride.

Once these sources of variation are eliminated, the clinician must still contend with variation due to day-to-day fluctuations in lipids. Although in some patients, little day-to-day variation is observed, in others, total and LDL cholesterol levels may vary by 10 to 40 mg per dL per day; HDL cholesterol levels, by 4 to 8 mg per dL per day; total triglyceride levels, by 50 to 150 mg per dL per day. To avoid errors in classification, the mean of several measurements should be used to diagnose a lipid disorder, and trends in lipid levels should be followed to assess the success of intervention.

Common patterns of dyslipidemia seen in a lipoprotein profile are listed in Table 2. The clinician should establish whether there is a family history of lipid disorders. Isolated hypercholesterolemia may be due to a genetic disorder such as familial hypercholesterolemia or polygenic hypercholesterolemia. Both genetic forms of isolated hypercholesterolemia are associated with premature coronary disease, and both require treatment. Isolated hypertriglyceridemia may be genetic or may be secondary to obesity or insulin resistance. Not all kindreds with familial hypertriglyceridemia have premature coronary disease; taking a family history will help establish the need for therapy. Less is known about the benefits of treating isolated hypertriglyceridemia because no clinical trials have been performed. Most lipid experts would consider triglyceride-lowering therapy (weight loss, alcohol restriction, statins, niacin or fibric acids) in patients with established disease and in patients with multiple risk factors.

Moderate or severe hypertriglyceridemia often is associated with glucose intolerance and hypothyroidism, and evaluation should include determinations of hemoglobin A_{1C} and thyroid-stimulating hormone. Mixed dyslipidemia may be an indicator of a modifiable condition such as poorly controlled diabetes or obesity or of familial combined hyperlipidemia or familial dysbetalipoproteinemia. Familial combined hyperlipidemia is an autosomal dominant disorder in which some family members have isolated hypertriglyceridemia, some have isolated hypercholesterolemia, and some have mixed dyslipidemia. Familial combined hyperlipidemia is associated with premature coronary disease and often requires drug therapy with two or more drugs such as statins and bile acid sequestrants, niacin and statins, niacin and fibric acids, or fibric acid and statins. Familial dysbetalipoproteinemia, also known as type III hyperlipoproteinemia, is an autosomal recessive disorder associated with palmar and tuberous xanthomas. Occasionally, dysbetalipoproteinemia can be the presenting manifestation of hypothyroidism, and thyroid hormone replacement therapy will be sufficient treatment for this disorder. Familial dysbetalipoproteinemia is associated with premature coronary disease. Effective treatment includes weight loss, a very-low-fat diet, and administration of niacin, statins, or occasionally fibric acids.

Isolated low HDL levels can be seen with excess body weight, physical inactivity, and genetic disorders. As with familial hypertriglyceridemia, some kindreds with low HDL do not have premature coronary disease. All lipid-lowering drugs have some effects on HDL, with niacin having the greatest effect. Whether patients with isolated

TABLE 3. **LDL Levels Indicating Need for Treatment of Hypercholesterolemia**

CHD Risk Status	LDL Criteria: *Diet Therapy*	LDL Criteria: *Drug Therapy*	LDL Target Level
Secondary Prevention			
Presence of CHD or other atherosclerotic disease	>100 mg/dL	≥130 mg/dL	≤100 mg/dL
Primary Prevention			
No CHD but two or more risk factors	≥130 mg/dL	≥160 mg/dL	≤130 mg/dL
No CHD and less than two other risk factors	≥160 mg/dL	≥190 mg/dL	≤160 mg/dL
No CHD, less than two other risk factors, and age less than 35 years for men or premenopausal for women	≥160 mg/dL	≥220 mg/dL	≤190 mg/dL
In children, familial dyslipidemias (notably familial hypercholesterolemia)	≥110 mg/dL	In children more than 10 years of age and LDL level of ≥190 mg/dL; consider if LDL level is ≥160 mg/dL in a child with family history of premature CHD or with two or more risk factors; bile acid sequestrants are the only drugs recommended for use in children	≤130 mg/dL

Abbreviations: CHD = coronary heart disease; LDL = low-density lipoprotein.

TABLE 4. **National Cholesterol Education Program Adult Treatment Panel Risk Factors for Coronary Disease Other Than LDL Cholesterol**

Positive Risk Factors

- Age:
  Male: ≥45 years
  Female: ≥55 years or premature menopause without estrogen replacement therapy
- Family history of premature CHD (definite myocardial infarction or sudden death before 55 years of age in father or other male first-degree relative, or before 65 years of age in mother or other female first-degree relative)
- Current cigarette smoking
- Hypertension (≥140/90 mm Hg, or on antihypertensive medication)
- Low HDL cholesterol (<35 mg/dL)
- Diabetes mellitus

Negative Risk Factor (if present, subtract one from above total)

- High HDL cholesterol (≥60 mg/dL)

Abbreviations: CHD = coronary heart disease; HDL = high-density lipoprotein; LDL = low-density lipoprotein.

low HDL will benefit from drug therapy is uncertain. The National Cholesterol Education Program (NCEP) Adult Treatment Panel has suggested that isolated low HDL levels be treated using hygienic measures such as weight loss and increases in physical activity.

The NCEP has identified LDL cholesterol levels as the target for therapy of dyslipidemias. Criteria for initiation of dietary therapy, drug therapy, and goals of therapy are detailed in Table 3. Patients with established atherosclerotic disease have a five- to sevenfold risk above that of the general population for a coronary event and accordingly have lower thresholds for the initiation of therapy. Some clinicians disagree with the guidelines and think that lipid-lowering drug therapy should be initiated in all patients with established disease. However, results from a large placebo-controlled secondary prevention trial suggests that patients whose initial LDL level was less than 124 mg per dL received little benefit from lipid-lowering therapy.

For patients without established disease, the presence and number of other cardiovascular risk factors (Table 4) define how aggressively lipid-lowering therapy should be pursued. Since children have lower cholesterol levels than adults, treatment guideline levels are appropriately reduced. In young adults with elevated LDL and no other risk factors, delay in the initiation of drug therapy is advised, because the immediate risk for disease is remote.

TREATMENT FOR DYSLIPIDEMIA

Diet and Lifestyle Changes

Diet and lifestyle modifications are fundamental treatments for all patients with dyslipidemia. Table 5 outlines each component of this approach with the expected effects on lipoproteins. A registered dietitian can be of invaluable help for patients and their families. Cholesterol-lowering diets have been classified as step I or step II diets. The step I diet, in which saturated fat is restricted to less than 10% of calories and dietary cholesterol to less than 300 mg per day, is appropriate for the population as a whole and as initial therapy for hypercholesterolemia. On average, a decrease in cholesterol levels by 3 to 10% can be expected. If the step I diet is ineffective at achieving goal or target levels, or if the patient has

TABLE 5. **Dietary and Lifestyle Modifications with Expected Effects on Lipoprotein Levels**

Lifestyle Factor	Treatment Goal	Expected Effect
Weight loss	If ideal body weight not attainable, weight loss of 5–10 lb	Weight loss of 5–30 lb can raise HDL 8–12 mg/dL and lower TG 80–200 mg/dL
Physical activity	Increase in physical activity, with athletic fitness as ultimate goal	2 h/wk of aerobic exercise can raise HDL 5–7 mg/dL and lower TG 80–200 mg/dL; regular exercise is associated with better long-term success on weight reduction diets
Restriction of dietary fat	<30% of calories	Very-low-fat diets (<25% of calories from fat) lower HDL 2–10 mg/dL and may also raise TG 40–100 mg/dL; by reducing input of chylomicrons, very-low-fat diets are appropriate treatment for patients with TG >2000 mg/dL
Restriction of saturated fat	<10% of calories; for those with high cholesterol, <7% is recommended	Saturated fat is the most potent dietary factor that raises serum cholesterol levels; a 3% reduction in calories from saturated fat will reduce LDL 6–40 mg/dL; saturated fat sources: fatty meats, whole milk dairy products, baked goods; lean beef is no more cholesterol-raising than chicken or fish
Restriction of dietary cholesterol	<300 mg/d; for those with high cholesterol, <200 mg/d is recommended	25 mg of dietary cholesterol has the cholesterol-raising potential of 1 gm of saturated fat
Alcohol	Current guidelines do not specifically recommend alcohol, but if alcohol is consumed, moderation is recommended	Alcohol, in a dose-dependent fashion, raises HDL cholesterol but also raises TG; 24 oz/d of wine can raise HDL 8–12 mg/dL, with nearly undetectable changes with consumption of 4 oz/d
Omega-3 fatty acids	Consider supplements as a treatment option for hypertriglyceridemia	6–12 gm/d of fish oil can lower TG 600–1200 mg/dL
Supplements including fiber, garlic, calcium, herbs	Current guidelines do not specifically recommend supplements	Most supplements have minimal if any effect on serum lipids; patients would be derive more benefit purchasing nutrient- and fiber-dense fresh produce

Abbreviations: HDL = high-density lipoprotein; LDL = low-density lipoprotein; TG = triglyceride.

TABLE 6. **Pharmacologic Treatment of Dyslipidemia**

Drug	Expected LDL Effect	Expected Effects on TG/HDL	Possible Combinations	Potential Contraindications
Bile acid sequestrants Cholestyramine (Questran) Colestipol (Colestid)	8–10 gm/d: decrease of 10–40 mg/dL	May increase TG 50 mg/dL; usually has 2–3 mg/dL HDL-raising effect	Can be used with any lipid-lowering regimen to augment LDL reduction	If baseline TG > 300 mg/dL, sequestrants will raise TG even further
Nicotinic acid	2.5–3.0 gm/d: decrease of 20–60 mg/dL	Lowers TG 200–500 mg/dL; raises HDL 5–10 mg/dL	Can be used with fibric acids for TG control; combinations with statins increase risk for myositis	May unmask glucose intolerance; may precipitate gout and raise uric acid levels
Statins Lovastatin (Mevacor) Pravastatin (Pravachol)	20 mg/d: decrease of 40–60 mg/dL	Statins lower TG 25–100 mg/dL, increase HDL 5–6 mg/dL	Statins can be used with any other lipid-lowering agent	Patients whose baseline values on liver function tests are >3 times normal may require limitation in use of statins
Simvastatin (Zocor)	10 mg/d: decrease of 40–60 mg/dL			Combinations with niacin or fibric acids increase risk for myositis; liver enzyme abnormalities more likely when combined with niacin
Fluvastatin (Lescol)	20 mg/d: decrease of 30–40 mg/dL			
Atorvastatin (Lipitor)	10 mg/d: decrease of 40–80 mg/dL			
Cerivastatin (Baycol)	0.3 mg/d: decrease of 30–40 mg/dL			
Fibric acids Gemfibrozil (Lopid) Clofibrate (Atromid-S)	1200 mg/d gemfibrozil 2 gm/d clofibrate: decrease or increase of 5–10 mg/dL	Fibric acids lower TG 100–800 mg/dL; raise HDL 2–10 mg/dL	Can be used with niacin to augment TG lowering	Renal insufficiency delays clearance and dose should be reduced
Estrogens	0.625 mg/d of conjugated estrogen (Premarin) or 2 mg/d of estradiol (Estrace): decrease of 20–30 mg/dL	Raise TG 50–100 mg/dL; increases far greater at higher doses	Can be used with any other lipid-lowering agent	If baseline TG > 300, some patients may experience 100–600 mg/dL further increases
Fish oil	May increase	6–12 gm/d lowers TG 600–2000 mg/dL; may raise HDL		May worsen glucose intolerance

Abbreviations: HDL = high-density lipoprotein; LDL = low-density lipoprotein; TG = triglyceride.

established disease, a step II diet with less than 7% of calories from saturated fat and less than 200 mg of dietary cholesterol is recommended; an additional 3 to 6% decrease may be achieved. Lifestyle changes such as regular physical activity and maintenance of ideal body weight are important aspects of therapy. Besides health clubs, home exercise equipment, and exercise training programs, clinicians should encourage patients to integrate physical activity into their daily routine such as walking the dog, taking the stairs, parking farther from the store and so on.

Drug Therapy

Table 6 presents the current lipid-lowering agents available and their expected effects on lipoprotein levels.

The cholesterol lowering achieved by diet should be continued even in patients who require drug therapy, as the effects of dietary therapy potentiate the benefits of drug therapy. Educating patients about compliance with diet and drug therapy as well as the need for lifelong therapy will maximize attainment of treatment goals. Once a drug is initiated, if the goal level is not reached, doubling the dose does not double the effect. For example, whereas a 20-mg dose per day of lovastatin lowers LDL 24%, a 40-mg dose lowers LDL only an additional 6%. An alternative to doubling the dose is to add another agent. For example, adding two scoops of bile acid sequestrants to the daily statin dose can achieve an additional 11% lowering.

Regarding risks of drug therapy, fibric acids and statins both rarely cause myositis. The risk for myositis is increased when the combination of fibric acids and statins is used. Monitoring creatine kinase (CK) levels during therapy is not a cost-effective way of screening for myositis, since transient increases in CK are common and appear unrelated to therapy. Niacin and statins can increase serum transaminase levels, which return to normal when the drug is discontinued. Niacin can cause hyperglycemia and hyperuricemia. Fibric acids increase the risk of cholelithiasis. Estrogens increase the rate of endometrial hyperplasia, and in women who have not undergone a hysterectomy, estrogens must be combined with a progestogen to mitigate this risk.

Regarding symptomatic side effects, statins are fairly well tolerated. Bile acid sequestrants are associated with gastrointestinal side effects of bloating and constipation, which most patients tolerate if the dose is 2 scoops or less per day. Niacin can cause flushing and heartburn; aspirin taken one half-hour before the niacin dose can eliminate flushing, and both flushing and heartburn symptoms diminish when niacin is given with meals.

Regarding benefits of drug therapy, placebo-controlled, randomized trials using bile acid resins, statins, and fibric acids have shown that LDL lowering reduces coronary event rates in patients with hypercholesterolemia. Prospective and case-control observational studies find estrogen therapy to be associated with lower coronary event rates. Niacin, bile acid sequestrants, and statins all have been shown to reduce coronary event rates in trials in patients with established disease.

OBESITY

method of
CHRISTOPHER D. STILL, D.O., M.Sc.
Penn State Geisinger Health Care System
Danville, Pennsylvania

and

GORDON L. JENSEN, M.D., Ph.D.
Vanderbilt University Medical Center
Nashville, Tennessee

Obesity is a chronic disease that affects millions of individuals worldwide. In the United States at least one in three adults is obese. According to the latest National Health and Nutrition Examination Survey (NHANES), the prevalence of obesity in the United States has increased from approximately 25 to 33% over the single decade ending in 1991, and obesity now affects nearly 26 million men and 32 million women. Unfortunately obesity does not spare children or adolescents. NHANES III data indicate that approximately 30% of children are overweight, which will translate to an even higher incidence of obesity in the adult population by the year 2001.

The magnitude of obesity differs widely among gender and ethnic groups. Findings demonstrate a marked prevalence of obesity among females of black and Mexican-American ethnic groups.

Obesity has major consequences to society. Health care providers need to have an appreciation of its complexity and the multiple co-morbid medical problems relating to it. This article reviews the epidemiology, definitions, and assessment of obesity, with emphasis on the clinical consequences of obesity, as well as for the most current techniques in evaluating and treating the obese patient.

INFLUENCES OF OBESITY

Obesity is a heterogeneous disease that encompasses genetic, environmental, socioeconomic, psychologic, and behavioral factors. Obesity is not caused simply by a lack of willpower: it is a complex disorder of appetite regulation and energy metabolism.

Studies with monozygotic twins suggested that resting metabolic rate thermogenesis, energy storage, energy expenditure, and body mass index (BMI) may all have significant genetic components. Other studies suggest, however, that genetic heritability accounts for only 34% of obesity, whereas environmental and behavioral factors make up 66%. It is important therefore to consider ethnic, socioeconomic status, education, and family behavioral patterns as having integral roles in the development of obesity. In addition, recent studies suggest that a child born to obese parents is more likely to develop childhood obesity.

FINANCIAL CONSEQUENCES

Obesity has profound financial consequences to society. Health care costs directly attributed to obesity account for

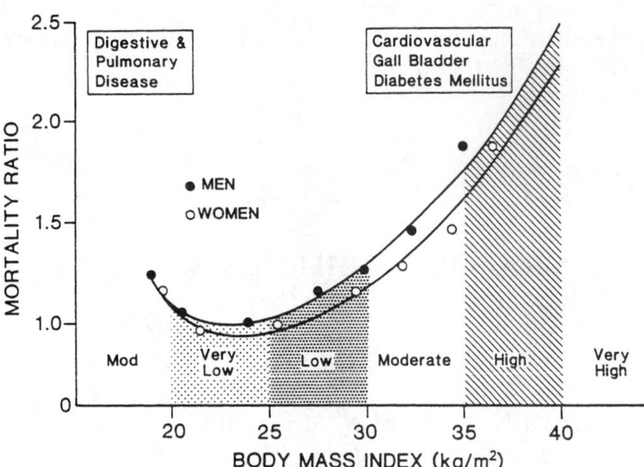

Figure 1. Correlation between mortality risk and increasing body mass index (BMI). As BMI increases to higher than 25, the risk for mortality from all causes increases. (From Gray DS: Diagnosis and prevalence of obesity. Med Clin North Am *73*:1, 1989.)

approximately $68 billion per year, corresponding to 6% of the total health care expenditures. Moreover, an additional $30 billion per year is spent on weight reduction programs and special foods. In recent years, obesity was the cause of an estimated 52 million days of lost productivity, costing employers nearly $4 billion. Job discrimination and higher insurance premiums further add to society's burden.

DEFINITION AND ASSESSMENTS

One of the difficulties with obesity treatment and management is determining who is actually obese. Determination of "ideal" body weight based on standard height/weight tables such as the Metropolitan Life Insurance tables has fallen out of favor. Most obesity experts recommend the use of a BMI. A BMI is defined as the ratio of body weight in kilograms to height in meters squared. The BMI correlates better with body fat as well as with morbidity and mortality (Figure 1). The BMI can also be calculated using a simple formula. Multiply the patient's weight (in pounds) by 705. Divide that product by the patient's height (in inches) and finally divide the result by height in inches a second time (Table 1).

Recent criteria define "overweight" as a BMI above 25 kg/m^2. Obesity begins at a BMI above 27.3 kg/m^2 for women and 27.8 kg/m^2 for men. Morbid obesity corresponds to a BMI of 39.0 kg/m^2 or higher. The BMI is a clinical tool to identify individuals at risk for developing co-morbid medical problems relating to their obesity. Individuals with a BMI of 30 kg/m^2 or higher or 27 kg/m^2 with co-morbid medical problems are at risk for developing increased morbidity and mortality due to their weight. Specific interventions should be considered in these individuals.

Another useful clinical tool in assessing the overweight patient is the waist/height ratio or simply waist circumference. A waist circumference, defined as the smallest area between the xiphoid process and the iliac crest, of more than 39 inches or a waist/hip ratio of more than 0.85 in women and 1.0 in men correlates with an upper body fat distribution. This upper body fat distribution puts one at greater risk for developing co-morbid medical problems (see later discussion).

Anthropometric measures are also commonly used in the office setting. However, in severely obese individuals, skinfold assessment is more poorly correlated with fat mass than weight, height, BMI, and circumferences. Skinfolds can be obtained by caliper measurements of the trunk and extremities. The ratio of skinfolds on the trunk to those on the extremities can be used to assess regional fat distribution. However, these measures require the availability of trained operators because of interobserver variations. Nonetheless, skinfold measurements are an easily attainable estimate of body fat in most individuals.

Many instrumental techniques and formulas are available to estimate body fat distribution more precisely; however, most are not practical or readily available for application in a physician's office.

DISTRIBUTION OF ADIPOSE TISSUE

Body fat distribution is a classification of obesity that has important clinical implications with regard to health risks. In addition to BMI determination, regional adipose tissue distribution as determined by waist/hip ratio or waist circumference is an important variable in determining increased morbidity and mortality associated with obesity.

Android or upper-body obesity (waist/hip ratio greater than 0.8 in females and greater than 1.0 in males, or waist circumference greater than 39 inches) is largely visceral adipose tissue and is associated with co-morbidities such as heart disease, lipid dyscrasias, insulin resistance, hyperinsulinemia, diabetes, and possibly cancer. In contrast, gynoid or lower-body obesity is mainly subcutaneous adipose tissue and is not associated with these adverse sequelae.

TABLE 1. **Clinical Use of the Body Mass Index (BMI)**

Definitions:

$$\text{BMI} = \frac{\text{weight in kilograms}}{(\text{height in meters})^2} \text{ or } \frac{\text{weight in pounds} \times 705}{(\text{height in inches})^2}$$

Obesity is defined as a BMI >27.8 (men) and >27.3 (women). If risk factors such as heart disease, hypertension, or elevated serum cholesterol levels are present, then intervention may be warranted for a BMI between 25 and 27.

Example 1: A 32-year-old asymptomatic woman desires weight reduction. Weight is 80 kg or 176 pounds, height is 157 cm or 62 inches, and she has a small frame.

$$\text{BMI} = \frac{80\text{ kg}}{(1.57\text{ m})^2} = 32.3\text{ kg/m}^2 \text{ or } \frac{176\text{ pounds} \times 705}{(62\text{ inches})^2} = 32.3\text{ kg/m}^2$$

The patient is obese and should be considered for a comprehensive weight management program.

ETIOLOGY AND PATHOPHYSIOLOGY OF OBESITY

Several etiologic factors provide additional means of classifying obesity. The first includes the neuroendocrine disorders: hypothalamic injury, Cushing's syndrome, polycystic ovarian syndrome, and gonadal failure. An underlying defect in energy metabolism is often detected in these syndromes leading to weight gain. The second group includes the rare single-gene deletion syndromes of obesity including Prader-Willi syndrome, Cohen's syndrome, Carpenter's syndrome, and the Bardet-Biedl syndrome.

Medications may also promote weight gain. These include phenothiazines, various antihistamines, antidepressants and antipsychotics, antiepileptics, corticosteroids, and certain antihypertensives. It is always important to take a thorough medication history to ensure that no medications, either prescription or over-the-counter, are prescribed that promote weight gain.

Advances continue on the molecular level of obesity research. The isolation of the mouse obese gene (ob) and identification of the gene product (leptin) occurred in the early 1990s. In genetically obese ob/ob mice, leptin was undetectable in their plasma. Leptin, when injected in the deficient ob/ob mouse, produced substantial weight loss, suggesting its importance in the regulation of body weight. Leptin was then identified in adipocytes in humans by radioimmune assay. Researchers found that plasma leptin concentrations in humans were not deficient but rather increased in direct proportion to body fat mass. However, because plasma leptin concentrations fall during hypocaloric intake, the administration of leptin might prove useful in promoting adherence to dieting regimens and maintenance of reduced body weight. Additional clinical trials are ongoing to evaluate leptin's efficacy in humans.

MEDICAL CONSEQUENCES OF OBESITY

Obesity is a chronic disease with multiple medical consequences that can be associated with profound increases in morbidity and premature mortality. With increasing BMI, there is an increased prevalence of insulin resistance, diabetes mellitus, lipid and cholesterol dyscrasias, hypertension, coronary artery disease, gallbladder disease, respiratory disease, degenerative joint disease, and cancer.

Insulin Resistance and Syndrome X

Insulin resistance, which is defined as decreased target tissue sensitivity and characterized by decreased glucose utilization, is a fundamental pathophysiologic defect that often leads to non–insulin-dependent diabetes mellitus (NIDDM). It is estimated that 25% of the population is insulin resistant. Hyperinsulinemia results from compensatory pancreatic cell hypersecretion, and hence serves as a biologic and laboratory marker of insulin resistance. After prolonged hypersecretion, the insulin secretory capacity of the beta cell diminishes, possibly owing to accumulation of amyloid deposits in the islet cells and eventually decompensation of insulin resistance to hyperglycemia. Hyperglycemia itself worsens insulin resistance. Obese patients often experience the Randall effect or insulin resistance that is due to high levels of fatty acids, which can be used by muscle at the expense of glucose. Other possibilities include a down-regulation of glucose transporters in skeletal muscle that can render beta cells insensitive to glucose. In addition, undetermined genetic factors and acquired factors such as aging, sedentary lifestyle, and obesity all contribute to insulin resistance.

Clinically, insulin resistance can be associated with abdominal obesity (android fat distribution), hypertension, hypertriglyceridemia, high-density lipoprotein (HDL)/low-density lipoprotein (LDL) abnormalities, hyperuricemia, fluid retention, polycystic ovarian syndrome, hypofibrinolysis, acanthosis nigricans, and skin tags. A condition termed syndrome X is commonly associated with a cluster of disorders including diabetes mellitus, abdominal obesity, hypertension, dyslipidemias, and atherosclerotic disease. Studies have shown that treatment options in this group of disorders favor complex carbohydrate modification, reduced fat intake, regular exercise, and possible use of medications that increase insulin sensitivity.

Diabetes Mellitus

The growing prevalence of NIDDM in the United States is undoubtedly associated with the increasing prevalence of obesity. Approximately 70 to 80% of patients with NIDDM are overweight. NHANES II data revealed a strong correlation between the relative risk of developing NIDDM and increasing BMI beyond 27 kg/m^2. For individuals who are severely obese (BMI >40 kg/m^2), there is a 10-fold increased risk for diabetes mellitus. In addition, a protracted duration of obesity also favors the development of insulin resistance and diabetes mellitus. The risk for the development of NIDDM also increases with a greater waist/hip ratio or android obesity. Individual risk factors for developing diabetes mellitus, regardless of sex, include increasing age, family history of diabetes mellitus, and android or central adipose distribution.

What should be emphasized, however, is that even a modest weight loss (5 to 10% of presenting weight) can have tremendous benefit on glycemic control and on curtailing development and progression of the multiple comorbidities associated with diabetes mellitus.

Lipid Dyscrasias

Obesity often leads to abnormalities in blood lipids. HDL cholesterol is lower in obese individuals and that has been associated with increased risk of coronary heart disease. Contrary to common beliefs, obese individuals routinely have normal or only slightly elevated total cholesterol or LDL cholesterol. However, because of the reduced level of HDL cholesterol, the ratio of HDL to LDL cholesterol is often elevated, leading to increased risk of atherosclerosis.

Unlike cholesterol, triglyceride levels are generally higher in obese individuals compared with those in normal weight individuals. Increased portal free fatty acid availability and hyperinsulinemia favor the hepatic synthesis of very-low-density lipoprotein. In addition, triglyceride clearance is delayed secondary to decreased lipoprotein lipase activity. Obese individuals often exhibit hyperlipoprotein class IV or V profiles, which may warrant pharmacologic intervention.

Hypertension

NHANES II data revealed a strong association between hypertension and obesity. In the United States, approximately 30 to 50% of hypertension is attributed to obesity. Although the relative risk of hypertension attributable to obesity decreases with age, adults 20 to 45 years of age with obesity have a fourfold to sixfold increase in hypertension. Interestingly, obesity exerts a greater effect on risk for hypertension in whites than in blacks, although hypertension is more prevalent in the black population.

As with diabetes management, a modest weight loss (5 to 10% of presenting weight) can have dramatic effects in lowering blood pressure as well as reducing left ventricular mass, which is often associated with long-standing hypertension.

Coronary Artery Disease

Although there is well-established association between obesity and elevated blood lipid levels, hypertension, and diabetes, the independent influence of obesity on the risk of coronary artery disease still remains controversial. The majority of studies suggest that obesity is an independent, long-term risk factor for cardiovascular disease. In addition, when other factors are present (i.e., hypertension, elevated LDL cholesterol, decreased HDL cholesterol, diabetes mellitus, and elevated serum triglyceride levels), obese individuals are at even greater risk for development of coronary artery disease.

Gallbladder Disease

Obese individuals have an increased prevalence of gallbladder disease. One proposed explanation is increased cholesterol production and secretion. Approximately 20 mg per day of cholesterol is produced for each additional kilogram of adipose tissue. Bile in turn is more saturated with cholesterol in obese patients as compared with nonobese persons. Women with a BMI greater than 30 kg/m^2 are at particular risk for the development of gallbladder disease.

Increased bile saturation and gallstone formation have been reported in obese individuals who have embarked upon aggressive weight reduction, such as extremely low-calorie diets and liquid diet preparations. In addition, a reduction in bile secretion occurs in association with weight reduction, causing a more lithogenic bile. This is a particular problem for obese patients who have rapid weight loss (i.e., very-low-calorie diets [VLCDs]). It has been suggested that a weight loss greater than 1.5 kg per week is associated with an increased risk of gallstone formation.

Depression

Depression, although not specifically caused by obesity, has an increased prevalence in the obese population. Studies suggest approximately 30% of obese individuals have clinical symptoms of depression by objective measures. Until the depression is treated, long-term weight loss maintenance is doubtful owing to the compulsive type eating pattern often seen in depressed, overweight individuals. It is speculated that increased complex carbohydrates trigger a release of serotonin in the brain, giving a temporary content, calming feeling. In obese patients with concomitant depression, treatment with a selective serotonin reuptake inhibitor may be a useful adjunct to a diet, exercise, and behavioral modification program. There have been limited studies supporting the appetite suppressant effects of fluoxetine (Prozac). However, indiscriminate use of serotonergic antidepressant medications for the sole purpose of appetite suppression is not indicated or recommended.

TREATMENT OPTIONS

Most successful weight management programs combine the use of modified diet plans, regular exercise, behavior modification, and the possible use of pharmacologic therapy. Programs that are not proportionately balanced or that require drastic dietary changes have high rates of recidivism. Following is a prudent approach to weight management in the primary care office setting.

Initial Evaluation

An initial thorough history and physical examination are crucial before initiating any weight loss program. Secondary causes of obesity such as Cushing's syndrome, hypothyroidism, and diabetes mellitus should be considered and ruled in or out by a thorough history and physical examination. Contraindications for weight reduction, such as pregnancy, lactation, unstable mental illness, unstable medical condition such as unstable angina or uncontrolled blood pressure, and anorexia nervosa, should all be screened before attempting weight loss. BMI and waist circumference should be determined to predict health risks and guide various treatment options (Table 2).

Initial blood work including complete blood count, lipid profile, thyroid stimulating hormone, and liver panel should be considered, as well as an electrocardiogram in appropriate individuals.

Diet

High rates of recidivism are likely to result from any diet that is viewed as a temporary drastic restrictive change in one's eating patterns. In the 1970s, VLCDs became popular because initial weight loss can be precipitous. VLCDs are highly limited in energy, usually between 600 and 800 calories per day, resulting in significant but usually short-term weight loss. There is no evidence to suggest that a diet less than 800 calories per day is of any additional benefit.

VLCDs have a role in weight management but should be reserved for severely obese patients or moderately obese patients with co-morbid medical problems. These individuals can protect their lean body mass much better than lean individuals. In a

TABLE 2. **Determination of Health Risk Based on BMI and Various Treatment Options**

BMI Category	Health Risk Based on BMI
<25	Minimal-low
25–<27	Low-moderate
27–<30	Moderate-high
30–<35	High-very high
35–<40	Very high-extremely high
>40	Extremely high
Health Risk	**Treatment Options**
Minimal and low	Healthful eating Increased physical activity Lifestyle changes
Moderate	All of the above plus low-calorie diet
High and very high	All of the above plus pharmacotherapy and very-low-calorie diet
Extremely high	All of the above plus surgical considerations

nonstressed state, obese individuals metabolize predominantly adipose tissue, whereas lean persons metabolize lean body mass. Therefore, some experts believe that VLCDs should be contraindicated for anyone less than 40% overweight or at a BMI less than 30 kg/m^2. Table 3 summarizes other contraindications to VLCDs.

Popular commercial liquid diet preparations contain 33 to 70 grams of protein, 30 to 45 grams of carbohydrate, and 1 to 2 grams of fat. Additional daily supplementation includes at least 1500 mL of water, multiple vitamins, calcium, magnesium, and potassium supplements.

A widely used food version VLCD is the protein-sparing modified fast (PSMF) diet. The PSMF provides 1.5 grams per kg ideal body weight as lean meat, fish, or poultry. Fat and carbohydrate sources are largely eliminated. As with the liquid diet preparations, multiple vitamins, minerals, and water are required daily. VLCDs should be prescribed only with medical supervision. Complications of VLCDs can be life-threatening and can include postural hypotension, arrhythmias, myocardial atrophy, electrolyte derangement, and sudden death. Insulin, oral hypoglycemic agents, and antihypertensive medications must often be carefully adjusted to avoid serious side effects.

Although weight loss on VLCDs is often dramatic and substantial (1.5 to 2.5 kg per week), gradual reintroduction of food over several weeks may produce greater recidivism with the liquid diets than with the PSMF. The liquid diets do not provide an opportunity for the patient to alter fundamental eating and lifestyle behaviors needed for sustained weight loss.

Another option for less drastic changes is a conventional balanced deficit diet. These provide approximately 1200 to 1800 calories per day, 20 to 30% of the calories from fat, 55 to 60% from carbohydrates, and 15 to 20% from protein. Conventional diets usually result in less dramatic but gradual weight loss. A conventional, balanced weight loss diet should result in 1 to 2 pounds of weight loss per week.

Although 1200 to 1500 calories in women and 1500 to 1800 calories per day in men should cause gradual weight loss, an alternative approach is to determine the individual's basal metabolic rate and then total daily energy expenditure (Table 4). One can then reduce the calories by 500 calories per day to promote approximately 1 pound of weight loss per week. An empirical approach for determination of energy expenditure is multiplying the patient's weight in pounds by 10 to 15 kcal per pound depending on the patient's activity level. For example, if a patient weighs 200 pounds and is moderately active, he or she should require approximately 13 calories per pound or 2600 calories per day to sustain current weight at his or her present activity level. By restricting intake to 2100 calories per day, one should lose approximately 1 pound per week or 4 pounds per month. This more moderate degree of restriction is often better tolerated, and long-term compliance may be superior to the more restrictive VLCDs.

TABLE 3. **Contraindications for Very-Low-Calorie Diets**

Recent myocardial infarction
Unstable angina
Malignant arrhythmias
Cardiovascular disease
Serious underlying disease: malignancy; liver or renal failure
Type I diabetes mellitus
Pregnancy
Certain medication therapies*: steroids, antineoplastics
Untreated metabolic cause of obesity
Hypothyroidism and other endocrine disorders
Cosmetic motivation: body weight <20% above ideal or a BMI <27 kg/m^2

*Medications such as insulin, oral hypoglycemics, and antihypertensives must be carefully monitored, and they are often tapered for patients enrolled in very-low-calorie diets.

TABLE 4. **Calculation of Daily Energy Requirements**

Daily Energy Requirement	=	**Resting Metabolic Rate**	+	**Gender Constant**
Men	=	10 × (weight in kg)	+	900
Women	=	7 × (weight in kg)	+	800

Activity Level	**Activity Factor**
Sedentary	1.2
Moderate	1.5
Heavy	1.7

Behavior Modification

With any of the diet plans, behavior modification must be an integral component of a successful weight management program. Controlled trials have demonstrated the effectiveness of behavioral techniques. The goal is to reinforce eating and physical activity habits that aid and/or maintain weight loss while discouraging adverse behaviors. For a busy practitioner, concise manuals that provide specific monthly goals, such as the *Learn Program for Weight Control* or the *Lifestyle Counsellor's Guide for Weight Control* from American Health Publishing Company in Dallas, Texas, are available. These provide excellent behavior modification goals for the patient to work through between office visits.

Exercise

Like behavior modification, exercise is also an integral component of a successful weight management program. Cardiovascular training, or aerobic activity, is most often recommended for weight management programs owing to the increased number of calories expended during its activity. In addition, adipose tissue is oxidized once a certain threshold of activity is reached. Resistance exercises are also important such as weight training to increase muscle mass and maintain metabolic rates, which often decrease with diet alone. The biggest difficulty with compliance in exercise prescriptions is unrealistic expectations for patients. In general, a minimum of 30 minutes of aerobic exercise at least 4 to 5 days per week is recommended. However, very few obese patients are able to sustain themselves for 30 minutes, so compliance precipitously drops. Several 10 minute or six 5-minute sessions of aerobic activity can be a reasonable starting point for obese individuals. This "occurrence" type of exercise increases compliance and is much better tolerated by the patient. Also, common everyday activities such as walking up stairs rather than taking the elevator, parking farther away from an entrance, or not using the television remote control can add up to small but meaningful periods of increased activity, thereby increasing energy expenditure. Studies have determined that if patients are able to progress up to 30 minutes of exercise, 5 days a week, they have a greater than 50% chance of achieving weight maintenance. It is important to explain to the patients that exercise promotes muscle mass, which in turn weighs more than adipose tissue. Patients become frustrated after diligently exercising daily for a week's time only to gain 1 or 2 pounds. Waist circumference and clothing sizes should continue to decline, however, during any exercise program.

Pharmacotherapy

In a comprehensive, office-based, weight management program, pharmacotherapy may be beneficial as an adjunct to the preceding diet, exercise, and behavior modification regimen. However, recent evidence of adverse patient reactions to fenfluramine (Pondimin) and dexfenfluramine (Redux), specifically valvular heart disease and primary hypertension (PPH), forced their withdrawal from the market in September 1997. Since this misfortune, development of drugs for the treatment of obesity has been intensified by the demand for safe and effective therapeutics.

Early in 1998, the Food and Drug Administration (FDA) approved the use of sibutramine (Meridia) for the treatment of obesity. Sibutramine is a selective re-uptake inhibitor of serotonin and norepinephrine, which promotes the sense of satiety. The initial starting dose is 10 mg daily.

The most common side effects associated with sibutramine include dry mouth, insomnia, anorexia, and constipation. In addition, tachycardia and hypertension (mean blood pressure increase of 2 to 3 mm Hg) have been reported. Therefore pulse and blood pressure should be monitored when initiating sibutramine. There have been no reports of valvular heart disease or PPH with the use of sibutramine. Efficacy studies revealed an approximate 8% weight loss at the end of 12 months when used in conjunction with diet.

Awaiting FDA approval is another antiobesity agent, orlistat (Xenical). Orlistat is a "statin" analogue that inhibits gastric and pancreatic lipase and may decrease fat absorption by up to 30%. Orlistat is not absorbed systemically after oral administration and inhibits lipases for approximately 90 minutes.

Certain adverse events can be predicted from the mode of action of orlistat including steatorrhea, oily spotting, flatus with discharge, fecal urgency, and incontinence. It has not, however, been demonstrated to cause diarrhea or malabsorption. Fat-soluble vitamins A, D, E, and K, as well as β-carotene may be somewhat decreased in individuals taking orlistat; therefore, multivitamin supplementation is recommended daily approximately 90 minutes after taking the medication.

The usual dosage of orlistat is 120 mg three times daily with meals. Efficacy studies after 2 years revealed an approximate 9% weight loss when used in combination with a mildly hypocaloric diet, exercise, and behavior modification.

Phentermine is an adrenergic medication that increases norepinephrine release. It has been available for years but was popularized in the early 1990s when Weintraub studied the efficacy of phentermine used in combination with fenfluramine or the "phen/fen" combination. Phentermine hydrochloride (Fastin, Adipex) or the resin (Ionamin) preparation is still available and indicated for short-term use. Potential side effects of phentermine include dry mouth, palpitations, tachycardia, hypertension, insomnia, or overstimulation.

The use of pharmacotherapy as an adjunct to diet and exercise is indicated for individuals with a BMI greater than 30 kg/m^2 or greater than 27 kg/m^2 with a co-morbid medical problem relating to their obesity such as diabetes, hypercholesterolemia, or hypertension. Pharmacotherapy alone is not indicated or recommended.

The popularity of serotonergic agents such as fluoxetine (Prozac) as appetite suppressant medications has been growing, especially among commercial weight loss programs. Fluoxetine, sertraline (Zoloft), fluvoxamine (Luvox), and paroxetine (Paxil) have not been found to be efficacious in obesity treatment and have significant side effects. Therefore, the use of these serotonergic medications for obesity treatment is not recommended. In addition, there have been no trials evaluating the use of a fluoxetine/phentermine combination, and therefore it is not recommended. Of note, fluoxetine has been beneficial in the treatment of binge eating disorders. Table 5 summarizes commonly prescribed medications for the treatment of obesity.

Bariatric Surgery

Bariatric surgery has evolved over the last several decades because of the generally limited long-term success of medical treatment for obesity. Obese patients can be considered for bariatric surgery if they are morbidly obese, manifest severe co-morbidities, and have already failed conventional medical treat-

TABLE 5. **Commonly Prescribed Medications for Obesity Treatment**

Class/Generic Name	Trade Name	Strengths Available (mg)	Typical Dose (mg)	Mode of Action
Noradrenergic				
Phentermine resin	Ionamin	15, 30	30 qd	Increase norepinephrine release
Phentermine HCl	Fastin, Adipex-P	15, 30, 37.5	30 qam	
Serotonergic/noradrenergic				
Sibutramine	Meridia	10, 15	10 qd	Inhibition of serotonin and norepinephrine reuptake
Lipase inhibitor				
Orlistat*	Xenical	120	120 tid	Inhibition of gastric and pancreatic lipase

*Pending FDA approval.

ment consisting of diet, behavior modification, and exercise.

The earliest procedure developed for obesity was the jejunoileal bypass, which was associated with serious sequelae, such as severe malabsorption and diarrhea; vitamin A, D, and B_{12} deficiencies; and occasional liver failure and cirrhosis. This procedure has since been abandoned. Two procedures were recommended at a recent National Institutes of Health (NIH) consensus conference on obesity: the vertical-banded gastroplasty and the Roux-en-Y gastric bypass operation. The vertical-banded gastroplasty is a procedure that creates a 15-mL stapled proximal stomach pouch, which limits the amount of food that can be taken at a single sitting. The opening between the pouch and the rest of the stomach is banded externally to create a narrowing of 1 cm to delay emptying (Figure 2). Complications of this procedure include staple line disruption, pouch distention, or erosion of the band. Other adverse outcomes include subsequent consumption of soft, calorically dense foods, which can curtail weight loss. Vomiting can occur from inadequate mastication and inappropriate intakes.

The Roux-en-Y gastric bypass is similar to the gastroplasty in the formation of a small gastric pouch and narrow outlet, but it also includes a bypass of the stomach, the duodenum, and the first portion of the jejunum (see Figure 2). Because of the interference with absorption resulting from the bypass, complications of this procedure are more likely to include iron, calcium, and B_{12} deficiencies. As in all bypass procedures, marginal ulceration can occur at the anastomosis.

Both the gastroplasty and the gastric bypass procedures are relatively safe in the hands of experienced surgeons, with an overall mortality rate of less than 2%, but the gastric bypass produces greater weight loss. Bariatric surgery improves diabetes mellitus, hypertension, hyperlipidemia, respiratory failure,

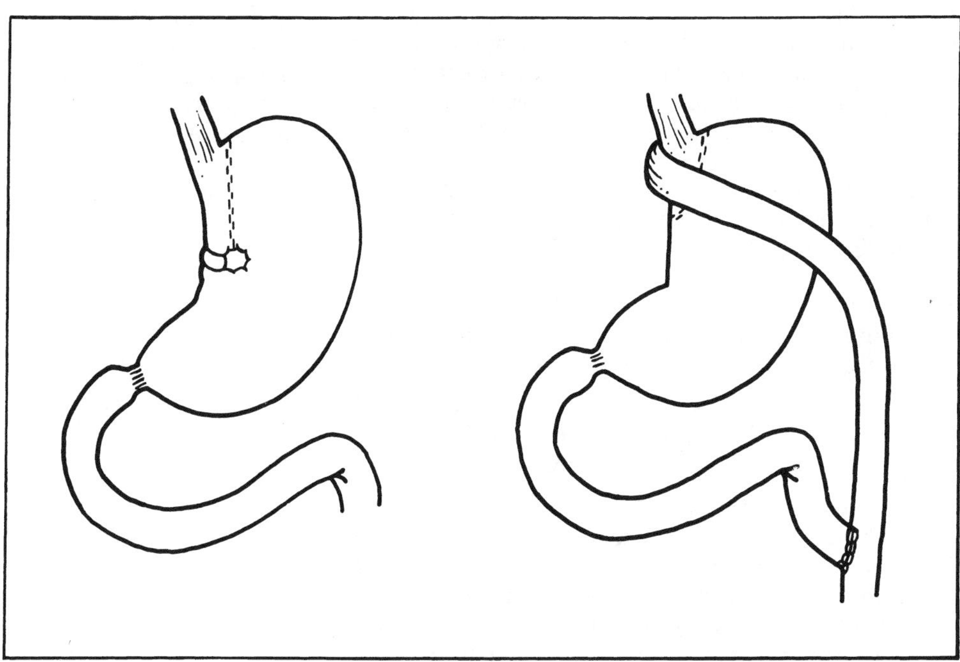

Figure 2. Clinically useful gastric surgical techniques include the vertical-banded gastroplasty *(left)* and the Roux-en-Y gastric bypass *(right)*. (From Apovian CM, Jensen GL: Overnutrition and obesity management. *In* Kirby DF, Dudrick SJ [eds]: Practical Handbook of Nutrition in Clinical Practice. 1994, p 43. Reprinted by permission of CRC Press, Boca Raton, FL.)

TABLE 6. **Contraindications for Bariatric Surgery***

Less than 100 lb (45 kg) overweight
Organic cause for obesity
Age older than 50 years
Serious underlying disease: cardiac, liver, or renal
Psychiatric disorder
Alcoholism or substance abuse
Endogenous depression
Misguided or ill-conceived motivation for surgery
Lack of support systems for follow-up and care
No history of failure of conventional medical therapy for obesity
History of gallstones or cholecystitis

*Many surgeons require proven medical complications of obesity before considering surgery; therefore, absence of these complications would be a relative contraindication.

and other co-morbidities in most patients who maintain weight loss for 5 years or more. Contraindications to bariatric surgery are listed in Table 6.

BENEFITS OF WEIGHT LOSS

It is obvious to most people that weight loss is beneficial to the obese individuals with co-morbid medical problems. However, what health care providers are not aware of is the tremendous benefit that even a modest (10 to 15%) weight loss can achieve. Several studies have demonstrated a significant benefit in blood pressure control, glucose control, and lipid management with modest weight loss of 10 to 12 kg. Although in many instances this modest weight loss still leaves patients obese by many practitioners' standards, there is tangible benefit in health risk reduction with the potential for decreased health care resource use.

REALISTIC GOALS

One of the most disturbing factors in weight management is setting unrealistic goals for overweight or obese patients. As discussed previously, modest weight loss can offer profound benefit in preventing or delaying the onset of co-morbid medical problems relating to obesity. For a patient weighing 300 pounds, it is unrealistic to expect a weight loss of 180 pounds to achieve an "ideal body weight." The patient is set up for failure. A more realistic goal is a 10 to 20% weight loss from the patient's presenting weight. This realistic goal keeps the patient focused and improves self-esteem and quality of life, as well as helping to manage any co-morbid medical problems associated with the obesity.

POSSIBLE FUTURE TREATMENT OPTIONS FOR OBESITY

As discussed in the pharmacotherapy section, any advances in the future treatment of obesity must be viewed as only an adjunct to diet, behavior modification, and exercise. However, great strides are being made in the treatment of obesity. In addition to leptin, there are multiple neurochemical mediators that affect food intake (Table 7). One neuropeptide that may have clinical benefit in the near future is neuropeptide Y. This peptide signals neuronal axons to affect energy intake and expenditure via endocrine, gastrointestinal, and central and peripheral nervous systems. Neuropeptide Y is a potent central appetite stimulant, which is increased by insulin and glucocorticoids and decreased by leptin and estrogen. Rodents injected with neuropeptide Y in the paraventricular nucleus increased food intake and increased lipoprotein lipase activity in white adipose tissue while decreasing sympathetic nervous system activity and thermogenesis in brown adipose tissue. Thus, neuropeptide Y antagonists are being studied for appetite suppressant effects.

Other potential targets of future adjunctive treatments for obesity include adipocyte transcription factors, which decrease differentiation of adipocytes from fibroblasts. Also under investigation are tumor necrosis factors, which interfere with insulin action and ameliorate insulin resistance by decreasing effects on skeletal muscle; GLP-1, a hormone which increases satiety; and butabindide, a compound that prevents the breakdown of cholecystokinin, a gut peptide, thereby reducing food intake 30% in mice. In addition, beta$_3$-receptor agonists have been studied to increase thermogenesis by increasing oxidative phosphorylation in white and brown adipose tissue.

CONCLUSION

Obesity is a chronic disease that affects nearly one third of individuals in the United States today. Health care providers can no longer view obesity as a social issue but rather a chronic medical condition requiring, in most cases, long-term treatment. A weight management program consisting of prudent dietary changes, behavior modification, and regular modest aerobic exercise with or without the adjunctive use of pharmacotherapy will provide patients with the best chance of weight loss and maintenance. Most important, realistic goals for attainable weight loss will be most rewarding not only for patients, but also for health care providers managing the co-morbid medical problems relating to obesity.

TABLE 7. **Various Neurochemical Mediators That Affect Food Intake**

Increase Feeding	Decrease Feeding
Neuropeptide Y	Leptin
Galanin	Serotonin
γ-Aminobutyric acid (GABA)	Dopamine
Opioids	Glucagon, GLP-1
Insulin	Bombesin
	Cholecystokinin
	Somatostatin
	Norepinephrine
	Cytokines

VITAMIN DEFICIENCY

method of
RICHARD S. RIVLIN, M.D.
Memorial Sloan-Kettering Cancer Center and New York Hospital–Cornell Medical Center
New York, New York

Before beginning to treat any suspected vitamin deficiencies, the physician must first consider all the factors that may have contributed to this condition and how they can be prevented in the future. Certain general considerations should be taken into account:

1. The impact of a poor diet is greatly intensified by the prolonged use of certain medications, such as laxatives and diuretics, particularly in older individuals.
2. Alcohol has specific and selective effects on vitamin metabolism that may become overt when the diet is also compromised.
3. The presence of so-called classic features of vitamin deficiency, such as the petechiae and curly hairs of scurvy, indicates that the disorder is far advanced and requires prompt intervention.
4. Vitamin deficiencies are rarely encountered singly; clusters of multiple deficiencies are usually the rule.
5. Deficiencies develop gradually, and symptoms may be nonspecific in their early stages.

When a poor dietary pattern develops, the deficiencies of the vitamins emerge in an ordered manner. Thus, water-soluble vitamin stores may be seriously depleted in a matter of weeks. Longer periods are needed for major depletion of fat-soluble vitamin stores (see the article on vitamin K deficiency). Several years of seriously inadequate vitamin B_{12} intake are necessary before there is clinically apparent deficiency of this vitamin.

In the process of correction of vitamin deficiency, the physician must remember that large doses of vitamins are in reality drugs, with a toxic/therapeutic ratio. Some vitamins, particularly A and D, have a real potential for causing untoward effects. Thus, both the prevention and treatment of vitamin deficiency require a knowledge of physiology and nutrition.

In recent years increasing attention has been directed toward detecting relative or marginal vitamin deficiency early in an effort to maximize the benefits of nutrition. For example, folic acid deficiency leads to elevated blood levels of homocysteine, an amino acid that is suspected of being a risk factor for cardiovascular disease. When serum levels of homocysteine are stratified according to the serum folic acid levels within the so-called normal range, individuals at the lower end of normal have been shown to have higher blood levels of homocysteine than persons at the higher end of normal. Possible health benefits may derive from elevating the lower levels of folic acid within the normal range through diet, food fortification, or supplementation.

DIETARY REFERENCE INTAKES

To enable the health professional to provide accurate and up-to-date information on prevention and treatment of vitamin deficiency, one must become familiar with the new nomenclature. In the latest report from the Food and Nutrition Board, National Academy of Sciences, the comprehensive term "dietary reference intake" (DRI) has been approved, which includes recommended dietary allowance (RDA), estimated average requirement (EAR), adequate intake (AI), and tolerable upper intake level (UL).

The RDA is used as a goal for healthy people. The RDA represents the average daily dietary intake that is sufficient to meet the nutrient requirements of nearly all (97 to 98%) healthy individuals in a particular age, gender, and pregnancy or lactation group.

THIAMINE DEFICIENCY (BERIBERI)

In the United States at present, overt thiamine deficiency is often encountered in the setting of chronic alcohol ingestion. Drinking portions of alcohol throughout the day prevents most of the dietary thiamine from being absorbed. It is for this reason that a proper clinical history tries to ascertain not only how much the patient drinks but also when the drinking occurs. It has been estimated that about one quarter of alcoholic patients admitted to hospitals in the United States show some evidence of thiamine deficiency. It is likely that alcohol has deleterious effects on thiamine metabolism as well as on its absorption. When alcohol abuse of long duration is superimposed on a dietary inadequacy of this vitamin, serious neurologic consequences may result.

Beriberi resulting from severe dietary thiamine deficiency is encountered more frequently in developing countries than in the United States, particularly where polished rice is a dietary staple. This food contains little thiamine. Whole-grain, unprocessed rice is much more nutritious. Thiamine deficiency may be encountered from time to time under conditions in which the metabolic requirement is increased, as in severe diabetes, far-advanced cancer, or pregnancy and lactation. Early features of the deficiency state are relatively nonspecific and include anorexia, irritability, weight loss, and weakness. Later there is prominent involvement of two major organ systems in the classic syndrome: (1) the cardiovascular system with beriberi heart disease, exhibiting high-output failure and features suggestive of thyrotoxic heart disease, and (2) the central and peripheral nervous systems, with peripheral neuropathy and the Wernicke-Korsakoff syndrome.

Prevention

With a diet containing adequate amounts of thiamine-rich sources, such as red meat, whole grains, legumes, and nuts, and with avoidance of milled or polished rice, beriberi should be preventable. Thiamine is unstable at alkaline pH and is also heat sensitive except under acidic conditions below a pH of 5. Thus, cooking may compromise thiamine sources to some degree.

The Food and Nutrition Board of the National Research Council, National Academy of Sciences, has established a DRI that ranges from 0.9 to 1.2 mg per day for males 9 years of age and older, and 0.9 to 1.1 mg per day for women, depending on age, with an increase to 1.4 mg during pregnancy and 1.5 mg during lactation. For infants the DRI is 0.2 to 0.3 mg per day and for children 1 to 8 years of age it is 0.5

to 0.6 mg per day. Such figures are intended to meet the needs of nearly all healthy persons and would need to be higher under conditions of increased metabolic requirements.

Treatment

The physician must keep a high index of suspicion in mind that thiamine deficiency may be present when heart disease or neurologic manifestations are prominently displayed in a patient who chronically abuses alcohol. In case of doubt the physician should err on the side of treatment, because little harm would result from thiamine injection when it is not needed. If thiamine deficiency is likely, prompt administration of 50 to 100 mg* intramuscularly or intravenously is indicated. Such large doses should be continued for 3 to 4 days, after which 5 to 10 mg can be given orally or intramuscularly.

As noted earlier, in far-advanced beriberi it is highly likely that other significant deficiencies in vitamins and minerals coexist and will also necessitate vigorous treatment. Continued alcohol abstinence is absolutely crucial to prevent recurrence, and the diet must be adequate in calories and nutrients.

Peripheral neuropathy in thiamine deficiency, manifested by numbness, tingling, and burning in the extremities, may be debilitating and responds poorly to analgesics. It is suggested that patients be kept active and that physiotherapy be instituted early. Recovery from the neurologic disorder may be quite prolonged, and patients are often discouraged by the slow rate of progress.

Cardiovascular symptoms of beriberi often resemble those of hyperthyroidism, as noted previously. Heart failure may develop and necessitate therapy with digitalis, diuretics, and other drugs. A brisk response to thiamine may obviate or reduce the need for diuretics. Thiamine alone may result in significant improvement in cardiovascular function, with a prompt diuresis in cases of heart failure, but the use of standard cardiac medications is generally required for an optimal response and full recovery. The possibility that other forms of heart disease, such as alcoholic cardiomyopathy, may be present as well must be considered, as they may be masked by the hyperkinetic state.

Rarely, one may encounter genetic disorders of thiamine metabolism, such as congenital lactic acidosis, Leigh's disease, and maple syrup urine disease, in which large doses of thiamine (100 to 500 mg) are necessary to achieve some benefit.

RIBOFLAVIN (VITAMIN B_2) DEFICIENCY

In understanding the pathogenesis and treatment of riboflavin (vitamin B_2) deficiency, it is essential to realize that the metabolic action of riboflavin resides largely in its role as a precursor of the coenzymes riboflavin-5′-phosphate (flavin mononucleotide [FMN]) and flavin adenine dinucleotide (FAD), and of flavins bound covalently to tissue proteins. All these derivatives of riboflavin are widely involved as coenzymes in intermediary metabolism. More recently, it has been suggested that riboflavin may provide antioxidant activity in its role as the precursor of FAD, the cofactor for glutathione reductase. This enzyme generates reduced glutathione, which is the substrate for glutathione peroxidase, a powerful enzyme that degrades reactive lipid peroxides.

Dietary deficiency of riboflavin is nearly always encountered in the setting of multiple deficiencies. It is important to remember that in addition to being caused by a poor diet, riboflavin deficiency may also result from the effects of hormones, drugs, or diseases that impair the body's utilization of this vitamin and its conversion to active derivatives. Phototherapy of newborn infants for elevated serum bilirubin concentrations may provoke riboflavin deficiency because the vitamin is light sensitive. Alcohol may also cause riboflavin deficiency by interfering with the digestion and absorption of the vitamin. There are conditions, such as severe burns, trauma, surgery, dialysis, and others, in which vitamin B_2 deficiency may also result from increased demands on tissue stores. Psychotropic drugs, antimalarial agents, and some cancer chemotherapeutic drugs impair the conversion of riboflavin into its active coenzyme derivatives.

Early in the course of riboflavin deficiency, the patient may exhibit burning and itching of the eyes and mouth as well as personality disturbances. Subtle manifestations of early deficiency, such as weakness and fatigue, may be difficult to distinguish from those of many other causes. Later on, angular stomatitis, seborrheic dermatitis, glossitis, and other epithelial abnormalities are found. Cheilosis and angular stomatitis are no longer believed to be specific for riboflavin deficiency. With further progression of the deficiency state, anemia and corneal neovascularization may develop.

Prevention

Riboflavin deficiency should be preventable if the diet contains an adequate supply of milk and dairy products, meat, and green, leafy vegetables. In the United States, dairy products are the most important sources of the vitamin, and the riboflavin nutritional status is generally correlated quite closely with that of calcium. Low-fat dairy products remain excellent sources of riboflavin as well as calcium. In developing countries, vegetable sources predominate. The DRI for riboflavin is 0.9 to 1.3 mg for males 9 years of age and older and 0.9 to 1.1 mg for women, with an increase to 1.4 mg during pregnancy and to 1.6 mg during lactation. The DRI for infants is 0.3 to 0.4 mg per day and that for children of ages 1 to 8 years is 0.5 to 0.6 mg per day.

*Exceeds dosage recommended by the manufacturer.

Treatment

Riboflavin deficiency can be treated with the previously mentioned food sources that are rich in this vitamin. Riboflavin can also be administered as a component of a multivitamin tablet. For rapid treatment of riboflavin-deficient patients, doses in the range of 10 to 15 mg per day are recommended. The poor solubility of riboflavin in aqueous solution limits its feasibility for intravenous administration and this formulation is seldom used.

NIACIN DEFICIENCY (PELLAGRA)

The well-described deficiency disease pellagra was quite common in the United States when corn was a dietary staple. Corn is relatively poor in tryptophan, the essential amino acid that serves as a precursor of niacin. At present, niacin deficiency in the United States largely results from prolonged alcohol abuse under conditions in which multivitamin deficits prevail. In rare instances, some degree of niacin deficiency may occur after the use of specific drugs that interfere with niacin metabolism, such as isoniazid (INH) or 6-mercaptopurine. In the malignant carcinoid syndrome, dietary tryptophan is diverted from the synthesis of niacin to that of serotonin, and some patients may exhibit signs of pellagra, particularly if they are also malnourished. In the autosomal recessive disorder Hartnup's disease, pellagra may develop because of a deficit in the absorption of tryptophan and other amino acids from the intestinal tract.

Prevention

Niacin deficiency is preventable by a diet that is high in proteins of animal origin, which have a high tryptophan content. Some vegetable proteins also have tryptophan but at lower amounts. The best sources of niacin besides meats are yeast, cereals, legumes, and seeds. Some newer varieties of corn have higher tryptophan and niacin concentrations than those prevalent earlier. Grain products often contain niacin but of relatively lower bioavailability. The DRI is expressed in terms of niacin equivalents; 60 mg of dietary tryptophan yields about 1 mg of niacin synthesized endogenously. Expressed in this manner as niacin equivalents, the DRI for niacin is 12 to 16 mg in males 9 years of age and older and 12 to 14 mg in females 9 years of age and older, with an additional 4 mg recommended during pregnancy and lactation. The DRI for infants is 2 to 4 mg per day, and for children of ages 1 to 8 years the DRI is 9 to 13 mg per day.

Treatment

Advanced pellagra is a serious life-threatening disorder, classically known by the four *d*'s: diarrhea, dermatitis, dementia, and death. Doses in the form of niacinamide (nicotinamide) in the range of 50 to 150 mg have generally been given to ill patients; marked clinical improvement is demonstrable within several days. Once these large doses have been administered, maintenance levels of several times the DRI together with satisfactory diet should be given to the patient. Other measures involved in supportive care include correction of acid-base imbalance, treatment of the skin disease, and recognition that the neurologic impairment may follow a prolonged course before recovery occurs.

Niacin in the form of nicotinic acid in much larger doses (3 to 6 grams per day) is a first-line drug for management of an elevated serum cholesterol level. Niacinamide, another form of niacin, does not cause the flushing symptoms associated with nicotinic acid, nor does it lower the serum cholesterol level.

PYRIDOXINE (VITAMIN B_6) DEFICIENCY

Vitamin B_6 is found in dietary sources primarily in three forms, as pyridoxal, pyridoxamine, and pyridoxine. Animal foods contain predominantly pyridoxal and pyridoxamine, whereas the predominant form in plants is pyridoxine. As an important coenzyme, pyridoxal phosphate participates in a wide range of reactions. Although best known for its involvement in transamination, pyridoxal phosphate also catalyzes decarboxylation, side chain cleavage, and dehydratase reactions. These functions are central to glucogenesis, lipid metabolism, central nervous system functioning, the immune system, nucleic acid synthesis, and endocrine function, as well as synthesis of certain other vitamins (e.g., niacin).

Dietary deficiency of pyridoxine occasionally occurs in the United States but almost never as an isolated entity. It is sometimes observed after prolonged therapy with certain pharmacologic agents, such as INH or cycloserine for tuberculosis, both of which are pyridoxine antagonists. Deficiency of pyridoxine occurs commonly in severe alcoholism in association with deficiencies of the other vitamins, as noted earlier.

Prevention

Deficiency of pyridoxine should be preventable by a diet that contains adequate amounts of meat, wheat, nuts, vegetables (particularly beans and potatoes), fruits, cereals, and grains. Some amount may be lost during pressure cooking and storage. The bioavailability of pyridoxine from food sources varies widely. The DRI for vitamin B_6 is 1.0 to 1.7 mg for males 9 years of age and older and 1.0 to 1.5 mg for women and is increased another 0.4 to 0.5 mg during pregnancy and lactation. The DRI for infants is 0.1 to 0.3 mg per day and that for children of ages 1 to 8 years is 0.5 to 0.6 mg per day.

Treatment

The dietary deficiency of pyridoxine can generally be treated with doses in the range of 2 to 10 mg per day. In more severe cases, particularly those occurring during pregnancy, doses in the range of 10 to 20 mg have generally been administered. In the event that deficiency has resulted from a drug inhibiting vitamin B_6 metabolism, somewhat higher doses may be needed, in some instances up to 50 to 100 mg per day. It is advisable to initiate pyridoxine therapy concomitantly when certain drugs are prescribed, a practice that is generally followed with INH treatment for tuberculosis but should be applicable more widely with vitamin B_6 antagonists. With respect to L-dopa, however, vitamin B_6 is generally not prescribed because it is believed by some authorities to interfere with therapeutic efficacy.

Rare cases of a pyridoxine-dependency syndrome, such as pyridoxine-responsive anemia, have been treated with doses in the 300- to 500-mg range. It is important to remember that peripheral neuropathy has been reported as a side effect of vitamin B_6 ingestion when 2 grams or more has been used in treatment. It is possible that lower doses, in the neighborhood of 200 to 500 mg, may also cause some degree of peripheral neuropathy.

FOLIC ACID DEFICIENCY

Folic acid and related compounds all have a pteroylglutamic acid structure and participate in many important reactions, including the synthesis of serine and methionine, purines, and thymidylate. Folic acid together with vitamin B_{12} is central to maintaining normal hematologic function. Attention has recently focused on folic acid as a methyl donor involved in the formation of methionine from homocysteine, the latter a compound associated with accelerated development of coronary, cerebrovascular, and peripheral vascular disease. The vital role of folic acid in the nervous system is exemplified by the association of its deficiency with formation of neural tube defects.

Dietary deficiency of folic acid occurs in people who do not consume adequate amounts of sources, such as meat, legumes and other vegetables, and fruits. The bioavailability of folates from food sources differs widely, and cooking destroys significant amounts. For individuals who shop infrequently and obtain out-of-date produce, there is some risk of folate deficiency because food folic acid is sensitive to processing, preparation, and storage. Alcohol intake damages the intestinal mucosa, and prolonged abuse, often of an episodic nature, is associated with folate deficiency. The first indication of folate deficiency is usually a macrocytic anemia, and later megaloblastosis may become more widespread throughout the gastrointestinal tract. Drugs that interfere with folate metabolism, the classic example of which is methotrexate, also produce manifestations of folic acid deficiency. Other important drugs causing folic acid deficiency are diphenylhydantoin and sulfasalazine.

Prevention

Because the bioavailability of folic acid in food sources is about 50% that of the synthetic form in supplements and fortified foods, a new unit has been approved for estimating folic acid intake: the dietary folate equivalent (DFE). One microgram of DFE can be derived from 1 μg of folic acid contained in food, 0.5 μg of folic acid taken on an empty stomach, or 0.6 μg of folic acid taken with a meal.

The current DRI for folic acid is 300 to 400 μg per day in males 9 years old and older and the same in females. Furthermore, it is recommended that during pregnancy and lactation, the DRI be increased to 600 and 500 μg, respectively. During pregnancy the blood volume is greatly increased and folate reserves may be strained, and for this reason folate intake should be greatly increased. For infants the DRI is 65 to 80 μg per day and for children of ages 1 to 8 years it is 150 to 200 μg per day.

A new dimension to the role of folic acid during pregnancy has been the recognition that the frequency of neural tube defects, such as spina bifida and anencephaly, may be reduced by daily consumption of 400 μg of folic acid. The folic acid must be consumed during the first 4 weeks of pregnancy to be effective, a period of time in which most women are unlikely to be aware of being pregnant. Furthermore, in the United States, approximately 50% of pregnancies are unplanned. With these considerations in mind, the Centers for Disease Control and Prevention recommended that "all women of childbearing age in the United States who are capable of becoming pregnant should consume 400 μg of folic acid per day for the purpose of reducing their risk of having a pregnancy affected with spina bifida or other NTDs [neural tube defects]."

Folic acid fortification of foods has been mandated in the United States beginning in 1998. Improvements in diet, food fortification, and the appropriate use of vitamin supplements should all help to prevent folic acid deficiency from becoming widespread. Increased folic acid intake, in turn, may be beneficial not only in the prevention of neural tube defects, but also possibly in diminishing the prevalence and severity of atherosclerosis in all of its manifestations. There is now evidence that folic acid may also have a protective role in preventing certain forms of cancer, such as those involving the epithelium of the uterine cervix, upper airway, breast, and colon.

Treatment

Folic acid deficiency can be treated by consistently adhering to a diet rich in folate-containing items, such as liver; yeast; green, leafy vegetables; legumes; and fruits. Care must be taken not to destroy food folates during food preparation and storage.

Therapeutic doses in the range of 1 to 2 mg per day can be administered to correct folate deficiency rapidly. In patients receiving anticonvulsant drugs, larger doses may be required to reverse the megaloblastic anemia that may result. One potential risk in administering excessive amounts of folic acid is that it may interfere with the diagnosis of vitamin B_{12} deficiency. At dose levels in excess of 1 mg per day, folic acid may correct the anemia from the deficiency of vitamin B_{12} but not delay the progression of neurologic deterioration. Thus, in cases in which combined vitamin deficiency is suspected, vitamin supplementation should include both vitamin B_{12} and folic acid.

VITAMIN B_{12} DEFICIENCY

Vitamin B_{12} deficiency is discussed in the treatment section in the article on pernicious anemia.

VITAMIN A DEFICIENCY

The best known function of vitamin A is in vision; a cascade of reactions involving vitamin A and its derivatives, particularly retinal, has been clearly defined. Vitamin A has important functions in other areas, including cellular differentiation, e.g., embryogenesis and spermatogenesis; sensations (taste); immunity; and growth.

Deficiency of vitamin A is of crucial importance as a worldwide nutritional problem because it is a cause of blindness in approximately half a million preschool children each year in the developing countries. In these areas the diet is composed primarily of such items as rice, wheat, maize, and tubers that contain far from adequate amounts of vitamin A precursors. The World Health Organization and other foundations and groups have made great efforts to plan programs to identify people at risk and to institute appropriate preventive measures on a broad scale.

Clinical deficiency of vitamin A may be overt or subclinical. In either instance, deficient children manifest increased incidence of serious and life-threatening infections and elevated mortality rates. It has been recognized that deficient vitamin A status is a risk factor for the maternal-to-fetal transmission of human immunodeficiency virus: the relative risk of transmission of this virus is fourfold greater in vitamin A–deficient than vitamin A–sufficient mothers.

Vitamin A deficiency in the United States is identified largely with certain risk groups: the urban poor; elderly persons, particularly those living alone; abusers of alcohol; patients with malabsorption disorders; and other persons with a poor diet. Vitamin A deficiency is generally found in a setting in which there are multiple vitamin and mineral deficiencies. Special attention must be paid to deficiency of zinc, a frequent finding in alcoholism, which interferes with the mobilization of vitamin A from its storage sites in liver. This effect is achieved by blocking the release of holo–retinol-binding protein from the liver.

The physician must keep in mind that deficiency of vitamin A in the United States may also develop after the long-term use of several medications. Drug-induced nutritional deficiencies in general, particularly those involving vitamin A, occur most frequently among elderly persons because they use medications in the largest number and for the most prolonged duration and may have borderline nutritional status to begin with. Among the drugs that are most relevant to compromising vitamin A status are mineral oil, which dissolves this nutrient; other laxatives, which accelerate intestinal transit and may diminish the rate of vitamin A absorption; cholestyramine and colestipol, which bind vitamin A; and, under certain conditions, neomycin and colchicine.

Prevention

Deficiency of vitamin A can be prevented by a diet high in carotenes, which serve as precursors to vitamin A. The carotenes, particularly β-carotene, are derived from plant sources, the richest of which are palm oil; carrots; sweet potatoes; dark-green, leafy vegetables; cantaloupe; oranges; and papaya. Vitamin A itself (preformed vitamin A) is derived from animal sources, such as dairy products, meat, and fish. The commercial preparations of fish oils are rich, sometimes too rich, as sources of preformed vitamin A.

The RDA for vitamin A is expressed in terms of retinol equivalents (RE): i.e., 1 RE is equal to 1 μg of all-*trans*-retinol or 6 μg of β-carotene.* The RDAs are 1000 μg RE for males and 800 μg RE for females from ages 11 to 51+ years. For infants the RDA is 375 μg RE and for children 1 to 10 years of age it is 400 to 700 μg RE. This standard nomenclature is nevertheless rarely found on vitamin bottles, on which the former system of IU is used. Expressed in this manner, the RDAs for vitamin A are 5000 IU for men and 4000 IU for women. Some authorities believe that because currently 1 IU of vitamin A is equal to 0.3 μg of all-*trans*-retinol, the RDA is actually 3333 IU for men and 2667 IU for women.

The nutritional value of dietary sources of vitamin A may be compromised when the food items are subject to oxidation, particularly in the presence of light and heat. Antioxidants, such as vitamin E, may prevent the loss of vitamin A activity.

Treatment

Vitamin A deficiency has been treated worldwide with single injections of massive amounts (100,000 to 200,000 IU) repeated at intervals of approximately 6 months to 1 year. Such doses have been effective and are associated with remarkably little toxicity, perhaps because body stores are so depleted at the time of therapy. These doses, however, may produce acute toxic symptoms in well-nourished persons.

Clinical vitamin A deficiency in the United States can be treated with either β-carotene, if there is normal body conversion to vitamin A, or vitamin A itself. Daily doses in the range of 25,000 IU of β-carotene are being consumed by many healthy individuals without apparent toxicity of any kind. The yellowish discoloration of the skin associated with prolonged use of β-carotene is not harmful. Vitamin

*These figures are based on the 1989 edition of the RDAs. At this writing the official RDIs for vitamin D have not been released.

A, in contrast, is quite toxic when ingested in amounts considerably higher than the RDA, especially for prolonged periods. It is probably advisable not to exceed two to three times the RDA for vitamin A in planning a treatment program. Congenital malformations, a particularly disturbing consequence of vitamin A overdosage, have been reported in women consuming 25,000 to 50,000 IU daily during pregnancy. The lowest dose of vitamin A that would be completely safe as a supplement for pregnant women is not known. Therefore, it is not a good idea for pregnant women to take supplementary vitamin A unless there are specific indications, such as malabsorption, or proven deficiency. Many advisory groups caution that the maximal intake of preformed vitamin A consumed during pregnancy should not exceed 10,000 IU.

At present, there is widespread interest in other therapeutic applications of vitamin A and its derivatives. Large doses of vitamin A have been found to reduce morbidity and mortality rates among children suffering from severe cases of measles. Certain forms of leukemia have been found to respond to derivatives of vitamin A. The therapeutic potential of this vitamin is being expanded greatly in studies of the chemoprevention and treatment of cancer. The toxicity of large doses of vitamin A itself places important limits on its feasibility in cancer prevention. Attention has turned to β-carotene and related agents, which in addition to their role as precursors of vitamin A have strong antioxidant activity and other effects as well.

Diminished prevalence of certain cancers has been found among people whose intake of fruits and vegetables is quite high; this finding has been attributable at least in part to the high content of carotenoids in the diet. Many phytochemicals have been found in fruits and vegetables that have potential health benefits. There is some evidence that a combination of antioxidants (i.e., vitamin E, vitamin C, and β-carotene) may be more effective than any of these agents singly. This area of research is innovative and exciting, but it is still too early to make firm recommendations for cancer prevention in the general public in the United States, particularly because prospective trials of β-carotene in cancer prevention have yielded disappointing results. Many other substances in fruits and vegetables appear to hold promise for cancer prevention.

VITAMIN D DEFICIENCY

Vitamin D occurs in two major forms, vitamin D_2 (ergocalciferol), a compound that is produced by irradiation of plant sterols, and vitamin D_3 (cholecalciferol), which is produced in the skin. Scientists are becoming increasingly aware of the important nutritional role of the skin in manufacturing vitamin D_3 under the influence of solar ultraviolet light.

Vitamin D_3 itself is relatively inert biologically and must be converted into active metabolites to exert its major effects. In the liver, vitamin D is converted to 25-hydroxyvitamin D_3, $25(OH)D_3$. Subsequently, in the kidneys, $25(OH)D_3$ is converted to 1,25-dihydroxyvitamin D_3, $1,25(OH)_2D_3$, the most important and active derivative. A less active vitamin D derivative, the 24,25-dihydroxy form, $24,25(OH)_2D_3$ is also produced from $25(OH)D_3$ in the kidney and other tissues. $1,25(OH)_2D_3$ is a secosteroid, and it has many properties of a steroid hormone. Indeed, vitamin D is considered to have hormonal properties.

There are three major sites of action of vitamin D in regulating calcium metabolism. Its best known action is to increase the absorption of calcium, both dietary and secreted, from the intestinal tract. At low doses of vitamin D, the amount of calcium absorbed is linear to the dose given. The second major site of action is bone, where together with parathyroid hormone it stimulates osteoclastic bone resorption. Under a wide variety of conditions, both physiologic and pathologic, the serum calcium level can be maintained within a narrow range at the expense of the calcium derived from bone. The third major site of action of vitamin D is the kidney tubule, where it increases the reabsorption of calcium.

Deficiency of vitamin D occurring in infancy and childhood is manifested as rickets, with severe developmental abnormalities. Vitamin D deficiency occurring during adult life is central to the pathogenesis of osteomalacia. In a general way, deficiency of vitamin D can result from inadequate intake from dietary sources; diminished synthesis in the skin; intestinal malabsorption, as occurs in a variety of diseases; accelerated catabolism, as caused by certain drugs; and defects in the conversion of vitamin D into its active derivatives. In a rare genetic disorder, vitamin D–resistant rickets, type II, the abnormality appears to reside not in the synthesis of the active derivatives but in target organ resistance to their action.

Prevention

Deficiency of vitamin D can be prevented by an adequate diet, conditions favorable to skin synthesis of the vitamin, or both. Studies suggest that exposure of small amounts of skin (e.g., the hands and face), for several minutes to the summer sun is enough to meet the nutritional needs of the body. Thus, prolonged exposure of the body to sunlight is not necessary to achieve optimal vitamin D synthesis. The goal of preventing skin cancer by avoiding excessive skin exposure to sunlight and consequent sunburn remains compatible with the goal of exposing enough skin to sunlight to achieve adequate synthesis of vitamin D. In northern cities, such as Boston, winter sun appears to be ineffective in promoting vitamin D synthesis in the skin. Furthermore, the ability of the skin to synthesize vitamin D is diminished with aging.

In the United States, where some foods, particularly milk, are fortified with vitamin D, sources of calcium and vitamin D often become consumed together. In children as well as in adults, having a quart of skim milk per day, with its 10 μg of cholecalciferol (400 IU), is a good way to ensure satisfactory vitamin D intake. If adequate amounts of dairy products are not consumed, a good case can be made, especially for older people, for the consumption of an additional 400 to 800 IU in the form of a supplement together with calcium.* With persons exposed to abundant sunlight, dietary sources become less important nutritionally, and it is difficult to set an RDA for vitamin D in such persons. Nevertheless, many conditions often prevail that limit the optimal synthesis of vitamin D in the skin. Air pollution and sunscreens prevent ultraviolet light from reaching the skin. Staying indoors or walking in shaded areas precludes any beneficial effects of sunlight. In addition, as noted previously, exposure to winter sun in northern cities does little to enhance vitamin D synthesis in skin. The amount of 10 μg of cholecalciferol has been set as the RDA in males from 6 months of age until the age of 24 years, after which 5 μg is advised. For females, similar recommendations are made except that all pregnant and lactating women are advised to consume 10 μg of cholecalciferol. For infants 0 to 6 months of age the RDA is 7.5 μg per day.

Treatment

The goal in the treatment of vitamin D deficiency is to restore bone structure and function to normal and to correct serum concentrations of calcium if inadequate. Rickets, the form of vitamin D deficiency in infants and children, as well as osteomalacia, the manifestation of vitamin D deficiency in adults, responds to the administration of vitamin D if calcium intake is also adequate. For this reason, the physician must first determine that calcium intake is at the level of 1 to 2 grams per day as elemental calcium, in the form of either food sources rich in calcium or supplementation.

The initial doses of vitamin D to be administered in either rickets or osteomalacia are in the general range of 400 to 4000 IU per day. Most authorities recommended 2000 to 4000 IU with supplementary calcium. As a frame of reference, a quart of milk is supplemented with 400 IU of vitamin D. Thus, consuming a diet high in milk and dairy products is a good way to treat vitamin D deficiency if continued consistently for an adequate time. Probably several months of treatment at these high doses is needed, after which daily doses in the range of 400 to 800 IU are generally adequate. During the treatment period, it is essential to provide exposure to sunlight and to encourage physical exercise of a weight-bearing nature that will facilitate the normal mechanisms of bone renewal.

In the event that the deficiency of vitamin D is complicated by intestinal malabsorption, larger doses of vitamin D in the range of 10,000 to 25,000 IU or higher may be required. Water-soluble preparations of vitamin D are now available and can be administered parenterally if necessary. More calcium, in the range of 2 to 3 grams per day, is also needed. An important consideration to keep in mind is that in some instances of hypocalcemia associated with malabsorption, the provision of supplementary magnesium renders the hypocalcemia more sensitive to treatment with calcium and vitamin D. If severe liver disease is present in association with vitamin D deficiency, larger doses of vitamin D are also needed because, as mentioned earlier, the initial conversion of vitamin D to $25(OH)D_3$ occurs in liver. If the patient requires certain drugs that bind bile salts (such as cholestyramine) or that increase vitamin D catabolism (such as phenytoin), larger doses are required for adequate therapy of the vitamin D deficiency.

Vitamin D deficiency complicated by renal disease is only poorly responsive to treatment with vitamin D, because the $1,25(OH)_2D_3$ derivative is formed inadequately from precursor in the renal parenchyma. For this reason, $1,25(OH)_2D_3$ (calcitriol [Rocaltrol]) must be given. Most patients respond quite satisfactorily to doses in the 0.5- to 1.0-μg range per day. A similar strategy of treatment is required in autosomal recessive vitamin D–dependent rickets, type I, in which there is a selective genetic defect in the conversion of $25(OH)D_3$ to $1,25(OH)_2D_3$. Much higher doses than these must be tried in the case of vitamin D–dependent rickets, type II, in which the defect is in the receptor response to $1,25(OH)_2D_3$. Patients with renal disease complicating the vitamin D deficiency also require other ancillary measures, such as phosphate restriction.

VITAMIN E DEFICIENCY

The most widely recognized role for vitamin E is as a scavenger of free radicals, and in this capacity it protects cell membranes from damage. It has many other properties as well. Vitamin E is essential for the immune system, particularly T lymphocytes, and has a role in DNA repair. Interest is growing in the effect of vitamin E on inhibiting oxidation of low-density lipoprotein (LDL): oxidized LDL is quite atherogenic. The neuromuscular system and the retina also require vitamin E for optimal function. The role of vitamin E as an antioxidant in health and disease is under intensive study at present.

Dietary vitamin E deficiency tends to be unusual under ordinary circumstances, as sources of vitamin E are widely available from the food supply. The recognizable cases of vitamin E deficiency tend to arise in debilitated patients who have had severe and prolonged periods of fat malabsorption. The reason is that vitamin E is incorporated into chylomicrons with other products of fat absorption. Any process that interferes with fat digestion and absorption also impairs absorption of vitamin E.

Other disorders in which symptomatic vitamin E deficiency may develop include cystic fibrosis, celiac disease, cholestatic liver disease, short-bowel syn-

*These figures are based on the 1989 edition of the RDAs. At this writing the official RDIs for vitamin D have not been released.

drome of any cause, and unusual genetic disorders mentioned later. Major abnormalities of neurologic function are observed in severe and prolonged vitamin E deficiency with evidence of involvement of the posterior column and spinocerebellar tract. Patients display areflexia, ophthalmoplegia, and disturbances of gait, proprioception, and vibration. In premature infants, vitamin E deficiency results in hemolytic anemia, thrombocytosis, edema, and intraventricular hemorrhage. There is increased risk of retrolental fibroplasia and bronchopulmonary dysplasia.

In hemolytic anemia, such as glucose-6-phosphate dehydrogenase deficiency and sickle cell anemia, vitamin E levels in blood tend to be decreased. Inborn errors of vitamin E metabolism have been identified. In one disorder, familial isolated vitamin E deficiency, there are severe neurologic abnormalities. Because of a genetically determined defect in incorporation of dietary vitamin E into the lipid transport protein very-low-density lipoprotein, vitamin E is cleared rapidly from plasma. In another genetic disorder, abetalipoproteinemia, there is a defect in the serum transport of vitamin E. A hallmark of this disease is the finding of an extremely low serum cholesterol level together with a very low serum level of vitamin E.

Prevention

Deficiency of vitamin E can be avoided by regular consumption of the many sources of this vitamin in the food supply. The richest sources of vitamin E in the U.S. diet are vegetable oils, including corn, cottonseed, safflower, and soybean oils, and the margarines and other products made from these oils. Green, leafy vegetables are also good sources of vitamin E. In evaluating the adequacy of any given dietary regimen, one should keep in mind that losses of the vitamin occur during storage, cooking, and food processing, particularly with exposure to high temperatures and oxygen.

Because vitamin E deficiency occurs as a result of severe intestinal malabsorption, it is essential to identify this condition early and to avoid measures that may intensify the degree of malabsorption. For example, cholestyramine (Questran) and colestipol (Colestid), resins used in the treatment of hypercholesterolemia, cause malabsorption of vitamin E and should be used only when strictly indicated.

The RDA for vitamin E has been set at 10 mg α-tocopherol equivalents (TEs) per day for males aged 11 years and older and at 8 mg α-TEs per day for females aged 11 years and older.* It is recommended that women consume 10 mg α-TEs per day during pregnancy and 11 to 12 mg α-TEs during lactation. The RDA for infants is 3 to 4 mg α-TEs per day and for children 1 to 10 years of age it is 6 to 7 mg α-TEs per day. The storage capacity of the body for vitamin E is quite considerable.

*These figures are based on the 1989 edition of the RDAs. At this writing the official RDIs for vitamin E have not been released.

There is a great deal of contemporary interest in the potential role of vitamin E in the prevention of heart disease, one mechanism of which may be the inhibition of LDL oxidation described previously. Studies are actively being pursued to determine whether vitamin E alone or in combination with other agents is effective not only in the prevention of heart disease, but also in the prevention of cataracts, cancer, and other disorders of aging.

Treatment

Vitamin E deficiency can be treated satisfactorily with oral preparations of the vitamin. There is a wide margin of safety in the therapeutic administration of the vitamin. Daily doses of vitamin E in the range of 100 to 800 mg can be given safely to nearly all deficient patients. This dose range can be used appropriately in those patients with vitamin E deficiency diagnosed in association with celiac disease, inflammatory bowel disease, or other chronic and prolonged forms of intestinal malabsorption. In such instances, many other nutrient deficiencies are likely to be found in association with that of vitamin E, and they too necessitate treatment.

In the genetic disorders of vitamin E metabolism, such as isolated vitamin E deficiency, higher doses of the vitamin, in the range of 800 to 1000 mg and higher, must be taken. Large doses of vitamin E given therapeutically can be quite safe. Some investigators have suggested that pharmacologic doses of vitamin E may possibly interfere with the intestinal absorption of vitamins A and K, but there are few data with which to evaluate this potential risk. There are reports that doses of vitamin E in excess of 1200 mg per day may interfere with the action of vitamin K and intensify the actions of anticoagulant drugs.

VITAMIN C DEFICIENCY (SCURVY)

Vitamin C is a powerful water-soluble antioxidant, and there is much contemporary interest in this action of the vitamin. Vitamin C is involved in lipid and vitamin metabolism, facilitates the intestinal absorption of nonheme iron, and is involved in collagen metabolism, biosynthesis of neurotransmitters, wound healing, immune function, and many other aspects of normal health. Vitamin C is a cofactor or substrate for eight known enzymes. Important physical properties of vitamin C include its sensitivity to prolonged storage and cooking at high temperatures, common events that greatly decrease biologic potency. As an antioxidant, vitamin C is destroyed by oxidation, as in exposure to air.

Vitamin C deficiency in its early stages gives rise to fatigue and lethargy, followed by petechiae and ecchymoses, follicular hyperkeratosis, and swollen and bleeding gums. Later there are arthralgias and joint effusions. Corkscrew hairs may be recognizable characteristics. Wounds heal poorly, and healed wounds have been observed to reopen.

Prevention

The best dietary sources of vitamin C are citrus fruits and green, leafy vegetables, particularly broccoli, green peppers, and cabbage. Tomatoes are also a good source. As noted earlier, care must be taken in proper food preparation and storage.

Vitamin C deficiency is common among urban poor persons, who may not be able to afford the fresh fruits and vegetables that constitute important sources. Vitamin C deficiency is also common among elderly persons, who may shop infrequently and allow produce to be stored longer than optimal. Food faddism, particularly the macrobiotic diet, adherents of which regularly subject food to pressure cooking, results in serious vitamin C deficiency. A "tea and toast" diet is virtually devoid of sources of vitamin C. Scurvy develops in alcoholic patients if their diet is deficient in food items containing vitamin C. Thus, much vitamin C deficiency could be prevented by making good dietary sources available to urban poor, elderly, and other persons on a subsistence economy; by ensuring that prolonged storage is avoided; by preventing alcohol abuse; and by learning proper food habits generally.

The RDA has been established at 50 to 60 mg per day in both males and females 11 years of age and older, at up to 70 mg per day in pregnancy, and at 90 to 95 mg per day during lactation.* These estimates are considered generally to be quite generous, as doses as low as 10 mg per day have been adequate in treating scurvy. It has been suggested that a new RDA of 200 mg per day more accurately reflects the amounts needed to saturate tissue stores. The RDA for infants is 30 to 35 mg per day and it is 40 to 45 mg per day for children 1 to 10 years of age.

Treatment

In approaching the treatment of scurvy, it is essential to recognize the nutritional deficiency before it becomes extreme. Early symptoms and signs, such as weakness, lethargy, and general malaise, are nonspecific. Pain in the bones and joints, perifollicular hemorrhages, and petechiae should alert the physician to the strong likelihood of scurvy. Swollen, bleeding gums indicate advanced disease, as does edema, oliguria, and peripheral neuropathy.

As noted earlier, as little as 10 mg per day of vitamin C can treat scurvy satisfactorily, but it is advisable to begin with larger amounts, in the range of 100 to 200 mg per day. Significant improvement should be noted within several days. A good diet is obviously crucial for recovery and for maintenance of health. Such doses should be safe to administer for weeks to months if necessary to restore health to normal.

Rare inborn errors of metabolism, including osteogenesis imperfecta, tyrosinemia, and Chédiak-Higashi syndrome, have in case reports been ameliorated by doses in the range of 50 to 200 mg per day. Further experience is needed in the management of these disorders before guidelines can be definitive. Vitamin C at the level of 0.5 to 2 or 3 grams per day has been used to acidify urine. In smaller amounts (40 to 100 mg), ascorbic acid is recommended to increase the intestinal absorption of nonheme iron. Patients following a strict vegetarian diet should be encouraged to consume orange juice with their meals, because the 40 to 50 mg contained in a glass of orange juice increases the bioavailability of iron from vegetable sources significantly. However, ascorbic acid decreases the absorption of copper. Care must be taken to avoid giving potentially toxic doses of vitamin C, and restricting therapeutic doses to the 1- to 2-gram range should minimize this possibility.

Inasmuch as vitamin C is widely used as a supplement by the general public, a word of caution is indicated. The gene for hemochromatosis is widely prevalent, and in individuals who have this gene, there may be a tendency to absorb excessive amounts of iron. Measurements of serum ferritin levels readily identify a state of excess iron stores.

There is great contemporary interest in the potential use of vitamin C alone or in combination with the other antioxidant vitamins, β-carotene and vitamin E, in the possible prevention of cancer, heart disease, certain manifestations of aging, and other conditions. This is an active area of research, and further investigations are necessary before recommendations for the general public as well as for the management of specific disorders can be advanced.

*These figures are based on the 1989 edition of the RDAs. At this writing the official RDIs for vitamin C have not been released.

VITAMIN K DEFICIENCY

method of
MARTIN J. SHEARER, Ph.D.
Haemophilia Centre, St. Thomas's Hospital, London, England

The parent structure of the vitamin K group of compounds is 2-methyl-1,4-naphthoquinone (common name, menadione). The naturally occurring K vitamins that are synthesized by plants and bacteria all share this naphthoquinone ring structure but differ in the structure of the side chain at the 3-position. In plants the only major form is phylloquinone (vitamin K_1) with a phytyl side chain. Bacteria synthesize a family of menaquinones (vitamin K_2) with side chains of repeating prenyl units, the number of units being given as a suffix (i.e., menaquinone-n [MK-n]). Menadione (vitamin K_3) is not a natural constituent of foods but does possess biologic activity in vertebrates because of their ability to add on a geranylgeranyl side chain at the 3-position to produce MK-4. Synthetic menadione, as a water-soluble salt, is widely used as a feed supplement in animal husbandry and, therefore, may enter the human food chain indirectly, either unchanged or as preformed MK-4.

The major dietary source of vitamin K is the plant form phylloquinone. Good sources are green vegetables such as kale, parsley, spinach, and cabbage (300 to 600 μg per 100 grams), broccoli, Brussels sprouts, and lettuce (100 to 200 μg per 100 grams), and certain vegetable oils such as soybean, rapeseed, and olive oils (50 to 200 μg per 100 grams). In the Western diet, the only significant dietary sources of menaquinones (10 to 20 μg per 100 grams) are cheeses (MK-8 and -9), animal livers (mainly MK-7 and MKs 10–13), and meat (MK-4).

Bacteria in the human intestine synthesize menaquinones (MKs 4–13), and long-chain menaquinones compose about 90% of human liver stores. The hepatic profile of menaquinones suggests that they originate from intestinal synthesis rather than the diet. However, the physiologic importance of this potentially large hepatic pool of menaquinones to vitamin K function and requirements remains uncertain.

Dietary vitamin K is absorbed from the proximal intestine after solubilization into mixed micelles composed of bile salts and the products of pancreatic lipolysis. In healthy adults, the efficiency of absorption of phylloquinone in its free form is about 80% but is less than 10% from green leafy vegetables such as spinach. Once absorbed, dietary vitamin K enters the circulation with chylomicrons and is cleared rapidly. After an overnight fast, more than half of the circulating vitamin K (mainly phylloquinone at concentrations of about 0.5 μg per liter) is still associated with triglyceride-rich lipoproteins. The bioavailability of the potentially large reservoir of intestinally synthesized menaquinones is low because the vast majority is bound to bacterial membranes, and even when free these highly lipophilic forms of menaquinones are poorly absorbed.

Vitamin K is metabolized extensively by the liver to side-chain–shortened metabolites that are excreted in the bile and urine. Approximately 60 to 70% of phylloquinone absorbed from a single meal is lost to the body by excretion within a few days, suggesting that the body stores are being replenished constantly. Further evidence for this rapid turnover of phylloquinone comes from the finding that hepatic reserves decline rapidly in surgical patients who have been placed on a low phylloquinone diet. In contrast, hepatic reserves of menaquinones seem more resistant to dietary restriction.

The only established role for vitamin K is as a cofactor for a post-translational modification in a diverse group of calcium-binding proteins, whereby selective glutamic (Glu) residues are transformed into γ-carboxyglutamic acid (Gla). The best characterized vitamin K–dependent proteins (also known as Gla-proteins) are listed in Table 1. They include the four classic vitamin K–dependent procoagulants (factors II, VII, IX, and X) and two feedback anticoagulants (proteins C and S), all synthesized by the liver.

Gla-proteins also occur in several other tissues. Osteocalcin, synthesized by the osteoblasts of bone, is one of the 10 most abundant proteins in the body and may play a role in regulating bone turnover. Matrix Gla-protein is more widely distributed, and there is now good evidence that this protein is an important inhibitor of calcification of arteries and cartilage. Gla residues provide efficient chelating sites for calcium ions that enable vitamin K–dependent proteins to bind to other surfaces (e.g., procoagulants to platelet and vessel wall phospholipids and osteocalcin to the hydroxyapatite matrix of bone). The carboxylation reaction is catalyzed by a microsomal vitamin K–dependent γ-glutamyl carboxylase, which requires the dietary quinone form of vitamin K to be first reduced to the active cofactor vitamin K hydroquinone (KH_2). The subsequent oxidation of vitamin KH_2 to vitamin K 2,3 epoxide (KO) provides the energy for the carboxylation. The epoxide metabolite thus generated is recycled back to vitamin K by a vitamin K epoxide reductase, thus conserving tissue stores of vitamin K. Oral anticoagulant drugs exert their effect by blocking the vitamin K epoxide reductase, resulting in the tissue accumulation of vitamin K epoxide. A second, warfarin-insensitive, vitamin K reductase activity provides an alternate, less efficient pathway for generating vitamin KH_2 from dietary vitamin K in the presence of oral anticoagulants. Therapeutic anticoagulation is dependent on achieving a balance between the inhibition of the recycling enzymes and the amount of dietary vitamin K that can enter the cycle to support carboxylation at a reduced efficiency.

TABLE 1. **Distribution and Roles of Vitamin K–Dependent (Gla) Proteins**

Gla-Protein	Tissue	Role
Prothrombin (factor II), factors VII, IX, and X	Liver (then plasma)	Procoagulants
Protein C	Liver (then plasma)	Anticoagulant
Protein S	Liver (then plasma), endothelium, bone	Anticoagulant role as cofactor for protein C Role in bone unknown
Osteocalcin (or bone Gla-protein)	Bone	Unknown, may be a matrix signal for osteoclasts
Matrix Gla-protein	Bone, cartilage, and most soft tissues	Unknown, may be a mineralization inhibitor

CAUSES OF VITAMIN K DEFICIENCY

Overt vitamin K deficiency in adults, resulting in clinical bleeding, is almost unknown except as a consequence of underlying disease, most commonly resulting from hepatointestinal disorders that lead to malabsorption by obstructing bile flow (e.g., common duct stones, carcinoma of the bile ducts and pancreas). Also at risk are hospitalized patients with a poor nutritional staus, particularly in the postoperative period when food intake may be absent or low and antibiotics are being given. Patients who have had gastrointestinal surgery or have renal failure are particularly susceptible to vitamin K deficiency. The traditional explanation for the effect of antibiotics is that they interfere with menaquinone production by the intestinal flora, but this is controversial. Certain antibiotics containing an *N*-methyl-thiotetrazole side chain (e.g., cefamandole, cefoperazone) have been shown to be inhibitors of vitamin K epoxide reductase, and although this coumarin-like antagonism is weak, it can precipitate bleeding in patients with marginal dietary intakes and impaired vitamin K status. Other drugs that may induce vitamin K deficiency in nutritionally compromised people are salicylates, anticonvulsants, and megadoses of vitamin E.

The use of oral coumarin anticoagulant drugs such as warfarin (Coumadin) in the prevention and management of thromboembolic disease is a special case of deliberately induced vitamin K deficiency with the aim of reducing the circulating levels of the vitamin K–dependent clotting factors to within a predetermined target range depending on the clinical condition. Accidental or deliberate poisoning with coumarin or indanedione anticoagulants, including the class of rodenticides known as "superwarfarins," is another possible cause of vitamin K deficiency.

BLEEDING IN INFANTS CAUSED BY VITAMIN K DEFICIENCY

Bleeding due to vitamin K deficiency may occur spontaneously in the first few months of life. This syndrome is traditionally known as hemorrhagic disease of the newborn or, more recently, vitamin K–deficiency bleeding (VKDB). The classification of VKDB, presenting features, and etiologic factors, when known, are listed in Table 2. Late VKDB has a peak incidence around the third to sixth week of life and remains a significant worldwide cause of infant morbidity and mortality because about half the patients present with intracranial hemorrhage. Reasons for the marginal vitamin K status of neonates include poor placental transfer, low concentrations in breast milk, and a sterile gut at birth that delays the nutritional impact of menaquinones. In some infants, late VKDB is the first sign of liver dysfunction and may reflect a previously undiagnosed hereditary disease. In others, VKDB may be triggered by a transient and self-correcting cholestasis.

LABORATORY TESTS

Routine screening tests for overt vitamin K deficiency are based on global coagulation assays such as the prothrombin time (PT) or activated partial thromboplastin time (APTT) that reflect a decreased activity of one or more of the four vitamin K–dependent procoagulants. Although simple to perform, such tests are neither specific nor sensitive. Inherent to the PT is its insensitivity, becoming prolonged only when the prothrombin concentration drops below 50%. Rarely, to rule out a single or combined congenital deficiency of the vitamin K–dependent factors, it may be necessary to perform individual assays for factors II, VII, IX, and X. The most useful confirmatory test of overt vitamin K deficiency is to show that the PT can be readily reversed by vitamin K administration.

The most sensitive tests of vitamin K deficiency or antagonism are based on the detection of circulating undercarboxylated (des-γ-carboxy) species of vitamin K–dependent proteins that are collectively known as PIVKA (proteins induced by vitamin K absence or antagonism). Enzyme immunoassays for des-γ-prothrombin (DCP or PIVKA-II) provide a powerful marker of subclinical vitamin K deficiency with respect to its coagulation role because undercarboxylated prothrombin species can be detected well before any changes occur in conventional clotting tests. The measurement of circulating undercarboxylated osteocalcin (ucOC) by immunoassay provides a sensitive marker of vitamin K sufficiency with respect to the carboxylation status of bone Gla-proteins. There is a growing body of evidence that an increase in ucOC has pathophysiologic significance for bone health insofar as ucOC measurements are predictive of both hip fracture risk and of bone mineral density in elderly women.

PREVENTION

The recommended dietary allowance (RDA) for the coagulation role of vitamin K is currently 1 μg per kg of body weight per day. Intakes of this order are sufficient to prevent the appearance of DCP in the circulation by the most sensitive assays. However, there is evidence that higher dietary intakes are needed to ensure the complete carboxylation of ostecalcin. The possible benefits of intakes above the current RDA to bone health and the amelioration of osteoporosis (or the prevention of arterial vascular calcification) are the subjects of ongoing research.

Patients who have poor oral intakes or are being fed parenterally (especially those on antibiotic therapy) should be given periodic intramuscular or intravenous injections of a drug formulation of phylloquinone (phytonadione). A dose of 10 mg of phytonadione (AquaMEPHYTON) given intravenously is protective for about 1 week. The intramuscular route may be advantageous in providing a depot store and gradual release.

The benefits of giving phytonadione at birth to prevent neonatal VKDB are now well established, but the route of administration is controversial because of an earlier epidemiologic study specifically linking the intramuscular route to childhood cancer. Several subsequent studies have not confirmed this association. A single dose of 1 mg of phytonadione given intramuscularly at birth is of proven efficacy against the late-onset form of VKDB, but repeated doses are necessary for full protection if given orally. This is especially relevant for those infants who may have a reduced efficiency of absorption owing to underlying and unrecognized cholestasis.

TREATMENT

The treatment of bleeding caused by vitamin K lack or antagonism depends on the site of bleeding, its severity, and, in the case of metabolic blockade, the potency of the causative agent. Nonemergency bleeding is readily correctable by giving phytonadione intramuscularly or, if there is a contraindication to intramuscular injection, by slow intravenous injection (1 mg for neonates, 5 to 10 mg for adults), after which the coagulation test results will normalize within a few hours. A regimen for the correction

TABLE 2. **Classification of Neonatal Vitamin K–Deficiency Bleeding (VKDB)**

VKDB Syndrome	Time of Presentation	Common Bleeding Sites	Etiologic Factors
Early	0–24 hours	Cephalohematoma, intracranial, intrathoracic, intra-abdominal	Maternal drugs (e.g., warfarin, anticonvulsants)
Classic	1–7 days	Gastrointestinal, skin, nasal, circumcision	Mainly idiopathic, breast-feeding (may be related to low milk intakes)
Late	1–12 weeks	Intracranial, skin, gastrointestinal	Mainly idiopathic, breast-feeding, some degree of cholestasis often present; may reflect underlying disease (e.g., biliary atresia, $alpha_1$-antitrypsin deficiency, cystic fibrosis)

of nonemergency bleeding during oral anticoagulant therapy must consider that too large a dose of vitamin K will result in a refractory period that may make the reestablishment of stable therapeutic anticoagulation difficult. For this group, 0.5 to 1.0 mg of phytonadione should be given intravenously. More serious bleeding may require fresh-frozen plasma (FFP) at doses of 10 to 20 mL per kg of body weight in addition to vitamin K. Depending on the degree of hemostatic correction achieved, a repeat dose or doses of phytonadione (10 mg) may be necessary; usually this may be given orally (Mephyton). A disadvantage of this FFP and phytonadione regimen is that the reversal of the hemostatic defect may take hours rather than minutes to achieve. Furthermore, the correction of factor IX levels by FFP may be especially poor and cannot be assessed from PT measurements alone. When immediate and complete correction is required, as in life- or limb-threatening hemorrhage, the use of clotting factor concentrates (containing factors II, VII, IX, and X), instead of FFP, is strongly indicated. Plasma products should be used with caution because of the risk of transmitting pathogenic viruses. Appropriate care and precautions should be taken when injecting vitamin K intravenously to minimize the small risk of anaphylactoid reactions from the solubilizing agent. The ingestion of "superwarfarins" presents special problems to patient management because of their high potency and tissue longevity. Treatment of the early phase of poisoning with these agents often requires FFP or factor concentrates and the repeated intravenous administration of 10 to 20 mg of phytonadione every few hours; thereafter, it may be necessary to give a daily dose of phytonadione for weeks or months to maintain a normal PT.

OSTEOPOROSIS

method of
J. C. GALLAGHER, M.D.
St. Joseph Hospital
Omaha, Nebraska

There has been increasing awareness of the importance of osteoporosis among the general population and also among health care professionals. This is because osteoporosis is a common disease that causes hip fractures in a third of all women and a fifth of all men and causes vertebral fractures in as many as 30 to 40% of women and half as many men. In addition, several other fractures are now recognized as osteoporotic, including fractures of the humerus, pelvis, ribs, and radius (Colles'). Approximately 1.3 million osteoporotic fractures occur annually; of these, about 250,000 are hip fractures. It appears that in several countries, including the United States and Canada, there is an increase in the age-adjusted incidence rates of these fractures, and because a larger proportion of men and women now survive past the age of 75 years, it means that many more persons will be at high risk for hip fractures in the future. In fact, the absolute number of hip fractures may quadruple during the next 30 years. Since the cost of a single hip fracture is close to $40,000, one can appreciate the large economic impact of the serious osteoporotic fractures, and the economic impact will become even more considerable in the next 30 years.

Most osteoporotic fractures occur because of a loss of bone from the fracture sites. In most cases, the fracture is associated with a traumatic fall, particularly with fractures of the hip, wrist, humerus, and pelvis. A traumatic fall is not usually reported in the history of vertebral fractures, which tend to be associated with bending and lifting, or to occur spontaneously.

Osteoporosis can be classified as either primary or secondary. Primary osteoporosis is due to the typical age-related loss of bone from the skeleton, and secondary osteoporosis is associated with well-known causes of bone loss such as corticosteroid therapy, anticonvulsant therapy, marked vitamin D deficiency, malabsorption syndromes, and hyperthyroidism. In various series of osteoporotic patients, secondary osteoporosis accounts for about 40% of the total number of osteoporotic fractures seen by a physician.

NUTRITIONAL REQUIREMENTS FOR CALCIUM AND VITAMIN D

Calcium given alone appears to be relatively ineffective in preventing bone loss during the early postmenopausal period. There is evidence that calcium is more effective in reducing the rate of bone loss in women 10 to 20 years past menopause. This suggests that there are factors operating in the early postmenopausal period that make inhibition of bone resorption more difficult to accomplish. Most studies of calcium supplements in the early postmenopausal period show continuing bone loss with intakes of 1500 to 2000 mg per day. Some of the results suggest that even in older women, calcium supplements are effective only if the calcium intake is low, i.e., less than 500 mg per day. This stresses the importance of having an adequate nutritional intake of calcium during the postmenopausal era since it suggests that the rate of bone loss may be increased in women whose calcium intake is extremely low. The National Osteoporosis Foundation has recommended that the calcium intake of postmenopausal women be 1500 mg daily. However, scientific support for this recommendation is not strong for women in the early postmenopausal period; in older women, it may reduce the rate of bone loss by 25 to 30%, although bone loss still continues. A significantly low calcium intake is found in 25% of the U.S. and Canadian female population. A common cause of low calcium intake in the general population is inadequate intake of dairy products. Inadequate intake is often related to the presence of varying degrees of lactose intolerance, so that the consumption of milk products is avoided; in addition, most people do not drink milk. In nutritional surveys, milk as a source of calcium accounts for about 30% of the total daily calcium intake. Thus, for ensuring an adequate calcium intake in the diet, all nutritional sources are important.

If calcium supplements are used, calcium preparations available include calcium carbonate, phosphate, citrate, lactate, and gluconate. These preparations are fairly similar in bioavailability of calcium, except for citrate, for which bioavailability is slightly higher. Calcium carbonate is one of the cheapest forms of calcium available. The two major side effects experienced with calcium carbonate supplementation are constipation and gaseous distention. If a patient develops symptoms from calcium carbonate, then calcium citrate (Citracal) is usually better tolerated. Use of calcium lactate or calcium gluconate is uncommon because the amount of elemental calcium in these preparations is relatively small, so that a large number of tablets must be consumed. The approximate amounts of elemental calcium per preparation are 40% for calcium carbonate, 33% for calcium phosphate, 25% for calcium citrate, 9% for calcium lactate, and 9% for calcium gluconate.

VITAMIN D SUPPLEMENTATION

Absorption of calcium from the intestine is normal in most women up to the age of 65. However, after age 65, there is a gradual decline in the intestinal ability to absorb calcium. Therefore, older women may benefit from additional supplements of vitamin D. Younger women obtain most of the required vitamin D from sunlight and milk (which is fortified with vitamin D in the United States and Canada). Older women who tend to stay indoors more and who do not drink milk are at a higher risk of vitamin D deficiency, and it is recommended that elderly persons take vitamin D, 400 to 800 IU per day. Any of several tablet combinations of calcium and vitamin D can be used. If it is suspected that a patient with osteoporosis also has osteomalacia, this should be confirmed by measurement of serum 25-hydroxyvitamin D. A value of less than 12 ng per mL is suspicious, and a value of less than 7 ng per mL is nearly always associated with osteomalacia. There is an increased risk for osteomalacia in persons who have had bowel surgery, take anticonvulsants, or avoid the sun and do not drink milk. Osteomalacia responds well to vitamin D, 400 IU daily.

PREVENTION AND TREATMENT OF OSTEOPOROSIS

Estrogen and Hormone Replacement Therapies

The mainstay for osteoporosis prevention in postmenopausal women is the use of estrogen replacement therapy (ERT) or hormone replacement therapy (HRT) using estrogen plus progestin. Several highly significant studies over the last decade show the effectiveness of HRT in the prevention of postmenopausal bone loss. In general, the effect on bone of a progestin added to estrogen is similar to the effect of estrogen only. There is some evidence that norethindrone,* which is a progestin not commonly used in North America, has an additional antiresorptive effect on the skeleton, resulting in an extra 2 to 3% increase in bone mineral density.

Table 1 summarizes the average doses of estrogen used to prevent postmenopausal bone loss. Although these doses are commonly referred to as minimal effective doses, this is in fact not the case. When the individual responses with the suggested doses are taken into account, 10 to 15% of women are found to actually lose bone, although probably the rate of bone loss is reduced. The minimal effective dose of estrogen also varies according to the number of years past menopause. Women who are within the first 5 years of menopause need an estrogen dose twice as large as women in their 70s or 80s to prevent bone loss. There is some evidence that when a calcium supplement is combined with ERT or HRT, there is a synergistic effect on bone mineral density (BMD), probably increasing BMD by another 1 to 2%. Typically, a woman within the first 5 years of menopause will show an increase in spine density of approximately 5% and an increase in femoral neck density of 2 to 3% on the doses of estrogen given in the table. In elderly women, aged 70 to 80 years, the increase in spine density is 7 to 8% and the increase in femoral neck density is 5 to 6%.

There are a number of options for the administration of estrogen to postmenopausal women. First of all, for women who have had a hysterectomy, it is necessary to treat only with estrogen. However, a significant proportion of women who have a uterus opt to take only estrogen therapy because they do not like the progestational side effects, and they need endometrial biopsies annually. For most women with a uterus, two common regimens are used. The first one is to administer estrogen for most days of the calendar month, together with cyclical progestins administered for the last 12 to 14 days of that cycle. It has been shown that the progestins given cyclically for only 10 days may still be associated with an increase in the risk of endometrial cancer. The other common regimen is the use of continuous combined HRT in which the estrogen and progestin pills are given every day of the year. A third regimen that has some popularity is to administer the estrogen every day but to give the cyclical progestin every third or fourth month.

So far as side effects are concerned, the two most common problems are fluid retention, which leads to bloating and breast tenderness, and the occurrence of

TABLE 1. **Minimal Effective Doses of Estrogen in Increasing Bone Mineral Density**

Preparation	Spine	Femur
Conjugated equine estrogens (Premarin)	0.625 mg	0.625 mg
Esterified estrogens (Estratab)	0.3 mg	0.3 mg
Estropipate (Ogen)	0.625 mg	1.25 mg
17β-Estradiol (Estrace)	1 mg	?
Transdermal estradiol (Estraderm)	50 μg	50 μg
Transdermal estradiol (Vivelle)	25 μg	25 μg

*Not FDA approved for this indication.

bleeding or spotting. For women who develop breast tenderness and fluid retention, we would usually use a diuretic such as hydrochlorothiazide, 25 mg, administered 3 to 4 days a week until symptoms have been relieved. Occasionally women with breast tenderness will need a reduction in the estrogen dose. Although some women attribute their breast tenderness to a progestin side effect, we have found that increasing the dose of progestin may lead to relief of breast tenderness. With regard to uterine bleeding, use of a cyclical regimen leads to regular monthly bleeding in 80 to 90% of the women, whereas continuous combined therapy causes spotting or bleeding in 30% of the patients; however, with the continuous regimen, the problem of spotting and bleeding tends to decrease over time, particularly after the first 6 months. Bleeding problems are more troublesome nearer the menopause, and some physicians opt to use cyclical therapy at that time because it causes predictable bleeding, whereas with continuous combined therapy, it is difficult to predict when spotting or bleeding may occur. Despite the high incidence of bleeding with a cyclical regimen or a continuous combined regimen, histologic examination of the endometrium shows no obvious cause. More than 95% of the patients show an atropic endometrium, and it is not clear why bleeding has occurred. Only rarely has a patient been found to have endometrial hyperplasia on either a 12-day cyclical or continuous combined regimen. It may be that in these cases, the cause of hyperplasia is not necessarily hormone-dependent.

The most common progestin used in North America to oppose the estrogen effect on the uterus is medroxyprogesterone acetate (Provera), either 2.5 or 5 mg daily. If the 5-mg dose is used for the cyclical regimen of 14 days, a small number of patients may still develop proliferative endometrium or hyperplasia, and a 10-mg dose may be safer. For the continuous regimen, the 2.5-mg dose appears to be effective in preventing hyperplasia of the endometrium when the progestin is used on a continuous basis. The other main type of progestin used is norethindrone. Although it is not commonly used in North America, it is quite widely used in Europe. The reason for the lack of use of norethindrone in this country has been its propensity to reduce HDL cholesterol levels.

Calcitonin

Like estrogen, calcitonin is another antiresorptive agent. In the last several years, we have seen the gradual replacement of calcitonin injections by nasal calcitonin (Miacalcin nasal spray). In studies of early postmenopausal women in North America, Miacalcin nasal spray has not been found to be effective in the prevention of early bone loss. However, in older women, Miacalcin nasal spray appears to be effective in the prevention of bone loss, and BMD generally increases by 1 to 2% at the spine and femur sites. Results of previous studies of the effect of nasal calcitonin in reducing fracture incidence in patients with established osteoporosis have been mixed, with some showing no effect and others showing significant effect. Unfortunately, all of these studies were small. There is a large ongoing multicenter study of Miacalcin nasal spray in osteoporotic patients in North America. An interim analysis after 3 years found that Miacalcin nasal calcitonin in a dose of 200 μg per day significantly reduced the incidence of new vertebral fractures. However, the other doses of 100 and 400 μg per day did not significantly reduce fracture incidence. The trial will continue for an additional two years, and these issues may become clearer at that time. My interpretation of the data is that calcitonin is probably effective in reducing fracture incidence on the 200-μg dose, and this can be safely used. Systemic side effects are minor. Facial flushing tends to decrease with time, and the major problem is difficulty in using the nasal spray in patients who have seasonal allergies.

Bisphosphonates

The first member of the bisphosphonate group, available for 20 years, is etidronate* (Didronel). This drug has been approved for the treatment of osteoporosis in several countries, including Canada, but not in the United States. This was because a pivotal trial of 400 osteoporotic patients showed that etidronate effectively increased BMD of the spine by 5% and of the femoral neck by 3% but failed to reduce fracture incidence significantly. On the other hand, subgroup analysis showed that the effect of etidronate in reducing fractures became significant if the analysis was conducted on patients with the lowest BMD. Cyclical administration of etidronate is easy to accomplish. Patients take etidronate, 400 mg daily, for 14 days every 3 months and during the intervening weeks take a calcium supplement of 1 gm per day. Etidronate should not be used on a long-term daily basis because it can produce osteomalacia in bone. There has been no evidence of osteomalacia in patients receiving cyclical etidronate therapy. The option of using etidronate creates a dilemma, because there is an increase in BMD but no clearly significant effect on fracture incidence, and it is not approved by the U. S. Food and Drug Administration (FDA). The most likely explanation for the lack of a clear-cut effect of etidronate in these studies is that the sample size in the trial was not large enough to allow detection of significant differences between treatment and placebo.

Alendronate (Fosamax) is a more potent bisphosphonate than etidronate and is approved by the FDA for the prevention and treatment of osteoporosis. Several studies conducted in early postmenopausal women (i.e., within 7 years of menopause) have shown that 5 mg of alendronate is the minimal effective dose for preventing postmenopausal bone loss, and the drug has been approved at this dose by the FDA. For older women, the minimal effective dose of

*Not FDA approved for this indication.

alendronate that prevents bone loss is 10 mg. It is interesting that this is exactly the opposite of the situation noted with estrogen, where higher doses are needed in early menopause and lower doses in the later postmenopausal years. Alendronate in a dose of 10 mg results in a gradual increase of bone mineral density of 5 to 7% in the spine and 3 to 5% in the femoral neck. Part of the increase in bone density occurs during the first year, and most of the increase occurs during the second year, with a slight increase in density in the third year. Some studies have shown a significant decrease in radial density and total body calcium, suggesting that in the first year of treatment, there is redistribution of calcium from cortical to trabecular areas of the skeleton. This decrease in total body calcium appears to be reversed at the end of the first year; however, the decrease in radial density continues during the second and third years, although the decrease is less than that seen with the placebo group. In all of these studies, alendronate was combined with a calcium supplement of 500 mg per day, and calcium may be an important adjunctive therapy for optimizing the effect of alendronate on bone. The major problem with alendronate is its low absorption, less than 1% of the dose, so that it is important to have the patient swallow the tablet first thing in the morning and then wait 30 to 45 minutes before having any food. The tablet must be taken with water and cannot be swallowed with orange juice, milk, or coffee since this reduces absorption even further. Surprisingly, most patients are tolerant of this restriction and quickly become used to the regimen. One of the more serious reported side effects has been the development of esophageal ulcers. Although there are trials showing no increased incidence of esophageal ulcers in the alendronate-treated versus placebo groups, nevertheless, many clinicians who treat osteoporotic patients find that esophageal ulceration is a distinct entity in alendronate-treated patients. It is probably important to reduce the risk by making sure that patients are not using concomitant nonsteroidal anti-inflammatory drugs (NSAIDs) for pain and do not have a history of peptic ulceration. Also, the presence of a hiatus hernia with reflux esophagitis may define a group that is at higher risk for developing esophageal irritation or ulceration. The manufacturer recommends that patients sit up or stand up for 30 minutes after taking the tablet.

Other bisphosphonates under evaluation include tiludronate (Skelid) and risedronate (Actonel). Although tiludronate has been shown to be effective in the treatment of Paget's disease, a recent phase III trial of several hundred osteoporosis patients was halted after analysis failed to show any significant change in bone density or reduction in vertebral fracture incidence in patients treated with tiludronate. Therefore, it is unlikely that this agent will be available for the treatment of osteoporosis in the near future. It has been suggested that the reason for the failure of tiludronate was that the dose used in the trial was too small. Risedronate is undergoing extensive clinical trials at the present time. Studies of the use of risedronate in women with low spine BMD have shown that risedronate exhibits a dose-response effect on bone density. A 2.5-mg dose increased spine density by approximately 3%, and a 5-mg dose increased spine density by almost 5%; similar dose-response effects were seen in the femoral neck and femoral trochanter. Similar studies also looked at the dose-response relation for risedronate in early and late postmenopausal women and found the increase in BMD to be twice as great in the older women as in the younger women when both received the lower (2.5-mg) daily dose of risedronate. On the 5-mg dose, the increase in BMD was slightly larger in the older women. Fracture efficacy studies are ongoing and may be expected to yield final results in 1998.

Another bisphosphonate that is undergoing investigation at the present time is ibandronate; phase III clinical studies on osteoporosis have just started. The drug is given as an intravenous push in the office every 3 months. On a theoretical basis, it appears to be a very potent bisphosphonate, but its clinical effect in fracture studies will not be elucidated for another 3 years.

Combination Therapy

Although many physicians ask about the concomitant use of estrogen and bisphosphonates, there are no substantial data at the present time on which one could pass judgment. Studies are under way and may be expected to provide an answer within two years.

Vitamin D Metabolites

The vitamin D metabolites 1,α-hydroxyvitamin D_3 and 1,25-dihydroxyvitamin D_3 are extensively used in Japan and other parts of Asia where they are the agents of first choice for the treatment of osteoporosis. They have had limited use in North America, apart from their administration to patients with chronic renal failure on dialysis. One of the largest osteoporosis studies to date, carried out in New Zealand, showed that 1,25-dihydroxyvitamin D_3 (Rocaltrol), 0.25 mg twice daily, significantly reduced the incidence of new vertebral fractures over a period of 3 years. The effect on BMD is relatively small, increasing spine density and total body calcium by 1 to 2%. Other studies have shown that 1,25-dihydroxyvitamin D_3 effectively reduces corticosteroid-induced bone loss. So far as side effects are concerned, there are very few, but theoretically, patients can develop hypercalcemia and hypercalciuria. These are uncommon clinical side effects and usually only occur if 1,25-dihydroxyvitamin D_3 is combined with a large calcium supplement. We recommend that 1,25-dihydroxyvitamin D_3 be used at a dose of 0.25 μg twice daily, and the calcium intake should not exceed 1000 mg daily. Most patients rarely exceed this limit unless they are given calcium supplementation.

Sodium Fluoride

Sodium fluoride has been used in the treatment of osteoporosis for many years, but its efficacy remains unclear. There is no doubt that sodium fluoride increases BMD quite remarkably. In our experience, about 70% of female patients and 95% of male patients show an average increase in BMD of the spine of 5% per year, or 20% over 4 years. Yet in two major studies, there was no decrease in the incidence of vertebral fractures in patients treated with fluoride despite an increase of BMD of 20% in the spine. The criticism of these studies was that the dose of fluoride used was 75 mg per day, which produced an osteomalacic change in bone. Lower doses of fluoride have been used—in particular, slow-release sodium fluoride, 25 μg twice daily. Like ordinary sodium fluoride, it increases BMD density 15 to 20% over 4 years and has been reported to reduce the incidence of vertebral fractures significantly. These studies are small in patient numbers, and the results need to be confirmed in a larger trial. When sodium fluoride is used, it must be combined with 1500 mg of elemental calcium daily to reduce the development of osteomalacia. It has been suggested that the risk of fluoride-related osteomalacia can be decreased by discontinuation of the fluoride for 2 months every year. Patients should receive fluoride plus calcium for 12 months, followed by calcium only for 2 months; then the cycle should be repeated. Some studies have reported an increase in peripheral fractures and hip fractures in patients on fluoride, but as suggested earlier, this could be due to the development of osteomalacia in bone.

Growth Hormone

There have been limited clinical trials that failed to show efficacy of growth hormone in increasing bone density or reducing fracture incidence. A fairly high incidence of side effects has been reported with growth hormone therapy.

Testosterone Therapy

One small study has shown that testosterone increases BMD 3 to 5% in the spine over a period of 2 years. This study was too small for a fracture study, so there are as yet no data on its efficacy in fracture prevention. Testosterone probably works like estrogen, mainly as an antiresorptive agent, and on theoretical grounds should be a suitable drug for men with osteoporosis. The problems with testosterone therapy are well known: An increase in prostate size and prostatic hyperplasia, sleep apnea, and polycythemia have been reported. More controlled studies need to be conducted on the use of testosterone therapy in men with osteoporosis.

Tibolone

Tibolone is a unique steroid hormone that has weak estrogenic, progestational, and androgenic side effects. It is approved for the treatment of osteoporosis in certain European countries and is presently finishing phase III clinical trials in the United States and Canada where it is being evaluated for the prevention of osteoporosis. There are no ongoing fracture studies at this time. In the European studies, tibolone was shown to increase BMD by 6%, with significantly better results than in the placebo group. Tibolone has a low incidence of side effects, and the drug appears to be well tolerated. Despite its partial estrogenic profile, it rarely causes endometrial stimulation and bleeding. This drug may have a potentially useful role as an alternative antiresorptive agent in older women who are unable to tolerate estrogens or bisphosphonate therapy.

FOLLOW-UP WITH TREATMENT FOR OSTEOPOROSIS

If the patient response to all medications were 100%, then follow-up of patients with osteoporosis would be fairly simple. However, that is not the case. For example, it has been estimated that BMD continues to decrease in 10 to 20% of patients on typical doses. Therefore, BMD should be monitored until there is a satisfactory response. We usually repeat BMD studies after 1 year and again after 2 years for the immediate response to therapy and then after 5 years to assess the long-term response. For various reasons, peripheral measurement of bone density (radius, metacarpals, phalanges, os calcis) may not always reflect the changes that occur in the spine and femur. Accurate measurement of standing height provides useful information on whether vertebral osteoporosis is being adequately treated. The average untreated patient with vertebral fracture loses height at the rate of 1 cm per year.

Another test that is undergoing evaluation as a marker of therapeutic response is the urine excretion of collagen crosslinks (assays by Metra, BS, or Ostex). This test is slightly more specific than hydroxyproline assay for measuring bone resorption. For monitoring therapeutic response, urine crosslinks can be remeasured at 6 and 12 months. Urine crosslinks should decrease into the lower quartile of the normal range to indicate a satisfactory antiresorptive effect. It should be noted that in untreated women, higher urine crosslinks do predict higher rates of bone loss and vice versa.

In summary, the use of BMD measurements or the response of urinary bone markers to therapy can allow the physician to assess the patient's response to therapy.

PAGET'S DISEASE OF BONE

method of
ROBERT D. TIEGS, M.D.
Mayo Clinic
Rochester, Minnesota

Paget's disease is a chronic skeletal disorder characterized by increased bone remodeling and abnormal bone architecture. The pathologic process is initiated by osteoclasts that are abnormal in morphology and function. In Paget's disease, osteoclasts are extremely large, containing up to 100 nuclei (a normal osteoclast contains 5 to 10 nuclei), and have increased bone-resorbing activity. The increase in resorption results in a compensatory increase in bone formation and accelerated bone turnover. Bone that is remodeled by this pathologic process is formed haphazardly and appears as a disorganized mosaic of woven and lamellar bone. Ultimately, pagetic bone becomes enlarged, mechanically weakened, and highly vascular.

The etiology of Paget's disease is unknown. Epidemiologic studies have documented a marked variation in the geographic distribution of the disease, suggesting a dominant influence of environmental and ethnic factors. Paget's disease is most common in western Europe (excluding Scandinavia), Australia, New Zealand, and North America. In contrast, Paget's disease is rare in Asia and most of Africa. In the United States, Paget's disease is believed to affect 2 to 3% of the population older than 60 years of age. A number of investigators have identified a familial aggregation of Paget's disease. From available data, it appears that familial cases are diagnosed earlier, have more extensive involvement, and probably have more aggressive disease.

A viral etiology for Paget's disease was first suggested by the presence of nuclear and cytoplasmic inclusions in pagetic osteoclasts. These inclusions resemble the paramyxovirus family of viruses and have been shown by immunohistochemical studies to contain measles virus, respiratory syncytial virus, and parainfluenza virus antigens. A variety of molecular techniques have been used to explore the role of viruses in Paget's disease and have produced conflicting results. Current epidemiologic data support the concept that Paget's disease may arise from an interaction of environmental factors, exposure to paramyxovirus, and genetic susceptibility.

CLINICAL FEATURES

Paget's disease usually develops after age 40 and is rarely diagnosed in individuals younger than 25 years of age. The disease may be monostotic or polyostotic with asymmetrical involvement. Although new sites rarely become involved after the initial diagnosis, the disease may progress at a given location. In long bones, the pathologic process may progress from one periarticular surface and eventually involve the entire bone. The pelvis, femur, spine, tibia, skull, humerus, and forearm are most frequently involved. Other commonly involved sites are the clavicle, scapula, ribs, and facial bones. The hands and feet are rarely affected.

Most patients with Paget's disease are asymptomatic. In symptomatic patients, bone pain is the most common symptom. The pain is typically characterized as dull and aching, is present at rest, and may be exacerbated by weight bearing if present in the back, pelvis, or lower extremity. Patients with skull involvement frequently complain of headache or a bandlike discomfort. Bone pain associated with Paget's disease is believed to be caused by mechanical factors (e.g., periosteal elevation and intraosseous pressure) and possibly by chemical stimulation of sensory receptors (nociceptors) by interleukin-6 or other mediators. Other causes of pain in Paget's disease include arthritis, fractures, and neural compression. Pagetic involvement adjacent to a joint predisposes to the development of secondary arthritis, which commonly affects the hips, knees, and ankles.

Deformity in patients with long-standing Paget's disease typically occurs in long bones and the skull. The spectrum of skeletal deformities includes bowing deformities of long bones, acetabular protrusion of the hips, frontal bossing, skull enlargement, kyphosis, and scoliosis. Fissure or stress fractures may occur along the convex surfaces of bowed long bones. These fractures may be asymptomatic or may cause focal discomfort.

Pathologic fracture is a common complication of Paget's disease. The most common sites for pathologic fracture are the femur and tibia. The spine and humerus are less frequently involved. Although the rate of healing is usually normal, healing may be complicated by delayed union.

The increased vascularity that is present in active disease is associated with increased skin temperature and may cause the patient discomfort. Increased vascularity of pagetic bone may also result in excessive blood loss during orthopedic surgery and may produce syndromes resembling myelopathy or radiculopathy on the basis of a vascular steal phenomenon. High-output cardiac failure can occur in patients with extensive skeletal involvement and increased cardiac output but probably only develops in individuals with underlying cardiac disease.

Involvement of the skull is associated with a mixed sensory and conductive hearing loss and less commonly with cranial nerve palsies. Severe, long-standing skull involvement may result in platybasia with basilar invagination. This deformity may be complicated by obstructive hydrocephalus, brain stem compression, or both. Involvement of the facial bones may result in dental, visual, and olfactory complications. Other neurologic complications include radiculopathy and spinal stenosis.

Malignant degeneration in Paget's disease probably occurs in less than 1% of patients. Most of the tumors are osteogenic sarcomas. Fibrosarcomas, chondrosarcomas, and malignant fibrous histiocytomas have also been reported. Malignant degeneration typically manifests as a change in symptoms (e.g., new pain, intensified pain, or pain that has changed in character) or as a pathologic fracture. On radiography, these lesions appear as areas of cortical destruction with an associated soft tissue mass. Diagnosis of these tumors is frequently delayed, and the clinical course is usually rapid and fatal. The most frequent sites of malignant degeneration are the pelvis, humerus, femur, and craniofacial bones.

Giant cell tumors are benign neoplasms that develop in patients with Paget's disease. These tumors usually occur in the skull or facial bones and occasionally in long bones, and they respond to glucocorticoid therapy.

DIAGNOSTIC STUDIES

Biochemical markers of bone turnover are useful for monitoring therapy. Although there is no ideal marker of bone turnover, there are disease-specific differences in the utility of these markers. Serum alkaline phosphatase is a marker of bone formation and in Paget's disease is an accurate indicator of bone turnover and disease activity. Bone-specific alkaline phosphatase has a slightly better diagnostic accuracy than the total serum alkaline phosphatase activity and should be used for evaluating and monitoring patients in whom the alkaline phosphatase may be affected by extraskeletal sources of the enzyme (e.g., patients with abnormal liver function tests).

Osteocalcin is a noncollagenous vitamin D–dependent protein of bone that is predominantly a marker of bone formation but, for reasons that remain unclear, is not a reliable indicator of pagetic activity. Urinary markers of bone resorption, such as hydroxyproline, pyridinium cross-links, and the *N*-telopeptide of type I collagen, are sensitive and early indicators of therapeutic response and can be used to monitor disease activity in patients with a predominantly lytic process and normal serum alkaline phosphatase levels. With the use of newer, more potent antipagetic agents, changes in markers of bone resorption can be detected in days, whereas the serum alkaline phosphatase nadir may lag for 3 months. Most patients can be monitored using a single variable of bone turnover.

The appearance of Paget's disease on routine bone radiographs is sufficient to establish the diagnosis in most cases. On radiographic examination, pagetic bone typically has a thick, coarse, trabecular pattern with mixed lytic and sclerotic areas. In addition, the bone is expanded with widening of the marrow cavity and thickening of the cortex. Early in the disease, patients may present with predominantly lytic disease characterized by an osteolytic wedge-shaped lesion advancing along a long bone or osteoporosis circumscripta involving the skull.

Radioisotope bone scanning is the most sensitive means of identifying sites of pagetic involvement. Clinicians should consider obtaining a bone scan at the time of presentation to define the extent of involvement. Because the findings on bone scan are nonspecific, plain bone radiographs are needed to confirm pagetic involvement in areas with increased isotope uptake.

Repeat bone scans and radiographs are usually unnecessary during follow-up but should be considered when (1) new symptoms develop; (2) current symptoms become significantly worse, suggesting the possibility of an impending fracture or, rarely, malignant degeneration; or (3) a fracture is suspected.

TREATMENT

The management of Paget's disease has benefited from the development of potent inhibitors of osteoclast-mediated bone resorption. Antiresorptive agents that can be used in the management of Paget's disease include calcitonin, bisphosphonates, plicamycin, and gallium nitrate.

When treating symptomatic patients, the clinician is challenged to identify patients who are likely to benefit from antiresorptive therapy. Patients with bone pain and increased warmth associated with hypervascularity respond well to antipagetic agents, whereas patients with arthritic pain may benefit from treatment with nonsteroidal anti-inflammatory drugs.

Treatment of asymptomatic patients who are at risk for developing complications has been proposed because of the progressive nature of the disease, the severity of its complications, and the observation that controlling the activity of the disease is associated with restoration of a more normal bone architecture. Individuals at risk for complications include patients with active disease (e.g., alkaline phosphatase levels two to three times the upper limits of normal) and involvement at sites where complications are likely to develop (e.g., skull, spine, long bones, areas near major joints). The serum alkaline phosphatase should not be used as an indication of disease activity in patients with predominantly lytic disease or in patients with limited skeletal involvement. Because the risk of complications is related to life expectancy, age and medical status also should be considered when deciding whether treatment is advisable.

The following indications for treatment have been proposed based on theoretical considerations and the clinical experience of experts in the field: (1) presence of symptoms likely to respond to antipagetic therapy (e.g., patients with bone pain, increased warmth, head discomfort related to skull involvement; selected patients with symptoms caused by neural compression); (2) prevention of local progression and future complications; and (3) preoperative treatment of patients scheduled for elective orthopedic surgery involving pagetic bone.

If the goal of treatment is to control disease activity in an attempt to prevent complications, the biochemical indices of bone remodeling should be maintained within the normal range whenever possible. Relapse has been defined arbitrarily as a 25% increase in the serum alkaline phosphatase (or other marker of bone turnover) above the prior nadir or above the upper limit of the normal range. If patients show evidence of recurrent disease activity, they can generally be retreated with the same drug regimen that induced the initial remission. Because there may be some loss of responsiveness with each successive cycle of therapy, clinicians should consider using a higher dose of the same drug or a different medication if the patient has a suboptimal response or does not respond to treatment.

In addition to periodic clinical assessment, biochemical indices of bone remodeling should be measured to determine the response to treatment and the need for retreatment. The frequency of follow-up testing depends on the severity of the disease and the presence of complications. When monitoring patients with active disease, clinicians should assess biochemical markers of bone remodeling at approximately 3- to 6-month intervals.

Calcitonin

Calcitonin is a polypeptide hormone secreted by C cells of the thyroid. In pharmacologic doses, calcitonin inhibits osteoclast-mediated bone resorption. Since its introduction in the early 1970s, calcitonin has been used extensively to treat Paget's disease. At present, the only form of calcitonin available in the United States is synthetic salmon calcitonin (Calcimar, Miacalcin) that has been formulated for parenteral and intranasal use. Human calcitonin was withdrawn from the market because of production problems. At this time, there are no plans to reintroduce this product.

The usual starting dose for salmon calcitonin is 100 units injected subcutaneously daily. Symptoms typically improve during the first few weeks of therapy. After a response has been achieved, the dose can be reduced in some patients to 50 to 100 units every other day or three times weekly with maintenance of the response. Patients with moderate or severe disease may require continuous treatment. A disadvantage of calcitonin is the relatively rapid loss of therapeutic effect after discontinuing treatment compared with bisphosphonates, which have the potential to induce a prolonged remission. Calcitonin and etidronate have similar response rates; a 50% lowering of the biochemical markers of bone turnover can be achieved in approximately two thirds of patients. Patients with severe disease are less likely to respond to initial treatment with calcitonin. Secondary failures occur after a variable period. In some patients, the loss of response is due to the development of neutralizing antibodies. These patients usually respond to human calcitonin (Cibacalcin), which is not currently available. When using nasal calcitonin (Miacalcin), 200 to 400 units daily are required to decrease bone turnover in Paget's disease. Nasal calcitonin is not approved for use in Paget's disease.

The most common adverse reactions associated with the use of calcitonin are flushing, especially of the face and upper body, and nausea. These symptoms occur less frequently with the nasal spray than with the injectable calcitonin and can be minimized or avoided by starting with a low dose and gradually titrating the dosage upward or by administering calcitonin at mealtime or bedtime. The nasal spray may cause rhinitis, epistaxis, or sinusitis.

There are no data to indicate that calcitonin is superior to the newer bisphosphonates for the treatment of acute neurologic complications, pain, fissure fractures, or osteolytic lesions.

Bisphosphonates

Bisphosphonates are synthetic analogues of inorganic pyrophosphate (P-O-P) in which oxygen has been replaced by a carbon atom (P-C-P) that has two side chains. Modification of the side chains alters the potencies of the various bisphosphonates. These agents have a strong affinity for calcium phosphate and are potent inhibitors of bone resorption. The intestinal absorption of bisphosphonates is poor (approximately 1%). After absorption, these drugs go primarily to bone and localize at the resorbing surfaces. The residual drug is rapidly excreted in the urine.

Patients with more severe disease, defined by the number of sites involved and the level of the serum alkaline phosphatase, are more resistant to therapy and require higher total doses. The duration of the therapeutic response depends on the degree of suppression of the serum alkaline phosphatase (or other marker of bone turnover). Prolonged remissions have resulted from suppressing the serum alkaline phosphatase into the lower portion of the normal range.

When using bisphosphonates, patient should have an adequate calcium intake to limit the increase in parathyroid hormone, because secondary hyperparathyroidism induced by bisphosphonate therapy may reduce their effectiveness.

Etidronate

The usual dose of etidronate (Didronel) for the treatment of Paget's disease is 5 mg per kg of body weight daily for 6 months administered as a single dose in the middle of a 4-hour fast. This regimen typically lowers the biochemical indices of bone turnover by 50% and results in symptomatic improvement in approximately two thirds of patients. Current recommendations are to treat for 6 months and then to withhold treatment for 6 months. Higher doses have been associated with an increased incidence of fractures and osteomalacia. In view of the potential to impair mineralization, etidronate should be avoided in patients who are planning to undergo orthopedic surgery, who have healing fractures, or who have osteolytic lesions in weight-bearing bones. Etidronate also should be avoided in patients with renal failure. Other adverse reactions include abdominal discomfort and diarrhea. With the emergence of newer bisphosphonates with substantially greater potency that do not impair mineralization at clinically effective doses, etidronate will probably have limited use in the treatment of Paget's disease.

Alendronate

Alendronate (Fosamax) is an orally administered aminobisphosphonate approved for the treatment of Paget's disease. Comparative trials in patients with Paget's disease have established that alendronate is considerably more potent than etidronate. Unlike etidronate, therapeutic doses of alendronate are not associated with abnormal mineralization. For treatment of Paget's disease, alendronate is prescribed at a dose of 40 mg per day for 6 months. The drug should be taken 30 to 60 minutes before the first food, beverage, or medication of the day. Taking alendronate with anything other than water will impair its absorption. To reduce the potential for esophagitis and esophageal ulceration, alendronate should be taken with 6 to 8 ounces of water; the patient should remain upright until food has been ingested; and the drug should be discontinued immediately if esophageal symptoms develop. In addition, alendronate should be avoided in patients with impaired swallowing or abnormal esophageal motility. Following the widespread use of alendronate for osteoporosis, a number of cases of severe esophagitis were reported. In these instances, esophagitis developed in patients who swallowed alendronate with little or no water, lay down after ingesting the drug, continued to take alendronate after the onset of symptoms, and had pre-existing esophageal disorders.

Tiludronate

Tiludronate (Skelid) was recently approved for use in the treatment of Paget's disease. This drug has been shown to be effective for treating Paget's disease when given orally at a dosage of 400 mg per day for 12 weeks. Tiludronate is to be taken as a single, 400-mg daily dose with 6 to 8 ounces of water and should not be taken within 2 hours of food, calcium, aspirin, indomethacin, or antacids. The drug has been shown to be more effective than etidronate; the therapeutic response was not compromised by the prior use of bisphosphonates. Bone biopsy data did not show evidence of impaired mineralization at the recommended dosage. The most common adverse reactions were nausea, vomiting, diarrhea, and dyspepsia.

Pamidronate

Pamidronate (Aredia) is an aminobisphosphonate that is available in the United States only as an intravenous preparation. The oral formulation was withdrawn from the United States market because it caused esophageal and gastric erosions. Intravenous pamidronate has been reported to be effective in a variety of therapeutic regimens and is approved for use in Paget's disease. Responses seem to correlate with total dose rather than with duration of infusion or interval between infusions. In general, patients with more severe disease require a higher total dose and frequently require multiple infusions to achieve maximal suppression of bone turnover. In patients with mild disease, a single 60-mg infusion may completely suppress disease activity, whereas patients with severe polyostotic involvement may require doses of 180 to 480 mg administered over several weeks or months. The dose must be individualized according to the clinical and biochemical response and the goals of therapy. A 60- or 90-mg dose can be administered over 4 hours as an outpatient treatment. Several studies have shown no evidence of impaired mineralization with cumulative doses of pamidronate of up to 2.5 grams. Although mineralization defects have been associated with doses of 180 to 360 mg delivered over 6 to 9 weeks in a small number of cases, the significance of this finding is uncertain. The potency of pamidronate and its rapid onset of action with intravenous administration make it an attractive agent for treating patients with neural compression syndromes.

Adverse reactions associated with intravenous pamidronate infusions are usually mild and include febrile reactions associated with influenza-like symptoms (e.g., fever, malaise, myalgia, headache), transient hypocalcemia, exacerbation of bone pain, venous irritation, uveitis and scleritis, and ototoxicity. Febrile reactions probably occur in 15 to 25% of patients, although higher estimates have been reported. Symptoms begin 1 to 48 hours after the infusion. If this reaction occurs with the initial infusion, it is usually less severe or absent with subsequent infusions.

Other Bisphosphonates Under Development

Residronate is a potent bisphosphonate that has been shown to be effective when administered orally to patients with Paget's disease, including patients refractory to other therapies. Zoledronate and ibandronate are new bisphosphonates that are effective at microgram doses. Clinical investigations are under way using these drugs as an intravenous injection and in a transdermal drug-delivery system. With emergence of more potent bisphosphonates, it should be possible to return bone markers to normal and restore normal new bone formation in most patients.

Plicamycin

Plicamycin (formerly mithramycin) is an antibiotic that has been shown to be effective in treating patients with Paget's disease when administered as a 4- to 8-hour infusion at doses of 15 to 25 μg per kg of body weight per day. Doses are repeated every 2 to 3 days as required. Because plicamycin may cause hepatic, renal, and bone marrow toxicity, its use is limited to patients with severe, refractory disease. Adverse reactions also include nausea and vomiting. The availability of potent new bisphosphonates should eliminate the need for plicamycin in the management of patients with Paget's disease.

Gallium Nitrate

Gallium, a group IIIa metal compound, is an inhibitor of bone resorption. It absorbs to calcium phosphate and localizes to sites of bone remodeling. Bone resorption is inhibited by the reversible inhibition of the adenosine triphosphate–dependent proton pump of osteoclasts. In a recent study, cyclic, low-dose, subcutaneously administered gallium nitrate was effective in reducing bone turnover in patients with Paget's disease. Although patients frequently experience minor discomfort at the injection site, no serious adverse reactions were observed. The role of gallium in the treatment of patients with Paget's disease is yet to be determined.

SUMMARY

With the availability of potent antipagetic agents capable of achieving and maintaining prolonged remissions, management of Paget's disease has undergone considerable change. Until outcome-based research is available, many questions related to the treatment of asymptomatic patients will persist. Based on the available data, the strategy of early treatment of patients with symptoms and asymptomatic patients at risk for complications is justified with the aim of maximally suppressing disease activity.

PARENTERAL NUTRITION IN ADULTS

method of
ELAINE B. TRUJILLO, M.S., R.D., and
DANNY O. JACOBS, M.D., M.P.H.
Harvard Medical School and Brigham and Women's Hospital
Boston, Massachusetts

In the last decade, the field of parenteral nutrition (PN) has matured in a number of ways. The initial excitement of being able to feed quantities of basic nutrients, vitamins, and trace elements intravenously has abated. This can now be done relatively safely and easily. We are now in a renaissance period in which the advent of molecular biologic engineering and other scientific advances are providing us with new tools for nutrition support. We may be able to do much more than just provide adequate nutrients for our patients. A patient's "metabolic" environment may be manipulated to his or her advantage, allowing the practitioner to actively intervene in a patient's recovery process. Therapies that will truly allow us to affect the patient's outcome, sense of well-being, speed of recovery, and rate of rehabilitation may not be available yet, but they are just around the corner.

INDICATIONS AND CONTRAINDICATIONS

Total parenteral nutrition is the provision of all nutrient requirements intravenously and is indicated when feeding through the gastrointestinal (GI) tract is not possible. It does reduce mortality and morbidity for severely malnourished, stressed, or catabolic patients; however, other evidence suggests that it may actually increase complications in patients who are not malnourished. It should be reserved for patients who either are already malnourished, defined as having 10% or more weight loss or 7 days or more of inadequate nutrient intake, or who have the potential for developing malnutrition and who are not candidates for enteral nutrition support. The published guidelines of the American Society of Parenteral and Enteral Nutrition (ASPEN) indicate that PN should be used when enteral feeding techniques have failed to provide some or all of the patient's nutrient requirements or in selected conditions when enteral nutrition support is contraindicated. These conditions include diffuse peritonitis, intestinal obstruction that prohibits use of the bowel, the early stages of short-bowel syndrome, intractable vomiting, paralytic ileus, and/or severe diarrhea that makes metabolic management difficult. Other conditions for which PN may be considered when enteral feeding is not indicated, depending on the clinical circumstances, include pancreatitis, enterocutaneous fistulae, and gastrointestinal ischemia (Figure 1).

In well-nourished patients, PN is not indicated unless the patient has had inadequate nutrient intake for at least 7 days. The body stores of well-nourished individuals are generally sufficient to provide the essential nutrients, resist infection, promote wound healing, and support other necessary physiologic functions within this period. Certain hypermetabolic states such as burn, trauma, and sepsis may warrant the early use of PN regardless of the current nutritional state of the patient. Parenteral feedings should be administered to hypermetabolic patients when enteral access cannot be obtained, when enteral nutrition support fails to meet nutritional requirements, or when feeding into the GI tract is contraindicated.

Parenteral nutrition support is unlikely to benefit a patient who will be able to take enteral nutrition within 4 to 5 days after the onset of illness or who has a relatively minor injury. There are four key steps to consider before initiating PN. These include assessing nutritional status, determining energy needs, evaluating GI function, and estimating the length of time a patient will require PN (Table 1).

NUTRITIONAL ASSESSMENT

Nutrient depletion is associated with increased morbidity and mortality. Given that the prevalence of malnutrition in hospitalized patients is approximately 50%, it is imperative, first, to identify patients who have, or are at risk of developing, protein-calorie malnutrition or specific nutrient deficiencies. The second goal of performing a nutritional assessment is to quantify a patient's risk of developing malnutrition-related medical complications. Finally, it is necessary to monitor the adequacy of nutritional therapy.

Nutritional assessment begins with a thorough history and physical examination in conjunction with selected laboratory tests aimed at detecting specific nutrient deficiencies in patients who are at high risk for future abnormalities. The nutritional assessment should establish whether the patient will need maintenance therapy or nutritional repletion and should assess the status of the patient's GI tract. The latter is important because, as mentioned previously, patients who have a GI tract that can be used safely are best served by enteral alimentation if nutritional support is needed.

The history should include an assessment of recent weight loss or gain, as well as dietary habits to determine whether there have been any significant changes in food intake. It should also be ascertained if there have been any GI symptoms that might preclude a normal food intake or be associated with abnormal losses through the GI tract (e.g., nausea, vomiting, colic, or diarrhea). Finally, the examiner should attempt to determine whether the patient has experienced any changes in his or her exercise tolerance or physical abilities that would indicate changes in functional capacity have occurred. During the physical examination, one looks for a loss of subcutaneous fat and muscle wasting, which are indicative of a loss of body energy and protein stores; edema and ascites, which are also important physical indications of altered energy demands or decreased energy intake; and signs of vitamin and mineral deficits such as dermatitis, glossitis, cheilosis, neuromuscular irritability, and coarse and easily pluckable hair.

The serum albumin concentration is the most widely used indicator of nutritional status and predictor of outcome. The serum albumin concentration differentiates hypoalbuminemic malnutrition from marasmic malnutrition. In marasmus, the serum albumin level should be above 3 grams per dL. Although severe undernutrition may contribute to hypoalbuminemia, the metabolic response to stress and illness is the most significant factor that contributes to depressed serum albumin levels. Although the serum albumin level cannot be restored to normal by

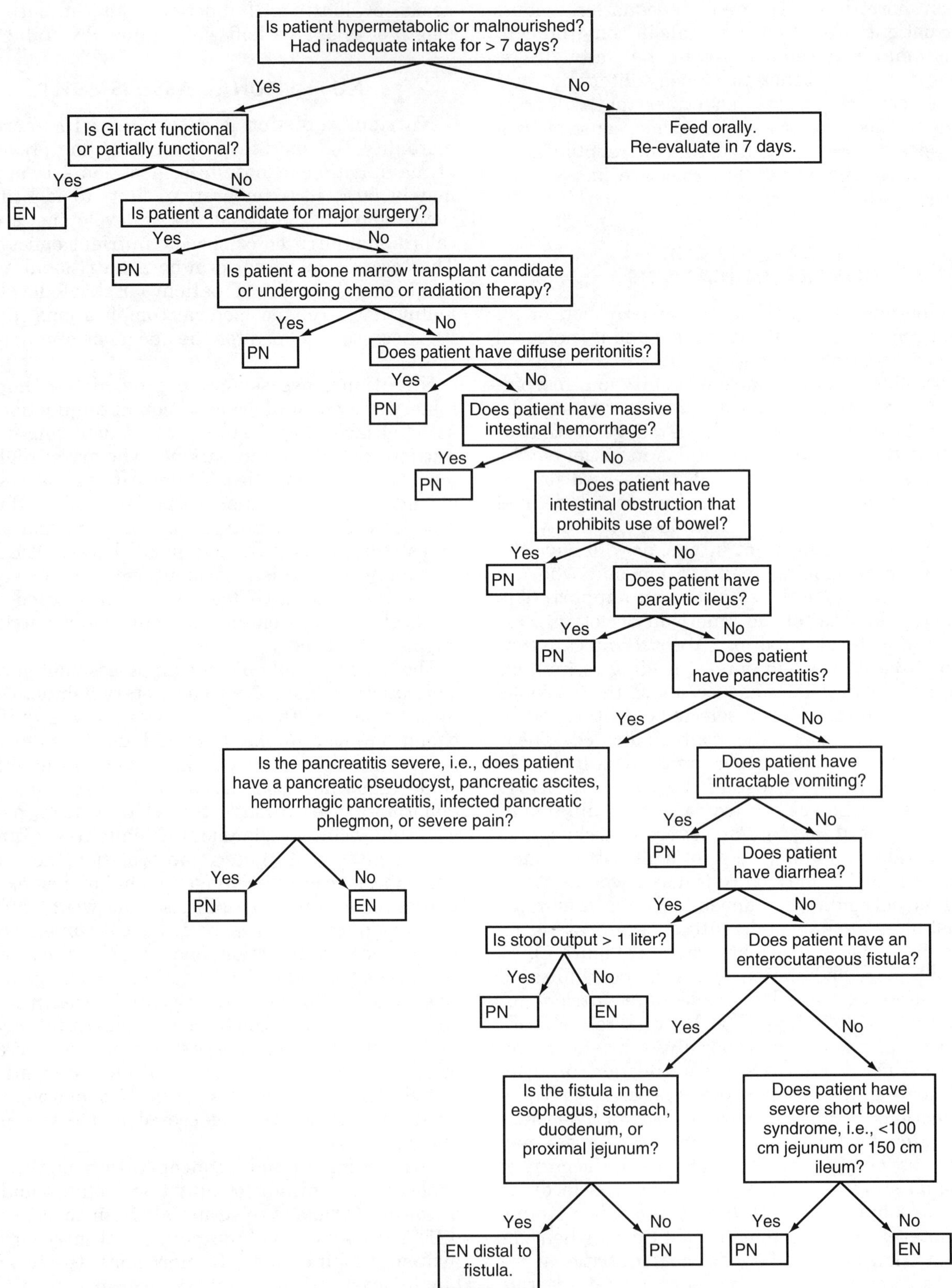

Figure 1. Indications for parenteral nutrition. *Abbreviations:* EN = enteral nutrition; PN = parenteral nutrition; GI = gastrointestinal.

TABLE 1. **Decision-Making Steps When Initiating Parenteral Nutrition**

Before considering parenteral nutrition support:

- Assess the patient's nutritional status. Parenteral nutrition should not be initiated in well-nourished patients unless they have received suboptimal intake for more than 7 days.
- Determine whether the patient has extreme energy needs (hypermetabolism) that warrant the early use of parenteral nutrition within 7 days of injury or illness. These are typically patients who have suffered severe burns or trauma. PN support is indicated until enteral access is established and the patient can be fed via this route.
- Evaluate the function of the gastrointestinal tract. If the gastrointestinal tract is intact and can be used safely, parenteral nutrition should be avoided.
- Estimate how long the patient will require parenteral nutrition support. If gastrointestinal function is expected to return within 5 days, there is no known benefit of initiating parenteral alimentation.

appropriate nutritional support in the presence of ongoing stress, often the level can be stabilized, and nutritionally related morbidity and mortality can be prevented or ameliorated. The long half-life of albumin (approximately 18 to 20 days) makes it a poor marker of short-term feeding in hospitalized patients.

Other serum proteins, such as prealbumin, transferrin, and retinol-binding protein have a rapid turnover rate and shorter half-lives and have been used as markers of nutritional status as well. However, these proteins are also affected by the metabolic response to stress/illness, as well as other conditions, including iron status (transferrin) and renal status (retinol binding protein, prealbumin). Serum transferrin and prealbumin correlate closely with nitrogen balance during nutrition therapy and, therefore, are sensitive indicators of the adequacy of nutrition support.

A simple and practical index of malnutrition is the degree of weight loss. Unintentional weight loss greater than 10% within the previous 6 months is indicative of protein-energy malnutrition and a good prognosticator of clinical outcome. However, the percentage of weight loss with respect to the usual weight is used most commonly and is the most reliable indicator. The percentage weight change with respect to the usual body weight is calculated as follows:

$$\%\ \text{usual body weight (UBW)} = (\text{actual weight} \times 100)/\text{UBW}$$

Another useful index is the percentage of recent weight change. This index is calculated using the following formula:

$$\%\ \text{of recent weight change} = (\text{UBW} - \text{actual weight} \times 100)/\text{UBW}$$

The results of these calculations can be used to estimate the severity of malnutrition (Table 2). Thus,

TABLE 2. **Weight Change as an Index of Malnutrition**

Percentage of Usual Body Weight		Percentage of Recent Weight Change
85–95%	Mild malnutrition	Significant weight loss is:
75–84%	Moderate malnutrition	>1–2% over 1 week
<74%	Severe malnutrition	>5% over 1 month
		>7.5% over 3 months
		>10% over 6 or more months

patients who are 75 to 84% of their usual body weight are moderately malnourished and candidates for nutrition support. Similarly, patients who have lost 5% of their usual weight over 1 month have experienced a significant weight loss.

Weight can also be compared to an "ideal" or "desirable" weight, or the body mass index (BMI) can be used to detect both undernutrition and overnutrition: BMI = weight (kg)/height $(m)^2$. This index is independent of height, and the same standards apply to both men and women. A BMI greater than 28 defines significant obesity, whereas a BMI of 20 to 25 is considered normal. Although the BMI is typically used to assess adiposity, it can also be used to define protein-energy malnutrition. If the BMI is 18 or less, malnutrition should be considered moderate: the lower the values, the greater the severity of malnourishment.

The Nutrition Risk Index (NRI) relies on the serum albumin concentration and the percent usual body weight to determine the severity of malnutrition (Table 3). Patients with an NRI of less than 83.7 are severely malnourished.

Another tool for evaluating nutritional status is the subjective global assessment (SGA) that encompasses historical, symptomatic, and physical parameters. The SGA technique determines whether (1) nutrient assimilation has been restricted because of decreased food intake, maldigestion, or malabsorption; (2) any effects of malnutrition on organ function and body composition have occurred; and (3) the patient's disease process influences nutrient requirements. The findings of the history and physical examination are subjectively weighted to rank patients as being well nourished, moderately malnourished, or severely malnourished and are used to predict their risk for medical complications (Table 4).

Muscle function tests represent a newer approach for evaluating nutritional status and include measuring grip strength, respiratory muscle strength, and

TABLE 3. **Calculation of the Nutrition Risk Index (NRI)**

	NRI = (15.9 × albumin [gm/dL] + (0.417 × % usual body weight)
NRI > 97.5	Well nourished
NRI 83.7–97.5	Mildly malnourished
NRI < 83.7	Severely malnourished

TABLE 4. **Subjective Global Assessment**

(Select appropriate category with a checkmark, or enter numerical value where indicated by "#".)

A. History

1. Weight change
   Overall loss in past 6 months: amount = # ____ kg; % loss = #____.
   Change in past 2 weeks: ________ increase, ________ non change, ________ decrease.
2. Dietary intake change (relative to normal)
   ____ No change
   ____ Change ____ duration = # ____ weeks.
   ____ type: ____ suboptimal solid diet, ____ full liquid diet, ____ hypocaloric liquids, ____ starvation.
3. Gastrointestinal symptoms (that persisted for >2 weeks)
   ____ none, ____ nausea, ____ vomiting, ____ diarrhea, ____ anorexia.
4. Functional capacity
   ________ No dysfunction (e.g., full capacity)
   ________ Dysfunction ____ duration = # ____ weeks.
   ____ type: ____ working suboptimally, ____ ambulatory, ____ bedridden.
5. Disease and its relation to nutritional requirements
   Primary diagnosis (specify) ________________
   Metabolic demand (stress): ____ no stress, ____ low stress, ____ moderate stress, ____ high stress.

B. Physical (for each trait specify: 0 = normal, 1+ = mild, 2+ = moderate, 3+ = severe).

#________ loss of subcutaneous fat (triceps, chest)
#________ muscle wasting (quadriceps, deltoids)
#________ ankle edema
#________ sacral edema
#________ ascites

C. SGA rating (select one)

________ A = Well nourished
________ B = Moderately (or suspected of being) malnourished
________ C = Severely malnourished

From Detsky AS, McLaughlin JR, Baker JP, et al: What is subjective global assessment of nutritional status? JPEN *11*:8–13, 1987.

the response of specific muscles to electrical stimulation. Starvation and refeeding alter the response of the adductor pollicis muscle to electrical stimulation. Changes in muscle function induced by malnutrition and refeeding occur rapidly, typically before there are measurable changes in body protein content. Although muscle function testing represents a promising approach, additional data and more widespread availability of the technology are needed before it can be incorporated into clinical practice.

ESTIMATING NUTRIENT REQUIREMENTS

Historically, PN often provided nutrients in excess of actual requirements. This was based on the assumption that patients requiring nutritional intervention were severely depleted and required aggressive repletion, hence the misnomer "hyperalimentation." It has since been apparent that such overfeeding is dangerous, and nutritional support should be titrated to match actual metabolic requirements.

Three major components are associated with daily energy expenditure. The first component is the basal metabolic rate (BMR), which is the amount of energy expended under complete rest, shortly after awakening and in a fasting state (12 to 14 hours). BMR varies with age, sex, and body size and correlates roughly with body surface area. It is proportional to the size of the fat-free mass, i.e., that portion of the body weight that is lean tissue and not fat. This relationship holds true even among individuals of different ages and sex. In contrast, resting metabolic rate or resting energy expenditure (REE) represents the amount of energy expended 2 hours after a meal under conditions of rest and thermal neutrality. However, although it is often used synonymously with BMR, the REE is typically 10% higher.

The second component of daily energy expenditure is the thermic effect of exercise or the energy used in physical activity. The thermic effect of exercise in a sedentary person accounts for 15 to 20% of daily energy expenditure. The contribution of this component increases markedly during intense muscular work. Admission to a hospital generally results in a marked decrease in physical activity. Hospital activity in a patient not confined to bed increases the BMR by approximately 20 to 30%.

The third component of energy expenditure is the increase in BMR that follows food intake. The digestion and metabolism of exogenous nutrients, whether delivered to the gut or vein, result in an increase in metabolic rate. This is known as dietary thermogenesis. The magnitude of this thermic effect of food varies depending on the amount and composition of the diet and accounts for approximately 10% of daily energy expenditure.

Illness adds an additional component to the daily energy expenditure. For example, a patient's metabolic rate increases by 10 to 30% after major fracture, from 20 to 60% with severe infection, and from 40 to 110% with a severe, third-degree burn. In addition, fever accelerates chemical reactions. For this reason, the BMR rises approximately 14% for each Celsius degree increase in temperature.

Thus, the first step of estimating calorie requirements is to estimate the BMR. This may be accomplished using predictive equations, nomograms, or body surface area (BSA) equations. The most commonly used method is based on the predictive equations reported by Harris and Benedict in 1909. The Harris-Benedict equations are:

$$\text{Men: } 66.47 + 13.75(W) + 5.0(H) - 6.76(A)$$
$$\text{Women: } 65.51 + 9.56(W) + 1.85(H) - 4.68(A)$$

where W = weight in kg, H = height in cm, and A = age in years.

Another method for determining BMR is based on the relationship between body BSA and BMR in which

$$\text{BMR} = \text{BSA} \times \text{kcal/m}^2\text{/h} \times 24 \text{ hours}$$

BSA can be determined using a nomogram (Figure 2) or from the following equation:

$$\text{BSA} = W^{.425} \times H^{.75} \times 71.84$$

where W = weight in kg and H = height in cm.

Kilocalorie/m² per hour can be obtained from standard (Fleisch) tables (Table 5) or by using the following equation:

$$\text{kcal/m}^2\text{/hour} = 55 - \text{age, for ages 0 to 19 years}$$
$$= 37 - (\text{age} - 20)/10\text{, for ages 20 or older}$$

After the BMR is calculated, the next step is to adjust the BMR for the level of stress induced by injury or the disease process (Figure 3). Some further adjustments are applied to compensate for the patient's physical activity. Activity factors for hospitalized patients are as follows:

Intubated—1.0–1.1
Confined to bed—1.2
Out of bed—1.3

Therefore, the patient's energy requirements are finally calculated: BMR × stress factor × activity factor = total energy expenditure.

However, using the Harris-Benedict equations to determine BMR multiplied by stress and activity factors often leads to overfeeding. Consequently, the

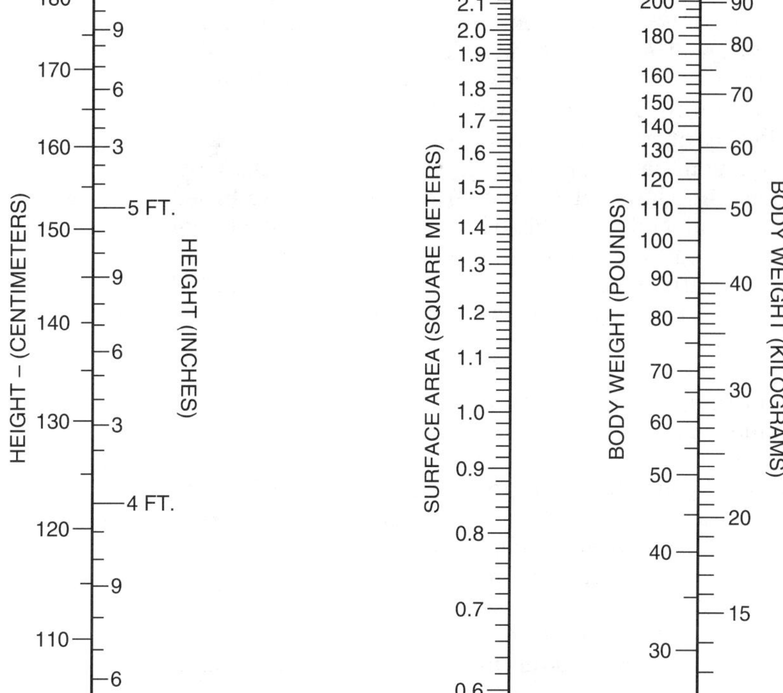

Figure 2. Surface area from height and weight. Connect the height on the left-hand scale to the weight on the right-hand scale with a straight edge to determine the body surface area on the middle scale.

TABLE 5. **Standard Metabolic Rates**

Age in Years	kcal/m²/hr		kJ/m²/hr	
	Men	**Women**	**Men**	**Women**
1	53.0	53.0	222	222
2	52.4	52.4	219	219
3	51.3	51.2	215	214
4	50.3	49.8	211	208
5	49.3	48.4	206	203
6	48.3	47.0	202	197
7	47.3	45.4	198	190
8	46.3	43.8	194	183
9	45.2	42.8	189	179
10	44.0	42.5	184	178
11	43.0	42.0	180	176
12	42.5	41.3	178	173
13	42.3	40.3	177	169
14	42.1	39.2	176	164
15	41.8	37.9	175	159
16	41.4	36.9	173	154
17	40.8	36.3	171	152
18	40.0	35.9	167	150
19	39.2	35.5	164	149
20	38.6	35.3	162	148
25	37.5	35.2	157	147
30	36.8	35.1	154	147
35	36.5	35.0	153	146
40	36.3	34.9	152	146
45	36.2	34.5	152	144
50	35.8	33.9	150	142
55	35.4	33.3	148	139
60	34.9	32.7	146	137
65	34.4	32.2	144	135
70	33.8	31.7	141	133
≥75	33.2	31.3	139	131

From Fleisch A: Le Metabolisme basal standard et sa determination su moyen du "metabocalculator." Helv Med Acta *18*:23, 1951.

Harris-Benedict equation is often used without the addition of stress and activity factors to determine energy needs. This is more commonly practiced in critically ill patients in whom overfeeding can have significant adverse effects (i.e., difficulty weaning from ventilator or hyperglycemia). Alternatively, some clinicians estimate energy requirements based on actual body weight. Thus, 20 to 25 kcal per kg body weight are administered to the critically ill intubated patient and 30 kcal per kg to nonventilated patients in whom excessive intake is not a major concern.

Other techniques may be used to measure energy requirements more accurately. In practice these techniques are rarely needed, but they may help to manage patients who continue to lose weight despite what appears to be an adequate caloric intake, who are critically ill, or who have rapidly changing needs. A more precise and individualized measurement of REE may be necessary in these situations. A technique that may be helpful is indirect calorimetry, which uses changes in oxygen consumption and carbon dioxide production to calculate the REE. Changes in substrate utilization can be determined from the respiratory quotient, which is equal to the carbon dioxide production divided by the oxygen consumption (VCO_2/VO_2) (Table 6). The indirect calorimeter uses either a preprogrammed formula to calculate the REE or a modification of the Weir equation.

The Weir equation can also be used to determine the REE of patients who are being mechanically ventilated because oxygen consumption and carbon dioxide production can be measured directly in these patients. The oxygen consumption and metabolic rate of patients who are not being ventilated can be measured using a spirometer, which is available in most pulmonary function laboratories. The Weir formula is:

$$\text{REE (kcal/day)} = [3.9(VO_2) + 1.1(VCO_2)]\ 1.44$$

If the oxygen consumption is known, then:

$$\text{Metabolic rate (kcal/h)} = VO_2(\text{mL/min}) \times 60\ \text{min/hr} \times 1\ \text{L}/1000\ \text{mL} \times 4.83\ \text{kcal/L}.$$

In a patient who has a Swan-Ganz catheter, oxygen consumption (and therefore the metabolic rate) can be calculated from simultaneously obtained measurements of cardiac output, mixed venous oxygen content ($C_{mv}O_2$), and arterial oxygen content (C_aO_2) according to:

$$VO_2\ (\text{mL/min}) = \text{cardiac output (L/min)} \times (C_aO_2)[\text{mL/L}] - C_{mv}O_2[\text{mL/L}]).$$

The use of a stress factor to account for injury or infection is not necessary when using these formulas because the measured energy expenditure accounts for the effects of disease state, stress, and trauma. However, because the measurement occurs at rest, it is necessary to multiply by an "activity" factor of 1.1 to 1.3 depending on whether the patient is intubated, at bed rest, or ambulatory, as discussed previously.

After the energy needs are determined, protein needs are calculated.* The recommended daily allowance of protein for most individuals is 0.8 gram of protein per kilogram body weight or about 60 to 70 grams of protein each day. The stressed, critically ill patient generally needs a higher dose in the range of 1.5 to 2.0 grams of protein per kilogram body weight per day. The calorie/nitrogen ratio for most PN solutions is approximately 150:1, with an acceptable range of 100:1 to 180:1. Nitrogen content is used as a marker for protein, and hence the two terms are used interchangeably. Usually, 6.25 grams of protein are equal to 1 gram of nitrogen. The conversion factor are slightly higher (6.4) for PN solutions, such as those with higher concentrations of crystalline amino acids. A 24-hour urinary urea nitrogen (UUN) measurement, which can be performed by all clinical laboratories, may be used to estimate nitrogen balance:

$$\text{Nitrogen balance} = \text{protein intake (grams)}/6.25 - \{24 - \text{hour UUN (grams)} \pm 4\}$$

*The contribution of protein to caloric intake is not usually included in estimates of caloric requirements.

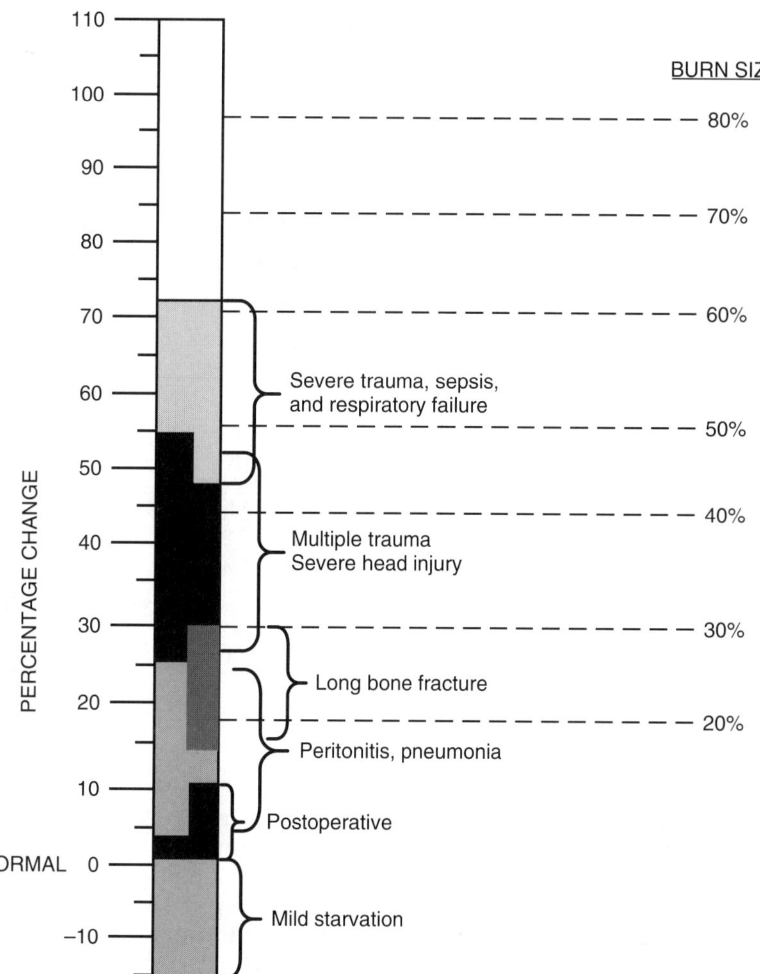

Figure 3. Percent change in metabolic rate due to injury. (Used with permission from Wilmore DW: The Metabolic Management of the Critically Ill. New York, Plenum Medical, 1977, p 36.)

Patients who are catabolic have a negative nitrogen balance, whereas patients who are anabolic have a positive nitrogen balance. Achieving a positive nitrogen balance is virtually impossible in critically ill patients but may be possible after the primary disease process is controlled or has resolved. Increasing protein intake beyond 2 grams per kg body weight per day is usually not beneficial. The provision of excessive protein does not enhance uptake and may lead to increased ureagenesis, which can cause renal injury in some patients.

Little is known about how vitamin and mineral requirements are changed by disease. In 1979, guidelines for parenteral vitamin and trace element administration were established by the Nutrition Advisory Group of the American Medical Association (AMA). The AMA's recommendations for daily intravenous intake, as well as the recommended daily allowances, are shown in Table 7. It is imperative that patients are provided adequate vitamins and trace elements while receiving PN.

TABLE 6. **Changes in Respiratory Quotient (RQ) According to Substrate Utilization**

Condition	Net RQ
Carbohydrate oxidation	1.00
Fat oxidation	0.70
"Mixed substrate" oxidation	0.85
Net lipogenesis during continuous nutrient infusions	1.00–1.20
During prolonged ketosis	0.68

Patients receiving a carbohydrate load are particularly susceptible to thiamine deficiency. In 1988, several deaths resulted from cardiac failure owing to thiamine deficiency when long-term PN patients did not receive vitamins for a few weeks. Megaloblastic anemia secondary to folate deficiency can occur in PN patients who do not receive folate for several weeks. Selenium is a trace element for which requirements have not been well established, but it should be added to solutions for patients receiving prolonged PN. Several cases of PN-associated selenium deficiency have manifested as cardiomyopathy. PN-associated deficiencies of copper, zinc, chromium, selenium, and molybdenum have also been reported. Iron deficiency with or without anemia is a common consequence of bleeding in many diseases for which parenteral alimentation is often indicated.

Some evidence indicates that in certain disease

TABLE 7. **Vitamin and Trace Element Recommendations for Adults**

Vitamin/Trace Element	Recommended Daily Allowance	Parenteral Requirements
Vitamin A	4000–5000 IU	3300.0 IU
Vitamin D	400 IU	200.0 IU
Vitamin E	12–15 IU	10.0 IU
Ascorbic acid (C)	60 mg	100.0 mg
Folic acid	400 μg	400.0 μg
Niacin	12–20 mg	40.0 mg
Riboflavin (B_2)	1.1–1.8 mg	3.6 mg
Thiamine (B_1)	1.0–1.5 mg	3.0 mg
Pyridoxine (B_6)	1.6–2.0 mg	4.0 mg
Cyanocobalamin (B_{12})	3 μg	5.0 μg
Pantothenic acid	5–10 mg	15.0 mg
Biotin	150–300 μg	60.0 μg
Zinc	15 mg	2.5–4 mg
Copper	2–3 mg	0.5–1.5 mg
Chromium	0.05–0.2 mg	10–15 μg
Manganese	2.25–5 mg	0.15–1.8 mg
Selenium	0.05–0.2 mg	
Iron	10–15 mg	
Iodine	150 μg	
Fluoride	1.5–4 mg	
Molybdenum	0.15–4 mg	
Cobalt	As part of B_{12} requirements	

states, vitamin and mineral requirements are altered, either owing to increased losses, greater utilization, or both. In most instances, vitamin supplementation is accomplished by using single vitamin preparations. For example, higher doses of vitamins A and C are indicated for wound healing; additional thiamine and folic acid are necessary in patients with alcoholism. Zinc is required in higher amounts when there are excessive gastrointestinal losses, i.e., massive diarrhea from short-bowel syndrome, inflammatory bowel disease, and malabsorption syndromes.

COMPOSITION OF CENTRAL AND PERIPHERAL VENOUS SOLUTIONS

The common macronutrients and their caloric densities and functions are presented in Table 8. In contrast to central parenteral nutritional alimentation solutions, peripheral alimentation solutions typically have a dextrose concentration of 5%. The number of calories that can be administered using this method is between 1000 and 1500 per day. The volume of fluid required to administer these calories is usually greater than 2 liters per day. In contrast to cases in which hypertonic dextrose solutions are administered through a central vein, and in which the substrate mixture is predominantly composed of carbohydrate, most of the calories from peripheral PN are derived from fat. Peripheral nutritional prescriptions typically provide 30% of calories as carbohydrate, 20% as protein, and 50% as fat (Table 9).

Peripheral PN is undesirable for several reasons. First, there is no evidence that it improves outcomes or significantly decreases nitrogen losses when it does not closely approximate a patient's energy needs. Second, the high fat content typically administered as part of peripheral PN regimens is associated with impaired reticuloendothelial system function. For these reasons, we limit the use of peripheral PN to situations in which it may be of value, such as to supplement nutritional intake for patients whose enteral intake is inadequate.

Central venous solutions, which are prepared by the hospital's pharmacy, typically combine 500 mL of 50% dextrose with 500 mL of a 10 to 15% amino acid mixture. Vitamins, electrolytes, and trace elements are added to the formulation as needed. Central PN solutions usually provide about 55 to 60% of calories as carbohydrate and 15 to 20% of calories as protein. Lipids contribute no more than 30% of the total calo-

TABLE 8. **Caloric Densities, Sources, and Functions of the Major Macronutrients**

Macronutrient (Caloric Density)	Common Sources	Functions
Carbohydrates (3.4 kcal/gm)	Dextrose	Essential fuels used by glycolytic tissues; normally the major or sole energy source for the central nervous system, peripheral nerves, red blood cells, and some phagocytes. During prolonged starvation, the glucose requirement of the brain decreases as adaptation to ketone oxidation occurs. Are used by tissues that oxidize fat (e.g., muscle) when carbohydrates are administered as the major fuel source. Maintain hepatic glycogen stores, which may protect hepatocytes during hypoxia or exposure to toxins.
Lipids (9 kcal/gm)	Polyunsaturated long chain triglycerides from soybean oil or a safflower/soybean oil mixture	The most concentrated forms of energy. Stabilize, support, and protect vital structures. Complex with fat-soluble molecules like some vitamins; are used as structural components in biologic membranes.
Proteins (4 kcal/gm)	Crystalline amino acids	Major structural component of the body. Some are essential (histidine, isoleucine, leucine, valine, methionine, cysteine, phenylalanine, tyrosine, threonine, tryptophan, and lysine) because they cannot be synthesized by the body. Others are nonessential because they can be made from carbon and nitrogen precursors. Act as peptide hormones, enzymes, and antibodies. May join with carbohydrates to form glycoproteins, to serve as plasma proteins and immune globulins and as components of connective tissue cell membranes and mucous secretions.

TABLE 9. **Central Versus Peripheral Nutrition**

	Central	Peripheral
Daily calories	2000–3000	1000–1500
Protein	Variable	56–87 gm
Volume of fluid required	1000–3000 mL	2000–3500 mL
Duration of therapy	≥7 days	5–7 days
Route of administration	Dedicated central venous catheter	Peripheral vein or multiuse central catheter
Substrate profile	• 55–60% carbohydrate • 15–20% protein • 25% fat	• 30% carbohydrate • 20% protein • 50% fat
Osmolarity	≈2000 mOsm/L	≈600–900 mOsm/L

ries administered (see Table 9). A typical prescription would administer 2 liters of this standard solution each day. Administration of 500 mL of a 20% fat emulsion 1 day each week is sufficient to prevent essential fatty acid deficiency. This method of administration is satisfactory if lipids are needed only as a source of essential fatty acids and are not needed as an additional source of calories. If additional calories are needed on a daily basis from lipids, they can be administered as a separate infusion or most commonly as part of a mixture of dextrose and amino acids. These three major nutrients are added together in a 3-liter bag in a technique known as triple mix or three-in-one. In this instance, the entire contents of a single bag are infused during a 24-hour period. With a mixed fuel system, the rate of infusion of lipid is constant over the infusion period. This increases the efficiency of fat utilization and minimizes the risk of decreased reticuloendothelial system function associated with infusion of lipids over the 10- to 12-hour period used for intermittent infusion protocols. However, the inclusion of intravenous fat emulsion into a PN admixture changes the conventional nutritional solution into an emulsion.

Various micronutrients can adversely influence emulsion stability. The higher the cation valence, the greater the destabilizing influence to the emulsifier. Therefore, trivalent cations such as the ferric ion (iron dextran) are more disruptive than divalent cations such as calcium or magnesium ions, which are more disruptive than monovalent cations such as sodium or potassium. Recent evidence demonstrates that there is no concentration of iron dextran that is safe in triple mix formulations. In-line filtration is necessary for all PN solutions, including triple mix solutions, as it is impossible to visually detect precipitates until they are grossly incompatible and unsafe for infusion.

Once the basic solution is created, electrolytes are added as needed (Table 10). Sodium or potassium salts are given as chloride or acetate according to the requirements of the individual patient. Normally, equal amounts of chloride and acetate are provided. However, if chloride losses from the body are increased, such as may occur in patients who have nasogastric tubes, then most of the salts should be given as chloride. Similarly, more acetate should be given to patients when additional base is required because acetate generates bicarbonate when it is metabolized. Sodium bicarbonate is incompatible with PN solutions and so cannot be added to the mixture. Phosphate may be given as the sodium or potassium salt. Lipid emulsions contain an additional 15 mmol per liter of phosphate.

Commercially available preparations of vitamins, minerals, and trace elements are added to the nutrient mix unless they are contraindicated. Both fat- and water-soluble vitamins should be given. Until recently, a standard 10 mL vial of a multivitamin-12 preparation that contained the doses of vitamins recommended by the AMA was routinely added to the PN solution. However, because of a national shortage of this standard preparation, various vitamin preparations are being introduced into the market. As alluded to earlier, the provision of adequate thiamine is essential for patients receiving PN and can be provided separately. Vitamin K is not a component of any of the vitamin mixtures formulated for adults. Maintenance requirements can be satisfied by adding vitamin K in the PN solution. Ten mg of vitamin K are given weekly to patients who are not receiving anticoagulants such as warfarin (Coumadin).

Trace element preparations that include zinc, copper, manganese, and chromium are added to the PN solution in amounts consistent with the AMA guidelines. We also add 60 μg of selenium daily to the

TABLE 10. **Electrolyte Concentrations in Parenteral Nutrition**

Electrolyte	Recommended Central PN Doses	Recommended Peripheral PN Doses	Usual Range of Doses
Potassium (mEq/L)	30	30	0–120 (CVL) 0–80 (PV)
Sodium (mEq/L)	30	30	0–150
Phosphate (mmol/L)	15	5	0–20
Magnesium (mEq/L)	5	5	0–16
Calcium (mEq/L) (as gluconate)	4.7	4.7	0–10
Chloride (mEq/L)	50	50	0–150
Acetate (mEq/L)	40	40	0–100

Abbreviations: CVL = central venous line; PV = peripheral vein.

solutions. Because copper and manganese are excreted by the biliary tract, their dosages should be modified or eliminated in patients with significant liver disease or biliary obstruction. In the absence of clear data in the literature, our practice is to withhold copper and manganese when the patient's serum bilirubin level exceeds 5 mg per dL. Ten to 15 mg per day of zinc are provided to patients with excessive GI losses. Iron is not a part of commercial additive preparations because it is incompatible with triple mix solutions and may cause anaphylactic reactions when it is given intravenously. Patients who need this trace element should have it administered orally or by injection. Iron is not given to the critically ill as hyperferremia can increase bacterial virulence, alter polymorphonuclear cell function, and increase host susceptibility to infection.

ADMINISTRATION AND ACCESS

With central venous nutrition, hypertonic nutrient solutions (>10% dextrose) are infused via a catheter inserted into a large central vein. Access to a large central vein is needed because these formulas are hyperosmolar (≥1900 mOsm per kg), and administration of the solutions into peripheral veins causes thrombophlebitis and venous sclerosis. When infused into the central venous system, the nutrients are rapidly diluted to near isotonicity and are then cleared from the bloodstream. Infusion of these solutions typically delivers between 2000 and 3000 kcal per day. The total volume of fluid administered is usually between 1 and 3 liters per day.

Typically, central PN solutions are administered into the superior vena cava. Access to this vein is usually accomplished by cannulation of the subclavian vein. Access can also be obtained via the internal or external jugular veins, but the location of the catheter exit site in the neck makes catheter care more difficult and renders it more susceptible to infection. Thus, the infraclavicular route is preferred unless the patient has a contraindication to this approach, i.e., abnormal or distorted anatomy, local irradiation, or trauma. Percutaneous insertion of the catheter on the right side avoids the possibility of injuring the thoracic duct. Peripherally inserted central venous catheters (PICC) that are typically inserted via an antecubital vein and advanced into the superior vena cava are being used more frequently for the provision of PN. PICC placement offers the advantage of central venous access while avoiding the risks of subclavian or jugular puncture.

Tunneled catheters or catheters with indwelling ports should be considered for patients who will need prolonged central venous nutrition. Patients who will be using their catheters solely for daily central PN and who require home intravenous feeding may be best served by a tunneled catheter rather than by an indwelling port. Tunneled catheters may be more easily manipulated and otherwise cared for, which may minimize the risk of infection.

Insertion of a dedicated line for the infusion of hypertonic glucose solutions requires strict aseptic technique, i.e., hat, mask, gown, and gloves must be worn. The position of the catheter tip in the superior vena cava is confirmed by chest roentgenogram before any concentrated solutions are administered. Once the position of the tip has been confirmed, the line should be used exclusively for the administration of the hypertonic nutrient solution. The drawing of blood, monitoring of central venous pressure, and the administration of medications through the dedicated lumen are prohibited because they markedly increase the risk of catheter infection.

Multiple-lumen central venous catheters are most commonly used. Whereas at least one lumen is dedicated to the infusion of the PN solutions, the other(s) may be used for monitoring, blood drawing, or medication. The rate of catheter sepsis associated with the use of multiple-port catheters is probably the same or slightly greater than the rate associated with the use of single-port catheters. However, multiple-port, percutaneously placed catheters are used to infuse PN solutions for a shorter time, which may minimize their inherent risk. In any case, if multiple-port catheters are used, they should be carefully maintained. Dressing changes should be performed according to an established protocol, the dedicated lumen should be carefully maintained, the other lumens should be handled carefully, and the catheter should be removed as soon as it is no longer needed.

Rarely, central venous access via the subclavian or jugular veins may be impossible or otherwise contraindicated. Furthermore, in very rare circumstances, it may be impossible or ill advisable to obtain or maintain a dedicated line. Our policy is to limit the dextrose concentration according to the type of line being used for alimentation and its exit site. Thus, whereas maximally concentrated solutions can be administered through a dedicated line where central access is obtained via the neck, upper torso, or upper extremities, concentrations less than or equal to 15% are appropriate for dedicated femoral lines. This is because of an increased risk of thrombosis owing to decreased flow rates in the femoral vein as compared with the superior vena cava. Because of the large number of skin bacteria and other pathogens in this area, if a femoral line is used, it should be replaced every 2 to 3 days. For multiuse (i.e., nondedicated, subclavian, jugular, or femoral) lines, a maximal dextrose concentration of less than or equal to 10% is indicated until dedicated access can be obtained because the risk of infection is probably higher when more concentrated dextrose solutions are used.

INITIATION AND MAINTENANCE OF INFUSION: PATIENT MONITORING

Typically, one initiates peripheral parenteral nutrition with 2 liters of the nutrient solution and 500 kcal as lipid. However, it is advisable to start with 1 liter of central PN and then to increase the volume as needed if the patient is metabolically stable. Blood sugar should be less than 200 mg per dL, and abnormal electrolyte levels should be corrected, especially potassium, phosphate, and magnesium, before starting or advancing to the goal solution. Obviously, patients with diabetes mellitus may need to be advanced more slowly to prevent severe glucose intolerance. Lipid can be infused as an alternative fuel source to fulfill energy requirements without increasing the glucose infusion rate. The solutions should be administered using a volumetric pump set at a constant rate. It is important not to modify the infusion rate during any given day to try to compensate for excess or inadequate administration of the PN solution (i.e., when the PN solution arrives later than expected). A cyclic schedule (8 to 16 hours per day) for patients requiring long-term PN can be initiated once the patient is metabolically stable. This should be done gradually, and the last hour of infusion should be tapered to one half the infusion rate to prevent rebound hypoglycemia.

Before central parenteral alimentation is discontinued, the rate of infusion should be decreased by half to avoid adverse effects that may occur secondary to relative hyperinsulinemia if the body is not allowed sufficient time to equilibrate. In emergency situations when the central PN solution must be suddenly discontinued, 10% dextrose should be given at the same infusion rate as was used for the PN unless there is severe hyperglycemia. When patients who are receiving PN require surgical operation, one can continue to administer the solution through the procedure, but the infusion rate should be reduced in half because circulating glucose and electrolyte levels are easier to control.

During the initiation of central PN, serum chemistries must be monitored frequently. Once the patient has stabilized on his or her individual nutritional prescription, blood samples should be obtained at least twice weekly to measure chloride, CO_2, potassium, sodium, blood urea nitrogen (BUN), creatinine, calcium, and phosphate levels, and once weekly for profile 20, magnesium, and triglyceride levels. Patients should be weighed each day on the same scale. Urine should initially be tested for sugar and acetone every 6 hours. Electrolytes and other medications should be added only by the pharmacist in preparation of the mixture.

PARENTERAL NUTRITION FOR PATIENTS WITH ABNORMAL ORGAN FUNCTION

Diabetes Mellitus

Control of blood glucose levels is important for all patients who receive PN. However, regulation may be especially difficult in patients who are known to have diabetes or in patients who develop insulin resistance in response to severe stress or infection. If blood glucose levels are not maintained lower than 200 mg per dL, leukocyte phagocytic function is inhibited and the patient may be at increased risk for infection. In the insulin-dependent patient, the same amount of insulin that would normally be taken is added to the PN solution on the first day. Because as much as one half of the insulin given binds to the container and intravenous tubing, the insulin given in this manner is almost always an underestimate of actual requirements. For example, if a patient's normal dose of regular insulin is 40 units per day for a 2000 kcal diet, then a PN solution of 1000 kcal should have 20 units added to it. Thereafter, blood glucose concentrations obtained by finger stick or blood sampling are determined every 6 hours, and a sliding scale for subcutaneous regular insulin is used to provide supplementary insulin doses as needed. For the next day, one half or all of the insulin given on the previous day according to the sliding scale is added to the PN solution, depending on the level of control that is required.

For nondiabetic patients who develop hyperglycemia, a similar procedure is used whereby a sliding scale estimates the amount of insulin that will be needed to maintain blood glucose levels lower than 200 mg per dL, and one half this amount is then added to the next day's PN orders.

Acute Renal Failure

In general, most patients with acute renal failure are catabolic with energy requirements of 50 to 100% greater than resting requirements. Calories should be provided in sufficient quantities to minimize protein degradation. Energy requirements can generally be met with the provision of 35 to 40 kcal per kg dry weight. Protein should be provided in the range of 1.2 to 1.5 gm per kg per day with a standard solution containing both essential and nonessential amino acids. Traditionally, formulas designed for renal failure contained predominantly essential amino acids. Although the theory may be reasonable, there are no conclusive data to show that special formulas containing only essential amino acids are superior to the less expensive standard formulations containing both nonessential and essential amino acids. Moreover, the provision of nonessential amino acids may enhance protein synthesis and nitrogen retention.

A balance of fat and carbohydrate should be provided. Lipid emulsions can be used as a source of concentrated energy in the patients who are fluid restricted. The contribution of fat to the total caloric intake should be no more than 30%, and the remainder of the caloric requirements is provided by glucose.

Fluid and electrolyte balance is often impaired in patients with acute renal failure. Potassium, phosphate, and magnesium levels must be monitored carefully and these minerals should be added to PN if blood levels fall. Acetate salts of potassium or sodium can be administered to help correct a metabolic acidosis. Standard doses of the water-soluble vitamins and additional folic acid (1 mg per day total) should be added to the solution of patients who are being dialyzed because these substances are lost from the body in the dialysate bath. The supplementation of fat-soluble vitamins is usually not required, especially in patients who are also eating, because excretion is reduced in renal failure. In anuric patients, trace elements are not added to the nutrient solutions; however, for prolonged PN, trace elements and fat-soluble vitamins should be replaced.

Hepatic Dysfunction and Liver Failure

Protein intake in patients with stable chronic liver disease depends on the patient's nutritional status and protein tolerance. Nutritionally depleted patients may require as much as 1.5 grams of protein per kg estimated dry weight. However, protein intake may need to be decreased in patients with liver failure and encephalopathy. Protein-sensitive encephalopathic patients should be given 0.5 to 0.7 grams protein per kg per day and increased gradually to 1.0 to 1.5 grams per kg per day if possible. These patients have deranged plasma amino acid profiles with increased concentrations of aromatic amino acids (phenylalanine, tyrosine, and tryptophan) and methionine and decreased branched-chain amino acids (valine, leucine, and isoleucine). Administration of solutions that contain high levels of branched-chain amino acids and no aromatic amino acids may be better tolerated than standard products and may allow a positive nitrogen balance or nitrogen equilibrium to be achieved in patients with hepatic insufficiency protein intolerance. These specialty products should be reserved for patients with disabling encephalopathy who do not tolerate standard proteins and who have not responded to other therapy (i.e., lactulose or neomycin administration).

Fluid restriction may be necessary in some patients with ascites and edema. In this instance, the concentration of dextrose can be increased to maintain the amount of calories administered as carbohydrate. The amount of sodium given is reduced as these patients excrete nearly sodium-free urine. Administration of trace elements is often contraindicated because a major route of excretion for these substances (e.g., copper and manganese) is via the biliary system. Zinc deficiency is common in cirrhotic patients, and supplementation of this mineral may be necessary, especially if there are excessive GI losses.

Other Conditions and Nutritional Treatments

Catabolism of major surgery, trauma, burn, and sepsis is characterized by a net breakdown of body protein stores to provide substrates for gluconeogenesis and acute-phase protein synthesis. The provision of adequate nutrition can attenuate whole body catabolism but rarely if ever prevents or reverses loss of lean body mass involving conventional management principles during the acute phase of injury. Several new strategies to accomplish this are under investigation. These include the administration of growth hormone and growth factors, and the provision of conditionally essential amino acids, such as glutamine.

Glutamine-supplemented PN solutions administered to traumatized or stressed patients may improve overall nitrogen balance, enhance muscle protein synthesis, improve intestinal nutrient absorption, decrease gut permeability, improve immune function, and decrease hospital stays and costs in some patient populations. A recent randomized controlled study suggests improved survival and reduced hospital costs in critically ill patients given glutamine-enriched PN. More and more data are accumulating on the metabolic effects of glutamine supplementation; however, glutamine-supplemented solutions should not yet be considered routine care. Patient groups that may benefit from glutamine-containing PN include patients with intestinal dysfunction requiring PN, such as those with short-bowel syndrome, mucosal damage following chemotherapy, and irradiation or critical illness; patients with immunodeficiency syndromes (i.e., AIDS, immune system dysfunction associated with critical illness and bone marrow transplantation); and patients with severe catabolic illness (i.e., major burns, multiple trauma, or other disease associated with a prolonged intensive care unit stay). Glutamine-containing PN should not be used in patients with significant renal insufficiency and in patients with significant hepatic failure.

Growth hormone administration to humans increases the rate of wound healing and decreases wound infection rates, decreases the catabolism and muscle wasting of critical illness, and decreases hospital stays in burned children and cholecystectomy patients. Because growth hormone is an expensive therapy, however, other agents such as oxandrolone (Oxandrin) are being pursued to induce positive nitrogen balance and enhance wound healing in critically ill patients. The use of growth factors should presently be reserved for patients with major burn and documented impaired healing, patients with large wounds and/or enterocutaneous fistulae who have impaired healing, and patients with muscle wasting and weakness associated with acquired immune deficiency syndrome and other “failure to thrive” conditions. In general, the use of adjuvant anabolic agents should be reserved for patients who have not responded to aggressive nutrition support but whose underlying disease processes are controlled.

COMMON COMPLICATIONS AND MANAGEMENT

Catheter Sepsis

Catheter sepsis is a serious complication associated with central venous alimentation. Primary catheter sepsis occurs when there are signs and symptoms of infection, and the indwelling catheter is the only anatomic focus of infection. Secondary catheter infections are associated with another focus or multiple infectious foci that cause bacteremia and seed the catheter.

Management of the patients with catheter infection depends on their clinical condition. Extremely ill patients with high fevers who are hypotensive or who have local signs of infection around the catheter site should have the catheter removed, its tip cultured, and peripheral and central venous blood cultures obtained. In the case of primary catheter sepsis, signs and symptoms can be expected to return to normal quickly. The organisms that grow from the catheter tip are the same as the ones that are identified in the peripheral blood culture. Typically, greater than 10^3 organisms are grown from cultures of the catheter tip.

Specific therapy should be initiated against the primary source in patients in whom a source of infection other than the catheter tip is present. Peripheral blood cultures are obtained. One should avoid taking blood cultures from the central venous catheter port dedicated for PN because this increases the risk of contaminating the line. If the infection resolves, central venous feedings can be continued. If a secondary source is not identified and the symptoms persist, the catheter should be removed and its tip cultured. If the catheter tip culture returns positive or if the index of suspicion is high, appropriate antibiotic therapy is initiated. Central venous feeding can be resumed, maintaining blood glucose levels below 200 mg per dL.

Occasionally, the situation arises in which a site of infection other than the catheter is identified, but signs and symptoms persist despite what is assumed to be adequate therapy. As before, if blood cultures are positive, the safest course of action may be to remove the catheter. If peripheral blood cultures are negative, the catheter may be changed over a guide wire and the catheter tip cultured to determine if it

TABLE 11. **Possible Etiologies and Treatment of Common Complications of Central Parenteral Nutrition**

Problem	Possible Etiology	Treatment
Glucose		
Hyperglycemia, glycosuria, hyperosmolar nonketotic dehydration, or coma	Excessive dose or rate of infusion; inadequate insulin production; steroid administration; infection	Decrease the amount of glucose given; increase insulin; administer a portion of calories as fat
Diabetic ketoacidosis	Inadequate endogenous insulin production and/or inadequate insulin therapy	Give insulin; decrease glucose intake
Rebound hypoglycemia	Persistent endogenous insulin production by islet cells after long-term high carbohydrate infusion	Give 5–10% glucose before total parenteral infusion is discontinued
Hypercarbia	Carbohydrate load exceeds the ability to increase minute ventilation and excrete excess CO_2	Limit glucose dose to 5 mg/kg/min Give greater percentage of total caloric needs as fat (up to 30–40%)
Fat		
Hypertriglyceridemia	Rapid infusion; decreased clearance	Decrease rate of infusion; allow clearance (≈12 hr) before testing blood
Essential fatty acid deficiency	Inadequate essential fatty acid administration	Administer essential fatty acids in doses of 4–7% of total calories
Amino Acids		
Hyperchloremia metabolic acidosis	Excessive chloride content of amino acid solutions	Administer Na^+ and K^+ as acetate salts
Prerenal azotemia	Excessive amino acids with inadequate caloric supplementation	Reduce amino acids; increase the amount of glucose calories
Miscellaneous		
Hypophosphatemia	Inadequate phosphorus administration with redistribution into tissues	Give 15 mm phosphate/1000 IV kcal; evaluate antacid and Ca^{2+} administration
Hypomagnesemia	Inadequate administration relative to increased losses (diarrhea, diuresis, medications)	Administer Mg^{++} (15–20 mEq/1000 kcal)
Hypermagnesemia	Excessive administration; renal failure	Decrease Mg^{++} supplementation
Hypokalemia	Inadequate intake relative to increased needs for anabolism; diuresis	Increase K^+ supplementation
Hyperkalemia	Excessive administration, especially in metabolic acidosis; renal decompensation	Reduce or stop exogenous K^+; if electrocardiogram changes are present, treat with Ca gluconate, insulin, diuretics
Hypocalcemia	Inadequate administration; reciprocal response to phosphorus repletion without simultaneous calcium infusion	Increase Ca^{2+} dose
Hypercalcemia	Excessive administration; excessive vitamin D administration	Decrease Ca^{2+} and/or vitamin D administration
Elevated liver transaminases or serum alkaline phosphatase and bilirubin	Enzyme induction secondary to amino acid imbalances or overfeeding	Re-evaluate nutritional prescription

TABLE 12. **Management of Parenteral Nutrition–Related Liver Dysfunction**

- Have the patient eat, if possible.
- Avoid administration of large amounts of glucose or protein calories.
- Lipid emulsions should be supplied (up to 30% of total calories).
- Cycle the parenteral nutrition administration, infusing for 8–12 h per day.
- Re-evaluate caloric needs; reduce caloric intake if liver dysfunction persists.

was contaminated. Central venous feedings can be continued during this interval if the patient is stable. If the catheter tip returns positive, a new catheter should be inserted at a different site. Changing the central venous catheter over a guide wire can also facilitate the diagnosis of primary catheter infections.

Other Complications

The common complications of central venous alimentation are usually related to excess administration or underadministration of the energy sources, electrolytes, or trace metals. Common complications, their etiologies, and treatment are outlined in Table 11.

Prolonged administration of PN may result in altered hepatic function tests and changes in liver pathologic conditions that can lead to liver failure. Initially (1 to 2 weeks after initiation of PN), there are elevations of transaminases, but they frequently resolve without any change in the composition or rate of PN administration. However,in patients receiving long-term PN (>20 days), prolonged elevations of serum transaminase levels may persist, even after discontinuation of therapy. Serum levels of alkaline phosphatase and bilirubin initially remain normal, but rise in many patients who receive long-term PN. Patients who do not receive lipids in the PN solution have more frequent and severe hepatic abnormalities. The provision of excess glucose increases insulin secretion, which stimulates hepatic lipogenesis and results in hepatic fat accumulation. Fatty infiltration is the initial histopathologic change; it is readily reversible and may not be accompanied by altered liver function tests. Longer PN therapy may be associated with cholestasis and nonspecific triaditis and may progress to active chronic hepatitis, fibrosis, and eventual cirrhosis. The management of PN-related liver dysfunction is summarized in Table 12.

Complications are minimized and nutritional therapy maximized when the care of patients who require specialized nutritional support is supervised by a nutrition support team. Ideally, the nutrition support team consists of a pharmacist, dietitian, nurse, and physician.

FLUID AND ELECTROLYTE ABNORMALITIES IN CHILDREN

method of
RAJEEV AGARWAL, M.B., B.S., and
RICHARD E. NEIBERGER, M.D., PH.D.
University of Florida College of Medicine
Gainesville, Florida

The management of fluid and electrolyte disturbances is a common and challenging therapeutic problem for physicians taking care of infants and children. These disorders are frequently associated with problems related to the gastrointestinal tract (e.g., vomiting, diarrhea). Dependence on adults for fluid and nutrition, limited renal concentrating and diluting capability, and relatively small reserves may complicate management. Infants and children differ from adults in their fluid requirements (corrected for body weight), relative fluid distribution, and renal concentrating ability; these differences necessitate special considerations in fluid and electrolyte management.

PHYSIOLOGY

Normal Volume and Normal Composition

Water accounts for as much as 80% of the total body weight in a premature infant. Total body water progressively decreases to 70% at birth and 60% at 1 year of age and beyond. Obese people and women have a lower percentage of body water because of a larger percentage of adipose tissue, which is 10% water, compared with muscle, which is 75% water.

The internal milieu can be visualized as two compartments separated by a semipermeable membrane, across which water moves freely to equilibrate the osmolality. These compartments are the intracellular fluid (ICF) and the extracellular fluid (ECF). The cell membrane has different permeabilities for solutes. Concentration gradients, differences in the hydrostatic and oncotic pressures, and electrical charge also affect the movement of ions across the cell membrane. Na^+,K^+-ATPase and other pump systems maintain concentration gradients on both sides of the membranes. Na^+,K^+-ATPase is primarily responsible for maintaining high intracellular K^+ concentration, high extracellular Na^+ concentration, and net intracellular electronegativity.

The ECF constitutes one third of the total body water, which as noted previously is 60% of the body weight after 1 year of age. It is divided into interstitial fluid, which accounts for three quarters of the ECF (15 to 20% of total body weight), and plasma (4 to 5% of total body weight). The interstitial fluid also contains the transcellular fluid (1 to 3% of total body weight). Transcellular fluid is kept separate from the rest of the interstitial fluid by a layer of epithelium and endothelium and consists of collections such as cerebrospinal fluid, synovial fluid, and pleural, peritoneal, and pericardial fluids; intraluminal fluid in the biliary, pancreatic, and hepatic system; and the vitreous and aqueous humors in the eye. Transcellular fluid is constantly secreted and reabsorbed and hence is in dynamic equilibrium with the other body fluids. In the ECF compartment, the principal cation is sodium and the principal anions are chloride and bicarbonate. The ECF compartment is in direct communication with the gastrointestinal system and the environment and hence is the route of exit for all acute losses. The fraction of the blood volume that perfuses the vital and regulatory organs such as the brain, heart, and kidneys is called the effective circulating volume and is kept in tight control by pressure and volume receptors.

The ICF constitutes two thirds of the total body water. The major cation in this compartment is potassium, and the major anions are proteins and phosphates. Because this fluid compartment is not in direct communication with areas of potential loss and has a much larger volume, it acts as a buffer in states of fluid and electrolyte loss. Fluid and electrolyte losses from the ICF are replenished over a longer period.

Under normal conditions, the osmolality of the ICF and ECF compartments ranges from 275 to 290 mOsm per kg H_2O. Water is freely permeable across biologic membranes and moves from hypo-osmolar compartment to hyperosmolar compartment.

Osmolality is dependent on the concentration of solute particles present. Solutes in the ECF are Na^+, Cl^-, glucose, blood urea nitrogen (BUN), K^+, Ca^{2+}, and Mg^{2+}. For clinical purposes plasma osmolality can be estimated as follows:

$$\text{Posm} = 2[\text{Na}^+]\,(\text{mEq/L}) + \text{BUN (mg/dL)}/2.8 + \text{glucose (mg/dL)}/18$$

Doubling the Na^+ concentration accounts for both Na^+ and its accompanying anions. The dissociation of sodium chloride (NaCl) is incomplete. The calculated result normally agrees within 10 mOsm per liter of the measured value. The divisors 2.8 and 18 for the BUN and glucose concentrations, respectively, convert from mg per dL to mEq per kg H_2O.

Na^+ is relatively impermeable across the cell membrane and is the major determinant of serum osmolality. Urea is permeable across membranes; thus, it does not contribute significantly to the difference in osmolality between intracellular and extracellular compartments.

Glucose is permeable across cell membranes in the presence of insulin. Therefore, it does not lead to a difference in osmolality between the ICF and the ECF. Insulin deficiency states can cause the ECF to become hyperosmolar, which leads to movement of water from cells, resulting in cellular dehydration.

Regulation of Cellular Fluid Volume and Composition

The osmolality of the ECF is monitored by osmoresponsive neurons in the hypothalamus that regulate the release of antidiuretic hormone (ADH) and control thirst. Although the osmolality of the ECF is determined by both the total body Na^+ and water, the response is to regulate the water content through thirst and ADH mechanisms. ADH is also regulated by volume status and blood pressure through receptors located in the carotid sinus, atria, and aorta. At times of hypovolemia, ADH is secreted even in the presence of hypo-osmolality, as seen in the clinical situation of hyponatremic dehydration. Effective circulating volume is kept under tight control through volume and pressure receptors in the central nervous system (CNS). The extracellular fluid volume is determined by the total body Na^+, which is regulated by renin-angiotensin-aldosterone, atrial natriuretic peptide, and other systems.

Physiologic Fluid Requirements

Maintenance water and electrolytes are required to provide for losses due to normal physiologic activities. These losses can be divided into insensible losses and urine output for excretion of renal solute load.

Numerous methods have been used to estimate the maintenance fluid requirement. The following three methods are widely used.

1. In the first method the daily fluid requirement is calculated according to the body surface area and is equal to 1500 mL per m^2. This method is cumbersome but gives good estimates. The body surface area (BSA) can be determined from standardized charts or can be roughly estimated from either of the following equations:

$$\text{BSA (in m}^2) = \sqrt{\frac{\text{weight (kg)} \times \text{height (cm)}}{3600}}$$

or

$$\text{BSA (in m}^2) = \frac{[\text{weight (kg)} \times 4] + 7}{\text{weight (kg)} + 90}$$

2. A second method divides the daily fluid requirement into insensible losses and urine output.

$$\text{Daily fluid requirement} = \text{insensible losses} + \text{urine output} = 400\ \text{mL/m}^2 + \text{urine output}$$

This technique is useful when urine output is marginal, as in acute renal failure, and the patient is at risk for fluid overload.

3. The third method is based on calorie intake, with 1 mL of water required for every kcal metabolized (Table 1).

Any of the three methods can be used to calculate fluid requirements; all give approximately the same values. Selection depends on the preference of the caregiver.

Roughly, the maintenance fluid requirement of 100 mL per kg per day can be divided into specific components reflecting fluid losses occurring by the various routes: 50 mL per kg for urine losses, insensible losses of 15 mL per kg through the lungs and 30 mL per kg through the skin, and 5 mL per kg lost in stool. It should be kept in mind that fever increases the fluid requirement by 12.5% for each 1°C elevation of body temperature above 37°C and by 7.5% for each 1°F above 99°F.

Obligatory urine output is the minimum volume of water required to excrete the daily solute load. The solute load is determined by the daily intake of solute and the rate of metabolism (rate of production of urea). The solute load depends on the kind of food ingested or intravenous fluid administered but is typically in the range of 10 to 40 mOsm per 100 kcal consumed. Each gram of dietary protein generates approximately 4 mOsm of urea, which adds to the renal solute load. The amount of water required to excrete a certain solute load depends on the renal concentrating ability, which ranges from 50 to 600 mOsm per liter in infants to 50 to 1200 mOsm per liter in an adult. A urine output rate of 50 mL per kcal permits the excretion

TABLE 1. **Estimates of Fluid Requirement in Children**

Body Weight (kg)	Daily Caloric Requirement	Fluid Requirement/24 h
3–10	100 kcal/kg	100 mL/kg
10–20	1000 + 50 kcal/kg	1000 + 50 mL/kg
>20	1500 + 20 kcal/kg	1500 + 20 mL/kg

of urine that is iso-osmolar with extracellular fluid and not maximally dilute or concentrated.

In basal conditions, two thirds of insensible water losses occurs through the skin and one third through the respiratory tract. These losses may vary depending on the water vapor tension, air movement, and respiratory rate and depth. It should be noted that sweat represents an additional water loss and is not accounted for in the evaporative losses through the skin. The water of insensible losses is electrolyte-free. Insensible water loss is dependent on the metabolic rate (and thus caloric expenditure) and on the ratio of surface area to body weight. It may account for as much as 50% of the daily requirement of an infant, whereas in an older child it may range from 35 to 50%.

Maintenance Electrolyte Requirements

The daily requirement of Na^+ is 3 mEq per 24 hours, and that of K^+ is 2 mEq per 24 hours, for every 100 kcal metabolized. For short-term therapy bicarbonate is not required because of intrinsic buffer systems. Chloride is the accompanying anion in parenteral fluids. Because of the large contribution by electrolyte-free insensible losses, maintenance fluids are hypotonic.

At least 20% of the daily requirement of calories is needed to prevent tissue breakdown and catabolism of proteins. For short term intravenous fluid therapy, the calorie requirement can be supplied by 5 grams of dextrose per 100 mL added to the intravenous fluid. A higher concentration of dextrose is required if long-term intravenous fluid therapy is planned.

Ongoing Losses

In some circumstances, ongoing losses may be considerable, and failure to replace them may result in dehydration. This is especially pertinent for children with gastroenteritis because of loss of gastric and intestinal contents through vomiting and diarrhea. After surgery, considerable amounts of electrolyte-rich body fluids may be lost through drains or stents. Table 2 gives the electrolyte composition of body fluids.

Sweating increases the fluid requirement by 5 to 25 mL per 100 kcal and the sodium requirement by 0.5 to 1 mEq of Na^+ per 100 kcal. In patients with cystic fibrosis, Na^+ replacement needs increase by 1 to 2 mEq per 100 kcal expended.

ABNORMALITIES OF VOLUME, COMPOSITION, AND OSMOLALITY

Hypovolemia (Dehydration)

Dehydration is caused by acute losses of body fluids and accompanying electrolytes or the inability to compensate for these losses. The most common cause of dehydration in infants and children is acute gastroenteritis. Diarrhea results in water and electrolyte losses. Accompanying vomiting complicates gastroenteritis further by increasing losses and an inability to compensate through ingestion. Other causes of dehydration include inadequate intake due to altered mental status or postsurgical states; increased renal losses as in diabetes insipidus, renal concentrating defects, or osmotic diuresis; and, rarely, increased insensible losses occurring with fever, burns, vigorous exercise, cystic fibrosis, or hyperventilation. Frequently, more than one factor is involved in clinical dehydration. The clinical presentation and laboratory values in a patient with dehydration result from the dynamic equilibrium between the volume and electrolyte composition of losses, replacement therapy, and renal function. All states of dehydration are accompanied by net loss of both water and electrolytes. The relative quantities of water and electrolyte loss (and replacements) determine whether hypotonicity, isotonicity, or hypertonicity (reflected by serum Na^+ concentration) results.

Fluid and electrolytes are lost directly from the ECF through gastrointestinal, urinary, respiratory, and skin routes. Losses from the ECF compartment are accompanied by contraction and subsequent loss of both water and electrolytes from the ICF. It has been estimated that in acute dehydration, 80% of fluid loss is from the ECF and 20% is from the ICF, with accompanying electrolytes to maintain osmotic equilibrium. With prolonged dehydration, losses are equal in both compartments. In both acute and chronic states the replacement fluids play an important role in determining clinical presentation and laboratory values.

TABLE 2. **Electrolyte Composition of Body Fluids**

	Electrolyte (mEq/L)			
Fluid	**HCO_3^-**	**Cl^-**	**Na^+**	**K^+**
Sweating, fever	0	50	50	0–15
Gastric juice	0	110	50	5–15
Pancreatic juice	110	75	140	5
Small bowel	30	110	140	5
Ileostomy	30	110	130	10
Diarrhea	15–50	55–100	50–140	5–15

Evaluation

For the purpose of the following discussion, it is assumed that the patient is *not* in a state of chronic malnutrition or congestive heart failure and does not have associated renal problems. The assessment of dehydration includes attention to (1) volume deficit; (2) osmolar disturbances; (3) acid-base disturbances; (4) potassium balance; and (5) renal function.

VOLUME DEFICIT

The best estimation of fluid loss is the acute loss of weight. Usually, however, the patient is being evaluated in an emergency setting, and the predehydration weight is not known. Sometimes the parents can supply this information. Rough estimate of weight may be obtained by plotting weight for height on the growth chart according to body habitus. If the preillness weight is known or can be estimated, then the percentage of dehydration may be obtained by the formula

$$\text{Degree of dehydration (\%)} = \frac{\text{preillness weight} - \text{weight at evaluation}}{\text{preillness weight}} \times 100\%$$

Dehydration is classified as mild, moderate, or severe depending on weight loss—up to 5%, 5 to 9%, or 10 to 15%, respectively. If preillness weight is not known, the degree of dehydration can be assessed by history and physical examination (Table 3). In general, infants and children have no manifestations with mild dehydration (except for thirst and possibly dry mucous membranes). If there is a history of decreased fluid intake or increased losses, it is reasonable to diagnose mild dehydration. A child with manifestations of dehydration on physical examination is approximately 5 to 10% dehydrated; with weight loss of 11 to 15% (severe dehydration), impending shock supervenes. In children 8 years of age or older and in adults, dehydration states with weight losses of 3%, 6 to 9%, and 10% or higher correspond to mild, moderate, and severe dehydration, respectively.

Clinical estimation of the degree of dehydration is imprecise at best because the clinical features are really signs of extracellular volume depletion. In addition, there may be significant intra- and inter-observer differences in the estimation of degree of dehydration. Decrease in urinary output reported by the parent is subjective and may reflect the parent's perception and the presence of multiple caregivers. Skin turgor and peripheral perfusion are the most reliable signs; lack of tears and dry mucous membranes may be misleading. "Tenting" produced by pinching the skin is indicative of severe dehydration. Peripheral perfusion is determined by noting the capillary refill time—i.e., the time required for recovery of blanching of color after light pressure is applied to the nail bed. Normally it is less than 2 seconds; any value exceeding 3 seconds is indicative of severe dehydration. The estimation of dehydration may be used to calculate the preillness weight.

Parenteral administration of fluid and electrolytes is indicated whenever the oral route is unavailable or contraindicated. The time period for which fluid therapy can be deferred depends on the age of the child, ranging from 2 hours in a premature infant to up to 12 hours in an adolescent. The fluid replacement required with mild dehydration is 50 mL per kg (or volume equal to loss in weight). Most affected children do not need parenteral fluid therapy and can be rehydrated enterally. With moderate dehydration, fluid requirement is 100 mL per kg, and with severe dehydration, it is 150 mL per kg. Maintenance requirements and those for ongoing losses have to be included in the fluid therapy. The total fluid administered should include fluid replacement, maintenance requirements (for the period of correction), and fluids for ongoing losses.

TABLE 3. **Estimate of Degree of Isotonic Dehydration by Physical Signs**

	Symptoms of Dehydration for Degree Shown		
Physical Sign	*<5%*	*5–9%*	*10–15%*
Skin turgor	Normal	Decreased	Tenting
Mucous membranes	Moist	Dry	Very dry
Eyes	Normal	Sunken	Very sunken
Fontanelle	Flat	Soft	Sunken
Central nervous system—mental status	Consolable	Irritable	Lethargic/comatose
Pulse	Normal	Orthostatic	Thready
Blood pressure	Normal	Normal/orthostatic	Impending shock
Capillary refill time	<2 s	2–3 s	>3 s

Note that with *hypotonic* dehydration, physical signs are accentuated; with *hypertonic* dehydration, physical signs are diminished, with "doughy" skin turgor.

OSMOLAR DISTURBANCE

Neither the history nor the physical examination can uncover accompanying osmolar disturbance associated with dehydration. In most cases the fluid lost from the body has a sodium concentration between 30 and 70 mEq per liter, except in cholera, in which the stool is almost iso-osmotic. Under normal circumstances, the primary determinant of serum osmolality is the serum Na^+ concentration. Serum osmolality (iso-, hypo-, and hyper-) corresponds closely to isonatremic, hyponatremic, and hypernatremic types of dehydration. Depending on the calculated osmolality, dehydration can be classified as hypo-osmotic (Posm of less than 275 mOsm per kg H_2O) or hyperosmotic (Posm of more than 295 mOsm per kg H_2O).

Isotonic (isonatremic) dehydration is the most common form of dehydration clinically (accounting for 80% of the cases). It represents iso-osmolar losses or compensation by iso-osmolar replacement fluid. The clinical picture is consistent with the degree of dehydration.

Hypotonic (hyponatremic) dehydration occurs when solute loss is in excess of the fluid loss and/or replacement fluids are hypotonic. Water moves from the relatively hypo-osmolar ECF to the ICF to equilibrate the tonicity, further decreasing the intravascular fluid volume. In this case, the extracellular fluid compartment loses fluid both to the external environment and to the intracellular fluid compartment. The clinical manifestations are exaggerated relative to the actual fluid loss. Patients present early with vascular instability, decreased blood pressure, and altered mental status (due to cerebral edema resulting from movement of water into cells). Urinary sodium level is low (less than 10 mEq per liter) because of avid reabsorption to maintain the intravascular volume and Na^+ concentration, and the urinary osmolality is high. Urine sodium concentration and osmolality are helpful in differentiating among the other causes of hyponatremia.

The net sodium loss can be divided into two components, an isotonic component responsible for the symptomatic ECF contraction and an additional net sodium loss. This additional sodium loss can be calculated as

$$Na^+ \text{ deficit (mEq)} = \text{body weight} \times 0.6 \times (135 - P_{Na})$$

The factor of 0.6 accounts for the percentage of body weight that is the total body water. The total body water is taken into consideration because water is freely permeable across the ECF and the ICF. P_{Na} is the plasma Na^+ concentration.

Hypertonic (hypernatremic) dehydration occurs when water loss is in excess of solute loss and/or hypertonic replacement fluids are used. Historically, this type of dehydration accounted for one third of the cases, but now its incidence has decreased remarkably, mainly because of discontinuation of the practice of using boiled skim milk for rehydration.

Hypertonic dehydration results in considerable morbidity and mortality because of delay in presentation and diagnosis and associated CNS complications. The clinical estimation of degree of dehydration is deceptively low because of movement of water from ICF to ECF, resulting in the preservation of ECF at the expense of ICF. Thus, in spite of severe dehydration, signs of shock may be absent. The child usually presents with CNS changes such as irritability and lethargy; the skin has a typical feel described as "doughy." ADH is maximally secreted because of a combination of hypovolemia and hyperosmolality. Because of high ADH levels, the urinary output is low and cannot be used as a measure of intravascular status or response to therapy.

In addition to the water lost in dehydration there is an additional free water loss that results in hypernatremia. It can be calculated from the formula

$$\text{Free water deficit} = \frac{0.6 \times \text{weight (kg)} \times \text{measured osmolality}}{\text{normal plasma osmolality}} - 0.6 \times \text{wt (kg)}$$

The factor 0.6 is the fraction of body weight that is water; measured osmolality can be approximated by $2 \times P_{Na}$; and normal plasma osmolality is 280 mOsm per kg H_2O.

ACID-BASE DISTURBANCES RELATED TO DEHYDRATION

The physiologic response of the body to severe dehydration is to maintain perfusion of vital organs at the cost of perfusion to peripheral organs, leading to anaerobic metabolism in muscle and subsequent lactic acidosis. These changes may be complicated by loss of bicarbonate-rich fluids as in diarrheal or ileostomy fluids and by reduced ability to excrete hydrogen ion, as seen in acute prerenal insufficiency. Venous blood gas values are adequate to evaluate the pH, bicarbonate level, and P_{CO_2} and can be used to differentiate between respiratory or metabolic acidosis or alkalosis.

In most cases mild metabolic acidosis is seen; this does not require treatment except fluid administration to restore adequate perfusion. Alkali administration may be required if the bicarbonate level is less than 8 mEq per liter, pH is less than 7.2, or a significant anion gap exists. In these situations, bicarbonate can be substituted for chloride as the accompanying anion. If bicarbonate administration is required, it is prudent to infuse it continuously rather than give it as a bolus (2.5 mEq of sodium bicarbonate per kg of body weight will increase the blood bicarbonate level by approximately 5 mEq per liter).

Metabolic alkalosis can develop with the loss of hydrogen ions occurring in patients on continuous nasogastric suctioning, or in infants with intractable vomiting, as classically seen in pyloric stenosis. In these cases, chloride losses also are high, resulting in hypochloremic metabolic alkalosis, frequently accompanied by hypokalemia. Other complex acid-base abnormalities may be present that require frequent determination of blood gases and serum and urine chemistries for evaluation and management.

POTASSIUM ABNORMALITIES

All types of dehydration are accompanied by significant potassium losses, especially when caused by gastric losses or intestinal drainage. Potassium is mainly an intracellular cation, occurring in a concentration of 150 mEq per liter (accounting for 98% of the body's total potassium), with a concentration of only 3.5 to 5.5 mEq per liter in the serum. Thus, large total body losses may occur before a significant change is seen in the laboratory values for potassium (because laboratory values reflect changes within the ECF). Moreover, acidosis raises the serum potassium level (even with total body potassium deficit), because hydrogen ions displace potassium ions within the cell. The deficit is further worsened by rapid excretion of the extracellular potassium.

Hyperkalemia associated with anuria or oliguria is indicative of acute renal failure. In children with dehydration, hypokalemia is even more common than hyperkalemia. Hyperkalemia occurs in association with metabolic acidosis. It is usually mild and does not require treatment. Children with hypokalemia are usually asymptomatic unless the abnormality is extreme (K^+ concentration of less than 2 mEq per liter), when muscle weakness, ileus, and electrocardiographic abnormalities such as occasional U waves and heart block are seen. Potassium supplementation is started after the child has voided. This precaution is to avoid giving K^+ if acute renal failure has already occurred. Potassium losses are gradually replaced over 3 or 4 days. Intravenous potassium is caustic to veins; therefore, the maximum concentration that can be given in a peripheral vein is 40 mEq per liter. If a bolus is required, then a small dose such as 0.5 mEq per kg over 1 to 3 hours usually suffices.

RENAL FUNCTION

The major concern in children with dehydration is differentiating oliguria due to prerenal azotemia from that occurring with progression to acute tubular necrosis. Most children with severe dehydration have enough ECF contraction to reduce the glomerular filtration rate (GFR); if correction is delayed, acute tubular necrosis and acute renal failure may result. If no urine is voided after the initial fluid therapy, the bladder should be catheterized to document urine production. The urine and serum chemistries should include creatinine and sodium levels to determine the fractional excretion of sodium (FE_{Na}).

$$FE_{Na} = \frac{U_{Na} / P_{Na}}{U_{Cr} / P_{Cr}} \times 100\%$$

U_{Na} and P_{Na} are urine and plasma concentrations of sodium, and U_{Cr} and P_{Cr} are urine and plasma concentrations of creatinine, respectively.

An FE_{Na} value of less than 1 to 2% indicates prerenal azotemia, which occurs as the tubules conserve sodium in an attempt to restore the circulating volume; an FE_{Na} value of 3% or greater suggests tubular damage and salt wasting, with impending acute renal failure. Persistent oliguria (urine output of less than 0.5 mL per kg per hour) with isotonic urine and increasing BUN and serum creatinine levels confirm the diagnosis of acute renal failure.

Treatment

There are three phases of management: (1) emergency fluid therapy; (2) replacement of deficit, maintenance, and ongoing losses; and (3) initiation of oral rehydration therapy.

EMERGENCY FLUID THERAPY

If the patient is severely dehydrated (loss of more than 10% of body weight) or has signs and symptoms of impending cardiovascular collapse, a bolus of an isotonic fluid (e.g., Ringer's lactate or normal saline), 10 to 20 mL per kg, should be given over 30 minutes through a large-bore intravenous line. If there is no improvement, the bolus may be repeated twice; if there is still no improvement, other causes of shock or fluid loss should be investigated. Usually the second and third fluid boluses need to be given over 1 to 2 hours, depending on the vital signs and perfusion status. Potassium supplementation should be withheld at this time. The majority of patients do not need emergency fluid therapy.

REPLACEMENT OF DEFICIT, MAINTENANCE, AND ONGOING LOSSES

The K^+ concentration in the ECF and the Na^+ concentration in the ICF are small and can be ignored for most calculation purposes. For fluid and electrolyte replacement, the ICF and ECF water deficit and the ECF sodium deficit should be calculated separately and then combined, so that an estimate of the volume and composition of the fluid required is obtained. Then the commercial fluid nearest in composition to the solute requirements should be used. Custom-made solutions for each patient are expensive and do not confer any advantage in clinical management except when renal function is compromised. Emergency replacement fluids are not included in these calculations.

Case Example

A previously healthy 1-year-old infant weighing 10 kg becomes dehydrated after an episode of vomiting and diarrhea. He is presented to the emergency room with a body temperature of 37°C, blood pressure of 80/60 mm Hg, and pulse rate of 160 per minute. On physical examination, the infant's mucous membranes are dry, his eyes are sunken, skin turgor is decreased, and capillary refill time is 2 seconds. He is estimated to be about 10% dehydrated. He is given a 10 mL per kg bolus of normal saline. Typical laboratory values are given in Table 4. As stated previously, it is useful to consider fluid and electrolyte losses separately. Calculations of fluid deficit and of replacement fluid composition for isotonic, hypotonic, and hypertonic types of dehydration are described in the following discussion.

Fluid deficit: With 10% dehydration the deficit is 100 mL/kg; therefore, 100 mL/kg × 10 kg = 1000 mL.

Solute deficit: Since the fluid loss is relatively rapid, 80% of this fluid loss is from the ECF and 20% from the ICF; therefore, the solute losses are

$$Na^+ \text{ loss} = 140 \text{ mEq/L} \times 0.80 \times 1 \text{ L} = 112 \text{ mEq}$$

$$K^+ \text{ loss} = 150 \text{ mEq/L} \times 0.2 \times 1 \text{ L} = 30 \text{ mEq}$$

If the fluid loss is chronic, then the fluid losses from both compartments are equal, and accompanying solute losses are

$$Na^+ \text{ loss} = 140 \text{ mEq/L} \times 0.5 \times 1 \text{ L} = 70 \text{ mEq}$$

$$K^+ \text{ loss} = 150 \text{ mEq/L} \times 0.5 \times 1 \text{ L} = 75 \text{ mEq}$$

Maintenance fluid for 24 hours: 100 mL/kg × 10 kg = 1000 mL

Maintenance solutes for 24 hours:

$$Na^+ \text{ requirement} = 2.5 \text{ mEq/kg} \times 10 \text{ kg} = 25 \text{ mEq}$$

$$K^+ \text{ requirement} = 2 \text{ mEq/kg} \times 10 \text{ kg} = 20 \text{ mEq}$$

Ongoing losses at the time of evaluation are not a factor but must be considered during the course of the therapy.

1. Isotonic Dehydration. Correction of the deficit is achieved over 24 hours; therefore, total fluid requirement for 24 hours = 2000 mL of fluid (i.e., 1000 mL deficit + 1000 mL maintenance).

TABLE 4. **Case Example: Solute Losses with Dehydration**

Dehydration Type	Weight (kg)	Solute Losses (mEq/L)			
		Na^+	K^+	Cl^-	HCO_3^-
1. Isotonic	10	140	4.0	105	20
2. Hypotonic	10	120	3.8	97	18
3. Hypertonic	10	164	5.0	129	18

$$Na^+ \text{ requirement} = 112 \text{ mEq (deficit)} + 25 \text{ mEq (maintenance)} = 137 \text{ mEq}$$

$$K^+ \text{ requirement} = 30 \text{ mEq (deficit)} + 20 \text{ mEq (maintenance)} = 50 \text{ mEq}$$

This can be corrected using 2 liters of fluid containing Na^+ 68.5 mEq per liter and K^+ 25 mEq per liter. For practical purposes, one-half normal saline (77 mEq of Na^+ per liter) with 20 mEq of K^+ per liter can be used. In isotonic dehydration the total fluid required is administered over 24 hours, half over the first 8 hours and the rest over the next 16 hours. Thus, one-half normal saline with 20 mEq of K^+ per liter is administered at 125 mL per hour for 8 hours, followed by 60 mL per hour for the next 16 hours.

2. HYPOTONIC DEHYDRATION. As this episode of gastroenteritis is fairly acute, the correction can be achieved over 24 hours.

Total fluid requirements are 1000 mL deficit and 1000 mL maintenance, as calculated previously. The laboratory values are shown in Table 4.

The sodium deficit is $10 \times 0.6 \times (135 - 120) = 90$ mEq (see section on hyponatremia); therefore, the total deficit is

$$Na^+ \text{ requirement} = 137 \text{ mEq (as calculated)} + 90 \text{ mEq} = 227 \text{ mEq}$$

$$K^+ \text{ requirement} = 50 \text{ mEq (as calculated)}$$

Thus, this can be corrected by using 2 liters of fluid containing Na^+ 113.5 mEq per liter and K^+ 25 mEq per liter. This is approximated by using three-fourths normal saline with 25 mEq of K^+ per liter at 125 mL per hour for the first 8 hours followed by 60 mL per hour for the next 16 hours.

3. HYPERTONIC DEHYDRATION. The correction in this case needs to be done over 48 hours. In hypernatremia the urine will be maximally concentrated because of maximal ADH secretion until the hyperosmolarity stimulus abates; thus, the maintenance requirements are decreased by about three fourths.

$$\begin{aligned} &\text{48-hour total water requirement} \\ &= \tfrac{3}{4} \text{ maintenance for 48 h} + \text{fluid deficit (as calculated)} + \text{free fluid deficit} \\ &= (2 \times \tfrac{3}{4} \times 1000) + 1000 + \left[\frac{0.6 \times 10 \times 2 \times 164}{280}\right] - 0.6 \times 10 \\ &= 1500 + 1000 + 1000 \text{ mL} \\ &= 3500 \text{ mL} \end{aligned}$$

$$Na^+ \text{ requirement} = 112 \text{ mEq} + (25 \times 2) \text{ mEq} = 162 \text{ mEq}$$

$$K^+ \text{ requirement} = 30 \text{ mEq} + (20 \times 2) \text{ mEq} = 70 \text{ mEq}$$

In this case the Na^+ deficit may be an overestimate and the K^+ deficit an underestimate because of proportionately larger losses from the ICF as compared with the ECF. Thus, 3.5 liters of fluid needs to be administered with Na^+ 46 mEq per liter, which is approximated by one-third normal saline, and with K^+ 20 mEq per liter. This is given at a rate of 73 mL per hour over 48 hours. Initial higher rates are usually not required because of stable cardiovascular status. Frequent monitoring is required to document that the fall in the sodium level occurs no faster than 0.5 mEq per hour and 12 mEq per day.

Oral Rehydration Therapy

The majority of patients with dehydration can be rehydrated through the enteral route. Contraindications to oral rehydration therapy (ORT) are altered consciousness, seizure activity, shock, persistent vomiting, and ileus. As most diarrheal diseases are self-limited, the use of ORT is particularly suited for use in Third World countries because of the decrease in the need for hospitalization and in the use of expensive parenteral solutions. A major advantage of ORT in the United States is its ready availability. Early use in the course of illness may prevent severe dehydration.

Glucose and sodium are absorbed in the small intestine through a cotransport mechanism. Water is absorbed with the sodium, and potassium is absorbed by solvent "drag." Thus, in spite of continued water and electrolyte losses in diarrheal fluid, net absorption occurs. The optimal composition of an oral rehydration solution is as follows: glucose, 2 to 2.5%; Na^+, 40 to 50 mEq per liter; K^+, 20 mEq per liter; and citrate, 30 mEq per liter. Potassium and citrate are added to prevent hypokalemia and acidosis. Higher concentrations can exacerbate diarrhea because of increased osmotic load. Volume for volume, sucrose (table sugar), glucose, and fructose are equivalent. However, fructose is not coupled with sodium transport. Therefore, in homemade oral rehydration solutions, twice the amount of sucrose is used to achieve the same efficacy. A larger volume of oral rehydration solution is recommended for rehydration than is used in parenteral therapy, because stool losses may increase with the use of ORT.

Various formulations of oral rehydration solution are available. Most such solutions are higher in sodium concentration than maintenance oral electrolyte solutions. The World Health Organization (WHO) formula contains 90 mEq of sodium per liter. This solution was made for rehydration in the presence of diarrhea with cholera, in which high concentrations of electrolytes are lost in stool. In the Western world, the infections causing diarrhea are associated with much lower concentrations of electrolytes lost in the stool. Thus, use of the WHO solution may result in hypernatremia. Commercial preparations are available with lower sodium concentrations, which may be used.

Rates of fluid replacement of 50 mL per kg over 4 hours and 100 mL per kg over 6 hours should be planned for mild and moderate dehydration, respectively. If vomiting limits the use of the prescribed

TABLE 5. **Recommendations for Oral Rehydration Therapy (ORT)**

1. Breast-feeding is continued through ORT.
2. Half-strength formula is started within 24 hours of beginning ORT.
3. ORT should not be given solely for more than 24 hours.
4. Full-strength formula is given within the first 36 to 48 hours.
5. Solid foods—low fat, high starch—are started in the first 24 hours. These include but are not limited to rice, potatoes, noodles, crackers, toast, bananas, dry cereal, cooked wheat cereal, shredded wheat, and oatmeal.

volumes, then small volumes of up to 30 mL can be given every 5 to 10 minutes, which can be slowly increased if tolerated. In case of hypernatremic dehydration, oral rehydration should be undertaken over 12 to 24 hours. After rehydration, more hypotonic solutions should be used. The oral rehydration solution can be combined with clear fluids or maintenance fluids in a 1:1 ratio. Such oral rehydration solutions should not be administered as the sole fluid for more than 24 hours. Parents should be cautioned to note an increase in the stool volume with refeeding, but this should not be a cause for major concern. The general practice has been to delay the reintroduction of lactose-containing foods and formulas. However, breast milk, which is high in lactose, is well tolerated and should be continued. See Table 5 for recommendations for use of ORT.

ABNORMALITIES OF SOLUTES

Sodium and Potassium

Sodium

HYPONATREMIA

The plasma fluid is composed of water, proteins, and lipids. Of the three components, only water serves as a solvent for Na^+. The Na^+ concentration in this water fraction is 150 to 155 mEq per liter. Proteins and lipids are devoid of Na^+. Normally, water constitutes 94% of the plasma volume. The laboratory quantifies the Na^+ content of the plasma water but reports it as the content of the whole plasma volume; generally, such measurements provide a good approximation of the plasma Na^+ level because of the relatively stable fractions of plasma constituents. In disorders causing hyperproteinemia or hyperlipidemia, however, the nonaqueous (non–Na^+-containing) fractions of the whole plasma are relatively increased, and correction for the presence of the excess proteins or lipids is necessary.

In factitious hyponatremia, osmotically active solutes in the ECF that are not transported across the cell membrane, such as mannitol and glucose (in insulin deficiency states), create an osmotic gradient. This osmotic gradient favors the movement of water from the ICF to the ECF. This water movement is not accompanied by Na^+ movement across the cell membrane. The net result is an increase in ECF water content with no change in ECF Na^+ content, which decreases the Na^+ concentration of the compartment. Osmotically active solutes such as urea and glucose (in the presence of insulin), which are freely permeable across the cell membrane, do not exert such osmotic forces and do not cause net movement of water.

The other causes of hyponatremia (Table 6) include the syndrome of inappropriate secretion of ADH (associated with an increase in weight, high urine sodium, and a urine osmolality that is inappropriately high for the hypotonic serum); congestive heart failure and nephrosis are associated with urinary findings similar to those for hyponatremic dehydration but are obviously associated with weight gain and edema. In water intoxication the urine is hypo-osmotic to serum although the urinary sodium level is low; similar findings associated with hyperkalemia suggest a diagnosis of adrenal insufficiency. Renal insufficiency or obstructive uropathy results in an inability to concentrate urine and a high urine sodium level (more than 50 mEq per liter).

The most common features of hyponatremia are CNS changes such as irritability, decrease in concentration, and seizures. If a patient presents with seizures due to hyponatremia, 3% saline can be given to rapidly raise the serum sodium concentration by 3 to 5 mEq per liter. Once the acute manifestations subside, the remainder of the solution is given slowly over 24 to 48 hours. During hyponatremia of more than 5 days' duration, there is a gradual reduction in the ICF of the brain cells. Rapid correction results

TABLE 6. **Hyponatremia: Etiologic Classification**

Isotonic hyponatremia (pseudo-hyponatremia): Posm = 275–295 mOsm/kg H_2O
- Hyperlipidemia (e.g., nephrotic syndrome)
- Hyperproteinemia (e.g., multiple myeloma)

Hypertonic hyponatremia (factitious hyponatremia): Posm > 295 mOsm/kg H_2O
- Hyperglycemia (e.g., diabetic ketoacidosis)
- Mannitol, glycerol

Hypotonic hyponatremia: Posm < 275 mOsm/kg H_2O
- Hypovolemic
  - Gastrointestinal—vomiting, diarrhea, tubes/fistulas
  - Renal losses—diuretic excess, salt-wasting nephropathy, osmotic diuresis, adrenal insufficiency, hypoaldosteronism, proximal renal tubular acidosis, metabolic alkalosis
  - Excessive sweating
  - Third spacing—burns, peritonitis/ascitis, pancreatitis, effusions, muscle trauma
- Euvolemic
  - Excess ADH—SIADH, drugs, nausea, pain
  - Glucocorticoid deficiency
  - Hypothyroidism
  - Water intoxication—intravenous therapy, psychogenic water drinking
  - Tap water enema
  - Reset "osmostat"
- Hypervolemic
  - Edematous states—congestive heart failure, cirrhosis, nephrotic syndrome
  - Renal failure—acute, chronic

Abbreviations: ADH = antidiuretic hormone; Posm = plasma osmolality; SIADH = syndrome of inappropriate ADH secretion.

in a fluid shift from hypo-osmolar ECF to hyperosmolar ICF, leading to brain edema and subsequent neurologic sequelae. In the therapy of chronic hyponatremia, serum sodium concentration should not increase by more than 24 mEq per 48 hours (0.5 mEq per hour), and it should not be higher than 135 mEq per liter after 48 hours. These guidelines have been formulated to prevent the development of central pontine myelinolysis. In children, most cases of dehydration are associated with acute gastroenteritis (of less than 5 days' duration), and deficits can be corrected over 24 hours.

HYPERNATREMIA

Considerations in the differential diagnosis for hypernatremia (Table 7) include increased free water loss as seen in diabetes insipidus or diabetes mellitus; increase in insensible losses as associated with strenuous exercise; water deficit in excess of sodium loss as in diabetes mellitus, obstructive uropathy, renal dysplasia, or osmotic diuresis; and high sodium intake, which may occur with improperly mixed formulas (this used to be the most common course) or may be iatrogenic, as with inappropriate supplementation in total parenteral nutrition.

Hypernatremia is usually associated with significant loss of fluid from the ECF and ICF compartments, resulting in cellular dehydration. As a protective mechanism against CNS cellular dehydration and subsequent decrease in brain volume, idiogenic osmoles are generated (taurine and other organic molecules). Rapid rehydration with hypotonic fluid causes acute disturbance in ECF osmolality relative to the ICF. This phenomenon is of clinical significance, because fluid shifts inside the brain cells may cause cellular swelling, resulting in brain edema, seizures, and even herniation and death. Hypernatremic dehydration should be corrected over at least 48 hours. Serum sodium concentrations of over 180 mEq per liter may be best reduced by dialysis. Hyperosmolality associated with hypernatremia interferes with insulin and parathormone release, resulting in hyperglycemia and hypocalcemia. These need to be kept in mind in tailoring therapy for affected children. The treatment of hyponatremia has been discussed in the preceding case example.

TABLE 7. **Hypernatremia: Etiologic Classification**

Primarily water deficit
- Diabetes mellitus
- Diabetes insipidus—central nephrogenic
- Increased insensible water loss (as in newborns with use of radiant warmer)
- Excessive sweating
- Inadequate access to water
- Central lack of thirst (adipsia)

Relative water deficit more than sodium loss
- Diarrhea
- Obstructive uropathy
- Renal dysplasia
- Osmotic diuretic
- Diabetes mellitus

Primarily sodium excess
- Improperly mixed formula or maintenance oral rehydration solution
- Iatrogenic in intravenous fluids, total parenteral nutrition, resuscitation
- Ingestion of sea water

TABLE 8. **Hypokalemia: Etiologic Classification**

Gastrointestinal losses
- Vomiting
- Diarrhea
- Laxative abuse
- Vasoactive intestinal polypeptide-secreting tumor

Renal losses
- Diuretics (non–potassium-sparing)
- Tubular diseases (drugs, cystinosis)
- Steroids (e.g., glucocorticoids, aldosterone)
- Nonreabsorbable anions (bicarbonate, penicillin)

Intracellular shift from extracellular compartment
- Alkalosis
- $Beta_2$-receptor agonists
- Insulin

Limited intake

Potassium

HYPOKALEMIA

The major causes of hypokalemia are listed in Table 8. In general, hypokalemia may be present with a total body potassium deficit or may be due to movement of potassium from the ECF compartment to the ICF compartment.

Hypokalemia affects growth and carbohydrate metabolism. Children with chronic hypokalemia as in Bartter's syndrome exhibit poor growth and have short stature. Hypokalemia can precipitate or worsen encephalopathy associated with hepatic failure. Hypokalemia also produces autonomic insufficiency manifesting as orthostatic hypotension, diminished neuromuscular excitability lending to muscular weakness, and adynamic ileus. In the kidney, hypokalemia causes an inability to maximally concentrate the urine and a phosphate-losing nephropathy. Acutely, hypokalemia causes electrocardiographic changes including flattened T waves, U waves, ST segment depression, and arrhythmias.

Treatment. Most of the manifestations of hypokalemia are not life-threatening, and thus the replacement can be done orally. Intravenous replacement is done for severe hypokalemia (K^+ concentration of less than 2.0 mEq per liter). Potassium can be given through the intravenous route at the rate of 0.5 mEq per kg over 1 to 3 hours by slow infusion. Potassium can be added to the peripheral intravenous solution for up to a maximum of 40 mEq per liter. Rarely, higher concentrations may need to be given through a central access line. Frequent monitoring for cardiac arrhythmia is required when high concentrations of potassium are used.

HYPERKALEMIA

Hyperkalemia is a medical emergency that occurs more frequently than hypokalemia. Hyperkalemia is defined as a serum potassium concentration above 6.0 mEq per liter in newborns and above 5.5 mEq per liter in older children and adults. Hyperkalemia usually does not imply an increase in the total body potassium but rather occurs with a shift of potassium from the ICF to the ECF and/or an inability to excrete potassium. The causes of hyperkalemia are listed in Table 9. Serum potassium is higher than plasma potassium by 0.5 mEq per liter because of release of potassium from cells during clotting. The most common cause of hyperkalemia is cell trauma incurred with an improper collection technique during phlebotomy. In the presence of normal renal function, large amounts of K^+ are tolerated without life-threatening hyperkalemia. Intravenous infusion rates higher than 0.5 mEq per kg per hour can cause fatal hyperkalemia even in patients with normal renal function.

Hyperkalemia causes neuromuscular abnormalities such as weakness and paralysis. It increases the serum aldosterone and insulin levels, increases the Na^+,K^+-ATPase activity in the renal cortex and medulla, and may lead to hyperchloremic acidosis. The most important and potentially fatal effects of hyperkalemia are on the heart. The electrocardiographic changes are peaked T waves, widened QRS complex, prolonged PR interval, decreased amplitude, and finally, disappearance of the P wave. In severe hyperkalemia the electrocardiographic complex is the classic sine wave. Ventricular arrhythmias and cardiac arrest may occur even before a sine wave is seen, leading to sudden death.

Treatment. Ca^{2+} has cardioprotective effects against hyperkalemia. Its effects are seen in a few minutes; however, it does not decrease the K^+ level, and multiple doses have to be given until definitive measures are taken to decrease the serum K^+ level. The dose of calcium gluconate is 100 to 200 mg per kg per dose intravenously (IV).

Potassium levels can be decreased by transcellular shifts. Glucose at 0.3 to 0.5 gram per kg per hour along with 1 unit of insulin per 4 grams of glucose decreases the K^+ level within 15 to 30 minutes. Sodium bicarbonate at a dose of 1 to 2 mEq per kg per dose also works through a similar mechanism.

Kayexalate is a polystyrene resin that exchanges Na^+ for K^+. It is given at a dose of 1 gram per kg orally (PO) or by retention enema. Time to onset of action is 1 hour by enema and 2 hours by the oral route. Furosemide causes loss of K^+ in the urine and can be given at a dose of 1 mg per kg per dose IV. In some cases, especially those complicated by renal failure, dialysis may be the modality of choice.

TABLE 9. **Hyperkalemia: Etiologic Classification**

Factitious
- Hemolysis, tissue trauma during blood draw (most common)
- Thrombocytosis (platelets >500,000/mm^3)

Shift from intracellular to extracellular compartment
- Acidosis
- Cell breakdown (trauma, rhabdomyolysis, chemotherapy)
- Succinylcholine
- Hypertonicity

Altered renal excretion
- Oliguria (acute and chronic renal failure)
- Drugs
  - Potassium-sparing diuretics
  - Angiotensin-converting enzyme inhibitors
  - Beta blockers
  - Cyclosporine, tacrolimus
  - Heparin
- Chronic hydronephrosis
- Renal tubular acidosis type IV

Adrenal insufficiency

Iatrogenic (intravenous fluids, total parenteral nutrition)

Increased intake (potassium-containing salt substitutes)

Calcium, Magnesium, and Phosphate

The most clinically relevant divalent ions are calcium, magnesium, and phosphate. There are some general similarities among these ions, and for each it is the ionized portion that is most important in physiologic regulation. Each is present in a relatively large quantity, but the major portion is sequestered, with only a small portion present in the ionized form. In each, the long-term regulation probably maintains total body content but the short-term (minute-to-minute) regulation of the ionized portion is the best understood and most important clinically. For each ion, the serum concentration does not correlate well with the total body content.

For each divalent ion the serum concentration is regulated by the net influence of four general processes: (1) increased or decreased exogenous intake, as in diet or intravenous fluids; (2) increased or decreased endogenous release into serum from body stores (e.g., calcium and phosphate release from bone); (3) increased or decreased uptake into body stores; and (4) increased or decreased excretion by the kidney and gut. Each of the divalent ions is in dynamic equilibrium with body fluids, and it is the net of uptake and release processes that move the ion concentration away from and then back toward the set range. Often, low serum concentration of any of the divalent ions is multifactorial, involving more than one of these four processes.

Calcium

Total serum calcium concentration is normally 2.2 to 2.6 mmol per liter. Ionized calcium concentration (clinically most important) ranges from 1.0 to 1.3 mmol per liter. The calcium concentration is affected by the calcium intake, serum albumin concentration, serum pH, parathyroid hormone, vitamin D metabolites, calcitonin, several other ions (e.g., Mg^{2+}, phosphate), a number of drugs, and renal excretion.

HYPERCALCEMIA

Hypercalcemia is best defined as a serum ionized calcium level of more than 1.3 mmol per liter. After the neonatal period, ionized calcium is maintained in a narrow range (1.0–1.3). In childen, hypercalcemia is caused by William's syndrome (infantile idiopathic hypercalcemia), vitamin D or A intoxication, granulomatous disorders, hyperparathyroidism, familial hypocalciuric hypercalcemia, thiazide diuretics, immobilization, malignancy, hypophosphatasia, subcutaneous fat necrosis, and oral dietary phosphate deficiency.

Several useful techniques can lower serum calcium. First, sodium diuresis can be produced by administration of normal saline at 2 to 3 times the normal fluid maintenance infusion rate (see Table 1). In some cases, this treatment will be sufficient. Addition of furosemide, 1 to 2 mg per kg given every 6 hours, may increase the effectiveness of diuresis. Children undergoing such diuresis must be monitored closely for urinary losses of water, sodium, potassium, phosphate, and magnesium during this therapy. Second, mobilization of the previously immobilized child can aid in reducing calcium. Third, decreasing calcium intake may be indicated. Fourth, prednisone administered at doses of 2 mg per kg per day, divided, every 6 hours may lower serum calcium. Fifth, agents that decrease the release of calcium from bone such as calcitonin (Calcimar), 4 to 8 units per kg per day IV, or etidronate disodium (Didronel), 7.5 mg per kg per day IV over 4 hours for 2 or 3 days, can be used.

With institution of urgent calcium-lowering therapy, testing should be initiated to determine the primary cause or causes of the hypercalcemia, and definitive therapy should be instituted if possible. A sixth technique to lower serum calcium, dialysis (peritoneal or hemodialysis) with low calcium bath, can produce net calcium removal in children with renal failure or in those in whom the preceding methods fail.

HYPOCALCEMIA

Hypocalcemia occurs when the serum ionized calcium falls below 1.0 mmol per liter. In children, hypocalcemia has many causes; some of these present only in certain age groups. Causative disorders or processes include critical illness, neonatal hypocalcemia, calcium deficiency, vitamin D deficiency, phosphate overload, hypoparathyroidism, DiGeorge's syndrome, chelation (with transfusion), hypomagnesemia, and pseudohypoparathyroidism.

Generally we try to treat symptomatic hypocalcemia with urgent intravenous calcium therapy and asymptomatic hypocalcemia with oral calcium and vitamin D supplementation. We treat acute hypocalcemia with intravenous infusion of elemental calcium in a dose of 4 mg (0.1 mmol) per kg per hour. This infusion may be repeated until symptoms cease. Administration of calcium chloride, calcium gluconate, or another calcium compound constitutes acceptable treatment. If magnesium deficiency is a significant contributor, magnesium replacement is given as described in the following section. When asymptomatic hypocalcemia is encountered, oral replacement of 75 to 100 mg of elemental calcium per kg per 24 hours can be administered as calcium carbonate, calcium citrate, or another form.

Magnesium

The serum magnesium concentration is maintained between 0.75 and 1.0 mmol per liter. Although serum magnesium is maintained within a narrow range, little is known about the regulatory mechanisms involved. Less than 1% of total body magnesium is in the ECF.

HYPERMAGNESEMIA

Hypermagnesemia is defined as a serum magnesium above 1 mmol per liter. Hypermagnesemia is rare in children. It may occur in children with acute or chronic renal failure. It may also occur in newborns whose mothers are given $MgSO_4$ in the perinatal period and infants or children given excessive amounts of magnesium-containing antacids or enemas.

The effects of excessive magnesium can be antagonized by calcium administration. The dosage and route of admission are described in the section on calcium. Magnesium can be removed by saline diuresis (saline infusion at 2 to 3 times maintenance). Furosemide, 1 to 2 mg per kg per dose IV every 6 hours, can increase urinary magnesium excretion. Magnesium can also be removed by hemodialysis or peritoneal dialysis.

HYPOMAGNESEMIA

Hypomagnesemia occurs when the serum magnesium is below 0.75 mmol per liter. Almost all cases of hypomagnesemia are caused by a combination of decreased magnesium intake and/or increased magnesium excretion. Causes of hypomagnesemia include drugs (e.g., cyclosporine [Sandimmune], cisplatin [Platinol]), Bartter's syndrome, starvation, decreased gastroenteral absorption, diuresis, hypercalcemia, and hyperaldosteronism.

As with calcium deficiency, severe symptomatic hypomagnesemia requires urgent intravenous treatment. Magnesium sulfate, 25 to 50 mg per kg every 4 hours, is given 3 to 4 times daily. The maximum single dose should not exceed 2 grams. When nonemergency treatment is appropriate, oral administration of magnesium sulfate (100 to 200 mg per kg per dose, four times daily) or magnesium oxide (65 to 130 mg per kg per 24 hours) is sufficient.

Phosphate

The majority of the total body phosphate is in bone or intracellular pools. A small portion is found in ECF. The normal value of serum phosphate varies with age. The normal value may be as high as 3.9 mmol per liter in early infancy to as low as 0.8 mmol per liter in an adult. The definitions of hyper- and hypophosphatemia are dependent on age.

HYPERPHOSPHATEMIA

Hyperphosphatemia is infrequent in children. It is recognized as the presence of a serum phosphate level above the age-related normal value. Causes in infants and children include (1) increased phosphate intake (diet, laxatives, or enemas), (2) decreased renal phosphate excretion (as in renal failure or parathyroid hormone deficiency), and (3) major shift of phosphate from ICF stores to ECF (as seen with rhabdomyolysis or tumor lysis syndrome).

Treatment is determined primarily by renal function but should include (in children with normal renal function) (1) oral phosphate restriction, (2) administration of an oral phosphate binder (e.g., calcium acetate or calcium carbonate* (given as elemental calcium in a dose of 25 mg per kg with meals), (3) solute diuresis with normal saline at 2 to 3 times maintenance and mannitol in a dose of 0.5 gm per kg every 6 hours, and if these measures do not give satisfactory results, or in patients with renal insufficiency, (4) hemodialysis or peritoneal dialysis may be required to remove phosphate.

*Not FDA approved for this indication.

HYPOPHOSPHATEMIA

The major causes of hypophosphatemia in children include decreased intake, excessive enteral loss, excessive renal loss, and cellular uptake. Hypophosphatemia is recognized when the serum phosphate concentration is less than the age-related normal value.

Phosphate replacement may be given PO or IV depending on the perceived urgency. Potassium phosphate or sodium phosphate (2 mg of elemental phosphate per kg) may be given IV and repeated. Once the serum phosphate concentration is above 2.5 mg per dL, replacement may be given PO.

Section 8

The Endocrine System

ACROMEGALY

method of
VIVIEN HERMAN-BONERT, M.D., and
GLENN D. BRAUNSTEIN, M.D.
Cedars-Sinai Medical Center and University of California, Los Angeles, UCLA School of Medicine
Los Angeles, California

Acromegaly, a chronic, insidious disorder, is due to excess growth hormone (GH) secretion. GH hypersecretion before epiphyseal fusion results in gigantism, whereas the syndrome of acromegaly results after the epiphyses have fused. The majority of GH-secreting pituitary tumors are sporadic, but they may be associated with multiple endocrine neoplasia (MEN-1), an autosomal dominant disorder resulting in neoplasms of the parathyroid glands, pancreas, and anterior pituitary gland. Acromegaly is a rare disorder, with a prevalence of 70 cases per 1 million and an incidence of three to four new cases per 1 million per year. Approximately 1000 new cases of acromegaly are diagnosed in the United States each year.

PATHOPHYSIOLOGY

Hypothalamic growth hormone–releasing hormone (GHRH) and somatotropin-release inhibiting factor (SRIF) or somatostatin interact to generate pulsatile GH secretion from the pituitary gland (Figure 1). GH binds to hepatic receptors stimulating insulin-like growth factor I (IGF-I) secretion from the liver. IGF-I is responsible for several of the peripheral effects of GH.

Ninety-eight percent of cases of acromegaly are due to GH-secreting tumors of the anterior pituitary gland, most likely due to an intrinsic pituitary genetic defect. Oncogene activation or deletion of a tumor suppressor gene has been implicated. A small percentage of GH-secreting pituitary tumors contain the *gsp* mutation, an amino acid substitution in the Gs protein, leading to constitutive activation of adenylyl cyclase and cyclic adenosine monophosphate and mimicking abnormal GHRH signaling. Two percent of cases of acromegaly are due to ectopic pituitary tumors (commonly in the sphenoid sinus), extrapituitary GH secretion (pancreatic islet cell tumors or carcinoids), excess GHRH secretion (hypothalamic hamartoma, carcinoid tumor, small cell lung cancer), or, rarely, the MEN-1 and McCune-Albright syndromes.

CLINICAL FEATURES

Clinical manifestations of acromegaly may be secondary to the local effects of a GH-secreting macroadenoma or may result from actions of excess GH and IGF-I (Table 1). Initially, the changes in physical appearance and metabolic consequences of GH excess are subtle, resulting in a delay in the diagnosis of acromegaly in the majority of cases. Average delay from onset of symptoms to the time of diagnosis is approximately 9 years. Retrospective analysis of serial old photographs can help establish the onset of acromegaly.

Because of the insidious onset of acromegaly, the diagnosis is often made by someone who has not seen the patient for several years and notices a dramatic change in physical appearance, by the dentist who is consulted for loosening of teeth or malocclusion, or by a chiropractor who is attempting to alleviate backache or painful joints caused by arthralgia.

Acral enlargement resulting from soft tissue and bony growth results in the characteristic appearance of acromegaly with frontal bossing, prognathism, maloccluded jaw and overbite, large fleshy nose, spadelike hands, and widened feet. Patients complain of increasing ring and hat size and progressive increase in shoe width.

Arthropathy and hyperhidrosis occur in 70% of patients. Large joints are usually affected, and joint pain may limit activity. Joint degeneration may be irreversible. A foul-smelling body odor may accompany hyperhidrosis and is usually reversible with treatment.

Hypertension and abnormal resting electrocardiograms are present in 50% of patients with active acromegaly. In addition to the cardiac effects of hypertension, a specific cardiomyopathy caused by excessive GH and IGF-I, which is responsive to lowering of the excess hormone levels, has been documented.

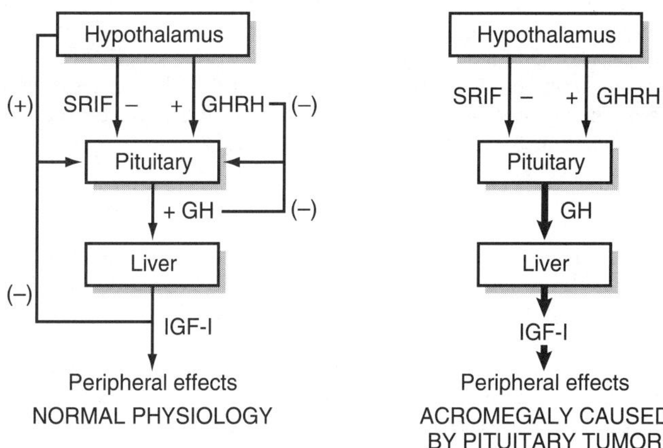

Figure 1. Hypothalamic-pituitary-peripheral feedback loop for control of somatic growth. Growth hormone–releasing hormone (GHRH) stimulatory and somatostatin inhibiting pulses interact to regulate pituitary growth hormone (GH) secretion. GH stimulates hepatic insulin-like growth factor (IGF)-I synthesis, which has a negative feedback inhibiting effect on pituitary GH secretion and a positive feedback effect on hypothalamic somatostatin secretion. GH exerts a negative autoregulatory feedback effect on pituitary GH secretion and hypothalamic GHRH secretion.

Abbreviation: SRIF = somatotropin-release inhibiting factor.

TABLE 1. **Clinical Manifestations of Acromegaly**

Symptoms

Pituitary Mass Effects

Headache
Visual impairment
Decreased libido and impotence

Effects of Growth Hormone Excess

Change in appearance
Loosening of teeth
Increased ring, shoe, and hat size
Carpel tunnel syndrome
Excessive perspiration
Arthralgia
Somnolence

Signs

Local Tumor Effects

Visual field defect, bitemporal hemianopia
Cranial nerve palsy III, IV, V, VI

Effects of Growth Hormone Excess

Skeletal changes: prognathism, overbite, malocclusion, spadelike hands, widened feet, frontal bossing, kyphosis
Skin tags
Acanthosis nigricans
Acne
Proximal myopathy
Cardiovascular: hypertension, left ventricular hypertrophy, congestive heart failure, arrhythmia
Visceromegaly: tongue, thyroid, liver, spleen, bones
Galactorrhea

Complications

Hypertriglyceridemia
Impaired glucose tolerance and diabetes mellitus
Sleep apnea
Colonic polyps
Neoplasms: colon, breast, stomach

Diabetes mellitus occurs in 20% of patients. An increased incidence of benign and malignant neoplasms has been reported in patients with acromegaly—specifically, colon polyps, colon cancer, and gastric cancer occur in 30 to 50% of patients. Colon polyps are frequently associated with the occurrence of skin tags. As GH and IGF-I are growth factors, acromegaly is also associated with an increased incidence of breast and esophageal malignancy.

DIAGNOSIS

Historically, random GH measurements have been used in the diagnosis of acromegaly. A random GH value less than 5 ng per mL or 10 mIU per liter was considered normal. However, as GH secretion is pulsatile, with intermittent secretory bursts, single random GH measurements are not confirmatory, and dynamic testing such as the oral glucose tolerance test is the preferred diagnostic tool. After an overnight fast, 75 to 100 grams of oral glucose will suppress serum GH levels to less than 2 ng per mL after 2 hours in normal people; however, levels will remain above 2 ng per mL in the majority of acromegalic patients, and in 10% of persons with acromegaly glucose may even stimulate GH levels.

Serum IGF-I levels are a good screening test for the presence of GH excess, as GH stimulates hepatic IGF-I synthesis. The IGF-I level reflects the integrated 24-hour serum GH secretion. The level of serum IGF-binding protein-3 (IGFBP-3), a glycoprotein that binds IGF-I and IGF-II in the circulation, is GH-dependent. Thus, IGFBP-3 levels are elevated in acromegaly.

The presence of an anterior pituitary tumor as the cause of GH hypersecretion can be confirmed by magnetic resonance imaging (MRI) with the administration of gadolinium, which enhances the tumor image. The absence of a pituitary mass on MRI suggests an ectopic GH- or GHRH-secreting tumor. This latter tumor manifests with elevated serum GHRH levels and may be identified in the chest or abdomen. GHRH-secreting tumors result in pituitary hyperplasia, demonstrable on pituitary MRI as an enlarged pituitary, without a focal mass. Chest and abdominal computed tomography (CT) scan or MRI can be used to confirm the anatomic location of ectopic GH- or GHRH-secreting tumors. In the case of very small ectopic neuroendocrine tumors, which cannot be visualized by MRI or CT scan, an octreoscan, using octreotide (Sandostatin) tagged with radiolabeled indium, can be helpful. Ectopic GH- or GHRH-secreting tumors have somatostatin receptors that bind the radiolabeled somatostatin. The octreoscan is very sensitive for the visualization of small tumors.

TREATMENT

The clinical goals of therapy for acromegaly are control of symptoms, reversal of GH and IGF-I hypersecretion, reduction of tumor mass, and prevention of recurrence, without causing hypopituitarism during the course of treatment.

Treatment modalities include surgery, radiation therapy, and medical management (Figure 2).

Surgery

Trans-sphenoidal surgery is the primary treatment of choice in acromegaly. Successful outcome is directly related to the surgeon's experience in the trans-sphenoidal removal of pituitary tumors; therefore, selection of a neurosurgeon with expertise in this technique is important. Surgery is curative in 90% of patients with intrasellar microadenomas (<

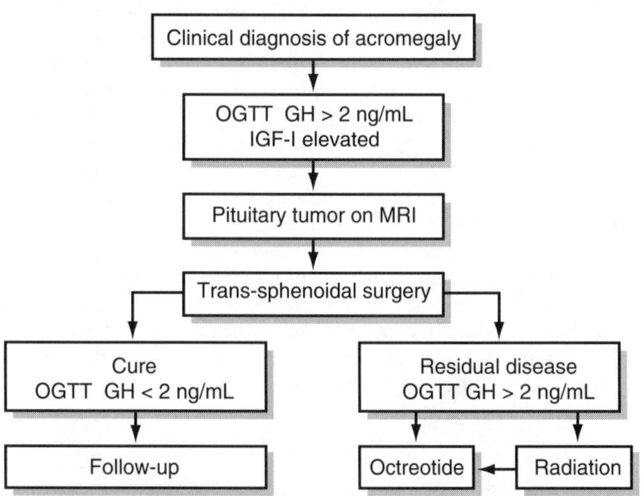

Figure 2. Algorithm for the management of acromegaly. *Abbreviations:* IGF-I = Insulin-like growth factor; OGTT = oral glucose tolerance test; GH = growth hormone; MRI = magnetic resonance imaging.

10 mm diameter) when performed by an experienced pituitary neurosurgeon. However, retrospective analysis of cure rates by trans-sphenoidal surgery, performed by all neurosurgeons (with various levels of expertise in trans-sphenoidal removal), indicates that only 60% of persons with acromegaly achieve cure. The size of the tumor and the preoperative GH level are the two factors that correlate best with surgical outcome in the hands of a competent surgeon. Smaller tumors and lower preoperative GH levels are associated with higher surgical cure rates and a lower incidence of hypopituitarism.

Well-encapsulated GH-secreting microadenomas confined to the sella can be removed by surgery with preservation of anterior pituitary function. However, invasive macroadenomas (> 10 mm diameter), extending beyond the sella into the cavernous sinus or suprasellar region, may require incomplete resection, resulting in continued postoperative GH hypersecretion, with a 20% incidence of new-onset hypopituitarism.

Complications of surgery include local effects (arachnoiditis, cerebrospinal fluid leaks), permanent diabetes insipidus, and new-onset hypopituitarism and development of secondary empty sella syndrome postoperatively.

Radiation Therapy

Radiation therapy has been used as adjuvant therapy in patients with incomplete tumor resection resulting in persistent GH hypersecretion postoperatively, for recurrent disease, or in patients who are medically unfit for surgery.

Conventional and proton beam radiation have been replaced more recently by stereotactic radiosurgery, which delivers a high dose of irradiation to a very localized area, sparing adjacent normal structures. GH reduction in response to radiation therapy is slow, and 20 years may elapse before 90% of patients achieve GH suppression. Conventional radiation results in 50% reduction in GH levels after 2 years and 75% reduction at 5 years. Furthermore, a high percentage of patients develop hypopituitarism. Other complications include cranial nerve damage (especially optic nerve), cognitive defects, and the development of secondary brain tumors in the radiation field several years later.

Drug Therapy

Bromocriptine (Parlodel),* a dopamine agonist, is effective in suppressing GH secretion in 15 to 20% of persons with acromegaly, as dopamine inhibits GH secretion in approximately 30% of patients with acromegaly. However, the suppressed GH secretion is not accompanied by reduction in tumor size. Furthermore, the low efficacy in acromegaly, as well as the high incidence of side effects incurred by the large dose required to suppress GH levels (up to 20 mg per day), has limited the use of bromocriptine in acromegaly. Common side effects include nasal stuffiness, postural hypotension, nausea, and vomiting. Cabergoline (Dostinex),* a longer-acting dopamine agonist, lowers plasma IGF-I into the normal range in about half of the patients with pretreatment IGF-I levels less than 2½ times above the normal range when given in weekly doses of 1.0 to 1.75 mg.

*Not FDA approved for this indication.

Octreotide, a long-acting somatostatin analogue, is a major advance in the medical management of acromegaly. Somatostatin, a hypothalamic peptide that inhibits pituitary GH secretion, has a very short half-life. Octreotide has a serum half-life of 2 hours and a potency 45 times that of native somatostatin in suppressing GH. It is administered subcutaneously in average doses of 100 to 200 μg three times a day, with a maximum dose of 1500 μg per day. Some patients may require continuous infusion to achieve adequate GH suppression. Ninety percent of patients with acromegaly respond to octreotide with significant suppression of GH and IGF-I levels. Somatostatin receptors, which recognize the octreotide molecule, can be demonstrated on the tumors of patients who are octreotide-responsive, whereas unresponsive patients are receptor-negative.

The clinical features of acromegaly respond to octreotide treatment shortly after initiation of therapy, with resolution of soft tissue swelling and improvement in fatigue, paresthesias, and joint pains. Headache dissipates within minutes after octreotide administration, suggesting a central analgesic effect of octreotide rather than hormone suppression. Reduction in tumor size, ranging from 20 to 80% in different studies, has been demonstrated in the first 4 months after initiation of therapy in 30% of patients.

Side effects of octreotide include transitory loose stools, abdominal pain, nausea, and flatulence, which usually subside after the initial 2 to 4 weeks of treatment. Octreotide rarely causes hypoglycemia or hyperglycemia; therefore, blood sugar levels must be monitored closely in diabetic acromegalic patients, who may require a reduction in the dose of insulin or antidiabetic drugs shortly after octreotide administration.

Twenty-five percent of patients with acromegaly develop ultrasonographically demonstrable gallbladder sludge owing to an octreotide-induced delay in gallbladder emptying and reduced contractility. However, an increased incidence of cholecystitis has not been demonstrated in acromegaly, and sludge disappears rapidly when the medication is discontinued.

New advances in the medical management of acromegaly include the development of a long-acting, slow-release intramuscular octreotide preparation that can be administered monthly. In addition, the safety and efficacy of a GH antagonist, Trovert,* with structural similarity to GH that competitively inhibits GH binding to hepatic receptors, are being investigated. This drug will be useful in patients whose tumors lack somatostatin receptors and are thus un-

*Not available in the United States.

responsive to somatostatin, as well as in patients who cannot tolerate the gastrointestinal side effects of octreotide.

ADRENOCORTICAL INSUFFICIENCY

method of
PAUL C. CARPENTER, M.D.
Mayo Medical School
Rochester, Minnesota

Adrenocortical insufficiency is a life-threatening disorder with a range of presentations, making it a sometimes difficult diagnostic problem. The potentially fatal outcome, along with high morbidity and mortality rates, makes awareness, accurate diagnosis, and timely management of this disorder critical. Treatment intervention produces prompt resolution of disabling symptoms with avoidance of fatal outcome. The fundamental physiologic issue in this disorder is the lack of adequate glucocorticoid (cortisol) and/or mineralocorticoid (aldosterone) to carry out many fundamental life maintenance processes.

ETIOLOGY

There are two fundamental etiologic divisions for the disease based on the site of the deficit in the hypothalamic-pituitary-adrenal axis. *Primary adrenal insufficiency* refers to the lack of cortisol or mineralocorticoid resulting from destruction or drug-mediated dysfunction of the adrenal cortex. *Secondary adrenal insufficiency* is caused by lack of adrenocorticotropic hormone (ACTH). This may be due to (1) damage to the anterior pituitary, (2) long-term hypothalamic-pituitary suppression from exogenous glucocorticoid administration, or (3) hypothalamic neuron destruction with resulting deficiency of corticotropin-releasing hormone (CRH). The last is sometimes termed tertiary adrenal insufficiency.

Primary Adrenocortical Insufficiency

Primary adrenocortical insufficiency (Addison's disease) has many potential causes (Table 1). The prevalence is estimated to be 40 to 60 cases per million, with a peak age at onset of 20 to 40 years. The most common cause is autoimmune destruction of portions or all of the adrenal cortex, accounting for 80% of cases in the western world; four times as many women as men are affected. Specific antibodies to the adrenal, particularly directed to the 21-hydroxylase antigen, have been identified. This type of autoimmune disease may occur as an isolated disorder, or it may be a component of broader autoimmune polyglandular failure, either type I (primary adrenal insufficiency, hypoparathyroidism, chronic mucocutaneous candidiasis, and pernicious anemia) or type II (primary adrenal insufficiency, type I diabetes mellitus, primary hypothyroidism, and vitiligo).

A variety of infections may damage the adrenals. Immune-based adrenal insufficiency is also found with other autoimmune diseases and at disproportionate frequency with sarcoidosis. Tuberculosis has seen resurgence in the past decade. Disseminated histoplasmosis is the next most common infectious cause. Overt or subclinical presentations of adrenal insufficiency are often seen in acquired immune deficiency syndrome (AIDS), particularly in patients with class III or IV disease as defined by the Centers for Disease Control and Prevention (CDC), and are usually associated with opportunistic infections, particularly tuberculosis and cytomegalovirus infection. Increased cognizance coupled with improvements in and more frequent use of imaging techniques has allowed detection of bilateral adrenal hemorrhage in seriously ill patients following trauma or with the use of anticoagulation therapy. Various medications may lead to partial or total cortical dysfunction via interference with steroid biosynthesis or acceleration of cortisol catabolism by induction of hepatic microsomal enzymes. Patients receiving corticosteroid replacement therapy have increased steroid requirements when also receiving agents with those effects, such as those listed in Table 1.

TABLE 1. **Etiology of Primary Adrenal Insufficiency**

Autoimmune adrenalitis (in 80% of cases in United States)
Infectious
- Tuberculosis
- Histoplasmosis
- AIDS-associated opportunistic infections (*Mycobacterium,* cytomegalovirus)
- Generalized bacterial sepsis (pneumococcosis, meningococcosis, *Haemophilus, Escherichia coli)*
- Blastomycosis
- Coccidioidomycosis
- Cryptococcosis

Bilateral adrenal hemorrhage—sepsis, hypotension, postoperative, anticoagulation
Metastatic or infiltrative malignancy—breast, lung, lymphoma, melanoma
Surgical—bilateral adrenalectomy
Infiltrative—sarcoidosis, hemochromatosis, amyloidosis
Congenital adrenal hyperplasia
Familial—adrenoleukodystrophy, adrenomyeloneuropathy, familial glucocorticoid deficiency
Drug effects
- Inhibition of cortisol biosynthesis: ketoconazole (Nizoral), metyrapone (Metopirone), mitotane (Lysodren), aminoglutethimide (Cytadren), etomidate (Amidate)
- Increase in steroid catabolism: rifampin (Rifadin), phenytoin (Dilantin), phenobarbital

Secondary Adrenocortical Insufficiency

The most common cause of secondary adrenocortical insufficiency is iatrogenic, related to the use and subsequent withdrawal of exogenous glucocorticoid preparations. Other causes are hypothalamic or pituitary destruction from neoplasms, infiltrative disorders, infection, trauma, autoimmune disease, or vascular insults. Therapeutic intervention for these disorders may also contribute to the ACTH deficiency (Table 2).

CLINICAL PRESENTATIONS

Adrenal insufficiency fundamentally presents in either a chronic or an acute mode. The *chronic* presentation is characterized by diverse and nonspecific symptoms and signs that too often extend the course until either an acute crisis occurs or the health care provider pinpoints the possibility and initiates appropriate testing. The health of affected patients declines over months and years, the hallmark symptoms being weakness, fatigue, and weight loss secondary to anorexia. Other findings aid in the recogni-

TABLE 2. **Etiology of Secondary Adrenocortical Insufficiency**

Exogenous glucocorticoid therapy
- Withdrawal of treatment or inadequacy of dosage levels owing to stress or illness in persons on long-term glucocorticoid treatment, independent of route of administration

Neoplasm
- Pituitary adenoma—functioning or nonfunctioning
- Metastases to pituitary-hypothalamus
- Craniopharyngioma

Head trauma

Vascular/ischemic
- Vascular thrombosis, embolic, Sheehan's syndrome (postpartum necrosis—may be autoimmune), intraneoplastic hemorrhage, anticoagulation

Surgical
- Pituitary adenoma removal, repair of aneurysm

Radiation
- To pituitary or regional neoplasm

Infiltrative
- Histiocytosis
- Sarcoidosis
- Hemochromatosis

Infectious
- Meningitis
- Encephalitis
- Tuberculosis

Autoimmune

Lymphocytic hypophysitis (postpartum in most cases)

Isolated ACTH deficiency (autoimmune origin likely)

Idiopathic

tion process. These include the development of hyperpigmentation, described by Thomas Addison as "a dingy or smokey appearance of various tints or shades of deep amber or chestnut brown." The pigment appears generalized, being more pronounced in body areas subject to abrasion, such as skin creases, elbows, knuckles, knees, buccal mucosa, and the vaginal orifice and in recent scars. The presence of vitiligo should increase suspicion. The patient with chronic adrenal insufficiency reports difficulty coping with minor illnesses. Depression and its related symptoms are very common among these patients. Unfortunately, some have spent considerable time under treatment for depression, generally with poor results. These presentations, along with hyperkalemia, hyponatremia, hypothyroidism, fasting hypoglycemia, and diminished insulin need in diabetics, promote diagnostic awareness and prevention of ongoing ill health, acute catastrophic adrenal crisis, and potential death.

The *acute* presentations of adrenal insufficiency often do not offer the assistance of long-term associated symptoms to guide diagnosis. It more often occurs in a setting of other severe illness or trauma, or perioperatively. Hyperpigmentation takes weeks to months to develop. Similarly, mood changes and weight loss are time-dependent. The acutely ill patient rapidly develops dehydration, hypotension, general cardiovascular collapse, and fever. This presentation is often confusing because of increasing signs of renal insufficiency, generally from prerenal causes. Intervention with plasma volume expansion, vasopressors, and other support measures temporarily improves the clinical state, often followed by further deterioration if the adrenal insufficiency goes unrecognized. In the setting of previous symptoms in keeping with adrenal insufficiency, findings such as those suggestive of adrenal hemorrhage, disseminated infections, blood loss with multiple transfusions, AIDS, and laboratory clues such as hypoglycemia, hyponatremia, or hyperkalemia should alert the provider to the possibility of adrenal insufficiency and often constitute adequate information to initiate therapy, leaving diagnostic testing to a time when the patient is more stable.

There is high variability in the degree of hypothalamic-pituitary suppression and in temporal recovery among patients who have received or are receiving exogenous glucocorticoids. Accordingly, definitive diagnosis of secondary adrenal insufficiency may be challenging. All patients with the disorders listed in Table 2 should be considered to have the potential for secondary adrenal insufficiency.

A variety of suggestive findings prompt the search for ACTH and secondary cortisol deficiency. These include the symptoms directly attributable to cortisol deficiency (fatigue, anorexia, hypotension, hypoglycemia) and those associated with other anterior or posterior pituitary hormone deficiencies. Decreased levels of thyroid-stimulating hormone (TSH), luteinizing hormone (LH), follicle-stimulating hormone (FSH), growth hormone (GH), or antidiuretic hormone (ADH) may lead to hypothyroidism, hypogonadism, growth failure, and diabetes insipidus. Pituitary hormone excess (as in acromegaly, Cushing's disease, or syndrome of inappropriate ADH secretion [SIADH]) may be associated with variable pituitary hormone deficiencies secondary to the mass effect of local tumor growth. Patients with gross cushingoid appearance due to effects of exogenous steroids may at the same time be cortisol-deficient if their steroid medication is withheld or discontinued. Other symptoms due to anatomic alterations, such as visual disturbances, cranial nerve palsies, or headache, can accompany growth of lesions.

DIAGNOSIS

The appropriate treatment of adrenocortical insufficiency is dependent on accurate diagnosis. The diagnosis is made combining precise medical-surgical history with detailed medication exposure history and appropriate testing. Careful history acquisition is sometimes needed to pinpoint exogenous glucocorticoid administration. This includes conventional therapy with oral glucocorticoid medications but also use of injectables for rheumatologic disorders, allergies or asthma, and epidural injections. Inhaled steroid medication use for asthma or chronic obstructive lung disease may also chronically suppress endogenous cortisol production. Surreptitious steroid use and its denial expose the patient to great risks when confronting major disease or surgical stress. Typical hyperpigmentation or vitiligo with hypothyroidism prompts diagnostic investigation. Secondary insufficiency should be suspected in patients with other pituitary hormonal losses or excesses in whom skin hyperpigmentation is lacking. Isolated ACTH deficiency is rare and usually of autoimmune origin and may be associated with pituitary enlargement as shown on imaging studies.

Laboratory testing for primary adrenal insufficiency, as well as interpretation of results, is usually straightforward. It is important that the clinician have knowledge of the quality of the laboratory assays used for these measurements and the potential for interference. For example, some blood cortisol assays will also detect glucocorticoids other than cortisol because of cross-reaction. The simultaneous measurement of blood cortisol and ACTH is usually diagnostic. The cortisol is low-normal to frankly low (usually less than 10 μg per dL), and the ACTH is elevated (greater than 150 pg per mL). It is desirable to obtain these samples in the acute phase of illness and before any treatment is initiated. Urgent treatment should not be withheld in severely ill patients if diagnostic suspicion is high and facilities for testing are not readily available.

Additional confirmatory testing is used when primary adrenal insufficiency is suspected in a patient who may have recently received exogenous glucocorticoid with its potential for ACTH suppression. For this test, synthetic ACTH (α^{1-24} - corticotropin, or cosyntropin [Cortrosyn]), 250 μg, is given intramuscularly (IM) or intravenously (IV) after pre-injection cortisol is obtained, and blood cortisol levels are drawn at 30 and 60 minutes after injection. A normal cortisol response is a peak value of 18 μg per dL or higher or a cortisol rise of 8 μg per dL or higher if the baseline cortisol might be exogenously suppressed to less than 5 μg per dL. If simultaneously measured, aldosterone will normally peak at 16 μg per dL or higher. Obviously, ACTH should not be measured after injection of cosyntropin. If a delay until ACTH stimulation testing is anticipated and the severity of symptoms warrants immediate initiation of therapy, the patient may be maintained with dexamethasone, 0.5 mg given orally (PO) once or twice daily (because it does not interfere with laboratory measurements) until testing is accomplished and results are available. Measurement of adrenal antibodies has become available.

In the patient with suspected secondary adrenal insufficiency who has received no glucocorticoid therapy, simultaneous blood cortisol and ACTH levels both will be low. Commonly, the ACTH level is near or below the lowest normal value for the assay and the cortisol level is less than 10 μg per dL. When the rapid cosyntropin ACTH stimulation test just described is used in patients with secondary adrenal insufficiency, the peak cortisol response is usually less than 18 μg per dL. A normal response excludes primary but not secondary adrenal insufficiency. Secondary adrenal insufficiency may be confirmed by insulin-induced hypoglycemia or metyrapone testing demonstrating the lack of cortisol response due to inadequate ACTH release. These tests pose some risks and should be performed only with appropriate precautions and controls. CRH may be used to differentiate primary from secondary adrenal insufficiency. The patient who has been receiving prolonged exogenous high-dose glucocorticoids poses special problems in diagnosis, and precise testing may not be possible until the glucocorticoids have been systematically withdrawn or at least lowered to doses deemed at or below those indicated for conventional replacement steroid therapy. The withdrawal protocol should emphasize use of single AM daily doses of short-acting steroid preparations.

Computed tomography (CT) or magnetic resonance imaging (MRI) of the adrenals may aid in the differential diagnosis of primary adrenal insufficiency. In autoimmune adrenal disease the adrenals are normal or reduced in size, while in essentially all other cases they are enlarged. With chronic granulomatous disease, old hemorrhage into the adrenal, or metastatic replacement, calcifications in the adrenal may be seen. Imaging of the adrenal is always indicated when the diagnosis of primary adrenal insufficiency has been made. MRI of the pituitary-hypothalamic area is useful for differentiating among causes of secondary adrenal insufficiency.

TREATMENT

Acute Adrenal Insufficiency

Acute adrenal insufficiency with associated cardiovascular collapse is a medical emergency; appropriate management, however, can give very rewarding results, including prevention of life loss. When the diagnosis is confirmed or even highly likely, treatment should begin with rapid plasma volume expansion with dextrose in normal saline and intravenous administration of 100 mg of hydrocortisone sodium succinate (Solu-Cortef) as a bolus, followed by similar doses of hydrocortisone every 6 hours. If intravenous access is not available, the intramuscular route may be used to give hydrocortisone in this dose schedule or other water-soluble, non-depot glucocorticoids such as methylprednisolone (Solu-Medrol), 40 mg; hydrocortisone sodium phosphate (Hydrocortone), 100 mg; or dexamethasone sodium phosphate (Decadron), 4 mg. The intramuscular route is less desirable and may be contraindicated if tissue perfusion is severely compromised. Mineralocorticoid is not necessary as the hydrocortisone has significant mineralocorticoid effects and the resuscitation fluid includes saline. After stabilization the patient may be started on oral replacement therapy. All instances of acute adrenal insufficiency should be thoroughly investigated to define, manage, or eliminate precipitating factors.

Chronic Adrenal Insufficiency, Primary or Secondary

Glucocorticoid Replacement

The use of glucocorticoid replacement is needed in both the primary and secondary types of chronic adrenal insufficiency. Management is directed at restoration of normal glucocorticoid-mediated physiology to maximize quality of life. Mineralocorticoid replacement may be needed in primary adrenal insufficiency but is needed only rarely in the secondary form.

Hydrocortisone (Hydrocortone) tablets may well be the most physiologic replacement agent. Hydrocortisone carries moderate mineralocorticoid properties, which may minimize the need for specific mineralocorticoid replacement. The standard dose is 12 to 15 mg orally per m^2 per day. In patients who are markedly cortisol-deficient there is ample evidence that twice-daily dosing leads to a better sense of well-being than do single AM doses. Some patients do best on a broader distribution of glucocorticoid over three doses. Avoiding late evening doses helps to minimize the absorbed burst of glucocorticoid, which will interfere with normal sleep mechanisms.

Alternative medications include cortisone acetate (Cortone-Acetate), given in an oral dose of 14 to 18 mg per m^2 per day, and prednisone (Deltasone), in a dose of 4 to 5 mg per m^2 per day. Oral doses are taken on arising in the morning and in late afternoon or at suppertime—for example, hydrocortisone, 20 mg AM and 10 mg PM; cortisone acetate, 25 mg AM and 10 mg PM; prednisone, 5 mg AM and 2.5 mg PM. Long-acting glucocorticoids such as dexamethasone (Decadron, Hexadrol) should be avoided because the potential for exogenously induced Cushing's syndrome is higher. In primary adrenal insufficiency mineralocorticoid replacement is given as fludrocortisone (Florinef Acetate), 0.2 to 0.5 mg orally once daily. The need for mineralocorticoid replacement is determined by demonstrating aldosterone deficiency at diagnosis or, commonly, by failure of full correction of hyperkalemia or hyponatremia after full glucocorticoid replacement and the patient is consuming an adequate amount of sodium in the diet. Elevated plasma renin levels in the same circumstances may also be a clue. Some patients increase their fludrocortisone dosage for very hot weather and intense physical activity.

The optimal treatment of adrenocortical deficiency and the hazards posed by conventional therapy have been the topics of ongoing discussion. Glucocorticoid administration, even when no deficiency is present, may deliver a sense of well-being. There is concern about the physiologic and psychologic addictive potential of glucocorticoids. Experienced physicians note that withdrawal from or even downward adjustment of glucocorticoid therapy to levels well within replacement range often precipitates symptoms of mood change, myalgias, diminished energy, and sleep disorders. Adequate blood cortisol levels may be shown at the same time. Conventional doses may potentiate bone mineral loss. Many patients, particularly those with secondary adrenal insufficiency, seem to maintain good quality of life with steroid doses below those used in conventional replacement therapy. Additionally, means of testing the adequacy of replacement steroid are very limited, so the practitioner must rely on indirect measures and the patient's testimony. Potentially helpful in the detection of hydrocortisone or cortisone acetate excess is the finding of 24-hour urinary free cortisol levels of more than 35 μg per day (on high-performance liquid chromatography assay for true cortisol). Absorbed oral hydrocortisone produces erratic plasma cortisol levels and generally produces higher urine cortisol levels than in those with comparable endogenous production. Subtle additional clues of excess are slow weight gain, increased insulin or oral hypoglycemic need in diabetic patients, relative lymphopenia, edema, and progressive osteopenia. Unlike the use of TSH measures in adjusting thyroxine therapy, glucocorticoid therapy in patients with continually suppressed or even normal ACTH levels may result in signs and symptoms of corticosteroid excess. An ideal timed-release glucocorticoid replacement preparation is not available.

Patient Education

Education is a critical component of therapy for patients with adrenocortical deficiency. It is our practice to thoroughly review aspects of normal pituitary-adrenal relationships to help the patient and other responsible family members understand the disease and its management. We stress the expectation of a normal life in terms of both quality and quantity of life if reasonable principles of treatment are followed. No activity, no matter how taxing, is proscribed.

Patients are advised to obtain a MedicAlert (MedicAlert Foundation International, Turlock, CA; 1-800-432-5378) or comparable bracelet or, preferably, necklace that details their need for cortisol. Patients must familiarize themselves with four therapy situations: (1) chronic maintenance therapy (as described in the preceding discussion), (2) treatment adjustment for minor stress, (3) emergency situation management, and (4) anticipated treatment during hospitalization for surgery or severe illness.

Minor Stress. Patients are instructed to double or (in febrile illnesses) triple their replacement corticosteroid for no more than 3 days without consulting their physician. Mineralocorticoid medication does not have to be altered. If the illness worsens in less than 3 days, they are directed to consult their physician. Such adjustments are unlikely to be needed more often than 3 or 4 times per year.

Emergency Management. Situations such as major trauma, myocardial infarction, severe body burns, or those involving nausea and vomiting create uncertainty about whether the necessary oral medications have been taken. For such cases, patients are provided with dexamethasone (Hexadrol) in 4-mg preloaded single-injection syringes. They are instructed to promptly inject the dexamethasone IM even if that day's medications might have been taken and then to seek medical attention immediately (i.e., "shoot first and ask questions later"). Any effort to consume fluids may also be helpful.

Hospital Treatment. At or before induction of general anesthesia we administer 8 to 10 times the patient's daily replacement equivalent of an aqueous glucocorticoid. The agent of choice is methylprednisolone (Solu-Medrol), in a dose of 40 mg IM given at anesthesia, and tapered rapidly, using 20 mg every 12 hours on the first postoperative day and 10 mg every 12 hours on the second day, and then in maintenance doses. The taper rate may be accelerated for less stressful procedures or extended if there are complications. For stressful diagnostic procedures such as colonoscopy or angiography, we advise patients to take double their morning glucocorticoid dose shortly before the procedure; alternatively, we may give methylprednisolone (Solu-Medrol), 10 mg IM. The parenteral route is used when it is anticipated that the procedure may be prolonged or that oral intake will be diminished for some time after the procedure. Conventional obstetrical delivery is managed in a similar manner.

CUSHING'S SYNDROME

method of
DIMITRIS A. PAPANICOLAOU, M.D., and
GEORGE P. CHROUSOS, M.D.
National Institutes of Health
Bethesda, Maryland

Cushing's syndrome (CS) results from prolonged exposure to high levels of glucocorticoid hormones. The cause can be exogenous (iatrogenic), owing to administration of glucocorticoids or adrenocorticotropic hormone (ACTH), or endogenous, as a result of autonomous secretion of ACTH or cortisol. Endogenous CS is classified as ACTH-dependent, which accounts for about 80% of endogenous cases, and ACTH-independent, which accounts for the remaining 20%. ACTH-dependent pituitary CS (Cushing's disease), which accounts for about 80% of the adult and 35% of the childhood cases, most commonly occurs during the third and fourth decades of life and is more common in females than males. It is most often caused by ACTH-secreting pituitary microadenomas (90%) or macroadenomas (10%). Rarely, diffuse corticotroph hyperplasia is found in association with ACTH hypersecretion, and corticotropin-releasing hormone (CRH) production by tumors of neuroendocrine origin can cause pituitary ACTH CS.

ACTH-dependent CS resulting from ectopic ACTH production accounts for about 20% of ACTH-dependent cases and is most often associated with bronchial carcinoid, small cell carcinoma of the lung, thymoma, medullary carcinoma of the thyroid, and pheochromocytoma.

ACTH-independent CS, which accounts for about 10% of adult cases and 65% of cases in children under 7 years of age, is usually the result of a benign cortisol-secreting adrenal adenoma or an adrenocortical carcinoma. Two rare forms of ACTH-independent CS are caused by bilateral adrenal disease: primary pigmented nodular adrenal disease and macronodular adrenal disease. The former is one of the manifestations of Carney's complex, which is an autosomal dominant disorder. Other manifestations of Carney's complex include myxomas, lentigines, acromegaly, and Sertoli tumors of the testis. In macronodular adrenal disease, the adrenal glands are often massively enlarged. Recently, a subcategory of this entity, food-induced CS, was recognized. It is characterized by abnormal increase in plasma cortisol levels after a meal; fasting cortisol levels are often low. The adrenals of these patients appear to respond to vasoactive intestinal peptide.

Pseudo-Cushing's syndrome (PCS) is a condition characterized by mild to moderate hypercortisolism in the absence of CS. PCS has been associated with several conditions, including depression, alcoholism, morbid obesity, and uncontrolled diabetes mellitus.

TABLE 1. **Evaluation of Hypercortisolism**

Diagnosis of Cushing's Syndrome

24-hour urinary free cortisol measurement
Midnight cortisol measurement
1-mg overnight dexamethasone suppression test
Dexamethasone-CRH test

Differential Diagnosis

Feedback Regulation of the Hypothalamic-Pituitary-Adrenal Axis

Basal plasma ACTH levels
8-mg overnight dexamethasone suppression test
CRH stimulation test
Measurement of other hormones or metabolites if multiple endocrine neoplasia or ectopic ACTH secretion is suspected (e.g., plasma calcitonin, gastrin, urinary 5-HIAA, catecholamines)

Localization Imaging Studies

Bilateral inferior petrosal sinus sampling combined with CRH stimulation
Pituitary MRI
Adrenal MRI-CT
Neck, chest, abdominal, and pelvic MRI-CT if ectopic ACTH secretion is suspected
Octreotide scan if ectopic ACTH-producing tumor is suspected
Iodocholesterol scan to examine bilateral or unilateral adrenal uptake or to localize functional adrenal tissue

Abbreviations: ACTH = adrenocorticotropic hormone; CRH = corticotropin-releasing hormone; 5-HIAA = 5-hydroxyindoleacetic acid; MRI = magnetic resonance imaging; CT = computed tomography.

DIAGNOSTIC EVALUATION

CS has a highly variable presentation. Common clinical features include truncal obesity, facial rounding and plethora (moon facies), easy bruising, purplish skin striae, acne, hirsutism, oligomenorrhea or amenorrhea, muscle weakness, emotional liability and/or depression, insomnia, memory loss, hypertension, peripheral edema, carbohydrate intolerance (frank diabetes mellitus is uncommon), and osteoporosis, mainly of the spine and femur. Patients may present with only a few or many of these features, depending to some extent on the severity and duration of hypercortisolism. In addition to the history and clinical evaluation, biochemical and imaging evaluation is necessary to establish the diagnosis and determine the cause.

The first step is to establish the presence of hypercortisolism (Table 1). Twenty-four-hour urinary free cortisol (UFC) measurement is the best single laboratory test for this purpose. However, hypercortisolism can be episodic. A single UFC measurement can be normal in as many as 10% of patients with proven CS; thus, at least four UFC measurements are necessary to exclude hypercortisolism. Further, in patients in whom periodic CS is suspected, measurement of UFC on a regular basis (weekly or monthly) often reveals hypercortisolism. In pediatric patients, UFC should be corrected per body surface area.

After hypercortisolism has been established, the differential diagnosis of CS versus PCS should be made. Isolated morning plasma ACTH and/or cortisol determinations are of no value, because both hormones are secreted episodically and their secretion is influenced by physical or emotional stress.

For the diagnosis of CS the following tests can be applied:

1. *Midnight cortisol measurement*: A single midnight plasma cortisol value can differentiate CS from PCS with a diagnostic accuracy of 95%. The patient should be resting in the recumbent position for at least 30 minutes after an intravenous line is placed for blood drawing. Because food intake and physical activity can normally raise plasma cortisol levels, the patient should not have anything to eat or drink after 9 PM and physical activity should be limited during this time as well. A plasma cortisol level more than 7.5 μg per dL is highly suggestive of CS. Salivary cortisol measurements can also be used.

2. *1-mg overnight dexamethasone suppression test*: Suppression of plasma cortisol levels below 3 μg per dL at 8 AM, after administration of 1 mg of dexamethasone orally at 11 PM. Patients with CS do not suppress plasma cortisol values to < 3 μg per dL. Even though the false-negative results are rare (~2%), the false-positive results are not uncommon (up to 20%), making a positive result less useful.

3. *Dexamethasone-CRH test*: This test is a modification of the classic Liddle's test. Dexamethasone, 0.5 mg, is given orally every 6 hours starting at noon for 2 days (total of 8 doses). The last dose is given at 6 AM. At 8 AM, CRH (1 μg per kg) is administered intravenously through an indwelling catheter. Plasma cortisol is measured at baseline and at 15 minutes after CRH administration. A plasma cortisol

value > 1.44 μg per dL is suggestive of CS, with a diagnostic accuracy of ~95%. The timing of the CRH injection is of great importance; it must take place 2 hours after the last dose of dexamethasone is given. Any delay may give false-positive results.

It should be mentioned that any test involving dexamethasone suppression may be falsely positive or falsely negative, depending on the metabolic clearance of dexamethasone. Certain medications (e.g., antiepileptics) can increase the hepatic clearance of dexamethasone, whereas hepatic or renal disease could lead to decreased clearance and thus prolonged effect. Therefore, it is important to obtain plasma dexamethasone levels, especially in the more difficult cases.

Even with the use of the aforementioned tests, the diagnosis of CS can be quite difficult, especially in cases of mild CS. Prolonged follow-up with repeated biochemical evaluation may be necessary in such cases. Unlike patients with PCS, patients with mild CS manifest a progression of their disease, and the deterioration of their clinical status makes the diagnosis clear.

Rarely, a patient with factitious CS is encountered. These individuals usually have CS with low levels of urinary free cortisol excretion because synthetic glucocorticoids, such as prednisone, prednisolone, or dexamethasone, are the most frequently abused agents. Specific plasma or urine assays for the steroids are usually necessary to confirm the diagnosis.

Once the diagnosis of CS has been confirmed, testing should be undertaken to determine the specific etiology of the syndrome (see Table 1).

1. *Plasma ACTH determination*: First, ACTH-independent CS should be excluded. A morning plasma ACTH level of < 5 pg per mL would make the diagnosis of ACTH-independent CS. Plasma ACTH levels of 5 to 15 pg per mL are indeterminate, and further diagnostic testing is required. Plasma ACTH > 15 pg per mL confirms the diagnosis of ACTH-dependent CS.

2. *8-mg overnight dexamethasone suppression test*: This test has replaced the high-dose Liddle's test because it is simpler and has a higher diagnostic accuracy. Blood is drawn at 8:30 AM for baseline plasma cortisol measurement, followed by dexamethasone administration orally at 11 PM, and finally a second plasma cortisol measurement at 9 AM. Patients with pituitary CS show suppression of cortisol levels more than 68% of baseline, whereas patients with ectopic ACTH production or primary adrenocortical disease show no or less suppression (specificity 100%, sensitivity 71%). This test carries the caveats discussed previously with regard to dexamethasone metabolism.

3. *CRH stimulation test*: Intravenous administration of CRH results in an increase in plasma ACTH and cortisol levels in patients with pituitary CS, but it has no effect in patients with ectopic ACTH production. Blood is drawn at 15 minutes and 1 minute before, and 15, 30, and 45 minutes after CRH administration (1 μg per kg). ACTH values at 15 and 30 minutes and cortisol values at 30 and 45 minutes are averaged. A 35% increase in the average ACTH value or a 20% increase in the average cortisol value over the average baseline value is suggestive of pituitary CS rather than ectopic ACTH production or primary adrenocortical disease (specificity 100%, sensitivity 93% for ACTH; specificity 88%, sensitivity 91% for cortisol). Even though ACTH measurements provide higher diagnostic accuracy than cortisol, cortisol measurements are much cheaper and require less expertise in sample handling and thus may be more practical.

4. *Inferior petrosal sinus sampling (IPSS)*: When the diagnosis of pituitary CS is uncertain, IPSS may be necessary. During this procedure, both femoral veins are catheterized by an interventional radiologist. The catheters are advanced to the two inferior petrosal sinuses, which drain the blood from the pituitary gland. A peripheral vein is cannulated as well. Blood is drawn at 15 minutes and 1 minute before and 3, 5, and 10 minutes after the test for plasma ACTH measurement. CRH is given intravenously through a peripheral line at time 0. A central peripheral ACTH level ratio of at least 3:1 strongly suggests pituitary CS (diagnostic accuracy >95%). Lateralization to either sinus does not appear to be useful with regard to the location of the adenoma.

5. *Magnetic resonance imaging (MRI) of the pituitary gland*: MRI of the pituitary should be performed on every patient with ACTH-dependent CS. The MRI should be of at least 1.5 Tesla. Enhancement with gadolinium can also be useful. Unfortunately, MRI fails to show the pituitary tumor in 40 to 60% of pituitary CS. Further, incidental findings suggestive of a pituitary adenoma can be seen in 10 to 15% of the population. Thus, the MRI of the pituitary should be interpreted by an experienced neuroradiologist. A positive MRI result should be considered diagnostic for pituitary disease only if indicated by the biochemical data. On the other hand, IPSS may be required to confirm the diagnosis of pituitary CS in a patient with a negative MRI result.

6. *Computed tomography (CT) scan of the adrenal glands*: CT scan of the adrenal glands should be performed only when ACTH-independent CS is suspected to establish the adrenal pathology (adenoma vs carcinoma vs bilateral adrenal disease). Adrenal CT scan is of no use in patients with ACTH-dependent CS (except for the detection of a pheochromocytoma causing ectopic CS). Even though ACTH-dependent CS is frequently accompanied by adrenal enlargement as seen on CT scan, there is significant overlap with the normal population, limiting the diagnostic use of this test. The presence of nodules of variable size on either adrenal can be seen in pituitary CS and in the normal population. However, any nodule greater than 5 cm is suspicious for adrenal carcinoma and should be further investigated.

7. *Imaging for the detection of a tumor causing ectopic ACTH CS*: If the patient's evaluation suggests the diagnosis of ectopic ACTH secretion, the primary tumor should be sought. More than 50% of these tumors are within the thorax (oat cell carcinomas, bronchial carcinoids, thymomas). Other ACTH-secreting tumors are found in the pancreas, the thyroid gland, and the adrenal medulla. Often these ectopic ACTH-producing tumors are occult and require extensive imaging, including CT scan with thin cuts (<1 mm) and MRI of the neck, chest, abdomen, and pelvis, as well as a whole-body octreotide scan. These tumors (especially the bronchial carcinoids) can be extremely small and easily mistaken for vessels. Thus, the concordance of at least two imaging studies may be required for the localization of the source of ectopic ACTH production. It may take 10 years or more for the source of ectopic ACTH production to be identified with repeated annual imaging. Finally, further biochemical tests may aid the diagnosis of ectopic ACTH production. For example, the presence of an occult medullary thyroid carcinoma producing ACTH can be suggested by elevated plasma calcitonin levels.

8. *Iodocholesterol scan*: This scan can be used to distinguish adrenocortical carcinomas from adenomas or ACTH-dependent macronodules. Carcinomas fail to be imaged with this technique, whereas benign adenomas and ACTH-

dependent macronodules concentrate iodocholesterol and, hence, produce an image.

TREATMENT

Therapy is indicated in all patients with CS. The treatment of choice depends on the specific cause of hypercortisolism, which must be established unequivocally (Table 2). Optimal treatment is the correction of hypercortisolism without permanent dependence on hormone replacement.

Cushing's Disease

Most cases of CS are caused by ACTH-secreting pituitary adenomas. These are usually benign and small (90% are < 10 mm in diameter) and cause no sellar enlargement. Currently, four therapeutic modalities are available for the treatment of these tumors: transsphenoidal adenomectomy, pituitary x-irradiation with concomitant therapy with the adrenolytic agent mitotane (*o,p'*-DDD) or the steroidogenic enzyme inhibitor ketoconazole, therapy with mitotane alone, and bilateral adrenalectomy.

Transsphenoidal Adenomectomy

Transsphenoidal adenomectomy is the treatment of choice for most cases of CS caused by pituitary microadenomas. If the presence of a pituitary microadenoma can be demonstrated preoperatively by imaging techniques or IPSS, transsphenoidal selective resection of the adenoma is indicated. If the microadenoma is not detected by radiographic techniques but typical diagnostic criteria for Cushing's disease exist and IPSS is positive, 90% of patients can be cured by hemihypophysectomy, even though in some patients the adenomas may not be identified at surgery. Successful surgery leads to cure of hypercortisolism with no need for permanent glucocorticoid replacement. The overall success rate of the operation exceeds 80 to 90% in the best series, with considerable variability. A small percentage of patients suffer recurrences. Current diagnostic methods appear to be improving results. The success rate of transsphenoidal operation is considerably lower (60%) in patients with recurrent Cushing's disease after a previously successful operation, or in patients with previously failed transsphenoidal operations or invasive macroadenomas.

Transient diabetes insipidus may occur during the early weeks after surgery. Permanent diabetes insipidus and cerebrospinal fluid rhinorrhea are uncommon complications but may occur more frequently in patients with repeated transsphenoidal surgery. Transient isolated hyponatremia is a well-recognized complication of transsphenoidal surgery that can occur on the fifth to eighth postoperative days. It is a self-limiting phenomenon, but it may require observation, fluid restriction, and rarely more aggressive treatment. The mortality rate is probably less than 1%, lower than that of bilateral adrenalectomy (approximately 4%). Treatment failures are most common in patients with pituitary macroadenomas. A CRH stimulation test has been used in the postoperative evaluation of patients cured of Cushing's disease by selective microadenomectomy. At the early postoperative period, these patients are hypocortisolemic with subnormal cortisol responses to CRH, presumably on the basis of suppression of the pituitary gland and/or hypothalamic CRH neurons, as a result of long-standing hypercortisolism. Normal cortisol levels and a normal response to CRH in this period may identify a subgroup of patients at risk for suboptimal resection and recurrence of disease.

Pituitary x-Irradiation

This is a reasonable alternative form of treatment following failure of transsphenoidal surgery or, rarely, as the first line of treatment in patients judged unsuitable for surgery. The most widely used dose of pituitary irradiation is 4500 rad total. High-voltage, conventional irradiation is given in 180 rad fractions over 5 weeks. This treatment cures only 10 to 15% of patients but markedly improves another 25 to 30% of untreated adult patients (responses are better in adults younger than 40 years of age) and about 80% of children younger than 18 years. Biochemical amelioration occurs with preservation of pituitary and adrenal function but is delayed by several months (6 to 18 months). Heavy particle beam

TABLE 2. **Therapy for Cushing's Syndrome**

Cushing's Disease (Pituitary)
Transsphenoidal microadenomectomy or hemopituitectomy
Pituitary x-radiation combined with medical therapy
Adrenolytic mitotane (low dose)
Steroid synthesis inhibitors, alone or in combination
Ketoconazole*
Aminoglutethimide
Metyrapone*
Trilostane
Bilateral adrenalectomy
Ectopic ACTH Secretion Syndrome
Removal of primary tumor and solitary accessible metastases
Adrenolytic mitotane (low dose)
Steroid synthesis inhibitors, alone or in combination
Ketoconazole*
Aminoglutethimide
Metyrapone*
Trilostane
Bilateral adrenalectomy
Palliative x-radiation
Somatostatin analogue SMS 201-995 (octreotide acetate)
Adrenal Cushing's Syndrome
Benign Adenomas or Micronodular Adrenal Disease
Unilateral or bilateral adrenalectomy
Adrenocortical Carcinomas
Surgery
Adrenolytic mitotane (high dose)
Steroid synthesis inhibitors
Ketoconazole*
Aminoglutethimide
Metyrapone*
Chemotherapy for solid tumors
Palliative radiotherapy for bone metastases

*Not FDA approved for this indication.

irradiation and Bragg peak proton irradiation therapy appear to be equally effective to conventional irradiation; however, the prevalence of postirradiation panhypopituitarism is higher with the former techniques. The side effects and the efficacy of therapy may be related to the dosage of radiation administered. Progressive anterior hypopituitarism, including growth hormone deficiency, hypothyroidism, and hypogonadism, occurs in 30 to 40% of patients. Radiation-induced atrophy of the brain also may be seen with high dosages. These complications may occur several years after radiotherapy. Usually, concomitantly with and after pituitary radiation, drug therapy (mitotane [Lysodren]) is given at low doses, ranging from 1 to 4 grams per day. Combined pituitary radiation and mitotane improve the success rate of either modality given alone. Ketoconazole has been shown to be a good alternative to mitotane as an adjuvant to radiation therapy. The results are as good as with mitotane, and ketoconazole is better tolerated and has fewer side effects than mitotane.

Drug Therapy

Drug therapy is rarely used alone to treat Cushing's disease except temporarily, before definitive treatment. Mitotane* is the only available pharmacologic agent that both inhibits biosynthesis of corticosteroids (inhibits 11-β-hydroxylase and cholesterol side chain cleavage enzymes) and destroys adrenocortical cells secreting cortisol, thus producing a long-lasting effect. Therapy with mitotane alone can be successful in 30 to 40% of patients with Cushing's disease. Addition of aminoglutethimide, up to 2 grams a day orally in four divided doses, or metyrapone, up to 2 grams a day in four divided doses, can improve the success rate. During treatment, the urinary free cortisol excretion should be monitored and the dosage of mitotane titrated to maintain urinary free cortisol excretion in the normal range. If adrenal insufficiency is suspected, oral hydrocortisone should be added.

Although mitotane is a selective inhibitor of the reticularis and fasciculata zones of the adrenal cortex, it may on occasion affect the zona glomerulosa, leading to hypoaldosteronism that requires replacement with oral fludrocortisone (Florinef), 50 to 300 μg per day. Because mitotane induces liver monooxygenases (cytochrome P-450 enzymes) that metabolize steroids and other drugs, an adequate dose of hydrocortisone and fludrocortisone may be higher than expected. Measuring urinary 17-hydroxysteroid excretion does not provide a reliable index of adrenal suppression by the drug, because an early fall in the urinary excretion of this metabolite occurs independent of the effect of the drug on cortisol secretion. This phenomenon is a result of mitotane-induced enhancement of liver 6-hydroxylase activity that results in side-tracking cortisol metabolism to 6-alpha-hydroxylated and related metabolites that are not detected by the Porter-Silber reaction, which detects 17-hydroxycorticosteroids.

*Not FDA approved for this indication.

Side effects with mitotane therapy include anorexia, nausea, vomiting, diarrhea, skin reactions, hyperlipidemia, hepatotoxicity and neurologic manifestations (primarily somnolence), lethargy, dizziness, and muscle weakness. All of the side effects can be reversed by reducing the dose of the drug or by discontinuing therapy.

Adrenal enzyme inhibitors—aminoglutethimide, metyrapone, trilostane, and ketoconazole—have been used alone or in combination with mitotane or each other to control some of the symptoms and metabolic abnormalities associated with the hypercortisolemia in Cushing's disease and the ectopic ACTH syndrome. Combinations are recommended because they most frequently alleviate breakthroughs that occur when the drugs are used alone. In addition, one can use moderate doses with fewer side effects.

Aminoglutethimide acts in the first step of steroid biosynthesis, in which it blocks the conversion of cholesterol to delta-5-pregnenolone in the adrenal cortex. As a result, the synthesis of cortisol, aldosterone, and androgens is inhibited. The drug has been used both in adults and children in doses of 0.5 to 2 grams daily. Aminoglutethimide alone is only transiently effective, as the inhibitory effect of the drug on cortisol synthesis is overcome by increasing plasma concentrations of ACTH. Aminoglutethimide has gastrointestinal (anorexia, nausea, vomiting) and neurologic (lethargy, sedation, blurred vision) side effects and can cause hypothyroidism in 5% of patients. A skin rash is frequently observed during the first 10 days of therapy, which usually subsides despite continuation of treatment.

Metyrapone (Metopirone), an 11-β-hydroxylase inhibitor, blocks the final step of cortisol biosynthesis by preventing the conversion of 11-deoxycortisol to cortisol. Treatment with metyrapone alone (250 mg twice daily to 2 grams divided four times daily) or in combination with mitotane or aminoglutethimide can result in biochemical and clinical remission in patients with Cushing's disease. Metyrapone causes hypertension and hypokalemic alkalosis, a result of blockade of 11-hydroxylase and accumulation of 11-deoxycorticosterone. It also produces gastrointestinal irritation, nausea, vomiting, and allergic rash and may worsen hirsutism. A combination of metyrapone and aminoglutethimide should lead to increased therapeutic effectiveness with decreased individual drug doses and fewer side effects.

Trilostane, which until recently was an investigational drug, inhibits the conversion of pregnenolone to progesterone, another critical step in cortisol biosynthesis. Trilostane at doses of 200 to 1000 mg daily has side effects similar to those observed with aminoglutethimide.

Ketoconazole (Nizoral), an antifungal agent, is a recent addition to our armamentarium of cortisol synthesis inhibitors. The drug can be given at 600 to 1200 mg a day in three or more divided doses. Amelioration of clinical and metabolic manifestations of hypercortisolism has been seen within 4 to 6 weeks of treatment. The drug is well tolerated but has some hepatotoxicity, primarily of the hepatocellular type. Ketoconazole can also cause nausea, vomiting, abdominal pain, and pruritus in 1 to 3% of patients. Etomidate, an imidazole-containing anesthetic agent, has also been found to inhibit cortisol secretion in a manner similar to that of ketoconazole. At the present time, etomidate has not been used for treatment of patients with CS in the United States.

Bilateral Adrenalectomy

The indications for adrenal surgery for Cushing's disease have been altered radically by the success and low morbidity of transsphenoidal surgery. Bilateral total adrenalectomy could be considered for adults who have failed selective pituitary adenomectomy or hypophysectomy and in whom ectopic ACTH secretion has been unequivocally ruled out. When performed properly, it leads to cure of hypercortisolism. The major disadvantages of bilateral adrenalectomy are that the individual after surgery is committed to lifelong daily cortisol and fludrocortisone replacement, that it fails to attack the cause underlying the hypersecretion of ACTH, and that relapses, although uncommon, can occur as a result of growth of adrenal rest tissue or an adrenal remnant. In addition, perioperative mortality is approximately four times higher than that associated with transsphenoidal surgery, although it can be minimized by careful perioperative preparation. Nelson's syndrome (large pituitary macroadenomas secreting great amounts of ACTH resulting in skin hyperpigmentation) may occur in approximately 10 to 15% of patients with Cushing's disease treated with bilateral adrenalectomy. Clinically apparent Nelson's syndrome may occur months or years after bilateral adrenalectomy. These ACTH-secreting macroadenomas may be locally invasive and extend above the diaphragma sellae, causing visual field defects. Rarely, they can metastasize locally in the brain, and distant hepatic metastatic nodules have been reported. Treatment for such ACTH-secreting macroadenomas is usually difficult and includes transsphenoidal surgery (if not too large) followed by 5000 rad of conventional pituitary irradiation.

The Ectopic ACTH Syndrome

Treatment of the ectopic ACTH syndrome is directed, if possible, at the primary tumor. If the tumor is totally excised, hypercortisolism is cured. Tumors secreting ACTH, however, are often occult or disseminated at the time of diagnosis, and other therapeutic options must be sought. Therapy, other than primary tumor excision, is directed toward the adrenal glands and at the glucocorticoid receptor level. Use of the adrenolytic mitotane and steroidogenic enzyme inhibitors, such as aminoglutethimide, metyrapone, and ketoconazole, is the first line of defense to control hypercortisolism and ameliorate the clinical manifestations of the syndrome. However, the very high ACTH levels usually present in the ectopic ACTH syndrome may rapidly overcome the suppressive effect of these drugs. Another drug, the long-acting somatostatin analogue SMS 201-995 (octreotide acetate [Sandostatin]), has been used successfully in the treatment of patients with the ectopic ACTH CS and probably could be valuable for the long-term medical management of such patients. SMS 201-995 may reduce ACTH secretion by occasional tumors but has no effect on tumor growth. The usual dose is 100 μg three times per day, subcutaneously. Bilateral adrenalectomy is indicated in a patient with CS caused by ectopic ACTH production when the patient is severely ill, the primary tumor is disseminated or not found, or medical therapy fails or is poorly tolerated.

Adrenocortical Tumors

Surgical resection is the treatment of choice for all primary adrenocortical tumors. Unilateral total adrenalectomy is recommended for the autonomous benign cortisol-secreting adrenal adenomas. Bilateral adrenalectomy is recommended for patients with micronodular or bilateral macronodular adrenal disease. Complete resection of the tumor is the treatment of choice for adrenal carcinoma. If complete resection cannot be achieved, however, as much of the tumor as possible should be removed. Solitary local recurrences or metastases of adrenocortical carcinoma should be removed surgically, if possible. Adrenal carcinomas causing CS are highly malignant neoplasms. Long-term remissions, however, have been reported following complete resection of adrenocortical carcinoma, and long-term remissions have followed surgical resection of hepatic, pulmonary, or cerebral metastases.

Once it is known that the patient does not have surgically curable disease, therapy with the adrenolytic agent mitotane is usually initiated. Mitotane given at maximally tolerated oral doses (up to 16 grams per day) has been the only drug that has some effectiveness in patients with metastatic adrenocortical carcinoma. Tumor regression or arrest of growth has been observed in as many as one third of patients, and the agent ameliorates the endocrine syndrome in approximately two thirds of these patients. Mean survival time, however, does not appear to be altered, although occasional patients with unresectable carcinomas achieve long-term survival.

The side effects of mitotane are dose dependent and have been previously mentioned. Starting with low doses of mitotane (250 to 500 mg four times a day) and gradually advancing to therapeutic levels (12 to 16 grams daily), one can minimize the side effects to some degree. Before initiation of therapy, a tumor mass should be defined, which can be followed objectively by radiologic procedures (usually CT or MRI) for monitoring therapeutic efficacy. Patients taking mitotane may develop hypocortisolism and hypoaldosteronism, and hydrocortisone or fludrocortisone should be added as needed. Occasionally, steroid synthesis inhibitors (aminoglutethimide, metyrapone, ketoconazole) can be given for the correction of hypercortisolism.

Postoperative Steroid Replacement

After a successful transsphenoidal operation for Cushing's disease or removal of an autonomous ACTH- or cortisol-secreting tumor, a period of adrenal insufficiency ensues, during which time glucocorticoids must be replaced. This abnormality of the hypothalamic-pituitary-adrenal axis can last as long as 1 year. Intraoperatively, and during the first 2 postoperative days, 100 mg per day of hydrocortisone or its equivalent is given intravenously. Once the patient has recovered from the surgical procedure, oral replacement doses of hydrocortisone, 20 to 30 mg (12 to 15 mg per m^2) per day, are initiated. Patients who are cured often complain of anorexia, somnolence, weakness, and lack of energy at these doses, a sign of successful surgery. The replacement dose of hydrocortisone is maintained for 3 months and then tapered, as the patient loses weight. Six months postoperatively the patient should be tested with a short ACTH stimulation test (cosyntropin [Cortrosyn], 250 μg intravenously, with cortisol measured at 60 minutes). When the response to this test becomes normal (plasma cortisol above 20 μg per dL), hydrocortisone therapy should be discontinued. If the result is subnormal, the therapy is continued for another 3 months and the test repeated. The majority of patients can discontinue glucocorticoid replacement within 9 to 12 months postoperatively. During this period, patients should be given extra glucocorticoids during stress. During minor stress (flu with fever above 38°C), the daily dose should be doubled until the illness is resolved. During major stress (surgery), they should be given 100 mg of parenteral hydrocortisone daily, beginning 1 day before surgery and tapered to normal replacement as rapidly as recovery allows. All patients should wear MedicAlert badges indicating that they are receiving glucocorticoid replacement and be prepared to use an emergency 100-mg hydrocortisone injection kit. This should be used when the patient has severe vomiting or diarrhea (i.e., when absorption by the gastrointestinal tract is impaired).

Exogenous Cushing's Syndrome

Exogenous CS is most commonly seen in patients with renal, autoimmune, hematologic, and neoplastic conditions that require chronic pharmacologic glucocorticoid therapy. Exposure to glucocorticoids for periods sufficient to produce symptoms and signs as those found in endogenous CS can be expected to produce hypothalamic-pituitary-adrenal axis suppression that may require up to 1 year for recovery. Therefore, every effort should be made to minimize the period during which steroids are given daily. Once the disease process has been controlled, the daily dose should be doubled and administered on alternate days. An alternate schedule of administration is crucial in children, in whom daily administration stunts growth. Many glucocorticoid-responsive diseases are now successfully controlled in this manner, whereas signs and symptoms of CS are diminished. Patients should be given extra glucocorticoids during stress (e.g., postoperative cured patients with CS).

DIABETES INSIPIDUS

method of
GEETHA NARAYAN, M.D., and
JAMES A. STROM, M.D.
Tufts University School of Medicine and St. Elizabeth's Medical Center of Boston
Boston, Massachusetts

Diabetes insipidus (DI) is a disorder of water balance in which there is an excessive urinary loss of solute-free water due to impaired renal concentration. The kidneys, through their normal capacity to vary urinary concentration from a low of 50 mOsm per kg H_2O to a high of 1200 mOsm per kg H_2O, permit large fluctuations or variations in water intake without causing net gain or loss of free water to the body fluids. The osmolality of body fluids is thus maintained within a narrow range of about 280 to 290 mOsm per kg H_2O.

PATHOGENESIS

The concentrating action of the kidneys is tightly regulated by the hypothalamic-pituitary axis. The sensitive osmoreceptors in the anterior hypothalamus respond to increases in plasma osmolality (Posm) of as little as 1% by stimulating the synthesis and release of vasopressin or antidiuretic hormone (ADH) through the posterior pituitary. The circulating ADH then acts on the renal collecting duct through specific V2 receptors to make the tubules more permeable to water, thereby promoting water reabsorption through osmotic equilibration with the hypertonic medullary interstitium. In humans, the release of ADH starts at Posm values of 275 to 280 mOsm per kg H_2O, and rises 5- to 10-fold at a Posm value of 295 mOsm per kg H_2O—levels that can sustain maximal urinary concentration of 800 to 1200 mOsm per kg H_2O. Above Posm of 290 mOsm per kg H_2O, thirst is stimulated, which aids in the restoration of plasma osmolality to normal.

It is the interruption of this hypothalamic-pituitary-renal mechanism of urinary concentration that leads to excessive free water losses as polyuria, which in turn can lead to hyperosmolality of body fluids, manifested as an increased concentration of plasma sodium, the main extracellular solute.

ETIOLOGY

There are two major etiologic categories of DI, central (CDI) and nephrogenic (NDI). The former results from decreased release of ADH from the hypothalamic-pituitary axis; the latter results from renal resistance to the action of normal circulating levels of ADH. The most common causes in each category are listed in Table 1.

TABLE 1. **Causes of Diabetes Insipidus (DI)**

Central DI

Idiopathic DI (possibly autoimmune)
Pituitary surgery
Trauma
Neoplastic disease—craniopharyngioma, metastatic carcinoma of lung or breast, lymphoma
Infiltrative disorders—sarcoidosis, histiocytosis, Wegener's granulomatosis
Vascular lesions—aneurysm, hypoxic/ischemic encephalopathy
Infection—encephalitis, meningitis
Familial

Nephrogenic DI

Drugs—lithium, demeclocycline, methoxyflurane, amphotericin, foscarnet
Electrolyte disorders—hypercalcemia, hypokalemia
Tubulointerstitial renal diseases—sickle cell nephropathy, Sjögren's syndrome, amyloidosis, sarcoidosis
Congenital

CLINICAL FEATURES

The clinical manifestations of DI are polyuria and hypernatremia. The clinical presentation, however, can vary, depending on the specific clinical setting. Since most persons with chronic DI have an intact thirst mechanism, they can adequately replace their (solute-) free water losses and thus maintain near-normal plasma osmolality and serum sodium concentration. In such alert ambulatory patients, polyuria and polydipsia are the primary symptoms, and the degree of polyuria corresponds to the severity of DI, which can be a complete or partial disorder in both the central and nephrogenic types. In contrast, patients with impaired thirst (e.g., patients with hypothalamic lesions, dementia, or cerebrovascular disease) or inability to drink water (e.g., feeble, bed-bound, or comatose patients) may present with progressive, even life-threatening hypernatremia requiring immediate correction. The accompanying cerebral dehydration can lead to symptoms of weakness, lethargy, irritability, confusion, and seizures, progressing to coma and death in severe cases.

A peculiar triphasic response may be seen in cases of severe DI following head trauma or surgery. There is an initial polyuric phase due to hypothalamic axonal injury with abrupt cessation of ADH release (at 2 to 4 days), followed by a period of uncontrolled release of stored ADH from dying neurons, leading to water retention and possible hyponatremia (at 5 to 7 days). In the final phase there is neuronal death and permanent DI. Most postsurgical or traumatic cases, however, are self-limited, with resolution over a period of days.

DIAGNOSIS

The first step in the diagnosis of polyuria is to distinguish between water diuresis (urine osmolality [Uosm] of less than 250 mOsm per kg H_2O) and solute diuresis (Uosm greater than 250 mOsm per kg H_2O). *Solute diuresis* is usually seen in the setting of uncontrolled diabetes, mannitol or diuretic therapy, or resolving acute renal failure. If the polyuria is secondary to *water diuresis*, the next step is to distinguish among its three major causes — namely, the two forms of DI (CDI and NDI) and primary polydipsia. A water deprivation test may be needed to confirm the diagnosis. Patients must be monitored carefully, because those with severe defects may become rapidly dehydrated. In general, water intake is restricted over a 4- to 12-hour period, with care taken to ensure that a maximal weight loss of 3 to 5% of body weight is not exceeded, and deprivation is not continued beyond the end points of a Posm value of 295 mOsm per kg H_2O and a stable Uosm value in two consecutive hourly specimens. At this point, exogenous ADH (usually 5 units of aqueous vasopressin [Pitressin] in a subcutaneous injection) is given, and after 60 minutes the urine osmolality is measured. A direct measurement of plasma ADH level can enhance the accuracy of the test. The expected responses are summarized in Table 2 and illustrated in Figure 1.

Partial NDI and primary polydipsia can usually be differentiated by a careful history combined with laboratory data, such as plasma sodium concentration, which tends to be low-normal to low in primary polydipsia and normal to high in DI.

TREATMENT

General Principles

The primary goals of therapy are correction of the water deficit and amelioration of polyuria. As mentioned earlier, in ambulatory patients with intact thirst, significant water deficits and resultant hypernatremia are uncommon, whereas polyuria and polydipsia are the most troubling symptoms. On the other hand, in sicker (usually hospitalized) patients with altered mental status, impaired thirst, or lack of access to water, varying degrees of hypernatremia can develop, demanding prompt attention. Since solute-free water readily equilibrates across all body fluid compartments, its loss is shared proportionately by the compartments, and thus only one twelfth of the total loss (e.g., 83 mL out of 1 liter) is borne by the intravascular space. As such, free water losses have little or no effect on intravascular volume status, unless the total body water (TBW) losses reach 4 to 6 liters, when signs of volume depletion (tachycardia and hypotension) may complicate the clinical picture.

TABLE 2. **Diagnosis of Diabetes Insipidus (DI)**

Disorder	Urine Osmolality After Dehydration (mOsm/kg H_2O)	Plasma ADH After Dehydration (pg/mL)	Urine Osmolality After Exogenous ADH (mOsm/kg H_2O)
Normal	>600–800	>2	No increase
Central DI			
Complete	<300	Undetectable	>50% increase
Partial	>300	<1.5	>10% increase
Nephrogenic DI			
Complete	<300	>5	<50% increase
Partial	>300	>2	<10% increase
Primary polydipsia	>500	>2	No response

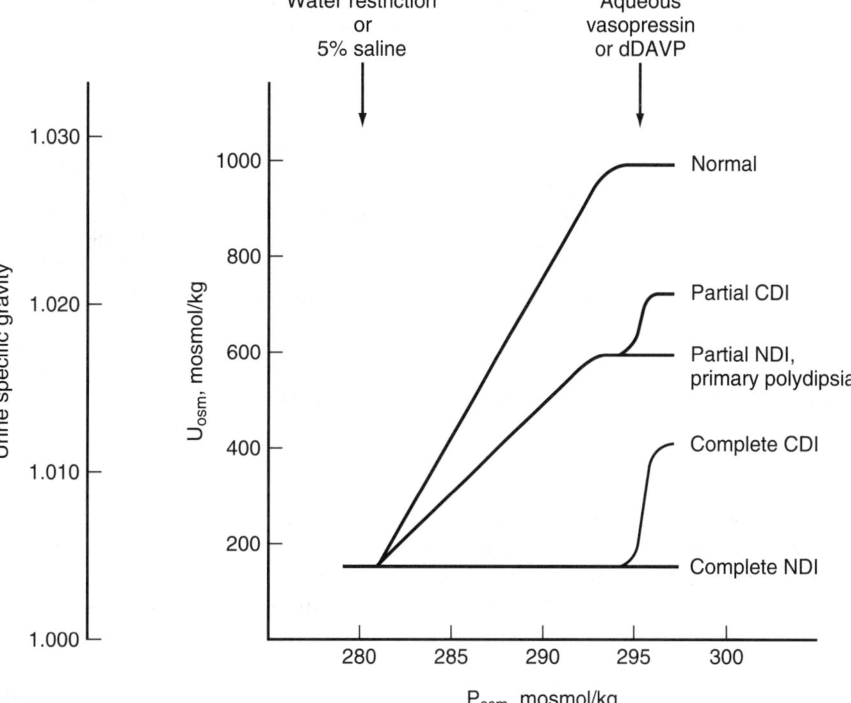

Figure 1. Schematic representation of typical responses to dehydration test. *Abbreviations:* CDI = central diabetes insipidus; NDI = nephrogenic diabetes insipidus. (From Rose BD: Clinical Physiology of Acid-Base and Electrolyte Disorders, 4th ed. New York, McGraw-Hill, 1994, p 717. Reproduced with permission of the McGraw-Hill Companies.)

Correction of Water Deficit

The treatment of hypernatremia is simply water replacement. The existing water deficit should be corrected and any ongoing free water losses replaced.

Estimation of Deficit

The water deficit may be estimated from the following formula:

$$\text{Water deficit} = 0.6 \times \text{body weight (kg)} \times [(\text{plasma Na}^{+} \div 140) - 1]$$

For example, the water deficit in a 60-kg woman with a plasma sodium level of 160 mEq per liter is $0.6 \times 60 \times (160/140 - 1)$, or 5.1 liters. Since the TBW is not always 60% of body weight, the preceding equation provides only an approximation of the water deficit for initiating therapy.

Rate of Correction

When hypernatremia develops acutely, the accompanying hyperosmolality results in transcellular movement of water out of the brain cells and intracerebral dehydration. On the other hand, in chronic hypernatremia, the brain cell has time to adapt to the hyperosmolar state with an increase in intracellular organic solutes ("idiogenic osmoles"). This allows water to shift back into the cell, thus restoring brain volume toward normal. Although such an adaptive response can mitigate the cerebral dehydration and render the patient relatively asymptomatic in chronic hypernatremia, it has serious adverse potential during therapy. Overly rapid correction of hypernatremia in the presence of now near-normal brain cell osmolality can lead to cerebral edema and neurologic deterioration. To minimize this risk, the current recommendation is that plasma sodium concentration be slowly lowered at a rate not exceeding 0.5 to 1 mEq per liter per hour, the total correction occurring over 48 hours or more. In addition to the estimated water deficit, the total volume of replacement should include concomitant daily losses.

Replacement Fluids

Enteral water administration (orally or via feeding tube) is always preferable, if this is feasible. Otherwise, a 5% dextrose solution is given as the intravenous replacement fluid of choice. An infusion of quarter-normal saline (0.225% saline) in 5% dextrose is preferable if salt depletion due to other causes is also a factor. Isotonic (0.9%) or half-normal (0.45%) saline should be used initially if the patient is hypotensive, even in the presence of hypernatremia, until volume is restored. Care should be taken to replace ongoing fluid losses as well.

Control of Polyuria

Control of polyuria is achieved through pharmacologic therapy directed at the underlying pathophysiologic derangement.

Therapy for Central Diabetes Insipidus
(Table 3)

Hormone replacement is the mainstay of therapy in CDI. Desmopressin (DDAVP), a synthetic analogue of arginine vasopressin, has essentially supplanted the use of earlier preparations such as L-arginine vasopressin (Pitressin) used as a parenteral injection, vasopressin tannate in oil used intramus-

TABLE 3. **Therapeutic Regimens for Diabetes Insipidus**

Disorder	Drug	Dose	Duration (h)
CDI			
Complete	Desmopressin (DDAVP)	5–20 μg intranasally qd or bid	8–12
		0.1–0.4 mg PO qd to tid	8–12
		1–2 μg IV or SC qd or bid	8–12
Partial	DDAVP	Same as above	Same as above
	Chlorpropamide (Diabinese)*	100–250 mg PO qd or bid	24–48
	Carbamazepine (Tegretol)*	100–600 mg PO bid	12–24
	Clofibrate (Atromid)*	500 mg PO tid to qid	12–24
NDI	Hydrochlorothiazide (HydroDIURIL)*	25 mg PO qd or bid	6–12
	Amiloride (Midamor)*	5–10 mg PO qd or bid	24
	Indomethacin (Indocin)*	25–50 mg PO bid or tid	6–8

Doses employed have varied widely outside the usual values shown. Dose and frequency must be titrated to desired response for each individual.
*Not FDA approved for this use.

cularly (IM), and lypressin (Diapid) used as a nasal spray. DDAVP has become the agent of choice because it has potent antidiuretic activity without the vasopressor effect of the other agents, has a substantially longer half-life, and is available in a convenient intranasal form in addition to the injectable form. A more convenient oral tablet form of DDAVP has become available in the United States and, like the nasal form, can be used in a once- or twice-a-day regimen. A safe approach is to start with just an evening dose (oral or nasal spray) to control the troubling nocturia and then introduce and titrate a daytime dose. This will minimize the risk of hyponatremia from therapy.

The short-acting aqueous form of vasopressin may be used in acute postoperative situations and in the dehydration test.

Other adjuvant agents may be of value in patients with an incomplete response to DDAVP, a drug that is also very expensive. These agents act by either increasing ADH release or enhancing the effect of ADH on the collecting duct. Since both actions require some endogenous ADH, these drugs are effective in partial CDI. Drugs such as chlorpropamide (Diabinese), an oral hypoglycemic agent, and carbamazepine (Tegretol), an anticonvulsant, may limit polyuria by potentiating the renal effect of ADH, while clofibrate (Atromid-S), a lipid-lowering drug, can lower urine output through an increase in ADH release. The use of these drugs is limited by their other pharmacologic as well as side effects.

Therapy for Nephrogenic Diabetes Insipidus
(see Table 3)

Therapy consists of correcting the underlying disorder where possible (e.g., hypercalcemia) or discontinuing the offending drug. Specific treatment options include use of diuretic agents, nonsteroidal anti-inflammatory drugs (NSAIDs), and a low-salt, low-protein diet, tried alone or in combination.

Thiazide diuretics such as hydrochlorothiazide (HydroDIURIL) act by inducing mild volume depletion, thereby enhancing proximal fluid reabsorption and diminishing water delivery to the distal nephron and thus reducing urine output. The diuretic amiloride (Midamor) is especially beneficial in reversing lithium-induced DI by blocking lithium uptake in the distal nephron, thus allowing continued lithium use in some patients.

NSAIDs, by inhibiting prostaglandin synthesis, block the antagonizing action of prostaglandins on ADH; that is, they potentiate ADH action on the collecting duct and increase the concentrating ability. Their actions may be additive to those of thiazide diuretics.

Last, a low-salt, low-protein diet may decrease urine output in NDI by decreasing net solute excretion, an effect independent of ADH action.

HYPERPARATHYROIDISM AND HYPOPARATHYROIDISM

method of
D. A. HEATH, M.B., CH.B.
Selly Oak Hospital
Birmingham, England

HYPERPARATHYROIDISM

Primary hyperparathyroidism is the autonomous oversecretion of parathyroid hormone (PTH) by the parathyroid glands. In 90% of cases, this is due to a single benign parathyroid tumor. In the majority of the remaining 10%, hyperplasia of all four parathyroid glands is seen. Occasionally, two adenomas are present, and parathyroid carcinoma is very rare. Secondary hyperparathyroidism is due to the expected stimulation of the parathyroid glands by hypocalcemia, typically occurring with renal failure or vitamin D deficiency. If persistent, this condition leads to parathyroid hyperplasia, and occasionally an autonomous tumor develops, leading to hypercalcemia—so-called tertiary hyperparathyroidism.

The actions of PTH are to increase calcium reabsorption in the renal tubule, to increase calcium reabsorption from the bone, and, by stimulating

1,25-dihydroxyvitamin D production by the kidney, to increase calcium absorption from the gut. All three actions will increase serum calcium.

The main factor regulating PTH secretion is the serum ionized calcium concentration. A calcium-sensing receptor is present in the parathyroid cell surface (and renal tubule) that detects the prevailing ionized calcium concentration and through this regulates PTH secretion. Genetic abnormalities of this sensor are the cause of familial benign or hypocalciuric hypercalcemia and familial hypocalcemia. In addition, drugs are now being developed that act on the sensor and alter PTH secretion, thus offering the potential for medical treatment of hyperparathyroidism.

Clinical Presentation of Primary Hyperparathyroidism

With the advent of biochemical screening, hyperparathyroidism has been found to be a much more common disorder than previously suspected, especially in older women. The female to male ratio of current series is around 3:1, most patients being over the age of 65 years. With the wider recognition of the disorder, up to half the patients now diagnosed appear to be completely asymptomatic; when symptoms do occur, the most common are increasing tiredness and lethargy. Other nonspecific symptoms include thirst, constipation, headaches, and muscular aches. Renal stones have occurred in less than 10% of the patients who have been identified by biochemical screening, and clinical bone disease is now extremely rare.

Diagnosis of Hyperparathyroidism

The advent of the newer immunoradiometric and immunochemiluminescence assays has greatly eased the diagnosis of primary hyperparathyroidism. These assays can detect PTH concentrations in all normal persons and some values that are below normal in cases in which PTH secretion is reduced. In primary hyperparathyroidism, PTH concentrations determined with these sensitive assays are usually above the upper limits of normal or at the very top of the normal range. Values in the middle or lower area of the normal range should not be interpreted as being inappropriately high in the presence of hypercalcemia. The combination of a high or high-normal PTH with hypercalcemia is sufficient to confirm the diagnosis of hyperparathyroidism unless familial benign hypercalcemia is considered a possibility (discussed later on). Indirect measurement of parathyroid function, by means of, e.g., serum phosphate or urinary phosphate and calcium determinations, is no longer indicated as routine.

Management of Hyperparathyroidism

Before the recognition of many asymptomatic patients it was considered that virtually all patients should be referred for parathyroid surgery. Many centers have now modified their practice and are prepared to consider conservative treatment in the asymptomatic older patient.

Surgical Treatment

Surgery is the treatment of choice for all symptomatic patients or those with complications of the disease. It should be performed only by a surgeon experienced in parathyroid surgery. Most experienced surgeons do not attempt to localize the lesion preoperatively, instead reserving such techniques for failed previous surgery. It is rarely necessary to give treatment, other than adequate hydration, to lower the calcium prior to surgery. At surgery, attempts should be made to visualize all four parathyroid glands. Any enlarged glands should be removed and their nature confirmed by frozen section. Normal-sized glands are best not biopsied because this increases the risk of permanent postoperative hypoparathyroidism. Following effective surgery, the serum calcium concentration should be normal within 24 hours except when the preoperative calcium level is very high. Mild hypocalcemia that usually does not require treatment may occur on the second or third postoperative day and usually corrects itself. Patients with more severe hypercalcemia preoperatively, especially in the presence of overt hyperparathyroidism-related bone disease, may develop more severe hypocalcemia that can last for a number of days or weeks. Such patients require intravenous calcium, often with vitamin D, until normocalcemia ensues.

Nonsurgical Management

Increasing numbers of older, asymptomatic patients are being managed conservatively. As a minimum, regular checks of well-being coupled with measurements of serum calcium and creatinine should be performed at monthly intervals of 6 or 12 months. The addition of regular abdominal radiographs and serial bone density measurements has not been proved to be necessary. Pharmaceutical interventions to lower the serum calcium level are usually not necessary and, while they may reduce the hypercalcemia, do not correct the hyperparathyroid state.

Differential Diagnosis for Hypercalcemia

Although there are many causes of hypercalcemia, most can be readily identified by clinical presentation or on initial investigation (Table 1). With hypercalcemia of malignancy, the malignant process is usually clinically apparent prior to the recognition of the hypercalcemia. PTH concentrations are suppressed. In most other hypercalcemic states, the serum PTH is suppressed. The condition most likely to be mistaken for primary hyperparathyroidism is familial benign hypercalcemia (FBH), in which PTH concentrations usually are normal but occasionally can be elevated. Once index cases are excluded, it appears that FBH in adults is truly a benign condition for which parathyroidectomy is ineffective and contrain-

TABLE 1. **Causes of Hypercalcemia**

Common
Hyperparathyroidism
Disseminated malignancy
Uncommon
Familial benign hypercalcemia
Thyrotoxicosis
Vitamin D therapy
Milk alkali syndrome—usually due to effervescent over-the-counter antacids
Sarcoidosis
Lithium } Both probably make underlying
Thiazides } hyperparathyroidism more apparent
Occult malignancy
Immobilization
Recovery phase of acute renal failure
Addison's disease

dicated. This condition must be ruled out wherever possible before any asymptomatic patients are referred for surgery, especially if the serum PTH is normal. At present the most conclusive investigation is to demonstrate a parent who is hypercalcemic. If parents are unavailable, the presence of hypercalcemia in a sibling or a child is again very suggestive of the condition, provided there are no other features of multiple endocrine neoplasia.

HYPOPARATHYROIDISM

By far the most common cause of hypoparathyroidism is postoperative, following surgery to the neck. Permanent hypoparathyroidism following a subtotal thyroidectomy or a parathyroidectomy is uncommon and occurs in less than 1% of operations. In these situations it is hard to imagine that all normal parathyroid glands were inadvertently removed, and the disorder is more likely to be due predominantly to infarction of the glands associated with the neck dissection. The operation associated with the highest incidence of postoperative hypoparathyroidism is pharyngolaryngectomy: the complication develops in 30 to 50% of cases. Symptomatic postoperative hypoparathyroidism usually develops acutely 2 to 4 days after neck surgery but occasionally develops insidiously many years after surgery. Very occasionally, hypoparathyroidism may occur after administration of radioactive iodine or local radiotherapy to the neck.

Idiopathic hypoparathyroidism is a rare condition sometimes associated with cutaneous moniliasis (candidiasis). Because of its rarity, care should be taken to exclude other conditions that can mimic the biochemical changes of hypoparathyroidism; these include vitamin D deficiency, hypomagnesemia, and familial hypocalcemia.

Transient hypoparathyroidism may occur in the neonatal period when the mother has been hyperparathyroid during pregnancy. This is, in fact, unusual and self-limiting. Rarely, congenital hypoparathyroidism occurs in association with a genetic disorder with various forms of inheritance: failure of the development of the third and fourth pharyngeal pouches leads to underdevelopment of the thymus, parathyroids, and heart abnormalities—the so-called DiGeorge syndrome.

Symptoms and Signs of Hypocalcemia

Initial manifestations of acute hypocalcemia include circumoral and pedal paresthesias progressing to painful cramps and contractions of the hands and feet, i.e., carpopedal spasm or tetany. In association with these symptoms, the patient is likely to demonstrate Chvostek's sign—contracture of the lower facial muscles following tapping of the facial nerve. Elicitation of Trousseau's sign, which is the precipitation of tetany by a sphygmomanometer cuff inflated to above systolic blood pressure, is a very painful procedure and should be abandoned. If the hypocalcemia worsens, seizures can occur. Symptoms of acutely developing hypocalcemia usually occur when the serum calcium concentration falls below 7.5 mg per 100 mL.

When hypocalcemia develops gradually, it is better tolerated and may not cause symptoms until serum calcium levels fall below 6 mg per 100 mL. In addition to the foregoing symptoms, tiredness and confusion may develop. Long-standing hypocalcemia may lead to the development of cataracts, papilledema, and intracerebral calcification.

Diagnosis of Hypoparathyroidism

The typical biochemical findings seen with hypoparathyroidism are hypocalcemia, hyperphosphatemia, a normal serum alkaline phosphatase, normal renal function and a low PTH. Occasionally, similar changes can occur in simple vitamin D deficiency, when the expected secondary hyperparathyroidism does not develop. Severe hypomagnesemia also produces the identical biochemical changes of hypoparathyroidism and must always be ruled out. Extensive small bowel dysfunction, chronic alcoholism, and a renal magnesium leak due to a primary defect or induced by drug therapy (e.g., aminoglycoside drugs, cisplatin) are the most likely causes. Failure to correct the hypomagnesemia makes the patient totally resistant to vitamin D therapy.

A familial form of hypocalcemia, due to a defect of the calcium-sensing receptor, has been identified. This was looked for initially as the mirror image of familial benign hypercalcemia, in which a low serum calcium is associated with hypercalciuria and a normal serum PTH. The postulate was that a genetic defect caused a resetting of the sensor whereby normal PTH concentrations were maintained by hypocalcemia. A number of cases were identified that initially had been diagnosed as familial hypoparathyroidism. Virtually all patients had been treated with large doses of vitamin D, and many had developed renal impairment and nephrocalcinosis, probably as a result of the treatment. Many persons may well have been asymptomatic. The likely explanation of the renal complications was that the intrinsic degree of hypercalciuria was made much worse by the vitamin D therapy.

Two cases have been described of what at first sight appeared to be idiopathic hypoparathyroidism with low PTH concentrations in which a defect of the calcium-sensing receptor was present. Such cases are analogous to those cases of familial benign hypercalcemia with elevated PTH concentrations. Because multiple defects of the calcium-sensing receptor have been reported, it is not possible at present to sequence the gene in all new index cases. An inappropriate degree of hypercalciuria should alert the practitioner to the possibility and lead to family screening.

Pseudohypoparathyroidism

An inherited resistance to PTH action produces a hypoparathyroid state but with elevated PTH concentrations. This is the condition of pseudohypoparathyroidism, sometimes associated with a series of phenotypic abnormalities including short stature, moon facies, mental retardation, and a short fourth metacarpal or metatarsal. Affected persons may have other hormone-resistant states leading to hypothyroidism and hypogonadism. Biochemical studies show a post-receptor defect of the Gsα component of the adenylate cyclase complex, leading to a generalized hormone-resistant state. Other patients with pseudohypoparathyroidism are phenotypically normal and appear to have an abnormality of only the PTH receptor mechanism.

The phenotypic features of pseudohypoparathyroidism may be seen with completely normal biochemistry and occasionally within different generations of families known to have pseudohypoparathyroidism. This is known as pseudopseudohypoparathyroidism; also, in such cases biochemical studies have demonstrated defects of the Gsα subunit.

Treatment of Hypoparathyroidism

Acute symptomatic hypocalcemia requires intravenous calcium therapy to control symptoms until oral vitamin D starts to be effective, which can take several weeks. An infusion of 100 mL of 10% calcium gluconate diluted with saline, given slowly over 24 hours, is effective, but great care must be taken to make sure that it does not extravasate outside the vein.

Treatment of significant hypoparathyroidism cannot be achieved with oral calcium supplements alone. Previously, treatment was with large doses of calciferol, on the order of 100,000 units or 2.5 mg per day. However, most patients are treated with one of the active vitamin D metabolites — 1α-hydroxycholecalciferol or 1,25-dihydroxycholecalciferol (calcitriol). Doses of 1 to 2 μg per day are usually required in adults. I do not prescribe concomitant calcium supplementation, because this increases the number of tablets taken per day and is associated with a significant risk of gastrointestinal side effects. With such therapies, hypercalcemia is always a risk, even in patients in whom the hypoparathyroidism has been under good control for a long time. Hence, lifelong monitoring is necessary. This risk can be reduced by deliberately maintaining the serum calcium around the lower limit of normal. In so-called idiopathic cases, it is now essential to consider a calcium-sensory defect; with this in mind it is necessary to monitor urinary calcium excretion and to perform regular renal ultrasound to look for evidence of nephrocalcinosis. Whether such cases can be managed by thiazide diuretics and much lower doses of vitamin D is not yet clear.

LOW-RENIN ALDOSTERONISM

method of
YORAM SHENKER, M.D.
University of Wisconsin–Madison Medical School and William S. Middleton Memorial Veterans Hospital
Madison, Wisconsin

Low-renin aldosteronism (LRA) is a syndrome characterized by a rate of aldosterone secretion that is high or inappropriately normal for volume expansion, causing hypervolemia, hypertension, and suppression of renin secretion. Most estimates of the prevalence of LRA range between 0.5 and 2% of all hypertensive patients. The importance of precise diagnosis of this syndrome and its subsets is that many cases of hypertension with LRA can be cured by surgery. In other cases, proper diagnosis can lead to effective medical treatment.

PHYSIOLOGY AND PATHOPHYSIOLOGY OF ALDOSTERONE SECRETION

Aldosterone secretion is regulated by at least three well established secretagogues: angiotensin II (A-II), adrenocorticotropic hormone (ACTH), and potassium. In LRA, aldosterone secretion is partially autonomous and leads to suppression of the renin–A-II system. Increased mineralocorticoid activity at the level of the renal tubule and collecting duct leads to increased reabsorption of sodium and water in exchange for potassium and hydrogen. This results in volume expansion, hypertension, hypokalemia, and metabolic alkalosis. The pathophysiologic causes of different subsets of LRA include malignant transformation of adrenal glomerulosa cells in aldosterone-producing carcinoma (APC), transformation of normal glomerulosa into adenoma in aldosterone-producing adenoma (APA), an abnormality of the chimeric gene that leads to production of aldosterone from the zona fasciculata under ACTH regulation known as glucocorticoid-suppressible aldosteronism (GSA), and, finally, an unknown pathophysiology that is presumably related to an as-yet unidentified aldosterone stimulator—idiopathic hyperplasia with aldosteronism (IHA).

CLINICAL PRESENTATION OF LOW-RENIN ALDOSTERONISM

Most patients with LRA have no symptoms at all. Hypokalemia can lead to functional nephrogenic diabetes insipidus with symptoms of nocturia, polyuria, and polydipsia. More severe hypokalemia (particularly in APC and APA) may have neuromuscular manifestations including weakness, cramping, paresthesia, and intermittent paralysis. In rare cases frank tetany occurs, attributable to a decrease in ionized calcium caused by alkalosis.

Signs of LRA are nonspecific. In many cases, hypertension is mild, but severe hypertension is not uncommon. Prolonged hypertension may lead to the usual funduscopic, renal, or cardiovascular sequelae. Trousseau's or Chvostek's sign may be occasionally present. Edema is extremely uncommon despite sodium and water retention because of the renal mineralocorticoid escape mechanism.

Routine blood tests show mild to severe hypokalemia. However, between 7 and 38% of patients with LRA may be normokalemic. A serum sodium level of 140 mEq per liter or higher and elevated serum bicarbonate levels are other features of LRA.

BIOCHEMICAL DIAGNOSIS OF LOW-RENIN ALDOSTERONISM

In most cases, the work-up to diagnose LRA is prompted by the presence of hypokalemia and hypertension. The most common cause of hypokalemia in hypertensive patients is treatment with diuretics. Thus, in patients who have discontinued the use of diuretics, spontaneous hypokalemia should be documented. Some patients are able to maintain normal potassium by adopting a low-sodium diet. In such patients, hypokalemia could be "unmasked" after several days on a high-sodium diet.

The screening tests for LRA are based on measurements of plasma renin activity (PRA) and 24-hour urinary aldosterone. Renin secretion is under beta-adrenergic stimulation, and treatment with beta blockers may result in false decreases in PRA. The presence of low PRA with high or sometimes inappropriately normal urinary aldosterone levels strongly suggests LRA. The definitive diagnosis is made by documenting high and nonsuppressible plasma aldosterone (PA). To suppress PA, a high-salt diet, mineralocorticoids, or captopril (Capoten) can be administered, or saline can be infused. To assess PA, the serum potassium level should be brought to at least 3 mEq per liter, because a low serum potassium concentration may lead to falsely low PA levels.

Another part of the diagnostic work-up should demonstrate low or unstimulatable PRA. This can be done by assessing the patient in an upright posture, with a low-salt diet or intravenous administration of furosemide (Lasix). Several researchers have found that an increased ratio of PA to PRA in random blood samples drawn after elimination of interfering medication is a reliable diagnostic indicator of LRA.

SUBSETS OF LOW-RENIN ALDOSTERONISM AND OTHER MINERALOCORTICOID EXCESS SYNDROMES

Close to two thirds of patients with LRA have APA. Production of aldosterone in APA is only partly autonomous; aldosterone no longer responds to A-II but does respond to ACTH. APA appears more often in the left adrenal gland. The average diameter of an adenoma is 1.8 cm; close to 20% of all adenomas are smaller than 1 cm.

The second most common cause of LRA is IHA. Patients with IHA have bilateral hyperplasia of the zona glomerulosa, which is frequently nodular. Bilateral adrenalectomy does not normalize blood pressure in this condition, and surgical treatment has been abandoned.

GSA, as mentioned previously, is due to a disease whereby a chimeric gene combines 11β-hydroxylase and aldosterone synthase activity, resulting in aldosterone secretion from the zona fasciculata under ACTH regulation. Many GSA patients are now identified by molecular biology techniques. Most of them seem to be normokalemic.

APC accounts for only about 1% of LRA cases. These tumors frequently secrete other steroids in addition to aldosterone. The biochemical abnormalities in APC are usually very severe, with potassium levels frequently below 2 mEq/L per liter and extremely high aldosterone levels.

Patients with hypokalemia, low PRA, and low aldosterone levels may have excess mineralocorticoid activity due to exogenous or endogenous steroids. For instance, some malignant tumors produce 11-deoxycorticosterone (DOC). Congenital adrenal hyperplasia with either 11β-hydroxylase or 17α-hydroxylase deficiency is also associated with increased DOC. Exposure to licorice may lead to an excess of mineralocorticoids because of inhibition of the enzymatic activity of the 11β-hydroxysteroid dehydrogenase, which protects the mineralocorticoid receptor from cortisol (cortisol has the same affinity for this receptor as that of aldosterone) by converting it to cortisone. A similar mechanism, by "overwhelming" this enzyme with high exposure to cortisol, may account for many cases of mineralocorticoid excess in Cushing's syndrome. Liddle's syndrome is another condition that closely mimics LRA, but aldosterone production is negligible. This syndrome is known to be the result of a mutation on the beta subunit of the epithelial sodium channel. Sodium transport inhibitors are effective in the treatment of this syndrome.

DIFFERENTIATION OF LOW-RENIN ALDOSTERONISM SUBSETS

The major thrust of differentiation of LRA subsets is to differentiate between APA, which should be treated surgically, and IHA, which should be treated medically.

Measurement of plasma aldosterone levels with the patient in the supine position through an indwelling catheter at 8:00 AM and then after four hours with the patient in an upright position, can differentiate between APA and IHA with 80 to 90% accuracy. Patients with IHA usually respond with at least a 33% increase in plasma aldosterone; patients with APA usually show no change or have decreased aldosterone levels.

Another biochemical test to differentiate between APA and IHA is to measure the plasma level of an immediate aldosterone precursor, 18-hydroxycorticosterone. Measurement performed at 8:00 AM using the supine position shows levels higher than 100 ng per dL in patients with APA; patients with IHA have levels lower than 100 ng per dL. The accuracy of this test is about 80%.

Computed tomography (CT) scanning shows most of the adenomas unless they are smaller than 7 mm in diameter. CT scanning in IHA usually shows normal glands or bilateral hyperplasia, but in some cases, large hyperplastic nodules may be misidentified as adenomas. The accuracy of a CT scan ranges between 70 and 90%. If the CT scan shows a lesion with a diameter greater than 3 cm, APC should be suspected.

Iodocholesterol or NP-59 scans in patients with LRA are done after 7 days of dexamethasone treatment. In APA, unilateral uptake is usually seen on day 3; in IHA, bilateral uptake is seen as early as day 3 or later, up to day 5. The diagnostic accuracy of this test is also around 70 to 90%.

Finally, the standard technique for localization is selective adrenal venous sampling. In this procedure, catheters are inserted into both adrenal veins, and blood samples are taken for aldosterone and cortisol. The ratio of aldosterone to cortisol on the side of the adenoma will be at least four times higher than on the other side. The accuracy of this test exceeds 95%.

Patients who have documented LRA, localization results suggestive of hyperplasia, and a family history of hypertension should be considered to have GSA and deserve a therapeutic trial of dexamethasone (Decadron), 0.5 to 2 mg daily. Such patients should achieve normalization of blood pressure and serum potassium within 2 to 3 weeks. The diagnosis of GSA can also be established using a molecular biology technique to demonstrate the presence of an abnormal chimeric gene for 11β-hydroxylase and aldosterone synthase.

TREATMENT OF LOW-RENIN ALDOSTERONISM

The cornerstone of treatment for APA is surgical removal of the adenoma. This results in cure in 60 to 70% of patients and significant improvement in blood pressure in another 30%. A unilateral posterior surgical approach assures a mortality rate of close to zero. Before surgery, patients should take spironolactone (Aldactone), a mineralocorticoid receptor antagonist, 200 to 600 mg daily, for at least 2 to 3 weeks to restore potassium reserves, normalize blood pressure, and bring the glomerulosa of the contralateral adrenal gland to normal function to prevent postoperative hypoaldosteronism.

Patients with IHA or APA who refuse or have contraindications to surgery should be treated with spironolactone. However, the antiandrogenic effects of this drug may result in intolerable side effects, including gynecomastia, decreased libido and impotence in males, and menstrual irregularities and breast soreness in women. If spironolactone is not tolerated, sodium transport inhibitors such as triamterene (Dyrenium) or amiloride (Midamor) can be used. Frequently, treatment with these agents alone will not control blood pressure, and addition of calcium channel blockers or potassium-sparing diuretic combinations may be required.

Some IHA patients show enhanced sensitivity to A-II and respond to angiotensin-converting enzyme (ACE) inhibitors.

Hypertension and hypokalemia in patients who ingest licorice disappear when this habit is discontinued. Patients with mineralocorticoid excess, suppressed PRA, and low levels of aldosterone should be evaluated for possible congenital adrenal hyperplasia by measuring DOC levels. If DOC levels are elevated, these patients should respond to treatment with dexamethasone. For long-term treatment with this agent, potassium-sparing diuretic therapy is indicated because the doses of dexamethasone required may lead to cushingoid complications. The same is true for GSA patients.

Patients with Liddle's syndrome have a primary renal defect in epithelial sodium channels, and they usually respond well to sodium transport inhibitors. Triamterene (Dyrenium), 25 to 100 mg daily, is effective in a majority of such patients.

HYPOPITUITARISM

method of
THOMAS P. JACOBS, M.D.
Columbia University College of Physicians and Surgeons
New York, New York

Hypopituitarism, the failure of the pituitary gland to secrete one or more of its trophic hormones in normal fashion, is most often caused by lesions in the pituitary or hypothalamus. The pituitary hormones are primarily secreted in response to humoral and neural signals from the hypothalamus. Destructive lesions of the hypothalamus, therefore, lead to reduced secretion of some or all of the hormones of the anterior pituitary. Prolactin is an exception, and its secretion is often increased in the setting of hypothalamic disease because of failure of tonic inhibition of prolactin secretion by the hypothalamus. Neurogenic diabetes insipidus (DI) results from failure of secretion of antidiuretic hormone (ADH) by the neurons of the posterior pituitary, whose cell bodies are located in the hypothalamus. Anterior pituitary dysfunction is more commonly caused by lesions of the pituitary itself: Pituitary adenomas are most common, but other causes include craniopharyngioma; metastatic tumor; other neural tumors such as meningioma, chordoma, and teratoma; autoimmune hypophysitis; pituitary hemorrhage (apoplexy); Sheehan's syndrome (postpartum pituitary ischemia); sarcoidosis; tuberculosis; histiocytosis; trauma; and as a late response to therapeutic ionizing radiation.

Pituitary trophic hormones are typically lost in a specific order in response to slowly destructive lesions such as a pituitary tumor: growth hormone (GH), follicle-stimulating hormone (FSH), and luteinizing hormone (LH) are lost first, followed by thyroid-stimulating hormone (TSH), and finally by adrenocorticotropic hormone (ACTH). ADH loss with resulting DI occurs rarely with pituitary lesions, and its presence usually implies hypothalamic damage.

DIAGNOSIS

Hypopituitarism must be suspected in order to be diagnosed. Common clinical settings that should prompt a search for reduced secretion of one or more pituitary hormones include unexplained growth failure in childhood, pubertal failure, amenorrhea or galactorrhea not explained by pregnancy, male sexual dysfunction, hypothyroidism accompanied by normal or reduced serum TSH levels, persistent or unexplained hyponatremia, weight loss, or hypercalcemia. Any visual symptoms accompanied by a chiasmal visual field deficit and any finding of an incidental pituitary or hypothalamic lesion on a computed tomography or magnetic resonance imaging scan of the head should prompt a search for hypopituitarism as well.

Testing to confirm suspected hypopituitarism is specific

to each trophic hormone: GH deficiency is usually of interest in children and is assessed by measuring GH response to two or more secretogogues (e.g., GH-releasing hormone, L-levodopa, glucagon, arginine, or insulin-induced hypoglycemia), serum IGF-I, and IGF binding protein-3. Amenorrhea is established as of pituitary origin when biologic indices of low estrogen effect (e.g., failure to menstruate after exposure to progestin, atrophic vaginal or uterine mucosa, absent ferning or spinnbarkeit of cervical mucus, absent breast development in puberty) are accompanied by low estradiol levels and LH-FSH levels in the low or inappropriately normal range. Whereas postmenopausal women will usually have elevated levels of LH and FSH, low or normal gonadotropin levels in patients of this age who are not severely ill with a nonendocrine disorder suggest a diagnosis of gonadotropin failure. Male hypogonadism is established by the presence of a low serum testosterone (or free testosterone if sex hormone–binding globulin protein levels are low) in the presence of low or normal levels of LH and FSH. Failure of ACTH secretion is often difficult to establish. Serum cortisol levels in blood drawn at 8 to 9 AM that are persistently below 10 μg per dL are suggestive, and in the appropriate setting sufficient evidence to initiate treatment. A Cortrosyn Stimulation Test (morning serum cortisol before and 1 hour after intramuscular [IM] or intravenous (IV) injection of 0.25 mg of synthetic 1-24 ACTH [cosyntropin (Cortrosyn)] will usually show a significant rise in cortisol despite low baseline levels (an increase over baseline of 7 μg per dL or more to a peak value of greater than 18 μg per dL), although if ACTH deficiency is long-standing, a subnormal or even "flat" response can be observed. Urine cortisol excretion is sometimes below normal but is often in the lower end of the normal range. Deficiency of ADH is established either with a classic dehydration test or by the timely observation of an inappropriately dilute urine in a patient whose serum osmolality is elevated, with maximal or near-maximal urine osmolality in response to administered ADH (5 units aqueous vasopressin [Pitressin]) given subcutaneously.

TREATMENT

An understanding of the natural history or post-treatment history of the various hormonal deficits in patients with hypopituitarism is a necessary adjunct to successful management of these patients. Most patients with hypopituitarism can expect little return of normal trophic hormone function, although in the setting of autoimmune hypopituitarism, pituitary hemorrhage, infundibulitis, and sarcoidosis, and after successful treatment of pituitary tumors with surgery or dopaminergic agents, some functional improvement in pituitary hormone secretion can occur. The specifics of treatment of the underlying cause of pituitary or hypothalamic dysfunction and the management of associated neurologic lesions are beyond the scope of this review. The patient must be educated about the lifelong need for hormonal replacement therapy, and should be encouraged to wear a MedicAlert identification tag, especially if hypoadrenalism or DI is present. The patient must be seen by the physician at regular intervals thereafter, both for detection of new deficits and adjustment of medications.

Hypoadrenalism resulting from ACTH deficiency can be treated with a glucocorticoid medication alone in most patients, as the intact renin-angiotensin axis makes mineralocorticoid or sodium supplements unnecessary. Prednisone can be given once daily and is the least expensive of the commonly used agents. Prednisone at doses of 3 to 7 mg daily, dexamethasone at doses of 0.5 to 1.0 mg daily, or cortisone acetate or hydrocortisone at divided daily doses of 10 to 30 mg daily is usually sufficient. Initial dosing should be at the upper end of the dose range, with an eventual attempt to reduce the dose downward to the lowest dose at which the patient maintains normal energy, weight, and sense of well-being. All patients must be reminded to at least triple their usual dose of glucocorticoid for a few days during physiologic stresses, such as fever, intercurrent viral illness, or minor trauma, and that "stress" doses of glucocorticoids (hydrocortisone 300 mg daily or its equivalent) must be administered during and after major surgery, infection, or trauma.

Therapy of secondary hypothyroidism is also subtly problematic in that the serum TSH is not useful as a guide to replacement therapy. Levothyroxine (Synthroid) in doses of 50 to 150 μg daily is usually sufficient, the exact dose determined by the presence or absence of symptoms or signs of hypothyroidism. The serum thyroxine (T_4) and triiodothyronine (T_3) resin uptake or its equivalent can be used to calculate a free thyroxine index as a guide to the appropriate thyroxine dosage. Patients discovered to have both adrenal and thyroid failure contemporaneously should be treated initially with glucocorticoids, as thyroid treatment alone may worsen symptoms of hypoadrenalism.

Replacement of gonadotropins or gonadal steroids is appropriate for most patients, but must be decided based on individual patient desire for fertility, libido, sexual potency, symptoms of estrogen-androgen lack, and risk of neoplasia in sex hormone–responsive organs (e.g., breast, uterus, prostate). Most males will require replacement of testosterone, which can be accomplished with either a number of preparations of testosterone for IM injection (e.g., testosterone cypionate), 200 to 300 mg given every 2 to 3 weeks, or transdermal testosterone (Testoderm, Androderm), 2.5- or 5-mg patches applied once daily for 24 hours. Males requiring fertility should receive human chorionic gonadotropin (hCG), the biologic activity of which is similar to LH, 1000 to 5000 IU given IM two to three times weekly. Those patients also may require either human menopausal gonadotropin, which contains both LH and FSH bioactivity, or a more purely FSH-like preparation (urofollitropin* [Metrodin] or recombinant FSH) given IM, 75 IU three times weekly. Once spermatogenesis has been established, it can usually be maintained by use of hCG alone. Males with isolated deficiency of gonadotropin-releasing hormone (GnRH) have been treated successfully with pulsatile parenteral administration of synthetic GnRH, but this remains a specialized

*Not FDA approved for this indication.

intervention best used in centers with broad experience in its application. Mature male patients should have a yearly digital prostate examination and, if appropriate, a determination of serum prostate-specific antigen. Those whose sexual dysfunction does not respond to androgen replacement should be referred to a urologist for consideration of oral sildenafil (Viagra), vacuum devices, intraurethral prostaglandin, intrapenile injections of vasodilators, or implantable prosthetic devices to achieve satisfactory erectile function.

Most premenopausal women and many women beyond the usual age of menopause should be treated with an estrogen (and a progestin if the uterus is intact) both to relieve symptoms of estrogen deficiency (e.g., hot flashes, vaginal dryness, insomnia) and to maintain long-term skeletal integrity and reduce coronary risk. Ovulation and pregnancy can often be achieved in younger women through the use of preparations containing LH and/or FSH (see previously), although discussion of the details of pregnancy induction should be sought in literature devoted to that topic. Androgen replacement in hypogonadal women is a topic of active investigation, although it is not routinely offered to women with hypopituitarism.

Administration of recombinant human growth hormone (somatropin [Humatrope]) to children with hypopituitarism and growth failure usually leads to significant acceleration of linear growth rates. Despite significant "catch-up" growth over the initial years of treatment, children usually will reach and maintain growth along a growth curve leading to an adult height that is less than predicted from parental heights. In short-term clinical studies, administration of GH to adults with documented GH deficiency led to predictable increases of lean body mass and extracellular fluid volume, to minor improvements in muscle strength, and to reduction in adipose tissue mass. Recombinant GH has recently been approved for use in GH-deficient adults, but because of the uncertainties concerning long-term effect of GH replacement on neoplasia, blood pressure, glucose tolerance, and longevity, and because of the major expense of growth hormone therapy, most endocrinologists outside the research setting do not currently initiate GH replacement in their adult patients with hypopituitarism.

Patients with DI whose thirst mechanisms are intact and who have access to water will drink sufficient fluid to replace excessive urine losses, although at the cost of interrupted sleep, inconvenience, and eventual gross enlargement of bladder capacity. In the perioperative period or in the setting of severe acute illness, uncontrolled DI can lead to serious hyperosmolality when consciousness is impaired or access to fluids is limited. These patients should be followed extremely carefully with body weights, electrolytes, urine volumes, and specific gravity determinations at the bedside. If urine volume becomes greater than 200 mL per hour and urine specific gravity is less than or equal to 1.005, aqueous vasopressin, 5 units, is administered IM or IV up to several times daily, and excessive urine water losses are replaced with 5% dextrose in water given IV. If a longer term antidiuretic effect is desired in these patients, a parenteral form of DDAVP (desmopressin) can be given at a dose of 1 to 2 μg subcutaneously once or twice daily. For ambulatory patients, DI is best controlled with intranasal DDAVP administered either by rhinotube or nasal spray, at a dose of 10 to 20 μg at bedtime with a daytime dose of 5 to 10 μg given either at a specific time or when thirst and polyuria appear. Some patients with mild partial DI are treated with a single daily dose of thiazide diuretic (e.g., hydrochlorothiazide, 50 mg). This drug likely lowers urine volume by inducing mild hypovolemia with reduced delivery of glomerular filtrate to the distal nephron. The appearance of severe hyponatremia in patients with DI usually signifies either that the patient is taking excessive doses of DDAVP or that untreated hypoadrenalism is present and should be treated with both fluid restriction and glucocorticoid administration if appropriate. Absent thirst mechanisms in some patients with more severe hypothalamic damage greatly complicates the therapy of DI, which must then be managed by prescription of constant daily fluid volume and DDAVP, frequent weighing, and determination of serum sodium levels, with adjustment in fluids or DDAVP as indicated.

HYPERPROLACTINEMIA

method of
MELISSA K. CAVAGHAN, M.D., and
DAVID A. EHRMANN, M.D.
University of Chicago Pritzker School of Medicine
Chicago, Illinois

Elevations in serum prolactin are among the most common abnormalities in endocrine testing. Not all hyperprolactinemia results from prolactinoma, however, and the clinical significance of minor elevations is not always obvious. The physiologic function of prolactin in humans is incompletely understood. The only established role is to initiate and maintain lactation, and prolactin deficiency has been implicated in some cases of lactation failure. Several characteristics of prolactin secretion are unique. Although control of prolactin secretion is complex, the most important regulator is the tonic inhibitory effect mediated by largely dopaminergic neurons emerging from the median eminence of the hypothalamus and traversing the pituitary stalk. This point is central to the understanding of hyperprolactinemia. While hyperprolactinemia is often explained by a pathologic increase in secretion, it more often results from a biochemical or physical interruption of these inhibitory pathways. When prolactin is elevated, gonadotropin-releasing hormone (GnRH) pulsatility is disrupted, either by reflex increases in dopamine or endogenous opiates or by a direct effect of prolactin itself. Decreased GnRH pulsatility begets alterations in levels of luteinizing hormone and follicle-stimulating hormone; the reduced end-organ stimulation results in hypogonadism.

CLINICAL PRESENTATION

Clinical manifestations of hyperprolactinemia are attributable to the elevated prolactin, to the mass effect of a space-occupying lesion, or to both. Thus, patients typically present with symptoms and signs of hypogonadism and/or with neurologic complaints such as headache, visual field defects from compression of the optic chiasm, or cranial neuropathies. Women classically present with oligo/amenorrhea and galactorrhea, but these signs are neither sensitive nor specific for hyperprolactinemia. Amenorrhea, and even galactorrhea, often occurs independent of elevations in prolactin. The prevalence of hyperprolactinemia is lowest in women with amenorrhea (15 to 20%), higher when galactorrhea is present alone (25 to 30%), and highest when they are present together (up to 75%). Patients also commonly note loss of libido and infertility. Bone mass is usually decreased in the setting of oligo/amenorrhea, a marker of hypoestrogenemia.

Men with hyperprolactinemia more often present with neurologic symptoms than with those attributable to endocrine dysfunction. Unlike females, in whom even modest degrees of hypoestrogenemia are clinically apparent, symptoms of hypogonadism in males are often not present until testosterone falls to much below the normal range. Since neurologic symptoms may be the first sign of disease, a tumor is more likely to be a macroprolactinoma than a microprolactinoma. Typical hormonal symptoms in males are loss of libido, impotence, gynecomastia, and infertility from oligospermia. Galactorrhea in males is uncommon due primarily to the lack of estrogen's priming effect on breast tissue.

ETIOLOGY

True pathologic elevation of prolactin must be distinguished from the numerous nonpathologic causes (Figure 1). Prolactin release is stimulated by thyrotropin-releasing hormone (TRH), food intake, physical and emotional stress, exercise, seizure, chest wall disease, nipple stimulation (breast feeding, breast examination), coitus or pelvic examination, pregnancy, various disease states, and numerous medications. The evaluation of modest elevations in prolactin (25 to 200 ng per mL) requires the recognition of the many secondary causes of hyperprolactinemia in order to avoid unnecessary diagnostic procedures. There is no absolute level below which one can confidently exclude a prolactin-producing neoplasm, and most experts suggest that a prolactinoma is the most likely cause of hyperprolactinemia only at levels as high as 200 to 250 ng per mL. Before adenoma is considered, any suspicion of primary hypothyroidism (prolactin secretion is stimulated by the compensatory rise in TRH), acromegaly (prolactin is cosecreted in up to 40% of cases), Cushing's syndrome (occasional), renal failure, or pregnancy must be pursued and these conditions ruled out. In the case of the incidentally discovered pituitary mass and no obvious symptoms, hypersecretion of all pituitary hormones must be excluded. Further, an exhaustive review of concurrent medications must be undertaken. The most common culprits in this category are neuroleptics, but numerous others have been implicated. These agents antagonize dopamine action, elevating prolactin by interference with inhibitory tone; prolactin levels up to 100 ng per mL are not infrequent. In these cases, there has rarely been evidence for tumor on systematic study.

Anatomic causes of hyperprolactinemia fall into two categories—"stalk effect" hyperprolactinemia and true adenomatous hypersecretion. Stalk-effect hyperprolactinemia results from partial or complete interruption of the dopaminergic signal to pituitary lactotrophs by compression of or damage to the pituitary stalk. Compression of the pituitary stalk can be caused by functioning or nonfunctioning pituitary adenomas, other primary brain tumors (e.g., meningioma, craniopharyngioma), metastatic disease, infiltrative or inflammatory disease, radiation, or autoimmune processes. Transection of the stalk, which may occur after head trauma, causes an immediate interruption of the dopamine signal. Empty sella syndrome, often found incidentally, can also be accompanied by hyperprolactinemia. In this condition, a congenital defect in the sellar diaphragm allows herniation of the arachnoid membrane into the sella turcica. Subsequent cerebrospinal fluid accumulation can exert enough pressure to compress the pituitary and stalk. True adenomatous hyperprolactinemia takes the form of microprolactinoma (<10 mm on magnetic resonance imaging [MRI]) or macroprolactinoma (>10 mm).

EVALUATION

Hyperprolactinemia is established when prolactin levels exceed 20 to 25 ng per mL on at least two occasions. Care must be taken to exclude physiologic and pharmacologic causes of prolactin elevation, as discussed previously. When no secondary causes of hyperprolactinemia can be identified, any persistent elevation in prolactin requires radiologic imaging to exclude not only micro- or macroadenoma, but other pituitary and peripituitary pathology as well. The imaging modality of choice is pituitary MRI with gadolinium infusion, although computed tomographic (CT) scanning can occasionally locate small focal lesions within the gland not seen on MRI. MRI permits better delineation of the gland and allows visualization of the optic chiasm and adjacent blood vessels, which may be involved by tumor growth. There is no role for plain skull radiography, which detects bony sellar deformity only after the tumor has become quite large and which is invariably followed by MRI. If there is a suggestion of a visual field abnormality on clinical examination and in every case of macroadenoma, formal visual field testing is mandatory. Although TRH stimulates prolactin secretion, the TRH stimulation test does not discriminate well between adenomatous and nonadenomatous causes of hyperprolactinemia and is not recommended. Evaluation of possible hypopituitarism is indicated in cases of macroadenoma and other significant pituitary pathology; it is usually appropriate to refer these cases to specialists in endocrinology.

MANAGEMENT

The goals of therapy for hyperprolactinemia are to relieve galactorrhea and restore gonadal function, to alleviate compressive symptoms, and to alter the natural history of the disease. In some cases, treatment is not required (see Special Considerations).

For documented prolactinoma, oral dopamine agonist therapy is the initial treatment of choice because of its effectiveness, safety, and long clinical experience. Of the dopamine agonists available in the

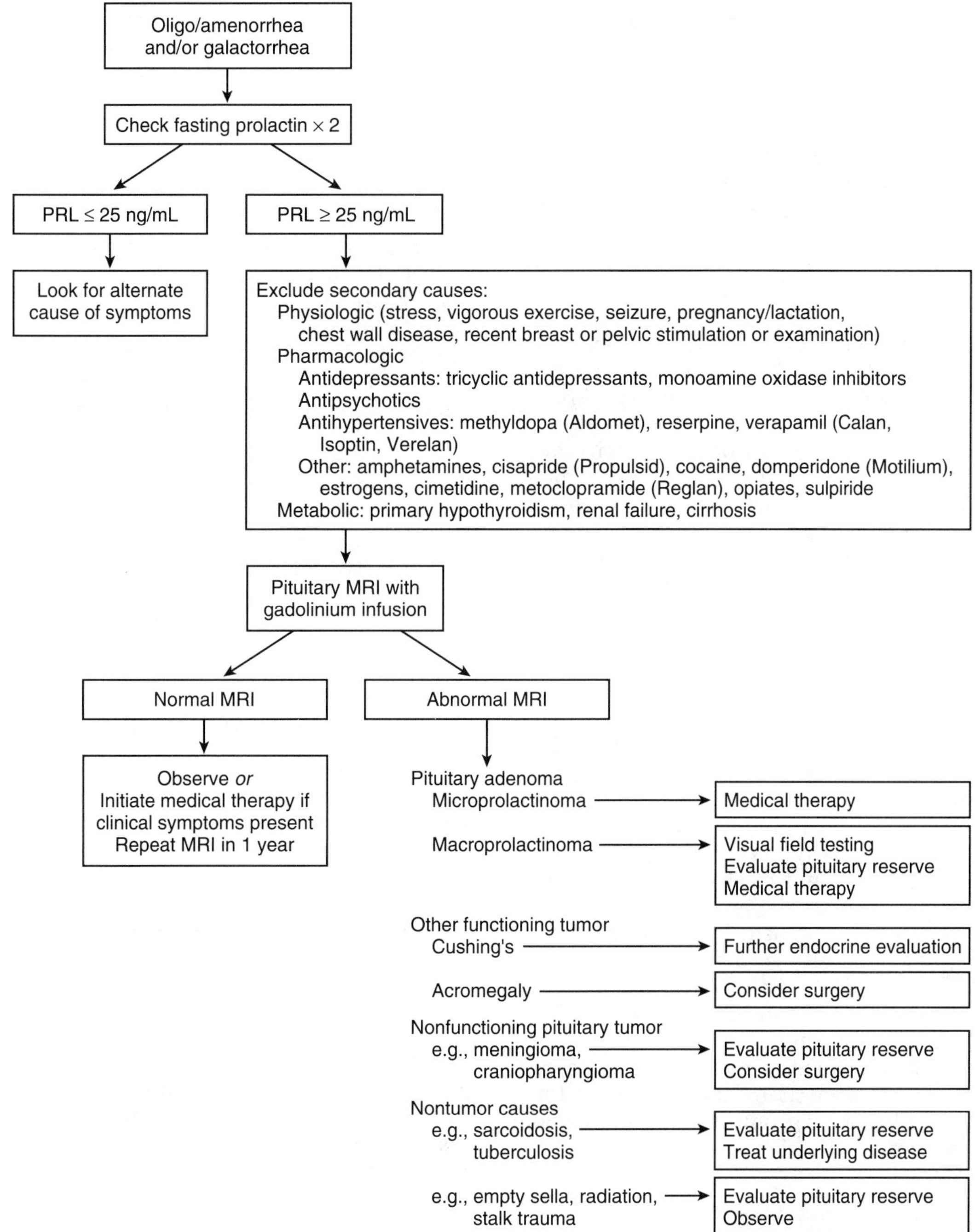

Figure 1. Algorithm for evaluation of hyperprolactinemia. *Abbreviations:* PRL = prolactin; MRI = magnetic resonance imaging.

United States (bromocriptine [Parlodel], pergolide [Permax], and cabergoline [Dostinex]), only bromocriptine and cabergoline are FDA-approved for treatment of prolactinoma. Pergolide has been demonstrated to be effective in small studies but is currently approved only for Parkinson's disease.

Clinical response should be expected in 70 to 90% of cases of microprolactinoma, resulting in tumor shrinkage and reduction of prolactin levels. In macroprolactinoma, the majority of tumors shrink by 25% but complete resolution is unusual. In women with amenorrhea, menstrual periods usually resume within 2 months, and most are ovulatory within 6 months, sometimes despite persistent mild elevations of prolactin. There is a variable improvement in galactorrhea, which in some cases may persist even after prolactin levels have become normal. Improvement in visual field testing can be seen within hours of the first dose. Because of the rapid response, initial therapy should be medical, even in patients with compressive neurologic symptoms from tumor effect, unless there is an immediate threat to vision, vascular structures, or in the setting of acute decompensation. Effectiveness of oral dopamine agonist therapy is occasionally limited by its side effects (i.e., nausea, lightheadedness, headache, and nasal congestion). Hypertension and hallucinations have also been described. Gastrointestinal side effects can be minimized by slow escalation of the dosing regimen. Tumor size is not predictive of dose requirement, and many patients can be controlled at submaximal doses. Bromocriptine should be started with half a 2.5-mg tablet once a day, at bedtime, with food. At 5 to 7 day intervals, or as side effects dictate, the dose can be increased by half-tablet increments. The prolactin level should be checked at 4 to 6 weeks with the patient taking a dose of 5 mg per day before increasing the dose further. Prolactin levels are typically checked every 3 months thereafter, and bromocriptine doses titrated to a maximum daily dose of 7.5 to 10 mg, in two to three divided doses with food. If bromocriptine therapy is not tolerated, cabergoline is an excellent alternative because it is given one to two times weekly, thus reducing the frequency of side effects. Cabergoline has been available in the United States only since 1997, but the early experience indicates that it is at least as effective as bromocriptine in both micro- and macroprolactinomas and is better tolerated. The recommended dose of cabergoline is half of a 0.5-mg tablet twice weekly, increased by 0.25 mg twice weekly at monthly intervals to a maximum dose of 1 mg twice weekly. Care should be taken when administering this drug to patients with hepatic dysfunction.

A drawback of medical therapy is the need for lifelong treatment in many cases. Dopamine agonist therapy is not curative, and most patients will experience a rebound increase in prolactin to pretreatment levels when it is stopped. In all patients with macroprolactinoma, despite good response to medical therapy, MRI (and visual field testing when indicated) should be performed within 6 to 12 months of diagnosis and annually thereafter. The natural history of microprolactinomas is not nearly as aggressive, and therapy is sometimes discontinued after 2 to 3 years to identify a subgroup of patients in whom the tumor will not recur.

Special Considerations

Observation

Not all hyperprolactinemia requires treatment. In men without significant hypogonadism and in women not desiring fertility, microprolactinomas may be observed by following prolactin levels and clinical signs of tumor progression and performing periodic imaging. Most of these lesions do not enlarge appreciably over several years of follow-up, and some may even spontaneously regress.

Bone Density

Particular attention must be paid to women with menstrual dysfunction, since the relative hypoestrogenemia is accompanied by rapid loss of bone mass. These women must receive estrogen replacement to prevent osteopenia and a progestational agent to ensure periodic shedding of the endometrium. Men with hyperprolactinemia and hypogonadism may also develop osteopenia; recovery of bone density occurs with reversal of the hyperprolactinemia or with testosterone replacement.

Pregnancy

Bromocriptine crosses the placenta and is not approved for use in pregnancy, although there have been no reports of adverse fetal outcomes in many years of its use. In all except the most aggressive macroprolactinoma, dopamine agonist therapy should be suspended for the duration of the pregnancy. The majority of patients with microprolactinomas (>95%) have no progression of tumor size despite pregnancy-associated estrogenic stimulation. Women with macroadenomas must be observed very carefully for any clinical sign of tumor enlargement. Visual field testing every 3 months is usually recommended. Treatment must be reinitiated if there are compressive symptoms, and occasionally, surgery may be necessary. Prolactin levels are physiologically elevated during pregnancy and lactation and therefore cannot be used to guide therapy.

Pharmacologic Hyperprolactinemia

In hyperprolactinemia due to medication, withdrawal of the offending agent will reverse the elevation. If this is not feasible, dopamine agonists may also be effective.

Surgery

Pituitary surgery is indicated when medical therapy has failed to reverse compressive symptoms and for the urgent relief of neurologic symptoms. Visual field defects at diagnosis, if chronic, do not require surgery and should respond quickly to medical therapy. Although surgery is usually performed using a transsphenoidal approach and carries low morbidity and mortality, it is not recommended as a primary mode of therapy, despite the possibility of definitive cure and relief from continuing treatment. Except in the best of hands, long-term recurrence rates can exceed 75% for macroprolactinomas and are up to 40% for microprolactinomas.

Radiation

Radiation is a last resort for patients who have failed medical and surgical therapies. Generalized pituitary irradiation can be effective but may require years before the full clinical effect is seen and is often complicated by panhypopituitarism. Newer, more precise delivery of pituitary radiation, the "gamma knife," is in its early stages of clinical experience and may become a reliable and available treatment modality.

SUMMARY

In summary, prolactin elevations are common, and treatment of most causes is relatively straightforward. Secondary causes of hyperprolactinemia must be understood in order to eliminate unnecessary radiologic evaluation. Medical therapy remains the initial treatment of choice to lower prolactin levels, relieve galactorrhea, normalize menstrual periods, restore libido and fertility, prevent loss of bone mass, and reduce tumor size, although therapy should be suspended during pregnancy. Surgery and radiation are reserved for emergencies and those failing medical therapy. Newer dopamine agonists are better tolerated and may improve compliance and overall outcome.

HYPOTHYROIDISM

method of
DANIEL N. BERGER, M.D., and
INDER J. CHOPRA, M.D.
UCLA Center for the Health Sciences
Los Angeles, California

Hypothyroidism is a clinical state in which the availability of thyroid hormone or its effect on peripheral tissues is diminished. At the tissue level, hydrophilic glycosaminoglycans such as hyaluronic acid aggregate along with water and lead to mucinous edema or myxedema. This process, in combination with a decrease in oxygen and substrate utilization by individual cells of the different organ systems, results in the protean clinical manifestations of hypothyroidism. Hypothyroidism is a very common and treatable disorder but is often overlooked and unrecognized owing to its nonspecific and insidious nature.

CAUSES OF HYPOTHYROIDISM

There are several causes of hypothyroidism (Table 1). Primary hypothyroidism refers to thyroid gland failure and accounts for nearly 99% of cases. Secondary or central hypothyroidism is due to a disorder of the pituitary, hypothalamus, or hypothalamic-pituitary portal circulation and accounts for the other 1% of cases. Extremely rare is the disorder of thyroid hormone resistance, in which the levels of thyroid hormone in the circulation are "normal" but the hormone does not have adequate effect on its target organs owing to a relative insensitivity to its actions. Although the specific signs and symptoms as well as the treatment for hypothyroidism may be essentially invariant, it is imperative to determine the underlying cause of the hypothyroidism, because other commonly associated disorders, such as autoimmune diseases or hypopituitarism, may warrant evaluation.

Primary hypothyroidism is a common entity, with a prevalence estimated at 0.8%. It is five to seven times more common in women than men and increases significantly in elderly women, with evidence of at least subtle thyroid failure in 10% of those over 50 years of age. Chronic autoimmune hypothyroidism (Hashimoto's disease, or lymphocytic thyroiditis) is the most common type, approximating 50% of cases, and involves cell-mediated and antibody-

TABLE 1. **Causes of Hypothyroidism**

Primary
Thyroiditis: chronic autoimmune (Hashimoto's disease), subacute, postpartum, external irradiation
Iatrogenic: Iodine 131 treatment or post thyroidectomy
Infiltrating disorders: infections, granulomatous disease, malignancy
Drugs: antithyroid agents, lithium, iodide, amiodarone, cytokines, perchlorate
Iodine deficiency
Congenital: thyroid dysgenesis, defects in thyroid hormone synthesis
Idiopathic: atrophy (probably autoimmune)
Secondary (central)
TSH deficiency due to pituitary disease: postpartum infarction, infiltration by tumor, granulomatous disease, hypophysitis, infection, irradiation, idiopathic
TRH deficiency due to hypothalamic disease: tumor (e.g., craniopharyngioma), irradiation; transiently occurring in nonthyroidal illness
Peripheral resistance to thyroid hormones

mediated destruction of the thyroid gland. Histologic changes in the thyroid include lymphocytic infiltration with follicular cell hyperplasia in the early stages and resultant fibrosis and atrophy later on. Ninety percent of patients will have either positive antithyroid peroxidase antibodies or antithyroglobulin antibodies; some 10% of the normal unaffected population may also have positive antibody status, however. It is not yet entirely clear whether these antibodies are actually pathogenic or mere bystanders to the autoimmune process. Other antibodies, including those directed at the thyroid-stimulating hormone (TSH) receptor, which inhibit TSH stimulation of the thyroid, and antibodies directed against the iodine transporter, which block thyroid uptake of iodine, have been implicated in autoimmune hypothyroidism as well. It may take several years of gradual thyroid destruction before the condition reaches clinical significance, and in the early stages, patients may have an enlarged thyroid goiter. Over time, the thyroid usually becomes atrophic, and physical examination may reveal only a small, firm thyroid. Once overt hypothyroidism is present biochemically, it is usually permanent. Autoimmune thyroiditis tends to have a genetic predisposition and can present in the very young as early as 1 or 2 years of age, but typically the condition is diagnosed later on in adulthood. Autoimmune thyroiditis may be associated with other autoimmune endocrinopathies including adrenal insufficiency, hypoparathyroidism, and insulin-dependent diabetes mellitus as well as other autoimmune conditions such as pernicious anemia and Sjögren's syndrome. Underlying autoimmune thyroid disease can also contribute to hypothyroidism from other causes, including long-term treatment with lithium carbonate, exposure to iodine-containing substances, or perhaps heavy tobacco use.

Next to thyroiditis, the most common cause of hypothyroidism is iatrogenic; this accounts for 30 to 40% of cases. Treatment of hyperthyroidism secondary to Graves' disease or toxic multinodular goiter with radioiodine, i.e., iodine 131(^{131}I), may result in hypothyroidism in up to 20% of patients within 1 year and in approximately 2 to 3% of patients per year subsequently. Surgery (subtotal thyroidectomy for hyperthyroidism or near-total thyroidectomy for thyroid cancer) is another common cause. External irradiation to the neck for conditions such as Hodgkin's lymphoma may also result in hypothyroidism in up to 30% of patients some 20 years later.

Although less common in the United States, either iodine deficiency (the most common cause worldwide) or iodine excess can result in hypothyroidism. Iodine excess inhibits iodide organification as well as thyroid hormone synthesis—i.e., the Wolff-Chaikoff effect. Although most persons who are exposed to excess iodine escape from this effect and remain euthyroid, a minority will not, especially if there is an underlying abnormality in the thyroid gland such as chronic thyroiditis. Many foodstuffs including kelp, seaweed, and shellfish, as well as medicinal products such as antitussive agents, health tonics, and some drugs, e.g., amiodarone, contain an abundant amount of iodine.

Another important although less common cause of primary hypothyroidism is drugs. These agents include the antithyroid medications (propylthiouracil and methimazole); phenytoin (Dilantin) and carbamazepine (Tegretol), which increase thyroid hormone metabolism and alter binding to carrier proteins in serum; lithium carbonate; and amiodarone. Furthermore, infections, e.g., tuberculosis, *Pneumocystis carinii* pneumonia, and infiltrative disorders, e.g., sarcoidosis, amyloidosis, hemachromatosis, may directly involve the thyroid and compromise its function.

Central or secondary hypothyroidism is relatively rare but when present necessitates a thorough work-up for other endocrine deficiencies. Causes include a pituitary mass lesion such as a primary adenoma, a metastatic infiltrative process, or hypophysitis. Other causes are trauma including that from surgery, irradiation of the pituitary, or, less commonly, developmental abnormalities. Idiopathic TSH or thyrotropin-releasing hormone (TRH) deficiencies can also rarely cause isolated secondary hypothyroidism.

Transient states of hypothyroidism may result from primary thyroid gland dysfunction, or they may be centrally related. Primary causes include subacute or postpartum thyroiditis, in which a state of hyperthyroidism may predate the hypothyroid phase. Hyperthyroidism is due to release of preformed thyroid hormone from an injured, inflamed gland. Subsequently, thyroid reserve is diminished, and the thyroid is unable to secrete adequate amounts of hormone. This situation may last from a few weeks to a few months, but then it resolves spontaneously in the majority of cases, although recurrences are not uncommon. A minority of patients (approximately 10%) may stay hypothyroid permanently and may thus require long-term treatment with levothyroxine. A transient form of central hypothyroidism may also occur in some forms of nonthyroidal illness (NTI), acute psychiatric disease, malnutrition, or administration of drugs that suppress release of TSH such as dopamine or high-dose glucocorticoids. In these conditions, the euthyroid state is restored if there is no underlying thyroid abnormality when the offending circumstance is resolved.

A very rare form of hypothyroidism is due to resistance to thyroid hormone. This results from a genetic mutation in the receptor to triiodothyronine that leads to the inability of thyroid hormone to exert its normal effects on gene transcription at the nuclear level.

CLINICAL FEATURES

The clinical manifestations of hypothyroidism are dependent on duration of disease, degree of insufficiency, and age at presentation. Because thyroid hormone plays a major role in growth and neurologic development, its deficiency early on can lead to growth and mental retardation. Greater than 95% of newborns show no clinical manifestations, but if hypothyroidism is severe, symptoms and signs include lethargy, respiratory distress, slowness of movement, hoarse cry, jaundice, and poor feeding. Fortunately, screening for hypothyroidism is the standard of care, and if the condition is diagnosed early and treated before 3 months of age, the consequences can be minimal. Hypothyroidism in childhood and adolescence may also be associated with growth and mental retardation as well as delayed dentition and bone maturation. Rarely, it is associated with precocious puberty.

In the adult population, the clinical manifestations of hypothyroidism are nonspecific and variable. Owing to the effects of thyroid hormone on virtually all organ systems, the signs and symptoms of hypothyroidism almost seem infinite. They result from a generalized slowing down of metabolic processes and from the accumulation of glycosaminoglycans and water in the interstitium. The clinical features tend to be more subtle and insidious, as the causative disease process often tends to be very gradual. Clinical features in the elderly mimic at times the normal aging process. Symptoms of hypothyroidism may include fatigue, generalized weakness, cold intolerance, dry skin, hair loss, myalgias, paresthesias, constipation, menometrorrhagia, sleep disturbances, mental confusion with cognitive decline, and weight gain. Signs often include bradycardia, diastolic hypertension, delayed relaxation of muscle reflexes, coarse skin, periorbital edema, hoarseness, macroglossia, and evidence of carpal tunnel syndrome. The cardiovascular effects of hypothyroidism can result in congestive heart failure via diminished cardiac output and decreased ventricular compliance, rhythm disturbances, and pericardial effusion.

DIAGNOSIS AND LABORATORY EVALUATION

Because the clinical features of hypothyroidism can be so nonspecific and subtle, the diagnosis often rests on biochemical confirmation or is commonly made during screening of an "asymptomatic" patient. The hallmark of overt hypothyroidism is a decreased concentration of peripheral thyroid hormone levels. In most situations, a free thyroxine (T_4) index is an acceptable measurement, but this can occasionally be inaccurate in the setting of marked abnormalities of thyroid-binding globulin (TBG) levels or thyroid function, as may be seen in liver disease, high estrogen or androgen states, or NTI. The reliability of the free T_4 index is also compromised in patients demonstrating circulating antibodies to thyroxine. We recommend measurement of free T_4 by equilibrium dialysis/radioimmunoassay as the preferred means of assessment of thyroid status except when a patient has been treated with intravenous heparin. Heparin administration may be associated with artifactual elevation of free T_4 measured by equilibrium dialysis.

Measurement of triiodothyronine (T_3) concentration is not helpful in the diagnosis of hypothyroidism. Serum total T_3 concentration may also be decreased in NTI when the patient is clinically euthyroid, and it may be clearly normal and sometimes even elevated in hypothyroid patients. Serum reverse T_3 (rT_3) levels will be low in hypothyroidism and elevated in most cases of NTI (except renal insufficiency) and thus may help to distinguish between the two.

With the advent of ultrasensitive radioimmunometric TSH assays, the measurement of serum TSH has become a very reliable test in the evaluation of hypothyroidism. Serum TSH is typically elevated in both overt primary hypothyroidism and subclinical primary hypothyroidism (the latter with normal serum T_4 concentration). It should be emphasized that the serum TSH may be low, normal, or slightly elevated in secondary hypothyroidism and is thus not very helpful in this circumstance. It is transiently suppressed during therapy with drugs such as dopamine, glucocorticoids, and somatostatin. It may be low, normal, or mildly elevated in patients with systemic illness or acute psychiatric illness. Thus, an awareness of the clinical setting is very important in using serum TSH levels for diagnosis.

Although the aforementioned tests establish the diagnosis of hypothyroidism and determine whether it is of a primary or secondary nature, they do not provide clear insight as to the underlying causative disorder. In this respect, the measurement of antithyroid peroxidase and antithyroglobulin antibodies is helpful. Positive results confirm the diagnosis of chronic autoimmune thyroiditis. These tests are also helpful in determining whether a patient receiving thyroid hormone replacement and a dubious history of hypothyroidism truly has underlying thyroid dysfunction. A positive antibody status supports a history of true underlying autoimmune thyroid disease, while a negative antibody status makes a diagnosis suspicious and thus warrants a trial of thyroid hormone withdrawal to evaluate whether the patient becomes hypothyroid when off thyroxine treatment.

Several other nonspecific laboratory abnormalities may be associated with hypothyroidism and may help the informed clinician to rule out other suspected diagnoses, or perhaps they may initiate an evaluation for hypothyroidism when obvious clinical evidence is lacking. These abnormalities include elevated cholesterol (LDL, HDL, triglycerides), creatine kinase, and carotene levels in hypothyroidism secondary to their decreased clearance and hyponatremia due to diminished free water excretion (from increased serum antidiuretic hormone levels). In summary, a thorough laboratory evaluation in hypothyroidism should include measurement of serum TSH, free T_4 by equilibrium dialysis/radioimmunoassay, antithyroid peroxidase and/or antithyroglobulin antibody levels, and occasionally reverse T_3 (in the setting of confounding systemic illness). When laboratory data are inconsistent or serum TSH is only mildly elevated to 15 to 20 mU/mL (normal 0.3–4.7 mU/mL), or when drug interference, systemic illness, or acute psychiatric disease is a consideration, it is prudent to wait 2 to 3 weeks and re-evaluate the patient's thyroid status before making a long-term commitment to treatment with thyroid hormone.

TREATMENT

Thyroid Hormone Replacement

The treatment of hypothyroidism remains the same independent of its cause. The aim of treatment is to achieve a euthyroid state. Potential treatment options for hypothyroidism include synthetic T_4 (levothyroxine [Synthroid, Levoxyl, Levothroid, Eltroxin]), synthetic T_3 (liothyronine [Cytomel]), and mixtures of T_4 and T_3, both synthetic (Thyrolar) and natural dessicated thyroid. In normal humans, approximately 100 μg of T_4 and 30 μg of T_3 are produced daily. Physiologically, the thyroid gland produces a disproportionate amount of T_4 relative to T_3 (the ratio of T_4 to T_3 in the thyroid approximates 15 to 20:1). Peripheral conversion of T_4 to T_3, most abundantly by the enzyme 5′-monodeiodinase type 1 (primarily found in the liver and kidney), accounts for close to 80% of T_3 production. Synthetic T_4 provides the closest approximation to this natural state and is thus the agent of choice (except for temporary treatment with synthetic T_3 in patients with differentiated thyroid carcinoma being prepared for radioiodine ablation). The other preparations do not merit a major role in chronic thyroid hormone replacement, as they lead to fluctuating serum levels of thyroid hormones and they cost more. During treatment with T_3, it becomes difficult to interpret follow-up thyroid function tests because the levels of T_4 will be low and those of T_3 variable. Finally, owing to the greater potency of T_3 with its approximately 10-fold higher binding affinity than that of T_4 for tissue nuclear receptors, overzealous treatment may more easily precipitate a cardiac event such as ischemia or tachyarrhythmia.

The mean replacement dose of T_4 for an adult male is 120 μg per day, with the usual daily dose ranging from 75 to 175 μg given once a day. Several important factors come into play in determining the dose of T_4 for an individual patient. The amount of T_4 required decreases with increasing age. Infants require approximately 100 μg per m^2 per day, and the average adult need is 1.6 μg per kg per day. In a normal adult, absorption from the intestine is 80 to 90%. The gastrointestinal absorption may be markedly decreased in malabsorptive syndromes or when the T_4 is ingested at or about the same time as other interfering substances or medications such as iron sulfate, cholestyramine, aluminum hydroxide, sucralfate, fiber, soybean products, and possibly calcium. For this reason, we generally advise patients to take their T_4 on an empty stomach at least 2 hours before or after from the aforementioned medications. Pregnant women with hypothyroidism may require 25 to 50% more T_4 during pregnancy to maintain a euthyroid state. Contributing factors may include increased serum TBG levels, transplacental passage of T_4 to the fetus, and increased metabolism of T_4 by the placenta. Other conditions that increase serum TBG including oral contraceptive use will also increase the requirement of T_4 dose in hypothyroidism. Drugs that increase metabolism of T_4, e.g., phenytoin (Dilantin), rifampin (Rifadin), phenobarbital, may increase the required dose of T_4 replacement in hypothyroidism. Finally, patients who have undergone thyroidectomy secondary to thyroid carcinoma are usually treated with higher doses of T_4 in an attempt to suppress TSH and thereby potentially reduce tumorigenesis.

In an otherwise healthy young patient recently diagnosed with hypothyroidism and without a cardiac history, T_4 replacement can be safely started at near-replacement doses (75 to 100 μg given once daily). In patients with a history of cardiac disease or with risk factors for cardiac disease or in the elderly, it is recommended to initiate therapy at smaller doses (25 to 50 μg given once daily). Higher doses may be associated with an adverse cardiac event such as angina pectoris, myocardial infarction, tachyarrhythmias, and/or congestive heart failure. The dose can be gradually increased (usually by 25 μg at monthly intervals if the therapy is well tolerated) until a euthyroid state is achieved. In some instances, the initiation of thyroid hormone replacement may unmask underlying adrenal insufficiency due to increased metabolism of hydrocortisone. If adrenal insufficiency is suspected, adrenal reserve can be evaluated by performing a cosyntropin (Cortrosyn) stimulation test. While awaiting the results, the patient can be started on hydrocortisone (20 mg in the morning and 10 mg in the evening). If adequate adrenal function is demonstrated, the hydrocortisone can then be discontinued. The initiation of thyroid hormone therapy may also have effects on medications that patients are already receiving. Thyroid hormone may potentiate the effects of sympathomimetic agents (e.g., epinephrine), tricyclic antidepressants (e.g., imipramine [Tofranil]), and anticoagulants (e.g., warfarin [Coumadin]). Doses of these drugs may thus have to be decreased. Rarely, allergic reactions have been reported to synthetic T_4; in such cases the reaction is most probably due to an allergy to a coloring dye in the tablet rather than to T_4 per se. If this occurs, the patient should not be switched to a different thyroid hormone preparation such as T_3 but rather should be given an alternative preparation of levothyroxine without the coloring dye.

Given that the half-life of levothyroxine is approximately 7 days, it will take approximately 6 weeks for serum levels of thyroxine to reach a steady state with a constant daily dose. However, most patients will experience symptomatic improvement within 2 to 3 weeks. Most if not all of the signs and symptoms of hypothyroidism in adults with mild to moderate disease should eventually resolve when a euthyroid state is reached. In primary hypothyroidism, the goal of therapy should be to normalize the serum TSH and serum free T_4 concentrations. Each time an adjustment in levothyroxine dose is made, it may take up to 6 to 8 weeks for the serum TSH to reach equilibrium. Thus, at the outset of therapy or after a dosage adjustment of levothyroxine in primary hypothyroidism, we measure serum free T_4 and TSH levels. When a patient has been on a stable dose of thyroid hormone replacement for primary hypothyroidism, then serum TSH alone may be monitored periodically (usually at 4- to 6-month intervals). Pregnant women with hypothyroidism should have their serum free T_4 and TSH levels monitored more frequently (every 8 weeks) because of the possibility of their increased requirements for thyroid hormone. We have noted that patients with primary hypothyroidism associated with amiodarone therapy often do not achieve normal serum TSH levels despite what should be an adequate replacement dose of levothyroxine. In these patients, we prefer to normalize the serum free T_4 levels while accepting a modestly elevated serum TSH. Patients with secondary hypothyroidism should be followed not with serum TSH levels, but rather serum free T_4 levels, with the goal to normalize the serum free T_4. Care must be taken to avoid overtreatment with thyroid hormone, as this may be associated with untoward cardiac events including tacharrhythmias (especially atrial fibrillation), cardiac ischemia, and, over a prolonged period, osteoporosis, especially in postmenopausal women not on estrogen replacement.

Evaluation of Hypothyroidism in Systemic Nonthyroidal Illness

Several conditions including infections, sepsis syndrome, trauma, burns, myocardial ischemia, chronic diseases, acute psychiatric illnesses, and malnutrition frequently result in transient alterations in thyroid hormone metabolism and thyroid function indices. The most common finding is a low serum T_3 state with normal serum T_4 and serum TSH. However, total serum T_4 may also be low, and serum TSH may be either low (usually in the acute stage of illness) or even high (usually in the recovery phase of illness). These possibilities may make interpretation of thyroid function tests difficult and confusing. For this reason, it is often wise not to measure thyroid function tests in the setting of systemic illness unless clinical findings suggest thyroid dysfunction. The serum reverse T_3 is a helpful parameter as it is elevated in NTI but less so or not at all in NTI patients with hypothyroidism. Furthermore, a serum TSH level greater than 20 μU per mL (normal, 0.35 to 4.7 μU per mL) is consistent with a diagnosis of true primary hypothyroidism. If the clinical picture is consistent with true hypothyroidism, then a trial of thyroid hormone replacement may be warranted, with re-evaluation of thyroid status at a later time when the patient's clinical status has improved. If the diagnosis of hypothyroidism is unclear, it is reasonable to wait 1 or 2 weeks after the patient's clinical status has improved and then re-evaluate thyroid function indices. There has been a controversy in treating severely ill patients with thyroid hormone replacement. Preliminary studies of T_3 treatment of hypothyroidism in cardiac patients with T_3 have been inconclusive with regard to benefit. At this time, we do not recommend routine treatment of NTI patients with thyroid hormone replacement unless there is a substantially clear indication of hypothyroidism.

Subclinical Hypothyroidism

Subclinical hypothyroidism is marked by normal serum levels of total and free T_4, normal total and free T_3 levels, and an elevated serum TSH level. The causes are the same as for overt primary hypothyroidism, and this entity can be thought of as a part of the continuum of primary hypothyroidism. If antithyroid antibody status is positive, the likelihood is high that overt hypothyroidism will eventually occur (in approximately 4% of cases per year over 20 years). Many patients with subclinical hypothyroidism will be asymptomatic, but others may demonstrate mild or vague symptoms of hypothyroidism. Some studies show that treatment with thyroid hormone results in moderation of symptoms (especially cognitive function), improvement in cardiac indices, and amelioration of dyslipidemia (lowering of cholesterol and triglycerides). Treatment is usually started with conservative doses of T_4 (50 to 75 μg) which are adjusted to achieve a normal serum TSH. If treatment is deferred, thyroid function indices should be repeated within 3 months and then at least twice a year, with initiation of therapy if the TSH continues to increase or the patient becomes increasingly symptomatic.

Surgery in Hypothyroidism

Surgery is relatively safe and not associated with increased perioperative risk in mild hypothyroidism. Thus, patients with mild hypothyroidism do not require aggressive thyroid hormone replacement prior to surgery. However, in moderate to severe hypothyroidism, there is an increased incidence of complications including congestive heart failure, cardiac arrhythmias, shock, respiratory compromise, hyponatremia, ileus, mental status changes, and increased sensitivity to anesthetic agents and narcotics. The stress of a surgical procedure may also precipitate myxedema coma in patients with severe underlying hypothyroidism. It is therefore advisable to make the patient at least close to euthyroid preoperatively, especially for an elective procedure. If surgery is urgent, then aggressive treatment with thyroid hormone is indicated.

Screening for Hypothyroidism

Screening for hypothyroidism is a somewhat controversial topic, as universal evaluation of thyroid function indices in asymptomatic patients would not be cost-effective. However, one target population in which screening may prove to be cost-saving is women greater than 60 years of age, as this segment of the population has the highest incidence of hypothyroidism. Other "asymptomatic" persons who may benefit from screening for hypothyroidism are those found to have nonspecific laboratory abnormalities, e.g., elevated cholesterol, creatine kinase, unexplained hyponatremia. Persons with nonspecific signs and symptoms of hypothyroidism would also benefit from screening. The single best test for screening for hypothyroidism in an outpatient population is the serum TSH, although uncommon cases of secondary hypothyroidism will be missed if a serum free T_4 is not also performed.

Myxedema Coma

Myxedema coma is the clinical manifestation of severe hypothyroidism and represents an endocrinologic emergency. The mortality rate is very high (30 to 40%). Myxedema coma may be the result of longstanding untreated hypothyroidism or may be precipitated by acute stress as in infection, myocardial infarction, trauma, surgery, or exposure to anesthetic drugs or narcotics. Severe cardiac dysfunction, respiratory failure, progressive lethargy and stupor, hypothermia, and hyponatremia may ensue. Treatment consists of aggressive replacement of thyroid hormone, with either (1) a 400- to 500-μg bolus of intravenous T_4 to replace the extrathyroidal pool of T_4, followed by 100 μg daily of intravenous T_4 until the patient has improved enough to tolerate oral T_4, or (2) 10 to 30 μg every 6 to 8 hours of T_3. Patients with myxedema coma are best managed in an intensive care setting, where close monitoring and attention to supportive measures can be given, including ventilatory assistance, management of fluid status, and use of blankets to diminish heat loss (active warming may result in shock secondary to peripheral vasodilation). Concomitant treatment with stress doses of hydrocortisone (approximately 150 mg per day) is recommended at least temporarily, owing to the association of underlying adrenal insufficiency, which may be overtly present or unmasked by the initiation of thyroid hormone treatment. Finally, evaluation and treatment of any precipitating factors must be undertaken.

HYPERTHYROIDISM

method of
PETER A. SINGER, M.D.
University of Southern California School of Medicine
Los Angeles, California

The term "hyperthyroidism" encompasses a heterogeneous group of disorders that have two features in common. First, all types of hyperthyroidism include a symptom complex of various degrees of severity and mediated by beta-adrenergic stimulation. Frequent symptoms include nervousness, heat intolerance, irritability, palpitations, and increased bowel motility, with more frequent bowel movements. Second, hyperthyroidism is associated with the catabolic effects of excess circulating levels of thyroid hormone; such effects may include weight loss, fatigue, muscle weakness, increased appetite, and bone loss. The symptoms and signs of hyperthyroidism depend on a number of variables, including levels of circulating thyroid hormone, duration of disease, the age of the patient, and concurrent illnesses.

CLASSIFICATION

Hyperthyroidism can be classified according to the capacity of the thyroid gland to trap radioactive iodine (Table 1). Disorders associated with increased radioiodine uptake have thyroid gland autonomy (with the exception of pituitary tumors that secrete thyroid-stimulating hormone [TSH]) and require specific treatment, while those associated with diminished radioiodine uptake include conditions that are usually self-limiting and may require only symptomatic treatment.

TABLE 1. **Causes of Hyperthyroidism**

Underlying Disorder*	Thyroid Findings on Palpation
Hyperthyroidism with Elevated RAIU	
Graves' disease	Diffuse enlargement
Toxic multinodular goiter	Multinodular
Toxic adenoma	Single nodule (usually >3 cm)
TSH-secreting pituitary tumor	Diffuse enlargement
Hydatidiform mole	Diffuse (usually mild) enlargement
Choriocarcinoma	Diffuse (usually mild) enlargement
Pituitary resistance to thyroid hormone	Diffuse enlargement
Hyperthyroidism with Low RAIU	
Factitious	Normal
Subacute granulomatus thyroiditis	Tender, usually nodular
Subacute lymphocytic (postpartum or sporadic)	Diffuse (usually mild) or absent
Amiodarone-induced thyroiditis	Diffuse (usually mild) enlargement
Iodine-induced hyperthyroidism	Usually multinodular
Radiation-induced thyroiditis	Tender, usually diffuse
Metastatic functioning follicular tumor	Normal
Struma ovarii	Normal

*Listed in probable decreasing order of frequency.
Abbreviation: RAIU = radioactive iodine uptake.

CLINICAL FEATURES

Physical examination of the hyperthyroid patient generally reveals a person who is somewhat anxious, with a rapid pulse (in the elderly, atrial fibrillation is common), widened pulse pressure, warm skin, and thyroid gland findings such as enlargement or nodularity (see Table 1) depending on the underlying causative disorder. Examination of the eyes in all types of hyperthyroidism may show eyelid retraction, which is mediated by beta-adrenergic stimulation. Infiltrative ophthalmopathy is seen almost exclusively in patients with thyrotoxic Graves' disease.

ESTABLISHING THE DIAGNOSIS

Since many of the symptoms of hyperthyroidism may be compatible with some non-thyroid disorders such as anxiety and with the perimenopausal state, persons in whom hyperthyroidism is suspected should have a sensitive assay of serum TSH, which is suppressed in hyperthyroidism. An exception is in patients with rare TSH-secreting pituitary tumors, in whom TSH levels may be normal or even slightly elevated. It should be noted that TSH levels may be suppressed in hospitalized individuals, especially those who are seriously ill, or who are receiving pharmacologic doses of glucocorticoids or dopamine, thus limiting the usefulness of serum TSH determination in such patients.

The presence of a suppressed TSH level in individuals suspected to have hyperthyroidism should be complemented with determination of a serum free thyroxine (T_4) level (or its estimate) to confirm the diagnosis. Patients with normal thyroid hormone levels and suppressed TSH concentrations have "subclinical hyperthyroidism," in which overt symptoms of hyperthyroidism are usually absent.

After the diagnosis of hyperthyroidism is confirmed, the underlying disorder should be determined by performing a radioactive iodine uptake scan of the thyroid. Patients with obvious Graves' disease (such as those with infiltrative ophthalmopathy or large goiters with bruits) may forgo the radioactive iodine uptake test. It is important, however, to differentiate between Graves' disease and conditions of low radioactive iodine uptake, which usually are self-limiting.

In addition to the radioactive iodine uptake test, a radioiodine scan may be helpful in establishing the diagnosis in patients with suspected toxic multinodular goiter, a condition encountered more frequently nowadays with increasing immigration into the United States from goiter-endemic regions.

TREATMENT OF HYPERTHYROIDISM

Since approximately 80% of patients with hyperthyroidism in the United States have thyrotoxic Graves' disease, most of the following comments pertain to that disorder. It should be noted that among individuals with hyperthyroidism associated with high radioactive iodine uptake, only Graves' disease may be associated with remission following the use of thionamide drugs.

Developing a Treatment Strategy

General Measures and Patient Education

Essential in the early management of Graves' hyperthyroidism is emphasizing to the patient that only with strict adherence to the treatment regimen will symptoms be promptly alleviated and health restored to the pre-thyrotoxic state. Individuals with hyperthyroidism frequently tend to be impatient, probably owing to their symptoms, and it must be stressed that compliance with prescribed treatment is essential for a successful outcome. If patients are seen in the company of family members or friends, it is helpful to familiarize them with the treatment plan as well.

Initial Treatment of Symptoms

Since many of the symptoms of hyperthyroidism are related to enhanced beta-adrenergic stimulation, I routinely employ beta-blocking drugs, although mild symptoms may not warrant their use. I prefer the use of propranolol (Inderal) even though it must be given approximately every 6 hours to be completely effective. I prefer this agent because of its relatively short half-life, as patients may learn to titrate their own medication depending upon their symptoms. As patients improve during the course of thionamide therapy (discussed subsequently), they are able to omit more doses of propranolol.

The usual starting dose of propranolol is between 20 and 40 mg orally approximately every 6 hours (or four times a day), with a target heart rate of approximately 80 beats per minute. Some physicians prefer the use of longer-acting beta blockers, such as atenolol (Tenormin), which may be given as a single daily dose. In individuals in whom compliance may be problematic, or in those who prefer once-a-day dosing, atenolol, 50 to 100 mg orally per day, is an excellent alternative. Other long-acting beta blockers are nadolol (Corgard) and metoprolol (Lopressor). Long-acting beta blockers are cardioselective and are not contraindicated in individuals with co-existing asthma.

In my experience, patients who are treated with adequate doses of beta-blocking drugs experience significant relief of symptoms within a few days after their initiation.

Reduction of Serum Thyroid Hormone Level

Unfortunately, there have been few advances in the management of hyperthyroidism in recent years. Treatment of hyperthyroidism basically consists of lowering the concentrations of serum T_4 and triiodothyronine (T_3), which is accomplished either with thionamide drugs or with ablative therapy, either radioiodine or surgery. In the United States, radioiodine ablation with ^{131}I is the preferred method of treatment of most practicing endocrinologists. In a survey of thyroid experts, 69% of respondents chose radioiodine ablation as the primary form of therapy for uncomplicated Graves' disease in a prototypical 43-year-old woman. Only 1% of the physicians recommended surgery, while 30% selected administration of thionamide drugs as the primary form of therapy. These responses were in sharp contrast to those of thyroid experts in both Europe and Japan, where a similar survey revealed that the majority of physicians favored administration of thionamide drugs as the primary form of therapy. The rationale provided by the U.S. physicians who selected radioiodine therapy was the fact that remission rates following 1 to 2 years of thionamide drugs were only approximately 30%.

Before a specific type of therapy for Graves' disease is recommended, it is essential that the patient be aware of the benefits and pitfalls of each type of treatment, as described in the following discussion.

Thionamide Drug Therapy

Initial Treatment

Currently, two thionamide drugs are available for clinical use in the United States: methimazole (MMI) (Tapazole), available in 5-mg and 10-mg tablets, and propylthiouracil (PTU), available in 50-mg tablets. Both agents inhibit synthesis of thyroid hormone by blocking organification of iodine. PTU also inhibits peripheral conversion of thyroxine to triiodothyronine, although clinically this may be more of a theoretical than a practical advantage.

I generally prefer MMI over PTU because of its longer biologic half-life and its potency. For uncomplicated hyperthyroidism, MMI may initially be given 2 to 3 times a day in a total dose of 20 to 30 mg, whereas PTU is usually administered 3 to 4 times a day in a total dose of 300 to 400 mg. When biochemical euthyroidism is achieved, usually after 6 to 8 weeks of therapy, MMI may be given once a day, or PTU twice a day, and the total dose may be halved. The relative simplicity of using MMI versus PTU may render it more suitable for persons in whom compliance may be difficult. It must be stressed to the patient that omitting medication doses may result in a rebound of the hyperthyroid state, since the intrathyroidal deficiency of iodine produced by thionamide drugs will result in more avid trapping of exogenous iodide.

In general, I obtain serum T_4 and T_3 levels about 6 to 8 weeks after initiation of thionamide drug therapy to ensure adequacy of treatment response. If there has been little clinical biochemical improvement, doses of medication are probably being omitted. A serum TSH level provides no additional information at this point, since TSH suppression is common for up to 3 or 4 months after euthyroidism has been achieved. Patients with very large goiters and fairly severe hyperthyroidism often take somewhat longer than 6 to 8 weeks to become euthyroid and may require larger doses of MMI (e.g., 40 mg per day) or PTU (e.g., 400 to 600 mg per day).

I stress to patients that any improvement with thionamide drugs may take several weeks, and I recommend that they defer, if possible, making definitive decisions regarding long-term thionamide versus ablative therapy until they have improved to the extent that they are better able to make more reasoned choices. I always discuss the various forms of treatment of hyperthyroidism with patients at our first encounter, however, and reiterate the options after they have improved.

Although the overall remission rate for patients receiving thionamide therapy is approximately 30%, some patients are more likely than others to go into remission. Patients with mild hyperthyroidism or small goiters and who have a negative family history for hyperthyroidism are more likely to go into remission, as are patients who respond quickly to thionamide drugs in terms of thyroid gland shrinkage and biochemical improvement. Conversely, patients with severe thyrotoxicosis and those with a strong family history of Graves' disease infrequently go into remission. Some clinicians have advocated the use of serologic markers, such as thyroid-stimulating immunoglobulin or anti-thyroperoxidase antibodies, in order to predict the likelihood of remission, but there has been no confirmation of their utility for such a purpose.

Continuing Treatment

I reevaluate patients taking thionamide drugs approximately every 3 months; in addition to the clinical examination, I obtain serum free T_4 (estimate) and TSH levels. If hypothyroidism occurs while the patient is on medication, I often add levothyroxine rather than reduce the dose of thionamide drug. Most patients can be maintained in a euthyroid state on 20 mg of MMI and 0.1 mg of levothyroxine, taken in a single daily dose. If PTU is employed, it usually must be given twice daily.

The use of combined thionamide and levothyroxine therapy was described by a Japanese group of researchers, who reported that 98% of patients taking both MMI and levothyroxine achieved remission. Serum TSH levels were maintained in the suppressed range; the researchers theorized that TSH inhibition with levothyroxine resulted in less stimulation of antigen release. Unfortunately, these findings have not been confirmed in subsequent studies, either in Japan or elsewhere. Nevertheless, some workers have reported improved remission rates following longer durations of thionamide administration, of up to 10 years. The practical aspects of such prolonged therapy however, are open to question.

Side Effects of Thionamide Drugs

The most common allergic effects of thionamide drugs range from mild maculopapular rashes to urticarial eruptions and occur in approximately 5% of patients. Allergic reactions usually do not occur until 2 to 4 weeks after initiation of therapy. Mild symptoms may be managed with the use of antihistamines, although in my experience complete amelioration of itching and rash is rare. Therefore, I routinely switch the patient from the type of medication causing problems (e.g., MMI) to PTU. Approximately 20% of patients will also be allergic to the other thionamide, preventing continued use of these drugs.

The most serious side effect of thionamide drugs is agranulocytosis, and although rare (occurring in 0.2 to 0.5% of patients), it is potentially fatal. Agranulocytosis usually manifests itself as fever and symptoms of infection, such as a severe sore throat. Patients must be instructed that if they develop fever and signs and symptoms of infection, they must stop the thionamide drug and call their physician immediately. A white blood cell count and differential must be performed; if agranulocytosis is diagnosed, hospital admission is required. Successful reversal of agranulocytosis, sometimes requiring the use of granulocyte colony–stimulating factor, should occur within a few days to a week.

Some physicians obtain periodic white blood cell counts, although this practice is probably unnecessary since the white count is not predictive of agranulocytosis. Nevertheless, before initiation of therapy with thionamide drugs, it is helpful to have a baseline white blood cell count, because leukopenia is frequent in patients with Graves' disease, and if a subsequent blood count is obtained, the baseline value would be useful for comparison.

Other potential side effects of antithyroid drugs include arthralgias and, rarely, hepatitis. The latter complication is also potentially fatal.

Stopping Antithyroid Drug Therapy

If therapy with thionamide drugs is used to induce remission, an end point of therapy should be determined. I usually treat for 12 to 18 months and then discontinue the thionamide agent. Patients are reevaluated approximately 4 to 6 weeks later and a serum TSH level is obtained. The presence of a suppressed serum TSH level in patients receiving thionamide drugs alone does not bode well for the likelihood of remission. However, if the patient is euthyroid at 4 to 6 weeks, the next visit is scheduled for approximately 3 months later, and at increasing intervals thereafter, but no further apart than yearly. Most relapses occur within the first year after stopping thionamide drugs but can occur at any time. If relapse occurs, a second course of thionamide drugs does not appear to increase the likelihood of remission, and ablation with radioiodine is then recommended. Some patients, however, prefer to take antithyroid drugs for several or even many years. A number of patients can be maintained on a very small dose of thionamide drug (e.g., 2.5 to 5 mg per day of MMI). Although such extended therapy is not my preference, there is no absolute contraindication to doing so. Patients on such a regimen need to be instructed that periodic follow-up, perhaps every 3 to 6 months, is necessary.

Radioactive Iodine Therapy

Ablative therapy with radioiodine (^{131}I) is the preferred method of treatment for hyperthyroidism among thyroid specialists practicing in the United States. Radioiodine ablation has distinct advantages: it is effective, relatively inexpensive, and predictable and appears to be free of side effects other than the development of hypothyroidism. Radioiodine ablation has been used for the treatment of hyperthyroidism for approximately 45 years in the United States. Careful follow-up has failed to show an increased incidence of cancer in persons who received this treatment for hyperthyroidism, or of genetic defects in offspring of patients who have received ^{131}I. Radioiodine is contraindicated during pregnancy, which should be ruled out in women of childbearing age before administration of the isotope. In addition, women who are breast-feeding should not receive radioiodine, because the isotope may recirculate in breast milk for up to several weeks after administration.

Selection of Radioiodine Dose

Some clinicians advocate administering a ^{131}I dose sufficient to control hyperthyroidism without resulting in hypothyroidism. Various strategies have been employed over the years in an effort to achieve this goal but generally have met with failure. Therefore, I prefer to administer a dose large enough to result in hypothyroidism, which will usually occur within 3 to 6 months after ^{131}I administration. A dose of 15 mCi of ^{131}I is usually sufficient to achieve this goal, but the appropriate dose is dependent on the radioactive iodine uptake and size of the thyroid gland. A 24-hour radioactive iodine uptake scan should be performed prior to administration of the treatment dose, to ensure that an adequate quantity of ^{131}I will be absorbed by the thyroid. A dose of 100 to 150 μCi per gram of thyroid tissue is generally an adequate ablative dose. Some patients are resistant to the initial dose of ^{131}I and may require a second or even third treatment. In my experience, patients of male gender and Asian patients appear to require larger or additional doses. If patients continue to be hyperthyroid 6 months following an initial treatment with radioiodine, a second dose is administered.

I usually advocate pretreatment with thionamide drugs until the patient is euthyroid, before radioiodine administration, because depletion of thyroid hormone from the thyroid prevents release of excess thyroid hormone from the gland, thereby avoiding exacerbation of hyperthyroidism. This is especially important for older patients or those with cardiovascular risk factors. Antithyroid drugs should be discontinued 3 to 5 days prior to radioiodine treatment.

Patients receiving ^{131}I who have not received pretreatment with antithyroid drugs (for example, those who are allergic to thionamides) benefit from administration of propranolol or other beta blockers after treatment, because their underlying hyperthyroidism may be transiently exacerbated by ^{131}I-induced thyroiditis.

Follow-up After Radioiodine Treatment

I usually evaluate patients approximately 6 weeks following radioiodine administration in order to assess the clinical and biochemical response. If the thyroid gland has not decreased in size by 6 weeks' time, the likelihood of a beneficial response to radioiodine is diminished. If patients are euthyroid at 6 weeks, they return 4 to 6 weeks later, and if they are hypothyroid by that time, levothyroxine therapy is begun. If patients are still euthyroid (or hyperthyroid) 3 months after therapy, they are reevaluated in another 3 months. As mentioned previously, nearly all patients are hypothyroid by 6 months after radioiodine treatment, and those who are still hyperthyroid require another treatment dose.

As experience with radioiodine has increased over the years, age limits for patients thought to be appropriate candidates for this treatment mode have decreased. It appears to be safe to treat teenagers with radioiodine, although I defer treatment in those who have not completed linear growth. There is little risk for developing thyroid nodularity in teenagers following ^{131}I treatment provided that ablative doses are administered.

Radioiodine Treatment and Ophthalmopathy

Some clinicians believe that the administration of ^{131}I to patients with Graves' ophthalmopathy may worsen the eye disease, and that administration of pharmacologic amounts of glucocorticoids for a period of a month to 6 weeks following radioiodine treatment will inhibit this occurrence. The data concerning efficacy of steroids are not conclusive. I recommend that patients with moderate symptoms and signs of eye disease be evaluated by an ophthalmologist with expertise in Graves' ophthalmopathy prior to administration of radioiodine. Indeed, it is often helpful to involve the ophthalmologist in the care of patients with ophthalmopathy, regardless of the type of treatment for hyperthyroidism.

Surgery

Surgery for Graves' hyperthyroidism is infrequently employed in the United States. Candidates for such treatment may include children and teenagers, especially those who have difficulty with compliance with antithyroid drugs. Other potential candidates may include patients with very large goiters, especially those likely to be resistant to radioiodine because of their mass. In addition, surgery is the only choice for patients who are allergic to thionamide drugs. Surgery for pregnant patients who are allergic to thionamide drugs is discussed subsequently. Finally, patients who have a coexistent thyroid nodule suspicious for cancer on fine needle aspiration should be managed surgically.

Prior to surgery, euthyroidism should be achieved, if possible, with thionamide drugs. Some surgeons prefer to administer exogenous iodides for 10 days prior to surgery. Exogenous iodides produce benefit both by inhibiting thyroid hormone release and by decreasing thyroid gland vascularity. Potassium iodide or Lugol's solution, 10 drops in a glass of water daily for 10 days, is sufficient.

Patients electing to undergo thyroidectomy should be made aware that permanent hypothyroidism will probably result, and that they will require the same type of follow-up as those treated with radioiodine ablation. If insufficient thyroid tissue is removed, persistent or recurrent hyperthyroidism will result, which then will necessitate radioiodine ablation.

Although surgery has the advantage of being rapidly curative, it also has potential complications of injury to the recurrent laryngeal nerve and the possibility of permanent hypoparathyroidism. In skilled hands, these complications occur in no more than 1 to 3% of cases, yet these potential risks must be explained fully to the patient beforehand.

Treatment of Other Forms of Hyperthyroidism

Toxic Multinodular Goiter. Toxic multinodular goiter increases in prevalence with increasing age. In elderly individuals it is a more common cause of hyperthyroidism than is Graves' disease. The diagnosis should be documented with a radioactive iodine uptake test and thyroid scan. Patients with toxic multinodular goiter will not go into remission on thionamide drugs, limiting definitive treatment to either radioiodine or surgery. Before radioiodine is employed in elderly individuals, thionamide drugs should be administered in order to minimize the risk of exacerbating hyperthyroidism. Radioiodine ablation is the treatment of choice for most individuals with toxic multinodular goiter, although surgery may be preferred for patients with especially large glands and/or with symptoms of compression who are good operative candidates. If radioiodine ablation is used for treatment of toxic multinodular goiter, the dose required is usually greater than that employed for treatment of Graves' disease.

Single Nodules. Single thyroid nodules producing hyperthyroidism occur much less often than toxic multinodular goiter and generally are seen in individuals younger than those with multinodular goiter. Although radioiodine ablation is commonly employed in such patients, surgery is usually recommended in individuals less than 25 to 30 years of age.

Special Problems

Hyperthyroidism and Pregnancy

Hyperthyroidism during pregnancy may lead to adverse outcomes for both mother and fetus. Adequate control of hyperthyroidism during pregnancy is essential. Although either MMI or PTU may be used during pregnancy, most clinicians favor the use of PTU, since it does not cross the placenta as easily as does MMI. For hyperthyroidism that is difficult to control, or if there is allergy to antithyroid drugs, thyroidectomy should be performed during the second trimester. Beta-blocking agents may be given safely during pregnancy to control symptoms.

Patients who continue to receive thionamide drugs during pregnancy should have a thyroid-stimulating immunoglobulin level drawn during the last trimester, in order to predict the possible occurrence of neonatal hyperthyroidism. Hyperthyroid pregnant individuals should be evaluated carefully at least every 4 to 6 weeks, and there should be close communication between the endocrinologist and the obstetrician. It is advisable to use a dose of thionamide drug as low as possible to maintain maternal euthyroidism.

Thyroid Storm

Thyroid storm (or crisis) is characterized by severe manifestations of hyperthyroidism, fever, and altered mental status. The disorder is usually precipitated by a concurrent illness.

Early recognition and treatment of thyroid storm are essential, because it is a life-threatening condition. Patients must be managed in the intensive care unit, and in addition to the usual supportive measures, treatment of any concurrent illness and aggressive pharmacologic management of the hyperthyroidism are necessary. Either MMI or PTU may be used, although as mentioned previously, PTU has a potential advantage of reducing production of T_3 from T_4. A dose of 150 mg of PTU every 6 hours, or 15 to 20 mg of MMI every 8 hours, is usually sufficient. For persons unable to take medication orally (PO), MMI may be crushed and given by nasogastric tube or may be prepared by the pharmacy as a rectal suppository.

In addition to thionamide drugs, exogenous iodides should be administered. I prefer iopanoic acid for this purpose, because it not only will inhibit thyroid hormone release but has the additional advantage of being a potent inhibitor of T_4 to T_3 conversion. A dose of 500 mg to 1 gram orally daily is sufficient. Alternatively, iodine can be administered in the form of Lugol's solution or saturated solution of potassium iodide, 10 drops in water three times daily, or sodium iodide, 500 mg intravenously every 12 hours. It is essential to administer the first dose of thionamide drug a few hours prior to administration of iodides, in order to prevent further organification of iodide with resultant additional thyroid hormone production. Some clinicians also use pharmacologic doses of glucocorticoids, in order to further inhibit T_4 to T_3 conversion, although their clinical efficacy has not been convincingly shown.

Beta-blocking agents, preferably propranolol, are essential in the management of thyroid storm, and may be given either PO or intravenously (IV). If the latter route is used, 1 mg every 5 to 10 minutes is given IV until the heart rate is below 100 beats per minute. Once adequate blockade is achieved, oral propranolol may be given, and doses of up to 160 mg or greater every 6 hours are not uncommon. Heart failure, which may be due in part to uncontrolled tachycardia, must be treated with adequate digitalization. If diuretics are used they must be administered very cautiously, because patients with thyroid storm have peripheral vasodilatation and may suffer vascular collapse if conventional doses of diuretics are given. Plasmapheresis has been described as a treatment for thyroid storm, although I have neither used it nor seen it employed for this purpose.

ACKNOWLEDGMENT

The author is grateful to Elsa C. Ahumada for her expert secretarial assistance.

THYROID CANCER

method of
ERNEST L. MAZZAFERRI, M.D.
Ohio State University College of Medicine
Columbus, Ohio

Thyroid cancer comprises only about 1% of all newly diagnosed malignancies in the United States, afflicting women more than twice as frequently as men and occurring at all ages. Its prevalence is high, however, because most patients do not die of the disease. In fact, it has the best survival rate of all cancers except skin cancer. Mortality rates are not uniformly low, however, and recurrence rates are paradoxically high, which causes considerable anxiety among patients, many of whom are very young at the time of diagnosis. In 1997, for example, more than 16,000 new cases were diagnosed, and about 10% of these were in people under age 30, while about 1200 people died of thyroid cancer, resulting in 5- and 10-year relative survival rates of around 95% and 90%, respectively. Although survival has improved significantly over that in years past, it varies substantially with different types of thyroid cancer.

The only known cause of thyroid cancer is head or neck irradiation. External beam radiation was widely used in the past to treat benign head and neck conditions in children and young adults, increasing the incidence of thyroid cancer as much as 100-fold for 30 years after the exposure. A major outbreak of thyroid cancer has occurred among the children of Belarus as the result of the 1986 nuclear reactor accident in Chernobyl. Occasionally, a predisposition to develop thyroid cancer is inherited as an autosomal dominant trait. Most patients with thyroid cancer, however, have no obvious predisposition to the disease.

CLASSIFICATION OF THYROID TUMORS

The current classification of thyroid tumors is shown in Table 1. Thyroid malignancies arise from distinctly different thyroid cells that have different embryologic origins, giving them different functional and clinical characteristics. Most tumors arise from thyroid follicular cells, which originate from the embryonic foregut, produce thyroglobulin (Tg), and concentrate iodine, features used in their diagnosis and treatment. A few cancers arise from thyroid C cells, which derive from the embryonic neural crest, produce calcitonin and other peptides, but do not concentrate iodine. Other cell types in the thyroid gland rarely give rise to malignancies such as sarcomas or thyroid lymphoma.

DIAGNOSIS OF THYROID CANCER

Early diagnosis of thyroid cancer is essential to its management because prognosis is significantly better when the tumor is identified at an early stage. Thyroid cancer usually is manifested as a thyroid nodule. Diagnosing cancer is problematic, however, because thyroid nodules are very common and most are benign. For example, palpable thyroid nodules increase in frequency from a prevalence of around 1% during the first 2 decades of life to about 5% after age 50. Many more are found when the thyroid is examined by ultrasound, which detects nodules in about half the general population. Most nodules so discovered are small benign nodules, referred to as "incidentalomas," that require no evaluation. This is why a palpably normal thyroid should not be imaged with ultrasonography in an asymptomatic patient.

Finding the few thyroid cancers among the many benign thyroid nodules is like finding a needle in a haystack. To make matters even more difficult, the prevalence of small (less than 1.0 cm in diameter), clinically insignificant papillary thyroid cancers (microcarcinomas) is estimated to be around 5% among the general population. Microcarcinomas pose no threat to life and never become apparent during life unless the thyroid gland is surgically removed for benign disease or they are discovered incidentally by ultrasonography, CT imaging, or MRI done for another reason.

Most thyroid cancers present as an asymptomatic thyroid nodule. However, any symptom that suggests tissue invasion, such as hoarseness, dysphagia, or hemoptysis, or any hint that a nodule is enlarging merits further investigation. A history of previous therapeutic head or neck irradiation or a family history of thyroid cancer is also important.

TABLE 1. **Classification of Thyroid Tumors**

	Benign	Malignant
Epithelial	Follicular adenoma	Follicular thyroid carcinoma (FTC)
	Simple (colloid)	Hürthle cell variant
	Fetal (microfollicular)	Papillary thyroid carcinoma (PTC)
	Oxyphil (Hürthle cell)	Pure papillary
	Embryonal cell	Papillary-follicular
	Atypical adenoma	Microcarcinoma
	Other adenomas	Tall cell variant
	Papillary	Columnar cell variant
	Signet ring cell	Solid variant
		Diffuse sclerosing
		Medullary thyroid carcinoma (MTC)
		Sporadic
		Familial
		Multiple endocrine neoplasia (MEN)
		Type 2A (MEN 2A)
		MTC
		Pheochromocytoma
		Hyperparathyroidism
		Type 2B (MEN 2B)
		MTC
		Pheochromocytoma
		Mucosal neuroma phenotype
		Familial MTC (FMTC) (without other tumors)
		Anaplastic thyroid carcinoma
Nonepithelial		Thyroid lymphoma
		Sarcomas
		Teratomas
Nonthyroidal		Metastatic cancer (e.g., breast)

Careful inspection and palpation of the neck usually reveal a thyroid nodule that moves upward with swallowing. Sometimes, however, a metastatic cervical lymph node is the only sign of cancer. A palpably hard or fixed thyroid nodule, or evidence that cancer is invading neck structures such as the recurrent laryngeal nerve, or the presence of large (greater than 2 cm) cervical lymph nodes, is almost always a sign of malignancy. Hoarseness due to vocal cord paralysis is an especially important sign. The likelihood of malignancy is well above 50% when one of these signs is present, although most cancers are asymptomatic without evidence of malignancy on examination.

A palpable thyroid nodule or one larger than 1.0 cm in diameter discovered by serendipity with ultrasound, *whether occurring in an otherwise normal gland or in a multinodular goiter*, should undergo biopsy. Fine-needle aspiration (FNA) biopsy is the first-line diagnostic test (Figure 1). It usually yields adequate material for cytologic diagnosis, which is categorized as benign, malignant, or indeterminate (suspicious). Papillary thyroid cancer is almost always identified correctly by FNA. Follicular cancer and adenoma usually cannot be differentiated from each other by FNA, however, and the cytology specimen is termed indeterminate or the tumor is designated as a follicular tumor. Distinction between the two requires examination of the tumor capsule and blood vessels for invasion by cancer cells. Other thyroid malignancies usually can be identified by FNA.

No further testing other than a serum thyroid-stimulating hormone (TSH) measurement is usually necessary. Thyroid ^{123}I scans provide no diagnostic information and are not obtained unless the cytology is indeterminate, because a hyperfunctional (hot) nodule is usually evidence of a benign follicular tumor. Computed tomography (CT) scanning or magnetic resonance imaging (MRI) is not done unless there is evidence of tumor invasion or substernal extension of the tumor.

Surgery is advised for all patients with thyroid cancer diagnosed by FNA and for those with an indeterminate cytology, because about 20% of the latter are follicular cancers unless the nodule is hyperfunctional.

PAPILLARY AND FOLLICULAR THYROID CANCER

The goal of therapy is to render the patient free of disease, an end point usually measured by serum Tg determinations and total body ^{131}I scans. When a cure of thyroid cancer is not possible, long-term palliation usually is achievable.

Prognostic Factors

Three main features determine prognosis: the patient's age at the time of diagnosis, the tumor stage (determined by primary tumor size, invasion of cancer into the surrounding tissues, and metastases), and effective treatment of the disease. Primary tumors smaller than 1.5 cm in diameter have a good prognosis, even with less than total thyroid ablation, while larger tumors are more likely to recur and cause death. Tumors that invade the soft tissues have an especially poor prognosis. Lymph node metastases are associated with high recurrence rates and increase cancer mortality rates when they are bilateral or involve mediastinal nodes. Histologic features such as the tall cell and columnar cell papillary variants and the Hürthle cell variant in follicular cancers worsen prognosis.

Prognosis becomes progressively worse in patients older than 40 years at the time of diagnosis. For this reason, some tumor prognosticating schemes use age and tumor stage to predict outcome. Although patients under age 40 have low cancer mortality rates,

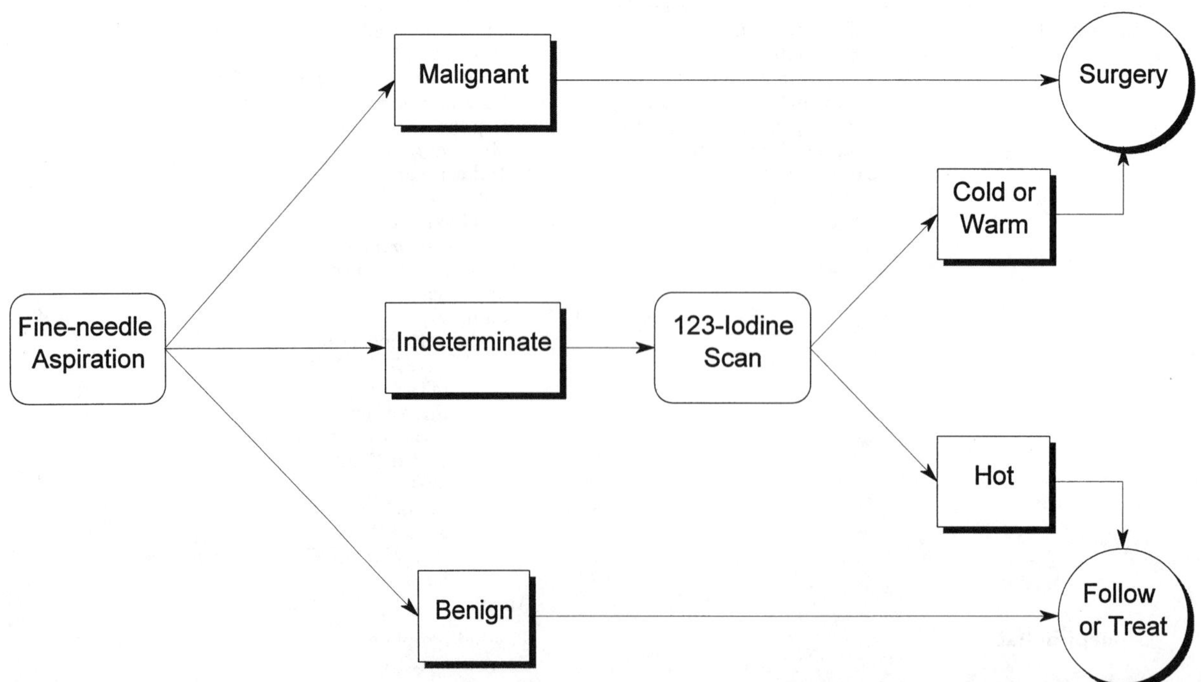

Figure 1. Algorithm showing the work-up of a thyroid nodule. A hot nodule concentrates most or all of the radioiodine, whereas a cold nodule concentrates none and a warm nodule traps iodine with the same avidity as normal thyroid tissue.

tumor recurrence rates are paradoxically high during the first two decades of life and after age 60. The tumor-node-metastasis (TNM) staging system and others that use age in predicting prognosis thus accurately predict cancer death but do not identify patients who are likely to have a recurrence, which leads to undertreatment of young patients with thyroid cancer.

Thyroid Surgery

The mainstay of initial treatment is surgery. When the diagnosis is known before surgery, regardless of the preoperative estimate of tumor stage, I recommend total or near-total thyroidectomy, whereby the surgeon leaves less than 2 grams of thyroid tissue. Some prefer less extensive thyroidectomy, which I do not advise. Involved lymph nodes in the central and lateral neck compartments are excised, but radical neck dissection is unnecessary unless tumor is invading the neck muscles and cannot otherwise be resected. When the diagnosis of thyroid cancer is uncertain, for example, with indeterminate FNA cytology, intraoperative frozen section diagnosis usually does not provide more accurate information, and a lobectomy is generally done. If follicular cancer is found on final pathologic examination, which happens in about 20% of cases with indeterminate cytology, completion thyroidectomy is performed within a few days. I generally advise completion thyroidectomy for tumors that are larger than 1.5 cm or are multicentric, or are invading soft tissues or accompanied by any metastases.

Radioactive Iodine

Radioactive iodine (^{131}I) is used to ablate normal thyroid remnant tissue and to destroy residual thyroid cancer that is not amenable to surgical removal.

RADIOACTIVE IODINE SCANS

Whole body radioiodine scans are done about 6 weeks after surgery and are most useful when there is little or no residual normal thyroid tissue. When large amounts of normal thyroid tissue remain in the neck, the serum TSH level often does not rise enough for performance of a scan and the test should be postponed until the remnant is destroyed. With a large thyroid remnant, the scan usually shows a starburst effect of high ^{131}I uptake in the neck, making visualization of uptake elsewhere impossible. A small amount of radioiodine uptake is seen in most patients after surgery.

For effective scanning with radioactive iodine, the serum TSH level must be above 30 μU per mL and the total body burden of iodine must be low. This is achieved with a low-iodine diet and by withdrawing thyroid hormone after 4 weeks. One method is to administer liothyronine (Cytomel), 1.0 μg per kg daily for 4 weeks after surgery. This is given as 25 μg orally two to three times a day,* depending upon the patient's age and general health. Lower doses are given to elderly patients or those with heart disease. Another way to raise the serum TSH level is to administer 50 μg of levothyroxine (Synthroid) daily for 4 weeks. After 4 weeks of liothyronine, the drug is discontinued for 2 weeks until the TSH rises above 30 μU per mL; with levothyroxine, the low dose may be continued until the scan day, provided the TSH rises above 30 μU per mL.

Scans are done with quantitative radiation dose estimates at 24, 48, and 72 hours after the oral administration of 2 mCi of ^{131}I. There has been concern about the "stunning" effect of such diagnostic scans, which impairs the uptake of therapeutic ^{131}I given shortly afterward. Some investigators now perform diagnostic scans with ^{123}I, although the optimal method for the use of this isotope has not yet been established.

RECOMBINANT HUMAN TSH

Recombinant human TSH (hrTSH) (Thyrogen) should soon be available for clinical use. In extensive studies in the United States and Europe, injection of hrTSH was almost as effective as withholding thyroid hormone in raising serum TSH concentrations and inducing ^{131}I uptake in normal and malignant thyroid tissues. Two daily injections of 10 units stimulates thyroid ^{131}I uptake in patients with low serum TSH concentrations almost as much as that seen with 2 or 3 weeks of thyroid hormone withdrawal. The side effects appear to be minimal. The initial studies were aimed at demonstrating the efficacy of hrTSH in ^{131}I scanning, and the drug has not yet been tested for use in treating patients with ^{131}I.

LOW-IODINE DIET

A low-iodine diet of about 50 μg daily can raise ^{131}I uptake and can double the rads per 100 mCi of ^{131}I administered, although total body radiation after therapeutic ^{131}I may be increased. This diet can be very tedious for the patient, but a daily iodine intake of 50 μg can be achieved by restricting the use of iodized salt, dairy products, eggs, and seafood. Patients should check the labels of prepared foods for algae derivatives and all breads for iodate, should avoid all red-colored foods and medicines, and should not eat in restaurants if possible. The diet should be started 2 weeks before ^{131}I scanning and continued for several days thereafter. More complex regimens that include diuretics can be used but are usually unnecessary.

RADIOIODINE ABLATION OF THYROID REMNANT TISSUE

Some thyroid tissue usually remains after surgery, regardless of the extent of thyroidectomy, which leaves the serum Tg detectable and a measurable uptake of radioiodine in the thyroid bed. Ablation of the thyroid remnant increases the sensitivity of serum Tg measurements and thyroid radioiodine scanning in the detection of cancer. Remnant ablation reduces the risk of cancer recurrence and lowers the mortality in high-risk patients, suggesting that it

*Exceeds dosage recommended by the manufacturer.

eradicates microscopic thyroid cancer. The thyroid remnant may be effectively destroyed with 30 mCi of ^{131}I, although some prefer larger doses.

RADIOIODINE TREATMENT OF THYROID CANCER

When thyroid cancer persists or recurs after initial therapy, surgical extirpation is the treatment of choice if the tumor is amenable to surgery. However, ^{131}I therapy is usually required preoperatively. Preparation for therapy is similar to that for postoperative scanning, although a scan may not be necessary before ^{131}I therapy. After thyroid ablation, the decision to treat with ^{131}I is largely based upon the serum Tg level (Figure 2). Doses of ^{131}I range from 30 to 200 mCi, although larger doses may be given. The main complications of ^{131}I therapy are intermittent parotid gland swelling, which may be suggestive of a Stensen's duct stone; transient glossitis and diminished taste; sudden tumor swelling, which may be a serious problem if it occurs in the brain or spinal cord; and gonadal damage. Leukemia may rarely occur when large cumulative doses of ^{131}I are given (usually over 800 mCi); however, studies show the risk of leukemia after ^{131}I is far less than of dying of thyroid cancer when ^{131}I is withheld. Although there is no upper dose limit for ^{131}I, treatment doses are usually less than 200 mCi and the cumulative dose is usually limited to 500 mCi in children and 800 mCi in adults, unless the patient has serious regional disease or distant metastases that continue to concentrate ^{131}I.

LITHIUM

Lithium* (Eskalith) may rarely be used to enhance tumor retention of ^{131}I, which it does by decreasing the release of iodine from both the thyroid and tumors. Lithium usually is unnecessary when the thyroid tumor concentrates ^{131}I well. Given at a dosage of 400 to 800 mg daily (10 mg per kg) for 7 days, lithium increases uptake in metastatic lesions while only slightly increasing ^{131}I uptake in normal tissue. It therefore is not useful in thyroid remnant ablation. Serum lithium concentrations should be measured daily and maintained between 0.8 and 1.2 nmol per L. The radiation dose to tumors in which the biologic half-life of iodine is short (less than 6 days) is maximized without increasing radiation to other organs.

Serum Tg Measurements

Thyroglobulin originates from only normal or neoplastic thyroid tissue and thus serves as a sensitive marker for cancer when all normal thyroid tissue has been ablated. Serum Tg is measured by radioimmunoassay (RIA) or immunometric assay (IMA). The lower limit of detection is around 1 to 3 ng per mL by RIA and about 0.5 ng per mL by IMA. Circulating serum anti-Tg antibodies, which are present in about 10 to 15% of patients, interfere with the measurement of thyroglobulin, falsely raising the serum Tg level in most RIAs and lowering it in most IMAs. Serum anti-Tg antibodies thus interfere sufficiently to make the serum Tg results quantitatively uncertain. Serum Tg levels rise in response to TSH stimulation. Depending upon the assay, serum Tg levels of less than 5 ng per mL by RIA or about 0.5 ng per mL by IMA usually indicate that the patient is free of disease. When the serum TSH concentration is raised by thyroid hormone withdrawal, serum Tg levels under 10 ng per mL usually indicate that the patient is free of disease, whereas higher levels usually indicate that residual thyroid tissue is present, either in the thyroid bed or elsewhere. Serum Tg levels above 40 ng per mL almost always indicate distant metastases. Serum Tg thus has assumed a central role in the management of papillary and follicular thyroid cancer (see Figure 2). In some instances, serum Tg is high, but x-ray studies, CT scans, and diagnostic scans are negative, and tumor is visualized only on scanning after large (100 mCi) treatment doses of ^{131}I have been administered. Distant metastases found in this way are usually associated with serum Tg levels above 40 ng per mL and have a high rate of cure.

*Not FDA approved for this indication.

MEDULLARY THYROID CARCINOMA

Medullary thyroid carcinoma (MTC) arises from the thyroid C cell, which secretes calcitonin. Most such cancers are unilateral sporadic tumors, but about 20% are bilateral familial tumors associated with C cell hyperplasia, a forerunner of MTC. This cancer occurs in four settings, each with its own clinical features and prognosis: (1) The most common is sporadic MTC. The three familial forms, which are transmitted as autosomal dominant traits caused by a mutation in the centromeric region of chromosome 10, are as follows: (2) MEN type 2A, comprising MTC, pheochromocytoma and hyperparathyroidism (HPT), which is the most common familial form; (3) MEN type 2B, comprising MTC, pheochromocytoma, and a mucosal neuroma phenotype that also can occur as a sporadic tumor; and (4) familial MTC (FMTC), which is the least common familial form.

Diagnosis

Screening patients with basal and provocative tests for serum calcitonin can identify C cell hyperplasia or MTC. Calcitonin release may be stimulated with pentagastrin (Peptavlon) and calcium, given alone or together, or by a rise in endogenous gastrin provoked with omeprazole (Prilosec), Calcitonin is usually measured before and at 2, 5, 7, 10, and 15 minutes after an intravenous bolus of pentagastrin* (0.5 μg per kg of body weight). Calcium (2 mg of elemental calcium per kg, infused over 60 seconds) can be given alone or may be followed by pentagastrin infusion. Endogenous gastrin is stimulated with oral omeprazole, 30 mg twice daily for 3 days.† Depending upon the calcitonin antibody used, the serum calcitonin level rises about fivefold in patients with MTC or C cell hyperplasia if the basal calcitonin

*Not FDA approved for this indication.
†Exceeds dosage recommended by the manufacturer.

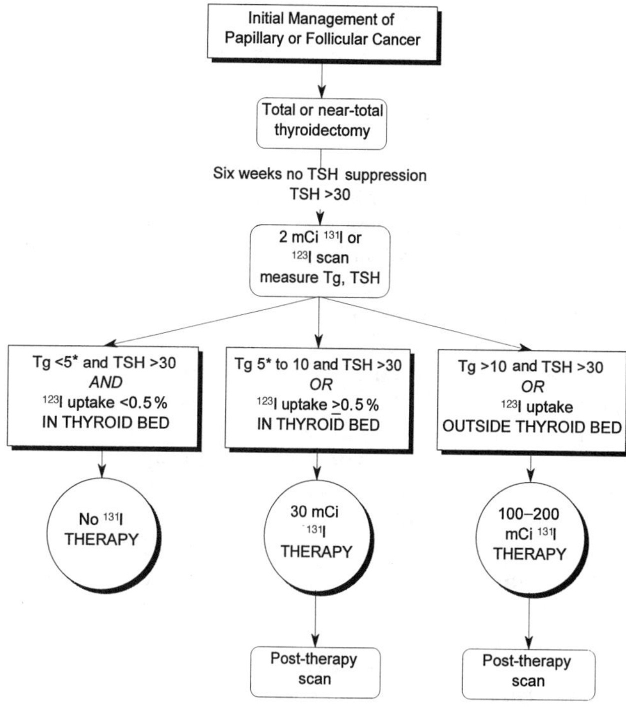

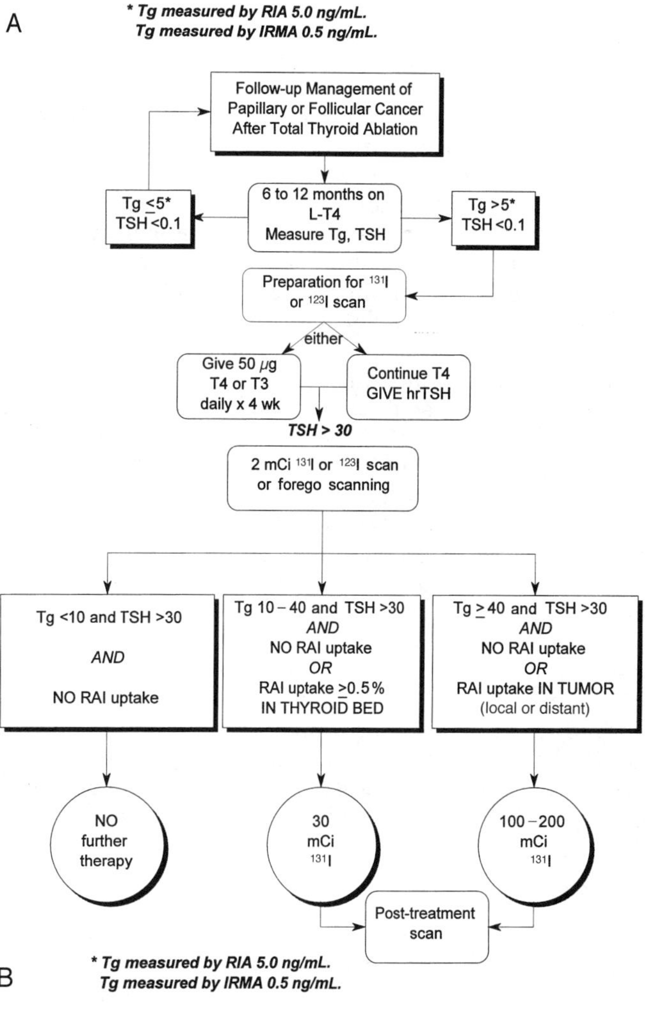

Figure 2. *A*, Algorithm showing the initial management of a patient with papillary or follicular thyroid cancer. Thyroglobulin may be measured by radioimmunoassay (RIA) or immunometric assay (IMA). *B*, Algorithm showing management of papillary and follicular thyroid cancer after the thyroid has been ablated with surgery and ^{131}I therapy. *Abbreviations:* L-T4 = levothyroxine; hrTSH = human recombinant thyroid–stimulating hormone; TSH = thyroid-stimulating hormone; Tg = thyroglobulin; RAI = radioactive iodine; RIA = radioimmunoassay.

level is minimally elevated. However, familial cases are now diagnosed by genetic screening.

Germline mutations in the *RET* proto-oncogene, which codes for a receptor tyrosine kinase, cause familial MTC and can be used to identify affected kindred members at an early age before MTC is manifested. Point mutations in one of five cysteine codons (609, 611, 618, and 620 in exon 10 and 634 in exon 11), which encode part of the extracellular cysteine-rich domain, are found in the majority of families with MEN 2A and FMTC. Mutations in two codons (768 in exon 13 and 804 in exon 14) within the intracellular tyrosine kinase domain of *RET* have been identified in FMTC. MEN 2B is associated with mutation of a single codon (918 in exon 16) that lies in yet another area of the tyrosine kinase domain. There is a statistically significant association between the presence of any mutation in codon 634 and the presence of pheochromocytoma and HPT. Other genotype-phenotype correlations coexist and may prove useful in management. When a mutation is identified and confirmed in a kindred member, thyroidectomy is done at an early age, usually at around age 5 years, before MTC has developed (Figure 3).

Prognosis

MTC is much more aggressive than papillary or follicular thyroid cancer and has a mortality rate of about 35% at 10 years. The survival is substantially worse in patients with sporadic tumors or in those with metastases at the time of diagnosis, in patients with MEN 2B phenotype, and in patients older than 50 at the time of diagnosis. Conversely, early detection and treatment have a profound impact on the clinical course of MTC: the 10-year survival rate in patients with MTC confined to the thyroid is similar to that in unaffected subjects, compared with about 45% in those with nodal metastases. Patients who undergo thyroidectomy during the first decade of life generally have no evidence of residual disease postoperatively, whereas MTC persists in about one third of patients operated on in the second decade, and the frequency of failed surgery gradually increases with age until the seventh decade, when about two thirds of patients have persistent disease after surgery. This is largely due to the clinical stage of the disease at the time of thyroidectomy. Before 1970, when calcitonin testing was not done, MTC was usually diagnosed in the fifth or sixth decade of life. With periodic calcitonin screening, affected patients in an MTC kindred are diagnosed at a much earlier stage, usually in the second decade or earlier, when they have C cell hyperplasia or microscopic cancer. With genetic testing, affected individuals now can be identified at birth.

Therapy

Surgery offers the only chance for cure and should be performed as soon as the disease is detected. Before thyroidectomy, however, pheochromocytoma must be carefully searched for and excised when detected. The treatment of MTC confined to the neck is total thyroidectomy, because the disease is often bilateral, even in patients with a negative family history, who are often unsuspected relatives or represent the index case of affected kindreds. Cervical lymph node metastases occur early in the course of the disease, adversely influencing survival, and the involved nodes should be dissected when they contain tumor, although routine radical neck dissection is not recommended.

Inoperable tumor is palliatively treated with external radiation therapy when the tumor is localized, and with doxorubicin or other chemotherapy combinations when tumor is widespread and life-threatening. Although it is not routinely given, ^{131}I has been reported to be effective in a few patients.

The response to therapy is assessed by measuring serum calcitonin levels, which may require up to 6 months to normalize. Persistent modest basal calcitonin elevation is often seen for years after surgery in patients, particularly those with MEN 2A who have no other evidence of disease. In those with extremely high serum calcitonin levels postoperatively, metastases can be localized by CT, radiolabeled octreotide, and venous catheterization studies.

ANAPLASTIC THYROID CANCER

Anaplastic thyroid cancer is distinguished by its rapid growth and poor prognosis. It comprises less than 5% of all thyroid cancers and has been declining in frequency, perhaps because of early diagnosis and treatment of benign tumors and well-differentiated thyroid carcinomas, which are often forerunners of anaplastic thyroid cancer. Its incidence peaks in the fifth decade of life, with both sexes being affected about equally. It is almost always manifested as a rapidly enlarging and symptomatic neck mass in a patient who may or may not have had an antecedent goiter. The trachea and other neck structures are often invaded and compressed, causing dyspnea and dysphagia. The tumor is typically hard, poorly circumscribed, and fixed to surrounding structures. Mortality rates are around 60% at 6 months, and few patients survive for more than a year.

Total or near-total thyroidectomy with resection of the involved neck tissues and cervical nodes should be done when possible. The airway is often compromised, and more than half the patients require a tracheostomy at some time during the clinical course. The best therapeutic results have been obtained when surgery, external irradiation, and chemotherapy, usually with doxorubicin, are combined.

THYROID LYMPHOMA

Primary thyroid lymphoma is an uncommon disorder comprising less than 5% of all thyroid malignancies, which has been increasing in frequency. It is a potentially life-threatening disorder that, unlike anaplastic thyroid cancer, may respond well to therapy. These tumors must be differentiated from small cell anaplastic thyroid cancers, most of which are

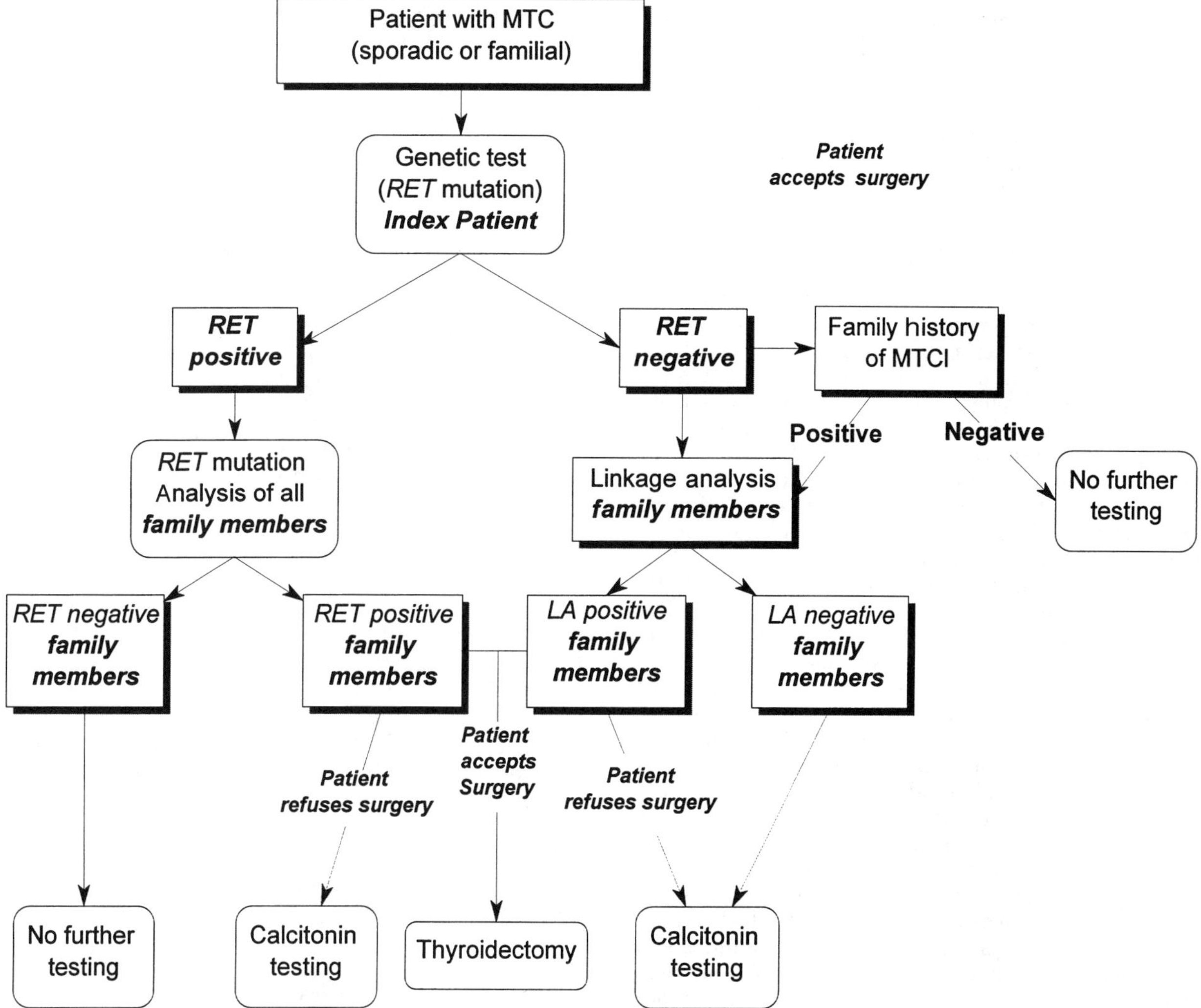

Figue 3. Algorithm for screening patients and family members of an affected kindred for medullary thyroid cancer (MTC). If *RET*-positive family members refuse surgery, they should undergo yearly calcitonin testing, although this is a less certain method than genetic testing for MTC.

actually misdiagnosed thyroid lymphomas. This is predominantly a disease of older women, possibly because it occurs in the setting of chronic lymphocytic thyroiditis. Its peak incidence is in the seventh decade, and most cases occur after age 50, usually with coexistent Hashimoto's disease, and sometimes with long-standing hypothyroidism. Prognosis depends upon tumor stage and grade.

The diagnosis should be suspected when a patient with Hashimoto's disease develops a rapidly enlarging goiter or a thyroid nodule, often in the face of long-standing hypothyroidism and thyroid hormone therapy. Patients typically have airway compromise, the diagnosis and treatment of which are urgent.

Open biopsy is performed to verify the diagnosis, with tracheostomy to protect the airway if necessary. Radiotherapy is the mainstay of treatment, often combined with chemotherapy. The latter is important because thyroid lymphoma is associated with recurrence rates as high as 50%. Most chemotherapy regimens consist of cyclophosphamide (Cytoxan), doxorubicin (Adriamycin), vincristine (Oncovin), and prednisone, with or without bleomycin (Blenoxane) (CHOP ± bleomycin). With this regimen, the overall 5-year survival and disease-free survival rates are about 70% and 65%, respectively.

PHEOCHROMOCYTOMA

method of
WILLIAM F. YOUNG, Jr., M.D.
Mayo Medical School and Mayo Clinic
Rochester, Minnesota

Pheochromocytoma is a tumor frequently sought and rarely found. It is associated with spectacular cardiovascular disturbances, and when correctly diagnosed and properly treated, it is curable; when undiagnosed or improperly treated, it can be fatal. Catecholamine-producing tumors that arise from chromaffin cells of the adrenal medulla and sympathetic ganglia are termed "pheochromocytomas" and "paragangliomas," respectively. However, the term "pheochromocytoma" has become the generic name for all catecholamine-producing tumors and is used in this article to refer to both adrenal pheochromocytomas and paragangliomas.

PRESENTATION

Prevalence estimates for pheochromocytoma range from 0.01 to 0.1% of the hypertensive population, with an incidence of 2 to 8 cases per million people per year. These tumors occur equally in men and women, manifesting primarily in the third through fifth decades. Patients harboring these tumors may be asymptomatic. However, symptoms usually are present and are due to the pharmacologic effects of excess circulating catecholamines. Episodic symptoms include abrupt onset of throbbing headaches, generalized diaphoresis, palpitations, anxiety, chest pain, and abdominal pain. These "spells" can be extremely variable in their presentation and may be spontaneous or precipitated by postural changes, anxiety, exercise, or maneuvers that increase intra-abdominal pressure. The pheochromocytoma spell may last 10 to 60 minutes and may occur daily to monthly. The clinical signs include hypertension (paroxysmal in half of the patients and sustained in the other half), orthostatic hypotension, pallor, grade I to IV retinopathy, tremor, and fever. Pheochromocytoma of the urinary bladder is associated with painless hematuria and paroxysmal attacks induced by micturition or bladder distention. Frequently, patients are diagnosed with possible pheochromocytoma before they are symptomatic because of genetic screening for hereditary endocrine syndromes or incidental discovery of adrenal masses on computerized abdominal imaging. These patients may harbor catecholamine-synthesizing neoplasms that are detected months or years before the onset of periodic hypersecretory states. Ten percent of the cases of benign sporadic adrenal pheochromocytoma that are diagnosed at the Mayo Clinic present as adrenal incidentalomas. In addition, in five separate reports and a total of 1488 patients with adrenal incidentalomas, the "clinically silent" adrenal pheochromocytomas constituted an average of 2.6% of cases studied.

DIAGNOSIS

The diagnostic approach to catecholamine-producing tumors is divided into two series of studies (Figure 1). First, the diagnosis of a catecholamine-producing tumor must be suspected and then confirmed biochemically by the presence of increased urine or plasma concentrations of catecholamines or their metabolites. Suppression testing with clonidine (Catapres) or provocative testing with glucagon, histamine, or metoclopramide (Reglan) is rarely needed. The differential diagnosis for pheochromocytoma spells is summarized in Table 1.

The next step is to localize the catecholamine-producing tumor to guide the surgical approach. Computer-assisted adrenal and abdominal imaging, by magnetic resonance imaging (MRI) or computed tomography (CT), is the first localization test. Approximately 90% of these tumors are found in the adrenals and 98% are in the abdomen. If results of the abdominal imaging studies are negative, then scintigraphic localization with [^{123}I]meta-iodobenzylguanidine (^{123}I-MIBG) is indicated. This radiopharmaceutical accumulates preferentially in catecholamine-producing tumors; however, this procedure is not as sensitive as was initially hoped (sensitivity 85%, specificity 99%). Computer-assisted chest, neck, and head imaging procedures are additional localizing modalities that can be used, although they are rarely required. Thorough discussions of the diagnostic investigation of catecholamine-producing tumors are found elsewhere.

PRINCIPLES OF TREATMENT

The treatment of choice for pheochromocytoma is surgical resection. Most of these tumors are benign and can be totally excised. However, the hypertension is usually cured by excision of the tumor. Careful preoperative pharmacologic preparation to reverse the chronic and acute effects of excess circulating catecholamines is crucial to successful treatment.

Preoperative Management

Combined alpha-adrenergic and beta-adrenergic blockade is required preoperatively to control blood pressure and to prevent intraoperative hypertensive crises. Alpha-adrenergic blockade should be started at least 10 days preoperatively to allow for expansion of the contracted blood volume. A liberal-salt diet is advised during the preoperative period. Once adequate alpha-adrenergic blockade is achieved, beta-adrenergic blockade is initiated (e.g., 3 days preoperatively). With this approach, only 7% of patients undergoing pheochromocytoma resection at the Mayo Clinic have needed postoperative hemodynamic management.

Alpha-Adrenergic Blockade

Phenoxybenzamine (Dibenzyline) is an irreversible, long-acting alpha-adrenergic blocking agent (Table 2). Approximately 25% of an oral dose of phenoxybenzamine is absorbed. Phenoxybenzamine is available as 10-mg capsules. The initial dosage of phenoxybenzamine is 10 mg orally (PO) two times daily; the dosage is increased by 10 to 20 mg every 2 to 3 days as needed to control the blood pressure and spells. The effects of daily administration are cumulative for nearly a week. The average dosage of phenoxybenzamine is 20 to 100 mg per day. Side effects include postural hypotension, tachycardia, miosis, nasal congestion, inhibition of ejaculation in men, diarrhea, and fatigue. Prazosin (Minipress), terazosin (Hytrin), and doxazosin (Cardura) are selective alpha$_1$-adrenergic blocking agents; because of the more favorable side effect profiles of these agents, they may be preferable to phenoxybenzamine when long-term pharmacologic treatment is indicated (e.g., for metastatic pheochromocytoma). However, phenoxybenzamine is the preferred drug for preoperative preparation because it provides alpha-adrenergic blockade of long duration. Effective alpha-adrenergic blockade permits expansion of blood volume, which usually is severely decreased as a result of excessive adrenergic vasoconstriction.

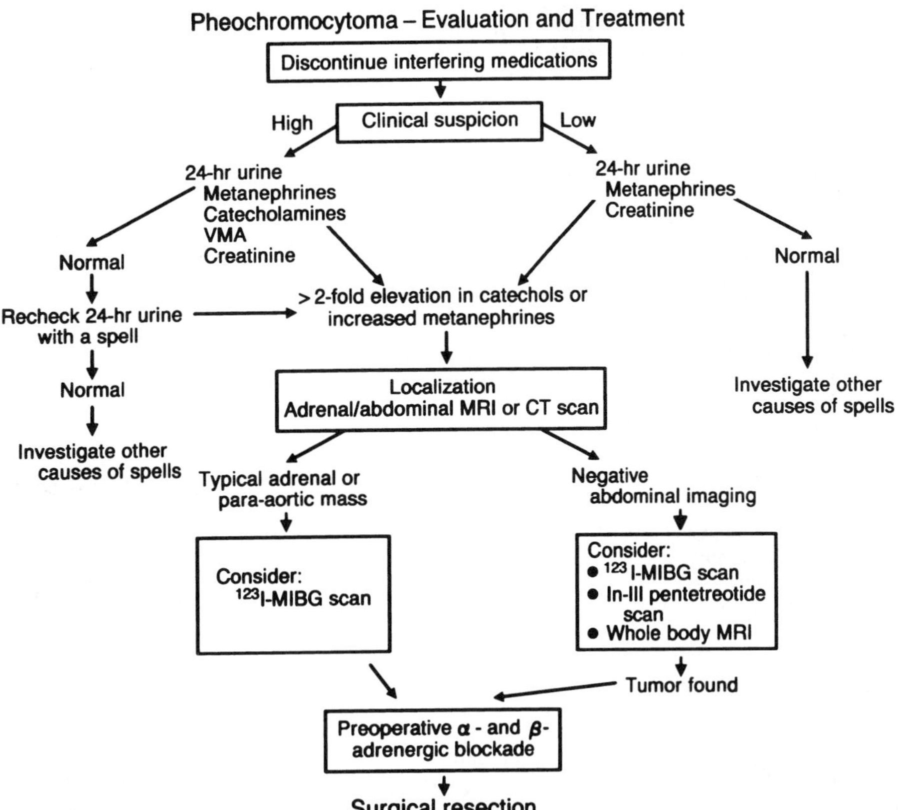

Figure 1. Evaluation and treatment of catecholamine-producing tumors. Clinical suspicion is triggered by the following: paroxysmal symptoms (especially hypertension); hypertension that is intermittent, unusually labile, or resistant to treatment; family history of pheochromocytoma or associated conditions; or an incidentally discovered adrenal mass. The details are discussed in the text. *Abbreviations:* VMA = vanillylmandelic acid; CT = computed tomography; MRI = magnetic resonance imaging; ^{123}I-MIBG = ^{123}I-meta-iodobenzylguanidine. (Modified with permission from Young WF Jr: Pheochromocytoma: 1926–1993. Trends In Endocrinology and Metabolism, Vol 4. New York, Elsevier Science, Inc., 1993, p 122).

Beta-Adrenergic Blockade

The beta-adrenergic antagonist should be administered only after alpha-adrenergic blockade has been effected, because beta-adrenergic blockade alone may result in more severe hypertension, owing to the unopposed alpha-adrenergic stimulation. Preoperative beta-adrenergic blockade is indicated to control the tachycardia associated with both the high circulating catecholamine concentrations and the alpha-adrenergic blockade. Caution is indicated if the patient is asthmatic or has congestive heart failure. Chronic catecholamine excess can produce a myocardiopathy, and beta-adrenergic blockade can result in acute pulmonary edema. Noncardioselective beta-adrenergic blockers such as propranolol (Inderal and Inderal LA) and nadolol* (Corgard) or cardioselective beta-adrenergic blockers such as atenolol* (Tenormin) and metoprolol* (Lopressor) may be used. When administration of the beta-adrenergic blocker is begun, the drug should be used cautiously and at a low dose. For example, propranolol is usually started at 10 mg orally every 6 hours at least 1 week after the initiation of alpha-adrenergic blockade. The dose is then increased as necessary to control the tachycardia.

Labetalol* (Normodyne, Trandate) exhibits both selective alpha$_1$-adrenergic and nonselective beta-adrenergic blocking activities in a ratio of approximately 1:3 (see Table 2). Some instances of paradoxical hypertensive responses in patients with pheochromocytoma treated with labetalol have been reported, presumably due to incomplete alpha-adrenergic blockade. Therefore, the safety of this agent for primary therapy is controversial. Its role in the therapy of pheochromocytoma may be in the chronic pharmacologic management of patients with metastatic disease.

Catecholamine Synthesis Inhibitor

α-Methyl-L-tyrosine (metyrosine) (Demser) inhibits the synthesis of catecholamines by blocking the enzyme tyrosine hydroxylase. It is rapidly absorbed from the gastrointestinal tract and most of it is excreted in the urine unchanged. Metyrosine is available as 250-mg capsules (see Table 2). The initial dosage is 250 mg orally four times daily. The dosage may be increased by 500 mg per day every 2 days to a maximum of 4 grams per day (1 gram four times per day) as needed for blood pressure control. Side effects include sedation, depression, diarrhea, anxiety, nightmares, crystalluria and urolithiasis, galactorrhea, and extrapyramidal manifestations. Therefore, this agent should be used with caution and only when other agents have been proved ineffective. The extrapyramidal effects of phenothiazines or haloperidol may be potentiated, and their use concomitantly with metyrosine should be avoided. High fluid intake to avoid crystalluria is suggested for any patient taking more than 2 grams daily. Although some centers have used metyrosine preoperatively, we have reserved it primarily for those patients in whom, for

*Not FDA approved for this indication.

TABLE 1. **Differential Diagnosis for Pheochromocytoma Spells**

Endocrine
Thyrotoxicosis
Primary hypogonadism (e.g., menopausal syndrome)
Pancreatic tumors (e.g., insulinoma)
Medullary thyroid carcinoma
"Hyperadrenergic" spells

Cardiovascular
Essential hypertension—labile
Angina and cardiovascular deconditioning
Pulmonary edema
Dilated cardiomyopathy
Syncope
Orthostatic hypotension
Paroxysmal cardiac arrhythmia
Aortic dissection
Renovascular hypertension

Psychologic
Anxiety and panic attacks
Somatization disorder
Hyperventilation
Factitious (e.g., drugs, Valsalva maneuver)

Pharmacologic
Withdrawal of adrenergic-inhibiting medications (e.g., clonidine)
Monoamine oxidase inhibitor treatment and concomitant ingestion of tyramine or a decongestant
Sympathomimetic ingestion
Illicit drug ingestion (e.g., cocaine, phencyclidine, lysergic acid diethylamide)
Gold myokymia syndrome
Acrodynia (mercury poisoning)
Vancomycin ("red man syndrome")

Neurologic
Postural orthostatic tachycardia syndrome (POTS)
Autonomic neuropathy
Migraine headache
Diencephalic epilepsy (autonomic seizures)
Cerebral infarction
Cerebrovascular insufficiency

Miscellaneous
Mastocytosis (systemic or activation disorder)
Carcinoid syndrome
Recurrent idiopathic anaphylaxis
Unexplained flushing spells

cardiopulmonary reasons, combined alpha- and beta-adrenergic blockade cannot be used.

Potential Alternative Agents and Approaches

An alternative approach that has been advocated includes the use of calcium channel antagonists for control of hypertension and expansion of intravascular volume with 2 units of whole blood 12 hours before the operation. In view of our experience with combined alpha- and beta-adrenergic blockade and its high degree of efficacy, we have not seen the need to pursue alternative strategies.

Acute Hypertensive Crises

Acute hypertensive crises may occur before or during operation and should be treated with nitroprusside (Nipride) or phentolamine (Regitine) administered intravenously (IV). Phentolamine is a short-acting, nonselective alpha-adrenergic blocker. It is available in lyophilized form in vials containing 5 mg. An initial test dose of 1 mg is administered and, if necessary, this is followed by repeat 5-mg boluses or a continuous infusion. The response to phentolamine is maximal in 2 to 3 minutes after a bolus injection and lasts 10 to 15 minutes. A solution of 100 mg of phentolamine in 500 mL of 5% dextrose and water can be infused at a rate titrated for blood pressure control. The use of nitroprusside is discussed below.

Anesthesia and Surgery

Extirpating a pheochromocytoma is a high-risk surgical procedure, and an experienced surgeon-anesthesiologist team is required. The last oral doses of alpha- and beta-adrenergic blockers can be administered early in the morning on the day of operation. Cardiovascular and hemodynamic variables must be monitored closely. Continuous measurement of intra-arterial pressure and heart rhythm is required. In the setting of congestive heart failure or decreased cardiac reserve, monitoring of pulmonary capillary wedge pressure is indicated. Premedication includes minor tranquilizers and barbiturates. Fentanyl and morphine should not be used because of the potential for stimulating catecholamine release from the pheochromocytoma. In addition, parasympathetic nervous system blockade with atropine should be avoided because of the associated tachycardia. Induction usually is accomplished with thiopental (Pentothal), and general anesthesia is maintained with a halogenated ether such as enflurane (Ethrane) or isofluorane (Forane). Hypertensive episodes should be treated with phentolamine (2 to 5 mg IV) or nitroprusside given in an intravenous infusion (0.5 to 5.0 μg per kg per minute; maximum dose should not exceed 800 μg per minute). Lidocaine (50 to 100 mg IV) or esmolol (Brevibloc) (50 to 200 μg per kg per minute IV) is used for cardiac arrhythmia.

In the past, an anterior midline abdominal surgical approach was usually used for adrenal pheochromocytoma. However, laparoscopic adrenalectomy is becoming the procedure of choice in patients with solitary intra-adrenal pheochromocytomas that are less than 8 cm in diameter. If the pheochromocytoma is in the adrenal gland, the entire gland should be removed. If the tumor is malignant, as much tumor as possible should be removed. If a bilateral adrenalectomy is planned preoperatively, the patient should receive glucocorticoid stress coverage while awaiting transfer to the operating room. Glucocorticoid coverage should be initiated in the operating room if unexpected bilateral adrenalectomy is necessary. Paragangliomas of the neck, chest, and urinary bladder require specialized approaches.

Hypotension may occur after surgical resection of the pheochromocytoma and should be treated with fluids and colloids. Postoperative hypotension is less frequent in patients who have had adequate alpha-adrenergic blockade preoperatively. If both adrenal

TABLE 2. **Orally Administered Drugs Used in Treatment of Pheochromocytoma**

Generic Name (Trade Name)	Dose (mg/day)* Initial	Dose (mg/day)* Maximum	Side Effects
Alpha-Adrenergic Blocking Agents			
Phenoxybenzamine (Dibenzyline)	20†	100†	Postural hypotension, tachycardia, miosis, nasal congestion, diarrhea, inhibition of ejaculation, fatigue
Prazosin (Minipress)	1	20‡	First-dose effect, dizziness, drowsiness, headache, fatigue, palpitations, nausea
Terazosin (Hytrin)	1	20†	First-dose effect, asthenia, blurred vision, dizziness, nasal congestion, nausea, peripheral edema, palpitations, somnolence
Doxazosin (Cardura)	1	20§	First-dose effect, orthostasis, peripheral edema, fatigue, somnolence
Combined Alpha- and Beta-Adrenergic Blocking Agent			
Labetalol (Normodyne, Trandate)	200†	1200†	Dizziness, fatigue, nausea, nasal congestion, impotence
Catecholamine Synthesis Inhibitor			
α-Methyl-ρ-L-tyrosine (Demser)	1000‡	4000‡	Sedation, diarrhea, anxiety, nightmares, crystalluria, galactorrhea, extrapyramidal symptoms

*Given once daily unless otherwise indicated.
†Given as two doses daily.
‡Given in three or four doses daily.
§Exceeds dosage recommended by the manufacturer.

glands were manipulated at operation, adrenocortical insufficiency should be considered as a potential cause of postoperative hypotension. Hypoglycemia can occur in the immediate postoperative period, and therefore blood glucose levels should be monitored, and the fluid given IV should contain 5% dextrose.

Blood pressure usually is normal by the time of discharge from the hospital. Some patients remain hypertensive for up to 8 weeks postoperatively. Long-standing, persistent hypertension has been noted postoperatively and may be related to accidental ligation of a polar renal artery, resetting of baroreceptors, established hemodynamic changes, structural changes in the blood vessels, altered sensitivity of the vessels to pressor substances, renal functional or structural changes, or coincident primary hypertension.

Approximately 2 weeks postoperatively, a 24-hour urine sample should be obtained for measurement of catecholamines and metanephrines. If the levels are normal, the resection of the pheochromocytoma can be considered to have been complete. In major centers the surgical mortality rate is less than 2%. At the Mayo Clinic the 30-day perioperative mortality rate in 110 patients operated on between 1980 and 1989 was 0.9%. The survival rate of patients who have undergone removal of a benign pheochromocytoma is nearly that of age- and sex-matched normal control subjects. The 24-hour urinary excretion of catecholamines should be checked annually for at least 5 years as surveillance for recurrence in the adrenal bed, metastatic pheochromocytoma, or delayed appearance of multiple primary tumors. Lifelong follow-up may be indicated if tumor DNA ploidy is abnormal.

The patient should be screened for MEN 2, von Hippel-Lindau syndrome, and familial pheochromocytoma during the first postoperative visit. Studies to be considered include *RET* proto-oncogene or pentagastrin stimulation test, ophthalmology consultation, head MRI scan, and 24-hour urinary metanephrines on all immediate family members.

Malignant Pheochromocytoma

The distinction between benign and malignant catecholamine-producing tumors cannot be made on the basis of clinical, biochemical, or histopathologic characteristics. Malignancy is confirmed by the finding of direct local invasion or disease metastatic to sites that do not have chromaffin tissue, such as lymph nodes, bone, lung, and liver. Although the 5-year survival rate is less than 50%, many patients have prolonged survival and minimal morbidity. Metastatic lesions should be resected if possible. Painful skeletal metastatic lesions can be treated with external radiation therapy. In initial studies, local tumor irradiation with ^{131}I-MIBG has been proved to be of limited therapeutic value. If the tumor is considered to be aggressive and the quality of life is affected, then combination chemotherapy may be considered. A chemotherapy program consisting of cyclophosphamide (Cytoxan, Neosar), vincristine (Oncovin, Vincasar), and dacarbazine (DTIC-Dome), given cyclically every 21 to 28 days, has been proved beneficial but not curative in these patients. Hypertension and spells can be controlled with combined alpha- and beta-adrenergic blockade.

Pheochromocytoma in Pregnancy

Pheochromocytoma in pregnancy can cause the death of both the fetus and the mother. The treatment of hypertensive crises is the same as for nonpregnant patients. Although there is some controversy regarding the most appropriate management, pheochromocytomas should be removed immediately if diagnosed during the first two trimesters of pregnancy. Preoperative preparation is the same as for the nonpregnant patient. If medical therapy is chosen or if the patient is in the third trimester, cesarean section and removal of the pheochromocytoma in the same operation are indicated. Spontaneous labor and delivery should be avoided.

THYROIDITIS

method of
NEENA NATT, M.B., B.CHIR., and
IAN D. HAY, M.B., PH.D.
Mayo Medical School and Mayo Clinic and Foundation
Rochester, Minnesota

The term "thyroiditis" encompasses a diverse group of diseases characterized by the histologic finding of inflammation associated with mononuclear infiltration and, rarely, thyroid fibrosclerosis. The precise etiology of many of these disorders remains unknown. As a result, classification into acute, subacute, and chronic types rests primarily on their relatively distinct clinical and pathologic characteristics.

ACUTE THYROIDITIS

Acute thyroiditis is a rare condition that results from bacterial, fungal, or, rarely, parasitic infection of the thyroid gland. Patients typically present with the abrupt onset of anterior neck pain and tenderness; erythema of the overlying skin; dysphagia, particularly with pharyngitis; fever associated with a leukocytosis; and other constitutional symptoms of infection. Thyroid hormone levels and radioactive iodine uptake are usually within the normal range. Fine needle aspiration of the thyroid gland provides confirmation of the diagnosis and identifies the causative organism. Treatment includes appropriate parenteral antimicrobial therapy and surgical drainage of any fluctuant areas or abscesses.

SUBACUTE GRANULOMATOUS THYROIDITIS

Subacute granulomatous thyroiditis is a spontaneously resolving inflammation of the thyroid gland that is presumed to be viral in origin. Patients often report a preceding respiratory infection or viral prodrome. The abrupt onset of anterior neck pain, associated with an elevated erythrocyte sedimentation rate (often greater than 80 mm per hour), and a low radioactive iodine uptake are characteristic of the disorder. Clinical manifestations of hyperthyroidism are present in approximately 50% of patients. Systemic symptoms are common, particularly malaise, fatigue, myalgia, and mild fever. The clinical picture of subacute granulomatous thyroiditis, however, can vary considerably and, in some cases, pain and tenderness may be relatively insignificant. A normal, or only slightly elevated, sedimentation rate virtually excludes the diagnosis. Thyroid dysfunction typically follows a triphasic pattern related to inflammatory changes within the gland. Early in the disease, patients are mildly thyrotoxic owing to the discharge of preformed thyroid hormone into the circulation. Later, as glandular hormone is depleted, the patient may pass through a transient hypothyroid phase, followed by full recovery of thyroid function within 4 to 6 months. Not all patients progress through all phases of thyroid dysfunction.

The treatment of subacute granulomatous thyroiditis is supportive. Nonsteroidal anti-inflammatory agents or coated aspirin, 650 mg every 6 to 8 hours, often relieve pain in mild disease. For more severe disease, corticosteroids are the preferred treatment. These agents typically produce dramatic amelioration of thyroid pain and constitutional symptoms within 24 to 48 hours. If the patient does not respond in this way, the diagnosis should be reconsidered. An effective regimen is prednisone in an initial dose of 40 to 60 mg per day for a week, followed by rapid tapering and withdrawal over 1 month. Pain recurs in approximately 20% of patients during tapering of steroids or shortly after discontinuation of therapy. If this occurs, treatment should be reinstituted at the lowest dose at which the symptoms were controlled and then tapered more slowly over another month.

Because thyrotoxic symptoms are usually mild and short lived, treatment may not be required. If symptoms are bothersome, a beta-adrenergic blocker, such as atenolol* (Tenormin), 50 to 100 mg per day, may provide relief. Antithyroid drugs are of no benefit because the thyrotoxicosis is due to release of preformed hormone by damaged follicles and not to increased synthesis of new hormone. For patients who enter a hypothyroid phase, short-term levothyroxine (Synthroid) therapy (50 to 75 μg per day) may be indicated by clinical symptoms until thyroid recovery occurs. As this is a temporary measure, it is not necessary to aim at suppressing serum thyroid-stimulating hormone (TSH) into the normal range. The clinician must remember to re-evaluate the patient's continued need for thyroid hormone replacement by discontinuing the drug for 6 weeks and measuring serum free thyroxine and TSH levels. Permanent hypothyroidism as a result of subacute granulomatous thyroiditis is rare.

*Not FDA approved for this indication.

SUBACUTE LYMPHOCYTIC THYROIDITIS

Subacute lymphocytic thyroiditis is a self-limiting form of thyroiditis that may occur spontaneously or in the postpartum period (10%). Its principal diagnostic features include mild to moderate thyrotoxicosis; a small, painless, nontender goiter; and a low radioactive iodine uptake. The clinical course of the disease closely parallels that of subacute granulomatous thyroiditis; patients characteristically progress from a thyrotoxic state, through a hypothyroid phase, before recovering normal thyroid function after about 4 to 6 months. Again, not all patients experience all phases of thyroid dysfunction. In particular, hypothyroidism may be the first manifestation of postpartum thyroiditis, the hyperthyroid phase having gone unrecognized. Clinically, it may be difficult to differentiate subacute lymphocytic thyroiditis from mild cases of Graves' disease, highlighting the diagnostic importance of measuring radioactive iodine uptake (increased in Graves' disease) in the evaluation of hyperthyroidism.

The treatment of subacute lymphocytic thyroiditis can often be limited to reassurance and observation. Symptomatic hyperthyroidism is best managed with a short course of beta-adrenergic blockers, such as atenolol, 50 to 100 mg per day. As with subacute granulomatous thyroiditis, antithyroid drugs are not indicated. Levothyroxine therapy (50 to 75 μg daily) may be helpful for hypothyroid symptoms and can often be discontinued, as in subacute granulomatous thyroiditis. Permanent hypothyroidism is rare, but recurrent episodes of hyperthyroidism may occur in as many as 10% of patients. Ablative radioactive iodine followed by levothyroxine therapy may be necessary in some patients after they recover from recurrent episodes of severe hyperthyroidism.

CHRONIC LYMPHOCYTIC THYROIDITIS

Chronic lymphocytic thyroiditis, or Hashimoto's thyroiditis, is an autoimmune disorder that is nearly always associated with the presence of antithyroid antibodies. It is the most common cause of spontaneous hypothyroidism, although, rarely, patients may develop hyperthyroidism (so-called hashitoxicosis). The disease is usually first detected as an incidental finding of a firm, "bosselated" goiter during routine physical examination. Most patients are asymptomatic at diagnosis; symptoms of hypothyroidism occur as initial manifestations of disease in approximately 20% of patients. When hypothyroidism exists, thyroid hormone replacement therapy with levothyroxine is indicated for life (mean replacement dose 1.6 μg per kg per day). The goal of therapy is to normalize serum TSH, correct hypothyroid symptoms and, in some cases, to reduce goiter size. Young patients with moderate to severe hypothyroidism may start immediately on near full replacement doses of levothyroxine, usually 75 to 100 μg per day with follow-up 6 to 8 weeks later for measurement of serum TSH. The dose can then be adjusted accordingly. Older patients, or those with known coronary artery disease, should start on a lower dose of levothyroxine (25 to 50 μg per day), with a stepwise increase of 25 μg every 8 weeks to full replacement dose, while carefully monitoring for symptoms and signs of unmasked cardiac disease. Treatment of hyperthyroidism associated with chronic lymphocytic thyroiditis is similar to that of Graves' disease and is addressed elsewhere in the text.

With the advent of highly sensitive TSH assays, patients with Hashimoto's thyroiditis and normal serum thyroxine values but elevated TSH levels are increasingly being recognized (so-called subclinical hypothyroidism). Many of these patients are asymptomatic, and the decision to treat them with thyroid hormone has been controversial. Left untreated, the incidence of symptomatic hypothyroidism in this group has been reported at the rate of 5 to 10% per year. Although this has led some to advocate treatment for all asymptomatic patients with subclinical hypothyroidism, we prefer the more conservative approach of observation and careful follow-up of such patients, particularly if the serum TSH is less than 10 mIU per mL. A therapeutic trial of levothyroxine may be justified in patients with nonspecific symptoms that may be related to thyroid hormone deficiency, or in those with significant thyroid enlargement that is cosmetically unacceptable or causing mild pressure symptoms. It should be recognized, however, that the goiter shrinkage effect of such therapy is often limited, particularly if the serum TSH is only mildly elevated. Surgery may be necessary in patients with large glands, particularly if associated with local symptoms of obstruction.

INVASIVE FIBROUS THYROIDITIS (RIEDEL'S THYROIDITIS)

Fibrous thyroiditis is an extremely rare disorder characterized by fibrosclerosis and inflammation of the thyroid gland that invariably extends beyond the thyroid capsule to involve surrounding structures. The disease frequently presents with painless enlargement of a pre-existing goiter and may gradually progress to produce symptoms of tracheal and esophageal obstruction. Clinically, the thyroid gland is strikingly hard on palpation and often fixed to adjacent tissues. Most patients are euthyroid unless extensive destruction of the gland occurs, resulting in hypothyroidism. Open surgical biopsy is essential to confirm the histologic diagnosis and to rule out carcinoma. Treatment is primarily directed toward relieving pressure symptoms. This can often be achieved by simple isthmectomy. More extensive surgery is not recommended because of obliteration of anatomic landmarks by the fibrosclerotic process. In some cases, corticosteroid therapy has been successful in reducing the size of the goiter, thus alleviating local pressure symptoms and avoiding the need for surgical intervention. Hypothyroidism, if present, should be treated with levothyroxine.

Section 9

The Urogenital Tract

BACTERIAL INFECTIONS OF THE URINARY TRACT IN MEN

method of
NAIEL N. NASSAR, M.D., and
JAMES W. SMITH, M.D.
Veterans Affairs Medical Center
Dallas, Texas

Urinary tract infection (UTI) in otherwise healthy adult men between the ages of 15 and 50 years is uncommon, and the difference in prevalence compared with women in the same age group is striking. This difference is thought to be secondary to the antibacterial activity of the prostatic fluid and the greater length of the male urethra. Invasive infections are most frequent in the very young (<3 months of age) or the elderly (>50 years of age). Identified risk for UTI in men include homosexuality, intercourse with an infected female partner, bladder outlet obstruction, and lack of circumcision. Local infection of the urethra is commonplace in young sexually active men.

The etiologic agents causing uncomplicated UTI in men are similar to those in women, with *Escherichia coli* being the predominant causative organism. *Staphylococcus saprophyticus* is rarely found. Rarely, hematogenous spread to the urinary tract occurs during bacteremic episodes, particularly with *Staphylococcus aureus* or *Candida albicans.*

Dysuria is common to UTI and urethritis. As in females, frequency, urgency, suprapubic pain, flank pain, or hematuria suggests UTI. Urethritis must be ruled out in sexually active men. Older men may present with symptoms of dysuria, frequent urination, and occasionally isolated hematuria. Up to half of elderly men with UTI have prostate infection as well; and localization of symptoms to the lower urinary tract, prostate, or kidney by clinical symptoms alone can be difficult. The scrotum should be examined because epididymo-orchitis may be a complication of urinary tract or prostatic infection. Bacterial infection is suspected if the urine leukocyte esterase test and the nitrite test for gram-negative bacteria are positive. The prevalence of asymptomatic bacteriuria in institutionalized elderly men varies with the underlying degree of disability and is reported to be from 15% to 35%. Asymptomatic UTI in institutionalized men is frequently (10 to 25%) polymicrobial; however, this has not been reported to be associated with an increased likelihood of long-term adverse outcomes, such as renal failure, genitourinary carcinoma, or shortened survival.

TREATMENT

Because penicillinase-producing *Neisseria gonorrhoeae* is found throughout the United States, uncomplicated gonococcal infections are best treated with ceftriaxone (Rocephin), 125 mg intramuscularly in a single dose. Alternatively, single oral dose regimens with either cefixime (Suprax), 400 mg; ciprofloxacin (Cipro), 500 mg; or ofloxacin (Floxin), 400 mg, can be given. All patients given these regimens, as well as those with nongonococcal urethritis, should be treated with doxycycline, 100 mg orally two times a day for 7 days. Alternative treatments for chlamydial urethritis include azithromycin (Zithromax), 1 gram orally in a single dose (a 2-gram single oral dose is effective against gonococcal and nongonococcal urethritis); alternatively, ofloxacin, 300 mg orally two times a day for 7 days, or erythromycin base, 500 mg orally four times a day for 7 days, can be administered. *Chlamydia trachomatis* may recur in patients who fail to comply with the treatment regimen or who are re-exposed to an untreated sex partner. Recurrent urethritis should be retreated with the initial regimen. In addition, a wet-mount preparation of a urethral swab specimen for *Trichomonas vaginalis* should be made and, if possible, metronidazole treatment should be offered. Another possible cause of recurrent urethritis is tetracycline-resistant *Ureaplasma urealyticum,* which responds to a 14-day course of erythromycin base at a dose of 500 mg orally four times a day.

Men with UTIs and temperatures lower than 39.6°C (102°F) can usually be managed as outpatients with trimethoprim-sulfamethoxazole (Bactrim, Septra), one double-strength tablet twice a day for 10 to 14 days (short-course therapy has not been studied in men). If the patient is allergic to sulfonamides, the quinolones such as ciprofloxacin, 500 mg twice daily; ofloxacin, 400 mg twice daily; or levofloxacin (Levaquin), 250 mg once daily are other effective oral medications. Because oral cephalosporins or penicillin derivatives are excreted rapidly, they have reduced response rates in comparison with trimethoprim-sulfamethoxazole and the quinolones. Nitrofurantoin should not be used in men with UTI because it does not achieve reliable tissue concentrations and would be ineffective for occult prostatitis or pyelonephritis.

Patients with severe upper UTIs and temperatures higher than 102°F, volume depletion, and/or change of mental status should be hospitalized and treated with intravenous trimethoprim-sulfamethoxazole, 160/800 mg every 12 hours, combined with gentamicin (Garamycin), 5 mg per kg per day; ceftriaxone, 1 gram daily, or an intravenous quinolone also could be given. A patient who responds to these drugs can be switched to an oral equivalent agent on the second or third hospital day to complete a 14-day course of therapy. One advantage of 2 to 3 days of parenteral aminoglycoside is that the aminoglycoside persists in the kidney for up to 1 month after administration, providing continuous synergistic activity with the other administered agents.

If the patient continues to have fever after 72 hours of therapy, however, a urine culture should be repeated, and ultrasonography or computed tomography (CT) should be performed to rule out an intrarenal infection such as a phlegmon (nephronia) or a perinephric abscess. A perinephric abscess is more likely to occur in patients who have spinal cord injury, diabetes mellitus, or continuous urinary catheterization. Nephronia occurs in approximately 5 to 10% of those with the clinical diagnosis of pyelonephritis (fever, flank pain, and UTI). Patients with this intrarenal process generally respond to parenteral antimicrobial therapy continued for more than 2 weeks, with some patients requiring up to 6 weeks of parenteral therapy. Patients with multifocal mass-like lesions on CT may require drainage, as this complication is associated with high mortality rates.

It is probably wise to obtain both pretreatment and post-treatment urine cultures routinely in all men with UTI. Early recurrence of cystitis or pyelonephritis with the same species suggests a prostatic or upper urinary tract source of infection and warrants a 4- to 6-week regimen of either trimethoprim-sulfamethoxazole or a quinolone. Urologic evaluation should consist of a careful history and physical examination to check for possible structural problems including kidney stones and clinically significant benign prosthetic hypertrophy. If the patient has signs or symptoms of urinary retention, an in-and-out bladder catheterization should be done to check for residual. Other voiding studies, such as an intravenous pyelogram, are not indicated unless evidence of other abnormalities is found during initial evaluation. After patients respond clinically with a decrease in temperature and symptoms, they can be observed on antimicrobial therapy. A urine culture 2 to 4 weeks after completing therapy can be done to check for recurrence or persistence of infection. If the follow-up urine culture result is positive, a 4- to 6-week course of antimicrobial treatment is indicated. However, subsequent courses of therapy for asymptomatic bacteria are not indicated.

Epididymitis can occur after infection of either the urethra or the urinary tract in sexually active men younger than 35 years of age, usually by infection with *N. gonorrhoeae* or *C. trachomatis*. Both urethral discharge and urine with cultures are obtained to determine the causative agent. In men older than 35 years, epididymitis follows UTI with gram-negative organisms such as *E. coli*. Antimicrobial therapy is determined by the antimicrobial susceptibility of the bacteria recovered from the urinary tract. For patients younger than 35 years of age, treatment with ceftriaxone, 250 mg intramuscularly, plus doxycycline, 100 mg twice a day for 10 days, is indicated; for older men, treatment should include trimethoprim-sulfamethoxazole, 160/800 mg twice daily for 14 days, or a quinolone. If serious systemic infection is present, a combination of a cephalosporin and aminoglycoside is indicated until the patient responds. In addition, supportive measures, including elevation of the scrotum, are indicated.

Most episodes of bacteriuria associated with short-term catheters are asymptomatic; however, fever or other symptoms of UTI occur in up to 30% of patients. Less than 5% of catheter-associated bacteriurias are associated with bacteremia. Most bacteriurias in short-term catherizations are of single organisms, *E. coli* being most frequent, but as many as 15% may be polymicrobial, and most have accompanying pyuria. Long-term catheterization, on the other hand, is associated with polymicrobial bacteriuria in up to 95% of cases. However, urine obtained from the catheter may not always reflect bladder urine, suggesting that organisms colonizing the catheter, perhaps under a biofilm, may not in all cases colonize the bladder itself. Condom catheters have been used widely for men with urinary incontinence, and some studies suggest a lower frequency of bacteriuria with condom catheters. In the individual patient with positive urine culture and nonlocalizing symptoms (fever), it may be impossible to determine whether this is symptomatic UTI, and individual judgment with respect to whether antimicrobial therapy is warranted seems reasonable. In elderly men with asymptomatic bacteriuria, antimicrobial therapy is indicated within 12 hours before an invasive procedure, such as cystoscopy or transurethral prostatic resection. Antibiotic selection is based on the infecting organism and susceptibilities.

BACTERIAL INFECTIONS OF THE URINARY TRACT IN WOMEN

method of
LISA D. CHEW, M.D., and
STEPHAN D. FIHN, M.D., M.P.H.
University of Washington School of Medicine and Harborview Medical Center
Seattle, Washington

Urinary tract infections (UTIs) are the most common bacterial infections in women. Approximately 20% of women will have a UTI during their lifetime, with 25% experiencing recurrent infections. The incidence rises quickly after beginning sexual activity and thereafter increases slowly. The cost of caring for women with UTIs probably exceeds $1 billion a year.

PATHOGENESIS

Uropathogenic bacteria from the fecal flora colonize the vaginal introitus and periurethral area, travel to the urethra and into the bladder, and, in some cases, ascend the ureters to cause pyelonephritis. Hematogenous and lymphatic spread, as well as direct extension of infection, is rare.

Factors such as host susceptibility and bacterial virulence, which predispose to bacterial colonization and enable organisms to ascend the urinary tract, are subjects of intense research. Sexual intercourse is a risk factor for UTI. In addition, contraceptive practices with spermicide and diaphragms or spermicide-coated condoms increase the risk of developing a UTI by altering the normal vaginal flora and possibly enhancing adherence of pathogens to the vaginal mucosa. Furthermore, women who have had a prior UTI are at increased risk for subsequent infections.

Bacterial strains with fimbriae or pili are more virulent because they have a higher degree of adherence. Other virulence factors include hemolysin, which degrades red blood cells, and aerobactin, which enhances iron uptake. These characteristics are more commonly found in *Eschericia coli* responsible for pyelonephritis and are usually absent in ordinary fecal isolates.

The most common causative organism is *E. coli* (80%), followed by *Staphylococcus saprophyticus* (10 to 15%). Other less common pathogens include gram-negative aerobic rods (e.g., *Proteus* and *Klebsiella* species) and *Enterococcus.*

CLINICAL SYNDROMES

In the female patient, UTIs can be broadly categorized as acute uncomplicated cystitis, acute uncomplicated pyelonephritis, recurrent uncomplicated UTI, complicated UTI, catheter-related UTI, pregnancy-associated UTI, and UTI in the elderly.

Acute Uncomplicated Cystitis

Acute cystitis, or lower UTI, results from a superficial bacterial infection of the bladder and/or urethra. Dysuria is the cardinal symptom of a lower UTI. Other symptoms include urinary frequency, urgency, hematuria, and suprapubic and pelvic pain. It is also important to consider other diagnoses with complaints of dysuria such as urethritis from *Chlamydia trachomatis, Neisseria gonorrhoeae,* herpes simplex virus, or vaginitis from *Candida* or *Trichomonas* species.

In evaluating a patient with a suspected lower UTI, a clinical distinction should be made between a lower and an upper UTI, which is suggested by fever (>38°C), flank pain, nausea, or vomiting.

Often, the history alone is sufficient to make a probable diagnosis of UTI, particularly in young women with a prior UTI. With an equivocal history, the diagnosis of a UTI is dependent on laboratory examination of a clean-catch midstream urine specimen, evaluating for bacteriuria and pyuria.

Quantitative urine for bacteriuria is the usual gold standard. Traditionally, patients with 10^5 or more bacteria per mL in the urine were considered to have significant bacteriuria and given the diagnosis of a UTI. However, this is an insensitive standard when applied to symptomatic women. A threshold of 10^2 or 10^3 bacteria per mL of urine provides a good combination of sensitivity (95%) and specificity (85%) for diagnosing acute cystitis. Microscopic evaluation of the urine on wet-mount or Gram's stain for bacteriuria is a specific screen for infection but is insensitive for low levels of bacteriuria ($<10^4$ per mL).

Pyuria is present in most women with acute cystitis. The most accurate way to detect pyuria is to examine unspun urine with a hemocytometer and/or microscopic evaluation. The presence of greater than 10 white blood count (WBC) per mL or 10 WBC/high-power field with bacteria is 90% sensitive for a UTI.

Urine dipsticks for leukocyte esterase (LE) and bacterially generated nitrite are useful substitutes if urine microscopy is not feasible. The LE test is a practical screening test, with sensitivities and specificities ranging between 75 and 96% and 94 and 98%, respectively. The nitrite dipstick has reported sensitivities between 35 and 85% and a specificity of 98%. The accuracy of these rapid tests is lower in infections associated with colony counts less than 10^4 bacteria per mL. Therefore, if both the LE and nitrite testing are negative and suspicion of a UTI is present, a urinalysis and culture should be performed.

Because the causative organism and the antimicrobial susceptibilities are predictable in women with uncomplicated cystitis, a urine culture is generally not necessary. Unless the history is strongly compatible with a UTI, an abbreviated laboratory work-up, either by direct microscopy or rapid detection methods for pyuria or bacteriuria followed by empiric therapy, is recommended. However, if pyuria is absent or atypical symptoms are present, a culture should be performed before therapy is started.

Traditionally, therapy for acute cystitis included antimicrobial therapy for 7 to 14 days (Table 1). Single-dose therapy is a reasonable alternative with the advantages of fewer side effects, lower cost, reduced emergence of resistant bacteria, and increased patient compliance. The major disadvantage of single-dose therapy is its failure to eradicate uropathogens from the vaginal reservoir, resulting in recurrent infections. To maintain the advantages of single-dose therapy but improve cure rates, 3-day courses of treatment have been advocated. With most antibiotics, a 3-day regimen appears optimal, with efficacy comparable to the 7-day regimen. Trimethoprim-sulfamethoxazole (TMP-SMZ) or trimethoprim can be used as first-line agents with reported cure rates of approximately 80%. Amoxicillin/clavulanate (cure rates 78 to 87%) and fluoroquinolones (cure rates 88 to 98%) are effective, although are more expensive, alternatives and may promote bacterial resistance. No follow-up visit or urine culture after treatment is necessary unless symptoms persist or recur.

Acute Uncomplicated Pyelonephritis

Acute pyelonephritis is an infection involving the kidney parenchyma and renal pelvis, with the most

TABLE 1. **Common Medications Used in the Treatment of Urinary Tract Infections in Women**

Clinical Syndromes	Antibiotic Medication	Dose*	Notes
Acute cystitis	TMP-SMZ (Bactrim, Septra)	1 DS (160/800) PO bid	Three-day therapy is adequate. Consideration should be given to 7- to 10-day therapy, if the patient is pregnant, older than 65 years of age, or is immunocompromised (e.g., diabetes). Single-dose therapy with TMP-SMZ (2 double-strength tablets) can be used but is associated with lower cure rates. Amoxicillin is not recommended owing to high rates of resistant *E. coli*.
	Trimethoprim	100 mg PO bid	
	Ciprofloxacin (Cipro)	250 mg PO bid	
	Norfloxacin (Noroxin)	400 mg PO bid	
	Ofloxacin (Floxin)	200 mg PO bid	
	Nitrofurantoin (Macrodantin)/(Macrobid)	100 mg PO qid/100 mg PO bid	
	Amoxicillin/clavulanate (Augmentin)	875 mg PO bid	
Acute pyelonephritis			
Outpatient management	TMP-SMZ (Bactrim, Septra)	1 DS (160/800) PO bid	Fourteen-day therapy should be given. Longer courses have not shown to have additional benefit even if blood cultures are positive.
	Ciprofloxacin (Cipro)	250–500 mg PO bid	
	Norfloxacin (Noroxin)	400 mg PO bid	
	Ofloxacin (Floxin)	200–400 mg PO bid	
	Amoxicillin/clavulanate (Augmentin)	875 mg PO bid	
Inpatient management	Ampicillin/gentamicin	1 g IV q 6 h/1 mg per kg q 8 h or 1 g IV q 6 h/5 mg per kg IV q 24 h	Therapy should be given for 14 days. Intravenous therapy can be switched to oral therapy once patient is afebrile. Pregnant patients should be admitted. Fluoroquinolones and TMP-SMZ should be avoided in pregnancy owing to potential teratogenicity.
	Ciprofloxacin (Cipro)	400 mg IV q 12 h	
	Ceftriaxone (Rocephin)	1–2 g IV q 24 h	
	Ampicillin/sulbactam (Unasyn)	1.5–3.1 g IV q 6 h	
	Ceftazidime (Fortaz, Tazidime)	1–2 g IV q 8–12 h	
	TMP-SMZ (Bactrim, Septra)	2 mg/kg IV q 6 h	
Recurrent urinary tract infections			
Continuous prophylaxis	TMP-SMZ (Bactrim, Septra)	1 SS (80/400) PO qhs or thrice weekly	Regimen is initiated after eradication of an acute infection. Patients are placed on continuous prophylaxis for 6 months and then observed for further infection. Factors that increase the risk of developing UTIs should be modified.
	Trimethoprim	100 mg PO qhs	
	Nitrofurantoin (Macrodantin)	50–100 mg PO qhs	
	Norfloxacin (Noroxin)	200 mg PO qhs	
	Cephalexin (Keflex)	250 mg PO qhs	
Postcoital prophylaxis	TMP-SMZ (Bactrim, Septra)	1 SS PO postcoitus	
	Nitrofurantoin (Macrodantin)	50–100 mg PO postcoitus	
	Cephalexin (Keflex)	250 mg PO postcoitus	
Pregnancy			
Asymptomatic bacteriuria	Amoxicillin	250 mg PO tid × 7 d or 3 gm single dose or 3 g PO followed by 3 g 12 h later	Single-dose therapy has lower eradication rates. Follow-up cultures should be obtained to ensure eradication of bacteriuria. Chronic suppressive antibiotic therapy is recommended if the patient has two or more episodes of recurrent bacteriuria.
	Nitrofurantoin (Macrodantin)	100 mg PO qid × 7 d 200 mg single dose 100 mg PO qid × 3 d	
	Amoxicillin/clavulanate (Augmentin)	250 mg PO tid × 7 d	

*Doses of drugs based on normal hepatic and renal function.
Abbreviations: DS = double strength; SS = single strength.

common pathogen being *E. coli* (>80%). Patients frequently present with the triad of dysuria, flank pain, and fever. Pyuria is nearly always present. Urine cultures should be obtained in all women suspected of pyelonephritis. Blood cultures should also be obtained in patients who are hospitalized because 15 to 20% are positive.

Patients with acute uncomplicated pyelonephritis can be stratified into those ill enough to require hospitalization and those able to be managed in the outpatient setting. Indications for admission include inability to maintain oral hydration or take oral medications, uncertain social situations, concerns about compliance, severe illness with high fevers, severe pain, and marked debility. Furthermore, in patients with co-morbidity such as diabetes, renal insufficiency, and immunosuppression, hospitalization should be strongly considered. Hospitalized patients should be started on intravenous antibiotics, usually ampicillin and gentamicin, a third-generation cephalosporin (e.g., ceftriaxone, ceftazidime), a broad-spectrum β-lactam (e.g., ampicillin/sulbactam), or a fluoroquinolone (see Table 1). When signs and symptoms improve or resolve, usually within 48 to 72 hours, the remaining treatment can be given orally. Evaluation of the upper urinary tract with ultrasound or computed tomography to detect nephrolithiasis, renal or perirenal abscess, or other complications should be considered if fever persists 72 hours after initiating treatment. If the patient qualifies for outpatient treatment, acceptable regimens include TMP-SMZ, fluoroquinolones, and amoxicillin/clavulanate (see Table 1). Antibiotic therapy for 14 days is adequate, even if blood culture results are positive. Cultures should be obtained 2 weeks after treatment to ensure eradication of the infection.

Recurrent Urinary Tract Infections

Approximately 20% of women with an initial episode of cystitis have a recurrent infection. Recurrent UTIs are classified as either a reinfection or a relapse. Reinfections account for 90% of recurrences and represent a new UTI following successful eradication of a previous infection. A relapse is defined as the recrudescence of a prior, partially treated infection with a persistent focus of infection usually in the upper tract. A relapse should be considered if the infection recurs within 2 weeks after antimicrobial therapy. The vast majority of women with recurrent uncomplicated cystitis have no anatomic or functional abnormality of the urinary tract and therefore do not need urologic evaluation.

There are three effective approaches to managing recurrent UTIs: continuous prophylaxis, postcoital prophylaxis, or intermittent self-treatment (see Table 1). Prophylaxis is advocated in women who experience three or more symptomatic UTIs over 12 months and should be instituted only after an existing infection has been eradicated. Women who report a temporal association between infection and sexual intercourse are candidates for the postcoital approach, whereas others should receive continuous prophylaxis. The most common medications used are TMP-SMZ and nitrofurantoin. Women who do not want to take continuous antibiotics can treat themselves with a single dose or 3-day regimen. It is important to alter those factors that may increase the risk of developing UTIs such as contraceptive practices with diaphragms and spermicide. A 6-month trial of prophylaxis is usually prescribed after which the patient is observed for further infection. If necessary, however, treatment can be continued for years without the emergence of resistance.

One clinical trial of topical intravaginal estrogen among postmenopausal women with recurrent UTIs demonstrated a decrease of recurrent UTIs. Lack of estrogen induces changes in the vaginal microflora, including loss of lactobacilli and increased colonization with *E. coli.* The effect of oral estrogen replacement on recurrent UTIs, however, is unknown.

Complicated Urinary Tract Infections

Complicated UTIs encompass those patients with a structural or functional abnormality of the urinary tract or underlying co-morbidity such as diabetes and immunosupression. Complicated UTIs are often caused by pathogens that are resistant to first-line antibiotics. Risk factors include indwelling bladder catheterization, recent urinary tract instrumentation, functional or anatomic abnormality of the urinary tract, diabetes mellitus, symptoms that last longer than 7 days, immunosuppression, recent antibiotic use, and hospital-acquired infection. Clinical presentations range from mild cystitis to life-threatening urosepsis.

Unlike the predictability of uropathogens in uncomplicated UTIs, a broader range of bacteria can cause complicated infections (e.g., *E. coli, Proteus* species, *Klebsiella* species, *Pseudomonas* species, *Staphylococcus* species). Urine cultures and susceptibility testing should be performed in all patients suspected of having a complicated infection. It is difficult to generalize the appropriate antibiotic regimen. Empirical therapy must take into account the setting, the medical history of the patient, the suspected organism, and any previous infecting organism and antimicrobial therapy. Usually a broad-spectrum antibiotic is administered for empirical therapy at least until resistance results are available. A 10- to 14-day course of therapy is usually necessary. Without correction of the underlying anatomic, functional, or metabolic defect, recurrent infections are common. Therefore, urine culture should be repeated 1 to 2 weeks after completion of therapy.

Catheter-Related Urinary Tract Infections

Catheterization is a risk factor for developing a UTI and is a common cause of nosocomial infections. The presence of a catheter in the bladder allows bacteria to adhere to the surface of the catheter and to initiate formation of biofilms that promote bacterial growth. Prevention is the best way to avoid morbidity and mortality from catheter-associated infection. Sterile insertion and care of the catheter, along with prompt removal, are effective preventive strategies.

Urine cultures from catheters that demonstrate bacterial growth higher than 10^2 colony-forming units per (cfu) mL are evidence of infection because these colony counts usually persist or increase within 48 hours. Systemic antibiotics prevent or delay the onset of bacteriuria but are not routinely recommended because of the cost and the emergence of antimicrobial resistance. Furthermore, there is little benefit in treating asymptomatic bacteriuria in chronically catheterized patients. Catheter-associated UTIs should be treated only if the patient shows signs or symptoms of a UTI (e.g., fever, hypotension, suprapubic pain, abdominal pain). Without removal of the catheter, prolonged or sequential courses of antibiotics for catheter-associated UTIs are usually unsuccessful.

Some authorities recommend giving a single dose of two double-strength TMP-SMZ tablets in women younger than 65 years of age who have persistent bacteriuria after catheterization for a week or less to prevent UTIs because many go on to have symptomatic UTIs.

Pregnancy-Associated Urinary Tract Infections

During pregnancy, hormonal and mechanical factors cause dilatation of the ureters and renal pelvis, referred to as hydroureter of pregnancy. The microbiology of pathogens is similar to that seen in nonpregnant women *(E. coli > Klebsiella > Enterobacter > Proteus >* Group B *Streptococcus).* The approach to the pregnant patient with a UTI differs from that to the nonpregnant patient in the following manner: Asymptomatic bacteriuria is aggressively sought and treated, drugs that can be used safely are limited, and follow-up of bacteriuria during pregnancy is more intense.

Asymptomatic bacteriuria affects 4 to 7% of pregnant patients and is defined as recovery of 10^5 cfu per mL on two consecutive urinary midstream clean catches. The risk of bacteriuria is highest between the ninth and the 17th gestational weeks. Untreated bacteriuria during pregnancy is associated with adverse effects in the mother (symptomatic UTI) and the fetus (premature delivery, fetal infection, and perinatal death). Pyelonephritis occurs in 20 to 40% of pregnant women with untreated bacteriuria. Treatment of asymptomatic bacteriuria reduces the incidence of pyelonephritis by 80 to 90%. The serious implications of untreated bacteriuria justify screening all pregnant patients and treating asymptomatic bacteriuria. Screening is performed in the first trimester and no later than the 16th week. Acceptable drugs include β-lactams (amoxicillin, amoxicillin/clavulanate, and oral cephalosporins) and nitrofurantoin (see Table 1). Single-dose therapies and 3- to 7-day treatment have been used. Regardless of the treatment regimen chosen, the important issue is not the length of therapy but the appropriate follow-up to ensure eradication of the bacteriuria. A follow-up culture should be performed 1 to 2 weeks after therapy. If short-course therapy fails to eradicate the infection, a 7- to 10-day regimen should be given. Recurrence of asymptomatic bacteriuria following two courses of antibiotics is an indication for suppression therapy.

Symptomatic UTIs develop in 1 to 2% of pregnancies without treatment of asymptomatic bacteriuria. The usual duration of treatment for lower UTIs is 7 to 10 days. Shorter courses (i.e., single-dose or 3-day) have a 20 to 40% failure rate. Management of acute pyelonephritis in a pregnant patient should consist of hospital admission with intravenous antibiotics, usually ampicillin and an aminoglycoside or a third-generation cephalosporin. Acute pyelonephritis is associated with prematurity, low birth weight, and increased perinatal mortality. Furthermore, bacterial sepsis is associated with worse outcomes in pregnancy, compared with the nonpregnant state. Duration of treatment for acute pyelonephritis is 14 days. Follow-up cultures should be obtained every 4 to 6 weeks to rule out recurrence. Some authorities recommend placing patients on antibiotic suppression therapy until delivery following an episode of pyelonephritis.

Urinary Tract Infections in Elderly Women

The prevalence of asymptomatic bacteriuria in women older than 65 years of age has been reported to be between 8 and 25%. The prevalence is highest in women living in nursing homes and in women who require intermittent catheterization and have incomplete bladder emptying. The elderly may present with atypical symptoms (e.g., fever, altered mental status, incontinence, abdominal pain) and are generally more difficult to treat because of the increased incidence of abnormal bladder function, vaginal or urethral atrophy, and intermittent catheterization. Lower UTIs should be treated with a 3- to 7-day course. Generally, elderly patients are admitted for treatment of upper UTIs.

The management of asymptomatic bacteriuria in the elderly, defined as urine cultures greater than 10^5 cfu per mL, is controversial. However, most authorities believe that treatment of asymptomatic bacteriuria in elderly patients without indwelling catheters is not beneficial.

BACTERIAL INFECTIONS OF THE URINARY TRACT IN GIRLS

method of
TIMOTHY P. BUKOWSKI, M.D.
University of North Carolina at Chapel Hill
Chapel Hill, North Carolina

In the first 11 years of life, 3% of girls will have symptomatic urinary tract infection (UTI), with a recurrence rate of 40% even with appropriate therapy. Typically, cystitis begins with colonization of the introitus by intestinal bacteria, with subsequent invasion of the bladder. Susceptibility to infection depends on a shift in the balance between host defense and bacterial virulence factors. Vesicoureteral reflux is also associated with UTI, and reflux nephropathy is a concern with untreated reflux.

DIAGNOSIS

Signs and symptoms in children with UTIs are often misunderstood. Neonates often present with irritability, temperature instability, lethargy, anorexia, emesis, and even jaundice. Failure to thrive represents a very important presenting symptom. In toddlers, screaming and irritability are common, as are diarrhea and vomiting. More specific signs and symptoms, such as malodorous or cloudy urine, hematuria, and urinary frequency, may become evident. Older children tend to present with specific manifestations that are similar to those expected in adults; frequency, urgency, urge incontinence, and dysuria become much more prominent. Evidence of infection outside the urinary tract does not eliminate the possibility of UTI. Respiratory or gastrointestinal symptoms are common in patients with UTI associated with fever.

A careful history to identify urinary and bowel symptoms, including the presence of constipation or encopresis, is important. Lower extremity symptoms such as pain, weakness, or incoordination should be sought, because the combination of lower extremity symptoms, bowel symptoms, and urinary symptoms may suggest a primary neurologic abnormality such as a tethered cord.

Physical Examination

Patients undergo a careful physical examination, with palpation of the abdomen to discover masses, fecal balls, or a distended bladder. The external genitalia are examined for diaper rash and other evidence of dermatitis. Girls should be examined for such lesions as vaginitis and labial fusion, which may potentiate the risk for infection. The normal female urethra is separate from the hymenal ring; female hypospadias may cause vaginal voiding with urinary trapping, increasing the risk for UTI. A limited neurologic examination of the perineum and anus is warranted. In addition, a spinal examination is necessary in order to fully assess the sacrum and overlying soft tissue structures. The presence of a cutaneous pit (other than pilonidal), lipoma, hair patch, or area of hyperpigmentation may indicate an underlying spinal anomaly, which may be associated with tethering of the spinal cord. In such cases, careful palpation over the bony sacrum may detect abnormalities or even absence of the sacrum.

Urinalysis

Microscopic examination of the urinary sediment may reveal white cells and bacteria. The presence of a white cell cast implies pyelonephritis. Hematuria is merely suggestive of infection. The finding of pyuria does not confirm UTI, as it may also be encountered with vaginitis, urinary calculi, chemical irritation of the perineum, diaper rash, gastroenteritis, trauma, and even viral immunization. The finding of nitrite and leukocyte esterase on a dipstick examination is highly suggestive of the presence of bacteria. Hydration status may affect urinalysis, with increased hydration leading to false-negative results due to dilution.

Culture

The administration of antibiotics to a child symptomatic for UTI without confirmation by urine culture is inappropriate. The most accurate urine samples are obtained by suprapubic aspiration or urethral catheterization. Positive culture of a urine sample obtained by the bag collection technique has only a 10% accuracy level; only negative results with such samples should be considered reliable. All positive bag specimen cultures must be confirmed by culture of a specimen obtained by catheterization.

Imaging Studies

Radiographic evaluation is necessary after the initial documented UTI. A renal ultrasound study is the best screening modality for evaluation of the upper tracts. The ultrasound scan may reveal hydronephrosis, irregularity suggesting previous pyelonephritis, or urolithiasis and is very helpful in assessing renal growth. The ureters can be evaluated, as can the bladder, to assess bladder wall thickness and other anatomic features, and the presence of ureteroceles, diverticula, calculi, and foreign bodies can be detected. Performing a voiding cystourethrogram requires use of a small catheter, contrast material warmed to body temperature, and a low infusion pressure in order to prevent false-positive results. Studies may be performed using a radioisotope technique, which has the proven advantage of lower radiation.

Dimercaptosuccinic acid (DMSA) scanning is currently the standard imaging technique to determine renal involvement; however, magnetic resonance imaging (MRI) and computed tomography (CT) scanning may allow similar accuracy in detection of parenchymal perfusion defects, with added anatomic differentiation. MRI has the added advantage of assessing differential blood flow to each kidney.

The ultimate goal of treatment is the prevention of renal injury from infection. It is often difficult to determine whether the UTI represents simple cystitis or potentially more damaging pyelonephritis. Not all cases of renal infection are associated with underlying vesicoureteric reflux, and not all patients with vesicoureteric reflux develop renal scarring. The risk for acquired renal scarring from reflux is directly related to the risk for acute pyelonephritis.

Although in vitro evidence suggests that injury from reflux occurs only with UTI and its attendant inflammatory response in the kidney, clinical review shows that renal injury can also occur prenatally with vesicoureteral reflux. Various studies have found that patients in whom reflux was detected antenatally have renal injury without infection, and a number of these patients develop new scars after infection. Is the incidence of end-stage renal failure related to reflux-mediated infection or to prenatal injury? Regardless, 10 to 20% of children with end-stage renal failure have reflux nephropathy.

Urodynamic studies are useful in children who have a significant voiding abnormality that fails to resolve after sterilization of the urinary tract. Radiographs of the lumbosacral spine (including antero-posterior and lateral views) should be obtained whenever a sacral abnormality is suspected. Formal spinal imaging using MRI should be considered if documented voiding dysfunction is associated with either significant bowel symptoms or lower extremity symptoms.

TABLE 1. **Common Antimicrobials for Pediatric Urinary Tract Infections**

Drug	Dosage	Frequency	Prophylaxis
Amoxicillin	20–40 mg/kg/d	q 8 h	10 mg/kg/d
Ampicillin	50–100 mg/kg/d	q 6 h	20 mg/kg/d
Nitrofurantoin	5–7 mg/kg/d	q 6 h	1–2 mg/kg/d
Sulfisoxazole	120–150 mg/kg/d	q 6–8 h	50 mg/kg/d
Trimethoprim-sulfamethoxazole	0.5 mL/kg/d*	q 12 h	0.25 mL/kg/d

*Suspension 40 mg TMP/200 mg SMX per 5 mL.

TREATMENT

The associated dysuria and irritative voiding symptoms with cystitis may be alleviated by increased hydration, administration of phenazopyridine (Pyridium), or having the child void in a tub of warm water. *Escherichia coli* is the most common cause of UTI in girls. Amoxicillin (Table 1) offers safe coverage in the newborn period but can be associated with diarrhea. The combination of trimethoprim-sulfamethoxazole offers good coverage, is inexpensive, and is selective for the urinary tract, with the possible complication of bone marrow suppression. Nitrofurantoin is very selective for the urinary tract, but the elixir may be bitter and cause gastrointestinal upset. Opening a capsule of the powder form and using the contents as "sprinkles" on food may suffice. The presence of acute pyelonephritis is an indication for hospital admission and parenteral antibiotic therapy. The use of oral antibiotics is considered after the child is afebrile for 48 hours, and a total therapeutic course of 10 to 14 days should be given. At this time fluoroquinolones are not acceptable for use in children with UTI.

Recurrent Urinary Tract Infection

Any patient with recurrent infections should keep a bladder and bowel diary, regardless of imaging results. Attention to hydration is helpful, as is a carefully instructed voiding program. This is especially important for the infrequent voider, who is best managed with a timed voiding regimen. In addition, most patients receive instructions on diet and bowel regimen, which usually includes milk of magnesia or mineral oil. If severe voiding dysfunction is suspected, urodynamic studies with a brief biofeedback session are performed. Anticholinergic therapy may be helpful. I prefer 6 months of low-dose antibiotics as an adjunct to the bowel and bladder program if a patient has more than two UTIs in a 3-month period.

Vesicoureteral Reflux

Reflux can be associated with UTI and may predispose the patient to renal scarring. Reflux is graded I to V on the basis of the cystogram findings. Spontaneous resolution with maturity of the bladder is possible, so administration of prophylactic antibiotics is typical first-line therapy. Resolution is most likely to occur with low-grade, unilateral reflux seen at a young age. Grade I or II reflux has an 80% chance of resolution, grade III a 50% chance, and grade IV a 20% resolution rate. Relative indications for surgical correction of reflux include breakthrough UTI in a child receiving prophylaxis, poor compliance or inability to tolerate medical therapy, and high-grade reflux.

CHILDHOOD ENURESIS

method of
BRENT W. SNOW, M.D.
University of Utah School of Medicine
Salt Lake City, Utah

Unintentional loss of urine occurring beyond the age of expected urinary control is called enuresis. *Nocturnal enuresis* refers to nighttime (sleep time) wetting; this term is generally reserved for patients who have this symptom after the age of 5 years. *Diurnal enuresis* refers to involuntary voiding occurring during the daytime while the child is awake. Differentiating nocturnal and diurnal enuresis is important because their etiologies are different and methods of treatment vary significantly. It is of great importance to recognize that enuresis is a symptom and not a disease. This realization helps physicians approach the disorder more appropriately.

NOCTURNAL ENURESIS

Infants void 20 times in a 24-hour period, and not until the age of 3 to 4 years are half of children dry both day and night. Approximately 15 to 20% of 5-year-olds still wet the bed. More boys have the symptom of nocturnal enuresis than girls. Approximately 15% of children achieve nighttime control each year, so that by age 15, only 1% still have a problem with nighttime wetting.

Some patients have a strong family history of enuresis. If both parents wet the bed as children, 77% of offspring do also. If one parent wet the bed, 44% of offspring are enuretic. If neither parent wet the bed, only 15% of their children are affected. In 25% of patients who have nocturnal enuresis, a significant period with dry nights preceded onset of the disorder, which is therefore called secondary enuresis. Enuresis is reported to be more frequent in populations of lower socioeconomic status, larger families, and socially stressed homes.

Etiology

Nocturnal enuresis has many proposed causes, including genetic and psychological factors, developmental delay, sleep disorders, maturational delay, and abnormality in antidiuretic hormone secretion.

Genetic Factors. As previously noted, nocturnal enuresis is associated with a strong family history. In a desmopressin study, 91% benefited from drug treatment if the family history was positive and only 7% did so if the family history was negative.

Psychologic Factors. Psychologic factors have been suggested as an underlying cause in many patients. It is known that children with psychologic disorders have more nocturnal enuresis than normal children, and children under stress have more episodes of nocturnal enuresis. It is generally thought that in only a minority of patients are psychologic factors the sole abnormality leading to enuresis.

Since one quarter of patients with nocturnal enuresis have secondary nocturnal enuresis, psychologic factors have been suggested; however, seldom are these factors proved as a cause. Psychologic therapy of these patients does not produce any great benefit, and patients with secondary enuresis respond to conventional treatments with similar degrees of success.

Developmental Delay. As studies on bladder development have shown, bladder capacity increases rapidly in toddlers. At this stage of growth, bladder volume is proportionately greater than the volume of urine produced. As the youngster learns to sense bladder filling, voluntary control of the striated urinary sphincter follows, and learning to exert volitional control over the spinal micturitional reflex is necessary to set the stage for urine control. It has also been noted that daytime urine control generally comes before nighttime urine control. Thus, when nighttime urine control is delayed, a developmental cause can be invoked.

Maturational Delay. The spontaneous cure often seen with enuresis suggests that as affected patients grow older, maturation occurs and dryness follows. One of the most consistent urodynamic findings is that the functional daytime bladder capacity correlates well with nighttime bladder capacity. Therefore, patients who still void in frequent, small quantities, as occurs in infants, are not as successful as their normal counterparts with nighttime control. The absolute bladder capacity in these patients is normal as tested under anesthesia, but the functional daytime volume is diminished and presumably increases as maturation occurs.

Sleep Disorder. Sleep disorders have long been thought to be an underlying cause of nocturnal enuresis. Parents are convinced that these children sleep more deeply and are more difficult to arouse. Deep sleep and arousal may be two separate problems. Urodynamic studies done simultaneously with sleep studies suggest that sleep patterns in these patients are no different from those in patients with normal urinary control. Enuretic patients void at any stage of sleep when the bladder is full.

Antidiuretic Hormone Secretion Pattern. Data suggest that patients with nocturnal enuresis do not have a normal diurnal pattern of secretion of antidiuretic hormone (ADH). Thus, urine is not concentrated during the sleeping hours, and urine output overwhelms bladder volume to cause nighttime wetting. In some patients, ADH secretion follows this pattern; however, most patients with nocturnal enuresis do not have abnormalities of ADH secretion. The explanation of why patients with ADH abnormalities spontaneously resolve their nighttime wetting has not been forthcoming.

Evaluation

When a patient presents with the symptom of enuresis, a limited evaluation should be pursued to detect daytime enuresis, urinary urgency and frequency, poor urinary stream, straining to void, abnormal bowel habits, and history of urinary tract infections; family history and psychosocial history should also be reviewed. Physical examination of the abdomen, genitalia, and lower spine is appropriate. Observing the patient walking is often the best way to evaluate lower spinal cord function. A urinalysis looking for evidence of urinary tract infection, glucosuria, and proteinuria is helpful. Urine specific gravity should be noted; if dilute urine is found, a first-voided, early-morning specimen should be obtained to evaluate concentrating defects. If the history and physical findings are unremarkable, radiographic evaluation of the urinary tract is not warranted. If history, physical, and laboratory findings indicate, an ultrasound scan of the kidneys and bladder, both full and empty, is an adequate screening study for most enuretic patients.

Infections. Since nocturnal enuresis is a symptom, infections can be a common treatable cause. In one study, 16 of 56 patients with nocturnal enuresis and urinary tract infections became dry with the treatment of their urinary tract infections. Obviously, if infection is discovered, appropriate x-ray studies of the bladder and an ultrasound scan of the kidneys should follow.

Treatment

Treatment for nocturnal enuresis is based on the suspected cause. Enuretic alarms are designed as biofeedback to enhance bladder sensation and overcome sleep arousal difficulties. Medications have been used in attempts to increase bladder capacity and to alter sleep patterns. Desmopressin has been used to lessen the volume of urine made at night so that bladder capacity is not exceeded.

Enuretic Alarms. Wetting alarms are devices that trigger a loud alarm when the underwear becomes wet. This treatment is based on conditioning therapy. Wetting alarms require a motivated patient and parents. The alarm sounds in the middle of the night, and the parent often needs to help the child to get out of bed, go to the bathroom, return, and reset the alarm. This can happen many times a night, and since conditioning is involved, this needs to last for many months before the alarm can be discontinued successfully. Wetting alarm therapy is quite successful, with initial cure rates in the 80% range. As with all enuretic patients in whom the disorder recurs after an initial cure, a second treatment can recover nighttime urine control. Wetting alarms enjoy the best long-term cure rate and lowest relapse rate of enuresis treatment.

Pharmacologic Treatment

IMIPRAMINE. Imipramine (Tofranil) is a tricyclic antidepressant that has been used for many years in the treatment of bed wetting. Its mechanism of action for the enuretic child is unknown. It does have a mild anticholinergic effect and seems to cause mild alterations in arousal and sleep patterns. Initial success rates in patients receiving imipramine can be expected to be in the 50% range. Some patients have relapses when they stop taking the drug. With prolonged treatment, the effects may wane. It is suggested that the medication be gradually withdrawn rather than stopped abruptly to avoid relapses. Imipramine can have side effects including anxiety, insomnia, dry mouth, nausea, and personality changes. Imipramine overdose is of great concern because it can cause fatal cardiac arrhythmias and conduction blocks that are untreatable. This is sufficiently important that all parents should be warned to keep this medication in a safe place.

DESMOPRESSIN. Desmopressin (DDAVP) is an analogue of vasopressin and mimics the urine-concentrating activity of vasopressin without its vasopressor activity. It is given by nasal spray. Oral preparations have been formulated. The effect is dose-dependent; 20 μg per day is the starting dose for the nasal spray, which can be increased to up to 40 μg per day as necessary. When desmopressin therapy is successful, it can be used on an as-needed basis. If the family history is strong, desmopressin therapy may be more likely to be efficacious. Initial response to desmopressin can be expected in approximately two thirds of patients, although complete success in terms of dryness is closer to 40%. Relapse occurs regularly after discontinuation of therapy. A longer course of treatment may be necessary. Desmopressin can cause electrolyte changes, but this seldom occurs in children. The most common side effects are nasal irritation and headaches.

ANTICHOLINERGICS. Oxybutynin (Ditropan)* is the most common anticholinergic drug used for enuresis. For patients who only have nighttime enuresis without diurnal enuresis, oxybutynin shows no benefit compared with placebo. However, for patients with both daytime and nighttime enuresis, it is more effective than placebo.

*Not FDA approved for this indication.

DIURNAL ENURESIS

Diurnal enuresis is the term for daytime or awake loss of urine after toilet training. The most common history is successful toilet training followed by a few years of good urine control and then the onset of occasional daytime "accidents." Patients report not knowing that a bladder contraction was imminent. Affected girls "dance" or squat on the heel (Vincent's curtsey) or hold their genitalia; boys just pinch their penis. The parents describe these children as lazy, because they are often found outside playing, or indoors near the bathroom, with wet spots on their pants but seldom with puddles on the ground or floor. The physician should explain to the parents that the child has a developmental delay in bladder maturation: some bladder contractions produce cortical awareness, but the abnormal contractions do not. The child's first clue that urination is beginning is urethral distention and dampening of the underwear. The child promptly contracts the external sphincter and begins posturing to assist in urine control. The parents note this behavior and encourage the child to go to the bathroom. If the child is moved while engaged in posturing, often further leakage occurs. Many times, after such posturing controls the urge to void and the contraction subsides, the child no longer feels the need to urinate. This leaves the child with a post-voiding residual, which predisposes to the development of urinary tract infections. Because affected children throughout the day exert extraordinary effort in external sphincter contraction to control urination, they also have a tendency to develop constipation. This frequently leads to mild encopresis, manifested as staining of underwear. Urinary tract infections are more common in these patients, especially girls.

Estimates suggest that between 5 and 10% of children have diurnal enuresis. The first step in evaluation is a careful voiding and bowel history, including a social history. Physical examination should include examination of the lower back as well as the urinary tract. Radiologic evaluation is reserved for children with urinary tract infections and includes a voiding cystourethrogram and renal ultrasound scan.

Treatment of diurnal enuresis is most successful when all aspects of the problem are addressed. A timed voiding regimen is helpful to avoid the unstable bladder contractions; depending upon the age of the patient, voiding should be done at between 1- and 2-hour intervals. The interval should be short enough that the child can be successful. Anticholinergic medications are helpful. Oxybutynin (Ditropan)* is the most common at a dose of 0.2 to 0.5 mg per kg per day. Other anticholinergics such as propantheline bromide (Pro-Banthīne)* or hyoscyamine (Levsin)* may be beneficial. For patients with urinary tract infections, prophylactic antibiotics are essential since good bladder control is difficult when the bladder is infected. Patients with mild encopresis should have anticonstipation treatment. Generally an initial clean-out followed by a regimen of mineral oil or milk of magnesia is sufficient. Care of these patients can be taxing, and frequent follow-up visits may be necessary, yet two thirds to three quarters of the patients show benefit with this multidirectional approach. If a specific treatment fails initially, a subsequent trial may be successful. In patients in whom these therapies produce no benefit, urodynamic studies of the bladder may be indicated.

Almost all children outgrow the unstable bladder of childhood. It is important to emphasize to the parents that their child is normal, and that their relaxed approach toward the wetting problem helps the child adjust until the diurnal enuresis resolves.

Two special groups of patients require special consideration. For patients with recurrent urinary tract infections, a very careful voiding history should be taken. A significant number of these patients have diurnal enuresis, and treating both the recurrent infections and the diurnal enuresis allows for the best results.

*Not FDA approved for this indication.

Occasionally, little girls will have wetting within 5 to 10 minutes after urination. Even those who void incompletely generally cannot empty more of the residual urine after voiding; therefore, the source of this "leakage" must be urine pooled elsewhere. These girls reflux some urine into their vagina (vaginal voiding) when perching on the edge of the toilet to void. Then, when they race off to play upon completion, the vagina drains, dampening the underwear. This daytime enuresis can easily be treated by repositioning the patient on the toilet. Generally, having the child sit on the back half of the toilet seat while leaning against the tank, and then either counting to 100 or perhaps reading a story before leaving the bathroom, allows the vagina to drain, thereby alleviating the problem.

URINARY INCONTINENCE

method of
KENNETH M. PETERS, M.D.,
JAY B. HOLLANDER, M.D., and
ANANIAS C. DIOKNO, M.D.
William Beaumont Hospital
Royal Oak, Michigan

Urinary incontinence is defined as involuntary loss of urine sufficient to constitute a problem. It affects approximately 13 million Americans, and the direct cost associated with treating urinary incontinence is more than $15 billion per year. The prevalence of urinary incontinence increases with age, but it is not a normal part of the aging process. Among noninstitutionalized persons more than 60 years of age, the prevalence of urinary incontinence ranges from 15 to 35%, with twice as many women affected as men. Over the past 10 years, urinary incontinence in men has increased secondary to a sharp rise in local treatment for prostate cancer. In nursing homes, the prevalence of urinary incontinence is greater than 50%.

Urinary incontinence results in a loss of self-esteem and decreases the ability to maintain an independent lifestyle. The quality of life of persons with incontinence is greatly diminished, and incontinence is under-reported and undertreated.

TYPES OF INCONTINENCE

Urge Incontinence. Urge incontinence is an involuntary loss of urine due to a sudden urge to void secondary to detrusor overactivity. The disorder may be idiopathic or neurogenic or secondary to outlet obstruction, or it may be due to bladder infection or carcinoma.

Stress Incontinence. Stress incontinence is an involuntary loss of urine due to coughing, sneezing, straining, or physical activity and may be secondary to a sphincter abnormality such as hypermobility or intrinsic sphincter deficiency. Such abnormalities may be neurogenic or caused by pelvic floor relaxation, or may follow urethral, bladder, or pelvic surgery.

Mixed Incontinence. Mixed incontinence is a combination of both urge and stress incontinence and is often associated with multiple etiologic factors.

Continuous/Unconscious Incontinence. Continuous/unconscious incontinence is due to an involuntary loss of urine not associated with stress or urge symptoms. It may be secondary to intrinsic sphincter deficiency, or it may represent overflow incontinence or extraurethral incontinence such as that due to a vesicovaginal fistula.

EVALUATION OF INCONTINENCE

History

A complete history is the most important aspect of the urologic evaluation for incontinence. The clinician must attempt to define the type and degree of incontinence. The patient should be asked if leakage of urine is due to a sudden urge to void (urge incontinence) or if the leakage occurs with coughing, sneezing, or straining (stress incontinence). If both urge and stress types of incontinence are identified, the predominant type should be noted. In addition, the degree of leakage should be assessed. The number of pads per day used should be determined, and patients should be asked if they ever have episodes of complete incontinence in which urine soaks the clothing. The frequency of voiding during the day and at night should be assessed; an accurate account can be determined by having the patient complete a voiding diary. Fluid intake as well as caffeine and alcohol consumption should be assessed and quantified.

Pertinent past medical history includes a review of neurologic conditions such as stroke, Parkinson's disease, myelodysplasia, lumbar disk disease, diabetes, multiple sclerosis, and previous spinal cord injury. Previous surgical procedures such as vaginal surgery, anti-incontinence bladder surgery, or radical prostatectomy may suggest sphincter or bladder dysfunction. Radiation therapy may lead to a small, contracted bladder or radiation cystitis. A previous abdominal and perineal bowel resection or radical hysterectomy may result in nerve injury to the bladder and sphincter, leading to incontinence. A rapid method for determining the type and degree of incontinence and for obtaining pertinent medical history is completion of an incontinence questionnaire by the patient before the office visit, which can be reviewed during the clinical evaluation. An example questionnaire is presented in Table 1; it has been validated in epidemiologic surveys on urinary incontinence conducted in Washtenaw County, Michigan, over a period of 7 years.

Physical Examination

Women. The patient voids before the examination, and a urine specimen is obtained for analysis. An abdominal examination is performed to rule out masses or a distended bladder. The patient is placed in the lithotomy position, and the external genitalia, vaginal mucosa, and urethral meatus are examined and sensation is tested. A provocative test is performed by having the patient cough and determining if leakage occurs per urethra. Next, after a povidone-iodine (Betadine) swab is used to cleanse the meatus, a small catheter is placed in the bladder, and a postvoiding residual volume is obtained and recorded. Next, one half of a disposable speculum is used to determine if a urethrocele, cystocele, or rectocele is present. The degree of pelvic relaxation is assessed. A bimanual examination is performed to rule out pelvic masses and uterine prolapse. In women with a previous hysterectomy, the presence of vaginal vault prolapse or enterocele is determined. The urethral region is palpated during a Valsalva maneuver to assess the degree of urethral mobility and to determine if a urethral diverticulum may be present.

TABLE 1. **Urine Loss Questionnaire**

MESA* Uncontrolled Urine Loss Questionnaire

1. Over the past 12 months, have you had urine loss beyond your control? ___ Yes ___ No
2. How long ago did your urine loss start? ___ Years ___ Months ___ Days
3. When does the urine loss usually occur? ___ Daytime only ___ Nighttime only ___ Both

Urge Symptoms

4. Some people receive very little warning and suddenly find that they are losing, or are about to lose, urine beyond their control. How often does this happen to you? ___ Often ___ Sometimes ___ Rarely ___ Never
5. If you can't find a toilet or find that the toilet is occupied, and you have an urge to urinate, how often do you end up losing urine and wetting yourself? ___ Often ___ Sometimes ___ Rarely ___ Never
6. Do you lose urine when you suddenly have the feeling that your bladder is very full? ___ Often ___ Sometimes ___ Rarely ___ Never
7. Does washing your hands cause you to lose urine? ___ Often ___ Sometimes ___ Rarely ___ Never
8. Does cold weather cause you to lose urine? ___ Often ___ Sometimes ___ Rarely ___ Never
9. Does drinking cold beverages cause you to lose urine? ___ Often ___ Sometimes ___ Rarely ___ Never

Stress Incontinence Symptoms

10. Does coughing gently cause you to lose urine? ___ Often ___ Sometimes ___ Rarely ___ Never
11. Does coughing hard cause you to lose urine? ___ Often ___ Sometimes ___ Rarely ___ Never
12. Does sneezing cause you to lose urine? ___ Often ___ Sometimes ___ Rarely ___ Never
13. Does lifting things cause you to lose urine? ___ Often ___ Sometimes ___ Rarely ___ Never
14. Does bending over cause you to lose urine? ___ Often ___ Sometimes ___ Rarely ___ Never
15. Does laughing cause you to lose urine? ___ Often ___ Sometimes ___ Rarely ___ Never
16. Does walking briskly or jogging cause you to lose urine? ___ Often ___ Sometimes ___ Rarely ___ Never
17. Does straining, if you are constipated, cause you to lose urine? ___ Often ___ Sometimes ___ Rarely ___ Never
18. Does getting up from a sitting to a standing position cause you to lose urine? ___ Often ___ Sometimes ___ Rarely ___ Never

---

19. Have you lost urine while at rest and without urgency or warning? ___ Often ___ Sometimes ___ Rarely ___ Never
20. Do you constantly and uncontrollably dribble or leak urine throughout the day? ___ Often ___ Sometimes ___ Rarely ___ Never
21. Do you use anything for protection against leaked urine? ___ Yes (go to next question) ___ No (skip next question and go to #23)
22. On average, how many of each of these do you use for protection? (please write the number used and check each day or each week)

	Number Used	
Sanitary napkins	______	___ each day or ___ each week
Pads like those placed on furniture (such as blue pads)	______	___ each day or ___ each week
Adult wetness control garments (such as Depends)	______	___ each day or ___ each week
Toilet paper or facial tissues	______	___ each day or ___ each week
Something else (please list):		
____________________	______	___ each day or ___ each week

---

23. While awake, when you are having urine loss problems, how much would you say you lose without control EACH TIME?
    ___ less than ½ teaspoon ___ ½ teaspoon to less than 2 tablespoons
    ___ 2 tablespoons to ½ cup ___ ½ cup or more
24. Over the course of an ENTIRE DAY (24 hours) how much urine in total would you say that you lose without control when you are having problems?
    ___ less than ½ teaspoon ___ ½ teaspoon to less than 1 tablespoon
    ___ 1 tablespoon to less than ¼ cup ___ ¼ cup or more
25. When you lose urine, how much wetness usually occurs?
    ___ Just creates some moisture ___ Wets your underwear
    ___ Trickles down your thigh ___ Wets the floor
26. Generally, how many times do you usually urinate from the time you wake up to the time before you go to bed? ___ times
27. Generally, how many times do you usually urinate after you have gone to sleep at night? ___ times

*MESA: Medical Epidemiologic and Social Aspect of Aging.

From Diokno A, Yuhico M Jr: Preference, compliance and initial outcome of therapeutic options chosen by female patients with urinary incontinence. J Urol *154*:1727–1731, 1995.

A rectal examination can be performed to assess voluntary control and anal sphincter tone and to rule out fecal impaction. In addition, a retroverted uterus can be better assessed via a bimanual examination with a finger in the rectum.

Men. An abdominal examination is performed to rule out masses and a distended bladder. The external genitalia are examined, and while in the upright position, the patient is asked to strain, and leakage is assessed. A digital rectal examination is performed to assess sphincter tone and prostate size and consistency. Postvoiding residual volume is determined by either ultrasound visualization or catheterization.

Laboratory Studies

Urinalysis/Urine Culture. A urinary tract infection can lead to incontinence by causing urinary frequency and urgency. If an infection is present, it should be treated and incontinence reassessed. In addition, if microscopic hematuria is present without infection, this requires further work-up, with urine cytology, cystoscopy, and upper tract imaging to rule out carcinoma, which can cause urinary urgency and urge incontinence.

Urodynamic Testing. In cases in which the underlying cause of the incontinence is unknown such as in patients with previous anti-incontinence procedures or with mixed incontinence, urodynamic evaluation can be performed. A cystometrogram can be performed to measure the volume at first sensation, bladder capacity, and intravesical pressure. A provocative stress test can be performed when the bladder is full. The leak-point pressure can be measured to determine the integrity of the urethral sphincter. The presence of uninhibited bladder contractions can be determined. When outlet obstruction is suspected, a pressure-flow study can be performed to simultaneously measure detrusor contraction and its associated urinary flow. Incontinence can be caused by bladder outlet obstruction, leading to urinary retention and overflow incontinence.

Cystoscopy. Cystoscopy can be used to visualize the internal surface of the urethra and bladder. This will allow assessment for urethral stricture disease, prostatic enlargement, and bladder calculi or tumors.

Imaging Studies. A lateral stress cystogram can be performed with the patient straining and nonstraining to assess for hypermobility and urethral funneling. Videofluoroscopy can be performed with the patient voiding to assess for bladder and urethral abnormalities and to determine the site of obstruction and degree of pelvic relaxation. Bladder ultrasound scans can be obtained to measure post-voiding residual volume, which obviates the need for catheterization.

TREATMENT

Urge Incontinence

Urge incontinence is caused by an overactive detrusor muscle. Patients should avoid overhydration and are instructed to limit fluid intake to 6 to 8 eight-ounce glasses of liquid per day. Caffeine and alcohol consumption should be limited. Patients should void by the clock, at routine intervals, prior to feeling the urge to void. By preventing the bladder from reaching the critical capacity that stimulates the strong urge to void, the ability to maintain continence can improve. Postmenopausal women with atrophic vaginitis may benefit from estrogen replacement therapy.

If these measures do not give satisfactory results, anticholinergic medication can be initiated. Common anticholinergics include tolterodine tartrate (Detrol), 1 to 2 mg by mouth (PO) twice daily; oxybutynin (Ditropan), 2.5 to 5 mg PO two to four times a day; propantheline bromide (Pro-Banthīne),* 7.5 to 15 mg PO three to four times a day; and hyoscyamine sulfate (Levsin),* 0.125 mg PO four times a day (qid). Potential side effects of anticholinergic therapy include visual blurring, nausea, constipation, tachycardia, drowsiness, confusion, and dry mouth. Anticholinergic therapy is contraindicated if narrow-angle glaucoma is present.

Imipramine hydrochloride (Tofranil),* 10 to 25 mg PO three times a day (tid) or qid, is a tricyclic antidepressant with anticholinergic and alpha-stimulating properties. It has been shown to facilitate urine storage by decreasing bladder contractility and increasing outlet resistance. This agent has synergistic properties when used in conjunction with standard anticholinergic medications to treat urinary urgency. In the elderly, half the standard dose should be given.

*Not FDA approved for this indication.

In refractory cases, correction by various surgical techniques such as a bladder augmentation along with intermittent catheterization may be beneficial. In addition, implantation of sacral nerve stimulators, a newer method to modulate the spinal reflex, can lead to significant improvement in ability to maintain continence.

Stress Incontinence

Hypermobility

Hypermobility is caused by relaxation of the pelvic musculature in women. Treatments include surgical and nonsurgical modalities. Conservative therapy should be initiated as a first-line treatment. Obese patients should be encouraged to begin a weight loss program, and postmenopausal women may benefit from estrogen replacement therapy. A pelvic muscle exercise program should be implemented to strengthen the pelvic floor; this may be done in conjunction with biofeedback techniques. Patients should be instructed to empty the bladder at defined intervals to prevent overfilling of the bladder. Short-term improvement with behavioral modification occurs in 50 to 85% of cases. Behavioral techniques work best in motivated patients with mild incontinence.

The bladder neck and proximal urethra contain a large number of alpha-adrenergic receptor sites that, when stimulated, produce smooth muscle contraction. Alpha-adrenergic agonists such as phenylephrine,* 50 mg PO tid, or phenylpropanolamine in a long-acting preparation such as Entex LA,* one tablet one or two times per day, are effective in some patients in treating stress incontinence.

Other nonsurgical options include use of the Introl Bladder Neck Support Prosthesis (UroMed Corp., Needham, Massachusetts). This is a silicone device similar to a pessary and is available in 25 different sizes. The device is fitted by a physician and must be removed and cleaned every 24 hours. A second nonsurgical therapy is use of a urethral plug called the Reliance Urinary Control Insert (UroMed Corp.). This device is placed by the patient within the urethra and treats incontinence by obstructing the urethra. The patient removes the device when she wants to void, and a new plug is then inserted. Another noninvasive device for mild to moderate stress incontinence is the Impress (UroMed Corp.). This is a soft patch with a hydrogel coating that adheres to the urethral meatus, promoting continence. The patch is removed when the patient wishes to void, and a new patch is placed by the patient. The three devices are best used as temporary solutions prior to definitive treatment or by those patients unwilling or unable to undergo surgery.

Surgery constitutes standard treatment for ure-

*Not FDA approved for this indication.

thral hypermobility and associated stress urinary incontinence. A bladder neck suspension can be done either transvaginally, laparoscopically, or through an open incision. The best long-term success rate has been attained using the open Burch colposuspension. There has been a current trend to treat stress incontinence with the vaginal sling procedure, described later on. Although this procedure is very effective for correction of intrinsic sphincter deficiency, long-term results with its use for pure stress incontinence are not available.

Intrinsic Sphincter Deficiency

Intrinsic sphincter deficiency is characterized by sphincter injury either due to previous surgery or of neurogenic origin. In female patients this can be treated by several modalities. First, periurethral bulking can be performed using glutaraldehyde cross-linked bovine collagen (Contigen; Bard Corp., Covington, Georgia). The collagen is placed using a cystoscope and needle after local anesthesia has been achieved. The success rate is variable but reported to be about 60%. Newer injectables are currently under investigation. A second treatment for sphincteric injury includes the transvaginal sling procedure. This procedure entails placing a piece of fascia or artificial sling material under the urethra near the bladder neck, which is secured with sutures to the suprapubic region. The support provided by the sling increases the resistance of the urethra, thus increasing continence. This approach is a very effective treatment in women. A specialized procedure in women is to place an artificial urinary sphincter around the bladder neck. This approach is very effective in treating incontinence; however, implantation procedures are technically demanding, and potential complications including infection, erosion, and mechanical failure present significant challenges.

Sphincteric insufficiency in men is most often due to surgical treatment for prostate disease. The incontinence may be associated with Valsalva maneuvers or may present as continuous leakage. The incontinence can be managed with protective pads or penile clamps. The use of periurethral bulking agents has not been successful in men. The most effective treatment is placement of an artificial urinary sphincter at the level of the bulbous urethra. This device remains in the closed position until the patient wishes to void. A pump, positioned in the scrotum, is used to open the sphincter and allow normal voiding. The sphincter automatically cycles to a closed position after 2 to 3 minutes.

Mixed Incontinence

Mixed incontinence is a combination of both urge and stress incontinence. Multimodality therapy can be instituted using anticholinergic medications and suspension procedures to treat this type of incontinence.

Overflow Incontinence

Overflow incontinence is caused by incomplete emptying of the bladder and may be secondary to a decompensated detrusor or to outlet obstruction from prostate hypertrophy or stricture disease. Surgical correction of outlet obstruction can allow for complete bladder emptying. However, if the detrusor is atonic secondary to chronic obstruction or to neurologic problems such as diabetic neuropathy, multiple sclerosis, or lower motor neuron lesions, the incontinence can be treated by clean intermittent catheterization (CIC). Since first introduced by Lapides in 1972, CIC has revolutionized the management of patients with detrusor failure. The technique can be taught on an outpatient basis and requires nothing more than clean catheters and lubricant. Catheterization intervals are adjusted to maintain bladder volumes sufficient to prevent leakage.

Refractory Incontinence

For patients who fail treatment and remain incontinent or those too ill for treatment, protective pads and garments can be used. These can be either disposable or washable. For men, external collection devices such as condom catheters can be used. In chronically ill patients with limited mobility, an indwelling Foley catheter or suprapubic tube can be placed. Tubes and catheters need to be changed monthly, and the catheter should be cleaned daily to prevent encrustation. In addition, patients with chronic catheters should undergo cystoscopy annually to rule out stone or cancer formation.

EPIDIDYMITIS

method of
STEPHEN N. ROUS, M.D., M.S.
Dartmouth Medical School
Hanover, New Hampshire
Dartmouth-Hitchcock Medical Center
Lebanon, New Hampshire
Veterans Affairs Medical Center
White River Junction, Vermont

Epididymitis is an inflammatory condition of the epididymis that is almost always caused by a bacterial infection but may, on infrequent occasion, be secondary to direct trauma to the epididymis. It is characterized by moderate to severe scrotal pain and is an extremely common problem bringing male patients to both the primary care physician and the urologist as well.

ETIOLOGY AND PATHOGENESIS

In younger men (under age 40), the usual route of bacterial infection is an ascending one from a focus of sexually transmitted infection in the urethra that is most often chlamydial, although *Neisseria gonorrhoeae* or any of the other sexually transmitted organisms may be the etiologic agent. The bacteria travel from the urethra in retrograde fashion through the ejaculatory ducts and the vas deferens and then to the epididymis. In these patients, a careful history may elicit the presence of a urethral discharge prior to or concurrent with the scrotal pain. Another and much smaller group of patients (of any age) may have noted a distant source of infection in places such as the oral cavity including the teeth, the ears, or the skin, and in these patients the route of spread of infection to the epididymis may be hematogenous. In older men, the infection usually begins in the bladder and is due to bladder outlet obstruction. The bacteria are carried in the urine during voiding to the prostatic urethra, the ejaculatory ducts, the vas, and the epididymis. Rarely, a focus of infection within the prostate itself (either acute or chronic bacterial prostatitis) may be the source of the infecting bacteria, which then follow the same route into the epididymis.

Uncommon causes of epididymitis include tuberculosis, as in patients with human immunodeficiency virus (HIV) infection. In the younger man or in the pediatric age group, an ectopic ureter emptying into a seminal vesicle can be the cause of recurrent epididymitis.

CLINICAL FEATURES

The primary symptom of acute epididymitis is gradually increasing pain, usually over a period of hours to days, that is usually noticed within the scrotum but may be noted initially in the groin or lower abdomen. If onset is in the abdomen, the pain rapidly shifts and localizes to the scrotum. When fully developed, the pain can be quite severe and may be accompanied by a low-grade fever (temperature rarely over 101°F). If the vas is also involved in the inflammatory process, the pain may include the cord and may even extend upward into the lower abdomen on the affected side. There may be some dysuria if there has been an antecedent infective process in the urethra. Not infrequently, the inflammatory process spreads to the adjacent testis producing an epididymo-orchitis. This is different from a pure orchitis, which is almost always viral in origin, being usually caused by an enterovirus (such as mumps virus), and in which the epididymis is normal and not involved in the inflammatory process.

PHYSICAL, LABORATORY, AND IMAGING FINDINGS

In the initial stages, the epididymis is very tender to palpation and may be slightly enlarged and indurated. When the inflammatory process is fully developed, the epididymis can be up to five or even 10 times its normal size and it is usually exquisitely tender to palpation. If the vas is also inflamed, the cord may feel somewhat thickened and may be tender to the touch. When the patient is in the dorsal recumbent position, elevation of the scrotum with the examining hand may relieve the pain somewhat; this can be an important point in the differential diagnosis for acute testicular torsion, in which elevation of the scrotum exacerbates the pain (because it is effectively pulling on the cord). The testis feels normal to palpation in the early phases of epididymitis unless or until a condition of epididymo-orchitis exists. In such cases it is not usually possible to palpate the epididymis separately, and the scrotal contents on the affected side present as one large, firm, and very tender mass about the size of a plum or a small lemon.

Urinalysis often discloses white blood cells and possibly even bacteria if the process originated with a nonspecific urethritis or any infection in the lower urinary tract. The white blood count may on occasion show a leukocytosis with a shift to the left but is more often normal. X-ray studies of the scrotum are not helpful, but ultrasonography with Doppler flow studies is most helpful both in suggesting the diagnosis of epididymitis (by an increased blood flow to the inflamed epididymis) and in differentiating this condition from torsion of the testis, which classically shows a decreased blood flow to the epididymis and testis.

DIFFERENTIAL DIAGNOSIS

It is absolutely critical to bear in mind that torsion of the spermatic cord can at times mimic epididymitis in its onset. Typically, torsion occurs in the first two decades of life and is very rare after age 25. Epididymitis tends to occur in a somewhat older age group. Physical examination is often helpful in making this distinction, and a Doppler ultrasound scan may help the clinician to the right diagnosis. Nevertheless, referral of the patient to a urologist is always in order unless torsion can be positively ruled out. Finally, the presenting sign with cancer of the testis can be a secondary epididymitis; this latter condition can often prevent the clinician from doing an adequate examination of the testis itself. The rule of thumb here is follow-up evaluation of the patient at intervals of 1 to 2 weeks, with one or more ultrasound examinations of the scrotum performed as needed. If the epididymitis has not resolved within about 3 weeks to the point that the testis can be adequately palpated and felt to be normal, and/or if the ultrasound scan of the testis suggests the possibility of a tumor, then surgical exploration should be considered.

TREATMENT

Symptomatic treatment consisting of elevation of the scrotum, usually with an athletic supporter, provides some degree of pain relief, as will administration of a nonsteroidal anti-inflammatory drug such as ibuprofen, 400 to 800 mg three times a day for 1 or 2 weeks. If the process is caught early before much swelling of the epididymis occurs, a spermatic cord block with bupivacaine (Marcaine) may prevent any severe discomfort. Antibiotics are indicated if fever is present and/or if a bacterial infection (as opposed to trauma) is thought to be etiologic. Appropriate cultures should be initiated, but antibiotic therapy may begin before culture results are available and then changed as indicated. If a sexually transmitted organism in the urethra is thought to be responsible, doxycycline (Vibramycin), in a loading dose of 200 mg orally and then 100 mg given twice daily (bid) for 2 weeks, is the agent of choice. If gonorrhea is thought also to be present, then ceftriaxone (Rocephin), 250 mg administered intramuscularly (IM) in a single dose, is given in addition to the doxycycline. Alternative antibiotic therapy for a gonorrheal infection is administration of one of the fluoroquinolones such as ciprofloxacin (Cipro), 500 mg orally in a single dose, combined with spectinomycin (Trobicin), 2 grams IM in a single dose. Alternative therapy for a chlamydial infection is administration of tetracycline, 500 mg by mouth (PO) four times daily for 2 weeks.

For an infection from a source in the bladder or prostate, or from one spread hematogenously, one of the fluoroquinolones, such as ciprofloxacin (Cipro), 500 mg orally bid for 10 days, or trimethoprim-sulfamethoxazole (Bactrim; Septra), one double-strength tablet bid for 10 days, should be used. If chronic bacterial prostatitis is diagnosed, the therapy should continue for 6 to 10 weeks. Chronic epididymitis, with continuous or recurring pain in the scrotum, is a sequela in some men. Epididymectomy may be indicated in these patients although this does not always resolve the problem.

It must be remembered that in immunocompromised patients with HIV infection, any infectious or inflammatory process is not likely to heal rapidly.

PRIMARY GLOMERULAR DISEASES

method of
SEAN F. LEAVEY, M.B., B.CHIR., and
ROGER C. WIGGINS, M.B., B.CHIR.
University of Michigan Medical School
Ann Arbor, Michigan

The primary care physician has a central role in the prevention of end-stage renal disease (ESRD). The enormous personal and economic costs of ESRD are shown in Table 1. The goal is to prevent or retard progression to ESRD, the underlying concept being that if the physician can delay progression to ESRD for even 1 year she or he will have saved $50,000 and 15% of a life. The opportunities to prevent progression to ESRD can be distilled down to three critical factors: (1) early recognition of disease; (2) aggressive management of blood pressure, proteinuria, lipids, and diet, and (3) judicious use of disease-specific therapies (Figure 1). Glomerular diseases are classified on the basis of histology and on the basis of being either "primary" (idiopathic and renal-limited) or "secondary," where there is an identifiable underlying systemic process.

Progression of a primary glomerular disease is the result of processes that lead to the irreversible replacement of normal renal tissues by scar tissue and eventually to a shrunken, scarred, nonfunctioning kidney. Progression to ESRD can take as little as 2 weeks or as long as 20 years. Rapid progression (a characteristic of the syndrome of rapidly progressive glomerulonephritis [RPGN]) can be halted by early diagnosis and emergent institution of disease-specific treatment, thereby preserving useful renal function. Even when this is done successfully and the underlying primary disease remains in remission, however, many of these patients still tend to progress to ESRD by mechanisms shown in Figure 1. In doing so, they join the even larger group of patients with other primary glomerular diseases that display a pattern of slow progression. In contrast to RPGN, with chronic progression there is a wider window of opportunity time for active intervention. Equally the window of opportunity for nonsustained intervention and poor compliance, which too often compromise the renoprotective effort, is also wide. Risk factors for progression, shared by all glomerular diseases, are shown in Table 2. The most important of these are hypertension and proteinuria. Whether the primary disease is active or in remission, the damaged glomerulus remains highly susceptible to further damage by systemic and glomerular hypertension (see Figure 1). Sustained aggressive blood pressure management represents the single greatest opportunity to prevent or delay the development of ESRD in these chronic diseases.

The following recommendations relate to the treatment of adults with primary glomerular diseases (Table 3). Although general principles are the same, blood pressure goals, drug dosing, dietary, and fluid prescriptions may differ in pediatric populations.

TABLE 1. **Personal and Economic Costs of Progression to ESRD**

Mortality ~ 15% per y
Decreased quality of life
Direct cost ~ $50,000/patient/y

Abbreviation: ESRD = End-stage renal disease (~250,000 cases in United States, 1995).

TABLE 2. **Risk Factors for Progression to ESRD**

1. Systemic hypertension
2. Persistent proteinuria
3. Impaired baseline renal function at diagnosis
4. Interstitial fibrosis on renal biopsy

TABLE 3. **Priorities in the Management of Glomerular Disease**

Recognition and Diagnosis
- Early recognition of chronic disease (hematuria, proteinuria, edema, hypertension, renal dysfunction)
- Early recognition and emergent management of RPGN
- Renal biopsy and exclusion of secondary etiologies

Risk Assessment for Progression (see Table 2)

Global Treatment Strategies (see Figure 1)
- Aggressive blood pressure control *for all:* target 120 mm Hg systolic, 80 mm Hg diastolic; prioritize ACE inhibition, patient education, patient involvement
- Antiproteinuric therapy with ACE inhibition for proteinuric patients (hypertensive or normotensive)
- Lipid-lowering therapy
- Avoid excess dietary protein and maintain adequate nutritional status

Disease-Specific Treatment Strategies
(see Figure 1 and text)

Longitudinal Follow-up/Chronic Care Plan
- Sustained aggressive blood pressure management *for all*
- Patient involvement: self-monitoring, diary, education
- Monitor urinary protein excretion, serum creatinine, underlying disease
- Monitor for treatment toxicities of specific therapies

Abbreviations: RPGN = rapidly progressive glomerulonephritis; ACE = angiotensin-converting enzyme.

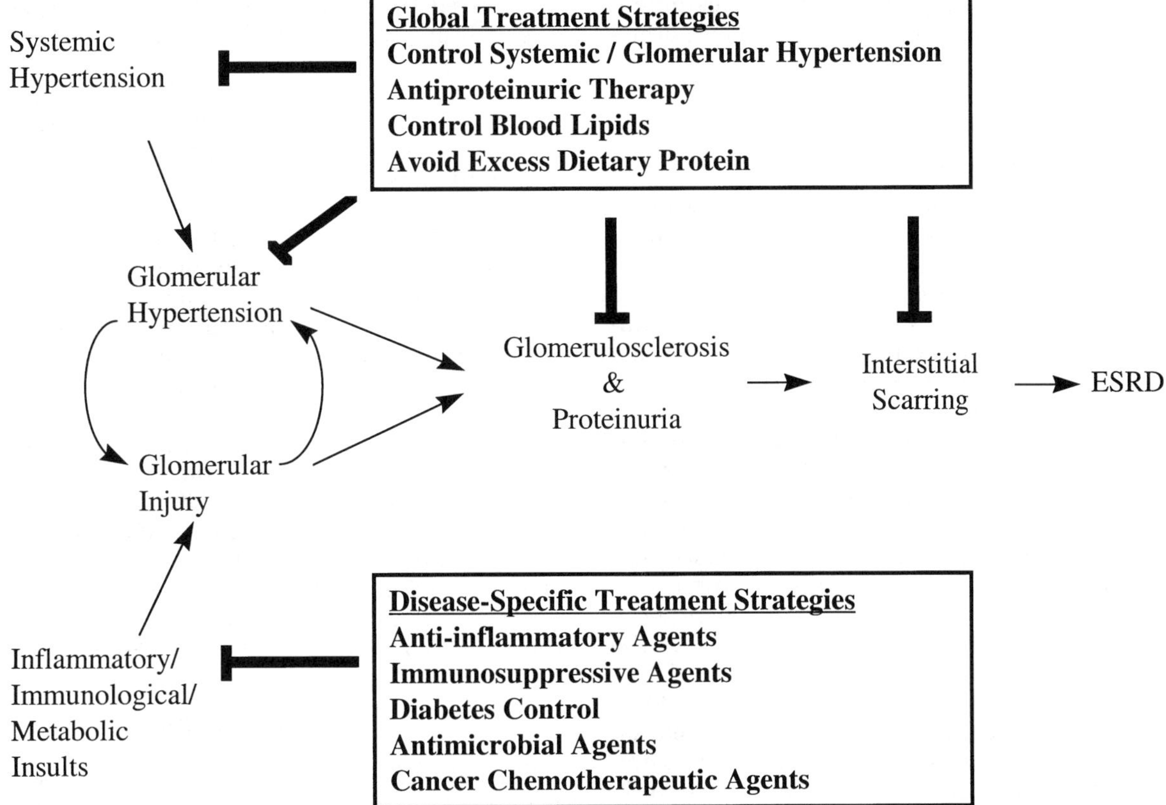

Figure 1. Progression of glomerular disease and opportunities for intervention.

RECOGNIZING GLOMERULAR DISEASE

For all its functional complexity, the normal glomerulus serves simply to elaborate, at a rate of approximately 125 mL per minute, an ultrafiltrate of plasma that is free of cellular components and all but a small amount of protein (<150 mg per 24 hours). Diseased glomeruli provide for a limited repertoire of clinical presentations that include some combination of reduced glomerular filtration rate (GFR), hematuria, leukocyturia, proteinuria, salt and water retention, hypertension, and metabolic derangement. Common clinical presentations are shown in Table 4. Elevated concentrations of the serum creatinine and blood urea nitrogen (BUN) are late, insensitive markers of a reduced GFR. Far too many cases of glomerular disease are diagnosed (some with ESRD) when these markers are substantially elevated and irreversible scarring has occurred. Early recognition of disease depends on astute integration of findings from the history, physical examination, and urinalysis.

Urinalysis and Serum Chemistries: When Should They Be Performed?

Symptoms and signs, both directly and indirectly referable to the urinary tract, that should prompt urinalysis (and usually serum chemistries) include loin pain, macroscopic hematuria, dysuria, frequency of micturition, nocturia, polyuria, frothy urine, malodorous urine, hypertension, edema, new heart murmur, allergic or vascular skin rash, arthralgias or arthritis, and a history of diseases known to injure the kidney. Sometimes an abnormal screening urinal-

TABLE 4. **Common Clinical Syndromes and Presentations**

Nephrotic syndrome	Proteinuria (>3.5 gm/1.73 m^2/day), hypoalbuminemia, edema, hypercholesterolemia, hypercoagulability, susceptibility to infections
Acute nephritic syndrome	Hypertension, hematuria, edema, reduced GFR
Chronic glomerulonephritis	Presentation with advanced disease, difficult diagnosis (biopsy and urinary protein excretion may not be helpful)
Persistent proteinuria and hematuria with normal GFR	Suggest intrarenal pathology
Persistent isolated asymptomatic proteinuria with normal GFR	Orthostatic proteinuria or intrarenal pathology
Isolated asymptomatic microscopic hematuria with normal GFR (>1 occasion)	Nonglomerular causes common (infection, stones, trauma, malignancies, hereditary) Glomerular causes (IgAN, thin GBM disease) less likely

Abbreviations: GFR = glomerular filtration rate; IgAN = IgA nephropathy; GBM = glomerular basement membrane.

ysis in a routine insurance/work physical examination can be the harbinger of underlying renal pathology.

Urinalysis, Urinary Protein Excretion, and Their Interpretation

Reagent strip testing of urine provides key information. Urine microscopy allows a diagnosis to be made.

In leukocyturia, the presence of white blood cells (WBCs) in the urine indicates urinary tract inflammation. The cause of inflammation may be infection or immune processes such as systemic lupus erythematosus (SLE), vasculitis, or other diseases.

White cells and red cells may enter the urine anywhere along the urinary tract, but their presence within casts or in association with tubular epithelial cells and cellular and granular casts points to renal parenchymal disease. Red blood cell (RBC) casts indicate glomerular disease but are by no means necessary for this diagnosis. Heme positivity alone does not increase urinary protein concentrations until the urine appears pink or frankly bloody.

In proteinuria, the persistent presence of 100 to 500 mg per dL proteinuria on dipstick examination is suggestive of parenchymal disease. Significant proteinuria (100 mg per dL and higher, or persistent 30 mg per dL proteinuria) should be quantitated either in a 24-hour urine sample along with creatinine measurement or by the calculation of a urine protein/creatinine ratio. Normally, less than 150 mg of protein is excreted per day. The protein/creatinine ratio is a reasonable estimate of 24-hour urinary protein, although it is subject to variations in muscle mass/creatinine generation. In tubular disease, less efficient absorption and catabolism of low-molecular-weight proteins that traverse healthy glomeruli can lead to 1 to 2 grams of proteinuria per day. In glomerular diseases, alterations in the filtration barrier can allow larger quantities of albumin and higher-molecular-weight proteins to enter the filtrate. Greater than 2 grams of proteinuria generally signifies underlying glomerular disease, and nephrotic-range proteinuria (>3.5 gm per 1.73 m^2 per day) is pathognomonic for its presence. Urine protein electrophoresis is useful to qualitatively describe proteinuria as glomerular or tubular in type. Urine immunoelectrophoresis may characterize gram quantities of immunoglobulin light chains in the urine as monoclonal or polyclonal in origin.

RECOGNIZING RAPIDLY PROGRESSIVE GLOMERULONEPHRITIS

RPGN is a clinical syndrome characterized by a rapid decrease in renal function that causes a rise in the serum creatinine over days or weeks. This is associated with signs and symptoms of fluid retention (hypertension, edema) and evidence of inflammation of the glomerulus detectable in the urine as manifested by the presence of protein, RBCs (some of which may be dysmorphic), leukocytes, and cellular and granular casts. The urine may even be frankly bloody. Diagnosis and treatment of RPGN syndromes is a medical emergency, because when diagnosed early and treated urgently, they are treatable and considerable renal function can be preserved.

RPGN should be suspected in any individual with an unexplained rise or newly diagnosed elevation in the serum creatinine, as well as blood and protein in the urine. Sometimes the same pathologic processes that give rise to RPGN can be more indolent, causing progression over many months, and may masquerade as chronic renal failure associated with other causes of renal failure such as hypertensive nephrosclerosis. In patients with persistent and unexplained symptoms such as fatigue, lethargy, flu, anorexia, malaise, gastrointestinal upset, dyspnea, and weight loss, serum creatinine measurement and a urinalysis should be performed. An unexplained elevation in the serum creatinine and blood and protein in the urine may be the clues to a treatable systemic disease.

RENAL BIOPSY

Cost-effectiveness issues mandate subspecialty nephrologic consultation. Kidney biopsy is often necessary because of considerable variation in both clinical presentations and disease-specific treatments, not just between but also within histologic variants of glomerular disease.

EXCLUSION OF SECONDARY CAUSES OF GLOMERULAR DISEASES

Exclusion of secondary causes of glomerular diseases is required because of differences in treatment and prognosis. History and physical examination may suggest underlying causes including drugs, infections, malignancies, and collagen vascular diseases. Chest radiography, stool guaiac testing (and/or sigmoidoscopy), prostate-specific antigen assay, mammography, and cervical smears are basic screening tools for occult cancers in adults with glomerular disease. Serologic tests in diagnosing glomerular disease may include any combination of assays for antistreptolysin-O antibodies, hepatitis B and hepatitis C antibodies, antinuclear and anti-DNA antibodies, complement levels, antineutrophil cytoplasmic antibodies (ANCA), anti–glomerular basement membrane antibodies (anti-GBM), cryoglobulins, and, where appropriate, human immunodeficiency virus (HIV) antibody. Low complement levels in glomerular disease narrow the differential diagnosis to acute postinfectious glomerulonephritis, primary and secondary causes of membranoproliferative glomerulonephritis, and SLE. Blood cultures, echocardiography, and abdominal imaging are sometimes indicated to look for deep-seated infections. Unexplained reductions in GFR in the over-40 age group require a serum protein electrophoresis and urine immunoelectrophoresis to screen for multiple myeloma.

The rapidity with which investigation should take place is dictated by clinical presentation. Insights into the acuity or chronicity of the presentation from old records and from ultrasound measurements of kidney size are helpful. Most glomerular diseases have a slow indolent course, but if there is a possibility of an RPGN, rapid diagnosis (within 24 to 48 hours of presentation) and rapid treatment (empirically within 24 hours of presentation if suspicion is high) are needed to preserve renal function.

AGGRESSIVE BLOOD PRESSURE CONTROL FOR ALL: TARGET 120/80

The modification of diet in renal disease (MDRD) study showed that patients with a mixture of nondiabetic renal diseases benefit from aggressive control of blood pressure and that the degree of benefit is positively correlated with the extent of proteinuria at baseline. Time must be spent educating patients regarding the importance of the role blood pressure control plays in preventing progression to ESRD. Patient involvement in measuring and recording home blood pressures to bring to the clinic is encouraged. The importance of compliance with medical regimens is emphasized. Reinforcing this education is important over the long term, as this is when the development of noncompliance and consequent avoidable progressive renal injury is often seen.

First-Line Strategies: Angiotensin-Converting Enzyme Inhibitors and Angiotensin II Receptor Blockers

The first-line antihypertensive agent in glomerular disease is an angiotensin-converting enzyme (ACE) inhibitor. A combination of experimental, clinical trial, and meta-analysis data has suggested superior renoprotective effects of ACE inhibitors over other antihypertensive agents at equivalent levels of blood pressure control. Together with the newer angiotensin II receptor blockers, this class of drug is associated with a predictable initial decline in GFR. The decline in GFR is the hemodynamic consequence of a reduction in the angiotensin II–mediated postglomerular arteriolar constriction that is almost universally present in patients with glomerular disease, chronic renal insufficiency, or decreased true or effective circulating blood volume. The early decline in GFR is desirable, as it is an immediate indicator of a successful reduction in glomerular hypertension, one of the mechanisms by which ACE inhibitors slow subsequent progressive declines in GFR (see Figure 1). A decline in GFR, therefore, *should not* prompt cessation of the ACE inhibitor unless it is also associated with problematic hyperkalemia or azotemia. Azotemia is generally a problem only when ACE inhibition is attempted in patients with advanced chronic renal failure (creatinine >4 mg per dL) or severe baseline prerenal azotemia. Holding a few diuretic doses in those with prerenal azotemia, or instituting a potassium-restricted diet (2 gm potassium) and a loop diuretic (or stopping potassium-sparing diuretics and potassium supplements) in patients with less severe baseline chronic renal insufficiency (creatinine <4 mg per dL) allows effective institution of ACE inhibition in most patients. Modest hyperkalemia (potassium <5.5 mEq per liter) may be managed with these approaches, sometimes without stopping or necessitating only temporary cessation of the medication.

Severe baseline renal failure and baseline hyperkalemia are limiting factors to the use of these agents. Acute renal failure may rarely complicate the use of ACE inhibition because of renal infarction. This occurs in patients with severe renovascular disease in whom abrupt hypotensive effects of ACE inhibition can drop the perfusion pressure across a tight renal artery stenosis and precipitate complete occlusion. Caution in using these agents is required in patients with suspected severe renal artery stenosis. A final caveat relates to women of childbearing age who should be counseled regarding the risks of ACE fetopathy. When it is desirable to use these medications in women of childbearing age, the use of effective birth control is required, and patients should report any pregnancy immediately, after which the drugs are discontinued.

In most patients we use a longer-acting ACE inhibitor from the start (enalapril [Vasotec], orally 5 to 20 mg twice daily, or lisinopril [Zestril, Prinivil], orally 10 to 40 mg once daily). The initial doses are always once daily at the lower end of the dosage scale but can be titrated upwards on a weekly basis as needed. After institution of an ACE inhibitor and with each dose escalation, we recommend checking potassium, creatinine, and BUN levels at 3 days and 1 week later. We do not stop the drug for asymptomatic changes in the BUN or serum creatinine. In patients with baseline azotemia, we prefer to initiate ACE inhibition with a short-acting ACE inhibitor initially at a low dose (captopril [Capoten], orally 12.5 mg twice daily). We switch to a longer-acting preparation to improve compliance if the short-acting medication is well tolerated. Patients who are prerenal or have heart failure should also start on a short-acting agent initially at half the initial doses recommended here.

If the kinin-mediated side effects of cough or angioedema preclude the use of ACE inhibitors, our next choice of medications are angiotensin II, class 1-receptor blockers (losartan [Cozaar], 25 to 100 mg orally once daily, or valsartan [Diovan], 80 to 320 mg orally once daily). The recommendations for chronic renal impairment, prerenal states, and for women of childbearing age also apply to these medications.

Second Line: Volume Control in Hypertensive Patients with Kidney Diseases

Often ACE inhibition alone fails to achieve the target set for aggressive blood pressure control because of intravascular volume expansion. The addition of sufficient loop diuretic to restore a normovolemic state usually makes the difference. When it is obvious that the patient is volume expanded, it is important to waste little time in the addition of a loop diuretic, as rapid and effective blood pressure control builds patient confidence. Furosemide ([Lasix], 40 mg orally once or twice daily), in an individual with good renal function is usually effective. Higher doses of loop diuretics with addition of metolazone (Zaroxolyn), 2.5 to 10 mg orally once daily, may be required in patients with advanced renal failure. This strategy applies to both edematous and nonedematous patients, because intravascular volume can be expanded in the absence of edema. The combination of an ACE inhibitor and a diuretic can be expected to cause an increase in the serum creatinine concentration, reflecting reduced glomerular hyperfiltration. This is usually associated with reduced proteinuria. Potassium supplements are usually not required because the ACE inhibitor causes reduced potassium excretion. Volume control in nephrotic syndrome is discussed elsewhere.

Beta Blockers, Alpha-Adrenergic Receptor Blockers, and Others

Additional antihypertensive medications are often required to achieve blood pressure goals. We use beta blockers (metoprolol [Lopressor, Toprol]) and/or alpha$_1$-receptor blockers (terazosin, [Hytrin]) or the combined agent (labetalol [Normodyne, Trandate]) next and subsequently either extended release preparations of non-dihydropyridine calcium channel blockers or the centrally acting drug clonidine (Catapres). Accelerated hypertension, which is beyond the scope of this discussion, may be managed with combinations of ACE inhibitors and injectable medications including labetalol, hydralazine [Apresoline], or sodium nitroprusside.

ANTIPROTEINURIC THERAPY WITH ACE INHIBITORS

In addition to their salutary effects on hypertension, ACE inhibitors and angiotensin-receptor blockers lead to a reduction in proteinuria, which may be independently beneficial. As with the predictable decline in GFR, the reduction in proteinuria may also be, at least initially, the result of the desired intrarenal hemodynamic effect of these treatments, namely, reduced glomerular hypertension. Over time, however, a sustained reduction in proteinuria may indicate reduced progressive glomerular injury. We use ACE inhibition in all proteinuric patients irrespective of the presence or absence of hypertension. They are introduced at low doses as discussed previously. The same side effects and caveats exist. We increase the dose gradually toward the same maximum doses. In the proportion of patients normotensive at onset, the dose level tolerated is generally determined by the onset of hypotension. This indication for ACE inhibition ceases in normotensive patients with normal renal function, whose disease is in complete remission. However, we continue the following groups on ACE inhibitors even when their disease is in remission: frequent relapsers with idiopathic nephrotic syndrome, normotensive patients with impaired renal function, and all hypertensive patients with renal disease. Nonsteroidal anti-inflammatory drugs also have been proposed as potential agents for reducing proteinuria; however, there are little data to support their prolonged use for this indication.

PROTEIN INTAKE AND MAINTENANCE OF AN ADEQUATE NUTRITIONAL STATE

We strongly discourage excessive protein intake (>1 gram per kg per day), prescribe all patients a protein intake of 0.8 gm per kg per day, and assess initially and longitudinally total dietary intake and nutritional status. These recommendations are based on the general literature and the MDRD clinical trial.

The MDRD clinical trial attempted to evaluate the role of protein restriction in preventing progression by comparing either "normal" 1.3 grams per kg per day or low 0.6 gram per kg per day dietary protein prescriptions in those with moderate renal impairment, and either a low or a very low (amino acid–supplemented) protein diet in patients with severe renal impairment. Although the intention-to-treat analysis failed to show a benefit, the study suffered from a number of major limitations: the low protein diet interventions resulted in an early decline of GFR (both predictable and desirable [consider the similar effect of ACE inhibition]); follow-up was too short; and in advanced renal disease the effect of a nonprotein-restricted diet was not assessed. A later analysis of study data on actual (not prescribed) protein intake concluded that the progression of advanced renal disease was retarded by an actual daily protein intake of 0.6 gram per kg per day. MDRD showed that protein restriction need not compromise overall nutritional status. This is important because patients who reach ESRD malnourished are at a significantly increased risk for mortality.

LIPID-LOWERING THERAPY

Hypercholesterolemia in primary glomerular disease warrants treatment not just for the primary prevention of coronary artery disease, but also because of experimental data suggesting that dyslipidemias enhance progressive renal injury. In nephrotic syndrome, hypercholesterolemia is understood to occur as a result of secondary up-regulation of biosynthetic pathways in the liver, the rate-limiting step in cholesterol synthesis being catalyzed by beta-hydroxy-methyl-glutaryl coenzyme A (HMGCoA) reductase. In sustained hypercholesterolemic states use of any of the "statin" class of medications (HMGCoA reductase inhibitors) can effectively lower both serum total and low-density lipoprotein cholesterol levels. The newly available medication atorvastatin (Lipitor) 10 to 40 mg orally once daily, appears to be particularly effective. These drugs are given once a day in the evening and are generally well tolerated. Myopathy/rhabdomyolysis (manifested by an elevated creatine kinase) and transaminasemia are rare complications. Increased vigilance for rhabdomyolysis is necessary when cyclosporine is being used concomitantly. In idiopathic nephrotic syndromes complete remission can remove the need for lipid-lowering intervention.

ANTICOAGULATION IN THE NEPHROTIC SYNDROME

Most patients with the nephrotic syndrome do not require anticoagulation. However, a hypercoagulable state in nephrotic syndrome, resulting from an imbalance in circulating procoagulants and anticoagulants secondary to urinary losses of proteins such as antithrombin-III and proteins S and C, is associated with an increased incidence of thrombosis. Immobilization secondary to swelling may also predispose to stasis and clotting. Lower extremity deep venous thrombosis, pulmonary embolism, and renal vein thrombosis are seen. Renal vein thrombosis may present classically with flank pain, hematuria, and an increase in the serum creatinine. More often, however, it is clinically silent and its presence, or that of a lower extremity venous thrombosis, is heralded by symptomatic pulmonary embolism. Diagnosis of a thrombotic or thromboembolic complication requires anticoagulation treatment with heparin, followed by warfarin, which should be continued as long as the patient is nephrotic, or for 3 months after the nephrotic syndrome has entered remission.

PROPHYLAXIS AND TREATMENT OF INFECTIONS IN NEPHROTIC SYNDROME

Urinary loss of immunoglobulin proteins, impaired humoral and cellular immunity, and defective opsonization and phagocytosis within the reticuloendothelial system are all seen in nephrotic patients. Spontaneous bacterial peritonitis with pneumococcus is a classic complication. It underlines a more general susceptibility to infections not just with encapsulated organisms, but also with opportunistic pathogens and a propensity for more severe disease in patients exposed to common viral pathogens such as varicella zoster. In general, infections are managed as per standard procedures in non-nephrotic patients. Exposure to varicella, however, in a nonimmune host requires immediate prophylaxis with zoster immune globulin. Live attenuated virus vaccines should only be used when the disease is in remission. Administration of pneumococcal and *Haemophilus influenzae* B vaccines is also most effective when the disease is in partial or complete remission because response rates are likely to be poor if the disease is not in remission.

EDEMA MANAGEMENT IN NEPHROTIC SYNDROME

In edematous patients, the goal is to establish a net negative salt and water balance to ameliorate swelling, and when this has been achieved, to maintain an even balance. However, it is usually not possible, nor is it desirable, to get rid of edema completely in severe nephrotics. The first steps are dietary salt restriction (a 2-gram sodium diet is prescribed) and a diuretic. A loop diuretic is used (furosemide, 20 mg orally twice daily) doubling the initial dose as necessary to achieve a natriuresis. Patients resistant to 200 mg orally twice daily of furosemide may be helped by the addition of metolazone, 2.5 mg orally once daily, increased in increments of 2.5 mg to a maximum of 10 mg to achieve an effect. Potassium supplements may not be necessary if an ACE inhibitor is used concomitantly to reduce protein loss in the urine. Throughout the diuresis, patients maintain a weight chart and are given weight reduction targets (in general 1 to 4 pounds per day is sought in adult patients). Some individuals have severe refractory edema and by admitting these patients and using large doses of loop diuretics (administered intravenously) and oral metolazone, we usually achieve a diuresis and natriuresis. Thigh-high elastic stockings may be helpful in some patients. On rare occasions it is necessary to use salt-poor albumin (Buminate), 25 grams intravenously in 100 mL together with an intravenous diuretic. Such albumin infusions cannot be used in the long term but can be given three times daily for a few days, under careful medical supervision, in situations where other treatment strategies are being adopted.

DISEASE-SPECIFIC TREATMENT STRATEGIES

General Principles

Two basic goals of disease-specific therapeutic interventions are the following:

1. To switch off the underlying immune process driving glomerular injury (e.g., production of anti-GBM antibodies or immune complexes). This applies to all situations in which we use disease-specific therapies.
2. To halt glomerular inflammation. This goal applies particularly to clinical presentations of RPGN but also to other inflammatory forms of glomerulonephritis.

Two basic overriding considerations of treatment are that (1) the expected benefit in terms of preventing progression to ESRD must be greater than the risk of treatment and (2) painstaking and continuous monitoring for treatment toxicities of immunosuppressive therapies is mandatory.

Commonly Used Therapeutic Agents

Glucocorticoids

Glucocorticoids are used both to suppress primary immune processes and to halt severe glomerular inflammation. In the latter instance, high doses must be given intravenously to achieve sufficient active concentrations at the site of injury. When using pulse intravenous steroids, care must be taken to administer them slowly over 20 to 30 minutes, as rapid infusions have been known to precipitate arrhythmias. The side effects of oral steroids are related to the duration of use and the total cumulative dose. Prolonged usage can lead to diabetes, osteoporosis, hypertension, cataracts, poor growth, increased susceptibility to infections, aseptic necrosis, myopathy, and muscle wasting. Frequent dose-related side effects that typically improve as the steroid doses are lowered include facial swelling, weight gain, acne, depression, and mood lability. If long-term glucocorticoids are to be used, they must be used at low doses. If higher doses are required, a steroid-sparing adjunctive agent (e.g., azathioprine* [Imuran], or mycophenolate mofetil* [CellCept]) must be added to the steroid regimen to allow the glucocorticoid dose to be reduced to a nontoxic level.

Cyclophosphamide

The alkylating agent cyclophosphamide* (Cytoxan) is an important adjunct to glucocorticoids in certain presentations of primary renal disease. Oral cyclophosphamide is used to achieve and maintain a WBC of approximately 5000 per mm^3. In taking the responsibility to use cyclophosphamide, one must recognize the potential side effects and take steps to prevent them. All side effects are dose related and include leukopenia leading to infection and death, induction of malignancy (primarily of skin, bladder, or lymphoproliferative type), loss of hair, ovarian failure (more commonly in the over-30 age group); azoospermia, and fibrotic and hemorrhagic cystitis.

Most reported series of prolonged cyclophosphamide use include infectious deaths from complications of cyclophosphamide treatment. Thus careful monitoring of the WBC count is mandatory. This is done twice per week for the first 4 weeks, so that trends of WBC declines can be detected, and the dose can be modified before onset of severe leukopenia. If the WBC count is falling rapidly, or it is less than 5000 per mm^3, cyclophosphamide is held temporarily until the WBC count stabilizes and is then reintroduced at a lower dose as needed. Once a dose has been established, the WBC count should be monitored weekly. When using cyclophosphamide, the following important caveats must be kept in mind:

1. The effect of cyclophosphamide on the bone marrow takes 2 weeks to be seen in the peripheral WBCs. A declining WBC count, therefore, must induce a change in dose of cyclophosphamide before severe leukopenia is present.
2. In individuals with impaired renal function, the half-life of cyclophosphamide and its active metabolites, and therefore the lag time between dose changes and an effect, are even longer.
3. Glucocorticoids are marrow-protective against cyclophosphamide. Therefore, as the dose of glucocorticoid is reduced, the dose of cyclophosphamide required to maintain the WBC count at 5000 per mm^3 is reduced.
4. Over time the marrow appears to become more sensitive to cyclophosphamide so that a dose required to maintain WBC levels at 2 months may be more than is required at 6 months.
5. The drug should always be given in the morning and copious fluids taken throughout the day to reduce the concentration and exposure time of the bladder epithelium to toxic metabolites.

The risks of leukopenia and hemorrhagic cystitis accompany all courses of cyclophosphamide therapy. Gonadal failure and induction of malignancy are not a major concern for the 8-week course of this drug in some presentations of idiopathic nephrotic syndrome. They become a concern in the treatment of crescentic glomerulonephritides and systemic diseases for which immunosuppressive treatment is maintained for at least 6 months, and may be continued for 1 to 2 years if evidence of disease activity or recurrence of disease occurs. Thus, the sooner cyclophosphamide treatment can be safely reduced or stopped the better. The risk of gonadal failure is dependent on the age and sex of the patients, as well as on the total cumulative dose. In adult men it can become a problem after only 100 mg per kg of total drug exposure. Prepubescent males and adult females begin to show a risk after 200 to 300 mg per kg and prepubescent females after 400 mg per kg. Risks of developing cancer later become substantial as cumulative doses rise above 30 grams.

Intravenous pulse treatment is less likely to cause bladder injury (inflammation/malignancy) because of shorter times of interaction between metabolites in the urine and the bladder wall, lower cumulative doses, and probably a protective effect of mesna (Mesnex) given at the time of the pulse. However, the effects (as well as the side effects) of cyclophosphamide are dose related, and sometimes it may be possible to gain control of a disease with oral cyclophosphamide when this cannot be achieved by monthly intravenous cyclophosphamide.

Cyclosporine

Cyclosporine* (Sandimmune, Neoral) is used in steroid-resistant, frequently relapsing, or steroid-dependent nephrotic syndromes. Side effects include hirsutism, gingival hypertrophy, hypercholesterolemia, hypertension, and cyclosporine arteriolopathy. Cyclosporine can lead to arteriolar hyalinosis within

*Not FDA approved for this indication.

*Not FDA approved for this indication.

the kidney and predispose to chronic renal injury secondary to ischemia. We dose cyclosporine (Neoral) orally twice daily and aim for trough blood levels of 100 ng per mL by high-performance liquid chromatography assay. These cyclosporine blood levels are lower than we use in transplantation and are associated with less toxicity. Kidney function is monitored carefully in all patients on cyclosporine. We do not perform protocol kidney biopsy after a course of cyclosporine.

Plasma Exchange

Plasma exchange is performed in anti-GBM disease at presentation for the purpose of removing pathogenic antibodies. Regimens use albumin to exchange for plasma in 4-liter exchanges. Plasma exchange is usually done daily for 3 to 5 days and then every other day for a total of 10 to 14 exchanges. The clinical level of disease, particularly lung hemorrhage, as well as the level of anti-GBM antibody, is measured as a guide to the need for further exchanges. Plasma exchange also removes creatinine, resulting in artificial lowering of this and other parameters of renal function.

Other Immunosuppressive Agents

Mycophenolate mofetil and azathioprine are occasionally used in primary glomerular diseases but are not discussed here.

Disease-Specific Therapies in Individual Glomerulopathies

A synopsis of the natural history of each disease and disease-specific therapies applicable to primary glomerulopathies follows. Readers are referred to general textbooks for a broader discussion. The common terminology that pertains to the management of idiopathic nephrotic syndromes is shown in Table 5.

Minimal Change Disease (MCD). This accounts for more than 85% of cases of nephrotic syndrome in children and 15% of cases in adults in the United States. It occurs predominantly in children between the ages of 2 and 8 years, but may occur at any age. Secondary etiologies include Hodgkin's lymphoma and nonsteroidal anti-inflammatory drugs. The exact pathologic basis of the disease is unclear. Environmental triggers such as allergens or infections may provoke onset of disease. Histologically, it is characterized by diffuse epithelial cell foot process effacement and the absence of immune complex deposition, proliferation, or inflammation within the glomerulus. True MCD is not associated with progression, but in a percentage of patients, intravascular volume depletion and renal edema cause the BUN and creatinine to be transiently elevated at presentation. Spontaneous remissions can occur but may take many months. The risks of pneumococcal peritonitis or pneumonia, other infections, and thromboses and the expectation of steroid sensitivity justify disease-specific therapies in MCD.

It is standard to forego biopsy in children with nephrotic syndrome between the ages of 1 and 8 years and assume the presence of MCD, but atypical features such as resistance to steroids, azotemia, hematuria, or hypertension may indicate need for a renal biopsy. Response is typical within 2 to 8 weeks for children but can take up to 12 weeks in adults. In 80% of children (and 40% of adults) relapse occurs at least once; some relapse more frequently, and some become steroid-dependent. Steroid resistance occurs in 10 to 15% of adults. The initial episode is managed with steroids (Prednisone 1 mg per kg per day [up to a maximum of 60 mg]), orally until 1 week after remission (up to 12 weeks). The prednisone is weaned to zero over 4 to 6 weeks. The first two relapses are also managed with steroids, but the third episode is managed with a slower taper. For frequent relapses and steroid-dependent cases, a short course of cyclophosphamide*, orally 1.5 mg per kg per day for 8 weeks, can achieve sustained remission in up to 75% of patients. It is least successful in steroid-resistant patients. Cyclosporine can be used as a third-line agent (or sometimes second-line agent in place of cyclophosphamide) in MCD. We use a 3-month trial of therapy. In patients who respond to cyclosporine (approximately 70% of steroid-dependent patients), the drug is weaned slowly over several months. Relapse after withdrawal is common but may be lessened by slow, deliberate tapering of the drug. All patients are maintained on ACE inhibitors.

Primary Focal and Segmental Glomerulosclerosis (FSGS). This accounts for 20 to 25% of nephrotic syndrome cases in adults. It describes a sclerosing glomerulopathy of obscure etiology that on light microscopy is both focal and segmental (initially involving the glomerular tufts segmentally in some but not all glomeruli). Immunofluorescence can show glomerular IgM and C3 in a mesangial and subendothelial distribution. As with MCD, diffuse foot process effacement is seen and glomerular inflammation is minor. Secondary causes of FSGS are myriad and

TABLE 5. **Frequent Terminology in Idiopathic Nephrotic Syndromes**

Complete remission	Negative or trace protein on 3 or more consecutive days (<300 mg/d)
Partial remission	Less than 2 gm/d proteinuria on 3 or more consecutive days (but >300 mg/d)
Relapse	Recurrence of 100 mg/dL or greater proteinuria by dipstick (>2 gm/d) on 3 consecutive days in a patient previously in remission
Frequent relapses	More than two relapses in 6 months or more than three relapses in a year
Steroid-responsive	Induction of a complete remission within 8 to 12 weeks
Steroid-dependent	Relapses occur during or within 2 weeks after steroid withdrawal
Steroid-resistant	Absence of a remission despite 8 or 12 weeks of therapy

*Not FDA approved for this indication.

include heroin nephropathy, HIV nephropathy (collapsing variant of FSGS), obesity, malignancy, reduced renal mass from another cause, obstructive uropathy, and advanced stages of other primary glomerulopathies. These candidates should be excluded, as none is expected to respond to disease-specific treatment.

FSGS presents typically with the nephrotic syndrome, but one third of patients may have subnephrotic range proteinuria and most have coexisting hematuria. Renal function may be normal or impaired. The natural history is to progress and spontaneous remissions are rare. Renal survival at 10 years is 85 to 90% in non-nephrotic patients versus 30 to 55% in nephrotic patients. Attainment of a sustained complete or partial remission improves the renal prognosis at 10 years to approximately 90%. Hypertension, impaired renal function, heavy proteinuria, and interstitial fibrosis at baseline portend a bad prognosis. Low-risk patients with non-nephrotic proteinuria are managed with general treatment strategies alone (see Figure 1). For others, longer courses of steroids can produce remission (up to 50% of adults). Steroid toxicity limits use of high-dose steroids beyond 3 months. Cyclophosphamide for 8 to 12 weeks is second-line therapy for patients who relapse. Cyclosporine may also be useful in relapses as a second- or third-line drug. In steroid-resistant patients, cyclosporine achieves a further 20% response rate while alkylating agents are generally not useful for these patients. For all these medications, we use the same doses as in MCD noted previously and maintain ACE inhibitor treatment to keep the blood pressure in the low-normal range and minimize proteinuria.

Membranous Glomerulonephritis (MGN). This is present in less than 5% of children but in approximately 25% of adults with nephrotic syndrome, increasing to 35% in the over 50-year age group. MGN is characterized by subepithelial accumulation of immune complexes. Membrane thickening (owing to laying down of new basement membrane) is accompanied by foot process effacement and dysfunction of the filtration mechanism so that high level proteinuria occurs. Secondary causes of MGN include drugs (e.g., gold, penicillamine), adenocarcinomas, infections (e.g., hepatitis B), and collagen vascular disease (e.g., SLE).

Childhood MGN has a high rate of spontaneous remission and a good prognosis for renal survival. In adults, 25% of cases have spontaneous complete remissions; another 20 to 25% may have spontaneous partial remissions. If this occurs in the first 3 years and a stable serum creatinine level is maintained, the long-term prognosis is excellent. However, 50% of patients have persistent nephrotic syndrome, and up to a half of these patients progress to ESRD and commence dialysis within 5 to 10 years of their diagnosis. Male gender, advanced age, renal insufficiency, and interstitial fibrosis at the time of diagnosis are predictors for progression. Non-nephrotic range proteinuria has a good prognosis, whereas persistent heavy proteinuria greater than 10 grams per day portends a poor prognosis.

The specific therapy for primary MGN is an area of great controversy. Selecting patients who stand to benefit from therapy is not as clear cut as in other glomerular diseases. Non-nephrotic patients have a good prognosis and are not treated. All other nephrotic patients are initially optimized with the global treatment strategies shown in Figure 1. Asymptomatic patients, whose edema is controlled on diuretics and ACE inhibition, are monitored over time to evaluate remission, stability, or progression. High-risk patients (those with interstitial fibrosis, renal insufficiency, or particularly heavy proteinuria) and those who are progressing despite general treatment measures receive disease-specific therapy. We use a 6-month trial of cyclophosphamide, 1.5 mg per kg per day orally, and prednisone (1 mg per kg per day up to a maximum of 60 mg initially). Steroids are weaned after 6 weeks to lower doses. The role of cyclosporine in high-risk patients with MGN remains uncertain.

Membranoproliferative Glomerulonephritis. This is an immune complex–mediated-disease that can present with a nephrotic, nephritic, or a mixed presentation. Many cases previously thought to be primary were in fact secondary to hepatitis C virus infection and are known to respond to specific antiviral therapy with recombinant interferon-α. General treatment strategies in addition to interferon treatment are the mainstay of management for this disease. Non-nephrotic patients generally have a good prognosis. Approximately 50% of the nephrotic patients reach ESRD within 5 years of diagnosis.

Mesangial Proliferative Glomerulonephritis—IgA Nephropathy (IgAN) or Berger's Disease. IgA immune complexes in a subendothelial/mesangial distribution cause variable mesangial matrix expansion and mesangial cell proliferation and glomerulosclerosis. Typical IgAN presentations include synpharyngitic (within 1 to 2 days) or exercise-related macroscopic hematuria, microhematuria, loin pain, or non-nephrotic proteinuria, with greater than 3 grams of proteinuria in only 10% of cases. Rarely, it presents as a rapidly progressive glomerulonephritis. Secondary causes include liver disease, celiac disease, and inflammatory bowel disease. Up to 30% of cases of IgAN develop ESRD over a 20-year period. There are no accepted disease-specific treatments of proven benefit. Risk factors for progression are noted in Table 2. The main focus of treatment is ACE inhibition and control of proteinuria, blood pressure, lipids, and diet.

Rapidly Progressive Glomerulonephritis/Crescentic Glomerulonephritis. This is a form of severe glomerular inflammation in which Bowman's space becomes occupied by cells and extracellular matrix materials. The correlated clinical presentation is RPGN. In RPGN, this inflammatory reaction to the underlying disease can cause severe, rapid scarring. The glomeruli are "ripped to pieces" by the inflammatory process. Recognition of RPGN has been dis-

TABLE 6. **Utility of the Renal Biopsy in Severe Glomerulonephritis (RPGN)**

1. Proportion of glomeruli with crescents
2. Type of underlying immune process (e.g., anti-GBM, pauci-immune, immune complex)
3. Potential for reversibility (degree of glomerular and interstitial scarring)

Abbreviations: RPGN = rapidly progressive glomerulonephritis; GBM = glomerular basement membrane.

cussed previously. The underlying pathogenic mechanisms of immune complex disease (40%), anti-GBM diseases (15%), or pauci-immune, so-called small vessel vasculitis (45%) are distinguished by immunofluorescence on a renal biopsy (Table 6).

Immune complex–mediated RPGN can be renal-limited (a crescentic presentation of one of the other primary glomerulopathies) or part of a systemic disease (SLE, cryoglobulinemia, Henoch-Schönlein purpura, infection). A wide variety of infections can cause immune complex glomerulonephritis. Infections involving lines, abscesses, shunts, cardiac valves, and other sites are all potential causes. The best recognized infection-associated glomerulonephritis is "postinfective glomerulonephritis" caused commonly by streptococci infecting the throat or skin. However, severe glomerular inflammation following streptococcal infection is unusual, and RPGN requiring urgent renal biopsy associated with postinfective glomerulonephritis is rare.

RPGN associated with anti-GBM antibody is usually rapid, severe, and often irreversible. As a general rule, if the serum creatinine is low (<2 mg per dL) and pulmonary hemorrhage absent then glucocorticoids and cyclophosphamide alone may suffice. For serum creatinine values between 2 and 7 mg per dL, plasma exchange and immunosuppressive strategies are warranted. If the serum creatinine is greater than 7 mg per dL, it is unlikely that useful renal function will be recoverable. However, these guidelines should be considered in association with the potential for recovery as determined from the renal biopsy. For example, acute tubular necrosis induced by dye or other factors may be superimposed on the glomerulonephritis and thereby obscure potential for recovery as assessed from functional studies alone. Associated alveolar hemorrhage should always be treated with plasma exchange.

Pauci-immune RPGN is characteristic of small vessel vasculitides. Although these are systemic diseases, a presentation that clinically appears renal-limited is not uncommon. Response to immunosuppression is excellent, whereas untreated disease is usually fatal within a year. Unlike with anti-GBM disease, patients with small vessel vasculitis on dialysis can recover useful renal function and dialysis independence.

Emergent treatment of crescentic nephritis, guided by the renal biopsy, is the key. If the underlying etiology is infection, use surgery, drainage, removal of an infected foreign body, and antibiotics as appropriate. In all other cases, we use aggressive immunosuppression when recovery of renal function is likely, keeping in mind that allowing progression to ESRD is associated with 15% mortality per year and direct costs of $50,000 per patient per year. Thus preservation of 15 to 20% of renal function for even 1 year is preferable to dialysis. High-dose pulse glucocorticoids (Solu-Medrol) 1 gram per day intravenously for 3 days, are used to suppress inflammation. This is followed by prednisone, 1 mg per kg per day, for 2 to 4 weeks until inflammation is reduced and the disease is in remission as assessed by function, circulating antibodies, and urine sediment (WBC count and granular casts). The glucocorticoid dose is then reduced to zero over 3 to 6 months (dependent on evidence for lack of ongoing activity of the underlying disease process). Oral cyclophosphamide, 2 mg per kg per day, is used from the onset to reduce further immune attack and scar formation according to the guidelines for cyclophosphamide use outlined previously. In primary renal diseases, we aim to stop cyclophosphamide after 3 to 6 months if the disease is in remission but in systemic vasculitis or SLE, longer periods of treatment are needed. In many cases, azathioprine or mycophenolate mofetil can be substituted for cyclophosphamide in an effort to reduce long-term toxicity. Plasma exchange is reserved for removing anti-GBM antibodies.

PYELONEPHRITIS

method of
JEANNE S. SHEFFIELD, M.D., and
SUSAN M. COX, M.D.
University of Texas Southwestern Medical Center at Dallas
Dallas, Texas

Pyelonephritis is broadly defined as infection of the renal parenchyma and the pelvicalyceal system. The majority of these infections are bacterial in etiology and include the Enterobacteriaceae as the main group of organisms. The clinical syndrome involves fever, flank pain, and pyuria. Urine culture is diagnostic, and treatment is empirical in nature.

PYELONEPHRITIS IN WOMEN

Urinary tract infections are common in women but are generally limited to asymptomatic bacteriuria (ASB) or acute cystitis. It is estimated that 1 to 2% of teenagers have ASB and that this incidence increases by 1% per decade of adult life. Urinary tract infections are much more common in women than in men, secondary to a short urethra and the close proximity of the urethral meatus to the anus and the bacterial flora of the rectum and vaginal vestibule. Although ASB is common in young women, the majority do not develop pyelonephritis. In fact,

TABLE 1. **Common Clinical Findings in Pyelonephritis**

Fever:temperature >38°C
Chills
Costovertebral angle tenderness
Nausea and vomiting
Lower tract symptoms

in patients who do develop acute pyelonephritis, urinary tract abnormalities, urolithiasis, and other conditions are frequent contributing factors. Additional risk factors include onset of sexual activity, which is more commonly associated with acute cystitis, and the use of barrier contraceptive methods such as the diaphragm. The most important risk factor for the development of pyelonephritis in a woman is pregnancy.

The clinical findings in pyelonephritis are listed in Table 1. The diagnosis is based not only on clinical features but also on the finding of greater than 10^2 colonies per mL of a single uropathogen in a catheterized urine specimen. The most common uropathogens are listed in Table 2. Therapeutic agents, as listed in Table 3, include cephalosporins, broad-spectrum penicillins, sulfa drugs, and monobactams, as well as the fluoroquinolones. Women with uncomplicated pyelonephritis outside of pregnancy, or with recurrent episodes of urinary tract infection, deserve urologic evaluation including renal ultrasonography, cystoscopy, intravenous pyelography (IVP), and other indicated tests.

PYELONEPHRITIS IN PREGNANCY

Symptomatic urinary tract infections, including acute pyelonephritis, complicate 1 to 3% of all pregnancies. Pyelonephritis, a serious medical complication necessitating hospitalization, frequently develops in women with untreated ASB and may be associated with significant maternal and fetal morbidity and mortality.

Up to 2% of all pregnancies are complicated by antepartum pyelonephritis. This incidence varies depending on the patient population and the prevalence of ASB. Pyelonephritis is more likely to occur during the last two trimesters because of increasing obstruction of the urinary tract with resulting stasis as pregnancy progresses. This is secondary to (1) mechanical obstruction of ureters due to the enlarging uterus and (2) hormonal effects secondary to increased progesterone in pregnancy.

TABLE 2. **Organisms Causing Acute Pyelonephritis**

Common	Rare
Escherichia coli	*Pseudomonas aeruginosa*
*Proteus mirabilis**	*Staphylococcus epidermidis*
Klebsiella pneumoniae	*Serratia marcescens*
Enterococcus faecalis	*Ureaplasma urealyticum*
	Mycobacterium hominis
	Staphylococcus aureus

*Associated with struvite calculi.

Affected women have fever, chills, flank pain, nausea, and vomiting (i.e., very similar complaints to those in nonpregnant women who present with pyelonephritis). Pregnant women may also complain of lower tract irritative symptoms. Physical examination reveals fever (with temperatures frequently greater than 38.3°C) and costovertebral angle tenderness (CVAT), manifesting predominantly on the right side. During pregnancy the uterus is dextrorotated, and the descending colon confers a protective effect on the left ureter. This accounts for the predominance of right-sided pyelonephritis in pregnancy.

Diagnosis is made by quantitive urine cultures yielding greater than 10^5 colonies per mL of a single uropathogen. Blood cultures are positive in approximately 15% of cases. Organisms of species in the family Enterobacteriaceae are the most commonly isolated pathogens, with *Escherichia coli* seen in greater than 70% of all cases (see Table 2). Microscopic examination of an uncentrifuged urine specimen will confirm bacteriuria and pyuria, with or without leukocyte casts. The identification of bacteria on a slide of an uncentrifuged specimen correlates well with a positive urine culture. Positive results on rapid diagnostic tests, such as the Griess test for nitrites, may increase the clinical suspicion of pyelonephritis. These and other test kits such as Microstix-3 have high sensitivity and specificity for detecting counts greater than 10^5 organisms per mL.

Acute pyelonephritis during pregnancy can be a devastating disease for both the mother and her fetus. Complications of pyelonephritis are listed in Table 4. Among women with severe infection, 25% will have evidence of multiple-system derangements secondary to the effects of endotoxemia. As many as 15% of women with severe antepartum pyelonephritis will have bacteremia, but fortunately septic shock is rare. Hypotension and diminished perfusion secondary to the consequences of endotoxemia must be differentiated from hypotension caused by dehydration from nausea, vomiting, and fever. Affected women generally respond to rapid fluid resuscitation, and cardiac output is usually restored without the use of vasopressor drugs. Of women who have pyelonephritis, 25% have seriously diminished renal function as defined by a creatinine clearance of less than 80 mL per minute corrected for body surface area. This renal dysfunction is transient in nature, and normalization occurs within several days after the therapy for pyelonephritis is begun. As many as 25% of patients who are admitted with pyelonephritis will develop anemia, as defined by a hemoglobin of less than 10 grams per dL. Furthermore, it is not unusual for the hemoglobin to be as low as 8.2 grams per dL, with evidence of hemolysis based on positive haptoglobins, erythrocyte morphology, and an increase in serum lactate dehydrogenase (LDH). These effects are also secondary to endotoxemia and are not due to alterations in erythropoietin production.

TABLE 3. **Pharmacologic Treatment Options for Acute Pyelonephritis**

Drug	Dosage	Frequency
Outpatient (duration of treatment: 10–14 d)		
Ciprofloxacin (Cipro)	500 mg PO	q 12 h
Levofloxacin (Levaquin)	250 mg PO	q 24 h
Ofloxacin (Floxin)	200 mg PO	q 12 h
Norfloxacin (Noroxin)	400 mg PO	q 12 h
Enoxacin (Penetrex)	400 mg PO	q 12 h
Cefixime (Suprax)	400 mg PO	q 24 h
Cefpodoxime proxetil (Vantin)	200 mg PO	q 12 h
Trimethoprim-sulfamethoxazole (Bactrim)	160/800 mg PO	q 12 h
Hospitalized Patients		
Ceftriaxone (Rocephin)	1–2 gm IV	q 12–24 h
Ciprofloxacin (Cipro)	200–400 mg IV	q 12 h
Ofloxacin (Floxin)	200–400 mg IV	q 12 h
Gentamicin	3–5 mg/kg/d IV	
Aztreonam (Azactam)	1–2 gm IV	q 6–8 h
Ampicillin (add if suspected pathogens include enterococci)	2 gm IV	q 6 h
Pregnancy		
Ceftriaxone (Rocephin)	2 gm IV	q 24 h
Gentamicin/ampicillin	80 mg IV/2 gm IV	q 8 h/q 6 h
Mezlocillin (Mezlin)	3–4 gm IV	q 4–6 h
Aztreonam (Azactam)	1–2 gm IV	q 6–8 h
Cefazolin (Ancef)	1 gm IV	q 6–8 h

Of women with severe pyelonephritis, 2% will develop respiratory insufficiency. Endotoxin alters alveolocapillary membrane permeability, and clinically the pulmonary injury is similar to that seen in other variants of adult respiratory distress syndrome (ARDS). These women will respond to oxygen delivered by face mask and only occasionally require intubation. Close monitoring of blood pressure, pulse rate, and urinary output is required, in addition to monitoring the respiratory rate for tachypnea and subsequent symptoms of dyspnea. This ARDS-like picture is also transient in nature, and with prompt diagnosis and aggressive therapy these patients generally do well. Cardiac effects secondary to endotoxemia have been reported and include a decrease in total peripheral resistance and increase in cardiac output.

Patients with acute antepartum pyelonephritis should be admitted to the hospital for close observation, because they frequently have severe nausea, vomiting, and anorexia combined with pyrexia, which leads to significant dehydration. Most of these women are unable to tolerate oral medications; therefore, hospitalization becomes necessary. Treatment is directed at restoration of the contracted blood volume and administration of intravenous antibiotics. The choice of antimicrobial agent is empirical; however, reports suggest that a regimen using broad-spectrum cephalosporins such as cefazolin (Ancef), ceftriaxone (Rocephin), or a combination of ampicillin and gentamicin is necessary (see Table 3).

In general, women who have antepartum pyelonephritis will respond to therapy within 48 to 72 hours. If by 96 hours the patient is still febrile without clinical evidence of improvement, then evaluation to rule out perinephric abscess, phlegmon, or urolithiasis must be undertaken. Work-up for these patients includes a renal ultrasound scan to look for hydroureter and hydronephrosis and possibly a plain film of the abdomen coupled with a single-shot intravenous pyelogram to look for urolithiasis.

TABLE 4. **Complications of Pyelonephritis**

Renal papillary necrosis	Adult respiratory distress syndrome (ARDS)*
Renal abscess	Hemolytic anemia
Perinephric abscess	

*Seen in pregnancy.

PYELONEPHRITIS IN MEN

Pyelonephritis is a rare finding in an otherwise healthy, normal man. In the absence of prior surgeries, intrinsic or hematologic sources should be investigated by culture and radiographic techniques. Overall, the incidence of pyelonephritis in young man is thought to be about 0.1%. This low rate may be due to multiple factors including a greater distance of the urethral meatus from the anus, as well as factors such as the antibacteriostatic properties of the prostatic fluid. Importantly, the incidence may increase after age 50 secondary to prostatic disease such as benign prostatic hypertrophy or cancer, as well as uncomplicated prostatitis. Additional risk factors include heterosexual contact with women who are vaginally colonized with *E. coli,* homosexual contact in which Enterobacteriaceae organisms from the rectum colonize the urethral meatus, neurogenic bladder, and obstructive lesions of the bladder. There may be a decreased risk for pyelonephritis in men who are circumcised.

Diagnosis is based on clinical findings coupled with a positive urine culture. Clinical findings in the male are similar to those in the female (see Table 1). Patients generally appear quite ill, with fever, tachycardia, and CVAT. Laboratory diagnosis is based on the presence of pyuria and bacteriuria and possible leukocyte casts and glitter cells on an uncentrifuged urine specimen. Culture reveals greater than 10^3 colonies per mL of a single uropathogen in a clean-catch midstream urine specimen. The most common organisms isolated are similar to those identified in women (see Table 2). Less common organisms found in men but not generally found in women include *Candida albicans, Staphylococcus epidermidis, Ureaplasma urealyticum, Mycoplasma hominis, and Staphylococcus aureus.*

Treatment for men with pyelonephritis has changed dramatically in the last several years. In the past, male patients were hospitalized and managed aggressively with hydration and antimicrobial therapy. Now pyelonephritis in men is more commonly treated on an outpatient basis with a multitude of different antibiotic regimens (see Table 3). In complicated cases the oral antibiotics are continued for a 14-day period if the patient is stable. If intravenous antibiotics are needed, they can be given by home therapy teams.

In the patient who is not responding to antibiotic therapy or who has been admitted to the hospital and has had aminoglycoside therapy started, it is important to check pretherapy renal function, i.e., serum creatinine level, and to monitor serial creatinine and/or aminoglycoside levels. Alternative agents to the aminoglycosides include the broad-spectrum quinolones and third-generation cephalosporins.

It is important to remember that a man who presents with acute pyelonephritis deserves a complete urologic work-up. The patient can be managed initially by a primary care physician but should be referred to the urologist for renal ultrasonography and IVP, as well as catheter studies, cystoscopy, and other indicated procedures.

TRAUMA TO THE GENITOURINARY TRACT

method of
RICHARD J. MACCHIA, M.D.
State University of New York Health Science Center at Brooklyn College of Medicine
Brooklyn, New York

and

THOMAS M. SCALEA, M.D.
University of Maryland School of Medicine
Baltimore, Maryland

The approach to the patient with suspected urologic injury must be part of an overall diagnostic and treatment scheme that identifies immediately life-threatening injuries for urgent care and assigns management priorities for other significant but less serious injuries. Urologic injuries in themselves are rarely fatal, but inadequately treated, they can cause substantial and lingering morbidity and disability. The magnitude of force required to produce major injury to the urologic organs is considerable. Thus, all patients with urologic injuries must be considered to be polytraumatized.

Urologic injury rarely produces exsanguinating hemorrhage. Thus, complete diagnostic evaluation and therapeutics may need to be delayed until other, life-threatening injuries have been controlled. Fortunately, a delay of several hours does not affect long-term outcome or increase the rate of complications. Urologic injury can often be suggested by the particulars of a thorough history including the mechanism of injury. Physical manifestations of injury, if present, add to the clinician's suspicion. Unfortunately, symptoms and signs may be absent until late in the course. Laboratory evaluation is also nonspecific. Hematuria, perhaps the most common laboratory finding, unfortunately may be absent in up to 50% of patients with serious injuries, particularly vascular or ureteral injuries. The mainstay of diagnostic evaluation is radiography, particularly in blunt trauma.

KIDNEY INJURIES

Blunt Trauma

Virtually any serious blunt trauma can cause renal injury. The most common mechanisms, however, are high-speed vehicular crashes, falls from a substantial height, and direct trauma to the flank. Renal injuries can be divided into two types: parenchymal and vascular. Parenchymal and vascular injuries generally result from injury that causes compression of the kidneys against the spine or posterior ribs. In addition, deceleration injuries, either vertical or horizontal, may cause stretch injuries with intimal disruption, thrombosis, and ischemia. Renal vascular injury can also involve transmural disruption and blood loss.

The clinical presentation of the patient generally reflects the magnitude of the renal injury. Symptoms include flank pain, but patients also complain of abdominal or lower chest pain. Occasionally, symptomatology is referable to blood loss, with complaints of dizziness, chest pain, or shortness of breath. Physical findings may include either flank or upper abdominal tenderness and ecchymoses. Occasionally, there is fullness in either the upper abdomen or the flank. Few patients exhibit all of the symptoms or signs, however, and many patients are completely asymptomatic. In patients with significant injuries such as a femur fracture or chest wall injury, symptoms referable to the kidney may go unnoticed. Urine output is extremely nonspecific and should not be used to make the diagnosis. Patients with bilateral renal arterial injuries will be anuric.

If hematuria is present, its degree does not necessarily correlate with the magnitude of the renal injury, although hemodynamically stable patients with minimal hematuria have a low incidence of clinically important renal injuries. In such patients, observation and selective imaging studies constitute appropriate management. Patients with gross hematuria require urgent diagnostic evaluation.

Computed tomography (CT) scanning, particularly "helical" CT, has largely replaced intravenous urography in the evaluation process. This technique allows complete imaging of the retroperitoneum, renal vasculature, parenchyma, kidney, abdomen, and chest with one bolus of intravenous contrast agent.

In the past, arteriography was the standard imaging technique to make the diagnosis of renal pedicle injury. This also has largely been replaced by CT scanning.

Management strategies depend on the degree and architecture of renal damage and the patient's hemodynamic status. In general, patients with relatively minor injuries can be managed nonoperatively. Extravasation within Gerota's fascia and perinephric hematoma are not absolute indications for surgery. Patients with more severe injuries can often also be managed nonoperatively. However, the risk of rebleeding is much higher. Thus, it is wise to perform diagnostic angiography. Advances in interventional radiology have greatly improved the techniques of nonoperative management. Pseudoaneurysms and/or other arterial injuries can be managed nonoperatively with transcatheter embolization techniques. Angiographic techniques should substantially decrease the rate of late blood loss. However, the emergence of worsening symptomatology or physical findings or evidence of ongoing blood loss must prompt laparotomy.

Occasionally, the diagnosis of renal injury is made at the time of emergency exploratory laparotomy for other injuries. Most often, the surgeon encounters a large retroperitoneal hematoma. If the hematoma is not expanding, there is no indication to explore the kidney. Such injuries can be managed expectantly, but all patients should undergo imaging studies postoperatively to ascertain the architecture of the renal damage and to rule out the presence of urinary extravasation. In these patients, angiographic embolization helps to preserve renal parenchyma. A rapidly expanding perinephric hematoma must be explored. It is wise to gain vascular control before directly exploring the kidney. Surgical options are defined by the extent of damage of the kidney but include suture repair, heminephrectomy, and nephrectomy.

The diagnosis of arterial renal thrombosis must be made quickly. The kidney tolerates 6 hours of warm ischemia time without significant long-term damage. The diagnosis can be made on the basis of helical CT study. CT scanning followed by angiography often is too time-consuming to allow renal salvage. Unfortunately, the diagnosis often is made late in polytraumatized patients. Thus, the success rate of renal revascularization is low.

Despite optimal care, complications of severe renal trauma do occur. Blood loss occurs early, and sepsis from infected or infarcted parenchyma or urinary extravasation can occur up to a few weeks after injury. Patients should be followed for hypertension secondary to parenchymal ischemia.

Penetrating Trauma

Renal injuries occur in approximately 10 to 15% of cases of penetrating abdominal injury. Because all patients with injuries involving a transabdominal wound trajectory require operation, the diagnosis is usually made at the time of laparotomy. Although observation may suffice for a small perinephric hematoma, large hematomas require exploration. Injuries are managed on the basis of operative findings. Simple repair or partial nephrectomy is appropriate in many patients. Patients with gunshot wounds to the kidney, particularly those with hypotension, often require a nephrectomy. Stable patients with stab wounds to the flank and back can be managed expectantly. The diagnostic test of choice, once intra-abdominal injury is excluded, is contrast-enhanced CT enema. Relatively small injuries without evidence of significant urinary extravasation can be managed by either observation or the use of angiographic techniques. Large injuries or those with uncontrolled urine leak require exploration and repair.

URETERAL INJURIES

Ureteral pelvic disruption is most often seen in children following severe blunt trauma, but it is occasionally seen in adults. Anatomic abnormalities of the kidney or ureter predispose to this injury.

Early on, symptomatology from ureteral injury is subtle if present at all. Full-thickness injuries leak urine. Patients with obstruction will present with pain, fever, and other signs of urinary infection, whereas those with unrecognized urinary extravasation may present with abdominal distention or ileus. Most often, hematuria is absent; if present, it is likely to be only microscopic.

Ureteral injury should be considered in postoperative patients who have had retroperitoneal exploration. In penetrating trauma, the diagnosis is usually made at the time of exploration of the transperitoneal wound trajectory. Contrast-enhanced CT enema may demonstrate free urinary extravasation from the ureter and/or formation of a urinoma.

If the diagnosis is in question, percutaneous aspiration of a suspected urinoma or paracentesis should be carried out. The fluid should be sent for determination of blood urea nitrogen and serum creatinine as well as gram staining and culture. Occasionally, cystoscopy and retrograde imaging of the ureters are helpful.

Most ureteral injuries can be treated either with primary repair or with débridement and anastomosis over a double-J stent. Very distal ureteral injuries are best treated with ureteroneocystostomy. If necessary, a psoas hitch is useful.

If the diagnosis is made late or if there is superimposed infection and azotemia, immediate ureteral reconstruction is ill advised. Several options exist. One is simply to stent the ureter. This may be done via a retrograde or antegrade approach. Urinomas may then be drained percutaneously, obviating the need for immediate surgery. Nephrostomy may help promote ureteral healing.

Complications include anastomotic leak with urinary extravasation, superimposed infection, and late stenosis.

BLADDER INJURIES

The most critical element in care of bladder injuries is differentiating intraperitoneal from extraperitoneal bladder rupture. Intraperitoneal bladder rupture generally occurs when a full bladder is subjected to a sudden increase in intraluminal pressure. Extraperitoneal bladder rupture occurs almost always from shear forces in conjunction with pelvic fracture and/or direct puncture from displaced fracture fragments. Symptoms of bladder rupture are usually due to associated intra-abdominal or pelvic injury.

The mainstay in diagnostic evaluation of bladder injury is the cystogram. A Foley catheter is inserted, and the bladder is distended by instilling at least 250 mL of radiopaque contrast by gravity drip. The bladder is then emptied and washed out with saline. Plain films including anteroposterior and oblique views are then obtained. With intraperitoneal rupture, loops of bowel are outlined by the contrast, and/or the contrast pools in the pericolic gutters. If the patient requires CT scanning for other purposes, the cystogram can be done under CT control.

Treatment of intraperitoneal bladder rupture requires laparotomy and direct repair. The injury is usually located in the dome of the bladder, which is closed in two layers. Extraperitoneal bladder rupture can almost be managed nonoperatively with Foley catheter drainage for 10 to 14 days. Healing can be confirmed by cystography. Patients with open pelvic fractures and/or severe crush injury may have complex bladder injuries, often occurring in concert with external genitourinary, vaginal, and/or rectal injuries. These require operative repair. Management must be individualized, as surgical entry of a contained retroperitoneal hematoma with a pelvic fracture can produce exsanguinating hemorrhage.

The diagnosis for penetrating bladder injury is often made at the time of laparotomy for exploration of other transabdominal or missile wound trajectories. In general, these should be treated as for intraperitoneal bladder rupture. The dome of the bladder can be opened, and injuries located deep in the bladder can be repaired from the inside. The dome of the bladder is then closed. Suprapubic cystostomy is not mandatory. Small extraperitoneal bladder injuries from knife or bullet wounds can be managed expectantly with Foley catheter drainage if there is no other indication for surgery.

URETHRAL INJURIES IN MEN

When urethral injury is suspected, catheterization is contraindicated. A retrograde urethrogram should be performed, if at all possible. Although false-negative results are possible, this test is highly reliable and will help to define the location and extent of the injury. For partial disruptions of the urethra, we usually treat with placement of a suprapubic tube only.

For total anterior urethral disruptions, primary surgical reanastomosis is desirable, if this can be done without removing an amount of urethral tissue that will produce a chordee upon erection. Total posterior urethral disruptions are a challenge even to the most experienced of surgeons. However, primary realignment without traction can give an excellent outcome. A urethral stricture frequently results but can usually be handled by minimal dilatation. A wide gap between the ends of the urethra is evidenced by a very high-riding prostate on rectal examination or a “pie-in-the-sky” bladder on imaging studies. If this lesion is managed with use of a suprapubic tube only, a prohibitively large gap may remain after resolution of the pelvic hematoma, making definitive repair extremely difficult. In this case, delayed primary exploration of the pelvis with realignment of the urethra is desirable. Minimal dissection should be undertaken.

PENILE INJURIES

A penile “fracture” during intercourse is a relatively frequent occurrence. The penis is usually so edematous as to preclude meaningful physical examination. As urethral injury may occur, we advocate a retrograde urethrogram. We do not advise cavernosography. We explore these injuries with a degloving incision, evacuate the hematoma, and repair any tears in the tunica.

PROSTATITIS

method of
PAUL O. MADSEN, M.D., PH.D.
University of Wisconsin School of Medicine
Madison, Wisconsin

The types of prostatitis currently recognized and their clinical features are outlined in Table 1, with approximate clinical incidence of the various types. A better term for nonbacterial prostatitis and prostatodynia may be “idiopathic prostatitis,” reflecting our very limited understanding of these types of prostatitis, and the uncertainty concerning the presence of actual infection.

For proper diagnosis, voided urine and prostate secretions are cultured in segmented specimens (Figure 1). Specimens must be obtained with care to prevent bacterial contamination, which may lead to misinterpretation of the results. The diagnosis of prostatic infection is confirmed when the bacterial

TABLE 1. **Clinical Features of Different Forms of Prostatitis**

Syndrome	UTI	Abnormal Rectal Exam	Excessive WBCs in EPS	Positive Culture of EPS	Common Causative Organisms	Response to Antimicrobials	Approx. Clinical Incidence
Acute bacterial prostatitis	+	+	+	+	Coliform bacteria	+	5–10%
Chronic bacterial prostatitis	±	±	+	+	Coliform bacteria	+	5–10%
Nonbacterial prostatitis	–	–	+	–	None ? *Chlamydia* ? *Ureaplasma*	±	40%
Prostatodynia	–	–	–	–	None	–	40%
Nosocomial prostatitis	–	+	±	+	Coliform bacteria	+	?
Rare types	±	+	±	±	Fungi Tubercle bacilli Parasites	±	?

Abbreviations: UTI = urinary tract infection; WBC = white blood cells; EPS = expressed prostatic secretion.

colony count for the prostatic secretion specimen significantly exceeds those of urethral and bladder specimens. These examinations frequently have to be repeated and are often cumbersome and expensive, and in the case of cystitis, sterilization of the urine, e.g., with nitrofurantoin, before this work-up may be necessary to obtain valid results.

Despite an extensive literature discussing diagnosis and treatment of the various types of prostatitis, understanding of the etiology of these conditions is limited, and information regarding incidence and the role of reoccurrence is lacking or controversial.

ACUTE BACTERIAL PROSTATITIS

Acute bacterial prostatitis is a well-established clinical entity. Affected patients present with signs and symptoms of an acute septic process, including irritative and obstructive voiding symptoms.

Since prostatic massage is contraindicated because of the possibility of sepsis, the diagnosis depends solely on the results of urine culture and physical examination of the prostate without the benefit of direct microscopic examination of prostatic fluid.

Acute bacterial prostatitis is treated with antibacterial agents according to sensitivity studies of urine cultures. No drug has been proved superior, but the favored treatment is with trimethoprim (Proloprim), trimethoprim-sulfamethoxazole (Septra; Bactrim), or a fluoroquinolone (ciprofloxacin [Cipro], ofloxacin [Floxin], norfloxacin [Noroxin], levofloxacin [Levaquin]) containing drugs. If gram-positive organisms are present (rare), one of the macrolide antibiotics (erythromycin [Erythrocin Stearate], rosaramicin, or azithromycin [Zithromax]) is indicated. These drugs all concentrate in the prostate by diffusion owing to their chemistry. Drug therapy should probably continue for a few weeks in order to prevent recurrence or development of chronic bacterial prostatitis.

CHRONIC BACTERIAL PROSTATITIS

Chronic bacterial prostatitis, in contrast to the acute form, is difficult to diagnose and treat and can

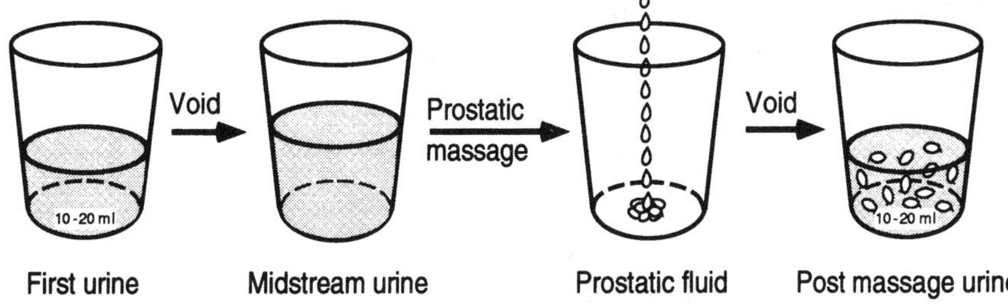

Cultures				Diagnosis:
+	–	–	–	Urethritis
±	–	+	+	Prostatitis
+	+	±	+	Cystitis
–	–	–	–	Idiopathic Prostatitis

Figure 1. Urine and prostatic secretions must be cultured in serial specimens to make an accurate diagnosis.

vary widely in its clinical presentation. This form of prostatitis is a confusing and frustrating clinical entity for physicians and patients. It is a common cause of relapsing urinary tract infections. Irritative voiding symptoms (dysuria, urinary urgency, and frequency) may or may not be present. Perineal, testicular, and low back pain are frequent complaints. Rectal examination discloses no characteristic findings, but on palpation the prostate sometimes feels spongy and may be slightly tender.

The organisms responsible for chronic bacterial prostatitis are usually gram-negative bacteria. The role of gram-positive organisms is uncertain and controversial.

Therapy for chronic bacterial prostatitis consists usually of several weeks' treatment with antibacterial agents that concentrate well in the prostate, such as trimethoprim, trimethoprim-sulfamethoxazole, or a fluoroquinolone (ciprofloxacin, ofloxacin, norfloxacin, or levofloxacin) or, in the case of gram-positive organisms, a macrolide antibiotic (erythromycin, rosaramicin, or azithromycin). The treatment is often unsatisfactory, and recurrence is frequent (about 50%).

IDIOPATHIC PROSTATITIS (NONBACTERIAL PROSTATITIS AND PROSTATODYNIA)

When the patients with acute and chronic bacterial prostatitis are excluded, an ill-defined group of patients—and probably the largest group—remains. Clinically, they have a wide variety of symptoms referable to the lower back, genitalia, perineum, and rectum. Quite often, symptoms related to the urinary tract, such as irritative and obstructive symptoms, are predominant. According to localization studies (see Figure 1), idiopathic prostatitis can be divided into two distinct disorders: nonbacterial prostatitis and prostatodynia. Possible etiologic and pathogenetic factors associated with these entities remain essentially unknown.

The treatment of these patients represents a very frustrating problem, and results are often unsatisfactory. Many, mostly unproven, modes of therapy have been recommended.

Nonbacterial Prostatitis

The main criterion used to distinguish patients with nonbacterial prostatitis from those with prostatodynia is the finding of white blood cells and lipid-laden macrophages (of unknown significance) on microscopic examination of the prostatic fluid. Findings on rectal examination are normal.

The patient coming to the urologist for treatment of this entity has usually received previous pharmacologic therapy with many different drugs. An initial approach by the urologist will be to administer one of the aforementioned antibacterial agents in case an infection has been overlooked. Many other modes of therapy will usually be tried by the urologist, such as repeated prostatic massage, warm sitz baths, administration of allopurinol* (Zyloprim) (changing the chemical composition of the urine and possibly diminishing the effect of refluxing urine into the prostate), hormone replacement with testosterone* as well as estrogens,* use of a 5α-reductase inhibitor (finasteride [Proscar]*, transrectal or transurethral microwave therapy (proved effective in prospective, controlled, randomized studies), or therapy with pollen extracts (Cernilton), smooth muscle relaxants such as a benzodiazepine* (Valium; Versed), or an alpha blocker* (Hytrin; Cardura); if all else fails, and if the symptoms are serious enough, an incision of the prostate (probably best performed at the 6 o'clock position) may be tried on an empirical basis.

Prostatodynia

Patients with prostatodynia present with multiple complaints, commonly including some combination of pain in the perineum, lower back, and suprapubic area as well as pain on ejaculation. Dysuria and frequency are generally absent. Findings on rectal examination of the prostate are normal. The diagnosis is made by finding no evidence of inflammation on microscopic examination of prostatic fluid. Because evidence of inflammation is lacking, some studies have indicated that the condition may be caused by detrusor sphincter dyssynergia. Other investigators have shown that prostatodynia may be caused by overactivity of pelvic sympathetic nerves acting at the level of the external urethral sphincter. It should be noted that accurate and reproducible urodynamic studies are difficult to perform in this group of often very anxious men.

The treatments are usually the same as for nonbacterial prostatitis, and results are just as unsatisfactory, but certainly treatment with alpha blockers should be tried, because several studies have shown efficacy in these patients. Since many patients with prostatodynia have associated psychiatric disturbances, it is possible that some of the therapeutic benefits may represent a placebo effect.

*Not FDA approved for this indication.

BENIGN PROSTATIC HYPERPLASIA

method of
DANIEL J. CULKIN, M.D., and
BRADLEY W. ANDERSON, M.D.
University of Oklahoma Health Sciences Center
Oklahoma City, Oklahoma

Benign prostatic hyperplasia (BPH) is a histologic as well as a clinical diagnosis. The incidence of histologic BPH is actually higher than that of the clinical form. According to the Bureau of Statistics there are 30 million men in the United States older than 50 years of age. Approximately 30% of these men suffer from symptoms related to BPH, also known as prostatism or bladder outlet obstruction (BOO), as summarized in Table 1. Because of the fear of being diagnosed with cancer or of developing surgical complications such as impotence and incontinence, many men will not freely offer the history of prostatism. Other men believe BOO to be part of the natural process of aging.

A process of education regarding BPH is ongoing through industry advertisements and medical lay publications, which encourage visits to the primary care physicians who subsequently identify affected men. Also, the percentage of men older than 50 years of age is expected to increase from 30 to 39% by the year 2000 as "baby boomers" age and survival statistics improve. These numbers speak to the socioeconomic implications of BPH in the United States. Recognition of these issues by pharmaceutical and technology companies has resulted in the development of several new medical and surgical treatments.

CLINICAL PRESENTATION

The clinical presentation of BPH is quite variable. Most commonly the patient will complain of a series of obstructive and irritative symptoms. Obstructive symptoms include decreased urinary flow rate, hesitancy, an intermittent voided stream, the need to strain to urinate, and the sensation of incomplete emptying. Irritative symptoms of BPH include urgency, frequency, nocturia, and dysuria. These symptoms vary in intensity, and they cause a significant reduction in quality of life. Other presentations include signs or symptoms of bladder stones, hematuria, recurrent urinary tract infections (UTIs), overflow incontinence, and complete urinary retention. Although the man who presents to the emergency department with symptoms of heart failure, profound azotemia, hydronephrosis, and a postvoid residual urine of greater than a liter is much less common today, these presentations still do occur. Just as the presentation is variable, the natural history of BPH is likewise variable and often unpredictable: about a third will remain the same, another third will improve, and a third will worsen.

To evaluate BPH initially and follow the clinical course of the disease, a self-administered questionnaire has been developed by the American Urological Association (AUA), presented in Table 2. This questionnaire elicits information on the presence of obstructive and irritative symptoms (i.e., urgency, frequency, weak stream, intermittent stream, incomplete emptying, hesitancy, and nocturia), which are graded in severity from 1 to 5. These scores are added to yield a composite symptom score of 0 to 35. Scores for mild symptoms are 0 to 8; moderate, 9 to 19; and severe, 20 to 35. Although treatment decisions cannot be made solely on the basis of the AUA symptom score, it is a reliable method for detecting BPH, selecting treatments, and monitoring disease and treatment progression.

PHYSICAL EXAMINATION

Physical examination centers on the genitourinary system. Abdominal examination may reveal a distended bladder resulting from a large postvoiding volume of urine. Costovertebral angle tenderness may indicate an associated pyelonephritis. Abnormal neurologic findings, especially lower extremity signs or abnormal rectal tone, raise the suspicion that symptoms may be from a neurogenic bladder rather than outlet obstruction. Digital rectal examination is most important in detecting other conditions such as prostate cancer (hard, rocklike, or gritty nodule), prostatitis (soft, boggy prostate that is very tender to palpation), severe fecal impaction, or a large rectal cancer. The palpated size of the prostate gland is of much less importance, because size of gland does not correlate reliably with symptoms or degree of urethral obstruction and because estimations of prostate volume obtained during digital rectal examination correlate poorly with objective (radiologic or surgical) findings, even for experienced examiners. Finally, a simple in-and-out catheterization after having the patient empty his bladder as much as possible gives a useful postvoid residual (PVR) urine volume. A PVR of greater than 60 mL is abnormal, and a PVR of greater than 150 mL is the sign of a significant problem. Patients presenting with urinary retention may have volumes of greater than 1 to 2 liters. Many urologists now have hand-held ultrasound machines that can in seconds measure a PVR without the discomfort and risk of introducing infection involved in a catheterization.

There are very few useful diagnostic tests and studies in the evaluation of BPH. A urinalysis (UA) should be performed to detect microscopic hematuria and to rule out a UTI, which can mimic or be caused by BOO. A urine culture should be performed if results of UA are suggestive of UTI. A prostate-specific antigen (PSA) level should be determined in all patients over the age of 40 years as a screening test for prostate cancer. Patients suspected of having associated prostatitis or UTI should receive appropriate antibiotic therapy before determination of PSA level. BPH can cause mild to moderate PSA elevations, especially when retention or significant obstruction is present, but even in these cases, serial measurements should be obtained because of the risk of coexistent prostate cancer. Serum creatinine determination is a good screening test to assess renal function. A complete blood count is necessary only in the face of a suspected severe infection or significant bleeding. Measurement of serum electrolytes is necessary only if a high serum creatinine level or heavy proteinuria suggests renal dysfunction.

Urologists commonly perform a uroflow test on patients with BPH since it is readily available to them and very inexpensive. The urinary flow rate and the duration of voiding are useful objective measurements that can be repeated for ongoing evaluation during medical or after surgical therapy. The voiding pattern also gives the urologist clues regarding possible bladder dysfunction that may be mimicking or complicating the BOO. Full urodynamic evaluation is not necessary in the vast majority of patients with BOO due to BPH. Patients in whom history, findings on physical examination, or results of uroflow studies are suspicious for bladder dysfunction (rather than obstruction) should, however, usually undergo urodynamic studies before surgical procedures are considered.

TABLE 1. **Symptoms of Benign Prostatic Hyperplasia**

Obstructive	Irritative
Weak urinary stream	Urgency
Hesitancy	Frequency
Intermittency	Nocturia
Straining to void	Dysuria
Sensation of incomplete emptying	

DIFFERENTIAL DIAGNOSIS AND ASSOCIATED CONDITIONS

Many conditions can mimic prostatism or BOO (Table 3). Prostate cancer can cause obstruction of the prostatic urethra. Anatomic obstruction can occur at locations other than the prostate, i.e., with meatal stenosis, urethral stric-

TABLE 2. **American Urological Association Symptom Index for Benign Prostatic Hyperplasia**

	Not at All	Less than 1 Time in 5	Less than Half the Time	About Half the Time	More than Half the Time	Almost Always
1. Over the past month, how often have you had a sensation of not emptying your bladder completely after you finished urinating?	0	1	2	3	4	5
2. Over the past month, how often have you had to urinate again less than 2 hours after you finished urinating?	0	1	2	3	4	5
3. Over the past month, how often have you found you stopped and started again several times while you urinated?	0	1	2	3	4	5
4. Over the past month, how often have you found it difficult to postpone urination?	0	1	2	3	4	5
5. Over the past month, how often have you had a weak urinary stream?	0	1	2	3	4	5
6. Over the past month, how often have you had to push or strain to begin urination?	0	1	2	3	4	5
7. Over the past month, how many times did you most typically get up to urinate from the time you went to bed at night until the time you got up in the morning?	none	1 time	2 times	3 times	4 times	5 or more times
		Symptom score = sum of questions 1–7 = __________				

Adapted from McConnell JD, Barry MJ, Bruskewitz RC, et al: Benign prostatic hyperplasia: Diagnosis and treatment. Clinical Practice Guideline, No. 8. AHCPR Publication No. 94-0582. Rockville, MD, Agency for Health Care Policy and Research, Public Health Service, U.S. Department of Health and Human Services, 1994.

ture disease, or bladder neck contracture. Other conditions that can cause irritation of the lower urinary tract are ureteral calculus, cystitis, carcinoma in situ of the bladder, prostatitis, urethritis, bladder cancer, and urethral cancer. In addition to such causes of anatomic obstructions and lower urinary tract irritation, neuromuscular diseases can also mimic BOO symptoms.

TABLE 3. **Differential Diagnosis for Signs and Symptoms of Bladder Obstruction**

Anatomic Lesions

Bladder neck contracture
Urethral stricture
Meatal stenosis
Anterior urethral diverticulum
Urethral polyp
Urethral carcinoma
Phimosis
Prostate cancer

Neurologic Disorders

Cerebrovascular accident
Brain tumor
Arteriovenous malformation
Parkinson's disease
Spinal cord injury
Amyotrophic lateral sclerosis
Multiple sclerosis
Diabetic neuropathy
Postsurgical neuropathy or bladder denervation

Muscular Disorders

Diabetic myopathy
Postsurgical changes
Fibrosis from recurrent UTIs
Myopathy from chronic obstruction

COMPLICATIONS OF BPH

The most serious complications of BPH include recurrent gross hematuria, renal failure, hydronephrosis, recurrent infection, urosepsis, bladder stone formation from stasis of urine, and destruction of the contractile properties of the detrusor muscle from the muscular damage of chronic distention (Table 4). Less serious complications are reduction in the quality of life from the inconveniences of urinary incontinence, nocturia, recurrent cystitis, and prolonged micturition. Also, chronic fatigue associated with frequent awakening due to nocturia can be quite debilitating.

TREATMENT

There are basically three categories of treatment: watchful waiting, medical treatment, and surgical treatment. Selection of the treatment modality is based largely on the severity of symptoms, changes

TABLE 4. **Complications of Benign Prostatic Hyperplasia**

Severe	Urinary retention Gross hematuria Recurrent urinary tract infection Urosepsis Renal failure Hydronephrosis Bladder calculus Loss of detrusor muscle contractility
Moderate	Urinary incontinence "Nagging symptoms" Sleep deprivation
Mild	Moderate to mild symptomatology

to the urinary tract (both upper and lower), and the patient's perceived change in quality of life. Indications for surgery include complete urinary retention, impending detrusor muscle decompensation, upper urinary tract dysfunction, bladder stones, refractory gross hematuria, recurrent cystitis, and urosepsis.

Surgical Treatment

Surgical treatments include transabdominal, transperineal, and transurethral approaches (Table 5). All of the surgical approaches involve removing ("enucleating") most or all of the adenoma that affects the transitional (periurethral) and central (near the posterior bladder neck) zones of the prostate; the peripheral zone of prostate tissue remains. The "open" surgical procedures are reserved for glands that are so large that troublesome intraoperative complications such as bleeding and electrolyte abnormalities are likely with a transurethral approach. Open prostatectomy effectively reduces the urethral resistance but also destroys part of the patient's continence mechanism, i.e., the bladder neck musculature, and the smooth muscle contractile force of the internal sphincter. Maintenance of continence requires the integrity of the pudendal nerve and the external sphincter. The side effects and risks of surgery include incisional pain and need for blood transfusion in up to 35% of patients. In terms of both short-term and long-term relief of voiding symptoms, open prostatectomy is the most successful of any form of treatment, with 98% of patients having subjective and objective (based on urodynamic studies) improvement. Subsequent reoperation is required in less than 1% of cases per year.

The other forms of surgical therapy involve transurethral delivery of energy to the prostatic urethra to ablate prostatic adenoma. Transurethral resection of the prostate (TURP) is the procedure most commonly performed for BPH. In the standard TURP, a wire loop electrode operated through a large cystoscopic sheath is used to resect the adenomatous tissue from the inside out under direct cystoscopic visualization. TURP requires a great deal of training and skill to perform effectively and safely. The procedure can be performed with the patient under general or spinal anesthesia. The symptomatic improvement rate with TURP is 88%, with only a 2% reoperation rate per year. The major surgical risks are bleeding and electrolyte disturbances from prolonged irrigation flow into open vascular channels. Rates of erectile dysfunction reported following TURP are less than 10%, and rates of incontinence are even lower (<2%). As with open prostatectomy, nearly all patients experience retrograde ejaculation following TURP and are thus essentially infertile; however, this is usually not an issue in the older BPH population.

TABLE 5. **Surgical Procedures for Treatment of Benign Prostatic Hyperplasia**

Open Surgical
Transperineal
Transabdominal
Suprapubic
Retropubic
Transurethral
Transurethral resection (TURP)
Transurethral incision (TUIP)
Transurethral vaporization (TUVP)
Transurethral needle ablation (TUNA)
Transurethral microwave therapy (Prostatron)

Another transurethral approach is electrovaporization of the prostate using a "roller ball"–type electrode and very high levels of electric current. Transurethral incision of the prostate involves use of an electric cutting knife to incise the prostate and bladder neck in one or two places. Both electrovaporization and incision are associated with lower rates of bleeding but have been found to be useful primarily only in patients with smaller glands. Laser procedures can be effective but are associated with high morbidity, because the treated tissue has to slough off over the month or so following the procedure. Prostate stents are effective in promoting bladder emptying, but a high incidence of severe irritative voiding symptoms has limited the use of these devices for now. Microwave therapy, cryotherapy, thermal therapy, newer laser techniques, and various other procedures have been or are being proposed, tested, and marketed. None of these techniques has been proved to match the effectiveness of TURP.

Medical Treatment

Medical treatment of BPH includes the use of alpha blockers and the 5α-reductase inhibitor finasteride (Proscar). The alpha blockers include terazosin (Hytrin), doxazosin (Cardura), and the "prostate-selective" alpha blocker tamsulosin (Flomax). The less selective alpha blockers have crossover effects on other receptors that can affect the venous and arterial receptors; therefore, these agents can produce systemic side effects such as orthostatic hypotension, syncope, dizziness, somnolence, nasal congestion, and nausea.

The alpha blockers cause relaxation of the smooth muscles at the bladder neck and the prostatic urethra, which can effectively reduce urethral resistance and ameliorate symptoms. The less selective alpha blockers doxazosin and terazosin are administered in slowly escalating doses over a 4- to 5-week period up to 4 and 5 mg, respectively. At these doses, 70% of the patients can be expected to have a 30% improvement in the AUA symptom score. This form of therapy is ineffective in the remaining 30%. Another dose escalation—to 8 mg for doxazosin and 10 mg for terazosin—may provide further symptomatic improvement in some patients. Above these levels, toxicity outweighs benefits. Tamsulosin is a prostate-selective alpha blocker that does not require dose titration. Postural and orthostatic hypotension are very rare with this drug, and onset of effect is within 2 weeks of initiating therapy. Its relative effectiveness in comparison with that of doxazosin or terazosin has yet to be established, however.

Finasteride produces its effect by blocking the conversion of testosterone to dihydrotestosterone, the most potent androgen. Early studies showed that 50% of patients could expect a 50% rate of symptomatic improvement. A Veterans Affairs cooperative clinical trial, however, has questioned the efficacy of finasteride. Perhaps the best candidate for this agent is a patient with BOO symptoms and a very large prostate.

Watchful Waiting

It should be emphasized that watchful waiting is not an absence of treatment but constitutes a treatment plan in itself. Watchful waiting for BPH involves yearly digital rectal examination (DRE), measurement of prostate-specific antigen (PSA), urinalysis, and monitoring of AUA scores. Complications are treated as they arise, and treatment (surgical or medical) is initiated as needed for symptom progression. Up to 30% of patients managed with watchful waiting experience symptomatic improvement. The patients who get better with watchful waiting, however, tend to be those with mild symptoms of a relatively recent onset, so patient selection for this treatment option is important.

Review of Management Options

Benign prostatic hyperplasia and its accompanying bladder outlet symptoms are significant causes of morbidity in the older male patient population. A variety of medical and surgical therapies of proven safety and effectiveness are available for treatment of this condition. The challenge facing clinicians today is in properly applying the sometimes bewildering array of treatment methods to their individual patients.

These choices can be guided by some basic principles. First, the severity of a patient's symptoms needs to be determined with some precision, especially the extent to which these symptoms interfere with daily activities and bother the patient. Second, the patient's expectations and hopes regarding treatment must also be identified. Third, the benefits, risks, and cost of each therapy need to be considered and discussed with the patient. Patients with minimal or moderate symptoms, for example, may be very happy with only modest improvement. Patients with severe symptoms, on the other hand, may not be satisfied by merely advancing to a less severe or moderate symptom category.

As previously described, 30% of patients will show some improvement with watchful waiting, but this is usually minimal improvement. With medical therapy, 50 to 70% of patients can be expected to show a 30% improvement in symptoms. With standard transurethral resection of the prostate, about 90% of patients can expect to experience minimal or no BPH symptoms after the initial recovery period.

In summary, then, patients with minimal symptoms are usually best served by watchful waiting or medical therapy. Patients with moderate symptoms are best initially managed with medical therapy, but clinicians must promote realistic expectations by articulating the high expense of the medications, the very real possibility of troublesome side effects, the degree of potential symptomatic improvement, and the 30% possibility of achieving little or no relief at all. Patients with severe symptoms usually need surgical therapy at some point in their clinical course if they hope to achieve significant relief. Here, too, realistic expectations need to be conveyed regarding the possibilities of surgical complications and inadequate symptomatic improvement.

Although therapeutic trials have helped clarify the proper use of these treatments, clinical experience applied attentively to the patient's specific symptoms, expectations, and overall health status remains the cornerstone of care in BPH.

ERECTILE DYSFUNCTION

method of
MANISH N. DAMANI, M.D., and
CULLEY C. CARSON III, M.D.
University of North Carolina School of Medicine
Chapel Hill, North Carolina

Erectile dysfunction (impotence) is the inability to achieve or sustain a firm erection of an appropriate duration for satisfactory sexual activity. In the United States, an estimated 20 to 30 million males, or 1 in 10 men, are affected by erectile dysfunction. In the past, a loss or decrease in erectile function was accepted as a normal attribute of the aging process. However, with the acquisition in the past two decades of new knowledge in the pathophysiology and neuropharmacology of the erectile process, as well as improvements in technology, impotence should no longer be ignored by the patient or the physician.

ERECTILE PHYSIOLOGY

The process of penile erection is a multifactorial one involving a delicate balance of androgen excretion, neurologic stimulation, arterial influx, and venous outflow. The paired internal pudendal arteries, from which the central corporal cavernous artery is derived, are the main source of blood supply to the penile erectile tissue. Venous drainage originates in the small vessels immediately beneath the tunica albuginea (subtunical venules), leading eventually to the paired internal pudendal veins and periprostatic plexus. The key to the erectile process lies with the numerous sinusoids within the tunica and the interwoven cavernous smooth musculature. With relaxation of these smooth muscles controlled by neurotransmitters as well as increased arterial flow from dilation, compression of subtunical venous plexuses, and stretching of the tunica albuginea to capacity, the rigid penile erection is obtained. Nitric oxide (NO), produced by the conversion of L-arginine by the enzyme nitric oxide synthase is the principal neurotransmitter producing corpus cavernosum smooth muscle relaxation through cyclic guanosine monophosphate (GMP).

CLASSIFICATION OF ERECTILE DYSFUNCTION

Erectile dysfunction can be divided into two broad categories: the more common organic causes and the less common psychogenic (nonorganic) causes (Table 1). Psychogenic impotence can be separated into primary psychogenic impotence, affecting men from sexually repressive or religiously orthodox backgrounds, and secondary impotence. The secondary form is poorly understood but involves emotional, familial, cultural, cognitive, maturational, and affective factors. The causes of psychogenic impotence can be divided more simply into desire inhibition, marital conflict, sexual deviation, and excitement inhibition, known as performance anxiety.

On the other hand, organic processes for erectile dysfunction include neuropathic dysfunction, endocrine-mediated dysfunction, arteriogenic impotence, venogenic impotence, surgical traumatic disorders, and drug-associated erectile dysfunction. Peripheral neuropathy as seen with diabetes mellitus, spinal cord lesions, and lesions of the cerebral hemispheres are the common sources of neuropathic dysfunction. Arteriogenic impotence or poor inflow states, usually caused by atherosclerosis, can be secondary to disease of the terminal aorta (Leriche's syndrome) or of the hypogastric, pudendal, or penile arteries. Perineal trauma from straddle injury in young men can also decrease arterial flow. Venogenic impotence is secondary to abnormal venous outflow, deficiency of the tunica albuginea, functional impairment of the erectile smooth muscle tissue (corporovenous leakage), or inadequate outflow restriction leading to short-lived erections. Endocrine disorders are caused by abnormalities in the hypothalamic-pituitary-gonadal axis, resulting in low levels of testosterone, which is intricately involved in maintaining male libido and potency. Such disorders include hypogonadotropic hypogonadism (Kallmann's syndrome), Cushing's syndrome, hypergonadotropic hypergonadism (Klinefelter's syndrome), hyperprolactinemia, thyroid abnormalities, and increased prolactin levels resulting from renal failure. In addition, trauma to the lower urinary tract, urethral or prostatic surgery, and bowel surgery can also lead to erectile dysfunction. Furthermore, 25% of all cases of impotence are drug-induced, resulting in a change in libido, diminished erectile ability, or ejaculatory dysfunction. These situations are often created by psychotropic drugs, antihypertensives, antidepressants, alcohol, tobacco, marijuana, and narcotics (Table 2).

TABLE 1. **Etiology of Erectile Dysfunction**

Nonorganic
Psychogenic impotence
Organic
Neuropathic dysfunction
Endocrine disorders
Arteriogenic impotence
Venogenic impotence
Surgical/traumatic disorders
Drug-associated impotence

TABLE 2. **Drugs Causing Erectile Dysfunction**

Major tranquilizers
Phenothiazines (e.g., fluphenazine, chlorpromazine, promazine, mesoridazine)
Butyrophenones (e.g., haloperidol)
Thioxanthines (e.g., thiothixene, chlorthixene*)
Antidepressants
Tricyclics (e.g., nortriptyline, amitryptiline, desipramine, doxepin)
Monoamine oxidase inhibitors (e.g., isocarboxazide,* phenelzine, tranylcypromine, pargyline, procarbazine)
Anxiolytics
Benzodiazepines (e.g., chlordiazepoxide, diazepam, chlorazepate)
Anticholinergics
Atropine, propantheline, benztropine, dimenhydrinate, diphenhydramine
Luteinizing hormone–releasing hormone agonists
Leuprolide acetate, goserelin acetate
Antiandrogens
Nilutamide, flutamide, bicalutamide
Antihypertensives
Diuretics (e.g., thiazides, spironolactone)
Vasodilators (e.g., hydralazine)
Central sympatholytics (e.g., methyldopa, clonidine, reserpine)
Ganglion blockers (e.g., guanethidine, bethanidine*)
Beta blockers (e.g., propranolol, metoprolol, atenolol)
Angiotensin-converting enzyme inhibitors (e.g., enalapril)
Calcium channel blockers (e.g., nifedipine)
Psychotropic drugs
Alcohol, marijuana, amphetamines, barbiturates, nicotine, opiates
Miscellaneous
Cimetidine, clofibrate, digoxin, estrogens, indomethacin, others

*Not available in the United States.

DIAGNOSIS OF ERECTILE DYSFUNCTION

History and Physical Examination

The history and physical examination constitute the most important elements in the initial evaluation of the patient with erectile dysfunction. The history helps to define the actual problem, to identify the occurrence of erections, and to determine whether the patient is able to achieve penetration and maintain the erection until orgasm and ejaculation. Assessment should begin with a detailed medical and surgical history, including a list of medications (see Table 2), and a review of urologic, neurologic, and vascular systems, as well as sexual and psychosocial evaluations. Noting key disease processes such as diabetes mellitus, hypertension, and spinal cord injury in addition to vascular and neurologic complications of surgical procedures is paramount. However, an accurate sexual history to determine maximal rigidity, sustaining capability, and the presence and occurrence of nocturnal erections, masturbation, and coital erections, as well as the duration and onset of the erectile dysfunction, is the most crucial aspect of the evaluation.

A thorough physical evaluation is essential in identifying obvious causes of erectile dysfunction. Inspection of the genitalia to exclude congenital and acquired abnormalities, such as Peyronie's plaques, microphallus, and penile curvature (chordee), as well as a rectal examination to evaluate the prostate, should be performed. The physical examination should also include an assessment of secondary sexual characteristics, with identification of gynecomastia and neck anomalies to rule out endocrine dysfunction. It is necessary to perform both a complete cardiovascular examination, including palpation of peripheral pulses, and a complete neurologic examination, to assess perineal sensation, anal tone, and presence of the bulbocavernosus reflex.

Laboratory Evaluation

Unlike in other disease processes, no one laboratory study is exclusively diagnostic of erectile dysfunction. Baseline hematologic and biochemical tests can be done to exclude significant disease processes such as diabetes mellitus, hyperlipidemia, hepatic and renal insufficiency, and anemia of various causes. Also, an underlying endocrine cause for erectile dysfunction can be discovered through determination of testosterone level, thyroid function tests, and measurement of serum prolactin, follicle-stimulating hormone, and luteinizing hormone. There is a wide variation in testosterone levels in normal men (greater than 250 ng per dL), with higher values noted in the morning, and thus this measurement should be obtained before noon. Free testosterone levels, although controversial, may identify those men with reduced levels of bioavailable testosterone.

Other Diagnostic Studies

After performing a thorough history and physical examination for erectile dysfunction, several other diagnostic studies may be necessary to identify the source of impotence. Although the history is often indicative, monitoring for nocturnal penile tumescence can be very helpful in identifying men suffering from a psychogenic cause of erectile dysfunction. For this study, sleep-associated erections are monitored over 3 days' time; the normal male has three to five erections per night, each lasting approximately 30 minutes, during the rapid eye movement (REM) cycle of sleep. Therefore, psychogenic impotence will be represented by a normal study, whereas organic impotence is discovered by impaired or absent erectile activity.

Diagnosis of a specific organic cause, however, can range from a simple office procedure to more complicated, highly invasive testing. A practical office procedure involves intracavernous injection with papaverine or alprostadil (Caverject) to obtain an erection. The lack of a full, rigid erection most likely rules out a psychogenic cause and suggests an underlying organic process. The next step is a combination of intracavernous injection with duplex Doppler technology to differentiate an arteriogenic from a venogenic cause. This technique, which allows the penile arteries to be visualized, measures blood flow and vessel diameter before and after intracavernosal injection of vasoactive substances. Mean peak flow velocity greater than 25 cm per second assures adequate arterial supply to the penis. In patients with abnormal results on Doppler study of the penile arteries, penile angiography represents the next step, specifically in young trauma patients who are candidates for surgical revascularization of the penis.

Erectile dysfunction secondary to venous leakage may be difficult to diagnose as well as to rectify. A venogenic cause of erectile dysfunction is suggested in a patient who quickly achieves a partial erection but loses rigidity rapidly after intracavernosal injection of vasoactive agents. In such cases, arterial inflow is often adequate, and thus pharmacocavernosometry and pharmacocavernosography are useful in evaluation. After intracavernous vasoactive agent administration, pharmacocavernosometry involves saline infusion into the corpora to generate an artificial erection, with simultaneous measurement of maintenance flow and pressure. Abnormal venous leakage is suggested by flow greater than 30 mL per minute to maintain an intracavernous pressure greater than 90 mm Hg or a fully rigid erection. Pharmacocavernosography provides additional information by infusing contrast material into the corpus cavernosum and radiographically identifying the area of venous leak.

TREATMENT OF ERECTILE DYSFUNCTION

As with other disease processes, there is as yet no cure for erectile dysfunction, but any of several modalities, both medical and surgical, can enhance existing erectile status. Once the etiology and pathophysiology of erectile dysfunction are understood, the therapeutic options are easily comprehended (Table 3).

Medical Management

Psychogenic erectile dysfunction can often be successfully treated with psychosexual therapy. In se-

TABLE 3. **Treatment of Erectile Dysfunction**

Medical Management	
Psychosexual therapy	As directed by therapist
Yohimbine (Yocon)	5.4 mg PO tid.
Trazodone (Desyrel)	50–100 mg PO 2–3 h prior to sexual activity
Sildenifil (Viagra)	1 tablet PO 1 h prior to sexual activity
Apomorphine (Spontain)	1 tablet PO 30–60 min prior to sexual activity
Alprostadil (Caverject)	5–20 μg of solution (0.1–1.0 mL) injected intracavernosally 10–20 min prior to sexual activity
Papaverine	30 mg/mL (0.1–1.0 mL) injected intracavernosally 10–20 min prior to sexual activity
Phentolamine (Regitine)	1 mg/mL injected intracavernosally 10–20 min prior to sexual activity
Alprostadil (MUSE)	125–1000 μg as suppository delivered via urethra 10–20 minutes prior to sexual activity
Vacuum constriction device	To be used as directed by manufacturer
Surgical Management	
Placement of semirigid rod prosthesis	
Placement of inflatable penile prosthesis	
Penile arterial revascularization	
Venous ligation	

vere or resistant cases, however, additional pharmacologic or other nonsurgical modalities will be necessary to functionally restore erectile capacity. For those patients with an endocrine dysfunction, such as hypogonadism, androgen replacement may be the treatment of choice. The two effective options include intramuscular testosterone injection and transdermal testosterone skin patches, with the latter preferred owing to fewer side effects and ease of use.

Oral pharmacologic agents such as yohimbine (Yocon, Yohimex) and trazodone* (Desyrel), as well as the newer drugs sildenifil (Viagra), apomorphine* (Spontain), and oral phentolamine* (Vasomax), are useful primary therapeutic agents for erectile dysfunction. Yohimbine, an alpha$_2$-adrenoceptor blocking agent, and trazodone, which is a central dopamine agonist with some peripheral alpha-blocking activity, produce a positive response in approximately 30% of patients, but studies demonstrate no significant improvement over placebo. The newer agent sildenifil, a phosphodiesterase type 5 inhibitor, prevents the intracorporeal breakdown of cyclic GMP, the second messenger of nitric oxide (NO), and thus enhances erectile function in approximately 70% of men. Administration of apomorphine, a centrally acting oral agent, also has significant effect as a precoital treatment.

Intracavernous pharmacotherapy has provided a significant breakthrough in the treatment of erectile dysfunction. Drugs formerly used for intracavernous injection therapy—papaverine, a smooth muscle relaxant, and phentolamine† (Regitine), a nonselective adrenoceptor-blocking agent—have been replaced by the Food and Drug Administration (FDA)–approved alprostadil (Caverject), which contains prostaglandin E_1 (PGE_1) and has fewer side effects. Alprostadil is injected intracavernosally at the base of the penis, as directed by trained personnel; following dose titration, an erection occurs within 15 minutes and is maintained for approximately 1 hour. Adverse side effects include priapism, hematoma formation, pain on injection, and fibrous plaque formation. Contraindications to this therapy include sickle cell trait or disease, leukemia, anticoagulation, and immunocompromising infectious diseases.

The harmful side effects of self-injection can be avoided by the use of intraurethral therapy, although this modality provides lower intracavernosal levels of PGE_1. With intraurethral therapy, known as Muse (medicated urethral system for erection), alprostadial in suppository form is absorbed into the cavernosal tissue via the urethra, to produce erections. Dosages include 125 μg, 250 μg, 500 μg, and 1000 μg. The usual initial dosage is 250 to 500 μg.

Another effective method to treat erectile dysfunction is with use of a vacuum constriction device. Via a pump mechanism, this device creates a negative pressure of at least 100 mm Hg when placed over the penis, trapping blood in both its intracorporeal and extracorporeal compartments. The artificially induced erection is then maintained by a constriction ring placed at the base of the penis for up to 30 minutes. Similar contraindications exist as for intracavernosal and intraurethral therapies, with side effects including penile numbness, difficult ejaculation, hematoma, and altered orgasm.

*Not yet approved for use in the United States.
†Not FDA approved for this indication.

Surgical Treatment

Surgical treatment modalities are generally reserved for use in patients in whom nonsurgical therapy for erectile dysfunction has failed. The most commonly used surgical device is the penile prosthesis. The two types of prostheses include the semirigid rod prosthesis and the inflatable penile prosthesis. The semirigid rod prosthesis is the simplest to implement and consists of paired silicone rubber cylinders with a central metal wire allowing flexibility to mimic erection. However, the inflatable penile prostheses are cosmetically more pleasing and sexually satisfying to patients and their partners. There are three different types of inflatable penile prostheses: the self-contained penile prosthesis, the two-piece inflatable penile prosthesis, and the three-piece inflatable penile prosthesis, the last providing the most increased length and girth. Three-piece prostheses are composed of paired penile cylinders with a suprapubic reservoir to provide fluid and a scrotally placed control pump. The mechanical malfunction rate for any of the penile prostheses is approximately 5% over 3 years, with similar rates of infection, necessitating replacement of part or all of the prosthesis.

For young trauma patients with arteriogenic impotence, penile arterial revascularization rather than placement of a penile prosthesis should be considered. With a variety of revascularization procedures available, the main objective is to use the inferior epigastric artery to provide arterial flow to the penis, usually via the dorsal artery. Success rates vary depending on the procedure chosen and patient selection, in many series reaching greater than 70%. On the other hand, results of surgical correction of venogenic impotence are less than adequate. Venous ligation procedures to increase venous outflow resistance based on pharmacocavernosography are successful approximately 40% of the time, often necessitating subsequent penile prosthesis placement.

ACUTE RENAL FAILURE

method of
DGANIT DINOUR, M.D.
Chaim Sheba Medical Center
Tel-Hashomer, Israel

Acute renal failure (ARF) is a clinical syndrome characterized by rapid deterioration of renal function that occurs within days (as opposed to weeks or months in subacute, or years in chronic renal failure). The principal feature of ARF is an abrupt decline in glomerular filtration rate (GFR), resulting in the retention of nitrogenous wastes such as urea and creatinine (azotemia). Other kidney functions including tubular handling of water and electrolytes, maintenance of acid-base balance, and metabolic and endocrine functions are disturbed to variable degrees in different types of ARF.

The incidence of ARF depends on the definition and the population studied. In the general adult population, 170 to 200 cases of severe ARF per million occur annually. ARF is present in approximately 1% of patients presenting to emergency departments and affects about 5% of hospitalized patients. Certain populations are especially at risk; the incidence of ARF is 15 to 30% in intensive care units or after cardiovascular surgery.

Accurate and rapid etiologic diagnosis of ARF is critical, because it may be possible in many cases to stop the injurious process and prevent further progression of renal insufficiency. ARF may have a multitude of causes, but an approach to the patient suffering from ARF by categorizing it as prerenal, intrarenal, and postrenal facilitates the diagnostic process.

Prerenal failure is a functional, rapidly reversible reduction in GFR, caused by renal hypoperfusion without any parenchymal damage to the kidney. Correction of the underlying cause promptly reverses kidney function to baseline within 24 to 72 hours. Prerenal failure is the most common cause of acute azotemia both in the community and in the hospital, accounting for 55 to 70% of cases of ARF. Renal hypoperfusion can result from true hypovolemia, decreased effective blood volume, or renal vasoconstriction (Table 1). Common causes of prerenal failure in the community are volume depletion resulting from gastrointestinal loss (vomiting, diarrhea) or overdiuresis and reduced renal perfusion owing to congestive heart failure or the use of drugs such as diuretics, nonsteroidal anti-inflammatory drugs (NSAIDs), or angiotensin-converting enzyme (ACE) inhibitors in high-risk patients. Additional frequent causes of prerenal failure in hospitalized patients include blood loss, sepsis, third spacing, burns, and cirrhosis.

Intrarenal ARF is the general term used to describe ARF accompanied by tubular, interstitial, glomerular, or vascular renal tissue damage (Table 2). The major type of intrarenal ARF in hospitalized patients is acute tubular necrosis (ATN), which results from ischemic or toxic renal insult. ATN is most often multifactorial, typically occurring in patients subjected to endogenous or exogenous nephrotoxins in the setting of renal hypoperfusion. In ATN, as opposed to prerenal failure, the abrupt decline in GFR is accompanied by tubular dysfunction and is not immediately reversible on removal of the inciting factor. Acute interstitial nephritis is an important form of intrarenal ARF following drug use, various infections, and malignancies. Persons with glomerular disease and vasculitides usually present with the nephritic or nephrotic syndromes and subacute or chronic renal insufficiency. However, some persons with glomerular and vascular diseases, such as rapidly progressive glomerulonephritis, lupus nephritis, hemolytic-uremic syndrome, and atheroembolic renal disease, may present with ARF.

Postrenal ARF, resulting from complete or partial obstruction of the urinary collection system (Table 3), is an important cause of severe ARF in the community. Common etiologies include prostatic hypertrophy, prostate or uri-

TABLE 1. **Major Causes of Prerenal Acute Renal Failure**

Intravascular Volume Depletion

Hemorrhage
Gastrointestinal loss: vomiting, diarrhea, gastrointestinal drainage
Renal loss: diuretics, osmotic diuresis (diabetes mellitus), diabetes insipidus, salt wasting nephropathy, hypoadrenalism
Third space sequestration: pancreatitis, ileus, hypoalbuminemia
Insensible loss: sweat, burns, respiratory loss

Decreased Cardiac Output

Congestive heart failure: ischemic heart disease, cardiomyopathy, valvular or pericardial disease
Pulmonary hypertension, massive pulmonary embolism

Decreased Renal Perfusion with Normal/High Cardiac Output

Sepsis
Cirrhosis
Drugs: nonsteroidal anti-inflammatory agents, angiotensin-converting enzyme inhibitors, alpha-adrenergic agonists, cyclosporine, radiocontrast agents

Renovascular Obstruction

Renal artery: embolism, thrombosis, dissecting aneurysm, atherosclerosis
Renal vein: thrombosis

TABLE 2. **Major Causes of Intrarenal Acute Renal Failure**

Acute Tubular Necrosis (ATN)

Ischemia: septic, hypovolemic or cardiogenic shock, major surgery
Exogenous toxins: aminoglycosides, radiocontrast agents, amphotericin B, cisplatin, foscarnet, heavy metals, ethylene glycol, acetaminophen intoxication
Endogenous toxins: hemoglobin (hemolysis), myoglobin (rhabdomyolysis), proteins (myeloma)

Tubulointerstitial Nephritis

Allergic interstitial nephritis: beta lactams, sulfonamides, trimethoprim, diuretics, nonsteroidal anti-inflammatory drugs, rifampin
Infectious: bacterial, tuberculosis, human immunodeficiency virus
Infiltration: lymphoma, leukemia, sarcoidosis
Radiation

Rapidly Progressive Glomerulonephritis

Immune complex mediated: postinfectious, lupus nephritis, membranoproliferative, cryoglobulinemia, IgA nephropathy
With vasculitis: Wegener's granulomatosis, microscopic polyarteritis
Anti–glomerular basement membrane disease

Vascular

Thrombotic microangiopathy: hemolytic-uremic syndrome, preeclampsia, disseminated intravascular coagulation, thrombotic-thrombocytopenic purpura
Atheroembolic disease
Malignant hypertension, scleroderma crisis

Renal Allograft Rejection

TABLE 3. **Major Causes of Postrenal Acute Renal Failure**

Prostatic hypertrophy
Neoplasm: prostate, bladder, cervix, colorectal
Nephrolithiasis
Neurogenic bladder
Papillary necrosis
Retroperitoneal fibrosis

nary tract malignancies, ureteral calculi, and neurogenic bladder. Typical features of the common forms of ARF are outlined in Table 4.

In addition to the pathophysiologic classification for patients with ARF, another category is based on urine output. Anuric patients have no urine output, oliguric patients produce less than 400 mL urine per 24 hours, and nonoliguric patients have a urine output of more than 400 mL per 24 hours. Patients with oliguric or anuric ARF are harder to manage than patients with nonoliguric ARF and have a more severe renal disease and a worse prognosis.

DIAGNOSIS

History

Outpatients with ARF may present with nonspecific complaints such as malaise, weakness, loss of appetite and nausea, and/or symptoms of fluid retention and decreased urine output. In hospitalized patients, the most common presentation is a rise in blood urea nitrogen (BUN) and creatinine. In both cases, careful history taking and a thorough chart review are necessary to confirm the presence of acute versus chronic renal failure, and to determine its cause.

Recent bleeding or fluid loss (diarrhea, vomiting, excessive diuresis) or the presence of severe congestive heart failure, extensive myocardial ischemia, arrhythmias, or liver disease suggests prerenal failure. Sepsis, major surgery, or prolonged hypotension usually indicates ATN. Records of fluid intake and output, vital signs, and weights may contribute substantially to the diagnosis of prerenal azotemia and ATN. A detailed drug history is essential and should include a review of the medication administration record and the timing and dosage of radiocontrast. In patients with a history of cancer, nephrolithiasis, or prostatism, postrenal failure should always be suspected. Recent vascular procedures suggest an atheromboembolic (cholesterol emboli) etiology. Purpura, hemoptysis, arthralgia, rash, and hematuria imply an immune complex disease or vasculitis.

Physical Examination

The diagnostic evaluation of ARF must always include a detailed physical examination. Vital signs and assessment of volume status are critical. Orthostatic hypotension, tachycardia, and dry mucous membranes suggest prerenal failure. Hypotension with fever or hypothermia implies sepsis. Edema, elevated jugular venous pressure, a third heart sound, and evidence of pulmonary congestion or pleural effusion indicate congestive heart failure or volume overload. New or worsening hypertension may suggest acute glomerulonephritis or atheroembolic disease.

An enlarged prostate or palpable bladder raises the possibility of obstruction. The presence of flank tenderness is nonspecific and may reflect obstruction, renal vein throm-

TABLE 4. **Typical Features of Major Forms of Acute Renal Failure**

Etiology	History	Physical Examination	Laboratory and Radiology Findings
Prerenal failure			
Volume depletion	Bleeding; vomiting, diarrhea; diuretics; oliguria	Orthostatic hypotension; tachycardia	↑ plasma BUN/Cr; ↓ urine Na and FE_{Na}; ↑ urine osmolality; benign urine sediment; normal kidney size and morphology
Low effective blood volume	Heart failure; cirrhosis; nephrotic syndrome	Normal or low blood pressure; pulmonary and/or peripheral edema; ascites	
Acute tubular necrosis	Nephrotoxic drugs; volume depletion; rhabdomyolysis; sepsis, multiorgan failure	Normal or low blood pressure; other findings depend on underlying disorder	↑ urine Na and FE_{Na}; isosthenuria; urine sediment granular casts and tubular cells and casts
Hepatorenal syndrome	Liver disease; recent hospitalization; oliguria; no response to volume repletion	Signs of liver failure; ascites	↓ ↓ urine Na and FE_{Na}; benign urine sediment; normal kidney size and morphology
Allergic interstitial nephritis	New drug	Fever; rash	Eosinophilia; urine sediment: WBCs, RBCs, eosinophils
Atheroembolic disease	Hypertension; systemic vascular disease; vascular procedures (surgery, angiography)	Elevated blood pressure, peripheral emboli (blue toes, retinal or cerebral emboli)	Eosinophilia; ↑ ESR; benign urine sediment or mild hematuria
Rapidly progressive glomerulonephritis	Recent infection; respiratory symptoms, pulmonary hemorrhage	Pulmonary rales; rash; arthritis; serositis	Nephritic urine sediment; anemia; echogenic, normal-sized kidneys
Thrombotic microangiopathy	Pregnancy; sepsis; diarrhea; certain drugs	Paleness, purpura	Microangiopathic anemia; ↑ LDH thrombocytopenia
Obstructive nephropathy	Prostatism; malignancy; nephrolithiasis; anuria or polyuria	Palpable bladder, enlarged prostate, abdominal mass, flank tenderness	Normal urine sediment, pyuria or hematuria; hydronephrosis on renal ultrasound

Abbreviations: BUN = blood urea nitrogen; Cr = creatinine; Na = sodium; FE_{Na} = fractional excretion of sodium; WBCs = white blood cells, RBCs = red blood cells; ESR = erythrocyte sedimentation rate; LDH = lactate dehydrogenase.

bosis, renal infarction, or pyelonephritis. Bilateral flank tenderness may accompany acute interstitial nephritis or glomerulonephritis. A careful evaluation of the skin may reveal rash in allergic interstitial nephritis or vasculitis, purpura in vasculitis or thrombotic microangiopathies, and blue toes in cholesterol embolization. The ophthalmic examination should not be neglected. Uveitis may be found in vasculitis or sarcoidosis, Roth's spots suggest endocarditis, and papilledema indicates malignant hypertension.

Laboratory Studies

The laboratory studies required for the evaluation of ARF include blood chemistry (BUN, creatinine, electrolytes, uric acid, albumin, globulin, liver function tests, lactate dehydrogenase [LDH] and creatine phosphokinase [CPK]), complete blood count and smear, blood gases, urinalysis, and urine electrolytes.

Blood Chemistry. Serum creatinine and BUN are elevated per definition owing to reduced GFR. Because tubular reabsorption of BUN is enhanced in prerenal states, an elevated BUN/creatinine ratio often implies prerenal azotemia (Table 5). Other conditions that increase BUN include a high-protein diet, gastrointestinal bleeding, and tetracyclines and glucocorticoid treatment, whereas malnutrition and liver disease decrease BUN. Serum creatinine is a more specific indicator of GFR and usually rises by 0.5 to 1.5 mg per dL per day in severe ARF. However, as ARF is a non–steady-state situation, GFR cannot be predicted by the absolute value of serum creatinine. Some conditions affect serum creatinine by mechanisms other than reduction of GFR; an isolated nonprogressive rise in creatinine may result from impaired tubular secretion owing to administration of drugs such as cimetidine or trimethoprim, and a marked elevation of serum creatinine without a parallel elevation of BUN may suggest rhabdomyolysis.

Hyperuricemia, a common finding in ARF, is more pronounced in prerenal failure. Hypokalemia may be secondary to gastrointestinal loss or diuresis. Hypercalcemia is seen in multiple myeloma, other malignancies, sarcoidosis, and the milk-alkali syndrome and may contribute to the development of ARF. The combination of hyperkalemia, hyperphosphatemia, hypocalcemia, and hyperuricemia is typical for tissue damage as in tumor lysis syndrome or rhabdomyolysis. Elevated CPK levels are highly suggestive of rhabdomyolysis, whereas elevated LDH levels suggest hemolysis. Hypoalbuminemia may indicate the nephrotic syndrome, liver failure, or malnutrition. Hyperglobulinemia may be the clue to the diagnosis of multiple myeloma.

TABLE 5. **Laboratory Tests to Distinguish Prerenal Azotemia from Acute Tubular Necrosis**

Test	Prerenal Azotemia	Acute Tubular Necrosis
BUN/plasma creatinine	>20:1	10–15:1
Urine specific gravity	>1.020	<1.010
Urine osmolality	>500 mOsm/kg	<350 (isosthenuria)
Urine sodium	<20 mEq/L	>40 mEq/L
Fractional excretion of sodium (FE_{Na})*	<1%	>1%
Urine sediment	Normal, hyaline casts	Granular casts, tubular cells

*FE_{Na} = sodium clearance/creatinine clearance = urine Na × plasma Cr/plasma Na × urine Cr.

Blood Count. Leukocytosis may support the diagnosis of sepsis, and eosinophilia may accompany allergic interstitial nephritis, vasculitis, or atheroembolic disease. Thrombocytopenia, anemia, and schistocytes indicate a microangiopathic hemolytic disease. Blood gases usually disclose a metabolic acidosis. The presence of metabolic alkalosis in the setting of ARF suggests volume depletion owing to vomiting or diuresis. Lactic acidosis implies septic, cardiogenic, or hemorrhagic shock; and combined metabolic and respiratory acidosis characterizes multiorgan failure or the pulmonary-renal syndrome.

Urinalysis. Urinalysis is a crucial part of the diagnostic evaluation of ARF. A normal urine sediment with only 0 to 2 red blood cells per high power field, 0 to 2 white blood cells, and a few hyaline casts is expected in prerenal failure and can also be found in postrenal failure and ARF of vascular etiology. Brown, coarse, granular casts; tubular epithelial cells; and tubular cell casts are the typical features of ATN. Leukocyturia, white blood cell casts, eosinophiluria (using Hansel's stain), and hematuria suggest allergic interstitial nephritis, although leukocyturia is also a feature of pyelonephritis and glomerulonephritis, and eosinophiluria may sometimes be seen in atheroembolism. Hematuria may reflect trauma (most often from a Foley catheter), nephrolithiasis, neoplasm, or a bleeding diathesis. Dysmorphic red blood cells and red blood cell casts indicate a glomerular lesion and are usually accompanied by some degree of proteinuria. Mild proteinuria (<1 gram per day) is common in ATN and up to 3 grams per day may be seen in other tubulointerstitial diseases. Nephrotic range proteinuria (>3.5 grams per day) suggests glomerulonephritis but may be found less commonly in other conditions, such as severe preeclampsia, malignant hypertension, and the hemolytic-uremic syndrome. When the sulfosalicylic acid test for protein is positive in the face of a negative dipstick for albumin, the presence of nonalbumin proteins such as Bence-Jones protein should be sought.

Urine Indices. In prerenal failure, the kidney responds to hypoperfusion by avid sodium and water reabsorption. In contrast, tubular damage in ATN impairs the kidney's ability to concentrate the urine and absorb sodium efficiently. These differences may be helpful in the differentiation between prerenal failure and ATN. A high specific gravity (SG >1.020) and a high urine osmolality (>500 mOsm per kg) reflect an efficient urine-concentrating mechanism and usually indicate prerenal failure. In contrast, low specific gravity (SG <1.010) and urine osmolality that is similar to plasma osmolality (isosthenuria) are typical of ATN (see Table 5). Likewise, low urine sodium, and particularly low fractional excretion of sodium (FE_{Na}), indicate prerenal failure, whereas high urine sodium and FE_{Na} support the diagnosis of ATN (see Table 5). The diagnostic role of these urinary indices, however, should not be overestimated, as a significant overlap may exist. ATN secondary to contrast nephropathy is typically associated with low urine sodium and FE_{Na}. Early interstitial nephritis and glomerulonephritis, as well as early postrenal failure, may present with urinary indices suggestive of prerenal failure. The lowest urine sodium and FE_{Na} are seen in hepatorenal syndrome. On the other hand, in patients with underlying chronic renal failure or under diuretic treatment, isosthenuria and high urine sodium and FE_{Na} may be present in prerenal states. Therefore, the urine indices should be interpreted in the context of the overall clinical picture.

Other Laboratory Tests. In some circumstances, further studies are required to establish the diagnosis of ARF. If multiple myeloma is suspected, serum and urine should be sent for immunoelectrophoresis. Low complement levels in ARF with a nephritic urinary sediment will limit the differential diagnosis to postinfectious glomerulonephritis, endocarditis, lupus nephritis, and cryoglobulinemia. Positive antinuclear factor and anti-DNA antibodies support the diagnosis of lupus nephritis, positive antineutrophil cytoplasmic antibodies (p-ANCA or c-ANCA) indicate small vessel vasculitis, and anti–glomerular basement membrane antibodies in a patient with the pulmonary-renal syndrome are specific for Goodpasture's syndrome. A skin biopsy may be helpful in the diagnosis of vasculitis or atheroembolic disease and may obviate the need for a renal biopsy.

Imaging

In most patients with ARF, a renal ultrasound study is indicated. A rapid, noninvasive test, it can be performed even at the bedside with minimal discomfort to the patient. Renal ultrasound is particularly important to rule out obstruction. It is highly sensitive for dilatation of the urinary tract after 24 to 48 hours of obstruction and may reveal anatomic anomalies and asymmetry, tumors, stones, or enlarged prostate. Ultrasound may also be used to estimate kidney size, an important clue to the differentiation between chronic and acute renal failure. Small, contracted, hyperechoic kidneys or large polycystic kidneys indicate chronic renal disease. Doppler ultrasonography or magnetic resonance imaging may be used to assess the patency of renal arteries and veins. A renal radionuclide scan is rarely helpful when GFR is significantly decreased (GFR <25 mL per minute). Finally, imaging modalities that require radiocontrast, such as intravenous pyelography and computed tomography, should be avoided in ARF because of their potential nephrotoxicity.

Biopsy

Renal biopsy plays a limited role in the diagnosis of ARF. Prerenal azotemia, postrenal failure, and most cases of ATN are diagnosed clinically. One exception is the transplanted kidney, in which it is often difficult to distinguish ATN from acute rejection without a biopsy. The etiology of acute intrinsic renal failure is evident from the history and clinical findings not only in ATN but also in many cases of interstitial nephritis, cholesterol emboli, and thrombotic microangiopathies. Renal biopsy is indicated in cases of ARF in which the diagnosis has not been ascertained and a pathologic diagnosis may affect treatment. These are usually cases of intrinsic ARF with a clinical presentation of rapidly progressive glomerulonephritis, where the suspected diseases are Wegener's granulomatosis, Goodpasture's syndrome, microscopic polyarteritis or lupus nephritis, and some ambiguous cases of interstitial nephritis, thrombotic thrombocytopenic purpura, and atheroembolism. With the use of automated biopsy needles and direct ultrasound guidance, the risks of renal biopsy are minimized, and it can be performed even in acutely ill patients. Hypertension and bleeding diathesis should be controlled before the procedure is performed.

TREATMENT

Prevention

Prevention is of paramount importance, because despite major advances in renal replacement therapy and supportive care, ARF still accounts for a remarkable rate of morbidity and mortality. ARF is often iatrogenic and many cases can be prevented by avoiding nephrotoxic medications, unnecessary invasive procedures, and the use of contrast agents in high-risk patients, as well as by prompt correction of volume depletion states. As insults are synergistic, it is imperative to avoid combinations of risks, such as ischemic and toxic injuries. The physician must be aware of the contraindications, interactions, and side effects of all medications and procedures prescribed. The use of contrast agents should be limited to conditions with a clear clinical indication, where noncontrast imaging methods are insufficient, and with consideration to the benefit/risk ratio. If contrast must be used in high-risk patients (chronic renal failure, diabetic nephropathy, multiple myeloma), a nonionic agent should probably be preferred and the minimal dose administered. Aminoglycosides can often be replaced by other, less nephrotoxic antibiotics (quinolones, cephalosporins, β-lactams). When aminoglycosides are prescribed, the doses should be adjusted to the estimated GFR, and blood levels carefully monitored. NSAIDs and ACE inhibitors should be avoided in patients with reduced effective blood volume.

Hydration and salt loading have been the cornerstone of prophylactic treatment against ATN for many years. Several clinical studies have confirmed the role of fluid loading as well as cisplatin, amphotericin, and contrast toxicity in preventing postoperative ARF. The protective effect of mannitol in rhabdomyolysis remains controversial, but no additional benefit of mannitol use over adequate hydration has been shown in preventing postoperative or contrast-induced renal failure. In fact, mannitol can itself induce ARF. Likewise, there is no convincing evidence to support the use of loop diuretics, low-dose dopamine, or calcium blockers to prevent ARF in high-risk patients. Moreover, in some circumstances, mannitol, furosemide, and dopamine may have deleterious effects and therefore should be avoided as routine prophylactic agents.

A few specific measures are available to protect the kidney from injury owing to specific toxins. These include *N*-acetylcysteine in acetaminophen overdose, the use of dimercaprol in heavy metal intoxication, and the use of volume diuresis plus alkalinization of the urine to reduce the toxicity of methotrexate, uric acid, and myoglobin.

Immediate Care

Most patients suspected to have ARF should be hospitalized to allow the best monitoring and care. Patients with mild renal failure with an obvious, easily corrected cause can sometimes be managed as outpatients. Hypovolemic prerenal failure is readily reversible with appropriate fluid replacement. Isotonic saline should be administered to replace urinary or gastrointestinal losses in hemodynamically unstable patients, and blood loss should be corrected with packed red blood cells or whole blood. Patients with postrenal failure should have a Foley catheter placed, when appropriate, and a urologist should be consulted quickly for the optimal means of relieving higher obstruction. Profuse diuresis is common following relief of obstruction, and special care should be taken to avoid volume and electrolyte depletion. Treatment of potentially dangerous complications of ARF, such as hyperkalemia, severe metabolic acidosis, pericarditis, and pulmonary edema (Table 6), should not be deferred until the diagnostic evaluation is completed and may necessitate an emergency dialysis.

Supportive Care

Supportive care consists of careful monitoring, maintenance of adequate fluid balance, modification of diet, avoidance of potential nephrotoxic drugs, and adjustment of medication doses to the estimated degree of renal impairment.

Monitoring

Provision of adequate hydration and the maintenance of effective blood volume are paramount in maintaining adequate renal perfusion and GFR. Maintenance of urine output is not an appropriate goal, because it is an inaccurate index of renal perfusion. Instead, the goal should be to improve cardiac output, avoid vasoconstriction, and optimize renal blood flow. Careful assessment of volume status should be obtained by physical examination, including daily weights, and by strict monitoring of fluid input and output. Hemodynamic monitoring may aid in the assessment of critically ill patients. Measurement of central venous pressure, pulmonary wedge pressure, cardiac index, and systemic vascular resistance are particularly helpful in the management of ARF associated with sepsis, cardiac dysfunction, and multiorgan failure. However, the overall benefit of invasive monitoring in terms of morbidity and mortality has not been proven.

Fluid Balance and Diuretics

Salt and fluid restriction is usually warranted in intrinsic ARF to match fluid input and output (urinary, gastrointestinal, drainage, and insensible losses). In patients with oliguric renal failure and volume overload, especially when pulmonary congestion and respiratory decompensation are present, diuretics and low-dose dopamine are often required to increase urine output. Furosemide (Lasix) may be given in repeated intravenous boluses of 40 to 120 mg every 4 to 6 hours, or as a continuous infusion of 5 to 20 mg per hour. A cumulative daily dose of greater than 500 mg adds little benefit and carries a high risk of ototoxicity. An alternative, probably less ototoxic, loop diuretic is bumetanide (Bumex, 2 to 10 mg intravenously [IV]). The relative potency of bumetanide to furosemide is 40:1 in normal kidney function, but near 20:1 in ARF. When loop diuretics alone fail to induce adequate diuresis, the addition of chlorothiazide (Diuril, 500 mg IV, every 12 hours) may be helpful. Metolazone (Zaroxolyn, 2.5 to 10 mg, orally, every 12 hours) is a potent diuretic, even in patients with marked renal insufficiency. Finally, low-dose dopamine (0.5 to 3 μg per kg per minute) may increase urine output in some patients who remain oliguric despite high-dose diuretics.

It should be emphasized, however, that the indication for diuretic administration in ARF is fluid overload. There is *no* evidence to support the routine use of either furosemide, mannitol, or "renal-dose dopamine" in ARF. Despite promising results in experimental models of ARF, none of these agents has been shown to improve outcome in patients. Moreover, even low doses of dopamine may cause severe complications, such as tachyarrhythmias and myocardial and peripheral ischemia. Increased urine output secondary to aggressive diuretic use may detract from the main goal of maintaining effective intravascular volume and lead to volume depletion.

TABLE 6. **Complications of Acute Renal Failure**

Volume overload	Pulmonary edema, peripheral edema, anasarca
Uremic manifestations	Loss of appetite, nausea, vomiting, hiccups
	Altered mental status
	Pericarditis
	Anemia
	Bleeding diathesis
Electrolyte and mineral imbalance	Metabolic acidosis
	Hyperkalemia
	Hyperphosphatemia
	Hypocalcemia
	Hypermagnesemia
Infections	

Nutritional Support

Diet should be modified to minimize sodium (2 grams per day), potassium (2 grams per day), and phosphate (800 mg per day), while providing enough calories (at least 35 kcal per kg per day). The optimal protein intake is not known. On the one hand, protein restriction to 0.6 to 0.8 gram per kg per day will reduce urea formation and uremic symptoms. On the other hand, nitrogen balance is extremely negative in ARF and is associated with a high protein catabolic rate. Previous studies on the impact of high protein intake (hyperalimentation, total parenteral nutrition) on outcome in ARF did not substantiate a beneficial effect. However, the role of parenteral nutrition should probably be re-evaluated in view of the recent advances in renal replacement therapies. Currently, most nephrologists believe that nutritional support should not be withheld to minimize azotemia and delay dialysis, and up to 1 to 1.5 grams per kg per day of high biologic value protein is usually prescribed to critically ill patients with ARF.

Management of Complications

Fluid Overload

Cardiac failure, pulmonary edema, and anasarca may develop in ARF owing to fluid overload (see

Table 6). Hypertension is rare in ATN but may be a major concern in patients with acute glomerulonephritis or atheroembolism. The maintenance of fluid balance and diuretic use have already been discussed. In addition, inotropic agents, vasodilators, and antihypertensive medications should be instituted as needed. Pulmonary edema unresponsive to conservative measures and intractable anasarca are indications for ultrafiltration with or without dialysis.

Metabolic Acidosis

Combined hyperchloremic and anion gap metabolic acidosis resulting from reduced acid excretion is common in ARF. In addition, ketoacidosis may be present in diabetic or alcoholic patients, severe hyperchloremic acidosis may complicate diarrhea, and lactic acidosis may develop in shock. The main hazards of metabolic acidosis include respiratory fatigue, decreased myocardial contractility, and increased susceptibility to cardiac arrhythmias. Therefore, bicarbonate repletion should be considered when blood pH falls below 7.2. Bicarbonate must be administered cautiously, however, as it may induce symptomatic hypokalemia, hypocalcemia, metabolic alkalosis, and volume overload. A practical approach is to add 2 to 3 ampules of 7.5% sodium bicarbonate (44.6 mEq per ampule) to 1000 mL of 5% dextrose solution, and give the infusion over 3 to 4 hours, with frequent assessment of volume and acid-base status and electrolyte levels. Usually, only a small rise in plasma bicarbonate is required to raise plasma pH to 7.2, and no attempt should be made to further elevate the pH. Dialysis is indicated in unresponsive metabolic acidosis, or in cases of volume overload or hypernatremia that preclude the use of bicarbonate therapy.

Hypokalemia and Hyperkalemia

Hypokalemia typically complicates nonoliguric cisplatin or amphotericin nephrotoxicity. Prerenal failure may also present initially with hypokalemia secondary to urinary or gastrointestinal losses. However, the major potassium disturbance in ARF is hyperkalemia owing to impaired potassium excretion resulting from reduced GFR. Oligoanuric patients are expected to have a daily rise in serum potassium of at least 0.5 mEq per liter. Tissue damage as in rhabdomyolysis, hemolysis, tumor lysis, and the postoperative state increases potassium load and aggravates hyperkalemia. Medications such as potassium-sparing diuretics, potassium salts, ACE inhibitors, spironolactone, trimethoprim, and beta blockers may lead to severe hyperkalemia even in nonoliguric patients with moderately reduced GFR.

Mild hyperkalemia (<6 mEq per liter) can be treated with dietary restriction and the potassium-binding resin sodium polystyrene sulfonate (Kayexalate), which exchanges potassium for sodium in the gut. Oral doses of 15 to 30 grams may be given one to four times daily in sorbitol. If oral administration is not feasible, a retention enema can be given as 30 to 50 grams resin in 100 mL aqueous solution, and repeated at 6-hour intervals as needed. Adverse side effects include nausea, vomiting, hypernatremia, volume overload, calcium and magnesium depletion, and rarely intestinal necrosis.

Symptoms of hyperkalemia are frequent when the serum potassium concentration exceeds 8.0 mEq per liter but may occur at a level between 6.5 and 8.0 mEq per liter. As serum potassium increases, electrographic changes evolve from peaked T waves to prolongation of the PR interval with bradycardia and heart block, then to widened QRS complex, and finally to a full blown sine wave pattern that can lead to ventricular fibrillation and asystole. Arrhythmias of hyperkalemia are exacerbated by concurrent hyponatremia, hypocalcemia, and acidosis, all common in ARF. Neuromuscular manifestations of hyperkalemia include paresthesias and weakness and eventually paralysis and respiratory failure.

Emergency reduction in serum potassium concentration is indicated when neuromuscular symptoms have occurred, when cardiac arrhythmias or electrocardiographic changes are present, or when serum potassium level is more than 7.0 mEq per liter. Emergency measures are directed to antagonize cardiac toxicity of hyperkalemia and to drive potassium into cells (Table 7). Calcium administration does not reduce serum potassium but immediately antagonizes the adverse cardiac and neuromuscular abnormalities. Calcium gluconate (10 mL of a 10% solution) should be given intravenously over 2 to 5 minutes. The dose can be repeated after 5 minutes if no response occurs. Further doses are unlikely to be of benefit unless hypocalcemia is present. Bicarbonate rapidly drives potassium into cells and is especially effective in acidemia. One to three ampules of 7.5% sodium bicarbonate (44.6 mEq bicarbonate per ampule) can be given intravenously over 5 minutes each. Bicarbonate should not be given in the same intravenous solution as calcium because an insoluble precipitate forms. Insulin also promotes an extracellular to intracellular potassium shift and is usually used with glucose to prevent hypoglycemia. Ten units of regular insulin can be added to 500 mL of 10% glucose solution and infused intravenously over 1 hour. Alternatively, 10 units of insulin may be given with 50 mL of 50% glucose solution over 5 minutes. Glucose should not be used as a sole agent because it may cause hyperglycemia and hyperosmolality and exacerbate the hyperkalemia. The use of beta agonists, such as nebulized albuterol (Ventolin, 10 to 20 mg), has been shown to effectively and rapidly redistribute potassium to the intracellular space. However, potential precipitation of tachyarrhythmias and myocardial ischemia is a concern in hemodynamically unstable patients.

Emergency measures should generally be followed by measures to remove potassium from the body. Administration of potassium exchange resins should not be delayed. If GFR is only moderately reduced, rapid and efficient potassium removal can be achieved with a loop diuretic such as furosemide (40 to 160 mg). However, diuretics may lead to volume

TABLE 7. **Emergency Treatment of Hyperkalemia**

Modality	Mechanism of Action	Onset	Duration	Prescription
Calcium	Antagonizes cardiac toxicity	1–2 minutes	1 hour	Calcium gluconate 10% 10 ml IV over 2–5 minutes, repeated once if needed
Bicarbonate	Potassium shift into cells	15–30 minutes	1–2 hours	Sodium bicarbonate 1–3 ampules (44–132 mEq) IV
Insulin	Potassium shift into cells	15–60 minutes	4–6 hours	Regular insulin 10 units IV in 50 mL glucose 5%, or in 500 mL glucose 10%
Beta agonist, albuterol	Potassium shift into cells	30 minutes	Several hours	Nebulized albuterol, 10–20 mg

depletion and a further lowering of GFR, so they should be used cautiously in ARF. Intractable hyperkalemia is an indication for dialysis treatment.

Hyperphosphatemia

Hyperphosphatemia resulting from impaired phosphate excretion develops rapidly in ARF and is most severe when renal failure results from rhabdomyolysis or tumor lysis syndrome. Symptoms of hyperphosphatemia are generally attributable to secondary changes in plasma calcium concentration and ectopic deposition of phosphorus with calcium. In addition to dietary phosphate restriction, phosphate binders are usually required. Aluminum hydroxide containing antacids such as Basaljel or Amphojel, 15 to 30 mL with each meal, should be used when phosphate level is above 7 mg per dL and the calcium phosphorus product exceeds 70 mg per dL. Once the phosphate level is controlled, calcium carbonate (Caltrate) or calcium acetate (PhosLo) should be substituted as phosphate binders. A dose of 600 to 1200 mg given thrice daily *with* meals is usually necessary, even in patients treated with intermittent hemodialysis. In contrast, continuous hemofiltration is so effective in removing phosphate that phosphate supplementation may be required.

Hypocalcemia

Mild hypocalcemia is frequently observed in ARF and should be treated with oral supplement. Symptomatic hypocalcemia, with tetany and convulsions, may complicate ARF associated with acute pancreatitis or rhabdomyolysis, or may be precipitated by rapid correction of acidosis with bicarbonate infusion or dialysis. Immediate treatment consists of intravenous administration of 10 to 20 mL of 10% calcium gluconate over 5 to 10 minutes, followed by continuous infusion of 10 to 15 mg per kg over 4 to 6 hours.

Hypermagnesemia

Hypermagnesemia in ARF results from decreased excretion. Moderate hypermagnesemia may cause lethargy, nausea, muscle weakness, hypotension, and arrhythmias. Severe hypermagnesemia (>10 mg per dL) can lead to coma and cardiac arrest. Ingestion of magnesium-containing compounds, therefore, should be avoided in ARF. In severe symptomatic cases, 10 to 20 mL of calcium gluconate should be infused intravenously over 10 minutes to rapidly antagonize the cardiac and neuromuscular effects of magnesium. If renal function is present, magnesium secretion can be promoted with saline infusion and loop diuretics. When GFR is severely depressed, however, hemodialysis is the definitive treatment.

Hyperuricemia

Hyperuricemia is common in ARF. Markedly elevated uric acid levels are most often a marker of prerenal failure, rarely cause acute gouty arthritis or renal stones, and therefore rarely warrant treatment. Massive uricosuria contributes to the development of ARF in the tumor lysis syndrome. Preventive measures include allopurinol (Zyloprim) and adequate hydration and alkalinization of urine.

Uremic Manifestations

Mild uremic symptoms such as anorexia, nausea, vomiting, and lethargy occur frequently in ARF and are often hard to distinguish from manifestations of the underlying disease. Protein dietary restriction and oral or intravenous metoclopramide (Reglan) may temporarily ameliorate gastrointestinal symptoms. However, if renal failure is not readily reversible, dialysis is needed. Pericardial effusion may present with chest pain, pericardial friction rub, and tamponade, or as an enlarged heart on chest radiograph. Uremic pericarditis is an indication for intensive dialysis with minimum anticoagulation. Cardiac tamponade necessitates an emergent pericardiocentesis. Manifestations of uremic encephalopathy range from somnolence or agitation through stupor, asterixis, behavioral changes, and psychosis to seizures and coma. Emergency dialysis is the only effective treatment. Because the combination of bleeding diathesis and acute stress in ARF predisposes to gastrointestinal bleeding, prophylactic use of H_2 blockers is justified. Interim measures to control uremic bleeding include intravenous administration of deamino-D-arginine vasopressin (DDAVP, 0.3 μg per kg in 50 to 100 mL saline over 15 to 30 minutes), conjugated estrogens (0.6 mg per kg per day for 5 days), or cryoprecipitate (1 to 2 units per kg per day). Uncontrollable bleeding mandates dialysis treatment.

Infection

Infection is a major complication of ARF and a leading cause of death. The high rate of infection (up to 50 to 90%) is attributed to the combination of prolonged hospitalization, the performance of invasive procedures, and the presence of multiple indwelling catheters in an immune-compromised host owing to uremia. Catheters should be frequently changed and removed whenever possible. High level of suspicion, frequent physical evaluation, and frequent culturing of body fluids are critical for the early diagnosis of infection. When infection is suspected, empirical antibiotic treatment should be initiated without delay.

Dialysis

Indications

Indications for renal replacement therapy in ARF are usually divided into two categories: the volume status of the patient or the need for ultrafiltration, and the need for solute clearance. The latter category includes symptomatic uremia and intractable hyperkalemia and acidosis. Considerable clinical judgment is required to assess volume status and the need for solute clearance. The indications for dialysis must be individualized by nephrologic consultation, and important factors such as the etiology of renal failure, rate of deterioration in renal function, and prospect for recovery must be considered.

Dialysis Dose

The appropriate frequency and duration of dialysis treatment are unknown, because the ideal delivered dose of dialysis in ARF has not been determined. Convincing evidence to support the early institution of renal replacement therapy or the benefit of intensive dialysis is still lacking. Currently, intermittent dialysis is usually prescribed to control uremic symptoms and electrolyte disturbances and to maintain predialysis BUN less than 80 to 100 mg per dL.

Dialysis Membrane

One adverse effect of the interaction between blood and dialysis membranes is complement activation. Experimental and clinical evidence suggests that dialysis membrane biocompatibility may have a significant impact on the rate of renal recovery in ARF and, perhaps, also on patient survival.

Modality of Renal Replacement Therapy

Renal replacement therapies include acute intermittent hemodialysis, acute intermittent ultrafiltration, peritoneal dialysis, and various modes of continuous renal replacement therapies (CRRTs): continuous arteriovenous and venovenous hemofiltration (CAVH, CVVH), and continuous arteriovenous and venovenous hemodiafiltration (CAVHD, CVVHD).

Acute intermittent hemodialysis allows the efficient removal of solutes and fluids over a short time. It is performed via a temporary double lumen catheter inserted into a central vein. Frequent occurrence of hemodynamic complications is the major drawback. Furthermore, several studies have supported the view that recurrent hypotension during dialysis may perpetuate renal injury and adversely affect outcome in ARF.

Acute intermittent ultrafiltration is sufficient when only fluid removal is needed. The procedure is similar to that of hemodialysis, except for the lack of dialysate, and it is better tolerated hemodynamically.

Peritoneal dialysis has been generally abandoned as a mode of acute dialysis in many centers, except in children. The efficiency of peritoneal dialysis is too low to provide adequate solute and fluid control in critically ill, hypercatabolic patients; but it has the advantage of being a relatively simple and nonexpensive modality.

In continuous hemofiltration, solutes are removed by convective flow, and appropriate replacement fluid is administered. CAVH and CAVHD involve the cannulation of the femoral artery and a central vein, whereas CVVH and CVVHD require a double lumen intravenous catheter and blood pump. In CAVHD and CVVHD, continuous slow dialysis is added to continuous ultrafiltration. CRRT offers the advantages of slow and controlled ultrafiltration with a more favorable hemodynamic response, and an excellent solute clearance and electrolyte titration. It can be used in unstable, critically ill, pressor-dependent patients and allows the administration of large volumes of nutritional support and blood products as needed. CRRT is a promising new technique with many theoretical benefits, but a favorable impact on outcome of patients with ARF remains to be proven. Major disadvantages include high cost, need for continuous supervision in an intensive care unit, and the need for continuous anticoagulation.

The choice of renal replacement modality should be tailored by the nephrologist for each patient and may depend on facility-specific issues such as nursing resources and technical proficiency.

Experimental Therapies

Studies to evaluate the clinical use of atrial natriuretic factors, growth factors, and antiadhesion therapies are in progress. These promising agents have all been shown to afford some protection in a variety of animal models of ARF. However, benefit in clinical ARF is not proven, and their use has not been approved. The studies completed so far have failed to demonstrate beneficial effects of either anaritide, a synthetic atrial natriuretic factor, or recombinant insulin-like growth factor I in critically ill patients with ATN. Additional work is needed in this potentially important area of investigation.

OUTCOME

Overall outcome in ARF is poor. Despite technical advances in critical care and in renal replacement therapy, the mortality rate in ARF is still 40 to 60%. It is at least partly related to the increased age of patients with ARF and the increasing number and severity of co-morbid conditions. The presence of co-morbid conditions is the major determinant of survival. Mortality rate increases from 7% in prerenal azotemia to more than 90% in critically ill patients with multiorgan failure. Among survivors of ARF, up to 30% require long-term dialysis, and about 45% have normal renal function 5 years later.

CHRONIC RENAL FAILURE

method of
DOUGLAS SHEMIN, M.D.
Brown University Medical School and Rhode Island Hospital
Providence, Rhode Island

and

JOSEPH A. CHAZAN, M.D.
Brown University Medical School and Artificial Kidney Centers of Rhode Island
East Providence, Rhode Island

The availability of dialysis for patients with end-stage renal disease (ESRD) together with its subsequent funding through Medicare since 1973 resulted in more than 250,000 patients being on dialysis in 1997. The annual mortality rate is about 20%, and approximately 5000 transplants are performed per year; therefore, more than 300,000 patients are treated annually. Chronic renal failure (CRF) is more prevalent in older age groups, and with the aging of the population, the number of patients with ESRD can be expected to continue to grow annually.

The average cost per patient per year is approximately $50,000. In the United States, the total expenditure for health care is in the range of $12 billion per year. This substantial expenditure is receiving increasing attention, and attempts to control these costs are being explored. Undoubtedly, resources for management of patients with chronic renal failure will be affected.

DIAGNOSIS OF CHRONIC RENAL FAILURE

Patients with CRF characteristically have a progressive, slow decline in the glomerular filtration rate (GFR) over time. Although the GFR is most accurately diagnosed by measuring inulin clearance or with radionuclide studies, these techniques are unwieldy and expensive and not practical in the clinical setting.

The blood urea nitrogen, which is affected by nonrenal factors such as volume status, protein intake, liver function, and medications, is not a useful guide to GFR. The rate of creatinine clearance does closely approximate the GFR but requires measurement of the serum creatinine and the collection of 24-hour urine volume in measuring urinary creatinine excretion.

The normal creatinine clearance is between 100 and 125 mL per minute (serum creatinine level of 1.0 mg per dL) in adults. Although the serum creatinine level is clearly abnormal when the creatinine clearance falls below 50 mL per minute (serum creatinine level of 2.0 mg per dL), intermediate values may be difficult to interpret. Creatinine clearance is also affected by age and lean muscle mass, and the calculated creatinine clearance (the Cockroft equation),* although not perfect, may be useful in taking these variables into account.

Because symptoms of uremia (Figure 1) do not occur until the GFR falls below 25 mL per minute (approximate serum creatinine level of 3 to 6 mg per dL), and dialytic intervention is not needed until the GFR is less than 10 mL per minute (serum creatinine of 8 to 10 mg per dL), subtle changes in GFR seen with early, mild renal failure are of more prognostic than therapeutic use.

CAUSES OF CHRONIC RENAL FAILURE

Patients with CRF characteristically have a progressive, slow linear decline in GFR and may have some nonspecific signs and symptoms (Table 1).

CRF can occur in systemic diseases affecting the kidneys such as diabetes or systemic lupus erythematosus or may be due to primary renal diseases affecting the glomeruli, the renal vasculature, the renal tubules, or the interstitium, which may either be inherited or acquired. Common causes of CRF leading to ESRD are listed in Table 2.

Many patients with advanced CRF present with small, scarred kidneys. At this point in the clinical course, renal pathologic findings are nonspecific; therefore, a renal biopsy would be of neither diagnostic nor therapeutic value. As a result, these patients do not have biopsies and generally are characterized as having chronic glomerulonephritis, hypertensive nephrosclerosis, or simply small, shrunken kidneys of questionable cause.

Because the symptoms, clinical manifestations, and treatment of CRF seem to be the same regardless of the underlying disease, it is not always critical to identify the underlying cause of the renal disease. However, it is still important in some cases to define the primary renal diagnosis because therapy in a subsequent transplant patient may vary.

For example, patients with focal sclerosis and other primary glomerulonephritides may have recurrences of their disease and respond to immunologic therapy even in an advanced stage of renal failure. Patients with polycystic kidney disease have a high incidence of intracranial aneurysms. Both polycystic kidney disease and hereditary glomerulonephritis are important to consider in the differential diagnosis because they have genetic implications. Patients with focal sclerosis, who have a high incidence of recurrence in renal transplantation, are not always considered optimal transplant candidates, but if the disease recurs in the transplant, plasmapheresis may be of benefit in some cases.

THERAPY: SLOWING THE RATE OF PROGRESSION OF CHRONIC RENAL FAILURE

Once CRF (of whatever cause) develops, it usually progresses to ESRD requiring supportive therapy. The progresssion tends to occur even if the underlying pathophysiologic abnormality is controlled or corrected. It is not certain why this phenomenon occurs,

---

$$\text{*Creatinine clearance (mL/min)} = \frac{(140 - \text{age} \times \text{ideal body weight) (kg)}}{\text{serum creatinine (mg/dL)} \times 72}$$

In women, a factor of 0.85 is included in the numerator to adjust for relatively less lean muscle mass.

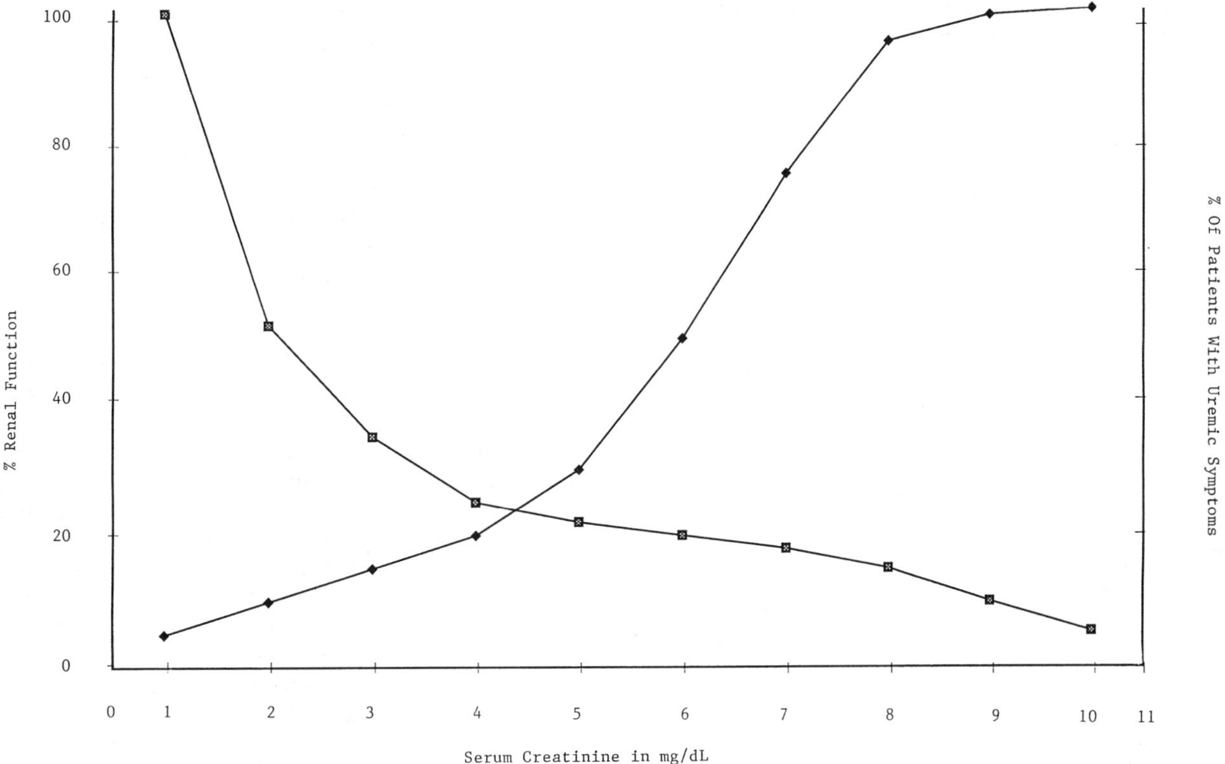

Figure 1. The serum creatinine is geometrically related to creatinine clearance, that is, a doubling of serum creatinine results in a halving of creatinine clearance. Symptoms of uremia rarely occur when creatinine is below 3 to 4 mg/dL and are almost always present when creatinine is above 8 to 10 mg/dL.

but in some cases, it it is thought that once a significant number of glomeruli is irreversibly damaged by a disease process such as diabetes mellitus, vascular disease, or polycystic kidney disease, an adaptive vasodilatation occurs in the remaining functioning glomeruli that is associated with increased hydrostatic pressure and hyperfiltration in the glomerulus. The combination of these factors leads to progressive scarring in the remaining functioning glomeruli with progression of the renal failure. Although progressive ESRD is likely once CRF develops, the rate of progression may be slowed by various therapeutic maneuvers. In addition, patients with CRF may develop acute reversible renal failure at any time. These acute causes should be considered and excluded in each case (Table 3).

TABLE 1. **Features Consistent with Chronic Renal Failure**

Examination	Finding
Physical examination	Pallor
	Short stature (in children)
	Skin excoriations
	Neuropathy
Urinalysis	Broad casts
Laboratory tests	Normocytic normochromic anemia
	High parathyroid hormone level
	History of high levels of serum creatinine and blood urea nitrogen
Renal ultrasound scan	Small kidney size (less than 9 cm in length)
	Increased echogenicity
	Attenuated cortices
Skeletal x-ray films	Subperiosteal bone resorption (especially in distal clavicles and radial margins of phalanges)

Control of Hypertension

Severe hypertension may exacerbate renal failure and, in the case of malignant hypertension, may actually be the cause of the renal failure. The renal failure in severe and malignant hypertension is due to an elevation in the arterial pressure that is transmitted to glomerular capillaries, causing capillary wall damage, inflammation, and scarring, which subsequently results in the decreasing of GFR. Studies show that limiting arterial blood pressure to below 140/90 mm Hg may delay the progression of renal failure caused by a variety of underlying disorders.

As the GFR decreases, hypertension may become more severe, perhaps related to up-regulating the renin-angiotensin axis. Antihypertensive agents of any class can lower the blood pressure in almost all patients with CRF, but angiotensin-converting enzyme (ACE) inhibitors are more effective in delaying the progression of CRF to ESRD. ACE inhibitors are particularly effective in patients with diabetic renal disease or nephrotic-range proteinuria because these agents have a salutary effect on the intraglomerular hydrostatic pressure. All ACE inhibitors probably

TABLE 2. **Causes of Chronic Renal Failure**

Cause	Percent of Cases
Diabetic nephropathy	30–35%
Hypertensive nephrosclerosis	25–30%
Glomerulonephritis Focal segmental glomerulosclerosis Membranous glomerulonephritis Membranoproliferative glomerulonephritis	10–15%
Polycystic kidney disease	5–10%
Interstitial nephritis	1–5%
Obstructive uropathy	1–5%
Collagen-vascular diseases Systemic lupus erythematosus Scleroderma Wegener's granulomatosis Polyarteritis nodosa	1–5%
Malignant diseases Multiple myeloma Renal cell cancer Renal lymphoma	1–5%
Metabolic diseases Amyloidosis Oxalosis Cystinosis Glycogen storage diseases	<1%
Goodpasture's syndrome	<1%
HIV nephropathy	<1%
Other/unclassified causes	5–10%

have equivalent renal-protective effects, but clinical studies have mostly involved enalapril (Vasotec), or captopril (Capoten). Most ACE inhibitors are renally excreted and, with the exception of captopril, have a long enough duration of action in renal failure to be given once daily. It should be cautioned that when CRF is significant, especially when caused by renal vascular stenosis, ACE inhibitors may exacerbate or worsen renal function and may also cause hyperkalemia. Therefore, it is imperative to monitor serum creatinine and potassium levels immediately after the inception of ACE inhibitor therapy.

There is some evidence that a blood pressure of less than 125/75 mm Hg (mean blood pressure of 92 mm Hg) has a greater effect on slowing the rate of progression of CRF than blood pressure of 140/90 mm Hg (mean 107 mm Hg). A lower blood pressure target has special beneficial effects in patients with proteinuria or diabetic nephropathy and in African-American patients. Because ACE inhibitors alone are

TABLE 3. **Reversible Causes of Renal Failure**

Obstruction
Volume depletion
Congestive heart failure
Hypercalcemia
Malignant hypertension

unlikely to achieve this degree of blood pressure control in many patients with renal failure before hyperkalemia supervenes, other agents should be added.

A diuretic is the ideal second-line agent, especially since patients with renal failure are commonly volume-overloaded. In addition, ACE inhibitors and diuretics are synergistic in effecting decrease in blood pressure. The details of diuretic use in renal failure are discussed subsequently. Calcium channel blockers are also effective. Among antihypertensive agents other than ACE inhibitors, diltiazem (Cardizem) has the most consistent effect on decreasing proteinuria and should be added to the regimen of nephrotic patients, especially when this syndrome is caused by diabetes.

Nifedipine (Procardia) has been shown to be preferable to adrenergic antagonists in delaying the progression of nondiabetic renal disease in refractory patients who do not achieve a low target blood pressure goal on an ACE inhibitor, diuretic, and calcium channel blocker. The potent vasodilator minoxidil (Loniten, Rogaine) is effective when started at a dose of 2.5 mg twice daily, which is then titrated upward, although side effects such as congestive heart failure and pericardial infusion may occur and have to be watched for carefully.

Protein Restriction

Before dialysis was uniformly available, dietary protein restriction was used symptomatically for patients with CRF. In the 1940s, the Kempner diet, limited to rice, fruit, and sugar and containing 20 grams of protein per day, was used in patients with malignant hypertension and renal failure with some success. In the late 1960s, and the 1970s, the Giordano-Giovanetti diet, also very low in protein and high in fats and carbohydrates, was used in uremic patients while they awaited dialysis, also with moderate success. Experimental evidence supports the conclusion that a dietary protein intake of less than 0.6 gram per day in rats decreases the rate of progression of renal disease. Clinical studies are less convincing, but it appears that limiting protein intake may delay or alleviate the onset of GI symptoms but may not necessarily prevent progression of renal failure.

To meet caloric requirements and avoid malnutrition, a diet consisting of less than 0.6 gram of protein per kg per day may be inadequate. Patients require careful follow-up to ensure that malnutrition does not occur. In view of the availability of dialysis, the value of protein restriction once symptomatic renal failure occurs is of some question.

In addition to the foregoing measures, specific treatment of the underlying renal disease, which may slow the progression of CRF, is always indicated. For example, in patients with diabetic nephropathy, hyperglycemia should be controlled and ACE inhibitors utilized. In patients with hypertensive nephrosclerosis, an aggressive antihypertensive regimen with a targeted blood pressure well below 140/90 mm Hg should be instituted, and patients with chronic obstructional reflux nephropathy should undergo frequent bladder decompression to limit intravesical pressure.

Correction of Volume Overload

The intravascular volume tends to increase as renal function deteriorates because excretion of sodium and water is retarded. The most common manifestation of volume overload in CRF is hypertension, but other features include weight gain, pulmonary vascular congestion, ascites formation, and peripheral edema. Volume overload should be treated initially with dietary sodium restriction to less than 88 mEq of sodium (2 grams of sodium daily) and diuretic therapy. Unfortunately, most patients do not respond when CRF has progressed. Diuretics include furosemide (Lasix) or other loop diuretics, which are most effective in renal failure.

A reasonable starting dose of furosemide is 80 mg daily; however, patients with advanced renal failure and severe volume overload may require as much as 400 mg per day. Occasionally, the addition of metolazone (Zaroxolyn), a thiazide-like diuretic (in a dose of 5 to 10 mg per day), potentiates the effects of loop diuretics. However, if volume overload becomes symptomatic or life-threatening and is not responsive to salt restriction and diuretics, dialysis should be instituted. Once chronic dialysis begins, volume overload can be managed with ultrafiltration at dialysis, and diuretics should be discontinued.

Hypertension, which is extremely common in CRF, is due to a large extent to volume expansion, secondary to sodium retention, although activation of the renin-angiotensin system and an augmented sympathetic tone also contribute. Since hypertension may contribute to accelerated cardiovascular and cerebrovascular mortality, and control of blood pressure may decrease these complications as well as slow the progression of renal disease, its treatment is imperative. Once dialysis is initiated, ultrafiltration alone may effectively lower the blood pressure, and antihypertensive agents may be decreased quantitatively and qualitatively and can frequently be completely withdrawn.

Correction of Hyperkalemia

Hyperkalemia (serum potassium levels of greater than 5.5 mEq per liter) is common in CRF, especially in patients with decreased urine output, those with renal tubulointerstitial disease, those with diabetic nephropathy (hyporeninemic hypoaldosteronism), and those with severe volume depletion. Hyperkalemia can be exacerbated with the use of ACE inhibitors, which decrease GFR and distal tubular potassium secretion, or of beta blockers, which decrease intracellular potassium uptake, and in metabolic acidosis and hyperglycemia, which shift potassium from intracellular locations.

Treatment of increased potassium should be determined by its influence on the electrocardiogram. In patients without ECG changes, hyperkalemia does not constitute a therapeutic emergency, whereas the need for urgent treatment in those with loss of P waves and widening QRS complexes is quite obvious. Treatment includes insulin and glucose, and sodium bicarbonate in the presence of metabolic acidosis to redistribute potassium from the extracellular space to the intracellular space, or calcium infusion to stabilize the transmembrane effect of potassium in life-threatening emergencies.

To remove potassium from the body, sodium polystyrene sulfonate (Kayexalate), a cation exchange resin in the sodium cycle, can be given by mouth. Sodium polystyrene sulfonate is usually given in 30- to 60-gram doses, which should remove between 30 and 50 mEq of potassium. In extreme cases with life-threatening ECG changes, intravenous calcium may be needed to offset the transmembrane effect of the increased potassium. In the presence of severe anuria, dialysis may be required immediately.

Correction of Metabolic Acidosis

Metabolic acidosis with an elevated anion gap commonly occurs in patients with CRF. The serum bicarbonate concentration is usually only mildly reduced, to 19 to 22 mEq per liter, until renal failure is very advanced, or until other complications such as diarrhea intervene, because of extensive acid buffering by bone. Patients with primary tubulointerstitial disease tend to have lower bicarbonate levels with lesser degrees of renal failure because of the disproportionate impairment of tubular hydrogen ion secretion and bicarbonate generation.

Patients with moderate renal failure and metabolic acidosis should receive treatment with sodium bicarbonate or sodium citrate (in starting dose of 0.5 mEq per kg per day) in an attempt to raise the bicarbonate level to approximately 18 mEq per liter or greater, thereby decreasing bone titration. In children and adolescents, in whom bone disease may be more severe and duration of renal failure more prolonged, the serum bicarbonate level should be raised to approximately 22 mEq per liter.

The use of sodium salts may be associated with edema formation, high blood pressure, and hypervolemia. Once dialysis is begun, alkali can be discontinued, because dialysate contains relatively large amounts of bicarbonate.

Therapy for Anemia and Uremic Bleeding

Anemia in CRF is primarily due to the decreased production of erythropoietin by the kidneys along with some degree of bleeding due to abnormalities in the clotting mechanism induced by renal failure. The availability of human recombinant erythropoietin (Epogen) has dramatically changed the treatment of patients with CRF. Previously, blood transfusions with all their inherent complications were used as temporary mollifiers of the symptoms of uremia. Now, the early use of erythropoietin in patients with modest renal failure can ameliorate virtually all their

TABLE 4. **Immunosuppressive Agents for Renal Transplantation**

Medication	Mechanism of Action	Dose	Side Effects
Prednisone (Deltasone)	Multiple anti-inflammatory effects	10 mg/day	Cataracts, Cushingoid features, glucose intolerance, osteoporosis, psychiatric disorder, proximal myopathy, infection risk
Mycophenolate mofetil (CellCept)	Bone marrow suppressant	1–2 gm/day	Anemia, leukopenia, thrombocytopenia, gastrointestinal complaints
Cyclosporine (Neoral, Sandimmune)	Inhibition of T cell–mediated immune response	3–5 mg/kg/day	Renal insufficiency, hypertension, gingival hypertrophy, hirsutism, hyperuricemia, tremor, drug interactions

symptoms, including fatigue, anorexia, weakness, nausea, and vomiting.

Erythropoietin must be given parenterally. It should be started at 50 to 100 units per kg per week when the hematocrit is below 30%. The reticulocyte count increases within 2 weeks, and the hematocrit rises within 2 to 6 weeks. The dose should be increased at 4- to 6-week intervals until the hematocrit approaches 35%. Virtually the only side effect is hypertension, due to increased peripheral vascular resistance, but this is uncommon and, if it occurs, can usually be managed with an increase in antihypertensive agents. Failure to respond to erythropoietin is either dose-related or due to iron deficiency. The transferrin saturation should be checked prior to initiation of therapy and frequently thereafter. Iron deficiency with a serum ferritin level of less than 100 ng per mL and a transferrin saturation below 20% requires treatment with parenteral iron, because absorption of oral iron is rarely adequate.

Some patients with CRF exhibit a bleeding tendency. The mechanism is primarily decreased platelet adherence to endothelial cells. The platelet count, prothrombin, and partial thromboplastin times are normal, but the bleeding time is prolonged. Patients typically demonstrate easy bruisability and ecchymosis. When epistaxis and gastrointestinal (GI) bleeding occur, anemia can be acutely and significantly exacerbated. In patients who are actively bleeding, the use of cryoprecipitate containing von Willebrand multimers improves the bleeding time, but there is an increased risk of transmitting viruses. Intravenous desmopressin acetate (1-deamino-8-D-arginine-vasopressin [DDAVP])* in a dose of 0.3 μg per kg transiently improves the bleeding time. Estrogens,* given either orally (PO) at a dose of 50 mg daily for 10 days or intravenously (IV) at a dose of 0.6 mg per kg per day for 5 days, are effective in normalizing the bleeding time; the mechanism is unknown, however.

Management of Hyperphosphatemia, Hypocalcemia, and Renal Osteodystrophy

Hyperphosphatemia (a serum phosphorus level of greater than 5 mg per dL) occurs when GFR falls below 25 mL per minute. Both hyperphosphatemia and progressive renal scarring decrease renal hydroxylation of 1,25-dihydroxycholecalciferol, the active form of vitamin D, which enhances GI absorption of calcium. These factors lead to a fall in serum calcium level. The fall in serum calcium stimulates parathyroid hormone release, which increases bone osteoclastic activity.

In its most severe form, hyperparathyroidism can cause bone erosion, cystic bone lesions, and bone marrow fibrosis. Other forms of renal osteodystrophy include osteomalacia, due to decreased vitamin D absorption, and adynamic bone disease, which historically was associated with excessive aluminum ingestion but is now observed even in the absence of aluminum exposure or deposition.

Patients with hyperphosphatemia should initially be treated with phosphate binders, preferably calcium carbonate. Aluminum-containing agents should not be given owing to risks of aluminum absorption because it has been shown that elevated aluminum blood levels are associated with increased mortality. The starting dose of calcium carbonate is one 500-mg tablet with each meal; alternatively, 667 mg of calcium acetate can be given. The dose is titrated upward as needed.

When the phosphorus level is controlled, calcitriol or hydroxylated vitamin D, should be given at a dose of 0.25 to 0.5 μg daily. It increases calcium absorption from the gut, inhibits PTH release, and may stimulate bone growth. Calcitriol can cause hypercalcemia and hyperphosphatemia; therefore, blood calcium and phosphate levels need to be checked frequently, and the dose adjusted accordingly.

Therapy for Other Uremic Symptoms

GI side effects including anorexia, nausea, and vomiting are common and may be treated with antiemetics and a low-protein diet. In some cases, treatment of concomitant anemia results in relief of the GI symptoms. If symptoms become severe or are poorly tolerated, dialysis should be initiated.

Pruritus, localized or diffuse, occurs frequently. Its presumed causes include intradermal deposition of uremic solutes, calcium phosphate crystals, secondary precipitation, and secondary hyperparathyroidism. In all patients, calcium and phosphorus levels should be normalized by the use of phosphorus binders with or without calcitriol.

Antihistamines and analgesics may provide short-term relief, but skin lubrication with emollients may be most effective. A variety of neuromuscular symp-

*Not FDA approved for this indication.

toms including muscle cramps, neuromuscular irritability, involuntary myoclonic jerks, or restless legs may occur in patients with advanced CRF, and dialysis is usually indicated.

Pericarditis may occur with or without pericardial effusion in advanced CRF and may necessitate aggressive supportive treatment with dialysis.

Dialysis and Renal Transplantation

A full discussion of dialysis and renal transplantation is beyond the scope of this article; however, it is noted here that chronic dialysis has been extraordinarily successful in sustaining meaningful quality of life in thousands of patients over the past 25 to 30 years. Neither chronic hemodialysis nor peritoneal dialysis is without difficulties—primarily, access-related problems and a restricted schedule in patients on hemodialysis, and peritonitis and daily commitment to therapy in patients on peritoneal dialysis. Each mode of dialysis provides advantages and disadvantages that need to be discussed on an individual basis, with the patient's preference being the major determining factor of the modality instituted.

Renal transplantation is the treatment of choice for ESRD in all patients without serious medical conditions that preclude the risk of surgery and the use of immunosuppresion. Living related transplants have the best results, with graft survivals of greater than 90% at 1 year and patient survival rate of virtually 100%. However, cadaveric and/or living unrelated transplants have excellent but somewhat less successful results (Table 4).

MALIGNANT TUMORS OF THE UROGENITAL TRACT

method of
JUDD W. MOUL, M.D., and
RAYMOND A. COSTABILE, M.D.
Walter Reed Army Medical Center
Washington, D.C.
Uniformed Services University of the Health Sciences
Bethesda, Maryland

and

JAMES BRANTLEY THRASHER, M.D.
Madigan Army Medical Center
Tacoma, Washington
Uniformed Services University of the Health Sciences
Bethesda, Maryland

KIDNEY TUMORS

Renal Cell Carcinoma

Renal cell carcinoma (RCC) is the third most common genitourinary malignancy, with 27,000 cases diagnosed per year. RCC occurs most often in the fifth and sixth decades of life but can be found in all age groups. There is a strong genetic component to renal cell carcinoma. Gene deletions leading to a loss of tumor suppressor genes have been localized at several positions on the short arm of chromosome 3 and on chromosome 17. Von Hippel–Lindau disease is a disorder with autosomal dominant inheritance associated with a high incidence of RCC. Gene deletions associated with von Hippel–Lindau disease have been identified at several positions on chromosome 3. RCC is also associated with long-term dialysis, autosomal dominant polycystic disease, and tuberous sclerosis.

The opinions and assertions contained herein are the private views of the authors and are not to be construed as reflecting the views of the U.S. Army or the Department of Defense.

Presentation and Diagnosis

With the increased utilization of abdominal computed tomography (CT), ultrasonography (US), and magnetic resonance imaging (MRI), most renal masses (60%) are incidentally discovered. The most common presenting symptom of RCC is hematuria. The triad of flank pain, mass, and hematuria is exceedingly rare. Over 30% of patients with RCC have metastatic disease at the time of diagnosis associated with systemic symptoms. RCCs produce a variety of hormonally active compounds that can cause a paraneoplastic syndrome comprising erythrocytosis, hypertension, hypercalcemia, pyrexia, and anemia. Diagnostic evaluation should include a complete blood count (CBC), determination of serum calcium and alkaline phosphatase, liver function tests, abdominal CT, and chest radiography. A bone scan is indicated for patients with bone pain and/or elevated alkaline phosphatase. MRI or arteriography is useful to define the extent of tumor thrombus in the renal vein, vena cava, or right atrium. Tumor-node-metastasis (TNM) staging for renal cell adenocarcinoma is shown in Table 1.

Management

Localized Disease. The treatment for RCC is surgical excision, as these tumors respond poorly to ex-

TABLE 1. **American Joint Committee on Cancer Staging of Renal Cell Carcinoma**

T1	Confined to renal capsule, <2.5 cm in diameter
T2	Confined to renal capsule, >2.5 cm in diameter
T3	Extends into veins or outside kidney but not beyond Gerota's fascia
T3a	Tumor in perinephric fat or adrenal gland but confined by Gerota's fascia
T3b	Tumor in renal vein or vena cava below the diaphragm
T3c	Tumor extends into supradiaphragmatic vena cava
T4	Tumor extends beyond Gerota's fascia
N0	No regional node metastasis
N1	Single node, 2 cm or less in diameter
N2	Single node, 2–5 cm in diameter
N3	Single or multiple nodes, >5 cm in diameter
M0	No distant metastasis
M1	Distant metastasis

Modified from Seigne JD, Grossman HB: Malignant tumors of the urogenital tract. *In* Rakel RE: Conn's Current Therapy 1997. Philadelphia, WB Saunders Co, 1997, p 714.

ternal beam irradiation or conventional chemotherapy. Surgical excision is indicated for localized tumors, including lesions with tumor thrombus in the renal vein, vena cava, or right atrium. For patients with distant metastases or extensive adenopathy, surgical excision confers no improvement in survival. Surgery in patients with metastatic disease is indicated only for palliation of pain, bleeding, or significant paraneoplastic symptoms. An extensive lymphadenectomy is not indicated for patients with RCC. Partial nephrectomy is indicated for patients with bilateral tumors, renal insufficiency, or tumor in a solitary kidney. The disease-free survival rate in patients undergoing partial nephrectomy equals that with radical nephrectomy (80% at 5 years). Patients with a solitary metastasis to lung or soft tissue may also benefit from complete surgical excision, with a disease-free survival rate of 70% at 5 years.

Prognostic factors for patients with RCC include tumor stage, Furman nuclear grade, and presence or absence of vascular invasion. Most RCCs are of proximal tubule origin. Tumors of collecting duct or medullary origin have a poorer prognosis than classic adenocarcinoma. Sarcomas and sarcomatoid tumors of the kidney account for less than 5% of renal carcinomas.

Metastatic Disease. Median survival in patients with metastatic disease is 6 months. Unfortunately, RCC responds poorly to conventional chemotherapy. Vinblastine (Velban) is the most effective chemotherapeutic agent, with combined response rates of 10 to 15%. Radiation therapy can be useful to relieve pain due to metastases. Therapeutic embolization of the renal artery or a branch of the renal artery can help control bleeding or paraneoplastic syndrome.

The most effective therapy for metastatic RCC is biologic immune response modifiers. High-dose continuous-infusion therapy with interleukin-2 (IL-2) is the only immunotherapy for RCC approved by the Food and Drug Administration (FDA). Unfortunately, high-dose IL-2 therapy is extremely toxic, with significant cardiopulmonary and neurologic side effects. Combined partial and complete response rates are between 15 and 25%. Additional protocols using low or intermediate doses of subcutaneous IL-2 demonstrate similar response rates, with a significant improvement in toxicity. Interferon (IFN-α and IFN-β) has also demonstrated some efficacy in the treatment of metastatic RCC, as has combination therapy with IL-2 and 5-fluorouracil. Immunotherapy utilizing lymphokine-activated killer cells (LAK) or tumor-infiltrating lymphocytes (TIL) combined with IL-2 has been variably successful.

Renal Oncocytoma

Renal oncocytoma accounts for 5 to 7% of all solid renal masses. These tumors have a typical gross and histologic appearance and usually behave in a benign fashion. Grossly, the tumors are well encapsulated and tan in color and classically have a central scar. Histologically, they consist of large cells with intensely eosinophilic granular cytoplasm. Although a central scar on a CT scan and a spoke-wheel pattern on an arteriogram have been associated with oncocytoma, preoperative differentiation between these tumors based on imaging studies is extremely difficult. Oncocytomas may invade local structures, despite their benign origin. Partial nephrectomy is usually curative for small lesions.

Angiomyolipoma

Angiomyolipomas account for less than 5% of solid renal lesions. Angiomyolipomas are hamartomas consisting of smooth muscle, blood vessels, and mature adipose tissue. Angiomyolipomas occur in 40 to 80% of patients with tuberous sclerosis. In most cases these tumors arise spontaneously, without associated genetic disorders. There is an 8:1 female to male ratio, and presentation is usually in the fifth through seventh decades of life. Patients may present with flank pain or hematuria. Between 10 and 25% of patients present with acute retroperitoneal hemorrhage and shock. Abdominal CT scanning is usually diagnostic. Angiomyolipomas are solid tumors that contain areas of fat with a density of between 10 and −80 Hounsfield units. Lesions that are smaller than 4 cm in diameter are unlikely to bleed and can be monitored with annual renal ultrasonograms. Lesions greater than 4 cm in size in women of childbearing age are at increased risk for hemorrhage and should be managed by partial nephrectomy. Acute hemorrhage can be controlled with selective angioinfarction.

Wilms' Tumor

Wilms' tumor is the most common renal malignancy of childhood but can occur rarely in adults. Most Wilms' tumors occur in children under the age of 5 years. Wilms' tumor may occur spontaneously or in association with aniridia, hemihypertrophy (Beckwith-Wiedemann syndrome), or genitourinary or chromosomal abnormalities. Gene deletions on the short arm of chromosome 11 associated with the lack of tumor suppressor are found in patients with Wilms' tumor.

Presentation and Diagnosis

A palpable abdominal mass is the most common presenting sign of Wilms' tumor, with few systemic complaints. Hematuria occurs in 25% of affected children. Diagnostic evaluation should include abdominal US or CT, chest radiography, and CBC. Prognostic factors associated with Wilms' tumor include histologic findings, tumor anaplasia, tumor stage, and age at presentation. Anaplastic tumors occur in less than 10% of patients with Wilms' tumor and are associated with an extremely poor prognosis.

Management

Treatment of Wilms' tumor involves a multimodality approach, as shown in Table 2. The 2-year disease-free survival rate for patients with stage I or

TABLE 2. **Staging and Management of Wilms' Tumor (National Wilms' Tumor Study IV)**

Stage	Description	Treatment
I	Tumor confined to kidney and completely resected; focal hyperplasia and anaplasia	Surgical excision and chemotherapy (18 weeks): actinomycin D, vincristine
II	Tumor extension beyond the kidney but tumor completely resected; focal hyperplasia and anaplasia	
II–IV	Diffuse anaplasia	Chemotherapy as for stage I + doxorubicin, cyclophosphamide, and etoposide (24 weeks) + radiation therapy
III	Residual nonhematogenous tumor confined to the abdomen (nodes, peritoneal implants), focal hyperplasia and anaplasia	Chemotherapy as for stage I + doxorubicin (24 weeks) and radiation therapy, 1080 cGY
IV	Hematogenous metastatic disease	Chemotherapy* and surgical excision
V	Bilateral Wilms' tumor at diagnosis	Chemotherapy* and surgical excision

*Doxorubicin, vincristine, dactinomycin, cyclophosphamide.

Modified from Seigne JD, Grossman HB: Malignant tumors of the urogenital tract. *In* Rakel RE: Conn's Current Therapy 1997. Philadelphia, WB Saunders Co, 1997, p 715.

II Wilms' tumor is 90%. The disease-free survival rate for patients with favorable histology and stage I disease is 78%. The National Wilms' Tumor Study (NWTS) IV is presently evaluating a reduction in adjuvant therapy to limit the side effects of multimodality therapy. Bilateral Wilms' tumor is treated initially by chemotherapy to initiate tumor shrinkage. Partial or radical nephrectomy is performed to remove residual tumor after maximum benefits have been obtained with chemotherapy. Survival of patients with bilateral disease and favorable histology is excellent.

ADRENAL TUMORS

Adrenocortical Carcinoma

Adrenal cancers are rare tumors that occur with an incidence of 1 per 1.7 million population. Most adrenocortical carcinomas produce biologically active adrenal hormones that result in a variety of disorders, including hypertension, Cushing's syndrome, virilization, feminization, and hyperaldosteronism. Adrenocortical carcinoma has a slight female preponderance and occurs in all age groups, with a higher incidence after the age of 40 years. With the increased use of abdominal US, CT, and MRI, most adrenal masses are discovered incidentally. Adrenocortical carcinomas tend to be larger than adenomas. Adrenal masses greater than 8 cm in diameter are highly likely to represent carcinoma.

Endocrine evaluation of a patient with an adrenal mass should include determination of serum and urine cortisol, androgens, estrogens, catecholamines (epinephrine and norepinephrine), vanillylmandelic acid (VMA), and metanephrins. Radiologic imaging should include CT or MRI. Metaiodobenzylguanidine (MIBG [iobenguane sulfate I 123]) nuclear scintigraphy is indicated for metastatic or extra-adrenal pheochromocytoma. MRI or venacavography may also be useful to evaluate potential tumor thrombus in the vena cava. Metastatic evaluation should include chest radiography, liver function tests, and determination of serum alkaline phosphatase.

Management

The primary therapy for adrenocortical tumors is surgical resection. Unfortunately, 70% of patients with adrenocortical carcinomas present with metastatic disease that is surgically unresectable. With the increasing use of abdominal imaging, earlier diagnosis may decrease the incidence of metastatic disease. Metastatic disease responds poorly to conventional chemotherapy, but treatment with mitotane (Lysodren) can control paraneoplastic symptoms associated with adrenal hormone production. Radiation therapy is indicated for management of painful or symptomatic metastatic lesions.

Pheochromocytoma and Neuroblastoma

Pheochromocytomas are rare tumors of paraganglionic chromaffin cells. Over 90% of pheochromocytomas are benign. Malignant pheochromocytomas are typically discovered after distant metastases or invasion of adjacent structures has occurred. Treatment of solitary pheochromocytoma is surgical excision. Catecholamines produced by these tumors cause hypertension, which can be sustained or paroxysmal. Additional symptoms of flushing, headaches, sweating, and palpitations are also common. Diagnosis is confirmed by abdominal CT or T2-weighted MRI and measurement of serum and urine catecholamines. Ten percent of pheochromocytomas are extra-adrenal. Extra-adrenal pheochromocytomas occur more often in children and can occur along the sympathetic chain, urinary bladder, or organ of Zuckerkandl.

Neuroblastomas are the most common solid tumors of children and occur principally in the adrenal gland. Neuroblastomas can arise anywhere along the sympathetic chain. Most children present with symptoms of metastatic disease and a large palpable abdominal mass that spans the midline. More than 70% of patients present with metastatic disease. Diagnostic evaluation should include determination of serum and urine catecholamines, chest radiography, bone scan, and bone marrow aspiration. Treatment of stage I or II disease is surgical excision, with adju-

TABLE 3. **Staging of Neuroblastoma and Related Treatment Regimens**

Stage	Description	Treatment
I	Confined to organ of origin	Surgical excision
II	Extends beyond organ of origin but not across the midline	Surgical excision and chemotherapy
III	Extends across the midline	Radiation therapy and chemotherapy
IV	Metastatic disease	Radiation therapy and chemotherapy
V-S	Local stage I or II with metastases confined to the bone marrow, skin, and liver	Symptomatic treatment Spontaneous regression

S = "special"—for confined metastases.
Modified from Seigne JD, Grossman HB: Malignant tumors of the urogenital tract. *In* Rakel RE: Conn's Current Therapy 1997. Philadelphia, WB Saunders Co, 1997, p 713.

vant chemotherapy for stage II disease. Advanced disease is treated with combination therapy (external beam irradiation and chemotherapy). Staging of neuroblastoma and related treatment regimens are outlined in Table 3.

UROTHELIAL TUMORS

Bladder Cancer

The bladder is the most common site of cancer in the urinary tract. Approximately 54,500 new cases of the disease were diagnosed in 1997, with 11,700 mortalities. The male-to-female ratio of bladder cancer is 2.5 to 3.0:1. It is the fourth most common cause of cancer in men (5%) and occurs twice as frequently in white men as in black men. Bladder cancer is uncommon in Asians, Hispanics, and American Indians. Transitional cell carcinoma is the most common histologic type in the United States (75 to 90%), followed by squamous cell carcinoma (2 to 15%) and adenocarcinoma (0.5 to 2%). A multitude of carcinogens have been implicated in the etiology of bladder cancer. Cigarette smoking has been the most commonly associated risk factor, causing 25 to 60% of bladder cancer in industrialized countries. Occupational exposure to certain chemical carcinogens has been documented to produce an increased incidence of bladder cancer. Workers in the aromatic amine, rubber, paint, aluminum, textile, and printing industries are at increased risk. Additionally, drugs such as phenacetin and cyclophosphamide as well as chronic urothelial irritants have been shown to increase the risk for bladder cancer.

Presentation and Diagnosis

Patients with bladder carcinoma usually present with gross or microscopic hematuria and/or irritative voiding symptoms (e.g., frequency and dysuria). After urinary infection has been ruled out, voided urine is obtained for cytologic studies, and intravenous urography (IVU) is performed to exclude upper tract (kidney and ureter) lesions. Renal US is an alternative that is more sensitive than IVU in detecting parenchymal tumors but less sensitive in detecting transitional cell carcinomas. The IVU is followed by cystoscopy to evaluate the lower urinary tract. The advantage of performing the IVU prior to cystoscopy is that if the upper urinary tracts are not visualized adequately during IVU, retrograde ureteropyelograms can be performed at cystoscopy. Exfoliative cytology is an important adjunct, especially in patients with irritative symptoms, since such symptoms may be the only presenting manifestation of carcinoma in situ. Additionally, no cystoscopic evidence of a lesion in conjunction with a positive cytologic result would lead the clinician to search for either carcinoma in situ or an unidentified lesion elsewhere in the urinary tract.

The cystoscopic demonstration of bladder cancer or cytologic abnormalities with normal findings on IVU lead to transurethral resection of the bladder tumor and/or multiple biopsies with the patient under anesthesia. Bimanual examination while the patient is under anesthesia will aid in staging muscle-invasive tumors. Additional preoperative studies should include electrocardiography, chest radiography, serum creatinine determination, liver function tests, and, if the tumor is large or appears muscle-invasive, abdominopelvic CT scanning. Patients with an elevated serum alkaline phosphatase level should undergo a technetium 99m bone scan to complete staging. Bladder tumors are staged using the American Joint Committee on Cancer (AJCC) system (Table 4).

Management

Bladder cancers can be divided into two groups with regard to treatment: (1) superficial disease (Ta, T1, Tis), accounting for 75 to 85% of bladder tumors, which usually requires local therapy and has a good prognosis; and (2) invasive disease (T2 through T4), accounting for 15 to 25% of bladder tumors, which usually requires aggressive surgical treatment and

TABLE 4. **American Joint Committee on Cancer Staging of Bladder Cancer**

T0	No evidence of primary tumor
Ta	Noninvasive papillary tumor
Tis	Carcinoma in situ; "flat tumor"
T1	Tumor invades subepithelial connective tissue
T2	Tumor invades superficial muscle (inner half)
T3	Tumor invades deep muscle or perivesical fat
T3a	Tumor invades deep muscle (outer half)
T3b	Tumor invades perivesical fat
T4	Tumor invades prostate, uterus, vagina, pelvic wall, or abdominal wall
T4a	Tumor invades prostate, uterus, vagina
T4b	Tumor invades pelvic wall or abdominal wall
N0	No regional node metastasis
N1–3	Regional node metastasis
M0	No distant metastasis
M1	Distant metastasis

Modified from Seigne JD, Grossman HB: Malignant tumors of the urogenital tract. *In* Rakel RE: Conn's Current Therapy 1997. Philadelphia, WB Saunders Co, 1997, p 716.

has a poorer prognosis. Many urologists now consider stage T1 disease as minimally invasive and treat these cancers (representing 30% of the cases of superficial disease) more aggressively than the usual superficial disease.

Superficial Disease. The treatment for superficial bladder cancer is transurethral resection. Although the risk of recurrence is 70 to 75%, only 10 to 15% of cases will progress to muscle-invasive disease. However, regular follow-up with cystoscopy and cytology every 3 months for 2 years, every 6 months for 2 years, and annually thereafter is necessary. Patients with high-grade disease, associated carcinoma in situ, multiple tumors at presentation, or frequent recurrences are candidates for intravesical chemotherapy. Chemotherapy agents such as thiotepa, mitomycin C, and doxorubicin have all been used effectively at a concentration of 1 mg of agent per 1 mL of normal saline, with a total volume of 50 to 60 mL. The instillations are begun 1 or 2 weeks after transurethral resection, with 6 weekly instillations given for 2 hours. However, bacille Calmette-Guérin (BCG), a live attenuated tuberculosis bacterium, has proved to be the most effective intravesical agent tested to date for treatment of carcinoma in situ and the superficial tumor with a high risk for muscle invasion. We use weekly doses for 6 weeks, commencing 1 or 2 weeks after transurethral resection (depending on when the urine clears), of lyophilized BCG solubilized in 50 mL of saline retained intravesically for 120 minutes. Intravesical BCG can reduce recurrence rates and progression to muscle invasion, with a second course of BCG noted to be effective in 35 to 75% of patients in whom disease recurs after an initial 6-week protocol. Additional maintenance therapy with doses once a week for 3 additional weeks may decrease recurrence rates if given every 3 months for 3 years. BCG, however, can cause significant side effects. Irritative voiding symptoms can occur in 90% of patients receiving BCG, although they are usually self-limited. For systemic symptoms, such as fever with temperatures higher than 38.5°C that do not respond to antipyretics or that last longer than 24 hours, a 3-month course of isoniazid (300 mg daily) is indicated. Patients who are critically ill should also receive rifampin*, 600 mg; ethambutol,* 1200 mg; cycloserine,* 500 mg bid; and, initially, prednisolone, 40 mg IV. BCG should *never* be administered if there is difficulty with catheterization or a traumatic catheterization; deaths have been documented in such instances.

Minimally Invasive Disease. Bladder cancer invading the lamina propria can be cured with transurethral resection alone, but progression rates average 29% overall and 40% in patients with high-grade disease. BCG therapy after transurethral resection has been shown to decrease progression rates by more than 10%, but patients with lesions that are recalcitrant to 1 or 2 cycles of BCG therapy should undergo cystectomy.

Invasive Disease. Radical cystectomy consisting of removal of the pelvic lymph nodes, bladder, and prostate in men and the uterus, urethra, and anterior vaginal wall in women with urinary diversion remains the treatment of choice for patients with clinically localized disease (T2, T3, and T4a). Contemporary series report 5-year survival rates of 80%, 70%, 30%, and 5% for pathologic (p) stage T2, T3a, T3b, and node-positive tumors, respectively. The operative mortality rate is less than 5%, and the risk of pelvic recurrence is 5 to 10%. The use of transurethral resection alone, laser therapy alone, or radiation therapy alone is associated with high recurrence rates and poor survival and is usually considered in patients whose medical condition precludes surgery. A bladder-sparing approach using transurethral resection, chemotherapy, and radiation therapy has been investigated in patients with T2 disease but remains investigational owing to the lifelong risk of recurrence when the bladder is left in place.

Following cystectomy, the urinary tract can be reconstructed either by creating a urinary conduit into an external collection device or by constructing a reservoir using a large piece of bowel. Traditionally, the conduit is created by anastomosing the ureters to the isolated segment of ileum brought to the abdominal wall as a stroma that drains into an external collection device. There is a growing experience with the use of reconstructive techniques that reconfigure a segment of isolated large or small bowel into a pouch. The pouch can be attached to the urethral stump to create a neobladder (allowing voiding per urethra) or brought to the abdominal wall as a continent, catheterizable stoma. Nocturnal incontinence is a problem in 20 to 30% of patients with neobladders. Continent diversions are associated with complication rates as high as 25% and a reoperation rate of approximately 15%.

Follow-up after cystectomy should consist of chest radiography, liver function tests, and serum chemistries including blood urea nitrogen (BUN) and creatinine performed every 6 months for 2 years and annually thereafter. In patients whose urethra was left in place, cytologic examination of urethral washings should also be performed. Patients with continent diversions should have vitamin B_{12} levels monitored as well. We perform an upper tract imaging study (IVU or "loopogram" in patients with ileal conduits) within the first 2 to 3 months and then annually for 5 years and every 2 years thereafter.

Metastatic Disease. Currently, the most effective chemotherapeutic regimen is methotrexate, vinblastine, doxorubicin, and cisplatin (MVAC). Overall response rates range from 40 to 70%, with complete response rates of 15 to 30%. Most responses are short-lived, with a median survival of approximately 13 months. New agents being investigated are gallium nitrate,* ifosfamide,* and paclitaxel.* MVAC and other combination regimens for metastatic bladder cancer have significant toxicities.

*Not FDA approved for this indication.

*Not FDA approved for this indication.

Carcinoma of the Ureter and Renal Pelvis

Renal pelvic tumors account for 5% and ureteral tumors for approximately 1% of all urothelial cancers. Most ureteral tumors occur in the distal ureter (73% of cases); the proximal ureter is least commonly affected (3% of cases). Bilateral involvement (synchronous or metachronous) occurs in 2 to 5% of upper tract tumors. Synchronous or metachronous bladder tumors occur in 30 to 75% of patients with upper tract cancers. The most common presentation of upper tract tumors is gross hematuria (75%), often with the passage of vermiform clots in the urine. Other signs and symptoms include flank pain, an incidental filling defect on IVU, and, rarely, a palpable mass or systemic symptoms of advanced disease. Initial evaluation should include IVU, retrograde pyelography, and cytologic examination of ureteral washings. Flexible or rigid ureteroscopy, abdominal and pelvic CT scanning, and brush biopsies of suspicious lesions are often necessary. Tumors are staged by the AJCC system (Table 5).

The multifocal nature of these tumors, the high rate of ipsilateral recurrence in any ureter left in place, and the low incidence of contralateral upper tract involvement are reasons why nephroureterectomy (including a 2-cm cuff of bladder) is the preferred treatment for most upper tract urothelial cancers. Low-grade and low-stage distal ureteral tumors can be treated by segmental resection and reimplantation of the ureter. When upper tract tumors occur in a solitary kidney or in association with a compromised contralateral kidney, endoscopic resection and laser tumor ablation are treatment options. Adjuvant therapy with the instillation of mitomycin C, BCG, or thiotepa to prevent recurrences has been used in a fashion similar to intravesical therapy, and when it is performed following strict protocol, complications remain low. The stage-specific 5-year survival rates are 100% for pTa, 96% for pT1, and 33% for pT2 or pT3 cancers. Patients with nodal or metastatic disease are treated with MVAC chemotherapy and rarely survive 5 years.

TABLE 5. **American Joint Committee on Cancer Staging of Renal Pelvis and Ureteral Cancers**

T0	No evidence of primary tumor
Ta	Papillary noninvasive carcinoma
Tis	Carcinoma in situ
T1	Tumor invades subepithelial connective tissue
T2	Tumor invades muscularis (ureter only)
T3	Tumor invades beyond muscularis into peripelvic fat or renal parenchyma (ureter only)
T4	Tumor invades adjacent organs or through the kidney into paranephric fat
N0	No regional node metastasis
N1–3	Regional node metastasis
M0	No distant metastasis
M1	Distant metastasis

Modified from Seigne JD, Grossman HB: Malignant tumors of the urogenital tract. *In* Rakel RE: Conn's Current Therapy 1997. Philadelphia, WB Saunders Co, 1997, p 717.

TABLE 6. **American Joint Committee on Cancer Staging of Urethral Cancer (Male and Female)**

T0	No evidence of primary tumor
Ta	Noninvasive papillary, polypoid, or verrucous carcinoma
Tis	Carcinoma in situ
T1	Tumor invades subepithelial connective tissue
T2	Tumor invades corpus spongiosum or prostate or periurethral muscle
T3	Tumor invades corpus cavernosum or beyond prostatic capsule or the anterior vagina or bladder neck
T4	Tumor invades other adjacent organs
N0	No regional node metastasis
N1–3	Regional node metastasis
M0	No distant metastasis
M1	Distant metastasis

Modified from Seigne JD, Grossman HB: Malignant tumors of the urogenital tract. *In* Rakel RE: Conn's Current Therapy 1997. Philadelphia, WB Saunders Co, 1997, p 718.

FEMALE URETHRAL CANCER

Urethral carcinoma is the only shared genitourinary malignancy more common in women than in men. The female urethra averages 4 cm in length. The lymphatic drainage of the distal third is to the inguinal lymph nodes, while the proximal two thirds drain into the deep pelvic nodes. The most common histologic types are squamous cell carcinoma (55%), transitional cell carcinoma (17%), and adenocarcinoma (16%). The most common presenting signs and symptoms are urethral bleeding or spotting, irritative or obstructive voiding symptoms, pain, and a palpable mass. Diagnosis requires cystoscopy and biopsy. Staging requires a careful bimanual examination and assessment of inguinal lymph nodes, abdominopelvic CT scan, chest film, liver function tests, and bone scans as indicated. Tumors are staged by the AJCC system (Table 6). Treatment depends on the location, stage, and grade of the tumor. Tumors of the distal urethra are usually superficial and can be managed by local excision with transurethral resection, laser therapy, or radiation therapy. Prognosis is excellent. Tumors of the proximal two thirds of the urethra are usually of higher stage and grade and frequently necessitate cystourethrectomy. Inguinal lymphadenectomy should be performed only in patients with palpably enlarged lymph nodes. The prognosis for women with proximal urethral tumors is poor (with a 13% 5-year survival rate), because most patients present with advanced disease.

MALE URETHRAL CANCER

The male urethra averages 21 cm in length. It is divided into the prostatic, membranous, bulbar, and pendulous (penile) portions. The lymphatic drainage of the penile skin is to the superficial inguinal nodes. The lymphatic drainage of the pendulous urethra, glans, and corpus spongiosum is to the deep inguinal nodes. The route for drainage of the bulbous, membranous, and prostatic (posterior) urethra is as follows: (1) the external iliac nodes, (2) the obturator and internal iliac nodes, and (3) the presacral nodes.

The bulbomembranous urethra is the most frequent location for tumors; most are squamous cell carcinoma (80% of cases), followed by transitional cell carcinoma (15%) and adenocarcinoma (5%). Approximately 50% of anterior urethral carcinomas are locally advanced at presentation, and almost 90% of posterior carcinomas present in advanced stages. Therefore, presentation is usually because of obstruction, a palpable mass, or periurethral abscess. Diagnosis requires cystoscopy and biopsy. Staging requires a careful bimanual examination and assessment of inguinal lymph nodes, abdominopelvic CT scan, chest film, liver function tests, and bone scans as indicated. Tumors are staged by the AJCC system (see Table 6). Treatment depends on the location, stage, and grade of the tumor. Most anterior urethral tumors can be managed by partial penectomy as long as a 2-cm tumor-free margin can be obtained. The expected 5-year survival rate for patients with anterior urethral tumors is 50%. Proximal urethral cancers frequently require total penectomy and radical cystoprostatectomy. Inguinal lymphadenectomy should be performed only in patients with palpably enlarged nodes. Prognosis is poor despite aggressive therapy. Transitional cell carcinoma of the prostatic urethra is usually associated with concurrent transitional cell carcinoma of the bladder. Treatment usually consists of radical cystoprostatectomy with total urethrectomy. Patients who have stromal involvement of the prostate by transitional cell carcinoma have a poor prognosis.

PROSTATE CANCER

Prostate cancer is the most common tumor and second most common cause of cancer deaths in men in the United States, with approximately 184,000 new cases diagnosed in 1998. Because of the impact of public awareness and screening with the prostate-specific antigen (PSA) blood test, the incidence peaked at 317,000 cases in 1996 and then declined to more steady-state levels. Prostatic tumors spread to the regional pelvic lymph nodes and via the bloodstream to the bones, where they classically cause osteoblastic metastases in the axillary skeleton; however, with the advent of screening, fewer cases of metastatic disease have been identified in the late 1990s. Thirty percent of men older than the age of 50 years have histologic evidence of prostate cancer. However, only one-fourth of these cancers are estimated to be clinically significant. The average age of patients diagnosed with clinical prostate cancer is approximately 66 years. The high incidence of incidental tumors combined with the older age at presentation of men with prostate cancer dictates a selective approach to treatment. Determining which cancers require treatment depends on the patient's physiologic age and the grade and stage of the tumor.

Prostate-Specific Antigen

The diagnosis and treatment of prostate cancer have been revolutionized by the discovery of PSA. PSA is a serine protease that is produced by prostatic epithelial cells, the function of which is to liquefy semen. The serum PSA level represents not only PSA produced by the normal prostate but also PSA produced in conditions such as benign prostatic hyperplasia, prostatitis, prostatic trauma, and cancer. Gram for gram, prostatic carcinoma produces approximately 10 times as much serum PSA as that produced in benign prostatic hyperplasia. Therefore, as the PSA level increases, the likelihood that the PSA elevation is caused by prostate cancer increases. With normal findings on digital rectal examination, approximately 2.5%, 33%, and 66% of patients with PSA levels of less than 4, between 4 and 10, and greater than 10 ng per mL, respectively, will have prostate carcinoma. To compensate for the increased prevalence of benign prostatic hyperplasia as men become older, an age-specific reference range for serum PSA can be used; PSA reference ranges are further categorized by race (Table 7). African-American men, in general, have higher PSA values, but their reference ranges are adjusted downward to improve cancer detection because they constitute a high-risk group. Before therapy, PSA is a useful prognostic marker. After treatment, progressive elevation of the PSA level indicates recurrent disease.

Presentation and Diagnosis

Prostate cancer does not usually cause symptoms unless the tumor is relatively advanced. In this case, the most frequent symptoms are those of hematuria, bladder outlet obstruction, and vesical irritation caused by local tumor growth. Occasionally, patients may present with symptoms of metastatic disease, especially bony metastases. Increasingly, patients come to medical attention because of an incidentally discovered elevated serum PSA level or a palpable abnormality on digital rectal examination. Approximately 30% of patients with a nodule on digital rectal examination will have prostate cancer. Prostatic biopsy is indicated for patients in whom a diagnosis of prostate cancer is suspected owing to elevated serum PSA level and/or abnormal findings on digital examination. Transrectal ultrasound (TRUS)–guided biopsy can be performed as an office procedure with minimal patient discomfort and risk. The complications of prostate cancer biopsy are infection and bleeding, which occur in less than 1% of the cases. The prostate is visualized with a TRUS probe, and any ultrasonically suspicious areas are biopsied. A

TABLE 7. **Age- and Race-Adjusted Prostate-Specific Antigen (PSA) Reference Ranges**

Age Range (y)	PSA Reference Range (ng/mL)		
	Asians	Blacks	Whites
40–49	0–2.0	0–2.0	0–2.5
50–59	0–3.0	0–4.0	0–3.5
60–69	0–4.0	0–4.5	0–4.5
70–79	0–5.0	0–5.0	0–6.5

Adapted from Richardson TD and Oesterling JE, Urol Clin North Am *24*:339, 1997.

minimum of six systemic prostate biopsies are then performed at the apex, midgland, and base of both right and left lobes of the prostate. Some urologists also perform additional biopsies of the transition zone of the prostate, which is in the anterior periurethral area. If findings on the initial biopsy specimens are negative and there is a high suspicion of cancer, another biopsy should be performed, because 15% of such patients will be found to have cancer.

If at presentation the PSA level is less than 10 ng per mL and the patient has no symptoms suggestive of metastatic disease, no other radiologic staging studies are generally necessary. If the PSA level is greater than 10 ng per mL, a radionuclide bone scan should be performed. Pelvic CT scanning is rarely indicated because of its low sensitivity and specificity in the detection of nodal metastases. Prostate cancer is staged by the AJCC system (Table 8). Prostate cancers are graded 1 to 5, depending on the architecture of the tumor, using the Gleason grading system. Grading is commonly reported as a Gleason score of 2 to 10, which is the sum of the Gleason grade of the major and minor patterns within the tumor. A Gleason score of 2 is the best differentiated and 10 is the most poorly differentiated tumor.

Management

ORGAN-CONFINED TUMORS (T1 AND T2 DISEASE)

The management options for patients with clinically organ-confined disease (T1 and T2 disease) include observation, radiation therapy, and radical prostatectomy. The choice of therapy depends on the tumor stage, Gleason score, patient's physiologic age, and patient preference. Patients with low-grade (Gleason score of less than 5) and low-stage (T1a) tumors are unlikely to experience tumor-related complications for 10 years or more. These patients are particularly suitable for observation unless they have a very long life expectancy. Patients with higher-stage (T1b and higher) and high-grade tumors (Gleason score of 6 or more) are likely to have symptoms of local progression and/or metastasis in a shorter time frame and are suitable candidates for definitive therapy.

TABLE 8. **American Joint Committee on Cancer Staging of Prostate Cancer**

T0	No evidence of primary tumor
T1	Impalpable tumor, not visualized on TRUS
T1a	Incidental tumor, <5% of tissue resected at prostatectomy
T1b	Incidental tumor, >5% of tissue resected at prostatectomy
T1c	Tumor identified by needle biopsy alone (performed because of elevated PSA level)
T2	Tumor confined within prostate
T2a	Tumor involves less than half of one lobe
T2b	Tumor involves more than half of one lobe
T2c	Tumor involves both lobes
T3	Tumor extends through prostatic capsule
T3a	Unilateral extracapsular tumor
T3b	Bilateral extracapsular tumor
T3c	Tumor involves seminal vesicles
T4	Tumor fixed to adjacent structures, e.g., bladder neck or pelvic wall
N0	No regional node metastasis
N1–3	Regional node metastasis
M0	No distant metastasis
M1	Distant metastasis

Abbreviations: PSA = prostate-specific antigen; TRUS = transrectal ultrasound.

Modified from Seigne JD, Grossman HB: Malignant tumors of the urogenital tract. *In* Rakel RE: Conn's Current Therapy 1997. Philadelphia, WB Saunders Co, 1997, p 719.

Observation and Delayed Hormone Therapy. Several retrospective studies have reported excellent 10-year survival rates (85 to 90%) with observation (also called "watchful waiting") and delayed hormonal therapy (delayed until symptoms develop or the PSA rises to a worrisome level, i.e., >20 mg per mL) for clinically localized prostate cancer. However, a significant proportion of men treated in this fashion will experience local progression (75%), and some will develop metastatic disease (20%). Therefore, it appears that given sufficient time, most prostate cancers will become symptomatic. Observation is recommended for patients who are likely to die of other causes before their prostate cancer progresses.

Radical Prostatectomy. This should be reserved for healthy men with clinically localized prostate cancer and a projected survival of greater than 10 years. The operation consists of removal of the prostate, ampulla of the vasa deferentia, and seminal vesicles, with reanastomosis of the bladder neck to the membranous urethra. The operation can be performed equally effectively via the retropubic (abdominal) and perineal approaches. Several series indicate that 15-year survival rates of 85 to 93% can be achieved in patients with clinically localized disease (T2 or less). Operative morbidity is low, with a mortality rate of less than 0.5% in most centers. Intraoperative complications include blood loss, necessitating a transfusion in 5 to 10% of patients, and rectal injuries, occurring in less than 1% of cases. The major long-term complications are urinary incontinence, impotence, and bladder neck contracture. Bladder neck contracture requiring dilation of internal urethrotomy occurs in 3 to 12% of patients. Eighty to 90% of patients are continent of urine 1 year after radical prostatectomy. Of the remaining 10 to 20%, most experience stress urinary incontinence that requires the use of a protective pad. Approximately 4% of patients have more severe or total incontinence that may require the placement of an artificial sphincter. The cavernosa nerves, which control erectile function, travel in neurovascular bundles alongside the prostate. The neurovascular bundles can be preserved by performing a nerve-sparing prostatectomy. Unilateral nerve-sparing prostatectomy can preserve potency in up to 50% of patients and bilateral nerve sparing preserves potency in 50 to 80% of men depending on their age and starting erectile function. Removal of the cavernosa nerves does not affect penile sensation or the ability to achieve orgasm. Therapeutic options for the impotent patient include the vacuum erection device, intracorporeal injection therapy, intraurethral vasoactive suppositories, penile prosthesis placement, and medication.

Radiation Therapy. External beam photon therapy delivered by a linear accelerator has been used extensively in the treatment of clinically localized prostate cancer. The best results have been achieved with delivery of a radiation dose of approximately 70 cGy to the prostate bed in 200-cGy daily increments over 7 weeks. Fifteen-year disease-specific survival rates of up to 85% have been reported for clinically localized (T1 and T2) disease. Complications are minor, with 30 to 40% of patients experiencing transient gastrointestinal symptoms. Approximately 10% of patients have prolonged gastrointestinal (chronic diarrhea and rectal bleeding) and genitourinary (urinary frequency, urgency, and hematuria) symptoms. Impotence occurs in approximately 50% of patients, and urinary incontinence in 3 to 5% of patients.

Interstitial radiation therapy, also called brachytherapy or seed implantation, using gold 198 and iodine 125 seeds had fallen into disfavor because variable seed placement resulted in uneven radiation delivery, causing an unacceptably high rate of local recurrence. Recent technologic advances, including the development of new isotopes, seed stabilization, and TRUS-guided seed placement, have led to a resurgence of interest in this treatment. Intermediate-term results at 5 to 7 years in carefully selected patients from experienced treatment centers show disease-free survival equivalent to that with radical prostatectomy. Although many investigators now consider brachytherapy a standard treatment option, others cite the need for long-term follow-up studies and the lack of results with widespread use and recommended that it be assigned investigational status.

Cryotherapy. Transperineal prostatic freezing has recently gained some popularity as a treatment of clinically localized prostate cancer. Early results suggest that cryotherapy results in effective local tumor control with moderate side effects. No long-term results are available, and many authorities consider this treatment still investigational.

Follow-up of Organ-Confined Tumors. Follow-up of patients with clinically localized prostate cancer includes measurement of PSA level every 3 months for 1 year, every 6 months for the next 2 to 3 years, and yearly thereafter. The PSA level should be undetectable at 6 weeks after radical prostatectomy. Any subsequent rise in the PSA level indicates a recurrent tumor. The PSA level should drop to less than 1 ng per mL by 12 to 18 months after radiation therapy. If the PSA level fails to drop below 1 ng per mL or starts to rise, there is a high probability of residual or recurrent tumor.

LOCALLY ADVANCED (T3) TUMORS

Many patients with locally advanced tumors have occult metastatic disease at diagnosis. There is little evidence to suggest that most patients whose tumors have spread beyond the prostate can be cured by more aggressive surgery or radiation therapy alone. Although the optimal treatment of T3 prostate cancer has not been completely defined, a combination of external-beam radiation therapy and neoadjuvant and/or adjuvant hormonal therapy has been shown to be effective in a number of clinical trials. This reversible hormonal therapy consists of luteinizing-hormone–releasing hormone (LH-RH) agonist injections with or without oral antiandrogen agents.

NODE-POSITIVE (N1 TO N3) DISEASE

Patients who are discovered to have positive pelvic lymph nodes at exploration before radical prostatectomy are unlikely to be cured by performing an extended lymph node dissection combined with surgical removal of the prostate. Several treatment options are advocated, including hormonal therapy alone, radical prostatectomy combined with hormonal therapy, and radiation therapy combined with hormonal therapy. Although there are no definitive data supporting combination therapy, early experience with local irradiation to control the primary tumor combined with androgen ablation to treat the metastatic disease may be beneficial in selected patients.

METASTATIC DISEASE (M1)

The observation by Huggins that most prostate cancers are androgen-dependent and regress after androgen withdrawal led to the development of hormonal therapy. Androgen ablation is the primary treatment for patients with metastatic prostatic carcinoma, 85% of whom will have a response to this modality. There previously was a debate as to whether hormone therapy should be administered at the time of diagnosis of metastatic disease or withheld until the patient becomes symptomatic. There is now evidence suggesting that early hormone therapy prolongs survival and decreases cancer-related morbidity including that due to spinal cord compression and bladder outlet obstruction. Although the majority of the androgen supply comes from the testes, a small but significant amount is derived from the adrenal secretion of androstenedione and peripheral conversion to testosterone. Standard hormonal therapy has been targeted at the elimination of testicular androgens by orchiectomy or LH-RH injections. Several studies have suggested that combined androgen blockage directed at the testicular and adrenal sources of androgens results in a modest prolongation of survival. Limited data suggest that patients with low-volume metastatic disease may derive the most benefit from combination therapy. Nevertheless, the use of combined androgen blockage remains controversial, especially in men who choose orchiectomy rather than LH-RH injections.

Testicular androgens can be eliminated by surgical castration (orchiectomy, an outpatient procedure), or by medical castration with estrogens or LH-RH agonist. Diethylstilbestrol used to be a commonly used estrogen but had cardiovascular side effects and caused gynecomastia, and this agent is no longer sold in the United States. LH-RH agonists initially result in an increase in testosterone production; this increase is followed by a decrease to castrate levels. An antiandrogen should be administered with LH-RH agonist when androgen ablation is initiated, to prevent a "flare" of the prostate tumor associated with the initial stimulation of androgen production. There are three FDA-approved antiandrogen medications: flutamide (Eulexin), 250 mg three times daily; bicalutamide (Casodex), 50 mg once daily; and nilutamide (Nilandron), 300 mg once daily for the first month and then 150 mg once daily thereafter. Most clinicians continue the antiandrogen medications as combination hormonal therapy; however, some continue the antiandrogen only for several weeks or months to combat the "flare." LH-RH agonist can be administered as depot injections (leuprolide [Lupron] or goserelin [Zoladex]). These depot injections are available as 1-, 3-, and 4-month formulations. Side effects include hot flushes, which can be treated with megestrol acetate (Megace)* at 20 mg twice daily, and diminished muscle mass, libido, and sexual potency. The median survival of patients with metastatic prostate cancer treated with androgen ablation is approximately 3 years, although there is wide variation depending on the severity of metastatic disease. Patients starting on a course of antiandrogen therapy should have blood drawn at the initiation of therapy and during the first few months of treatment to monitor the serum alanine aminotransferase level, as rare hepatic toxicity (in less than 1% of cases) may occur.

A decline in the PSA level indicates a response to therapy. In patients who do not respond to initial hormonal therapy, the level of serum testosterone should be measured to ensure that it is indeed at the castration level. A subsequent increase in the PSA level is an indicator of tumor progression. If the PSA level rises during combined hormonal therapy, the antiandrogen should be withdrawn, because up to 75% of patients will show another, usually short response.

Adenocarcinoma of the prostate is resistant to most chemotherapeutic regimens, but trials of single-agent and multiple-agent chemotherapy for hormone-refractory prostate cancer are ongoing. Mitoxantrone (Novantrone),* a chemotherapeutic agent similar to doxorubicin, is FDA-approved for hormone-refractory prostate cancer in combination with prednisone or hydrocortisone and is effective in palliation of bone pain, although a survival benefit has not been demonstrated. Current trials are focusing on ketoconazole, estramustine phosphate, paclataxol, etoposide alone and in combination, and mitoxantrone in combination with other agents.* There is a push to identify patients earlier in their course of hormone refractory disease to improve response rates and affect survival with these newer agents. Symptomatic treatment of bone metastasis can be achieved with palliative local irradiation or intravenous chemotherapy with strontium chloride Sr 89 (Metastron) or sumarium (Quadramet).

*Not FDA approved for this indication.

SCREENING FOR PROSTATE CANCER

No curative treatment is available for advanced prostate cancer. However, radical prostatectomy is a potentially curative treatment for organ-confined cancer. Early detection has the potential to affect the mortality rate for this cancer by identifying organ-confined tumors before the development of extracapsular and metastatic disease. A combination of annual PSA determination and digital rectal examination appears to be the most effective method for the early detection of prostate cancer and is recommended by the American Cancer Society and the American Urological Association for all men over the age of 50 years. African-Americans and men with a family history of prostate cancer are at increased risk and should be screened from the age of 40 years. Men who have a life expectancy of less than 10 years are unlikely to benefit from early detection and therefore should not be screened. Screening for prostate cancer remains controversial, because no study has demonstrated a decrease in the prostate cancer mortality rate as a result of screening. Such studies are under way, but the results will not be available for many years. These pros and cons should be discussed with patients, and they should at least have the option of yearly testing.

PENILE CANCER

Penile cancer is an uncommon tumor, with an incidence of 1 to 2 per 100,000 population. The majority of these tumors are squamous cell carcinomas. The peak incidence is in the sixth decade, but tumors can occur in men as young as 30 years of age. Phimosis and poor hygiene play a role in the development of penile cancers.

Presentation and Diagnosis

Penile cancer presents as a lesion on the glans or prepuce. Frequently, patients present late with fungating masses. However, in early cases the presenting lesion may be a red irritative area that resembles local inflammation. Diagnosis is established by performing a biopsy. Careful attention should be paid to evaluating the regional lymph nodes (inguinal nodes) for metastatic disease. Tumors are staged by the AJCC system (Table 9).

TABLE 9. **American Joint Committee on Cancer Staging of Penile Cancer**

Tis	Carcinoma in situ
Ta	Noninvasive verrucous carcinoma
T1	Tumor invades subepithelial connective tissue
T2	Tumor invades corpora spongiosa or corpus cavernosum
T3	Tumor invades urethra or prostate
T4	Tumor invades other adjacent structures
N0	No regional node metastasis
M0	No distant metastasis
M1	Distant metastasis

Modified from Seigne JD, Grossman HB: Malignant tumors of the urogenital tract. *In* Rakel RE: Conn's Current Therapy 1997. Philadelphia, WB Saunders Co, 1997, p 722.

Management

T1 lesions of the foreskin can be treated by circumcision. T1 and small T2 lesions of the glans penis can be treated by local excision using Mohs' microsurgery or CO_2 laser ablation. Larger T2 and T3 lesions require excision of the tumor with a 2-cm margin. Tumor excision can be performed by partial penectomy if a sufficient portion of the penis will remain for the patient to stand to void. Otherwise, total penectomy with perineal urethrostomy is performed.

In addition to treatment of the primary tumor, all patients require continued assessment of the inguinal nodes. Enlarged inguinal nodes may result from infection or neoplasm. Enlarged nodes may be immediately evaluated with aspiration cytology. Alternatively, patients can be given 6 weeks of antibiotics therapy followed by re-evaluation. Patients with persistent nodal enlargement should undergo bilateral inguinal node dissection. Patients whose primary tumor is poorly differentiated or invades the corpora spongiosa or cavernosa should undergo prophylactic node dissection, because 78% will have nodal metastasis. Prognosis is excellent for patients with T1 or T2 tumors and negative inguinal nodes. Patients who undergo immediate node dissection and have less than two positive nodes have a 5-year survival rate of 10 to 30%. Close follow-up is essential and consists of clinical examination every 3 months for 2 years and every 6 months thereafter. Patients with metastatic disease are treated with combination chemotherapy (bleomycin, methotrexate, and cisplatin).

UNUSUAL TUMORS

Sarcomas, melanomas, lymphomas, and Kaposi's sarcomas all occasionally occur on the penis. Treatment depends on tumor type and the stage of disease. Up to 20% of acquired immune deficiency syndrome (AIDS) patients with Kaposi's sarcoma have genital involvement. Kaposi's sarcoma responds well to low-dose irradiation.

TESTICULAR CANCER

Testicular cancer is the most common tumor of young adult males, with an incidence of 3.7 per 100,000 population. The tumor is uncommon in African-Americans. A history of cryptorchidism increases the risk of testis cancer between 3 and 48 times. The increased risk of testis cancer is not eliminated by orchidopexy. However, orchidopexy is valuable in preserving testicular function and permits easy examination of the testicle. Germ cell tumors are the most common malignant tumors of the testis and for therapeutic purposes can be divided into seminomas and nonseminomatous germ cell tumors (NSGCTs).

Presentation and Diagnosis

The most common presenting feature is a testicular mass that may be first recognized after minor trauma. Physical examination usually reveals a firm testicular mass. Occasionally the tumor may be obscured by a reactive hydrocele. A testicular ultrasonogram is useful if the diagnosis is unclear. All patients with suspected testicular tumors should have blood drawn for measurement of beta-human chorionic gonadotropin (β-hCG), alpha-fetoprotein (AFP), and lactate dehydrogenase (LDH). Ten percent of patients with seminoma will have an elevated β-hCG level. Fifty to 90% of patients with NSGCT will have an elevated level of either or both β-hCG and AFP. Patients with a primary tumor that is histologically a pure seminoma but who have an elevated level of AFP are classified for treatment purposes as having NSGCT. Testicular tumors spread through both the lymphatic and vascular systems. The lymphatics of the left testicle primarily drain to the left para-aortic retroperitoneal nodes; those of the right testicle, to the interaortocaval group. The most common site of hematogenous metastasis is in the lung. Surgical exploration of a possible testicular tumor should be performed through an inguinal incision to permit early control of the spermatic cord and to prevent contamination of the inguinal lymphatics. After the testicle has been removed, metastatic work-up should be performed consisting of an abdominal CT scan to evaluate the para-aortic nodes and a chest x-ray film to rule out pulmonary metastases. Patients with retroperitoneal metastasis should also have a chest CT scan; however, if the abdominal CT scan does not show metastases, a chest film constitutes sufficient study of the chest for staging. The staging system for testis cancer is shown in Table 10. Treatment depends on histologic tumor type and stage of disease.

Management

Seminomas. The treatment of stage I and stage IIa seminomas is radical orchiectomy combined with 25 to 30 cGy of radiation delivered to the retroperitoneum. Prognosis is excellent, with a greater than 95% 5-year survival rate. Historically, stage Ib and stage III tumors were treated with abdominal and mediastinal irradiation. Currently, cisplatin-based chemotherapy is curative for most patients and is the treatment of choice. Prognosis is excellent, with more than 90% of patients achieving long-term survival. Adjuvant radiation therapy is indicated only for bulky lesions that do not respond adequately to chemotherapy. Follow-up consists of a physical examination and chest radiograph every 6 months. Patients should be taught testicular self-examination, because up to 5% of testicular tumors are bilateral.

TABLE 10. **Staging of Testicular Cancer**

Stage	Description
I	Tumor confined to the testis
II	Nodal metastases
IIA	Limited nodal metastases
IIB	Bulky nodal metastases
III	Tumor involving lymphatics above the diaphragm
IV	Hematogenous metastases

Modified from Seigne JD, Grossman HB: Malignant tumors of the urogenital tract. *In* Rakel RE: Conn's Current Therapy 1997. Philadelphia, WB Saunders Co, 1997, p 722.

Nonseminomatous Germ Cell Tumors. The treatment of patients with stage I NSGCT is controversial. Twenty to 25% of patients with clinical stage I disease will have occult retroperitoneal nodal metastasis. These patients can be identified and potentially cured by retroperitoneal lymph node dissection (RPLND). However, to identify the 20 to 25% of patients who have occult metastasis, 75% of the patients have to be subjected to an unnecessary operation. The major long-term complication of RPLND is failure of antegrade ejaculation from injury to the lumbar sympathetic chain. The use of template dissection and nerve-sparing surgery has decreased the frequency of this complication. An alternative approach to RPLND for patients with clinical stage I disease is observation with tumor marker assays and chest radiography monthly for 1 year, every 3 months for 1 year, and then every 6 months thereafter. Abdominal CT scanning is performed every 3 months for the first year and then every 6 months for two additional years. The potential for rapid undetected tumor growth on observation protocols underscores the need for close follow-up. Early treatment in the case of recurrence is important because prognosis is related to tumor volume. The presence of vascular invasion and a higher amount of the embryonal carcinoma component in the primary tumor are associated with a higher risk of metastasis, and patients bearing tumors with these features are not suitable candidates for observation protocols and should undergo RPLND. Patients who are discovered to have lymph node metastasis at the time of RPLND and who receive two cycles of postoperative cisplatin-based chemotherapy have a tumor recurrence rate approaching zero. The long-term survival rate associated with both methods (observation and initial RPLND) is greater than 95% at 5 years.

Patients with higher stages of disease (stages II, III, and IV) should undergo primary chemotherapy (bleomycin, etoposide, and cisplatin), with resection of residual tumor masses after chemotherapy. We continue chemotherapy until maximum tumor shrinkage has been achieved and then resect any residual masses. The most common site for residual disease is in the retroperitoneum. However, patients should undergo resection of residual masses in other organs, e.g., lung or liver, if tumor stabilization and normalization of tumor markers are achieved by chemotherapy. Residual masses represent fibrous scar in 40% of patients, benign teratoma in 40%, and viable tumor in 20%. RPLND after chemotherapy is technically more demanding than a primary dissection because residual masses are often adherent to the surrounding structures, including the aorta and vena cava. Occasionally aortic replacement and vena caval resection are necessary to achieve clear margins. Post-chemotherapy RPLND is associated with a greater likelihood of complications, including intraoperative blood loss, chylous ascites, pancreatitis, and failure of ejaculation. Prognosis depends on tumor volume, with 95% of patients with low-volume disease achieving long-term survival. With the use of modern multidisciplinary approaches, long-term survival is possible in 70 to 80% of patients, even those who have massive metastatic disease.

SCROTAL TUMORS

Squamous cell carcinoma of the scrotum became the first cancer known to be caused by an industrial carcinogen when it was identified as a disease of chimney sweepers by Pott in 1775. Scrotal cancer exhibiting other than squamous histology is rare. Scrotal cancers metastasize via the lymphatics to the inguinal nodes. Treatment is similar to that for penile carcinoma, with local excision and management of the regional nodes. Prognosis is good, with 50 to 70% 5-year survival rates in the absence of positive nodes.

Malignant intrascrotal tumors (excluding testicular cancer) are rare, and most are sarcomas.

GENITOURINARY SARCOMAS

Sarcomas are rare tumors of diverse histologic types that can arise from any mesenchymal tissue in the body. The percentage of patients presenting with local disease depends on the histologic type and organ of origin. Sarcomas are staged by careful physical examination, MRI of the affected organ (MRI defines tumor margins more accurately than CT), and CT of the chest. Careful pathologic review by an experienced pathologist is important to determine the histologic type and tumor grade. The mainstay of therapy for clinically localized tumors is wide local excision. The roles of pre- or postoperative irradiation and chemotherapy are unknown. Patients with clinically localized tumors less than 5 cm in diameter and of low histologic grade have a 3-year relapse-free survival rate of 89%. Locally advanced and metastatic tumors are treated with combination chemotherapy (doxorubicin, dacarbazine, and cyclophosphamide), followed by surgical excision and postoperative irradiation. The 3-year relapse-free survival rate in this group of patients is less than 25%.

Retroperitoneal Sarcomas

Retroperitoneal sarcomas account for 10 to 15% of all sarcomas. Liposarcoma is the most common histologic type. Most tumors present late as a large retroperitoneal mass that should be differentiated from retroperitoneal lymphoma. Surgical excision is the primary therapy. The 5-year survival rate is 50% after complete local excision. However, more than 90% of patients will develop local recurrence at 10 years of follow-up.

Renal Sarcomas

Sarcomas constitute 1 to 2% of all renal tumors. Leiomyosarcomas are the most common type. Three-year survival is dismal even after complete resection. Chemotherapy and radiation therapy are ineffective.

Bladder and Prostatic Sarcomas

Sarcomas account for 0.5% of all bladder and prostate tumors. Sarcomas should be differentiated from benign spindle cell nodules, which can occur after transurethral surgery. Rhabdomyosarcomas are the most common histologic type and occur primarily in children. Modern approaches using combination chemotherapy and irradiation permit an organ-sparing approach in 35% of these patients. Long-term survival is achieved in 75%. Leiomyosarcomas are the most common histologic type in adults. The survival rate is worse for adults than it is for children.

Paratesticular Sarcomas

Rhabdomyosarcomas of the paratesticular tissues are the most common paratesticular tumor of children and are treated by orchiectomy, retroperitoneal node dissection, and combination chemotherapy. Radiation therapy is administered to patients who have residual disease after surgery. Prognosis is good, with 60% of patients achieving long-term survival. Leiomyosarcomas are the most common tumor type in adults.

URETHRAL STRICTURES

method of
RAUL C. ORDORICA, M.D.
University of South Florida College of Medicine and James A. Haley Veterans Affairs Hospital
Tampa, Florida

A urethral stricture is the narrowing of the urethral lumen secondary to scarring and fibrosis. It can form anywhere along the entire length of the urethra and can vary markedly between patients. When significant, the resultant decrease in urinary flow causes signs and symptoms consistent with bladder outlet obstruction. It can be found at any age, and while it can occur in women, it is predominantly found in men.

The urethra acts as a conduit for the passage of urine and ejaculate. It extends from the bladder neck to the meatus. It traverses the prostate where it forms an integral part of the gland, with the ejaculatory and prostatic ducts emptying into the urethral lumen. Immediately at the apex of the prostate is the membranous sphincter, which surrounds the urethra and is made up of nonfatiguing slow-twitch striated muscle fibers. This is one of the continent mechanisms and can be compromised by both the stricture itself or by its subsequent therapy. Distal to this is the bulbar urethra, extending from the membranous sphincter to the suspensory ligaments of the penis. At this portion it is surrounded by the corpus spongiosum, a highly vascularized supportive stroma that can also be involved with the stricture disease. The corpus spongiosum extends from the bulbar urethra to the meatus, where it is continuous with the glans penis. Surrounding the bulbar urethra are the paired bulbospongiosus striated muscles. These contract with ejaculation, which results in the emission of semen and ejaculatory fluid. They can also contract voluntarily with voiding to assist in drainage of the urethra to prevent pooling of urine in what is the widest portion of the urethral lumen. Distal to the suspensory ligaments is the pendulous urethra where the urethra narrows slightly from the bulbar segment. The lumen then remains constant until the fossa navicularis, which is the junction at which two embryologically separate tissues meet to form a continuous urethral lumen. Distal to this is the urethral meatus.

The epithelium of the urethra is formed by transitional cells in its proximal portion, followed by pseudostratified columnar epithelium along the pendulous urethra, with nonkeratinizing squamous epithelium at its most distal segment. Throughout its length it is impervious to urine. The proximal bulbar urethra is penetrated by the paired Cowper's glands, and the remaining urethra is lined by the glands of Litre, which are multiple small glands along its length. The distal urethra, along with the dorsally adjacent paired corpora cavernosa, is surrounded by the fibrous Buck's fascia, followed by the loosely adherent dartos fascia, and then skin.

The blood supply to the urethra is derived both proximally and distally. Proximally the corpus spongiosum of the bulbar urethra is perforated with the bulbar arteries. Distally, the glans penis is in continuity with the dorsal artery of the penis. Both groups of vessels are branches of the pudendal arteries. The venous drainage is through emissary veins in communication with common drainage of the corpora cavernosa of the penis.

ETIOLOGY

Urethral strictures are most commonly due to trauma, infection, or inflammation. Congenital narrowing can be seen in the distal urethra at the fossa navicularis or meatus. Traumatic injuries most often affect the proximal portion of the urethra, where the membranous or bulbar portions are relatively fixed in position and more vulnerable to injury. In the case of pelvic fracture, the prostate, secured by the puboprostatic ligaments, is torn away from the remaining urethra at its membranous portion. Direct blows to the perineum, as in the case of straddle injuries, can result in the crushing of the bulbar urethra against the pubic symphysis. It is not uncommon for patients to present with strictures of the bulbar urethra, with poor recollection of an injury that might have occurred in the distant past. Although less common, trauma can also involve the distal urethra, such as in the case of penile fracture in which the corpora cavernosa are torn due to buckling in the erect state during forceful intercourse. The adherent pendulous urethra is sheared by the disruption of the adjacent corpora. Incomplete healing can result in subsequent stricture formation, as it can in any form of direct urethral injury. Iatrogenic urethral injury can be caused by extensive endoscopic manipulation, as in the case of transurethral resection. These most often occur in the fossa navicularis, where the urethral lumen is relatively narrow, or at the junction between the bulbar and pendulous urethra, where the suspensory ligament limits urethral mobility.

Urethral infections that classically result in stricture disease are gonococcal urethritis. With the advent of nongonococcal urethritis, this must also be considered as a source, although it is often missing from the history owing to the absence of significant symptoms. The strictures caused by urethritis can be extensive, involving significant lengths of the urethra, at times its entirety. Urethral inflammation can occur with chronic indwelling catheter placement. Latex catheters incite the greatest degree of urethral inflammation. In all cases of urethral stricture, with the exception of pelvic fracture, the inciting event may be far removed by many years from the development of symptoms.

SIGNS AND SYMPTOMS

The presenting signs and symptoms of urethral stricture disease are similar to those of other forms of bladder outlet obstruction. Patients may note a decrease in their force of stream, with a prolonged time necessary to void to completion. This can also be accompanied by the requirement to forcefully strain to empty the bladder. As the bladder compensates for the increased resistance caused by the narrowed lumen, bladder irritability may result with increased frequency and nocturia. If the lumen narrows further, retention may ensue. With urinary stasis, urinary tract infections may result. Urine extravasation can occur proximal to the stricture with urinoma formation and possible urosepsis. Infections of other segments of the urinary tract, such as epididymo-orchitis or pyelonephritis, can also be the presenting signs of urethral stricture.

DIAGNOSIS

As with any lower urinary tract pathology, diagnosis requires careful history and examination. Symptoms may be consistent with urinary tract obstruction and infection. Of note, many patients with a chronic urethral stricture may not realize that their voiding habits are in fact abnormal. Any history of genital trauma or urethritis should be elicited. Physical examination should include the abdomen, pelvis, penis, scrotum, and rectum and may demonstrate bladder distention, prior trauma, scarring, local infection, urine extravasation, abscess formation, urethral diverticula, fistula, prior surgeries, or benign prostatic hypertrophy (BPH). Urinalysis should be obtained to rule out the presence of infection or to determine the presence of hematuria. Serum creatinine can be measured to screen for obstructive uropathy. Bladder obstruction, including that caused by urethral stricture, should be ruled out in any male with urinary tract infection. A screening test may include measurement of urinary flow rate and postvoid residual as performed by basic urodynamic testing. Peak urinary flow rate is decreased in the case of urethral stricture, although this is a nonspecific finding also noted with other forms of bladder outlet obstruction such as BPH or with decreased detrusor contractility. Attempts to pass a catheter to measure postvoid residual volume can indicate the presence of a urethral stricture. Initial diagnosis is often made with the inability to pass a catheter, as the stricture is relatively fixed and rigid; in contrast, in BPH catheter passage can typically be accomplished. The length that the catheter can be passed may also give some indication of the location of the stricture.

Much information can be gained by the determination of the exact length and number of strictures present using radiographic techniques. The radiographic procedure of choice is the retrograde urethrogram. By any number of methods, contrast is instilled from the distal urethra flowing proximally to display the full length of the urethra, captured on static radiographic images. Additional studies are required if areas of the urethra proximal to the stricture are not well visualized because of inadequate distention with contrast. This can include a voiding cystourethrogram provided by either the retrograde trickling of contrast into the bladder through the urethra, the placement of a small lumen catheter beyond the stricture, or the percutaneous placement of a suprapubic catheter. This study is typically of higher quality than an intravenous pyelogram followed by patient voiding.

Cystoscopy can be helpful to identify and calibrate the diameter of a given stricture. Often the quality of the tissue can be assessed by its relative pallor. The use of ultrasound remains investigational in the evaluation of urethral strictures. Information can be gained regarding the depth of spongiofibrosis (scarring of the corpus spongiosum), which may indicate potential recalcitrance to minimally invasive therapies.

MANAGEMENT

Little is known about the natural history of patients who have asymptomatic minor narrowings of the urethra. For patients who present with symptoms related to the stricture, however, the tendency is for the stricture to either remain stable or progress. Therefore, there is little role for observation, and intervention is typically pursued.

Patients who present with urinary retention require bladder decompression. This requires either some form of manipulation of the urethral stricture or placement of a suprapubic tube. This often involves dilatation of the urethra with use of either Van Buren sounds, filiforms and followers, or Amplatz dilators over a guide wire. This can be a relatively blind procedure, which may cause further injury to the urethra with marked bleeding and discomfort. If these procedures cannot be performed easily, it is best to abandon them early rather than risk further trauma. Providing the bladder is full, placement of a percutaneous suprapubic tube allows for bladder decompression, removes the risk for further urethral inflammation, and allows for patient evaluation at a nonurgent interval.

Urethral dilatation typically requires the progressive passage of instruments of increasing diameter. This can result in a repeated shearing effect of the urothelium. It is unclear whether this hypothetical disadvantage has any significant impact. Balloon dilatation addresses this disadvantage, but its benefit over other standard methods remains unclear. Significant strictures that extend below the urothelium do not actually stretch with dilatation, but are torn apart at multiple foci. After this tearing, healing of the defect with minimal scarring is required for good long-term results. This can occur if the exposed bulbar spongiosum can epithelialize before collagen deposition, contraction, and dense scar formation.

Rather than allow the tissue to tear in a random fashion, the stricture can be incised under direct vision. This provides control over the location, number, and depth of the incisions, minimizing the potential for false passages. However, these strictures tend to recur over months to years and require continued vigilance and possibly alternative treatment. Results are not sufficiently altered with either variations in technique (direction and number of incisions), technology (use of electrocautery, laser), or ancillary methods (postoperative intermittent catheterization, steroid injection) to allow designation of any single endoscopic method as clearly superior.

Stents can be used to attempt to alter the course of stricture healing and recurrence. A metallic stent for permanent placement is currently available in the United States as a Food and Drug Administration–approved device. Placed after dilatation or incision of stricture, it is meant to control the ingress of scar tissue that would otherwise occlude the urethral lumen. It is best for proximal strictures in older non–sexually active patients owing to potential discomfort when in the distal urethra or with erection. Failure rate may be higher in patients with dense extensive scarring of the corpora spongiosa with obliteration of the stented lumen. Temporary stents may provide relief of symptoms and may alter the long-term course of recurrence, although they are not currently available in the United States. Investigations continue into the use of absorbable stents, some of which may promote the epithelialization of the urethral defect either by the inherent nature of the stent material, the use of growth factors, or the implantation of autologous epithelium.

Despite these minimally invasive maneuvers, open surgical techniques are necessary for many patients with recurrent urethral strictures or extensive scarring on initial diagnosis. Basic techniques involve either the excision of the defect with primary anastomosis of the urethral margins, or the transfer of healthy tissue to replace the damaged urethra. Primary anastomosis is reserved for strictures of the proximal urethra. Long defects of up to 6 cm involving distraction injuries of the membranous urethra can be repaired with excellent results. This requires the anastomosis of healthy tissue, for if any scarred tissue remains, the stricture will recur regardless of the amount of scarred urethra removed. Smaller defects of the bulbar urethra of up to 2 cm can be repaired in a similar fashion without tethering of the penis.

Tissue transfer techniques involve the use of either epithelial grafting or the transfer of a vascularized pedicle flap. Grafted epithelium has included both penile and nonpenile skin, vein, bladder mucosa, and buccal mucosa. Of all these choices, it is perhaps buccal mucosa that combines ease of harvesting, graft success, impermeability to urine, and long-term result that make it the tissue of choice in regard to urothelium replacement within the urethra. However, despite the advantages of buccal mucosa, limitations in the host bed may compromise the "take" of the graft and limit the success of this procedure. Therefore the most reliable method for tissue replacement is to ensure the blood supply, as with the use of the vascularized pedicle flap.

Vascularized flaps for urethral replacement have been taken from all areas of genital skin, including prepuce, penile shaft, scrotum, and perineum. The skin of the prepuce and penile shaft is better suited to be constantly exposed to urine because of its relatively impermeable nature. Scrotal skin has a tendency to break down over time, form diverticula, and be hair bearing, with the formation of urethral bezoars. Depending on the presence of foreskin, penile shaft length, and skin redundancy, the entire urethra can be replaced. The procurement of such flaps and the assurance of their viability requires more exacting techniques than all other therapies for urethral stricture management.

For those patients without adequate penile skin, a combination of both graft and flap techniques can be used. As an initial stage, the strictured urethra is opened along its length. Split-thickness skin grafts harvested from the leg are then placed alongside the opened urethra supported by the adjacent tissue. After complete healing, these grafted areas are rotated in to form the new urethral lumen. This obviously requires a two-stage approach, which otherwise has been widely replaced with the aforementioned techniques of tissue transfer.

Alternative therapy must be sought for patients in whom extensive reconstruction is ill advised owing to either age or debility, and who do not desire continued endoscopic management in the form of urethral dilatations, incisions, and catheterizations. For patients who are otherwise continent, a perineal urethrostomy can be formed, which bypasses the stricture. For patients who cannot undergo surgery or who have intractable incontinence, a suprapubic catheter can be placed. Given our current armamentarium of surgical techniques, however, it is only in rare cases that urethral reconstruction cannot be performed by a skilled physician for the motivated patient.

URINARY STONE DISEASE

method of
NOAH S. SCHENKMAN, M.D., and
MARSHALL L. STOLLER, M.D.
University of California, San Francisco, School of Medicine
San Francisco, California

Urinary calculi have plagued humans for centuries. The diagnosis and treatment of urinary stones have advanced significantly since the Egyptians' use of diamond-tipped reeds to fragment bladder stones. New endourologic techniques have replaced open surgery in most cases and continue to improve patient care. New diagnostic techniques are making it simpler and safer to evaluate patients with urolithiasis.

CLINICAL PRESENTATION

Patients typically present with colicky flank pain. The pain may radiate to the ipsilateral groin, testis, or labia and it may be associated with nausea, vomiting, and gross hematuria. Colic can be severe and is characterized by writhing as the patient tries to find a comfortable position, in contrast to intraperitoneal processes, in which the patient tends to lie still. Irritative voiding symptoms are frequent when a stone is lodged in the distal ureter. The stone may cause dysuria and marked urinary frequency and urgency. Clinical presentations can vary, ranging from asymptomatic, incidentally noted calculi to frank urosepsis.

EVALUATION

Urinalysis and urine culture may help direct therapy. Microhematuria will be absent in up to 15% of patients presenting with renal colic. Pyuria may be a clue to associated infection. Urine pH may be helpful in predicting stone type: a pH of less than 5.5 is associated with uric acid calculi; a pH of more than 7.0 is associated with struvite (magnesium ammonium phosphate) infection stones. Crystalluria may be a helpful finding if struvite, uric acid, or cystine crystals are present. The ubiquitous nature of calcium oxalate crystals in urine makes their presence nondiagnostic.

A complete blood count is warranted if the patient presents with fever or the diagnosis is in doubt. Measurements of serum electrolytes and creatinine should be obtained. After the acute stone episode has resolved and the diagnosis of urolithiasis is confirmed, an evaluation with determination of serum calcium, phosphorus, uric acid, and parathormone is performed to rule out obvious medical causes of urolithiasis such as gout, renal tubular acidosis, and hyperparathyroidism.

A plain abdominal radiograph—namely, a kidney-ureter-bladder film (KUB)—constitutes the best initial imaging study. (In female patients, pregnancy status should first be ascertained.) This study helps pinpoint the location of the calculus, as 85 to 90% of urinary tract calculi are radiopaque. Common sites of stone obstruction include the ureteropelvic junction, as the ureter crosses over the iliac vessels (overlying the sacroiliac joint seen on x-ray film), and the ureterovesical junction.

Intravenous pyelography (IVP) is the standard technique for imaging calculi, evaluating renal anatomy, and obtaining a gross estimate of renal function. It is readily available and is relatively safe and rapid. However, anaphylactic reactions to iodinated contrast material occur in approximately 1 in 10,000 patients. In addition, pregnancy, renal insufficiency, diabetes mellitus, and dehydration are relative contraindications to the use of IVP. Inexperienced technicians, uncooperative patients, and inadequate bowel preparation can result in a suboptimal study.

Renal ultrasonography is useful in patients in whom IVP is unavailable or contraindicated and is the examination of choice in pregnant women. It is quick and noninvasive and avoids ionizing radiation. However, usefulness is operator-dependent and may be limited by body habitus, especially in the obese patient. Doppler techniques can be used to improve diagnostic accuracy by measuring the renal artery resistive index and identifying the presence of ureteral jets. Overall, ultrasound and Doppler techniques are best used in conjunction with a scout KUB radiograph and clinical history to help direct the examination.

Noncontrast helical computed tomography (CT) scanning, where available, is rapidly replacing other modalities and will probably become the diagnostic study of choice in acute renal colic. It is safe and rapid and has shown 97% sensitivity and 96% specificity in detecting ureteral calculi. Advantages include the avoidance of iodinated contrast and improved cost-effectiveness in dedicated centers compared with that for IVP. It also can help diagnose nonrenal causes of abdominal pain.

Contrast CT scans should be reserved for defining renal anatomy when planning a surgical approach. A follow-up KUB film obtained after a contrast CT scan can help further delineate anatomy. Renal scintigraphy may be useful to estimate relative renal function, but caution should be used in the presence of unrelieved obstruction. Magnetic resonance imaging is not useful for evaluating urinary calculi.

TREATMENT

Initial treatment should be directed at hydration to a euvolemic state, pain relief using analgesics, and confirmation of stone passage by straining the urine for calculi (Figure 1). Overhydration inhibits ureteral wall coaptation and weakens the efficiency of ureteral peristalsis. Furthermore, the increased urine production with overhydration results in elevated ureteral and renal pressures, which exacerbates pain. A euvolemic state should be the goal; overhydration does not push calculi down the ureter.

Opiate analgesics are effective in relieving colicky pain. The most commonly used parenteral agents are morphine sulfate and meperidine. These agents have no effect on ureteral peristalsis or on intrarenal pressures. A nonsteroidal anti-inflammatory drug, ketorolac, has the advantage of lowering intrarenal pressures by decreasing renal plasma flow. It is effective in relieving renal colic without the sedative side effects associated with opiates. This medication is inappropriate for those patients with underlying renal disease, advanced age, and pregnancy.

Most patients respond to hydration and analgesics and can be managed expectantly on an outpatient basis while awaiting stone passage. Patients with intractable pain unresponsive to parenteral analgesics, with persistent nausea and vomiting, or with fever should be admitted to the hospital. Adequate urinary drainage from the obstructed renal unit must be obtained in patients with fever and signs of systemic infection using a ureteral catheter or percutaneous nephrostomy tube.

Most calculi less than 6 mm in greatest dimension will pass spontaneously. Symptomatic stones that do not pass spontaneously may necessitate surgical intervention. Surgical treatment depends upon stone location, size, and composition, as well as underlying renal anatomy. Most renal calculi less than 2.5 cm across can be managed with extracorporeal shock wave lithotripsy (ESWL). These focused shock waves are used to fragment stones. Small fragments usually pass spontaneously and uneventfully. Lower pole renal calculi greater than 1 cm and other renal calculi greater than 2.5 cm are best managed with percutaneous nephrostolithotomy. Ureteral stones may be managed with in situ ESWL or with ureteroscopy and extraction. Endoscopic procedures allow a variety of fragmentation devices, including the ultrasonic, electrohydraulic, pneumatic, and laser lithotrites, to be used. Open surgical treatment is rarely required today and is reserved for patients with un-

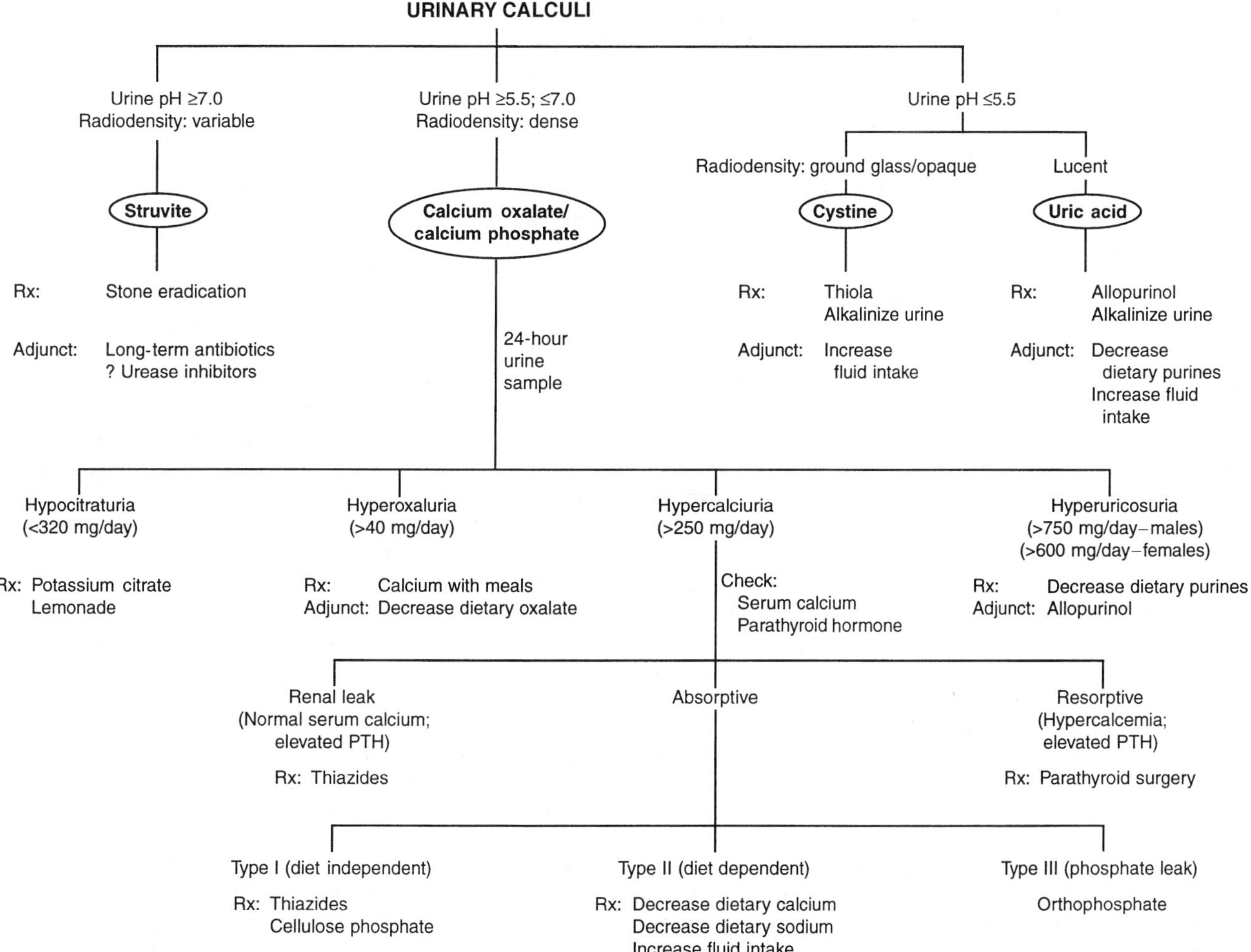

Figure 1. Decision tree for urinary stone disease.

usual anatomy in whom less invasive treatments have failed.

LONG-TERM MANAGEMENT

After the acute episode has resolved and the patient has passed a calculus or has had it surgically extracted, a thorough medical evaluation should be initiated. The stone should be sent for laboratory analysis. Serum levels of routine electrolytes, creatinine, calcium, phosphate, uric acid, and parathyroid hormone (PTH) should be obtained. A 24-hour urine collection should measure urine volume, pH, specific gravity, calcium, creatinine, citrate, oxalate, phosphate, uric acid, and sodium. Results of laboratory tests and stone analysis will guide subsequent medical therapy.

Medical Therapies

Calcium Urolithiasis

Stone analysis indicating calcium phosphate should raise suspicion of distal renal tubular acidosis (RTA) or primary hyperparathyroidism. Distal RTA can be confirmed by hypokalemia, low serum bicarbonate, and a fasting urinary pH of greater than 5.5. Hyperparathyroidism can be confirmed with increased PTH, increased serum calcium, and decreased serum phosphorus levels.

In approximately 75% of cases, stone analysis will reveal calcium oxalate. These stones develop owing to a variety of underlying metabolic defects, which are divided into hypercalciuric and normocalciuric states.

HYPERCALCIURIC STATES

Absorptive hypercalciuria is subclassified into three types: diet-independent (type I), diet-dependent (type II), and renal phosphate "leak" (type III). All three states are associated with hypercalciuria (defined as the presence of more than 250 mg of calcium in a 24-hour urine specimen). Type I patients have hypercalciuria during both low and high dietary calcium intake. Serum calcium is normal, and PTH is low or normal. Fasting urinary calcium is normal, but urine calcium levels increase with an oral calcium load. Treatment is usually effective with thiazide diuretics (hydrochlorothiazide, 50 mg twice daily). Oral cellulose phosphates may be used to bind calcium in the gut, rendering it insoluble, thus decreasing urinary calcium levels.

Type II absorptive hypercalciuria patients exhibit hypercalciuria only during periods of increased calcium dietary intake. Therapy is directed at decreasing dietary intake of calcium by 50%, sodium restriction, and hydration adequate to produce 2 liters of urine per day.

Type III absorptive hypercalciuria is characterized by high urinary phosphate levels due to a renal phosphate "leak." Serum phosphate concentration is usually less than 2.5 mg per dL. The hypophosphatemia results in increased levels of 1,25-dihydroxyvitamin D_3. This compound stimulates intestinal phosphate and calcium absorption and renal excretion of calcium. Type III hypercalciuria is treated by adding dietary phosphate in the form of neutral orthophosphate (250 mg three times a day) and titrating the dosage until urinary calcium levels normalize.

Resorptive hypercalciuria is due to primary hyperparathyroidism. Renal calculi can be the initial manifestation of this disorder. The hypersecretion of PTH results in bone resorption and increased intestinal absorption of calcium, leading to hypercalcemia, hypercalciuria, and hyperphosphaturia. Treatment of this disease is surgical removal of the parathyroid adenoma.

Renal phosphate leak hypercalciuria is characterized by impaired renal tubular absorption of filtered calcium. The reduced serum calcium stimulates production of PTH, leading to subsequent stimulation of 1,25-dihydroxyvitamin D_3. This results in normal serum calcium with normal or increased PTH levels and hypercalciuria. This is effectively treated over the long term with thiazides.

Hydrochlorothiazide will correct secondary hyperparathyroidism in all of the hypercalciuric metabolic states except resorptive hypercalciuria. This is a clinically useful method of differentiating secondary from primary hyperparathyroidism in patients presenting with urinary stone disease.

NORMOCALCIURIC STATES

When the 24-hour urine collection reveals normal calcium levels (less than 250 mg per day), one or more of three metabolic defects is responsible: hyperuricosuria, hypocitraturia, and hyperoxaluria.

Hyperuricosuria is found in up to 20% of patients with calcium oxalate stones. It is characterized by urinary uric acid levels greater than 750 mg per day in men and greater than 600 mg per day in women. It may be seen in patients with primary gout, myeloproliferative states, glycogen storage diseases, and malignancy. Purine overproduction more frequently occurs owing to dietary overindulgence. Monosodium urates may act as a nidus for precipitation of calcium oxalate owing to heterogeneous nucleation. Monosodium urates may also bind urinary inhibitors of calcium stone formation. Treatment involves limiting dietary purines; if this is unsuccessful, administration of allopurinol may be tried.

Hyperoxaluria is caused by three mechanisms: primary overproduction, dietary overindulgence, and increased intestinal absorption. The most common of these is increased absorption, also known as enteric hyperoxaluria. A variety of bowel disorders such as inflammatory bowel disease and short gut syndrome and the decreased absorption in patients who have undergone intestinal bypass may result in fat malabsorption. Fat saponifies dietary calcium and results in increased levels of free intestinal oxalate, which normally binds with calcium. Free oxalate is readily absorbed. A small increase in absorbed oxalate is more significant in stone formation than a small increase in absorbed calcium. Restricting dietary intake of oxalate-rich foods is usually unsuccessful. Effective treatment is directed at binding dietary oxalate with calcium supplements at mealtime. Mild cases will respond to intake of calcium-rich foods, such as milk and cheese, at mealtimes. More severe cases may require use of calcium-containing antacids at mealtimes.

Citrate is a potent inhibitor of calcium stone formation. Hypocitraturia has been noted in up to 40% of calcium stone formers, often in combination with other disorders. Patients with citrate levels of less than 320 mg per day should be treated with citrate supplements. The simplest and most palatable regimen for many patients is lemonade therapy. Patients are directed to add 4 ounces of lemon juice concentrate to one-half gallon of water and sweeten to taste. The lemonade is consumed over the course of the day. This treatment has resulted in significant increases in urinary citrate levels. For patients unable to consume the lemonade, supplementation with potassium citrate, 60 to 120 mEq per day in divided doses, is recommended.

Presence of Non–Calcium-Containing Stones

Uric acid stones account for about 10% of all cases of urolithiasis. Uric acid stones are relatively radiolucent but may contain variable amounts of calcium. Uric acid stones, in contrast to calcium stones, are treatable by dissolution with medical therapy. The dissociation constant of uric acid is 5.75; above this pH, the solubility increases rapidly. If a lucent calculus is noted radiographically, alkalinization therapy using potassium citrate is initiated to raise the urinary pH to 6.5 to 7.0. In addition, patients are encouraged to void more than 2 liters of urine per day and to decrease dietary purines. Progress with therapy can be monitored using ultrasound or noncontrast CT. Approximately 1 cm of uric acid stone seen on imaging studies can be dissolved in 4 to 6 weeks. Dissolution rapidly increases after performance of ESWL, as the stone surface area dramatically increases with fragmentation.

Patients with hyperuricosuria or hyperuricemia should receive allopurinol. Those with no serum or urinary uric acid excess should be treated with urinary alkalinization, such as administration of potassium citrate, to keep urinary pH at greater than 6.5.

Stones containing magnesium ammonium phosphate (struvite) or carbonate apatite are most commonly associated with infection. Struvite calculi occur only in the presence of urease-producing microorganisms, which cleave urea to ammonia, resulting in an alkaline urinary milieu. Precipitation of the struvite occurs in urine with a pH of greater than 7.19. *Proteus mirabilis* is the most common organism associated with these stones, but *Pseudomonas, Providencia,* staphylococci, *Serratia,* and *Mycoplasma* may also produce the urease responsible for stone formation. The key to therapy is complete stone removal. These stones frequently fill the renal collecting system with a "staghorn" configuration. The large stone size makes ESWL a poor choice for stone eradication; percutaneous nephrostolithotomy is often needed for complete stone removal. Antibiotic therapy will be unable to sterilize urine in the presence of residual calculi. Frequently, the extensive nature of the condition dictates that several percutaneous procedures, supplemented with ESWL, are needed for complete stone removal. After stone removal patients should be monitored closely for urinary tract infections and stone recurrence.

Cystine stones account for about 1% of cases of urolithiasis. Persons with cystinuria have an autosomal recessive disorder affecting the transport of dibasic amino acids. This results in high urinary levels of cystine, which is insoluble at normal urinary pH. The solubility of cystine increases rapidly above pH 7.5. Diagnosis of cystinuria is made on the basis of 24-hour urine analysis; most heterozygotes will excrete more than 200 mg of cystine per day.

The goal of therapy is to keep patients well hydrated with urine production at more than 2 liters per day and urine pH at 7.0 to 7.5, using an alkalizing agent such as potassium citrate. Specific therapy is also aimed at reducing urinary cystine levels to less than 100 mg per day, using agents that increase cystine solubility by creating a mixed disulfide. Penicillamine has been used in the past, but its association with frequent side effects, including gastrointestinal upset, nephrotic syndrome, dermatitis, and pancytopenia, has limited its usefulness. Tiopronin, i.e., α-mercaptopropionylglycine (Thiola), which also works by increasing disulfide bonds, has fewer side effects and is currently the drug of choice at a dose of 0.5 to 1 gram per day in divided doses.

Other Stones

Stones may be composed of a variety of other substances, including matrix, xanthine, triamterene, and indinavir. Indinavir calculi have recently been cited as a common complication of therapy directed at HIV infection with the protease inhibitor indinavir. Management of these calculi generally consists of temporary cessation of medication with aggressive hydration.

General Dietary Measures

Patients with stones often require dietary manipulation in addition to specific medical therapy. General guidelines include maintaining euvolemia with approximately 1.5 to 2 liters of urine output per day; there is little evidence to support the common recommendation of vigorous overhydration. In addition, table salt should be restricted to less than 2 grams per day, because sodium exacerbates hypercalciuria. Furthermore, a low-protein diet (protein intake of less than 65 grams per day) is recommended to prevent the metabolic acidosis with subsequent mobilization of calcium from bone that occurs after protein-rich meals.

CONCLUSION

Management of urinary stone disease is often frustrating for both the patient and the physician. A recurrence rate of up to 50% in 5 years is noted with no metabolic intervention. Although renal failure is rarely due to recurrent stone disease, the morbidity and inconvenience for patients are substantial. Many of these episodes can be prevented with a thorough metabolic work-up and directed therapy for specific defects.

Section 10

The Sexually Transmitted Diseases

CHANCROID

method of
DAVID H. MARTIN, M.D.
Louisiana State University Medical School
New Orleans, Louisiana

Chancroid, caused by the gram-negative bacillus *Haemophilus ducreyi,* may be the most important cause of genital ulcer disease worldwide. In the United States, the disease had nearly disappeared by the 1970s. However, beginning in the early 1980s, isolated outbreaks began to appear once again. The disease initially occurred primarily among migrant workers and was associated with door-to-door prostitution, but by the mid-1980s, the disease established itself endemically in a number of urban centers such as Dallas, the New York–Philadelphia metroplex, and Miami. Subsequently, the disease appeared in many other cities, especially in the South. In 1988, 5001 cases were reported to the Centers for Disease Control and Prevention (CDC) in Atlanta, Georgia. Epidemiologic research established that the rise in cases during the late 1980s and early 1990s was related to sexual behavior associated with crack cocaine abuse.

Since 1987, the number of reported cases has gradually declined to the point that the disease appears to have disappeared in many locations once again. Only 609 cases were reported to the CDC in 1995. The reasons for the decline in incidence are unclear because there is no evidence that crack cocaine use has diminished significantly. The important lesson learned in the last 10 years is that health care providers in the United States can never completely discount *H. ducreyi* as a cause of genital ulcer disease.

The major public health problem associated with chancroid is that it has been shown to be an important cofactor for the heterosexual transmission of the human immunodeficiency virus (HIV). The number of heterosexual HIV infections attributable to chancroid in the last 10 years is unknown but is likely to have been high.

Classically, chancroid presents as multiple, painful ulcers that have a purulent base and ragged, undermined borders. Because lesions are usually not indurated, they are often referred to in the older literature as "soft chancre." Fifty to 60% of men with chancroid will develop inguinal lymphadenopathy, which is usually unilateral. In a small proportion of cases, the inguinal node mass, or bubo, becomes fluctuant and may rupture, resulting in a draining abscess. Despite the distinctive features of "classic" chancroid, it is clear that there is considerable overlap among this disease, syphilis, and genital herpes, which makes accurate clinical diagnosis difficult.

For reasons that are not clear, the ratio of male to female chancroid cases ranges from 3:1 to 25:1. In part, this may be because internal lesions in women often go unnoticed, as is the case in primary syphilis. However, the male/female ratio for chancroid cases is higher than that for primary syphilis, suggesting that there may be other reasons for this phenomenon, such as an asymptomatic carrier state in women.

Laboratory confirmation of the diagnosis of chancroid is difficult because *H. ducreyi* has special in vitro growth requirements. Most clinical laboratories cannot successfully cultivate this slow-growing organism. New tests based on DNA amplification technology have been developed, and they appear to be more sensitive than culture. However, it appears that these tests will not become available commercially; they will be used by a few research laboratories to support epidemiologic studies. Therefore, in clinical practice, the diagnosis continues to be one of exclusion. Unfortunately, this approach is not helpful in guiding therapy at the time of the initial encounter with the patient, especially when darkfield microscopy is not available, as is often the case. Therefore, by necessity, treatment is empirical and should be guided by knowledge of the incidence of chancroid in a given area. A useful clue to the presence of the disease is the observation of primary syphilis "treatment failures" resulting from *Treponema pallidum* and *H. ducreyi* co-infection as well as from misdiagnosis of chancroid as syphilis. Another clue is an increased frequency of patients presenting to local acute care facilities for the treatment of painful inguinal buboes. If there is reason to suspect that *H. ducreyi* is present in a given community, then all genital ulcer cases not obviously caused by herpes simplex virus should be treated empirically for both syphilis and chancroid.

TREATMENT

Although increasing resistance to some of the older drugs used to treat chancroid has been observed in the last 10 years, there remain a number of drugs both old and new that have good activity against *H. ducreyi.* Ceftriaxone (Rocephin), 250 mg as a single intramuscular dose, is effective for both ulcers and buboes. The only drawbacks to this approach are the inconvenience of intramuscular administration and the relatively high cost of the drug.

As with ceftriaxone, there has been no evidence of development of erythromycin resistance among *H. ducreyi* strains worldwide. The standard dose of erythromycin is 500 mg orally four times daily for 7 days. One study has suggested that as little as 500 mg three times a day for 5 days may also be effective.

Sulfonamide resistance among *H. ducreyi* strains has steadily increased worldwide, and more recently, trimethoprim resistance has become a problem in both Thailand and Africa. At one time, a single high dose of trimethoprim/sulfamethoxazole (Bactrim, Septra) was widely used for chancroid. Whereas increased treatment failure rates were first reported with single-dose therapy, failures have been noted in the Far East and Africa with the multiple-dose regimens as well. Although in vivo and in vitro experience with trimethoprim-sulfamethoxazole in the United States is limited, this drug should probably not be used any longer in view of the availability of effective alternatives.

A number of the more recently developed broad-spectrum oral antibiotics have promise in the therapy for chancroid. Among the quinolones available in the United States, ciprofloxacin (Cipro) has been studied most extensively. Studies have shown that a single 500-mg dose is effective, although a failure rate of 26% was reported in HIV-positive Rwandan patients. In the United States, 500 mg twice daily for 3 days is the currently recommended dose. Fleroxacin, a newer quinolone not available in the United States, has also been found to cure most cases when it is given as a single dose.

Almost all *H. ducreyi* strains produce β-lactamase and therefore are resistant to amoxicillin alone, but amoxicillin-clavulanate (Augmentin), in a dose of 500 mg of amoxicillin plus 125 mg of clavulanate three times daily by mouth for 7 days, is effective. Finally, studies in both Africa and the United States have shown that cure rates for the new macrolide azithromycin (Zithromax) given as a single 1-gram oral dose* are equal to those for intramuscular ceftriaxone. Azithromycin is available in a 1-gram powdered formulation specifically designed for treating sexually transmitted diseases. This dose form is less expensive than four 250-mg capsules.

Studies from Kenya have suggested that chancroid in HIV-infected individuals is more difficult to treat than those without HIV infection. Treatment failure rates of 20 to 50% have been reported among these patients after single doses of a number of the drugs discussed, although this experience has not been reproduced in South Africa or in Rwanda. Thus, some experts believe that patients with chancroid who are known to be HIV-infected should be treated with one of the multiple-dose regimens. Clearly, HIV-infected patients require close follow-up for evidence of an appropriate therapeutic response regardless of the therapeutic regimen employed.

Given the difficulty of clinically distinguishing between syphilis and chancroid, and because the two diseases may coexist in 10 to 20% of cases, patients suspected of having chancroid who have not had a negative result on darkfield examination should also receive treatment for primary syphilis unless adequate follow-up can be ensured. An important point to remember is that all recent sexual contacts of patients suspected of having chancroid should receive treatment as well.

*Not FDA approved for this indication.

Fluctuant buboes should be drained to prevent rupture. Insertion of an 18-gauge needle into the center of the lesion through normal skin at the margin of inflammation is the simplest approach. However, patients may require one or more repeated aspirations. Treatment by incision and drainage is also acceptable, as clearly demonstrated by a randomized study comparing this approach with needle aspiration. Large node masses may become fluctuant after treatment with effective antibiotics. This development should not be taken as evidence of treatment failure, because the pus aspirated from these lesions is usually sterile.

GONORRHEA

method of
JOHN S. MORAN, M.D., M.P.H.
Centers for Disease Control and Prevention
Atlanta, Georgia

Gonorrhea is the second most frequently reported infectious disease in the United States; only *Chlamydia trachomatis* infection is reported more often. It is primarily a disease of adolescence and young adulthood, with 60% of reported infections occurring among persons 15 to 24 years of age. Rates peak among females in the 15- to 19-year age group at 757 per 100,000 population and among men in the 20- to 24-year age group at 522 per 100,000. Overall incidence fell by 73% during the past 21 years to 125 per 100,000 population in 1996. As its incidence has fallen, gonorrhea has become less widespread in the United States and is now distributed more focally, with most infections occurring in poor communities.

Gonorrhea control has received new attention in recent years as evidence mounts that human immunodeficiency virus (HIV) transmission may be facilitated by gonococcal infection. One landmark study in Africa showed a 40% reduction in the incidence of HIV infection in communities offered enhanced sexually transmitted disease (STD) treatment services; another showed a marked decrease in HIV shedding in men treated for gonococcal urethritis. This evidence is strong enough to make gonorrhea control an important strategy for reducing HIV transmission in areas where both infections are prevalent.

CLINICAL MANIFESTATIONS

Neisseria gonorrhoeae infects mucosal surfaces to which it is spread by direct contact or fresh secretions. Genital infection is almost always a result of sexual contact; primary infection of other sites (e.g., the eye) most often occurs during birth.

Men are more likely to be symptomatic than women but are less likely to suffer sequelae. Among men, uncomplicated urethritis is the most common manifestation, with dysuria and urethral discharge developing 2 to 3 days after infection. Symptoms are severe enough and common enough to cause most affected men to seek treatment, but an estimated 1 to 3% remain asymptomatic.

Women are especially susceptible to complications because early infection often goes unrecognized. In women, the most common site of primary infection is the endocervix, causing a cervicitis that produces symptoms (e.g., vaginal discharge, lower abdominal discomfort, dyspareunia) only half the time. Like symptoms, signs of infection are often absent. Signs of gonococcal cervicitis include cervical edema, erythema, friability, and mucopurulent discharge. The frequent lack of readily discernible signs or symptoms of infection of the cervix means that many infections go unrecognized and untreated. In an estimated 10 to 20% of cases, infection spreads to the fallopian tubes and ovaries, causing pelvic inflammatory disease (PID). PID, like cervicitis, may be symptomatic or silent. Even when promptly treated, PID can result in tubal scarring with an increased risk of subsequent subfertility and ectopic pregnancy.

Women as well as men may develop gonococcal urethritis, and either sex may suffer rectal infection. Among men, rectal infection is a result of penetration by an infected penis and is followed by symptomatic proctitis in half of the cases. Symptoms are mucopurulent discharge, tenesmus, and constipation. Among women, rectal infection is found in 5 to 10% of those with cervical infection and is assumed to be due most commonly to contamination by fluids from the introitus. Rectal infection is usually asymptomatic among women.

Gonococcal infection of the pharynx results from oral exposure to infected genitalia, usually to an infected penis. Pharyngeal infection is often asymptomatic, but affected persons may present with manifestations of pharyngitis indistinguishable from pharyngitis caused by more banal organisms.

Infection of the eye occurs most often at birth. Among older children and adults, most eye infections are due to sexual exposure, poor hygiene, or the home medicinal use of contaminated urine.

In a few patients (less than 0.5%), gonococci spread from the primary site of infection through the bloodstream to cause the syndrome of disseminated gonococcal infection (DGI). Characteristic findings in DGI are fever, monoarticular or oligoarticular septic arthritis, pustular rash, arthralgia, and tenosynovitis. Very rarely the meninges or the endocardium may become infected.

DIAGNOSIS

Gonococcal urethritis in males does not usually pose a diagnostic challenge; infections elsewhere often do. Urethral infection classically causes marked dysuria with a purulent discharge that may stain the underclothing. Less typically, signs and symptoms are more mild and indistinguishable from the typical presentation of chlamydial urethritis. In all such cases, gonorrhea can be ruled in or ruled out with reasonable confidence by microscopy using Gram's stain, which has greater than 90% sensitivity and specificity for symptomatic urethritis in men. However, no sign, symptom, or combination of signs and symptoms can be used to reliably distinguish between women with sexually transmitted cervicitis (i.e., cervicitis caused by *N. gonorrhoeae* or *C. trachomatis* or both) and those without. Microscopy adds little because it is only 30 to 50% sensitive for detecting gonococci and useless for detecting chlamydial organisms. It is, however, highly specific for gonorrhea: the finding of gram-negative intracellular diplococci in a smear of cervical secretions is 90% specific for gonococcal infection.

Definitive diagnosis at both genital and extragenital sites is usually best done by culture on selective media followed by specific tests for *N. gonorrhoeae*. Culture is also useful for screening asymptomatic persons for gonococcal infection. Screening is recommended for certain high-risk populations (e.g., young women attending family planning or prenatal clinics in communities in which gonorrhea prevalence is high). For screening and for diagnosis of urogenital infection, alternative, nonculture methods including DNA probe, ligase chain reaction, and polymerase chain reaction have become available. They are generally more expensive than culture but can be much more sensitive when the viability of specimens taken for culture cannot be preserved during transport. Nonculture methods should not be used for specimens from sites for which they have not been approved.

TREATMENT

Criteria for Selecting Treatment Regimen in Uncomplicated Infections

Despite the notorious ability of gonococci to develop resistance to antibiotics, numerous safe and effective therapeutic choices remain. Choosing an appropriate regimen requires attention to the following criteria:

1. *One hundred percent efficacy.* To prevent complications in infected persons, to interrupt transmission, and to obviate the need for follow-up cultures, only regimens proven to be close to 100% effective in clinical trials should be used. To ensure that the treatment is as effective in clinical use as in trials, the following precautions are important:
   a. Minimizing the danger of noncompliance. Fortunately, compliance can be assured by using a single-dose antibiotic regimen so that therapy can be completed during the initial visit.
   b. Avoiding treatment failure due to antibiotic resistance. Routine susceptibility testing of *N. gonorrhoeae* isolates is performed by few clinical laboratories, so clinicians rarely know the susceptibility of the strain they are treating. To choose appropriate antibiotic regimens, they must be aware of patterns of resistance in the community. The U.S. Public Health Service maintains a surveillance network to monitor the antimicrobial susceptibility of *N. gonorrhoeae* in about 25 U.S. cities. This system tests isolates from more than 1% of all gonococcal infections reported among males in the United States. With this surveillance system it is possible to monitor trends in antimicrobial susceptibility and to predict clinical treatment failure before it becomes widespread. Data from this system are used by the Public Health Service in formulating its STD treatment recommendations.
2. *Co-treatment of concurrent chlamydial infection.* Treating gonorrhea patients presumptively for chlamydial infection has been recommended since it was observed in the 1980s that co-infection was common. At that time, testing for *Chlamydia* was

often unavailable, expensive, time-consuming, and not highly sensitive; co-treatment with a tetracycline was safe and inexpensive. Since then, testing for *Chlamydia* has become more widely available, more affordable, quicker, and more sensitive, and *Chlamydia* prevalence has dropped in some populations. Nevertheless, *Chlamydia* is still found among 10 to 30% of patients with gonorrhea in many clinics, leading most experts and the Public Health Service to continue to recommend routine co-treatment.

Routine co-treatment with an antibiotic regimen effective against *Chlamydia* has two other theoretical benefits: (1) it may inhibit the development of antibiotic resistance among gonococci because the recommended antichlamydial regimens are highly active against more than 90% of gonococcal strains circulating in the United States; and (2) the treatment may cure unrecognized incubating syphilis (this was a much greater concern during the syphilis epidemic of 1990 than today, when incubating syphilis is rare among gonorrhea patients).

Specific Therapies

Uncomplicated Urogenital and Rectal Infections

The following recommendations for the treatment of uncomplicated gonococcal infections are based on a systematic review of the results of clinical trials conducted by the Centers for Disease Control and Prevention (CDC), with input from practicing physicians (Table 1). Criteria for recommendation are safety and effectiveness. To be recommended for the treatment of urogenital and rectal infections, a regimen must have been proved to be at least 95% effective in eradicating urogenital and rectal infections.

Ceftriaxone (Rocephin), in a dose of 125 mg, cured 99.1% of evaluable infections in clinical trials. Its disadvantage is that it must be given by injection. Cefixime (Suprax), 400 mg, is an oral alternative to ceftriaxone for the treatment of uncomplicated infections; it has cured 97.1% of evaluable urogenital and rectal infections. Two oral fluoroquinolone regimens are also recommended: ciprofloxacin (Cipro), 500 mg, which has cured 99.8% of urogenital and rectal infections in published studies, and ofloxacin (Floxin), 400 mg, which has cured 98.4%.

TABLE 1. **Treatment of Uncomplicated Urogenital and Rectal Gonorrhea in Adults and Adolescents**

Ceftriaxone (Rocephin), 125 mg IM in a single dose OR
Cefixime (Suprax), 400 mg PO in a single dose OR
Ciprofloxacin (Cipro), 500 mg PO in a single dose OR
Ofloxacin (Floxin), 400 mg PO in a single dose
PLUS
Doxycycline (Vibramycin), 100 mg PO twice daily for 7 days OR
Azithromycin (Zithromax), 1 gm PO in a single dose

Abbreviations: IM = intramuscularly; PO = by mouth.

Other third-generation cephalosporin and fluoroquinolone regimens have also been shown to be safe and effective and are listed as alternatives by the CDC. However, none has any advantage over the four more highly recommended regimens listed previously.

Gonococcal therapy should include presumptive treatment for chlamydial infection unless the patient is known to be free of chlamydial infection. For patients who can take neither doxycycline (Vibramycin) nor azithromycin (Zithromax), erythromycin may be substituted (e.g., erythromycin base, 500 mg by mouth four times daily for 7 days).

Pharyngeal Infections

Pharyngeal infections are more difficult to cure and are less well studied than urogenital or rectal infections. Few regimens have been proved to be more than 80% effective against them. Recommended regimens are ceftriaxone, 125 mg, which has cured 93.7% in clinical trials, and ciprofloxacin, 500 mg, which has cured 97.2%. Routine treatment with a regimen effective against *C. trachomatis* is advisable for the aforementioned reasons, although the prevalence of chlamydial infection is lower among homosexual men with gonorrhea than it is among heterosexuals.

Disseminated Gonococcal Infection

No studies of the treatment of DGI have been published in more than 10 years; the CDC's treatment recommendations are based on expert opinion. The CDC recommends ceftriaxone, 1 gram intramuscularly (IM) or intravenously (IV) every 24 hours, continued for 24 to 48 hours after symptomatic improvement begins, followed by cefixime, 400 mg by mouth twice daily, or ciprofloxacin, 500 mg by mouth twice daily, or ofloxacin, 400 mg by mouth twice daily, to complete 7 days of therapy. Treatment for chlamydial infection should be given unless testing rules out infection. Treatment failures have not been reported.

Special Situations

Gonorrhea in Pregnancy. Because fluoroquinolones and tetracyclines are contraindicated in pregnancy, a cephalosporin regimen or spectinomycin (Trobicin) in a single 2-gram intramuscular injection should be given with either azithromycin (Zithromax) or erythromycin to cover chlamydial infection unless testing rules it out. Routes and dosages are the same as for men and nonpregnant women.

Gonorrhea in HIV-Infected Persons. Antimicrobial regimens effective against uncomplicated gonococcal infections in HIV-negative persons appear to be equally efficacious in HIV-positive persons, so any of the foregoing regimens can be used in patients with HIV infection. However, special care must be taken to ensure that these patients are appropriately educated and counseled, because acquisition of a gonococcal infection is evidence of the recent practice of "unsafe sex."

Imported Gonorrhea. Quinolone-resistant strains of *N. gonorrhoeae* are becoming common in some Asian countries, and sporadic cases have been reported in several countries in Europe as well as in the United States and Canada. It would therefore be prudent to give therapy with a cephalosporin or with spectinomycin to persons who may have been infected by a person who was infected in Asia.

Allergy. Persons who can tolerate neither cephalosporins nor quinolones should receive therapy with spectinomycin.

PUBLIC HEALTH MANAGEMENT ISSUES

Referral of Sex Partners. Patients found to be infected with *N. gonorrhoeae* should be strongly encouraged to refer their recent (over the past 30 days) sex partners for examination and treatment. If they are reluctant to do so, the local health department may be able to assist by notifying the partner in confidence without naming the patient. Partners presenting for examination should generally be presumed to be infected and treated for gonorrhea on the spot. They should also be examined and tested for gonorrhea and other STDs. The purpose of testing sex partners for gonorrhea just before they are presumptively treated is to guide further partner notification efforts.

Reporting. Gonorrhea is reportable in all states. Clinicians should not assume that reports from laboratories make reports from clinicians superfluous.

Other STDs. Infection with one STD is prima facie evidence of a high risk of exposure to other STDs. Therefore, all patients who contract gonorrhea should be offered screening for other STDs including chlamydial infection, syphilis, and HIV infection.

Counseling. As its prevalence in the general population has declined, gonococcal infection has become a better marker for unprotected sexual contact with a member of a population potentially at risk of HIV infection. Any patient diagnosed as having gonorrhea must be counseled about his or her risk of HIV infection and other STDs and must be educated about practical means that can be used to lower that risk.

NONGONOCOCCAL URETHRITIS

method of
HEATHER SELMAN, M.D., and
PHILIP HANNO, M.D.
Temple University Hospital
Philadelphia, Pennsylvania

Urethritis is defined as an inflammation of the urethra, usually manifested by burning on urination, urethral discomfort or itching, meatal erythema, and mucoid or purulent urethral discharge. In some cases, the presence of urethral discharge may be evident only before the first morning void as meatal crusting or staining of the underwear. Asymptomatic infections occur as well. Urethritis is one of the most common problems in ambulatory medicine. Risk factors include unprotected intercourse with multiple sexual partners and change of sexual partners within 3 months. Sexual partners are often not examined and treated, because nongonococcal infections are infrequently reported to health authorities. For this reason, the incidence of nongonococcal urethritis (NGU) continues to rise.

NGU urethritis is defined as urethral inflammation not caused by *Neisseria gonorrhoeae.* Causes in men include infections with *Chlamydia trachomatis* in 23 to 55% of patients, *Ureaplasma urealyticum* in 20 to 40%, and *Trichomonas vaginalis* in 2 to 5%. Symptoms usually appear between 1 and 5 weeks after unprotected intercourse with a partner infected with these organisms. Herpes simplex virus and human papillomavirus have been implicated as well, as has yeast. Postgonococcal urethritis is defined as NGU occurring after effective treatment for gonococcal urethritis while simultaneous infection with *C. trachomatis* has been missed. A noninfectious form of urethritis can result from foreign bodies, soaps, shampoos, vaginal douches, spermicidal agents, catheters, urethral instrumentation, and manual stimulation. A cause is not always found.

NGU may be seen in the systemic diseases Stevens-Johnson syndrome and Wegener's granulomatosis. Reiter's syndrome, with arthritis and uveitis, follows 1 to 4% of cases of NGU. Epididymitis is another possible complication. Transmission of the human immunodeficiency virus (HIV) is increased two- to fivefold in association with other sexually transmitted diseases, and testing for HIV infection and syphilis should be recommended to patients with NGU. Female partners of patients with chlamydial infections are at risk for pelvic inflammatory disease, with possible subsequent ectopic pregnancies or infertility secondary to fallopian tube scarring.

Urethritis in women may be caused by *N. gonorrhoeae* or *C. trachomatis.* Although a urethral discharge is not often present in women, dysuria may occur. The physician will often incorrectly presume the presence of a bladder infection. Urinalysis may show pyuria, but cultures for routine urinary pathogens will be negative.

DIAGNOSIS

NGU is diagnosed by the presence of 5 or more polymorphonuclear leukocytes per oil immersion field on a gram-stained smear of the urethral discharge, an intraurethral swab specimen, or the first 10 mL of the patient's voided urine. The diagnosis of infectious urethritis is made by positive culture of these samples, although sampling of the urethral epithelium specifically (from 2 to 4 mm inside the urethra) must be performed to diagnose chlamydial infection. Preliminary results become available within 2 to 3 days. The inflammation is shown to be localized to the urethra by the presence of a significantly greater number of white blood cells in the first voided urine sample compared with a midstream urine specimen or that obtained after prostatic massage. The patient should be examined in the morning before voiding if urethral inflammation is suspected but cannot be detected.

TREATMENT REGIMENS

Both the patient and any sexual partners should receive treatment. Sexual partners should be treated if they were last exposed to the symptomatic patient within 30 days of the onset of symptoms or within 60 days of diagnosis in the asymptomatic patient. The most recent sexual partner should be treated if the last sexual intercourse preceded these times. Patients and partners should abstain from sexual intercourse during treatment and until both are free of symptoms and signs.

Any of the following drugs can be used as a first-line agent: doxycycline, 100 mg twice a day (bid) by mouth for 7 days, or azithromycin (Zithromax), 1 gram by mouth in a single dose, or tetracycline, 500 mg by mouth four times daily for 7 days. As alternative agents, erythromycin ethylsuccinate, 800 mg by mouth four times daily for 7 days (or 400 mg four times daily for 14 days); erythromycin base, 500 mg by mouth four times daily for 7 days (or 250 mg by mouth four times daily for 14 days); or ofloxacin (Floxin), 300 mg by mouth twice daily for 7 days, may be used. Erythromycin is the agent of choice during pregnancy and lactation. Treatment recommendations remain the same for patients with HIV infection.

FOLLOW-UP CARE

Patients should return if their symptoms persist or recur after therapy. They should be re-treated with the original regimen if they did not comply initially or if they were reinfected by an untreated sex partner. Otherwise, a wet mount of a urethral swab should be performed and the specimen sent for culture for *T. vaginalis.* If results are positive, definitive treatment consists of metronidazole (Flagyl), 2 grams by mouth in a single dose, or clotrimazole suppositories, 100 mg per vagina daily for 2 weeks during pregnancy. If results are negative, an alternative regimen is used for 14 days to treat possible infection with tetracycline-resistant *U. urealyticum,* which occurs in 6 to 10% of cases. Evaluation of sexual partners may help identify an underlying infectious cause of the urethritis.

Physical examination and a diminished urinary flow rate may suggest clinically significant structural abnormalities as the cause of chronic urethritis in approximately 10% of patients. Such abnormalities can be further evaluated by endoscopy of the lower urinary tract. They include urethral strictures, urethral diverticula, meatal stenosis, condyloma, foreign bodies, and periurethral abscesses. Bacteriuria and prostatitis may also cause chronic urethritis and may necessitate longer courses of therapy (4 to 6 weeks).

GRANULOMA INGUINALE
(Donovanosis)

method of
YEHUDI M. FELMAN, M.D.
State University of New York Health Science Center at Brooklyn College of Medicine
Brooklyn, New York

Granuloma inguinale is a chronic, mildly communicable, slowly progressive granulomatous anogenital infection caused by a gram-negative rod, *Calymmatobacterium granulomatis.* It is rare in the United States but endemic in Papua New Guinea, the Caribbean, and parts of Africa and Southeast Asia. The incubation period ranges from 8 to 80 days. The primary lesions are red papules, which then enlarge to form painless indurated ulcers or hypertrophic or verrucous lesions elevated above the skin surface; the inguinal and perianal areas are most often involved, both by direct extension and by autoinoculation. Often lesions become granulomatous and coalesce, forming elevated borders. Granuloma inguinale does not produce inguinal adenopathy (buboes).

Diagnosis is made by microscopic examination of crush preparations, obtained by punch biopsy of the margins of active lesions, and stained with Wright's or Giemsa stain. The *C. granulomatis* organism, found in mononuclear cells, is bright red and resembles a closed safety pin. No reliable culture or serologic tests are available.

TREATMENT

The treatment of choice is administration of doxycycline (Vibramycin), 100 mg orally (PO) twice a day for 21 days. I have occasionally treated severe or recalcitrant cases with doxycycline 300 mg daily*; liver function should be monitored with this dose. Other recommended drugs include trimethoprim-sulfamethoxazole (Bactrim DS), 180 mg of trimethoprim and 800 mg of sulfamethoxazole, PO twice a day for 21 days; minocycline, 100 mg PO twice a day for 21 days; and erythromycin,* 500 mg PO four times a day for 21 days (this drug is somewhat less effective but is useful in pregnant women). Patients often require treatment for up to 6 weeks to obtain complete resolution of the infection. Scarring often remains. Azithromycin† (Zithromax) has been shown to be helpful when given in a dose of 500 mg daily for 2 weeks.* Ceftriaxone† (Rocephin), 1 gram given intramuscularly daily for 2 weeks, has been shown to be effective in Australia.

*Exceeds dosage recommended by the manufacturer.
†Not FDA approved for this indication.

LYMPHOGRANULOMA VENEREUM

method of
YEHUDI M. FELMAN, M.D.
State University of New York Health Science Center at Brooklyn College of Medicine
Brooklyn, New York

Lymphogranuloma venereum is a systemic sexually transmitted disease that is uncommon in the United

States. The incidence is greatest in Southeast Asia, Africa, Central and South America, and the Caribbean. It is caused by *Chlamydia trachomatis* serovars L-1, L-2, and L-3.

The primary lesion, a small painless papule, appears within 10 to 30 days of exposure, but only 10% of patients have such a lesion at presentation, as it heals quickly. The second stage of the disease, occurring 2 to 6 weeks later, consists of painful inguinal lymphadenopathy, usually unilateral. Lymphadenopathy occurring both above and below the inguinal ligament produces the "sign of the groove," seen in approximately one third of all patients. Acute lymphogranuloma venereum is often associated with fever and leukocytosis. Late complications include strictures and fistulas involving the penis, urethra, and rectum, and elephantiasis and ulcerations of the genitalia (esthiomene).

Diagnosis is made in the appropriate clinical setting by a complement fixation antibody titer of greater than 1:64.

TREATMENT

Treatment consists of oral administration of either tetracycline, 500 mg four times a day for 21 days; doxycycline (Vibramycin), 100 mg twice daily for 21 days; trimethoprim-sulfamethoxazole (Bactrim DS),* 160 mg of trimethoprim and 800 mg of sulfamethoxazole, twice daily for 21 days; minocycline (Minocin), 100 mg twice a day for 21 days; or erythromycin, 500 mg four times daily for 21 days (a good choice for pregnant women). Azithromycin* (Zithromax), although effective in other chlamydial infections such as nongonococcal urethritis, has not been shown to be effective in lymphogranuloma venereum. Buboes requiring surgical treatment should be aspirated, rather than excised and drained, to avoid fistula formation.

SYPHILIS

method of
MICHAEL F. REIN, M.D.
University of Virginia Health Sciences Center
Charlottesville, Virginia

There is no evidence that the spirochete of syphilis has become resistant to penicillin. Virulent *Treponema pallidum* is killed at the maximum rate by concentrations of penicillin G as low as 0.1 μg per mL. Penicillin G remains the treatment of choice for all forms and stages of syphilis in patients who are not allergic to the drug. Clinical and laboratory data support the value of relatively long duration therapy for the successful treatment of syphilis.

CONTACTS TO INFECTIOUS SYPHILIS

One third to one half of the sexual partners of patients with primary or secondary syphilis will contract the infection. Clinical and serologic evidence of infection may develop as late as 90 days after exposure, although it usually becomes manifest by about 21 days, and patients exposed during the previous 90 days should be treated as if they had early syphilis. Treating the patient before the development of lesions prevents spread of infection to other sexual partners, and adequate treatment given before a patient's nontreponemal serologic test becomes reactive usually prevents seroreactivity.

Treatment of gonococcal or chlamydial infection with a standard regimen, other than with a fluoroquinolone, may mask the signs of syphilis without curing the infection. Treatment of gonococcal or chlamydial infection with a fluoroquinolone has no effect on incubating syphilis.

EARLY SYPHILIS

For therapeutic and epidemiologic purposes, early syphilis is defined as primary or secondary syphilis or latent syphilis of less than 1 year's duration. This diagnosis can be made on clinical grounds, by a nonreactive serologic test within the last year, or by finding early syphilis in a current sexual partner.

The regimen of choice, because of its efficacy and convenience, is benzathine penicillin G (Bicillin, Permapen), 2.4 million units by intramuscular injection.

Patients allergic to penicillin may be treated with doxycycline (Doxy, Doryx, Vibramycin), 100 mg twice daily by mouth for 15 days. Doxycycline should be taken with meals but not with antacids that contain divalent cations. One can use an older regimen, tetracycline hydrochloride (Achromycin, Panmycin, Robitet, Sumycin, Tetralan), 500 mg four times daily by mouth for 15 days, but patients must be cautioned to take the drug on an empty stomach (at least 1 hour before or 2 hours after eating) and not with milk or antacids.

Patients who are allergic to penicillin for whom tetracycline is also contraindicated (late pregnancy, hypersensitivity, gastrointestinal intolerance) and whose penicillin allergy is not of the immediate type may be treated with ceftriaxone (Rocephin), 250 mg intramuscularly daily for 10 days. Treatment of patients with immediate hypersensitivity to the β-lactams and who cannot tolerate tetracyclines is controversial. Their history of penicillin allergy should be evaluated carefully, and these patients should be managed in consultation with an expert; desensitization may be required. Unfortunately, treponemal resistance to erythromycin has been documented and renders the drug unreliable.

More than half the patients treated for early syphilis experience a Jarisch-Herxheimer reaction. Usually beginning within 6 hours of treatment, the reaction consists of fever, transient exacerbation of skin lesions and adenopathy, occasional arthralgias, and, rarely, transient hypotension. The reaction is usually mild and abates within 24 hours. It can be managed with an antipyretic and reassurance.

*Not FDA approved for this indication.

LATE LATENT, CARDIOVASCULAR, AND LATE BENIGN SYPHILIS

It is generally held that syphilis of longer duration requires therapy of longer duration. This may be because more spirochetes are present, they are reproducing more slowly, or they may be residing in microenvironments relatively protected from antibiotics. Antibiotics often fail to reverse the pathology of cardiovascular syphilis.

From the standpoint of efficacy and convenience, the regimen of choice is benzathine penicillin G, 2.4 million units intramuscularly at each of three weekly visits. Far less acceptable to patients is procaine penicillin G (Pfizerpen-AS, Wycillin), 600,000 units intramuscularly, administered daily for 15 days.

No published clinical data adequately document the efficacy of drugs other than penicillin for syphilis of more than 1 year's duration. Thus, a history of penicillin allergy should be carefully established before alternatives to penicillin are used. In this setting, skin testing for immediate hypersensitivity to penicillin may be particularly useful. Patients allergic to penicillin might be treated with doxycycline, 100 mg twice daily by mouth for 30 days. The drug should be taken with meals but should not be taken with antacids.

Neurologically asymptomatic patients with syphilis of undetermined duration should undergo an examination of the cerebrospinal fluid (CSF) to rule out asymptomatic neurosyphilis if they have serologic evidence of treatment failure with a previous regimen (see later), other clinical evidence of active syphilis (e.g., aortitis), or a positive human immunodeficiency virus (HIV) antibody test.

SYMPTOMATIC OR ASYMPTOMATIC NEUROSYPHILIS

Optimal therapy for syphilis of the central nervous system is controversial. Published data on the efficacy of benzathine penicillin G are limited. Many patients treated with benzathine penicillin G have undetectable penicillin levels in CSF, and there are anecdotal reports of patients who failed to respond to benzathine penicillin G but who apparently responded to subsequent treatment with higher dose regimens.

The treatment of choice for patients with documented neurosyphilis is crystalline penicillin G (potassium or sodium), 20 million units intravenously per 24 hours by continuous infusion or in divided doses every 3 to 4 hours for 15 days.

Alternatively, one might administer procaine penicillin G, 2.4 million units intramuscularly daily for 15 days along with probenecid, 500 mg by mouth four times daily.

The treatment of neurosyphilis with drugs other than penicillin is empirical. Patients whose allergy does not involve anaphylaxis and who have negative penicillin skin tests might be treated with ceftriaxone, 2 grams intravenously every 24 hours for 15 days. The patient with immediate hypersensitivity to the β-lactams is a major therapeutic problem, and desensitization is probably required. The neurosyphilitic who has had an anaphylactic reaction to penicillin and who cannot be desensitized, might, on theoretical grounds, be treated with chloramphenicol (Chloromycetin), 500 mg orally four times daily for 30 days. Chloramphenicol penetrates well into the central nervous system, but the drug has been associated with fatal aplastic anemia, and hematologic parameters should be followed closely. Alternatively, but with very few supporting data, one might consider the administration of doxycycline, 200 mg twice daily by mouth for 30 days. Careful clinical and laboratory follow-up is crucial in the post-treatment management of neurosyphilis. Antibiotic therapy often fails to reverse the pathology of neurosyphilis.

SYPHILIS IN PREGNANCY

The pregnant woman should be treated with a penicillin regimen appropriate to her stage of syphilis. Such regimens are highly effective in preventing the stigmata of congenital syphilis in the infant. The old teaching that the fetus was protected against infection until 16 weeks of gestation is incorrect.

Because the efficacy of nonpenicillin drugs in preventing congenital syphilis is not adequately established, careful documentation of penicillin allergy in pregnant women is important. A pregnant woman who is allergic to penicillin and whose allergy is not manifested by anaphylaxis can be treated with ceftriaxone in doses appropriate to her stage of syphilis. The pregnant woman with immediate hypersensitivity to the β-lactam antibiotics is a candidate for careful desensitization. The Jarisch-Herxheimer reaction can precipitate labor.

Pregnant women who have been treated for syphilis should have monthly quantitative nontreponemal serologic tests for the remainder of the current pregnancy. Women showing a fourfold rise in titer should be retreated. After delivery, follow-up is the same as that for nonpregnant patients.

FOLLOW-UP

Adequate therapy for any stage of syphilis is suggested by a fourfold drop in the titer of a quantitative nontreponemal test (Venereal Disease Research Laboratory [VDRL] test, rapid plasma reagin [RPR] test, automated reagin test [ART], reagin screen test [RST], toluidine red unheated serum test [TRUST], unheated serum reagin [USR] test) for syphilis. Patients treated for syphilis should return for nontreponemal serologic tests every 3 months until a fourfold drop in the titer is observed. Failure of the titer to drop fourfold by 6 months after adequate therapy is unusual (except in neurosyphilis) and mandates careful re-evaluation. Thereafter, patients should return for serologic testing every 6 months until the quantitative nontreponemal test has become nonreactive or the titer has remained stable for 12 months.

TABLE 1. **Percentage of Patients Becoming Seronegative at Intervals After Adequate Treatment for Early Syphilis**

Stage of Syphilis	Serologic Test	12 Months	24 Months
Primary	VDRL	75	97
	RPR	44	60
	MHA-TP	8	9
	FTA-ABS	11	15
Secondary	VDRL	40	75
	RPR	22	42
Early latent	RPR	13	13

Abbreviations: VDRL = Venereal Disease Research Laboratory; RPR = rapid plasma reagin; MHA-TP = microhemagglutination assay— *Treponema pallidum*; FTA-ABS = fluorescent treponemal antibody absorption.

Documentation of the patient's lowest post-treatment titer is important, because a subsequent fourfold rise strongly suggests relapse or reinfection. The same nontreponemal test must be used in following a patient's course. Titers obtained with the RPR test and the ART are frequently higher than those obtained with the VDRL test, and comparing results from different tests may be confusing. The relative sensitivities of some of the newer nontreponemal tests have not been well defined, especially in late syphilis, and direct comparison of titers across tests may also be misleading.

After adequate treatment for primary syphilis, some patients achieve seronegativity with the nontreponemal tests, and very few eventually become seronegative with the treponemal tests (Table 1).

If initially manifesting a pleocytosis, the CSF should be examined every 6 months after completion of therapy for syphilis until it returns to normal. If the CSF cell count has not decreased after 6 months or returned to normal after 2 years, retreatment should be considered. After adequate treatment, 60 to 80% of patients no longer show CSF pleocytosis within 3 months. CSF protein levels usually return to normal within 6 months, and the VDRL titer in CSF generally shows a fourfold drop within 6 months. Patients treated for neurosyphilis should be followed for several years.

SYPHILIS AND HIV INFECTION

The coprevalence of syphilis and HIV infection is high. A diagnosis of syphilis obligates testing for HIV infection. Patients with early syphilis should be retested for HIV about 3 months later. The management of syphilis in the presence of HIV infection is controversial because of limited experience. Coincident infection may make the serodiagnosis of syphilis problematic, may increase the frequency and rate of progression to neurosyphilis, and may make therapy more difficult. Approaches vary widely among experts.

The recommended treatment of early syphilis in patients with HIV infection is the same as for other patients. Limited data suggest a higher rate of treatment failure, and careful follow-up is therefore critical. It is our practice to examine CSF in patients with any stage of syphilis and HIV infection, but it must be remembered that the spinal fluid formula in neurosyphilis may be identical to that in HIV infection. A reactive CSF VDRL mandates treatment for neurosyphilis, but the presence of a low level, lymphocytic pleocytosis or low-grade elevation in the CSF protein is often difficult to interpret. We tend to err on the conservative side and treat with regimens effective for neurosyphilis all syphilitic patients with CSF abnormalities. Nontreponemal serologic tests should be followed every 3 months for 1 year after treatment. The use of doxycycline for the treatment of syphilis in the HIV-infected patient has been criticized on the theoretical ground that the drug is bacteriostatic rather than bactericidal and may fail in the setting of impaired host defenses.

Section 11

Diseases of Allergy

ANAPHYLAXIS AND SERUM SICKNESS

method of
MICHAEL A. KALINER, M.D.
Institute for Asthma and Allergy at Washington Hospital Center
Washington, D.C.

Nothing is as frightening to physicians as the occurrence of sudden and life-threatening anaphylaxis in a patient who has just received a therapeutic injection. Within minutes, an otherwise healthy person may be suddenly prostrate, unconscious, gasping for breath, hypotensive, and in immediate danger of death.

Portier and Richet coined the word "anaphylaxis" to describe the fatal reaction induced by the introduction of minute amounts of antigen into dogs that had been previously sensitized to that antigen. The dramatic and unexpected fatal response was the opposite (Greek *ana*: back, backward) of protection (Greek *phylax*: guard). Anaphylaxis is the syndrome elicited in a hypersensitive subject upon subsequent exposure to the sensitizing antigen. The components of the anaphylactic response are (1) introduction of a sensitizing antigen, usually administered parenterally; (2) an IgE-class antibody response resulting in systemic sensitization of mast cells (and basophils); (3) reintroduction of the sensitizing antigen, usually systemically; (4) mast cell degranulation with mediator release and/or generation; and (5) production of a number of responses by the mast cell–derived mediators and manifested as anaphylaxis. Because the mediators that are released or generated by mast cells cause anaphylaxis, any event associated with mast cell activation may produce the same clinical features. *Anaphylaxis* usually refers to IgE-mediated, antigen-stimulated mast cell activation, while *anaphylactoid reactions* denote other, non–IgE-mediated responses such as may be produced by chemical agents capable of causing mast cell degranulation (e.g., radiocontrast media or opiates).

CAUSES OF ANAPHYLAXIS

IgE-Mediated Reactions

IgE-mediated anaphylaxis has been implicated in untoward reactions elicited by many drugs, chemicals, insect stings, foods, preservatives, and environmental factors. Common antigens that can cause anaphylaxis include, among others, allergenic extracts used for immunotherapy of allergic diseases, insulin, Hymenoptera venom, foods, seminal plasma, L-asparaginase, chymopapain, and latex proteins (Table 1). Latex is a milky sap produced by the rubber plant, *Hevea brasiliensis.* Latex-related allergic reactions may occur in patients undergoing procedures such as surgery (from latex gloves) or barium enema (from the latex catheter tip). Systemic reactions as well as asthma and rhinitis have been documented in medical personnel after they have donned latex gloves. Patients with spina bifida or congenital urologic abnormalities may be at increased risk because of frequent exposure to urinary catheters.

TABLE 1. **Causes of Anaphylaxis/Anaphylactoid Reactions**

IgE-mediated reactions
Antibiotics and other drugs
Foreign proteins (insulin, seminal proteins, chymopapain)
Foods
Immunotherapy
Hymenoptera stings
Exercise plus food ingestion
Complement-mediated reactions
Blood, blood products
Non-immunologic mast cell activators
Opiates (narcotics)
Radiocontrast media
Vancomycin (red man syndrome)
Dextran
Modulators of arachidonic acid metabolism
Nonsteroidal anti-inflammatory drugs
Tartrazine (possible)
Sulfiting agents
Idiopathic causes
Exercise
Catamenial anaphylaxis
Idiopathic recurrent anaphylaxis

Haptens are molecules that are too small to elicit immune responses; however, haptens may bind to serum proteins and become antigenic. The most important haptens are penicillin and related antibiotics. The majority of IgE-mediated anaphylactic deaths occurring in the United States (some 400 to 800 annually) are related to penicillin exposure (Table 2). Penicillin is metabolized to a major determinant, benzylpenicilloyl, and a series of minor determinants. These haptens circulate bound to serum proteins and produce IgE antibodies that can be detected by skin testing. Among patients with initially positive skin tests

TABLE 2. **Incidence of Anaphylactic Reactions and Frequency of Anaphylactic Deaths in the United States**

	Incidence of Reactions		
Agent	*Mild*	*Severe*	**Deaths/y**
Penicillin	1:100–200	1:2500	400–800
Hymenoptera venom	1:200	1:2000	40 or more
Contrast media	1:20	1:1000	250–1000

after their last course of penicillin, results on retesting revert to normal at a rate of 10% of patients per year. Therefore, a patient with a history of penicillin reactions is almost certainly at no appreciable risk 10 years later.

One to 2% of the courses of penicillin therapy in the United States are complicated by systemic allergic reactions, and 10% of these reactions are serious or life-threatening. Of those patients with histories suggestive of penicillin allergy, 14 to 20% of adults and less than 10% of children will have positive skin tests. If the patient has a positive skin test, there is a 50 to 60% risk for occurrence of an anaphylactic reaction upon subsequent challenge. Skin testing detects about 95% of persons who will react adversely. However, the majority of serious anaphylactic reactions occur in persons in whom no history of hypersensitivity to the drug is suspected and no skin testing is performed. Although serious reactions occur about twice as frequently after systemic administration, oral penicillin administration may also be associated with anaphylaxis and death. It is interesting that atopy is not a risk factor for the development of penicillin allergy.

Other beta-lactam–containing antibiotics may act as haptens in their own right or may cross-react with penicillin. About 8% of penicillin-sensitive persons will react to cephalosporins, and penicillin-sensitive persons are four times more likely than normal persons to have an allergic reaction to cephalosporins. However, the overall risk for a reaction to cephalosporins in a person with a history suggestive of penicillin allergy is low, less than 2%.

Venoms of Hymenoptera insects (bees, yellow jackets, hornets, wasps, and fire ants) contain enzymes such as phospholipases and hyaluronidases that are capable of eliciting an IgE antibody response. Between 0.5 and 4.0% of the population experience a systemic reaction after being stung, and at least 40 persons die annually as a result.

Ingested foods are a rich source of antigens that may cause anaphylaxis in sensitive individuals. Foods that are frequent offenders include peanuts (which are actually legumes), tree nuts, fish, and eggs. Some persons exhibit such extreme sensitivity that even exposure limited to the opening of a jar of peanut butter or inhaling the odor of cooked fish may cause a systemic response. Other less frequently implicated foods include milk, shellfish, chocolate, grains (particularly wheat and corn), fruits, and vegetables.

Immunotherapy for allergic diseases is probably the most frequent trigger of mild anaphylaxis, in that this treatment involves giving progressively increasing doses of antigens to sensitive individuals. A survey has identified 45 fatalities due to immunotherapy or skin testing since 1945. Of the 30 patients for whom sufficient data were available, 24 deaths occurred during immunotherapy and 6 during skin testing.

Complement-Mediated Reactions

Anaphylactic responses have been observed after the administration of whole blood or its products, including serum, plasma, fractionated serum products, and immunoglobulins. One of the mechanisms responsible for these reactions is the formation of immune complexes resulting in the activation of the complement cascade. Of the active by-products generated by complement activation, the anaphylatoxins, C3a, C4a, and C5a, are capable of causing mast cell (and basophil) degranulation, mediator release and generation, and consequent systemic reactions. In addition, the anaphylatoxins may directly induce vascular permeability and contract smooth muscles.

Persons who are congenitally deficient in certain serum proteins may become sensitized to the missing factors when they are provided in blood products. For example, patients with selective IgA deficiency (1 in 500 to 600 of the general population) have a greater chance of developing anaphylaxis when repeatedly given blood products, owing to the formation of anti-IgA antibodies (probably IgE–anti-IgA).

Cytotoxic reactions can also cause anaphylaxis, via complement activation. Antibodies (IgG and IgM) against red blood cells, as occur in a mismatched blood transfusion reaction, activate complement. This reaction causes agglutination and lysis of red blood cells and perturbation of mast cells, which results in anaphylaxis.

Non-immunologic Mast Cell Activators and Anaphylactoid Reactions

Mast cells may degranulate when exposed to neuromuscular blocking agents, opiates and other narcotics, radiocontrast media, dextrans, and a myriad of low-molecular-weight chemicals. Mild adverse reactions are experienced by about 5 percent of persons receiving radiocontrast dyes. Severe systemic reactions occur in 1 in 1000 exposures, with death in 1 in 10,000 to 40,000 exposures. In 1982, there were 10 million injections of contrast media in the United States, and it is estimated that from 250 to 1000 deaths resulted. Iodinated contrast media may cause mast cell degranulation by their hyperosmolarity, and by activation of the complement, clotting, and coagulation systems. The hyperosmolar iodinated contrast media are responsible for the bulk of adverse reactions, but reactions also occur in persons receiving the newer nonionic contrast media. Documentation of elevated urine histamine levels in patients experiencing adverse reactions lends additional support to the concept that this adverse reaction is an anaphylactoid response.

Narcotics and neuromuscular-relaxing agents are recognized mast cell activators capable of causing elevated plasma histamine levels and anaphylactoid reactions, observed most commonly by anesthesiologists. Reactions to local anesthetic agents appear to be largely non–IgE-mediated. IgE-dependent hypersensitivity to local anesthetics is well documented but probably accounts for less than 1% of the total number of adverse reactions to these agents, the majority of reactions being due to vasovagal, toxic, or idiosyncratic responses. Skin tests for sensitivity to some local anesthetics are useful in identifying affected persons. Alternative drugs can then be selected if sensitivity is proved. In contrast, reactions to muscle relaxants, especially succinylcholine, appear to be largely IgE-dependent. Although most such reactions occur on the first known exposure, prior sensitization to muscle relaxants may occur through exposure to cross-reacting quaternary ammonium groups in more commonly encountered chemicals.

Modulators of Arachidonic Acid Metabolism

About 5 to 10% of persons with asthma react to nonsteroidal anti-inflammatory drugs (NSAIDs)—such as aspirin, ibuprofen, and indomethacin—with rhinorrhea, bronchorrhea, bronchospasm, and, rarely, vasomotor collapse. Clinical indicators of the aspirin sensitivity are chronic sinusitis, nasal polyposis, and asthma; eosinophilia may also be present. In persons who do not have asthma, NSAIDs may cause urticaria and angioedema and, rarely, vasomotor collapse.

Sulfiting Agents

Sulfiting agents (sodium and potassium sulfites, bisulfites, metabisulfites, and gaseous sulfur dioxide) are added to foods as preservatives, to prevent discoloration. Before restrictions were placed on their use by the Food and Drug Administration (FDA), sulfites were added in high concentrations to leafy salad greens at salad bar restaurants and are still added to light-colored fruits and vegetables (particularly dried fruits, such as apples or golden raisins, and instant potatoes); wine and beer; dehydrated soups, fish, and shellfish (particularly shrimp); and rapidly perishable foods such as avocados. Sulfites are also used as preservatives in a variety of medications. Ingestion of sulfites may produce asthma and anaphylactoid reactions in susceptible persons. The mechanism involves conversion of the sulfites in the acid environment of the stomach to sulfur dioxide and sulfurous acid, which are then inhaled. Asthmatics react with bronchospasm to concentrations of SO_2 below 1 ppm.

Exercise-Induced Response

Strenuous exercise may lead to anaphylaxis in susceptible subjects. This reaction can be differentiated from exercise-induced asthma by the frequency with which the response follows exercise (in the asthmatic, exercise *regularly* causes asthma) and the symptom complex is initiated. The response induced by exercise resembles anaphylaxis in every respect, including elevated urine and plasma histamine levels. The syndrome often requires both exercise and ingestion of foods to which the subject is sensitive. This reaction should be suspected in any person who collapses after exercise, particularly if flushing, urticaria, and angioedema are evident. Most affected persons are not aware of concomitant food sensitivity, as the implicated food does not cause symptoms unless exercise occurs within 2 to 6 hours of its ingestion.

Idiopathic Recurrent Anaphylaxis

A group of subjects who recurrently experience anaphylaxis due to no recognized cause has been identified. Affected persons commonly experience flushing (100%), tachycardia (100%), angioedema (96%), upper airway obstruction (76%), urticaria (72%), bronchospasm (48%), gastrointestinal complaints (32%), and syncope or hypotension (28%). The diagnosis is based upon the spectrum of clinical signs and symptoms, evidence of elevated urine histamine, and an exhaustive search for causative factors.

An unusual cause of repeated episodes of anaphylaxis is *catamenial anaphylaxis,* a syndrome of hypersensitivity induced by endogenous progesterone secretion. Some but not all patients with catamenial anaphylaxis exhibit a cyclical pattern of attacks that intensifies during the luteal phase of the menstrual cycle. These patients develp anaphylaxis in response to provocation with medroxyprogesterone, develop systemic reactions to infusions of luteinizing hormone–releasing hormone (LHRH) (which causes endogenous progesterone secretion), and respond favorably to ovarian suppression with LHRH agonists or oophorectomy.

CLINICAL FINDINGS IN ANAPHYLAXIS

The primary anaphylactic shock organs in humans are the cutaneous, gastrointestinal, respiratory, and cardiovascular systems (Table 3). Characteristically, patients describe immediate onset of a sense of impending doom, coincident with flushing, tachycardia, and often pruritus (either diffuse, localized to the palms and soles, and/or noted particularly in the genital and inner-thigh areas). The initial signs and symptoms rapidly evolve to include urticaria, angioedema, rhinorrhea, bronchorrhea, nasal congestion, asthma, laryngeal edema, abdominal bloating, nausea, vomiting, cramps, arrhythmias, faintness, syncope, prostration, and death. The organ systems involved in these responses have two features in common: they are exposed to the external environment, and they contain the largest numbers of mast cells.

Involvement of the respiratory and cardiovascular systems is the most significant in terms of mortality. The most common causes of death are cardiovascular collapse and asphyxiation secondary to laryngeal edema. In most cases, laryngeal edema is preceded by a sensation of "a lump in the throat," hoarseness, changes in voice quality, and difficulty in breathing. Hypotension due to anaphylactic shock is usually preceded by diffuse flushing, urticaria, lightheadedness, faintness, and syncope. Anaphylactic deaths following immunotherapy are most commonly due to severe asthma, probably reflecting the specific predisposition of persons receiving immunotherapy for the development of asthma.

In the usual clinical course, symptoms begin within minutes of exposure to the inciting agent and peak within 15 to 30 minutes; recovery is complete within hours. Some subjects have spontaneous recrudescence of anaphylaxis 8 to 24 hours later. For this reason, individuals who have experienced a significant episode of anaphylaxis may require admission for overnight observation.

PATHOGENESIS

When mast cells degranulate, pre-formed and rapidly generated mediators are released into the connective tissue along with the molecules that constitute the granular matrix. Although many of these mediators induce dramatic local effects, few mediators other than histamine are capable of entering the circulation in an active state. Thus, the symptoms of anaphylaxis can be attributed primarily to

TABLE 3. **Clinical Findings in Anaphylaxis and Anaphylactoid Reactions**

System	Signs	Symptoms
Cutaneous	Flushing, urticaria, angioedema	Flushing, pruritus
Cardiovascular	Tachycardia, hypotension, shock, syncope, arrhythmias	Faintness, palpitations, weakness
Gastrointestinal	Abdominal distention, vomiting, diarrhea	Bloating, nausea, cramps, pain
Respiratory	Rhinorrhea, laryngeal edema, wheezing, bronchorrhea, asphyxiation	Nasal congestion, shortness of breath, difficulty breathing, choking, cough, hoarseness, "lump in throat"
Other	Diaphoresis, fecal or urinary incontinence	Feeling of impending doom, conjunctivitis, genital burning, metallic taste

TABLE 4. **Differential Diagnosis for Anaphylaxis and Anaphylactoid Reactions**

- Anaphylaxis
  - IgE-mediated
  - Complement-mediated
  - Non-immunologic mast cell degranulation
  - Idiopathic
  - Exercise-related
  - Sulfiting agents
  - Idiopathic causes
- Nonsteroidal anti-inflammatory drug reaction
- Vasovagal collapse
- Hereditary angioedema
- Serum sickness
- Systemic mastocytosis and urticaria pigmentosa
- Pheochromocytoma
- Carcinoid syndrome
- Panic reactions

the local actions of the many mast cell mediators and the circulating effect of histamine. Infusion of histamine into normal subjects causes the following signs and symptoms (which can be diminished by antagonists of specific histamine receptors, as noted): flushing (H_1 plus H_2), hypotension (H_1 plus H_2), headache (H_1 plus H_2), tachycardia (H_1), pruritus (H_1), rhinorrhea (H_1), and bronchospasm (H_1). Tryptase, an enzyme found in mast cell granules, can also be detected in the serum following generalized anaphylaxis. Since it persists for hours, plasma tryptase may be a useful marker of mast cell–mediated reactions.

DIFFERENTIAL DIAGNOSIS (Table 4)

The diagnosis of anaphylaxis is not difficult, given the constellation of an acute exposure to a provocating condition followed within minutes by the evolution of multisystem manifestations, including flushing, urtication, pruritus, and angioedema. Anaphylaxis is most easily confused with a vasovagal reaction. The manifestations of vasovagal reactions, however, are pallor, extreme diaphoresis, and bradycardia or normal sinus rhythm; tachycardia, flushing, urticaria, angioedema, pruritus, and asthma, as seen in anaphylaxis, are notably absent.

The correct diagnosis is much more difficult in a syncopal or sedated patient. The usual considerations in the differential diagnosis include cardiac arrhythmias, myocardial infarction, pulmonary embolism, seizures, asphyxiation, hypoglycemia, and stroke. In the syncopal patient, anaphylaxis should be considered if flushing, urticaria, angioedema, or asthma is present or if the history suggests an acute exposure to conditions associated with anaphylaxis (e.g., Hymenoptera sting). If the reaction occurs during a medical procedure, it is important to consider a possible reaction to latex or to anesthetic or other drugs.

If laryngeal edema is the presenting problem, hereditary angioedema (HAE) must be considered. This disorder is usually inherited and is accompanied by painless (and pruritus-free) angioedema, gastrointestinal cramps and distention, recurrent attacks, and usually a family history of similar attacks and/or sudden death. HAE is not associated with flushing, asthma, or urticaria; is of slower onset; and, in the absence of severe airway obstruction, is not a cause of hypotension.

Serum sickness is characterized by fever, lymphadenopathy, maculopapular and urticarial rashes, arthralgias and arthritis, myalgias, and, less frequently, nephritis and neuritis. Serum sickness generally develops 5 to 10 days after exposure to antigens (usually in medications or serum such as antilymphocytic serum for treatment of aplastic anemia) and may persist for 2 to 3 weeks. Hypotension and tachycardia are not features of this disease, and the clinical picture is usually much less acute. The syndrome is usually self-limited and treated either symptomatically or with corticosteroids if nephritis develops.

Systemic mastocytosis is a generalized disorder of mast cells that may represent an isolated overgrowth of mast cells. Urticaria pigmentosa is a generalized overgrowth of mast cells, characterized by the formation of salmon-colored freckle-like lesions. In either disease, it is possible for the mast cells to degranulate, generally producing local or systemic effects resembling anaphylaxis. Degranulation of mast cells can occur after exposure to NSAIDs, alcohol, narcotics, and other non-immunologic mast cell degranulating agents. The diagnosis should be suggested by the recognition of the classic reddish brown macular to low papular skin lesions that urticate on application of traumatic stimuli (Darier's sign), flushing attacks, evidence of bone involvement (pain, abnormalities on bone scans and x-ray studies), gastrointestinal pain and peptic ulcers, histaminuria, histaminemia, and increased urinary prostaglandin D_2 metabolites. Bone marrow or skin biopsy is usually diagnostic.

Other conditions to consider in the differential diagnosis include medication overdose, cold urticaria, cholinergic urticaria, pheochromocytoma, carcinoid tumors, and sulfite or monosodium glutamate ingestion in sensitive persons.

TREATMENT OF ACUTE ANAPHYLAXIS

Anaphylaxis is an acute medical emergency requiring prompt and appropriate attention (Table 5). If possible, the source of antigen should be removed or

TABLE 5. **Treatment of Acute Anaphylaxis in the Adult**

1. When possible, apply a tourniquet to obstruct the draining blood flow from the source of the antigen or inciting medication. When possible, remove the stinger from the site of an insect sting. Release the tourniquet every 15 minutes.
2. Place patient in recumbent position, elevate lower extremities, keep warm, and provide O_2.
3. Give aqueous epinephrine 1:1000, 0.3–0.5 mL SC; inject epinephrine 1:1000, 0.1–0.2 mL, mixed in 10 mL saline, slowly IV in cases of severe hypotension.
4. Give diphenhydramine (Benadryl), 25–50 mg IM or IV.
5. Give cimetidine* (Tagamet), 300 mg IV, or ranitidine* (Zantac), 50 mg IV, over 3–5 min.
6. Establish and maintain airway; administer racemic epinephrine by metered dose inhaler or epinephrine 1:1000 by wall-driven nebulizer, to closed airway if laryngeal edema is present.
7. Maintain blood pressure with fluids, volume expanders, or vasopressors: dopamine hydrochloride, 2–10 μg/kg/min, or norepinephrine bitartrate, 2–4 μg/min.
8. If wheezing is a problem, administer aminophylline, 5.6 mg/kg over 20 min, with maintenance dose of 0.9 mg/kg/h thereafter.
9. For prolonged reactions, repeat epinephrine every 20 min for total of 3 doses; give hydrocortisone (Solu-Cortef), 100 mg IV every 6 h.

*Not FDA approved for this indication.

its systemic circulation retarded. If a bee sting is responsible, the stinger should be carefully removed, a venous tourniquet applied to the extremity, and aqueous epinephrine (1:1000), 0.1 to 0.2 mL, injected directly into the site of the sting in order to reduce the local circulation. Aqueous epinephrine (1:1000), 0.3 to 0.5 mL given subcutaneously, is the mainstay of the treatment plan. This drug maintains the blood pressure, antagonizes many of the adverse actions of the mediators of anaphylaxis, and reduces the subsequent release of mediators.

In moderate to severe cases in which administration of epinephrine alone is not adequate therapy, both H_1 and H_2 antihistamines—diphenhydramine (Benadryl), 25 to 50 mg by the intramuscular route, and cimetidine* (Tagamet), 300 mg intravenously, or ranitidine (Zantac),* 50 mg intravenously (slowly, over 3 to 5 minutes)—are administered. If upper airway obstruction is evident ("lump in the throat," hoarseness, stridor), the patient should spray epinephrine from a metered dose inhaler or wall-driven nebulizer against a closed glottis in order to try to reduce the local swelling. If the obstruction is progressing, *immediate* tracheal intubation or tracheostomy is indicated. Once laryngeal edema has developed, tracheal intubation may become impossible.

Blood pressure should be maintained with fluid, plasma expanders, and vasopressors, as needed. Asthma should be treated with aminophylline, in a loading dose of 5.6 mg per kg every 20 minutes, followed by maintenance doses of 0.9 to 1.0 mg per kg per hour, and inhaled beta$_2$-adrenergic agonists. Corticosteroids have no immediate effect but should be administered to prevent prolonged or recurrent reactions. The usual dose is 100 mg of hydrocortisone every 6 hours.

Treatment of anaphylaxis may be complicated by the effects of beta-adrenergic blocking agents (e.g., for headaches, tremor, hypertension, cardiac arrhythmias, glaucoma). In this setting, if initial treatment with epinephrine is ineffective, glucagon, 5 to 15 μg per minute IV, should be infused.

PREVENTION AND PROPHYLAXIS OF ANAPHYLAXIS

Persons with known sensitivity should be cautioned to avoid re-exposure to causative agents. It is important for any person who has had systemic anaphylaxis to obtain an emergency treatment kit (an Epipen or other preparation of injectable epinephrine). Immunotherapy against Hymenoptera venom should be recommended, as this effectively reduces anaphylactic responses.

When a medication is required despite possible reactivity, the patient should receive prophylactic treatment with oral H_1 and H_2 antihistamines and oral corticosteroids—for example, fexofenadine (Allegra)*, 60 mg; ranitidine, 150 mg; and prednisone, 30 mg—three doses of each, administered at 24 hours, 12 hours, and 1 hour before exposure. Addition of ephedrine, 25 mg given 1 hour prior to the procedure, may provide some additional protection. Antibiotics such as β-lactam–containing antibiotics can be administered in progressively larger doses given orally or parenterally in order to desensitize the patient.

*Not FDA approved for this indication.

ASTHMA IN ADOLESCENTS AND ADULTS

method of
RICARDO A. TAN, M.D.
Antelope Valley Allergy Medical Group
Palmdale, California

and

SHELDON L. SPECTOR, M.D.
University of California, Los Angeles, UCLA School of Medicine
Los Angeles, California

Asthma is now widely recognized as a chronic inflammatory condition. Whereas therapy in the past emphasized reversal of acute bronchospasm with bronchodilators, the hallmark of current asthma therapy is the amelioration of chronic airway inflammation. Despite better understanding of the pathophysiology of asthma and the introduction of potent anti-inflammatory therapy, morbidity and mortality from asthma continue to rise, especially in the inner cities. To counter this trend and assist practitioners, several useful treatment guidelines have been developed, including the latest recommendations from the National Institutes of Health's (NIH) National Asthma Education and Prevention Program. Most guidelines advocate a comprehensive approach to therapy that includes avoidance of triggers, preventive measures, and long-term stepwise pharmacologic therapy based on the severity of asthma.

PATHOGENESIS

Asthma is characterized by chronic airway inflammation, bronchial hyperresponsiveness, and reversible airway obstruction. Genetic and environmental factors determine the appearance of asthma. Chronic airway inflammation results from complex interactions of inflammatory cells and their products, including mast cells, eosinophils, macrophages, neutrophils, the TH$_2$ subtype of T cells, and the proinflammatory cytokines interleukin (IL)-4 and IL-5. Inflammatory mediators such as histamine, leukotrienes, and prostaglandins are produced by inflammatory cells in response to allergen and other stimuli and produce bronchoconstriction, increased vascular permeability, edema, mucus production, and infiltration of inflammatory cells, with disruption of airway epithelium and injury.

DIAGNOSIS

History

Persons with asthma complain most commonly of episodic shortness of breath, wheezing, chest tightness, and cough in response to allergens such as pollen or animal dander, irritants such as cigarette smoke or perfume, exercise, or viral and bacterial respiratory tract infections. Typically, pollen sensitivity has seasonal manifestations, whereas symptoms from animal or dust mite exposure are present year-round. Many asthmatics have constant symptoms despite avoidance of precipitating factors. A subgroup of patients may have cough-variant asthma, with cough as their sole complaint. Allergic rhinitis and atopic dermatitis may be associated with asthma. A family history of atopy is usually present.

Physical Examination

In between asthma exacerbations, physical examination is often normal. A rapid respiratory rate, labored breathing, flaring of the nostrils, and retractions of the intercostal muscle are common findings during an acute attack. Pulsus paradoxus, a difference in systolic and diastolic blood pressure of more than 12 mm Hg, is a sign of decreased intrathoracic pressure in asthma. On auscultation, expiratory wheezes can be heard diffusely over the lung fields. In severe asthma with impending respiratory failure, auscultation may reveal no wheezes owing to the diminished air entry into the lungs. Hypoxia may be manifested by confusion and cyanosis.

Diagnostic Procedures

The peak flow monitor is a simple means to assess for airway obstruction in the office. Readings done at home at least once a day are useful in following patients' status, especially those with decreased symptom awareness. Instructions on when to use medications based on peak flow readings are helpful in such patients.

Computerized office pulmonary function testing can be used for diagnosis and monitoring of asthma and has the added advantage of better characterizing the location of the obstruction. The diagnosis of asthma can be confirmed by demonstrating an increase in forced expiratory volume in 1 second (FEV_1) of 15% or more from baseline after an inhaled $beta_2$-agonist treatment. If a patient has normal spirometry results but asthma is still suspected, a bronchial challenge with inhaled methacholine or histamine can be performed.

Skin testing for allergens is helpful in identifying allergenic triggers for asthma. Both scratch and intradermal testing correlate better clinically than serum radioallergosorbent testing (RAST) for specific IgE antibodies to allergens. Antihistamines block the wheal and flare response and should be stopped 48 to 72 hours, and sometimes longer, before skin testing. RAST can be performed if patients refuse skin testing, when there is extensive skin disease such as eczema, or if antihistamines or other medications that can affect test interpretation have been taken by the patient.

Differential Diagnosis

Dyspnea, wheezing, and cough may be seen in various conditions that should be differentiated from asthma such as vocal cord dysfunction, foreign body aspiration, congestive heart failure, allergic bronchopulmonary aspergillosis, bronchiolitis obliterans, bronchopulmonary dysplasia, chronic bronchitis, emphysema, and cystic fibrosis.

TREATMENT

Control of Aggravating Factors

Allergens

The most common allergenic stimuli for asthma include pollen, animal dander, dust mites, and molds. Pollen from trees, grass, and weeds is responsible for most seasonal symptoms. Trees generally pollinate in the spring, grasses in the summer, and weeds in the fall, with less pollination in the winter. Local pollen counting bureaus provide specific pollen count and distribution information. It is helpful to keep windows closed at home and in the car to minimize pollen exposure. Keeping the air conditioner on and the windows closed minimizes pollen entry in the summer.

Cat and dog dander is a common source of allergenic proteins. Because most patients are unable to give up their pets, keeping the pets out of the bedroom may help ameliorate symptoms. Animal dander has been detected in rooms up to 6 months after removal of the animals, so carpets should be steam cleaned, walls washed, and sheets cleaned in hot water to take out as much allergen as possible. Cockroach allergy is an important trigger, especially in inner cities.

Dust mite allergy is primarily due to two species: *Dermatophagoides farinae* and *Dermatophagoides pteronyssinus*. Because dust mites thrive in pillows, mattresses, and upholstered furniture, especially those containing feathers, one effective control measure is to use impermeable covers for pillows and mattresses. Indoor humidity should be kept low, as dust mites thrive in high humidity. Occasionally, it may be necessary to remove carpets and install hardwood floors to lessen the dust mite population.

Different species of fungi or mold predominate indoors and outdoors. Mold allergy is a major problem in humid climates. Bleach solutions may be used to wash off visible mold on bathroom walls. Old carpets should be removed if there are patches of mold underneath.

Air cleaners with high efficiency particulate air (HEPA) filters can help remove pollen and animal dander but not dust mites, which are usually not airborne. Tannic acid solutions may be used to neutralize allergenic proteins in carpets and upholstered furniture.

Immunotherapy has been shown to be effective in improving chronic asthma in patients allergic to such allergens as ragweed, dust mite, cat dander, grass, and *Alternaria*. The mechanism of immunotherapy is still unclear, but IgG "blocking antibodies" are thought to prevent the effects of specific IgE antibodies. Immunotherapy is usually given for at least 3 to 5 years. Injections should be given in a medically supervised setting with resuscitation equipment available. The possibility of having systemic reactions without proper emergency treatment available makes home self-injection an unacceptable risk. Although recent studies suggest that immunotherapy may be unnecessary if proper avoidance and pharmacologic therapy are observed, many specialists still believe that immunotherapy is a beneficial adjunct to asthma management.

Allergic Rhinitis

There is growing evidence that treatment of upper airway inflammation in allergic rhinitis leads to better control of asthma. Intranasal steroids such as beclomethasone (Vancenase), fluticasone (Flonase), and mometasone (Nasonex) are effective in long-term control of symptoms in chronic allergic rhinitis and should be used regularly, especially if there is concomitant asthma.

Sinusitis

Acute sinusitis and chronic sinusitis both produce purulent discharge and trigger asthma. Chronic sinusitis can easily be missed because it manifests with nonspecific symptoms such as cough or postnasal drip. Limited computed tomography (CT) scans of the sinuses provide more information than the conventional sinus series x-ray films, often at the same cost. Acute sinusitis may respond to 2 weeks of antibiotics, but chronic sinusitis usually requires a prolonged course of up to 4 to 6 weeks.

Exercise

Exercise can be the sole trigger in some patients. Exercise-induced asthma (EIA) is defined as a drop in FEV_1 of 10 to 15% or more after 10 to 15 minutes of exertion. Symptoms usually peak after exercise. The exact mechanism of EIA is unclear, but the two main hypotheses suggest that (1) loss of water due to increased ventilation leads to increased osmolarity, causing mast cell degranulation, or (2) rapid rewarming after exercise causes vasodilatation and edema in the airways. A refractory period for up to 3 hours after exercise during which repeat exercise does not cause recurrence of symptoms has been observed. This refractory period can be used by asthmatic athletes to their advantage by warming up before exercise and gradually increasing the intensity of exertion. In general, maintaining good long-term control of asthma with anti-inflammatory therapy diminishes EIA. Prophylactic use of inhaled β_2-agonists, cromolyn (Intal) or nedocromil (Tilade) 30 minutes to 1 hour before exercise is also effective.

Aspirin and Nonsteroidal Anti-inflammatory Agents

Asthma may be part of the syndrome that includes nasal polyps, sinusitis, and sensitivity to aspirin and nonsteroidal anti-inflammatory agents. The mechanism of aspirin sensitivity is non–IgE-mediated and most commonly attributed to excessive production of leukotrienes from the lipoxygenase pathway because of blockage of the cyclooxygenase pathway of arachidonic acid metabolism. The effectiveness of antileukotriene agents in blocking aspirin-induced bronchospasm supports this mechanism. Desensitization with increasing doses of aspirin has been shown in some studies to improve asthma.

Gastroesophageal Reflux Disease

Gastroesophageal reflux disease can precipitate asthma attacks if acid reflux spills over to the upper or lower airway. Patients with refractory asthma should be asked about symptoms of heartburn or epigastric pain. Esophageal pH monitoring may occasionally be needed if the diagnosis is not clear. Elevating the head during sleep and not lying down for up to 3 hours after meals can prevent reflux. H_2-blockers such as ranitidine (Zantac), 150 mg twice daily, or proton pump inhibitors such as omeprazole (Prilosec), 20 mg daily, can decrease acid production.

Infections

Viral respiratory tract infections are common precipitating factors for acute asthma, especially in children. Bacterial infections should be recognized promptly and treated with antibiotics if necessary. Pneumococcal and annual influenza vaccinations are recommended for persons with chronic asthma.

Air Pollution and Occupational Exposures

Ozone, nitrogen dioxide, sulfur dioxide, and total suspended particulates are air pollutants that have been implicated as bronchial irritants. Persons with occupational asthma have symptoms primarily in the work place. Examples of occupational allergens include *Bacillus subtilis* enzymes for detergent workers and soybean dust for farmers. Removal of the person or the offending agent from the workplace is the treatment for this condition.

Pharmacologic Therapy

Beta$_2$-Agonists

The short-acting beta$_2$-agonists act selectively on beta$_2$-adrenergic receptors to produce bronchodilatation and are the treatment of choice for fast relief of bronchospasm. Albuterol (Ventolin), terbutaline, and metaproterenol (Alupent) are most commonly used. Beta$_2$-agonists are available in oral, nebulized, and metered-dose inhaler preparations. A long-acting (up to 12 hours) beta$_2$-agonist, salmeterol (Serevent), is effective for long-term control but should not be used for acute attacks. The use of beta$_2$-agonists only as needed is now recommended, as some studies have shown increased morbidity and mortality associated with chronic regular use. Whether the regular use of beta$_2$-agonist is the cause or effect of worsening asthma is still unclear.

Anticholinergic Agents

Ipratropium bromide (Atrovent) is relatively free of side effects, unlike older preparations such as atropine. It is useful in patients with incomplete relief from beta$_2$-agonists or who have concomitant chronic obstructive pulmonary disease.

Cromolyn and Nedocromil

Cromolyn and nedocromil stabilize the mast cell membrane and prevent degranulation and release of inflammatory mediators. Both diminish the early- and late-phase response to allergenic stimuli. Cromolyn and nedocromil are effective prophylactically before allergen exposure and exercise. They are also effective nonsteroidal alternatives for anti-inflammatory therapy.

Theophylline

Theophylline and aminophylline are methylxanthines that have been part of asthma treatment for decades. Both improve diaphragmatic contraction and may have anti-inflammatory properties as well. The need for regular monitoring of serum levels to avoid overdosage and adverse events such as seizures has lessened the use of theophylline over the years. Theophylline is currently recommended as additional long-term treatment for patients not controlled on inhaled steroids. Certain patients may respond favorably to intravenous aminophylline in acute asthma.

Inhaled Steroids

Inhaled corticosteroids are the most potent anti-inflammatory agents available. Corticosteroids improve asthma symptoms by decreasing the chemotaxis of inflammatory cells such as eosinophils, the production of proinflammatory cytokines, and the release of inflammatory mediators. Studies show that beclomethasone (Vanceril), triamcinolone (Azmacort), flunisolide (AeroBid), fluticasone (Flovent), and budesonide (Pulmicort) can all improve pulmonary function and clinical symptoms if used regularly. Unlike systemic steroids, the inhaled steroids have a good safety profile, and the benefits currently outweigh concerns about osteoporosis, growth retardation, cataracts, or hypothalamic-pituitary axis suppression. Local side effects include hoarseness and oral thrush, both of which can be avoided by proper inhaler technique. Oral thrush can be avoided by rinsing of the mouth after inhalation.

Antileukotrienes

The antileukotriene agents are the first new category of asthma drugs introduced in the last two decades. Leukotrienes are released by mast cells and eosinophils in response to stimuli and cause bronchoconstriction, increased vascular permeability, edema, mucus production, and influx of inflammatory cells. The two types of antileukotriene agents are leukotriene synthesis inhibitors and leukotriene receptor antagonists. Leukotriene synthesis inhibitors can be either 5-lipoxygenase inhibitors or 5-lipoxygenase activating protein inhibitors. Zafirlukast (Accolate), leukotriene receptor antagonists, and zileuton (Zyflo), a 5-lipoxygenase inhibitor, are currently available and pranlukast may be introduced in the future. Studies show improvement of both spirometry results and clinical symptoms with regular use of antileukotrienes in chronic asthma. Although antileukotrienes are recommended mainly for long-term control of mild asthma at this time, recent studies suggest their usefulness can be expanded to all categories of asthma severity. Both types of antileukotrienes have been shown to be safe and well tolerated in studies. Mild, reversible elevation of liver enzyme levels has been seen with zileuton.

New or Alternative Treatments

Other treatments that have been studied in asthma include troleandomycin,* methotrexate,* gold,* cyclosporine,* and hydroxychloroquine.* Promising new treatments include intravenous immunoglobulin* and intravenous anti-IgE antibodies, which have shown efficacy in patients with severe, refractory asthma.

Metered Dose Inhalers

Proper technique is of crucial importance in ensuring delivery of the drug to the lower airways. Patients who have difficulty with technique should be given spacers or chambers that improve delivery. Nonchlorofluorocarbon propellants are replacing chlorofluorocarbon propellants, which have been shown to damage the ozone layer of the atmosphere. No differences in effectiveness have been seen.

Approach to Acute Asthma

Persons having acute asthma symptoms of wheezing and shortness of breath should first take 2 puffs every 4 to 6 hours of a metered dose inhaler with a beta$_2$-agonist, such as albuterol or metaproterenol. For more severe symptoms, two puffs from a metered dose inhaler may be taken every 30 minutes to 1 hour up to three times a day. A nebulizer machine delivers more medication and may be used for more persistent symptoms. Oral steroids should be started if there is only partial relief of symptoms.

In the emergency room, nebulized beta$_2$-agonist treatment should be given at frequent intervals or continuously until improvement is seen. Subcutaneous epinephrine may also be effective. Anticholinergic agents can be helpful in selected patients. Oxygen via nasal cannula or face mask should be given to keep O_2 saturation at greater than 90%. Patients who respond poorly to treatment should be admitted for hospital care and started on intravenous methylprednisolone (Solu-Medrol), 40 to 60 mg every 4 to 6 hours. The usefulness of intravenous aminophylline continues to be debated. Respiratory failure can develop rapidly and should be anticipated in patients who have deteriorating mental status, show signs of respiratory fatigue, or have a P_{CO_2} of higher than 42 mm Hg. These patients should be intubated and started on mechanical ventilation as soon as possible to avoid respiratory or cardiac arrest.

Approach to Chronic Asthma

Anti-inflammatory therapy is the cornerstone of chronic asthma therapy. The 1997 NIH Guidelines classify asthma as being mild intermittent, mild persistent, moderate persistent, or severe persistent according to various criteria.

Short-acting beta$_2$-agonists used as needed are the medication of choice for quick relief of symptoms in all categories. Mild intermittent asthmatics do not require regular daily medication. For long-term con-

*Not FDA approved for this indication.

trol, mild persistent asthmatics should be started on daily anti-inflammatory therapy with inhaled steroids; cromolyn, 2 to 4 puffs three to four times daily; or nedocromil, two to four puffs two to four times daily. The antileukotrienes zafirlukast, 20 mg twice daily; montelukast (Singulair), 10 mg in the evening; and zileuton, 600 mg four times daily; or sustained-release theophylline, daily or twice daily, are alternatives. Both moderate and severe persistent asthma should be treated with daily inhaled steroids, with the dose increased according to the severity. Long-acting bronchodilators such as long-acting inhaled beta$_2$-agonists (salmeterol, two puffs twice daily), oral beta$_2$-agonists, or sustained-release theophylline should be added if control of moderate to severe asthma is not complete with the inhaled steroids.

Risk Factors for Fatal Asthma

Risk factors associated with death from asthma include poorly controlled asthma, previous intensive care admissions or intubations, use of systemic steroids, poor patient perception of asthma severity, concomitant systemic diseases, psychiatric disorders, low socioeconomic status, illegal drug abuse, and allergy to *Alternaria*. Recognition and close monitoring of patients with these risk factors can prevent unfortunate outcomes.

Asthma in Pregnancy

Inhaled or nebulized beta$_2$-agonist therapy may be used for rapid relief of symptoms throughout pregnancy. Terbutaline is preferred, although other beta$_2$-agonists can be used. Regular use of inhaled cromolyn, inhaled beclomethasone, or oral theophylline for chronic asthma has been shown to be safe in pregnancy. Systemic steroids and intravenous aminophylline may be used for asthma exacerbations. All these medications may be used at the same dosages as in nonpregnant patients. Immunotherapy should not be started or increased during pregnancy, as a systemic reaction would be harmful to the fetus. Maintenance immunotherapy may be continued through the pregnancy.

Referral to Subspecialists

The Joint Task Force on Practice Parameters representing the American Academy of Allergy, Asthma and Immunology and the American College of Allergy, Asthma, and Immunology recommends evaluation by an asthma specialist (1) in patients with severe, unstable or poorly controlled asthma; (2) when identification of allergens is needed, or if immunotherapy is being considered; (3) for patient education; or (4) when the diagnosis of asthma is in doubt. The primary care practitioner and the asthma specialist should work together to achieve the best possible control of asthma.

Patient Education

Education and participation of patients and their families in their care are important in achieving maximum control of asthma. Patients should be encouraged to learn how the medications work and to help formulate plans for home treatment and for avoiding precipitating factors. With proper instructions on the use of medications, regular physical activity and sports can be encouraged, especially for adolescents.

ASTHMA IN CHILDREN

method of
MARTHA V. WHITE, M.D.
Institute for Asthma and Allergy at Washington Hospital Center
Washington, D.C.

Asthma is one of the most common chronic illnesses of childhood, affecting 5 to 10% of children younger than 20 years. In the United States, asthma and its attendant allergies are the leading cause of time lost from school and work and sick child visits to the physician. Americans spend more than $1 billion each year on asthma, and as many as 50% of asthma patients spend more than 18% of their family income on asthma therapy.

Fortunately, our understanding of the pathophysiology of asthma has improved dramatically in the last 2 decades. We now know that asthma is due to a combination of smooth muscle contraction, excessive secretion of mucus, mucosal edema, and inflammation. Pulmonary autopsy tissue taken from patients who died of asthma reveals epithelial denudement, thickening of the basement membrane, infiltration of the lamina propria by eosinophils and neutrophils, and smooth muscle, goblet cell, and glandular hyperplasia. Airway luminal secretions are excessive and copious and contain increased numbers of eosinophils, neutrophils, mast cells, Creola bodies, Curschmann's spirals, and Charcot-Leyden crystals. These changes were previously thought to occur only in severe asthma, but airway biopsies obtained from patients with mild asthma also demonstrate epithelial denudement, eosinophil and neutrophil infiltration, edema, basement membrane thickening, and mast cell hyperplasia with evidence of degranulation.

Typical asthma attacks consist of an early, short-lived bronchoconstrictive response to an asthma trigger and a late phase reaction (LPR). The LPR consists of inflammatory events occurring 5 to 12 hours after the inciting trigger and is characterized by wheezing that is poorly responsive to bronchodilators. The LPR last hours to days and can render the patient's airways hyper-reactive to additional asthma triggers for prolonged periods. Further exposure to asthma triggers during this hyper-reactive period can initiate an escalating cycle of acute asthma, LPR, and increased hyper-reactivity, which can culminate in a prolonged, recalcitrant asthma attack requiring hospitalization and intravenous corticosteroid administration.

The bulk of evidence suggests that the airway inflammation observed in asthma is caused by mast cell–initiated LPR. Antigen-stimulated mast cells release chemotactic factors, vasoactive factors, and inflammatory leukotrienes and prostaglandins. Mast cells can also induce epithelial cell expression of leukocyte adhesion molecules, such as the vascular cell adhesion molecule, which selectively recruit eosinophils to the site of the allergic reaction. Thus, mast cell–induced up-regulation of adhesion molecule expression may enhance airway inflammation in asthma. Antigen-stimulated mast cells synthesize and release a number of inflammatory cytokines, including interleukin (IL)-3, IL-4, IL-5, IL-8, tumor necrosis factor, and interferon-γ. Activated T cells and macrophages release a similar pattern of cytokines as well as IL-10 and IL-11. The pattern of lymphocyte cytokines produced during the allergic response differs from that of other inflammatory disorders. In most inflammatory diseases studied thus far, IL-2 and interferon-γ, but not IL-4, IL-5, and IL-10, are produced. However, in allergic disorders, IL-4, IL-5, and IL-10 are preferentially produced. These cytokines are important in IgE production as well as eosinophil chemotaxis and survival and thus promote the allergic response. The interleukins and tumor necrosis factor enhance mast cell growth and up-regulate IgE production. Through cytokine production, mast cells may regulate their own function and growth, regulate airway inflammation, and ultimately regulate airway hyper-reactivity.

The degree of airway hyper-reactivity to nonspecific stimuli, such as histamine and methacholine, correlates closely with asthma severity. Furthermore, airway hyperreactivity increases during the allergy season and during rhinovirus infections. In previous years, bronchodilators, such as theophylline and beta-adrenergic agonists, were used as first-line asthma therapies. Specialists now agree that the primary focus of asthma management should be the reduction and prevention of airway hyper-reactivity and late phase inflammatory reactions. Indeed, guidelines for the management of asthma, which stress the importance of anti-inflammatory medications, have been published through the National Institutes of Health and other world agencies. Consequently, allergen avoidance coupled with inhaled cromolyn sodium (Intal) or inhaled corticosteroids is increasingly being used as a primary form of therapy, and bronchodilators are being used as second-line symptomatic drugs.

Despite improvements in our understanding of asthma and in delivery systems for asthma medications, the incidence of asthma and of deaths owing to asthma is rising. The reason for this is unclear; however, it has been suggested that pollution, passive exposure to tobacco smoke, excessive reliance on symptomatic medications (e.g., bronchodilators) in lieu of lesion-reversing measures (e.g., allergen avoidance, corticosteroid or cromolyn sodium therapy, and immunotherapy) to treat asthma, excessive indoor allergen exposure (e.g., cockroaches, cats, dust mites), and restricted access to long-term follow-up care may be contributing factors. Whatever the reason, asthma must be regarded as a potentially life-threatening disorder. Even in extremely mild cases, disruption of family dynamics, school attendance, and social interactions can be significant. The goals of therapy should be to reduce or eliminate symptoms while normalizing daily activities. This can usually be accomplished with minimal or no side effects. With optimal management, the activities of most children should be unrestricted, allowing a normal lifestyle and reducing the risk of emotional repercussions from asthma.

DIAGNOSIS

Asthma is a disease characterized by episodic wheezing or cough, responsive to defined asthma management protocols, for which other causes have been eliminated. It can present as recurrent cough, especially at night; a cough or wheeze associated with exercise or infections; or frank episodic wheezing, usually with recognizable triggers. The spectrum of severity ranges from a few mild episodes in a lifetime to daily debilitating symptoms. A careful history and a physical examination are the most useful diagnostic aids; and special attention should be given to the timing of symptoms, potential triggers, family history, and exposure to environmental allergens, such as cats, cockroaches, and dust mites, and irritants, such as tobacco smoke. A diagnosis of asthma can be confirmed by a postbronchodilator increase of 12% in the forced expiratory volume in 1 second, or 20% in forced expiratory flow ($FEF_{25\%-76\%}$). If spirometry is normal, it may be necessary to perform an exercise challenge to establish the diagnosis. A simple exercise challenge, which can be performed in the office, is supervised running in place or up and down the stairs until the patient feels too tired to continue. Bronchial constriction usually occurs about 10 minutes after the challenge.

Some children normally perform as much as 40% above predicted normal levels for spirometry. These children may have "normal lung functions" during an asthma attack but improve with bronchodilators. Alternatively, if the child has a history of wheezing that cannot be confirmed by physical examination, a diagnosis can be reached by using a peak flow meter at home and at school, especially during asthma attacks and after bronchodilator use. Children as young as 4 years are capable of performing a peak flow maneuver. For children too young to cooperate, a trial with asthma therapy is warranted.

If a more definite diagnosis is required, a methacholine or histamine challenge can be performed to demonstrate airway hyper-reactivity, the hallmark of asthma. An antigen challenge can also be diagnostic of antigen-induced asthma, but it carries the risk of inducing an LPR. These tests are time-consuming, require precision, and are best left to physicians trained in these techniques.

Although it is true that not all that wheezes is asthma, asthma is common, and the other causes of wheezing are rare. The differential diagnosis includes tracheobronchomalacia, cystic fibrosis (particularly in children with nasal polyps or histories of meconium ileus), bronchial stenosis, mass lesions such as lymphomas, foreign bodies (particularly in wheezing of sudden onset), congenital and acquired structural lung disorders such as vascular rings, and many infections such as tuberculosis and infection with *Mycoplasma* or respiratory syncytial virus.

TREATMENT

Environmental Control

Most asthmatic children develop allergies. The development of allergies and the severity of existing allergies depend on the level of exposure to a given allergen. Allergies to foods emerge during infancy, followed somewhat later by allergies to cockroaches, indoor pets, and house dust mites, which are present all year but peak in the winter. Pollen allergies generally develop after three or more seasons of exposure. Children younger than 4 years rarely test positive for pollens.

The diagnosis of allergic triggers can be made by allergy skin testing combined with a temporal pattern of symptoms consistent with the skin test results. Optimization of asthma therapy is difficult without rigorous avoidance of allergic triggers. Exposure to high levels of house dust mites or cockroaches during infancy increases the atopic child's risk of developing asthma by fourfold in some studies. House dust mite avoidance is accomplished by the use of plastic, allergen-proof encasings on all mattresses, box springs, and pillows in the child's bedroom and removal of all venetian blinds and rugs wherever possible. Simplification of the bedroom to eliminate feather bedding (unless enclosed), clutter, stuffed furniture, and other dust collectors is also important. Book-shelves should be enclosed or moved to a different room, closet doors closed, and stuffed animals kept to a minimum. Mites in the stuffed animals may be killed by placement in the hot air cycle of the dryer for 10 to 15 minutes or in the freezer overnight. The entire house should be dusted and vacuumed at least weekly, and the bedroom should be cleaned more often. Cockroaches are often carried into the home in paper grocery bags. Mold exposure can be reduced by eliminating potted plants, especially in the bedroom. Persons allergic to outdoor allergens should keep the doors and windows closed during the pollen season (trees in early spring; grass in late spring and early summer; weeds in late summer and early fall; molds in fall). Bathing and dressing for bed after coming indoors for the day eliminate exposure to pollens on clothing and hair.

Animal fur picks up outdoor allergens. Thus, the family pet may be an additional source of pollen exposure. In cases of animal allergy, family pets should be given away. The presence of cats in the house during infancy raises an atopic child's chances of developing asthma by 10-fold. If the family refuses to eliminate the pet, the pet should be kept outside, if possible, and definitely out of the allergic child's bedroom, and the child should be instructed to avoid the animal's saliva.

Passive smoke inhalation is unequivocally deleterious to the pulmonary functions of normal and asthmatic children. In some studies, smoking atopic mothers were four times as likely to have an asthmatic child as nonsmoking atopic mothers. Smoking should not be permitted in the asthmatic child's house.

Immunotherapy

The efficacy of immunotherapy in allergic rhinitis is well documented. Demonstration of the efficacy of immunotherapy in asthma is more difficult because of the etiologic complexities of the disease. However, carefully performed trials of single agents used to treat well-defined allergic asthmatic patients (e.g., cat- or birch pollen–induced asthma) have documented that immunotherapy reduces symptoms and prevents the increases in airway reactivity normally seen during the allergy season. If allergen exposure cannot be completely eliminated, immunotherapy can be helpful in asthmatic patients with known allergic triggers. Although the exact mechanism by which immunotherapy works is unclear, it reduces late asthmatic responses to allergens and, over time, can reduce bronchial reactivity. To be successful, the immunotherapy prescription must contain all relevant allergens, and improvement occurs gradually over 2 or more years. Injections are given once or twice weekly in increasing doses until an optimal dose is achieved. Thereafter, injection intervals are gradually lengthened to monthly.

Severity Assessment

To gauge the success of therapy, it is necessary to determine the maximal lung functions achievable by the patient, often after a therapeutic trial of cromolyn or inhaled corticosteroids plus bronchodilators, as needed. Patients may report fewer symptoms than they are actually experiencing because they have not learned to recognize milder, more chronic pulmonary symptoms of asthma. A daily peak flow graph, filled out thrice daily, is quite helpful, both for the assessment of severity and to help patients recognize asthma symptoms and triggers. Patients soon learn to think of their peak flow meter as their "asthma thermometer." The frequency of bronchodilator use (if used as needed) and nighttime awakenings owing to asthma is also a good yardstick for measuring asthma severity.

Cooperative Management

As with diabetes, optimal management of asthma cannot be achieved with crisis care alone. It requires a maintenance program designed to prevent asthma flares and early intervention when flares do occur. Patients and parents should be taught to listen to chest sounds and to monitor peak flow readings, trigger exposure, and symptoms to facilitate physician-patient communication and the early identification of asthma flares. The family and school should be provided with a written medication plan for handling flares based on peak flow readings and response to therapy, including instructions about when to call the physician.

Pharmacologic Management

Pharmacologic products useful in the treatment of asthma can be divided into two groups: (1) anti-inflammatory medications, which heal and prevent airway inflammation that leads to airway hyper-reactivity, and (2) bronchodilators, which relax smooth muscle, thus relieving the acute symptoms of asthma. The anti-inflammatory medications are disease-altering medications that work slowly and do not produce immediate relief of symptoms. Thus a patient's compliance with these products is poor unless their role in asthma management and their expected benefits are clearly outlined for the patient.

Mast Cell Stabilizers

Mast cell stabilizers are probably the safest drugs available for the treatment of asthma. Disodium cromoglycate (Intal) and nedocromil sodium (Tilade) prevent early- and late-phase allergic reactions. They are not bronchodilators and do not reverse acute symptoms. They work preventively to inhibit inflammation and antigen-induced increases in airway hyper-reactivity. A single dose (2 puffs) inhibits the asthmatic response to exercise or allergen exposure if given 10 to 20 minutes in advance. Maintenance therapy requires 3 or 4 daily doses, and it can take as long as 4 weeks for an effect to be appreciated. Both drugs are provided as metered-dose inhalers. Cromolyn is also provided in a nebulizable form (frequently used in combination with beta agonists). Nedocromil nebulizer solution is in clinical trials. Discontinuation of cromolyn or nedocromil during an asthma attack is counterproductive and not indicated.

Corticosteroids

Corticosteroids are extremely potent antiasthma agents. They reduce inflammation, edema, and mucus secretion and restore $beta_2$-adrenergic responsiveness. Corticosteroids inhibit increases in airway responsiveness and can reverse the baseline airway hyper-responsiveness characteristic of asthma. Several topical formulations delivered by metered-dose inhalers are available (beclomethasone [Vanceril, Beclovent], flunisolide [AeroBid], triamcinolone [Azmacort], and fluticasone [Flovent]). Budesonide (Pulmicort) and fluticasone (Flovent) are also available as dry powder inhalers. These potent topical agents are quickly metabolized and rarely cause any of the side effects of oral corticosteroids. In asthmatic patients requiring daily bronchodilator therapy despite cromolyn use, the addition of or substitution with these agents can lead to dramatic clinical improvement. In unstable asthma, best results are obtained after the symptoms are stabilized with oral corticosteroids, followed by maintenance inhaled corticosteroids. From 100 to 200 μg twice daily is the usual dose; however, higher doses may be necessary in more refractory asthma. Nebulized budesonide is used in doses of 250 to 1000 μg per day in one or two divided doses. In the most difficult cases, maintenance oral corticosteroids may be required. Alternate-day dosing is associated with fewer systemic side effects than daily dosing and is the oral regimen of choice.

The key to proper management with oral steroids is to use doses sufficient to cause a dramatic improvement in pulmonary functions and to continue them until pulmonary functions (including $FEF_{25\%-76\%}$) normalize. The patient is then weaned as quickly as possible off oral corticosteroids, and the effect is maintained with inhaled corticosteroids. If a prolonged course of oral corticosteroids is required, the patient may need to be weaned to alternate-day oral corticosteroids before ceasing to take oral steroids completely. Inhaled corticosteroid doses should be increased early during asthma exacerbations. If this fails, a short course of oral steroids should be instituted before the patient's condition deteriorates to the point of requiring emergency intervention.

Pulmonary delivery of any inhaled medication by metered-dose inhaler is enhanced by the use of spacer devices (AeroChamber, InspirEase). The AeroChamber may be ordered prefitted with a child's face mask to facilitate delivery of inhaled medications to young children, although nebulization provides superior drug delivery in small children. Inhaled corticosteroids and cromolyn sodium are best given 10 minutes after inhaled beta-adrenergic agonists, because beta agonists cause bronchodilatation and facilitate penetration of subsequent inhaled medications. Gargling or rinsing the mouth with a few sips of water after steroid inhalation is usually sufficient to avoid thrush, the major side effect of inhaled corticosteroids.

Beta-Adrenergic Agonists

Beta agonists are bronchodilators and are effective in treating and preventing early asthmatic responses, but they are less effective in reversing LPRs (Table 1). They are excellent for preventing exercise-induced asthma when given 10 minutes before exercise. Both nonselective (e.g., isoproterenol) and $beta_2$-selective (e.g., metaproterenol, albuterol, terbutaline, bitolterol, and pirbuterol) beta-adrenergic agonists are available. The selective drugs are preferred because they have selective pulmonary effects and fewer cardiac side effects. These preparations are available as metered-dose inhalers, nebulizer solutions, oral preparations, and parenteral preparations.

Delivery by inhalation targets the medication to the lungs and produces fewer systemic effects, such as tremor, nervousness, and palpitations. Nebulizer treatments, often combined with cromolyn or budesonide, are particularly useful in young asthmatic patients and in older children during acute exacerbations of asthma. Ideally, the family should possess a nebulizer for home use and a portable battery-operated unit for travel (which could be rented). There are several lightweight battery-operated models with adapters for plugging into automobile cigarette lighters. In general, the nonportable air compressors have more power than the portable units.

Metered-dose inhalers, preferably operated with

TABLE 1. **Dosing Guidelines for Theophylline, Oral $Beta_2$-Adrenergic Agonists, and Corticosteroids**

Theophylline		
Dose to achieve serum concentrations of 5–15 mg/mL		
Albuterol		**Prednisolone**
(0.1–0.15 mg/kg q 4–6 h)		Pediapred (5 mg/5 mL)
Ventolin (2 mg/5 mL)		Prelone (15 mg/5 mL)
Proventil (2 mg/5 mL)		**Prednisone**
Metaproterenol		Liquid Pred (5 mg/5 mL)
(0.3–0.5 mg/kg q 4–6 h)		
Alupent (10 mg/5 mL)		
Age (y)	**Beta Agonist**	**Prednisone**
<2	¼–½ tsp tid or qid	5–7.5 mg bid
2–6	½–1 tsp tid or qid	7.5–10 mg bid
6–12	1–1½ tsp tid or qid	10–15 mg bid
>12	1–2 tsp tid or qid	10–20 mg tid

spacer devices, can be used by older children. The availability of an AeroChamber fitted with a pediatric mask has made the use of metered-dose inhalers possible even in infants, although good studies comparing the two inhalant delivery systems in this age group are lacking. Oral beta$_2$-adrenergic agonists are useful for treating mild asthma, especially in infants, and as adjuncts to inhaled corticosteroids and inhaled beta-adrenergic agonists. In more resistant asthma, the slow-release oral preparations (e.g., albuterol extended release [Proventil Repetabs]) or long-acting inhaled preparations (salmeterol [Serevent]) are excellent alternatives to theophylline (e.g., Theo-Dur) for nighttime coverage, or to four-times-daily dosing with short-acting beta agonists. Systemic preparations are reserved for office and hospital use, with the exception of epinephrine (EpiPen), used as self-administered emergency treatment for anaphylaxis caused by insect stings, food allergens, or drug reactions.

Theophylline

The use of methylxanthines by asthma specialists has decreased steadily in the last several years, partly because of its side effects and as a result of an improvement in our understanding of the pathogenesis of asthma. It was originally thought that theophylline worked by inhibiting phosphodiesterase; however, other mechanisms, including inhibition of adenosine, are more important. Theophylline, a bronchodilator, is useful in the symptomatic treatment of acute asthma, but it has little effect on the inflammatory component and does not reverse airway hyper-reactivity. It is an effective oral bronchodilator, can be used with twice-daily or once-daily dosing, and is easy to administer; compliance can be ascertained through serum theophylline levels (see Table 1).

Theophylline, at levels slightly above recommended therapeutic levels (5 to 15 μg per mL), is associated with several unpleasant side effects, including a short attention span in predisposed individuals, nausea and vomiting, and behavioral and sleep alterations in some children. Serious theophylline toxicities (e.g., seizure, arrhythmias, death) generally do not occur below 40 μg per mL; however, in rare cases, a seizure can be the first symptom of theophylline toxicity. With the availability of improved delivery systems and toxicity profiles for the beta-adrenergic agonists, the side effects of theophylline have limited the usefulness of the drug.

Leukotriene Modifiers

The leukotriene modifiers represent the first new class of antiasthma medications to be licensed in 20 years. These oral medications are effective bronchodilators that also inhibit airway hyper-reactivity. There are three types of leukotriene-modifying drugs; two work by inhibiting the production of leukotrienes C_4, D_4, and E_4 (5-lipoxygenase inhibitors and 5-lipoxygenase-associated protein [FLAP] inhibitors) and the third blocks the binding of leukotriene D_4 to its receptor. Zafirlukast (Accolate) and montelukast (Singulair), leukotriene D_4 antagonists, and zileuton (Zyflo), 5α-lipoxygenase inhibitor, have been approved for use in the treatment of chronic asthma in the United States. Leukotriene modifiers are generally well tolerated, although zileuton, but not zafirlukast or montelukast, causes reversible liver toxicity in about 4% of patients. They are appropriate first-line controlled medications in mild persistent asthma or as adjuncts to inhaled corticosteroids in moderate or severe asthma.

Anticholinergics

Anticholinergics act as bronchodilators in most asthmatic patients. Ipratropium bromide (Atrovent), a quaternary isopropyl derivative of atropine, is poorly absorbed and has few of the systemic side effects of atropine, making it the anticholinergic of choice. Although it is not approved by the Food and Drug Administration (FDA) for use in children younger than 12 years, many younger children benefit from its use. It can prolong the effectiveness of concomitantly administered beta-adrenergic agonists and is useful in asthma induced by cold air, irritants, or emotion. Atropine is administered by nebulization, and ipratropium is available as a metered-dose inhaler; both can be used three or four times each day.

Antihistamines

Some data suggest that high-dose nonsedating antihistamines offer statistically, but probably not clinically relevant, benefits in asthma. Previous concerns about the mucus-drying effects of H_1 antihistamines have also proved to be clinically irrelevant. Although antihistamines are probably not much help in asthma, they should not be withheld in children who require them for other reasons, such as allergic rhinitis or eczema.

Antibiotics

The routine use of antibiotics for asthma is not warranted; however, children with frequent asthma attacks often have sinusitis exacerbating their asthma. All asthmatic patients with frequent or difficult asthma, especially those requiring hospitalization, should be evaluated for sinusitis. Chronic sinusitis can be indolent and generally requires 3 to 6 weeks of therapy with appropriate antibiotics. Amoxicillin-clavulanate (Augmentin), cefuroxime axetil (Ceftin), and clarithromycin (Biaxin) are frequently successful. Amoxicillin (Amoxil), erythromycin (E-Mycin), cefaclor (Ceclor), and trimethoprim-sulfamethoxazole (Septra, Bactrim) are less effective because of the emergence of drug-resistant strains of bacteria.

Management Strategies

No single asthma management strategy is successful for all patients. Each person has a unique mix of triggers and baseline airway reactivity, necessitating individualization of asthma therapy. However, the following guidelines have been adopted by the National Institutes of Health and apply to most patients.

Occasional mild asthma can be effectively managed with bronchodilators alone. They should be administered by inhalation (2 puffs) because the onset of action is more rapid and side effects are lower by this route. Patients with exacerbations of their asthma symptoms more than twice a week should receive bronchodilators as needed, coupled with daily prophylactic therapy designed to inhibit inflammation and reverse airway hyper-reactivity. Cromolyn is remarkably safe and is an effective prophylactic agent in many children. An adequate trial requires at least 4 weeks of daily administration (2 puffs or 1 nebulization four times a day). If successful, the patient can be weaned to the lowest daily dose giving normal pulmonary functions and adequate protection from symptoms. Children who respond to disodium cromoglycate will probably also respond to nedocromil, particularly children with cough-variant asthma. In the event of cromolyn failure, inhaled corticosteroids should be instituted. Beclomethasone has been used most extensively in children and has a high topical/systemic ratio. Four puffs twice daily is a reasonable starting dose. If this fails to provide adequate control, a more potent corticosteroid, such as triamcinolone, budesonide, or fluticasone, could be tried. Flunisolide is also an excellent choice, although the taste is prohibitively objectionable to some children. After pulmonary functions have normalized, the dose of inhaled steroids can be reduced to the minimum required to maintain good control. The frequency of bronchodilator use should be monitored as an index of success of prophylactic therapy. Leukotriene modifiers should be added if bronchodilators are required frequently to reverse symptoms. Although the exact role of leukotriene modifiers is still being determined, it may be reasonable to use leukotriene modifiers as first-line anti-inflammatory prophylactic agents.

In cases of moderate to severe asthma with daily debilitating symptoms, the institution of inhaled corticosteroid therapy is often insufficient to achieve adequate control, and a course of oral corticosteroids, administered in divided doses concomitant with inhaled steroids, should be considered. The dose of prednisone required is highly individual, but in general, infants and preschoolers require about 15 to 20 mg per day, whereas school-aged children require 30 mg per day. Occasionally, a steroid-dependent asthmatic adolescent may require up to 60 mg per day to effect a remission. The dose should be sufficient to cause a marked improvement in pulmonary functions within a week, and the steroid therapy should be continued until optimal improvement has been achieved. In most patients, complete control can be achieved within 7 to 10 days, but some need longer treatment. The key to success is to use a high enough dose for a sufficient time to maximize lung functions. After control is achieved, the patient should be weaned from the oral steroids as rapidly as is practical and safe.

Patient Education

It is often not difficult to achieve good control. However, maintaining control requires the cooperation of a knowledgeable patient or parent who has been taught to recognize triggers and early signs of asthma. Knowledge is a powerful combatant to the fear, confusion, frustration, and desperation experienced by many families attempting to deal with the seemingly unpredictable nature of asthma and its effects on the quality of life and family dynamics.

Patients should be directed to appropriate resources and support groups. Several organizations provide plentiful resources and support for the patient. Allergy and Asthma Network/Mothers of Asthmatics (Fairfax, Virginia; telephone 800-385-4403) publishes a monthly newsletter filled with practical information and numerous educational and practical resources. They also publish a reference list of asthma resources entitled *Team Work.* Local chapters of the American Lung Association sponsor lectures by physicians and paramedics for asthmatic patients and their families, and local Asthma and Allergy Foundation of America chapters sponsor allergy support groups. In addition, the Food Allergy Network publishes helpful information for patients with food allergies, including notices about contamination of commercial foods with possible food allergens.

Patients and their families must be taught to monitor peak flow readings and to record any possible events that may lead to decreases in peak flow. The physician can use this information to help the patient identify triggers and recognize early signs of asthma exacerbations. On the basis of this information, the physician should instruct the patient about avoidance of allergens and other triggers. The patient should also be provided with a written asthma management plan, including a maintenance medication prescription and details of expected medication effects and common side effects. The asthma management plan should detail additional medications that are to be taken when peak flow readings begin to drop or when known triggers, such as an upper respiratory infection, are encountered. It should also give instructions about when to contact the physician. Graded asthma management plans must be individualized, but Figures 1 and 2 can be used as guidelines. Asthmatic patients whose condition deteriorates quickly usually require early intervention with oral corticosteroids to prevent complete deterioration and the need for emergency care.

Emotional Considerations

Parents must be encouraged to expect comparable behavior and, within reason, comparable achievements from their asthmatic and nonasthmatic children. Care must be taken to avoid sibling jealousies over attention given to the asthmatic child. An attitude of achievement and well-being can replace an attitude of defeat if the patient and parent are made

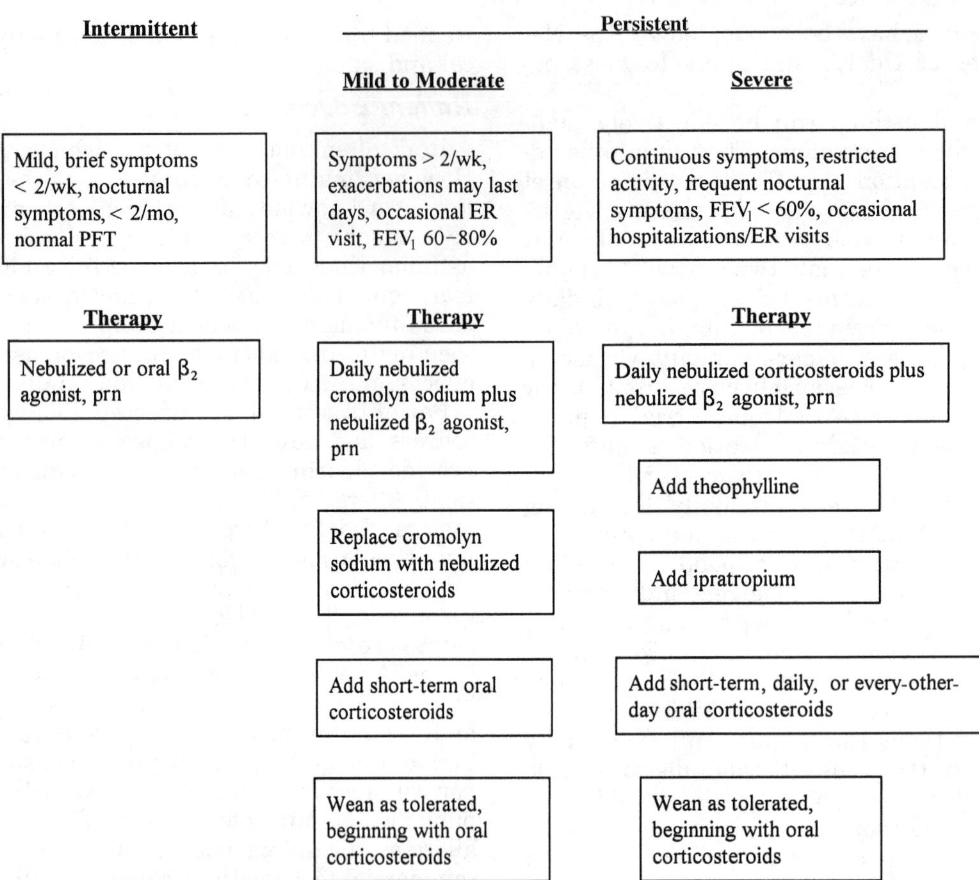

Figure 1. Treatment of asthma in infants and toddlers.
Abbreviations: PFT = pulmonary function test; FEV_1 = forced expiratory volume in 1 second; ER = emergency room.

to realize that they can control the asthma rather than having the asthma control them. With proper management, most asthmatic children can lead normal lives with normal activities as long as they take their regular medications and premedicate appropriately.

Age Considerations

Relevant asthma triggers and the therapeutic agents available to treat children vary with age.

INFANTS AND TODDLERS

Close monitoring of the asthmatic infant is a challenge, because typical wheezing may be difficult to detect. Parents should pay particular attention to cough and labored breathing, especially labored exhalation that occurs after hard play, nursing, or crying, particularly in association with respiratory infections. Cough and noisy breathing at night should also be monitored. The primary caregiver's observations, recorded in a symptom diary, can be an invaluable aid to the physician.

There are two major types of asthmatic infants: those who wheeze only with infections and frequently improve with age and those who wheeze continuously and experience considerable difficulty. Overlap exists between the two groups, and it is impossible to predict which infants will enter remission.

Response to therapy in infancy is often poor. Milder symptoms can be treated with oral beta-adrenergic agonists; more moderate symptoms may respond to nebulized beta-adrenergic agonists (0.2 to 0.3 mL of 5% solution) diluted in cromolyn (2 mL). In more severe cases in which the combination of beta agonists and cromolyn fail to control symptoms, nebulized budesonide should be given prophylactically in place of cromolyn. Acute severe symptoms unresponsive to beta agonists may necessitate treatment with oral corticosteroids (5 to 7.5 mg of prednisone or prednisolone twice daily). In difficult cases, oral theophylline may also be administered if additional bronchodilation is required (see Figure 1). Prescriptions for infants and toddlers should be dispensed in duplicate form when indicated so that day care providers can have their own supply. Written asthma management plans complete with medication side effects should also be made available to day care providers.

THREE- TO SIX-YEAR-OLD CHILDREN

Many 3-year-old and most 4-year-old children can perform peak flow maneuvers. This information adds a whole new dimension to the asthma management plan. For instance, in cases with a mild exercise component, the decision about premedicating before moderate exercise can be based on the peak flow

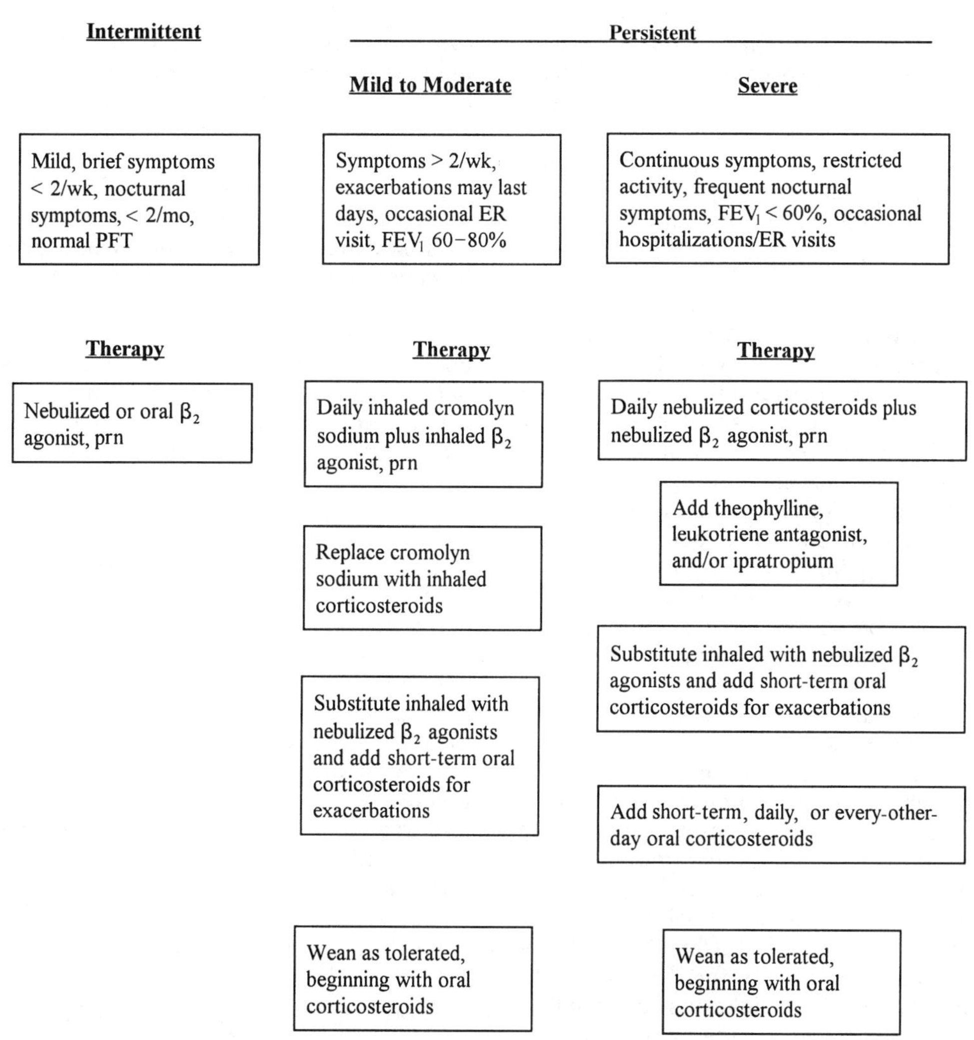

Figure 2. Treatment of asthma in children 4 years old to adolescents.
Abbreviations: PFT = pulmonary function test; FEV_1 = forced expiratory volume in 1 second; ER = emergency room.

reading. Peak flow readings can provide information about airway reactivity, because the differences in peak flow readings before and after bronchodilator use, as well and morning to evening peak flow variability, seem to correlate positively with airway hyper-reactivity. However, peak flow readings do not reflect small airway disease, which takes the longest to resolve. Although peak flow readings are a valuable and inexpensive tool, they cannot take the place of complete pulmonary function testing.

Most preschoolers can use metered-dose inhalants delivered through spacer devices. There are many available choices (InspirEase, Inhal-Aid, AeroChamber). The InspirEase is compact and provides excellent aerosol delivery to the lungs. Because the bag collapses as the child inhales, it provides excellent visual feedback for the child and confirmation for the parent that the child actually inhaled through the mouth. It is important to take a slow deep breath and hold it to maximize aerosol delivery. Most spacers contain whistles that blow when the inhalation is too rapid.

Occasional symptoms are best treated with two inhalations of a beta-adrenergic agonist (e.g., albuterol [Ventolin], metaproterenol [Alupent]). For more persistent symptoms, inhaled cromolyn (2 puffs four times each day) or a leukotriene-receptor antagonist should be administered daily for reversal of airway hyper-reactivity, and bronchodilators should be continued as symptomatic medications. As with the younger group, inhaled corticosteroids are substituted in the event of a therapeutic failure, and more severe cases may require a short course of oral steroids (10 to 20 mg twice daily) to achieve control. In difficult cases, cromolyn or a leukotriene modifier and inhaled corticosteroids should be used concomitantly. Oral beta-adrenergic agonists, ipratropium bromide (Atrovent), 2 puffs four times a day as needed or oral theophylline may be added as additional bronchodilators. Ipratropium bromide is especially useful if cholinergic mechanisms are involved (e.g., those evoked by emotion or cold weather). This age group is also particularly susceptible to exacerbations with upper respiratory tract infections, and inhaled prophylactic medications (cromolyn or corticosteroids) should be increased or instituted at the first sign of an infection in susceptible patients (see Figure 2). Prescriptions for preschool-aged children should be dispensed in duplicate form when indicated, so that day care providers can have their own supply. Written asthma management plans complete with medication side effects and a peak flow meter should also be given to day care providers.

SIX- TO TWELVE-YEAR-OLD CHILDREN

Children in this age group should take increasing responsibility for their asthma. Younger children should be encouraged to guess their peak flow readings and should record the actual values. It has been demonstrated that the regular use of a peak flow meter results in improved perception of airway obstructions and more accurate early recognition of impending exacerbations. As children mature, they should be taught the names of their medications and encouraged to use their peak flow readings to identify their asthma triggers. These children, especially the older ones, can also be given some responsibility (with careful supervision) for keeping their rooms free of clutter and dust and for taking their own medications. A flow-chart on which children can record medications taken, symptoms, and peak flow reading can help to teach self-management skills. Prescriptions for school children should be dispensed in duplicate form so that school nurses can have their own supply. Written asthma management plans complete with medication side effects and a peak flow meter should also be provided for school nurses.

The medication scheme outlined for the 3- to 6-year-old group is also appropriate for this group. If, however, administration of medications at school is undesirable, inhaled corticosteroids or leukotriene modifiers should be given instead of cromolyn, because they are frequently more effective than cromolyn if twice-daily administration is necessary. Inhaled beta-adrenergic agonists are the bronchodilators of choice, especially if needed for exercise asthma. These agents should always be available for symptom reversal. If bronchodilators are required several times daily despite inhaled corticosteroid use, a long-acting bronchodilator, such as salmeterol or extended-release albuterol, can be added, or theophylline or a leukotriene modifier could be prescribed. Some specialists prescribe a morning dose of salmeterol given before school to protect against exercise asthma during the school day.

ADOLESCENTS

It is during adolescence that asthma frequently becomes a battleground between parent and patient. All too often, this results in poor asthma control. The need for continual education cannot be overemphasized. Adolescents must understand that they have control over their disease and that disruption of their lifestyles and the need for additional medications can be reduced if they monitor themselves closely and follow their asthma management plans. It is preferable to allow adolescents to self-medicate at school; however, if school policy does not permit this, duplicate prescriptions, asthma management plans complete with medication side effects, and a peak flow meter should be made available to the school nurse.

The agents of choice for reversing inflammation and hyper-reactivity are inhaled corticosteroids, because compliance with four-times-daily dosing of cromolyn is often a problem. Inhaled beta-adrenergic agonists are preferred for symptomatic treatment; however, slow-release albuterol is a good alternative. Ipratropium bromide, oral theophylline, and leukotriene modifiers are also acceptable choices. Some adolescent girls experience monthly asthma exacerbations immediately before menses. These episodes can be anticipated and should be treated with increased medications as the peak flows dictate.

TREATMENT OF EXACERBATIONS

A 20% fluctuation in peak flow readings is normal. A fall of more than 20%, however, is often a harbinger of an asthma attack and should be the trigger for instituting the backup asthma management plan. Treatment of an asthma exacerbation depends on how quickly the pulmonary functions usually fall. Most children's condition deteriorates slowly over several days or weeks, allowing the physician to take a conservative approach. Others deteriorate rapidly and require hospitalization within 24 to 48 hours. These children must be aggressively managed if hospitalization is to be avoided. In either case, triggers of asthma, such as otitis and sinusitis, or allergen exposure, should be sought and dealt with.

Management of Children Subject to Slow Deterioration

In children subject to slow deterioration, occasional peak flow readings between 70 and 80% of predicted can be treated with an additional dose of an inhaled beta-adrenergic agonist. Nebulized treatments should be used if the response to metered-dose inhalers is poor. Infants with occasional symptoms may also be treated with oral or nebulized beta-adrenergic agonists. However, infants with continual symptoms or children with peak flow readings that stay between 70 and 80% for several days despite four-times-daily bronchodilators should begin taking or increasing their dose of inhaled corticosteroids to reverse the airway hyper-reactivity. Oral beta-adrenergic agonists, ipratropium bromide, or theophylline can be added to give additional symptomatic relief.

If the peak flow readings drop to between 50 and 70% of predicted values or fail to improve on the described regimen, a short course of oral prednisone is probably needed to reverse the attack. The sooner this is instituted, the less is required. I usually prescribe prednisone thrice daily and continue until the peak flows have been normal for 2 days. Prednisone given for 7 days or less can be stopped abruptly. If longer administration is required, the afternoon prednisone dose may be discontinued after improvement has been steady for a few days. Thereafter, prednisone may be slowly discontinued, taking care not to stop prednisone completely until after the peak flows have normalized. Ideally, these children should have pulmonary function tests done before steroids are discontinued to be sure that the small airways have normalized. The effectiveness of corticosteroids seems to be determined by the incremental dose prescribed. Thus, children taking maintenance oral prednisone may require a higher dose of prednisone during an exacerbation than those not receiving corticosteroids. If peak flows fall below 50% of predicted, the need for hospitalization is likely in the absence of intervention, and oral corticosteroids should be instituted immediately. Precipitating factors, such as sinusitis or otitis, should be sought and treated aggressively.

Management of Children Subject to Rapid Deterioration

Children who require hospitalization within 24 hours of an exacerbation should be managed very aggressively. At the first sign of a likely trigger, such as an upper respiratory tract infection, inhaled corticosteroids should be instituted or increased, and beta-adrenergic agonists should be administered as needed, via nebulization if necessary. If, despite these precautions, peak flow readings drop below 75% of predicted, oral corticosteroids and nebulized beta-adrenergic agonists should be started immediately. Oral beta-adrenergic agonists, ipratropium bromide, or theophylline can be added for additional symptomatic relief. The family should have a supply of prednisone at home, and reliable parents should be given permission to start prednisone on their own if the peak flow readings are down and the patient cannot be seen right away, or if the physician does not return their phone call within a stated period.

For children who do not require hospitalization as often or who tend to deteriorate over 24 to 48 hours, the decision about starting prednisone can be more relaxed. Peak flow readings that are dropping in the morning can be treated with inhaled steroids and nebulized beta-adrenergic agonists. However, it is often wise to begin prednisone if peak flow readings are falling in the late afternoon. It usually takes at least 6 to 8 hours for prednisone to start producing an effect. Because asthma is usually worse in the middle of the night and early morning, the patient's condition can be expected to deteriorate rapidly in the middle of the night, and this is the time when the parents' awareness and the physician's availability are at a low point. Early administration of oral corticosteroids to patients with histories of rapid deterioration can significantly reduce the need for hospitalizations and the cumulative dose of prednisone required.

Exacerbations at School

Occasionally, asthma is worse during the week than on the weekend. The pattern can be confirmed with frequent peak flow readings taken at home and at school. In such cases, antigen exposure at school may be a problem. The best solution is antigen elimination at school, but often, the problem is more complex and difficult to correct. In these cases, frequent administration of cromolyn (every 2 hours) while at school may solve the problem. Although administration of cromolyn more often than four times daily is not FDA approved, cromolyn is extremely safe. A lethal dose is unobtainable in animal models, and adverse effects are not seen below several grams (300 mL) per kg per day of inhaled cromolyn sodium.

STATUS ASTHMATICUS

Children presenting with acute severe asthma require both beta$_2$-adrenergic agonists and corticosteroids. Unless the asthma is a component of anaphylaxis, there is little need to use injected epinephrine. Nebulized albuterol, terbutaline, or metaproterenol should be administered every 20 minuets three times (as long as the heart rate remains below 80% of predicted maximum) or until a satisfactory increase in the peak flow reading has been obtained. Methylprednisolone (Solu-Medrol), 2 mg per kg, should be administered intravenously early in the course of treatment. Oxygen therapy is frequently required and when needed can improve the response to beta$_2$-adrenergic agonists.

A sinus radiograph is probably the most useful screening test in status asthmaticus. Radiographic evidence of sinusitis is found in approximately 50% of children hospitalized in status asthmaticus. Often the infection is silent, but proper antibiotic therapy can cause marked improvement in asthma symptoms. Arterial blood gas measurements are also helpful, because the hypoxic lung is poorly responsive to beta$_2$-adrenergic agonists. A chest radiograph is helpful if a pneumothorax or pneumonia is suspected or if other causes for wheezing are sought, and serum theophylline levels should be obtained in patients receiving theophylline.

If hospitalization is necessary, particular attention should be paid to oxygenation, adequate hydration, and expulsion of mucus. Chest percussion should be performed every 4 hours as long as mucus plugging persists. Nebulized beta$_2$-adrenergic agonists and intravenous methylprednisolone are usually required every 4 hours; however, in difficult cases, beta$_2$-adrenergic agonists can be administered more frequently as long as the heart rate remains acceptable. If the patient is receiving cromolyn or theophylline, these agents should be continued. Little added benefit is derived from the addition of these agents during status asthmaticus, and theophylline given acutely can cause numerous unpleasant side effects.

In cases of respiratory failure, the child should be admitted to the intensive care unit for an albuterol drip and possible ventilatory support. The need for either procedure is rare, and both involve risk to the patient. Therefore, if respiratory failure is anticipated, it is advisable to refer the child to a physician specifically trained to treat respiratory failure in asthmatic patients.

The adequacy of the discharge plan is as important as the acute treatment. Patients who are not already monitoring peak flow readings should be given a peak flow meter and educated in its use. Unless pulmonary functions have normalized, discharged patients should receive a short course of oral corticosteroids to avert a relapse. Because crisis care alone is inadequate for optimal asthma management, patients not currently receiving long-term follow-up care should receive appropriate referrals. Children not previously evaluated for allergies should also receive appropriate referrals. Following these guidelines can reduce subsequent hospitalizations.

ALLERGIC RHINITIS CAUSED BY INHALANT FACTORS

method of
JOHN W. GEORGITIS, M.D.
Wake Forest University Baptist Medical Center
Winston-Salem, North Carolina

Allergic rhinitis affects between 15 and 20% of the U.S. population, thereby qualifying it as one of the most common chronic diseases. Even though the disorder can develop at any age, two thirds of patients report symptoms before the age of 30 years, with a peak incidence in childhood and adolescence. Rhinitis has a significant impact on public health from missed days from school and work, reduced school and work performance, and the cost of treatment. Complications of chronic rhinitis include chronic and recurrent sinusitis, chronic cough, otitis, nasal polyposis, and sleep disturbance. There is also convincing evidence that untreated allergic rhinosinusitis worsens asthma. Allergic rhinitis is associated with a genetic predisposition for atopic disease. Persons with one atopic parent have a 30% chance of developing allergic rhinitis. If both parents have allergies, this increases to 50%.

PATHOPHYSIOLOGY

Atopic patients following adequate allergen exposure produce excessive amounts of IgE antibodies against the allergens. IgE binds to high-affinity receptors on the surface of mast cells and basophils. With allergen re-exposure, cross-linkage of the IgE receptors on the mast cell takes place and triggers cell activation. This is followed by the release of a number of inflammatory mediators, including histamine, prostaglandin D_2, and leukotriene C_4. These mediators act on the nasal tissue (nerve endings, blood vessels, and mucous glands), resulting in the symptoms of sneezing, pruritus, congestion, and rhinorrhea, which occur promptly after allergen exposure.

The mast cell–dominated immediate reaction can be demonstrated in the laboratory using nasal allergen challenge. Both the acute symptoms and the release of mediators subside after approximately 30 to 45 minutes. In about 50% of patients with allergic rhinitis, the acute response is followed by a late phase 3 to 12 hours later. This is accompanied by the release of most but not all of the acute phase mediators. More importantly, there is an influx of eosinophils, neutrophils, lymphocytes, and basophils. Cellular activation results in a subacute inflammatory reaction, which can last for a longer period. Changes in the function of the nasal mucosa take place, the most important being the development of hyperreactivity. This hyperreactivity of a nonspecific nature (reactivity against nonallergenic environmental stimuli) explains why patients with allergic rhinitis also complain of symptoms when exposed to irritants such as tobacco smoke, chemicals, and perfumes. Mucosal changes lower the threshold for subsequent allergen activation (priming effect), causing symptoms at lower doses of allergen. This may explain why patients continue to have symptoms at the end of the pollen season, when pollen counts are significantly decreased. The major allergens responsible for the symptoms of allergic rhinitis are shown in Table 1.

TABLE 1. **Major Inhalant Allergens in Allergic Rhinitis**

Outdoor Allergens
Pollens
- Trees (e.g., oak, birch, alder, cedar)
- Grasses (e.g., timothy, orchard, Bermuda, June rye)
- Weeds (e.g., ragweed, plantain, Russian thistle, sage)

Fungi
- Molds (e.g., *Alternaria, Cladosporium*)

Indoor Allergens
Dust mites (*Dermatophagoides pteronyssinus, Dermatophagoides farinae*)
Cat
Dog
Cockroach
Molds (e.g., *Aspergillus, Penicillium*)
Laboratory animals (rat, mouse)
Indoor pets (gerbil, guinea pig, hamster)

DIAGNOSIS

The diagnosis is usually established by a thorough history and can be confirmed with either allergen skin testing or blood tests such as the radioallergosorbent test (RAST). Physical examination is important in evaluating complications of allergic rhinitis. Table 2 shows a number of conditions that can produce symptoms that mimic allergic rhinitis.

TABLE 2. **Causes of Chronic Nasal and Sinus Symptoms**

Allergic rhinitis (seasonal, perennial)
Nonallergic, noninfectious, chronic rhinitis
Nonallergic rhinitis with eosinophilia syndrome (NARES)
Sinusitis
Allergic fungal sinusitis
Infectious rhinitis (bacterial, fungal)
Rhinitis medicamentosa (caused by topical decongestants)
Drug-induced rhinitis (aspirin, oral contraceptives, beta blockers, reserpine)
Anatomic abnormalities (septal deviation, septal spurs, concha bullosa)
Obstructive lesions (polyps, hypertrophic adenoids, tumors)
Endocrine causes (hypothyroidism, pregnancy, menses)
Granulomatous diseases (Wegener's granulomatosis, sarcoidosis)

History

The patient usually presents with nasal congestion, clear rhinorrhea, recurrent sneezing, and pruritus of the upper respiratory passages (nose, ears, throat, and oral mucosa). Most patients also have associated ocular symptoms such as tearing, redness, and pruritus of the eyes. Less common symptoms include ear "popping," posterior nasal drainage, throat clearing, and chronic cough. In fact, rhinitis is considered the most common cause of chronic cough in adults. Chronic rhinitis sufferers may complain of malaise and fatigue. Pruritus and sneezing are the most characteristic symptoms of allergic rhinitis and are helpful findings in the differential diagnosis of other rhinitic syndromes.

The interviewer should clarify whether the patient's symptoms are perennial and/or seasonal and how they are affected by seasonal changes. In seasonal allergic rhinitis (hay fever or rose fever), there is a temporal relationship between exposure to particular antigens, usually grass or ragweed pollen and/or molds, and the occurrence of symptoms. The age at onset and the severity and progression of symptoms are important elements of the history. Early onset of rhinitis indicates a very high probability of allergic etiology. Of patients whose chronic rhinitis begins before the age of 10 years, 90% have allergic disease. In contrast, of patients whose rhinitis begins after age 40, a nonallergic etiology is diagnosed in close to 60%.

Exacerbating factors such as cutting grass, raking leaves, weather changes, animal contact, and dust exposure should be identified. An assessment of the home and work environments and of the school environment for children is also important. The patient should be asked about his or her living conditions, the type of mattress and pillow used, including protective covering, and the décor in the bedroom. The presence of pets in the house, especially in the bedroom, should also be assessed. Exposure to animal material, indoor dust, and molds at the workplace or school can be important. Any changes in the environment that relate to the onset or worsening of symptoms should be noted. When the problem is related to pets, the patient often denies any symptomatic association.

Past medical history as well as medications currently in use or used in the past should be evaluated, as this information can provide important diagnostic clues. Some forms of nonallergic rhinitis can be caused by pharmacologic agents (topical decongestant sprays, some antihypertensives) or by systemic illnesses, including autoimmune disease or vasculitis and granulomatous disorders. Family history of any atopic disease should be elicited. This enhances the confidence of a history-based diagnosis. The most important elements of the history in the differential diagnosis for allergic rhinitis are summarized in Table 3.

TABLE 3. **Diagnostic Clues to Differentiate Allergic from Nonallergic Rhinitis**

- Temporal relationship between symptom onset, duration, and seasonal or environmental changes (moving to a new location, acquiring a pet) is suggestive of allergic rhinitis
- Sneezing, nasal pruritus, and associated conjunctival symptoms are characteristic of allergic rhinitis
- Allergic triggers (pollen, dust, molds, pets) suggest allergic rhinitis; nonspecific irritants (perfumes, tobacco smoke, cold or dry air) suggest nonallergic disease
- Age at onset: The earlier the onset, the more likely that allergies are involved
- Personal or family history of rhinitis, asthma, or eczema: more likely to identify patients with allergic rhinitis

Diagnostic Testing

To confirm the diagnosis of allergic rhinitis, laboratory tests can be performed, with the goal of establishing the presence of specific IgE antibodies against suspected allergens on the patient's skin tissue or in the serum. The standard diagnostic technique is allergen skin testing. Because serum IgE is in equilibrium with the clinically important mast cell-and-basophil–bound IgE, serum testing is a viable alternative, but it is expensive. When skin testing or serum testing is performed, careful selection of the material to be tested is needed to include all relevant allergens, depending on the geographic location and the patient's environment. The interpretation of allergy tests should take into account the patient's history. For example, if the patient does not complain of food-related symptoms, testing with food allergens is of no use.

There are two types of skin tests: puncture (prick) and intradermal. It is safer to start with puncture and then perform intradermal testing if the puncture tests give negative results. The combination of negative skin test results and a history of nonspecific aggravating factors such as tobacco, strong odors, paint, or solvents is diagnostic for nonallergic rhinitis. In a general practitioner's office, skin testing is not an option, and the patient must be referred to an allergy specialist because of the risk of anaphylaxis. However, serum-specific IgE detection tests (in vitro allergy tests) can be used to partially fulfill the same purpose. The most common such test is the radioallergosorbent test (RAST). RAST is less sensitive and more expensive than skin tests; in addition, results are not available for several days after the evaluation. However, a screen RAST panel including a major tree pollen (e.g., oak for the northeastern United States), a common grass (e.g., June), a ragweed, a dust mite, cat and/or dog, cockroach, and possibly a mold (e.g., *Alternaria*) may offer a rough idea of the atopic status of the patient. A referral to an allergy specialist and skin testing may be required if, despite negative or equivocal results on the RAST panel, the suspicion of allergic rhinitis based on the patient's history is high, or if management with detailed environmental control and/or immunotherapy is indicated. In the latter situation, testing needs to be more extensive, and the sensitivity of the procedure should be optimal. Even in the allergist's practice, in vitro testing may be the only option in patients with skin diseases such as severe eczema or dermatographism, or in those who are being treated with antihistamines and cannot discontinue treatment for the required 2- to 5-day period, or in those who have received astemizole (Hismanal) for the prior 2 months (astemizole is a nonsedating antihistamine with a very long half-life).

Nasal smears have been used to detect local eosinophilia (greater than 5 eosinophils per high-power field). This finding is suggestive but not diagnostic for allergic rhinitis, since eosinophils can be seen in the nonallergic rhinitis with eosinophilia syndrome (NARES). However, nasal eosinophilia predicts a favorable response to treatment with topical intranasal corticosteroids. The presence of neutrophilia without eosinophils in the nasal secretions should point away from allergic rhinitis, because this finding tends to be indicative of bacterial sinus infection. The presence of blood eosinophilia and total serum IgE levels are not useful in the diagnosis of allergic rhinitis, since they are neither specific nor sensitive. Some patients may have significant levels of specific IgE to a particular allergen (or to a small group of allergens) with normal or even low levels of total serum IgE.

Physical Examination

Normal findings on physical examination do not preclude the diagnosis of allergic rhinitis. Certain features, however, are classic. Examination of the eyes shows mildly hyperemic conjunctivae, with tearing or the presence of a gelatinous exudate. On routine anterior rhinoscopy, the nasal mucosa typically is pale or has a slightly bluish discoloration with boggy and edematous turbinates. Various amounts of watery, clear secretions can be observed. Erythematous mucosa with thick yellowish mucus should raise suspicion for other causes of rhinitis. Anterior rhinoscopy can offer further information regarding the presence of polyps or tumors, as well as anatomic lesions such as septal spurs or septal deviation. If the mucosa is severely swollen with the inferior turbinates touching the septum, topical decongestant sprays (Afrin, Neo-Synephrine) can shrink the mucosa to allow visualization of the posterior structures. Nasal endoscopy (using either a rigid or a flexible rhinopharyngoscope) can be even more helpful in this regard. In children, darkening under the eyes due to chronic venous pooling (allergic shiners) can sometimes be observed. Also, because of frequent rubbing of the nose upward (the allergic salute), a characteristic nasal crease may be seen in both adults and children.

MANAGEMENT

Allergen Avoidance

Avoidance is the first step that should be initiated after identification of the offending allergens. Complete avoidance of pollens is difficult; however, minimizing outdoor activities during the peak season of a particular allergen can be helpful. Air conditioning and keeping the windows closed can effectively reduce pollen levels inside the house. Use of high-efficiency particulate air (HEPA) filters in the main ventilation system can further reduce indoor pollen.

If the patient is allergic to pets, the obvious and most effective environmental control is to remove the pet from the indoor environment. If this is not an acceptable option, the pet should be kept out of the bedroom to minimize allergen accumulation on the bedding and the floors. In addition, pet allergen levels can be reduced by washing the animal weekly or on alternate weeks. Removal of carpeting—a major reservoir for most indoor allergens—may be of significant help. Also, transfer of pet allergen into the bedroom can be minimized by removing shoes and possibly clothing prior to entering the room and by frequent carpet vacuuming using a vacuum cleaner equipped with HEPA filters. Obviously, any close contact between the patient and the pet should be minimized. The patient should also be informed that it takes from several weeks to several months after an animal is removed for the indoor allergens to fall to substantially lower levels. This is well documented in the case of cat allergens but should be considered for other pets as well.

Both indoor and outdoor molds can be inducers and triggers of allergic rhinitis. Outdoor molds, most commonly *Alternaria* and *Cladosporium,* are present in higher numbers in the fall, as the decaying leaves and rotting vegetation provide an excellent material for fungal growth. Patients should avoid activities such as raking leaves, cutting grass, and working in barns or with compost. If this is not possible, wearing a paper mask or a scarf may provide some protection. *Penicillium* and *Aspergillus,* the most common indoor molds, are more prevalent in basements and damp areas. Limiting indoor relative humidity to 50% or less is an effective way to decrease mold growth. Adequate ventilation and repair of water leaks, as well as care not to overwater indoor plants, help keep humidity under control. In very humid environments (such as in waterfront residences), dehumidifiers can be useful.

Dust mites constitute the most common source of indoor allergen for patients with perennial allergic rhinitis. The gastrointestinal tracts of the two species of house dust mites, *Dermatophagoides farinae* and *Dermatophagoides pteronyssinus,* produce allergenic glycoproteins that are released into the environment through the fecal material. Since dust mites feed on the dead skin that humans continually shed, they tend to congregate in mattresses, pillows, carpets, and places where people generally sit or lie. Dust mites also thrive in high-humidity areas such as inside old organic materials. Placing plastic mite-proof covers over the mattresses, box springs, and pillows can result in a significant reduction in dust mite exposure. Patients should avoid using feather pillows and having upholstered furniture in the bedroom. Stuffed animals are a high-level dust mite reservoir in children's bedrooms and should be removed. Washing the bed sheets, blankets, pillowcases, and comforters in hot water (120° to 140°F) every week is an effective way to kill dust mites. Maintaining an indoor humidity of 50% or less can also slow dust mite growth. Acaricides (benzyl benzoate), substances that kill dust mites, and allergen-denaturing chemicals (tannic acid) are relatively effective but only temporarily. Air filtration devices are not particularly useful in eliminating dust mites, because the allergens are relatively heavy and settle quickly on the floor.

Cockroach sensitivity has been recognized as a significant problem in populations of lower socioeconomic status who live in inner-city areas. The most common species in the United States are the German cockroach *(Blattella germanica)* and the American cockroach *(Periplaneta americana).* Although several studies have found a significant association between cockroach sensitivity and asthma, the relationship is less clear in allergic rhinitis. Since these conditions often coexist, an attempt to decrease exposure to cockroach allergens should be encouraged. Helpful measures include reducing access to food material and water sources, spraying cockroach runways with 0.5 to 1% diazinon or chlorpyrifos, blowing boric acid powder into inaccessible areas, and setting out bait stations containing hydramethylnon (Combat).

Pharmacologic Intervention

Antihistamines

Antihistamines are effective in reducing pruritus, sneezing, tearing, and rhinorrhea, but not nasal congestion. These agents complete with histamine for the H_1 receptors on specific target cells. They can be used on an as-needed basis, although they have a better effect if taken before symptoms develop or on a daily basis. The use of the older compounds (first-generation antihistamines) has been limited because of unwanted side effects, mainly sedation. These agents, owing to their lipophilic structure, are able to cross the blood-brain barrier and cause central nervous system (CNS) suppression (histamine is an excitatory CNS neurotransmitter). The sedative effect often lessens after continued use for 1 to 2 weeks. Another important side effect is the prolongation of voluntary reaction time, which affects the performance of motor tasks such as driving, job performance, and schoolwork. These drugs also have side effects due to their anticholinergic action, including dry mouth, constipation, blurry vision, and difficulty in urination. They should be avoided in elderly people, especially those with symptomatic benign prostatic hypertrophy, bladder neck obstruction, and narrow angle glaucoma.

A new generation of antihistamines was introduced about 10 years ago. These low-sedating antihistamines have relatively poor CNS penetration, and the incidence of sedation is no different from that of placebo (Table 4). They also show no interference with the performance of motor tasks and have no anticholinergic side effects. There is evidence that these compounds have a broader mechanism of action.

A still newer class of antihistamines has a slightly higher incidence of sedation but not as high as that seen with the older antihistamines. These antihistamines have the ability to inhibit the release of inflammatory mediators from a variety of cells. Several of the newer antihistamines have longer half-lives and active metabolites, which also prolong their action. This allows them to be administered once or twice daily, thus enhancing patient compliance. The active metabolite of astemizole, methylastemizole, has a half-life of 10 to 12 days.

Astemizole (Hismanal), loratadine (Claritin), and terfenadine (Seldane) are metabolized by the hepatic P-450 cytochrome system. This mechanism can be inhibited in the same P-450 hepatic cytochrome system by antifungals—ketoconazole (Nizoral), fluconazole (Diflucan), itraconazole (Sporanox)—and by macrolide antibiotics—erythromycin, clarithromycin (Biaxin), troleandomycin (Tao). Thus, concomitant administration of these two types of agents may elevate serum levels of the antihistamine. This increase can result in side effects involving the cardiac muscle such as QT interval prolongation as seen on the electrocardiogram, which could then lead to more serious cardiac adverse effects, including ventricular tachyarrhythmias (torsades de pointes) and sudden death. Cardiovascular side effects have been reported with both astemizole and terfenadine. Loratadine and cetirizine (Zyrtec) have not been associated with QTc abnormalities. Increased awareness of such potential cardiac effects and patient education have been very successful in substantially controlling this

TABLE 4. **Antihistamines Used for Allergic Rhinitis**

Agent	Dosage		
	Adult or Child >12 y	*Child 6–12 y*	*Child <6 y*
Oral—High Sedation			
Chlorpheniramine (Chlor-Trimeton)	4 mg 4–6 times a day 8 mg tid 12 mg bid	2 mg qid	1 mg qid
Clemastine (Tavist)	1.34–2.68 mg bid	0.5 mg bid	—
Diphenhydramine (Benadryl)	25–50 mg qid	5 mg/kg/day in divided doses	
Tripelennamine (pyribenzamine [PBZ])	25–50 mg qid or 100 mg bid		
Cyproheptadine (Periactin)	4 mg tid	4 mg bid	2 mg bid
Hydroxyzine (Atarax)	50–100 mg qid	10–25 mg qid	10 mg qid
Oral—Low Sedation			
Astemizole (Hismanal)	10 mg qd		
Loratadine (Claritin)	5–10 mg qd	10 mg qd	—
Terfenadine (Seldane)	60 mg bid	—	—
Fexofenadine (Allegra)	60 mg bid	—	—
Oral—Moderate Sedation			
Cetirizine (Zyrtec)	10–20 mg daily	5–10 mg daily	—
Acrivastine (Semprex*)	8 mg qid	—	—
Nasal Antihistamines			
Azelastine (Astelin)	137 μg/spray: 2 sprays bid each nostril	—	—

*Available only with pseudoephedrine.

problem. It is important to mention that the dose needs to be reduced in patients with hepatic dysfunction, in those who receive medication affecting the QT interval (procainamide), or in those with cardiac dysrhythmias affecting repolarization. Terfenadine is now replaced by fexofenadine (Allegra), which is the major metabolite of terfenadine. Cardiovascular events noted with terfenadine have not been reported with fexofenadine. Seasonal and perennial allergic rhinitis symptoms have been effectively controlled with use of fexofenadine. Azelastine nasal spray (Astelin) is now available as an alternative mode of administering an antihistamine. Through topical delivery, the antihistamine works both locally and systemically to block histamine receptors. More commonly, antihistamines are given in combination with oral decongestants (discussed subsequently). The beneficial effects of both agents effectively relieve the majority of mild to moderate symptoms seen with allergic and nonallergic rhinitis. In addition, the newer, nonsedating antihistamine loratadine, combined with pseudoephedrine (Claritin-D 24 Hour), can be given once a day for rhinitis.

In conclusion, antihistamines are a reasonable choice for use as first-line agents in the treatment of intermittent or mild symptoms of allergic rhinoconjunctivitis. In moderate or severe disease, they can be useful adjunctive agents in therapy with topical corticosteroids or cromolyn sodium (Nasalcrom).

Sympathomimetics (Decongestants)

Decongestants belong to the alpha-adrenergic agonist family and are effective in the treatment of mucosal congestion, as they can constrict the blood vessels and reduce blood flow to the nasal tissues. They have no significant effects on the other symptoms of rhinitis. Decongestants exist in topical preparations as well as oral forms.

Topical forms include oxymetazoline (Afrin, Nōstrilla), naphazoline (Privine), and phenylephrine (Neo-Synephrine) sprays. Patients should be cautioned not to use these preparations for more than 3 to 5 days, because prolonged use may lead to rhinitis medicamentosa (tolerance, rebound nasal congestion, and hyperemic nasal mucosa). In the occasional patient who presents with severe nasal swelling, intranasal administration of a topical decongestant for the first few days can facilitate the administration of other sprays such as topical corticosteroids or cromolyn. Topical decongestants are also used to allow visualization of the posterior nasal passages during diagnostic rhinoscopy and to help patients sleep when they experience severe nasal blockage.

Oral decongestants such as pseudoephedrine hydrochloride (Sudafed) and phenylpropanolamine hydrochloride (Entex) can be taken for longer periods than recommended for topical preparations, because they do not cause rhinitis medicamentosa. However, alpha-adrenergic agonists can stimulate the CNS, causing nervousness and insomnia. For some patients, it is advisable to avoid these agents at night. Decongestants can elevate blood pressure, and persons with hypertension or borderline high blood pressure should use them cautiously. Also, decongestants should be avoided in patients with coronary artery disease or hyperthyroidism, in those taking monoamine oxidase inhibitors, and in those with seizure disorders.

Oral decongestants are often combined with antihistamines. Given the ineffectiveness of antihistamines in relieving nasal congestion, these preparations are superior to the individual compounds. The usual adult dose of pseudoephedrine hydrochloride is 60 mg taken every 6 hours. Children 6 to 12 years old should take half of this dose, and those between 2 and 5 years old should take only a quarter of the dose (15 mg) every 6 hours.

Guaifenesin

Guaifenesin (Humibid L.A.), originally an expectorant used in preparations intended for management of lower respiratory tract problems, is currently an ingredient of numerous prescription and over-the-counter preparations for the treatment of rhinitis. It is formulated either as a single agent or in combination with antihistamines and decongestants. Its mode of action is believed to be the loosening of respiratory secretions by increasing their water content. It is therefore thought to facilitate mucociliary clearance of secretions from the sinus and the nasal mucosa.

The recommended dose of guaifenesin for upper respiratory tract therapy is 1200 mg twice a day. The clinical effect of this compound is quite subtle. Whether it is beneficial in allergic rhinitis is not clear. However, guaifenesin administration can be tried as adjuvant therapy in rhinitis patients with concomitant chronic sinus complaints and/or posterior nasal drainage of secretions that is refractory to other treatment. Guaifenesin has an excellent safety record.

Ipratropium Bromide

Intranasal ipratropium bromide (Atrovent Nasal Spray 0.03%) is now available for use in allergic rhinitis. This anticholinergic preparation is not absorbed into the circulation, and atropine-like systemic side effects are minimal to nonexistent. Ipratropium should be used mainly to control nasal secretions in selected cases in which rhinorrhea is not responding to other preparations. It does not affect the other symptoms of allergic rhinitis. The recommended dose is 2 sprays per nostril two to three times a day. Adjusting the dose can prevent nasal dryness, which is the main side effect. The higher-dose formulation (0.06%) is effective in reducing secretions seen with upper respiratory tract infections.

Cromolyn Sodium

Cromolyn sodium (Nasalcrom) is used as a 4% topical spray for the treatment of allergic rhinitis. Its mode of action is claimed to be through the stabilization of mast cells in the nasal mucosa. However, studies on human mast cells do not strongly support this mechanism. When the drug is taken properly (1 to 2 sprays in each nostril four to six times a day), its efficacy is similar to or better than that of antihistamines. In addition to the symptomatic relief, cromolyn appears to have various anti-inflammatory properties that could be beneficial chronically. This agent works better if used preventively a couple of weeks before seasonal symptoms begin. Because of its anti-inflammatory action, the effect of cromolyn takes some time to become obvious. Cromolyn is not very useful when taken on an as-needed basis. Nasal application is usually well tolerated, and except for mild, transient stinging, no major side effects have been reported. Cromolyn is a pregnancy category B agent; therefore, it is used frequently in pregnant or lactating women. An ophthalmic preparation of cromolyn (Crolom) is available to be used for the treatment of allergic conjunctivitis. This form also needs frequent dosing—1 or 2 drops in each eye four to six times per day.

Ophthalmic Preparations for Allergic Conjunctivitis

Patients frequently report bothersome conjunctivitis during seasonal exacerbations of their allergic rhinitis. This conjunctivitis is only partially responsive to oral antihistamines and decongestants or nasal anti-inflammatory agents. Therefore, topical ophthalmic preparations are often given concomitantly with other rhinitis medications. Cromolyn ophthalmic solution (Crolom) may be given as 1 or 2 drops in each eye every 4 to 6 hours. Lodoxamide (Alomide), also a mast cell stabilizer, may be given as 1 or 2 drops four times a day for up to 3 months. Alternatively, ketorolac (Acular), a nonsteroidal anti-inflammatory drug, can be given to relieve the ocular itching of allergic rhinitis; long-term use (for more than 1 week) has not been fully investigated. Topical antihistamine-sympathomimetics such as pheniramine-naphazoline (Naphcon-A) may be given as 1 or 2 drops four times a day for the ocular itching and redness.

Saline Nasal Sprays

Occasionally, a rhinitis patient may have severe thickened secretions or extremely dry nasal mucosa. Simple saline nasal sprays (Ayr, NaSal, Ocean, Salinex) can be administered two to four times a day to loosen the secretions and add some moisture back to the mucosa. The only risk is bacterial contamination of the spray bottle with chronic use; patients should be warned about this possibility.

Corticosteroids

The most effective agents for the treatment of allergic rhinitis are corticosteroids. Owing to the significant side effects with systemic administration, topical preparations are highly preferred. If systemic corticosteroids are needed, their use should be limited to the occasional patient who presents with complete nasal obstruction. Because complete obstruction can cause significant discomfort, with eustachian tube dysfunction and sleep disturbance, a short course of oral corticosteroids (e.g., 40 mg of prednisone for 5 days) is recommended. This type of management is meaningful, however, only when it is offered in parallel with the initiation of therapy with a topical corticosteroid preparation. Oral corticosteroids should not be used as a substitute for topical preparations.

The potency of topical corticosteroids is higher than that of any other treatment modality. In fact, topical application is as effective as systemic treatment and is not associated with systemic side effects, because the dose is small and the absorption minimal. The number of available topical corticosteroids is increasing (Table 5), and their share of the allergic rhinitis prescription market has risen from 8 to 20% within the past 10 years. The mode of action of corticosteroids at the cellular level is not fully understood. However, their anti-inflammatory activity in allergic rhinitis has been clearly demonstrated. Topical application of nasal steroids for 1 week inhibits not only the late inflammatory sequelae of acute exposure to allergen (cellular infiltration, increased nasal reactivity to nonallergic stimuli, nasal priming to allergen) but also, surprisingly, the symptoms and the release of inflammatory mediators of the immediate allergic reaction. The latter effect is believed to be secondary to the ability of local glucocorticoids to reduce the number of mucosal mast cells. This effect is not obtained with systemic steroid treatment.

Patients should be informed that therapy with nasal corticosteroids does not result in the rapid responses seen with antihistamines or decongestants and that the drug must be used for at least a few days before significant effects are noticed. Patients should be instructed to place the tip of the drug delivery apparatus in the middle of the nasal passages and to avoid aiming toward the septum or the inferior turbinate. After each puff is administered, they should sniff slightly to facilitate distribution to other parts of the nasal mucosa. In addition, the newer corticosteroids (fluticasone and mometasone) produce symptom relief within the first few days of use.

After a few weeks of treatment, these preparations should provide excellent results in the majority (more than 80%) of patients with allergic nasal symptoms.

TABLE 5. **Nasal Glucocorticosteroid Preparations**

Drug	Dosage
Beclomethasone dipropionate (Vancenase, Beconase)	1–2 puffs or sprays bid
Budesonide (Rhinocort)	2–4 puffs qd
Flunisolide (Nasarel)	2 sprays bid
Fluticasone (Flonase)	2 sprays qd
Triamcinolone acetonide (Nasacort)	2–4 puffs qd or 2–4 sprays qd
Mometasone (Nasonex)	1–2 sprays qd

At that point, the dose can be adjusted according to the patient's clinical picture. Once-a-day or alternate-day dosing, even below insert recommendations, is often enough to control the disease.

Local side effects are minimal and usually involve irritation of the nasal mucosa. About 10% of patients using intranasal steroids may complain of burning or sneezing after local application. Epistaxis (blood-tinged secretions) or, rarely, hemorrhage has been observed in about 2% of patients. Discontinuing the medication for 2 to 3 days and applying a topical ointment on the nasal mucosa usually resolve this problem. Septal perforation, although rare, has been reported; the mechanism for this adverse event is unknown. It is important that rhinoscopy be performed prior to the initiation of treatment to rule out the pre-existence of septal mucosal ulcerations that might contraindicate the use of corticosteroids. Prolonged administration of topical corticosteroids has been studied and appears to be a safe option. In one study, administration of beclomethasone (Beconase, Vancenase) for 5 years did not cause nasal atrophy in mucosal biopsy specimens. These compounds very rarely are associated with nasal candidiasis.

Preparations are available in both aqueous and aerosol forms. The decision to use one versus the other is more a matter of patient preference. Aerosol preparations may be more irritating to the nasal mucosa, whereas aqueous preparations may drip into the throat, resulting in reduced deposition of active medication in the nasal mucosa.

Some practitioners use intramuscular or intranasal injections of long-acting corticosteroid preparations. Because of the prolonged half-life, these preparations can ameliorate the symptoms of allergic rhinitis during the entire pollen season. However, the risk of side effects—e.g., adrenal suppression—makes these practices potentially hazardous.

Immunotherapy

Immunotherapy is the only therapy for allergic rhinitis that entails the theoretical cure. This involves the administration of specific allergens in escalating doses until a target dose (maintenance) is reached. Administration is usually subcutaneous. Approximately 80% of patients have symptomatic improvement with immunotherapy. It is not clear, however, what this percentage is among patients who have failed all other treatments.

The mechanism of action in immunotherapy is still unknown, although several immunologic changes have been observed. Increased serum-specific IgG antiallergen antibodies (which are thought to block the allergen binding with mast cell–bound IgE) and the generation of antigen-specific suppressor T cells have been reported. Recently, several studies reported a reduction in "pro-allergic" cytokine (interleukin-4 and interleukin-5) production by lymphocytes and other cells of the immune system and/or promotion of the "antiallergic" (TH_1) phenotype of T lymphocytes. TH_1 cells characteristically produce interferon-γ and interleukin-2 upon activation.

Several placebo control trials have documented the efficacy of immunotherapy with a variety of allergens. Immunotherapy using high doses of allergen extracts is considered better than therapy with antihistamines and decongestants and probably than topical corticosteroid therapy. However, low-dose immunotherapy is no better than placebo and should be avoided. Allergen immunotherapy is a proven treatment modality only when subcutaneous injections are used, and other methods (oral) have not been found to be efficacious or practicable. It has been suggested that sublingual or intranasal immunotherapy may be an effective form of treatment, but more studies are needed to confirm this. Immunotherapy starts at extremely low concentrations of allergen, and injections are given once or twice weekly for 4 to 6 months until a maintenance dose is reached, and then every 2 to 4 weeks. Therapy should be offered for 1 year before a firm evaluation of efficacy is performed. If therapy has been successful, at least 3 to 5 years of treatment is recommended. After that, a decision whether to discontinue treatment has to be made. Unfortunately, this decision can be based only on intuition rather than on scientific evidence, because there is no way to predict the outcome of immunotherapy discontinuation. The beneficial effects can be sustained for a long time in some patients, but in others, symptoms recur soon after discontinuation of the injections.

Immunotherapy should be reserved for patients not responding to pharmacologic therapy or those who have significant side effects from the drugs. Some patients may have a preference for immunotherapy because of its appealing "natural" form of treatment. The risks and benefits of this treatment must be clearly explained to all patients. Although local reactions at the site of injection are frequent, they are easily controlled. Systemic reactions occur

TABLE 6. **Summary of Recommended Pharmacologic Regimens for Allergic Rhinitis**

Aspect of Disease	Pharmacologic Regimen
Mild disease	Antihistamines and decongestants, as needed
Moderate disease	Continuous cromolyn or topical corticosteroids; antihistamines and decongestants, as needed
Severe disease	Continuous topical corticosteroids; immunotherapy; antihistamines and decongestants, as needed
Thick secretions	Guaifenesin
Difficult-to-control rhinorrhea	Ipratropium bromide

infrequently and may require the use of epinephrine and intravenous fluid support. Adjustment of the allergen dose in patients with even mild systemic reactions is important, and only practitioners trained in the management of anaphylaxis should administer immunotherapy.

Table 6 summarizes our recommendations with respect to available therapies in allergic rhinitis.

ALLERGIC REACTIONS TO DRUGS

method of
LEMAN YEL, M.D., and
MICHAEL S. BLAISS, M.D.
University of Tennessee, Memphis
Memphis, Tennessee

An adverse drug reaction is an unintended and undesired response to an appropriate drug administered for diagnostic, therapeutic, or prophylactic benefit. Most adverse reactions do not have an allergic basis; only 6 to 10% are true allergic drug reactions. The risk of an allergic reaction is 1 to 3% for most drugs. Adverse drug reactions occur in 15 to 30% of hospitalized patients and in a substantial number of outpatients with various acute or chronic diseases. Drug-attributed deaths occur in 0.01% of surgical inpatients and in 0.10% of medical inpatients. Because of the morbidity and mortality resulting from adverse drug reactions, the proper evaluation and prevention of these reactions are of prime importance for the success, efficiency, and cost of patient care.

CLASSIFICATION OF DRUG REACTIONS

Adverse drug reactions can be divided into two major groups: predictable and unpredictable (Table 1). Approximately 80% of reactions are predictable. These are usually dose-dependent and are related to the pharmacologic drug action. *Toxicity* or *overdosage* is directly due to an excessive amount of the given drug above the threshold level. *Side effects* develop from therapeutically undesirable pharmacologic actions of the drug. A *drug interaction* is manifested by an unusual reaction occurring when two or more drugs are administered simultaneously. *Secondary* or *indirect effects* are consequences of the primary drug action, such as development of mucocutaneous candidiasis due to altered normal microbial microenvironment with prolonged antibiotic administration. Unpredictable drug reactions are usually dose-independent and unrelated to the pharmacologic action of the drug in a susceptible person. *Intolerance* occurs as a result of a lowered threshold to the normal pharmacologic action of the drug (e.g., tinnitus experienced at normal or small doses of aspirin). An *idiosyncratic reaction* is an unexpected response different from the drug's known pharmacologic actions in a genetically susceptible population, such as hemolytic anemia encountered in glucose-6-phosphate dehydrogenase deficiency after administration of an oxidant drug. *Allergic reactions* are immune-mediated, relatively rare responses in which drug-specific antibodies and/or sensitized T lymphocytes are involved. Previous exposure to the same drug is necessary for sensitization. Immediate reactions occurring within minutes often include manifestations of anaphylaxis such as urticaria, angioedema, hypotension, and respiratory distress. Allergic reactions can be clinically classified on the basis of the involved organ systems (Table 2). *Pseudoallergic reactions* refer to clinical manifestations similar to those seen in allergic reactions that are not triggered by immune mechanisms.

TABLE 1. **Adverse Drug Reactions**

Predictable	Unpredictable
Toxicity or overdose	Intolerance
Side effects	Idiosyncrasy
Drug interaction	Allergy (hypersensitivity)
Secondary (indirect effects)	Pseudoallergy

Coincidental and psychogenic reactions that are not related to drug effects may also be encountered. *Coincidental reaction* is the incorrect attribution of a manifestation to a drug, although it is actually caused by the primary illness. For example, a viral exanthem during a course of antibiotic therapy is freqently misdiagnosed as a drug allergy. Similarly, *psychogenic reactions* that are actually of psychologic etiology, such as hyperventilation after administration of a drug, can be attributed to the given drug.

RISK FACTORS FOR DRUG ALLERGY

Several factors related to the drug itself, concurrent disease or medication, or patient characteristics affect the expression of immune responses and clinical reactions to drugs. For instance, macromolecular drugs such as insulin are more likely to cause a drug reaction. Angiotensin-converting enzyme inhibitors can cause isolated angioedema. Vancomycin (Vancocin), radiocontrast media, and opiates can pharmacologically activate mast cells, resulting in immediate hypersensitivity type reactions. In general,

TABLE 2. **Clinical Classification of Allergic Reactions to Drugs**

Systemic Reactions	Single Organ Reactions
Anaphylaxis (IgE-mediated reactions)	Dermatologic reactions
Anaphylactoid reactions (IgE-independent reactions)	Urticaria and angioedema
Vasculitis	Macular and papular exanthems
Serum sickness	Vasculitis
Drug fever	Fixed drug eruption
Drug-induced autoimmune diseases	Toxic epidermal necrolysis
Complex multisystem reactions	Stevens-Johnson syndrome
	Erythema multiforme
	Exfoliative dermatitis
	Contact dermatitis
	Photoallergic reactions
	Pulmonary manifestations
	Asthma
	Pulmonary infiltrates with eosinophilia
	Fibrotic reactions
	Hematologic reactions
	Eosinophilia
	Cytopenias
	Hepatic inflammation
	Hepatocellular
	Cholestatic
	Nephritis
	Nephrotic syndrome
	Acute interstitial nephritis
	Carditis

topical administration is the most sensitizing route, followed by intramuscular, intravenous, and oral administrations. Frequent intermittent therapy courses with the same drug are more likely to result in sensitization than rare therapy courses. A drug taken continuously for long periods of time is less likely to cause a reaction. Beta-adrenergic blocking agents increase the likelihood and severity of anaphylaxis and interfere with the effect of epinephrine for therapy. Atopic patients do not have increased risk of drug allergy. However, they develop pseudoallergic reactions, especially to radiographic contrast media.

DIAGNOSIS

A detailed history is the cornerstone of the diagnosis of adverse drug reaction. The first step is considering the possibility of a drug reaction, followed by making a complete list of all drugs taken recently by the patient. In most cases, allergic reactions to a drug occur within at least 1 week after initiation of treatment unless there is a previous exposure. Differentiating a predictable reaction such as a side effect from an allergy prevents incorrect labeling and unnecessary avoidance of the drug itself or the same drug class.

In vivo and in vitro diagnostic tests are of limited value and should be used only when clinically indicated.

In Vivo Tests. Epidermal (prick) and intradermal skin tests may be useful in the diagnosis of immunoglobulin E (IgE)-mediated drug reactions. For large-molecular-weight agents such as foreign antisera, insulin, or enzymes, a positive wheal and flare reaction suggests an increased risk of anaphylaxis. However, skin tests are of limited value with low-molecular-weight drugs such as penicillin or sulfonamides, because without binding to carrier proteins, such drugs cannot achieve IgE antibody cross-linking on the mast cell surface, a phenomenon required for mediator release in an allergic reaction.

Patch or photopatch tests can be used for identification of delayed-hypersensitivity reactions such as contact dermatitis.

Provocative test dosing is done by starting with an initial dose of generally 1% of the therapeutic dose and increasing the dose by increments of two- to 10-fold every 15 to 30 minutes until a therapeutic dose is achieved. It is the most reliable method of diagnosis. However, it is potentially dangerous and requires a setting appropriate to treat anaphylaxis. It is not a desensitization method.

In Vitro Tests. Radioallergosorbent tests (RASTs) for identification of drug-specific IgE antibodies are rarely helpful in clinical practice, because there are few available antigens and most of the drug reactions are not IgE-mediated. Determination of drug-specific IgG and IgM antibodies, e.g., by Coombs' test, is used in diagnosis of drug-induced immune cytopenias.

TREATMENT

The treatment of choice is withdrawal of the suspected drug. In case of absolute need for continuation of the drug, introducing anti-allergy medication, i.e., antihistamines and corticosteroids, and close monitoring of the symptoms for progression can be considered to complete the recommended course of treatment.

In general, drug-induced anaphylaxis and anaphylactoid reactions, urticaria, angioedema, and asthma symptoms are treated symptomatically, as described elsewhere in this text.

Penicillin and Other Beta-Lactam Antibiotics

Beta-lactam antibiotics are the most common cause of anaphylactic reactions to drugs (80% of cases). Anaphylaxis and death due to anaphylaxis have been reported to occur in 0.01% to 0.05%, and 0.0015 to 0.002% of treatment courses, respectively. The overall prevalence of β-lactam allergy is around 2% of treatment courses. The most frequent manifestation is a morbilliform and urticarial rash.

Reactions to penicillins are classified as type 1, or immediate, reactions: IgE-mediated and potentially life-threatening reactions seen within the first hour after administration of the drug; type 2, or accelerated, reactions: usually IgE-mediated, rarely severe urticaria-angioedema reactions occurring 1 to 72 hours after drug administration; and type 3, or delayed or late, reactions: often IgE-independent, benign morbilliform skin eruptions that appear after 3 days of administration. Exfoliative dermatitis and Stevens-Johnson syndrome may also be encountered. All β-lactam antibiotics cause similar reactions. Anaphylaxis is more common with natural penicillins than with penicillinase-resistant penicillins (methicillin, nafcillin, dicloxacillin), aminopenicillins (ampicillin, amoxicillin), broad-spectrum penicillins (carbenicillin, ticarcillin, mezlocillin, azlocillin, piperacillin), and the cephalosporins. A non–IgE-mediated rash is commonly seen with use of ampicillin or amoxicillin. It is usually a nonpruritic and maculopapular rash that starts on the elbows and knees and spreads symmetrically to the body after at least 1 week of therapy. Ampicillin treatment in the presence of infectious mononucleosis classically results in a more severe rash, occurring in 90% of cases. The incidence of rash also increases in HIV infection, cytomegalovirus infection, chronic lymphocytic leukemia, and hyperuricemia.

All β-lactam antibiotics (penicillins, cephalosporins, monobactams, carbapenems, oxacephems, clavams, carbacephems) contain the main four-member β-lactam ring linked to a second five- or six-member ring, except for monobactams, which lack the second ring. Cross-reactivity between penicillins and carbapenems (imipenem, meropenem) is significant. Although less cross-reactivity has been reported with cephalosporins (occurring in 10% of treatment courses with first-generation drugs and in 1 to 3% with third-generation drugs), they should be administered cautiously in penicillin-allergic patients. Aztreonam (Azactam) is weakly immunogenic and may be given safely to patients allergic to other β-lactam antibiotics. Ceftazidime (Fortaz) and aztreonam share an identical side chain, and ceftazidime should be generally avoided in patients with aztreonam allergy.

Metabolites of penicillin and rarely the penicillin itself cause penicillin allergy. Ninety-five percent of penicillin is metabolized to penicilloyl, which is the major determinant. It is commercially available for

TABLE 3. **Beta-Lactam Antibiotic Skin Tests**

Skin Test Reagents	Route	Drug Test Concentration	Skin Test Volume
Benzylpenicilloyl-polylysine (Pre-Pen; 6×10^{-5} M)	Prick Intradermal	Full strength Full strength	1 drop 0.02 mL
Penicillin G potassium (fresh–1 week old)	Prick Intradermal Serial (optional)	10,000 U/mL 10,000 U/mL 10, 100, 1000 U/mL	1 drop 0.02 mL 0.02 mL
Penicillin minor determinant mixture* (10^{-2} M)	Prick Intradermal Serial (optional)	Full strength Full strength 10, 100, 1000 U/mL	1 drop 0.02 mL 0.02 mL
Cephalosporins and other penicillins†	Prick Intradermal Serial 10-fold dilutions (optional)	3 mg/mL 3 mg/mL	1 drop 0.02 mL
Aztreonam† (Azactam)	Prick Intradermal Serial 10-fold dilutions (optional)	3 mg/mL 3 mg/mL	1 drop 0.02 mL
Imipenem† (Primaxin)	Prick Intradermal Serial 10-fold dilutions (optional)	1 mg/mL 1 mg/mL	1 drop 0.02 mL

*Reagents available at some medical centers.
†Testing not validated. Negative results do not rule out a possible reaction.
Modified from DeSwarte RD, Patterson R: Drug allergy. *In* Patterson R, Grammer LC, Greenberger PA (eds): Allergic Diseases, 5th ed. Philadelphia, Lippincott-Raven Publishers, 1997, pp 317–412.

skin testing. Other metabolites including benzyl penicillin, penicilloate, and penilloate are named as minor determinants and are responsible for most of the penicillin anaphylactic reactions. A commercially standardized solution of these metabolites is not available for skin testing. Skin testing with both major determinant and fresh benzyl penicillin can identify approximately 95% of patients at risk for anaphylactic reactions. Ninety-nine percent of patients with negative skin test results to major and minor determinants may be given penicillin safely. Skin test reagents of other β-lactam antibiotics have not been standardized and remain investigational for now.

Penicillin skin testing should be done only when the patient has a history suggesting penicillin allergy and administration of the drug is essential. It is contraindicated with a history of Stevens-Johnson syndrome, toxic epidermal necrolysis, or exfoliative dermatitis. The patient should not take any antihistamines for at least 48 hours before skin testing. Three penicillin reagents, a positive control (histamine), and a negative control (saline or diluent) are used for testing (Table 3). When a minor determinant mixture is not available, test dosing can be performed in case of history of penicillin allergy and negative results on skin tests to major determinant and penicillin G, or when the questionable drug is a β-lactam antibiotic other than penicillin (Table 4). An antibiotic dose of 0.001 mg is administered by mouth or the intravenous route, and subsequent doses are given if no symptom develops. Results of the test are considered positive if a reaction occurs with any test dose. At this point, desensitization can be considered. The basic principle is starting with an initial dose of 1/10,000 of the recommended dose and then doubling the dose every 15 to 20 minutes until a full therapeutic dose can be achieved. In case of allergic reaction during desensitization, symptomatic treatment is given, and the protocol is continued from one dose below the point of reaction. After administration of the first therapeutic penicillin dose upon completion of desensitization, it is necessary to continue the treatment course without interruption. Any dose interval longer than 12 hours may cause the patient to return to his or her baseline allergic state.

TABLE 4. **Beta-Lactam Antibiotics**

Penicillins	Cephalosporins
Penicillin G	Cephalothin (Keflin)
Penicillin V (Pen Vee K)	Cefazolin (Ancef)
Methicillin (Staphcillin)	Cephalexin (Keflex)
Oxacillin (Prostaphlin)	Cephradine (Velosef)
Cloxacillin (Tegopen)	Cefadroxil (Duricef)
Nafcillin (Unipen)	Cefaclor (Ceclor)
Ampicillin (Omnipen)	Cephalexin (Keflex)
Amoxicillin (Amoxil)	Cephalothin (Keflin)
Carbenicillin (Geocillin)	Cefamandole (Mandol)
Ticarcillin (Ticar)	Cefuroxime (Zinacef)
Mezlocillin (Mezlin)	Cefonicid (Monocid)
Piperacillin (Pipracil)	Cefpodoxime proxetil (Vantin)
	Cefprozil (Cefzil)
Clavams	Cefotetan (Cefotan)
Clavulanic acid	Cefotaxime (Claforan)
Monobactams	Ceftixozime (Cefizox)
Aztreonam (Azactam)	Ceftriaxone (Rocephin)
	Cefoperazone (Cefobid)
Carbapenems	Ceftazidime (Fortaz)
Imipenem (Primaxin)	Cefixime (Suprax)
Meropenem (Merrem)	
	Oxacephems
Carbacephems	Moxolactam (Moxam)
Loracarbef (Lorabid)	

TABLE 5. **Sulfa Drugs**

Sulfonamide antibiotics
- Sulfamethoxazole (with trimethoprim: Bactrim, Septra)
- Sulfisoxazole (Gantrisin, Pediazole)
- Sulfacetamide (Sultrin cream, Blephamide eye drops)
- Sulfadoxine (Fansidar)
- Sulfasalazine (Azulfidine)
- Sulfinpyrazone (Anturane)

Oral hypoglycemics
- Glyburide (Diabeta, Micronase)
- Glipizide (Glucotrol)
- Chlorpropamide (Diabinese)
- Tolbutamide (Orinase)
- Acetohexamide (Dymelor)
- Tolazamide (Tolinase)

Diuretics
- Hydrochlorothiazide (Hydrodiuril, Esidrix)

Antihypertensive
- Diazoxide (Hyperstat)

Carbonic anhydrase inhibitor
- Acetazolamide (Diamox)

Sulfonamides and Other Antibiotics

Trimethoprim-sulfamethoxazole (TMP-SMX) (Bactrim, Septra) is the most commonly used sulfonamide antibiotic (Table 5). It is the best drug for prophylaxis and treatment of *Pneumocystis carinii* pneumonia in human immunodeficiency virus (HIV)-infected patients. It is also used as a prophylactic agent for *Toxoplasma gondii* infection in the same population. The most common reaction is a generalized maculopapular rash that develops 7 to 12 days after initiation of the treatment at a rate of 3% in the general population, 12% in immunodeficient patients, and 29 to 70% in HIV-infected patients. Most of these reactions are IgE-independent. Sulfa drugs can also be associated with erythema multiforme, Stevens-Johnson syndrome, and toxic epidermal necrolysis. When treatment with TMP-SMX is essential, as in HIV-infected patients with low $CD4^+$ cell counts, a desensitization protocol can be selected (Table 6). Because most of the protocols take several days, delayed reactions can be encountered and treated with antihistamines and corticosteroids. Sulfasalazine (Azulfidine) is effective in the treatment of ulcerative colitis; approximately 2% of patients develop maculopapular rash, fever, or both. A desensitization protocol can be used for such instances.

TABLE 6. **Trimethoprim-Sulfamethoxazole (TMP-SMX) (Bactrim, Septra) Desensitization Protocol**

Day	TMP-SMX Dose (mg)
1	0.4/2
2	0.8/4
3	1.6/8
4	3.2/16
5	8/40
6	16/80
7	32/160
8	64/320
9	80/400
10	160/800

Vancomycin (Vancocin) is an alternative antibiotic for treatment in severe staphylococcal and streptococcal infections. "Red man syndrome," characterized by pruritus, erythema or flushing on the face, neck, and upper trunk, and hypotension, results from rapid infusion of vancomycin (1 gram given over 1 hour). This represents a nonimmunologic release of histamine. Slower infusion of the drug over 2 hours or longer and pretreatment with hydroxyzine (Atarax) or diphenhydramine (Benadryl) may prevent the reaction. Vancomycin (Vancocin) can also cause an IgE-mediated rash. In such cases, readministration of the drug may cause exfoliative dermatitis.

Rare cases of skin rashes and pruritus have been reported with ciprofloxacin (Cipro). An alternative antibiotic should be substituted.

Aspirin and Nonsteroidal Anti-inflammatory Drugs

Adverse reactions to aspirin typically include urticaria, angioedema, asthma, chronic rhinosinusitis, and nasal polyps in sensitive patients. These reactions are not IgE-mediated. They probably result from inhibition of cyclooxygenase and subsequent increased production of leukotrienes. Because the sensitivity persists for life, management entails strict avoidance. Acetaminophen (Tylenol, Excedrin) is the most recommended drug as an alternative. Salsalate (Disalcid), choline salicylate–magnesium salicylate (Trilisate), and propoxyphene hydrochloride (Darvon) are the other drugs that can be chosen. All nonsteroidal anti-inflammatory drugs may cross-react with aspirin to varying degrees. Desensitization can be considered in aspirin-sensitive patients with respiratory disease.

Insulin

Reactions to insulin include local or systemic allergic reactions and insulin resistance. Although human recombinant DNA insulin appears to be less antigenic than bovine-type insulin, it can cause allergic reactions. Local reactions are the most common and are generally encountered during the first 1 to 4 weeks of therapy. They are usually IgE-mediated and consist of mild erythema and swelling, burning, and pruritus at the injection site. These local reactions usually disappear in 3 to 4 weeks with continued administration of insulin. Dividing the insulin dose into two or more sites or switching to a different preparation is generally helpful. If not, antihistamines may be given until the reaction disappears. Local reactions may precede anaphylactic reactions. Therefore, epinephrine (EpiPen auto-injector) should be made available to these patients. Systemic reactions include urticaria, angioedema, bronchospasm, and hypotension. Most of these reactions occur upon re-starting of insulin after an interruption in insulin therapy. In treatment of the systemic reactions, it is important not to discontinue insulin. If the last dose is given within 24 hours, the next dose should be decreased by one third and then subsequently increased slowly by 2 to 5 units per dose until the diabetes is under control. If it has been more than 24 hours since onset of the systemic reaction, a serious reaction with readministration of insulin is more probable. The least allergic insulin is selected by skin testing using several kinds of insulin, and desensitization is done in an intensive care unit (Table 7).

Radiographic Contrast Media

Immediate generalized reactions, most commonly urticaria, are encountered in 0.5 to 3% of patients receiving radiographic contrast media (RCM). These reactions are not IgE-mediated but probably involve mast cell activation with release of histamine and other mediators. Use of nonionic, lower-osmolarity agents reduces the risk of reaction; however, their use is limited because of higher expense. In patients who receive beta-adrenergic blocking agents, the reactions may be more severe and less responsive to treatment. There is no association between reaction to RCM and topical iodine solution or shellfish allergy.

The risk of subsequent reactions is substantially reduced by using pretreatment regimens of corticosteroids, antihistamines, and adrenergic agents and low-osmolarity nonionic RCM. Pretreatment medications include prednisone, 50 mg orally, administered 13, 7, and 1 hour(s) before the procedure; diphenhydramine, 50 mg orally or intramuscularly, given 1 hour prior to the procedure; and albuterol (Ventolin), 4 mg orally, or ephedrine, 25 mg orally, given 1 hour before the procedure in the absence of cardiac risk factors such as angina or arrhythmia.

Local Anesthetics

IgE-mediated reactions to local anesthetics are extremely rare. The adverse reactions usually take the form of vasovagal or hyperventilation episodes, toxic reactions, or epinephrine side effects. The preservatives in local anesthetics, sulfites and parabens, may be responsible for allergy-type reactions. In case of reaction, the suspect anesthetic should be replaced with a different agent (Table 8). A prick test is done with the undiluted local anesthetic, which does not contain epinephrine. If the result of the test is negative, graded subcutaneous injections of diluted and full-strength local anesthetic are given at 15-minute intervals. The tolerated agent is reported to the referring physician.

TABLE 7. **Insulin Desensitization Protocol**

Day	Time	Type	Dose (units)	Route
1	7:30 AM	Regular	0.00001	Intradermal
	Noon	Regular	0.0001	Intradermal
	4:30 PM	Regular	0.001	Intradermal
2	7:30 AM	Regular	0.01	Intradermal
	Noon	Regular	0.1	Intradermal
	4:30 PM	Regular	1.0	Intradermal
3	7:30 AM	Regular	2.0	SC
	Noon	Regular	4.0	SC
	4:30 PM	Regular	8.0	SC
4	7:30 AM	Regular	12.0	SC
	Noon	Regular	16.0	SC
5	7:30 AM	NPH/Lente	20.0	SC
6	7:30 AM	NPH/Lente	25.0	SC
≥7	7:30 AM	NPH/Lente	↑ 5 U/day until therapeutic level attained	SC

Abbreviation: SC = subcutaneous.
Modified from DeSwarte RD, Patterson R: Drug allergy. *In* Patterson R, Grammer LC, Greenberger PA (eds): Allergic Diseases, 5th ed. Philadelphia, Lippincott-Raven Publishers, 1997, pp 317–412.

TABLE 8. **Local Anesthetics**

Group 1: Benzoic Acid Esters	Group 2: Amide or Miscellaneous
Benzocaine	Bupivacaine (Marcaine)
Butamben picrate (Butesin Picrate)	Dibucaine (Nupercaine)
Chloroprocaine (Nesacaine)	Dyclonine (Dyclone)
Procaine (Novocain)	Etidocaine (Duranest)
Proparacaine (Ophthaine)	Lidocaine (Xylocaine)
Tetracaine (Pontocaine)	Mepivacaine (Carbocaine)
	Pramoxine (Tronothane)
	Prilocaine (Citanest)
	Ropivacaine (Naropin)

Heterologous Sera

Anaphylaxis and serum sickness may result from injection of heterologous antisera. Anaphylaxis is less common and occurs in atopic patients with preexisting IgE antibodies to the corresponding animal dander. Serum sickness is more common and is dose-related. Before administration of heterologous antisera to any patient, regardless of history, skin testing must be performed. Prick tests are done by using antisera diluted 1:10 with normal saline. If the result of the test is negative, intradermal skin testing with 1:100 dilution of antisera is performed. A negative result on skin testing rules out the possibility of significant anaphylactic reaction. In case of serum sickness, treatment with antipyretics, analgesics, antihistamines, and corticosteroids may be required.

Tetanus Toxoid

Minor reactions such as local swelling are common after tetanus toxoid or diphtheria–tetanus toxoid vaccinations. True IgE-mediated reactions are rare. When a patient with a history of a previous adverse reaction needs tetanus toxoid, a skin test–graded challenge may be performed. If the result of a prick test with undiluted aqueous tetanus toxoid is negative, 0.1 mL of tetanus toxoid is given subcutane-

TABLE 9. **Doses for Gradual Tetanus Toxoid Administration (Prick Test–Positive)**

Tetanus Toxoid Dilution*			Undiluted Tetanus Toxoid
1:1000	*1:100*	*1:10*	
0.05 mL	0.05 mL	0.05 mL	0.05 mL
0.10 mL	0.10 mL	0.10 mL	0.10 mL
0.20 mL	0.20 mL	0.20 mL	0.20 mL
0.30 mL	0.30 mL	0.30 mL	0.30 mL
0.50 mL	0.50 mL	0.50 mL	

*Stronger dilutions are used after injections from a given dilution are completed by incremental dose. Injections are administered subcutaneously every week or every other week.

TABLE 10. **Gradual Influenza Vaccine Administration (Prick Test–Positive)***

Dilution	Dose (mL)
1:100	0.05
1:10	0.05
Undiluted	0.05
Undiluted	0.10
Undiluted	0.15
Undiluted	0.20

*Intramuscular injections are administered at 15- to 20-minute intervals.

ously. In the absence of local reaction in 30 minutes, the rest of the vaccine dose is injected. If results on prick testing are positive, the steps in Table 9 are followed.

Avian-Derived Vaccines

MEASLES-MUMPS-RUBELLA (MMR). Currently available measles and mumps vaccines are derived from chick embryo fibroblast tissue cultures and do not contain significant amounts of egg cross-reacting proteins. Although immediate reactions occur following administration of MMR, in most cases they appear to be due to other vaccine components such as gelatin or neomycin. Therefore, the American Academy of Pediatrics recommends that children with egg allergy may routinely be given MMR, measles, or mumps vaccine without prior skin testing, and that the vaccine be given in one injection rather than in a series of increasing doses.

INFLUENZA AND YELLOW FEVER. Currently available yellow fever and influenza vaccines also contain egg proteins and on rare occasions may induce immediate allergic reactions. Skin testing with yellow fever vaccines is recommended for individuals with a history of systemic anaphylactic symptoms after egg ingestion. In adults with such a history who are to receive influenza vaccine, skin testing is recommended. In case of positive results on prick or intradermal testing, the decision to give the vaccine may be reassessed. If vaccination is essential, gradual administration at 15- to 20-minute intervals is preferred (Table 10). The American Academy of Pediatrics suggests that children with severe anaphylactic reactions to eggs should not receive influenza vaccine in view of the reaction risk, the likely need for yearly vaccination, and the availability of chemoprophylaxis against influenza A infection. Less severe or localized manifestations of allergy to egg or to feathers are not contraindications to yellow fever or influenza vaccines and do not warrant skin testing.

ACKNOWLEDGMENT

We would like to thank Philip Lieberman, M.D. for his review of the manuscript.

INSECT STING HYPERSENSITIVITY

method of
RICHARD F. LOCKEY, M.D.,
KEVIN P. ROSENBACH, M.D., and
ROBERT P. NELSON, JR., M.D.
University of South Florida College of Medicine
Tampa, Florida

Stinging insects include many different species and are responsible for significant morbidity and mortality. Insects of the order Hymenoptera account for most instances of insect sting hypersensitivity. Three taxonomic families are commonly involved: Apidae, which includes the honeybees (genus *Apis*) and bumblebees *(Bombus)*; Vespidae, which includes the wasps *(Polistes)*, yellow jackets *(Vespula* and *Dolichovespula)*, and hornets *(Vespa)*; and Formicidae, which includes the imported fire ants *(Solenopsis)* and harvester ants *(Pogonomyrmex)*.

The incidence of insect hypersensitivity is estimated at between 0.4 and 4% of the general population in the United States and may be higher in persons with a history of atopic disease or a family history of atopic disease. There is a 2:1 male/female ratio, and reactions are more common in rural populations and in the younger age group. The number of deaths attributed to Hymenoptera stings is estimated to be 40 per year in the United States (published in 1973). A 10-year survey of 460 venom-related fatalities in the United States, including snake bites, revealed that stinging insects caused the greatest number of deaths. A third study of 2606 insect sting–hypersensitive persons in the United States found yellow jackets incriminated most often, honeybees second, and wasps third. A study of persons in whom death had been attributed to unknown causes suggests that insect-related fatalities occur more frequently than had previously been reported. Some of the subjects, who had high postmortem serum titers of venom-specific IgE, probably died secondary to an insect sting.

The incidence of allergic reactions to each insect species varies with its geographic distribution; however, hymenopterans are found throughout the world. Affected persons usually alter their lifestyles, work patterns, and leisure activities because of the fear of having another insect sting reaction, particularly if they experienced a systemic reaction. Large local reactions and systemic allergic reactions can occur, with the most serious of the IgE-mediated reactions being anaphylaxis.

It is often possible to identify a specific stinging hymenopteran by its nesting characteristics; e.g., wasps build open paper nests under the eaves of homes and other buildings, in bushes, and in shrubbery around the homes. Yellow jackets build their nests in concealed locations, either underground, in wall cavities, or in decaying logs or stumps. Hornets usually build their nests in trees or bushes or on buildings, although some hornets build large paper nests and attach them to limbs of a tree. The honeybee is found throughout the United States in large hives, with up to 65,000 bees per colony. Most honeybee colonies live within man-made hives and are commercially managed for honey production and pollination. There are several genera of stinging ants, the most important of which are *Solenopsis* (imported fire ants) and *Pogonomyrmex* (harvester ants). The *S. invicta* and *S. richteri* species are most commonly incriminated in sting-induced anaphylaxis. *S. invicta* and *S. richteri* or a hybrid are found in various regions of the south central and southeastern United States. These ants build large subterranean nests and are difficult to eradicate with pesticides. Harvester ants are primarily but not exclusively found in the southern and western United States.

CLINICAL MANIFESTATIONS

Local Cutaneous Reaction

The normal response to an insect sting is a localized cutaneous reaction characterized by erythema and edema that may be associated with pain. Local cutaneous reactions and envenomation are nonallergic and are caused by the trauma inflicted by the stinger or the toxin injected by the insect. The local reaction may be mild and transient, lasting several hours, or the sting site may become erythematous and indurated, these effects persisting over 48 hours. This represents a toxic response to the venom. *Solenopsis* stings leave a characteristic sterile pustule that begins as a clear vesicle but becomes cloudy in 24 hours. The pustule is usually umbilicated and surrounded by a large erythematous, slightly painful area. If undisturbed, the pustule remains for 3 to 10 days before rupturing and resolving with subsequent crust formation. Pigmented macules, residual fibrotic nodules, or small scars may form at the site. *Pogonomyrmex* stings result in a wheal and flare reaction similar to a honeybee sting.

Large Local Reaction

Allergic local reactions are more extensive and persistent than nonallergic local reactions. Sensitization leading to large local reactions occurs in 17% of persons experiencing Hymenoptera stings and 30 to 50% of those experiencing imported fire ant stings. These reactions are presumed to be due to an IgE mechanism, although the pathogenesis is not understood. A large local reaction is manifested clinically by an extended area of warmth that may be painful or tender, pruritus, edema, and erythema at the sting site. It usually evolves over 24 to 72 hours and may last up to 5 days and involve an entire extremity. This type of reaction rarely becomes infected, although it is not uncommon for physicians to institute inappropriate treatment in these persons, whom they suspect to have cellulitis. Large local reactions do not predispose to systemic reactions, even though the majority of persons who experience such a reaction have positive results on skin testing and/or in vitro testing with Hymenoptera vaccines.

Systemic Reactions

Most systemic reactions (anaphylaxis) begin within the first 100 minutes following a sting, although they typically begin within the first 2 to 30 minutes. Some reactions can begin several hours following a sting. Generalized urticaria, pruritus, and erythema are the most common clinical manifestations. Angioedema of the lips, periorbital areas, tongue, ears, and other cutaneous organs; laryngioedema; asthma; abdominal cramps and diarrhea; and hypotension secondary to vascular collapse (anaphylactic shock) can also occur. Such reactions in their most severe form cause death.

Sustained anaphylactic reactions may persist for 24 hours or more, despite appropriate therapy. Rarely, delayed reactions involving the central nervous system develop 24 to 96 hours after the sting and may not be associated with a preceding immediate-type reaction. Neurologic manifestations such as encephalitis are possible. Other infrequent and late reactions include serum sickness, vasculitis, acute glomerulonephritis with renal failure, and nephrotic syndrome. The cause of these late reactions is not understood; however, they appear to be mediated by immunologic or toxic responses to venom. Reports concerning fatal toxic reactions to multiple bee stings and from Africanized "killer" bees have been published. Localized infections and septicemia may also occur, especially following imported fire ant stings. Fatalities following insect sting reactions most commonly result from upper and lower airway obstruction, acute vascular collapse, and hemorrhagic reactions. Deaths most often occur within 1 hour and are more common in older subjects, particularly in the presence of underlying disease such as coronary artery disease or generalized atherosclerosis. Occasional deaths have been reported several days after the sting, associated with sustained or delayed systemic reactions.

DIAGNOSIS

Hymenoptera venom vaccines are used to diagnose and treat honeybee, wasp, yellow jacket, and hornet systemic reactions; whole-body vaccines are used to diagnose and treat imported fire ant systemic reactions. Vaccines containing only ant venoms are not available for diagnosis and treatment of imported fire ant hypersensitivity. However, experimental evidence indicates that most commercial imported fire ant whole-body vaccines contain the allergens responsible for the hypersensitivity reaction. Skin testing is the most sensitive method of diagnosis, although in vitro techniques are also reliable methods for determining clinical sensitivity.

TREATMENT

Large Local Reactions

Ice packs applied to the sting site are beneficial. Topical corticosteroids are used extensively in clinical practice, although no convincing scientific evidence demonstrates their efficacy. Antihistamines and analgesics are useful to relieve the pruritus and painful swelling. Systemic corticosteroid therapy may benefit large painful reactions, although most local reactions resolve over a few days or a week and do not require treatment. The sting sites should be kept clean and intact, and scratching should be avoided to prevent secondary infection. This is especially true for imported fire ant stings.

Generalized Systemic Anaphylactic Reactions

Pharmacotherapy for Acute or Anaphylactic Reactions

(Table 1)

Treatment for any anaphylactic reaction is the same regardless of the cause. Aqueous epinephrine 1:1000 (0.1% or 1 mg/mL), 0.3 to 0.5 mL, subcutaneously (SC) or intramuscularly (IM), should be administered immediately in adults. Children experiencing anaphylaxis require 0.01 mL of epinephrine per kg of body weight, not to exceed 0.3 mL per dose. Epinephrine 1:1000, 0.1 to 0.3 mL, may also be injected directly into the sting site to delay absorption of

TABLE 1. **Treatment of Anaphylaxis**

I. Immediate measures
   a. Aqueous epinephrine 1:1000, 0.3 to 0.5 mL (0.01 mL/kg in children, maximum dose of 0.3 mL), given SC or IM; repeat as necessary (up to two times) every 15–20 minutes to control blood pressure and symptoms.
   b. Aqueous epinephrine 1:1000, 0.1 mL in 10 mL of normal saline (1:100,000), given IV over several minutes; repeat as necessary for anaphylaxis not responding to therapy. A 1:10,000 dilution may be necessary for intravenous use.

II. General measures
   a. Place patient in recumbent or Trendelenburg position and elevate lower extremities.
   b. Establish and maintain airway (endotracheal tube or cricothyrotomy may be required).
   c. Give oxygen.
   d. Give normal saline IV for fluid replacement and venous access. If severe hypotension exists, rapid infusion of volume expanders (colloid-containing solutions or saline) is necessary.
   e. Place a venous tourniquet above the reaction site to decrease absorption of the antigen.

III. Specific measures
   a. Aqueous epinephrine 1:1000, 0.1 to 0.3 mL, injected at the reaction site will delay antigen absorption.
   b. Diphenhydramine (Benadryl), 50 mg PO or IM given q 4–6 h, with a maximum daily dose of 400 mg in adults. In children, 1 mg/kg up to 50 mg PO or IM q 4–6 h.
   c. For asthma, give a nebulized beta$_2$ agonist such as albuterol (Ventolin or Proventil), 2.5–5 mg in adults in saline to a volume of 3 mL; 0.05 mg/kg in children continuously over 20-minute intervals.
   d. Aminophylline or ipratropium bromide should be given if patient is not responding to inhaled beta$_2$ agonist.
      Aminophylline: 6 mg/kg IV given over 20 minutes (adjust dose depending on age and concurrent illnesses or medications)
      Ipratropium: 0.5 mg in 3 mL normal saline given every 30 minutes up to three times, then every 2 to 4 h (0.25 mg in children).
   e. If hypotension persists, give dopamine, 400 mg in 500 mL of D5W, IV; adjust rate to maintain normal blood pressure.
   f. Cimetidine (Tagamet),* 300 mg (adults), or ranitidine (Zantac),* 150 mg (adults) IV given over 5 minutes; ranitidine 0.75–1.25 mg/kg IV or IM every 8 h (children).
   g. Glucagon, 1 mg or unit, SC, IM, or IV for adults or children weighing more than 20 kg; for children weighing less than 20 kg, give 0.5 mg or unit or a dose equivalent to 20–30 µg/kg.
   h. A corticosteroid, e.g., methylprednisolone (Solu-Medrol), 1 to 2 mg per kg for 24 hours, is usually not helpful in acute anaphylaxis but may be useful in delayed-onset or protracted anaphylaxis.

Abbreviations: D5W = 5% dextrose in water; IM = intramuscularly; IV = intravenously; SC = subcutaneously.
*Not FDA approved for this indication.

venom. Additional doses for protracted symptoms should be given as necessary or every 15 to 20 minutes. All patients, especially those with a history of cardiac disease, should be carefully monitored. Intravenous epinephrine, 1:100,000 (0.001%, or 0.1 mg in 10 mL of normal saline) given slowly, is indicated for anaphylactic shock not responding to standard therapy. Parenteral antihistamines should be used for persistent urticaria, angioedema, or laryngeal edema in patients who are not responding to epinephrine. Diphenhydramine hydrochloride (Benadryl) is administered in divided doses: adults receive 50 mg per dose, with a maximum dose of 400 mg per 24 hours, and 1 mg per kg per dose is given in children, with a maximum dose of 50 mg orally (PO) or IM every 4 to 6 hours.

Asthma should be treated with inhalational nebulized beta$_2$ agonists (albuterol, 5 mg per mL, 2.5 to 5.0 mg in adults, 0.05 mg per kg in children) given every 20 minutes up to three times or, when necessary, by continuous inhalation. If necessary, additional bronchodilation can be effected with intravenous infusion of aminophylline (6.0 mg per kg) administered over 20 minutes initially, with maintenance of therapeutic serum levels by continuous infusion. Ipratropium bromide (Atrovent), 0.5 mg in adults and 0.25 mg in children, is an effective adjuvant therapy and may be used with albuterol, particularly in patients with severe airflow obstruction. Oxygen therapy and maintenance of airway patency are essential, and intubation or cricothyrotomy is indicated for severe upper airway edema not responding to therapy. Intravenous fluid replacement, e.g., with saline or colloid-containing solutions, is necessary to correct persistent hypotension. Vasopressor agents should be administered if shock persists, and systemic corticosteroids, if given early, may reduce the risk of protracted or delayed anaphylaxis. Histamine H$_2$ blockers may be useful for the treatment of hypotension refractory to usual therapy. Glucagon, 2 to 5 units given intravenously (IV) over 2 minutes, may be useful in protracted anaphylaxis, especially when beta blockers complicate treatment.

Venom Immunotherapy

Venom immunotherapy reduces the risk of re-sting anaphylaxis from 40 to 60% to less than 5% in persons who have experienced systemic reactions. If anaphylaxis occurs after maintenance venom therapy has been instituted, it is almost always less severe than that which occurred before such therapy. Immunotherapy is not recommended for persons in whom severe, large local reactions have occurred. Adult subjects (16 years of age or older) who have experienced systemic reactions to honeybee, yellow jacket, hornet, and wasp stings should have appropriate venom skin or in vitro testing. If results of the tests are positive, venom immunotherapy should be initiated.

Fatal reactions from stinging insects rarely occur in children 3 to 16 years of age. Most reactions in this age group are mild (with cutaneous symptoms only), and re-sting usually does not result in a reaction or results in a mild reaction, despite positive results on skin testing. Venom immunotherapy is not indicated in this group, although it is recommended for children and young adults with a history of a severe systemic reaction and positive skin or in vitro tests (Table 2). There is some evidence that systemic reactions limited to the skin may not place the adult patient at risk for a more severe systemic reaction or death.

Physicians trained to care for persons with allergic diseases should institute appropriate therapy in those who have had a systemic reaction to Hymenoptera stings, especially those who are most likely to be re-stung or have altered their lifestyle to avoid being stung. In some centers throughout the world, no patient, regardless of age, receives venom immunotherapy without first having a positive sting test challenge. A study of 75 persons from the Netherlands with yellow jacket sensitivity found no relationship between the risk of relapse on sting challenges and the duration of venom immunotherapy, gender, age, severity of field sting reaction, skin test reactivity prior to immunotherapy, or changes in IgG4 level. The risk of relapse sting reaction was greater among patients with high levels of venom-specific IgE before and after immunotherapy. Specific IgE decreases with immunotherapy, and this decrease persists 3 years after the immunotherapy has been discontinued. Patients without detectable specific IgE did not experience relapse sting reactions to field stings or insect challenge stings. However, the IgE level need not be undetectable for protection against relapse. Patients with detectable IgE were also protected if their specific IgE decreased with immunotherapy. Another study compared the degree of venom skin test reactivity and the severity of a subsequent sting reaction. Persons who experienced asymptomatic field sting reactions but remained venom skin test–positive were at a higher risk (17%) of developing an allergic response to subsequent stings than venom skin test–negative persons or patients receiving venom immunotherapy (2%). The decision to initiate venom immunotherapy based on sting test challenge reactivity is controversial. Therefore, persons with a history of systemic reactivity to insect venom should receive venom immunotherapy if their RAST or skin test results are positive.

METHOD

Increasing increments of honeybee, wasp, yellow jacket, and hornet venom vaccines or whole-body vaccines for imported fire ant–induced anaphylaxis are administered in a series of weekly injections until the subject can tolerate a venom dose equivalent to one or more insect stings. Once a maintenance dose is reached and after 1 year of monthly injections, the interval can be increased to every 6 weeks. In most persons receiving vaccine therapy, various immunologic parameters are altered, among which are a decrease in venom-specific IgE and an increase in venom-specific IgG or blocking antibody. Treatment occasionally fails, particularly in yellow jacket–hypersensitive persons and those who do not achieve adequate levels of venom-specific IgG. The maintenance venom dose for these persons should be increased to 200 μg from the usual maintenance dose of 100 μg. The commonly used venom protocols take

TABLE 2. **Selection of Patients for Hymenoptera Venom Immunotherapy**

Sting Reaction in Children and Adults	Skin Test and/or RAST	Venom Vaccine (Honeybee, Wasp, Yellow Jacket, or Hornet)	Whole-Body Vaccine (Imported Fire Ant or Harvester Ant)
Children (1–16 years old)			
Systemic cutaneous reaction: non–life-threatening; immediate; generalized urticaria, angioedema, erythema, pruritus	+ or −	No	Yes*
Systemic generalized reaction: life-threatening; cutaneous lesions and either respiratory symptoms (laryngeal edema or bronchospasm) and/or cardiovascular symptoms (hypotension or shock)	+	Yes	Yes*
Adults			
Systemic reaction (cutaneous or generalized)	+ −	Yes No†	Yes* No†
Children and Adults			
Large local reaction (>2 inches in diameter, duration of >24 h)	+ or −‡	No	No
Normal reaction (<2 inches in diameter, duration of <24 h)	+ or −	No	No

Abbreviation: RAST = radioallergosorbent test.
*Only if results of skin test or RAST are positive for ant whole-body vaccine.
†The subject should be skin-retested, with reconstituted vaccine, in 4 to 6 weeks. If results are still negative, RAST should be repeated to confirm the negative result on skin testing. The opposite is true for a RAST-negative subject, in whom the skin test should confirm negative RAST results.
‡Subjects with large local reactions should not be skin-tested.
Modifed from Graft DF: Venom immunotherapy: Indications, selection of venom, techniques and efficacy. *In* Levine MI, Lockey RF (eds): Monograph on Insect Allergy. Milwaukee, American Academy of Allergy, Asthma and Immunology, 1995, p 77.

14 weeks to achieve a target maintenance dose of 100 μg and 6 weeks using the modified "rush" protocol. Rapid venom immunotherapy protocols can achieve this level safely in 3 weeks, and "rush" venom immunotherapy protocols can achieve a maintenance dose in 1 to 3 days.

Although venom vaccines have replaced whole-body vaccines for most hymenopterans, whole-body vaccines are still used for imported fire ant and harvester ant immunotherapy. Experimental evidence exists to support the use of whole-body vaccines for ant hypersensitivity, but blinded studies have not been done. Various species of ants can cause sting-induced systemic reactions. The venoms from four species of *Solenopsis* found in the United States (*S. invicta, S. richteri, S. xyloni*, and *S. aurea*) are highly cross-reactive, particularly allergens Sol 1 (phospholipase AB) and Sol 3 (antigen 5 family). Sol 1 and Sol 3 are similar to allergens found in wasp venom, and Sol 1 cross-reacts with vespid wasp venom phospholipase. *S. invicta* whole-body extract is sufficient to treat and diagnose reactivity to any ant species in the genus *Solenopsis*. Persons who have experienced systemic reactions to fire ant stings should be tested with serial dilutions of whole-body vaccine and started on immunotherapy at the dilution of the vaccine to which they did not react. The dose should be increased to the highest tolerated dose or to 0.5 mL of a 1:10 weight-to-volume preparation. When maintenance therapeutic doses are reached, the interval between injections can be gradually increased to 6 weeks over several months.

TABLE 3. **Measures for Prevention of Hymenoptera Stings and Bites**

What to do:	What not to do:
Know the stinging insects	Don't use lotions or perfumes that attract insects.
Know nesting and foraging behaviors.	
Remove or destroy nearby nests and hives; have professionals do this.	Don't provoke the insects or disturb a nest or hive.
Wear clean, light-colored, smooth-finished clothes; cover the body as much as possible and be practical.	Don't wear wool, leather, or suede.
Wear ankle socks and ankle-high shoes.	Don't go barefoot.
Keep outdoor activity area clean and free of food refuge and garbage.	Don't leave garbage cans uncovered.
Insect repellents are useless for stinging insects.	
For biting insects, midges, flies, and mosquitoes, use DEET*-containing repellents on clothes and skin, or apply Avon Skin-So-Soft.	

*N,N-diethyl-3-methylbenzamide. Most insect repellents contain this chemical. It is the only chemical insect repellent currently approved by the U.S. Food and Drug Administration.

Modified from Graft DF: Venom immunotherapy: Indications, selection of venom, techniques and efficacy. *In* Levine MI, Lockey RF (eds): Monograph on Insect Allergy. Milwaukee, American Academy of Allergy, Asthma and Immunology, 1995, p 97.

DURATION

Venom immunotherapy can be discontinued when results of repeated skin tests become negative. Venom vaccine immunotherapy can be safely discontinued after 5 years in all persons except those in whom the level of venom sensitivity has not declined. There appears to be a late-onset, non–IgG-mediated mechanism for the long-term suppression of allergic sensitivity by prolonged high-dose venom immunotherapy. Venom immunotherapy may be discontinued after 5 years regardless of skin test results, particularly in persons who have experienced mild to moderate systemic reactions, because the beneficial effects of venom immunotherapy appear to occur after a relatively short course of therapy. Sensitivity, even without treatment, is self-limited in up to 40% of affected persons. A duration of 3 to 5 years of venom immunotherapy is associated with a low risk of relapse after the immunotherapy has been discontinued. The study of 75 yellow jacket–sensitive persons in the Netherlands suggests immunotherapy can be safely discontinued if the specific IgE is undetectable, without regard to duration of immunotherapy. The converse is true for persons with a history of serious systemic reactions, loss of consciousness, or severe respiratory distress, in whom results of skin testing remain positive; immunotherapy should be continued for a more prolonged period.

POTENTIAL RISKS

Immunotherapy and venom skin testing is not without risk. A study of 1410 Hymenoptera-sensitive persons demonstrated venom immunotherapy to be safe, but systemic reactions did occur and could not be predicted by historical or diagnostic criteria. The systemic reactions were most likely to occur at doses between 1 and 50 μg and at maintenance doses, and honeybee and wasp venoms were most likely to produce a systemic reaction. Patients placed on immunotherapy are hypersensitive, and systemic reactions have been reported as a result of the therapy itself. Therefore, Hymenoptera vaccines should be used only by physicians experienced in immunotherapy and only when adequate means for treating systemic reactions are available. Patients should be informed of the possible risk for a systemic reaction and closely observed for at least 20 minutes after each injection. Initiating venom immunotherapy during pregnancy, especially during the first trimester, must be considered carefully. Anaphylaxis from an insect sting can cause fetal loss and maternal morbidity, whereas venom immunotherapy has been shown to be safe for use during pregnancy.

PROTECTION AND PREVENTION

Persons who have a history of insect hypersensitivity should carry an emergency insect sting kit containing aqueous epinephrine in a pre-filled syringe, at least until maintenance doses of immunotherapy have been attained. Several devices are available in the United States, including the EpiPen, EpiPen Jr., Epi E-Z and the Ana-Kit; other brands of injectable epinephrine are available in different parts of the world. The commercially available EpiPen and Epi E-Z Pen are syringes activated by a pressure mechanism that automatically injects epinephrine, 0.15 or 0.3 mL (0.15 or 0.3 mg); the Ana-Kit includes a self-injecting syringe that contains two 0.3-mL (0.3-mg) doses of epinephrine.

A Medic-Alert bracelet or medallion (Medic Alert, Turlock, CA) should be worn by persons who may be exposed to stings and have experienced insect-induced anaphylaxis. They should also be instructed on how to avoid being stung (Table 3). Scented hair oils, perfumes, and dark or floral-patterned clothing should be avoided. Persons at risk should wear shoes and avoid insect-populated areas.

Section 12

Diseases of the Skin

ACNE VULGARIS AND ROSACEA

method of
ZOE DIANA DRAELOS, M.D.
Bowman Gray School of Medicine of Wake Forest University
Winston-Salem, North Carolina

ACNE VULGARIS

Acne vulgaris is a disease with a bimodal age distribution, affecting adolescents as well as men and women 35 to 50 years of age. Treatment is aimed at minimizing lesions and scarring; thus, control is possible, while cure is not. Acne progresses through several well-defined stages, each of which requires accurate lesion recognition to initiate effective therapy (Table 1).

Initially, acne begins at about age 12 in girls and age 14 in boys, when the first signs of puberty are apparent. The lesions consist of closed comedones ("blackheads") and open comedones ("whiteheads") prominent on the nose, medial cheeks, central forehead, and middle chin. This distribution has been referred to as the T zone and corresponds to the facial areas containing the largest sebaceous glands. When sex hormone production begins in both genders, sebaceous glands begin to secrete into the duct connected to the follicular unit, which has not previously functioned with such vigor. The ducts become plugged with keratinous debris containing *Propionibacterium acnes* organisms, which produce lipases that degrade the sebum into irritating free fatty acids, stimulating hyperproliferation and further abnormal keratinization. This leads to development of microcomedones, which eventually enlarge the follicular ostia to yield open and closed comedones.

This stage of comedonal acne is treated with keratolytics and/or retinoids. Keratolytics such as benzoyl peroxide and salicylic acid chemically digest the keratin plug and follicular debris to allow sebaceous secretions to flow freely onto the skin surface. Benzoyl peroxide also has antibacterial properties, decreasing the number of *P. acnes* organisms available to degrade sebum. Retinoids (tretinoin [Avita, Retin-A], adapalene [Differin]) act to normalize follicular keratinization. Optimal therapy is obtained by combining both mechanisms of treatment, i.e., a keratolytic in the morning followed by a retinoid in the evening. Further keratolytic treatment can be obtained by using benzoyl peroxide– or salicylic acid–containing soaps, cleansers, or astringents. The next stage of acne is characterized by pustules in addition to open and closed comedones in the T zone distribution. Pustular acne develops when the follicular wall ruptures high in the dermis and minimal inflammation ensues. The use of keratolytics in addition to topical antibiotics (benzoyl peroxide with topical erythromycin [Benzamycin]) in the morning with retinoids in the evening constitutes effective treatment. Fortunately, this stage of acne is nonscarring, unless lesions are manipulated.

Follicular rupture and extrusion of the contents deeper into the dermis causes a foreign body–type inflammatory reaction resulting in production of an inflammatory papule. These papules are erythematous, tender, indurated, slow-healing lesions on the forehead, cheeks, and chin. Healing usually takes 3 to 6 months, but the postinflammatory hyperpigmentation may last longer, especially in darker-skinned persons. Scarring may occur if the lesion induces sufficient dermal damage.

Inflammatory acne requires a combination of topical keratolytics, retinoids, and oral antibiotics for

TABLE 1. **Acne Treatment**

Type of Acne	Characteristic Acne Lesion*	Treatment Options
Comedonal	Open and closed comedones	Benzoyl peroxide, salicylic acid, tretinoin (Avita, Retin-A), adapalene (Differin)
Pustular	Pustules	Topical antibiotics: erythromycin (E-Mycin), clindamycin (Cleocin T), sulfa drugs and sulfur (Sulfacet-R, Novacet), azelaic acid (Azelex)
Inflammatory	Erythematous papules	Oral antibiotics: tetracycline (Sumycin), doxycycline (Vibramycin, Monodox), minocycline (Minocin, Dynacin), erythromycin (E-Mycin), trimethoprim-sulfamethoxazole (Septra, Bactrim), ciprofloxacin (Cipro), cefadroxil (Duricef), oral contraceptives and spironolactone (Aldactone) (female patients only)
Cystic	Deep-seated inflammatory cysts with scarring	Oral isotretinoin (Accutane)

*Acne lesions of several types may be present, requiring selection of treatment options from several categories.

resolution (see Table 1). The keratolytics act as comedolytics, and the retinoids prevent microcomedo formation by inhibiting follicular hyperproliferation and normalizing follicular keratinization. Oral antibiotics are necessary to decrease inflammation and reduce the number of *P. acnes* organisms. Usually, tetracycline (Sumycin), 500 mg twice a day (bid), and erythromycin (E-Mycin), 500 mg bid, are used as first-line oral antibiotics, followed by trimethoprim-sulfamethoxazole (Bactrim, Septra), one tablet bid, and doxycycline (Vibramycin), 50 mg bid, with minocycline (Minocin), 50 mg bid, ciprofloxacin (Cipro), 250 mg bid, and cefadroxil (Duricef) 500 mg by mouth (PO) daily (qd) reserved for refractory inflammatory acne owing to the expense of these agents. Twice-daily administration provides a more consistent blood level, resulting in a better anti-inflammatory effect.

Some women who require both contraception and acne treatment may benefit from the use of oral contraceptives. Only the estrogen-containing birth control pills (Demulen) are effective. Low-dose estrogen pills and progesterone-only pills may actually worsen or induce acne in some women. Sometimes effective acne therapy in women is as simple as selecting another oral contraceptive. For other women who cannot or will not take birth control pills, administration of spironolactone (Aldactone)* 75 to 200 mg qd, offers another hormonal therapy, which acts by suppressing adrenal androgen production. Spironolactone is particularly useful in women who have other signs of androgen excess such as increased facial hair, female pattern hair loss, and increased body hair. Spironolactone is usually best administered with oral contraceptives because it can cause more frequent, irregular menses as well as feminization of a male fetus should conception occur during therapy with this agent. Thus, the drug is best used in mature women who are past their childbearing years. It also requires periodic potassium level monitoring because spironolactone is a potassium-sparing diuretic. In some cases, inflammatory acne is resistant to the aforementioned therapy and must be treated like cystic acne, discussed next.

The most serious form of acne is characterized by cysts and nodules, which result from deep dermal inflammation and may lead to prominent scarring. Cystic acne should be treated aggressively with topical keratolytics, retinoids, and oral antibiotics. If improvement is not obtained with 6 to 8 weeks of minocycline or another third-line acne antibiotic, a dermatologist should be consulted and the use of oral isotretinoin (Accutane) considered (0.5 to 1 mg per kg, divided into two daily doses, if possible). Oral isotretinoin is the only acne medication that can alter the acne course beyond the 16-week period it is administered. Successful treatment with oral isotretinoin requires an extraordinarily compliant patient who is willing to experience dry skin, eyes, and mucous membranes in addition to possible muscle pains and joint aches. Blood work is also required, including blood chemistry with liver function studies, hematology profile, and a negative serum pregnancy test in the female. Female patients must be carefully counseled to avoid pregnancy, through either abstinence or highly effective contraception (i.e., oral contraceptives, intrauterine device, medroxyprogesterone [Depo-Provera]), while on oral isotretinoin, because it is a potent teratogen.

Patients are exposed to much popular press regarding acne treatment. Certainly, the skin is a reflection of a healthy diet, but no well-controlled medical studies exist to demonstrate that basic acne is worsened by consuming chocolate, nuts, greasy foods, milk products, and so forth. Nevertheless, anecdotal reports abound. It is worth mentioning, however, that topical application of animal and vegetable oils or fats does cause comedonal acne. Thus, the face should be thoroughly washed following a greasy meal.

Much has also been made of the selection of "noncomedogenic" and "nonacnegenic" skin and hair care products, but testing methods are erratic, and these words constitute primarily marketing claims. The incidence of comedogenesis compared with that of acnegenesis from topical products is low. Acnegenesis from cosmetics and hair products probably represents a follicular irritant phenomenon. The use of products containing silicone oils (cyclomethicone, dimethicone, amodimethicone) instead of heavier mineral and vegetable oils has benefit for the acne patient.

ROSACEA

Rosacea is a form of adult acne seen in fair-skinned middle-aged and elderly men and women of Celtic genetic background; however, predisposition to development of the disease can be seen in younger individuals who flush easily with persistent redness. The complete features of rosacea develop with time if the condition goes untreated. Initially, patients demonstrate prolonged facial redness provoked by dietary, environmental, or physical factors (Table 2). This erythema is due to vasodilatation triggered by genetically inherited vasomotor instability and is best managed by avoiding triggering factors. Next, telangiectasias develop, especially on the nose and adjacent malar area. Sun protection is useful in preventing additional solar-induced telangiectasias, but only prevention of vasodilatation can reduce the chances of developing rosacea-related telangiectasias. The tetracyclines are somewhat helpful in reducing vasodilatation and consequent erythema, but the telangiectasias require surgical treatment with either electrocautery or laser.

After development of erythema and telangiectasia, inflammatory pustules and/or papules develop—hence the name acne rosacea. At this stage, ocular rosacea may also develop, with conjunctival injection and stye formation. Topical and oral antibiotics are useful in controlling the inflammatory aspects of ro-

*Not FDA approved for this indication.

TABLE 2. **Major Factors Contributing to Rosacea**

Major Dietary Factors

All alcoholic beverages (especially red wine and beer)
Aged foods (especially aged cheeses and meats)
Spicy foods (curry, chili peppers, black pepper)
Caffeine-containing foods (tea, coffee, chocolate, cola soft drinks)
Hot foods (soups, hot beverages)

Environmental Factors

Sun
Wind
Cold weather
Hot weather

Physical Factors

Exercise
Emotional stress
Menopause

sacea (Table 3), which have been attributed to *Demodex folliculorum* and *Helicobacter pylori*. Usually, combined oral and topical antibiotics are administered twice daily until control is achieved, and then maintenance therapy with topical antibiotics applied once or twice daily is continued as needed.

If the inflammatory papules persist, granulomatous rosacea results, with large, tender nodules appearing on the nose and cheeks. This condition necessitates treatment with oral antibiotics and possibly isotretinoin. Failure to treat granulomatous rosacea may result in the formation of rhinophyma, which is an unsightly enlargement of the nose resulting from tissue overgrowth and sebaceous hyperplasia. Rhinophyma may be treated by scalpel or laser removal of the exuberant tissue. It is important to recognize rosacea early and provide effective treatment to prevent progression to the more severe and disfiguring later stages of the disease.

The erythema of rosacea can also be minimized by recommending a simple skin care maintenance routine, with avoidance of cutaneous irritants (Table 4). Judicious use of camouflaging cosmetics may also be of psychological benefit in some patients.

A combination of good dermatologic care, awareness of the importance of a careful diet, and good hygiene can yield excellent results for rosacea patients. Further patient information can be obtained from the National Rosacea Society, 220 South Cook Street, Suite 201, Barrington, IL 60010.

TABLE 3. **Rosacea Treatments**

Topical Treatments

MetroGel or MetroCream (metronidazole)
Novacet (sulfacetamide and sulfur)
Sulfacet-R (pigmented sulfacetamide with sulfur)
Erythromycin (Emgel, Erygel, T-Stat, Erycettes)
Clindamycin (Cleocin T lotion, gel, or pledgets)

Oral Treatments

Tetracycline (Sumycin)
Doxycycline (Vibramycin, Monodox)
Minocycline (Minocin, Dynacin)
Trimethoprim-sulfamethoxazole (Bactrim, Septra)
Erythromycin (PCE, E-Mycin)
Isotretinoin (Accutane)

TABLE 4. **Skin Care Recommendations for Rosacea**

1. Mild, nonirritating cleanser to remove oils, dirt, and bacteria without drying skin (Oil of Olay Beauty Bar, Procter & Gamble; Aquanil Lipid-free Cleanser, Person & Covey; Neutrogena Non-drying Cleanser, Neutrogena).
2. Daily sunscreen-containing moisturizing lotion to provide sun protection and smooth skin scale (Oil of Olay Daily UV Defense Moisturizer SPF 15, Procter & Gamble; Eucerin for Face SPF 25, Biersdorf; Neutrogena Moisture SPF 15, Neutrogena; Purpose Facial Moisturizer SPF 15, Johnson & Johnson).
3. Eliminate rapidly evaporating products such as rubbing alcohol and astringents.
4. Avoid products containing ingredients that may sting the skin such as glycolic acid, lactic acid, salicylic acid, menthol, peppermint oil, cinnamon oil, witch hazel, and eucalyptus oil.
5. Consider cosmetics to cover redness such as brown facial foundations or green undercover products (Undercover primer, Estee Lauder) to blend red facial tones.

HAIR DISORDERS

method of
DIRK M. ELSTON, M.D.
Wilford Hall Air Force Medical Center
San Antonio, Texas

The evaluation of hair disorders requires an organized approach. Haphazard history taking and laboratory tests are time-consuming and expensive and seldom result in satisfaction for either the patient or the physician. A systematic approach will assist the clinician in conducting an orderly, cost-effective evaluation.

When confronted with a patient with hair loss, the clinician must first establish whether there is increased shedding or progressive thinning without increased shed. Next, the evaluation is directed at establishing whether there is hair shaft fracture or shedding at the root. Last, the patient is examined for the presence of scarring and for signs or symptoms of associated systemic disease.

PATTERN ALOPECIA

The first question to be answered is whether there is increased shedding of hair or gradual thinning without increased shed. Patients refer to both as "hair loss," but the two suggest different disorders.

Males who enter the accelerated stage of pattern hair loss during young adulthood will notice both

The views expressed are those of the author and are not to be construed as official or as reflecting those of the Department of Defense, the Army Medical Department, or the U.S. Air Force.

increased shedding and thinning. This is because the hair cycle, which usually lasts 3 to 5 years, has shortened to as little as several months. Hairs within the evolving area of alopecia have a thin shaft diameter and never have the opportunity to grow more than a few inches before they are shed. This accounts for the "flat top" noticed by men with evolving pattern alopecia.

Women with pattern alopecia generally experience a much more gradual hair loss involving the apical scalp but sparing the frontal hair line. Temporal recession is seldom present in female pattern alopecia. When temporal recession is present in a female with alopecia, it may be associated with frank virilization resulting from an ovarian or adrenal tumor.

Women with gradual onset of pattern alopecia experience hair thinning but no increased hair shedding. Follicular density on the apical scalp is decreased, and the "part" is widened.

It is important to differentiate pattern alopecia from diffuse alopecia areata (see later on). Diffuse alopecia areata may mimic both male and female pattern alopecia.

Treatment of Pattern Alopecia in Men

Treatment of pattern alopecia in males includes finasteride (Propecia) and topical minoxidil (e.g., Rogaine). Some physicians prescribe topical tretinoin (Retin-A, Avita) once weekly to nightly as tolerated, to decrease the thick cornified layer of scalp skin and to increase penetration of minoxidil. This is, of course, an "off-label" use of tretinoin. Rogaine extra strength may be of greater benefit in males than regular strength Rogaine.

Finesteride is the first and only oral medication approved for the treatment of male pattern alopecia. The dose is 1 mg daily and is generally well tolerated. The drug inhibits 5-alpha reductase, an enzyme that plays a critical role in converting testosterone to the much more potent dihydrotestosterone. Side effects in males may include a small risk of impotence, but this appears to be reversible when the drug is discontinued. Finesteride can feminize a male fetus. Therefore, any exposure to crushed tablets or ingestion of the drug is contraindicated in women who are or may become pregnant.

Evaluation and Treatment of Pattern Alopecia in Women

Women with iron deficiency, thyroid disease, or connective tissue disease frequently develop an accelerated pattern alopecia. Women should be asked about heavy or frequent periods, surgical blood loss, weight change, heat or cold intolerance, constipation, tremor, arthralgia, rash, and photosensitivity.

In general, an iron/total iron-binding capacity (TIBC) and thyroid-stimulating hormone (TSH) determinations are low-cost, high-yield tests for the evaluation of women with pattern alopecia. They should be performed in the presence of any historical clue or physical sign suggesting anemia or thyroid disease.

Women with pattern alopecia should be questioned about signs of virilization and menstrual irregularity. Women with facial hirsutism and pattern alopecia frequently have elevated androgen levels. Those with hirsutism of recent onset or virilization should be evaluated for an adrenal or ovarian tumor. Those with hirsutism of gradual onset and a strong family history generally do not require an endocrinologic evaluation.

When a hormonal evaluation is deemed necessary, total serum testosterone and dehydroepiandrostenedione sulfate (DHEA-S) measurements are the minimum requirement. Tumors are generally associated with significant elevations in testosterone, but even minor elevations in DHEA-S may be a sign of an adrenal tumor. Magnetic resonance imaging (MRI) of the adrenal is the standard technique for evaluating the presence of an adrenal tumor in a suspected case. In patients with irregular menses, galactorrhea, or infertility, serum prolactin level should be determined. If there are signs of Cushing's syndrome, a 24-hour urine cortisol should be collected. If late-onset adrenogenital syndrome is suspected, a stimulated 17-hydroxyprogesterone test is appropriate. If poycystic ovarian syndrome is suspected, a pelvic ultrasound examination should be performed.

Treatment of female pattern alopecia includes the correction of any underlying anemia or thyroid disorder and topical minoxidil. Women with pattern alopecia who choose to use an oral contraceptive should choose one that is estrogen-dominant or has a progestin with less androgenic effect (Ortho Tri-Cyclen, Ortho-Cept, Desogen, Demulen 1/50). Women taking estrogen and progesterone replacement therapy should take the lowest dose of progesterone that results in monthly bleeding. Frequently, 2.5 mg of medroxyprogesterone acetate (Provera) daily for the last 10 days of the cycle is all that is needed.

Antiandrogen therapy with spironolactone (Aldactone), 100 mg twice daily, can be helpful in some women with pattern alopecia. This is an "off-label" use of the drug. Finesteride, recently marketed for males with pattern alopecia, is currently being evaluated as a treatment for females. The drug is teratogenic for a male fetus. Rogaine extra strength appears to be of no greater benefit than the 2% regular strength solution.

TELOGEN EFFLUVIUM

Telogen effluvium presents as markedly increased shedding of scalp hair. The hairs are telogen hairs (characterized by a nonpigmented hair root and the lack of a gelatinous sheath surrounding the hair root).

The telogen (resting) phase of the hair cycle normally lasts 3 to 5 months. At the end of that time, the telogen hair is shed, and a new anagen (growing) hair begins its cycle. Normally, up to 100 telogen hairs are shed each day. During periods of stress, such as a febrile illness, crash diet, childbirth, or surgery, the body converts many anagen hairs to telogen (resting) hairs. Three to 5 months later, the individual experiences a massive shed of telogen hair. The loss may last for several months, but gradually the lost hairs are replaced by new anagen hairs.

Individuals with increased telogen shed and no obvious precipitating event should be evaluated for iron deficiency, thyroid disease, and connective tissue disease. In this setting, iron/TIBC and TSH determinations are low-cost, high-yield studies.

HAIR SHAFT DISORDERS

The next question that must be answered is whether the hair is breaking or falling out at the root. Hair that is breaking suggests a hair shaft disorder. These disorders are common, especially in black patients. If large areas of hair are broken off short, the diagnosis is usually obvious. However, more commonly, the breakage is diffuse and subtle. The patient simply complains of hair "loss."

Scalp biopsies and blood tests are generally useless. The diagnosis is made by microscopic examination of the broken hair shafts. A useful technique is to hold a white 3-inch by 5-inch card behind a tuft of hair. Fracture sites can generally be seen against the light background.

Patients frequently bring in a bag or envelope of hair, in an effort to demonstrate the seriousness of their hair loss. When confronted with such a hair ball, the physician may feel impelled, after conveying an appropriately sympathetic attitude, to throw it in the trashcan at the first opportunity. Not so fast! Instead, the ball of hair should be placed on a piece of white paper and then tossed like spaghetti. As it is tossed, smaller, broken hairs will fall onto the paper. These can easily be collected and placed in a drop of immersion oil on a glass slide for microscopic examination. This method is fast and efficient and can enable the clinician to establish a diagnosis within seconds.

Trichorrhexis nodosa is by far the most common hair shaft abnormality. It is an acquired disorder, frequently associated with overprocessing of the hair. Fractured ends have a broom-like appearance. Patients must be instructed to refrain from permanents, tight hair styles, and the use of metal combs or brushes. They must use liberal protein conditioner and treat the hair gently to minimize breakage until a length of new healthy hair grows.

Lifelong hair shaft abnormalities are frequently associated with systemic disease, ranging from aminoaciduria to neuroectodermal defects. Specific systemic disorders are associated with specific shaft abnormalities.

ALOPECIA AREATA

Alopecia areata is an extremely common disorder characterized by patchy hair loss with or without nail pitting. Hair loss typically occurs in smooth circular patches but may be diffuse and mimic pattern alopecia. In cases of diffuse alopecia areata, the correct diagnosis may be suggested by the presence of nail pits, more typical patches of alopecia, shedding of pigmented hairs with sparing of white hair, "exclamation point" hairs, tapered fractures (fractured hair shaft with tapered proximal end), and a history of periodic regrowth or response to therapy for alopecia areata. When diffuse alopecia areata is suspected, a scalp biopsy may be of help.

Alopecia areata, an autoimmune disorder, is sometimes associated with other autoimmune disorders, including vitiligo, diabetes, thyroid disease, and pernicious anemia. Individuals with alopecia areata should be asked about symptoms of these disorders. Screening blood tests are justified only in the presence of signs or symptoms of disease. The one exception to this rule is a screening test for syphilis reagin (RPR). Syphilis may closely mimic alopecia areata. I draw an RPR in any adult with new-onset alopecia areata.

Self-limited patches of alopecia areata may not require treatment. When required, treatment for small patches is best accomplished with intralesional injections of triamcinolone, beginning at a concentration of 3 mg per mL. Some patients respond to fluorinated topical steroids, topical anthralin, topical contact sensitizers, or topical psoralens with ultraviolet A (PUVA). Individuals with a history of periodic massive shedding and relatively rapid regrowth may be treated with short (3-week) courses of prednisone to prevent the massive shed.

TINEA CAPITIS

Children with inflammatory alopecia or patches of black-dot alopecia, short broken hair, or scale should be evaluated for tinea. Tinea is much less common in adults but does occur. Short broken hairs should be collected for potassium hydroxide examination or culture. The best method is to rub the scalp gently with a moist 4-inch by 4-inch gauze pad. The short hairs that stick to the gauze are then examined or cultured. In cases of very inflammatory tinea capitis (kerion), a Sabouraud's agar plate may be pressed gently directly against the lesion to inoculate the plate.

Most cases of tinea capitis in the United States are caused by *Trichophyton tonsurans*. This organism does not fluoresce under a Wood's lamp. Infected hairs demonstrate large round spores in chains within the hair shaft (large-spore endothrix). This appearance is diagnostic.

Treatment of tinea capitis requires oral antifungal drugs. Griseofulvin (Gris-PEG, Grifulvin V suspension) should be given with a fatty meal. In children, the griseofulvin suspension may be given at a starting dose of 5 mg per pound of body weight. Higher doses are frequently needed. Gris-PEG tablets may be ground and added to ice cream. In children, Gris-PEG should be used at a beginning dose of 3.3 mg per pound of body weight. Headache is the most frequent side effect and responds to a temporary reduction in dose. Newer alternatives include itraconazole (Sporanox)* and terbinafine (Lamisil).* Itraconazole has been used at a dose of 100 mg per day in children. Studies of safety, efficacy, and optimal dosing regimens are ongoing. Itraconazole interacts with many drugs, and physicians should consult the *Physicians' Desk Reference*, the *United States Pharmacopeia Drug Information* directory, or a pharmacist. Shedding of fungal spores can be dramatically reduced by shampooing the hair and scalp with selenium sulfide (Selsun).

SCARRING ALOPECIA

Patients with lupus erythematosus, lichen planopilaris, sarcoidosis, and many other conditions may present with scarring alopecia. A new patch of alopecia may also be the presenting sign of a metastatic cancer. The diagnosis of scarring alopecia is generally made by scalp biopsy. Tissue is generally submitted for histologic examination and direct immunofluorescence testing. The combination of vertical and transverse histologic sections can increase the diagnostic yield. Special arrangements should be made with the laboratory.

I generally do two 4-mm punch biopsies. The biopsy punch should be inserted parallel to the direction of hair growth to avoid transecting hairs. In persons with curly hair, the punch is placed square against the scalp. The first biopsy specimen is bisected vertically. Half is submitted in an appropriate transport medium for direct immunofluorescence testing. The other half is placed in a formalin bottle for histologic examination. The second specimen is bisected transversely, about 1 mm above the junction of the fat and dermis. The two halves of the second specimen are added to the half of the vertically bisected specimen in the formalin bottle. All three pieces are submitted together in one bottle, and the laboratory will embed them together in a single paraffin block. This increases the diagnostic yield and reduces the cost of the histologic examination.

*Not FDA approved for this indication.

CANCER OF THE SKIN

method of
PHILIP L. BAILIN M.D., and
S. TERI McGILLIS, M.D.
Cleveland Clinic Foundation
Cleveland, Ohio

Nonmelanoma skin cancers are the most common neoplasms affecting humans. It is estimated that approximately 1 million Americans will develop skin cancer in 1998. There are two major types of nonmelanoma skin cancer: basal cell carcinoma (BCC), which accounts for approximately 80% of cases, and squamous cell carcinoma (SCC), which accounts for 15% or more. Both types share a number of etiologic factors. The most prominent are genetic predisposition (light skin, eyes, hair color; inability to tan easily) and excessive chronic cumulative exposure to ultraviolet radiation (UVA/UVB). Other etiologic factors include remote exposure to ionizing radiation; chronic exposure to industrial chemicals such as tar, coal, and fuel oils; and chronic immunosuppression. Patients with chronic scarring, ulcers, or burn scars may develop SCC in the scar bed (Marjolin's ulcers). Certain human papillomavirus subtypes such as types 16, 18, 31, 33, and 35 have been implicated in genital, oral, and periungual SCCs. Basal cell carcinomas have an extremely low metastatic potential (< 0.01%) but may be locally aggressive. Squamous cell carcinomas arising in sun-damaged skin have a very low metastatic rate (< 5%), whereas those arising in ulcerations or on mucous membranes have a considerably higher metastatic potential.

Despite their potential for morbidity, early detection and treatment lead to high cure rates. Therapeutic options for these cutaneous malignancies are multiple. For primary BCC, the overall cure rate is approximately 95%, whereas for primary SCC, the cure rate is approximately 80%. Certain clinical or histologic features are associated with reduced cure rates. Among these are large size (> 2 cm), location in the midfacial triangle or around the ears, infiltrative histologic subtypes (e.g., morpheaform BCC), and recurrence after any of the standard recognized therapies. This group of "high-risk" tumors has a cure rate that declines to the 50 to 60% range with conventional therapy. Therefore, complete eradication of the tumor at the outset greatly decreases eventual total morbidity.

The first step of any therapeutic program for these tumors includes a biopsy of the lesion. The biopsy not only confirms the diagnosis, but also identifies tumor subtype (e.g., distinguishes morpheaform BCC from a superficial BCC, where ultimate treatment choices may differ). Although an excisional biopsy may be performed, it is usually more prudent to initially obtain a tissue sample with a shave or punch biopsy. Either of these options provides an adequate specimen for diagnosis (and subtyping) while leaving the remainder of the lesion clearly visible for later definitive treatment. The appropriate treatment choice depends on the characteristics of the specific lesion, the particular patient, and the physician's preferences and skills. All patients with suspected invasive SCC should have regional lymph nodes palpated.

SURGICAL THERAPIES

Electrodesiccation and Curettage

This method relies on the relative difference in palpable texture between tumor tissue and normal dermis. The palpable or visible borders of the tumor are marked and the area infiltrated with local anesthetic. The lesion is then scraped with a surgical curette, which removes the softer gelatinous tumor tissue. When normal dermal tissue is encountered, it is palpably firmer and grittier, and often the surgeon can actually hear a rough scraping sound. The base is then lightly electrocoagulated. This sequence is normally repeated three times (each time with a successively smaller curette) to complete the procedure.

This technique offers no histologic margin control. It is best used for low-risk tumors, such as those on the trunk and those with superficial histologic patterns. It should be avoided for infiltrating histologic types, midfacial lesions, or recurrent lesions. If the surgeon encounters subcutaneous adipose tissue as curetting is carried out, the procedure should be abandoned and another modality chosen, because the tactile difference between normal and malignant tissue is no longer valid. Healing of the coagulated wound base proceeds by second intention over several weeks. This technique frequently leaves a depigmented irregular scar, so cosmesis is often less than optimal.

Surgical Excision

Standard elliptical excision is a common therapeutic choice. It provides a complete specimen for pathologic examination (including traditional margin control) and results in a sutured wound that usually gives acceptable cosmetic results in any area. However, the surgeon must decide preoperatively on the size of the surgical margin. A margin of at least 0.4 cm should be taken. This is a problem with poorly defined lesions or where the lesion resides on irregular tissue planes. There is little tactile feedback as the surgeon cuts, so infiltrating lesions are likely to be incompletely removed. Also, if the lesion is large, a local flap or skin graft may be required for closure. If this is done and the pathology report subsequently identifies residual tumor, the reconstruction may have to be sacrificed.

Mohs Micrographic Surgery

Mohs surgery is a specialized excisional technique named after Dr. Frederic Mohs. The technique involves sequential excision of the tumor followed by immediate horizontal frozen section analysis. After initial debulking of any grossly visible tumor, the cancer is excised as thin segments of tissue that are color coded and recorded on a map. The map is a drawn illustration demonstrating the exact orientation and location of the tissue that has been removed. The tissue is carefully sectioned horizontally (in contrast to the vertical sections performed by most laboratories) and examined microscopically. Horizontal sections allow the entire base and all peripheral margins to be completely viewed. Any residual tumor is outlined on the map and then removed from that specific area. This allows for complete margin control, with maximum conservation of uninvolved tissue.

Mohs surgery, however, is time and resource intensive and, therefore, is reserved for high-risk skin cancers. Those may be defined as recurrent tumors or those involving old scars, tumors of the midfacial triangle or periauricular area, infiltrating histologic subtypes, lesions with clinically indistinct margins, or tumors larger than 2.0 cm in diameter. It is also reserved for any lesion occurring in areas where tissue sparing is necessary. Mohs surgical technique provides the highest cure rates for primary and recurrent tumors. Cure rates approach 98% for primary BCC and 90% for primary SCC. For recurrent tumors (which have only a 50 to 60% cure rate by conventional methods), Mohs surgery yields an 85 to 90% cure rate.

NONSURGICAL THERAPIES

Cryotherapy

Freezing tumors with liquid nitrogen drops their temperature to lethal levels, thus halting cellular activity. Tumor cells are more sensitive to cryogenic injury compared with healthy tissue. Tumors must reach a temperature of at least −20°C for optimal effect. This is usually done during a double freeze-thaw cycle. To ensure the degree of freezing, special thermocouple electrodes can be placed beneath the tumor for monitoring temperature. This technique causes local edema and necrosis, which usually heals with a soft but hypopigmented scar. It is indicated in patients who are poor surgical candidates. It is not effective on the scalp (too vascular for adequate freezing) or on the lower extremities (commonly delayed healing). Because the procedure does not result in a pathologic specimen, the completeness of removal cannot be documented. Therefore, an ample margin must be clinically selected both peripherally and in depth. Further, this technique should not be performed in patients with known cold sensitivities, dysglobulinemias, or tumors that overlie nerves.

Radiation Therapy

Although ionizing radiation is a well-recognized cause of skin cancer, it is also a most effective therapeutic option in certain circumstances. Patients who are elderly, debilitated, or are not surgical candidates for various reasons may be treated with either orthovoltage or electron beam. By fractionating the total dose (4500 to 6000 rads) over several weeks, the tumor may be adequately treated without the acute side effects frequently associated with radiation therapy. Late secondary changes in the skin may still occur (atrophy, telangiectasia, discoloration, malignant transformation) after 15 to 20 years, so most physicians do not use this modality in patients younger than 60 years of age. Radiation is often used as palliative treatment in those with extensive tumors, or as adjunctive therapy in those in whom perineural or lymphatic involvement is noted.

Chemotherapy/Immunotherapy

Topical chemotherapy with 5-fluorouracil (5-FU) is very effective for premalignant lesions such as actinic keratosis or Bowen's disease. It is not as reliable for the treatment of skin cancer. The agent does not penetrate deeply enough into the skin to ensure destruction of aggregates of cells within the dermis or along adnexal epithelium. Recently there has been some enthusiasm regarding the efficacy of 5-FU intradermal implants, but these are still investigational.

Immunotherapy with intralesional interferon-α has been reported to be effective in small solid or nodular variants of basal cell carcinoma. It is given several times weekly for courses of varying lengths and is associated with minor flulike side effects. However, it has been disappointing in larger tumors or those with an infiltrative pattern.

Laser Therapy

The carbon dioxide laser has been used to vaporize cutaneous carcinomas and is most suited to those that are superficial in nature such as superficial BCC and in situ SCCs. A 0.5 cm margin should be vaporized around the visible tumor. As with the electrodesiccation and curettage technique, laser vaporization does not provide a tissue specimen, and wounds are left to heal by second intention. Because the laser seals small vessels, bleeding is reduced. This technique is useful for patients with pacemakers (because there is no electric current), those on anticoagulant therapy, and those with multiple superficial lesions. When used in the cutting mode, the carbon dioxide laser acts as an excision tool and can be used to excise or perform Mohs surgery.

Photodynamic Therapy

Photodynamic therapy is a rapidly evolving area. It involves the administration of a potent photosensitizing agent, either intravenously or topically, to the target tumor or tumors. Malignant cells preferentially absorb and retain the agent while it is cleared from uninvolved tissues. A high intensity light source or specialized laser light is then used to activate the photosensitized tumors. This combination causes cytotoxic changes by the production of lethal singlet oxygen at the cellular level, which leads to tumor destruction. This therapy is still investigational for cutaneous tumors (there has been much success with bladder and pulmonary carcinomas) but has proven of great value for individuals with multiple tumors or those deemed noncandidates for conventional treatments.

CUTANEOUS T CELL LYMPHOMA

method of
BIJAN SAFAI, M.D., D.Sc., and
PAMELA SCHUTZER, M.D.
New York Medical College
Valhalla, New York

Cutaneous T cell lymphomas (CTCLs) are primarily lymphomas of the skin that encompass a heterogeneous group of skin disorders (Table 1). They are wildly disparate in clinical presentation, course of disease, and prognosis. Consequently, the choices and indications for treatment and the response rates are quite different. The appropriate medical management and the selection of therapeutic modalities, therefore, should be based on the clinical presentation and the natural course of the disease in each of the subgroups. Practicing physicians are encouraged to properly classify the CTCL in a given patient by using the clinical and laboratory findings before choosing the appropriate and effective therapeutic modalities.

This article presents basic information about this group of lymphomas and provides a summary of the currently utilized therapeutic modalities.

CLINICAL PRESENTATION

Mycosis Fungoides. The classic form of CTCLs was initially described by Alibert in 1806 in a patient who had a desquamating eruption that evolved into "mushroom-like" tumors. Mycosis fungoides manifests initially as erythematous scaly patches on the skin that later become more infiltrated and form raised plaques. In the late stages of the disease, large nodules and tumors appear that may break down and manifest with ulcerated fungating masses. Secondary infections are quite common. In the tumor stage, the disease may manifest as involvement of lymph nodes and/or other internal organs. It is noteworthy that the patch stage of the disease may last for many years. With proper treatment, this stage may not progress to the plaque and tumor stage.

Parapsoriasis (Premycosis Fungoides). Before the patch stage of CTCL, some patients may present with skin eruption that lacks the clinical and histologic criteria denoting mycosis fungoides. This stage is variably called parapsoriasis or premycosis fungoides. The literature contains descriptions of patients with parapsoriasis or premycosis fungoides who have lived 30 to 50 years without progressing to the classic mycosis fungoides. A definitive diagnosis of mycosis fungoides in such cases is quite diffi-

TABLE 1. **Clinical Subtypes of Cutaneous T Cell Lymphoma**

Mycosis fungoides
Parapsoriasis en plaque
Tumor d'emblée
Exfoliative erythroderma
Poikiloderma atrophicans vasculare
Follicular mucinosis
Pagetoid reticulosis
Granulomatous mycosis fungoides
Sézary syndrome
Adult T cell leukemia-lymphoma
Lymphomatoid papulosis

cult, and clinicohistopathologic correlation is recommended.

Tumor d'emblée. Mycosis fungoides d'emblée was first described by Vidal and Brocq in 1885. It manifests as sudden (d'emblée) development of skin tumors without the patch and plaque stages. This form of the disease has a worse prognosis.

Exfoliative Erythroderma. Desquamation and generalized erythrodermas are the presenting manifestations in exfoliative erythroderma. Patients do not show the classic progressive stages from patch to plaque and to tumors. The prognosis of this type of T cell lymphoma is much better, and patients usually live a long time. The clinician should note the similarity in clinical presentation between this form and the more severe form of CTCL, the Sézary syndrome. The differential diagnosis of this subtype includes atopic dermatitis, psoriasis, contact dermatitis, and drug eruption.

Poikiloderma Atrophicans Vasculare. Although poikiloderma atrophicans vasculare is characterized by hypopigmentation, hyperpigmentation, telangiectasia, and atrophy, pruritus may also be a prominent symptom. Ulceration may occur on the dry, atrophic skin. Poikilodermatous skin lesions may be seen as part of the clinical presentation of other medical illnesses such as dermatomyositis, lupus erythematosus, acrodermatitis chronica atrophicans, xeroderma pigmentosa, poikiloderma congenitale, dyskeratosis congenital, and arsenicum.

Follicular Mucinosis (Alopecia Mucinosa). Follicular mucinosis manifests as grouped follicular papules devoid of hair with or without signs of inflammation. The disease may regress spontaneously but may be followed by remissions and exacerbations and subsequent development of plaques and tumors of mycosis fungoides.

Pagetoid Reticulosis (Woringer-Kolopp Disease). Pagetoid reticulosis manifests as solitary patches that resemble patch stage of mycosis fungoides clinically and histologically. The course of the disease, however, is more chronic and indolent.

Granulomatous Mycosis Fungoides. The granulomatous form of mycosis fungoides is characterized by papular and nodular lesions resembling the tumor stage that resolves into a poikilodermatous presentation. This condition is associated with long survival.

Sézary Syndrome. Initially described by Sézary and Bouvrain in 1838, this syndrome manifests with generalized erythroderma, enlarged lymph nodes, pruritus, thickening of the palms and soles with fissures, loss of hair, nail dystrophy, ectropion, edema of the skin, and infiltrated lesions on the face (leonine face). Presence of large abnormal mononuclear cells with cerebriform (folded) nuclei is one of the hallmarks of this condition; these cells are present in skin lesions of patients with Sézary syndrome and mycosis fungoides and have proved to be of the helper T cell subset of lymphocytes. On the basis of the presence of these cells in the skin and peripheral blood, mycosis fungoides and Sézary syndrome are considered to be part of a broader spectrum of CTCLs. Thus, it is believed that Sézary syndrome is the leukemic form of mycosis fungoides. Patients with Sézary syndrome have a shorter survival and a worse prognosis than those with other forms of CTCL.

Adult T Cell Leukemia/Lymphoma (ATL). This form of CTCL was first described in Japan in 1977. It has a different geographic distribution from that of mycosis fungoides; it is limited to clusters in southern Japan, the West Indies, and the southern part of the United States. In most cases, the course of the disease is acute, with skin lesions appearing in patch, plaque, or tumor stages separately or one after the other and with rapid progression and shorter survival. Other features are circulating abnormal lymphocytes and hypercalcemia. The ATL cells are reported to be TAC-positive in most cases. In rare cases of ATL, the abnormal T cells in skin and peripheral blood have been reported to be of the suppressor T subset rather than the helper T subset usually seen in mycosis fungoides and Sézary syndrome. It has been well documented that ATL is one of the clinical manifestations of infection with the human T cell lymphotropic virus type I. More than two thirds of patients with ATL have skin involvement in the form of patches, plaques and/or nodules, generalized erythroderma, and poikiloderma.

Lymphomatoid Papulosis. Characterized by recurrent self-healing papules and nodules, lymphomatoid papulosis histologically shows features of a malignant lymphoma but clinically follows a benign course. Ten to 20% of cases, however, are reported to progress to aggressive lymphoma. The cells of this disease are Ki-1 positive. The cell involved in lymphomatoid papulosis is the T cell; therefore, this entity is also classified as one of the CTCLs.

Histologic variants of CTCL include (1) subcutaneous CTCL with troposin to the sweat gland, (2) spongiotic CTCL, (3) bullous CTCL, (4) angiotropic CTCL, (5) immunoblastic large cell lymphoma, (6) anaplastic large cell lymphoma (Ki-1 +), and (7) peripheral T cell lymphoma. The last two have been incorporated in the recent revised European/American lymphoma classification.

EXTRACUTANEOUS INVOLVEMENT

In patients with CTCL, occurrence of extracutaneous disease is uncommon except in late or terminal stages of the disease. Several autopsy reports, however, suggest that extracutaneous involvement is common. These reports support the clinical and laboratory findings noted during the late stages of the disease. However, in the early stages, internal involvement is quite rare.

Enlarged lymph nodes are usually seen in the tumor stage of mycosis fungoides and the early course of Sézary syndrome. Postmortem data demonstrate lymph node involvement in 60%, spleen in 50%, and liver and lung in 40% each. Bone marrow involvement in mycosis fungoides is rare: 2% of all patients and 5% of erythrodermic patients have positive results on bone marrow biopsies. Bone marrow is commonly reported to be involved in Sézary syndrome. Skeletal involvement is rarely reported in CTCL; but when it does occur, osteolytic lesions, osteoblastic lesions, and diffuse osteoporosis may be seen. Involvement of the oral cavity is also rare and usually occurs during dissemination of the disease. The most commonly reported intraoral site is the tongue; the lesions are usually indurated and ulcerated nodules.

STAGING CLASSIFICATION

Staging classification is helpful in the management of most human cancers including lymphomas and leukemias. With CTCL, however, staging classification seems to be less effective for management, mostly because of the heterogeneous presentation. At least five different staging classifications have been suggested. The clinical staging classification is based on the TNM nomenclature, in which *T* represents the skin stage, *N* represents the peripheral lymph nodes, and *M* represents visceral organ involvement. Another variable, *B*, represents peripheral blood involvement. However, because it is not clear whether peripheral blood is an independent prognostic variable unre-

TABLE 2. **TNM Classification for Cutaneous T Cell Lymphoma**

Skin (T)	
T0	Clinically and/or histologically suspicious lesions
T1	Limited plaques, papules, or eczematous patches covering less than 10% of skin surface
T2	Limited plaques, papules, or eczematous patches covering 10% or more of skin surface
T3	Tumors (one or more)
T4	Generalized erythroderma
Lymph Nodes (N)	
N0	No clinically abnormal peripheral lymph nodes; pathologic findings not CTCL
N1	Clinically abnormal peripheral lymph nodes; pathologic findings not CTCL
N2	No clinically abnormal peripheral lymph nodes; pathologic findings positive for CTCL
N3	Clinically abnormal peripheral lymph nodes; pathologic findings positive for CTCL
Peripheral Blood (B)	
B0	Atypical circulating cells not present (less than 5%)
B1	Atypical circulating cells not present (5% or more)
Visceral Organ (M)	
M0	No visceral organ involvement
M1	Visceral involvement (must have pathologic confirmation)

Modified from Bunn PA, Lamberg SI: Report of the Committee on Staging and Classification of Cutaneous T-Cell Lymphoma. Cancer Treat Rep *63:*725–728, 1979.

lated to node and/or visceral involvement, the B has not been incorporated into the staging classification for this disorder (Tables 2 and 3). Staging systems based only on skin involvement and lymph nodes have been recommended for general use because the information needed is readily available, requiring only thorough physical examination of the patient (Table 4).

DIAGNOSTIC PROCEDURES

To confirm the diagnosis of CTCL and identify the subtype as well as the stage of the disease, the following procedures should be performed. The information yielded enables the physician to select appropriate treatment modalities for a given patient.

Clinical Examination. The physical examination should include a total skin examination and lymph node palpation. From these clinical findings, one can easily identify the subtype as well as the stage of the disease.

TABLE 3. **Staging Classification for Cutaneous T Cell Lymphoma**

Stage	Skin	Lymph Nodes	Visceral Involvement
IA	T1	N0	M0
IB	T2	N0	M0
IIA	T1, T2	N1	M0
IIB	T3	N0, N1	M0
III	T4	N0, N1	M0
IVA	T1–T4	N2, N3	M0
IVB	T1–T4	N0–N3	M1

Modified from Lamberg SI, Bunn PA Jr: Cutaneous T-cell lymphomas. Summary of the Mycosis Fungoides Cooperative Group–National Cancer Institute Workshop. Arch Dermatol *115:*1103–1105, 1979. Copyright 1979, American Medical Association.

TABLE 4. **Clinical Staging Classification for Cutaneous T Cell Lymphoma**

Clinical Stage	T Category (Skin) +	No. Clinically Enlarged Nodal Sites
1	T0–T1	0–1
2	T0–T1	2–8
	or	
	T2	0–1
3	T2	2–8
	or	
	T3	0–8
4	T4	0–8

Modified with permission from Lamberg SI, Green SB, Byar DP, et al: Clinical staging for cutaneous T-cell lymphoma. Ann Intern Med *100:*187–192, 1984.

Histopathologic Examination. The diagnosis of CTCL is based on a combination of clinical and histopathologic findings. In most cases, multiple skin biopsies are preferred, because they increase the chance of detecting the characteristic histopathologic findings. In the patient with Sézary syndrome or erythrodermic mycosis fungoides, the histopathologic diagnosis of the skin lesions may not be as easy and helpful as it is in the patient with mycosis fungoides. One of the essential features in the histologic diagnosis is the presence in the epidermis of atypical lymphocytes with large, hyperchromatic, convoluted nuclei and scanty cytoplasm, which are known as mycosis fungoides cells.

In the early stages of mycosis fungoides (parapsoriasis and premycosis fungoides), it is usually difficult to establish a histopathologic diagnosis. If clinical suspicion of mycosis fungoides cannot be corroborated, close regular follow-up with repeated biopsies is warranted.

In the plaque stage of mycosis fungoides, the epidermis usually shows acanthosis and elongation of the rete ridges. Mycosis fungoides cells are seen in the epidermis or dermis. Epidermotropism and Pautrier's microabscesses are prominent, and the dermis shows a patchy bandlike infiltrate of lymphocytes and histiocytes and occasional eosinophils and plasma cells.

In the tumor stage, the epidermis may show ulceration secondary to an extensive infiltrate, consisting mainly of mycosis fungoides cells, which occupies much of the dermis and penetrates into the subcutis.

In Sézary syndrome, Pautrier's microabscesses are rarely present in the epidermis. The upper dermis shows a dense infiltrate of lymphocytes, histiocytes, and Sézary cells (see next section). The latter cells are indistinguishable from the mycosis fungoides cells seen in the plaque stage of mycosis fungoides.

Peripheral Blood Smear. Examination of a peripheral blood smear enables detection of presence of circulating Sézary cells, which are large mononuclear cells with folded and cerebriform nuclei. The presence of more than 15% of Sézary cells in peripheral blood is a minimal requirement for the diagnosis of Sézary syndrome, although this is not uniformly agreed on by all experts. In the case of mycosis fungoides, circulating Sézary cells are found only in rare instances and in a low percentage. In a few case reports, small Sézary cells are observed that are not identifiable by light microscopy. For this reason, electron microscopic examination has been performed and found to be useful.

With the leukemic form of CTCL, the higher the number of atypical cells, the worse the prognosis.

Immunologic Studies. These assays are not usually helpful in confirming the diagnosis of CTCL or its subtype. Most patients have normal numbers of T and B cells and normal immune reactivity, even in the late stages of the disease.

Nuclear Contour Index. Quantitative determination of the nuclear hyperconvolution of mycosis fungoides cells using morphometry (nuclear contour index) reveals that the atypical lymphocytes in mycosis fungoides have greater nuclear indentation and higher nuclear contour index values than those seen in benign skin diseases. The nuclear contour index is obtained by examining electron micrographs, measuring the length of the nuclear membrane of a suspected cell and then dividing this value by the square root of the cross-sectional area. This test has not been used routinely, and its prognostic value is not as yet confirmed.

Cytophotometry (DNA Histogram Study). In more than 65% of patients with suspected mycosis fungoides in whom light microscopy studies were not definitive, DNA histograms of lymphoid cells are abnormal. It is believed that with this technique, one might predict which patients would subsequently develop typical histologic changes of CTCL. The prognostic value of this test needs to be further substantiated.

Cytogenetic Studies. Various studies for CTCL have shown a wide range of heteroploidy. No specific pattern of chromosomal abnormalities is seen. In one report, chromosome abnormalities were frequently detectable before morphologic changes became apparent. In addition, cytogenetic findings supported the impression that CTCL is a disease in which various clinical manifestations represent a chronologic sequence, with the cytogenetic findings paralleling the clinical symptoms. In other words, patients with minimal chromosomal changes had the best survival, and those with more extensive chromosome abnormalities had more advanced stages of the disease. Those patients who developed clonal abnormalities had a poorer prognosis and a shorter survival.

Computer-Assisted Studies. Two new computerized techniques, laser flow microfluorimetry (studying DNA content and structure) and automated image analysis (studying chromatin dispersion), promise additional refinement in detecting aneuploid cell populations in the blood of patients suspected of having CTCL.

T Cell Receptor Gene Rearrangement. Lymphocytes express antigen recognition molecules, that is, immunoglobulin (Ig) in B cells and T cell receptors (TCRs) in T cells. Genes for Ig and TCRs share certain homologies, including similar nucleotide segments and rearrangements to become functionally active during early B or T cell development. Therefore, analysis of the Ig and TCR alpha and beta chain gene rearrangements has become useful for determining the lineage and clonality of lymphoid neoplasms. A third gene that rearranges in T cells, designated the T cell gamma gene, also exhibits sequence similarity with Ig gene segments and undergoes rearrangement in both suppressor/cytotoxic and helper T cells. Using methods to detect T cell receptor gene rearrangements for beta and gamma chain on 30 patients with adult ATL and 17 patients with non-ATL T cell neoplasms, Matsuoka and colleagues reported T beta gene rearrangement in all 47 cases; T gamma gene rearrangement was seen in all but one ATL patient. Other studies have used these advances to obtain strong evidence that some CTCL precursors, variants, or early lesions are clonal in nature. Wood and associates reported a case of pagetoid reticulosis in which the atypical cells were deficient in multiple T cell antigens. Rearranged bands of beta and gamma T cell receptor genes were noted in DNA from lesional skin. The rearranged bands did not represent inherited DNA polymorphism, because DNA extracted from peripheral blood that was concurrently obtained lacked these bands. This lack also indicated that the clonal population identified in the skin was not circulating in the blood. These findings suggest the biologic potential to evolve into a more aggressive form of the disease.

Computed Tomography. Computed tomography is not considered clinically useful in the early plaque phase of CTCL. During the nodal phase, it is useful for determining lymph node involvement.

Lymphangiogram. Lymph node involvement in CTCL is an important determinant of extracutaneous involvement. Although the lymphangiogram is rarely used today, it can determine the extent of lymph node involvement in this disease.

TREATMENT

Once a diagnosis of CTCL has been established, the extent of disease involvement should be assessed. Regardless of the extent of the disease, symptomatic care is warranted. Liberal use of emollients and moisturizers to treat the dry, scaly, pruritic eruption is suggested. Topical steroids and oral antihistamines may be helpful and should be added to the regimen. If skin infections are seen, topical or systemic antibiotics, or both, are recommended.

For patients in stage IA disease, options for treatment vary from periodic examination with no treatment except for lubrication and occasional use of topical steroids and ultraviolet B (UVB) exposure, to continuous topical treatment with corticosteroid. However, if progression is noted, or if the disease manifests beyond this early stage, topical chemotherapy, the combination of PUVA (psoralen plus ultraviolet A), or electron beam therapy should be considered.

Topical Chemotherapy

Mechlorethamine hydrochloride (nitrogen mustard, HN2)* has been used as a topical cutaneous medication for mycosis fungoides since the 1950s. It is a proven regimen for control of early stage CTCL, with 94% complete remission in stage IA and 59% in stage IB. The exact mechanism of action is not known. A 10-mg vial of nitrogen mustard is dissolved in water (120 mL or more); the solution is then applied daily to the entire skin surface including all uninvolved areas. Limitations of this treatment modality include relapses occurring steadily over the years, a high rate of hypersensitivity reactions, the need for continuous daily application, lack of effectiveness in the tumor stage of the disease, and high cost. Long-term use of nitrogen mustard could cause severe aggressive squamous cell carcinomas.

Another modality is the topical use of carmustine

*Not FDA approved for this indication.

(BCNU), an alkylating agent with the ability to inhibit DNA repair. In one report, complete remission was achieved in 84% of stage IA and 52% of stage IB in patients with mycosis fungoides.

Psoralen and Ultraviolet A

In the presence of UVA (longwave ultraviolet light of wavelengths 320 to 400 nm), methoxsalen (Oxsoralen), a photosensitizing furocoumarin compound with an action spectrum centered at 340 to 360 nm, produces photoadducts with thymine in the DNA of mammalian cells. This effect has been shown to inhibit DNA synthesis in human epidermal cells and fibroblasts. Use of PUVA in CTCL has demonstrated clinical clearing, especially in early-stage lesions.

Limitations of this modality include many relapses if PUVA is not maintained continuously or even during the maintenance period. In addition, the risk of developing skin cancers, including malignant melanoma, and the degree of carcinogenicity of PUVA therapy remain to be fully determined.

Radiotherapy

More than 30 years ago, conventional x-ray therapy was the most effective palliative treatment for CTCL. Since the 1950s, however, electron beam therapy has been utilized. In contrast to x-rays, electrons with appropriate energies penetrate only the upper dermis. Thus, the skin alone can be treated without systemic effects.

Any of the several multiple-field techniques for delivering electron-beam therapy are acceptable, including four-, six-, or rotational-field techniques; the choice of technique depends on the equipment and expertise available at each institution. One protocol involving once weekly radiation for 6 consecutive weeks resulted in disappearance of all skin lesions and median duration of remission of more than 1.5 years. Another recent study showed a 24% 5-year disease-free survival.

Limitations of electron beam therapy include its expense and availability. In addition, uniform exposure of the entire skin surface is technically, dosimetrically, and physically difficult. Adverse local cutaneous effects include alopecia, atrophy of skin, damage to sweat glands, radiodermatitis, and edema of the skin.

Systemic Chemotherapy

Because PUVA, electron beam therapy, and topical chemotherapeutic agents penetrate only the epidermis and upper dermis, systemic chemotherapy is necessary to treat any visceral or lymph node involvement by CTCL. Single agents, inducing systemic mechlorethamine, methotrexate, high-dose methotrexate with L-leucovorin rescue, bleomycin,* doxorubicin (Adriamycin),* and VP-16,* produced complete but short-term remissions. However, single agents have not been shown to cure any patients with internal CTCL. Combination chemotherapy used in CTCL includes the following regimens: (1) mechlorethamine, vincristine, prednisone, and procarbazine*; (2) bleomycin and methotrexate; (3) cyclophosphamide, doxorubicin, vincristine, and prednisone; and (4) chlorambucil and prednisone. The number of patients treated with any one regimen is small, and as yet there are no convincing data that any one regimen is better than the others. Moreover, some investigators believe that combination chemotherapy may actually reduce survival.

Cyclosporine

A profound immunosuppressive agent, cyclosporine (Sandimmune)* blocks antigen-specific T cell proliferation, possibly by decreasing expression of interleukin-1 (IL-1) and IL-2 receptors on T cells, thus down-regulating their activation. Cyclosporine has been utilized in selected refractory cases of CTCL, with a temporary response at the expense of profound immunosuppression and renal toxicity.

Purine Nucleotide Analogues

Purine nucleotide analogues have shown promising results in patients with advanced CTCL. Fludarabine (Fludara),* cladribine (Leustatin),* and pentostatin (Nipent)* have all yielded a response rate of 30 to 40%. Toxicity includes bone marrow and immune suppression, as well as neurologic dysfunction.

Retinoids

Retinoids (vitamin A analogues), including etretinate* (Tegison), and isotretinoin* (Accutane), have demonstrated antiproliferative and antineoplastic activity. In a study involving patients with extensive mycosis fungoides, retinoid therapy achieved a 44% objective clinical response rate. Doses of 1.5 to 2.0 mg per kg per day of retinoid were used and lymph node remissions were reported. A later study using combined systemic chemotherapy (cyclophosphamide, bleomycin, and prednisolone) with oral retinoids in 20 patients with progressive tumor-stage disease showed no further disease progression with treatment. In addition, long-term retinoid therapy may prolong remission after systemic chemotherapy is terminated. Retinoids have also been used in combination with interferon, but without increase in complete response rate. Combination of retinoids and total skin electron beam (TSEB) is reported to be safe but without beneficial effects.

Combined Therapeutic Modalities

Combined therapy employing electron beam irradiation with systemic chemotherapy (single agents

*Not FDA approved for this indication.

*Not FDA approved for this indication.

such as mechlorethamine or combinations) has shown some promising results. One study reported good results with a protocol of total body electron beam therapy, followed by six monthly cycles of chemotherapy (doxorubicin once monthly and cyclophosphamide daily for 14 days). In 50 patients with stages I or II mycosis fungoides, such treatment achieved complete clinical remission with a follow-up period of up to 75 months in some cases. Despite the good response, all patients continued to show karyotypic abnormalities in circulating lymphocytes.

Leukapheresis

Leukapheresis involves passage of anticoagulated whole blood from a catheter placed in one antecubital vein through a continuously operating centrifuge and back into the body. As the blood components separate, the lymphocyte-enriched buffy coat is selectively removed, thus reducing the circulating "leukemic" T cells. It is believed that this procedure causes disequilibrium of T cells between the soft tissues and intravascular compartment, with subsequent migration of cells from the skin to the blood.

Photopheresis

In photopheresis, extracorporeal anticoagulated whole blood is subjected to PUVA photochemotherapy. One study showed that the combination of UVA and methoxsalen caused an 88% loss of viability of target lymphocytes, whereas the drug alone was inactive; 27 of 37 patients in this study who had otherwise resistant CTCL responded to the treatment. Clinical complete response rates ranged from 15 to 25%. Erythrodermic patients may be the best candidates for this approach. Partial response is reported to improve when combined with interferon, methotrexate, TSEB, PUVA, and others. There is no consensus that photopheresis can increase survival of CTCL patients. Treatment is quite costly.

Antibodies

Polyclonal anti–T cell globulin administered intravenously has been shown to bind to essentially all normal blood mononuclear cells, as well as the malignant cells of CTCL. With the advent of monoclonal antibodies, this form of therapy with more specific and selective antibodies against CTCL cells may prove to be extremely rewarding. Antithymocyte globulin (Atgam)* and IL-2 antibodies are currently undergoing trial.

Interferon

The largest series of patients with CTCL treated with interferon showed a 50% response rate. Whether interferon works because of its antiviral, antiproliferative, or immunomodulatory properties remains unanswered. Further documentation of this work is obviously needed. Inteferon alfa-2a (Roferon-A) and alfa-2b (Intron A) have been used with dosages as high as 12 million units three times weekly. Toxicity is dose dependent and includes fevers, chills, myalgia, malaise, anorexia, and even bone marrow suppression. Median time to optimal response is reported to be 4 to 6 months, which is quite long, and treatment has to be continued in responding patients for years. Interferon has been used in combination with photopheresis, PUVA, and retinoids. Even complete responses are reported with the combination therapy.

*Not FDA approved for this indication.

IL-2 Fusion Toxin (DAB389IL2)

A chimeric protein, IL-2 fusion toxin contains diphtheria toxin and IL-2 gene. It targets those cells bearing IL-2 receptors and releases the toxin fragment intracellularly after internalization of the ligand-receptor complex. It is reported that 30 to 40% of those patients whose T cells have IL-2 receptors have responded to this approach. Obviously more detailed trials are needed before the final results can be determined.

Thymopentin

A pentapeptide similar to the thymopoietin, thymopentin* has been used in some cases of Sézary syndrome with up to 60% response rates. Further studies are under way. A clinical response correlated with a rise in CD8$^+$ and natural killer cells, suggesting immunomodulatory activity in treated patients.

Autologous Bone Marrow Transplantation

In the treatment of CTCL, autologous bone marrow transplantation may be helpful.

SELECTION OF APPROPRIATE TREATMENT FOR A GIVEN SUBTYPE OF CUTANEOUS T CELL LYMPHOMA

For early-stage disease, a nonaggressive approach should be taken. First, emollients, gentle skin care, topical antipruritics, and moderate exposure to sunlight should be used, as this regimen tends to produce substantial improvement. High-potency topical steroids (class 1 to 3), along with antineoplastic treatment should be avoided at this time. UVB seems to work by reducing the number of proliferated epidermal Langerhans' cells as well as the thymus-like cytokines. For disease of plaque stage, more aggressive topical treatments should be used, consisting of aqueous topical nitrogen mustard, topical carmustine (BCNU), and PUVA. Some authorities suggest that extracorporeal photopheresis is needed at this point.

In the tumor phase, more aggressive systemic ther-

*Investigational drug in the United States.

apy is necessary. Total body electron beam therapy, chemotherapeutic regimens, and the experimental treatments discussed earlier have been used. Other potential therapies are autologous bone marrow transplantation, adenosine analogues, pentostatin, fludarabine phosphate, antithymocyte globulin, and δ-aminolevulinic acid photodynamic therapy.

Alopecia mucinosa (follicular mucinosis) is treated with diaminodiphenylsulfone.* Poikiloderma atrophicans vasculare should be treated aggressively to prevent progression to mycosis fungoides plaque and tumor stages. It has been treated with topical mechlorethamine, three times a week, but one case study reported the development of melanoma and dysplastic nevi after such treatment. Generalized erythroderma (exfoliative dermatitis) is secondary to underlying benign or malignant causes, which can be treated by determining the true cause. PUVA and photopheresis have been used with success for this disease. Pagetoid reticulosis (Woringer-Kolopp disease) is optimally treated by low-dose radiotherapy or topical nitrogen mustard; however, controversy exists as to whether this is a benign disease that can be treated with intralesional steroids. Granulomatous mycosis fungoides tends to be resistant to current treatments.

Lymphomatoid papulosis has been treated successfully with low-dose methotrexate, from 5 to 25 mg orally, which decreases the risk of transformation into a malignant process. It is also treated with PUVA but has been shown to have a high rate of relapse upon discontinuance of treatment. Interferon alpha has also been tried, although it also was shown to have a high rate of relapse. Hexadecylphosphocholine is an experimental topical treatment that has been shown to be effective.

Mycosis fungoides d'emblée requires more aggressive treatment than earlier stages. The recommended treatment is a combination of topical and systemic therapy. One study obtained good results with a combination protocol of TSEB irradiation (30 cGy), followed by six monthly cycles of systemic chemotherapy of either mechlorethamine or cyclophosphamide with vincristine, procarbazine, and prednisone. Topical immunotherapy, with mechlorethamine hydrochloride as the immunogen, was also shown to create prolonged remission. In primary CD30 CTCL, the prognosis is excellent, with more than 90% of patients so treated alive and disease free after 5 years. This stage of disease has been successfully treated with methotrexate at doses of 25 mg or less given every 1 to 4 weeks.

Treatment of Sézary syndrome consists of photochemotherapy in addition to a cytotoxic drug. The most common cytotoxic drug used is low-dose chlorambucil. Systemic corticosteroids are also used. In ATL the first-line treatment is with total body irradiation at 100 to 150 cGy. This form of the disease has been treated successfully with a combination chemotherapy called the RCM (response-oriented cyclic multidrug) protocol.

*Not available in the United States.

PAPULOSQUAMOUS DISEASES

method of
WILLIAM ABRAMOVITS, M.D., and
ALAN MENTER, M.D.
Baylor University Medical Center
Dallas, Texas

Papulosquamous diseases are a group of skin disorders characterized by scaly papules and plaques and mostly unrelated in their etiopathogenesis. Their histopathologic features, while subtle, are usually readily distinguishable by dermatopathologists. Included in this group of diseases are psoriasis, pityriasis rubra pilaris, lichen planus, seborrheic dermatitis, and pityriasis rosea.

PSORIASIS

Psoriasis affects approximately 2% of the population of the United States. With the exception of scattered foci of lesser prevalence in some ethnic groups, a similar rate of occurrence is accepted worldwide. Of an estimated 5 million persons with psoriasis in the United States, over 500,000 seek attention for their condition every year; about 3 million psoriasis-related visits are made to physicians or health care facilities, incurring a burden of $1.6 to $3.2 billion per year. In severe cases, the cost of annual care may exceed $10,000. Psoriasis has no cure; symptoms and physical manifestations may progress with age, or the condition may wax and wane, sometimes lessening in severity in the elderly.

The lesions may cause functional impairment, disfigurement, and distress that may be disproportionate to their extent, having a deleterious impact on social and family life, work performance, and overall quality of life. Occasionally the condition may be life-threatening, especially in the erythrodermic or pustular forms, from complications such as infections and cardiovascular and renal effects. Suicide is not unknown.

The Committee on Guidelines of Care and the Task Force on Psoriasis of the American Academy of Dermatology define psoriasis as "a chronic skin disease that is classically characterized by thickened, red areas of skin covered with silvery scales. The extent of skin involvement can range from discrete, localized areas to generalized body involvement. The joints, nails and mucous membranes may also be affected with the disease."

More than 60% of patients develop their first evidence of psoriasis before the age of 35 years. Less than 10% present during childhood, and occasionally the condition may be manifested initially in infancy, as severe "cradle cap" or diaper dermatitis. About 30% of patients have a family history of psoriasis.

Many have associated autoimmune disorders such as diabetes mellitus, thyroid disease, or inflammatory bowel disease. Initial episodes or recurrences may be precipitated by infections (particularly streptococcal in children), physical trauma, metabolic or emotional stress, and drugs such as chloroquine, alpha-interferon, lithium, beta blockers, and systemic glucocorticosteroids.

Morphologic variants include vulgaris or plaque-type, guttate, inverse or flexural, erythrodermic, palmar-plantar, and pustular (localized or generalized), as well as nail psoriasis.

Classic lesions of psoriasis vulgaris are discoid or nummular (coin-shaped) but may be annular, linear, or geographic. Lesions are erythematous, raised, indurated, and scaly (typically silvery or micaceous), ranging in size from a few millimeters in diameter (papules) to several centimeters across (plaques). These are located on the elbows, knees, and knuckles, as well as on the scalp, back (particularly the sacral area), buttocks, abdomen, chest, and genitalia.

Gentle lifting of the scale reveals a base prone to pinpoint bleeding (Auspitz's sign). Trauma may trigger the development of psoriatic lesions (the idiomorphic effect, or Koebner's phenomenon). Guttate lesions are typically papules (less than 1 cm) scattered over the trunk and extremities and usually present in a "shower" of sudden onset. Flexural lesions, mostly seen in the inframammary, abdominal, axillary, groin, and buttock folds, are usually moist and nonscaly and may be complicated by candidiasis. Erythrodermic forms cover more than 80% of the body surface and may progress to a diffuse exfoliative dermatitis (in some cases associated with high-output cardiac failure, hypoalbuminemia, and renal failure, particularly in the elderly).

Palmar-plantar psoriasis is characterized by hyperkeratotic scaly plaques, usually more inflammatory and severe at the mid-palms or sole arches, or by diffuse hyperlinearity and fissuring. Pustular forms usually are localized to the palms and soles, with 1- to 2-mm-diameter sterile pustules. Less commonly seen are tiny pustules studding extensive and usually highly inflammatory plaques, often associated with fever, arthralgias, leukocytosis, and occasionally hypocalcemia.

The nails in psoriasis may be affected independently or in association with classic lesions; the presence of more than 20 pits per nail plate is said to be pathognomonic, but distal onycholysis (loosening), crusting under the free edge, and an oil drop pattern under the nail plate are seen more commonly. Arthritis of the affected finger or toe is a not uncommon association.

Etiopathogenesis

The theory that psoriasis is primarily a focally proliferative disorder of the skin has been challenged by the concept of the disease as a genetically inherited autoimmune disorder involving abnormal activation of T lymphocytes.

The study of the human genome has led to the discovery of genes responsible for psoriasis on chromosomes 1, 4, 16, and 17. Of interest is that the locus on 16 is adjacent to a locus for Crohn's disease. On chromosome 6, at the site of the human lymphocyte antigen (HLA), the locus *HLACW6* has been associated with the development of disease before the age of 40 years. The immediate future of psoriasis therapy lies in the manipulation of the interaction of keratinocytes and dendritic epidermal cells with specific populations of helper T lymphocytes and, later, in genetic engineering.

Therapy

We utilize a three-tier approach: topical preparations, phototherapy, and systemic medications. A single agent or a combination of these options is selected, and treatments are individualized for each patient. Topical preparations include glucocorticoids, tar, anthralin, calcipotriene, and retinoids. Phototherapy is delivered as ultraviolet B (UVB), ultraviolet A (UVA), or combinations of the two or, most recently, narrow-band UVB, which promises less risk of actinic damage, including skin cancers. Photochemotherapy utilizing systemic psoralens with UVA (PUVA therapy) is highly effective.

As a rule, topical therapy alone is useful in patients with localized forms of psoriasis covering less than 20% of the body surface (one palm constitutes 1% of the body surface). Topical glucocorticoids work by a direct antiproliferative as well as an anti-inflammatory effect. A glucocorticoid of ultra-high potency in an ointment, gel, or cream base is selected to reduce the thickness of the plaques in areas except the face, genitalia, and flexural areas, in which the skin is particularly susceptible to atrophy. No more than 50 grams of the ultra-high-potency topical steroid should be used each week, and no more than 10% of the body surface should be treated at one time to avoid systemic effects or rebound upon discontinuance. The face and flexural areas may be treated with low-potency topical steroids, usually in a lotion or cream vehicle. Ultra-high-potency topical steroids should be tapered after 2 to 3 weeks either by switching to so-called pulse therapy (weekend use only) or by substituting with lower-potency preparations, calcipotriene, or topical retinoids. Topical glucocorticoids in solution, oil, or gel vehicles are useful for scalp psoriasis. Palmar-plantar psoriasis or extremely thick plaques often require occlusive therapy.

Tars have antimitotic effects and have been used in psoriasis therapy for over 75 years. Crude coal tar in concentrations of up to 20% may be compounded in yellow paraffin and in up to 10% concentrations may be found in commercially available creams, oils, and shampoos. Liquor carbonis detergens, a refined derivative with less smell and color, may be compounded in 5 to 15% concentrations in vehicles including those already containing glucocorticosteroids. Folliculitis is the most likely side effect of tar use.

Tars may sensitize the skin to ultraviolet A and B and are commonly used in conjunction with the latter.

Anthralin (Anthra-Derm, Dithocreme) is a synthetic analogue of a tree bark extract. Application of this agent in paste form in 0.5 to 8% concentrations daily over thick lesions for periods of 10 minutes to 4 hours per day causes resolution in approximately 4 weeks. Irritation and staining are major drawbacks. Over the past few years, more elegant preparations with less staining potential in cream formulations have become available.

Calcipotriene (Dovonex) is a vitamin D_3 analogue that induces cellular differentiation, inhibits epidermal proliferation, and produces anti-inflammatory effects. It is equipotent to mid-potency steroids but does not cause atrophy. It has a slower onset of action (of up to 4 to 6 weeks), with skin irritation as the most common side effect. Calcium levels may need monitoring if more than 100 grams of this cream is used weekly.

Tazarotene (Tazorac) is a synthetic retinoid that normalizes differentiation, inhibits proliferation, and decreases the expression of inflammatory markers in the epidermis. Its potency is comparable to that of fluocinonide (Lidex), a high-potency steroid. Tazarotene has a rapid onset of action and sustained therapeutic effects. Side effects are those of all topical retinoids, i.e., skin irritation, usually seen surrounding the plaques, sometime with moderate pruritus, burning, erythema, and desquamation. Like other retinoids, it must be avoided during pregnancy.

Phototherapy with UVB is utilized as monotherapy or combined with tars (the Goeckerman regimen) and, less often, with anthralin (the Ingram regimen). It is administered to tolerance with specialized equipment in dermatology offices or programmable home units.

Phototherapy with UVA is usually administered with extreme caution in specialized centers in combination with methoxsalen, in a dose based on weight, taken orally 1 hour before exposure. Prolonged UVA exposure at tanning salons has minimal effect. Psoralens such as methoxsalen remain in the lens for up to 24 hours after ingestion; eye protection with special wrap-around sunglasses is thus essential. Burns and fatalities may occur from added exposure to sunlight or improper dosing. Premature skin aging and increased epithelial and melanocytic skin tumor formation are long-term risks with high accumulated doses of PUVA.

Patients with mild or localized psoriasis are managed initially with topical therapy. Use of tazarotene or calcipotriene as monotherapy, or with additional topical steroids, is the first choice for convenience and effectiveness. The steroid should quickly be tapered to its minimal effective dose, i.e., twice weekly. Calcipotriene or tazarotene is suitable for long-term control and maintenance programs.

For unresponsive cases or more extensive involvement, UVB phototherapy is recommended. PUVA is selected for cases unresponsive to UVB or for more widespread indurated disease. Either may be aided by topical or systemic medications. Yearly evaluation for skin cancers and pigmented lesions and, with PUVA, ophthalmologic evaluation are advised.

When phototherapy fails or is impracticable, or the accumulated dose reaches unsafe levels, a systemic drug is prescribed. Methotrexate* is an ideal choice in the absence of liver disease or history of alcohol abuse or hematologic disorders. Tests to monitor liver function and hematologic parameters are performed frequently, and a liver biopsy is done with every 1.5 grams of accumulated dose. Sulfasalazine (Azulfidine) may be an alternative if there is no history of allergy to sulfa and if glucose-6-phosphate dehydrogenase (G6PD) levels permit. Hydroxyurea (Hydrea)* may also be chosen with close monitoring of hematologic parameters. These two preparations are generally less effective than methotrexate.

Cyclosporine (Neoral)* is particularly suitable for severe cases such as extensive plaque-type, erythrodermic, or pustular psoriasis. The nephrotoxic and immunosuppressive effects of this agent limit its use to interventional therapy or for periods up to 1 year of treatment. Frequent monitoring of blood pressure and urinary protein and creatinine levels is imperative, and tests of glomerular filtration or creatinine clearance should be performed every 3 months and at the first evidence of nephrotoxicity. Rotating patients between different systemic therapies and PUVA helps minimize the occurrence of individual toxic effects.

The psychosocial impact of this disease should not be overlooked. Support from psychiatric and social work arenas as well as support groups should be offered to the patient.

PITYRIASIS RUBRA PILARIS

Pityriasis rubra pilaris (PRP) is an infrequently occurring skin disease affecting both genders and all races equally. This chronic skin disorder is characterized by reddish-orange scaly plaques with prominent follicular papules. The extent of skin involvement ranges from localized to generalized with characteristic sparing of small islands of healthy skin.

The classic adult form of PRP starts on the head, neck, or upper trunk as a reddish-orange macule, followed by the development of multiple follicular erythematous lesions with a keratotic top. These coalesce into groups and are later surrounded by interfollicular erythema that spreads caudally. The face becomes red and scaly, and ectropion develops frequently. The scalp shows erythema covered by "branny" scales. The palms and soles develop keratoderma, i.e., a yellow-orange thick stratum corneum. The nails also thicken. PRP is occasionally associated with hypothyroidism, myasthenia gravis, leukemia, and the eruption of multiple seborrheic keratoses.

The classic juvenile form resembles the classic adult form, usually following an infection, and spon-

*Not FDA approved for this indication.

taneously resolves in 1 to 2 years. A circumscribed juvenile variant affects mostly the elbows and knees and palms and soles, with a few macules on the trunk. An atypical childhood form may present at birth or in the first few years of life, with features suggestive of ichthyosis but with follicular papules and keratoderma.

Etiopathogenesis

The assumption that PRP results from a vitamin A deficiency has not been borne out. Recent findings of T cell impairment and the expression of abnormal keratin patterns are supportive of an immunologic basis.

Treatment

In spite of a usually benign, even self-limited course for most forms of PRP, many cases defy the clinician's best efforts. Topical steroids may be of help for circumscribed or limited forms. These agents, in conjunction with alpha-hydroxy acid creams or topical retinoids, may be of value on hyperkeratotic areas such as the palms and soles.

For extensive involvement, rest and bland emollients may be recommended in addition to systemic therapy. This therapy involves the use of retinoids such as natural vitamin A at doses of up to 300,000 units a day over several months, with careful monitoring of liver enzymes as well as for signs of pseudotumor cerebri or other manifestations of neurotoxicity. Synthetic retinoids (acitretin [Soriatane] or 13-*cis*-retinoic acid [isotretinoin; Accutane]) in doses up to 1 mg per kg per day are more effective and may be used with similar precautions.

If retinoids fail to effect improvement, methotrexate, given as for psoriasis (as described previously), or even cyclosporine is frequently beneficial.

LICHEN PLANUS

Lichen planus accounts for 1 to 2% of dermatology visits and 5% of patients attending oral medicine skin and oncology clinics combined. Worldwide prevalence varies between 0.1 and 0.8%. Most affected persons are between 30 and 60 years of age, and the gender and race distributions are even.

HLA A associations suggest a genetic predisposition. The pathogenesis may involve antigen presentation by dendritic to helper T cells.

Classic lesions are *p*ruritic, *p*urplish, *p*olygonal, *p*lanar (flat-topped) *p*apules with a translucent scale, creating a network of white lines (Wickham's striae), usually on the ventral aspect of the wrist and forearms, legs, thighs, and at the waist. Oral lesions may be present in more than 50% of patients, and genital lesions are likewise common. The isomorphic effect (Koebner's phenomenon) may also be present. Resolution leads to striking hyperpigmentation, which may persist indefinitely.

Linear (zosteriform) or annular lesions may also occur. Nail and follicle involvement may affect up to 10% of patients. Appearance on regular and immunofluorescence histologic examination is usually characteristic.

The cutaneous lesions of drug-induced eruptions as well as of those in graft-versus-host disease may also be lichen planus-like.

Treatment

If a causative link can be identified, it should be treated or eliminated. Possible causative factors include drugs, rheumatoid arthritis, lupus erythematosus, primary biliary cirrhosis, inflammatory bowel disease, herpetic infections, hepatitis C (with increasing frequency), and dental metal compounds.

Limited forms of the disease may be treated with potent topical steroids. Occlusion or intralesional corticosteroids may be added for localized hypertrophic lesions. If lesions are pruritic, topical doxepin or systemic antihistamines may be tried. Diphenhydramine (Benadryl) elixir helps anesthetize the buccal mucosa to allow eating. If the lesions are extensive, inflammatory, symptomatic, or ulcerative, short-term systemic steroids may be required. A steroid-sparing effect may be obtained with azathioprine.

Cyclosporine, at a dose of 3 mg per kg per day, is very useful, particularly for treatment of mucosal erosive forms or extensive cutaneous disease. Topical preparations of cyclosporine as well as triamcinolone and fluocinonide in adhesive pastes are useful for treatment of mucosal disease. Acitretin, in a dose of 0.25 to 0.5 mg per kg per day, has been successful in controlling eczematous, nail, palmoplantar, and ulcerative forms.

Hydroxychloroquine,* dapsone,* metronidazole,* alpha-interferon* and the combination of tetracycline with nicotinamide may be of value in selected variants. PUVA is particularly useful for the treatment of lichenoid graft-versus-host reactions and extensive forms of the disease.

Erosive lesions contaminated with *Candida* improve symptomatically and objectively with systemic azole antifungals.

SEBORRHEIC DERMATITIS

Seborrheic dermatitis is a very common skin condition and may occur at any age. In infancy, it appears as cradle cap and diaper rash. The usual form affects men 20 to 50 years old, or it may develop in older patients with Parkinson's disease, with a prominent facial component. It is particularly severe in patients with human immunodeficiency virus (HIV) infection. Seborrheic dermatitis results from the interplay of *Pityrosporum ovale* and the immune system in genetically predisposed patients, with some effect attributed to emotional, climactic, nutritional, neural, and sebum composition factors.

Classic lesions of seborrheic dermatitis are thin

*Not FDA approved for this indication.

erythematous papules covered by a yellowish crust that is sticky and fissured. The scalp may be affected diffusely or by discrete discoid patches. Scalp lesions around the hairline may be most noticeable on the forehead and behind the ears. The face may be affected at the brows, glabella, lid margins, butterfly area, and moustache, chin, and beard areas. The ear canals are frequently affected with pruritic scaly lesions, and the collar and presternal areas, umbilicus, axillae, groins, and genital and inframammary folds may also be involved. A red scrotum is not uncommon.

Therapy

Antimycotic treatment is a recent welcome addition to available therapeutic modalities. Shampoos or creams containing an azole antifungal, ciclopirox or piroctone olamine, zinc pyrithione, selenium sulfide, or tars are helpful. Ketoconazole shampoo applied twice weekly, with lathering for 4 minutes, is convenient and elegant. Creams with ketoconazole (Nizoral) or terbinafine (Lamisil) may be preferred for facial and other body lesions, alone or in combination with low-potency corticosteroids.

For stubborn scalp dermatitis, a stronger steroid in solution or gel is recommended. A dexamethasone-containing ophthalmic ointment may be used very sparingly on blepharitis that fails to respond to mild cleansers and emollients such as baby shampoo, Cetaphil, or Occu-Soft wipes.

Systemic therapy is rarely necessary, but oral antimycotics, antiandrogens, and retinoids to modify sebum composition or decrease the amount of scaling may be considered for particularly severe cases, or those associated with HIV infection. Persistent cradle cap in children may be safely treated with borage oil and topical azole antifungals.

PITYRIASIS ROSEA

The cause of pityriasis rosea, common in healthy young adults, is unknown. Because it often appears in mini-epidemics with season change, is self-limiting, and seldom recurs, an infectious etiology is presumed. It classically presents with a single oval scaly macule, often on the trunk, resembling a ringworm lesion (herald patch). This is followed within 1 to 2 weeks by a rapidly spreading scaly, erythematous rash on the trunk and proximal extremities, with individual lesions smaller than the herald patch. Lesions often follow rib lines. The rash is usually only mildly pruritic and is self-limiting, with resolution in approximately 2 months.

Therapy

No therapy is usually required. If the condition is symptomatic, topical steroids and antihistamines may be used. Cautious use of natural sunlight or UVB phototherapy may be helpful in widespread, symptomatic cases.

CONNECTIVE TISSUE DISORDERS
(Systemic Lupus Erythematosus, Dermatomyositis, and Scleroderma)

method of
VICTORIA P. WERTH, M.D., and
JOAN VON FELDT, M.D.
University of Pennsylvania
Philadelphia, Pennsylvania

SYSTEMIC LUPUS ERYTHEMATOSUS

Systemic lupus erythematosus (SLE) is a multisystem, potentially fatal autoimmune disease that can involve the skin, joints, muscles, heart, lung, kidneys, peripheral nerves, central nervous system (CNS), and blood. The severity is largely determined by which organs are involved, patients with CNS or renal involvement often having the most serious disease. The diagnosis of SLE is made if patients fulfill at least 4 of the 11 criteria designated by the American College of Rheumatology, but these need to be used with caution because many patients may not fulfill strict criteria for SLE at presentation but acquire additional features of the disease over time to allow a more definitive diagnosis later on.

Constitutional Features

Constitutional symptoms are frequent in patients presenting with SLE, especially fatigue, which is reported by 80 to 100% of patients. Fever and weight loss occur in more than 60% of patients as well. Lymphadenopathy is a common manifestation of SLE.

Skin Manifestations

Some patients with lupus erythematosus (LE) have only skin disease and no evidence of systemic disease. Numerous different cutaneous eruptions may be seen in LE, including the typical malar rash seen in acute LE, and defining the specific type of cutaneous LE can give prognostic information about the likelihood of SLE. Discoid lupus erythematosus (DLE) lesions are scarring and occur either alone or in association with SLE. Subacute cutaneous LE (SCLE) includes two types of lesions: psoriasiform and annular polycyclic. These lesions are nonscarring and are often photodistributed, and ultraviolet light is often a significant trigger. Acute cutaneous LE normally includes confluent photodistributed erythematous patches and, occasionally, bullous or toxic epidermal necrolysis (TEN)–like lesions. Skin biopsy usually helps confirm a diagnosis of LE, but clinical-pathologic correlation is extremely important because dermatomyositis and LE look similar histologically.

Treatment of LE is dependent on whether the disease is cutaneous or systemic and, if systemic, which organs are affected. Localized skin lesions can be treated with topical or intralesional steroids. Ointments usually work best, and starting with a potent fluorinated steroid such as clobetasol propionate (Temovate) for a couple of days, with a taper to fluocinonide (Lidex) and then hydrocortisone, is often effective. Prolonged use of potent topical steroids on the face needs to be avoided because of the potential for atrophy and withdrawal (rebound) rosacea. Sunscreens with a skin protection factor (SPF) of 30 or higher plus a Parsol 1789–containing sunscreen (which blocks ultraviolet A [UVA] better than other chemicals) and sun avoidance are important. In general, chronic cutaneous LE, including DLE, panniculitis, papulomucinous LE, and SCLE, are best treated with antimalarials. Hydroxychloroquine (Plaquenil)* should be used at a dose of 200 to 400 mg per day (up to 6.5 mg per kg per day), with complete blood counts, liver function tests, and eye examinations performed every 6 months. Chloroquine phosphate (Aralen)* can be substituted for hydroxychloroquine at a dose of around 250 mg per day (up to 3.5 mg per day), although eye examinations should be done every 4 months. For severe skin disease, prednisone at a dose of 20 to 40 mg per day can be used during the 6 to 8 weeks while antimalarials are becoming effective, although usually prednisone is not very effective and should be avoided.

Musculoskeletal Manifestations

Musculoskeletal manifestations are common. Acute arthritis, typically involving the small joints of the hands, wrists, and knees, is usually episodic and symmetrical in distribution. Avascular necrosis (AVN) is seen in 5% of SLE patients, affecting the hip most commonly but also the shoulder, knee, and ankle. The duration of treatment as well as higher doses of corticosteroids correlates with the development of AVN.

Cardiac Manifestations

The most common cardiac presentation in SLE is pericarditis, with an incidence of 20 to 30% in most large series. Clinical findings at presentation usually include precordial chest pain and a pericardial rub. Myocarditis presenting as dysrhythmias and/or cardiomegaly is a less common manifestation but may be more life-threatening. Libman-Sacks endocarditis, with sterile verrucous vegetations on the mitral valve, is less common, but prophylactic antibiotics during surgical and dental procedures are advisable if the diagnosis is suspected. Premature atherosclerosis is a major cause of morbidity and mortality in SLE. Both renal disease and chronic corticosteroid use may play an important role in pathogenesis.

Renal Manifestations

Renal disease is a common finding on kidney biopsy in most patients with SLE and can be asymptomatic until there's advanced disease. SLE patients with active disease should have screening urinalyses done regularly. The excretion of more than 500 mg of urinary protein per 24 hours (or greater than 3+ proteinuria on dipstick testing), the presence of casts (including red blood cells [RBCs], hemoglobin, granular, tubular, or mixed), hematuria (more than 5 RBCs per high-power field) or pyuria (more than 5 white blood cells [WBCs] per high-power field), or an elevated serum creatinine level is evidence of renal disease and should prompt the clinician to a more thorough investigation of renal status and referral to a specialist.

The World Health Organization (WHO) classification of lupus nephritis is the standard by which most lesions are classified and can prognosticate survival of the kidney. In one series of 148 patients with SLE, only 3 patients had a normal renal biopsy result. About 40% of the patients had mesangial abnormalities (WHO class II), 20% had focal glomerulonephritis (class IIIA and class IIIB), 40% had diffuse proliferative glomerulonephritis (class IV), and less than 10% had a predominant membranous lesion (class V). Class I and class II lesions require no treatment. Class III lesions can undergo transition to a more proliferative and diffuse process, necessitating treatment. The consequences of nephrotic syndrome, hypertension, hyperlipidemia, and hypercoagulability, seen with both class IV and class V lesions, can increase mortality in these patients. Class V (membranous) lesions usually have a slowly progressive course, and treatment varies, including steroids or immunosuppressives, neither of which have been shown to alter the course of the disease. Class IV (diffuse proliferative) lesions affect more than 50% of the glomeruli, with progression to renal failure in most cases.

Treatment to preserve renal function usually includes corticosteroids at 1 mg per kg and intravenous cyclophosphamide (Cytoxan).* The NIH (National Institutes of Health) protocol for lupus nephritis is cyclophosphamide 500 to 1000 mg per m^2 of body surface every month for 6 months, followed by an every-3-month dosing schedule for 18 months. Relapses can occur during treatment or after 2 years, and the monthly cycle is reinstituted at that time. Immediate toxic effects of cyclophosphamide include hemorrhagic cystitis, now mostly obviated with the use of prehydration and mesna (Mesnex) during the cyclophosphamide infusion, and nausea and vomiting, usually controlled with pretreatment use of ondansetron hydrochloride (Zofran). Immunosuppression is significant and the WBC counts are usually lowest (3000 to 4000 per mm^3) at about 10 days. Late toxic effects of cyclophosphamide include infertility in 50% of women less than 30 years of age and in 100% of women older than 30, premature ovarian failure, and gynecologic and lymphoproliferative malignancies. Newer immunosuppressive agents and biologic agents are being studied to prevent some of these sequelae.

*Not FDA approved for this indication.

*Not FDA approved for this indication.

Pulmonary Manifestations

The pulmonary manifestations of SLE are numerous and include pleuritis, pulmonary alveolar hemorrhage, pneumonitis, pulmonary infiltrates, chronic interstitial lung disease, shrinking lung syndrome, pulmonary hypertension, and pulmonary embolism. Acute pneumonitis frequently responds to corticosteroids (1 mg per kg per day). Pulmonary alveolar hemorrhage is a rare but serious manifestation and carries a high mortality. Very aggressive treatment is required for improved survival, and cytotoxic agents or plasmapheresis may be necessary.

Patients with chronic interstitial lung disease can present with typical symptoms of restrictive lung disease, including nonproductive cough, dyspnea on exertion, and basilar rales on physical examination. Pulmonary hypertension may be a finding in many of the collagen-vascular diseases and occurs in 1 to 2% of SLE patients. Pulmonary hypertension can present insidiously with progressive exertional dyspnea, and early disease can be detected by an abnormal carbon monoxide diffusing capacity (DLCO) on pulmonary function testing. Pulmonary embolus is a serious potential complication of antiphospholipid (APL) antibody syndrome (discussed later) in patients with SLE. Pleuritic chest pain in an SLE patient cannot be assumed to be due to SLE serositis. In an SLE patient with a normal chest film, pulmonary embolus must be excluded.

Gastrointestinal Manifestations

Abdominal pain, anorexia, nausea, and vomiting are common gastrointestinal manifestations of SLE. Serositis is the most common underlying causative disorder and frequently responds to moderate doses of corticosteroids. The presenting manifestation of mesenteric vasculitis can be lower abdominal pain accompanied by frank or occult rectal bleeding, and perforation of the bowel can result. If the diagnosis of mesenteric vasculitis is suspected, intensive investigation should be undertaken, with appropriate treatment with high doses of steroids. Acute pancreatitis can occur in SLE patients, manifesting as abdominal pain, nausea, vomiting, and elevated serum amylase.

Neuropsychiatric Manifestations

Neuropsychiatric SLE (NP-SLE) is a significant cause of morbidity, mortality, and disability in SLE patients. Diffuse manifestations are the most common CNS presentation in NP-SLE patients (60% of cases). Headaches occur in 30 to 50% of patients. Some patients with refractory headaches respond to nonsteroidal anti-inflammatory drugs (NSAIDs) or corticosteroids. Frank psychosis is seen in 5 to 15% of patients. Serum antiribosomal P antibodies have been associated with this manifestation. Major depression or dementia can also be a manifestation of the disease secondary to NP-SLE activity; a reactive depression secondary to a chronic devastating illness is also possible. In addition, dementia can be a sequela of multiple infarctions secondary to APL antibody syndrome or other vasculopathy.

Seizures are a common manifestation of NP-SLE and can be caused by a number of factors, including focal infarct or ischemia from vasculitis or APL antibody syndrome, embolic phenomenon or hemorrhage, or brain-reactive antibodies. Focal manifestations such as strokes occur in the minority of CNS SLE patients (10 to 35% of cases). These stroke syndromes can affect any area of the brain and are usually caused by thrombosis from vasculopathy or by emboli from cardiac valvular lesions. New understanding of APL-associated disease has helped in the diagnosis and management of thrombotic strokes.

The most common histologic finding in the brain of SLE patients is a vasculopathy, with associated microinfarcts. True vasculitis is rare. The evaluation of an SLE patient with CNS manifestations includes cerebrospinal fluid (CSF) evaluation for routine studies, antineuronal antibodies (seen in patients with diffuse manifestations), quantitative CSF immunoglobulins, and oligoclonal bands (elevations commonly seen in active CNS SLE disease). Magnetic resonance imaging (MRI) can sometimes demonstrate small, high-signal-intensity vascular lesions but cannot define active disease.

Treatment of the diffuse manifestations may include administration of antiseizure drugs or antipsychotics but usually requires high-dose steroids (1 mg per kg per day) or pulse high-dose steroids (1 gram per day for 3 days). Refractory cases sometimes respond to intravenous cyclophosphamide, plasmapheresis, or a combination of these. Focal manifestations seen in association with APL antibodies are treated with anticoagulation, in addition to the aforementioned medications.

Cranial neuropathies can be transient, resolving with corticosteroid therapy. They are frequently associated with APL antibody syndrome and are presumed to be of thrombotic origin. Movement disorders such as chorea are rare. Transverse myelitis is an infrequent but devastating manifestation of NP-SLE and can frequently be the presenting manifestation of SLE. Reports in the literature associate the presence of APL antibodies with transverse myelitis. Characteristic findings include an elevated CSF protein (in 82% of cases), CSF pleocytosis (in 70%), and a low (less than 30 mg per dL) CSF glucose (in 50%). Owing to the poor prognosis with transverse myelitis, early diagnosis and aggressive therapy are important. Mononeuritis multiplex secondary to small vessel vasculitis can also be seen in SLE.

Hematologic Manifestations

Cytopenias, including anemia, leukopenia, lymphopenia, and thrombocytopenia, are frequent findings in SLE. Hemolysis in SLE is usually Coombs'-positive owing to the presence of antibodies directed against RBC antigens. Leukopenia (2500 to 4000

WBCs per mm^3) in an SLE patient suggests active disease, although other causes of leukopenia such as infection or drugs must be excluded. Neither leukopenia nor lymphopenia (less than 1500 WBCs per mm^3) predisposes to infection, because the bone marrow is usually normal. Thrombocytopenia (platelet counts of less than 100,000 per mm^3) in an SLE patient is common but, like anemia, requires that other possible causes such as infection or drug effect be excluded. Most thrombocytopenic patients with SLE are asymptomatic, but in some patients, the platelet counts can drop quite low and predispose to bleeding, requiring aggressive management with high-dose steroids, cytotoxic drugs, intravenous immune globulin, and very rarely, splenectomy. A subset of SLE patients with thrombocytopenia have associated APL antibody syndrome and are predisposed to thrombotic events.

Malignancy

Malignancy continues to increase in SLE patients with increasing use of alkylating agents. Over 100 cases of non-Hodgkin's lymphoma have been reported, and there is an increased frequency of gynecologic cancers. In one series, the mean time from onset of treatment to cancer was only 4.1 years. Frequent surveillance, including Papanicolaou smears and mammograms, is important.

Pregnancy and SLE

Patients with SLE should have their disease controlled before becoming pregnant. The frequency of flares in pregnant patients is similar to that in nonpregnant patients. The chances of a normal pregnancy are reduced because of increased spontaneous abortions, prematurity, and intrauterine death. Neonatal lupus in the fetus can be seen in some mothers who have anti-SSA or anti-SSB antibodies in their blood. SLE patients with a history of late miscarriages should be checked for the presence of APL antibodies. SLE patients should be followed by obstetricians experienced in the management of high-risk cases.

The diagnosis of lupus flares in pregnancy can be difficult, because preeclampsia and eclampsia can appear similar clinically. The presence of other features of SLE, as well as elevated anti-dsDNA and depressed complement levels, may be helpful.

Drug-Induced Disease

A number of drugs can cause a lupus-like syndrome. Commonly associated drugs include procainamide, hydralazine, anticonvulsants, chlorpromazine, and isoniazid. Symptoms include fever, arthritis, and serositis but not renal or CNS disease and normally resolve in 6 to 8 weeks after the drug is stopped. In 90% of the cases an anti-histone antibody can be identified. Specific skin manifestations, particularly those of SCLE, may also be associated with use of thiazides, diltiazem, griseofulvin, sulfonylureas, and carbamazepine.

Antiphospholipid Antibodies

A variety of clotting abnormalities have been reported in SLE, including the presence of the lupus anticoagulant, manifested as a prolonged activated partial thromboplastin time (APTT) that does not normalize with mixing studies. Patients with the lupus anticoagulant, a false-positive result on VDRL testing, or a high titer of anticardiolipin antibodies fall under the umbrella term of "APL antibody–positive" and are predisposed to thrombotic events. The APL antibody syndrome describes the association of these APL antibodies with arterial and venous thrombosis, recurrent fetal loss, and immune thrombocytopenia. Management of SLE patients with APL antibodies who have never had a thrombotic event is usually with low-dose aspirin therapy. Once patients have had a thromboembolic event, lifelong anticoagulation with warfarin is established, with an INR (International Normalized Ratio) of 3.0, to prevent recurrent events. Recurrent fetal loss is managed with initiation of heparin therapy at the onset of pregnancy, because the fetal loss is presumed secondary to placental insufficiency. Low-molecular-weight heparin is being used more commonly and obviates the need for frequent PTT monitoring.

DERMATOMYOSITIS

Patients with dermatomyositis can have disease affecting only muscles (polymyositis), skin (amyopathic dermatomyositis), or both muscles and skin. The disease can evolve over time. The findings on skin biopsy resemble those seen with LE, so clinical-pathologic correlation is essential. It is important to document muscle involvement with muscle enzymes (creatine kinase, aldolase), electromyogram, or MRI, followed by a muscle biopsy of an involved muscle group, because treatment varies according to whether there is skin and/or muscle disease. Other causes of myopathy need to be considered, such as SLE, Sjögren's syndrome, hypothyroidism, viral infections (hepatitis, influenza, human immunodeficiency virus [HIV]), trichinosis, bacterial infections, and drugs (lovastatin [Mevacor], clofibrate [Atromid-S], cimetidine [Tagamet]).

Dermatologic findings in dermatomyositis, often quite characteristic, include Gottron's papules, which are lesions located over the extensor joints, and Gottron's sign, the presence of erythema in the same distribution as that of the papules. Other features that are common but not pathognomonic include a heliotrope, which is the presence of erythema and edema in a periorbital distribution, periungual telangiectasias, dystrophic cuticles, a violaceous erythema in a photodistribution that commonly also involves the upper back ("shawl sign"), and erythematous scaly patches on the palms—"mechanic's hands." The mechanic's hands are seen in association with the anti-Jo-1 antibody, found in a subset of patients with dermatomyositis with increased risk of interstitial lung disease.

Treatment is determined by whether the patient has muscle disease. If muscle disease is present, then prednisone at a dose of about 1 mg per kg per day should be given for several months, followed by a slow taper of 5 mg every 2 to 3 weeks if the patient has responded. If disease flares occur with the taper, the steroid dose should be increased again. Undertreatment results in incomplete resolution of the disease and prolongation of steroid therapy. Patients who do not respond to prednisone or who experience disease flares with attempted slow tapering of dose should be given steroid-sparing therapy with methotrexate,* 7.5 to 30 mg per week, or azathioprine (Imuran), 3 mg per kg per day, along with the prednisone. Careful monitoring of complete blood counts and liver function tests is essential. Patients with dermatomyositis or polymyositis, particularly those more than 60 years of age or experiencing resistant disease or relapses, should be screened for potential underlying malignancies, most commonly lung, breast, or ovary. Patients with amyopathic dermatomyositis or resolved myositis with residual skin disease can be given hydroxychloroquine* at a dose of 400 mg per day. Frequently, adding quinacrine,* 100 mg per day, or switching to chloroquine,* 250 mg per day, adds additional therapeutic benefit. Administration of methotrexate, 7.5 to 30 mg per week, is an alternative therapy for skin disease. Prednisone is not necessary to treat the skin disease.

SCLERODERMA

Scleroderma comprises a spectrum of sclerosing conditions, including morphea (skin only), limited cutaneous scleroderma, and diffuse cutaneous scleroderma (progressive systemic sclerosis). Most patients with morphea have atrophic, indurated plaques that early on can have erythematous inflammatory borders, but lesions can be linear, localized, or generalized over much of the skin. These patients nearly all have purely cutaneous disease that will not progress. Limited cutaneous scleroderma begins with more acral and facial skin involvement with edema, followed by sclerosis, and features can include those in the CREST association (calcinosis, Raynaud's phenomenon, esophageal dysmotility, sclerodactyly, and telangiectasias), as well as pulmonary hypertension. The disease progresses more slowly than diffuse cutaneous scleroderma, and renal disease and pulmonary fibrosis are rare. Diffuse cutaneous scleroderma involves both acral and proximal skin and is associated with scleroderma renal crisis and pulmonary fibrosis. The anti-topoisomerase I (anti-scl 70) antibody, when present, is found mainly in patients with diffuse cutaneous disease, and the anti-centromere antibody is much more prevalent in patients with limited cutaneous disease. Raynaud's phenomenon, due to vasospasm of the digital arteries, is usually precipitated by exposure to cold.

*Not FDA approved for this indication.

Treatment of scleroderma is mostly directed at symptoms, because there is no cure for the disease. Cold avoidance, including wearing warm gloves, is essential. Smoking can exacerbate the Raynaud's symptoms. Calcium channel blockers such as nifedipine (Procardia XL), 30 mg per day, can be given to decrease vasospasm. This dose can be increased as tolerated, with monitoring of the blood pressure. Any skin erosions or ulcers can be treated with Polysporin and DuoDerm semi-occlusive dressing. Early morphea lesions can be treated with potent topical steroids, and hydroxychloroquine,* 400 mg per day, can also occasionally be helpful. Arthralgias and myalgias are treated with NSAIDs.

The most common gastrointestinal symptoms are dysphagia, esophageal reflux, diarrhea, and malabsorption. Hypomotility of the small intestine is associated with bacterial overgrowth, malabsorption, and steatorrhea, for which antibiotic therapy is given. Rectal and colonic hypomotility lead to constipation, and formation of wide-mouth diverticula of the colon can occur. Dysphagia and esophageal reflux can be treated with metoclopramide hydrochloride (Reglan) or cisapride (Propulsid), each at a dose of 10 mg 30 minutes before eating and at bedtime. Esophageal reflux is treated with histamine H_2 blockers or omeprazole (Prilosec), 20 mg per day. Patients with reflux should be monitored by endoscopy for Barrett's esophagus, because there is an associated increased risk of malignancy. Any strictures should be dilated.

Cardiac disease is common; manifestations include pericarditis, myocardial fibrosis, and arrhythmias. Pericarditis can be treated with NSAIDs or prednisone. Pulmonary disease is frequent in scleroderma. Pulmonary fibrosis is seen mainly with diffuse cutaneous scleroderma, and pulmonary hypertension is mostly seen with limited scleroderma. Pulmonary function tests, including diffusion capacity, should be assessed when lung disease is suspected. The chest film commonly shows pulmonary fibrosis in the lower half of both pulmonary fields, and high-resolution computed tomography (CT) scan of the chest can help in assessing active inflammatory disease. Treatment includes use of prednisone and pulse therapy with intravenous cyclophosphamide.*

Renal disease is associated with severe arterial hypertension and renal insufficiency. The onset of malignant hypertension is associated with high plasma renin, arterial sclerosis, and rapid progression to renal failure. Other findings in renal disease include microscopic hematuria and proteinuria. Treatment of renal disease with angiotensin-converting enzyme (ACE) inhibitor drugs has decreased the high mortality that was previously associated with scleroderma renal disease.

*Not FDA approved for this indication.

CUTANEOUS VASCULITIS

method of
JEFFREY P. CALLEN, M.D.
University of Louisville
Louisville, Kentucky

The term "cutaneous vasculitis" may refer to a number of syndromes. Leukocytoclastic vasculitis is a specific histopathologic entity. This pattern is observed in many of the vasculitic syndromes that affect the small vessels of the skin. Although circulating immune complexes are involved in the pathogenesis of many of the vasculitic syndromes, the exact pathogenetic mechanisms have not been fully elucidated. However, even when the skin is seemingly the only system organ involved, vasculitis should be thought of as a systemic process.

Syndromes that can involve the small cutaneous vessels include hypersensitivity vasculitis, Henoch-Schönlein purpura, vasculitis associated with paraproteinemias, vasculitis as part of a collagen-vascular disorder, and hypocomplementemic (or urticarial) vasculitis. In addition, many patients with Wegener's granulomatosis, microscopic polyarteritis, and other vasculitides involving small to medium-sized vessels have cutaneous small-vessel disease. Therefore, prior to any pharmacologic therapy, a thorough evaluation should be performed.

EVALUATION

Evaluation of the patient with cutaneous vasculitis is useful in determining possible etiologic factors or associated processes, in assessing for the presence of systemic disease, and in formulating a prognosis. Historical information can reveal the presence of a pre-existing disorder or disease, medications taken prior to the onset of the vasculitis, the presence of infection, and symptoms suggestive of systemic involvement. On physical examination, both the type of cutaneous lesion and the extent of disease are of prognostic importance. Purpura, livedo reticularis, subcutaneous nodules, and ulcerations may be manifestations of noninflammatory vascular compromise such as in hypercoagulable states, scurvy, left atrial myxoma, atheromatous emboli, or calciphylaxis; these conditions should be ruled out. Immunofluorescence microscopy is helpful when the possibility of Henoch-Schönlein purpura is considered, particularly in adults. Tissue confirmation of vasculitis is almost always necessary, and biopsy should be performed on an early lesion (less than 48 hours old) if possible. A complete laboratory evaluation is also helpful and should include a complete blood count, urinalysis, cryoglobulin determination, serum protein electrophoresis, hepatitis B surface antigen test, hepatitis C antibody test, antinuclear antibody test and possibly an anti-Ro (SS-A) test, tests of renal function, and a chest film. The presence of cytoplasmic antineutrophil cytoplasmic antibody (c-ANCA) has been closely associated with Wegener's granulomatosis and may be predictive of the activity of the disease. Perinuclear ANCA (p-ANCA) may be present in other vasculitic syndromes such as polyarteritis nodosa and microscopic polyarteritis, but may also be present in nonvasculitic states such as Sweet's syndrome, pyoderma gangrenosum, and/or ulcerative colitis.

TREATMENT

General Measures

If an associated condition or etiologic factor is present, its removal or therapy can result in a cure of the process. Identification and treatment of an infection, discontinuation of offending medicaments or other ingestants, and therapy directed against the production of an abnormal protein are most important. An open-label trial in Italy studied the effect of an elimination diet on five patients. With reintroduction of foods and food dyes, the offending agent was identified and sustained control of the disease was possible. Dietary restriction has been of limited value in my practice. Because lesions are more frequent or more severe in the skin overlying dependent areas and on cooler acral regions of the body, frequent turning, compression stockings, elevation, and a warm environment are helpful.

Disease-Specific Considerations

Hypersensitivity vasculitis and Henoch-Schönlein purpura are often self-limited, and only symptomatic therapy may be required. Polyarteritis nodosa, Wegener's granulomatosis, and systemic necrotizing vasculitis are potentially life-threatening conditions, and without treatment, patients may die from renal or central nervous system involvement. Thus, aggressive therapy is often necessary. Urticarial vasculitis may be a chronic condition with a benign course or, in the presence of hypocomplementemia, may be complicated by chronic obstructive pulmonary disease. The chronic nature of the process necessitates continual suppressive therapy. Manifestations of vasculitis complicating rheumatoid arthritis, systemic lupus erythematosus (SLE), or Sjögren's syndrome range from benign palpable purpura to severe life-threatening disease, and therapy should be based on the severity of the process. In patients with paraproteinemias, therapy required for suppression of the abnormal protein may be more aggressive than that needed for the cutaneous vasculitis. It has been recognized that many patients with cryoglobulinemia-associated vasculitis also have hepatitis C virus infection. Currently available antiviral agents are not effective, but there may be agents available in the near future that will effectively suppress hepatitis C viral replication. At this time, for patients with hepatitis C–associated vasculitis/vasculopathy, the use of oral prednisone, 1 mg per kg per day, followed by subcutaneous interferon alfa,* 3 million units three times per week, may be effective.

Nonimmunologic Drug Therapy

Administration of antihistamines has often been suggested as a first line of therapy, based on the observation that injected histamine allows deposition of immune complexes in the vessel walls with the

*Not FDA approved for this indication.

eventual development of leukocytoclastic vasculitis. In patients with palpable purpura, antihistamines have rarely if ever been effective in my practice. However, in patients with urticarial vasculitis, I generally begin therapy with a nonsoporific agent such as astemizole (Hismanal)* or loratadine (Claritin) each morning and a histamine H_1 inhibitor in the evening. An agent such as doxepin (Sinequan),* may have both H_1- and H_2-inhibiting effects and is preferable in some cases.

Various nonsteroidal anti-inflammatory drugs (NSAIDs) have been used in the treatment of vasculitic syndromes. In particular, patients with urticarial vasculitis may respond to ibuprofen or indomethacin. The therapeutic benefit of NSAIDs comes from their effect on prostaglandins and leukotrienes and possibly on platelet aggregation. In my experience, NSAIDs have not been particularly effective in any vasculitic syndrome.

Pentoxifylline (Trental)* has been reported to be useful in some patients. In particular, those patients with evidence of an occlusive vasculopathy such as livedo vasculitis may respond. I have not found it to be of benefit in any of my patients.

Antimalarials, such as hydroxychloroquine (Plaquenil)* and chloroquine (Aralen),* have been used for some patients with vasculitis. Although they are effective for the cutaneous lesions of SLE, they have not been effective for vasculitis, even in my patients with SLE.

Diaminodiphenylsulfone (DDS), i.e., dapsone,* has received some recent attention. It is effective in dermatitis herpetiformis, a disease characterized by neutrophilic papillitis, and has various effects on leukocytes. It is the agent of choice for treatment of the rare cutaneous vasculitic syndrome of erythema elevatum diutinum. In selected patients it has been effective in controlling the manifestations of palpable purpura in doses of 100 to 200 mg per day. A recent report suggested that there may be a synergistic effect between pentoxifylline and dapsone.

Colchicine* has been reported to be effective in open-label trials for cutaneous vasculitis as manifested by palpable purpura or urticarial lesions. Colchicine is an alkaloid derived from a crocus-like plant, *Colchicum autumnale.* Its effects in vasculitis may be related to a blockade of disease expression. Colchicine inhibits leukocyte chemotaxis, blocks the release of lysosomal enzymes, inhibits DNA synthesis and cell proliferation, and may inhibit the effects of prostaglandins. Of the more than 50 patients I have treated and observed, colchicine has been effective in about 35, nonevaluable in about 5, and ineffective in the remaining 10 patients. The only double-blind placebo-controlled trial failed to demonstrate a positive benefit; however, the colchicine-treated group included all the dapsone failures, and thus there may have been some inadvertent selection bias. I use a dose of 0.6 mg given orally twice daily. If this dose is tolerated, effects are usually observed within 7 to 14 days. In patients with associated arthralgias or arthritis, colchicine may also be of benefit. Immune complexes are unaffected by the drug, and this leads to my belief that the mechanism of action is a suppression of disease expression. Long-term effective usage (up to 10 years) has been possible in some of my patients without serious side effects. These patients should be regularly monitored with complete blood counts.

Corticosteroids

Systemic corticosteroids are useful in most patients with vasculitis, but because of multiple potential toxic effects, their use should be limited to patients with severe disease or cases in which the use is expected to be short-term. The absolute indications for systemic corticosteroids include a rapid progressive course, neurologic involvement, renal involvement with loss of function, carditis or coronary vasculitis, and severe pulmonary disease with cavitation or infiltration. Among the relative indications are chronic cutaneous disease unresponsive to other agents, peripheral neuropathy, chronic lung disease, weight loss, and fever.

Corticosteroids should be given in moderate to high daily dosages. I use prednisone; when there are strong indications for its use, a starting dose of 60 to 80 mg per day is given in divided doses. Divided doses are clinically more effective than a single morning dose, even in equivalent milligram-for-milligram doses. However, in addition to the greater clinical efficacy, the divided dosage schedule has more chance of toxicity. Prednisone is continued until the signs and symptoms of vasculitis have been controlled. At this point a switch to a single morning dose should be attempted, and the drug can then be slowly tapered. Tapering should take place over a period of about twice the length of the active treatment phase. If reactivation of the disease occurs, the original dosage should be reinstituted, followed by a slow taper.

Intravenous administration of methylprednisolone in high doses (1 gram per day for 5 days) has been used in patients with acute fulminating vasculitis. This therapy is not without risk: sudden electrolyte shifts, cardiac arrhythmias, and cardiac arrests have been reported. The patient should be carefully monitored throughout the therapy. This approach constitutes a stop-gap measure for management of severe disease, and other means of disease suppression are necessary for long-term control of the vasculitic process.

Corticosteroid therapy, as mentioned, is frequently accompanied by side effects. Careful monitoring for diabetes mellitus, hypertension, peptic ulcer disease, osteoporosis, cataract formation, and glaucoma is important. Also, reactivation of *Mycobacterium tuberculosis* infection is possible, and attempts to identify the patient at risk should be made at the onset of therapy. It has been pointed out that reliable purified protein derivative skin testing can be done during the first few days to weeks of therapy with systemic

*Not FDA approved for this indication.

corticosteroids, and thus the patient in need of rapid treatment need not wait for the result of the skin test prior to initiation of therapy.

Immunosuppressives

Patients who fail to respond to systemic corticosteroids, who develop steroid-related side effects, or in whom the disease is severe may be given an immunosuppressive agent. The agents most often used in vasculitis are alkylating agents such as cyclophosphamide (Cytoxan)* and chlorambucil (Leukeran),* antimetabolites such as azathioprine (Imuran),* the folate antagonist methotrexate (Rheumatrex),* and cyclosporine (Sandimmune, Neoral).* Earlier studies suggested that cyclophosphamide was the agent of choice in conditions such as severe necrotizing vasculitis and Wegener's granulomatosis, but later reports have suggested that methotrexate may be equally effective in the management of Wegener's granulomatosis. Cyclophosphamide has been used in a daily oral dose of 1 to 2 mg per kg. It is administered in the morning, and the patient is given adequate hydration throughout the day to prevent hemorrhagic cystitis. This agent should not be given during pregnancy. Its beneficial effects are often delayed, beginning within 4 to 6 weeks. Recently, cyclophosphamide has been administered in intermittent intravenous pulses. This method avoids some of the potential long-term toxicity, but hemorrhagic cystitis remains a possibility. Chlorambucil is an agent with presumably a similar mechanism of action, without associated bladder toxicity, but it has been much less well studied. Both cyclophosphamide and chlorambucil have been linked to an increased risk of neoplasia—in particular, lymphoreticular malignancies (both agents), skin cancer (chlorambucil), and bladder cancer (cyclophosphamide).

Azathioprine has been reported to be useful in patients with severe refractory cutaneous vasculitis and in patients with rheumatoid vasculitis. It has also been used in severe necrotizing vasculitis, polyarteritis nodosa, and Wegener's granulomatosis but is probably less effective than cyclophosphamide in these conditions. It is administered in a single oral dose of 1 to 2 mg per kg. The primary toxic effects that occur are drug-induced fever, pancreatitis, hepatitis, and bone marrow toxicity. The onset of its action is also delayed, occurring within 4 to 6 weeks. Long-term toxic effects such as potential neoplasia have been studied in patients with rheumatoid arthritis, and the risk of subsequent malignancy was no greater in the patients receiving azathioprine than in those with similar disease levels who were not given azathioprine.

Low-dose weekly methotrexate (7.5 to 15 mg) has been used to treat patients with Wegener's granulomatosis, rheumatoid vasculitis, and cutaneous polyarteritis nodosa. Methotrexate can be administered orally, intramuscularly, or intravenously. Renal function should be carefully assessed prior to initiating methotrexate therapy, because inability to excrete the drug increases the potential for severe toxicity. Initial monitoring of patients receiving methotrexate should include frequent complete blood counts and liver function tests. Patients receiving long-term therapy will need periodic liver biopsies to monitor for potential fibrosis and/or cirrhosis.

Cyclosporine is a relatively new agent developed to prevent transplant rejection. The mechanism of its action is unknown. It is administered in doses of 3 to 8 mg per kg per day, with effects and side effects closely linked to one another. Nephrotoxicity is a limiting factor, and careful monitoring of renal function and blood pressure is necessary. Blood levels (trough) can be obtained, but it is not clear how meaningful they are in terms of toxicity or effect. Clinical experience with cyclosporine therapy of vasculitis is anecdotal.

*Not FDA approved for this indication.

Plasmapheresis

Plasma exchange can be an adjunct to therapy for severe diseases characterized by circulating immunoreactants, such as vasculitis. A number of exchanges are required, and the procedure must be performed in a hospital setting. This therapy can protect patients through a severe flare of disease, although systemic therapy with corticosteroids and/or immunosuppressives is required for long-term control of the disease process.

DISEASES OF THE NAILS

method of
J. ANDRÉ, M.D., and N. LATEUR, M.D.
Brussels Free University
C.H.U. Saint Pierre
Brussels, Belgium

The nail is a plate of hard keratin embedded in the tissues of the fingertip, separated from them by proximal, lateral, and distal nail grooves. It is produced by the nail matrix, which is partly covered by the proximal nail fold (PNF). It grows towards the end of the fingertip, sliding along the nail bed, to which it is firmly attached. The hyponychium represents the thickened distal part of the nail bed, and the cuticle is the horny portion of the free margin of the PNF. These two structures play an important role as seals between nail plate and nail bed at one end and between nail plate and nail matrix at the other end.

Appropriate treatment requires an accurate diagnosis. The presence of a diseased nail should prompt a search for disease in other nails, skin, and mucosae (e.g., mycosis of the folds, psoriasis, lichen planus). Evaluation should include a complete medical history that identifies any drugs taken by the patient. In many cases, complementary investigations are necessary: culture for bacteria and fungi, radiography, and biopsy.

In addition to specific treatment, some general measures are important in the management of ungual pathology:

- The nail must be preserved. Affected parts of the nail can be removed using files, clippers, or partial surgical avulsion. Unnecessary avulsion should be avoided, as the procedure may damage the nail matrix, often leading to the regrowth of a more abnormal nail.
- The avoidance of microtrauma is essential and should be emphasized to the patient. Nails should be cut short, and manicures performed gently. This is particularly important in onycholysis (detachment of the nail plate from the nail bed) of any cause, in which the condition can be aggravated by overzealous cleaning of the distal nail groove. The patient should be advised to wear protective gloves or low-heeled shoes with rounded tips, as appropriate.
- Affected nails should be regularly disinfected to avoid secondary infection in cases of onycholysis or with small periungual wounds.
- Patience is also essential. The normal fingernail grows 3 mm per month, and for toenails the growth rate is only 1 mm per month. This explains why, even with effective treatment, several months (up to 12 months for the big toenail) is necessary for the full regrowth of a nail.

NAIL INFECTIONS

Onychomycosis

Onychomycosis, or fungal nail infection, occurs frequently: it represents 30% of all onychopathies. Classification of onychomycosis is based on the type of pathogen (dermatophyte, yeast, or mold) and the clinical findings. In our laboratory, dermatophytes were identified as the causative agent in onychomycosis in 77.6%, yeasts in 14.1%, and molds in 5.5% of the cases. Mixed infections were observed in 2.8%.

In onychomycosis due to dermatophytes, *Trichophyton rubrum* and *T. interdigitale* are the main pathogens worldwide. Dermatophytic onychomycosis affects men and women equally and is observed most often in toenails, mainly the big toenail. Dermatophytes invade the nail at sites of diminished resistance: the distal and lateral nail grooves, in which infection is termed distal and lateral subungual onychomycosis (DLSO); the proximal nail groove, in which infection is called proximal subungual onychomycosis (PSO); and the surface of the nail plate, in which infection is called superficial white onychomycosis (SWO). In DLSO, which is the most common form, a distal or lateral yellowish discoloration is accompanied by subungual pachyonychia (thickening of the subungual keratin) or by onycholysis. In PSO, yellowish-white patches appear from under the proximal nail fold. In SWO, opaque punctiform white spots appear on the nail surface. Total dystrophic onychomycosis (TDO) represents the most advanced form of all three types, especially DLSO. TDO is characterized by invasion and progressive destruction of the nail plate itself. The yellow to brown nail becomes fragile and gradually crumbles.

In onychomycosis due to yeasts, *Candida albicans* is often isolated. This type is more frequent in women and affects mainly the fingernails. It usually starts as a paronychia or an onycholysis and then extends to the nail plate.

In onychomycosis due to molds, *Scopulariopsis brevicaulis, Scytalidium dimidiatum, Fusarium* species, and *Aspergillus* species are among the most frequently isolated pathogens. Clinical aspects are similar to those described for onychomycosis due to dermatophytes.

Clinical diagnosis must always be confirmed by laboratory tests to avoid unjustified therapies. Laboratory studies are performed on affected keratin taken with nail clippers as close as possible to the healthy portion of the nail. This sample is sent, without fixation, to the laboratory for direct microscopy, culture, and, if possible, histologic examination of the keratin.

Treatment

The treatment of onychomycosis takes several months and requires regular and conscientious care. Its principles are identical for the different forms of onychomycosis and include the following measures.

Elimination of Infected Keratin. Removal of infected keratin can be achieved using nail clippers or files. In some cases, chemical or surgical avulsion is required. A paste of 40% urea* containing 1% bifonazole (Amycor, Onychoset)* can be used. Urea produces onycholysis in 1 to 3 weeks, which allows the cutting away of diseased keratin. Surgical avulsion is rarely necessary and should be performed only locally to remove affected parts of the nail. Total avulsion should be avoided.

Use of Oral Antimycotics. We prefer itraconazole (Sporanox) and terbinafine (Lamisil), which have a high affinity for keratinized tissues. Short-term therapy with these agents yields good therapeutic results, with a good safety profile. Terbinafine is mainly active against dermatophytes and is particularly effective in onychomycosis due to *T. rubrum*. Itraconazole has a broader spectrum of action, being effective against dermatophytes, yeasts, and some molds. It is useful in fingernail onychomycosis, which is mainly caused by yeasts, and in cases of mixed infection and those in which molds are pathogenic.

Itraconazole must be given at the end of a meal and can be prescribed in a regimen of either continuous therapy (200 mg per day for 2 to 3 months) or pulse therapy (200 mg twice daily for 1 week, followed by a 3-week rest period). We prefer the latter because it is cheaper and there is no need for blood tests. For fingernail infections, two pulses are sufficient. Three pulses are necessary for toenail infec-

*Not available in the United States.

tions. The most frequent side effects of itraconazole therapy are gastrointestinal complaints and headaches, but skin rashes have also been reported. In patients receiving other pharmacologic agents, possibility of drug interactions should be considered: itraconazole is contraindicated with terfenadine (Seldane), astemizole (Hismanal), cisapride (Propulsid), midazolam (Versed), triazolam (Halcion), and lovastatin (Mevacor).

Absorption of terbinafine is not influenced by timing of meals. In adults, the drug is given in a dose of 250 mg daily for 6 weeks, to treat fingernail infections, or for 12 weeks, to treat toenail infections. Side effects of terbinafine therapy are similar to those reported with itraconazole. Changes in the sense of taste, which are reversible on cessation of therapy, are characteristic. Fewer drug interactions have been reported than with itraconazole. We advise performing a complete blood cell count and liver function tests before beginning therapy and again 1 month later. At the start of terbinafine therapy, we also check creatinine and urea.

Use of Topical Antimycotics. Topical antimycotics enhance therapeutic results and reduce the relapse rate when combined with oral agents. They can be used alone at the onset of DLSO, in SWO, or when systemic antimycotics are contraindicated or refused by the patient. These agents are of no benefit when used alone for the treatment of infections involving the nail matrix. The most suitable products are the recently developed medicated nail polishes such as amorolfine 5% (Loceryl)* and ciclopirox 8% (Loprox). These agents are used twice a week until cure is complete.

Paronychia

Paronychia, or inflammation of periungual tissues, can be acute or chronic. Acute paronychia generally affects a single finger. The most common pathogenic agents are *Staphylococcus aureus* and streptococci, but gram-negative bacteria and herpes simplex virus may also be identified. The entry lesion may be minor.

In bacterial paronychia, erythema, edema, and throbbing pain are present before pus accumulation occurs. In paronychia due to *Pseudomonas aeruginosa*, the nail exhibits a greenish color. The pathogenic agent is identified by direct examination and culture.

Chronic paronychia is a condition of multifactorial origin, often involving several fingers. It is most commonly seen in women and is due to repeated exposure to water, detergents, and foodstuffs handled in meal preparation. It can be also seen in thumb-sucking children. Chronic paronychia may be infectious, with mostly mixed flora (such as aerobic and anaerobic bacteria, or yeasts and bacteria), or noninfectious (as in eczema and psoriasis).

Clinically, the periungual region becomes deformed owing to painless erythematous swelling, and the cuticle disappears, which allows further penetration of organisms as well as food and detergents, which in turn will aggravate the inflammation. The nail plate exhibits transverse striations, and sometimes the lateral edges become brown-green in color owing to *Candida albicans* invasion.

Treatment

Acute Paronychia. The lesion should be incised and drained as soon as possible to avoid transient or permanent nail dystrophy. Antiseptic baths with hexamidine or povidone-iodine and penicillinase-resistant antibiotics should be prescribed. When necessary, antibiotic treatment should be adjusted in accordance with results of antibiotic sensitivity testing.

Chronic Paronychia. Treatment consists of a number of ancillary measures in addition to specific therapy. Patients should be advised to

- Keep their nails clean but avoid overzealous manicure, which disrupts the nail seals
- Avoid contact with water and irritants, dry the hands carefully every time, and wear cotton gloves under rubber or vinyl gloves when using detergents, preparing food and vegetables, or handling "do-it-yourself" products
- Wear leather or other weatherproof gloves in cold and windy conditions

Specific therapy consists of taking bacterial and fungal swabs, treating the infection topically with povidone-iodine, and the use of broad-spectrum antimycotics with antibacterial activity. Possible candidiasis of the nail should be treated with two pulses of itraconazole.

Warts

Periungual and subungual warts are contagious, firm keratotic papules, of variable size, due to human papilloma virus. They particularly affect school-aged children, and trauma (nail biting or picking) and moisture (hyperhidrosis and finger-sucking) are predisposing factors. More than 65% of warts will disappear spontaneously after 2 to 5 years. The diagnosis is essentially clinical, but in long-standing lesions in adults, Bowen's disease should be ruled out by biopsy.

Treatment

Treatment is often painful and frustrating, periungual and subungual warts being more recalcitrant than warts in other locations. Therapy can be withheld in many cases, but measures such as reducing moisture and avoiding nail biting and picking are essential. When the patient demands treatment or intervention is deemed necessary owing to multiplication of the warts, nail plate deformation, or pain caused by fissuring, the practitioner should keep in mind that aggressive therapy applied to the proximal nail fold can damage the nail matrix and lead to transient or permanent alterations to the nail plate.

---

*Not available in the United States.

The nail plate should be cut away prior to treating subungual warts.

As many therapeutic options as authors have been published. None guarantees the cure or the absence of recurrences.

Chemical Treatments. When several nails are affected, we recommend a daily massage with an ointment containing 12% urea and 0.03% retinoic acid. If only a few warts are present, salicylic acid, either in equal parts with lactic acid (Duofilm) or at a concentration of 40% in an ointment base, can be applied nightly under occlusion. Warts should be abraded twice a week before reapplication. Scarification with bleomycin (Bleomycin), at a concentration of 1 mg per mL, should be considered only for recalcitrant warts in adults.

Physical Treatments. Physical treatments carry the risk of damaging the matrix. Cryotherapy with liquid nitrogen is efficient but painful. Curettage, electrodessication, or carbon dioxide laser vaporization can be considered for management of recurrent warts in adults.

THE NAIL IN DERMATOLOGIC DISEASES

Psoriasis

Psoriasis frequently affects the nails, particularly the fingernails. In cutaneous psoriasis, the nails are involved in 10 to 55% of the cases.

Psoriasis can affect the matrix, causing pitting (small punctate depressions of the nail surface) and more severe alterations of the nail plate. Nail bed involvement gives rise to salmon-colored spots, splinter hemorrhages (filiform longitudinal hemorrhages), subungual hyperkeratosis, or onycholysis. Proximal nail fold involvement can mimic chronic paronychia.

Clinical diagnosis is possible in the presence of cutaneous psoriasis, involvement of several nails, combination of suggestive signs such as pitting and onycholysis, and/or subungual hyperkeratosis. Diagnosis is difficult when nail involvement occurs as an isolated finding or when only one nail is affected. Ungual biopsy is then often necessary.

Treatment

Treatment of nail psoriasis is long and tedious, often with disappointing results. It should be considered only if the patient is very motivated. In all cases, nails must be cut short to avoid precipitation of Koebner's phenomenon (ocurrence of the disease at sites subjected to microtrauma), and secondary onychomycosis should be ruled out. In women, nail polish will frequently conceal the nail changes; however, the use of artificial nails is not recommended.

Pitting does not respond well to treatment. More severe nail plate dystrophies can benefit from application of high-potency corticosteroid lotion under the proximal nail fold; clobetasol propionate (Temovate) can be used once daily initially and then once every 2 days thereafter. Although they are painful, steroid injections in the matrix can be used in severe involvement limited to a few fingers (as described for lichen planus).

Distal subungual onycholysis can benefit from daily application of a high-potency corticosteroid. Regular disinfection is mandatory to prevent secondary infection. Local photochemotherapy with ultraviolet A and a psoralen (PUVA) can also be tried.

In subungual hyperkeratosis, we advocate application of a high-potency corticosteroid ointment containing 3% salicylic acid (Diprosalic),* alternating with calcipotriene ointment (Daivonex).* Use of 1% 5-fluorouracil cream (Efudex)† can also be tried.

Ungual psoriasis does not justify the use of systemic treatment with oral methotrexate, cyclosporine, or retinoids. The nails sometimes improve when these treatments are prescribed for severe cutaneous psoriasis.

In children, treatment should be withheld.

Lichen Planus

Ungual lichen planus merits definitive diagnosis because it can cause permanent loss of the nail. Nail involvement occurs in 10% of cases of cutaneous lichen planus and can take various clinical forms. Nail plate thinning with longitudinal striation and distal splitting is characteristic. The destruction of the matrix can progress to dorsal pterygion (adhesion of the PNF to the nail bed). Clinical diagnosis is possible when cutaneous or mucous lesions are associated; nail biopsy is necessary when the nail involvement is isolated.

Treatment

Most cases of lichen planus affecting the nail are of moderate severity, with a good prognosis. Treatment is unnecessary except for possible topical application of corticosteroids. Severe, progressive, scarring lichen planus affecting several nails justifies the use of oral prednisolone, 0.5 mg per kg per day for 3 weeks, followed by gradual tapering over a period of 3 weeks. If only a few fingernails are affected, intramatrix injections, once a month for 3 to 6 months, can be prescribed. Less than 0.3 mL of an aqueous solution of dexamethasone acetate, 2.5 to 5 mg per mL, should be injected per finger.

Alopecia Areata

In 7 to 66% of cases of alopecia areata, nail changes can be observed. The disease mainly affects the matrix, giving rise to nail plate alterations. The most frequent finding is regular and superficial pitting or trachyonychia, i.e., nail roughness due to superficial longitudinal striations, with loss of luster. Diagnosis sometimes requires biopsy. Histology shows a spongiotic dermatitis, which can also be observed in eczema.

---

*Not available in the United States.

†Not FDA approved for this indication.

Treatment

In alopecia areata, nail alterations usually regress and do not require any treatment. In very motivated adult patients, topical application of a corticosteroid lotion under the PNF can be prescribed.

Twenty-Nail Dystrophy Syndrome

The twenty-nail dystrophy syndrome is characterized by involvement of the 20 nails without any cutaneous lesions. This condition is mainly observed in children. The nails show trachyonychia. Biopsy reveals either a spongiotic dermatitis or, more rarely, psoriasis or lichen planus. The syndrome usually regresses after a few years and does not require any treatment.

TRAUMATIC INJURIES OF THE NAIL

Acute Trauma

Acute trauma most often leads to a painful subungual hematoma. A small hematoma can be drained through a small hole burned into the nail plate with a red-hot paper clip or by delicately removing successive thin nail layers with a scalpel blade.

If the hematoma involves 40 to 50% of the nail area, a radiograph is mandatory to rule out an associated bone fracture. Severe matrix and nail bed injury should also be suspected, and surgical nail avulsion is therefore indicated to explore the tissues. Lacerating wounds necessitate meticulous repair by a specialized hand surgeon.

Chronic Finger Trauma

In the fingers, the nails are submitted to daily trauma related to occupational, housework, and recreational activities. Self-inflicted injuries are also frequent (from overzealous manicure, nail biting, habit of pushing back the cuticle with a adjacent fingernail).

Nail brittleness is a common presenting complaint, mainly among women. It is often accompanied by splitting of the distal nail edge or presence of thin longitudinal furrows in the nail plate. Causes of nail brittleness are numerous; it can be due to disease of the nail, such as onychomycosis or psoriasis, but, more often, it results from repeated microtrauma acting on a favorable ground.

Treatment

It is important to explain to the patient that the ungual alterations are due to or favored by trauma. Possible sources of trauma, particularly self-inflicted trauma, should be highlighted. For brittle nails, in addition to treatment of possible underlying nail disease, the most useful approach involves the following considerations:

- Limiting microtrauma by filing the nails very short, gentle manicure, and the wearing of protective gloves for household work
- Everyday, regular application of moisturizing cream on the nail apparatus and the wearing of nail polish 5 days a week; however, the use of "therapeutic" polish containing formaldehyde or acrylic derivatives should be avoided
- Although the efficacy of oral treatments is questionable, biotin 2.5 mg and cysteine 2 grams daily for several months can be useful

Chronic Toe Trauma

In the toes, footwear-induced trauma predominates as the mechanism of injury and is frequently responsible for various commonly seen nail disorders: onycholysis, leukonychia, brown-black discoloration due to melanin or hematoma, nail thickening, pincer nail, ingrown nail, and subungual horn.

Pincer nail is characterized by the presence of a transverse overcurvature that increases along the longitudinal axis of the nail and reaches its greatest magnitude at the distal part. It mainly affects the big toe in elderly women and can be very painful.

Ingrown nail is a nail that grows into the lateral nail fold. It is mainly observed in the big toe in male adolescents or young adults in whom sport trauma acts on a nail plate that is too wide for its bed. It can be followed by edema, secondary infection, and the formation of granulation tissue. Distal nail embedding is rarer and usually follows nail shedding; the nail regrowth is impaired by a hypertrophied distal wall.

Clinical diagnosis of footwear-induced nail disorders is usually possible, but sampling to exclude onychomycosis is often necessary.

Treatment

Wearing proper footwear as well as regular filing and trimming of the nails should be emphasized to the patient. Big toenails should be cut straight across, 1 mm beyond the distal groove. Correction of orthopedic abnormalities should also be considered.

Pincer nail can benefit from orthonyx (mechanical correction) performed by a podiatrist. Surgical treatment is indicated in later stages and is best achieved with phenolization of the lateral horns of the matrix and resection to correct possible subungual hyperostosis.

With ingrown nail, surgical avulsion is not advisable. In early stages, disinfection of the affected nail with povidone-iodine, with interposition of a small piece of povidone-iodine gauze between the nail and the lateral nail groove, is beneficial. Silver nitrate can be applied on the granulation tissue. If there is a nail spicule that penetrates the periungual fold, it should be removed, usually necessitating the use of local anesthesia. In more advanced stages, phenolization of the lateral horn of the matrix with granulation tissue curettage is indicated.

In distal nail embedding, an acrylic "sculptured" nail can be anchored on the stump nail when the hypertrophied distal wall cannot be reduced by regular massage.

TUMORS OF THE NAIL APPARATUS

It is easy to recognize a tumor in the presence of an exophytic mass partially destroying the nail, but other, less clear-cut clinical presentations are possible. A longitudinal lesion of the nail plate, in the form of either a groove, a hyperpigmentated area, or a yellowish thickening, can represent a matrix tumor; a circumscribed discoloration, onycholysis, or subungual hyperkeratosis can be due to a nail bed tumor, or a chronic paronychia can be due to a PNF tumor.

The possibility of an ungual tumor should always be kept in mind in the presence of a chronic lesion affecting a single nail. In case of doubt, a radiograph should be obtained and a biopsy performed.

Treatment

Complete surgical excision constitutes appropriate treatment for most ungual tumors. This approach allows accurate diagnosis and prevents recurrences. Surgery is best performed by a physician with good knowledge of nail anatomy in order to avoid long-term serious dystrophies.

Complete removal of the tumor is also the treatment for epidermoid carcinoma. Excision should be limited and amputation of the phalanx avoided because of possible polydactylous involvement and the relatively good prognosis with this tumor.

LONGITUDINAL MELANONYCHIA AND MELANOMA

Longitudinal melanonychia (LM) is a brown-black longitudinal band due to the presence of melanin in the nail plate; the source of the melanin is the matrix melanocytes. The causes of LM are numerous: it can be due to melanocytic activation, which can be racial, inflammatory, iatrogenic, or traumatic, or to a localized increased number of matrix melanocytes as in lentigo, nevus, or melanoma.

Early matrix melanoma should always be ruled out in presence of LM in an adult patient. Clinical signs evocative of a melanoma are

- LM affecting a single digit, especially the thumb, index finger, or big toe
- LM observed in a patient aged 60 years or more, or at increased risk of developing a melanoma (e.g., with a history of melanoma or dysplastic nevus syndrome)
- LM that develops abruptly or becomes suddenly darker or wider
- LM that is accompanied by periungual pigmentation and/or dystrophy of the nail plate
- LM with blurred borders or presenting as a wide, dark, heterogeneous band

However, an apparently stable pale LM can also be a melanoma, and biopsy of every monodactylic LM wider than 2 mm occurring in an adult is recommended.

Benign lesions do not require treatment. Intraepidermal melanoma (Clark level I) necessitates total excision of the nail apparatus. In invasive melanoma, amputation of the distal phalanx is indicated.

In children, a wait-and-see policy can be followed, because ungual melanoma is extremely rare, and clinical presentation as an LM has never been documented.

KELOIDS

method of
MARLENE S. CALDERON, M.D., and
WARREN L. GARNER, M.D.
University of Michigan Medical Center
Ann Arbor, Michigan

Keloids are abnormal overgrowths of connective tissue, usually occurring at the site of skin trauma. They are distinct from hypertrophic and other scars and are characterized by their propensity to extend beyond the boundary of the original injury. Keloid scars rarely regress and can become disfiguring and pendulous. They occur most often in dark-skinned persons and demonstrate a familial predisposition. Areas of skin tension, such as those overlying the presternum and deltoid muscles, are commonly affected. Other sites of skin injury on the earlobes and upper arms, from piercing and vaccination, can also develop keloids.

ETIOPATHOGENESIS

The etiopathogenetic mechanism for keloid scars is unknown. Histologically, keloids demonstrate the presence of excessive, broad eosinophilic collagen fibers and overabundant mucinous ground substance, with low fibroblast density. Biochemically, increased procollagen and messenger RNA synthesis by keloid fibroblasts correlates with increased collagen synthesis. Collagenase activity is also increased, but the rate of collagen synthesis exceeds the rate of degradation, with resultant net collagen deposition. Many growth factors, such as transforming growth factor β, epidermal growth factor, and platelet-derived growth factor, have been implicated in the pathogenesis of keloid scars, but other factors such as wound tension, chronic inflammation, and immune response also probably play a role. The precise mechanism at the cellular and molecular levels continues to be investigated.

TREATMENT

No consistently effective treatment for keloid scars exists. Prevention is best. Unnecessary procedures in susceptible persons should be avoided. Currently, the treatment of keloids can be divided into three types: nonsurgical treatment, surgical treatment, and combination treatment.

Nonsurgical Treatment

Corticosteroids

Intralesional corticosteroid injection is the most common treatment for keloids. The specific mechanism of action is unknown, but the clinical result is decreased collagen and inflammation. Used alone, intralesional corticosteroids provide effective relief of signs and symptoms, such as redness and pruritus, in most patients. The effect on size and appearance of the scars is variable. The technique is useful for the treatment of isolated earlobe keloids. The injections, using triamcinolone acetonide (Kenalog) in a 50:50 mixture with 1% lidocaine, are often quite painful. The dense composition of the keloid scar makes the injection difficult. Side effects including tissue atrophy and hypopigmentation can be minimized with careful injection within the scar to avoid extravasation of the solution into adjacent normal tissues. Systemic response is rare and can be avoided by timing injections at 4- to 6-week intervals.

Silicone Gel Sheeting

Silicone gel sheeting is a simple, painless, and easy treatment, with few side effects. It is especially useful in children, who often cannot tolerate the pain of steroid injections. The mechanism of action is unclear, but wound hydration, temperature, and occlusion may be important factors in its effectiveness. Most lesions demonstrate lessening of hardness, elevation, and itching with use of silicone gel sheeting. The sheeting is cut 1 to 2 cm larger than the involved area, and the dressing is applied directly to the scar and worn for 12 to 24 hours per day. This treatment continues for 3 to 6 months or until the desired change in appearance is achieved. From 80 to 85% of keloids treated with this modality will demonstrate significant improvement.

Interferon

Intralesional injection of interferon gamma-1b (Actimmune)* has been studied as a treatment for keloid scars. This lymphokine down-regulates collagen synthesis and theoretically can moderate the development of abnormal and excessive scars. The treatment is expensive, and the dosing regimens have yet to be standardized, but the results with limited trials are encouraging. Few local side effects have been demonstrated, but occasional systemic effects such as headache, muscle ache, and malaise have been reported at high doses. This promising new therapy continues to be investigated.

Surgical Treatment

Primary Excision

Surgical excision alone is complicated by recurrence rates of from 50 to 80%. Surgical excision as a primary treatment without adjuvant radiation, pressure, or steroids has a limited role. Strict adherence to gentle surgical technique, avoidance of wound tension, and limited usage of subcutaneous absorbable sutures helps to minimize the rate of recurrence. Carbon dioxide laser ablation creates less local tissue trauma and less bleeding than "sharp" surgical excision. However, no data suggest that this technique is more effective than standard excision.

*Not FDA approved for this indication.

Cryoablation

Cryosurgery with hand-held liquid nitrogen sprays is most effective on new keloids, i.e., less than 2 years old. Keloid scars are treated with two or three freeze-thaw cycles per session, and the treatments are repeated at 1-month intervals. Side effects include hypopigmentation and skin atrophy.

Combination Treatment

Surgery with Steroids

Many studies have demonstrated the effectiveness of intraoperative and postoperative intralesional corticosteroid injections for the treatment of recalcitrant keloids. Triamcinolone acetonide is injected into the wound prior to wound closure, followed by serial intralesional injections for up to 6 months postoperatively. Although effective, this protocol is not well tolerated by patients. As many as two thirds of patients will drop out owing to the inconvenience and pain of frequent follow-up injections. Recurrence rates range from 10 to 50% with this modality.

Surgery with Irradiation

The role of irradiation in the treatment of keloid scars is primarily as a postoperative adjuvant. Postoperative irradiation has been reported to be as successful in treating recurrent keloid scars as intralesional steroid injections. Radiotherapy is much better tolerated and requires fewer follow-up visits. A single postoperative dose of 1000 cGy has decreased the recurrence rate to 12.5%. Hyperpigmentation is seen in as many as two thirds of patients. There is a theoretical risk of malignancy, but the actual incidence of carcinogenesis in several large series is zero.

Surgery with Pressure

The use of pressure earring devices used following excision of earlobe keloids have been reported to be an effective treatment. Pressure earrings must be worn continuously for 6 to 12 months to be effective. Pressure therapy in other anatomic locations has not been as effective for preventing keloids.

SUMMARY

Currently, the best approach to the treatment of severe keloids uses surgical excision with steroid injections or low-dose radiation therapy. Combination therapy demonstrates better response rates and lower recurrence rates than with other treatment modalities alone, but no therapy is consistently effective. Results with use of agents such as interferon-γ that specifically target collagen synthesis are encouraging. As research clarifies the mechanisms of abnormal wound healing, new treatments will be investigated, and a cure for keloid scars may be discovered.

WARTS

method of
KARL R. BEUTNER, M.D., PH.D.
Solano Dermatology Associates and University of California, San Francisco
San Francisco, California

Warts are the most common clinical manifestation of infection with human papillomavirus (HPV). There are at least 100 genotypes of HPV, which have been further classified on the basis of the infection at different anatomic sites. In the immunocompetent host, when HPV infection is clinically noted, it is seen in the form of warts. The development of squamous cell carcinoma in warts is extremely rare in immunocompetent patients but is a frequent complication in immunosuppressed patients, particularly in sun-exposed skin. Warts can be classified on the basis of anatomic location or morphologic type. The two major morphologic types of common warts are verrucae vulgaris and flat warts. Verrucae vulgaris are keratotic papules. Warts are confined entirely to the epidermis. Wart thickness is determined by the thickness of the infected epidermis. Flat warts are slightly raised, flat-topped, papular lesions that are rarely more than a few millimeters in diameter. Warts can also be classified anatomically; the major classifications are periungual, plantar, and facial. Warts can be found on any cutaneous surface.

The differential diagnosis of verrucae vulgaris, or common warts, includes molluscum contagiosum, Gottron's papules of dermatomyositis, acrochordon, perforating granuloma annulare, acrokeratosis verruciformis, lichen nitidus, lichen planus, seborrheic keratosis, actinic keratosis, and squamous cell carcinoma. The differential diagnosis of a flat wart would include freckles, lichen planus, or appendigeal tumors. The differential diagnosis of plantar warts includes clavus (corn), acquired digital fibrokeratoma, callus, and foreign body. The diagnosis of warts is established predominantly by physical examination, but it can be histologically confirmed.

Warts appear to be most common in children. Patients with atopic dermatitis show a predilection to cutaneous infections, including viral warts. Individuals who do wet work or have hyperhidrosis have warts more frequently, which are also more extensive and difficult to treat. If the environmental conditions can be modified, treatment can be facilitated. In addition, warts that occur in areas that are shaved, such as the face of men and legs of women, tend to be spread by this hair removal process. Extensive cutaneous warts appear to be a complication of chronic immunosuppression. Warts on sun-exposed skin of immunosuppressed patients frequently become squamous cell carcinoma. What appears to be an inflamed wart in immunosuppressed patients may turn out to be a squamous cell carcinoma. About one half to two thirds of warts will resolve in immunocompetent patients within 1 to 2 years.

Reasons to treat warts, in addition to their cosmetic appearance, include that depending on their location, warts can be painful, are susceptible to trauma, can present mechanical problems, and are a source of infection to others.

Currently available treatments include surgery, cryosurgery, scissors excision, curettage, blunt dissection, electrosurgery, laser surgery, and infrared coagulation; trichloroacetic acid, bichloroacetic acid, and the keratolytic salicylic acid; and contact sensitization with dinitrochlorobenzene, diphencyprone, or squaric acid. The selection of treatment, in part, is dictated by the anatomic location of the warts, the number of warts, the previous treatment, the patient's preference, and the clinician's experience.

CRYOTHERAPY

Cryotherapy is most often performed with liquid nitrogen applied by the spray technique, with a large loosely wound piece of cotton on a wooden stick, or with a cryoprobe. Cryotherapy cannot be done effectively with a small, tightly wound cotton-tipped applicator, which simply cannot hold an adequate amount of liquid nitrogen to effectively freeze a wart.

Cryotherapy is moderately painful and highly dependent on the operator's experience. The extent of the freeze is determined by the thickness of the wart and the anatomic location. Inadequate freezing results in poor efficacy; excessive freezing results in greater pain, scarring, and, in rare instances, damage to nerves and nail beds. Clinicians should not undertake cryotherapy without proper training and/or supervision.

SURGERY

The surgical approach requires achieving local anesthesia. This is most commonly obtained with an injection of lidocaine. Once anesthesia is obtained, surgery should be painless with only mild pain in the postoperative period. Surgical approaches that can be used are scissors excision, curettage, blunt dissection, electrodesiccation, laser vaporization, or coagulation with an infrared coagulator. The blunt dissection is most commonly achieved with plantar warts. With the surgical approach, scarring may be more common, particularly on the hands and feet.

CAUSTIC AGENTS

Bichloroacetic acid has been used for sequential treatment of warts, particularly in the plantar areas. Availability of this treatment approach varies considerably.

KERATOLYTICS

Keratolytics, predominantly in the form of various salicylic acid preparations, have been a mainstay of home treatment of warts for decades. Unlike trichloroacetic acid or bichloroacetic acid, salicylic acid is not caustic. It appears to work by drawing water into the wart and allowing it to be easily pared away. The solid dosage form is 40% salicylic acid plasters. The liquid forms consist of various concentrations of salicylic acid in either acrylic or flexible collodion. Salicylic acid plasters for the treatment of plantar warts should be applied to the wart and a small area of surrounding tissue and held in place by a cloth type of adhesive tape. The plaster can be left on for 2 to 3 days. After removal, the area should be pared with a scalpel blade or with coarse sandpaper or a pumice stone. This process is continued until the wart is gone as indicated by the return of normal dermatoglyphics. This approach should never produce bleeding and should not result in pain. If either of these occurs, the patient should be instructed to stop therapy.

The liquid keratolytics are applied most commonly after the patient soaks the area in warm to hot water. The area is lightly dried, and the keratolytic is applied as film. This is repeated daily until the wart resolves.

MISCELLANEOUS TREATMENTS

A variety of treatments, such as topical 5-fluorouracil cream (Efudex),* tretinoin (Retin-A),* and tretinoin creams, have sometimes been used. The scientific basis for the use of these drugs is not clear.

CONTACT SENSITIZER

The current theory is that patients who are infected with HPV and do not develop warts, or patients who develop warts that resolve spontaneously, do so because the body makes an adequate immune response. The theory of immunotherapy for warts is the elicitation of low-grade delayed-type hypersensitivity reaction in the vicinity of the wart. This local immune response results in recruitment not just of cells specific to the contact sensitizer but of cells that are able to recognize a wide variety of epitopes. By stimulating this response, the hope is to accelerate the host's immunologic recognition of the wart infection. Common contact sensitizers that have been used for this include dinitrochlorobenzene and squaric acid. Unfortunately, no standardized preparations or protocols are available for these agents.

TREATMENT BY ANATOMIC SITE

Whereas a variety of factors influence the treatment of warts, anatomic site may be the major determinant.

Warts on the Face

Two major types of warts are seen on the face most commonly. The major therapeutic challenge of the face is the removal of the warts without significant scarring in the form of hypopigmented or hyperpigmented macules. Although there is little proof of its efficacy, topical tretinoin is frequently used for multiple flat warts on the face. Alternative treatment would include light electrocautery or cryotherapy. With cryotherapy or other surgical approaches to multiple warts, people with olive-skinned complexions or darker should be cautioned that they may have significant hyperpigmented or hypopigmented macules. For filiform warts on the face, particularly in men who shave, light cryotherapy is effective. These warts often have a base of less than 1 mm and when frozen properly will rarely result in significant scarring.

*Not FDA approved for this indication.

Warts on the Hands

Care should be taken with ablative and surgical modalities on warts on the proximal nail fold. Overaggressive treatment in this area can result in damage to the nail matrix and transient or permanent nail dystrophies. The current mainstay of treatment of warts on the hands is cryotherapy. The second line of therapy would be a surgical approach, but again caution patients about scarring.

Overaggressive surgical treatment on the hands can result in damage to the nerves that run along the lateral aspect of the digits.

Plantar Warts

Keratolytics in the form of salicylic acid plasters are ideal for the feet. Deep plantar warts sometimes can be anesthetized and bluntly dissected with little or no bleeding and good wound healing. The problem is that other ablative modalities result in pain; having a sore hand is one thing, but having a surgical site or wound on the foot can result in much more disability than the same procedure performed on the hand. For this reason, the use of a keratolytic is the preferred method. Salicylic acid plasters, when used properly, will alleviate this wart-related pain by softening the area and not producing additional therapeutically induced pain.

CONCLUSION

In the treatment of warts, patients should have reasonable expectations of therapies, and these would include induction of a wart-free period. Patients should be told prospectively that recurrences do happen. A treatment no worse than the disease is also desired. Patients should also be warned that ablative modalities in active wart infection can sometimes result in koebnerization of the warts or an increase in the number and size of warts. Sometimes in this case, the central area where the wart had originally been treated is clear and is surrounded by a rim of wart tissue referred to as a "doughnut" wart. Although warts are clearly transmitted from person to person, there is no clear interventional method available to prevent transmission to household or other social contacts.

CONDYLOMATA ACUMINATA

method of
LIBBY EDWARDS, M.D.
Carolinas Medical Center
Charlotte, North Carolina

Genital warts are benign tumors produced by a form of the human papillomavirus (HPV) that is usually sexually transmitted. Visible warts occur in about 1% of adults between the ages of 18 and 45 years. However, sensitive testing by the polymerase chain reaction technique shows evidence of HPV in up to 40% of sexually active people even when the skin appears normal.

Genital warts have varying appearances. Warts may be filiform with acuminate, keratotic tips. They may be lobular, resembling raspberries. Occasionally, genital warts are pedunculated and attached by a narrow stalk. At other times, genital warts are flat. In addition, genital warts tend to be grouped, and they may be skin colored, pink, or brown. When they occur on moist skin, the surface is often white. Warts that are flat or hyperpigmented are more likely than warts of other morphologic appearances to exhibit histologic dysplasia and carcinogenic HPV types.

TREATMENT

The management of warts requires sensitive and informative education so that patients can both resolve personal issues and become prepared for the often lengthy treatment process. First, patients should understand that there are currently no specific, effective antiviral agents for HPV. Therefore, eradication of warts is often difficult. Because the virus cannot be selectively destroyed, most wart therapies function by destroying the skin harboring the virus. This is generally painful, slow, and/or expensive. Second, warts can live in a latent form in the skin, so that recurrences soon after therapy are usual. Even after apparently effective treatment, warts sometimes recur months or years later, especially during illness or immunosuppression. Third, because of this latency, the apparent incubation period from exposure to the appearance of clinical warts can vary enormously, from weeks to years. This, as well as the nearly ubiquitous nature of subclinical HPV, makes contact tracing difficult or impossible. Because this is usually a sexually transmitted disease, warts can be passed from one partner to another. Therefore, avoidance of intercourse is the only sure way to prevent spreading genital warts.

Condoms can help minimize transmission, however, and those patients with a stable relationship have already exposed their partner. Also, the length of time required to eliminate clinical warts is so long as to make abstinence impractical for most people. Finally, elimination of the visible wart does not signify elimination of the virus, so that a (smaller) risk of transmission remains after therapy. However, patients need to understand that genital warts are usually a nuisance only and most often do not cause significant symptoms or produce important medical disease. Still, the presence of a sexually transmitted disease, especially a chronic one, often produces significant damage to self-esteem and to intimate relationships. Some HPV types are also carcinogenic, producing dysplasia within the warts of the external genitalia and, more important, predisposing the patient to invasive squamous cell carcinoma. This transformation occurs primarily on the areas where squamous epithelium and glandular epithelium meet, such as the cervix and anus.

A second important aspect of management of condylomata acuminata is an evaluation for vaginal and cervical involvement and, if perianal warts are present, for rectal disease. For most women with genital warts, yearly Papanicolaou (Pap) smears are adequate for the early detection of cervical dysplasia. Anoscopy for those patients with perianal disease is generally sufficient to evaluate for the presence of warts within the anal canal. However, patients with flat warts, and particularly those with pigmented flat warts, should be assessed especially carefully because this morphologic form is most often associated with those HPV types known to carry a higher risk for dysplasia and squamous cell carcinoma. A small skin biopsy of one of these warts can be performed, and if it shows changes of dysplasia, the patient (if female) or the female partner can be regarded as high risk for squamous cell carcinoma of the cervix. Any significantly abnormal Pap smear results should be evaluated more fully with colposcopy. Patients with external warts showing dysplasia on a biopsy specimen but having normal cervical Pap smear results should have Pap smears performed twice yearly.

Finally, the wart tumor should be eliminated when possible (Table 1). This is usually performed by chemical, physical, or surgical destruction. A comparison of the effectiveness of these methods is difficult, be-

TABLE 1. **Comparison of Current Therapies**

Therapy	Elimination Rates (%)	Recurrence Rates (%)	Advantages	Disadvantages
Podophyllin	22–80	30–60		Slow, sometimes erosive
Podofilox	45–88	35–60	Home use	Slow, somewhat irritating
Trichloroacetic acid, dichloroacetic acid	<80	30–60		Slow, irritating
Imiquimod	40–77	13	Home use	Slow, mildly irritating
Interferon	36–62	21–25	No erosions, no irritation	Slow, expensive, requires multiple injections
Cryotherapy	69–79	45	Faster than chemotherapy	Painful, occasional dyspigmentation
Excision	100	12	Fast	Painful, scarring
Hyfrecation	100	9	Fast	Painful, scarring
Laser	100	9–72	Fast	Painful, expensive

cause various studies are not comparable. Different end points, different numbers of applications of medication, and different follow-up periods produce widely varying results.

Podophyllin at a concentration of 20% in benzoin is a time-honored therapy that slowly eliminates many warts when it is applied once every 1 to 2 weeks in the office. This therapy has been largely replaced by the home application of podofilox (Condylox), a much milder, purified form of podophyllin. Podofilox is applied by the patient to the warts twice a day for 3 consecutive days each week until visible warts are eliminated. Other chemical modalities often used in an office setting include trichloroacetic acid and dichloroacetic acid preparations. These medications are most useful for flat warts. Trichloroacetic acid (Tri-Chlor) and dichloroacetic acid (Bichloracetic Acid) are reapplied as soon as erosions from the previous application have healed, usually every 2 to 4 weeks.

Fluorouracil cream 1% (Fluoroplex)* is a medication that is indicated for the removal of actinic keratoses, but it has been shown to be effective for the treatment of genital warts. It is applied once or twice daily to the warts until a brisk inflammatory response eliminates the visible wart. Erosion, exudation, and pain are usual. Unlike the other therapies, this medication is sometimes used in the vagina for internal warts. An applicatorful is inserted into the vagina once a week. This therapy is limited by the erosive vaginitis that can occur and by its teratogenic potential in a sexually active population that is generally of childbearing potential.

The application of liquid nitrogen is effective for the treatment of genital warts. This destructive therapy is faster than the application of chemicals, but it is generally more painful. Temporary white or dark areas on the skin can occur after healing, especially on the penile shaft.

The most common surgical therapies include hyfrecation (an electric needle), laser therapy, and snipping exophytic warts. The advantages include the elimination of all visible wart during one office visit, but the primary disadvantage is pain. Even these therapies are often followed by recurrence, because latent wart virus can be detected in normal surrounding skin.

A recent addition to the armamentarium of wart therapies is imiquimod 5% cream (Aldara), a topical interferon inducer. This agent does not remove warts by destruction of skin; rather, it provokes an immune response. Patients apply this medication to warts overnight three times a week, with the most common side effect being mild to moderate local irritation. In addition, preliminary data from clinical trials suggest that warts cleared by imiquimod may have a lower recurrence rate.

Recurrence is common with all of these therapies. The usual course of genital warts is recurrence and re-treatment until warts finally disappear when the virus is eliminated by the patient's immune response or the virus becomes latent.

*Not FDA approved for this indication.

NEVI

method of
VICTOR D. NEWCOMER, M.D.
Santa Monica, California

Nevi, or moles, are the most common tumors in humans and represent the single strongest risk factor for the development of melanomas. The greater the number of moles present, the greater the risk. Detailed knowledge regarding the appearance and behavior of nevi is important so that early changes that have the potential to progress to malignancy, as well as those pigmented lesions considered to be precursors of malignant melanoma, can be recognized for appropriate early treatment. Nevi can be separated into two groups, acquired and congenital.

ACQUIRED MELANOCYTIC NEVI

Acquired nevi (common moles) are categorized as junctional, intradermal, or compound nevi, depending upon whether the nests of nevus cells are located in the epidermis, dermis, or both areas. These nevi are not present at birth but begin to appear shortly thereafter. Peaks in appearance occur in young children 2 to 3 years of age and in older children 11 to 18 years of age; however, new lesions may appear at any age. Excessive sun exposure appears to stimulate their development. Pigmented nevi tend to disappear spontaneously with advancing age, and few can be found on individuals in their 80s. Caucasian adults normally have from 10 to 40 nevi, whereas African-Americans average only 2 to 8. The common distribution is to the head, neck, trunk, and upper and lower extremities and only rarely to the scalp, breasts, or buttocks. Nevi vary considerably in their appearance and may be flat, slightly elevated, verrucoid, polypoid, dome-shaped, sessile, or papillomatous. Their color ranges from black through all shades of brown to colorless. Individual nevi are normally of uniform color and round in shape, with a sharp, clear-cut border and a diameter of usually less than 5 mm.

Treatment

It is physically and economically impossible to remove all acquired melanocytic nevi. The vast majority are harmless and can be left alone if they have a benign gross appearance and stable growth pattern. Some of the reasons for removal of nevi include suspicion of melanoma, repeated infection, inflammation, irritation, cosmetic appearance, and patient anxiety. Whenever malignant melanoma is a possible diagnosis, complete excision is recommended for pathologic examination.

Clinically benign lesions may be removed by the scalpel shave technique, which removes the raised portion of the lesion, followed by desiccation of the base. However, if the nevus has a hairy component, it should be excised, because nevus cells located around the follicle tend to migrate to the skin surface, resulting in recurrence of the lesion. Removed tissue should always be sent for histologic examination. Destructive methods such as electrodesiccation, liquid nitrogen freezing, and acid or laser therapy do not yield a pathologic specimen and are not recommended.

A history of a pre-existing pigmented lesion at the site of a primary cutaneous melanoma may be elicited in 18 to 85% of patients. Therefore, it is extremely important to recognize the early changes suggestive of malignancy:

1. Disarray in the pattern of pigmentation (the most helpful feature in the early diagnosis of cutaneous melanoma); darkening of the lesion or color variation from one area to another with shades of tan, brown, or black, or areas of pink, red, or blue; blue, gray, red, or white coloration is not a typical feature of benign nevi
2. Appearance of a new pigmented lesion
3. Enlargement, either horizontally or vertically, of an existing pigmented lesion
4. Decrease in size and disappearance of a previously existing pigmented lesion
5. Development of an irregular, scalloped, or poorly circumscribed border
6. Persistent itching of a pigmented lesion
7. Development of crusting or bleeding in a pigmented lesion
8. Darkly pigmented lesions on the palms, soles, or mucous membranes
9. Pigmented streaks of the nail bed if enlarging and spreading onto the nail fold, which should receive immediate attention

Moles may change as the result of nonmalignant causes such as following sun exposure or with steroid therapy, puberty, or pregnancy. Under these conditions, all moles appear to be in phase with each other; however, early melanoma presents as a single changing mole.

The prevention and cure of malignant melanoma depend on early recognition and total excision of the lesion while it is still localized. Individual judgment is necessary to determine whether a given lesion should be removed. Until improved diagnostic techniques are available, it is better to be on the safe side and promptly perform an excisional biopsy of any lesion that has features suggestive of a melanoma. Although a complete excision is optimal for microscopic examination, incisional biopsy for cosmetically difficult locations will not adversely affect the prognosis even if the lesion is a melanoma.

Halo Nevus

The halo nevus is characterized by a pigmented lesion of any type, but usually compound or intradermal, and is surrounded by a zone of nonerythematous depigmentation. The lesion is seen most frequently on the backs of children and adolescents. No treatment is indicated, as the central nevus gradually disappears within several months and repigmentation eventually occurs over several months or years.

Epithelioid or Spindle Nevus

The epithelioid or spindle nevus (Spitz's nevus) is a variant of the compound nevus and is characterized by a raised, round papule that is usually reddish-brown in color. The spindle nevus generally appears as a rosy papule on the face during early childhood through the first 20 years of life. The lesion must be differentiated from pyogenic granuloma, juvenile xanthogranuloma, and even melanoma. Full excision is advisable for histologic confirmation.

PREDISPOSING FACTORS AND PIGMENTED LESIONS AT RISK FOR DEVELOPMENT OF MALIGNANT MELANOMA

Sun Exposure

Melanomas appear to preferentially affect individuals who have a light complexion, blue eyes, and blond or red hair (associated with a two- to fourfold increased risk) and those who freckle and sunburn easily and tan poorly. Individuals who develop relatively persistent erythema after acute ultraviolet radiation and those whose lifestyles involve periodic excessive exposure resulting in severe sunburn and blistering appear to be more vulnerable. For example, excessive sun exposure in the first 10 to 15 years of life may increase the risk of melanoma by threefold. Persons at risk should be advised to wear appropriate sun-protective clothing and sunscreens throughout the year, and sunbathing should be strongly discouraged.

The average person has approximately 30 nevi, the presence of which does not appear to increase the melanoma risk. The presence of more than 30 nevi or of atypical nevi increases the risk significantly. Individuals with 50 moles or more located solely on the arms and back have five times the increased risk of developing melanoma.

Dysplastic Nevus Syndrome

The dysplastic nevus serves as an indicator that identifies specific family members who are at increased risk for melanoma. These lesions occur in two settings, congenital and acquired. An increased risk for melanoma in the general population occurs in approximately 1 in 84 persons. Dysplastic nevus syndrome occurs as an autosomal dominant trait, and it is estimated that 50,000 individuals in the

United States have congenital dysplastic nevi. Familial dysplastic nevus syndrome accounts for 5% of all melanoma cases in the United States. In families whose members have dysplastic nevi and in which two or more first-degree members have malignant melanomas, the lifetime melanoma risk approaches 100%. As many as 4.6 million persons in the United States have one or more acquired dysplastic nevi, and even one such lesion is a significant risk factor, conferring a twofold increased risk for melanoma, while 10 or more lesions confer a 12-fold increased risk.

Clinical Features

Patients who have dysplastic nevi typically have dozens or even hundreds of lesions. The gross features of dysplastic nevus syndrome in children may not be significantly evolved enough to establish a diagnosis; however, the presence of scalp nevi and an increased number of normal nevi are early diagnostic clues. The lesions of the dysplastic nevus syndrome vary in their distinguishing features, exhibiting mixtures of colors such as tan, brown, black, red, and pink in a single mole. The borders are irregular and notched, and the color may fade gradually into the color of normal skin. Many are 5 to 10 mm or more in diameter. They are found not only on the sun-exposed areas but may also involve the buttocks and, in females, the breasts, which are areas rarely involved by commonly acquired melanocytic nevi. The only available method to confirm the clinical diagnosis of dysplastic nevus syndrome is biopsy of the entire lesion including a 2- to 3-mm margin of normal skin.

Treatment

The wholesale prophylactic removal of these nevi is not necessary, because the chance of any one lesion's becoming malignant is quite small, with the exception of hidden lesions such as those on the mucous membranes and the hair-bearing scalp. Nevi that develop blue-black color changes or changes in size, shape, sensation, consistency, or any other changes that raise the suspicion of a possible transformation to a malignant melanoma should be completely removed for histologic examination. Patients should undergo follow-up examination every 3 to 4 months and should be educated regarding the recognition of early signs of melanomas and the importance of examining their own skin. Patients with dysplastic nevus syndrome should undergo an ophthalmoscopic examination for possible ocular nevi. All bloodline members of melanoma-prone families should be encouraged to avoid excessive sun exposure, because sunlight may induce the development of dysplastic nevi and may cause them to become malignant melanomas.

Congenital Nevomelanocytic Nevus

Congenital nevomelanocytic nevi are pigmented lesions of the skin that are apparent at birth. They have arbitrarily been divided according to their largest diameter into small nevi, less than 1.5 cm in diameter; intermediate, 1.5 to 20 cm; and giant, 20 cm or greater. The lifetime melanoma risk with giant congenital nevi is estimated to be at least 6.3%; about half of the melanomas occur during the first 3 to 5 years of life, and 60% occur during the first decade of life. One-step excision of a very large congenital nevus should be considered as soon as the lesion is recognized, because the nonepidermal origin of this lesion in two thirds of the cases makes early recognition in a curable state difficult. Such definitive surgery, however, may not be possible owing to technical, cosmetic, and functional considerations.

Small congenital nevi are present in 1% of newborn infants in the United States. Some physicians believe that congenital nevi are not associated with an increased risk of melanoma, while others believe they carry a lifetime risk of 5%. Until the potential of these moles is better defined, it is best to take the safest approach and excise the lesion prior to puberty, because the incidence of malignant melanoma rises sharply after that age. Any atypical-appearing congenital nevi should be considered for immediate prophylactic excision.

Lentigo Maligna and Lentigo Maligna Melanoma

Lentigo maligna characteristically develops on sun-damaged skin of adults as a progressive, enlarging, pigmented, and irregularly-shaped macule. The average age at onset is 47 years. Lentigo maligna is important because of its developmental relationship with cutaneous melanoma, and particularly because these lesions are readily identifiable and usually curable if treated in an early phase of development. The median age at diagnosis of lentigo maligna melanoma is approximately 70 years. Lentigo maligna melanoma accounts for 4% of cutaneous melanomas, and it is estimated that the lifetime risk of melanoma for individuals with lentigo maligna may not exceed 5%. Surgical excision offers the most reliable method of removing a lentigo maligna, although advanced age or poor health may justify no therapy other than close observation.

Acral Lentiginous Nevi

Lentiginous nevi may appear as light or dark brown or black macules on the palms and soles, on the mucous membranes, at the mucocutaneous junctions, and as linear pigmented bands in the nails. Darkly pigmented lesions in these areas should be considered as potential precursors of melanoma. Pigmented nail plate bands are commonly observed in African-Americans and Native Americans but rarely in Caucasians. In any adult, however, the finding of widening pigmented nail plate bands or pigmented extension into the adjacent paronychial tissue necessitates removal of affected tissue for histologic examination.

Acral lentiginous and unclassified melanomas account for approximately 10% of all melanomas. In the United States, melanomas arising from these types of lesions are most frequently observed in African-Americans and Asians but may also occur in Caucasians. In the final analysis, whenever there is doubt in the physician's mind, it is appropriate to biopsy any suspicious lesion.

MALIGNANT MELANOMA

method of
FADI F. HADDAD, M.D., and
DOUGLAS S. REINTGEN, M.D.
H. Lee Moffitt Cancer Center
Tampa, Florida

Malignant melanoma is becoming more common. Its incidence is increasing rapidly and faster than any other human cancer. Although the risk of developing melanoma in 1935 was 1 in 1500 persons, this ratio has increased dramatically to be 1 in 125; it is projected that it will increase to 1 in 75 by the year 2000. The National Cancer Institute's Surveillance, Epidemiology and End Results (SEER) program estimated 41,600 new cases of invasive malignant melanoma and 21,000 new cases of melanoma in situ in the United States in 1998; it is also estimated that 7300 deaths will occur from melanoma in 1998. Although many causes for this drastic increase in incidence are yet to be elucidated, it is believed that an increase in sun exposure (i.e., ultraviolet B [UVB] irradiation) is in part responsible. No other major environmental factors have been identified as contributing substantially to the increase in incidence. Moreover, the genetically inherited susceptibility in a subpopulation of individuals may play a role in the etiology of familial melanoma. Of interest, the majority of melanomas currently seen have become thinner, less invasive, less frequently ulcerated, and subsequently more curable. An increase of extremity melanomas and a decrease of head and neck melanomas have been observed. No change in the incidence was noted for trunk tumors. Table 1 summarizes the risk factors for the development of malignant melanoma.

TABLE 1. **Risk Factors for the Development of Malignant Melanoma**

1. a. >120 nevi between 1 and 5 mm
   b. >5 nevi between 5 and 10 mm
   c. One atypical nevus
2. Freckling tendency
3. ≥3 atypical or dysplastic nevi > than 5 mm
4. History of severe blistering sunburn, 3 or more episodes (propensity to sunburn)
5. History of nonmelanocytic skin cancer
6. Time spent outdoors from the age of 10 to 24
7. Family history of melanoma
8. Individuals with a fair complexion and light skin
9. A changing mole
10. History of actinic lentigines
11. Previous personal history of melanoma

SIGNS AND SYMPTOMS

Melanoma can be located anywhere on the body, but it most commonly occurs on the lower extremities in women and the back in men. Although melanoma may have a variety of clinical appearances, the most common denominator is its changing nature; therefore any pigmented lesion that undergoes a change in size, configuration, or color should be considered suspicious for melanoma and should undergo biopsy. The ABCD paradigm is often used in the description of suspicious lesions; an *a*symmetrical lesion greater than 6 mm in *d*iameter with irregular *b*order and *c*olor variation is highly suggestive of melanoma.

GROWTH PATTERNS

A convenient way to categorize melanomas is by their growth patterns; these patterns are distinct pathologic entities with unique clinical features. Four major patterns are noted. *Superficial spreading melanoma* (SSM) constitutes the majority of melanomas (~70%). The lesions generally arise in pre-existing nevi. SSM can occur at any age after puberty. A typical SSM first appears as a deeply pigmented area in a brown junctional nevus. The second most common pattern is the *nodular* type (15 to 30%). Nodular melanomas (NMs) are more aggressive tumors and usually develop more rapidly than SSMs. They begin usually in uninvolved skin and occur mainly in middle-aged patients. They are more common over the face, neck, and trunk. Men tend to have more NMs than women, whereas the opposite is true for SSMs. *Lentigo maligna melanomas* (LMMs) constitute a small percentage of melanomas (4 to 10%) and are typically located on the face in older white women. They have a low potential for metastasis and rarely occur before the age of 50 years. Finally, the *acral lentiginous melanomas* (ALMs) characteristically occur on the palms or soles or beneath the nailbeds of elderly patients. ALMs occur in 2 to 8% of white patients but in 35 to 60% of dark-skinned patients, such as blacks, Asians, and Hispanics.

STAGING

Table 2 shows the American Joint Committee on Cancer (AJCC) melanoma staging system. The histologic depth (Clark's classification) and the tumor thickness (Breslow's classification) are used; when conflict arises between both systems, the least favorable indicator is retained. However, it has been shown that the total number of positive nodes is more significant and useful than the size of the nodal mass by physical examination or the size of the largest node by pathology. Hence, this staging system is currently being revised to include the prognostic factors that are better predictors of survival, namely the total number of positive lymph nodes, sex, ulceration of the primary, race, and anatomic location. Because lymph node status is the most powerful predictor of recurrence and survival, the detection of submicroscopic metastatic lymph node disease, using the reverse transcription and double round polymerase chain reaction (RT-PCR) to detect the presence of messenger RNA, may play a major role in staging patients. Data from the Moffit Cancer Center (MCC) show that patients whose tumor stage was increased with the RT-PCR assay had a worse outcome when compared with those whose nodes were histologic and RT-PCR negative. These findings will be tested in the Sunbelt Melanoma Trial (SMT), a national multicenter study.

TABLE 2. **American Joint Committee on Cancer 1988 Melanoma Staging System**

Primary Tumor	
Tx	Cannot be assessed
T0	No primary tumor identified
Tis	In situ melanoma, Clark I
T1	≤0.75 mm, Clark II
T2	0.76–1.5 mm, Clark III
T3	1.6–4.0 mm, Clark IV
T4	>4.0 mm, ± satellitosis, Clark V
Regional Nodes	
Nx	Cannot be assessed
N0	No regional node metastases
N1	Regional node metastases <3 cm in diameter
N2	Regional node metastases >3 cm in diameter and/or intransit metastases
Distant Metastases	
Mx	Cannot be assessed
M0	No distant metastases
M1	Distant metastases

Stage Grouping

Stage 0	Tis	N0	M0
Stage I	T1-2	N0	M0
Stage II	T3-4	N0	M0
Stage III	any T	N1-2	M0
Stage IV	any T	any N	M1

PROGNOSTIC FACTORS

The 10-year survival rates for patients with AJCC stages I, II, III, and IV are 85%, 60%, 30%, and 5%, respectively. However, the single most important prognostic factor in predicting survival in stages I and II is the thickness of the melanoma tumor. The thicker the tumor, the worse the prognosis. Similarly, the presence of ulceration was associated with poorer survival rate. Other factors analyzed by a multifactorial regression that emerged as important variables overall or within selected subgroups were sex, race, patient age, tumor diameter, level of invasion (Clark level), anatomic site, cell types, microscopic satellites, mitotic activities, and DNA content. Once the patient develops metastatic melanoma, prognostic factors based on the primary melanoma contribute little to the overall survival rate. Hence, as for most solid tumors, the most powerful predictor of survival and recurrence is the presence or absence of nodal metastasis. As previously discussed, the number of positive nodes plays a major role in the prognosis. The 3-year survival rates of patients with one positive node, two to four positive nodes, and five or more positive nodes were 40%, 26%, and 15%, respectively. Finally, the site of first relapse is an important prognostic variable. The median survival is 18 months for patients with skin, subcutaneous tissue, and regional node disease; 11 months for patients whose first relapse is confined to the lung; and 6 months for patients with brain, bone, or liver metastases.

DIAGNOSIS

Biopsies for melanomas can be either excisional or incisional. Whichever technique is used, full-thickness biopsy into the subcutaneous tissue must be performed to permit microstaging of the lesion (for thickness and level of invasion). Shave or curette biopsies are absolutely contraindicated for lesions suspected of being melanomas, because true tumor thickness cannot be ascertained with these biopsy techniques, which invariably give a positive deep margin.

An excisional biopsy is indicated for a suspicious lesion that is not large (i.e., < 1.5 cm in diameter) and is situated so that the amount of skin excised is not critical (e.g., on the trunk). The lesion should be excised with an elliptical incision, including a narrow margin (2 mm) of normal-appearing skin. The direction of the biopsy incision is important, as a biopsy that is not oriented properly may necessitate a skin graft when an elliptical incision and primary closure might have been possible. The biopsy incision should be oriented so that it can be re-excised with optimal skin margins and minimal skin loss if the lesion proves to be malignant. For extremity lesions, the recommendation is for orienting the biopsy axis in the same direction as the axis of the extremity. Punch biopsies may be performed if the entire lesion can be encompassed with the punch; the largest available punch biopsy is 6 mm. Care should be taken to perform this biopsy into the subcutaneous fat, so that the evaluation of tumor thickness is not compromised. Incisional biopsies should be performed when the amount of skin removed is critical (e.g., face, hands, or feet). They may also be indicated for large lesions, for which an excisional biopsy would be a formidable procedure. An incisional biopsy can be made with a scalpel, but usually a 6 mm punch biopsy is preferred to take a full-thickness core of skin and subcutaneous tissues from the most raised or irregular area of the lesion. The biopsy specimen should not be taken at the periphery of the lesion unless there are areas of raised nodularity at this location. No decrease in survival rates or increase in local recurrence rates has been observed with the incisional biopsy approach. Moreover, an incisional biopsy is a simple, expedient office procedure and, if taken properly, provides representative tissue for diagnosis.

TREATMENT

Management of the Primary Lesion

Local control of a primary melanoma requires wide local excision (WLE) of the tumor or biopsy site with a margin of normal-appearing skin. The reason for a WLE is that approximately 5% of primary melanomas have a satellite focus of melanoma separated from the main lesion. The risk of local recurrence correlates more with tumor thickness than with the margins of surgical excision. Therefore, it is recommended that the biopsy site of an in situ melanoma be excised, usually with a 0.5 to 1 cm margin of skin. For thin melanomas (< 1.00 mm thick), the standard of care is a 1.0 cm WLE. For intermediate thickness melanomas (1.0 mm to 4.0 mm), a 2.0-cm WLE is indicated. The risk of local recurrence may exceed 10 to 20% for those melanomas over 4 mm thick, and no study has addressed the proper WLE margin for thick melanomas. However, our practice is to achieve a 2-cm WLE on these lesions whenever technically feasible. The overall expected local recurrence rate after surgery is 4%.

The WLE is usually elliptical (the length is three times the width) and oriented along the lines of skin tension, to prevent the formation of "dog ears." We always attempt a primary closure of the defect; however, if this is not feasible, rotational flaps and split-thickness skin grafts are acceptable alternatives.

A melanoma located on the skin of a digit or beneath the fingernail must be removed by a digital amputation. A melanoma on the plantar surface often involves a sizable defect in a weight-bearing area. If possible, a portion of the heel or ball of the plantar surface should be retained to bear the greatest burden of pressure. Where possible, the deep fascia over the extensor tendons should be preserved as a base for the skin coverage. Free flap coverage may be indicated for the weight-bearing part of the foot. For a small suspicious lesion of the helix, the preferred initial procedure for diagnosis is excisional biopsy followed by a wedge re-excision if the diagnosis of melanoma is confirmed. A partial amputation may be necessary for larger lesions. A total amputation of the ear should be restricted to patients with widespread local disease or those with recurrence after partial amputation. Facial lesions usually cannot be excised with more than 1-cm margin because of adjacent vital structures. In these cases, the surgeon should use best judgment based on the width and thickness of the melanoma and its exact location on the face.

Elective Lymph Node Dissection (ELND)

Despite all the retrospective studies and prospective trials, a great deal of controversy persists as to the role of ELND. The results of the Intergroup Melanoma Surgical Trial showed no overall added benefit from ELND. However, on subset analysis, a small group of patients was identified that benefited from ELND. The group includes patients who are 60 years of age or younger and whose melanomas are 1.1 to 2 mm thick.

Lymphatic Mapping and Sentinel Lymph Node (SLN) Biopsy

Several studies have demonstrated an orderly progression of melanoma nodal metastases. Based on these findings, a new procedure has been developed to assess the status of the regional lymph nodes more accurately while decreasing the morbidity and expense to the health care system of a complete ELND. Morton initially proposed the "intraoperative lymphatic mapping and selective lymphadenectomy" technique consisting of a preoperative lymphoscintigraphy to identify basins at risk for disease, followed by intraoperative lymphatic mapping using a vital blue dye (Isosulfan Blue). With the addition of the intraoperative technetium-labeled sulfur colloid mapping, investigators at MCC were able to render this technique more reliable and more widely applicable. With lymphatic mapping, we are able to identify intransit areas of nodal collections, as well as all nodal basins at risk for metastatic melanoma, especially when the primary lesion involves watershed areas of the body such as the trunk or head and neck regions.

Several investigators showed that the histology of the first draining lymph node, known as the SLN, reflected the histologic status of the rest of the nodal basin. Once the SLN is harvested, a detailed examination is then performed using serial sectioning of the node, immunohistochemical (IHC) staining with specific monoclonal antibodies, and RT-PCR determination. The value of the latter is currently being evaluated by the Sunbelt Melanoma Trial. The status of the SLN can then be used as a prognostic factor to identify patients who require a complete node dissection. If the SLN is positive either by routine histology or IHC, a complete nodal dissection is warranted. However, if the SLN is negative, the patient is observed. Of interest, the rate of skip metastasis, defined as involvement of the nodal basin at a higher level while the SLN is negative, is low, approximately 0.5%.

Therapeutic Lymph Node Dissection

If a patient presents with clinically enlarged lymph nodes, a preoperative confirmation of metastatic disease is warranted. This can be achieved either through a fine-needle aspiration and cytologic examination or by an excisional biopsy. Once the diagnosis of regional disease is obtained, a complete basin nodal dissection is performed. The recommendation for the axilla is a level I, II, and III dissection; for the groin, a superficial inguinal dissection associated with iliac dissection only if either a positive Cloquet's node or four or more positive nodes are harvested; for cervical nodal metastasis, a modified radical neck dissection; and for parotid nodal disease, a superficial parotidectomy associated with either a suprahyoid neck dissection or a modified radical neck dissection. These same guidelines are used if an SLN harbors metastatic disease.

Local Recurrences

A local recurrence is defined as any tumor that occurs within 5 cm of the scar of a previously excised melanoma. They are distinct from satellites and in transit metastases that are intralymphatic in origin and occur between the primary tumor site and the regional lymph nodes. Risk factors for the development of local recurrences are the following: (1) a tumor 4 mm or greater in thickness, (2) the presence of ulceration, and (3) location over the foot, hand, scalp, or face. Of interest, the most common site for relapse is usually in the vicinity of the primary tumor site. This is usually a solitary soft tissue recurrence for which we would recommend a 2 cm wide excision only. Patients with local recurrent disease confined to one extremity, presenting either as multiple local recurrences (simultaneous or sequential) or a single local recurrence of a primary lesion that has poor prognostic factors (thickness >4 mm, ulceration), may be considered for hyperthermic isolated limb perfusion (ILP) using phenylalanine mustard (melphalan [Alkeran]) with or without recombinant tumor necrosis factor (rTNF-α). ILP with melphalan resulted in an approximately 50% complete response rate, compared with a 91% response rate with the combination. For patients with extremity lesions on whom ILP has failed or is not available, intra-arterial infusion of dacarbazine or cisplatin can be considered.

If local recurrent disease is too extensive for surgical excision and ILP is not an option, effective local control can be achieved with radiation therapy. Wide fields and the use of an electron beam of 6 to 9 MeV with an appropriate bolus to encourage skin sparing are recommended.

Intransit Metastasis

Intransit metastases are located between the primary melanoma and the first station regional nodal basin. They probably originate from melanoma cells trapped in lymphatic channels. Although they may occur in deeper lymphatics, intransit metastases are usually observed as either subcutaneous or intracutaneous metastases (i.e., satellitosis). The treatment for intransit metastases is not standardized. Surgery may be considered for one or a few lesions. Amputation of an extremity is rarely indicated, and then only when other treatments have failed and the patient is quite symptomatic with pain, bleeding, or odor. As in the case of multiple local recurrences, ILP is the treatment of choice for most patients with several intransit metastases involving extremity and no sign of systemic disease. For patients who are not candidates for ILP and have extensive disease, surgical resection with radiation therapy is used. Other treatment options in such a condition would be electroporation, intralesion injections of chemotherapy, laser vaporization, and intra-arterial injection of chemotherapy.

Distant Metastatic Disease

Melanoma can metastasize to almost every major organ and tissue. The majority of patients die with disseminated disease. The cause of death is often the result of a respiratory or brain complication. Solitary metastases or regional nodal disease should be surgically resected with the expectation of long-term survival and cure in approximately 5 to 10% of patients. Surgical excision of metastatic melanoma probably gives the patient the best and longest lasting palliation. In cases of solitary visceral metastases, we recommend 4 to 6 months of systemic therapy before surgery. This regimen allows one to assess the tumor response to treatment. If a partial or no response is obtained and the disease remains solitary, then surgical ablation is indicated.

Systemic chemotherapy for stage IV patients remains palliative. Patients with metastatic disease should generally be considered for enrollment in investigational studies. The best-studied single agents, dacarbazine and nitrosoureas, induce a 10 to 20% objective response. Several ongoing studies involving a combination of triple chemotherapy (carmustine, cyclophosphamide, cisplatin, melphalan, ifosfamide) induced a 50% overall response rate. This was accomplished at the expense of substantial toxicity, mortality, and absence of improvement in the fraction of patients with cure.

Biochemotherapy, a treatment modality that combines the use of triple chemotherapeutic agents along with interlukin-2 (IL-2) and IFN-α has been under extensive investigation. The early results have been promising, with response rates around 60% and durable complete response rate of 10%. A phase III comparative study of concurrent biochemotherapy versus triple chemotherapy treatment has been initiated to ascertain the superiority of the former.

ADJUVANT TREATMENT

Patients with nodal disease or tumors greater than 4 mm thick, who have no evidence of distant metastasis, represent a poor prognostic group; they are at a higher risk for relapse and adjuvant therapy should be considered. High-dose IFN-α-2b (Intron A) was found to prolong the relapse-free interval and overall survival in a prospective randomized trial. This treatment led to the increment in median disease-free survival from 1.0 to 1.7 years and overall survival from 2.8 to 3.8 years. It is associated with a 42% improvement in the fraction of patients who remain disease-free after the treatment. However, of note, the toxicity of this treatment was significant but yet tolerable by the majority of patients. On the other hand, chemotherapy has no role in an adjuvant setting. Radiation therapy may be administered in a clinical setting to patients with either extranodal extension of their disease or a melanoma with desmoplastic features, particularly in the head and neck areas. Several vaccines are being investigated, but randomized trials have not shown a survival benefit.

FOLLOW-UP

The evaluation of stage I and II patients includes a chest radiograph, complete blood profile, and a careful physical examination. Patients with resected stage III disease may require a computed tomography scan of the abdomen and pelvis to rule out distant metastasis. An extensive radiographic evaluation of patients with AJCC stage I, II, or III who are free of disease rarely reveals metastases. Hence, in the absence of symptoms, signs, or abnormal blood test results, no radiographic work-up is recommended.

PREMALIGNANT LESIONS

method of
LEONARD H. GOLDBERG, M.D.
Baylor College of Medicine
Houston, Texas

The commonly occurring cancers of the skin are basal cell carcinoma (BCC), squamous cell carcinoma (SCC), and malignant melanoma (MM). Less common cancers are dermatofibrosarcoma protuberans (DFSP), microcystic adnexal carcinoma (MAC), and Merkel cell carcinoma (MCC). In the following discussion, only premalignant lesions of the common cancers are included, as there are as yet no agreed-upon premalignant lesions for DFSP, MAC, or MCC.

The basis of the formation of the common skin cancers is the genetic makeup of the affected person, carcinogenic influences on the skin, and time. Sunlight is the most prevalent carcinogen, even though we do not understand the exact mechanisms or ultraviolet-wavelength dosages and incubation periods.

Patients with BCC or SCC invariably have evidence of the long-term influence of sunlight on the skin. This will be in the form of elastosis, wrinkles, freckles, yellowing or graying of the skin, telangiectasias and venous lakes, hyperpigmented and hypopigmented macules, and, eventually, actinic keratosis and skin cancer. On the hands and the arms the skin will be thinned, with exaggerated veins, a tendency to easy bleeding (ecchymosis) in the dermis, easy tearing, and multiple linear scars. These clinical features are always seen in sun-exposed skin but are absent in non–sun-exposed skin. When sun-exposed skin is examined under the microscope, the epidermis is seen to contain numerous microscopic actinic keratoses and can be considered in its entirety to be premalignant. The clinical premalignant lesion, the actinic keratosis, is a precursor for SCC and a marker of skin that is so badly sun-damaged that the formation of BCC and SCC is imminent. A patient who has developed a skin cancer is at increased risk for the development of another tumor, so that a skin cancer is also a marker for a severely damaged epidermis and the imminent development of other cancers. Patients with basal cell nevus syndrome do not have these skin changes, because they have a strong genetic predisposition for BCC. The main genetic predisposing factor in the development of skin cancer is poorly functional melanin, which is manifested as freckles, light-colored skin and eyes, red or blond hair, easy sunburning, and a family history of skin cancer. Poor repair of DNA-induced sun damage as found in xeroderma pigmentosum and in some individuals also predisposes to the development of skin cancer. Other carcinogenic influences are radiation therapy, chemotherapy, trauma to the skin, oral steroid therapy, and any diseases (such as lymphoma, leukemia, chronic viral infections, and connective tissue disease) that incur a perturbation of the immune system.

ACTINIC KERATOSIS

The clinically detectable actinic keratosis is a precursor for SCC and should be removed, but more important, its presence is a sign that the sun-exposed skin of the affected person contains numerous microscopic actinic keratoses and can be considered premalignant. Management should be directed at sun avoidance, removal of the individual actinic keratosis, and treatment of the entire sun-exposed skin area.

Individual actinic keratoses are most easily, quickly, and cost-effectively frozen with liquid nitrogen. This treatment method causes the least morbidity, is environmentally safe, and can also be used at the same time to freeze wider areas of adjacent skin (liquid nitrogen peel) and so prevent the formation of skin cancers in severely damaged epidermis. Other treatment methods widely employed are curettage and electrodesiccation, electrodesiccation, chemical destruction using topical application of 35% to 50% trichloroacetic acid (TCA), thin shave biopsy/excision, formal elliptical excision, and laser ablation with the carbon dioxide (CO_2) laser.

I do not use topical 5-fluorouracil (5-FU; Efudex) application by choice. The reasons for this are as follows:

1. Topical creams are active only to the depth of the epidermis in which they are absorbed. They are not effective in the dermis, and thus the premalignant actinic keratoses, which penetrate the dermis as basilar budding, are not effectively treated by topical 5-FU.
2. When topical 5-FU is used to treat a BCC or SCC, the superficial improvement obtained gives the impression of adequate treatment, while in fact the tumor continues to grow unabated in the dermis beneath an apparently healthy epidermis.
3. There is a category of usually male patients who, when given a tube of 5-FU to take home and use at their own discretion, will treat any skin lesion with the cream, including skin cancers, and thus delay the definitive treatment of these tumors, which have in the meantime grown to a considerable size. In these cases, adequate treatment is thus broad and complicated in scope and associated with much morbidity.
4. The morbidity associated with an adequate and successful course of 5-FU is considerable and often associated with numerous phone calls between the patient and the physician's office, and even numerous patient visits. Patients often do not like physicians who cause them undue morbidity.

I treat all actinic keratoses preferably with liquid nitrogen and examine the patient at regular follow-up visits to check for skin cancer and to treat new keratoses. I encourage patients who have had a BCC or SCC to consider a chemical peel, liquid nitrogen peel, or laser ablation to the sun-exposed skin of the head and neck as a means of prevention of skin cancer.

Hypertrophic Actinic Keratosis

Hypertrophic actinic keratosis is a thickened keratotic papule less than 1 cm in diameter usually found on the dorsum of the hands or the arms. On biopsy, 50% of these lesions can be found to have either SCC or BCC as a component; therefore, these lesions should be treated as early malignancies. I perform deep shave excision, with re-excision if there is visible tumor at the base of the biopsy specimen, and application of 35% TCA for 60 seconds with a cotton-tipped applicator. Then I freeze to 4 mm beyond the width of the papule and to the full thickness of the dermis in depth, being careful not to freeze the tendons on the hand.

Proliferative Actinic Keratosis

Proliferative actinic keratosis is an actively enlarging actinic keratosis that is resistant to standard treatments for actinic keratosis and is often found to have infiltration of the dermis leading to formation of SCC. Some think that this lesion is already a SCC and should be treated as such. Certainly, if it recurs after standard therapy, it should be biopsied and excised with frozen section control (Mohs' micrographic surgery).

Cutaneous Horn

The cutaneous horn is a distinctive clinical lesion that fits into the same category as for the hypertrophic actinic keratosis in that it has a malignant basis—usually SCC in 50% of the cases. I excise these lesions either by deep shave biopsy or by elliptical excision and closure. If the pathologic examination indicates inadequate excision, the lesion must be re-excised.

Sebaceous Nevus

It is said that 10% of persons with sebaceous nevi develop a BCC or SCC during their lifetime. My advice is to excise these congenital lesions at the convenience of the patient. If a change, especially a nodule or ulceration, develops within this lesion, it should be biopsied. If the biopsy specimen contains a BCC component, as much of the lesion should be excised as is cosmetically feasible.

Bowen's Disease

Bowen's disease (BD) is an SCC in situ and should be treated as a skin cancer. It is considered by some to be premalignant for SCC. In fact, it is already SCC while still in the pre-invasive stage. However, 50% of these lesions infiltrate down the hair follicles and the sweat ducts and will not respond to topical or superficial treatments. I excise these lesions with microscopic control.

Leukoplakia of the Lip

Leukoplakia of the lip is the mucosal equivalent of actinic keratosis. I treat the whole lip with liquid nitrogen initially and, if the lesion recurs, with CO_2 laser or excision of the sun-exposed mucosa and repair with a mucosal advancement flap from within the mouth.

Bowenoid Papulosis

Bowenoid papules are premalignant lesions of the genital regions and should be treated. Patients must be informed of the viral origin of these lesions (caused by human papillomavirus types 16, 18, and 31) and the possibility of transmission of the viral infection to sexual partners. Conservative first-line treatments include application of podophyllin, podofilox (Condylox), or TCA. Resistant lesions may be treated with liquid nitrogen, curettage and desiccation, or CO_2 laser ablation.

MALIGNANT MELANOMA

The increase in incidence and mortality from malignant melanoma (MM) continues unabated. Because melanoma is easily seen owing to its color and location on the skin, there is no reason why all tumors cannot seen early, biopsied, and excised before metastasis has occurred and the disease becomes fatal. The American Academy of Dermatology has instituted an annual "Skin Cancer Awareness Week" during which free skin cancer screening clinics are held and patient education materials are given out in an effort to educate the public about this unnecessarily fatal killer disease. The clinically stable premalignant lesions of MM are the clinically atypical mole (CAM) and the giant congenital nevus (GCN). However, the majority of melanomas occur on sun-damaged, otherwise normal-appearing skin, without a specific premalignant lesion.

Prevention and Early Diagnosis

The secret to a reduction in the incidence and mortality of MM lies in pubic education about sun avoidance and protection and safe sun habits and lifestyles. Fair-skinned people with light-colored eyes, blond or red hair, freckles, and a tendency to burn easily in the sun are prone to develop MM. These and other susceptible persons should be taught self-examination and should be examined monthly by spouses and as needed by physicians. Suspicious lesions must be biopsied and treated as early as possible.

Biopsy of Pigmented Lesions

It is so easy to safely biopsy pigmented lesions that there is no reason to incur risk by watching a lesion that is possibly a melanoma. A deep shave or punch biopsy is quick, easy, and safe. The pathologist's report rules out any doubt in the mind of the patient or the physician about the malignant nature or potential of the pigmented lesion.

Melanoma Families

Persons with a first-degree relative who has had MM are at risk for the development of MM. There is a strong genetic component in both animal species and humans in the predisposition to develop MM. All family members of patients with MM should be examined and then particularly well educated about the danger of developing MM. Thereafter they should be examined monthly by a spouse and by a physician when necessary.

Lentigo Maligna

Lentigo maligna is melanoma in situ, although it has no metastatic potential per se and is considered by some to be premalignant for MM. It is a destabilized lesion in the superficial lateral growth phase and inevitably invades the dermis as a MM. On careful serial sectioning, an area that has already invaded the dermis may be seen. Lentigo maligna is already a malignant lesion and should be treated as such by excision with frozen section control, Mohs' micrographic surgery, or excision with 5-mm margins of normal-appearing skin after examination with a Wood's light in the dark.

Giant Congenital Nevus

The diagnosis of giant congenital nevus is obvious because of the distinct clinical features of one or many pigmented, usually hairy plaques covering large areas of the body. The major considerations in the management of these cases is the cosmetic appearance and the potential to develop into MM. The lesions may be too large for excision or may be accompanied by other small and medium-sized pigmented nevi. These may penetrate the subcutaneous tissues or the muscle and, when present over the spine, may be associated with spina bifida and central nervous system lesions and pigmentation. The malignant potential of each giant congenital nevus is of the order of 5 to 10% over a lifetime, and MM may develop in childhood. Excision when possible is the treatment of choice; otherwise, careful observation with palpation at regular intervals is mandatory. Any localized change must be biopsied (excised) without delay.

Clinically Atypical Mole (Dysplastic Nevus)

The CAM, or dysplastic nevus, is the most common premalignant lesion and marker for MM. It is present in 5 to 10% of the population. A CAM is a larger-than-usual mole and has atypical features that suggest the diagnosis of MM (asymmetry, irregular, ill-defined or notched borders, variegated color, greater than 0.5 cm in diameter, and often an erythematous hue).

Although individual CAMs have a very low malignant potential, the malignant potential increases with the number of CAMs, their presence on non–sun-exposed areas, and a history of a previous MM, or of CAMs and MM in the family. The diagnosis of a CAM usually necessitates a biopsy to rule out the possibility that the lesion is a MM. When multiple CAMs are present, it is prudent to biopsy 3 or 4 of the most atypical-looking lesions. This process can be repeated at subsequent office visits. Patients with a family history of CAMs and MM need to be examined frequently for changing lesions that may represent early MM.

BACTERIAL DISEASES OF THE SKIN

method of
BRYAN D. HARRIS, M.D., and
KENNETH J. TOMECKI, M.D.
Cleveland Clinic Foundation
Cleveland, Ohio

IMPETIGO

Impetigo is a common contagious, superficial cutaneous infection that occurs mainly in children. The usual causative organism is *Staphylococcus aureus*, or occasionally *Streptococcus pyogenes*; or the infection may be due to a combination of staphylococcal and streptococcal species. Classically, non-bullous impetigo is characterized by erythematous papules and, later, vesicles or pustules, which may rupture to form adherent, honey-colored crusts, usually located on exposed areas of the face or extremities. Facial involvement is often periorificial. Impetigo is usually asymptomatic, but pruritus may occur. Some patients have tender regional lymphadenopathy, and leukocytosis is common. Predisposing factors include hot, humid environments, minor trauma, and poor hygiene. Bacterial cultures are generally unnecessary.

Bullous impetigo is a toxin-mediated disease caused by *S. aureus,* phage II, group 71; the bullous variant accounts for less than 30% of all cases of impetigo. The presence of vesicles or bullae on an erythematous base is the early sign of disease, although these lesions easily rupture, leaving a thin, brown, lacquer-like crust. Unlike in non-bullous impetigo, lymphadenopathy and leukocytosis are uncommon.

Cellulitis may be a complication of impetigo; less commonly, septic arthritis, osteomyelitis, and pneumonia may occur. Poststreptococcal glomerulonephritis may occur after impetigo, invariably with certain strains of *S. pyogenes,* after a latency of about 3 weeks. Treatment of impetigo may halt the progression of epidemics but does not alter the likelihood of glomerulonephritis. Rheumatic fever is not a sequela of impetigo.

Treatment

The use of topical antibiotics constitutes adequate and appropriate therapy in most patients. The agent of choice is mupirocin ointment (Bactroban), applied three times daily (tid) to affected areas for 10 days, which is just as effective as oral erythromycin for the treatment of localized disease. Adjunctive therapy should include the application of warm compresses, applied for 10 to 15 minutes tid or four times daily (qid), which helps to débride crusts. For extensive or resistant disease, oral antistaphylococcal antibiotics such as dicloxacillin may be necessary (Table 1). Since approximately 20% of staphylococcal strains are resistant to erythromycin, the use of penicillin alone is no longer efficacious, owing to drug resistance. Mupirocin nasal ointment (Bactroban Nasal), 0.5 gram to each nostril twice daily (bid) for 5 days, is effective treatment for both nasal carriage of *S. aureus,* which may promote flares of disease in some patients, and for household contacts who may be *Staphylococcus* carriers. Lesions of impetigo usually heal without scarring.

Bullous impetigo is usually self-limited, and treatment is the same as for non-bullous impetigo: antibiotic therapy aimed at staphylococci (see Table 1). Occasionally, severe, exfoliating bullous impetigo may require the administration of an intravenous β-lactamase–resistant penicillin such as oxacillin or nafcillin.

Treatment failures with systemic or topical antibiotics should suggest the possibility of antibiotic-resistant organisms. In such cases, results of bacterial culture and sensitivity testing may guide the selection of appropriate antimicrobials. Preventive measures include good hygiene, topical antibiotics (e.g., Polysporin ointment) for minor skin trauma, and the identification of asymptomatic *S. aureus* carriers, especially in outbreaks of impetigo in schools and day care settings.

TABLE 1. **Systemic Medications for Staphylococcal and Streptococcal Skin Infections***

Medication	Dosage (Adult)	Comments
Cephalexin (Keflex)	250 mg qid or 500 mg bid	For patients with penicillin allergy
Ciprofloxacin (Cipro)	500 mg bid	For patients with drug allergies or resistant disease
Dicloxacillin (Dynapen)	250 mg qid	Preferred initial agent for impetigo
Erythromycin	250 mg qid or 500 mg bid	For penicillin-allergic patients
Nafcillin (Nafcil, Unipen)	500 mg IV qid	For severe, life-threatening infections, followed by oral therapy (with clinical improvement)
Oxacillin (Bactocill, Prostaphlin)	500 mg IV qid	See nafcillin
Penicillin G	1.2 million units IM	Single monthly dose for recurrent cellulitis
Penicillin V	250 mg qid	One week per month for recurrent cellulitis
Vancomycin (Vancocin)	1 gm IV bid	For methicillin-resistant *Staphylococcus aureus*

*Duration of therapy is 7 to 10 days, unless noted otherwise.

ECTHYMA

Ecthyma resembles impetigo, but infection extends deeper, with shallow ulcerations that usually heal with scarring. Usually caused by strains of *Staphylococcus* or *Streptococcus* or both, ecthyma occurs most commonly on the legs and primarily affects children and the elderly. The skin exhibits pustules or vesicles, which progress to ulcerations, often with a "punched-out" appearance, with surrounding erythema and thick, adherent crusts. Ecthyma may mimic ecthyma gangrenosum, which follows *Pseudomonas* septicemia. Treatment for ecthyma is administration of systemic antibiotics effective against *Staphylococcus* and *Streptococcus,* which may be necessary for several weeks (see Table 1).

CELLULITIS/ERYSIPELAS

Cellulitis, an infection of the skin and subcutaneous soft tissues (but not muscle), is commonly caused by streptococci, usually group A organisms but also group G, C, and B organisms. Typically, a reddened, warm plaque with irregular, well-demarcated margins occurs, occasionally with vesicles and exudate. Cellulitis commonly occurs on the calf and resembles erysipelas, because both exhibit tender plaques with fever, lymphadenopathy, and leukocytosis. Predisposing factors for cellulitis include chronic lymphedema, eczema, trauma, stasis ulcerations, and tinea pedis. When caused by *S. aureus,* the cellulitic plaque is commonly more circumscribed, usually occurring in association with cutaneous abscesses or ulcerations. Facial cellulitis due to *Haemophilus influenzae* still occurs mainly in children but has become less common since the advent of the *H. influenzae* type b (HIB) conjugate vaccine. The agent of choice for *H. influenzae* cellulitis is a second-generation cephalosporin such as cefaclor (Ceclor), 20 mg per kg per day in divided doses, or amoxicillin-clavulate (Augmentin), 20 to 40 mg per kg per day for 7 to 10 days. Perianal cellulitis, with its persistent erythema and fissuring, occurs primarily in children; the infection is usually caused by group A streptococci, and administration of erythromycin, 20 to 30 mg per kg per day in divided doses for 7 to 10 days, is the treatment of choice. In diabetics, polymicrobial cellulitis, often with gram-negative organisms, or pneumococcal cellulitis may occur.

Needle aspiration for culture is unrewarding, yielding causative organisms in only about 10% of cases; tissue culture is helpful in only 20% of cases. An antistreptolysin O (ASO) titer and measurement of antiDNAse B titer are unnecessary.

Compared with cellulitis, erysipelas is a more superficial infection, with more sharply delineated erythema and edema. Classically, it occurs on the cheeks of the elderly, often accompanied by pain and itching. Erysipelas has therefore often been considered a facial disease, but most episodes actually involve the legs and feet.

Treatment

Elevation of the affected extremity and the use of cold compresses help to reduce tissue edema and symptoms of burning and pruritus. For mild to moderate disease, treatment is the administration of oral antibiotics directed against staphylococci and streptococci (see Table 1). For more severe disease, for erysipelas, and for patients with diabetes, administration of intravenous oxacillin or nafcillin for 2 to 3 days (see Table 1), followed by a 7- to 10-day course of oral antibiotics (see Table 1), is the treatment of choice. For diabetic patients and those with foot or leg ulcers, administration of ticarcillin-clavulanate (Timentin), 3.1 grams intravenously (IV) every 4 to 6 hours, is the empirical treatment of choice, followed by an aminoglycoside. If tinea pedis is present, treatment with a topical antifungal is also necessary.

During the first 2 days of therapy with antibiotics, patients often appear to worsen, with fever and increasing erythema, owing to the release of bacterial enzymes including streptokinase and DNAse.

For recurrent cellulitis, prophylactic intramuscular benzathine penicillin, 1.2 million units monthly, or penicillin or erythromycin given orally (PO) for 1 week each month may be necessary (see Table 1).

STAPHYLOCOCCAL SCALDED SKIN SYNDROME

Staphylococcal scalded skin syndrome (SSSS) is a toxin-mediated manifestation of infection with staphylococci (usually phage group II), typically occurring in infancy or early childhood. Acute fever, skin tenderness, and a scarlatiniform erythema are harbingers of SSSS. Flaccid bullae and erosions develop in 1 or 2 days, followed by desquamation, leading to a "scalded" appearance of the skin. Areas prone to mechanical stress are frequently denuded.

Treatment

Patients with SSSS should be hospitalized. Treatment should include fluid and electrolyte management and administration of nafcillin or methicillin, 100 mg per kg per day IV every 6 hours for several days, followed by dicloxacillin (Dynapen), 50 mg per kg daily for 10 days. For penicillin-allergic patients, the antimicrobial of choice is a cephalosporin such as cephalexin (Keflex), 25 to 50 mg per kg per day, given after a test dose, or clindamycin (Cleocin), 8 to 25 mg per kg per day.

Systemic antibiotics should be coupled with topical mupirocin ointment or silver sulfadiazine ointment, applied to denuded areas bid or tid. Medical personnel should maintain strict antiseptic techniques, including regular hand washing using antibacterial solutions. To minimize the likelihood of epidemics in the hospital or in daycare settings, *Staphylococcus* carriers must be identified and treated with dicloxacillin, 250 mg qid for 10 days.

NECROTIZING FASCIITIS

Necrotizing fasciitis (streptococcal gangrene) is an infection of subcutaneous tissues, including fascia, caused by group A streptococci ("flesh-eating bacteria"), although most cases are probably polymicrobial, including species of the family Enterobacteriaceae and *Bacteroides.* Young children, the elderly, and persons with underlying medical conditions such as diabetes and peripheral vascular disease are at increased risk for infection. Necrotizing fasciitis often follows minor cuts and burns, varicella, and trauma.

Affected patients initially develop diffuse swelling, usually of an extremity, which may progress to bullae, accompanied by fever and tenderness localized to the underlying muscle group. Without therapy, rapid evolution to frank necrosis or gangrene may occur, often followed by shock and multisystem organ failure. The mortality rate approaches 30 to 40%.

Differentiating cellulitis from necrotizing fasciitis may be difficult. Cellulitis usually responds to antibiotics; necrotizing fasciitis requires débridement. If the diagnosis is suspected, computed tomography (CT) or magnetic resonance imaging (MRI) may help to define the extent of disease but should not delay therapy. Deep incisional biopsies with frozen section pathology help to confirm the diagnosis. Measurements of muscle compartment pressures may also aid in the decision for surgical exploration and débridement.

Treatment

Surgical débridement of necrotic tissue is essential, coupled with administration of vancomycin, 500 mg IV every 6 hours, and clindamycin, 900 mg per day IV in divided doses for anaerobes. For type 1 infection (characterized by mixed bowel flora), an aminoglycoside such as gentamicin, 3 mg per kg per day IV in divided doses, should be given. For type 2 infection (due to *S. pyogenes*), penicillin G, 24 million units per day IV, and clindamycin, 900 mg per day IV for anaerobes, should be effective. Intravenous erythromycin with clindamycin may be an effective substitute regimen in type 2 infection. Adjuvant therapy with hyperbaric oxygen may be helpful.

FOLLICULITIS

Folliculitis is an inflammation of the epithelium of the hair follicle, secondary to follicular occlusion by keratin, overhydration, or bacterial or fungal inflammation. Most often due to *S. aureus* infection, folliculitis is characterized by small pustules at follicular orifices on the scalp, trunk, or extremities. A deeper folliculitis may occur in the bearded area of men (sycosis barbae).

Folliculitis unresponsive to antistaphylococcal therapy may represent infection due to gram-negative organisms, which may occur after chronic use of oral antibiotics for acne. *Klebsiella pneumoniae* and Enterobacteriaceae species are frequent causative organisms in gram-negative folliculitis.

Patients with human immunodeficiency virus (HIV) infection often develop eosinophilic folliculitis, a chronic, pruritic follicular dermatitis on the chest and face, characterized by edematous, urticarial follicular papules (rather than pustules). A biopsy helps to confirm the diagnosis. Use of topical corticosteroids such as clobetasol propionate (Temovate) is the treatment of choice for eosinophilic folliculitis, though therapy with ultraviolet (UV) light (UVB or psoralen plus UVA [PUVA]) or itraconazole may be helpful.

"Hot tub folliculitis" occurs in persons exposed to *Pseudomonas aeruginosa* in the warm, alkaline water of a hot tub or whirlpool. Pruritic erythematous papules and pustules develop on the buttocks, hips, and flanks and occasionally in the axillae, usually 6 hours to 5 days after exposure. Spontaneous resolution usually occurs within 3 to 5 days.

Treatment

For localized folliculitis, topical treatment with either 2% erythromycin solution or 1% clindamycin solution or gel (Cleocin T), applied twice daily, is effective, coupled with the use of an antibacterial soap or chlorhexidine (Hibiclens) wash.

For more extensive involvement, preferred treatment is administration of dicloxacillin, 250 mg qid, or erythromycin, 250 mg qid, for 10 days. For refractory disease and infection due to gram-negative organisms, results of bacterial cultures with drug sensitivity testing should direct treatment. Amoxicillin-clavulanate (Augmentin), 500 mg bid, or ciprofloxacin (Cipro), 500 mg bid, or trimethoprim-sulfamethoxazole (Bactrim DS), 1 tablet bid is often effective. Administration of trimethoprim-sulfamethoxazole, 1 tablet bid or ciprofloxacin, 500 mg bid, is the treatment for erythromycin- or methicillin-resistant disease. Some patients may benefit from a course of isotretinoin (Accutane), 1 mg per kg per day for 16 to 20 weeks, if all else fails.

Nasal carriage of staphylococci may be a factor in recurrent folliculitis; if such carriage is present, it merits treatment with mupirocin ointment, 0.5 gram to each nostril bid, for 5 days. Adjunctive treatment for folliculitis includes daily use of an antibacterial soap or chlorhexidine, wearing of loose-fitting cotton clothes, and application of astringent solutions such as aluminum chloride (Xerac AC).

FURUNCLES AND CARBUNCLES

A furuncle, or boil, is a cutaneous abscess, usually a result of *S. aureus* infection, that invades tissue more deeply than folliculitis. The typical lesion is an inflammatory nodule with an overlying pustule. Furuncles occur most often on the hairy areas of the legs, trunk, neck, buttocks, and face. A carbuncle, also usually caused by *S. aureus*, represents inflammation, with abscess formation, of more than one follicular unit. Carbuncles typically occur on the back of the neck, most often in diabetic patients. Other predisposing factors for carbuncle formation include chronic hemodialysis and intravenous drug abuse.

Treatment

Application of moist, warm compresses generally constitutes sufficient treatment for small furuncles. Larger furuncles and carbuncles may require incision and drainage, especially if they are fluctuant. Systemic antibiotics are generally unnecessary. For localized cellulitis, the treatment is administration of dicloxacillin, 250 to 500 mg qid, for 10 to 14 days. Adjunctive measures, especially for buttock involvement, include the use of loose, cotton clothing and absorbent powder (Zeasorb). Staphylococcal nasal carriage, if present, merits treatment with mupirocin ointment, 0.5 gram to each nostril bid, for 5 days. Recurrent staphylococcal furunculosis may indicate immunologic deficiency or phagocyte dysfunction.

PARONYCHIA

Paronychia is an infection of the proximal and lateral nail folds, characterized by erythema, edema, and tenderness. Acute paronychia, usually secondary to infection with *S. aureus,* group A streptococci, or *Pseudomonas*, may follow minor trauma to the nail fold. Chronic paronychia, characterized by edema and erythema and retraction of the proximal nail fold, is usually insidious in onset and often secondary to infection with *Candida.* Exacerbating factors include repeated hydration or dehydration and trauma. Chronic paronychia in the absence of wet work suggests diabetes.

Treatment

For acute paronychia, incision and drainage may be necessary, coupled with Gram stain, culture, and potassium hydroxide preparation of the fluid to identify the causative organisms. For bacterial paronychia, administration of dicloxacillin, 250 mg qid, or erythromycin, 500 mg bid, for 7 to 10 days is the treatment of choice. For candidal paronychia, usually associated with wet work, aeration and use of a topical antiyeast preparation such as clotrimazole 1% lotion (Lotrimin) bid usually constitute adequate treatment, coupled with avoidance of overhydration of the nail, use of cotton gloves inside any rubber gloves, and lubrication of the cuticle; for onycholysis, trimming the nail plate to the point of attachment is helpful. Adjunctive therapy includes painting the nail fold and surrounding nail plate with tincture of iodine or 3% thymol (mixed with equal parts of 70% isopropyl alcohol), once or twice a day.

VIRAL DISEASES OF THE SKIN

method of
ANGELA YEN MOORE, M.D., and
JESSICA L. SEVERSON, M.D.
University of Texas Medical Branch
Galveston, Texas

HUMAN HERPESVIRUS INFECTIONS

Infections Due to Herpes Simplex Virus Types 1 and 2

Etiology and Epidemiology

Herpes simplex viruses (HSVs) belong to the family Herpesviridae and the subfamily Alphaherpesvirinae. Herpes labialis and genital herpes are the two most common diseases caused by herpes simplex virus type 1 (HSV-1) and herpes simplex virus type 2 (HSV-2), respectively. HSV-1 seropositivity is greater than 85% worldwide, but only 20 to 40% of people infected with HSV-1 have a history of lesions. The prevalence of HSV-2 infection has increased by 30% since 1976. Between 1988 and 1994, 45 million people were estimated to be HSV-2–seropositive. This corresponds to 1 out of every 5 persons over the age of 12.

Pathogenesis

HSV is spread by direct contact with active lesions, saliva, semen, or cervical secretions, even in patients without active disease, in whom subclinical or asymptomatic viral shedding occurs. During a primary infection, the virus enters nerve endings underlying the lesion and ascends through peripheral nerves to the dorsal root ganglion, where it enters a latent stage lasting for days to years. Latent virus has been recovered from trigeminal, sacral, and vagal ganglia both ipsilateral and contralateral to the clinical lesion. Reactivation of latent infection occurs in the presence of humoral and cell-mediated immunity. Reactivation of the virus to descend through sensory nerve axons to the skin occurs spontaneously but may be triggered by physical or emotional stress, fever, exposure to ultraviolet light, skin damage such as chapping or abrasion, immune suppression, menses, or fatigue.

Clinical Manifestations

Most herpes simplex infections are subclinical. When present, however, classic HSV infection consists of a prodrome followed several days later by the development of erythema, papules, vesicles, ulcers or erosions, crusting, loss of crust, and then re-epithelialization. In the moist genital region, crusts may not form. Prodromal symptoms and signs include localized pain, tingling, burning, tenderness, mild paresthesias, lymphadenopathy, headache, generalized aching, and fever. About 25% of recurrences abort or fail to progress beyond a prodrome or a papule stage. Lesions typically heal within 7 to 10 days without scarring. Orolabial herpes is the most common manifestation of HSV infection. Primary infection with HSV can present as herpetic gingivostomatitis in children and young adults, although those affected are most commonly between the ages of 2 and 5 years. Sore throat and fever develop, as well as painful vesicles and ulcers on the tongue, palate, gingiva, buccal mucosa, and lips. First-episode primary genital herpes is defined as the first infection with HSV in a seronegative patient. First-episode nonprimary genital herpes is defined as the first symptomatic episode in a seropositive patient. These episodes are milder and shorter in duration than in primary genital herpes.

Although HSV infections are primarily oral or genital, the virus may infect any area of the body. Herpetic whitlow was common among health care workers when their fingers were exposed to patients' oral mucosa without glove protection. Herpes gladiatorum occurs in contact sports such as wrestling, when direct skin-to-skin contact occurs with an athlete with active skin lesions. Lumbosacral herpes is often misdiagnosed as shingles until recurrence becomes apparent from the patient's history. Herpetic sycosis of the beard area and folliculitis have been reported in which painful follicular vesicles are unresponsive to antibacterial or antifungal treatment. Eczema herpeticum is a widespread infection with HSV in a person with an underlying skin disorder such as atopic dermatitis. Erythema multiforme, classically presenting as erythematous papules that develop into target lesions and mucosal ulcerations, can appear with each recurrent episode of herpes. Herpes infections in immunocompromised patients are more severe, with HSV recurrences often resulting in chronic and nearly continuous ulcerations.

Neonatal herpes mostly results from intrapartum acquisition of HSV, which can lead to death or severe neurodevelopmental disability. The incidence of neonatal infection is 2 to 13.8 cases per 100,000 live births. Twenty-five percent of infants who contract herpes at delivery will develop disseminated herpetic infection, which has a 40% mortality rate despite antiviral therapy.

Diagnosis

Besides an adequate history and physical examination, multiple laboratory techniques may be used to diagnose HSV infection. Viral culture is the standard method of diagnosis. Positive culture results may be obtained using scrapings obtained from vesicular lesions for up to 5 days. Culture differentiates between HSV-1 and HSV-2 with high sensitivity. The Tzanck smear, which can be used to identify multinucleated giant cells in vesicular fluid, does not differentiate among HSV-1, HSV-2, and varicella-zoster virus (VZV) but is rapid and easily performed. On biopsy, ballooning or multinucleated keratinocytes are seen in the sample; sensitivity and specificity are similar to those of Tzanck smears. Fluorescent antibody staining (FAS) of vesicle base scrapings is 95% diagnostic in infection with HSV-1 and HSV-2. The indirect method is less specific than the direct because cross-reactivity with VZV is more difficult to identify. Enzyme-linked immunosorbent assay (ELISA) and complement fixation are readily available serologic techniques that detect circulating antibodies with 90% sensitivity and 50% specificity. Western blot, another serologic technique, distinguishes between HSV-1 and HSV-2 with high sensitivity and specificity (greater than 99%) but is not always available.

Treatment (Table 1)

Acyclovir was first approved in 1985, but owing to its low bioavailability (15 to 20%), intracellular half-life of only 1 hour, and necessity of frequent dosing (5 times per day), newer agents were developed. Valacyclovir is the L-valyl ester of acyclovir and has a bioavailability of 65%. Famciclovir is the oral prodrug of penciclovir. Famciclovir has a 77% bioavailability and an intracellular half-life of 10 to 20 hours in HSV-1/HSV-2–infected cells. Acyclovir and penciclovir are competitive inhibitors of viral DNA polymerase, acting to effect termination of viral replication. Acyclovir, valacyclovir, and famciclovir are extremely well tolerated. In fact, the side effect profiles match that of placebo. Headache, nausea, vomiting, and diarrhea are the most common complaints.

Oral acyclovir has shown efficacy in healing the lesions of herpes labialis, although use of topical acyclovir cream has yielded inconsistent results and further studies are being conducted. Topical penciclovir is currently the only FDA-approved antiviral for treatment of herpes labialis in immunocompetent persons. Lesions, pain, and viral shedding resolve more quickly, with the side effects being comparable to those with placebo.

In genital herpes, acyclovir, valacyclovir, or famciclovir therapy results in decreased duration of illness, pain, and viral shedding. Suppressive therapy reduces clinical outbreaks and asymptomatic viral shedding. Vaccines are currently being investigated for suppression of herpes simplex recurrences and prevention of HSV infection.

TABLE 1. **Antiviral Drugs**

Viral Disease	Drug	Dosage
Herpes Simplex Virus Infection		
Orolabial herpes	Penciclovir (Denavir)	1% cream applied q 2 h for 4 d
Genital herpes		
First episode	Acyclovir (Zovirax)	400 mg PO tid or 200 mg PO 5 times/d for 7 to 10 d
	Valacyclovir (Valtrex)	1 gm PO bid for 7 to 10 d
Recurrence	Acyclovir	400 mg PO tid for 5 d
	Valacyclovir	500 mg PO bid for 5 d
	Famciclovir (Famvir)	125 mg PO bid for 5 d
Chronic suppression	Acyclovir	400 mg PO bid
	Valacyclovir	500 mg PO bid
	Famciclovir	250 mg PO bid
Immunocompromised status	Acyclovir	5 mg/kg IV q 8 h for 7 to 14 d OR 400 mg PO 5 times/d for 7 to 14 d
Neonatal	Acyclovir	10 mg/kg IV q 8 h for 10 to 21 d
Varicella-Zoster Virus Infection		
Varicella	Acyclovir	20 mg/kg (800 mg maximum) PO qid for 5 d
Herpes zoster	Acyclovir	800 mg PO 5 times/d for 7 to 10 d
	Valacyclovir	1 gm PO tid for 7 d
	Famciclovir	500 mg PO tid for 7 d
Adult		
Immunocompromised status	Acyclovir	10 mg/kg IV q 8 h for 7 d
Pediatric		
Immunocompromised status	Acyclovir	500 mg/m² IV q 8 h for 7 to 10 d

Infection Due to Human Herpesvirus Type 3 (Varicella-Zoster Virus)

Etiology and Epidemiology

Varicella-zoster (VZV) is the third human herpes virus. It is the cause of varicella, more commonly known as chickenpox, and its reactivation results in zoster, also known as herpes zoster and shingles. Greater than 90% of the population has been infected with VZV. Twenty percent of those infected with VZV will develop shingles. Incidence and severity increase with age.

Pathogenesis

Initial infection with VZV is spread by respiratory droplets and contact with vesicular fluid. A person is considered contagious until the last vesical crusts. A person with zoster cannot infect another with zoster but can infect another with chickenpox if the susceptible individual comes into direct contact with vesicular fluid. Everyone infected with VZV has the potential to develop zoster. VZV, similar to HSV, has the capacity to invade and replicate in the central nervous system and establish latency in the dorsal root ganglion. The stimulus for reactivation is similar to that for HSV as well. Immunologic suppression and stress, both emotional and physical, are often linked to the development of zoster.

Clinical Manifestations

Chickenpox consists of a generalized exanthem of pruritic macules, papules, vesicles, and crusts occurring simultaneously. The lesions are located centrally and on the proximal extremities. A low-grade fever and malaise are typical. Secondary bacterial infection is the most common complication of varicella in children. In adults, pneumonia may develop, with a 10 to 30% mortality rate. Zoster patients often have prodromal symptoms of pain, numbness, tingling, and/or itching prior to the appearance of classic vesicles with an erythematous base. Pain can be severe enough to prompt such misdiagnoses as myocardial infarction or surgical abdomen. Pain is described as burning, aching, and/or lancing. The outbreak typically follows a unilateral dermatomal distribution. The outbreak is bilateral in 4% of patients, and recurrences in immunocompetent patients occur in 1 to 5% of cases, with 50% of these recurring in the same dermatome. Occasionally, cutaneous dissemination, defined as involvement of 20 or more vesicles outside primary or adjacent dermatomes, may occur. Other complications of zoster include postherpetic neuralgia (PHN), ophthalmic zoster, motor paralysis, secondary bacterial infection, pneumonitis, encephalitis, and hepatitis. PHN, which is pain after the rash resolves, increases with age, and the pain may continue for months or even years. Zoster has a 20% to 70% chance of involving the eye; ophthalmic zoster may cause problems ranging from conjunctivitis to blindness.

Diagnosis

The same diagnostic techniques used for HSV infection can be used for VZV infection, but often a careful history and physical examination are all that is needed. A history of recurrences is important, because shingles on the buttocks that keep coming back are caused by HSV until proven otherwise. This distinction affects treatment (i.e., dosage) and patient counseling regarding spread of the infection.

Prevention

Varicella virus vaccine (Varivax) was approved in the United States in March of 1995 and is recommended by the American Academy of Pediatrics for all children 12 months of age or older. One dose is recommended for children 12 months to 13 years of age, and two doses, with a 4- to 8-week interval, for those older than 13. In children, seroconversion after one dose of the Varivax vaccine occurs in 97% of cases, and it gives 95% protection against severe disease. Use of this live attenuated vaccine is contraindicated in immunocompromised persons, those with a family history of immunodeficiency, those with anaphylaxis to neomycin, and pregnant women. Side effects include injection site tenderness in 20 to 30% of patients, a transient rash in 5 to 10%, and, rarely, fever with a temperature of 102°F or greater. Studies are in progress to determine if a "booster" immunization 4 to 6 years after the primary vaccine is necessary. Also, the vaccine is being tested in older persons to boost their natural immunity to VZV and to prevent zoster.

Varicella-zoster immune globulin (VZIG) is recommended for passive immune prophylaxis of the immunocompromised patient if exposure to the virus occurs without previous varicella infection or vaccination. VZIG should also be considered in neonates whose mothers develop varicella 5 days before delivery until 2 days after delivery and in susceptible pregnant women exposed to VZV.

Treatment (Table 1)

Antiviral treatment for varicella is usually not necessary in healthy children, but acyclovir may be used in immunocompromised patients and adults. Early treatment is vital for shingles, however. By the time vesicles are seen on the skin, active replication of the virus is occurring. Acyclovir, valacyclovir, or famciclovir treatment results in decreased duration of pain and healing time of cutaneous lesions. Use of valacyclovir and famciclovir also decreases the duration and severity of PHN. Multiple treatments are available for PHN. Patients should be treated early with an antiviral to decrease the severity and duration of pain. Other treatment options for PHN include therapy with analgesics, narcotics, amitriptyline, or capsaicin and nerve blocks.

Infection Due to Human Herpesvirus Type 4 (Epstein-Barr Virus)

Human herpes virus 4 (HHV-4), or Epstein-Barr virus (EBV), is associated with such diseases as infectious mononucleosis (IM), African Burkitt's lymphoma, nasopharyngeal carcinoma, oral hairy leukoplakia in patients with acquired immune deficiency syndrome (AIDS), lymphoma and lymphoproliferative diseases in immunocompromised patients, and chronic fatigue syndrome. In IM, the virus is spread by saliva, giving it the name the "kissing disease." Clinical symptoms consist of a prodrome of headache, malaise, and fever for 3 to 5 days before the onset of a sore throat and posterior cervical lymphadenopathy. Other findings may include a gray-white exudative tonsillitis, red petechiae at the border of the hard and soft palate, splenomegaly, and hepatomegaly. An exanthem that is macular, maculopapular, morbilliform, urticarial, vesicular, petechial, or erythema multiforme–like develops on the trunk and upper extremities in 3 to 16% of patients. If patients have been given a penicillin derivative such as ampicillin for suspected bacterial pharyngitis, the likelihood of the rash is increased fivefold. The rash may last 1 week, followed by desquamation. Patients may tolerate ampicillin after the EBV infection has cleared. Initially, granulocytopenia occurs, followed in 1 week by a lymphocytic leukocytosis with atypical lymphocytes. A positive result on a Monospot test or increased titers of heterophil antibodies (greater than 1:112) may be detected by 4 weeks after onset of the illness. Ten percent of patients are heterophil-negative, and children under 4 years of age have a high false-positive rate, so EBV-specific antibodies are needed for a definitive diagnosis. Treatment is symptomatic.

Infection Due to Human Herpesvirus Type 5 (Cytomegalovirus)

Most people are infected with human herpes virus 5, or cytomegalovirus (CMV). It remains in a latent stage and is typically symptomatic only in neonates or immunocompromised persons. The virus is found in urine, tears, breast milk, feces, semen, cervical secretions, blood, and saliva. After initial reactivation, viremia occurs, followed by infection of the vascular endothelium, with an exanthem, vasculitis, and ulcerations. Relative sparing of epithelium occurs because the virus prefers endothelial and ductal cells. The presence of basophilic intranuclear inclusions, or "owl's eyes," is a pathognomonic finding on urine, blood, and throat cultures.

Congenital CMV is the major infectious cause of mental retardation and deafness in the United States. The term "blueberry muffin baby" used to describe affected infants refers to the purpuric macules and papules present. Immunocompromised patients may have multiple skin lesions as well as CMV retinitis, colitis, and esophagitis. Cidofovir (Vistide), foscarnet (Foscavir), and ganciclovir (Cytovene) are approved for treatment of CMV infections.

Infection Due to Human Herpesvirus Type 6

Human herpesvirus type 6 (HHV-6) infection is also called exanthem subitum, roseola infantum, and sixth disease. HHV-6 causes a mild, self-limited disease, usually occurring in children 6 months to 2 years of age. High fever for 3 to 5 days is followed by the appearance of 2- to 3-mm discrete rose-pink macules or maculopapules that blanch and may be tender. The trunk is affected first, followed by the neck and extremities. Treatment is symptomatic.

Infection Due to Human Herpesvirus Type 7

Human herpesvirus type 7 (HHV-7) was isolated in 1990. Primary infection occurs during childhood, but its association with human disease has not been definitive. Some cases of roseola infantum have been linked to HHV-7. In addition, HHV-7 DNA has been found in patients with pityriasis rosea during an outbreak but not after recovery or in controls.

Infection Due to Human Herpesvirus Type 8

The eighth human herpesvirus (HHV-8) is postulated to be a latent virus that is associated with the occurrence of Kaposi's sarcoma (KS) lesions during immunosuppressed states. HHV-8 DNA has also been found in patients with carcinomas, lymphomas, pemphigus vulgaris, and pemphigus foliaceus.

HUMAN PARVOVIRUS B19 INFECTION

A benign childhood exanthem, erythema infectiosum or fifth disease is caused by a single-stranded DNA virus, parvovirus B19, in the family Parvoviridae. The virus is transmitted through respiratory secretions, with infection occurring mainly in 4- to 15-year-olds. The peak incidence is in the spring and winter. Headache, chills, and mild constitutional symptoms are followed 7 days later by a "slapped-cheek" appearance, manifested as a bright red rash on the cheeks with circumoral pallor. At 1 to 4 days later, an erythematous maculopapular rash with a lacelike reticular pattern may be seen on the proximal extremities. Treatment is symptomatic.

INFECTIONS DUE TO POXVIRUSES

Molluscum contagiosum virus is a DNA virus of the poxvirus family. It affects children, sexually active adults, and immunocompromised persons. It is mostly a benign, asymptomatic disease but can be troublesome in 5 to 18% of cases of human immunodeficiency virus (HIV) infection. The virus is spread by direct person-to-person contact as well as by fomites. Molluscum contagiosum manifests as dome-shaped papules with an umbilicated center, which can be found anywhere on the body. Curdlike material from the papules can be extracted, stained, and observed under the microscope; the presence of Henderson-Patterson bodies—large intracytoplasmic inclusion bodies—aids in the clinical diagnosis. Multiple treatments are available, including tretinoin,* cantharidin, excision, curettage, electrodessication, oral griseofulvin,* topical fluorouracil,* acyclovir ointment,* carbolfuchsin, cryotherapy, cimetidine,* topical mupirocin,* oral isotretinoin,* intralesional interferon,* 30% trichloroacetic acid peel, topical and systemic psoralens with UVA, and electron irradiation. Topical and intravenous therapy with cidofovir,* which has broad-spectrum antiviral DNA activity, has resulted in significant improvement in HIV-infected patients. Further studies are being conducted.

Orf, or ecthyma contagiosum, is a zoonotic infection endemic in sheep and goats. Infection causes nodules on the mouth and nose of animals and can spread to humans. The virus is quite hardy, living on fomites for extended periods of time. In humans, the infection typically involves the right index finger with single to multiple 1.5- to 5.0-cm papules or nodules. The infection heals slowly in about 35 days after proceeding through papule, target, regenerative, papillomatous, and finally regression stages. Diagnosis is by history and physical examination. Treatment is symptomatic.

Milker's nodule is a zoonotic infection that is endemic among cows, in which it is termed pseudocowpox. When transmitted to humans, it causes macules on the finger, hand, or forearm, which progress to papules and then to targetoid papulovesicles that erode and crust. The lesions are asymptomatic and heal in approximately 4 weeks. Again, diagnosis is by history and physical examination, and treatment is symptomatic.

COXSACKIEVIRUS INFECTIONS

Hand-foot-and-mouth disease (HFMD) is associated with several coxsackieviruses, especially A16, in

*Not FDA approved for this indication.

the family Picornaviridae. The infection is spread by the oral or fecal-oral route. A prodrome of malaise, low-grade fever, anorexia, abdominal pain, or respiratory symptoms is followed by the appearance of painful oral lesions. Red macules progress to 1- to 3-mm to 2-cm vesicles with an erythematous base. Soon thereafter, shallow yellow-gray ulcerations surrounded by a red halo develop on the hard palate, tongue, and buccal mucosa. On the extremities, an exanthem of macules and papules develops into gray vesicles with an erythematous base. Healing occurs in about 1 week. Diagnosis is by physical examination, and treatment is symptomatic.

PARASITIC DISEASES OF THE SKIN

method of
AMY D. KLION, M.D.
National Institutes of Health
Bethesda, Maryland

Involvement of the skin and soft tissues is a common feature of many parasitic diseases. Although most parasitic infections are geographically restricted to tropical regions of the world, recent increases in international travel, immigration, and immunosuppressive disorders have led to an upsurge in the number of cases of parasitic infection being seen by primary care physicians in more temperate regions, including the United States. Since dermatologic manifestations appear relatively early in the course of many parasitic infections, recognition of characteristic cutaneous lesions may provide the earliest clue to the correct diagnosis and appropriate therapy. Table 1 summarizes the cutaneous manifestations of parasitic infections.

PROTOZOAN INFECTIONS

Amebiasis

Skin involvement in *Entamoeba histolytica* infection (amebiasis cutis) is a rare consequence of direct contact with the organisms (from feces or abscesses or other cutaneous lesions). The characteristic lesion is a painful, solitary, irregularly shaped ulceration with a purulent exudate located in the perineal area or on the abdomen. Organisms can be demonstrated by direct microscopic examination of the ulcer base. Therapy is with metronidazole (Flagyl and others), 750 mg orally (PO) three times a day for 10 days, followed by a luminal agent such as iodoquinol, i.e., diiodohydroxyquinoline (Yodoxin), 650 mg orally three times daily for 20 days, to eradicate the intestinal source.

Leishmaniasis

Transmitted by the bite of an infected sandfly, *Leishmania* infections are an important cause of chronic nonhealing skin ulcers in many areas of the world, including portions of Asia, Africa, the Middle East, and Latin America. Other cutaneous manifestations of leishmaniasis include erythematous plaques, most commonly seen on the ear at the site of a previous scar (chiclero ulcers); erythematous papules (lupoid leishmaniasis); diffuse nodularity of the skin (disseminated cutaneous disease); and destructive lesions of the oral, nasal, or pharyngeal tissues (mucocutaneous leishmaniasis). Diagnosis is usually made by culture or visualization of the organism in smears from a skin biopsy specimen.

Although many cutaneous lesions resolve spontaneously or in response to local therapy (heat, cryotherapy, or topical paromomycin, i.e., aminosidine [Humatin]), systemic therapy with intravenous pentavalent antimony, i.e., sodium stibogluconate (Pentostam),* at a dose of 20 mg per kg intravenously or intramuscularly per day for 20 days, should be considered for potentially disfiguring lesions and is essential in *Leishmania brasiliense* infection because of the risk of subsequent destructive mucocutaneous disease. Intravenous administration of amphotericin B (Fungizone) may be necessary for refractory lesions.

Trypanosomiasis

In as many as 50% of patients with African trypanosomiasis (sleeping sickness), the earliest sign of infection is a painful erythematous nodule, 2 to 5 cm in size, surrounded by a white halo, at the site of a tsetse fly bite. The nodule, or trypanosomal chancre, generally appears within 5 to 15 days of the bite and may persist for several weeks. The appearance of an evanescent macular rash with central clearing on the trunk, thighs, and shoulders after fever of 1 to 7 days' duration is another common cutaneous manifestation of infection and may occur weeks *(Trypanosoma brucei rhodesiense)* to months *(Trypanosoma brucei gambiense)* after exposure.

Because the stage of infection is an important determinant of the response to therapy in trypanosomiasis, recognition of these early cutaneous manifestations in a patient with an appropriate travel history is essential. Central nervous system (CNS) involvement and death are inevitable in untreated infection. For *T. b. gambiense* infection, eflornithine, i.e., difluoromethylornithine (Ornidyl),† at a dose of 400 mg per kg per day intravenously (IV) in four divided doses for 14 days followed by 300 mg per kg per day PO for 3 to 4 weeks is effective in both early and late disease. Alternatively, suramin sodium* (a 100- to 200-mg test dose followed by 1 gram IV on days 1, 3, 7, 14, and 21) can be used to treat either *T. b. gambiense* or *T. b. rhodesiense* infection if CNS penetration has not occurred. For *T. b. rhodesiense* infection

*Available from the CDC Drug Service, Centers for Disease Control and Prevention, Atlanta, GA (404) 639-3670.

†Available only from the World Health Organization, Geneva, Switzerland.

TABLE 1. **Dermatologic Manifestations of Parasitic Disease**

Class	Organism	Geographic Distribution	Dermatologic Manifestations	Treatment*
Protozoa	*Entamoeba histolytica*	Worldwide	Amebiasis cutis	Metronidazole (Flagyl), 750 mg q 8 h PO for 10 d, followed by iodoquinol
	Leishmania spp.	Africa, Asia, the Middle East, Central and South America	Cutaneous leishmaniasis	Observation, local measures, or pentavalent antimony (Pentostam),† 20 mg Sb/kg/d IV for 20 d
	Trypanosoma cruzi	Central and South America	Chagas' disease (Romaña's sign, chagoma)	Nifurtimox (Lampit),† 8–10 mg/kg/d in 4 doses for 120 d
	Trypanosoma brucei rhodesiense and *T. b. gambiense*	Africa	Trypanosomal chancre (acute), macular rash (subacute)	Eflornithine,‡ suramin,† or melarsoprol,† depending on stage of infection and species
Helminths	Animal hookworm spp.	Worldwide	Cutaneous larva migrans	Ivermectin, 200 μg/kg PO (Stromectol)
	Dracunculus medinensis	Asia, Africa, and the Middle East	Guinea worm	Surgical removal ± metronidazole, 250 mg PO bid for 10 d
	Loa loa	West and Central Africa	Calabar swellings	Diethylcarbamazine‡ (Hetrazan), 8 mg/kg/d for 21 d
	Onchocerca volvulus	Africa, Central and South America	Onchodermatitis	Ivermectin, 150 μg/kg PO yearly
	Schistosoma spp.	Africa, Asia, the Middle East, South America, and the Caribbean	Cercarial dermatitis (swimmer's itch)	Praziquantel (Biltricide), 20 mg/kg PO bid or tid on 1 day, depending on species
	Strongyloides stercoralis	Worldwide	Larva currens, urticaria	Ivermectin 200 μg/kg PO
	Wuchereria bancrofti and *Brugia* spp.	Asia, Africa, South America, and the Caribbean	Lymphatic filariasis	Diethylcarbamazine,‡ 6 mg/kg/d PO for 6–12 d
Ectoparasites	*Diptera* larvae/*Tunga penetrans*	Worldwide	Myiasis/tungiasis	Surgical removal
	Pediculus humanus and *Phthirus pubis*	Worldwide	Head, body, and pubic lice	1% permethrin (Nix Creme Rinse) applied for 10 min, repeated in 1 wk
	Sarcoptes scabiei	Worldwide	Scabies	5% permethrin cream (Elimite) or ivermectin, 200 μg/kg PO

*Refer to text for details and alternate regimens.
†Available in the United States only from the Centers for Disease Control and Prevention, Atlanta, GA.
‡Available in the United States only from the manufacturer.

with CNS involvement, melarsoprol (Arsobal),* a highly toxic derivative of arsenic, is the only available therapy.

Inflammation at the site of initial infection also occurs in American trypanosomiasis (Chagas' disease) but is clinically inapparent in a majority of cases. When present, Romaña's sign (unilateral lacrimal sac inflammation, conjunctivitis, and eyelid edema) or the development of a chagoma (an indurated erythematous subcutaneous nodule) is characteristic. Diagnosis is confirmed by the demonstration of *Trypanosoma cruzi* trypomastigotes in the blood. If the condition is untreated, the acute symptoms resolve, but chronic disease, including cardiomyopathy and gastrointestinal involvement, may develop years later. Nifurtimox (Lampit),* 8 to 10 mg per kg per day in four divided doses for 120 days, is the therapy of choice for acute Chagas' disease and may prevent the development of antibodies and chronic disease in some patients. There is no effective therapy once chronic infection is established.

*Available from the CDC Drug Service, Centers for Disease Control and Prevention, Atlanta, GA (404) 639-3670.

HELMINTHIC INFECTIONS

Cutaneous Larva Migrans

Cutaneous larva migrans is a reactive dermatitis produced by the migration of a variety of animal hookworms (most commonly dog or cat hookworm) in human skin. Infections are most common in regions with warmer climates, beaches, and sandy soil, including the southeastern United States. Presence of the extremely pruritic, painful, erythematous, serpiginous tracts is pathognomonic, and biopsy is generally not indicated for diagnosis. Use of single-dose ivermectin (Stromectol), 200 μg per kg PO, or albendazole (Albenza), 200 mg PO twice a day for 3 days, has been the best-studied therapy and appears to be effective, although neither of these has been approved by the Food and Drug Administration (FDA) for this purpose.

Dracunculiasis (Guinea Worm Infection)

The emergence of an adult worm through a vesicular lesion in the skin of the lower extremity is characteristic of infection with *Dracunculus medinensis* (or guinea worm). The commonly used method of slowly winding the exposed worm onto a stick is inexpensive but time-consuming and may result in intense local inflammation or anaphylaxis if the worm is accidentally ruptured. Administration of metronidazole, 250 mg PO three times daily for 10 days, decreases inflammation and facilitates worm removal.

Filariasis

Dermatologic manifestations are a major component of filarial infection in humans. In onchocerciasis (river blindness), pruritic dermatitis and subcutaneous nodules are characteristic, and microfilariae may be demonstrable in skin snips. Therapy with ivermectin at a dose of 150 μg per kg PO given every 6 or 12 months is effective against the microfilarial stage of the parasite and helps to control the progression of disease and prevent blindness. Since adult worms are unaffected by ivermectin and have a lifespan of up to 15 years, prolonged therapy is necessary.

Migratory angioedema (or Calabar swellings) and/or subconjunctival migration of adult worms are the hallmark of infection with *Loa loa*. Treatment with diethylcarbamazine (DEC) (Hetrazan),* 8 mg per kg PO per day in three divided doses for 21 days, rapidly kills the blood-borne microfilariae and is also effective against adult worms, although several courses of therapy may be necessary.

Lymphatic filariasis is characterized by a range of cutaneous manifestations including nonpitting lymphedema, lymphangitis, and elephantiasis. The recommended treatment for lymphatic filariasis is high-dose therapy with DEC, 6 mg per kg per day in three divided doses for 12 days in infection due to *Wuchereria bancrofti* or for 6 days in *Brugia malayi* infection. Potential alternative regimens for asymptomatic microfilarial carriers include yearly ivermectin (400 μg per kg),† ivermectin and DEC (6 mg per kg), and albendazole and DEC, although large comparative studies are lacking. For symptomatic patients, intensive local hygiene and prompt treatment of bacterial or fungal superinfection of edematous limbs should be instituted as well.

Schistosomiasis

Penetration of schistosomes into the epidermis provokes a local hypersensitivity response (cercarial dermatitis or swimmer's itch) consisting of intensely pruritic erythematous papules that last 5 to 7 days. The cutaneous manifestations are worse with repeated exposure to nonhuman schistosome species, which undergo arrested development in the human. Recommended therapy for infection with any of the human schistosome species is administration of praziquantel (Biltricide), 20 mg per kg PO for two (*Schistosoma mansoni* and *Schistosoma haematobium*) or three (*Schistosoma japonicum* and *Schistosoma mekongi*) doses in a single day. Infection with the nonhuman species is self-limited and requires no therapy.

*Available in the United States only from Wyeth-Ayerst, Philadelphia, PA.

†Exceeds dosage recommended by the manufacturer.

Strongyloidiasis

Strongyloides stercoralis is a common cause of intestinal infection, with 50 to 100 million people affected worldwide. Most prevalent in the tropics and subtropics, strongyloidiasis is also endemic in the southeastern United States. Infection occurs when larvae penetrate the skin of the host from fecally contaminated soil. Larvae shed intermittently in the stool may also penetrate the skin of the host and provoke a transient linear or serpiginous urticarial rash, most commonly seen on the buttocks, thighs, or perineum. This form of infection is called larva currens because of the rapid rate of migration of the larvae (up to 15 cm per hour). Intermittent maculopapular or urticarial rashes frequently occur in patients with chronic strongyloidiasis, and rashes may persist for years if untreated because of the autoinfective cycle. In immunocompromised patients, dissemination of infection, known as the hyperinfection syndrome, may occur. Ivermectin in a single oral dose of 200 μg per kg has replaced thiabendazole (Mintezol) as the drug of choice for strongyloidiasis, owing to its increased efficacy and lower incidence of side effects. Albendazole* has also been used in chronic infection with good results.

ECTOPARASITIC INFECTION

Worldwide in their distribution, ectoparasites (parasites that live on or in the skin) are an important cause of cutaneous disease in humans.

Scabies

More than 300 million people worldwide are infected with *Sarcoptes scabiei* (scabies). Although transmission is most common during intimate personal contact, live mites have been recovered from bed linens, furniture, and other fomites for up to 36 hours, and epidemics do occur, particularly in institutional settings.

Infected persons typically complain of intense pruritus, worse at night. The characteristic dermatologic findings are erythematous papules and elevated linear scabies burrows in the interdigital web spaces, wrists, ankles, axillae, and periumbilical and genital areas. Vesicles may also be present, especially in children. In some cases, excoriations and/or second-

*Not FDA approved for this indication.

ary bacterial infection may be the predominant clinical findings. Norwegian (crusted) scabies is a clinical variant that is most common in immunosuppressed or debilitated persons, including patients with AIDS, and presents as thick-crusted hyperkeratotic plaques full of mites. Patients with this form of infection are highly contagious and should be isolated. Secondary bacterial infection is common and may lead to fatal septicemia.

Microscopic examination of skin scrapings is usually adequate to demonstrate the mites, confirming the diagnosis of scabies. The recommended therapy for adults and children older than 2 months of age is topical application of permethrin 5% cream (Elimite) to all skin surfaces from chin to toes. The cream should be washed off after 8 to 10 hours. In Norwegian scabies, multiple applications are usually necessary. Administration of ivermectin,* 200 μg per kg PO in a single dose, is an effective alternative therapy but has not been FDA-approved for this purpose. Scabies in children under 2 months of age and in pregnant women can be treated with 6 to 10% precipitated sulfur in petrolatum applied daily for 3 days. This therapy should also be used in all household members and close contacts. Regardless of the mode of therapy, nails should be trimmed and all clothing and bed linens used during the 3 days preceding therapy washed in hot water and dried in the hot cycle of the dryer. Itching may persist for several weeks after successful therapy owing to persisting mite antigens. Topical steroids, calamine lotion, and antihistamines generally provide symptomatic relief.

Pediculosis

Head lice *(Pediculus humanus capitis)* are transmitted by close personal contact or the sharing of hats, combs, or hair brushes. Head lice infect persons from all socioeconomic backgrounds, and infections may occur in epidemics. The predominant symptom is intense pruritus of the scalp, and excoriation may lead to secondary bacterial infection. Adult lice may be difficult to see, but nits (eggs firmly attached to hair shafts) are readily apparent. Application of 1% permethrin (Nix Creme Rinse) for 10 minutes, repeated at 1 week, constitutes effective and nontoxic therapy. Nits should be removed with a fine-toothed comb dipped in vinegar. Antihistamines and topical corticosteroids may be useful for symptomatic treatment of pruritus.

Body lice *(Pediculus humanus corporis)* are associated with conditions of overcrowding and poor sanitation and may transmit rickettsial diseases. Cutaneous findings include pruritic, erythematous macules and papules primarily on the trunk. Long-standing infection can lead to hyperpigmentation and lichenification. Since the lice infest the seams of clothing and bedding rather than the skin, patients with body lice do not need specific treatment. Clothing and other contaminated items should be discarded or laundered at high temperature and ironed to eliminate the lice.

*Not FDA approved for this indication.

Although pubic lice *(Phthirus pubis)* are usually confined to the pubic hair, the eyelashes, axillary or truncal hair, and, rarely, the scalp may be affected. Since transmission is predominantly through sexual contact, patients with pubic lice should be evaluated for other sexually transmitted diseases. Intense pruritus and an erythematous maculopapular rash are typical. Small blue-gray macules (maculae ceruleae) may also be present on the trunk, thighs, and upper arms. Therapy is identical to that used for pediculosis capitis, except when the eyelids are involved. Eyelid infestation should be treated with a thick layer of petrolatum applied twice a day for 8 days.

Myiasis/Tungiasis

Myiasis, penetration of the skin by larvae of Diptera (two-winged flies), is most common in the tropics and subtropics, although cases have been reported from more temperate regions. When fly eggs are deposited on the skin, the larvae hatch and burrow into the adjacent tissue. Serpiginous lesions similar to those of cutaneous larva migrans may be seen at this stage. As the larva grows, an erythematous pruritic papule with a central punctum develops and becomes indurated and painful. Lesions may become secondarily infected. Therapy is generally surgical, although occluding the central opening with petroleum jelly may cause the larva to emerge to avoid suffocation.

The flea *Tunga penetrans* may cause dermatologic manifestations very similar to the furuncular lesions of myiasis when the female flea burrows into the skin during egglaying. Distinguishing features include the location of lesions (usually on the feet) and presence of a central black dot corresponding to the posterior abdomen of the flea. Treatment is generally surgical, although niridazole (Ambilhar)* has been used in severe infections.

*Not available in the United States.

FUNGAL DISEASES OF THE SKIN

method of
JOHN THORNE CRISSEY, M.D.
University of Southern California School of Medicine
Los Angeles, California

USEFUL ANTIFUNGAL AGENTS: AN OVERVIEW

Topical Antifungals

Older antifungal topicals—Whitfield's ointment, sulfur preparations, and the like—have largely been supplanted by azole and allylamine creams (Table 1). All appear to be effective against cutaneous dermato-

TABLE 1. **Modern Topical Antifungals**

Azoles
Ketoconazole (Nizoral)
Clotrimazole (Lotrimin)
Econazole nitrate (Spectazole)
Oxiconazole nitrate (Oxistat)
Sulconazole nitrate (Exelderm)
Miconazole nitrate (Micatin)
Allylamines
Naftifine hydrochloride (Naftin)
Terbinafine (Lamisil)

phyte infections, and I have no preferences among them. Selection is dictated by formularies of various treatment facilities more often than not. For cutaneous candidosis, clotrimazole cream (Lotrimin) is a good choice.

Systemic Antifungals

Griseofulvin, for many years the sole systemic medication available for the treatment of dermatophyte infections, has been joined now by azole and allylamine antifungals, which have superseded the older drug in many clinical situations. The systemic azoles I prefer are itraconazole (Sporanox) and fluconazole (Diflucan). The allylamine I prescribe is terbinafine (Lamisil).

Itraconazole is a relatively safe antifungal, but it has been involved in a significant number of dangerous drug interactions. Co-administration of itraconazole with terfenadine, astemizole, cisapride, triazolam, or midazolam is contraindicated.

Because the systemic azoles and allylamines are relatively new and under continued evaluation, practitioners are advised to consult the latest information available on drug interactions and untoward effects before prescribing them.

DERMATOPHYTE INFECTIONS

Tinea Pedis and Tinea Manus

Acute vesiculobullous forms respond well to saline or Burow's solution compresses. Large bullae are best incised. The use of topical azole or allylamine creams applied twice daily will shorten the course. Secondary staphylococcal and streptococcal infections, which are common, should be treated promptly with appropriate antibiotics.

Chronic forms respond to topical azole or allylamine creams applied twice daily. For refractory cases, griseofulvin (microsize) (Grifulvin V) by mouth is indicated. A single daily dose of 500 mg for 4 to 8 weeks produces satisfactory results.

Recurrences can be minimized by foot care designed to reduce sweating and maceration. The wearing of cotton socks or openwork footwear and the use of drying powders such as Zeasorb-AF are helpful measures.

Tinea manus, which often occurs in association with tinea pedis, is resistant to topical treatment. The condition usually responds to a single daily dose of griseofulvin, 500 mg by mouth, for 4 to 8 weeks.

Tinea Unguium (Dermatophytic Onychomycosis)

Management is similar for all clinical forms of dermatophytic nail infections. Treatment should not be started until the presence of the fungus in the nail or nail bed has been confirmed by potassium hydroxide (KOH) examination or culture. Topical treatment is futile. Results with griseofulvin by mouth have been disappointing, but response to newer antifungals has been excellent. Itraconazole (Sporanox) and terbinafine (Lamisil) are the agents of choice. The following dosage schedules are recommended for itraconazole: for toenail infection with or without fingernail involvement, 200 mg (two capsules) by mouth (PO) daily for 12 consecutive weeks; for fingernail infections only, two treatment pulses, each consisting of 200 mg (two capsules) PO twice daily for 1 week. Pulses should be separated by 3 weeks with no itraconazole. Itraconazole should be taken with a full meal. *The possibility of drug interactions, as described previously, must be considered in prescribing this medication.*

Terbinafine in tablet form is an effective alternative. The recommended dosage schedule for fingernail infections is 250 mg (one tablet) daily by mouth for 6 weeks; for toenail infections, 250 mg daily for 12 weeks. Pulsed dosage is equally effective: 500 mg by mouth once daily for the first 7 days of each month for 3 months. Compliance rates are higher with the pulsed regimen.

Tinea Corporis (Ringworm)

Whether caused by contact with infected animals or associated with tinea capitis or tinea cruris, tinea corporis responds well to thrice-daily application of topical azole or allylamine cream. Unusually extensive eruptions or bizarre presentations may indicate concomitant disease, particularly diabetes mellitus.

Tinea Capitis

"Gray patch" tinea capitis (TC), contracted from infected animals (usually kittens), and "black dot" TC, a person-to-person contagious infection restricted to humans, continue to occur with regularity in the United States. Both clinical forms are readily manageable, but treatment should not be started until the presence of the fungus in or on the hair shaft has been confirmed by KOH examination or culture.

Griseofulvin (microsize) remains the medication of choice for both types of TC. An effective adult dose in my experience is 250 mg twice daily for 6 to 12 weeks. Some cases, especially black dot infections, require 250 mg three times a day. The dose for children is 5 mg per pound of body weight for the same length of time. When ultra-microsize griseofulvin (Grisactin Ultra) is used, doses can be reduced by about 30%. Itraconazole and terbinafine are effective alternatives but are not yet approved for this purpose in the United States.

A successful management strategy for gray patch TC includes treatment or removal of infected animal contacts. In black dot cases, a search for human carrier contacts is essential, along with elimination of fomites such as shared combs, brushes, and hair rollers.

CANDIDAL INFECTIONS

Among the localized forms of candidosis, perlèche, erosio interdigitalis blastomycetica, candidal intertrigo (adult and infantile), balanitis, and pruritus ani respond well to topical antifungals. Clotrimazole cream (Lotrimin) is the agent I routinely prescribe. Candidal vulvovaginitis also responds to topical clotrimazole preparations (vaginal creams or tablets), but the treatment is messy. Most women prefer systemic treatment; a single oral dose of fluconazole (Diflucan), 150 mg, will usually suffice.

Topical antifungal agents by themselves are ineffective in the treatment of candidal paronychia, onychia, and onycholysis, pseudomembranous candidosis (thrush), and candidal esophagitis. For these conditions I prescribe fluconazole, 200 mg PO on the first day, followed by 100 mg daily for at least 2 weeks. When thrush and esophagitis are associated with acquired immune deficiency syndrome (AIDS), as they often are, treatment may need to be continued indefinitely.

Candida infections are enhanced or caused by conditions producing maceration or debilitation, such as intercurrent disease (particularly diabetes mellitus), immune defects, pregnancy, immersion in water, the presence of indwelling catheters, vascular stasis, obesity, and the like. Prolonged regimens of antibacterial antibiotics may also result in candidosis. Successful treatment depends on the elimination or amelioration of as many of these factors as possible.

PITYRIASIS VERSICOLOR (TINEA VERSICOLOR)

Pityriasis versicolor (PV) responds well to topical treatment. Topical azoles (Nizoral cream, Exelderm, many others) are effective. Ciclopirox cream (Loprox) and selenium sulfide lotion (Selsun, Exsel) are also useful. The selenium preparations are less expensive than other topicals, but the unpleasant odor that accompanies their use often results in noncompliance, and agents containing selenium are contraindicated in pregnancy. Topical treatments for PV should be continued for 2 to 3 weeks. Results can be improved by extending the applications well beyond the visible areas of involvement.

Recurrences are common. The disease also responds readily to short courses of oral itraconazole and fluconazole. These medications have not been approved for the treatment of PV, and I do not personally prescribe them for this purpose. Griseofulvin is ineffective.

DISEASES OF THE MOUTH

method of
CATHERINE M. FLAITZ, D.D.S., M.S.
University of Texas Health Science Center at Houston
Houston, Texas

Categorizing oral diseases according to their primary clinical appearance is a practical method for determining a reasonable differential diagnosis and management approach. In the following discussion, selected symptomatic conditions and the most common premalignant and malignant diseases are divided into the following groups: white, white and red, red, and ulcerative lesions. Because many diseases have more than one clinical presentation, the lesions are described under their classic appearance.

WHITE LESIONS

Frictional Keratosis

The lesion of frictional keratosis is an asymptomatic white plaque with a rough, adherent surface, caused by persistent low-grade irritation. When it presents as a white scalloped line along the occlusal plane of the buccal mucosa it is referred to as *linea alba.* Chronic cheek and tongue chewing is a common habit that gives the mucosal surface a shaggy appearance. Other common causes include trauma from sharp tooth surfaces, dental appliances, and masticatory function. Typically, the most common sites of involvement are the buccal and labial mucosa, lateral tongue, and alveolar ridge. This lesion is reversible when the source of the irritation is removed or the habit is discontinued. Frictional keratosis is not a precancerous condition; however, it is important to differentiate this lesion from leukoplakia.

Smokeless Tobacco Keratosis

The habit of chewing or holding cut tobacco in the vestibule of the mouth results in formation of an adherent white patch with a corrugated, thickened surface. This lesion is termed smokeless tobacco keratosis. Other oral manifestations of smokeless tobacco use include gingival recession, extrinsic staining of the teeth, and halitosis. A low-grade malignancy, verrucous carcinoma, is specifically associated with this carcinogenic habit, but the overall risk of transformation is less than 1% over a lifetime. Discontinuing the habit results in reversal of the condition after 2 weeks. If a white patch persists, then a biopsy is indicated.

Nicotine Stomatitis

The lesion of nicotine stomatitis is a white keratotic patch of the hard palate associated with long-term tobacco use, especially with cigar and pipe smoking. Nicotine stomatitis appears to develop more in response to the heat that is generated than as a reaction to the tobacco product. Typically, the hard palate becomes white and wrinkled, with numerous papules containing punctate red centers. These papules represent inflamed minor salivary glands. This lesion is reversible with discontinuation of the habit, and malignant transformation is rare. At times this entity may appear erythematous and must be differentiated from the denture-induced lesion papillary hyperplasia or erythroplakia.

Hairy Leukoplakia

Hairy leukoplakia manifests as white vertical streaks or plaques with a shaggy surface that does not rub off. The most common site of involvement is the lateral border of the tongue, usually with a bilateral distribution. Hairy leukoplakia is a marker for immunosuppression, in particular, human immunodeficiency virus (HIV) infection, but has been noted in immunocompetent persons. The Epstein-Barr virus is associated with this entity, and there is frequently a superimposed candidal infection. Although no treatment is necessary, tenderness, dysgeusia, and cosmetic concern may justify therapy. The use of systemic acyclovir,* 2000 to 4000 mg per day is effective, but the lesions recur when the drug is discontinued. Topical management with 1 or 2 applications of 25% podophyllum* resin, 1 week apart, is effective, but the bad taste is not well tolerated. This lesion is not precancerous and tends to wax and wane over time. Many tongue diseases mimic hairy leukoplakia, such as frictional keratosis, lichen planus, leukoplakia, hyperplastic candidiasis, and benign migratory glossitis.

Hairy Tongue

Diffuse elongation of the filiform papillae results in a tan to black matted coating on the dorsal surface of the tongue with hairlike projections. Predisposing factors associated with hairy tongue include tobacco use, antibiotics, oxidizing mouth rinses, poor oral hygiene, xerostomia, and overgrowth of fungal and bacterial organisms. Dysgeusia, halitosis, and cosmetic concerns are common complaints. Treatment usually involves brushing the tongue, increasing the amount of moisture in the mouth, and eliminating the contributing factors, if possible.

Leukoplakia

Leukoplakia is the most common oral precancer, with a malignant transformation rate of 4 to 6%.

*Not FDA approved for this indication.

However, as many as 20% of these white lesions show evidence of dysplasia or carcinoma at first clinical recognition. The most important etiologic factor in the development of leukoplakia is tobacco use, while alcohol intake has a strong synergistic effect when used concurrently. Ultraviolet radiation is the primary etiologic factor when the lower lip vermilion is involved. Leukoplakia affects about 3% of the adult population, with a predilection for men older than 40 years of age. The most common sites of occurrence include the lip vermilion, buccal mucosa, and floor of the mouth. However, lesions that are most likely to exhibit evidence of dysplasia or carcinoma are found on the tongue and floor of the mouth.

Clinically, leukoplakia varies in size, thickness, and surface irregularity, depending on the stage of the disease. Early and mild lesions present as slightly elevated, translucent white plaques with well-demarcated borders and a slightly wrinkled surface. These mild cases of leukoplakia do not show evidence of dysplasia and may spontaneously resolve. The intermediate-stage lesion demonstrates increased thickness, intense whiteness, numerous fissures, and irregular margins. Although the majority of the lesions persist in this stage, about one third will regress, while a small percentage will become more severe. This later stage is characterized by extensive lesions with rough surface irregularities and occasional papillary projections. The overall malignant transformation rate for this latter group is as high as 15%.

Excision is the treatment of choice for most lesions that exhibit dysplasia. The use of 13-*cis*-retinoic acid (isotretinoin [Accutane]),* 1 to 2 mg per kg per day, leads to temporary remission of leukoplakia in some cases, but significant side effects are reported in a high percentage of patients. Other antioxidants, such as beta carotene alone or in combination with ascorbic acid and/or alpha tocopherol, lack the side effects but require further clinical trials to document their effectiveness.

WHITE AND RED LESIONS

Candidiasis

Candidiasis is the most common oral fungal infection, which is typically caused by *Candida albicans.* Predisposing conditions associated with this opportunistic infection include xerostomia, the use of broad-spectrum antibiotics and corticosteroids, chemoradiotherapy, poor oral hygiene, prosthetic oral appliances, diabetes mellitus, and immunosuppressive diseases, such as HIV infection.

Candidiasis has a variety of clinical presentations that tend to overlap. *Pseudomembranous candidiasis* is the most recognizable form of the disease and is characterized by nonadherent, creamy, white papules and plaques with an underlying normal or erythematous mucosal base. *Erythematous candidiasis* pre-

*Not FDA approved for this indication.

sents as a generalized or patchy redness with either a smooth or granular surface. *Hyperplastic candidiasis* (candidal leukoplakia) consists of diffuse, adherent, white, wrinkled or stippled plaques. Focal areas of erythema are often associated with this chronic form. Although candidiasis may be asymptomatic, a burning sensation and a foul taste are common complaints.

When the clinical diagnosis is questionable, exfoliative cytologic studies or fungal cultures are recommended. If lesions do not respond to antifungal therapy, then a biopsy is recommended to exclude a superimposed candidal infection associated with epithelial dysplasia, squamous cell carcinoma, or lichen planus.

Several antifungal treatments are available for the management of this oral mucosal disease. Topical antifungals include nystatin (Mycostatin, Nilstat) oral suspension, 100,000 units per mL, used as a rinse of 2 to 5 mL every 6 hours for 2 minutes and then swallowed or amphotericin B (Fungizone) oral suspension, 100 mg per mL, used as a rinse of 1 mL for 2 minutes and then swallowed. Nystatin pastilles, 200,000 units, or clotrimazole troches (Mycelex), 10 mg, are slowly dissolved in the mouth five times a day. When topical therapy is not practicable or is ineffective, then systemic fluconazole (Diflucan), 100 mg daily for 2 weeks, is recommended. Nystatin ointment may be applied to the inner surface of a removable dental prosthesis to treat the adjacent mucosa after each meal.

Median Rhomboid Glossitis

Median rhomboid glossitis, another variant of candidiasis, usually presents as a depapillated oval patch in the central middle third of the dorsal surface of the tongue. It may occur as a solitary lesion or in combination with other clinical forms of candidiasis. Although this lesion is most frequently red and smooth, it may appear fissured or ulcerated or as a white rough plaque with focal erythema. A faint red palatal blush may accompany this entity, owing to repeated contact of the tongue against the palate. Median rhomboid glossitis may mimic erythema migrans or a traumatic erosion. Antifungal medications are recommended for management (as discussed previously for candidiasis).

Erythema Migrans

Erythema migrans is a common benign condition that primarily affects the tongue (geographic tongue) but may occur at other mucosal sites. Although the cause of this lesion is unknown, a hypersensitivity reaction is suspected in some patients. Typically, erythema migrans presents as multiple well-defined foci of erythema, surrounded by a white, serpentine border. The erythematous patches on the dorsal surface of the tongue represent atrophy of the filiform papillae. The distribution and pattern of the lesions change over time. Most cases are asymptomatic; however, sensitivity to hot or spicy foods is a common complaint when lesions are widespread. To relieve the periodic discomfort, the use of topical anesthetics may be beneficial, such as an equal mixture of diphenhydramine syrup (Benylin) or elixir (Benadryl), 12.5 mg per 5 mL, with instructions to rinse with 1 teaspoonful every 2 hours and expectorate, in combination with Kaopectate or unflavored Maalox. Some patients may benefit from the use of topical corticosteroids (as described for lichen planus later on), alone or in combination with topical antifungal agents (as described for candidiasis).

This common condition may be similar in clinical appearance to median rhomboid glossitis, lichen planus, and erythroplakia. Persistent lesions of the ventral or posterior lateral surface of the tongue require a biopsy to exclude erythroplakia or squamous cell carcinoma.

Lichen Planus

Lichen planus is a relatively common mucocutaneous disease that appears to be immunologically mediated. Lichen planus occurs usually in middle-aged adults, with a predilection for women. Oral involvement is more common than skin lesions, with a prevalence as high as 2%. Several clinical patterns are associated with this disease, but the majority are categorized as reticular or erosive variants. The classic reticular lesions appear as interlacing white lines, or Wickham's striae, with focal erythema; however, white papules and plaques may be present. Although the typical lesion distribution involves the posterior buccal mucosa bilaterally, multiple sites may be affected concurrently. The reticular form of lichen planus is mildly symptomatic, with occasional burning or irritation on ingestion of acidic or spicy foods and beverages and with use of certain dental hygiene products. In contrast, the erosive form of the disease is painful and manifests as multifocal erythematous patches with areas of ulceration and surrounding striations. The posterior buccal mucosa, gingiva, and tongue are the most frequent sites of involvement. All variants of lichen planus are characterized by periods of exacerbation and remission.

Incisional biopsy may be necessary for the diagnosis of lichen planus, especially when the patient presents with the erosive variant or when a unilateral or isolated distribution pattern exists. It is important to distinguish lichen planus from a drug-induced lichenoid reaction, erythroleukoplakia, contact stomatitis, and lupus erythematosus. Periodic monitoring of patients with lichen planus is recommended because of the potential for malignant transformation.

Asymptomatic reticular lichen planus usually does not require treatment. The presence of a burning sensation suggests a superimposed candidal infection. If symptoms persist, then topical corticosteroids, either alone or in combination with antifungal agents, are recommended. Fluocinonide (Lidex) gel or ointment 0.05% or clobetasol propionate (Temovate) gel or ointment 0.05% is applied to the lesions after each meal and before bedtime. For prolonged adherence of these topical agents, Orabase paste may be added in equal parts to the topical steroids. Rinsing for 2 minutes with 1 teaspoonful of dexamethasone (Decadron) elixir, 0.5 mg per 5 mL, and then expectorating, after meals and before bedtime may be effective when lesions are widespread. In severe cases, systemic prednisone, 40 to 60 mg a day for 10 days, may be required, followed by topical corticosteroids for maintenance. Proper oral hygiene combined with periodic professional prophylaxis has been shown to reduce the severity of the disease.

RED LESIONS

Erythroplakia

Although less common than leukoplakia, erythroplakia exhibits dysplasia or invasive carcinoma at the time of diagnosis in approximately 90% of the cases. The lesion of classic erythroplakia is a persistent red velvety or granular plaque. More frequently, a variegated red and white plaque is observed, which is referred to as erythroleukoplakia. This lesion is usually asymptomatic and has a predilection for the floor of the mouth, ventrolateral tongue, and soft palate. Excisional biopsy is recommended, in addition to long-term follow-up and the discontinuation of carcinogenic habits, especially tobacco use. These lesions may be difficult to distinguish from lichen planus, candidiasis, and traumatic erosions.

Angular Cheilitis

Angular cheilitis is another form of candidiasis that occurs at the angles of the mouth and is characterized by localized erythema, scaling, fissuring, and ulceration. Constant moistening of the lips and a decreased vertical dimension, which causes wrinkling of the skin and pooling of saliva, are common predisposing factors. *C. albicans,* either alone or in combination with *Staphlococcus aureus,* is associated with the majority of cases. When this lesion occurs unilaterally, it may resemble herpes labialis. If the lips exhibit multiple fissures with generalized scaling, exfoliative cheilitis or a contact allergy should be excluded.

Topical combination agents, such as triamcinolone acetonide–nystatin (Mycolog-II) ointment or 1% hydrocortisone-iodoquinol (Vytone) cream, applied after meals and at bedtime are most effective. Concurrent intraoral antifungal treatment (as described previously for candidiasis) may be indicated.

Plasma Cell Gingivitis (Atypical Gingivostomatitis)

Plasma cell gingivitis represents an idiopathic or a peculiar allergic reaction. Numerous allergens, including chewing gum, toothpaste, mint candy, and pepper, have been implicated. The enlarged and brightly erythematous lesions of the gingiva are tender and of sudden onset. Depapillation of the tongue and/or crenations of the lateral border of the tongue, together with chapped lips and angular cheilitis, may also be present. Elimination of the allergen is the treatment of choice. For those patients in whom the offending agent cannot be identified, topical corticosteroids have variable effectiveness (as described previously for lichen planus). Diagnosis is made by clinical presentation and supported by an incisional biopsy. Pregnancy gingivitis, erosive lichen planus, cicatricial pemphigoid, erythematous candidiasis, and leukemic gingival infiltrates may mimic this condition.

Xerostomia

Oral dryness, or xerostomia, does not represent a specific disease but rather is a sign of salivary gland dysfunction. A number of factors are associated with persistent xerostomia, including aging, salivary gland agenesis, Sjögren's syndrome, mouth breathing, dehydration, medication effects, and therapeutic radiation to the head and neck. Drug effects are the most common cause of oral dryness in the adult; antihistamines, decongestants, antidepressants, antipsychotics, antispasmodics, and antihypertensives have been implicated. Patients with xerostomia frequently complain of a generalized burning sensation, difficulty speaking and swallowing, abnormal taste, and sticking of the lips to the teeth and of the tongue to the palate. Clinically, the saliva is foamy or ropy and pooled in the buccal vestibule. In general, the oral mucosa has a thin, erythematous appearance. The dorsal tongue is red, fissured, and devoid of filiform papillae, and the lips are chapped. Xerostomia increases the risk for candidiasis, dental caries, periodontal disease, and traumatic ulcers.

The treatment for xerostomia is challenging and often is only partially effective. Conservative management includes restricting the intake of caffeinated drinks and alcoholic beverages and avoiding mouth rinses that contain alcohol. Slowly sipping water or crushed ice during the day is frequently necessary for patient comfort. In addition, artificial salivas and oral moisturizing gels are commercially available. Sugarless candy and chewing gum help to mechanically stimulate the salivary flow. Good oral hygiene is required in order to prevent dental caries and periodontal disease. Topical fluoride therapy, such as the application of neutral sodium fluoride gel 1% (PreviDent, Thera-Flur-N) in a custom mouth tray for 5 minutes daily, is an important preventive measure. Residual functional salivary glands may be stimulated with pilocarpine hydrochloride (Salagen) tablets, 5 mg three times a day. If medications are the primary cause for the oral dryness, then drug substitutions or dose modifications may be needed. Management of secondary candidal infections may decrease the burning sensation.

The most important disease to exclude in patients with persistent xerostomia is Sjögren's syndrome, which is characterized by xerostomia, xerophthalmia, and rheumatoid arthritis. Biopsy of the lower lip salivary glands is a useful test for making this diagnosis.

ULCERATIVE LESIONS

Acute Necrotizing Ulcerative Gingivitis

Acute necrotizing ulcerative gingivitis (ANUG) is a painful gingival condition that is associated with stress, cigarette smoking, poor nutritional status, and inadequate oral hygiene. Furthermore, this condition may be observed in patients with HIV infection and infectious mononucleosis. Fusiform bacteria and spirochetes have been implicated in this disease. ANUG is characterized by a fetid odor, severe pain, spontaneous gingival bleeding, necrosis, and ulceration, especially of the interdental papillae. Lymphadenopathy, fever, and malaise may accompany the oral lesions. The most important treatment is local débridement of the tissues. Rinsing with warm alkaline saline (salt-bicarbonate) solution or chlorhexidine gluconate 0.12% (Peridex, PerioGard) may be beneficial. Systemic antibiotics, such as metronidazole (Flagyl) or penicillin, are reserved for severe cases that have concurrent constitutional signs and symptoms.

Recurrent Aphthous Ulcers

Recurrent aphthous ulcers are common oral mucosal lesions that affect about 30% of the general population. Although the pathogenesis of this condition is unclear, either a primary immunodysregulation or a localized antigenic response is the most commonly attributed cause. There are three clinical variants of aphthous ulcers: the minor, major, and herpetiform types. The *aphthous minor ulcer* presents as a solitary, oval ulcer measuring less than 10 mm in diameter. This painful ulcer develops almost exclusively on the nonkeratinized or thin movable lining of the mouth. Lesion resolution occurs in 3 to 14 days, with a variable recurrence rate. *Aphthous major ulcers* are larger than 1 cm in size and have a multifocal pattern. These deep ulcers with irregular margins often persist from 3 to 6 weeks and heal with extensive scarring. The most common sites of occurrence are the labial mucosa, soft palate, and tonsillar pillar region. *Herpetiform aphthous ulcers* consist of numerous small, punctate lesions, ranging from 1 to 3 mm in diameter. Clusters of these lesions may coalesce to form large, irregular ulcers. There is a predilection for the nonkeratinized mucosa, and recurrences are common.

The minor and herpetiform variants may be differentiated from recurrent herpes simplex virus by their site predilection for the nonkeratinized mucosa. The persistent aphthous major ulcer may mimic factitial lesions, deep mycotic infections, and ulcerative squamous cell carcinoma. In addition, aphthous-like ulcerations may be seen with Behçet's syndrome, Crohn's disease, celiac disease, cyclic neutropenia, and HIV infection.

Recurrent aphthous ulcers are best treated with topical corticosteroids, if the antigenic stimulus cannot be identified. Examples of topical corticosteroids include 0.05% fluocinonide gel or ointment or 0.05% clobetasol propionate gel or ointment, applied after meals and before bedtime. Mixing the gels or ointment with an occlusive dressing, such as Orabase, in equal portions promotes adhesion of the medications and may provide more symptomatic relief. If multiple widespread ulcers are present, rinsing with 1 teaspoonful of dexamethasone elixir, 0.5 mg per 5 mL, after meals and before bed for 2 minutes and then expectorating is more practicable. In severe cases, systemic corticosteroids, such as prednisone, 40 to 60 mg per day for 5 to 10 days, may be necessary.

Herpes Simplex Infection

Acute herpetic gingivostomatitis represents a symptomatic primary oral infection, usually caused by herpes simplex virus type 1 (HSV-1). This disease is characterized by an abrupt onset of cervical lymphadenopathy, fever, malaise, excessive drooling, and vesicular eruptions of the vermilion border of the lips and oral mucosa. In all cases, the gingiva is enlarged, painful, and brightly erythematous. Self-inoculation of the fingers and eyes may occur, especially in the young child. Lesion resolution occurs within 7 to 14 days; however, the virus remains in a latent state in the trigeminal ganglion.

Reactivation of the virus may produce clustered vesicular lesions in up to 40% of the population. Triggering factors for recurrent HSV infection include ultraviolet light, stress, trauma, systemic diseases, menstruation, and immunosuppression. Prodromal signs and symptoms frequently occur several hours prior to lesion formation, such as burning, itching, and a tingling sensation. The most common site of recurrence is the vermilion of the lip and perioral skin; this form of infection is referred to as *herpes labialis.* Intraorally, these lesions are limited to the keratinized tissues, especially the attached gingiva and the hard palatal mucosa. The lesions begin as localized, erythematous macules with clusters of vesicles that ulcerate. Healing occurs within 7 to 10 days without scarring. Chronic herpetic infections may develop in immunocompromised patients and involve any oral mucosal site.

Diseases that may resemble acute herpetic gingivostomatitis include erythema multiforme and ANUG. Recurrent intraoral herpetic lesions may mimic traumatic ulcers, recurrent aphthous ulcers, and herpes zoster. Although most cases are diagnosed by clinical history and appearance, laboratory confirmation by viral culture, cytologic smears, or tissue biopsy may be indicated for severe or atypical cases.

Management of primary herpetic gingivostomatitis usually involves symptomatic relief. Topical anesthetics may provide temporary comfort, such as an equal mixture of diphenhydramine syrup or elixir, 12.5 mg per 5 ml, with instructions to rinse with 1 teaspoonful every 2 hours and expectorate, in combination with Kaopectate or unflavored Maalox. For children who can expectorate and adults, 1 ounce of dyclonine hydrochloride (Dyclone), 0.5% or 1%, may be added to the suspension for greater anesthetic efficacy. In some patients, systemic acyclovir (Zovirax) suspension, 200 mg per 5 ml, with instructions to rinse and swallow, five times a day for 7 days may be useful. Regular fluid intake and management of the fever are important for preventing dehydration in the young child with this infection.

Recurrent HSV lesions are treated with variable success with 5% acyclovir ointment or 1% penciclovir (Denavir) cream, applied every 2 hours during waking hours. Patients with multiple, severe recurrences or immunocompromised persons are best managed with systemic acyclovir, 200 mg, five times a day. Increased dosages may be indicated for some patients, especially immunocompromised persons. Lip balms, lotions, and gels with a skin protection factor (SPF) of 15 or higher are useful for preventing herpes labialis when recurrence is triggered by excessive sunlight exposure.

Cicatricial Pemphigoid

Cicatricial pemphigoid (benign mucous membrane pemphigoid) is a chronic, autoimmune blistering disease that usually affects older women. Oral lesions are diagnosed in most patients, but the conjunctival, nasal, esophageal, and vaginal mucosa and the skin may be involved. These painful lesions typically involve the gingival tissues and present as vesicles and bullae that ulcerate. A complication of cicatricial pemphigoid is ocular involvement, which may result in blindness.

It may be difficult to distinguish this condition from other mucocutaneous diseases including erosive lichen planus, lupus erythematosus, pemphigus vulgaris, allergic gingivostomatitis, and chronic ulcerative stomatitis. Definitive diagnosis requires a perilesional biopsy and direct immunofluorescence studies to detect immunoglobulins and complement.

The oral lesions are usually controlled by the use of potent topical corticosteroids. In particular, 0.05% flucinonide gel or ointment, placed into a customized soft acrylic mouthguard for 15 minutes twice daily, is effective until the lesions are controlled. Widespread refractory lesions may be managed with systemic corticosteroids, often in combination with immunosuppressive drugs, such as azathioprine.* Good oral hygiene is important for reducing the severity of the disease. Baseline and periodic evaluations by an ophthalmologist are recommended.

Squamous Cell Carcinoma

Squamous cell carcinoma is the most common form of oral cancer, accounting for more than 90% of all oral malignancies. In general, this form of oral cancer has a predilection for men over the age of 40 years, with tobacco use as a primary risk factor. The most common intraoral site of involvement is the tongue, in particular the posterior lateral and ventral surfaces, followed by the oropharynx, lower lip, and floor of the mouth. In most cases, squamous cell carcinoma presents as a persistent erosion, indurated ulcer, or fixated mass with a variegated red and white, granular, stippled, or papillary surface. Many early lesions are nontender to mildly irritative, while more advanced cancers are painful. Other signs and symptoms include prolonged hoarseness, sudden tooth mobility, paresthesia or dysesthesia of the tongue and lip, dysphagia, trismus, otalgia, and firm, fixed lymph nodes. Diagnosis requires histopathologic examination of the biopsied lesion, followed by clinical staging of the disease.

Treatment of intraoral squamous cell carcinoma depends on the clinical stage of the disease and the accessibility of the lesion to surgical management. In general, wide surgical excision, radiation therapy, or a combination of these two modalities is used. Adjunctive chemotherapy is instituted in patients with recurrent or widespread metastatic disease. The overall 5-year survival rate for intraoral carcinoma is about 50% but is significantly higher with localized disease, at 80 to 90%. Owing to the well-documented phenomenon of "field cancerization," approximately 25% of patients are at risk for developing a second upper aerodigestive tract malignancy.

Long-term follow-up is required for patients because of the increased risk for a second cancer and for the prevention and management of treatment complications. The permanent radiation side effects of salivary gland hypofunction may contribute to the development of dental caries, candidiasis, and mucosal atrophy. Management options for this treatment side effect are as described previously for xerostomia. The most serious complication of head and neck irradiation is osteoradionecrosis. To decrease this risk, teeth of questionable prognosis should be removed prior to initiation of therapy, as should dental implants in involved areas and root fragments or other bony lesions in the field of radiation. Management of osteoradionecrosis is difficult and usually involves the use of hyperbaric oxygen in combination with antibiotic therapy and surgery.

*Not FDA approved for this indication.

VENOUS ULCERS

method of
ROBERT S. KIRSNER, M.D.
University of Miami School of Medicine
Miami, Florida

Venous insufficiency is the most common cause of leg ulcers. Although venous ulcers are sometimes referred to as stasis ulcers, this is in fact a misnomer because there is increased blood flow in the affected area. Venous ulcers account for approximately 70% of all leg ulcers. An additional 20% are seen in combination with arterial insufficiency. All told, venous ulcers affect about 1 to 2% of the population. The classic venous ulcer occurs on the medial aspect of the lower leg near the ankle and is associated with fibrosis and pigmentation of the surrounding skin (lipodermatosclerosis) as well as varicose veins in the leg.

Venous ulcers are thought to result from venous hypertension, which is defined as sustained elevated venous pressures during ambulation. These elevated venous pressures cause vascular changes that have been hypothesized to cause adherence of white blood cells to endothelial cells, leading to capillary permeability and deposition of fibrin and other macromolecules around blood vessels. Additionally, these changes may cause local binding of important growth factors. Patients with venous disease may also have systemic alteration in fibrinolysis contributing to the aforementioned processes.

Several factors portend a poorer prognosis for patients with leg ulcers, including the size of the ulcer, how long the ulcer has been present, and the presence of lipodermatosclerosis around the ulcer. In addition, although the majority of ulcers heal with conservative therapy, prevention of recurrence is difficult, especially among patients of lower socioeconomic status.

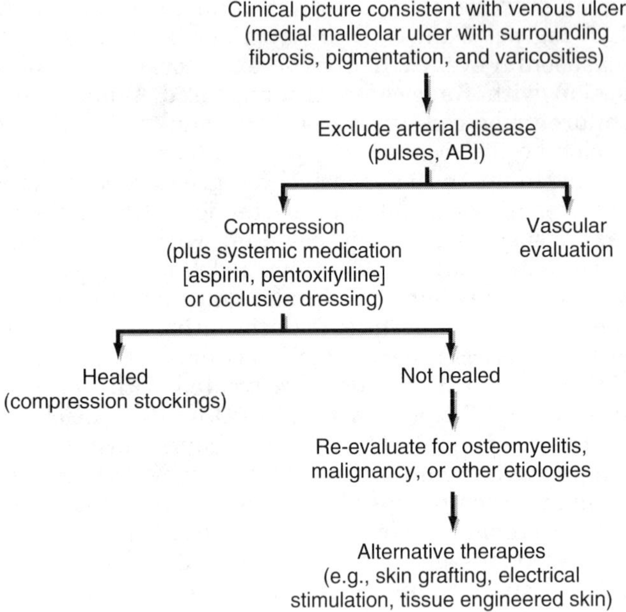

Figure 1. Simplified algorithm for the diagnosis and treatment of patients with venous ulcers.
Abbreviation: ABI = ankle/brachial index.

TREATMENT

As more than 20% of patients with venous ulcers have associated arterial insufficiency, arterial disease should be ruled out by the measurement of arterial pulses. In the presence of diminished or nonpalpable arterial pulses, a simple noninvasive measurement is the ankle/brachial index (ABI), which is calculated by dividing the systolic pressure in the ankle by that in the arm (Figure 1). An ABI of less than 0.7 indicates moderate arterial insufficiency and may be an independent risk factor for coronary artery disease as well. Patients with an ABI of less than 0.7 should undergo further vascular evaluation. Care must be taken in diabetic or elderly patients, who may have a falsely negative ABI.

Once arterial disease has been excluded, reversal of the effects of venous hypertension through the use of compression bandages and leg elevation constitutes the standard management approved. A variety of compression bandages or devices are available; they may be either elastic or inelastic. The Unna boot (a zinc oxide–impregnated bandage) is probably the most commonly employed, followed by an elastic compression bandage (Coban). However, other compression bandage systems such as a four-layered compression wrap or a legging orthosis may have advantages. The overall goal is to provide graded compression of 30 to 40 mm Hg. These bandages are applied circumferentially from the toes to the knees (involving the heel) with the foot dorsiflexed. Patients with associated lymphatic damage resulting in lymphedema may also benefit from pneumatic compression. Additionally, compression bandages plus either pentoxifylline (Trental) or aspirin may be superior to compression bandages alone with regard to rate of healing.

Local care of the wound is best accomplished with occlusive dressings. Occlusive dressings provide a moist environment for healing, and although their use may result in higher bacterial counts, they do not cause infection and are not associated with higher infection rates. Topical antiseptics and cleansing agents should be used only with caution as they may prolong healing. A variety of occlusive dressings are available in five general categories: hydrocolloids, hydrogels, alginates, foams, and films. The location of the wound and the amount of exudate are important determinants in choosing a specific dressing.

Wounds that persist for longer than 3 months, that do not fit the typical clinical picture, or that have exposed tendon or bone should be evaluated for osteomyelitis, malignant changes, or other potential nonvenous causes of the ulcer. Obtaining radiographs and performing biopsy for histology and culture are appropriate first steps.

A subset of venous ulcers are slow to heal and may require other treatment options. Alternative therapies include the use of split-thickness skin grafts, electrical stimulation, and, possibly tissue engineered skin (skin substitutes grown in the laboratory).

As mentioned previously, once healing has occurred, patients are at risk for recurrence. The lifelong use of elastic compression stockings (30 to 40 mm Hg) is the mainstay of therapy, but early intervention after recurrence is also critical.

PRESSURE ULCERS

method of
LAWRENCE CHARLES PARISH, M.D.
Jefferson Medical College of Thomas Jefferson University
Philadelphia, Pennsylvania

and

JOSEPH A. WITKOWSKI, M.D.
University of Pennsylvania School of Medicine
Philadelphia, Pennsylvania

A pressure ulcer represents a defect in the skin and the underlying structures. The destruction of skin, subcutaneous tissue, and even bone and muscle are the result of pressure or shearing force injury leading to vascular occlusion. Pressure is applied vertically, with shear stress being applied tangentially to the skin surface, which occurs when the skin is dragged across the deeper and more rigid tissues.

Because the pathophysiology of pressure ulcer is still incompletely understood, the terminology cannot be exact. The terms "decubitus ulcer," "pressure ulcer," or "bedsore" can be used interchangeably.

PRESSURE ULCER PATHWAY

To treat an ulcer appropriately, the caregiver needs to understand the decubitus ulcer pathway (Figure 1). The initial sign of a decubitus ulcer is blanchable erythema; the area has reversible redness following finger pressure. Nonblanchable erythema indicates that the area remains red following pressure. Decubitus dermatitis shows redness, scaling, and even bullae. The formation of a superficial or deep ulcer reflects a further compromised localized circulation. Finally, there may be full destruction with gangrene and eschar formation.

DIAGNOSIS

The diagnosis of a pressure ulcer is made clinically. Because the lesions occur over areas that are compressed against a firm area such as bony prominences, the bedbound patient may develop ulcerations over the sacrum, trochanters, and heels, whereas the chair-bound patient will most often have involvement of the ischial tuberosities. The extent of the destruction may be quantified by using the following simple staging method:

- Stage 1 nonblanchable erythema
- Stage 2 ulceration of the epidermis and dermis
- Stage 3 destruction to the subcutaneous fat level
- Stage 4 defect extending to bone, tendon, and/or joint capsule

ETIOLOGY

Many factors contribute to the development of pressure ulcers including nutritional status, age, medical status, edema, fever, vascular status, and anatomic defects. These augment the problem created by the exertion of pressure beyond a timed threshold. In addition, inactivity, immobility, and sensory perception loss add to the problem. A clear cause of pressure ulcers has not been identified.

IDENTIFYING THE HIGH-RISK PATIENT

Several scales are used to identify the patient who may develop a decubitus ulcer. These include the Braden and Norton scales.

A clinical assessment of the high-risk patient can be readily accomplished by observing the amount of inactivity, immobility, sensory deprivation, hypotension, malnutrition, and incontinence.

The greatest risk for the development of ulcers occurs during the first 10 days of being immobilized. The concept of skin failure also needs to be understood because the skin and subcutaneous tissue can fail just as the heart or kidneys can.

PREVENTION

Bed- or chair-bound patients or others who are not able to reposition themselves adequately are prone to pressure effects on the skin. Such patients are prime candidates for deterioration of the skin. Assessments on admission to a facility or when an underlying problem occurs are helpful in determining the course of events. Assessments may then be made at regular intervals.

There is no question about the necessity of adequate nutrition to preserve tissue integrity and assist in wound healing. Good intake, feeding assistance, nutritional supplements, or even parenteral feeding are all theoretically important. Unfortunately, we cannot yet determine the utilization of nutrients at the cellular level, and skin failure can ensue.

The skin needs to be kept clean but not scrubbed. Fecal and urinary contamination may cause breakdown. Moisture barrier creams, underpads, and even urinary catheters may help prevent further deterioration of the skin by decreasing skin maceration.

Friction can be minimized by keeping the skin dry, using a lubricant, and applying a film or hydrocolloid dressing over pressure points. Further reduction of friction can be accomplished by proper positioning, turning, and application of linens and lifting devices. Shearing can be reduced by keeping the bed elevated less than 30 degrees.

Eliminating or decreasing pressure is more complicated, as there is no such thing as suspended animation. Periodic turning is helpful, but the frequency is highly variable; the order "turn every 2 hours" is purely arbitrary. Use of pillows and foam wedges may be helpful, as are support systems. Completely immobilized patients should have heels raised from the bed, but all of the pressure should not be transferred to the sacrum and ischial tuberosities.

Despite these preventive measures, some patients will still have skin failure and develop decubitus ulcers.

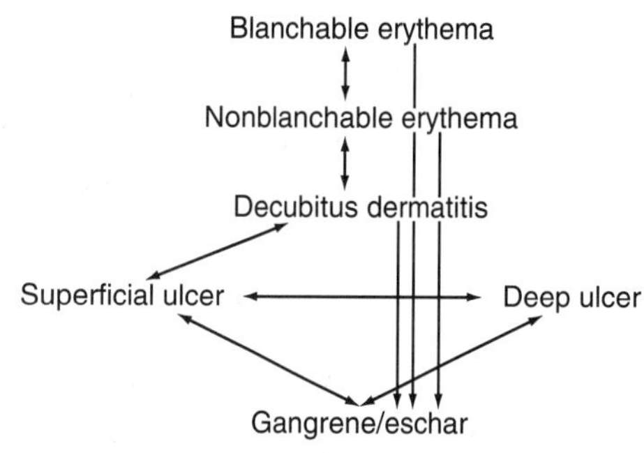

Figure 1. Decubitus ulcer pathway.

SUPPORT SYSTEMS

Support systems vary considerably and should be selected according to whether prevention, treatment, and/or comfort are the goals. They can be nonpowered, static and powered, or dynamic. They can utilize air, foam, water, or gel and be mattresses or overlays. These systems must be checked for bottoming out (i.e., the patient slips down in the bed).

Powered surfaces range from low air-loss overlays, mattresses, and beds to air-fluidized beds. Pulsating systems are helpful in patients with compromised circulation, and oscillating beds are recommended for patients with pulmonary disease so that pulmonary secretions can be mobilized and ventilation promoted.

MEDICAL MANAGEMENT

The prime concern is treatment of an identifiable condition that immobilized the patient and allowed the skin failure. Adequate nutrition should be maintained, whether by oral intake, assisted feeding, enteral administration, or parenteral delivery. Generally, 30 to 35 calories per kg per day are needed. This should include 1.25 to 1.50 grams of protein per kg per day and 500 mg to 1 gram of ascorbic acid (vitamin C) daily. Hemoglobin above 10 grams per dL and plasma protein levels about 6 grams per dL are desirable. A transthyretin (prealbumin) level less than 10 mg per dL suggests the need for nutritional therapy.

Although most patients with decubitus ulcers have absent to diminished pain sensation, those demonstrating discomfort may obtain relief by covering the ulcer with an occlusive dressing. Patients with spinal cord injury or other neurologic diseases leading to spasticity may require diazepam, 2 to 10 mg three to four times a day, or dantrolene sodium (Dantrium), 25 to 100 mg two, three, or four times a day.

The decubitus ulcer is generally colonized by a variety of bacteria, making the use of routine cultures unnecessary. Bacterial infection is diagnosed by observing redness, induration, and warmth. There may be tenderness, and the ulcer may contain purulent material. Anaerobic infection is suggested by a foul odor, crepitus, and a sanguinous exudate. Systemic signs of fever, leukocytosis, and elevated sedimentation rate may not always be present. Cultures of the infected ulcer, both aerobic and anaerobic, are indicated, as are blood cultures. Serious swabbing of the area, curetting, punch biopsying, or aspiration may be used to obtain the material for cultures. Until microbiologic confirmation is obtained, treatment may be initiated with ceftazidime (Fortaz), 1 gram every 12 hours intravenously, or a quinolone such as ciprofloxacin (Cipro), 500 mg every 12 hours intravenously or orally, or trovafloxacin (Trovan), 200 mg orally once daily. When an anaerobic infection is suspected, metronidazole (Flagyl), 1 gram every 12 hours orally, may be added. An infectious disease consultation is indicated for serious infections.

LOCAL MANAGEMENT

Early Phases

Blanchable erythema can be treated with pressure relief only. The patient should be moved off the area, if possible, or rotated to various other positions.

Nonblanchable erythema may be treated with 2% nitroglycerin ointment. One half to 1 inch of the ointment is placed on the lesion and occluded with an impermeable plastic wrap. To avoid development of tolerance, it should be applied only for 12 hours daily. For the deep red or purple nonblanchable erythema, a thin hydrocolloid dressing may be used. Alternative therapies include the application of zinc oxide paste (Lassar's paste) every shift or a fluorinated steroid gel every shift.

The treatment of decubitus dermatitis should be addressed as in any other dermatitides. Burow's 1:40 compresses and/or fluorinated steroid gel should be applied every shift. Alternative regimens include the use of silver sulfadiazine (Silvadene) cream every shift or a hydrocolloid dressing.

Débridement

When there is significant necrotic tissue, débridement is indicated. The dead tissue can be separated from the viable tissue by applying to the borders 5-fluorouracil cream (Efudex)* every shift for several days. Elimination of dead tissue can also be accomplished by using wet to dry dressings every shift. A damp sponge is applied to the tissue; when it dries, it is removed along with the debris. (A wet to dry dressing is not a wet dressing covered by a dry dressing.)

Surgical débridement can be accomplished by removing a small amount of tissue daily, using a forceps, scissors, or scalpel. If local anesthetic is needed, it can be applied under plastic wrap occlusion 1 hour before débridement by the application of a eutectic mixture of lidocaine and prilocaine (Emla) cream. Lidocaine can also be injected into the borders. Mild bleeding can be controlled by applying absorbable gelatin sponge, a calcium alginate dressing, or pressure. More serious débridement should be done in the operating room.

Débridement may cause transient bacteremia, which may be treated with antimicrobial agents. Elimination of necrotic tissue may reveal bone or joint capsules. Consideration should then be given to the diagnosis of osteomyelitis, and appropriate radiographic studies should be ordered.

Clean Ulcers

Clean ulcers may be treated by the use of hydrocolloid dressings. The ulcer is cleaned with water (sterile water is unnecessary). The area is damp dried and the ulcer covered with the dressing. The dressing

*Not FDA approved for this indication.

needs to be changed when the seal breaks and may stay in place for up to 7 days. Generally, an order to change every 3 days is appropriate.

Initially, there may be much drainage, for which a hydrocolloid paste may be used to absorb the fluid. Undermined areas or deep ulcers may also benefit from the use of such paste or beads. Occasionally, a calcium alginate pad or rope may be used.

The most important consideration in treating decubitus ulcers is not to injure the viable tissue. Povidone-iodine and hydrogen peroxide compresses should be avoided, as they interfere with wound healing, as do irrational combinations of agents.

Eschar/Gangrene

The hard, even mushy, necrotic tissue may be removed medically or surgically. There is no hurry. In fact, some of the tissue may separate by itself.

SURGICAL MANAGEMENT

Excellent plastic surgical procedures are available to cover ulcers. The techniques include rotational flaps and grafts. These repairs should be limited to patients who have an appropriate quality of life and an adequate life expectancy. Spinal cord patients and patients with some neurologic diseases are candidates. Elderly and infirm patients ordinarily should not be subjected to such surgery. Making the ulcer clean may be all that is indicated.

ATOPIC DERMATITIS

method of
SETH R. STEVENS, M.D.
Case Western Reserve University/University Hospitals of Cleveland, and Cleveland Veterans Affairs Medical Center
Cleveland, Ohio

Atopic dermatitis (AD) is an exceptionally common condition, affecting 10 to 20% of individuals and accounting for 4% of pediatric emergency department visits and more than 80% of occupational skin disease. The tendency is for familial clustering of AD, asthma, and allergic rhinitis, comprising the atopic triad.

Edematous papules and vesicles and ill-defined, erythematous, scaling patches are characteristic. Pruritus is a unifying feature, and excoriations are common. Chronic scratching and rubbing cause lichenification. Before infants begin to crawl, their lesions are characteristically on the face and scalp but may be seen anywhere. Once crawling begins, extensor surfaces (knees and elbows) become affected. During childhood, features evolve toward those seen in adults. Chronic drier lesions become more common. Some children retain extensor-dominated distribution. The norm is for flexural (characteristically antecubital and popliteal fossae) and neck involvement to become prominent.

The diagnosis is based on characteristic lesion appearance, personal or family history of atopy, and pruritus. Differential diagnosis includes cutaneous T cell lymphoma, seborrheic dermatitis, contact dermatitis, scabies, dermatophytosis, nutritional or metabolic inadequacy, and immunodeficiency syndromes. Secondary infection is a common complication owing to diminished cell-mediated immune responses and reduced barrier function of involved skin. Common bacterial pathogens are *Staphylococci aureus* and group A beta-hemolytic streptococci. Viral infections with human papillomavirus and herpes simplex virus are common, and eczema herpeticum is most commonly seen in patients with AD.

MANAGEMENT

The most critical element to the management of AD is education of the patient and/or parent. The key educational points are avoidance of trigger factors; proper skin care, particularly bathing regimens; judicious use of topical steroids; and recognition and treatment of secondary infection.

Trigger Factor Avoidance

The relative role of allergy in AD is controversial. For a small selected group of patients, the difficult task of identifying and eliminating food and aeroallergens can be helpful, albeit difficult to accomplish in a real-world setting. Scrupulous housekeeping and elimination of surfaces that harbor aeroallergens (e.g., upholstery, curtains, stuffed animals) are required. Ventilating bathrooms and kitchens and reducing houseplants can lessen mold exposure. Spring or summer exacerbation suggests a possible role for pollens. One must always critically assess whether allergen reduction is useful for an individual patient; success will be the exception, not the rule. Contact allergy (nickel and topical medicaments, e.g., topical steroids) or urticaria (latex, foods) should be considered as aggravating factors in some patients with AD.

Reduction of nonspecific irritants that occurs concomitantly with meticulous housekeeping can be helpful. Limited exposure to furry and feathered pets can help. Breeds with short hair and minimal dander are preferred. Avoidance of other irritants is also imperative. Wool and nylon next to the skin, harsh chemicals such as cleansers, hair colorants, and permanent wave preparations commonly trigger flares. Adequate rinsing out of laundry detergent is essential; the use of fabric softeners should be discouraged. Vocations (e.g., housekeeping, laundry work, dishwashing, hairdressing) that require frequent contact with water or irritating chemicals should be avoided. Evaporation from the skin leads to dryness and can flare AD. Thus, after swimming, exercise, or bathing the skin should be patted dry and a moisturizer applied immediately.

These recommendations should not be construed as meaning that AD patients should not participate fully in life. Rather, because AD is chronic and chronically relapsing, the habits of trigger avoidance and proper skin care need to be ingrained at an early age and practiced throughout life. Children need not be kept from participation in outdoor activities, swimming, or other sports. Excessive dietary manipulation can lead to malnourishment, which likewise needs to be avoided.

Skin Care

Bathing need not be prohibited. Bathing hydrates the skin. To take advantage of this hydration, moisturizer must be applied within 3 minutes to prevent evaporation from the skin and resulting dryness. Generally, lotions are insufficient for patients with AD. Petrolatum is the gold standard. Myriad ointments are available and acceptable, including Aquaphor and Crisco. For modest dryness, creams (e.g., Nivea, Cetaphil, Eucerin) can be adequate and more acceptable to patients. Products containing hydroxy acids, phenol, or urea can ameliorate scaling and dryness but can also sting inflamed skin and should be used with caution. Mild superfatted soaps such as Dove and Oil of Olay are recommended. Soap substitutes such as Cetaphil are also acceptable. Bubble baths and scented bath salts and oils can be irritating, although unscented products help; a nonskid rubber mat in the tub is recommended to prevent injury. Scalp care should include a bland shampoo (Dupinol). Tar shampoo (DHS), baths (Balnetar), and topical cream or lotion (5 to 10% liquor carbonis detergens) are helpful. Baths, Burow's soaks, or compresses can ameliorate crusted, infected, eczematous patches. Cotton clothing, washed to remove finishing (often formaldehyde-containing or -releasing), is preferred.

Topical Corticosteroids

Trigger factor avoidance and skin care are often inadequate, and topical steroids may be needed to control pruritus and inflammation. Ointments are preferred except in markedly humid environments. Creams are generally second choice, usually when compliance is an issue. Skin penetration is improved if topical steroids are applied immediately after bathing. A balance needs to be found between the desire to reduce the risks of side effects and the desire to quickly gain control of a flare with more potent preparations. Chronic use of inadequately potent topical steroids may pose more risk of side effects than does brief use of more potent agents that allow rapid taper to bland emollients. Potent topical steroids should be avoided in areas most susceptible to steroid-induced atrophy: face, intertriginous areas (groins, axillae, inframammary folds), and under diapers.

For these susceptible areas, 0.5 to 1% hydrocortisone (Cortaid, Hytone) or 0.05% desonide (DesOwen) ointments are appropriate. For the rest of the body, triamcinolone acetonide 0.1% ointment (Aristocort A), a moderately potent preparation, in 1-pound jars, is a good value. Other midpotency preparations such as fluocinolone acetonide (Synalar) and betamethasone valerate (Valisone) are also useful. For lichenified plaques, 0.05% fluocinonide (Lidex) and desoximetasone 0.25% (Topicort), which are more potent ointments, are useful. Flurandrenolide (Cordran) tape helps prurigo nodularis lesions because it also physically protects the area from scratching. For scalp lesions, fluocinolone acetonide 0.01% solution (Synalar, Fluonid) is often adequate, but more potent solutions such as 0.05% fluocinonide (Lidex) may be required. Sprays such as triamcinolone acetonide 0.1% (Kenalog) may be preferred. Blacks may prefer creams or ointments for the scalp to reduce matting that can occur with solutions.

Antimicrobials

AD skin is virtually always colonized with *S. aureus*; superinfection is common. For localized disease, mupirocin 2% ointment (Bactroban) should be used. For more extensive disease, oral antistaphylococcal therapy, such as cephalexin (Keflex), 25 to 50 mg per kg per day, is required. Some find such treatment useful for lesions that are not frank cellulitis, perhaps by reducing superantigens. Eczema herpeticum should be treated with oral or intravenous therapy as detailed elsewhere.

Control of Pruritus

Typically, nonsedating antihistamines are inadequate for treating AD pruritus. Oral agents such as hydroxyzine (Atarax) or diphenhydramine (Benadryl), 2 to 5 mg per kg per day, can help, particularly at bedtime. Topical doxepin (Zonalon) can help but can likewise be sedating. Measures to reduce inflammation outlined previously are the best ways to reduce pruritus. Also, addressing psychologic factors, such as stress, secondary gain, or boredom, can assist in pruritus reduction.

Advanced Therapy

Numerous phototherapy regimens exist, including ultraviolet B (UVB), combined ultraviolet A (UVA)/UVB, narrow-band UVA, psoralen photochemotherapy, and photopheresis. Systemic corticosteroids are rarely indicated because of risks of side effects and rebound exacerbation after cessation. Immunosuppression can help: methotrexate,* 10 to 25 mg weekly; azathioprine* (Imuran), 50 to 200 mg per day; and cyclosporine* (Sandimmune), 5 mg per kg per day tapered to 3 mg per kg every other day. Promising therapeutic approaches include interferon gamma-1b* (Actimmune), topical FK506* (Tacrolimus [Prograf]), photopheresis,* and Chinese herbal medicine.

---

*Not FDA approved for this indication.

ERYTHEMA MULTIFORME

method of
DARLENE S. JOHNSON, M.D.
Harvard Medical School

and

KENNETH ARNDT, M.D.
Harvard Medical School and Beth Israel Deaconess Medical Center
Boston, Massachusetts

Erythema multiforme (EM) is a term used to describe a spectrum of inflammatory cutaneous and mucocutaneous eruptions of variable form. Multiple classifications have been proposed based on morphology of lesions and extent of involvement. Erythema multiforme minor is described as a sudden onset of target (iris) lesions with a symmetrical, primarily extensor, and sun-exposed distribution, which may have no or one mucous membrane involved with erosions. EM minor affects otherwise healthy young adults and has no race or sex predilection. It is self-limited, resolving within 2 to 4 weeks, often leaving residual hyperpigmentation. Erythema multiforme major is a possibly life-threatening condition often manifesting with a prodrome of constitutional symptoms: fever, cough, sore throat, myalgias, and malaise. It is more generalized than EM minor, with prominent truncal lesions, involvement of two or more mucosal surfaces, and association with systemic toxicity (lung, liver, kidney). It occurs primarily in children and young adults. EM major has been divided into five categories: bullous erythema multiforme, Stevens-Johnson syndrome (SJS), overlap SJS–toxic epidermal necrolysis (TEN), TEN with discrete lesions, and generalized TEN. Whether this represents a continuum of disease or independent diseases is unknown. This chapter does not address TEN.

TREATMENT

The treatment of these entities is directed at removing possible antigenic stimuli to which an inflammatory response has been mounted. It was originally thought that EM was a result of circulating antibody-antigen (AB-Ag) complexes. However, histologic sections are suggestive of a delayed type of hypersensitivity reaction showing lymphocyte and basophil infiltrates with fibrin deposition. Recent studies demonstrated an increased expression of intercellular adhesion molecule 1 (ICAM-1), up-regulation of VPF/VEGF mRNA, and their receptors flt-1 and KDR in lesional skin, further emphasizing the inflammatory nature of these lesions. Infections, medications, chemical exposures, and systemic diseases have all been implicated as triggers (Table 1). The work-up listed in Table 2 is suggested to evaluate for possible etiologic agents, as well as extent of systemic involvement.

For EM minor, especially recurrent or persistent EM minor, a preceding herpes simplex virus (HSV) infection is the most common cause. HSV has been detected in EM lesional skin and lesion-resolved skin, implying the significance of clinical and subclinical infections. Sun avoidance with the use of sunscreens (SPF 15+), protective clothing, and avoidance of the midday sun (10 AM to 3 PM) is the most basic care to prevent future flares. Ultraviolet radiation exposure has been shown not only to trigger HSV infection but also to independently increase ICAM-1 expression, perhaps accounting for the photodistribution of EM minor. Acyclovir, 400 mg twice a day for 6 months, has been shown in a double-blind, placebo-controlled trial to decrease recurrent eruptions of EM. The dose should be titrated to effect after 6 months and intermittently discontinued to determine necessity of treatment. Newer antiviral agents should also be effective (Valtex, 500 mg daily by mouth; Famvir, 250 mg orally twice daily). Because of the inflammatory nature of EM, numerous anti-inflammatory agents have been used anecdotally to suppress the inflammatory reaction until the activating agent has been eliminated. For recurrent EM not responsive to acyclovir, anecdotal reports include the use of hydroxychloroquine, dapsone, colchicine, azathioprine, and potassium iodine. When these drugs fail, thalidomide, 100 mg orally every day (subsequently titrated to effect), has been prescribed. One must closely monitor the patient for changes on electromyography and peripheral neuropathy with thalidomide use. For oral EM lesions, a double-blind cross-over trial of 14 patients showed that levamisole, 100 to 150 mg orally (with meals) every day for 3 consecutive days each week at first appearance of a lesion, decreased severity, duration, and frequency of attacks at a 2-year follow-up.

The etiologic agent for EM major most commonly is a medication. Trimethoprim-sulfamethoxazole (Bactrim, Septra), carbamazepine (Tegretol), phenobarbital, phenytoin (Dilantin), valproic acid (Depakene, Depakote), allopurinol, and oxicam nonsteroidal anti-inflammatory agents are the most commonly implicated medications. Stopping all nonessential medications is imperative, and implicated agents should be avoided permanently. Of note, carbamazepine (Tegretol), phenobarbital, and phenytoin (Dilantin) have cross-sensitization. Therefore, if an anticonvulsant needs to be continued, valproic acid (Depakene, Depakote) could be an alternative (nevertheless, this agent also carries its own increased relative risk of EM). If infectious agents such as *Mycoplasma pneumoniae* are thought to be present, they must be treated.

Care should be individualized depending on the needs of the patient and the extent of disease. Most fundamental is the need for meticulous skin and wound care to minimize risk of secondary infection. Pruritic or painful skin lesions may be treated for symptomatic relief with a topical moisturizer that does not contain possible allergens such as lanolin, fragrances, or preservatives (hydrated petrolatum twice daily full body); systemic antihistamines (hydroxyzine [Atarax, Vistaril]), 25 to 50 mg orally or intramuscularly every 4 to 6 hours; or analgesics (acetaminophen [Tylenol]), 500 mg orally every 6 hours, preferably not nonsteroidal anti-inflammato-

TABLE 1. **Possible Etiologic Agents for Erythema Multiforme***

- Medications
  - Antimicrobials
    - Aminopenicillamines
    - Ciprofloxacin (Cipro)
    - Dideoxycytidine (ddC)
    - Erythromycin
    - Griseofulvin (Fulvicin)
    - Minocycline (Minocin)
    - **Nitrofurantoin**
    - Pyrazinamide
    - Sulfa derivatives
      - pyrimethamine-sulfadoxine (Fansidar)
      - **trimethoprim-sulfamethoxazole (Bactrim, Septra)**
    - Terbinafine (Lamisil)
    - Tetracycline/Doxycycline (Vibramycin)
    - Vancomycin
  - Anticonvulsants
    - **Carbamazepine (Tegretol)**
    - **Phenobarbital**
    - **Phenytoin (Dilantin)**
    - **Valproic acid (Depakene, Depakote)**
  - Antimetabolites
    - 9-Bromofluorene
    - Cyclophosphamide (Cytoxan)
    - Cyclosporine (Sandimmune)
    - Methotrexate
    - Nitrogen mustards
  - Miscellaneous
    - Acetazolamide (Diamox)
    - **Allopurinol (Zyloprim)**
    - Amlodipine (Norvasc)
    - Cimetidine (Tagamet)
    - Clofibrate (Atromid-S)
    - Corticosteroids
    - Danazol (Danocrine)
    - Dapsone
    - Diltiazem (Cardizem)
    - Etoposide (VP-16, VePesid)
    - Etretinate (Tegison)
    - Fenbufen (Cinopal)
    - Furosemide (Lasix)
    - Glucagon
    - GM-CSF (Leukine)
    - Intravenous immunoglobulin
    - Lithium
    - Nifedipine (Procardia, Adalat)
    - Progesterone
    - Ritodrine (Yutopar)
    - Theophylline (Slo-Phyllin, Elixophyllin)
    - Tocainide (Tonocard)
- Infectious
  - Bacterial
    - Bacterial endotoxin (lipopolysaccharide)
    - *Haemophilus influenzae*
    - *Pseudomonas*
    - Psittacosis
    - Tularemia
    - *Vibrio parahaemolyticus*
  - Viral
    - Adenovirus
    - EBV
    - Hepatitis B and C
    - HIV
    - Human Orf
    - HSV
    - Parvovirus B19
  - Other
    - Dermatophytosis
    - Histoplasmosis
    - *Mycoplasma pneumoniae*
    - *Trichomonas*
- Immunizations
  - BCG
  - dT
  - Hepatitis B
- Chemicals
  - Arsenic
  - Budesonide
  - Capsicum
  - Epoxy sealant
  - Hair dyes
  - Insecticide spray
  - Isopropyl-p-phenylenediamine of rubber
  - Nickel and cobalt contact
  - Reaction to patch testing
  - Rhus antigen
  - Sesquiterpene lactone in herbal medicine
- Neoplasms
  - Renal cell carcinoma
  - T cell lymphoma
- Systemic disorders
  - Lymphatic obstruction
  - Inflammatory bowel disease (Crohn's, ulcerative colitis)
- Miscellaneous
  - Deep radiation therapy
  - Salmon berries

*Inclusive, but not exhaustive, list of medical literature since 1978.
Bold notation for agents with increased crude relative risks in case-control studies.
Abbreviations: EBV = Epstein-Barr virus; HIV = human immunodeficiency virus; HSV = herpes simplex virus; BCG = bacille Calmette-Guérin; dT = diphtheria and tetanus.

ries. For oozing and crusted erosive skin lesions, frequent wet-to-damp compresses may be used (sterile water/or Domeboro compresses mixed as directed, applied for 30 to 60 minutes, three to four times a day). Because of possible cross-sensitization with etiologic sulfa-containing agents (trimethoprim-sulfamethoxazole [Bactrim], furosemide [Lasix]), silver sulfadiazine (Silvadene) should be avoided. Blood, urine, and wounds should be cultured frequently, as well as during fever spikes, to monitor for possible infection. The use of indwelling catheters and lines should be minimized. With signs of infection or sepsis, broad-spectrum antibiotics should be started and tailored to results of culture sensitivities (avoid the use of drugs etiologically associated with EM [e.g., sulfonamides and penicillins]).

If more than 20% of body surface area is involved with total skin thickness sloughing, treatment in a burn unit is optimal. Patients must be monitored closely for fluid and electrolyte abnormalities, protein losses, compromise of major organ function, sufficient caloric intake for increased metabolism, and special needs of wound care (use of biologic dressings, allografts, or porcine xenografts). For oral lesions,

TABLE 2. **Laboratory Evaluation for Erythema Multiforme**

Complete blood count with differential
Erythrocyte sedimentation rate
Urinalysis
Chest radiography
Serologic studies for *Mycoplasma* infection
Cultures of skin, blood, urine

mouthwashes (chlorhexidine gluconate [Peridex]) or irrigations (hydrogen peroxide and water 1:1 three times a day swish and spit) should be used to minimize infection. For anesthetic relief, 2% viscous lidocaine, or a mixture of 2% viscous lidocaine, Kaopectate, and diphenhydramine (Benadryl) (1:1:1) may be used. A liquid, soft diet, nasogastric feedings, or parental nutrition may be needed to ensure adequate intake. Ocular manifestations carry possible long-term complications of lid deformities, adhesions, and blindness. Early evaluation by an ophthalmologist is recommended to direct proper irrigations, tear replacement, adhesion lysis, surveillance cultures, and topical antibiotic uses.

The use of systemic immune modulatory agents is considered imperative in some studies and contraindicated in others. No controlled trials regarding the use of oral steroids in the treatment of severe erythema multiforme have been carried out, and their use remains controversial. The addition of steroids may further increase the risk of infection and, therefore, mortality rates. However, some case series, in both adult and pediatric literature, argue that early use of corticosteroids reduces the period of acute eruption, reduces the period of fever, and yields milder signs of prostration. A prospective study of 41 patients advocated the use of early oral prednisone (1 to 2 mg per kg per 24 hours until stabilization and/or improvement), or intravenous methylprednisolone (Solu-Medrol), 4 mg per kg per day, to minimize visceral organ involvement, a treatment considered life-saving for some cases. The addition of cyclophosphamide* (Cytoxan), 150 mg over 1 hour every 24 hours, to oral prednisone, 15 mg orally every 6 hours, is reported to have dramatic improvement and reversal of EM major. In HIV-infected patients with EM, major use of intravenous immunoglobulin* (Gamimune), 400 mg per kg per 24 hours for 3 to 5 days, may prevent or shorten hospitalization.

*Not FDA approved for this indication.

BULLOUS DISEASES

method of
LUIS A. DIAZ, M.D., and
SHARON A. FOLEY, M.D.
Medical College of Wisconsin
Milwaukee, Wisconsin

PEMPHIGUS SYNDROMES

Pemphigus encompasses a group of autoimmune blistering diseases characterized by flaccid, thin-walled, easily ruptured bullae resulting in large areas of denuded skin. In some clinical variants, especially pemphigus vulgaris, before the introduction of corticosteroids, mortality was 50%. Currently, the mortality rate in treated patients is approximately 10%. This is largely a result of steroid and immunosuppressant therapy complications. There are five recognized clinical variants, which include pemphigus vulgaris and its localized variant pemphigus vegetans, foliaceus, erythematosus, drug-induced, and paraneoplastic. Each is characterized by the presence of tissue-bound autoantibodies to specific desmosomal protein antigens. It is thought that these autoantibodies lead to separation of keratinocytes and resultant intraepidermal blisters.

Pemphigus Vulgaris

Pemphigus vulgaris (PV) is the most common form of pemphigus, generally seen in the fourth or fifth decade of life. It rarely affects children. The blisters typically affect the scalp, face, trunk, groin, and axilla. The individual lesions are tender and when ruptured can coalesce into large patches of denuded skin, which become partially covered with crusts. If the area is extensive, patients can be quite debilitated. Initially only a few innocuous bullae may occur, but typically the disease evolves into a more generalized and extensive eruption within weeks. The lesions heal slowly and leave residual hyperpigmentation and hypopigmentation, although scar formation is rare. Because of the lack of cohesion between keratinocytes, with minimal pressure the upper layer of the epidermis can be made to slip laterally. This results in extension of the bullae, known as the Nikolsky sign. Although characteristic, this sign is not pathognomonic of PV, as it can also be seen in toxic epidermal necrosis and *Staphylococcus* scalded skin disease.

Approximately 50 to 60% of patients present with oral lesions, which can precede cutaneous disease by several months. The appearance of a desquamative gingivitis is common. Erosive mucosal involvement can extend from mouth to esophagus, causing severe pain, especially with ingestion of food. Other involved areas include the nasal mucosa, conjunctiva, larynx, vagina, cervix, and anus. PV has been reported to be associated with other autoimmune diseases, most commonly myasthenia gravis and thymoma, as well as systemic lupus.

Early blisters are the best to select for biopsy. The characteristic histologic finding is the presence of suprabasilar bullae. This results from the characteristic loss of normal adhesion between epidermal keratinocytes (acantholysis). Many of the acantholytic cells lie in clusters within the bullae. Usually there is little inflammation.

Direct immunofluorescence (IF) is a reliable diagnostic test for PV and is positive in almost 100% of cases, even in the very early stages of disease. Unfixed frozen sections of perilesional or uninvolved skin are used. A positive test results in fluorescent staining of the intercellular spaces (ICS) of the epidermis. IgG is almost always present, and in 50% there are also deposits of IgA, IgM, or C3.

Indirect IF is positive in 80 to 90% of patients demonstrating antiepidermal ICS autoantibodies. The autoantibody titer roughly correlates with disease activity and should be monitored during therapy. IgG is the most frequent autoantibody demonstrated, and occasionally IgA autoantibodies are seen. It is well established that PV autoantibodies are pathogenic (i.e., they reproduce the classic clinical, histologic, and immunologic features of PV when passively transferred to experimental animals). It is postulated that these autoantibodies may impair the adhesive function of desmoglein 3, the desmosomal antigen recognized by these antibodies. Epidermal cell detachment and blister formation may result from this antigen-antibody reaction. Complement is not required in this model.

Skin lesions can be painful in advanced cases of PV, and patients frequently are treated similarly to burn patients. Electrolytes and fluid status should be monitored closely. Silver sulfadiazene (Silvadene) is an effective topical antimicrobial agent. Wet dressings such as 1:40 aluminum acetate (Burow's) solution can be applied for 15 to 20 minutes two to three times a day. Although of limited value, topical fluorinated steroids can be applied to perilesional inflamed skin. Many patients are started on prophylactic antibiotics owing to an increased risk for sepsis. Painful oral ulcers can be treated with viscous lidocaine or topical triamcinolone acetonide in an adherent base (Kenalog in Orabase).

Although PV tends to be a chronic disease, treatment can result in long-term remission in some patients. The disease behaves differently for each patient, so treatment plans must be designed to suit an individual's requirement. The majority of patients ultimately require immunosuppressive therapy.

The initial treatment of choice is prednisone. Patients typically respond to prednisone at doses of 1 to 2 mg per kg per day given as a single dose each morning. Response to therapy is adequate if patients develop only one to two new blisters a week, and if existing lesions heal progressively quicker. If the disease is well controlled at 1 mg per kg per day for 6 to 8 weeks, a fairly rapid taper of 5 mg per week can be started until the patient reaches 40 mg per day. Prednisone is then further tapered by 2.5 mg every other day each week until a dose of 25 mg every other day is obtained. It is then tapered by 2.5 mg every other day every 2 weeks until discontinued. The autoantibody titer is a good indicator of disease activity and should be checked every 2 months. Initially controlling the disease with higher doses of prednisone (200 to 400 mg per day) has been advocated (although in our practice doses > 100 mg per day have rarely been used), but this can increase the risk of life-threatening infection.

Additional immunosuppressants are often required for disease control or for their steroid-sparing effects. A variety of immunosuppressant agents have been used. Azathioprine* (Imuran), cyclophosphamide* (Cytoxan), and methotrexate* (Rheumatrex) are the most beneficial. Because these agents can take 4 to 6 weeks to take effect, they are not the treatment of choice for acute phase PV. They are typically begun once the prednisone is tapered to 40 mg per day.

Azathioprine (Imuran) is the most widely used agent in doses of 1 to 2 mg per kg per day. Bone marrow suppression, hepatotoxicity, and increased risk of malignancy are the major adverse effects. A chemistry profile and complete blood count (CBC) should be routinely monitored, initially every 2 weeks, and once safety is established, every 4 to 6 weeks.

Cyclophosphamide (Cytoxan) is an effective alternative to azathioprine. Doses of 1 to 3 mg per kg per day are typically used. Significant adverse effects include bone marrow suppression, sterility, and increased long-term risk for malignancy, as well as bladder fibrosis, bladder cancer, and hemorrhagic cystitis. Patients must have routine monitoring of CBCs and microscopic urinalysis. Cystitis can be reduced by taking the drug early in the morning and increasing fluid intake. Some reports have claimed good therapeutic response with the use of intravenous (IV) Cytoxan in PV patients.

Less often, methotrexate (Rheumatrex) has been used as adjunctive therapy, at doses of 10 to 30 mg per week. Patients should be monitored for leukopenia, thrombocytopenia, and hepatotoxicity. Concomitant administration of folic acid 1 mg per day can decrease the incidence of gastrointestinal distress and stomatitis. Routine CBC and chemistry is necessary, and some advocate a baseline liver biopsy and repeat biopsy at a cumulative dose of 1.5 grams.

Intramuscular gold sodium thiomalate (Myochrysine) and gold thioglucose (Solganal) have both been used successfully as steroid-sparing agents. A test dose of 10 mg intramuscularly (IM) is followed by 25 mg 1 week later, then 50 mg each week. Response is slow, with beneficial effect first seen at 500 mg to 1 gram. Maintenance therapy then consists of 50 mg IM every 2 to 4 weeks. Approximately 40% of patients experience adverse effects. These include nitroid reactions, mucocutaneous eruptions, nephritis, leukopenia, and thrombocytopenia. A CBC and urine microanalysis are obtained before each IM dose.

*Not FDA approved for this indication.

There is no evidence that oral gold therapy is beneficial in the management of patients with pemphigus.

Plasma exchange has been used sparingly in the management of steroid-resistant widespread PV. It may be useful in bringing acute disease under control, particularly in patients with high-titer autoantibodies. Concomitant corticosteroids and immunosuppressive agents must always be used to prevent a rebound in autoantibodies.

Any patient with widespread skin disease on high-dose steroids and immunosuppression is at risk for opportunistic infection. This is a major cause of mortality in pemphigus.

Pemphigus vegetans is a localized variant of PV in which flaccid bullae develop, primarily in the intertriginous regions, which erode and heal with papillomatous proliferation. Large coalescing verrucous vegetations are not uncommon. The histologic findings are identical to PV, with the exception of increased papillary proliferation and marked epidermal hyperplasia. Otherwise the pathogenesis, laboratory findings, and treatment are similar to those of PV.

Pemphigus Foliaceus

Pemphigus foliaceus (PF), is a less aggressive, chronic variant of PV, with lower morbidity and mortality. It is characterized by superficial blisters occurring high in the epidermis. Therefore, intact blisters are rarely seen, and crusts and erosions tend to dominate the clinical picture. The disease most commonly occurs in adults between the ages of 30 and 40. Common areas of involvement include the face, scalp, upper chest, and back, although it can be generalized. Oral involvement is not seen. Patients generally are not severely ill but can experience pain, burning, and pruritus. Histologic findings are similar to those in PV; epidermal bullae and intercellular acantholysis are seen. However, the acantholysis is more superficial, occurring in the upper epidermis usually in the granular layer. Direct IF demonstrates intercellular IgG throughout the epidermis. Indirect IF is usually positive, demonstrating circulating autoantibodies directed against the epidermal ICS. Treatment, although less vigorous, is similar to that for PV.

Fogo selvagem, a variant of PF, is endemic in Brazil and other South American countries. Clinically, cutaneous involvement is similar to that for PF, with lesions found primarily in seborrheic areas of the face and trunk. However, it occurs in younger adults, primarily women, and children. One third of cases occur before age 20 and two thirds by the age of 40. The lesions frequently cause a painful burning sensation. The etiology, although not yet fully determined, is thought to be secondary to an environmental agent unique to the endemic areas of Brazil.

Pemphigus Erythematosus

Pemphigus erythematosus (Senear-Usher syndrome) is a less severe variant of pemphigus that shares the same clinical and serologic features as PF. In addition, patients with pemphigus erythematosus possess a lupus-associated serology and in rare cases the clinical manifestations of lupus (i.e., nephritis). The skin eruption occurs primarily on the face, scalp, upper chest, and back. Facial involvement may occur in a characteristic butterfly distribution similar to lupus erythematosus. Thickly crusted erythematous lesions are typical, but atrophy is not commonly present. Direct IF from perilesional skin reveals intercellular staining with IgG and C3. In addition, the lupus band test is present in 60% of patients. Antinuclear antibodies are also demonstrated in approximately 30%. Treatment is similar to that of PF; however, the disease is controlled with lower doses of prednisone.

Drug-Induced Pemphigus

Drug-induced pemphigus is a disease with clinical and immunologic features suggestive of pemphigus but is induced by drugs. It occurs most commonly with D-penicillamine (Cuprimine), inducing features most reminiscent of PF. Other drugs that have been implicated include captopril (Capoten), penicillin, and rifampin (Rifadin).

Paraneoplastic Pemphigus

Paraneoplastic pemphigus is a recently recognized mucocutaneous blistering disease associated with specific antiepidermal autoantibodies that are unique to this syndrome. A severe mucositis and skin erosions are typical findings. It is associated with underlying malignancy, usually lymphoproliferative in origin. The mortality rate is high.

BULLOUS PEMPHIGOID

Bullous pemphigoid (BP) is an autoimmune, subepidermal blistering disease occurring primarily in middle-aged and elderly people. It is characterized by the development of tense bullae on inflamed skin, typically in flexural areas such as the groin, axilla, and antecubital and popliteal fossae. In contrast to PV, large denuded areas of skin typically do not occur, lesions heal spontaneously without scarring, and there is no increase in mortality. Prednisone is the primary therapeutic agent, although immunosuppressants may be required.

BP is a disease of the elderly, with the average age of onset between 65 and 75, although it can occur in younger people and children. Males and females are equally affected, and there is no human leukocyte antigen (HLA) association. Although the classic feature is a tense, dome-shaped bullae on normal or erythematous skin, the clinical presentation can vary, and erythematous patches and urticarial plaques may also occur. Pruritus may be intense and can warn of an ensuing BP eruption. Mucous membrane involvement is infrequent and asymptomatic. Oral lesions may occur in 20% of patients. The bullae are tough and can last intact for days; when they rupture, they leave erosions that heal rapidly with minimal postinflammatory changes. Although a mild leukocytosis can accompany the eruption, patients in general feel well. Peripheral eosinophilia may occur in 50% of patients.

BP has occasionally been associated with other diseases such as rheumatoid arthritis, ulcerative colitis, myasthenia gravis, and thymoma. In general it is not thought to be an indicator or a manifestation of underlying malignancy. BP has been induced by several drugs, including furosemide (Lasix) and ibuprofen (Motrin).

Biopsy results are fairly characteristic when taken from early bullae arising on erythematous skin. The earliest histologic feature is cleft formation at the dermoepidermal junction. Subepidermal bullae are then seen in association with a superficial dermal infiltrate. The amount of infiltrate is variable. When "cell rich," it consists of extensive accumulations of eosinophils intermingled with mononuclear cells and scattered neutrophils typically in close approximation to the epidermis. The inflammatory cells can extend into the bulla cavity. Eosinophilic spongiosis may precede these more classic findings.

Direct IF is positive in close to 100% of patients. Unfixed frozen sections of the patient's perilesional skin are used. The IF staining produces a linear pattern along the basement membrane zone (BMZ). IgG is found in 80% of patients, and C3 is detectable in all patients. Occasionally, early in the disease, only C3 is found and IgG is absent. IgA and IgM are each present in 25% of cases.

Indirect IF is positive in 70% of cases, demonstrating circulating anti-BMZ autoantibodies that are always of the IgG class. Unlike with PV, there is no correlation between the titer and the disease activity. Even patients with long-standing active disease may not have circulating autoantibodies. The finding of anti-BMZ autoantibodies is not specific to BP and has also been reported in some patients with burns, *Staphylococcus* scalded skin syndrome, psoriasis, leg ulcers, and eczema.

BP serum contains two populations of autoantibodies that recognize hemidesmosomal antigens: the BP230 antigen and a transmembrane glycoprotein named the PB180 antigen. The ectodomain of the BP180 antigen contains a cluster of epitopes that are recognized by all patients as demonstrated by enzyme-linked immunosorbent assay (ELISA) technique. Experimentally produced antibodies to the BP180 antigen are pathogenic when transferred to experimental animals. They reproduce the clinical, histologic, and immunologic features of BP in these animals. The lesion in BP is the result of recruitment and activation of neutrophils by complement activation. We have recently shown that neutrophil elastase is the major culprit in inducing the subepidermal blisters in this experimental model of BP.

Oral corticosteroids are the mainstay of therapy for BP. The majority of patients respond to 1 mg per kg per day given as a single morning dose. It usually takes a week for new blister formation to stop and bullae to heal. The prednisone is then tapered slowly over months as previously outlined. Unlike with PV, corticosteroid-sparing immunosuppressants are required in a minority of cases. Azathioprine* (Imuran), 1 mg per kg per day, appears to be effective and has been the most widely used agent for BP. Other alternative agents include cyclophosphamide* (Cytoxan) and methotrexate* (Rheumatrex). Their dosing schedules and significant adverse side effects were noted previously under the treatment of PV. A small percentage of patients with BP (10%) may respond to dapsone (50 to 150 mg per day) or sulfapyridine. These patients tend to be younger and have a predominantly neutrophilic infiltrate on histopathology. Dapsone is particularly effective in patients with localized oral disease. Occasionally, localized disease may be treated with topical corticosteroids alone. A mid- to high-potency preparation is usually necessary. Tetracycline 1.5 to 2.0 grams daily, alone or in combination with niacinamide, 1.5 grams daily, has also been reported to be effective in some cases of limited disease. In general, prolonged clinical remission is the usual outcome in BP patients.

CICATRICIAL PEMPHIGOID

Cicatricial pemphigoid (CP) is an uncommon chronic subepidermal blistering disease involving the mucous membranes and resulting in permanent scarring of affected areas.

CP can occur at any age, although middle age is most frequent. The female/male ratio is 2:1. The oral mucosa is almost always involved (90% of cases). In the mouth, small vesicles or bullae are seen, which can remain intact for long periods and are slow to heal. Eventually extensive erosions can develop over the palate and buccal mucosa, resulting in a reticulate scarring similar to that of lichen planus. Conjunctival lesions are also common and seen in 66% of cases. Involvement is usually bilateral and associated with erythema and flaccid vesicles, which result in fibrous adhesions (symblepharon) and scarring. Vesicles and inflammation with scarring can also occur in the pharynx, larynx, esophagus, nose, anus, and vagina. Although the general health of the patient is rarely affected, it can be debilitating, with resultant mutilation. Unlike in BP, remissions are rare; the disease extends over many years, with periods of activity followed by quiescence every several months.

Histologically, CP is indistinguishable from BP. It shows subepidermal blisters, but usually with fewer eosinophils than in BP. Fibroblasts can be seen at a later stage, resulting in fibrosis and scarring in the upper dermis. Direct IF studies of perilesional tissues show features identical to those of BP, with IgG and C3 deposition in a linear pattern at the BMZ in 80 to 90% of cases. Less commonly, IgA and IgM are present. However, indirect IF reveals circulating IgG

*Not FDA approved for this indication.

antibodies in only a small number of patients (20%) and usually in low titer. As with BP, the titer does not correlate with disease activity.

Therapy for CP depends on the severity of the disease and the organs involved. Prednisone is administered in a fashion similar to that for BP at doses of 1 mg per kg per day. Because of the scarring nature and risk for blindness with ocular involvement associated with CP, immunosuppressants are commonly required. Cyclophosphamide* (Cytoxan) and azathioprine* (Imuran) are the most frequently used immunosuppressants. Unfortunately, some patients with severe CP receive only partial benefit from such combined therapy. Dapsone* (50 to 150 mg per day) may be of benefit, especially for patients who have exclusive intraoral disease.

HERPES GESTATIONIS

Herpes gestationis (HG) is a rare, pruritic subepidermal nonscarring bullous disease with onset during pregnancy. It is estimated to occur in 1/10,000 to 1/60,000 pregnancies. It has several clinical, histologic, and immunopathologic features similar to those of BP.

HG typically begins during the second or third trimester of pregnancy, with average onset at 21 weeks of gestation. It can also occur around the time of delivery, or in the immediate postpartum period. Although the disease is generally self-limited and remits spontaneously, it can recur with subsequent pregnancies, menstrual periods, or the taking of oral contraceptives. Intense pruritus is the hallmark of the disease. The eruption consists of urticarial plaques and papules that develop around the umbilicus and then spread to the abdomen, trunk, and thighs. The oral mucosa, face, and scalp are usually spared. Tense vesicles and bullae may occur in a polycylic or annular configuration.

Maternal health is usually not affected, but there is some controversy as to whether fetal survival is adversely affected. In less than 5% of cases, infants may experience a transient urticarial, vesicular, or bullous eruption during the first several weeks.

Histology reveals subepidermal bullae with eosinophils. The bullae occur secondary to basal cell necrosis. Early urticarial lesions have epidermal and papillary dermal edema, with occasional foci of eosinophilic spongiosis. Differentiation of HG from other subepidermal blistering diseases can be difficult.

Indirect IF reveals circulating IgG anti-BMZ autoantibodies in only 10 to 20% of patients, usually in low titer. However, in nearly 75% of patients, a complement-fixing IgG autoantibody (the "herpes gestationis factor") can be demonstrated by complement-enhanced IF. Direct IF studies show strong linear staining of C3 at the cutaneous BMZ.

Treatment typically involves symptomatic relief. Prednisone (1 mg per kg per day) is the initial drug of choice and typically can be used safely throughout the remainder of the pregnancy. The dose is titered to the minimum amount necessary to control blister formation and pruritus. Antihistamines are also occasionally required. Rarely plasmapheresis is needed for severe cases. The disease generally subsides within 6 months.

*Not FDA approved for this indication.

DERMATITIS HERPETIFORMIS

Dermatitis herpetiformis (DH) is a rare, chronic, recurrent papulovesicular disease characterized by intense pruritus. The eruption is symmetrical and pleomorphic, with papular, papulovesicular, vesiculobullous, bullous, or urticarial lesions. The majority of patients have a gluten-sensitive enteropathy, suggesting that DH is a systemic disease.

DH occurs mainly between the ages of 20 and 55 years, with the median age of onset in the third decade. The male/female ratio is 2:1. The onset may be acute or chronic, with pruritus frequently manifesting as the heralding sign. Once present, the disease is lifelong, characterized by periods of exacerbation and quiescence. Spontaneous remission is rare. The typical lesions are erythematous papules or groups of small 3- to 6-mm vesicles; bullae are rare. Frequently, the only manifestation is the presence of excoriations due to pruritus. The eruption is characteristically symmetrical, primarily on extensor surfaces such as the knees, elbows, buttocks, sacrum, and natal cleft. Lesions can heal with hypopigmentation and hyperpigmentation, but scarring is rare. The mucous membranes are rarely involved.

Direct IF of noninvolved skin reveals granular IgA deposition at the BMZ and the dermal papilla. Although deposition of IgA and C3 is the most common and characteristic finding, IgM and IgG may also be found in association with IgA.

A variety of autoantibodies have been detected in DH patients; their pathophysiologic significance is unknown. These include antithyroid, antigluten, and antireticulin autoantibodies. An IgA autoantibody against endomysium, a smooth muscle component, has also been identified in 70% of patients. This autoantibody is almost never seen in other diseases. The actual target of autoimmunity in DH is unknown.

Thyroid disorders are increased in patients with DH and include Graves' disease and Hashimoto's thyroiditis and idiopathic hypothyroidism. Antithyroglobulin and antimicrosomal antibodies are also seen. There is an increased incidence of malignancy, primarily small bowel lymphoma. The association of achlorhydria, atrophic gastritis, and pernicious anemia is well established. There have also been sporadic associations with other autoimmune diseases, including rheumatoid arthritis, systemic lupus, ulcerative colitis, and Sjögren's disease.

Small bowel disease similar to that seen in adult celiac disease, characterized by jejunal atrophy, can occur. Patients with this condition appear to be antigenically stimulated by gluten, with the formation of IgA antibodies, and resultant gastrointestinal and cutaneous changes. Although deficiencies of folate, vitamin B_{12}, and iron can occur secondary to malabsorption, less then 5% have symptoms of steatorrhea. The patchy jejunal involvement can improve with a gluten-free diet.

Cutaneous histology reveals a lymphohistiocytic perivascular infiltrate in the papillary dermis with nuclear dust. Neutrophils then accumulate in the dermal papillae and form micro abscesses, which are pathognomonic. These abscesses then produce papillary edema, which results in a subepidermal blister. Gastrointestinal histopathology reveals a mononuclear cell infiltrate in the lamina propria with villous atrophy.

Dapsone is the treatment of choice for DH. The disease responds rapidly, usually within 3 days of starting therapy. Although dapsone controls the disease, it does not cure it or lead to remission, and discontinuance of therapy causes prompt relapse. Typical starting doses vary from 50 to 100 mg per day. The most common side effects are hemolysis and methemoglobinemia resulting from the oxidizing ability of dapsone. Other less common adverse effects include leukopenia, peripheral neuropathy, toxic hepatitis, and, rarely, fatal agranulocytosis. Reduction of hemoglobin by 2 to 3 grams is to be expected with a compensatory reticulocytosis. Most patients tolerate the decrease in hemoglobin and methemoglobinemia well, but those with cardiopulmonary disease need to be closely monitored. Because patients with a glucose-6-phosphate dehydrogenase (G-6PD) deficiency can experience severe hemolysis, this level should be checked before starting therapy. A baseline CBC and chemistry profile should also be obtained. A CBC should be followed weekly for the first month, then monthly for 5 months, and semiannually thereafter. Liver and renal function should be monitored periodically.

Sulfapyridine is an alternate drug that may be used in patients who do not tolerate dapsone, but it is less effective in controlling the disease. The starting dose is 500 mg two to four times daily. On the average 1.5 grams is needed for maintenance.

In the majority of patients, a gluten-free diet will improve the enteropathy, as well as decrease the dapsone requirement. However, the patient must be highly motivated because gluten is ubiquitous, and the diet must be followed for 6 to 12 months before a benefit is seen.

EPIDERMOLYSIS BULLOSA ACQUISITA

Epidermolysis bullosa acquisita (EBA) is a rare, acquired mechanobullous disease occurring in the elderly population, with distinct clinical and pathologic manifestations.

The clinical manifestations are variable and mimic a number of bullous dermatoses. In general, patients suffer with chronic trauma-induced subepidermal blistering. Blisters, which can be serous or hemorrhagic, tend to be localized to extensor surfaces. Involved skin heals with scarring, milia formation, and hyperpigmentation. The skin is characteristically fragile. Mucosal involvement is variable; but involvement of the mouth, larynx, and esophagus has been reported. The etiology is unclear, but EBA has been reported in association with several diseases such as amyloid, inflammatory bowel disease, multiple myeloma, lymphoma, and sarcoid.

On histopathologic examination, the lesions show subepidermal bullae, with neutrophils predominating over eosinophils, aligned linearly along the dermoepidermal junction.

Direct IF reveals linear IgG along the BMZ in 100% of cases. C3 deposition is reported in most cases. IgA and IgM are seen more frequently in EBA than in BP.

Indirect IF is positive in 50% of cases and is similar to that of BP, revealing circulating anti-BMZ autoantibodies. These autoantibodies are directed against type VII collagen present in anchoring fibrils in the sublamina densa. The pathogenic role of these anti-type VII collagen autoantibodies in blister formation is unknown.

The diagnosis is made primarily by excluding other bullous diseases. Certain features can mimic those of mild dystrophic epidermolysis bullosa (EB), porphyria cutanea tarda (PCT), or BP. Dystrophic EB can be eliminated by lack of family history and PCT ruled out by normal porphyrin analysis. However, to distinguish EBA from BP one must use NaCl split skin for indirect IF. In EBA, autoantibodies stain the roof of the split, and in BP they stain the floor. EM reveals cleavage beneath the basal lamina and IgG deposition in the dermis.

Unfortunately, treatment for EBA is generally unsatisfactory and is primarily supportive. Local wound care involves application of topical antimicrobials such as silver sulfadiazine (Silvadene) or mupirocin (Bactroban). Dressings should be nonadherent such as Telfa, for adhesive tapes and tightly applied dressings will mechanically induce further blistering. Chronic ulcerations may ultimately require skin grafts or other surgical intervention. A few patients with inflammatory lesions may respond to corticosteroids. In general, no systemically administered drugs have been beneficial in the treatment of EBA.

CONTACT DERMATITIS

method of
JOHN E. WOLF, JR., M.D.
Baylor College of Medicine
Houston, Texas

The skin is, among many other things, a barrier—an interface between a person's internal and external environments. It is generally an effective barrier but is thus exposed to many noxious agents, both physical and chemical. These agents may cause contact dermatitis, an inflammation of the skin first described by Pliny the Younger in the first century AD.

There are two general types of contact dermatitis—irritant and allergic—and these, in turn, like any other form of dermatitis (eczema), may be acute, subacute, or chronic. The management of contact dermatitis must account for these variations and must be prefaced by careful description and accurate diagnosis.

Irritant contact dermatitis results from exposure of the skin to inherently injurious chemicals or toxins and does not require allergic sensitization. Examples include dermatitis caused by detergents, household or industrial cleansers, or the sting of the Portuguese man-of-war *Physalia physalis.* On the other hand, allergic contact dermatitis follows exposure to a substance capable of sensitizing the skin; subsequent re-exposure may elicit a contact dermatitis. The classic illustration is *Rhus* contact dermatitis (poison ivy).

AVOIDANCE AND PHYSICAL PROTECTION

With either form of contact dermatitis, a critical component of proper management is identification of the inciting agent followed by careful avoidance of that substance. In the case of irritant contact dermatitis, this information is generally obtained by a probing history of the patient, sometimes combined with a careful examination of the home or work place. Evaluation of allergic contact dermatitis may also include open or closed patch testing.

Once an inciting or provocative agent has been identified, the patient must make every effort to avoid further contact with that substance, which may be difficult. A bricklayer with a contact allergy to chromates may be unable to avoid contact with chromate-containing cement. Seemingly ubiquitous substances such as nickel may also be difficult to avoid. Short of outright avoidance, the use of protective clothing such as gloves, boots, masks, and long-sleeved shirts may help. Barrier creams, especially in an industrial setting, may also be useful.

TREATMENT

Acute Contact Dermatitis

Acute contact dermatitis, irritant or allergic, is usually a weeping, oozing, exudative process, which is often accompanied by vesicles or bullae and is sometimes complicated by secondary bacterial infection. The application of cool or tepid soaks or compresses may be both soothing and drying; tap water or Burow's solution (Domeboro) may be used. Colloidal oatmeal (Aveeno) baths may also be comforting. Itching is often intense and may be controlled by antihistamines such as diphenhydramine (Benadryl) or hydroxyzine (Atarax) or one of the newer, less sedating antihistamines such as cetirizine (Zyrtec), loratadine (Claritin), astemizole (Hismanal), and fexofenadine (Allegra). Astemizole has been associated with rare cases of serious cardiovascular adverse events.

Most cases of acute contact dermatitis require the use of topical and/or systemic corticosteroids for effective management. Systemic steroids, used for the more severe cases, may be administered either orally (as prednisone, 40 to 60 mg daily for 7 to 14 days) or intramuscularly (as triamcinolone acetonide [Kenalog] or betamethasone acetate [Celestone]). Oral steroids are generally tapered during a 1- to 2-week period, whereas intramuscular preparations may persist for 1 week (betamethasone) to 3 weeks (triamcinolone). The well-known contraindications for the use of systemic corticosteroids must, of course, be considered when deciding whether to use them in the treatment of acute contact dermatitis.

For an acute contact dermatitis, topical corticosteroids are most often prescribed in the form of a lotion, cream, or solution. Solutions are particularly useful for hair-bearing areas or for sites such as the ears or interdigital spaces, whereas lotions may be spread easily over larger areas of affected skin; creams may be ideal for hands, feet, or smaller patches of contact dermatitis. In any format, topical corticosteroid preparations may be mild (hydrocortisone), moderate (hydrocortisone valerate [Westcort], desonide [Tridesilon], hydrocortisone butyrate [Locoid]), potent (desoximetasone [Topicort], fluocinonide [Lidex], amcinonide [Cyclocort]), or superpotent (augmented betamethasone dipropionate [Diprolene], diflorasone diacetate [Psorcon], halobetasol propionate [Ultravate], clobetasol propionate [Temovate]) formulations. Milder preparations should be used on the face, breasts, groin, and axillae. With the potent or superpotent preparations, local (atrophy, telangiectasia, striae) or even systemic (adrenal axis suppression) side effects are potential problems. The superpotent steroids must be used with special caution.

Chronic Contact Dermatitis

In the chronic form, allergic or irritant contact dermatitis generally produces thickening, lichenification, and fissuring, often intermixed with acute or subacute manifestations of the eczematous process. As with acute contact dermatitis, secondary infection may be a problem and necessitate the use of topical antibiotics such as mupirocin (Bactroban) or systemic antibiotics such as penicillin, erythromycin, tetracycline, or cephalosporins. The dry, cracked, thickened skin of chronic contact dermatitis is generally treated with the application of moisturizing or emollient lotions, creams, and ointments, rather than with the baths, soaks, and compresses that are most helpful in acute forms of the disorder. Likewise, when topical corticosteroid preparations are used, creams or ointments are generally favored over the less emollient lotions and solutions. Because a chronic disease process predicts a prolonged therapeutic course, the physician must be especially vigilant when using the more potent topical corticosteroid preparations. Certainly the same caveat applies to systemic corticosteroids, which should be used carefully and infrequently to control severe flare-ups of chronic contact dermatitis. Pruritus is, indeed, a problem here, as with the acute process, and oral antihistamines may provide at least temporary relief.

PATCH TESTING

The complete evaluation of patients when a diagnosis of contact dermatitis is suspected will generally include patch testing. The birth date of modern patch testing may be traced to a presentation of Jadassohn in 1895. Whereas patch testing does require training and experience, especially in the interpretation or "reading" of tests, its use has been greatly facilitated by the development of a new standardized system (allergen patch test, TRUE Test) in which materials are already incorporated in easy to apply test strips. Only when a causative agent is identified can contact dermatitis be optimally managed.

SKIN DISEASES OF PREGNANCY

method of
SARAH A. MYERS, M.D.
Duke University Medical Center
Durham, North Carolina

Certain skin diseases occur exclusively during pregnancy. Multiple confusing terms have been published delineating dermatoses with pregnancy, but recently three specific pregnancy-associated dermatoses have been described: herpes gestationis, polymorphic eruption of pregnancy, and prurigo of pregnancy.

HERPES GESTATIONIS

Herpes gestationis is an autoimmune blistering disorder that occurs during pregnancy. The incidence is between 1 in 3000 and 1 in 50,000, with higher incidence usually cited in referral populations. Herpes gestationis may occur during any pregnancy and tends to recur in subsequent pregnancies. Clinical manifestations typically appear in the second and third trimesters of pregnancy. The initial presentation is pruritus, often severe. The eruption consists of erythema and urticarial plaques, which may develop tense vesicles and bullae. Most cases appear on the abdomen near and within the umbilicus, and many progress to involve the extremities including the palms and soles. Facial and mucosal involvement is rare. The clinical course is highly variable, but generally patients proceed from pruritus to bullae within weeks after the onset of pruritus. Exacerbation at delivery is common, and some patients may present with onset of disease at parturition. Postpartum onset is uncommon. Patients may have recurrence with subsequent pregnancies, menstruation, or oral contraceptive use.

Histology is not specific and reveals subepidermal bullae with spongiosis and a perivascular lymphohistiocytic infiltrate rich in eosinophils. The diagnosis of herpes gestationis is confirmed by direct immunofluorescence of normal-appearing perilesional skin. This demonstrates linear deposition of C3 (100%) and IgG (30 to 50%) at the basement membrane zone. Immunoreactants bind to the epidermal aspect of the lamina lucida of split-skin specimens. Using conventional indirect immunofluorescence, only 25% of patients have circulating anti-basement membrane zone (BMZ) antibodies. Using complement fixation techniques, however, a circulating IgG1 antiepidermal BMZ antibody ("HG factor") can be detected in 50 to 75% of patients. The herpes gestationis antigen is a 180-kilodalton protein, which appears to be a transmembrane protein as determined by immunoelectron microscopy. The binding of the IgG1 autoantibody to this protein activates complement by the classic pathway, leading to subsequent inflammation and tissue damage.

Five to 10% of infants born to mothers with herpes gestationis may be born with a vesiculobullous eruption owing to transplacental passage of maternal IgG1 antibodies. Lesions generally resolve within weeks to months as the maternal antibodies are cleared, and there appears to be no evidence for increased risk of long-term sequelae in these children. Much has been written regarding increased fetal morbidity and mortality associated with herpes gestationis. Several studies have reported increased frequency of placental insufficiency, low birth weight, and prematurity; but increased risk of spontaneous abortions and stillbirths has not been found consistently.

Mild cases may be treated with topical fluorinated steroids and oral antihistamines. Cyproheptadine (Periactin), 4 mg three to four times daily, or diphenhydramine (Benadryl), 25 to 50 mg every 4 to 6 hours, can be helpful, and both are believed to be relatively safe in pregnancy. The newer nonsedating antihistamines, including astemizole (Hismanal), loratadine (Claritin), and terfenadine (Seldane), are contraindicated in pregnancy because no formal trials for their use have been performed. Moderately potent topical steroids such as fluocinonide 0.05% cream (Lidex) or amcinonide 0.1% cream (Cyclocort) can be effective and may need to be applied three to five times per day to the affected area to be successful. Ultrapotent steroids such as clobetasol propionate 0.05% (Temovate) should be restricted to short-term use only.

Most refractory cases of herpes gestationis generally require oral prednisone, 40 mg per day, until improvement is noted and then the dosage may be decreased to 10 mg per day for maintenance. Prednisone dosages are adjusted according to clinical course, and occasionally patients require maintenance dosage until parturition. In addition, the dosage often needs to be increased in anticipation of postpartum flare. Although steroid usage during pregnancy may contribute to the development of gestational diabetes, hypertension, and fetal adrenal insufficiency, the perinatal mortality rate is not increased in herpes gestationis patients treated with systemic steroids.

Plasmapheresis has been described as a useful treatment in herpes gestationis but has limited use owing to expense and inconvenience. Gold, methotrexate, and dapsone are other options with less promising results and are limited to postpartum (nonlactating) use, as they are all contraindicated during pregnancy.

POLYMORPHIC ERUPTION OF PREGNANCY

Polymorphic eruption of pregnancy (PEP), previously termed pruritic urticarial papules and plaques of pregnancy (PUPPP), is a common dermatosis of pregnancy, with a reported incidence of 1 in 250 pregnancies. PEP usually presents in primigravidas late in the third trimester or rarely in the postpartum period. Lesions begin on the lower abdomen, sparing the umbilicus, and usually involve the striae. Erythematous papules and urticarial plaques associated with intense pruritus are the most common findings. Coalescing polycyclic wheals, erythema multiforme–like target lesions, and small papulovesicles may also be present, but bullae are not observed. The eruption may spread to involve thighs, buttocks, and arms. No known systemic symptoms or laboratory abnormalities have been reported. In general, the eruption clears spontaneously with delivery or within the first week postpartum. Postpartum flare or recurrences with subsequent pregnancies, in contrast to herpes gestationis, do not generally occur. Fetal skin involvement has been reported rarely. There is no increase in fetal morbidity, malformations, stillbirths, or prematurity.

Diagnosis is made by clinical presentation. Histologic examination of involved skin is not specific and demonstrates variable dermal edema, a perivascular lymphocytic infiltrate with varying numbers of eosinophils, plus or minus epidermal spongiosis with mild acanthosis and parakeratosis. Direct and indirect immunofluorescent studies are characteristically negative.

Symptomatic treatment is often all that is required. Moderately potent topical steroids including fluocinonide 0.05% cream (Lidex) and triamcinolone acetonide 0.1% cream (Aristocort A) applied to the affected areas three to four times per day are often effective. Oral antihistamines (as described for herpes gestationis) can be used adjunctively for pruritus. Recalcitrant cases may require oral prednisone beginning at 40 mg per day with gradual dose reduction. Increased doses are not needed postpartum, as PEP usually resolves spontaneously after delivery without sequalae.

PRURIGO OF PREGNANCY

Prurigo of pregnancy is a common condition of pregnancy affecting 1 in 300 pregnancies. The onset is after the 25th week of gestation and can persist several months postpartum. The eruption consists of small excoriated papules, generally on the extensor extremities, abdomen, and shoulders. No vesicles or bullae have been reported and the lesions appear nonspecific. The etiology is unknown, but many patients have an atopic diathesis. Although laboratory examinations are normal, liver function tests and total serum bile salts should be obtained to exclude cholestasis of pregnancy (which usually manifests as pruritus without a primary skin eruption). Treatment of prurigo of pregnancy is symptomatic with the use of topical fluorinated steroids and oral antihistamines to help control inflammation and pruritus. No associated risk to mother or fetus has been reported. For cholestasis of pregnancy, cholestyramine may be tried to reduce serum bile salts. Dosages of 4 grams two to three times a day have produced a reduction in serum bile acid levels and relief from pruritus in some patients. Symptoms generally resolve with delivery. Increased fetal distress has been reported with this condition.

PRURITUS ANI AND VULVAE

method of
MARILYNNE McKAY, M.D.
Emory University School of Medicine
Atlanta, Georgia

Acute-onset perineal itching is most often due to one of the following: *Candida* infection, irritant and contact dermatitis, urinary tract infection, hemorrhoids, pinworms, and condylomata. Fecal contamination of the anus can be extremely irritating, as can overcleansing; contact dermatitis may develop after application of medications such as neomycin, benzocaine, or those containing preservatives such as ethylenediamine. Cleanliness, the use of bland emollients, and treatment of infection or infestation will generally resolve perineal itching that has been present for a few days to a few weeks.

Diagnostic tests for acute itching should specifically rule out infection, and examination of the female patient should include a vaginal smear for *Candida, Trichomonas,* and bacterial vaginosis (*Gardnerella*). Even though bacterial vaginosis is not typically itchy, the characteristic odor often induces patients to overcleanse or douche with irritating solutions. Recurrent candidiasis is common; culture specimens for *Candida* should be taken from the vagina, and anal culture should be considered in both sexes. Risk factors for *Candida* infection include antibiotics for sinusitis, urinary tract infections, or acne; steroids or other immunosuppressants; human immunodeficiency virus infection; and estrogen therapy (oral contraceptives, estrogen replacement). Itching resulting from estrogen deficiency may be important in perimenopausal women, because dry mucosal epithelium is easily irritated. Systemic disorders that may be associated with itching include diabetes, uremia, and hepatitis.

Chronic perineal itching is more difficult to evaluate than itching of recent onset, because the likelihood of discovering an underlying cause is significantly diminished when itching has persisted for months. With chronic pruritus, repeated episodes of itching and scratching cause local thickening of the skin called lichen simplex chronicus (LSC). LSC is identified by a leathery scaly texture with accentuation of normal skin lines. Irritable nerve endings in LSC lesions trigger an "itch-scratch-itch" cycle that typically continues long after the initial insult has resolved. LSC is secondary to rubbing and scratching, and this chronic skin change must be treated separately from the usual primary causes of acute perineal itching. Lichen sclerosus is an entirely different condition that may itch or burn; this dermatosis typically presents with thin, pale, friable skin around the anus and/or vulva.

If there are visible skin changes, a biopsy should be considered to differentiate LSC from other genital dermatoses such as psoriasis, lichen planus, or lichen sclerosus, as well as to rule out malignant neoplasms such as intraepithelial neoplasia (carcinoma in situ) or extramammary Paget's disease. A 3- to 4-mm punch biopsy specimen should be taken from the thickest areas of any lesions (plaques, scarring, thickening). Acetowhitening (application of vinegar or 3 to 5% acetic acid for 1 to 2 minutes) can be used to highlight thickened areas if there is a history of genital warts (human papillomavirus [HPV]). If HPV infection is found on the vulva, colposcopy of the vagina and cervix is recommended; if on the anus, proctoscopy. Biopsy of multifocal lesions, typical of HPV-associated intraepithelial neoplasia, should be done.

THERAPY

As mentioned before, the etiology of acute-onset perineal itching is most likely to be discovered by diagnostic testing. Therapy for infections should reduce itching within a few days, but *Candida* may be especially recalcitrant. Women with a tendency for recurrent candidiasis may need to use vaginal creams such as clotrimazole (Gyne-Lotrimin) or terconazole (Terazol) once a week for several months. An effective *Candida* suppression regimen is oral fluconazole (Diflucan), 150 to 200 mg weekly for 2 months, tapering to every 2 weeks for 2 months, then monthly. For relatively mild itching, 1% hydrocortisone cream is effective, especially when it is mixed with pramoxine, a mild anesthetic (Pramosone, Zone-A).

Proper cleansing is the single most important factor in management of perineal itching. After each bowel movement or possible soiling, the patient should cleanse gently with Tucks pads, Balneol or Cetaphil lotion, or a mild soap (Neutrogena, Purpose) followed by cool-water rinses. Plain white unscented toilet tissue is recommended, but Tucks cloth pads are probably better. The patient should be advised to pat the skin gently, because rubbing can be irritating. Tight or occlusive garments should be avoided; this includes plastic-backed panty shields, which can contribute to maceration—perfumes in these products can be irritating as well. Cotton underwear and the avoidance of fabric softeners are often helpful.

There is debate over whether spicy or caffeine-containing foods contribute to pruritus ani; probably the best course is to advise the patient to adopt a bland diet at first and then add back one or two items a week to see whether symptoms are exacerbated. Some patients already realize that certain foods worsen their problem. Food allergens are another possible factor, and an elimination trial of milk, tomatoes, corn, and nuts should be considered.

Older patients who complain of burning or stinging rather than itching (and who usually have minimal skin change as a result) may actually suffer from a cutaneous dysesthesia. Low-dose tricylic antidepressants such as amitriptyline (Elavil)* or nortriptyline (Pamelor)* are especially effective. Begin with 10 to 20 mg at bedtime and increase by 10 mg weekly to a dose of 30 to 50 mg per day. It may take 4 to 6 weeks to reach an adequate therapeutic dose. Once improvement has been maintained for a month or two, the dosage can gradually be tapered.

For LSC, the mainstay is topical steroid therapy. Caution is always advised in using fluorinated topical steroid preparations in intertriginous areas; side effects include skin thinning, striae formation, and rebound erythema and burning. On the other hand, nonfluorinated class VII preparations such as hydrocortisone are unlikely to be effective in severe thickened LSC. Short-term application of a high-potency class I steroid ointment such as betamethasone dipropionate 0.05% (Diprolene) or clobetasol propionate 0.05% (Temovate) can be extremely effective; I prescribe twice-daily applications for 3 to 4 weeks, then once daily for 3 to 4 weeks. Evaluation of the patient at 6 to 8 weeks almost always reveals significant improvement, sometimes for the first time in years. At this point, the potency and/or frequency of application should be decreased, using only the strength necessary to control symptoms. Triamcinolone acetonide 0.1% (Kenalog, Aristocort) may be used as a short-term stepdown to maintenance therapy with 1% hydrocortisone. Fluorinated steroids are recommended for use only on LSC or severe lichen sclerosus; they are contraindicated for erythema and burning, both of which can be worsened by their use. Overuse of potent topical steroids on vulvar skin will cause steroid rebound dermatitis with burning and erythema; perianal skin is more likely to develop thinning and telangiectasia.

It often takes 3 or 4 weeks for a topical steroid to begin to affect well-established LSC, and itching typically flares from time to time during the healing process. The patient must be told that this does not mean that the medication is not working, especially if symptom-free intervals indicate that treatment is progressing satisfactorily. The patient's anxiety is often a significant factor in episodic itching, and reassurance is an important part of therapy.

*Not FDA approved for this indication.

URTICARIA AND ANGIOEDEMA

method of
ELYSE S. RAFAL, M.D., and
TARA L. KAUFMANN, B.S.
Stony Brook Medical Center
Stony Brook, New York

Urticaria, which is a common skin disorder, is characterized by transient wheals of varying sizes. The prevalence of urticaria is high, with a 20% lifetime incidence. A related and sometimes associated condition, angioedema, is easily recognized by the presence of large subcutaneous swellings of the skin and/or mucous membranes, often involving the eyelids, lips, tongue, hands, and genitalia. Urticaria can be provoked by a number of agents, including foods, drugs, infections, malignancies, physical agents, inhalants, and contactants. Discovering and avoiding the causative agent are the most practical approaches to preventing the signs and symptoms. However, the precipitating factor cannot be easily identified in the majority of patients, especially those with chronic urticaria. The goal of treatment, in most cases, is to decrease the effects of various mediators such as histamine, which play an important role in triggering the urticarial reaction.

EVALUATION: ACUTE URTICARIA

Acute urticaria is defined as lesions of less than 6 weeks' duration; chronic urticaria refers to lesions lasting more than 6 weeks. The clinical features of acute urticaria are pruritic, edematous wheals of various sizes and shapes. The individual wheals are evanescent, usually lasting less than 4 hours, but can remain for up to 24 hours. Urticaria can present itself on any cutaneous surface with crops of lesions, which can be generalized or localized.

The most common causes of acute urticaria are foods and medications. If an episode of hives can be attributed to a specific ingestant, that particular substance should be avoided. Some of the most allergenic foods are chocolate, fish, shellfish, nuts, eggs, strawberries, milk, and tomatoes. Occasionally, an elimination and addition diet, in which there are at least 2 to 3 days between each elimination or addition, can be effective in the identification of food allergies. Medications, especially penicillin and other antibiotics, can trigger hives by an IgE-dependent process. Opiates, polymyxin B, curare, and radiocontrast media can degranulate mast cells and directly cause urticarial symptoms. Aspirin and nonsteroidal anti-inflammatory agents can precipitate urticaria by altering arachidonic acid metabolism. Patients intolerant to aspirin can experience cross-sensitivity to food additives, notably azo dyes and benzoic acid. Food additives are an important provoking factor for acute and chronic urticaria.

Physical and contact urticarias compose a smaller portion of the acute cases. Causes of physical urticaria include cold, trauma, sunlight, heat, water, pressure, stress, and exercise. Contact urticaria may occur after direct contact with foods, drugs, animals, plants, and substances such as latex. Patch testing may be a useful means of ascertaining the causative agent.

Evaluation of patients with acute urticaria should include a thorough history, with special emphasis on the possible precipitating factors, as well as a complete physical examination. Any suspected causes should be identified and removed. Most patients do not require any laboratory studies.

Angioedema is characterized by the sudden onset of diffuse localized subcutaneous edema, which is usually unilateral. In general, there is no erythema or pruritus. The most common sites are the lips, eyelids, and genitalia. Swelling can persist for up to 3 days. It is often preceded by trauma such as dental extraction. Angioedema usually accompanies urticaria, but it may occur alone. Angioedema may be hereditary or acquired. Hereditary angioedema is a rare autosomal dominant condition caused by a quantitative or functional deficiency of C1-esterase inhibitor. These patients have low C4 levels, which is the most reliable diagnostic test. Laryngeal involvement can occur and may be life-threatening. Acquired angioedema is a nonhereditary deficiency of C1-esterase inhibitor triggered by lymphoproliferative disorders, systemic lupus erythematosus, hypereosinophilia, drugs, cold, exercise, and sunlight. This acquired form of angioedema can be differentiated from the hereditary form by the decreased levels of the first component of complement, which is present in normal amounts in hereditary angioedema.

EVALUATION: CHRONIC URTICARIA

When urticaria persists for more than 6 weeks, it is classified as chronic. In the vast majority of patients with chronic urticaria, no trigger can be found. Although laboratory results rarely identify the etiology, the initial workup may include a complete blood count with differential, chemistry profile, erythrocyte sedimentation rate, urinalysis, and serologic test for syphilis. Eosinophilia may suggest allergic disorders or drug reactions, lymphocytosis may indicate an infection, and an elevated erythrocyte sedimentation rate may be consistent with urticarial vasculitis. Further diagnostic studies should only be performed based on the findings elicited by history, physical examination, and screening tests. A stool examination may show ova and parasites, and the presence of antinuclear antibodies may uncover systemic lupus erythematosus. Urticarial vasculitis is characterized by individual wheals that persist for more than 24 hours.

THERAPEUTIC APPROACH

Acute Urticaria

Ideally, a careful history and physical examination will identify the cause of acute urticaria. Therefore, treatment can focus on avoidance or removal of the particular substance. However, the provoking factor often cannot be discovered, necessitating the use of other treatment methods. In a severe acute reaction involving anaphylaxis, subcutaneous epinephrine (0.3 to 0.5 mL of 1:1000), supplemental oxygen, intravenous diphenhydramine (Benadryl), 50 to 100 mg, and systemic corticosteroids may be necessary.

In acute urticaria, administration of the H_1 class of oral antihistamines, which include the traditional sedating and nonsedating antihistamines, usually decreases the signs and symptoms. The problem with the traditional H_1 antagonists is that they often induce sedation. Some of the traditional H_1 antagonists include diphenhydramine (Benadryl) (25 to 100 mg three to four times daily),* hydroxyzine (Atarax) (10 to 50 mg three to four times daily), and cyproheptadine (Periactin) (4 mg four times a day). Cyproheptadine is the drug of choice for essential cold urticaria. A side effect of cyproheptadine is increased appetite and weight gain. Chlorpheniramine (Chlor-Trimeton), 8 to 12 mg twice daily, causes less sedation, but stimulation of the central nervous system is a side effect.

Nonsedating antihistamines such as loratadine (Claritin), 10 mg daily, and astemizole (Hismanal), 10 mg daily, have emerged that are effective in the management of urticaria. A relatively new medication, fexofenadine (Allegra), a metabolite of terfena-

*Exceeds dosage recommended by the manufacturer.

dine (Seldane), appears to be promising. Fexofenadine has replaced terfenadine and the dosage is 60 mg twice daily. Cetirizine (Zyrtec), 10 mg daily, is an H_1 receptor antagonist but also has a unique property of inhibiting the influx of eosinophils in the late phase allergic response. A combination of a sedating antihistamine at night with a nonsedating antihistamine during the day is sometimes needed to control urticarial symptoms. When these therapeutic interventions are unsuccessful, oral prednisone, starting with 40 to 60 mg every morning with 2 to 3 week taper, can be prescribed.

The treatment of choice for hereditary angioedema is danazol (Danocrine), 400 to 600 mg daily, or stanozolol (Winstrol), 2 to 6 mg daily. It is important to note that oral antihistamines, corticosteroids, and adrenergic drugs are ineffective. Trauma, intense physical exercise, and dental and surgical procedures should be avoided because they can trigger angioedema. Patients with angioedema not controlled by oral antihistamines and who have severe laryngeal edema should be given adrenaline. If adrenaline does not abort the attack, intravenous hydrocortisone and antihistamines should be administered.

Chronic Urticaria

Traditional antihistamines include diphenhydramine, chlorpheniramine, and brompheniramine (Dimetapp). Although relief of symptoms can be achieved with the traditional H_1 antagonists, they commonly induce sedation. Patients must be warned not to drive or operate machinery. Therefore, the nonsedating H_1 antihistamines such as astemizole, fexofenadine, and loratadine are often useful in treating chronic urticaria. Certirizine is also effective for long-standing urticaria. Dosing is similar to that for acute urticaria. The simultaneous administration of H_1 and H_2 blockers can result in a better response in some patients; cimetidine (Tagamet),* 400 mg four times daily, can be effective.

Tricyclic antidepressants such as doxepin (Sinequan), 10 mg three times daily, are the most potent antihistamines known, and they block the H_1 and H_2 receptors. Beta-adrenergic agonists such as terbutaline* (Brethine), 2.5 mg three times daily, increase mast cell intracellular cyclic adenosine monophosphate (cAMP) by stimulating membrane-bound adenylate cyclase, thus inhibiting histamine release from mast cells. Calcium channel blockers such as nifedipine* (Procardia), 10 mg three times daily, also interfere with mast cell degranulation and can be an effective treatment. Colchicine* (ColBenemid), 0.6 mg twice daily, or dapsone*, 100 mg to 150 mg twice daily, with an H_1 blocker may be effective. A short course of oral corticosteroids may be required to supplement these treatments.

*Not FDA approved for this indication.

PIGMENTARY DISORDERS

method of
CHRISTY A. LORTON, M.D.
Perrysburg, Ohio

The four pigments primarily responsible for normal skin color are oxygenated hemoglobin, reduced hemoglobin, carotenoid, and melanin. Of these, melanin is the major determinant of skin color. Disorders of pigmentation can be caused by at least three mechanisms: (1) an enhanced or diminished production of melanin by the melanocyte, (2) an increase or decrease in the number of melanocytes, and (3) an abnormal location of melanin and/or melanocytes within the dermis. The clinical result is either decreased pigment (hypopigmentation) or increased pigment (hyperpigmentation).

HYPERPIGMENTATION

Ultraviolet Light–Induced Hyperpigmentation (Suntan)

The constitutive or baseline skin color is genetically determined. It is independent of extrinsic factors such as exposure to sunlight. Facultative skin color is the inducible darkening of the skin that most often follows exposure to ultraviolet radiation. Suntan results from two different mechanisms. Longwave ultraviolet light (type A [UVA], 320 to 400 nm) causes immediate darkening of pigment. This occurs within 15 to 30 minutes after exposure and disappears within hours. It is probably caused by an oxidative change in the pre-existing melanin molecules. Immediate tanning is responsible for the bronzing of the skin that most individuals observe after intense exposure to summer sunlight.

Shortwave ultraviolet light (type B [UVB], 290 to 320 nm) produces sunburn and delayed tanning. Delayed tanning is often much darker than the immediate type and is caused by proliferation of melanocytes, as well as enhanced production of melanin. It takes 3 to 4 days to develop and lasts for many weeks.

Both longwave ultraviolet light and shortwave ultraviolet light contribute to photoaging, and both increase the risk of developing skin cancers. Both types of ultraviolet light are responsible for the mottled hyperpigmentation and wrinkling that are observed on heavily exposed areas of the skin such as the face, neck, and dorsum of the hands. Exposure to ultraviolet radiation in tanning parlors also hastens the process of photoaging and wrinkling and possibly increases the risk of developing skin cancers.

Treatment

The patient must recognize that sun-induced pigmentation can be reversed only by avoiding exposure of the skin to all forms of ultraviolet light. Many physical sun blocks are available that reflect ultraviolet light and protect the skin well. Clothing such as tightly woven outerwear or hats, which can be very elegant, are excellent protectants. Physical sun blocks such as zinc oxide, calamine, talc, titanium dioxide, and kaolin are opaque and act to scatter and reflect light. Most preparations, which are available commercially in skin tints to match the complexion or in microsized dispersions that rub in easily, are now cosmetically and socially acceptable. For individuals who are unusually sensitive to sunlight and who desire to enjoy outdoor activities, these sun blocks are essential. Chemical sunscreens function in a different way. They absorb ultraviolet light in the UVB and/or UVA range. Para-aminobenzoic acid (PABA), PABA esters, salicylates, and cinnamates absorb radiation in the UVB range. Although PABA esters are used extensively in sunscreens, the use of PABA has been limited because of its potential to cause allergic reactions. Benzophenone derivatives absorb radiation mainly in the UVA range. The ideal broad-spectrum sunscreen contains an agent that absorbs UVB and an agent that absorbs UVA.

Two factors should be considered when choosing a sunscreen: the skin protection factor (SPF) and the substantivity. The SPF is the ratio of the minimal sunburn (UVB) dose of sunlight on chemically protected skin to that on unprotected skin. At the beginning of summer (June 21) the average unprotected person burns after 15 to 20 minutes of direct exposure to the sun at noontime. A sunscreen with SPF 2 absorbs half of the UVB striking the skin. Therefore, it takes twice as long to burn the treated skin (30 to 40 minutes of exposure on June 21). An SPF of 15 to 30 (which requires 15 to 30 times more UVB to burn the skin) is considered to be adequate protection against UVB radiation.

The substantivity of the sunscreen is its ability to withstand sweating and water immersion. Table 1 gives examples of current commercially available sunscreens with SPFs equal to or greater than 15 that also have good to excellent water and sweat resistance. Ideally, all sunscreens should be reapplied after prolonged swimming or heavy sweating.

TABLE 1. **Partial List of Sunscreens That Have Good to Excellent Substantivity**

Brand Name Sunscreens (SPF)	Active Ingredients
PreSun (15 or 29)	Octylmethoxycinnamate, oxybenzone, octylsalicylate
Solbar (15 or 50)	Octylmethoxycinnamate, oxybenzone, octrocrylene (SPF 50)
Coppertone Sport (15 or 30)	p-Methoxycinnamate, oxybenzone, ethylhexyl salicylate
Neutrogena Sunblock (25)	Octylmethoxycinnamate, oxybenzone, octylsalicylate
Water Babies (45)	p-Methoxycinnamate, oxybenzone, ethylhexyl salicylate, homosalate
Banana Boat Ultra (30)	p-Methoxycinnamate, oxybenzone, ethylhexyl salicylate

TABLE 2. **Common Causes of Postinflammatory Hyperpigmentation**

Exanthems	Acne
Drug eruptions	Tinea versicolor
Lichen planus	Cutaneous lupus
Atopic dermatitis	Psoriasis
Trauma, burns	Lichen simplex chronicus
Herpes zoster	Pityriasis rosea
Ashy dermatosis	Fixed drug eruption

Postinflammatory Hyperpigmentation

A variety of inflammatory conditions and infections (Table 2) cause hyperpigmentation of the skin, usually called *postinflammatory hyperpigmentation.* The dyschromia follows the pattern and distribution of the original disease, but its intensity is not necessarily related to the degree of the previous inflammation. Postinflammatory hyperpigmentation is common and rather persistent in darkly pigmented people. It is caused by stimulation of melanocytes to produce excessive amounts of melanin. If the melanin remains in the epidermis, the color of the skin appears to be deep tan to dark brown. Often the inflammation is associated with disruption of the dermal-epidermal barrier. Melanin is then deposited in the upper dermis. When brown melanin is located in the dermis, its color appears to be slate gray or bluish.

Treatment

Epidermal forms of hyperpigmentation may respond to treatment with bleaching agents. Dermal hyperpigmentation does not respond to any medical treatment and usually is permanent. It is important, therefore, to determine whether the pigmentation has mainly an epidermal or a dermal component. Examination of the patient with a Wood lamp (black light) in a totally dark room can facilitate this evaluation. Epidermal melanin turns almost black when viewed with the Wood lamp. In contrast, dermal pigmentation, when observed with a Wood lamp, is not visible to the examiner, and the blemishes on the patient's skin disappear.

Optimal management of the primary underlying skin problem is essential for treatment and prevention of further hyperpigmentation. If the hyperpigmentation is primarily epidermal, the patient may benefit from various topical modalities, which are discussed in the following section along with treatment for other disorders of epidermal hyperpigmentation.

Melasma (Chloasma)

Melasma ("mask of pregnancy") is a common patchy, irregular, tan to brown pigmentation that is usually located on the face of women. It occurs in women who are taking oral contraceptives or who are pregnant. It usually fades slowly after the termination of either event and is exacerbated by exposure to sunlight. It also occurs in women who are not taking birth control pills or whose last pregnancy occurred many years earlier. Occasionally, it occurs in men. Melasma is caused by increased epidermal melanization, although in some patients there is a moderate amount of dermal pigment as well. In these latter individuals, treatment can never return the skin entirely to its normal appearance.

Freckles (Ephelides)

Freckles first appear in childhood in individuals who have fair complexions and who are genetically of Celtic or northern European ancestry. Freckles fade in the winter and become more prominent after exposure to sunlight. Middle-aged and older adults usually lose some or all of their freckles.

Solar Lentigines

Solar or senile lentigines are dark brown macules, usually 1 to 3 cm in diameter, that occur on the chronically sun-exposed surfaces of elderly individuals, especially on the dorsum of the hands or on the face. They are commonly misnamed "liver spots." In contrast to freckles and melasma, they do not fade in the winter but persist throughout the calendar year. They must be distinguished from lentigo maligna or seborrheic keratoses.

Treatment

Patients with these sun-induced pigmentary disorders must avoid further unprotected exposure to sunlight. This should be stressed as the most important part of their therapy. Sunscreens or sunblocks help to prevent further pigmentary abnormalities.

There is considerable individual variation in the response to treatment, but in general, most patients will respond to one or a combination of preparations. Most bleaching medications must be applied conscientiously, often for 6 to 12 months, to achieve optimal results.

Various bleaching medications are available that contain hydroquinone, either in an over-the-counter 2% concentration (Esoterica, Porcelana) or a 3% (Melanex) or 4% (Eldopaque Forte, Solaquin Forte) strength by prescription. Hydroquinone suppresses pigmentation, probably by blocking the activity of tyrosinase, the enzyme primarily involved in melanin synthesis. Side effects from hydroquinone are rare but include mild skin irritation. At higher concentrations, colloid milia, dermal pigmentation, or both have been reported. The addition of a mild corticosteroid cream (hydrocortisone 1 to 2.5%) increases the effectiveness of the hydroquinone and possibly reduces the frequency of skin irritation. Caution must be exercised when prescribing corticosteroids for prolonged periods. On the face, steroids can cause telangiectasia, atrophy, or acneiform lesions. The more potent fluorinated corticosteroids should not be used on the face except under special circumstances. On the arms and trunk, potent topical steroids can cause striae. These are irreversible.

Tretinoin cream (Retin-A, Renova)* can also be used in conjunction with hydroquinone and/or mild corticosteroids to decrease epidermal hyperpigmentation. There has been a great deal of interest in the use of tretinoin alone to remove pigmentation associated specifically with photoaging. Tretinoin can be irritating to the skin and can cause erythema, desquamation, and soreness. To minimize the side effects, the following approach is suggested. Therapy should be initiated with 0.025 or 0.05% tretinoin applied at bedtime twice weekly for 1 to 2 weeks, then three times weekly for a few more weeks, followed by nightly applications. Thereafter the concentration of the cream can be increased to 0.1% if tolerated by the patient. Alternatively, the patient can begin nightly with Renova, which is tretinoin in an emollient cream.

The application of alpha-hydroxy acids (AHAs) can be used to improve hyperpigmentation, whether postinflammatory, melasma, or lentigines. Glycolic acid and lactic acid are the two most common agents used in products, most of which are available over-the-counter. AHAs appear to work by altering corneocyte cohesion, which results in desquamation and dispersion of melanin granules. Clinical lightening of the skin is observed after several weeks of application of skin lotions or creams containing 8 to 15% concentration of AHA. In higher concentrations, glycolic acid is used in serial skin peel systems to treat hyperpigmentation.

Topical 20% azelaic acid cream (Azelex)* causes skin lightening, possibly by inhibition of hyperactive melanocytes and by interfering with tyrosinase. The effect of tretinoin with azelaic acid is additive. A good combination approach would be to use a tretinoin cream at night and azelaic acid cream in the morning.

There are other modalities for treating localized pigmented spots such as freckles or solar lentigines. Gentle freezing with liquid nitrogen can decrease the amount of color. Melanocytes are particularly susceptible to destruction by this treatment. One must avoid causing necrosis of the skin or blistering. Dark-skinned patients should not have lesions frozen except in special circumstances because of the risk of permanent depigmentation.

Trichloroacetic acid (TAC) is another agent that is effective for solar lentigines or other localized patches of pigmentation but is generally not useful in dark-skinned individuals. Aqueous TAC in strengths ranging from 15 to 75% is used as a peeling agent alone or in combination with Jessner's solution (resorcinol, lactic acid, and salicylic acid in an ethanol solution). An alternative to the aqueous solution is the TAC masque, which is a chelated TAC in a creamy clay formula. TAC must be used with extreme caution because it is a highly reactive chemical that can cause epidermal necrosis, delayed healing, and

*Not FDA approved for this indication.

TABLE 3. **Systemic Causes of Hyperpigmentation**

Metabolic Conditions	Drugs and Metals
Hemochromatosis	Mercury
Porphyria cutanea tarda	Silver
Addison's disease	Arsenic
Vitamin B deficiency	Gold
Pellagra	Antimalarial agents
Scleroderma	Minocycline
Acanthosis nigricans	Phenothiazines
Pregnancy	Beta carotene

scarring. In the hands of the experienced physician, these peels can be done safely and effectively to improve dyschromia.

Systemic Causes of Hyperpigmentation

Generalized hyperpigmentation is associated with many systemic disorders. Usually the color is due to melanin, for example, in Addison's disease. Metabolic, nutritional, or endocrine disorders should be considered in patients with widespread or diffuse hyperpigmentation. Generalized hyperpigmentation can also be caused by drugs or heavy metals. A partial list of these disorders and drugs is given in Table 3.

Treatment

Treatment for hyperpigmentation caused by systemic disorders is directed at correcting the underlying disease or discontinuing the medication.

HYPOPIGMENTATION

Vitiligo

Vitiligo is a common acquired depigmenting disorder that occurs in about 1% of the general population. It is characterized by white (depigmented) patches on the skin. Only about 5% of affected individuals have a positive (primary family) history of vitiligo. About 15% of patients with vitiligo have thyroid disease, and 5% have diabetes mellitus. Rarely, the patient with vitiligo has Addison's disease, pernicious anemia, or other endocrine disorders.

There are two types of vitiligo. In the generalized form, the white patches are spread over the body. In the second form, segmental vitiligo, the patches are limited to localized areas (e.g., one half of the face, an entire arm, or one leg). Segmental vitiligo usually does not follow dermatomes. In either type of vitiligo, the white patches generally appear spontaneously without a pre-existing rash. The depigmented areas are completely devoid of epidermal melanin and melanocytes. The cause of vitiligo is not known. Although it is commonly assumed to be an autoimmune disease, depigmentary disorders in several animal models that resemble human vitiligo suggest that the disorder may have a biochemical basis.

Treatment

The physician should be aware of the strong psychosocial impact that vitiligo has on the patient and should be prepared to provide reassurance, explanation, and appropriate referral to support groups, consultants, or psychiatrists as needed. For most people, vitiligo is a devastating disfigurement.

For certain individuals, the use of cosmetics or stains to conceal the more apparent vitiligo is all that is desired. Cover Mark and Dermablend are two opaque types of makeup that some patients find helpful. Stains or self-tanning products that contain dihydroxyacetone can be used to tint the depigmented areas so that they are less obvious.

Judicious use of broad-spectrum sunscreens is recommended for three reasons. First, the areas of vitiligo burn more easily than normal skin when exposed to sunlight. Second, sunburn injury can extend the depigmentation, a process called Koebner's phenomenon. Third, exposure to sunlight induces darkening of the surrounding normal-appearing skin and causes accentuation of the cosmetic disfigurement.

Repigmentation requires regrowth of melanocytes into the white epidermis. Unfortunately, melanocytes do not migrate more than a few millimeters from the edge of a lesion. Thus, successful repigmentation requires the presence of hair bulbs from which melanocytes can be stimulated to migrate into the surrounding white skin. Skin on the dorsa of the hands or distal to the ankles repigments poorly because this skin lacks sufficient numbers of hair bulbs.

The most effective method of treatment for vitiligo is photochemotherapy. It requires a motivated patient who is committed to prolonged therapy. It is intended for patients older than 10 years of age who are neither pregnant nor lactating. There must be no history of a photosensitivity disorder. If a collagen vascular disorder is suspected, an antinuclear antibody level and other evaluations should be obtained before starting photochemotherapy.

Psoralen (available as 8-methoxypsoralen [Oxsoralen-Ultra]) is a potent photosensitizer in combination with UVA (PUVA). PUVA therapy for vitiligo takes 6 to 24 months and must be given two times a week in gradually increasing dosages. The patient must be given careful instruction in the proper use of protective glasses that block out UVA, which might damage the eyes and lead to cataract formation. The patient must also avoid unprotected sunlight exposure for 24 hours after taking the psoralen because of the increased photosensitivity.

Topical PUVA is intended for the treatment of limited areas of vitiligo. Skin treated with topical psoralen is extremely sensitive to sunlight and UVA. Even inadvertent exposure of the treated skin through car windows for a few minutes can cause painful second-degree burns. Topical psoralen should be used only by physicians thoroughly acquainted with its safe use.

Topical mild steroid creams such as hydrocortisone, 2.5% applied once daily, often treat vitiligo successfully. The medication must be applied for 6 to 12 months. The patient should be observed carefully to prevent damage to the skin from steroids. Caution must be used when applying steroids around the eyes. Patients with vitiligo probably should have a baseline eye examination that is repeated yearly if they are receiving PUVA or applying steroids around the eyes.

For patients with extensive (more than 50%) vitiligo, careful consideration should be given to total depigmentation of the remaining pigmented skin. This is accomplished by application of 20% monobenzyl ether of hydroquinone twice daily for a period of weeks to years. The medication is applied until depigmentation is complete. This medication causes irreversible destruction of melanocytes. This procedure should be done only after the patient gives careful consideration and consent. Patients need to understand that the depigmentation is permanent. They will always be sensitive to sunlight. However, the cosmetic result is gratifying.

Postinflammatory Hypopigmentation

Many of the same inflammatory disorders or infections that cause postinflammatory hyperpigmentation can also cause hypopigmentation. The most common causes are eczema, atopic dermatitis, tinea versicolor, secondary syphilis, chickenpox, and psoriasis. Pityriasis alba is a mild form of dermatitis that is common in children. It is characterized by hypopigmented patches with fine scales. Although most commonly noted on the face, it can also affect the arms, thighs, or trunk.

Treatment

Unlike postinflammatory hyperpigmentation, postinflammatory hypopigmentation usually resolves slowly over time. Hydrocortisone, 2.5% in a cream or lotion applied twice daily, may accelerate repigmentation.

Idiopathic Guttate Hypomelanosis

This common condition is characterized by hypopigmented, confetti-like macules on the extremities. These macules can also occur on the trunk and, rarely, on the face. The condition occurs in all races but is more noticeable in darker skinned or tanned people. It must be distinguished from vitiligo. The cause of idiopathic guttate hypomelanosis is not known, although sunlight is thought to be a contributing factor. There is a reduction in the number of melanocytes in the pale macules.

Treatment

The patient should always apply a broad-spectrum sunscreen and avoid excessive sun exposure. This prevents further sun damage and avoids accentuating the hypomelanosis by darkening the surrounding skin.

SUNBURN

method of
WARWICK L. MORISON, M.D.
Johns Hopkins University School of Medicine
Baltimore, Maryland

Sunburn is a common problem, particularly for fair-skinned whites, caused by excessive exposure to ultraviolet (UV) radiation from sunlight or artificial sources such as sunlamps. When induced by sunlight, it is mainly due to UVB (280 to 320 nm) radiation plus a smaller contribution from UVA (320 to 400 nm) radiation. Erythema appears 3 to 4 hours after exposure, reaches a maximum at 12 to 18 hours, and usually settles after 72 to 96 hours. In severe reactions with blistering, complete resolution may take a week or more. Sunburns are graded as pink, red, and blistering. The classification by degree (first, second, and third) used for thermal burns should not be applied to sunburns because thermal burns have quite different sequelae, such as scarring and death, which are extremely rare consequences of a sunburn. Keratoconjunctivitis or ocular "sunburn" can also be caused by UV radiation and follows a similar time course.

There are two facets to management of sunburn: prevention and treatment. Because there is no effective treatment for an established sunburn, most emphasis should be placed on prevention.

PREVENTION

Skin color and the capacity of an individual to tan determine how important it is for an individual to take preventive measures. However, even dark-skinned people can sunburn if the exposure dose is sufficiently high. Skin color, past history of sunburn, and likely exposure should be used as a guide in advising people about protection.

Avoidance of Exposure

Simple avoidance of excessive exposure to a threshold dose of UV radiation is often the best advice for fair-skinned people. Scheduling outdoor activities for before 10 AM and after 3 PM will avoid the peak UV irradiance period and still permit enjoyment of the outdoors. This advice for people should be accompanied by several warnings. Sitting in the shade or under a beach umbrella reduces exposure by only about 70%. A cloudy day is often the setting for the worst sunburns, as even complete white cloud cover reduces UV exposure by only about 50%. Clothing is not always an effective protector. If it is possible to see through a fabric, UV radiation can also penetrate to a significant extent. Finally, the geographic location of exposure must be considered, as UV radiation may be twice as intense at the equator compared with much of continental North America.

Sunscreens

Many sunscreens are commercially available that contain numerous active ingredients. If this is not enough to cause confusion, some are not even labeled as sunscreens: Sunblocks and tanning lotions are other terms. However, the informed physician need know only four properties of a sunscreen: the skin protective factor (SPF), the spectrum of protection, the base, and whether it is waterproof.

The SPF is an index of the amount of protection provided

by the sunscreen. For example, a fair-skinned individual who normally begins to sunburn after a 10-minute exposure to sunlight should be able to tolerate up to 150 minutes of exposure after application of an SPF 15 sunscreen. There are several caveats for this statement. To provide the stated protection, a sunscreen must be applied 10 minutes before exposure to allow binding to skin proteins to occur, and it must be applied in an adequate amount. Several studies have shown that under ideal circumstances in which sunscreen is supplied free and the subject observed while making the application, most people use only half the required amount. Ordinary use probably provides much less protection. As a rough guide, 1 ounce of sunscreen is necessary to cover a 70 kg adult in a bathing suit; in other words, a 4 ounce bottle of sunscreen provides only four applications.

Sunscreens vary in the amount of the solar spectrum for which they provide protection. All sunscreens provide good protection against UVB radiation and the shorter end of UVA radiation. Some sunscreens contain avobenzone and provide good protection across the whole of the UVA band. Sunblocks or so-called nonchemical sunscreens provide protection against UVB, UVA, and visible radiation and usually contain titanium dioxide.

The base of a sunscreen is also important because it often determines whether a sunscreen will be used. Men usually prefer alcohol-based lotions because they dry quickly and leave a dry, nongreasy film. Women usually prefer lotions or creams because they give a moisturizing feel to the skin.

Finally, a sunscreen may be labeled water-resistant or waterproof. Because almost all outdoor pastimes involve perspiring or contact with water, a waterproof sunscreen should be selected.

A fair-skinned individual should always use a sunscreen with an SPF 15 or higher. People who tan well and never burn are probably adequately protected with an SPF 8 to 10. People with black or brown skin probably do not need sunscreens except for extreme occupational or social exposure.

A few myths should be dismissed. There is no effective oral sunscreen. Many have been tested and all have failed. Self-tanning preparations are not sunscreens. They do provide the appearance of a tan and are safe to use, but they provide no protection against UV radiation.

Protective Tanning

The proliferation of suntan parlors has generated much interest in protective tanning, with misinformation provided by the commercial interests involved. Little scientific information is available to provide a guide as to whether protective tanning is of any value in preventing the long-term hazards of excessive exposure to sunlight, namely skin cancer and premature aging of the skin. Certainly, preventive tanning by using multiple suberythemal doses of UV radiation can prevent sunburn, but the cost in terms of chronic damage is unknown.

Most suntan parlors claim to use only UVA radiation in their tanning beds, but this claim is false. All so-called UVA tanning beds emit some UVB radiation, the most damaging wavelengths; in addition, UVA radiation, especially in large doses, can produce the same damaging effect as UVB radiation. Furthermore, a UVA-induced tan is not very protective and at most has an SPF 6 to 8. A person who tans well and never burns may gain some protection from sunlight by preventive tanning without incurring too much damage. However, the benefit/risk ratio for people who do sunburn is probably very unfavorable.

TREATMENT

When a person has a sunburn, general supportive measures are the only approach to treatment. Cold compresses and cool baths with bath oil provide some relief. Frequent application of moisturizing creams helps alleviate dryness. Blistering of the skin may lead to secondary infection and require use of an antibiotic cream. Rarely, an extremely severe sunburn may necessitate hospitalization and management as a thermal burn.

Topical corticosteroids reduce erythema by causing vasoconstriction, but this effect is temporary and does not reduce epidermal damage. Systemic corticosteroids, even in large doses, do not alter the course of a sunburn. Nonsteroidal anti-inflammatory drugs, if given at the time of exposure or beforehand, reduce the degree of erythema over the first 24 hours but do not change epidermal damage. Of course, few people lying on the beach anticipate an excessive exposure, so they are unlikely to embark on such preventive measures.

Section 13

The Nervous System

ALZHEIMER'S DISEASE

method of
RACHELLE SMITH DOODY, M.D., PH.D.
Baylor College of Medicine
Houston, Texas

AGING, DEMENTIA, DELIRIUM, AND DEPRESSION

Alzheimer's disease (AD) is an abnormal condition characterized by unique neuropathologic changes in brain tissues and a clinical syndrome of memory loss, difficulty with other thought processes, and behavioral changes. Memory and thinking abilities change with age, but it is not normal to lose the ability to remember new information. The normal changes consist of some word-finding difficulties (particularly for proper nouns), slowing of thought processes, and the need for more exposures to learn new information. People who begin to forget recent information, lose track of time (temporal disorientation), get lost (spatial disorientation), and experience other subtle failures of cognition are almost always experiencing dementia.

Dementia is defined as memory loss with at least one other impaired area of cognition, such as language ability, orientation, attention and concentration, frontal executive function (self-monitoring, judgment, and problem solving), praxis (the ability to perform previously acquired motor skills), or activities of daily living (finances, using appliances, bathing, toileting). It is progressive when due to Alzheimer's disease, but there are more static forms of dementia as well, such as some cases of cerebrovascular disease. The dementias are associated with insidious onset and progression. Patients may or may not be aware of the cognitive problem, and the presence or absence of insight, once thought to differentiate AD from other forms of dementia, does not aid in defining the type of dementia. Delirium and depression must always be ruled out before making a diagnosis of dementia. Delirium, a form of acute encephalopathy, has diverse causes such as metabolic disturbances, central nervous system infections, and intoxications. Patients with an underlying dementia are more prone to delirium, but the delirium needs to be properly diagnosed and treated before a diagnosis of dementia can be made. Treatment of the delirium is also necessary before the severity of the underlying dementia can be estimated, a critical step in recommending treatment.

The relationship between depression and dementia is complex, and is a significant reason that patients with dementia may experience a delay in diagnosis and treatment. Depression without dementia can cause demonstrable changes in cognition, such as slow thinking, poor test performance, and lack of self-confidence. Although the cognitive profile of depression is usually identifiable on neuropsychologic testing, it takes considerable skill to be able to rule out dementia in a patient who is severely depressed. When depression is the sole cause of a patient's cognitive difficulty, the patient usually functions better than the test scores predict and is somewhat inconsistent in test performance, and the cognitive deficit gets better with treatment of the depression. However, patients with dementia can also be depressed. Sometimes the depression is an appropriate response to the patient's awareness of declining cognitive ability. Sometimes the dementia causes symptoms that fall short of a major depressive disorder (e.g., lack of interest in former activities) but are incorrectly perceived as depression. More rarely, major depression is a direct neuropsychiatric manifestation of the underlying dementia. Although the major depression responds to antidepressants, the dementia will continue to get worse and should be treated separately. Patients who have depressive features and cognitive problems require frequent reassessment of the cognitive difficulties, and the possibility of an alternate or additional diagnosis of dementia should be suspected.

CLINICAL FEATURES

Patients with Alzheimer's disease vary in their presentation, but they do have several features in common that should suggest the diagnosis. There is the insidious onset of memory difficulty, which may take the form of repeating information or repeating questions, forgetting information, and/or misplacing objects. Eventually, patients have trouble estimating time frames (e.g., how long ago something happened) and keeping appointments because they have difficulty keeping up with the date, day of the week, or month. All of these symptoms of mild AD can occasionally occur in normal individuals, but they become a pattern in AD patients. This mild stage of AD may or may not include personality and behavior changes or obvious problems with judgment. Mild AD is often missed entirely by patients, their families, and physicians because it does not necessarily preclude carrying out everyday tasks.

As AD progresses, patients develop worsening of the memory loss and temporal disorientation as just described. Most develop spatial disorientation, such as difficulty navigating to unfamiliar, then even to familiar, places. Language problems, initially limited to dysnomia (coming up with words), begin to be obvious and may affect the patients' ability to comprehend explanations as well as the ability to express themselves in words. Some patients lose personal information, such as their age, and may give their birth year or make a joke when asked to give their age. As the disease becomes moderate, patients are no longer able to carry out the complex activities of daily life such as shopping (efficiently), handling finances, and maintaining their households and their hobbies. Many patients develop behavior changes: apathy, anxiety, depression, or even agitation or psychosis. Unfortunately, most patients are not diagnosed until they reach this moderate stage of dementia.

As AD becomes severe, all of the problems described here worsen, and patients are not able to function independently in even the most basic tasks, such as maintaining their personal appearance or making sure that they are adequately nourished. Some patients reach this severe level of dementia before diagnosis, often because they lack insight and caregivers are unwilling or unable to face up to the problem. Patients who reach severe stages after having been diagnosed early may do much better than patients who do not obtain medical attention until this point. In those who were diagnosed early, there has been a chance for constructive adaptation, the use of support services, and medications for cognition and behavioral management. In those who reach this point before obtaining medical care, there is often severe injury to the family structure and caregiver stress or illness, and the patient may be out of reach, no longer able to respond socially. There is a strong argument for early diagnosis of AD.

Formerly, most AD patients with profound levels of dementia lived in institutions and required total nursing care. Most were not ambulatory, wheelchair-bound at best and curled up into the fetal position at worst. A growing number of profoundly demented people now live successfully at home. These individuals are usually mute and do not participate in any of their self-care. They are usually able to ambulate with assistance and some have maintained other motor skills as well, such as the ability to throw and catch a ball, to ride an exercise bicycle, or to hit tennis balls. They require total assistance with eating, dressing, and personal hygiene. Not all families are able to take care of such individuals at home, but with adequate (full-time) caregiving help, increasing numbers are taking advantage of this alternative to long-term placement.

DIAGNOSIS AND DIFFERENTIAL DIAGNOSIS

After ruling out delirium and depression and establishing a clinical picture that is consistent with AD (see previously), diagnostic accuracy can be further enhanced by seeking other disturbances that could cause or contribute to dementia. Table 1 lists several conditions that should be considered, including a number of neurodegenerative disorders. The list of neurodegenerative disorders that can be distinguished from AD is growing, and again argues for early diagnosis, as many of these are diagnosed by variations in the onset or early course of the dementia. In their latest stages, most dementias overlap clinically and psychometrically.

The work-up for dementia remains a controversial topic, with economics fueling the controversy. Every patient should have a thorough work-up at least once in the course of the disease to rule out contributory or alternative diagnoses. As shown in Table 2, this thorough evaluation always includes an imaging study (preferably magnetic resonance imaging), neuropsychologic testing, blood work, a chest radiogram, and electrocardiogram. In special cases, such as a rapid onset or decline within 1 year, or concurrent delirium and dementia, electroencephalogram and lumbar puncture are also indicated. Clinical circumstances may dictate the need for even more specialized tests, such as serum ammonia levels (hepatic dysfunction), amino acid screens (young patients with unusual neurologic findings), or overnight sleep studies (suspected sleep apnea).

TABLE 1. **Differential Diagnosis of Alzheimer's Disease**

Systemic and Brain Conditions	Neurodegenerative Disorders
Depression	Parkinson's disease
Multiple strokes	Lewy body dementia
Alcohol or drugs	Progressive supranuclear palsy
Vitamin deficiencies	Frontotemporal dementias
Hormonal disturbances	(e.g., Pick's disease, primary
Neoplasm	progressive aphasias)
Subdurals	Cortical-basal degeneration
Infections	Hippocampal sclerosis
Vasculitis	Subcortical gliosis

TREATMENT

General Issues

At one time, Alzheimer's disease was referred to as a "nontreatable dementia" to contrast it with other forms of dementia. This distinction was probably incorrect, because the behavioral disturbances of AD have always been amenable to therapy, and it is especially incorrect now because the Food and Drug Administration (FDA) has approved options for treating the cognitive disturbance as well. The currently marketed treatments for AD and many drugs under development are designed to counter the profound cholinergic transmitter deficiency that occurs in this disease. The loss of cholinergic cells is probably a "downstream" event in AD, making it likely that cholinergic treatments are primarily symptomatic and that their effects will be self-limited over time, as critical numbers of cells continue to be lost, despite bolstering of transmitter activity. Still, the degree of symptomatic improvement can be significant, and the duration of such effects, although not rigorously studied, may be years.

Before discussing cholinergic therapies, it is important to realize that other potential therapies are simultaneously being explored in highly publicized clinical trials, and to examine the rationale for some of these potential therapies. Table 3 lists putative risk factors and proposed neuroprotective factors thought to be important for the development of AD based on epidemiologic studies. Clearly, the etiologic link between these factors and AD is relatively weak because most of the studies are retrospective or involve small numbers of AD cases. Probably the best-studied approaches include the use of antioxidants, especially vitamin E and selegiline* (Eldepryl), as possible agents to slow the progression of AD (the data for Gingko Biloba are much weaker), but trials are under way to assess the probability that estrogen and various anti-inflammatory agents can slow the progression of AD. Until such studies are complete, these agents should not be prescribed as therapies, with the possible exception of vitamin E, which appears to be safe in the doses studied (1000 units orally twice daily).

Ultimately, truly disease-modifying therapies for

*Not FDA approved for this indication.

TABLE 2. **Diagnostic Tests in the Evaluation of Demented Patients**

Basic Studies	Clinical Implications
Complete blood cell count	B_{12} or folate deficiency; anemia; polycythemia
Chemistry battery (electrolytes, glucose, liver function tests, calcium, creatinine, blood urea nitrogen)	Hyponatremia; hyperglycemia; chronic renal or liver failure; hyperparathyroidism
Thyroid-stimulating hormone (thyrotropin), T_3	Hypothyroidism; hyperthyroidism
Serum cyanocobalamin (vitamin B_{12})	B_{12} deficiency
Antinuclear antibody	Systemic lupus erythematosus
Venereal Disease Research Laboratory test	Syphilis
Brain imaging: Computed tomography or magnetic resonance imaging	Structural lesions (subdural hematoma; hemorrhage; tumor; infarcts; normal pressure hydrocephalus)
Ancillary Studies	
Human immunodeficiency virus	Acquired immune deficiency syndrome dementia
Cerebrospinal fluid analysis	Meningitis; encephalitis; vasculitis
Electroencephalogram	Creutzfeldt-Jakob disease; seizure disorder
Overnight sleep study	Sleep apnea
Research Studies (Unproven Diagnostic Value)	
Cerebrospinal fluid markers (β-amyloid, τ protein)	
Apolipoprotein E genotype	
Positron emission tomography	
Single-photon emission tomography	

AD will likely be based on an understanding of what causes the tissue changes, such as neurofibrillary tangles, senile plaques, and the recently described new lesion, AMY plaques in the brains of AD patients. Laboratory studies and transgenic mouse models of AD, based on rare genetic forms of AD that occur in humans, are providing the strategies for future medications that could potentially stop the progression of AD.

Treating the Cognitive Disturbance

The FDA has approved two medications for the specific treatment of AD: tacrine (Cognex) was approved in 1993 and donepezil (Aricept) was approved in 1997. Both are cholinesterase inhibitors, which block the normal breakdown of acetylcholine in brain and peripheral tissues. Yet the two drugs have very different chemical structures, toxicities, and pharmacokinetics. Tacrine, an aminoacridine, has been associated with reversible hepatotoxicity, and the FDA recommends monitoring of alanine aminotransferase (ALT) levels every 2 weeks until a stable dose is achieved, and then every 3 months thereafter. The starting dose is 10 mg orally four times a day, and the dose is increased by 10 mg per dose every 6 weeks until adverse effects occur or until a dose of 40 mg orally four times a day has been reached. Dosage escalation is recommended because treatment effects are dose-related. Common side effects include nausea, diarrhea, other gastrointestinal (GI) complaints, and anorexia, sometimes leading to significant weight loss. As many as 60% of patients have been unable to tolerate the higher doses of this drug in clinical trials.

TABLE 3. **Proposed Risk and Protective Factors**

Risk Factors	Neuroprotective Factors
Family history of Alzheimer's disease	Anti-inflammatory use
	Antioxidants
APO E genotype (ϵ_4)*	Postmenopausal estrogen use
Aging and estrogen deficiency	APO E genotype (ϵ_2)
Head injury	High education
Low education	Linguistic complexity (as a reflection of early brain development)

*The type of apolipoprotein E (APO E) is a risk factor for late-onset familial and sporadic forms of AD. Those who inherit one or more ϵ_4 alleles (as opposed to ϵ_2 or ϵ_3) are at greater risk.

Donepezil is a piperidine class compound not associated with hepatotoxicity. No laboratory monitoring is required. In contrast to tacrine, donepezil is about 1200 times more selective for acetylcholinesterase, the cholinesterase common in the brain, as compared to butyrylcholinesterase, the cholinesterase found in peripheral tissues such as the GI tract. This selectivity is believed to account for the low incidence of GI side effects with donepezil (less than 8%) and the good tolerability even at the highest dose. The starting dose is 5 mg orally at bedtime, which can be increased to 10 mg orally at bedtime after 4 weeks. Both doses were effective in clinical trials, but the average percentage of acetylcholinesterase inhibition achieved with the 10-mg dose is higher than with the 5-mg dose, arguing for increasing the dose if the patient is not experiencing side effects.

Both of these cholinesterase inhibitors were approved because they showed benefits for the drugs on group mean psychometric test scores (the Alzheimer's Disease Assessment Scale [ADAS]) and in an independent assessment made by the clinician (the Clinician's Interview-Based Impression of Change [CIBIC]). The ADAS is a test of memory, learning, language, orientation, construction, and praxis that does not lend itself to an office setting. On average, the treated groups scored about 3 points better on this 70-point scale, but individual patients often improved much more than 3 points. On average, then, the effect is modest as assessed by this scale. It is also interesting to note that in the donepezil studies, more patients on the drug improved compared with those on placebo, there were greater degrees of response in drug-treated patients, and more patients on the drug than on placebo "stabilized" or did not change during the studies. Also, fewer patients (half as many compared with placebo) got worse. These findings suggest that an individual patient may benefit from donepezil by improving, staying at the same level longer, or getting worse at a slower rate. However, all of these effects are likely to wear off over time.

When should a physician prescribe these drugs, how should they be monitored, and when should the therapeutic trial be considered a failure or the drug be stopped because it has lost its effects? Research studies have not been performed to answer these questions. Donepezil and tacrine are officially indicated for mild to moderate AD patients because these are the only levels of severity that have been studied so far. Although future studies of donepezil will answer questions of whether it benefits severe patients, empirical trial of these drugs in severe AD patients may be justified. When is the disease too severe to consider using the drugs? This is a quality of life issue to be decided be the clinician and the family: if there is no meaningful function to preserve and nothing to be gained by slowing the disease in an individual subject, it should not be used.

How long will the symptomatic effects last? We can find this out only by conducting long, placebo-controlled trials, which are now unethical because there is a treatment that works. Clinicians and families are again left to make the determination that an individual's condition has progressed sufficiently to justify discontinuation of the drug when they perceive that there is no good quality of life. Tacrine must be tapered slowly because a delirium-like withdrawal effect may occur. This effect has not been described with donepezil.

Finally, how should the clinician monitor for symptomatic improvement and/or deterioration? The CIBIC used in the clinical trials was a comprehensive interview with the patient and caregiver that involved mental status testing of the patient, assessment of behavior, and discussion of the activities of daily living tasks at home. A clinician's assessment taking these areas into account should be used at intervals, either during a clinic visit or by combining a clinic visit with testing information performed by another clinician. Most communities contain at least one person, a neuropsychologist, general psychologist, counselor, or social worker, who can aid busy clinicians in gathering information to make these assessments.

Treating Behavioral Disturbances

Some patients with AD experience disturbances of behavior as part of their illness, whereas others do not. The prevalence of such disturbances depends on how they are defined; for example, apathy will occur almost universally by the time the disease is severe, but some studies do not count this as a behavioral disturbance. It is essential to realize that altered behavior comes about in AD for several reasons, and that successful treatment requires a combination of nonpharmacologic and pharmacologic approaches (Table 4). A few minutes spent assessing the circumstances, details, and triggers for the behavior will

TABLE 4. **Recommended Therapies by Indication**

Sleep/Anxiety
Nonpharmacologic
Daytime stimulation
Adequate supervision
Avoidance of napping
Respite care
Counseling for caregiver
Pharmacologic
Chloral hydrate, 500 to 1000 mg po prn (up to 2/d or 10/wk)
Zolpidem (Ambien), 5 to 10 mg po hs prn
Lorazepam (Ativan), 0.5 to 1 mg po prn (up to 2/d or 10/wk)
Buspirone (Buspar), 5 to 10 mg po tid for short-term (few weeks)
Trazodone (Desyrel), 50 mg po hs, may increase gradually to 50 mg po bid or tid
Possibly melatonin, 1 to 2 mg po hs prn (investigational)
Depression
Nonpharmacologic
Appropriate levels of activity (not too hard or too easy)
Support group for patient
Support group for caregiver
Pharmacologic
Fluoxetine (Prozac), 20 to 40 mg po q AM
Paroxetine (Paxil), 20 to 40 mg po q AM
Sertraline (Zoloft), 50 to 100 mg qd
Agitation/Psychosis
Nonpharmacologic
Identify patterns
Remove triggers
Decide on target symptoms
Treat hallucinations only if they bother the patient
Pharmacologic
Thioridazine (Mellaril), 10 to 25 mg po tid
Olanzapine (Zyprexa), 5 to 10 mg qd
Risperidone (Risperdal), 0.5 to 2 mg qd or bid
Haloperidol (Haldol), 0.5 to 2 mg po bid
Cognition
Nonpharmacologic
Preserve activities through use when possible
Maintain social contacts
Pharmacologic
Donepezil (Aricept), 5 mg po qd for 1 month, then 10 mg po qd
Tacrine (Cognex), 10 mg po qid; increase by 10 mg/dose every 6 weeks to a maximum of 40 mg po qid; must check ALT every other week until highest stable dose for 6 weeks, then check every 3 months
Possibly vitamin E, 1000 IU po bid (investigational)

save time and costs later by reducing the prescription of unneeded or ineffective drugs.

Depression, discussed previously, is usually due to a mismatch between the patient's cognitive abilities and level of functioning. A patient doing too much becomes frustrated and depressed by failures; a patient doing too little is depressed by feelings of worthlessness. Counseling patients and caregivers with solid recommendations (e.g., volunteer work for the patient, change of living circumstances to provide more supervision, day center activities) usually obviates the need for drugs. Certain patients who seem to have a more biochemically based depression (often with premorbid history of depression) may require drugs, and I recommend the selective serotonin-reuptake inhibitors to avoid the anticholinergic side effects seen with some of the other antidepressants. Similarly, sleep disturbance is usually caused by a disrupted sleep routine, such as daytime napping or going to bed too early. Daytime stimulation, such as a day center, with a regular bedtime and regular routine at bedtime (to compensate for the patient's temporal disorientation) are usually more effective than medications. Sometimes the patient is unable to fall asleep, and intermittent hypnotics may be useful, but if used daily, they will lead to other sleep disturbances. If nocturnal agitation is keeping the patient awake on a regular basis, a sedating antidepressant such as trazodone (Desyrel) or a neuroleptic may become necessary.

Anxiety occurs frequently and should be distinguished from agitation, with its potential to harm the patient or someone else. Many anxious patients are reflecting the feelings of their caregiver, or expressing their discomfort with insufficient structure or supervision. Respite care should be suggested, and caregivers may require outside counseling to help them identify options such as (1) regular scheduled "time-off" during which a friend or family member stays with the patient, (2) hired respite aids, and (3) day center or overnight admissions. Anxiety in AD patients should be treated with medication only if it is likely to be short term, for example, after the hospitalization or death of a caregiver.

True agitation (as opposed to anxiety) and psychosis with delusions and disturbing hallucinations may require neuroleptics. The trade-off is always some loss of cognition and possibly some loss of mobility if these agents are used. It is critical to determine the agitated or psychotic behaviors, so that these can be targeted for treatment and so that the family knows what is and what is not being treated. It is equally critical to ensure that the agitation is not just a triggered response to an event or a person in the environment, which would be better treated by removing the trigger. For example, one patient was agitated only when a hired caregiver washed her genitalia, although her behavior was described as "obstructive" before further questioning revealed this pattern. Other patients are agitated in the shower, but respond calmly to a bath. If neuroleptics are used, they should be reassessed at least every 6 months, as their use is not necessary indefinitely. When such agents become necessary, the physician should also initiate (or refer the family for) a discussion of long-term care options in case the drugs are not sufficient to control the target behaviors.

INTRACEREBRAL HEMORRHAGE

method of
ADRIAN J. GOLDSZMIDT, M.D.
Sinai Hospital
Baltimore, Maryland

and

LOUIS R. CAPLAN, M.D.
Beth Israel Deaconess Medical Center
Boston, Massachusetts

Intracerebral hemorrhage (ICH) affects nearly 40,000 Americans yearly. ICH accounts for 10 to 15% of strokes in the United States, and these patients have a poorer prognosis than those with ischemic stroke. Mortality from ICH is 35 to 50% at 30 days, and only 10 to 20% of patients resume independent living. Diagnosis and treatment of ICH are important components of neurologic practice.

ETIOLOGY

Half of spontaneous ICH is attributable to arterial hypertension. Hypertensive hemorrhages typically occur in specific areas: the putamen, thalamus, subcortical white matter, cerebellum, and pons. Two mechanisms are responsible: (1) rupture of small penetrating arteries damaged by chronic hypertension and aging and (2) sudden blood pressure increases causing rupture of arterioles unaccustomed to high blood pressure. Congenital or acquired vascular anomalies such as aneurysms and arteriovenous malformations account for 25% of ICH. Cerebral amyloid angiopathy is a leading cause of ICH, particularly in older patients. Amyloid angiopathy is seen in 10% of people at age 70, but in 60% of people older than 90. Bleeding diathesis, tumors, vasculitis, and drugs (especially cocaine and amphetamines) are other frequent causes (Table 1). Aging, African-American heritage, previous strokes, anticoagulation, coronary artery disease, alcohol abuse, and diabetes mellitus increase the risk for ICH.

CLINICAL FEATURES

Neurologic signs and symptoms vary depending on the location and size of the hemorrhage. About 50% of patients have headache, nausea, and vomiting. Most patients present with focal neurologic deficits, with smoothly progressive deterioration over minutes to hours; in 33%, the deficit is maximal at onset without further progression. Most ICH occurs during routine daily activities. Only 10% of patients note symptoms on awakening, which is less often than occurs in ischemic stroke. In another 10%, ICH is associated with physical or emotional stress.

Depressed level of consciousness may be found in 50% of patients with ICH, and coma is a sign of poor prognosis. Coma occurs in about 20% of patients at presentation. In pontine or thalamic hemorrhage, coma is caused by

TABLE 1. **Etiologies of Spontaneous Intracerebral Hemorrhage**

Arterial Hypertension

Aneurysms

Saccular
Infective
Traumatic
Neoplastic

Vascular Malformations

Arteriovenous malformations
Capillary telangiectasias
Cavernous angiomas
Venous malformations

Bleeding Diatheses

Leukemia
Thrombocytopenia
Disseminated intravascular coagulation
Polycythemia
Hyperviscosity
Hemophilia
Hypoprothrombinemia
Afibrinogenemia
Clotting factor deficiencies
von Willebrand's disease
Sickle cell anemia
Anticoagulant therapy
Thrombolytic therapy

Cerebral Amyloid Angiopathy

Arteritis/Arteriopathies

Infective vasculitis
Multisystem vasculitis
Isolated central nervous system angiitis
Moyamoya disease

Drug-Related

Amphetamines
Cocaine
Phenylpropanolamine
Pentazocine (Talwin)-pyribenzamine
Phencyclidine
Heroin
Monoamine oxidase inhibitor

Intracranial Tumors

Primary malignant or benign
Metastatic

Cerebral Venous Occlusion

Miscellaneous

After carotid endarterectomy
After neurosurgical procedures
After spinal anesthesia
Postmyelography
Cold related
Lightning stroke
Heat stroke
Fat embolism
After painful dental procedures
Protracted migraine
Methanol intoxication

Adapted from Biller J, Shah MV: Intracerebral hemorrhage. In Rakel RE (ed): Conn's Current Therapy 1997. Philadelphia, WB Saunders Co, 1997, p 877.

involvement of the reticular activating system. In lobar hemorrhage, depressed consciousness is due to midline shift from mass effect.

Seizures occur in less than 10% of ICH, but are much more common with lobar hemorrhage, approaching 25% of patients. Overall, seizures are much more likely with supratentorial hemorrhages. Patients who do not have seizures at onset are unlikely to develop seizures.

COMMON SYNDROMES

The most common site for ICH is the putamen, accounting for 33% of all hemorrhages. Typical signs include contralateral hemiplegia with sensory impairment, hemianopia, contralateral gaze paresis, and aphasia (dominant hemisphere) or neglect (nondominant hemisphere). Enlarging putaminal hemorrhages can spread medially into the internal capsule, caudate nucleus, and lateral ventricle, or laterally into the insula.

Lobar hemorrhages are usually due to hypertension or amyloid angiopathy. They occur in the subcortical white matter, and the clinical syndromes resemble those seen with ischemic infarction in the involved territory. Seizures are common.

Thalamic hemorrhages account for 20% of ICH. Posterolateral thalamic hemorrhages are most common, and patients present with sensory deficits and mild hemiparesis. Small hemorrhages in the anterior thalamus can disrupt frontal lobe connections resulting in abulia, with impaired memory, hemiparesis, and minimal sensory loss. Vertical gaze palsy is due to pressure on the adjacent midbrain tectum. Aphasia may be seen in dominant hemisphere thalamic ICH, whereas nondominant lesions produce neglect. Medial thalamic ICH produces markedly depressed level of consciousness, with subsequent abulia and difficulty making new memories.

Cerebellar hemorrhage occurs in 8% of patients. The hemorrhages are usually in the dentate nucleus. Vermian hemorrhages are less frequent. Compression or extension into the fourth ventricle is common. Patients may be drowsy, with nuchal rigidity and headache. Ipsilateral ataxia and hypotonia are present, but hemiparesis and hemisensory loss are absent. Conjugate gaze palsy or sixth nerve palsy and ipsilateral facial weakness may be seen. Pupils tend to be small and reactive. Rapid clinical deterioration from brain stem compression may occur. Death may result from medullary compression by cerebellar tonsillar herniation. Mortality is higher for patients who are comatose at presentation; however, decreased responsiveness may be due to hydrocephalus and can be reversed with prompt ventricular drainage.

Pontine hemorrhages are nearly as common as cerebellar hemorrhages, usually at the junction of the basis pontis and tegmentum. This area receives blood from paramedian pontine perforating vessels from the basilar artery. The hematoma can extend rostrally into the midbrain, or rupture into the fourth ventricle. Findings include quadriplegia, pinpoint pupils, horizontal gaze palsies, and coma. Weakness may initially be asymmetrical before progressing to quadriplegia. Respiratory abnormalities, including Cheyne-Stokes respirations, are common. Lateral pontine tegmental hemorrhages, which occur in areas supplied by penetrators from short circumferential branches of the basilar artery, produce crossed hemisensory loss, ataxia, and oculomotor deficits, as well as ipsilateral cranial nerve signs. The pupils may be asymmetrical, with ipsilateral meiosis.

Caudate hemorrhages account for 4% of ICH. These can rupture into the ventricle, dissect laterally into the internal capsule and putamen, or inferiorly into the diencephalon. With intraventricular spread, there is headache, vomiting, and mental status changes with few motor or sensory signs. Hemorrhages that dissect posterolaterally may be difficult to distinguish from primary putaminal hemorrhages. Those that dissect posteroinferiorly cause a Horner's syndrome from hypothalamic involvement and vertical gaze paresis from thalamic involvement.

DIAGNOSIS

Thorough history taking and examination are important to diagnosis. History of hypertension, drug and alcohol ingestion, systemic diseases, and coagulopathies should be sought. Unenhanced computed tomography (CT) scanning remains the safest, most sensitive method available to identify and localize ICH (Table 2). CT findings of subarachnoid or intraventricular hemorrhage, abnormal intracranial calcification, and prominent vascular structures should prompt further evaluation for an underlying structural abnormality. Younger patients, especially those without hypertension, should also be further studied. Magnetic resonance imaging is an important tool for identifying vascular malformations and tumors and may be better than cerebral angiography in detecting cavernous angiomas. Angiography may reveal an aneurysm, moyamoya disease, vasculitis, or an arteriovenous malformation.

MEDICAL TREATMENT

Despite the morbidity associated with ICH, there are no good studies documenting widespread efficacy for medical or surgical treatment modalities; therefore, there is tremendous variability in treatment. All patients should be admitted to the hospital, ideally to an intensive care or stroke unit, where blood pressure monitoring and frequent neurologic assessment can occur. Immediate assessment of ventilation is important, with intubation for obtunded patients who are at increased risk for aspiration.

Coagulation defects should be corrected. For patients receiving warfarin, subcutaneous vitamin K (10 mg), and fresh-frozen plasma, 20 mL per kg should be administered. For patients receiving heparin, protamine (1 mg intravenously for each 100 units of heparin infused in the previous 2 hours, but no more than 50 mg per 10 minutes) should be infused. Patients with hemophilia require therapy with factor VIII to achieve a level of 80 to 100% of normal; immediate neurosurgical evaluation may also be needed. Patients with thrombocytopenia require platelet transfusion. Thrombolytic-associated bleeding requires administration of 10 units of intravenous cryoprecipitate. Fresh-frozen plasma, 20 mL per kg, may also be needed. Aminocaproic acid (Amicar), 5 grams over 30 to 60 minutes followed by 1 gram per hour intravenously, may be used for continued bleeding.

Blood pressure management is crucial. Maintaining adequate blood pressure prevents ongoing or recurrent bleeding, while preserving cerebral perfusion. Patients with systolic pressures greater than 180 mm Hg or mean arterial pressure (MAP) greater than 130 mm Hg should be treated. The goal is to maintain cerebral perfusion pressure at 70 to 100 mm Hg, which can be achieved with a MAP of 100 to 130 mm Hg. Antihypertensive agents should have rapid effects, be easily adjustable, and not have adverse effects on cerebral blood flow or intracranial pressure. For moderate blood pressure elevations, intravenous labetalol (Normodyne), 10 to 20 mg intravenously, may be used, with repeated doses given until an effect is achieved. For severe blood pressure elevations, nitroprusside 0.2 μg per kg per minute; titrated up or down every 5 to 10 minutes by similar increments, is recommended.

Patients with neurologic deterioration, signs of herniation, or respiratory depression should be intubated. Some patients may require intracranial pressure monitoring for optimal management. Hyperventilation (lowering the P_{CO_2} to 25 to 30 mm Hg) is the fastest way to decrease intracranial pressure. Hyperosmolar therapy is with mannitol, 1 gram per kg over 20 to 30 minutes, followed by 0.25 to 0.5 gram per kg every 4 to 6 hours. Serum osmolality should be monitored. Head elevation (15 to 30 degrees) promotes venous drainage. Hypo-osmolar solutions increase edema and should be avoided. Corticosteroids are associated with increased complications without clear benefit and are not recommended.

Prophylactic anticonvulsants should be considered for cases of lobar hemorrhage. Phenytoin (Dilantin), 18 mg per kg intravenously at a maximum of 50 mg per minute, or fosphenytoin (Cerebyx), 18 mg per kg phenytoin equivalents at a maximum of 150 mg per minute, may be given. Patients with ICH are also at risk for deep venous thrombosis, and pneumatic compression stockings are recommended. Frequent turning and variable pressure mattresses reduce the risk of decubitus ulcers.

TABLE 2. **Laboratory and Radiologic Evaluation in Intracerebral Hemorrhage**

All Patients

1. Complete blood count with platelet count
2. Prothrombin time, international normalized ratio, partial thromboplastin time
3. Erythrocyte sedimentation rate
4. Blood glucose
5. Serum alkaline phosphatase, glutamic oxaloacetic transaminase, calcium, blood urea nitrogen, creatinine
6. Urinalysis
7. Chest roentgenogram
8. Electrocardiogram
9. Unenhanced cranial computed tomography (CT)

Selected Patients

1. Blood cultures
2. Drug screen
3. Antinuclear antibodies assay
4. Sickle cell screen
5. Hemoglobin electrophoresis
6. Serum fibrinogen, fibrin split products, serum viscosity
7. Thrombin time, reptilase time, bleeding time
8. Type and screen
9. Human immunodeficiency virus antibody
10. Contrast-enhanced cranial CT
11. Magnetic resonance brain imaging
12. Cerebral angiography

Adapted from Biller J, Shah MV: Intracerebral hemorrhage. In Rakel RE (ed): Conn's Current Therapy 1997. Philadelphia, WB Saunders Co, 1997, p 879.

SURGICAL TREATMENT

Indications for surgical treatment of ICH remain controversial, without data to support clear indications for surgery. Patients with massive hemorrhage who are in a coma are not likely to benefit. Patients with putaminal hemorrhages that rupture into the ventricle also do poorly regardless of treatment modality; for deteriorating patients with moderate ICH, without ventricular spread, surgery should be considered. Young patients with lobar hemorrhage who deteriorate during observation should also be considered for surgery. Patients with thalamic hemorrhage rarely need surgery, except ventricular drainage for hydrocephalus. Patients with small ICHs who are fully conscious do best with medical therapy.

Patients with cerebellar hemorrhage greater than 3 cm in diameter, or those with smaller hemorrhages and deterioration, should be treated surgically. Brain stem compression and ventricular obstruction may be rapidly fatal, but completely reversible with early surgery.

Research is under way to evaluate whether early surgical intervention, or newer, less invasive modalities such as stereoscopic or endoscopic surgery may be beneficial in some cases. Stereotactic irrigation with thrombolytic agents is also being investigated.

ISCHEMIC CEREBROVASCULAR DISEASE

method of
PIERRE B. FAYAD, M.D.
Yale University School of Medicine
New Haven, Connecticut

The management of stroke has dramatically evolved over the last decade in parallel with an improvement in epidemiology and diagnostic techniques and the increased availability of newer medications and treatment strategies. Effective stroke management avoids lumping together all strokes or treating them equally, but rather targets treatments to the specific pathology identified while balancing the prognostic profile and the risks of therapy. The opportunities for stroke prevention have become more specific and effective with agreement on diagnostic strategies that distinguish between stroke subtypes and various prognostic categories. Acute stroke therapy has become more scientifically tested, and massive research efforts are ongoing to provide effective therapies. This article summarizes the latest advances in the acute treatment and prevention of ischemic stroke.

ACUTE STROKE MANAGEMENT

The care for acute stroke is changing rapidly as results from clinical trials become available. With shorter hospital stays, the evaluation and treatment must be more efficient and goal directed.

Acute Stroke Is an Emergency

Acute stroke is an emergency that requires immediate attention. In the past, this was not the standard of treatment. "Time Is Brain." Time is critical if any ischemic brain is to be salvaged by the approved or investigational therapies. This puts pressure on the primary care physicians, emergency teams, and the neurologists to organize the care of stroke in response to those needs. Patients at risk and their families should be educated about the signs and symptoms of stroke. They should also be instructed to call 911, activating the emergency system, when these symptoms are experienced or observed to achieve the fastest arrival to the emergency department and receive appropriate treatment without delay.

Stroke Care Is Managed by a Team

Involvement of a multidisciplinary team of physicians (primary care, neurology, physical medicine, emergency medicine, radiology, and surgery) and other medical and paramedical staff (nurses; social workers; physical, occupational, and speech therapists) mandates a close coordination to focus and render more efficient the care of stroke patients.

Good stroke care begins by establishing clear management goals and adopting strategies to achieve them in a timely fashion. The major goals for care can be categorized as shown in Table 1. Providing supportive care and preventing complications are as important as pharmacologic therapy for improving patient outcome.

SUPPORTIVE CARE

The basic clinical care of stroke requires early and close attention to details. The overwhelming majority (>90%) of deaths in the first week after a stroke are caused by associated medical complications. The primary goal of supportive care is to acknowledge the risks and provide strategies to prevent those complications. The following is a description of the main complications, those at risk for experiencing them, and ways to prevent them.

There is increasing evidence that mild changes in temperature can significantly influence stroke outcome. Thus any fever in the setting of stroke should be lowered aggressively short of masking an infection. Patients are generally placed on bed rest for a few hours, because of common gait and balance impairment, which may place them at risk for falling, until their safety evaluation is initiated by physical therapists. A few patients may also develop worsening of their neurologic deficits when they stand. Maintaining adequate nutrition is a challenge because of acquired swallowing difficulties. Nutrition therapy

TABLE 1. **Goals of Acute Stroke Care**

1. Rapid triage and identification of stroke (exclude other nonvascular causes)
2. Determine stroke type: ischemic or hemorrhagic
3. Determine the eligibility for "acute stroke therapy"
4. Determine size, location, and vascular territory (carotid vs vertebrobasilar)
5. Establish plans for efficient management and discharge
6. Stabilize and prevent complications
7. Determine etiology and mechanism (e.g., large-vessel, cardioembolic)
8. Initiate secondary stroke prevention strategies
9. Initiate rehabilitation assessment and therapy

should be started as soon as possible, through a nasogastric tube if there are concerns about dysphagia, to prevent loss of muscle mass or strength and the ability to ambulate. Often patients with stroke suffer from dehydration, but fluid supplementation with isotonic saline solutions should be used cautiously because of the potential for concomitant cardiac or renal disease. Hypotonic solutions should be avoided because they can worsen cerebral edema.

PREVENTING COMPLICATIONS

The brain's ability to regulate cerebral blood flow is impaired acutely. Thus decreases in systemic blood pressure are reflected as decreased brain perfusion to the area of the stroke resulting in neurologic deterioration.

Hypertension is found in more than two thirds of all patients acutely and is considered reactive, probably on a compensatory basis, as it resolves spontaneously over the first few days. Therefore, no antihypertensive therapy is advocated to avoid worsening the cerebral ischemic damage. However, hypertension should be treated when end-organ damage such as heart or kidney failure or hypertensive encephalopathy becomes evident. Treatment should be initiated when systolic blood pressure is greater than 220 mm Hg and diastolic blood pressure is greater than 120 mm Hg. Tighter treatment parameters are used when alteplase (Activase) is given to lower the risk of hemorrhage. When immediate blood pressure lowering is indicated, agents with smooth effects (e.g., labetalol, enalapril, nicardipine) are preferred. Antihypertensive agents with rapid action (sublingual nifedipine) are contraindicated because of potential worsening of the neurologic deficits.

Urinary tract infections are common in patients with acute stroke and contribute to several negative effects by prolonging hospital stay, producing fever, worsening the neurologic deficits, and delaying recovery. Most urinary tract infections are related to indwelling urinary catheters, which should be avoided and replaced by condom catheters if necessary.

Dysphagia occurs in 25% of hemispheric strokes and 60% of brain stem strokes and increases the risk of aspiration pneumonia, which is responsible for most stroke-related deaths. The presence of brain stem infarctions, multiple or bilateral strokes, large hemispheric stroke, buccal apraxia, aphasia, and dysarthria or depressed level of consciousness should mandate more careful evaluation for swallowing ability to prevent aspiration. A swallowing evaluation by a speech pathologist in patients at risk can be helpful. Patients with severe dysphagia generally require a gastrostomy tube for enteral feeding.

Deep venous thrombosis (DVT) is found in 50% of paralyzed legs. Immobilized patients or those paralyzed are at highest risk for developing DVT. With proper attention to activity and early mobilization, its incidence can be reduced. Low-dose and subcutaneous heparin or a low-molecular-weight heparin can help further reduce the risk of DVT. Although uncommon with proper care, pulmonary embolism is the most life-threatening result of DVT.

Cytotoxic edema occurs with ischemic stroke and becomes maximal within 3 to 5 days from onset, precipitating brain herniation in large infarctions. Unfortunately, there is no effective strategy to decrease the edema. Corticosteroids that are effective in vasogenic edema (i.e., tumors) have no role in the treatment of cytotoxic edema and increase the risk of infections. Mannitol and hyperventilation that can decrease edema have a short-lived effectiveness and are used only with impending herniation, but are ineffective for a longer period. Surgical resection of the infarcted brain tissue and/or lifting an area of the skull can be used to prevent death from the mass effect; this procedure should be used emergently for cerebellar infarctions compressing the brain stem (Table 2).

MEDICAL THERAPY

The medical strategies can be divided into antithrombotic, thrombolytic, and neuroprotective therapy groups.

Antithrombotic Therapy

The goal of antithrombotic therapy is to improve outcome by preventing progression and recurrence of cerebral thromboembolism and to prevent systemic thromboembolic complications (myocardial infarction, deep venous thrombosis, and pulmonary embolism).

Aspirin should be started as soon as possible after an ischemic stroke if no thrombolytic therapy is considered. When started within 48 hours in the Chinese acute stroke trial, it significantly decreased the risk of death, with a trend toward lowering the risk of recurrent stroke. When the results were analyzed along with other aspirin trials, however, a benefit in reducing the risk of stroke recurrence became significant, despite a small increase in hemorrhagic stroke.

Acute full anticoagulation is losing favor in the treatment of acute stroke after completion of recent trials. Even subcutaneous heparin should be used only in patients with hemiplegia or those who are bedridden for DVT prophylaxis. Whatever the benefit may be, it appears small compared with an increased risk for symptomatic cerebral hemorrhage. A major recent trial, the International Stroke Trial using high-dose unfractionated heparin (UFH) (12,500 units twice daily), low-dose UFH (5000 units twice daily), or aspirin, started within 48 hours from symptoms, failed to show any significant benefit in improving overall stroke outcome. Despite a small reduction of recurrent ischemic stroke, the benefit was outweighed by an increase in the risk of hemorrhagic stroke. Similar results were found in another trial using ORG 10172 (danaparoid) (a low-molecular-weight heparin) in acute stroke, where no improvement in outcome was seen. Only subgroup analysis suggested some benefit in preventing stroke recurrence related to large artery occlusive disease.

Thrombolytic Therapy

Thrombolytic therapy is aimed at restoring blood flow to the brain by dissolving the clot responsible for the stroke, thereby preventing further ischemic damage. From a flurry of clinical trials investigating thrombolytic agents for acute stroke, only one study, the National Institutes of Neurologic Disease and Stroke (NINDS) r-tPA (Activase) study, demonstrated its effectiveness. A 30% increased chance of being minimally impaired or without deficits was demon-

TABLE 2. **Surgical and Endovascular Interventions for Stroke**

Intervention	Description	Indications	Status
Acute Stroke Therapy			
Intra-arterial thrombolysis	Placing microcatheter in clot and infusing thrombolytic agent	Acute large vessel occlusion, basilar thrombosis, sinus venous thrombosis	Investigational
Suboccipital craniectomy	Removing part of cranium and infarcted cerebellum	Cerebellar infarct with brain stem compression	The only emergency surgery for acute stroke
Craniotomy and temporal lobectomy, strokectomy	Removing part of skull and infarcted brain	Only as a life-saving measure in large infarcts with pending herniation	Life-saving measure only
Stroke Prevention			
Carotid endarterectomy	Resection of plaque with or without venous patch	Symptomatic carotid stenosis >70%, severe asymptomatic carotid stenosis	Well investigated, results pending for symptomatic 30–69% stenosis
Carotid angioplasty and stenting	Endovascular balloon inflation followed by expanding stent	Inoperable or high-risk symptomatic carotid stenosis	Investigational

strated above placebo 3 months after the stroke. The dose used is lower than the one for acute myocardial infarction (AMI) (0.9 mg per kg to a maximum of 90 mg, given as 10% bolus with the rest infused over 1 hour) and should be started intravenously within 3 hours from the onset of symptoms.

The concerns are mainly of intracerebral bleeding (6% absolute risk), which is frequently fatal when it occurs. Despite the increased bleeding risk, death was not increased in the treated group, but rather a lower mortality trend was found at 3 months. To obtain the beneficial results, patients need to be selected and monitored carefully according to the criteria set in the trial.

Other thrombolytic trials using doses similar to those for AMI and a wider time window failed to show a benefit while increasing the risk of intracranial hemorrhage. Still other ongoing trials will help refine thrombolytic therapy's applications with wider time windows, intra-arterially with r-prourokinase (Prolyse), or in combination with neuroprotective agents. Currently, only r-tPA is approved by the Food and Drug Administration (FDA) for the treatment of acute ischemic stroke.

Neuroprotective Therapy

Neuroprotective agents are aimed at antagonizing different biochemical and molecular processes that are triggered by cerebral ischemia and are responsible for progressive cerebral damage. These include an excessive release of excitatory neurotransmitters (e.g., glutamate, aspartate), activation of ion channels (e.g., Na^+, Ca^{2+}, and postsynaptic receptors NMDA and AMPA), free radical accumulation, excessive entry of calcium and free water into the cells, preprogrammed cell death, and destruction of cell membrane and organelles. The trials that are closest to conclusion involve two agents: lubeluzole (Prosynap) (blocks nitric oxide–mediated pathway of glutamate toxicity) and citicoline (a phospholipid that enhances the restoration of damaged cellular membranes).

STROKE PREVENTION

Prevention of stroke is key in reducing the burden of this disease from both human and financial aspects. A well-established fact is that stroke is preventable. Major information has been gained from epidemiologic studies and randomized trials that allows the identification of several risk factors and the persons at highest risk. Any judicious stroke prevention starts by identifying the risk factors and modifying them (Table 3). Thus, stroke prevention can begin even before any symptoms are evident (primary prevention) with guidelines summarized in Figure 1. Stroke prevention becomes even more important after a transient ischemic attack (TIA), transient monocular blindness (TMB), or stroke (secondary prevention), all of which offer unique opportunities for identifying patients at high risk for imminent stroke. Guidelines for secondary prevention are summarized in Figure 2.

The pharmacologic agents available for stroke prevention are limited (Table 4). Antiplatelet agents are overwhelmingly used in most patients without cardioembolic risk. Low-dose aspirin (81 to 325 mg daily) is the first line drug because of low cost, good tolerability, once-a-day dose, and large cardiovascular prevention experience. Patients who are intolerant of aspirin or who develop recurrence of TIA or stroke are switched to ticlopidine (Ticlid). Other agents with proven efficacy for stroke prevention could become alternatives once they are approved by the FDA.

Determining the pathology that predisposes patients to stroke whether in primary or secondary prevention is essential to improve treatment effectiveness. Figure 3 presents a suggested algorithm for determining the pathophysiology of stroke or TIA.

TABLE 3. **Risk Factors for Stroke**

Risk Factor	Relative Risk	Treatment	Modification Effect
Hypertension	6X	Antihypertensives	Beneficial, proven
Smoking	2X	Stop smoking	Beneficial, proven
Diabetes mellitus	2–4X	Tight control	Beneficial, unproven
Atrial fibrillation	3X	Warfarin	Beneficial, proven
Coronary artery disease	2–6X		Beneficial, unproven
Recent transient ischemic attack or stroke	10X	Treatment by mechanism	Beneficial, proven

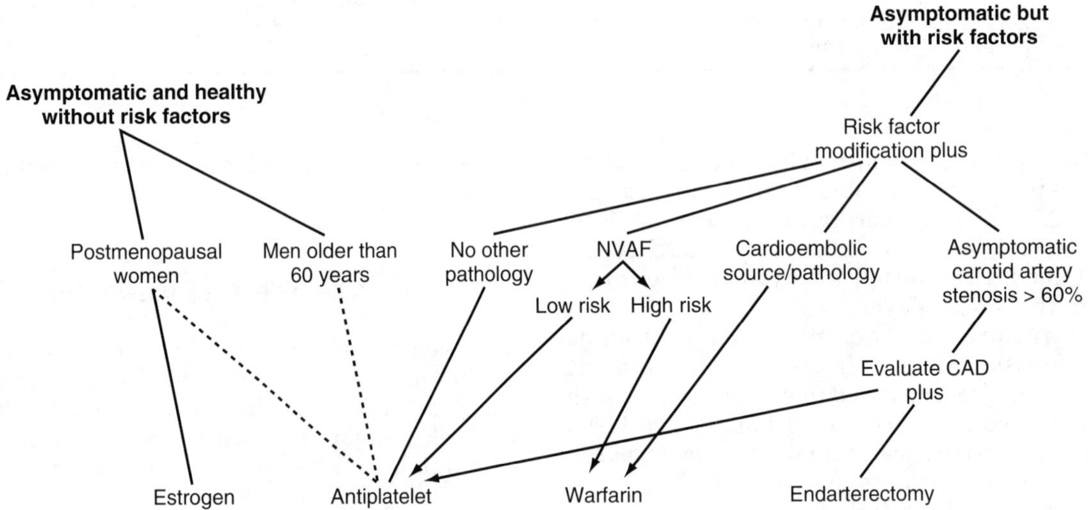

Figure 1. Primary stroke prevention. *Abbreviations:* NV AFib = nonvalvular atrial fibrillation; CAD = coronary artery disease; solid arrow = highly recommended indication; solid line = commonly used indication, but not exclusive; broken line = possible but uncommonly recommended indication. (Adapted from Fayad PB: Advances in stroke prevention. J Cardiovasc Diagn Proc *12*:35–42, 1994.)

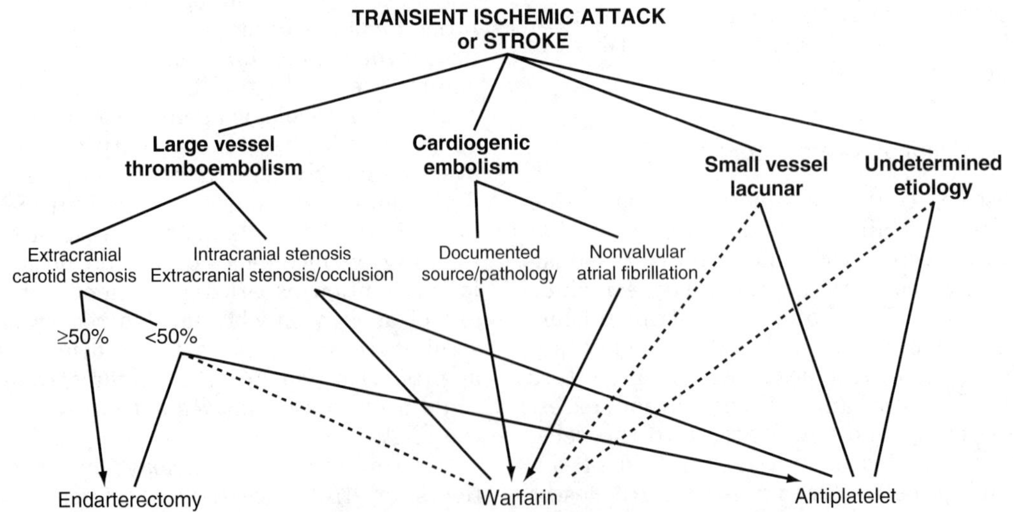

Figure 2. Secondary stroke prevention. *Abbreviations:* Solid arrow = highly recommended indication; solid line = commonly used indication, but not exclusive; broken line = possible but uncommonly recommended indication. (Adapted from Fayad PB: Advances in stroke prevention. J Cardiovasc Diagn Proc *12*:35–42, 1994.)

TABLE 4. **Medical Therapies for Stroke**

Name	Mechanism of Action	Daily Dose	Administration	Major Adverse Effects	Indications	Status
Aspirin	Antiplatelet, CO pathway inhibitor	81–1200 mg	81–325 mg PO qd, 325–650 mg PO bid-tid	GI upset, bleeding	AIS, stroke prophylaxis	Approved
Ticlopidine (Ticlid)	Antiplatelet, ADP pathway inhibitor	500 mg	250 mg PO bid	Diarrhea, rash, neutropenia (CBC q 2 w × 6)	Stroke prophylaxis, I/F other antiplatelets	Approved
Dipyridamole-ASA combination, slow-release	Antiplatelet, PDE and CO pathway inhibitor	ASA 50 mg + DP 400 mg	ASA 25 + DP 200 PO bid	Headache, diarrhea, GI irritation	Stroke prophylaxis, I/F other antiplatelets	Not yet approved
Clopidogrel (Plavix)	Antiplatelet, ADP pathway inhibitor	75 mg	75 mg PO qd	Rash, diarrhea, GI irritation	Stroke prophylaxis, I/F other antiplatelets	Approved
Warfarin (Coumadin)	Anticoagulant, limits gamma-carboxylation of factors II, VII, IX, X and proteins C and S	Adjusted dose	PO adjusted dose to INR target	ICH, systemic bleed, drug interactions	Stroke prophylaxis, INR 2–3 most cardioembolism, INR 3–4.5 prosthetic valves	Approved
Heparin, unfractionated, high dose	Anticoagulant, catalyst for thrombin-antithrombin binding	Adjusted 1000 IU/h infusion, no bolus	Adjusted IV infusion, target PTT 1½–2 X control	ICH, systemic bleeding, immune thrombocytopenia	AIS with large vessel stenosis or cardioembolism	Approved
Heparin, unfractionated, low-dose	Anticoagulant, catalyst for thrombin-antithrombin binding	10,000 IU	5000 IU SC bid	Bleeding	DVT prophylaxis	Approved
r-tPA (Activase)	Thrombolytic, plasminogen activator	0.9 mg/kg (max 90 mg)	10% dose IV bolus, 90% dose IV infusion × 1 h	ICH, systemic bleeding	AIS ≤3 h onset	Approved

Abbreviations: ADP = adenosine-diphosphate; AIS = acute ischemic stroke; ASA = aspirin; CBC = complete blood count; CO = cyclooxygenase; DP = dipyridamole; DVT = deep venous thrombosis; GI = gastrointestinal; ICH = intracerebral hemorrhage; I/F = intolerance/failure; INR = international normalized ratio; PDE = phosphodiesterase; PTT = partial thromboplastin time.

Large Vessel or Atherothromboembolic Stroke

Large vessel narrowing, extracranially (in the neck) or intracranially, from atherosclerotic plaque produces artery-to-artery embolism or hemodynamic perfusion failure. Higher risk factors for intracranial stenosis include diabetes and being African-American or Hispanic. Most commonly, carotid duplex ultrasound screening is used, but is limited to the cervical carotid artery segment. Investigating the rest of the vascular tree requires magnetic resonance angiography or transcranial Doppler. Catheter cerebral angiography, which is the gold standard for imaging the whole vascular tree, is also the most accurate at measuring the degree of stenosis, which correlates with clinical outcome. Management can be planned based on the presence and degree of stenosis. When carotid endarterectomy (CEA) is considered, knowledge of the surgeon's rate of complications from previous surgeries is essential to maximize the benefit to the patients (Table 2).

In the setting of symptomatic extracranial carotid stenosis (associated with ipsilateral TMB, TIA, or minor stroke), the risk of stroke becomes distinctly high. It has been well demonstrated through NASCET (North American Symptomatic Carotid Endarterectomy Trial) that the risk of stroke is high (26% over 2 years) and proportional to the degree of stenosis in patients with stenosis between 70% and 99% as measured by catheter angiography according to NASCET criteria. The relative stroke risk reduction from CEA in this subgroup reaches 80%. The risk of stroke associated with TMB (16%) is less than that for hemispheric TIA (43%). The results from NASCET for CEA on carotid stenoses of 30 to 69% have not been published. When the carotid narrowing is below 30% but associated with ipsilateral symptoms, CEA did not reduce the future stroke risk in the European Carotid Surgery Trial.

The risk of stroke is substantially lower (3 to 4%) yearly in asymptomatic extracranial carotid stenosis. Although the Asymptomatic Carotid Artery Study demonstrated that CEA reduced the risk of stroke by 55% in patients with carotid stenosis of at least 60%, the absolute stroke risk reduction, from 12% to 5% over 3 years, is considered too small to systematically adopt CEA for asymptomatic patients. Patients with higher degrees of stenosis, 80% or higher by angiography, and those with multiple vascular risk factors are selected for surgery because of their higher risk of stroke.

The subset of patients with intracranial carotid or vertebral or basilar stenosis has not been studied as well as those with extracranial carotid stenosis. Stroke prophylaxis in this situation is mainly medi-

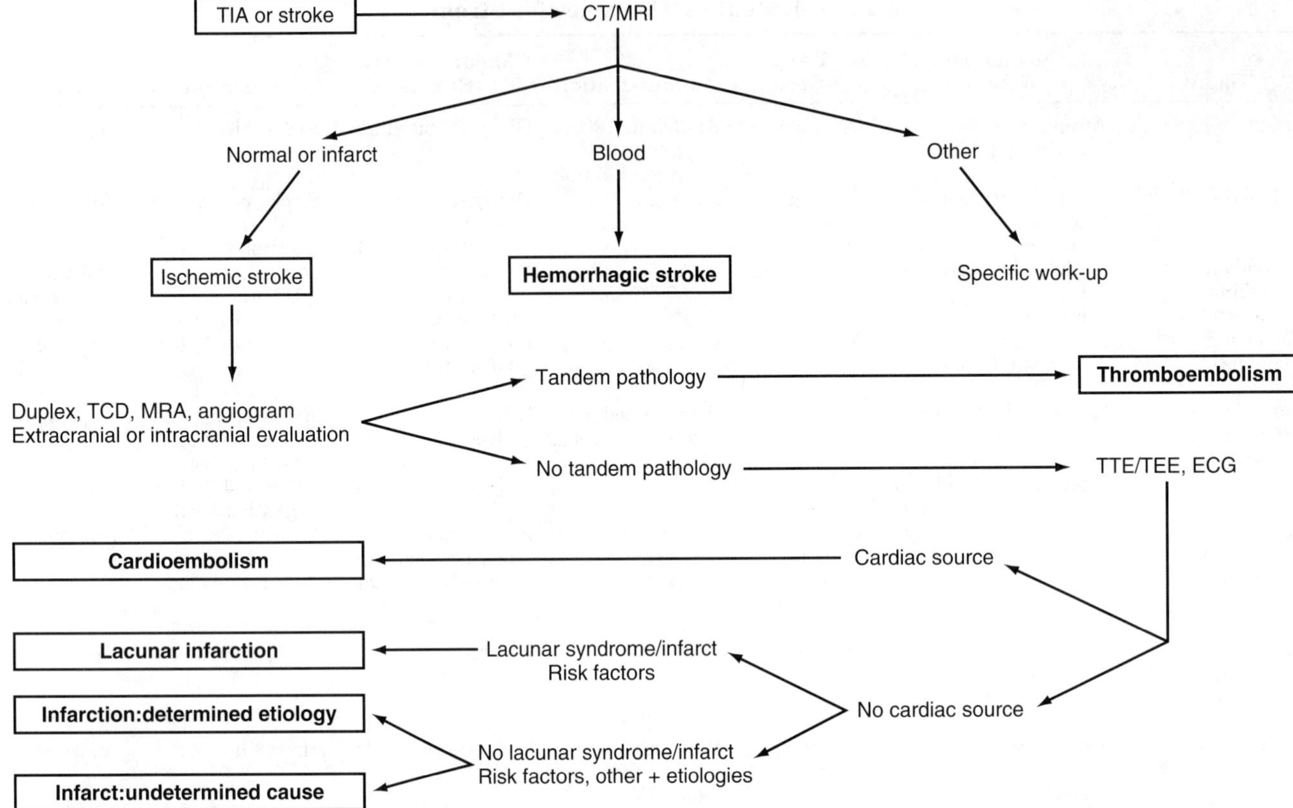

Figure 3. Suggested algorithm for stroke subtype and pathophysiology determination. *Abbreviations:* TIA = transient ischemic attack; CT = computed tomography; MRI = magnetic resonance imaging; TCD = transcranial Doppler; MRA = magnetic resonance angiography; TTE = transthoracic echocardiography; TEE = transesophageal echocardiography; ECG = electrocardiography. (Adapted from Fayad PB: Advances in stroke prevention. J Cardiovasc Diagn Proc *12*:35–42, 1994.)

cal. Although antiplatelet agents are widely used, warfarin is sometimes indicated in patients with recurrent cerebral ischemic events and those with vertebrobasilar stenosis. Surgery is not indicated in this setting, but endovascular therapy with angioplasty and stenting are being investigated and may play a role in the coming years if proven useful.

Cardioembolism and Stroke

Cardioembolic stroke is caused by an embolus originating from a well-documented cardiac source or condition (e.g., thrombus, artificial valve, atrial fibrillation) in the absence of significant proximally occlusive cerebrovascular disease. Warfarin (Coumadin) is the drug of choice in preventing cardioembolic stroke. The dose is adjusted to the International Normalized Ratio (INR) with low-intensity anticoagulation (INR = 2 to 3) for most conditions, and high-intensity (INR = 3 to 4.5) for prosthetic valves.

Despite a low annual risk of cerebral infarction (5%) in patients with nonvalvular atrial fibrillation (NVAF), its high prevalence makes it responsible for more than 50% of all cardioembolic strokes. Several studies have established the superiority of warfarin to aspirin or no treatment in reducing stroke risk (60 to 80% relative risk reduction). The risk of stroke is dramatically increased in patients with NVAF who have already suffered a stroke, and in such patients warfarin is even more effective than in patients who did not have a stroke. The most serious complication of warfarin is intracranial hemorrhage, which is most common in elderly patients. Lone atrial fibrillation (in young patients and no other associated conditions or valvular disease) does not require any treatment.

Small or Penetrating Vessel Disease and Lacunar Stroke

Small or penetrating vessel disease is generally associated with hypertension and diabetes mellitus. Typically, lipohyalinosis or microatheromas obstruct these end vessels that supply the subcortical white matter, basal ganglia, and brain stem. Less commonly, occlusion of these vessels is caused by microemboli. Lacunar stroke presents clinically as one of the classically described lacunar syndromes (pure motor, pure sensory, pure sensory motor, dysarthria-clumsy hand, ataxic hemiparesis) and is associated on computed tomography or magnetic resonance imaging with a small subcortical or brain stem lesion corresponding to a single perforating vessel occlusion. To qualify as a lacunar stroke, the patient needs also to have risk factors for lacunar disease (e.g., hypertension, diabetes).

Lacunar strokes generally have a better prognosis

than other strokes, although the tendency to have multiple and recurrent strokes in these patients could worsen the outcome significantly. Even with a lacunar stroke presentation, it is often necessary to exclude the presence of large vessel intracranial stenosis that could also worsen outcome. Antiplatelet agents are overwhelmingly used for stroke prevention because of the favorable prognosis.

Stroke of Other Determined Etiology

Although stroke caused by other conditions, including dissection, hypercoagulable state, aortic atheroma, and sinus venous thrombosis, forms a small percentage of the population at risk for stroke, it is responsible for a large number of strokes in young adults (< 35 years old). The therapy is generally directed at the underlying mechanism or cause.

Stroke of Undetermined Etiology

A stroke is classified in this category when none of the preceding categories applies despite adequate diagnostic evaluation. It is one of the largest categories, representing 20 to 30% of all strokes. Because no mechanism or etiology can be determined, antiplatelet agents are most commonly used for secondary stroke prevention. The best therapy for stroke prevention in this category is not known. A large trial sponsored by the National Institutes of Health is comparing the effectiveness of aspirin and warfarin in secondary stroke prevention.

REHABILITATION OF THE STROKE PATIENT

method of
ARTHUR M. GERSHKOFF, M.D.
MossRehab Hospital and Temple University School of Medicine
Philadelphia, Pennsylvania

With approximately 400,000 survivors each year, stroke is the leading cause of acquired disability in adults in the United States. The total number of stroke survivors exceeds 3 million, most of whom have been able to return to reasonably satisfying and productive lives through rehabilitation. Breakthroughs have recently occurred in the management of thrombotic stroke (thrombolytic therapy), intracranial hemorrhage, and increased intracranial pressure. These have led not only to greater numbers of stroke patients achieving full recovery, but also to greater numbers of severely disabled victims who survive. Thus, the need for rehabilitation services has not diminished. This article explores impairment and disability following stroke, as well as the specific rehabilitation interventions that can help reduce the morbidity associated with this devastating disease.

STROKE SYNDROMES, RECOVERY, AND PROGNOSIS

Stroke syndromes (Table 1) are usually vascular in origin; 92% of strokes are embolic or thrombotic in origin, and 8% are hemorrhagic. For thromboembolic strokes, neurologic deficits usually reflect infarction of brain tissue subserved by the occluded arteries.

Approximately 50% of strokes involve occlusion of the main trunk or branches of the middle cerebral arteries (MCA). Large-vessel MCA occlusions can cause substantial infarctions of the outer posterior frontal, parietal, and temporal lobes. The effects of this include contralateral hemiplegia, hemisensory deficit, and often homonymous hemianopsia. Ninety-three percent of patients have their dominant hemisphere on the left, and for those patients a major left MCA stroke typically causes aphasia, usually with expression more severely affected than comprehension. Nondominant hemisphere strokes cause more impaired spatial orientation and posture and some form of visual or tactile neglect of stimuli, usually on the left. Involvement of the dominant posterior parietal area, particularly the angular gyrus, is associated with visuospatial and reading deficits.

Intracerebral hemorrhage often affects the basal ganglia, thalamus, pons, or cerebellum. The severity of the symptoms—usually hemiparesis—is related to the size and location of the bleed and complications, including associated cerebral edema, herniation, and need for surgical decompression. Thalamic hemorrhage frequently affects the neighboring midbrain, leading to severe dysconjugate gaze, dysarthria, dysphagia, and other brain stem signs, as well as contralateral sensory deficits. Damage may sometimes be severe with little recovery, but many patients regain substantial function as blood resorbs and edema resolves over several weeks.

Subarachnoid hemorrhage (SAH), associated with a ruptured aneurysm, affects the anterior circulation (anterior and middle cerebral, internal carotid, and anterior communicating arteries) 85% of the time, leading to severe irritation and dysfunction of the frontal and parietal lobes. Additional severe focal damage frequently occurs from subsequent vasospasm of intracranial arteries. SAH can be devastating, but with prompt surgical treatment and postsurgical monitoring, most patients survive and can recover substantially. Patients often have good sensorimotor recovery, but suffer persistent memory and cognitive deficits.

Lacunar strokes involve occlusion of small arterioles, often those that feed the basal ganglia or periventricular white matter. Most single lacunae are silent; however, ongoing multiple lacunar strokes eventually become clinically apparent. Multiple bilateral lacunae in these areas can lead to severe motor rigidity, suggestive of Parkinson's disease, and severe cognitive deficits.

Motor recovery of the hemiplegic patient usually follows a characteristic pattern, starting with gross multijoint movement patterns ("synergistic") involv-

TABLE 1. **Common Stroke Syndromes: Common Impairments**

Stroke Syndrome	Common Impairments
Middle cerebral artery (MCA) infarct (either side)	Contralateral hemiparesis (arm and face weaker), hemisensory deficits, and visual loss. Uninhibited bladder and bowel with incontinence. Dysphagia
Dominant MCA (main/upper branch)	Aphasia (usually global or expressive)
Dominant MCA (lower branch)	Aphasia (receptive)
Nondominant MCA	Spatial disorientation, contralateral neglect
Anterior cerebral artery infarct	Contralateral hemiparesis (leg weaker), hemianesthesia, grasp reflex, cognitive deficits (abulia; object use problems, memory, attention, and concentration deficits), uninhibited bowel and bladder with incontinence
Posterior cerebral artery infarct	Contralateral homonymous hemianopsia, spatial orientation and balance problems
Thalamic infarction	Contralateral hemianesthesia and dysesthetic or spontaneous sensations (sometimes painful)
Thalamic hemorrhage	Contralateral hemianesthesia, dysesthetic or spontaneous sensations (sometimes painful), and hemiparesis, upward or downward gaze paresis, balance dysfunction, and dysphagia
Basal ganglia infarct or hemorrhage	Contralateral hemiparesis. (If large enough): speech and cognitive dysfunction
Lacunar stroke of posterior limb internal capsule	Contralateral hemiparesis (no other deficits)
Brain stem infarct or hemorrhage	
Midbrain, pons	Contralateral hemiparesis, and limb/body hemisensory deficit, ipsilateral hemfacial sensory loss, severe dysarthria and eye gaze deficits, incontinence, and dysphagia (severe aspiration risk)
Lateral medulla	Contralateral limb/body hemianesthesia, ipsilateral facial hemianesthesia, hoarseness, ipsilateral ataxia, balance disturbance
Cerebellar (lobe or peduncle)	Ipsilateral hemiataxia, balance disturbance

ing flexors in the upper extremity and extensors and plantarflexors in the lower extremities. Proximal muscles often regain strength earlier. Eventually, most patients regain isolated movement at individual joints. Permanent moderate to severe deficits remain in 20 to 25% of stroke survivors. At any stage of recovery, the existing motor function in a limb is the best predictor of ultimate return. If the arm has been rendered plegic, fine motor coordination of the hand returns only rarely. Overall, most patients can learn to compensate for residual motor deficits; about 80% achieve independence in ambulation, and 60% achieve independence in self-care. Patients able to compensate for motor deficits tend to be younger and more cognitively intact. Most patients are also able to achieve bowel and bladder continence and improvement in speech to allow for some useful communication. Almost all patients eventually swallow food safely.

Neurologic recovery is usually complete by 3 months; exceptions include severe motor deficits; hemorrhagic strokes, especially of the brain stem or thalamus; cognitive deficits; and speech deficits. All of these can have recovery lasting 6 to 12 months, sometimes even longer. Younger patients can also have a more prolonged recovery. Other patients may show significant functional improvement after 3 months, despite minimal further neurologic gains. During the period of recovery, patients need to be monitored regularly by a physiatrist or other rehabilitation professional, who can assess if further therapy is indicated to achieve new goals.

A variety of factors predict outcome. Strokes that are multiple, bilateral, or large in overall volume are likely to have a poorer outcome than single, small strokes. Young patients usually have a tremendous potential to regain neurologic function, but most older patients will also respond to rehabilitation. Patients who are incontinent or who have major cognitive deficits are less likely to return to the community. Other factors that portend a poorer overall outcome include major proprioceptive deficits, severe depression, and poor sitting balance.

SETTINGS FOR REHABILITATION AND SELECTION OF PATIENTS

Virtually all stroke patients respond to rehabilitation services; it is imperative, therefore, that all patients with persistent neurologic deficits and significant disability be considered for rehabilitation. According to the Post-Acute Stroke Care Guidelines developed by the Agency for Health Care Policy and Research, the Public Health Service, and Health and Human Services (1995), it is recommended that patients with significant disabilities in more than one category (Table 2) be referred to an *interdisciplinary* setting for rehabilitation (Table 3). This implies that all therapists and other providers who treat the patient will meet together, usually weekly or biweekly, to discuss progress, coordinate efforts, and troubleshoot problems. Settings in which such interaction does not occur are termed *multidisciplinary* or *unidisciplinary.* For stroke patients with multiple disabilities, interdisciplinary rehabilitation is much more effective at achieving maximal potential recovery.

TABLE 2. **Disabilities Resulting from Stroke**

Disability Category	Specific Deficits	Essential Discipline(s)
Mobility	Bed mobility, transfers, sitting or standing balance, and ambulation on levels, steps, and uneven surfaces	PT
ADLs	dressing, bathing, grooming, toileting (perineal hygiene), feeding, toilet transfers, and tub transfers	OT
Communication	Aphasia or dysarthria	ST
Swallowing	Dysphagia, with or without aspiration	ST
Bowel and bladder control	Incontinence of bowel and/or bladder. Urinary retention, fecal impaction	RN, MD/DO
Cognition	Memory, judgment, attention and concentration, orientation, executive function (planning, sequencing, and carrying out activities)	NP
Emotional functioning	Severe depression, severe anxiety, severe disinhibition of emotion	NP, MD/DO
Pain management	Limitation in mobility, self-care, or toleration of exercise resulting from pain	MD/DO

Abbreviations: ADL = activities of daily living; PT = physical therapy; OT = occupational therapy; ST = speech therapy (speech/language pathology); NP = neuropsychology; RN = rehabilitation nursing; MD/DO = physician with appropriate skill and training to evaluate and treat deficits.

In the acute-care hospital setting immediately following a stroke, rehabilitation interventions should *not* be delayed in order to complete all diagnostic neurologic tests. Within 24 hours of the stroke, patients should be screened for dysphagia by a speech therapist (or provider with equivalent skills). Physical therapy evaluation needs to occur as soon as the patient is neurologically stable and able to get out of bed, usually within 24 hours. Patients with upper extremity weakness who will be discharged home without home services should be checked by an occupational therapist.

Patients with minimally or mildly severe deficits who have sufficient family support can be discharged home with home or outpatient therapies. Alternatively, such patients usually respond well to therapies provided in skilled care or subacute rehabilitation facilities. Patients who are debilitated or who suffer from medical or surgical problems (such as fractures) that interfere with therapy may need to recuperate in a skilled care setting before starting more intensive therapy. Such patients need to be followed closely to determine the appropriate time for transfer to an interdisciplinary rehabilitation setting. Patients with complex cognitive, communication, or perceptual deficits may respond poorly to a skilled care setting and should be transferred to interdisciplinary units that can handle their specific needs.

Patients able to participate in therapy who have (1) mild deficits and potentially unstable medical problems or (2) moderate to severe deficits (regardless of medical stability) should be considered for transfer to an interdisciplinary setting, usually an acute intensive rehabilitation hospital or unit. Such patients are often referred to subacute rehabilitation

TABLE 3. **Settings for Rehabilitation**

Settings	Intensity of Services	Comments
Inpatient settings		
Intensive inpatient	3–5 h/d, 5–7 d/wk PT, OT, ST, TR, NP. 24-h RN available	Interdisciplinary. The most expensive setting. Needed for the most complex deficits
Subacute	2–3 h/d, 5–7 d/wk PT, OT, ST, TR, NP(?) 24-h RN available	Interdisciplinary. Some services (ST and NP) may not be as available.
SNF	1–1.5 h/d, 5 d/wk PT, OT, ST. Nursing may not have extensive rehab training	Multidisciplinary.*
Outpatient/home settings		
Day hospital	3–5 h/d, 5 d/wk PT, OT, ST, TR, NP. Nursing available during hours of program	Interdisciplinary. Same intensity as intensive inpatient, but the patient goes home at night. Not covered by Medicare
Day treatment/CORF	2–3 h/d, 3–5 d/wk PT, OT, ST, NP. Limited nursing available in some programs	Interdisciplinary
Intensive home therapy	3 h/d, 5 d/wk PT, OT, ST, RN, NP (?)	Interdisciplinary. Limited availability at present.
Standard home therapy	1–2 h/d, 2–5 d/wk PT, OT, ST, RN	Unidisciplinary/Multidisciplinary.*
Standard outpatient therapy	1–2 h/d, 2–5 d/wk PT, OT, ST, Psychology	Unidisciplinary/Multidisciplinary.*

*There may be limited interdisciplinary interaction in some settings or agencies.
Abbreviations: PT = physical therapy; OT = occupational therapy; ST = speech therapy (speech/language pathology); NP = neuropsychology; RN = rehabilitation nursing; TR = therapeutic recreation; CORF = comprehensive outpatient rehabilitation facility.

units, but individual patient needs must be matched with the ability of the facility to deliver therapy. For example, it is inappropriate to refer a patient with major speech and swallowing problems to a facility with minimal or intermittent speech therapy availability. Patients with major cognitive or behavioral problems need rehabilitation settings where nursing and therapy staff are capable of recognizing and handling such needs, and where a neuropsychologist is integrated into the therapeutic team.

At any level of care, therapy services are selected to meet specific realistic goals for the patient. For example, it is realistic for most patients, even those with severe lower extremity weakness, to learn to walk. If the patient was nonambulatory before the stroke, however, ambulation after the stroke is usually not realistic. Patients who are likely to need 24-hour supervision or assistance, but who lack any social supports, may require placement in a skilled care facility that can offer long-term custodial services. If the patient improves, intensive rehabilitation to achieve independence and return home alone could be considered.

Transfer to rehabilitation can occur as soon as the patient is sufficiently medically stable to tolerate the therapy offered. Optimally, the neurologic evaluation and imaging studies are completed first, but transfer need not be delayed if the patient is deemed stable and the rehabilitation facility can arrange to complete the studies. Thus, patients may be ready for transfer as early as 48 to 72 hours poststroke. Consultation with a physiatrist or other rehabilitation physician can sometimes help establish realistic goals, select an appropriate facility to meet the patient's needs, and determine the earliest time when the patient is stable for transfer.

Currently, programs exist to accredit rehabilitation facilities and evaluate the quality of care delivered to patients. Commonly accepted standards of care include collection of functional assessment data on patient responsiveness to rehabilitation in each facility. In selecting settings for stroke patients, clinicians may seek information verifying the accreditation status for particular facilities and comparing outcomes and cost of care with regional and national data.

REHABILITATION PROCESS

Patients with motor deficits require motor retraining for optimal recovery. About six schools of therapy offer different approaches to this; none has ever been proven superior to the others. Physical and occupational therapists work to facilitate early motor recovery and promote improved balance and mobility. Hands-on sensory and postural feedback offered by the therapists is crucial; there is no machine or technological innovation that can substitute. As soon as possible, the clinician should order nursing staff to assist or supervise the patient during ambulation and transfer activities on the nursing unit. Similarly, nursing personnel need to reinforce activities of daily living (ADL) skills learned in occupational therapy. Lack of carryover of therapy activities to the nursing floor can slow down progress in inpatient settings.

Patients and families should be taught range of motion (ROM), strengthening exercises, and self-care and mobility activities to perform when the patient is not receiving therapy. This regimen becomes the home exercise program (HEP), which needs to be performed regularly. Only through hands-on training can families develop confidence and competence in mobilizing the patient. In the inpatient setting, this training should start early and becomes increasingly important as the time for discharge home approaches. Social work communicates with families and often coordinates this training. Compliance with home exercise and activity programs is a major factor in patients achieving optimal recovery. Noncompliance with home exercise programs can lead to complications, especially shoulder contractures, and suboptimal overall outcome.

Patients with lower extremity weakness often benefit from ankle-foot orthoses (AFOs). If possible, the patient should use a training brace to start. With the pressure from insurance companies for short inpatient lengths of stay, it is important to order and fabricate orthoses early. Most patients, even those with severe knee weakness, can ambulate with an AFO, which usually can stabilize the knee by blocking motion at the ankle. If there is any voluntary ankle movement or the likelihood of significant further recovery, the clinician should order an orthosis with adjustability. Spasticity may mandate the need for a more rigid orthosis. Orthoses may be metal, attached to shoes, or custom-molded plastic. The last, molded ankle foot orthoses (MAFOs), are lightweight, cosmetically more acceptable to patients, and can be worn with different footwear.

At any stage of rehabilitation, clinicians assess progress and continued benefit from therapy based on attainment of the functional goals set previously. Progress can usually be identified weekly for inpatients and semimonthly or monthly for outpatients. If the patient demonstrates progress toward the established goals, therapy should continue. If progress stops before attaining the goals, the clinician needs to re-evaluate the patient to determine whether the goals are indeed feasible, or if impediments exist that limit progress. Impediments include intercurrent illnesses, excessive or inadequate intensity of therapy, severe co-morbid conditions (such as cardiac, respiratory, or arthritic limitations), family noncompliance with the HEP, or poor patient motivation.

The transition from inpatient to outpatient rehabilitation can be complex. Safe discharge home often requires one or more of the following before discharge: identifying vendors for equipment and orthoses, obtaining and checking out equipment, obtaining and checking out the orthosis, family training, identifying follow-up physicians, communicating with outpatient or home care agencies for providing further therapy, and identifying a pharmacy for filling medication prescriptions. Many insurance policies have limitations for therapy and equipment. The team social worker is essential to clarifying all of these issues to make the transition home as smooth as possible.

After discharge from inpatient programs, most patients receive home or outpatient therapies. A major goal for outpatient therapy is independence in community mobility and other activities. As early as possible (starting with inpatient treatment), patients should be encouraged or trained to participate in community-oriented activities. Occupational therapy can evaluate and train patients in instrumental ADLs (e.g., kitchen/homemaking, money management, shopping) and vocationally related skills. Therapeutic recreation works to identify feasible avocational activities for patients. Stroke support groups in the community offer the opportunity for stroke survivors to meet and share information in order to further enhance their quality of life.

Stroke frequently leaves the patient with actual or threatened catastrophic disability. Virtually all patients react emotionally. Adjustment disorders with emotional features, usually depressed mood, are common. A variety of disciplines offer support in the rehabilitation environment. The psychologist can offer counseling and evaluation to rule out more serious psychopathology. The social worker helps patients and families confront and untangle the myriad of complexities they need to address before discharge. Chaplains help patients cope through prayer and pastoral counseling.

COMPLICATIONS AND ASSOCIATED CONDITIONS

Heart disease is the second most common killer of stroke patients (behind the stroke itself) in the first 30 days after stroke, and the most common cause of death thereafter. Most patients with thrombotic strokes have, or are at risk for, coronary artery disease. It is essential for rehabilitation providers to know the cardiac status of stroke patients under their care and to maintain vigilance for cardiac symptoms during progressive exercise programs. Suspicious symptoms warrant cessation of vigorous exercise and aggressive, definitive investigation and intervention. Stroke patients with myocardia ischemia or infarction need to have their rehabilitation programs adjusted, so that the rise in pulse and blood pressure with exercise or activity is limited.

All stroke patients are at risk for deep venous thromboses (DVT) and pulmonary emboli (PE). Definitive prophylaxis includes warfarin (Coumadin). Adequate prophylaxis includes subcutaneous heparin or intermittent pneumatic compression boots, each of which cuts the risk by about 50%. Some advocate screening all patients for DVT on admission, but this is expensive and tends to uncover many calf clots that may be nonpropagating, and therefore non–life-threatening if they embolize. The clinician should maintain a high index of suspicion and should investigate all cases of persistent swelling with color duplex ultrasound. Symptoms and signs suggestive of hypoxia or PE warrant ventilation-perfusion lung scans. Once the diagnosis is made, patients should receive therapeutic anticoagulation. If DVT is above the midthigh, or if anticoagulation is contraindicated, the clinician should consider inferior vena cava filter placement. Patients should remain at bed rest until anticoagulation has been therapeutic for 24 hours, after which they can be mobilized.

Patients with brain stem strokes, bilateral strokes, or the most severe hemiplegia are at greatest risk of severe dysphagia and aspiration pneumonia. Acutely, speech therapy evaluation can help analyze if thickened liquids, pureed, or mechanical soft foods are adequately tolerated. Patients who have a strong cough reflex are relatively protected from aspiration pneumonia. If the patient has a persistent wet vocal quality, suggesting pooling of secretions or food, or if the cough reflex is weak or absent, the patient should take nothing by mouth. A three-textured barium video swallow, ideally performed in the presence of the speech therapist, will help identify solid and liquid consistencies that the patient can manage safely. During subsequent rehabilitation, speech therapy training can be used to teach the patient to manage thinner liquids and more complex food textures safely. The clinician needs to examine the lungs regularly during this period; any sign of congestion or pneumonia should be followed up with chest radiography and vigorous pulmonary treatment or antibiotics when indicated.

Dysphagic and obtunded patients are at risk for malnutrition. Intravenous fluids may be appropriate for 24 to 48 hours after the stroke, but are inadequate for longer times. Patients unable to take sufficient oral foods warrant nasogastric tube placement within 24 to 48 hours. If this is poorly tolerated or problematic, percutaneous enterogastrostomy or gastrostomy tube placement is indicated, as early as 5 days poststroke. Full daily caloric intake to meet metabolic needs is necessary for the patient to progress in rehabilitation.

Stroke patients are at risk for peptic ulcer, and most are given prophylaxis with H_2 blockers. In rehabilitation, these agents can usually be tapered off, at least by the completion of inpatient treatment.

Achieving adequate bladder emptying is critical. Indwelling catheters should be removed as soon as possible after beginning rehabilitation. The clinician should measure postvoid residual volume, ideally noninvasively with a portable ultrasound device (Bladderscan). High residual volumes or incontinence warrants investigation for infection with urinalysis and culture and treatment of infection if present. Incontinent patients with low volumes are likely to have an uninhibited bladder, which often responds to timed voiding by nursing and therapy staff and low-dose anticholinergic agents. Patients with superimposed problems, such as prostatic hypertrophy or diabetic-origin neurogenic bladder, warrant urodynamic studies and possibly urologic consultation. Postvoid residual volumes should be rechecked any time anticholinergic medication (including antidepressants) is started. Double voiding, standing or sitting while voiding, and elimination of anticholinergic medications may improve emptying. Patients with persistent inadequate emptying may need intermittent catheterization or permanent indwelling catheters.

Peristalsis tends to slow down with reduced activity following stroke; severe constipation or impaction occurring during rehabilitation needs to be treated aggressively. For ongoing prevention, stool softeners such as docusate (Colace) or bulk agents are helpful, but only if the patient can take adequate oral fluids. Incontinent patients usually respond to timed defecation, achieved by administering a small cathartic enema (Fleet Bisacodyl Enema) or suppository (Dulcolax) immediately after breakfast or dinner, then placing the patient on the toilet or commode. Oral cathartics need to be used cautiously, as they can increase fecal urgency and incontinence in some patients.

Immobile stroke patients, or those with severe hemisensory deficits, are at risk for skin ulceration. Preventive measures include heel-relieving ankle splints, repositioning of patients every 2 hours while in bed, and alternating pressure mattresses when repositioning is not possible. Thick air or water mattresses may impede bed mobility and transfer training. Severely immobile patients also may need weight shifts every 20 to 30 minutes, while sitting for prolonged periods in a wheelchair.

Recurrent stroke is an ever-present risk that needs to be addressed; its occurrence during rehabilitation not only causes further disability, but also necessitates painful reassessment of all goals of the rehabilitation team and expectations of the patient and family. Warfarin is usually definitive prophylaxis of recurrent thrombosis, when indicated. The incidence of hemorrhagic complications of warfarin for patients in supervised intensive rehabilitation settings is surprising low; the risk of falling usually should not limit the use of warfarin while the patient undergoes inpatient rehabilitation. Aspirin, clopidogrel (Plavix), and ticlopidine (Ticlid) have at best modest effects. Recurrent stroke or transient ischemic attack mandates assessment of cerebral and extracranial circulation, with re-analysis of the potential risks and benefits of surgical or antithrombotic interventions.

Spasticity is usually minimal in the first several days after the stroke but gradually increases thereafter in most patients. The primary treatment is regular range of motion (at least twice daily) by staff and/or family. Organ system problems that can increase tone (fecal impaction, bladder infection, pelvic or lower extremity infections, decubitus ulcers) must be ruled out or addressed. Patients with severe tone may require splints that keep the extremity stretched during sleep. Spastic contractures may require serial casting to stretch out. Medications such as dantrolene sodium (Dantrium), baclofen (Lioresal), tizanidine (Zanaflex), and diazepam (Valium) may reduce tone but often have systemic adverse effects in stroke patients.

Motor point (MP) blocks of overactive muscles are indicated for problematic focal spasticity. Ideally, specific muscles are identified by multichannel electromyographic analysis during rest, gait (for lower extremities), or functional activities (for upper extremities). Practically, most clinicians select muscles based on patient history (how activities are limited) and physical examination (testing of tone during passive ROM and observation of active limb movement). For the standard treatment, aqueous solutions of phenol or alcohol are injected into the MP of target muscle. This technique is painful, tedious, and requires electrical stimulation of the muscle to locate exactly the MP (point of maximal muscle excitation with minimal electricity), but offers instantaneous reduction of tone when successful. A newer alternative is botulinium toxin (Botox*) injection. This can be injected with a smaller needle (helpful for a patient on warfarin), does not require finding the MP, and is less painful; however, reduction of tone develops only gradually over 1 to 2 weeks, the toxin is very expensive, and antibodies to the toxin can develop. For both substances, spasticity of injected muscles usually returns in 3 to 6 months and may require reinjection.

Shoulder pain is extremely common after stroke. Potential causes with suggested interventions are listed in Table 4. Subluxation itself usually does not cause pain, but indicates loss of protective muscle tone and an increased risk of injury from trauma owing to falls or overstretching. Rehabilitation staff must range the flaccid extremity carefully, supporting the shoulder in the socket at all times. When repositioning a patient with hemiparetic shoulder in bed or chair, it is better to pull the patient up by a bed sheet or by the leg than to pull up by the flaccid arm. Functional electrical stimulation of the supraspinatus and deltoid probably helps to facilitate early return of at least minimal tone. Slings are helpful if the subluxed arm is more painful when unsupported and if the dangling arm interferes with ambulation; however, the arm still needs to be removed from the sling for twice daily ROM. When the patient is sitting in a wheelchair, the arm should be supported by an arm trough, pillows, or lap board.

Persistent pain, progressive intolerance of ROM, and distal swelling or temperature changes of an extremity indicate the presence of reflex sympathetic dystrophy. This disturbing complication, of unknown origin, is diagnosed clinically. Triple phase bone scan is sometimes helpful in clarifying the diagnosis in patients with borderline signs. Treatment includes frequent ROM, along with oral steroids (prednisone 80 mg/day or equivalent, tapering over 10 to 14 days) or sympathetic blocks. Prompt early recognition and treatment (within days, if possible) are essential to prevent chronic pain, contractures, and tissue atrophy that can occur in later stages. Symptoms sometimes recur after treatment and warrant re-treatment.

---

*Investigational drug in the United States.

TABLE 4. **Some Causes of Shoulder Pain in Stroke and Their Management**

Etiology	Management
Adhesive capsulitis	Aggressive passive stretching while the joint is heated with ultrasound.
Impingement syndrome	Range of motion to promote external rotation, then flexion and abduction within a relatively pain free functional range. Steroid injection may be appropriate.
Glenohumeral subluxation	Sling if reduction of subluxation (during upright posture) is associated with reduction in pain. Functional electrical stimulation of supraspinatus and deltoid.
Rotator cuff tendinitis/subacromial bursitis	Steroid injection of subacromial area.
Bicipital tendinitis	Steroid injection of bicipital tendon sheath.
Trigger point of subscapularis	Trigger point injection, followed by stretching.
Brachial plexus injury	Avoidance of overstretching. Treatment of neuropathic pain (see discussion of central poststroke pain).
Central poststroke pain	(See discussion of central poststroke pain.)
Reflex sympathetic dystrophy	Aggressive passive stretching, while treating syndrome (see discussion on reflex sympathetic dystrophy).
Spasticity	Stretching of tight muscles. Motor point block of spastic muscles.

When the thalamus, sensory tracts, or sensory cortex is damaged, central poststroke pain can be a challenging problem that seriously complicates the disability from motor deficits. Typically, pain occurs in a bodily part with absent or severely reduced sensation. All patients with central poststroke pain warrant attempts at sensory and proprioceptive retraining. Transcutaneous electrical stimulation is worth trying. Medications of benefit include tricyclics (nortriptyline* [Pamelor] or amitriptyline* [Elavil]), and anticonvulsants (carbamazepine [Tegretol] or gabapentin* [Neurontin]). Narcotics often do not help and must be used cautiously. It is important to differentiate central pain from bothersome but nonpainful spontaneous sensations; the latter warrant patient education more than active pain intervention. In either case, keeping the patient active psychologically and physically is critical. Symptoms often improve over time.

Depression occurs in as many as 50% of stroke patients and can seriously impede progress in rehabilitation. Patients with dominant frontal lesions are at particularly high risk for major depressive disorders. The diagnosis may be challenging, as patients with language impairment will have difficulty expressing depressed thoughts, whereas depressed patients with nondominant hemisphere lesions may have blunted or inappropriately disinhibited affect. Severe symptoms that prevent participation in therapy, psychotic symptoms, or suicidal ideation warrant urgent psychiatric consultation.

Depression usually responds to oral antidepressants. Selection of agents often depends on side effects to be encouraged or avoided. As examples, trazodone (Desyrel) or paroxetine (Paxil) at bedtime is helpful for patients with insomnia, whereas methylphenidate (Ritalin) can help patients with lassitude or daytime somnolence. In general, drugs with anticholinergic effects should be used cautiously in patients at risk for urinary retention.

*Not FDA approved for this indication

ACKNOWLEDGMENT

I thank John Melvin, M.D., for his critical review of this article.

EPILEPSY IN ADOLESCENTS AND ADULTS

method of
MARK A. GRANNER, M.D.
University of Iowa College of Medicine
Iowa City, Iowa

Epilepsy has been recognized since the dawn of recorded history, but even today it is misunderstood. Few conditions carry with them the social stigma associated with the diagnosis of epilepsy. Part of this is undoubtedly the result of the complexities of epilepsy itself, for epilepsy is not a single disease, nor even a single syndrome, but rather a collection of syndromes, each with their own unique pathophysiology and natural course. Thus, no two patients with epilepsy are exactly alike, and the effective management of epilepsy requires particular attention to the manifestations of the epilepsy syndrome in the context of that individual's life. A systematic approach to the management of the patient with epilepsy begins with an understanding of the cardinal manifestation of epilepsy, the seizure. It also mandates a quest for the underlying cause of the seizure, an accurate classification of the type of seizure, and an assessment of the risk of subsequent seizures.

EPIDEMIOLOGY OF EPILEPSY

One of 10 Americans will have at least one seizure at some time in his or her life. Only 40% (4% of the total) will have a subsequent seizure. A single seizure, therefore, is most often a solitary event. Large epidemiologic studies have estimated the lifetime risk of epilepsy in the United States at approximately 3%, and the point prevalence at 0.6%. Epilepsy most commonly begins in the first few years of life or after the age of 65, but can potentially present at any age. Thus, epilepsy is the most common serious

TABLE 1. **Classification of Seizures**

Partial (Focal, Local) Seizures
Simple partial seizures
Complex partial seizures
Partial seizures evolving to secondarily generalized seizures
Generalized Seizures
Absence seizures
Myoclonic seizures
Clonic seizures
Tonic seizures
Tonic-clonic seizures
Atonic seizures
Unclassified Seizures

Modified from Commission on Classification and Terminology of the International League Against Epilepsy: Proposal for revised clinical and electroencephalographic classification of epileptic seizures. Epilepsia *22*:489–501, 1981.

neurologic condition that affects people of all ages. The majority of patients with epilepsy are initially evaluated and treated in the primary care setting, making a basic knowledge of epilepsy mandatory for all physicians.

DEFINITIONS

A seizure is a paroxysmal event involving a transient disturbance in the excitability of a population of neurons, associated with some clinical change. The electrical component of a seizure, measured on the electroencephalogram (EEG), may be generalized or focal. The location of this activity will determine the associated clinical manifestations. For example, a seizure arising from somatosensory cortex will produce a contralateral change in sensation, whereas a seizure arising from motor cortex will produce movement. The brain can be provoked into a seizure by either extrinsic or intrinsic causes. Those of extrinsic nature, owing to a variety of insults to an otherwise normal brain, are known as acute symptomatic seizures. Those owing to intrinsic dysfunction of the brain constitute epilepsy, defined as the tendency to have recurrent, unprovoked seizures.

CLASSIFICATION

Seizures are classified on electrophysiologic and clinical grounds. Seizures originating simultaneously from both cerebral hemispheres are referred to as generalized and those arising from a focal region of the brain are called partial. Generalized seizures are subclassified as tonic (manifesting as a generalized increase in muscle tone), atonic (a sudden, generalized decrease in muscle tone; often referred to as a "drop attack"), clonic (repetitive muscle jerks), tonic-clonic (a tonic phase, followed by a clonic phase), myoclonic (a single, sudden diffuse muscle jerk), or absence (brief staring and unresponsiveness). By definition, consciousness is impaired during a generalized seizure. Partial seizures are subclassified as simple if consciousness is not impaired, or complex if it is. Partial seizures that subsequently spread to both cerebral hemispheres are referred to as partial seizures with secondary generalization. Seizures that do not readily fit into this classification scheme may be considered unclassified. Older terms such as "petit mal," "grand mal," or "psychomotor," although more familiar to some patients, are nonspecific and their use is discouraged. The classification of seizures is summarized in Table 1.

An epilepsy syndrome is determined by the type or types of seizures, the underlying cause of the seizures, the age of onset, the presence of a family history of epilepsy, findings on examination, results of the EEG, and the natural history of the condition. Epilepsy syndromes are classified as generalized if the patient has generalized seizures, or localization-related if the seizures arise from a focal area. Subclassification is based on the underlying cause; idiopathic (or primary) syndromes are largely genetically based, symptomatic syndromes are acquired, and cryptogenic syndromes are of presumed, but unknown, cause. Epilepsy syndrome classification and some specific syndromes are listed in Table 2. Accurate classification of the epilepsy syndrome carries with it some prognostic information regarding the likelihood of seizure control and chance for eventual remission.

APPROACH TO THE FIRST SEIZURE

The first seizure may be encountered in the emergency department, on the inpatient ward, or in the clinic. The fundamental principles of evaluation do not differ significantly among these settings. A logical and thorough approach will enhance diagnostic accuracy and lead to more effective treatment.

History

The single most valuable source of diagnostic information is the history. The patient should be queried about the event itself, including the presence of any precipitating factors or prodromal symptoms, level of awareness during the episode, and the presence of any aftereffects. However, episodes that affect consciousness require the perspective of an eyewitness. The witness should be asked about the

TABLE 2. **Modified International Classification of Epilepsies and Epileptic Syndromes**

Classification	Subclassification	Example
Localization-related (focal, partial)	Idiopathic	Benign Rolandic epilepsy
	Symptomatic	Post-traumatic epilepsy
	Cryptogenic	
Generalized	Idiopathic	Childhood absence epilepsy
	Symptomatic	Early myoclonic encephalopathy
	Cryptogenic	Lennox-Gastaut syndrome
Undetermined whether focal or generalized		Landau-Kleffner syndrome
Special syndromes		Febrile convulsions

Modified from Commission on Classification and Terminology of the International League Against Epilepsy: Proposal for revised classification of epilepsies and epileptic syndromes. Epilepsia *30*(4):389–399, 1989.

first visible signs of the event, its duration, the level of awareness or responsiveness during and after the event, and the presence of involuntary movements (ranging from subtle automatic movements of the face or limbs, called automatisms, to frank convulsive movements). Observations about the frequency, amplitude, distribution, symmetry, and synchrony of movements may prove valuable. The presence of tongue biting or urinary or fecal incontinence may be a helpful sign. If more than one episode has been witnessed, the degree of homogeneity between events may be informative.

The history should also include factors that may have predisposed to seizures. Remote risk factors include the presence of childhood febrile (if prolonged or focal) or afebrile seizures, infection of the central nervous system (meningitis or encephalitis), and significant head injury (complicated by depressed skull fracture or intracranial hemorrhage, or followed by unconsciousness or amnesia lasting longer then 30 minutes). The family history should be explored for epilepsy (particularly idiopathic epilepsy). Besides acute head injury and central nervous system infection, other recent risk factors include sleep deprivation (a common precipitant of new onset seizures in college students), alcohol and other drug intoxication or withdrawal, and systemic illness. Although it has received attention in recent years, exposure to flashing lights (e.g., with some video games) is a rare cause of seizures in a person otherwise not predisposed.

Examination

The general physical examination should focus on evidence of systemic metabolic, toxic, or infectious illness, with an eye not only toward those conditions that can cause seizures, but those that can produce episodes mimicking a seizure. Specific attention should be paid to the vital signs (for signs of postural hypotension or cardiac arrhythmia), the cardiac examination, and the skin examination (for the cutaneous stigmata of systemic disease and the manifestations of neurocutaneous syndromes such as neurofibromatosis and tuberous sclerosis). Asymmetry of limb growth or facial features may be a clue about injury to the brain early in life.

The neurologic examination may provide evidence of either diffuse or focal cerebral dysfunction. Global developmental delay may be an important clue, as the incidence of epilepsy in this population is relatively higher. Focal signs immediately after a seizure (e.g., asymmetry of the tendon stretch reflexes, a Babinski sign, or postictal hemiparesis) may point to a partial-onset seizure. Focal signs persisting hours or more after a seizure should prompt an investigation into a possible structural lesion of the brain.

Electroencephalography

The EEG records regional voltage potential changes from the superficial layers of the cerebral cortex and is therefore an electrophysiologic measure of the brain's function. Possible EEG abnormalities include generalized slowing (indicating diffuse cerebral dysfunction, usually of a nonspecific nature), focal slowing (implying focal cerebral dysfunction, although not necessarily a tendency toward seizures), generalized paroxysmal activity (often spike or spike-wave in morphology, implying a tendency toward generalized seizures), or focal paroxysmal activity (usually sharp waves or spikes, suggesting a tendency toward partial seizures). The EEG is of greatest value when it supports an already strong clinical suspicion based on the history and examination. For example, a history suggestive of complex partial seizures with an EEG showing occasional temporal spikes strongly supports the diagnosis of localization-related (focal) epilepsy. On the other hand, if the history is more indicative of syncope and the EEG is normal, the diagnosis of epilepsy is less likely. However, a normal EEG result does not exclude the diagnosis of epilepsy, and an abnormal EEG result (unless a seizure itself is recorded) does not prove it.

Neuroimaging

Computed tomography (CT) and magnetic resonance imaging (MRI) provide a structural complement to the electrophysiologic measure of the EEG. Neuroimaging is therefore of more value in assessing the underlying reason for seizures than it is in determining whether a seizure occurred. In general, MRI is the preferred imaging modality, as its resolution is superior to that of CT. MRI is indicated in all adults with new onset seizures not attributable to other readily explainable extrinsic causes. The MRI may show changes consistent with neoplasm, stroke, vascular malformation, abscess, cortical malformation, cortical atrophy, or mesial temporal sclerosis. An imaging protocol that includes a sequence perpendicular to the long axis of the hippocampus will optimize the resolution of this important temporal lobe structure. Often, however, the MRI is normal.

CT should be performed emergently after a first seizure if elevated intracranial pressure, infection of the central nervous system, or intracerebral hemorrhage is suspected. On the other hand, if recovery to baseline occurs shortly after the seizure, with no evidence of unexplained encephalopathy or focal neurologic deficits, emergent CT can be deferred as long as MRI can be performed within days.

Laboratory Studies

The main purpose of laboratory studies is to exclude systemic metabolic, toxic, or infectious causes of seizures. A general chemistry screen is helpful in looking for evidence of hypoglycemia, hyponatremia, uremia, or hepatic dysfunction. A complete blood count may reveal leukocytosis as a sign of infection, or anemia if the differential diagnosis includes syncope. A urine toxicology screen should be obtained if drug intoxication is a reasonable suspicion. A lumbar puncture is usually optional in the evaluation of the first seizure, but should be performed in the setting of unexplained fever, meningismus, or persistently altered mental status.

PUTTING IT ALL TOGETHER

The following four questions should be answered based on the information described previously. These answers serve as the foundation of subsequent management.

Was the Event a Seizure?

The differential diagnosis of a seizure is broad and includes a variety of systemic, psychiatric, and other neurologic conditions. In general, states of transient alteration in consciousness, sensation, or movement are most often confused for seizures. Common conditions that mimic a seizure are listed in Table 3.

TABLE 3. **Differential Diagnosis of a Seizure**

Systemic
Syncope
Hypoglycemia
Psychiatric
Anxiety attack
Conversion disorder
Malingering
Factitious disorder
Neurologic
Migraine
Transient ischemic attack
Narcolepsy/cataplexy
Paroxysmal nocturnal dystonia

Some disturbances of systemic metabolic, endocrine, or hemodynamic function may pose as seizures. Attacks of hypoglycemia can often be distinguished from seizures by the history. Hypoglycemia is often accompanied by prodromal symptoms of nausea, diaphoresis, and tremor. Although the level of alertness may be affected, frank unresponsiveness or unconsciousness usually requires a profound degree of hypoglycemia. The symptoms of hypoglycemia usually last longer than a typical seizure. Hypoglycemia can be evaluated by serum determination of glucose (especially during an episode) or, in cases of suspected reactive hypoglycemia, with a glucose tolerance test. Syncope, caused by transient failure of adequate cerebral perfusion, may range from the relatively benign (vasovagal syncope) to the malignant (cardiac arrhythmia). Syncope is usually preceded by a prodrome of light-headedness ("presyncope"), then produces a sudden loss of consciousness associated with muscle atonia. Syncope is usually brief and is rarely accompanied by overt motor activity, although some minor limb movements may be seen. Syncope of a suspected benign nature may require nothing more than an assessment of postural pulse and blood pressure. When cardiac arrhythmia is suspected, however, a more extensive cardiac evaluation may be warranted.

Psychiatric conditions frequently present as "spells" and are often misdiagnosed as seizures. These can range from the involuntary (anxiety attacks or conversion reactions) to the volitional (malingering or factitious disorder). Anxiety attacks are diagnosed by the presence of a set of hallmark symptoms, including tachycardia, palpitations, diaphoresis, tachypnea, and a sense of overwhelming doom or foreboding. Frank unresponsiveness is unusual during an anxiety attack, which typically lasts longer than a seizure. Other episodic attacks of psychiatric cause are commonly referred to as pseudoseizures, a term sometimes misunderstood to imply that the patient is "faking" the episodes. In fact, most pseudoseizures occur on an involuntary or subconscious basis, often as a manifestation of conversion disorder. Less often, patients are found to be frankly malingering or falsely reporting their symptoms. Pseudoseizures are often misdiagnosed as seizures because they can manifest with apparent unresponsiveness and involuntary limb movements, occasionally even convulsive in appearance. Although often appearing clinically similar, pseudoseizures lack the electrophysiologic concomitant of seizures; the EEG during a pseudoseizure is normal. The diagnosis of pseudoseizures can be suspected when episodes begin in an adult without apparent physical precipitant, include reports of unusual or bizarre activity, and are accompanied by a significant psychiatric history. Within a given patient, pseudoseizures are less likely to be uniform in their length and clinical features than seizures. However, recent reports have pointed out that bizarre clinical features once felt to be a hallmark of pseudoseizures (such as pelvic thrusting and asynchronous limb movements) are just as likely to occur in complex partial seizures of frontal lobe origin. It is because of this apparent clinical similarity that pseudoseizures are so often misdiagnosed as seizures, leading to the inappropriate use of anticonvulsant medication, which ultimately proves ineffective. The diagnostic "gold standard" for pseudoseizures consists of prolonged video-EEG monitoring, usually carried out on a specialized diagnostic unit. The ability to visually examine the episodes and correlate them with the presence or absence of EEG change is most helpful. If pseudoseizures are confirmed, unnecessary antiepileptic medication can be stopped and appropriate psychiatric care obtained.

A number of other neurologic conditions can masquerade as seizures. Migraine headaches are occasionally associated with transient neurologic symptoms such as visual field defects, aphasia, and abnormal sensations. Amnesia may rarely accompany a migraine, but unresponsiveness should not. The presence of an associated unilateral, pounding headache with nausea and photophobia is a clue to the diagnosis of migraine. Transient ischemic attacks produce episodic neurologic symptoms, although they usually consist of a loss of function rather than a gain of function as with a seizure. Transient ischemic attacks should not affect the level of consciousness to the degree that seizures might. Cerebral ischemia and seizures are both relatively common in the elderly, and the distinction often requires video-EEG monitoring. The pathologic tendency to fall asleep seen in narcolepsy may mimic a seizure, but the distinction between sleep attacks and seizures can usually be made by the history. A polysomnogram and mean-sleep latency test may be required for confirmation. Cataplexy, a feature of narcolepsy consisting of sudden muscle atonia with some degree of preserved consciousness, may also be mistaken for a seizure, but is usually triggered by an emotional stimulus and often lasts longer than the average seizure. Some movement disorders, particularly paroxysmal nocturnal dystonia, can be mistaken for seizures. Video-EEG monitoring may be necessary to distinguish these from complex partial seizures of frontal lobe origin.

Why Did It Occur?

Once the diagnosis of a seizure is made, the underlying cause should be sought. Seizures can be divided into those that occur in a normal brain because of some acute provocation (acute symptomatic seizures) and those that occur more or less spontaneously from an injured brain (epileptic seizures).

A variety of insults can produce seizures in the otherwise normal brain. Metabolic causes of seizures include hypoglycemia, hyponatremia, and acute uremia. A number of prescription medications have been associated with seizures, as have recreational drugs such as stimulants. A seizure can be precipitated by both intoxication and withdrawal from alcohol, as well as by rapid withdrawal from sedative medications such as benzodiazepines and barbiturates. An overwhelming systemic illness can be accompanied by a seizure, as can cerebral anoxia. Prolonged sleep deprivation may also provoke a seizure.

The brain can be injured in a variety of ways, and if that injury is severe enough, epilepsy can result. The likely causes of epilepsy vary according to the age of the patient, reflecting the relative prevalence of certain conditions at these times in life. While genetic-based epilepsy commonly presents in childhood and adolescence, it is unlikely to begin after the age of 25. Adolescents and young adults are most likely to develop acquired epilepsy as the result of a head injury, and somewhat less likely as a consequence of encephalitis or meningitis. Cerebral tumors, both primary and metastatic, are the leading cause of epilepsy later in adult life. The elderly, in whom epilepsy is more prevalent than at any other time in adult life, most often develop epilepsy following a stroke, and less often from degenerative conditions such as Alzheimer's disease. Evidence of these conditions should be sought in all adults with new-onset seizures not explained by an acute precipitant. However, the underlying cause of adult epilepsy often remains elusive.

Are Seizures Likely to Recur?

The direction of subsequent management depends on whether seizures are likely to recur. Because the majority of people having a single seizure will never have a subsequent seizure, treatment with an antiepileptic drug (AED) is not always warranted. Although we can never answer this question with absolute certainty, the basic investigation described previously will yield some information about prognosis. The risk of seizure recurrence, and the risks and benefits of treatment, should be discussed thoroughly.

Acute symptomatic seizures may recur if the provoking cause persists. For example, if a seizure occurs because of encephalitis or intracerebral hemorrhage, the likelihood of subsequent seizures is fairly high. In addition, the consequences of a subsequent seizure in an ill patient may be severe. In this setting, treatment may be considered. On the other hand, a seizure in the setting of alcohol withdrawal is less likely to recur, and treatment with an AED can often be deferred. In any event, treatment with an AED long after the insulting illness has resolved is not indicated, and any use of an AED in this setting should be of limited duration. Although no consensus exists on the optimal duration of treatment in this setting, the AED can usually be withdrawn within weeks or months of the resolution of the illness.

When no acute precipitating cause is evident after the first seizure, the risk of a subsequent seizure can be estimated from the information gathered in the evaluation. Studies have found that a family history of epilepsy, an abnormal neurologic examination, and an abnormal EEG are each independent factors associated with higher risk of subsequent seizures. One study found a 50% risk of a subsequent seizure over 3 years if the EEG was abnormal. The absence of a family history of epilepsy, a normal neurologic examination, and a normal EEG carries about a 30% risk of a subsequent seizure over the next several years. The risk of a recurrent seizure must be balanced against the consequences of a subsequent seizure and the cost and risks of AED treatment. For example, a person who depends on seizure-freedom to maintain employment may opt for treatment even if the risk of recurrence is relatively low. On the other hand, an individual in a chronic care facility on many other medications can often be observed until the second verified seizure, as the risks of treatment may outweigh the benefits.

How Should It Be Treated?

A number of medications are marketed in the United States for the prophylactic treatment of epileptic seizures, with four (phenytoin, ethosuximide, carbamazepine, and valproic acid) considered standard monotherapy agents. Two barbiturates, phenobarbital and primidone, have found extensive use over the years but are less favored now because of their potential cognitive toxicity. Five new AEDs (felbamate, gabapentin, lamotrigine, topiramate, and tiagabine) have been released in the United States since 1993, and several more are likely to be approved by the Food and Drug Administration (FDA) within the next few years. The new AEDs are currently indicated as add-on therapy, but studies verifying their effectiveness in monotherapy are being completed. Clinical practice suggests that each can be used effectively as a single agent in some patients. Selected pharmacologic and clinical properties of these AEDs are contained in Table 4.

Because the goal of therapy is complete seizure control with no adverse effects, an AED should be chosen with both efficacy and toxicity in mind. The following treatment principles can help achieve this goal:

- *Choose an AED likely to be effective against the type or types of seizures the patient has.* First- and

TABLE 4. **Selected Properties of Standard and New Antiepileptic Drugs (listed in order of release to U.S. market)**

AED	Formulations	Titration Rate	Dosing Frequency	Usual Daily Dose (Adult)	Usually Effective Plasma Concentration	Common Drug Interactions: AED Effect On	Common Drug Interactions: Affects AED Level	Adverse Effects: Neurologic	Adverse Effects: Systemic	Relative Cost*
Phenobarbital (PB)	PO 15 mg, 30 mg, 100 mg tablet; 100 mg/5 mL elixir IV various concentrations available	Gradual. Loading dose possible	qd-bid	90–180 mg	10–30 μg/mL	↑ metabolism of PHT, CBZ, VPA, warfarin, oral contraceptives, theophylline, cyclosporine	↓ PB: VPA, acetazolamide. PHT may ↑ or ↓ PB level	Sedation Impaired cognition Hyperactivity	Rash	$
Phenytoin (PHT) (Dilantin)	PO 30 mg, 100 mg capsule; 50 mg tablet; 125 mg/5 mL suspension IV 250 mg/5 mL IM 250 mg/5 mL (fosphenytoin)	Rapid. Loading dose possible	qd-bid	200–400 mg	10–20 μg/mL	↑ metabolism of CBZ, VPA, PB, oral contraceptives, quinidine, theophylline, cyclosporine	↑ PHT: FBM, cimetidine, isoniazid, fluconazole ↓ PHT: CBZ, PB, antacids	Ataxia Nystagmus Slurred speech	Rash Gingival hypertrophy Hypertrichosis Osteomalacia Lymphadenopathy Hepatic enzyme elevation Blood dyscrasias (rare)	$
Ethosuximide (ESM) (Zarontin)	PO 250 mg capsule; 250 mg/5mL suspension	Gradual	tid	1000–2000 mg	40–100 μg/mL	? Effect on PHT, CBZ, oral contraceptives	VPA may ↑ or ↓ ESM level	Dizziness Fatigue	Nausea, vomiting, rash Blood dyscrasias (rare)	$$$
Carbamazepine (CBZ) (Tegretol, Tegretol XR)	PO 100 mg, 200 mg tablet; 100 mg, 200 mg, 400 mg sustained-release tablet (XR)	Gradual	tid bid (XR)	600–1200 mg	6–12 μg/mL	↑ metabolism of PHT, warfarin, oral contraceptives, theophylline	↑ CBZ: cimetidine, erythromycin ↓ CBZ: PHT, PB	Diplopia Sedation Dizziness	Rash Nausea Hyponatremia Blood dyscrasias (rare)	$$
Valproic acid (VPA) (Depakene, Depacon) Sodium divalproex (Depakote)	PO 125 mg, 250 mg, 500 mg tablet; 125 mg capsule ("sprinkles"); 250 mg/5 mL syrup IV 500 mg/5 mL	Gradual	tid-qid	1000–3000 mg	50–120 μg/mL	↓ metabolism of LTG, PB, FBM	↑ VPA: cimetidine, salicylates ↓ VPA: PB, PHT, CBZ	Tremor	Nausea Weight gain Alopecia Thrombocytopenia Hepatic failure (rare)	$$$$
Felbamate (FBM) (Felbatol)	PO 400 mg, 600 mg tablet; 600 mg/5 mL suspension	Gradual	tid	1800–3600 mg	Not established	↑ level of PHT, free VPA, CBZ epoxide	↑ FBM: VPA ↓ FBM: PHT, CBZ	Insomnia Headache	Anorexia Aplastic anemia Hepatic failure	$$$$
Gabapentin (GBP) (Neurontin)	PO 100 mg, 300 mg, 400 mg capsule	Rapid	tid-qid	900–3600 mg	Not established Clinical response may occur with level 4–16 μg/mL	None	Antacids ↓ absorption	Sedation	Weight gain	$$$$
Lamotrigine (LTG) (Lamictal)	PO 25 mg, 100 mg, 150 mg, 200 mg tablet	Slow, especially if on VPA	bid tid if on PHT, CBZ qd if on VPA	100–1000 mg	Not established Clinical response may occur with level 2–20 μg/mL	None	↑ LTG: VPA ↓ LTG: PHT, CBZ	Ataxia Dizziness Diplopia	Rash (rarely severe; more likely with rapid titration in presence of valproate) Nausea	$$$$
Topiramate (TPM) (Topamax)	PO 25 mg, 100 mg, 200 mg tablet	Slow	bid	200–400 mg	Not established	May ↑ PHT level	↓ TPM: PHT, CBZ	Cognitive slowing Sedation Behavioral changes	Renal calculi	$$$$
Tiagabine (TGB) (Gabitril)	PO 4 mg, 12 mg, 16 mg, 20 mg tablet	Slow	tid	20–60 mg	Not established	None	↓ TGB: PHT, CBZ	Cognitive slowing Asthenia Nervousness	Nausea Pharyngitis	$$$$

*Cost (per month): $, less than $20; $$, $21–50; $$$, 51–100; $$$$, greater than $100.
†Low doses (100–200 mg/d) required if on valproate. Higher doses (600–800 mg/d) often required if on carbamazepine or phenytoin.

second-line AEDs for various types of seizures are listed in Table 5.

- *Use one AED at a time.* If the first AED fails, substitute another before combining two or more together.
- *Use the dose of medication that controls the seizures without adverse effects.* By definition, this is the "therapeutic dose" for a given patient.
- *Use the AED plasma concentration as a guideline.* Blood levels are especially useful when noncompliance is suspected, when evaluating possible adverse effects, or to establish a baseline when the patient is doing well. However, the plasma concentration should never be the sole determinant of a dose change. For example, a patient who is seizure-free and without adverse effects with a phenytoin concentration of 23 μg per mL (usual therapeutic range, 10 to 20 μg per mL) does not need a dose adjustment. In fact, a decrease in dose may increase the risk of a breakthrough seizure.

ISSUES IN ONGOING MANAGEMENT

Intractable Seizures

About 30% of patients with epilepsy continue to have seizures despite medical management. When faced with uncontrolled seizures, the following actions should be taken:

- *Rethink the diagnosis.* Nonepileptic episodes will not respond to AEDs. Review the history and diagnostic information, and re-evaluate the differential diagnosis. Further diagnostic testing or referral to a specialized center for prolonged video-EEG monitoring may be necessary.
- *Reassess the seizure type.* Different seizure types may produce similar clinical features, yet respond dramatically differently to AEDs. For example, both generalized absence and complex partial seizures may manifest as blank staring and unresponsiveness. Whereas ethosuximide is the treatment of choice for the former, it will be ineffective for the latter. If further differentiating historical information is lacking, options include an empirical trial of another AED or video-EEG monitoring to record and accurately classify the seizures.
- *Determine compliance.* The best AED will be ineffective if left in the bottle. Reasons for poor compliance are varied and include issues of cost, dosing frequency, toxicity, ignorance about the proper use of the medication, and occasionally even downright defiance.
- *Consider alternative treatments.* Several nonpharmacologic treatments can be considered for medically intractable seizures. The FDA recently approved the vagal nerve stimulator, a pacemaker-type device implanted subcutaneously that delivers low-current electrical stimulation to the vagus nerve in the neck. Although its mechanism of action is still uncertain, it has been shown to reduce seizures in some patients, although it rarely offers complete seizure control. Epilepsy surgery refers to a variety of operative techniques designed to either remove the area of tissue producing seizures or interrupt routes of seizure propagation. Temporal lobectomy, the most commonly performed epilepsy surgery, is effective in completely controlling seizures in up to 80% of patients with seizures of discrete temporal lobe origin. Many patients remain on some medication after surgery, although numbers and doses of AEDs can usually be significantly reduced.

Medically intractable seizures should prompt consideration of referral to an epilepsy center where specialized diagnostic units, trials of experimental AEDs, and epilepsy surgery are available.

TABLE 5. **Recommended Antiepileptic Drug Therapy of Seizures**

	First Line	Second Line
Partial Seizures		
(including simple partial, complex partial, and secondarily generalized seizures)	Carbamazepine Phenytoin Valproic acid	Felbamate Gabapentin Lamotrigine Phenobarbital Topiramate Tiagabine
Generalized Seizures		
Tonic-clonic	Valproic acid	Phenytoin Carbamazepine Phenobarbital Lamotrigine Felbamate Topiramate
Myoclonic	Valproic acid Lamotrigine	Felbamate Clonazepam
Atonic	Valproic acid Lamotrigine	Felbamate
Absence	Ethosuximide	Valproic acid Lamotrigine

Status Epilepticus

Status epilepticus is defined as frequently recurrent seizures without intervening return to normal consciousness, or a single prolonged continuous seizure. Most seizures stop spontaneously in less than 5 minutes, and those that last longer than 5 to 10 minutes should be treated aggressively. Convulsive status epilepticus is a medical emergency that requires a prompt and accurate clinical diagnosis, and treatment that simultaneously supports the ventilatory and hemodynamic status of the patient and provides for the termination of the seizure (Table 6). A recent study has estimated that more than 125,000 cases of status epilepticus occur in the United States each year, with a mortality rate of 22%. Outcome depends in large part on the underlying cause, but the age of the patient and the duration of status epilepticus also independently influence outcome.

A minority of status epilepticus cases are nonconvulsive. Absence status epilepticus does not seem to

TABLE 6. **Status Epilepticus Treatment Timeline**

Minutes	Action
0–1	Assess airway, breathing, circulation Diagnosis status epilepticus on clinical grounds
2–5	IV access Labs (CBC, general chemistry screen, arterial blood gas, urine toxicology, AED levels) Continuous ECG monitoring, frequent BP and respiratory monitoring. Intubate as needed
5–10	Thiamine 1 mg/kg IV, glucose 1 gm/kg IV Lorazepam (Ativan) 0.05–0.2 mg/kg IV at 2 mg/min, up to 8 mg
10–40	Phenytoin (Dilantin) 20 mg/kg IV, no faster than 50 mg/min *or* fosphenytoin (Cerebyx) 20 mg/kg (phenytoin-equivalent) IV up to 150 mg/kg
40–	Options: Pentobarbital 12 mg/kg IV loading dose, followed by 5 mg/kg/h initial infusion rate, or Midazolam 0.2 mg/kg IV loading dose, followed by 0.1 mg/kg/h initial infusion rate, or Propofol 3–5 mg/kg IV loading dose, followed by 1 mg/kg/h initial infusion rate All three require bedside EEG monitoring to determine suppression-burst pattern and complete control of seizures. Titrate infusion rate as needed. Hold infusion after 12 hours and reassess for presence of seizures on EEG

Abbreviations: CBC = complete blood count; AED = antiepileptic drug; ECG = electrocardiography; BP = blood pressure; EEG = electroencephalography.

carry the same risk of morbidity and mortality as convulsive status epilepticus, and does not require treatment as aggressive as outlined in Table 6. Still, it should be treated urgently with AEDs effective against absence seizures. Complex partial status epilepticus may carry with it a risk of permanent neuronal injury; some advocate treating it aggressively (see Table 6).

Pregnancy

Pregnancy issues should be discussed with all epileptic women of childbearing age, preferably long before conception is planned. Relevant issues include the effect of AEDs on contraception, the effect of pregnancy on a woman's seizure frequency, and the teratogenic effects of AEDs.

Medications that induce hepatic enzyme activity (including phenobarbital, phenytoin, and carbamazepine) will reduce the potency of oral contraceptives, rendering a woman more prone to conception. If midcycle bleeding is noted, a contraceptive pill with higher estrogen content or alternative means of birth control should be pursued.

Seizure frequency may either increase or decrease during pregnancy, but usually remains close to the woman's baseline. Factors for increased seizure frequency can include the effects of sleep deprivation and general stress. However, altered physiology is often primarily responsible. During pregnancy, AED volume of distribution and metabolism tend to increase, producing a decline in steady state plasma concentration. On the other hand protein binding tends to decrease, resulting in a relative increase of unbound medication. Because the unbound fraction is the active fraction, toxicity may result despite a decrease in the total AED concentration. Plasma concentrations should be followed more closely during pregnancy and determination of the free concentration may be necessary, especially when seizure frequency increases or toxicity occurs. Similarly, the dose may need to be readjusted after delivery as the woman's physiology returns to baseline.

The risk of a pregnancy complication is doubled in women with epilepsy, and the risk of fetal malformation is increased in women with epilepsy who take an AED compared to those who do not. However, more than 90% of pregnancies in women with epilepsy are uneventful and result in a healthy infant. The following guidelines should be observed to minimize the risks of epilepsy in pregnancy:

- *If a woman has been seizure-free for several years, rethink the need for continued AED treatment.* Ideally, this should be done before conception.
- *Use a single AED whenever possible, at the lowest effective dose.* Polytherapy increases the risk of fetal teratogenicity.
- *Use a prenatal vitamin with 2 to 4 mg folate per day.* This should be started before conception.
- *Perform a fetal ultrasound around week 16 to 18.* If suspicious for fetal malformation, perform amniocentesis.
- *Give the mother vitamin K_1, 20 mg a day, starting 3 weeks before the due date.* This may reduce the risk of fetal hemorrhage.

The decision to breast-feed is a personal one, and the pertinent risks and benefits should be discussed with the mother. The concentration of an AED in breast milk will approximate that of the mother's free plasma concentration. Therefore, AEDs that are highly protein bound will not appear in significant concentrations. Other AEDs, such as phenobarbital, which are largely unbound may appear in the baby's blood and can occasionally cause toxicity in the form of somnolence or poor suck. On balance, however, the nutritional, immunologic, and psychologic benefits of breast-feeding usually outweigh the risks.

Epilepsy in the Elderly

Treating the older adult with epilepsy poses a number of challenges not present in younger patients. The prevalence of epilepsy increases dramatically after the age of 65, largely owing to cerebrovascular disease. The diagnosis of epilepsy in the elderly is often more difficult because relatively common things such as transient ischemic attacks, medication effects, and syncope enter the differential diagnosis. AED pharmacokinetics are also significantly altered in the elderly. Decreases in absorption, volume of distribution, protein binding, hepatic metabolism, and renal clearance result in the net effect of higher total and free plasma AED concentrations at a given dose, compared with younger adults. The elderly are more susceptible to the cognitive and motor effects of AEDs, and are more likely to be taking multiple other medications, resulting in a greater chance of drug interactions. The following guidelines should be observed in treating the elderly epilepsy patient:

- *Avoid AEDs with significant cognitive effects.* In particular, the use of barbiturates (phenobarbital, primidone) and benzodiazepines is discouraged.
- *Use the lowest effective AED dose.* Compared with younger adults, the elderly require a lower AED dose to achieve a similar plasma concentration.
- *Avoid polytherapy.* Use one AED whenever possible. Re-evaluate the need for other medications, especially antihypertensive, sedative, and anticholinergic agents.
- *When faced with toxicity despite a "therapeutic" total plasma concentration, consider measuring the free concentration (phenytoin, valproate) or metabolite concentration (carbamazepine epoxide).*

Driving

Few privileges are as central to the American identity as the right to operate a motor vehicle. Conversely, the loss of this privilege is one of the great burdens of epilepsy. Given the need to ensure the safety of the individual and society as a whole, all states have laws restricting driving by people with poorly controlled epilepsy. The laws are far from uniform, however, with mandated seizure-free periods before driving ranging from 3 months to 2 years. Most states do not require the physician to report drivers directly to the state, but require that the physician apprise patients of their legal responsibilities. Most states also allow for an appeal process and some offer exceptions in cases of strictly nocturnal seizures, simple partial seizures, or seizures occurring in the setting of a physician-supervised medication adjustment. Because of the potential legal and safety implications, driving laws should be reviewed in detail at the first visit, and at least annually thereafter.

Medication Withdrawal

With the exception of epilepsy syndromes unlikely to remit, it is appropriate to consider withdrawal of AED therapy after a 2- to 3-year period of complete seizure control. Although absolute prognosis cannot be determined, normal developmental status, a normal neurologic examination, no family history of epilepsy, and a normal EEG suggest an approximately 30% risk of a recurrent seizure off medication over the subsequent 3 years. The risk of a recurrent seizure is greatest in proximity to the period of medication withdrawal and decreases thereafter. The consequences of a recurrent seizure (including its impact on driving, work, and safety) and the consequences of ongoing AED therapy (including toxicity, potential teratogenicity, and cost) should be thoroughly discussed. The optimal rate of AED withdrawal is a matter of individual preference. Most physicians agree that barbiturates and benzodiazepines should be tapered slowly (e.g., over 6 to 8 weeks) to minimize the risk of inducing a physiologic withdrawal seizure. Although withdrawal seizures probably do not occur with other AEDs, most physicians also prefer a gradual taper (e.g., over 3 to 4 weeks). Driving should be limited during the withdrawal period and for a brief time after the medication has been discontinued.

EPILEPSY IN INFANTS AND CHILDREN

method of
GREGORY L. HOLMES, M.D.
Children's Hospital and
Harvard Medical School
Boston, Massachusetts

Epilepsy is commonly defined as a condition in which there have been two or more seizures during normal physiologic conditions. The latter portion of the definition is important. A child who has seizures during abnormal physiologic conditions such as fever, hypoglycemia, or an intracranial infection is not considered to have epilepsy. Epilepsy is far more common in children than in adults, and in childhood, it has the highest incidence in the first decade.

The first task of the physician when evaluating a patient with a suspected seizure is to determine whether the patient actually has seizures. Many disorders can be confused with seizures. These disorders include breath-holding attacks, pallid infantile syncope, spasmus nutans, night terrors, somnambulism, syncope, rage attacks, migraines, cardiac arrhythmias, and pseudoseizures. It is a serious mistake to inappropriately label a child as having epilepsy because the social consequences and risks of antiepileptic drugs (AEDs) are significant. If a firm diagnosis cannot be established through history and diagnostic testing, it is generally preferable to closely follow the child until the diagnosis is firmly established.

The next priority when evaluating a child with epileptic seizures is to determine seizure type. Seizures are classified into two basic groups, partial and generalized (Table 1). Partial seizures involve only a portion of the brain at the onset. They can be further divided into those not involving impairment of consciousness (simple partial) and those with impaired consciousness (complex partial). Both types of partial seizures can spread, resulting in generalized tonic-clonic seizures. Primary generalized seizures are those in which the first clinical changes indicate initial involvement of both hemispheres. There is usually impairment of consciousness during generalized seizures, although some seizures, such as myoclonic, may be so brief that impairment of consciousness cannot be assessed.

After identification of the epileptic seizure type, it is important for the clinician to determine whether the patient has an epileptic syndrome, which is defined as a cluster of signs and symptoms customarily occurring together. Identification of an epileptic syndrome may allow the physician to determine genetic risk (i.e., certain epileptic syndromes are associated with specific genotypes). In addition, syndrome identification helps determine appropriate therapy and prognosis. Table 2 lists some common syndromes.

TABLE 1. **Classification of Epileptic Seizures**

I. Partial Seizures
  A. Simple partial seizures
    1. With motor signs, such as focal clonic activity
    2. With somatosensory or special-sensory symptoms, such as lateralized numbness, tingling, visual or auditory hallucinations, abnormal odors, or smells
    3. With autonomic symptoms or signs such as tachycardia, diaphoresis
    4. With psychic symptoms such as fear, anxiety, déjà vu, jamais vu, confusion
  B. Complex partial seizures
    1. With simple partial seizures (aura) at onset
    2. With impairment of consciousness at onset
  C. Partial seizures evolving to secondarily generalized seizures
II. Generalized Seizures
  A. Absence seizures
  B. Myoclonic seizures
  C. Clonic seizures
  D. Tonic seizures
  E. Tonic-clonic seizures
  F. Atonic seizures

DIAGNOSTIC EVALUATION OF THE CHILD WITH EPILEPSY

The history and neurologic examination remain the cornerstone of neurologic diagnosis. They are the most important factors in determining whether the patient has epilepsy, and if so, what type. After a diagnosis of epilepsy has been made, the clinician must determine the underlying or precipitating cause of the seizure. The initial workup is partly determined by the way in which the patient presents. The patient who arrives to the emergency department in status epilepticus or coma or who is febrile is approached differently from the patient who has totally recovered from the seizure by the time he or she presents to the clinician. In the former conditions, there is an urgency to determine whether the patient has a cause for the seizures, such as infection or metabolic disturbance. Likewise, the neurologic examination is important in diagnostic investigations. A child with focal neurologic findings usually requires neuroimaging as part of the evaluation.

TABLE 2. **Classification of Epileptic Syndromes**

I. Localization-related (focal, local, partial) epilepsies and syndromes
  A. Idiopathic
    1. Benign rolandic epilepsy
    2. Benign occipital epilepsy
  B. Symptomatic
II. Generalized epilepsies and syndromes
  A. Idiopathic, age-related
    1. Benign neonatal familial convulsions
    2. Benign idiopathic convulsions
    3. Benign myoclonic epilepsy in infancy
    4. Childhood absence epilepsy
    5. Juvenile absence epilepsy
    6. Juvenile myoclonic epilepsy
    7. Epilepsy with grand mal seizures on awakening
  B. Idiopathic and/or symptomatic
    1. Infantile spasms (West syndrome)
    2. Lennox-Gastaut syndrome
    3. Epilepsy with myoclonic-astatic seizures
    4. Epilepsy with myoclonic absences
  C. Symptomatic: early myoclonic encephalopathy
III. Epilepsies and syndromes undetermined as to whether they are focal or generalized
  A. Neonatal seizures
  B. Severe myoclonic epilepsy in infancy
  C. Epilepsy with continuous spike waves during slow-wave sleep
  D. Acquired epileptic aphasia (Landau-Kleffner syndrome)

Electroencephalography

Because the electroencephalogram (EEG) is noninvasive, benign, and relatively inexpensive, it is reasonable to obtain at least one EEG on any patient with seizures or suspected seizures. An awake and sleep recording is desirable. Hyperventilation and photic stimulation frequently activate generalized discharges and may occasionally elicit abnormalities in patients with partial seizures.

The EEG is only suggestive of epilepsy and is rarely diagnostic of the disorder. The primary exception to this rule is absence seizures. It is quite likely that in untreated patients, hyperventilation, photic stimulation, or sleep will result in generalized spike-and-wave activity on the EEG. For practical purposes generalized spike-and-wave activity lasting longer than 3 seconds can be considered a seizure.

Neuroimaging

Computed tomography (CT) and magnetic resonance imaging (MRI) have now been shown to be superior to the clinical examination, EEG, and routine skull radiographs in the diagnosis of structural lesions of the central nervous system. Identification of benign and malignant tumors, focal cerebral dysgenesis, sclerosis, and vascular malformations has been aided greatly by improved anatomic neuroimaging. Because the MRI is more sensitive than the CT scan, it is now the preferred test in the evaluation of most patients with epilepsy. However, CT still has a role in the acute evaluation of patients with seizures. CT detects most tumors and is useful when looking for calcified lesions or hemorrhage.

Not all children with seizures require neuroimaging. Children with benign syndromes such as benign rolandic epilepsy, juvenile myoclonic epilepsy, the absence syndromes, and febrile seizures do not typically require neuroimaging. Abnormal scans are most frequent in patients who have partial seizures, abnormal neurologic findings, and focal paroxysmal discharges or slowing on the EEG.

TREATMENT PLAN

As noted previously, epilepsy is a condition characterized by recurrent seizures. It is not always necessary to treat the first seizure. In prospective studies of children presenting with their first seizure, approximately 30 to 40% will have a second seizure. If the child has a second seizure, the risk for continued seizures increases substantially. Therefore, it is quite reasonable to wait for a second seizure in a child presenting with a partial or generalized tonic-clonic seizure before embarking on a course of AED therapy. Patients presenting with absence or myoclonic seizures or infantile spasms are usually seen after the child has had many seizures. Unless there is some question about the diagnosis, treatment should begin immediately.

Once the diagnosis is established and the physician decides to treat, the next decision is to deter-

TABLE 3. **AEDs of Choice in the Treatment of Seizures**

AED	Partial Seizures: *Simple*	Partial Seizures: *Complex*	Generalized Seizures: *GTC*	Generalized Seizures: *Absence*	Generalized Seizures: *Myoclonic*	Generalized Seizures: *Clonic*	Generalized Seizures: *Tonic*	Generalized Seizures: *Atonic*
First Choice	Carbamazepine Phenytoin Valproic acid*	Carbamazepine Phenytoin Valproic acid*	Carbamazepine Phenytoin Valproic acid	Ethosuximide Valproic acid	Valproic acid	Valproic acid*	Valproic acid*	Valproic acid*
Second Choice	Gabapentin Lamotrigine Phenobarbital Tiagabine Topiramate	Gabapentin Lamotrigine Phenobarbital Tiagabine Topiramate	Gabapentin Lamotrigine* Phenobarbital Topiramate*	Lamotrigine	Clonazepam Phenobarbital	Phenobarbital	Carbamazepine Lamotrigine* Phenytoin Topiramate*	Lamotrigine* Topiramate*

*Not FDA approved for this indication.
Abbreviation: GTC = generalized tonic-clonic.

mine which antiepileptic drug to use. This decision is based on efficacy and possible toxicity. Tables 3 and 4 list the AEDs used in the various seizure types and syndromes. Tables 5 and 6 provide summary information on the older or established AEDs and the recently released AEDs.

Treatment should always be initiated with a single AED and the dosage slowly increased until the seizures are controlled or until clinical toxicity ensues. If the first AED does not work, the drug should be slowly tapered while a second AED is introduced. AEDs should never be stopped abruptly unless there is a severe side effect. Although it is sometimes difficult to avoid polytherapy, the goal should be to have the patient on a single AED. This is likely to result in higher blood levels, fewer side effects, and better control.

Serum AED levels are useful guides in assessing therapy. In general, patients with blood levels that are within the therapeutic range have a higher likelihood of seizure control than when the level is below the therapeutic range. Likewise, patients that have blood levels exceeding the upper therapeutic range are more likely to experience side effects than when the levels are therapeutic. Phenytoin (Dilantin), phenobarbital, carbamazepine (Tegretol), and primidone (Mysoline) levels are most useful, correlating better with seizure control and toxicity than valproic acid (Depakote, Depakene), ethosuximide (Zarontin), gabapentin (Neurontin), lamotrigine (Lamictal), tiagabine* (Gabitril), and topiramate (Topamax) levels. Far more can be learned by reviewing the history and examining the patient than strictly guiding therapy by the blood level. If seizures are continuing and the patient is tolerating the medication well, the dosage should be increased. Conversely, if the patient has persistent side effects, the dosage should be reduced regardless of the level. Each patient has an individualized "therapeutic" level.

Many children with epilepsy will eventually achieve remission. The likelihood of this depends on many factors. Children with benign syndromes such as benign rolandic epilepsy or childhood absences have a high likelihood of eventual remission while children with Lennox-Gastaut syndrome rarely can be successfully weaned from AEDs. Patients with a symptomatic etiology for their seizures, such as central nervous system infections, trauma, and brain malformations, have a lower likelihood of remission than children with idiopathic etiologies. Nevertheless, some children with severe neurologic disorders can eventually be weaned from drugs, and it is important for the physician to reassess the situation periodically in all children with epilepsy.

TABLE 4. **AEDs of Choice in the Treatment of Epilepsy Syndromes**

Syndrome	First Choice	Second Choice
Benign rolandic epilepsy	Carbamazepine Gabapentin Phenytoin Valproic acid	Gabapentin Lamotrigine Topiramate
Benign occipital epilepsy	Carbamazepine Gabapentin Phenytoin Valproic acid	Gabapentin Lamotrigine Topiramate
Childhood absence	Ethosuximide	Lamotrigine Valproic acid
Juvenile absence	Valproic acid	Lamotrigine
Infantile spasms	Vigabatrin (not approved in the United States)	Adrenocorticotrophic hormone Valproic acid
Lennox-Gastaut	Valproic acid	Lamotrigine Tiagabine Topiramate

Simple and Complex Partial Seizures

The last few years have seen a rapid growth in number of AEDs available for the treatment of partial seizures. The established AEDs carbamazepine, phenobarbital, phenytoin, and valproic acid have been joined by gabapentin, lamotrigine, tiagabine, and topiramate. The new AEDs all received approval from the Food and Drug Administration (FDA) for add-on therapy for partial seizures in adults. Unfortunately they were released with little information on dosage, efficacy, and side effects in children. How the new drugs will compare with the established AEDs in childhood onset partial seizures remains to be determined.

*Investigational drug in the United States.

TABLE 5. **Summary of Commonly Used AEDs (Established Drugs)**

AED	Indications	Maintenance Dosage	Starting Dosage	Half-Life (h)	Therapeutic Range	Common Side Effects	Serious Idiosyncratic Side Effects
Carbamazepine (Tegretol)	1. Partial 2. Partial with 2° general. 3. 1° general. tonic-clonic	10–20 mg/kg/d	5–10 mg/kg/d	8–25	8–12 μg/mL	Diplopia Lethargy Blurred vision Ataxia	Rashes Hepatic dysfunction Pancreatitis Aplastic anemia Leukopenia
Ethosuximide (Zarontin)	1. Absence	15–40 mg/kg/d, most children require 15–20 mg/kg/d	<6 y: 10 mg/kg/d >6 y: 250 mg/d	25–40	40–100 μg/mL	Gastrointestinal distress Hiccoughs Lethargy	Rashes Leukopenia Pancytopenia Systemic lupus erythematosus
Phenobarbital	1. Partial 2. Partial with 2° general. 3. 1° general. tonic-clonic	<1 y: 3–5 mg/kg/d >1 y: 2–4 mg/kg/d Teenagers, adults: 2–3 mg/kg/d	Same as maintenance	40–70	15–40 μg/mL	Irritability Hyperactivity Lethargy	Rashes
Phenytoin (Dilantin)	1. Partial 2. Partial with 2° general. 3. 1° general. tonic-clonic	5 mg/kg/d (may need higher doses in children <5–6 y)	Same as maintenance	Dependent on concentration	10–20 μg/mL	Lethargy Dizziness Ataxia Gingival hypertrophy Hirsutism	Rashes Hepatic dysfunction Lymphadenopathy Blood dyscrasias
Primidone (Mysoline)	1. Partial 2. Partial with 2° general. 3. 1° general. tonic-clonic	12–25 mg/kg/d	<6 y: 50 mg qhs <12 y: 100 mg qhs >12 y: 150 mg qhs	5–8 (phenobarbital 40–70)	5–12 μg/mL	Irritability Hyperactivity Lethargy Nausea	Rashes
Valproic Acid (Depakote)	1. Partial 2. Partial with 2° general. 3. 1° general. tonic-clonic 4. Absence 5. Myoclonic 6. Tonic 7. Atonic	15–60 mg/kg/d	15 mg/kg/d; increase by 10–15 mg/kg/d every 2 weeks	4–14	50–150 μg/mL	Lethargy Weight gain or loss Hair loss Tremor	Hepatic dysfunction Pancreatitis Anemia Thrombocytopenia

Abbreviations: 1° = primary; 2° = secondary.

TABLE 6. **Summary of Commonly Used AEDs (New Drugs)**

AED	Indications	Maintenance Dosage	Starting Dosage	Half-Life (h)	Therapeutic Range	Common Side Effects	Serious Idiosyncratic Side Effects
Felbamate (Felbatol)	1. Partial 2. Partial with 2° general. 3. Tonic 4. Atonic	30–45 mg/kg/d	15 mg/kg/d, increase in 10 mg/kg increments to 60 mg/kg, if necessary	13–24	Not established	Anorexia Insomnia Somnolence	Aplastic anemia Hepatotoxicity
Gabapentin (Neurontin)	1. Partial 2. Partial with 2° general.	20–60 mg/kg/d	10 mg/kg/d, increase in 5 mg/kg increments	5–8	Not established	Lethargy Dizziness	None
Lamotrigine (Lamictal)	1. Partial 2. Partial with 2° general. 3. Absence	5–15 mg/kg/d; dosage dependent on other drugs used; if on enzyme inducers use 10–15 mg/kg/d, if on valproate use 5 mg/kg/d	12.5–25 mg/d, increase slowly, be cautious if patient is on valproate	15–60 (highly dependent on concomitant AEDs)	Not established	Rashes Lethargy Irritability	Rashes
Tiagabine (Gabitril)	1. Partial 2. Partial with 2° general.	0.5–1.0 mg/kg/d; dosage dependent on other drugs used; if on enzyme inhibitors use 0.7–1.5 mg/kg/d, if on no enzyme inhibitors use 0.3–0.4 mg/kg/d	0.1 mg/kg/d; increase weekly by 0.1 mg/kg/d	3–8	Not established	Lethargy Confusion Mental dullness Difficulties with concentration	None
Topiramate (Topamax)	1. Partial 2. Partial with 2° general.	5–10 mg/kg/d	1–2 mg/kg/d; increase weekly by 1 mg/kg/d	12–30	Not established	Irritability Hyperactivity Mental dullness Weight loss	None

Abbreviations: 1° = primary; 2° = secondary.

Carbamazepine is widely used for the treatment of partial seizures with and without secondary generalization. Initiating treatment with small multiple doses followed by incremental adjustments over 1 to 2 weeks reduces the risk of toxicity and encourages patient compliance. An extended release formulation is now available (Tegretol-XR), and a twice daily dosage schedule can be used for children that can swallow a tablet. A liquid preparation is also available.

Carbamazepine produces no adverse cosmetic effects and interferes only minimally with cognitive function. However, mild side effects are common with carbamazepine use. Visual disturbances may be the most troublesome clinically and can usually be correlated with elevated serum concentrations. Some individuals note recurrent diplopia or blurred vision several hours after each dose of carbamazepine. Reduction of dosage or adjustment of dosage intervals may be necessary. Aplastic anemia and serious liver toxicity are rare reactions. Hematologic and liver function monitoring is recommended.

Phenobarbital is the most commonly used barbiturate in epilepsy. Introduced in 1912, the drug is effective in the treatment of generalized tonic-clonic and partial seizures. Although recently physicians have been avoiding phenobarbital in favor of other anticonvulsants, it remains an inexpensive, effective, and generally safe medication. Because of the long half-life, it takes 2 to 3 weeks for phenobarbital to reach a steady-state therapeutic level. Twice daily dosing is typically used in infants; in older children once daily dosing is adequate.

In young children the most common side effects of the barbiturates include irritability, hyperactivity, sleep disorders, and cognitive abnormalities. Other side effects such as rash or allergic manifestations occur in less than 1 to 2% of patients. Frequent routine laboratory monitoring is not necessary with phenobarbital.

Phenytoin, like the barbiturates, has been used as a first-line AED for many years. Since its introduction in 1934, phenytoin has been one of the major AEDs used in the treatment of partial seizures. However, the drug is difficult to use because of the nonlinear elimination kinetics. Because metabolism of phenytoin is linear only at low serum levels, once the therapeutic range is approached, a small increase in phenytoin dose can lead to a marked increase in blood level. Patients with toxic levels of phenytoin have half-life values longer than patients with levels near the therapeutic range.

Side effects include gingival hypertrophy and hirsutism in a small percentage of patients. These cosmetic changes resolve when phenytoin is discontinued. With toxic levels, behavioral changes, cognitive dysfunction, nausea, emesis, nystagmus, ataxia, and lethargy may be present. More serious side effects include Stevens-Johnson syndrome, lymphadenopathy, and rare hematologic abnormalities such as thrombocytopenia, anemia, and leukopenia.

Valproic acid was used initially in generalized seizures (absence, myoclonic, and tonic-clonic) but has proven effective as well in partial seizures. The drug comes in convenient dosing forms for children, with both a liquid and sprinkle preparation.

Valproic acid is usually well tolerated by children. The drug has minimal effects on cognitive function. Side effects of valproic acid include mild sedation, nausea, vomiting, and anorexia. These side effects may occur at the beginning of therapy, but are usually transient or may respond to a slight decrease in dosage. Tremor, weight gain, and hair loss may also occur. The major serious adverse reaction is severe hepatic dysfunction. The highest risk group for hepatotoxicity is children under the age of 2 years who are in polytherapy. Fatal hepatic dysfunction associated with valproic acid does not appear to be a dose-related phenomenon. It is essential that a serum transaminase (serum glutamic-oxaloacetic transaminase, serum glutamate-pyruvate transaminase) be obtained before initiation of treatment and at regular intervals while the child is on the medication. Transient, mild elevation of liver enzymes occurs commonly and may return to normal with decreases in the dosage. Children with elevations of a transaminase two or more times the upper limit of normal for that test, or with clinical symptoms of hepatic dysfunction, should discontinue the medication.

Rare cases of leukopenia and thrombocytopenia have been reported; thus, routine monitoring of complete blood count and platelets is necessary. Prolonged bleeding times owing to abnormal platelet adhesion can occur with valproic acid and should be measured before undertaking any surgical procedure. Thrombocytopenia is more likely to be encountered with high levels of valproate, particularly if the child develops a viral illness. In addition, rare cases of fatal pancreatitis have also been reported; serum amylase levels should be drawn when clinically indicated.

Gabapentin is an amino acid structurally related to γ-aminobutyric acid and which readily passes through the blood-brain barrier. Despite the molecular structure, the mechanism of gabapentin is not clear. In studies of primarily adults with partial seizures with and without secondary generalization, gabapentin used as adjunctive therapy was superior to placebo.

Adverse effects with this drug appear to be quite rare and typically consist of somnolence, fatigue, dizziness, nausea, unsteadiness, and weight gain. Most of the side effects are transient. In children, an escalation of behavioral problems, such as obstreperousness, aggressiveness, or hyperactivity can be seen. One of the major advantages of this drug is that it is relatively free of interactions with other drugs. Unlike other AEDs, gabapentin is not metabolized by the liver, does not induce hepatic enzymes, and is not protein bound. It is almost completely eliminated by renal excretion of the parent compound. Gabapentin does not affect the concentrations of other AEDs.

Lamotrigine was released in 1994. In animal studies, the drug has a profile similar to phenytoin. As with gabapentin, toxicity in animal studies has been low. Controlled clinical trials have shown lamotrigine to be effective as add-on therapy in refractory epilepsy for both partial and tonic-clonic seizures. Adverse effects are relatively infrequent and usually consist of diplopia, drowsiness, ataxia, and headache. Rashes have been a significant problem in both children and adults. Although in some patients the rashes are mild and transient, in other patients the severity of the rash has been significant enough to require withdrawal of the drug. The drug must be started at low doses and slowly increased, especially if the patient is also taking valproic acid. The drug should be stopped immediately if a rash occurs.

Lamotrigine does not appear to affect the pharmacokinetics of other AEDs to any major degree. However, carbamazepine and phenytoin will increase metabolism of lamotrigine, whereas valproate will inhibit metabolism. Smaller dosages of lamotrigine are required when patients are taking valproate concurrently than when they are taking phenytoin or carbamazepine.

Topiramate and tiagabine were released in 1997. In small clinical trials, the drugs have been determined to be superior to placebo in partial seizures in children. Based on limited information, the drugs appear to be well tolerated. No serious adverse events have been described with either drug to date, although the experience in children is quite limited.

Absence Seizures

Absence seizures are the major seizure type in two syndromes in childhood: childhood absence epilepsy and juvenile absence epilepsy. Childhood absence seizures occur in children between the ages of 3 years and puberty, who are otherwise normal. The absences are frequent, occurring multiple times daily, and tend to cluster. Juvenile absence epilepsy begins around puberty and differs from childhood absences primarily in that the seizures are more sporadic. Children with juvenile absence epilepsy are at higher risk for generalized tonic-clonic seizures than children with childhood absences. Both syndromes are characterized by bilateral, synchronous symmetrical 2.5 to 3.5 cycles per second spike-and-wave discharges on the EEG.

Ethosuximide and valproic acid are most commonly used to treat absence seizures. Because ethosuximide is not useful in the treatment of generalized tonic-clonic seizures, valproic acid is usually used when the child has both generalized tonic-clonic and absence seizures. Lamotrigine appears to have considerable promise in the treatment of absence seizures.

Generalized Tonic-Clonic Seizures

Most children with generalized tonic-clonic (GTC) seizures have partial seizures that secondarily generalize. These seizures respond to the same group of drugs used to treat partial seizures. Primary GTC seizures, in which the seizure is generalized from onset respond to valproate and lamotrigine.

Infantile Spasms

Infantile spasms typically consist of sudden flexion of the head, abduction and extension of the arms, and simultaneous flexion of the knees. The seizures usually occur in clusters. An abnormal EEG pattern, hypsarrhythmia, is characteristic of the disorder. In many children, onset of the seizures is associated with a slowing of development. Although vigabatrin (Sabril) is an effective medication for this disorder, the drug has not yet been approved for use in the United States. The drug of choice in the United States is ACTH (adrenocorticotrophic hormone), given intramuscularly for several months.

Lennox-Gastaut Syndrome

The Lennox-Gastaut syndrome consists of a mixed seizure disorder, in which the most common seizure type is tonic, an EEG pattern showing a slow spike-and-wave pattern, and mental retardation. The syndrome begins in early childhood, sometimes evolving from infantile spasms. The disorder is difficult to treat and many children become toxic because of the multiple drugs used to try to stop the seizures.

Felbamate (Felbatol) was released in the United States in 1993 as adjunctive therapy in the treatment of partial and generalized seizures associated with Lennox-Gastaut syndrome in children. Unfortunately, the drug has been linked to aplastic anemia and hepatic toxicity. At this time, the drug is recommended only for patients with very severe epilepsy, not controlled with other AEDs. Valproate, lamotrigine, and topiramate have shown some limited efficacy in the treatment of this syndrome.

Although the ketogenic diet is one of the oldest methods of treating childhood epilepsy, it is a reasonable therapy for children with seizures refractory to standard AED therapy. The diet consists of a high proportion of fats and small amounts of carbohydrate and protein with a fat/carbohydrate and protein ratio of 4:1. Although it is clear that the child must remain in a state of ketosis for the diet to be effective, the basis of the therapeutic effectiveness of the ketogenic diet remains uncertain.

The ketogenic diet improves seizure control in a significant number of children with medically intractable epilepsy. One third to one half of the children appear to have an excellent response to the ketogenic diet in terms of a marked or complete cessation of seizures or reduction in seizure severity. Another one third have a partial reduction in seizure frequency or severity; the remaining children have no appreciable benefit from the diet. Improvement in alertness and behavior is often seen when the child is placed on the diet. It is not clear whether this improvement is secondary to withdrawal of AEDs, reduction in seizure frequency, or a direct result of the diet.

Neonatal Seizures

Neonatal seizures are one of the most common, yet ominous, neurologic signs in newborns. Because seizures may be the first and only sign of a central nervous system disorder, their recognition is extremely important. Despite advances in obstetrics and perinatal care, seizures continue to be a significant predictor of poor neurologic outcome.

Most neonatal seizures are secondary to an acute etiology such as hypoglycemia, infection, or hypoxic-ischemic event. The most important therapy in neonatal seizures is a search for the cause of the seizures and prompt treatment. With recurrent seizures, treatment consists of phenobarbital or phenytoin, both given as an intravenous loading dose of 20 mg per kg.

Febrile Seizures

A febrile seizure is a seizure disorder that occurs in children between 6 months and 5 years of age, in association with a fever but without evidence of intracranial infection. Febrile seizures are differentiated from epilepsy, which is characterized by recurrent, afebrile seizures. Patients with epilepsy, however, are often more susceptible to seizures during fever. Unfortunately, when a child has a seizure with fever, there is no definitive way to determine whether the seizure is secondary to the fever or is the first manifestation of epilepsy.

Febrile seizures are associated with a very low mortality rate. When deaths do occur, they are usually secondary to the agent causing the fever or an antecedent neurologic disorder. In addition, there is a low incidence of acquired motor or intellectual abnormalities after a febrile seizure.

Although relatively few children who experience febrile seizures develop epilepsy, recurrences of febrile seizures are commonplace. Approximately one third of the children have at least one recurrence, and half of those who have one recurrence have an additional attack. Recurrence risk is not uniform for all children with febrile seizures. The most important factor appears to be age of onset at the first febrile seizure. The younger the child at the first attack, the more likely are further febrile seizures. Three fourths of recurrences take place within 1 year of the first febrile seizure, and 90% within 2 years.

The physician must first identify whether there is an underlying illness that requires immediate, specific treatment. The most urgent diagnostic decision is whether to do a lumbar puncture. One of the earliest signs of meningitis may be a seizure, which like a febrile seizure, is usually short and GTC in type. Although meningitis usually results in meningismus, in patients under the age of 2 years, clinical signs of meningitis may be minimal or absent.

Although prophylactic use of phenobarbital was often recommended for children with recurrent febrile seizures, the large number of side effects of the drug coupled with the benign nature of febrile seizures has significantly curtailed this practice. Oral or rectal diazepam (Valium), in a dose of 0.5 mg per kg every 8 hours during febrile illnesses, has also been used. However, a significant number of children will have side effects with this medication. In addition, parents may not recognize the child has a fever until after the seizure has occurred. For that reason prophylactic therapy for febrile seizures is usually not recommended.

Surgical Therapy

The possibility of surgery should always be considered for a child with intractable epilepsy. Success rates in children with regard to control of seizures are equal to, and possible greater than, the success rates for comparable surgery in adults. In addition, because of the more plastic nature of the immature brain, recovery from surgery is often better and quicker in children than in adults. Surgical resection of the epileptic focus has the potential of "curing" the epilepsy as opposed to trying to suppress the seizures with either drugs or diet.

Several varieties of surgical procedures are now offered. Children with partial seizures with or without generalization can have focal resection of the epileptic tissue. Children who have discrete lesions on MRI or a well-delineated focal onset of seizures during EEG monitoring are the most likely to benefit from the surgery. Children with severe unilateral hemispheric disease, such as Sturge-Weber syndrome, Rasmussen's encephalitis, and cerebrovascular accidents often have miraculous outcomes after total removal of the hemisphere. Corpus callosotomy, which interrupts the spread of seizures from one hemisphere to another, may be useful in children with bilateral EEG abnormalities. This surgery can be particularly helpful in children who fall during their seizures.

ATTENTION DEFICIT HYPERACTIVITY DISORDER (ADHD)

method of
LOUISE S. KIESSLING, M.D.
Memorial Hospital of Rhode Island and Brown University School of Medicine
Providence, Rhode Island

Attention deficit hyperactivity disorder (ADHD) is one of the most common neurobehavioral disorders of childhood. It is characterized by problems with attention and distractibility, as well as elements of motor impersistence and impulsivity. A significant component of ADHD is disinhibition, the inability to inhibit extraneous activity, thoughts, or emotions. The current Diagnostic and Statistical Manual of Mental Disorder (DSM-IV) discriminates three categories: ADHD, inattentive type; ADHD, impulsive/hyperactive type; and ADHD, combined type. Table 1 lists the characteristics from the DSM-IV manual.

More recently, the Diagnostic and Statistical Manual–Primary Care has been developed. The impetus for this

TABLE 1. **Diagnostic and Statistical Manual-IV Criteria for Diagnosis of Attention-Deficit/Hyperactivity Disorder**

A. Either (1) or (2):
  (1) six (or more) of the following symptoms of inattention have persisted for at least 6 months to a degree that is maladaptive and inconsistent with developmental level:
  Inattention
    (a) often fails to give close attention to details or makes careless mistakes in schoolwork, work, or other activities
    (b) often has difficulty sustaining attention in tasks or play activities
    (c) often does not seem to listen when spoken to directly
    (d) often does not follow through on instructions and fails to finish homework, chores, or duties in the workplace (not due to oppositional behavior or failure to understand instructions)
    (e) often has difficulty organizing tasks and activities
    (f) often avoids, dislikes, or is reluctant to engage in tasks that require sustained mental effort (such as schoolwork or homework)
    (g) often loses things necessary for tasks or activities (e.g., toys, school assignments, pencils, books, or tools)
    (h) is often easily distracted by extraneous stimuli
    (i) is often forgetful in daily activities
  (2) six (or more) of the following symptoms of hyperactivity-impulsivity have persisted for at least 6 months to a degree that is maladaptive and inconsistent with developmental level:
  Hyperactivity
    (a) often fidgets with hands or feet or squirms in seat
    (b) often leaves seat in classroom or in other situations in which remaining seated is expected
    (c) often runs about or climbs excessively in situations in which it is inappropriate (in adolescents or adults, may be limited to subjective feelings of restlessness)
    (d) often has difficulty playing or engaging in leisure activities quietly
    (e) is often "on the go" or often acts as if "driven by a motor"
    (f) often talks excessively
  Impulsivity
    (g) often blurts out answers before questions have been completed
    (h) often has difficulty awaiting turn
    (i) often interrupts or intrudes on others (e.g., butts into conversations or games)

B. Some hyperactive-impulsive or inattentive symptoms that caused impairment were present before age 7 years.
C. Some impairment from the symptoms is present in two or more settings (e.g., at school [or work] and at home).
D. There must be clear evidence of clinically significant impairment in social, academic, or occupational functioning.
E. The symptoms do not occur exclusively during the course of a Pervasive Developmental Disorder, Schizophrenia, or other Psychotic Disorder and are not better accounted for by another mental disorder (e.g., Mood Disorder, Anxiety Disorder, Dissociative Disorder, or a Personality Disorder).

Code based on type:
  314.01 Attention-Deficit/Hyperactivity Disorder, Combined Type: if both Criteria A1 and A2 are met for the past 6 months
  314.00 Attention-Deficit/Hyperactivity Disorder, Predominantly Inattentive Type: if Criterion A1 is met but Criterion A2 is not met for the past 6 months
  314.01 Attention-Deficit/Hyperactivity Disorder, Predominantly Hyperactive Type: if Criterion A2 is met but Criterion A1 is not met for the past 6 months.

From American Psychiatric Association: Diagnostic and Statistical Manual of Mental Disorders, 4th ed. Washington, DC, American Psychiatric Association, 1994, pp 63–65.

manual is to provide a way of categorizing childhood neurobehavioral disorders in primary care. One of the characteristics of DSM-PC is the levels of severity. The first level is Developmental Variation: V65.49 Hyperactive Impulsive Variation. The next is Problem: V40.3 Hyperactive/Impulsive Behavior problem; and the third is Disorder: 314.01 Attention Deficit/Hyperactivity Disorder, which is subdivided into the three types. There are three levels of care; only at the third level does the syndrome become a disorder.

EPIDEMIOLOGY

Previous studies at multiple sites around the world have suggested a prevalence of about 6% for ADHD using earlier definitions. Studies from the United States, Sweden, and China support this percentage. The criteria and labeling changed a bit from the early 1960s when the first DSM-II was published through DSM-III-R, but there was a fair amount of congruence between them. The current criteria, as published in DSM-IV, may be identifying an increased number of children as ADHD, particularly boys. A study done in Germany and then replicated in Tennessee suggested that somewhere between 11 and 17% of all boys in an elementary school at the fifth grade level might meet criteria for ADHD under DSM-IV criteria based on teacher ratings. These figures seem excessive. A number of people are concerned that the current criteria are overidentifying ADHD.

Given that background, a recent study from Australia is quite interesting. Investigators studied twins and siblings where at least one child was previously diagnosed with ADHD based on DSM-III-R criteria, which included the Inattentive Type and the Hyperactive Impulsive Type. This study suggests that the criteria are all on a continuum of behavior. Genetic studies determined that the trait was prominent. The data are consistent with the approach of DSM-PC, as opposed to a categoric approach (i.e., the disorder is present or absent). Given this study as well as the previous information on the DSM-IV criteria, one can see that in making this diagnosis, the physician must consider the total child. The criterion that the symptoms must be present in at least two environments, e.g., home and school, home and office, school and office, is clearly essential. These data make it clear that we need to ensure that we are not misdiagnosing children with language disorders, seizure disorders of the absence type, children with significant obsessive-compulsive symptoms, or children from dysfunctional, disorganized families with ADHD. It is also important to identify the different levels of severity; some children may have subtle problems with attention that will respond to structured environmental manipulation, whereas others may not respond adequately to environmental changes and require active medication.

HISTORY

At the turn of the century, Little, one of the founders of pediatrics, was well aware of youngsters who were active and impulsive. The modern history for ADHD begins at Bradley Hospital in East Providence, Rhode Island, in the 1930s when Dr. Charles Bradley (no relation to hospital founder) and his successors Drs. Maurice Laufer, Eric Denhoff, and Gerald Solomons began to systematically study a group of children with inattention, distractibility, impulsivity, poor persistence, and disinhibition. The group used names such as "minimal brain dysfunction" and then "hyperkinesis," which were incorporated into DSM-II, to describe behavior now grouped under the disorders of ADHD.

Bradley was the first to use stimulant medication with this population. The first compound used was racemic amphetamine (Benzedrine), followed by dextroamphetamine (Dexedrine) and then in the mid-50s methylphenidate (Ritalin). Early research by Stewart and colleagues in Iowa showed a familial tendency toward ADHD with those with a family history for externalizing behavior, such as alcoholism and criminal behavior, forming a subgroup. This differentiation has continued. Work from our unit at Brown University by Julie Wilson, Ph.D., has shown that children diagnosed with ADHD in a pediatric referral population have less co-morbidity than is reported from psychiatric evaluation units. Thus, the site of referral affects the co-morbidities reported. Familial characteristics are also important when one considers ADHD and associated learning disabilities. There tends to be similarity in families. The parental phenotype, namely whether they have ADHD plus learning disabilities or only ADHD, as well as whether there is a tendency toward externalizing behavior, persists in successive generations.

GENDER

Numerous studies have shown that girls are underidentified for ADHD. They tend to present with primarily the inattentive type or the inattentive-impulsive type without the extremes of hyperactivity that one sees in the male probands. However, there is some suggestion that girls who have been so identified may have an increased incidence of learning disabilities as a co-morbidity. This may simply be a factor of ascertainment bias because girls are referred far less often than boys. In our own practice, approximately the same percentage of girls referred for ADHD as boys are identified, but the actual number of girls referred is much fewer. It is important to assess the inattentive, disorganized side carefully. Girls are more likely to present with fidgetiness rather than overhyperactivity. The net result is that girls have often been underidentified. Conversely, there is a higher likelihood of boys with associated comorbidity of conduct disorder being identified as having ADHD. In fact, the externalizing scales really are more often identifying elements of conduct disorders than strictly impulsive-hyperactive states. This may be the area where the DSM-IV criteria are overidentifying ADHD.

MANAGEMENT

One of the most important elements in management is to ensure that one has diagnosed the child completely. Table 2 outlines the elements necessary for evaluation.

The mainstay of management of ADHD remains stimulant medication. In addition, treatment for any learning disabilities, family support, and help for parents on limit setting and structure at home, along with counseling where indicated, are mandatory. The child who has a subtle problem with ADHD that is having minimal impact on schoolwork and functioning in the community may be able to be managed by a combination of appropriate structure and support, but the child who has a significant problem such that schoolwork and relationships with other children and adults are impaired, should be treated fully.

Table 3 shows the stimulant medications currently available with a description of the usual dosages. Our mainstay is methylphenidate (Ritalin) because it produces the fewest side effects and the least loss of appetite. Its effect is also immediate. The majority of children respond to methylphenidate, variously estimated from different studies as between 67 and 96%. In our own practice approximately 75 to 85% of children respond to methylphenidate immediately. We start with 0.3 mg per kg per dose and may increase to as much as 0.6 mg per kg per dose, but rarely above that level. A dose covering after school homework or to prevent rebound is usually one half the morning or noon dose. For children with a weight between even doses, two strategies are available. A higher dose can be given in the morning and a lower one at noon, so they average 0.3 mg per kg. Alternately, the physician can prescribe in half pills (or in one fourth pill for dextroamphetamine saccharate [Adderall]). For example, for a child weighing 25 kg (55 pounds), the dose is methylphenidate 10 mg with breakfast, 5 mg with lunch, and one half of 5 mg if needed after school. The alternative approach is to prescribe methylphenidate, 5 mg, 1.5 tablets with breakfast and lunch and one half of 5 mg for after school. The incidence of side effects, namely adventitious movements, such as choreiform movements and tics, increases rapidly after a dose of 0.6 mg per kg. Also the presence of an overfocused or "zombie" state becomes more apparent at the 0.75 to 1 mg per kg per dose level. At one time, many people recommended 1 mg per kg dose per dose for "behavior control." The purpose of the stimulant medication is not behavior control. It is to enhance the ability to inhibit and focus and to diminish distractibility and impulsivity.

We use the long-acting methylphenidate with children once they have attained a weight of approximately 60 to 70 pounds (30 kg). A subgroup of children do not metabolize this medication well because it is in a wax matrix, and apparently some children do not dissolve the wax evenly. Thus, a child who did well on a dose of 10 mg morning and noon and 5 mg at 3:00 PM and suddenly does not respond at all to the 20-mg sustained-release tablet is probably not metabolizing it properly. In that case, we shift to dextroamphetamine, 5-mg spansule, as being roughly equivalent. We move toward dextroamphetamine with adolescents also. With children under the age of 6, we are likely to start with methylphenidate or dextroamphetamine as a medication of choice. Dextroamphetamine saccharate plus three other amphetamines is a recently reconstituted medication that was used for weight loss under another name. It is similar to dextroamphetamine, but is made up of several other amphetamine congeners. Like dextroamphetamine, it also has a longer half-life than methylphenidate and has the potential for less frequent dosing. However, it also promotes more anorexia, as does dextroamphetamine. The pills for dextroamphetamine saccharate are also scored such that they can be quartered. Recently a 5-mg dose has also been developed. The usual dose for dextroamphetamine is about half of that of methylphenidate, although the equivalence has never really been fully scientifically established.

TABLE 2. **Elements of Evaluation**

I. History
   A. Problem: Obtain a detailed history of the symptoms from the earliest age.
   B. Family—maternal and paternal
      1. Attention-deficit/hyperactivity disorder in parents or siblings.
      2. Co-morbidities of anxiety, obsessive-compulsive behavior, tics and Tourette's syndrome.
      3. Conduct disorder in family members.
      4. Learning disabilities, types, and outcomes in family members.
      5. Other externalizing problems, such as alcoholism.
      6. Often clarifying question: "Does this child remind you of any family member?"
   C. Social
      Educational level, jobs, antisocial behavior of relatives, etc. Child's ability to relate to family and peers. Involvement in community activities.
   D. Developmental
      Document the child's development with delays or acceleration noted, attainment of motor and language milestones, readiness skills.
   E. Sleep history
      Snoring, apneic episodes, nightmares, other parasomnias, enuresis, episodes of daytime sleepiness.
   F. School history
      Attendance, relationship to faculty and students, retention or promotion, discipline problem or star pupil.
   G. Medical history
      History of language delay, seizures or seizure-like activity, prematurity, traumatic head injury, growth delay, any chronic medical problems, such as frequent ear infections or asthma for which they are currently being treated.
II. Child Assessment
   A. School
      1. Assessment for learning disabilities.
         What is the child's current academic and intellectual functioning? If you don't have the current data, request it. Review the Individual Educational Plan (IEP) or 504 plan if available. Refer for evaluation if a question of learning disability is present.
      2. Behavior/Attention: Have current teacher rating scales for baseline. Examples of a useful one is the Conners' 48 Item Teacher Questionnaire or the DuPaul DSM-IV scale. Request a brief narrative from the teacher on school concerns. Questionnaires such as the Teacher Form of the Child Behavior Checklist give additional information on other behavior. Russell Barkley, Ph.D., has a DSM-IV Teachers Questionnaire available.
      B. Medical–Physical examination including looking for skin stigmata of neurofibromatosis or tuberous sclerosis, plotting growth, assessing for thyromegaly, neurologic assessment for reflex asymmetries as well as "soft" or "subtle signs" using the Pediatric Assessment for Soft or Subtle Signs (PANESS) codified by Martha Denckla, M.D.
   C. Child Interview/Assessment to assess for anxiety and depression; get the child's perception of the problem. In young children, use drawings of a person and family "doing something together." In older children and adolescents, instruct them to "write a one page story with a beginning, a middle, and an end." Children with ADHD typically write briefer stories or use run-on sentences and poor punctuation, grammar, and spelling. However, they have good, creative, age-appropriate themes. In older children, use a self-report questionnaire, such as that devised by Barkley as well as the self-report form of the Child Behavior Checklist to assess for other behavioral concerns.
   D. Parent interview and questionnaire such as the Conners' items. Assess the family structure and feelings about the child, their ability to cope with behavior, their knowledge of treatment. Use of the Child Behavior Checklist–Parent Form gives information on other emotional behavioral issues. Barkley again has a new parent DSM-IV keyed questionnaire available.

Pemoline (Cylert) is used much less frequently because of recent liver function warnings, although the data on hepatic deaths are not recent. Although pemoline acts biochemically like methylphenidate, the effect is slower and daily dosing is necessary. Regular blood tests to check for liver abnormalities are also necessary.

Nonstimulant Medication

onstimulant medications have recently been suggested as potential treatments for ADHD. The tricyclic antidepressants have been used the longest. Research suggests that desipramine* (Norpramin) can be an effective medication, particularly in adolescents. Because of at least five published case reports of sudden death in prepubescent children from taking desipramine, many people are not prescribing this medication for prepubescent children with ADHD. This is a source of considerable disagreement and debate among various experts. Other antidepressants, including amitriptyline* (Elavil), nortriptyline* (Pamelor), and imipramine* (Tofranil) have also been used. Only desipramine has shown consistent effectiveness for ADHD in well-designed studies. Dosages are listed in Table 3. Monitoring of electrocardiograms (ECGs) is essential. It is theorized that the deaths have been related to prolonged QT syndrome. Baseline ECGs to assess for congenital prolonged QT syndrome are essential, as are ECGs 5 to 7 days after dosage changes.

More recently, a group of alpha-adrenergic blocking agents usually used to treat hypertension in adults have come into use, particularly for the elements of impulsivity noted in children with ADHD. These include clonidine* (Catapres) or guanfacine* (Tenex). Clonidine 0.1 mg has been used most extensively. It is effective in post-traumatic stress disorder, but must be used cautiously, with slow advancement of the dose at one half to one fourth pill every 3 to 4 days, and slow discontinuation because with sudden omission of the doses, the child can develop rebound

*Not FDA approved for this indication.

*Not FDA approved for this indication.

TABLE 3. **Commonly Used Medications for ADHD**

Medication	Dosage Range	Side Effects/Remedy	Effectiveness
Methylphenidate (Ritalin) 5, 10, 20 mg	0.3 mg/kg–0.6 mg/kg per dose Short-acting	Loss of appetite, brief. Rebound, adjust dose. Sleep difficulty, adjust dose.	67–96%
Methylphenidate (Ritalin) 20 mg sustained release	Long-acting 0.6 mg/kg/dose–1.2 mg/kg/dose	Overfocused state, tics rarely. Lower dose. Same as above; more complaints of stomach upset.	Not as effective sometimes (return to short-acting). Advantage: no dose in school; therefore better compliance.
Dextroamphetamine (Dexedrine) 5, 10 mg	0.15 mg/kg/dose–0.3 mg/kg/dose	More loss of appetite More overfocused. Some children do better with it empirically.	Similar to methylphenidate, more side effects. Longer acting, may need only AM dose even if short-acting.
spansules 5, 10, 15 mg	Long-lasting		
(Dextrostat) 5 mg	Same	Same	Less expensive; short-acting
Pemoline (Cylert)	18.75–75 mg	Same as above. Some data suggest may trigger more tics. Liver function abnormalities	Similar to methylphenidate but not in school doses, taken daily.
Desipramine* (Norpramin)	25–100 mg	Cardiac in prepubertal, prolonged QT; get baseline ECG and at intervals in all patients.	Can be effective; may be drug of choice for some adolescents.
Clonidine* (Catapres)	0.1–0.4 mg, usual 0.1–0.3 mg	Sleepiness or sleep disturbance, hypotension, dizziness	Can be helpful adjunct, especially for impulsivity, tics
Guanfacine* (Tenex)	0.1–0.4 mg	Similar to clonidine, sleep said to be less of a problem	Similar to clonidine, longer half-life
Dextroamphetamine saccharate and sulfate; amphetamine aspartate and sulfate (Adderall)	0.15 mg/kg/dose–0.3 mg/kg/dose	Similar to Dexedrine	See Dexedrine

*Not FDA approved for this indication.

hypertension. The main side effects from this medication are sedation and hypotension with dizziness. The data on its effectiveness for all elements of ADHD are not strong, but it is commonly used as an adjunct in children who are impulsive or who have a concomitant sleep disorder. Clonidine is particularly helpful in inducing sleep in some children. It has to be used cautiously because some children develop nightmares or a sleep disorder while taking it. In children who have developed tics, sometimes clonidine is preferred by some providers. Guanfacine 1 mg is longer acting and can be taken less often during the day. It is also less sedating. It appears to have some beneficial effects on the impulsivity and aggression seen in some children with ADHD.

Finally, some of the newer antidepressants, specifically, bupropion* (Wellbutrin), have been used with children with anxiety and ADHD successfully. The dosage for this medication is usually started with 75 mg once a day and then gradually advanced up to a maximum of 300 mg per day depending on the size of the child. One must wait 4 to 6 weeks for maximum effect, so choosing an appropriate dose takes time. Buspirone* (BuSpar) has also been suggested as useful, particularly for children with anxiety. Bupropion can be an effective medication if anxiety and ADHD are co-morbid. A sustained-release form is also available. Another method for handling the child with ADHD who is anxious is to first treat with a stimulant medication and, if the anxiety persists, add an additional medication. Most commonly we have used paroxetine* (Paxil), starting with 10 mg and gradually advancing after 3 to 6 weeks to 20 mg, and occasionally 30 mg daily.

*Not FDA approved for this indication.

The data on the use of the other selective serotonin reuptake inhibitor compounds as treatment for ADHD are not strong. They do not help with increasing the ability of the child to inhibit, to be organized, to maintain motor persistence, or to focus. They are effective for obsessive-compulsive symptoms and depression, but may cause activation or aggression in some individuals. We do not use them for ADHD. For children whose primary care provider feels unsure of treatment, referral to a behavioral/development pediatrician, pediatric neurologist, or child psychiatrist experienced in the diagnosis and treatment of ADHD is appropriate.

*Not FDA approved for this indication.

GILLES DE LA TOURETTE SYNDROME

method of
JOSEPH JANKOVIC, M.D.
Baylor College of Medicine
Houston, Texas

Gilles de la Tourette syndrome (TS) is a chronic, childhood-onset neurologic disorder manifested by motor and vocal tics and often accompanied by neurobehavioral problems such as obsessive-compulsive disorder (OCD), attention-deficit/hyperactivity disorder (ADHD), and lack of impulse control. Once considered a rare psychiatric curiosity, TS is now recognized as a relatively common neurologic and behavioral disorder. Because the clinical criteria are not well defined, the prevalence rates have been estimated to vary between 0.1 and 1%.

The cause of TS is yet unknown, but the disorder appears to be inherited in nearly all patients. The clinical expression of this genetic defect may be different in various family members. The clinical heterogeneity, marked fluctuation severity, and bizarre nature of some of the symptoms are some of the reasons why the disorder is often not recognized or is misdiagnosed. Educational efforts directed to physicians, educators, and the general public have increased the awareness about TS. Many patients, however, still remain undiagnosed, or their symptoms are wrongly attributed to "habits," "allergies," "hyperactivity," "nervousness," and many other conditions.

Tics, the clinical hallmark of TS, consist of relatively brief and intermittent movements (motor tics) or sounds (phonic tics). Currently accepted criteria require both types of tics to be present for the diagnosis of TS. Motor tics are usually abrupt in onset and rapid (clonic tics), but they may be slower, causing a briefly sustained abnormal posture (dystonic tics) or an isometric contraction (tonic tics). *Simple motor tics* involve only one group of muscles, causing a brief, jerklike movement or a single, meaningless sound. Examples of simple clonic motor tics include blinking, nose twitching, and head jerking; simple dystonic tics include blepharospasm, oculogyric movements, bruxism, sustained mouth opening, torticollis, and shoulder rotation; and tensing of abdominal or limb muscles is an example of a tonic tic. *Complex motor tics* consist of coordinated, sequenced movements resembling normal motor acts or gestures that are inappropriately intense and timed. They may be seemingly nonpurposeful, such as head shaking or trunk bending, or they may seem purposeful, such as touching, throwing, hitting, jumping, and kicking. Additional examples of complex motor tics include gesturing "the finger" (copropraxia) or imitating gestures (echopraxia). *Simple phonic tics* typically consist of sniffing, throat clearing, grunting, squeaking, screaming, coughing, blowing, and sucking sounds. *Complex phonic tics* include linguistically meaningful utterances and verbalizations, such as shouting of obscenities or profanities (coprolalia); repetition of someone else's words or phrases (echolalia); and repetition of one's own utterances, particularly the last syllable, word, or phrase in a sentence (palilalia).

Most motor and phonic tics are preceded by premonitory feelings or sensations, such as "a burning feeling" in the eye before an eye blink, "a tension or a crick in the neck" relieved by stretching of the neck or jerking of the head, a "feeling of tightness or constriction" relieved by arm or leg extension, "nasal stuffiness" before a sniff, "dry or sore throat" before throat clearing or grunting, and "itching" before a rotatory movement of the scapula. The sensations or feelings that often precede motor tics usually occur out of a background of relative normality and are clearly involuntary, even though the movements (motor tics) or noises (phonic tics) that occur in response to these premonitory symptoms may be regarded as semivoluntary or involuntary. Many patients report that they have to repeat a particular movement to relieve the uncomfortable urge and until "it feels good." The "just right" feeling has been associated with compulsive behavior, and as such the involuntary movement may be regarded as a compulsive tic. Some complex motor tics may be difficult to differentiate from compulsions, but compulsions are often preceded by or associated with a feeling of anxiety or panic, as well as an irresistible urge to perform the movement or sound because of a fear that if it is not promptly or properly executed something "bad" will happen.

In addition to motor and phonic tics, patients with TS often exhibit a variety of behavioral symptoms, particularly ADHD and OCD. These co-morbid conditions often interfere with learning, academic and work performance, social adjustment, and psychosocial development. A common link between the motor and behavioral manifestations of TS is a loss of impulse control. Indeed, many of the behavioral problems, such as uncontrollable temper outbursts, seen in patients with TS can be attributed to poor impulse control. Some TS patients exhibit inappropriate sexual aggressiveness and antisocial, oppositional, violent, and self-injurious behavior. Conduct disorders and problems with discipline at home and in school are among the most frequently discussed topics during an office visit.

Although the pathogenetic mechanisms of TS are still unknown, the weight of evidence supports organic rather than psychogenic origin. Sleep studies have provided additional evidence that tics are truly involuntary, in that tics are often present in all stages of sleep. Quantitative magnetic resonance imaging studies have found subtle, but possibly important, reductions in the volume of caudate nuclei in patients with TS. In contrast, the corpus callosum has been found to be larger in children with TS than in normal control subjects. Positron emission tomography (PET) has shown variable rates of glucose utilization in the basal ganglia of TS patients compared with those of control subjects, but fluorodopa uptake and the density of dopamine receptors, as determined by PET studies, have demonstrated no significant abnormalities. An alteration in the amounts of central neurotransmitters has been suggested, chiefly because of relatively consistent responses to modulation of the dopaminergic system. Dopamine antagonists and depletors generally have ameliorating effects on tics, whereas drugs that enhance central dopaminergic activity exacerbate tics. Other biochemical abnormalities in postmortem brains include low serotonin levels, low glutamate levels in the globus pallidus internum, and low cyclic AMP levels in the cortex.

The most intriguing hypothesis, supported by increased ^{3}H-mazindol binding in postmortem brains and by increased binding of the dopamine transporter ligand 2β-carboxymethoxy-3β-4(^{123}I)iodophenyl trepane demonstrated by single photon emission computed tomography, suggests that TS represents a developmental disorder resulting in dopaminergic hyperinnervation of the ventral striatum. This portion of the basal ganglia is anatomically and functionally linked to the limbic system. The link between the basal ganglia and the limbic system may explain the frequent association of tics and complex behavioral problems. A disturbance in sex hormone levels and activity and certain excitatory neurotransmitters that normally influence the development of these structures may be ultimately expressed as TS. This hypothesis may explain the remarkable sex difference in TS, with males outnumbering females by 3 to 1, the exacerbation of symptoms at the time of puberty and during the estrogenic phase of the menstrual cycle, the characteristic occurrence of sexually related complex motor and phonic tics, and a variety of behavioral manifestations with sexual content. According to this hypothesis, the gene defect in TS results in an abnormal production of gonadal steroid hormones and increased trophic influence exerted by the excitatory amino acids, causing disordered development and increased innervation of the striatum and the limbic system. Further studies are needed to test this hypothesis.

Finding a genetic marker, and ultimately the gene, has been the highest priority in TS research during the past decade. Unfortunately, despite a concentrated effort by many investigators, the TS gene has thus far eluded this intensive search. Assuming that genetic heterogeneity is not an important factor in TS, more than 95% of the genome has already been excluded. Linkage disequilibrium has been demonstrated between the D4 receptor locus (on chromosome 11) and TS. Current concepts of the genetics of TS support a sex-influenced autosomal dominant mode of inheritance with a nearly complete penetrance for males and 56% penetrance for females when only tics are considered and 70% when OCD is included. Common bilineal transmission may lead to frequent homozygosity and the high density of TS observed in some families. Furthermore, because this type of transmission violates the standard principle of one-trait–one-locus, it may hinder linkage studies and may explain why a gene marker has not yet been identified for TS despite intense collaborative research efforts. Twin studies, showing 89% concordance for TS and 100% concordance for either TS or chronic motor tics, provide strong support for the genetic etiology of TS.

DIAGNOSIS

Without a specific biologic marker, the diagnosis depends on a careful evaluation of the patient's symptoms and signs by an experienced clinician. To aid in the diagnosis of TS, the Tourette Syndrome Classification Study Group (TSCSG) formulated the following criteria for definite TS: (1) both multiple motor and one or more phonic tics have to be present at some time during the illness, although not necessarily concurrently; (2) tics must occur many times a day, nearly every day, or intermittently throughout a period of more than 1 year; (3) the anatomic location, number, frequency, type, complexity, or severity of tics must change over time; (4) the onset must be before the age of 21 years; (5) involuntary movements and noises must not be explained by other medical conditions; and (6) motor and/or phonic tics must be witnessed by a reliable examiner directly at some point during the illness or be recorded by videotape or cinematography. Probable TS type 1 meets all the criteria except 3 and/or 4, and probable TS type 2 meets all the criteria except 1; it includes either a single motor tic with phonic tics or multiple motor tics with possible phonic tics. In contrast to the criteria outlined by the *Diagnostic and Statistical Manual of Mental Disorders,* fourth edition (DSM-IV), the TSCSG criteria do not include a statement about "impairment." There is considerable controversy about the DSM-IV criteria, which require that "marked distress or significant impairment in social, occupational or other important areas of functioning" be present.

TREATMENT

The first step in the management of TS is proper education of the patient, parents and other family members, teachers, and other individuals who interact with the patient about the nature of the disorder. School principals, teachers, and students can be helpful in implementing the therapeutic strategies. In addition, the parents and the physician should work as partners in advocating the best possible school environment for the child. This may include preferential seating; assignment sheets; shorter writing assignments; one-on-one tutoring; extra break periods and a refuge area to "allow" the release of tics; waiving time limitations on tests; and other measures designed to relieve stress. National and local support groups can provide additional information and can serve as a valuable resource for the patient and the family.*

Not all patients require pharmacologic therapy; counseling may be sufficient for those with mild symptoms. Medications, however, may be considered when symptoms begin to interfere with peer relationships, social interactions, academic or job performance, or activities of daily living. Because of the broad range of neurologic and behavioral manifestation and varied severity, therapy of TS must be individualized and tailored specifically to the needs of the patient. The most troublesome symptoms should be targeted first. Medications should be instituted at low doses and titrated gradually to the lowest, but effective, dosage and tapered during nonstressful periods (e.g., summer vacations). Another important principle of therapy in TS is to give each medication and dosage regimen an adequate trial. This approach avoids needless changes made in response to variations in symptoms during the natural course of the disease.

Tics

The goal of treatment should not be to completely eliminate all the tics, but to achieve a tolerable suppression. Of the pharmacologic agents used for tic suppression, the dopamine-receptor–blocking drugs (neuroleptics) are clearly the most effective (Table 1). Although haloperidol (Haldol) has frequently been recommended in the past and pimozide (Orap) is the only neuroleptic actually approved by the Food and Drug Administration for the treatment of TS, I prefer fluphenazine (Prolixin) as the first-line anti-tic pharmacotherapy. If fluphenazine fails to adequately control tics, I substitute pimozide. Both fluphenazine and pimozide are started at 1 mg at bedtime and increased by 1 mg every 5 to 7 days. If these drugs fail to adequately control tics, I then try haloperidol, risperidone (Risperdal), thioridazine (Mellaril), trifluoperazine (Stelazine), molindone (Moban), or thiothixene (Navane). Risperidone, a neuroleptic with both dopamine- and serotonin-blocking properties, has been shown to be effective in reducing tic frequency and intensity in some patients. It is not clear whether some of the new atypical neuroleptics, such as olanzapine (Zyprexa), will be effective in the treatment of tics and other manifestations of TS. Tetrabenazine, a monoamine-depleting and dopamine-receptor–blocking drug, is a powerful anti-tic drug, but regrettably it is not readily available in the United States.

---

*Tourette Syndrome Association, 42–40 Bell Boulevard, Bayside, NY 11361–2857.

TABLE 1. **Pharmacology of Tourette's Syndrome**

Drugs	Initial Dosage (mg/d)	Clinical Effect
Dopamine receptor blockers		Tics
Fluphenazine	1	+ + +
Pimozide	2	+ + +
Haloperidol	0.5	+ + +
Risperidol	0.5	+ +
Thiothixene	1	+ +
Trifluoperazine	1	+ +
Molindone	5	+ +
Dopamine depleters		Tics
Tetrabenazine	25	+ +
CNS stimulants		ADHD
Methylphenidate	5	+ + +
Pemoline	18.75	+ +
Dextroamphetamine	5	+ +
Amphetamine mixture	10	+ +
Noradrenergic drugs		Impulse control and/or ADHD
Clonidine	0.1	+ +
Guanfacine	1.0	+ +
Serotonergic drugs		OCD
Fluoxetine	20	+ + +
Clomipramine	25	+ + +
Sertraline	50	+ + +
Paroxetine	20	+ + +
Fluvoxamine	50	+ + +
Venlafaxine	25	+ + +

Abbreviations: CNS = central nervous system; ADHD = attention-deficit/hyperactivity disorder; OCD = obsessive-compulsive disorder.

The side effects associated with neuroleptics, such as sedation, depression, weight gain, and school phobia, seem to be somewhat less frequent with fluphenazine than with haloperidol and the other neuroleptics. The most feared side effects of chronic neuroleptic therapy include tardive dyskinesia and hepatotoxicity. In addition, pimozide may prolong the QT interval, and therefore patients treated with this drug must have an electrocardiogram (ECG) before starting therapy. I obtain another ECG about 3 months later and once a year thereafter. Tardive dyskinesia, usually manifested by stereotypic involuntary movements, is only rarely persistent in children. Tardive dystonia, a variant of tardive dyskinesia most frequently encountered in young adults, however, may persist and occasionally progresses to a generalized and disabling dystonic disorder. Other movement disorders associated with neuroleptics include bradykinesia, akathisia, and acute dystonic reactions. Therefore, careful monitoring of the patients is absolutely essential, and whenever possible the dosage should be reduced or even discontinued during periods of remission or during vacations. Tetrabenazine has a major advantage over other neuroleptics in that it does not appear to cause tardive dyskinesia.

Of the non-neuroleptic drugs, clonazepam (Klonopin)* is sometimes useful, particularly in patients with clonic tics. Motor tics can be ameliorated by local injections of botulinum toxin.* By preventing the release of acetylcholine from the nerve terminal, the toxin causes focal chemodenervation, and the resulting weakness may be partly responsible for its beneficial effects. Another mechanism by which botulinum toxin improves tics is its effect on the local premonitory sensations. Presumably by lessening the "tension" in the muscles, botulinum toxin prevents the urge to perform a tic. In addition to ameliorating motor tics, botulinum toxin injections have been useful in the treatment of phonic tics, including severe coprolalia. In addition to pharmacologic therapy, behavioral and muscle relaxation techniques, such as stress management and biofeedback, may play an important ancillary role.

*Not FDA approved for this indication.

Behavioral Symptoms

Attention-Deficit/Hyperactivity Disorder

Behavioral modification, school and classroom adjustments, and other techniques described previously may be useful in some selected patients for the management of behavioral problems associated with TS, but in my experience these approaches are rarely effective and at best play an ancillary role. Such behavioral strategies, however, may provide important emotional support for the patient and the family members and may be helpful in raising self-esteem and improving motivation.

When these measures are insufficient to maintain good academic performance and to allow a satisfactory adaptation, pharmacologic therapy may need to be employed. I use clonidine (Catapres),† a presynaptic alpha$_2$-adrenergic agonist used as an antihypertensive because it decreases plasma norepinephrine levels, in mild cases of ADHD and impulse control problems. Although initially thought to be effective in controlling tics, clonidine has been shown to be ineffective as an anti-tic agent. However, the drug is quite useful in controlling a variety of TS-related behavioral symptoms, particularly ADHD and problems with impulse control. The usual starting dose is 0.1 mg at bedtime, and the dosage is gradually increased up to 0.5 mg per day in three divided doses. The drug is also available as a transdermal patch (TTS-1, TTS-2, TTS-3, corresponding to 0.1, 0.2 and 0.3 mg) that should be changed once a week, using a different skin location. Side effects include sedation, lightheadedness, headache, dry mouth, and insomnia. Although the patch can cause local irritation, it seems to cause fewer side effects than oral clonidine. Another drug increasingly used in the treatment of ADHD and impulse control problems is guanfacine (Tenex),† available as 1- or 2-mg tablets. Pharmacologically similar to clonidine, guanfacine may be effective in patients in whom clonidine failed to control the behavioral symptoms. Guanfacine may have some advantages over clonidine in that it has a

*Not yet approved for use in the United States.
†Not FDA approved for this indication.

longer half-life, it appears to be less sedating, and it produces less hypotension. It also seems to be more selective for the alpha$_2$-noradrenergic receptor. Although both clonidine and guanfacine appear to be effective in the treatment of attention deficits with and without hyperactivity, they appear to be particularly useful in the management of oppositional, argumentative, impulsive, and aggressive behavior. Although less effective than methylphenidate (Ritalin), the drugs have an advantage over methylphenidate in that they do not increase tics. The most frequently encountered side effects of the two drugs include sedation, dry mouth, itchy eyes, postural hypotension, and headaches. The beneficial effects may not be appreciated for several weeks after the initiation of therapy, and the symptoms may markedly intensify if the medications are withdrawn abruptly. We have found deprenyl or selegiline (Eldepryl),* a monoamine oxidase B inhibitor, to be effective in controlling the symptoms of ADHD without exacerbating tics. It is not clear how deprenyl improves symptoms of ADHD, but the drug is known to metabolize into amphetamines. Other drugs frequently used in relatively mild cases of ADHD include imipramine (Tofranil),* nortriptyline (Pamelor),* and desipramine (Norpramin).* Because of potential cardiotoxicity, ECG or cardiologic evaluation may be needed before the initiation of desipramine therapy, and follow-up ECGs should be obtained every 3 to 6 months.

A central stimulant, methylphenidate, although clearly effective in the treatment of ADHD, may exacerbate or precipitate tics in 25% of patients. If, however, the symptoms of ADHD are troublesome and interfere with a patient's functioning, it is reasonable to use this, or other central nervous system stimulants such as an amphetamine mixture (Adderall), pemoline (Cylert), or dextroamphetamine (Dexedrine) and titrate the dosage to the lowest effective level (see Table 1). The initial dose for methylphenidate is 5 mg in the morning, and the dose can be gradually increased to 20 to 30 mg per day. Besides the possible development of tolerance, other possible side effects of these stimulant drugs include nervousness, insomnia, anorexia, and headaches. The dopamine-receptor–blocking drugs can be combined with the central nervous system stimulants if the latter produce unacceptable exacerbation of tics.

Obsessive-Compulsive Disorder

Although imipramine and desipramine have been reported to be useful in the treatment of OCD, the most effective drugs are the selective serotonin reuptake inhibitors (SSRIs). These include fluoxetine (Prozac), fluvoxamine (Luvox), paroxetine (Paxil),* sertraline (Zoloft),* and venlafaxine (Effexor).* No comparative study has been performed of the various agents in patients with TS and OCD, but clomipramine, fluvoxamine, and fluoxetine seem to be particularly effective. The initial dosage of clomipramine is 25 mg at bedtime, and the dosage can be gradually increased up to 250 mg per day, using 25-, 50-, or 75-mg capsules after meals or at bedtime. Fluoxetine and paroxetine should be started at 20 mg after breakfast, and the dosage can be increased up to 80 mg per day. In contrast to fluvoxamine, the other SSRIs should be started as a morning, after-breakfast dose. In addition to the SSRIs, anxiolytics, such as alprazolam and clonazepam, have been used with modest success. Likewise, monoamine oxidase inhibitors, trazodone, and buspirone have limited efficacy in the treatment of OCD. In patients with extremely severe and disabling OCD, in whom optimal pharmacologic therapy has failed, psychosurgery, either limbic leucotomy or cingulotomy, may be considered as a last resort. Although stereotactic operations creating infrathalamic lesions can improve OCD and even tics, such procedures can be complicated by severe disturbances in speech, swallowing, and gait.

*Not FDA approved for this indication.

HEADACHES

method of
ALEXANDER MAUSKOP, M.D.
New York Headache Center
New York, New York

TENSION-TYPE HEADACHES

Nonpharmacologic Treatment

Biofeedback is one of the most effective treatments for both tension and migraine headaches. Meditation, yoga, and other mental exercises can help, but biofeedback is a more direct and most time-efficient approach. Well-trained staff and patient compliance are essential for achieving a high success rate. Follow-up studies indicate up to 80 to 90% improvement 5 years after completion of a biofeedback training course. This course usually consists of 6 to 10 weekly 30-minute sessions. Children can learn to rid themselves of headaches in as few as three to four sessions.

Acupuncture can provide fast relief for tension headaches. Acupuncture has a solid scientific basis but lacks large clinical studies proving its efficacy. Acupuncture can stop an acute headache or relieve a chronic one with a series of treatments.

Regular aerobic exercise is an excellent way to reduce adverse effects of stress on the body, and it usually prevents headaches. Aerobic exercise can even relieve an acute attack.

Pharmacologic Treatment

Abortive Therapy

Occasional attacks of severe tension-type headaches may respond to analgesics. Nonsteroidal anti-inflammatory drugs (NSAIDs) such as ibuprofen (Motrin, Advil) or naproxen (Naprosyn, Anaprox) have proven effective. Hydrocodone (Vicoprofen, Vicodin) or even stronger opioids may be required in a patient with occasional severe attacks. Long-term use of opioid analgesics in the treatment of headaches should be avoided. Drug combinations are effective for infrequent use. Combination of acetaminophen or aspirin with caffeine and a short-acting barbiturate such as butalbital is very popular with many patients (Fiorinal, Fioricet, Esgic, Medigesic). Isometheptene, a sympathomimetic amine with vasoconstrictive properties, is available in combination with dichloralphenazone, a mild sedative and acetaminophen (Midrin, Isocom). This combination can be effective in many patients. Drowsiness is a potential side effect. A limit of 15 to 20 tablets a month is placed on combination drugs or strong analgesics. If a patient takes more than that amount, the medication may begin to worsen the headache through a rebound mechanism. Such patients require prophylactic treatment.

Prophylactic Therapy

Pharmacologic treatment of severe persistent headaches begins with nortriptyline* (Pamelor) or another tricyclic antidepressant (TCA). Among the TCAs, amitriptyline* (Elavil) has been studied most extensively, but nortriptyline, imipramine* (Tofranil), and desipramine* (Norpramin) are effective as well and may have fewer anticholinergic side effects. If one TCA is ineffective or produces unacceptable side effects, another one should be tried. The starting dose for any TCA is 25 mg in a young or middle-aged individual and 10 mg in an elderly person. The average effective dose, however, is 50 to 75 mg taken once a day in the evening. I explain to patients that antidepressants are used for chronic painful conditions even if there is no associated depression. Warning patients about possible side effects such as dryness of the mouth, drowsiness, and constipation tends to improve their compliance. Some of the contraindications for the use of TCAs include concomitant use of monoamine oxidase inhibitors, recent myocardial infarction, cardiac arrhythmias, glaucoma, and urinary retention. An electrocardiogram should be obtained before the initiation of treatment in all elderly patients and those with risk factors for heart disease.

Antidepressants that are selective serotonin reuptake inhibitors (SSRIs), such as fluoxetine (Prozac), sertraline (Zoloft), and paroxetine (Paxil), can be effective with fewer side effects. These drugs lack the analgesic effect of TCAs but may help indirectly by reducing anxiety and depression. Young women, who constitute the majority of headache sufferers who seek help, often prefer the latter group because these drugs, unlike TCAs, do not have a potential for weight gain and can even help them reduce weight. Recent reports indicate that the SSRIs cause a very high incidence of sexual dysfunction, most commonly, loss of libido; I have been using more of bupropion (Wellbutrin) and nefazodone (Serzone), which do not cause sexual dysfunction. Despite the fact that stress and tension are major causes of tension headaches, use of tranquilizers should be avoided. Long-term use of these drugs can lead to addiction and worsening of headaches.

*Not FDA approved for this indication.

MIGRAINE HEADACHES

Nonpharmacologic Treatment

Occasionally, dietary changes can stop migraine headaches completely, but in many patients they only reduce the frequency of attacks. Some of the foods that can provoke migraine headaches include yogurt, bananas, dried fruit, beans, aged cheese, pickled and marinated foods, and buttermilk. Monosodium glutamate and aspartame should be avoided. Among the alcoholic beverages, red wine and beer are more likely to induce a migraine headache than vodka. Biofeedback, acupuncture, relaxation techniques, and regular aerobic exercise are as effective for prevention of migraine headaches as they are for preventing tension headaches.

Pharmacologic Treatment

Abortive therapy alone is used when the attacks are not very frequent. NSAIDs, mentioned earlier, can be effective for migraine headaches as well. Rapid onset of action can be achieved by using an effervescent form of aspirin (Alka-Seltzer). Combination medications listed in the section on tension headaches can be very effective. Ergots alone (Ergostat, sublingual) and with caffeine (Cafergot suppositories, Wigraine tablets) are quite effective. These drugs can sometimes worsen or cause nausea. Reducing the dose, particularly of Cafergot suppositories, to one quarter or one half of a suppository can prevent nausea and provide effective and rapid relief. Ergots are contraindicated in patients with cardiac or peripheral ischemia and in pregnant women. Dihydroergotamine (D.H.E. 45, Migranol) is effective for abortive treatment of migraines. This ergot derivative can be given subcutaneously, intramuscularly, intravenously, and intranasally (Migranol). In an injection, a dose of 1 mg is sufficient for most patients, but some may require 2 or 3 mg. The starting dose should be 0.5 mg repeated in 45 minutes, if necessary. Once a total effective dose is established for a patient, that amount is given for future attacks. If the headache is accompanied by nausea, the author gives an injection of an antiemetic such as prochlorperazine (Compazine) or metoclopramide (Reglan), 10 mg intramuscularly. These medications can be given with D.H.E. 45 if the latter consistently produces nausea.

Sumatriptan (Imitrex) is a "designer" drug specifically developed to bind to 5-HT 1B/1D serotonin receptors, which are operational in the pathogenesis of migraine headaches. Sumatriptan relieves both the pain and the nausea and allows the patient to return to normal functioning within 10 to 20 minutes. Sumatriptan is available in a 6-mg injection, which is easy to self-administer by the patient, in 25- and 50-mg tablets, and as a 5- and 20-mg nasal spray. The usual starting oral dose is 50 mg; some patients require 25 or 100 mg, with a maximum daily dose of 200 mg. The nasal spray dose for an adult is 20 mg. Side effects are more common with injection and include a flushed sensation, paresthesias, and injection site pain. Sumatriptan is contraindicated in patients with uncontrolled hypertension, ischemic heart disease, and complicated migraines (migraines that are accompanied by a transient neurologic deficit). Sumatriptan and ergots should not be given on the same day. Naratriptan (Amerge), zolmitriptan (Zomig), and rizatriptan (Maxalt) are new oral 5-HT 1B/1D drugs that should become available in 1998. They are similar to sumatriptan, but some may work when sumatriptan fails and may have faster onset of action, longer duration, or fewer side effects.

Intranasal administration of butorphanol (Stadol NS) offers a rapid onset of action. The limitation of this drug is that it has a high incidence of central nervous system side effects, including severe sedation, confusion, and hallucinations. Butorphanol is a partial agonist-antagonist drug with a lower potential for addiction; however, addiction does occur. It should not be given to patients who are maintained on opioids that are pure agonists of the morphine type, because the antagonist properties of butorphanol can induce a withdrawal reaction.

Prophylactic Therapy

Tricyclic and other antidepressants can be as effective for migraine headaches. Propranolol (Inderal LA), timolol (Blocadren), and other beta blockers are good prophylactic drugs. The effective dose for propranolol can be as low as 40 mg daily but is usually 80 to 240 mg. Contraindications for the use of beta blockers include bronchial asthma, sinus bradycardia, greater than first-degree heart block, congestive heart failure, and diabetes. In some patients who do not respond to either a TCA or a beta blocker alone, the use of these two drugs together may stop the headaches. No clinical trials have been published, however, to prove the efficacy of this combination. Divalproex sodium (Depakote) can effectively relieve migraine headaches. Most migraine patients respond to 250 mg twice a day, but some need 500 mg twice a day. Potential side effects include nausea, asthenia, and somnolence. Weight gain is not a very frequent side effect, but the potential for this side effect is often of great concern to young women, who constitute the majority of migraine sufferers. Menstruating women must use an effective mode of contraception because of the teratogenicity of this drug. Calcium channel blockers are sometimes effective for migraines but are more likely to benefit patients with cluster headaches. Long-acting NSAIDs can be given prophylactically with good results. Long-term use of opioid analgesics in noncancer patients is becoming somewhat more accepted, although it remains controversial. In my experience, opioid maintenance is less effective in chronic headache patients than it is in patients with other pain syndromes. However, a small number of headache patients can also benefit from long-term opioid therapy. I obtain a verbal informed consent from such patients, warning them about the risk of addiction, see them every month, have a single physician prescribe all opioid drugs, and frequently have the patient followed by a psychologist.

CERVICOGENIC HEADACHES

Elderly Patients

Cervicogenic headaches are very common in elderly patients owing to arthritic changes in the cervical spine. Pain described as radiating from the neck or pain that is occipital in location suggests this diagnosis. Pain of cervical spine origin, however, can sometimes be felt only in the front of the head. Loss of sensation over the occipital area, often on one side, can accompany occipital neuralgia. Neck muscles are tender, frequently in spasm, and their movement can aggravate the pain. In many patients, immobilization using a soft cervical collar during the night combined with a NSAID and regular neck exercises will provide relief. Local heat application, transcutaneous electrical nerve stimulation (TENS), and acupuncture may also help. If the headache is occipital and has a burning or lancinating quality, greater occipital neuralgia is the likely cause. Blockade of that nerve by a local anesthetic is relatively easy to perform and may provide lasting relief. A successful block of this nerve does not have any diagnostic significance, as many types of headaches, including cluster and migraine, may improve as well. TCAs also have a good potential to relieve the pain of occipital neuralgia. The starting dose should be only 10 mg every night because of the higher incidence of side effects in elderly patients.

Whiplash Injuries

Another frequent cause of cervicogenic headaches is a whiplash injury commonly sustained in car accidents. Treatment should include a soft cervical collar, which the patient wears only at night. Wearing the collar during the day for any length of time may cause atrophy of the neck muscles, which may in turn delay the recovery. If pain is severe, the collar can be worn around the clock for the first few days. An active exercise program is started as soon as the patient tolerates it. Providing good analgesia allows an early start for such exercises. Opioid analgesics such as hydrocodone (Vicodin, Vicoprofen) or oxycodone (Roxicodone, Percocet, Percodan), local heat, trigger point injections, acupuncture, and TENS are effective as a part of the treatment of acute neck pain and the associated headache. When muscle spasm is prominent, a short course (1 to 2 weeks) of diazepam

(Valium), 5 to 10 mg every 8 hours, is very effective. Diazepam can be combined with an opioid analgesic when a single drug does not relieve the pain. I reassure patients that a short course (1 to 2 weeks) of these medications carries almost no risk of addiction.

POST-TRAUMATIC HEADACHES

In many patients post-traumatic headaches subside in a few weeks or months without any treatment. However, chronic post-traumatic headaches in many patients are notoriously hard to treat regardless of whether litigation is pending. Biofeedback, TCAs, SSRIs, beta blockers, and acupuncture are effective in some patients. A supportive and understanding attitude is important in treating this condition because of the frequent ineffectiveness of treatment and because of the associated neurologic and psychiatric symptoms (memory impairment, dizziness, anxiety, and depression).

CLUSTER HEADACHES

Cluster headaches are accompanied by most intense pain, leading some patients to thoughts of suicide. Headaches occur in clusters, frequently during the same season each year, with each episode lasting for several weeks or months. The pain often wakes the patient from sleep, sometimes at the same time every night and usually lasts for 30 to 90 minutes. Such regular occurrence, however, is not always present. The pain is described as retro-orbital and unilateral and is associated with agitation, nasal congestion, conjunctival injection, and lacrimation.

Abortive Treatment

Treatment of cluster headaches begins with measures designed to reduce the pain of each attack while prophylactic drugs take effect. The most benign and frequently effective treatment is inhalation of oxygen. It is done through a mask (not nasal prongs), using 100% oxygen at a high flow of 8 to 10 liters per minute. It should be used for patients who get most of their attacks at home. If headaches occur during the day and if practical, patients can store another oxygen tank at work. Ergotamine can abort a cluster headache in up to 75% of patients. It is best given by a suppository or sublingually to provide rapid onset of action. Dihydroergotamine is given by injection or nasal spray (Migranal) and can be self-administered by the patient. Self-administered sumatriptan injection is very effective in most patients and has few side effects.

Prophylactic Treatment

A short course of prednisone will frequently stop the cluster headaches. Dosage is started at 60 to 80 mg daily and then is tapered down over a period of 2 weeks. Calcium channel blockers are suggested for patients not responding to a course of prednisone. Nifedipine* (Procardia), 40 to 120 mg daily, or verapamil* (Calan, Isoptin), 120 to 360 mg daily, can prevent cluster headaches in some patients. Methysergide (Sansert) in a dosage of 2 mg three or four times a day is recommended for patients who are not helped by prednisone and calcium channel blockers. Fibrotic complications are less likely to occur because clusters rarely last for more than a few months. However, some reports suggest that this complication is more likely to be idiosyncratic than dose-related. Divalproex sodium (Depakote), 500 to 2000 mg daily in two divided doses, can provide relief for some patients. Lithium carbonate,* 300 mg two to four times a day, is effective within 1 to 2 weeks of beginning therapy. It can work for both episodic and chronic forms of cluster headaches, sometimes transforming chronic into episodic. Adding 2 to 4 mg of ergotamine a day to lithium may produce remission in patients who do not respond to lithium alone. Ergotamine in a dose of 2 mg can provide good relief if taken 2 hours before the expected attack. Regular intake of 1 to 2 mg of ergotamine three times a day has been reported to be effective in some patients. TCAs may also help both the pain and the accompanying reactive depression.

HEADACHES ASSOCIATED WITH SUBSTANCES OR THEIR WITHDRAWAL

Many prescription medications can cause headaches. The most common offenders are nitrates, appetite suppressants, oral contraceptives, estrogens, and antihypertensive medications. Foods can also cause headaches, specifically, those containing nitrites, monosodium glutamate, tyramine, and aspartame. Other factors that can lead to headaches include excessive intake of caffeine, analgesics, and ergot preparations. The treatment of a patient who is dependent on analgesics, caffeine, or ergot preparations can be very difficult. In such patients the headaches, to a great extent, are due to an ongoing withdrawal or rebound from these substances. An abrupt and complete discontinuation temporarily worsens the pain, and some patients prefer to get off these drugs gradually. Withdrawal headaches can be treated with self-administration of sumatriptan, dihydroergotamine, or ketorolac (Toradol). Admission to a hospital is occasionally necessary because of uncontrollable pain. While in the hospital, dihydroergotamine taken intravenously, opioid analgesics, and prochlorperazine or chlorpromazine (Thorazine) will provide relief or, at least, will sedate the patient for the period of withdrawal. Prophylactic drugs are started after the withdrawal is completed. The medications that were ineffective while the patient was overusing abortive drugs can become effective once the offending drugs are stopped.

---

*Not FDA approved for this indication.

BENIGN INTRACRANIAL HYPERTENSION (PSEUDOTUMOR CEREBRI)

Weight loss in overweight patients is highly effective in reducing intracranial pressure but is difficult for many patients to achieve. Acetazolamide* (Diamox) is an effective drug in many patients. It is available in a sustained-release preparation. The dose ranges between 250 and 1500 mg daily. For patients with severe persistent headaches, lumbar punctures can be performed while other treatments are being tried. These can also be performed during pregnancy. In pregnant women this condition often subsides after the delivery. Beta blockers and TCAs can sometimes provide relief of headaches. Prednisone is useful in reducing intracranial pressure from a brain tumor, but its efficacy in pseudotumor cerebri remains controversial. Regular visual field testing is paramount in the management of benign intracranial hypertension. Patients with progressive visual loss should undergo optic nerve sheath fenestration. This operation is the treatment of choice for patients with visual impairment, but it is not consistently effective for the relief of headaches. A lumbar-peritoneal shunt is more appropriate for patients with intractable headaches, but it should be used as a last resort because of possible complications.

POST–LUMBAR PUNCTURE HEADACHE

The use of a thin or conical spinal needle reduces the incidence of post–lumbar puncture headaches. Contrary to popular belief, bed rest following a lumbar puncture does not prevent these headaches. When a patient does develop headaches, bed rest, good hydration, and analgesics usually provide relief. Most patients improve within a few days on this regimen. Those who do not improve should receive a "blood patch." This procedure involves withdrawing 15 to 20 ml of the patient's venous blood and injecting it into the epidural space at the same level that the lumbar puncture was performed. This supposedly stops the leakage of cerebrospinal fluid that is causing the headache.

*Not FDA approved for this indication.

EPISODIC VERTIGO

method of
TERRY D. FIFE, M.D.
University of Arizona and Barrow Neurological Institute
Phoenix, Arizona

Vertigo is the illusion of motion, particularly rotational motion or spinning. This symptom indicates localization to the labyrinth or central vestibular pathways. One of the first challenges of evaluating patients with dizziness, therefore, is determining whether they have vertigo or another nonvestibular form of dizziness. Table 1 outlines a general classification of dizziness because episodic vertigo is only one type of episodic dizziness.

Episodic vertigo can be classified as being of peripheral, central, or unknown origin. Vertigo is of peripheral origin when the dysfunction is related primarily to the labyrinth or vestibulocochlear nerve. Central vertigo is caused by dysfunction of vestibular structures within the central nervous system (CNS) such as the vestibular nuclei or cerebellum. Vertigo of unknown origin applies to conditions with vestibular symptoms but unclear localization. Success in treating or managing dizziness is highly dependent on determining the mechanism and cause of the disorder.

VERTIGO OF PERIPHERAL ORIGIN

Peripheral vestibular disorders cause most cases of episodic vertigo. These conditions can affect the inner ear itself or the vestibulocochlear nerve. Some conditions such as vestibular neuritis and labyrinthitis can affect both the labyrinth and the nerve simultaneously.

Benign Paroxysmal Positional Vertigo (BPPV). BPPV is the most common cause of episodic vertigo seen in general practice. BPPV results in attacks of spinning usually brought on by such activities as lying back or getting out of bed, turning in bed, looking up, or straightening up after bending over. The episodes of vertigo last 10 to 30 seconds and are not accompanied by any additional symptoms except nausea in some patients. The degree of nausea, pallor, diaphoresis, or even diarrhea depends on the patient's inherent tolerance to vertigo as well as on the severity of the BPPV. Patients who are prone to motion sickness may feel queasy and lightheaded for hours after the attack of vertigo, but most patients feel well between episodes of vertigo. If the patient reports spontaneous episodes of vertigo lasting more than 1 or 2 minutes or if episodes never occur in bed, then one should question the diagnosis of BPPV.

The diagnosis of BPPV is confirmed by eliciting paroxysmal positional nystagmus during the Dix-Hallpike maneuver. The Dix-Hallpike maneuver is performed by moving the head rapidly from an upright to a head-hanging position with one ear 45 degrees to the side. In Figure 1, movement from position A to position B constitutes the Dix-Hallpike maneuver testing of the right ear. In those with typical BPPV affecting the posterior semicircular canal, the Dix-Hallpike maneuver results in torsional upbeating nystagmus corresponding in duration to the patient's subjective vertigo and occurring only after Dix-Hallpike positioning on the affected side. A presumptive diagnosis can be made by history alone, but paroxysmal positional nystagmus confirms the diagnosis.

BPPV is a mechanical disorder of the inner ear caused by calcium carbonate crystals inappropriately

TABLE 1. **Classification of Dizziness**

Type	Common Description	Example
Vertigo	Spinning, tilting, whirling, toppling, free falling	Vestibular neuritis, benign positional vertigo, Meniere's disease, brain stem ischemia
Presyncope	Lightheadedness, near-faintness, fading out	Orthostatic hypotension, vasovagal near-syncope
Dysequilibrium without vertigo	Imbalance only when standing or walking; unsteadiness	Sensory ataxia from diabetic neuropathy, cerebellar ataxia
Cryptogenic dizziness	Chronic rocking, floating, fatigue, wafting, nausea, others	Postconcussive dizziness, migraine-associated
Psychiatric dizziness	Chronic rocking, floating, fatigue, wafting, nausea, others	Panic disorder, generalized anxiety, depression, phobias
Physiologic dizziness	Motion sickness, nausea, queasiness, disorientation	Seasickness, carsickness, airsickness, hyperventilation, visual vertigo*

*Visual vertigo is dizziness evoked by seeing objects in motion such as ceiling fans, moving traffic, motion picture scenes, and optokinetic stimulation from grocery store aisles or the motion of people in crowds.

located in one of the semicircular canals of the inner ear. The most commonly affected semicircular canal is the posterior canal; it accounts for approximately 90% of cases of BPPV. The calcium debris originates from the utricular statoconia that may break off following trauma, viral infection, or simply degeneration. While supine, loose calcium debris from the utricle may become trapped in the semicircular canal, where it produces endolymph fluid movement during certain head movements. This stimulates the cupula, causing vertigo.

THERAPY. Treatment of BPPV is illustrated in Figures 1 and 2. Figure 1 depicts the canalith repositioning maneuver, or Epley maneuver, and Figure 2 depicts the liberatory maneuver sometimes referred to as the Semont maneuver. Both maneuvers and variations of them are designed to clear calcium debris from the posterior semicircular canal by moving it back into the utricle. This is achieved by the effect of gravity because calcium sinks in the endolymphatic fluid. Once it is back in the utricle, it is generally absorbed or eliminated within a period of days in most patients through mechanisms yet to be determined. If properly done, the canalith repositioning maneuver eliminates BPPV immediately in more than 90% of patients. Similar success has been reported with the Semont maneuver. Patients who do not respond to canalith repositioning have calcium particles that are immobile or that are attached to the cupula. BPPV that is disabling and refractory to all positioning treatments can be managed surgically, though this is rarely necessary.

Meclizine (Antivert) and other vestibular suppressants can be effective for patients with severe motion sickness but are generally not useful for BPPV because the episodes are so brief and because the therapeutic maneuvers are so immediate and effective. BPPV is a mechanically produced disorder best managed with a mechanical solution. Occasionally the anterior or horizontal canals are affected and positioning maneuvers are somewhat less effective for BPPV involving these canals. Fortunately, most cases involving the horizontal or anterior canal clear spontaneously within weeks to a few months.

Features distinguishing typical BPPV of the posterior semicircular canal from central positional vertigo include (1) the direction of the nystagmus, (2) the tendency of vertigo and nystagmus to fatigue (lessen with each successive Dix-Hallpike maneuver), and (3) the response to canalith repositioning treatment. A latency of several seconds between positioning and the onset of nystagmus as well as the partial suppression of the nystagmus by visual fixation are associated with BPPV but are not as useful. Typical BPPV results in transient torsional nystagmus with the top pole of the eye beating with fast phases toward the ground and undermost ear. This torsional nystagmus is admixed with an upbeating component. Nystagmus straying from this pattern should raise suspicions for central positional nystagmus.

Acute Unilateral Loss. Sudden unilateral loss of peripheral vestibular function produces acute vertigo that lasts from days to weeks. The most common cause is viral neurolabyrinthitis. *Vestibular neuritis* refers to acute vestibular loss due to a virus in which hearing is spared. *Labyrinthitis* indicates unilateral loss of both hearing and vestibular function due to viral infection. Other causes of acute vestibular loss include vestibular nerve sectioning and labyrinthectomy, ischemia, trauma, inflammation, or other infections. Herpes zoster oticus sometimes leads to vertigo due to unilateral vestibular loss in addition to painful herpes zoster vesicles deep in the external ear canal or occasionally behind the ear. When accompanied by ipsilateral Bell's palsy, the syndrome is referred to as Ramsay Hunt syndrome.

The onset of vestibular neuritis and labyrinthitis is characterized by rapidly increasing vertigo, nystagmus, and nausea over a period of 30 minutes to several hours. Vertigo is present in all head positions but is aggravated by head motion and gradually abates in the ensuing days to weeks. The nystagmus has fast phases directed away from the injured ear, which is more intense during gaze in the direction of the fast phase and absent or less intense but in the same direction with gaze opposite the direction of the fast phase. This is referred to as Alexander's law

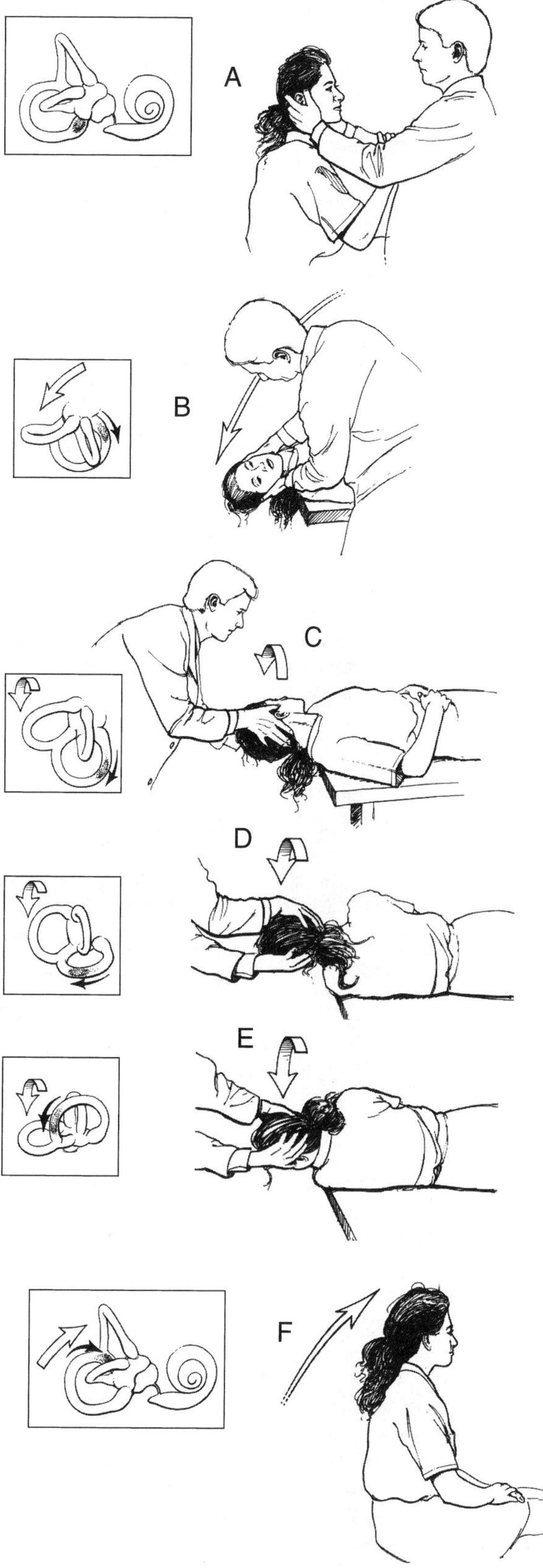

Figure 1. Canalith repositioning maneuver for right-sided benign paroxysmal positional vertigo. *A,* With the patient sitting up and the head turned 45 degrees to the right, the patient is positioned rapidly to the head-hanging position, *B.* This constitutes the Dix-Hallpike maneuver, and vertigo and nystagmus develop usually within seconds. After all nystagmus has subsided, the head is turned 90 degrees toward the unaffected left ear, as in *C.* Additional turns of 60 degrees are done stepwise in *D* and *E.* Canalith debris is thereby moved toward the common crus and eventually into the utricle as depicted in semicircular canal figures. Finally, the patient is moved up from *E* to the sitting position *(F).* The maneuver is then repeated until positioning from *A* to *B* results in no further nystagmus. (With permission from Barrow Neurological Institute.)

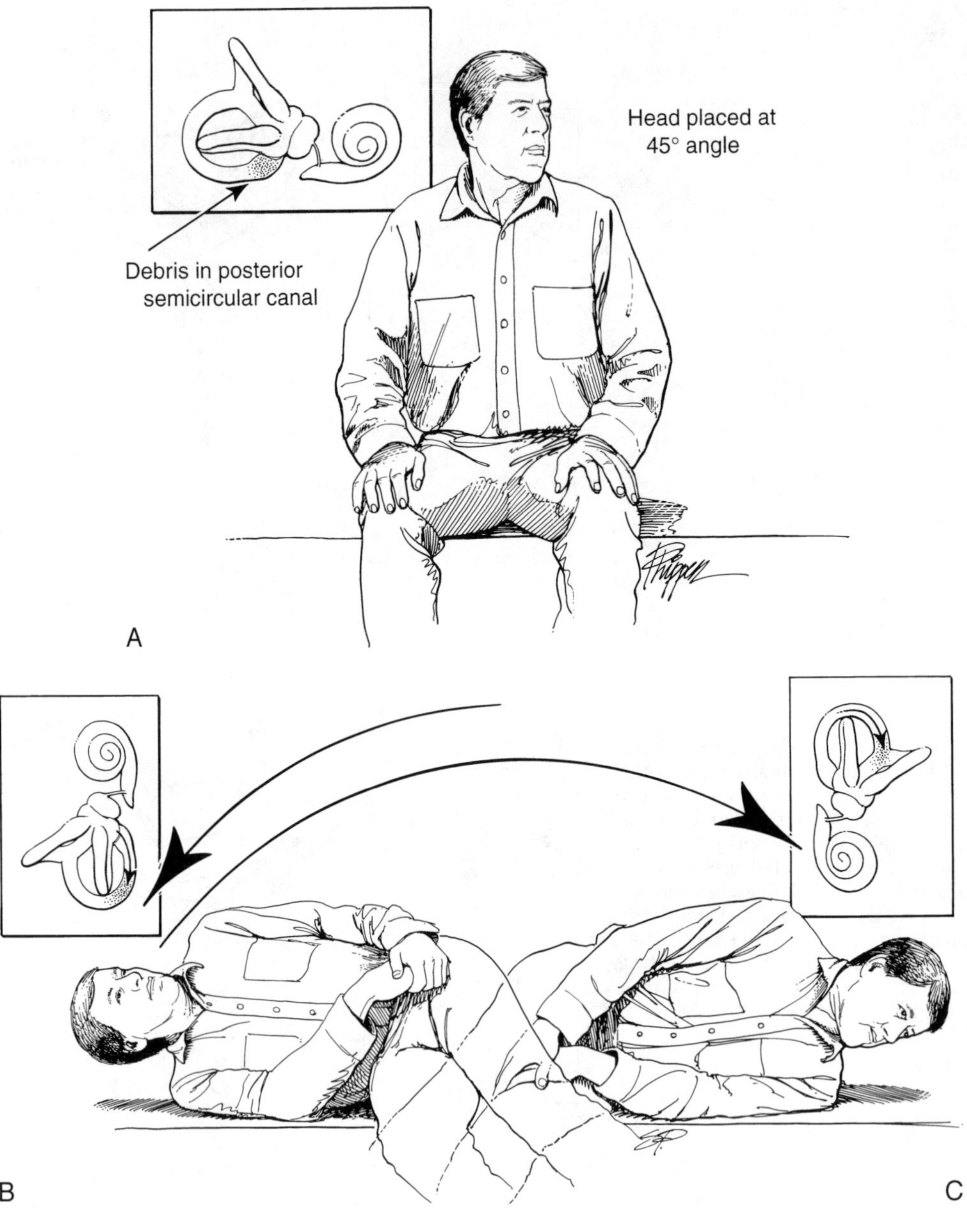

Figure 2. Liberatory maneuver of Semont for right-sided benign paroxysmal vertigo. *A,* The head is turned 45 degrees away from the affected ear (yaw plane). *B,* The patient is then taken to the side without turning the head. This will produce vertigo and nystagmus. After 1 minute in position *B,* the patient moves to position *C* rapidly without turning the head. Subsequently the patient may sit up. Canalith debris is moved from the posterior canal to the utricle as illustrated. (With permission from Barrow Neurological Institute.)

and is characteristic of acute peripheral vestibular nystagmus.

THERAPY. In the acute situation, vestibular suppressants are often helpful in easing the vertigo and nausea (Table 2). Once nausea has subsided, the vestibular suppressants should be used more sparingly or eliminated because these medications may delay or limit CNS adaptation to the acute vestibular loss. Initially, patients should begin moving their heads from side to side, extending the activity each day until they are capable of undergoing a full battery of vestibular exercises such as those outlined in Table 3. Eventually, the patient can adapt to unilateral vestibular loss and make a complete or nearly complete recovery. Vestibular rehabilitation is effective in accelerating adaptation by repeated exposure to head motion. Studies in primates and humans indicate that vestibular exercises can accelerate the recovery from a unilateral vestibular loss and improve overall balance function.

Bilateral Peripheral Vestibular Loss. Symmetrical bilateral loss of vestibular function does not usually manifest with prominent complaints of vertigo. Patients more commonly report dysequilibrium that is more prominent during head motion. In severe peripheral vestibular loss the vestibulo-ocular reflex can result in blurring or bouncing of vision (oscillopsia) during head motion. Bilateral vestibular loss is not easily detected at bedside, so quantitative vestibular testing by electronystagmography or rotary chair testing is often necessary to confirm the diagnosis. The most well-recognized cause of bilateral peripheral loss is aminoglycoside (especially gentamicin) ototoxicity. Some patients with end-stage renal disease on hemodialysis or peritoneal dialysis develop vestibulotoxicity because gentamicin levels are

TABLE 2. **Vestibular Suppressant and Anti–Motion Sickness Medications**

Generic Drug	Brand Name	Form and Dosage	Sedative	Antiemetic	Precautions
Meclizine	Antivert, Bonine	12.5–50 mg PO qid	+ +	+	Prostate hypertrophy, glaucoma
Dimenhydrinate	Dramamine	50 mg PO qid	+	+	Prostate hypertrophy, glaucoma
Promethazine	Phenergan	25–50 mg PO or IM q 4–6 h; 50-mg suppos PR qid	+ + +	+ +	Patients with seizures
Diazepam	Valium	2.0–7.5 mg PO qid	+ +	+	Dose-related sedation
Lorazepam	Ativan	0.5–2 mg PO tid	+ +	+	Dose-related sedation
Clonazepam	Klonopin	0.25–0.5 mg PO tid	+ + +	+	Dose-related sedation
Scopolamine	Transderm Scop	Patch 1 q 3 d	+	+	Prostate hypertrophy, glaucoma
Metoclopramide	Reglan	10–20 mg PO q 4–6 h; 10–20 mg IV q 6 h	+	+ + +	Extrapyramidal effects
Prochlorperazine	Compazine	10 mg PO q 6 h; 10 mg q 6 h IM; 25-mg suppos PR q 6 h	+	+ + +	Extrapyramidal effects

not monitored as closely given that renal function is not in jeopardy. Other causes include luetic otitis, Lyme disease, bilateral vestibular neuritis, bilateral Meniere's disease, and idiopathic vestibular loss.

THERAPY. Minor spontaneous recovery may be possible in some cases, but in general, the vestibular function that is lost is gone forever. Treatment of bilateral vestibular loss therefore consists of teaching patients to balance using visual and somatosensory signals, which are still intact. That is, balance exercises such as those in Table 3 are employed to promote a retraining of balance so that joint position sensation and vision become the dominant and most relied-on methods of balance maintenance. The goal in such cases is to improve balance and reduce the risk of falling, although probably the oscillopsia and the feeling of dysequilibrium with rapid movements may not be eliminated. Vestibular suppressants (e.g., meclizine, diazepam) should be avoided in patients with bilateral vestibular loss because they suppress vestibular function further and may cause sedation.

Meniere's Disease. This condition produces episodic vertigo lasting 1 to 8 hours with nausea, vomiting, and often with concurrent unilateral roaring tinnitus, worse hearing, and ear fullness. Eventually, unilateral low-frequency hearing loss and vestibular loss develop in the affected ear. This is discussed further in the article on Meniere's disease.

TABLE 3. **Habituation Exercises for Recovering from Vestibular Loss**

1. *Thumb tracking test, side-to-side.* Turn head quickly from right to left, then left to right, then up and down while focusing on your thumb held out directly in front of you. As your head turns, your focus should be fixed on your thumb, and you should move your thumb along with your head so it is always directly in front of your eyes. Repeat this for 90 seconds at a time for a total of four times per day. This helps improve your ability to focus on things while your head is moving side to side.
2. *Head shaking.* Practice slowly turning the head from side to side while standing with your feet shoulder-width apart. Gradually increase the speed of head movements. The head turning can include side-to-side and up-and-down movements rapidly and repetitively with eyes open and in good lighting. This helps you become more used to rapid movements of the head, which are often a source of momentary imbalance.
3. *Lie to stand test.* Practice getting up from the lying down position to standing as quickly (but carefully) as possible. This may be done on a sofa or bed. Practice getting up toward the left and toward the right side. Be careful not to fall. Get up quickly five times to each side; gradually try to increase the quickness but avoid falling. This trains the brain to coordinate quick movements of the head and body.
4. *Tightrope exercise.* Walk heel to toe as though walking a tightrope. This can be done in a hallway or corridor where there is something to hold on to if needed. Gradually try to achieve 10 steps (heel touching toe) without holding on or sidestepping. This trains the cerebellum in standing balance.
5. *Standing balance test.* Stand with feet together (touching); try to maintain the position for 15 seconds. Once you accomplish that, try closing your eyes with someone nearby to keep you from falling. Try to be able to stand with feet together and eyes closed for 8 seconds. This trains you to keep your balance using ankle sensation and inner ear signals. If you are able to do this for 8 seconds, then practice standing on one leg (eyes open) or while standing on a foam pillow. Eventually try to stand for 10 seconds on foam with eyes closed and to stand on one leg for 12 seconds.
6. *Pick-up exercise.* Place 5 pennies on a saucer on the floor. Rapidly bend over, pick up one penny each time, and place it on a nearby counter or table and retrieve the next penny. Do this twice. Time yourself and try to gradually increase your speed while avoiding falling, and be careful if bending over bothers your back. This improves your balance with quick bending.
7. *Walk and turn test.* Walk 10 steps down in a corridor or hallway and then turn right; walk back to the starting point. Do this five times turning to the right, then five times turning toward the left. Time how long it takes you and try to improve your speed, being careful to avoid falling. This helps walking balance and balance with turns.
8. *Walking.* Each day try to walk at least 20 minutes. This can be around your neighborhood or wherever is convenient for you. This helps general conditioning and cardiovascular status but also improves balance.
9. *Ball toss exercise.* Toss a tennis ball at least 3 feet above your head and catch it. This can be done while you sit or stand. Practice for 5 to 10 minutes each day, eventually practice while walking. This improves eye-hand coordination, visual tracking, and reflexes.

Otolithic Vertigo. Spinning is a vestibular symptom often attributable to a disturbance of the semicircular canals. Tilting, flipping, pulling to one side, free falling, and translational sensations represent symptoms that suggest otolithic dysfunction. The otoliths are structures in the utricle and saccule that detect changes in the gravity vector and translational acceleration. Otolithic vertigo may occur after motor vehicle accidents and trauma, but there is no adequate clinical testing method of otolith function. Generally, one must rely on caloric or rotational vestibular testing to determine whether there is a peripheral vestibular disorder, although these techniques test horizontal semicircular canal function and may not reveal abnormalities limited to the otolith organs. When the central otolithic pathways are affected, skew diplopia may accompany the dizziness. Recovery may be incomplete with lesions of the central otolith pathways, but peripheral otolithic disorders often improve with rehabilitation and habituation exercises that include head rolling (counter-rolling) (see Table 3).

Perilymph Fistula. A perilymph fistula represents an abnormal opening, often between the oval or round windows, that allows the transfer of pressure from the middle ear to the receptors of the inner ear vestibular system. As a result, patients report momentary vertigo or illusions of movement with sneezing, lifting, or straining. A fistula test consists of applying pressure to the external ear canal by insufflation to see whether it can be transmitted across the middle ear to produce vertigo and nystagmus. A positive result on a fistula test is helpful, but some fistulas are not detected by this test. Many perilymph fistulas occur in the aftermath of otologic surgery; however, some occur as a result of trauma or extreme straining. The patient should be instructed to avoid straining and heavy lifting. Perilymph fistulas often heal with time, but those that do not heal generally require surgery. A careful history should be sought and as much corroborative evidence as possible should be obtained before recommending surgical exploration.

Acoustic Neuroma. Acoustic neuromas are benign schwannomas, usually arising from the vestibular portion of the vestibulocochlear nerve. They gradually produce loss of vestibular and hearing function and usually manifest with a progressive unilateral hearing loss, perhaps with a history of intermittent dysequilibrium or dizziness. Although a brain stem–evoked potential may be helpful in detecting an acoustic neuroma, a magnetic resonance imaging (MRI) scan of the brain with contrast more reliably confirms or rules out an acoustic neuroma. Acoustic neuromas can be treated with surgical excision, and often residual hearing can be preserved with smaller acoustic neuromas. Gamma knife radiotherapy has been employed with success in patients who were deemed poor surgical candidates because it does not require general anesthesia or craniotomy.

Other Causes. Basilar meningitis, including inflammatory, infectious, and neoplastic processes affecting structures in the posterior fossa near the prepontine cistern, can irritate or damage the vestibulocochlear nerves that pass through the subarachnoid space and can lead to vertigo worsened by any head motion. Treatment is directed at the underlying cause. Neurovascular compression is a controversial diagnosis said to account for "disabling positional vertigo" caused by pulsating vessels abutting the vestibulocochlear nerve on one or both sides. This condition has vague diagnostic criteria and should be viewed with cautious skepticism before subjecting a patient to a craniotomy and microvascular decompressive surgery. Such patients should have a thorough neuro-otologic evaluation, one that checks for refractory benign positional vertigo, uncompensated vestibular neuritis, and vestibular migraine, all of which could produce persistent vertigo worsened by position changes. If neurovascular compression is still strongly suspected, patients should undergo a trial of carbamazepine* (Tegretol), 200 mg three times a day (tid), or gabapentin* (Neurontin), 300 to 400 mg tid, on a trial basis. Surgery is the last resort for treatment.

VERTIGO OF CENTRAL ORIGIN

Vascular Causes

Transient Ischemic Attacks (TIAs). Transient ischemia of the brain stem or cerebellum may produce episodic vertigo or dysequilibrium usually lasting 1 to 15 minutes. Vertigo may be an isolated symptom of vertebrobasilar insufficiency, but a history of additional symptoms of brain stem ischemia such as diplopia, dysarthria, ataxia, or clumsiness of the extremities should be sought to bolster the diagnosis. Vertebrobasilar ischemic attacks manifesting as isolated episodes of vertigo are usually related to vascular occlusion in the distal segments of the vertebral arteries between the posterior and anterior inferior cerebellar arteries (PICA and AICA). Both central and peripheral vestibular structures are supplied by this segment of vasculature, including vestibular nuclei, the cerebellum, flocculus, nodulus, and the labyrinth itself, which is supplied by a branch off of the AICA. Therapy for TIAs thought to cause episodic vertigo may include aspirin, 81 to 650 mg daily, ticlopidine, 250 mg twice a day (bid), or systemic anticoagulation with heparin or warfarin (see "Ischemic Cerebrovascular Disease"). Clopidogrel (Plavix), 75 mg once daily, is a newer platelet aggregation inhibitor that may be used in those who are intolerant of aspirin. In confirmed cases with continuing episodes while on therapeutic doses of warfarin, daily aspirin may be added along with warfarin provided there are no contraindications.

Cerebral Infarction: PICA Syndrome. The posteroinferior cerebellar artery supplies the lateral medulla and the posterior and inferior cerebellum. Occlusion of this vessel leads to vertigo, nystagmus, and ataxia. An infarct of the lateral medulla is called a Wallenberg stroke. MRI is the imaging procedure of

*Not FDA approved for this indication.

choice in detecting this infarct because it is typically missed on even high-resolution head computed tomography (CT) scans. An evaluation for the cause should include a search for sources of embolism or vertebral artery dissection, depending on the patient's age and risk factors for vascular disease. The most common cause of this type of stroke is intrinsic atherosclerotic disease in the vertebral arteries.

THERAPY. If the infarct is less than 3 hours old, thrombolytic therapy with intravenous tissue plasminogen activator (alteplase [Activase]), 90 to 100 mg, can be considered (see "Ischemic Cerebrovascular Disease"). Acute management of vertigo following a brain stem or cerebellar stroke includes minimization of movement and use of vestibular suppressants such as promethazine (Phenergan) and diazepam (Valium) for the first 12 to 24 hours. As soon as the nausea subsides, these medications should be withdrawn and head movements resumed and increased as rapidly as the patient can tolerate it without becoming too nauseated. Early exposure to vestibular stimuli may promote more rapid and complete CNS adaptation. Balance training exercises under the guidance of physical and occupational therapists are usually indicated.

AICA Syndrome. The AICA supplies some crucial vestibular structures, including the flocculus and other anterior portions of the cerebellum that are important for ocular motor control; portions of the lateral pons and pontomedullary junction; and the inner ear itself. An occlusion of the AICA may produce an isolated cerebellar stroke or a lateral pontine stroke, or both. When the lateral pons is affected, ipsilateral hearing loss and peripheral facial paresis can be seen. Treatment for this is similar to that for PICA syndrome.

Nonvascular Causes

Nonvascular causes of episodic vertigo can include space-occupying lesions, such as tumor or abscess, which produce a gradual unsteadiness and imbalance rather than discrete episodes of dizziness. Demyelinating or inflammatory disorders can also produce vertigo, by affecting either the peripheral cranial nerve fascicles or the vestibular or cerebellar nuclei. Acute vertigo due to multiple sclerosis may improve with high-dose methylprednisolone (Solu-Medrol), 1 gram intravenously daily for 3 to 5 days (see "Multiple Sclerosis"). Familial periodic ataxia is a rare dominantly inherited condition associated with *episodes* of vertigo and ataxia that may respond to oral acetazolamide* (Diamox), 250 to 500 mg bid. Rarely, epileptic vertigo manifests as isolated episodes of vertigo, although most vertigo associated with epilepsy occurs in patients with known epilepsy that affects the vestibular cortex. Treatment for epileptic vertigo calls for the same treatment indicated for the seizures in general.

*Not FDA approved for this indication.

VERTIGO OF UNKNOWN ORIGIN (CRYPTOGENIC DIZZINESS)

Vestibular Migraine. Vestibular migraine can manifest with episodes of spinning vertigo lasting minutes to hours at a time. The majority of patients do not have a migraine headache at the same time as the vertigo. Some patients with migraine also experience chronic dizziness, often described as a rocking or an oscillating sensation associated with motion sickness. A family history of migraine headaches, visual phenomena, motion sickness, or unexplained vertigo is common. The mechanism underlying vertigo in migraine is not known. Although some cases may be due to vasospasm of the posterior circulation, recent evidence suggests that migraine-associated dizziness has a more complex mechanism related to neurotransmitter or ion channel disturbances.

THERAPY. For episodes occurring infrequently, antivertiginous medications (see Table 2) can be used during the episodes to improve comfort. Treatment should also include attempts to control dietary triggers, stress, and lifestyle factors when appropriate. When the episodes are frequent or interfering with daily functions, a migraine prophylactic such as verapamil* (Calan), 180 to 360 mg daily, imipramine* (Tofranil), 50 to 100 mg daily, atenolol* (Tenormin), 100 mg daily, venlafaxine* (Effexor), 37.5 to 75 mg bid, or acetazolamide*, 250 mg bid or tid, can be used.

Post-traumatic Dizziness. Post-traumatic dizziness, like postconcussive syndrome in general, is a difficult and perplexing problem. One of the challenges is disentangling vague, nonobjective symptoms such as dizziness, pain, and headache from secondary gain associated with litigation. However, there is a common story reported by many patients, including those who have no evident secondary gain. Constant rocking or floating dizziness and motion-related dysequilibrium are common. Benign positional vertigo should always be excluded because it is fairly common in the aftermath of trauma. Migraine headaches and dizziness can sometimes follow head injury and should be considered as well. Finally, partial vestibular loss or otolithic vertigo can occur after trauma, so vestibular habituation exercises may be helpful (see Table 3).

PSYCHIATRIC DIZZINESS

Dizziness associated with a psychiatric diagnosis is fairly common and is usually not the focus of therapy rendered by the treating psychiatrist, whose attention is commonly directed at the behavioral and affective components of these disorders. Patients with panic syndrome frequently experience a floating, rocking dizziness that occurs separately from panic attacks. Medications that could be effective for this include imipramine*, 50 to 150 mg per day; nortriptyline* (Pamelor), 50 to 150 mg daily, or paroxetine* (Paxil), 20 to 40 mg daily. I generally avoid amitriptyline (Elavil) except in those with insomnia

*Not FDA approved for this indication.

because it is quite sedating and can be difficult for patients to tolerate at higher doses. Other useful medications include venlafaxine*, 75 to 225 mg daily; sertraline* (Zoloft), 50 mg daily; and intermittent use of alprazolam* (Xanax), 0.25 mg tid. Except for alprazolam, most of the medications used for panic disorder and associated dizziness take several weeks to have any effect. Symptoms gradually lessen in frequency and intensity over time, but it requires some patience and perseverance for both patient and physician during the first few weeks of treatment.

Other psychiatric conditions associated with dizziness include generalized anxiety, somatoform illnesses, and factitious disorder. Some phobias such as agoraphobia, with or without panic attacks, and acrophobia are associated with dizziness. Patients with these phobias may respond to behavioral therapy or tricyclic amines such as imipramine, 50 to 200 mg daily.

PHYSIOLOGIC VERTIGO

Physiologic vertigo is dizziness that can be experienced by anybody, even though in some patients it becomes a pathologic symptom.

Motion Sickness. Motion sickness is usually described as a floating lightheadedness or drunken sensation associated with nausea, pallor, diaphoresis, and hypersalivation. Motion sickness develops with exposure to passive motion, such as in a car (carsickness), in an airplane (airsickness), or on water (seasickness). The actual mechanism on a molecular basis for this condition is not known, although it is attributed to maladaptation to visual and vestibular signals not in congruence with one another and to predicted responses based on prior motion experiences. For example, while sitting in a van with no windows the surroundings are mostly stationary, but the vestibular signals detect motion. Certain exposures are more likely to evoke motion sickness than others: riding in the back seat of a car or bus, traveling on a winding road while reading, and riding in a boat on choppy water with large wave swells are strong stimuli. Driving the car rarely produces motion sickness, in part because of improved visualization in the front of the car and because of the predictability and control associated with driving. Motion sickness may occur in nearly anyone with normal vestibular function given sufficient exposure, but some people are more susceptible, possibly owing to inherited factors.

THERAPY. Prevention and avoidance is the first line of defense. When travel or motion activity is necessary, preemptive use of vestibular suppressants before motion exposure is more effective than using the same medications after motion sickness has begun. Table 2 lists the medications that are most effective as vestibular suppressants. When these medications are too sedating, pemoline* (Cylert), 19 to 37 mg, can be taken once in the morning to counteract their sedating effects. Hence, in patients with severe motion sickness, a regimen of diazepam*, 4 mg; meclizine, 25 mg; and, if needed to avert sedation, Cylert may be taken 1 hour before exposure to motion. At the first hint of increasing motion sickness, promethazine, 25 to 50 mg, can be added. Patients should be warned in advance that this combination of medications may temporarily impair alertness or on-the-job performance.

*Not FDA approved for this indication.

Visual Vertigo. Visual vertigo, like motion sickness, is not completely understood and is attributed to reduced tolerance of mismatch between moving visual stimuli and stationary somatosensory and vestibular signals and brain stem expectations related to prior motion experience. Dizziness and nausea develop from seeing objects in motion, even though the person is not moving. Many, but not all, patients with visual vertigo also have a tendency to experience motion sickness. This symptom complex can be seen in some patients with acute vertigo, vestibular migraine, some forms of psychiatric dizziness, or as a lifelong isolated trait. Sometimes it can be severely disturbing, such that a patient cannot see others in motion and cannot be exposed to environments with visual commotion. Situations often reported as disturbing include grocery store aisles; crowded places such as malls or theaters; and watching moving ceiling fans, traffic, merry-go-rounds, or motion pictures. This syndrome should be distinguished from agoraphobia, although some patients with panic attacks may have both. If symptoms begin to intrude on daily activities, treatment with clonazepam* (Klonopin), 0.25 to 1 mg daily, or imipramine*, 75 mg daily, may be effective.

Hyperventilation. It is normal to develop lightheadedness during hyperventilation: it is a physiologic form of lightheadedness caused in part by hypocapnia and cerebral vasoconstriction. Some patients are pathologic hyperventilators and are not fully aware of it. Generally, however, if they are made aware of it they can manage their symptoms quite adequately. Hyperventilation has been reported to cause vertigo in a large percentage of patients with dizziness in some earlier studies. Many patients previously diagnosed as having hyperventilation have also had panic attacks or general anxiety, and their dizziness was probably due more to the anxiety disorder than to overbreathing. Treatment should include management of the underlying anxiety disorder in addition to the overbreathing.

*Not FDA approved for this indication.

MENIERE'S DISEASE

method of
CHARLES M. LUETJE, M.D.
Otologic Center, Inc.
Kansas City, Missouri

The cause of Meniere's disease remains unknown. The endolymphatic space of the inner ear becomes hydropic, with pressure imparted on the organ of Corti, Reissner's membrane, and throughout the vestibular system. Contributing factors to this abnormality include things as simple as dietary habits with excessive salt and caffeine, use of nicotine and inhalants, and food allergies. There is growing indication that in almost a third of the cases the endolymphatic hydrops may be immune mediated. Thus, many of the cases of Meniere's disease have short-term, or perhaps even long-term, responses to steroids.

The mainstay of treatment for Meniere's disease is dietary management with salt restriction and elimination of nicotine and caffeine. With dietary modifications supplemented by medicine and at times by appropriate surgery, the symptoms of Meniere's disease can usually be controlled.

The salient features of Meniere's disease are fluctuating hearing loss with distortion of sound and speech discrimination; roaring or seashell type tinnitus in the affected ear; whirling and incapacitating vertigo, nausea, and vomiting; and fullness and pressure in the ear. These attacks are episodic and usually last from 1 to a few hours. Spontaneous recovery of the vertigo occurs within hours to a day, although the hearing may still be depressed.

When all of the symptoms are present, including the whirling vertigo, the attack of Meniere's disease is called *definitive*. If no whirling vertigo is evident and only symptoms of unsteadiness with some tinnitus and perhaps fluctuation of hearing are present, the attacks are *adjunctive*.

Initially, it is not uncommon for the early symptoms to be that of fluctuation of hearing, with fullness and pressure and tinnitus without the vertigo. Patients may have a warning that the attack of vertigo is going to occur because of the hearing symptoms. On rare occasions, the symptoms of vertigo can be present with minimal symptoms related to hearing. Occasionally tinnitus or fullness in the ear without hearing loss is the only symptom that occurs with the acute definitive spell of vertigo.

In Meniere's disease, it is more common to have hearing symptoms without vertigo than to have vertigo without the hearing symptoms. Usually they all occur together, but in the early stages, hearing symptoms usually precede the vertigo spells.

MANAGEMENT

The management of patients with Meniere's disease consists of dietary control, medical management, and selective surgical procedures. Salt restriction is important. The goal should be limitation of sodium to approximately 1200 grams per day. Elimination of nicotine and caffeine is mandatory.

Management of the Acute Attack

An acute attack of Meniere's disease is an urgent matter. Patients exhibit violent vertigo, nausea, vomiting, and marked nystagmus. Otoscopic examination will rule out acute otitis media or an obvious infection. A brief neurologic examination is indicated.

Every attempt should be made to have the patient lie as quietly as possible with the eyes closed. Intravenous diazepam (Valium) can be given slowly and titrated until the acute symptoms of vertigo diminish. If patients are not in a position to receive intravenous diazepam, such as in an emergency department, a rectal suppository of prochlorperazine (Compazine), 25 mg, can be used. Many patients keep these on hand. These can be used at 6-hour intervals.

Management Following an Acute Attack

The diagnosis of Meniere's disease is made by history. It is not made by other methods of testing; however, audiometric data indicating a low tone sensorineural hearing loss, electrocochleography, and vestibular testing can be helpful. When the diagnosis of Meniere's disease is suspected, the patient should be referred to an otolaryngologist or otologist for definitive diagnosis.

Having established the diagnosis of Meniere's disease, and in some instances ruling out other disease with gadolinium-enhanced magnetic resonance imaging, a low-sodium diet should be instituted. Allergy evaluation with food allergy testing may also be indicated. Patients generally respond well to a vasodilator such as papaverine hydrochloride (Pavabid), 150 mg three times daily; a parasympathetic blocker such as propantheline bromide (Pro-Banthīne), 15 mg daily; and symptomatic treatment with an antivertiginous medication such as meclizine (Antivert) or dimenhydrinate (Dramamine). Some otologists prescribe diuretics.

Long-Term Management

Most individuals respond favorably to medical treatment and dietary control. However, medical management is unsuccessful in some individuals. Surgical decompression of the endolymphatic sac through the mastoid should be considered in all patients with Meniere's disease. The timing of this surgical decompression should be relatively early in the course of Meniere's disease before the distention of the endolymphatic system is so great that it is stretched beyond repair. This surgical procedure can be accomplished on an outpatient basis, with the chances of further hearing loss from surgery being less than 5%.

There is some evidence to indicate that perfusion of the round window membrane with steroids injected into the middle ear may be of some benefit. This treatment method is relatively new and requires long-term follow-up.

A more definitive operative procedure is to cut the vestibular nerve leading from the affected ear to the brain stem. This can be accomplished through a middle cranial fossa approach or a retrolabyrinthine approach, and the hearing can be preserved. If hearing is not a high priority, a destructive labyrinthectomy or labyrinthectomy and vestibular nerve section can be accomplished. The cochlear nerve can be saved, or if tinnitus is loud, the cochlear nerve can also be sectioned. Chemical labyrinthectomy may be performed in some individuals by placing an ototoxic antibiotic into the middle ear and allowing it to diffuse through the round window membrane. This usually is reserved for patients who may need a surgical labyrinthectomy but who want to avoid surgery. The early results of chemical labyrinthectomy treatment are favorable. However, the extent and precision with which the vestibular system is ablated and hearing preserved are unpredictable.

In some individuals in whom an immunologic abnormality is suspected, a favorable response to prednisone may lead to periodic use of steroids.

SUMMARY

Patients with Meniere's disease should be referred to otolaryngologists and otologists or neurotologists for definitive care. Meniere's disease should be treated aggressively to minimize the symptoms of vertigo and try to preserve hearing. Some patients may develop Meniere's disease in their other ear. This becomes one of the most challenging treatment problems for those who specialize in treating Meniere's disease.

Advances in immunology of the inner ear have provided considerable understanding of the treatment of bilateral cases of Meniere's disease. It is in these situations that steroids and other immunologically active drugs such as cyclophosphamide (Cytoxin)* and methotrexate* are useful.

The cornerstone of treatment of Meniere's disease over the years has been dietary and medical management. However, with new and improved surgical techniques that are nondestructive in nature, early combined medical and surgical treatment renders the best chance for elimination of the disabling symptoms of vertigo and stabilization of hearing.

*Not FDA approved for this indication.

VIRAL MENINGITIS AND ENCEPHALITIS

(Meningoencephalitis)

method of
RICHARD B. TENSER, M.D.
Pennsylvania State University College of Medicine
Hershey, Pennsylvania

Viral meningitis and encephalitis (meningoencephalitis) are included in the category of nonpurulent, or aseptic, meningitis. Viral infection may manifest primarily as meningitis or as encephalitis. The term "nonpurulent aseptic meningitis" indicates nonbacterial meningitis, and aseptic meningitis implies viral infection. Neoplastic and fungal meningitis are other categories of meningitis. Because of the importance of appropriate antibacterial therapy, it is most important initially to rule out bacterial meningitis and to consider fungal meningitis. Partially treated bacterial meningitis may manifest with cerebrospinal fluid (CSF) abnormalities similar to those of viral meningitis. Typical CSF findings in viral meningoencephalitis include a moderate increase in white blood cells (WBCs) (usually mononuclear cells), a moderate increase in protein, and normal glucose (Table 1). Similar CSF findings may also be noted with cerebral abscess and other illnesses. Increased CSF polymorphonuclear cells and red blood cells (RBCs) and decreased glucose may be seen with herpes simplex virus (HSV) encephalitis (see Table 1). Viral meningoencephalitis caused by multiple agents is discussed later. Viruses that cause acquired immune deficiency syndrome (AIDS) encephalopathy (human immunodeficiency virus [HIV]) and that occur as complications of AIDS (e.g., progressive multifocal leukoencephalitis) are considered only for comparative purposes (see Table 1). These viral infections are causes of viral encephalitis but are usually chronic infections with little inflammation, unlike the acute-subacute presentation of infections to be discussed later. However, HIV may also cause an acute viral meningitis typically at the time of initial infection. This is usually mild to moderate in severity and clears with supportive conservative therapy.

CLINICAL PRESENTATION

Typical presenting symptoms of viral meningitis include headache, malaise, fever, photophobia, and anorexia (Table 2). Headache may be worse when supine and may cause nausea and vomiting. Encephalitic symptoms may manifest with impaired memory and judgment, altered personality, and abnormal taste or smell sensation. The last occurs because of prominent temporal lobe involvement in HSV encephalitis. Epilepsy and focal neurologic signs may also occur with encephalitis. Increased intracranial pressure may result in papilledema.

SEASONAL OCCURRENCE

Meningoencephalitis is most common in the July to October period or may be seasonally sporadic. The latter is the case for HSV encephalitis. Mosquito- and tick-transmitted diseases are typically summer and early fall illnesses. These may occur in epidemics or may be endemic in an area. Mosquito-borne illnesses may be particularly prominent when summers have been rainy and in places where water facilitates mosquito breeding.

RNA VIRUSES

Among RNA virus infections are summer and early fall infection by arthropod-borne viruses (arboviruses) including togaviruses and *Bunyavirus*. The former include eastern, western, and Venezuelan equine encephalomyelitis viruses (EEE, WEE, VEE); St. Louis encephalitis (SLE) virus; and California encephalitis (CE) virus. Arbovirus is not a taxonomic classification but rather indicates the vector of transmission. The previously named viruses are transmitted by mosquitoes, whereas other arboviruses are transmitted by ticks. SLE, usually in epidemics, and CE are probably the most important arbovirus infections in the United States.

SLE virus is a well-documented cause of meningoencephalitis (e.g., in Houston) with particular central nervous system (CNS) involvement of the thalamus, basal ganglia, and brain stem. Mortality after CNS involvement is approximately 20 to 25%. CE has been most frequent in the upper Midwest. Usually, infections are not life-threatening. Infection by EEE, WEE, and VEE viruses varies from frequently severe disease caused by EEE virus, usually over the eastern seaboard, to mild disease generally caused by VEE virus. All of these viral infections may manifest as meningitis or encephalitis, with encephalitis being more common with severe disease (e.g., EEE). Subclinical infec-

TABLE 1. **Typical Cerebrospinal Fluid Abnormalities in Meningitis-Encephalitis**

	Cells/mm³		Protein (mg/dL)	Glucose (mg/dL)
	Lymphs	Polys		
Bacterial meningitis	+ to ++	++ to ++++	+ to +++	+ to ++
HSV	+ to ++	+ to ++	+ to ++	N to +
Enterovirus	+ to ++	N to +	N to ++	N
Arbovirus*	+ to +++	N to +	N to +++	N to +
HIV meningitis	+ to ++	N	+ to ++	N
HIV encephalitis (AIDS)	N to +	N	N to +	N
Progressive multifocal leukoencephalopathy	N to +	N	N to +	N
Tuberculous meningitis	+ to +++	N to ++	++ to ++++	+ to +++

*Infection by arboviruses may be very mild or very severe.
Abbreviations: Lymphs = lymphocytes; polys = polymorphonuclear leukocytes; N = normal; HSV = herpes simplex virus; HIV = human immunodeficiency virus; AIDS = acquired immune deficiency syndrome; *Cells:* + = 5–50; ++ = 100; +++ = 1000; ++++ = 5000; *Protein:* + = 50–75; ++ = 100; +++ = 500; ++++ = 1000; *Glucose:* + = <60; ++ = <40; +++ = <20.

tion may occur with any of the arboviruses, and positive serology may be the only evidence of prior infection. Supportive therapy but not specific therapy is available for patients with arbovirus meningitis-encephalitis.

The enteroviruses including poliovirus, coxsackievirus, and the echoviruses are small RNA viruses and are part of the picornavirus group. These are the most frequent causes of summer-fall viral meningitis. The proportion of infected individuals developing encephalitis is low. Meningitis due to these agents is most common in the July to October period and in many ways is the prototype of human viral meningitis. The disease course is generally self-limited and relatively benign. However, newborns and individuals with agammaglobulinemia may develop lethal enterovirus infections. Spread of enterovirus infection is by contact with infected individuals who may be symptomatic or asymptomatic. Poor sanitary conditions, particularly contaminated water, and the occurrence of oral-fecal spread are particular epidemiologic factors.

TABLE 2. **Evaluation of the Patient with Suspected Viral Meningitis-Encephalitis**

Typical symptoms
- Headache, photophobia, malaise, confusion, inappropriate behavior, personality change, anorexia, impaired memory, nausea, vomiting, lethargy, seizure

Typical signs
- Fever, neck stiffness, skull tenderness, impaired memory, confusion, photophobia, obtundation, focal neurologic findings with more severe illness

Important history
- Recent viral immunization in family (e.g., polio)
- Season of occurrence, epidemic or endemic viruses reported in area
- Medications that may produce CSF abnormalities typical of aseptic meningitis: NSAIDs, IGIV, OKT3
- Other illnesses that may produce CSF abnormalities typical of aseptic meningitis: neoplastic meningitis, intracranial hypotension, partially treated bacterial meningitis, brain abscess, subdural or epidural infection, vasculitis

Laboratory evaluation
- Routine chemistries, CBC
- Brain CT scan with enhancement—rule out intracranial mass; look for meningeal enhancement
- EEG—helpful when it is unclear whether the patient has a psychiatric illness or an infectious-metabolic illness
- CSF—if no evidence of intracranial mass; record opening pressure; polymerase chain reaction for HSV DNA; attempt isolation of enterovirus
- Brain MRI—if CT scan results are normal; may be abnormal in HSV encephalitis; look for meningeal enhancement

Abbreviations: CSF = cerebrospinal fluid; NSAID = nonsteroidal anti-inflammatory drug; IGIV = intravenous immune globulin; OKT3 = monoclonal antibody to CD3 T cell antigen; CBC = complete blood count; CT = computed tomography; EEG = electroencephalogram; HSV = herpes simplex virus; MRI = magnetic resonance imaging.

Meningitis, with or without mild myelitis, may be caused by poliovirus (three types are known), although disease is presently uncommon because of immunization. Some cases may occur in vaccine recipients or their family members after immunization with live attenuated polio vaccine. The term "poliomyelitis" indicates gray matter (i.e., polio) and spinal cord inflammation (i.e., myelitis). Infection of the nervous system by a nonpolio enterovirus (e.g., echovirus) generally only causes meningitis, but myelitis may occur. Generally, one or several of these enteroviruses are the causal agents of viral meningitis in a specific locale during a particular period of time. Coxsackie type A viruses (23 types) are less common causes of viral meningitis than coxsackie type B viruses (6 types); of the latter, coxsackievirus types B2 to B5 are most commonly associated with meningitis. The most common causes of enteroviral meningitis, however, are the echoviruses (29 types), particularly types 4, 6, 9, and 11. Most instances of pharyngeal and intestinal enterovirus infection do not proceed to meningitis, and asymptomatic infection is common. Many individuals are seropositive for enterovirus without having had meningitis. In addition, few cases of meningitis proceed to encephalitis. Supportive therapy is available for patients with enterovirus meningitis, and gammaglobulin is of some value in neonates or agammaglobulinemic individuals.

Meningoencephalitis may occur with low frequency after infection by other RNA viruses, including rubella, mumps, and measles. Influenza A virus may cause meningitis or myositis, the latter with significantly elevated serum creatine kinase. Unlike infection with the viruses discussed previously, infection with these viruses is most common in the winter and spring. Of these infections, rubella meningoencephalitis is the least common. It is reported to occur in 1 in 5000 cases of rubella, with approximately a 20% mortality rate. Measles meningoencephalitis occurs with a frequency of approximately 1 per 1000 cases of clinical measles, and in patients with CNS disease the mortality rate is approximately 10%. An additional 50% of patients have severe residual morbidity. Approximately 50% of all children with clinical measles have been reported to have abnormal electroencephalograms, which may be taken to indicate frequent mild encephalitis. In patients with mumps infection, asymptomatic CSF pleocytosis may be present (50% or more of patients). Clinical meningitis may occur in up to 10% of patients and encephalitis in approximately 1 per 1000 patients. However, mortality is low. Vaccines have greatly decreased the occurrence of this group of illnesses. Most important is the decrease in measles.

POSTINFECTIOUS ENCEPHALOPATHY

Brain–spinal cord immune-mediated inflammation rather than direct infection may occur in the postinfectious period, particularly after measles virus infection. Infectious virus is not present, and disease is caused by the inflammatory response. It may be difficult to differentiate between infectious and postinfectious disease, because the latter may closely follow an infectious period. Meningitic symptoms are less common than spinal cord (myelitis) or brain symptoms. Immunosuppressive treatment may be of value, although care needs to be exerted because of the possibility of infectious virus being present. Other postinfectious syndromes of the CNS include optic neuritis and cerebellitis. CSF abnormalities may be similar to those of viral meningoencephalitis, although usually less inflammatory.

DNA VIRUSES

Chickenpox due to infection by varicella-zoster virus (VZV) results in meningoencephalitis, with a frequency of approximately 5 per 10,000 cases, and the mortality rate in these patients is approximately 20%. VZV also causes shingles (herpes zoster) after reactivation of virus that had been maintained in a latent state in dorsal root and trigeminal ganglia. VZV myelitis and meningoencephalitis may occur as a result of infection in immunosuppressed or otherwise normal patients. Immunosuppressed children without a history of primary chickenpox who are exposed to VZV may be treated with zoster immune globulin, and recently immunization of such children with a live virus vaccine has been shown to be useful. The usefulness of antivirals for patients infected with VZV will be noted later (see treatment of HSV infection). Postinfectious inflammation of the nervous system may occur after chickenpox infection, the most well-described syndrome being cerebellar inflammation in children. This cerebellitis is usually readily reversible without specific treatment. Herpes zoster of the face in adults (trigeminal distribution zoster) may cause carotid artery arteritis and subsequent stroke.

Epstein-Barr virus (EBV) is the usual cause of infectious mononucleosis and may occasionally cause encephalitis or myelitis. The latter may be an autoimmune postinfectious syndrome. EBV encephalitis is usually not severe and usually improves without specific treatment.

Of the viral meningoencephalitides, infection by the herpesviruses, particularly HSV types 1 and 2 (HSV-1, -2), has been of greatest interest in recent years, in part because of the development of new antivirals. HSV-2 meningoencephalitis is generally seen in newborn infants and is the result of infection during the birth process. For this reason, it is suggested that infants of women who are shedding HSV at the time of planned parturition be delivered by cesarean section. Vaginal delivery is appropriate if active shedding of HSV-2 is not occurring. HSV-2 meningoencephalitis may occur in adults, and this virus may also cause radiculopathy of the lower extremities with viral meningitis. The latter syndrome is most likely to occur with genital reactivation episodes. HSV-1 is likely to be the etiologic agent of HSV meningoencephalitis in adults and in children past the newborn period.

DIAGNOSIS OF HERPES SIMPLEX VIRUS ENCEPHALITIS

In the past, brain biopsy was the only reliable means to readily establish the diagnosis. For that reason, many patients with suspected HSV encephalitis, based on the occurrence of various combinations of confusion, headache, photophobia, nuchal rigidity, periodic electroencephalogram, abnormal magnetic resonance imaging (MRI) scan, and abnormal CSF results (see Table 2), were treated with acyclovir (Zovirax) without brain biopsy. Specific diagnosis is now facilitated by polymerase chain reaction testing of CSF for HSV DNA.

TREATMENT

Treatment of viral meningoencephalitis can be divided into three parts: (1) supportive therapy, (2) therapy for cerebral effects of disease, and (3) specific treatment of viral infection.

Supportive Therapy. Therapy includes that used in the treatment of patients with other neurologic illnesses. An adequate airway is necessary, and this may require tracheostomy. Depending on the patient's level of consciousness, suctioning may be necessary to prevent airway obstruction. Adequate hydration, particularly in febrile patients, is necessary, although the potential for development of the syndrome of inappropriate antidiuretic hormone (SIADH) needs to be considered. Fluid restriction is usually sufficient to treat SIADH, but administration of hypertonic saline may be necessary. Serum osmolality measurements are useful in following patients in whom fluid abnormalities may have developed. Elevated temperatures should be treated with appropriate antipyretics, and if necessary an external cooling apparatus should be used to decrease, but not necessarily eliminate, fever.

Depending on severity of disease, vital signs including pupillary responsiveness should be measured, initially at 1- to 2-hour intervals and subsequently at longer intervals. Determination of the patient's level of consciousness by checking the appropriateness of responses to specific questions should be made. In lethargic or comatose patients, extraocular muscle function should be tested by employing the doll's head maneuver or ice water caloric testing. Obtunded and comatose patients should have their urinary bladders catheterized, and comatose patients should be placed on an air mattress and turned at 1- to 2-hour intervals to prevent pressure sores. Responsive patients will often request that their room be darkened to reduce photophobia. Patients should be kept on bed rest and on analgesics, including acetaminophen or other analgesics for headache. Sedating medication should be minimized to permit accurate testing of mental status. Supportive therapy is appropriate for patients with viral meningoencephalitis from any cause.

Therapy for Cerebral Effects of Disease. This type of therapy largely refers to eliminating or diminishing the development of epileptic seizures and methods to decrease intracranial pressure. Patients with encephalitis (although not those with meningitis) should be treated with phenytoin (Dilantin) at a dose of 200 mg three times a day, orally or intravenously, for 2 to 3 days and then should be placed on maintenance therapy of 300 to 400 mg daily. Patients presenting with a single seizure episode should be treated more vigorously with phenytoin, with three doses of 300 mg orally or intravenously given three times over approximately 12 hours and then started on maintenance therapy. Patients presenting with multiple seizures or developing status epilepticus should be treated with diazepam (Valium), 10 mg intravenously over 3 to 5 minutes, and phenytoin, 20 mg per kg intravenously, at a rate not to exceed 50 mg per minute. Respirations and cardiac function should be monitored carefully during this therapy. Patients who develop seizures secondary to meningoencephalitis should be maintained on anticonvulsants for at least 1 year, the duration in part based on electroencephalogram status.

Treatment of increased intracranial pressure may be necessary in patients with cerebral edema, including those with meningoencephalitis. Dexamethasone, 10 mg intravenously and then 4 mg at 6-hour intervals, should be started. It is unlikely that this will depress host defenses and enhance virus replication. With further evidence of cerebral edema and possible cerebral herniation, mannitol (25% solution) should be given intravenously (1.0 to 1.5 grams per kg over 25 to 30 minutes). Fluid input and output should be monitored carefully. Mannitol can be repeated, but efficacy is diminished when serum osmolality exceeds 320 mOsm per liter, and with repeated use, rebound and increased intracranial pressure may result. Hyperventilation to maintain the P_{CO_2} mm Hg may also be a valuable means of decreasing intracranial pressure. Neurosurgically inserted dural monitoring devices are useful for following intracranial pressure and determining appropriate times for the administration of medications such as mannitol. These devices are of particular importance in sedated patients who are pharmacologically paralyzed and in whom neurologic examination is therefore difficult. These therapies are appropriate for patients with meningoencephalitis caused by any virus.

Specific Treatment of Viral Infections. Treatment has improved markedly in recent years, particularly for HSV encephalitis. The present medication of choice is acyclovir given intravenously, 10 mg per kg, or in children, 500 mg per m^2, every 8 hours for at least 10 days. The recommended treatment period is 10 days, but some patients are best treated for 12 to 14 days. Acyclovir should be administered over 1 hour at a concentration of 7 mg per mL or less. Elevation of serum creatinine or blood urea nitrogen may occur, and the dosage of acyclovir should be decreased in patients with renal impairment. An important factor in estimating the long-term prognosis of the patient is mental status at the onset of drug treatment; early treatment is clearly indicated.

In immunocompromised adults and children infected with VZV, intravenous acyclovir treatment is also indicated. Dosage is as for HSV encephalitis. Efficacy in nonimmunocompromised patients with VZV encephalitis is not yet clear but can be considered in appropriate clinical situations. A new drug, famciclovir (Famvir), is approved for the treatment of herpes zoster and may prove useful in the treatment of VZV encephalitis.

Acyclovir and famciclovir are both inactive against HSV and VZV until the drugs are specifically phosphorylated by viral enzymes (i.e., viral-encoded thymidine kinase) to the active antiviral form. Therefore, the drugs are inactive against mutant virus that is lacking viral thymidine kinase activity. Such mutant virus is seen clinically only in immunocompromised patients treated with these antiviral drugs. In these patients, rare, spontaneous viral thymidine kinase mutants that develop are not inhibited by the drugs, whereas wild-type virus that expresses thymidine kinase is inhibited. Mutant virus replicates because it is not inhibited by the drugs, whereas standard wild-type virus is inhibited. From a clinical point of view, mutant virus may be of significance in causing cutaneous infection in immunocompromised patients, but meningitis-encephalitis is not probable.

MULTIPLE SCLEROSIS

method of
HOWARD L. WEINER, M.D., and
LYNN STAZZONE, R.N.
Harvard Medical School and Brigham and Women's Hospital
Boston, Massachusetts

Multiple sclerosis (MS) is an inflammatory disease of the central nervous system (CNS) that affects CNS myelin. Although the cause and pathogenesis of MS are unknown, the most commonly held view is that it is an autoimmune disease related in some way to a viral infection. The inflammatory response in the CNS consists predominantly of activated T lymphocytes and macrophages accompanied by a local immune reaction with the secretion of cytokines and the synthesis of oligoclonal immunoglobulin within the CNS. In addition, immune abnormalities have been described in the peripheral blood of MS patients, including the loss of suppressor function, the presence of activated T cells, alterations of T cell populations, and increased secretion of inflammatory cytokines. The two major hypotheses to explain CNS inflammation are either a cell-mediated autoimmune attack against myelin antigens or the presence of a persistent virus or infectious process within the nervous system against which the inflammatory response is directed. Despite many attempts, an infectious agent has not been identified in MS.

Therapy of MS can be divided into three categories: (1) treatment to prevent the ongoing destruction of nervous system tissue by inflammatory cells, (2) symptomatic treatment to allow a damaged nervous system to function at a higher level, and (3) treatment designed to repair damaged CNS myelin. If the destructive inflammatory process in the CNS could be arrested at an early stage, the accumulation of neurologic disability could be prevented. Symptomatic treatments are also available for MS patients, for example, those that relieve spasticity, improve bladder function, or help fatigue. Treatment to repair damaged myelin remains in the research stage. The clinical features of the disease make therapy difficult, because MS is a chronic, relapsing-progressive disease with an unpredictable clinical course that generally spans 10 to 20 years, during which time neurologic disability accumulates.

Despite these difficulties, significant progress is being made in understanding the disease and devising therapy. Advances in two areas have made an impact on developing therapy for MS: (1) magnetic resonance imaging (MRI) and (2) understanding how the immune system functions and how it is regulated. MRI has shown MS to be a much more chronically active process than can be discerned clinically and MRI has become an important outcome measure in clinical trials. Also as the function of the immune system has become better understood, the ways in which it can be manipulated and monitored have expanded greatly. Although MS has not been proven formally to be a cell-mediated autoimmune disease directed against CNS myelin, most disease-modifying therapeutic strategies are based on this hypothesis.

CLINICAL COURSE OF MULTIPLE SCLEROSIS

1. *Relapsing-remitting:* Patients have discrete motor, sensory, cerebellar, or visual attacks that come on over a 1- to 2-week period and resolve over a 4- to 8-week period with or without corticosteroid treatment. Patients in this category return to their preattack baseline.

2. *Relapsing-remitting progressive (transitional):* Patients have attacks but do not return to their baseline and accumulate stepwise disability. This category is a transitional stage between relapsing-remitting and progressive. It has also been recently classified as a more severe form of relapsing-remitting disease.

3. *Progressive:* Patients have progressive worsening with no periods of stability. The progressive form may be secondarily progressive, that is, develop in patients who began with relapsing-remitting disease, or be primary progressive, in which the pattern is progressive from the outset. The primary progressive form may be a subcategory that is less responsive to immune therapy. Some patients with the progressive form of the disease have superimposed attacks.

4. *Stable MS:* Patients have had no clinical disease activity and report no subjective worsening in their condition over the previous 12 months.

PRINCIPLES OF IMMUNOTHERAPY FOR MULTIPLE SCLEROSIS

We believe the following principles are important for the immunotherapy of MS and can serve as a framework from which to view the various treatment modalities that are currently being used and tested (Table 1). In essence, a hierarchy of treatments is given, with the least toxic therapy given first. Our approach to the treatment of MS is an aggressive one, aimed at preventing the accumulation of neurologic disability.

TABLE 1. **Principles of Immunotherapy for Multiple Sclerosis**

First-line "nontoxic" therapy
Intravenous steroids for relapses
Plasmapheresis for refractory fulminant central nervous system demyelination
Second-line immunosuppression to halt refractory, transitional, or progressive disease
Reinstitution of first-line therapy
Combination and pulse therapy
Disease monitoring: magnetic resonance imaging, immune measures

1. *First-line, "nontoxic" therapy.* Currently available treatments are interferon beta-1b (Betaseron), interferon beta-1a (Avonex), and glatiramer acetate (Copaxone).

2. *Intravenous steroids for relapses.* Based on what is currently known about interferon beta and other relatively nontoxic drugs that can be given early in the disease course, it is expected that patients will continue to have relapses. Thus, short courses of intravenous (IV) methylprednisolone are given when a significant relapse occurs to speed recovery and, given what was reported in the optic neuritis study, perhaps to have a salutory effect on the disease course. In rare cases of fulminant CNS demyelination, plasmapheresis may be given.

3. *Second-line immunotherapy to halt refractory or progressive disease.* Although some patients may respond to first-line treatments, it is expected that others will be refractory to therapy or enter the progressive stage. In these instances, more potent immunotherapy or immunosuppression may be warranted depending on the individual case. Drugs in this category are classified as second- or third-line treatment depending on the risk-benefit ratio of the therapy. Second- or third-line therapy may be useful even if such treatment is only given on a short-term basis as rescue therapy if such treatment allows reinstitution of first-line therapy.

4. *Reinstitution of first-line therapy.* One of the principles of second- or third-line therapy is to induce a remission, after which first-line, nontoxic therapy is instituted to maintain the remission. The degree to which subsequent first-line therapy will be effective is unknown.

5. *Combination and pulse therapy.* Until the pathogenesis of MS is precisely understood, it is unlikely that a single treatment will be effective in all patients. The principle of combination therapy has found utility in cancer treatment and is likely to be an important principle for the therapy of MS and other autoimmune diseases. Pulse steroids or relatively nontoxic immunomodulation may find utility in conjunction with antigen-specific forms of therapy. Furthermore, because MS appears to be more chronically active as viewed by MRI than can be evident clinically and because some forms of therapy cannot be given on a long-term basis, intermittent pulse therapy with drugs that affect the immune system

may become an important principle for MS therapy. This principle is currently being tested in our center using pulse methylprednisolone and pulse cyclophosphamide.

6. *Disease monitoring.* The major problem confronting therapy of MS remains its unpredictable course and the length of time over which disability accumulates. Even for treatments that have proven to be efficacious, it may be difficult to determine in an individual patient whether the treatment is having a therapeutic effect unless the disease becomes truly quiescent clinically or the patient improves with therapy. In some instances it is clear that a patient is either a responder or a nonresponder to a particular treatment. We have occasionally seen such positive clinical effects in younger patients with rapidly progressive, steroid-unresponsive disease who were treated with pulse cyclophosphamide. The hope is to find a surrogate marker that is linked to the underlying disease process that will allow a more rational approach to assessing therapy, apart from clinical assessment. MRI has provided such a surrogate marker and was one of the major factors in approval of interferon-beta for the treatment of relapsing-remitting MS. Even though MRI is not a perfect correlate of disease activity, it may ultimately serve as the best objective measure of ongoing disease in the nervous system, given that it is now known that MS is chronically active even when clinical activity is not present. However, apart from formal clinical trials, MRIs are costly and impractical to perform on a frequent basis in a general neurology practice.

Apart from formal studies, the treating neurologist must decide on therapy based on clinical assessment and accumulation of disability. Furthermore, a decision must be made as to whether a person has responded to therapy or whether additional treatment should be given. These decisions are generally made based on the frequency with which the patient is having attacks, the level of progression, and the MRI results (lesion burden and presence of gadolinium-enhancing lesions). In addition, we have constructed a simple disease steps scale that classifies MS patients according to functional changes that impinge on a patient's lifestyle and can be easily recognized by physician and patient (Table 2). Movement from one step to another can be used as a guide to assess the effectiveness of therapy and when to intervene with additional treatment.

TABLE 2. **Disease Steps Scale**

0	*Normal:* Functionally normal; no limitations on activity or lifestyle
1	*Mild disability:* Minor, but noticeable symptoms and/or signs; normal gait
2	*Moderate disability:* Main feature is a visibly abnormal gait
3	*Early cane:* Use of a cane for greater distances but can walk 25 feet in 20 seconds or less without a cane
4	*Late cane:* Unable to walk 25 feet without a cane or unilateral support
5	*Bilateral support:* Requires bilateral support to walk 25 feet
6	*Wheelchair:* Essentially confined to a wheelchair, although may be able to take one or two steps

DISEASE-MODIFYING THERAPY IN MULTIPLE SCLEROSIS (Table 3)

Therapy for Relapsing-Remitting Disease

Acute attacks are either not treated or treated with a short course of corticosteroids. Indications for treatment of a relapse include functionally disabling symptoms with objective evidence of neurologic impairment. Thus, mild sensory attacks are typically not treated. In the past adrenocorticotropic hormone (ACTH) and oral prednisone were primarily used. Now, physicians treat with short courses of IV methylprednisolone (Solu-Medrol). We treat with a 5-day course of IV methylprednisolone (1000 mg/day) without a prednisone taper. Optic neuritis may occur during the course of MS or be one of the initial symptoms. A trial of optic neuritis demonstrated that patients treated with oral prednisone alone were more likely to suffer recurrent episodes of optic neuritis compared with those treated with methylprednisolone followed by oral prednisone. These results now make IV methylprednisolone the primary treatment for optic neuritis and lend support to its use for major attacks. Furthermore, as part of the optic neuritis study, it was found that treatment with a 3-day course of high-dose methylprednisolone reduced the rate of development of MS over a 2-year period. The protective effect was most apparent in patients at highest risk for MS, those with multiple focal brain MRI abnormalities. Although these results need to be confirmed in a larger series of patients, they support the use of high-dose IV methylprednisolone for acute MS attacks. As described later, we also use monthly pulses of IV methylprednisolone for the treatment of transitional (relapsing-remitting progressive) and progressive MS. High-dose IV methylprednisolone appears to be accompanied by relatively few side effects in most patients, although mental changes, unmasking of infections, gastric disturbances, and increased incidence of fractures have occasionally been observed. Patients treated with pulse IV methylprednisolone need to be monitored for decreased bone density. Anaphylactoid reactions and arrhythmias may also occur.

Plasma exchange in conjunction with corticotropin (ACTH)* and oral cyclophosphamide* (Cytoxan) enhanced recovery from acute attacks in patients with relapsing-remitting disease in a double-blind study, although no long-term benefit was seen and it is not known the degree to which IV methylprednisolone would have produced similar effects. Nonetheless, an open study of plasmapheresis in acute episodes of fulminant CNS inflammatory demyelination showed marked improvement in patients who failed a course of high-dose IV methylprednisolone. Plasmapheresis

*Not FDA approved for this indication.

TABLE 3. **Disease-Modifying Therapy in Multiple Sclerosis**

Stage or Course of Disease	Treatment
Optic neuritis	IV methylprednisolone, 1000 mg for 5 days without oral taper
Relapsing-remitting with fewer than 2 attacks per year with low MRI activity*	IV methylprednisolone, 1000 mg for 5 days without oral taper
Relapsing-remitting with more than 2 attacks per year and/or high MRI activity	IV methylprednisolone for attacks plus Avonex, 30 μg IM weekly, *or* Betaseron, 1 mL SC qod, *or* Copaxone, 20 mg SC qd
Relapsing-remitting (Interferon beta/glatiramer acetate nonresponders)	Add monthly IV methylprednisolone†
Relapsing-remitting with accumulating disability (Steroid interferon beta, glatiramer acetate nonresponders)	IV cyclophosphamide-methylprednisolone pulse therapy‡
Rapid progressing disability	IV cyclophosphamide-methylprednisolone induction followed by pulse therapy
Fulminating disability	Plasma exchange
Secondary progressive	IV methylprednisolone monthly boosters IV cyclophosphamide-methylprednisolone pulse therapy Methotrexate weekly given with or without IV methylprednisolone boosters§
Primary progressive	IV methylprednisolone monthly pulse therapy Methotrexate weekly given with or without IV methylprednisolone boosters§

*Some treat these patients with interferon beta or glatiramer acetate.
†Depending on severity, cyclophosphamide-methylprednisolone pulse therapy may be given. Some may treat with IGIV.
‡Other options include IGIV, methotrexate, cladribine, mitoxanthrone.
§Other options include IGIV, cladribine.

appears to be an important therapeutic option for this rare subset of patients.

Prevention of Relapses

Interferon Beta. Two forms of recombinant interferon beta, 1a and 1b, are approved for the treatment of relapsing-remitting MS. Interferon beta-1b is a nonglycosylated recombinant bacterial cell product in which serine is substituted for cysteine at position 17. Interferon beta-1a is a glycosylated recombinant mammalian-cell product with an amino acid sequence identical to that of natural interferon beta. Interferon beta-1b given subcutaneously in every-other-day injections was shown to decrease the relapse rate by 31%, increase the proportion of patients who were relapse free, and reduce the number of patients who had moderate and severe relapses. There was no difference in proportions of patients whose disability increased or in changes in disability scores among treatment groups. However, MRI progression, as measured by new MRI lesions and T2-weighted area were reduced in interferon beta-1b–treated patients. Interferon beta-1a is given as a weekly intramuscular injection and demonstrated in a multicenter trial that the length of time to progression of disability was improved in patients treated compared with placebo patients. In addition, patients treated with interferon beta-1a had fewer gadolinium-enhancing lesions on MRI. Side effects of interferon beta include injection site reactions, influenza-like symptoms, and worsening of pre-existing depression. The choice between the different interferon preparations depends on the patient and individual physician. Interferon beta-1a is often prescribed as it requires only a weekly injection, appears to be better tolerated, and affects progression of disability.

Glatiramer acetate (Copaxone) is a mixture of random synthetic peptides synthesized initially as a compound to mimic myelin basic protein, a long-studied autoantigen in multiple sclerosis. Glatiramer acetate was effective in the animal model of MS (EAE), and in a double-blind trial of relapsing-remitting MS its use decreased relapse rate. Treatment consists of daily subcutaneous injections of 20 mg. The most common side effects are mild reactions at the injection site and in some patients unexplained reactions involving episodes of flushing, chest tightness, shortness of breath, and palpitations.

The choice of beginning a relapsing-remitting patient with interferon beta versus glatiramer acetate has not been resolved. Patients with depression, those very early in their course, or those who cannot tolerate interferon beta are often preferentially treated with glatiramer acetate. Patients who are nonresponders to beta interferon or glatiramer acetate may be treated with the other medication depending on how active the disease has become (see later discussion).

*Azathioprine** (Imuran) has been the subject of a large number of studies in MS, and meta-analysis of the results of all published blind, randomized, controlled trials showed a statistically significant benefit in reducing frequency of relapses over a 3-year period but minimal effect on disability. Although not commonly used in the United States, and not in our center, it is a therapeutic option for patients with relapsing-remitting disease.

*IGIV** has been used in immune disorders of the nervous system such as demyelinating polyneuropathies, and recent studies suggest it may have benefit in relapsing-remitting MS.

*Not FDA approved for this indication.

Rescue Therapy for Interferon Beta/ Glatiramer Acetate Nonresponders

A major challenge facing treatment of MS are relapsing-remitting patients who do not respond well to the approved drugs for relapsing-remitting MS and who begin to have increasing attacks or accumulate disability (transitional) or begin to enter the progressive stage. In patients with relapsing-remitting disease without accumulating disability one can switch from interferon beta to glatiramer acetate or vice versa, although increasing attacks are usually associated with disability. In addition, we add pulses of methylprednisolone given on a monthly basis to stabilize patients. However, stronger treatment is often needed, and we use short-term rescue therapy with immunosuppressive agents in these nonresponder patients. We favor short-term rescue therapy with 6 to 12 months of pulses of methylprednisolone or pulses of cyclophosphamide-methylprednisolone. Patients are then treated again with drugs for relapsing-remitting disease. Our center is therapeutically aggressive in our approach to the illness, and we have found that pulse cyclophosphamide has the most profound effect on disease in relapsing-remitting progressive-type patients—patients who are in a transitional phase from relapsing-remitting to progressive disease. Other options at this stage include the use of azathioprine,* methotrexate,* IGIV,* cladribine,* or mitoxanthrone.*

Therapy for Progressive Multiple Sclerosis

Treatment directed at the progressive phase is the most difficult, as the disease may be harder to affect once the progressive stage has been initiated. Cyclophosphamide,* total lymphoid radiation, cyclosporin,* methotrexate* and 2-chloro-2′-deoxyadenosine* (CdA), and mitoxanthrone* have shown some positive clinical effects in progressive disease. Depending on the type of progressive disease and how long the patient has been progressive, our drug of choice is cyclophosphamide. Recently, interferon beta-1b has shown positive MRI and clinical effects in secondary progressive patients. The effectiveness and use of interferon beta-1b in clinical practice remains to be determined. Of note is that many patients who enter the progressive phase have already failed interferon therapy. It may be useful for patients who have been stabilized by immunosuppressive therapy.

Cyclophosphamide. We have investigated the use of cyclophosphamide to treat progressive MS over the past 15 years based on reports of European investigators. Our initial study demonstrated a positive effect in patients treated with a 2-week course of cyclophosphamide-ACTH compared with patients that received ACTH alone. However, within 1 to 3 years, most patients began to reprogress. These findings led to the study of the Northeast Cooperative Treatment Group, a randomized single-blind trial that tested the efficacy of every-2-month outpatient cyclophosphamide pulses in 236 patients who received an initial cyclophosphamide-ACTH induction. The results demonstrated a modest positive clinical effect in patients receiving pulses compared with those who did not. Most striking was the finding that younger patients (under 40 years of age) tended to respond to therapy, whereas older patients did not. We have subsequently investigated 95 patients treated with pulse cyclophosphamide following methylprednisolone-only induction and found that the factor most closely linked to response is the length of time in the progressive phase, independent of age. We found that patients with progressive disease for more than 2 years do not respond as well. In addition, we found that primary progressive patients do not respond as well as patients with secondary progressive disease. These findings are consistent with what is being learned about progressive MS. Specifically, primary progressive may be a different form of the disease, and with time axonal loss may make patients nonresponsive to immunotherapy.

We have different regimens for the use of cyclophosphamide depending on the stage of illness (Table 4). Our most commonly used regimen involves induction with 5 days of IV methylprednisolone followed by monthly pulses of cyclophosphamide-methylprednisolone designed to produce a leukopenia. Pulses are given monthly for a year, every 6 weeks in the second year and every 2 months in the third year. This regimen produces hair thinning but not hair

*Not FDA approved for this indication.

TABLE 4. **Cyclophosphamide (Cytoxan) Dosing**

Inpatient Induction (8 days)

IV methylprednisolone, 1000 mg daily for 8 consecutive d
IV cyclophosphamide, 600 mg/m^2 on days 1, 2, 4, 6, 8

Outpatient Induction (5 days)

IV methylprednisolone, 1000 mg daily for 5 consecutive d
IV cyclophosphamide, 800 mg/m^2 on day 5

Pulse Therapy (1 day)

IV methylprednisolone, 1000 mg
IV cyclophosphamide, 800 mg/m^2

Booster Dosing: Intermittent Pulse Therapy Given Every 4–8 wk*

Cyclophosphamide dose is dependent on white blood cell (WBC) count on day 8, 11, and 14 after previous cyclophosphamide dose and WBC count before treatment.
- Total WBC nadir should be 1500–2000/mm^3
  - If nadir <1500, dose is decreased by 100–200 mg/m^2
  - If nadir >2200, dose is increased by 200 mg/m^2
- Total WBC count before cyclophosphamide dose should be >4000/mm^3
  - If 3000–4000, 75% of dose is administered
  - If 2000–3000, 50% of dose is administered
  - If <2000, booster is not given and WBC count is checked in 1 wk

*IV methylprednisolone-cyclophosphamide boosters are begun 1 mo after induction and are given monthly for 1 y, every 6 wk for 1 y, every 2 mo for 1 y, then discontinued if the patient is stable. Pulse therapy may be given for shorter periods of time (e.g., 6–12 mo) when used as rescue therapy for interferon beta failures.

loss and can be given solely on an outpatient basis. We are also using this regimen for a 6- to 12-month period as rescue therapy in interferon beta and glatiramer acetate nonresponders. In some patients, we begin with pulse therapy without a methylprednisolone induction. In patients with rapidly progressive disease, we induce with cyclophosphamide given over an 8-day period, a regimen that produces alopecia. A Canadian study did not find positive clinical effects treating patients with only a 2-week course of cyclophosphamide and prednisone. The lack of response to cyclophosphamide in that study most likely relates to the use of a different treatment regimen, treatment of primary progressive patients, and treatment of patients with progressive disease for longer than 2 years.

The toxicities of cyclophosphamide are well known and make the use of the drug appropriate only for carefully selected patients with actively progressive disease. By using outpatient pulse therapy in a fashion analogous to its use in lupus nephritis, the therapy is tolerated reasonably well. Side effects include loss of menstrual periods, risk of bladder cancer, and secondary malignancies. It is important that adequate hydration is given with treatment, and treatment is best given by an oncologist or physician familiar with the use of the drug. Ondansetron (Zofran) is very important as it helps to control the nausea associated with treatment. In patients with progressive disease who have not had an adequate trial of steroids, we treat with methylprednisolone induction followed by methylprednisolone monthly pulses before initiating cyclophosphamide therapy.

Methotrexate. This drug, 7.5 mg per week orally, has been reported to positively affect upper extremity function in progressive MS, although lower extremity function as measured by ambulation and disability scales was not affected. Methotrexate has been useful in treating rheumatoid arthritis and has a known side effect profile. We treat relapsing-progressive and some progressive patients with oral methotrexate (7.5 to 15 mg) or with weekly injections of methotrexate at a dose of 20 mg either alone or in combination with pulse steroids. We do not find methotrexate as effective as cyclophosphamide. Some patients have been treated for more than 2 years with no toxicity as measured by blood screening and liver biopsies.

CdA (Cladribine). This potent immunosuppressive agent, useful in the treatment of hairy cell leukemia, has been reported to be of benefit in treating progressive MS. Treated patients had improvement of disability, no increase in brain MRI lesions, and decreased cerebrospinal fluid oligoclonal bands. Side effects include herpes zoster and persistently lowered CD4 counts. Cladribine is given subcutaneously every month for 1 week over a 4- to 6-month period. If patients stabilize, they begin reprogressing after 12 months and one re-treatment can be given. Because of persistently low CD4 counts, treatment with other agents may not be possible.

Mitoxanthrone. European investigators have reported that mitoxanthrone helps treat progressive MS. It can be given for only a 2-year period because of potential cardiac toxicity.

Other Therapy. Total lymphoid irradiation has potent immunosuppressive effects, and a double-blind study of lymphoid irradiation reported benefit in patients with progressive MS. The absolute lymphocyte count appeared to be a crude indication of therapeutic efficacy, with greater efficacy in patients with lower counts. Many patients began reprogressing after initial therapy, and a major limitation of the use of total lymphoid irradiation is that it may preclude the use of other treatments that affect the immune system at a subsequent time for those who reenter the progressive phase despite radiation therapy. A large multicenter trial of cyclosporine in the United States and a trial in London indicate that cyclosporine has a beneficial, albeit modest, effect in ameliorating clinical disease progression, but it has not found clinical use because of the narrow benefit-to-risk ratio.

SYMPTOMATIC TREATMENT

A number of symptomatic treatments may help MS patients, although they do not affect the progression of the disease.

1. *Fatigue* affects up to 80% of patients and can be severe and disabling. The pathophysiology of fatigue in MS is unknown, although it may relate to the release of inflammatory cytokines in the brain. Treatments include periodic rest, energy conservation, routine exercise programs, and medications such as amantadine and pemoline. Unfortunately, these drugs are only effective in a minority of patients, and even in responders, the effects are not dramatic. More recently, approaches include selegiline and fluoxetine.
2. *Spasticity* typically affects the lower extremities most severely in MS patients. There may also be superimposed extensor spasms, particularly at night. Patients with moderate to severe paraparesis may rely on extensor tone for ambulation, and aggressive treatment of spasticity in these patients may lead to functional worsening. Physical therapy and regular passive muscle stretching are simple nonpharmacologic approaches to decreased muscle tone. Medications include oral baclofen (Lioresal), benzodiazepines, dantrolene (Dantrium), and tizanidine (Zanaflex). Occasionally, these drugs need to be used in combination to overcome troubling spasticity. For more severely affected patients, procedures including nerve root blocks, rhizotomy, tenotomy, or myotomy are sometimes used. A more recent approach involves intrathecal baclofen, administered using an implantable, programmable pump.
3. *Tremor* is a particularly difficult symptom to manage. Drug therapy may be helpful occasionally, but typically the effects are short lived. Agents include gabapentin (Neurontin),* isoniazid,* benzodi-

*Not FDA approved for this indication.

azepines, primidone (Mysoline)*, and propranolol (Inderal).* Weighted bracelets are often the most practical approach. Surgical thalamotomy has been tried in some cases with reduction in tremor but often without significant functional improvement.

4. *Bladder dysfunction* is common and may be difficult to manage. It has been shown that one cannot predict the mechanism of bladder dysfunction based on symptoms alone. Thus, patients with troublesome bladder symptoms should be referred to a urologist for urodynamic testing. The most common pattern of bladder dysfunction in MS is detrusor-sphincter dyssynergia (DSD). Detrusor muscle hyper-reflexia can be managed with anticholinergic agents, including oxybutynin (Ditropan), propantheline (Pro-Banthine), imipramine (Tofranil), and hyoscyamine (Levsin). These drugs will lessen symptoms of frequency, nocturia, urgency, and incontinence, but one must guard against subsequent urinary retention and resultant urinary tract infection, especially because with DSD, the external sphincter fails to relax appropriately. Monitoring for and treating urinary tract infections are very important. Acidification of the urine with ascorbic acid (vitamin C) or cranberry juice may protect against gram-negative infections. Long-term antibiotic therapy may lead to resistant organisms. Often, patients require intermittent self-catheterization to ensure complete bladder emptying. Indwelling catheterization carries the risk of increased infection. Surgical procedures are sometimes necessary. Constipation is not uncommon in MS, especially in more severely affected, wheelchair-confined patients. Bowel urgency and incontinence are much less common. Most patients benefit from increased fluid and roughage in their diet. Metamucil or glycerin suppositories are often helpful. Cathartics should be used only as a last resort.

6. *Sexual dysfunction*. Erectile dysfunction is quite common in patients with spinal cord involvement. Patients should be referred to a urologist. Approaches include sildenafil (Viagra), intracorporeal papaverine,* phentolamine* or prostaglandin injections, or, at times, penile prostheses.

7. *Paroxysmal tonic seizures* usually last 1 to 2 minutes and occur several times per day. They consist of paresthesias or pain in the face or a limb, followed by painful tonic contraction. Another paroxysmal symptom consists of dysarthria and ataxia, usually unilateral limb ataxia, although gait may also be affected. These episodes are also short lived (often less than 1 minute) and can occur several times per hour. Paroxysmal phenomena typically subside after a period of weeks. They are likely caused by ephaptic transmission of nerve impulses at sites of previous disease activity. Low doses of carbamazepine, phenytoin, gabapentin, or baclofen* are usually effective and can be tapered after several weeks.

8. *Potassium channel blockers*,† including 4-aminopyridine and 3,4-diaminopyridine have been shown to improve MS symptoms, especially in heat-sensitive patients. These agents enhance conduction through demyelinated nerves. Studies are in progress to further establish clinical efficacy and evaluate toxicity.

Other symptoms requiring long-term management include chronic pain that may develop in some patients and cognitive and emotional dysfunction.

*Not FDA approved for this indication.
†Investigational drug in the United States.

MYASTHENIA GRAVIS

method of
ROBERT M. PASCUZZI, M.D.
Indiana University School of Medicine
Indianapolis, Indiana

Myasthenia gravis (MG) is an autoimmune disorder of neuromuscular transmission involving the production of autoantibodies directed against the nicotinic acetylcholine (ACh) receptor. ACh-receptor antibodies are detectable in the serum of 80 to 90% of patients with MG. The prevalence of MG is about 1 in 10,000 to 20,000. Women are affected about twice as often as men. Symptoms may begin at virtually any age, with a peak in women in the second and third decades, whereas the peak in men occurs in the fifth and sixth decades. Associated autoimmune diseases such as rheumatoid arthritis, lupus, and pernicious anemia are present in about 5% of patients. Thyroid disease occurs in about 10%, often in association with antithyroid antibodies. About 10 to 15% of MG patients have a thymoma, and thymic lymphoid hyperplasia with proliferation of germinal centers occurs in 50 to 70% of cases. In most patients the cause of autoimmune MG is unknown. However, there are three iatrogenic causes for autoimmune MG. D-Penicillamine (Cuprimine) (used in the treatment of Wilson's disease and rheumatoid arthritis) and interferon alfa therapy are both capable of inducing MG. In addition, bone marrow transplantation is associated with the development of MG as part of graft-versus-host disease.

CLINICAL FEATURES

The hallmark of MG is fluctuating or fatigable weakness. The presenting symptoms are ocular in half of all patients (25% of patients present initially with diplopia, 25% with ptosis), and by 1 month into the course of illness, 80% of patients have some degree of ocular involvement. Presenting symptoms are bulbar (dysarthria or dysphagia) in 10%, leg weakness (impaired walking) in 10%, and generalized weakness in 10%. Respiratory failure is the presenting symptom in 1% of cases. Patients usually complain of symptoms from focal muscle dysfunction, such as diplopia, ptosis, dysarthria, dysphagia, inability to work with arms raised over the head, or disturbance of gait. In contrast, patients with MG tend not to complain of "generalized weakness," "generalized fatigue," "sleepiness," or muscle pain. In the classic case, fluctuating weakness is worse with exercise and improved with rest. Symptoms tend to progress and become more pronounced later in the day. Many different factors can precipitate or aggravate weakness, such as physical stress, emotional stress, infection, or exposure to medications that impair neuromuscular transmission (perioperative succinylcholine, aminoglycoside antibiotics, quinine, quinidine).

DIAGNOSIS

The diagnosis is based on a history of fluctuating weakness with corroborating findings on examination. There are several different ways to validate or confirm the diagnosis.

Tensilon Test. The most immediate and readily accessible confirmatory study is the edrophonium (Tensilon) test. To perform the test, choose one or two weak muscles to judge. Ptosis, dysconjugate gaze, and other cranial deficits provide the most reliable end points. Use a setting in which hypotension, syncope, or respiratory failure can be managed, as patients occasionally decompensate during the test. If the patient has severe dyspnea do not perform the test until the airway is secure. Start an intravenous line. Have intravenous atropine, 0.4 mg, readily available in the event of bradycardia or extreme gastrointestinal (GI) side effects. Edrophonium, 10 mg (1 mL), is drawn up in a syringe and 1 mg (0.1 mL) should be given as a test dose while checking the patient's heart rate (to ensure that the patient is not supersensitive to the drug). If no untoward side effects occur after 1 minute, another 3 mg is given. Many MG patients will show improved power within 30 to 60 seconds of giving the initial 4 mg, at which point the test can be stopped. If after 1 minute there is no improvement, give an additional 3 mg; if there is still no response 1 minute later, give the final 3 mg. If the patient develops muscarinic symptoms or signs at any time during the test (sweating, salivation, GI symptoms), one can assume that enough edrophonium has been given to see improvement in strength and the test can be stopped. When a placebo effect or examiner bias is of concern, the test is performed in a double-blind placebo-controlled fashion. The 1-mL controlled syringe contains either saline, 0.4 mg atropine, or nicotinic acid (10 mg). Improvement lasts for just a few minutes. When improvement is clear-cut, then the test is positive. If the improvement is borderline, it is best to consider the test negative. The test can be repeated several times. Sensitivity of the edrophonium test is about 90%. The specificity is difficult to determine, as improvement following intravenous edrophonium has been reported in other neuromuscular diseases, including Lambert-Eaton syndrome, botulism, Guillain-Barré syndrome, motor neuron disease, and lesions of the brain stem and cavernous sinus.

Acetylcholine Receptor Antibodies. The standard assay for receptor-binding antibodies is an immunoprecipitation assay using human limb muscle for ACh-receptor antigen. In addition, assays for receptor-modulating and receptor-blocking antibodies are available. Binding antibodies are present in about 80% of all myasthenic patients (50% of patients with pure ocular MG, 80% of those with mild generalized MG, 90% of patients with moderate to severe generalized MG, and 70% of those in clinical remission). By also testing for modulating and blocking antibodies, the sensitivity improves to 90% overall. Specificity is outstanding, with false positives exceedingly rare in reliable laboratories. If blood is sent to a reference laboratory, the test results are usually available within a week.

Electromyography (EMG) (Electrophysiologic Testing). Repetitive stimulation testing is widely available and has variable sensitivity depending on the number and selection of muscles studied and various provocative maneuvers. However, in most laboratories this technique has a sensitivity of about 50% in all patients with MG (lower in patients with mild or pure ocular disease). Single-fiber EMG is a highly specialized technique, usually available in major academic centers, with a sensitivity of about 90%. Abnormal single-fiber results are common in other neuromuscular disease, and therefore the test must be used in the correct clinical context. The specificity of single-fiber EMG is an important issue in that mild abnormalities can clearly be present with a variety of other diseases of the motor unit, including motor neuron disease, peripheral neuropathy, and myopathy. Disorders of neuromuscular transmission other than MG can have substantial abnormalities on single-fiber EMG. In contrast, receptor antibodies are not present in non-MG patients. In summary, the two highly sensitive laboratory studies are single-fiber EMG and receptor antibodies; nonetheless, neither test is 100% sensitive.

PROGNOSIS

Appropriate management of the patient with autoimmune MG requires an understanding of the natural course of the disease. The long-term natural course of MG is not clearly established other than being highly variable. Several generalizations can be made. About half of MG patients present with ocular symptoms, and by 1 month 80% have eye findings. The presenting weakness is bulbar in 10%, limb in 10%, generalized in 10%, and respiratory in 1%. By 1 month symptoms remain purely ocular in 40%, generalized in 40%, limited to the limbs in 10%, and limited to bulbar muscles in 10%. Weakness remains restricted to the ocular muscles on a long-term basis in about 15 to 20% (pure ocular MG). Most patients with initial ocular involvement tend to develop generalized weakness within the first year of the disease (90% of those who develop generalized weakness do so within the initial 12 months). Maximal weakness occurs within the initial 3 years in 70% of patients. In the modern era, death from MG is rare. Spontaneous long-lasting remission occurs in about 10 to 15% of patients, usually in the first year or two of the disease. Most MG patients develop progression of clinical symptoms during the initial 2 to 3 years. However, progression is not uniform, as illustrated by 15 to 20% of patients whose symptoms remain purely ocular and those who have spontaneous remission.

TREATMENT

First-Line Therapy: Mestinon

Cholinesterase inhibitors (CEIs) are safe, effective, and first-line therapy in all patients. Inhibition of acetylcholinesterase (AChE) reduces the hydrolysis of ACh, increasing the accumulation of ACh at the nicotinic postsynaptic membrane. The CEIs used in MG bind reversibly (as opposed to organophosphate CEIs, which bind irreversibly) to AChE. These drugs cross the blood-brain barrier poorly and tend not to cause central nervous system side effects. Absorption from the GI tract tends to be inefficient and variable, with an oral bioavailability of about 10%. Muscarinic autonomic side effects of GI cramping, diarrhea, salivation, lacrimation, diaphoresis, and, when severe, bradycardia may occur with all of the CEI preparations. A feared potential complication of excessive CEI use is skeletal muscle weakness (cholinergic weakness). Patients receiving parenteral CEIs are at the greatest risk for cholinergic weakness. It is uncommon for patients receiving oral CEIs to develop significant cholinergic weakness even while experiencing muscarinic cholinergic side effects. Commonly available CEIs are summarized in Table 1.

Pyridostigmine (Mestinon) is the most widely used CEI for long-term oral therapy. The onset of effect is within 15 to 30 minutes of an oral dose, with peak effect within 1 to 2 hours. It wears off gradually 3 to 4 hours after the dose is given. The starting dose is 30 to 60 mg three to four times per day depending on symptoms. Optimal benefit usually occurs with a dose of 60 mg every 4 hours. Muscarinic cholinergic side effects are common with larger doses. Occasional patients require and tolerate more than 1000 mg per day, dosing as frequently as every 2 to 3 hours. Patients with significant bulbar weakness will often time their dose about 1 hour before meals to maximize chewing and swallowing. Of all the CEI preparations, pyridostigmine has the fewest muscarinic side effects. Pyridostigmine may be used in a number of alternative forms to the 60-mg tablet. The syrup may be necessary for children or for patients with difficulty swallowing pills. Sustained-release pyridostigmine, 180 mg (Mestinon Timespan), is sometimes preferred for nighttime use. Unpredictable release and absorption limit its use. Patients with severe dysphagia or those undergoing surgical procedures may need parenteral CEIs. Intravenous pyridostigmine should be given at about 1/30 of the oral dose. Neostigmine (Prostigmin) has a slightly shorter duration of action and slightly greater frequency of muscarinic side effects. Ambenonium (Mytelase) has shown no significant advantages over the other CEIs but has been suggested to be of greatest use in treating appendicular weakness. Headache is an additional occasional side effect.

For patients with intolerable muscarinic side effects at CEI doses required for optimal power, a concomitant anticholinergic drug such as atropine sulfate (0.4 to 0.5 mg orally) or glycopyrrolate (Robinul) (1 mg orally) on an as needed basis or with each dose of the CEI may be helpful. Patients with mild disease can often be managed adequately with CEIs. However, patients with moderate, severe, or progressive disease usually require more effective therapy.

Thymectomy

Association of the thymus gland with MG was first noted at the turn of the century, and thymectomy has become standard therapy over the past 50 years. Prospective controlled trials have not been performed for thymectomy. Nonetheless, a thymectomy is generally recommended for patients with moderate to severe MG, especially for those inadequately controlled on CEIs, and those younger than 55 years. All patients with suspected thymoma undergo surgery. About 75% of MG patients appear to benefit from a thymectomy. Patients may improve or simply stabilize. For unclear reasons, the onset of improvement tends to be delayed by a year or two in most patients (some patients seem to improve 5 to 10 years after surgery). The majority of centers use the trans-sternal approach for thymectomy with the goal of complete removal of the gland. The limited transcervical approach has been largely abandoned owing to the likelihood of incomplete gland removal. Some centers perform a "maximal thymectomy" to ensure complete removal. The procedure involves a combined trans-sternal-transcervical exposure with en bloc removal of the thymus. Because a sternal splitting thymectomy is a rugged procedure that results in a modest amount of temporary pain, an inability to work, and a cosmetically significant scar, newer approaches using thoracoscopy are becoming increasingly popular. If a thymectomy is to be performed, an experienced surgeon and anesthesiologist and a center with a good track record should be chosen and the patient should insist that they remove the entire gland.

Which patients do not undergo thymectomy? Patients with very mild or trivial symptoms do not have surgery. Most patients with pure ocular MG do not undergo thymectomy, although there has been some reported benefit in selected patients. Thymectomy is often avoided in children owing to the theoretical possibility of impairing the developing immune system. However, reports of thymectomy in children as young as 2 to 3 years of age have shown favorable results without adverse effects on the immune system. Thymectomy has been largely discouraged in patients older than 55 because of expected increased morbidity, latency of clinical benefit, and frequent observation of an atrophic, involuted gland. Nonetheless there are older patients reported to benefit from thymectomy. Major complications from thymectomy are uncommon as long as the surgery is performed at a center with anesthesiologists and neurologists familiar with the disease and perioperative management of MG patients. Common though less serious

TABLE 1. **Cholinesterase Inhibitors**

	Unit Dose	Average Dose
Pyridostigmine bromide tablet (Mestinon)	60 mg tablet	30–60 mg every 4–6 h
Pyridostigmine bromide syrup	12 mg/mL	30–60 mg every 4–6 h
Pyridostigmine bromide timespan (Mestinon Timespan)	180 mg tablet	1 tablet twice daily
Pyridostigmine bromide (parenteral) (Mestinon)	5 mg/mL ampules	1–2 mg every 3–4 h (1/30 of oral dose)
Neostigmine bromide (Prostigmin)	15 mg tablet	7.5–15 mg every 3–4 h
Neostigmine methylsulfate (parenteral)	0.25–1.0 mg/mL ampules	0.05 mg every 3–4 h
Ambenonium chloride (Mytelase)	10 mg, 25 mg tablets	2.5–5.0 mg every 4–6 h

aspects of thymectomy include postoperative chest pain (which may last several weeks), a 4- to 6-week convalescent period, and a cosmetically displeasing incisional scar.

Corticosteroids

No controlled trials document the benefit of corticosteroid* use in MG. However, nearly all authorities have personal experience with the virtues and complications of corticosteroid use in MG patients. In general corticosteroids are used in patients with moderate to severe disabling symptoms that are refractory to CEI therapy. Patients are commonly hospitalized to initiate therapy owing to the risk of early exacerbation. Opinions differ regarding the best method of administration. For patients with severe MG, it is best to begin with high-dose daily therapy of prednisone, 60 to 80 mg per day orally. Early exacerbation occurs in about half of patients usually within the first few days of therapy and typically lasting 3 or 4 days. In 10% of cases the exacerbation is severe, requiring mechanical ventilation or a feeding tube (thus the need to initiate therapy in the hospital). Overall about 80% of patients show a favorable response to steroids (with 30% attaining remission and 50% marked improvement). Mild to moderate improvement occurs in 15%, and 5% have no response. Improvement begins as early as 12 hours and as late as 60 days after beginning prednisone, but usually the patient begins to improve within the first week or two. Improvement is gradual, with marked improvement occurring at a mean of 3 months and maximal improvement at a mean of 9 months. Of those patients having a favorable response, most maintain their improvement with gradual dosage reduction at a rate of 10 mg every 1 to 2 months. More rapid reduction is usually associated with a flare-up of the disease. Although many patients can eventually be weaned off steroids and maintain their response, the majority cannot. They require a minimum dose (5 to 30 mg, alternate days) to maintain their improvement. Complications of long-term high-dose prednisone therapy are substantial, including cushingoid appearance, hypertension, osteoporosis, cataracts, aseptic necrosis, and the other well-known complications of chronic steroid therapy. Older patients tend to respond more favorably to prednisone. An alternative prednisone regimen involves low-dose alternate-day therapy, gradually increasing the schedule in an attempt to avoid the early exacerbation. Patients receive 25 mg of prednisone every other day, which is increased by 12.5 mg every third dose (about every fifth day) to a maximum dose of 100 mg every other day, or until sufficient improvement occurs. Clinical improvement usually begins within 1 month of treatment. The frequency and severity of early exacerbation is less than that associated with high-dose daily regimens. High-dose intravenous methylprednisolone (1000 mg daily for 3 to 5 days) can provide improvement within 1 to 2 weeks, but the clinical improvement is temporary.

*Not FDA approved for this indication.

Alternative Immunosuppressive Drug Therapy

Azathioprine (Imuran).* This drug is a cytotoxic purine analogue frequently used for immunosuppressive treatment of MG. Experience with azathioprine in treating MG is extensive but largely uncontrolled and retrospective. The starting dose is 50 mg orally daily, with complete blood count and liver function tests weekly in the beginning. If the drug is tolerated and if the blood work results are stable, the dose is increased by 50 mg every 1 to 2 weeks, aiming for a total daily dose of about 2 to 3 mg per kg per day (about 150 mg per day in the average-sized adult). When azathioprine is first started, about 15% of patients will have intolerable GI side effects (nausea, anorexia, abdominal discomfort) sometimes associated with fever, leading to discontinuation. Bone marrow suppression with relative leukopenia (white blood cell [WBC] count 2500 to 4000) occurs in 25% of patients but is usually not significant. If the WBC count drops below 2500 or the absolute granulocyte count falls below 1000, the drug is stopped (and the abnormalities usually resolve). Macrocytosis is common and of unclear clinical significance. Liver enzyme elevation occurs in 5 to 10% of patients but is usually reversible, and severe hepatic toxicity occurs in only about 1%. Infection occurs in about 5%. There is a theoretical risk of malignancy (based on observations in organ transplant patients), but this increased risk has not been established clearly in the MG patient population. About half of MG patients improve on azathioprine, with onset about 4 to 8 months into treatment. Maximal improvement takes about 12 months. Relapse after discontinuation of azathioprine occurs in more than half the patients, usually within 1 year.

Cyclosporine* (Sandimmune). This drug is used in patients with severe MG who cannot be managed adequately with corticosteroids or azathioprine. The starting dose is 3 to 5 mg per kg per day given in two divided doses. Cyclosporine blood levels should be measured monthly (aiming for a level of 200 to 300) along with electrolytes, magnesium, and renal function (in general, serum creatinine should not exceed 1.5 times the pretreatment level). Blood should be sampled before the morning dose is taken. More than half of patients improve on cyclosporine. The onset of clinical improvement occurs about 1 to 2 months after beginning therapy, and maximal improvement occurs at about 3 to 4 months. Side effects include renal toxicity and hypertension. Nonsteroidal anti-inflammatory drugs and potassium-sparing diuretics are among the drugs that should be avoided while on cyclosporine. For patients on corticosteroids, the addition of cyclosporine can lead to a reduction

*Not FDA approved for this indication.

in steroid dosage (although it is usually not possible to discontinue prednisone).

Cyclophosphamide (Cytoxan).* This drug is a nitrogen mustard antimetabolite occasionally used in severe refractory MG. A dose of 150 to 200 mg (3 to 5 mg per kg per day) oral cyclophosphamide or 5 days of 250 mg intravenous cyclophosphamide (followed by long-term oral therapy) is generally used. About half the patients improve beginning at about a month or two. Maximum improvement occurs by 6 months. The drug is discontinued if significant leukopenia or other major side effects occur. Alopecia, nausea, vomiting, anorexia, and infection are additional complications.

Plasma Exchange

Plasma exchange (plasmapheresis) removes ACh receptor antibodies and results in rapid clinical improvement. The standard course involves removal of 2 to 3 liters of plasma every other day or three times per week until the patient improves (usually a total of five or six exchanges). Improvement begins after the first few exchanges and reaches maximum within 2 to 3 weeks. The improvement is moderate to marked in nearly all patients but usually wears off after 4 to 8 weeks owing to the reaccumulation of pathogenic antibodies. Vascular access may require placement of a central line. Complications include hypotension, bradycardia, electrolyte imbalance, hemolysis, infection, and access problems (e.g., pneumothorax from placement of a central line). Indications for plasma exchange include any patient in whom a rapid temporary clinical improvement is needed.

High-Dose Intravenous Immunoglobulin

High-dose intravenous immunoglobulin (immune globulin intravenous [IGIV])* administration is associated with rapid improvement in MG symptoms. The mechanism is unclear but may relate to down-regulation of ACh-receptor antibody production or to the effect of anti-idiotype antibodies. The usual protocol is 2 grams per kg spread over 5 consecutive days (0.4 grams per kg per day). Different IGIV preparations are administered intravenously at different rates (contact the pharmacy for guidelines). The majority of MG patients improve, usually within 1 week of starting IGIV. The degree of response is variable, and the duration of response is limited, like plasma exchange, to about 4 to 8 weeks. Complications include fever, chills, and headache, which respond to slowing down the rate of the infusion and administering diphenhydramine. Occasional cases of aseptic meningitis, renal failure, nephrotic syndrome, and stroke have been reported. Also, patients with selective IgA deficiency can have anaphylaxis, which is best avoided by screening for IgA deficiency ahead of time. The treatment is relatively expensive, comparable to plasma exchange.

*Not FDA approved for this indication.

GUIDELINES FOR MANAGEMENT

1. Be certain of the diagnosis.
2. Provide patient education. Give the patient information about the natural course of the disease (including its variable and somewhat unpredictable course). Briefly review the treatment options outlined earlier, pointing out effectiveness, time course of improvement, duration of response, and complications. Provide the patient with educational pamphlets prepared by the Myasthenia Gravis Foundation or the Muscular Dystrophy Association.
3. Know when to hospitalize the patient. Patients with severe MG can deteriorate rapidly over a period of hours. Therefore, those having dyspnea should be hospitalized immediately in a constant observation or intensive care setting. Patients with moderate or severe dysphagia or weight loss and those with rapidly progressive or severe weakness should be admitted urgently. This will allow close monitoring and early intervention in the case of respiratory failure and will also expedite the diagnostic work-up and initiation of therapy.
4. Be familiar with the signs and symptoms of a myasthenic crisis. Myasthenic crisis (Table 2) is a medical emergency that is characterized by respiratory failure from diaphragm weakness or severe oropharyngeal weakness leading to aspiration. Crisis can occur in the setting of surgery (postoperative), acute infection, or following rapid withdrawal of corticosteroids (although some patients have no precipitating factors). Patients should be placed in an intensive care unit setting and have forced vital capacity (FVC) and forced expiratory volume in 1 second checked every 2 hours. Changes in arterial blood

TABLE 2. **The Acutely Deteriorating Myasthenic Patient**

Myasthenic Crisis
Respiratory failure
Respiratory arrest
Cyanosis
Increased pulse and blood pressure
Diaphoresis
Poor cough
Inability to handle oral secretions
Dysphagia
Weakness
Improves with edrophonium
Cholinergic Crisis
Abdominal cramps
Diarrhea
Nausea and vomiting
Excessive secretions
Miosis
Fasciculations
Diaphoresis
Weakness
Worse with edrophonium

gases occur relatively late in neuromuscular respiratory failure. There should be a low threshold for intubation and mechanical ventilation. Criteria for intubation include a drop in the FVC below 15 mL per kg (or below 1 liter in an average-sized adult), severe aspiration from oropharyngeal weakness, or labored breathing regardless of the measurements. If the diagnosis is not clear-cut, it is advisable to secure the airway with intubation, stabilize ventilation, and only then address the question of the underlying diagnosis. If the patient has been taking a CEI, the drug should be discontinued temporarily to rule out the possibility of "cholinergic crisis."

5. Screen for and correct any underlying medical problems such as systemic infection, metabolic problems (e.g., diabetes), and thyroid disease (hypo- or hyperthyroidism can exacerbate MG).

6. Know the drugs to avoid in MG. Avoid using D-penicillamine, interferon alfa, chloroquine, quinine, quinidine, and procainamide. Aminoglycoside antibiotics should be avoided unless they are needed to combat a life-threatening infection. Neuromuscular blocking drugs such as pancuronium (Pavulon) and D-tubocurarine can produce marked and prolonged paralysis in MG patients. Depolarizing drugs such as succinylcholine can also have a prolonged effect and should be used by a skilled anesthesiologist who is well aware of the patient's MG status.

GUIDELINES FOR SPECIFIC THERAPIES

Treatment for MG must be individualized (Table 3). Mild diplopia and ptosis may not be disabling for some patients, but for a pilot or neurosurgeon mild intermittent diplopia may be critical. In similar fashion, some patients may tolerate side effects better than others.

1. Mild or trivial weakness, either localized or generalized, should be managed with a CEI (pyridostigmine).

2. Moderate to marked weakness, localized or generalized, should be managed initially with a CEI. Even if symptoms are adequately controlled, patients younger than 55 undergo thymectomy early in the course of the disease (within the first year). In older patients, thymectomy is usually not performed unless the patient is thought to have a thymoma. Thymectomy is performed at a center with experienced personnel with the clear intent of complete removal of the gland. All patients with suspected thymoma (by chest scan) should have a thymectomy, even if their myasthenic symptoms are mild. Unless a thymoma is suspected, patients with pure ocular disease are usually not treated with thymectomy.

3. If symptoms are inadequately controlled with a CEI, immunosuppression is used. High-dose corticosteroid therapy is the most predictable and effective long-term option. If patients have severe, rapidly progressive, or life-threatening symptoms, the decision to start corticosteroids is clear-cut. Patients with disabling but stable symptoms may instead receive azathioprine, especially if there are particular concerns about using corticosteroids (i.e., the patient is already overweight, diabetic, or has cosmetic concerns). Patients who respond poorly or have unacceptable complications on steroids are started on azathioprine.

4. Plasma exchange or IGIV are indicated in the following circumstances:

- Rapidly progressive, life-threatening, impending myasthenic crisis or actual crisis, particularly if prolonged intubation with mechanical ventilation is judged hazardous.
- Preoperative stabilization of MG (such as before thymectomy or other elective surgery) in poorly controlled patients.
- Disabling MG refractory to other therapies.

5. If the previously listed options fail, use cyclosporine.

6. If the patient's condition remains poorly controlled despite treatment as mentioned earlier, then perform a repeat chest computed tomography scan looking for residual thymus. Some patients improve after "repeat thymectomy." Check for other medical problems (diabetes, thyroid disease, infection, and coexisting autoimmune diseases).

7. Referral to a neurologist or center specializing in neuromuscular disease is advised for all patients with suspected MG and can be particularly important for complicated or refractory patients.

TABLE 3. **Treatment of Myasthenia Gravis**

Mild weakness: cholinesterase inhibitors
Moderate-marked localized or generalized weakness:
  Cholinesterase inhibitors, and
  Thymectomy for patients younger than age 55 (complete removal)
If symptoms are uncontrolled on cholinesterase inhibitors, use immunosuppression
  Prednisone if severe or urgent
  Azathioprine if
    Prednisone contraindicated
    Prednisone failure
    Excessive prednisone side effects
Plasma exchange or intravenous immune globulin (IGIV)
  Impending crisis, actual crisis
  Preoperative boost (if needed)
  Chronic disease refractory to drug therapy
If the above fails:
  Search for residual thymus tissue
  Cyclosporine
  High-dose IGIV (monthly)
  Referral to neuromuscular specialty group

OTHER ISSUES

Transient Neonatal Myasthenia. This condition occurs in 10 to 15% of babies born to mothers with autoimmune MG. Within the first few days after delivery, the baby has a weak cry or suck, appears floppy, and on occasion requires mechanical ventilation. The condition is caused by maternal antibodies that cross the placenta late in pregnancy. As these maternal antibodies are replaced by the baby's own antibodies the symptoms gradually disappear, usually within a few weeks, and the baby is normal thereafter. Infants with severe weakness are treated with oral pyridostigmine, 1 to 2 mg per kg every 4 hours.

Congenital Myasthenia. This represents a group of rare hereditary disorders of the neuromuscular junction. The patients tend to have lifelong relatively stable symptoms of generalized fatigable weakness. These disorders are nonimmunologic, without ACh-receptor antibodies, and therefore patients do not respond to immune therapy (steroids, thymectomy, plasma exchange). Most of these patients improve with CEI use.

Lambert-Eaton Syndrome (LES) (Myasthenic Syndrome). This syndrome is a presynaptic disease characterized by chronic fluctuating weakness of proximal limb muscles. Symptoms include difficulty walking, climbing stairs, or rising from a chair. In LES there may be some improvement in power with sustained or repeated exercise. In contrast to MG, ptosis, diplopia, dysphagia, and respiratory failure are far less common. In addition, LES patients often complain of myalgias, muscle stiffness of the back and legs, distal paresthesias, metallic taste, dry mouth, impotence, and other autonomic symptoms of muscarinic cholinergic insufficiency. LES is rare compared with MG, which is about 100 times more common. About half to two thirds of LES patients have an underlying malignancy that is usually small cell carcinoma of the lung. In patients without malignancy, LES is an autoimmune disease and can be associated with other autoimmune phenomena. In general, patients older than 40 are more likely to be men and have an associated malignancy, whereas younger patients are more likely to be women and have no neoplasm. LES symptoms can precede detection of the malignancy by 1 to 2 years.

The diagnosis is confirmed with EMG studies, which typically show low amplitude of the compound muscle action potentials (CMAP), and a decrement to slow rates or repetitive stimulation. Following brief exercise, there is marked facilitation of the CMAP amplitude. At high rates of repetitive stimulation, there may be an incremental response. Single-fiber EMG results are markedly abnormal in virtually all patients with LES. The pathogenesis involves autoantibodies directed against voltage-gated calcium channels at cholinergic motor nerve terminals. These IgG antibodies also inhibit cholinergic synapses of the autonomic nervous system. More than half of LES patients demonstrate these antibodies to voltage-gated calcium channels in serum, providing another useful diagnostic test. In patients with associated malignancy, successful treatment of the tumor can lead to improvement in the LES symptoms. Symptomatic improvement in neuromuscular transmission may occur with the use of CEIs such as pyridostigmine. Guanidine has shown some benefit, but its use has been limited by bone marrow, renal, and hepatic toxicity. Guanidine increases the release of ACh by increasing the duration of the action potential at the motor nerve terminal. 3,4-Diaminopyridine (DAP) increases ACh release by blocking voltage-dependent potassium conductance and thereby prolonging depolarization at the nerve terminal and enhancing the voltage-dependent calcium influx. 3,4-DAP has been shown to clearly improve the condition of most patients with LES with relatively mild toxicity and is becoming increasingly available, such that it represents first-line symptomatic therapy for LES.

Immunosuppressive therapy is used in patients with disabling symptoms. Long-term high-dose corticosteroids, azathioprine, plasma exchange, and IGIV have all been used with moderate success. In general, the use of these therapies should be tailored to the severity of patients' symptoms.

TRIGEMINAL NEURALGIA

method of
KIM J. BURCHIEL, M.D., and
DEON LOUW, M.D.
Oregon Health Sciences University
Portland, Oregon

CLINICAL PRESENTATION

Trigeminal neuralgia (tic douloureux) is typically described as fleeting, lancinating pain lasting seconds to minutes that occurs in the sensory distribution of the trigeminal nerve. The pain commonly strikes the third (mandibular) division of the nerve along the jaw or lower teeth or tongue; less commonly, it affects second (maxillary) and first (ophthalmic) divisions. Frequently, more than one distribution is affected, and the pain seemingly radiates from one division to the other. The pain is almost always unilateral, although very rarely, bilateral trigeminal neuralgia can be seen. The typical pains are always paroxysmal, often described as "electrical" in quality by patients.

There is usually a perioral trigger zone in the second or third division. Triggering stimuli often include talking, eating, oral hygiene activities such as toothbrushing, and wind or cold temperatures on the face. Light tactile, nonnoxious stimulation of the trigger zone produces the typical neuralgic pains commonly seen. Frequently, the pain occurs spontaneously either from environmental stimuli or without apparent trigger. Because of the triggerability of the pain, patients often do not groom the affected side of the face during acute episodes and may not eat or even swallow oral secretions.

The disorder is often characterized by pain-free intervals, which can last from months to even years. After a pain-free interval, the pain returns exactly as before the hiatus. Neurologic examination in the typical case reveals no deficit. Sensory loss, even minimal, in the area of the pain or of the trigger zone suggests structural pathology or severe compression of the nerve in the posterior fossa.

This disorder primarily affects older patients (60 years and older), but individuals from their teens to older than 90 years can be affected. There is a slight predominance of females to males with the disorder, and the pain is slightly more common on the right side of the face.

Atypical trigeminal neuralgia combines features of typical idiopathic trigeminal neuralgia, i.e., brief, lancinating, unilateral, electrical pains, with a constant background pain that is usually described as either aching or burning. These pains are likewise unilateral, and facial sensory loss is more common.

Secondary trigeminal neuralgia represents approximately 2% of cases of trigeminal neuralgia, and atypical pain is more common. There is always a sensory loss, and patients are found to have tumors or vascular lesions that cause compression of the nerve. The age range is usually lower than that for typical idiopathic trigeminal neuralgia, and male and female incidences are about equal.

Symptomatic trigeminal neuralgia occurs in association with multiple sclerosis and may manifest as either typical or atypical pains. Approximately 1% of patients with multiple sclerosis develop trigeminal neuralgia, which in rare cases is the presenting complaint. Thirty to 35 years is the average age at presentation for symptomatic trigeminal neuralgia.

Post-traumatic trigeminal neuralgia occurs approximately 5 to 10% of the time after facial trauma or oral surgery. It is reported to be seen in between 1 and 5% of patients after removal of impacted teeth. The painful episodes are sharp and episodic and are often triggered, like the pain of typical trigeminal neuralgia. Superimposed is a background of dull, throbbing, or burning pain like that of atypical trigeminal neuralgia. These post-traumatic pain problems may represent either trigeminal "neuroma" or deafferentation pain, i.e., pain after *loss* of nervous system input. This diagnosis overlaps substantially with atypical facial pain.

Atypical facial pain may be included with a number of disorders that come under the rubric pain of psychologic origin in the head and face. There is no known physical cause or pathophysiologic mechanism for this type of pain. Once other causes of the pain are ruled out, such as sinus disease and migrainous neuralgia, the diagnosis of atypical facial pain should be considered. Usually, there is also proof of contributing psychologic factors, and the characteristics of this group of patients overlap those in the American Psychiatric Association definition of psychogenic pain disorder. The pain is usually described as diffuse or nonanatomic in the orofacial region. There is a steady, often burning or aching quality. Atypical facial pain may mimic other syndromes. There is often obvious psychopathology, including delusions, hallucinations, and multiple physical complaints. There may also be conversion or pseudoneurotic symptoms and signs. Psychologic evaluation reveals signs of somatization, depression, and illness behaviors. Patients typically exhibit excessive treatment- or medication-seeking behavior. Neurologic examination is almost invariably normal, although there may be poorly localized tenderness and vague, nonreproducible sensory loss.

DIAGNOSIS

The diagnosis of typical trigeminal neuralgia is usually not difficult if it is considered. Again, a patient with unilateral, fleeting, lancinating, electric shock–like facial pains in the trigeminal sensory distribution generally has trigeminal neuralgia. The pains are alleviated by carbamazepine (Tegretol), which in itself is a diagnostic test, because no other orofacial pain responds to this anticonvulsant. The diagnosis of the overlap syndrome, atypical trigeminal neuralgia, may be more problematic, but again, fleeting pains are the hallmark of the disorder. Patients with constant pain only (atypical facial pain) should be treated nonsurgically and not without thorough diagnostic evaluation, in most cases including psychologic evaluation.

Although the diagnosis of trigeminal neuralgia is generally made from clinical criteria, computed tomography or magnetic resonance imaging of the head should be performed to rule out the uncommon instance of intracranial pathology. The latter may be preferable because of its superior imaging of the posterior fossa and of demyelinating disease.

ETIOLOGY

The underlying cause of trigeminal neuralgia is still debated. In typical trigeminal neuralgia, considerable evidence suggests that cross-compression of the nerve at its entry into the pons by an artery or vein may be the inciting event. Demyelination may occur at this point of cross-compression. Some autopsy results in patients with trigeminal neuralgia and multiple sclerosis indicate that demyelination within the descending tract of the trigeminal nerve or within the nerve itself can be correlated with the disorder. As mentioned previously, other structural lesions, such as tumors, aneurysms, and arteriovenous malformations, rarely can cross-compress the nerve and produce quite typical pain.

TREATMENT

Medical Management

The medical treatment of typical idiopathic trigeminal neuralgia is usually quite rewarding. Carbamazepine is started in doses of 100 mg twice daily and then increased by 200 mg per day every 2 to 3 days, until a final daily dose in the range of 800 to 1000 mg is reached. Under unusual circumstances, experienced clinicians have prescribed up to 2000 mg per day.

Before this medication is started, a baseline white blood cell (WBC) count is obtained, because not uncommonly, mild leukopenia can occur during medical treatment. Rarely, a non–dose-dependent and idiosyncratic bone marrow suppression (aplastic anemia) can occur early in treatment, which must be watched for diligently. The WBC count is typically repeated a week after therapy is begun, approximately 3 to 4 weeks later, and then every several months while the patient is taking the drug. Most typical cases of trigeminal neuralgia respond to carbamazepine to some extent. In fact, as mentioned previously, this response is a powerful and reliable diagnostic confirmation of trigeminal neuralgia.

Limitations of carbamazepine treatment are hypersensitivity reactions that preclude use of the drug and, at higher doses, symptoms of drowsiness, mental dullness, subjective dizziness, and ataxia. These latter, common symptoms can be quite troublesome in elderly patients.

A newer agent, gabapentin (Neurontin)* may be as effective as carbamazepine. Gabapentin seems to be better tolerated, although it also can produce drowsiness, dizziness, and mental dullness at higher

*Not FDA approved for this indication.

doses. It is typically begun at 300 mg per day and the dose is increased by 300 mg every 2 to 3 days until relief is achieved. Some patients can tolerate as much as 4000 to 6000 mg per day, but most experience side effects at 1500 to 1800 mg per day. Alternatively, baclofen (Lioresal)* may be substituted with good effect. This drug is started at 5 mg twice daily and then increased by 5 to 10 mg every 2 to 3 days to a maximal dose of 80 mg per day. Baclofen is not usually helpful in patients who are otherwise able to take carbamazepine or gabapentin but who continue to have neuralgic pains at high doses and are intolerant of the side effects. The anticonvulsant phenytoin can also be used but is rarely of additional benefit when the other drugs have failed. Should any of these agents prove to be ineffective, patients should be weaned gradually to prevent withdrawal seizures. A typical regimen is dose reduction by a single tablet on alternate days.

In general, about 70% of patients respond at least initially to medical management. However, as time goes on, the drugs become ineffective in many patients, and the pain "breaks through" the pharmacologic therapy. In fact, for most patients followed up carefully for many years, medical management eventually fails.

Surgical Management

The surgical approach to trigeminal neuralgia is likewise highly effective. The procedures can generally be considered in two groups, percutaneous procedures and microvascular decompression. Dozens of other operations have been developed in the past 5 or 6 decades, but these two surgical approaches seem to hold most of the surgical attention and promise at present.

Percutaneous procedures are generally performed on an outpatient basis or with, at most, a brief stay in the hospital. In general, the risks of the procedures are minimal, and for this reason, they are generally thought to be more appropriate for the elderly (older than 65 years) or debilitated patient. The risk of death from these operations is close to zero, and morbidity is usually minimal or acceptable.

Currently, three main percutaneous procedures are performed: percutaneous radiofrequency trigeminal gangliolysis (PRTG), percutaneous retrogasserian glycerol rhizotomy (PRGR), and percutaneous balloon microcompression (PBM). In all these procedures, with the patient under local or brief general anesthesia, a needle or trocar is inserted from a point on the cheek just lateral to the corner of the mouth, and then, under fluoroscopic guidance, the needle is introduced into the ipsilateral foramen ovale. The position of the needle is fluoroscopically verified in the lateral position, and then the gangliolysis is performed.

The PRTG procedure uses radiofrequency (RF) heating of the tip of an electrode to produce a thermal lesion in the ganglion, with the production of appropriate facial numbness in the area of pain or the trigger zone as the end point. RF lesions are produced using brief general anesthesia with a short-acting intravenous anesthetic.

The PRGR procedure is likewise performed using a spinal needle, until cerebrospinal fluid (CSF) from the trigeminal cistern is encountered. With the patient in the sitting position, a trigeminal cisternogram is obtained using radiopaque, water-soluble contrast material. After the contrast dye is removed, anhydrous glycerol (approximately 0.3 mL) is instilled into the cistern. The patient remains in the seated position with the neck flexed slightly forward for 2 hours to obtain the maximal neurolytic effect.

The PBM procedure uses a trocar placed into the region of the trigeminal ganglion, whereupon a balloon catheter is inserted into this region and is inflated for 2 minutes. The PRGR and PBM procedures do not routinely produce facial numbness, which therefore is not used as an end point. Sporadically, considerable numbness can be produced by the glycerol procedure, although it is reportedly rare with the balloon compression technique.

The alternative procedure, which is more commonly applied to younger (younger than 65 years) and healthy patients with typical or atypical trigeminal neuralgia, is the microvascular decompression procedure. With the patient under general anesthesia, a small incision is made behind the ear. A 2.5- to 3-cm craniectomy is performed, the dura is opened, and the cerebellum is microsurgically retracted, revealing the trigeminal nerve. Typically, an artery or other vascular cross-compression of the nerve is identified at the pontine entry area of the nerve; the vascular structure is padded away from the nerve with polytetrafluoroethylene (Teflon) felt. This operation has a low but nonzero mortality rate, between 0.1 and 0.5% in most series. It does not ordinarily produce numbness, but complications involving hearing loss, dizziness, cerebellar syndrome, CSF leaks, meningitis, and diplopia have been seen in a few patients. Serious morbidity probably averages between 1 and 5%. An alternative surgical treatment is gamma-knife radiosurgery. However, patient volume and follow-up are not as extensive with this modality.

Results of Surgical Therapy

The best way to compare the outcome of pain-relieving procedures such as these is to look at the point at which 50% of patients can be statistically expected to experience return of pain. Initial efficacy for these surgical procedures is quite good. Most series report that more than 90% of patients are pain free after any of the procedures previously described. If the pain recurs, a percutaneous procedure can be repeated, and by that means, almost all patients can be successfully treated. If microvascular decompression initially fails to relieve the pain, a percutaneous procedure can be performed after an appropriate recovery interval and is also highly likely to result in a pain-free state.

*Not FDA approved for this indication.

For the PRGR procedure, the expected pain-free interval is approximately 1.5 to 2 years, and similar results have been seen with the PBM technique. The PRTG procedure produces about twice the pain-free interval, or about 3 to 4 years; for microvascular decompression, the pain relief can be expected to last an average of 15 years.

OPTIC NEURITIS

method of
ANDREW G. LEE, M.D.
Baylor College of Medicine
Houston, Texas

and

PAUL W. BRAZIS, M.D.
Mayo Clinic—Jacksonville
Jacksonville, Florida

Optic neuritis (ON) is an immune-mediated, demyelinating (idiopathic or associated with multiple sclerosis [MS]) disease of the optic nerve, which typically manifests with the following clinical profile:

1. Acute, usually unilateral (but may be bilateral) loss of visual acuity, color vision, and/or visual field that usually progresses over 7 days or less and begins to improve over the following 30 days.
2. An afferent pupillary defect in unilateral or bilateral but asymmetrical cases.
3. Periocular pain, especially with eye movement, in 90% of patients.
4. Usually normal (i.e., retrobulbar) in 65% but sometimes swollen (i.e., papillitis) optic nerve head in 35% of patients, with eventual optic disk atrophy after 4 to 6 weeks.
5. Often a young adult female (but may affect patients of any age and either gender).
6. Transient visual loss with exercise or increased body temperature (Uhthoff's phenomenon).
7. Objects traveling in a straight line (e.g., a pendulum swinging back and forth) may appear to follow a curved trajectory (the Pulfrich phenomenon) owing to an asymmetrical conduction time between normal and abnormal optic nerves.

We consider the following features to be atypical manifestations of ON:

1. Bilateral simultaneous onset of ON in an adult patient (although bilateral onset may be present in children).
2. Lack of pain (although may be painless in 10% of patients).
3. Greater than minimal vitreous cell reaction (although pars plana inflammation and/or retinal periphlebitis may be present).
4. Presence of macular exudate (star figure).
5. Lack of significant improvement after 30 days.
6. Age older than 50 years.

The Optic Neuritis Treatment Trial (ONTT) was a randomized, controlled clinical trial sponsored by the National Eye Institute that enrolled 457 patients at 15 clinical centers in the United States between the years 1988 and 1991. The ONTT entry criteria included the following:

1. Patients who were between the ages of 18 and 46 years.
2. Patients who had an afferent pupillary defect and a visual field defect in the affected eye consistent with the clinical diagnosis of ON.
3. Patients who were examined within 8 days of the onset of visual symptoms of a first attack of acute unilateral ON.

Patient exclusion criteria included the following:

1. Previous episodes of ON in the affected eye.
2. Previous corticosteroid treatment for ON or MS or systemic disease other than MS that might be a cause for the ON.

The patients were assigned randomly to one of three treatment arms in the study:

1. Intravenous (IV) methylprednisolone sodium succinate (Solu-Medrol) (250 mg every 6 hours for 3 days) followed by oral prednisone (1 mg per kg per day for 11 days).
2. Oral prednisone (1 mg per kg per day for 14 days).
3. Oral placebo for 14 days. Each oral regimen was followed by a short oral taper consisting of 20 mg on day 15 and 10 mg on days 16 and 18.

In the ONTT, all patients underwent testing for collagen vascular disease (e.g., antinuclear antibody [ANA]), serologic testing for syphilis (e.g., FTA-ABS), and a chest radiograph for sarcoidosis. A lumbar puncture was optional. The ANA test results were positive in a titer less than 1:320 in 13% of patients, and 1:320 or greater in 3% of patients. Only one patient was eventually diagnosed with a collagen vascular disease. Visual and neurologic outcomes in these patients were no different from those in the other ONTT patients. The FTA-ABS test results were positive in six patients (1.3%), but none had syphilis. A chest radiograph did not reveal sarcoidosis in any patient. Lumbar puncture did not produce any additional unsuspected diagnoses in the 141 patients undergoing cerebrospinal fluid analysis.

TESTING

We follow the management recommendations of the ONTT study group for patients with typical acute ON:

1. Laboratory testing. Chest radiograph, laboratory tests (e.g., syphilis serology, collagen vascular disease, serum chemistries, complete blood counts), and lumbar puncture are not necessary for patients with typical ON.
2. Neuroimaging. Magnetic resonance (MR) imaging of the brain should be considered to assess the risk of future neurologic events of MS and for treatment decision-making.
3. Patients with atypical ON should undergo laboratory testing, including consideration for a lumbar puncture, depending on the results of a thorough history and examination for evidence of syphilis or other sexually transmitted disease, underlying collagen vascular disease, or sarcoidosis. Patients with optic disk edema and a macular star ("neuroretinitis") should undergo a more directed evaluation (e.g., syphilis serology, cat-scratch titer, Lyme titer).

TREATMENT

Although corticosteroids have been the mainstay of therapy for acute ON, well-controlled data to support their treatment efficacy have been lacking until recently. The ONTT was subsequently developed to evaluate the efficacy of corticosteroid treatment for acute ON and investigate the relationship between ON and MS. The major conclusions of the ONTT related to treatment are summarized as follows:

1. High-dose IV corticosteroids followed by oral corticosteroids accelerated visual recovery but provided no long-term benefit to vision.
2. "Standard dose" oral prednisone alone did not improve the visual outcome and was associated with an increased rate of new attacks of ON.
3. IV corticosteroids followed by oral corticosteroids reduced the rate of development of clinically definite MS during the first 2 years, particularly in patients with signal abnormalities on brain MR imaging, but by 3 years the treatment effect had subsided.

Based on these results, the ONTT study group recommended that treatment with oral prednisone in standard doses be avoided in ON and that treatment with IV methylprednisolone be considered in patients with abnormal brain MR imaging results or a particular need (e.g., a monocular patient or one with an occupational requirement) to recover visual function more rapidly. Although brain MR imaging may not be necessary for diagnosis of ON, neuroimaging may be valuable for prognostic purposes. In the ONTT, patients with multiple signal abnormalities on MR imaging most clearly benefited from IV corticosteroid therapy in terms of the development of MS, but the rate of development of MS was too low in the patients with normal MR imaging results to assess treatment benefit in this group.

PROGNOSIS

Although most patients with idiopathic or demyelinating ON recover visual function within 30 days, some patients do not experience complete recovery. Other patients, despite 20/20 Snellen visual acuity, complain of subjective visual loss that may correspond with persistent defects of color vision, contrast sensitivity, depth perception, visual field, or motion perception. In the ONTT, visual acuity was 20/40 or better in 93% of patients at 12 months, but 3% of patients had 20/200 or worse visual acuity. Patients with idiopathic ON (especially those with multiple periventricular white matter abnormalities on MR imaging) are at risk for the development of MS. The rate of development of MS following ON is quite variable in the literature but may be as high as 75% after 15 years in some series.

GLAUCOMA

method of
TODD W. PERKINS, M.D.
University of Wisconsin
Madison, Wisconsin

Glaucoma is an eye disease that is related to elevated intraocular pressure (IOP), which causes progressive damage to the optic nerves and leads to loss of peripheral vision that can be detected with visual field testing. Glaucoma is the third leading cause of blindness in the United States overall and the leading cause in African-Americans. However, probably less than 10% of appropriately treated glaucoma patients become blind; half of the patients who are blind in one eye became so because of undiagnosed disease. Most glaucoma is difficult to detect because no symptoms occur until very late in the disease.

Although the management of glaucoma is mainly within the purview of ophthalmologists and some optometrists, primary care physicians can play an important role in the diagnosis and concomitant medical care of patients with glaucoma. Approximately half of the patients with glaucoma in the United States do not know that they have the disease, and many of these patients see primary care physicians for other health problems. It is important that these patients be screened for glaucoma with ophthalmoscopy in the course of routine physical examination. Patients with optic nerve cupping that creates a cup to disk ratio of 0.7 or greater require a work-up that includes measurement of IOP, automated visual field analysis, and photographic and scanning laser images of the optic nerves. Patients with a family history of glaucoma in a parent or sibling should also receive a baseline examination.

Approximately 90% of patients with glaucoma in the United States have primary open-angle glaucoma (POAG). A closely related form of glaucoma that may occur in adults younger than 40 years old is juvenile open-angle glaucoma (JOAG), which is largely genetic in origin. The other major form of glaucoma is acute angle-closure glaucoma (AACG). A rare form of glaucoma—congenital glaucoma—affects infants.

PRIMARY OPEN-ANGLE GLAUCOMA

POAG is generally treated medically. The number and variety of medications used in glaucoma treatment has expanded greatly in the past 2 years, and the place of many of the newer medications in the therapeutic decision tree has not been well established.

It is essential that primary care physicians recognize that all of the medications used in glaucoma treatment may cause systemic side effects that may not be connected by the patient to their eye drops. Drugs delivered as eye drops still achieve significant systemic blood levels. The general approach to drug therapy for POAG is similar to that used for systemic hypertension. Treatment is started with the medication least likely to cause side effects yet potent enough to bring the IOP down below a target level set for each patient. In glaucoma, however, the target pressure is slightly different for each patient, depending on the stage of the disease and the IOP at which previous damage occurred. Generally, a level of 15 to 18 mm Hg is chosen, or a reduction of 25 to 30% below pretreatment levels. A list of medications and their common systemic side effects is given in Table 1.

The usual first-line drug for treatment of POAG is a nonspecific beta blocker. Beta blockers typically result in a 25% reduction in IOP. One formulation of timolol uses a gel vehicle (Timoptic-XE) that allows

TABLE 1. **Glaucoma Medications**

Medication	Dose	Systemic Side Effects
First-Line Drugs		
Beta-adrenergic antagonists		Bronchospasm, bradycardia, depression
Nonselective		
Timolol maleate gel (Timoptic-XE)	0.5% qd	
Timolol maleate (Timoptic, Betimol, generic)	0.5% bid	
Levobunolol hydrochloride (Betagan)	0.5% bid	
Carteolol hydrochloride (Ocupress)	1% bid	
Metipranolol (Optipranolol)	0.3% bid	
Selective (beta$_1$)		
Betaxolol hydrochloride (Betoptic)	0.25–0.5% bid	Rare bronchospasm, bradycardia
Prostaglandin agonist		
Latanoprost (Xalatan)	0.005% qhs	Few
Second-Line Drugs		
Alpha agonist		
Brimonidine (Alphagan)	0.2 tid	Dry mouth, tiredness
Carbonic anhydrase inhibitor		
Dorzolamide (Trusopt)	2% bid–tid	Metallic taste
Third-Line Drugs		
Alpha agonist		
Apraclonidine (lopidine)	0.5% tid	Dry mouth, tiredness
Cholinergic agonist		Rare gastrointestinal upset, cardiac symptoms at high doses
Pilocarpine hydrochloride (Isopto Carpine, Pilocar, generic pilocarpine)	1–4% qid	
Pilopine HS gel	4% qhs	
Ocusert Pilo membrane	20, 40 μg/h	
Oral carbonic anhydrase inhibitors		Malaise, gastrointestinal upset, diarrhea, potassium depletion
Methazolamide (Neptazane)	50 mg tid	
Acetazolamide (Diamox)		
Sequels	500 mg qd–bid	
Tablets	250 mg qid	
Nonspecific adrenergic agonists		
Dipivefrin (Propine)	0.1%	Rare tachycardia, hypertension
Epinephrine (Glaucon, Epifrin)	1%	Tachycardia, hypertension

once-daily administration. The other preparations are usually given twice daily. This class of drug is contraindicated in patients with reactive airway disease or high degrees of heart block. With these limitations in mind, side effects are relatively uncommon but include all the effects of systemic beta blockers, including depression and impotence. The relatively selective beta$_1$ agent betaxolol (Betoptic) poses much less risk of systemic side effects but is slightly less effective as well.

An exciting new class of drug that is potent at very low concentrations and has extremely rare systemic side effects is a prostaglandin agonist. Preliminary work has shown the first of these, latanoprost (Xalatan), to be more effective than a beta blocker and to have fewer side effects. It has two interesting ocular side effects: hazel-colored irides become more brown, and eye lashes become longer, darker, and thicker. It is used once a day at bedtime. Currently a first-line drug, more widespread use will determine whether other presently unknown deleterious effects will change its position.

Second-line agents include two newer agents that have few side effects but that are slightly less efficacious than the first-line drugs and require twice to thrice daily use. The first is brimonidine (Alphagan), an alpha agonist. When used three times a day, this drug is probably almost as effective as a beta blocker. The major ocular side effect is local allergy (10%), and systemic effects include tiredness and dry mouth. The other second-line agent is dorzolamide (Trusopt), a topical carbonic anhydrase inhibitor. This drug is less effective than a beta blocker, although it has few side effects other than causing a metallic taste in the mouth.

Third-line agents include several drugs that were recently considered first-line agents but have side effects that make them much less attractive than the newer agents. Apraclonidine (lopidine) is an alpha agonist similar to brimonidine, although its use is limited by a high incidence of local allergy (10 to 30%) and a question of tachyphylaxis. Pilocarpine (Pilocar) is limited by four times a day usage and pupillary constriction that causes decreased vision and headaches. Alternative delivery systems are available such as a nighttime gel and a membrane that releases the drug slowly over a week, but these vehicles are variably tolerated by patients. Oral carbonic anhydrase inhibitors are limited by side effects of malaise and gastrointestinal upset. Potassium loss is common, particularly in patients receiving hydrochlorothiazide diuretics. Dipivefrin (Propine) is limited by a 25% incidence of redness and irritation of the eye.

Medications are generally started in one eye (a monocular trial) for 1 month. The IOP is measured and compared with that in the untreated eye, and any side effects are noted. If effective, the medication is started in the other eye. Additional medications are added until the target IOP is reached. Medications causing troublesome side effects are generally discontinued and others substituted. Not uncommonly, medications cause no side effects until much later during use. Patients may report systemic symptoms that are related to glaucoma medications to their primary care physician that they do not connect to their eye drop use. For example, a family member may note that an elderly parent is increasingly fatigued and "not herself," a not uncommon side effect of brimonidine.

An alternative to medication for treatment of POAG, and about as effective as a beta blocker, is the use of argon laser trabeculoplasty. Laser treatment is tolerated well by patients. This mode of treatment may be especially useful for patients who cannot be relied on to comply with a regimen of drops or who have side effects from the medications.

When medications and laser have both failed to control IOP, a surgical procedure, trabeculectomy, may be performed. This procedure creates another outflow tract for fluid to leave the eye, thus lowering the IOP. In the United States, most physicians exhaust medical options before recommending trabeculectomy because its effectiveness is about 80% and it carries an approximately 5 to 10% risk of diminished vision or the need for reoperation for complications.

JUVENILE OPEN-ANGLE GLAUCOMA

A form of glaucoma indistinguishable from POAG except for the age of onset is JOAG. JOAG is a rarer form of glaucoma that represents only 2 to 3% of patients; it may manifest in the third and fourth decade of life. Almost all patients with JOAG have a genetic abnormality and a strong family history of the disease. Treatment is the same as for POAG except that many patients with JOAG respond very poorly to medication and often require surgery to control their disease.

ACUTE ANGLE-CLOSURE GLAUCOMA

In contrast to POAG, AACG manifests with dramatic symptoms of blurred vision with colored halos around lights, pain, redness, and often nausea and vomiting related to the pain. The diagnosis is based on findings of a mid-dilated and unreactive pupil, a cloudy cornea obscuring the view inside the eye, and a vastly elevated IOP (40 to 80 mm Hg). When the primary care physician is seeing such a patient in the emergency department and local ophthalmologic care is unavailable, initial medical treatment is often commenced by the primary care physician before referral of the patient owing to the acute nature of this disease. Delay in treatment may result in development of a chronic severe glaucoma that is resistant to all treatment, permanent vision loss, or even blindness.

Treatment of AACG requires prompt lowering of the IOP, typically with hyperosmotic agents. In the emergency department setting, the easiest approach is to use intravenous (IV) mannitol, 1 to 2 grams per kg of body weight. The solution is given as quickly as the patient's medical condition allows, usually 500 mL over 15 to 20 minutes. In an office setting, where placement of an IV line may be delayed, an oral solution of isosorbide 45% (Ismotic), 1 to 2 grams per kg, can be given with orange juice and ice chips. Another alternative is glycerin 50% (Osmoglyn), 1 to 2 grams per kg, although this solution has enough calories to be a problem for diabetic patients. At the same time, topical pilocarpine 2% is given to constrict the pupil and to "break the attack," although the pilocarpine will not be effective until the IOP is reduced below approximately 50 mm Hg. Other topical drugs are also given to assist lowering the IOP. A nonspecific beta blocker such as timolol, an alpha agonist such as apraclonidine, and oral acetazolamide (Diamox), 500 mg tablets, are all typically given. If such a regimen is given, almost all attacks will be broken unless there has been a delay of a number of hours in treatment.

The mainstay of treatment is a yttrium aluminum garnet (YAG) laser peripheral iridotomy, which may be performed as soon as the cornea is clear enough to pass laser energy (1 to 12 hours). An argon laser peripheral iridoplasty may also be performed almost immediately and may more rapidly break the attack by pulling the iris out of the drainage tract of the eye. An attack of AACG is not considered treated until a peripheral iridotomy is in place and the drainage angle of the eye is visibly open on examination by gonioscopy.

Patients with AACG treated within a few hours of an attack can be effectively cured of their disease. A prophylactic laser treatment is performed on the other eye to prevent a similar attack. Patients who have had a delay of treatment of more than several hours may present particular difficulties in management. Medical and laser treatment may fail and necessitate surgical intervention and lifetime management of chronic angle-closure glaucoma.

Patients may be screened for a predisposition to AACG by examining the depth of the anterior chamber angle using a slit lamp. Patients with so-called occludable angles who are at risk for an attack of AACG can receive laser peripheral iridotomy to prevent an attack.

CONGENITAL GLAUCOMA

Congenital glaucoma is a rare disease that typically manifests within the first 6 months of life with hazy corneas, tearing, and light sensitivity. Management is primarily surgical.

ACUTE IDIOPATHIC FACIAL PALSY
(Bell's Palsy)

method of
MANUEL MAÑÓS-PUJOL, M.D., PH.D.
Ciutat Sanitària Universitària de Bellvitge
Barcelona, Spain

Bell's palsy is an acute peripheral paralysis of the face produced by a viral immune-mediated disease. Until a few years ago, Bell's palsy was considered of idiopathic origin and was a diagnosis exclusion disease. Now, we know that Bell's palsy is a different disease entity, with characteristic symptoms and signs, and diagnosis is not made by exclusion but by clinical history and physical examination. To establish a correct and early diagnosis and treatment plan, it is mandatory to know some aspects of its incidence, etiology, pathogenesis, diagnosis, and treatment.

INCIDENCE

Among the more than 90 causes of facial paralysis, Bell's palsy is the most frequent. Its incidence varies between 15 and 40 per 100,000 population per year, without evidence of racial predilection. The incidence of Bell's palsy increases with age. Between the ages of 10 and 19 years, Bell's palsy is twice as common in women, whereas after the age of 40 years, it is 1.5 times more common in men. Pregnant women have 3.3 times more risk than nonpregnant women in the same age group. Diabetic patients are 4.5 times more likely to develop Bell's palsy. In 10% of the patients, a positive family history of Bell's palsy is also present.

ETIOLOGY AND PATHOGENESIS

Bell's palsy is the result of a viral infection produced by the reactivation of the herpes simplex virus. After a primary infection, the virus subsides to latency in the cranial and spinal sensory ganglia. When an immunodepressed state is produced, the virus is reactivated and replicates within the ganglion cells, where it is protected from any response of the the immune system, and produces local damage. The clinical result is hypoesthesia of the face, pharynx, head, and neck. Then the virus passes up and down to the axons, where it produces some changes on the antigens of the Schwann cell membranes that induce an inflammatory response from the immune system: antibody and lymphocytic infiltration. The final result is a segmental demyelination clinically presented as nerve paralysis. Once the infection and the immune-mediated response resolve, remyelination follows and muscle innervation is restored. The degree and rate of recovery are directly related to the degree and rate of nerve damage.

CLINICAL COURSE

Bell's palsy is characterized by a sudden onset, a viral prodrome, and a previous immunodepressed period. The full extent of the paralysis is normally reached within 1 to 14 days in Bell's palsy patients and within 1 to 21 days in herpes zoster oticus patients. In the early phase, the symptoms and signs are retroauricular pain, facial numbness, epiphora, parageusia, decreased tearing, and hyperacusis. The physical findings are facial paresis or paralysis, hypoesthesia or dysesthesia of cranial nerves V and IX and cervical nerves II to VI, motor paresis of cranial nerves IX and X, and papillitis of the tongue. The clinical picture of Bell's palsy is that of a mononeuritis multiplex. Bell's palsy is usually unilateral; however, 10% of cases are bilateral. When severe retroauricular pain is present, a frustrée type (herpes sine herpetae) of Ramsay Hunt syndrome has to be ruled out.

DIAGNOSIS

Bell's palsy is diagnosed when a facial paralysis is presented as peripheral in origin, with a sudden onset, without evidence of systemic disease, and with concomitant cranial polyneuritis evident. Also, the diagnosis of Bell's palsy has to be questioned in any total facial paralysis with no evidence of regeneration in 4 to 6 months or in any facial paresis that does not resolve in 3 to 6 weeks; then a second ear, nose, and throat and neurologic evaluation is mandatory, including serologic testing and imaging of the complete course of the seventh nerve by computed tomography (CT) scan and/or magnetic resonance imaging.

PROGNOSIS

The difficulty in making an accurate prognosis in the early stages of facial paralysis is still one of the most challenging problems with Bell's palsy, although a complete recovery rate of about 60 to 80% is accepted. The clinical evaluation and the electrodiagnostic test results help us make a prognosis.

Clinical evaluation prognostic factors are as follows:

1. Age: The younger the patient, the better the prognosis.
2. Completeness of palsy: Incomplete paralysis almost always leads to a complete recovery.
3. Time of recovery: When recovery begins between days 10 and 21, a satisfactory result is obtained.
4. The association with systemic diseases (e.g., diabetes): Such association is related to a higher chance of unsatisfactory recovery.

Electrodiagnostic tests attempt to predict a prognosis by determining the physiologic extent of nerve damage and the need for possible changes in the previous treatment given (e.g., the need for surgery or neuromuscular retraining). The most widely used and the most sensitive tools are the maximal stimulation test (MST), evoked electromyography (EEMG), and electroneurography (ENOG). The goal is to determine the degree of distal axonal degeneration. However, those tests are not the best tests for patient selection because they can only detect denervation 3 days after the damaging lesion has been produced and they cannot be used to monitor reinnervation. So currently, electrical tests are helpful only if the clinician will make changes in the treatment schedule on the basis of the results of the tests.

TREATMENT

Some authors recommend not treating Bell's palsy because between 73 and 84% of patients recover completely. However, I reject this view because it is not

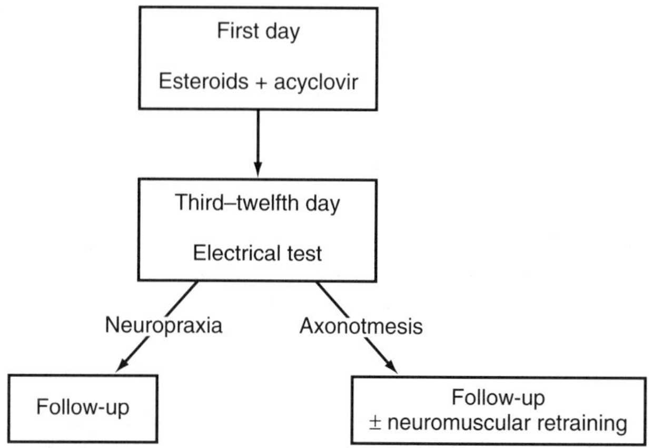

Figure 1. Schedule for Bell's palsy treatment.

possible at present to predict which patients will progress to a severe form of Bell's palsy and because the early and correct administration of treatment will relieve the pain and will reduce significantly the rate and degree of denervation (Figure 1).

Drug Therapy

The association of acyclovir and prednisone produces better results than prednisone and placebo.

Corticosteroids. These are an excellent treatment for immune-mediated demyelinating diseases. Although there is a debate about the efficacy of steroids for the treatment of Bell's palsy, there is also strong support in the literature for the use of cortisone. Steroids relieve pain and reduce denervation. The dosage suggested of prednisone is 1 mg per kg of body weight daily for 15 days, tapering to 0 during the next 5 days.

Acyclovir* (Zovirax). Its antiviral action has been proved. It reduces pain and degree of denervation and heals the vesicles. The dosage schedule advised for Bell's palsy is 200 mg orally five times per day for 10 days.

Eye Care

Drying keratitis and foreign bodies are some of the sequelae of Bell's palsy. To avoid them, it is important to instill artificial tears five times per day and to tape the eye closed during sleep.

Neuromuscular Retraining

Neuromuscular retraining is the treatment of choice for the sequelae of Bell's palsy. The abnormal pattern produced by the facial nerve lesion may be modified: the brain's plasticity has the capacity to modify its organization, resulting in lasting functional changes. This capacity explains the acquisition of new motor behaviors after spontaneous recovery has been completed. Facial muscles are different from most other skeletal muscles: they lack muscle spindles, the motor units are small, they receive volitional and emotional neural inputs, and they are slower to degenerate. The principles consist of the practice of slow and little movements to reach symmetry. Neuromuscular retraining candidates must have innervation to the facial musculature, they must be motivated to ensure follow-through, and they must have an adequate attention span and cognitive abilities for practice of the program. Each treatment program is different, is based on the individual's level of function, and lasts for 1 to 3 years.

There are two treatment techniques: (1) Visual feedback (mirror feedback), using a mirror to change the motor facial pattern and to reinforce proper responses, and (2) biofeedback or surface electromyography feedback, which reinforces the proper movement pattern and demonstrates the presence of muscle activity to the patient. The patient increases the activity of the weak muscles and decreases the activity of the hyperactive muscles so that the coordination between the different muscular groups is better.

*Not FDA approved for this indication.

Surgical Decompression

Bell's palsy is a viral immune-mediated demyelinating disease that is longitudinal, not perpendicular, to the facial canal. Therefore, surgical decompression cannot benefit this viral disease. Today, there is no place for surgical decompression in the treatment of Bell's palsy.

PARKINSON'S DISEASE

method of
STANLEY VAN DEN NOORT, M.D.
University of California, Irvine
Irvine, California

Parkinson's disease is a common degenerative disorder of the aging brain. The prevalence is 100 per 100,000 persons, but it comes to affect several percent of the elderly population. It is a progressive disorder that until the last few decades caused total disability and death within less than 10 years. Today many patients achieve nearly normal lifespans with good quality of life owing to effective treatment. Rates of progression are quite variable. More rapid progression is seen in patients with an older age of onset. Although age of onset is most common after the age of 65 years, onset in the early forties is not rare.

PATHOGENESIS

The pathogenesis of Parkinson's disease remains obscure. There is a predominant loss of dopaminergic neurons in the substantia nigra causing disordered control of movement marked by bradykinesia, tremor, rigidity, and loss of postural reflexes. Most cases are sporadic, but a percentage are familial. Genetic and environmental factors interact to influence the longevity of nigral neurons, which cannot reproduce themselves. Other system degenerations can appear. Transitions to amyotrophic lateral sclerosis or Alzheimer's disease are rarely seen.

DIAGNOSIS

Classic Parkinson's disease with its stooped posture, soft rapid speech, lack of blinking, drooling, loss of arm swing, impaired mimicry, resting tremor, festinating movements, progressive micrographia, and slowness of movement is relatively easy to recognize. Difficulty turning over in bed may be an early symptom. Symptoms are often unilateral at first. Tremor may be subtle or absent, leading to diagnostic error.

There is a paucity of spontaneous movement. The glabella reflex is released. Blepharospasm may emerge with efforts to examine the eyes. Tremor is usually observed as a rhythmic 4 per second movement of the hand at rest, and it is briefly ameliorated by any spontaneous voluntary movement of the affected limb. Resting tremor may be evident in lips, tongue, or legs. Tremor may be observed and facilitated by walking or by gripping with the opposite hand. Passive movement reveals rigidity on passive manipulation of a plastic or cogwheeling character. "Plastic" in this context is a consistent "lead pipe" rigidity as opposed to phasic or brief changes in muscle resistance. Rigidity is often enhanced by having the patient use the opposite hand for a movement such as patting the knee.

Observation of walking is important and shows the stooped posture, flexed arms, and reduction of normal arm swing. There may be an increase in the speed of walking over a distance. Turning is broken up into several hesitating maneuvers. Festination is the increase in the frequency of repetitive movements while the amplitude of these movements is reduced. This results in progressive micrographia, increased speed and decreased volume of speech, and a tendency to run after walking.

DIFFERENTIAL DIAGNOSIS

Several less common illnesses manifest in a fashion resembling Parkinson's disease but do not respond well to treatment. There are patients with atypical features who respond poorly to treatment. We often seem to diagnose Parkinson's disease when a person has a typical response to treatment, and we call the failures "parkinsonism" or "Parkinson's plus."

Iatrogenic parkinsonism due to phenothiazines and kindred drugs such as metoclopramide (Reglan) is common and is best treated by withdrawal of the offending drug. Familial parkinsonism and familial dystonias overlap each other. Some patients with these disorders have excellent and protracted responses to low doses of medication. Parkinsonism that is less responsive to medication may be progressive supranuclear palsy (impaired vertical eye movements and easy falling), multisystem atrophy (orthostatic hypotension, dysarthria, ataxia), or corticobasal degeneration (impaired position sense in one hand and alien hand syndrome). Parkinsonism also is seen in strionigral degeneration, anoxic brain injury, trauma, manganese intoxication, viral infections, and idiosyncratic responses to a variety of drugs.

Making a distinction between Parkinson's disease and essential tremor is critical. The latter is an action tremor that quiets at rest and is unaccompanied by rigidity or bradykinesia. But Parkinson's disease sometimes evolves from a background of essential tremor. In essential tremor, handwriting is usually large and shaky. The voice is often tremulous. A "no" tremor of the head may be seen. This is usually a benign familial disorder that may appear in young or old alike. Alcohol in small doses relieves the tremor briefly.

DIAGNOSIS

Confirmation of the diagnosis of Parkinson's disease is best achieved by a visit to the office of an experienced neurologist. The only objective test is positron emission tomography, which has limited value and is very expensive, although it is an invaluable research tool.

TREATMENT

Without treatment, the quality of life for patients with Parkinson's disease declines progressively. Serious falls with injury are a major hazard. Dependence for dressing, feeding, and activities of daily living is increased. The optimal time to initiate treatment is controversial, with a majority of physicians feeling that delay is desirable. But too much delay may lead to injury with fixed disability or death. There is now evidence that some forms of therapy may have a degree of neuroprotection, which would argue for early treatment.

Pharmacologic Approaches

The finding of effective treatment with dihydroxyphenylalanine (DOPA; levodopa) by Cotzias in 1964 was a great milestone in therapeutics. People who had been bedridden for years got up and walked. Use of levodopa alone required doses of up to 8000 mg every day (qd) because so much levodopa was decarboxylated in the bloodstream. This resulted in the development of carbidopa (CD), which inhibits DOPA decarboxylase in the bloodstream, but this agent, unlike levodopa, cannot pass the blood-brain barrier. Hence, we arrived at carbidopa-levodopa (Sinemet), which can do the job with less than 1000 mg of levodopa and 400 mg of carbidopa per day.

Initial treatment is now leaning toward agents that, although therapeutic, also display some evidence of neuroprotection. The oldest of these is tocopherol (vitamin E), for which evidence is meager. Nonetheless, many physicians urge the ingestion of several thousand units of vitamin E per day. A second agent is selegiline (Eldepryl), 5 mg twice a day (bid), given before afternoon. A third group is the dopamine agonists. Pergolide (Permax) and bromocriptine (Parlodel) have been available for some years. The newly released agent pramipexole (Mirapex) may be more effective and have fewer side effects. A just-released agent, ropinarole (Requip), may have similar value. Usually these are started in lower doses of 0.125 mg three times a day (tid) and slowly increased to therapeutic levels, which may require several milligrams or more per day. In high dosages these agents may produce nausea, hallucinations, and/or psychosis. In early cases and in younger patients, it may be best to use tocopherol, selegiline, and a mild dose of a dopamine agonist for months or years before increasing agonists or adding Sinemet. In older patients, even small doses of dopamine agonists may be poorly tolerated owing to hallucinations.

Tolcapone (Tasmar) is an inhibitor of catechol *O*-methyltransferase, which prolongs the presence of dopamine in the synapse. The dose is 100 or 200 mg tid. Side effects are minimal. It will allow moderately lower doses of Sinemet and may reduce the frequency of Sinemet-induced dyskinesia.

When the previously mentioned agents are poorly tolerated or ineffective, it is appropriate to initiate the carbidopa-levodopa combination Sinemet. Sinemet is now available in slow-release forms, which minimize side effects in early treatment but are more expensive than short-acting forms. Medication costs can be prohibitive for many patients who would be well advised to use short-acting Sinemet at intervals of 2 to 3 hours rather than long-acting Sinemet at intervals of 4 to 6 hours. When starting therapy, it is often desirable to give medicine after food to prevent nausea, but absorption is better when it is given before food. A very slowly graded increase of dosage over many weeks is often helpful. The nausea is a central phenomenon and is uninfluenced by stomach medicines. The addition of carbidopa (Lodosyn) can be effective in reducing nausea. The absorption of levodopa is from the small bowel, and gastric emptying may be a problem. Use of polycarbophil (Fiber Con) with each dose may be helpful. When using short-acting Sinemet, even a cracker or two to slow absorption may help to reduce nausea. Cisapride (Propulsid) has been used with indifferent results. For the carbidopa element of Sinemet to exercise its full effect, about 100 mg a day are necessary.

In the early treatment of Parkinson's disease, effects are often smooth and morning doses last well into the day. As the disease advances, fluctuations in responses become more evident with end-of-dose stiffness, end-of-dose dystonia, and peak dose dyskinesia. Dyskinesia is a major problem. Many patients prefer moderate dyskinesia to the bradykinesia that attends lower doses. Families and physicians find the dyskinesia disturbing and advocate lower doses. Best results are usually achieved by lower doses of Sinemet, more frequent dosing (sometimes hourly), variation in dosing through the day, use of polycarbophil (FiberCon) to promote gastric emptying, and, particularly, increased reliance on dopamine agonists. These now require tight timing of doses. Use of controlled-release Sinemet minimizes motor fluctuations. In refractory patients, a reduction of daytime protein intake may be desirable. Because dihydroxyphenylalanine shares transfer mechanisms with other amino acids, absorption is best without competition. The use of nighttime medication is variable. It is desirable to minimize nighttime medication to permit receptor recovery and limit nightmares, but many patients require around-the-clock dosing. If dopamine agonists have not been initiated before Sinemet, it is well to add them before pushing the dosage limits of Sinemet. Individualized treatment schedules should and do vary widely from one patient to the next and change in the course of the illness. Tolcapone promises to be a valuable adjunct to reduce fluctuations in therapeutic effects.

Usually a combination of selegiline, 5 mg qd or bid, pramixapole, 0.5 mg tid, or another dopamine agonist and Sinemet CR, 50/200 mg tid or qid, is optimal. Tremor is often stubbornly resistant to treatment. Although patients complain of tremor, its contribution to disability is usually moderate, and overtreatment is unwise. Amantadine (Symmetrel), 100 mg tid, may help tremor. The addition of benztropine (Cogentin), 0.5 to 1.0 mg, or trihexyphenidyl (Artane), 2 to 6 mg, may help tremor but must be used with great caution in the elderly. Propanolol (Inderal) and/or primidone (Mysoline), 50 to 100 mg tid, may be useful adjuncts. The effectiveness of amantadine (Symmetrel) has been highly unpredictable in my experience. Occasionally it is extraordinarily effective in atypical cases. Orthostatic hypotension is common in Parkinson's disease and is often aggravated by Sinemet. The release of midodrine (ProAmatine), 5 to 10 mg tid, has been a step forward for treatment of this symptom. Immobility often produces ankle edema, which is best relieved by elevation of the legs above the level of the heart. Some edema is often an internal "elastic hose," which curtails orthostatic hypotension. Diuresis may provoke orthostatic symptoms. This hypotension is usually not attended by pallor due to failure of vasoconstriction; usually the pulse is fixed as well. Orthostatic hypotension needs to be frequently assessed by measurement. Falls due to syncope are a substantial hazard.

Another major problem with the use of Sinemet and dopamine agonists is the emergence of nightmares, restless legs, hallucinations, paranoid ideation, and depression. The emergence of depression often requires discontinuation of selegiline if one is to use antidepressants. Hallucinations are often visual and bland without agitation. The recently released olanzapine (Zyprexa), 2.5 to 10 mg qd, is a major advance in the management of these symptoms. Clozapine (Clozaril) has similar benefit but is subject to bone marrow depression and requires a complete blood count weekly. Strict avoidance of all phenothiazines and inhibitors of dopamine receptors is essential. This includes most antinausea medicines such as metoclopramide and some antihistamines such as promethazine (Phenergan). Ondansetron (Zofran) is safe for nausea in Parkinson's disease and has the added benefit of reducing visual hallucinations. Restless legs and myoclonus respond nicely to clonazepam* (Klonopin) and to valproic acid* (Depakote).

In a minority of patients, usually those with severe Parkinson's, a state of anxiety is commonly present, which responds to regular divided doses of lorazepam (Ativan) tid. In other patients, lethargy is a common problem, and methylphenidate (Ritalin), 5 mg tid, may be helpful and have independent beneficial effects on Parkinson's disease. Again, selegiline should

*Not FDA approved for this indication.

be stopped for some weeks before methylphenidate (Ritalin) is introduced.

Because this is an illness of the elderly, it is often necessary to use these medicines in the context of other illnesses. Glaucoma may worsen with anticholinergic agents. I am struck by the paucity of coronary disease in patients on Sinemet. Stroke is infrequent. Hypertension is more common. Diabetes may occur. There has been concern that Sinemet may contribute to the development of malignant melanoma, but this is certainly rare. Avoidance of excessive sun exposure is prudent. Sinemet in large doses has been associated with arrhythmias in some patients. Obstructive sleep apnea is not uncommon in this population. Stubborn constipation is the rule, and it resists common management with psyllium, docusate sodium (Colace), and enemas or bisacodyl (Dulcolax). Lactulose syrup (Cephulac), ½ to 2 ounces a day, is often invaluable. Both early and late in Parkinson's disease shoulder and hip pain are commonly due to bursitis, probably potentiated by gait changes and reduced arm swing. Bladder dysfunction is common, and it is hard to distinguish neurogenic bladder dysfunction from prostatism in males or stress incontinence in women. Surgical approaches may increase incontinence. The use of anticholinergics, e.g., flavoxate (Urispas), 100 mg every 8 hours, may help, and the use of an alpha-adrenergic antagonist such as terazosin* (Hytrin) may reduce detrusor-sphincter dyssynergia. The new antispastic bladder remedy tolterodine (Detrol), 1 to 2 mg every 12 hours, may be helpful.

The advent of dementia is common in elderly Parkinson's disease patients. Concurrent Alzheimer's disease and similar states may occur. There is an uncommon dementia with early confusion and hallucinations and with cellular inclusions that are also seen in Parkinson's disease (Lewy body disease). Some evidence of subcortical dementia, marked by a slowness in solving problems, is quite common. Insomnia is a widespread problem; 50 mg of diphenhydramine (Benadryl), 1000 mg of chloral hydrate, or a benzodiazipine or 50 to 100 mg of trazodone* (Deseryl) may be helpful.

All of these treatments depend on a healthy upper gastrointestinal tract. Late in Parkinson's disease, swallowing defects are common, and the need for gastrostomy may arise. I have seen advantages and disadvantages to surgical, gastrointestinal, and radiologic approaches to gastrostomy. The radiologists have quite good results, but replacements are easier in cases with the surgical approach. It is very important that Sinemet not be withdrawn abruptly for fear of triggering neuroleptic malignant syndrome with rhabdonecrosis, myoglobinuria, and renal failure. The absence of convenient parenteral preparations is an obstacle to treatment.

Nonpharmacologic Approaches

When quality of life cannot be sustained by medications, surgical alternatives should be considered. Although grafts hold promise for the future, they are very expensive and difficult and have variably acceptable results. Medial pallidotomy has become increasingly popular as an adjunct to medical treatment. Treatment responses are often bilateral, gratifying, and persistent for years. Medial pallidotomy is particularly effective for dyskinesia, rigidity, and tremor. The placement of electrodes in striatum, subthalamic nucleus, and/or the thalamus now offers promise for the individualization of bilateral treatment approaches, which can be adjusted. At present, these procedures are done at the relatively few centers that have the expertise and equipment. The development of techniques to remove progenitor nerve cells that can be manipulated in culture to multiply and produce neurotransmitters is a promising future direction.

The atypical parkinsonian syndromes generally do not respond well to dopamine agonists and the previously mentioned schedules. Nonetheless, a needed temporary improvement may be achieved in some cases of progressive supranuclear palsy, corticobasal degeneration, and multisystem atrophy.

Great attention to nonpharmacologic approaches is very desirable. Occupational and physical therapy have much to offer in the preservation of walking and independence in activities of daily living. Large-wheel walkers with handbrakes and a seat are often helpful. Falls and fractures remain major hazards to patients with Parkinson's disease and often spell the end of independence. Often these patients develop high degrees of dependence on caregivers who are only a little less frail than themselves. The unexpected demise of a caregiver whose own health has been ignored is a very common event. Other caregivers may be unable to carry on without respite, and insurance does not usually cover home care.

Examples of Progressive Treatment

Eliminate all medicines that may inhibit dopamine receptors

Tocopherol, 1000 units tid
Selegiline (Eldepryl), 5.0 mg bid (before 1:00 PM)
Pramipexole (Mirapex), 0.25 mg
  Week 1: ½ tid
  Week 2: 1 tid
  Week 3: 1½ tid
  Week 4: 2 tid
  Week 5: 3 tid
  Titrate to higher doses as required up to 4 mg qd

Other dopamine agonists may be equally effective, and individuals may respond better to one or another dopamine agonist.

Carbidopa-levodopa (Sinemet CR 25/100)
  Week 1: bid
  Week 2: tid
  Week 3: qid

Then consider an increase in Sinemet to CR 50/200 with a similar schedule; doses of 2 tablets

*Not FDA approved for this indication.

qid may be required; tolcapone may reduce the need for higher doses.

or

Sinemet 25/100
- Week 1: ½ bid after meals (pc) or after a few crackers
- Week 2: ½ tid pc
- Week 3: ½ qid pc
- Week 4: 1½ qid pc
- Week 5: add tolcapone 100 mg tid
- Week 6: 1½ qid before meals (ac)
- Week 7: 2 qid ac or increase tolcapone to 200 mg tid
- Dosage intervals of every 2 hours may be required.

As required:
- Midodrine (Proamatine), 5 to 10 mg tid
- Olonzapine (Zyprexa), 2.5 to 10 mg qd or bid
- Benztropine (Cogentin), 0.5 mg qd
- Propanolol LA (Inderal), 60 qd

ACKNOWLEDGMENTS

I wish to thank Janet Chance, M.D., for review and individual comments.

PERIPHERAL NEUROPATHIES

method of
PHILIP G. MCMANIS, M.D.
University of Sydney
Sydney, Australia

The peripheral nervous system has afferent (sensory) and efferent (motor) components. Most peripheral nerves consist of mixed motor and sensory nerve fibers (axons) that can be affected in isolation or together. Nerve fibers that make up the peripheral nerves are of various diameters and can be classified into large myelinated, small myelinated, and small unmyelinated fibers. Most motor axons are large myelinated fibers, but sensory axons can be of any of the types mentioned. Large-diameter sensory axons carry information about vibration and joint position, whereas small-diameter sensory axons transmit information about pain and temperature. The autonomic nerves consist of small unmyelinated fibers. Disorders of the peripheral nervous system may affect some or all of these fiber types. If involvement is selective, a distinctive clinical syndrome results (Table 1).

A useful way of approaching peripheral neuropathies is to place patients into one of several diagnostic categories based on the distribution of nerves affected, the type of nerve fiber involved, and the time course of the disease (see Table 1). This allows a problem-based approach to the evaluation of peripheral neuropathies and minimizes unnecessary testing. The process is not dependent on the results of laboratory testing of the peripheral nerves and begins with a careful and thorough history, paying particular attention to other illnesses, toxin exposures, habits, and medications. The types of motor, sensory, and autonomic symptoms require careful documentation. The findings on clinical examination supplement this information, which then allows the classification of the type of peripheral neuropathy. When approaching the problem in this way, it is important to remember that diabetes can cause any of these categories of neuropathy.

TABLE 1. **Diagnostic Categories of Peripheral Neuropathies**

Distal symmetrical sensorimotor neuropathy ("glove and stocking")
Polyradiculoneuropathy
Mononeuritis multiplex
Large-fiber sensory neuropathy
Small-fiber sensory and autonomic neuropathy
Motor neuropathy

DISTAL SYMMETRIC SENSORIMOTOR NEUROPATHY

Sometimes called "glove and stocking" neuropathy, this is the most commonly encountered form of peripheral neuropathy. Many different conditions produce this pattern of distal muscle wasting and weakness with decreased or absent tendon reflexes and loss of sensation. In general, these are "dying back" or "axonal" neuropathies, but some demyelinating neuropathies manifest in the same way. If the cause of the neuropathy is found, the treatment is directed toward curing the underlying disease or eliminating the offending drug or toxic agent.

About 60% of patients with this clinical syndrome will be found to have diabetes mellitus or an inherited neuropathy. In a further 30% the cause cannot be identified.

Hereditary Neuropathies

As many as 30% of undiagnosed neuropathies are eventually found to be familial, and it is important to look for the clues to hereditary neuropathies before undertaking an expensive diagnostic work-up. The presence of pes cavus, clawed toes, and scoliosis together with a youthful age at onset or very longstanding symptoms are strongly suggestive of hereditary neuropathy. If possible, family members should be examined and sometimes tested with electromyography to attempt to identify subclinical neuropathy in relatives. The inherited neuropathies may be axonal or demyelinating and are sometimes associated with other abnormalities of the nervous system (Table 2).

Patients can be given genetic counseling regarding the likelihood of their progeny developing the disor-

TABLE 2. **Inherited Peripheral Neuropathies**

Hereditary motor and sensory neuropathies (Charcot-Marie-Tooth disease)
Type I (demyelinating; three subtypes)
Type II (axonal)
Type III (severe demyelinating; Dejerine-Sottas disease)
Type IV (Refsum's disease; phytanic oxidase deficiency)
Type V (with spastic paraplegia)
Type VI (with optic atrophy)
Type VII (with retinitis pigmentosa)
Fabry's disease
Hepatic porphyrias
Giant axonal neuropathy
Neuroaxonal dystrophy
Neuropathies associated with central nervous system myelin disorders
Adrenomyeloneuropathy
Metachromatic leukodystrophy
Krabbe's disease

der. They can also be informed about the prospective severity of their disease and counseled about suitable employment. Treatment can be offered to a few patients with inherited neuropathies; some of them have a peculiar predisposition to developing pressure palsies, and measures can be taken to avoid situations likely to produce these and to treat them if they occur. This disorder has been shown to be due to a deletion in the gene of a peripheral myelin protein (PMP-22). Another group may inherit a polyradiculoneuropathy and have elevated cerebrospinal fluid protein levels. This group obtains considerable benefit from prednisone therapy.

Neuropathies with Predominant Axonal Degeneration

Most distal sensorimotor neuropathies are caused by primary axonal degeneration. At times the same clinical picture can be produced by a demyelinating neuropathy, and nerve conduction studies may be very helpful in differentiating between these groups. In axonal degeneration the amplitude of the evoked motor or sensory response will be low (or absent), whereas conduction velocities will be relatively unaffected. In demyelinating neuropathies there is a prominent reduction in nerve conduction velocities, sometimes with conduction block, together with marked prolongation of distal latencies and F wave latencies, but amplitudes are relatively spared.

Metabolic and Endocrine Disorders

Diabetes Mellitus. In this condition the neuropathy may be predominantly axonal, demyelinating, or angiopathic. Some diabetics will present a picture of mononeuritis multiplex, whereas others will present with predominant involvement of either large or small nerve fibers (see later). The most common form of diabetic neuropathy is a mild to moderate distal sensorimotor neuropathy, which is almost invariably present in patients with long-standing non–insulin-dependent diabetes. This is frequently asymptomatic, although patients may admit to mild distal tingling or numbness.

The aim of treatment is to obtain the best possible control of the blood sugar level. If this cannot be achieved with diet alone or with oral hypoglycemic agents, then insulin therapy may be indicated. However, caution should be exercised when first beginning insulin treatment, as rapid normalization of blood glucose may cause the acute onset of severe painful tingling and hypersensitivity of the extremities. Thus, a gradual reduction in the elevated blood sugar levels may be preferable to a rapid change.

It has been shown that pancreas transplantation is beneficial for diabetic peripheral neuropathy, even when strict glycemic control has failed to help.

Uremia. The neuropathy associated with renal failure follows a pattern typical of distal neuropathies, with distal loss of strength and sensation and decreased reflexes. One notable feature, however, is that unpleasant sensory symptoms are pronounced; patients complain of unpleasant pulling or drawing sensations in their legs together with burning or tingling discomfort in the feet. Frequent cramps and restless legs may appear during the development of the neuropathy.

Uremic neuropathy occurs only in end-stage renal failure. Treatment of the neuropathy depends on correction of the chronic metabolic abnormalities, but hemodialysis is generally not effective in improving the symptoms and may even fail to prevent progression. On the other hand, renal transplantation is almost always followed by a significant improvement in the neuropathy. This may influence the choice of treatment in patients with severe uremic neuropathy.

Other Metabolic Disorders. A peripheral neuropathy may be seen in acromegaly. In this condition, nerves are edematous and are susceptible to compression. Patients may present with carpal tunnel syndrome or ulnar nerve compression at the elbow. In the absence of focal compressions, the neuropathy is usually mild. A dramatic improvement in symptoms may be seen after hypophysectomy.

Distal sensorimotor neuropathy may also occur in rare disorders such as porphyria and recurrent hypoglycemia secondary to an insulinoma. Both of these are predominantly motor neuropathies and tend to affect the upper extremities before the lower. Porphyric neuropathy may produce greater weakness in proximal muscles than in distal muscles and is characteristically associated with autonomic disturbances, abdominal pain, and neuropsychiatric symptoms. Again, the treatment is directed at the underlying disease process.

Drugs and Toxins

Drugs. Many drugs are known to cause a peripheral neuropathy. Some medications do this only rarely, whereas peripheral neuropathy is expected when other agents are used (Table 3). The pattern of disease is variable: some agents produce a mild distal sensory neuropathy, whereas others lead to a gener-

TABLE 3. **Drugs Causing Peripheral Neuropathy**

Drugs frequently causing neuropathy
Amiodarone (Cordarone)
Isoniazid
Misonidazole*
Platinum antineoplastic drugs
Megadose pyridoxine
Thalidomide
Vinca alkaloids
Drugs occasionally causing neuropathy
Chloramphenicol
Chloroquine
Colchicine
Dapsone
Disulfiram
Phenytoin (Dilantin)
Nitrofurantoin (Macrodantin)
Metronidazole (Flagyl)
Gold salts

*Not available in the United States.

alized motor neuropathy, sometimes affecting proximal and upper limb muscles more than distal lower limb muscles (e.g., chloroquine). Megadose pyridoxine causes a severe and often irreversible dorsal root ganglionopathy. It is essential that a careful drug history be taken from any person with neuropathy so that suspect drugs can be discontinued.

Toxins. Toxins that cause peripheral neuropathy are predominantly heavy metals (lead, mercury, arsenic, thallium), hexacarbons (e.g., *n*-hexane, methyl *n*-butyl ketone), and industrial agents (e.g., acrylamide monomer, carbon disulfide, methyl bromide, trichloroethylene, organophosphates). Most toxic agents produce a typical pattern of neuropathy: symptoms are very symmetrical and begin in the feet, with the severity and rate of proximal progression being dose-related. Upper limbs are affected later in the course. Sensory nerves are more affected than motor fibers. The patient complains of distal burning and tingling together with prominent hypersensitivity. Examination reveals impaired sensation. The sensory deficit may be very mild relative to the symptoms in milder cases. Weakness is not a prominent feature early in the course or in mild to moderate toxic neuropathy. Exceptions to this pattern include glue sniffer's neuropathy, which is due to the long-term inhalation of *n*-hexane, and lead neuropathy. Both produce predominantly motor abnormalities. In addition, lead intoxication may result in a mononeuritis multiplex picture and often preferentially affects the upper extremities.

Treatment of these neuropathies is dependent on the identification of the toxin. Recovery generally follows the withdrawal of the causative agent but is slow and frequently incomplete. Specific therapy is available for metal poisoning (arsenic, lead, mercury, thallium); this is best and most safely treated with D-penicillamine. The usual dose is 250 mg four times daily, and therapy should continue until urinary excretion of the metal returns to the normal range.

Lead. In adults, lead intoxication generally causes an axonal neuropathy, whereas in children it usually causes a demyelinating neuropathy in association with encephalopathy and anemia. Although lead is ubiquitous in the environment, lead neuropathy is now a rare disease because of the awareness of the toxic nature of lead and the institution of effective precautions to minimize lead exposure. Nevertheless, lead neuropathy may still occur in certain groups exposed to high lead concentrations, especially those in lead-working industries. Children with pica may ingest lead-containing paint from old houses, but lead-intoxicated children usually present with the encephalopathy rather than the neuropathy.

The clinical picture is one of a motor neuropathy mainly affecting upper limbs, often in the pattern of a mononeuritis multiplex. Wrist drop is a prominent feature, but sensory symptoms are virtually absent. Lead-poisoned children are more likely to have a symmetrical distal motor neuropathy. A hypochromic microcytic anemia with basophilic stippling of red blood cells is almost always present. The optimal method of treatment is controversial, but, as with other metal intoxications, most cases of lead neuropathy can be treated safely and effectively with oral D-penicillamine.

Vitamin Deficiencies and Alcohol

Alcoholic Neuropathy. Alcoholics frequently develop a sensorimotor neuropathy characterized by distal muscle wasting and weakness with prominent sensory symptoms. Hypersensitivity and burning discomfort in the soles of the feet are frequent complaints, and calf tenderness is often present. Examination reveals distal lower limb weakness with absent ankle jerks and mild to moderate reduction of all sensory modalities. The upper extremities are relatively spared. The skin over the legs is often thin, pigmented, and shiny. Although a direct toxic effect of alcohol on nerve cannot be completely excluded, it is more likely that the nerve damage is due to nutritional deficiencies, especially a lack of thiamine and other B group vitamins. Alcoholic neuropathy occurs in the setting of grossly abnormal dietary intake; heavy drinkers who maintain a satisfactory diet rarely develop peripheral neuropathy. For these reasons, treatment of the neuropathy consists of a balanced high-protein diet with B vitamin supplements. The recommended daily vitamin doses are 100 mg of thiamine, 50 mg of pyridoxine, 100 mg of niacin, 10 mg of riboflavin, and 10 mg of pantothenic acid. Abstinence from alcohol should be encouraged, as this is likely to lead to an improvement in diet.

Vitamin B_{12} Deficiency. In contrast to the vitamin deficiency syndromes seen in alcoholics and others, lack of vitamin B_{12} is not caused by reduced dietary intake. In most cases the condition is due to an inability of the gut to absorb the vitamin, resulting from an autoimmune disease that reduces the production or blocks the action of intrinsic factor or other forms of malabsorption. This substance is essential for the absorption of vitamin B_{12}. Examination of patients with vitamin B_{12} deficiency reveals prominent loss of vibration and joint position sense in the lower limbs. This often results in a sensory ataxia. Because weakness and reflex changes appear later in the course, the presence of neuropathy may be masked by a concurrent myelopathy. Treatment consists of intramuscular injection of B_{12} and must be continued indefinitely. The usual dose is 1000 μg five times the first week followed by the same dose once a month.

Other B Group Vitamin Deficiencies. Other nutritional neuropathies are rarely due to a single vitamin deficiency. Patients with neuropathy due to poor diet usually have other evidence of malnourishment, such as loss of fat and muscle bulk. These patients have clinical signs similar to those seen with alcoholic neuropathy and should be treated the same way, with a balanced diet and supplementary vitamins.

Pellagra is a vitamin deficiency syndrome consisting of diarrhea, dermatitis, and dementia. These symptoms respond to treatment with niacin. On occasion a peripheral neuropathy occurs in conjunction with the classic triad, but it is rarely responsive to niacin supplementation. In these cases the neuropathy will improve with pyridoxine and other B group vitamins. In the United States pellagrins are usually alcoholics, and vitamin supplements should be given in doses similar to those recommended for alcoholic neuropathy except that the niacin dose should be increased to 100 mg three times daily.

Deficiency of three other B group vitamins—thiamine, pantothenic acid, and pyridoxine—is also thought to produce a peripheral neuropathy. As a rule, these are seen only as part of a general nutritional deficiency except for pyridoxine. This substance may be specifically deficient in some patients during treatment with the antituberculous drug isoniazid. The deficiency causes a neuropathy characterized by a symmetrical numbness and tingling in the feet followed by burning pains and calf tenderness. It has been shown that the neuropathy results from markedly increased excretion of pyridoxine and that it can be prevented by the administration of pyridoxine in a dose of 50 to 100 mg daily.

Patients with peripheral neuropathy of unknown cause rarely benefit from the indiscriminate use of vitamins. In particular, large doses of B_6 (pyridoxine) can cause a very severe sensory neuropathy that responds only slowly (if at all) to withdrawal of the vitamin. Dorsal root ganglion cells may be irreversibly damaged. Patients taking vitamin supplements should be advised to adhere to recommended dosage regimens.

Neoplasms

Neoplasia is associated with several different neuropathic syndromes, including large-fiber sensory neuropathy, acute pandysautonomia, subacute neuropathy resembling the Guillain-Barré syndrome, and other demyelinating neuropathies. However, the most common form is a mild, chronic, distal sensorimotor peripheral neuropathy. This can be detected in many cancer patients if specifically sought but does not often cause significant symptoms, partly because it commonly appears during the terminal stages of cancer. Improvement with treatment of the underlying neoplasm has not been documented except in the case of solitary plasmacytomas of bone and osteosclerotic myeloma. Irradiation of these tumors may result in improvement of the neuropathy.

Infections

Although uncommon in the United States, the most frequent cause of peripheral neuropathy worldwide is leprosy. It is the lepromatous, rather than the tuberculoid, form of the disease that causes neuropathy. Because the organism (*Mycobacterium leprae*) grows best at temperatures lower than body core temperature, it is the cooler parts of the body that are most affected, such as fingers and toes and cheeks and the tip of the nose.

Most patients with human immunodeficiency virus (HIV) infection develop a peripheral neuropathy. This is most commonly a small-fiber neuropathy, although some patients have Guillain-Barré syndrome, often at the time of seroconversion. Lyme disease may cause a polyradiculoneuropathy or mononeuritis multiplex. Cytomegalovirus infections are associated with a painful lumbosacral plexopathy or polyradiculopathy similar to that caused by diabetes.

Neuropathies with Predominant Demyelination

Neuropathies with primary demyelination of the peripheral nerves commonly manifest with the clinical pattern of polyradiculoneuropathy. The prototypes of this pattern are acute and chronic inflammatory demyelinating polyradiculoneuropathy (see later discussion). In these conditions proximal and sometimes trunk and cranial muscles are weak. Less commonly, some patients with a distal sensorimotor neuropathy are found to have primary demyelination or mixed demyelination and axonal degeneration on pathologic examination of the nerves. The clinical symptoms and signs may be indistinguishable from those of distal sensorimotor neuropathies with primary axonal degeneration. However, electromyography may be very helpful, as outlined previously, and the cerebrospinal fluid protein is more likely to be elevated in demyelinating neuropathies.

Acromegaly

In this condition the distal sensorimotor neuropathy is frequently accompanied by entrapment neuropathies, particularly median nerve compression in the carpal tunnel. The nerves are edematous and often palpably enlarged. Hypophysectomy is followed by a rapid and complete recovery from the neuropathy.

Hypothyroidism

Hypothyroid patients may develop a severe demyelinating neuropathy that mainly affects large sensory fibers. Clinically there is distal sensory loss, particularly of proprioception and vibration, whereas loss of strength is minimal. There may be an associated proximal myopathy, and cerebellar degeneration may combine with the proprioceptive loss to produce severe ataxia. Cerebrospinal fluid protein level is usually elevated. Treatment with thyroid hormone replacement leads to a complete resolution of the neuropathy.

Paraproteinemia

Patients with paraproteinemias who develop neuropathy may present with a distal sensorimotor neuropathy or with a polyradiculoneuropathy. Most patients with an abnormal serum protein have a monoclonal gammopathy of undetermined significance (MGUS) and only a minority have myeloma, amyloidosis, or Waldenström's macroglobulinemia. About 10% of MGUS patients develop neuropathy, and it is thought that the paraprotein contains antibodies directed against peripheral nerve myelin in these cases, especially myelin-associated glycoprotein (MAG) and P zero. Most of these antibodies are IgM immunoglobulins, which tend to produce a demyelinating peripheral neuropathy. Occasionally IgG and IgA paraproteins occur, and these are more likely to cause axonal degeneration. The neuropathy in patients with myeloma and macroglobulinemia is often associated with amyloid deposits in nerves. The clinical picture in these cases is of a dominantly sensory peripheral neuropathy, unlike primary amyloidosis, which causes a small-fiber neuropathy with prominent autonomic dysfunction.

An unusual form of myeloma with osteosclerotic bone lesions (osteosclerotic myeloma) has a strong association with neuropathy, either the distal sensorimotor form or a polyradiculoneuropathy. Patients with this form of neuropathy also have a high incidence of endocrine abnormalities such as hirsutism, hypogonadism, gynecomastia, and skin pigmentation. Bony lesions may be solitary or multiple and either sclerotic or mixed lytic and sclerotic. The acronym POEMS is used to describe this condition (Peripheral neuropathy, Organomegaly, Endocrine disturbances, M-protein, and Skin changes).

Treatment of the paraproteinemic neuropathies seen with macroglobulinemia or multiple myeloma is difficult, as there is no therapy available for amyloid infiltration. The treatment of the underlying disorder with prednisone and melphalan or chlorambucil may help if the paraprotein itself is neurotoxic. On the other hand, the neuropathy of osteosclerotic myeloma often improves with excision or irradiation of the bony lesions. The response is not as good in patients with widespread disease. The treatment of the neuropathy of MGUS is still being evaluated in clinical trials, but prednisone, immunosuppressive agents, intravenous infusions of high-dose immunoglobulins (IGIV),* and plasma exchange all hold promise. The relative safety and efficacy of plasma exchange and IGIV suggest that these modalities should be tried as initial therapy. Some groups recommend prednisone in the high doses used to treat chronic inflammatory demyelinating polyradiculoneuropathy (120 mg and 7.5 mg on alternate days, gradually tapering to a low maintenance dose over several months). Others use a combination of prednisone with melphalan or chlorambucil* (Leukeran) and treat those who fail to respond with plasma exchange or IGIV.

*Not FDA approved for this indication.

Other Demyelinating Neuropathies

Diabetes may result in demyelination of peripheral nerves as already discussed. Sarcoidosis can produce a demyelinating distal sensorimotor neuropathy but more commonly manifests with the picture of mononeuritis multiplex or polyradiculoneuropathy. Lead causes a demyelinating neuropathy in children. Multifocal conduction block motor neuropathy (see later discussion) and hereditary neuropathy prone to pressure palsies are associated with focal areas of demyelination.

POLYRADICULONEUROPATHY

The next major group of peripheral neuropathies consists of disorders that produce a clinical picture of a polyradiculoneuropathy. These may be acute, subacute, or chronic. Although sensory and motor fibers are usually involved together, weakness is much more prominent than sensory complaints. Nerve roots and proximal portions of nerves are frequently affected, resulting in proximal limb, trunk, and cranial nerve involvement. Weakness may be severe and life-threatening. Tendon reflexes are universally hypoactive or absent. Minor abnormalities of sensation can often be detected. Examination of the cerebrospinal fluid usually reveals a high protein level with normal cell counts, and nerve conduction studies show marked slowing of conduction in most cases.

Acute Inflammatory Demyelinating Polyradiculoneuropathy

Often known as Guillain-Barré syndrome, this neuropathy is abrupt in onset and rapidly progressive. There is often a precipitant such as preceding viral infection, vaccination, or bee sting, and the syndrome may be seen in association with diseases such as infectious mononucleosis, *Campylobacter jejuni* and HIV infections, viral hepatitis, sarcoidosis, lymphoma, and leukemia. The clinical picture is of a rapidly ascending weakness of all four extremities, which frequently progresses to involve respiratory, facial, and bulbar muscles. Sphincter muscles are invariably spared. Sensory loss is usually mild but in some patients may be the dominant feature of the illness. Autonomic neuropathy may be present and in some cases may be severe and life-threatening with sustained or paroxysmal tachycardia or hypertension.

The most important aspect of treatment for this

*Not FDA approved for this indication.

disorder is early diagnosis and admission to the hospital, because mild weakness may progress to respiratory failure within hours. The respiratory function and pulse rate must be monitored closely, and assisted ventilation should begin if the vital capacity falls below 1 liter. Meticulous pulmonary hygiene must be maintained. Physical therapy to prevent contractures should begin early, and great care should be taken to avoid complications of prolonged bed rest such as decubitus ulcers and hypostatic pneumonia. If tachycardia or sustained hypertension develops, propranolol should be given. Paroxysmal fluctuations in blood pressure generally require a combination of alpha and beta blockers.

Recovery often begins 1 to 3 weeks after onset, and in these cases the prognosis for recovery is good. Patients whose illness continues to progress for more than 6 weeks are more likely to have a chronic or relapsing course. Some patients will have a severe axonal (instead of demyelinating) neuropathy and may have a very prolonged illness with incomplete recovery after months or years. This syndrome has been called acute motor axonal neuropathy (AMAN).

Specific therapy is now available for Guillain-Barré syndrome. Steroids are no longer used, as studies show no benefit from corticosteroids or adrenocorticotropic hormone, and one trial documented a slower recovery in patients treated with prednisone. Steroids also reduce the patient's resistance to respiratory and urinary infection. Most physicians use either plasmapheresis (2 to 3 liter exchanges, two to three treatments for mild disease or 4 to 5 treatments for more severe disease), or IGIV* (0.4 g per kg per day for 5 days) in the management of this condition. Treatment is based on the proposal that weakness is caused by demyelination and conduction block produced by circulating antibodies. If this is so, plasma exchange should be effective because the antibodies would be removed by the procedure. High-dose IGIV works by bulk displacement of pathogenetic antibodies from myelin. Patients undergoing plasma exchange or given IGIV improve more rapidly and have shorter hospital stays than untreated patients. Problems in the use of these therapies are the expense, the inconvenience to the patient, and the potential for anaphylactic reactions to the products used to replace the serum. There is a risk of viral infection with the use of pooled blood products. Treatment is not recommended for the patient with mild or improving neuropathy.

Chronic Inflammatory Demyelinating Polyradiculoneuropathy

In this disorder the initial rate of progression is slower than that in Guillain-Barré syndrome. The time to maximum disability is greater than 6 weeks in most cases and may be a year or more in some. There is rarely a history of an antecedent illness or other precipitating factor. Other features differentiating the two disorders include nerve thickening, more prominent sensory symptoms, and a more protracted course, sometimes with spontaneous remissions and relapses, in chronic inflammatory polyradiculoneuropathy. Clinical symptoms and signs are otherwise similar; evidence of a generalized neuropathy with proximal weakness is essential to the diagnosis of both. The cerebrospinal fluid protein is elevated, and nerve conduction velocities are slowed in both disorders, although these abnormalities are more common and more marked in the chronic form.

*Not FDA approved for this indication.

Despite the apparent similarities, it is important to distinguish chronic inflammatory demyelinating polyradiculoneuropathy from the Guillain-Barré syndrome because the response to treatment is different. Evidence strongly suggests a definite benefit from prolonged prednisone therapy in the chronic form. For moderate to severe disease, a trial of at least 3 months is indicated. Prednisone is given in doses of 120 mg and 7.5 mg on alternate days initially. If a response occurs, the doses are slowly tapered over 9 months, but if there is no beneficial effect after 2 months the prednisone is reduced more rapidly. For patients with less severe disease, the potential benefit must be weighed against the risks of long-term corticosteroid therapy such as infection, cataracts, and elevated blood sugar level. Plasmapheresis has been shown in a double blind sham-controlled clinical trial to be beneficial. It therefore should be considered in the management of patients with severe disease unresponsive to conventional treatment. Similarly, IGIV* is effective in inducing and maintaining a remission in the disorder. An occasional patient is unresponsive to all conventional therapy but improves with a combination of plasmapheresis and IGIV.

Before making a diagnosis of chronic inflammatory polyradiculoneuropathy, certain conditions that mimic this disorder must be excluded. A similar clinical picture with increased cerebrospinal fluid protein may be seen in diabetes, sarcoidosis, various neoplastic disorders (especially lymphoma, POEMS, and other paraproteinemic neuropathies), and some of the hereditary neuropathies. These diseases should be sought by careful clinical examination, including testing of relatives and appropriate laboratory tests.

MONONEURITIS MULTIPLEX

This distinctive pattern of peripheral nerve disease is characterized by marked asymmetry of limb involvement and is the result of damage of individual peripheral nerves rather than diffuse disease. The nature and distribution of symptoms are determined by the nerves that are affected.

Mononeuritis Multiplex of Gradual Onset

The most common cause of a slowly progressive mononeuritis multiplex is entrapment or pressure

*Not FDA approved for this indication.

palsies of multiple nerves. Many of the peripheral nerves are vulnerable at well-known sites, such as the median nerve in the carpal tunnel, the ulnar nerve at the elbow, the radial nerve in the upper arm, and the peroneal nerve at the fibular head. When these nerves are chronically compressed, symptoms can be alleviated in most cases by surgery and avoidance of activities known to compress these nerves. However, if damage to axons has been severe, recovery will be slow and incomplete.

Several medical conditions predispose to the development of pressure palsies. In rheumatoid arthritis, bony deformities may result in chronic nerve compression, and surgery may be necessary to correct the deformity or move the nerve to a less vulnerable site. Hypothyroidism and acromegaly are associated with multiple focal neuropathies, and correction of the hormonal abnormalities leads to rapid symptomatic relief. Amyloidosis may cause local pressure palsies by infiltrating tight compartments. This is most common in the carpal tunnel. Surgical decompression relieves the compressive neuropathy, but there is currently no effective treatment for amyloidosis. Mononeuritis multiplex is also one of the most common manifestations of sarcoidosis involving the nervous system and is often seen in association with large areas of sensory loss over the trunk. This probably represents involvement of thoracic nerve roots. Nerve lesions in sarcoidosis tend to worsen slowly and then recover gradually, but prednisone therapy is usually warranted, as it is believed to abbreviate the course of neuropathy and to prevent new lesions from appearing. The recommended dose is 60 mg daily with gradual tapering to 15 mg daily. This dosage should be maintained for several months and then withdrawn slowly.

Lead neuropathy is currently a rare disorder but typically manifests as a mononeuritis multiplex with a predilection for the radial nerves. Treatment is discussed in the section on demyelinating neuropathies.

Mononeuritis Multiplex of Abrupt Onset

When a patient develops a flurry of individual nerve lesions, with each one evolving almost overnight, the underlying process is usually a vasculitis. Typically, the onset of paralysis is preceded by severe pain and paresthesias, which are often more distressing than the weakness that follows. The clinical picture is easily recognized, but the diagnosis can be confirmed by sural nerve biopsy. Even if this nerve is not involved clinically, the pathologic changes of the underlying angiopathy can almost always be demonstrated. Nerve tissue has low metabolic demands and a richly anastomotic blood supply, so angiopathic changes must be extensive before nerve infarction develops.

Many diseases are known to produce this pattern of disease: polyarteritis nodosa and the Churg-Strauss syndrome, rheumatoid arthritis, systemic lupus erythematosus, Sjögren's syndrome, diabetes, Wegener's granulomatosis, cryoglobulinemia, and cranial arteritis. With the exception of diabetes and cryoglobulinemia, these conditions are treated with high doses of prednisone, 60 to 100 mg daily for 2 weeks, then 100 mg on alternate days. Disease progression sometimes occurs on this schedule, so cyclophosphamide (Cytoxan), 2 mg per kg, is often added (this use not listed by maker). A high fluid intake is recommended to avoid hemorrhagic cystitis, and regular checks of the blood count and platelet count, blood sugar level, and blood pressure are essential on this drug regimen. The use of cyclophosphamide may permit a lower corticosteroid dose than would otherwise be necessary, and weaning from steroids can often be started earlier.

The management of diabetic mononeuritis multiplex is essentially the same as for other types of diabetic neuropathy discussed previously. Cryoglobulinemia causes nerve infarction by occluding vessels with proteins that precipitate on exposure to cold. Essential (idiopathic) cryoglobulinemia is best dealt with by simple avoidance of cold exposure, but cryoglobulins produced in plasma cell dyscrasias as paraproteins often require more aggressive treatment. This is usually directed toward the cause of the paraprotein, but in some cases plasma exchange can be of great benefit in decreasing the total amount of the cryoglobulin.

LARGE-FIBER SENSORY NEUROPATHY

Some peripheral neuropathies cause selective dysfunction of the largest nerve fibers. This produces an easily recognizable clinical syndrome resulting from the loss of proprioceptive sense that travels in these large fibers. Patients with this disorder have a severe sensory ataxia in darkness or with eyes closed. Examination shows disproportionate loss of vibration and joint position sense with relative preservation of pain, temperature, and touch sensations. The inability to sense the position of the joints may cause pseudoathetosis or "searching" movements of fingers and toes, particularly when the individual is attempting to maintain a specified posture.

Neoplastic Sensory Neuropathy

In some patients with carcinoma, a slowly progressive large-fiber neuropathy occurs and may antedate the diagnosis of the cancer by up to 3 years. The associated malignancy is almost always an oat cell carcinoma of the lung, but occasional instances of other primary lung neoplasms or carcinoma of the cecum or esophagus are found. The usual symptoms are peripheral numbness and tingling associated with clumsiness and falls due to the sensory ataxia. Treatment of the neoplasm does not appear to influence the course of this neuropathy. In most cases the symptoms are due to disease of the dorsal root ganglia ("paraneoplastic sensory neuronopathy").

Drug-Associated Sensory Neuropathy

The long-term abuse of nitrous oxide can produce a large-fiber neuropathy with sensory ataxia. This is usually found in medical personnel with ready access to the drug but has also been reported with the inhalation of nitrous oxide from canisters used to prepare whipped cream. Cessation of the abuse is generally followed by improvement, but a residual deficit may persist. Large doses of pyridoxine (vitamin B_6) can lead to a severe large-fiber sensory neuropathy. Clioquinol, a drug once commonly used for travelers' diarrhea, is thought to be the cause of a degenerative disorder of spinal cord and optic nerves known as subacute myelo-optic neuropathy. An associated large-fiber neuropathy has been described but not clearly documented.

Other Large-Fiber Neuropathies

Some of the classic causes of this syndrome have already been discussed in earlier sections. These include hypothyroidism, which is associated with a demyelinating large-fiber neuropathy that is exquisitely responsive to replacement therapy, and diabetes mellitus, which can cause selective damage to large sensory fibers as well as other types of peripheral neuropathy. Vitamin B_{12} deficiency produces a large-fiber neuropathy, but the peripheral abnormalities are often overshadowed by the presence of myelopathy. IgM paraproteinemia is sometimes associated with a large-fiber neuropathy, and treatment rarely leads to improvement. Idiopathic subacute sensory neuronopathy may affect the upper limbs more than the lower limbs and can be difficult to distinguish from neoplastic sensory neuropathy. The treatment of these disorders is described in the appropriate sections.

SMALL-FIBER SENSORY AND AUTONOMIC NEUROPATHY

Patients with this type of neuropathy can sometimes cause diagnostic confusion because pain and discomfort may be severe in the absence of the usual clinical signs of neuropathy. The main complaints are of intense pricking, tingling, and burning pains in the feet and sometimes in the hands. Symptoms of autonomic nervous system dysfunction are also common and consist of postural dizziness, bloating, diarrhea, and impotence in males. Severe autonomic neuropathy may cause urinary and fecal incontinence. Examination reveals normal distal strength and reflexes, whereas sensory testing shows marked impairment of pain and temperature sensation with preserved joint position and vibration sense. Electromyography is often completely normal in the beginning but may show mild abnormalities with progression.

Diabetes

This form of neuropathy is seen most commonly in insulin-dependent juvenile diabetics. Adult diabetics whose blood sugar level is normalized rapidly with insulin may also develop a neuropathy with prominent positive sensory symptoms that may be associated with a less severe dysautonomia. The prognosis for recovery from the painful symptoms is good with satisfactory control of the blood glucose, but recovery from autonomic neuropathy is unusual.

Amyloidosis

The next largest group of patients with small-fiber neuropathy consists of patients with primary amyloidosis. These patients are usually middle-aged or elderly males with postural syncope, impotence, constipation, bladder disturbances, and impaired sweating. Examination shows decreased pain and temperature sensation. About 90% have an abnormal protein band on immunoelectrophoresis of serum and urine. Amyloid deposits can also be found in abdominal fat, in peripheral nerves, and in rectal neurons. There is no effective treatment available at present for this condition, though the use of colchicine has been described. Amyloidosis secondary to myeloma, macroglobulinemia, or chronic inflammation does not often produce this type of neuropathy.

Other Small-Fiber Neuropathies

Occasionally, small-fiber neuropathy occurs in patients with lung cancer. In these cases the autonomic failure may be severe with complete anhidrosis and marked postural hypotension, and peripheral nerve symptoms may be absent. Treatment of the malignancy has been reported to improve the autonomic function. Rare hereditary neuropathies such as Fabry's disease, Tangier disease, and hereditary sensory neuropathy type 1 can manifest with dysautonomia and the sensory symptoms. Autonomic function may be prominent in acute inflammatory demyelinating polyradiculoneuropathy.

MOTOR NEUROPATHY

Acute motor axonal neuropathy has been described earlier. A syndrome of selective motor axonal neuropathy associated with multiple conduction blocks on nerve conduction studies has been recognized in the last few years. Affected patients may have fasciculations and severe proximal and distal wasting and weakness, resembling amyotrophic lateral sclerosis. In some instances the tendon reflexes are preserved or brisk, making it difficult to separate the two disorders on clinical grounds. This problem emphasises the need for careful nerve conduction studies in patients with peripheral nerve disease.

Lead intoxication, the hepatic porphyrias (acute intermittent, variegate, and coproporphyria), and diphtheria can all cause selective motor peripheral neuropathies. Some patients with IgM paraproteinemia have a purely motor syndrome.

TREATMENT OF PERIPHERAL NEUROPATHY

In many instances there is no specific treatment for a particular type of neuropathy. It is important to keep in mind the value of general supportive measures in alleviating symptoms. Range-of-motion exercises to prevent joint contractures, and braces and splints for weakened muscle groups are often invaluable in maintaining mobility. Patients with severe lower extremity weakness or sensory loss often derive considerable benefit from the stability provided by a cane. The importance of protection and care of insensitive feet, particularly in the patient with diabetes, cannot be overemphasized. Patients should be instructed to trim their toenails with great care and to be fastidious about foot hygiene. Any fungal or bacterial infection requires prompt medical attention. The need for well-fitting shoes should also be emphasized. In addition, patients should be warned that the lack of sensation makes their feet more susceptible to damage from frostbite in winter.

Patients with peripheral neuropathy severe enough to confine them to bed (e.g., Guillain-Barré syndrome) are at risk for deep vein thrombosis and respiratory complications. Care should be taken to prevent these complications or to treat them promptly if they arise.

TREATMENT OF PAINFUL NEUROPATHIES

Pain is a prominent feature in some peripheral neuropathies and can be the most distressing part of the disease. The quality of the pain is usually an intense burning or pricking sensation and is often associated with marked hypersensitivity to light touch. Some patients complain of deep-seated aching and pulling sensations or tightness. Certain neuropathies are more prone to produce these sensations than others: the worst offenders are generally axonal degenerations, particularly alcoholic and uremic neuropathies; metal intoxications; and the small-fiber neuropathies of diabetes and Fabry's disease. Pain is often severe in nerve infarction resulting from angiopathy and in the neuropathy produced by some drugs, such as gold and vincristine (Oncovin). In addition, some patients with very little clinical evidence of neuropathy complain of prominent positive symptoms but do not have the marked loss of pain and temperature sensation and the dysautonomia that characterize small-fiber neuropathies. These patients probably have an idiopathic minimal sensory neuropathy.

Treatment of these symptoms can be challenging, as they often do not respond well to conventional analgesics, and there is a real risk of drug dependence developing. Mild symptoms can be relieved by soaking the extremities in cool tap water (about 15°C) for 20 minutes. If this is done late in the evening and combined with 600 to 900 mg of aspirin orally, the patient may be able to sleep undisturbed. When more severe symptoms are present, phenytoin* (Dilantin) or carbamazepine* (Tegretol) can be tried in standard anticonvulsant doses. Amitriptyline* (Elavil), 25 mg in the morning and 50 mg at night, sometimes provides very effective relief, although anticholinergic drugs should be used with caution in the elderly, in whom there is a significant risk of inducing delirium and autonomic side effects. Mexiletine* (Mexitil), 300 to 900 mg daily in divided doses, is effective in some patients. An electrocardiogram should be obtained to avoid giving this drug to patients with heart block or myocardial disease. Capsaicin creams (0.025% or 0.075%), applied sparingly 3 or 4 times a day, often relieve pain after the initial burning wears off. Transcutaneous nerve stimulation is often effective at the outset, but the benefit is often transient.

*Not FDA approved for this indication.

ACUTE HEAD INJURIES IN ADULTS

method of
DONALD W. MARION, M.D.
University of Pittsburgh Medical Center
Pittsburgh, Pennsylvania

Traumatic brain injury remains a common cause of death and disability in the United States. Approximately 180 to 220 persons per 100,000 per year suffer a head injury, and 14 to 30 persons per 100,000 die each year as a result. Ten percent of these victims have severe injuries that render them comatose, 20% have moderate neurologic deficits but are still conscious, and 70% have mild injuries. Most victims of head injury are between the ages of 15 and 24 years, and men are two to three times more likely to suffer a head injury as women. A positive blood alcohol level is detected in 50 to 60% of head-injured patients. The most common causes of traumatic brain injury are motor vehicle accidents, falls, and assaults. In the country as a whole, motor vehicle accidents account for the majority of head injuries, but in large urban areas, assaults and gunshot wounds are a more common cause. In the elderly, falls may be a more common cause than motor vehicle accidents.

PATHOPHYSIOLOGY OF HEAD INJURIES

Neurologic outcome after traumatic brain injury is a result of damage to the brain that occurs at the time of the trauma (primary brain injury) and of delayed neurochemical and metabolic changes that occur during the first few hours and days after the injury (secondary brain injury). Primary injuries to the skull and brain are a result of impact, translational, and rotational forces applied to the head. The types of skull and brain injuries that occur depend on the type of force applied. For example, direct impact to the head, such as a blow to the head with a rigid object, is far more likely than a motor vehicle accident to result in a skull fracture and intracranial hematoma. High-speed motor vehicle accidents cause severe rotational forces to the head, diffuse brain injuries, and brain swelling, and less commonly, intracranial hematomas. Primary injuries include skull fractures, subdural and epidural hematomas, contusions, and diffuse axonal injuries.

Secondary injury occurs during the first few hours and days after the trauma. Several pathophysiologic abnormalities exacerbate brain tissue injury and lead to brain swelling. Early after the injury, cerebral blood flow is typically less than half of normal values, the blood-brain barrier is disrupted, and cerebrovascular autoregulatory mechanisms responsible for modulating normal cerebral blood flow are disrupted. In some cases, these changes may exist for several days after the injury. The abrupt decrease in cerebral blood flow and the inability of the cerebrovasculature to maintain an adequate blood supply to damaged areas of the brain result in ischemia. Focal and, in some cases, global cerebral ischemia leads to the release of high levels of excitotoxic amino acids, lactate, and oxygen free radicals. Disruption of the blood-brain barrier and other factors result in an intense inflammatory response around contusions and underlying subdural hematomas. All of these conditions increase brain tissue injury, swelling, and ischemia.

The challenge for the contemporary neurotraumatologist is to intervene early after traumatic brain injury to prevent as much secondary injury as possible. On the basis of our current understanding of the pathophysiologic abnormalities associated with secondary brain injury, the treatment of these patients should focus on enhancing cerebral blood flow, avoiding therapies that can exacerbate ischemia, and identifying and applying therapies that effectively reduce the production of oxygen free radicals and suppress the inflammatory response.

TREATMENT

Mild Head Injuries

The majority of patients with head injuries have only a brief period of loss of consciousness, followed by several minutes of amnesia for the event. In more severe cases, retrograde amnesia for several minutes may occur. On evaluation, victims may be neurologically normal or somewhat confused or disoriented. An estimated 2 million people per year suffer head injuries, but only 400,000 require hospitalization. The challenge is to identify patients who are at risk for the development of intracranial mass lesions or brain swelling and delayed neurologic deterioration. Risk factors include mechanism of injury, age, predisposing medical conditions (e.g., use of anticoagulants), duration of loss of consciousness, and duration of pre- or post-traumatic amnesia (Table 1). If any of these risk factors exist, the patient should be taken to an emergency department and undergo a thorough evaluation, in most cases including computed tomography (CT) of the head. The patient should be observed with serial neurologic examinations for a minimum of 1 hour. Neurologic assessment should include cranial nerve, motor, and sensory function, as well as the more subtle neuropsychologic and cognitive functioning. If any abnormality persists, the patient should be admitted for observation for 24 hours and closely monitored for neurologic deterioration. In most cases, those patients with post-traumatic lesions identified by CT should also be hospitalized and have an additional CT examination within 12 to 24 hours to rule out enlargement of intracranial mass lesions. When discharged from the hospital or the emergency department, the patient and family members should be carefully informed, both verbally and with written instructions, about the symptoms and signs of delayed brain injury and whom to contact if these symptoms occur. The significance of increasing headaches, lethargy, nausea or vomiting, or new onset of focal neurologic deficits should be emphasized.

TABLE 1. **Risk Factors for Delayed Neurologic Deterioration After Head Injury**

Mechanism
High-speed motor vehicle accident
Fall of more than 8 ft
Injury that causes significant damage to other areas of the body
Age greater than 65 y
Medical conditions
Long-term anticoagulation therapy
Presence of cerebrovascular malformation
Duration of loss of consciousness more than 5 min
Pre- or post-traumatic amnesia for longer than 10 min

Moderate to Severe Head Injuries

Prehospital Management

The first priority in the initial evaluation of the patient with moderate to severe head injury is to restore and/or maintain normal oxygenation and blood pressure. Most severely head-injured patients who are rendered comatose benefit from early endotracheal intubation and controlled ventilation. Portable pulse oximetry should be used to verify arterial oxygen saturations of greater than 96%, and supplemental oxygen should be provided to achieve this level. A ventilatory rate of 10 to 12 breaths per minute (arterial P_{CO_2} of 35 to 40 mm Hg) is recommended. In larger patients, higher ventilatory rates may be required to provide adequate minute ventilation. Patients who suffer neurologic deterioration while being observed are at high risk for the development of intracranial mass lesions and may also benefit from higher ventilatory rates until the mass lesion is removed. Hypotension is aggressively treated by placement of several large-bore intravenous catheters and administration of isotonic crystalloid or colloid solutions as necessary to restore a mean blood pressure of 90 to 100 mm Hg.

After the airway is secured, normal oxygenation is ensured, and the blood pressure is stabilized, a rapid assessment of injuries is conducted. A rigid cervical spine collar is applied, and the patient is placed on a back board. Any points of active bleeding are tamponaded with external dressings. The neurologic status is assessed in terms of the Glasgow Coma Scale score (Table 2). Any asymmetry in motor functioning or eye opening is noted, and pupil size and reactivity to light are documented.

At this point, the patient is transported rapidly to

TABLE 2. **Glasgow Coma Scale Scoring***

Measure	Score
Eye Opening	
Spontaneously	4
To verbal command	3
To painful stimuli	2
None	1
Verbal Response	
Oriented and converses	5
Disoriented and converses	4
Inappropriate words	3
Incomprehensible sounds	2
No audible sounds	1
Motor Response	
Follows verbal commands	6
To painful stimuli	
Purposeful localization	5
Withdraws from stimulus	4
Flexor posturing	3
Extensor posturing	2
No response	1

*Total score equals eye opening + verbal response + motor response; scores range from 3 to 15.

a trauma center capable of definitive neurosurgical intervention. For transport times longer than 15 to 20 minutes, serial neurologic assessments should be documented every 10 to 15 minutes. Early contact by telephone or radio should be made with the trauma center, and medications given to the patient should be coordinated through the neurosurgeons and other health care providers at the trauma center.

Emergency Department Management

Transfer of the severely head-injured patient to a trauma center certified by the American College of Surgeons or state trauma certification systems is highly recommended. Such trauma centers typically have a trauma surgeon in house 24 hours a day and a neurosurgeon available within 10 minutes of notification. The patient is initially evaluated according to the guidelines of the Advanced Trauma Life Support protocol of the American College of Surgeons. The primary survey is conducted to identify all life-threatening injuries and to assess the level of consciousness of the patient. Life-threatening chest or abdominal injuries are identified immediately and treated. Cervical spine radiographs are obtained to rule out cervical spine instability. A diagnostic peritoneal lavage or diagnostic abdominal ultrasound scanning is done to rule out significant intra-abdominal hemorrhage. The patient is taken to the CT suite and has CT of the head to identify any surgical intracranial mass lesions. If abdominal ultrasound scanning or diagnostic peritoneal lavage has not been performed, most comatose head-injured victims also have CT of the abdomen and, if thoracic hemorrhage is suspected, CT of the chest.

If the blood pressure is difficult to control, or the diagnostic peritoneal lavage is positive, the patient may be taken immediately to surgery without CT of the head. In these cases, an intraoperative air ventriculogram can be obtained to detect large intracranial mass lesions.

Once CT of the head is done, whether a craniotomy is indicated is determined by the size and location of intracranial hematomas or hemorrhagic contusions. Approximately 20% of comatose head-injured patients have one or more hemorrhagic contusions, and 20% have an acute subdural hematoma. In most cases, lesions larger than 25 to 30 mL, particularly those within or adjacent to the temporal lobes, should be evacuated. In addition to the size and location of the mass lesion, the decision to operate is based on the patient's neurologic status, change in the neurologic status, presence or absence of pupil abnormalities, and age. For example, an 80-year-old patient who is admitted with a fixed and dilated pupil and a Glasgow Coma Scale score of 3 or 4 is not likely to have a functional recovery, even though he or she may have a large subdural hematoma that can be evacuated. In such cases, the decision is often made not to intervene surgically.

Intensive Care Management

Once all life-threatening and surgical issues are resolved, the patient with severe to moderate head injury is transferred to an intensive care unit staffed by nurses familiar with the management of patients with head injuries. An intracranial pressure monitor is placed for continuous intracranial pressure monitoring in all patients who are unable to follow commands and have post-traumatic intracranial abnormalities at CT. I prefer a ventriculostomy catheter placed into the right lateral ventricle and fluid-coupled to a transducer; this device permits intermittent cerebrospinal fluid drainage as a potential treatment for raised intracranial pressure.

Every attempt is made to normalize the patient's physiologic and hemodynamic parameters. The mean arterial blood pressure is kept at 100 ± 10 mm Hg. The central venous pressure is kept at 6 to 15 cm H_2O, the arterial P_{CO_2} at 35 ± 2 mm Hg, and the arterial P_{O_2} higher than 98 mm Hg. In addition, the core body temperature is maintained at 37 ± 5°C. The head is kept in the midline, and compression of the soft tissues of the neck is avoided. For the first 24 hours after injury, I keep the head of the bed flat to enhance cerebral perfusion. Cerebral perfusion pressure (mean arterial pressure minus intracranial pressure) is maintained above 70 mm Hg with the use of vasopressor agents if necessary. A 20-gauge Silastic catheter is inserted into the internal jugular vein with its tip in the jugular bulb, usually on the right, and frequent assessments of the arterial jugular venous oxygen content difference are obtained. My goal is to maintain these values at less than 7 vol%. The hemoglobin is maintained at 10 to 12 mg per dL, sodium and potassium values are normalized, partial thromboplastin time and prothrombin time are normalized, and any other hematologic or electrolyte abnormalities are corrected.

The presence or absence of cervical spine instability must also be determined early after injury. Good quality lateral, anteroposterior, and open-mouth odontoid radiographs of the cervical spine, when properly interpreted, will identify more than 99% of unstable cervical spine injuries. The lateral view must include the C7–T1 interspace. The most common reasons for missed cervical spine injuries are inadequate radiographs or improper interpretation of the radiographs. In patients who are alert and awake and have neck pain, flexion and extension films are recommended.

Phenytoin (Dilantin) is administered to all patients who have post-traumatic parenchymal injuries, such as contusions, subdural hematomas, and diffuse brain swelling. Therapy is discontinued after 7 days unless the patient has delayed post-traumatic seizures, in which case the therapy is continued for 6 months to 1 year. An H_2 blocker is given to lower the risk of stress ulcers. Sequential pneumatic compression devices are applied to the lower extremities. Nutritional supplementation, preferably enteral, is begun within 48 to 72 hours after the injury, and the goal is to reach 2000 to 2500 kcal per day.

Management of Elevated Intracranial Pressure

Brain swelling occurs after most severe traumatic brain injuries. A primary goal of the critical care of severely head-injured patients is to prevent elevated intracranial pressure. Normal intracranial pressure is less than 12 to 15 mm Hg. Most studies find a significant increase in mortality and morbidity when intracranial pressure exceeds 20 mm Hg for prolonged periods.

I use a stepwise approach to the management of elevated intracranial pressure (Table 3). Therapies are added only when the previous one fails to reduce intracranial pressure. If there is an abrupt increase in intracranial pressure after the pressure had previously been well controlled, CT of the head is performed immediately. In addition, follow-up CT of the head is routinely performed within 12 to 24 hours after the patient is admitted, particularly for those patients in whom small contusions or subdural or epidural hematomas were documented at the initial CT. Approximately 20 to 30% of such lesions are found to be larger at follow-up CT.

When intracranial pressure remains below 20 mm Hg for 24 to 48 hours without treatment, the ventricular catheter is removed. Shortly thereafter, most patients can be weaned from mechanical ventilation. Patients who remain comatose for longer than 5 to 10 days usually benefit from the placement of a tracheostomy and feeding jejunostomy tube for long-term care. During the second week after injury, physiatry personnel should be involved with care on a day-to-day basis to coordinate a routine of bedside physical therapy and occupational therapy. Long-term anticoagulation therapy should be considered for patients who have little or no spontaneous extremity movement.

TABLE 3. **Stepwise Approach to Management of Elevated Intracranial Pressure**

All physiologic and hemodynamic parameters normalized

- P_{CO_2} 35 ± 2 mm Hg
- P_{O_2} > 98 mm Hg
- Mean arterial pressure 100 ± 10 mm Hg
- Central venous pressure 6–15 cm H_2O
- Core temperature 37 ± 5°C

Systemic neuromuscular paralysis (vecuronium or pancuronium)
Narcotic sedation (morphine or fentanyl)
Intermittent CSF drainage
Mannitol (25–50 gm q 3–4 h)

- Not used if serum osmolality exceeds 315 mOsm
- Urine output replaced milliliter per milliliter with isotonic saline solution

Furosemide (40 mg q 4 h)

- Not used if serum osmolality exceeds 315 mOsm

Pentobarbital to achieve electroencephalographic burst suppression
Moderate hypothermia (32–33°C for 24 h)

Abbreviation: CSF = cerebrospinal fluid.

Complications

The most common complications that occur early after severe traumatic brain injury are infectious, pulmonary, and gastroenterologic. Pneumonia occurs in 30 to 50% of intubated head-injured patients in the intensive care unit. These infections are usually treated with broad-spectrum antibiotics until the organism and antibiotic sensitivities are identified, at which point antibiotic coverage is adjusted. Atelectasis and pneumothorax are also common complications. The most common gastroenterologic complications are paralytic ileus and gastrointestinal hemorrhage from stress ulcers. I start all severely head-injured patients on H_2 blockers on admission to the intensive care unit. Other less common complications are pituitary insufficiency as a result of damage to the hypothalamus, pituitary stalk, or pituitary gland. Within 4 to 5 days after admission, the comatose head-injured patient should have a screening endocrine battery, including cortisol, prolactin, growth hormone, and thyroid function studies.

Longer term complications include post-traumatic hydrocephalus, heterotopic ossification, decubitus ulcers, malnutrition, and spastic contractures. Many of these complications are prevented or limited with aggressive daily physical therapy routines. The risk of deep venous thrombosis or pulmonary embolism is lowered with the use of anticoagulant therapy.

PROGNOSIS

Mild Head Injuries

Most patients who suffer mild head injuries have a complete recovery by 3 months after injury. However, some studies have found that as many as two thirds of mildly head-injured patients may have significant neurobehavioral deficits, memory problems, and headaches until then. A few studies have found that two thirds of mildly head-injured patients remain unemployed after 3 months. Patients with mild traumatic brain injury are particularly at risk for postconcussive syndrome, which manifests as headaches, dizziness, and reduced energy levels. As many as 47% of victims of mild head injury complain of headaches 3 months after injury.

Severe Traumatic Brain Injury

The prognosis for patients with severe traumatic brain injury has changed a great deal in the last 10 to 15 years. In 1985, mortality rates for patients who suffered closed head injury were 36 to 40%, and the rate of functional recovery was 20 to 30% at 1 year after the injury. Several more recent studies have found a mortality rate of approximately 20% and good recovery rates of 35 to 45% at 1 year after injury. This improved outcome is attributed to the focus on enhancing cerebral perfusion and avoiding therapies that may exacerbate early cerebral ischemia. A prospective randomized trial of the use of therapeutic moderate hypothermia has demonstrated even further improvement in outcomes for those patients who are treated with cooling to 32 to 33°C for 24 hours early after injury.

PEDIATRIC HEAD INJURY

method of
FERNANDO STEIN, M.D., and
JOSE A. CORTES, M.D.
Texas Children's Hospital and
Baylor College of Medicine
Houston, Texas

Typically head trauma in children is closed and mild to moderate. Head injury is a frequent problem encountered by primary care physicians. After a child is injured, the caregivers usually contact the physician by telephone first.

The majority of cases of head injury in children do not require any diagnostic imaging and even less hospitalization. The emphasis of this chapter is on mild to moderate head injury, because most cases of pediatric head trauma fall into this category.

Head injury has been classified as mild, moderate, and severe.

1. Mild head injury is divided in two categories.

Low risk: Glasgow Coma Scale (GCS) score of 15 without acute radiologic abnormality

High risk: GCS score of 13 to 14 or GCS score of 15 with acute radiologic abnormality, both with a period of unconsciousness of less than 20 minutes

2. Moderate head injury is defined as a GCS score of 9 to 12 or a GCS score of 13 to 14 with a mass effect or lesion on computed tomography (CT) scan.
3. Severe head injury is defined as a GCS score of less than 8.

The classic criteria have been based on the GCS score (Table 1). However, other elements of judgment such as the degree of concussion or the time of loss of consciousness have been used (Table 2). The GCS score has not been validated for children younger than 5 years old.

TABLE 1. **Glasgow Coma Scale Score**

Eye Opening Response	**Score**
Spontaneous	4
To verbal command	3
To pain	2
None	1
Motor Response	
Obeys verbal commands	6
Localizes pain	5
Withdraws to pain	4
Decorticate posture	3
Decerebrate posture	2
None	1
Verbal Response	
Oriented	5
Confused	4
Inappropriate words	3
Incomprehensible sounds	2
None	1

In the simplest analysis, mild to moderate head injury is any head trauma that did not cause coma.

EPIDEMIOLOGY

Each year an estimated two per 1000 children sustain a head injury. Common causes are falls, sporting accidents, and child abuse.

At all ages, the male to female ratio is 2:1 for head trauma. In children younger than 2 years of age, falls and abuse are responsible for the majority of injuries. Motor vehicle–related injuries are more common in older children.

Eighty percent of children who sustain a head injury are not hospitalized. Close to 12% of children are hospitalized for fewer than 3 days, and only about 8% who are considered to have severe head injury are hospitalized for more than 3 days. Mild to moderate head injuries account for 93% of all hospital admissions for head injury, whereas severe head injuries account for only 7%.

PATHOPHYSIOLOGY

Brain injury occurs in two phases: primary and secondary. The primary injury is the damage sustained at the

TABLE 2. **Classification of Concussion**

Grade	Symptoms
0	Not stunned or dazed. Later headache and difficulty in concentration.
1	Stunned or dazed. No loss of consciousness or amnesia. Sensorium clears in less than 1 minute.
2	Clouding, not loss of consciousness, tinnitus, amnesia. Confused or dizzy.
3	Loss of consciousness for less than 1 minute, never comatose.
4	Loss of consciousness for more than 1 minute, without coma. Hyperexcitable, confused, or dizzy afterward.

Adapted and modified from Nelson WE, Glieck JH, Jane JH, Hawthorne P: Athletic head injuries. J Natl Athletic Trainers Assn *19*:95–102, 1984.

time of impact. It is proportional to the magnitude, duration, and velocity of the applied mechanical force. The brain may become distorted, leading to axonal injuries.

Secondary injury is the neuronal damage caused by the pathophysiologic consequences of the primary injury such as decreased cerebral blood flow, cerebral hypoxia, brain swelling, and uncoupling of energy-substrate ratios. Systemic complicating factors that include hyperthermia and hypotension also aggravate secondary injury. The main goal of therapy is to limit secondary injury to allow maximal functional recovery.

EVALUATION

The majority of children sustain mild to moderate head injury and are not hospitalized. Normally, the family calls the physician first, inquiring whether the child with the injured head should be examined. This is the first decision that has to be made. Of the patients who are examined by a physician, more than 75% receive only a physical examination and require no imaging. Strict office policies on what to ask and what answers to give to parents or caregivers during the initial telephone contact need to exist so that there can be a consistent and disciplined approach to the evaluation of the child with head trauma.

The initial telephone interview will determine whether the child needs to be examined, whether the child can be transported safely by the parents to the office or to an emergency center, and whether the child needs to be transported to an emergency center by an ambulance. In determining who should be examined, it is necessary to establish as clearly as possible the mechanism of the injury. If the injury involves the generation of high velocity, the child should be examined.

A child should be examined by a physician if any of the following is present:

- History of loss of consciousness for more than 1 minute
- Vomiting more than twice
- Lethargy lasting more than 30 minutes
- Severe persistent headache, confusion, weakness, incoordination, abnormal gait, or slurred speech
- Swelling over a body part other than the head
- Fall from height greater than an adult waist
- High-velocity injury (bicycle, skateboard)
- High-velocity projectile injury with loss of consciousness (baseball, softball, stone)
- Blood coming from the ear or bruising behind the ear
- Loss of a previously mastered developmental milestone
- Parental desire to have the child examined

If the child is not evaluated in the office, specific instructions must be given regarding what to look for and when to call. Obviously, the availability of a telephone has to be ascertained. No analgesics other than acetaminophen or ibuprofen should be used.

If no imaging studies were indicated following the child's evaluation, a "head injury sheet" should be given to the family. The physician should determine whether the family has a reliable form of transportation immediately available.

IMAGING IN HEAD INJURY

The most important objective in the patient evaluation after head trauma is to identify whether the child has sustained an intracranial injury as opposed to a skull fracture.

Skull Films

This technique is useful only in identifying skull fractures or radiopaque lesions. Patients who present with low-risk criteria such as headache, scalp hematoma, or scalp laceration have been studied systematically with skull radiograph and CT of the head. In 7035 cases out of 31 hospitals, no intracranial injuries were discovered in any low-risk patient. Therefore, no intracranial pathology would have been missed by excluding the skull radiograph.* Skull fractures can be identified by CT scan of the head.

Computed Tomography

A CT scan of the head is the imaging modality of choice and is recommended in all head trauma patients who exhibit the following:

- A GCS score lower than 14
- Persistent vomiting after 1 hour of injury
- Loss of consciousness for more than 1 minute
- Deteriorating mental status, focal neurologic deficit, and seizure
- High-velocity injury with history of loss of consciousness for an undertermined amount of time
- Depressed skull fracture
- Penetrating head injury
- Unwitnessed head injury (relative indication)

CT is not indicated in minor injuries when there is a GCS score of 15, without loss of consciousness, without focal neurologic signs, and without clinical evidence of a depressed skull fracture.

The CT scan without contrast is an important tool to define any surgical lesion that should be treated promptly. This technique allows visualization of epidural and subdural hematomas, intraventricular and subarachnoid hemorrhage, skull fractures, and cerebral edema.

Magnetic Resonance Imaging

Magnetic resonance imaging (MRI) is superior for visualizing diffuse axonal injury and subarachnoid hemorrhage and for detecting traumatic hematomas of varying ages. It is not the imaging modality of choice in emergencies, because it is time consuming and it requires heavy sedation in younger children and uncooperative adolescents.

MANAGEMENT

The patient should be admitted to a hospital that can offer definitive care. The hospital should offer pediatric intensive care services and, ideally, neurointensive care for the patient who needs neurosurgical interventions. Although initially the child may show few or no symptoms, a neurosurgeon must be available with the necessary support services if an intracranial bleed or an increase in intracranial pressure (ICP) develops. These services include a 24-hour blood bank, anesthesia, clinical laboratory, and neuroimaging availability. The reason for this is obvi-

---

*(N Engl J Med *316*:84–91, 1987.)

ous: transporting a patient with these symptoms to another hospital once a problem has developed increases morbidity and mortality. An interhospital transport should be provided by medical personnel trained in pediatric intensive care with experience in the care of critically ill and injured children. If the mentioned services are not available, the transport should take place as soon as possible.

Mild to Moderate Head Injury

The child who sustained a mild head injury and who did not require hospitalization will need close observation from a responsible adult for 24 to 48 hours. During this time the caregiver should keep the child at home in a quiet environment. The child must be prohibited from working or playing hard, from riding a bicycle or skateboard, and from driving any vehicle. The child should be awakened every 2 hours and checked for arousal abnormalities for the first night. If during the observation period, the child develops one or more of the "signs of danger" (Table 3), the observer must call a physician or the emergency center immediately for further recommendations. If the child does not develop any of the symptoms in Table 3 during the first 24 hours after head injury, the child can be allowed to return to normal activities.

If the decision was made to hospitalize a child with mild to moderate head injury the anticipation should be that some interventions may become necessary such as intensive monitoring and/or care. The hospitalization purpose is to watch closely for the need of interventions, and therefore services such as those mentioned under "Management" must be available.

Severe Head Injury

In children who sustained severe head injury defined as a GCS score of 8 or less, the following five items are crucial for brain protection.

1. Maintaining adequate oxygenation and ventilation
2. Maintaining adequate blood pressure and perfusion (remember that a single episode of hypotension following head injury worsens prognosis significantly)
3. The prevention and treatment of cerebral edema
4. The adequate monitoring and general supportive care (probably the single most effective group of interventions)
5. Immediate availability of neurosurgery, anesthesia, neuroimaging, and full laboratory and intensive care capabilities

TABLE 3. **Signs of Danger Requiring Immediate Call**

The child does not wake up as usual.
The child is sleepy at unusual times.
The child has seizures.
The child vomits more than six times in 24 hours.
The child has problems with coordination.
The child has a bad headache that does not go away.
The child experiences a change in the visual pattern.
The child seems confused and does not act normally.
When the observer thinks that the child's condition has changed.

Securing the airway and providing appropriate oxygenation as well as ventilation is universally accepted. The provision of prophylactic hyperventilation has not been proven scientifically as beneficial for the prevention of cerebral edema. The liberal use of osmotic diuretics without regard to the circulating blood volume of the child may prove hazardous, although it is frequently necessary to use these agents for the treatment of cerebral edema. The prevention of hypotension is considered paramount to avoid further neurologic injury. Well-documented studies show that elevation of body temperature more than 102°F is detrimental and therefore meticulous attention should be paid to the prevention of fever in this type of children. From the surgical standpoint the most frequently needed interventions are the drainage of hematomas and elevation of fractures.

Intracranial Pressure Measurements

Children who have traumatic brain injury with brain swelling generally need to be monitored for increases in ICP. The most commonly used devices are the intraventricular cannula and the intraparenchymal monitors. Intradural and epidural monitors are still used in some institutions. Patients who sustain ICP elevations have impairment of cerebral blood flow and therefore worsening of neurologic injury.

The cerebral perfusion pressure should be maintained above 50 mm Hg in younger children and above 70 mm Hg in adolescents and young adults.

Published clinical experience indicates that ICP monitoring and control may improve outcome and help determine prognosis and that ICP can be reduced by drainage of cerebrospinal fluid. ICP monitoring can help in the early detection of an expanding intracranial mass lesion.

Barbiturate therapy is effective in the setting of uncontrollable ICP refractory to all other conventional medical and surgical treatments. This kind of therapy should be provided in the critical care unit with the appropriate systemic monitoring.

Nutritional support of the head-injured patient should be instituted as early as possible, because poor nutrition worsens outcome.

PROGNOSIS AND COMPLICATIONS

Few criteria allow us to predict the clinical outcome in a head-injured patient. However, the GCS score carries a relationship with recovery, disability, and mortality. There is direct correlation in the degree of disability and duration of coma following head injury (Figure 1).

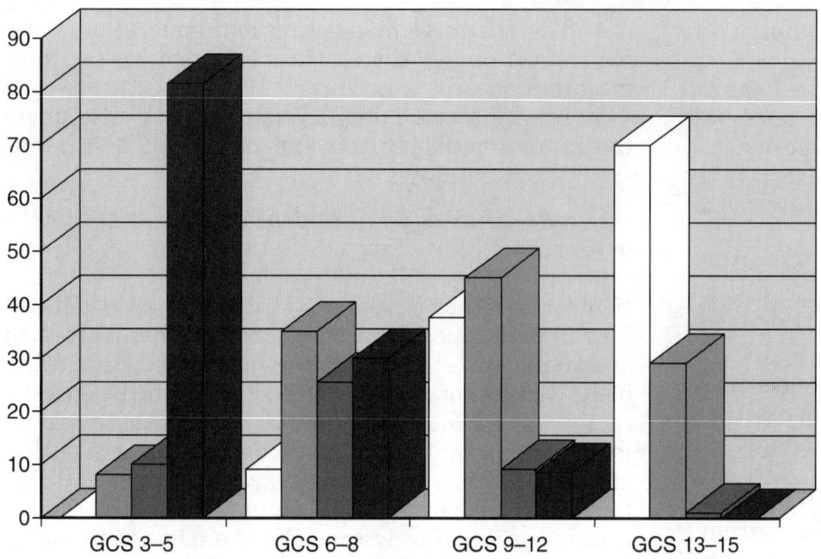

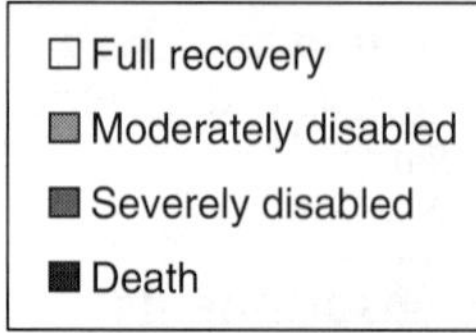

Figure 1. Outcome related to Glasgow Coma Scale (GCS) score.

Postconcussion Syndrome

Postconcussion syndrome is a combination of affective, somatic, and cognitive complaints that follow head injury. Although the literature has questioned its existence, well-controlled studies have shown that more than 50% of the patients blindly interviewed reported symptoms (Figure 2). Most of the somatic complaints tend to decrease or disappear within 3 months of the injury, whereas the affective and cognitive complaints tend to remain for a longer period of time. This period of time for the majority of cases seems to be 6 to 9 months.

Post-traumatic Epilepsy

Post-traumatic epilepsy (PTE) is a condition of recurrent seizures that occur without cause other than an enduring physiologic abnormality of the brain, which is the result of trauma. Ninety percent of post-traumatic seizures occurred within the first 2 years

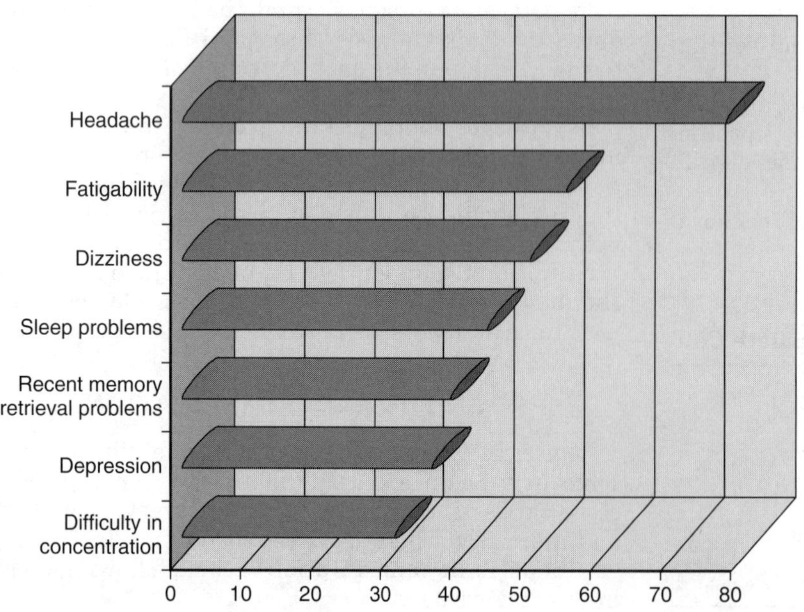

Figure 2. Associated symptoms of postconcussion syndrome.

after the injury. PTE has been classified into early PTE (occurring within 7 days after the event) and late PTE (occurring more than 7 days after the event). Immediate seizures (PTE that occurs during the first 24 hours) are 50 to 80% of all early PTE.

The pathogenesis of PTE has been associated with pathophysiologic findings of bruised parenchyma with leptomeningeal thickening and the subsequent deposition of hemosiderin. Gliosis, neuronal loss, and microglial reaction determine the formation of scars that act as a focus for seizures. A single seizure at the time of injury increases the risk of post-traumatic epilepsy 10-fold.

Treatment Guidelines

1. A generalized seizure at the time of injury should be treated with a long-acting anticonvulsant.
2. The prophylactic administration of anticonvulsant has been proved in double-blind and placebo-controlled studies to be ineffective in prevention of PTE.
3. The current recommendation is that patients with mild to moderate head injury who have had a seizure at the time of injury or are considered at risk for PTE should receive diphenylhydantoin for the first 7 days after injury. Treatment is then stopped and the patient kept on seizure precautions. If seizures develop, appropriate medication should be started.

There are no reliable objective tests (electroencephalogram, CT, MRI) that can predict the development of PTE.

COGNITIVE AND BEHAVIORAL DEFICITS

It is well known that apparent intact survivors of severe head injury may have minor neurobehavioral and learning disabilities that require special evaluation and therapy.

The younger the child, the more likely that injury will be permanent. Incompletely myelinated neurons are more susceptible to injury. Early head injuries impair the ability for new learning.

In older children the best predictor of cognitive problems is amnesia after injury for longer than 7 days.

The indications for neuropsychiatric evaluation are patients who suffered from intracranial hemorrhage, patients with post-traumatic amnesia of more than 24 hours, patients with postconcussion syndrome of more than 3 months, and patients with PTE.

The most common language problem is word retrieval, in which the child is unable to name an object. Other language problems include difficulty writing from dictation, problems with organizing thoughts, difficulty understanding multiple-step commands, and decreased speed with information processing. Cognition problems include lack of attention and concentration, distractibility, short-term memory impairment, and difficulty with logical reasoning. The problems tend to improve over time. Persistent neurobehavioral deficits for moderately and severely injured children improve over 3 years of follow-up, with a rapid rate of improvement during the first year and then a negligible rate of change.

REHABILITATION

Children of school age who sustain a moderate head injury that keeps them from being able to attend school for a period of time longer than 3 to 4 weeks have an interruption of social life and an interruption of academic life. Frequently there are unrealistic expectations and poor understanding on the part of the parents and teachers about the consequences of brain injury of this magnitude, and there is a very high frequency of academic and social failure. A negative behavioral response is displayed by the child, and when coupled with the misinterpretations of teachers, parents, and friends that this response represents a behavioral issue, many of these children fail academically.

These children are not mentally retarded. What they need is a mainstream experience in a creative mix. This includes a learning disabilities resource room at the school or individual tutoring according to their needs. Appropriate ancillary services such as speech, physical, and occupational therapy are highly recommended as well as counseling for both parents, teachers, and friends.

BRAIN TUMORS

method of
DANIEL H. LACHANCE, M.D.
Medical Associates Clinic
Dubuque, Iowa

and

PETER K. DEMPSEY, M.D.
Lahey Hitchcock Medical Center
Burlington, Massachusetts

The general concept of brain tumors refers loosely to a group of neoplasms that may arise from diverse cellular structures in the cranium and may affect the function of the central nervous system (CNS). Although glial tissue neoplasms constitute the most commonly encountered and most feared tumors, neoplastic transformation can occur in neurons, the meninges, vasculature, primitive notochord, primitive neuroectoderm, choroid, ependyma, pineal, pituitary, cranial nerves, and primary or metastatic lymphocytes. Neoplasms metastasic from other sites are also among the most common brain tumors. Clinical presentations are, therefore, diverse and depend primarily on the age of the patient and the primary histology and location of the tumor. Management generally employs a limited number of modalities, but treatment plans are highly specific and heavily depend on the age of the patient and tumor histology and location.

CLASSIFICATION AND PRESENTATION

A general approach to brain tumors considers lesions as extra-axial, intra-axial (within brain or spinal cord) but well demarcated, or intra-axial and infiltrative.

Extra-axial tumors are usually well circumscribed with benign histology. Clinical presentation is directly related to the nervous system structures immediately adjacent to the lesion. In childhood, craniopharyngioma and pineal region tumors are most common, whereas in adulthood meningioma accounting for 18 to 20% of all cranial tumors and acoustic neuroma are commonly encountered. Craniopharyngioma arises from remnants of squamous epithelium in the region of the sella. Growth failure, hypothalamic and pituitary failure, visual loss, and, less commonly, hydrocephalus are the major management issues. Pineal region tumors arise from primary pincocytes, primitive germ cells, primitive neuroectoderm, and, rarely, glial cells. Presentation varies with histology but includes obstructive hydrocephalus, dorsal midbrain dysfunction, and meningeal seeding with cranial nerve, spinal cord, and nerve root dysfunction. Meningiomas are generally benign tumors arising from cells within the arachnoid layer of the meninges. They can occur anywhere along the neuroaxis but commonly appear over the convexities or at the skull base. Meningiomas are often encapsulated, making separation from the surrounding brain and surgical resection possible. Involvement of anatomic structures such as blood vessels or cranial nerves can cause problems. Approximately 7% of meningiomas have malignant features with substantial invasiveness and potential for metastasis. Subtypes of meningiomas may have receptors for estrogen or progesterone, which may explain the slight female predominance of these tumors. Acoustic neuromas are more properly called vestibular schwannomas, as they arise from Schwann cells on the vestibular portion of cranial nerve VIII. These tumors usually manifest with hearing loss, although tinnitus and disequilibrium occur. Surgical resection is the treatment of choice, and with present microsurgical techniques, facial nerve function can be preserved nearly 100% of the time.

Intra-axial, well-circumscribed tumors are usually also of very different histologies in adults and children. Although most of these lesions are radiographically distinct, few are so well circumscribed as to lend themselves to complete microscopic surgical excision, and adjunctive therapy is often necessary depending on malignant growth potential. A typical example is ependymoma. This tumor often occurs in childhood. It arises from ependyma in the fourth ventricle and has a tendency to recur at the primary site and along cerebrospinal fluid (CSF) pathways. A childhood tumor with low growth potential arises from astrocytes. Juvenile pilocytic astrocytoma is an easily identifiable histologic subtype of glial tumor that, unlike all its other glial counterparts, is primarily noninfiltrating. In young children, the cerebellum is the likely site of occurrence; in older children and younger adults, the diencephalon around the third ventricle and, less commonly, brain stem are usual locations. Presentation is often heralded by the effects of large cystic structures on nearby regions of the brain.

The most common well-circumscribed intraparenchymal lesion is a metastasis. Spread to the brain is usually hematogenous. Incidence is primarily in adults. Location in the cortex is often at the junction of gray matter and white matter, but any area of the neuroaxis, including the pituitary and spinal cord, may be affected and frequency of occurrence in any one particular region is generally proportional to the size of that region. Presentation is directly related to the particular CNS region affected. The mass lesion itself does not usually cause symptoms directly except as may be related to its proclivity to cause seizures by way of particular location (temporal and frontal lobes) or hemorrhage by way of particular histologies (melanoma, choriocarcinoma, renal cell carcinoma). Usually, symptoms relate primarily to the sometimes-massive extent of edema in adjacent brain tissue. Dysfunction is most often directly related to the size and location of brain affected and to the extent to which mass effect compresses nearby structures, occupies intracranial space, and effects increase in intracranial pressure. Primary lung tumors and tumors metastatic to lung frequently herald brain metastasis, which presumably is related to direct access to systemic arterial circulation. Besides primary lung tumors, melanoma and breast, renal, and colorectal carcinomas account for 85% of metastasis.

A few, less common, intra-axial, well-circumscribed lesions in adults deserve special mention, as accurate diagnosis and direct surgical management are extremely important to long-term outcome. Central neurocytoma and colloid cysts are lesions that may occur in the region of the foramen of Monro and may manifest with the sudden development of potentially life-threatening hydrocephalus. Neurocytoma is a monomorphic clear cell lesion with no anaplastic features that appears to be of neuronal origin. Colloid cysts are nonenhancing cystic structures composed of primitive neuroepithelial cells with minimal growth potential. Another lesion of primary neuronal origin is the ganglioglioma. Discovered mainly in frontal and temporal lobes, it may be responsible for years of medically refractory epilepsy in some patients. Other uncommon entities such as dysembryoplastic neuroepithelial tumor and pleomorphic xanthoastrocytoma may be similarly responsible for years of poorly controlled seizures. Complete surgical excision of these lesions is sometimes possible, often resulting in dramatic improvement in seizure frequency. Hemangioblastoma is a highly vascular, angioblastic, nonanaplastic lesion often associated with large cysts primarily in the cerebellum and, less commonly, in the spinal cord. When occurring in an individual younger than 50, 10 to 40% may be associated with von Hippel–Lindau disease, an autosomal dominant disorder with incomplete penetrance associated with retinal angiomas, renal and pancreatic cysts, and, most important, hypernephroma.

Infiltrative neoplasms of the CNS are primarily of primitive neuroectodermal (PNET) or glial origin. Medulloblastoma and brain stem astrocytomas occur primarily in children, whereas supratentorial gliomas occur mainly in adults. Astrocytic and PNET tumors behave very differently, and management principles are accordingly very different. In medulloblastoma, histologic subtyping is of no prognostic significance, but the extent of local and meningeal disease at diagnosis, extent of surgical resection, patient age, and local and craniospinal axis radiation dose are major determinants of survival. Glial neoplasms are usually of astrocytic or oligodendrocytic origins. On occasion, the two cell types may be mixed in a single lesion. Survival depends on a number of factors, but tumor grade is most important. The grading system of glial tumors can often cause confusion. The two most commonly accepted systems use either a three- or four-tiered scale, with grade I tumors being more indolent with longer survival and the highest grade tumors (grade III/III or grade IV/IV), commonly known as glioblastoma multiforme (GBM), being most aggressive. Middle-grade tumors—anaplastic astrocytoma (AA) and anaplastic oligodendroglioma (AO)—have fewer malignant histologic features with a more favorable prognosis than that of glioblastoma. In most classification systems, the degree of anaplasia and the presence or absence of vascular proliferation and necrosis are the main determinants of grade and prognosis.

Brain stem gliomas are almost always of astrocytic origin. Histologic subtype seems to vary with location. Dorsal midbrain and medullary lesions are usually low grade and can often be excised from the medullary region or watched, with the possible exception of surgical management of hydrocephalus, in the case of a dorsal midbrain lesion. Pontine and ventral midbrain astrocytomas are almost always highly anaplastic and uniformly fatal. Recent intensive accelerated and hyperfractionated radiotherapy schemes have been of no benefit.

In adults, survival with astrocytic tumors is highly dependent not only on histology, but also on age and general and neurologic performance status (Table 1). In general, low-grade and anaplastic tumors occur in younger adults. Glioblastoma may occur at any age but is predominant in older adults. Low-grade tumors progress by increasingly extensive infiltration, often with minimal clinical symptoms. With time, dedifferentiation to a more aggressive histology is the main determinant of survival. Anaplastic astrocytoma and glioblastoma manifest clinically with the effects of destruction of brain parenchyma; infiltration of surrounding brain, often at a distance of several centimeters; and, most significantly, extensive associated edema. The size of the tumor and the extent of associated edema often generate significant mass effect. Seizures may be a presenting or secondary feature of each histologic grade but may be the only clinical consequence of low-grade lesions. Recent observations suggest that anticonvulsants do not prevent the development of seizures that occur in up to 25% with GBM.

DIAGNOSIS

Computed Tomography

The advent of computed axial tomography (CT) in the mid-1970s revolutionized diagnosis and treatment of CNS neoplasms. Late generation CT scans not only show parenchymal lesions, but are also capable of delineating vascular structures. Three-dimensional volumetric reconstructions of the brain are possible with newer scanners. CT remains the initial radiographic tool in the management of most patients with brain tumors. The speed and ubiquity of CT scanners allow for any patient with signs or symptoms of neurologic compromise to be evaluated quickly. The administration of intravenous iodinated contrast allows for demonstration of blood-brain barrier breakdown. The neovascularity of rapidly growing tumors results in permeable vascular membranes, allowing the contrast agent to "leak" out into the parenchyma, showing up as an increased density on the image.

TABLE 1. **Glioma Survival Statistics**

	Median (months)	2 Years	5 Years	10 Years
AA, age <50, KPS = 100, no neurologic deficit	58	76%	20–30%	?
GBM, age <50, KPS = 90–100	18	35%	5–6%	?
GBM, age >50, KPS = 90–100	11	15%	? 0	
GBM, age >50, KPS <70, neurologic deficit	5	4%	? 0	
Low-grade astrocytoma	60			25–30%
Oligodendroglioma, age 20–59			56%	32%

Abbreviations: AA = anaplastic astrocytoma; GBM = glioblastoma multiforme; KPS = Karnofsky performance status.

Magnetic Resonance Imaging

Magnetic resonance imaging (MRI) has further expanded the visualization of the structure and function of the brain. Often after establishing the presence of a neoplasm on CT, MRI is employed to better define the lesion. Valuable data regarding anatomic location and proximity to neural and vascular structures can be obtained with MRI. Later generation scanners also provide information regarding function of the brain. Perfusion imaging indicates blood flow to regions of the brain and can often distinguish between areas of necrosis versus tumor growth. Functional MRI can localize motor, visual, and speech regions of the brain and can be used in preoperative planning.

TREATMENT

Despite imaging advances, the first step in the management of most patients with CNS neoplasms is to obtain tissue for diagnosis.

Surgery: Craniotomy

As outlined previously for extra-axial or intra-axial well-circumscribed lesions, surgery is not only diagnostic but definitive therapy. Surgery appears to have a clear role in the treatment of symptomatic, superficially located, solitary metastatic tumors. A distinct benefit has been measured in patients who underwent surgical resection followed by radiation therapy as opposed to those undergoing radiation alone. Craniotomy for resection of infiltrative glial tumors is usually reserved for superficially located tumors with evidence of mass effect. Debulking the tumor mass is often helpful in both providing a histologic diagnosis and relieving symptoms of elevated intracranial pressure (headache, nausea, and vomiting). Debate exists over the value of cytoreduction in the treatment of these lesions. Proponents believe that reducing the tumor burden will allow for greater success using subsequent radiation and chemotherapy. Risks of craniotomy are generally quite low and include bleeding, infection, neurologic injury (coma, stroke, death), and the generation of seizures. These risks, not to mention additional hospitalization, may not be justified by the potential benefit. Surgical resection is not an ideal treatment for an infiltrative neoplasm. It is difficult, if not impossible, to detect where the tumor margin ends and normal tissue begins. In addition, tumor cells may migrate several centimeters along white matter pathways, including the corpus callosum, making complete resection impossible.

Surgery: Image Directed

For deep-seated tumors in eloquent areas of the brain, stereotactic biopsy has been a valuable technique. Commonly, this is done with a guiding device (stereotactic frame) attached to the outer table of the skull using pins and local anesthesia. Imaging with CT or MRI is obtained; a target is selected and its location measured relative to this frame. The frame then serves as a platform for guiding a biopsy needle to the selected target. This can usually be accomplished under local anesthesia, using a small burr hole. Diagnostic samples are obtained more than 90% of the time. The limitation of stereotactic biopsy comes from small sample size. This can occasionally lead to sampling error, in which a portion of the tumor with less aggressive histologic features is obtained, leading to a diagnosis of a lower grade neoplasm. In addition, stereotactic biopsy does not allow for treatment of mass effect. However, in poor surgical risk patients, stereotactic biopsy is preferred.

Techniques have been developed that allow stereotactic guidance to be used during a conventional craniotomy. This allows the surgeon to have imaging information during the procedure and helps to improve localization and resection. Several centers have incorporated intraoperative MRI scanners, which provide real-time imaging during the surgery. The cost of these units as well as the necessary modifications to the surgical and anesthesia equipment is prohibitive for most institutions at this time.

Radiation Therapy

Photon irradiation from linear accelerators is derived from an accelerated beam of electrons striking tungsten and emitting photons. These particles create free radicals and can disrupt cellular functions, damage DNA, and induce apoptosis. Mitotically active cells are most prone to radiation injury. Normal cells are capable of repair processes that can restore cell integrity after damage by radiation. Tumor cells are often deficient in such repair mechanisms. The efficacy of radiotherapy lies in the exploitation of this difference, mainly through fractionation (the daily delivery of small doses of radiation), which allows normal cells to repair while tumor cells are unable to do so.

Radiation therapy is generally well-tolerated by patients. The most noticeable side effects are alopecia and fatigue. Women usually have return of hair growth after treatment, whereas hair growth in men is more variable. Fatigue often occurs toward the end of radiotherapy and can persist for several weeks. Late effects of radiation including necrosis, memory dysfunction, loss of higher cognitive functions, and hypothalamic failure can occur months to years after treatment and are generally irreversible. The risk of the most serious consequence of standard radiotherapy, radiation necrosis, is about 5%.

Radiation treatment protocols are determined by tumor type. Malignant gliomas are usually treated using a dose approaching 6000 centigray (cGy). Initially, the tumor and a generous margin are covered, with the treatment volume focusing to the tumor location as the cumulative dose increases. The daily fraction is usually 200 cGy, administered over a 5- to 6-week period. In contrast, metastatic tumors to the brain are treated with whole brain radiation to a typical dose of 3000 cGy, usually in a smaller number of fractions.

Stereotactic Radiosurgery

Stereotactic radiosurgery is a single session radiation treatment in which a small, well-defined, intracranial target is treated. Either a gamma knife or a modified linear accelerator is used. Both methods are similar in that the tumor is localized using stereotactic techniques and the radiation is precisely delivered to the specified target. Due to the high degree of accuracy in targeting and the rapid fall-off of radiation dose, a tumoricidal dose can be delivered to the lesion, while normal brain structures a few millimeters away are spared. The two techniques differ in that gamma radiation from 201 sources of radioactive cobalt is used in the gamma knife and conventional photon radiation is used in the linear accelerator. The gamma unit is devoted solely to the treatment of brain lesions, whereas the linear accelerator is more versatile. The major limitation of this technique is the volume of the tumor that can be irradiated. If the lesion is larger than 3.5 to 4 cm in maximal diameter, irradiation of surrounding structures becomes too great, with potentially severe radiation injury to normal brain structures a result.

Radiosurgery can be used either as a boost to conventional, fractionated radiation or as a single treatment. Tumors often resistant to conventional radiation, such as melanoma, seem to be particularly sensitive to single-treatment radiosurgery. Gliomas, with no well-defined margin, are not ideally treated with radiosurgery. Nevertheless, radiosurgery in addition to fractionated radiation may offer some benefit in slowing the rate of local recurrence in small-volume gliomas.

Chemotherapy

Chemotherapy for brain tumors has been generally considered adjunctive therapy for highly aggressive and infiltrating neoplasms. Scattered small series have been reported for meningioma with agents such as actinomycin (Cosmegen), tamoxifen (Nolvadex),* and mifepristone (RU486†). Carboplatin* has been used with some success in juvenile pilocytic astrocytoma. Medulloblastoma, germ cell tumors, and lymphomas have proved to be highly sensitive to a variety of chemotherapeutic agents with significant survival impact. Alkylating agent chemotherapy probably produces a small increase in the number of

---

*Not FDA approved for this indication.

†Not yet approved for use in the United States.

1-year and 18-month survivors in GBM and may have a somewhat greater impact for AA. BCNU (carmustine), or a combination of procarbazine (Matulane), CCNU (lomustine), and vincristine (Oncovin) (PCV), is a standard therapy. In the last few years, the distinction of oligodendroglioma with both low-grade and anaplastic histologies has taken on major importance as 75 to 80% of lesions appear to be chemosensitive to a variety of drugs, especially variants of PCV. It remains yet to be determined how this affects survival.

Unfortunately, a great deal of time and effort in therapeutic trials of a number of agents over 20 years since the first published report of the impact of BCNU on survival in malignant glioma has produced little therapeutic advance. Promising avenues in current clinical trials include the placement of polymer waivers impregnated with chemotherapeutic agents intraoperatively, a variety of gene therapy approaches, new approaches to blood-brain barrier disruption, new chemotherapeutic agents such as topoisomerase inhibitors, and metabolic pathway inhibitors such as merimistat and tamoxifen.

Treatment of Symptoms

Day-to-day therapeutic issues are no less important in the management of brain tumor patients. Neurologic deficits can have major impact on quality of life, and standard rehabilitation strategies may play a major role in maximizing performance. The need to address spiritual and psychosocial concerns is often of paramount importance in developing a specific treatment program. Social service input is invaluable. Some patients derive tremendous help from each other in organized support groups. Depression is often a significant problem, and appropriate pharmacotherapy should be offered early. Fatigue is common, especially during and after radiotherapy. Stimulants such as pemoline (Cylert) and protriptyline (Vivactil*) may be useful.

A number of specific medical issues are important in patient management. Seizures may present significant morbidity. Special concerns in brain tumor patients include propensity for adverse drug interactions and a higher incidence of postictal neurologic deficit. The proper and reserved use of corticosteroids cannot be overemphasized. Lowest effective doses for management of associated brain edema should be monitored constantly. Cushingoid side effects and steroid myopathy can sometimes become severe. Many patients with brain tumors, especially those with neurologic deficit and immobility, are at risk for deep vein thrombosis and pulmonary emboli. Recent reports have suggested that the risk of tumor bleeding with anticoagulants is not as high as was once feared, and anticoagulants should be considered in appropriate cases.

Finally, the process of death and dying should not be ignored. Hearing patients' fears and concerns and responding to them can be of great value to patients, their families, and caregivers. Hospice groups are available in many locations and can be exceedingly helpful in managing the final phase of illness in many patients with malignant brain tumors.

---

*Not FDA approved for this indication.

Section 14

The Locomotor System

RHEUMATOID ARTHRITIS

method of
LEE S. SIMON, M.D.
Harvard Medical School and Beth Israel Deaconess Medical Center
Boston, Massachusetts

Arthritis is one of the most common afflictions in humans. In 1994 the Centers for Disease Control and Prevention (CDC) reported that by the year 2020 arthritis will have the largest increase in numbers of new patients of any disease in the United States. Arthritis is not one disease but is a generic term that describes more than 100 different conditions. The most common condition is osteoarthritis, which affects at least 16,000,000 Americans, typically those older than 60 years of age. It is one of the more expensive and debilitating of all diseases in the United States. Rheumatoid arthritis, a systemic, chronic, progressive inflammatory disease, is far less common, affecting about 2,400,000 Americans.

BACKGROUND

The joint consists of bone, cartilage, and connective tissue. The subchondral bone is covered by hyaline or articular cartilage, which consists of type II collagen, chondrocytes, proteoglycans, and high-molecular-weight glycoproteins that allow the cartilage to retain water to provide for increased resiliency. The collagen fibrils are arranged in arcade fashion to provide tensile strength, with the proteoglycans providing distensibility by retaining adequate hydration. There is a synovial cell layer, which is typically two cells thick and lacks a basement membrane. It produces a highly viscous lubricating fluid, the synovial fluid, for the joint. Outside of the synovial membrane is a tight joint capsule and ligaments and tendons. In strategic spots outside the joint proper are bursae, providing a smooth surface for muscle, tendon, and ligaments to pass over roughened bone surfaces. The joint components serve to provide motion and allow for load bearing across nearly frictionless surfaces. Any or all of these joint components are involved in the arthritic process, depending on the extent of the disease.

EPIDEMIOLOGY

Rheumatoid arthritis is a destructive and commonly a debilitating disease initially of the tissues surrounding the joint, beginning in the synovium. It typically affects women more frequently than men, has a peak incidence between the ages of 20 and 50, and a prevalence of 1 to 2% of adults, ranging from 0.3% of the population younger than 35 years old to about 10% of those older than 65. It is a chronic autoimmune disorder characterized by symmetrical synovitis of the joint and typically affects small and large diarthrodial joints, leading to their progressive destruction. It is heterogeneous in nature with a variable disease expression and is associated with the formation of serum rheumatoid factor in 90% of patients sometime during the course of the illness. The rheumatoid factor is an antibody to the Fc portion of a second antibody forming immune complexes.

ETIOPATHOGENESIS

Some patients have extremely mild disease associated with spontaneous remissions whereas others suffer an unremitting destructive course. The disease begins in the synovium, but as it progresses major systemic manifestations may develop, including fever, weight loss, thinning of skin, multiorgan involvement, scleritis, corneal ulcers, and the formation of subcutaneous or subperiosteal nodules. In addition to these extra-articular manifestations, rheumatoid arthritis may lead to premature death. The etiology of this disease remains unknown. Possibilities include various viral or bacterial infections such as Epstein-Barr virus or infection with certain *Mycobacterium* species. One possible explanation for the events leading to this disease is an environmental exposure or infection, perhaps viral particles or bacterial proteins, that stimulates an immune response in the appropriate genetic host, which subsequently leads to an host immune response that begins to cross-react with similar antigens in the host and localizes in joint tissue. This molecular mimicry in association with an activated immune system may subsequently lead to the cataclysmic events of rheumatoid arthritis. The great majority of patients have a genetic susceptibility associated with increased activation of class II major histocompatibility complex molecules on monocytes and macrophages, which act as antigen-presenting cells, presenting antigen to similarly activated T cells bearing receptors for these class II molecules. The human leukocyte antigen DR subtypes Dw4, Dw14, and Dw 15 are highly conserved among patients with rheumatoid arthritis who have very severe disease.

Once the appropriate monocytes and macrophages are activated and interacting with and presenting antigen to the appropriate T cells, a cascade of events ensues that leads ultimately to the further activation of more monocytes and macrophages, more T cells, B cell activation, and endothelial cell activation. This activation increases the synthesis of adhesion molecules, leading to increased margination of even more mononuclear cells and now polymorphonuclear cells, which are attracted to the inflamed joint by the elaboration of multiple cytokines, some of which act as chemoattractants, leading to the increased delivery of inflammatory cells to the synovium and synovial fluid. Cytokines such as interleukin (IL)-1α or β, IL-4, IL-8, IL-10, tumor necrosis factor (TNF)-α, platelet-derived growth factor (PDGF), fibroblast growth factor (FGF), granulocyte-macrophage colony-stimulating factor (GM-CSF), interferon (IFN)-γ, transforming growth factor (TGF)-β, IL-2, and IL-6 all lead to increased activation of fibroblast-like cells in the synovium, chondrocytes as well as macrophages, which release increased amounts of prostaglandins, neutral proteinases such as collagenases, transin/stromelysin, and lead to the recruitment of osteoclast precursors, which culminates in the destruction of bone and cartilage by the invading proliferative synovium. As the cartilage is damaged, there is increased thinning of this tissue, leading to a cycle characterized by decreased proteoglycan synthesis, leading further to decreased cartilaginous load-bearing capacity. The chondrocyte responds initially by attempting to repair, but as it is overwhelmed there is increased release of neutral metalloproteinases such as collagenase, gelatinase, and stromelysin and lysosomal proteases, leading to further thinning and ultimately increasing the destructive cascade.

CLINICAL MANIFESTATIONS

Clinically, rheumatoid arthritis as a systemic inflammatory disease of younger people manifests with a multitude of symptoms and signs and can at times be a difficult diagnostic and management problem. Patients with rheumatoid arthritis may present with pain, swelling, warmth, and tenderness of various joints and may have gel phenomenon. They typically suffer morning stiffness that may last several hours or fill the entire day. Many patients suffer from afternoon fatigue and may require enforced rest for about 1 hour each day. Fever and/or weight loss are not uncommon. Extra-articular manifestations can affect any organ system. Symmetrical involvement of small and large joints is typical. Progressive destruction of the joint leading to loss of typical mechanical function and consequent inability to perform even the essential activities of daily living is the rule in the unresponsive or untreated patient.

DIAGNOSIS

The diagnosis of rheumatoid arthritis is primarily dependent on the history and physical examination of the patient. The history of a chronic, progressive, systemic inflammatory disease in the presence of significant soft tissue joint swelling, the synovitis, along with warmth and tenderness and at times large synovial effusions characterized by large numbers of polymorphonuclear (PMN) cells (about 20,000 to 50,000 white blood cells with usually between 50 to 70% PMN cells), some mononuclear cells, poor viscosity, and no crystals is typical. Subcutaneous or subperiosteal nodules on extensor surfaces or pressure points are evidence of a rheumatic process. Further laboratory evidence includes elevation of acute phase reactants such as an elevated erythrocyte sedimentation rate or C-reactive protein and a progressive normocytic (or less commonly microcytic) anemia of chronic inflammatory disease. A falling serum albumin is a poor prognostic sign and usually suggests evidence of end-stage disease or emerging vasculitis. Other laboratory tests suggestive of extra-articular organ involvement may be noted. More than 90% of patients have evidence of rheumatoid factors in their blood and generalized polyclonal hypergammaglobulinemia. Thrombocytosis may be prominent.

The radiographic abnormalities are highly time dependent and variable. Early in the disease there may be evidence of juxta-articular osteoporosis due to local inflammation and disuse, but only by special magnetic resonance imaging studies can small early erosions be appreciated. Subsequently, even the comparatively imprecise traditional radiographs will reveal progressive marginal joint erosions, cartilage loss as evidenced by joint space narrowing, and lack of attempts at repair. When these changes affect symmetrically the wrists, the metacarpophalangeal (MCP) joints, and the proximal interphalangeal (PIP) joints, with sparing of the distal interphalangeal (DIP) joints, then the likely diagnosis is rheumatoid arthritis or one of its variants.

Unfortunately, although there has been a significant increase in our knowledge about the pathophysiology of rheumatoid arthritis, there has not been as much progress in the development of improved diagnostic tools for this disease. We still lack definitive biologic markers for diagnosis as well as progression of the illness. Perhaps further development of biochemical markers such as cartilage breakdown or synthetic by-product markers or markers of bone resorption might be useful in diagnosing or monitoring the progressive destruction mediated by rheumatoid arthritis. For now, however, we remain dependent on the previously described procedures.

THERAPY

In the development of effective therapy for rheumatoid arthritis, it is important to determine either the as yet unknown etiologic agent or event or the identity of one specific site in the cascade of increasing inflammation that will shut off the progress of the disease before too much destruction has been achieved.

There is now clear information from both longitudinal observational studies and epidemiologic trials to provide guidelines for the therapy of rheumatoid arthritis. These guidelines are based on data that demonstrate the importance of early diagnosis, identification of biologic signs and events that bear significance regarding prognostic outcome, and early aggressive therapy. Attempts at earlier diagnosis and assumed earlier appropriate therapy are believed to prevent irreversible joint damage. Poor prognostic features include the early onset of active severe synovitis with functional limitations; the presence of joint erosions (joint damage); extra-articular manifestations such as pleurisy, pericarditis, myositis, or neurologic or vascular disease; positive measures of serum rheumatoid factors; and a family history of severe rheumatoid arthritis. It is now also clear that joint destruction begins early and is quite pronounced in the first 2 years of disease. Therefore, some clear guidelines emerge and are presented after each type of pharmacologic therapy has been reviewed. The knowledge that this disease requires early aggressive therapy has led to an understanding that physicians who care for rheumatoid arthritis patients require considerable experience with a multidisciplinary approach and significant experience using drugs that are known to alter the natural history of the disease but also have known potential toxic reactions.

The discussion of therapy is in three parts. The first part discusses the issues of nonpharmacologic therapies. The next part is a discussion regarding the most frequently used drugs to treat rheumatoid arthritis, the nonsteroidal anti-inflammatory drugs (NSAIDs). The last section deals with therapies that are thought to have some disease modifying effects, the disease-modifying antirheumatic drugs (DMARDs). Although the NSAIDs are typically used first as drugs that decrease pain and inflammation, their known and relatively common toxic effects may require the caregiver to give pause before prescribing them. Table 1 describes the relative toxicity of the various drugs used in this disease and places them in the context of the level of disease activity.

Nonpharmacologic Therapies

Therapy for arthritis of almost any type includes nonspecific nonpharmacologic measures such as rehabilitation therapy, education, and support. The establishment of an effective patient-physician relationship is crucial for effective therapy. Patients need to become educated consumers of medical care. They need to understand the importance of adequate rest and judicious exercise in conjunction with appropriate pharmacotherapy. In addition, they need to understand the importance of compliance with the medical regimen. Patients also need to be enlisted by their physicians so that they become empowered and do not feel victimized by the disease or its therapy. The physician-patient relationship becomes stronger, and as patients learn about their disease and its therapy they can be more of a participant in the process.

Pharmacologic Therapies

Nonsteroidal Anti-inflammatory Drugs

The first-line pharmacologic therapy includes simple analgesics and NSAIDs (Table 2). Although NSAIDs are considered analgesics and anti-inflammatory drugs, little evidence has accumulated to date that proves that these drugs modify the natural history of the diseases for which they are prescribed. However, these drugs are quite successful at relieving pain and decreasing inflammation. The toxicities of these drugs are often due to their main mode of action, the inhibition of prostaglandin synthesis. Table 3 reviews the potential toxic reactions. The available NSAIDs come in various classes, and all of these agents have similar modes of action; however, some of the effects are unique to specific classes or drugs. The toxic reactions can at times be minimized. This is particularly true of effects on the kidneys or gastrointestinal tract. Patients who are at risk for an adverse kidney effect when treated with a NSAID include patients with severe hemodynamic compromise such as serious hemorrhage, significant congestive heart failure, a problem of overdiuresis, or a problem of cirrhosis and/or ascites. Patients with intrinsic kidney disease and older patients are also at some risk.

NSAIDs bear the common property of inhibiting cyclooxygenase, the enzyme that catalyzes the synthesis of cyclic endoperoxides from arachidonic acid to form proinflammatory and other forms of prostaglandins. In the gastric mucosa, prostaglandins promote the generation of a protective barrier of mucus and bicarbonate; decrease the synthesis of gastric acid; stimulate glutathione production, which acts to scavenge superoxides; and promote adequate blood flow to meet the needs of the cells of the gastric mucosa. In the kidney, prostaglandins act to modulate intrarenal plasma flow and electrolyte balance. The ability to inhibit cyclooxygenase varies among the different NSAIDs; however, there are no studies relating the degree of cyclooxygenase inhibition with anti-inflammatory efficacy in individual patients. Two isoenzymes of cyclooxygenase have been identified and are referred to as COX-1 and COX-2. COX-1 acts as a constitutive enzyme in the gastric mucosa, renal parenchyma, and platelets as well as other tissues. Inhibition of COX-1 activity is considered a major cause of the gastrointestinal toxic effects of NSAIDs. COX-2, although present in most tissues in minute amounts and particularly in brain and in the kidney in certain areas, is highly inducible at sites of inflammation. Theoretically, the ideal NSAID would inhibit COX-2 activity and exert no effect on COX-1.

TABLE 1. **Activity of Disease as a Function of Potential Drug Toxicity**

Level of Toxic Effect	Disease Severity			
	Mild	*Moderate*	*Severe*	*Refractory*
Low	Hydroxychloroquine (Plaquenil) Sulfasalazine (Azulfidine) Auranofin (Ridaura)	Hydroxychloroquine Sulfasalazine Glucocorticoids (short course)	Glucocorticoids (short course)	Glucocorticoids (short course)
Moderate	NSAIDs	NSAIDs Parenteral gold Methotrexate Azathioprine (Imuran) Combination DMARDs	NSAIDs Parenteral gold Methotrexate Azathioprine Combination DMARDs	NSAIDs Parenteral gold Methotrexate Azathioprine Combination DMARDs
Moderate to high		Cyclosporine (Sandimmune)	Daily glucocorticoids Cyclosporine Penicillamine	Daily glucocorticoids Cyclosporine Penicillamine Cyclophosphamide

Abbreviations: NSAIDs = nonsteroidal anti-inflammatory drugs; DMARDs = disease-modifying antirheumatic drugs.

From Simon LS: Rheumatoid arthritis. *In* Kliipel JH (ed): Primer on the Rheumatic Diseases, 11th ed. Atlanta, GA, Arthritis Foundation, 1997, pp 168–174. Copyright 1997. Used by permission of the Arthritis Foundation. For more information, please call the Arthritis Foundation's information line 1-800-283-7800.

TABLE 2. **The Nonsteroidal Anti-inflammatory Drugs (NSAIDs)**

NSAID	Trade Name	Usual Dose	Approved Use*
Carboxylic Acids			
Aspirin (acetylsalicylic acid)	Multiple	2.4–5 g/24 h in 4–5 divided doses	RA, OA, AS, JCA, ST
Buffered aspirin	Multiple	Same	Same
Enteric-coated salicylates	Multiple	Same	Same
Salsalate	Disalcid	1.5–3.0 g/24 h bid	Same
Diflunisal	Dolobid	0.5–1.5 g/24 h bid	Same
Choline magnesium trisalicylate	Trilisate	1.5–3 g/24 h bid-tid	RA, OA, pain, JCA
Propionic Acids			
Ibuprofen	Motrin, OTC	OTC: 200–400 mg qid Rx: 400, 600, 800 max 3200 mg/24 h	RA, OA, JCA
Naproxen	generic, Naprosyn, enteric,	250, 375, 500 mg bid	RA, OA, JCA, ST
Fenoprofen	Nalfon	300–600 mg qid	RA, OA
Ketoprofen	Orudis	75 mg tid	RA, OA
Flurbiprofen	Ansaid	100 mg bid-tid	RA, OA
Oxaprozin	Daypro	600 mg; 2 tabs q day 1200 mg/24 h	RA, OA
Acetic Acid Derivatives			
Indomethacin	Indocin, Indocin SR	25, 50 mg tid or qid SR: 75 mg bid; rarely >150 mg/24 h	RA, OA, G, AS
Tolmetin	Tolectin	400, 600, 800 mg; 800–2400 mg/24 h	RA, OA, JCA
Sulindac	Clinoril	150, 200 mg bid (some inc. to tid)	RA, OA, AS, ST, G
Diclofenac	Voltaren	50, 75 mg bid	RA, OA, AS
Etodolac	Lodine	200, 300 mg b-t-qid max: 1200 mg/24 h	OA, pain
Fenamates			
Meclofenamate		50–100 mg tid-qid	RA, OA
Mefenamic acid	Ponstel	250 mg qid	RA, OA
Enolic Acids			
Piroxicam	Feldene	10, 20 mg q day	RA, OA
Phenylbutazone	Butazolidin	100 mg tid up to 600 mg/24 h	G, AS
Naphthyl-alkanones			
Nabumetone	Relafen	500 mg bid up to 1500 mg/24 h	RA, OA

*FDA approved.
Abbreviations: RA = rheumatoid arthritis; OA = osteoarthritis; AS = ankylosing spondylitis; G = gout; JCA = juvenile chronic polyarthritis; ST = soft tissue injury.

Several non–prostaglandin-mediated mechanisms of action have recently been implicated to explain the effects of NSAIDs in experimental models. NSAIDs have been shown to reduce the expression of L-selectin, thus affecting a critical step in the migration of granulocytes to sites of inflammation. In addition, NSAIDs in vitro inhibit inducible nitric acid synthetase, which has been associated with increasing inflammation. The clinical significance of non–prostaglandin-mediated processes in inflammation is unknown, however. Of note, nonacetylated salicylates are weak inhibitors of cyclooxygenase, but clinically they appear to inhibit inflammation as effectively as some traditional NSAIDs. Non–prostaglandin-mediated effects may help to explain these observations.

PHARMACOKINETICS

NSAIDs appear to be absorbed completely. Most have negligible hepatic metabolism, are tightly bound to albumin, and have small volumes of distribution. Half-lives of the various NSAIDs vary, but, in general, can be divided into "short" (less than 6 hours) and "long" (more than 6 hours). Patients with low serum albumin as measured in cirrhosis, nephrotic syndrome, or active rheumatoid arthritis may have higher free concentration of drug. Protein binding is usually saturable in the normal dosage range of NSAIDs. Of clinical relevance, maximum therapeutic response for a given NSAID depends on the time needed to reach the steady state plasma concentration, which is roughly equal to three to five half-lives of the drug.

CLINICAL USE

Indications

NSAIDs are typically prescribed as first-line therapy for rheumatologic diseases. They are both effective and appropriate treatment for the pain and inflammation due to rheumatoid arthritis. Unfortu-

TABLE 3. **Adverse Reactions of the NSAIDs**

System	Effects
Gastrointestinal	Nausea, vomiting, dyspepsia, diarrhea, constipation
	Gastric mucosal irritation, superficial erosions, peptic ulceration, increased fecal blood wasting
	Major gastrointestinal hemorrhage, penetrating ulcers,
	Small bowel erosions, induction of "diaphragm" development in small bowel, large bowel
	Hepatotoxicity, hepatitis, fulminant hepatic failure
Renal	Glomerulopathy, interstitial nephritis, alterations in renal plasma flow leading to fall in glomerular filtration rates; interference with naturesis induced by diuretics; inhibition of renin release; induction of edema
	Alterations in tubular functions
Central nervous	Headaches, confusion, hallucinations, depersonalization reactions, depression, tremor
	Aseptic meningitis, tinnitus, vertigo, neuropathy, toxic amblyopia, transient transparent corneal deposits
Hematologic	Anemia, marrow depression, Coombs' positive anemia, decreased platelet aggregation
Hypersensitivity	Asthma, asthma/urticaria syndrome, urticaria, rashes, photosensitivity, Stevens-Johnson syndrome
Other	Drug interactions such as displacement of oral hypoglycemics and warfarin from protein binding sites and from sites of metabolism
	Interference with the actions of beta blockers and some diuretics

nately, although powerful anti-inflammatory drugs and analgesics, they do not appear to alter the natural history of diseases such as rheumatoid arthritis. With the current trend toward using disease-modifying agents or second-line agents earlier in rheumatoid arthritis as well as in other systemic inflammatory arthropathies, requirements for NSAIDs may decrease in this particular patient population.

NSAID Selection

The selection of a particular NSAID is typically based on several qualities: efficacy, regimen, safety, availability, and cost. At equipotent doses, the efficacy of the different NSAIDs is similar across patient populations; however, responsiveness of individual patients to a specific NSAID clearly differs. For a given patient, lack of response to a particular NSAID does not preclude response to another. The determinants of individual patient responsiveness to NSAIDs are not understood. Possibilities to explain these effects include variable absorption and bioavailability; patient compliance with the prescribed regimen; other biologic effects of the NSAIDs, which may be variably expressed; and metabolism and excretion of the active agent. The biologic effects once prostaglandins are inhibited are also not well understood. As awareness of adverse effects of NSAIDs, particularly those on the gastrointestinal (GI) tract, has grown, safety issues have become central in the selection of a NSAID. Various studies have attempted to demonstrate that specific NSAIDs are more likely to cause an ulcer or its complications. This is very difficult to prove because the drugs are used at various doses and have different effects on COX-1 and COX-2 activities, and patients are variously at risk. In addition, there has been renewed interest in the nonacetylated salicylates because of their lower toxicity rating compared with that of other NSAIDs. All these factors need to be considered and may affect prescription practice, as do physician and patient preferences. Although acetylsalicylic acid (ASA) is inexpensive, its frequent dosing makes it inconvenient, and patients often complain of gastric upset with its use. Enteric-coated aspirin may alleviate some symptoms of local gastric irritation, but it does not provide greater protection from ulcers and it is more costly than traditional ASA. Traditional use of specific NSAIDs often influences physicians' selection of NSAIDs, for instance, the historical experience with indomethacin for gout and ASA for rheumatoid arthritis. Individual patient characteristics may also require the selection of a particular NSAID. For example, in patients with a history of asthma, nasal polyps, and aspirin sensitivity, nonacetylated salicylates have been shown to be safer and may be used. Close monitoring, however, is still required because of the potential for cross-sensitivity.

Pharmacologic variables of the various NSAIDs may also influence prescription practices. NSAIDs with short half-lives are best suited for treatment of acute musculoskeletal pain, such as athletic injuries and gouty attacks, to allow for rapid onset of action, whereas NSAIDs with longer half-lives are more appropriate for long-term use in patients with rheumatoid arthritis. NSAIDs with extended half-lives allow for more successful treatment in chronic conditions because of improved compliance as a result of more convenient dosing regimens. However, once-daily NSAID preparations should be used with caution in the elderly and in patients with hepatic or renal impairment. To summarize, as a result of these issues physicians and patients together must review the various qualities of the available NSAIDs and find the best fit.

TOXICITY

Gastrointestinal

GI side effects due to NSAIDs are frequent and often interfere with treatment. GI symptoms due to NSAIDs may include dyspepsia, nausea, and, infrequently, vomiting, which may but more frequently will not herald the onset of significant toxic events such as the formation of significant gastric ulcers with their attendant potential complications. These effects tend to be dose related; for this reason, the lowest effective dose of the NSAID should be used. Taking the medication with food or antacids may alleviate such symptoms. However, one recent study has shown that there may be little validity in this advice with regard to ulcer prevention.

Less than half of NSAID users with GI symptoms have erosions or ulcers at endoscopy, and the point prevalence for true endoscopic ulcers is 15 to 31%. This discrepency between symptoms and ulcers unfortunately creates a situation that provides no guide to help determine decisions about who should receive diagnostic studies or procedures, ulcer treatment or prophylaxis, and/or who can be symptomatically treated. GI side effects of NSAIDs are common, and serious complications such as bleeding, perforation, and death affect between 1 to 2% of users per year. The ubiquitous use of NSAIDs, however, results in a significant number of individuals affected by such events. A recent meta-analysis of pooled data showed a relative risk of adverse GI effects in NSAID users that was threefold that of the nonusers. In a univariate analysis of 2400 rheumatoid arthritis patients, a hazard ratio for hospitalization (more significant problems than those that could be approached in an outpatient setting) due to adverse GI effects was identified that was sevenfold greater in NSAID users than in nonusers. NSAID-induced ulcers are more often asymptomatic in the elderly, who tend to present with anemia, hemorrhage, or perforation rather than abdominal pain. Perhaps for this reason, the elderly more frequently require emergency surgical intervention and have an increased mortality rate.

Unfortunately, no individual patient is completely free of the risk of NSAID-induced gastric or duodenal damage. Investigators have identified groups of patients who seem to be at increased risk for developing NSAID-induced ulcers; and it is in these groups that NSAIDs should be avoided or prophylaxis should be considered. Definite risk factors proven by cross-sectional analysis and more recently by prospective analysis for the development of NSAID-induced ulcer and its complications include age older than 60 years, prior history of ulcer disease of any cause, prior history of GI bleeding, presence of significant co-morbid illnesses such as cardiovascular disease, increased underlying disability caused by the inflammatory disease, and concomitant glucocorticoid therapy. In a meta-analysis of 16 studies, the relative risk ratio of NSAID-induced ulcer was 5.5 in persons over the age of 60. Concomitant use of glucocorticoid therapy and NSAID may increase the risk for ulcer disease as much as fourfold. Although it is prudent to dissuade patients from ingesting alcohol or smoking tobacco while taking NSAIDs, there are few data to suggest an increased risk for peptic ulcer disease in NSAID users who smoke or drink. The presence of infection with *Helicobacter pylori* does not appear to increase the risk for peptic ulcer disease induced by NSAIDs; however, patients may complain of more GI distress if they are on NSAIDs and are infected with *H. pylori*.

All NSAIDs possess the potential to cause GI adverse events, but their relative risks differ. Nabumetone and etodolac, two newer NSAIDs, have been heralded as safer, perhaps because of their relatively selective COX-2 effects. In vivo nabumetone has been demonstrated to have a sevenfold greater effect on COX-2 than on COX-1. Similarly, in vitro low-dose etodolac had a 10-fold greater effect on COX-2 than on COX-1, but at high dose these effects were mitigated. In contrast to these studies, other studies using human models failed to demonstrate COX selectivity with either of these agents. Manufacturers are currently studying highly selective COX-2 inhibitors with a 400-fold or more effect on COX-2 over COX-1, thus offering the beneficial anti-inflammatory effects yet avoiding the undesirable COX-1 effect on gastric prostaglandin synthesis at physiologically efficacious drug levels. Whether the projected effects of highly selective COX-2 inhibitors will be clinically significant remains to be demonstrated.

Because dyspeptic symptoms and fecal occult blood testing are poor predictors of ulcer and its complications, they are not particularly helpful in the decision of whom to pursue with interventional studies. Arguments can be made to treat the majority of patients empirically according to symptoms because the presence of endoscopic lesions does not predict serious complications such as bleeding or perforation. The argument in favor of pursuing diagnostic imaging or endoscopy is localization of the mucosal lesions, which has therapeutic implications. A moderate approach would be to strongly consider diagnostic studies in patients with dyspeptic symptoms who fall into a high-risk category for NSAID-induced gastric or duodenal damage or in those in whom iron-deficiency anemia develops.

PROPHYLAXIS

Preventing GI complications of NSAIDs is the goal of physicians but is problematic, as currently available gastroprotective agents are not completely effective. Whenever possible, NSAIDs should be avoided in patients at high risk for ulcer and its complications. There are no studies that demonstrate that antacids and histamine antagonists prevent serious GI complications. Recently published data showed that patients on NSAIDs taking antacids or H_2 antagonists prophylactically had a higher risk of serious GI complications than those who did not take these medications. Misoprostol, a synthetic prostaglandin analogue, has been shown to be effective in both the treatment and the prevention of endoscopically defined gastric and duodenal ulceration and their complications in patients taking NSAIDs. In a randomized, multicenter placebo-controlled trial, a 40 to 50% reduction in serious gastrointestinal complications was demonstrated, including upper GI ulceration, perforation, and obstruction in rheumatoid arthritis patients on NSAID therapy treated with misoprostol compared with placebo. The incidence of hematemesis, however, was comparable in both groups. Using linear regression analyses on data from the same study, it was shown that patients at highest risk have even further benefited from misoprostol co-therapy. Patients with more significant rheumatoid arthritis as defined by a standardized health assessment questionnaire, with a prior history of peptic ulcer disease or with a history of GI bleeding, had their risk for a poor GI outcome reduced by up to 87% using concomitant misoprostol therapy. Unfortunately, treatment with misoprostol may be limited by diarrhea, which is dose-related and may occur in as many as 30 to 40% of patients receiving 200 μg four times daily (qid). In one study, approximately 8% of patients discontinued misoprostol because of intolerable diarrhea and abdominal pain. Recently, twice and three times daily dosing of misoprostol was studied, and less diarrhea occurred while clinical efficacy defined by endoscopic changes was reasonably preserved.

Histamine-2 blockers (H_2 antagonists) taken concomitantly with NSAIDs have been shown to prevent duodenal but not gastric ulcers or their complications in most studies. One study reported that treatment with high-dose famotidine (40 mg orally [PO] twice a day [bid]), an H_2 antagonist, in patients with arthritis (rheumatoid or osteoarthritis) receiving long-term NSAID therapy reduced the incidence of both gastric and duodenal ulcers defined by endoscopy. In their 24-week study of 285 patients, the cumulative incidence of gastric ulcers in the placebo group was 20% compared with 8% in the high-dose famotidine group ($P = 0.03$). This reduction in endoscopically defined gastric ulcers is similar to that seen in misoprostol endoscopy studies. In contrast to misoprostol, these high doses of famotidine were well tolerated for the study period. The study, however, excluded patients who were at high risk for developing a NSAID-induced gastric or duodenal ulcer. Thus, the patients studied may behave biologically in a different manner from patients defined at greatest risk for serious GI events. If, as the authors suggest, high-dose famotidine has similar effects on ulcer complications, it may be a more feasible prophylactic agent than misoprostol, given the reported side effects. Unfortunately, we do not know the long-term effects of high-dose H_2 antagonists in these patients. Table 4 reviews a series of suggestions with our present knowledge regarding prophylaxis of a potential NSAID-induced GI toxic event.

Renal

At this time, no NSAID can be considered completely safe with regard to kidney effects. The adverse renal effects appear to be both prostaglandin and nonprostaglandin mediated. Prostaglandins play a central role in renal hemodynamics, glomerular filtration, and sodium, potassium, and water metabolism. Patients at highest risk for renal failure from NSAIDs are those with diseases in which normal renal function is dependent on intrarenal production of prostaglandins. These disorders include clinically significant congestive heart failure, cirrhosis with or without attendant ascites, and intrinsic renal diseases such as nephrotic syndrome. In patients with these disorders, NSAIDs should be avoided. If substitution is not an option, nonacetylated salicylates may be used at the lowest dose possible for the shortest acceptable period. Nonacetylated salicylates as weak inhibitors of prostaglandin synthesis may offer a theoretical advantage over traditional NSAIDs. To date, however, there is no documented clinical evidence to suggest that patients treated with nonacetylated salicylates have a lower incidence of adverse renal effects; however, there are few studies documenting clear increased risk with these drugs. Patients should be hemodynamically improved as much as possible before initiating therapy.

In patients with normal renal function, a course of NSAIDs for 1 to 2 weeks can be given safely. Even patients older than 60 with mild renal insufficiency (mean creatinine clearance between 50 and 60 mL per minute) have been shown to tolerate a 2-week course of naproxen (750 mg per day) without renal compromise. However, for patients older than 60 who have pre-existing renal or hepatic disease or congestive heart failure or who are on concomitant diuretic therapy, close follow-up and monitoring are essential. Baseline electrolytes, blood urea nitrogen (BUN), and creatinine should be performed, and repeat measurements should be taken within 1 to 2 weeks and then every 3 to 6 months while being treated with NSAIDs.

Papillary necrosis, also referred to as "analgesic nephropathy," remains the most common non–prostaglandin-mediated cause of NSAID-related renal failure. Phenacetin is the most common offender, but other NSAIDs, including meclofenamate, fenoprofen, phenylbutazone, and aspirin, have all been implicated. Allergic interstitial nephritis is another potential non–prostaglandin-mediated complication associated with the use of NSAIDs. Pre-existing renal insufficiency does not predispose to its development. Onset typically occurs within 2 weeks of NSAID initiation and is not necessarily associated with eosinophiluria, fever, or rash. Complete return to previous renal function is usually the rule, although interim hemodialysis and at times glucocorticoid therapy may be required for severe cases.

Insofar as prostaglandins help to regulate vascular tone, there is some evidence that NSAIDs interfere with beta blockers, angiotensin-converting enzyme (ACE) inhibitors, and loop and thiazide diuretics in the management of hypertension. In a meta-analysis, a clinically significant rise in blood pressure was seen in patients on NSAID therapy. The mean increase was 5 mm Hg, but the variance was large and effects were greatest in patients taking antihypertensive agents. Blood pressure should be checked at baseline and within 1 to 2 weeks of initiation of NSAID treat-

TABLE 4. **Prophylaxis Algorithm**

1. Identify the high-risk patient.
2. Use non-NSAID analgesics or nonacetylated salicylates or the lowest possible dose of NSAIDs.
3. In the high-risk patient, if NSAIDs are necessary treat with misoprostol (Cytotec).
4. If misoprostol side effects are intolerable, use H_2 blockers or omeprazole (Prilosec).
5. If patients are not in high-risk group, do not treat with misoprostol, H_2 blockers, or omeprazole.

ment in hypertensive patients, particularly those on therapy.

Hepatic

Infrequently, elevations of serum transaminases are associated with NSAID use. Diclofenac has been reported to cause clinical hepatitis and has been associated with several reported incidences of hepatic death. Duration of therapy and total daily dosage have been noted to be determinants of transaminase elevations. In a retrospective cohort study, it was noted that sulindac conferred a significantly higher risk of acute liver injury than other NSAIDs. However, the liver injury associated with sulindac and the other NSAIDs in this study was generally mild and reversible. Liver function test abnormalities due to NSAIDs may be disease specific. For example, naproxen more commonly causes liver function test abnormalities in osteoarthritis patients than in rheumatoid arthritis patients. Similarly, aspirin seems to cause elevated serum transaminase values in 40% of patients with active juvenile rheumatoid arthritis. NSAIDs should be discontinued when the transaminases rise more than three times the upper limit of normal, when there is a fall in serum albumin suggestive of a synthetic defect induced by the drug, or when the prothrombin time is prolonged. Clinically, symptomatic hepatitis is quite rare.

Central Nervous System

The central nervous system (CNS) side effects of NSAID use that have been reported have included aseptic meningitis, psychosis, and cognitive dysfunction. Psychosis and cognitive impairment are more prevalent in elderly patients, particularly with indomethacin use. In the elderly, indomethacin should be prescribed judiciously and mental status examinations followed.

Tinnitus is a common problem with patients who are prescribed high-dose salicylates, but it can be a problem with all of the available NSAIDs as well. Tinnitus is typically reversible and is a good warning sign to identify patients who are developing high blood levels of the drug; however, it may not be evident in patients at the extremes of age.

Ocular manifestations are typically unimportant clinically. They include the deposition of drug crystals in the cornea and, rarely, the development of corneal edema. The latter is reversible but when present may affect vision. Rare idiosyncratic and anecdotal events including optic nerve insults whose biology remains poorly understood have also been reported.

Hematologic

The antiplatelet effects of NSAIDs are well recognized. The use of aspirin for coronary artery disease is based on these antiplatelet effects. NSAIDs should be avoided in patients who have platelet defects, as in uremia and von Willebrand disease, or thrombocytopenia (platelet count less than 50,000). Nonacetylated salicylates are a safer therapeutic alternative in such patients. Doses of nonacetylated salicylates should remain, however, within recommended dosage ranges to avoid any possible inhibition of platelet cyclooxygenase, which may be observed at the highest dosage levels. In patients about to undergo surgery, NSAIDs should be withheld preoperatively at a time that takes into consideration the half-life of the particular drug. Because acetylsalicylic acid (ASA) irreversibly inhibits platelet cyclooxygenase and platelets lack the machinery to produce new cyclooxygenase, patients should stop taking ASA a week before a planned surgical procedure to allow for the body to repopulate the platelet pool with platelets that have not been exposed to the drug. New highly selective COX-2 inhibitors may have no effect on the platelet because COX-2 activity has not been found in the platelet. Anticoagulants are not a risk factor for gastroduodenal erosive disease but may predispose to increased hemorrhage once a mucosal break is induced. Rarely, idiosyncratic bone marrow effects may occur in association with NSAID use.

Pregnancy and Lactation

For various reasons, NSAIDs are best avoided altogether in pregnancy. The safety of NSAIDs has not been evaluated extensively in controlled studies in pregnant women. In animal models, NSAIDs have been shown to increase the incidence of dystocia and postimplantation loss as well as to delay parturition. The prostaglandin inhibitory effects of NSAIDs may result in premature closure of the ductus arteriosus and other harmful effects to the fetus. Although ASA has been associated with smaller babies and neonatal bruising, the drug has been used for years in patients requiring NSAID therapy while pregnant. Studies in rhesus monkeys have not demonstrated ASA to be a teratogen. In a recently published prospective study, a cohort of 88 pregnant patients with inflammatory rheumatic disease were divided into two groups: 45 were treated with NSAIDs during pregnancy and 43 were not. No difference in pregnancy outcome, duration of labor, complications at delivery, or neonatal health were found. NSAIDs are excreted in breast milk but in very small amounts. It is generally agreed that salicylates in normally recommended doses are not harmful to nursing infants. Misoprostol causes increased uterine contractility and thus is considered an abortifacient agent. In women of childbearing potential who take misoprostol, appropriate caution and contraceptive methods are essential.

Drug Interactions

Drug interactions with NSAIDs are common. The prevalence and incidence of NSAID-related adverse drug interactions has not been satisfactorily assessed, however. Clinicians need to be aware of the potential interactions (Table 5) and should review medication lists before prescribing NSAIDs. Given the availability and frequent use of over-the-counter NSAIDs, physicians need to inquire about use of nonprescription medications to avoid duplicate prescribing. Combination NSAID therapy cannot be rationalized given the increased toxicity and lack of improved efficacy.

Glucocorticoids

These are very potent anti-inflammatory drugs that clearly inhibit the translation of COX-2 but also

TABLE 5. **Nonsteroidal Anti-inflammatory Drug Interactions**

Anticoagulants: co-administration with NSAIDs may prolong prothrombin time; also consider NSAID effects on platelet function and gastric mucosa.
Probenecid: may increase plasma concentration of NSAIDs and possibly their toxicities.
Thiazide and loop diuretics: may reduce diuretic effects except sulindac, which may enhance the effects of thiazides.
Antihypertensives: their effects may be blunted by NSAIDs.
Digoxin: NSAIDs may elevate serum levels.
Methotrexate: NSAIDs may increase the risk of toxicity including stomatitis and bone marrow suppression.
Lithium: NSAIDs may elevate serum levels and toxicity (except sulindac, which may have no effect or may decrease serum levels).
Cyclosporine: combined use with NSAIDs may increase drug level.
Phenytoin: NSAIDs may increase serum levels and thus toxicity.

have many other effects. A placebo-controlled trial demonstrated that the use of low doses of these drugs (less than 7.5 mg per day of prednisone orally) for 2 years was associated with the onset of fewer erosions than those seen in the placebo-treated patients. Clearly, there have been significant other studies demonstrating the lack of positive long-term effects of even low doses of glucocorticoids when balanced against their known long-term toxic effects. However, short courses of these drugs may be useful (10 to 20 mg per day of prednisone, then tapered over 5 to 7 days) and may be effective in controlling significant flare-ups of the disease. If control cannot be achieved, then every attempt should be made to try to use these drugs on an every-other-day basis at the lowest possible dose. Intra-articular injections of long-acting glucocorticoids can be especially useful in controlling oligo- or monoarticular flares. Rarely should these be done more than three times per year, and care should be followed in the methodology to reduce the incidence of complications such as infection. In addition, rarely pulse methylprednisolone (250 to 1000 mg intravenously over 1 hour every day for 1 to 3 days) might be helpful in life-threatening vasculitis or in particularly difficult cases. Toxic reactions such as septicemia or osteonecrosis are important complications of such interventions.

Disease-Modifying Antirheumatic Drugs or Slow-Acting Antirheumatic Drugs

Second-line agents are drugs that may modulate the natural history of the disease. These drugs may be referred to as DMARDs or as slow-acting antirheumatic drugs (SAARDs). These are a heterogeneous group of drugs that vary in their chemical structure and in their modes of action. In addition, their toxic profiles also tend to define their place within the treatment algorithm. To be in this category a drug must have shown that it can alter the course of the disease for at least 1 year, leading to sustained improvement in physical function, decrease in the synovitis, and fundamental slowing of the destructive joint damage. All presently available drugs have been demonstrated in standard short-term trials to have been better than placebo or equal to the effects of another DMARD for less than 1 year in randomized controlled trials. Most often clinicians choose to use these drugs in their order of potential toxic reactions, choosing first drugs that have been demonstrated to be effective with less risk for toxicity and, if these fail, then potentially more dangerous drugs as the next step in therapy.

Clinical observations have demonstrated that most commonly used DMARDs for rheumatoid arthritis are not continued long term. At 2 years of therapy about 50% of patients have discontinued treatment and at 5 years less than 25% of patients are still using these drugs. Methotrexate has been the most successful DMARD to date with about 50% of patients still taking drug 5 years after starting. These data are likely due to both lack of effectiveness of these therapies and in some cases particular relationships with toxic reactions. These dismal results have led some investigators to try combinations of these drugs. Some of the better studied combinations are hydroxychloroquine, methotrexate, and sulfasalazine and azathioprine, hydroxychloroquine, and cyclophosphamide.* The latter combination has been shown to be useful in refractory rheumatoid arthritis but is impossible to use long term because of its potential toxic reactions. One series of observations suggests that combination therapy with methotrexate and cyclosporine might be useful in refractory cases.

In general, hydroxychloroquine is considered one of the best tolerated of the disease-modifying drugs, but it is often only a useful adjunct to other therapeutic approaches and rarely is effective enough to be used alone. The usual dose is 200 mg bid to start, and then the dose is decreased to once daily. The major toxicity is retinal, and the patient needs ophthalmologic examination about every 6 months to ensure that there is no increased pigmentation in the retina, which may lead to blindness. The pigmentation is stimulated by the antimalarial agent. Discontinuing the drug early on if pigmentation develops allows the process to reverse, whereas continued therapy can lead to permanent blindness. Often loss of color vision precedes extensive retinal damage.

Methotrexate, either as an oral or a parenteral therapy, is considered one of the more effective agents, although there have not been remissions reported in patients treated with it over the short or the long term. Patients are often better relatively quickly, and the once-a-week regimen is quite attractive. The average dose tends to be between 7.5 and 15 mg per week. Toxicity is relatively rare, and except for untoward pulmonary events can be monitored effectively. The most common toxic reactions are nausea and mouth sores. The mouth sores can be inhibited effectively by the concomitant use of folic

*Not FDA approved for this indication.

acid at a dose of 1 mg per day. Other relatively frequent adverse events include drug-induced hepatitis and macrocytic changes in the red blood cells. Liver function test results must be monitored regularly, and if the serum glutamic-oxaloacetic transaminase and serum glutamic-pyruvic transaminase levels are elevated consistently above normal for 4 to 6 months after the first 6 months of therapy, a liver biopsy needs to be considered. The patients should be instructed to not drink any alcohol while taking this drug. Unfortunately, the sedimentation rate and anemia often improve but rarely return to normal despite ongoing therapy, and once therapy is discontinued a flare of the disease usually follows within 1 month. Over time it is not unusual to require more therapy to maintain the same response.

Despite some recent negative reports, parenteral gold therapy has remained one of the few agents associated with true remissions. However, this event is quite rare, and more than 40% of the patients do not tolerate the therapy owing to its toxic effects. The weekly dosing is attractive, and there were older reports demonstrating healing of joint erosions. Toxic reactions are not uncommon and include heavy metal damage to the kidneys consisting of proteinuria and an active urinary sediment. A blood sample and a urinalysis are required regularly before each injection. If the drug works, the onset of positive effects may be between 3 and 6 months after initiation of therapy. Oral gold therapy has been demonstrated to work in only a few studies. The delay in onset of effect may approach 9 to 10 months, and more than 25% of patients suffer intolerable diarrhea. Sulfasalazine is quite popular in Europe, but studies in the United States demonstrate only a moderate effect. The dose is typically 2 to 4 grams in divided doses initially, with maintenance therapy at about 2 grams per day. The drug interferes with folate metabolism, and the clinician needs to be cautious when prescribing this drug in concert with methotrexate.

Other drugs include D-penicillamine, which has been described to be as effective as parenteral gold therapy by some investigators. It is even more toxic, however, which diminishes its appeal. The immune modulating drugs such as azathioprine and cyclophosphamide are important drugs for the patient with very severe disease. The risk of malignancy with both agents but particularly with cyclophosphamide lessens enthusiasm for their use. Cyclosporine is a very effective agent at a dose somewhere between 5 and 10 mg per kg as an older formulation, but potential toxicity, especially on the kidney, has limited its use. Interesting data have been accumulating regarding combination chemotherapy such as methotrexate in combination with cyclosporine. As further work is done delineating the biology of rheumatoid arthritis, it is hoped that it will point to agents that interrupt the inflammatory process more effectively and with less risk for toxicity and a better outcome.

Azathioprine is a drug typically used to treat patients with disease refractory to other drugs or patients who suffer rather severe extra-articular manifestations of the disease. It does cause the patient to be immunocompromised, although not to a great degree, but its use may lead to an increased risk for bone marrow compromise or susceptibility to infections. There is a small risk for tumor development with long-term use of this drug. Typically the dose is 100 to 150 mg per day.

Penicillamine has been shown to be a useful drug to treat patients with rheumatoid arthritis, but its toxicity has precluded general use. Thus, it has been relegated for use in patients who have marked refractory disease with prominent extra-articular manifestations such as vasculitis. It is recommended to begin at low doses with small incremental increases over weeks to months to achieve a top dose no greater than 750 mg per day. The side effects are many and include renal disease, bone marrow effects, and unique problems such as altering the immune system. Its use has been associated with precipitating Sjögren's syndrome, alveolitis, and systemic lupus erythematosus.

A new formulation of cyclosporine became available in 1997. This version provides a more predictable drug bioavailability and thus better control of its use. It has been shown to be efficacious and is becoming a more popular therapeutic choice for patients with severe, progressive disease that has been refractory to other interventions. The new formulation should not be used at doses higher than 3 mg per kg per day to start, and maintenance should be less. Irreversible renal damage and hypertension remain the major problems with its use. Patients should have their blood pressures checked regularly and health care providers should perform regular urinalyses and serum kidney function tests.

Cyclophosphamide has remained the drug of last resort for patients with severe, unremitting disease with vasculitis and other life-threatening extra-articular manifestations of rheumatoid arthritis. Although highly effective, it has become increasing unpopular because of its high toxicity profile, including its oncogenic potential, particularly in long-term oral use (bladder and transitional cell carcinomas), bone marrow toxicity (as well as leukemias), and infertility.

There has been increasing interest in combination chemotherapeutic interventions. As noted, these have included myriad drugs, and it is reasonable to believe that in such a complicated disease as rheumatoid arthritis that combinations of drugs with multiple effects may be important. More important, with the advent of new information regarding the use of biologic agents such as the soluble receptor to tumor necrosis factor-α (sTNF-α), induction therapies with later switching to other therapies during the course of treatment may become popular. Research will indicate which of these new therapeutic interventions will be of some use. In addition, there is increasing evidence that certain antibiotics specifically derived from minocycline may be useful in the treatment of rheumatoid arthritis. This is not due to an antibacterial effect but instead is likely due to its effects on inhibiting collagenases, important enzymes in the destructive cascade produced by the cells involved in rheumatoid arthritis. Clinical trials have shown some mild effects of standard, presently available tetracycline-derived drugs. In the future, newly developed metalloproteinase inhibitors that inhibit the activity of the collagenases as well as other neutral proteases will be of interest.

There is some older information about the utility of omega-3 fatty acids found in fish oils that may provide benefit for pain and inflammation approximately equivalent to that seen with NSAIDs with fewer potential toxic effects. Unfortunately, the beneficial effects may take up to 9 months to become evident.

The use of the drugs described previously necessitates an understanding about their risks and benefits. The knowledge of the effects of the drug has to be balanced against the state of the disease. Thus, practitioners should be quite experienced in the care of all types of rheumatoid arthritis patients. If they are not, then early referral to a specialist such as a rheumatologist is imperative. Patients with mild disease who show a lack of poor prognostic indicators should be treated less aggressively than patients with evidence of early destruction and lack of good functional status, significant evidence of early erosions, positive serum rheumatoid factor, or increasing debility. Treatment for the more mild version of disease includes NSAIDs along with nonpharmacologic therapies such as education and physical and occupational therapy. DMARDs with low risk such as hydroxychloroquine, sulfasalazine, or the two in combination should be considered. Before initiation of NSAID therapy, it should be determined whether the patient is at risk for a poor renal or GI outcome with these drugs. If so, precautions should be taken. Prophylaxis should be started if the patient is at increased risk for a NSAID-induced GI toxic event.

The patient with moderately severe disease should have all of the above instituted; however, the DMARD choice might be methotrexate or parenteral gold. In addition, early use of low-dose glucocorticoids (e.g., prednisone, less than 7.5 mg per 24 hours) for a short while followed by an appropriate taper may be reasonable. If glucocorticoids are contemplated, then steps should be taken to decrease the risk of bone loss.

If, however, the patient suffers from disease with a significantly poorer prognosis, then a far more aggressive approach should be adopted. First, an absolutely appropriate diagnosis must be achieved. Then an extensive program of education and physical and occupational therapy should be instituted. Along with a NSAID, and the appropriate risk analysis for the potential for a NSAID-induced toxic event, a DMARD such as methotrexate or parenteral gold should be started. Also the use of early combination therapy with low-dose glucocorticoid may be appropriate. Hydroxychloroquine or sulfasalazine may be considered. If these interventions fail, then earlier use of azathioprine and cyclosporine, in combination or alone, should be considered.

If there is clear lack of improvement or if toxicity with any particular regimen ensues, then a reappraisal is warranted and is extremely important. Patients require very close monitoring by individuals who understand the implications of the use of these potentially very toxic drugs. Ultimately, when all else fails and the patient is increasingly debilitated by pain both day and night or mechanical joint failure, then joint replacement may be appropriate. Consultation with surgeons even early in the disease may be useful because there are operative procedures that may serve to enhance pharmacologic success and improve functional outcomes without resorting to total joint replacements.

JUVENILE RHEUMATOID ARTHRITIS

method of
ROBERT W. WARREN, M.D., PH.D., M.P.H.
Baylor College of Medicine
Houston, Texas

Juvenile rheumatoid arthritis (JRA) is a chronic disease of joints and other tissues that affects approximately 250,000 children in the United States. JRA is subdivided into three major subgroups, based on the clinical course in the first 6 months of illness. These subgroups are (1) systemic, characterized by spiking fevers, evanescent rash, and other extra-articular disease; (2) pauciarticular, with four or fewer affected joints; and (3) polyarticular, with five or more affected joints. Only a small minority of JRA patients have an illness like adult rheumatoid arthritis (RA); unlike adults with RA, the majority of children who are treated appropriately recover from JRA without significant disability. The mortality rate in the United States is less than 1%.

JRA must be differentiated from arthritis of other causes. Indeed, more likely causes of childhood arthritis include trauma and infectious and postinfectious etiologies. Whereas these processes usually resolve over days to weeks, the arthritis of JRA persists in at least one joint for a minimum of 6 weeks. The formal diagnosis of JRA also requires age at onset younger than 16 years and exclusion of other inflammatory joint diseases. There are no diagnostic laboratory tests; antinuclear antibody (ANA) and rheumatoid factor assist in subclassification of JRA, but not its diagnosis.

GENERAL MANAGEMENT

There is no specific cure for JRA. No medication safely and totally quells the inflammation of JRA. Continuing or recurrent inflammation produces secondary phenomena, including joint destruction, soft tissue contractures, and growth abnormalities, with accompanying psychologic trauma.

MEDICAL FOLLOW-UP

Excellent home- and community-based care is critical for the child with JRA, but every child with active

JRA should also be evaluated periodically by a health care team that specializes in the care of children with arthritis. The frequency of such visits depends on the diagnosis and the problems of specific patients but should be no less frequent than annually. A systemic JRA flare or acutely increased joint symptoms in any JRA patient should command immediate medical attention.

EDUCATION AND COUNSELING OF FAMILY AND PATIENT

The family's understanding and commitment to the care of the child with JRA is the most critical element in management. Common family concerns are physical deformity and the possible dangers of physical therapy and aspirin therapy. The physician's role in education of the patient and family should be supplemented by literature on diseases and medication, family support groups (such as those sponsored by the parent-run American Juvenile Arthritis Organization), and professional assistance by rheumatology nurses, social workers, and child psychologists.

Family anxieties and concerns are normal. On the other hand, the JRA-provoked psychosocial dysfunction in the patient and family may far outstrip and outlast active or even residual joint disease. The need for psychosocial intervention must be periodically assessed.

MEDICATIONS

Nonsteroidal Anti-inflammatory Drugs

Nonsteroidal anti-inflammatory drugs (NSAIDs) remain first-line medical therapy for all forms of JRA. Responses to NSAID therapy generally occur within weeks. Despite the fact that no one NSAID has proved to be more efficacious than the others, there are differences in chemical structure and unpredictable differences in a patient's response; thus, changing to another NSAID is reasonable in therapeutic failures. On the other hand, the rare child with aspirin allergies should not be given any other NSAID. Although anecdotally successful, the simultaneous use of two NSAIDs has not been carefully studied in JRA, nor is the practice approved by the Food and Drug Administration, because of the risk of significant additive side effects.

Used for decades for children with JRA, aspirin is inexpensive and efficacious; no other NSAID is clearly superior. Compliance with aspirin therapy is much easier to measure than that with other drugs, although more difficult to obtain because of the frequency of administration and parental worries about aspirin's efficacy and about Reye's syndrome. Aspirin is often begun in doses as low as 80 mg per kg per day to decrease the chance of toxicity, but 90 to 100 mg per kg per day (to a maximum of 4 grams per day) divided three or four times daily is usually required for a therapeutic serum salicylate level of 20 to 30 mg per dL. Illnesses affecting gastrointestinal absorption, low serum albumin levels, other medications, and aspirin coating can influence the obtained level. Levels should be reached 7 to 10 days after the initiation or any change of therapy, including the institution or withdrawal of other drugs, or with the advent of any signs of salicylate toxicity (e.g., tinnitus, hyperpnea).

A number of prescription salicylate derivative drugs are marketed, including choline magnesium trisalicylate (Trilisate), which is approved for use in children. Potential advantages include twice-daily dosing, a liquid form (500 mg per 5 mL), less gastrointestinal intolerance, and the lack of an effect on platelet function. Disadvantages include higher cost and the lack of a chewable, small children's tablet. Dose ranges are identical to those of aspirin.

Many other NSAIDs are used by pediatric rheumatologists in the care of children with JRA, although only tolmetin (Tolectin) and naproxen (Naprosyn) are currently approved for use in children from 2 to 14 years of age. Tolmetin is available in 200-mg tablets and 400-mg capsules, and therapy should be initiated at 20 mg per kg per day divided into 3 doses and increased to 30 mg per kg per day (maximum 1.6 grams per day) if well tolerated. Tolmetin bioavailability is decreased by food and milk. Naproxen is available in 250-, 375-, and 500-mg tablets as well as a suspension of 125 mg per 5 mL. Naproxen may be given on a twice-daily schedule, with doses of approximately 15 mg per kg per day (maximum 1 gram per day). Other commonly used NSAIDS include ibuprofen (Motrin), 40 mg per kg per day in three or four divided doses (maximum 2.4 grams per day); diclofenac (Voltaren), 2 to 3 mg per kg per day in two divided doses; and indomethacin (Indocin),* 1.5 to 3 mg per kg per day, in two to four divided doses depending on form (maximum 150 mg daily). Indomethacin is often considered the most potent NSAID, but its usefulness is sometimes limited by dosing schedules and side effects, particularly those affecting the central nervous system. Physicians should be aware that the lower dose, over-the-counter versions of naproxen, ibuprofen, and other NSAIDS may be more appropriate and less expensive.

Potential adverse effects of NSAID therapy include gastrointestinal symptoms, such as vomiting, abdominal pain, gastritis, ulcer disease, and constipation. Parents should report complaints of abdominal pain, vomiting, and hematochezia. Although children seem less likely to develop these problems than adults, they are not exempt and should thus take NSAIDs with meals or snacks. Buffered products offer little additional protection. Antacids, sucralfate (Carafate), and H_2 blockers such as ranitidine (Zantac) are used with variable effect, and misoprostol (Cytotec) is occasionally used. A hemoglobin level or hematocrit and red blood cell indices should be obtained at least every 4 months to assess occult blood loss. Mild liver function abnormalities sometimes occur in chil-

*Not FDA approved for this indication.

dren taking NSAIDs; rarely, children develop significant hepatitis or even liver failure, which is generally rapidly reversible. Liver function studies should be obtained within 1 month of beginning or changing therapy and thereafter, if values are normal, as indicated by careful physical examination. Liver function should be monitored more closely and NSAID therapy decreased if serum transaminase values consistently exceed twice normal. Therapy should be discontinued temporarily with significant transaminase elevation and then restarted at a lower dose after recovery. NSAIDs, and particularly salicylates, should be temporarily discontinued when there is a presumed increased risk for Reye's syndrome (e.g., after exposure to influenza or chickenpox).

Renal effects of NSAIDs include hematuria and decreased creatinine clearance. Urinalysis should be performed every 3 to 4 months, and blood urea nitrogen and serum creatinine levels every 6 months. Some nephrologists recommend that creatinine clearance be checked yearly. Finally, significant central nervous system symptoms (e.g., hallucinations) are rare adverse effects of aspirin and other NSAIDs that necessitate discontinuance of the drug.

Other Agents

In most patients, NSAIDs alone will not control the polyarticular arthritis of systemic or polyarticular JRA, as judged by clinical examination and evidence of progressive, erosive joint disease by diagnostic imaging. Therapy with other medications is then indicated, and NSAIDs are often continued. Given the natural history of polyarticular JRA, many subspecialists begin aggressive second-line medication early in the treatment program in the hope of preventing permanent joint changes.

For such children, the medication of choice is usually methotrexate,* typically in an oral dose of approximately 10 mg per m^2, once weekly. If this dose is ineffective, higher doses are sometimes used, and the medication may be given intramuscularly, subcutaneously, or intravenously as appropriate. Although methotrexate is generally well tolerated, parents are often hesitant about the use of a chemotherapeutic drug; indeed, although the risks of secondary malignancy and decreased fertility are apparently quite small, they merit discussion. Teenagers should be particularly counseled about the risks of pregnancy, given the reported teratogenic effects of methotrexate, and birth control should be advised, as appropriate. Teenagers taking methotrexate should also be warned about the increased risk of liver damage with alcohol ingestion. Patients taking methotrexate should be monitored for liver and bone marrow toxicity with blood counts and chemistry profiles at least every 1 to 2 months. Renal function should also be studied periodically. Treatment with folic acid daily (0.5 to 1.0 mg orally) or folinic acid weekly the day after methotrexate administration (1.25 to 5 mg orally) may help limit side effects of methotrexate. Sulfasalazine* is also an appropriate second-line agent, particularly for patients with aggressive spondyloarthropathy, although it is generally considered not as potent as methotrexate. Dosage is 40 to 50 mg per kg per day in two divided doses, reaching the maximal dose with increments over 1 to 2 months with close monitoring for bone marrow toxicity in particular. The coated preparation (Azulfidine EN-tabs) may be better tolerated in terms of nausea. As with methotrexate, laboratory monitoring is essential.

Children who do not respond well to methotrexate and NSAID therapy are sometimes treated with steroids (see later), but experimental combination therapy is also sometimes used by pediatric rheumatologists. Methotrexate therapy is typically continued and used with hydroxychloroquine (Plaquenil), sulfasalazine, cyclosporine (Sandimmune), or other agents. Azathioprine (Imuran) may also be used. Other experimental therapies include cyclophosphamide and intravenous immunoglobulin infusions. The efficacy of biologic agents for JRA is unknown, but preliminary studies suggesting the efficacy of agents such as anti–tumor necrosis factor in RA are encouraging. Of note, although approved for use in children, intramuscular gold is now only rarely used to treat children with JRA, because of a poorer benefit/risk ratio compared with methotrexate. Oral gold preparations are ineffective in children. Similarly, penicillamine is now an unusual therapy for children with JRA.

Corticosteroids

Systemic steroids are rarely used in the treatment of JRA. Intravenous steroids are indicated in the therapy of acutely ill children with systemic JRA and polyarticular JRA patients, who require hospitalization. Methylprednisolone (Solu-Medrol) may then be given intravenously, 0.25 to 0.5 mg per kg every 6 hours. Methylprednisolone may also be given in crises as pulse intravenous therapy, generally 30 mg per kg per dose, to a maximum of 1 gram. In addition, systemic oral steroids are occasionally needed to control chronic symptoms in systemic JRA, such as severe anemia and rheumatoid lung disease. They may also rarely be necessary to control extremely active, severe polyarticular arthritis that is unresponsive to other medications. In these circumstances, oral prednisone is given daily or preferably every other day, in as low a dose as possible for therapeutic effect. Systemic steroids have no place in the therapy of pauciarticular JRA, except for severe uveitis. Possible benefits of systemic steroids must always be balanced against the well-described major short- and long-term risks, and these should be discussed in detail with the family.

Intra-articular steroid injections of triamcinolone hexacetonide (Aristospan) are now often used in the therapy of JRA. Intra-articular steroid injections have a role in pauciarticular JRA, as well as in flares

*Not FDA approved for this indication.

of single and few joints in polyarticular disease. The recommended dosage is 5 to 40 mg of triamcinolone (depending on the age of the child and on the particular joint), which can be mixed with preservative-free lidocaine; this should be injected no more than twice a year per joint. Activity of the joint should be limited for 1 to 3 days after the injection. Although most patients respond well, there are potential problems associated with intra-articular injections. These include minimal or brief overall response, postinjection arthritis flare, and the psychologic trauma of intra-articular injection. Risks of bleeding, damage to joint cartilage, and infection should be minimal. Some systemic absorption of the drug may occur, and therefore brief adrenal suppression is theoretically possible. Secondary poor bone growth and weakness of surrounding structures near the injected joints have not been confirmed.

Topical steroids are used in the eye for treatment of uveitis (discussed later).

PHYSICAL AND OCCUPATIONAL THERAPY

Physical therapy and occupational therapy are essential elements in the treatment of JRA. The goals of therapy are to maintain and improve the range of motion, strength, and function. Specific guidelines and components for physical therapy for JRA include the following:

1. A home-, school-, and community-based exercise program should be planned and supervised by a licensed physical and/or occupational therapist. Normal activities that accomplish the desired joint motions should be strongly encouraged. Swimming and bicycle and tricycle riding are excellent activities for the child with JRA.
2. Splinting is used for many purposes in JRA, including reducing pain, protecting joints, improving contracture and muscle strength, and increasing function. Night splinting is a highly successful and standard technique for reducing peripheral joint contractures, particularly at the wrist and knees. On the other hand, daytime use of immobilizing splints should at most be only a temporizing measure while other therapies are being instituted. Dynamic splints, which hold joint position and yet encourage specific joint motions against resistance to increase strength, are sometimes used in JRA patients. Shoe inserts and other orthotic devices such as metatarsal bars and pads, as well as comfortable, well-supported shoes, reduce pain. Serial casting is a technique occasionally used to reduce joint contractures unresponsive to physical therapy and splinting.
3. Localized therapy, and sometimes mild pain relievers such as acetaminophen, can be extremely useful in decreasing joint stiffness and discomfort. Warm baths, local application of moist heat, and frequent changes of position can combat joint stiffness. "Icing" a joint can temporarily decrease discomfort and is used as an adjunct in serial casting.

SURGERY

Orthopedists should see children with severe leg length discrepancy, cervical spine disease, and subluxed and/or extremely restricted joint movement or severe pain. However, surgery is not a cure for JRA; in fact, synovectomy may worsen the disease. On the other hand, surgery can be extraordinarily valuable as a reconstructive modality. Unilateral epiphyseal stapling can improve leg length discrepancy in the growing child with asymmetrical pauciarticular arthritis. Specific operations to be considered in the child with severe deforming polyarticular arthritis include soft tissue releases, metatarsal head resection, pin traction for joint subluxation, and cervical spine stabilization. Selective joint replacement may be considered for the older adolescent and young adult patient.

PREVENTION AND TREATMENT OF EYE DISEASE

JRA is a major cause of blindness in children. Chronic, occult iridocyclitis is most common in ANA-positive pauciarticular JRA and less common in systemic and polyarticular JRA. The risk for eye disease does not correlate with the activity of arthritis. Eye pain and photophobia are uncommon complaints, and ophthalmoscopic examination rarely suggests uveitis until significant eye damage has occurred. Thus, slit-lamp examination must be done as frequently as every 6 weeks in the young, female, ANA-positive, new pauciarticular JRA patient; in the older patient with systemic or polyarticular JRA, the examination should be performed at least annually. The consulting ophthalmologist should direct any needed therapy for iritis, which generally includes topical steroids and a mydriatic agent.

ANKYLOSING SPONDYLITIS

method of
MUHAMMAD ASIM KHAN, M.D.
Case Western Reserve University School of Medicine
Cleveland, Ohio

Ankylosing spondylitis (AS) is a chronic systemic inflammatory rheumatic disorder that affects the axial skeleton primarily, and sacroiliac joint involvement (sacroiliitis) is its hallmark. Involvement of the limb joints other than hips and shoulders is uncommon. The disease is strongly associated with a genetic marker HLA-B27 and may show familial aggregation. The inflammatory process involves the synovial and cartilaginous joints as well as the osseous attachments of tendons and ligaments, frequently resulting in fibrous and bony ankylosis. The disease may occur in association with reactive arthritis (Reiter's syndrome), psoriasis, or chronic inflammatory bowel disease ("secondary" AS), but most patients have no evidence of these associated diseases ("primary" or "pure" AS).

CLINICAL FEATURES

Clinical manifestations of the disease usually begin in late adolescence or early adulthood. The disease can begin in childhood, but onset after age 40 is uncommon. The disease is three times more common in men than in women, and its clinical and roentgenographic features seem to evolve more slowly in women. The diagnosis is based on clinical features; the best clues are offered by the patient's symptoms, the family history, the articular and extra-articular physical findings, and the roentgenographic evidence of bilateral sacroiliitis. The most common and characteristic early complaint is chronic low back pain of insidious onset, dull in character, difficult to localize, and felt deep in the gluteal or sacroiliac region. The pain may be unilateral or intermittent at first; however, within a few months, it generally becomes persistent and bilateral, and the lower lumbar area becomes stiff and painful. Pain in the lumbar area rather than the more typical buttock-ache may be the initial symptom in some patients. The second common early symptom is back stiffness, which is worse in the morning and is eased by mild physical activity or hot shower. Prolonged periods of inactivity worsen back pain and stiffness; the patient often experiences considerable difficulty in getting out of bed in the morning. At times, the pain may awaken the patient from sleep; some patients have difficulty sleeping well or find it necessary to wake up at night to move about or exercise for a few minutes before returning to bed. The back symptoms may be absent or mild in an occasional patient, whereas some may complain only of back stiffness, fleeting muscle aches, or musculotendinous tender spots. These symptoms may be worsened on exposure to cold or dampness, and such patients may occasionally be misdiagnosed as having "fibrositis."

Extra-articular or juxta-articular bony tenderness may be an early feature of the disease and is due to enthesitis (inflammatory lesions of entheses) at costosternal junctions, spinous processes, iliac crests, ischial tuberosities, or heels. Involvement of the costovertebral and the costotransverse joints and occurrence of enthesitis at costosternal areas may cause chest pain that may be accentuated on coughing or sneezing. Some patients may complain of inability to expand the chest fully on inspiration. Stiffness and pain in the cervical spine and tenderness of the spinous processes may occur in early stages of the disease in some patients, but generally this tends to occur after some years. The reported frequency of hip joint involvement varies from 17 to 36%; it is usually bilateral, insidious in onset, and potentially more crippling than involvement of any other joint of the extremities. Some degree of flexion contractures at the hip joints is not uncommon at later stages of the disease, giving rise to a characteristic, rigid gait with some flexion at the knees to maintain erect posture. Involvement of peripheral joints, other than hips and shoulders, is quite infrequent in primary AS; it is rarely persistent or erosive and tends to resolve without any residual joint deformity. For example, intermittent knee effusions may occasionally be the presenting manifestation of AS of juvenile onset. Involvement of the temporomandibular joint with resultant pain and local tenderness may occur in about 10% of patients. Mild constitutional symptoms, such as anorexia, malaise, or mild fever, may occur in some patients in early stages of their disease and may be observed relatively more commonly among patients with juvenile onset.

A thorough physical examination, particularly of the axial skeleton, is critical in making an early diagnosis of AS; there is often some limitation of motion of the lumbar spine, most easily recognized on hyperextension, lateral and forward flexion, or rotation. The ability of a patient to touch the floor with fingertips, keeping the knees fully extended, should not be solely relied on for evaluation of spinal mobility because a good range of motion of the hip joints can compensate for considerable loss of mobility of lumbar spine. Direct pressure over the inflamed sacroiliac joints frequently elicits pain, but sometimes the sacroiliac tenderness may be absent because these sacroiliac joints are surrounded by strong ligaments that may allow only minimal motion or in late stages of the disease when inflammation is replaced by fibrosis and bony ankylosis. The chest expansion becomes restricted, the breathing becomes primarily diaphragmatic, and the abdomen becomes protuberant. The entire spine becomes increasingly stiff after many years of disease progression, with progressive flattening of lumbar spine and gentle thoracic kyphosis. Involvement of the cervical spine results in progressive limitation of neck motion and a forward cervical stoop. The diagnosis is readily apparent at this advanced stage because of the characteristic gait and posture and the way the patient sits or rises from the examining table. Spinal ankylosis develops at a variable rate and pattern; sometimes the disease may remain confined to one part of the spine. Typical deformities tend to evolve after 10 or more years.

The most common extraskeletal involvement is acute anterior uveitis (acute iritis), and it occurs in 25 to 30% of patients at some time in the course of their disease. The eye inflammation is typically unilateral and has an acute onset; symptoms include pain, increased lacrimation, photophobia, and blurred vision. Rare extra-articular involvements or complications include aortitis (leading to slowly progressive aortic valve incompetence and conduction abnormalities, sometimes requiring a pacemaker), apical pulmonary fibrosis and cavitation, amyloidosis, and IgA glomerulonephropathy. There is a lack of convincing evidence for involvement of skeletal muscles; the marked muscle wasting seen in some patients with advanced disease results from disuse atrophy. Neurologic involvement may occur owing to fracture-dislocation, atlantoaxial subluxations, or cauda equina syndrome. The spinal fracture can follow a relatively minor trauma in patients with ankylosed spine; it usually occurs in the lower cervical spine; and the resultant quadriplegia is the most dreaded complication, with a high mortality rate.

DIAGNOSIS

The absence of a known cause of AS provides a hurdle to its early diagnosis; one has to depend primarily on the patient's clinical history and the clinical and roentgenographic findings. Low back pain and stiffness are the most common presenting symptoms, although a variety of other presentations may antedate back symptoms in some patients. Restriction of spinal mobility and a decreased chest expansion further support the diagnosis. There are no diagnostic or pathognomonic laboratory tests. An elevated erythrocyte sedimentation rate is seen in up to 75% of patients, and a mild to moderate elevation of serum IgA concentration is also frequently observed. There is no association with rheumatoid factor and antinuclear antibodies, and the synovial fluid or synovial biopsy does not show markedly distinctive features as compared with other inflammatory arthropathies.

The characteristic radiographic changes of AS may evolve slowly over many years but are usually present by the time the patient seeks medical attention. They are primarily seen in the axial skeleton, especially in the sacroiliac joint. Radiographic evidence of sacroiliitis is required for diagnosis and is the most consistent finding (Table 1). A simple anteroposterior roentgenogram is usually sufficient for its detection. The changes are bilateral and symmetrical and consist of blurring of the subchondral bone plate, followed by erosions (similar to postage stamp serration) and sclerosis of the adjacent bone. These are first noted and are more prominent on the iliac side of the joint, later progressing to "pseudowidening" followed by gradual narrowing owing to interosseous bridging and ossification. Ultimately (usually after many years) there may be complete bony ankylosis of the sacroiliac joints and resolution of the juxta-articular bony sclerosis.

The inflammatory lesions in the vertebral column affect the superficial layers of the anulus fibrosus at their attachment to the corners of vertebral bodies, resulting in reactive bone sclerosis, seen roentgenographically as highlighting of the corners and subsequent bone resorption (erosions). This leads to "squaring" of the vertebral bodies and gradual ossification of the superficial layers of the anulus fibrosus that form intervertebral bony "bridging" called syndesmophytes. There are often concomitant inflammatory changes resulting in ankylosis of the apophyseal joints and ossification of the spinal ligaments, ultimately resulting in a virtually complete fusion of the vertebral column ("bamboo spine") in patients with severe AS of long duration. Spinal osteoporosis is also frequently observed, in part as a result of ankylosis and lack of spinal mobility. In patients with early disease in whom standard roentgenography of the sacroiliac joints may show normal or equivocal changes, computed tomography appears to be more sensitive but equally specific when compared with conventional roentgenography but is rarely needed. Magnetic resonance imaging can produce excellent but costly imaging without ionizing radiation and is especially useful in cauda equina syndrome. Quantitative radioactive scintigraphy may be too nonspecific to be useful.

HLA-B27 typing can occasionally be used as an aid to the diagnosis of AS, but an overwhelming majority of patients with AS can be readily diagnosed clinically on the basis of history, physical examination, and roentgenographic findings, and they do not need the B27 test. It is not a routine, diagnostic, confirmatory, or screening test for AS in patients with back pain, even though the test in some ethnic and racial groups is highly sensitive for AS (90% sensitivity among whites compared with 50% among African-Americans). HLA-B27 is present in 8% of the normal population (2% of African-Americans).

TABLE 1. **Modified New York Diagnostic Criteria for Ankylosing Spondylitis (AS)**

Clinical Criteria
Low back pain for >3 months improved by exercise and not relieved by rest
Limitation of lumbar spine movement in the frontal and sagittal planes
Reduced chest expansion (corrected for age)
Radiologic Criteria
Bilateral sacroiliitis, grades 2–4
Unilateral sacroiliitis, grades 3–4
AS is diagnosed if either radiologic criterion plus any clinical criterion is present.

Modified from Wright V, Helliwell PS: Ankylosing spondylitis. *In* Rakel RE (ed): Conn's Current Therapy 1997. Philadelphia, WB Saunders Co, 1997, p 1005.

NATURAL HISTORY

The course of AS is highly variable, characterized by spontaneous remissions and exacerbations, but it is generally favorable; earlier studies suggesting a generally unremitting course primarily involved patients with severe disease studied in hospitals. It has become apparent in the last decade that a number of HLA-B27–positive individuals, not previously recognized as having AS, manifest clinical features that are often relatively mild or self-limited. Good functional capacity and the ability to work are maintained in most patients, even in cases of protracted disease. Although it is difficult to predict the ultimate prognosis for an individual patient, those with hip involvement or completely ankylosed cervical spine with kyphosis are more likely to be disabled. Fortunately, the results of total hip arthroplasty in recent years are gratifying in preventing partial or total disability. Some studies have suggested a slightly reduced life expectancy of patients with AS, but because of the selection bias for severe disease inherent in those studies, it is likely that patients with relatively milder disease have normal life expectancy.

MANAGEMENT

There is currently no preventive measure or cure for AS, but most patients can be well managed. A concerned physician providing continuity of care can be most valuable. Patient education is crucial for successful management. The patient should thoroughly understand that although pain and stiffness can often be well controlled by appropriate use of nonsteroidal anti-inflammatory drugs (NSAIDs), regular therapeutic exercises to minimize and prevent deformity and disability are the single most important measure in medical management. The patient should walk erect; do back extension exercises regularly; and sleep on a firm mattress, without a pillow if possible. It is better to sleep on the back or in a prone position with an extended and stretched back and avoid sleeping curled up on one side. The patient should avoid cigarette smoking and do regular deep breathing exercises to preserve normal chest expansion. Swimming is the best over-all exercise for patients with AS, and use of snorkel and face mask may permit even those with considerable cervical flexion deformity to do freestyle swimming under observation.

Aspirin seldom provides an adequate therapeutic response. Phenylbutazone (Butazolidin) is probably the most effective NSAID for AS patients and offers good symptomatic relief, but because of its potentially greater risk of bone marrow toxicity, other NSAIDs are used, such as indomethacin (Indocin), naproxen (Naprosyn), diclofenac (Voltaren), or sulindac (Clinoril) (Table 2). There are additional NSAIDs that may be equally effective in AS, but they may not be currently approved by the U.S. Food and Drug Administration for such clinical use. Some patients may respond better to one NSAID than another.

TABLE 2. **Nonsteroidal Anti-inflammatory Drug (NSAID) Therapy in Ankylosing Spondylitis**

Indomethacin (Indocin), diclofenac (Voltaren), naproxen (Naprosyn), or sulindac (Clinoril) in a full dose is usually most effective, although any tolerated NSAID will help
Avoid combinations of NSAIDs
Slow-release preparations give better overall control and compliance. They may be more effective in relieving morning stiffness
Co-prescribe a gastroprotective agent if there is a history of dyspepsia or peptic ulcer
Provide information to the patient regarding the mode of action and potential side effects of drugs

Modified from Wright V, Helliwell PS: Ankylosing spondylitis. *In* Rakel RE (ed): Conn's Current Therapy 1997. Philadelphia, WB Saunders Co, 1997, p 1006.

These drugs should be used in full therapeutic anti-inflammatory doses during the active phase of the disease. The patient should be informed about this because otherwise he or she may use the NSAID for its analgesic effect only.

Sulfasalazine may be effective for peripheral arthritis in some AS patients whose symptoms are not adequately controlled by NSAIDs; because of its efficacy in inflammatory bowel disease as well, it would appear to be especially useful in enteropathic AS or for those intolerant to NSAIDs. D-Penicillamine is not effective, and antimalarial drugs and immunosuppressants have not been well studied in AS. A few patients unresponsive to NSAIDs and sulfasalazine have responded to oral methotrexate therapy. Oral corticosteroids have no therapeutic value in the long-term management of the musculoskeletal aspects of AS because of their potential for serious side effects, and they do not halt the progression of the disease. Recalcitrant enthesopathy and persistent synovitis may respond quite well to a local corticosteroid injection, and therapeutic contribution of injection into the sacroiliac joints is being evaluated.

Acute anterior uveitis can be well managed with dilatation of the pupil and use of corticosteroid eye drops. Systemic steroids or immunosuppressants may be needed for rare patients with severe refractory uveitis. Cardiac complications may require aortic valve replacement or pacemaker implantation. Apical pulmonary fibrosis is not easy to manage; surgical resection may rarely be required. It is the general consensus that radiotherapy has no role in the modern management of patients with AS because of the high risk of leukemia and aplastic anemia. Splints, braces, and corsets are generally not helpful in the management of AS. There is no special diet, and there is no evidence that any specific food has something to do with the initiation or exacerbation of AS. Pregnancy usually does not affect the symptoms, and fertility and childbirth have been reported to be normal.

In extreme cases in which the disease has progressed to a severe stage, surgery is helpful. Total hip replacement gives good results and prevents partial or total disability from severe hip disease. Vertebral wedge osteotomy may be needed for correction of severe kyphosis in some patients, although it carries a relatively high risk of paraplegia.

Many patients may have difficulty driving because of the impaired neck mobility, and special wide-view mirrors can be helpful for such patients. Similarly, special prism glasses can help improve vision in those rare patients who are so kyphotic that they cannot look ahead while walking. There are many AS patient support groups in various countries that, in addition to enlisting enthusiastic cooperation of the patients, also provide useful pamphlets and information about the disease and its management and advice about life and health insurance, jobs, working environment, wide-view mirrors, and other useful items. They are accessible on the internet at http://www.spondylitis.org or at http://web.ukonline.co.uk/members/nass/.

TEMPOROMANDIBULAR DISORDERS AND CRANIOFACIAL PAIN

method of
RICHARD OHRBACH, D.D.S., PH.D.
State University of New York at Buffalo
Buffalo, New York

and

JEFFREY BURGESS, D.D.S., M.S.D.
University of Washington
Seattle, Washington

Temporomandibular disorders (TMD) and craniofacial pain are two major groups of disorders that include pain in the oral, facial, or head regions as the primary complaint. TMD is a collection of conditions that affect the muscles of mastication, the temporomandibular joints (TMJs), or both. The primary presenting symptom of a TMD is pain, which is localized most often in the muscles of mastication or in the preauricular area. Pain symptoms may also be associated with the ear, head, or cervical muscles. The other major presenting symptoms include limitation in jaw functioning (e.g., restriction in range of motion, difficulty with mastication) or noises or altered functioning in the TMJ. In contrast, craniofacial pain disorders are a group of pain disorders that are *not* typically associated with alterations in mandibular function and that extend diagnostically across the disciplines of neurology, otolaryngology, psychiatry, and dentistry. The pain complaint is located primarily within the orofacial area, but the distribution may extend beyond the orofacial area in either a caudal or a cephalad direction. Diagnostic distinctions between TMDs and craniofacial pain disorders are generally clear and made by taking a careful history. This chapter discusses clinical evaluation, the characteristics of the major disorders, and treatments.

EPIDEMIOLOGY

The TMDs are relatively common; estimated prevalences within the United States are about 12% for TMD-related pain (6-months' duration) and about 5% for a diagnosed TMD requiring treatment. Any of the three major characteristics of a TMD (pain, limitation in motion, joint noise) occurs in 5 to 50% of the population, and treatment seeking appears to be related to the severity of pain and limitation in jaw functioning. The modal patient is 18 to 45 years old, and females present for treatment at a rate of four to seven times greater than that for males, whereas the population prevalence of TMDs is only about twice as high for females as for males. The prevalence is much lower for late adolescents, the middle-aged, and elderly. There are no other presently known risk factors regarding the development of a TMD. Emerging evidence suggests that hormonal factors may account for the gender disparity in prevalence, but an explanatory mechanism remains absent.

The craniofacial pain conditions, excluding toothache and sinusitis, are much less common. The facial migraine variants are probably less common than migraine headache, but they are also probably underdiagnosed at present so their true prevalence remains to be determined.

CLINICAL ASSESSMENT

The clinical assessment format for both groups of disorders is similar. Although the central role of psychosocial factors in the diagnostic process and in treatment has been amply demonstrated for the TMDs, psychosocial factors are also presumed to play a role in the management of the craniofacial pain disorders when they have become chronic (i.e., at least 3 to 6 months in duration) and refractory to initial treatment approaches. Thus, a dual axis approach that includes both biomedical and biobehavioral aspects is highly recommended.

Biomedical Evaluation

History. The pain history is critical in evaluation of a TMD or craniofacial pain disorder. It includes assessment of pain location, referral patterns, quality (e.g., ache, throb, burning, electrical), duration (e.g., brief, hours, days, months), temporal characteristics (e.g., intermittent, paroxysmal, recurrent, constant), patterning (e.g., morning, evening, during sleep), ameliorating and exacerbating factors (e.g., cold, chewing, head or body movement), and associated symptoms (e.g., dysesthesia, photophobia, or phonophobia). A pain description that appears atypical should not be discounted but approached with scrutiny, as it may reflect multiple diagnoses or etiologies: central (e.g., intracranial), nonfacial (e.g., cardiac, oncologic, neck), or biobehavioral etiology.

A past or present history of TMJ noises such as clicking, popping, or crepitus is important in TMD. A distinct click or pop occurring in the TMJ suggests possible anterior disk displacement with reduction (i.e., internal derangement). However, nonpainful TMJ noise is considered to be benign, self-limiting, and not needing intervention. Significant TMJ dysfunction includes that occurring during mid to late opening with pain and/or catching, coupled with intermittent or persistent locking for longer than 24 hours. Crepitus suggests degenerative disease. A history of intermittent joint noise (click or pop) followed by sudden opening limitation, pain, absence of noise, and severe opening deviation suggests nonreducing disk displacement. Chronic nonreducing disk displacement, ruled out by imaging via magnetic resonance imaging (MRI) or arthrogram, may or may not be symptomatic and is characterized by a history of acute opening limitation with subsequent slow increase in opening; the patient usually reports a continued limitation in opening.

Orofacial trauma involving jaw fracture or TMJ intracapsular injury is often associated with a patient report of acute malocclusion and severe pain at the fracture site or in the TMJ when the teeth are brought together. Condylar fracture may also be associated with limited jaw opening and lateral movement while the patient may be able to occlude the teeth partially. Complaint of progressive change in the bite, such as an opening between the posterior or anterior teeth, may indicate the presence of significant joint (e.g., rheumatoid or degenerative) or endocrine (e.g., acromegaly) disease. A perceived malocclusion (in the absence of objective evidence of such) coupled with facial or head pain suggests the presence of a myofascial or biobehavioral condition.

Physical Examination. Examination of the patient should include vital signs, general inspection of the head, and cranial nerve and otologic examination. Palpation of the neck, including the musculature, is also recommended, as pain can be referred from this region to the cranium. Lack of published criteria for performing neck muscle palpation may limit its reliability and validity, and results should be interpreted cautiously, particularly in the absence of accompanying history. It is generally accepted that if pain in the head is being caused by the neck musculature, repeated palpation of identified trigger points should reproduce the phenomena. With respect to TMD, there is little scientific support for a causal relationship between masticatory muscle conditions and TMJ and neck abnormality, although referred pain may produce overlap.

The use of a standardized examination (e.g., the Research Diagnostic Criteria, RDC) has become the norm in assessing patients for TMD. Although initially intended as a research instrument to provide improved assessment reliability, the RDC is also time efficient in the clinical setting. The use of a nonstandardized examination format invites overdiagnosis of TMDs.

For palpation, about 2 pounds of pressure should be applied to the facial and extraoral masticatory muscles and about 1 pound to the TMJs and the intraoral masticatory muscles. Jaw opening is measured with a millimeter ruler. Although female jaw opening is less than that of males, less than 35 mm is generally considered limited; normally an individual should be able to place three fingers vertically between the front teeth. Jaw opening is evaluated for deviation and for disk movement by the application of light pressure over the joints. False-positive results may occur with the use of a stethoscope. The teeth, mucosa, and posterior pharynx should always be evaluated. Excessive tooth wear indicates past or present parafunctional behavior. Although TMD is not generally associated with malocclusion, malocclusion may be significant in certain circumstances.

Head and face imaging and laboratory and serologic assessment are needed for evaluation of selected craniofacial pain patients, depending on history and examination findings. Panography provides an initial screening examination for maxillomandibular pathology or TMJ degenerative disease and may be the only imaging necessary for most patients. Plain film radiography or computed tomography is useful for confirming the diagnosis and extent of disease with suspected developmental abnormalities, neoplasm, trauma/fracture, sinus pathology, degenerative disease, chronic infection (e.g., osteomyelitis), and TMJ ankylosis. For degenerative disease, conventional TMJ tomography permits a more accurate segmental assessment of the extent of disease. TMJ intracapsular disease is best visualized via MRI or arthrogram, although the latter is invasive. Single photon emission computed tomography

(SPECT), although not specific, can be helpful with suspected inflammatory disorders.

Biobehavioral Evaluation

From a biobehavioral perspective, chronic TMD is similar to other chronic pain conditions such as headache and back pain in terms of psychophysiologic mechanisms, coping processes, behavioral manifestations, and personal impact; attention must be directed toward these aspects for both diagnosis and treatment. In contrast, it is believed that the diagnosis and management of the acute TMDs require less consideration of these aspects. For the chronic intermittent or acute craniofacial pain problem, these aspects may not be important for diagnosis but may be needed for treatment when the craniofacial pain disorder has become more enduring, persistent, or refractory. Then, biobehavioral aspects become highly salient at both diagnostic and management phases.

TMD characteristics shared with other chronic musculoskeletal pain disorders include (1) poor correspondence between subjective complaints of pain and suffering and the identifiable pathophysiology; (2) impact of psychosocial stress in effecting nonfunctional increases in muscle activity, such as oral parafunctional habits; (3) greater reporting of distressing emotions and situations, implying greater difficulty in coping, which may be either a premorbid style or a style that has emerged from conditions of chronic pain and associated distress; (4) possible presence of clinically diagnosable depression, anxiety, and/or somatization, the latter referring to the reporting of multiple somatic problems simultaneous with significant life disarray; (5) disruption in usual performance at home, work, or school; and (6) frequent health care visits, often characterized by previous treatment successes that are no longer effective, medication abuse, seeking treatments that are exclusively somatic, and avoiding consideration for biobehavioral treatments.

These similarities inform the following considerations for the biobehavioral portion of the assessment. Specifically, we suggest that the following four domains be evaluated.

Subjective Aspects of the Condition. The *pain complaint* should be evaluated for (1) its relationship to relevant anatomy and physiology, (2) which factors (physical, psychosocial) alter it, and (3) what activities have been altered due to it. *Treatment history* should be evaluated with respect to (1) which types of treatments were successful and unsuccessful, (2) whether there was a preponderance or avoidance of any particular type (e.g., medications, behavioral treatment), (3) whether there was premature abandonment of a treatment, and (4) what factors were involved with resuming treatment when prior treatment seeking was intermittent. These areas provide information about the patient's compliance style, explanatory model, and expectations regarding treatment. The patient's *explanatory model* should also be explored regarding (1) the origin of the problem, (2) the meaning of the symptoms, and (3) the role of physical and psychologic treatments, with respect to etiology, maintenance, and exacerbation of the problem. The explanatory model provides an excellent context for introducing the use of broad-based treatment, including the potential need for referral for biobehavioral treatment, instead of waiting until all physical diagnostic or therapeutic approaches have been tried and then referring the patient to a psychologist or psychiatrist. That latter approach to intervention gives the implicit message that the pain was initially real but, with the failure of treatment, has become imaginary. A patient with a rigid explanation that the problem is completely of physical origin is often highly reluctant, perhaps even resistant, to consider an alternative model that incorporates a biobehavioral perspective. Such views are often a consequence of repeated evaluations that are very somatically focused and that have excluded the biobehavioral domain.

Behaviors. The primary consideration is oral parafunctional behaviors (nocturnal or diurnal). These behaviors are often indicative of psychosocial stress responding, masticatory muscle abuse, or both. Other muscle groups are also often similarly involved, most notably the cervical muscles, contributing to the overall pain problem and perhaps indicating how extensive the pattern of stress responding may be. Other potentially important behaviors, such as whether pain intensity follows certain home or work-related situations, also should be addressed. This is often best done when supplemented by a self-report diary containing columns for the desired information coupled with specific instructions and follow-up by the physician. For example, a patient who reports no linkage of symptoms to daily events (especially when the pain is daily and reported as unchanging) may, after maintaining a diary for a week, report a very different symptom picture. The power of empirical data should not be underestimated.

Psychological Status. The primary areas to be assessed include depression, anxiety, and somatization. These can be assessed through standard clinical interview, structured clinical interview (e.g., SCID), or standardized questionnaires such as the SCL-90R. Other measures can be used for depression and anxiety, but the SCL-90R is perhaps the best current tool for formal assessment of somatization as a continuum. Regardless of the approach used, all patients with these pain problems should receive the same evaluation, thereby avoiding one of the common difficulties of targeting only the patient for whom it seems appropriate, which then leads to that patient somehow feeling singled out, which then leads to defensiveness. The question is not whether biobehavioral aspects are involved, but to what degree or extent and in what specific ways do they manifest in this particular patient and contribute to the suffering associated with the pain. The primary purpose of this part of the assessment is screening: whether to refer the patient for more specialized evaluation, generally through referral to a clinical psychologist or psychiatrist who specializes in the evaluation of chronic pain. Depression is common in the TMD population, often co-morbid with elevated anxiety, and is responsive to treatment (either pharmacologic or behavioral), which often alters the reported pain as well. Somatization as a formal disorder is less common but as a continuum is present surprisingly often, and when present it may influence treatment outcome significantly and increase doctor shopping and treatment-seeking behavior.

Psychosocial Status. Questions are posed regarding interference in psychosocial function (activities of daily living, mastication and speech, social interaction, oral intimate behaviors) and health care utilization. Prognosis is typically worse when there is high interference, avoidance of responsibilities, and deactivation coupled with pain rated as severe.

Diagnostic Integration

For the TMDs, a dual axis system has been in use for about 10 years. Axis I contains the physical diagnosis. Axis II contains the summary from the biobehavioral assessment and implies specific areas for other aspects of treatment. We suggest that this formulation is also applicable to craniofacial pain disorders. One common practice is to escalate diagnostic testing for the axis I aspects of the disorder without equal consideration of the axis II domain; we suggest that both areas be investigated equally from the outset.

TEMPOROMANDIBULAR DISORDERS

The most common TMDs are described in Table 1. Note that some potential disorders that are not yet described consistently in the literature and that do not have clear inclusion criteria are not included in this table: muscle contracture, spasm, splinting, inflammatory disease (synovitis), and ligamentous injury (perforation, tearing).

CRANIOFACIAL PAIN DISORDERS

Craniofacial pain differential diagnosis is confounded by the complexity of the region and potential for noncranial referral. In patients with chronic craniofacial pain the diagnosis may be further complicated by multiple overlapping diagnoses and emergence of biobehavioral factors.

Facial pain conditions to be considered in the differential are presented in Table 2. Of the many intracranial problems causing facial pain, cerebellar pontine angle meningioma (versus neuralgia or pulpal pathology) should be considered when there is paroxysmal pain plus patient description of dysesthesia (i.e., tingling or numbness) confirmed by cranial nerve examination. Other conditions associated with neuralgia-like pain presentation include cranial tumor (e.g., epidermoid, metastatic, and brain stem glioma), acoustic neuroma, nasopharyngeal carcinoma, vascular lesions (e.g., arteriovenous malformation), scleroderma, and Paget's disease. Neuralgia-like pain may also follow orthognathic and third-molar surgery in a small number of cases. Neurovascular problems presenting diagnostic difficulty include the atypical migraine variants, paroxysmal hemicrania, cluster-tic syndromes, temporal arteritis, carotodynia, and chronic cluster, in which pain may be perceived in the midface, cheek, or temple.

In differentiating among these conditions the clinician

TABLE 1. **Temporomandibular Disorders: Diagnostic Criteria**

Condition	Essential Diagnostic Features
Group I: Muscle Disorders	
Ia. Myofascial pain (pain in the muscles of mastication)	1. Pain or ache, at rest or during function, in the jaw, temples, face, preauricular area, inside the ear; plus 2. Palpation pain in at least 3 of 20 muscle sites (posterior, middle, anterior temporalis; origin, body, insertion of masseter; stylohyoid, digastric, lateral pterygoid, temporalis tendon). Palpation pain must be at least present on the side of pain complaint
Ib. Myofascial pain with limited opening	1. Myofascial pain, as defined above; plus 2. Pain-free unassisted mandibular opening of less than 40 mm; plus 3. Maximum assisted opening at least 5 mm greater than pain-free unassisted opening
Group II: Disk Displacements	
IIa. Disk displacement with reduction	1. Reciprocal clicking in the temporomandibular joint (TMJ) (click on both opening and closing, or a click on either opening or closing and click during lateral or protrusive excursions)
IIb. Disk displacement without reduction, with limited opening	1. Report of significant limitation of mandibular opening; plus 2. Maximum unassisted opening ≤35 mm; plus 3. Passive stretch increases opening 4 mm or less beyond unassisted opening; plus 4. Contralateral excursion <7 mm and/or uncorrected deviation to the ipsilateral side on opening; plus 5. Absence of joint sounds, or presence of joint sounds not meeting criteria for disk displacement with reduction
IIc. Disk displacement without reduction, without limited opening	1. Report of significant limitation of mandibular opening; plus 2. Maximal unassisted opening >35 mm; plus 3. Passive stretch increases opening at least 5 mm; plus 4. Contralateral excursion ≥7 mm; plus 5. Presence of joint sounds not meeting criteria for disk displacement with reduction; plus 6. If joint imaging is requested, it should image the disk in closed and open mouth positions with arthrography or MRI
Group III: Arthralgia, Arthritis, Arthrosis	
IIIa. Arthralgia (pain in the joint)	1. Pain in one or both joint sites during palpation; plus 2. One or more self-reports of pain in the region of the joint, pain in joint during maximum unassisted or assisted opening, or lateral excursions; plus 3. Absence of coarse crepitus
IIIb. Osteoarthritis of the TMJ (inflammatory changes in the joint)	1. Arthralgia (see above); plus 2. Coarse crepitus in the joint or joint imaging showing erosions, sclerosis or condylar head or articular eminence, or flattening of the joint surfaces
IIIc. Osteoarthrosis of the TMJ (remodeling of the articulating surfaces)	1. Absence of arthralgia; plus 2. Coarse crepitus or joint imaging showing joint changes

Modified from Dworkin SF, LeResche L. Research diagnostic criteria for temporomandibular disorders: Review, criteria, examinations and specifications, critique. J Craniomandib Dis Facial Oral Pain 1992;6:301–355.

TABLE 2. **Craniofacial Pain Disorders: Characteristics and Differential Diagnosis**

Condition	Pathognomonic Pain Characteristics	Pathognomonic Nonpain Characteristics	Differential Diagnosis
Intracranial			
Cerebellar pontine angle tumor	Constant ache exacerbated by head movement or coughing; or neuralgia-like	Dysesthesia, paresthesia	Trigeminal neuralgia, odontogenic pathology
Aneurysm	Throb with rapid increase in severity worsened with exertion	Neurologic signs, gastrointestinal upset	Odontogenic pathology, temporomandibular disorder (TMD), sinus disease, Tolosa-Hunt syndrome, migraine
Neurovascular	(Throbbing, midface or temporal)		
Migraine variant*	Pain intensity exacerbated by physical activity; triggered by stress or alcohol	Autonomic dysfunction, somatosensory hyperesthesia	Common migraine, Chiari malformation, Tolosa-Hunt syndrome, Raeder's syndrome
Chronic paroxysmal hemicrania	3–5 minute paroxysms 5–20 episodes/day, pain-free intervals between paroxysms; no known trigger (unremitting form: daily at least for 1 year) (remitting form: daily for days to months, with remissions and recrudescence)	Responsive to indomethacin	Cluster, neuralgia, sinusitis, odontogenic
Cluster†	Burning/sharp, unilateral, eye region	Nocturnal episodes, Horner's facial flushing, tearing, conjunctival injection	Atypical cluster, cluster-tic syndrome,† sinusitis, odontogenic, atypical migraine, chronic paroxysmal hemicrania (remitted form)†
Atypical cluster†	Throbbing, bilateral, noneye region	Non-nocturnal, infrequent ocular/ nasal signs	[same as cluster], chronic paroxysmal hemicrania (unremitted form)†
Temporal arteritis	Burning, associated claudication pain	Scalp allodynia, hyperesthesia, pain in maxillary teeth, positive sedimentation rate	Migraine, sinusitis, odontogenic, TMD
Neurogenic			
Neuralgia (trigeminal, glossopharyngeal)	Stabbing or electrical quality, paroxysmal triggered by trivial sensation in associated distribution, duration of seconds with complete remission between episodes	Absence of sensory or reflex deficit by neurologic testing	Tumor (epidermoid, metastatic), brain stem glioma, acoustic neuroma, nasopharyngeal carcinoma, vascular lesion, connective tissue disease, Paget's syphilis, toxins, multiple sclerosis
Postherpetic	Distribution of V3, burning/ache with allodynia (cold), dysesthesia	Preceded by vesicular disease	Odontogenic pain, post-trauma, jaw surgery
Odontogenic Pathology	(Pain in jaw, teeth, midface) Pain with chewing, intraoral hot/ cold	Caries, exposed cementum/ dentin, mucosal swelling, acute malocclusion	Neurogenic, neurovascular pain, TMD, sinusitis
Stylohyoid Process Syndrome†	Deep throbbing pain (mandible or throat region) evoked by swallowing or head turning or by palpation of stylohyoid ligament or carotid trunk	Dizziness	TMD, glossopharyngeal neuralgia, carotid arteritis, tonsillitis, parotitis, osteomyelitis
Salivary Disease	(Pain in cheek, inferior mandible) Pain with introduction of food or drink, sour	Associated swelling in region of gland with resolution/ recrudescence	TMD, odontogenic pathology
Sinus Pathology	(Pain in midface) Constant or intermittent ache aggravated by postural change involving head movement; maxillary tooth pain	Facial flushing, positive imaging	Migraine variants, odontogenic pathology, TMD

*Classic and common migraine should also be considered in the differential when TMD or craniofacial pain is located in or refers to the temporal region.
†Per taxonomy from Merskey H, Bogduk N, eds. Classification of Chronic Pain: Descriptors of Chronic Pain Syndromes and Definition of Pain Terms, ed 2. Seattle, WA: IASP Press, 1994.

should be familiar with the epidemiology and pay particular attention to precipitating factors and associated symptoms. For example, patients with nonchronic cluster are typically males aged 18 to 40, and ipsilateral nasal discharge, lacrimation, conjunctival injection, and facial flushing occurs with pain. Patients with temporal arteritis, in contrast, are typically older men or women who report pain and feeling ill, and the pain location and scalp hyperpathia in conjunction with muscle palpation tenderness could be misdiagnosed as a TMD. Atypical neurogenic conditions, including the neuralgias and deafferentation syndromes, can be confused with pain of odontogenic as well as intracranial etiology as previously described. Craniofacial pain associated with TMD must be differentiated from tension headache; the migraine variants; odontogenic pain from pulpal or periapical pathology (abscess); neurovascular or inflammatory headache with facial involvement; lesions of the parotid, ear, nose, and pharynx; and pain referred from the cervical musculature. When a TMD is present, it is not uncommon to have multiple TMD and non-TMD pain conditions. With traumatic injury, there is often extensive overlapping of multiple conditions causing pain, and differential diagnosis can be problematic.

TREATMENT

Biomedical Treatment

The treatment of craniofacial pain is predicated on the identified pathology, clinical diagnosis, and extent and duration of the problem, which, if chronic, includes biobehavioral as well as biomedical components. For most craniofacial pain conditions not involving frank disease, initial therapy is pharmacologic with the proper drug, dosage, and frequency of administration dependent on the specific problem. Specific therapies, including drug protocols, are outlined in the chapters detailing individual conditions (e.g., migraine, cluster, migraine variants, neuralgia, odontogenic disease, inflammatory and tension headache, disease of the mucosa, sinus, parotid, ear, nose and throat) and are not reviewed here. Adjunctive therapy may also include biobehavioral, nutritional, and preventive treatment, and, in limited cases, surgery.

The management of TMD varies depending on the identified problem, pain duration, and presence of biobehavioral factors but generally consists of treatments used in the management of other musculoskeletal conditions. Normally, TMD is self-limiting, and symptoms can be reduced effectively with assurance, accurate information regarding the disease and prognosis, instructions regarding behavior modification, and short-term use of medications. If parafunctional behaviors such as nail biting, daytime tooth clenching, gum chewing, or habitual jaw popping are identified, they should be managed. Because habitual behavior is often stress-related, patients may also benefit by exploring the environmental factors that initiate or perpetuate the activity.

Pharmacologic management includes use of analgesics, nonsteroidal anti-inflammatories, anxiolytics, muscle relaxants, and occasionally corticosteroids. Antidepressants, specifically the tertiary tricyclics (e.g., amitriptyline,* nortriptyline*), are especially useful for TMD because in addition to analgesic activity, they improve sleep and can suppress nocturnal bruxism; dosages are typically in the range of 10 to 25 mg at bedtime. In contrast, the selective serotonin reuptake inhibitor (SSRI) antidepressants* have been linked to increased nocturnal bruxism and could aggravate TMD unless combined with sleep medication. Although controversial, narcotic analgesics are discouraged in cases other than trauma because other approaches are generally available. Nonsteroidal anti-inflammatory drugs (NSAIDs) are particularly effective for managing joint and muscle pain; dosages generally range to the maximum recommended dose for each drug. If one drug is ineffective, an additional trial (or trials) with another is appropriate. To prevent abuse, muscle relaxant medication such as carisoprodol (Soma) or cyclobenzaprine (Flexeril) or anxiolytics such as diazepam (Valium) should be prescribed using a time-dependent protocol. Therapeutic benefit may be increased by coupling these drugs with physical medicine intervention and/or a treatment contract. In the patient with severe joint inflammation, pain relief can be achieved with corticosteroid (dexamethasone) delivered via iontophoresis, injection (0.5 mg per session with a maximum dose of 3 mg delivered over six sessions) or by mouth (40 to 60 mg tapered over 7 to 10 days). If trigger points are identified in the masticatory muscles, 0.5% procaine in isotonic saline or isotonic saline alone can be delivered via local injection. Dry needling of trigger points may also be efficacious.

Physical therapy can reduce symptoms in TMD but should be prescribed carefully to avoid dependence. The main modality with proven efficacy is repetitive active or passive jaw exercises; ultrasound is commonly used, but efficacy data are absent. A home program in which the patient opens slowly in the midline 10 times, four times a day, coupled with thermal agents may be as useful in reducing pain as professional physical therapy. Active jaw stretching is contraindicated with acute nonreducing disk displacement. Continuous passive jaw movement may be helpful following TMJ surgery and in cases of chronic nonreducing disk displacement and osteoarthritis.

Intraoral appliances (splints, orthotics, nightguards) have been used historically by dentists to treat TMD. Constructed of soft or hard acrylic, they fit over maxillary or mandibular teeth and may protect the joint or joints in cases of trauma or TMJ injury or assist in controlling nocturnal bruxism. No additional benefit is gained with the appliance by repositioning the jaw. Intraoral appliances are an active treatment that can alter the occlusion; hence, this treatment should be used only by a knowledgeable clinician. Orthodontics, dental reconstruction, and bite adjustment are unlikely to cause greater symptom reduction than reversible treatment, are expensive, and create additional risk that may out-

*Not FDA approved for this indication.

weigh any long-term benefit; they are appropriate therapies only when symptoms are confounded by dental pathology or significant tooth loss.

TMJ surgery can improve jaw function and reduce symptoms associated with disk displacement without reduction or severe osteoarthritis. Arthrocentesis involves corticosteroid medication injected into the joint in conjunction with joint lavage and may be performed on an outpatient basis at minimal cost. Arthroscopic surgery, in addition to irrigating the joint, allows visualization of the superior synovial space, débridement of minor adhesions, and biopsy. It is not useful for changing disk position in cases of locking, but it may increase associated hypomobility. Arthrotomy or open joint surgery may be helpful for fibrous ankylosis, suspected neoplasm, chronic nonreducing disk displacement, and severe osteoarthritis. The published criteria for defining the need for surgery include failure of medical management, identifiable disease, and increasing disability. Regardless of potential need for surgery, refractory pain warrants additional medical (e.g., neurosurgical, neurologic) and biobehavioral assessment and potential referral to a multidisciplinary pain clinic.

Biobehavioral Treatment

Although treatment of acute craniofacial pain disorders may appropriately rely on a medical management model, chronic craniofacial pain disorders as well as both acute and chronic TMDs are best managed, like all chronic pain conditions, using a rehabilitation approach. In this approach, more reliance is placed on the patient acquiring self-management skills, as described previously, and including useful pain-coping behaviors, cognitive skills, and responses to emotional states, coupled with a re-evaluation of the role of medications and provider-mediated therapies.

Although it is not clear what contributes to the efficacy of a biobehavioral approach, there is substantial agreement that such approaches are safe, noninvasive, and effective; whereas the gain is often modest initially compared with that obtained by more direct physical forms of therapy, at 1-year follow-ups the biobehavioral approaches are either as effective or more so. Almost all chronic pain treatment programs use these approaches as an integral part of the treatment model, and although such approaches are seen less often in the treatment of craniofacial pain disorders and the TMDs, current evidence indicates that they should nevertheless be used.

The most commonly used biobehavioral approaches include biofeedback, relaxation, hypnosis, education, and cognitive-behavioral treatments, all based on cognitive and behavioral principles. These approaches are based on two fundamental aims: change the perception of the pain and modify the accompanying suffering and psychosocial dysfunction. Psychodynamic and psychoanalytic approaches to pain treatment remain unvalidated but promising.

Similar to its impact in back pain and headache, a single psychoeducational session (group or individual) for TMD pain can remain effective for reducing pain-related interference at 1-year follow-up. Relaxation, biofeedback, and hypnosis all have clear beneficial effects in both reducing the psychophysiologic activation generally present with TMD pain and in promoting general self-regulation. Often, however, premorbid psychosocial characteristics influence the degree to which the individual will effectively use these three methods, and these characteristics often become the focus of the biobehavioral therapy. In that case, biobehavioral therapy focuses on the interactions among emotional reactivity, pain, suffering, and coping, and rapid improvement in general functioning as well as in pain relief can be observed in as few as six sessions when the patient is motivated. Motivation, on the other hand, is often influenced by the nature of the referral and the quality of the relationship that the patient has with his or her primary provider. Nevertheless, these approaches appear to be capable of significant and enduring benefits compared with those from the usual clinical treatment for TMD. Given the current emphasis on providing conservative and noninvasive treatments as the general overall treatment approach, the biobehavioral treatments outlined here incorporate many of the critical elements found in the typical clinical treatment: relaxation, education, habit management, self-control, and the like.

For both biomedical and biobehavioral domains, very little is known about which aspect of treatment is responsible for change in clinical symptoms. Thus, multimodal approaches are common and currently recommended because which patient will respond to which treatment is presently not understood. A multimodal approach has the potential to maximize the clinical benefits from a conservative noninvasive approach. Before escalating either diagnostic intervention or treatment within the biomedical domain, we strongly advocate that at the outset the biobehavioral domain be included and that its diagnostic or treatment escalation be simultaneous with that in the biomedical domain. In contrast, treatment for TMD is generally driven by the physical diagnosis alone without addressing the psychosocial impact of the pain and disability or the coping patterns of the patient. These latter issues affect not only the course of the condition but also how the individual responds to biomedical treatment. Outcome assessment has almost exclusively been focused on physical parameters and not psychosocial ones. We suspect that failure to attend to the biobehavioral domain results in the necessity for further treatment bouts and increased invasiveness of treatment in certain individuals.

For craniofacial pain disorders, the role of the biobehavioral treatments has been little studied or utilized clinically. As stated at the outset, their role is likely small for the acute craniofacial pain disorder; however, we suspect that the biobehavioral approaches as outlined for TMD are likely just as useful when craniofacial pain disorders become chronic or refractory to the standard biomedical treatments.

BURSITIS, TENDINITIS, MYOFASCIAL PAIN, AND FIBROMYALGIA

method of
THOMAS W. JAMIESON, M.D.
Uniformed Services University of the Health Sciences
Bethesda, Maryland

BURSITIS

Bursae are subcutaneous spaces lined with synovial membranes that secrete fluid to allow smooth and nearly frictionless motion among muscles, ligaments, tendons, bones, and skin. Some bursae are present at birth and are constant throughout life, whereas others are "formed" in response to repetitive physical pressure (e.g., bursae under metatarsal heads that may occur in rheumatoid arthritis). Although there are approximately 150 bursae in the body, most are not likely to be of pathologic significance. Bursal inflammation may be a clinical problem, however, in a few predictable anatomic sites: the subacromial bursa of the shoulder, olecranon bursa at the elbow, iliopsoas bursa near the hip, trochanteric-subtrochanteric bursae below the hip, gastrocnemiosemimembranous bursa of the knee, and retrocalcaneal bursa of the heel.

Subacromial bursitis is usually secondary to inflammatory lesions of the rotator cuff or bicipital tendon, both of which are anatomically contiguous to the bursal floor. Subacromial bursitis causes severe pain in all planes of movement but usually is worse with abduction and internal-external rotation movements. Subacromial bursitis should be distinguished from the more frequently encountered tendinitis problems of the shoulder, as the latter are more indolent and longer tolerated by patients. Subacromial bursitis causes prompt and severe pain and is distinguished on physical examination from the tendinitis overuse syndromes.

The olecranon bursa overlies the distal portion of the triceps tendon and the olecranon of the ulna. With inflammation, swelling is seen at the point of the elbow and pain may be present. If so, it occurs most typically with resisted extension of the arm (i.e., with increased tension in the adjacent triceps tendon). If pain is present, particularly with accompanying skin erythema, suspicion of an infection or a crystal-induced process is heightened and a bursal aspiration is indicated. Presumably, bacteria can access the olecranon bursa through the skin even without a visible skin wound. Typically, septic olecranon bursitis is seen in manual laborers and in alcohol abusers; chronic obstructive pulmonary disease patients may also be disproportionately affected. Hemorrhagic olecranon bursitis may be seen in uremic patients undergoing dialysis.

The iliopsoas bursa overlies the hip capsule (lateral to the femoral blood vessels, between the iliopsoas muscle and the anterior surface of the hip joint). The iliopsoas bursa is large (about 6 x 3 cm) and may communicate with the hip joint in select patients. Most often the iliopsoas bursa becomes symptomatic in a patient with predicate hip pathology (often osteoarthritis) and may manifest as an enlarging inguinal mass with pressure on adjacent tissues. These protruding bursae may be confused with a hernia, hydrocele, adenopathy, or psoas abscess. Computed tomography or magnetic resonance imaging scan is diagnostically useful and will demonstrate a well-defined water density mass in the appropriate anatomic site, often with a concurrent hip joint effusion.

The trochanteric bursae, several in number, overlie the lateral hip region. The largest and most important structure lies between the gluteus maximus and the tendon of the gluteus medius muscles. Patients usually complain of a deep, dull, aching pain in the lateral hip area, but half also describe anterolateral proximal lower extremity pain radiating to the knee, often worsening with activity and sometimes disturbing sleep. Differential diagnostic considerations here may include herniated nucleus pulposus of L3–4 (i.e., with symptoms in the L-4 nerve root distribution), spinal stenosis, or an entrapment neuropathy (namely, meralgia paresthetica).

Distention of the gastrocnemiosemimembranous bursa (Baker's cyst) often is a subclinical finding. Baker's cysts may be present and not palpable and may be palpable but not of clinical significance. In inflammatory knee conditions there is usually communication with the knee joint and a one-way synovial fluid flow into the bursa. If dissection or rupture of a Baker's cyst occurs, differentiation from deep vein thrombophlebitis can be difficult ("pseudo-thrombophlebitis"). Diagnostic ultrasonography is sensitive in detecting the presence of an intact Baker's cyst, but it becomes less reliable when bursal dissection or rupture into the calf occurs. Associated thrombophlebitis must be definitively excluded by venography or reliable, noninvasive means before accepting knee cyst–related phenomena as the sole cause of calf-foot pain and swelling.

Between the calcaneus bone and the Achilles tendon lies the retrocalcaneal bursa. Symptoms in the area of this bursa may be mistaken for Achilles tendinitis, and care should be taken to differentiate these conditions. A swollen retrocalcaneal bursa commonly will show bulging on the medial and lateral sides of the Achilles tendon. The swollen bursa may be extremely sensitive to pressure on direct palpation and with dorsiflexion of the foot. (Caution regarding the introduction of corticosteroid agents in the vicinity of the Achilles tendon is discussed in the treatment section later.)

TENDINITIS

Common sites of tendon inflammation are the frequently used tendons of the upper extremities where they pass over bony prominences. Although the rotator cuff refers generically to a collection of four muscles about the shoulder, it is specifically the supraspinous muscle that is most commonly involved in tendinitis, perhaps owing to the stress resulting from humeral impingement against the coracoacromial arch. Patients note pain subacromially and laterally over the shoulder with abduction of the arm. Bicipital tendinitis affects the long head of the biceps muscle and characteristically causes shoulder pain anteriorly and over the bicipital groove (particularly with flexion of the shoulder against resistance, elbow extended, and forearm supinated).

Lateral epicondylitis at the elbow ("tennis elbow") results from inflammation and degeneration of extensor tendons of the forearm, particularly the extensor carpi radialis brevis, with eventual fibrous adherence to the capsule of the lateral elbow. Contracture of the wrist extensor muscles then chronically pulls on the capsule, producing pain about 2 cm distal to the lateral epicondyle. Medial epicondylitis ("golfer's elbow") similarly produces pain at the origin of the flexor muscles of the wrist, distal to the medial epicondyle.

The dorsum of the wrist contains six compartments through which numerous tendons glide. Although an inflammatory process may affect any of these, inflammation of the abductor pollicis longus and extensor pollicis brevis tendons in the first compartment (i.e., most radial) may result in a lack of smooth excursion of the enclosed tendons, a condition known as de Quervain's disease (stenosing tenosynovitis). Patients describe pain at the radial aspect of the wrist, especially with pinch gripping. Palpation of the tendons in the anatomic "snuff box" area may reveal swelling compared with the uninvolved side.

TREATMENT OF BURSITIS AND TENDINITIS

Immobilization of an inflamed musculoskeletal part, whether partial or complete, is an important adjunct in management and helps to expedite and optimize chances for recovery. The exception to this general rule is with tendinitis or bursitis of the shoulder, where immobilization may foster development of a "frozen" shoulder and, except for brief periods (e.g., 24 to 48 hours), should be avoided. Splints are especially useful in epicondylitis of the elbow ("elbow band") and in de Quervain's disease of the thumb. Ice during the acute phase and moist heat during the chronic phase are useful, and nonsteroidal anti-inflammatory drugs (NSAIDs) are helpful in many cases. The choice of a specific NSAID is not critical, but all such agents should be given in ample doses and with food (ideally in the middle of a meal) to lessen the risk of gastropathy. An enteric-coated aspirin preparation, 975 mg every 6 to 8 hours; naproxen (Naprosyn), 250 to 500 mg twice daily; and oxaprozin (Daypro), 1200 mg once a day, are representative examples. For patients with a bleeding diathesis, persons on warfarin (Coumadin) therapy, or those otherwise unable to tolerate the standard NSAIDs, possible treatment options include a nonacetylated salicylate (e.g., Trilisate or Disalcid) or a course of a centrally acting synthetic analgesic such as tramadol (Ultram), 50 to 100 mg every 6 hours as needed.

Physical therapy, ultrasound, or hydrotherapy has application in many cases but is most important in shoulder tendinitis or bursitis, in which there is greater risk of permanent compromise in range of motion. Acute tendinitis or bursitis may render such severe pain, however, that physical therapy intended to augment range-of-motion function becomes impractical or ignored. In such a clinical setting selective local anesthetic-corticosteroid injections are often valuable. The anatomic area is cleaned with povidone-iodine (Betadine) and alcohol, and an ethyl chloride spray may be applied as a topical anesthetic. Selection of corticosteroid is based on the extent of symptoms and, for practical reasons, the relative depth of involved tissue pathology owing to the potential for soft tissue atrophy (especially likely with synthetic fluorinated preparations such as triamcinolone). Consideration should be given to the relative solubility and potency when selecting a corticosteroid preparation (or combination) for soft tissue injection. Medium-potency agents include prednisolone sodium phosphate and prednisolone tebutate; these agents are useful at superficial injection sites. A high-potency fluorinated corticosteroid, such as triamcinolone hexacetonide (Aristospan Intra-articular, slow onset but prolonged duration of action) should be used only for injection of deep structures or for intra-articular injections, to minimize the danger of leakage to the skin with resultant atrophy and/or depigmentation of skin. Ideal technique favors injection near the affected tendon but not directly into the structure itself. A frequently used narrow tendon, such as the bicipital tendon, may be prone to rupture with direct injection; the Achilles tendon and surrounding areas should not be directly exposed to corticosteroid agents because this structure is inherently weak and prone to tear. Although more than a single corticosteroid injection may not be necessary to modify a soft tissue pain syndrome, caution should be taken not to exceed three injections in the same anatomic site over a 12-month period. Under sterile conditions, the incidence of iatrogenic infection with soft tissue injection is extremely low. A patient with glucose intolerance may have a transient effect from local corticosteroid injection. A period of reduced activity of 24 to 48 hours is best to optimize therapeutic results.

Surgical attention is seldom necessary in tendinitis or bursitis, but with structural rupture or recalcitrance to full conservative measures, surgical excision or repair may become a consideration.

Patients with recurrent symptoms must be instructed to avoid provocative or aggravating activities that strain susceptible anatomic structures by overuse. Warm-up and stretching exercises should always precede aerobic conditioning activities.

MYOFASCIAL PAIN

In the nomenclature of soft tissue pain syndromes, "myofascial pain" infers regional discomfort, often with a discernible soft tissue focus palpable on physical examination and radiating pain with modest pressure (4 kg) ("trigger zone"). The development of an anatomic trigger zone may result from trauma (of even minimal severity) or from overuse. Although often post-traumatic, or ostensibly autonomous, myofascial pain may also occur in systemic illnesses. The lack of gross "swelling" should not mislead the physician to conclude that the patient has no "sensation of swelling." The importance of a careful and "hands-on" physical examination cannot be overstated in this setting. Documentation of palpable soft tissue abnormalities is obviously important, but assessment of joint range of motion (passive and active), possible joint hypermobility, and subtle synovial warmth and/or thickening is useful whether any abnormalities are, in fact, present.

Myofascial pain appears to be distinct from the condition of fibromyalgia. Unlike the generalized pain and fatigue of fibromyalgia, and the disproportionate female preponderance of fibromyalgia patients, the condition of myofascial pain shows negligible gender variation, stiffness that is regional rather than generalized, and pain that is more focused and less whole bodied.

FIBROMYALGIA

Fibromyalgia is a common pain amplification syndrome characterized by generalized chronic pain (longer than 3 months in duration), stiffness, gelling, and fatigue. Typically, patients are women of middle age with predictable tender points on physical examination and a disturbed sleep pattern such that they awaken nonrefreshed from sleep (a nonrestorative sleep pattern). The most frequently affected anatomic sites in fibromyalgia include (bilaterally) at the occiput, low cervical region, midpoint of the trapezius, supraspinatus at the medial border of the scapula, second ribs at costochondral junctions, 2 cm distal to the lateral epicondyles of the elbow, gluteal area in the upper-outer quadrants of the buttocks, 2 cm posterior to the greater trochanter, and at the medial fat pads of the knees proximal to the joint line. Predictable features of fibromyalgia (100% incidence) include generalized pain for at least 3 months and widespread local tenderness at 11 or more of the aforementioned 18 anatomic sites; characteristic features (greater than 75% incidence) are fatigue, sleep disturbance, and morning stiffness; common features (greater than 25% incidence) may be headache, paresthesias, psychologic abnormality, subjective swelling, and functional disability.

The diagnosis of fibromyalgia is based on a characteristic history, the exclusion of systemic diseases that may cause musculoskeletal pain (e.g., rheumatoid arthritis, systemic lupus erythematosus, inflammatory muscle disease, polymyalgia rheumatica, and hypothyroidism), the finding of nonarticular tender points with an essentially normal joint examination, and a normal laboratory profile (i.e., complete blood count, acute phase response, and thyroid functions). Occasionally, a low titer of antinuclear antibody is found but in the absence of an obvious cause such as connective tissue disease or a drug-induced effect.

The pathophysiology of fibromyalgia is not well understood, although an association with psychologic abnormalities has been suggested. There may be a subgroup of fibromyalgia patients with significant coexisting psychologic problems, especially depression, and there appears to be an increased incidence of depression in first-degree relatives of fibromyalgia patients. Most patients with fibromyalgia, however, are not depressed.

The most characteristic sleep abnormality in fibromyalgia is the loss of "slow-wave" deep sleep with a relative loss of the restorative phase of sleep. Sleep apnea may be seen disproportionately in male patients with fibromyalgia, and polysomnography is a reasonable consideration in selected patients. The natural history of fibromyalgia is not established definitively. Although symptoms may be chronic, perhaps lasting 10 to 15 years or longer, a majority of patients show symptomatic improvement when fully informed and optimally managed.

Fibromyalgia may occur following motor vehicle accidents or other trauma. Although some have suggested that no scientific data support a causality link between soft tissue trauma and the development of fibromyalgia, it seems presumptuous to rule out completely any possible linkage between trauma and fibromyalgia when so little is definitively understood about the latter condition itself. Patients who develop neck, upper back, or upper extremity pain after automobile trauma may have experienced sudden extreme movements of the cervical spine ("whiplash") and may stretch an individual nerve root with impingement or a herniated disk. Some patients may continue to complain of soft tissue pain a year or more after traumatic injury yet have no objective evidence of neurologic pathology or radiographic abnormalities. A diagnostic-prognostic paradigm is not easily applied to the work-up, disposition, or compensatory claims of post-traumatic nonarticular pain patients. Although doubtlessly there are self-serving motives in some cases, it would seem reckless to categorically discount or dismiss the potential problems patients may encounter in the post-traumatic setting.

Treatment

Proper management of fibromyalgia must begin with a definite diagnosis and assurance regarding the noncrippling nature of the process. Physician-patient dialogue is essential for the initiation of an effective treatment program, and printed educational material, including that from the Arthritis Foundation, often is also useful. Pharmacologic intervention is used most effectively in attempting to rectify the underlying sleep abnormality. Favorable results often are seen by instituting amitriptyline* (Elavil), 10 mg 2 hours before bedtime with increments of 10 mg every 2 weeks if necessary, not to exceed 50 mg total dose. These are not, of course, antidepressant dosages of amitriptyline, and depression is usually not the pathologic focus of managing fibromyalgia. A concurrent morning dose of a selective serotonin reuptake inhibitor such as paroxetine (Paxil), 20 mg, may be useful in depressed patients. The improvement of sleep pattern with the resulting attenuation or amelioration of pain symptoms is the single most important application of pharmacology in fibromyalgia. Cyclobenzaprine* (Flexeril), 10 mg at bedtime, may also be useful in improving sleep patterns. Owing to their similar side effects, though, antidepressants and muscle relaxants should not be prescribed concurrently. NSAIDs sometimes are helpful as analgesics but not as the sole drug used to alleviate the symptoms of fibromyalgia. Generally, NSAIDs should

*Not FDA approved for this indication.

be minimally utilized. In selected patients, tender point injections with corticosteroids or lidocaine may be useful. A reasonable injection regimen is 2 mL of 1% lidocaine, or the same amount of lidocaine plus a corticosteroid. The total amount of corticosteroid administered (to all sites in total) should not exceed 40 mg of methylprednisolone or the equivalent, and tender points should not be injected more than once a month or three times a year. Synthetic fluorinated corticosteroid agents are not recommended for soft tissue injection owing to the potential atrophy of subcutaneous tissues and depigmentation of skin at the injection site. Nonpharmacologic modalities, including meditation, relaxation techniques, and biofeedback, may be useful in lessening tension. Physical fitness training resulting in cardiovascular conditioning is beneficial. Patients should select the aerobic activity of their choice (walking, running, swimming, bicycling) and commit themselves to incorporate such activity into their routine daily schedules three to five times per week. Patients must start slowly and advance their workouts gradually, and exercise periods should not become an "inner competition" but remain relaxing and not unduly stressful. A caring physician can provide important psychologic support for most patients, but in a few select cases the help of a psychologist or psychiatrist may be necessary.

OSTEOARTHRITIS

method of
JOEL A. BLOCK, M.D.
Rush–Presbyterian–St. Luke's Medical Center
Chicago, Illinois

and

THOMAS J. SCHNITZER, M.D., PH.D.
Northwestern University
Chicago, Illinois

Osteoarthritis (OA), also known as osteoarthrosis or degenerative joint disease (DJD), represents the clinical manifestations of a series of degenerative processes that affect the articular structures and result in pain and diminished function. The incidence of OA increases with age, and evidence of OA involvement can be detected in some joint in the majority of the population by age 65. OA is therefore the most common arthritic condition, and the number of patients with symptomatic disease may be expected to rise dramatically with the aging of the general population. Although it is not a rapidly debilitating disease, the sheer number of symptomatic patients makes the economic impact of OA enormous in terms of loss of work and direct costs of medical care. The aggregate societal costs of OA dwarf the costs of the other arthritides; calculations based on the National Health Interview Survey have yielded estimates that the impact of OA is more than 30-fold greater than that of rheumatoid arthritis, the most common inflammatory form of arthritis.

Rather than a single disease, OA likely represents the final common pathway of joint destruction resulting from a number of different processes; although the pathophysiology is principally degenerative, it is typically accompanied by a local inflammatory component that may accelerate joint destruction. Although it is not established that the primary insult is to the articular cartilage, OA is characterized by disruption of the smooth articulating surface of cartilage, followed by formation of clefts and fibrillation, and ultimately by the full-thickness loss of the cartilage. Coincident with the cartilaginous changes are alterations of the periarticular bone. These include the development of bony sclerosis in the areas subjacent to the cartilage and the growth of osteophytes. During the progression of the degenerative process, periods of local inflammation may accelerate cartilage loss and result in exacerbation of pain.

The osteoarthritic diseases have classically been categorized as primary and secondary. Primary OA refers to the clinical spectrum of degenerative joint diseases for which no underlying etiology has been determined. Typically, the joints involved include the interphalangeal joints of the hands as well as the first carpometacarpal joints, the hips, the knees, the spine, and some joints in the midfoot; curiously, other large joints, such as the ankles, elbows, and shoulders, tend to be spared in primary OA. Several variants of primary OA have been defined. Inflammatory or erosive OA has a predilection for the distal interphalangeal joints of the hands and typically involves a destructive arthropathy leading to ankylosis of the joints. Diffuse idiopathic skeletal hyperostosis (DISH) has been classically described as flowing osteophytosis bridging at least four vertebral bodies; it is frequently asymptomatic and is commonly detected incidentally on radiographic examination. In contrast to primary OA, secondary OA occurs as a result of defined insults. Common associations include *metabolic diseases* such as hemochromatosis and alkaptonuria; *developmental abnormalities* such as developmental dysplasia of the hips (formerly congenital dislocation of the hips) and limb-length discrepancies; and long-term sequelae of *significant articular derangements*, including trauma, inflammatory arthritides such as rheumatoid arthritis or gout, septic arthritis, and neuropathic arthritis. Calcium pyrophosphate dihydrate deposition in degenerative hyaline and fibrocartilage results in chondrocalcinosis and may present as pseudogout or as typical OA.

CLINICAL PRESENTATION

OA is frequently identified as an incidental finding during radiographic procedures performed for other indications; in cases of asymptomatic disease, there is almost no reason for further evaluation or treatment. The initial clinical presentation of *symptomatic* OA usually consists of local pain at involved joints, typically with onset after use; with disease progression, OA pain may evolve to a continuous aching sensation and may wake the patient at night. In addition to pain, local discomfort frequently accompanies disease progression. At times, the principal complaint may be of cosmetic alterations, especially in the fingers. As OA is not a systemic inflammatory disease, one does not expect systemic symptoms to be associated with disease progression. When constitutional symptoms are present, such as malaise or weight loss, a search for another underlying pathology is required.

There are characteristic physical findings in OA. Osteophytes are often palpable as bony enlargements at the joint margins; when these occur in the distal and proximal interphalangeal joints of the hands, they are referred to as Heberden's nodes and Bouchard's nodes, respectively.

Crepitus is palpable on passive range of motion of affected joints and is diagnostic of cartilage abnormalities. Cartilage damage tends to be asymmetric within each involved joint; thus, the external appearance of OA joints is often deformed. For example, when the medial compartment of the knee is disproportionately affected relative to the lateral compartment, a varus abnormality of the leg results. With advancing disease, range-of-motion limitations become significant.

Except for radiography, the use of the laboratory in the evaluation of OA is principally to exclude other sources of pain. The characteristic radiographic appearance of OA includes osteophytes, sclerosis of the subchondral bone, and asymmetric joint space narrowing. However, it should be remembered that the correlation between radiographic severity and symptomatic disease is poor; hence, the routine use of radiography for the diagnosis of OA is probably unnecessary. There are no specific abnormalities in hematologic and laboratory chemistry evaluations. When joint effusions are present, they are usually noninflammatory; the total leukocyte count is typically less than 1000 cells per mm^3, and there is a lymphocyte predominance. Subtle laboratory markers of inflammation as well as direct visualization via arthroscopy have demonstrated that local synovitis frequently accompanies painful flares in OA; however, this is not detectable with routine laboratory markers.

THERAPY

Mature cartilage is a nonhealing tissue; hence, rather than attempting to arrest or reverse the course of OA, therapeutic approaches until recently have been directed at palliating pain and at maintaining articular function. This involves both pharmacologic intervention and multidisciplinary efforts to optimize the function of the entire joint, including the musculature and the subchondral bone. Before initiating or changing therapy, however, the correct diagnosis must be established and the pain must be determined to be OA-related. As discussed previously, a large proportion of asymptomatic adults may have evidence of OA; therefore, merely identifying the presence of radiographically abnormal joints in a patient with pain ought not necessarily imply a causal relationship to OA. A careful history and physical examination directed at identifying whether the pain arises intra-articularly or from the periarticular soft tissues, such as the myofascial pain of fibromyalgia, are therefore the first steps of the therapeutic approach. If the symptoms do arise from the joints, it is important to exclude inflammatory and infectious etiologies. In contradistinction to OA, the inflammatory arthritides are associated with systemic symptoms such as malaise and prolonged morning stiffness. Once the presence of symptomatic OA is confirmed, coexisting alternative sources of pain, such as trauma or malignancy, need to be ruled out.

Analgesics. Fundamentally unchanged for decades, the mainstay of OA therapy remains pharmacologic pain palliation, typically with pure analgesics and nonsteroidal anti-inflammatory drugs (NSAIDs). As OA is not considered to be primarily an inflammatory disease, and the NSAIDs may be associated with significant morbidities, it is appropriate to initiate therapy with a trial of pure analgesics, such as acetaminophen (Tylenol) or tramadol (Ultram). It is common, however, for these agents to provide either inadequate or only short-term pain relief, and a trial of NSAIDs should then be given. The anti-inflammatory activities of the NSAIDs have not been shown to positively affect the OA process; hence, their chief advantage in OA therapy appears to be their potent analgesic properties. Treatment should therefore begin at the lowest therapeutic doses and be advanced as necessary. A variety of NSAIDs are available (Table 1), both by prescription and over the counter. The currently available NSAIDs all have comparable analgesic potency at full therapeutic dosage; moreover, although some NSAIDs may have lower overall gastrointestinal, renal, or hepatic toxicity, the onset of adverse reactions is unpredictable among individual patients. Thus, the selection of a particular NSAID with which to initiate therapy should usually be made based on dosing convenience, physician and patient comfort, and price. It is not unusual for several different NSAIDs to be tried before a suitably effective and well-tolerated agent is identified.

TABLE 1. **Currently Available Nonsteroidal Anti-inflammatory Drugs (NSAIDs)**

Class	Usual Doses	Maximum Daily
Heteroarylacetic Acids		
Diclofenac (Voltaren)	50–75 mg bid*	225 mg
Tolmetin (Tolectin)	200–600 mg tid	1800 mg
Diclofenac/misoprostol (Arthrotec)	50/200 bid-qid or 75/200 bid	
Indoleacetic Acids		
Etodolac (Lodine)	200–400 mg bid-tid*	1200 mg
Indomethacin (Indocin)	25–50 mg bid-tid*	200 mg
Sulindac (Clinoril)	150–200 mg bid	400 mg
Naphthyl-alkanones		
Nabumetone (Relafen)	500–1000 mg bid/ 750–1500 mg q d	2000 mg
Oxicams		
Piroxicam (Feldene)	20 mg q d	20 mg
Propionic Acids		
Fenoprofen (Nalfon)	300–600 mg tid-qid	3200 mg
Flurbiprofen (Ansaid)	50–100 mg bid-tid	300 mg
Ibuprofen (Motrin)	400–800 mg tid-qid	2400 mg
Ketoprofen (Orudis)	50–75 mg tid-qid*	300 mg
Naproxen (Naprosyn)	250–500 mg bid*	1500 mg
Oxaprozin (Daypro)	600–1200 mg q d	1800 mg
Salicylates		
Aspirin	500–1000 mg qid	4000 mg
Choline magnesium trisalicylate (Trilisate)	1000–1500 mg bid/750 mg tid	3000 mg
Diflunisal (Dolobid)	500 mg bid	1500 mg
Salsalate (Disalcid)	750–1500 mg bid/1000 mg tid	3000 mg

Agents unavailable in the United States or restricted to short-term use, such as ketorolac and mefenamic acid, are not listed.

*Extended release forms are available for less frequent dosing.

NSAIDs should not be combined concurrently, as this practice increases the risk of toxicity without a concomitant increase in efficacy; however, NSAIDs may be used in conjunction with acetaminophen or acetaminophen-codeine (e.g., Tylenol No. 3) when each agent alone proves insufficient. For patients with more than intermittent NSAID use, evaluations of renal and hepatic function should be considered after a few weeks.

The adverse gastrointestinal effects of NSAID use, including dyspepsia, gastric erosions, and peptic ulcers, are well known and are typically treated by neutralization of gastric acid. This may be accomplished by H_2-antagonists, proton-pump inhibitors, or classic antacids. The NSAIDs exert their anti-inflammatory activity by inhibiting cyclooxygenase activity and thereby diminishing prostaglandin synthesis. A synthetic prostaglandin, misoprostol (Cytotec), has been shown to be protective of the gastric and duodenal mucosa during NSAID use; a combination preparation of misoprostol and diclofenac (Arthrotec) has recently become available in the United States and is already one of the most widely used NSAIDs outside of the United States. An alternative strategy to minimize the adverse effects of the NSAIDs is to identify specific inhibitors of the isoform of cyclooxygenase that is induced in inflammation (COX-2) while not affecting the cyclooxygenase responsible for the protective prostaglandins (COX-1). Several COX-2 inhibitors are currently in advanced phase clinical trials in the United States and may be available by the time of publication. They appear in clinical trials to offer comparable analgesic effects to the classic NSAIDs and are expected to have markedly diminished renal and gastrointestinal toxicities. If these findings are borne out, the COX-2 inhibitors may offer a significant treatment advantage in OA.

Topical and Injectable Medications. Capsaicin (Zostrix), the active ingredient in chili peppers, is available both by prescription and over the counter for topical application; regular usage may provide relief to some patients with OA, presumably via local depletion of substance P. Patients who use capsaicin should be cautioned to wash their hands carefully after application, as contact with mucous membranes is highly irritating. Intra-articular injections of glucocorticoids may provide short-term palliation of OA flares in isolated joints. Typically, the frequency of such injections should be limited to no more than every 3 to 4 months per joint. The most commonly injected glucocorticoids are triamcinolone (Kenalog) and methylprednisolone (Depo-Medrol), and they are usually mixed with injectable lidocaine to provide immediate relief. Hyaluronic acid, or hyaluronan, an unsulfated glycosaminoglycan prevalent in cartilage matrix and synovial fluid, represents another class of injectable pharmaceutical that has become available for analgesia in OA. In the form of Synvisc or Hyalgan, it may be injected weekly, for three to five times, respectively, into affected joints and may provide significant relief for several months in some patients.

Adjunctive Measures. Pharmacologic pain relief alone is insufficient therapy for OA; supportive adjunctive therapy is essential to improve functional adaptation and to diminish pain. Measures such as patient education about the disease process and regular reinforcement by telephone contact have been shown to be effective in reducing the symptoms of OA. Weight loss, if sustained, may be beneficial. Ice may be helpful in reducing the local inflammatory component associated with OA; hence, patients with a flare of their OA pain should apply ice to the affected joint before and immediately following increased activity of that joint as well as a few times each day. Conversely, there is no demonstrated harm from therapeutic heat for patients who have felt that they derive more symptomatic relief from heat than from ice. Muscle conditioning and rehabilitation in supervised nontraumatic regimens is effective in improving functional parameters and pain in OA. The periarticular musculature normally absorbs a large percentage of transmitted forces during joint loading; strengthening of these muscles may therefore substantially reduce the loading forces across degenerative joints. This may be particularly helpful in mild to moderate OA, in which patients are asymptomatic at rest but have pain with weight bearing. Assistive devices such as canes and walkers are especially useful in lower extremity OA. Biomechanical studies have demonstrated that simple measures such as walking with a cane provide significant unloading of the weight-bearing joints and thereby result in symptomatic relief. The cane should be held in the hand contralateral to the painful lower extremity. Among patients with unsteady stance or unstable gait, walkers are more effective at unloading the joints and may provide additional stability. Short-term use of splints may be quite effective in certain circumstances. For example, splinting of the thumb for a few weeks in refractory OA of the first carpal-metacarpal joints typically results in resolution of symptoms. However, there is no evidence that prolonged splinting is beneficial; in fact, it may be detrimental if it results in deconditioning of the periarticular musculature.

Interventional Options. As a result of dramatic improvements in prosthetic biomaterials and in surgical techniques, joint replacement surgery (arthroplasty) has become an excellent alternative for many OA patients who have refractory pain or disability. Patients who are not ready for surgical intervention may be offered temporizing measures, such as tidal joint lavage or arthroscopic lavage; each of these procedures improves pain in some OA patients, but the appropriate subpopulations likely to respond to these techniques have not yet been clarified. Finally, if patients with advanced OA are not surgical candidates, attention must be directed at maintaining the patient's mobility and independence; this may often be accomplished by the use of motorized scooters or wheelchairs.

Disease-modifying Anti-OA Agents. Although there are no pharmacologic agents that have been demonstrated to interrupt or reverse the natural history of OA, many potential candidates are under investigation and may be available in the next several years. One approach that may be effective would be to arrest articular cartilage degeneration by inhibiting the proteolytic degradation of the cartilage extracellular matrix. A number of proprietary compounds that specifically inhibit matrix metalloprotease activity are currently in either preclinical or clinical trials and may turn out to be effective "chondroprotective" agents. The tetracyclines have been shown to inhibit proteolytic degradation in cartilage and are currently being evaluated for efficacy in OA but should not yet be considered for routine use.

There is a great deal of interest among patients in several carbohydrates that are marketed in the media as disease-modifying agents for OA. Glucosamine and chondroitin sulfate are both precursor carbohydrates of cartilage proteoglycans. Neither has been demonstrated to alter the natural history of OA, and the issue of whether they offer analgesic benefit remains controversial. The preparations available over the counter, however, are not currently regulated by the Food and Drug Administration; hence, their purity and composition are not ensured. Bovine tracheal-derived glycosaminoglycan preparations that have been chemically oversulfated to form so-called GAG-polysulfates (GAG-PS) represent another category of complex carbohydrates that have been used both intramuscularly and intra-articularly in veterinary practice as well as clinically outside of the United States and appear to have protease inhibitory activity; true therapeutic effects have not been consistent, however.

In conclusion, OA is a common and painful disease for which therapeutic approaches are geared toward alleviating pain and optimizing functional adaptation. This requires a multidisciplinary approach involving medication, patient education, and adjunctive therapeutic modalities. Although it is not yet possible to interfere with the natural history of the disease, several experimental approaches may permit actual disease modification in the near future.

POLYMYALGIA RHEUMATICA AND GIANT CELL ARTERITIS

method of
EDWIN A. SMITH, M.D.
Medical University of South Carolina
Charleston, South Carolina

POLYMYALGIA RHEUMATICA

Polymyalgia rheumatica (PMR) is a syndrome experienced almost exclusively by individuals older than 50 years of age. The primary symptom is pain in the neck, shoulders, low back, and hips along with prominent morning stiffness. The erythrocyte sedimentation rate (ESR) is almost always elevated and may be greatly so. Accompanying findings may include low-grade fever, mild synovitis, weight loss, anemia, and mild elevations of hepatic transaminases. Although the patients may interpret the pain as weakness, muscle strength testing and the serum creatine phosphokinase level are normal. Included in the differential diagnosis are cervical and lumbar spondylosis, fibromyalgia, myositis, and rheumatoid arthritis. A diagnostic challenge is presented by the patient with an elevated ESR and limited physical findings, and chronic infection and neoplasia (particularly plasma cell dyscrasia) must be considered. In addition, symptoms of giant cell arteritis (GCA) (see later discussion) must be sought because treatment is different for that associated syndrome.

Treatment of PMR is often very gratifying for both patient and physician because the symptoms usually improve within 1 week and often overnight. Lack of this prompt response requires a re-evaluation of the diagnosis. Treatment is initiated with 15 mg of prednisone (Deltasone) every morning for 1 month. The ESR usually becomes normal within several weeks and can be used as a guide to therapy. Prednisone is tapered to 12.5 mg per day for another month, then to 10 mg per day after another month. Tapering should then proceed more gradually, at a rate of 1 mg per day per month. If at any time or any prednisone level symptoms recur and the ESR becomes elevated, the prednisone dose is returned for a time to the previous higher dose. If symptoms remain quiescent but the ESR rises somewhat, the prednisone dose is maintained at the current dose and the ESR is checked again in 1 month. If there is no recurrence of symptoms and the ESR elevation is only moderate and also stable, tapering of prednisone dose may be continued. Patients with PMR may be able to discontinue steroids by following this tapering method, but many are taking some small dose of prednisone as long as 5 years after the diagnosis.

Patients with PMR should be informed of the symptoms of GCA (see later discussion) and should contact the physician immediately if any occur, because higher doses of prednisone must be initiated.

In all patients, and particularly in postmenopausal women with PMR, coexistent osteoporosis must be sought and treated appropriately, as prednisone at any dose is likely to accelerate bone loss.

GIANT CELL ARTERITIS

Temporal arteritis is one of two types of GCA (the other being Takayasu's arteritis) but is commonly called GCA. The pathologic basis of GCA is an arteritis of the large and medium-sized arteries, most commonly the arteries of the head, but in some cases the pulmonary, coronary, subclavian, axillary, hepatic, renal, mesenteric, or aortic vaso vasorum arteries are involved. GCA occurs in 15 to 25% of persons with

PMR but may occur without musculoskeletal symptoms.

The symptoms of GCA directly attributable to inflammation of cephalic arteries include either unilateral or bilateral frontotemporal region headache, jaw or tongue claudication on chewing, amaurosis fugax, sudden and complete unilateral blindness, cranial neuropathies, and transient ischemic attacks. Involvement of other vessels may produce Raynaud's phenomenon, angina pectoris or myocardial infarction, extremity claudication, dissection of the aorta, or pulmonary hemorrhage. Constitutional symptoms may include fever, sweats, weight loss, and depression.

There are few physical findings in GCA, although there may be tenderness or nodularity along the temporal artery. As with PMR, the ESR is nearly always elevated.

Because blindness, a result of involvement of the ophthalmic artery, may be permanent and occur without suggestive visual symptoms, the diagnosis and treatment of GCA must be pursued vigorously. Treatment of GCA is initiated as soon as the diagnosis is suspected with a prednisone dose of 1 mg per kg of body weight per day in three divided doses (usually 20 mg three times a day [tid]). Within 1 week of starting steroids, one should biopsy both temporal arteries to confirm the diagnosis. Because the classic histologic picture (internal elastic lamina disruption by a mononuclear cell infiltrate, which contains multinucleated giant cells) occurs in discrete areas along the arteries, long portions of both temporal arteries should be harvested and examined by extensive serial sectioning. In a clinical setting compatible with the diagnosis of GCA, evidence of previous internal elastic lamina disruption without current inflammation should be accepted as evidence of current disease and treated as such. Indeed, when the clinical findings cannot be explained by some other process, treatment is warranted even in the presence of histologically normal temporal arteries.

After a few weeks of therapy, the symptoms of GCA have usually abated and the ESR has returned to normal. The total daily prednisone dose is consolidated to a single morning dose and continued for 1 month. As with PMR above, tapering of the prednisone dose is done while monitoring for both return of clinical symptoms and elevation of the ESR. Elevation of the ESR without a worsening of symptoms should cause the physician to stop tapering the dose but by itself should not prompt a return to the higher dose. A return of symptoms accompanying such an elevation should, however, cause a return to the initial high and divided dose to avoid the possible tragic and preventable consequence of irreversible blindness.

Tapering of the prednisone dose in the face of no symptoms and normal ESR should proceed at 10 mg per day per month to a level of 30 mg, then 5 mg per day per month to 15 mg, then 2.5 mg per day per month to 10 mg, then 1 mg per day per month. As with the treatment of PMR, several years may be required to discontinue glucocorticoids.

Concern for adverse effects of high-dose glucocorticoids (hypertension, diabetes mellitus, osteoporosis, and ischemic osteonecrosis) must be maintained throughout therapy. When glucocorticoid dose tapering proves difficult, either azathioprine (Imuran)* (up to 3 mg per kg per day) or methotrexate (Rheumatrex)* (up to 20 mg per week) may be used as a steroid-sparing agent. Neither of these drugs can be used as primary therapy, however, because their onset of action is delayed compared with that of the glucocorticoids.

*Not FDA approved for this indication.

OSTEOMYELITIS

method of
TONI DARVILLE, M.D., and
RICHARD F. JACOBS, M.D.
Arkansas Children's Hospital
Little Rock, Arkansas

GENERAL CONCEPT OF OSTEOMYELITIS

The difficult reputation of osteomyelitis arises from the tendency toward chronic, recurrent infection. In patients with compromised immune status or other co-morbidities such as vascular insufficiency and/or diabetes mellitus, clinical infection can indeed become extremely chronic or episodes of inflammation can occur unpredictably at variable intervals. Chronic osteomyelitis infections are the most difficult to treat, often requiring multiple surgical débridements and prolonged antimicrobial therapy. The acute versus chronic character of osteomyelitis in a patient is likely one of the most important issues that affects treatment course and outcome. Acute disease manifests as suppurative infection accompanied by edema, vascular congestion, and small vessel thrombosis. In early acute disease, the vascular supply to the bone is compromised by infection extending into the surrounding soft tissue. When both the medullary and periosteal blood supplies are compromised, areas of dead bone (sequestra) may be formed. The sequestrum acts as a foreign body, providing a nidus for continued bacterial colonization. This necrotic bone is poorly vascularized, leading to poor penetration of antibiotics and host inflammatory cells. Bacteria adhering to the necrotic bone produce a biofilm that protects them from host defense mechanisms and antibiotics. Clinically, acute osteomyelitis evolves into chronic disease. The infection can extend beyond the bone to include adjacent soft tissue abscesses and sinus tracts.

Bacteria are introduced into the bone from the hematogenous route, by extension from a contiguous focus of soft tissue infection, or by direct inoculation from the environment in trauma-related injury. The source of the infection, its extent and duration, and the age and status of the host are all important to consider when treating a patient with osteomyelitis.

HEMATOGENOUS OSTEOMYELITIS

Hematogenous Osteomyelitis in Children. Hematogenous osteomyelitis characteristically is a disease of children. Although the infection can occur in any bone, it usually affects the metaphyses of the most rapidly growing bones, especially the long bones of the lower extremity. During growth, there is steady formation of new metaphyseal capillaries, which are fenestrated, allowing escape of red blood cells and other blood elements into the extravascular space. The normal ability of endothelial cells to phagocytose particles is deficient in the metaphyseal capillary loops. Thus, during transient bacteremia, bacteria may escape into this region of relative phagocytic deficiency and establish infection. In addition, the physometaphyseal junction is a zone of great metabolic activity that offers opportunities for specific bacterium-substrate adhesion.

Staphylococcus aureus is the organism responsible for more than 90% of cases of acute hematogenous osteomyelitis in otherwise normal children. Other causative organisms are *Streptococcus* species, Enterobacteriaceae, *Salmonella* (in patients with sickle cell disease), and *Haemophilus influenzae*. Before the introduction of antibiotics, hematogenous osteomyelitis was an urgent and serious disease, with a mortality approaching 20% and a morbidity of approximately 60%. With the availability of prompt diagnosis and treatment, however, mortality in the industrialized world is negligible, and the complication rate is approximately 5%.

The usual child with acute hematogenous osteomyelitis presents with a history of bone pain of 1 to several days' duration. The hallmark of pain caused by infection is its constant nature. The level of pain may fluctuate, but it never disappears. The onset is gradual (over a few hours or days). The pain usually is severe enough to seriously limit the use of the involved extremity. On physical examination, point tenderness and well-localized pain suggest the diagnosis. The classic signs of inflammation (redness, warmth, and swelling) do not appear unless the infection is allowed to progress and extend through the metaphyseal cortex into the subperiosteal space. The bacteremic phase of hematogenous osteomyelitis may be recognized by malaise and low-grade fever, may be entirely subclinical, or may be characterized by severe constitutional symptoms and a temperature as high as 40°C.

Hematogenous Osteomyelitis in Newborns. In newborns with hematogenous osteomyelitis, pseudoparalysis of a limb often is the first sign to call attention to the affected extremity. Systemic signs may be minimal, or there may be signs of sepsis and subtle local findings. Multiple sites of infection are not uncommon. The relatively thin cortex and loosely applied periosteum are poor barriers to the spread of infection. Consequently, the purulence may rupture into the surrounding muscular tissue, producing a deep soft tissue abscess. The limb may be red, swollen, and discolored at presentation. Because the epiphyseal-metaphyseal junction frequently is within the joint capsule, contiguous septic arthritis is frequent, especially with the long tubular bones. Group B streptococci and *S. aureus* are the most common etiologic agents; gram-negative bacilli cause a minority of cases.

Vertebral Osteomyelitis. Vertebral osteomyelitis is also hematogenous in origin but has a more indolent clinical course. Although vertebral osteomyelitis is occasionally seen in children, it is much more common in the elderly. *S. aureus* is the most commonly isolated organism in both of these patient populations. Users of illicit intravenous drugs are also predisposed to infection, with *Pseudomonas aeruginosa* being the most common isolate from these patients. The segmental arteries supplying the vertebrae usually bifurcate to supply two adjacent bony segments. Therefore, infection usually involves two adjacent vertebrae and the intervertebral disk. Localized pain and tenderness is present in 90% of the cases. Young children may refuse to walk or to sit upright. The pain is usually insidious and progresses over weeks to months. Posterior extension of the infection may lead to epidural and subdural abscesses resulting in motor and sensory neurologic defects in 6 to 15% of cases.

CONTIGUOUS FOCUS OSTEOMYELITIS

Contiguous Focus Osteomyelitis Without Vascular Insufficiency. These bone infections arise from inoculation of organisms into the bone at the time of trauma, during operative procedures, or from extension of an adjacent soft tissue infection. Common predisposing factors include surgical reduction and internal fixation of fractures, prostheses, open fractures, and chronic soft tissue infections such as infected pressure sores. In contrast to hematogenous osteomyelitis, these infections are often polymicrobial. *S. aureus* remains the most commonly isolated organism, but gram-negative bacilli and anaerobes are also frequently found. The patient usually presents within 1 month of the inoculation incident with low-grade fever, pain, and drainage. Loss of bone stability, bone necrosis, and soft tissue damage are frequent, making this infection difficult to treat. Open fracture is probably the most common predisposing factor leading to chronic osteomyelitis. The risk of bone infection is related to the degree of soft tissue infection that accompanies the fracture. In fractures with soft tissue damage so severe that closure of the wound over the fracture is not possible, the incidence of infection may exceed 30%.

Nosocomial neonatal osteomyelitis may occur secondary to infection of heel puncture sites, arterial cannulae, cut-down sites, and cephalohematomas. Blood and bone cultures are necessary to establish the organism and antibiotic susceptibilities. *S. aureus* is the most common organism isolated, but *Staphylococcus epidermidis* and nosocomially acquired gram-negative bacilli may be present. These infections may also be polymicrobial.

Contiguous Focus Osteomyelitis with Vascular Insufficiency. The majority of these patients have diabetes mellitus, with the small bones of the feet being most commonly affected. Multiple organisms are usually isolated, including coagulase-positive and coagulase-negative staphylococci, *Streptococcus* species, *Enterococcus* species, gram-negative bacilli, and anaerobes. Fever and systemic toxicity are infrequent. Recurrent infection is common even with adequate treatment.

DIAGNOSIS

The diagnosis of osteomyelitis relies primarily on clinical suspicion. A patient who presents with localized bone pain and fever can be presumed to have osteomyelitis until proved otherwise. Laboratory tests that can be helpful include erythrocyte sedimentation rate (ESR), blood culture, and bone or joint culture. Radiographic studies that aid in diagnosis include plain radiographs, bone scintigraphy, and, in some cases, ultrasonography, computed tomography (CT), and magnetic resonance imaging (MRI).

The complete blood count may be normal in more than 50% of patients with osteomyelitis, but the ESR is elevated in the majority of cases, making it a useful sensitive test. Serum C-reactive protein (CRP) is also sensitive and tends to normalize more rapidly than the ESR in uncomplicated cases, making it perhaps more useful than the ESR for following the patient's response to therapy.

Specific identification of the pathogen or pathogens involved is an important goal in the assessment of osteomyelitis. Blood cultures will be positive in 50% of patients with acute hematogenous long bone osteomyelitis, and these can direct antibiotic therapy. Cultures from the bone or from a contiguously infected joint are likewise helpful but are positive in only 40% of cases of acute hematogenous osteomyelitis. Because 90% of cases of acute hematogenous osteomyelitis in children are due to *S. aureus*, empirical therapy can be undertaken despite negative blood cultures without pursuit of a bone culture.

Blood cultures are almost always negative in chronic osteomyelitis, and a culture from the infected bone is necessary. Sinus tract cultures are not reliable for predicting the pathogens responsible for an underlying bone infection. In most cases, antibiotic treatment should be based on meticulous cultures taken at débridement surgery or from deep bone biopsies and on antibiotic susceptibilities. Both aerobic and anaerobic cultures should be performed, and in selected cases, cultures for *Mycobacterium* species, fungi, or other unusual pathogens may be indicated.

Plain radiographs are useful in diagnosing osteomyelitis in patients with prolonged symptoms. Abnormal findings include lytic lesions, periosteal elevation, osteoporosis, and deep soft tissue swelling. Deep soft tissue swelling can be seen at 1 week, but bone changes are not evident until at least 7 to 14 days after symptoms develop.

For patients with earlier presentation and normal plain radiographs, a technetium bone scan can be very helpful. In cases of osteomyelitis, there will be increased bone uptake over the course of the study, resulting in "hot spots" over the area of acute infection. A newer modality that can be used to aid diagnosis of acute osteomyelitis is ultrasonography. There are three typical abnormal findings: (1) thickening of the periosteum, giving the appearance of a sandwich; (2) elevation of the periosteum by more than 2 mm, indicative of subperiosteal pus; and (3) swelling of overlying muscle or subcutaneous tissue, particularly that nearest to the bone, with altered echogenicity of the tissue. Sonographic changes produced by osteomyelitis in contiguous soft tissues can be detected as early as the first 24 hours after the onset of symptoms. Technetium bone scanning has been shown to have variable accuracy in neonates, making early diagnosis particularly difficult in this age group. In an institution with quality ultrasonography available, reasonable indications would be in neonates and in patients who may present late in the evening when bone scanning is unavailable to localize an abscess amenable to drainage.

Determining the extent of disease may sometimes be difficult. There may be more than one site of bone involvement, especially in vertebral osteomyelitis. The CT scan provides excellent visualization of cortical abnormalities and can depict intraosseous gas, which is an infrequent but reliable sign of osteomyelitis. In recalcitrant infection, the CT scan may assist in identifying the surgical approach and augment débridement. MRI is now recognized as a useful modality for diagnosing and determining the scope of musculoskeletal infections. The spatial resolution of MRI makes it useful in differentiating between bone and soft tissue infection. The typical appearance of osteomyelitis is a localized area of abnormal marrow with decreased signal intensity on T1-weighted images and increased signal intensity on T2-weighted images. Because differentiation of neoplasm, fracture, or bone infarct from osteomyelitis may be difficult using MRI, clinical and radiologic confirmation are necessary. Imaging studies with gallium or indium-labeled white blood cells may be considered in selected cases but have not proved to be of value in the routine evaluation of osteomyelitis.

TREATMENT

The components of osteomyelitis treatment include evaluation of host factors, assessment of source and extent of disease, identification and sensitivity of microorganisms, administration of antibiotics, débridement surgery, dead space management, and, if necessary, stabilization of the bone.

Acute Hematogenous Osteomyelitis. Children with acute hematogenous long bone osteomyelitis with no evidence of abscess or septic arthritis clinically and on radiographic studies can be treated medically. Blood cultures should always be obtained. Otherwise healthy children with acute hematogenous long bone osteomyelitis secondary to *S. aureus* or those who are culture negative with up-to-date *H. influenzae* type b immunization status (fully immunized) can be divided into two groups. Patients with less than 72 hours of symptoms before initiation of antibiotics who have a good clinical response within 48 hours of starting parenteral therapy are treated with 1 week of parenteral antistaphylococcal antibiotics and then given 3 weeks of an appropriate oral antibiotic. If patients have more than 72 hours of symptoms before initiation of antibiotics or a poor response to parenteral therapy, 2 to 3 weeks of parenteral antibiotics are given followed by 1 to 3 weeks of oral therapy. Clinical follow-up together with measurement of ESR or CRP can be used to aid in the determination of length of therapy. The minimal total duration of therapy should be 4 weeks (Figure 1). Patients can be discharged home on either home intravenous therapy or oral therapy only after compliance is ensured by the family. The highest recommended dosages of intravenous and oral antibiotics should be given (see Figure 1). Weekly follow-up by an infectious disease specialist and close orthopedic follow-up are mandatory as long as the patient remains on therapy and after that less frequently to monitor for long-term complications.

Neonates may have inadequate absorption of oral antibiotics and therefore require parenteral therapy for 4 to 6 weeks. Patients with sickle cell anemia may have areas of poorly perfused bone and need longer parenteral therapy to ensure higher levels of antibiotic in the bone. Patients with compromised immunity also may need prolonged parenteral therapy. Surgical intervention is indicated if the patient has not responded to specific antimicrobial therapy within 48 hours or has evidence of soft tissue, periosteal, or bone abscess at diagnosis.

Vertebral Osteomyelitis. In adult patients, although *S. aureus* remains the most commonly isolated organism, biopsy and débridement cultures should dictate the choice of antibiotics, as the infection can be seeded from multiple sources including the genitourinary tract, skin and soft tissue infections, respiratory tract, endocarditis, dental infection, and unknown sources. In otherwise healthy

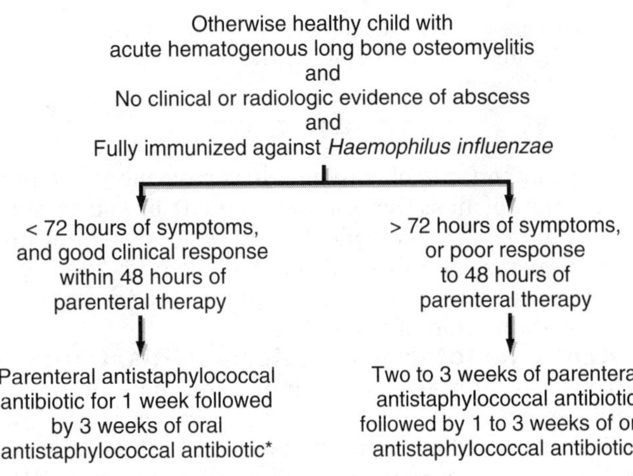

*Appropriate agents and dosages:

Antibiotic	*Route*	*Dosage*†	*Frequency*
Nafcillin (Nafcil)	IV	200 mg/kg/d	q 6 h
Cefazolin (Ancef)	IV	100 mg/kg/d	q 8 h
Clindamycin (Cleocin)	IV/PO	40 mg/kg/d	q 8 h
Vancomycin (Vancocin)	IV	40 mg/kg/d	q 6 h (based on levels)
Cephalexin (Keflex)	PO	100 mg/kg/d	q 6 h
Cefadroxil (Duricef)	PO	100 mg/kg/d	q 12 h

†One must consider child's weight and maximum total dose of drug given per day to select optimal therapy.

Figure 1. Treatment of acute hematogenous long bone osteomyelitis in otherwise normal healthy children.

children with vertebral osteomyelitis, empirical coverage for *S. aureus* is acceptable. Blood cultures should be obtained, although they are frequently negative. A CT or MRI scan should be obtained in all patients with vertebral osteomyelitis to establish the extent of vertebral disease and to assess for epidural or paravertebral abscess. The neurologic status of the patient should be monitored closely. Surgical fusion of the involved vertebrae is usually not required, as spontaneous bony fusion occurs in 1 to 12 months following appropriate antibiotic therapy. Antibiotics are given for 4 to 6 weeks, and the ESR can be used to follow response to therapy.

Osteomyelitis Secondary to Contiguous Focus Infection or Chronic Osteomyelitis. In contiguous focus and chronic osteomyelitis, the first and most important objective is to obtain adequate surgical débridement. Any nidus of infected necrotic bone remains a source of continued contamination. However, thorough débridement is not always easily accomplished, for débridement of all the affected bone and tissue may threaten the stability and function of the limb, as well as leave poorly vascularized dead space at risk for further infection. If possible, antibiotics should not be initiated until the results of bone bacterial cultures and sensitivities are known. However, if clinically necessary, empirical broad-spectrum antibiotics can be started and then tailored when the results of débridement cultures are available.

The majority of patients should be treated with 4 to 6 weeks of parenteral antimicrobial therapy dated from the last major débridement surgery. This can be administered on an outpatient basis when the patient has clinically responded. It is likely that the duration of antibiotic therapy required is inversely proportional to the adequacy of débridement. In selected patients with milder disease, sequential parenteral-oral therapy has been used successfully. It is recommended that a minimum of 2 weeks of parenteral therapy be administered to any patient with contiguous focus osteomyelitis before switching to an oral agent. Agents with excellent bioavailability that can be considered for oral therapy once the organism has been proved susceptible include amoxicillin, oral first-generation cephalosporins, clindamycin, metronidazole, quinolones in adults, and trimethoprim-sulfamethoxazole. The maximum recommended dose of the antibiotic should be administered (see Figure 1). The patient's clinical status and ESR or CRP level should be followed weekly while on therapy to assess for continued steady improvement.

Appropriate management of any dead space created by débridement surgery or the initial trauma itself is essential to arrest disease. Dead bone and scar tissue should be replaced with durable vascularized tissue as much as possible. Secondary intention healing is discouraged; complete wound closure should be attained whenever possible. Local tissue flaps or free flaps may be used to fill dead space. Antibiotic-impregnated beads may be used to sterilize and temporarily maintain dead space. The beads are usually removed in 2 to 4 weeks and replaced with a cancellous bone graft.

Any fractures present must be stabilized. Stability may be achieved with plates, screws, rods, and/or an external fixator. The Ilizarov external fixation method uses distraction or compression histogenesis, a process of bone regeneration to fill bone defects. This method is reserved for cases in which extensive involvement of bone requires segmental resection. The presence of a fixation device impedes the clearance of infection, but the infection will not heal in the face of an unstable fracture. Thus, in some situations, suppressive antibiotics are given to keep the infection under control, and then once the fixator device is removed, definitive antibiotic therapy is administered. This can require the administration of several months of antibiotics, which may be given in sequential parenteral-oral fashion as long as patient compliance is ensured.

Contiguous Focus Osteomyelitis with Vascular Insufficiency. These infections are often insidious and may manifest beyond the time for salvage of the bone. The patient may be managed with local débridement surgery and antibiotic therapy if good tissue oxygen perfusion can be established. If not, some type of ablative surgery may be required.

COMMON SPORTS INJURIES

method of
RUSSELL D. WHITE, M.D.
Bayfront Medical Center
St. Petersburg, Florida

Sports injuries result from either of two mechanisms—macrotrauma or microtrauma. *Macrotrauma* is an acute injury with immediate impairment of function, for instance, collision, fall, and twisting. Examples include acute anterior cruciate ligament rupture, distal radius fracture, and ankle sprains. *Microtrauma* is due to repetitive overload (overuse) and subsequent inflammation, for example, plantar fasciitis, supraspinatus tendinitis, or stress fractures.

The components of evaluating and treating an injury include (1) history of injury or provocative factors, (2) examination, (3) special studies, and (4) management. The detailed history of an acute injury often determines the diagnosis. The examination includes location of pain and radiation, warmth, erythema, effusion, range of motion, weakness (strength testing), and provocative tests. Special studies include plain radiographs, computed tomography (CT) scans, bone scans, and magnetic resonance imaging (MRI) scans. The management of injuries depends on the severity of the injury and the desires of the athlete. Basic treatment of an acute injury includes PRICES—*p*rotection, *r*est, *i*ce, *c*ompression, *e*levation, and *s*upport. Most injuries are treated by the primary care physician, but some require interventional surgery by the orthopedist.

UPPER EXTREMITY

Shoulder Injuries

The shoulder joint is a complex structure consisting of the rounded humeral head rotating on the saucer-shaped glenoid fossa. The four rotator cuff muscles and tendons (supraspinatus, infraspinatus, teres minor, subscapularis) serve as dynamic stabilizers for the shoulder because this joint must function in different positions. The three functions performed by these four muscles are elevation (supraspinatus), internal rotation (subscapularis), and external rotation (infraspinatus, teres minor). Pain with strength testing suggests tendinitis, whereas weakness suggests tearing of the muscle components. Historical facts are important in delineating shoulder injuries. One must determine whether symptoms are due to an acute traumatic injury or chronic activity. The timing of pain (nocturnal occurrence in bursitis) may point to a diagnosis. Specific movements, such as overhead activity of throwing a baseball, may suggest subluxation, tendinitis, or impingement.

Impingement syndrome is a common cause of discomfort and suggests injury or inflammation producing restriction in the subacromial space. This may be associated with subacromial bursitis, rotator cuff tendinitis, or degenerative osseous changes. Impingement signs are noted in Table 1. A positive impingement test result is the resolution of pain following a subacromial bursa injection of lidocaine. The normal range of shoulder motion is listed in Table 2. The painful arc of impingement refers to pain noted at 60 to 120 degrees of abduction. (Table 3 lists strength testing of shoulder muscles.) Shoulder instability refers to subluxation, often with apprehension, on movement. Table 4 contains common maneuvers for evaluating shoulder instability.

TABLE 1. **Shoulder Impingement Signs (Maneuvers)***

Hawkin's sign	Arm is forward flexed 90 degrees; elbow is flexed 90 degrees; shoulder is slowly internally rotated.
Neer's sign	Arm is completely pronated; shoulder is moved into complete forward flexion (overhead position)

*Pain produced by maneuvers indicates impingement.

Other shoulder injuries include *acromioclavicular sprains* (shoulder separation), which are due to direct trauma to the shoulder or falling on an outstretched hand. Typical symptoms are localized pain to palpation and discomfort with shoulder movement. *Adhesive capsulitis* is common in diabetics and older athletes. Chronic shoulder pain with marked decrease in range of motion is common. *Referred shoulder pain* from ischemic heart disease or intra-abdominal pathology must always be considered.

Elbow Injuries

Medial epicondylitis ("golfer's elbow") is due to microtrauma to the wrist flexors at their insertion at the medial epicondyle. Symptoms include tenderness to palpation at the medial epicondyle, pain on resistance to wrist flexion or pronation, and relative weakness. Treatment focuses on rest or avoidance of inciting activity, use of nonsteroidal anti-inflammatory drugs (NSAIDs), steroid injection (avoid neurovascular structures), or iontophoresis.

A *sprain of the ulnar collateral ligament* occurs in throwing and racquet sports. The chronic valgus strain produces medial elbow pain. This problem usually responds to rest and NSAID use. Surgical reconstruction is indicated in those with persistent pain or valgus insufficiency.

Little leaguer's elbow involves repetitive stress on the growth plate before its closure. This valgus stress

TABLE 2. **Normal Range of Motion of Shoulder***

Forward flexion	180 degrees
Extension	60 degrees
Abduction	180 degrees
Adduction	60 degrees
External rotation	90 degrees
Internal rotation	90 degrees

*All motions in the plane of the body.

TABLE 3. **Tests of Rotator Cuff Muscles***

Muscle	Test Method
Supraspinatus	Arm extended completely Arm at 30-degree forward flexion and 70-degree abduction Thumb pointing to floor ("empty soda can position") *Arm is elevated against resistance*
Infraspinatus and teres minor	Arm held at side of torso Elbow flexed to 90 degrees Forearm in neutral position with thumbs pointed upward *Arm is externally rotated against resistance*
Subscapularis	Arm held at side of torso Elbow flexed to 90 degrees Forearm in neutral position with thumbs pointed upward *Arm is internally rotated against resistance*

*Pain or weakness denotes injury.

produces stretching of the medial compartment and compression of the lateral compartment. Evaluation includes examination and radiographs. If only stress reaction is found, then rest for 3 weeks followed by no throwing for 6 to 8 weeks will suffice. Ice massage twice daily, NSAIDs, and elbow support are often beneficial. If a fracture is confirmed (<5-mm displacement), treat with cast immobilization for 3 to 4 weeks, followed by gradual return to activity. No hard throwing or pitching is allowed for 12 weeks. If valgus instability is confirmed or a 5-mm or greater fracture displacement is found, open repair is indicated.

Lateral epicondylitis (tennis elbow) is due to chronic repetitive stress to the forearm and wrist extensors at their attachment to the lateral epicondyle. Typically, this is diagnosed in racquet players whose racquet handle is too small or whose racquet strings are set with excessive tension. The problem is accentuated when the ball strikes the racquet off-center in the backhand position, increasing the torque and transmitted force. Examination reveals lateral epicondyle tenderness, which is increased with resisted dorsiflexion of the wrist. Pain over the lateral epicondyle is found on applying resistance against an extended long finger, with grasping a heavy textbook in the supine position and rotating to the pronated position, or with lifting a cup of coffee (Conrad's sign). Radiographs may show calcific deposits in chronic cases. Treatment includes rest, correction of faulty equipment (racquet), NSAIDs, cock-up wrist splint, steroid injection, and a counterforce elbow brace. Recalcitrant cases require surgery. *Posterior interosseous nerve (PIN) compression syndrome* (radial tunnel syndrome) is a "look-alike" that may mimic or coexist with lateral epicondylitis. PIN compression syndrome is a neuropathy due to entrapment of the posterior interosseous branch of the radial nerve. Symptoms include aching elbow pain radiating into the forearm more distal than that seen with lateral epicondylitis. This motor loss produces extensor weakness of the wrist and fingers. Treatment consists of rest, activity modification, NSAIDs, cross-friction massage, phonophoresis, and sometimes surgery.

TABLE 4. **Tests of Glenohumeral (Shoulder) Instability/Apprehension**

Anterior	Place the patient in supine position (may be done sitting or standing). Abduct and externally rotate the shoulder. Place patient's shoulder in 90-degree abduction with elbow at 90-degree flexion. Grasp the glenohumeral joint and palpate the humeral head anteriorly with thumb and posteriorly with fingers. Slowly lever the humeral head anteriorly—noting any anterior laxity, subluxation, or apprehension. *Abnormal movement or apprehension suggests dislocation or subluxation.* *Pain suggests rotator cuff injury or tear of glenoid labrum.*
Posterior	Place the patient in supine position (or sitting). Place elbow in 90-degree flexion. Place shoulder in 90-degree forward flexion; then rotate shoulder into 90-degree internal rotation. (The hand/wrist should now be directly over the face.) Axially load the humerus and attempt to sublux the humeral head posteriorly. *Abnormal movement, pain, or apprehension suggests subluxation or dislocation.*
Inferior	Place the patient in supine position (or sitting). Place the shoulder in 0 degrees of adduction and elbow at 0-degree flexion. Apply caudal traction to the arm. *Feel for inferior subluxation or observe for a "sulcus sign" (sulcus or space between acromion and humerus).*

Wrist and Hand Injuries

Carpal tunnel syndrome is produced by entrapment of the median nerve as it passes through the wrist joint. It is common in athletes who use their hands in repetitive motion. Symptoms typically include nocturnal wrist, hand, and finger pain and numbness. Occasionally, retrograde pain produces shoulder symptoms. Sensory loss is found in the radial 3½ fingers. History of nocturnal paresthesias relieved by shaking the hand over the side of the bed or walking the floor is typical. Examination may reveal a tingling sensation secondary to a positive Tinel's sign (percussion of the median nerve at the carpal tunnel) or Phalen's sign (volar flexion of the wrist for 60 seconds). Atrophy of the abductor pollicis brevis may occur. Diagnosis is made clinically along with electrodiagnostic tests. Treatment includes wrist splinting, NSAIDs, steroid injection, and surgical decompression.

De Quervain's syndrome is stenosing tenosynovitis of the abductor pollicis longus and extensor pollicis brevis in the first dorsal compartment. This exquisite tenderness (proximal to radial styloid) is due to repetitive movement of the thumb. Examination reveals swelling and inflammation and a positive Finkelstein's test result (pain on having the patient tuck the thumb beneath the folded fingers and placing the fist into ulnar deviation). Treatment includes phonophoresis or steroid injection followed by immobilization in a thumb spica splint.

A *scaphoid fracture* must be considered with wrist trauma producing pain in the "anatomic snuffbox." One should immobilize the wrist and repeat radiographs in 10 to 14 days to avoid missing an occult fracture on initial evaluation.

LOWER EXTREMITY

Foot Injuries

Plantar fasciitis may result from either microtrauma or macrotrauma. Three ligamentous bands (the medial, central, and lateral) originate on the anterior portion of the calcaneus. Microtrauma (overuse) injuries are common and typically produce heel or foot pain following rest (early morning) and a nagging medial heel and plantar pain. The average duration of symptoms is 1 year. Diagnosis is by careful history and examination. Radiographs may be necessary to rule out stress fractures or foreign bodies. The "heel spur" seen on radiographs is a reaction to chronic stress and is not the cause of the pain. Treatment includes relative rest, stretching, noninflammatory medicines, taping, orthotics, and injection. Therapeutic modalities include ice in the acute phase followed by ultrasound or electrical stimulation when pain improves. Surgery is rarely indicated.

Turf toe results from hyperextension of the first metatarsophalangeal joint. Exquisite pain occurs in those who wear flexible shoes on firm, synthetic surfaces. Treatment includes taping, rest, anti-inflammatory medications, and the use of a shoe with rigid support to prevent hyperextension.

Tarsal tunnel syndrome is due to compression or traction of the posterior tibial nerve as it passes behind the medial malleolus. Medial foot pain is common in runners. Examination reveals reproduction of symptoms with pressure over the nerve and a positive Tinel's sign. Treatment consists of relative rest, NSAIDs, orthotic correction of hyperpronation, and pad taping over the flexor retinaculum.

Common foot fractures occur in the digits (secondary to direct trauma) or in the metatarsals (secondary to either direct trauma or overuse). Diagnosis is made by typical history and examination and is confirmed by radiographs. Digital fractures are treated by buddy-taping and protection. Metatarsal stress fractures may go undiagnosed, and confirmation may require bone scans. There is often pain on plantar palpation of the foot. Treatment with a firmly laced boot or a short leg walking cast will allow healing without pain. A *Jones fracture* occurs at the base of the fifth metatarsal. This transverse fracture is prone to poor healing and may require surgical repair. It must be distinguished from the common (peroneal) *avulsion fracture* of the fifth metatarsal.

Ankle Injuries

Ankle injuries, mainly sprains, account for 10 to 30% of musculoskeletal injuries. Inversion (lateral) injuries account for 85% of ankle sprains. The remainder are medial (5%) and combined (10%). Lateral injuries involve the anterior talofibular, calcaneofibular, or posterior talofibular ligaments. Less common medial sprains (eversion) involve the wide, thick deltoid ligament. History of the injury, examination, and radiographs (when indicated) yield the diagnosis. Instability maneuvers include the talar tilt test and anterior drawer sign. Because the ankle is constructed as a circle, any stress on one area will be transferred to an opposite portion. Tenderness with compression of the proximal fibula may suggest a fracture produced by cephalad transmission of energy from an ankle sprain. The treatment of ankle sprains includes PRICES.

Knee Injuries

Patellofemoral stress syndrome (PFSS) is a common source of pain, particularly in adolescent females. This syndrome encompasses patellar subluxation, chondromalacia patellae, patellofemoral pain syndrome, and patellofemoral tracking syndrome. Symptoms include anterior knee pain, patellar popping (crepitus), exquisite pain on descending stairs, and a positive "theater sign" (pain after sitting with knees flexed). Symptoms are often bilateral, and any history of bilateral knee pain in an adolescent female suggests this problem. Examination may reveal a small effusion, peripatellar tenderness, a positive Clarke compression test, a positive lateral apprehension sign, an increased Q angle, genu valgus deformity, and hyperpronation of the feet. Radiographs may reveal an abnormal patella position, or they may be normal and may differentiate other diagnoses such as osteochondral fracture, bone tumor, or osteochondritis dissecans. Treatment consists of orthotics, quadriceps strengthening, patella bracing or taping, deep friction massage, hamstring stretching, and NSAIDs.

Osgood-Schlatter disease is common in male adolescents. Pain, localized to the anterior tibial tubercle, is due to repetitive microtrauma of the patellar tendon at the attachment to the tibial tuberosity. History includes chronic localized pain that is made worse by direct trauma, running, and descending stairs. Examination of the anterior tibial tuberosity reveals enlargement and exquisite tenderness with direct palpation or resisted knee extension. Radiographs show nonclosure (not avulsion fracture) of the growth center. Treatment consists of restriction of activity, knee pads to prevent direct trauma, NSAIDs, ice packs, quadriceps strengthening, and stretching exercises. The process resolves when the growth center closes, although an occasional case will persist into adulthood.

Anterior cruciate ligament (ACL) injuries usually occur with a varus force, hyperextension of the knee,

TABLE 5. **Knee Examination**

Maneuver/Sign/Test	Description	Significance
Anterior drawer sign	Knee is flexed to 90 degrees; foot is stabilized; anterior translation of tibia on femur.	Anterior tibial translation denotes ACL injury. Not sensitive.
Clarke compression test	Knee is extended; direct pressure applied to distal quadriceps tendon; quadriceps is contracted.	Pain produced by loading of patella onto knee joint denotes PFSS.
Lachman's test	Knee is flexed 20 degrees; distal femur is stabilized with one hand; tibia is translated anteriorly with other hand.	Excessive anterior movement of tibia or lack of firm end point denotes ACL injury. Most sensitive test.
Lateral apprehension sign	Patella is subluxed laterally with/without flexion of knee.	Pain/apprehension denotes subluxating patella or PFSS.
McMurray's test	Flex knee maximally; internally rotate tibia (lateral meniscus); fully extend knee. (Flex knee maximally; externally rotate tibia [medial meniscus]; fully extend knee.)	Palpable bulge or pop with/without pain over lateral joint line denotes lateral meniscal injury (or medial meniscal injury over medial joint line).
Pivot-shift test	Knee is fully extended; internally rotate foot and tibia; valgus stress then applied to knee which is slowly flexed.	Observe/feel for anterior translation of lateral tibia on femur. Denotes ACL injury. Most specific test.
Posterior drawer sign	Knee is flexed to 90 degrees; foot is stabilized; posterior translation of tibia on femur.	Posterior tibial translation denotes PCL injury.

Abbreviations: ACL = anterior cruciate ligament; PCL = posterior cruciate ligament; PFSS = patellofemoral stress syndrome.

and internal rotation of the tibia. Practically, this occurs when a runner suddenly stops, plants the foot, and turns. Symptoms include a loud pop, immediate swelling (hemarthrosis), and instability. Positive examination evidence of an ACL injury includes a positive anterior drawer sign, positive Lachman's test, or positive pivot-shift test (Table 5).

Posterior cruciate ligament (PCL) injuries occur with either a valgus or a varus force with the knee in full extension. In addition, a direct force to the anterior proximal tibia (e.g., falling onto a playing surface with the knee flexed 90 degrees) may produce this injury. Examination reveals minimal swelling and a posterior drawer sign (see Table 5).

A *medial collateral ligament (MCL) injury* occurs with a lateral force to the knee. This injury often coexists with other knee injuries. Examination reveals tenderness over the MCL and pain with laxity on valgus stressing of the knee.

Lateral collateral ligament (LCL) injuries are less common and occur with a varus or twisting force. History consists of knee instability with pivoting or cutting. Examination reveals pain over the lateral knee and pain with laxity on varus stressing of the knee.

Medial meniscal injuries are due to twisting and flexing of the knee. History includes swelling (if the peripheral vascular area is involved), joint line pain, and a locking sensation of the knee. Examination reveals effusion, joint line tenderness, and a positive McMurray's test (see Table 5). In young, active persons surgical repair is recommended. In mild cases involving those less active, one may consider conservative management with rehabilitation. *Lateral meniscal injuries* are less common and cause less swelling but sometimes produce more pain. Examination and management are similar to medial meniscal injuries. Because of difficulty in localizing pain, some patients with a lateral meniscal injury will manifest medial joint line tenderness.

Pes anserine bursitis may manifest as knee pain and must be differentiated from other injuries.

Hip Injuries

Large muscles surround the hip joint, and either muscle strains or avulsion fractures are common. Both injury types occur with inadequate warm-up and stretching. *Muscle strains* manifest as a "pop" or "snap" with sudden bursts of speed. Common examples include hamstring or quadriceps strains. Examination shows tenderness, swelling, and ecchymosis. Treatment includes initial ice and relative rest, followed by stretching and muscle strengthening. Return to activity must be avoided until complete healing has occurred. Examples of *avulsion injuries* include ischial spine avulsions by the hamstrings in sprinters, avulsion of the iliac crest by the abdominal oblique muscles, and anterior inferior iliac spine avulsions by the quadriceps (rectus femoris).

Greater trochanteric bursitis occurs with direct trauma to the lateral hip or secondary to other gait-altering injuries. NSAIDs, iontophoresis, or steroid injection resolves this inflammation. *Lumbar disk disease* and *pyriformis syndrome* are causes of persistent hip pain. Careful evaluation of hip injuries is necessary to differentiate localized hip pain from referred back pain.

Any vague pain in the hip made worse with activity should suggest a *stress fracture* of the pubis or femur. These fractures are common in distance runners. Diagnosis is confirmed by plain films or bone scans. Management consists of no weight bearing until the pain is resolved. Aquatic aerobic exercises may be substituted during the non–weight-bearing period. Surgical intervention may be warranted.

Section 15

Obstetrics and Gynecology

ANTEPARTUM CARE

method of
PAUL J. WENDEL, M.D., and
J. GERALD QUIRK, M.D., PH.D.
University of Arkansas for Medical Sciences
Little Rock, Arkansas

Prenatal care is designed to maximize the probability that every pregnancy produces a healthy baby without compromising the health of the mother. To achieve this goal, prenatal care should be thought of as encompassing evaluations and interventions before conception (preconceptual care) and after pregnancy has been diagnosed. In 1991, the U.S. Department of Health and Human Services released the recommendations of their expert panel convened to review the content of prenatal care in the United States. The panel concluded that a significant portion of maternal conditions (i.e., medical and behavioral) that can potentially lead to poor pregnancy outcomes could be identified and altered before conception.

PRECONCEPTUAL CARE

Significant anatomic, physiologic, and psychosocial changes occur throughout the course of pregnancy. As a consequence, various underlying maternal conditions may be affected both positively and negatively by the pregnancy. Thus, addressing these issues and conditions before conception allows the greatest potential for a favorable outcome. The key components of preconceptual care, as defined by the American College of Obstetrics and Gynecology, are listed in Table 1.

TERMINOLOGY

The mean duration of a normal pregnancy is calculated from the first day of the last normal menstrual period. A normal pregnancy lasts approximately 280 days, or 40 weeks, from the first day of the last menstrual period. An estimate of the expected date of delivery is arrived at by adding 7 days to the date of the first day of the last normal menstrual period and counting back 3 months (Nägele's rule). It has become customary to divide pregnancy into three equal trimesters of approximately three calendar months each. All subsequent prenatal care is based on the precise knowledge of the age of the fetus; therefore, for ideal obstetric management, it is imperative to know the gestational age at any given time during pregnancy. Thus, early prenatal care makes it possible to assign gestational age through an accurate history of the last menstrual period and physical assessment of uterine size.

THE INITIAL PRENATAL VISIT

The initial prenatal visit is perhaps the most important visit of this care sequence. At this time, the relationship between the patient and the health care provider is established. It is the time to establish the goals of assessing the health of both the mother and the fetus, establishing the gestational age of the fetus, and initiating a plan for continuing obstetric care. To do this, a comprehensive medical and obstetric history must be obtained. The medical history should inquire about any prior hospitalizations, surgical procedures, underlying medical conditions, or current diseases that are being followed by a medical caregiver. Any family history of birth defects, mental retardation, or developmental delays should be obtained. The obstetric history should document the number, duration, and outcomes of all prior pregnan-

TABLE 1. **Components of Preconceptual Care**

Systematic identification of preconceptional risks through assessment of reproductive, family, and medical histories; nutritional status; drug exposures; and social concerns of all fertile women
Provision of education based on risks
Discussion of possible effects of pregnancy on existing medical conditions for both the prospective mother and the fetus and introduction of interventions, if appropriate and desired
Discussion of genetic concerns and referral, if appropriate and desired
Determination of immunity to rubella and immunization, if indicated
Determination of hepatitis status and immunization, if desired
Laboratory tests as indicated
Nutritional counseling on appropriate weight for height, sources of folic acid, and avoidance of vitamin oversupplementation; referral for in-depth counseling, if appropriate and desired
Discussion of social, financial, and psychological issues in preparation for pregnancy
Discussion regarding desired birth spacing and real and perceived barriers to achieving desires, including problems with contraceptive use
Emphasis on importance of early and continuous prenatal care and discussion of how care may be structured based on the woman's risks and concerns
Recommendation for women to keep menstrual calendar

From Cunningham FG, MacDonald PC, Gant NF, et al: Williams Obstetrics, 20th ed. Norwalk, CT, Appleton & Lange, 1997, p 228.

cies, including infant weights, delivery methods, and pregnancy complications. Any prior abdominal surgeries should be investigated, and the uterine scar type of any prior cesarean section should be documented to determine whether the patient is a candidate for a subsequent vaginal birth.

A complete physical examination should be performed on the patient at the first prenatal visit. Any examination should include a routine evaluation of all the major organ systems, with special attention to be paid to the genital tract. A pelvic examination should include assessment of the vulva and any associated physical findings, evaluations of the vagina and cervix, as well as a Papanicolaou (Pap) smear. Ideally, any early examination should include a bimanual examination to determine the patency, length, and consistency of the external cervix, as well as the uterine size. This examination also helps to confirm the gestational age of the pregnancy. In addition to the Pap smear, a gonorrhea culture should be obtained. Any findings suggestive of other sexually transmitted diseases may prompt the culturing for *Chlamydia or Trichomonas*.

The first prenatal visit is an ideal time to obtain a host of laboratory tests, which include a hemoglobin and hematocrit with platelets; a urinalysis, including a microscopic examination and culture; blood group and D typing; indirect Coombs; syphilis serology; hepatitis B serology; and voluntary human immunodeficiency virus (HIV) testing. Selective populations should undergo testing for sickle cell anemia, diabetes, hemoglobinopathies, and tuberculosis.

Knowledge gathered from a history and physical examination allows the caregiver to provide a risk assessment program for each patient. Typically, pregnancies that include underlying pre-existing medical illness or previous poor pregnancy performance may be categorized as high risk and may be referred on for consultation.

SUBSEQUENT PRENATAL CARE

Traditionally, women with pregnancies at low risk for adverse outcomes have been seen on a monthly basis until 28 weeks, then every 2 weeks until 35 weeks and weekly thereafter. If prenatal care is initiated early, this typically results in 13 to 15 visits. One of the recommendations of the expert panel on prenatal care was to modify this schedule. It was their belief that a woman should be seen early in pregnancy to be screened for underlying conditions. She should return at 10 to 12 weeks to be offered chorionic villus sampling and electronic identification of fetal heart tones. The next visit should occur in the interval from 16 to 20 weeks, when maternal serum screening and an ultrasound may be performed. The next important visit is at 26 to 28 weeks, during which time the diabetes screen, complete blood count, and Rh screen could be repeated, along with RhoGAM administration, if necessary. Finally, visits in the third trimester could be performed every 2 weeks to monitor fundal height growth, fetal activity, and blood pressure. The clinician should remain flexible in the assigning of subsequent visits depending on the performance of the pregnancy and underlying conditions or complications that may arise.

PRENATAL SURVEILLANCE

Follow-up visits are designed to determine the well-being of both the mother and the fetus. Therefore, information that is especially important to obtain from the fetal aspect is heart rate, size of the fetus (actual and rate of change), amount of amniotic fluid, presenting part and station (late in pregnancy), and fetal activity. From the maternal standpoint, the following information should be obtained: blood pressure, weight, general well-being, and distance to the uterine fundus from the symphysis pubis. Late in pregnancy, a pelvic examination provides potentially important information regarding confirmation of the presenting part, station of the presenting part, clinical assessment of the pelvis in relation to the fetus, and the consistency effacement and dilatation of the cervix.

GENERAL GUIDELINES DURING PREGNANCY

In addition to the physical examination and medical history obtained at the first prenatal visit, information should be provided to the patient regarding a host of topics to optimize the potential for a successful pregnancy performance.

Nutrition

In general, a well-balanced diet in pregnancy provides the majority of the Food and Drug Administration (FDA) recommended daily allowances of dietary requirements. The Institute of Medicine concluded that iron was the only nutrient whose dietary requirement during pregnancy could not be met by diet alone. It is recommended that 30 to 60 mg of elemental iron be supplied on a daily basis. In the preconceptional period, the Centers for Disease Control and Prevention recommends dietary supplementation of 0.8 mg of folic acid for approximately 4 weeks before and 3 months after conception for all women in an effort to prevent neural tube defects, (NTD); for women who previously conceived a fetus with an NTD, this should be increased to 4.0 mg. Importantly, additional nutritional supplements are unnecessary and indeed could be harmful; certain minerals and vitamins (including zinc; selenium; and vitamins A, B_6, C, and D) may produce toxic effects in excess amounts.

Weight Gain

In 1990, a committee from the National Academy of Science published its recommendations for weight gain during pregnancy. It recommended weight gains of 28 to 40 pounds for underweight women, 25 to 35 pounds for normal-weight women, and 15 to 25 pounds for overweight women. These categories were based on body mass index (weight [kg] divided by height [m^2]), defined by prepregnancy weight. Underweight women had an index less than 19.8 kg/m^2, and overweight women exceeded 26 kg/m^2.

Exercise

As a rule, it is not necessary for the pregnant woman to limit exercise, provided that she does not become excessively fatigued or risk injury to herself or her fetus. The American College of Obstetricians and Gynecologists recommends that women who are accustomed to aerobic exercise before pregnancy should be allowed to continue this during pregnancy; however, caution should be taken against starting new exercise programs or intensifying training efforts during pregnancy. Women should avoid exercises that are performed in the supine position.

Employment

As with exercise, pregnant women should be encouraged to work throughout their pregnancy up until the time of delivery. Care should be taken to provide a healthy working environment, free from excessive physical exertion, prolonged standing, and exposure to occupational hazards. Limitations on employment and hours worked should be individualized to the patient, depending on the health of the mother.

Travel

In low-risk pregnancies, there is no reason to limit travel for a pregnant woman, as long as she has access to medical care. There is essentially no risk to the fetus in a pressurized cabin of an airplane. Whether traveling by car, train, or airplane, women should be encouraged to walk at least every 2 hours. Travel in a car should be the same as in the nonpregnant state; passengers should be restrained with three-point seat belts. The lap belt portion of the restraining belt should be placed under the abdomen and across the upper thighs, the upper shoulder belt should be snugly applied between the breasts. International travel should be limited only by the access to medical care and exposure to areas with endemic diseases. Those patients requiring vaccines for international travel should consult their physician regarding the nature of the vaccine because of the potential for harmful effects from live attenuated virus vaccines.

Sexual Activity

Whenever a threatened abortion or preterm labor is present, any erotic stimulation should be avoided, since it may produce uterine contractions. Otherwise, it has generally been accepted that in healthy pregnant women, sexual activity usually does no harm. Although uterine activity may transiently increase following erotic stimulation, this is usually self-limited. In pregnancies complicated by placenta previa and threatened preterm delivery, coitus should be avoided.

Smoking

In general, smoking leads to decreased birth weight by an average of 200 grams; consequently, smoking should be discouraged for all pregnant patients. Nicotine replacement therapies, such as patches and chewing gums have been reported to be effective in achieving smoking cessation in pregnancy.

Alcohol

Because alcohol use during pregnancy may be harmful to the fetus, the Surgeon General recommends that women who are pregnant or considering pregnancy abstain from using any alcoholic beverages.

Caffeine

The Fourth International Caffeine Workshop concluded that there was no evidence that caffeine increases teratogenic or reproductive risk. Most studies on human pregnancy report no association between caffeine consumption and early pregnancy wastage, birth defects, or low birth weight. Patients should be encouraged to take a common-sense approach in their daily intake of caffeine in pregnancy.

COMMON COMPLAINTS IN PREGNANCY

Nausea and Vomiting

Nausea and vomiting are very common in the first half of pregnancy. Typically, they have a self-limited course and begin to subside after the 14th to 16th week of pregnancy. The etiology continues to be unclear. Supportive therapy with oral and rectal antiemetics usually proves beneficial. Promethazine, 25 to 50 mg orally or rectally every 6 to 8 hours, proves helpful in most cases. The restriction to clear liquids and the addition of metoclopramide (Reglan) orally may be of benefit in some recalcitrant cases. Intravenous feeding and hospitalization may be necessary in unusual cases.

Back Pain

Low back pain is very common, especially as pregnancy progresses. Significant movement of the skeleton and softening of the fibroelastic cartilages are hormonally mediated. Women should be instructed on proper body mechanics when lifting, rising, and lying down. Occasionally, supportive braces and physical therapy may be of some benefit.

Constipation

Constipation is a result of delayed gastric emptying and increased intestinal transit time, which are both hormonally and mechanically mediated. Both processes result in greater resorption of water from the gastrointestinal tract, resulting in hard stools and constipation. Typically, constipation responds well to increasing fluid intake and eating smaller, more frequent meals. The addition of bulk to the diet, through either high-fiber foods or supplements, usually proves helpful. Stool softeners may prove beneficial.

Hemorrhoids

Hemorrhoids are varicosities of the rectal veins; they may appear for the first time during pregnancy. Their development or aggravation is undoubtedly related to the increased pressure in the rectal veins caused by the obstruction of the venous return by the enlarging uterus. Constipation typically promotes their development or makes them more symptomatic. Pain and swelling are usually relieved by topically applied anesthetics, warm soaks, and stool softeners. Occasionally, thrombosis of the rectal vein may require excision under topical anesthesia.

Heartburn

Heartburn is probably the most common complaint in pregnant women. It is caused by reflux of gastric contents into the lower esophagus, made worse by the upward displacement of the stomach and compression of the uterus against the lower esophageal sphincter. Antacid preparations of aluminum hydroxide and magnesium hydroxide usually provide considerable relief. H_z blockers should be reserved for mothers who fail oral antacids.

PRENATAL DIAGNOSIS

Approximately 3 to 5% of all newborns are delivered with some form of birth defect, whether it is major or minor. Only about 25 years ago, a fetal anomaly was first diagnosed in utero. With the development of increasingly sophisticated imaging technology, especially ultrasonography, fetal anomalies are diagnosed regularly. At present, however, no authoritative body recommends the use of routine ultrasonographic examination for population-based screening of congenital anomalies. As maternal age increases, there is an increasing risk of delivering a baby with an autosomal trisomy such as Down syndrome. The current standard of care is to offer amniocentesis for fetal karyotype to all women who will be 35 years of age or older at the time of delivery. All women who are older than 35 should be offered an amniocentesis. Maternal serum screening programs have been developed in attempts to identify fetuses at risk of neural tube defects, trisomies, and abdominal wall defects. Neural tube defects are usually seen in 1 to 2 of 1000 infants in the United States and 1 to 2 of 100 in Great Britain. An elevated maternal serum alpha-fetoprotein (MS-AFP) identifies patients at risk for delivering an infant with neural tube defects or abdominal wall defect, i.e., greater than 2.5 multiples of the median (MoM).

Shortly after the initiation of MS-AFP screening in the United States, it was noted that low MS-AFP values, (i.e., < 0.5 MoM) may identify as many as 30% of mothers at risk of delivering a fetus with an autosomal trisomy. Recently, the addition of human chorionic gonadotropin and unconjugated estriol to the MS-AFP have made it possible to identify as many as 60 to 70% of fetuses with chromosomal abnormalities. This program has proven extremely beneficial to the roughly 80% of women in the United States who deliver chromosomally abnormal babies without known risk factors. Unfortunately, the positive predictive value of these serum screens is low; as a result, only 1 in 60 to 70 abnormal screens result in identification of a trisomic fetus. Universal application of maternal screening for fetal anomalies and trisomies would result in 5 to 10% of all pregnant women undergoing amniocentesis.

The advent of genetic testing has now increased the number of diseases that can be potentially identified through prenatal testing. Currently, more than 500 genetic diseases can be identified, either through direct gene mapping or linkage testing. Consultation with a geneticist is important, as the list of potentially identifiable genetic diseases continues to increase on a rapid basis.

ULTRASONOGRAPHY

Ultrasound is perhaps the most revolutionary development in prenatal care during this century. The advantages of routine ultrasonographic screening include less-frequent labor inductions for post-term pregnancy, earlier detection of fetal growth restriction, and identification of malformed fetuses. No clear-cut guidelines exist that define which women should receive an ultrasound or how many should be performed during a pregnancy. However, Table 2 lists the components of a basic ultrasound examination according to the trimester of the pregnancy in which it is performed. Regardless of the controversy, in general, the earlier the ultrasound is performed, the greater the accuracy in determining gestational age. Information obtained at less than 18 weeks' gestational age typically has a margin of error less than 10 days. Studies performed in the third trimester may have a margin of error of roughly 3.5 weeks.

VAGINAL BLEEDING IN PREGNANCY

The significance of vaginal bleeding depends on the trimester in which it occurs. First-trimester vaginal bleeding can be from a variety of sources, including eversion of the endocervical canal, threatened abortion, and fetal death. Infectious etiologies, such as gonorrhea or chlamydial infections, may cause in-

TABLE 2. **Components of Basic Ultrasound Examination According to Trimester of Pregnancy**

First Trimester
1. Gestational sac location
2. Embryo identification
3. Crown–rump length
4. Fetal heart motion
5. Fetal number
6. Uterus and adnexal evaluation
Second and Third Trimester
1. Fetal number
2. Presentation
3. Fetal heart motion
4. Placental location
5. Amnionic fluid volume
6. Gestational age
7. Survey of fetal anatomy
8. Evaluation for maternal pelvic masses

Modified from Cunningham FG, MacDonald PC, Gant NF, et al: Williams Obstetrics, 20th ed. Norwalk, CT, Appleton & Lange, 1997, p 1024.

flammatory cervicitis, which produces bleeding. Second-trimester vaginal bleeding may be a sign of continued threatened abortion or missed abortion. Other causes that require investigation include preterm cervical dilatation and cervical incompetence, as well as preterm labor producing cervical change. A placenta previa may also be a cause of mid-trimester vaginal bleeding. It is usually described as painless vaginal bleeding that may or may not be associated with uterine activity. An ultrasound should be performed to identify the location of the placenta before performing a pelvic examination. Again, careful speculum examination will identify signs of cervical infections, trauma, or neoplasms. Third-trimester vaginal bleeding is a common event. Placenta previa needs to be excluded and other causes sought. Cervical dilatation and labor should be ruled out as a sign of any bleeding. Finally, bright red bleeding associated with increased uterine tone and pain may be a sign of placental abruption. Placental abruption is usually associated with hypertensive diseases, trauma, and illicit drug use, especially cocaine.

TERATOGENS AND RADIATION EXPOSURE

A teratogen is any agent or factor that produces a permanent alteration in form or function of an organism when exposure to the agent or factor occurs in the embryonic or fetal period. Pregnancy is divided into the ovum period (from fertilization to implantation), the embryotic period (from the second through the eighth week) and the fetal period (from 8 weeks until term). Typically, agents that affect the ovum produce an all-or-nothing phenomenon. The major impact of teratogens occurs during the embryotic period. The factors that affect whether a drug has teratogenic effects depend on whether the fetus is exposed in quantities sufficient to cause it developmental anomalies. Many factors play a role in the accumulation of the drug or its metabolites to potentially toxic levels in the fetal compartment. These include the degrees of maternal absorption and metabolism, protein binding and storage, molecular size, electrical charge, and lipid solubility, all of which affect the degree of placental transfer. Any drug given to pregnant women should be thoroughly researched by the caregiver before exposing the woman and her fetus to it. As with all medications in pregnancy, the potential to be gained from maternal exposure should be weighed against the potential side effects to the fetus. Medications with known fetal effects should be used only after consultation with medical specialists and with clear indications.

Unfortunately, radiologic procedures often are performed during early pregnancy prior to the time that pregnancy is diagnosed. As with medications, radiologic procedures may have defined specific risks based on the fetal dose of radiation. When calculating the dose of ionizing radiation from x-rays, it is important to consider: the type of study, the type and age of the equipment, the distance of the organ in question from the source of radiation, the thickness of the body part penetrated, and the method or technique employed in the study. Current evidence suggests that there is no increased risk to the fetus with regard to congenital malformation, growth restriction, or abortion from ionizing radiation at a dose less than 5 rads to the fetus. (A standard chest x-ray has a dose exposure of >0.05 rads.) Currently, no single diagnostic procedure results in a radiation dose significant enough to threaten the well-being or development of an embryo or fetus.

INFECTIONS IN PREGNANCY

Varicella Virus

Varicella infection in adults tends to be more severe than in children. There is evidence that the infection may be especially severe in pregnancy. Serious sequelae, such as the development of pneumonitis in the mother may occur. Maternal chickenpox may infect the fetus by transplacental infection. In early pregnancy, infection may result in severe congenital malformations, including chorioretinitis, cerebral cortical atrophy, and limb defects. Administration of varicella zoster immune globulin (VZIG) may prevent or attenuate the varicella infection in mothers if given within 96 hours of exposure. The dose is 125 units per 10 kg, given intramuscularly. The maximum dose is 625 units intramuscularly. If practical, maternal varicella IgG titers should be assessed before VZIG administration.

Parvovirus

Human parvovirus B19 causes erythema infectiosum or fifth disease. The maternal infection is usually associated with a rash, accompanying arthralgias and many nonspecific symptoms. However, maternal infection may also be associated with adverse pregnancy outcomes, including abortion and fetal death. Diagnosis is confirmed by serologically demonstrating the presence of IgM parvo-specific antibodies. If fetal hydrops develops, fetal transfusion may be considered. Currently, there is no known maternal treatment for the disease.

Cytomegalovirus

Cytomegalovirus (CMV) is the most common cause of perinatal infection and may be found in as many as 2% of all neonates. Maternal CMV infection is characterized by fever, pharyngitis, lymphadenopathy, and polyarthritis. A risk of seroconversion among susceptible women during pregnancy is roughly 1 to 4%. Immunity from prior infection can be demonstrated in as many as 85% of pregnant women. Congenital CMV infection causes a syndrome that includes low birth weight, microcephaly, intracranial calcifications, chorioretinitis and mental retardation. This syndrome is seen more commonly in mothers with primary infection in pregnancy and may be present in as many as 20% of infants whose mother demonstrates primary infection during pregnancy. Recurrent infection in the mother is rarely associated with clinical sequelae. No effective therapy for maternal infection is presently known. Primary infection is diagnosed by a fourfold increase in IgG titers in paired acute and convalescent serum or by the identification of IgM CMV antibody in maternal serum. Recurrent infection is usually not accompanied by IgM antibody production.

Toxoplasmosis

Toxoplasmosis gondii infection is transmitted by the eating of infected raw or undercooked meat or through contact with infected cat feces. Maternal immunity is usually protective against intrauterine infection. Maternal infection is characterized by fatigue, muscle pain, and lymphadenopathy, although subclinical infection may be present. At birth, affected infants usually have evidence of generalized disease with low birth weight, and hepatosplenomegaly, along with various neurologic complications. The presence of toxoplasma IgG antibody confers immunity for the mother. The most accurate method of diagnosis currently is a polymerase chain reaction (PCR). There is some evidence that maternal treatment with spiramycin* may be effective in preventing fetal infection and/or modifying its severity. Treatment has also been demonstrated to be effective with pyrimethamine (Daraprim), plus sulfadiazine.

Syphilis

Syphilis is a treponemal infection that can produce profound effects on the pregnancy by causing an endarteritis that results in preterm labor, fetal death, and neonatal infection by transplacental or perinatal infection. Fortunately, syphilis is highly preventable and very susceptible to therapy. Diagnosis is made by serologic screening via such tests as the Venereal Disease Research Laboratory or the rapid plasma reagin, usually at the first prenatal visit. (This screen is required by law in most areas.) Positive findings should be confirmed by fluorescent treponemal antibody absorption or a microhemagglutination assay–*Treponema pallidum* preparation. Penicillin remains the treatment of choice. Intramuscular penicillin G cures early maternal infection and prevents neonatal syphilis in 98% of cases. Primary and secondary syphilis should be treated with 2.4 million units of benzathine penicillin G intramuscularly each week for 2 weeks. Syphilis of more than 1 year's duration should be treated with three sequential doses. Women with penicillin allergies should be referred for therapy.

Gonorrhea

In most cases of new gonococcal infection in pregnancy, the infection is limited to the lower genital tract. Acute salpingitis rarely develops because of obliteration of the uterine cavity after 8 weeks' gestational age. However, there is some evidence that pregnancy may place the patient at an increased risk for systemic infection. There is an association between gonococcal infection, septic abortion, preterm delivery, premature rupture of membranes, chorioamnionitis, and postpartum infection. Treatment of uncomplicated gonococcal infection includes ceftriaxone (Rocephin), 125 mg intramuscularly, or cefixime (Suprax), 400 mg orally in a single dose. Patients with a positive gonorrhea culture should be screened for other sexually transmitted diseases.

Chlamydial Infections

Genital infection with *Chlamydia trachomatis* is the most common sexually transmitted bacterial disease in women of reproductive age. Cultures are positive in as many as a quarter of pregnant women. PCR testing of cervical secretions is now the detection method of choice. The role of routine screening for *C. trachomatis* during pregnancy remains unclear. However, there appears to be some evidence that this organism is linked to preterm delivery, premature rupture of membranes, and chorioamnionitis. Current treatment guidelines include erythromycin base 500 mg orally four times per day for 7 days, or the new macrolide antibiotic azithromycin (Zithromax), 1 gram orally as a single dose.

Herpes Simplex Virus

The management of herpes simplex virus (HSV) infection in pregnancy continues to evolve. The distinction between type I and type II herpetic infections has become blurred. Both virus types may produce maternal genital and neonatal infection. Most serious sequelae result from primary or first-episode

*Not available in the United States.

infection in pregnancy. Primary infection is typically associated with more significant maternal symptoms, along with greater potential for vertical transmission to the fetus. A primary herpetic outbreak in pregnancy may be associated with a 25 to 40% transmission rate to the infant if delivered over an active lesion, whereas recurrent lesions typically produce neonatal infection in only 3 to 5% of cases. Current management schemes continue to advocate cesarean delivery if herpetic vesicles or ulcers, whether primary or recurrent, are present at the time of rupture of membranes or labor. In the absence of a clinical lesion or prodromal symptoms, vaginal delivery is usually allowed. Diagnosis of a herpetic lesion should be confirmed by a tissue culture. Recent development of PCR assay for herpes simplex virus shows promise. New strategies for viral suppression with oral acyclovir (Zovirax), after 36 weeks may prove helpful in preventing recurrent lesions and may decrease viral shedding.

Human Immunodeficiency Virus

HIV infection rates among young women of reproductive age are increasing more than among any other subgroup population because of transmission via heterosexual contact. As a consequence, all pregnant women should be counseled regarding HIV infection and offered screening. A positive enzyme-linked immunosorbent assay test should be repeated and, if positive a second time, confirmed with a Western blot analysis. A confirmatory finding on the Western blot indicates current infection. Protocols for the treatment of HIV-positive women in pregnancy have demonstrated decreased vertical transmission from the mother to the infant by greater than 68%. Current recommendations include starting zidovudine (ZDV) (Retrovir), 500 mg orally, daily after 14 weeks until the patient presents in labor. Women are then administered ZDV (2 mg per kg) intravenously over 1 hour, followed by 1 mg per kg intravenously throughout labor. Once the infant is delivered, the infant receives oral zidovudine syrup, 2 mg per kg for 6 weeks postpartum. Infants should be monitored and referred to a pediatrician for follow-up. Mothers with a viral load of greater than 10,000 copies or a CD4 count of less than 200 should be referred to a specialist for consideration for multiple-drug regimens.

Gestational Diabetes

Gestational diabetes is defined as carbohydrate intolerance of variable severity, with onset or first recognition during pregnancy. Undoubtedly, some women with gestational diabetes have previously unrecognized overt diabetes. There is neither agreement as to the most appropriate diagnostic criteria for gestational diabetes nor consensus regarding the most appropriate women to be screened for this disorder. Whether universal screening or screening based on maternal risk factors is employed, any program should be instituted between the 24th and 28th weeks of gestational age. Screening programs involving risk factors should include age over 30, family history of diabetes, prior macrosomic fetus, infant malformed or stillborn, obesity, hypertension, or glycosuria. Those patients undergoing screening should be given a 50-gram oral glucose tolerance test between the 24th and 28th weeks, without regard to the time of day or last meal. A plasma value at 1 hour exceeding 140 mg per dL is used as the cutoff for a positive test. The diagnosis of gestational diabetes is made using a 100-gram, 3-hour oral glucose tolerance test. Women with a previous history of gestational diabetes may benefit from earlier screening. If screening is performed early in pregnancy and yields a normal value, subsequent screening should still be performed at 24 to 28 weeks. If a 100-gram, 3-hour oral glucose tolerance test is performed, it should be done after an overnight fast. Typically, the cutoff values for a positive 3-hour glucose tolerance test are plasma values as follows (mg per dL): fasting, 105; 1 hour, 190; 2 hour, 165; 3 hour, 145. A positive test is defined as two or more values that are abnormal. Importantly, because women with gestational diabetes may not have fasting hyperglycemia during the time of organogenesis, the fetus may not be at any increased risk for fetal anomalies as are women with overt diabetes. Similarly, whereas pregnant women with overt diabetes are at a greater risk for fetal death, this danger does not appear to be apparent in those women with postprandial hyperglycemia only (gestational diabetes class A1).

Current management strategies for the treatment of gestational diabetes are primarily aimed at preventing macrosomia and the associated risks for birth trauma due to shoulder dystocia. Fetuses of diabetic mothers are anthropometrically different from other large-for-gestational-age infants. Typically, the infants of diabetic mothers have excess fat deposition on the shoulders and trunk, thus predisposing them to shoulder dystocia. These processes are consequences of maternal hyperglycemia, resulting in fetal hyperinsulinemia, which in turn stimulates excessive somatic growth. To this end, women who exhibit fasting plasma glucose levels of over 105 mg per dL or a 2-hour postparanoidal value of over 120 mg per dL may benefit from dietary counseling and the addition of insulin. Those women with a diagnosis of gestational diabetes should initially be started on the American Diabetes Association diet of 30 to 35 kcal per day as determined by the patient's ideal body weight. Any decision to add insulin should be undertaken after the initiation of this diet and monitoring of fasting values and 2-hour postprandial values.

The decision on whether to perform antenatal fetal testing to prevent fetal losses should be individualized according to the patient. There is no evidence that antenatal fetal testing is required in gestational diabetics who are diet controlled. Expert opinion is divided on whether fetuses born to mothers who require insulin require fetal testing in the third trimester. It is currently our practice not to include fetal testing as a part of their management if glucose levels are well controlled and there is no suspicion of fetal macrosomia. Additionally, there is no evidence to support the fact that fetuses born to mothers with gestational diabetes have delayed lung maturity. As a result, amniotic fluid testing for lung maturity is not required in gestational diabetics prior to delivery. Management in labor should include control of maternal blood sugar using intravenous insulin if needed to decrease the risk of fetal hypoglycemia in the neonatal period.

The consequence of gestational diabetes on future outcome is important. It has been estimated that 50% of women with gestational diabetes will develop overt diabetes within 20 years of delivery. As a result, women should be evaluated with a 75-gram oral glucose tolerance test within 3 months of delivery. In addition, the recurrence of gestational diabetes in subsequent pregnancies has been documented to be as high as 20 to 30%.

Hypertensive Disorders in Pregnancy

Hypertensive disorders complicating pregnancy are common and form one component of the deadly triad that includes hemorrhage and infection, which are responsible for the majority of maternal deaths. Because of the potentially severe sequelae of this diagnosis, the development of hypertension in a previously normotensive pregnant woman should and must be considered potentially dangerous to both the mother and the fetus. Pregnancy-induced hypertension (PIH) is divided into three categories: hypertension alone, preeclampsia, and eclampsia. The diagnosis of PIH is made when the blood pressure is 140/90 mm Hg or greater. The diagnosis of preeclampsia has traditionally required the identification of PIH plus proteinuria or generalized edema. However, because generalized edema is such a common finding, its presence should not validate, nor should its absence exclude, the diagnosis of preeclampsia. Proteinuria is defined as more than 300 mg of protein in a 24-hour period or 100 mg per dL on two random urine specimens collected 6 hours apart. The degree of proteinuria may fluctuate widely over 24 hours; thus, a single random sample may fail to demonstrate significant proteinuria. Chronic hypertension in pregnancy is defined as the presence of hypertension (≥140/90 mm Hg) either preceding pregnancy or detected before 20 weeks of pregnancy. The presence or absence of other associated symptoms and/or the identification of abnormalities in specified laboratory tests is used to assess the severity of PIH or preeclampsia. The key indicators that differentiate mild from severe preeclampsia are listed in Table 3. Management of PIH should be individualized on a patient-to-patient basis. Management of preeclampsia should take into account the severity of the disorder as assessed by the presence or absence of other conditions, identified in Table 3, the duration of the gestation, and the condition of the cervix. When the diagnosis of severe preeclampsia is made, hospitalization and prompt delivery should be undertaken in almost all cases. Unless the pregnancy is at the extreme limits of prematurity or the disease has not met severe criteria, expectant management and careful surveillance of the mother may prove beneficial to obtain greater fetal maturity.

TABLE 3. **Pregnancy-Induced Hypertension: Indications of Severity**

Abnormality	Mild	Severe
Diastolic blood pressure	<100 mm Hg	≥110 mm Hg
Proteinuria	Trace to 1+	Persistent 2+ or more
Headache	Absent	Present
Visual disturbances	Absent	Present
Upper abdominal pain	Absent	Present
Oliguria	Absent	Present
Convulsions	Absent	Present (eclampsia)
Serum creatinine	Normal	Elevated
Thrombocytopenia	Absent	Present
Hyperbilirubinemia	Absent	Present
Liver enzyme elevation	Minimal	Marked
Fetal growth restriction	Absent	Obvious
Pulmonary edema	Absent	Present

Modified from Cunningham FG, MacDonald PC, Gant NF, et al: Williams Obstetrics, 20th ed. Norwalk, CT, Appleton & Lange, 1997, p 695.

Unfortunately, drug therapy for early mild preeclampsia and/or severe preeclampsia has been disappointing. Almost universally, the addition of antihypertensive agents fails to treat the underlying cause of the PIH and has failed to show improvements in mean pregnancy prolongation, gestational age at delivery, or birth weight. It is important to keep in mind that preeclampsia is a multisystem disorder that includes hypertension; it is not, strictly speaking, merely a hypertensive disorder with accompanying edema and/or proteinuria. Consequently, enthusiasm for the treatment of preeclampsia through pharmacologic agents has not been great. As part of any treatment plan for patients with PIH, intramuscular glucocorticoids to enhance fetal lung maturity and prevent intracranial hemorrhage should be used. These glucocorticoids do not seem to affect the cause of maternal hypertension. During labor, women with PIH or preeclampsia should be given intravenous magnesium sulfate to prevent seizure activity. The usual dose is 4 grams intravenously as a loading dose over 20 minutes, followed by a continuous intravenous maintenance dose of 2 grams per hour. As long as urinary output is adequate (i.e., >30 mL per hour with a serum creatinine of <1.2), serum magnesium levels need not be measured. Preeclamptic patients managed expectantly should have their blood pressure, proteinuria, creatinine, liver functions, and platelet counts monitored closely. Additionally, some form of fetal surveillance should be performed on a regular basis to avoid potential perinatal morbidity or mortality. In women whose pregnancies are between 32 and 34 weeks' gestational age, testing for fetal lung maturity may be appropriate as an indication of whether to deliver.

After 34 weeks' gestational age, PIH with complications usually is best remedied by delivery. In the postpartum period, magnesium sulfate therapy should be continued for 24 hours. Intravenous hydralazine may be given intermittently as needed for diastolic blood pressures over 110 mm Hg or systolic values over 170 mm Hg. Patients may be discharged when there is evidence that severe hypertension is showing a downward trend or laboratory values begin to normalize. Follow-up should be individualized according to the severity of the disease.

Preterm Delivery

Premature birth in the United States is defined as any delivery prior to 37 weeks, and low birth weight is defined as any baby weighing less than 2500 grams at birth. The great majority of mortality and serious morbidity from preterm birth occurs before 34 weeks. Approximately 8 to 10% of all live births in the United States are low birth weight. The underlying etiology of preterm labor and preterm birth is poorly understood; consequently, interventions to prevent it have been disappointing. Associated maternal conditions, such as low socioeconomic status, nonwhite race, poor nutrition, multiple gestation, maternal smoking and alcohol use, as well as poor prenatal care attendance have been linked to preterm labor and birth. It is now thought that ascending genital tract infections may be an etiologic factor in some cases of preterm labor. Current interventional strategies at this time are now being aimed at the early mid-trimester. It is during this time that patients are being offered screenings for vaginal infections. It is theorized that intravaginal infections, such as chlamydia, bacterial vaginosis, gonorrhea and mycoplasma, may be responsible for ascending infections that tip off a biochemical cascade, which produces uterine activity. Whether these strategies will prevent preterm delivery will be answered with time. Clinical interventions to treat these infections are beginning to show promise but should be considered investigational at this time.

Programs designed to identify patients at risk for preterm delivery generally use scoring systems that identify predisposing factors. Although they may be useful for identification purpose, interventions to prevent preterm delivery based on these factors have been disappointing. Additionally, programs designed to identify early uterine activity through either self-palpation or electronic monitors have been disappointing. Although these methods are good at identifying uterine activity, there still are very few interventions that can prevent this uterine activity from resulting in a preterm delivery.

Once uterine activity has begun, efforts must be made to determine the underlying cause. In as many as 50% of cases, no significant underlying etiology is identified. Strategies to determine an infectious etiology include vaginal cultures, as well as amniocentesis. Debate continues on whether treatment of intrauterine amniotic infection will prevent preterm delivery. However, if intrauterine infection is identified, intravenous antibiotics should be considered. Typically, women will initially be started on intravenous fluids and given intravenous sedation as necessary. If this therapy proves ineffective, the decision of whether to include an intravenous tocolytic agent should be undertaken. Currently, the tocolytic agents include betasympthomematics (i.e., ritodrine [Yutopar] and terbutaline [Brethine]*), nonsteroidal anti-inflammatory agents (i.e., indomethacin [Indocin]*), calcium channel blockers (i.e., nifedipine [Procardia]*), and magnesium sulfate. Although data have failed to prove conclusively that tocolytic therapy arrests labor for more than 48 to 72 hours, it should not be misconstrued as a reason not to treat the patient. This 48- to 72-hour delay makes it possible to institute intramuscular corticosteroid treatment, thus decreasing the incidence of hyaline membrane disease, intraventricular hemorrhage, and necrotizing enterocolitis.

New strategies that show promise in the prediction of preterm delivery include the identification of fetal fibronectin in the cervix and vagina and measurement of cervical length by vaginal ultrasound. As with identification and treatment of infections in the genital tract, these methods are not yet proven to decrease the rate of preterm birth and should therefore continue to be considered investigational.

*Not approved by the Food and Drug Administration for this indication.

ECTOPIC PREGNANCY

method of
MARK X. RANSOM, M.D.
St. Joseph's Hospital and Medical Center
Paterson, New Jersey

Whereas mortality due to ectopic pregnancy has declined, the incidence of the disease continues to rise. In the United States from 1970 to 1989, case-fatality rates dropped from 35.5 deaths per 10,000 ectopic pregnancies to 3.8, and overall rates rose from 4.5 cases per 1000 reported pregnancies to 16.0. Curiously, although pelvic inflammatory disease is often cited as the principal etiologic factor for ectopic pregnancy, its incidence has not kept pace. The basis for the rise in ectopic gestations is likely multifactorial and includes increased clinician suspicion, increased recognition and reporting, increased utilization of assisted reproductive technologies, and increased use of conservative tubal surgery.

Direct visualization of the ectopic gestation, either by laparoscopy or laparotomy, has been the longtime standard for diagnosis. As reliable and rapid hormonal assays have become available, coincident with improved ultrasonographic technology, the diagnosis is now more commonly made nonsurgically and prior to the patient becoming symptomatic. A variety of diagnostic algorithms relying on hormonal measurement and sonographic findings have been described that have enabled earlier and earlier detection.

With earlier diagnoses have come unique approaches to the management of this condition. Once exclusively a surgical disease, medical treatment is quickly becoming the first line of treatment for ectopics suspected so early that even direct visualization might not reveal the tiny gestation. Medical treatment offers the possibilities of lower-cost management, faster recovery, and subsequent fertility rates comparable to those with traditional surgery.

DIAGNOSIS

The ectopic trophoblast produces β-human chorionic gonadotropin (β-hCG), which can be detected by serum assay. A single quantitative value does offer some diagnostic clues when ruling out an ectopic gestation. The "discriminatory zone" has been described as the hCG level at which ultrasonographic identification of an intrauterine sac is possible. Expectations to visualize an intrauterine sac predicted by a serum level must be correlated to the method of sonography. For example, an intrauterine sac may be seen transabdominally at hCG levels between 6000 and 6500 IU per liter but transvaginally at levels of only 1500 to 3000 IU per liter. To conclusively diagnose an intrauterine gestation, it is important to identify a yolk sac or fetal pole within the sac, as ectopic pregnancies may have a "pseudosac" present and confuse interpretation. Observing these correlations between hCG level and sonogram findings, 94% of normal gestations will be seen when hCG levels are above the discriminatory zone.

Other than as a reference for sonographic interpretation, a single hCG level provides little information with regard to diagnosing an ectopic pregnancy. More helpful than a single hCG is the pairwise hCG measurements taken 48 hours apart. Failure of a 66% or greater rise in hCG will identify 87% of ectopics and incorrectly label 15% of normal gestations as ectopic. Parenthetically, it is critical that the two samples are assayed in the same laboratory. Values can markedly differ from laboratory to laboratory, depending on what method of assay is utilized and what standard is referenced.

Progesterone production is also decreased in ectopic gestations and has been used as a marker for abnormal pregnancies. Low progesterone levels may signal an abnormal gestation before hCG levels reach the discriminatory zone for ultrasound evaluation. Progesterone levels below 5 ng per mL have been correlated absolutely to nonviable gestations (intrauterine and extrauterine). Progesterone levels less than 15 ng per mL are present in 81% of ectopics, 93% of abnormal gestations, and only 11% of normal intrauterine gestations. Levels above 25 ng per mL are seen in fewer than 2% of ectopics. The interpretation of progesterone is obfuscated, however, when considering the patient who conceives by clomiphene or menotropins. Because these cycles are as a rule multifollicular and, consequently, multi–corpora luteal, their progesterone levels may be elevated, even when an abnormal gestation is present.

Creatine kinase (CK), an intracellular metabolic enzyme that catalyzes adenosine triphosphate (ATP), is important for both contractile and transport systems. CK levels are highest in skeletal muscle, myocardium, and brain. Initial reports of levels over 45 IU per liter as predictive of ectopic pregnancy resulting from the gestation's damage to smooth muscle within the fallopian tube have been disputed. These discrepancies may be caused in part by the populations studied by each author. That is, when CK levels are measured among symptomatic patients, the levels are truly elevated. When asymptomatic patients are compared with control patients, no differences can be identified. Quite possibly, the worth of the CK measurement may be limited to the patient with abdominal pain of unclear etiology, where ultrasound findings are inconclusive and only qualitative hCG levels are available.

MANAGEMENT

Surgery

Since 1884, salpingectomy has been the traditional approach to the patient with ectopic pregnancy. Laparoscopy has obviated the need for laparotomy in many cases, and also provided the patient with a shorter hospital course and faster recovery time. Additionally, both salpingectomy and salpingosotomy may be performed through the laparoscope, the latter procedure indicated for cases of ampullary gestation. This more conservative approach is particularly valuable for the younger patient, in whom future fertility is a concern.

There is a 5 to 10% risk of a "persistent" ectopic pregnancy following salpingostomy. This entity exists because the trophoblastic tissue was incompletely removed at the time of the initial surgery. The villi continue to grow, and the patient classically becomes symptomatic 10 to 20 days following the primary surgery. It is therefore critical that following any conservative surgical procedure for ectopic pregnancy, hCG levels be monitored in the patient postoperatively until they become negative. In the case of persistent ectopic pregnancy, a second surgical procedure may be performed to remove the tube, or the patient may be treated medically with methotrexate.

Medical

Although a variety of medical agents have been employed to treat ectopic pregnancy (e.g., actinomycin-D,* prostaglandins, RU486, hyperosmolar glucose, potassium chloride), methotrexate* has been used most often. As a folic acid antagonist, methotrexate inhibits the synthesis of purines and pyrimidines, thereby interfering with DNA synthesis and cell division. Multidose regimens along with a citrovorum (leucovorin [Wellcovorin]) rescue were soon abandoned in favor of a single-dose approach. The single dose offered safe and effective treatment for patients with unruptured ectopic pregnancies and virtually eliminated chemotherapeutic side effects, which occurred in as many as 10 to 50% of those receiving the multidose regimen (Table 1).

The standard dose of methotrexate is 50 mg/m^2 intramuscularly, where the calculation of body surface area is made by obtaining the height and weight of the patient and referring to a nomogram. The leucovorin "rescue" is not administered. Patients are asked to abstain from alcohol, nonsteroidal anti-inflammatory drugs, intercourse, folic acid–containing substances (prenatal vitamins), and sun exposure because of photosensitivity.

---

*Not approved by the Food and Drug Administration for this indication.

TABLE 1. **Protocol for Treatment of Unruptured Ectopic Pregnancy**

Day 0:	CBC with platelets, SGOT, BUN, serum creatinine, blood type and Rh (within 1.5 times normal values) hCG, progesterone level
Day 1:	Methotrexate administered
Day 4:	hCG
Day 7:	hCG, CBC, SGOT Monitor hCG titers biweekly until hCG levels < 15 IU/L

A decline in hCG levels by at least 15% between consecutive measurements is necessary to document success. The 15% figure represents the typical hCG assay variation present, and a change in value of less than that number cannot reliably document response. A second identical dose of methotrexate may be given if the values plateau or begin to rise. Transient pelvic pain is common 3 to 7 days following the administration of methotrexate and may persist for 4 to 12 hours. This pain is believed to represent tubal abortion and resolution. Following resolution of the ectopic pregnancy and disappearance of hCG titers, the patient is advised to avoid pregnancy for 2 months and may use either barrier or oral contraception.

A serum progesterone taken prior to methotrexate administration has value with regard to prediction for success of medical management. That is, among a group of non-progesterone supplemented pregnancies, a progesterone level of 10 ng per mL or less predicted success among all patients, whereas less than half of patients with progesterone values over 10 ng per mL responded.

Overall, approximately 96% of properly selected patients treated with methotrexate will not require surgery. The mean time to resolution is 36 days. Only 3.3% of patients will require a second dose of methotrexate.

Reproductive performance after methotrexate treatment is comparable to that after traditional surgical methods. Follow-up hysterosalpingography results in one large series of methotrexate-treated women demonstrated an 84.5% patency rate on the involved side, and subsequently 89.2% pregnancies were intrauterine and 10.8% recurrent ectopics.

VAGINAL BLEEDING BEYOND THE FIRST TRIMESTER OF PREGNANCY

method of
HUNG N. WINN, M.D., and
JOSEPH B. SHUMWAY, M.D., M.P.H.
St. Louis University School of Medicine
St. Louis, Missouri

Vaginal bleeding is one of the common complications occurring during the last two trimesters of pregnancy. Maternal and perinatal mortality and morbidity depend on the prompt diagnosis and treatment of the condition. Vaginal bleeding from abruptio placentae is usually associated with abdominal pain, whereas that associated with placenta previa or vasa previa is usually painless. This chapter addresses the three most common causes of vaginal bleeding beyond the first trimester: abruptio placentae, placenta previa, and vasa previa.

ABRUPTIO PLACENTAE

Abruptio placentae is the most frequent cause of acute decompensated disseminated intravascular coagulation in the obstetric patient. The incidence of abruptio placentae varies from 0.2 to 2.4% of all pregnancies. The etiology of abruptio placentae is usually unknown. Risk factors include a history of severe abruptio placentae in a previous pregnancy, high parity, hypertensive disease of the mother, cigarette smoking, cocaine use, and external trauma. The role of other proposed causes, such as polyhydramnios, a short umbilical cord, uterine anomalies, and folate deficiencies remains obscure and is not likely to be significant.

The clinical manifestations of abruptio placentae depend on the site of placental implantation, the degree of separation, the amount of blood lost, and the presence of disseminated intravascular coagulation. Women with extensive placental separations usually present complaining of abdominal pain and vaginal bleeding. It must be remembered that the amount of vaginal bleeding is not a reliable indicator of the degree of placental separation. Significant amounts of blood can be concealed within the uterus until delivery. When fetal death occurs, maternal blood loss commonly amounts to 2500 mL and may exceed 5000 mL. Maternal complications include anemia, hypovolemic shock, acquired consumptive coagulopathy, renal failure, postpartum hemorrhage, and the sequelae of ischemic damage to distant organs. The uterus is often tetanically contracted, and fetal heart tones may be absent. In the case of significant abruptio placentae (> 30% of placenta is separated from the uterine wall), an ultrasound examination usually reveals a retroplacental sonolucent mass representing a blood clot. Ultrasound examination may not detect mild abruptio placentae or a marginal separation of a normally implanted placenta.

The occurrence of disseminated intravascular coagulation seems to be related to the degree of placental separation and retroplacental bleeding. The greater the separation, the higher the likelihood of significant bleeding and acquired coagulopathy. Disseminated intravascular coagulation with fibrinogen concentrations of less than 100 mg per deciliter complicates one third to one fourth of the cases. It has been postulated that thromboplastic material is introduced through the maternal venous sinuses and that activation of the extrinsic mechanism of blood coagulation results in disseminated intravascular coagulation. It must be stressed that the bleeding diathesis associated with abruptio placentae is due not only to fibrinogen consumption but also to depletion of other coagulation factors, such as factors V and VIII, and to the anticoagulant effects of fibrin degradation products. The clinical course and laboratory findings of the coagulopathy of abruptio placentae are those of decompensated acute disseminated intravascular coagulation.

The fetal mortality rate in abruptio placentae has been reported to be over 50%, and a significant number of perinatal deaths occur prior to hospital admission. The fetal complications in this disorder are related to hypoxemia and anemia. Hypoxemia results from maternal hypovolemia, anemia, and reduction of the available placental interface for fetal-maternal exchange. When fetal anemia occurs, it is probably caused by bleeding from lacerated villi.

The management of individual cases of abruptio placentae depends on gestational age, fetal status, severity of the abruption, feasibility of vaginal delivery, and the presence of shock and disseminated intravascular coagulation. In the cases of severe abruptio placentae, as evidenced by such conditions as coagulopathy, hypotension from hypovolemia or fetal distress, delivery is indicated. If the fetus is previable or dead, every effort should be made to accomplish vaginal delivery because this imposes less-severe demands on the hemostatic system than hysterotomy or cesarean section. If fetal distress is present in a viable infant, delivery should be accomplished in the most expeditious way; cesarean section is likely to improve perinatal salvage. If fetal distress is not present, vaginal delivery may be attempted, provided fetal assessment, anesthesia, blood products, and operating room access are readily available. Induction of labor should begin with amniotomy if it is feasible. The loss of amniotic fluid decreases intrauterine volume and allows more effective hemostasis at the placental site. Following delivery, control of uterine bleeding depends on myometrial contraction, which constricts the severed vessels at the placental implantation site. This mechanism cannot operate efficiently in abruptio placentae because the uterine cavity remains distended by the presence of the fetus. Because the maternal venous sinuses are opened, thromboplastic material can be infused into the maternal circulation. Oxytocin administration by intravenous infusion may be started immediately following the amniotomy.

A patient with mild or moderate abruptio placentae whose condition is stable and whose fetus is immature may be managed expectantly. Tocolysis may be attempted to prolong the pregnancy. Close monitoring of fetal well-being and fetal growth is important because fetal distress and fetal growth retardation may occur because of placental insufficiency.

PLACENTA PREVIA

Placenta previa is classified as complete, partial, or marginal depending on whether the placenta completely, partially, or marginally covers the internal cervical os. It is important to note that the lower uterine segment undergoes significant growth during the later half of the pregnancy. As a result, most cases of complete, partial, or marginal placenta that are commonly seen during the first and second trimesters resolve by the third trimester. The incidence of placenta previa is estimated at 0.5% of all live births. Epidemiologic risk factors include advanced maternal age (>35 years), increased parity (three pregnancies or greater), and previous cesarean delivery. The risk of placenta previa increases proportionally with each additional cesarean delivery.

Placenta previa typically presents with painless vaginal bleeding. Twenty-five percent of patients also have uterine contractions. Placental disruption secondary to the development of the lower uterine segment in preparation for labor is probably the mechanism for bleeding in placenta previa. As the lower uterine segment thins in the second half of the pregnancy, the abnormally implanted placenta previa bleeds as its implantation site is disrupted. Complete placenta previa is more likely to cause a significant maternal bleeding than partial or marginal placenta, and the hemorrhage can be brisk and life threatening.

Diagnostic ultrasound evaluation is usually definitive in diagnosing placenta previa and thus makes a "double-setup" examination rarely necessary. In the presence of an obese patient or posterior previa, transvaginal or transperineal ultrasound examination may be necessary to clearly visualize the placenta in relation to the internal cervical os.

If a double-setup examination is necessary, there should be full capability to proceed to emergency cesarean delivery, because massive vaginal bleeding may occur. Preparation may include a stand-by anesthesiologist, typing and screening for packed red blood cells, and ready intravenous access. Digital examination of the vaginal fornices for fullness and cautious examination of the internal cervical os for placenta may be attempted by an experienced physician.

The management of placenta previa depends on many factors, such as the gestational age, the extent of persistent hemorrhage, presence of uterine contractions, status of fetal well-being as demonstrated by real-time ultrasound evaluation and fetal heart rate monitoring, and fetal lie within the uterus.

Once the vaginal bleeding stops and preterm labor is controlled, outpatient management is acceptable for those whose fetuses are immature. Proximity to the hospital and a highly motivated patient are essential ingredients for success. If significant recurrent vaginal bleeding recurs, hospitalization is recommended. Amniocentesis may be considered in patients at 34 to 36 weeks of gestation to determine fetal lung maturity prior to delivery.

The mode of delivery depends on the type of placenta previa, gestational age, and fetal status. Vaginal delivery may be attempted in the cases of: (1) a marginal or partial placenta previa with minimal vaginal bleeding and reassuring fetal well-being during labor and delivery or (2) complete placenta previa with intrauterine fetal demise, lethal fetal malformations or previable gestations (<22 weeks). Appropriate backup emergency capabilities should be available. Cesarean section is indicated in the presence of complete previa, fetal distress, or severe vaginal bleeding.

At the time of delivery, several caveats must be remembered. In the presence of a prior cesarean section delivery or other uterine surgery, there is an increased risk not only for placenta previa but also for excessive postpartum bleeding from placenta accreta, increta, or percreta. These represent abnormally firm attachment of the placenta to the uterus. The potential for cesarean hysterectomy should be discussed with the patient prior to delivery because it is likely to be necessary in two thirds of patients with placental accreta or increta. Various conservative surgical measures such as packing the lower segment, use of argon beam photocoagulation of the raw uterine/placental bed, and angiographic embolization of pelvic vessels have been attempted with success.

VASA PREVIA

An important and rare cause of third-trimester painless vaginal bleeding is vasa previa. In vasa previa, velamentous insertion of the umbilical cord into the placenta places those fetal vessels at risk of bleeding on rupture of the fetal membranes. Velamentous and marginal insertions of the umbilical cord are common in placenta previa and in multiple gestations (particularly in monochorionic, diamniotic twin gestation). Fetal exsanguination can occur rapidly, and fetal mortality rates in this condition approach 50%.

The combination of significant vaginal bleeding, fetal distress, and rupture of membranes is pathognomonic of vasa previa. Fetal tachycardia or a sinusoidal pattern on the fetal heart rate monitor may be the earliest sign of a vasa previa in the presence of significant vaginal bleeding. Fetal survival depends on timely diagnosis and intervention. Diagnosis of this condition can be made by demonstrating fetal red blood cells in the blood passing vaginally using the Apt test (sodium hydroxide elution testing). As adult oxyhemoglobin is less resistant to alkali than fetal oxyhemoglobin, fetal blood appears pink, and adult blood appears as a brownish supernatant after being oxidized. Alternatively, fetal blood can be diagnosed by measuring the mean corpuscular volume using the Coulter machine. Fetal red blood cells have higher mean corpuscular volume than maternal red blood cells. Once the diagnosis is made, prompt delivery by cesarean section is necessary to reduce the perinatal mortality and morbidity.

GENERAL MANAGEMENT

A patient with significant uterine bleeding during the third trimester should be cared for in the labor and delivery unit. The initial management involves obtaining a maternal medical history, performing a physical examination including an ultrasound examination of the uterus and the fetus, and establishing intravenous access. Relevant and important maternal history includes maternal blood type, prior vaginal bleeding, the amount of bleeding, trauma to the abdomen or genital area, bleeding diathesis, presence of abdominal pain, leakage of fluid, fetal movement, gestational age, and results of prior ultrasound examinations. Physical examination may include recording of vital signs, a speculum examination of the vagina and cervix to determine the amount and source of vaginal bleeding, and the existence of any apparent cervical or vaginal lesions. An ultrasound examination of the uterus and the fetus is helpful in assessing the fetal anatomy, the amount of amniotic fluid, the status and location of the placenta, and the location of the umbilical cord. A secure intravenous route for administration of blood and fluid should be started by using a 16- or 18-gauge cannula, and blood for baseline studies (hematocrit, platelet count, fibrinogen, prothrombin time, partial thromboplastin time, fibrinogen split products) should be obtained. It is important to initiate continuous monitoring of uterine contractions to detect preterm labor and fetal heart rates to assess fetal well-being.

If there are signs of circulatory collapse from severe bleeding associated with placenta previa or severe abruptio placentae, rapid-volume replacement is necessary to prevent acute renal failure. Replacement with Ringer's lactate solution is initiated pending availability of blood products. In the case of abruptio placentae with a fetal demise, a maternal deficit of at least 1000 to 2000 mL of blood can be estimated. A central venous pressure line may be necessary to assess the effectiveness of intravascular volume replacement. The average central venous pressure in the third trimester is about 10 cm H_2O, which can be used as a guide to follow the progress of fluid replacement.

Disseminated intravascular coagulation may occur in the setting of severe abruptio placentae or deficiency of coagulation factors from severe bleeding. Fresh-frozen plasma can be used to replace the hemostatic components consumed in disseminated intravascular coagulation, such as fibrinogen, factor V, factor VIII, and antithrombin III. Cryoprecipitate is the most volume-efficient form of fibrinogen replacement. Its use is indicated when fibrinogen concentrations are below 100 mg per dL. Each unit of cryoprecipitate contains approximately 250 mg of fibrinogen and raises the fibrinogen concentration by approximately 5 mg per dL. Once the fibrinogen level is above 100 mg per dL, volume replacement therapy can be given as packed red cells and fresh-frozen plasma or crystalloid solutions. The best combination is packed red cells and fresh-frozen plasma, because it provides more labile coagulation factors than whole blood and avoids crystalloid-induced dilution of circulating coagulation factors.

Expectant management for patients with mild

bleeding from placenta previa or abruptio placentae between 24 to 35 weeks is usually successful. The psychologic health of the mother should be frequently assessed, as prolonged bed rest and disruption of usual routines is a significant source of stress. However, all patients with active bleeding will need continuous fetal monitoring, preferably in the setting of an obstetric unit. Transfusion of packed red blood cells may be necessary to maintain maternal hematocrit of 27 to 30%. Each unit of packed red blood cells can be expected to increase the maternal hemoglobin by 1 to 1.5 grams per dL and the hematocrit by 3%. All Rh-negative mothers (in whom the Rh of the fetus is unknown) require RhoGAM administration to prevent Rh isoimmunization. A Kleihauer-Betke acid elution test of maternal blood can be used to determine the amount of fetal blood in the maternal circulation. One 300-μg vial of RhoGAM protects against 30 mL of fetal red cells in the maternal circulation from fetomaternal hemorrhage.

Expectant management of placenta previa and abruptio placentae may include the judicious use of tocolytic therapy if preterm labor also occurs. Maternal administration of corticosteroids may be given to accelerate fetal pulmonary maturity to fetuses who have immature lungs or are less than 34 gestational weeks if delivery is anticipated within 48 hours. There is no ideal choice for tocolytic agent, as both beta mimetics and intravenous magnesium have untoward effects. Magnesium sulfate is preferable to beta mimetics because the latter have more cardiovascular effects (hypotension, tachycardia), which may worsen the maternal hemodynamics. Magnesium can be given as a bolus of 4 to 6 grams over 20 minutes and then at the maintenance infusion dose of 1 to 3 grams per hour to control the uterine contractions. The solution is prepared by mixing 40 grams of magnesium sulfate in 1000 mL of 0.45 normal saline solution. Close monitoring of the patient for signs of toxicity by physical examination is essential. Serum level of magnesium may be helpful in diagnosing magnesium toxicity and may be ordered when the clinical situation indicates. Side effects include maternal flushes, hyporeflexia, muscle weakness, and, in toxic levels, respiratory depression, pulmonary edema, and cardiovascular collapse. Intravenous magnesium sulfate should be used with caution in patients with impaired renal function, because renal secretion is the main route of elimination. Magnesium sulfate should also be used with caution in patients with a history of recent myocardial infarction. Magnesium sulfate is contraindicated in the presence of myasthenia gravis because of its suppression of motor end-plate transmission. Overdose of $MgSO_4$ may be treated with 1 gram of calcium gluconate given by intravenous push with excellent results.

HYPERTENSIVE DISORDERS OF PREGNANCY

method of
LINE LEDUC, M.D.
Sainte-Justine Hospital
Montréal, Québec, Canada

Hypertensive disorders in pregnancy remain one of the major causes of fetal and maternal morbidity and mortality. Hypertensive pregnant women are at risk for abruptio placentae, cerebrovascular accidents, end-organ failure, and disseminated intravascular coagulation, and the fetuses are at risk for prematurity, intrauterine growth retardation, and death.

There are currently no uniform guidelines for the management of hypertension in pregnancy because of insufficient information on the necessity of pharmacologic intervention and how to initiate it. The pharmacologic treatment of hypertension remains a clinical challenge for the clinician, who must consider the benefits and risks of acute and long-term therapy for both the mother and the fetus.

BLOOD PRESSURE CHANGES IN NORMAL PREGNANCY

Blood pressure is highest when the patient is seated and lowest when she lies on her side. Furthermore, there is a 10- to 12-mm Hg difference in blood pressure between the superior and inferior arms in the lateral recumbent position, the superior arm having the lower pressure. This emphasizes the need for consistency when measuring blood pressure in pregnancy.

Peripheral vascular resistance falls during pregnancy, resulting in a progressive decrease in systemic arterial blood pressure during the first 24 weeks of gestation, with a nadir between 16 and 20 weeks, at which time systolic pressure declines on average by 5 to 10 mm Hg, and diastolic pressure drops by 10 to 15 mm Hg. After 24 weeks of gestation, systolic and diastolic pressures rise gradually and return to nonpregnant levels by term. Acknowledgement of these physiologic changes is important because chronic hypertension may be masked by the fall in blood pressure in mid-pregnancy, and a diagnosis of pre-eclampsia may be made erroneously in the third trimester on the basis of increments in blood pressure if no consideration has been given to it in the first and second trimesters.

CLASSIFICATION

The most widely used classification is the one proposed by the American College of Obstetrics and Gynecology in 1972 and endorsed by the National High Blood Pressure Education Program Working Group Report in 1990. This consensus has classified hypertension associated with gestation in four categories: chronic hypertension, pre-eclampsia, pre-eclampsia superimposed on chronic hypertension, and transient hypertension.

Chronic Hypertension

Essential or secondary chronic hypertension is defined as blood pressure of 140/90 mm Hg or greater before or after pregnancy or before the 20th week of gestation. Mild or moderate chronic hypertension usually has an uncomplicated course during pregnancy. The severe form of the disease is associated with certain fetal morbidity and mortality.

Pre-eclampsia

Pre-eclampsia, a disorder unique to pregnancy, is characterized by a triad of hypertension, proteinuria, and edema. It occurs in 2 to 7% of all pregnancies after the 20th week of gestation. The exact etiology is still unknown, but mounting evidence implicates endothelial dysfunction and vasospasm as being responsible for many clinical manifestations of the disease. Traditionally, hypertension is defined as blood pressure of 140/90 mm Hg or greater. Readings exceeding 140/90 mm Hg, particularly those exceeding 160/110 mm Hg, have been linked with adverse maternal and neonatal outcomes, especially in the presence of new-onset proteinuria. The second sign, proteinuria, is consistently defined in the literature as the excretion of proteins in urine in excess of 300 mg in 24 hours (0.3 gram per day). A 24-hour urine collection remains the most reliable method of measurement. Commercially available dipsticks permit simple and rapid testing, but the results are unreliable; positive results (+1 or greater) warrant further evaluation with 24-hour urine collection, and negative results do not necessarily rule out proteinuria. The third clinical sign, edema, must be interpreted with caution, because edema of the face or hands is reported in 64% of normotensive women, whereas as many as 40% of women with eclampsia have no edema before the onset of convulsions.

This multisystemic disease can be mild or severe; it can develop slowly or acutely. When other organs are involved, it is automatically classified as severe. End-organ failure can result. There are alterations in liver function and integrity with elevated alanine aminotransferase, aspartate transaminase, and hematologic disorders such as thrombocytopenia, seen in 17 to 35% of cases. Microangiopathic intravascular hemolysis can occur with the presence of schistocytes, elevated lactate dehydrogenase, and heightened indirect bilirubin levels. Disseminated intravascular coagulation with both prolonged prothrombin time and partial thromboplastin time is rare. A differential diagnosis must be made at this point with the hemolysis, elevated liver enzymes, and low platelets (HELLP) syndrome, acute fatty liver, hemolytic uremic syndrome, and thrombotic thrombocytopenic purpura.

In the kidney, reversible glomerular damage is noted with the presence of proteinuria. When oliguria turns to anuria, we need to rule out acute tubular necrosis or, in the worst cases, cortical necrosis.

Pre-eclampsia Superimposed on Chronic Hypertension

Once a patient is affected by vascular disease, there is an associated risk of subsequent pre-eclampsia during pregnancy in 15 to 25% of cases. A differential diagnosis between deterioration of the hypertension versus the onset of pre-eclampsia is sometimes difficult to make. A rapid increase in 24-hour proteinuria or laboratory signs suggesting organ changes, such as elevated liver enzymes or thrombocytopenia, can help in diagnosing pre-eclampsia.

Transient Hypertension

This disorder is characterized by the onset of isolated hypertension at the end of pregnancy or in the early puerperium. It usually disappears by 10 days post partum.

Transient hypertension usually recurs in later pregnancies and often predicts ultimate chronic hypertension. It is most often latent essential hypertension unmasked by pregnancy.

HEMODYNAMIC CHANGES AND INVASIVE MONITORING

Major hemodynamic changes occur during pregnancy with a fall in systemic vascular resistance and mean arterial pressure and an increase in cardiac output and plasma volume. With the onset of pre-eclampsia, the hemodynamic settings are different: systemic vascular resistance rises, mean arterial pressure is elevated, and cardiac output can vary from an increase to normal or a decrease.

In the presence of persistent oliguria unresponsive to volume therapy, pulmonary edema of unclear etiology, or cardiac failure, it may be appropriate to centrally monitor the patient with a Swan-Ganz catheter for appropriate management. Left atrial diastolic pressure, i.e., pulmonary postcapillary wedge pressure (PCWP) rather than only central venous pressure (CVP), should be documented because no direct or indirect linear correlation exists between CVP and PCWP.

MANAGEMENT: WHEN TO DELIVER

Delivery is the definitive treatment of choice. When severe pre-eclampsia or eclampsia presents, the patient needs to be delivered, regardless of gestational age. However, in pregnancies of less than 32 weeks, conservative management is possible in selected cases with severe disease. These cases should be confined to a hospital setting, preferably a tertiary care center with daily maternal and fetal monitoring and where high-risk obstetrics and neonatal intensive care expertise are available. Some centers have reported excellent results with home management of selected patients. Outpatient surveillance appears reasonable when daily maternal and fetal monitoring is provided. Worrisome signs, such as persistent severe headache, blurred vision, high blood pressure uncontrolled with antihypertensive medication, thrombocytopenia with a platelet count less than 100,000/mm^3, liver enzyme levels greater than 3 SD above the mean, oliguria (< 500 mL/24 hours), or rising creatinine with progressive renal insufficiency, pulmonary edema, eclampsia or the HELLP syndrome will dictate delivery.

Sometimes, close monitoring of patients with severe preeclampsia may be undertaken over 48 hours to allow time for betamethasone to enhance fetal pulmonary maturity. This close observation can only be provided in a tertiary care center.

NONPHARMACOLOGIC TREATMENT

Nonpharmacologic approaches are of uncertain benefit. They may be an option, depending mainly on blood pressure, the specific hypertensive disorder, its degree of severity, and other maternal and fetal risk factors.

Bed Rest

Bed rest is the most often prescribed treatment for hypertensive disorders in pregnancy. However, there is no evidence offered by well-designed controlled trials to support its effectiveness. Meta-analysis comparing the effect of hospital admission with or without bed rest in the management of hypertension in pregnancy with proteinuria was done in two clinical research trials (CRTs) involving a total of 145 women. No significant differences were found in any of the outcomes measured. Therefore, we cannot recommend strict bed rest in patients with hypertensive disorders.

Volume Therapy

Meta-analysis of the effect of plasma volume expansion in the treatment of hypertension in pregnancy involved a total of 42 women. It reported no beneficial effect. Further studies are needed before this approach can be supported.

PREVENTION OF PRE-ECLAMPSIA

Calcium Supplementation

The results of 13 CRTs and several meta-analyses have suggested that calcium supplementation (2 grams per day) reduces the incidence of pre-eclampsia. The most recent CRT on this topic, involving 4589 healthy nulliparous women, revealed in 1997 that pre-eclampsia occurred in 6.9% of cases in the calcium group versus 7.3% in the placebo group. There were nonsignificant differences between the two groups in the prevalence of pregnancy-associated hypertension without pre-eclampsia (15.3% vs. 17.3%) or of all hypertensive disorders (22.2% vs. 24.6%). Mean systolic and diastolic blood pressures during pregnancy were similar in both groups. Calcium did not reduce the numbers of preterm deliveries, small-for-gestational age cases, or fetal or neonatal deaths, nor did it increase urolithiasis during pregnancy. The utility of calcium supplementation in patients at high risk of pre-eclampsia needs to be confirmed with further well-designed studies.

Low-Dose Acetylsalicylic Acid Therapy

Initial interest in the use of acetylsalicylic acid (ASA) (60 to 80 mg per day) therapy in the prevention of pre-eclampsia arose because of the finding of an increase in in vitro placental imbalance in the production of vasoactive prostaglandins (thromboxane A_2 [TXA_2]) and prostacyclin (PGI_2) leading to platelet activation and arteriolar vasoconstriction. PGI_2 produced in the vascular endothelium induces inhibition of platelet aggregation and is an active vasodilator. TXA_2, synthesized predominantly by platelets, has opposite effects, with activation of platelet aggregation and vasoconstriction.

Low-dose ASA selectively suppresses the synthesis of platelet TXA_2. Meta-analysis of all trials has revealed a 25% odds reduction in pre-eclampsia, with a modest decline in the incidence of preterm delivery (19.8% to 18.3%) and low birthweight (8.7% to 7.9%) but no significant decrease in perinatal mortality. However, ASA is not beneficial once pre-eclampsia is clinically evident. It appears to be safe for use in pregnancy. No significant maternal or fetal bleeding has been observed, even during epidural anesthesia. Up to now, it seems reasonable to give ASA daily to patients at high risk of pre-eclampsia, such as women with previous severe preterm pre-eclampsia (<34 weeks) and women with chronic hypertension. However, some concerns have been raised regarding the efficacy of ASA in preventing of pre-eclampsia since the publication of a study in 1997. In this study, 2503 women were grouped into four high-risk categories: diabetes, multiple gestations, previous pre-eclampsia, and chronic hypertension. Each was randomized to receive either ASA, 60 mg, or placebo. Low-dose ASA did not reduce the incidence of pre-eclampsia in these high-risk patients, and the medication had no effect on proteinuric hypertension, preterm birth, or fetal growth. Thus, ASA efficacy is questioned, but a consensus will be needed before this preventive approach is changed.

A role for ASA can be maintained in cases with the antiphospholipid syndrome. Anticardiolipin antibodies are known to be associated with an increased risk of arterial and venous thrombotic disorders. Antiphospholipid syndrome is characterized by recurrent fetal loss, fetal growth retardation, and severe early-onset pre-eclampsia. The most recent therapeutic regimen proposed consists of low-dose ASA in addition to heparin.

TABLE 1. **Antihypertensive Medication in Acute, Severe Hypertension in Pregnancy**

		Dose	Onset of Action	Side Effects
First-Line Drugs	Hydralazine (Apresoline)	5 mg IV/IM, then 5–10 mg q 20–40 min	IV 10 min IM 10–30 min	Tachycardia, flushing headache, nausea/vomiting
	Labetalol (Trandate, Normodyne)	20 mg IV, then 20–80 mg IV q 20–30 min—max 300 mg	5–10 min	Flushing, nausea, vomiting, tingling of scalp
	Nifedipine (Adalat)	5–10 mg PO, then in 30 min if necessary, followed by 10–20 mg PO BID, QID	10–15 min	Headache, flushing, tachycardia, nausea, myometrial relaxation
Special Indications (Patient Refractory to First-Line Drugs)	Diazoxide (Hyperstat)	30–50 mg IV q 5–15 min	2–5 min	Severe hypotension, hyperglycemia, myometrial relaxation, fluid retention with repeated doses
	Na^+ nitroprusside (Nipride)	0.5–10.0 U/kg/min IV	Instantaneous	Severe hypotension, fetal cyanide toxicity, nausea/vomiting

ANTICONVULSANT THERAPY

Magnesium sulfate ($MgSO_4$) has been the subject of considerable debate in the last few years because of its use as an anticonvulsant for prophylaxis or treatment. Prophylactic anticonvulsant therapy is recommended for all women with high blood pressure and proteinuria. There is one CRT reported in the literature that concludes that $MgSO_4$ is superior to phenytoin for the prevention of eclampsia. $MgSO_4$, phenytoin (Dilantin), and diazepam (Valium) have been compared in women with pre-eclampsia. This large trial, a multicenter randomized study, included 1680 women. $MgSO_4$ was the best anticonvulsant in patients who had seizures, with a 52% lower risk of recurrent seizures than those receiving diazepam and a 67% lower risk than those given phenytoin.

The major side effects of $MgSO_4$ are caused by overdosage in cases of renal insufficiency. This agent can cause hot flushes and dyspnea, as well as transient burning at the intravenous site. It may also cause hypotension or neuromuscular blockade when used concomitantly with nifedipine or in women with muscular dystrophy. It may decrease short- and long-term fetal heart rate variability.

The optimal regimen of $MgSO_4$ dosing has not yet been determined. One way to administer it is to give 4 grams intravenously over 10 minutes followed by a constant infusion of 1 to 2 grams per hour. There is no consensus on whether to administer it to all pre-eclamptic women or only to those with severe cases.

PHARMACOLOGIC TREATMENT OF ACUTE HYPERTENSION

Pregnant women with systolic blood pressure of 170 mm Hg or higher or diastolic pressure of 110 mm Hg or higher or both should receive pharmacologic treatment to prevent maternal intracerebral hemorrhage. For women with lower readings, there is a lack of consensus in the literature on what is appropriate management. In most studies, the treatment goal was to decrease diastolic blood pressure to 90 to 100 mm Hg. Table 1 summarizes the antihypertensive medication choices available. Hydralazine (Apresoline) has been traditionally the first choice to decrease blood pressure in pre-eclampsia. Labetalol and nifedipine, administered intravenously or sublingually, have been demonstrated to be safe and effec-

TABLE 2. **Antihypertensive Medication in Chronic Hypertension in Pregnancy**

		Dose	Side Effects
First-Line Drugs	Methyldopa (Aldomet)	250 mg up to 3 g/d divided in 2–4 doses	Sedation
Second-Line Drugs	Labetalol (Trandate, Normodyne)	200–1200 mg/d divided in two to three doses	None reported
	Pindolol (Visken)	5–30 mg bid	Fetal bradycardia and hypoglycemia may occur
	Oxprenolol (Trasicor)	20 mg tid—max 480 mg/d	Same as pindolol
	Metoprolol (Lopressor)	50–200 mg bid	Fetal bradycardia may occur
	Nifedipine (Adalat)	10–20 mg bid, qid—max 120 mg/d	Myometrial relaxation
	Hydralazine (Apresoline)	25 mg bid, qid—max 300 mg/d	No serious side effects
	Clonidine (Catapres)	0.05–0.4 mg bid	Limited data
Third-Line Drugs	Clonidine + hydralazine; metoprolol + hydralazine; methyldopa + beta blockers or hydralazine		

tive. However, neuromuscular function and blood pressure should be closely watched when using nifedipine and $MgSO_4$ because respiratory depression has been reported. Fetal heart rate should be monitored during acute treatment. Diazoxide is rarely required. It may cause severe hypotension. Sodium nitroprusside must be used with caution and at the lowest dose because it may elicit fetal cyanide toxicity.

PHARMACOLOGIC TREATMENT OF CHRONIC HYPERTENSION

Chronic treatment of hypertension is appropriate in the presence of pre-existing hypertension or in preterm pregnancy complicated by pre-eclampsia when the pregnancy is to be prolonged. No data have been found to determine the optimal blood pressure that is to be attained with antihypertensive treatment. Nevertheless, the incidence rates of perinatal death and intrauterine growth retardation (IUGR) increase with elevation of blood pressure with or without proteinuria. When specified in the trials, the aim of treatment is usually to lower blood pressure to below 90 mm Hg. There is no established blood pressure threshold at which pharmacologic treatment may be started. However, according to the National High Blood Pressure Education Program Working Group, diastolic pressure of higher than 99 mm Hg is the threshold for treatment initiation.

Table 2 summarizes the specific agents that can be used for chronic treatment of hypertension. In cases of pre-existing hypertension, methyldopa has been shown to be effective in preventing severe hypertension. This is our first drug choice because it has been well studied during pregnancy, and its short- and long-term effects have been well documented. Atenolol, labetalol, nifedipine, oxprenolol,* pindolol, or combined treatment with metoprolol and hydralazine but not diuretics is as effective as methyldopa in preventing severe hypertension. Angiotensin-converting enzyme (ACE) inhibitors are contraindicated because of adverse effects on fetal and neonatal renal function, IUGR, and fetal loss. Angiotensin II receptor antagonists are also contraindicated because of theoretical concerns that their side effects could be similar to those of ACE inhibitors. No antihypertensive medication has proven to be effective in preventing pre-eclampsia in women with pre-existing hypertension.

We usually refrain from giving antihypertensive medication in the first and second trimesters to patients with mild to moderate hypertensive disorders because a physiologic fall occurs in blood pressure in the first half of pregnancy. However, for the patients with severe disease, we need to obtain good control of blood pressure with medication to prevent fetal and maternal complications associated with hypertension, such as abruptio placentae, IUGR, and cerebrovascular accidents.

*Not available in the United States.

FUTURE PROJECTIONS

Severe early-onset pre-eclampsia appears more and more to be associated with certain disorders that are likely to provoke an arterial thrombotic process by impairing normal endothelial cell-platelet interactions. Therefore, patients with a history of severe early-onset pre-eclampsia should be screened for protein S deficiency, activated protein C resistance, hyperhomocysteinemia, and anticardiolipin antibodies, because these results may have an impact on pharmacologic management in future pregnancies.

OBSTETRIC ANESTHESIA

method of
BRADLEY E. SMITH, M.D.
Vanderbilt University Medical Center
Nashville, Tennessee

A CENTURY OF PROGRESS IN OBSTETRIC ANESTHESIA

At the beginning of the 20th century, maternal mortality in the United States was incredibly high by today's standards and neonatal mortality was even worse. Most normal labor and birth occurred at home, and cesarean section was very rare. Most women received no anesthesia at all for normal obstetric labor. A form of sedation including morphine and scopalamine called *dammerschlaffe* (twilight sleep) became an almost universal sedative analgesic during most of the first half of the century. This resulted in excited, uncontrollable laboring mothers with no memory of the labor or delivery of the baby. Anesthesia for the occasional instrumented vaginal delivery and for cesarean section was almost entirely by inhalation of ether, chloroform, or cyclopropane. Spinal anesthesia was used in some institutions, but it was not in great favor owing to mixed opinions concerning its potential serious complications.

By the mid-20th century, there had been a remarkable decrease in both maternal and perinatal mortality largely because of better obstetric knowledge, better blood banking techniques, and beginning effectiveness of antibiotics. At the end of the century, maternal mortality has declined to approximately 1 per 10,000 in the United States, and perinatal mortality is below 10 per 1000 live births. Although the forerunner of today's most frequent labor analgesia, lumbar epidural analgesia, was introduced by Robert Hingson in 1942 as caudal epidural anesthesia, it was rarely used until after 1960. "Saddle block" (low spinal) was introduced by John Adriani and John Parmley in 1946, but it met great resistance until the mid 1950s, when for a time it became the most frequent anesthetic for both vaginal and cesarean deliveries.

During the era when general anesthesia held sway, explosions were a constant threat from these agents, but their greatest danger was depression of the respiration of the newborn baby, aspiration of vomitus by the mother, and airway obstruction of the mother during anesthesia. In fact, during that period, 3 to 10% of all maternal mortality was due to complications of general anesthesia. Attention to the effects of obstetric sedation and anesthesia on both babies and mothers was finally focused in 1953 by Virginia Apgar with publication of her famous "Apgar score." However, the use of heavy medication and general anesthesia persisted in many hospitals and regions of the United States, even into the 1980s. By 1999, inhalation anesthesia has almost disappeared in obstetrics as have these complications.

At the end of this century of progress almost every obstetric hospital maintains a qualified staff of highly skilled and trained anesthesia personnel who largely administer only regional block analgesia during obstetric labor and delivery. These highly trained personnel are required because regional anesthesia, despite its marvelous pain-relieving qualities, retains the potential to cause some very serious complications. These include maternal convulsions, "total spinal block," hypotension, and rarely, even paraplegia.

CHOICE OF ANESTHESIA AND ANALGESIA IN NORMAL PREGNANCIES

Pain Relief During Labor

Psychologic Management of Labor Pain

Grantly Dick Read had published his famous treatise entitled "Childbirth Without Fear" only 6 years before the first *Conn's Current Therapy.* His methods, along with related techniques such as natural childbirth, psychoprophylaxis, Lamaze, and medical hypnosis, were slow to gain popularity. Even today, psychologic preparation for labor is a great benefit to most pregnant patients and should not be neglected even when use of continuous epidural analgesia techniques is anticipated. Psychologic support helps the mother relax and better endure the discomfort and reduces the total quantity of necessary sedatives and pain relievers.

Sedative and Narcotic Management of Labor Pain

Heavy prepartum use of narcotic and sedative drugs has almost entirely disappeared from American obstetric practice owing to recognition of their detrimental effects on the infant. However, some centers still use small intravenous doses of these drugs in the prepartum period for reassurance and comfort. A popular method is the use of fentanyl (Sublimaze) 25 μg given intravenously in single bolus doses no more frequently than twice per hour. Some experts may add 0.5 to 1 mg diazepam (Valium) at 1-hour intervals, but I do not because of demonstrated effects on the newborn baby. Additional sedation such as promethazine (Phenergan) or propiomazine (Largon) are used in some centers, but these may also lead to oversedation of the mother and respiratory depression in the newborn baby.

Paracervical Block

Paracervical block, properly administered, delivers major pain relief during cervical dilatation and descent of the head, particularly in multiparous women. When used along with pudendal block, it may be sufficient pain relief for spontaneous or outlet forceps delivery. It is established by infiltration of approximately 10 mL of 1% lidocaine (Xylocaine) in the submucosal tissue of the cervix at 4 and 8 o'clock positions, with a delay between the injections. Careful fetal heart rate monitoring should be carried out during and immediately after each injection. A fetal heart rate of less than 100 along with fetal acidosis can develop immediately after this block. It is recommended that the block be abandoned immediately if fetal bradycardia develops. If fetal bradycardia does develop, alert, expectant waiting will usually be rewarded by return of the fetal heart rate to normal, but persistence of fetal bradycardia may indicate fetal deterioration or imminent fetal demise. However, the incidence of this serious complication is low. The use of bupivacaine (Marcaine) for this block has ceased in many centers because of suggestions that it may cause a higher incidence of fetal bradycardia.

Continuous Lumbar Epidural Analgesia During Labor

The general trend has been toward reduction in concentration of the local anesthetic used in this block. The addition of small doses of opioids in the epidural space improves pain relief and allows such small concentrations of local anesthetic to be used that little or no voluntary muscle paralysis occurs. There is some suggestion that epidural analgesia may slow labor, cause maternal fever, or increase the incidence of forceps or cesarean delivery. Nonetheless, epidural analgesia remains popular because it is effective.

Technique. A large epidural needle is inserted into the epidural space by any of a variety of techniques. A thin plastic catheter is then advanced about 3 cm beyond the needle tip. Immediately, a test to determine whether the catheter tip is epidural, intrathecal, or intravascular is carried out by injection of 3 mL of 1.5% lidocaine with 1:100,000 epinephrine. Signs of excitement, convulsions, respiratory impairment, or tachycardia may indicate intravascular placement, whereas the rapid onset of muscle weakness may indicate intrathecal placement. In the absence of these signs, an initial dose of local anesthetic can be given. One of several acceptable medication schemes is the use of a mixture of 8 to 10 mL of 0.125% bupivacaine and 5 μg per mL of fentanyl. Analgesia can usually be maintained with an infusion of 8 to 12 mL per hour of 0.125% bupivacaine with 5 μg per mL of fentanyl. Bolus doses of up to 4 mL each may be needed if the analgesic level is inadequate.

Combined Spinal-Epidural Analgesia During Labor

Combined spinal-epidural (CSE) analgesia is rapidly superseding the older epidural analgesia techniques for labor. In this method, "spinal" injection of opioids and local anesthesia combined with epidural analgesia vastly relieves early labor pain almost immediately and usually allows the laboring woman to walk about if she chooses.

Technique. CSE analgesia is also sometimes called the "double-needle technique." An epidural needle is initially inserted into the epidural space, followed by placement of a second thin intrathecal needle placed through the first needle. With the patient in the sitting position, many experts inject 10 μg of sufentanil or 25 μg of fentanyl along with 2.5 mg of bupivacaine and 0.2 mg of epinephrine diluted with preservative-free saline to a total volume of 2 to 3 mL of solution.

Anesthesia During Vaginal Delivery

Pudendal Block for Vaginal Delivery

Pudendal block is a useful option, particularly in multiparous women, to establish surgical anesthesia of the perineum. It has no effect on the course of labor and is administered by the obstetrician at the time of birth. Many women may be comfortable during episiotomy, vacuum extraction of the fetus, or even outlet forceps delivery. It is executed by placing 10 mL of 1% lidocaine on each pudendal nerve at the origin of the sacrosciatic ligament. Complications are possible with inadvertent administration of as little as 3 mL of 1% lidocaine into a vein or into a highly vascular area or 300 mg in the less vascular tissues.

Spinal Anesthesia (Saddle Block) for Vaginal Delivery

In the primiparous patient, saddle block anesthesia is usually administered when the infant's head is at about +2 to 3 station late in second stage, but it may be established earlier in the multiparous patient. Hypotension occurs in approximately 18% of patients who receive saddle block anesthetics, so blood pressure should be monitored carefully. Saddle block provides complete pain relief and pelvic relaxation for low forceps and midforceps delivery and fetal rotation or perineal surgery virtually without pain for the mother and does not affect uterine contractions.

Technique. After subarachnoid puncture with the smallest possible needle (25 to 27 gauge) (many now prefer the Sprotte design to avoid spinal headaches), a dose of about 0.5 mL of 0.75% bupivacaine in dextrose, diluted to 1.5 to 2 mL with cerebrospinal fluid, should produce anesthesia to about T-10, if the patient sits erect about 30 seconds after the injection. Some controversy has arisen of late concerning an alleged elevated incidence of radicular pain in the legs associated with the use of 5% lidocaine for this purpose. If lidocaine is to be used because of its more rapid onset, 0.8 to 1 mL (40 to 50 mg) of 5% lidocaine may be diluted to 3 mL with preservative-free 5% glucose.

Inhalation Analgesia for Vaginal Delivery

Inhalation of anesthetic vapors in concentrations too low to produce surgical anesthesia can be a safe and simple form of effective analgesia for vaginal delivery. This technique can allow the mother to remain conversant, alert, and cooperative and self-controlled without danger to the infant. Constant inhalation of 40 to 50% nitrous oxide and oxygen, 0.25 to 0.4% isoflurane (Forane), or 0.5 to 1.0% sevoflurane (Ultane) is effective in producing analgesia and amnesia in approximately 75% of patients. All of these agents demonstrate essentially no effects on the fetus at these low-dose concentrations.

General Anesthesia for Vaginal Delivery

General anesthesia is now almost never used in vaginal delivery except under special circumstances. When it is needed, the dose, depth, and duration of anesthesia before delivery should be minimized. Mixing of all intravenous and inhalational anesthetics with the fetal blood begins almost immediately after administration. Induction of general anesthesia (not "inhalation analgesia") usually calls for endotracheal intubation to avoid aspiration of gastric contents or loss of patency of the airway.

INHALATION ANESTHETIC AGENTS

These anesthetics pass the placenta immediately, and in anesthetic concentrations they can all produce significant respiratory and neurologic depression in the newborn. All but nitrous oxide can lead to postpartum uterine bleeding. Although they are of great help in certain obstetric complications (e.g., tetanic uterine contractions), their routine obstetric use is not recommended because of their ability to "make the infant sleepy." Inhalation of sevoflurane 4 to 6% in 100% oxygen, with reduction to 3% when stable anesthesia is reached, can result in surgical anesthesia in about 3 to 4 minutes but includes a danger of aspiration. More frequently, intravenous induction, a muscle paralysant, and immediate endotracheal intubation are to be preferred.

THIOPENTAL

Thiopental may cause depression of newborn breathing. A dose of 3.5 mg of thiopental (Pentothal) per kg intravenously is commonly used. The shortest interval practical between induction and delivery of the infant is safest for the infant. High-risk or premature infants are even more susceptible to respiratory depression of the newborn.

KETAMINE

Although much slower in onset, intravenous ketamine (Ketalar) in small doses (up to 0.75 mg per kg) is recognized as a reasonable alternative to thiopental for induction in obstetrics. Both immediate and delayed newborn alertness appear better than with thiopental, and the blood pressure of both mother and newborn are better supported. However, neurologic complications and respiratory depression may be caused by ketamine doses greater than 0.75 mg per kg. Rarely, maternal hallucinations may occur during emergence from ketamine, but they can be prevented or treated by 2 mg of intravenous diazepam.

PROPOFOL

This new induction agent is notable for its antinausea qualities and prompt, pleasant emergence. For either vaginal or cesarean delivery, induction with 1.5 to 2.5 mg of propofol (Diprivan) per kg intravenously is pleasant, appears to suppress hypertension due to endotracheal intubation, and has been reported to be no more depressant to the fetus than thiopental.

Anesthesia During Cesarean Section

Major regional analgesia is favored for cesarean section today. The mother is alert and able to participate in and remember the birth, and serious respiratory depression of the infant caused by anesthetics, narcotics, and sedatives is avoided.

Technique of Epidural Block for Cesarean Section

After an infusion is started with a large intravenous catheter, 800 to 1500 mL of intravenous lactated Ringer's solution without dextrose (to avoid responsive neonatal hypoglycemia) is administered to help prevent hypotension. The epidural catheter is placed and tested for safety as outlined earlier. After the test dose, medication for cesarean section under epidural block could include 15 to 22 mL of bupivacaine 0.5% mixed with 100 μg of fentanyl, administered in three divided doses. Later, if discomfort develops, 50 to 75% of the original dose of the same solution may be added about every hour, provided that a pinprick test verifies a safe block level. If some discomfort persists, intravenous analgesics and tranquilizers may be used in reduced doses.

Ketamine in doses of 5 to 10 mg intravenously is used by many experts as a supplemental analgesic-sedative during surgery, and it does not depress respiration in these small doses. However, narcotics and benzodiazepines synergize their respiratory depressant effects when used together, particularly during high regional block analgesia, and therefore extreme alertness for respiratory depression of the mother should always be exercised. Fentanyl in 25-μg intravenous boluses with midazolam (Versed) in 0.5-mg boluses is a common combination used for supplemental analgesia as well.

Technique of Spinal Anesthesia for Cesarean Section

Bupivacaine 0.75% in doses of 8 to 13 mg along with 15 to 20 μg of fentanyl or 0.2 to 0.3 mg of "spinal morphine" (Duramorph) mixed with 0.2 mL of 1:1000 fresh epinephrine is often used for subarachnoid block for cesarean section. After injection, the patient is placed supine with her head on a pillow, and the table is tilted 15 degrees to the left. A pillow, balloon, or wedge is placed under the right hip to displace the uterus away from the vena cava and aorta. Arterial blood pressure is monitored at least every 60 seconds. If the systolic pressure falls 30% below the preanesthesia level or below 100 mm Hg, the left uterine displacement is increased, the Trendelenburg position is steepened, the rate of intravenous infusion is increased, oxygen by face mask is administered, and 12.5 mg of ephedrine or 0.5 to 1 μg of phenylephrine per kg may be used.

Technique of General Anesthesia for Cesarean Section

Before anesthesia is induced, neutralization of acid stomach contents with 30 mL of oral sodium bicitrate (Bicitra) is useful. Some also administer 20 mg of intravenous famotidine (Pepcid) and/or 10 mg of intravenous metoclopramide (Reglan) to reduce production of stomach acid and to promote expulsion of acid into the duodenum. The dangers of aortocaval compression are present during general as well as regional anesthesia. The patient is placed on the operating table in left lateral recumbent position until the start of the skin preparation, then elevated to the left on a pillow, or the uterus should be manually deflected to the left during cesarean section under general as well as regional anesthesia.

Premedication is usually omitted because of its effect on the infant. An intravenous infusion is started with use of a large catheter. During "prepping," the patient is preoxygenated for 3 minutes. When the surgeon is ready, 0.6 mg of scopolamine (for amnesia and protection against vagal cardiovascular reflexes) and 0.3 mg of pancuronium are given about 3 minutes before induction followed by thiopental, 3.5 mg per kg, or ketamine, 0.75 mg per kg. After unconsciousness, intravenous succinylcholine (Anectine), 2 mg per kg, followed by a continuous drip of 0.2% succinylcholine is added. (Some experts prefer the use of a nondepolarizing muscle relaxant such as vecuronium [Norcuron] at a dose of 0.05 mg per kg, but I do not because I strongly believe succinylcholine is safer for the infant.) Cricoid pressure should be instituted and maintained by someone other than the anesthetist as soon as consciousness is impaired. The trachea is intubated and ventilation is checked in both lungs with a stethoscope before the incision is permitted.

Even these limited doses of drugs may result in reduction of alertness or depression of the respirations of the newborn, and therefore preparations for newborn resuscitation should be made in advance. After tracheal intubation, many elect to administer only nitrous oxide 4 liters per minute and oxygen 4 liters per minute until the cord is clamped. In this case, the level of anesthesia can be deepened with thiopental and/or narcotics and/or potent inhalation agents immediately when the cord is clamped. The continuing use of succinylcholine drip (or vecuronium) should be monitored with a nerve block stimulator. Some experts advocate addition of a small dose of fentanyl, sufentanil, or alfentanil (Alfenta) and/or a limited concentration of a potent inhalation anesthetic agent such as 0.5% isoflurane (Forane) before birth of the infant to reduce maternal stress response and the possibility of memory. However, the possibility of respiratory depression in the newborn after administration of these drugs cannot be disregarded.

POSTPARTUM PAIN CONTROL

Control of Postpartum Pain After Vaginal Delivery

The intensity of pain in the postpartum period after vaginal delivery is rarely as severe as in cesarean section. A variety of oral analgesic agents are commonly employed for this purpose (see later), and rarely, a few doses of common parenteral opioid agents are used. Oral and parenteral opioids or even milder oral analgesics such as oxycodone, 5 mg, and acetaminophen, 325 mg orally (Percocet), every 6 hours, often in conjunction with antiprostaglandins (e.g., ibuprofen [Motrin] 400 mg orally every 6 hours), have become standard in treating this type of pain. Research has shown many deficiencies in this method, including “peaks and valleys” in the intensity of pain due to the varying blood levels achieved by intermittent intramuscular injection. On the other hand, this method is by far the least costly of all those that are described here and may be expedient and sufficient in many patients. In the occasional patient with a large episiotomy or perineal lacerations, it may be anticipated that the pain will be severe enough to warrant use of techniques described in conjunction with cesarean section. I do not use ketorolac (Toradol) in obstetric patients.

Patient-Controlled Analgesia After Cesarean Section

Although the concept of patient-controlled analgesia (PCA) is more than 25 years old, its popularity has surged in the past few years. Numerous studies verify that eliminating the peaks and valleys of analgesia along with the undefinable psychologic comfort of knowing that the patient can instantly treat her own pain clearly results in overall administration of a lesser total dose of analgesic agent over any given time. Although many narcotics are in use for PCA, a typical basic plan for PCA might be an initial intravenous bolus of 2 mg of morphine followed by patient-controlled injections of 1 mg of morphine on demand no more frequently than every 10 minutes with a maximal total dose of 14 mg in any 4 hours. Unexpected apnea from the respiratory depressant effects of the opioids has been reported, but it is not as frequent as after intrathecal or epidural use of opioids. This should be anticipated by standing orders for stat intravenous injection of 200 μg of naloxone (Narcan) if the nurse suspects respiratory depression.

CHOICE OF ANESTHESIA AND ANALGESIA IN COMPLICATED PREGNANCIES

Forceps

Forceps are rarely used in modern obstetrics but still have some indications. During the use of forceps or vacuum extraction devices, a relaxed perineum and a quiet patient aid in preventing maternal vaginal lacerations and extension of the episiotomy and help minimize trauma to the infant’s head. These conditions are provided by spinal and epidural blocks, which also allow the mother to participate in the birth.

Breech Presentation

Many experts advocate epidural analgesia for vaginal breech births. An alternative choice consists of good psychologic support supplemented by minimal narcotics and tranquilizers, a paracervical block in the first stage, and a quick induction of general endotracheal anesthesia, including succinylcholine, when the infant’s umbilicus becomes visible.

Multiple Births

The second infant may be delivered under pudendal or local anesthesia in some cases. If the second infant is to be delivered by means of version and breech extraction, endotracheal general inhalation anesthesia may be used to relax the uterus, in which case preparations for active resuscitation of the infant should be made in advance.

Tetanic Contractions

Regional anesthesia does not relax the uterus. The older standard method of rapid relaxation of the uterus during tetanic contractions required endotracheal inhalation anesthesia. A new faster anesthetic, sevoflurane, at 3 to 4% for 3 to 5 minutes is preferable to halothane (Fluothane), which may cause hypotension, or isoflurane, which is slower and may also cause hypotension. Intravenous “beta-stimulator” catecholamines do not work as completely or as rapidly. Intravenous nitroglycerin (in 100- to 300-μg boluses) may relax the uterus but often causes dangerous maternal hypotension.

Fetal Distress

When fetal distress exists, further depression of the newborn by potent anesthetics given to the mother should be avoided. Some experts advocate spinal anesthesia in fetal distress, but if it is used, no time should be wasted, nor should hypotension be tolerated.

Antepartum Hemorrhage

Sudden antepartum bleeding leading to maternal hypotension is detrimental to the fetus, and hypovolemia adds risk to the mother from anesthesia of any type. All forms of major regional block are frequently contraindicated in this emergency, because the resulting sudden sympathetic blockade paralyzes the compensatory mechanisms ordinarily required to maintain the mother’s blood pressure during hemorrhage. Management by local anesthesia, pudendal block, or subanesthetic inhalation analgesia is recommended when applicable, but with all choices, maternal vascular volume should be restored as rapidly as possible with an appropriate fluid. Vasopressors should *not* be used in place of adequate volume replacement. Potent inhalation anesthetics are avoided because they may accentuate the hypotension caused by hypovolemia.

Pregnancy-Induced Hypertension (Toxemia of Pregnancy)

In a toxemic pregnancy, maternal liver and kidney function may be poor, convulsions may be encountered, severe maternal hypertension and increased sensitivity to vasopressors frequently exist, and the infant is often born prematurely and is undernourished. Some obstetricians still believe that hypotension develops more easily during epidural analgesia. Care should be taken to evaluate and correct the hypovolemia frequently seen in toxemia before any regional block is placed. In managing general anesthesia during toxemia, efforts to attenuate the hypertensive response to endotracheal intubation are important. For this, nitroglycerin, 100 to 300 μg, by intravenous bolus is sometimes used. Intravenous magnesium sulfate synergizes with anesthetic muscle relaxants and may contribute to newborn drug depression.

Prematurity

In premature newborns, respiratory and cardiovascular depression can result from pain or anesthetic drugs given to the mother. Continuous epidural analgesia is the method of choice during the first and second stages of labor. Saddle block is excellent for delivery but is not suitable for labor. Pudendal block is not dangerous in prematurity but does not relax the birth canal sufficiently to minimize head trauma to the premature infant.

Diabetes

Major regional analgesia is desirable when practical. Insulin and glucose control should be meticulous and should be monitored frequently during labor and the induction of anesthesia. Most experts restrict maternal intravenous glucose, which may stimulate insulin release by the infant, leading to hypoglycemia.

Cardiac Disease

Less than 2% of pregnant patients suffer from severe heart disease, which is less than half the incidence noted 40 years ago, but an increasing proportion of pregnant cardiac patients today suffer from complicated congenital heart defects. Continuous epidural analgesia is popular for patients with a wide variety of acquired or congenital heart lesions. Great caution should be exercised in regard to the potential of regional anesthesia to precipitate heart failure or intracardiac reversal of shunt by causing a sudden decrease in peripheral systemic resistance. There should be continuing consultation with the cardiologist.

Sickle Cell Disease

Sickle cell disease remains a grave threat to women with the SS hemoglobin configuration and to their infants. Although stasis in the peripheral vascular bed and possible coagulation problems at the needle site have been theoretical objections to the use of major regional analgesia in sickle cell disease, no objective evidence has ever been offered to support these theories. Inhalation anesthesia has not been followed by sickle cell crisis, and there are reports that it may protect against sickling for several hours.

COMPLICATIONS OF ANESTHESIA

Airway Obstruction

Less than 20 years ago, 11 obstetric patients were reported to have died in New York City in one 2-year period because of failure to achieve and maintain ventilation of the lungs during induction of general anesthesia for obstetric delivery. Before induction of general anesthesia, it is essential that the obstetrician and the anesthetist agree on the steps to be taken should intubation of the trachea prove impossible. These will vary according to the condition of the mother and the infant. This "failed intubation" protocol should be instituted skillfully.

Aspiration of Gastric Contents

Aspiration of stomach contents is a major hazard during heavy sedation, under general anesthesia, or even under major regional anesthesia. Until recently, reports from Great Britain demonstrated that 35% of all anesthetic-related obstetric deaths were directly caused by inhalation of stomach contents. However, aspiration of gastric contents is now reported to be fatal in less than 10% of aspirations by obstetric patients in reporting university hospitals. Treatment of aspiration pneumonia should be based on the principles of immediate establishment of airway and ventilation, suppression of transudation by positive end-expiratory intratracheal pressure, and careful monitoring for inadequate ventilation or the delayed development of bacterial pneumonia. Although steroid therapy after aspiration into the trachea has been advocated by many, evidence from animal research indicates that it is ineffective. The combination of famotidine, (Pepcid) 20 mg, and metoclopramide, 10 mg, given orally 90 minutes before surgery as prophylaxis against acid aspiration is helpful.

COMPLICATIONS OF SPINAL AND EPIDURAL ANESTHESIA

Hypotension and Circulatory Failure During Spinal or Epidural Anesthesia

Hypotension and circulatory failure may account for 34% of all maternal deaths due to anesthesia and are also a hazard to the fetus. The most frequent cause of maternal death is the aortocaval compression syndrome complicated by blockade of the sympathetic nervous system incidental to spinal or epidural anesthesia. This syndrome can be diagnosed by the presence of hypotension, dyspnea, and acute apprehension, often with tachycardia. It is treated by lifting the uterus to the left or placing the patient on her left side or tilting the patient to the left with a pillow. Further treatment of hypotension includes position change, vigorous fluid infusion, and, if necessary, a bolus injection of intravenous ephedrine, 5 to 12.5 mg, or phenylephrine, 0.5 to 1 μg per kg.

Seizures Due to Local Anesthetics During Epidural Anesthesia

Convulsions due to local anesthetic drugs may account for about 11% of all disastrous complications of regional anesthesia. Unexpected neurologic events ranging from disorientation to tonic-clonic convulsions after the injection of a local anesthetic drug should be assumed to be due to the local anesthetic until proved otherwise, even in pregnant patients. Local anesthetic-induced convulsions are rarely due to allergy but most often result from elevated blood concentrations of the local anesthetic. Subarachnoid (spinal) anesthesia almost never results in convulsions because of the small dose of local anesthetic. With prompt therapy, lidocaine-induced convulsions have relatively benign neurologic and cardiovascular sequelae; however, seizures due to bupivacaine are much more ominous for cardiovascular collapse. Emergency treatment of local anesthetic convulsions consists of skillful support of cardiovascular function and prompt ventilation. The injection of a small bolus dose (100 mg of thiopental or 5 mg of diazepam) intravenously along with succinylcholine, 40 to 80 mg followed by intermittent positive-pressure breathing, is useful.

Subarachnoid Instillation of Local Anesthetic ("Total Spinal")

Unintended total spinal anesthesia is still a frequent problem during both intended spinal and epidural anesthesia and may occur in as many as 1 in every 1000 attempted epidural blocks. The epidural catheter can "migrate" into the subdural space from the epidural space some hours after original institution of the block, leading to a total spinal after a reinjection. When this occurs during establishment of spinal block, the duration of both respiratory and cardiovascular embarrassment can be expected to be relatively shorter than the planned duration of the intended subarachnoid block. Total spinal anesthesia resulting from subarachnoid injection of local anesthetic that was intended for the epidural space is a greater emergency because the dose of local anesthetic injected is usually much greater than is used for intentional spinal anesthesia. Patients experiencing this unfortunate situation should be adequately sedated immediately until the complete return of spontaneous vital functions. Respiratory and cardiovascular support usually prevents the otherwise fatal outcome of this complication.

Inadvertent Dural Puncture During Attempted Epidural Block

Even a skilled anesthetist may puncture the dura in up to 0.5 to 2% of attempts. A second attempt at an epidural in an adjacent interspace is routine in this event, but extreme care should be taken to administer and observe test doses at every subsequent injection into the epidural catheter. Because postpartum headaches occur in 25 to 75% of patients who have experienced inadvertent dural puncture by the epidural needle, immediate precautions against headache may be desirable. Immediate postpartum instillation of large volumes (up to 60 mL) of normal saline has been 75% successful in preventing headache. Persistent spinal headaches are often eliminated by injections of autologous blood (10 mL) in the epidural space no sooner than the third postpartum day.

Hazards of Obstetric Anesthesia to the Newborn

Three main factors may contribute to anesthesia-related morbidity in newborns: (1) sedatives, analgesics, and anesthetics administered to the mother during labor; (2) trauma of labor and delivery; and (3) asphyxia due to impaired exchange of respiratory gases during labor and delivery. Obstetric factors such as toxins from amnionitis, muscle depression due to magnesium sulfate, and other factors cannot be disregarded. A newborn is more susceptible than an adult to anesthetic overdose because the undeveloped brain is more susceptible to these drugs. Modern practice attempts to minimize the use of prepartum sedatives by encouraging the use of psychologic techniques such as prepared childbirth, regional analgesia techniques, and concurrent use of synergistic but less depressant drugs.

POSTPARTUM CARE

method of
TONY WEN, M.D.
University of Texas Health Science Center at San Antonio
San Antonio, Texas

The postpartum period, or puerperium, has been defined as the first 6 weeks after the delivery of infant and placenta. During this period, the woman undergoes physiologic reversal toward the nonpregnant state and emotional adjustments associated with having a newborn(s). During the immediate puerperium—the first 24 hours—and early puerperium—24 hours to 7 days—the surveillance is focused on the detection of infection, bleeding, and complications associated with anesthesia and delivery in a hospital setting. During the late puerperium—7 days to 6 weeks—these conditions are managed in an outpatient setting, with a focus on breast-feeding and contraceptive issues. In the United States, the maternal mortality rate is 9.1 per 100,000 live births, and most of these deaths (61 to 72%) occur within the postpartum period. The causes of maternal death include pulmonary embolism (31.8%), pre-eclampsia complications (27.9%), hemorrhage (25.7%), and infection (9.4%).

IMMEDIATE PUERPERIUM

Recovery. The patient should be observed closely in the recovery room for 1 hour after vaginal delivery (VD) and for 2 hours after cesarean section (CS) or until the return of motor function after epidural anesthesia. During this period, the vital signs are monitored closely, and the uterine fundus is palpated for contractility and degree of vaginal bleeding. Intravenous crystallized fluid with oxytocin (10 to 20 U per liter) is infused to prevent uterine atony and postpartum hemorrhage (PPH). Subsequently, the parturient is transferred to the postpartum floor, where the vital signs are monitored every 4 to 6 hours; the fluid status is also monitored in the CS patient until she is able to take oral fluids. The day after delivery, hematocrit is drawn to ensure the patient's hemodynamic stability.

Diet and Activity. After VD, the patient may be placed on a regular diet. After CS, she should be placed on ice chips and advanced to clear liquids with active bowel sounds and regular diet with passage of flatus. Ambulation is encouraged after VD. The woman may need assistance initially if an epidural was used or if delivery was complicated by PPH. The CS patients may sit up in a chair on postpartum day (PPD) one and be encouraged to ambulate by PPD two.

Postpartum Hemorrhage

The blood loss from normal VD and CS is 500 mL and 1000 mL, respectively. Postpartum hemorrhage occurs in 5% of deliveries, and its causes include uterine atony (50%), lower genital tract injury (20%), uterine or placental anomalies (20%), and subinvolution or retained placenta (10%). At term, the uterine blood flow is 500 mL per minute; thus, early recognition and intervention (intravenous [IV] fluid and blood product replacement) are important. The birth canal is examined carefully, with special attention to the episiotomy site, cervix, and consistency of the uterus, which should be contracted to the level of the umbilicus.

If uterine atony is unresponsive to fundal massage, oxytocin (Pitocin) infusion, and the emptying of bladder, then pharmacologic agents should be administered to increase uterine tone: (1) oxytocin at 20 to 40 U per liter of intravenous fluid (at 10 mL per minute); (2) methylergonovine (Methergine) or ergonovine (Ergotrate) maleate at 0.2 mg intramuscularly (IM) (contraindicated for cardiac disease or hypertension); (3) prostaglandin 15 methyl-F2-alpha, 250 μg IM (contraindicated for asthma), with the dosage repeated every 15 to 90 minutes, for up to eight doses, with a success rate of 95%.

Persistent PPH requires further evaluation for laceration, coagulopathies, and retained placental fragments, with continuing hemodynamic resuscitation. Large blood clots or placental tissue requires uterine evacuation manually or with large bovine curettage. Uterine packing may be used to achieve hemostasis. In selected stable patients with a bleeding site not easily accessible, angiographic embolization may be useful.

Tears and hematoma may develop during a rapid labor, an instrumental delivery, or with the use of a needle for anesthesia. After delivery, adequate visualization of the cervix, with special attention to the 3- and 9-o'clock positions, where the descending branch of the uterine artery and vein are located, is necessary. Cervical lacerations are the most common complication, but they are rarely severe. Transvaginal reapproximation of the defect is performed with a 2-0 or 3-0 absorbable suture incorporating the apex. More commonly, vaginal and vulvar lacerations occur along the lower and mid-vagina as a sidewall or sulcus tear with generalized venous oozing. Occasional lacerations at the fornix may extend into the cul-de-sac. Interrupted absorbable sutures are placed in the deep portion, followed by running, locking sutures for hemostasis. Some lacerations are better treated with gauze packing in the deep lacerations, followed by counterpacking of the vagina for 24 to 36 hours.

The location and size of the hematoma determine the ease of diagnosis and the severity of hemorrhage. Vulvar hematoma (below the pelvic diaphragm) is least problematic, with the exception of severe vulvar pain. Vaginal hematoma (above the pelvic diaphragm but below the cardinal ligament) is less common and more difficult to diagnose, with vague pelvic pain. Pelvic examination reveals a mass distortion of the mid-vagina, often penetrating deeply, resulting in a large hematoma that may lead to hypovolemic shock. Subperitoneal hematoma (above the cardinal ligament) is the rarest, but because of its location, it can expand into a large potential space of broad ligament and retroperitoneum. Generally, subperitoneal hematoma presents with late symptoms of pelvic pain, hypovolemia, and shock. One needs to be suspicious of any unexplained significant drop in the hematocrit. Most hematomas need exploration and evacuation because of the pain and the possibility of extension. A linear incision is placed over the point of maximal distention or in the hymenal ring, with the blood clot evacuated and the bleeding vessels sutured. The anatomic planes are identified, and the sutures are carefully placed to avoid injury to the ureter, bladder, and bowel. The small cavity may be sutured closed, but the large cavity recovers better with cavity packing and vaginal counterpacking for 12 to 24 hours.

If the patient is hemodynamically stable, occasionally one may follow the stable subperitoneal hematoma with serial ultrasound and allow it to resolve over time. Otherwise, many will require aggressive blood and fluid replacement with laparotomy. The O'Leary stitch (suturing through the broad ligament around the ascending uterine arteries and myometrium) is a rapid method to reduce uterine hemorrhage or to correct a cesarean incisional extension. Bilateral ligation of the hypogastric artery (the pelvic sidewall retroperitoneal space is open, and hypogastric arteries are located for placement of two permanent ligatures) will reduce the pulse pressure by 85%; this method has a success rate of 40%. If other methods have failed to achieve hemostasis or if the patient is hemodynamically unstable, hysterectomy may be the better approach. Any coagulation abnormalities will require blood product replacement.

Puerperal Infection

Endometritis is the most frequent postcesarean complication. It occurs in 30 to 40% of unscheduled cesareans, 5 to 15% of scheduled cesareans, and 2 to 3% of vaginal deliveries. The responsible pathogens are part of the normal vaginal flora and include aerobic and anaerobic streptococci, aerobic and anaerobic gram-negative bacilli, and facultative anaerobic organisms. Endometritis manifests with fever, tachycardia, pelvic peritonitis, malodorous lochia, and uterine and adnexal tenderness 24 to 48 hours after CS. Patients are examined for noninfectious febrile morbidity (breast engorgement, atelectasis, and wound seroma) and other sources of infection (pyelonephritis, pneumonia, pelvic cellulitis, and wound infection). Laboratory evaluation should include complete blood count, urine analysis and culture, and blood culture to identify the seriously ill patient, who will need prolonged parenteral antibiotic therapy. Endometrial culture is difficult to obtain without contamination; however, it may be of value in the patient who does not respond to therapy. Parenteral broad-spectrum antibiotics should be administrated until the patient is afebrile and asymptomatic for 24 to 48 hours. The recommended regimen includes the following: clindamycin (Cleocin), 900 mg every 8 hours, with gentamicin (Garamycin), 1.5 mg per kg every 8 hours, or clindamycin with aztreonam (Azactam), 1 to 2 grams every 8 hours, or metronidazole (Flagyl), 500 mg every 6 hours, with penicillin, 5 million units, with gentamicin or cefoxitin (Mefoxin), 2 grams every 6 hours, or cefotetan (Cefotan), 2 grams every 6 hours,* or piperacillin-tazobactam (Zosyn), 3.375 grams every 6 hours, or ticarcillin-clavulanic acid (Timentin), 3.1 grams every 6 hours, or ampicillin-sulbactam (Unasyn), 3 grams every 6 hours, or imipenem-cilastatin (Primaxin), 500 mg every 6 hours. Oral antibiotics are not indicated in cases of uncomplicated endometritis.

Failure of initial treatment is uncommon and most often is related to resistant organisms, which require additional antibiotics for broader coverage (clindamycin or metronidazole with penicillin or ampicillin with gentamicin). Other causes of persistent fever despite adequate therapy include abdominal wound infection (treatment includes incision, drainage, and débridement), mastitis, pelvic abscess (evidence of clinical deterioration and acute peritonitis, which requires surgical intervention or percutaneous drainage), and septic pelvic vein thrombophlebitis (treatment includes 7 to 10 days of therapeutic heparin therapy and administration of broad-spectrum antibiotics).

Perineal Care and Pain Control

If repair of episiotomy or vulvar laceration is required, the parturient should be taught front-to-back vulvar cleansing and how to use sitz baths. The application of ice packs or cold sitz baths and topical anesthetic sprays offer much pain relief. Nonsteroidal anti-inflammatory drugs (e.g., ibuprofen) have been shown to be superior in the relief of episiotomy pain and uterine cramping. Acetaminophen, codeine, or propoxyphene (Darvon) also has achieved some pain relief. For women whose delivery was complicated by a third-degree or fourth-degree extension of episiotomy, stool softeners are prescribed. Women with parturient complaints of severe perineal pain should be examined for possible angioedema, necrotizing fasciitis, or perineal cellulitis.

EARLY AND LATE PUERPERIUM

Late Hemorrhage

During the puerperium, vaginal bleeding becomes scantier, as lochia rubra, lochia serosa, and lochia alba; however, many parturients experience a transient increase in uterine bleeding between PPDs 7 and 14 secondary to eschar sloughing. Serious vaginal bleeding late in the puerperium is associated with the retention of placental fragments or subinvolution at the placental site. The initial management should be medical therapy with methylergonovine or prostaglandins. If the bleeding persists, then surgical curettage for the retained placental fragments should be done, and some recommend a course of antibiotics to reduce uterine synechiae. However, if subinvolution is the underlying cause, curettage may iatrogenically cause more profuse bleeding.

---

*Exceeds dosage recommended by the manufacturer.

Breast-Feeding

Breast-feeding should be encouraged to promote mother-child bonding, to meet the infant's nutritional needs, and to augment the infant's immune system. Although the transmission rate of most viruses (e.g., hepatitis B, rubella, herpes simplex) via breast milk is low, breast-feeding is discouraged for women with human T-cell lymphocyte virus and cytomegalovirus infection. The risk of transmission of human T-cell lymphocyte virus to newborns through breast-feeding is 29%.

The mother should expect initial breast engorgement on PPDs two through four, and this may be relieved by 24-hour demand feedings. In stubborn cases, the use of hot compresses or nasal oxytocin (Syntocinon) to augment milk letdown is helpful. During late puerperium or beyond puerperium, the woman may develop lactation failure. Decreasing the interval between feedings will enhance letdown, and a course of metoclopramide (Reglan),* 10 mg three or four times a day, will enhance lactation.

Another common complaint is nipple soreness, which can be relieved by alternating nursing from each breast and changing infant position every 5 minutes, avoiding irritating soaps and wet nursing pads, allowing the nipple to air dry, and temporarily using a nipple shield. Mastitis manifests with high fever, malaise, localized erythema, and breast tenderness and should be treated with antistaphylococcal penicillin or cephalosporin. If one suspects a breast abscess, then surgical drainage is indicated.

During breast-feeding, the parturient should be encouraged to compensate with a protein-rich diet and an additional 600 calories per day. Increasing oral hydration will also improve the breast milk production. For women who do not desire to breast-feed for personal or medical reasons, breast engorgement may be alleviated by breast support, ice packs, and analgesic medication. Bromocriptine (Parlodel) is no longer approved for lactation suppression by the Food and Drug Administration, secondary to its rare association with puerperal stroke, seizures, and myocardial infarction.

Postpartum Laboratory Tests and Immunization

Reactive Protein Reagent (RPR) and Human Immunodeficiency Virus. Many states require evaluation for syphilis and offer human immunodeficiency virus testing on admission for labor and delivery. Counseling and treatment are needed for those with evidence of such infection.

Rhesus Immune Globulin. The unsensitized Rh(D)- negative parturient who has delivered an Rh-positive infant must receive 300 μg RhoGAM within 72 hours of delivery. When there is a high suspicion of excessive fetomaternal hemorrhage (e.g., with placenta previa, placenta abruption, multiple gestation), the blood bank may advise administration of more than 1 unit of RhoGAM, based on a routine quantification in the maternal circulation via Kleihauer-Betke.

Rubella. Six to eleven percent of postpubertal women remain immunologically seronegative for rubella; thus, some institutions have chosen the postpartum period to begin vaccination against rubella, hepatitis B, mumps, and measles.

Depression

The puerperium is an emotionally exciting and stressful period, with a new infant in the family, changes in parental role, postpartum physiologic reversal, and absence from the routine of work. Maternity blues inflict 50 to 70% of parturients, with transient states of tearfulness, insomnia, anxiety, confusion, restlessness, exhaustion, and elation. These symptoms may manifest around PPDs three to five; they generally self-resolve by day 10. Maternity blues do not require any medical treatment—only reassurance and support.

Postpartum depression inflicts 8 to 15% of parturients, with depressed mood or anhedonia and other common features of depression. Postpartum psychosis (schizophrenia, schizoaffective, and bipolar disorders) does manifest with increased frequency in the puerperium and generally lasts 2 to 3 months, with a more favorable prognosis than nonpuerperial psychosis. Postpartum depression and psychosis require inpatient care from a psychiatrist for the initial evaluation and the institution of therapy (i.e., tricyclic antidepressants, anxiolytics, or selective serotonin reuptake inhibitors and neuroleptics, lithium carbonate, or electroconvulsive therapy). There is a high rate of recurrence of postpartum depression in subsequent pregnancies (50 to 100%). The postpartum period is also associated with an increased risk of developing autoimmune thyroiditis and hypothyroidism; thus, evaluation for postpartum depression should include screening for these conditions.

Contraception

Contraception counseling should be initiated during prenatal care and in the early puerperium, because the average times to return of ovulation among non–breast-feeding and breast-feeding women are 45 plus or minus 3.8 days and 189 plus or minus 14.7 days, respectively. Most women resume intercourse by 3 months. Generally, combination oral contraceptive pills (OCPs) are started at 2 to 3 weeks after delivery to avoid the period of increased risk for thromboembolism. Some studies have found a suppressive effect on lactation with the 50-μg estrogen and the low-dose combination OCPs. Progestin-only OCPs do not demonstrate this suppression. The efficacy of depot medroxyprogesterone acetate (Depo-Provera), 150 mg IM every 3 months, exceeds 99%; this drug may be given prior to discharge. The intra-

*Not approved by the Food and Drug Administration for this indication.

uterine contraceptive device (ParaGard, Progestasert) can be inserted immediately after the delivery; however the rate of expulsion or uterine perforation is higher than if the placement is at the postpartum examination at 4 to 6 weeks. The barrier methods (diaphragm and condom) and vaginal spermicides (nonoxynol-9) are advised among those who are delaying a decision on sterilization or OCPs until the postpartum visit.

FOLLOW-UP CARE

The follow-up examination at 1 to 2 weeks post partum should be scheduled for pregnancies with medical or obstetric complications. The CS patient is examined for evidence of wound infection or seroma. This is also a good time to discuss and initiate contraception. The visit at 4 to 6 weeks includes a complete physical examination, along with a Pap smear. Again, contraceptive issues, including their side effects, may be addressed.

RESUSCITATION AND STABILIZATION OF THE NEWBORN

method of
JAMES M. ADAMS, M.D.
Baylor College of Medicine
Houston, Texas

The depressed neonate represents a true medical emergency. The primary physician may encounter this situation in the delivery room, the nursery, the emergency department, or even the office environment. In trained hands, effective resuscitation can be accomplished in any setting using a simple approach that requires minimal equipment and personnel.

The American Academy of Pediatrics and the American Heart Association have developed guidelines for neonatal resuscitation. These are contained in the training modules of the Neonatal Resuscitation Program (American Academy of Pediatrics, 141 Northwest Point Blvd., Elk Grove, IL.), which emphasize several important concepts: (1) the anticipation of problems in high-risk infants, (2) the availability of a designated resuscitation area and the presence of two trained care providers at every live birth, and (3) the use of a simple approach based on basic physiology. These concepts form the basis for the recommendations outlined in this article.

ANTICIPATION OF THE DEPRESSED INFANT

Most newborns requiring resuscitation have respiratory failure. This may occur in utero (failure of the placenta or fetal circulation) or in the postnatal environment (failure of the lung or control of breathing). Many of the conditions leading to such circumstances can be anticipated. Table 1 lists high-risk conditions that may result in respiratory depression or perinatal asphyxia. Placental insufficiency and umbilical cord accidents may be associated with abnormal fetal heart rate patterns during fetal monitoring. When such conditions exist, arrangements should be made for the availability of personnel able to provide immediate care of the neonate in the delivery room and the possibility of a critically ill infant should be anticipated.

TABLE 1. **Perinatal Conditions Predisposing to a Depressed Neonate**

Placental Insufficiency
Maternal diabetes
Toxemia
Chronic hypertension
Postmaturity
Maternal hyperventilation
Maternal hypotension
Maternal cigarette smoking
Uterine tetany
Umbilical Cord Accidents
Cord compression
True knot in cord
Cord laceration
Anomalous insertion with disruption at birth
Postnatal Depression
Narcotics, sedatives, anesthetics
Infection
Cardiopulmonary disease
Congenital anomalies
In these circumstances fetal acid base balance is often normal at birth but derangements occur when lung function is inadequate to replace the detached placenta.
Other Etiologies of Bradycardia
Head compression during terminal labor
Local anesthetic toxicity
Postnatal Respiratory Failure
Acute pulmonary disease
Infection
Congenital anomalies

PHYSIOLOGY OF ASPHYXIA

The lung is the organ of respiration for the neonate while the placenta is that for the fetus. Both are simple gas exchange organs serving to facilitate diffusion of oxygen and removal of carbon dioxide. Carbon dioxide tension, in turn, acutely regulates extracellular pH. Failure of either of these respiratory organs leads to a typical sequence of metabolic events. In the absence of adequate gas exchange, hypoxemia and hypercarbia develop rapidly, accompanied by acute respiratory acidosis. If such circumstances persist for a more prolonged period, or if circulatory failure coexists, tissue hypoxia will develop, accompanied by the appearance of metabolic (lactic) acidosis. During the early course of these events, heart rate and circulatory function are maintained at the expense of vasoconstriction and diversion of blood flow away from noncritical organs. If the process continues, however, heart rate will fall and even essential organ perfusion will fail.

Experimentally, the course of perinatal asphyxia has been described in three clinical phases: primary apnea, gasping, and secondary (terminal) apnea. These represent progressive stages of asphyxia with increasingly severe metabolic derangements. The phases are useful in understanding the progression of clinical and metabolic events in the asphyxiated infant.

1. Primary apnea
   Metabolic derangements mild
   Heart rate above 80 beats per minute

Blood pressure normal or increased (palpable pulses)
Response to tactile stimuli
"Gasp before pink" response
Apgar usually 4 or greater

2. Gasping respirations
Indicative of serious acidemia and need for resuscitation with positive pressure ventilation. Without such intervention the infant will soon enter phase of secondary apnea.
3. Secondary apnea
Metabolic derangements severe
Heart rate below 80 beats per minute
Blood pressure low (pulses poor or absent)
No response to tactile stimuli
Resuscitation requires positive-pressure ventilation
"Pink before gasp" response
Apgar may be 3 or less

In the clinical setting, however, primary and secondary apnea may be indistinguishable, and the criteria listed are not adequately sensitive to guide intervention. *When faced with an apneic infant, secondary apnea should always be assumed and positive pressure ventilation initiated with mask and bag without delay for clinical staging.*

The Apgar score has been used widely to assess the overall state of reactivity of infants at birth. Although still useful in delivery room evaluation, the Apgar score neither detects nor excludes perinatal asphyxia. It frequently correlates poorly with the underlying acid-base status at birth and is not useful for decision-making at initiation of resuscitation. In a depressed infant, intervention should not be delayed for assignment of a 1-minute Apgar score. Evaluation of the infant should begin at birth, and the need for resuscitation is assessed most accurately by evaluation of respiratory activity, heart rate, and color.

Establishment of effective alveolar ventilation is the primary step in newborn resuscitation. Adequate ventilation should be accompanied by a prompt increase in heart rate followed by progressive improvement in oxygenation and respiratory acidosis. Additional intervention is rarely necessary. Maintenance of intact circulatory function during asphyxia, however, is a critical factor determining survival and outcome. Ischemia has a more profound effect on tissue oxygenation than low blood oxygen content alone. Cardiac output and blood flow in the newborn are heart-rate related; thus, persistent bradycardia may be accompanied by a profound fall in cardiac output. Closed chest cardiac massage is the central tool in maintenance of circulatory function in the face of persistent bradycardia during resuscitation.

Because hypoxemia and acidosis may depress myocardial function, drugs have historically been used as an ancillary means of improving circulatory status during resuscitation. Epinephrine is the primary agent used for this purpose. It increases heart rate, augments cardiac contractility and induces peripheral vasoconstriction, which may help sustain coronary blood flow. The use of buffer agents such as sodium bicarbonate remains controversial. Early animal studies demonstrated improved circulatory function and survival after bicarbonate administration. If alveolar ventilation is inadequate, however, bicarbonate administration will exacerbate acidosis and may be accompanied by a fall in cardiac output, as well as increased lactic acid production by the gut. The role of sodium bicarbonate appears to be secondary at present, reserved for circumstances of prolonged resuscitation with documented metabolic acidosis.

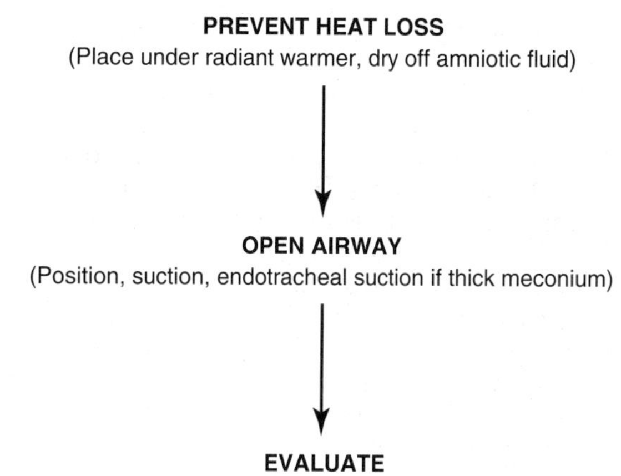

Figure 1. Resuscitation-stabilization, phase 1 (all deliveries).

RESUSCITATION-STABILIZATION PROCEDURE

Neonatal resuscitation requires the combined efforts of two trained individuals. The procedure is carried out in two phases, the first of which is performed on every newborn at birth (Figure 1). The need for intervention (Figure 2) is determined by evaluation of respirations, heart rate, and color.

Phase 1

The following steps should be carried out in all newborns immediately following delivery:

1. *Prevent heat loss.* Place infant under a radiant warming device and dry off amniotic fluid.
2. *Open the airway.* Position the infant with neck slightly extended and gently suction first the mouth then the nose. If mechanical suction is used, limit negative pressure to 100 mm Hg. (Intubation and direct tracheal suctioning should be performed at

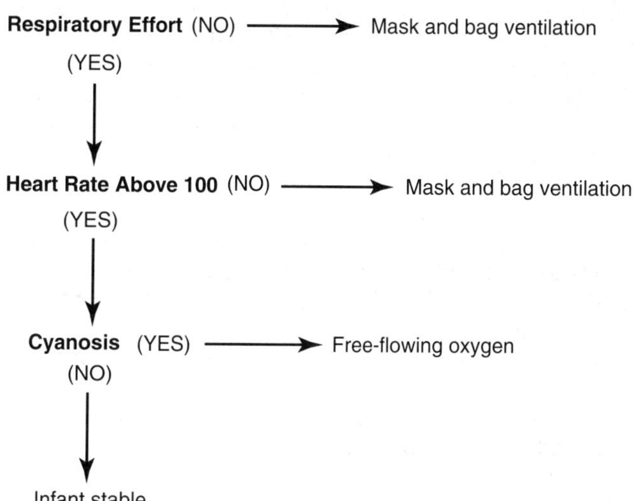

Figure 2. Resuscitation-stabilization, phase 2 (evaluation-based intervention).

this point on infants having thick meconium staining as discussed later.) Avoid prolonged suctioning, which may induce apnea or bradycardia.

3. *Stimulate the infant.* Drying and suction both provide tactile stimulation, which may help induce spontaneous respirations. If initial respiratory activity is poor, additional stimulation may be provided by briefly flicking the soles of the feet or rubbing the infant's back. If respiratory activity remains depressed, or the infant is apneic, mask and bag ventilation should be initiated.

4. *Evaluate the infant.* Is respiratory effort present? Is the heart rate higher than 100 beats per minute? Is the infant cyanotic?

Phase 2

The following definitive steps should be taken if phase 1 evaluation reveals apnea or inadequate respirations, heart rate below 100 beats per minute, or the presence of cyanosis. The response to each step is the key to the next step in the sequence. The basic tools in this sequence are mask and bag ventilation and closed chest cardiac message. Mask and bag ventilation is the basic skill for newborn resuscitation because it can be mastered and used by all caregivers, both physician and nonphysician. This technique alone will resuscitate most depressed infants adequately.

1. If the infant is apneic or has inadequate respirations, provide mask and bag ventilation with 100% oxygen at a rate of 40 to 60 breaths per minute until heart rate is above 100 beats per minute and effective spontaneous respirations are established. If the technique is adequate, the heart rate should rise above 100 beats per minute within 30 seconds, to be followed by improvement in color and return of spontaneous breathing.

2. If the infant is breathing but the heart rate is below 100 beats per minute, provide mask and bag ventilation until the heart rate is stable above 100 and spontaneous respiratory activity has returned. If the heart rate is less than 80 beats per minute or remains below 100 per minute and does not rise despite adequate ventilation, begin cardiac compressions. This should be done at a rate of 90 per minute in conjunction with a ventilation rate of 30 per minute. Ventilation and compressions should be coordinated in a ratio of 1:3.

3. If cyanosis is present but the infant is breathing spontaneously with a heart rate above 100 beats per minute, deliver free-flowing oxygen at 5 liters per minute directly from oxygen tubing attached to an infant mask or held directly one-half inch from the nose.

4. If an infant requires mask and bag ventilation and endotracheal intubation is indicated for ongoing care, this can be carried out under controlled conditions once the heart rate is stable above 100 beats per minute and color has been improved using the mask and bag ventilation.

MEDICATIONS

Medications are rarely needed in newborn resuscitation because effective ventilation with 100% oxygen usually reverses the metabolic consequences of respiratory failure. Medications are indicated, however, for infants who do not improve with ventilation and chest compressions. The umbilical vein is the preferred route for administration of drugs in the delivery room, but epinephrine and naloxone may also be given via the endotracheal tube (ET). In older infants, peripheral veins can be used but may be difficult to access during resuscitation. The following medications are currently recommended for use in newborn resuscitation:

1. *Epinephrine (1:10,000)* increases heart rate, stimulates cardiac contractility, and increases peripheral vascular resistance. It should be administered when the heart rate remains below 80 beats per minute despite adequate ventilation and chest compressions or if the heart rate is zero. *Dose*: 0.1 to 0.3 mL per kg given intravenously or by the ET tube. May be repeated every 3 to 5 minutes if necessary. If vascular access is unavailable or if the neonate does not respond to standard doses, 1 to 2 mL per kg may be given via the ET tube.

2. *A volume expander* may be considered if the heart rate remains below 100 beats per minute and there is evidence suggesting acute blood loss with signs of hypovolemia. *Dose*: 10 mL per kg of 5% albumin-saline, normal saline, or Ringer's lactate solution.

3. *Sodium bicarbonate* may be useful in buffering metabolic acidosis, but adequate ventilation must precede and accompany its use. Although not a primary drug, it may be indicated in circumstances of prolonged resuscitation with documented metabolic acidosis and incomplete response to the primary resuscitation maneuvers. *Dose*: 2 mEq per kg given intravenously using a solution containing a concentration of 0.5 mEq per mL.

4. *Naloxone hydrochloride* may be indicated if there is severe respiratory depression accompanied by a history of maternal narcotic administration within 4 hours of delivery. Effective ventilation must be initiated and maintained. The duration of action of naloxone is 1 to 4 hours, but the duration of action of the offending narcotic agent may be longer. As a result, repeat dosing may be necessary, and infants receiving this agent should be monitored closely for return of respiratory depression for 8 to 12 hours after use. Administration of naloxone to an infant of a narcotic-addicted mother may result in abrupt appearance of withdrawal symptoms or seizures. *Dose*: 0.1 mg per kg given intravenously or via the ET. The intramuscular route can be used, but onset of action will be delayed and response variable.

MANAGEMENT OF THE MECONIUM-STAINED INFANT

The presence of thick or particulate meconium in the amniotic fluid is associated with increased perinatal morbidity and mortality. This includes a risk of meconium aspiration into the lungs, which can result in severe respiratory distress accompanied by a high incidence of complications such as pneumothorax. Thick meconium staining is also associated with persistent pulmonary hypertension and progressive postnatal hypoxemia.

The presence of thick meconium-stained fluid necessitates a combined obstetric and pediatric approach. When the head of the infant appears on the perineum, the mouth and hypopharynx should be quickly but gently suctioned by the delivering physician. Once delivery has been accomplished, the trachea of the infant should be intubated for removal of any meconium present by direct suctioning. This is done by applying suction directly to the endotracheal tube using a regulated suction source limited to a maximum of 100 mm Hg and connected via one of the commercial adapters now available. The suction is applied while withdrawing the tube from the trachea. If no meconium is present, proceed with the usual stabilization sequence. If meconium is present, evaluate the heart rate.

If the heart rate is greater than 80 beats per minute, repeat intubation if needed to remove any further meconium. Then administer free-flowing oxygen, observe color, and monitor for signs of respiratory distress. If the heart rate falls below 80 beats per minute after initial suctioning, ventilate with mask and bag until the heart rate is stable above 100 beats per minute and then proceed with repeat suctioning if necessary. Suctioning should be done via ET directly. Thick meconium is not effectively removed by passing a suction catheter into the ET. Saline lavage of the trachea should be avoided, as this may hasten peripheral deposition of meconium. Tracheal suctioning is not necessary in the presence of thin meconium staining of amniotic fluid.

It is important that optimal conditions be provided following suctioning to promote normal postnatal fall in pulmonary vascular resistance. Deliver oxygen initially and withdraw it stepwise rather than abruptly. If any cyanosis or respiratory distress is present, continue oxygen in amounts adequate to achieve good color until blood gas analysis or pulse oximetry can be done to provide more definitive information. The dangers of meconium aspiration syndrome with persistent pulmonary hypertension cannot be overemphasized.

Following suctioning of a meconium-stained infant, the physician will be faced with one of three circumstances:

1. No meconium in the airway and no distress. The infant can be transferred to routine level 1 nursery care.
2. Meconium in airway, no distress, and no oxygen requirement. The infant may go to a level 1 or level 2 nursery to be observed closely for 6 hours. If any symptoms develop, chest radiograph and further evaluation are indicated.
3. Meconium in the airway with respiratory distress or an oxygen requirement present. These infants should be transferred to a level 3 nursery (neonatal intensive care unit).

POSTRESUSCITATION PROCEDURE

Following resuscitation, infants should remain in a heat-conserving environment and receive whatever support is necessary to maintain adequate ventilation with a stable heart rate above 120 beats per minute, a pink color, and a temperature in the normal range. Ongoing care may require biochemical monitoring, such as pH, blood gases, hematocrit determination, or blood glucose screening. Patients requiring intubation should not be extubated until transported to a final destination, where continued observation and biochemical monitoring demonstrate recovery. Many such infants will continue to have respiratory distress. (An exception is the infant intubated for suctioning of meconium who has no meconium in the trachea and no symptoms.) Adequate alveolar ventilation and circulatory support, if needed, must be ensured during transport. After stabilization, infants requiring resuscitation should have a source of intravascular glucose provided to prevent the occurrence of hypoglycemia. The peak period of risk for this metabolic disturbance in the compromised neonate occurs in the first 30 minutes to 2 hours of life.

CARE OF THE HIGH-RISK NEONATE

method of
AMIR KHAN, M.D., and
SUSAN E. DENSON, M.D.
University of Texas Health Science Center at Houston
Houston, Texas

Almost 4 million infants are born each year in the United States, and a significant number of these will require special attention in the neonatal period owing to maternal, fetal, or socioeconomic factors. To ensure optimal outcomes for these infants, one must anticipate the need for this special care and implement the necessary interventions either prenatally, intrapartum, or as soon as possible after delivery. Anticipation requires recognition of risk factors (Table 1), which can surface prenatally, intrapartum, or postnatally, and appropriate responses to these risk factors. The majority of high-risk infants can be recognized before delivery, and as a result their delivery can occur at a site that can provide the appropriate level of care. Regionalization of perinatal care in the 1970s resulted in delivery of high-risk infants, particularly those of low birth weight, those with prenatally diagnosed problems, and those with known anomalies or surgical problems, at centers capable of providing the necessary treatments. This approach, along with improvements in perinatal and neonatal care, led to improved outcomes for many infants. The 1990s have brought new issues to bear on the delivery of perinatal health care, as there has been an increase in the number of uninsured, an epidemic of drug abuse, a contin-

TABLE 1. **Maternal, Fetal, and Neonatal Risk Factors**

	Antepartum	Intrapartum	Postnatal
Maternal conditions	Diabetes Pregnancy-induced hypertension Maternal drug use Rh isoimmunization Poor reproductive history	Maternal fever Abruptio placentae Placenta previa Prolonged rupture of membranes Premature labor	
Fetal/neonatal conditions	Congenital anomalies Abnormalities of growth Multiple gestation Discordant twin Polyhydramnios Oligohydramnios	Fetal distress Meconium-stained amniotic fluid Pulmonary immaturity by amniocentesis Perinatal depression	Respiratory distress Cyanosis Congenital anomalies Prematurity Postmaturity Large for gestational age Small for gestational age Anemia Infection Polycythemia Hypoglycemia Hypothermia Hypotension

ued increase in the incidence of prematurity, and the advent of managed care, which has changed traditional referral patterns. To maintain the improved outcomes seen over the past 2 decades, we must develop integrated delivery systems that will continue to respond to the high-risk pregnancy and high-risk infant. The Committee on Perinatal Health in the document "Toward Improving the Outcome of Pregnancy: The 90s and Beyond" has provided guidance in accomplishing these goals. All services need to reassess their capabilities and determine their role in this integrated system as basic perinatal centers, specialty perinatal centers, or subspecialty perinatal centers (Table 2). With this system in place, decisions can be made regarding the appropriate sites for delivery and ongoing care of high-risk neonates.

INITIAL EVALUATION AND ASSESSMENT

The medical history for the newborn would appear to be brief because of its recent entry into this world; however, it is as complex as the mother's history and encompasses perinatal events as well. The history is often obtained in stages in many high-risk situations, with as much information as possible being obtained before delivery and the remainder obtained following stabilization and after discussion with the family. The complete newborn history includes an extensive maternal history, including previous pregnancies and outcomes, prenatal laboratory test results (blood type and Rh, rapid plasma reagin [RPR] or Venereal Disease Research Laboratory [VDRL], hepatitis B, human immunodeficiency virus [HIV], gonorrhea, *Chlamydia*, group B streptococcus), medications, complications and events during this pregnancy, and maternal illnesses that may affect this infant. A social history should be obtained about maternal drug, alcohol, and tobacco use as well as insight into the family structure and support systems. The family history should include information about family illnesses, genetic disorders, and consanguinity. A complete review of the labor and delivery includes information about the onset of labor, length of rupture of membranes, medica-

TABLE 2. **Levels of Inpatient Perinatal Care**

Basic Perinatal Center	Specialty Perinatal Center	Subspecialty Perinatal Center
Function Includes	*Function Includes*	*Function Includes*
Management of newborns with uncomplicated conditions and those requiring emergency resuscitation and/or stabilization for transport. Risk assessment to identify need for consultation/referral. Capability to resuscitate and stabilize infants in the delivery room and/or nursery with formal education in resuscitation such as the NRP. Continuing education consistent with patient population served.	Management of newborns with selected complicated conditions. Expanded capabilities could include: • Moderately ill newborns with problems expected to resolve rapidly. • Extremely ill newborns requiring stabilization before transfer. • Recovering infants who can be transferred from a perinatal center. • Consultation and/or referral to subspecialty center for infants requiring ventilation for >6 h. • Risk assessment with consultation and referral based on guidelines. Continuing education consistent with patient population served.	Management of normal newborns, moderately ill newborns, and extremely ill newborns. Neonatal intensive care unit staffed and equipped to treat critically ill neonates with sufficient intermediate care area for convalescing and moderately ill neonates. Provision of continuing education relative to neonatal care and stabilization.

Additional guidelines apply to the obstetrical services and the support services. This table addresses only inpatient neonatal services.
Adapted from Toward improving the outcome of pregnancy: The 90s and beyond. March of Dimes Birth Defects Foundation, 1993.

tions during labor, fever or other complications during labor, method of delivery, anesthesia, Apgar scores, umbilical cord blood gas results, and steps required in resuscitation.

The infant should have a gestational age assessment with weight, length, and head circumference plotted on an appropriate growth curve. With this tool, infants can be assessed as premature (less than 38 weeks' gestation), full term (38 to 42 weeks' gestation), or postmature (more than 42 weeks' gestation) and as large for gestational age (LGA) (greater than the 90th percentile), appropriate for gestational age (AGA) (10th to 90th percentile) or small for gestational age (SGA) (less than the 10th percentile). This classification helps to determine levels of risk, as infants who are premature or postmature and/or SGA or LGA are at greater risk than infants who are born full term and/or AGA.

The initial physical examination is important for determining immediate status, recognizing certain risk factors, and identifying congenital abnormalities. The extent of the initial examination is dependent on the status of the infant after birth and initially may be more narrowly focused. The first step is visual inspection, including general appearance, color (pale, plethoric, cyanotic, pink), respiratory status (grunting, flaring, retracting, tachypneic), activity (nonresponsive, jittery), and any apparent abnormalities. Examination of the head includes assessment of size and shape, anterior fontanelle (size, tenseness), sutures (overlapping, separated), eyes (red reflex, anterior vascular capsule in prematures for gestational age assessment), ears (position, shape, size), nose (patency, philtrum), and mouth (shape, size, palate, tongue). Examination of the chest includes chest movement, the lungs (symmetry, character of breath sounds, air movement), and the heart (murmurs, pulses). Examination of the abdomen should include palpation (masses) and auscultation (bowel sounds). Genitalia are examined for gender identification and to determine any abnormalities. The extremities are examined for symmetry, and the hips are evaluated for dislocation. The neurologic examination includes observation of responses, muscle tone, reflexes, and activity level. This examination is completed during the stabilization period and may require updates if the initial examination is limited owing to the infant's status.

STABILIZATION

In utero, the fetus is dependent on the placenta for transfer of fluids and nutrients, exchange of critical gases including oxygen and carbon dioxide, acid-base balance, removal of wastes, and temperature support. At the time of delivery, the infant must establish effective gas exchange, establish adequate cardiac output, obtain nutrients from an external source, and maintain body temperature. Initial stabilization of the high-risk infant requires attention to multiple factors simultaneously as the physician assesses how well the infant has made the transition from intrauterine to extrauterine life.

Respiratory

At birth the lung must replace the placenta as the organ of gas exchange. This occurs successfully in most infants, but in the infant with respiratory distress at birth, the physician's priorities are to achieve adequate oxygenation and ventilation and to make a diagnosis. If the infant has adequate respiratory effort and does not require immediate ventilation, an oxygen hood can be used to deliver the appropriate amount of oxygen. Assessment of adequate oxygenation requires monitoring. Initially, this can be accomplished with the measurement of oxygen saturation with pulse oximetry. This technique is helpful in assessing an infant who has transitional respiratory distress, but if respiratory distress persists, or is moderate to severe, measurement of arterial blood gas samples will be required to assess ventilatory and oxygen requirements. An arterial blood gas sample can be obtained from a peripheral arterial line or from an umbilical artery catheter. Capillary blood gas samples are less useful in the immediate stabilization period because although they may accurately reflect pH and P_{CO_2}, they are not accurate for Pa_{O_2}. Pulse oximetry has limitations in that it is more helpful with the assessment of hypoxemia, but as changes in saturation are small as the oxygen dissociation curve flattens, hyperoxia may be difficult to detect. A chest radiograph should be considered in the stabilization period of an infant with respiratory distress as it can often make the diagnosis.

Cardiovascular

Stabilization of blood pressure is essential in the infant's transition. Failure to recognize and treat hypotension puts the infant at increased risk for morbidity and mortality. Infants who are born prematurely, those with infection, those with blood loss in utero or at delivery, and those with perinatal depression are at risk for hypotension. Blood pressure can be measured either directly with an arterial line or with noninvasive techniques. There are multiple sources available for blood pressure values in the newborn infant, but a reasonable guideline during stabilization is a mean arterial pressure approximately equal to the infant's gestational age. If the blood pressure is low, heart rate elevated, and perfusion poor with decreased capillary refill, the infant should be given a trial of volume expansion. This can be done initially with normal saline or 5% albumin as an infusion of 10 mL per kg over 10 minutes. This can be repeated one to two times while assessing further the cause. If the cause is blood loss and is associated with a low or falling hematocrit, the infant may require transfusion of blood. If the hypotension is due to perinatal depression and therefore due to myocardial depression, pharmacologic intervention may be necessary. Dopamine can be started intravenously at 5 μg per kg per minute and increased in increments of 2.5 to 5 μg per kg per minute to 20 μg per kg per minute until there is a response. Most infants will respond to these steps, but some will require more aggressive volume management.

Temperature

Immediate attention to temperature support is equally important. At delivery, the infant is at highest risk as he or she is wet and immediately loses heat to the environment by multiple mechanisms including radiation, convection, conduction, and evaporation. If not dried well and if the head is not covered with a cap, the infant will be brought to the nursery with a rapidly falling temperature. The consequences of cold stress at this time include hypoglycemia, metabolic acidosis, central nervous system depression, and, if extreme, can result in apnea, bradycardia, and pulmonary hemorrhage. The infant should initially be placed on a preheated radiant warmer, which is servocontrolled to the infant's abdominal skin temperature (set point at 36.5°C). The extremely-low-birth-weight infant may benefit from the use of a plastic wrap to insulate the warmer and decrease the heat loss. This should be used only in an intubated infant, and the head should not be covered. The infant may need additional heat from a heated blanket. Hot water bottles or intravenous bottles heated in the microwave should not be used, as they can result in burns.

Metabolic

A normal glucose level is essential for the high-risk newborn, as it is the principle energy source at this age. In utero, the fetus has received a continuous infusion of glucose along with amino acids, lactate, ketone bodies, and free fatty acids, which are utilized for growth and energy stores. Glucose is stored in the liver and the myocardium as glycogen in increasing amounts near term. These glycogen stores serve as the major source of glucose in the first few hours of life. If the infant is born prematurely and hepatic glycogen stores have not yet developed or if the infant is stressed by perinatal depression or cold stress and glycogen stores have been depleted, the infant is at high risk for hypoglycemia. Glucose levels must be monitored in the immediate stabilization period. Glucose screening tests may be helpful, but true blood glucose levels should be sent if the glucose screen is in the lower range. The glucose level should be maintained at a level of higher than 40 mg per dL. To accomplish this and to avoid hypoglycemia, most high-risk infants will require intravenous fluids. A glucose infusion rate of at least 5 to 7 mg per kg per minute (D10W at a rate of 80 to 100 mL per kg per day) will usually be adequate to maintain a normal glucose level. If hypoglycemia occurs, a bolus of 2 mL per kg of D10W will correct most glucose levels, but this must be followed with a continuous infusion of glucose. If the glucose remains low, the glucose infusion rate should be gradually increased to a level at which the glucose remains higher than 40 mg per dL. This is initially accomplished by increasing the rate of the infusion. If the infant requires more glucose despite an increase in fluids up to 140 to 160 mL per kg per day, the glucose concentration can be increased. If more than D12.5W is required, a central line will be needed.

Hematologic

Measurement of the hematocrit should be obtained, as abnormalities in either direction may interfere with stabilization. The infant with anemia (hematocrit lower than 45) may have increased difficulty during transition, and the cause of the anemia must be clarified. If it is secondary to hemolytic disease (ABO or Rh incompatibility), this has implications for further care, and if it is due to blood loss, it may have more impact on the cardiovascular system. The need for treatment with packed red blood cell transfusion depends on presentation and etiology. Acute anemia causing cardiovascular compromise requires transfusion, but a chronic anemia may be better tolerated and not require transfusion. In polycythemia (venous hematocrit higher than 65), there may be increased respiratory distress and the infant may require a partial exchange transfusion with fresh-frozen plasma to correct the hematocrit if symptoms are significant.

CONTINUING CARE

Fluids, Electrolytes, and Nutrition

After achieving a normal glucose in the stabilization period, the focus of fluid management is initially hydration and then nutrition. The initial fluid requirement of the newborn is a function of the amount of fluid necessary to meet insensible water loss, including that lost through the skin and respiratory tract, and measurable losses, including urine output and gastrointestinal losses. It is affected by the degree of prematurity, with increasing transepithelial water loss with decreasing gestational age, and the environment in which the infant is cared for, with losses greater in a radiant warmer than in an incubator. Fluid requirements can be met in most infants with 80 to 100 mL per kg per day of fluid, and D10W is appropriate unless hyperglycemia or hypoglycemia develops. This is increased each day by 20 mL per kg up to 140 to 160 mL per kg per day. The amount is modified if measurement of electrolytes shows increasing sodium levels (increase fluid intake depending on sodium level), if the infant requires phototherapy (increase by 20 mL per kg), or if excessive weight loss occurs. Rarely, this amount may need to be decreased in the presence of renal dysfunction to avoid fluid overload. Monitoring of fluid therapy includes accurate intake and output records and daily weights.

Electrolytes are usually added on the second day of life, but this depends on renal function and degree of prematurity. The extremely-low-birth-weight infant may not need sodium added for the first few days of life to minimize the risk of hypernatremia. The larger premature infant and the full-term infant with normal renal function usually require 2 to 4 mEq per kg per day of sodium and 1 to 2 mEq per kg per day of potassium in the first few days of life. The addition of 2 mEq per kg per day of calcium is often done in premature infants but is not usually necessary in term infants. Electrolyte panels should be obtained on the smaller premature infant every 12 hours until electrolytes are stable and then decreased to daily measurements. The larger premature infant and the full-term infant can be managed with daily electrolyte measurements until a stable intake is reached.

The role of nutrition in the high-risk infant is critical, as body stores of nutrients are limited and are depleted rapidly even in the full-term infant. As a result, total parenteral nutrition (TPN) should be initiated no later than the second day of life in the high-risk infant in whom early feeding is not anticipated. This can be initiated with 1 to 2 grams per kg per day of protein of a neonatal amino acid solution and 0.5 gram per kg per day of intravenous fat emulsion along with electrolytes, vitamins, and trace elements. These can be advanced as tolerated over the first few days of life to a maximum of 3 to 4 grams per kg per day of protein and 3 grams per kg per day of fat. This amount can be given initially through a peripheral intravenous line, but if prolonged TPN is anticipated, a central line (percutaneous or surgically placed) should be considered to allow for advancing glucose concentrations. Parenteral nutrition is not without risks, and appropriate preparations and electrolyte concentrations are necessary to minimize both short-term and long-term complications. If nursery personnel are not familiar with these preparations, consultation should be obtained.

The goal in neonatal nutrition is to maximize enteral intake to establish growth. When the infant is stable and ready for enteral feeding, the optimal preparation for the full-term and the premature infant is human milk, but if this is not available, a commercial infant formula can be used. If the mother chooses not to breast-feed, a 20-calorie per ounce whey-predominant infant formula for premature infants is preferable for initial feedings. The method of feeding depends on the condition of the infant and the gestational age. More mature infants may be able to tolerate nipple feeding if their respiratory status is stable (respiratory rate < 60 per minute and no distress). Infants less than 33 to 34 weeks' gestational age require tube feedings, either by the intermittent or the continuous method. Feeding tolerance is determined by monitoring the physical examination for any signs of abdominal distention and by checking gastric residuals before each feeding. In the smaller premature infant, feedings can be initiated at 20 to 30 mL per kg per day. If this is tolerated, the feedings can be increased by 20 to 30 mL per kg per day until the infant is on 150 mL per kg per day. As the feedings are advanced, the intravenous fluids are decreased to maintain a total intake of 150 to 160 mL per kg per day. When the infant is tolerating 100 mL per kg per day of enteral feeding, most can have intravenous fluids discontinued as feedings continue to advance. When the infant is tolerating approximately 150 mL per kg per day of feedings, the expressed breast milk can be supplemented with one of the commercially available breast milk fortifiers or the formula can be changed to a 24 calories per ounce premature formula. This will give 120 calories per kg per day, which is adequate for growth in most premature infants. Growth should be monitored in these infants with daily weights and weekly length and head circumference measurements, which can be charted on appropriate growth curves.

Temperature Support

Older studies have demonstrated that a warm environment can decrease neonatal mortality in low-birth-weight infants, but temperature support is essential in infants of all weights and ages. During stabilization and during the acute phase of illness when more intervention is necessary, a radiant warmer may be optimal for care. When the infant is stable, the larger infant can be placed in an open crib and the smaller infant into an incubator. If the infant is requiring frequent interventions while in the incubator, the temperature may need to be managed by servocontrol to the infant's abdominal skin temperature with the set point at 36.5°C. When less intervention is necessary, the smaller infant will benefit from being placed in an incubator set to provide a neutral thermal environment (NTE). NTE, that temperature at which oxygen consumption is minimized, can be determined from standard charts based on weight and postnatal age. The infant should remain in the incubator until weight gain is established and the infant is able to maintain his or her temperature in an open crib and still gain weight.

Environment

Historically, neonatal critical care units have been brightly lit and often chaotic with constant activity 24 hours a day. Newer concepts appear to benefit the infants, their parents, and the nursery staff. Although no studies have been performed to determine the optimal level of lighting in a neonatal unit, many units, including our unit, are minimizing light exposure. The lights are kept dim throughout most of the day and individual incubators are covered with quilted coverlets to minimize light exposure. When an infant is on an open warmer the eyes can't be shielded in the same way as an infant in an incubator, but they can be covered when the examination light is turned on for procedures and achieve the same effect. In addition to reducing light exposure, reduction of noise exposure appears to be of benefit as well. This is accomplished by reducing conversations at the bedside; by being aware of environmental noises, including closing of incubator doors, opening and closing of garbage cans, and ringing telephones; and by removing radios from the nursery. Other important changes in infant care include individualizing care plans for infants that minimize their handling, clustering care tasks to increase quiet time, and positioning the infant so that he or she is "nested" rather than left unconstrained. Parental contact is encouraged, and even the smallest infant on a ventilator is usually able to tolerate being held with the use of "kangaroo care" techniques. This skin-to-skin contact with the parent maintains temperature better than older methods of swaddling with blankets. Implementation of these techniques requires commitment on the part of medical and nursing staff and consultation with individuals experienced with these techniques.

NEONATAL DISORDERS

Respiratory Distress

Respiratory distress is the most common admitting diagnosis to a neonatal critical care unit. Although some causes are similar in pathology to disorders in older children and adults, such as pneumonia, others manifest only in the newborn period because they are the result of disruption in development of the respiratory system. Some represent congenital anomalies that are due to disruption of anatomic development in utero, whereas others result from interruption of biochemical development because of premature delivery. The cause of respiratory distress needs to be determined to institute appropriate therapy. The premature infant, depending on risk factors, is more likely to have respiratory distress syndrome (RDS) or infection, whereas the full-term infant, depending on risk factors, is more likely to have meconium aspiration syndrome, transient tachypnea of the newborn, or sepsis. A thorough history, physical examination, laboratory studies, and chest radiograph will help clarify the cause.

Respiratory Distress Syndrome

RDS due to surfactant deficiency is the most common cause of respiratory distress among premature infants and before the introduction of exogenous surfactant was the single leading cause of death in newborns. The diagnosis is made on the basis of risk factors, clinical presentation, and chest radiograph findings. Risk factors in the history include an overall risk of 10% if born prematurely that increases with decreasing gestational age, a risk of approximately 90% if there was a sibling with RDS, and an increased risk in infants born to diabetic mothers at every gestational age. The clinical presentation is with respiratory distress, as progressive atelectasis results in impaired oxygenation and ventilation and the chest radiograph has a reticulogranular pattern with air bronchograms. Arterial blood gas samples show a falling pH and $Pa{O_2}$ and a rising $Pa{CO_2}$. Before the availability of exogenous surfactant therapy and in the larger infant whose disease is not severe enough to qualify for surfactant therapy, the clinical course is one of increasing severity of respiratory symptoms for 48 to 72 hours followed by improvement in the uncomplicated patient. The course can be complicated by the development of pulmonary air block, especially pneumothorax. With surfactant replacement therapy, the course can be different, with a decreased oxygen requirement, decreased ventilation requirement, and earlier extubation. Management is determined by the severity of the disease. Goals include maintaining the pH at 7.25 to 7.40, the $Pa{O_2}$ at 50 to 80, and the $Pa{CO_2}$ at 40 to 60. Some infants with mild RDS may require only supportive care (temperature support, fluids, and nutrition) and oxygen therapy, but the majority require some form of respiratory assistance either as continuous positive airway pressure or mechanical ventilation.

An infant requiring mechanical ventilation with a moderate oxygen requirement ($Fi{O_2}$ higher than .40) is a candidate for surfactant replacement therapy. This treatment is best administered in a setting in which the physicians, nursing staff, and respiratory therapists are familiar with the results of the treatment. The infant with severe RDS may not tolerate the dose and may require aggressive ventilation after administration, and when the infant responds to the surfactant, the rapidly changing lung compliance requires rapid ventilator and oxygen changes to avoid complications. In addition, surfactant replacement addresses only one aspect of the care of a premature infant. Its availability should not change the criteria for referral of a mother in premature labor or the neonatal transport of a premature infant to the appropriate level of care.

Bronchopulmonary Dysplasia

Bronchopulmonary dysplasia (BPD) is a form of chronic lung disease that affects at least 75% of infants who weigh less than 1000 grams. The diagnosis is made if the oxygen requirement persists beyond the 28th day of life and the chest radiograph shows signs of chronic lung disease. These infants may require oxygen therapy for variable periods of time up to several months. The course can be complicated by reactive airway disease, pulmonary edema, and the development of cor pulmonale. Bronchodilators, including albuterol nebulizer treatments, may be beneficial for treating bronchospasm in neonates with BPD, and pulmonary edema may require the use of diuretics. As recovery depends on lung growth, nutrition is perhaps the most important treatment for infants with BPD. Because of the increased work of breathing, these patients may require higher caloric intake to grow and because they may not tolerate an increased fluid volume, they may require manipulation of their diet to 27 to 30 calories per ounce by the addition of carbohydrate or medium chain triglycerides. Consultation with a dietitian is often necessary to optimize their nutrition.

Persistent Pulmonary Hypertension

Persistent pulmonary hypertension of the neonate (PPHN) occurs because of the failure of the pulmonary vascular system to adapt to the extrauterine environment. In utero the pulmonary vascular resistance is elevated, blood is shunted right to left across the patent ductus arteriosus, and only approximately 15% of the cardiac output goes to the lung. After birth with expansion of the lungs, the pulmonary artery pressure decreases, the ductus arteriosus closes, and there is redistribution of blood flow to the lungs. If this decrease in pulmonary artery pressure fails to occur, a persistent right to left shunt across the ductus and across the foramen ovale can occur that results in systemic hypoxemia. Factors that exacerbate this pulmonary hypertension include hypoxemia and acidosis. PPHN can be the primary diagnosis, or it can complicate other respiratory disorders including meconium aspiration syndrome (MAS), sepsis, and diaphragmatic hernia. The presentation is with severe respiratory distress, and the chest radiograph reflects the findings of the underlying disorder. Management of PPHN focuses on improving oxygenation. In milder cases supplemental oxygen may be adequate, but the infant usually needs to be intubated and placed on mechanical ventilation. These infants can deteriorate rapidly and may require aggressive ventilator strategies, including high-frequency ventilation, and treatment with extracorporeal membrane oxygenation (ECMO). Because of the high mortality in this disorder and difficulty in management, early recognition and transfer of infants with PPHN is encouraged.

Meconium Aspiration Syndrome

MAS has been associated with a death rate as high as 28%. This disorder can occur when an infant passes meconium in utero, often as a sign of fetal distress, and aspirates in the perinatal period. At delivery, if meconium is present in the mouth or pharynx, it may be aspirated when the infant takes the first breath. This condition is further aggravated if the infant is asphyxiated and requires resuscitation and the infant is bagged before the airway is suctioned. The combined pediatric and obstetric approach to prevention of MAS involves suctioning of the mouth, nose, and pharynx when the head is on the perineum, followed by intubation and suction of meconium after delivery if the meconium is thick or the infant is depressed. This technique decreases the risk for MAS in most infants. If aspirated in utero or postnatally, meconium causes a chemical pneumonitis and may cause airway obstruction. This chemical pneumonitis can lead to difficulty in oxygenation and ventilation, the airway obstruction increases the risk of pneumothorax, and the course is frequently complicated by PPHN. The infant presents with meconium staining and respiratory distress. The chest radiograph shows patchy infiltrates with areas of hyperinflation. Therapy in this disorder is aimed at improving oxygenation and ventilation and minimizing PPHN. These infants often require aggressive ventilator management including high-frequency ventilation. In some infants, respiratory failure progresses and they become candidates for ECMO. Early referral to a subspecialty perinatal center capable of providing high-frequency ventilation and/or ECMO should be considered.

Transient Tachypnea of the Newborn

Transient tachypnea of the newborn (TTN) is the most common cause of respiratory distress in the term or near-term infant. It results from delayed clearance of lung fluid after birth, which alters lung compliance and leads to respiratory distress. The presentation is with tachypnea, and the chest radiograph shows hyperinflation with perihilar streaky densities. TTN is a self-limited disease that responds to oxygen therapy and usually resolves in 24 to 72 hours.

Air Block

Another cause of respiratory distress in the newborn is air block or collections of air in the chest that are outside the lung. This includes pneumothorax, pneumomediastinum, and pulmonary interstitial emphysema. These events can occur either spontaneously at birth or in association with mechanical ventilation for lung disease. Pneumothoraces can be responsible for respiratory distress in an otherwise well infant and may occur in up to 0.8% of full-term deliveries. The infant usually presents with tachypnea and may require oxygen therapy. A chest radiograph demonstrates the presence of the pneumothorax. These spontaneous pneumothoraces usually resolve without intervention, but the infant should be monitored, with frequent vital signs, and treated with oxygen if required until the pneumothorax resolves. The infant who develops a pneumothorax on mechanical ventilation may acutely deteriorate and require decompression with needle aspiration and/or placement of a chest tube to suction.

Tracheoesophageal Fistula

Tracheoesophageal fistula, usually accompanied by esophageal atresia, results in respiratory distress secondary to aspiration of secretions or feedings. The diagnosis is suspected with a history of polyhydramnios, increased secretions in the infant, and respiratory distress with feedings if not recognized early. The presumptive diagnosis is made when an orogastric tube is passed and meets obstruction, and the definitive diagnosis is made when the radiograph demonstrates the orogastric tube curled in the proximal esophageal pouch. Once the diagnosis is made, management consists of preventing aspiration of secretions from the upper pouch and gastric secretions from the lower pouch. This is done by keeping the infant in an upright position to prevent aspiration from below and by placing a double lumen tube in the pouch to suction to keep it empty. Surgery is performed as soon as the infant is stable. This disorder always alerts one to search for associated anomalies including vertebral or vascular anomalies, imperforate anus, and renal or radial anomalies in addition to the tracheoesophageal fistula and esophageal atresia.

Diaphragmatic Hernia

Diaphragmatic hernia results when the diaphragm fails to complete its development, which allows the abdominal contents to be displaced into the chest. As a result of this constraint, lung growth is impaired and the lung is hypoplastic on the side of the defect and decreased in size on the contralateral side. The clinical presentation depends on the severity of the lung hypoplasia, and the diagnosis is suspected in an infant with respiratory distress, asymmetrical breath sounds, and a scaphoid abdomen. The diagnosis is made by radiograph with abdominal contents, usually intestines, seen in the chest. The course in most of these infants is complicated by PPHN and respiratory failure. The treatment is with immediate intubation and aggressive ventilation, including high-frequency ventilation, and infants failing this treatment are candidates for ECMO. Surgery is no longer done immediately in most of these infants but is delayed to allow for resolution of the PPHN. In spite of these therapies, mortality rates remain high in this diagnosis.

Cardiac Lesions

Cyanotic Congenital Heart Disease

Cyanotic congenital heart disease, including transposition of the great vessels, tetralogy of Fallot, and tricuspid atresia, must be in the differential diagnosis for respiratory distress. The infant with heart disease, although cyanotic and often tachypneic, is not usually in respiratory distress unless in congestive heart failure with an obstructive left-sided lesion. An infant with cyanosis who does not respond with an increase in $Pa{O_2}$ when the oxygen concentration is increased is likely to have cyanotic heart disease. The diagnosis can usually be clarified by the use of an echocardiogram, which can rule in or out the major causes of cyanotic heart disease. If the infant is critically ill and the presumptive diagnosis of ductal-dependent cyanotic heart disease has been made, treatment with a continuous infusion of prostaglandin E_1 (Prostin VR Pediatric) may be indicated. Complications of this therapy, including apnea, must be anticipated. If the infant is thought to have cyanotic heart disease, consultation should be obtained and transfer to a subspecialty perinatal center should be arranged.

Patent Ductus Arteriosus

Premature infants are at increased risk for presenting with a symptomatic patent ductus arteriosus (PDA), and approximately 15% of those weighing less than 1700 grams have this complication. The development of a significant left to right shunt is associated with widening pulse pressures, pulmonary edema, metabolic acidosis, and worsening of the respiratory status. A murmur is usually present, and peripheral pulses, including palmar pulses, are prominent. The diagnosis is confirmed by echocardiogram, and treatment decisions are made based on clinical status. Many infants respond to indomethacin therapy if it is not contraindicated. Surgical ligation may be indicated in infants who fail to respond to indomethacin and in whom the PDA is hemodynamically significant.

Infection

Infection is a major contributor to neonatal mortality and morbidity, as the newborn infant is exquisitely susceptible to infection as a result of immaturity in the immune defense system. To avoid and/or fight infection effectively requires an intact immune system at several levels, including an efficient host barrier, an adequate population of white blood cells that migrate to the site of inflammation and phagocytose and destroy bacteria, and specific immunoglobulins. In the newborn, the host barrier is disrupted in routine care, the cellular response to infection is limited by a reduced and inefficient population of leukocytes, and specific antibody is usually absent.

Sepsis

Although gram-negative infection, particularly from *Escherichia coli*, continues to occur, the most common organisms in neonatal sepsis for almost 3 decades have been group B streptococci. The mode of transmission is vertical from maternal genital tract to infant by one of two routes: either by ascending infection through ruptured membranes or by contact with organisms in the birth canal at the time of vaginal delivery. Group B streptococcal disease (GBS) manifests in a bimodal distribution of early-onset disease and late-onset disease. Early-onset disease manifests in the first 5 days of life with 60 to 70% of cases appearing in the first 6 hours of life. Obstetric complications including premature labor, prolonged rupture of membranes, twin gestation, and maternal infection are found in approximately 60% of cases. The presenting sign is respiratory distress in about 90% of the cases, with chest radiographic findings indistinguishable from those of RDS in approximately 50%; infiltrates are seen in approximately 30%, and the remainder look like TTN or are normal. Laboratory evaluation includes a complete blood count with differential, which may show neutropenia and/or thrombocytopenia; blood cultures (optimally two separate cultures); and a lumbar puncture to rule out meningitis. The course is variable. Some infants rapidly wean to room air and have a benign course, whereas others progress to require ventilation and have courses complicated by severe respiratory distress with pulmonary hypertension. Early transfer of these infants to a subspecialty perinatal center may be indicated because they may need more than supportive therapy. Therapy for group B streptococcal disease is both supportive and specific. Antibiotics are obviously important in specific therapy. The initial therapy is usually ampicillin and gentamicin, as in any newborn with possible sepsis. The organism continues to be susceptible to ampicillin, and although resistant to gentamicin, there appears to be synergism when the two are used in combination. Supportive therapy includes ventilatory support, management of hypotension often requiring pressor agents, and careful monitoring of fluids and electrolytes. Some infants require ECMO, as sepsis

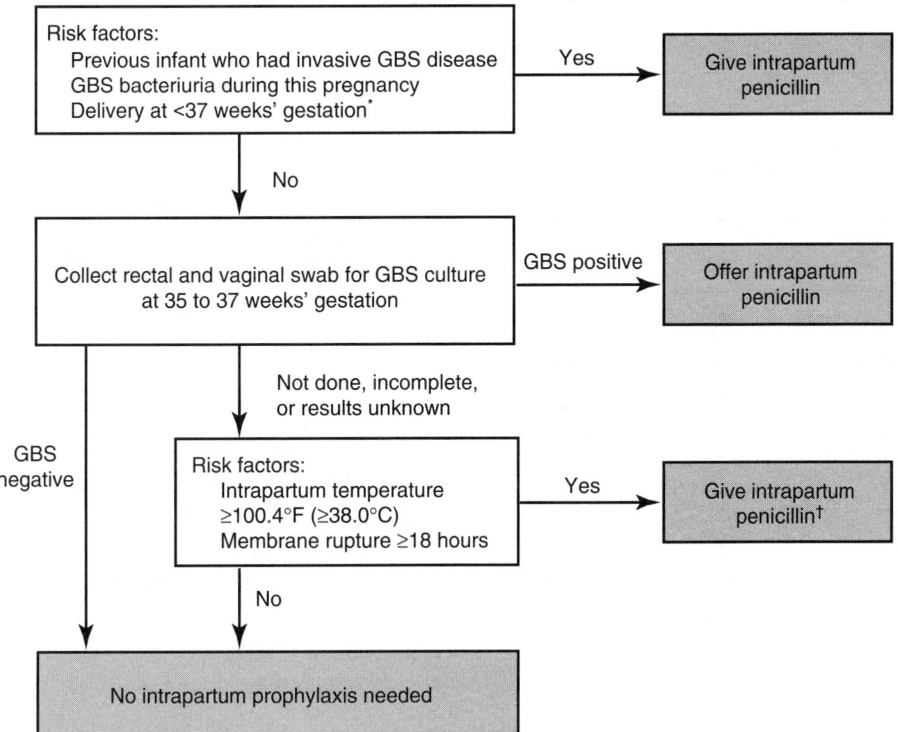

*If membranes ruptured at <37 weeks' gestation and the mother has not begun labor, collect group B streptococcal culture and either (a) administer antibiotics until cultures are completed and the results are negative or (b) begin antibiotics only when positive culture results are available. No prophylaxis is needed if culture results obtained at 35 to 37 weeks' gestation were negative.
†Broader spectrum antibiotics may be considered at the physician's discretion, based on clinical indications.

Figure 1. Algorithm for prevention of early-onset group B streptococcal (GBS) disease in neonates, using prenatal screening at 35 to 37 weeks' gestation. (From Prevention of perinatal group B streptococcal disease: A public health perspective. MMWR *45*:16, May 31, 1996.)

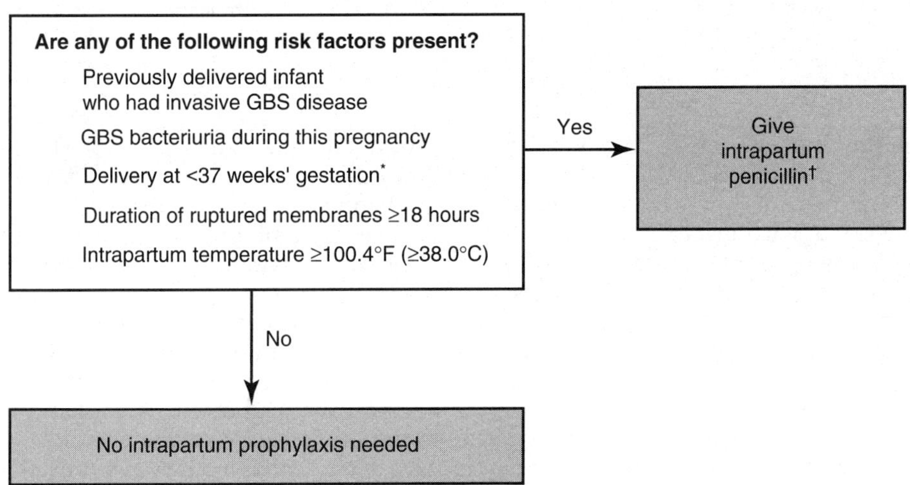

*If membranes ruptured at <37 weeks' gestation and the mother has not begun labor, collect group B streptococcal culture and either (a) administer antibiotics until cultures are completed and the results are negative or (b) begin antibiotics only when positive culture results are available.
†Broader spectrum antibiotics may be considered at the physician's discretion, based on clinical indications.

Figure 2. Algorithm for prevention of early onset of group B streptococcal (GBS) disease in neonates, using risk factors. (From Prevention of perinatal group B streptococcal disease: A public health perspective. MMWR *45*:19, May 31, 1996.)

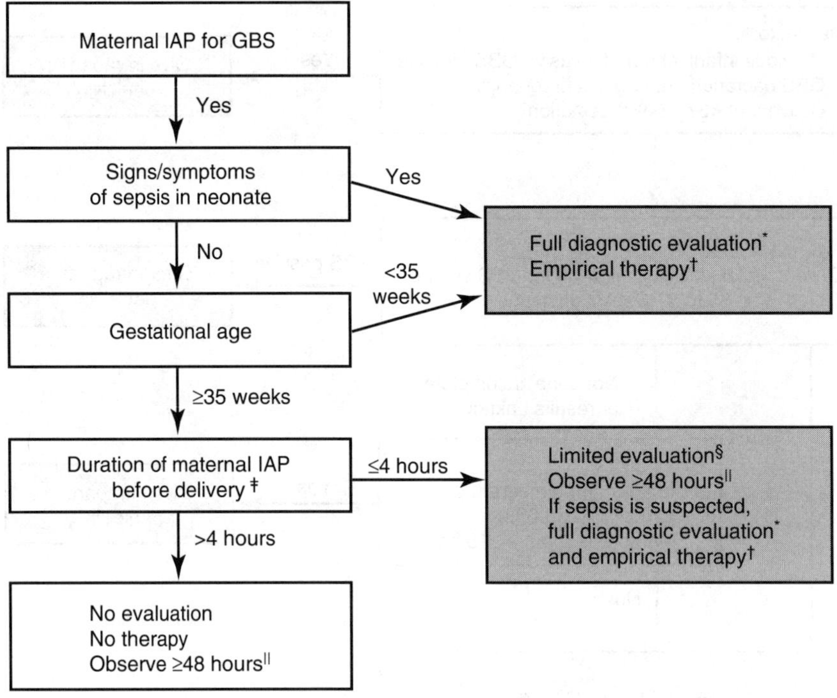

This algorithm is not an exclusive course of management. Variations that incorporate individual circumstances or institutional preferences may be appropriate.

* Includes a complete blood count (CBC) and differential, blood culture, and chest radiograph if neonate has respiratory symptoms. Lumbar puncture is performed at the discretion of the physician.

† Duration of therapy varies depending on blood culture and cerebrospinal fluid (CSF) results and the clinical course of the infant. If laboratory results and clinical course are unremarkable, duration of therapy may be as short as 48 to 72 hours.

‡ Duration of penicillin or ampicillin chemoprophylaxis.

§ CBC and differential and a blood culture.

|| Does not allow early discharge.

Figure 3. Algorithm for management of a neonate born to a mother who received intrapartum antimicrobial prophylaxis (IAP) for prevention of early-onset group B streptococcal (GBS) disease. (From Prevention of perinatal group B streptococcal disease: A public health perspective. MMWR *45*:20, May 31, 1996.)

is the second leading cause of respiratory failure requiring ECMO.

Because of the high mortality, morbidity, and difficulty in treating patients with group B streptococcal sepsis, prevention is the optimal approach. The Centers for Disease Control and Prevention has published prevention guidelines based on two prevention strategies, one using intrapartum antibiotic prophylaxis to mothers screened at 35 to 37 weeks and found to be positive for group B streptococcus and the other for women who develop one or more risk conditions at the time of labor or rupture of membranes. These guidelines also offer suggestions for management of the infant. It is anticipated that many of the current cases of GBS sepsis in the newborn can be avoided by following these guidelines (Figures 1 to 3).

Nosocomial Infection

High-risk infants who remain hospitalized are at risk for acquiring infections later in their course. They continue to be at risk because of their impaired immune system, their need for invasive lines and multiple procedures, and perhaps because of multiple courses of broad-spectrum antibiotics altering their flora. The age at which this occurs is variable, and the presenting signs are usually worsening respiratory status including increased apnea and bradycardia and increasing oxygen and ventilatory requirements, temperature instability, lethargy or irritability, and often glucose intolerance. The most common causes vary from unit to unit depending on the dominant flora but are more commonly *Staphylococcus aureus, Enterococcus, Candida*, and gram-negative organisms including *Pseudomonas* and *Enterobacter*. The initial evaluation includes a complete blood count with differential, which may show a high or low white blood cell count with a left shift; blood cultures (preferably two separate sites and from any indwelling lines); urine culture (preferably catheterized specimen or suprapubic tap); and a lumbar puncture. Antibiotic therapy is usually initiated with vancomycin (Vancocin) and tobramycin (Nebcin) and is adjusted to single therapy when an organism is identified.

Necrotizing Enterocolitis

Necrotizing enterocolitis is a disorder of multifactorial etiology seen primarily in premature infants and is the major gastrointestinal cause of neonatal mortality and morbidity. Although the cause is not clearly understood, it is most likely related to bowel ischemia, bacterial or viral colonization, and feedings. Inflammatory mediators including platelet-activating factor and tumor necrosis factor have an emerging importance as possible contributors to this disorder. The clinical presentation is with feeding intolerance, usually displayed by the presence of gastric residuals, abdominal distention, and usually guaiac positive or grossly bloody stools. These infants consistently have acute respiratory deterioration and may develop blood pressure instability. Evaluation includes abdominal films, which show dilated bowel and may show intramural air (pneumatosis intestinalis), free peritoneal air, and/or portal venous air. Aggressive medical management is indicated and includes placement of a double-lumen orogastric tube on continuous suction, broad-spectrum antibiotics (after cultures are obtained), intravenous fluids, and blood pressure support, which may require vasopressors. Surgical intervention is often required, and consultation should be done when this diagnosis is made and transfer to a subspecialty perinatal center considered. These infants should be followed with frequent abdominal films to detect perforation (kidney and upper bladder and left lateral decubitus every 6 to 8 hours); complete blood count with differential and platelet count to detect neutropenia and thrombocytopenia, which are frequent complications; and blood gas and electrolyte panels to follow for the development of metabolic acidosis. Bowel perforation is an absolute indication for surgical intervention (laparotomy or placement of a drain), whereas evidence of dead or dying bowel with thrombocytopenia unresponsive to platelet transfusions and progressive metabolic acidosis may be a relative indication for surgical intervention.

Human Immunodeficiency Virus Exposure

Treatment of HIV infection during pregnancy has been shown to significantly decrease the transmission of infection to the infant. Treatment must be continued in the infant, and consultation with a pediatric infectious disease specialist is recommended for the current protocol for prevention.

NORMAL INFANT FEEDING

method of
NANCY HURST, M.S.N., R.N., and
WILLIAM J. KLISH, M.D.
Texas Children's Hospital and Baylor College of Medicine
Houston, Texas

GROWTH AND DEVELOPMENT

Growth is the standard by which infant nutrition is judged. Birth weight triples and length increases by 50% during the first year. Growth is especially rapid during the first few months of life when the infant gains about 200 grams in weight and 1 cm in length weekly. Brain growth is profound, tripling in size during infancy to reach 90% of adult size at 2 years of age. Scientific evidence is emerging that different diets in early infancy can have long-term consequences. This so-called nutritional imprinting or programming affects metabolism, development, and disease processes later in life.

Human milk has the distinct capability of providing not only energy to fuel growth, but unique properties benefiting the infant's immune system and health status. Immune properties, most specifically secretory IgA, present in human milk, protect the infant from infection. Studies comparing morbidity rates among feeding types found fewer incidences of otitis media and respiratory and gastrointestinal infections in breast-fed versus formula-fed infants. Furthermore, breast milk has a direct effect on the infant's own immune system. These observations may explain the evidence that breast-feeding protects against some chronic diseases, such as diabetes, rheumatoid arthritis, malignant lymphoma, and atopy conditions. Recently, the content of long-chain polyunsaturated fatty acids, such as docosahexaenoic acid (DHA), present in human milk but not in formula, have received a significant amount of investigation. It has been determined that the presence of these fatty acids affects the composition of cell membranes in the brain and retina and might also affect development of visual acuity in the infant.

In terms of infant growth, what are the optimal patterns that infants should achieve? The growth charts that are used to monitor the individual infant's growth patterns should not be considered to define normal but should be used only as reference standards. Charts currently used throughout the world are based on the U.S. National Center for Health Statistics reference data from 1977. For the first 2 years, these data are based on the Fels Longitudinal Study, conducted in Yellow Springs, Ohio, from 1929 to 1975. These data have come under scrutiny because (1) the incidence of breast-fed infants in the cohort was low, (2) the measurement intervals were too infrequent to capture adequate patterns of growth, and (3) the reference group used was not a representative sample.

It has been demonstrated in several studies that the growth patterns of breast-fed infants differ from those in the NCHS reference data. An explanation commonly given for this difference is that the majority of infants in the NCHS cohort were formula-fed. In longitudinal studies continuing throughout the first year, breast-fed infants showed as rapid or more rapid weight gains as formula-fed infants during the first 2 to 3 months. In contrast, evidence from these data show formula-fed infants are heavier during the later months of the first year. As a result of these findings, The World Health Organization

(WHO) completed a comprehensive review in 1995 of the uses and interpretation of the "growth standards" currently in use. They concluded that the current NCHS reference is inadequate and recommended that a new international growth reference for infants was needed to reflect the population and current health recommendations more accurately. However, given the differences in growth patterns based on feeding mode, there is concern that a growth reference constructed to be representative of a whole population may be less useful for judging the growth of either breast- or formula-fed infants. WHO has concluded that a multicountry growth study designed specifically to develop an alternative growth reference is necessary. The new reference sample should be based on breast-fed infants living in healthy environments that do not limit their genetic growth potential. In addition, measurements should be taken frequently to provide proper data for developing growth patterns and the sample size should be large enough to ensure that centile curve estimation is stable.

Until new growth references are available, health care providers need to take into account these differences in growth rates based on feeding mode. Clinicians need to make appropriate recommendations when observing deviations from the NCHS reference. Misinterpreting growth patterns of healthy breast-fed infants and advising mothers to supplement unnecessarily or to stop breast-feeding altogether have profound public health significance.

ENERGY

Energy requirements for growth, metabolism, and activity are met by the macronutrients, primarily fat and carbohydrates. Protein may also provide energy, but its most important function in growth is to provide the amino acids necessary for synthesis of body proteins and the hormones and enzymes that regulate metabolism. Most of the data on total energy expenditure and balance have been defined from measurements of intake rather than determinations of energy need. Indirect calorimetry has been the most common technique used. This procedure measures energy production through the assessment of oxygen consumption and carbon dioxide production. Direct calorimetry, which directly measures heat loss from the infant, has also been used to assess expenditure but with far less frequency. A newer approach for assessing total energy expenditure is the doubly labeled water stable isotope technique. Validation studies have shown good correlation between double-labeled water and more conventional approaches to total energy expenditure.

Because the composition and quantity of human milk consumed by infants vary, absolute requirements cannot be determined, but normal ranges can be estimated. The current recommendations for energy requirements for the breast-fed infant are 95 kcal and 84 kcal per kg from birth through 6 months and 6 months through 12 months, respectively. These revised estimates reflect more accurately what healthy infant populations receiving human milk ingest.

PROTEIN

The amount of total energy intake utilized for growth is higher during the first 2 months of life than at any other time. During this most rapid period of postnatal growth, breast-fed infants may use 60% of the protein they consume in producing new tissue. About 45% of the dietary protein intake of human milk–fed infants comes as essential amino acids. In contrast, adults need only about 13 to 20% of their recommended protein intake in the form of essential amino acids.

There are significant differences between the digestibility and quality of human milk proteins and those of bovine milk–based formulas. The proportion of whey (supernatant) and casein (curd) in human milk is of interest. Human milk is more whey-dominant, with a ratio of approximately 70:30 compared with 18:82 in bovine milk. In general, the whey fraction is soluble protein (does not form curd), which is more easily digested and more rapidly emptied from the stomach. However, as with many of the constituents of human milk, composition varies with the stage of lactation.

The type of proteins contained in the whey fraction differs between human and bovine-derived formulas. The major human whey protein is alpha-lactalbumin, a nutritional protein for the infant and a component of mammary gland lactose synthesis. Lactoferrin, lysozyme, and secretory immunoglobulin A (sIgA) are specific human whey proteins involved in host defense that are present only in trace amounts in bovine-derived formulas. The major whey protein in bovine milk is beta-lactoglobulin, which has been implicated in bovine milk protein allergy.

FAT

The fats in human milk provide approximately 50% of the calories of the milk. The lipid profile consists of 98% triglycerides, 1% phospholipids, and 0.5% cholesterol and cholesterol esters. In addition, fats are an integral part of all cell membranes, provide fatty acids necessary for brain development and are the sole vehicle for fat-soluble vitamins and hormones in milk. The total fat content of human milk is approximately 3.5 to 4.5%; however, it is the most variable component of milk, varying in content throughout lactation and within and between feedings. The fat content of human milk increases markedly during a single feed from a breast, with the concentration of hind-milk (milk produced toward the end of a nursing interval) typically being twice that in fore-milk. In addition, fat content rises during the day, early morning milk having the lowest fat content. Total fat content increases gradually from colostrum (2.0%) through transitional milk (2.5 to 3.0%) to mature milk (3.5 to 4.5 %).

In addition to the diurnal variations seen in human milk, differences exist in the lipid profile compared with that in infant formulas. Whereas human milk contains very-long-chain fatty acids, formulas are absent of fatty acids greater than C18 and contain only traces of cholesterol, compared with an average amount of 10 to 15 mg per dL of cholesterol in human milk. Recently two of these very-long-chain fatty acids, arachidonic acid (AA) (C20) and DHA (C22), have received a significant amount of investigation, specifically their role in the developing retina and brain. These fatty acids are components of phospholipids found in brain and red blood cell membranes. AA and DHA have been implicated in growth and development as well as cognition and vision.

Human milk fat digestion and absorption are facilitated by the complex organization of the human milk fat globule, the pattern of fatty acids, their distribution on the triglyceride molecule, and the presence of bile salt–stimulated lipase. These features are especially important for the preterm infant. Because lipid deposition and accretion of specific lipids occur in the last trimester of intrauterine development, very-low-birth-weight infants are deficient both in specific metabolites as well as in the enzymes needed for fat digestion and metabolism.

Normal fat requirements for newborn infants are 3.3 to 6.0 grams per 100 kcal, which represents 30 to 54% of calories. It is interesting to note that several studies have shown that the fatty acid composition of the human milk lipid system is affected by maternal diet. For example, vegan mothers consuming no animal products subsequently have lower levels of DHA in their breast milk.

CARBOHYDRATE

Carbohydrates provide substrates for fetal and neonatal metabolism, supplying both immediately usable and stored energy as well as carbon skeletons for macromolecule synthesis and tissue accretion. Approximately half of the glucose utilized is oxidized during normal metabolic processes, and the remainder is used in nonoxidative pathways, such as glycogen and fat synthesis. The neonatal brain is the major consumer of glucose, relying almost exclusively on glucose for its metabolism.

Lactose is the principal carbohydrate in human milk and provides approximately 50% of the energy content. The dietary lactose that resists hydrolysis by intestinal enzymes is the main source of carbon and energy for colonic bacteria. *Lactobacillus bifidus*, a strain of bifidobacteria, requires oligosaccharides from human milk for growth in the infant colon. This bifidobacteria represents 99% of total bacterial counts in most exclusively breast-fed infants by the end of the first week of life. Lowering the pH in the gut aids in excluding other enteropathic bacteria such as *Escherichia coli*. The fecal flora of the bottle-fed infant, on the other hand, resembles that of older children and adults, with less than 70% bifidobacteria and a higher intestinal pH.

Approximately half of the oligosaccharides present in human milk are sialylated. Animal studies have revealed a significant proportion of this monosaccharide in the developing brain. Decreased concentrations of sialic acid in the brain during early development were found to be associated with impaired learning behavior in these animals. A high concentration of sialic acid is present in human milk in the first week of lactation, coinciding with a time of rapid synthesis of brain sialylated glycoproteins. In addition, lactose is a readily available source of galactose, which is essential to the production of the galactolipids, including cerebroside. These galactolipids are essential to CNS development.

WATER AND ELECTROLYTES

Water represents the constituent in the largest quantity in human milk, providing approximately 89 mL of preformed water in each 100 mL of milk consumed. Water is required by the infant to replace evaporative losses of water from skin and lungs and in feces and urine. The first priority for water expenditures is for evaporative loss and the second for urinary water necessary for the excretion of solute. In the case of healthy full-term infants receiving adequate milk volume, supplemental water is not necessary.

Estimates of requirements for sodium, chloride, and potassium are based on estimates of what is needed for growth and for replacement of obligatory losses. These amounts depend on the rate at which extracellular fluid volume expands, a rate which varies with age. The concentration of sodium in human milk varies from 36 to 104 mg per liter, chloride concentrations are 360 to 420 mg per liter, and potassium concentrations most commonly are 400 to 500 mg per liter. A breast-fed infant consuming 750 mL of milk a day is provided with approximately 78 mg of sodium, 250 mg of chloride, and 300 mg of potassium per day. These intakes are well above the requirement.

MINERALS

Calcium (Ca), phosphorus (P), and magnesium (Mg) homeostasis in the newborn involves hormonal influences that regulate the concentrations of these minerals in the infant. Most of the body's mineral content is in tissues, and less than 1% of Ca, P, and Mg is in the circulation. However, serum concentrations are useful because fluctuations from "normal ranges" are often associated with clinical symptoms.

Blood Ca concentration is maintained within very narrow limits by the interplay of several hormones (1,25-dihydroxycholecalciferol, parathyroid hormone, calcitonin, estrogen, and testosterone), which control Ca absorption and excretion, as well as bone metabolism. The 1% of Ca not found in the bone is essential in nerve conduction, muscle contraction, blood clotting, and membrane permeability. These extraskeletal levels of Ca are maintained at the expense of bone in the face of inadequate Ca intake or absorption. In the event of such circumstances, there is the resultant demineralization of bone and reduction in strength.

Ca homeostasis is closely linked with that of P and Mg. Longitudinal studies measuring Ca and P in human milk and maternal and infant sera show progressive increases in infant serum Ca in association with decreasing P content in breast milk and infant serum. In addition, progressive increases in serum magnesium level were seen in the breast-fed infants in association with decreasing P content of the milk. Ca and P decrease over time during lactation. Human milk provides optimal Ca, Mg, and P content for the bone mineralization of term newborns. Cow's milk–based formulas generally have higher Ca content than human milk to compensate for the poorer absorption rates with the formulas. Infants receive an average of 240 mg of Ca from 750 mL of human milk, of which they retain approximately two thirds. The retention of Ca from formulas based on cow's milk is less than one half. Therefore, the recommendation for formula-fed infants is 400 mg per day for the first 6 months; and 600 mg per day from 6 to 12 months. The P content of human milk is 14 mg per 100 grams, which is adequate to meet the full-term infant's needs. The recommended daily allowance (RDA) for formula-fed infants is 300 mg per day for the first 6 months and 600 mg per day from 6 to 12 months. It should be noted that the premature infant has increased needs for these minerals and may require supplementation.

TRACE ELEMENTS

Iron, zinc, copper, manganese, selenium, molybdenum, chromium, and iodine are generally considered to be the essential trace minerals. Whereas the macronutrients (protein, fat, carbohydrate, and major minerals) are essential components of body structure and energy sources, micronutrients do not serve as energy stores and contribute to body structure. Their function, for the most part, is in providing protection against oxidative damage during cellular metabolism.

Iron is a powerful oxidant and a constituent of hemoglobin, myoglobin, and a number of enzymes and therefore is an essential nutrient for the infant. Owing to stored iron, the term infant can maintain satisfactory hemoglobin levels from human milk without other iron sources during the first 4 months of life. The RDA from 6 months to 3 years of age is set at 10 mg per kg per day for healthy infants.

Zinc is essential as a component of a large number of enzymes and plays a role in cellular immune function. Because exclusively breast-fed full-term infants rarely show signs of zinc depletion, maternal milk levels must satisfy zinc requirement. During the first month of life, breast-fed infants consume an average of 2 mg of zinc per day. The dietary zinc requirement of infants consuming formula is higher than that of breast-fed infants because of lower zinc availability in the formula. Assuming an intake of 750 mL per day of formula, the recommended intake for formula-fed infants is 5 mg per day of zinc.

The remaining trace elements have received less investigation but are no less important in the body's enzymatic activity. One consistent finding from studies of trace element levels in human milk is their variability among individuals and stages of lactation.

WATER-SOLUBLE VITAMINS

The water-soluble vitamins (C and B vitamins) are, for the most part, present in the serum and, as its name implies, the fluid compartments of the body. With the exception of vitamin B_{12}, these vitamins can be excreted in urine easily if their blood concentration rises too high.

Vitamin C (ascorbic acid) functions primarily as an antioxidant and a reducing agent. As a reducing agent, vitamin C serves as a cofactor for a number of essential enzymatic reactions. In addition, vitamin C enhances iron absorption from the gastrointestinal tract. Human milk is a rich source of vitamin C, containing approximately 43 mg per 100 mL. Concentrations of ascorbic acid in milk are generally considered to average approximately seven times those in plasma.

Thiamine primarily serves as a cofactor for three enzyme complexes involved in carbohydrate metabolism. Daily allowances for thiamine are based on the mean thiamine concentration in human milk plus two standard deviations, which is 0.3 mg per liter, or 0.4 mg per 1000 kcal.

Riboflavin serves as an essential component of flavoproteins, which function as hydrogen carriers in a number of critical oxidation-reduction reactions such as energy metabolism, glycogen synthesis, erythrocyte production, and the conversion of folate to its active coenzyme. Requirements for riboflavin are related to nitrogen intake. The riboflavin intake of an infant consuming 750 mL per day of human milk is approximately 250 μg per day, an intake that probably exceeds requirement.

Niacin is converted in the liver to the active cofactors that play central roles in body metabolism in a wide range of oxidation-reduction reactions including glycolysis, electron transport and fat synthesis. Human milk contains approximately 1.5 mg of niacin and appears to be adequate to meet the niacin needs of the infant.

Vitamin B_6 serves as a cofactor for a large number of reactions involved in the synthesis, interconversion, and catabolism of amino acids and neurotransmission. Most of the vitamin B_6 in human milk is in the form of pyridoxal. There is 12 to 15 μg per 100 mL of vitamin B_6 in human milk and 64 μg per 100 mL in cow's milk. The recommended daily intake for infants is 0.3 mg per day from birth to 4 months and 0.6 mg per day from 4 months to 1 year.

Folates function metabolically as coenzymes that transport single carbon fragments from one compound to another in amino acid metabolism and nucleic acid synthesis. Both human and cow milk contains about 50 μg of folate per liter. The needs of infants are adequately met by milk from humans and cows.

Vitamin B_{12} functions as an enzyme in amino acid metabolism. The recommended minimum daily requirement for infants is 0.3 μg per day in the first year of life, when growth is rapid. In breast-fed infants, vitamin B_{12} deficiencies occur most commonly in those whose mothers are strict vegetarians and vegans. To avoid deficiencies, it is advisable to supplement the lactating woman, as well as the infant, with up to 4 mg per day of vitamin B_{12}.

FAT-SOLUBLE VITAMINS

Vitamins A, D, E, and K are the fat-soluble vitamins, differing from the water-soluble vitamins in several ways. They are found in the fat component of milk and other foods and tend to move into the liver and adipose tissue and remain there, rather than be excreted, as in the case of the water-soluble vitamins.

Vitamin A is essential for vision, growth, cellular differentiation, reproduction, and the integrity of the immune system. The vitamin A content of human milk is reported as retinal equivalents. A breast-fed infant consuming 750 mL of milk per day is provided with 450 μg, which is considered to be at or above the requirement.

Vitamin D is essential for proper formation of bone and mineralization. The metabolite of vitamin D, 1,25-dihydroxyvitamin D, in concert with parathyroid hormone, is responsible for the mobilization and absorption of calcium, thereby promoting mineralization of the skeleton. Vitamin D is unique from the other nutrients because the body can synthesize it with exposure to sunlight. The level of 40 IU per 100 mL or 1.0 μg per 100 mL in human milk should provide adequate amounts in the fully breast-fed infant to meet the requirements of 40 IU or 10 μg per day. The exception is breast-feeding infants and their mothers who are not exposed to adequate sunlight. It is recommended that these infants receive a daily supplement of 5 to 7.5 μg.

Vitamin E is an antioxidant similar in function to vitamin C, but it is fat-soluble. Its primary function is as a scavenger of free radicals, thereby protecting cellular membranes against oxidative destruction. Because the requirement for vitamin E is closely related to the intake of polyunsaturated fatty acids, the recommendation for infants from birth to 6 months of age (3 mg) is based on the tocopherol concentration of human milk.

Vitamin K is a group of compounds essential for the formation of prothrombin and other proteins involved in the regulation of blood clotting. Owing to the low concentrations of vitamin K reported in human milk (2 μg per liter), it is recommended that exclusively breast-fed infants receive a supplement at birth. In addition, infant formulas should contain 4 μg of vitamin K per 100 kcal.

BREAST-FEEDING AND HUMAN MILK FEEDING

As previously stated, breast-feeding and human milk feeding is the optimal choice of infant feeding by all major societies and agencies, including the American Academy of Pediatrics, American Dietetics Association, and WHO. These groups base their recommendations on the strong scientific evidence of decreased infant mortality in developing countries and decreased morbidity in developed countries seen in exclusively breast-fed infants compared with those fed human milk substitutes.

Whereas lactation is a complex physiologic process under

neuroendocrine control, breast-feeding is the technical process by which milk is transferred from the maternal breast to the infant. Understanding the difference in these two interrelated processes is important when counseling the mother and her infant. Most lactation and breast-feeding problems are preventable and with proper knowledge and technical skills can be overcome.

THE PHYSICIAN'S ROLE IN INFANT FEEDING DECISION-MAKING

Prenatal visits should include discussion on infant feeding issues. This provides the parents an opportunity to make an informed choice by gaining information. Allowing for this open discussion of the facts helps diffuse guilt because lack of knowledge or support from a physician about breast-feeding causes guilt. Studies have demonstrated that prenatal education, breast-feeding support from family and friends, and especially support from the infant's father are associated with mother's choice of breast-feeding regardless of maternal age, ethnic group, educational level, or marital status. Prenatally, mothers are intensely focused on readiness for the birth experience; therefore, breast-feeding instruction and information will need to be reviewed following delivery. The office and clinic environment can send a strong message to parents about the priorities of the clinician and staff. An office replete with formula advertisements in the form of posters, pads, and pencils gives a subtle message that may undermine any verbal "lip service" paid to breast-feeding. A thorough history and breast examination should be performed during the prenatal period. History of previous breast surgery and previous breast-feeding experiences should be obtained. Previous breast surgery is not a contraindication to breast-feeding; however, the type of surgery (augmentation versus reduction) and surgical technique utilized (periareolar versus submammary) might affect lactation performance and must be considered during progression of lactation. An assessment of nipple type will allow for early intervention when appropriate. Flat and inverted nipples are not always of concern because the infant latches to the areola and not the nipple. Breast care beyond normal daily hygiene is not necessary. Practices such as "toughening of the nipples" are not recommended and can actually damage breast tissue.

INITIATION OF BREAST-FEEDING

Breast-feeding is enhanced by early initiation. It is ideal to place the infant at breast immediately following birth. Test feedings of water are not necessary to assess suck and swallow. Subsequent feedings are usually sporadic depending on the use of maternal medication during labor and delivery but should not go more than 3 to 4 hours apart. Frequent feedings provide the necessary hormonal stimulation needed for establishment of an adequate maternal milk volume. To allow for adequate milk transfer to the infant, proper positioning and latch-on at the breast are important. This is facilitated with "hands-on" instruction provided by knowledgeable nursing or medical staff. Breast-feeding books and videos are helpful but should not be used as a replacement for supportive assistance. Hospital policies that support rooming-in options and avoidance of water and glucose feedings after breast-feeding send a clear message to breast-feeding mothers. Controlled studies have demonstrated clearly that infants who are given water, glucose water, or formula instead of human milk exclusively in the first week lose more weight, regain it more slowly, and have higher bilirubin levels, and fewer stools.

Early feedings should not be timed to some predetermined duration. Infants are individual in their feeding behavior and especially in the first few days may be too sleepy to nurse for long durations. Feeding duration may range from 3 to 20 minutes at each breast. Improper positioning and latch-on at the breast rather than length of feeding is associated with degree of nipple soreness. Both breasts are usually offered at each feed; however, some infants may fall asleep before taking the second breast. An understanding that the fat content in the milk increases as the breast is emptied further validates the importance of not limiting feeding duration. This change in milk fat content also explains why the infant can get an adequate volume and caloric intake by nursing one breast at a feed.

Frequent feedings allowing time for complete breast emptying are associated with adequate maternal lactogenic hormone levels and increased milk volume. Most infants will drive their mothers' milk volume by waking for 10 to 12 feeds in a 24-hour period. Some infants may sleep for one extended duration of 4 hours in a 24-hour period and as a result cluster those 10 or so feedings in a tighter period. Given these variations in infant behavior and the move to shorter hospital stays, instruction regarding breast-feeding should be kept simple and as uncomplicated as possible. Discharge information regarding breast-feeding should be kept simple with emphasis on what to expect in terms of breast changes with the increase in milk flow, frequency and duration of feedings, and signs of adequate milk intake including stooling and urination patterns.

EARLY BREAST-FEEDING MANAGEMENT AND FOLLOW-UP

With the change to shorter hospital stays following delivery, breast-feeding mothers are discharged with little instruction before the transition from colostrum to transitional and subsequent mature milk. Most mothers will experience increased breast fullness during the first few days following delivery. However, a distinction should be made between breast fullness and engorgement. Breast fullness is a normal transitory state during which the breast tissue remains compressible, allowing the infant to suck efficiently and comfortably. Engorgement can result from improper positioning and/or delay or restriction of feeding frequency and duration. It manifests as generalized swollen rigid tissue, resulting in a taut, shiny appearance to the breast. Given this tightness, the infant finds it difficult to grasp the breast, causing increased milk stasis and maternal discomfort. Prompt intervention is needed to promote milk flow and reduce swelling. An electric *intermittent* minimum pressure breast pump along with warm compresses may need to be utilized to facilitate milk flow. Providing the primipara mother with information on these breast changes, emphasizing the importance of frequent feedings, significantly reduces the chances of severe engorgement.

Another result of early hospital discharge is the loss of the opportunity by the physician to observe the establishment of successful breast-feeding. To compensate for this, a mechanism for early postpartum follow-up is essential to ensure breast-feeding success. A visit to the office on the third day post partum allows the physician to assess the infant's positioning at the breast, passing of meconium stool, urination patterns, and maternal breast changes. On postpartum day 6, a follow-up phone call is helpful to document feeding frequency and duration, to check urine and stool frequency, and to offer support and information. This should be followed by a clinic (or home) visit at 2 weeks to check infant weight gain. Follow-up allows monitoring of the mother's and infant's progress and early intervention when necessary. Exclusively breast-fed infants receiving adequate milk intake usually follow the pattern described in Table 1.

Inadequate infant weight gain may be due to infant or maternal factors. An assessment of the breast-feeding mother-infant dyad is necessary to make a thorough assessment. Treating only one member of this dyad is not sufficient if breast-feeding is to be preserved. The most common cause of inadequate milk supply is improper instruction to the mother. Maternal stress and fatigue can result in a faulty milk ejection (letdown) reflex. When supplemental feeding is necessary, the mother should continue breast stimulation via mechanical breast pumping to maintain milk volume. If milk volume is maintained, exclusive breast-feeding can again resume once the infant's weight gain improves.

When mothers complain of sore nipples, the first step is to observe the infant latching to the breast. Infants should latch on the soft tissue of the areola, not at the base of the nipple. For this reason, mothers with flat or even inverted nipples may not experience a problem breast-feeding because the infant sucks the areola and not the nipple. If the physician is not experienced in observing breast-feeding, an *experienced* individual should be consulted.

TABLE 1. **Signs of Adequate Milk Intake in the Exclusively Breast-Fed Infant**

Nurses approximately 8–10 times/24 h; may cluster feeds
Has at least 6 (paper) to 8 (cloth) wet (pale yellow urine) diapers in 24 h
Transition from meconium (tarry) to milk stool (yellow, seedy) by day 4 postpartum; may have as many as 5–10 stools/day during the first month, less often after 4 wk
Initial weight loss not exceeding 10% of birth weight
Regain birth weight by the second week of life with an average weight gain of 30 gm/d thereafter

BREAST-FEEDING AND MATERNAL EMPLOYMENT

Many women return to work outside the home following delivery. Continuation of breast-feeding is possible during work but requires some planning and support. It has been shown that employees who delay returning to their work and those who work part-time tend to breast feed longer. When that is not possible, a gradual return to full-time employment may facilitate the development of feeding and pumping schedules. The mother will need to express her milk during the workday to maintain hormonal levels and milk volume. A variety of electric and battery-operated breast pumps are available for purchase and rent. Expressed breast milk should be refrigerated and fed to the infant within 48 hours. Glass or hard plastic is ideal for milk storage. When using soft plastic bags it is best to double-bag to prevent leakage during storage. Mothers should be informed that it is normal to see a decrease in expressed milk volume during a 5-day work week. Breast-feeding exclusively on the weekend will restore the lowered volume.

Many companies have seen a decrease in employee absenteeism due to infant illness when mothers can continue breast-feeding. Some companies provide facilities to allow privacy while pumping. Enabling a mother to continue this breast-feeding relationship following her return to work makes the transition from full-time mother to working mother less stressful.

MATERNAL FEVER

Maternal fever *is not* a contraindication to breast-feeding. The maternal ability to manufacture secretory IgA specific to the infection her infant is exposed to and excrete it in her milk provides her infant with a unique and potent protection from infection. Cessation of breast-feeding during this time will prevent this elegant protective cycle from occurring.

CONTRAINDICATIONS TO BREAST-FEEDING

Some Maternal Medications

Breast-feeding is contraindicated during maternal use of drugs of abuse (i.e., heroin, cocaine). There are few other drugs that are contraindicated during breast-feeding. Up-to-date references are important to keep current with recommendations. The *Physicians' Desk Reference* is a poor resource for information on excretion of drugs in breast milk.

Breast Cancer

A mother with breast cancer should not nurse her infant to allow immediate definitive treatment. Prolactin levels remain very high during lactation, and prolactin may advance mammary cancer.

Human Immunodeficiency Virus (HIV)–Positive Mother

The Centers for Disease Control and Prevention and the Public Health Service recommend that women who test positive for HIV antibody should be counseled to avoid breast-feeding.

Active Tuberculosis

It is safe to breast-feed if the mother and infant are allowed to have contact and both are receiving treatment. Because mother and infant are usually treated with isoniazid concurrently, consideration should be made regarding accumulation of the drug in the infant as isoniazid does pass into the breast milk.

COMMERCIAL INFANT FORMULA

No commercially processed infant formula has been developed that reproduces the immunologic properties, nutrient bioavailability, digestibility, and trophic effects of human milk. The composition of infant formulas, however, has improved tremendously in the last 50 years as a result of a greater understanding of infant nutrient requirements, absorption, and metabolic activities. Continued research is under way to qualitatively enhance infant formulas.

When used as the sole source of infant nutrition, infant formula must meet all the energy and nutrient requirements for the healthy term infant for the first 6 months of life. The American Academy of Pediatrics Committee on Nutrition develops infant formula standards. The Food and Drug Administration regulations for infant formula are based on these standards. In addition, the Infant Formula Act mandates adherence to standards and quality control and requires that quantitative label declaration be made for 38 nutrients. Amounts of each nutrient are added in formulas at higher concentrations than those in human milk to compensate for the lower bioavailability of nutrients from infant formula.

Commercially available infant formulas fall into several categories which include (1) standard cow's milk–based formulas; (2) soy-based lactose-free formulas; (3) elemental, hydrolyzed protein formulas; (4) premature infant formulas; and (5) specialty infant formulas, including those for infants with metabolic disorders. These formulas come as powder, concentrate, or ready to feed. Health care providers should make sure that parents understand how to mix these formulas correctly. If using a ready-to-feed formula after the infant is 6 months of age or if living in an area with nonfluoridated water, a fluoride supplement may be required.

INTRODUCTION TO SOLID FOODS

Solid foods can be introduced to infants at 4 to 6 months of age depending on development as well as social, cultural, and economic consideration. The feeding of solids before 4 months of age offers no nutritional or developmental benefits and may result in excessive weight gain. Up until about 4 months of age the feeding of solids by spoon is difficult because of the presence of the extrusion reflex. When food is placed on the anterior half of the tongue, this protective reflex causes the tongue to move forward pushing food from the mouth. Mothers attempt to stay ahead of this reflex by scraping the food from the chin and pushing it back in. There is no need to feed with a spoon until this reflex spontaneously disappears at 4 to 5 months of age. At 6 months of age, an infant's iron stores may be diminished, so the introduction of solids to supplement this nutrient is desirable.

When solid foods are introduced, single-ingredient foods should be selected and introduced one at a time in no less than 3-day intervals to permit the identification of food intolerance if present. Infant cereal is the optimal first supplemental food because it not only contains additional energy but is fortified with iron. Cereal should be fed by spoon and not added to the nursing bottle except for medically indicated reasons such as gastroesophageal reflux.

The order in which solid foods have traditionally been introduced has been cereal, fruit, yellow vegetables, green vegetables, meats, and desserts. There is no physiologic reason why this order of introduction is necessary. After cereals, the food that is introduced can be at the discretion of the mother.

Commercially prepared strained foods or those prepared at home are both acceptable. If infant foods are prepared at home, precaution should be taken to avoid highly seasoned food or food salted to adult taste. The salt content of commercially prepared U.S. baby food is low. Honey should not be fed to infants younger than 12 months of age owing to its association with infant botulism.

The amount of water needed by infants to replace their losses and provide for growth is available in both human milk and infant formula during the nursing period. Healthy infants require little or no supplemental water except in hot weather. When solid foods are introduced, additional water is required because the renal solute load is high in solid foods owing to their higher protein and salt content. Infants should be offered water to allow an opportunity to fulfill fluid needs without an obligatory intake of extra calories. Fruit juice is not a good choice as a water substitute because it may introduce poor eating habits by emphasizing the sweet flavor. If placed in a bottle, which an infant is allowed to drink from over prolonged periods, fruit juice increases the risk of dental caries.

VITAMIN SUPPLEMENTS

Vitamin K is effective in preventing hemorrhagic disease of the newborn because it prevents or minimizes the postnatal decline of the vitamin K–dependent coagulation factors II, VII, IX, and X. Vitamin K is given as a single, intramuscular dose of 0.5 to 1 mg or an oral dose of 1.0 to 2.0 mg. Large doses of water-soluble vitamin K analogues can produce hyperbilirubinemia.

Questions still exist regarding whether breast-fed infants require any vitamin or mineral supplements before the introduction of solid foods at 6 months of age. The vitamin D content of human milk is low and rickets can occur in breast-fed infants who are deeply pigmented and have an inadequate exposure to sunlight. Therefore, vitamin D supplementation is recommended for these breast-fed infants at a dose of 400 IU per day. There is no evidence that vitamin A or E is needed for healthy breast-fed term infants.

Fluoride supplementation at 0.25 mg per day should be started once the teeth erupt if the infant does not receive an adequate source of fluoridated water. Parents may contact their local water service to check the fluoride levels in their community.

In conclusion, infancy is a period of rapid growth and development during which adequate nutrition is essential. Breast milk remains the feeding choice for the infant for the first year of life, enhancing immunity and cognitive development. Formulas are available but have yet to mimic all the important attributes found in mother's milk.

DISEASES OF THE BREAST

method of
ROGER S. FOSTER, Jr., M.D.
Emory University
Atlanta, Georgia

Breast cancer is the most important of all breast diseases. For the average woman, the cumulative probability of developing breast cancer by the age of 90 years is about 9%. Of the women who do develop breast cancer, 20 to 30% can be expected to die of breast cancer. Death from breast cancer currently reduces the life expectancy of the average woman in North America by approximately 0.5 year. The risk of death from breast cancer can be reduced by both earlier detection and effective primary treatment. Chemoprevention reduces the incidence of breast cancer in high-risk women.

SCREENING FOR BREAST CANCER

In the screening of asymptomatic women for breast cancer, breast palpation and mammography are the two techniques of proven value. There are no convincing data to establish the worth of thermography, transillumination, or sonography as screening procedures.

Mammographic screening of asymptomatic women aged 50 to 74 years has been demonstrated in several controlled trials to reduce breast cancer deaths by about one third. The benefits of screening mammography for average-risk women younger than 50 years are less and are the subject of considerable debate. The density of normal breast tissue makes imaging more difficult in younger women, and faster tumor growth rates may make it more difficult to get a screening benefit, particularly if mammograms are performed at intervals longer than annually. Nevertheless, there is increasing evidence of a benefit from the screening of women aged 40 to 49 years. The American Cancer Society and the National Cancer Institute recommend that mammographic screening of average-risk women begin at the age of 40 years.

Factors that place a woman at increased risk for breast cancer include family history, early menarche, late menopause, nulliparity, first full-term pregnancy after the age of 30 years, and exposure to ionizing radiation. The two most important risk factors, however, are female sex and increased age. Less than 1% of all breast cancers occur in women younger than 30 years, 2% occur in women younger than 35 years, and 70% occur in women older than 50 years. No factors can define a set of women older than 40 years who are not at significant risk of breast cancer; therefore, breast cancer screening is important in all women. It is estimated that 5 to 10% of breast cancers in the United States occur in women who have inherited a strong genetic susceptibility. A positive family history of breast cancer is of particular significance when the patient's mother, aunt, or daughter has had breast cancer diagnosed before the age of 50 years or when a relative has had bilateral breast cancer.

Genetic screening for inherited mutations that put patients at high risk for breast cancer is becoming available. A decision to order such testing is complex. Genetic testing should not be ordered until there has been informed counseling of the patient about the many issues involved with genetic testing. These issues include the psychologic impact of the information on the individual tested, as well as on any relatives; how the information will be used in clinical management; and confidentiality of the information relative to potential health, disability, and life insurance and/or work place discrimination.

On the basis of currently available data, the breast cancer screening program that I recommend is as follows:

1. Women aged 20 to 39 years with no personal or significant family history of breast cancer: breast self-examination (BSE) monthly and clinical breast examination (CBE) every 2 to 3 years.
2. Women aged 40 to 49 years: BSE monthly, CBE yearly, and mammography yearly. For women younger than 50 years who decide to have mammographic screening, I advise annual mammograms, rather than every-other-year mammography, because of the more rapid growth rate and shorter time to reach a palpable size in younger women.
3. Women aged 50 to 65 years: BSE monthly, CBE yearly, and mammography every year.
4. Women aged 65 years and older: BSE monthly, CBE yearly, and mammography every 1 to 2 years. (Medicare guidelines permit payment for screening mammograms only every 2 years in the absence of symptoms or a personal history of breast cancer.)
5. Women aged 75 years and older: CBE yearly, monthly BSE if they are capable. Any mammography screening should be restricted to those in general good health with a long life expectancy, because the benefits of screening probably take 5 or more years to become evident.
6. Women with a strong family history of breast cancer, or of premenopausal breast cancer: BSE monthly, CBE yearly, and mammography yearly beginning at the age of 35 years.
7. Women who have been treated for one breast cancer should have yearly follow-up mammograms.

BREAST CANCER CHEMOPREVENTION

The antiestrogen drug tamoxifen has been shown to reduce the incidence of invasive breast cancer by 45%. There is a similar reduction in the incidence of noninvasive breast cancers. At this writing, the initial results of a large U.S. trial of women at increased risk of breast cancer have just been released. Women taking tamoxifen also benefit from lower rates of the osteoporosis-related fractures of the hip, wrist, and spine. However, tamoxifen also has negative health effects, particularly in women older than 50 years. The tamoxifen-treated women have more than a twofold increase in endometrial cancer; almost all of the endometrial cancers are readily treatable stage 1 cancers. There is an increased rate of venous thrombosis and thromboembolic disease, with approximately a threefold increase in the rates of life-threatening pulmonary embolus in tamoxifen-treated women. Tamoxifen also has non life-threatening toxicities, such as hot flashes, vaginal discharge, and irregular menses.

The decision to recommend tamoxifen for the prevention of breast cancer in individual patients requires multiple considerations. A history of deep vein thrombosis is a relatively strong contraindication. Women who might be considered particularly strong candidates for chemoprevention with tamoxifen include any patient with a prior diagnosis of invasive breast cancer who has not been treated with a course of tamoxifen as systemic adjuvant therapy; patients with ductal carcinoma in situ (DCIS) or lobular carcinoma in situ (LCIS); patients who have had a breast biopsy showing atypical lobular or ductal hyperplasia; and women who, on genetic testing, have been found to be positive for abnormal *BRCA1* or *BRCA2* genes, a Li-Fraumeni P-53 gene mutation, or Cowden's syndrome (multiple hamartoma syndrome). Among the patients with a previous diagnosis of invasive breast cancer, the women least likely to have been treated with tamoxifen therapeutically in the past will be those whose first breast cancer was estrogen receptor negative or was under the size of 1 cm; it appears that there is a lower rate of contralateral breast cancer with tamoxifen, both when the first tumor was estrogen receptor positive and when it was estrogen receptor negative.

Although the women described in the previous paragraph probably have the strongest indications for tamoxifen chemoprevention, there are many other risk factors that may contribute toward a decision to take tamoxifen as breast cancer prevention. Because only the preliminary results of the U.S. trial are available at this writing, further analysis of the risks and benefits will undoubtedly aid in better guideline formation regarding the net benefit for women at lower risk. Age is a major risk factor, and 30% of the women in the U.S. Breast Cancer Prevention Trial were eligible simply because they were older than 60 years. In fact, many who entered the trial had risk factors in addition to age older than 60. Additional breast cancer risk factors include early menarche, nulliparity, or having one's first child at a later age, late menarche, and first-degree relatives with breast cancer, particularly premenopausal breast cancer. Tables are available to aid in calculating the absolute risk of breast cancer when the various relative risk factors are added together.

When used for breast cancer prevention, the dose and duration of treatment with tamoxifen are the same as when tamoxifen is used as systemic adjuvant therapy: 20 mg daily for 5 years. No additional therapeutic benefit has been seen in the adjuvant therapy trials when tamoxifen was given beyond 5 years, and the reduction in risk of contralateral breast cancer has persisted even after the tamoxifen has been stopped. Multiple new breast cancer chemoprevention trials are being planned to compare tamoxifen with other antiestrogen compounds, such as toremifene and raloxifene, and the results of ongoing trials of retinoids as possible breast cancer prevention agents are awaited.

BENIGN BREAST PROBLEMS

The most important aspect of the management of benign breast problems is to exclude the possibility of malignancy.

Physiologic Nodulation and Fibrocystic Breast Disease

The breasts of premenopausal women undergo repeated cyclical hormonal stimulation, and physiologically induced breast nodulations (or lumpiness) develop in many women. Such nodulations typically increase during the premenstrual period and regress afterward. Accompanying symptoms are variable, but for some women there may be fairly severe premenstrual pain, swelling, and tenderness. The term "fibrocystic breast disease" for a condition that occurs to some degree in the majority of women is inappropriate and frightening. There is no increased risk for breast cancer associated with fibrocystic breast changes unless there are pathologic findings of epithelial proliferation, such as ductal or lobular hyperplasia (slightly increased risk) or atypical hyperplasia (moderately increased risk). Treatment of the patient with physiologic breast nodulation and moderate discomfort is careful physical examination (best performed during the postmenstrual interval) and reassurance, with the suggestion that analgesics such as aspirin be used if the symptoms interfere with physical or sexual activity.

The degree of breast nodulation is probably not related to the ingestion of methylxanthines (caffeine, theophylline, theobromine), but in some women the degree of breast tenderness may be related. For the rare patient whose problem does not respond to simple measures, there is a limited role for treatment with antiestrogen medication such as tamoxifen (Nolvadex); bromocriptine (Parlodel), which inhibits pituitary prolactin; or an impeded androgen such as danazol (Danocrine), which inhibits the release of pituitary gonadotropins. Attempts at treating these patients with subcutaneous mastectomies have resulted in symptomatic failures and complications, and such treatment is inappropriate.

Women with asymmetrical areas of breast nodulation may require additional investigation. Breast imaging may be obtained as appropriate for the patient's age: ultrasonography for women younger than 35 years and mammography with or without ultrasonography for older women. Fine-needle aspiration biopsy (to be described) of such areas occasionally demonstrates malignant cells even in the absence of a distinct mass or a mammographic or ultrasonographic abnormality. If the fine-needle aspiration biopsy demonstrates an adequate number of normal ductal cells, there is considerable reassurance that the area is benign, and open breast biopsy is not necessary.

Gross Cysts

In contrast to physiologic breast nodulations, true breast masses, which are distinguished as being discrete, dense, dominant, and different from the rest of the breast tissue, should receive surgical attention. Most palpable true breast masses are aspirated with a fine needle (e.g., 21 gauge). Gross cysts, which can occur in patients of any age but are most common in the 15 years before menopause, are completely evacuated, and the fluid is discarded if it is typical cyst fluid (tawny to grayish or dark green opalescent fluid). Cytologic examination and further evaluation of the patient are necessary if the fluid is bloody.

Fibroadenomas

Fibroadenomas are benign fibroepithelial neoplasms that occur most commonly in women younger than 30 years. Fibroadenomas tend to be quite firm, mobile, nontender, and well delineated, and some resistance to withdrawal of the needle occurs after attempted aspiration. Cytologic examination is obtained on material aspirated with a fine needle from any solid lesion in which malignancy is deemed a possibility. Fibroadenomas and other true discrete breast masses may be excised on an outpatient basis, usually with local anesthesia.

An alternative to removing benign breast masses is observation after a negative "triple test." A negative triple test consists of physical examination consistent with a benign lump, a breast image (ultrasonogram or mammogram) consistent with a benign lump, and a needle biopsy result consistent with a benign lump.

Nipple Discharges

Nipple discharge is of clinical significance only if it is spontaneous. Self-induced nipple discharges have no importance, and patients should be taught not to squeeze the nipples as part of BSE. Spontaneous serous and bloody discharges are most commonly caused by an intraductal papilloma, but mammographic evaluation followed by excision of the distal duct or ducts is necessary to rule out the possibility of a carcinoma. Nonlactational milky discharge should be evaluated with a test for serum prolactin because of the possibility of a pituitary adenoma.

Infection

Most of the infections that occur in other areas of the body can occur in the breast. Infections from *Staphylococcus aureus, Staphylococcus epidermidis,* and *Streptococcus* species are particularly common in lactating breasts, and if the lesion is cellulitis and not an abscess, it can usually be managed with antibiotics; breast-feeding can be continued during treatment. A nipple shield or breast pump may be used if a nipple fissure makes breast-feeding painful. If a breast abscess is present, the abscess should be drained. Alternative drainage techniques are needle aspiration, catheter drainage (e.g., placed under ultrasound guidance), or open surgical drainage. Recurrent periareolar abscess in nonlactating women is commonly caused by squamous metaplasia of the lactiferous ducts. Treatment is by surgical excision of the abnormal distal duct or ducts, usually after the acute process has been controlled by drainage of the abscess and antibiotics.

Noninfectious Breast Inflammations

Trauma to the breast can cause a breast mass that may mimic the clinical characteristics of carcinoma. Sometimes the clinical history and mammographic appearance are sufficiently convincing to permit management by observation only, but most commonly biopsy is required to exclude a malignancy.

Thrombosis of a superficial vein in the breast (Mondor's disease) can cause skin retraction that mimics the Cooper ligament retraction caused by a breast cancer. The linear cord of the thrombosed vein can usually be palpated. Sometimes the thrombosis occurs after a surgical procedure or after a blow to the breast, but frequently there is no evident cause. Once breast cancer has been excluded, no specific treatment is required.

Localized breast erythema of unknown cause occurs occasionally. The process may last days to months. Such patients need to be examined by an experienced clinician and may require a biopsy to exclude inflammatory carcinoma or infection.

COSMETIC SURGERY

Cosmetic surgery may be desired by women who have asymmetrically sized breasts, whose breasts have not developed to an acceptable size or have involuted after pregnancy, or whose breasts have developed to an abnormally large size. The augmentation mammoplasty operation involving the use of a submusculofascial Silastic bag implant is relatively simple and usually provides good cosmetic results, but there has been controversy about safety. Reduction mammoplasty for excessively large and heavy breasts is a more complex procedure in which the breast is resized and the nipple-areolar complex is repositioned. When the volume of breast tissue is satisfactory but stretching of skin has led to marked ptosis, a mastopexy operation, in which excess skin is removed and the nipple-areolar complex is repositioned, can be performed.

PRIMARY BREAST CANCER

Diagnosis and Staging of Breast Cancer

The diagnosis of a palpable breast cancer can be established by fine-needle aspiration biopsy, by core-cutting needle biopsy, by open incisional biopsy, or by excisional biopsy. Fine-needle aspiration biopsy is of particular value because it can be performed as an office procedure. Although this procedure is conceptually a simple technique, the operator must be able to obtain an adequate sample, and the cytopathologist must be experienced in providing reliable interpretation. The diagnosis of nonpalpable breast cancers that are detectable only by mammography is made either by needle biopsy or by open biopsy. Open biopsy is performed after the area to be biopsied is localized by the mammographic placement of a needle at the site from which the specimen is to be taken. Fine-needle aspiration biopsy and core needle biopsy of mammographic lesions may be done with ultrasound guidance or with a stereotactic mammography technique.

Excisional biopsies of lesions known or suspected to be cancer should be performed as formal partial mastectomies—that is, a small margin of apparently normal breast tissue surrounding the lesion is also excised, and the pathologist paints the external surface with ink before sectioning—so that it can be established that there are tumor-free margins. If tumor-free margins are obtained and the patient's definitive treatment is to be partial mastectomy, no further resection of breast tissue is needed; the cosmetic results are better than when a second resection of breast tissue must be performed after an excisional biopsy.

The histologic type of breast cancer has a bearing on both the prognosis and the management. The most important distinction in terms of biologic behavior is between invasive breast cancer, which has a relatively high likelihood of systemic metastases, and noninvasive or in situ cancer, in which there should be no systemic metastases. Unfortunately, the noninvasive cancers are much less common than the invasive cancers; they are, however, being increasingly recognized with screening mammography.

The two different types of noninvasive breast cancer are (1) ductal carcinoma in situ (DCIS, or intraductal carcinoma), which usually affects only one breast, and (2) lobular carcinoma in situ (LCIS), sometimes referred to as lobular neoplasia, which commonly affects both breasts. With the passage of time, noninvasive intraductal carcinomas frequently, but not inevitably, develop into invasive cancer. A coexistent invasive carcinoma has been reported in about 20% of patients whose predominant lesion is a DCIS. In 15 to 20% of patients with small areas of DCIS who have undergone only a limited biopsy, invasive ductal carcinoma develops in the same site over a median interval of 10 years. In about 25% of patients with LCIS who have undergone only biopsy, invasive carcinoma develops over a median interval of 20 years and the risk is relatively even for both breasts and is not specifically related to the site at which the LCIS was biopsied. Patients with LCIS and DCIS are candidates for chemoprevention therapy.

Invasive ductal carcinoma is the most common type of invasive breast carcinoma, accounting for about 70% of these cancers. Invasive ductal carcinomas frequently cause a productive fibrosis, which is responsible for much of the hardness that is felt on palpation and the grittiness that is felt when the tumor is cut with a knife or entered with a needle. Lobular invasive carcinoma accounts for 5 to 10% of invasive cancers. The biologic behavior and prognosis of lobular carcinoma are similar to those of invasive ductal carcinoma. Medullary carcinomas account for 5% of invasive cancers, and it has been suggested that they carry a somewhat more favorable prognosis. Their biologic behavior is not much different from that of invasive ductal carcinoma. Colloid, tubular, adenocystic, and papillary carcinomas are relatively rare types and generally carry much better prognoses than do the more common types of invasive carcinoma.

Once a diagnosis or even strong presumptive diagnosis of breast cancer has been made, the clinical stage, or extent of disease, should be established. Clinical TNM (tumor, node, metastases) staging is based on the size of the primary cancer and any invasion of skin or underlying muscle or chest wall, clinical evidence of involvement of regional nodes (axillary, supraclavicular, or infraclavicular), and any evidence of more distant metastases. In addition to physical examination, the clinical evaluation of all patients with invasive breast cancer should include a chest radiograph and liver enzyme assays to screen for hepatic involvement. Routine bone scans, liver scans, and computed tomographic scans are not indicated unless the patient is symptomatic, has evidence of locally advanced disease on physical examination, or has an elevated liver enzyme level.

Pathologic staging of breast cancer is more definitive than clinical staging. For surgically operable invasive breast cancers, the presence or absence of histologically documented regional node metastases (axillary nodes) and the determination of the absolute number of nodes involved by metastases may provide the most important information for prognosis and for decision-making in relation to the use of systemic adjuvant chemotherapy. The levels of estrogen and of progesterone receptor proteins in the tumor provide additional prognostic and management information; high levels of receptor proteins indicate both a slightly more favorable prognosis and a greater likelihood of response to hormonal therapy when there are metastases.

Treatment

Local and/or Regional Treatment

The majority of patients are probably candidates for breast-conserving surgery; in the United States, however, the most common local and/or regional treatment for surgically operable carcinoma of the breast is total mastectomy and axillary dissection with preservation of the chest wall muscles (modified radical mastectomy). For most patients with stage I or II breast cancer, radiotherapy to the regional lymph nodes after mastectomy and axillary dissection does not improve survival and increases morbidity. Breast-conserving surgery (lumpectomy or partial mastectomy and radiotherapy) is increasingly being used.

In my practice, most patients with primary invasive cancers less than 4 to 5 cm in diameter are treated by partial (segmental) mastectomy followed by radiotherapy (5000 rad to the breast delivered through tangential ports with or without a radiation boost to the tumor bed); either a sentinel node biopsy or an axillary dissection is usually performed through a separation incision. This technique has been demonstrated by the National Surgical Adjuvant Breast Project studies and six other studies to provide 10-year survival rates similar to those obtained with modified radical mastectomy and to permit preservation of the breast in most of the patients. A small percentage of patients treated by partial mastectomy demonstrate recurrence of tumor in the breast and subsequently require a total mastectomy. In many patients older than 70 years, it is my practice to omit breast irradiation after partial mastectomy, as in-breast recurrence rates are much lower without irradiation than they would be in younger patients.

Most women whose disease is unsuited to partial mastectomy are offered either immediate or delayed breast reconstruction. In some patients, the breast is appropriately reconstructed with a submuscular tissue expander and a Silastic implant; many patients are better served by procedures that transfer the abdominal or latissimus dorsi muscle with overlying fat and skin.

Patients with noninvasive DCIS may present particular difficulties in relation to the amount of breast tissue that needs to be removed. In contrast to most invasive cancers, many intraductal carcinomas involve the breast so diffusely that they cannot be excised by partial mastectomy, and thus many women with these prognostically favorable tumors are treated by total mastectomy, which may be followed by reconstruction. Patients with localized intraductal carcinoma may be treated by a combination of partial mastectomy and breast irradiation, or occasionally partial mastectomy without irradiation. Chemoprevention with tamoxifen is recommended for most DSIC patients.

Appropriate management of LCIS is even more poorly defined; because this disease is diffuse and bilateral, any management policy should be the same for both breasts. Most patients with LCIS are managed with a conservative policy of chemoprevention and repeated physical and mammographic examinations; selected patients may elect bilateral total mastectomy and breast reconstruction.

Systemic Adjuvant Treatment

Although in 95% of patients the disease is apparently localized to the breast and regional nodes at the time of initial treatment, systemic metastases develop during a 10-year period in approximately one third of the patients receiving only local regional therapy (surgery with or without radiotherapy). In the era before systemic adjuvant therapy, 75% of the patients with metastases to the axillary nodes had recurrences and were dead at 10 years. Patients with palpable tumors but without axillary node metastases have a recurrence rate of more than 40% at 10 years. For axillary node–negative patients with invasive tumors 1 cm or less in diameter, which are frequently detected by screening mammography, 90% are expected to be free of recurrence at 10 years. For patients with noninvasive cancers, who should be recurrence free if resection is complete, the 10-year systemic recurrence rate is 1 to 2%, presumably because an invasive component was present and missed at pathologic diagnosis.

It has been shown that systemic adjuvant therapy can produce modest but quite meaningful reductions in recurrence and improvements in survival in both premenopausal and postmenopausal patients with breast cancer. Benefit has been seen in both node-positive patients and in those node-negative patients who are higher risk. The relative magnitude of the benefits of systemic adjuvant therapy are similar in high-risk and low-risk patients. Because a higher proportion of the low-risk patients are destined never to have a recurrence, the absolute benefits of systemic therapy are less for them. A larger proportion of the lower risk patients bear the cost and toxicity of treatment without benefit. Outside the context of a formal clinical trial, systemic adjuvant therapy is not recommended for patients with invasive tumors less than 1 cm in diameter or for patients with the smaller pure tubular, papillary, or colloid histologic findings, and it is not recommended for noninvasive cancers. Systemic adjuvant therapy is given to almost all patients with primary breast cancer with metastases to the regional nodes and to most patients with tumors 3 cm in diameter and larger.

Patients with node-negative tumors in the 1- to 3-cm range are problematic; overall, recurrences can be expected in approximately 30% of these patients. The ability to distinguish the majority of patients who will not benefit from chemotherapy from the minority who will is imperfect. Most patients with node-negative 1- to 3-cm cancer are treated with systemic adjuvant treatment.

When premenopausal patients are treated with systemic adjuvant therapy, a cytotoxic chemotherapy protocol is most often used; there is added benefit from tamoxifen in patients with hormone receptor–positive tumors. Postmenopausal patients whose breast cancer hormone receptor assays are negative also have improved survival rates with cytotoxic chemotherapy. Postmenopausal patients with hormone receptor–positive tumors are most commonly treated with the antiestrogen tamoxifen (Nolvadex). Many clinicians prescribe cytotoxic chemotherapy in addition to tamoxifen for postmenopausal women with receptor-positive tumors, particularly for higher risk patients.

METASTATIC BREAST CANCER

Metastatic breast cancer is rarely cured, which is the reason for the emphasis on systemic adjuvant therapy given at the time of diagnosis of the primary tumor. There has been an attempt to cure metastatic breast cancer in younger women with the use of intensive cytotoxic chemotherapy programs that require special support of the bone marrow through transplantation of bone marrow cells, peripheral blood progenitor cells, or both along with the administration of blood cell growth factors. The preliminary data from the uncontrolled reports are encouraging, but the favorable results may be related to the screening and the selection of patients rather than the treatment. The data from the controlled trials currently under way are not yet available.

The common sites for breast cancer metastases include bone, the liver, the lungs, the brain, and the chest wall. Although a limited number of patients remain free of disease after resection of solitary lung, brain, or cutaneous metastases, treatment of metastatic breast cancer is, for the most part, palliative. Therapy for metastatic breast cancer includes both cytotoxic chemotherapy and hormonal manipulations, as well as site-specific local therapy.

Patients with oncologic emergencies such as hypercalcemia, central nervous system metastases, unstable bone metastases, or pleural effusion need prompt therapy specific for the problem. Hypercalcemia usually responds to intravenous hydration and furosemide-induced diuresis. Brain and spinal cord metastases should be treated with high doses of corticosteroids, and immediate neurosurgical and radiotherapy consultations should be obtained. Patients with hip and leg pain should undergo bone scan and radiographic evaluations to determine whether lesions that may lead to pathologic fracture are present; impending fractures can be prevented by radiotherapy with or without insertion of a metal prosthesis as indicated. Large pleural effusions can be treated by insertion of a chest tube to evacuate the effusion, after which a sclerosing agent can be injected to create an adherence between the parietal and visceral pleura (pleurodesis).

About 50% of breast cancer patients are estrogen- or progesterone-receptor–positive. Hormonal manipulations are preferred over cytotoxic chemotherapy in many receptor-positive and receptor-unknown patients because the response durations tend to be longer and side effects are fewer. Older patients and patients with well-differentiated tumors are more likely to be receptor-positive. Initial hormonal therapies include antiestrogens, such as tamoxifen; progestational agents; and, for premenopausal patients, oophorectomy or agents that suppress pituitary gonadotrophins. The median duration of an endocrine response is about 12 to 18 months. After initial response to hormonal therapy and then further progression of disease, additional responses may be obtained by secondary hormonal manipulations. Patients whose disease is unsuited for hormonal manipulations or is no longer responsive are treated with combination cytotoxic chemotherapy. Response to current first-line combination chemotherapy occurs in 50 to 75% of patients, with a median duration response of 6 to 12 months. Response to second-line chemotherapy regimens tends to be less.

ENDOMETRIOSIS

method of
AGNETA BERGQVIST, M.D., PH.D.
Huddinge University Hospital
Huddinge, Sweden

Endometriosis is a complicated disease that includes several pathophysiologic mechanisms. It sometimes may develop for several years before the symptoms motivate the woman to see a physician to get help. The cause of the disease is not known, so a specific causal treatment is not available. However, the pathophysiologic process is partly characterized, which is of the greatest importance, because it is only by interrupting this process that we may give some relief to the patients. This fact makes the treatment design complicated but also exciting.

Before discussing different therapeutic approaches, the process should be clarified. During menstruation, the shedded endometrial fragments follow the blood out through all open channels, including the tubes, into the peritoneal cavity. This is a normal process, and all strange cells or substances that enter the pelvic cavity are normally attacked by the immune system, in this case mainly the natural killer (NK) cells that present the antigens for macrophages that clear the cells away. Women with endometriosis have been found to have lower levels of NK cells in their peritoneal fluid, and their cytotoxic activity is decreased. The explanation for this is not known. The macrophages are hyperactivated because of their duty to rid the pelvis of the explants, but for some unknown reasons they are not successful. This hyperactivation leads to an increased secretion of different inflammatory and growth factors, such as cytokines, which may further stimulate the growth of the endometriotic cells and thus enhance the disease. The cytokines also have different systemic effects, such as inducing fever and pain, as well as a varying effect on fertility. No therapy is yet available that normalizes the function of NK cells and macrophages.

Secondary activation of the humoral immune system has also been shown. This includes an increase of complement factors, factors that influence both general well-being and fertility.

The first question is why is there a defect in the defense system? There is a certain hereditary component in endometriosis. The heritage is probably polygenetic, and several studies are ongoing to further characterize the genetic aspects. Further, women with frequent and/or heavy menstrual bleeding that appeared early in life and was not interrupted by pregnancies run an increased risk. High-risk patients might be given health care information and if possible prophylaxis. Heredity and bleeding pattern might be two, but not the only, explanations for the disturbed defense in the pelvic cavity.

The endometrial cells may settle down on any surface, and as they do, they adhere and invade. Unlike normal intrauterine endometrium, endometriotic implants have the capacity to grow invasively, not always respecting organ or tissue limits. An increased proteolytic activity in endometriotic tissue compared with that in the woman's uterine endometrium has been shown. Furthermore, a significantly higher fibrinolytic capacity has been shown in endometriotic tissue and the endometrium in women with endometriosis compared with that in the endometrium of healthy controls. Some studies on adhesion molecules have shown that some of these are differently expressed in endometriotic tissue than in endometrium. Thus, the question has been raised regarding wether the primary disturbance is localized in the woman's uterine cavity instead of in the lesions. Is the endometrium in some women different, having the capacity to adhere to and invade other tissues more easily than that in women who do not develop endometriosis?

When discharged endometrial cells enter the pelvic cavity, they usually settle in the lowest parts like different pocket formations. For some reason they also often attach to elevated structures like the ovarian surfaces, the uterosacral ligaments, and the uterus. Some investigators claim that the attachments occur only to defects in the surface lining, making invasion possible. Early superficial implants may be seen through the laparoscope as minute red spots, but the initial lesions are not visible to the eye. Half of the biopsy specimens from the peritoneal surface regarded as normal in women with endometriosis have shown endometriotic implants.

The inflammatory process evoked results in the creation of fibrosis that to varying degrees surrounds and grows into the explant to extinguish it. The explant may react to circulating ovarian steroids like the endometrium and thus bleed at menstruation. However, when the fibrosis has covered the explant, the bleeding is included, giving the lesion a red-blue color. In time the red blood cells are broken down, leaving a brownish hemosiderin pigment behind, which is visible to the naked eye. The fibrosis grows into the stroma and replaces these cells but never the epithelial structures. When the fibrotic reaction has started, it may continue and spread as long as a stimulating factor remains. The volume of fibrosis will far exceed the volume of endometriotic tissue, and the lesion looks like a whitish spot or area. This is called "burned out endometriosis." However, although no endometriotic structures are visible to the eye, they can usually be found microscopically when such an area is sectioned and stained. During the fibrosis creation, endometriotic tissue may break through and invade behind, and sometimes it appears as if a war is being waged between the invasive endometriotic tissue and the defense system of fibrosis.

The fibrotic tissue is very tight and hard, and the adhesions created are different from adhesions created after infection or surgical trauma, which are usually loose, thin curtains or strings that leave the organ structures at each side undestroyed. Endometriosis fibrosis involves surrounding organs so tightly that cleavage between organs often is missing, making surgery technically difficult. Lesions surrounded by such hard fibrosis are often called deep lesions. They are usually located in the uterosacral ligaments, rectovaginal septum, or scars in the abdominal wall. In the bowel the fibrosis is different, containing more shiny, collagen-rich structures, radiating from the endometriotic foci in the serosa toward the mucosa without growing into this layer. However, also in this cell-free looking fibrosis, small endometriotic lesions are spread out microscopically, and they usually show a vital growth pattern. These lesions rarely respond to hormonal treatment, either clinically or morphologically. Other growth-stimulating factors probably regulate their growth. Although the endometriotic tissue is included in the fibrosis, the glands may remain in atrophy for a long time, and many have the capacity to respond by proliferation when exposed to estrogen again.

Endometriosis is extremely uncommon in women with amenorrhea. This fact led early to the idea that it is estrogen regulated. Comparative studies on estrogen and progesterone receptors have shown that the receptor levels are lower in endometriotic tissue than in endometrium from the same woman. The estrogen receptors in the endometriotic tissue do not show a pronounced cyclic variation according to the menstrual phase, whereas the progesterone receptors show a different cycle pattern. These results indicate that endometriotic tissue is regulated by the ovarian steroids in most cases but in a different way from the endometrium. The expression of steroids is influenced by other autocrine and paracrine factors, and the difference found in women with endometriosis between their intrauterine endometrium and extrauterine implants might be related to other regulators in the surrounding tissues. A different estrogen metabolism and even a local production of estrogen has been found in endometriotic lesions compared with endometrium. This might explain why not all cases of endometriosis, or not all lesions in any one woman, respond to hormonal treatment.

Thus, there are several indications that different factors regulate the growth of endometriotic cells. So far we have only hormonal treatment available to reduce and reverse the growth.

TREATMENT

Several aspects have to be taken into consideration when treatment of endometriosis is planned: cell biologic, immunologic, vascular, and menstrual, for example. In fact, because no direct treatment of the disease is available, it is extremely important to discuss the therapeutic alternatives with the patient and to consider her priorities. The age of the patient, fertility plans, localization and extent of lesions, involvement of different organs, previous surgery, previous experiences of hormonal treatment, other therapeutic requirements, bleeding pattern, sexual life, physical activity, other diseases, and the like have to be taken into consideration. Is a generalized treatment preferred or a local extirpation? Does the patient want a short-term or a long-term treatment;

a fertility-preserving treatment or a radical clearing of the pelvis, including the uterus and adnexes; surgical treatment or pharmacologic treatment orally, nasally, or by injection; pharmacologic forms with a short or a long half-life; or a combination of surgical and pharmacologic treatments? Generalized hormonal treatment resulting in down-regulation of the ovaries usually gives good symptomatic relief after a few weeks. Surgical treatment relieves symptoms only from the lesions extinguished.

For the choice between surgery and pharmacologic treatment, some guidelines are available. Deep lesions do respond weakly and often not at all to hormonal treatment. The lesions included in fibrosis seem to be regulated more by local growth factors than by circulating hormones that to a limited degree reach the lesions through the extensive fibrosis. Deep lesions often invade or in other ways disturb surrounding organs like the ureters or bowel, leading to defective functioning, and this type of lesion often produces heavy and often constant pain, which is why surgical extirpation usually is recommended. As the fibrosis sometimes surrounds the ureters, but less commonly invades them, they can usually be dissected free and left intact. Preoperative insertion of catheters in the ureters is really helpful, as the location of the ureters might be changed because of the structural derangement in the area. Bowel endometriosis probably originates from the serosal surface, invades the muscle layers, resulting in hypertrophy of the muscle layers, but it rarely affects the mucosa. Thus, small lesions might be extirpated without opening the bowel lumen. However, often the fibrosis more or less surrounds the bowel, which is why a resection has to be performed. The lesion is always distinctly limited and seldom longer than 10 cm. The margins of healthy tissue can be fairly small, 5 cm, which is why it is always possible to make an end-to-end anastomosis. The most common localization of bowel endometriosis is the rectal-sigmoid transmission or the proximal rectum, including the wall, or even to the proximal part of the vagina and the posterior part of the cervix. Surgery is complicated, but the lump can usually be excised, leaving a normal uterus. In these extensive cases, the fibrosis often reaches the lateral pelvic walls. It is important to remove all fibrosis, as endometriotic tissue otherwise might be left behind and give rise to new problems.

Endometriotic cysts also respond very slowly to hormonal treatment, which is why they have to be removed surgically. Using laparascopic surgery, this is a fast and effective procedure. Endometriotic cysts do not recur very often, and if no other endometriosis is visible during the operation, no other treatment is required. It also should be kept in mind that endometriotic tissue may develop into malignant forms, which is most common in the ovaries and the rectovaginal wall.

No long-standing effect on pelvic pain has been shown after surgical treatment of disseminated small peritoneal lesions. However, if the woman wants to become pregnant as soon as possible, this might still be the treatment of choice. A significantly higher pregnancy rate has been shown, both spontaneously and after in vitro fertilization. The explanation might be that the focus of the inflammatory process is removed, even if only for a limited period. The cytotoxic and gametotoxic environment might be cleared away. If the woman becomes pregnant, the inflammatory reaction will subside.

The pharmacologic treatments available today are hormonal and anti-inflammatory. All hormonal treatment is given mainly to down-regulate the ovarian steroid production, but some substances also have a direct effect on the lesions by binding to progesterone or androgen receptors, giving an antiestrogenic result. Gestagens have been used for decades and still have their definite place. Their combination of direct and indirect antiestrogenic effect might explain why the doses often can be kept low. Medroxyprogesterone acetate (Provera) is a weak gestagen, and the therapeutic range is wide, between 5 and 100 mg daily orally. The initial dose is normally 20 to 30 mg daily. Thereafter the patient often can learn to reduce the dose slowly by herself if the side effects are discouraging, until they are acceptable, or to increase the dose at least up to 50 mg daily if she has bleeding disturbances. A higher dose is very seldom indicated, although it has been used in clinical studies. If the woman is satisfied with medroxyprogesterone acetate, it can be administered in a 3-month depot formulation (Depo-Provera) for years if needed. Other gestagens used are lynestrenol* in a dose of 5 to 20 mg daily or norethindrone (Aygestin), 1 to 10 mg daily. Derivatives of testosterone have been used since the 1970s. Besides giving a better bleeding control, the effect on endometriosis symptoms or lesions is no better than that of other hormonal regimens. As the androgenic and anabolic side effects often are pronounced, the usage of danazol (Danocrine) and gestrinone* is decreasing.

A third therapeutic approach with steroids is the combination of estrogen and gestagen available in oral contraceptives. As a primary treatment, oral contraceptives have not been shown to be effective, but the combination might have some preventive effect on recurrences, probably because of the extinction of the high ovulatory estrogen levels and the reduction of bleeding volumes at menstruation. Local application in the uterine cavity of progesterone, loaded in an intrauterine device (Levonova),* might be useful. When the symptoms are weak or when prophylaxis for recurrences is needed, Levonova* has proved to be a good option.

Gonadotropin-releasing hormone (GnRH) agonists were introduced nearly 20 years ago, offering a more complete down-regulation of the ovaries than had previously been available. The treatment was named "medical oophorectomy," and the hope was that a complete extinction of the ovarian activity would result in a starvation and disappearance of endometrio-

*Not available in the United States.

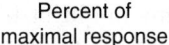

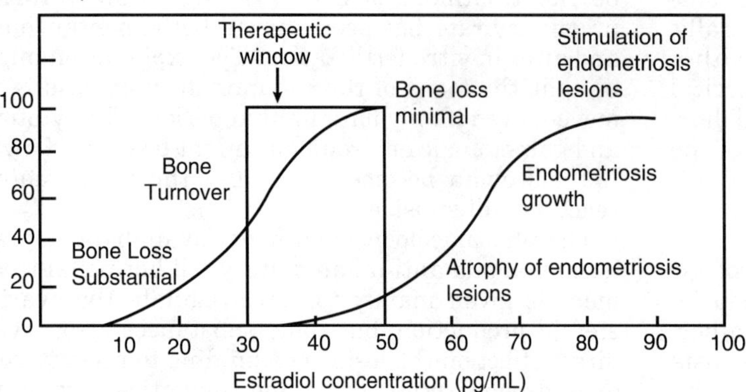

Figure 1. Estradiol therapeutic window. The concentration of estradiol required to cause growth of endometriosis lesions may be greater than the concentration required to stabilize bone mineral density. (From Barbieri R: Hormone treatment of endometriosis: The estrogen threshold hypothesis. Am J Obstet Gynecol *166*:740, 1992.)

sis. However, several comparative randomized studies have shown that the effect is not significantly better than that obtained by other hormones. However, although the hypoestrogenic side effects might be pronounced, with sweating, hot flashes, headache, and vaginal dryness, they are often better tolerated by the patient than those of gestagens or testosterone derivatives, giving such anabolic-androgenic side effects as mood changes, weight gain, acne, greasy skin, and muscle pain. The steroid metabolism loads the liver, sometimes resulting in elevated liver enzymes. It also influences the serum lipid pattern in an unfavorable way. This has to be compared with the hypoestrogenic effects that GnRH agonists have on the skeleton, reducing the bone mass median 6% during a 6-month period of treatment, which is reversed within another 6 months. The lipid balance is also unfavorably influenced when the estrogenic effect is reduced. GnRH agonists are available in daily nasal sprays (nafarelin, Synarel)* or monthly injectable depots (goserelin [Zoladex], leuprolide,† [Lupron], triptorelin, [Decapeptyl]).†

Thus, there are different hormonal regimens available, having no significantly different effect on the disease. The woman's choice regarding possible side effects and administration routes is important. The goal of the treatment is to give the woman as high a quality of life as possible. The late side effects are seldom of major importance for the standard initial treatment period of 6 months. However, when long-term treatment has to be considered, the side effects can become important.

In 1992 Barbieri very elegantly expressed what many people had thought before, namely, that a complete extinction of the ovarian function should not be the goal in controlling endometriosis, which massively had been shown when GnRH agonists had been compared with gestagens. Different tissues have their own sensitivity to, among others, estrogen. The endometrium is very sensitive, presenting morphologic changes day to day when the serum level is fluctuating, whereas the vaginal mucosa is comparatively insensitive, passing through degenerative changes after a fairly long period of estrogen deprivation. Endometriotic tissue and bone mass, for example, are in between. Thus, if we reduce the estrogen exposition so that the endometrium and the endometriotic tissue remain in a resting phase but no degeneration is obtained in the skeleton or vaginal mucosa, we are in the "therapeutic window," where we may keep the patient for a longer period than 6 months when needed because of recurrent problems (Figure 1). This therapeutic window may be reached by giving GnRH agonists to down-regulate the ovaries completely and thereafter give back as much estrogen as the woman needs to reach her therapeutic window. An attractive model is to add back both estrogen and a low dose of gestagen, the latter in a dose low enough not to give the undesired side effects but to give positive effects on the endometrium, skeleton, and endometriosis. All different estrogen and gestagen formulas have been tried, and no significant difference in effect has been shown. The role is to start with as low a dose as possible, for example, estradiol percutaneously 25 μg or 50 μg daily, or conjugated estrogens, 0.625 mg (Premarin) combined with medroxyprogesterone acetate, 5 to 10 mg, lynestrenol, 5 to 10 mg, or norethisterone, 0.2 to 1.2 mg daily. In some studies it has been recommended to start the treatment only with the GnRH agonist to obtain as fast an effect as possible and add the steroids after 3 months.

However, the combination of a GnRH agonist and steroids is costly and may seem to be illogical. Another option is to give a low dose of a GnRH agonist. This is possible only with the nasal sprays, nafarelin or buserelin,* as all injectables are available only in monthly depots. Nafarelin, which is usually given as 200 μg twice daily, that is, one spray twice daily, may be reduced to one spray daily with the same effect on the disease. Although bleeding control is less effective with the lower dose, the result is the same. Thus, just as the patient may learn to vary the dosage of gestagens according to side effects and symptoms, she can also learn to vary the dosage of the

*Not FDA approved for this indication.
†Not available in the United States.

*Not available in the United States.

nasal spray between one spray daily and two sprays twice daily. There are no indications that light bleeding during treatment reduces the therapeutic effect, but for the patient's benefit it should be avoided.

Beside hormones, few other pharmacologic substances have shown a therapeutic effect on endometriosis. Nonsteroidal anti-inflammatory drugs (NSAIDs) are often successful in the early stages in stopping the dysmenorrhea if the treatment is induced very early before the pain has become too great. The positive effect is probably related to the release of prostaglandins that is obtained as part of the acute inflammatory process. However, when the effect of the prostaglandins on the uterus is pronounced, with cramps in the uterine muscle, the pain reducing effect often fails to appear. It has been shown that the volume of bleeding is reduced by NSAID use, which to some degree may contribute to the effect.

When chronic pain has developed and no surgical procedure can relieve the pain, a substance that might decrease the pain sensitivity such as amitriptyline is often helpful. Whether central sensitization is developed is not quite clear yet, but different studies in this area are ongoing. To avoid development of chronic central sensitization, it is important to help the patient in early stages to interrupt a bad pain cycle.

The causal connection between endometriosis and infertility is not clear. In cases of mechanical destruction of the genital organs, there is no question about a relationship. Although this is not the case for most women with endometriosis, they have more difficulty becoming pregnant than women who do not have endometriosis. The inflammatory process that is stimulated over and over again in menstruating women, including the release of a cascade of inflammatory transmitters to the peritoneal fluid, influences the fertilization process in several ways. For example, tumor necrosis factor-α, interferon-γ, interleukin-1β, and other cytokines are gametotoxic. The macrophages, although unable to break down the endometrial cells, have the capacity to engulf the gametes. The cytokines and growth factors influence, and in different ways regulate, the process of follicular development, granulosa cell function, and corpus luteum development. The prostaglandins in different ways have an effect on the follicular rupture, tubal motility, and myometrial activity. But because the inflammatory process varies according to the bleedings, being retrograde or not, the intensity of the inflammatory process varies, and occasionally the whole complicated fertilization process is successful.

The most important prognostic factor for fertility is the duration of infertility. Today some couples with endometriosis are helped with in vitro fertilization, and the results are not significantly different from those in women with tubal disease. Interestingly, however, even if the number of oocytes retrieved is the same as in women with diseased tubes, the fertilization rate has been shown to be significantly lower in women with endometriosis. This difference remains even if intracytoplasmic sperm injection is performed. An explanation for this is not clear, although different studies are attempting to discover whether the development of the oocyte is disturbed in the toxic pelvic environment that might also influence the intrafollicular environment.

DYSFUNCTIONAL UTERINE BLEEDING

method of
ANDREW E. GOOD, M.D.
Mayo Medical School
Rochester, Minnesota

Dysfunctional uterine bleeding (DUB) is abnormal bleeding from a cause other than a structural or a systemic one. It arises from abnormalities in the normal menstrual cycle, usually from disorders in ovulatory functioning. Because the uterus is the end organ for a series of complex hormonal interactions, changes in these hormonal signals result in abnormal bleeding.

The key to the treatment of DUB is to realize that the condition results from an alteration in normal physiology and that it is often only a temporary change. In other words, if nothing is done, the condition is often self-limited. If treatment is required, it is usually needed only for a short duration.

"Normal" menstruation occurs every 21 to 40 days. The amount of bleeding can range from spotting to heavy and can last up to 10 days. Problems with quantifying the amount of blood loss limit accurate assessment of "heavy" flows. Self-reports of the amount of flow are inaccurate because each woman has her own idea of normal, depending on her previous menstrual pattern.

There are classic definitions of abnormal flow patterns, however. Menorrhagia is defined as *regularly* occurring flows that are heavier or longer than normal. Metrorrhagia is bleeding that occurs in an irregular fashion. Logically, then, menometrorrhagia is irregular bleeding that is heavier and longer than normal.

COMMON VARIETIES

Anovulatory Bleeding. This is probably the most common cause of abnormal bleeding. It results from a failure of ovulation in a given cycle. The bleeding pattern is one in which the onset of menstruation is at the appropriate time but the duration is longer. Typically, the patient complains of a menses that does not stop, with lighter bleeding after the first 5 to 7 days.

Ovulatory Bleeding. This bleeding usually occurs at the midcycle, around the time of suspected ovulation. It results from the temporary lowering of estrogen levels that occurs after ovulation. Usually, ovulatory bleeding is of short duration, lasting from hours to several days, and is not very heavy.

These two categories of DUB often occur as isolated episodes, and the factors that cause them are infrequent. Diagnosis is best made with a menstrual calendar. With accurate plotting of the onset and duration of menses, patterns emerge that are characteristic.

OTHER CAUSES

Bleeding that is different from the occasional long anovulatory bleed or the midcycle ovulatory spotting is more problematic. Examples are instances of menorrhagia that can cause anemia or cases of metrorrhagia that can cause major inconvenience and disruption for the patient. The physiology of bleeding is not as simple as in the anovulatory-ovulatory types. One theory is that the endometrium becomes dysynchronous, with different sections being in differing stages of maturation. Thus, when one part is breaking down and shedding, another is proliferating, only to shed several weeks later. These changes are frequently seen in the perimenopausal period, as the ebb and flow of hormonal signals becomes less orderly.

DIAGNOSIS

The purpose of diagnosis in DUB is to rule out other, nonphysiologic causes of bleeding. Endocervical or endometrial polyps, fibroids, cervical cancer, or endometrial or uterine pathology can all create bleeding pictures that are similar to those in DUB. These are the most common causes of non-DUB bleeding and should be considered first in the diagnosis. Other rarer causes such as coagulation disorders, renal or hepatic disease, or thyroid problems should be considered only if the cause of bleeding cannot be explained by one of the more common causes.

A basic step in diagnosing DUB is with a menstrual calendar, by documenting the duration and amount of flow. These records can be as simple as marking in a pocket calendar or as precise as using a calendar designed for the purpose. If an uncomplicated, self-limited cause is not uncovered, then other diagnostic tools should be employed. These include endometrial biopsy, ultrasound and sonohysteroscopy, office or operative hysteroscopy, or, as a last resort, a dilatation and curettage (D & C).

Office endometrial biopsy is helpful in ruling out endometrial hyperplasia or cancer. It is convenient, being done at the time of the patient's visit, inexpensive, and has a diagnostic accuracy equal to that of a D & C. It is limited in that it cannot easily diagnose fibroids or endometrial polyps.

Ultrasound, especially the transvaginal approach, is useful for determining the presence of fibroids and thickening of the endometrial stripe. Hyperplasia and endometrial cancer have not been reported in an endometrial stripe thinner than 5 mm (measuring both sides of the endometrium). Ultrasound does not provide a view of the endometrial cavity, missing potential causes such as intracavitary fibroids or endometrial polyps. If 10 mL of saline are instilled at the time of ultrasound, a sonohysterogram is obtained. This separates the uterine walls with a sonolucent medium and allows an accurate diagnosis of any endometrial thickening or intrauterine masses such as polyps.

Office hysteroscopy, using a fiberoptic cable and carbon dioxide distention, provides a direct look at the endometrium, making directed biopsies possible. This method requires specialized equipment and is more expensive than either ultrasound or biopsy.

D & C is a blind method of assessment and should be done in conjunction with hysteroscopy. Although expensive, it can sometimes provide relief from DUB.

TABLE 1. **Diagnosis and Treatment Options for Dysfunctional Uterine Bleeding**

Diagnosis
Time and menstrual calendar
Endometrial biopsy
Ultrasound with sonohysterography
Hysteroscopy
Dilatation and curettage (D & C)

Treatment
Time and menstrual calendar
Progestins: single course of therapy
  Medroxyprogesterone acetate (Provera, Cycrin), 10 mg daily × 5
  Norethindrone acetate (Aygestin), 10 mg, daily × 5
  Micronized progesterone (Prometrium), 100 mg, daily × 5
Progestins: repetitive courses
  Same doses as above, used for 10 days, in the second half of the cycle
Oral contraceptives
Antiprostaglandins (e.g., Advil, Motrin), 400 mg q 4 h during menses
Progesterone intrauterine device (Progestasert)
D & C, with or without hysteroscopy
Endometrial ablation
Hysterectomy

TREATMENT

Treatment should be considered in cases in which spontaneous resolution of the DUB does not occur after a cycle or two. Therapy should attempt to recreate the normal physiologic milieu for the endometrium, allowing regular, orderly shedding.

DUB can be caused by the temporary progesterone deficiency created by anovulation. Thus, one of the mainstays of treatment is progestin. Medroxyprogesterone acetate (Provera, Cycrin) is the most common progestin used in the United States. Treatment consists of 10 mg taken daily for 5 or 10 days. A 5-day course is usually adequate to correct the isolated episode of anovulatory bleeding. The longer routine may be necessary to correct more serious alterations of the endometrial cycle because 10 days are necessary to bring about normal induction of receptors in the endometrium.

When using progestins, there may be immediate resolution of the bleeding. However, depending on endogenous ovarian hormone activity and the effects of the progestin, there may be another menses within 7 to 10 days after stopping the medicine. The patient should be warned about this possibility.

In some cases, progestins are used in a monthly regimen, attempting to supplement the ovarian signal. In these cases, the progestin should be started in the second half of the cycle, around day 17, to coordinate with the baseline hormonal levels.

If menstrual flow is not controlled by "supplementation" of the existing ovarian hormones, it will be necessary to eliminate these endogenous signals. Then, oral contraceptives are the treatment of choice. These suppress ovarian activity and substitute an ordered ebb and flow of hormones. They are particularly useful in perimenopausal women (as long as they do not smoke).

There are also reports of menorrhagia being improved by up to 50% with the use of antiprostaglandins such as ibuprofen* (Motrin) and mefenamic acid* (Ponstel). These are used during the menses

*Not FDA approved for this indication.

and perhaps work by improving vasoconstriction of the spiral arteries of the endometrium.

Progesterone-containing intrauterine devices (IUDs)(Progestasert) can reduce the amount of menstrual bleeding and are appropriate in select cases of menorrhagia. This type of IUD has a disadvantage of yearly replacement and thus becomes somewhat expensive.

If hormonal therapy is not effective or is contraindicated, surgery should be considered. Surgery should be considered only after other anatomic possibilities such as polyps and fibroids or unusual medical conditions are eliminated.

Ablation of the endometrium during hysteroscopy using wire loops, electrified roller balls, or computer-controlled heating elements provides a 90% rate in reducing or stopping bleeding.

D & C is the traditional choice for surgical treatment. It stops heavy bleeding and, in selected cases, effects a long-term cure. It should be done, if possible, in conjunction with hysteroscopy.

In refractory cases of bleeding or in cases of uterine prolapse or pelvic relaxation, hysterectomy is definitive treatment. A summary of diagnosis and treatment options is listed in Table 1.

AMENORRHEA

method of
STEPHEN M. SCOTT, M.D., and
WILLIAM D. SCHLAFF, M.D.
University of Colorado Health Sciences Center
Denver, Colorado

Amenorrhea is an abnormal physical sign defined as the failure to menstruate by 16 years of age (primary amenorrhea) or cessation of previous menses for more than 6 months (secondary amenorrhea). In contrast, normal menstruation is a visual marker reflecting cyclic sloughing of endometrial tissue if conception fails to occur after ovulation. Menstruation is a complex event requiring coordination between hormonal signals from the brain and ovary, responsive endometrial tissue within the uterine cavity, and a patent outflow tract. If one or more of these organs do not develop or function properly, normal menstruation will not occur, resulting in amenorrhea. Review of the function and development of female genitalia, hormone production, and stimulation of end-organ tissue will aid physicians in understanding different etiologies of amenorrhea.

PHYSIOLOGY

In the early fetus there is the potential for either male or female genital development. The presence of a Y chromosome prevents the formation of female internal genitalia and stimulates growth of male internal and external genitalia through the production of antimüllerian hormone (AMH), testicular development, and androgen production. The absence of AMH allows the müllerian ducts to persist and develop into fallopian tubes, uterus, and upper vagina. Without androgen stimulation, male genital ducts regress and female external genitalia form. A female genotype 46XX influences gonadal transformation to an ovary and organization of granulosa and theca cells around individual ovum. Once ovarian gonadal tissue and female phenotype are established, the remaining stages required for menstruation remain dormant until puberty.

Puberty initiates a second process, hormone production. Once coordinated, the hormones produced in the hypothalamus, pituitary, and ovary establish cyclic buildup followed by removal of uterine endometrium. During early puberty, the hypothalamus begins to secrete gonadotropin-releasing hormone (GnRH) in a pulsatile fashion stimulating the pituitary to initially secrete follicle-stimulating hormone (FSH) followed by luteinizing hormone (LH). Ovarian granulosa and theca cells begin their respective production of estrogens, leading to breast development, and androgens, which stimulate secondary sexual hair growth. Early ovarian function does not lead to ovulation.

Eventually a single follicle establishes dominance each cycle with its ability to produce estradiol under FSH stimulation. Because of its high quantity of FSH receptors and preferential blood supply, this follicle is able to increase estradiol production despite decreased FSH secretion from the pituitary. Once serum estradiol reaches a critical level, pituitary inhibition ceases and the LH surge occurs. Ovulation and conversion of the follicle to a corpus luteum soon follow. LH receptors on the corpus luteum initiate progesterone production after ovulation. The corpus luteum has a limited life span, and progesterone levels fall within 2 weeks after ovulation if conception does not occur.

Cyclic endometrial stimulation is the final process in normal menstruation. In preparation for a possible pregnancy implantation, the functionalis layer of endometrium increases mitotic activity under the influence of estrogen. Endometrial thickness can increase 10-fold during the follicular phase. Underlying spiral arteries become prominent and tortuous during this time. Progesterone limits mitosis of endometrial cells and stabilizes tissue structure by decidualization. A fall in progesterone level initiates a cascade of prostaglandins and lytic enzymes, leading to vasospasm of the spiral arteries and endometrial cell ischemia distal to the basal layer. The necrotic tissue and associated debris become menstrual flow. During menstruation the basal layer of endometrium begins regenerating a healthy functional layer under the influence of estrogens produced in the next follicular phase. This cycle repeats until interrupted by pregnancy or dysfunction.

DIFFERENTIAL DIAGNOSIS

With the normal development and function of the hypothalamus, pituitary, ovary, and genital tract as a guide, the physician may point to a specific organ dysfunction leading to amenorrhea. A physical examination is key to determining the etiology of amenorrhea in an adolescent patient who has never menstruated. Specific evaluation for breast development (signifying estrogen stimulation) and female internal genitalia (requiring normal female genotype 46XX) aids in categorization.

PRIMARY AMENORRHEA

Patients with no breast or internal genital development are very rare. All have a male karyotype with previous AMH production causing regression of müllerian structures. Low male testosterone levels are noted owing to the "vanishing testes syndrome" or the enzyme deficiencies—17-alpha-hydroxylase or 17,20 desmolase—leading to a block in sex steroid production. Without androgen influence female external genitalia will form, but breasts will remain infantile because of estrogen deficiency. Elevated FSH and LH levels occur from lack of sex steroid inhibition on the pituitary.

Two possible etiologies exist when breast development is present but female internal genitalia are absent. Androgen insensitivity syndrome occurs in genotypic males. Their müllerian structures regress in the presence of AMH; however, insensitivity to androgens and peripheral conversion of androgens to estrogens lead to female external genitalia and secondary breast development. Pubic and axillary hair growth is underdeveloped in the absence of androgen sensitivity. Patients with uterine or uterovaginal agenesis have a 46XX female genotype and normally functioning ovaries. It is unclear what specifically leads to regression of müllerian structures in these patients. Patients with uterovaginal agenesis have normal (female) secretory patterns and normal receptors. Therefore, they will have normal pubic and axillary hair. Thus, normal male testosterone levels, a lack of pubic or axillary hair growth, and an XY karyotype distinguish androgen insensitivity syndrome from uterine agenesis.

Gonadotropin levels help to define two broad categories of amenorrhea when breast development is absent in the presence of normal female internal genitalia. If FSH and LH levels are below normal, i.e., hypogonadotrophic hypogonadism, the dysfunction is located within the hypothalamus or pituitary. Space-occupying lesions, previous infections, or irradiation in either the hypothalamus or pituitary may destroy GnRH- or FSH/LH-producing cells, respectively. Ovarian stimulation and estrogen production will not occur without these hormones. Endocrinologic disruption of the GnRH pulse can also lead to amenorrhea. This is seen in hyperprolactinemia, hypothyroidism, and stress states described later. Gonadotropin stimulation narrows the source of the dysfunction to the hypothalamus or the pituitary. Increasing FSH/LH levels following exogenous pulses of GnRH agonist point to the hypothalamus.

Initially high gonadotropin levels, i.e., hypergonadotrophic hypogonadism, in an estrogen-deficient patient with developed female internal genitalia point to ovarian failure as the origin of amenorrhea. Typically these cases are due to isolated or familial deletions in all or part of an X chromosome leading to absent or diminished ovarian tissue and follicles. Features consistent with 45XO Turner's syndrome may be present, including short stature, depending on the area of X chromosome deletion. Complete gonadal agenesis in a 46XX or 46XY genotype could result in a similar phenotype without Turner's features. Genotypic females who lack the 17-alpha-hydroxylase enzyme will have infantile secondary sexual development owing to lack of steroid conversion to estrogens. Figure 1 shows the differential diagnosis path for causes of primary and secondary amenorrhea.

SECONDARY AMENORRHEA

Once a patent vagina is visualized, a patient with normal müllerian structures and secondary sexual development is assumed to have functioning organs. Assessment is similar to one who has previously menstruated. Each organ is evaluated for possible dysfunction. A history of cervical trauma including birth or D and C may indicate cervical stenosis, whereas a history of vigorous uterine curettage, especially in the presence of infection, may be suspicious for Asherman's syndrome. This syndrome describes the replacement of functioning endometrial tissue with unresponsive scar tissue. Ovarian hormone production and ovulation occur in both situations leading to cyclic moliminal symptoms and often cyclic pelvic pain in the case of cervical stenosis. A serum progesterone level of greater than 5 ng per mL during the expected luteal phase also confirms ovulation.

Some patients who previously ovulated may be prone to loss of ovarian follicles and early ovarian failure. Etiologies include genetic predisposition, autoimmune disease, infection, chemotherapy, or irradiation. If premature ovarian failure occurs before age 35, a karyotype is warranted to rule out XX/XO or XX/XY mosaicism. A positive antinuclear antibody and/or serum antithyroid and antimicrosomal antibodies can indicate an autoimmune etiology.

Pituitary lesions may interfere with gonadotropin release. Damage to gonadotropin-producing cells as noted previously may halt their release of hormones. Sheehan's syndrome is a specific cause of pituitary cell compromise. During pregnancy the pituitary is highly vascularized. A sudden decrease in blood flow to the pituitary may follow a severe postpartum hemorrhage. Hypotensive ischemia and subsequent cell necrosis result in a loss of gonadotrophic and other pituitary hormone production. Space-occupying tumors can compress pituitary cells and compromise FSH/LH secretion. The most common pituitary tumors secrete prolactin that feeds back to disrupt hypothalamic function.

Pulsatile release of GnRH within the hypothalamus is essential for normal pituitary and ovarian hormone production. Norepinephrine stimulates GnRH production, whereas dopamine inhibits its pulsatile release. Increased prolactin levels from a pituitary tumor and/or specific medications interfere with GnRH secretion. Thyroid-releasing hormone (TRH) also increases prolactin secretion. Hypothyroidism resulting from decreased thyroid hormone production results in high TRH levels and prolactin stimulation. Cases of severe emotional stress, weight loss, and exercise also inhibit GnRH secretion. Stressful situations produce increased opiate endorphins and stimulate conversion of estrogens to catechol-estrogens. Both substances increase dopamine activity in the hypothalamus.

Polycystic ovarian (PCO) syndrome results from a spectrum of defects that alter the ratio of FSH/LH secretion. Relatively high tonic levels of LH inhibit formation of a dominant follicle, resulting in multiple androgen-secreting follicles. This leads to anovulation and amenorrhea. Hirsutism, acne, and weight gain can result from hyperandrogenemia. Androgens also convert to estrogens in the periphery, which may stimulate endometrial cell division. Chronic mitotic activity without the protective effects of progesterone increases the risk of endometrial hyperplasia and/or cancer.

A small number of women with amenorrhea and hyperandrogenemia have a partial 21-hydroxylase enzyme deficiency. Insufficient conversion of progesterone to cortisol leads to increased adrenal stimulation by adrenocorticotropic hormone (ACTH) and higher sex steroid levels. The high androgen state increases the LH/FSH ratio, suppressing ovulatory function and leading to amenorrhea. Primary testosterone-secreting tumors are another rare cause of hyperandrogenemia.

At times no underlying defect is found to account for hypothalamic dysfunction. Functional hypothalamic hypogonadism is diagnosed in these cases.

DIAGNOSIS

A systematic approach in each case of amenorrhea allows a physician to diagnose a specific dysfunction and

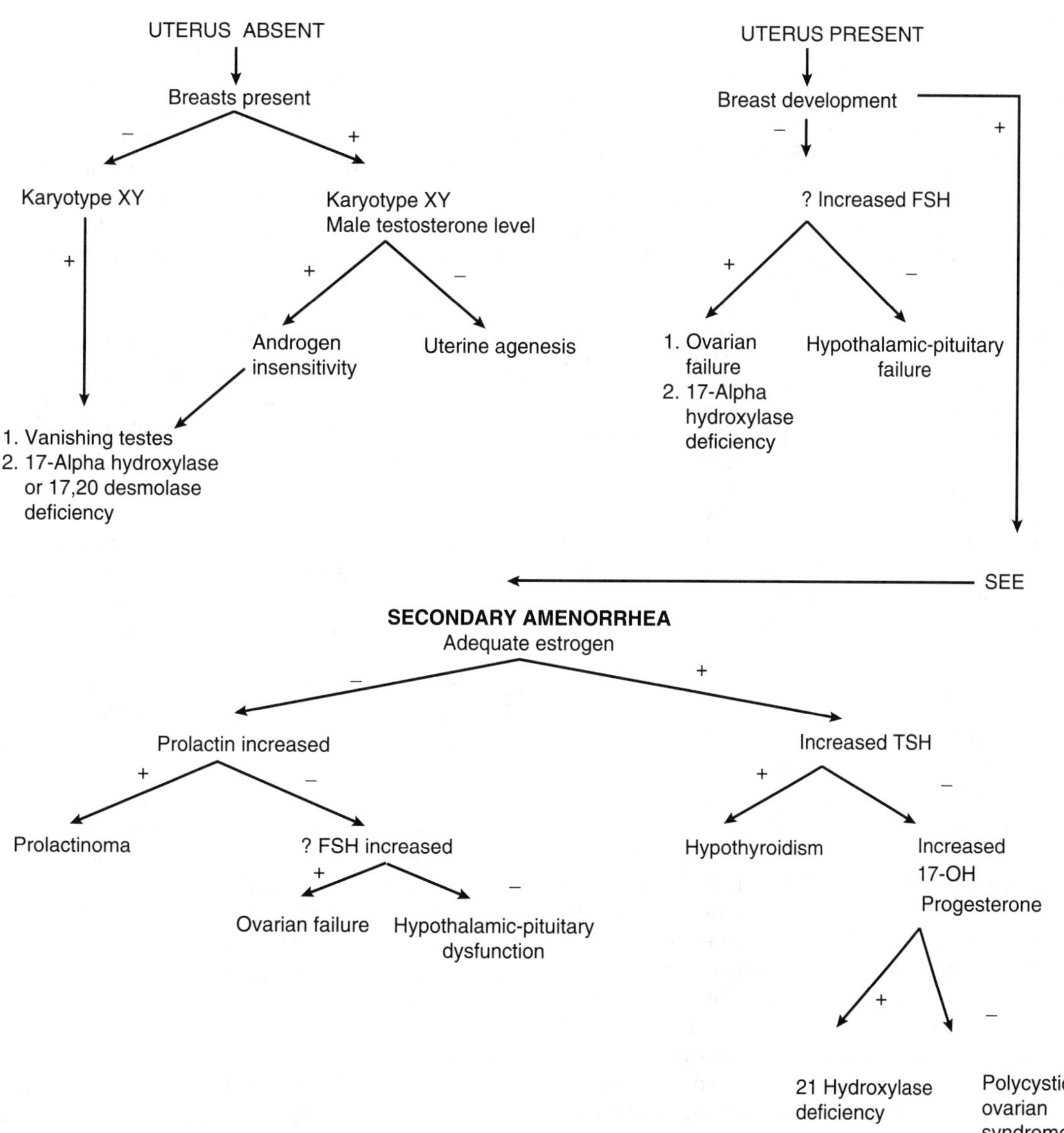

Figure 1. Amenorrhea. *Abbreviations:* FSH = follicle-stimulating hormone; TSH = thyroid-stimulating hormone.

begin treatment more efficiently. If müllerian structures are absent on physical examination a karyotype is required to confirm the presence of a Y chromosome. Male gonadal tissue present intra-abdominally has an increased rate of degeneration to malignant dysgerminoma and must be removed surgically. Surgery for patients with androgen insensitivity should be delayed until after puberty. In these cases testicular production of androgens leads to peripheral estrogen conversion and aids the patient in achieving full secondary sexual development.

Patients who appear to be ovulating and give a history of uterine instrumentation may benefit from a pelvic ultrasound. Hematocolpos is consistent with cervical stenosis. A fluid contrast ultrasound or hysterosalpingogram may suggest Asherman's syndrome. Patients with these conditions should be referred to an experienced gynecologist for surgical therapy. Consultation is also suggested in the absence of a patent vaginal canal. Perineal ultrasound can aid in differentiating between an imperforate hymen and a transverse vaginal septum.

All other patients with secondary amenorrhea are divided into two categories: estrogen deficient and estrogen sufficient with anovulation. Assessment of estrogen levels does not require the time-consuming and cumbersome progestin withdrawal test. Abundant cervical mucus with thin consistency and increased elasticity that ferns on drying is seen in the presence of estrogen. Vaginal cytology on Papanicolaou (Pap) smear will reveal at least 20% superficial cells with estrogen stimulation. Finally, an endometrial stripe less than 5 mm on ultrasound is associated with estrogen deficiency, whereas a stripe greater than 6 mm is consistent with adequate estrogen.

Patients in a hypoestrogenic state have either severe hypothalamic-pituitary axis dysfunction, ovarian failure, or hyperprolactinemia. Fasting serum prolactin and FSH determine the specific etiology. Elevated prolactin levels are most consistent with a prolactin-secreting pituitary tumor when associated with estrogen deficiency or a serum prolactin level exceeding 60 ng per mL. TRH stimulation of prolactin can determine the cause of hyperprolactinemia in the face of intermediate values. If prolactin fails to triple in value after TRH stimulation, a prolactinoma is suggested. Computed tomography or magnetic resonance imaging (MRI) of the pituitary can locate the lesion. A normal prolactin level narrows the focus to ovarian or hypothalamic-pituitary origin. An elevated FSH suggests ovarian failure, whereas a normal or low FSH indicates hypothalamic-pituitary dysfunction. A TSH level may diagnose hypothyroidism but is unlikely to be positive when clinical signs are absent and prolactin levels are normal.

Estrogen-sufficient patients who appear anovulatory, have a normal prolactin, and have no history of uterine instrumentation most likely have chronic androgenized anovulation. A testosterone level less than 2 ng per mL or a dehydroepiandrosterone value less than 7000 ng per mL makes an androgen-secreting tumor unlikely. 17-Hydroxyprogesterone levels greater than 800 ng per dL or a significantly increased value after ACTH stimulation diagnoses 21-hydroxylase deficiency. Most patients will not have these abnormalities, suggesting the diagnosis of polycystic ovarian syndrome. All other causes of amenorrhea must be excluded before making this diagnosis.

TREATMENT

Amenorrhea itself does not adversely affect patient health; however, its underlying etiology can create problems if not addressed. Identification of its cause leads to specific treatment for each dysfunction.

Osteoporosis and coronary artery disease can result from long-term estrogen deficiency. When ovaries fail to develop or premature ovarian failure occurs, estrogen replacement is essential to prevent these long-term problems. Conjugated estrogens (Premarin), 0.625 mg, or estradiol (Estrace), 1 mg, given daily will supplement low estrogen levels and reduce the risk of bone loss and heart disease. If a uterus is present, medroxyprogesterone acetate (Provera), 2.5 mg per day, should be added to prevent endometrial hyperplasia.

Patients with severe hypothalamic-pituitary axis dysfunction also have ovarian suppression. When hyperprolactinemia is the cause, return of ovulation occurs with treatment to normalize prolactin levels. Treatment involves medical, surgical, or radiation therapy. Bromocriptine (Parlodel) is a dopamine agonist. Observations suggest dopamine to be the prolactin-inhibiting factor on prolactin-secreting cells in the anterior pituitary. Daily use restores physiologic levels of prolactin. Side effects, including nausea, vomiting, headaches, and dizziness, occur with bromocriptine. Using the lowest effective dose minimizes side effects. Bromocriptine, 5 mg per day, when no adenoma is seen on MRI, or 7.5 to 10 mg per day in the presence of an adenoma, successfully lowers prolactin levels in most cases. Menses resumes within 6 to 10 weeks of therapy. Ninety percent of patients treated with bromocriptine for 2 years maintain normal prolactin levels. When an adenoma is present, periodic observation by MRI is needed to ensure no increase in tumor size. Failure of bromocriptine suppression or intolerance to its side effects requires an alternative therapy.

Surgical treatment of an adenoma involves removal of tissue through the trans-sphenoid route. This technique achieves a success rate of 50 to 80% in tumors less than 1 cm and 10 to 30% in larger tumors. Significant morbidity and a recurrence rate of 50% after 5 years make surgical treatment a second line therapy. Radiation also has limited treatment value. Delay in resumption of menses and a higher rate of pituitary and hypothalamic damage make radiation therapy less appealing.

In less severe cases of hyperprolactinemia, the ovaries may produce estrogen. If an adenoma is absent or less than 1 cm, then observation with a periodic MRI is acceptable. Cyclic withdrawal using medroxyprogesterone acetate, 10 mg per day on days 1 to 14 each month, protects against endometrial hyperplasia.

Chronic androgenizing anovulation states not only have high androgens, but abundant estrogen levels because of peripheral androgen conversion. Morbidity includes virilizing signs such as acne, weight gain, hirsutism, and in severe cases, clitorimegaly and deepened voice. Androgens also adversely alter LDL/HDL cholesterol ratios, increasing the risk of coronary artery disease. Finally, without the protective effect of ovulatory progesterone, chronic estrogen stimulation of the endometrium increases the risk of endometrial hyperplasia and cancer.

Primary androgen-secreting tumors require surgical treatment. Medical therapy is indicated in other androgenized states. Replacing corticosteroids in patients with 21-hydroxylase deficiency reduces ACTH stimulation and sex steroid levels.

Treatment of polycystic ovarian syndrome includes endometrial protection from hyperplasia, reversal of hirsutism, and ovulation induction if desired. Oral contraceptive pills (OCPs) or cyclic medroxyprogesterone acetate administration introduces progestins to the endometrium and affords protection against hyperplasia. OCPs are also first line therapy in hirsutism treatment. Their suppression of ovarian androgen production and stimulation of sex hormone–binding globulin lead to decreased absolute and active androgen levels. Additional therapy may include spironolactone (Aldactone), 200 mg per day initially followed by a taper to 25 to 50 mg per day. Spironolactone blocks dihydrotestosterone binding to hair follicle receptors. Progression of villus to terminal hair is slowed but not reversed. Noticeable changes with either therapy require at least 6 months of treatment. Ovarian suppression by progestins may give limited benefit if OCPs are contraindicated.

Ovulation induction can also be achieved with medical therapy if pregnancy is desired. Clomiphene citrate (Clomid), 50 mg per day on days 5 to 9 after a withdrawal bleed, blocks estrogen inhibition on the pituitary. Increased serum FSH levels follow and a dominant follicle is often produced. Ovulation occurs

6 to 8 days after ingestion of the final clomiphene pill. Dosage may be progressively increased by 50 mg per day on days 5 to 9 if a follicle does not respond. If conception fails on 150 mg per day, additional causes of infertility should be explored. Pure FSH can be used to induce ovulation if clomiphene fails.

The impact of hyperandrogenemia on coronary artery disease makes nongynecologic therapies important in PCO treatment. Good nutrition, regular exercise, and stable glucose control are essential in lowering the risks of coronary artery disease.

DYSMENORRHEA

method of
CHRISTINE W. JORDAN, M.D.
Lakeside Hospital
Metairie, Louisiana

and

ANDREW M. KAUNITZ, M.D.
University of Florida Health Science Center/ Jacksonville
Jacksonville, Florida

Primary dysmenorrhea is defined as menstrual discomfort occurring in ovulatory women without pelvic pathology. Usually, the pain is colicky, midline lower abdominal pain that may radiate to the thighs and lower back. It typically begins just before the onset of menstrual flow, peaks in less than 24 hours, and resolves within 3 days. It may also be associated with systemic symptoms, such as headache, nausea/vomiting, diarrhea, and backache. Primary dysmenorrhea affects over half of postpubescent females, generally within 6 months to 1 year after menarche, as regular ovulation starts. Without treatment, 10% of women with this condition are disabled for up to 3 days each month. Some women experience improvement of symptoms after childbirth. The great majority of women with primary dysmenorrhea can be managed effectively by primary care providers.

Secondary dysmenorrhea is menstrual pain related to pelvic pathology and frequently begins later in reproductive life. Conditions most frequently associated with secondary dysmenorrhea include uterine leiomyomata ("fibroids"), endometriosis, adenomyosis, pelvic inflammatory disease/chronic salpingitis, and cervical and endometrial polyps. Other causes of secondary dysmenorrhea include congenital and acquired müllerian anomalies resulting in outflow tract obstruction, and use of an intrauterine device. The pain of secondary dysmenorrhea, usually noted to be midline plus one or both lower quadrants, starts before menstrual flow, continues throughout menstruation, and persists after the flow has ceased. Dyspareunia, which may worsen with menses, commonly accompanies this condition. The pelvic examination of a patient with secondary dysmenorrhea may reveal uterine and/or adnexal tenderness, fixed uterine retroflexion, uterosacral nodularity, or a pelvic mass. In contrast, the pelvic examination of a patient with primary dysmenorrhea should not demonstrate tenderness, masses, or any other pathologic changes.

In ovulatory women, endometrial production of prostaglandin $F_{2\alpha}$ ($PGF_{2\alpha}$) increases in the late luteal phase. Release of $PGF_{2\alpha}$ causes sensitization of myometrial nerve endings, uterine contractions, and local ischemia. Prostaglandin-synthetase inhibitors reduce the synthesis of $PGF_{2\alpha}$ by inhibiting cyclooxygenase, the enzyme that converts arachidonic acid to cyclic endoperoxides. Thus, a reasonable first approach to treating dysmenorrhea is to advise use of the nonsteroidal anti-inflammatory drug (NSAID) ibuprofen, which is the least expensive of all the NSAIDs and available over the counter. Ibuprofen reduces menstrual pain by decreasing the $PGF_{2\alpha}$ levels in the menstrual fluid and reducing intrauterine pressure. The fenamates are the most effective class of NSAIDs for treating menstrual pain, with 90% of patients reporting excellent pain relief. Fenamates not only inhibit prostaglandin synthetase, but also decrease the activity of already synthesized prostaglandins. Continuous, rather than "as needed" use of NSAIDs, beginning with the onset of symptoms, may treat dysmenorrhea more effectively. See Tables 1 and 2 for a complete listing of drugs effective in treating dysmenorrhea.

TREATMENT

In patients desiring pregnancy, NSAIDs are the mainstay of therapy for dysmenorrhea. In patients

TABLE 1. **Prescription NSAIDs for Dysmenorrhea**

Drug (by Class)	Brand Name	Dosage
Anthranilic Acid		
Mefenamic acid	Ponstel	500 mg stat, then 250 mg q 6 h
Meclofenamate*	**Meclomen**	**100 mg q 8–12 h**
Phenylpropionic Acid		
Ibuprofen*†	**Motrin**	**400 mg q 4 h/800 mg q 8 h**
Ketoprofen*	Orudis	50 mg q 6–8 h
Oxaprozin	Daypro	600–1200 mg q 24 h
Arylacetic Acid		
Naproxen sodium*	**Anaprox**	**550 mg stat, then 275 mg q 6–8 h**
Naproxen†	**Naprosyn**	**500 mg stat, then 250 mg q 6–8 h**
	Naprelan	375 mg and 500 mg controlled-release tabs, 2 tabs PO q 24 h
Fenoprofen	Nalfon	200–600 mg q 6 h
Phenylalkanoic Acid		
Flurbiprofen	Ansaid	100 mg q 8–12 h
Phenylacetic Acid		
Indomethacin†§	Indocin	25–50 mg q 6–8 h
Diclofenac potassium	Cataflam	50–100 mg stat, then 50 mg q 8 h
Pyranocarboxylic Acid		
Etodolac	Lodine	300 mg q 6–8 h‡
Oxicam		
Piroxicam§	Feldene	20 mg q 24 h
Salicylates§		
Salsalate	Salflex	500–1000 mg q 8 h
Choline magnesium trisalicylate†	Trilisate	1 gm q 8 h
Diflunisal	Dolobid	500 mg q 12 h

Most commonly used drugs are listed in **bold.**
*Peak in 30 to 60 minutes; most commonly used because of faster pain relief.
†Available in suspension form.
‡Exceeds dosage recommended by the manufacturer.
§Piroxicam, indomethacin, and salicylates are not considered first-line agents because of high incidence of gastrointestinal (GI) upset, diarrhea, and GI bleeding.

TABLE 2. **Over-the-Counter NSAIDs for Dysmenorrhea**

Drug (by Class)	Brand Name	Dosage
Phenylpropionic Acid		
Ibuprofen*	**Advil, Motrin IB, Nuprin, Haltran, Midol IB, generic**	**200 mg, 1–2 tablets q 4–6 h**
Ketoprofen*	Actron, Orudis KT	12.5 mg, 1–2 tablets q 4–6 h
Arylacetic Acid		
Naproxen sodium*	**Aleve, generic**	**220 mg, 2 tablets stat, then 220 mg q 8–12 h**
Salicylates		
Aspirin	Bayer, Bufferin, Ecotrin, generic	650 mg q 4 h

Most commonly used drugs are listed in **bold.**
*Fast onset of action.

who do not wish to conceive, combination oral contraceptive pills (OCs) and depot medroxyprogesterone acetate (DMPA) (Depo-Provera) provide highly effective pain relief and, if desired, protection from pregnancy. Both of these agents suppress ovulation, preventing the late luteal phase increase in prostaglandin production. The use of these contraceptive agents also results in much decreased menstrual flow. Three consecutive cycles of OCs use are necessary before determining their effectiveness. Initially combining NSAIDs with OCs is appropriate, as the NSAIDs typically provide relief during the initial cycle of use. Any low-dose (less than 50 μg estrogen) combination OC should be acceptable if no contraindications to OC use are present. Recent studies have shown that prolonging the interval between cycles by extending the duration of active OC use (i.e., 42 or 63 consecutive active OC tablets) effectively decreases the frequency of dysmenorrhea and other menstruation-related problems.

DMPA (150 mg every 3 months) suppresses ovulation and endometrial growth. Most women bleed or spot intermittently after the first injection or two, but then develop oligomenorrhea or amenorrhea with continued use. Over half of all women using DMPA for 1 year (4 injections) experience amenorrhea. The irregular bleeding associated with DMPA tends to be very light and is typically not associated with significant dysmenorrhea. Patients counseled about these expected menstrual changes tend to be more compliant with continued therapy. DMPA is an excellent choice for the patient with contraindications to use of OCs, including smokers over age 35, as well as those with a history of thromboembolism, active liver disease, or coronary artery disease. Patient noncompliance with daily OC use or nausea is not encountered with DMPA use. Patients desiring fertility should be counseled about DMPA's prolonged duration of action, with ovulation returning on average 9 to 10 months after the last injection.

Patients unable to achieve relief from their dysmenorrhea after a 6- to 12-month trial of OCs with or without concomitant use of NSAIDs or a trial of DMPA should be referred to a gynecologist to further investigate for possible pelvic pathology and to consider the need for diagnostic laparoscopy and hysteroscopy. In 20% of such women, no evidence of pelvic pathology is noted. If such women have completed childbearing, hysterectomy can be considered.

PREMENSTRUAL DYSPHORIC DISORDER

method of
LISA S. WEINSTOCK, M.D., and
MARGARET MOLINE, PH.D.
Cornell University Medical Center
New York, New York

Premenstrual syndrome (PMS) refers to a set of physical and emotional symptoms occurring in a cyclical fashion, during the luteal phase of the menstrual cycle. While many women experience mild discomfort in the days preceding menstrual flow (breast tenderness, fatigue, cramping, or bloating), in most cases symptoms are not severe and do not interfere with daily functioning. However, a small percentage of women experience more distressing emotional and physical symptoms premenstrually and find that these symptoms interfere with social or occupational functioning. These women may suffer from premenstrual dysphoric disorder (PMDD), a more severe form of PMS that requires evaluation and treatment by a health professional.

DIAGNOSIS

Many women who present to their gynecologist or primary care physician complaining of PMS have other disorders that worsen premenstrually. Many medical and psychiatric disorders worsen during the luteal phase of the menstrual cycle (Table 1). Women suffering from depression or anxiety often present to their doctors complaining of symptoms that worsen premenstrually, but are not aware that they are symptomatic throughout the men-

TABLE 1. **Medical and Psychiatric Disorders Exacerbated During Luteal Phase**

Migraine headaches	Depression
Allergies	Anxiety
Asthma	Bulimia
Seizures	Substance abuse
Genital herpes	Mania
	Psychosis

strual cycle. The American Psychiatric Association diagnostic criteria for PMDD require that symptoms occur only during the luteal phase of the menstrual cycle and remit during the follicular phase. At least one symptom must be emotional (depressed mood, irritability, mood lability, or anxiety), and a woman must have at least 5 of 11 symptoms. Symptoms must interfere with social or occupational functioning and must not merely be an exacerbation of another disorder (Table 2). To confirm a diagnosis of PMDD, women are asked to rate symptoms prospectively for 2 months using a daily rating scale. If symptoms occur throughout the entire menstrual cycle, a diagnosis of premenstrual worsening of an underlying disorder is more accurate than a diagnosis of PMDD.

ETIOLOGY

Because PMDD symptoms occur cyclically as levels of estrogen and progesterone fall during the end of the menstrual cycle, researchers have proposed that PMDD may result from abnormal levels of circulating ovarian steroid hormones. However, most studies have failed to document abnormalities at any level of the hypothalamic-pituitary-gonadal axis in women with PMDD. It appears more likely that women with PMDD may have abnormalities in some of the neurotransmitters implicated in the etiolgy of mood and affective disorders. Estrogen, progesterone, and progesterone metabolites have been shown to alter the function of neurotransmitters such as norepinephrine, serotonin, and γ-aminobutyric acid (GABA). Women with PMDD have diminished whole blood serotonin and platelet serotonin uptake. Abnormalities in norepinephrine function also have been reported. Women with PMDD also may have abnormalities in their sleep cycle. Further research is necessary to accurately delineate the relationship between PMDD and neurotransmitter function.

TABLE 2. **Research Criteria for Premenstrual Dysphoric Disorder**

A. In most menstrual cycles during the past year, five (or more) of the following symptoms were present for most of the time during the last week of the luteal phase, began to remit within a few days after the onset of the follicular phase, and were absent in the week postmenses, with at least one of the symptoms being either (1), (2), (3), or (4).
   (1) markedly depressed mood, feelings of hopelessness, or self-deprecating thoughts
   (2) marked anxiety, tension, feelings of being "keyed up" or "on edge"
   (3) marked affective lability (e.g., feeling suddenly sad or tearful or increased sensitivity to rejection)
   (4) persistent and marked anger or irritability or increased interpersonal conflicts
   (5) decreased interest in usual activities (e.g., work, school, friends, hobbies)
   (6) subjective sense of difficulty in concentrating
   (7) lethargy, easy fatigability, or marked lack of energy
   (8) marked change in appetite, overeating, or specific food cravings
   (9) hypersomnia or insomnia
   (10) a subjective sense of being overwhelmed or out of control
   (11) other physical symptoms, such as breast tenderness or swelling, headaches, joint or muscle pain, a sensation of "bloating" weight gain

B. The disturbance markedly interferes with work or school or with usual social activities and relationships with others (e.g., avoidance of social activities, decreased productivity and efficiency at work or school).

C. The disturbance is not merely an exacerbation of the symptoms of another disorder, such as Major Depressive Disorder, Panic Disorder, Dysthymic Disorder, or a Personality Disorder (although it may be superimposed on any of these disorders)

D. Criteria A, B, and C must be confirmed by prospective daily ratings during at least two consecutive symptomatic cycles. (The diagnosis may be made provisionally prior to this confirmation.)

From American Psychiatric Association. Diagnostic and Statistical Manual of Mental Disorders, 4th ed. Washington DC, American Psychiatric Association, 1994. Copyright 1994, American Psychiatric Association.

PREVALENCE

PMDD is estimated to affect between 3 and 8% of women in the reproductive years. While anecdotally many women report worsening of symptoms with age, some studies do not support the finding of increased prevalence at older ages. There does appear to be an association between PMDD and depression. Women with PMDD have higher rates of prior depression and higher rates of prior postpartum mood disorder than women without PMDD.

TREATMENT

Psychotropic Agents

Selective Serotonin Reuptake Inhibitors

Selective serotonin reuptake inhibitors (SSRIs) are considered to be first-line treatment for PMDD. Originally designed as antidepressants, SSRIs are used for a number of different psychiatric disorders including obsessive-compulsive disorder (OCD), panic disorder, and bulimia, all of which are thought to stem from abnormalities in brain serotonin function. Given the data regarding abnormalities in serotonin function in patients with PMDD, it is not surprising that SSRIs have been shown to be effective in treating PMDD.

A number of double-blind, placebo controlled studies have demonstrated the efficacy of fluoxetine* (Prozac) in the treatment of PMDD. At a dose of 20 mg per day, given throughout the entire menstrual cycle, fluoxetine has demonstrated significant efficacy in treating PMDD symptoms. Although dose ranges for fluoxetine are between 20 and 80 mg per day, most women respond to a 20 mg dose. For women who have trouble tolerating an initial dose of 20 mg, treatment can be initiated at a dose as low as 5 mg per day and gradually increased as tolerated. Some women note a response at doses as low as 5 or 10 mg per day.

Two other SSRIs, sertraline* (Zoloft), and paroxetine* (Paxil), have also demonstrated efficacy in the treatment of PMDD. Typical dosing of sertraline ranges from 50 to 200 mg per day, and paroxetine dosing typically ranges from 20 to 60 mg per day.

The most common side effects of SSRIs include headache, insomnia or agitation, gastrointestinal disturbance, and sexual dysfunction. Side effects are experienced in approximately 15% of patients taking SSRIs, and in approximately 5% of patients side ef-

*Not FDA approved for this indication.

fects are severe enough to require discontinuing the medication. Most patients, however, are able to tolerate the medication without significant complaints.

Anecdotal reports have suggested that fluoxetine given only during the luteal phase of the cycle, from day 14 until end of menses, may be helpful to some women. This regimen may minimize side effects as well. Additional research is needed to validate this treatment regimen.

Anxiolytics

Some double-blind studies have suggested that luteal phase administration of alprazolam (Xanax) may be helpful in treating PMS symptoms, although not all studies have shown effectiveness. The usual starting dose of alprazolam is 0.25 mg three times a day, with an increase up to a maximum dose of 4 mg per day, given during the luteal phase of the menstrual cycle. Side effects of alprazolam include sedation, which has been described in up to 40% of patients. In many patients, sedation decreases after a few weeks on the medication. Starting at a lower dose, such as 0.125 mg and increasing more slowly may also minimize problems with sedation. Other frequent side effects include hypotension and lightheadedness. The most serious side effect of luteal phase alprazolam treatment is risk of withdrawal symptoms on discontinuation of the medication. Withdrawal symptoms from benzodiazepines include tremor, anxiety, insomnia, nausea, and muscle cramps. Seizures, although rare, can occur as a result of rapid withdrawal from benzodiazepines. Therefore, patients on high-dose alprazolam during the luteal phase may require tapering of the medication each month to prevent withdrawal symptoms.

No other benzodiazepines have shown efficacy in double-blind, placebo-controlled studies. However, given the similar mechanism of action of all benzodiazepines, other benzodiazepines have been prescribed for the treatment of PMS. Further research is required to demonstrate efficacy of these agents in controlled studies.

Buspirone (BuSpar), a nonbenzodiazepine anxiolytic, has been described as an effective treatment for PMS in one study. Dosage was 10 mg three times per day. Further studies are needed to confirm this finding.

Hormonal Treatments

Gonadotropin-Releasing Hormone Agonists

In women with severe PMDD, inducing a medical menopause through the administration of a gonadotropin-releasing hormone (GnRH) agonist,* can cause significant improvement of symptoms. GnRH agonists act on the pituitary gland to cause down-regulation of GnRH receptors, and lead to decrease in pituitary luteinizing hormone (LH) and follicle-stimulating hormone (FSH) secretion. This leads to a decrease in ovarian production of estrogen and progesterone, and levels of these hormones are similar to levels seen in postmenopausal women.

*Not FDA approved for this indication.

GnRH analogues can be administered either through daily subcutaneous injections, depot monthly intramuscular injections, or through a nasal spray administered two to three times per day.

Although treatment with GnRH agonists has been shown to improve severe PMDD, they have a number of drawbacks. Side effects are due to hypoestrogenism and mimic the symptoms of menopause. Hot flashes are common. In addition women may notice emotional lability, insomnia, vaginal dryness, and urinary tract infections. The most serious side effects of GnRH-agonist treatment are risks of osteoporosis and cardiovascular disease. For this reason, it is recommended that use of GnRH agonists for the treatment of PMDD not exceed 6 months.

To minimize side effects and risk of bone loss, some clinicians have combined GnRH agonists with postmenopausal doses of estrogen and progesterone. There is some evidence that this "add back" regimen can treat PMDD effectively while decreasing the negative side effects associated with GnRH agonist therapy.

Danazol

Danazol* (Danocrine), is a synthetic testosterone derivative that also suppresses ovulation. At a dose of 600 to 800 mg per day, it causes amenorrhea and has been reported to be helpful in the treatment of PMDD; however, it has a high rate of side effects. Androgenic side effects include acne, weight gain, and masculinization (clitoromegaly and deepening of the voice). Antiestrogenic side effects include vaginal dryness, hot flashes, mood lability, and adverse effect on lipid profiles. Hepatotoxicity is also a potential side effect. Because of these adverse side effects, danazol is not commonly used to treat PMDD.

Oral Contraceptives

Although a small minority of women report improvement of PMDD symptoms while on oral contraceptives, most studies have not shown them to be effective in treating PMDD. In fact, some women note that symptoms worsen while on oral contraceptives. Thus, they are not a first-line treatment for PMDD.

Progesterone

In the past, progesterone by vaginal or rectal suppository was a common treatment for PMS. However, a number of recent double-blind, placebo-controlled studies have shown that progesterone is not effective in the treatment of PMDD. Therefore it is not currently recommended.

*Not FDA approved for this indication.

Vitamins

Although vitamin B_6 is commonly used to treat PMDD, most studies fail to show its efficacy above placebo levels. At doses higher than 500 mg per day, vitamin B_6 can cause peripheral neuropathy. In addition, there is no good evidence to suggest that women with PMDD are vitamin B_6 deficient. Therefore, vitamin B_6 is not recommended to treat PMDD.

Vitamin E has also been suggested as a treatment for PMDD. However, data do not suggest that it is effective in treating symptoms of PMDD.

Dietary and Behavioral Changes

Although elimination of caffeine or chocolate is often suggested to women who have PMDD, there is little evidence to support this recommendation. Decreasing sweet or salty food intake has also not been demonstrated to be effective in treating PMDD. Dietary supplements such as evening primrose oil or magnesium also have not proved helpful in the treatment of PMDD.

Researchers are beginning to examine the effect of exercise, relaxation therapy, and other behavioral interventions on PMDD. Although women anecdotally report improvement of symptoms with such changes, further studies are required to examine the efficacy of such interventions.

Treatments for Specific Symptoms

Several treatments are helpful for women who complain of one particular symptom premenstrually, but do not fit criteria for PMDD. For example, spironolactone (Aldactone), is used to treat premenstrual fluid retention, bromocriptine* (Parlodel), has been reported helpful in the treatment of mastalgia, and nonsteroidal anti-inflammatory drugs are useful in the treatment of cramps.

Pharmacologic Considerations

Women should be advised that currently no pharmacologic treatment for PMDD has been approved by the Food and Drug Administration for such use. They should also be advised of the risks and benefits of any pharmacologic intervention. The physician must ensure that a patient is using adequate contraception while on pharmacotherapy and should discuss with the patient the potential risks of in utero exposure of any pharmacologic agent that is prescribed.

*Not FDA approved for this indication.

MENOPAUSE

method of
LILA E. NACHTIGALL, M.D.
New York University School of Medicine
New York, New York

and

LISA B. NACHTIGALL, M.D.
Tufts University School of Medicine
Boston, Massachusetts

We entered the 1990s with 43 million women over the age of 50 in the United States, and it is estimated that in the year 2000 there will be 50 million. The last menstrual period occurs at an average age of 51.4, meaning that many of those 43 million women are past menopause, and more than 30 million of these women will live half their lives postmenopausally. In addition, 1.9% of women will have premature menopause (defined as menopause before 40 years of age) and will live more than half of their lives after menopause. All these statistics imply that menopause has become a major health issue.

The question of whether menopause is a physiologic occurrence or whether it is an endocrine deficiency state has been discussed for at least the 50 years that hormone replacement therapy has been available. A lack of true scientific data had kept us from a consensus. However, during the last decade many controlled scientific studies have been completed that help to answer this question. Each woman must be evaluated individually, as with any endocrinopathy, to determine whether therapy is indicated.

The most common and universal symptom of menopause is the "hot flush," or "hot flash." This symptom is part of a complex of vasomotor symptoms that also includes paresthesias, formication, irritability, sweats, sleep disturbances, and occasionally even cold chills. The pathogenesis of this vasomotor instability has been poorly understood, and only since 1983 have researchers been searching for answers. The relationship of the high follicle-stimulating hormone (FSH) level (pathognomonic of menopause) and peaks of luteinizing hormone (LH) level to the flush has been studied but discounted. The best theory appears to be that estrogen receptors, normally present in varying numbers in the hypothalamus of women, play a major role in temperature control and catecholamine release. This explains both the variation in symptoms among women and the reason no other medication is as effective as estrogen in relieving these vasomotor symptoms. Therefore, unless there is an absolute contraindication to its use, estrogen replacement should be given to any woman with flushes, insomnia, irritability, or difficulty with temperature control. Treatment for this type of instability is usually short term (2 to 5 years) and can be withdrawn gradually with no return of symptoms. In cases in which a patient cannot or will not take hormone replacement therapy, alternative treatment includes clonidine in doses of 1 to 2 mg daily, which is effective in less than 50% of women, or megestrol (Megace), 40 mg daily, which is an antimitotic progesterone and the only progesterone approved for women who have had breast cancer. Unfortunately, the newly approved specific estrogen receptor modulators (SERMs) not only do not decrease vasomotor symptoms, but seem to increase them. Of the women who started with no flushes, 30% developed flushes during the 2-year trial.

During the last 2 decades, data have been accumulated that indicate that natural or surgical menopause is directly related to bone loss. The 1984 National Institutes of Health Consensus Conference on Osteoporosis noted the high risk of fractures in postmenopausal white women and suggested that these women are candidates for hormone replacement therapy for the prevention of osteoporotic fractures. Trabecular bone osteoporosis, which leads to reduced height, spinal compression fractures, and "dowager's hump," is familiar to most women. However, the more serious osteoporosis of cortical bone, which leads to fracture of the hip, affects one of three women over the age of 85, has a 20% mortality rate, and a 50% permanent incapacitation rate. Therefore, because no treatment for osteoporosis exists once it occurs, a serious attempt must be made at prevention.

Effective prevention requires assessment of risk factors, which are listed in order of importance in Table 1. Any woman having two or more risk factors should be considered for treatment with hormone replacement therapy. To prevent bone loss, therapy should begin within 3 years from the last menstrual period and should continue somewhere between 10 and 15 years, depending on the patient's age at menopause and the degree of risk. Adequate calcium intake, preferably in the diet, should be encouraged as well. Women who are either producing or receiving estrogen require about 1000 mg of calcium daily. A study by Ettinger and colleagues demonstrated that women continued to lose bone when calcium was given without estrogen but increased bone density when they were given in combination. Estrogen replacement therapy [ERT] started any time after menopause stabilizes bone density but does not increase it once 3 years have elapsed from the last menstrual period. Alternate therapy includes calcitonin (Calcimar), to which patients become refractory and which has to be given parenterally. Calcitonin is now available by intranasal spray (Miacalcin), which is more acceptable to patients but is less effective for cortical bone. Fluorides, which stimulate bone formation but can lead to fluorosis and gastrointestinal disturbances, has recently been approved in a timed-release form reported to have many fewer side effects. Recently bisphosphates such as etidronate or alendronate (Fosamax) have been shown to halt the progression of osteoporosis and prevent fractures; they were approved for this purpose in 1997. In addition, in early 1998, the first SERM, raloxifene, was approved to prevent bone loss and increase bone density.

TABLE 1. **Risk Factors for Osteoporosis**

Menopause before age 40
Family history of osteoporosis
Family origin in British Isles, northern Europe, China, or Japan
Heavy cigarette smoking (½ pack or more per day)
Loss of height, especially in upper body
Fracture with no known cause
Hyperparathyroid disease
Uremia
Increased cortisone production or previous long-term cortisone ingestion
Vitamin D deficiency state
Very fair skin
Small bones
Consumption of more than 5 ounces of alcohol per day or known liver disease
Diet low in calcium
Lactase deficiency
Malabsorption problem
Hyperthyroidism
Underweight
Sedentary lifestyle
Previous high-protein, low-carbohydrate diet for more than 1 year in adulthood

From Nachtigall LE, Heilman J: Estrogen: The Facts Can Change Your Life, 2nd ed. New York, Harper Collins, 1995.

Urogenital atrophy, almost entirely related to estrogen deficiency, will eventually occur in all untreated postmenopausal women. The time of occurrence is extremely variable, with a range of between 1 and 15 years. As a result of estrogen deprivation, the vagina loses its rugae, and its cornified epithelium becomes thin and nonelastic. This leads to diminution in vaginal lubrication, resulting in dyspareunia and eventually total inability to have intercourse. The lack of cornification leads to increased incidence of bacterial, fungal, or trichonomonal vaginitis. The lack of cornification around the urethra leads to increased incidence of urethritis and cystitis. Fortunately, all urogenital atrophy can be reversed by estrogen replacement therapy given orally, transdermally, parenterally, or intravaginally. An approved low-dose estradiol timed-release vaginal ring is now available, marketed under the brand name Estring. The ring stays in place for 3 months and releases only 2 mg over that time. Reversal of atrophy can be accomplished even many years postmenopausally.

Cardiovascular disease, a major cause of death in the United States, accounts for 355,000 deaths per year in women. The possible role of estrogen in decreasing the cardiovascular disease mortality has been assumed, but is still controversial. Certainly the epidemiology of cardiovascular disease points to a protective effect of endogenous estrogen. The male/female ratio is 4:1 at age 35 and still is 3:1 at the time of menopause. In addition premenopausal oophorectomy is associated with the increased risk of cardiovascular disease. Of dozens of case-control and cohort studies of estrogen replacement of the cardiovascular system, all but one show a decreased mortality rate in women on ERT as opposed to women on no replacement. The one study in which there was an increased incidence of cardiovascular disease in women on ERT was confounded by an exceptionally high evidence of cigarette smoking. Originally, the sole explanation for the beneficial effect of estrogen on cardiovascular risk was the favorable alteration of lipids. The median high density lipoproteins (HDLs) are 10% higher in estrogen users, and the median low density lipoproteins (LDLs) are 11% lower. It now appears that this accounts for about 30% of the benefit. The other factors are the estrogen antioxidant effect and increased cardiac output with decreased peripheral resistance.

An epidemiologic study from the Netherlands actually showed a 12% incidence of atherosclerosis in untreated postmenopausal women as compared with a 3% incidence in women of the same age on hormone replacement. ERT appears to be useful for both primary and secondary prevention of coronary ischemic disease. Several studies have revealed ERT to be effective in women with previous myocardial infarction (MI), with repeat MI occurring 40% less frequently than in nontreated women. Treadmill exercise tolerance testing in anginal menopausal women showed a 30% increase in exercise tolerance with the administration of sublingual estradiol. This result indicates a vasodilator effect. Angioplasty patency was 28% greater in women on ERT compared with non–hormone-replaced menopausal women at 1 year follow-up. Figure 1 illustrates the significant improvement in 10-year survival of women with coronary artery disease on ERT.

It is now generally accepted that postmenopausal hormone replacement with estrogen alone raises high-density lipoprotein (HDL) and lowers low-density lipoprotein (LDL), resulting in a favorable lipid profile. Whether the addition of progestogens changes this profile or if there are differences with doses, preparations, and duration of use is still being actively debated. For the most part, studies using low-dose medroxyprogesterone acetate (Provera), micronized progesterone, and megesterol (Megace), show little change in the beneficial effect derived from estrogen alone.

For now, women who develop an unfavorable lipid pattern after menopause or have a strong family history of ischemic heart disease or atherosclerosis should be given hormone replacement.

After considering the multiple benefits of treatment for specific indications in the menopausal and postmenopausal woman, it is necessary to examine the risks. The strong association of unopposed estrogen and development of endometrial cancer is well known. Progestogens protect the endometrium against excessive estrogen-induced stimulation, and an inverse relation exists between the proliferative features under microscopy and progesterone dose. Because of lipid pattern alteration in high doses and adverse symptomatic effects, the minimum dosage that leads to consistent endometrial transformation should be used. Daily low doses of estrogen combined with daily micronized progesterone (100 to 200 mg) have been shown to give minimal side effects, total symptomatic improvement, an improved lipid profile, and amenorrhea without endometrial hyperplasia in all menopausal patients in one clinical trial. However, any oral progestin can be poorly tolerated for its side effects of depression, edema, and breast tenderness. For this reason, a new vaginal natural progesterone has been developed in a polycarbophil base, which allows it to avoid absorption into the circulation. Instead it enters the endometrium through the cervical lymph system and in the early studies has been effective. It is marketed for use in infertility patients as Crinone 8%, but for any

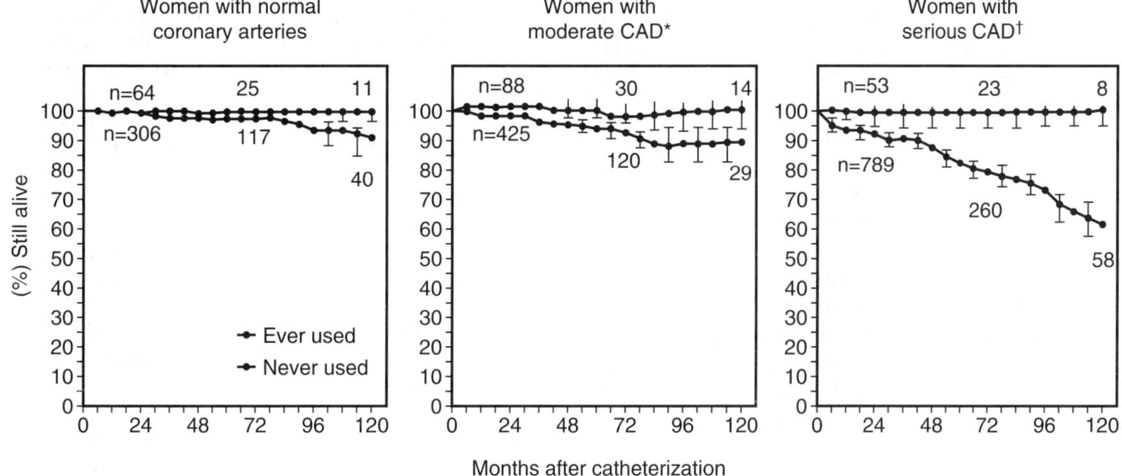

Figure 1. Effect of estrogen replacement therapy on 10-year survival. *Abbreviations:* CAD = coronary artery disease. (From Sullivan JM, Vander Zwaag R, Hughes JP, et al: Estrogen replacement and coronary artery disease. Effect on survival in postmenopausal women. Arch Intern Med *150*:2557, 1990. Copyright 1990, American Medical Association.)

secondary amenorrhea, including menopause, it is marketed in 4%.

The epidemiologic literature on breast cancer and estrogen replacement therapy is confusing. Although most studies have found little or no increase in breast cancer risk, a study done in Sweden seems to show a slightly increased risk in certain subgroups, even though they represented small enough total numbers to be related to chance only. The follow-up nurse's health study report indicated a significant increase in risk ratio to 1.4 after 10 years of ERT. However, the overall cancer mortality was decreased to a risk ratio of 0.8. The current thinking is that estrogen is not a carcinogen for breast cancer, but can be a growth accelerator factor, and for this reason it is important for women to have a careful breast examination as well as a mammogram to rule out early malignancy before beginning ERT. Breast examination and mammography should be performed annually thereafter.

This leads to the conclusion that menopausal women need to be carefully evaluated. If they have vasomotor instability, a high risk for development of osteoporosis, vaginal or urogenital atrophy, high risk of ischemic or atherosclerotic heart disease, or premature ovarian failure, they should begin hormone replacement therapy. This is usually accomplished with a dose of conjugated estrogen, 0.625 mg daily or its equivalent, but can be up to 1.25 mg daily in patients who have had surgical menopause or early menopause with severe symptoms. Women who have not had hysterectomies should receive medroxyprogesterone, 10 mg daily for 10 days a month or its equivalent, but an individual dose can be determined with an endometrial biopsy after therapy is instituted. Recent studies have shown low-dose progesterone (i.e., medroxyprogesterone [Provera] 2.5 mg or megestrol [Megace] 10 mg on a daily basis) to be successful.

Although the oral route is the most common form of estrogen replacement therapy, the transdermal route has the advantage of avoiding the first hepatic pass, which is beneficial in women with previous liver disease, and also prevents the concentration of gallbladder disease associated with the oral medication. If urogenital atrophy is the only symptom being treated, vaginal conjugated estrogen creams of 1 gram 1 to 2 times per week are most effective. However, vaginal routes are notorious for their absorption variability. The vaginal ring, because of its extremely low daily dose, is almost never absorbed.

Four retrospective large studies show not only evidence of Alzheimer's disease being prevented in women who took estrogen, but also cognitive improvement in women who already had Alzheimer's disease and were placed on estrogen. This issue will become clearer as the prospective studies are completed and apply more to older women than to women at the time of menopause. However, a study of the National Institute of Aging showed continual improvement of memory and mentation in women over 40 who were on ERT compared with women who were on no therapy over a 10-year period. Consideration will have to be given to this issue when weighing risks and benefits.

Women with previous breast cancer usually should not be given hormone replacement therapy. At one time, the same was said for women with previous endometrial cancer. However, the feeling now is that if the cancer was Stage 0 or Stage 1 and 2 years have passed without sequelae, these patients can be treated. The new SERMs are not contraindicated in women with previous breast or endometrial cancer.

VULVOVAGINITIS

method of
SEBASTIAN FARO, M.D., PH.D.
Rush–Presbyterian–St. Luke's Medical Center
Chicago, Illinois

The most common gynecologic complaint addressed by the physician rendering ambulatory care to the female patient is vulvovaginitis, which may be due to an allergic reaction, infection, or lack of hormones. The three most common causes of vaginitis are bacteria, *Candida albicans,* and *Trichomonas vaginalis.* Although a variety of bacteria may cause vaginitis, the two most common types of bacterial vaginitis are *Gardnerella vaginalis* infection and anaerobic vaginitis (bacterial vaginosis). The latter is a polymicrobial infection due to an overgrowth of anaerobic bacteria but may also involve *G. vaginalis.* In addition to *T. vaginalis,* other parasites may cause vulvovaginitis.

Vulvovaginitis due to a lack of estrogen is referred to as atrophic vaginitis, whereas inflammation due to the application of an external irritant is referred to as contact vulvovaginitis. The differentiation of microbial and nonmicrobial vulvovaginitis can be established by performing colposcopically directed biopsy of the vulva and a macroscopic as well as a microscopic examination of the vaginal discharge. The vaginal discharge reflects the status of the lower genital tract environment. In an asymptomatic or healthy or normal vagina, the discharge has a pH of 3.2 to 4.2, is white to slate gray, and does not have an odor. Microscopic examination reveals squamous epithelial cells that are estrogenized and not covered with bacteria, thus obliterating the nucleus and cell membranes. There is not an abundance of white blood cells (WBCs). The bacteria seen in the surrounding milieu are usually not clumped together and consist mainly of bacilli.

The examination of a patient complaining of vaginal burning, discomfort, dyspareunia, or abnormal vaginal discharge should begin with a detailed history. It is often helpful to show the patient a photograph or diagram of the vulva, vestibule, introitus, and vagina and then ask her to indicate on the diagram where her symptoms are located. Frequently, the patient states she has vaginal itching when in reality the inflammation is localized to the introitus. Questions should be asked as to whether she douches; if so, how often, and with which agent? Does the douching agent contain perfume? Is the patient utilizing a new soap or a new laundry detergent? Questions should be asked regarding her sexual habits. Is she using a new form of birth control? For example, has she begun to use a spermicidal cream or jelly or a coital lubricant? Does she practice cunnilingus, which may lead to excessive moisture on the vulva and clitoris, thus resulting in maceration of the tissue and inflammation?

CONTACT VAGINITIS

Patients with contact vaginitis present with complaints of itching or burning that involves the vulva but usually does not involve the vagina. The vagina is affected only if the inflammatory agent is introduced into the vagina. The tissues appear erythematous and excoriated. Inspection of the vulva with the aid of a colposcope does not reveal any discrete lesions. The vagina commonly has a normal pH, unless the patient has been douching repeatedly with either an acidic or an alkaline solution.

Elimination of the suspected agent often results in resolution of the symptoms. In some instances, a topical steroid ointment or cream may be required. The patient should be advised to apply the cream lightly and rub it into the affected area thoroughly. It should not be applied for longer than 10 days, because prolonged administration of a topical steroid may result in thinning of the tissues and thus in continuing symptoms.

ATROPHIC VAGINITIS

Postmenopausal patients not receiving estrogen replacement therapy often develop atrophic vaginitis. The hallmark of this condition is regression of the genital structures; the labia become less prominent, the vaginal mucosa becomes smooth owing to the loss of the rugae, and the epithelium thins. The pink color gives way to a pale pink to white. The pH often is above 4.5 and may be as high as 7.5. There is a change in the bacterial flora, with the lactobacilli no longer being dominant. The patient commonly complains of burning, dyspareunia, and vaginal spotting. In addition, the patient may complain of urinary incontinence and burning when she urinates. The latter complaint is due to the passage of urine over the atrophic tissue.

Pelvic examination reveals the vulva to be smooth with loss of definition of the external genitalia, especially loss of the labia minora. The vagina is as described previously. The vaginal discharge is scant and appears gray. The pH is between 5.0 and 7.5. Microscopic examination of the discharge reveals few epithelial cells; those present tend to be elliptical to round and are referred to as parabasal cells. The bacteria tend to be few in number, and numerous WBCs may be present. If a specimen of the vaginal discharge is cultured for aerobes and anaerobes, there will be a noticeable decrease in or absence of lactobacilli as well as an increase in anaerobic colonization. It is important to remember that the same presentation is found in patients who have had a total hysterectomy with bilateral salpingo-oophorectomy.

It is extremely important in patients with vaginal bleeding or spotting that the origin of the bleeding be determined. The etiology of the bleeding should be established before estrogen therapy is instituted. If the patient has a uterus, an endometrial biopsy should be performed. Other possible sites of origin are the lower urinary tract and rectum, which should be investigated.

Treatment for this condition is not systemic or topical antibiotics but hormonal replacement. This can be accomplished by applying topical estrogen cream or oral estrogen or a combination of both. If topical estrogen cream is utilized after the acute phase has been corrected, the patient may require a maintenance program of once-weekly or as-needed use of the estrogen cream.

MICROBIAL VAGINITIS

The physician attempting to treat the patient with complaints of vaginal itching, burning, or discomfort must be familiar with the normal status of the healthy or asymptomatic vagina. The symptomatic vagina has a pH of greater than 4.5 and usually above 5. The discharge is usually a cream color, green, yellow, or dirty gray. The odor is usually offensive and described as fishlike or foul (fetid). The discharge is frequently frothy, that is, it appears to contain air bubbles. The amount of discharge may vary from scant to copious, depending on the phase of the menstrual cycle, the concentration of estrogen and progesterone influencing the vagina, and the number of growing microbes present.

The lower genital tract has an endogenous microflora made up primarily of aerobic and anaerobic bacteria. The predominant bacterium of an asymptomatic vagina is *Lactobacillus.* This bacterium may play a pivotal role in maintaining the equilibrium of the healthy vagina by maintaining a pH of 3.8 to 4.2 through the production of lactic acid. This pH is not favorable to the growth of other more pathogenic bacteria, such as the facultative and obligate anaerobes. In addition, it is theorized that the ability of lactobacilli to produce hydrogen peroxide may also play a role in suppressing the growth of anaerobic bacteria. Thus, when a patient is found to have vaginitis, the pH is often above 5 and there is a marked reduction in the number of lactobacilli.

Before examining the patient, the physician should ask questions focusing on factors that may influence the normal vaginal environment. The patient should attempt to describe the characteristics of the initial episode and how the episodes have changed over time. Has she used antibiotics? Have they been used for maintenance or therapeutic indications? Does the patient douche? If so, how often and with what agent? Questions regarding sexual habits should be asked. How many sexual partners does she have? Does she know whether her partner has sexual contact with others? Does she practice cunnilingus, fellatio, or rectal intercourse? The patient should be asked to localize her symptoms, that is, are they located at the opening of the vagina or in the vagina proper? Finally, she should be asked to characterize her discharge with regard to color, consistency, and odor.

HUMAN PAPILLOMAVIRUS VESTIBULITIS

The examination should begin with the external genitalia. Attention should be paid to the medial aspect of the labia minora and majora, especially the area of the vestibule and introitus. Patients often complain of itching or burning and dyspareunia in this area. Examination often reveals a horseshoe-shaped area of erythema, which is commonly painful or tender to palpation. Examination under magnification reveals the presence of glistening papules. Application of 5% acetic acid turns this epithelium white, which is characteristic of human papillomavirus (HPV) infection. It is best to refer the patient for further evaluation to a gynecologist specializing in infections of the genital tract. Colposcopically directed biopsies are required to establish a diagnosis. Treatment is usually initiated with laser ablation of this area followed by intravaginal application of 5-fluorouracil cream. The patient should undergo colposcopic examinations of the vulva, vagina, and cervix every 3 to 4 months for the next 2 years to determine whether there is a recurrence. The patient's partner requires a similar examination to determine whether there are HPV lesions present on his penis.

YEAST VAGINITIS

Typically, yeast favors a pH of 4.5 or lower, but not always. WBCs are usually present, and the number of free-floating bacteria is usually reduced. The discharge is white and tends to be pasty but may be liquid. Classically, the discharge is cottage cheese–like and clings to vaginal epithelium. The microscopic picture may be that of elliptical yeast cells, budding cells, cells with germ tubes present, or long strands of pseudohyphae. These different forms of the yeast can easily be seen when the vaginal discharge is mixed with potassium hydroxide (KOH). It is not necessary to culture routinely for yeast, except when the patient's symptoms suggest a yeast infection but no fungal forms are seen microscopically.

Atypically, the patient may have a vaginal pH above 4.5 and there may be an increase in the number of bacteria seen in a wet preparation of the vaginal discharge. The physician should rely on a wet preparation mixed with KOH to rule out the presence of yeast.

Initial treatment should be with an intravaginal cream, ointment, or suppository such as clotrimazole (Lotrimin, Gyne-Lotrimin, Mycelex G), miconazole (Monistat), terconazole (Terazol), or nystatin. These are all beneficial in treating yeast vulvovaginitis. There are different dosing regimens ranging from a single dose to 3-day and 7-day courses. A patient with an initial infection may do well with a short treatment schedule if the precipitating factors can be established. Patients with recurrent infection require longer treatment regimens and the possible use of maintenance therapy. Some patients benefit from gentian violet applied as a vaginal paint or tampon. In addition, consideration should be given to examination and treatment of the patient's sexual partner. Ketoconazole (Nizoral) has been used in single doses of 400 mg with good results. However, hepatic and renal toxicities have been reported, and use of ketoconazole for vaginal yeast infection has not been encouraged.

BACTERIAL VAGINOSIS

The vagina houses a complex ecosystem. One component consists of a large number and variety of bacteria. The endogenous bacterial flora comprises gram-positive and gram-negative aerobic, facultative, and obligate anaerobes. The bacteriology of a healthy vaginal ecosystem is dominated by *Lactobacillus acidophilus.* This bacterium appears to exert its influence by maintaining the pH between 3.8 and 4.2, resulting in the suppression of the potentially pathogenic bacteria. This pH range also favors the growth of lactobacilli as well as other commensal bacteria, such as *Corynebacterium,* diphtheroids, and other nondescript streptococci.

These bacteria, as well as others, may act synergistically with one another, whereas others, such as lactobacilli and facultative and obligate anaerobes, may act antagonistically. Some strains, such as *L. acidophilus,* produce hydrogen peroxide, which is toxic to anaerobic bacteria; because they lack the enzyme catalase, anaerobic bacteria cannot convert hydrogen peroxide to oxygen and water. Other mechanisms by which bacteria, such as lactobacilli, inhibit the growth of other bacteria are the production and secretion of lysozyme and bacteriocins. It is important to note that the equilibrium of the vaginal ecosystem is extremely delicate and can easily be disrupted. Once the equilibrium is significantly disturbed, the growth of lactobacilli is retarded. This, in turn, may result in a decrease in the hydrogen ion concentration or an increase in pH. The alteration in pH causes a further decline in the growth of lactobacilli and greater growth of the potentially pathogenic bacteria.

The initial insult or factor that begins the change in the ecosystem is not known. However, if this alteration favors the growth of *G. vaginalis,* a further decrease in hydrogen ion concentration occurs. When the pH reaches a value of 5 or greater, facultative anaerobic bacterial growth occurs. Growth of *G. vaginalis* and the facultative anaerobes results in a progressive decrease in the oxygen concentration, favoring growth of obligate anaerobic bacteria. This causes the condition known as bacterial vaginosis (BV). Another organism that can alter the ecosystem in a similar manner is *T. vaginalis.* This protozoan favors a more alkaline pH (>4.5), which favors growth of the facultative and obligate anaerobic bacteria.

TABLE 1. **Characteristics of the Vaginal Ecosystem**

Characteristic	Healthy Ecosystem	Bacterial Vaginosis
Discharge	White to slate gray	Dirty gray
pH	3.8–4.2	>4.5
Clue cells	Absent	Present
White blood cells	Rare	Rare
Whiff test	Negative	Positive

BV is characterized by a vaginal pH greater than 4.5, the presence of clue cells, and a fishlike odor. This odor is typically manifested when a drop of vaginal discharge is mixed with a drop of concentrated KOH, releasing catecholamines (whiff test). The patient may also complain of a copious, dirty gray vaginal discharge with a foul or fishy odor. This odor may also be noted by the patient's sexual partner. However, approximately 50% of patients with BV are asymptomatic and are diagnosed because they are being examined for another reason.

BV is not an infection but should be viewed as a disturbance in the vaginal ecosystem. This disturbance in the endogenous vaginal microflora is significant, because it has been linked to postpartum endometritis, posthysterectomy pelvic infection, and preterm labor. Therefore, many obstetrician-gynecologists recommend that pregnant and preoperative patients be screened for BV. The differences between a healthy vaginal ecosystem and BV are listed in Table 1.

The color of the vaginal discharge is not a reliable characteristic with regard to establishing a diagnosis. However, any color other than white or slate gray should be considered abnormal. The key characteristics that can be utilized during the pelvic examination to assist in establishing an accurate diagnosis are pH, the presence of a fishlike odor when the vaginal discharge is mixed with KOH, and the presence of clue cells.

The pH can be determined easily and inexpensively by placing a ColorpHast pH strip on the lateral vaginal wall and comparing the wall's color with the accompanying chart. A pH lower than 4.5 essentially rules out the presence of BV. A pH higher than 4.5 does not establish, but is strongly suggestive of, the diagnosis of BV. A microscopic examination of the vaginal discharge must be performed to determine whether clue cells are present and whether there is an absence of a dominant bacterial morphotype. Evaluation of the vaginal discharge can be of assistance in differentiating among a variety of causes of vaginitis (Table 2). Although the conditions are presented as pure entities in Table 2, it should be understood that any of these conditions can be present simultaneously. The noticeable presence of WBCs (>5 per high-power field) indicates that an inflammatory response has been triggered. Women with pure BV do not have WBCs in their vaginal discharge.

A specimen of the vaginal discharge should be collected by swabbing the lateral vaginal wall with a cotton-tipped applicator. The applicator is immersed in 2 to 3 mL of normal saline and vigorously agitated to dilute the specimen. A drop of the resulting solution should be placed on a glass slide, covered with a glass coverslip, and examined with the assistance of 40× magnification.

The microscopic picture of BV is characterized by the presence of numerous individual free-floating bacteria, the absence of a dominant bacterial morphotype, the presence of clue cells, and the relative absence of WBCs. Clue cells are defined as squamous epithelial cells that have numerous bacteria adherent to their cytoplasmic membrane. If a Gram stain is performed, clue cells are seen to have gram-negative bacteria adherent to the cytoplasmic membrane. This is characteristic of *G. vaginalis* infection. The whiff test is performed by placing a drop of vaginal discharge on a glass slide and mixing in a drop of concentrated KOH; if there is a significant concentration of anaerobic bacteria present, a fishlike odor is detected.

Typically, in uncomplicated BV, WBCs are not present in the vaginal discharge. The presence of an obvious leukorrhea should alert the physician to the possible existence of an associated condition, i.e., a sexually transmitted disease (STD). The frequency of recurrent BV is linked to the frequency of sexual intercourse. Patients who experience recurrent episodes of BV should be queried as to their sexual practices. The presence of vaginal leukorrhea should alert the physician to the possible existence of pelvic inflammatory disease (PID). Therefore, the patient presenting with BV and leukorrhea should be evaluated for PID, trichomoniasis, cervical gonorrhea, and chlamydial infection.

TABLE 2. **Evaluation of the Vaginal Ecosystem**

Characteristic	Healthy	Bacterial Vaginosis*	Trichomoniasis*	Candidiasis
pH	3.8–4.2	≥5	≥5	<5
Squamous cells	Estrogenized	Clue cells +	Clue cells ±	Estrogenized
KOH (whiff test)	Negative	Fishlike odor +	Fishlike odor ±	No odor
KOH preparation	Destruction of all cellular constituents			Hyphae remain
Dominant bacterial morphotype	Bacilli	None	None	Bacilli
White blood cells	Rare	Rare	Positive	Positive

*The + indicates present; ± indicates present or absent.

Individuals found to be positive for an STD should also be evaluated for syphilis, hepatitis B, and human immunodeficiency virus. If there is strong suspicion that gonorrhea or *Chlamydia* (or both) is present, appropriate treatment should be instituted. In the patient found to be culture-positive for the gonococcus and/or *Chlamydia,* cultures should be repeated within 1 to 2 weeks after completion of therapy. She should also be encouraged to refrain from sexual intercourse during this period. If this is not possible or practical, the patient should insist that her partner wear a condom. Patients treated for PID should be re-evaluated within 72 hours after beginning antibiotic therapy to determine whether there has been a positive response. Patients failing to demonstrate improvement should be re-evaluated for having either more advanced PID or other pelvic diseases.

Patients found to have BV may be treated with one of the regimens listed in Table 3.

The patient should be re-evaluated 7 and 30 days after the completion of therapy to ensure that the condition has resolved. She should be advised to either refrain from intercourse or have her partner wear a condom. This practice should continue throughout the follow-up period.

Individuals who have recurrent or persistent BV should be treated as described earlier and, when found to be free of BV, should be considered for maintenance therapy. There are no good data available with regard to maintenance therapy, but two factors that may contribute to recurrent BV are (1) the vaginal ecosystem is cleared of clue cells, and there is now a high-density mixture of bacteria, but noticeable lactobacilli are lacking, and (2) the vaginal pH remains above 4.5. A patient with both these factors is likely to have a relapse in a short time, and unless the pH is restored to a range of 3.8 to 4.2, lactobacilli will not resume a place of dominance in the vaginal ecosystem. Thus, a healthy vaginal ecosystem will not become re-established, and the BV cycle is likely to begin again.

Unfortunately, there are no specific medications or treatments for restoring the vaginal pH to a range of 3.8 to 4.2. However, acid gel can be administered twice daily for 10 to 14 days in an attempt to lower the pH of the vagina. One week after the completion of therapy, the patient should be re-evaluated to determine whether a healthy vaginal ecosystem has been restored. Failure of the patient to respond to therapy is an indication for referral to a specialist with an interest in vulvovaginal disease.

TABLE 3. **Antibiotic Regimens for the Treatment of Bacterial Vaginosis**

Clindamycin (Cleocin) vaginal cream, 2%, one applicator administered intravaginally, qhs × 7 nights
Metronidazole vaginal gel (MetroGel), 0.75%, one applicator bid × 7 d
Metronidazole (Flagyl), 250 mg orally bid × 7 d or 375 mg orally bid × 5 d
Clindamycin (Cleocin), 300 mg orally bid × 7 d
Amoxicillin-clavulanate (Augmentin), 500 mg orally tid × 7 d

PARASITIC VULVOVAGINITIS

The most common agent of parasitic genital infection is *T. vaginalis.* Other common but less frequent parasites are *Phthirus pubis, Sarcoptes scabiei,* and *Enterobius vermicularis.*

P. pubis, commonly referred to as "the crabs," is one of three species of lice that infect humans; the others are *Pediculus humanus corporis,* the body louse, and *Pediculus humanus capitis,* the head louse. Lice are transmitted by person-to-person contact. Although the pubic louse is most commonly transmitted via sexual contact, cases have been documented in which transmission has occurred from toilet seats, bed linen, and infected loose hairs. The incidence of infection is highest among individuals with gonorrhea and syphilis. The affected patient presents with itching, evidence of excoriation, erythema, irritation, and inflammation. Patients who have a large number of bites may even develop a mild elevation in body temperature, malaise, and irritability.

The diagnosis is established by taking a detailed history and carefully examining the patient. The adult crab louse and nits (eggs) can be seen by the naked eye. A simple magnifying glass facilitates examining the pubic area. The pubic lice may appear as scabs; however, when the scab is removed and examined microscopically, the crab louse becomes easy to identify. If no adults are present, the eggs or nits can be identified.

Treatment must be effective against both the adult lice and the nits. The partner of the infected patient must also be examined, as should other household members. Several agents are available, including preparations with pyrethrins and piperonyl butoxide (RID [liquid and shampoo]; Triple X Kit [liquid and shampoo]; and Barc [liquid]), lindane (Kwell [lotion, shampoo, and cream]), crotamiton (Eurax [cream and lotion]), 20% benzyl benzoate, and 10% sulfur ointment. The pediculicide should remain in contact with the infected area for at least 1 hour to be ovicidal. Kwell is probably the most commonly used pediculicide. The proper use of this agent requires the patient to shower before applying the Kwell (1% γ-benzene hexachloride), which then remains on the body surface for 8 hours. This process should be followed for three applications of Kwell, and each 8-hour application is followed by a shower. The patient should wash thoroughly with soap and water to remove the Kwell. After the final shower, no further treatment should be necessary.

Kwell is absorbed, especially if the skin has been severely excoriated, and may cause neurotoxicity. This agent should not be used on children or pregnant women.

The patient's clothing and fomites should also be treated for adult lice and nits. Clothes should be washed in hot water (125°F), and nonwashable items should be dry cleaned; either process will kill adult lice, nymphs, or nits. Inanimate or nonwashable items that cannot be processed by dry cleaning can be treated with disinfectants containing pyrethrin and piperonyl butoxide.

Sarcoptes scabiei is the causative agent of scabies, which is transmitted via close personal contact. The organism is transmitted by sexual and nonsexual contact. The hands and feet are initially infected. The female breast may have lesions resembling those of Paget's disease. Infection may occur in skin folds such as the umbilicus, the groin, and where the buttocks meet the thigh. The characteristic lesion is a burrow. Most sites are erythematous and excoriated, as is most commonly seen in the web between the fingers.

The infection can be diagnosed by taking skin scrapings and examining them microscopically for the presence of the mite. Other diagnostic modalities are needle extraction of a mite from a burrow; epidermal shave biopsy of a burrow or papule; covering the burrow with ink and wiping with alcohol (if a mite is present, it will be stained by the ink); scraping the burrow, mixing the scrapings with mineral oil, and examining microscopically; punch biopsy; and placing topical tetracycline on the infected area, wiping, and then examining under ultraviolet light for fluorescence.

Treatment of scabies is best accomplished with topical agents such as 1% γ-benzene hexachloride (lindane cream or lotion, Kwell, or Scabene), crotamiton (Eurax), or sulfur.

DISEASE CAUSED BY *Trichomonas vaginalis*

T. vaginalis is a protozoan with five flagella, four located anteriorly and one located in an undulating membrane. The organism has the ability to adhere to epithelial cells. The hallmark of *T. vaginalis* infection is vaginal discharge, which may vary in color from a dirty gray to a yellow-green. The discharge appears frothy owing to the presence of gas bubbles. The pH of the discharge is usually greater than 5. The patient may complain of dyspareunia, dysuria, pruritus, and a foul vaginal odor. She also may note an exacerbation of symptoms shortly after her menses.

Pelvic examination may reveal the vulva to be erythematous, slightly edematous, and excoriated. Petechiae may be present on the cervix and vaginal walls. A urine specimen may also reveal the presence of trichomonads. One or two drops of the vaginal discharge mixed with 1 to 2 mL of normal saline and examined microscopically typically shows numerous bacteria, WBCs, and mobile trichomonads. However, if no protozoans are seen, it would be beneficial to inoculate a medium designed for the growth of *T. vaginalis* (e.g., Diamond's medium), because this is a more sensitive method of detecting *T. vaginalis* than microscopic examination of vaginal discharge.

Treatment should be instituted with metronidazole, 250 mg given orally three times daily for 7 days or 375 mg orally twice a day for 7 days. I prefer this regimen over intravaginal suppositories, because the organism commonly infects extravaginal sites, such as the bladder, urethra, or periurethral glands. I have found that the single 2-gram dose is not well tolerated by the patient because of gastric upset. The male partner should be treated to achieve a cure in the female patient. Condoms should be utilized during the treatment period. The patient should be reexamined to determine whether the organism has been eradicated and the vaginal environment restored to a healthy state.

CONCLUSION

Patients who present to the physician with vulvovaginitis of microbial etiology should be considered to have an STD. Consideration should be given to obtaining a culture specimen to test for the presence of *Neisseria gonorrhoeae* and *Chlamydia trachomatis*. In addition, serologic study for syphilis should be performed. These recommendations should be followed especially for the patient who is between the ages of 15 and 30 years, unmarried, and sexually active.

TOXIC SHOCK SYNDROME

method of
ROBERT L. DERESIEWICZ, M.D.
*Harvard Medical School and Brigham and Women's Hospital
Boston, Massachusetts*

Staphylococcal toxic shock syndrome (TSS) is an acute, severe, febrile illness characterized by fever, hypotension, rash, multiorgan dysfunction, and convalescence-stage desquamation. It results from intoxication by any of several related *Staphylococcus aureus* exotoxins, most commonly TSS toxin type 1 (TSST-1). A related and clinically indistinguishable illness, toxic shock–like syndrome (TSLS), may follow infection by toxigenic strains of *Streptococcus pyogenes*.

TSS was first described in a pediatric population but became widely known in 1980 after the occurrence of a large outbreak among young, menstruating women, the overwhelming majority of whom were tampon users. Menstrual cases presently account for about half of TSS cases reported in the United States. The remainder occur in association with staphylococcal colonization or superinfection at diverse body sites, and among patients of either sex and any age. With prompt recognition and proper management, the outcome in most cases is good; the principal challenge, as with many rare and severe diseases, is to recognize the illness and intervene promptly.

ETIOLOGY AND PATHOGENESIS

Virtually all menstrual TSS cases and about 60% of nonmenstrual cases are caused by TSST-1. Most of the remainder are caused by staphylococcal enterotoxin B

(SEB), and a small fraction by enterotoxin C. Coagulase-negative staphylococci do not produce TSS toxins and are not capable of causing TSS. The TSS toxins are encoded by *variable genetic elements*, meaning that the genetic capability to produce one or more of the toxins is present in only a subset of strains. About 10 to 20% of human *S. aureus* isolates produce TSST-1 and 7 to 14% produce SEB.

Necessary steps in the pathogenesis of TSS are as follows: colonization of a nonimmune host by a toxigenic strain, toxin production, toxin absorption, and intoxication. About 4 to 10% of people harbor toxigenic staphylococci at any site at any given time, including approximately 1 to 4% of postmenarcheal women who carry TSST-1–producing staphylococci vaginally. Protective levels of antibodies to TSST-1 and SEB are acquired by most people during youth and adolescence, presumably in response to benign staphylococcal colonization or infection. By adulthood, more than 90% of people are immune to each toxin.

Toxigenic staphylococci that have the genetic capability to produce a TSS toxin actually do so only at limited times. The risk of TSS associated with the use of tampons and certain surgical dressings likely derives from changes that these products effect in the local microenvironment and the stimulus to toxin production resulting therefrom. For example, tampon use introduces oxygen into the normally anaerobic vagina; oxygen is required for TSST-1 synthesis, at least in vitro. Once produced, TSST-1 is rapidly transported across the vaginal mucosa.

The TSS toxins are *superantigens*—V_β-restricted T-cell mitogens—whose toxicity for humans is thought to derive, at least in great part, from their ability to stimulate certain immune cells, and thereby to provoke exuberant, dysregulated cytokine release. How, exactly, that cytokine release culminates in the various manifestations of TSS remains uncertain. One of the important sequelae, however, is the development of capillary leak syndrome, which may be principally responsible for the hypotension and end-organ damage that occurs in TSS.

EPIDEMIOLOGY

As noted, TSS cases are classified as menstrual or nonmenstrual. By definition, menstrual cases begin during menses; their peak incidence is between the third and fifth days of menstruation. The vast majority are in tampon users. Nonmenstrual cases include those related to colonization or infection of the female genitourinary tract (e.g., puerperal cases and cases associated with barrier contraceptive use, septic abortion, and nonobstetric gynecologic surgery); those associated with skin or soft tissue infections (including both primary staphylococcal infections, such as folliculitis, cellulitis, and furunculosis, and secondary infections, such as those of burns, bites, varicella lesions, and surgical wounds); and those related to infections of the respiratory tract (e.g., staphylococcal pharyngitis, tracheitis, sinusitis, or pneumonia), the musculoskeletal system (e.g., osteomyelitis, septic arthritis), or rarely, the bloodstream. In postoperative cases, the illness may manifest within hours of the surgical procedure or may be delayed until days or weeks later.

The number of TSS cases reported annually to the Centers for Disease Control and Prevention (CDC) has dropped considerably since the early 1980s (Figure 1). The drop is attributable partly to the impact of safer tampons and tampon usage practices, but likely also to substantial under-reporting. The true frequency of menstrual TSS is

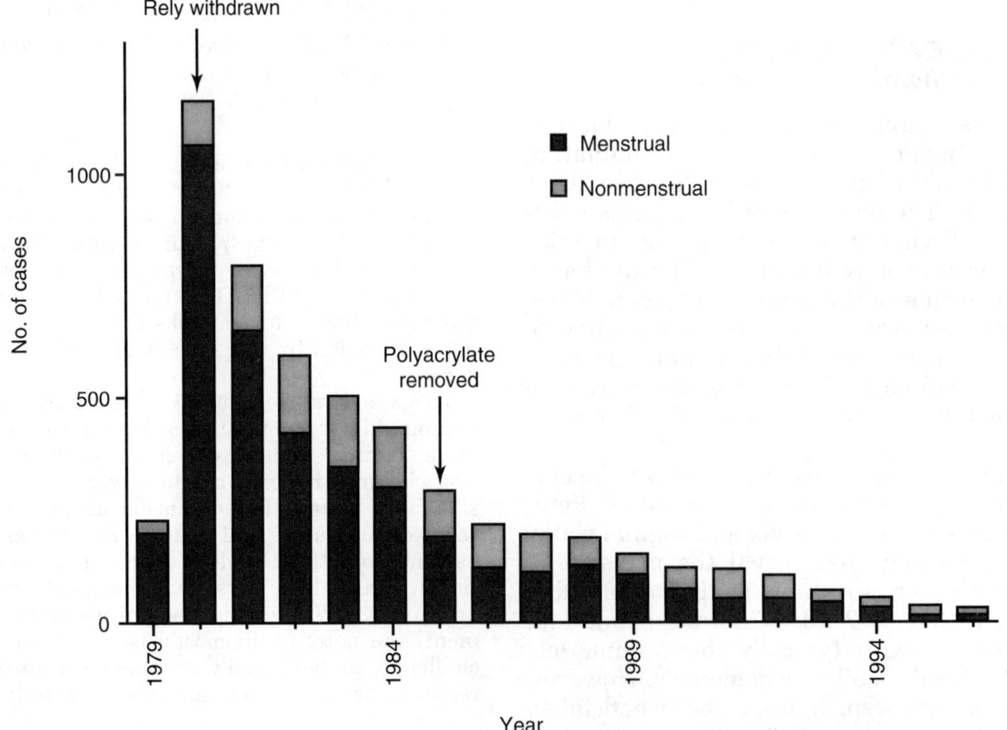

Figure 1. Toxic shock syndrome cases reported to the Centers for Disease Control and Prevention (CDC), by year and menstrual status. The dates of withdrawal or reformulation of certain tampon products are indicated by arrows. (Data kindly provided by Dr. Rana Hajjeh, National Center for Infectious Diseases, CDC, Atlanta, GA. Figure modified from Deresiewicz RL: Staphylococcal toxic shock syndrome. *In* Leung DYM, Huber BT, Schlievert PM [eds]: Superantigens: Molecular Biology, Immunology, and Relevance to Human Disease. New York, Marcel Dekker, 1997, pp 435–479. Modified by courtesy of Marcel Dekker, Inc.)

probably at least 1 case per 100,000 women per year, and is likely even higher among menstrual women in their teens and early twenties. According to a recent study, the incidence of postoperative (nonmenstrual) TSS is 3 cases per 100,000 patients.

Mortality also appears to have diminished over time. For the most recent 10-year period for which data are available (1987-1996), the minimum case fatality rate for definite and probable menstrual cases reported to the CDC was 1.8%; for nonmenstrual cases the minimum rate was 5.5%.

CLINICAL MANIFESTATIONS

Mild, prodromal flulike symptoms occur in a minority of patients. The acute illness begins precipitously, with high fever, chills, headache, severe myalgias, muscle tenderness, abdominal pain, nausea, vomiting, and profuse, watery diarrhea. Oral, conjunctival, and/or vaginal mucosal irritation also typically occurs. Orthostasis or hypotension and the characteristic macular erythroderma develop over the next 2 days. The erythroderma is usually generalized, often intense, and blanches with pressure. However, it may be locally distributed, mild, or fleeting and may be subtle, particularly in the presence of severe hypotension. On admission, patients appear toxic, with hypotension, tachycardia, and oliguria. Examination may reveal conjunctival suffusion; tender, beefy-red oral or vaginal mucosa; and strawberry tongue. Peripheral cyanosis and edema are common, as is diffuse abdominal tenderness. Rales may be present. The liver, spleen, and lymph nodes are usually unremarkable. Encephalopathy, as evidenced by confusion, disorientation, agitation, or somnolence, is also common, but the neurological examination is typically nonfocal. The site of staphylococcal toxin production may be purulent or erythematous, or it may appear entirely benign. Laboratory studies reflect multiorgan dysfunction. Frequent findings include leukocytosis, thrombocytopenia, coagulopathy, azotemia, transaminitis, hypoalbuminemia, hypocalcemia, hypophosphatemia, and pyuria. Disseminated intravascular coagulation is not a common feature of TSS.

Like many other toxin-mediated diseases, TSS follows a somewhat predictable course. The early manifestations of fever, erythroderma, gastrointestinal distress, and blood chemistry abnormalities resolve within the first few days of illness. In severe cases, hypotension may persist and may be complicated by myocardial dysfunction, pulmonary edema, severe rhabdomyolysis, hepatic damage, renal failure, or peripheral gangrene.

Desquamation is a late event in TSS. Superficial flaking of the skin of the trunk and extremities begins about a week after the onset of illness. The characteristic full-thickness desquamation of the palms, soles, and digits follows in the second week and may continue for up to 1 month. Late sequelae of TSS include postfebrile telogen effluvium (reversible hair and nail loss), prolonged fatigue and weakness, memory loss, emotional changes, and impaired ability to concentrate. Fatalities typically occur within the first few days of illness, most commonly from refractory shock, respiratory failure, or cardiac arrhythmias.

Although not accounted for by the case definition of TSS, mild systemic intoxications by the TSS toxins probably occur. Such cases lack two or more criteria for TSS, but have certain epidemiologic or clinical features particularly suggestive of the diagnosis (e.g., erythroderma, severe gastrointestinal disturbance, and/or convalescent desquamation). The occurrence of such an illness during menses in a young tampon user should prompt a search for evidence of TSST-1 involvement, particularly if the illness is recurrent. Compatible findings include the isolation of TSST-1–producing *S. aureus* from the vagina, and the demonstration of a nonprotective titer of serum anti–TSST-1 antibodies. Although such findings do not prove that an illness was TSST-1–related (indeed, most perimenstrual flulike illness is certainly not attributable to TSST-1), they should nevertheless prompt discontinuation of tampon use until seroconversion has been documented. An attempt to eradicate vaginal staphylococcal carriage in such circumstances is also reasonable.

DIAGNOSIS

The diagnosis of TSS rests exclusively on clinical grounds (Table 1). A host of possibilities other than TSS should be considered in the patient acutely ill with fever, rash, and hypotension. These include severe group A streptococcal infections (scarlet fever, necrotizing fasciitis, streptococcal TSLS), Kawasaki syndrome (particularly in children under 4 years of age), staphylococcal scalded skin syndrome, Rocky Mountain spotted fever, leptospirosis, meningococcemia, exanthematous viral syndromes, and severe allergic drug reactions.

In menstrual TSS cases, particularly when a purulent vaginal discharge is present, the diagnosis may be readily apparent. The challenge is to recognize subtle cases, including nonmenstrual cases and cases in which the rash is evanescent. A careful history with attention to past health,

TABLE 1. **Staphylococcal Toxic Shock Syndrome: Case Definition**

I. Fever: temperature ≥ 102°F (38.9°C)
II. Rash: diffuse macular erythroderma ("sunburn" rash)
III. Hypotension: systolic blood pressure ≤ 90 mm Hg (adults) or < 5th percentile for age (children under 16 years of age), or orthostatic hypotension (orthostatic drop in diastolic blood pressure ≥ 15 mm Hg, orthostatic dizziness or orthostatic syncope)
IV. Involvement of at least three of the following organ systems:
   A. Gastrointestinal: vomiting or diarrhea at onset of illness
   B. Muscular: severe myalgias, or serum creatine phosphokinase level at least twice the upper limit of normal
   C. Mucous membranes: vaginal, oropharyngeal, or conjunctival hyperemia
   D. Renal: blood urea nitrogen or creatinine at least twice the upper limit of normal, or pyuria (≥ 5 leukocytes per high-power field), in the absence of a urinary tract infection
   E. Hepatic: total serum bilirubin or transaminase level (alanine aminotransferase or aspartate aminotransferase) at least twice the upper limit of normal
   F. Hematologic: thrombocytopenia (platelets ≤ 100,000 per μL)
   G. Central nervous system: disorientation or alteration in consciousness but no focal neurologic signs at a time when fever and hypotension are absent
V. Desquamation: 1 to 2 weeks after the onset of illness (typically palms and soles)
VI. Evidence against an alternative diagnosis: If obtained, negative cultures of blood, throat, or cerebrospinal fluid;* absence of a rise in antibody titers to the agents of Rocky Mountain spotted fever, leptospirosis, or rubeola

*Blood culture may be positive for *S. aureus*.
From Reingold AL, Hargrett NT, Shands KN, et al: Toxic shock syndrome surveillance in the United States, 1980 to 1981. Ann Intern Med *96*(Part 2):875–880, 1982.

possible infectious exposures, travel, vocation, avocation, vaccination status, menstrual status, and medication usage often narrows considerably the etiologic possibilities. Backdrops particularly suggestive of TSS include the menstruating or postpartum female, the female who uses barrier contraceptive methods, the postoperative patient, the patient with varicella-zoster infection, and the patient with chemical or thermal burns.

Laboratory evaluation should include a complete blood count and differential; serum electrolytes; calcium, phosphate, and albumin; liver and renal function tests; creatine phosphokinase level; prothrombin and partial thromboplastin times; and urinalysis. A chest x-ray film and electrocardiogram should also be obtained. In females vaginal culture should be performed. Blood, urine, and respiratory cultures should also be obtained, as should cultures of all wounds, regardless of how benign they may appear. The laboratory should be instructed to speciate any staphylococci isolated from mucosal sites. *S. aureus* isolates (mucosal or otherwise) should be referred for TSST-1 testing, if possible.

Acute and convalescent sera should be tested for antibody to TSST-1, particularly in suspected menstrual cases. The absence initially of a protective titer to TSST-1 supports the clinical diagnosis of TSS, and seroconversion, if it occurs, confirms it. The majority of patients, however, do not seroconvert following TSS; such patients, menstrual cases in particular, are at risk for recurrent disease.

TREATMENT

With prompt treatment, the serious consequences of TSS (organ failure, limb loss, death) can often be avoided. Treatment involves four components: decontamination of the site of toxin production, administration of antistaphylococcal antibiotics, fluid resuscitation, and general supportive care.

The nidus of toxin production should be carefully sought. If present, vaginal tampons or other types of foreign bodies should be removed. Purulent foci should be drained and debrided, and cutaneous lesions copiously irrigated. Thorough lavage lowers the burden of organisms and potentially slows toxin accretion. For TSS occurring in the postoperative period, the surgical wound *must* be explored, even if it appears uninfected.

Antibiotic administration offers a second opportunity to interrupt intoxication. While β-lactamase–resistant semisynthetic penicillins or first-generation cephalosporins have historically been given for TSS, growing evidence suggests that clindamycin (Cleocin), is superior. Under conditions of saturating growth, staphylococci express only low levels of penicillin-binding proteins, the molecular targets of β-lactam antibiotics. β-lactams are relatively ineffective against such cells, but TSST-1 is essentially only produced under those saturating conditions. Organisms producing TSST-1, therefore, are likely to be relatively resistant to β-lactams. In addition, β-lactam levels fluctuate widely during dosing and may fall below the minimum inhibitory concentration for *S. aureus* toward the end of each dosing interval. Subinhibitory concentrations of β-lactams actually enhance TSST-1 production, at least in vitro.

Clindamycin, on the other hand, is a protein synthesis inhibitor; its antistaphylococcal activity is independent of growth phase. Moreover, clindamycin potently suppresses TSST-1 production in vitro, even at concentrations insufficient to inhibit staphylococcal growth. The great majority of *S. aureus* strains causing TSS, particularly menstrual TSS, remain susceptible to clindamycin (and to methicillin). I prescribe clindamycin, 900 mg intravenously every 8 hours, for suspected cases of TSS. In the critically ill patient in whom clindamycin- or methicillin-resistant infection is a concern, it is reasonable to coadminister vancomycin (Vancocin), 1 gram intravenously every 12 hours, until microbiologic data are available. If the diagnosis of TSS is initially uncertain, broader empiric coverage is prudent. Antibiotics should be administered for at least 10 days but can be given orally once the patient has stabilized.

Aggressive fluid resuscitation should be initiated to reverse hypotension and forestall end-organ damage. Adult patients may require up to 10 liters of crystalloid over the first 24 hours of treatment to maintain adequate cardiac filling. The principal mechanism of hypotension in TSS is believed to be capillary leak syndrome; fluid therapy therefore is typically complicated by massive weight gain and peripheral edema. Pressors and central hemodynamic monitoring may be used in cases of refractory hypotension, particularly if oxygenation is impaired.

In addition to the specific interventions outlined previously, intensive care should be provided, with attention to correcting metabolic abnormalities and monitoring closely for complications. A final therapeutic option for refractory cases or cases associated with an undrainable focus of infection is pooled human immunoglobulin (IVIG; Sandoglobulin, Gamimune N).* All commercial preparations contain levels of anti–TSST-1 sufficient to generate a protective titer after a single intravenous dose of 400 mg per kg. Evidence supporting this therapy in humans is strictly anecdotal; high cost precludes its routine use except in severe cases.

*Not FDA approved for this indication.

Chlamydia trachomatis INFECTION

method of
SEBASTIAN FARO, M.D., PH.D.
Rush–Presbyterian–St. Luke's Medical Center
Chicago, Illinois

Chlamydia trachomatis is a true bacterial parasite. The organism requires adenosine triphosphate (ATP), which is derived from the host, to carry on its metabolic processes and reproduction. This species is responsible for trachoma and two major sexually transmitted diseases (STDs), lymphogranuloma venereum (LGV), and infection of the lower and upper genital tract. Serovars L1, L2, and L3 cause LGV. Serovars A through K are responsible for infection of the lower and upper genital tract. The latter infection includes urethritis, Bartholin's gland abscess, cervicitis, endometritis, and salpingitis. These serovars have also been implicated as a possible cause of preterm labor, premature rupture of amniotic membranes, septic abortion, and postpartum endometritis.

The significance of *C. trachomatis* is not because of the infection of the lower genital tract, but to the upper genital tract and the resultant sequelae. Upper genital tract infection, salpingitis, can result in partial damage of the ciliated endothelial cells found in the fallopian tubes, which inhibits migration of a fertilized ovum and results in ectopic pregnancy. Damage can result in complete blocking of the fallopian tubes at the proximal and distal ends, rendering the patient infertile. Unique to this organism is that pelvic infection is usually asymptomatic. Therefore, the infection is undetected and treatment is not administered. It is up to the physician and other health care providers to consider the presence of this infection in patients who are sexually active, especially those in the reproductive age group.

Some investigators recommend screening all patients of reproductive age for the presence of *C. trachomatis*. This practice would have a poor yield and would not be cost effective. Perhaps a more productive approach is to obtain a detailed history to determine whether a patient is at risk for contracting an STD (Table 1). This determination is extremely important because it encourages the physician to look for clues that this patient is at risk for an STD. The risk can be strengthened by finding vaginal trichomoniasis, bacterial vaginosis, herpetic ulcerations, chancre, and condyloma acuminata.

During the pelvic examination, the physician should examine the vaginal discharge microscopically to determine whether the patient has a leukorrhea and/or trichomoniasis. The presence of leukorrhea may suggest that the patient has pelvic inflammatory disease (PID), but this finding is not pathognomonic of salpingitis. The presence of trichomoniasis indicates that the patient is at risk for other STDs. There is a tendency for an STD to travel in the company of other STDs; for example, *Neisseria gonorrhoeae* and *C. trachomatis* are found to co-infect an individual in approximately 60% of cases.

Another physical clue of the possible presence of *C. trachomatis* is the presence of endocervical mucopus. This characteristic is usually detected by placing a Dacron-tipped applicator into the endocervical canal and rotating it 360 degrees for approximately 30 seconds. A purulent exudate on the tip of the applicator is highly suggestive of the presence of *C. trachomatis*. The specimen should be processed for the isolation and identification of *C. trachomatis* by one of the following methods: culture, fluorescent antibody-antigen detection, DNA or RNA probes, antibody-antigen detection (enzyme-linked immunosorbent assay), polymerase chain reaction, or ligase chain reaction. The specimen should also be processed for the detection of *N. gonorrhoeae* and it should be gram-stained. The presence of white blood cells and the absence of bacteria would suggest, and be compatible with, infection with *C. trachomatis*. The presence of white blood cells containing gram-negative diplococci is highly suggestive of infection with *N. gonorrhoeae*.

Other physical clues include a cervix that bleeds briskly when gently touched with a cotton- or Dacron-tipped applicator, pain on palpation, and movement of the cervix and uterus. Pain also may be elicited when the adnexa are palpated. The patient may complain of dysuria and/or urinary frequency. A urine analysis may reveal the presence of pyuria and the absence of bacteria. This should encourage the physician to obtain a urethral specimen for the isolation of *C. trachomatis* and *N. gonorrhoeae*.

TABLE 1. **Historic Risk Factors for Contracting *Chlamydia trachomatis* Infection**

1. Multiple sexual partners
2. History of a sexually transmitted disease (STD)
3. Having a partner with an STD
4. First sexual intercourse at an early age
5. History of having used an intrauterine device
6. Previously treated for pelvic inflammatory disease
7. Recent onset of:
   a) postcoital bleeding or spotting
   b) dyspareunia
   c) vague lower abdominal pain
   d) irregular uterine bleeding
   e) breakthrough bleeding if the patient uses oral contraceptive pills

TREATMENT

Individuals with evidence of chlamydial infection should start on appropriate treatment. A test in which the answer cannot be obtained within 30 minutes is too long to wait to begin treatment. Remember, infection of the genital tract is typically asymptomatic; therefore, discovery is based solely on the investigational procedures of the physician. Because the infection may have been in place for a prolonged period of time, it may have already ascended to the upper genital tract. Any further delay may result in increased damage to the fallopian tubes. Administration of appropriate treatment should commence immediately. If cultures do not support the diagnosis, treatment can be interrupted. Patients who are culture positive should be counseled as to the significance of such an infection, specifically, the possibility of the patient's potential risk for infertilities associated with the number of episodes of PID. Individuals who experience a single episode of PID have a 13% risk of being infertile, two episodes are associated with a 35% risk, and those who have had three episodes of PID have approximately a 75% risk of infertility.

Treatment of urethritis is based on whether gonococci are present. In the absence of gonococci, treatment is directed against *C. trachomatis* (23 to 55%), *Ureaplasma urealyticum* (20 to 40%) and *Trichomonas vaginalis* (2 to 4%). Treatment regimens for chlamydial infection in the absence of other STDs are listed in Tables 2 and 3.

Patients whose symptoms persist should return for re-evaluation to determine whether (1) they were compliant in taking their medicine, and (2) they refrained from sexual intercourse to avoid reinfection. A repeat swab should also be performed, not only to determine if reinfection has occurred, but to see whether *T. vaginalis* is present. If trichomonads are detected, the patient should be treated with metronidazole (Flagyl), 250 mg orally, three times daily for 7 days. If the patient does not have trichomoniasis and was treated with doxycycline, a second course of

TABLE 2. **Treatment Regimens for Uncomplicated Chlamydial Infection in Nonpregnant Women**

1) Doxycycline (Vibramycin), 100 mg orally bid × 7 d
2) Erythromycin base, 500 mg orally qid × 7 d
3) Erythromycin ethylsuccinate, 800 mg orally qid × 7 d
4) Erythromycin base, 250 mg orally qid × 14 d
5) Erythromycin ethylsuccinate, 400 mg orally qid × 14 d
6) Azithromycin (Zithromax), 1 gm orally in a single dose
7) Amoxicillin, 500 mg orally tid × 7 d
8) Amoxicillin-clavulanate (Augmentin), 500 mg orally tid × 7 d
9) Ofloxacin (Floxin), 300 mg orally bid × 7 d
10) Trovafloxacin (Trovan), 200 mg orally qd × 7 d

doxycycline could be instituted, or one of the alternate choices listed in Table 2 could be chosen.

Patients with endocervical mucopus should be treated as being infected with both *C. trachomatis* and *N. gonorrhoeae*. It is difficult to determine the appropriate treatment regimen because it is not known if the infection is confined to the cervix or has begun to ascend to the upper genital tract. If there is no evidence or suggestion of upper tract involvement, then standard treatment of ceftriaxone (Rocephin), 125 mg once intramuscularly, and doxycycline, 100 mg orally, twice daily for 7 days, is acceptable. Individuals whose infection is confined to the cervix can be treated with ceftriaxone, 125 mg, once intramuscularly, and azithromycin (Zithromax), 500 mg, twice daily for 1 day. The patient should be advised not to engage in sexual intercourse during the management phase. The patient should be educated on prevention of reinfection. The patient's partner, and anyone else she has had sexual contact with, must be treated as well.

The patient with endometritis should have an endometrial biopsy, and the specimen should be divided into two portions. One specimen should be sent for the isolation and identification of *N. gonorrhoeae, C. trachomatis*, aerobic, facultative, and obligate anaerobic bacteria. The other specimen should be processed for histologic evaluation. The presence of plasma cells strongly suggests that the infection has involved the fallopian tubes. Treatment for this level of infection is best carried out with broad-spectrum antibiotics (Table 4).

Ofloxacin (Floxin) has been demonstrated to be as effective as ceftriaxone for the treatment of gonorrhea and as effective as doxycycline for treating chlamydial infection. The combination of an anaerobic agent such as metronidazole or clindamycin with ofloxacin offers a regimen with activity against the nonsexually transmitted agents that are endogenous to the lower genital tract and may be involved in the infectious process. Trovafloxacin (Trovan), a fluoroquinolone, has activity against both gonococci and chlamydiae, as well as the gram-negative and gram-positive facultative and obligate anaerobic bacteria. Therefore, trovafloxacin can be used alone for the treatment of *N. gonorrhoeae* and *C. trachomatis* infection, and PID.

TABLE 3. **Treatment Regimens for Uncomplicated Chlamydial Infection in Pregnant Women**

1) Erythromycin base, 250 mg orally qid × 14 d
2) Erythromycin ethylsuccinate, 800 mg orally qid × 7 d
3) Erythromycin ethylsuccinate, 400 mg orally qid × 14 d
4) Amoxicillin, 500 mg orally tid × 10 d

TABLE 4. **Oral Antibiotic Regimens for the Treatment of Ambulatory Patients with a Diagnosis of Endometritis and/or Salpingitis**

Metronidazole (Flagyl), 500 mg bid × 7 d, plus ofloxacin, 300 mg bid × 7 d
Clindamycin (Cleocin), 300 mg tid × 7 d, plus ofloxacin, 300 mg bid × 7 d
Amoxicillin-clavulanate (Augmentin), 500 mg tid × 7 d

Patients suspected of having PID and requiring hospitalization must also receive antibiotic regimens that are effective against the commonly involved STDs, as well as the aerobic, facultative, and obligate anaerobic bacteria. The hospitalized patient can receive any one of the regimens listed in Table 5.

The pregnant patient with cervical infection can be treated with azithromycin, 500 mg orally, twice daily for 1 day. She should *not* receive doxycycline or quinolones. The Centers for Disease Control and Prevention recommends erythromycin; however, this antibiotic is not well tolerated by pregnant women. Another alternative is amoxicillin, 500 mg orally, three times daily for 7 days. This agent is not effective against penicillinase-producing *N. gonorrhoeae*, but is effective against non–penicillinase-producing strains.

The patient who is positive for an STD should also be screened for hepatitis B, human immunodeficiency virus (HIV), and syphilis. Pregnant patients found to be positive for *N. gonorrhoeae* or chlamydial infection should be screened in each trimester for reinfection as well as for syphilis, hepatitis B, and HIV.

TABLE 5. **Parenteral Antibiotic Regimens for the Treatment of Hospitalized Patients with a Diagnosis of Pelvic Inflammatory Disease**

1) Cefoxitin (Mefoxin), 2 gm intravenously q 6 h, plus doxycycline, 100 mg (may be given orally) q 12 h
2) Cefotetan (Cefotan), 2 gm q 12 h, plus doxycycline, 100 mg q 12 h
3) Ceftizoxime (Cefizox), 2 gm q 8 h, plus doxycycline, 100 mg q 12 h
4) Ampicillin/sulbactam (Unasyn), 3 gm q 6 h
5) Piperacillin/tazobactam (Zosyn), 3.375 gm q 6 h
6) Metronidazole (Flagyl), 500 mg q 8 h, plus ofloxacin, 300 mg q 12 h
7) Clindamycin (Cleocin), 900 mg q 8 h, plus gentamicin, 2 mg/kg of body weight (loading dose) followed by 1.5 mg/kg administered q 8 h
8) Ofloxacin (Floxin), 300 mg q 8 h
9) Trovafloxacin (Trovan), 200 mg orally qd × 7 d

Patients treated for uncomplicated PID typically respond to antibiotic therapy within 48 hours. Patients not improving after 48 hours of antibiotic therapy should be re-evaluated to determine whether the infection has progressed (e.g., the development of a tubo-ovarian abscess).

The partner of a patient known to have an STD should be referred to a physician who specializes in the treatment of STDs. This is essential in controlling the spread of the diseases. It is important to educate both the patient and her partner as to the method of transmission and the significant morbidity associated with *C. trachomatis* infection.

PELVIC INFLAMMATORY DISEASE

method of
PAMELA D. BERENS, M.D.
University of Texas Health Science Center at Houston
Houston, Texas

Pelvic inflammatory disease (PID) has a major economic and social impact on female health. PID is usually the result of a sexually transmitted infection affecting the upper genital tract, which may present as endometritis, salpingitis, pelvic peritonitis, and/or tubo-ovarian abscess formation. Women with a history of PID are at risk for sequelae including tubal factor infertility, ectopic pregnancy, and chronic pelvic pain. Accurate and prompt diagnosis is important in successful management.

Risk factors for developing PID are similar to those for acquiring any sexually transmitted infection. Multiple sexual partners increases the potential exposure to pathogens. Having a partner with a sexually transmitted infection or history of multiple partners also increases risk. Young age positively correlates with the risk of PID. This is thought to be multifactorial. Younger women may be more likely to experiment sexually. The cervical ectropion, an area of columnar epithelium, which is everted onto the ectocervix, is also more pronounced in younger women. *Chlamydia trachomatis* and *Neisseria gonorrhoeae* adhere readily to this type of epithelium. Adolescents may also be less likely to use contraceptives, and certain forms of contraception may be protective against PID. Barrier methods such as condoms and diaphragms can reduce the incidence of sexually transmitted diseases (STDs). Use of spermicide also reduces transmission owing to its bactericidal properties. This method acts by reducing the incidence of the etiologic organisms associated with PID. Oral contraceptive pills (OCPs) also reduce the incidence of PID. The mechanism of action involves altering the cervical mucous plug, thereby reducing the ability of organisms to ascend and cause an upper genital tract infection. Additionally, there is typically reduced menstrual flow, which would provide less culture medium if the organisms ascend. The form of contraception associated with a potential increase in the incidence of PID is the intrauterine device (IUD). This increase is noted primarily around the time of insertion and is likely associated with the introduction of causative organisms during the insertion procedure.

Any procedure that introduces lower genital tract organisms to the upper tract could also increase the risk of PID. Factors that have been implicated in increasing the risk of PID include menstruation, prior PID, uterine instrumentation, and alterations in the normal vaginal flora. Douching negatively influences the vaginal floral hemostasis and increases the ability of the organisms to ascend. Bacterial vaginosis has been found to increase the risk for PID.

Symptoms of PID include lower abdominal pain, adnexal tenderness, and cervical motion tenderness. However, these symptoms are nonspecific, and often the disease may present atypically. Irregular vaginal bleeding may also occur. The implications for both overdiagnosis and underdiagnosis of this disease are far reaching. In an attempt to make the diagnosis more specific, one or more of the following additional criteria are suggested. Routine criteria include oral temperature greater than 38°C, leukocytosis greater than 10,000/mm^2, abnormal cervical or vaginal discharge, or evidence of *N. gonorrhoeae* and/or *C. trachomatis* by laboratory testing. Some authors include an elevated erythrocyte sedimentation rate or C-reactive protein among these criteria, although they are nonspecific and of limited clinical utility. More elaborate criteria for diagnosis include a pelvic mass by ultrasound or other radiographic testing consistent with tubo-ovarian abscess or pyosalpinx, purulent material in the peritoneal cavity by culdocentesis or laparoscopy, or histopathologic evidence of endometritis (plasma cell infiltrate) on endometrial biopsy. Approximately two thirds of women with a clinical diagnosis of PID have laparoscopic findings confirming the diagnosis. Although laparoscopy is considered the standard for the

TABLE 1. **Guidelines for Treatment of Pelvic Inflammatory Disease**

Treatment	Regimen A	Regimen B
Inpatient Requires discharge medication for a total course of 14 days of either doxycycline (Vibramycin), 100 mg orally twice daily or clindamycin, 450 mg orally 4 times daily.	1. Cefoxitin (Mefoxin) 2 g IV every 6 h or cefotetan (Cefotan) 2 g IV every 12 h plus 2. Doxycycline (Vibramycin) 100 mg orally or IV every 12 h	1. Clindamycin (Cleocin) 900 mg IV every 8 h plus 2. Gentamicin 2 mg/kg load IV or IM followed by 1.5 mg/kg every 8 h
Outpatient	1. Cefoxitin (Mefoxin) 2 g IM with probenecid (Benemid) 1 g orally or ceftriaxone (Rocephin) 250 mg IM or another third-generation cephalosporin plus 2. Doxycycline (Vibramycin) 100 mg orally 2 times daily for 14 d	1. Ofloxacin (Floxin) 400 mg orally 2 times daily for 14 d plus 2. Clindamycin (Cleocin) 450 mg orally 4 times daily or metronidazole (Flagyl) 500 mg orally 2 times daily for 14 d

diagnosis of PID, it is important to remember that 10 to 30% of women with negative laparoscopic findings have an endometrial sampling consistent with endometritis. These considerations reveal the difficulty in accurately diagnosing PID. Ectopic pregnancy should be ruled out by pregnancy test. A thorough sexual and gynecologic history can narrow the remaining differential diagnosis, which also includes ovarian cysts, torsion, endometriosis, appendicitis, irritable bowel syndrome, and gastroenteritis.

The etiologic organisms most commonly involved with initiation of PID include *N. gonorrhoeae* and *C. trachomatis*. The percentage of patients with these organisms depends on the specific population and anatomic site studied. These organisms are more frequently found from endocervical sampling; however, endocervical sampling for other organisms is not useful. Cultures taken from the fallopian tubes and pelvic cavity indicated that PID is often a polymicrobial infection. Commonly found organisms include facultative aerobes such as *Escherichia coli, Gardnerella vaginalis*, streptococci including enterococci, and *Haemophilus influenzae*; anaerobes such as *Bacteroides* species, *Peptostreptococcus*, and *Actinomyces*; and *Mycoplasmas* such as *Mycoplasma hominis* and *Ureaplasma urealyticum*. In up to 25% of cases of PID, only anaerobes and facultative aerobes are found. This is referred to as *nongonococcal, nonchlamydial* PID. PID initiated by gonorrhea typically has a more abrupt and dramatic onset, whereas that initiated by chlamydia is typically more indolent and therefore more likely to go undiagnosed.

TREATMENT

Treatment for PID can be either inpatient or outpatient depending on various patient characteristics. Treatment guidelines suggested by the Centers for Disease Control and Prevention were published in 1993 (Table 1). Factors suggesting the need for inpatient treatment include adolescent age, inability to tolerate oral medication, suspected pelvic abscess, severe illness (temperature > 101°F, white blood cell count > 15,000/mm^2, and/or sepsis), unclear diagnosis, pregnancy, human immunodeficiency virus (HIV) infection, IUD, history of uterine instrumentation, failed outpatient therapy, or suspected noncompliance with follow-up at 72 hours. Inpatient therapy is continued for 48 hours after patient improvement, and the patient is discharged on oral therapy for 14 days. If inpatient therapy has not resulted in significant improvement by 48 to 72 hours, consideration should be given to diagnostic laparoscopy. Operative laparoscopy may be used for diagnosis, lysis of adhesions, abscess drainage, and irrigation. Laparotomy is recommended for suspected ruptured tubo-ovarian abscess or severe PID refractory to medical management. At laparotomy, the decision to proceed with total abdominal hysterectomy and bilateral salpingo-oophorectomy versus more conservative surgery focusing on abscess drainage depends on the extent of disease and patient wishes for future fertility.

Long-term sequelae from PID are estimated to occur in 25% of patients. It is estimated that the risk for tubal-factor infertility after one episode of PID is 8%, increasing to nearly 20% and 40% for two and three episodes of PID, respectively. Women with a history of PID have a 6 - to 10-fold increased risk for ectopic pregnancy. The risk for developing chronic pelvic pain has been reported to be 18%. Other sequelae include Fitz-Hugh-Curtis syndrome (perihepatic adhesions), recurrent PID, worsened dysmenorrhea, dyspareunia, and chronic pyosalpinx.

In addition to providing prompt treatment for the woman, it is important to refer her sexual partner for testing and treatment as well. I also recommend testing the patient for other sexually transmitted diseases such as syphilis, hepatitis, and HIV. The patient should be counseled regarding contraception and prevention of further STDs.

UTERINE LEIOMYOMATA

method of
MALCOLM L. MARGOLIN, M.D.
University of Southern California School of Medicine and Cedars-Sinai Medical Center
Los Angeles, California

Uterine leiomyomata are the most common female pelvic neoplasm. It has generally been stated that they occur in 20 to 30% of women, but the incidence is probably much higher. Some studies suggest that the incidence of clinically occult leiomyomata is as high as 75%. Most leiomyomata are found in patients in the reproductive age group as single or multiple tumors. Recent epidemiologic reviews have shown that they occur from the early twenties to mid eighties, with 75% being found in the premenopausal and perimenopausal patient.

The etiology of leiomyomata has not been definitely established, but the cells of a single leiomyoma are identical, suggesting that each individual tumor probably arises from a single neoplastic smooth muscle cell that underwent mutation. Chromosome analysis of individual tumors demonstrates abnormal karyotypes of several chromosomes. Many abnormalities have been found, including translocations and deletions.

Leiomyoma growth may be affected by a multitude of factors. Epidermal growth factor and insulin-like growth factor I (IGF-I) as well as estrogen and progesterone can alter their growth patterns. Estrogen and progesterone receptors have been found in leiomyomata, and a hypoestrogenic state is often associated with leiomyoma tumor shrinkage. These tumors vary greatly in growth potential and basic biology. They may undergo changes resulting in hemorrhage, infarction, calcification, ulceration, infection, torsion, abortion, or large growth. It is these changes along with their location that result in the majority of the symptoms associated with leiomyomata. Myomas may be located completely or partially within the myometrium (intramural), projecting into the endometrial cavity (submucosal) or projecting from the uterus into the pelvic or abdominal cavities (subserosal). They may be on pedicle (pedunculated) or become attached to adjacent structures (parasitic).

Leiomyosarcoma etiology is controversial. Some authors believe their origin to be degenerative from benign leiomyomata, whereas others believe they have a distinctively different origin from benign leiomyomata. They occur at an incidence of approximately 0.5% of all leiomyomata and their diagnosis is based on cytology containing more than 10 mitosis per 10 consecutive high-power fields. The symptoms of rapid growth and hemorrhage often associated with these sarcomas require making the correct diagnosis imperative when these symptoms persist.

SYMPTOMS

Most fibroids are asymptomatic, but when symptoms occur they are usually related to menstrual or sexual dysfunction, tumor enlargement, pressure on bowels or bladder, or reproductive complications. The symptoms include menorrhagia, dysmenorrhea, dyspareunia, urgency, frequency, urinary obstruction, constipation, rectal pain, abdominal cramping, and pelvic or abdominal pain. The pain symptoms may vary from mild to severe and range from dull aching pressure to the sharp or acute type pain associated with myoma degeneration or torsion of a pedunculated myoma. These symptoms may be accompanied by signs of uterine tenderness and peritoneal irritation and be associated with symptoms of nausea, vomiting, fever, and chills. Menometrorrhagia can result in anemia with its associated symptoms of weakness and fatigue. Tumor enlargement can lead to abdominal distention, the sensation of bloating, and/or the recognition of an abdominal mass. Reproductive complications include symptoms associated with spontaneous abortion, premature labor, dysfunctional labor, dystocia, or infertility.

DIAGNOSIS

Diagnosis is usually made by physical examination, but a multitude of procedures and techniques are used for evaluation of the tumors depending on their number, location, and associated symptoms. Ultrasonography is a mainstay along with sonohysterography for identifying intracavitary lesions. Hysteroscopy, hysterosalpingography, magnetic resonance imaging, barium enema, and intravenous pyelogram have all been used to clarify the location and diagnosis of the lesions.

These techniques have been especially useful in differentiating an abdominal or pelvic mass that is a leiomyoma from an ovarian neoplasm. Laparoscopy or laparotomy may be necessary in the unusual case when less invasive procedures do not provide an accurate diagnosis.

TREATMENT

Leiomyomata are benign tumors and do not require therapy unless they cause symptoms or undergo rapid growth. The major reasons for any therapy are uncontrollable bleeding, pressure on adjacent organs, pain, rapid change in size or consistency, or the development of reproductive function disorders. Therapy varies greatly depending on the symptoms resulting from the tumors, the size and location of the tumors, the patient's age, parity, or her desire to keep her uterus. In an asymptomatic individual with slow-growing leiomyomata, observation is the appropriate management. Symptoms may often be controlled in the patient with menometrorrhagia, dysmenorrhea, or pelvic pain or pressure by a therapeutic trial of an antiprostaglandin or oral contraceptive. The following regimens have been successful: ibuprofen (Motrin), 800 mg orally at onset of bleeding or pain, followed by additional doses of 200 to 400 mg every 4 to 6 hours; naproxen sodium (Anaprox/Anaprox DS), 550 mg every 12 hours or an initial dose of 550 mg followed by 275 mg every 6 to 8 hours; cyclic progestin therapy of medroxyprogesterone acetate (Provera), 10 mg for 10 to 14 days each month; continuous progestin therapy, norethindrone ([Micronor]), 0.35 mg per day); low-dose combined oral contraceptive therapy containing 20 to 50 μg of estrogen combined with a progestational agent (e.g., Loestrin, Levlen, Lo/Ovral, Demulen).

No controlled studies have demonstrated an increased risk of increased growth of leiomyomata in women using low-dose oral contraceptives. Gonadotropin-releasing hormone agonists (GnRHag) have been used to produce a hypoestrogenic state. Although the individual response has been variable, GnRHag therapy has consistently resulted in a reduction in uterine volume and myoma size. The maximum reduction in size occurs after 12 weeks of therapy, with little to no further reduction occurring after that. Rapid regrowth of the tumors occurs after discontinuance of GnRHag therapy. Because of the adverse sequelae of the hypoestrogenic state, such as decreased bone density and vasomotor symptoms, continuous GnRHag therapy, alone, for more than 6 months is not recommended. Recent regimens, however, are utilizing an "add back" technique of cyclic or continuous estrogen and or progesterone following the initial 12 weeks of therapy. Add-back therapy consists of conjugated estrogens (Premarin), 0.625 mg, and medroxyprogesterone acetate (Provera), 2.5 mg daily.

The current most frequently used regimen of GnRHag therapy consists of leuprolide acetate (Depot Lupron), 3.75 mg intramuscularly per month for 3 months before surgery. This regimen is used to decrease uterine total volume to possibly allow for the conversion of an abdominal to a transvaginal or hysteroscopic surgical approach. It is also used to decrease blood loss, before and during surgery.

In the symptomatic patient who does not improve with conservative management, operative therapy should be considered. Hysteroscopic resection or ablation of submucous myomata provides a surgical approach to control menorrhagia that is less extensive than a laparotomy. For the patient desiring to maintain her reproductive potential, myomectomy is a therapeutic option. Indications for myomectomy include persistent pain, pressure or bleeding, a rapidly expanding mass, recurrent abortion, or long-standing infertility. Because as many as one fourth of patients undergoing myomectomy later require an additional procedure, a hysterectomy might be the treatment of choice if the patient has completed her childbearing and does not have a specific desire to keep her uterus. Indications for hysterectomy are similar to those for myomectomy. The route of surgery may be abdominal, vaginal, laparoscopic, or a combination of laparoscopic and vaginal, depending on uterine size, location of tumors, pelvic dimensions, and operator expertise.

CANCER OF THE ENDOMETRIUM

method of
ANDREW BERCHUCK, M.D.
Duke University Medical Center
Durham, North Carolina

Endometrial cancer is the most common gynecologic malignant neoplasm in the United States, and the median age at presentation is 60 years. The majority of cases are diagnosed when endometrial biopsy is performed to investigate the cause of abnormal uterine bleeding. Because most endometrial adenocarcinomas are confined to the uterus at diagnosis, hysterectomy is the cornerstone of therapy, and 70 to 80% of patients with this disease are cured.

PRIMARY THERAPY

Most patients are suitable candidates for primary surgical therapy, but in cases in which surgery is considered unacceptably risky, curative treatment can often be accomplished with radiation therapy. For patients with cancer confined to the uterus, the cure rate with radiation therapy is only about 50 to 60%, compared with 80 to 90% with surgery. Patients in whom neither surgery nor radiation can be accomplished are best treated with progestin therapy. Many patients respond well to progestin therapy with megestrol acetate (Megace), 40 to 80 mg orally twice daily, as evidenced by cessation of bleeding, and progestin therapy may be curative in some cases.

Because many women with endometrial cancer are obese and have accompanying medical conditions such as diabetes mellitus and hypertension, a careful preoperative evaluation should be performed. Medical problems should be optimized before surgery in hopes of avoiding perioperative complications. In addition to a history and physical examination and routine preoperative blood tests, a chest radiograph is performed to exclude the presence of lung metastases. Additional radiographic studies and other diagnostic procedures should be employed selectively in the minority of patients who have signs or symptoms of metastatic disease.

Thrombophlebitis leading to pulmonary embolus is the most common cause of death after surgery for endometrial cancer. Therefore, either minidose heparin (5000 to 8000 units subcutaneously every 8 to 12 hours, starting the evening before surgery) or intermittent pneumatic compression devices are used for prophylaxis. In addition, because the vagina is heavily colonized by bacteria, prophylactic antibiotics such as cefazolin (Ancef), 1 gram intravenously every 6 hours, are administered perioperatively (4 doses total starting 1 hour before surgery) to decrease the frequency of pelvic infection. Finally, before surgery, the patient's bowel is prepared with oral magnesium citrate and enemas.

The majority of endometrial adenocarcinomas can be cured by performing abdominal hysterectomy and removal of the fallopian tubes and ovaries. Surgical exploration is performed through a midline lower abdominal incision to allow access to the upper abdomen. The abdominal organs are carefully palpated, with special attention paid to the omentum and peritoneal surfaces. After exploration, a self-retaining retractor is placed in the incision and the bowel is packed into the upper abdomen. Approximately 100 mL of normal saline is instilled into the pelvis, aspirated, and submitted for cytologic examination. Extrafascial hysterectomy and bilateral salpingo-oophorectomy are then performed. After the specimen has been extirpated, the uterus is opened and the cavity is inspected. The location of the cancer and gross depth of invasion into the uterine wall are noted. In many cases, frozen section is performed to define the depth of invasion intraoperatively. In addition, a sample of tumor is submitted for determination of estrogen- and progesterone-receptor levels.

The majority of endometrial adenocarcinomas are either well or moderately differentiated, and these cancers are usually confined to the inner part of the uterine wall. Because minimally invasive cancers have a low incidence of occult metastases, further staging beyond gross inspection and palpation is not usually productive. If the cancer is poorly differentiated or is noted to invade into the outer half of the uterine wall or to involve the cervix, however, further surgical staging is performed. This includes sampling of the regional lymph nodes in the pelvic and aortic areas, which are the most common sites of occult metastases. Approximately 10% of apparent early-stage cases are found to have occult lymph node metastases. In addition, 5 to 10% of patients with endometrial cancer will be found to have visible extrauterine disease at surgical exploration. The most common sites of grossly apparent metastases are the ovaries, peritoneal surfaces, and lymph nodes. In these cases, attempts are usually made to remove the extrauterine metastases.

Most patients with endometrial cancer have stage I or II disease that appears to be confined to the uterus (Table 1), and survival rates for this group are excellent with surgery alone. Because 10 to 20% of these patients will develop recurrent cancer, adjuvant therapy is often prescribed for patients at high risk for recurrence. External pelvic radiation has been employed frequently as adjuvant therapy, but an unequivocal survival benefit has not been demonstrated. In the past, as many as 30 to 40% of patients with early-stage disease have been considered candidates for adjuvant pelvic radiation on the basis of prognostic factors such as poor histologic grade, deep myometrial invasion, and cervical involvement. More recently, selective lymph node sampling has been used to identify patients who actually have evidence of early metastatic disease and are likely to benefit from adjuvant radiation. With use of this selection

TABLE 1. **International Federation of Gynecology and Obstetrics (FIGO) Staging of Endometrial Carcinoma***

Stage I: Confined to the Uterus	
IA	No myometrial invasion
IB	Inner half myometrial invasion
IC	Outer half myometrial invasion
Stage II: Cervical Involvement	
IIA	Endocervical gland involvement
IIB	Cervical stromal invasion
Stage III	
IIIA	Positive peritoneal cytology result, adnexal metastases, uterine serosal involvement
IIIB	Vaginal metastases
IIIC	Pelvic or aortic lymph node metastases
Stage IV	
IVA	Bladder or rectal involvement
IVB	Distant metastases

*Note: Within each stage, the histologic grade also is recorded (G1 = well differentiated, G2 = moderately differentiated, G3 = poorly differentiated).

process, only 10 to 20% of patients receive pelvic radiation. In addition, if aortic lymph nodes are involved, the radiation field can be tailored to include this area, which is not part of the standard pelvic field. Thus, with surgical staging, more patients are spared the potential morbidity of radiation, whereas radiation fields can be planned accurately for patients who are most likely to benefit from adjuvant therapy.

Approximately 10 to 15% of patients with early-stage endometrial cancer are found to have malignant cells in pelvic peritoneal washings obtained at laparotomy. Most series have shown that a positive result on cytologic examination is associated with an increased risk for recurrence even when there is no other evidence of metastatic disease. When a positive cytologic result is the only evidence of extrauterine spread, I have instilled radioactive phosphorus ^{32}P intraperitoneally 5 to 7 days postoperatively using a small plastic catheter that is inserted at the time of surgery. Survival of these patients has been better than that of a historical control group. When both positive cytologic results and lymph node metastases are found, I do not combine ^{32}P and external radiation, however, because an unacceptably high proportion of patients treated in this fashion subsequently have developed small bowel obstruction.

TREATMENT OF RECURRENT DISEASE

Although postsurgical surveillance has not been proved to improve outcome in patients who have undergone treatment for early-stage endometrial cancer, I continue to encourage patients to return for periodic examinations. Eighty-five percent of patients who develop recurrence do so within 3 years of primary therapy. Patients are seen every 4 months for the first 2 years and every 6 months the third through fifth years. Detection of recurrences in the vagina is the primary focus of my examination, because approximately half of patients with localized vaginal recurrence can be salvaged with radiation and/or surgery. A chest radiograph is ordered on a yearly basis to detect recurrent disease in the lungs, but the utility of this practice is dubious because pulmonary metastases cannot be treated effectively.

Endometrial cancer initially recurs locally in the pelvis in 50% of patients, at distant sites in 25% of patients, and both locally and at distant sites in 25% of patients. A significant proportion of pelvic recurrences are confined to the vagina and can be cured with radiation therapy. Other pelvic recurrences are also usually treated with radiation, but salvage rates are much poorer. Treatment of distant metastases is either with progestin therapy or cytotoxic chemotherapy. Approximately 25% of patients with metastatic disease will have a significant response to progestins such as megestrol acetate (40 to 80 mg orally twice daily), and some of these responses are prolonged. A favorable response to progestins usually occurs in well-differentiated cancers that express steroid receptors. I use the receptor status of the tumor to determine whether progestin therapy is appropriate. If tumor from the site of recurrence cannot be obtained to measure estrogen- and progesterone-receptor levels, I use the receptor status of the primary tumor to guide therapy.

Patients with metastatic or recurrent cancers that do not express steroid receptors are treated with cytotoxic chemotherapy. The most frequent regimen employed includes doxorubicin (Adriamycin),* 50 mg per m² intravenously, and cisplatin (Platinol),* 50 mg per m² intravenously, administered every 3 weeks. Although a substantial proportion of patients have objective responses, few are cured. Thus, although cure rates are excellent after surgery in patients with early-stage disease, further improvement in survival for patients with endometrial cancer awaits the development of effective treatment for metastatic disease.

*Not FDA approved for this indication.

CARCINOMA OF THE UTERINE CERVIX

method of
PHYLLIS A. LEVINE, M.D.
Lenox Hill Hospital
New York, New York

In 1999, it is expected that approximately 14,000 women in the United States will be diagnosed with invasive carcinoma of the cervix. The previously observed trend showing a continuous decline in disease incidence has recently reversed, with a slight rise in incidence noted. As cervical cancer is thought to result from the progression of preinvasive lesions through a continuum ending in invasion, the previously noted decline in incidence is most likely attributable to the detection of lesions in an earlier premalignant state through increased screening for cervical neoplasia with Papanicolaou (Pap) smears. Case-control studies have reported relative risks between 0.2 and 0.7 associated with screening.

Epidemiologically, several risk factors are thought to be associated with the development of cervical cancer. Included in this list are the presence of human papillomavirus (HPV), most notably types 16, 18, 31, and 45; exposure to sexually transmitted genital infections such as herpes simplex virus 2 (HSV-2); multiparity; excessive cigarette smoking; the use of oral contraceptives; lower socioeconomic status; early age at first coitus; and multiple sexual partners. Among these contributing factors, the presence of HPV is likely the most significant, with the integration of the HPV genome into the host DNA noted. The pivotal role that HPV plays in cervical carcinogenesis is also supported by the demonstration of proteins generated from E_6 and E_7 promoter regions interacting with the regulatory gene products p53 and retinoblastoma protein.

DIAGNOSIS

A majority of patients diagnosed with cervical cancer present with abnormal vaginal bleeding. However, some patients seek consultation for an abnormal Pap smear result, whereas those with advanced disease may complain of a malodorous discharge or weight loss or display signs and symptoms of obstructive uropathy. If a suspicious lesion is detected by inspection and/or palpation of the uterine cervix, a diagnosis can be made by a simple punch biopsy. If the patient presents with an abnormal Pap smear result and does not have a gross lesion, the physician needs to perform a thorough colposcopic examination with generous use of biopsies and endocervical curettage to make a definitive diagnosis. In the presence of cervical carcinoma, not all Pap smears reveal carcinoma; some may merely be suggestive of intraepithelial neoplasia or may have atypical cells present. Therefore, the level of expertise of the colposcopist is important in preventing an invasive cancer from being missed. Colposcopic findings indicative of invasion include abnormal blood vessels, surface patterns, and color tone changes. Adenocarcinomas of the cervix may be more difficult to diagnose, as the Pap smear is less reliable for screening and there is no specific colposcopic appearance.

Once a pathologic diagnosis has been made, patients are staged according to the guidelines established by the International Federation of Gynecology and Obstetrics (FIGO) (Table 1). The procedures allowed by FIGO include clinical examination of the pelvis and lymph nodes, intravenous pyelogram, barium enema, chest radiograph, skeletal radiograph, cystoscopy, proctoscopy, and computed tomography (CT) assessment of the ureters and kidneys. Although cervical cancer remains a cancer with clinical staging, the clinical stage alone does not always dictate optimal therapy. To determine the treatment that will result in the greatest likelihood of cure for each patient, optional studies, including CT, lymphangiography, ultrasonography, magnetic resonance imaging, and radionuclide scanning, with fine needle aspiration of detected abnormalities, as well as surgical staging, are often performed. In addition, human immunodeficiency virus (HIV) counseling and testing is currently offered to at-risk individuals. It must be remembered that information obtained from these modalities cannot be used to change FIGO stage, although it may guide management and, therefore, affect prognosis and survival.

TABLE 1. **International Federation of Gynecology and Obstetrics Staging of Cervical Carcinoma**

Preinvasive Carcinoma		
Stage	0	Carcinoma in situ; intraepithelial carcinoma
Invasive Carcinoma		
Stage	I*	Carcinoma strictly confined to cervix (extension to corpus should be disregarded)
Stage	Ia	Invasive cancer identified only microscopically. All gross lesions even with superficial invasion are stage Ib cancers Invasion limited to measured stromal invasion with maximum depth of 5.0 mm and no wider than 7.0 mm
	Ia1	Measured invasion of stroma no greater than 3.0 mm in depth and no wider than 7 mm
	Ia2	Measured invasion of stroma greater than 3 mm and no greater than 5 mm and no wider than 7 mm
Stage	Ib†	Clinical lesions confined to the cervix or preclinical lesions greater than stage Ia
	Ib1	Clinical lesions no greater than 4 cm in size
	Ib2	Clinical lesions greater than 4 cm in size
Stage	II	Carcinoma extends beyond cervix onto either vagina or parametrium but not to lower third of vagina and not to pelvic wall
	IIA	No obvious parametrial involvement
	IIB	Obvious parametrial involvement
Stage	III	Carcinoma extends either to lower third of vagina or to pelvic wall; if hydronephrosis or nonfunctioning kidney, unless known to be due to another cause, must allocate to stage IIIB
	IIIA	Involvement of lower third of vagina; no extension to pelvic wall
	IIIB	Extension to pelvic wall or hydronephrosis or nonfunctioning kidney
Stage	IV	Carcinoma extends beyond true pelvis or involves mucosa of bladder or rectum; if bullous edema, assignment to stage IV not permitted
	IVA	Spread to bladder or rectum
	IVB	Spread to distant organs

*Changed in 1995.

†The depth of invasion should not be more than 5 mm taken from the base of the epithelium, either surface or glandular, from which it originates. Vascular space involvement, either venous or lymphatic, should not alter the staging.

TREATMENT

After the patient with cervical cancer has been staged, treatment must be initiated in a timely fashion. Therapeutic modalities may include surgery, radiation therapy and chemotherapy, aimed at treating the primary lesion, as well as documented and potential metastases. For patients with stage IA1 carcinoma, who have undergone complete excision of their lesions and in whom stromal invasion is less than 3 mm, the presence or absence of lymphvascular space involvement (LVSI) will determine therapy. When there is no LVSI, patients can be treated with simple abdominal or vaginal hysterectomy. If preservation of fertility is desired, therapeutic conization alone is considered adequate treatment as long as continued careful follow-up is instituted. When LVSI is present or if the carcinoma is stage IA2, the risk of pelvic lymph node involvement is sufficiently significant to warrant treatment with modified radical hysterectomy and pelvic node dissection. Those patients who are not surgical candidates can be treated effectively with radiation therapy.

Definitive radiation therapy and radical hysterectomy with pelvic node dissection are both effective treatments for stage IB and IIA carcinoma of the cervix and provide comparable cure rates. The decision to select one approach over the other depends on variables such as individual physician choice, institutional bias, age of the patient, and the desire to preserve ovarian function and sexual activity. Another variable that may affect treatment decisions is the size of the lesion. Although patients with lesions greater than 4 cm in diameter can be treated with radical hysterectomy, in general, these patients should initially be treated with pelvic radiation. Several studies have suggested a survival advantage if radiation is followed by extrafascial hysterectomy, whereas others have demonstrated improved local control, but with no improvement in overall survival. These findings have prompted many centers to perform extrafascial hysterectomy at completion of radiation therapy. The inclusion of surgery in the treatment of these patients provides the benefit of a surgical evaluation of the para-aortic lymph nodes, which may be positive and often cannot be accurately assessed radiologically. Knowing that metastatic carcinoma is present in these lymph nodes allows for subsequent treatment with additional radiotherapy, with the potential for improved survival.

Recently, the use of neoadjuvant chemotherapy in patients with bulky carcinomas has been investigated. Patients were treated with one to three cycles of cisplatin-based therapy followed by radical hysterectomy with promising short-term results. A randomized clinical trial is still needed to assess the true efficacy of this approach.

After radical hysterectomy, the risk of recurrence and death is increased by the presence of tumor metastases in lymph nodes, large tumor size, deep stromal invasion, LVSI, and involvement of paracervical tissues. On review of the final pathology, if two or more pelvic lymph nodes are positive or if a surgical margin or the parametrium is invaded, postoperative therapy is indicated. In the past, pelvic radiation therapy has been the standard, although it remains to be demonstrated that this therapy improves 5-year actuarial survival. Because many recurrences develop outside of standard radiation fields, attention recently has been directed at systemic adjuvant therapy. It appears that cisplatin-based postoperative therapy may be as effective as radiation therapy with significantly lower morbidity. A multicenter randomized study is needed to definitively resolve this issue.

Treatment for patients with stage IIB and III carcinomas is primarily radiation therapy. External teletherapy is expected to shrink the primary tumor and treat the regional lymph nodes, whereas brachytherapy provides additional control of the primary site. Many physicians administer cytotoxic agents such as cisplatin, 5-fluorouracil, mitomycin-C, and hydroxyurea at the time of radiation to obtain a radiosensitizing effect. The goals of such combined therapies are to improve response rates, and long-term survival. A randomized trial comparing concomitant use of irradiation with cytotoxic agents and optimally maximized doses of irradiation alone has yet to be performed. Therefore, it is not known if one approach is truly advantageous. Patients with stage IVA disease can be treated with either pelvic exenteration if the pelvic disease is central and a tumor fistula is present, or more typically with radiation therapy. Patients with stage IVB disease or patients with lower clinical stages of disease in whom radiologic evaluation has detected significant extrapelvic disease may be offered palliative systemic therapy.

With current surgical techniques, acute complications after radical surgery, including ureterovaginal fistula, vesicovaginal fistula, pulmonary emboli, small-bowel obstruction, and pelvic hemorrhage, occur in less than 2% of patients. The acute side effects of radiotherapy include nausea, diarrhea, urinary frequency, and intestinal spasm. Long-term complications, occurring months to years after completion of therapy, include urinary and gastrointestinal fistulas, small-bowel obstruction, proctosigmoiditis, and strictures. These complications are observed in as many as 8% of patients.

POST-TREATMENT SURVEILLANCE

Most recurrences develop during the first 2 years after the completion of therapy. During this high-risk period, patients should be evaluated every 3 months. The visit should include physical examination of the pelvic, abdominal, inguinal, and supraclavicular regions, as well as the taking of a Pap smear. The follow-up visits can then be spaced to twice yearly for 3 years, with annual evaluation performed thereafter. Radiologic evaluation may not be necessary for all patients, but for patients at high risk for recurrence, an accepted schedule would be a semiannual CT scan of the abdomen and pelvis for 3 years and a yearly chest radiograph. Any abnormality detected requires biopsy for pathologic evaluation.

In contrast to ovarian cancer in which early recurrences are often difficult to diagnose clinically and the first suspicion of recurrent disease may be a rising CA 125 level, recurrent cervical carcinoma can often be detected by simple physical examination. Therefore, there has been a lag in the use of tumor markers in patients with cervical cancer. It is now recognized that pretreatment levels may determine prognosis, extent of disease, and propensity for lymph node metastases, and that sequential levels may be used to monitor response to therapy and to detect recurrences approximately 5 months before they may be clinically evident. The most useful markers in cervical cancer are SCC, UGF, CA 125, and IAP. Levels of SCC are considered elevated if serum concentrations exceed 1.5 to 2.5 ng per mL. However, false elevations can be seen in patients with extensive benign skin diseases, such as psoriasis and eczema.

RECURRENT CERVICAL CARCINOMA

After a diagnosis of recurrent cervical cancer has been made, some patients can still be managed with additional therapies. For patients with postsurgical locoregional recurrences, treatment consists of a combination of external and intracavitary radiation. In general, radiation therapy is no longer an option for patients who have previously been exposed to curative doses. For these patients, surgery is the only option for cure. If evaluation reveals the combined findings of unilateral leg edema, sciatic pain, and ureteral obstruction, it is likely that the recurrence is unresectable. However, if assessment reveals that the recurrence is limited to the pelvis without fixation to the sidewall, pelvic exenteration can be performed with en bloc removal of the pelvic viscera. The procedure includes radical hysterectomy, pelvic lymph node dissection, and removal of the rectum for posterior exenteration, the bladder for anterior exenteration, or both if total exenteration is deemed necessary to adequately excise all recurrent diseases. Urinary and gastrointestinal diversions are then performed as indicated.

In the past, this procedure has been extremely difficult for the patient, from both a physical and a psychologic perspective. However, recently with increased usage of continent urinary diversion, vaginal reconstruction, and low-rectal anastomosis, the procedure has become less morbid and less disfiguring. Many patients no longer require any external appliances, as permanent colostomy often can be avoided and a continent urinary diversion can simply be covered with a single gauze pad without leakage, as long as periodic self-catheterization is performed. Survival after exenteration is reported to be between 25 and 60%. The other group of patients who may receive curative treatment are those with isolated late lung metastasis. With surgical resection, 5-year survival for these patients is approximately 25%.

Unfortunately, little in the way of effective therapy remains for patients who cannot be cured with surgery or radiation therapy, either primarily or at the time of recurrence. Although chemotherapy is typically offered to patients with initially advanced systemic disease or recurrent disease not amenable to radiotherapy or surgery, the intent is palliation, not cure. Agents that have demonstrated activity in the treatment of cervical cancer include cisplatin, carboplatin, ifosfamide, methotrexate, 5-fluorouracil,* doxorubicin, bleomycin,* mitomycin-C,* vincristine,* chlorambucil, and melphalan.*

PREGNANCY

Fortunately, most patients with cervical cancer during pregnancy have stage I disease. When a diagnosis is made, therapy must be individualized based on presenting stage, duration of gestation, and the patient's desire to continue the pregnancy. As it has not been demonstrated that the pregnant state negatively affects disease outcome, patients with early stage disease may choose to delay treatment, with the understanding that their decision may be associated with a slight increase in risk, until fetal viability can be documented by amniocentesis. Definitive therapy is decided by a process similar to that used in the nonpregnant patient. Modalities may include simple or radical surgery and radiation therapy. If the patient is to be treated with radiotherapy, a classic cesarean section is first performed when the fetus is viable. Before viability, external radiation is started with the expectation of spontaneous abortion.

INADEQUATE SURGERY

When invasive cancer is treated with simple hysterectomy, additional therapy is usually required if disease more significant than microinvasive carcinoma is found. Therapy should be initiated without any significant delay to optimize prognosis and survival. Patients with stage I disease, in particular young patients who desire preservation of ovarian function, can be offered reoperation with removal of parametrial tissue, cardinal ligaments, uterosacral ligaments, vaginal cuff, and pelvic lymph nodes. For the remainder of patients, radiation therapy is indicated. Of note is that the expected complication rate after combined therapy is higher than after treatment with either modality alone.

HORMONE REPLACEMENT THERAPY

Treatment of premenopausal patients with cervical cancer often results in cessation of ovarian function. Other patients with this disease are already menopausal at the time of presentation. Therefore, a majority of patients with cervical cancer may benefit from hormone replacement therapy. It is well known that hormone replacement therapy has the potential to prevent osteoporosis, cardiovascular disease, vasomotor symptoms, and significant vaginal stenosis. Although both estrogen and progesterone receptors have been identified in the cells of the normal epithelium of the uterine cervix, as well as in carcinomas of the cervix, no evidence exists that either estrogen or progesterone stimulates the growth of cervical carcinoma. As a result, hormone replacement therapy is considered both safe and effective in this group of patients. Some controversy exists regarding which hormones to administer. It has been demonstrated that endometrial activity may persist after radiation therapy for cervical cancer. This finding has led some investigators to suggest that progesterone supplementation to estrogen is necessary. However, others claim that the use of progesterone to supplement estrogen is not warranted if the uterus has decreased in size in response to irradiation, which occurs in a majority of cases, and if no withdrawal bleeding in

*Not FDA approved for this indication.

response to cyclic hormone therapy has been observed.

NEOPLASMS OF THE VULVA

method of
IRA R. HOROWITZ, M.D.
Emory University School of Medicine
Atlanta, Georgia

Vulvar neoplasias are the fourth most common genital tumor in women, accounting for 3 to 5% of genital tumors and 0.3% of all female malignancies. The majority of patients present in the sixth decade of life. Unfortunately, vulvar disease and its treatment have altered the psychosocial well-being of women. The surgery is frequently disfiguring and is fraught with complications such as leg edema, vaginal stenosis, dyspareunia, wound separation, and lack of a cosmetic vulva. Recent changes in treatment protocols have helped to decrease the procedural morbidity and improved the patient's self-image.

PREINVASIVE LESIONS

The Ninth Congress of the International Society for the Study of Vulvar Disease (ISSVD) in 1987, in conjunction with the International Society of Gynecological Pathologists (ISGYP), changed the nomenclature for preinvasive vulvar disease (Table 1). *Non-neoplastic epithelial disorders of the skin and mucosa* is the new term for vulvar dystrophies. Hyperplastic dystrophy is classified as squamous cell hyperplasia, and atypical hyperplastic dystrophy is categorized as vulvar intraepithelial neoplasia (VIN) (Table 2). Mixed dystrophies will be reported as lesions containing both lichen sclerosus and squamous cell hyperplasia.

NON-NEOPLASTIC EPITHELIAL DISORDERS

On gross examination, lichen sclerosus and squamous cell hyperplasia manifest as white plaques (leukoplakia), the former being an atrophic lesion with the microscopic appearance of a thin squamous epithelium and flattened rete ridges. In squamous cell hyperplasia, microscopically the squamous epithelium has a thick superficial layer of parakeratosis or hyperkeratosis and elongated rete ridges. Mixed lesions demonstrate the histologic features of both lesions. Occurring in 20% of non-neoplastic epithelial disorders, mixed lesions are more difficult to treat. Early studies have suggested that mixed lesions have a predisposition to transform into vulvar malignancies. However, this issue continues to be debated and should not alter treatment protocols.

TABLE 1. **Non-neoplastic Epithelial Disorders of the Skin and Mucosa**

Old Terminology	New Terminology (ISSVD 1987)
Lichen sclerosus et atrophicus	Lichen sclerosus (LS)
Hyperplastic dystrophy (without atypia)	Squamous cell hyperplasia (SCH)
Mixed dystrophy	LS and SCH

Abbreviations: ISSVD = International Society for the Study of Vulvar Disease–1987.

TABLE 2. **Vulvar Intraepithelial Neoplasia (VIN)**

Old Terminology	New Terminology (ISSVD 1987)
Mild atypia (dysplasia)	VIN I
Moderate atypia (dysplasia)	VIN II
Severe atypia (dysplasia)	VIN III
Carcinoma in situ	VIN III

Abbreviations: ISSVD = International Society for the Study of Vulvar Disease–1987.

Diagnosis

Patients with non-neoplastic epithelial disorders frequently present with pruritus and vulvodynia. Often, patients are treated by practitioners for atrophic vulvitis and/or monilial vulvitis, only to have their symptoms persist. The hallmark to making a correct diagnosis is a thorough medical history followed by a comprehensive inspection of the genitalia, including the cervix, anus, and vagina. Non-neoplastic epithelial disorders and intraepithelial neoplasia are multifocal and may be present on all anogenital mucosal surfaces. On completing visual and digital examination, 3% acetic acid is placed on the vulva, anus, vagina, and cervix, and a colposcopic evaluation is performed. Raised white plaques and increased vascularity, punctation, and mosaicism should be biopsied to identify histologic changes. If colposcopy is not available or additional diagnostic tests are warranted, the vulva and anus are painted with a 1% aqueous solution of toluidine blue, which is allowed to stain for 3 minutes. The epithelium is then decolorized with 1% acetic acid for 1 minute. Surface nuclei of dysplastic or anaplastic lesions will retain the blue stain and should be biopsied. Biopsies are easily performed using 1% lidocaine injected circumferentially around the lesion with a 25-gauge needle. A Keyes punch enables the physician to circumscribe the lesion and incise the epidermis. Forceps and scissors are then required to free the remainder of the specimen from the underlying tissue. The vagina and cervix also can be evaluated with Schiller's or Lugol's solution, which will not stain intraepithelial neoplasia.

Treatment

Lichen sclerosus is treated primarily with high-potency topical steroids such as betamethasone dipropionate (Diprosone), 0.05% daily for 1 month, then twice weekly as needed. In the past, testosterone or progesterone creams were first-line treatment. Two percent testosterone propionate cream is made by adding testosterone propionate, 3 mL of 100 mg per mL in sesame oil, with 12 mg of petroleum. The cream is applied to the vulva three times daily for 6 to 8 weeks, followed by a daily application for 1 week and then weekly application. Testosterone's androgenic side affects such as clitoromegaly, hirsutism, voice changes, acne, and dermal hypertrophy may not be accepted by all patients. Alternatively, 1% or 2% progesterone cream has been substituted in patients who could not tolerate testosterone. Results have been comparable but without the androgenic side affects. Seventy-five to 90% of patients treated with either regimen have reported symptomatic relief.

Squamous cell hyperplasia is best treated with medium potency topical steroids such as triamcinolone acetamide 0.1% (Aristocort) and desoximetasone 0.25% (Topicort) twice daily for 1 month or when symptoms decreased. The patient is then weaned to daily, twice weekly, and as needed administration. Non-neoplastic epithelial disorders frequently recur and require chronic administration of topical agents as described previously. Surgical procedures such as laser vaporization, ultrasonic surgical aspiration, loop excision, simple lesion excision, and cryotherapy have also been utilized in treating non-neoplastic epithelial disorders but should be reserved as second-line therapy after the patient has failed treatment with topical compounds. Unless all conservative measures have failed, vulvectomy and skinning vulvectomy should be avoided in these patients because of the recurrence rate and disfiguring secondary to the procedure. The pruritus and vulvodynia that plague patients with non-neoplastic epithelial disorders can be controlled by administering benzocaine or lidocaine ointment topically during the initial steroid therapy. Patients with more severe and recalcitrant disease can be given palliative treatment with triamcinolone diacetate (Aristocort) injections in a grid distribution on the vulva. Intradermal alcohol injections were previously used in recalcitrant cases. Recent advances in treating these patients with topical medium- and high-potency steroids have essentially eliminated the use of intradermal alcohol injections.

GRANULAR CELL TUMORS

Granular cell tumors (GCTs) were initially described in 1854. Over a 31-year period, 20 patients presented with GCT of the vulva at my institution. Two patients presented with additional lesions not on the vulva. Patients with localized disease were treated successfully with wide local excision. Although benign, GCT may resemble an invasive lesion grossly and histopathologically to the untrained eye. If surgical margins are positive, additional resection is required. A minimum of 1- to 2-cm margins are required to decrease the risk of recurrence.

VULVAR INTRAEPITHELIAL NEOPLASIA

Mild and moderate dysplasias of the vulvar epithelium are designated VIN I and II. Bowen's disease, erythroplasia of Queyrat, and carcinoma simplex have been classified as VIN III, which also includes in situ disease and severe dysplasia. VIN is multifocal, with 50% of the patients presenting in the third and fourth decades of life. An association has been found between VIN and human papilloma virus (HPV) subtypes 6, 11, 16, 18, 31, 33, 35, 45, 51, 52, 56, 58, and 61. HPV 16 and 18, however, are responsible for the majority of VIN III and invasive neoplasias. Patients presenting with atypical or flat condylomata acuminata should have their lesions biopsied before conservative chemical desiccation to rule out intraepithelial neoplasia. Twenty to 30% of patients with VIN III also have associated genital tract neoplasias, with the preponderance being intraepithelial neoplasia of the anus, vagina, and cervix, followed by cervical, vaginal, and endometrial carcinoma. The diagnostic evaluation of VIN is identical to that described for non-neoplastic epithelial disorders of the skin and mucosa.

Treatment

Small focal lesions of VIN may be treated with local excision, cryotherapy, ultrasonic surgical aspiration, loop excision, or laser vaporization. Extensive and multifocal lesions, however, are best treated with laser vaporization, skinning vulvectomy, or simple vulvectomy. Laser vaporization is performed under regional or general anesthesia with a carbon dioxide laser attached to a colposcope and microslad. The laser is set with a 2.0-mm spot size, power of 20 to 30 watts superpulse, and vaporization performed to a depth of 2 to 3 mm. On completing vaporization of the lesion, the operative field is dressed with 1% silver sulfadiazine (Silvadene) cream and 5% lidocaine mixture. Ample quantities of analgesic medications must be prescribed postoperatively, as the patient may experience excruciating discomfort. Unfortunately, many physicians frequently forget that laser vaporization results in a third-degree burn and requires special care. Ultrasonic aspiration of these lesions does not result in a third-degree burn and heals faster without much discomfort.

Skinning vulvectomy may be partial or complete; unlike with laser vaporization, a specimen can be sent for histologic evaluation. Unfortunately, this procedure carries increased morbidity when compared with laser therapy. Split-thickness skin grafts are also required on completion of the skinning vulvectomy. Carbon dioxide laser vaporization, ultrasonic surgical aspiration, electroloop excision, and skinning vulvectomy offer cosmetic and functional results without mutilation of the female genitalia. Hair dryers and heat lamps provide valuable assistance in keeping the surgical field dry after either procedure.

Local chemotherapeutic regimens such as 5% fluorouracil cream* (Efudex), bleomycin sulfate* (Blenoxane), and interferon* have met with limited success.

PAGET'S DISEASE

Paget's disease of the breast was first described by James Paget in 1874. Its manifestation on the vulva was reported in 1901 by W. Dubrewilh. Twenty percent of patients with Paget's disease of the vulva have an underlying adenocarcinoma versus more than 90% of patients with a Paget's breast lesion who have occult carcinomas. Grossly, Paget's has an eczematoid scaly appearance, is well demarcated, and frequently presents as a raised velvety lesion. The most common symptoms, as with most vulvar lesions, are pruritus and vulvodynia. It is imperative to obtain a vulvar biopsy to make a definitive diagnosis. Microscopically, cells are large and round with abundant cytoplasm, few mitotic figures, and hyperchromatic or vesicular nuclei.

Treatment

After diagnosis is confirmed, a thorough evaluation should be made to rule out breast, vaginal, cervical, bladder, or gastrointestinal adenocarcinoma. Wide local excision with 2- to 3-cm margins is suggested in treating Paget's disease. This affords the surgeon the opportunity to evaluate the surgical specimen for an underlying adenocarcinoma. In addition, Paget's disease spreads laterally beyond the lesion and requires extensive resection with 2- to 3-cm margins. As a result of this lesion's behavior, its mode of spread, and the frequency of occult carcinomas, Paget's disease should not be treated primarily with laser vaporization or ultrasonic surgical aspiration. Recent studies using monoclonal cytokeratin antibodies have enabled pathologists to distinguish Paget's disease of the vulva from Bowen's disease (VIN-III) and superficial spreading melanoma (Table 3).

Follow-up

All patients treated for preinvasive disease of the vulva require a minimum follow-up 1 month postoperatively, quarterly for 1 year, and then semiannual evaluations. Patients with procedure morbidity or recurrence require more comprehensive and frequent evaluations.

*Not FDA approved for this indication.

TABLE 3. **Cytokeratin Expression**

Histology	54 kDa	57 kDa	66 kDa
Paget's disease	Positive	Variable	Negative
Bowen's disease (VIN III)	Negative	Positive	Positive
Melanoma	Negative	Negative	Negative

Modified from Shah KD, Tabibzadeh SS, Germa MA: Immunohistochemical distinction of Paget's disease from Bowen's and superficial spreading melanoma with the use of monoclonal cytokeratin antibodies. Am J Clin Pathol *88*:689–695, 1987.

TABLE 4. **TNM Classification for Vulvar Carcinoma (FIGO October 1988)**

Primary tumor		
	TIS	Vulvar intraepithelial neoplasia III
	T1	Confined to vulva and/or perineum, diameter < 2 cm
	T2	Confined to vulva and/or perineum, diameter > 2 cm
	T3	Adjacent spread to urethra and/or vagina and/or anus
	T4	Infiltration of upper urethral mucosa and/or bladder mucosa and/or rectal mucosa and/or fixed to the bone
N	Regional lymph nodes	
	N0	No nodes palpable
	N1	Unilateral lymph node metastasis
	N2	Bilateral lymph node metastasis
M	Distant metastasis	
	M0	No clinical metastasis
	M1	Distant metastasis (including pelvic node metastasis)

Abbreviations: FIGO = International Federation of Gynecology and Obstetrics.

Modified from FIGO News: Int J Gynecol Obstet *28*:189, 1989, with permission from Elsevier Science.

INVASIVE CARCINOMA OF THE VULVA

Vulvar carcinoma accounts for 3 to 5% of all female genital cancers, with approximately 90% being squamous cell carcinoma. The most common presenting signs and symptoms are pruritus and pain, followed by vulvar lesions, bleeding, and dysuria. The International Federation of Gynecology and Obstetrics (FIGO) clinical staging for vulvar carcinoma is based on the TNM classification (Tables 4 and 5). This system evaluates lesion size, location, and inguinal node spread and metastasis. Clinical staging includes physical examination, chest radiograph, vulvar biopsy, node biopsy, serum chemistries, hematologic profile, intravenous pyelogram, cystoscopy, and sigmoidoscopy (the last three if required by location

TABLE 5. **FIGO Clinical Staging**

Stage	T	N	M
Stage 0		TIS	
Stage I	T_1	N_0	M_0
Stage II	T_2	N_0	M_0
Stage III	T_3	N_0	M_0
	T_1	N_1	M_0
	T_2	N_1	M_0
	T_3	N_1	M_0
Stage IV A	T_1	N_2	M_0
	T_2	N_2	M_0
	T_3	N_2	M_0
	T_4	N_2	M_0
	T_4	N_0	M_0
	T_4	N_1	M_0
Stage IV B	T_x	N_x	M_1
	X = Any T and/or N		

Abbreviations: FIGO = International Federation of Gynecology and Obstetrics.

Modified from FIGO News: Int J Gynecol Obstet *28*:189, 1989, with permission from Elsevier Science.

of the lesion). Additional studies obtained but not used for staging are magnetic resonance imaging (MRI), computed tomography (CT), ultrasound, and lymphangiography. Lymphangiography has not proven efficacious in vulva disease, with a sensitivity of less than 20% and specificity of less than 70%. DNA hybridization has revealed the presence of HPV 6, 11, 16, 18, 31, 33, 35, 45, 51, 52, 56, 58, and 61 in VIN and invasive carcinoma.

The majority of the anaplastic lesions are HPV subtypes 16, 18, 31, 33, 35, 45, 51, 52, 56, 58, and 61. Traditional treatment for vulvar carcinoma had been en bloc resection of the vulva, including the clitoris and a bilateral superficial and deep inguinal femoral lymphadenectomy. This has been replaced with vulvectomy and lymphadenectomy through separate incisions. In the past, more extensive lymph node dissections including pelvic lymphadenectomy were performed in patients with positive inguinal lymph nodes. Presently radiation therapy rather than lymphadenectomy is the preferred therapy to treat the pelvic nodes, as demonstrated by a recent Gynecologic Oncology Group study. Inguinal femoral lymphadenectomy is evaluated surgically. Primary radiation of groins is not as efficacious. Some surgeons report up to a 90% incidence of wound separation in patients undergoing an en bloc resection of the vulva and inguinal nodes. Recent modifications advocate a radical vulvectomy or radical hemivulvectomy with inguinal femoral lymphadenectomy through separate incisions. This has resulted in decreased wound separations, infections, and hospital stays. The number of positive inguinal nodes is a prognostic factor in determining survival (Table 6). Radiation therapy, however, has been successful in obtaining local control in advanced disease. Surgery is more efficacious than primary radiation in the treatment of vulvar carcinoma. Radical vulvectomy and bilateral inguinal femoral lymphadenectomy have resulted in 5-year survivals of 60 to 65% versus 25 to 30% in patients treated with definitive radiation therapy. Teletherapy and iridium needle placement in large tumors have been used to decrease tumor burden and permit a less radical procedure. This has helped to decrease the number of exenterations for lesions extending into the urethra and/or anus. The vulva unfortunately has a poor tolerance to high doses of radiation, and therefore this results in marked skin toxicity, especially in the menopausal patient.

TABLE 6. **Correlation of Positive Inguinal Lymph Nodes and Survival**

Positive Lymph-Node N	Estimated 2-Year Survival
>4	27%
2–3	66%
1	80%

Modified from Homesley HD, Bundy BN, Sedlis A, Adcock L: Radiation in therapy versus pelvic node resection for carcinoma of the vulva with positive groin nodes. Obstet Gynecol *68*:733, 1986, with permission from the American College of Obstetricians and Gynecologists.

Stage I and II Lesions

Stage I lesions are defined as being less than or equal to 2 cm in largest diameter with no inguinal nodes palpable. Several studies have not found positive inguinal nodes in patients with less than 1 mm of invasion, and therefore many gynecologic oncologists have advocated not doing lymphadenectomies in patients with less than 1 mm of invasion. Superficial lymphadenectomy in patients with less than 5 mm of invasion carries a nodal positivity of 10 to 30%. This has enabled us to alter therapy by performing radical local excisions of the primary lesion to the inferior fascia of the urogenital diaphragm and ipsilateral superficial inguinal lymphadenopathies. The lymph nodes are then sent for frozen section, and, if positive, a more thorough dissection of the deep femoral lymph nodes below the cribriform fascia and adjacent to the femoral vessels is performed. Superficial lymphadenectomy consists of the removal of the nodal tissue above the cribriform fascia and adjacent to the greater saphenous and superficial epigastric veins.

Recently treatment protocols have been modified in patients with lateralizing lesions 2 cm or less in greatest diameter. Radical hemivulvectomy and ipsolateral inguinal femoral lymphadenectomy are performed rather than a complete vulvectomy and bilateral inguinal femoral lymphadenectomy. This modification has markedly decreased the morbidity of wound separation and bilateral lymphedema. In addition, a hemivulvectomy frequently preserves the clitoris, thereby improving sexual function postoperatively. Midline and stage II lesions (>2 cm) are treated with a radical vulvectomy and bilateral inguinal femoral lymphadenectomy through separate incisions to decrease morbidity. The perineal defects can be closed in a multitude of fashions, including primary closure, secondary granulation, Z-plasty (rhomboid flap), gracilis myocutaneous graft, and tensor fascia lata myocutaneous graft. If two or more nodes are positive, the patient should receive radiation therapy to the ipsilateral groin, ipsilateral pelvis, and contralateral groin. Alternatively, the patient can choose to have a radical vulvectomy and bilateral inguinal femoral radiation consisting of 45 to 50 cGy over a 5-week interval rather than lymphadenectomy. In addition, radiation therapy is used to provide a perineal boost in patients with positive surgical margins. Complications of a radical inguinal femoral lymphadenectomy can be divided into immediate postoperative and delayed complications (Table 7).

Stage III and IV Vulvar Disease

Stage III tumors can be lesions of any size with adjacent spread to the urethra, anus, or vagina (T3 lesions) and/or unilateral lymph node metastasis

TABLE 7. **Complications of Radical Vulvectomy and Inguinal Lymphadenectomy**

Immediate	%	Delayed	%
Wound separation infection	85	Leg edema	69
Urinary tract infection	18	Lymphangitis, phlebitis, cellulitis	13
Thromboembolic disease	9	Vaginal stenosis	13
		Pelvic relaxation	11
		Stress urinary incontinence	11
		Hernia	5

Modified from Podratz KC, Symmonds RE, Taylor WF, Williams TJ: Carcinoma of the vulva: Analysis of treatment and survival. Obstet Gynecol *61*(1):63–74, 1983, with permission from the American College of Obstetricians and Gynecologists.

(N1). Patients with T1 or T2 lesions with N1 nodes are treated as described previously with a radical vulvectomy and bilateral inguinal femoral lymphadenectomy. As with stage I and II lesions, the patient undergoes pelvic radiation if inguinal nodes are positive. Stage III lesions with minimal spread to organs adjacent to the vulva can be treated by extending the surgical margins of the vulvectomy to include the distal one third of the urethra, distal vagina, or anus as long as the lesion does not involve the anal sphincter. For extensive T3 lesions and T4 (stage IV lesions) invading the bladder or bowel mucosa, treatment consists of an exenterative procedure, radiation, or a combination of radiation and surgery. Recent studies have advocated the combination of chemotherapy and teletherapy to treat cervical and vulvar carcinomas.

Recurrence

Recurrence and survival are directly correlated with lesion size and the number of positive lymph nodes. Table 8 summarizes the gynecologic oncology literature for the last 2 decades, as well as the 1985 FIGO Annual Report. Small local recurrences can be treated with wide local excision or radiation therapy. Extensive recurrences, however, require exenterative procedures and/or a combination of radiation therapy and extensive resection of the perineum. Chemotherapy thus far has limited use in the treatment of vulvar carcinoma. Chemotherapeutic agents such as doxorubicin* (Adriamycin), cisplatin* (Platinol), ifosfamide* (Ifex), bleomycin sulfate* (Blenoxane), methotrexate,* mitomycin-C* (Mutamycin), 5-fluorouracil,* and etoposide* (VePesid) have had minimal success in controlling recurrent or systemic disease.

*Not FDA approved for this indication.

TABLE 8. **5-Year Survival in Patients Treated for Vulvar Carcinoma**

FIGO Stage	5-Year Survival
I	70–90%
II	45–80%
III	30–50%
IV	10–20%

Abbreviations: FIGO = International Federation of Gynecology and Obstetrics.

VERRUCOUS CARCINOMA

Unlike invasive squamous cell carcinoma of the vulva, verrucous carcinoma is an indolent, locally invading, cauliflower-like tumor that rarely metastasizes. The verrucous lesion is frequently mistaken for a giant condyloma of Buschke-Lowenstein; therefore it is imperative that the surgeon obtain multiple biopsies to ensure the diagnosis. Treatment consists of radical local excision for small lesions and radical vulvectomy for larger lesions. In light of the tumor's indolent nature, lymphadenectomy is rarely required unless palpable and suspicious lymph nodes are present. If lymph nodes are positive on frozen section, the patient should undergo a radical vulvectomy and bilateral inguinal femoral lymphadenectomy. Radiation therapy may transform this lesion into a more anaplastic lesion and is contraindicated in its treatment.

MELANOMAS OF THE VULVA

Melanomas are the second most common vulvar malignancy. Two thirds of the patients presenting with melanomas are postmenopausal and fair skinned. There are three histologic types of melanomas: superficial spreading, lentigo maligna, and nodular. The most aggressive is the nodular melanoma. Unlike squamous lesions, melanomas are not staged by the FIGO classification but by the depth of invasion (Table 9). Preoperative evaluation should include a chest radiograph and a CT or MRI of the abdomen and pelvis to rule out retroperitoneal, hepatic, or pelvic disease.

Treatment

Treatment is tailored to the depth of invasion. Melanotic level I or II lesions (<1 mm) can be treated with wide local excision without lymphadenectomy. No studies have reported level I or II lesions with positive inguinal lymph nodes. Patients with level III small lateralizing lesions can be treated with a radical hemivulvectomy and ipsilateral inguinal femoral lymphadenectomy. Larger lesions and level IV and V lesions require radical vulvectomy and bilateral inguinal femoral lymphadenectomy. Occasionally large lesions necessitate perineal resection, vaginectomies, or exenterations to adequately resect the tumor. Poor results have been obtained using radiation and chemotherapy to control this disease. Responses to tamoxifen citrate (Nolvadex) have been reported but require prolonged administration as long as the patient's condition is stable. The prognosis of melanoma patients depends on the depth of

*Not FDA approved for this indication.

TABLE 9. **Staging Systems for Vulvar Melanoma**

Level	Clark	Breslow	Chung
I	Intraepithelial	<0.76 mm	Intraepithelial
II	Into papillary dermis	0.76–1.50 mm	<1 mm superficial penetration
III	Filling dermal papillae	1.51–2.25 mm	1–2 mm into subepithelial tissue
IV	Into reticular dermis	2.26–3.0 mm	Penetration >2 mm
V	Into subcutaneous fat	>3 mm	Into subcutaneous fat

invasion, tumor volume, and lymph node metastasis, with an overall 5-year survival rate of 30%.

BARTHOLIN'S GLAND CARCINOMA

Bartholin's gland carcinomas account for 3 to 5% of all vulvar carcinomas, with a mean age of 57 years and a range of 14 to 85 years of age. Ninety percent of the histologic cell types are equally divided between adenocarcinoma and squamous cell carcinoma, with the remaining 10% consisting of adenoid cystic, transitional, and mixed cell types.

Treatment

Treatment consists of radical hemivulvectomy or radical local excision and an ipsilateral inguinal femoral lymphadenectomy. Postoperative pelvic and contralateral groin irradiation should be performed if ipsilateral groin nodes are positive. If the tumor is adherent to the pubic ramus, preoperative radiation may permit future surgical resection. Occasionally large Bartholin's gland carcinomas invading the rectum require exenterative procedures to obtain adequate surgical margins.

BASAL CELL CARCINOMA

Basal cell carcinoma accounts for approximately 2% of all vulvar lesions and usually presents with vulva pruritus and/or ulceration. This tumor is locally invasive and is treated with a wide local excision of the lesion. Basal cell carcinomas rarely metastasize to lymph nodes and therefore do not require lymphadenectomy unless suspicious lymph nodes are palpated.

VULVAR SARCOMAS

Vulvar sarcomas account for 1 to 3% of all vulvar malignancies. The most common histologic type is leiomyosarcoma, which occurs in the third and fourth decades of life. The patient frequently presents with a rapidly growing tumor. Prognostic features include lesion size, contour, and mitotic figure index.

Treatment

Treatment consists of a radical local excision, with lymphadenectomy required only if a suspicious lesion is present. Recurrences are treated with a wide local excision. More aggressive rhabdomyosarcomas can also manifest on the vulva. Treatment consists of radical local excision followed by chemotherapy with VAC (vincristine sulfate [Oncovin], actinomycin D [Dactinomycin], and cyclophosphamide [Cytoxan], with or without doxorubicin [Adriamycin]). In patients with positive surgical margins, nodal metastasis, and recurrence, radiation therapy can be helpful in controlling central disease.

NONGYNECOLOGIC METASTASIS TO THE VULVA

Although rare, several nongynecologic primary tumors have been reported to metastasize to the vulva. They include non-Hodgkin's lymphoma and melanoma as well as breast, pulmonary, gastric, and renal carcinomas. The primary tumor is treated and the metastatic lesions are excised.

CONTRACEPTION

method of
LUIGI MASTROIANNI, JR., M.D.
Hospital of the University of Pennsylvania
Philadelphia, Pennsylvania

Contraceptive services include not only pregnancy prevention, but consideration of the side effects and health benefits of contraceptive modalities, the impact of disease processes on contraceptive choice, and the overall evaluation of general health status. Contraceptive choice affects the lives of both men and women, but the impact on women is obviously substantially greater. Two thirds of American women have at least one unintended pregnancy, and more than half of all pregnancies are unintended. Contraceptives are the most effective means of abortion prevention. The factors behind this surprisingly high incidence of accidental pregnancy must be factored into the equation as contraceptive choices are outlined and suggested. Although choices reviewed herein offer substantial options, there is still a need for additional methods, and there continues to be a lag in the development of new contraceptives. Contraceptive research and development have been the subject of two Institute of Medicine–National Academy of Sciences studies, the most recent of which was completed in 1996.

Unintended pregnancy is the result either of failure to use a contraceptive or failure of the method itself. In discussions of contraceptive choices, the characteristics of the ideal contraceptive are often referred to as safe, effective, convenient to use, and inexpensive. Although today's choices include methods that approach the ideal for some individuals, a number of factors must be considered before a given method is earmarked for use. For example, a method may be ideal for spacing pregnancy but may not necessarily be appropriate for the person who wishes to avoid childbearing completely, or for someone in whom additional childbearing would pose an inordinate medical or psychologic risk. Those who are having intercourse sporadically, and, hence, are in need of only occasional contraception are in a vastly different category from those who are having intercourse with some frequency. Because coitus is associated with the potential of transmitting a sexually transmitted disease (STD), risk factors in that sphere must be considered. In 1997, acquired immune deficiency syndrome (AIDS) was the third leading killer of women of reproductive age, and in two thirds of these, the condition was sexually transmitted. Other factors that must be considered include the ability of an individual, perceived or real, to use a given method, the overall impact of an unintended pregnancy, and the acceptability of the method within the social and religious framework of the individual.

HEALTH BENEFITS OF CONTRACEPTIVE METHODS

Every effective method is obviously associated with the health benefit of preventing an unintended pregnancy. This benefit is modulated by the level of effectiveness when used in the field. Some methods are associated with substantial positive effects on overall health including protection against STDs. The male condom and the female condom both provide some protection. Diaphragm, cervical cap, and spermicides also are partially effective. The contraceptive implant (Norplant), medroxyprogesterone acetate (Depo-Provera), and the progestin-only pill provide some protection against the ascent of bacteria from the cervix to the upper reproductive tract and, hence, against pelvic inflammatory disease. These contraceptives are associated with decreased total blood loss and decreased incidence of dysmenorrhea, and long-term studies suggest a decreased risk of ovarian and endometrial cancers. The combined oral contraceptive is also associated with a decreased incidence of endometrial and ovarian cancer, pelvic inflammatory disease, benign breast disease, ectopic pregnancies, and dysmenorrhea. The cycles are more regular and menstrual periods are lighter. Hence, there is a positive effect on blood iron and on iron deficiency anemia, especially among women whose diets are iron deficient.

The contraceptive effectiveness of a given method is clearly influenced by its ease of use. Its intrinsic effectiveness is a function of its mechanism of action. Issues of user reliability play a major role in contraceptive choice. For example, a barrier method might be the method of choice, but it may prove difficult to convince the partner that it should be used each time intercourse occurs. When a permanent method or a method with a prolonged contraceptive effect is considered, plans for future fertility need to be thoroughly explored. Individuals who find themselves in uncertain circumstances with less than reliable partners should consider a method associated with the least possible risk of STD transmission, perhaps in concert with a method of greatest effectiveness (e.g., a combination barrier and combined oral contraception).

STERILIZATION PROCEDURES

Sterilization is a widely used option in the United States. Vasectomy is increasingly popular and is selected by at least one third of couples opting for permanent sterilization. Vasectomy techniques have been improved in recent years. By and large, vasectomy is performed with the patient under local anesthesia in an outpatient setting and is associated with minimal risk. Following vasectomy, the distal male reproductive tract still contains active spermatozoa, and alternative contraception is recommended until one is assured that the ejaculate is sperm free. Although vasectomy is considered to be a permanent method of sterilization, vas reversal procedures are available. In expert hands, microsurgical repair of the vas is associated with pregnancy rates of up to 80%. The potential for success depends on the status of the remaining portions of the vas, the presence or absence of antisperm antibodies, and the skill of the surgeon. Modern techniques of assisted reproductive technology provide ability to produce pregnancies, using spermatozoa recovered from the proximal vas or even from the testis, in combination with intracytoplasmic injection of spermatozoa (ICSI) for in vitro fertilization. These procedures are complicated and expensive but nevertheless provide options for the couple whose vas is irreparably damaged. Vasectomies rarely fail, with a first-year failure rate estimated at 0.15%.

Female sterilization is carried out by ligation or coagulation of the fallopian tubes. The procedures themselves are associated with relatively low risk. The failure rate is in the range of 0.4%, but there is a continued possibility of pregnancy in time resulting from inexplicable recanalization of the fallopian tubes. There is potential for a tubal ectopic pregnancy, and this diagnosis must always be considered and ruled out in any patient who conceives after tubal sterilization. Tubal sterilization can be reversed using microsurgery, with success rates up to 80%, depending on the amount of tube available for anastomosis. Laparoscopic approaches to tubal sterilization reversal have recently been developed, obviating a major abdominal procedure. In vitro fertilization is also an option in most cases.

LONG-ACTING REVERSIBLE METHODS

Long-acting methods include the levonorgestrel implant (Norplant), intrauterine device, and the injectable medroxyprogesterone (Depo-Provera). These have in common the complete absence of day-to-day intervention and provide duration of action ranging from 3 months for Depo-Provera to up to 5 years for Norplant. This characteristic offers considerable advantage and is particularly important when there is need for contraceptive protection but absence of consistent motivation.

Long-Acting Levonorgestrel Implant (Norplant)

Introduced in 1991, the Norplant system was the first new contraceptive brought to market in the United States since the introduction of oral contraception more than 3 decades earlier. It involves the subcutaneous introduction of six Silastic rods into the upper arm. The rods are responsible for the slow release of levonorgestrel. Therapeutic levels occur shortly after the capsules are introduced and are maintained for up to 5 years. The method provides remarkably efficient pregnancy protection either through inhibition of ovulation and/or modification of the cervical mucus to impede sperm transport. The most common side effect is irregular bleeding. Some patients also complain of bloating but this usually disappears in time. Headache, weight gain, and acne are also occasional side effects. Insertion of Norplant is a relatively straightforward procedure but does require training and attention. In many large clinics the nurse practitioner routinely does insertions with few, if any, problems. In a few cases, difficulties have been encountered during removal, mainly the result of improper insertion in the first place. Norplant became widely accepted after it was introduced, but enthusiasm waned, principally as a result of highly publicized litigation. The implants are particularly effective among previously pregnant teens who find it difficult to use other methods effectively. The method is often considered by women who are in their late reproductive years for whom the alternative would be surgical sterilization. Modification to require insertion of only two rods with an effective life of 3 years is under consideration and single rod, progestin-releasing systems have been tested and are now marketed abroad. The unintended pregnancy rate for levonorgestrel subdermal implants is 0.9%. The method's long-term effectiveness and low unintended pregnancy rate must be weighed against the inconvenience of having to undergo a minor surgical procedure to remove the implants.

The Intrauterine Device

Intrauterine devices (IUDs) have been among the mainstays of contraception worldwide for several decades. The earlier devices have been modified by the inclusion of copper or progesterone, which is released slowly over the life of the device. Insertion of the intrauterine device is a relatively simple procedure, which, as with Norplant, can be carried out by a well-trained nurse practitioner or physician's assistant. The two devices available in the United States are the Copper T 380A (CUT380 or ParaGard), and the progesterone-containing device, Progestasert.

The CUT380 has contraceptive effectiveness of at least 10 years. It has a failure rate in the 0.6 to 0.8% range and hence has an effectiveness equivalent to that of sterilization. Earlier devices were associated with excessive bleeding and abdominal pain, but these side effects are rarely experienced with the new models. The CUT 380A is marketed with extensive informed documents and is recommended only for couples who are in a monogamous relationship. After exposure to organisms such as *Chlamydia* or gonococcus, with infection of the lower genital tract, there is a greater likelihood of pelvic inflammatory disease. In the absence of exposure to this risk, as in a monogamous relationship, pelvic inflammatory disease is not an issue. Hence, the lifestyle of the couple must be considered before the IUD is recommended.

The progesterone-containing T-shaped intrauterine device is associated with decreased flow during menstruation and relief of dysmenorrhea. The unintended pregnancy rate with the progesterone T 380A IUD is in the 1.5 to 2% range. It presents a slightly greater incidence of tubal ectopic pregnancy, probably the result of the effect of progesterone on tubal transport mechanisms. The progesterone T device requires removal and reinsertion on an annual basis.

Long-Acting Injectable Provera (Depo-Provera)

Injectable provera was not approved for use in the United States until 1992. Before then it had been used extensively in more than 90 countries. It is administered intramuscularly in a dose of 150 mg at 3-month intervals. It can be used in lactating women. Its principal side effect is menstrual irregularities, and some women complain of headache and weight gain. Although the effective contraceptive action of a single injection is 3 months, there is a variable interval beyond that point before fertility is regained. Depo-Provera was recently extensively evaluated by the World Health Organization and its safety and effectiveness confirmed. It does require a medical visit at 3-month intervals and unless that timetable is adhered to, its low unintended pregnancy rate of only 0.3% cannot be guaranteed.

ORAL CONTRACEPTION

The pill was introduced more than 4 decades ago in the United States and has maintained its position as the most popular method of birth control. Oral contraception involves the administration of estrogen combined with a progestational agent. One product, norethindrone (Micronor), involves a progestin-only approach. The typical regimen involves the ingestion of the active ingredients for 21 days of each month. The mechanism of action involves suppression of ovulation, changes in cervical mucus, and changes in the endometrium. Because ovulation is almost invariably suppressed, the incidence of ectopic pregnancy is diminished. For the typical pill user, the unintended pregnancy rate is in the 3% range, but this is reduced with perfect and consistent use to 0.1% with the combined pill. Oral contraceptives are available in various formulations. In some packages, the ratio of progestin and estrogen is phased during the course of the cycle. The alternative approach, daily administration of a single dose of estrogen progestational agent from cycle day 5 through 25, was used originally and continues to be widely prescribed today, although the dose has been dramatically reduced. Side effects of oral contraception include breast tenderness, weight gain, and headaches. A major but rare complication of oral contraception has been cardiovascular events such as stroke, heart attack, thrombophlebitis, and hypertension. Their incidence has been markedly diminished as the dose level has been reduced over time. There is evidence that the risk of these complications is increased significantly in women older than 35 who smoke more than 15 cigarettes per day. Overall, there is growing evidence that the health benefits of oral contraception for healthy, nonsmoking women, regardless of age, substantially outweigh the risks. In epidemiologic studies, oral contraception has been shown to provide protection against ovarian and endometrial cancer, pelvic inflammatory disease, fibrocystic breast disease, iron deficiency anemia, dysmenorrhea, and ovarian cysts. When taken consistently, it provides truly efficient protection against unintended pregnancy, and this effectiveness is, in large measure, responsible for its popularity.

Breakthrough bleeding is a commonly encountered problem with standard oral contraceptive use, occurring in up to 30% of women during the first month of use and falling to less than 10% in the third month. Because breakthrough bleeding is likely to resolve, it is important not to change the pill formulation unless the symptoms are extreme. Breakthrough bleeding is often the result of missed pills.

Drug interactions should be considered when prescribing oral contraceptives. Medications that may reduce oral contraceptive efficacy include the antituberculosis agent rifampin and some of the antifungals, such as griseofulvin. Some anticonvulsants such as phenytoin, ethotoin, mephenytoin, phenobarbital, primidone, carbamazepine, and ethosuximide are also suspect. It has been suggested that some antibiotics (tetracycline, doxycycline, penicillin, ampicillin) decrease contraceptive efficacy, but confirmatory studies on this relationship are not available. The activity of some drugs may be modified by oral contraceptives, and larger doses may be required. These include acetaminophen, aspirin, and morphine. The action of some antidepressants, such as imipramine, and tranquilizers, such as diazepam and benzodiazepines, may be enhanced. The same applies to some bronchodilators and antihypertensives.

The progestin-only oral contraceptive can be used during lactation. The pregnancy rate with the progestin-only pill is somewhat greater than with the combined pills, and there is less protection against ectopic pregnancy. Breakthrough bleeding is observed more frequently with the progestin-only pill.

BARRIER METHODS

This category of contraception functions to prevent the passage of spermatozoa through the cervix and beyond during coitus. Physical barriers include condoms, both male and female, the diaphragm, and the cervical cap. Chemical barriers that contain a spermicide are also available. Nonoxynol 9, a surfactant, nonionic detergent that immobilizes and kills spermatozoa is the agent used in most of these products. Physical and chemical barriers are commonly used in concert. The male condom is often packaged with a lubricant, which is spermicidal, but it is the physical barrier capability of the condom that provides its principal contraceptive action. The standard male condom is made of latex. A polyurethane condom (Avanti) was approved by the Food and Drug Administration in 1994. Experience with the Avanti in the field uncovered a high incidence of rupture and presently it is being redesigned. The female condom (Reality) is a latex product with an inner ring that is placed within the vagina and an outer ring that is located outside the introitus. It transfers the control of contraception to the woman, and its importance lies in its potential for prevention of transmission of STDs including the AIDS virus. The male condom provides contraceptive protection in the 3% range when used perfectly, but up to 12% overall. In contrast, the female condom in typical use is associated with a pregnancy rate of more than 20%. Because reuse is not advised, cost is one major issue.

The diaphragm was, until the introduction of the pill, the only method that provided female autonomy. The diaphragm must be fitted to size. It is used with a contraceptive cream or gel containing Nonoxynol 9. The diaphragm with spermicide is associated with a pregnancy rate in the 18% range with typical use but when used consistently and appropriately, the pregnancy rate drops to 6%. The effectiveness of barrier methods is, of course, heavily dependent on the motivation of the couple using them. Spermicides may be used alone, but their unintended pregnancy rate is estimated at between 6 and 21%. A cervical cap, which is placed over the cervix and is used with a spermicide, is available. It must be measured for size and fitted by a health care professional. The cap is associated with failure rates of 12 to 18%. All barrier methods provide some protection against STDs but may create vaginal irritation, which obviates some of this protection.

TABLE 1. **Currently Available Reversible Contraceptive Options**

Method	Mode of Action	Typical Use	Perfect Use	Advantages	Adverse Effects	Dangers
Female Hormonal Methods						
Oral contraceptives (combined)	Suppression of ovulation, changes in cervical mucus and endometrium	3%	0.1%	Protection against ovarian/endometrial cancer, PID, fibrocystic breast disease, ovarian cysts, iron deficiency anemia, dysmenorrhea; prevention of ectopic pregnancy	Nausea, headaches, dizziness, spotting, weight gain, breast tenderness	Cardiovascular stroke, heart attack, blood clots (risk substantially reduced with newer low-dose formulations), hypertension; depression, hepatic adenomas
Oral contraceptives (progestin only)	Changes in cervical mucus and endometrium, possible ovulation suppression	4%	0.5%	Protection against PID, iron-deficiency anemia, dysmenorrhea	Menstrual irregularities	Unknown
Implants—levonorgestrel subdermal implants (Norplant)	Similar to progestin only	0.09%	0.09%	Effective for 5 years	Site tenderness, removal problems, menstrual irregularities, headache, weight gain, acne	Infection at implant site after insertion
Injectables—depomedroxy-progesterone acetate	Suppression of ovulation, changes in cervical mucus and endometrium	0.3%	0.3%	Effective for 3 months Reduced risk of endometrial cancer, PID	Menstrual irregularities, headache, weight gain, delayed return to fertility	None proven
Intrauterine Devices (IUDs)						
Progesterone T (Progestasert)	Inhibition of sperm migration, fertilization, and ovum transport (progesterone is responsible for primary mode of action)	2%	1.5%	Diminished menstrual blood loss and relief of dysmenorrhea	Increased risk of pregnancy if not removed and reinserted annually; increased cramping and menstrual flow	Increased risk of ectopic pregnancy
Copper T 380A	Copper is responsible for primary mode of action	0.8%	0.6%	Protection against ectopic pregnancy; 10-year useful approved life	Increased menstrual blood loss, cramping, spotting, dysmenorrhea	Uterine perforation (rare), increased PID risk limited to 20–30 days postinsertion; anemia
Barrier Methods						
Spermicide alone	Inactivation of sperm	21%	6%	May protect against bacterial STDs	Vaginal irritation	None proven
Cervical cap with spermicide	Mechanical barrier; inactivation of sperm	18%	11.5%	Protection against STDs	Cervical irritation, vaginal discharge, pelvic pressure, Pap-smear abnormalities	Toxic shock syndrome
Diaphragm with spermicide	Mechanical barrier; inactivation of sperm	18%	6%	Protection against STDs	Cervical irritation	Toxic shock syndrome, urinary tract infections
Condom (male)	Mechanical barrier	12%	3%	Protection against STDs	Latex allergies	None
Condom (female)	Mechanical barrier	21%	5%	Protection against STDs includes external genitalia	Difficult to insert	None

NATURAL METHODS OF FAMILY PLANNING

It has long been recognized that fertility is impaired during lactation. The association of suckling with ovulatory arrest has been suggested as an effective means of pregnancy prevention for a limited interval after delivery. The method requires consistent suckling with no regular food or liquid supplements and is useful for no more than 6 months postpartum. In carefully supervised studies, the pregnancy rate is exceedingly low, estimated at 0.1% with perfect use, and a 6-month rate of 1 to 2%. It should be remembered that these studies are carried out with highly motivated women who have the advantage of frequent counseling.

Methods have been suggested to modify what was referred to in earlier times as the "rhythm method" of family planning. This involves periodic abstinence during the ovulatory phase of the menstrual cycle. Unfortunately, spermatozoa are capable of surviving in the female reproductive tract for several days after coitus. Intercourse at any time before ovulation is associated with some risk of pregnancy. Because the egg is not fertilizable beyond 36 hours, coitus in the luteal phase of the cycle, when it can be properly

TABLE 1. **Currently Available Reversible Contraceptive Options** *Continued*

Method	Mode of Action	Typical Use	Perfect Use	Advantages	Adverse Effects	Dangers
Non–Commodity-Based Methods						
Lactational amenorrhea method	Based on enhancement of lactational physiology and identification of period of lactational infertility using three criteria	1–2% (6-mo rate)	0–1%	No commodities necessary; enhances breast-feeding practices	Markedly decreased effectiveness begins 6 months postpartum	Provides no protection against STDs
Periodic abstinence methods	Avoidance of coitus during days when fertilization might occur	20%	0–9%	No commodities necessary; enhances breast-feeding practices	Prolonged intervals of abstinence required	Provides no protection against STDs
Coitus interruptus	Withdrawal of the penis from the vagina before ejaculation	18%	4%	No commodity necessary, no advance planning or charting		Provides no protection against STDs
Emergency Contraception						
Emergency contraceptive pills (combined oral contraceptive pills containing combination of estrogen and progestin)	2 Ovral pills initially, 2 more 12 h later; *or* 4 Lo/Ovral, Nordette, or Levlen initially, 4 more 12 h later; *or* 4 Triphasil or Tri-Levlen (yellow only), 4 more 12 h later		75%	Medications relatively easy to obtain	Nausea, vomiting	

Abbreviations: PID = pelvic inflammatory disease; STD = sexually transmitted disease.
Modified with permission from Harrison PF, Rosenfield A (eds): Contraceptive Research and Development: Looking into the Future. Washington DC, Academy of Sciences. National Academy Press, 1996, pp 96–101. Copyright 1996 by the National Academy of Sciences. Courtesy of the National Academy Press.

defined and identified, is entirely safe. Methods to identify this "safe" interval have included careful recording of the menstrual calendar supplemented by the basal body temperature, and observations on characteristics of the cervical mucus. Except in the most motivated of couples, the pregnancy rate is high. Coitus interruptus can also be used to affect sperm transport adversely, but, in typical use, this approach is associated with an estimated 18% failure rate.

POSTCOITAL METHODS

The physician/health care provider advising on contraception needs to be aware that pregnancy prevention methods are available when coitus has occurred without contraception or when a method may have failed (e.g., ruptured condom). The pharmacologic method for emergency contraception available in the United States is the combined contraceptive pill. Two standard dose or four low-dose oral contraceptives are taken as soon as possible after unprotected intercourse. An additional two or four tablets are given 12 hours later. Nausea is the most commonly experienced side effect. No product is marketed for emergency contraception, but the combined pills are readily available. When these pills are given before ovulation, ovulation is delayed. An alternative mechanism of action involves a modifying effect on the endometrium to prevent implantation. The antiprogestin, mifepristone (RU486), has been extensively studied as a postcoital contraceptive with a very high success rate and few side effects. Mifepristone is not yet available in the United States.

Contraceptive choices are wide and varied. Table 1 provides a listing of the methods available in the United States. A brief rundown on their mode of action, advantages and disadvantages, side effects, and serious health issues is provided. Estimated pregnancy rates observed with typical and with "ideal" usage are also included.

Section 16

Psychiatric Disorders

ALCOHOLISM

method of
STEPHEN M. JURD, M.B., B.S.
Royal North Shore Hospital and University of Sydney
Sydney, New South Wales, Australia

In a substantial proportion of all patients presenting for medical treatment, alcohol is a causal factor or a coexisting health risk. One of every six patients in family practice and one of five in hospital practice is at risk. Community statistics indicate that lifelong prevalence of alcohol abuse among men is in the range of 19 to 30%. Usual estimates of point prevalence of serious drinking problems (alcohol dependence) range from 3 to 5% of the adult male population. Women have approximately half the risk of men.

THE PHYSICIAN'S ROLE

There is no doubt that much alcohol-related illness goes undiagnosed. Therefore, the physician's principal role is that of case identification and provision of information to the patient. The usual situation is that neither physician nor patient has considered behavioral change as a health strategy. The next stage depends on the severity of the presenting problem and the patient's willingness to accept treatment.

LEVELS OF SEVERITY

There are essentially three levels of severity that require clinical attention: hazardous, harmful, and dependent drinking. The first two levels have been defined from epidemiologic studies that have indicated an increased risk for a variety of disorders once these limits are exceeded. A standard drink is a 1-ounce (30-mL) shot of whiskey, a 2-ounce (60-mL) glass of fortified wine, a 4-ounce (120-mL) glass of table wine, and a 10-ounce (300-mL) glass of beer.

Women are more sensitive to the effects of alcohol than are men. There are three reasons for this: women are, overall, smaller than men; women have a lower percentage lean body mass (alcohol is poorly distributed to adipose tissue); and women have lower levels of gastric alcohol dehydrogenase. For these reasons, women have higher blood levels per standard drink consumed.

Hazardous Drinking

Drinking more than four standard drinks (40 grams of alcohol) daily in men or more than two standard drinks (20 grams of alcohol) a day in women confers a significant risk for alcohol-related problems. To maintain low-risk drinking, there should be two or three alcohol-free days each week and no episodes of drinking more than six drinks on one occasion.

Harmful Drinking

This exists when known alcohol-related harm, such as any of the problems listed in Table 1, occurs in the presence of hazardous drinking.

Alcohol Dependence Syndrome

This syndrome is a complex biopsychosocial disorder that has internationally accepted major features:

1. Subjective awareness of compulsion to drink, usually manifested by multiple attempts to control, cut down, or abstain
2. Stereotyped, narrowed pattern of drinking, i.e., the drinking predicts the social life rather than vice versa
3. Increased importance of drinking over other activities, eroding work, family, and personal responsibilities
4. Pharmacologic tolerance resulting in an increased capacity to drink without showing signs of intoxication
5. Repeated withdrawal symptoms (e.g., nausea, tremor, irritability, and anxiety, especially in the morning)
6. Relieving or preventing withdrawal by drinking
7. Reinstatement of pathologic drinking after a period of abstinence

These features, as in any syndrome, tend to predict each other's presence, but not always. In general, the presence of three features is required for a diagnosis of alcohol dependence syndrome, although the presence of any feature is relevant. Dependence ranges from the mildest degree to the most severe. Severe dependence is usually complicated by multiple problems. The presence of dependence does not mean that affected individuals will experience serious withdrawal, but the more severe the dependence, the more likely it is that clinically significant withdrawal will occur.

ALCOHOL-RELATED PROBLEMS

An attempt to summarize the many complications of excessive drinking is made in Table 1. The ubiquity of excessive drinking means that many of these problems present in relative isolation, leading alcohol to be considered the modern "great imitator" of other diseases.

FAMILY PROBLEMS

Every problem drinker seriously affects the lives of at least four other people. The family disruption may result in the development of psychiatric symptoms in family members. Domestic violence commonly coexists with alcohol problems and cannot be managed without dealing with the alcohol problem. Some family members are assisted by Al-Anon, a worldwide self-help group for relatives of problem drinkers. This group is available to families regardless of whether the drinker accepts treatment.

TABLE 1. **Alcohol-Related Problems**

Trauma	**Psychiatric Problems**	**Neurologic Problems**
Motor vehicle accidents	Suicide	Peripheral neuropathy
Falls	Parasuicide	Subdural hematoma
Fractures	Depression	Wernicke-Korsakoff psychosis
Head injuries	Paranoia	**Muscle Problems**
Drownings	Dementia	Myopathy
Domestic fires	Alcohol withdrawal delirium	Rhabdomyolysis
Social Problems	Anxiety	**Hematologic Disorders**
Financial problems	Phobias	Macrocytosis
Marital conflict	Panic attacks	Anemia
Absenteeism	**Gastrointestinal Disorders**	Thrombocytopenia
Unemployment	Gastritis	Leukopenia
Drunk driving	Ulcers	**Metabolic Disorders**
Convictions	Reflux esophagitis	Obesity
Assault	Esophageal varices	Gout
Homicide	Diarrhea	Hyperlipidemia
Domestic violence	Vomiting	Diabetes
Indirect Presentations*	Fatty liver	Impotence
Spouse	Mallory-Weiss syndrome	Gynecomastia
Injury	Cirrhosis	**Obstetric Problems**
Depression	Pancreatitis	Low birth weight
Psychosomatic illness	**Cardiovascular Problems**	Fetal alcohol syndrome
Children	Hypertension	Second-trimester abortion
Abuse	Arrhythmias	**Oncologic Problems**
Depression	**Respiratory Problems**	Oropharyngeal cancers
Anxiety	Lung abscess	Esophageal cancers
School refusal	Sleep apnea	
	Tuberculosis	

*Indirect presentations occur when family members display problems consequent to the drinking of their relative.

DIAGNOSIS

The high frequency of alcohol problems in clinical practice and the low diagnosis rate indicate a need for a much higher index of suspicion. Meticulous assessment is required wherever one of the problems listed in Table 1 presents.

History of Alcohol Use

An attitude of nonjudgmental acceptance of heavy drinking as a common human behavior should pervade all history-taking efforts. One technique that emerges from this attitude is the "top-high" technique, in which one deliberately overestimates the amount consumed and places the onus of denial on the patient, for example, "I bet you could drink two bottles of whiskey in a day." A variant of this technique can be used in taking a daily drinking estimate by asking whether a patient has the first drink of the day before or after breakfast. This having been ascertained, the clinician builds up a picture of the typical drinking that occurs in a day. This eventually allows the clinician to estimate how many standard drinks (10 grams of alcohol) are consumed during an average day. The perceived benefits and the social setting of the drinking should also be elicited.

Physical Examination

During the physical examination, the physician looks for the following signs:

1. Signs of trauma
2. Signs of liver disease—tender hepatomegaly, spider nevi, secondary lunulae, palmar erythema, bruising, parotid enlargement, ascites
3. Conjunctival injection, facial telangiectasia, tongue and hand tremors
4. Hypertension, obesity
5. Withdrawal features, commonly anxiety, sweating, and tachycardia
6. Evidence of intoxication—alcohol on the breath, ataxia, disinhibition

Clinical Investigations

These are used to confirm the suspected diagnosis. Because all tests have a low sensitivity, negative test results cannot exclude alcohol problems.

1. Liver function tests show some abnormality in about 50% of cases; the γ-glutamyltransferase measurement is the most sensitive.
2. The mean corpuscular volume is elevated.
3. Blood alcohol levels may be detected, especially in emergencies. Apparent sobriety with a substantial blood alcohol level may clarify the situation.
4. Screening devices such as the Alcohol Use Disorders Identification Test (AUDIT) (Figure 1) can assist in identifying individuals who need more detailed assessment. This instrument is in the public domain and does not require permission for reproduction. Each question is scored on a scale of 0 to 4, the left column scoring 0, the right column 4. A score below 8 indicates nonhazardous drinking. A score of 8 to 15 indicates hazardous or harmful drinking. A score above 15 indicates probable dependence.

World Health Organization

AUDIT

Please place a mark in the box next to your answer. One standard drink equals approximately one 12-oz glass of beer; one 4-oz glass of wine; one 2-oz glass of sherry or port; or one ounce of spirits. *Note:* the average light beer is about half the strength of normal beer.

1 How often do you have a drink containing alcohol?
☐ never (0) ☐ monthly or less (1) ☐ 2 to 4 times a month (2) ☐ 2 to 3 times a week (3) ☐ 4 or more times a week (4)

2 How many standard drinks containing alcohol do you have on a typical day when you are drinking?
☐ 1 or 2 (0) ☐ 3 or 4 (1) ☐ 5 or 6 (2) ☐ 7 to 9 (3) ☐ 10 or more (4)

3 How often do you have six or more drinks on one occasion?
☐ never (0) ☐ less than monthly (1) ☐ monthly (2) ☐ weekly (3) ☐ daily or almost daily (4)

4 How often during the last year have you found that you were not able to stop drinking once you had started?
☐ never (0) ☐ less than monthly (1) ☐ monthly (2) ☐ weekly (3) ☐ daily or almost daily (4)

5 How often during the last year have you failed to do what was normally expected from you because of drinking?
☐ never (0) ☐ less than monthly (1) ☐ monthly (2) ☐ weekly (3) ☐ daily or almost daily (4)

6 How often during the last year have you needed a drink in the morning to get yourself going after a heavy drinking session?
☐ never (0) ☐ less than monthly (1) ☐ monthly (2) ☐ weekly (3) ☐ daily or almost daily (4)

7 How often during the last year have you had a feeling of guilt or remorse after drinking?
☐ never (0) ☐ less than monthly (1) ☐ monthly (2) ☐ weekly (3) ☐ daily or almost daily (4)

8 How often during the last year have you been unable to remember what happened the night before because you had been drinking?
☐ never (0) ☐ less than monthly (1) ☐ monthly (2) ☐ weekly (3) ☐ daily or almost daily (4)

9 Have you or someone else been injured as a result of your drinking?
☐ no (0) ☐ yes, but not in the last year (2) ☐ yes, during the last year (4)

10 Has a relative, a friend, a doctor or other health worker been concerned about your drinking or suggested you cut down?
☐ no (0) ☐ yes, but not in the last year (2) ☐ yes, during the last year (4)

Figure 1. (Adapted from Babor TF, De La Fuente JR, Saunders J, Grant M: The Alcohol Use Disorders Identification Test: Guidelines for use in primary health care. WHO Publication no. 89.4. Geneva, World Health Organization, 1989; and Saunders JB, Aasland OB, Babor TF, De La Fuente JR, Grant M: Development of the Alcohol Use Disorders Identification Test [AUDIT]; WHO Collaborative Project on Early Detection of Persons with Harmful Alcohol Consumption-II Addiction, *88*:791–804, 1993. All rights to this questionnaire are reserved by the World Health Organization. However, this questionnaire may be freely reproduced or translated but not for sale or use in conjunction with commercial purposes.)

TREATMENT

Brief Intervention

After a thorough assessment as just outlined, patients whose alcohol use is hazardous or harmful but not dependent should receive a brief (10- to 15-minute) intervention along the following lines.

Feedback. Explain why alcohol is relevant to the patient, providing details about any abnormal test results and never explaining away minor abnormalities if they fit the clinical situation. Indicate to patients who have no clinically apparent harm how their drinking behavior puts them at risk.

Listen. Pay careful attention to the way in which the patient responds to the information provided. Defensiveness may interfere with communication and requires clarification, without argument.

Outline Benefits. Provide an account of the future prospects, outlining the benefits to the patient if drinking behavior is altered.

Set Goals. Inform the patient of the limits of low-risk drinking. If harm is manifest, a brief (1- to 3-month) period of abstinence may be indicated.

Set Strategies. Provide suggestions about altering behaviors, e.g., start with a nonalcoholic drink, avoid heavy drinking parties, resurrect an old hobby, engage in physical fitness activities, alternate alcoholic and nonalcoholic drinks, avoid buying rounds of drinks.

Evaluate. Encourage each patient to return for a review of his or her progress with attempts at behavioral change. Exceeding the drinking goals set should not be seen as a failure but as part of a learning process.

If clinically significant medical problems are present, closer follow-up is indicated, with regular monitoring of any abnormal test results. Despite all efforts by clinicians, some people who are dependent will not disclose their symptoms, so prolonged inability to change drinking behavior should indicate a need to consider a diagnosis of alcohol dependence.

ALCOHOL DEPENDENCE

If patients are physically dependent, they will experience some withdrawal symptoms. These can be a potent stimulant to return to drinking. An inpatient detoxification program is often necessary to allow the patient to withdraw safely from alcohol. Sedatives such as chlordiazepoxide (Librium) or diazepam (Valium) may occasionally ease withdrawal, but great care should be taken to taper the dose to ensure that the sedative is stopped before discharge. At least relative malnutrition is the rule in alcohol dependence, so multivitamins, particularly vitamin B_1 (thiamine), should be prescribed.

Regular contact with the clinician, especially early in the abstinence period, can be helpful, as can referral to a counselor skilled in drug and alcohol problems. Difficulties with personal relationships and family situations commonly require attention. Patients with more severe or complicated problems or continual relapses may benefit from an inpatient rehabilitation program. These exist in a variety of forms, and the clinician should attempt to match the patient to the appropriate program.

The seventh feature of alcohol dependence is a return to pathologic use after a period of abstinence. The more severe the dependence, the more inevitable the return to damaging drinking habits. Under these circumstances, the only solution is lifelong total abstinence. This is a tall order for those who value alcohol highly and is why members of Alcoholics Anonymous (AA) say they do it "one day at a time." AA is a worldwide self-help organization founded in 1935 in Akron, Ohio, that has more than 1.5 million members. It is based on spiritual principles and encourages altruistic endeavor but makes no demands of its members apart from a desire to stay sober. AA can be an invaluable source of support for patients who espouse abstinence as a goal.

In the last few years anticraving drugs (naltrexone [ReVia] and acamprosate*) have been shown to decrease relapse in alcohol dependence. These drugs offer the first hope that pharmacologic treatments may be able to moderate desire to drink and hence relapse.

LONG-TERM FOLLOW-UP

It is rare for patients to change ingrained habits without a struggle. Maintenance of a nonjudgmental stance and positive expectations despite a relapse are useful. Patients often learn from a relapse and are better able to pursue complete recovery. Experience indicates that even the most profoundly damaged patients can attain long-term sobriety.

*Not available in the United States.

DRUG ABUSE

method of
LESLIE K. JACOBSEN, M.D., and
THOMAS R. KOSTEN, M.D.
Yale University School of Medicine
New Haven, Connecticut

Abuse of and dependence on illicit substances are among the most prevalent psychiatric disorders. The 1996 National Institute on Drug Abuse Household Survey estimated that 13 million people in the United States were current illicit drug users. The 1988 Surgeon General's Report indicated that relapse rates for abusers of most substances range between 80 and 90%. Those who are able to remain abstinent for long periods usually do so only after many failed attempts at quitting. Thus, substance abuse and addiction are pervasive and tenacious problems.

With the third revised and fourth editions of the *Diagnostic and Statistical Manual of Mental Disorders*, emphasis has shifted toward loss of control over substance use and disruption of normal activities in defining all addictions. Tolerance, or reduction in drug effect with repeated use, and symptoms and signs of a characteristic withdrawal syndrome on abrupt cessation of drug use are no longer required for the diagnosis of addiction. Treatment must focus beyond initial detoxification and address relapse prevention, bearing in mind that successful treatment often is preceded by multiple failures. Often referral to specialized clinics or treatment facilities is required. Although some medications reduce craving and/or abuse of some substances, postdetoxification treatment programs generally also include a psychosocial component geared toward helping addicts shift from the drug-abusing lifestyle and culture toward being constructive members of their families and society. Vigorous treatment of co-morbid psychiatric conditions, including mood, anxiety, and psychotic disorders, is also a key component of relapse prevention.

An important cornerstone of both emergency department management and postdetoxification treatment of substance abuse is accurate drug testing. Abusers of substances may not be willing or able to reliably inform caregivers of the identity of the substances they have used. Furthermore, in some individuals, abuse of certain substances can trigger symptoms that mimic other psychiatric disorders, such as schizophrenia. Although blood drug levels are more closely related to brain levels and represent stronger evidence of recent use, urine is usually the preferred biofluid for drug detection, as drug levels are higher in urine than in blood. For Department of Health and Human Services Substance Abuse and Mental Health Services Administration certification, laboratories are required to screen samples for amphetamines, cannabinoids, cocaine, opioids, and phencyclidine. Additional substances commonly screened for include barbiturates, benzodiazepines, methadone, propoxyphene, methaqualone, and ethanol. Substances usually not screened for include lysergic acid diethylamide (LSD), fentanyl, psilocybin, methylenedioxymethamphetamine (MDMA), methylenedioxyamphetamine (MDA), and other designer drugs.

COCAINE

The 1996 National Institute on Drug Abuse Household Survey estimated that 1.75 million people in the United States currently use cocaine. Cocaine is taken intransally ("snorting"), intravenously (when combined with heroin this is referred to as "speed bailing"), or by smoking of cocaine freebase or "crack" cocaine (freebase prepared with sodium bicarbonate). Although substance abuse is generally more common in males, this male dominance is less for crack cocaine, in part owing to the frequent use of crack in drugs-for-sex exchanges. An association between cocaine abuse and human immunodeficiency virus (HIV) infection has been observed.

Because cocaine is a stimulant, its acute subjective effects include intense euphoria and alertness, grandiosity, and anxiety. These effects rapidly give way to dysphoria as the drug is metabolized and excreted, leading to the binge pattern of usage that is commonly seen, where the drug is used repeatedly until either the supply or the user is exhausted. Intense usage can lead to pervasive anxiety states, which can be treated with lorazepam (Ativan), 2 mg orally or 1 mg intramuscularly (IM), and psychotic symptoms, including paranoid ideation and auditory, visual, or tactile hallucinations. These latter symptoms can be treated with haloperidol (Haldol), 5 mg orally or 2.5 mg IM. Large doses of cocaine can lead to atrial and ventricular arrhythmias, hypertension, myocardial infarction, cerebrovascular accidents, and seizures.

Withdrawal from cocaine after heavy, prolonged use may involve dysphoric mood, vivid dreams, insominia or hypersomnia, increased appetite, and psychomotor retardation. This constellation of symptoms may be accompanied by suicidal ideation, which should prompt close observation and formal psychiatric consultation.

Common therapeutic goals of all treatment approaches for cocaine abuse include keeping the abuser in treatment, disrupting the binge cycle, and preventing relapse. Crack and freebase abusers tend to drop out of treatment at a higher rate than abusers of other forms of cocaine. Psychosocial rehabilitation, including behavioral treatment that reinforces cocaine-free urine tests, can be effective in preventing relapse and, when relapse occurs, reducing its severity. Given the rapidity with which cocaine is metabolized, use of a sensitive assay for screening urine samples is important.

The tricyclic antidepressants and serotonin re-uptake inhibitors have been shown to be effective in some, but not all, double-blind studies in initiation of abstinence and reduction of craving for cocaine. Depressed cocaine abusers may be especially responsive to desipramine (Norpramin).* Because there may be a 2- to 3-week delay before patients experience a reduction in target symptoms from antidepressants, dropout rates are high. Both of the dopamine-agonist agents amantadine (Symmetrel)* and bromocriptine (Parlodel)* have been found to be effective in reducing craving and cocaine abuse, although not consistently. Amantadine has fewer side effects than bromocriptine. Mood stabilizing agents, such as lithium and carbamazepine (Tegretol), have not been found to be effective in the treatment of cocaine abuse.

AMPHETAMINES AND DESIGNER STIMULANT DRUGS

Amphetamines, which include dextroamphetamine (Dexedrine), methylphenidate (Ritalin), and pemoline (Cylert), are not as frequently abused as cocaine; but rates of abuse of these substances are increasing. These drugs are usually taken orally; however the methamphetamine ("ice") form of amphetamine can be taken intravenously, intranasally, or by smoking. The effects of methamphetamine in particular are similar to those of cocaine, except that they are approximately 10 times longer in duration. Acute clinical management and postdetoxification treatment are also similar. Hyperpyrexia is a serious complication of methamphetamine overdose that can develop from the resulting vasoconstriction, hepatic metabolism of fat and glucose, agitation, and muscle rigidity. This can be managed with hydration, infusion of ice cold saline, and external cooling with ice packs, sponging, and cooling blankets. If the drug has been ingested, gastric lavage and activated charcoal can be administered. Ipecac should not be used because of the risk of inducing seizures, arrhythmias, or hypertensive hemorrhages. Cardiac monitoring for arrhythmias in the setting of stimulant (cocaine or amphetamine) overdose is necessary. Significant stimulant-induced hypertension should be carefully controlled with antihypertensive agents. As with cocaine intoxication, psychotic symptoms and agitation may develop and can be treated with haloperidol; however, because of the longer half-life of methamphetamine, these symptoms may persist longer.

Transplacental exposure to stimulants, including cocaine, is associated with intrauterine growth retardation, preterm labor and premature birth, fetal distress, placental hemorrhage, decreased head circumference, neonatal anemia, and postnatal developmental abnormalities. The withdrawal syndrome associated with amphetamines is similar to that associated with cocaine.

MDMA ("Ecstasy," "E," "Adam"), MDA, and the less commonly abused methylenedioxyethamphetamine (MDME; "Eve") are amphetamine analogues with many of the effects of amphetamine and are most popular among adolescents and college students. Physiologic toxicity is relatively common at

*Not FDA approved for this indication.

high doses of MDMA and can include cardiac arrhythmias, seizures, hyperthermia, renal failure, intracerebral hemorrhage, metabolic acidosis, and disseminated intravascular coagulation.

OPIOIDS

Opioids include natural substances, such as opium, heroin, and morphine, and synthetic substances, such as meperidine (Demerol), fentanyl (Sublimaze; "China White"), methadone (Dolophine), 1-methyl-4-phenyl-1,2,3,6-tetrahydropyridine (MPTP), and 1-methyl-4-phenyl propionoxy-piperidine tetrahydropyridine (MPPP). These drugs can be taken orally, intravenously, intranasally, or by smoking them. The 1996 National Institute on Drug Abuse Household Survey estimated that 216,000 Americans currently use heroin. Although many believe that current patterns of heroin usage in the United States are endemic, Drug Abuse Warning Network data have recently shown marked increases in heroin-related emergency department visits, made chiefly by older chronic heroin users.

Opioid intoxication is associated with euphoria, analgesia, drowsiness, respiratory depression, and pinpoint pupils. Opioid overdose is associated with respiratory arrest and death. Meperidine overdose is also often associated with seizures. Treatment involves providing a patent airway and mechanical ventilation as needed and administering the opioid antagonist naloxone (Narcan). Overdoses with synthetic or longer acting opioids, such as methadone, require higher and repeated doses of naloxone, which is relatively short acting.

Onset and course of opioid withdrawal are determined by the pharmacokinetics of the particular opioid used. Subjective symptoms include restlessness, insomnia, drug craving, and anxiety. Objective signs include myalgia, vomiting, lacrimation, rhinorrhea, meiosis, diarrhea, sweating, and chills. Although opioid withdrawal is very uncomfortable, it is not associated with serious medical complications except in pregnancy, where it can precipitate spontaneous abortion or preterm labor and premature birth later in pregnancy.

The choice of treatment referral for opioid addiction should involve consideration of the extent and severity of previous opioid abuse and past treatment history. Patients with a relatively recent onset of opioid abuse and no previous treatment are optimally referred for rapid opioid detoxification, which typically involves naltrexone (ReVia), and clonidine (Catapres), or for drug-free treatment. Patients with a long history of opioid abuse and multiple previous treatment attempts are best referred for treatment with methadone or *l*-α-acetyl-methadol (LAAM), another long-acting opioid. In all cases, concomitant random urine drug screening and psychosocial treatments focused on helping patients shift away from the drug-abusing lifestyle are essential. In addition, screening for HIV, hepatitis B, and tuberculosis should be offered to all intravenous drug abusers.

Pregnant heroin addicts in methadone treatment are less likely to experience withdrawal, receive better prenatal care and nutrition, and have lower rates of prematurity, low birth weight, and infant mortality relative to pregnant heroin addicts not receiving methadone. Thus, all pregnant heroin addicts should be referred for methadone maintenance. Sixty percent of methadone-exposed neonates experience a withdrawal syndrome within 72 hours of birth, which is often treated with paregoric. No long-term sequelae of prenatal methadone exposure have been noted.

SEDATIVE HYPNOTICS AND ANXIOLYTICS

The sedative hypnotics and anxiolytics include the benzodiazepines, barbiturates (e.g., secobarbital; [Seconal]), the barbiturate-like hypnotics (e.g., methaqualone), and the carbamates (e.g., meprobamate; [Equanil]), all of which are taken orally. These agents are available through prescription and illegal sources, are brain depressants, and in high doses can be lethal, particularly when combined with alcohol. These drugs may be used by individuals to promote sleep after abuse of cocaine or other stimulants.

Patients taking prescription sedative hypnotics or anxiolytics can become physiologically dependent such that a withdrawal syndrome is elicited on abrupt medication discontinuation, which can include sweating; tremor; autonomic hyperactivity; insomnia; nausea; vomiting; psychomotor agitation; anxiety; transient visual, tactile, or auditory hallucinations or illusions; generalized seizures; and life-threatening delirium. Physiologic dependence in the absence of unauthorized dose escalation, drug-seeking behavior, or other behavioral signs of addiction does not merit a formal diagnosis of addiction. Timing of the onset of the withdrawal syndrome after drug cessation is determined by the pharmacokinetics of the specific drug used. Shorter-acting medications, such as lorazepam (Ativan) and oxazepam (Serax), produce withdrawal symptoms within 6 to 8 hours, which peak in intensity by the second day and improve substantially by the fourth or fifth day. With longer-acting medications, such as diazepam (Valium) and chlordiazepoxide (Librium), withdrawal symptoms may not develop for a week, peak during the second week, and improve by the third or fourth week. Severity of withdrawal is determined by the amount of drug routinely taken. Severe withdrawal is treated with long-acting benzodiazepines (e.g., diazepam; [Valium] or chlordiazepoxide; [Librium]) and anticonvulsants such as carbamazepine (Tegretol) or valproate (Depakote).

Symptoms of sedative hypnotic or anxiolytic intoxication are similar to those associated with alcohol intoxication and include behavioral disinhibition, slurred speech, nystagmus, incoordination, unsteady gait, memory or attentional impairments, and stupor or coma. Overdose may necessitate intubation and mechanical ventilation. Benzodiazepine overdose can be treated with flumazenil (Romazicon), a benzodiazepine antagonist. Postdetoxification treatment of sedative hypnotic abuse and addiction is primarily psychosocial.

PHENCYCLIDINE

Phencyclidines or phencyclidine-like substances include phencyclidine (PCP), ketamine (Ketalar, Ketaject), and 1-[1-2-thienyl-cyclohexyl]piperidine (TCP). These substances can be taken orally or intravenously, or they can be smoked. Phencyclidine is the most commonly abused substance of this group and is usually mixed with tobacco or marijuana and smoked. Phencyclidine abuse is most common among individuals between 20 and 40 years of age and is more common among males.

Phencyclidine intoxication is associated with rapid onset of impulsive, unpredictable behavior, psychomotor agitation, impaired judgment, and assaultiveness. In addition, nystagmus, hyperacusis, ataxia, hypertension, tachycardia, hyperthermia, dysarthria, muscle rigidity, seizures, psychotic symptoms, or coma can be seen. Although a withdrawal syndrome has not been observed in humans, dependent individuals may take phencyclidine as often as two or three times per day, despite clear social and medical sequelae of ongoing use. Heavy users do report experiencing craving for phencyclidine. Patients presenting to the emergency department with phencyclidine intoxication are often brought there by the police because of their aggressive behavior. Restraints are often necessary, along with haloperidol, 2 mg intramuscularly, and lorazepam, 1 mg intramuscularly. Because intoxicated patients may experience brief lucid periods only to return to an agitated and aggressive state, restraints should be maintained until consistent lucidity and impulse control are demonstrated.

HALLUCINOGENS

The hallucinogens include lysergic acid diethylamide (LSD), mescaline (peyote), and psilocybin mushrooms, all of which are usually taken orally. A 1996 Substance Abuse and Mental Health Services Administration household survey found that 2% of individuals over the age of 12 years had used hallucinogens in the previous month. LSD use is most prevalent in individuals between the ages of 18 and 25 years. The different hallucinogens produce similar intoxication syndromes consisting of significant anxiety or depression, ideas of reference, paranoid ideation, impaired judgment, illusions, vivid visual hallucinations, depersonalization, derealization, pupillary dilation, tachycardia, diaphoresis, blurred vision, tremor, and incoordination. Tolerance develops to the psychedelic and euphoric effects of hallucinogens, but not to their autonomic effects. Cross-tolerance has been observed between LSD and other hallucinogens. However, no withdrawal syndrome has been demonstrated for the hallucinogens.

Management of hallucinogen intoxication is generally conservative; however, lorazepam, 1 to 2 mg orally or intramuscularly, and/or haloperidol, 2 mg orally or intramuscularly, can be administered in cases of significant agitation or distress. Hallucinogen persisting perception disorder (flashbacks) may develop in some hallucinogen users and consists of transient recurrence of perceptual disturbances experienced during previous episodes of hallucinogen intoxication in the absence of current hallucinogen intoxication. These episodes may remit after several months, although in some cases they have persisted for years. Persistent psychotic symptoms may develop after LSD use, although this appears to occur primarily in individuals predisposed to psychosis (e.g., by virtue of previous episodes of psychosis in the absence of drug use, family history of psychosis). Such cases merit formal psychiatric consultation and referral for psychiatric treatment.

INHALANTS

Inhalants are a heterogenous group of psychoactive substances found in gasoline, adhesives, spray paints, cleaning fluids, typewriter correction fluid, and lighter fluids. These agents are taken only by inhalation, usually by "sniffing" an open container or "huffing" a rag soaked in the substance. Because of their low cost, ease of concealment, and easy availability, inhalants are often the first psychoactive substance used by young people. In 1989 it was estimated that 7% of high school seniors had used inhalants during the previous year. In addition, evidence suggests that the prevalence of inhalant abuse among 9- to 12-year-olds is increasing. Inhalant abuse may be more common among impoverished ethnic minorities, with the exception of African-Americans.

Inhalant intoxication resembles alcohol intoxication, with stimulation and disinhibition followed by depression at higher doses. In addition, dizziness, nystagmus, incoordination, slurred speech, lethargy, decreased reflexes, tremor, generalized muscle weakness, blurred vision or diplopia, and stupor or coma may be seen. An odor of the inhalant used, as well as burns resulting from the flammability of these substances, may be present. Treatment of acute intoxication is generally supportive. Physical complications of inhalant abuse include cardiac arrhythmias, which can lead to sudden death; cerebellar disease, including cerebellar atrophy; cranial neuropathies; generalized cerebral atrophy and demyelination; distal renal tubular acidosis, glomerulonephritis; hepatic disease; chemical pneumonitis; and bone marrow suppression. Thus, thorough medical evaluation is warranted.

Prenatal exposure to toluene, present in most volatile adhesives, has been associated with craniofacial and limb abnormalities, developmental delay, and behavioral deficits. Tolerance to the effects of inhalants has been reported. A withdrawal syndrome consisting of sleep disturbance, nausea, tremor, diaphoresis, abdominal and chest discomfort, and irritability developing within 24 to 48 hours of cessation of use and lasting 2 to 5 days has been observed in some chronic users. Currently, there are no efficacious medications for the treatment of inhalant abuse and addiction. Psychosocial approaches have had limited success, except when treatment occurs in a residential setting and/or is court mandated.

CANNABINOIDS

Cannabinoids, specifically marijuana, are the most widely used of illegal drugs and are often the first drugs used by all cultural groups in the United States. The 1996 National Insitute on Drug Abuse Household Survey estimated that there are 10.1 million regular marijuana users in the United States. Derived from the cannabis plant, marijuana consists of the dried tops and leaves of the plant, whereas hashish consists of exudate from the leaves. These substances are usually smoked, but can be ingested, such as when mixed with food. Heavy users are predominantly males between the ages of 18 and 30 years. The component primarily responsible for the psychoactive properties of cannabis is δ-9-tetrahydrocannabinol (THC).

Intoxication can be associated with euphoria, anxiety, impaired coordination, impaired judgment, sensation of slowed time, social withdrawal, conjunctival injection, increased appetite, dry mouth, and tachycardia. High doses of cannabinoids can be associated with effects similar to those of hallucinogens, including paranoid ideation, delusions, hallucinations, depersonalization, and derealization. A withdrawal syndrome associated with cannabinoid use has not been reliably demonstrated. However, a dependence syndrome consisting of compulsive use despite disruption of family, work, social, psychological, and physical functioning does occur. Few cannabinoid users seek treatment for intoxication or dependence. Conservative treatment of intoxication is indicated. Psychosocial treatments of marijuana dependence may be associated with reduction in the frequency of marijuana use.

ANTICHOLINERGICS

Abused anticholinergics include antihistamines, such as diphenhydramine (Benadryl) and benztropine (Cogentin), and tricyclic antidepressants, such as amitriptyline (Elavil) and doxepin (Sinequan). Intoxication is associated with euphoria, delirium, visual hallucinations, mydriasis, tachycardia, hypertension, arrhythmias, increased temperature, and seizures. Treatment involves maintaining an airway and administering charcoal and a cathartic. This should be done even if a number of hours have transpired since ingestion, as anticholinergics markedly decrease gastrointestinal motility. Physostigmine can be administered for arrhythmias that do not respond to beta blockers; however, physostigmine can produce seizures, bradycardia, bronchospasm, and laryngospasm and so must be used with caution and only if the potential benefits outweigh the risks.

ANABOLIC STEROIDS

Anabolic steroid abuse has become an increasing problem among adolescent and young adult competitive sports participants and body builders. Both natural (e.g., testosterone) and synthetic (e.g., stanozolol, metandienone, I17-beta-methyl-5 beta-androst-1-ene-3 alpha, 17 alpha-diol, and 18-nor-17, 17-dimethyl-5 beta-androsta-1, 13-dien-3 alpha-ol) anabolic androgenic steroids are abused. Anabolic steroids are typically injected. These substances have recently been placed on the Food and Drug Administration's list of controlled substances because of the adverse effects seen in athletes taking these drugs. Symptoms of anabolic steroid abuse include weight gain, irritability, major mood disturbance, personality disorders, and self- and other-directed aggressive behavior. Occasionally, anabolic steroid abuse has been associated with severe, aggressive criminal behavior, including homicide. Anabolic steroid abusers are more likely than nonabusers to also use alcohol, tobacco, marijuana, cocaine, hallucinogens, sedatives, opiates, amphetamines, and designer drugs. Medical complications of anabolic steroid abuse include liver neoplasms, gynecomastia, severe coronary artery disease leading to myocardial infarction, activation of the hemostatic system (which may contribute to acute vascular events), and renal cell carcinoma. In addition, a significant proportion of anabolic steroid abusers share needles, thus increasing the risk of HIV and hepatitis B transmission.

Detection of anabolic steroid abuse is most reliably accomplished by analysis of urine specimens using gas chromatography-mass spectrometry, or high-resolution mass spectrometry. Educational programs that emphasize adverse anabolic steroid effects, strength training alternatives to anabolic steroid abuse, and drug refusal role play may reduce established anabolic steroid abuse and reduce the number of nonabusers who begin to abuse anabolic steroids.

NICOTINE

Approximately 37% of the general population in the United States currently uses nicotine-containing products, with 30% of this group smoking cigarettes. Between 50% and 80% of persons who currently smoke are addicted to nicotine, as manifested by their smoking to avoid withdrawal symptoms, avoidance of situations where smoking is restricted, smoking more than intended, inability to quit smoking, and continuing to smoke despite having tobacco-related illnesses such as chronic obstructive lung disease or cancer. The addiction produced by nicotine is extremely difficult to treat, with long-term abstinence rates among smokers receiving treatment for nicotine addiction being the poorest of any drug of abuse. Most alcoholics and cocaine and heroin addicts who also smoke experience greater difficulty with smoking cessation than with achieving abstinence from other addicting substances.

Nicotine acutely produces both stimulant (increased alertness) and depressant (muscle relaxation) effects. Symptoms of nicotine withdrawal develop within 24 hours of cessation of nicotine use and include dysphoric or depressed mood, insomnia, irritability, anxiety, difficulty concentrating, restlessness, decreased heart rate, and increased appetite and weight gain. These symptoms peak within 1 to 4 days and last for 3 to 4 weeks. Tobacco use also increases the risk of lung, oral, and other cancers; chronic obstructive lung disease; ulcers; cardiovascular and cerebrovascular disease; and maternal and fetal complications, including intrauterine growth retardation.

There is evidence that at least part of the drive to use nicotine-containing products is to maintain a certain blood level of nicotine. Consistent with this, nicotine replacement therapies (nicotine gum or patch) appear to help with the first phase of treatment of nicotine addiction. However, although most nicotine users are able to achieve abstinence, within 6 months most resume smoking. There appears to be a small advantage of the nicotine patch over placebo that persists for 6 to 12 months. Abstinence rates at 12 months are typically in the range of only 20%. Efforts to improve these abstinence rates include combining nicotine replacement therapy with behavioral therapy. Antidepressant therapy may be helpful when smoking cessation is accompanied by depression.

ANXIETY DISORDERS

method of
NAOMI M. SIMON, M.D., and
MARK H. POLLACK, M.D.
Massachusetts General Hospital
Boston, Massachusetts

Anxiety is common in the medical setting. It may represent a transient response to concerns about medical illness, be a symptom of a medical syndrome, emerge as a side effect of medication, or be due to use of, or withdrawal from, alcohol or other abused substances (Table 1). Primary anxiety disorders may also be present in patients in the medical setting but may manifest primarily with somatic symptoms. Anxiety may worsen the presentation and experience of medical illness, increase utilization of medical services, decrease compliance with prescribed regimens, and be a significant source of distress and disability.

Although the common presence of anxiety or fear in the medical setting may lead to its dismissal as "normal," it is important to recognize pathologic anxiety. Pathologic anxiety is distinguished by four criteria: autonomous distress not clearly due to an external cause, high intensity of symptoms, persistence over time, and the development of harmful behavioral strategies (e.g., avoidance, compulsions) that impair function.

Anxiety disorders are among the most common psychiatric disorders in the general population, with almost one in four people in the United States experiencing pathologic anxiety over his or her lifetime, as reported by the National Comorbidity Survey. Patients with panic and other anxiety disorders typically present first to their primary care doctors, emergency rooms, or other medical settings; and many high utilizers of medical service have anxiety or affective disorders. Appropriate diagnosis and treatment are critical to optimize utilization of medical services and improve the patient's quality of life and overall outcome.

TABLE 1. **Common Medical Causes of Anxiety**

Medical Conditions	Substances
Cardiovascular and Respiratory	Intoxication
Arrhythmia	Amphetamines
Cardiac ischemia	Antidepressants
Congestive heart failure	Antiparkinsonian agents
Hypoxia (i.e., in COPD)	Caffeine
Pulmonary embolus	Chemotherapy
	Cocaine
Endocrine and Metabolic	Corticosteroids
Adrenal dysfunction	Digitalis
Acute intermittent porphyria	Neuroleptics
Electrolyte abnormalities	Sympathomimetics
Hyperparathyroidism	Theophylline
Hypoglycemia	Thyroid hormone
Pheochromocytoma	Withdrawal
Thyroid dysfunction	Alcohol
	Narcotics
Neurologic	Sedative hypnotics
Brain tumor	
Cerebral anoxia	
Delirium (toxic, metabolic, infectious)	
Epilepsy (especially complex partial seizures)	
Migraines	
Vestibular dysfunction	

Abbreviation: COPD = chronic obstructive pulmonary disease.

DIAGNOSIS AND ASSESSMENT

Diagnosis of anxious patients in the medical setting must include consideration of organic factors, reactive or situational distress, and primary psychiatric disorders. All patients should undergo a thorough medical evaluation, including history, and relevant physical and neurologic examination. A careful substance abuse history should be taken to consider both current abuse (e.g., caffeine, cocaine) and withdrawal (e.g., alcohol, benzodiazepines) as contributing factors. Prescribed medications must also be considered for their potential anxiogenic potential (e.g., bronchodilators). Although many medical and neurologic illnesses may underly or contribute to anxiety symptoms (see Table 1), the extent of the work-up varies by patient age, associated symptoms and health status, medical history, and the nature of the anxiety. Physical examination and laboratory studies should be targeted to the major locus of symptomatology (e.g., prominent respiratory or cardiac symptoms).

Several factors may help distinguish an organic anxiety syndrome (i.e., anxiety secondary to a medical illness or substance) from a primary anxiety disorder, including (1) onset of anxiety symptoms after age 35, (2) absence of personal or family history of anxiety disorders, (3) absence of childhood anxiety difficulties, (4) absence of life stressors precipitating or contributing to the anxiety symptoms, (5) absence of avoidance behavior, and (6) poor treatment response to anxiolytic medications. Any identified medical illness or organic factor should be treated, though associated anxiety symptoms may persist and require additional specific anxiolytic interventions.

PRIMARY ANXIETY DISORDERS

Primary anxiety disorders include adjustment disorder with anxiety, panic disorder with or without agoraphobia (see page 1147), generalized anxiety disorder, social phobia, specific phobia, obsessive compulsive disorder, post-traumatic stress disorder, simple phobias, and anxiety disorder not otherwise specified.

Adjustment Disorder with Anxiety

Reactive or situational anxiety, diagnosed in DSM-IV as Adjustment Disorder with Anxiety, involves nervousness or anxiety as a response to a situational stressor that occurs within three months of the onset of the stressor and causes clinically significant marked distress or impairment in social or occupational functioning.

Treatment of adjustment disorders may include psychosocial interventions, including provision of general support, psychotherapy, or specific environmental interventions targeted to the stressor (e.g., public assistance programs). Anxiety symptoms may also require symptomatic relief with anxiolytic or antidepressant medications. Although adjustment disorders are sometimes dismissed by clinicians and family members as expected reactions to distressing situations, symptomatic treatment may greatly improve the patient's quality of life and prevent the development of more severe symptomatology.

Panic Disorder (with or Without Agoraphobia)

Panic disorder is characterized by recurrent panic attacks, which initially may occur spontaneously or "out of the blue" and, over time, may develop in a number of agoraphobic situations (i.e, situations in which the patient has previously experienced a panic attack or one in which escape may be difficult or help not readily available). The symptoms associated with a panic attack usually peak within a few minutes and may last 30 minutes or more. They include a number of physical symptoms of autonomic arousal such as cardiac, respiratory, neurologic, and gastrointestinal. The patient may experience a sense of terror or fear associated with a panic attack, including concerns about dying, going crazy, or losing control. Behaviorally, the patient may feel the need to flee the setting in which the attack occurred to a more safe and familiar place or person. Agoraphobic situations include crowds, shopping malls, public transportation, bridges, tunnels, open spaces, or being at home alone. Panic disorder has its typical onset in adolescence through the third and fourth decade of life and tends to occur more frequently in women than in men. Panic disorder can be associated with marked emotional and physical disability and is associated with high rates of medical utilization, making it a critical disorder to recognize and treat in the medical setting.

Treatment (Table 2) includes the use of the antidepressants, particularly the serotonin reuptake inhibitors (SSRIs) (e.g., fluoxetine* [Prozac], paroxetine* [Paxil], or sertraline* [Zoloft]), tricyclic antidepressants (TCAs) (e.g., imipramine* [Tofranil]), and monoamine oxidase inhibitors (MAOIs) (e.g., phenelzine* [Nardil]), or high potency benzodiazepines (e.g., alprazolam [Xanax], clonazepam [Klonopin]). Cognitive-behavioral therapies are also effective.

*Not FDA approved for this indication.

Generalized Anxiety Disorder

Generalized anxiety disorder (GAD) is defined in DSM-IV as excessive anxiety or worry that is difficult to control and occurs disproportionate to any situational factors. It should be present for a majority of days over a 6-month period and is associated with fatigue, poor concentration, restlessness or inability to relax, irritability, muscle tension, and insomnia. Although generalized anxiety symptoms may fluctuate in response to life stressors, patients with GAD are described as persistent "worriers" in contrast to patients with more episodic attacks of panic disorder or situationally related phobic symptoms. GAD usually occurs co-morbid with other affective disorders. Clinicians should be particularly alert to the common presence of depressive symptoms in patients with generalized anxiety, as this would indicate the need for treatment with an antidepressant rather than with anxiolytics such as a benzodiazepine or buspirone alone.

Treatment (see Table 2) includes benzodiazepines, buspirone, antidepressants, and cognitive behavioral therapy.

Social Phobia

Social phobia is defined in DSM-IV by marked or persistent fear of embarassment or humiliation in response to situations in which the person is exposed to possible scrutiny by others. The social or performance situations nearly always bring on anxiety and possibly situational panic attacks, resulting in avoidance or marked distress that interferes with social or occupational function. Social phobia may be generalized to many social situations (i.e., meeting new people, speaking to authority figures) or occur solely in response to performance situations such as public speaking. Although "performance anxiety" is common, symptoms occurring in these situations must be intensely distressing or cause impairment to warrant a diagnosis of social phobia. Social phobia may be diagnosed in children and often presents initially in adolescence, with persistence of symptoms into adulthood.

Treatment (see Table 2) includes high potency benzodiazepines (e.g., clonazepam), SSRIs, MAOIs, beta blockers, and cognitive behavioral therapy. MAOIs have typically been used for social phobia and are generally more effective than the tricyclics (e.g., imipramine) but, given ease of use, side effect profile, and efficacy, SSRIs are now first-line pharmacotherapy. Beta blockers are useful for performance anxiety but are not as effective for the generalized type of social phobia.

Specific Phobia

DSM-IV differentiates specific phobias from less significant, though more common fears, by the excessive distress and impairment associated with the anxious response to the phobic stimulus (i.e., heights, blood/injection, airplanes, animals). Phobias frequently begin in childhood or during the middle twenties varying by type, or may occur at any time in response to a traumatic event (e.g., being attacked by a dog). Predisposing factors include related

*Not FDA approved for this indication.

TABLE 2. **Standard Medication Treatment for Anxiety Disorders**

Medication	Initial Dose (mg)	Dose Range (mg)	Main Limitations	Indication
SSRIs				
Fluoxetine (Prozac)	5–10	10–80	SSRI side effects	PDAG, OCD,* PTSD, SP, GAD
Sertraline (Zoloft)	25	25–200	SSRI side effects	PDAG,* OCD,* PTSD, SP, GAD
Paroxetine (Paxil)	10	10–50	Sedation, SSRI side effects	PDAG,* OCD,* PTSD, SP, GAD
Fluvoxamine (Luvox)	50	50–300	SSRI side effects	PDAG, OCD,* PTSD, SP, GAD
TCAs				
Clomipramine (Anafranil)	25	25–250	Weight gain, sedation, TCA side effects	OCD,* PTSD, GAD, PDAG, ?SP
e.g., Desipramine (Norpramin) Imipramine (Tofranil)	10–25	150–300	TCA side effects, jitteriness	GAD, PTSD, PDAG, ?SP
MAOIs				
e.g., Phenelzine (Nardil)	15–30	45–90	Drug and diet interactions, MAOI side effects	OCD, PTSD, SP, PDAG, ?GAD
Novel Antidepressants				
Venlafaxine (Effexor)	37.5	75–300	Jitteriness, GI distress	PDAG, ?GAD, ?PTSD, ?SP, ?OCD
Nefazodone (Serzone)	50	300–550	Sedation, GI distress	?PDAG, GAD, ?OCD, ?PTSD, ?SP
Buspirone (BuSpar)	5 tid	15–60/d	Dysphoria	GAD*
Beta Blockers				
e.g., propranolol (Inderal)	10–20	10–160/d	Depression, sedation	SP (esp. performance), PDAG (adj), GAD (adj)
Benzodiazepines				
Alprazolam (Xanax)	0.25 qid	2–10/d	Memory impairment, abuse risk, sedation discontinuation difficulties, interdose anxiety (shorter acting agents)	PDAG,* PTSD, GAD, SP, ?PS
Clonazepam (Klonopin)	0.25 qhs	1–5/d		PDAG,* PTSD, GAD, SP
Lorazepam (Ativan)	0.5 tid	3–12/d		GAD, SP, PS, PDAG

*FDA approved.
Abbreviations: GAD = generalized anxiety disorder; PDAG = panic disorder and agoraphobia; PTSD = post-traumatic stress disorder; SP = social phobia; PS = specific phobia; BDZ = benzodiazepine; MAOI = monoamine oxidase inhibitor; SSRI = serotonin reuptake inhibitor; TCA = tricyclic antidepressant; adj = adjunctive.

traumatic events, unexpected panic attacks associated with the phobic stimulus, or transmission of information by media or from others (i.e., dramatic newspaper reports or parental warnings). In addition, there may be familial transmission by type of phobia.

Although benzodiazepines may be used on an as needed basis to help patients tolerate the feared stimulus on a short-term basis, behavior therapy (i.e., exposure and desensitization) is generally more definitive treatment.

Obsessive-Compulsive Disorder

Obsessive-compulsive disorder (OCD) is characterized by persistent, intrusive, anxiety provoking thoughts or images (obsessions) (e.g., contamination fears) and/or driven, repetitive behaviors (compulsions) that are aimed at decreasing anxiety (e.g., handwashing, checking). The obsessions or compulsions must cause significant distress, take more than 1 hour daily, or significantly interfere with the patient's normal functioning to warrant a diagnosis of OCD. OCD is typically chronic with onset in childhood or adolescence for males and during the twenties for females. OCD occurs in 1 to 2% of the population and has been associated with Tourette's syndrome and other tic disorders.

Treatment for OCD includes serotonergic antidepressants (i.e., SSRIs), clomipramine (Anafranil), and cognitive-behavioral therapy, including exposure and response prevention to extinguish obsessive thoughts and compulsive behaviors.

Post-traumatic Stress Disorder

To meet DSM-IV criteria, patients with post-traumatic stress disorder (PTSD) must have experienced an event involving serious injury or death, or a threat to physical integrity, to which they responded with fear, helplessness, or horror. Traumatic events may vary from a single disaster (i.e., earthquake) to more chronic, repetitive traumas (e.g., combat, childhood physical abuse). Patients persistently re-experience the trauma in some way (e.g., nightmares, flashbacks), and experience marked physiologic arousal or psychologic distress to cues that remind them of the traumatic event. In addition, they have at least three psychologic symptoms, including numbing, detachment, decreased pleasure and interest, avoidance of reminders of the trauma, amnesia for the trauma, or a sense of a foreshortened future, and at least two symptoms of hyperarousal, including insomnia, irritable outbursts, poor concentration, hypervigilance, and easy startle. This syndrome may be acute or chronic and is quite heterogeneous in presentation. For example, some patients show more prominent depressive symptoms and withdrawal, whereas others are more angry, agitated, and suspicious.

Symptoms usually present within 3 months of the trauma but may have a delayed onset. Some patients develop chronic symptoms, although about half remit within 3 months. Population assessments have reported the lifetime incidence of PTSD ranging from 1 to 14%, but rates are higher in populations exposed to serious trauma (e.g., disaster victims, combat veterans).

Pharmacologic treatment is generally directed at relief of predominant symptoms (i.e., antidepressants for depression or anxiety, anticonvulsants for agitation). The Food and Drug Administration has not indicated a specific medication for PTSD. SSRIs are often used because of their broad spectrum of activity against a range of mood, anxiety, and impulsive symptoms. Psychotherapy, including cognitive behavioral therapy, may also be helpful.

TREATMENT CONSIDERATIONS

Explanation of the diagnosis and education provided in a supportive, informative manner can in itself be quite reassuring for many patients. Therapeutic options, including pharmacotherapies and cognitive behavioral therapy, should be reviewed. Patients started on medication should be followed closely initially in person and/or by telephone. Treatment with antidepressants or benzodiazepines should be initiated with low dose and gradually titrated upward tc minimize side effects and maximize compliance. Patients with complex symptoms (often patients with PTSD, OCD, or co-morbidity) or poor initial response to medication may benefit from psychiatric referral. Anxious patients should be carefully observed for the development or presence of depressive symptoms, necessitating the administration of an antidepressant to avoid the common scenario of incomplete treatment with a benzodiazepine alone.

SSRIs are now used as first-line therapy for many anxiety disorders because of their broad spectrum of activity against most mood and anxiety disorders and their relatively favorable side effect profile. SSRIs are better tolerated than older classes of antidepressants (e.g., tricyclic antidepressants [TCAs]), yet may be associated with transient or persistent adverse effects, including nausea, gastrointestinal distress, headaches, sexual dysfunction, and sleep disturbance. SSRIs are usually administered in the morning to minimize insomnia, with the exception of paroxetine, which may be more sedating. Patients with anxiety disorders may experience an initial increase in anxiety when SSRIs are initiated. To minimize this, patients initially receive lower doses (e.g., 5 to 10 mg fluoxetine*), 25 mg sertraline*, 10 mg paroxetine*, 25 mg fluvoxamine [Luvox]) than are indicated for depression, but generally acclimate to dose increases within a week. Therapeutic levels appear similar to those for depression, although higher doses (e.g., fluoxetine 60 to 80 mg/d) may be necessary for patients with OCD and PTSD. Another technique to reduce initial increased anxiety associated with antidepressants in anxious patients is coadministration of benzodiazepines (e.g., lorazepam [Ativan], clonazepam). Benzodiazepines also provide more rapid anxiolysis during the 2- to 6-week therapeutic lag for SSRI effects. For some patients, benzodiazepines may be tapered after a few weeks when the antidepressant becomes effective, but many patients benefit from combined treatment without significant adverse effects.

*Not FDA approved for this indication.

Other newer agents, including venlafaxine* (Effexor), nefazodone* (Serzone), and mirtazapine* (Remeron), appear to be effective for anxious patients in clinical practice, although there is relatively little systematic data for these indications. Venlafaxine and nefazodone may cause jitteriness or anxiety during treatment initiation, and thus, as with the SSRIs, should be initiated at low doses (i.e., venlafaxine, 18.75 to 25 mg per day, nefazodone 50 mg per day) with gradual titration to therapeutic levels. Limited data suggest that buproprion and trazodone may not be as reliably anxiolytic as other antidepressants.

Other antidepressants, such as the TCAs and MAOIs, may be useful but have a more aversive side effect profile than the newer agents. TCAs (i.e., desipramine* [Norpramin], imipramine*) are effective for panic disorder and generalized anxiety disorder, but less so for social phobia, and are, with the exception of clomipramine, ineffective for OCD. The TCAs are also effective for depressive and anxiety symptoms associated with PTSD. Side effects of the TCAs include anticholinergic effects (e.g., dry mouth, constipation), cardiac conduction disturbance, orthostatic hypotension, weight gain, and sexual dysfunction. In addition, the TCAs, unlike the SSRIs, may be fatal in overdose. MAOIs (i.e., phenelzine* [Nardil] and tranylcypromine* [Parnate]) are broadly effective for the treatment of panic disorder, social phobia, agoraphobia, OCD, PTSD, generalized anxiety, and depression. The MAOIs are less likely to cause increased anxiety at treatment initiation than are the other antidepressants, but over time may be associated with a variety of side effects, including weight gain, insomnia, edema, sexual dysfunction, and myoclonus. In addition, patients on MAOIs must maintain a strict diet free of tyramine and avoid sympathomimetic agents (e.g., pseudoephedrine) to prevent hypertensive reactions. In addition, all physicians should be aware that MAOI-treated patients should not receive meperidine (Demerol) because of a potentially fatal interaction. Because of the higher risks associated with their use, the MAOIs are generally reserved for patients who are refractory to other interventions and are typically prescribed by psychiatrists or others experienced in their use.

Because many anxiety disorders are effectively treated with either antidepressants or benzodiazepines, the choice of initial medication involves consideration of the risks and benefits of each class of agents. Benzodiazepines act more rapidly than antidepressants, but carry a greater abuse potential, and may cause sedation, psychomotor impairment, ataxia, physical dependence, and disinhibition. They should generally be avoided in patients with organic brain impairment; elderly patients in general should be dosed cautiously and are at increased risk for adverse effects, including falls, disinhibition, and oversedation. Respiratory depression is rare, but is a concern in overdose, when benzodiazepines are combined with alcohol or other sedatives, and in patients

*Not FDA approved for this indication.

with chronic obstructive pulmonary disease or sleep apnea. Depression, frequently co-morbid with anxiety disorders, is usually poorly responsive and may be worsened by benzodiazepines.

Pharmacokinetic properties may be used to guide benzodiazepine selection. All benzodiazepines are effective for generalized anxiety and insomnia; however, panic disorder may be more responsive to high potency benzodiazepines (e.g., alprazolam, clonazepam). Rapid-onset, short-acting agents (e.g., alprazolam) can provide acute anxiolysis, but may have higher addictive potential, require frequent dosing, and may be associated with interdose rebound anxiety. Longer acting agents (e.g., clonazepam) provide more consistent anxiolysis and require less frequent dosing. A short-acting agent free of liver metabolites (e.g., lorazepam) can minimize drug accumulation and oversedation, particularly in the medically ill. Benzodiazepines should be initiated at low doses (e.g., alprazolom, 0.5 mg two to three times daily; clonazepam, 0.25 to 0.5 mg at bedtime) to minimize initial sedation and increased every 3 to 4 days as tolerated until therapeutic effects are achieved. Although tolerance to the anxiolytic effects of benzodiazepines is rare, patients do become physically dependent after being maintained on benzodiazepines for a few weeks. Benzodiazepine discontinuation may be difficult, and the drug should be tapered slowly to minimize rebound or withdrawal symptoms.

Buspirone (BuSpar) is an azapirone anxiolytic with effects on serotonin and dopamine receptors. As a nonbenzodiazepine, it lacks sedative properties and abuse potential. It is primarily indicated in generalized anxiety disorder and is not effective alone for the treatment of panic disorder. Experience with buspirone in clinical practice has been variably effective, particularly in patients with prior exposure to benzodiazepines. It is not yet clear if this is due to inadequate dosing or to the lag time (several weeks) for therapeutic response.

Beta blockers are primarily indicated for "performance anxiety," (e.g., propranolol [Inderal], 10 to 40 mg per day as needed 1 to 2 hours before a performance situation) and may reduce peripheral autonomic symptoms of anxiety. They are poorly effective in preventing cognitive and affective symptoms (e.g., worry or fear) associated with anxiety, although they may be useful adjunctively to reduce physical symptoms of arousal. Atenolol (Tenormin), 25 to 100 mg per day, is also effective and may cause fewer side effects to the central nervous system, such as dysphoria and fatigue, than propranolol because it is less lipophilic.

BULIMIA NERVOSA

method of
DAVID C. JIMERSON, M.D.
Beth Israel Deaconess Medical Center and Harvard Medical School
Boston, Massachusetts

Bulimia nervosa, which is frequently associated with depression and other psychiatric disorders, can result in psychosocial difficulties and significant medical complications. Some patients show marked improvement with short-term treatments, while others may have a chronic course in spite of intensive therapeutic interventions. Initial patient assessment in a primary care setting is generally followed by consultation with a mental health professional regarding a more detailed psychiatric evaluation and treatment planning.

CLINICAL CHARACTERISTICS

Bulimia nervosa is a psychiatric disorder characterized by recurrent binge eating episodes. In addition, patients manifest preoccupation with body shape and weight, which unduly influences their self-evaluation and self-esteem, and employ stringent compensatory weight control measures. Bulimia nervosa was identified as a syndrome distinct from anorexia nervosa in the late 1970s. Table 1 summarizes current diagnostic criteria for bulimia nervosa based on the *Diagnostic and Statistical Manual of Mental Disorders*, Fourth Edition (DSM-IV), published by the American Psychiatric Association in 1994.

Characteristic differences between bulimia nervosa and

TABLE 1. **DSM-IV Criteria for Bulimia Nervosa**

A. Recurrent episodes of binge eating. An episode of binge eating is characterized by both of the following:
   (1) eating, in a discrete period of time (e.g., within any 2-hour period), an amount of food that is definitely larger than most people would eat during a similar period of time and under similar circumstances
   (2) a sense of lack of control over eating during the episode (e.g., a feeling that one cannot stop eating or control what or how much one is eating)
B. Recurrent inappropriate compensatory behavior in order to prevent weight gain, such as self-induced vomiting; misuse of laxatives, diuretics, enemas or other medications; fasting; or excessive exercise.
C. The binge eating and inappropriate compensatory behaviors both occur, on average, at least twice a week for 3 months.
D. Self-evaluation is unduly influenced by body shape and weight.
E. The disturbance does not occur exclusively during episodes of Anorexia Nervosa.

Specify type:
   Purging Type: during the current episode of Bulimia Nervosa, the person has regularly engaged in self-induced vomiting or the misuse of laxatives, diuretics or enemas
   Non-purging Type: during the current episode of Bulimia Nervosa, the person has used other inappropriate compensatory behaviors, such as fasting or excessive exercise, but has not regularly engaged in self-induced vomiting or the misuse of laxatives, diuretics or enemas

anorexia nervosa are apparent by comparing the DSM-IV criteria for the disorders (Tables 1 and 2). In contrast to individuals with anorexia nervosa, patients with bulimia nervosa are generally in a normal weight range, although recurrent fluctuations in weight are frequently reported. A history of previous low-weight episodes of anorexia nervosa is not uncommon. It should be noted that recurrent binge eating is not unique to bulimia nervosa, in that approximately half of low-weight patients with anorexia nervosa report binge eating or purging episodes (i.e., DSM-IV Binge-Eating/Purging Type). Additionally, up to a third of obese individuals in some treatment settings may have recurrent binge eating associated with the recently described syndrome of binge eating disorder.

Epidemiologic surveys indicate that bulimia nervosa has a typical age of onset of 18 years. The prevalence in adolescent and young adult women is approximately 2%, while in young men the disorder is thought to be only approximately one tenth as frequent.

Specific etiologic factors in bulimia nervosa have not been identified, although family and twin studies suggest the presence of biologic and environmental risk factors. For many patients, the onset of the disorder is preceded by a history of dieting behavior. Psychosocial stressors, as well as biologic changes in neurotransmitter systems modulating mood and ingestive behaviors, are likely to play a role. For example, recent clinical investigations suggest that decreased efficiency in central nervous system serotonin function may contribute to diminished postingestive satiety and mood fluctuations in bulimia.

CLINICAL ASSESSMENT

Symptom Patterns. Because of the stigma and shame associated with eating disorders, patients are often reluctant to reveal the presence or extent of symptoms. Additionally, symptoms tend to vary over time and patients may have difficulty estimating average frequency of binge eating and purging behaviors. It is often useful for the clinician to inquire about examples of typical binge eating episodes, e.g., duration of a binge, and type and quantity of foods consumed. Patterns of dieting, fasting, and exercise should be reviewed. Pertinent information regarding methods of purging includes the extent to which the patient uses self-induced vomiting, laxatives, diuretics, or syrup of ipecac. Additional informative aspects of symptom history include age of onset of dieting, binge eating, and purging behaviors; desired weight; previous high and low adult weight; and recent changes in body weight. Previous treatments for eating disorder symptoms and outcome should be noted, including the nature of any past psychotherapy or nutritional counseling, hospitalization, and psychopharmacologic treatments.

Given that bulimia nervosa is associated with an increased prevalence of other serious psychiatric disorders, it is useful to inquire specifically regarding current and past symptoms of depression, substance use disorders, obsessive-compulsive disorder and other anxiety disorders, and DSM-IV Axis II personality disorders. Any current or past suicidal ideation should be assessed with regard to patient safety. In general, co-occurrence of other major psychiatric symptomatology is likely to significantly influence initial treatment approaches.

Psychosocial and Family History. The initial evaluation includes an assessment of psychosocial adjustment and resources at home, school, and work. Factors associated with an increase or decrease in symptom frequency should be noted (e.g., examination periods or school vacations). Particularly for younger patients, it is useful to assess family awareness and attitudes toward the eating disorder. Studies have shown an increased frequency of eating disorders as well as mood disorders in family members of patients with bulimia nervosa. Family history of obesity and other medical disorders should be reviewed.

Medical History. Patients with bulimia nervosa may report symptoms of lethargy associated with poor nutrition or anemia. Symptoms potentially related to purging behaviors include dehydration and lightheadedness, constipation or diarrhea, or blood-tinged vomitus. Irregular menstrual cycles or secondary amenorrhea is experienced by some female patients, although the possibility of unanticipated pregnancy should be considered in the context of a recently missed menstrual period.

It is important to assess whether abnormal eating patterns or marked weight fluctuations may be related to an occult medical disorder. Rare medical or neurologic disorders (e.g., Klein-Levin syndrome) may contribute to appetite dysregulation. Additionally, the presence of an eating disorder may complicate treatment of another medical disorder, such as diabetes, that involves specific dietary guidelines.

Physical Examination. A full physical examination is important for identifying physiologic alterations associated with bulimia nervosa, as well as other medical problems that may influence the medical management of the patient. As noted, patients with bulimia nervosa are typically in a normal weight range for height. Conversely, a diagnosis of anorexia should be considered for a young woman with symptoms of an eating disorder, amenorrhea, and a body mass index (BMI) of less than approximately 18.5 kg per m^2. Similar considerations apply to a male patient with unexplained weight loss. Consumption of a low-calorie diet with attendant weight loss may contribute to bradycardia, while exaggerated orthostatic pulse and blood pressure changes may reflect dehydration. Examination of the

TABLE 2. **DSM-IV Criteria for Anorexia Nervosa**

A. Refusal to maintain body weight at or above a minimally normal weight for age and height (e.g., weight loss leading to maintenance of body weight less than 85% of that expected; or failure to make expected weight gain during period of growth, leading to body weight less than 85% of that expected).
B. Intense fear of gaining weight or becoming fat, even though underweight.
C. Disturbance in the way in which one's body weight or shape is experienced, undue influence of body shape and weight on self-evaluation, or denial of the seriousness of current low body weight.
D. In postmenarcheal females, amenorrhea, i.e., the absence of at least three consecutive menstrual cycles. (A woman is considered to have amenorrhea if her periods occur only following hormone, e.g., estrogen, administration.)

Specify type:

Restricting Type: during the episode of Anorexia Nervosa, the person has not regularly engaged in binge-eating or purging behavior (i.e., self-induced vomiting or the misuse of laxatives, diuretics or enemas).

Binge-Eating/Purging Type: during the current episode of Anorexia Nervosa, the person has regularly engaged in binge-eating or purging behavior (i.e., self-induced vomiting or the misuse of laxatives, diuretics or enemas).

mouth may reveal subtle erosion of the dental enamel from recurrent vomiting. Calluses on the dorsal surface of the hands can result from manually induced vomiting.

Laboratory Assessment. The extent of the initial laboratory assessment should be based on current symptoms, medical history, physical examination, and treatment setting (e.g., outpatient versus inpatient). A complete blood count (CBC) may reflect an anemia related to nutritional deficiency. Serum electrolyte abnormalities may occur in approximately 25% of outpatients with bulimia nervosa, depending on symptom severity and nutritional status. Hypokalemia can have serious adverse effects on cardiac conduction. Binge eating with associated purging practices and variations in fluid intake can result in hypochloremia, hyponatremia, and elevated or decreased serum bicarbonate. Other common tests may include serum BUN/creatinine levels and urinalysis. An electrocardiogram may help to detect abnormalities in cardiac rhythm including bradycardia, as well as signs of hypokalemia or ipecac-induced myopathy.

More comprehensive laboratory testing is generally considered for the severely symptomatic or significantly malnourished patient. Additional serum chemistry measurements to be considered include calcium, magnesium, phosphorus, and liver function tests. Hyperamylasemia, with elevation of the salivary isoenzyme, has been reported in some patients. Endocrine hormone changes can include decreased thyroid hormone levels, most likely to reflect effects of prolonged dieting. Serum cortisol may be elevated as a consequence of weight loss or in association with concurrent depression. More detailed studies related to menstrual abnormalities have shown variability in estrogen and progesterone regulation. Although brain imaging and bone mineral density studies are usually not conducted, abnormalities can be anticipated in the context of poor nutrition.

TREATMENT CONSIDERATIONS

Psychotherapy

Controlled trials have demonstrated that cognitive behavioral therapy or interpersonal therapy results in a significant decrease in frequency of binge eating and purging symptoms for a majority of patients with bulimia nervosa. Patients participating in these studies often report having approximately ten episodes of binge eating per week at assessment, and typically achieve a decrease of 60 to 80% in symptom frequency by the end of treatment. Controlled clinical trials have generally been based on detailed treatment manuals, with duration ranging from 16 to 20 weeks.

Cognitive behavioral therapy for bulimia nervosa focuses on restructuring of cognitions related to eating behavior and body shape and weight. Interventions are employed to interrupt binge eating and purging patterns, and efforts are made to restructure beliefs, attitudes, and values that maintain the disorder. Common components include self-monitoring, dietary intake journals, education related to eating patterns and body weight, introduction of problem-solving techniques, and response prevention approaches. Interpersonal therapy focuses more specifically on improved relationships in family, social, school, and work settings.

In addition to individual treatment, group psychotherapy may also be beneficial. Psychodynamically oriented therapy may be helpful in exploring the relationship among current psychosocial stresses, previous life experiences, and symptoms of an eating disorder, although outcome data from controlled trials are limited.

There has been recent interest in developing treatment algorithms based on progressive hierarchical or "stepped care" approaches. Thus, for a patient with a low frequency of binge eating and purging behaviors, relatively recent onset of symptoms with no previous treatment interventions, and minimal psychiatric comorbidity, there may be significant improvement with less intensive outpatient approaches such as psychoeducational interventions and nutritional counseling. Given that there has been limited research on selection criteria for these approaches, for most patients an initial trial of short-term psychotherapy is recommended.

Psychopharmacology

Controlled trials have shown that antidepressant medications decrease symptoms in bulimia nervosa. In some of the larger studies, evaluation of the selective serotonin reuptake inhibitor fluoxetine (Prozac) showed significant efficacy at a dose of 60 mg per day, administered in the morning, in trials of 8 to 16 weeks in moderate to severe bulimia nervosa. Controlled trials with other antidepressant medications such as desipramine have shown significant decreases in symptom frequency, although in general these studies have included smaller numbers of patients and have been of relatively short duration (e.g., 8 weeks). Product labeling based on Food and Drug Administration (FDA) review provides an important source of updated information on medication indications, recommended dosage, and side effects.

Indications favoring early treatment with an antidepressant medication include concurrent depression, obsessive-compulsive disorder, and presence of symptoms not previously responsive to psychotherapy. It is of note that in patients with concurrent depression, improvement in bulimic symptoms is not necessarily correlated with improvement in depressive symptoms. Patients with eating disorders may be at increased risk for side effects of antidepressants and other medications. Patients should be given a detailed explanation of potential medication-related side effects.

Although controlled trials have generally shown significant decreases in frequency of binge eating and self-induced vomiting during administration of antidepressant medications, only a minority of patients achieved complete absence of symptoms during short-term treatment. Treatment nonresponse needs to be evaluated on an individualized basis. An important first step is to assess the possibility of poor compliance with the prescribed medication protocol. It is important to make sure that the patient is not taking the medication immediately prior to episodes of self-induced vomiting. Switching to a different class of antidepressants may be useful, although the status of the medication should be reviewed with respect to potential side effects, and allowance should be made for appropriate dose reduction or discontinuation of one medication before switching to another. There are few published data on addition of a second medication to potentiate antidepressant treatment response in bulimia nervosa. Case reports and preliminary open trials suggest that other classes of medications may be helpful in some patients, but these more experimental interventions should be evaluated on an individualized basis by a psychopharmacologist experienced in the treatment of eating disorders.

Inpatient/Day Hospital

Hospitalization is usually reserved for the severely symptomatic patient with medical problems requiring intensive monitoring, active suicidal ideation, or impaired capacity for self care. Patients may benefit from a specialized inpatient treatment program that uses cognitive and behavioral protocols, with monitoring for self-induced vomiting and other covert purging behaviors. Another option for the severely symptomatic patient is referral to a day treatment program, which provides a structured but less restrictive setting than inpatient care. Staff are available to monitor symptomatic behaviors (e.g., during group meals), and to initiate cognitive, behavioral, and other psychotherapeutic interventions.

Follow-Up Studies

Some evidence suggests that approximately one third of patients treated for more severe symptoms of bulimia nervosa experience one or more symptomatic relapses. The limited data available indicate that one half or more of patients are in full remission from bulimia nervosa when contacted 3 to 10 years following treatment, while 10 to 15% still meet criteria for the disorder. There is preliminary evidence that patients with the Purging Type of the disorder may have a more complicated course than patients with the Non-purging Type.

Consultation and Collaborative Care

Identification of bulimia nervosa in a primary care setting is often enhanced by the clinician's alertness to a patient's preoccupation with weight and shape. The assessment requires a careful psychiatric and medical evaluation. Given the complexity of symptom patterns, likelihood of psychiatric comorbidity, and specialized nature of current treatment approaches, consultation with a mental health professional is generally recommended. Although some patients achieve a sustained response following short-term intervention, individuals with more severe symptoms and concurrent psychiatric disorders may require extended treatment. Patient compliance with treatment is enhanced by effective communication and collaboration among members of the multidisciplinary caregiving team.

DELIRIUM

method of
SUE LEVKOFF, Sc.D.
Harvard Medical School
Boston, Massachusetts

Although the diagnostic criteria for delirium have changed over the years, the core features have remained relatively unchanged. Diagnostic criteria, as identified in the Diagnostic and Statistical Manual of Mental Disorders, Fourth Edition (DSM-IV), include (1) disturbance of consciousness (i.e., reduced clarity of awareness of the environment) with reduced ability to focus, sustain, or shift attention; (2) a change in cognition (such as memory deficit, disorientation, language disturbance) or the development of a perceptual disturbance that is not better accounted for by a pre-existing, established, or evolving dementia; (3) rapid onset (usually hours to days) and fluctuations during the course of a day; and (4) evidence from the history, physical examination, or laboratory findings that the disturbance is caused by the direct physiologic consequences of a general medical condition.

Prevalence rates of delirium in hospitalized elderly medical patients range from 10 to 30%, with incidence rates ranging from 4 to 55%. As the numbers of elderly individuals increase, clinicians can expect to encounter delirium more frequently. Clinicians are not typically well-trained in the diagnosis, work-up, and management of delirium. This omission in training is significant, given that substantial research has documented the poor clinical outcomes associated with the syndrome, including longer hospital lengths of stay, increased risk of institutionalization upon discharge, and poorer physical function up to 6 months post–hospital discharge. Moreover, the fact that large numbers of hospitalized patients have been found to be discharged with symptoms of delirium that persist for up to 6 months past hospital discharge has implications for discharge planners, who are responsible for ensuring a safe environment for patients on their return home from hospital.

CLINICAL FEATURES

Delirium has several subtypes: the hyperactive variant, the hypoactive variant, and the mixed variant, which demonstrates features of both clinical subtypes. Research has found no differences among these groups with respect to age, sex, or presence of dementia. It is important that clinicians recognize these different subtypes, because the hyperactive patient who develops the florid subtype with its accompanying psychomotor overactivity, hyperresponsiveness to stimuli, hallucinations, fear, and irritability is more likely to be diagnosed and treated than the hypoactive patient with reduced levels of psychomotor activity, alertness, and vigilance.

While studies of the phenomenology of delirium in the elderly do not exist, it is believed that the core features of the syndrome are consistent across all age groups. Because of age-related biologic changes in the central nervous system, the elderly have a reduced reserve capacity and reduced ability to compensate for insult to homeostasis. As a result, the elderly brain is likely to show impaired function in response to stress. The symptoms of delirium can develop more insidiously in the elderly because the added impairment is superimposed on pre-existing limitations, and symptoms typically subside more slowly following treatment.

CLINICAL COURSE

The onset of delirium is rapid and occurs over a few hours or days. Often a patient first experiences symptoms during the night, after waking from a dream. The patient may become confused, inattentive, and disoriented. The patient's awareness of his or her surroundings and ability to communicate can become extremely impaired. Many patients develop olfactory and gustatory hallucinations and paranoid delusional ideas. Often, patients experience reversal of sleep patterns, being drowsy and difficult to arouse during the day and confused and agitated during the night. While it has generally been assumed that delirium resolves within 1 to 2 weeks, research has found that symptoms can persist for up to 6 months after hospital discharge.

DIAGNOSTIC WORK-UP

Because delirium often has multiple etiologies, the work-up should include a thorough search for all potential contributing factors. Knowledge of a patient's baseline cognitive function is crucial, as the more impaired the patient, the fewer the stressors needed to precipitate delirium. Table 1 provides an overview of the known contributing factors. Medications are the most common reversible causes of delirium, with benzodiazepines, narcotics, and medications with anticholinergic side effects the most common offenders. A careful review of all medications, including both prescription and nonprescription drugs, and attention to recent additions, dose changes, and discontinuations is important. A work-up should include a careful history with the patient (when possible) and family, physical examination (including the Mini-Mental Status Examination), and medication review. Additional diagnostic testing may be necessary, depending on findings from the initial work-ups: for example, laboratory-examination for complete blood count (CBC), electrolytes, glucose, calcium, magnesium, phosphate, renal function, hepatic function, and oxygen saturation; infection work-up (urinalysis, chest film, additional cultures); and selected additional testing (dementia profile, serum drug levels, toxicology, arterial blood gases, electrocardiogram, brain imaging, cerebrospinal fluid).

Table 2 demonstrates how important knowledge of a patient's prior cognitive status is to distinguish delirium from dementia. The central diagnostic feature of delirium is inattention, which can be assessed formally by forward and backward digit span or reciting the months of the year backwards. Additional key diagnostic elements for delirium are an abnormal level of consciousness (comatose, drowsy, hyperalert) and disorganized thinking (rambling, incoherent speech), which should be evident from taking a basic history. Another feature is a fluctuating course over minutes to hours. An acutely ill, hospitalized elderly patient with an acute change in mental status, inattention, and disorganized thinking or an abnormal level of consciousness with fluctuations almost certainly has delirium. The Confusion Assessment Method (CAM) is an easy-to-use diagnostic algorithm for clinicians (Table 3).

TABLE 1. **Contributing Factors in Delirium**

Therapeutic drug intoxication/withdrawal
Psychoactive drugs
Toxic levels of drugs
Any drug with appropriate time course of initiation, change, withdrawal
Disorders of inadequate cerebral oxygenation
Hypoxia
Anemia
Hypotension or low cardiac output
Arteriovenous shunting states (sepsis)
Metabolic disorders
Hypo/hypervolemia
Electrolyte disorders (especially hyponatremia, hypercalcemia)
Glucose disorders
Hypercapnia
Renal/hepatic failure
Infection and/or fever
Pneumonia
Urinary tract infection
Soft tissue infections
Others
Cardiovascular disorders
Congestive heart failure
Arrhythmia
Acute myocardial infarction
Brain disorders
Stroke
Trauma
Infection
Tumors (primary and metastatic)
Severe pain
Postoperative states
Terminal states
Sensory deprivation/alteration
Blindness and/or deafness
Severe isolation
Environmental change/loss of cues
Alcohol intoxication/withdrawal
Urinary retention/fecal impaction

MANAGEMENT

Management of the delirious patient requires a thorough search for and correction of all contributing factors. While some factors, such as an offending medication, can be rectified immediately, others, such as underlying medical problems, may take longer to correct. Even with prompt reversal of contributing factors, rapid resolution of delirium does not always occur, due to the existence of new exacerbants.

Since delirium may not reverse quickly even with appropriate intervention, delirious patients should be managed by an interdisciplinary team of physi-

TABLE 2. **Delirium Versus Dementia**

Delirium	Dementia
Develops abruptly	Develops slowly
Reversible	Progressive
Short duration	Present for many months or years
Fluctuating consciousness	Rarely altered consciousness
Precise time of onset	Uncertain date of onset

TABLE 3. **Confusion Assessment Method (CAM) Diagnostic Algorithm**

Feature 1: Acute Onset and Fluctuating Course

This feature is usually observed by a family member or nurse and is shown by positive responses to the following questions: Is there evidence of an acute change in mental status from the patient's baseline? Did the (abnormal) behavior fluctuate during the day (that is, tend to come and go) or increase and decrease in severity?

Feature 2: Inattention

This feature is shown by a positive response to the following question: Did the patient have difficulty focusing attention (for example, being easily distracted) or have difficulty keeping track of what was being said?

Feature 3: Disorganized Thinking

This feature is shown by a positive response to the following question: Was the patient's thinking disorganized or incoherent, such as rambling or irrelevant conversation, unclear or illogical flow of ideas, or unpredictable switching from subject to subject?

Feature 4: Altered Level of Consciousness

This feature is shown by any answer other than "alert" to the following question: Overall, how would you rate this patient's level of consciousness? (alert [normal], vigilant [hyperalert], lethargic [drowsy, easily aroused], stupor [difficult to arouse], or coma [unarousable].

The diagnosis of delirium by CAM requires the presence of features 1, 2, and either 3 or 4.

From Inouye SK, Viscoli CM, Horwitz RI, et al: Clarifying confusion: The confusion assessment method. Ann Intern Med *113*:941–948, 1990.

cians, nurses, family members, and anyone else who comes into contact with the patient. Table 4 lists the delirious patient's vulnerabilities and proposes management strategies.

The best way to manage delirium is to prevent it. Very old patients (>80 years of age); patients with sensory, cognitive, and functional impairments; and those with multiple chronic medical problems and medications are at greatest risk. Especially in these high-risk patients, clinicians must attempt to prevent problems that precipitate delirium by recognizing and treating illnesses early, minimizing medicines, providing appropriate treatment environments, and attending to nutrition and mobility. In effect, the clinician should treat the delirium before it begins. It is only by understanding delirium—its clinical features, course, diagnosis, and management—that the clinician can hope to prevent it, which may be the best way of avoiding its adverse clinical, functional, and economic sequelae.

TABLE 4. **Management of the Delirious Patient**

Vulnerability	Management
Agitated behavior	Obtain a sitter Allow family to stay in room
Medication side effects	Carefully review and discontinue medications
Deconditioning	Mobilize patient to chair, and even ambulate, with assistance
Malnutrition	Feed patient, if necessary by hand
Failure to rehabilitate	Work with patient as tolerated, using simple repetitive tasks
Sensory deprivation	Use glasses, hearing aids Provide adequate (soft) lighting Provide clocks, calendar, radio Socialize as tolerated Allow patient to sleep when possible
Nosocomial complications	Re-evaluate carefully for Cardiac decompensation Infections, especially lung, urinary tract Aspiration
Incontinence/retention/ obstipation	Toilet frequently Careful perineal hygiene Monitor output carefully Fecal disimpaction, if necessary Administer gentle laxatives
Severe pain	Administer round-the-clock: Acetaminophen Local/regional analgesia Low-dose narcotics

MOOD DISORDERS

method of
ELLIOTT RICHELSON, M.D.
Mayo Clinic–Jacksonville
Jacksonville, Florida

Depression is a relatively common disease that is vastly undertreated and largely treatable. It is thought to result ultimately from biochemical changes in the brain. Aside from the risk of suicide in untreated depression, this disease significantly modifies outcome for other diseases. For example, in the months after myocardial infarction, death is much more likely to occur in patients who are depressed. Pharmacologic treatment of depression is the focus of this article; however, other modalities (psychotherapy and electroconvulsive therapy [ECT]) are briefly discussed.

In most cases, depression can be effectively treated in an outpatient setting, with inpatient treatment being reserved for the more severely ill, such as those patients who are actively suicidal. In either case, the treatment modality is most likely to involve a pharmacologic agent alone or in combination with some form of psychotherapy. ECT is usually used for the patient who has failed to respond to other types of treatment (treatment-resistant patient), for the patient who is very debilitated due to lack of nourishment, or for the patient with an overwhelming desire to commit suicide.

There are 20 drugs approved by the Food and Drug Administration (FDA) for use as antidepressants in the United States, and if one goes outside the approved indication, two other drugs can be added to the list. This discussion aims to simplify the selection of an antidepressant by providing information on their pharmacologic properties.

EPIDEMIOLOGY

Depression afflicts about 5% of the adult population in the United States at any given time. In addition, about 1 to 2% of the adult population has acute manic-depressive (bipolar) illness. About 30% of the adult population will suffer from at least one episode of depression at some point in their lives. Also, the lifetime probability of death by suicide in major depressive disorder has been estimated to be as high as 25%. Studies suggest that more than 50% of patients who committed suicide saw a physician during the month before death; however, these patients were not diagnosed as being depressed. Data on suicide in the United States from 1991 show that there were 30,000 reported suicides in that year. It is the eighth leading cause of death in the United States, which ranks 24th in the rate of suicide worldwide.

The risk of depression is two to three times higher among women than among men. In addition, depression is two to three times higher in first-degree relatives of depressed individuals. Days lost from work (disability days) for persons with major depression are nearly five times higher than for individuals who are not depressed. Thus, depressive illness can have major economic impact.

Depression unfortunately is underdiagnosed and undertreated. Surveys done by the National Institute of Mental Health (NIMH) show that about 70% of depressed patients do not get treatment for their disease even though about 85 to 90% can be treated successfully.

About 70% of patients respond to antidepressant drug therapy and can enjoy a complete recovery from their depression. ECT can help those patients who are refractory to antidepressants (about another 20%). About 10% of depressed patients are resistant to all known forms of therapy.

DIAGNOSIS

The diagnosis of depression rests on the identification of core signs and symptoms. These include depressed mood, diminished pleasure or interest in activities, significant change in appetite or weight, alterations in sleep (insomnia or hypersomnia), psychomotor agitation or retardation, fatigue or loss of energy, inability to concentrate, indecisiveness, and thoughts of death, dying, or suicide. The clinician's index of suspicion should also be raised if a patient presents with a chief complaint of fatigue, pain, sleep disturbances, anxiety, irritability, or gastrointestinal problems. If a physical reason for these complaints is not found, the clinician should evaluate the patient for depression.

Other psychiatric disorders, such as schizophrenia, schizoaffective disorder, and anxiety disorders, may also have features of depression, which can coexist with another disorder. Many nonpsychiatric disorders can present with complaints of fatigue, insomnia, and difficulty concentrating. The differential diagnosis includes endocrinopathies (hypothyroidism, hyperparathyroidism, Cushing's and Addison's diseases), subcortical dementias (Huntington's and Parkinson's diseases), frontal lobe disease, right hemisphere stroke, occult tumors outside the brain, and infections of the brain. In addition, anemia, hypoglycemia, and hyperglycemia may simulate depression.

TREATMENT

Antidepressant Drugs

Classification

Treatment of depression is largely pharmacologic, usually in combination with some form of limited, supportive psychotherapy. The antidepressants available in the United States today include two drugs classified as monoamine oxidase inhibitors (MAOIs) (phenelzine [Nardil]; tranylcypromine [Parnate]) and 18 others (see Table 1). Until several years ago, the so-called tricyclic antidepressants (for example, amitriptyline [Elavil], desipramine [Norpramin]) were the first-line drugs. However, with the introduction of newer compounds with more favorable side effect profiles and low toxicity in overdose, the older drugs are being prescribed less often (although the economics of healthcare may reverse this trend).

Until the 1970s, antidepressants approved for use in the United States could be classified into two groups: tricyclic antidepressants and MAOIs. This classification mixed structural (tricyclic) and functional (inhibition of monoamine oxidase) criteria; a classification based upon either structure or activity would be better. With the introduction of some of the newer compounds (e.g., mirtazapine [Remeron]), drugs could be divided into multiple classes, complicating the picture. A simplified classification for the purpose of this review divides the antidepressants into those that are inhibitors of monoamine oxidase and those that are not (the majority) (see Table 1). This functional classification eliminates the confusion in the literature from the incorrect usage of terms such as heterocyclic, tricyclic, and tetracyclic. Classifying antidepressants as either tricyclic or heterocyclic is not correct. For example, doxepin [Adapin, Sinequan] is correctly classified on the basis of its structure as a heterocyclic, tricyclic antidepressant.

Clinical Pharmacology

The clinical effects of antidepressants generally do not appear until the first week or two after the start of therapy. This time lag for the onset of therapeutic effects may relate to changes in sensitivity of certain neurotransmitter receptors. As a clinical rule of thumb, an adequate trial constitutes at least 6 weeks of treatment at an adequate dosage, which is often difficult to know. The wide interindividual variation in the absorption, distribution, and excretion of antidepressants may explain why dosages for specific antidepressants may vary widely. In addition, drug clearance generally declines with increasing age.

Table 1 outlines the usual daily doses and projected optimal therapeutic plasma ranges of antidepressants currently available in the United States. Few antidepressants have rigorously defined therapeutic blood ranges. Nonetheless, one can use the *projected* ranges presented in Table 1 as a guide in clinical practice. For newer second-generation compounds (bupropion [Wellbutrin]; fluoxetine [Prozac];

TABLE 1. **Pharmacokinetics, Daily Doses, and Projected Therapeutic Plasma Ranges of Antidepressants**

Drug (Generic and Trade Names)	Individual Variation in Metabolism	Elimination Half-Life, $T_{1/2}$ (h)		Starting Dosage‡ (mg/day)	Usual Daily Dose for Adults (mg)	Usual Dose Range (mg/day)	Projected§ Optimal Therapeutic Plasma Range (ng/mL)
		Mean	*Range*				
Non–Monoamine Oxidase Inhibitor Antidepressants							
Amitriptyline (Elavil)‖	10-fold	21	13–36	50	150–200	50–300	80–250¶
Amoxapine (Asendin)		8	8–30**	50	200–300	50–400	200–600††
Bupropion (Wellbutrin)		9.8	3.9–23.1	200‡‡	300§§	100–450‖‖	
Bupropion SR (Wellbutrin SR)		21		150	150–300	100–400	
Citalopram (Celexa)		33		20	20–60	20–80	
Desipramine (Norpramin)‖	10-fold	21	12–30	50	100–200	50–300	125–300
Doxepin (Adapin, Sinequan)‖	10- to 15-fold	17	8–24	50	75–150	50–300	150–250¶¶
Fluoxetine (Prozac)		87	26–220	20	20–80	20–80	
Imipramine (Tofranil)‖	30-fold	28	18–34	50	75–150	50–300	150–250***
Maprotiline (Ludiomil)		43		50	100–150	50–225	200–600
Mirtazapine (Remeron)		30	20–40	15	15–45	15–60	
Nefazodone (Serzone)		3	2–4	200	300–600	200–600	
Nortriptyline (Pamelor)‖	30-fold	36	14–79	20	75–100	30–125	50–150
Paroxetine (Paxil)		21	4–65	10	20–50	10–50	
Protriptyline (Vivactil)‖	10- to 15-fold	78	55–127	10	15–40	10–60	70–260
Sertraline (Zoloft)		26		25	50–150	50–200	
Trazodone (Desyrel)		7	3–16	50	150–400	50–600	800–1600
Trimipramine (Surmontil)‖		13		50	100–200	50–300	150–250
Venlafaxine (Effexor)		5	2–7	37.5	75–225	75–375	
Venlafaxine XR (Effexor XR)		5		37.5	75–225	75–375	
Monoamine Oxidase Inhibitors							
Phenelzine (Nardil)		2.8	1.5–4	15	45–60	45–90†††	
Tranylcypromine (Parnate)	4-fold	2.4	1.5–3	10	30–40	30–60	

‡Dosage should be divided initially for all listed drugs, and elderly persons should be treated with about half of the usual dosage for adults. §Only amitriptyline, imipramine, nortriptyline, and desipramine have been significantly studied for blood level versus clinical response. ‖A classical tricyclic antidepressant. ¶Amitriptyline + nortriptyline. **Amoxapine, 8 hours; 8-hydroxyamoxapine, 30 hours. ††Amoxapine + 8-hydroxyamoxapine; of total drug measured, amoxapine ≈ 20%; 7-hydroxyamoxapine ≈ 15%; and 8-hydroxyamoxapine ≈ 65%. ‡‡Dose should be divided, 100 mg bid. §§The divided dose by fourth day of treatment. ‖‖Maximum recommended divided dose achieved if no response after 3 weeks at the lower dosage. ¶¶Doxepin + desmethyldoxepin. ***Imipramine + desipramine. †††1 mg/kg.

Updated and modified from Richelson E.: Antidepressants: Pharmacology and clinical use. *In* Karasu TB (ed): Treatments of Psychiatric Disorders. A Task Force Report of the American Psychiatric Association, Washington, DC Vol 3, pp. 1773–1787, 1989, and reproduced with permission from the publisher.

mirtazapine [Remeron]; nefazodone [Serzone]; paroxetine [Paxil]; sertraline [Zoloft]; and venlafaxine [Effexor]), projecting a therapeutic range at this time is not possible. Two drugs listed in Table 1, clomipramine (Anafranil) and fluvoxamine (Luvox) are presently approved in the United States for treatment of obsessive-compulsive disorder but are marketed elsewhere as antidepressants.

Therapeutic drug monitoring is most readily available for the tricyclic compounds. Reasons for monitoring these drugs include assessing compliance, maximizing response, avoiding toxicity, reducing cost for the patient, and avoiding medical-legal problems.

There is a substantiated 10- to 30-fold variation in individual metabolism for some of these tricyclic compounds (Table 1). This variation requires specific attention to individualization of drug dosages and emphasizes the need to monitor drug plasma levels to achieve an appropriate therapeutic response, particularly in the elderly patient.

The idea of a therapeutic window (i.e., a blood level range below and above which the drug is ineffective) has been thoroughly evaluated only for nortriptyline (Pamelor). Protriptyline (Vivactil) and nortriptyline in comparison with other tricyclic antidepressants, have increased potency (see Table 1). Therefore, a smaller mean daily dose of these drugs should be prescribed. The longer elimination half-life ($T_{1/2}$) for protriptyline may in part explain the requirement for a lower dosage.

The mean elimination half-lives of most of the antidepressants listed in Table 1 are in the 15- to 30-hour range. The half-lives of maprotiline (Ludiomil), protriptyline, and fluoxetine, however, are much longer. Consequently, these drugs not only require a longer time to achieve a steady state after initiation of treatment, but also need a longer period of observation of complications after ingestion of an overdose. Based upon pharmacokinetic considerations, a rational dosing interval for an antidepressant drug is equal to its elimination half-life (Table 1). In practice, a single daily dose is appropriate for those drugs with half-lives of around 15 hours or greater. It is also reasonable to consider prescribing the very long half-life compounds—protriptyline, fluoxetine, and maprotiline—less frequently, especially in the elderly patient. Bupropion and venlafaxine are now available in a sustained-release and extended-release form, respectively (Wellbutrin SR and Effexor XR), allowing less frequent (once or twice daily) dosing than is required for the immediate-release formulations.

A pharmacokinetic rule of thumb is that it takes about four to five times the elimination half-life with a constant dosing interval to achieve steady-state levels. Another pharmacokinetic rule of thumb based on the elimination half-life is that it takes about four to five times this number to have greater than 90% of the drug eliminated from the body after stopping the medication. Abrupt discontinuation of drugs with elimination half-lives of around 24 hours or less can result in a withdrawal syndrome.

These agents are highly lipid soluble and therefore have a high volume of distribution. Most are also strongly bound to plasma proteins. Changes in body fat and plasma proteins with aging, therefore, can have effects on the clearance of a drug and its potency.

Basic Pharmacology (Table 2)

For the pharmacodynamic effects of antidepressants, the site of action that may be especially relevant clinically is the synapse. By blocking transport of neurotransmitters, blocking certain neurotransmitter receptors, or inhibiting the mitochondrial enzyme monoamine oxidase, antidepressants alter the effects of neurotransmitters at synapses.

Neurons use neurotransmitters to communicate with one another and with other cell types. These small molecules, usually amino acids or their derivatives, are released from the nerve ending to interact with specific receptors on the outside surface of cells. Receptors are highly specialized proteins, which have often been molecularly cloned by researchers. These receptors are very selective in their ability to bind neurotransmitters. When the chemical messenger stimulates its receptor, the receiving neuron is changed electrically and biochemically because of the coupling of the complex of neurotransmitter and receptor to other components of the membrane in which the receptor resides. However, some receptors (e.g., nicotinic acetylcholine receptor) are ion channels, which open upon binding the neurotransmitter. Thus, this class of receptors requires no other membranal component to activate the receiving cell.

Neurons can also regulate their own activity by feedback mechanisms involving receptors on the nerve ending (autoreceptors). An example of an autoreceptor is the α_2-adrenergic receptor on noradrenergic nerve endings that modulate release of norepinephrine. When stimulated, this presynaptic receptor inhibits further release of norepinephrine.

Some biogenic amine neurotransmitters (e.g., norepinephrine, serotonin, and dopamine) are taken back into the nerve ending after release (a process called uptake, reuptake, or simply, transport). Reuptake occurs through transport proteins (transporters), which have been molecularly cloned from human and other species. This transport is a mechanism that prevents overstimulation of receptors in the synapse. Neurotransmission can be enhanced acutely by blocking this uptake with a drug. However, the blockade of uptake can ultimately diminish neurotransmission as the receptor undergoes

TABLE 2. **Some Pharmacodynamic Effects of Antidepressants**

	Potency of Blockade of Transporters				**Potency of Blockade of Neurotransmitter Receptors**			
Drug	*5-HT*	*NE*	*DA*	**Transporter Selectivity (5-HT/NE)***	*Histamine H_1*	*Muscarinic*	*α_1-Adrenergic*	*Dopamine D_2*
Amitriptyline (Elavil)	++++	+++	+	+++	++++	++	++	+/−
Amoxapine (Asendin)	+++	+++	+	−−−	++	+/−	++	+
Bupropion (Wellbutrin)	0	0	++	+++	0	0	0	0
Citalopram (Celexa)	++++	0	0	+++++++	+/−	0	0	0
Clomipramine† (Anafranil)	++++++	+++	+	++++	++	++	++	+
Desipramine (Norpramin)	+++	++++	+	−−−−	+	+	+	0
Doxepin (Adapin, Sinequan)	+++	+++	0	−−−	++++++	+	++	0
Fluoxetine (Prozac)	++++	++	+	++++++	0	0	0	0
Fluvoxamine† (Luvox)	++++	+	0	+++++++	0	0	0	0
Imipramine (Tofranil)	++++	+++	0	++++	+++	+	+	0
Maprotiline (Ludiomil)	0	++++	++	−−−−−	++++	+/−	+	+/−
Mirtazapine (Remeron)	0	0	0	−−−−	+++++++	+/−	+/−	0
Nefazodone (Serzone)	++	++	++	+++	++	0	++	+/−
Nortriptyline (Pamelor)	+++	++++	+	−−−	+++	+	++	+/−
Paroxetine (Paxil)	+++++++	+++	++	++++++	0	+	0	0
Phenelzine (Nardil)	0	0	0		0	0	0	0
Protriptyline (Vivactil)	+++	++++	+	−−−−	++	++	+	0
Sertraline (Zoloft)	++++++	++	+++	+++++++	0	+/−	+/−	0
Tranylcypromine (Parnate)	0	0	0		0	0	0	0
Trazodone (Desyrel)	++	0	0	++++	++	0	++	0
Trimipramine (Surmontil)	++	+	+	++++	++++++	++	++	+
Venlafaxine (Effexor)	++++	+	0	++++	0	0	0	0

*Ratio of potency of 5-HT transport blockade to potency of NE transport blockade: +++++++ means very selective for 5-HT and −−−−− means very selective for NE.

†Not marketed in the United States as an antidepressant.

Data can be compared both vertically and horizontally to find the most potent drug for a specific property and to find the most potent property for a specific drug.

a compensatory change and becomes less sensitive (desensitizes) to the neurotransmitter. Antidepressants of many types, probably acting by different mechanisms, can desensitize certain receptors for catecholamines and serotonin. These effects are the basis of one hypothesis of their mechanism of action. On the other hand, the therapeutic effects of the new antidepressant mirtazapine may be caused by direct blocking of presynaptic α_2-adrenergic receptors.

By blocking the postsynaptic receptor with an antagonist, the effects of the neurotransmitter can be selectively and acutely abolished. Very often with chronic blockade, the receptor undergoes another type of compensatory change and becomes more sensitive (supersensitive) to the neurotransmitter. Supersensitivity may be the mechanism of adaptation to some receptor-related side effects of certain drugs. This process may also be related to the development of tardive dyskinesia following chronic treatment with neuroleptics that block dopamine receptors. This adaptive process may also be involved in causing the withdrawal effects that sometimes occur with abrupt cessation of some antidepressants.

Most antidepressants can block uptake of biogenic amine neurotransmitters and antagonize certain receptors. In addition, a few antidepressants inhibit the activity of monoamine oxidase, a ubiquitous enzyme that is important in the degradation of catecholamines, serotonin, and dopamine. Since this enzyme is present in mitochondria, which are found in most cells and in the nerve ending, its inhibition results in an elevation in the concentration of neurotransmitter available for release at the synapse.

Blockade of Neurotransmitter Transport

Most antidepressants are more potent at blocking transport of serotonin than transport of norepinephrine at the human transporters (see Table 2). Newer antidepressants are generally more selective and more potent than the older compounds at blocking transport of serotonin over norepinephrine (selective serotonin reuptake inhibitors, or SSRIs) (Figure 1). In addition, some antidepressants (e.g., bupropion, mirtazapine) very weakly block transport of norepinephrine, serotonin, and dopamine. Bupropion is the only antidepressant more selective in blocking uptake of dopamine (see Table 2) than other neurotransmitters. However, bupropion is more noradrenergic than dopaminergic, due to the effects of a metabolite that is present in much higher concentrations than the parent compound. Sertraline is the most potent of the antidepressants at blocking transport of dopamine, being about as potent as methylphenidate (Ritalin). Paroxetine is the most potent blocker of uptake of serotonin, while the soon to be marketed citalopram (Celexa), is the most selective.

Selectivity cannot be equated with potency, since selectivity is derived from a ratio of potencies. In the foregoing example, citalopram is more selective (i.e., more specific) at blocking transport of serotonin than paroxetine but only about one-tenth as potent as paroxetine.

Blockade of Some Neurotransmitter Receptors

Most of the newer, second-generation antidepressants are weaker than the older compounds (especially, tricyclic antidepressants) at blocking receptors for neurotransmitters. This fact predicts a side effect profile for these compounds that is different from that for older drugs.

Overall, the most potent interaction of antidepressants, especially the classical tricyclic drugs, is at the histamine H_1 receptor (see Table 2). Histamine is considered a neurotransmitter in the brain where, as elsewhere in the body, it causes its effects by acting at three types of receptors, histamine H_1, H_2, and H_3. The most recently discovered histamine receptor, H_3, affects the presynaptic synthesis and release of histamine and other neurotransmitters. Histamine H_2 receptors are present in the brain, but classically these receptors are involved with gastric acid secretion. Outside the nervous system, histamine H_1 receptors are involved in allergic reactions. Some antidepressants are exceedingly potent histamine H_1 antagonists (see Table 2), being more potent than all of the newer generation histamine H_1 antagonists marketed in recent years in the United States. As a result, clinicians are using them to treat allergic and dermatologic problems.

The next most potent effect of antidepressants is at the muscarinic acetylcholine receptor, which is the predominant type of cholinergic receptor in brain. In that organ they are involved with memory and learning, among other functions. In addition, some evidence suggests that these brain receptors are involved with affective illness. Antidepressants have a broad range of effectiveness at blocking human brain muscarinic receptors (see Table 2). The most potent is amitriptyline. The SSRI paroxetine is unique among the newer compounds for having appreciable antimuscarinic potency (similar to that for imipramine) (see Table 2). Studies with the molecularly cloned human muscarinic receptors, of which there are five, show that paroxetine has the highest affinity for the m3 subtype of this receptor, which is found predominantly in brain, glandular tissue, and smooth muscle. Overall, antidepressants vary little in their affinities for the five subtypes of the human muscarinic receptor.

The most potent compounds, although a little weaker than the antihypertensive drug phentolamine, are likely to have clinical effects at alpha$_1$-adrenergic receptors (Table 3). Antidepressants are also weak competitive antagonists of dopamine (D_2) receptors (see Table 2). The most potent compound, amoxapine (Asendin), is a demethylated derivative of the neuroleptic loxapine (Loxitane).

MAOIs have negligible direct effects on transporters and receptors (see Table 2).

Clinical Relevance of Synaptic Pharmacology

Because all of the pharmacologic effects of these drugs occur shortly after ingestion, most of the possi-

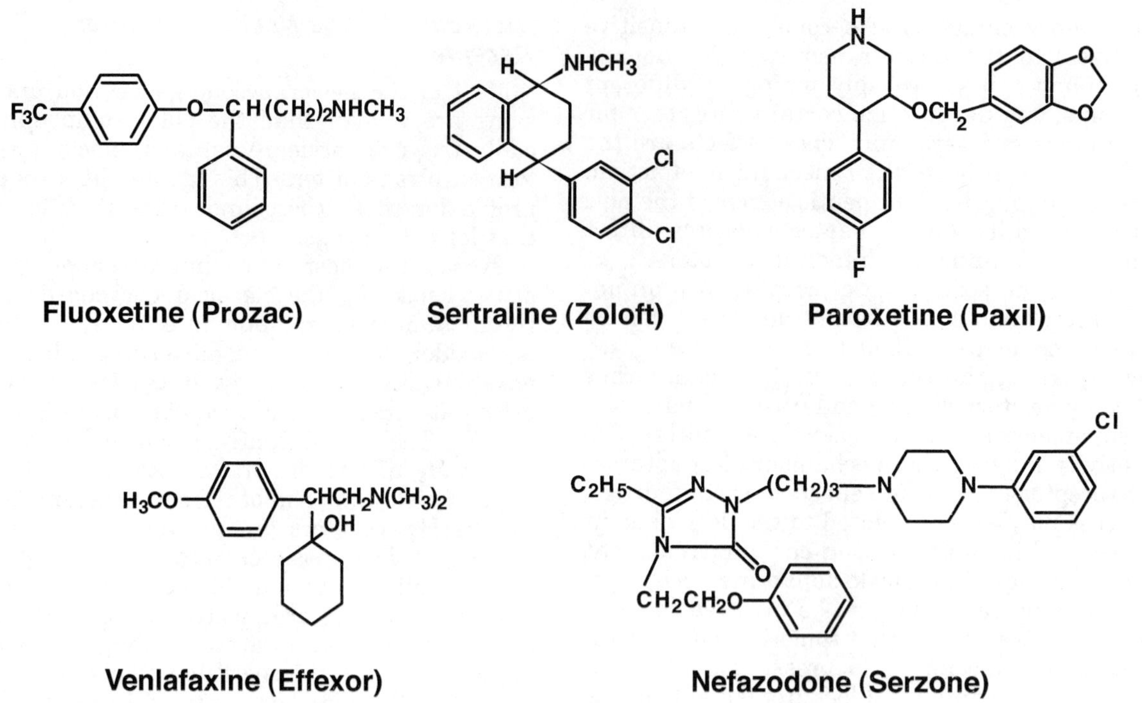

Fluoxetine (Prozac) Sertraline (Zoloft) Paroxetine (Paxil)

Venlafaxine (Effexor) Nefazodone (Serzone)

Figure 1. Some selective serotonin reuptake inhibitors (SSRIs).

ble clinical effects discussed below occur early in treatment. However, with chronic administration of the drug, changes may occur that can result in adaptation to certain side effects, the development of new side effects, and the onset of therapeutic effects. Table 3 lists the pharmacologic properties of various antidepressants and their possible clinical consequences. The clinician should keep in mind that the more potent the drug for a given property, the more likely it is to cause the associated effect (see Table 2).

Evidence to date suggests that the efficacy of antidepressants is not related to selectivity or potency

TABLE 3. **Pharmacologic Properties of Antidepressants and Their Possible Clinical Consequences**

Property	Possible Clinical Consequences
Blockade of norepinephrine uptake at nerve endings	Tremors Tachycardia Erectile and ejaculatory dysfunction Blockade of the antihypertensive effects of guanethidine (Ismelin and Esimil) and guanadrel (Hylorel) Augmentation of pressor effects of sympathomimetic amines
Blockade of serotonin uptake at nerve ending	Gastrointestinal disturbances Increase or decrease in anxiety (dose-dependent) Sexual dysfunction Extrapyramidal side effects Interactions with L-tryptophan and monoamine oxidase inhibitors
Blockade of dopamine uptake at nerve ending	Psychomotor activation Antiparkinsonian effect Aggravation of psychosis
Blockade of histamine H_1 receptors	Potentiation of central depressant drugs Sedation drowsiness Weight gain
Blockade of muscarinic receptors	Blurred vision Dry mouth Sinus tachycardia Constipation Urinary retention Memory dysfunction
Blockade of α_1-adrenergic receptors	Potentiation of antihypertensive effect of prazosin (Minipress), terazosin (Hytrin), doxazosin (Cardura), labetalol (Normodyne) Postural hypotension, dizziness Reflex tachycardia
Blockade of dopamine D_2 receptors	Extrapyramidal movement disorders Endocrine changes (including hyperprolactinemia, which can lead to sexual dysfunction in males)

for norepinephrine, serotonin, or dopamine transport blockade. These data are from clinical studies and basic studies that show the wide range of potencies of antidepressants at blocking this transport (see Table 2). On the other hand, clinical data suggest that potent transport blockade of serotonin is necessary for treatment of certain anxiety disorders including obsessive-compulsive disorder.

Transport blockade of neurotransmitters by antidepressants likely relates to certain adverse effects of these drugs and to some of their drug interactions (see Table 3). For example, serotonin transport blockade likely is the property that causes sexual side effects, seen more commonly with the SSRIs. This same property underlies the serious consequences that occur when an MAOI is combined with an antidepressant (serotonergic syndrome). In addition, researchers have reported adverse interactions between L-tryptophan, the precursor of serotonin, and fluoxetine. St. John's wort, which has become popular recently, has some monoamine oxidase activity and therefore should not be combined with an antidepressant that is a potent blocker of serotonin transport (see Table 2).

There are reports of adverse effects of fluoxetine (and other SSRIs), including extrapyramidal side effects, anorgasmia and other sexual problems, paranoid reaction, and intense suicidal preoccupation. The extrapyramidal side effects are not due to blockade of dopamine receptors, because these SSRIs are very weak at this binding site (see Table 2). Serotonin receptor antagonists (e.g., cyproheptadine [Periactin]) have been useful in treating all these side effects.

Potentiation of the effects of central depressant drugs, which cause sedation and drowsiness, is a pharmacodynamic drug interaction of antidepressants related to histamine H_1 receptor antagonism. This antagonism is probably responsible for the side effects of sedation and drowsiness. Sedation, however, may be a desired effect in patients who are agitated as well as depressed. This property may also be responsible for weight gain.

Muscarinic receptor blockade by these antidepressants may be responsible for several adverse effects (see Table 3). The relatively high affinity of paroxetine for these receptors distinguishes it from the other newer, second-generation compounds. In addition, it may explain the common complaint of dry mouth and constipation reported in some published clinical trials with paroxetine. Because elderly patients are more sensitive to the antimuscarinic side effects of drugs (see Table 3), it is best to select antidepressants that are weak in this property (see Table 2).

α_1-Adrenergic receptor blockade by antidepressants may be responsible for orthostatic hypotension, the most serious common cardiovascular effect of these drugs, which can cause dizziness and a reflex tachycardia. In addition, this property of antidepressants results in the potentiation of several antihypertensive drugs that potently block α_1-adrenergic receptors (see Table 3).

Antidepressants are weak competitive antagonists of dopamine (D_2) receptors (see Table 2). The most potent compound, amoxapine, is a demethylated derivative of the neuroleptic, loxapine (Loxitane). It is very likely that this property of amoxapine explains its extrapyramidal side effects and its ability to elevate prolactin levels. Because of this dopamine receptor blocking property, amoxapine should be reserved for patients with psychotic depression.

Antidepressants also block α_2-adrenergic receptors and 5-HT_{1A} and 5-HT_{2A} receptors. Usually, the blockade is weak; the exceptions are trazodone (Desyrel) and nefazodone (Serzone), which are relatively potent at these three receptors, and mirtazapine, which is relatively potent at α_2-adrenergic and 5-HT_{2A} receptors.

Pharmacokinetic Drug Interactions

Drug interactions for antidepressants can be divided into two groups: pharmacokinetic and pharmacodynamic. Pharmacokinetic interactions occur when one drug affects the metabolism or protein binding of another drug. Pharmacodynamic interactions occur when one drug affects the mechanism of action of another drug. These pharmacodynamic interactions relate to the synaptic effects of antidepressants discussed previously.

The important pharmacokinetic interactions of antidepressants relate to their effects on the cytochrome P450 system. Although we lack complete knowledge of the metabolism of many of the antidepressants, available data show that antidepressants can be substrates or inhibitors of more than one enzyme of the cytochrome P450 system, which consists of many isozymes coded for by distinct genes. The inhibition of cytochrome P450 2D6 enzyme by fluoxetine and its metabolite norfluoxetine is now well established. This enzyme is involved with the aromatic 2-hydroxylation of imipramine (Tofranil) and the biotransformation of many other drugs. Inhibition of cytochrome P450 2D6 likely underlies the many reports of elevations in blood levels of other drugs used in combination with fluoxetine.

Pharmacokinetic drug interactions of antidepressants are a potential rather than a certain problem. These interactions are more likely to occur with high-risk drugs such as nefazodone at CYP 3A4; fluoxetine and paroxetine at CYP 2D6; and fluvoxamine at CYP 1A2. They are less likely to occur with low-risk drugs, such as venlafaxine, sertraline, and probably bupropion and mirtazapine. Therefore, the clinician needs to be vigilant.

Cytochrome P450 3A4 metabolizes many drugs, including the prodrug antihistamines terfenadine (Seldane) and astemizole (Hismanal) and active compounds, such as triazolam (Halcion) and alprazolam (Xanax). Combinations of these antihistamines with potent inhibitors of this enzyme (e.g., ketoconazole [Nizoral]) can lead to fatal arrhythmias. Antidepressants that inhibit this enzyme, such as nefazodone, are contraindicated with these antihistamines. However, terfenadine was recently removed from the market in the United States by the FDA because of its potential cardiotoxicity. The drug's manufacturer is now promoting the noncardiotoxic metabolite of terfenadine, fexofenadine (Allegra).

Drugs metabolized by cytochrome P450 2D6 include tricyclic antidepressants, neuroleptics, antiarrhythmics, and beta blockers. Cytochrome P450 1A2 metabolizes some antidepressants and some neuroleptics, along with caffeine and theophylline (Aerolate and others).

Clinical Guidelines

The clinician should consider any concomitant medical disorder (Table 4), whether the patient is experiencing agitation or psychomotor retardation, and possible side effects when deciding on the appropriate choice of a drug in any particular clinical situation. Certain clinical guidelines exist for drug choice, dosage, duration, maintenance, termination, and alternatives to treatment with antidepressants (Table 5).

The first step is the appropriate choice of a drug. A history of a previous response by the patient or a family member to a particular antidepressant drug can sometimes be helpful. Starting anew, one usually chooses a more sedating drug (potent histamine H_1 antagonist) for patients with episodes of agitated depression and a less sedating one (weak histamine H_1 antagonist) for those with retarded depressive episodes. With the new antidepressant mirtazapine, sedation is usually more prominent at lower dosages, due to counteracting mechanisms occurring at the higher dosages.

The second important guideline is the appropriate dose of medication. Most patients tolerate treatment best if the beginning dose is one fourth of the maximal usual daily dosage for adults (see Table 1). The dosage should be increased in a stepwise, divided-dose fashion every 2 to 3 days until the maximal, usual daily dose has been achieved, if tolerated. For example, for sertraline the target dose is 100 mg per day. A patient could be started on sertraline, 25 mg every day for 2 days; then 25 mg twice a day for 2 days; then 50 mg in the morning, and 25 mg in the evening for 2 days; and finally, if no very troublesome adverse effects are present, 100 mg once per day.

After about 1 to 2 weeks of therapy at the target dosage, patients may take antidepressants with the longer elimination half-lives (around 15 hours or more; Table 1) once a day at bedtime, *except bupropion*. Elderly patients taking the older antidepressant compounds may benefit from continuation of the divided-dose schedule, so that high blood levels (possibly leading to the adverse effect of postural hypotension or difficulty urinating) do not occur during the night when the patient may arise to elimi-

TABLE 4. **Preferred Antidepressants When Specific Medical Disorders Coexist with Depression**

Cardiovascular Disorders
Congestive heart failure or coronary artery disease—bupropion (Wellbutrin or Zyban), citalopram (Celexa), fluoxetine (Prozac), mirtazapine (Remeron), sertraline (Zoloft), venlafaxine (Effexor)
Conduction defect—monoamine oxidase inhibitors, bupropion or fluoxetine, mirtazapine, sertraline, paroxetine (Paxil), venlafaxine
Hypertension treated with guanethidine (Ismelin and Esimil*) and guanadrel (Hylorel)—bupropion, trazodone (Desyrel), mirtazapine, citalopram, trimipramine (Surmontil)
Hypertension treated with prazosin (Minipress), terazosin (Hytrin), doxazosin (Cardura), labetalol (Normodyne)—venlafaxine, fluoxetine, bupropion, paroxetine, citalopram, mirtazapine
Hypertension treated with clonidine (Catapres), guanabenz (Wytensin), guanfacine (Tenex), or α-methyldopa (Aldomet)—venlafaxine, bupropion, paroxetine, fluoxetine
Untreated mild hypertension—monoamine oxidase inhibitor
Postural hypotension—venlafaxine, fluoxetine, bupropion, paroxetine, citalopram, mirtazapine, sertraline, protriptyline (Vivactil), desipramine (Norpramin). Avoid imipramine (Tofranil), amitriptyline (Elavil), and monoamine oxidase inhibitors.
Neurologic Disorders
Seizure disorder—monoamine oxidase inhibitor best, fluoxetine, secondary amine tricyclic (desipramine) better than tertiary amine (e.g., imipramine). Avoid maprotiline (Ludiomil), amoxapine (Asendin), trimipramine (Surmontil), bupropion.
Organic mental disorders—venlafaxine, trazodone, bupropion, nefazodone (Serzone), citalopram, fluoxetine
Chronic pain syndrome—amitriptyline, imipramine
Migraine headaches—nefazodone, trazodone, mirtazapine, doxepin (Sinequan or Adapin), amitriptyline, trimipramine
Psychosis—antidepressant plus neuroleptic, amoxapine
Parkinsonism—amitriptyline, protriptyline, trimipramine, doxepin, bupropion, or sertraline. Avoid amoxapine.
Tardive dyskinesia—bupropion, maprotiline, mirtazapine. Avoid amoxapine.
Allergic Disorders—mirtazapine, doxepin, trimipramine, amitriptyline, maprotiline
Gastrointestinal Disorders
Chronic diarrhea—amitriptyline, protriptyline, trimipramine, doxepin.
Chronic constipation—venlafaxine, trazodone, bupropion, nefazodone, citalopram, fluoxetine
Peptic ulcer disease—doxepin, trimipramine, amitriptyline, imipramine
Urologic Disorders
Neurogenic bladder—venlafaxine, trazodone, bupropion, nefazodone, citalopram, fluoxetine
Organic impotence—nefazodone, trazodone, bupropion
Ophthalmologic Disorders (angle-closure glaucoma)—venlafaxine, trazodone, bupropion, nefazodone, citalopram, fluoxetine

*Not available in the United States.
Updated and modified from Richelson, E: Antidepressants: Pharmacology and clinical use. *In* Karasu TB (ed): Treatments of Psychiatric Disorders. A Task Force Report of the American Psychiatric Association, Washington, DC, Vol. 3, pp 1773–1787, 1989, and reproduced with permission from the publisher.

TABLE 5. **Clinical Guidelines for Use of Antidepressants**

1. Appropriate choice: Select on the basis of the profile of side effects, particularly sedative effects in agitated patients or on the basis of previous response or family history of a response to a particular antidepressant
2. Adequate dose: Check blood level if toxicity ensues or if response is inadequate
3. Adequate duration: Administer for a minimum of 4 months after recovery
4. Adequate termination or maintenance: For first depressions, 4 to 5 months after recovery, taper dose gradually for 2 to 4 months and then discontinue therapy. For recurrent unipolar depression, maintain therapy with antidepressant
5. Adequate therapy: For almost all types of depression, a combination of psychotherapy (usually, brief supportive) and antidepressants may be slightly more effective than antidepressants alone
6. Adequate alternative: Change drug; add lithium carbonate; add thyroid hormone; add buspirone, or use electroshock therapy

Modified from Richelson E: Antidepressants: Pharmacology and clinical use. *In* Karasu TB (ed): Treatments of Psychiatric Disorders. A Task Force Report of the American Psychiatric Association, Washington, DC, Vol 3, pp 1773–1787, 1989, and reproduced with permission from the publisher.

nate. This will likely not be a problem with the newer second-generation drugs that can be given once per day (i.e., fluoxetine, sertraline, paroxetine, and mirtazapine).

Use of MAOIs requires special considerations. These are efficacious drugs for treating depression, are well tolerated by the elderly, and should be used when a patient fails to respond to antidepressants of other classes. However, these drugs are not suitable for all patients because of the need for the patient receiving an MAOI to avoid certain foodstuffs, especially those containing tyramine, and certain drugs, especially over-the-counter cold remedies containing sympathomimetics. The clinician must make the patient aware of these important precautions when prescribing an MAOI. A convenient way to ensure that the patient has all the information in hand is to give him or her a copy of the list of "foods to avoid" in the package insert. When a patient is not willing or able to comply with these restrictions, another type of antidepressant should be prescribed.

The two antidepressant MAOIs currently in use in the United States are irreversible inhibitors. This means that "washout" from the drug depends not on its pharmacokinetics but rather on the synthesis of new monoamine oxidase. Reversible MAOIs are under development that promise to pose less of a problem with tyramine-containing foodstuffs.

If the patient is taking a tricyclic antidepressant or another MAOI, then this drug should be stopped for 10 days before starting a new MAOI inhibitor. To be underscored in the list of drugs that should be avoided by patients taking an MAOI are meperidine (Demerol), imipramine, clomipramine (Anafranil), fluoxetine, sertraline, paroxetine, and venlafaxine. Because of the very long half-life of fluoxetine and the even longer half-life of its active metabolite, norfluoxetine, at least 5 weeks' washout is required before starting an MAOI. Some evidence suggests that this washout period should be longer.

Of the two MAOIs available in the United States (see Table 1), researchers have studied phenelzine most frequently. About 2 weeks are needed to achieve maximal inhibition of platelet monoamine oxidase when depressed patients are given phenelzine and about the same length of time is necessary to recover activity after the drug is stopped. Patients with 80% or greater inhibition of this platelet enzyme have a better antidepressant response than do those with less enzyme inhibition. Although laboratories are making measurement of platelet monoamine oxidase available, a clinically useful rule of thumb is to target a dosage of 1 mg per kg body weight per day for the patient to achieve this desired level of inhibition.

As with other antidepressants, MAOIs may be started slowly. For example, when starting a patient on phenelzine, the clinician may prescribe 15 mg the first day, 15 mg twice daily the second day, 15 mg thrice daily the third day, and so forth until the target dosage is achieved.

A treatment period of 2 to 4 weeks is usually necessary before the onset of therapeutic effects of any type of antidepressant. At the outset, the patient may need a thorough explanation of the side effects to be expected and encouragement to persist with treatment until some clinical response results. If the clinical response is inadequate after 3 to 4 weeks and the adverse effects are small, one should increase the dosage a step further. Underdosing is a common error with these drugs. As outlined previously for sertraline, one should increase the dosage another 25 to 50 mg per day; with phenelzine, increase the dosage another 15 mg per day. However, if poor response persists after 2 more weeks at the higher dosage or if toxicity supervenes, then plasma levels of the drug (if it is not an MAOI) may be obtained when available.

Although therapeutic plasma concentrations have been firmly established for only imipramine, nortriptyline, desipramine, and possibly amitriptyline, enough data are available for other antidepressants (other than MAOIs and the newer second-generation antidepressants bupropion, fluoxetine, nefazodone, paroxetine, sertraline, trazodone, venlafaxine, and mirtazapine) to decide whether a dosage of a drug is adequate for problem patients or elderly patients. The projected optimal therapeutic plasma ranges presented in Table 1 for the other antidepressants are to be used only as a very rough guide.

Elderly patients are likely to require about one half the usual daily dose recommended for a younger adult and may require a slower escalation of the dosage to the maximal level because of their increased sensitivity to the adverse effects of antidepressants. However, under-dosing can be a mistake in treating elderly patients, and plasma levels should be used more often with this group to determine proper dosage. Achievement of a steady state in these patients may take longer as well.

The third guideline is adequate duration of treatment. After a complete clinical response has been achieved, therapy should be continued for at least 4 to 5 months.

The fourth important clinical guideline involves stopping antidepressant therapy or maintenance therapy for patients with recurrent illness. Four to five months after complete recovery, the drug dose should be tapered gradually over 2 to 4 months and then stopped. A slow taper is essential, because abrupt withdrawal of medication can predispose the patient to relapse of depressive symptoms, to uncomfortable symptoms (for example, dysesthesias and severe sleep disturbance), or to a withdrawal syndrome. The evidence being gathered suggests that maintenance therapy with the same antidepressant *without lowering the dosage* should be used for those patients with recurrent unipolar depression.

The fifth clinical guideline is that adequate therapy for most types of depression should include some form of psychotherapeutic alliance between the patient and doctor at least to ensure compliance with the pharmacotherapy. This may be achieved through brief (10 to 20 minutes) supportive visits with the primary physician or, sometimes, more extensive psychotherapy. However, a combination of antidepressants and psychotherapy may be only slightly more effective than antidepressants alone.

Finally, adequate knowledge of alternative or adjunctive treatments for depression is important. This includes a change in the primary antidepressant drug to an antidepressant of a different chemical class; the addition of lithium carbonate in sufficient dosage to achieve a blood level of 0.6 to 1.0 mEq per liter; the addition of thyroid hormone (1-triiodothyronine, 25 to 50 μg per day); or the addition of buspirone.

Electroconvulsive therapy is still the most effective treament for refractory depression and may be the treatment of choice in certain situations in which antidepressants are contraindicated, in patients at extremely high suicidal risk, or in depression with psychotic features. In this latter case, the combination of an antidepressant with a neuroleptic may be superior to either drug alone. Psychostimulants (e.g., methylphenidate [Ritalin]) may also be useful to treat depression in certain medical and surgical patients, but their efficacy in more general cases of depression is not established.

Bipolar (Manic-Depressive) Illness

This disorder, which is much less common than unipolar illness, occurs in about 1% of the general population, affecting men and women equally. Modal age of onset is 30 years. It is more frequently diagnosed in higher social classes. In about 7% of cases, a first-degree relative is affected. Acute episodes of bipolar disorder recur about every 3 to 9 years.

For the bipolar patient in a depressive phase, decisions about choice and use of an antidepressant are the same as for the unipolar depressed patient, with at least two important exceptions. First, the bipolar patient is much more likely to switch suddenly into mania during this treatment. The literature is controversial regarding whether one type of antidepressant is less likely than another to cause this switch. However, tricyclic antidepressants may induce rapid cycling in some bipolar patients.

Another exception to the treatment of the bipolar depressed patient is that this patient will very likely be medicated with a mood stabilizer as well. Lithium carbonate (Eskalith, Lithobid, Lithonate), the only medication approved by the FDA for maintenance therapy of bipolar disorder, is a mood stabilizer. However, other types of medications, such as anticonvulsants, are being used, too, as mood stabilizers.

Lithium salts are effective in the treatment of acute mania and in the prophylaxis of mania and depression. In the prophylaxis of bipolar disorder, the efficacy of imipramine plus lithium carbonate is equal to that of lithium carbonate alone. In the prophylaxis of recurrent, unipolar depression, imipramine plus lithium carbonate has similar efficacy to imipramine alone.

Salts of lithium ion have similar physiologic effects to those of sodium and potassium. Lithium ion is readily assayed in biologic fluids by flame-photometric and atomic-absorption spectrophotometric methods. Traces are found in animal tissues. It is abundant in some mineral springs, which are thought to have medicinal properties.

There is no known physiologic role for lithium ion, i.e., the body appears not to require lithium ion for normal function. Lithium ion is readily absorbed in the gut and distributed throughout the body. It is concentrated in bone, thyroid, and brain. The majority is excreted in the urine. Therapeutic blood levels range from about 0.6 mEq per liter to 1.0 mEq per liter, beyond which serious toxic effects can occur. Side effects, which may not be dose-related, include tremor, edema, nausea, psoriasis, weight gain, acne, mental dulling, hypothyroidism, and nephrogenic diabetes insipidus/polyuria. Thus, prior to initiation of lithium therapy, patients need to have baseline laboratory tests of thyroid and kidney function, which are repeated, depending on the patient, every 4 to 6 months, during therapy.

Acute manic episodes are managed with antipsychotic drugs or divalproex sodium (Depakote), which is the only anticonvulsant drug that has received FDA approval for treatment of acute mania. Although not approved for this use by the FDA, it and other anticonvulsants (e.g., carbamazepine [Tegretol]) are being used for the prophylaxis of bipolar disorder in patients who are intolerant or nonresponsive to lithium salts. Sometimes these drugs are used in combination with one another and with lithium salts.

Acute mania can often be a very serious clinical situation, requiring hospitalization and occasionally

ECT. Compliance can often be a problem with bipolar patients, who prefer to have their mood elevated above the normal range.

SCHIZOPHRENIC DISORDERS

method of
ROBERT CANCRO, M.D., MED.D.SC.
New York University School of Medicine
New York, New York

The etiopathogenesis of the schizophrenic disorders is not known. In at least some cases, there is evidence of a genetically loaded vulnerability that predisposes the patient to a later psychotic decompensation. The vulnerability may reflect an abnormal gene or abnormal gene expression or may be the result of a statistically infrequent pattern of normal genes.

TREATMENT

Psychosocial Treatments

It is useful to make a distinction between psychosocial interventions and psychosocial treatments. Psychosocial interventions almost always have therapeutic benefits. Both the patient and the family require emotional support and education concerning the nature of the illness and the necessity for ongoing treatment. The denial presented by both patient and family can often be best managed by family physicians, because they have developed a reservoir of trust and confidence. Family education influences the way families respond to the patient's illness and plays a positive role in preventing relapse.

The actual psychosocial treatment of schizophrenia is highly specialized and is outside the usual resources available to the family physician. It can have individual, group, or family components and is best done by a facility that has the necessary expertise. This caveat is relevant to behavior modification as well, which can be helpful particularly in chronic cases in which specific symptoms create problems for the patient and/or the family.

Rehabilitation

Virtually all schizophrenic patients require both social and vocational rehabilitation in order to return to a meaningful role in society. Such forms of psychosocial rehabilitation require specialized facilities and specialized competencies.

Somatic Treatments

Pharmacotherapy

The antipsychotic drugs are not to be used as anxiolytics. They are powerful compounds that have major and diffuse effects on the central nervous system and must be used judiciously. A large number of antipsychotic compounds exist that are divided into traditional and newer or "atypical" antipsychotics clozapine (Clozaril), risperidone (Risperdal), and olanzapine (Zyprexa). It is most useful for the physician to master two or three traditional and one or two newer drugs, rather than to attempt to become proficient in a dozen or more. With the conventional drugs it is best to select compounds from different chemical groupings so that if the patient is not responsive to a particular drug, the next one selected is from a different chemical class. Frequently used agents are listed in Table 1.

Before instituting therapy with any antipsychotic, the physician should obtain baseline blood pressure measurements with the patient in both standing and reclining positions. Initial laboratory work should include a complete blood count, liver profile, and electrocardiogram (ECG) in older patients. These tests should be repeated at approximately 6-month intervals.

It is essential clinical practice to obtain a comprehensive drug history prior to initiating treatment. This history should include previous drugs taken and response to those medications, including side effects. The physician should identify target symptoms and goals so that the dosage can be titrated against a specific clinical response. After the maximum control of the target symptoms has been obtained, the patient experiencing the first episode of a schizophrenic disorder should be continued on the lowest effective dose of medication for at least 1 year.

It is good clinical practice to utilize only one antipsychotic agent at a time, rather than to practice polypharmacy. An adequate dose of one drug is to be preferred over only a homeopathic dose of two or more. The admixture of drugs merely increases the risk of untoward effects without increasing the potential benefit. There is no evidence that any of the traditional antipsychotic drugs are inherently superior to any other traditional compound. Clozapine has been demonstrated to be effective in patients resistant to conventional antipsychotic drug treatment. There is some evidence that olanzapine and risperidone are also superior to traditional antipsychotics in overall effectiveness in symptom management. In the absence of a history of a good response to a particular agent, drug choice should be based on the clinician's familiarity with the drug and its side effect profile and cost. The routine addition of antidepressive or antianxiety drugs to antipsychotic medication is to be discouraged.

Patients who show severe schizophrenic symptomatology should receive rapid drug treatment, with achievement of therapeutic doses in 3 to 7 days. Obviously, if the patient has a history of idiosyncratic drug effects, arrhythmia, or hypotension, more care is necessary. On those rare occasions when megadoses appear to be required, it is best to handle the patient in consultation with an experienced psychiatrist.

Antipsychotic drugs are best administered on a

TABLE 1. **Antipsychotic Drugs in Common Use**

Generic Name	Trade Name	Type	Daily Oral Dosage Range (mg)	Potency Equivalent	Comments
Chlorpromazine	Thorazine	Aliphatic	200–1200 mg*	1	High sedation, low EPS
Thioridazine	Mellaril	Piperidine	200–600 mg	1	High sedation, low EPS; a strong anticholinergic agent; inhibits ejaculation; Ca^{2+} channel blocker
Perphenazine	Trilafon	Piperazine	8–64 mg	10	Low sedation, high EPS including dystonia
Trifluoperazine	Stelazine	Piperazine	5–30 mg	20	Low sedation, high EPS including dystonia
Fluphenazine	Prolixin	Piperazine	5–20 mg	50	Low sedation, high EPS including dystonia, low hypotensive effect
Thiothixene	Navane	Thioxanthene	6–30 mg	20	High EPS including dystonia, low hypotensive effect
Haloperidol	Haldol	Butyrophenone	4–15 mg	50	High EPS including dystonia, low hypotensive effect
Clozapine	Clozaril	Dibenzodiazepine	200–750 mg	1.5	No EPS, high sedation
Loxapine	Loxitane	Dibenzoxazepine	50–100 mg	10	High EPS including dystonia, low hypotensive effect
Molindone	Moban	Dihydroindolone	20–250 mg	5	High EPS, lowest weight gain
Pimozide	Orap	Diphenylbutylpiperidine	1–10 mg	100	High EPS
Risperidone	Risperdal	Benzisoxazole	2–8 mg	100	Low EPS, high prolactin
Olanzapine	Zyprexa	Thienobenzodiazepine	5–20 mg	50	Low EPS, weight gain

Abbreviation: EPS = extrapyramidal side effects.
*Exceeds dosage recommended by the manufacturer.

once- or twice-a-day basis as soon as the initial symptoms are controlled. Occasionally, paradoxical reactions are possible—for example, the patient may become restless or have difficulty sleeping. Should this be the case, the bulk of the dose should be given in the morning. Most patients, however, who are placed on a twice-a-day schedule should receive the bulk of their dose at night. After habituation takes place, the patient can usually tolerate a full dose at bedtime. In this way, the patient obtains the benefits with the least awareness of side effects.

During hospitalization, it is frequently useful to use parenteral or liquid forms of antipsychotic medication. At least 20 to 25% of hospitalized patients do not actually take their oral medication. Urine and blood tests can be helpful in identifying which patients are actually taking drugs. In the case of intramuscular medication, it is important to remember that drugs given by this route are usually 2 to 4 times more powerful than the oral forms, and the dosage level must be corrected accordingly. Slow-acting fluphenazine and haloperidol decanoate are not useful for rapid control of psychotic symptoms. These agents take longer to have their initial effect. Their use is primarily in the management of patients who cannot be depended upon to take oral medication.

A 6- to 8-week trial on a particular drug is required before it can be considered to have failed in the case of acute schizophrenic disorders. Patients with chronic conditions may require 4- to 6-month trials before a particular drug should be discarded. These clinical realities pose major problems in an era of managed care. It is frequently necessary in the present climate to utilize anxiolytics and sedatives in addition to antipsychotic drugs so as to shorten the initial period of hospitalization.

The newer, so-called atypical antipsychotics have certain advantages over the traditional compounds. In general, they have modest to no extrapyramidal side effects (EPS). Some of the newer compounds do not raise prolactin levels. Clozapine has been shown to be significantly superior for cases resistant to traditional drug treatment. However, it causes bone marrow suppression, which can actually lead to death in as much as 1% of the cases. Clozapine therapy therefore requires careful monitoring and weekly blood counts. All of the newer antipsychotics are associated with significant weight gain, and this may pose a problem in patient acceptance.

Contraindications. Severe cardiovascular disease is a contraindication to antipsychotic medication. Caution is also warranted in the face of serious liver damage. The effects of these agents on pregnancy are not known. There is some evidence that they may reduce the risk of psychosis in the unborn fetus.

Side Effects. Drowsiness is a common side effect, particularly with the aliphatic and piperidine side chain compounds. The newer compounds are also associated with a degree of drowsiness. Tolerance is usually achieved reasonably rapidly, and after several weeks of therapeutic levels the drowsiness is diminished.

Some dermatologic side effects may also occur. Urticaria, contact dermatitis, and photosensitivity all have been reported.

Metabolic side effects are also common. Weight gain is a frequent side effect of all of these compounds and in particular, with the newer so-called atypical agents. Molindone is the drug of choice in patients in whom weight gain is a problem. Noncompliance can be a particular problem in young patients concerned with their appearance. Rigid dietary management is to be encouraged and the use of appetite suppressants avoided. Other metabolic changes include gynecomastia, galactorrhea, and amenorrhea.

Ocular changes may also occur. Pigmentation of the lens and cornea is frequently seen with chlorpromazine therapy, particularly when the drug is given in dosages in excess of 2500 mg per day.

Electrocardiographic changes occur in 2 to 3% of patients receiving traditional antipsychotics. The changes are usually seen as Q wave and T wave alterations. Dysrhythmias can also occur. Syncope is not uncommon and is related to the hypotensive effect of some of these drugs.

Jaundice is a possible side effect, and the medication must be discontinued if jaundice develops.

Hematologic changes may occur. Leukocytosis, leukopenia, and eosinophilia all are common with the traditional compounds. Agranulocytosis is a particular concern with clozapine.

Extrapyramidal signs are a frequent concomitant of traditional antipsychotic drug treatment. The newer compounds, because of their low incidence of EPS, have the benefit of not causing these side effects to the same degree. Extrapyramidal signs are particularly common in elderly patients, women, and persons with central nervous system disease. The treatment of choice for extrapyramidal signs is the use of anticholinergic drugs such as benztropine mesylate (Cogentin), 0.5 to 3 mg per day by mouth. Diphenhydramine (Benadryl) is also helpful for management of EPS.

Akathisia is a very common manifestation of extrapyramidal involvement and should not be confused with agitation. Most frequently it involves the lower limbs and takes the form of regular and rhythmic motor movements, e.g., tapping or rocking. The use of anticholinergic drugs or reduction in the dosage level of the antipsychotic medication is indicated in the presence of akathisia.

Dystonic reactions are also common and are usually manifested as torticollis and oculogyric crises. The treatment of dystonic reaction is to reduce the dosage of antipsychotic medication or to add anticholinergic drugs. Anticholinergic drugs should be given in divided doses because their action is short. They should not be given at bedtime because the extrapyramidal and dystonic effects cannot be observed while the patient is asleep. After 2 to 3 months of treatment it is often possible to eliminate the anticholinergic drug, and the majority of the patients who have shown EPS will not continue to do so.

Persistent tardive dyskinesia is a disorder involving primarily buccolingual movements. It is particularly common in elderly patients and women. Vitamin E in doses of up to 2 grams a day can be helpful in reducing this untoward effect.

Electroconvulsive Therapy

Electroconvulsive therapy (ECT) has been of limited use in the treatment of schizophrenic disorders since the advent of the antipsychotic drugs. Occasional patients, however, are resistant to medication and can benefit from a course of treatment with ECT. The usual course consists of 20 ECT procedures administered on a three-times-a-week basis. Electroencephalographic monitoring of the treatment is important to ascertain that a seizure of adequate depth has been induced. Patients who have been resistant to drug therapy are often more responsive to medication following a course of ECT.

No other somatic treatment has been demonstrated to be in fact helpful in these disorders.

PANIC DISORDER

method of
SMIT S. SINHA, M.D., and
JACK M. GORMAN, M.D.
Columbia University College of Physicians and Surgeons and New York State Psychiatric Institute
New York, New York

Panic disorder is a common and debilitating illness, affecting approximately 2 to 3% of the population and defined by the occurrence of spontaneous panic attacks. The illness is a serious one, associated with considerable morbidity; therefore, it has been the focus of vigorous scientific research over the past two decades, and promising advances have been made toward the development of effective treatment strategies to control symptomatology and improve clinical course.

The core clinical feature of panic disorder is the spontaneous panic attack, a rapid crescendo of intense fear lasting approximately 10 to 30 minutes and occurring with several somatic and cognitive symptoms. The patient experiences a sudden, massive outburst of autonomic activity with palpitations, shortness of breath, chest pain, trembling, diaphoresis, dizziness, and paresthesias. In addition, patients fear they will die, "go crazy," or lose control of themselves. The experience of panic is exceptionally frightening; patients often believe they are having a heart attack, stroke, or other condition constituting a medical emergency. A spontaneous panic attack by definition occurs "out of the blue," without any environmental or situational trigger. Panic attacks are common events that are also seen in a number of medical and psychiatric conditions as well as in a significant portion of the general population. However, for the diagnosis of panic disorder to be made, the patient must experience recurrent, unexpected panic attacks; following an attack, the patient must experience at least a 1-month period of fearing the occurrence or consequences of another attack. This persistent fear is known as anticipatory anxiety. Panic disorder usually begins in late adolescence to early adulthood, and is two to three times more likely to affect women than men.

Closely associated with panic disorder is the development of phobic avoidance, in which the patient's fear of experiencing future attacks leads to an avoidance of places or situations in which a panic attack occurred previously, such as while driving a car, riding the subway, or being inside an elevator. This avoidance can then become generalized to other situations and become so severe that the patient may be globally incapacitated, unable even to venture out of the house unless accompanied by a close friend or relative. This extreme form of avoidance behavior is known as *agoraphobia* and occurs in an estimated 50 to 60% of patients with panic disorder as a significant complication of the illness.

Panic disorder creates numerous impairments in lifestyle, and patients often find it inordinately difficult to function in regular work and social environments. Also, because intense physical symptoms dominate the clinical picture, patients with panic disorder routinely seek help from various medical specialists and are frequent users of medical emergency departments. It is necessary for the clinician to inquire about co-morbid psychiatric illnesses, as panic patients are at serious risk for the development of major depression and have an elevated attempted suicide rate. Furthermore, patients with panic disorder have a propensity toward self-medication with alcohol and nonprescription sedative hypnotics; the presence of a co-morbid substance use disorder thus needs to be ruled out, as this may preclude the use of certain treatments, particularly the benzodiazepines, in such cases.

DIFFERENTIAL DIAGNOSIS

Panic disorder has been referred to as the "great masquerader," because the vast array of intense somatic symptoms that characterize the illness can mimic a host of medical and psychiatric conditions. The clinician must be careful to rule out, through proper history, physical examination, and laboratory evaluation, any possible organic cause of the panic symptomatology. A number of conditions need to be excluded, as shown in Table 1.

TREATMENT

Successful treatment of panic disorder targets the spontaneous panic attack. Once the panic attacks are blocked, anticipatory anxiety decreases, with a subsequent reduction in phobic avoidance. Proper treatment involves utilization of specific pharmacologic therapy as well as cognitive-behavioral psychotherapeutic intervention. A good treatment strategy must be tailored to the needs of the individual patient and may involve drug treatment alone, cognitive-behavioral therapy alone, or a combination of the two modalities.

TABLE 1. **Common Organic Causes of Panic Symptomatology**

Condition	Diagnostic Tests/Considerations
Endocrine	
Hypothyroidism	Thyroid function studies
Hyperthyroidism	Thyroid function studies
Hyperparathyroidism	Serum calcium
Pheochromocytoma	24-hour urine collection for measurement of catecholamine metabolites
Cardiovascular	
Acute myocardial infarction	Electrocardiogram
Cardiac arrhythmias	Consider 24-hour monitor
Mitral valve prolapse	
Neurologic	
Temporal lobe epilepsy	Electroencephalogram
Vestibular disorders	Referral to otolaryngologist or neurologist
Substance withdrawal	
Alcohol, barbiturate, opiate	Urine and serum toxicologic studies
Acute intoxication	
Amphetamines, cocaine	Urine and serum toxicologic studies

Pharmacotherapy

Antidepressants

Antidepressants have long been known to block spontaneous panic attacks and induce clinical remission in most patients. The major advance in recent years in the treatment of panic disorder has been the advent of the selective serotonin reuptake inhibitors (SSRIs) and their recognition as powerful anti-panic drugs. The SSRIs act preferentially at serotonin receptors, blocking reuptake and enhancing availability of this neurotransmitter, and should now be considered as first-line agents for treatment of panic. Currently available SSRIs include fluoxetine (Prozac),* paroxetine (Paxil), sertraline (Zoloft), and fluvoxamine (Luvox).* These medications possess distinct advantages over the traditional antidepressants in that they maintain a much more favorable side effect profile while achieving comparable or often greater efficacy. SSRIs have little anticholinergic activity and are less likely to produce dry mouth, blurred vision, constipation, and urinary hesitancy. In addition, SSRIs have no significant cardiovascular effects and do not usually alter blood pressure or cardiac rhythm. Other problematic side effects such as weight gain and sedation are uncommon, and these medications are also relatively safe when taken in overdose. It is imperative that SSRIs be initiated at very low doses, as there is a risk of exacerbating anxiety and causing jitteriness early in treatment. Titration to higher doses should then be done gradually and cautiously. Dosages are shown in Table 2. Apart from the initial stimulatory effects, SSRIs can cause gastrointestinal distress, headache, sleep disturbance, sexual dysfunction, and hypomania. Typically, SSRIs exert their anti-panic effects after 4 weeks, with continued improvement evident through the first 3 months of drug treatment.

The tricyclic antidepressants (TCAs) also have the ability to block spontaneous panic and, before the introduction of the SSRIs, represented the standard pharmacologic treatment for panic disorder. If a trial of one or more SSRIs proves ineffective in a particular patient, implementation of therapy with a TCA is the next consideration in the treatment strategy. TCAs such as imipramine (Tofranil),* nortriptyline (Pamelor),* desipramine (Norpramin), and clomipramine (Anafranil)* are inexpensive, highly effective medications and achieve panic blockade in ap-

*Not FDA approved for this indication.

TABLE 2. **Medication Regimens for Panic Disorder**

Medication	Initial Dose	Target Dose
SSRIs		
Fluoxetine (Prozac)	5–10 mg/d	20–40 mg/d
Paroxetine (Paxil)	10 mg/d	20–40 mg/d
Sertraline (Zoloft)	25 mg/d	50–200 mg/d
Fluvoxamine (Luvox)	25 mg/d	75–100 mg/d
Tricyclic antidepressants		
Imipramine (Tofranil)	10 mg/d	100–300 mg/d
Nortriptyline (Pamelor)	10 mg/d	50–150 ng/ml (blood level)
Clomipramine (Anafranil)	10 mg/d	50–200 mg/d
Desipramine (Norpramin)	10 mg/d	100–300 mg/d
Monoamine oxidase inhibitors		
Phenelzine (Nardil)	15 mg/d	45–90 mg/d
Benzodiazepines		
Alprazolam (Xanax)	0.25–0.5 mg tid	2–6 mg/d total
Lorazepam (Ativan)	0.5 mg tid	1–2 mg/d total
Clonazepam (Klonopin)	0.25–0.5 mg bid	1–3 mg/d total

Abbreviation: SSRIs = selective serotonin reuptake inhibitors.

proximately 80% of patients. Unfortunately, they have a number of deleterious side effects, including those associated with a high degree of cholinergic blockade. They also adversely affect the cardiovascular system, with resultant tachycardia, orthostatic hypotension, and cardiac conduction delays. Weight gain and sedation also occur and can affect patient compliance. TCAs are potentially lethal in overdose. Panic patients are very sensitive to the effects of TCAs, and it is important that the starting dose be low and gradually increased to therapeutic levels. Typical dosages are shown in Table 2. Therapeutic effects are generally seen after approximately 8 to 12 weeks of treatment.

The monoamine oxidase inhibitors (MAOIs), such as phenelzine (Nardil),* are the third class of antidepressants with marked anti-panic activity. The major disadvantage of MAOIs is their risk of producing a hypertensive crisis due to inhibition of monoamine metabolism. To prevent this medical emergency, patients are required to follow a special tyramine-free diet. In addition, several medications, including most sympathomimetic amines, antihistamines, and meperidine, are contraindicated. Other side effects include orthostatic hypotension, weight gain, and sedation. Because of these limiting factors, MAOIs are utilized in panic disorder as third-line agents for therapy in patients refractory to the other treatments available.

*Not FDA approved for this indication.

Benzodiazepines

Therapeutic response to antidepressant treatment usually takes a minimum of 4 weeks or longer; however, it is often necessary to achieve anti-panic effects more quickly. High-potency benzodiazepines such as alprazolam (Xanax), clonazepam (Klonopin), and lorazepam (Ativan)* all have been shown to block spontaneous panic and to ameliorate anticipatory anxiety as well and generally produce their effects within the first week of treatment. These medications are thus extremely effective for rapid anxiolysis during the initiation phase of antidepressant therapy and can later be used intermittently to abort episodes of acute panic. Benzodiazepines are also useful for patients who have contraindications to using antidepressants or who cannot tolerate the unwanted side effects of those drugs. Sedation is the main side effect of the benzodiazepines, with ataxia, memory disturbance, and paradoxical disinhibition occurring infrequently. The major disadvantage of chronic benzodiazepine use is the likelihood of physiologic dependency. This can result in a serious withdrawal syndrome if the drug is abruptly discontinued, characterized by rebound anxiety, insomnia, and an increased risk of seizures. Slow, gradual tapering of the benzodiazepine dosage is thus recommended for all patients. Usual dosages are shown in Table 2.

Cognitive-Behavioral Therapy

Although psychotropic medications have been the mainstay of treatment for panic disorder, recent evidence shows that cognitive-behavioral therapy (CBT) is also a highly effective treatment. CBT for panic disorder involves four main components: (1) breathing retraining to decrease the tendency to hyperventilate; (2) cognitive restructuring to block catastrophic, anxiety-producing, and distorted thoughts; (3) interoceptive deconditioning to desensitize the patient to somatic sensations; and (4) exposure training to reduce phobic avoidance. A usual course of CBT lasts approximately 3 months, and ongoing research indicates that the combination of medication plus CBT may be more effective in treating panic than either modality alone.

*Not FDA approved for this indication.

Section 17

Physical and Chemical Injuries

BURNS

method of
STEVEN E. WOLF, M.D., and
DAVID N. HERNDON, M.D.
Shriners Hospital for Crippled Children, Galveston Burn Unit
Galveston, Texas

Burn injuries from flame, chemicals, hot liquids, and electricity affect more than 2 million people per year in the United States. Most of these injuries are minor and can be treated on an outpatient basis; however, nearly 70,000 patients have moderate to severe injuries and require hospitalization. Moderate to severe injuries by American Burn Association criteria include burns over 10% of the total body surface area (TBSA) or burns of the eyes, ears, face, hands, feet, or perineum. Burns in patients that meet these criteria; full-thickness burns in any area; electrical burns, chemical burns, burns associated with inhalation injury; or burns in patients with significant comorbid conditions or in patients with other trauma that has stabilized should be referred to a qualified burn unit with special resources and expertise to address these patients' unique needs (Table 1).

Mortality rates from burns have markedly decreased over the last four decades because of new treatment modalities derived from ongoing research. In 1952, a 50% TBSA burn was associated with a 50% mortality. Now, a young, previously healthy person can survive almost any size burn, even in the presence of complicating injuries such as inhalation injury or other trauma. This staggering improvement is due to improved understanding of the importance of resuscitation, early wound excision and closure, metabolic support after the injury, and control of infection. Further challenges for the future include better control of pain, restriction of hypertrophic scarring, improvement of cosmetic outcomes, and efficient rehabilitation for full return of occupation and vocation.

TABLE 1. **Definition of Burns Requiring Care in a Specialized Burn Unit**

- Partial-thickness burns >10% total body surface area (TBSA)
- Burns of the hands, face, feet, perineum, across major points
- Full-thickness burns in any age group
- Electrical burns (including lightning injury)
- Chemical burns
- Inhalation injury
- Burns in patients with significant co-morbid medical conditions
- Burns in patients with other traumatic injuries that have been stabilized

INITIAL EVALUATION AND MANAGEMENT

Treatment begins at the scene by controlling the burn process. This involves removing the patient from the source of heat in the case of thermal injury, from the caustic agent by rinsing in the case of chemical injury, or from the electricity source to which the victim is often gripped upon in tetanic agony. For flame burns, the patient should be placed on the ground and either rolled to extinguish the flames or wrapped in a fire-resistant material. After the fire has been extinguished, all remaining embers of charred clothing or other material involved should be removed. The patient is then covered with clean sheets and blankets. Application of ice or damp dressings to decrease the level of injury should be discouraged, as this can result in hypothermia. Every effort should be made to keep the patient warm. For chemical burns, all contaminated clothing should be removed, with care taken not to extend the burn area by placing tainted items on unburned areas of the patient's body, and to protect rescuers from contact with the chemical. The burned area should then be rinsed with copious quantities of water or saline (10 liters or more) to dilute the active chemical; care should be taken that diluent does not drain over normal skin, thus bringing the noxious agent to noninjured areas potentially extending the injury. Patients should also never be immersed in the irrigant, to avoid spreading the burn to previously nonexposed areas. Irrigation should continue during transport to the treating facility.

In all traumatic injuries including burns, airway patency is of primary concern. When inhalation injury is suspected, 100% O_2 should be administered as soon as possible by face mask. Smoke inhalation can cause severe upper airway hyperemia and the resulting irritation can induce dense bronchospasm, which will critically reduce gas exchange. At the slightest indication of impending airway loss, such as the development of stridor, inspiratory grunting, wheezing, or tachypnea, prophylactic intubation should be performed. If possible, a continuous oxygen saturation monitor should be used during transport and resuscitation of all burn patients; however, normal values should be interpreted with caution, because carbon monoxide (CO) in the blood will falsely elevate apparent oxygen saturation. CO has 280 times the affinity for hemoglobin as O_2, and it is present in high quantities in most smoke. Because CO binds hemoglobin at the O_2-binding site and turns the blood red, modern oxygen saturation monitors measure it as oxygen. Therefore, patients who are severely hypoxic because of CO poisoning will have normal oxygen saturation values. Because of the high affinity of CO for hemoglobin, the half-life of CO-bound hemoglobin is 4 hours under room air conditions. This can be reduced by increasing the partial pressure of O_2 with use of 100% O_2, thus increasing the gradient for O_2 binding. The unbound CO is then expelled through the lungs, where concentrations of CO are low because the patient has been removed from the smoke. Providing 100% O_2 will decrease the half-life from 4 hours to 45 minutes. If there is any question of critical CO poisoning, the safest course is endotracheal intubation with administration of 100% O_2. Patients with severe burns of the face and neck should also be intubated early, before the development of edema, which can make endotracheal access very difficult. Occasionally, a surgical airway through the cricothyroid membrane is required, particularly if stridor has already developed from near-occlusion of the vocal cords. Tracheal intubation in such circumstances is difficult at best, with laryngospasm occurring on contact with the tightened cords, which are resistant to local anesthesia with topical lidocaine.

Once the airway is established, intravenous resuscitation is the next priority. Fluids should be administered via peripheral larger-bore intravenous catheters, which are safely secured by suture ligation as soon as possible, because delays in resuscitation will adversely affect outcome. In patients in whom age, associated injury, or co-morbid medical conditions may complicate the resuscitation, central venous catheters should be considered before placement landmarks are lost owing to edema formation; however, peripheral venous catheters should be placed first to begin the resuscitation. If necessary, catheters can be placed through burned skin. Venous cutdowns using the saphenous vein at the ankle or in the groin are indicated if necessary. Any patient with moderate or severe burns or serious co-morbid conditions should have bladder catheters placed to monitor the progress of the resuscitation using urine output as a guide.

Patients do not expire from undressed wounds during the initial assessment but generally develop complications from loss of the airway, hypovolemia, or hypothermia; therefore, these issues must be addressed first. When the airway is secure and resuscitation has begun, attention to the wounds and other associated injuries can proceed at a more deliberate pace. Severe burns can cause alterations in gastrointestinal tract function; therefore, nasogastric tubes should be placed in patients with moderate and severe burns, initially for gastric decompression and later as feeding access. Early feeding within 6 to 8 hours of the injury has been shown to diminish the hypermetabolic response and to maintain intestinal integrity. Occasionally, transduodenal tubes may be necessary to achieve this goal because of gastric ileus. Initial laboratory studies should include determination of hemoglobin and platelet concentrations; measurement of serum electrolytes, serum osmolarity, blood urea nitrogen (BUN), and serum creatinine; and arterial blood gas analysis. Routine electrocardiographic monitoring and frequent temperature determinations should also be performed.

An initial rapid examination of the burn wound is made, as well as an assessment of distal extremity pulses and tissue compartment pressures. Full-thickness injuries produce a nonyielding eschar that will not expand with increasing edema formation. Generalized swelling that occurs after injury combined with localized edema under burned skin increases tissue pressures. First, venous outflow diminishes; then arterial inflow is compromised as the pressures further increase. With circumferential burns, an acutely diminished or absent pulse in an extremity with a normal central blood pressure indicates the need for escharotomies to relieve the pressure. Note, however, that it usually takes 3 to 8 hours for edema to develop sufficiently to increase pressure. The most common cause for lack of pulses in an extremity is hypovolemia with peripheral vasoconstriction. Measured pressures in a tissue compartment of greater than 40 mm Hg should also prompt intervention.

Escharotomies are generally performed on the medial and lateral aspects of the extremity and must extend the length of the constricting eschar to completely relieve the pressure. These incisions can be done with a scalpel blade with minimal bleeding, because the eschar is devascularized; however, an electrocautery device can also be used. A proper depth is assured by obvious release of edematous tissues. If the vascular compromise has been prolonged, reperfusion in an extremity after the escharotomy may result in a reactive hyperemia and edema of the compartment muscles, necessitating fasciotomies to completely restore perfusion. Systemic acidosis from reperfusion of ischemic areas can occur after escharotomies and fasciotomies; thus, resuscitation should be well under way to avoid hypotension when these interventions are performed. Bleeding can occur from these incisions as well and should be controlled with direct pressure to prevent further volume loss.

All burn patients have traumatic injuries, and physicians distracted by the burn may miss associated injuries. All patients should have a full secondary survey for other traumatic injuries as dictated by Advanced Trauma Life Support Program (ATLS) protocols during their initial assessment. Failure to respond to the calculated amounts of resuscitation fluid should increase an already high degree of suspicion for other injuries. Initial burn treatment may be superseded by management of other injuries if these are severe enough to warrant surgical intervention; however, the receiving burn center should be notified while this is taking place so that a timely burn treatment plan can be established.

Patients with burns of sufficient severity to require transfer to a burn center should be evaluated for airway patency, intravenous access, and other injuries prior to transfer while the transport arrangements are made. After these issues are appropriately addressed, the patient is ready for transfer. The burn wounds themselves should be covered with dry dressings without ointments or creams to avoid heat loss, allowing subsequent treatment with biologic dressings if necessary.

FLUID RESUSCITATION

The first step in effective resuscitation is a rapid clinical assessment of the extent and depth of the burn, as well as determination of the presence of associated injuries such as inhalation injury. An accurate estimation of the area and depth of the wound is essential. The commonly used "rule of nines" provides a quick assessment of the burn area in adults. However, in children it can overestimate the size of the burned area on the trunk and extremities, because in this age group, the head makes up a relatively larger area in proportion, especially in infants (Table 2). Age-appropriate diagrams of Lund-Browder charts can be used to accurately quantify burn size. Smaller burns and those of noncontinuous distribution can be quantitated using the size of the patient's palm, regardless of age, which is approximately 1% of the TBSA.

Once the burn surface area is established, the amount of resuscitation fluid can be estimated. Burn shock is caused by the formation of generalized edema, transvascular fluid shifts, and massively increased evaporative volume losses. Edema formation is maximal at 8 to 12 hours after injury for small burns and at up to 24 to 48 hours for large burns. The prime goal of resuscitation is to support this process and thus avoid hypovolemia and microvascular ischemia. Various formulas based on the total burn size and patient size have been devised, and all have been used with success. The Parkland formula, otherwise known as the Baxter formula, recommends administration of 2 to 4 mL of lactated Ringer's solution per kg of body weight for each percent of TBSA burned in the first 24 hours after burn, one half of which is given in the first 8 hours and the rest in the following 16 hours. This is the most commonly used formula and is very effective in estimating needs in adults; however, in children it underestimates the evaporative losses and maintenance needs. Calculations in children, therefore, should use estimates based on the body surface area in square meters instead of weight. The Galveston formula estimates 5000 mL of fluid per m^2 of TBSA burned plus 2000 mL per m^2, using 5% dextrose in lactated Ringer's solution, in the first 24 hours, again divided into one half in the first 8 hours and the rest in the subsequent 16 hours. Dextrose is used in resuscitation fluid in children to prevent hypoglycemia because of their relatively diminished glycogen stores. Smoke inhalation may require use of up to 33% more fluid volume because of edema formation within the injured lung. Delays in resuscitation can increase required volumes as well because of even further increases in obligatory edema.

Once resuscitation has been initiated, patients must be monitored closely for the effectiveness of the resuscitation efforts. All resuscitation formulas are only guidelines to volume requirements, and the adequacy of the resuscitation must be measured and changes implemented as appropriate to avoid over- or under-resuscitation. A urine output of 0.5–1.0 mL per kg per hour is a reasonable clinical indicator of vital organ perfusion and can be used to guide therapy. This must be tempered by the fact that burn patients can develop a high serum glucose with resultant glycosuria, causing an osmotic diuresis; therefore, frequent glucose measurements are necessary.

Hypertonic salt solutions are used by some centers to resuscitate burn patients; however, recent studies have not been able to demonstrate decreased fluid requirements or decreased percent weight gain with hypertonic saline compared with Ringer's solution. In fact, the rapid and dramatic increases in blood pressure induced by hypertonic saline have been suggested to do more harm than good. Some studies have shown an increase in renal failure in patients treated with hypertonic saline, and hyperchloremic metabolic acidosis is a potential effect of hypertonic saline that could potentiate the metabolic acidosis of hypovolemic shock. For these reasons, hypertonic saline is not currently recommended in the treatment of burns but may be useful in improved formulations in the future with further research.

TABLE 2. **Estimation of Body Surface Area: "Rule of Nines"**

	% of Total Body Surface Area	
Body Area	*Child*	*Adult*
Head and neck	18	9
Anterior torso	18	18
Posterior torso	18	18
Arm	9	9
Leg	14	18
Perineum	1	1

WOUND CARE

Current therapy for burn wounds can be divided into three stages: assessment, treatment, and rehabilitation. Assessment involves precise determination of the extent of injury, including location and depth of the burn. Accurate evaluation of the depth of the wound is essential in development of a successful treatment plan. Traditionally, burns have been divided into first-degree, second-degree, and third-degree burns, which correspond anatomically to epidermal burns, partial-thickness dermal burns with remaining viable dermis and epidermis, and full-thickness burns, respectively. Epidermal burns heal completely without scarring within a few days and require nothing more than symptomatic care. At our institution, aloe vera gel is used to relieve the discomfort of these wounds. Partial-thickness dermal burns usually heal within 3 weeks; however, the deeper of these may develop hypertrophic scarring once healed, and sometimes only a tenuous epithelial covering develops in the first several months after injury. Full-thickness burns have no remaining skin elements and can heal spontaneously only by migration of cells from the wound edge—a process that can take months to years without grafting. Determination of the type of wound that is present at the outset can provide the basis for timely treatment, because each type of wound is treated differently.

Burn wound depth is generally assessed by an experienced examiner and is based on the characteristics of the wound. First-degree wounds are erythematous and painful and have an intact skin barrier. Second-degree wounds differ according to the depth of injury within the dermis. Superficial wounds involving only the papillary dermis often develop blisters. After removal of this layer, the wounds are typically pink, wet, and hypersensitive to touch. Burns that are deeper and extend into the reticular dermis can develop blisters; however, the surface underneath may appear mottled pink and white, and capillary refill is slow. These wounds, however, remain sensate to pinprick. Full-thickness wounds often have a charred appearance with a firm leathery eschar that is completely insensate owing to loss of nerve fiber endings. These wounds do not blanch with pressure. Occasionally, a burn injury may have the appearance of a deep second-degree wound that is pink to red in color; however, on closer inspection, it will not blanch with pressure and is insensate. This is also a full-thickness injury, and it is particularly common with immersion scald as the mechanism. It should be emphasized that assessment by examination can be difficult because of the dynamic nature of the wound. Some burns that appear to be second-degree initially turn out to be full-thickness, and vice versa. Because the evaluation of depth is essential for effective management, numerous devices and techniques have been developed to assist the physician in the evaluation, including burn wound biopsy, vital dyes, ultrasound studies, fluorescein fluorometry, thermography, light reflectance, MRI, and laser Doppler flowmetry, all with varying measures of success. Laser Doppler and light reflectance have shown the most promise; however, these technologies are still in development and are not standard in everyday practice.

Once the extent of injury is established, an individualized management plan is formulated. After the wound is assessed, cleaned, and débrided by the primary care physician, an appropriate dressing should be placed. A dressing serves four functions: first, to protect the damaged epithelium; second, to splint the area into the desired position to maximize long-term function; third, to occlude the wound and reduce evaporative heat loss; and fourth, to provide comfort. The optimal burn dressing does all of these with relatively little effort by health care personnel. Most wounds are treated with some type of topical antibiotic salve on a cotton dressing that is reinforced by more dry cotton dressings, and affixed with elastic wrap bandages or surgical net–type stockings. In the case of second-degree wounds that have been cleaned and are without necrotic debris, biologic dressings such as cadaver allograft skin or pig xenograft skin can be used. These adhere to the wound and provide for all the functions of a dressing with minimal care and, in the case of cadaver allograft, provide some barrier to infection. Such dressings work best if put on soon after the injury in a noncolonized wound. Synthetic dressings such as Biobrane will perform in a similar fashion except that the immunologic properties of cadaver allograft are absent. Cadaver allograft does have the disadvantages of carrying donor antigens and of possible disease transmission, minimized by extensive testing of the donor skin; because of these drawbacks, it is recommended only for patients with large burns who are at greatest risk for acute infectious complications.

Topical antimicrobial agents are typically used over second-degree wounds until the wound is completely reepithelialized, to limit bacterial and fungal colonization in burn wounds. They can also be used over biologic or synthetic occlusive dressings. The three agents most commonly used are silver sulfadiazine (Silvadene), mafenide acetate (Sulfamylon), and 0.5% silver nitrate solution. Sulfamylon is also available in solution form. These agents should not be mixed. Topical nystatin can be added to any of these to inhibit fungal growth. Other agents such as bacitracin and polymyxin B are less effective for bacterial killing but are loss toxic to reepithelialization. Usage should be dictated by the typical flora, usually staphylococci, streptococci, and *Pseudomonas* species. When culture identifies other pathogens in the flora, the antibiotics can be changed as appropriate. The ultimate goal of topical antimicrobial therapy is to prevent invasive infection until the burn wound reepithelializes or can be excised and grafted.

An aggressive approach to burn wound excision and grafting is the standard of care for full-thickness wounds. Early excision of the entire wound with closure either by skin grafting with autograft taken from unburned areas on the patient or by cadaver allograft at the first operation, or both, has been shown to reduce mortality in patients with massive burns. All excisions, however, must be customized to the individual patient, to maximize cosmetic outcome in the most efficient fashion. Tangential excision with sequential shaving of the eschar until a viable grafting bed is reached gives a better cosmetic outcome by leaving some dermis and the subcutaneous fat; however, blood loss will be greater than that with fascial excisions. Tourniquets can be used on extremities, but then determination of the level of excision to viable tissue is more difficult. Other techniques such as subcutaneous injection of epinephrine and rapid excision with pressure application can also decrease blood loss in these situations. Blood loss despite these maneuvers can be estimated to be 0.5 to 1.0 mL per cm^2 of tissue excised. These techniques, however, should not be used in patients with deep full-thickness wounds who cannot tolerate significant blood loss owing to myocardial disease or other comorbid conditions. These patients may be better served with excision to the level of fascia with electrocautery to minimize blood loss.

After excision of the eschar, the wound must be closed. In burns of less than 30% TBSA, wound closure is usually completed in one operation with split-thickness skin grafts from unburned areas on the patient taken in sheets or meshed either 1:1 or 2:1. In burns larger than 40%, the skin grafts are meshed wider (3:1 or 4:1) and overlaid with cadaver allograft and applied until they run out. The remaining open areas are covered with cadaver allograft skin in preparation for grafting at a later staged procedure. The use of allograft, xenograft, or artificial coverings such as Integra or Dermagraft-TC is almost certainly necessary for burns over 40% TBSA. In these patients, all the available donor sites are used to provide autograft in the first operation. After the donor sites heal in 1 to 2 weeks, the patient is returned to the operating room for repeat grafting of areas temporarily covered with other coverings, using the same donor sites. Patients with greater than 90% burns may require up to 10 such cycles to completely close the wounds, and in these cases, tissue-cultured autologous skin may be useful.

Commercial products such as Integra are available to provide closure of the wound in large burns. When autograft is available, the silicone layer is removed and autograft is applied. This product provides the additional benefit of a neodermis that may provide some cosmetic and functional advantage by decreasing hypertrophic scar formation. One disadvantage to using this product for this purpose specifically is that it must be engrafted for 2 weeks prior to placement of autograft, so that patients with smaller burns whose wounds would be completely healed by that time will experience a delay in their rehabilitation. A product that provides a neodermis compatible with immediate placement of autograft is Alloderm, which is decellularized cadaver dermis; thus, all the alloantigens have been removed. This product, however, has the disadvantage of not providing wound coverage except with overlying autograft for persons in whom excision and grafting must be staged.

CRITICAL CARE

During the course of staged autograft coverage of major burns, organ dysfunction and failure associated with the systemic inflammatory response that occurs maximally with these injuries may occur. Particular attention should be paid to the respiratory and renal systems. Support of the hypermetabolic response with nutrition is also very important during the acute treatment phase.

Lung injury from smoke inhalation or acute lung injury from release of toxic inflammatory mediators associated with the open wounds may necessitate a course of ventilatory support. Every effort should be made to wean patients from the ventilator early in their course because an important aspect of management is clearing the bronchial secretions associated with airway inflammation, which the patient can do much more efficiently with coughing and pulmonary toilet in the absence of an endotracheal tube. When mechanical ventilation is necessary, however, pressure-controlled ventilation with lower airway pressures can be used to minimize barotrauma. The use of the more recently developed oscillating ventilator, which superimposes high-frequency oscillation onto conventional tidal volume breaths, also holds promise as a better method of ventilation after smoke injury. This technique reduces barotrauma and provides for vibratory air movement, which assists in removing airway casts, a hallmark of smoke inhalation. When the airway epithelium is injured, the ciliated cells slough into the lumen along with an inflammatory exudate that coalesces into casts. These casts can then set up a ball-valve effect by which airway pressures in the distal lung increase: air can flow past the cast when the airway is expanded during inspiration but cannot return when the airway collapses onto the cast during exhalation. Nebulized heparin inhalation treatments (5000 units in 10 mL of normal saline every 4 hours) also decrease plug formation by inhibiting fibrin clot formation in the airway.

Advances in early resuscitation have markedly decreased the incidence of renal failure occurring after burn injuries to the point that it is relatively rare. Also, advances in the care of patients with renal failure have decreased mortality by 50% for what was once a lethal complication after burn. In addition, the severity of acute tubular necrosis after burn injury has apparently diminished owing to improved complete care of these patients, so that this condition is relatively infrequent; among those who are affected, it is relatively less severe, with eventual recovery in most cases. The hallmarks of renal failure are an elevation in serum creatinine and a fall in creatinine clearance. Care must be taken to prevent the development of this complication with adequate resuscitation, judicious treatment of infection in the wound and other sites, and close surveillance of nephrotoxic drugs such as the aminoglycoside antibiotics, vancomycin, and loop diuretics. When complications of electrolyte or fluid balance problems from inadequate renal function intervene, dialysis may become necessary. We prefer peritoneal dialysis or continuous venovenous hemodialysis because of the lability of the electrolyte levels and fluid balance in these patients, and frequent changes as dictated by frequent monitoring are often necessary.

Patients with severe burns have metabolic rates that are 100 to 150% higher than normal. These patients have increased energy and protein requirements that must be satisfied in order to prevent impaired wound healing, cellular dysfunction, and altered resistance to infection. Early enteral feedings have been shown to decrease levels of catabolic hormones, improve nitrogen balance, maintain gut mucosal integrity, lower the incidence of diarrhea, and decrease the length of hospital stay. Total parenteral nutrition in burn patients has been associated with metabolic and immunologic complications, and its use should be limited to those with severe gastrointestinal dysfunction in this population of patients. The Curreri formula, based on body weight plus percent TBSA burned, is used to calculate estimated calorie and protein needs in adults, while formulas using only body surface area (e.g., the Galveston formula) are used in children (Table 3). In burn patients, enteral formulas based primarily on carbohydrate, which maximizes the endogenous insulin production for anabolic purposes, are preferred. Vitamin and mineral supplementation is recommended, particularly with vitamin A, vitamin C, and zinc to support wound healing. Omega-6 fatty acids, glutamine, arginine, and nucleic acids may also be recommended in the future.

The degree of metabolic alteration experienced by burn patients is directly related to the extent of injury. The decrease in cardiac output and metabolic rate experienced immediately after injury has been referred to as the "ebb phase." After successful resuscitation, cardiac output increases to supranormal levels, with a simultaneous increase in resting energy expenditure. This has been referred to as the "flow phase" of the response to injury. A severe burn can drive the metabolic rate to twice-normal, which can be blunted by 40% with use of occlusive dressings and increased ambient temperature. A true reset of central temperature to around 38°C occurs at 5 to 10 days after injury; central temperature remains elevated for up to 2 months in burns of greater than 60% TBSA. This change is due to direct stimulation of the hypothalamus by inflammatory mediators and various cytokines. Attempts to decrease the temperature to normal by external cooling only increase the metabolic rate as the body strives to compensate.

TABLE 3. **Estimations of Caloric Needs in Burns**

Formula	Age (y)	Daily Calorie Requirement
Curreri	Adults	25 kcal/kg + 40 kcal/% TBSA burned
Galveston	0–1	2100 kcal/m^2 + 1000 kcal/m^2 TBSA burned
	2–11	1800 kcal/m^2 + 1300 kcal/m^2 TBSA burned
	12–18	1500 kcal/m^2 + 1500 kcal/m^2 TBSA burned

Abbreviation: TBSA = total body surface area.

Amino acids are released in massive quantities from the lean muscle mass after injury. In fact, free concentrations of glutamine in the muscle, one of the primary amino acids released, are reduced by 50%. This decrease is caused by increased proteolysis of muscle protein and increased export of amino acids from the muscle cells. Effectors of this response are likely to be increases in the catabolic hormone cortisol and decreases in the anabolic hormones such as growth hormone and insulin. Growth hormone treatment improves protein metabolism and accelerates wound healing after burn. Other anabolic hormones such as dehydroepiandrosterone, insulin-like growth factor complexed with its binding proteins, oxandrolone and other synthetic androgens, and insulin itself are being studied to evaluate their effects when given to severely burned patients to determine if these substances have other beneficial effects, particularly better rehabilitation potential, greater strength, and shorter hospitalizations.

REHABILITATION

Once closure of the wound is achieved, the focus of treatment shifts to rehabilitation. Goals are full return of function first and cosmesis second. Better control of burn scarring is achieved with application of pressure garments to healed wounds, which reorients the collagen strands such that the scars remain smooth and flat and mature quicker. Timely application of proper splints that retain range of motion of affected joints is also helpful. When contractures develop that prohibit function, operative release with closure of the wound with local flaps or skin grafting may be necessary; however, the mainstay of treatment remains vigorous occupational and physical therapy beginning during the wound closure process.

ALTITUDE ILLNESS

method of
STEPHEN A. BEZRUCHKA, M.D., M.P.H.
University of Washington
Seattle, Washington

Diagnosis and treatment of altitude illness usually take place outside of any clinical facilities, sometimes under conditions as severe as any on the earth. Mechanized evacuation from the high-altitude locale may be impossible, and medical personnel may not be present. Much of the information presented here is supplied with the understanding that the clinician must educate the visitor to high-altitude regions in field diagnosis and treatment of altitude illness.

ALTITUDE ILLNESS SYNDROMES: CLINICAL FEATURES

Acute mountain sickness (AMS), with symptoms mimicking a hangover, occurs a few hours to days after exposure. Severe enough to limit normal activities, it is found in 15 to 30% of Colorado resort skiers, 50% of climbers on Denali, 70% of climbers on Mount Rainier, and 25 to 50% of trekkers to the base of Mount Everest. It is more common among persons who ascend quickly, those who are younger, and those with a past history of AMS. AMS is more likely in persons with mild infections, those who retain fluid at high altitudes, and those whose normal mode of breathing is relative hypoventilation. Intracranial pressure is elevated in severe AMS, which melds into cerebral edema.

Mild AMS is characterized by headache (usually frontal), anorexia, insomnia, nausea, and malaise. Moderate forms are manifested by vomiting, unrelieved headache, and decreased urine output. Features of severe AMS are altered consciousness, localized rales, cyanosis, and ataxia, which may be the most sensitive early sign and represents early high-altitude cerebral edema (HACE). Peripheral edema of the hands, face, and ankles is common at high altitudes, especially in persons with AMS, and occurs more frequently in female than in male subjects. Symptoms such as headache that come on during the day's climb may be more ominous than those that begin after a night's sleep.

Mild AMS resolves over a few days if the hypobaric stress is not increased by ascending. Severe AMS usually progresses unless treated aggressively.

High-altitude pulmonary edema (HAPE), a noncardiogenic pulmonary edema with a significant mortality rate, occurs in 5 to 10% of persons with AMS but can occur without previous symptoms. One to two percent of those traveling above 12,000 feet (3660 meters) are affected, and males predominate. HAPE often occurs on the second night after ascent to altitude. Relative hypoxemia and a low hypoxic ventilatory response are present. This condition is characterized by a lung leak, not a lung injury, because people who recover on temporary descent have gone back up to a higher altitude on the same trip. HAPE victims have extremely high pulmonary artery pressures compared with those in unaffected altitude control subjects. The edema fluid is very protein rich, as in adult respiratory distress syndrome.

Features of early HAPE include decreased exercise performance (the earliest symptom), dry cough, fatigue, tachycardia (above resting levels for that person at altitude), rales in the right middle lobe, and tachypnea. Later there are cyanosis, extreme weakness, productive cough, and dyspnea at rest. Mental obtundation, irrational behavior, and coma can be present. Fever with body temperature less than 38.3°C may be present and by itself is not a helpful sign. Subclinical HAPE manifested as rales is probably very common at altitude. A chest radiograph obtained at altitude can demonstrate HAPE before rales are heard, with the earliest findings in the right middle lobe.

Risk factors include rapid ascent, strenuous exertion on arrival, obesity, male gender, and a previous history.

High-altitude cerebral edema (HACE) is possibly an end stage of AMS and usually presents several days after the onset of mild AMS. Intracranial pressure is increased, perhaps owing to increased cerebrospinal fluid (CSF) volume, secondary to vasogenic edema from a leaky blood-brain barrier. Victims probably have poorly compliant brain tissue and adapt more slowly to the increased CSF volume. HACE is very uncommon below 10,000 feet (3050 meters). Rapid ascent to significant altitudes strongly predisposes to the development of HACE.

Clinical presentation includes impaired judgment and ability to make decisions, irrational behavior, severe headache, nausea and vomiting, truncal ataxia, severe lassitude, and progression to coma. HAPE often can accompany HACE, and vice versa. Hallucinations, hemiparesis, and other focal neurologic signs have been reported, but these may be due to thrombosis.

PREVENTION

Persons at risk for altitude illness include members of groups in which peer pressure, tight schedules, and little flexibility in waiting for acclimatization operate. Rapid ascent, especially by flying or driving to altitude, is also associated with high risk, as noted previously.

The physician can advise a person going on a commercial tour to high-altitude destinations to inquire about the availability of oxygen or a hyperbaric bag, the flexibility of the itinerary, and the availability of rescue. Travelers should also be advised to carry acetazolamide, dexamethasone, and nifedipine and be instructed in their use. In addition, they should be taught about the tandem walking test for ataxia. A small pocket manual written for the lay person, *Altitude Illness: Prevention and Treatment*,* is available as a helpful resource for use in the field.

Slow ascent is important, and the sleeping altitude in particular should rise gradually: "Climb high, but sleep low." Prudence suggests taking at least 2 days to get to a sleeping altitude above 10,000 feet (3050 meters). Thereafter, raising the sleeping altitude by more than 1000 feet a day should be avoided, and the slowest-adapting person should be accommodated. The use of sedatives and tranquilizers must be avoided at altitudes above 8000 feet (2440 meters), as they depress respiration.

Drinking plenty of fluids is routinely recommended, because the altitude environment is usually very dry and insensible losses are high. A high-carbohydrate diet may be beneficial. Iron supplementation can be advised for women with prolonged (more than 3 weeks) stay at altitude.

Strenuous overexertion is contraindicated for the first few days at high altitude. Hypothermia is synergistic with the deleterious effects of altitude. Conscious effort to increase the depth and frequency of breathing at high altitude is beneficial.

Acetazolamide (Diamox), by inhibiting carbonic anhydrase in the kidney and lung, promotes the excretion of bicarbonate, resulting in a slight metabolic acidosis. Acetazolamide reduces symptoms by speeding acclimatization and decreases susceptibility to AMS. It increases minute ventilation and oxygen saturation and decreases the periodic breathing at night. Use of acetazolamide can be considered for persons driving or flying to altitudes of 10,000 feet (3000 meters) or more but is also beneficial on slower ascent. It is recommended for those who have had significant symptoms in the past. The dose is 125 mg twice a day, or once at bedtime. This is adequate for adults, taken on the day of ascent and continued for 2 days upon arrival at altitude. Common side effects of this sulfa drug include polyuria, paresthesias, and, less commonly, nausea, myopia, and impotence.

Dexamethasone (Decadron) is also effective as a prophylactic for AMS but is not routinely recommended because of significant dysphoria and the likelihood of rebound altitude illness when it is discontinued. It does not facilitate acclimatization. Travelers can be advised to carry dexamethasone to treat cerebral symptoms, but not for prophylaxis. Those who need to ascend rapidly for rescue purposes can take dexamethasone 4 mg orally (PO) every 6 hours along with acetazolamide. Those who cannot take acetazolamide

*Bezruchka S: Altitude Illness: Prevention and Treatment. Seattle, WA, The Mountaineers, 1994.

and who have a history significant of altitude illness but who must be exposed to the hypoxia of altitude may also benefit. Dexamethasone therapy should not be stopped at altitude until there has been a considerable descent. Tapering may be necessary after use of this drug for 3 days or more. There may be an additive effect with use of acetazolamide and dexamethasone. Clinicians should be aware that dexamethasone is being used by climbers for rapid altitude ascents.

Nifedipine (Procardia), which decreases pulmonary artery pressures, appears to be an effective prophylactic for persons who are susceptible to HAPE. The dose is 20 mg (long-acting preparation) three times a day. It is not indicated for AMS.

DIAGNOSIS

Within the altitude environment, diagnosis is difficult because of judgment made worse by hypoxia. The physician advising persons going to heights must stress ways of determining that descent is needed, or that further ascent must not take place. A review of the ascent profile, and the signs and symptoms at various altitudes, is needed to diagnose altitude illness. Table 1 lists signs and symptoms helpful in field diagnosis of altitude illness by persons in the altitude environment.

DIFFERENTIAL DIAGNOSIS

Although an illness at high altitude is considered altitude illness until proven otherwise, the list of conditions that can mimic altitude illness is protean and can include migraine headache, subarachnoid hemorrhage, pulmonary embolus, newly symptomatic brain tumor, Guillain-Barré syndrome, panic attacks, and carbon monoxide intoxication from use of stoves in snow-covered tents or snow caves or igloos.

TREATMENT

Two protocols for treatment are described: one for use in the field, and one for use in clinical facilities after evacuation.

Acute Mountain Sickness

Mild forms of AMS can be treated by a stay of a day or two at the current altitude, with cautious ascent subsequently if symptoms have ameliorated. Symptomatic treatment includes administration of mild analgesics, acetazolamide (Diamox) in a dose of 125 or 250 mg two or three times daily (starting with a dose at bedtime), and prochlorperazine (Compazine) for nausea and vomiting. Significant signs or symptoms, such as a severe headache, that come on during the day's ascent may be a harbinger of more severe illness and constitute a reason to descend rather than to see what happens after a night's sleep.

Severe AMS calls for immediate descent to below the altitude at which any manifestations of altitude illness first occurred and administration of oxygen, dexamethasone (Decadron) in a dose of 4 mg PO given every 6 hours, and acetazolamide. One or two hours of simulated descent in the hyperbaric bag may be as effective as oxygen therapy. Longer periods are necessary for serious illness. Barotitis and claustrophobia are possible complications. Benefits obtained with use of the hyperbaric bag and acetazolamide may be synergistic; therefore, this approach represents an option of descent if impossible.

High-Altitude Pulmonary Edema

Treatment of HAPE relies on early recognition and must be expeditious to avoid death. The victim should be kept warm, given oxygen, and taken down from the high altitude, avoiding strenuous exertion. Descent to below the altitude at which any symptoms of altitude illness first occurred is mandatory. A 4- to 6-hour stay in the pressurized chamber can be used initially if available for those unable to descend on their own. Ten percent of HAPE victims who are

TABLE 1. **Symptoms and Signs That Suggest Significant Altitude Illness**

Self-monitoring
- Resting pulse above 110 per minute
- Ominous: An increase in pulse at altitude occurring some time after ascent to that altitude
- Marked shortness of breath at rest (after recovery from the activity, with a respiratory rate of more than 20 breaths per minute)
- Loss of appetite
- Great fatigue experienced during an activity, especially if it is increasing in comparison to the level observed in companions

Monitoring of companions
- Skipping meals and wanting to spend more time in the tent
- Change in behavior: a gregarious person may become quiet and retiring, or a quiet person may become quieter or suddenly boisterous
- Persistent somnolence
- The person having the most difficulty with the activity should be observed carefully, especially if this represents a change

Measures to confirm the presence of altitude illness in a person with suggestive manifestations
- Get the person breathing more oxygen, by
  1. having the person descend, or
  2. giving oxygen by mask, or
  3. placing the person in a hyperbaric bag

  and observing the response

Descent is the preferred option, and other possible causes for the observed changes are never made worse by descent.

- Wait at a specific altitude that is no higher than the previous night's sleeping altitude and see if the person gets better (this strategy is recommended only for someone suspected to have mild to moderate AMS or peripheral edema) orthopneic find it difficult to lie flat if the hyperbaric bag is used.

Pulmonary vasodilators improve gas exchange and relieve the symptoms of HAPE. Nifedipine (Procardia), 10 mg sublingually, can be tried. It is given acutely with 20 mg of the long-acting preparation and continued every 6 hours. Postural symptoms and signs should be monitored.

In serious cases of HAPE, dexamethasone (or another corticosteroid) should be given when CNS symptoms are present. Acetazolamide may be useful early on in HAPE. With the non-descent treatment modalities available today, there is a tendency to delay descent or to cancel evacuation plans when some improvement occurs. HAPE has recurred fatally in such situations. Descent remains the mainstay of treatment and should be undertaken along with hyperbaric, oxygen, and drug therapies.

After resolution of HAPE, some persons have re-ascended gradually without recurrence on that trip. Re-ascent should only be undertaken carefully, with responsible supervision. Slow-release nifedipine in a dose of 20 mg PO three times daily should be given. On Denali (in Alaska), where HAPE is common, victims who descend, recover, and rest for 4 days have re-ascended with only rare recurrences.

Protocols for treating HAPE in a clinical facility include pulse oximetry on room air (low readings after evacuation indicate severe disease); oxygen by mask or nasal canula to increase the saturation above 90% (if this cannot be accomplished, more aggressive intervention is warranted); chest radiograph (not routinely needed but in suspicious cases can demonstrate unexpected cardiomegaly and pleural effusion); and pulmonary vasodilators if needed, following the field treatment regimens.

People stricken with HAPE on a high-altitude vacation and given treatment at a facility at altitude may be eager to continue the climb or other planned activity. Those who remain confused must descend. If they are moderately sick and have no complications but need oxygen to maintain saturation, they should be observed overnight and, if better the next day, sent to a hotel to rest on oxygen and be re-evaluated again that day. Persons whose hypoxemia is easily corrected with low-flow oxygen can be sent to a hotel with a responsible companion and portable oxygen. If asymptomatic the next day, and with normal findings on physical examination, they may be able to resume activity after that day's rest, provided that medical care is easily accessible and the activity is carried out with a non-afflicted responsible companion. Persons presenting with very mild cases (oxygen saturation mildly depressed, a few rales on auscultation, and perhaps a small infiltrate on a chest radiograph) can be given nifedipine and sent to a hotel room without oxygen if attended by a companion, to be re-checked the next day.

High-Altitude Cerebral Edema

Key principles in therapy include descent to below the altitude at which any symptoms of altitude illness first occurred and the administration of oxygen and dexamethasone, 4 to 8 mg every 6 hours. If descent cannot be accomplished expeditiously, the use of loop diuretics can be considered. Response to treatment may be slow. If descent is not possible, use of the hyperbaric bag for 6 hours or more is indicated. Re-ascent in improved cases should not be considered. If the victim has descended to a clinical facility but neurologic deterioration continues, prompt investigation is warranted, as HACE usually resolves very quickly with descent. Mannitol as well as endotracheal intubation and hyperventilation can be used in severe cases. Re-ascent should not be undertaken.

DISTURBANCES DUE TO COLD

method of
DANIEL F. DANZL, M.D.
University of Louisville School of Medicine
Louisville, Kentucky

ACCIDENTAL HYPOTHERMIA

Accidental hypothermia occurs when the body's core temperature unintentionally drops below 35°C (95°F). At this temperature, the compensatory physiologic responses to conserve heat begin to fail. Primary hypothermia results from exposure in previously healthy patients, but the mortality is much higher when diseases or injuries result in secondary hypothermia, which is often under-reported. Cold-induced tragedies continue to afflict both military and civilian populations. Urban indoor and outdoor settings produce the most cases in the United States.

Pathophysiology

Humans are unable to generate sufficient heat to maintain thermoneutrality under a variety of conditions (Table 1). Significant cold exposure normally activates the preoptic anterior hypothalamus, which orchestrates thermoregulation. Physiologic responses to the cold include shivering thermogenesis as well as endocrinologic and autonomic nervous system activities. Adaptive behavioral responses include donning of more clothing and seeking a heat source. Radiation normally accounts for 55 to 65% of the heat loss. Conductive losses increase up to 5 times in wet clothing and 23 times in water. Compensatory responses to heat loss through radiation, conduction, convection, evaporation, and respiration eventually fail. As the core temperature continues to fall, the patient becomes poikilothermic and cools to the ambient temperature.

Each organ system is affected uniquely. Cerebral metabolism is depressed 6 to 7% per 1°C. Cerebrovascular autoregulation remains intact until below 25°C (77°F), which helps maintain cortical blood flow. The electroencephalographic activity is clearly not prognostic and silences around 19 to 20°C. The lowest

TABLE 1. **Factors Predisposing to Hypothermia or Frostbite**

Physiologic

Decreased Heat Production

Age extremes (infants, elderly)
Prior cold injury
Dehydration or malnutrition
Overexertion
Endocrinologic insufficiency
Trauma (multisystem or extremity)
Physical conditioning
Diaphoresis or hyperhidrosis
Hypoxia

Impaired Thermoregulation

Central nervous system trauma, disease
Spinal cord injury
Pharmacologic or toxicologic agents
Metabolic disorders
Sepsis

Psychologic

Mental status or attitude
Fear or panic
Peer pressure
Fatigue
Intense concentration on tasks
Hunger
Intoxicants

Environmental

Heat loss (conductive, evaporative, radiative, convective)
Ambient temperature or humidity
Duration of exposure
Wind chill factor
Altitude ± associated conditions
Quantity of exposed surface area

Increased Heat Loss

Vascular diseases
Shock
Poor acclimatization or conditioning
Dermatologic malfunction
Burns
Emergency resuscitation
Cold infusions

Mechanical

Inadequate insulation
Constricting or wet clothing or boots
Immobility or cramped positioning

temperature for a neurologically intact survivor of accidental hypothermia is 15.2°C, and of induced hypothermia, 9°C.

Cardiovascular effects are often pronounced. After the initial tachycardia, there is progressive bradycardia. The heart rate drops to half its normal rate at 28°C. Hypothermia also progressively depresses the mean arterial pressure and cardiac index. Core temperature "afterdrop" refers to the continual decline in core temperature after removal from the cold. This phenomenon results from temperature equilibration and reversal of circulatory arteriovenous shunting in the extremities.

All atrial arrhythmias are commonly encountered, have a slow ventricular response, and should be considered innocent. The clinical significance of ventricular arrhythmias is more difficult to assess, because suppressed pre-existent ectopy may reappear during rewarming. The decreased ventricular fibrillation threshold is a real hazard below 28°C. Cardiac cycle prolongation is pronounced, as reflected in the corrected QT interval on the electrocardiogram. A J wave, or an Osborn hypothermic hump, may be present at the junction of the QRS complex and ST segment.

Respiratory stimulation is followed by a progressive reduction in respiratory minute volume, which reflects the metabolic depression. Carbon dioxide production falls 50% for each 8°C drop in temperature. Although renal blood flow declines, there is a large initial paradoxical osmolar diuresis. Vasoconstriction in the extremities expands the capacitance vessels, temporarily producing a central hypervolemia.

Clinical Presentation

Historical circumstances suggest the diagnosis when exposure is obvious. More subtle presentations predominate in urban settings. In such cases, the clinician may misfocus on a solitary diagnosis of a medical, toxicologic, neurologic, traumatic, or psychiatric emergency. Symptoms are often vague, and physical findings nonspecific or deceptive. For example, if tachycardia is disproportionate for the temperature, the physician should consider a secondary cause of hypothermia, such as hypoglycemia, hypovolemia, or a drug overdose. Persistent hyperventilation suggests a central nervous system (CNS) lesion or an organic acidosis, such as lactic acidosis or diabetic ketoacidosis. A cold-induced ileus and rectal spasm mimic and mask an acute abdomen. When the level of consciousness is inconsistent with the temperature, an overdose or CNS trauma or infection should be suspected. Hypothermic areflexia can also obscure a spinal cord injury. Last, temporary psychiatric sequelae during hypothermia include maladaptive behavior such as paradoxical undressing, which is the inappropriate removal of clothes in response to cold stress.

Treatment

Hypothermia is confirmed with a core temperature (e.g., rectal, esophageal, tympanic) measurement, preferably from two sites. Further heat loss should be gently prevented, and cardiac monitoring initiated. Hypothermia adversely affects tissue oxygenation by numerous mechanisms, including the leftward shift of the oxyhemoglobin dissociation curve. Most patients are significantly dehydrated and will benefit from a bolus crystalloid administration.

Routine hematologic evaluations should include arterial blood gases uncorrected for temperature. An uncorrected pH of 7.4 and P_{CO_2} of 40 mm Hg reflect acid-base balance at any temperature. The hematocrit also increases 2% per 1°C drop in temperature, which can mask anemia. Leukopenia does not imply the absence of infection, because bone marrow suppression and white blood cell sequestration are common. Unfortunately, there is no safe predictor of the electrolyte status. For example, hyperkalemic electrocardiogram changes are obscured by hypothermia. Hypokalemia is more common in chronic hypothermia. Last, cold induces a renal glycosuria, which does not exclude hypoglycemia.

A full clotting screen is necessary, because cold hemagglutination and coagulation are aberrant. Platelet function is impaired. Cold also directly inhibits the enzymatic reactions of the coagulation cascade. This in vivo coagulopathy is not reflected by a deceptively normal prothrombin time, activated partial thromboplastin time, or International Normalized Ratio (INR); these tests are performed at 37°C in the laboratory.

Rewarming Strategies

Choosing passive versus active rewarming is the key clinical decision. Passive external rewarming is noninvasive and ideal for mild cases in previously healthy persons. The patient should simply be covered with insulating materials. Active rewarming should be considered in the following situations: core temperature below 32°C (90°F), age extremes, CNS dysfunction, endocrine insufficiency, and cardiovascular instability.

Active external rewarming can be accomplished with heating blankets, radiant heat sources, and immersion. Forced-air heating blankets are the safest. There is a potential for thermal injury to vasoconstricted skin with use of electric blankets. There are reservations about externally heating the extremities. Limiting heat application to the trunk minimizes many of the physiologic concerns with use of these techniques. For example, heating the extremities after the occurrence of the diuresis and fluid sequestration common to chronic hypothermia causes a core temperature afterdrop.

There are many techniques for delivering direct heat internally. Active core rewarming options include inhalation of heated, humidified oxygen; intravenous fluids and irrigation of the peritoneum, thorax, or gastrointestinal tract; hemodialysis; extracorporeal rewarming; and diathermy. Airway rewarming (40 to 45°C [104 to 113°F]) with a mask or endotracheal tube is a valuable adjunct in all cases, because the access is simple. Preoxygenation and gentle technique prevent intubation arrhythmias. The inhalation eliminates respiratory heat loss. During massive volume resuscitations, administration of heated intravenous fluid and blood is helpful. The use of countercurrent heat exchangers is the most efficient method for heating and delivering the fluid.

Peritoneal lavage is another option for severely hypothermic patients. Peritoneal dialysate at 40 to 45°C delivered by two catheters with outflow suction efficiently transfers heat. Thoracostomy tube irrigation with warm saline is also valuable. The sterile saline is warmed to 42°C, infused anteriorly, and then continuously drained from the efferent midaxillary tube. Finally, irrigation of the gastrointestinal tract is of limited value and should be reserved for use in combination with all available techniques in patients with cardiac arrest.

Extracorporeal rewarming is potentially indicated in patients with cardiac arrest, completely frozen extremities, or severe rhabdomyolysis. The standard circuit uses a mechanical pump with an oxygenator and heat exchanger. Other options are continuous arteriovenous, venovenous, and hemodialysis rewarming. Cardiopulmonary resuscitation is indicated unless (1) a do-not-resuscitate status is documented and verified, (2) obviously lethal injuries are present, (3) chest wall depression is impossible, (4) any signs of life are present, or (5) rescuers are endangered by evacuation delays or altered triage conditions.

The misdiagnosis of a cardiac arrest should be avoided. Palpation of peripheral pulses is difficult when an extreme bradycardia is coupled with peripheral vasoconstriction. The examiner should take a full minute to check for a central pulse, especially if no cardiac monitor is available. After one attempt to defibrillate with 2 watt-seconds per kg, active rewarming should be continued past 32°C. Successful re-establishment of flow below that temperature is rare.

Resuscitation pharmacology usually reflects substandard therapeutic activity while the patient is cold, which progresses to toxicity after rewarming. Drug protein binding increases, and metabolism and excretion are impaired. Manipulation of the vasoconstricted and depressed cardiovascular system must be avoided. Bretylium (Bretylol) is the only effective antiarrhythmic agent at low temperatures. During ventricular fibrillation, 10 mg per kg should be infused. The empirical use of levothyroxine and corticosteroids is hazardous.

Because hypothermia is a great masquerader, no rigid treatment protocol can be suggested. Clinical treatment should be predicated on the duration and extent of temperature depression and the severity of the predisposing factors. The caveat "No one is dead until he or she is warm and dead" is evolving. Indicators of grave prognosis include evidence of cell lysis (hyperkalemia with potassium levels greater than 10–12 mEq per liter), intravascular thrombosis (fibrinogen value below 50 mg per dL), a pH below 6.5, and a core temperature below 12°C.

PERIPHERAL COLD INJURIES

Peripheral local cold injuries include freezing and nonfreezing syndromes. Frostbite is the most common freezing injury. Trench foot and immersion foot are nonfreezing injuries resulting from exposure to wet cold. Nonfreezing injury after exposure to dry cold is called chilblain (pernio). With cold stress, the core temperature is maintained at the expense of vasospasticity and shunting, which prevent heat distribution to the extremities.

Pathophysiology

A unique aspect of peripheral cold injury is the pathogenesis of the freezing injury cascade. Tissue is initially damaged by the freeze-thaw insult and subsequently by progressive dermal ischemia. Before freezing, tissue cooling increases the viscosity of the vascular contents as the microvasculature constricts.

The freeze-thaw sequence begins during extracellular fluid crystallization. Water exits the cell, causing intracellular dehydration, hyperosmolality, cellular shrinkage, and collapse. Arachidonic acid breakdown products are then released from underlying damaged tissue into the vesicle fluid. Both prostaglandin $F_{2\alpha}$ and thromboxane A_2 produce platelet aggregation, leukocyte immobilization, and vasoconstriction. Endothelial cells are quite sensitive to cold injury, and the microvasculature becomes distorted and clogged.

After tissue thawing, there is progressive edema formation for 48 to 72 hours. Subsequent thrombosis and early superficial necrosis develop. This tissue eventually mummifies and demarcates, often more than 60 to 90 days later—hence the surgical aphorism "Frostbite in January, amputate in July."

The incidence and severity of peripheral cold injury are determined by the duration and intensity of cutaneous cold exposure. Factors predisposing to peripheral cold injuries are listed in Table 1.

Clinical Presentation

The initial presentation of frostbite is often deceptively benign. Unlike in burns, classification of frostbite by degrees is often prognostically inaccurate and therapeutically misleading. The physical findings at 24 to 72 hours after completion of rewarming are more reliably used to classify frostbite. Superficial or mild frostbite does not entail eventual tissue loss, but deep or severe frostbite does. "Frostnip" is a superficial cold insult producing transient numbness or tingling that resolves after rewarming.

All patients with frostbite have some initial sensory deficit in light touch, pain, or temperature. Acral areas and distal extremities are the usual insensate sites. Patients also complain of being clumsy or having a "chunk of wood" sensation in the extremity.

Deep frostbite may initially appear to be deceptively benign. However, tissues remaining frozen can appear mottled, violaceous, pale yellow, or waxy. Favorable presenting signs are warmth, normal color, and some sensation. If the subcutaneous tissue is soft and pliable or the dermis can be rolled over the bony prominences, the injury may be superficial.

Rapid rewarming produces an initial hyperemia, even in severe cares. A residual violaceous hue is ominous. Early formation of clear, large blebs is a more favorable sign than smaller, dark, hemorrhagic blebs, which imply cold damage to the subdermal vascular plexus.

Chilblain is a form of dry cold injury often developing after repetitive exposures. These "cold sores" typically involve facial areas and the dorsa of the hands and feet. Young women, especially those with a history of Raynaud's phenomenon, are at risk. Persistent vasospasticity and vasculitis result in pruritus, erythema, and mild edema. Plaques, blue nodules, and ulcerations eventually develop. Treatment of perniosis is difficult; the physician should consider using nifedipine (Procardia) at a dose of 20 to 60 mg daily.

Immersion (trench) foot is produced by prolonged exposure to wet cold at above-freezing temperatures. Feet often appear erythematous, edematous, or cyanotic. The bullae are indistinguishable from those seen in frostbite. However, this vesiculation proceeds to ulceration and liquefaction gangrene. In milder cases, hyperhidrosis, cold sensitivity, and painful ambulation persist for years.

Warm-water immersion foot affects the soles of the feet and results from waterlogging of the thick stratum corneum. This commonly occurs in persons wearing wet shoes for prolonged periods owing to a lack of shelter.

Ancillary diagnostic adjuncts continue to be investigated for peripheral cold injuries. Doppler ultrasonography, digital plethysmography, scintigraphy, routine radiography, and angiography do not consistently predict tissue loss at presentation. Delayed studies may guide subsequent therapy.

Treatment

Mills popularized rapid immersion rewarming after extensive experience with severe Alaskan frostbite cases. Before thawing, frozen parts should not be exposed to dry heat sources. Tissue refreezing is also disastrous; as an extreme example, it is preferable to ambulate to safety on frozen extremities. A treatment protocol is summarized in Table 2.

A circulating tank is ideal for rewarming the extremities, but a large container suffices for the hands and feet. Care should be taken to avoid thermal injury, which occurs if the water temperature exceeds 42°C. A common error is premature termination of rewarming, because the establishment of reperfusion is quite painful. Rewarming may take up to 1 hour.

Extreme caution should be exercised in treating patients with completely frozen extremities, because they are invariably hypothermic. Thawing produces significant core temperature, fluid, and electrolyte fluxes. Persistent cyanosis after a complete thaw should suggest raised fascial compartment pressures.

Management of frostbite vesicles also varies. Some physicians initially leave large, clear blisters intact; however, sterile aspiration or débridement seems preferable. The débridement of hemorrhagic vesicles, however, can extend the injury by allowing secondary desiccation of deep dermal layers. There are two strategies for inhibition of prostaglandins. Topical aloe vera (Dermaide) is a specific thromboxane inhibitor. Systemically, ibuprofen is preferable to the salicylates. Ibuprofen produces fibrinolysis in addition to

TABLE 2. **Treatment of Frostbite**

Before Thawing

1. Stabilize core temperature.
2. Address medical or surgical conditions.
3. Protect and do not massage frozen part.
4. Avoid partial thawing and refreezing.
5. Extricate from environment.

Thaw

1. Provide parenteral analgesia and hydration.
2. Rapidly rewarm entire part in 38–40°C circulating water until distal flush occurs (thermometer monitoring).
3. Requires 10–60 min with gentle motion of part by the patient without friction massage.

After Thawing

1. For clear vesicles: aspirate if intact; débride if broken.
2. For hemorrhagic vesicles: do not débride; may aspirate.
3. Apply topical aloe vera q 6 h.
4. Use ibuprofen, 400 mg orally q 12 h (12 mg/kg/d).
5. Administer tetanus and streptococcal prophylaxis.
6. Elevate part in protective cradle.
7. Use whirlpool hydrotherapy two or three times daily (37°C).
8. Avoid vasoconstrictors, including nicotine.

limiting the accumulation of inflammatory mediators.

Multiple experimental antithrombotic and vasodilatory treatment regimens have been proposed. There is no conclusive evidence of enhanced tissue salvage with administration of dextran, heparin, steroids, nonsteroidal anti-inflammatory drugs (NSAIDs), dimethylsulfoxide (DMSO),* nonionic detergents, dipyridamole (Persantine), calcium channel blockers, or hyperbaric oxygen. Pentoxifylline (Trental), 400 mg given orally every 8 hours, may facilitate small-vessel perfusion.

A long-acting alpha blocker, phenoxybenzamine (Dibenzyline),* 10 mg per day up to 60 mg per day, may decrease the refractory vasospasm during the clinical course in selected patients. Aggressive hydration is essential to minimize orthostatic hypotension. Sympathectomy, both pharmacologic (e.g., intra-arterial reserpine*) and surgical, can relieve painful vasospasm and decrease edema but has not been demonstrated to enhance tissue salvage.

Sequelae

Residual neuropathic symptoms are common and result from abnormal sympathetic tone and neuronal damage. Dermatologic findings include lymphedema, ulcerations, hair and nail deformities, and epidermoid or squamous carcinomas. Occult musculoskeletal injuries are most pronounced in children. Premature epiphyseal fusion and fragmentation are another concern. Amputation decisions should be deferred unless there is supervening sepsis or gangrene. The ultimate tissue salvage after a spontaneous slough usually far exceeds the most optimistic initial estimates.

*Not FDA approved for this indication.

DISTURBANCES DUE TO HEAT

method of
LAWRENCE E. HART, M.B.B.CH., M.SC.
McMaster University
Hamilton, Ontario, Canada

Hyperthermia is a state of thermoregulatory failure in which heat generation exceeds heat loss, causing heat retention within the body and a resultant increase in core temperature. Historic accounts of heat illness date back more than 2000 years, and since then there have been frequent and graphic descriptions of the impact of hyperthermia on athletes, military personnel, and civilian populations. Heatstroke, the most serious form of heat injury, is associated with significant morbidity and mortality. In the United States, for example, 5200 deaths from excessive heat exposure were recorded for the period 1979 to 1991. A heat wave in the summer of 1995 claimed an estimated 750 lives, with 500 deaths in Chicago alone. Of the 2912 spectators and staff members who required medical attention during the 1996 Olympic Games in Atlanta, 372 (12.8%) were treated for heat-related conditions.

TEMPERATURE REGULATION

Thermal homeostasis is controlled by the preoptic nucleus of the anterior hypothalamus. Under normal conditions, heat generation is a by-product of metabolic processes, and body temperature is maintained within a range of 36°C (96.8°F) to 37.5°C (99.5°F). When core temperature rises above normal, efferent fibers of the autonomic nervous system are activated to produce cutaneous vasodilation and increased sweating. Hyperthermia occurs when thermoregulatory mechanisms are overwhelmed by excessive metabolic production of heat, excessive environmental heat, or impaired heat dissipation.

MINOR HEAT ILLNESSES

Heat illness refers to a spectrum of disorders that vary in severity from mild forms of thermal disequilibrium to full-blown, often life-threatening heatstroke. Relatively minor conditions include heat edema, heat tetany, heat cramps, heat syncope, and miliaria rubra.

Heat edema is usually a benign, self-limited condition that affects unacclimatized persons who are exposed to hot environmental temperatures. Manifesting as mild edema, usually of the hands, feet, and ankles, it usually resolves spontaneously once acclimatization occurs.

Heat tetany refers to carpopedal spasm and paresthesias that probably result from the hyperventilation that may accompany heat exposure.

Heat cramps are characterized by intermittent, although severe, cramping of heavily exercised muscles, usually of the calves and thighs but also of the shoulders and abdomen. Common in athletes who train and compete in hot weather, this condition is attributed to inadequate salt intake during profuse sweating. Management should focus on cooling the athlete, stretching the affected muscles, and replacing salt (with commercially available sodium-containing electrolyte drinks, 1% salt solutions, or intravenous normal saline).

Heat syncope is a consequence of postural hypotension that is caused by peripheral vasodilation and volume depletion. After other possible causes of syncope are ruled out, treatment is aimed at restoring hydration.

Miliaria rubra, also known as prickly heat, lichen tropicus, or heat rash, is an erythematous maculopapular rash that is precipitated by keratin plugging of sweat gland pores. Secondary infection, most frequently with *Staphylococcus aureus*, is a usual consequence. This condition occurs on clothed parts of the body. Treatment includes decreasing time spent in hot environments, wearing loose-fitting clothes, and avoiding the use of talcum or baby powders. Antihistamines can be used to reduce itching, and either cleansing with chlorhexidine (Hibiclens) or applying the agent as a light cream or ointment has also been found to be helpful. A 1% solution of salicylic acid applied three times a day can be used to promote skin desquamation, although care should be taken to avoid salicylate toxicity when large areas of skin are involved. Oral antibiotics such as cephalexin (Keflex) may be required for management of the *S. aureus* infection.

HEAT EXHAUSTION

Caused by excessive water losses or electrolyte depletion (or both), heat exhaustion is distinguished from heat cramps by the additional presence of systemic symptoms such as fatigue, headaches, dizziness, nausea, vomiting, malaise, weakness, myalgias, and muscle cramps. Clinical features may include diaphoresis, orthostatic hypotension, and tachycardia. In more severe cases, heat exhaustion can be differentiated from overt heatstroke by the preservation of mental function and core temperatures that usually do not exceed 39°C (102.2°F).

Although it may be clinically challenging to determine whether the heat exhaustion is due primarily to dehydration or to salt depletion, it is far more practical to manage this condition as though both were present. After the patient has been moved to a cool environment, treatment should focus on judicious fluid replacement and should be guided by pulse and blood pressure and the presence of orthostatic signs and symptoms. For milder heat exhaustion, oral rehydration may be sufficient, while in more severe cases, intravenous saline solutions (0.9% or 0.45%) are required. The addition of a 5% dextrose solution with the first liter of intravenous fluid should also be considered. After such initial treatment, decisions on further electrolyte replacement can be guided by results of laboratory studies.

HEATSTROKE

Regarded as a medical emergency, heatstroke is a devastating condition that is characterized by rectal temperature elevations in excess of 40.5°C (105°F), cerebral dysfunction, and, in many cases, cessation of sweating. Two categories of clinical heatstroke have been described: exertional and classic.

Etiology

Exertional heatstroke usually occurs in otherwise healthy persons who work or exercise vigorously in hot, humid conditions. Among the more susceptible are miners, military recruits, and athletes. In these populations, added risk factors include the use of medications that impair heat loss, drugs of abuse (such as amphetamines or cocaine), poor physical conditioning, lack of acclimatization, obesity, recent diarrheal or febrile illnesses, dehydration, sleep deprivation, and the use of inappropriate clothing or protective gear.

Classic heatstroke, in contrast, typically presents in elderly or chronically ill patients in whom thermoregulatory function becomes compromised following prolonged exposure to high environmental temperatures. Among the most susceptible are persons who live in large cities under conditions of low airflow and lack of air conditioning. The prevalence of classic heatstroke also increases significantly during seasonal heat waves. A variety of chronic disabling illnesses predispose to the development of heatstroke. Among the more common are diabetes mellitus, cardiac disease, peripheral vascular disease, dementia, malnutrition, and skin conditions that impair sweating (e.g., miliaria, advanced scleroderma). Heatstroke can also be precipitated by alcohol abuse and by medications that may promote volume depletion (e.g., diuretics), sweating (e.g., anticholinergics), or reduced cardiac output (e.g., beta blockers).

Diagnosis

Although anhidrosis is generally considered one of the three primary criteria for diagnosing heatstroke and is invariably present in classic heatstroke, it may not be present in exertional heatstroke. Instead, active sweating may persist in the victim of exertional heatstroke. This results in a relatively cool, clammy skin, even when core temperature elevations are in excess of 44°C (112°F). Although tachycardia (pulse rate 120 to 160 beats per minute) is characteristic of exertional heatstroke, it is important to recognize that relative bradycardia (70 to 80 beats per minute) may be evident in highly conditioned distance runners with hyperthermia. Shock, arrhythmias, myocardial ischemia, and pulmonary edema tend to occur relatively early in classic heatstroke but as later (and ominous) features of exertional heatstroke. The neurologic manifestations of heatstroke include headaches, dizziness, and weakness. Mental confusion or euphoria may precede actual collapse. Coma, stupor, or combative delirium may become evident in severe cases, accompanied by pupillary abnormalities and generalized convulsions. Gastrointestinal features may include nausea, vomiting, diarrhea, stress ulceration, and frank hemorrhage.

The widespread organ damage that characterizes heatstroke is reflected in an array of laboratory abnormalities. Leukocytosis, a raised hematocrit, and thrombocytopenia are often reported, while prolongation of the prothrombin time, decrease in fibrinogen levels, and elevation of fibrin split products denote the presence of disseminated intravascular coagulation (DIC). Renal compromise, which may be severe, is manifested as hematuria, proteinuria, myoglobinuria, the presence of urinary casts, and raised blood urea nitrogen (BUN) and creatinine levels. Elevations in transaminase levels, reflecting hepatic injury, are common in heatstroke, while increases in bilirubin levels occur less frequently. Raised creatine phosphokinase and aldolase levels are markers of muscle damage. Respiratory alkalosis is the predominant acid-base disturbance in heatstroke, although lactic acidosis may also occur, especially in exertional heatstroke. Hypokalemia, hypophosphatemia, hypoglycemia, and hyperuricemia occur with variable frequency and severity.

Management

The successful management of heatstroke depends on the prompt recognition and early reversal of hyperthermia. Immediate cooling, careful rehydration, and appropriate attention to circulatory compromise are the cornerstones of effective care. Treatment is started at the site of collapse, with transfer of the patient to a cool setting, removal of clothing, fanning, bathing the skin with cool water, and placing ice packs at points of major heat transfer such as the groins, axillae, and chest. Basic first aid measures to maintain the patient's airway and breathing should be undertaken, and an intravenous line should be established as soon as possible. The preferred solution for initial fluid therapy is normal saline or half-normal saline with 5% dextrose. Once initial stabilization has been achieved, evacuation to a tertiary care facility should follow.

Rapid cooling is recommended until a core temperature of 39°C (102.2°F) is recorded. Ideally, core temperature should be monitored by a rectal probe or tympanic membrane thermistor. Various methods have been proposed to promote body cooling. Although controversial, ice water immersion is still frequently used. A major disadvantage of this technique is that it provokes cutaneous vasoconstriction, which could impede heat transfer from the body surface. Moreover, the practical difficulty of dealing with potentially combative or confused heatstroke patients, or those with seizures, vomiting, or diarrhea, needs to be considered in determining optimal treatment. Evaporative cooling using fans and the continuous spraying of tepid water onto the skin is also effective and is usually better tolerated by the patient. Other cooling modalities have included peritoneal, gastric, and colonic lavage, but none of these has gained wide acceptance as a useful alternative to surface cooling. Shivering may impair cooling and can be quickly treated by administering diazepam (Valium)* intravenously (IV) in 2- to 5- mg increments until a positive response is demonstrated. Because of its anticholinergic effects, chlorpromazine (Thorazine)* is no longer recommended for the management of shivering.

Profound hypotension may accompany heatstroke. An impairment of myocardial performance may precipitate this disturbance, but more often, it is caused by the transfer of blood volume to dilated superficial vessels, which occurs during the evolution of heatstroke. By inducing cutaneous vasoconstriction, cooling alone can restore the blood pressure to normal. Therefore, the administration of large volumes of intravenous fluid to raise blood pressure should be avoided in the early management of heatstroke. Indeed, if large volumes are infused while simultaneous cooling is returning blood to the central circulation, fluid overload may result, and pulmonary edema may occur. When cooling does not restore a normal blood pressure, 250 to 500 mL of normal saline can be rapidly infused. In advanced cases, dopamine (with hemodynamic monitoring) should be tried. Alpha-adrenergic agents should be avoided, because they promote vasoconstriction and impair cooling.

Patients with confirmed heatstroke should be hospitalized so that potential complications can be identified and managed accordingly. Renal function needs to be carefully monitored. Evidence of rhabdomyolysis or a urinary output of less than 30 mL per hour signals the need for treatment with volume replacement, mannitol (12.5 to 25.0 grams), and bicarbonate (44 mEq per liter in 0.45% normal saline) to induce an osmotic diuresis and urinary alkalization. Despite optimal management, renal failure has still been reported in 5% of patients with classic heatstroke and in 25% of those with exertional heatstroke. The presence of hypoglycemia and other metabolic abnormalities, seizures, DIC, hypoxemia, adult respiratory distress syndrome, aspiration pneumonia, hepatic injury, or congestive heart failure requires additional interventions.

PREVENTION OF HEAT ILLNESS

Guidelines for preventing heat illness can be summarized as follows:

- Identifying persons in high-risk populations and educating them in the principles of conditioning, acclimatization, and hydration. The elderly or infirm, in particular, should be advised about the use of air conditioning and electric fans, the advantages of loose and lightweight clothing, and the benefits

*Not FDA approved for this indication.

of cool showers or baths to combat the effects of oppressive heat.
- Minimizing strenuous work or exercise at the hottest times of day.
- Avoiding athletic competition in conditions of heat excess and/or high humidity. The wet bulb–globe thermometer index (WBGT), a composite measure of regular temperature, the effect of humidity on temperature, and wind speed, is an excellent indicator of environmental heat stress. In the presence of WBGT readings above 25°C (77°F), athletic events should be postponed or canceled.
- Ensuring that athletes, especially those in distance events, understand the importance of fluid intake during training and competition. Four hundred to 500 mL of fluid should be consumed prior to an event, as well as 200 to 300 mL at frequent intervals during the race itself.
- Teaching persons in potentially high-risk groups how to recognize the early symptoms of heat illness, i.e., dizziness, headache, nausea, stumbling or clumsiness, changes in mental status, and excessive sweating or lack of sweating.

HYPERTHERMIA WITHOUT HIGH AMBIENT TEMPERATURES

Hyperthermia in the absence of high environmental temperature is an intrinsic feature of various conditions.

The *neuroleptic malignant syndrome* (NMS), first described in 1968, is characterized by hyperthermia, hypertonicity of skeletal muscles, fluctuating consciousness, and evidence of autonomic dysfunction (pallor, diaphoresis, blood pressure instability, and cardiac dysrhythmias). NMS is usually precipitated by neuroleptic (antipsychotic) drugs such as phenothiazines, butyrophenones, and thioxanthines or by the sudden withdrawal of amantadine, levodopa, or other dopaminergic drugs used to treat Parkinson's disease. Temperatures of 41°C (105.8°F), or higher have been reported in this syndrome. Laboratory findings include electrolyte disturbances, metabolic acidosis, rhabdomyolysis, hemoconcentration, leukocytosis, and abnormalities in renal and hepatic function tests. Treatment includes cessation of the responsible neuroleptic agent, fluid replacement, correction of electrolyte imbalance, and support of cardiac, respiratory, and renal function. Dantrolene sodium (Dantrium),* amantadine (Symmetrel),* and bromocriptine (Parlodel)* all have been used in the management of NMS, but none has been rigorously evaluated in clinical trials. Physical cooling may be helpful in the acute phase of the syndrome.

Malignant hyperthermia of anesthesia (MHA) is an extremely rare, genetically mediated disorder that presents as muscle rigidity, fever, and autonomic dysfunction. It is precipitated by halogenated inhalation agents and depolarizing muscle relaxants used in anesthesia. Discontinuation of anesthesia, initiation of cardiopulmonary support, correction of metabolic abnormalities, physical cooling, and the intravenous administration of dantrolene sodium are integral to the management of this life-threatening condition.

Other rare causes of hyperthermia include (1) endocrine disorders such as thyroid storm and pheochromocytoma crisis, (2) drug-induced states (usually caused by cocaine, amphetamines, or phencyclidine, or aspirin toxicity in children), (3) neurologic disorders such as delirium tremens, generalized tetanus, and status epilepticus, (4) hypothalamic disorders, and (5) the serotonin syndrome, a condition that has been described following an increase in the dosage of potent serotonin agonists.

*Not FDA approved for this indication.

SPIDER BITES AND SCORPION STINGS

method of
FINDLAY E. RUSSELL, M.D., PH.D.
University of Arizona College of Medicine
Tucson, Arizona

Spiders and scorpions are arachnids, members of the class Arachnida, which consists of at least 10 orders, including the mites, ticks, whip scorpions, pseudoscorpions, solpugids, and others.

SPIDER BITES

Spiders are classified in the order Aranaea. Spider envenomation is known as *araneism*, although it is preferred to identify the specific genus or species involved, such as *latrodectism, loxoscelism, chiracanthism*, and so on, provided that positive identity of the offending culprit is established. In my experience over a 45-year period at the Los Angeles County General Hospital (now LAC/USC Medical Center), Loma Linda University Medical Center, and the University of Arizona Medical Center, at least 64% of all "spider bites" were eventually attributed to some other arthropod, principally fleas, ticks, bedbugs, biting flies, and mites. The remaining 15% were due to one of 20 other disease states, including erythema nodosum, lymphomatoid papulosis, purpura fulminans, and pyoderma gangrenosum. Unless the offending spider (not one from the garden) is captured and identified, the evidence, in both the medical and the legal senses, is circumstantial unless systemic manifestations demonstrate otherwise. Even then, the diagnosis of "spider bite" must be based on careful evaluation. It should be remembered that spiders are very reluctant to bite.

Approximately 100 of the 20,000 species of spiders so far examined have been shown to contain toxins within their venom or maxillary glands. Only two families appear not to have viable venom glands. In human cases, the principal characteristic of spiders capable of delivering a poisonous bite is the presence of fangs, or chilicerae, strong and stout enough to penetrate the skin. The filistatids (Filistatidae) and widow spiders (*Latrodectus* species) have relatively large venom glands and chilicerae for their size, while the jumping spiders (*Phidippus* species) have very large and powerful fangs. Some of the larger spiders, such as the wolf spiders, have proportionately smaller venom glands but strong chilicerae and stouter legs and thus are more able to control their prey. The relationships among fangs, chilicerae, venom glands, and spider size are well documented, and one can only say that nature has carried out the applicability very well. In the United States, fewer than 50 species have been definitely implicated in venom poisoning. In most instances, the reaction is restricted to local manifestations. In some bites the reaction appears allergic in nature, while in a few cases the reaction is definitely serious, evoking both local and systemic effects. The following discussion focuses on spiders known to cause venom poisoning, although some notice is addressed to other, potentially venomous species.

Latrodectus Species (Widow Spiders)

There are five species of widow spiders. The black widows are *L. mactans* in the east and *L. hesperus* in the west. *Loxosceles variolus* is found in the east and south into Florida and eastern Texas. The red widow, *L. bishopi*, is a colorful spider generally found in central and southeast Florida, and the imported species, *L. geometricus*, the brown widow, is sometimes found in southern Florida. All widow spiders are venomous, but only the black widows present a danger to humans. The males are venomous but too small to be a threat. Biochemical and pharmacologic studies indicate that the principal neurotoxic component is a high-molecular-weight polypeptide, alpha-latrotoxin, that provokes massive release of transmitter substances at the presynaptic junction, particularly in vertebrates. Its actions in the other phyla vary considerably, but at least in humans it can account for the greater part of the neuromuscular changes. The relationship between the toxin and Ca^{2+}-dependent and -nondependent binding proteins may account for its variable properties in the different phyla.

Most patients envenomated by widow spiders report a pinprick-like bite, although it may go unnoticed. There is some initial pain, often followed by a localized, sometimes numbing sensation. The bite area may show blanching of the skin with surrounding hyperemia, which may persist for up to several hours. Sensation in the immediate area is often altered, and perspiration and piloerection may be evident near the lesion. Edema is usually minimal; lymphadenitis has been recorded. Pain and cramping of the large muscle masses, particularly in the abdomen, shoulders, back, chest, and thighs, are common. Children may flex their legs, display an expiratory grunt, and be very restless, and they are often unable to remain sitting or standing in one position. Paresis is not unusual, and reflexes are often hyperactive. Nausea and vomiting are common. Other manifestations may include muscle fasciculations, headache, dizziness, ptosis, increased salivation, hypertension, opisthotonos, flushing of the face, rash, and arthralgia. Laboratory findings, including electrolyte levels, are usually normal, although a transient hyperglycemia has been reported.

The number of therapeutic agents that have been suggested for treatment of latrodectism is impressive. Today, antivenom, calcium gluconate, muscle relaxants, morphine, and diazepam, and nitroprusside for hypertension, appear to be the drugs most often used. Positive-pressure ventilation may be necessary. The commercially available antivenom antivenin (Latrodectus mactans), prepared in horses, must be used with great care and only following skin testing and with the shock cart at hand. In our practice we have restricted its use to children, pregnant women, and the most severe adult envenomations when all else has failed. Calcium gluconate, 10 mL, can be given intravenously (IV) but slowly and followed by another 10 mL in a drip of 250 mL of 5% dextrose in water (D5W). Even a third dose may be necessary. Morphine has been used successfully since the days of the Arab physician Avicenna (979–1037).

Loxosceles Species (Brown Spiders)

Loxosceles spiders are variously known as brown, fiddleback, and brown recluse spiders, although the last term should be restricted to the species *L. reclusa*. There are more than 10 species in the United States, including two imported species, *L. rufescens* and *L. laeta*. The true brown recluse spider, *L. reclusa*, is the most widely spread, ranging from near the East Coast to New Mexico, with scattered numbers being transported to Massachusetts, California, and elsewhere. In the West, the clinically important species are *L. deserta, L. arizonica, L. sabina*, and, possibly, *L. russelli*. The venom is complex, although the most toxic component is a sphingomyelinase, a protein of 35 kilodaltons that is apparently responsible for most of the complement-dependent hemolytic and dermal necrosis-inducing properties. Characteristic of the envenomation is the accumulation of polymorphonuclear cells at the bite site. Intravascular clotting and hemolysis leading to systemic changes, including hemolytic anemia, thrombocytopenia, hemoglobinuria, and renal failure, may occur.

Development of the local lesion is diagnostic. The bite produces pain, although children may be unaware of the injury. A localized burning sensation may develop and usually lasts for 10 to 30 minutes. Pruritus is often present. The area begins to appear red, with a small blanched area around the bite site. The hyperemic area enlarges during the subsequent 1 to 12 hours, often becoming irregular in shape and ecchymotic with petechial hemorrhages. A bleb or vesicle usually forms at the bite site, increases in size, and subsequently ruptures, with formation of a pustule. Necrosis of variable depth can occur at the lesion site.

Local measures should be avoided, as the development of the lesion is often diagnostic, particularly during the first 8 hours. If pain is severe, a piece of ice can be applied to the wound area. An antivenom for *L. reclusa* is available only in Tennessee. The antivenom produced in South America is of questionable value in North American *Loxosceles* bites. Dapsone has been used successfully when given in the early stages of poisoning. Corticosteroids have been used with equivocal results. Early excision of the bite area should be avoided. The usual precautions for infection must be taken. Specific measures for hemolytic anemia and renal failure may be warranted.

Other Spiders

Members of the genera *Phidippus* (jumping spiders), *Chiracanthium* (running spiders), *Lycosa* (wolf spiders), *Steatoda* (cobweb spiders), and *Aphenopelma* (tarantulas) appear to be the other spiders most frequently implicated in araneism. Rarely are their bites serious, and the application of a lotion or cream composed of hydrocortisone acetate 0.5%, diphenhydramine 2%, and tetracain 1% to the wound area is usually sufficient. This balm is available commercially as Itch Balm Plus.

SCORPION STINGS

Scorpions are also arachnids, of the order Scorpionida. Of the 800 or so species, only 50 are found in the United States. The most important medically is *Centruroides exilicauda*, common in Arizona but also found in neighboring areas of New Mexico and California, and transported elsewhere in the Southwest. Stings by scorpions of *Vejovis, Hadrurus, Uroctonus*, and *Pandinus* species, however, are reported and produce localized transient pain, minimal swelling, and, occasionally, paresthesia and tenderness. Paresis or muscle fasciculations may rarely be seen. The venom of *C. exilicauda* contains several short-chain neurotoxic fractions. Of particular importance are the cobatoxins, which block potassium channels; one such toxin has 28 amino acid residues with four disulfide bonds.

Patients stung by *C. exilicauda* experience some localized pain, with the affected area becoming hypersensitive or paresthetic. There is minimal edema. Children develop random head, neck, and shoulder movements, frequently with roving eye movements, nystagmus, and oculogyration. They become restless, tense, and weak. Opisthotonos is not rare, and tachycardia may be apparent. In adults, generally the restlessness and roving eye movements are absent, but random shoulder movements may be apparent. Fasciculations often occur in both children and adults, and hypertension is not uncommon, particularly in adults. Respiratory and heart rates are often increased early on, but respirations may be markedly reduced as a respiratory deficit sets in. Slurring of speech and increased salivation are common, and convulsions may occur.

Most patients require only mild sedation with diazepam and some analgesia. In children, assisted ventilation may be necessary but because of the child's often jerky movements this may be difficult. Propranolol (Inderal), a nonselective beta-adrenergic blocker, has been used for some foreign scorpion species stings to alleviate the hypertensive effect of the venom. The drug may have some central nervous system effect. Nitroprusside (Nipride) has also been used for treatment of severe hypertension. In Arizona, the monospecific antivenom for this species, prepared in goats, has enjoyed considerable success, with few serious immediate serum reactions (often caused by too rapid and undiluted administration) and very minor delayed serum reactions. The use of this agent should always be considered in children in whom there are severe neurologic signs and a respiratory deficit.

SNAKE VENOM POISONING

method of
BARRY S. GOLD, M.D.
Johns Hopkins University School of Medicine
Baltimore, Maryland

Snake venom poisoning is a complex type of poisoning that not only affects the bite site but may affect multiple organ systems either primarily or secondarily. An estimated 45,000 snakebites occur annually in the United States, of which about 8000 are venomous, averaging 5 to 6 deaths per year. The majority of deaths occur in children, the elderly, victims in whom antivenin was not administered or was delayed or given in insufficient quantities, or members of certain sects who handle snakes during their religious ceremonies. Most victims are young males, of whom 50% are intoxicated and deliberately handling or molesting the snake. Most bites occur between April and October, with the highest incidence in July and August. The most common bite site is on the extremities.

Only about 25 of the 120 species of snakes native to the United States are poisonous. At least one species of poisonous snake is found in every state except Alaska, Maine, and Hawaii. The majority of poisonous snakebites are caused by members of the family Crotalidae, or pit vipers, which includes rattlesnakes, copperheads, and cottonmouths. The coral snake (family Elapidae) is the only other native poisonous snake and accounts for fewer than 20 to 25 bites per year. About 100 bites per year occur from foreign or exotic species that are held in zoos or found in amateur and professional collections. Most deaths are due to bites of the Eastern diamondback rattlesnake *(Crotalus adamanteus)*, the Western diamondback rattlesnake *(C. atrox)*, various subspecies of the Western rattlesnake *(C. viridis)*, and the timber rattlesnake *(C. horridus)*. Deaths resulting from coral snake bite are rare. A small number of deaths occur from bites of exotic or foreign snakes imported illegally.

Pit viper venoms are complex proteins, many of which possess enzymatic activity. Although the enzymes contribute to the deleterious effects of the venom, the lethal components may be secondary to the smaller, low-molecular-weight polypeptides. The effects of pit viper venom cause local tissue damage, vascular defects, hemolysis, a disseminated intravascular coagulation (DIC)–like syndrome, and pulmonary, cardiac, renal, and neurologic defects. Coral snake venoms cause changes in neuromuscular transmission, with minimal local tissue damage.

DIAGNOSIS

A definitive diagnosis of snakebite poisoning requires identification of the snake along with signs and symptoms of envenomation. Usually the snake is not available for identification; therefore, accurate diagnosis and treatment depend on identifying symptoms and signs of snakebite poisoning. About 25% of all pit viper bites and 50% of all coral snake bites are "dry" and do not result in envenomation. Fear is the most commonly encountered reaction associated with any snakebite. Consequently, it is essential not to mistake autonomic reactions for systemic symptoms and signs from the bite, which could lead to unwarranted treatment. The primary local clinical findings with most pit viper bites occur within 30 to 60 minutes after the bite. These consist of single or multiple fang punctures, pain, and edema, erythema, or ecchymosis of the bite site and adjacent tissues. Single or multiple punctures and scratches are commonly seen. Pain initially follows envenomation, and edema appears within 10 minutes and is rarely delayed longer than 20 to 30 minutes. Rarely, bullae may be seen. There may be signs of lymphangitis, with tender regional lymph nodes. Frequent systemic manifestations include nausea, vomiting, perioral paresthesias, tingling of the fingertips and toes, fasciculations, lethargy, and weakness. Complaints of a rubbery, minty, or metallic taste in the mouth are frequent following bites by some species of rattlesnakes. More severe, systemic effects include hypotension, dyspnea, and altered sensorium. Coagulopathies are frequently seen following bites by rattlesnakes and may result in a DIC-like picture manifested by prolonged prothrombin time (PT) and activated partial thromboplastin time (aPTT), hypofibrinogenemia, thrombocytopenia, and abnormal fibrin degradation products. Pit viper venoms increase capillary membrane permeability, resulting in extravasation of electrolytes, colloid, and red blood cells into the envenomated site. This process may also occur in the lungs, kidneys, peritoneum, myocardium, and, rarely, the central nervous system. There may also be changes in the membranes of red blood cells, leading to hemolysis. Edema formation, hypoalbuminemia, and hemoconcentration occur initially. They are followed by pooling of blood and fluids in the microcirculation, resulting in hypovolemic shock. Renal failure may be secondary to decreased glomerular filtration rate, intravascular hemolysis, DIC, or the nephrotoxic effects of the venom components.

The ultimate severity of any venomous snakebite depends on the size and species of the snake, the amount and toxicity of venom injected, the location of the bite, first aid modalities performed, timing of definitive treatment, and underlying medical conditions in the victim, among other factors. Envenomations are graded as minimal, moderate, or severe. Minimal envenomations are localized to the bite site and demonstrate edema, erythema, or ecchymosis, unassociated with any systemic manifestations or coagulation or laboratory abnormalities. Moderate envenomations show progression beyond the bite site, significant symptoms and signs (e.g., nausea, vomiting, paresthesias, fasciculations) or mildly abnormal results of coagulation and laboratory studies. Severe envenomations show rapid progression of edema, erythema, or ecchymosis to involve the entire extremity. Systemic manifestations are severe and may include dyspnea, tachypnea, tachycardia, altered sensorium, and profound hypotension. Severe bleeding and markedly abnormal coagulation profile including PT, aPTT, hypofibrinogenemia, and thrombocytopenia (less than 20,000 cells per μL) and a DIC-like picture may result, in addition to other laboratory abnormalities.

Coral snake envenomations produce little or no pain after the bite. Occasionally, there is a delay of 8 to 24 hours prior to the onset of systemic manifestations. These are usually cranial nerve palsies manifested as ptosis, dysarthria, dysphagia, intense salivation, and respiratory depression.

FIELD TREATMENT

If the bite occurred within 60 minutes of a medical facility, the victim should be placed at rest, reassured, kept warm, and transported to the facility as quickly as possible. The injured part should be immobilized in a functional position below the level of the heart, and all rings, watches, and constrictive clothing removed. The use of ice, tourniquets, incision and suction, or electroshock is contraindicated. A Sawyer Extractor applied directly over the fang punctures may be of value when used within the first 5 minutes of the bite and kept in place for 30 to 40 minutes. Emergency medical personnel should be advised to establish an intravenous access line on the contralateral side and to administer oxygen.

EMERGENCY DEPARTMENT TREATMENT

A rapid, detailed history should include time of the bite, description of the snake, type of field therapy, and identification of co-morbid medical conditions, allergy to horse products, or prior history of snakebite and therapy. A complete physical examination should be performed, with special emphasis on the cardiovascular, pulmonary, and neurologic systems, followed by inspection of the bite site for fang punctures or scratches. If not previously done, a venous access site should be established in the contralateral extremity. A tourniquet or constriction band should not be removed until venous access has been established. Baseline laboratory tests should include a complete blood count with platelets, coagulation profile (PT, APTT, fibrinogen), electrolytes, blood urea nitrogen (BUN), serum creatinine, and urinalysis. These tests should be repeated every 4 hours for the first 12 hours and then on a daily basis. Additional tests such as blood typing and cross-match, measurement of creatine kinase, chest radiography, and electrocardiography should be performed for moderate or severe envenomations. The envenomation should be classified as minimal, moderate, or severe based on the most severe symptom, sign, or laboratory finding noted at that time. The patient should be continuously assessed, because a mild envenomation may progress rapidly to severe over a period of an hour in the absence of treatment. Circumferential measurements at several points above and below the bite site should be recorded every 15 to 20 minutes, and the advancing edge of the swelling should be marked with a pen.

Administration of antivenin is the only effective treatment for moderate to severe envenomations, along with aggressive life support in an intensive care setting. Its effectiveness is both dose- and time-related, with its greatest effect occurring during the first 4 hours. It is less effective after 12 hours but has been shown to reverse coagulopathies after 24 hours. A skin test for hypersensitivity to horse serum should be performed, according to the instructions in the package insert, *only* if antivenin is to be administered. A negative result on skin testing does not preclude the possibility of an immediate hypersensitivity reaction. If the skin test is positive and the envenomation is life- or limb-threatening, antivenin treatment must not be delayed, and the antivenin should be administered after consultation with a regional poison control center. The amount of antivenin (Crotalidae) polyvalent to be administered should be based on the severity and progression of local signs, systemic symptoms and signs, or results of coagulation studies. No antivenin is administered for trivial or minimal poisoning. Moderate cases require the use of 10 vials administered over 1 to 2 hours. Severe cases usually require the use of 15 vials or more. Those patients with profound circulatory collapse should initially receive 20 vials over 1 hour. Isotonic fluid administration followed by pressors is appropriate for severe hypotension. Antivenin dosage is usually lower for cottonmouth envenomations, and antivenin therapy is unnecessary in most cases of copperhead bites. Reconstituted antivenin should initially be diluted in 250 to 1000 mL of sterile 0.9% sodium chloride or 5% dextrose and given by intravenous drip. It should initially be administered slowly at 1 mL per minute for the first 15 to 20 minutes. If there is no reaction, the remainder can be infused over 1 to 2 hours. The amount of intravenous fluids given should be reduced in pediatric and geriatric patients, except when hypovolemia or shock occurs. The initial dose of antivenin should be re-administered every 1 to 2 hours until local and/or systemic symptoms or laboratory abnormalities no longer progress or are terminated. Antitetanus therapy should be administered when indicated. Antimicrobial should be given based on clinical signs of wound infection. Hypovolemic shock, often with concomitant lysis of red blood cells and platelet destruction, requires fluid and blood component replacement. Severe defects of hemostasis such as abnormal clotting or disturbance of platelets require replacement with fresh-frozen plasma or platelets.

Early reactions to antivenin are common and anaphylactoid (dose-related), generally resulting from too-rapid infusion of the antivenin. If this occurs, the antivenin infusion should be discontinued immediately. Epinephrine, diphenhydramine (Benadryl), and ranitidine (Zantac) (or other histamine H_2 blockers) should be administered. The benefit/risk ratio should be re-evaluated before antivenin therapy is continued. In most instances, antivenin administration can be resumed after further dilution, with administration at a slower rate. Mild sedation with diazepam is indicated in all severe cases of snakebite in which respiratory depression is not a problem. Codeine may be used for moderate pain and morphine for severe pain. Acetylsalicylic acid (ASA) should be avoided.

All victims of snakebite, whether venomous or nonvenomous, should be observed for at least 12 hours. Routine use of fasciotomy should be discouraged. It is usually unnecessary, and the presence of compartment pressure syndrome reflects a lack of or insufficient antivenin administration during the first 12 hours after the envenomation. Fasciotomy may be necessary when there is objective evidence of a compartment syndrome, as demonstrated by measurements of compartment pressures of greater than 30 mm Hg, that is unresponsive to limb elevation and administration of mannitol (1 to 2 grams per kg) and an additional 10 vials of antivenin. The wound should be cleansed and covered with a sterile dressing, and the injured extremity maintained in a functional position. The use of corticosteroids has no proven clinical efficacy in the acute phase of envenomation and is contraindicated except in treatment of delayed reactions. Follow-up care utilizing appropriate corrective measures and exercises can prevent contractures. Within 3 to 4 days after the bite, a complete evaluation should be instituted by a physiatrist, who should perform periodic assessments of joint motion and muscle strength and girth measurements. The most frequently recognized complication of venomous snakebite treatment is serum sickness, which occurs about 7 to 14 days following the administration of antivenin. The probability of serum sickness increases with the administration of more than 5 vials of antivenin. It is usually manifested as fever, arthralgias, rash, and lymphadenopathy and responds to a rapid tapering course of prednisone.

The same principles noted for management of pit viper envenomations should be followed for coral snake envenomations, with the exception of the recommended application of a pressure/immobilization splint to retard absorption of the venom. It should not be removed until antivenin administration has been begun or envenomation is excluded. The value of other first aid measures has not been established for coral snakebites. Five vials of North American coral snake antivenin, i.e., antivenin (*Micrurus fulvius*), should be administered when a possible coral snake envenomation has occurred. If symptoms evolve, an additional 10 to 15 vials should be administered. The patient's condition should be monitored in an intensive care unit because of the potential for respiratory paralysis. There is no antivenin for the Arizona coral snake, and treatment is symptomatic, because bites are rarely serious.

The local zoo is the initial place to call when a patient presents with a bite from an exotic venomous snake. All zoos maintain a list of consulting physicians, as well as the *Antivenin Index*,* which lists the location and number of vials of antivenin available for exotic snakes. Regional poison control centers also maintain listings for antivenin. In all envenomations, it is wise to consult with a regional poison control center, where trained physicians and specialists in the management and treatment of snakebite are available at all times.

*Boyer DM (ed): Dallas, Dept. of Herpetology, Dallas Zoo, 1994.

HAZARDOUS MARINE ANIMALS

method of
PAUL S. AUERBACH, M.D., M.S.
Stanford University School of Medicine
Stanford, California

The expanses of ocean that cover the earth are the greatest wilderness. Seventy-one percent of the earth's surface is composed of ocean, the volume of which exceeds 325 million cubic miles. Within the undersea realm exist four fifths of all living organisms. Some aquatic microorganisms, plants, and animals can be hazardous to humans. This chapter describes treatment for marine envenomations.

Naturally occurring aquatic zootoxins are designated as oral toxins (poisonous to eat; they include bacterial poisons and products of decomposition), parenteral toxins (venom produced in specialized glands and injected mechanically [by spine, needle, fang, fin, or dart]), and crinotoxins (venom produced in specialized glands and administered as slime, mucus, or gastric secretion).

FIRST AID

The physician should adhere to fundamental principles of medical rescue. Simultaneously with any specific interventions directed against a particular venom or poison the rescuer must be certain that the victim maintains a patent airway, breathes spontaneously or with assistance, and is supported by an adequate blood pressure. Because marine envenomations may afflict a scuba diver, the rescuer should anticipate near-drowning, immersion hypothermia, decompression sickness, or arterial air embolism. Conversely, any person rescued from the ocean should be thoroughly examined for external signs of a bite, puncture, or sting.

Anaphylaxis

An envenomation or administration of antivenin can elicit an allergic reaction. The signs and symptoms of anaphylaxis may occur within minutes of exposure and include hypotension, bronchospasm, tongue and lip swelling, laryngeal edema, pulmonary edema, seizures, cardiac arrhythmia, pruritus, urticaria, angioedema, rhinitis, conjunctivitis, nausea, vomiting, diarrhea, abdominal pain, gastrointestinal bleeding, and syncope. Most severe allergic reactions occur within 15 to 30 minutes of envenomation, and nearly all occur within 6 hours. Fatalities are related to airway obstruction or hypotension. Acute elevated pulmonary vascular resistance may contribute to hypotension that results from generalized arterial vasodilatation.

Decisive treatment should be instituted at the first indication of hypersensitivity:

1. Maintain the airway and administer oxygen.
2. Obtain intravenous access and administer crystalloid to achieve a systolic blood pressure of 90 mm Hg in an adult. If the reaction is severe or the victim is older than 45 years, apply a cardiac monitor.
3. Administer epinephrine. Begin with administration of aqueous epinephrine 1:1000 subcutaneously in the deltoid region. The dose for adults is 0.3 to 0.5 mL and that for children, 0.01 mL per kg. If the reaction is sustained, the initial dose may be repeated in 15 to 20 minutes. Aerosolized aqueous epinephrine is not adequate to abort systemic anaphylaxis. If the reaction is limited to pruritus and urticaria, there is no wheezing or facial swelling, and the victim is older than 45 years, administer an antihistamine and reserve epinephrine for a worsened condition.

If the reaction is life-threatening and there is no response to subcutaneous epinephrine, administer epinephrine intravenously. An adult should receive a 0.1 mg bolus of 1:1000 aqueous epinephrine (0.1 mL) diluted in 10 mL of normal saline (final dilution 1:100,000) infused over 10 minutes (10 μg per minute). A mixture for continuous infusion is prepared by adding 1 mg of 1:1000 aqueous epinephrine (1 mL) to 250 mL of normal saline to create a concentration of 4 μg per 1 mL. This infusion should be started at 1 μg per minute (15 minidrops per minute) and increased to 4 to 5 μg per minute if the clinical response is inadequate. In children and infants, the starting dose is 0.1 μg per minute up to a maximum of 1.5 μg per kg per minute; it should be noted that infusion rates in excess of 0.5 μg per kg per minute may be associated with cardiac ischemia and arrhythmias.

4. Relieve bronchospasm. Widely employed bronchodilators for inhalation are albuterol (Ventolin, Proventil), 0.5 mL, and metaproterenol (Alupent, Metaprel), 0.3 mL in 2.5 mL of normal saline administered by hand-held nebulizer. If a liquid $beta_2$-sympathomimetic agent is not available, micronized versions may be administered by a hand-held metered dose inhaler with spacer. Inhaled ipratropium may be added in refractory cases.
5. Administer an antihistamine. A mild reaction may be managed with diphenhydramine HCl (Benadryl), 50 to 75 mg given intravenously (IV), intramuscularly (IM), or orally (PO). The dose for children is 1 mg per kg. Nonsedating antihistamines, such as fexofenadine (Allegra), 60 mg PO, loratadine (Claritin), 10 mg PO, cetirizine (Zyrtec), 5 mg PO, or cimetidine (Tagamet), 300 mg, are adjuncts.

6. Administer a corticosteroid. If the reaction is severe or prolonged, or if the victim is regularly medicated with corticosteroids, administer hydrocortisone (Solu-Cortef), 200 to 300 mg, methylprednisolone (Solu-Medrol), 50 to 75 mg, or dexamethasone (Decadron), 10 to 25 mg IV, with a 7- to 14-day oral taper to follow. The parenteral dose of hydrocortisone for children is 2.5 mg per kg. If therapy is initiated by mouth, administer prednisone in a dose of 50 to 60 mg for adults and 1 mg per kg for children.

BACTERIOLOGY OF THE AQUATIC ENVIRONMENT

Wounds acquired in the aquatic environment are soaked in natural source water and sometimes contaminated with sediment. Penetration of the skin by spines or the razor-sharp edges of coral may inoculate pathogenic organisms, leading to a wound that heals slowly and with marked soft tissue inflammation. Such a wound may become infected, and the infection may be refractory to standard antimicrobial therapy. Indolent or extensive soft tissue infections develop in the normal or immunocompromised host. A clinician faced with a serious infection after an aquatic injury frequently needs to administer antibiotics before definitive laboratory identification of pathogenic organisms.

Ocean water provides a saline milieu for microbes. Although the greatest number and diversity of bacteria are found near the ocean surface, diverse bacteria and fungi are found in marine silts, sediments, and sand. Marine bacteria are generally halophilic, heterotrophic, motile, and gram-negative rod forms. Growth requirements vary from species to species with respect to utilization of organic carbon and nitrogen sources and requirements for various amino acids, vitamins and cofactors, sodium, potassium, magnesium, phosphate, sulfate, chloride, and calcium. Most marine bacteria are facultative anaerobes and are able to thrive in oxygen-rich environments. Few are obligatory aerobes or anaerobes. Some marine bacteria are highly proteolytic.

Numerous bacteria, microalgae, protozoans, fungi, yeasts, and viruses have been identified in or cultured from seawater, marine sediments, and marine life and from marine-acquired or marine-contaminated infected wounds or body fluids of septic victims (Table 1). In the setting of wound infection or sepsis, the clinician should alert the laboratory that a marine-acquired organism may be present, because special culture and identification techniques may be indicated.

The objectives for the management of infections from marine microorganisms are to recognize the clinical condition, culture the organism, and provide antimicrobial therapy. Management of marine-acquired infections should include therapy against *Vibrio* species. Third-generation cephalosporins (cefoperazone, cefotaxime, or ceftazidime) provide excellent coverage; first- and second-generation products (cefazolin, cephalothin, cephapirin, cefamandole, cefonicid, ceforanide,* or cefoxitin) appear to be less effective in vitro. Imipenem-cilastatin (Primaxin) is efficacious against gram-negative marine bacteria, as are trimethoprim-sulfamethoxazole (Bactrim, Septra), tetracycline, azlocillin (Azlin), mezlocillin (Mezlin), and piperacillin (Pipracil). Gentamicin, tobramycin (Nebcin), and chloramphenicol have tested favorably against *Pseudomonas putrefaciens* and *Vibrio* strains. Nonfermentative bacteria (such as *Alteromonas, Pseudomonas,* and *Deleya* species) appear to be sensitive to most antibiotics.

TABLE 1. **Bacterial and Fungal Species Isolated from Marine Water, Sediments, Marine Animals, and Marine-Acquired Wounds**

Achromobacter	*Pasteurella multocida*
Acinetobacter lwoffi	*Propionibacterium acnes*
Actinomyces	*Proteus mirabilis*
Aerobacter aerogenes	*Proteus vulgaris*
Aeromonas hydrophila	*Providencia stuartii*
Aeromonas sobria	*Pseudomonas aeruginosa*
Alcaligenes faecalis	*Pseudomonas beijerinckii*
Alteromonas espejiana	*Pseudomonas cepacia*
Alteromonas haloplanktis	*Pseudomonas iridescens*
Alteromonas macleodii	*Pseudomonas maltophilia*
Alteromonas undina	*Pseudomonas marinoglutinosa*
Bacillus cereus	*Pseudomonas nigrifaciens*
Bacillus subtilis	*Pseudomonas putrefaciens*
Bacteroides fragilis	*Pseudomonas stutzeri*
Branhamella catarrhalis	*Salmonella enteritidis*
Chromobacterium violaceum	*Serratia*
Citrobacter	*Staphylococcus aureus*
Clostridium botulinum	*Staphylococcus citreus*
Clostridium perfringens	*Staphylococcus epidermidis*
Clostridium tetani	*Streptococcus*
Corynebacterium	*Vibrio alginolyticus*
Deleya venustus	*Vibrio carchariae*
Edwardsiella tarda	*Vibrio cholerae*
Enterobacter aerogenes	*Vibrio damsela*
Erysipelothrix rhusiopathiae	*Vibrio fluvialis*
Escherichia coli	*Vibrio furnissii*
Flavobacterium	*Vibrio harveyi*
Fusarium solani	*Vibrio hollisae*
Klebsiella pneumoniae	*Vibrio mimicus*
Legionella pneumophila	*Vibrio parahaemolyticus*
Micrococcus sedentarius	*Vibrio pelagius II*
Micrococcus tegragenus	*Vibrio splendidus I*
Mycobacterium marinum	*Vibrio vulnificus*
Neisseria catarrhalis	

There is no advantage to quantitative wound culture before the appearance of a wound infection. Pending a prospective evaluation of prophylactic antibiotics in the management of marine wounds, the following recommendations are based on the indolent nature and malignant potential of soft tissue infections caused by *Vibrio* species:

1. Minor abrasions or lacerations (e.g., coral cuts or superficial sea urchin puncture wounds) do not require the administration of prophylactic antibiotics in the normal host. Persons who have a chronic disease (e.g., diabetes, hemophilia, or thalassemia) or are immunologically impaired (as in leukemia or acquired immune deficiency syndrome, or owing to on-

*Not available in the United States.

going chemotherapy or prolonged corticosteroid therapy), or who suffer from serious liver disease (e.g., hepatitis, cirrhosis, or hemochromatosis), particularly those with elevated serum iron levels, should immediately after the injury be given oral ciprofloxacin (Cipro), trimethoprim-sulfamethoxazole, or tetracycline therapy, as these persons appear to have an increased risk for serious wound infection and bacteremia. Preliminary experience suggests that cefuroxime (Zinacef) may be a useful alternative. Penicillin, ampicillin, and erythromycin are not acceptable alternatives. Other quinolones (ofloxacin, enoxacin, pefloxacin,* fleroxacin,* lomefloxacin) have not been extensively tested against *Vibrio,* so although they may be reliable alternatives, this awaits definitive evaluation. The appearance of an infection indicates the need for prompt antibiotic therapy. If an infection develops, antibiotic coverage should be chosen that will be efficacious against *Staphylococcus* and *Streptococcus,* as these are still the most common perpetrators of infection. In general, the fluoroquinolones, which are particularly effective for treating gram-negative bacillary infections, may become less and less useful against resistant staphylococci.

2. Serious injuries from an infection perspective include large, deep puncture wounds and those with retained foreign bodies. Examples are stingray spine wounds, deep sea urchin punctures, scorpaenid spine envenomations that enter a joint space, and full-thickness coral cuts. If the victim requires hospitalization and surgery for standard wound management, recommended antibiotics include gentamicin, tobramycin, amikacin, trimethoprim-sulfamethoxazole, cefoperazone, cefotaxime, ceftazidime, and chloramphenicol. There may be an increased tendency to seizures in patients who simultaneously receive imipenem or ciprofloxacin and theophylline.

If the victim is managed as an outpatient, the drugs of choice to cover *Vibrio* are ciprofloxacin, trimethoprim-sulfamethoxazole, and tetracycline. Cefuroxime (Ceftin, Zinacef), is an alternative. It is a clinical decision whether or not oral therapy should be preceded by a single intravenous or intramuscular loading dose of a similar or different antibiotic, commonly an aminoglycoside.

3. Infected wounds should be cultured for aerobes and anaerobes. Pending culture and sensitivity results, the patient should be managed with antibiotics as described previously. A person who has been wounded in a marine environment and who develops rapidly progressive cellulitis and/or myositis should be suspected of suffering from *Vibrio parahaemolyticus* or *Vibrio vulnificus* infection, particularly in the presence of chronic liver disease. If a wound infection is minor and has the appearance of a classic erysipeloid reaction (due to *Erysipelothrix rhusiopathiae*), penicillin, cephalexin, cephalothin, or ciprofloxacin should be administered.

*Investigational drug in the United States.

STONY CORALS

True (stony) corals exist in colonies that possess calcareous outer skeletons with pointed horns and/or razor-sharp edges. Snorkelers and divers frequently handle or brush against these living reefs, sustaining superficial cuts and abrasions on the extremities. Coral cuts are probably the most common injuries sustained under water. The initial reaction to a coral cut is stinging pain, erythema, and pruritus, most commonly on the forearms, elbows, and knees. Divers without gloves frequently receive cuts to the hands. A break in the skin may be surrounded within minutes by an erythematous wheal that fades in 1 to 2 hours. "Coral poisoning" describes these red, raised welts and local pruritus. Low-grade fever may be present and does not necessarily indicate an infection. With or without prompt treatment, this may progress to cellulitis with ulceration and tissue sloughing. These wounds heal slowly (3 to 6 weeks) and result in prolonged morbidity. In an extreme case, the victim develops cellulitis with lymphangitis, reactive bursitis, local ulceration, and wound necrosis.

Coral cuts should be promptly and vigorously scrubbed with soap and water and then irrigated copiously with a forceful stream of freshwater or normal saline to remove all foreign particles. It is occasionally helpful to use medicinal hydrogen peroxide to bubble out "coral dust." Any fragments that remain can become embedded and increase the risk for an indolent infection or foreign body granuloma. If stinging is a major symptom, there may be an element of envenomation by nematocysts. A brief rinse with diluted acetic acid (vinegar) or isopropyl alcohol 20% may diminish the discomfort (after the initial pain from contact with the open wound). If a coral-induced laceration is severe, it should be closed with adhesive strips rather than sutures if possible; preferably, it should be débrided for 3 to 4 days and closed in a delayed fashion.

There are a number of approaches to take with regard to wound care. The first (preferred) is to apply twice-daily sterile wet-to-dry dressings, using saline or a dilute antiseptic (povidone-iodine solution, 1 to 5%). Alternatively, a nontoxic topical antibiotic ointment (bacitracin or polymyxin B–bacitracin–neomycin [Neosporin]) may be used sparingly, the wound covered with a nonadherent dressing (Telfa), and secondary infections dealt with as they arise. A less often utilized approach is to apply a full-strength antiseptic solution, followed by a powdered topical antibiotic, such as tetracycline powder.* No method has been supported by a prospective trial.

Despite best efforts, the wound may heal slowly, with moderate to severe soft tissue inflammation and ulcer formation. All devitalized tissue should be débrided regularly using sharp dissection. This should be continued until a bed of healthy granulation tissue is formed. Wounds that appear infected should be

*Not available in the United States.

cultured and treated with antibiotics as previously discussed.

The patient who demonstrates malaise, nausea, and low-grade fever may be suffering from a systemic form of coral poisoning or be manifesting early signs of a wound infection. It is prudent at this point to search for a localized infection, procure wound culture or biopsy specimens as indicated, and initiate antibiotic therapy pending confirmation of the organisms. If the patient is started with antibiotic therapy and does not respond, a supplemental trial of systemic corticosteroids (prednisone 60 mg tapered over 2 weeks) is not unreasonable. In the absence of an overt infection, the natural course of the affliction is spontaneous improvement during a 4- to 12-week period.

SPONGES

Sponges are composed of elastic "skeletons" embedded with spicules of silicon dioxide or calcium carbonate. Two general syndromes, with minor variations, are induced by contact. The first is a pruritic dermatitis similar to plant-induced allergic dermatitis. A typical offender is the friable fire sponge *Tedania ignis.*

Within a few hours after skin contact, the reactions are characterized by itching and burning, which may progress to local joint swelling, soft tissue edema, vesiculation, and stiffness, particularly if small pieces of broken sponge are retained in the skin near the interphalangeal or metacarpophalangeal joints. The skin may become mottled or purpuric. Untreated, mild reactions subside within 3 to 7 days. With extensive skin surface area involvement, the victim may complain of fever, chills, malaise, dizziness, nausea, muscle cramps, and formication. Bullae may become purulent. Systemic erythema multiforme or an anaphylactoid reaction may develop 7 to 14 days after a severe exposure. In severe cases, surface desquamation of the skin may follow in 10 days to 2 months. No medical intervention can retard this process. Recurrent eczema and persistent arthralgias are rare complications.

The second syndrome is an irritant dermatitis and follows the penetration of small spicules into the skin. Most sponges have spicules; "toxic" sponges may possess toxins that enter microtraumatic lesions caused by the spicules.

Because it is usually impossible to distinguish clinically between the allergic and spicule-induced reactions, it is safest to treat for both. The skin should be gently dried. Spicules should be removed, if possible, using adhesive tape, a thin layer of rubber cement thinly applied and then peeled off, or a facial peel product. As soon as possible, dilute (5%) acetic acid (vinegar) soaks for 10 to 30 minutes three or four times daily should be applied to all affected areas. Although topical steroid lotions may help to relieve the secondary inflammation, they are of no value as an initial decontaminant. If they precede the vinegar soak, they may worsen the primary reaction. Delayed primary therapy or inadequate decontamination may result in the persistence of bullae, which may become purulent and require months to heal. Erythema multiforme may require the administration of systemic corticosteroids, beginning with a moderately high dose (prednisone 60 to 100 mg) tapered over 2 to 3 weeks. Other anecdotal remedies for the management of sponge envenomation that have been suggested without demonstration of efficacy include antiseptic dressings, broad-spectrum antibiotics, methdilazine (Tacaryl), pyribenzamine, phenobarbital, diphenhydramine, promethazine hydrochloride, and topical carbolic oil* or zinc oxide cream.

After the initial decontamination, a mild emollient cream or steroid preparation may be applied to the skin. If the allergic component is severe, particularly if there is weeping, crusting, and vesiculation, systemic corticosteroids (prednisone 60 to 80 mg, tapered over 2 weeks) may be beneficial. Severe itching may be controlled with an antihistamine. Frequent wound checks are important, because some patients develop significant infections.

Sponge-diver's disease is a stinging syndrome related to contact with the tentacles of anemones that attach to the base of a sponge. Treatment should include that for coelenterate envenomation.

COELENTERATES

Coelenterates are an enormous group, comprising approximately 10,000 species, at least 100 of which are dangerous to humans. Coelenterates hazardous to humans possess venom-charged stinging cells called nematocysts and include feather hydroids, fire coral, the Portuguese man-of-war, Indo-Pacific jellyfish, soft corals, and anemones. Seabather's eruption, commonly misnomered "sea lice," refers to a dermatitis that involves predominantly covered areas of the body and has been postulated to be caused by larvae of the thimble jellyfish *Linuche unguiculata* or the sea anemone *Edwardsiella lineata.* The larger jellyfish include the Portuguese man-of-war *Physalia physalis,* the deadly box jellyfish *Chironex fleckeri,* and the sea wasp *Chiropsalmus quadrumanus.* These creatures are armed with some of the most potent venoms in existence. An adult *Chironex* carries enough venom (in excess of 10 mL) to kill three adult humans. Sea nettles are considerably less lethal animals and can be found in both temperate and tropical waters, particularly in the Chesapeake Bay.

There is considerable phylogenetic relationship among all stinging species, such that the clinical features of the coelenterate syndrome are fairly constant, with a spectrum of severity.

Mild Envenomation

The stings caused by the hydroids and hydroid corals, along with lesser envenomations by jellyfish and anemones, result predominantly in skin irrita-

*Not available in the United States.

tion. There is usually an immediate pricking or stinging sensation, accompanied by pruritus, paresthesias, burning, throbbing, and radiation of the pain centrally from the extremities to the groin, abdomen, and axillae. The area involved by the nematocysts becomes red-brown-purple, often in a linear whiplike fashion, corresponding to "tentacle prints." Other features are blistering, local edema, and wheal formation, as well as violaceous petechial hemorrhages. The papular inflammatory rash is strictly confined to the areas of contact and may persist for up to 10 days. Areas of body hair appear to be somewhat more protected (from contact) than hairless areas. Seabather's eruption is manifested as a papular rash on bathing suit–covered areas.

If an envenomation is slightly more severe, then the aforementioned symptoms, which are evident in the first few hours, can progress over a course of days to local necrosis, skin ulceration, and secondary infection. This is particularly true of certain anemone stings.

Untreated, the minor to moderate skin disorder resolves in 1 to 2 weeks, with occasional residual hyperpigmentation for 1 to 2 months. Rubbing can cause lichenification. Local hyperhidrosis, fat atrophy, and contracture may occur. Permanent scarring may result. Persistent papules or plaques at the sites of contact may be accompanied by localized arthritis and joint effusion. Granuloma annulare, which is usually both a sporadic and a familial inflammatory dermatosis, has been associated with a *Physalia utriculus* envenomation.

Moderate and Severe Envenomation

The prime offenders in moderate and severe envenomations are the anemones, *Physalia* species, and Indo-Pacific jellyfish. The skin manifestations are compounded by the onset of systemic symptoms, which may appear immediately or be delayed by several hours:

1. Neurologic—malaise, headache, aphonia, diminished touch and temperature sensation, vertigo, ataxia, spastic or flaccid paralysis, mononeuritis multiplex, parasympathetic dysautonomia, plexopathy, radial-ulnar-median nerve palsies, delirium, loss of consciousness, convulsions, coma, and death
2. Cardiovascular—anaphylaxis, hemolysis, hypotension, small-artery spasm, bradyarrhythmias (including electromechanical dissociation and asystole), tachyarrhythmias, congestive heart failure, and ventricular fibrillation
3. Respiratory—rhinitis, bronchospasm, laryngeal edema, dyspnea, cyanosis, pulmonary edema, and respiratory failure
4. Musculoskeletal and rheumatologic—abdominal rigidity, diffuse myalgia and muscle cramps, muscle spasm, fat atrophy, arthralgias, reactive arthritis (seronegative symmetrical synovitis with pitting edema), and thoracolumbar pain
5. Gastrointestinal—nausea, vomiting, diarrhea, dysphagia, hypersalivation, and thirst
6. Ocular—conjunctivitis, chemosis, corneal ulcers, iridocyclitis, elevated intraocular pressure, synechiae, iris depigmentation, chronic unilateral glaucoma, and lacrimation
7. Other—acute renal failure, chills, fever, and nightmares

The extreme example of envenomation occurs with *Chironex fleckeri,* the dreaded box jellyfish. The sting is immediately intensely painful, and the victim usually struggles purposefully for only a minute or two before collapse. The toxic skin reaction may be quite intense, with rapid formation of wheals, vesicles, and a darkened reddish brown or purple whiplike flare pattern with stripes 8 to 10 mm in width. With major stings, skin blistering occurs within 6 hours, with superficial necrosis in 12 to 18 hours. On occasion, a pathognomonic "frosted" appearance with transverse cross-hatched pattern may be present. *Physalia* and anemone stings, although extremely painful, are rarely fatal. Death after *Physalia* stings has been attributed to anaphylaxis, primary respiratory failure, or cardiac arrhythmia.

A person recently stung by *P. physalis* may develop recurrent cutaneous eruptions for 2 to 3 weeks after the initial episode, without repeated exposure to the animal. This may take the form of lichenification, hyperhidrosis, angioedema, vesicles, large bullae, nodules that resemble erythema nodosum, granuloma annulare, or a more classic linear urticarial eruption. Acute regional vascular insufficiency of the upper extremity has been reported after jellyfish envenomation. It can be manifested by acral ischemia, signs and symptoms of compartment syndrome, and massive edema.

Treatment

Therapy is directed at stabilizing major systemic decompensation, opposing the venom's multiple effects, and alleviating pain. Generally, only severe *Physalia* and toxic jellyfish stings result in rapid decompensation. In both cases, supportive care is based on the presenting signs and symptoms. Hypotension should be managed with the prompt intravenous administration of crystalloid, such as lactated Ringer's solution. This must be done in concert with detoxification of any nematocysts (particularly those of *Chironex* or *Chiropsalmus*) that are still attached to the victim, to limit the perpetuation of envenomation. Hypotension is usually limited to very young or elderly victims who suffer severe and multiple stings, and it is worsened by fluid depletion that accompanies protracted vomiting. Hypertension is an occasional side effect of a jellyfish envenomation, such as that of *Carukia barnesi.* Excessive catecholamine stimulation is one putative cause, which has prompted clinical intervention with phentolamine (Regitine), an alpha-adrenergic blocking agent (5 mg IV as an initial dose). Bronchospasm may be managed as an allergic component. If the victim is in respiratory distress with wheezing, shortness of breath, or heart failure, pulse oximetry or arterial blood gas measurement may be used to guide supplemental oxygen administration. Seizures are generally self-limited but should be treated with intravenous diazepam (Valium) for 24 to 48 hours, after which they rarely recur.

All victims with a systemic component should be observed for a period of at least 6 to 8 hours, as rebound phenomena after successful treatment are not uncommon. All elderly victims should undergo electrocardiographic evaluation and continuous cardiac monitoring, with frequent checks for arrhythmias. Urinalysis demonstrates the presence or absence of hemoglobinuria, indicating hemolysis after the putative attachment of *Physalia* venom to red blood cell membrane glycoprotein sites. If this is the case, the urine should be alkalized with bicarbonate to prevent the precipitation of pigment in the renal tubules, while a moderate diuresis (30 to 50 mL per hour) is maintained with a loop diuretic (such as furosemide) or mannitol (0.25 gram per kg IV every 8 to 12 hours). In rare instances of acute progressive renal failure, peritoneal dialysis or hemodialysis may be necessary.

If there are signs of distal ischemia or an impending compartment syndrome, standard diagnostic and therapeutic measures apply. These include Doppler ultrasonography and/or angiography for diagnosis, regional thrombolysis for acutely occluded blood vessels, and measurement of intracompartmental tissue pressures to guide fasciotomy. Reversible regional sympathetic blockade may be efficacious if vasospasm is a dominant clinical feature. However, the vasospasm associated with a jellyfish envenomation may be severe and prolonged and refractory to regional sympathectomy and intra-arterial reserpine therapy.

A small child may pick up tentacle fragments on the beach and place them into his or her mouth, resulting in rapid intraoral swelling and potential airway obstruction, particularly in the presence of exceptional hypersensitivity. In such cases, an endotracheal tube should be placed before edema precludes visualization of the vocal cords. In no case should any liquid be placed in the mouth if the airway is not protected.

C. fleckeri produces the only coelenterate venom for which there is a specific antidote. If the reaction is severe, *Chironex* antivenin* should be administered IV as soon as possible. The intramuscular route is a less desirable alternative. The antivenin is supplied in ampules of 20,000 units. The dose is 1 ampule (diluted 1:5 to 1:10 in isotonic crystalloid; dilution with water is not recommended) administered IV over 5 minutes, or 3 ampules IM. Although the antivenin is prepared by hyperimmunizing sheep, the risk of anaphylaxis or serum sickness should be assumed to be the same as with use of equine hyperimmune globulin preparations. In addition to its lifesaving properties, the early administration of antivenin may markedly reduce pain and decrease subsequent skin scarring. Antivenin administration may be repeated once or twice every 2 to 4 hours until there is no further worsening of the reaction (skin discoloration, pain, or systemic effects). A large sting in an adult may require the initial administration of 2 ampules. The antivenin may also be used to neutralize the effects of a *Chiropsalmus* envenomation. The antivenin should be stored in a refrigerator at 2 to 10°C and must not be frozen. Concomitant administration of a corticosteroid (hydrocortisone 200 mg IV) is often recommended for its anti-inflammatory activity but is no substitute for the administration of antivenin.

Often, pain can be controlled by treating the dermatitis. However, if pain is excruciating and there is no contraindication (head injury, altered mental status, respiratory depression, allergy, profound hypotension), the administration of narcotics is often indicated. Severe muscle spasm may respond to 10% calcium gluconate (5 to 10 mL IV slow push), diazepam (5 to 10 mg IV), or methocarbamol (1 gram, infused no faster than 100 mg per minute through a widely patent IV line).

Coelenterate Dermatitis

If a person is stung by a coelenterate, the following steps should be taken:

1. In the case of a known or suspected box jellyfish envenomation, the victim must be rapidly assessed for the adequacy of breathing and supported with an airway and artificial ventilation if necessary. The victim should be moved as little as possible. It is absolutely essential to immediately apply acetic acid 5% (vinegar) liberally ("flooding" the skin) to any adherent tentacles before any attempt is made to remove them, to paralyze the nematocysts and avoid worsening the envenomation. One should not expect significant pain relief from this maneuver. Although most nematocysts cannot penetrate the thickened skin of the human palm, the rescuer should pay particular attention to his or her own skin protection. Isopropyl alcohol 40 to 70% should be used as a last resort. A number of authors recommend that isopropyl alcohol not be used, based upon in vitro observation of inefficacy and nematocyst discharge after the application of this detoxicant.

First aid at the scene should include the pressure-immobilization technique. If practicable by virtue of location of the sting, a cloth or gauze pad of approximate dimensions 6 to 8 cm by 6 to 8 cm by 2 to 3 cm (thickness) should be placed directly over the sting and held firmly in place by a circumferential bandage 15 to 18 cm wide applied at lymphatic-venous occlusive pressure. The arterial circulation should not be occluded, as determined by the detection of arterial pulsations and proper capillary refill. One hypothesis holds that the pressure-immobilization technique devascularizes the area immediately below the pad and prevents the distribution of venom into the general

*Not available in the United States.

circulation. The limb is then splinted in the position of function. The splint and bandage should be released after the victim has been brought to proper medical attention and the rescuer is prepared to provide systemic support.

2. For other coelenterate envenomations, the wound should be immediately rinsed with seawater, *not with freshwater.* The wound should not be rubbed with a towel or clothing to remove adherent tentacles. Freshwater and abrasion stimulate any nematocysts that have not already fired. The gross tentacles should be removed with forceps or a well-gloved hand.

Commercial (chemical) cold packs applied over a dry cloth have been shown to be effective when applied to mild to moderate *Physalia* stings. Whether or not the direct application of ice to envenomed skin and the resulting freshwater melt stimulates the discharge of nematocysts has not been determined.

Applications of hot packs or gentle rinses with hot water are not recommended, as they may worsen the envenomation or in repeated applications lead to lymphangitis. However, beach patrol members who have been stung by jellyfish (presumably Portuguese man-of-war) report that an immediate hot shower with a forceful stream of water relieves the pain. This observation implies that the benefits of applying a forceful jet of water that can dislodge tentacle fragments and nematocysts may supersede the deleterious effect caused by the hypotonicity of freshwater that leads to nematocyst discharge.

3. Acetic acid (vinegar) 5% is the treatment of choice to inactivate the toxin. An alternative is isopropyl alcohol (40 to 70%). Baking soda has been recommended for sea nettle envenomations. Perfume, aftershave lotion, and high-proof liquor are less efficacious and may be detrimental. The detoxicant should be applied continuously for at least 30 minutes or until there is no further pain. Other substances reputed to be effective as alternatives are organic solvents such as formalin, ether, and gasoline (all to be condemned); dilute ammonium hydroxide (household ammonia); olive oil; sugar; urine; and papain (papaya latex [juice], pads soaked with papain solution, or unseasoned meat tenderizer).

4. No systemic drugs are of verifiable use. Ephedrine, atropine, calcium, methysergide, and hydrocortisone have all been touted at one time or another, but there is no proof that they help. Antihistamines may be useful if there is a significant allergic component. The administration of epinephrine is appropriate only in the setting of anaphylaxis.

5. Immersing the area in hot water is generally not recommended, as the hypotonic solution causes nematocysts to fire.

6. Once the wound has been soaked with vinegar or the toxin(s) otherwise inactivated, the remaining nematocysts must be removed. The easiest way to do this is to apply shaving cream or a paste of baking soda (after first removing residual vinegar), flour, or talc and to shave the area with a razor or reasonable facsimile. If sophisticated facilities are not available, the nematocysts should be removed by making a sand or mud paste with seawater and using this to coat the victim's skin and then scraping with a sharp-edged shell or piece of wood. The rescuer must take care not to become envenomed; bare hands must be frequently rinsed.

7. Local anesthetic ointments (lidocaine HCl, 2.5%) or sprays (benzocaine, 14%) or mild steroid lotions (hydrocortisone 1%) may be soothing. Calamine with 1% menthol has been recommended for seabather's eruption.

8. Patients should receive standard antitetanus prophylaxis.

9. There is no need for prophylactic antibiotic therapy. The wounds should be checked for infection at 3 and 7 days after injury. Any ulcerating lesions should be cleaned three times a day and covered with a thin layer of nonsensitizing antiseptic ointment. A jellyfish sting to the cornea may cause a foreign body sensation, photophobia, and decreased (or "hazy") vision. Ophthalmologic examination reveals hyperemic sclera, chemosis, and irregularity of the corneal epithelium with stromal edema. Depending on the extent of the wound, the anterior chamber may demonstrate the inflammatory response of iridocyclitis ("flare" with or without cells). The patient should be referred to an ophthalmologist, who may prescribe a steroid-containing eye medication such as prednisolone acetate 1% with hyoscine 0.25%. It is not recommended that any traditional skin detoxicant be applied directly to the cornea, as it is likely to worsen the tissue injury.

Delayed Reaction

A delayed reaction in areas of skin contact similar in appearance to erythema nodosum may be accompanied by fever, weakness, arthralgias, painful joint swelling, and effusions. This may recur multiple times over the course of 1 to 2 months. The treatment is a 10- to 14-day taper of prednisone, starting with 50 to 80 mg. This may need to be prolonged or repeated with each flare of the reaction.

Persistent Hyperpigmentation

Postinflammatory hyperpigmentation is common after the stings of many jellyfish and other lesser coelenterates. A solution of hydroquinone 1.8% in a glycol-alcohol base (70% ethyl alcohol, *n*-propylene glycol mixed at a 3:2 ratio) twice a day as a topical agent for 3 to 5 weeks has been used successfully to treat hyperpigmentation that followed a *Pelagia noctiluca* sting.

ECHINODERMATA

Sea Urchins

The spines of sea urchins are often quite brittle and break off easily in the flesh, lodging deeply and making removal difficult. Pedicellariae are small and delicate seizing organs attached to the stalks scattered among the spines. The outer surface of each jaw is covered by a large venom gland, which is triggered to contract with the jaw on contact.

Venomous spines inflict immediately and intensely painful stings. The pain is initially characterized by burning, which rapidly evolves into severe local muscle aching with visible erythema and swelling of the skin surrounding the puncture site(s). Frequently, a spine lodges in the victim's flesh. Some sea urchin (e.g., *Diadema setosum* or *Strongylocentrotus purpuratus*) spines contain purplish dye, which may give a false impression of spines left in the skin. If a spine enters into a joint, it may rapidly induce severe synovitis. If multiple spines have penetrated the skin, particularly if they are deeply embedded, the victim may rapidly develop systemic symptoms, which include nausea, vomiting, paresthesias, numbness and muscular paralysis, abdominal pain, syncope, hypotension, and respiratory distress. The presence of a frank neuropathy may indicate that the spine has lodged in contact with a peripheral nerve. The pain from multiple stings may be sufficient to cause delirium. Secondary infections and indolent ulceration are common.

The stings of pedicellariae are often of greater magnitude, causing immediate intense and radiating pain, local edema and hemorrhage, malaise, weakness, paresthesias, hypesthesia, arthralgias, aphonia, dizziness, syncope, generalized muscular paralysis, respiratory distress, hypotension, and, rarely, death. In some cases, the pain may disappear within the first hour, whereas the localized muscular weakness or paralysis persists for up to 6 hours.

The envenomed body part should immediately be immersed in nonscalding hot water (upper limit 113°F, or 45°C) to tolerance for 30 to 90 minutes in an attempt to achieve pain relief. Any pedicellariae that are still attached to the skin must be removed by applying a shaving foam and gently scraping with a razor. Embedded spines should be removed with care, as they are easily fractured. After the spines are removed, black or purplish discoloration surrounding the wound may be seen; this is spine dye and of no consequence. Although some thin venomous spines may be absorbed within 24 hours to 3 weeks, it is best to remove those that are easily reached and leave the remainder for dissolution. All thick calcium carbonate spines should be removed because of the risk for infection, a foreign body encaseation granuloma, or a dermoid inclusion cyst. External percussion to achieve fragmentation may prove disastrous if a chronic inflammatory process is initiated in sensitive tissue of the hand or foot. If the spines have acutely entered into joints or are closely aligned with neurovascular structures, the surgeon should use an operating microscope to remove all spine fragments. The extraction should be performed as soon as possible after the injury. If the spine has entered into an interphalangeal joint, the finger should be splinted until the spine is removed to limit fragmentation and further penetration. This may also control the fusiform finger swelling that is commonly noted after a puncture in the vicinity of the middle or proximal interphalangeal joint. It is inappropriate to rummage about in a hand wound in the emergency department, virtually looking for a needle in a haystack. If there is a question about whether a spine is present, soft-tissue-density radiographic techniques (magnetic resonance imaging or mammography is best) for detecting a radiopaque foreign body may be diagnostic. Although the calcium carbonate is relatively inert, it is accompanied by slime, bacteria, and organic epidermal debris. Therefore, secondary infections are common, and deep puncture wounds are an indication for prophylactic antibiotics.

Some sea urchin spines are phagocytosed in the soft tissues and ultimately dissolve. The granulomas caused by retained sea urchin spine fragments generally appear as flesh-colored or dye-colored surface or subcuticular nodules 2 to 12 months after the initial injury. In thin-skinned areas, they are erythematous and rubbery, painless, and infrequently umbilicated. In thicker skinned areas (palms and soles, knees) that are frequently abraded, they develop a keratinized appearance. Although necrosis and microabscess formation may be evident microscopically, suppuration is unusual. If a spine cannot be removed and forms a nidus for cyst or granuloma formation, the lesion may be removed surgically. Intralesional injection with a corticosteroid (triamcinolone hexacetonide [Aristospan] 5 mg per mL) is less efficacious but may be successful. Systemic anti-inflammatory drugs may be minimally helpful but are not a substitute for removal of the spine. A diffuse delayed reaction consisting of cyanotic induration, fusiform swelling in the digits, and focal phalangeal bone erosion may be treated with systemic corticosteroids and antibiotics.

Starfish

The carnivorous *Acanthaster planci* is a particularly venomous species of starfish. The sharp, rigid, and venomous aboral spines of this animal may grow to 4 to 6 cm and can penetrate the hardiest of diving gloves. As a spine enters the skin, it carries venom into the wound, with immediate pain, copious bleeding, and mild edema. The pain is generally moderate and self-limited, with remission during a period of 0.5 to 3 hours. The wound may become dusky or discolored. Multiple puncture wounds may result in acute systemic reactions, which are manifested as paresthesias, nausea, vomiting, lymphadenopathy, and muscular paralysis. If a spine fragment is retained, a granulomatous lesion akin to that from a sea urchin puncture wound may develop. A victim who has been previously sensitized may suffer a prolonged (lasting weeks) reaction consisting of local edema and pruritus. Treatment is similar to that for a sea urchin puncture. Because of the stout nature of the spines, it is rare to retain a fragment.

STINGRAYS

The stingrays are the most commonly incriminated group of fishes involved in human envenomations. The venom organ consists of one to four venomous stings on the dorsum of an elongate, whiplike caudal appendage. Stingray "attacks" are purely defensive gestures that occur when an unwary human handles, corners, or steps on a camouflaged creature while wading in shallow waters. The tail of the ray reflexly whips upward and accurately thrusts the caudal spine(s) into the victim, producing a puncture wound or jagged laceration. The integumentary sheath covering the spine is ruptured, and venom is released into the wound, along with mucus, pieces of the sheath, and fragments of the spine. On occasion, the entire spine tip is broken off and remains in the wound.

Because of the retrorse serrated teeth and powerful strikes, significant lacerations can result. Secondary bacterial infection is common. Osteomyelitis may occur if the bone is penetrated. The lower extremities, particularly the ankle and foot, are involved most often. The envenomation causes immediate local intense pain, edema, and variable bleeding. The pain may radiate centrally, peaks at 30 to 60 minutes, and may last for up to 48 hours. The wound is initially dusky or cyanotic, with rapid progression to erythema and hemorrhagic discoloration, with rapid fat and muscle hemorrhage and necrosis. If discoloration around the wound edge is not immediately apparent, within 2 hours it will often extend several centimeters from the wound. Minor stings may simulate bacterial cellulitis. Systemic manifestations include weakness, nausea, vomiting, diarrhea, diaphoresis, vertigo, tachycardia, headache, syncope, seizures, inguinal or axillary pain, muscle cramps, fasciculations, generalized edema (with truncal wounds), paralysis, hypotension, arrhythmias, and death.

The success of therapy is largely related to the rapidity with which it is undertaken. Treatment is directed at combating the effects of the venom, alleviating pain, and preventing infection. The wound should be irrigated immediately with whatever cold diluent is at hand. If sterile saline or water is not available, tap water may be used. This removes some venom and mucus, provides mild anesthesia, and induces local vasoconstriction, possibly retarding the absorption of the toxin. In a rapid primary exploration of the wound, any visible pieces of the spine or integumentary sheath should be removed. Local suction, if applied in the first 15 to 30 minutes, may be of some value (this is controversial), as may application of a proximal constriction band (also controversial) that occludes only superficial venous and lymphatic return. This should be released for 90 seconds every 10 minutes to prevent ischemia.

As soon as possible, the wound should be soaked in nonscalding hot water to tolerance (upper limit 113°F, or 45°C) for 30 to 90 minutes. This attenuates some of the thermolabile components of the protein venom and relieves pain. There is no indication for the addition of ammonia, magnesium sulfate, potassium permanganate, or formalin to the soaking solution. In this circumstance, they are toxic to tissue, and/or they obscure visualization of the wound. During the hot-water soak, the wound should be explored and débrided of any readily visible pieces of the sting's integumentary sheath, which would continue envenomation. Cryotherapy is potentially disastrous, and there are no data to support the use of antihistamines or steroids.

Pain control should be initiated during the first débridement or soaking period. Narcotics may be necessary. Local infiltration of the wound with 1 to 2% lidocaine (Xylocaine) without epinephrine may be quite useful.

After the soaking procedure, the wound should be prepared in a sterile fashion, re-explored, and thoroughly débrided. Wounds should be packed open for delayed primary closure or sutured loosely around adequate drainage. Prophylactic antibiotic therapy is recommended because of the high incidence of ulceration, necrosis, and secondary infection. A victim who is to be given treatment and released should be observed for a period of at least 3 to 4 hours for systemic side effects.

Wounds that are not properly débrided or explored and cleansed of foreign material may fester for weeks or months. It is not at all uncommon for such wounds to appear infected, when in reality what exists is a chronic draining ulcer initiated by persistent retained organic matter. Exploration at this time may reveal erosion of adjacent soft tissue structures and the formation of an epidermal inclusion cyst or other related foreign body reaction. As with other marine-acquired wounds, indolent infection should prompt a search for unusual microorganisms.

SCORPION FISH

Distributed in tropical and less commonly in temperate oceans, several hundred species of scorpion fishes are divided into three groups typified by different genera on the basis of venom organ structure: (1) *Pterois* (zebra fish, lionfish, and butterfly cod), (2) *Scorpaena* (scorpion fish, bullrout, and sculpin), and (3) *Synanceja* (stonefish). Some species bury themselves in the sand, and most dangerous types lie motionless on the bottom. The 17 or 18 venom organs consist of 12 or 13 dorsal, 2 pelvic, and 3 anal spines, with associated venom glands. Stonefish venom has been likened in potency to cobra venom.

When any of these fish is removed from the water, handled, stepped on, or otherwise threatened, it reflexly erects the spinous dorsal fin and flares out the armed gill covers and the pectoral and anal fins. If provoked while still in the water, it will actually attack. The venom is injected by a direct puncture wound through the skin, which tears the sheath and may fracture the spine, in a manner analogous to that of a stingray envenomation.

Pain is immediate and intense, with radiation centrally. Untreated, the pain peaks at 60 to 90 minutes and persists for 6 to 12 hours. In the case of the stonefish, the pain may be severe enough to cause delirium and may persist at high levels for days. The wound and surrounding area are initially ischemic and then cyanotic, with more broadly surrounding areas of erythema, edema, and warmth. Vesicles may form. Rapid tissue sloughing and close surrounding areas of cellulitis, with anesthesia adjacent to peripheral hypesthesia, may be present within 48 hours. Systemic effects include anxiety, headache, tremors, maculopapular rash, nausea, vomiting, diarrhea, abdominal pain, diaphoresis, pallor, restlessness, delirium, seizures, limb paralysis, peripheral neuritis or neuropathy, lymphangitis, arthritis, fever, hypertension, respiratory distress, bradycardia, tachycardia, atrioventricular block, ventricular fibrillation, congestive heart failure, pericarditis, hypotension, syncope, and death. Pulmonary edema is a bona fide potential sequela. Resulting death in humans, which is extremely rare, usually occurs within the first 6 to 8 hours. The wound is indolent and may require months to heal, only to leave a cutaneous granuloma or marked tissue defect, particularly after a secondary infection or deep abscess. Mild pain may persist for days to weeks. After successful therapy, paresthesias or numbness in the affected extremity may persist for a few weeks.

First aid and emergency therapy are identical to those for a stingray envenomation. A stonefish antivenin* is manufactured by the Commonwealth Serum Laboratories, Melbourne, Australia. In cases of severe systemic reactions from stings of *Synanceja* species, and rarely from other scorpion fish, it is administered IV. The antivenin is supplied in ampules containing 2 mL (2000 units) of hyperimmune horse serum, with 1 mL capable of neutralizing 10 mg of dried venom. The antivenin should be diluted in 50 to 100 mL of normal saline and administered slowly IV. Although the product may be given IM before dilution, this route is not recommended in serious envenomations, as absorption may be erratic. As a rough estimate, 1 vial should neutralize one or two significant stings (punctures).

OCTOPUSES

Octopuses and cuttlefish are usually harmless and retiring. Octopus bites are rare but can result in severe envenomations. Fatalities have been reported from bites of the Australian blue-ringed (or "spotted") octopuses, *Octopus (Hapalochlaena) maculosus* and *O. (H.) lunulata.* These small creatures, which rarely exceed 20 cm in length with tentacles extended, are found throughout the Indo-Pacific area (Australia, New Zealand, New Guinea, Japan) in rock pools, under discarded objects and shells, and in shallow waters, posing a threat to curious children, tidepool visitors, fossickers, and unwary divers.

The venom apparatus of the octopus consists of the anterior and posterior salivary glands, salivary ducts, buccal mass, and beak. This complex, concealed by the tentacles, is fronted by two parrot-like, powerful and chitinous jaws (beak), which bite and tear with great force at food held by the suckers. The venom, normally released into the water to subdue crabs, may be injected into the victim with great force through the dermis down to the muscle fascia. The toxin contains at least one fraction identical to tetrodotoxin, which blocks peripheral nerve conduction by interfering with sodium conductance in excitable membranes. This paralytic agent rapidly produces neuromuscular blockade, notably of the phrenic nerve supply to the diaphragm, without any apparent direct cardiotoxicity. It has been estimated that enough venom may be present in one full-grown (25-gram) octopus to paralyze 10 adult humans.

Most victims are bitten on the hand or arm as they handle the creature. An octopus bite usually consists of two small puncture wounds produced by the chitinous jaws. The bite goes unnoticed or causes only a small amount of discomfort, described as a minor ache, slight stinging, or pulsating sensation. Occasionally, the site is initially numb, followed in 5 to 10 minutes by discomfort that may spread to involve the entire limb, persisting for up to 6 hours. Local urticarial reactions occur variably, and profuse bleeding at the site is attributed to a local anticoagulant effect. Within 30 minutes, there are considerable erythema, swelling, tenderness, heat, and pruritus. By far the most common local tissue reaction is the absence of symptoms, a small spot of blood, or a tiny blanched area. Within 10 to 15 minutes of the bite, the patient notices oral and facial numbness, rapidly followed by systemic progression. Voluntary and involuntary muscles are involved, and the illness may rapidly progress to total flaccid paralysis and respiratory failure. Other symptoms include perioral and intraoral anesthesia (classically, numbness of the lips and tongue), diplopia, blurred vision, aphonia, dysphagia, ataxia, myoclonus, weakness, a sense of detachment, nausea, vomiting, peripheral neuropathy, flaccid muscular paralysis, and respiratory failure that may lead to death. Ataxia of cerebellar configuration may occur after an envenomation that does not progress to frank paralysis. The victim may collapse from weakness and remain awake, so long as oxygenation can be maintained. When breathing is disturbed, respiratory assistance may allow the victim to remain mentally alert, although paralyzed. Cardiac arrest is probably a complication of the anoxic episode.

Treatment is based on the symptoms and is supportive. Prompt mechanical respiratory assistance has by far the greatest influence on the outcome. First aid at the scene should include the pressure-immobilization technique as described previously for the treatment of box-jellyfish sting. Respiratory failure should be anticipated early, and the rescuer should be prepared to provide artificial ventilation, including endotracheal intubation and the application of a mechanical ventilator. The duration of the intense clinical venom effect is 4 to 10 hours, after

*Not available in the United States.

which the victim who has not suffered an episode of significant hypoxia shows rapid signs of improvement. If there is no period of hypoxia, mentation may remain normal. Complete recovery may require 2 to 4 days. Residua are uncommon and are related to anoxia rather than venom effects.

Management of the bite wound is controversial. Some clinicians recommend wide circular excision of the bite wound down to the deep fascia, with primary closure or immediate full-thickness free skin grafts, whereas others advocate observation and a nonsurgical approach. Because the local tissue reaction is not a significant cause of morbidity, excision is putatively recommended to remove any sequestered venom.

SEA SNAKES

Sea snakes are probably the most abundant reptiles worldwide. The snakes are distributed in the tropical and warm temperate Pacific and Indian oceans, with the highest number of envenomations occurring along the coast of Southeast Asia, in the Persian Gulf, and in the Malay Archipelago.

The well-developed venom apparatus consists of two to four hollow maxillary fangs and a pair of associated venom glands. Fortunately, because the fangs are short and easily dislodged from their sockets, most bites do not result in significant systemic envenomation. The protein venom is quite toxic and includes stable peripheral neurotoxins more potent than those of terrestrial snakes. *Enhydrina schistosa* is considered to be the most dangerous sea snake. *E. schistosa* is the most widely distributed sea snake in the Arabian Sea.

Bites are usually the result of accidental handling of snakes snared in the nets of fishermen, or of wading and accidentally stepping on a snake. Nearly all

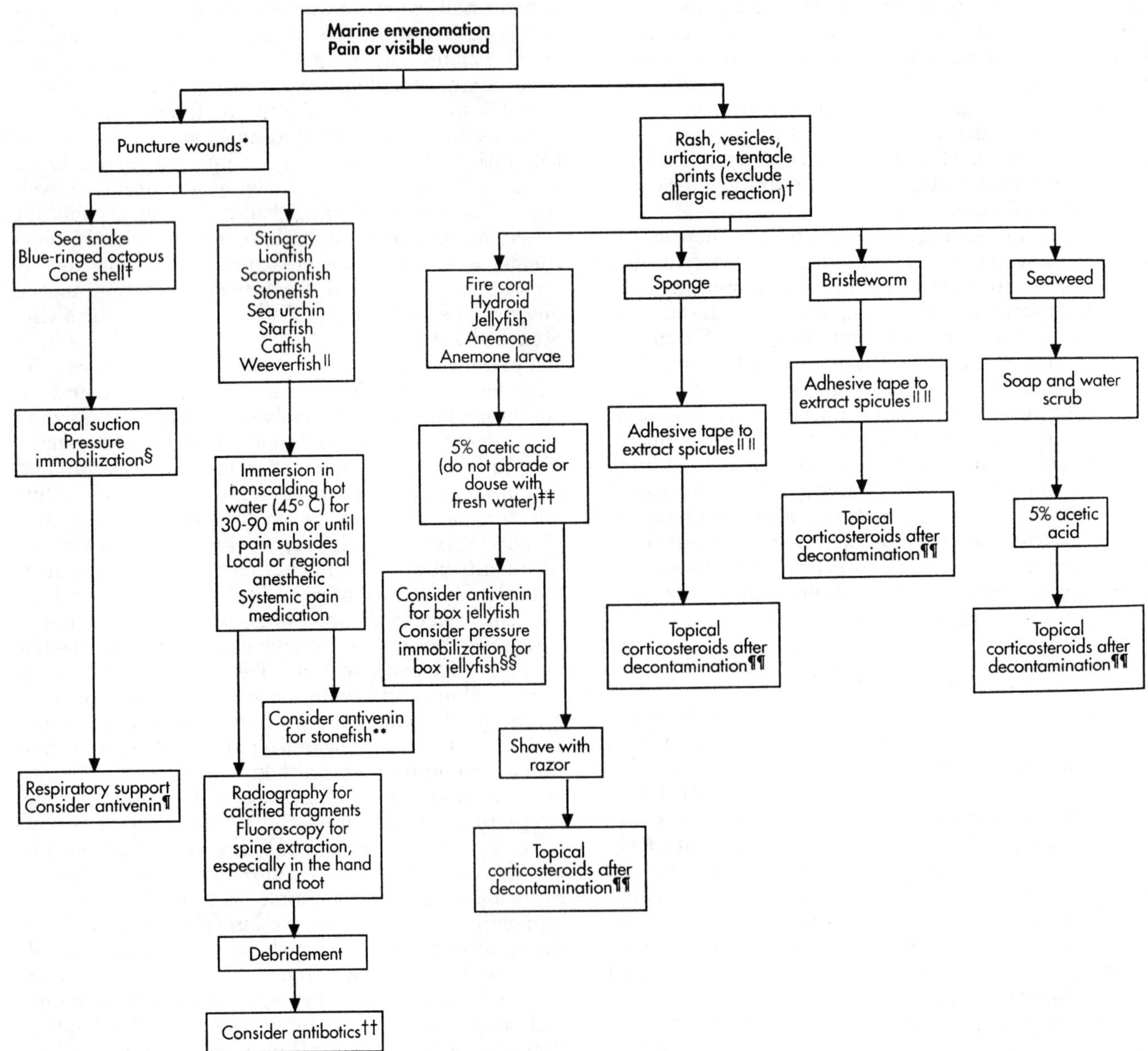

Figure 1 *See legend on opposite page*

bites involve the extremities. Initially, a sea snake bite does not cause great pain and may resemble only a pinprick. Fang marks are characterized by multiple pinhead-sized hypodermic-like puncture wounds, usually 1 to 4, but potentially up to 20. In some cases, particularly if a superficial injury has been perpetrated through the arm or leg of a neoprene wet suit, the fang marks may be difficult to find because of the lack of a localized reaction.

The onset of symptoms can be as rapid as 5 minutes or as long as 8 hours after the bite. Characteristic symptoms include painful muscle movement, lower extremity paralysis, arthralgias, trismus, blurred vision, dysphagia, drowsiness, vomiting, and ptosis. Neurotoxic symptoms are rapid in onset and usually appear within 2 to 3 hours. If symptoms do not develop within 6 to 8 hours, there has been no envenomation.

The first complaint may be one of euphoria, malaise, or anxiety. Over 30 to 60 minutes, classic muscle aching and stiffness (particularly of the bitten extremity and neck muscles) develop, along with a "thick tongue" and sialorrhea, indicative of speech and swallowing dysfunction. Within 3 to 6 hours, moderate to severe pain is noted with passive movements of the neck, trunk, and limbs. Ascending flaccid or spastic paralysis follows shortly, beginning in the lower extremities, and deep tendon reflexes diminish and may disappear after an initial period of spastic hyper-reactivity. Nausea, vomiting, myoclonus, muscle spasm, ophthalmoplegia, ptosis, dilated and poorly reactive pupils, facial paralysis, trismus, and the pulmonary aspiration of gastric contents are frequent manifestations. Occasionally, bilateral painless swelling of the parotid glands develops.

Severe envenomations are marked by progressively intense symptoms within the first two symptom hours. The skin becomes cool and cyanotic; the patient begins to lose vision and may lapse into coma. Failing vision is reported to be a preterminal symptom. If peripheral paralysis predominates, the victim may remain conscious if hypoxia is avoided. Leukocytosis may be significant, with more than 20,000 white blood cells per mm^3; elevated plasma creatine kinase levels are variable. An elevated aspartate aminotransferase level reflects hepatic injury. Pathognomonic myoglobinuria becomes evident about 3 to 6 hours after the bite and may be accompanied by albuminuria and hemoglobinuria. Cerebrospinal fluid is normal. Respiratory distress and bulbar paralysis, pulmonary aspiration–related hypoxia, electrolyte disturbances (predominantly hyperkalemia), and acute renal failure (attributed in part to myonecrosis and pigment load) all contribute to the ultimate demise of the victim, which can occur hours to days after the untreated bite. Preterminal hypertension may occur. The mortality rate is 25% in patients who do not receive antivenin and 3% overall.

The bitten limb should be immobilized and maintained in a dependent position while the victim is

---

Figure 1. Algorithmic approach to marine envenomation.

*A gaping laceration, particularly of the lower extremity, with cyanotic edges suggests a stingray wound. Multiple punctures in an erratic pattern with or without purple discoloration or retained fragments are typical of a sea urchin sting. One to eight (usually two) fang marks are usually present after a sea snake bite. A single ischemic puncture wound with an erythematous halo and rapid swelling suggests scorpion fish envenomation. Blisters often accompany a lionfish sting. Painless punctures with paralysis suggest the bite of a blue-ringed octopus; the site of a cone shell sting is punctate, painful, and ischemic in appearance.

†Wheal and flare reactions are nonspecific. Rapid (within 24 hours) onset of skin necrosis suggests an anemone sting. "Tentacle prints" with cross-hatching or a frosted appearance are pathognomonic for box jellyfish *(Chironex fleckeri)* envenomation. Ocular or intraoral lesions may be caused by fragmented hydroids or coelenterate tentacles. An allergic reaction must be treated promptly.

‡Sea snake venom causes weakness, respiratory paralysis, myoglobinuria, myalgias, blurred vision, vomiting, and dysphagia. The blue-ringed octopus injects tetrodotoxin, which causes rapid neuromuscular paralysis.

§If *immediately* available (which is rarely the case), local suction can be applied without incision using a plunger device, such as The Extractor (Sawyer Products, Safety Harbor, FL). As soon as possible, venom should be sequestered locally with a proximal venous-lymphatic occlusive band of constriction or (preferably) the pressure-immobilization technique, in which a cloth pad is compressed directly over the wound by an elastic wrap that should encompass the entire extremity at a pressure of 9.33 kPa (70 mm Hg) or less. A splint is then applied. Incision and suction are not recommended.

¶Early ventilatory support has the greatest influence on outcome. The minimal initial dose of sea snake antivenin is 1 to 3 vials; up to 10 vials may be required.

‖The wounds range from large lacerations (stingrays) to minute punctures (stonefish). Persistent pain after immersion in hot water suggests a stonefish sting or a retained fragment of spine. The puncture site can be identified by forcefully injecting 1 to 2% lidocaine or another local anesthetic agent without epinephrine near the wound and observing the egress of fluid. Do not attempt to crush the spines of sea urchins if they are present in the wound. Spine dye from already-extracted sea urchin spines disappears (is absorbed) in 24 to 36 hours.

**The initial dose of stonefish antivenin is 1 vial per two puncture wounds.

††The antibiotics chosen should cover *Staphylococcus, Streptococcus,* and microbes of marine origin, such as *Vibrio.*

‡‡Acetic acid 5% (vinegar) is a good all-purpose decontaminant and is mandated for the sting from a box jellyfish. Alternatives, depending on the geographic region and indigenous jellyfish species, include isopropyl alcohol, papain, bicarbonate (baking soda), ammonia, and preparations containing these agents.

§§The initial dose of box jellyfish antivenin is 1 ampule intravenously or 3 ampules intramuscularly.

¶¶If inflammation is severe, steroids should be given systemically (beginning with at least 60 to 100 mg of prednisone or its equivalent) and the dose tapered over a period of 10 to 14 days.

‖‖An alternative is to apply and remove a thin layer of rubber cement or commercial facial peel materials followed by topical soaks of 30 mL of 5% acetic acid (vinegar) diluted in 1 liter of water for 15 to 30 minutes several times a day until the lesions begin to resolve. Anticipate surface desquamation in 3 to 6 weeks.

(Adapted from Auerbach PS [ed]: Wilderness Medicine: Management of Wilderness and Environmental Emergencies, 3rd ed. St Louis, Mosby–Year Book, 1995, pp 1368–1369.)

kept as quiet as possible. The pressure-immobilization technique for venom sequestration described previously for box-jellyfish sting should be applied.

Incision and suction therapy for snakebite is highly controversial and rarely recommended. It should be employed only under the following conditions:

- if a mechanical suction extractor device is not available
- if the victim is seen within 5 minutes of the bite
- if the victim is elderly, chronically ill, or less than 32 kg in body weight
- if the snake is positively identified as venomous
- if clear puncture marks are seen
- if the pressure-immobilization technique cannot be employed
- if antivenin will be unavailable for 2 hours

Two longitudinal parallel incisions should be made directly through the fang marks for a length of 5 mm to a depth of 5 to 10 mm. Cruciate incisions are improper. Suction is better applied with a rubber suction cup or commercial plunger–type venom extraction device; the mouth should be used only as a last resort, as the introduction of oral cavity flora into the wound creates a contaminated human bite situation. Suction should be applied continuously for 30 to 60 minutes. A rescuer with denuded intraoral mucous membranes should take care to rapidly spit out the mixture of blood and venom. There is little clinical enthusiasm for the perpetuation of incision and suction therapy, which may soon be relegated to therapeutic history.

With any evidence of envenomation, polyvalent sea snake antivenin* should be administered after appropriate skin testing for equine serum hypersensitivity. If this is not available, tiger snake antivenin* should be used. The administration of antivenin should begin as soon as possible and is most effective if initiated within 8 hours of the bite. The minimal effective adult dose is 1 ampule (1000 units), which neutralizes 10 mg of *E. schistosa* venom. Depending on the severity of the envenomation, 3000 to 10,000 units (3 to 10 ampules) may be required. The proper administration of antivenin is clearly described on the antivenin package insert.

Sea snake envenomation may induce severe physiologic derangements that require intensive medical management. Urine output and measured renal function should be closely monitored, as hemolysis and rhabdomyolysis release hemoglobin and myoglobin pigments into the circulation, which precipitates acute renal failure. If hemoglobinuria or myoglobinuria are detected, the urine should be alkalized with sodium bicarbonate and diuresis promoted with a loop diuretic (furosemide) and/or mannitol. Acute renal failure may necessitate a period of peritoneal dialysis or hemodialysis. Hemodialysis offers an alternative therapy that may be successful if antivenin is not available.

Respiratory failure should be anticipated as paralysis overwhelms the victim. Endotracheal intubation and mechanical ventilation may be required until antivenin adequately neutralizes the venom effects. Serum electrolyte levels should be measured regularly to guide the administration of fluids and electrolyte supplements. Hyperkalemia related to rhabdomyolysis and renal dysfunction must be promptly recognized and treated.

If there is no early evidence of envenomation, the victim should be observed for 8 hours before discharge from the hospital.

*Not available in the United States.

SUMMARY

An algorithmic approach to marine envenomation can be taken when the causative agent cannot be positively identified, as summarized in Figure 1.

ACUTE POISONINGS

method of

HOWARD C. MOFENSON, M.D.,
THOMAS R. CARACCIO, PHARM.D., and
JOSEPH GREENSHER, M.D.
Long Island Regional Poison Control Center
Mineola, New York

COMMON ABBREVIATIONS

ABG	=	arterial blood gas
AC	=	activated charcoal
ALT	=	alanine aminotransferase
AST	=	aspartate aminotransferase
AV	=	atrioventricular
BDP	=	benzodiazepine
BUN	=	blood urea nitrogen
CDC	=	Centers for Disease Control and Prevention
CK	=	creatine kinase
CNS	=	central nervous system
ECG	=	electrocardiogram
EEG	=	electroencephalogram
FDA	=	Food and Drug Administration
GABA	=	γ-aminobutyric acid
GI	=	gastrointestinal
G6PD	=	glucose-6-phosphate dehydrogenase
HIV	=	human immunodeficiency virus
ICU	=	intensive care unit
MAOI	=	monoamine oxidase inhibitor
MDAC	=	multiple-dose activated charcoal
NAC	=	*N*-acetylcysteine
NIOSH	=	National Institute for Occupational Safety and Health
OSHA	=	Occupational Safety and Health Administration
$Paco_2$	=	arterial carbon dioxide tension
Pao_2	=	arterial oxygen tension
PEEP	=	positive end-expiratory pressure
PEG	=	polyethylene glycol
pK_a	=	negative logarithm of dissociation constant

PTZ = phenothiazine
SG = specific gravity
$t_{1/2}$ = half-life
Vd = volume of distribution
WBC = white blood cell

MEDICAL TOXICOLOGY (INGESTIONS, INHALATIONS, DERMAL AND OCULAR ABSORPTIONS)

Epidemiology

An estimated 5 million potentially toxic exposures occur each year in the United States. Poisoning is responsible for almost 12,000 deaths (including those caused by carbon monoxide) and more than 200,000 hospitalizations.

Poisoning accounts for 2 to 5% of pediatric hospital admissions, 10% of adult admissions, 5% of hospital admissions in the elderly population (older than 65 years), and 5% of ambulance calls. In one urban hospital, drug-related emergencies accounted for 38% of the emergency department visits. One evaluation of a medical intensive care unit (ICU) and step-down unit in a 3-month period indicated that 19.7% of admissions were for poisonings.

The largest number of fatalities resulting from poisoning are caused by carbon monoxide (CO). Most occur before arrival at the hospital. The mortality resulting from CO poisoning decreased from 600 deaths in 1989 to 500 in 1991. The other principal toxicologic fatalities in 1997 were due to analgesics, antidepressants, sedative hypnotics and antipsychotics, stimulants and street drugs, alcohols, cardiovascular drugs, and chemicals. Less than 1% of overdose cases reaching the hospitals result in fatality. However, patients presenting in a deep coma to medical care facilities have a fatality rate of 13 to 35%. The largest single factor in coma of inapparent cause is drug poisoning.

Pharmaceutical preparations are involved in 40% of poisonings. The number one pharmaceutical toxic exposure is to acetaminophen. The leading pharmaceuticals causing fatalities in 1994 were the analgesics, antidepressants, sedative hypnotics or antipsychotic drugs, stimulants and street drugs, cardiovascular agents, and alcohols.

The severity of the manifestations of acute poisoning exposures varies greatly with the intent of the victim.

Nonintentional (accidental poisoning) exposures make up 60 to 65% of all poisoning exposures. The majority are acute, occur in children younger than 5 years, occur in the home, and result in no or minor toxicity. Many are ingestions of relatively nontoxic substances that require minimal medical care.

Intentional (suicidal poisoning) exposures constitute 10 to 15% of exposures and may require the highest standards of medical and nursing care and the use of sophisticated equipment for recovery. Intentional ingestions are often of multiple substances and frequently include ethanol, acetaminophen, and aspirin. Suicides make up 60 to 90% of reported poisoning fatalities. About 25% of suicides are attempted with drugs. Sixty percent of patients who take a drug overdose use their own medication, and 15% use drugs prescribed for close relatives. The majority of drug-related suicide attempts involve a central nervous system (CNS) depressant, and coma management is vital to the treatment.

ASSESSMENT AND MAINTENANCE OF VITAL FUNCTIONS

The initial assessment of all medical emergencies follows the principles of basic and advanced cardiac life support. The adequacy of the patient's airway, degree of ventilation, and circulatory status should be determined. The vital functions should be established and maintained. Vital signs should be measured frequently and should include body core temperature. Evaluation of vital functions should include not only rate numbers but also effective function (e.g., respiratory rate and depth and air exchange) (Table 1).

The level of consciousness should be assessed by immediate AVPU signs (alert, responds to verbal stimuli, responds to painful stimuli, and unconscious). If the patient is unconscious, the severity is assessed by the Reed classification (Table 2) or the Glasgow Coma Scale (Table 3).

If the patient is comatose, management requires administering 100% oxygen, establishing vascular access, obtaining blood for pertinent laboratory studies, and administering glucose, thiamine, and naloxone (Narcan); intubation to protect the airway should also be considered. Pertinent laboratory studies include arterial blood gases (ABGs), electrocardiography, determination of glucose and electrolyte concentrations, renal and liver tests, and for all intentional ingestions determination of the acetaminophen plasma concentration (APC). Radiography of the chest and abdomen may be useful.

The severity of a stimulant's effects can also be assessed (Table 4). The assessment should be recorded to follow the trend.

Exposure: Completely expose the patient by removing clothes and other items that interfere with a full evaluation. Look for clues to etiology in the clothes, including the hat and shoes.

Prevention of Toxin Absorption and Reduction of Local Damage

Routes

Poisoning exposure routes include ingestion (80%), dermal (7%), ophthalmic (5%), inhalation (5%), insect bites and stings (2.7%), and parenteral injections (0.3%). The effect of the toxin may be local, systemic, or both.

Local effects (skin, eyes, mucosa of respiratory or gastrointestinal [GI] tract) occur in areas of contact with the poisonous substance. Local effects are nonspecific chemical reactions that depend on the chemi-

TABLE 1. **Important Measurements and Vital Signs**

Age	BSA (m^2)	Weight (kg)	Height (cm)	Pulse (bpm), Resting	Blood Pressure (mm Hg) *Hypotension*	*Hypertension* SIGNIFICANT	*Hypertension* SEVERE	RR (rpm)
NB	0.19	3.5	50	70–190	<40/60	>96	>106	30–60
1–6 mo	0.30	4–7	50–65	80–160	<45/70	>104	>110	30–50
6 mo–1 y	0.38	7–10	65–75	80–160	<45/70	>104	>110	20–40
1–2 y	0.50–0.55	10–12	75–85	80–140	<47/74	>74/112	>82/118	20–40
3–5 y	0.54–0.68	15–20	90–108	80–120	<52/80	>76/116	>84/124	20–40
6–9 y	0.68–0.85	20–28	122–133	75–115	<60/90	>82/122	>86/130	16–25
10–12 y	1.00–1.07	30–40	138–147	70–110	<60/90	>82/126	>90/134	16–25
13–15 y	1.07–1.22	42–50	152–160	60–100	<60/90	>86/136	>92/144	16–20
16–18 y	1.30–1.60	53–60	160–170	60–100	<60/90	>92/142	>98/150	12–16
Adult	1.40–1.70	60–70	160–170	60–100	<60/90	>90/140	>120/210	10–16

Abbreviations: bpm = beats per minute; BSA = body surface area; NB = newborn; rpm = respirations per minute; RR = respiratory rate.
Data from Nadas A: Pediatric Cardiology, 3rd ed. Philadelphia, WB Saunders Co, 1976; Blumer JL (ed): A Practice Guide to Pediatric Intensive Care. St Louis: CV Mosby, 1990; AAP and ACEP Respiratory Distress in APLS Pediatric Emergency Medicine Course, 1993, p 5; Second Task Force on blood pressure control in children—1987. Pediatrics *79*:1, 1987; and Linakis JG: Hypertension. *In* Fliesher GR, Ludwig S (eds): Textbook of Pediatric Emergency Medicine, 3rd ed. Baltimore, Williams & Wilkins, 1993, p 249.

cal properties (e.g., pH), concentration, contact time, and type of exposed surface.

Systemic effects occur when the poison is absorbed into the body and depend on the dose, the distribution, and the functional reserve of the organ systems. Complications resulting from shock, hypoxia, chronic exposure, and existing illness may also influence systemic toxicity.

Delayed Toxic Action

Most pharmaceuticals are absorbed within 90 minutes. However, the patient with exposure to a potential toxin may be asymptomatic at the time of presentation for several reasons: the substance may be nontoxic, an insufficient amount of the toxin may have been involved, or a sufficient amount may not yet have been absorbed or metabolized to produce toxicity.

Absorption may be significantly delayed for several reasons:

- A drug with anticholinergic properties is involved (e.g., antihistamines, belladonna alkaloids, diphenoxylate with atropine [Lomotil], phenothiazines [PTZs], cyclic antidepressants).
- Sustained-release and enteric-coated preparations, which have delayed and prolonged absorption, are involved.
- Concretions may form (e.g., with ingestions of salicylates, iron, glutethimide, or meprobamate) that can delay absorption and prolong the action.

Substances must be metabolized to a toxic metabolite or time is required to produce a toxic effect on the organ system (e.g., acetaminophen, *Amanita phalloides* mushrooms, acetonitrile, carbon tetrachloride, colchicine, digoxin, ethylene glycol, heavy metals, methanol, methylene chloride, monoamine oxidase inhibitors [MAOIs], oral hypoglycemic agents, parathion, paraquat).

Decontamination

Decontamination procedures should be considered for an asymptomatic patient if the exposure involves potentially toxic substances in toxic amounts.

Ocular exposure should be treated immediately

TABLE 2. **Classification of the Level of Consciousness**

Stage	Status	Conscious Level	Pain Response	Reflexes	Respiration	Circulation
0	Lethargic, able to answer questions and follow commands	Asleep	Arousable	Intact	Normal	Normal
I	Responsive to pain, brain stem and deep tendon reflexes intact	Comatose	Withdraws	Intact	Normal	Normal
II	Unresponsive to pain	Comatose	None	Intact	Normal	Normal
III	Unresponsive to pain, most reflexes absent, respiratory depression	Comatose	None	Absent	Depressed	Normal
IV	Unresponsive to pain, all reflexes absent, cardiovascular and respiratory depression	Comatose	None	Absent	Cyanosis	Shock

Modified from Reed CE, Driggs MF, Foote CC: Acute barbiturate intoxication: A study of 300 cases based on a physiologic system of classification of the severity of the intoxication. Ann Intern Med *37*:290, 1952.

TABLE 3. **Glasgow Coma Scale**

Scale	Adult Response	Score	Pediatric Response (0–1 y)*
Eye opening	Spontaneous	4	Spontaneous
	To verbal command	3	To shout
	To pain	2	To pain
	None	1	No response
Motor response			
To verbal command	Obeys	6	
To painful stimuli	Localized pain	5	Localized pain
	Flexion withdrawal	4	Flexion withdrawal
	Decorticate flexion	3	Decorticate flexion
	Decerebrate extension	2	Decerebrate extension
	None	1	None
Verbal response, adult	Oriented and converses	5	Cries, smiles, coos
	Disoriented but converses	4	Cries or screams
	Inappropriate words	3	Inappropriate sounds
	Incomprehensible sounds	2	Grunts
	None	1	Gives no response
Verbal response, child	Oriented	5	
	Words or babbles	4	
	Vocal sounds	3	
	Cries or moans to stimuli	2	
	None	1	

*From Seidel J: Preparing for pediatric emergencies. Pediatr Rev *16*:466–472, 1995.

Modified from Teasdale G, Jennett B: Assessment of coma and impaired consciousness. Lancet *2*:81–84, 1974; and Simpson D, Reilly P: Pediatric coma scale. Lancet *2*:450, 1982.

with water or saline irrigation for 15 to 20 minutes with the eyelids fully retracted. The use of neutralizing chemicals is contraindicated. All caustic and corrosive injuries should be evaluated with examination after instillation of fluorescein dye and by an ophthalmologist.

Dermal exposure is treated immediately with copious irrigation (not forceful flushing) for 30 minutes. Shampooing the hair; cleansing fingernails, navel, and perineum; and irrigating the eyes are necessary in an extensive exposure. The clothes should be specially bagged and may have to be discarded. Leather goods can be irreversibly contaminated and must be abandoned. Caustic (alkali) exposures can require hours of irrigation. Dermal absorption can occur with, for example, pesticides, hydrocarbons, and cyanide.

Injection exposures to drugs and toxins can involve envenomation. Cold packs and tourniquets should not be used, and incision is generally not recommended. Venom extractors may be used within minutes of envenomation, and proximal lymphatic constricting bands or elastic wraps may be used to delay lymphatic flow and immobilize the extremity.

TABLE 4. **Classification of Severity of Effects of Stimulants**

Severity	Manifestations
Grade 1	Diaphoresis, hyper-reflexia, irritability, mydriasis, tremors
Grade 2	Confusion, fever, hyperactivity, hypertension, tachycardia, tachypnea
Grade 3	Delirium, mania, hyperpyrexia, tachydysrhythmia
Grade 4	Coma, convulsions, cardiovascular collapse

Modified with permission from Espelin DE, Done AK: Amphetamine poisoning. Effectiveness of chlorpromazine. N Engl J Med *278*:1361–1365, 1968.

Inhalation exposure to toxic substances is managed by immediately removing the victim from the contaminated environment, by protected rescuers if necessary.

GI exposure is the most common route of poisoning. GI decontamination may be done by gastric emptying (induction of emesis, gastric lavage), adsorption by administering single or multiple doses of activated charcoal (AC), or whole-bowel irrigation. No procedure is routine; the procedure should be individualized on the basis of the patient's age, properties of the substance ingested, and time since the ingestion. If no attempt is made to decontaminate the patient, the reason should be clearly documented on the medical record (e.g., time elapsed, past peak of action, ineffectiveness, or risk of procedure).

Gastric Emptying Procedures. The procedure used is influenced by the patient's age and the procedure's effectiveness (the size of the orogastric tube used in a small child may not be large enough for adequate lavage, e.g., with iron tablets), time of ingestion (gastric emptying is usually ineffective more than 1 hour after ingestion), clinical status (asymptomatic time of peak effect has elapsed or the patient's condition is too unstable), formulation of substance ingested (regular release, sustained release, enteric coated), amount ingested, caustic action, and rapidity of onset of CNS depression or stimulation (convulsions). Most studies show that only 30% (19 to 62%) of ingested toxins are removed by gastric emptying under optimal conditions. It has not been demonstrated that the procedure improved the outcome.

A mnemonic for gathering information is SATS: substance, amount and age, time of ingestion, and symptoms.

The clinician should attempt to obtain ample information about the patient. A mnemonic for this is AMPLE: A for age and allergies; M for available medications; P for past medical history including pregnancy or psychiatric illnesses, substance abuse, or intentional ingestions; L for time of last meal, which may influence absorption and the onset and peak action; and E for events leading to the present condition. The intent should be determined.

The regional poison control center should be consulted for the exact ingredients and the latest management. The first-aid information on the labels of products is notoriously inaccurate, and product ingredients change.

Syrup of Ipecac–Induced Emesis. This is most useful for young children with a recent witnessed ingestion of a known agent. To be effective, vomiting should be induced immediately at the site (in the home). The poison control center should be called before emesis is induced.

Contraindications or situations in which induction of emesis is inappropriate include the following:

- Caustic ingestions
- Loss of airway protective reflexes—this can occur with substances that can produce rapid onset of CNS depression (e.g., ethanol, short-acting [SA] benzodiazepines [BZPs], SA barbiturates, SA nonbarbiturate sedative hypnotics, SA opioids, tricyclic antidepressants) or convulsions (e.g., beta blockers, camphor, calcium channel blockers, chloroquine, codeine, isoniazid, mefenamic acid, nicotine, propoxyphene, phencyclidine, organophosphate insecticides, strychnine, cyclic antidepressants)
- Ingestion of high-viscosity petroleum distillates (e.g., gasoline, lighter fluid, kerosene)
- Significant vomiting before presentation, or hematemesis
- Age younger than 6 months (no established dose, safety, or efficacy)
- Foreign bodies (emesis is ineffective and may lead to aspiration)
- Clinical conditions: pregnancy, neurologic impairment, hemodynamic instability, increased intracranial pressure, and hypertension
- Delay in presentation (more than 1 hour after ingestion)

The presence of factors such as oral injury may interfere with administration of AC or oral antidotes. The patient cannot tolerate oral intake for a mean of 2 to 3 hours after ipecac-induced emesis.

The dose of syrup of ipecac (SI) for the 6- to 9-month-old infant is 5 mL; for the 9- to 12-month-old, 10 mL; and for the 1- to 12-year-old, 15 mL. For children older than 12 years and adults, the dose is 30 mL. The dose may be repeated once if the child does not vomit in 15 to 20 minutes. The vomitus should be inspected for remnants of pills or toxic substances, and the appearance and odor should be documented. When SI is not available, 30 mL of mild dishwashing soap (not electric dishwasher detergent) may be used, although it is less effective.

Complications are rare but include aspiration, protracted vomiting, rarely cardiac toxicity with long-term abuse, pneumothorax, gastric rupture, diaphragmatic hernia, intracranial hemorrhage, and Mallory-Weiss tears.

Gastric Aspiration and Lavage. The contraindications are similar to those for ipecac-induced emesis. The procedure can be accomplished after the insertion of an endotracheal tube in CNS depression or controlled convulsions. The patient should be placed with the head lower than the hips in a left lateral decubitus position. The location of the tube should be confirmed by radiography, if necessary, and suctioning should be available.

Contraindications to gastric aspiration and lavage include the following:

- Caustic ingestions (risk of esophageal perforation)
- Uncontrolled convulsions, because of the danger of aspiration and injury during the procedure
- High-viscosity petroleum distillate products
- CNS depression or absent protective airway reflexes, which require insertion of an endotracheal tube to protect against aspiration
- Significant cardiac dysrhythmias, which should be controlled
- Significant emesis before presentation or hematemesis
- Delay in presentation (more than 1 hour after ingestion)

The best results with gastric aspiration and lavage are obtained with the largest possible orogastric tube that can reasonably be passed (nasogastric tubes are not large enough except for liquid ingestions). For adults, a large-bore orogastric Lavacuator hose or a No. 42 French Ewald tube is used. For children, a No. 22 to No. 28 French orogastric-type tube is used, but this is usually ineffective with solid ingestions (e.g., iron tablets).

The amount of fluid used for lavage varies with the patient's age and size. In general, aliquots of 50 to 100 mL per lavage are used for adults and 5 mL per kg up to 50 to 100 mL per lavage for children. Larger amounts of fluid may force the toxin past the pylorus. Many physicians add AC after the initial aspiration as a marker and many instill AC before removing the tube. Lavage fluid is 0.89% saline.

Complications are rare and may include respiratory depression, aspiration pneumonitis, cardiac dysrhythmias caused by increased vagal tone (e.g., with ingestions of beta-adrenergic blockers, calcium channel blockers, or digoxin overdoses), esophageal-gastric tears and perforation, electrolyte imbalance in young children, laryngospasm, and mediastinitis.

Activated Charcoal. Oral AC adsorbs the toxin onto its surface before GI absorption and interrupts enterogastric and enterohepatic circulation of toxic metabolites. AC is a stool marker, indicating that the toxin has passed through the GI tract.

AC does not effectively adsorb small molecules or molecules lacking carbon, as listed in Table 5. AC adsorption may be diminished by the concurrent presence in the stomach of ethanol, milk, cocoa powder, or ice cream.

There are a few relative contraindications to the use of AC:

- It should not be given before, concomitantly with, or shortly after oral antidotes unless it has been proved not to interfere significantly with their effectiveness. It does not interfere with the effectiveness of *N*-acetylcysteine (NAC) in acetaminophen overdose (although there is up to a 39% reduction in NAC), and it may contribute to vomiting.
- It does not effectively adsorb caustics and corrosives, may produce vomiting or cling to the mucosa, and may falsely appear as a burn at endoscopy.
- It should not be given if the patient is comatose without securing the airway.
- It should not be given if there are no bowel sounds (may form concretions or perforation).

The dose of AC is 1 gram per kg per dose orally (PO), with a minimum of 15 grams. Optimal dosage has not been established. Ideal therapy allegedly requires a 10:1 ratio of AC to toxin. The usual initial adult dose is 60 to 100 grams and the dose for children is 15 to 30 grams. It is administered PO as a slurry mixed with water or by nasogastric or orogastric tube. Caution: The clinician must be sure the tube is in the stomach. AC is usually administered initially with a cathartic in adults. Cathartics are not necessary in children.

MULTIPLE-DOSE ACTIVATED CHARCOAL. Repeated dosing with AC decreases the half-life and increases the clearance of phenobarbital, dapsone, salicylate, quinidine, theophylline, and carbamazepine. With multiple-dose AC (MDAC), subsequent cathartics should be given every 24 hours, not with each dose. No controlled studies have demonstrated that the use of MDAC or cathartics alters the clinical course of an intoxication. The MDAC dose varies from 0.25 to 0.50 gram per kg every 1 to 4 hours, and continuous nasogastric tube infusion of 0.25 to 0.5 gram per kg per hour has been used to decrease vomiting.

TABLE 5. **Substances Poorly Adsorbed by Activated Charcoal**

C—Caustics and corrosives, cyanide*
H—Heavy metals (arsenic, iron, lead, lithium, mercury)
A—Alcohols (ethanol, methanol, isopropyl) and glycols (ethylene glycol)
R—Rapid onset or absorption of cyanide and strychnine
C—Chlorine and iodine
O—Others insoluble in water (substances in tablet form)
A—Aliphatic and poorly absorbed hydrocarbons (petroleum distillates)
L—Laxatives, sodium, magnesium, potassium

*If cyanide is ingested, AC is given in large doses; 1 gm of AC adsorbs 35 mg of cyanide.

GI dialysis involves the diffusion of the toxin from the higher concentration in the serum of the mesenteric vessels to the lower levels in the GI tract mucosal cells and subsequently into the GI lumen, where the concentration has been lowered by adsorption by the intraluminal AC.

Complications of AC have been reported in at least a dozen cases. There are many cases of unreported pulmonary aspiration and "charcoal" lung, intestinal obstruction (three cases reported), empyema after esophageal perforation, and hypermagnesemia and hypernatremia, which have been associated with repeated concurrent doses of AC and saline cathartics.

Catharsis. Cathartics are used to hasten the elimination of any remaining toxin in the GI tract. No studies have demonstrated the effectiveness of a cathartic used alone. AC and cathartic have been shown to be more effective than AC alone in managing slow-release theophylline overdose. However, a cathartic with AC was less effective than AC alone in salicylate poisoning. A study using AC alone and magnesium citrate indicated no benefit when the cathartic was administered.

Cathartics are relatively contraindicated in the following circumstances:

- Ileus as indicated by absence of bowel sounds
- Intestinal obstruction or evidence of intestinal perforation
- Cases with pre-existing electrolyte disturbances
- Magnesium salts contraindicated in renal impairment
- Sodium salts in heart failure or diseases requiring sodium restriction

Magnesium sulfate or sodium sulfate is administered in doses of 250 mg per kg per dose as 20% solutions. The adult dose is 30 grams. Sorbitol is given at 2.8 mL per kg to a maximum of 200 mL of a 70% solution in adults. Sorbitol should not be used for children. It is best to avoid cathartics for pediatric patients because hyponatremia, hypocalcemia, hyperphosphatemia, and death have occurred.

Whole-Bowel Irrigation. In whole-bowel irrigation, bowel-cleansing solutions of polyethylene glycol (PEG) with balanced electrolytes are used to avoid changes in body weight or electrolytes.

Indications (not approved by the Food and Drug Administration [FDA]): Whole-bowel irrigation may be indicated with ingestions of substances that are poorly adsorbed by AC, such as iron and other heavy metals, lithium, and sustained-release preparations. The procedure has been studied and used successfully in iron overdose when abdominal radiographs revealed incomplete emptying of excess iron. There are additional implications in other ingestions, as in body packing of illicit drugs (e.g., cocaine, heroin). The procedure is to administer, PO or by nasogastric tube, the solution (GoLYTELY or Colyte), at 0.5 liter per hour in children younger than 5 years or 2 liters per hour in adolescents and adults for 5 hours. The end point is reached when the rectal effluent is clear or radiopaque materials can no longer be seen in the GI tract on abdominal radiographs.

Contraindications: These measures should not be used if extensive hematemesis, ileus, or signs of bowel obstruction, perforation, or peritonitis are present.

Animal experiments in which PEG was added to AC indicated that AC-salicylate and AC-theophylline combinations resulted in decreased adsorption and desorption of salicylate and theophylline and no therapeutic benefit over that obtained with AC alone. Polyethylene solutions are bound by AC in vitro, which decreases the efficacy of AC.

Dilution. Dilutional treatment is indicated for the immediate management of caustic and corrosive poisonings but is otherwise not useful. Administration of large quantities of diluting fluid—above 30 mL in children and 250 mL in adults—may produce vomiting, re-exposing the vital tissues to the effects of local damage, and possible aspiration.

Neutralization. Neutralization has not been proved to be safe or effective.

Endoscopy and Surgery. Surgery has been required in the management of body packer's obstruction, intestinal ischemia produced by cocaine ingestion, and local caustic action of iron.

Common Toxicologic Presentations

Table 6 shows the common clinical presentations in poisoning and the toxic agents and the underlying medical conditions most frequently involved. A mnemonic for miosis (as the presenting manifestation) is VCPOOP: valproic acid, clonidine, phencyclidine, organophosphates, opioids, phenothiazines. A mnemonic for mydriasis is SHAW: sympathomimetic, hallucinogens, anticholinergic, withdrawal.

Differential Diagnosis Based on Central Nervous System Manifestations of Poisoning

Neurologic parameters help in classifying and assessing the need for supportive treatment and provide diagnostic clues to the etiology. See Tables 7 through 10.

Guidelines for In-Hospital Disposition

Classification of the patient as being at high risk depends on clinical judgment. Any patient with the need for cardiorespiratory support or persistent altered mental status for 3 hours or more should be considered for intensive care.

Guidelines for admitting patients older than 14 years to an ICU, after 2 to 3 hours in the emergency department, include the following:

- Need for intubation
- Seizures
- Unresponsiveness to verbal stimuli
- Arterial carbon dioxide partial pressure ($Pa{CO_2}$) greater than 45 mm Hg
- Cardiac conduction or rhythm disturbances (any rhythm except sinus arrhythmia)
- Close monitoring of vital signs during antidotal therapy or elimination procedures
- Need for continuous monitoring
- QRS complex greater than 0.10 second in tricyclic antidepressant poisoning
- Systolic blood pressure less than 80 mm Hg
- Grade 3 or 4 stimulation or depression (see Tables 2, 3, and 4)
- Hypoxia, hypercapnia, acid-base disturbance, metabolic abnormalities
- Extremes of body temperature
- Progressive deterioration or significant underlying medical disorders

Use of Antidotes

Antidotes are available for only a relatively small number of poisons. An available antidote should be administered only after the integrity of vital functions has been established. Table 11 lists the toxins for which antidotes are available. Table 12 summarizes the commonly used antidotes, their indications, and methods of administration. The regional poison control center should be consulted for further information on these antidotes.

Enhancement of Elimination

The medical methods for elimination of absorbed toxic substances are diuresis, dialysis, hemoperfusion, exchange transfusion, plasmapheresis, enzyme induction, and inhibition. Methods of increasing urinary excretion of toxic chemicals and drugs have been studied extensively, but the other modalities have not been well evaluated.

In general, these methods are needed in only a minority of instances and should be reserved for life-threatening circumstances or when a definite benefit is anticipated.

Diuresis

Diuresis increases the renal clearance of compounds that are eliminated primarily by the renal route, are significantly reabsorbed in the renal tubules, and have a small volume of distribution (Vd) and low protein binding (PB). The risks of diuresis are fluid overload, with cerebral and pulmonary edema, and disturbances in acid-base and electrolyte balances. Failure to produce diuresis may imply renal failure. At present, the only effective diuresis used in the management of the poisoned patient is alkaline diuresis. Diuretics have been administered to maintain the diuresis.

Although acid diuresis may enhance the elimination of weak bases (e.g., amphetamines, fenfluramine [Pondimin], quinidine, phencyclidine, strychnine), it is not recommended because of adverse effects of metabolic acidosis with rhabdomyolysis (e.g., precipi-

TABLE 6. **Common Clinical Presentations and Etiologic Factors in Poisoning**

Clinical Presentation	Toxic Agents	Medical Diseases
Acidosis, metabolic	Alcohols and glycols Cyanide Iron Isoniazid Metformin Salicylates Toluene	Diabetes mellitus Convulsions GI losses Inborn errors of metabolism Lactic acidosis Shock Starvation Renal tubular acidosis Uremia
Bradycardia	Beta-adrenergic blockers Calcium channel blockers Central alpha agonists Cholinergic agents CNS depressants Digitalis (acute) Lithium Opioids Organophosphate insecticides Phenylpropanolamine (reflex) Quinidine Tricyclic or cyclic antidepressants	Increased ICP Structural heart lesions Conduction defects Hypothermia Sleep Athletes at rest Jaundice Stokes-Adams syndrome Carotid sinus syndrome Hypothyroidism
Bradypnea, hypoventilation, apnea	Botulism Cholinergic drugs Clonidine CNS depressants Colchicine Elapidae envenomation (coral snake, cobra) Ethanol Neuromuscular blockers Nicotine Organophosphate insecticides Paralytic agents (in shellfish, tetrodotoxin) Paralytic plants (poison hemlock) Sedative hypnotics Ticks	Vascular CNS disorders Neuromuscular disorders Guillain-Barré syndrome Myasthenia gravis Poliomyelitis Amyotrophic lateral sclerosis Muscle disorders Muscular dystrophy Polymyositis, dermatomyositis Myotonia Electrolyte abnormalities Hypokalemia Hypophosphatemia Familial paralysis
Coma	Alcohols Barbiturates Benzodiazepines Carbon monoxide Gases and fumes Neuroleptics Opioids Sedative hypnotics Tricyclic or cyclic antidepressants	Anoxia Diabetic ketoacidosis and nonketotic hyperosmolar coma Encephalopathies Epilepsy, postictal CVA Electrolyte disturbances Hepatic encephalopathy Hypertensive encephalopathy Infections (meningitis, brain abscess) Hypoglycemia Metabolic disorders Shock (septic, cardiogenic) Trauma Uremia
Convulsions	Alcohols or glycols Camphor Carbon monoxide Cyanide Heavy metals (lead, lithium) Hypoglycemia agents Isoniazid Mushroom (*Gyromitra*) Opioids (propoxyphene, meperidine) Phenothiazines Salicylates Strychnine Sympathomimetics (cocaine, amphetamines, PCP) Theophylline Tricyclic or cyclic antidepressants Withdrawal	Anoxia Febrile (child) Infections Metabolic or endocrine disorders (hypoglycemia, hyponatremia, hypocalcemia, inborn metabolic disorders) Neoplastic Traumatic Vascular (CVA) Idiopathic epilepsy
Dysrhythmias	Anticholinergic agents Antidysrhythmic agents Antihypertensive agents Beta-adrenergic blockers Calcium channel blockers Chloral hydrate Chloroquine Digitalis Lithium Neuroleptics Nonsedating antihistamines (terfenadine, astemizole) Opioids (propoxyphene) Sympathomimetics (cocaine, amphetamine, PCP, phenylpropanolamine, theophylline) Tricyclic antidepressants	Electrolyte disturbances Hereditary (e.g., prolonged QT interval) Hypoxia Idiopathic dysrhythmias Myocarditis Myocardial infarction Sick sinus syndrome Uremia

Table continued on following page

TABLE 6. **Common Clinical Presentations and Etiologic Factors in Poisoning** *Continued*

Clinical Presentation	Toxic Agents	Medical Diseases
Hypertension	Anticholinergic (T)* Clonidine (R) Hallucinogens (T) Lead encephalopathy (B) Licorice MAOI overdose and interaction Phenylephrine (R) Phenylpropanolamine (R) Sympathomimetics (T) (amphetamine, cocaine, PCP, theophylline) Thyroid (T) Vitamin A excess (B) Withdrawal (T)	Aldosteronism (primary) Acute porphyria Carcinoid syndromes Coarctation of aorta Congenital adrenal hyperplasia Essential hypertension Hyperthyroidism Increased ICP Pheochromocytoma Psychologic causes or anxiety Renal disease
Hypotension	Antihypertensive agents (T) Arsenic (T) Barbiturates (T) Beta-adrenergic blockers (B) Calcium channel blockers (B) Carbon monoxide (T) Caustics (T) Clonidine (B) Cyanide (T) Cyclic antidepressants (T) Digitalis (acute B, chronic T) Disulfiram reaction (T) Ethanol Heavy metals Iron (T) Opioids (B) Organophosphate insecticides (B) MAOI (T) Neuroleptics (T) Nitrites Sedative hypnotics (T) Theophylline (T) Vasodilators (nitrites) (T)	Adrenal insufficiency Anaphylaxis Anoxia Burns Cardiac causes (dysrhythmias, myopathy, pericardial disease, aortic aneurysm) Fluid sequestration (ascites, bowel obstruction) GI losses Heart failure Hemorrhage Hypothermia Hypovolemia or dehydration Sepsis Shock of any cause Spinal cord dysfunction
Hyperthermia (see "Disturbances Due to Heat" on page 1162)		
Hypothermia	Alpha-adrenergic antagonists Barbiturates Benzodiazepines Beta-adrenergic antagonists Carbon monoxide Ethanol Hypoglycemic agents Nitrites Opioids Phenothiazines Sedative hypnotics†	Adrenal insufficiency Cold blood or IV fluids Diabetic ketoacidosis Environmental factors Hypoglycemia Hypothalamic lesions Hypothyroidism Shock Spinal cord transection Uremia
Miosis	Clonidine Imidazoles Organophosphates Opioids—all except the following: meperidine, diphenoxylate with atropine (Lomotil), dextromethorphan (paralysis of iris) PCP Phenothiazines Cholinergic medications	Pontine lesions Aging Iritis Posterior synechiae Neurosyphilis
Mydriasis	Anticholinergic agents Botulism (delayed) Ethanol Hallucinogens Methanol (delayed) Opioids (meperidine, dextromethorphan, diphenoxylate [Lomotil]) Sedative hypnotics† Sympathomimetics Withdrawal	Midbrain lesions Ocular trauma Cranial trauma Increased ICP

TABLE 6. **Common Clinical Presentations and Etiologic Factors in Poisoning** *Continued*

Clinical Presentation	Toxic Agents	Medical Diseases
Organic brain syndrome (toxic psychosis)	Anticholinergic agents Ethanol Digitalis Hallucinogens Inhalants (solvents) Stimulants (cocaine, amphetamines, PCP) Withdrawal	Infections Metabolic disorders Psychosis
Pulmonary edema	Cardiac: antidysrhythmics, beta-adrenergic antagonists, calcium channel blockers, cyclic antidepressants Noncardiac: barbiturates, hydrocarbon aspiration, opioids, organophosphates, salicylates, toxic gases Irritant gases: smoke, chlorine inhalation Neurogenic: sympathomimetics	Aspiration Fluid overload Heart failure Hypoxia Near-drowning Shock
Tachycardia	Alcohols and glycols (early) Anticholinergics Antihistamines CNS stimulants Digitalis (chronic) Hallucinogens Nitrates and nitrites PCP Phenothiazines Plants Salicylates Sedative hypnotics (early)† Sympathomimetics (amphetamines, cocaine, theophylline) Thyroid Tricyclic or cyclic antidepressants Withdrawal	Fever Hyperthermia Hyperthyroidism Hypovolemia Shock Dysrhythmia PAT, atrial dysrhythmias Electrolyte imbalance Anxiety Carditis Heart failure
Tachypnea and hyperventilation	Acidosis (ethanol ketoacidosis, ethylene glycol, methanol, phenformin) Carbon monoxide CNS stimulants (camphor) Cyanide Dinitrophenol Salicylates Sympathomimetics (amphetamines, cocaine, theophylline) Withdrawal Inhaled gases Irritant gases	Temperature elevation Compensation metabolic acidosis Pneumonitis Other pulmonary conditions Heart failure Other cardiac conditions
Torsades de pointes	Amantadine (Symmetrel) Arsenic Antidysrhythmic agents of class IA, IB, IC, III Cocaine Erythromycin Fluoride Haloperidol (Haldol) Itraconazole (Sporanox) Maprotiline (Ludiomil) Nonsedating antihistamines (terfenadine, astemizole) Organophosphates Pentamidine Phenothiazines (e.g., thioridazine) Sotalol (Betapace) Thallium	Congenital long QT syndromes (Romano-Ward; Jervell and Lange-Nielsen) Electrolyte derangement (↓ magnesium, ↓ calcium) Coronary artery disease
Wheezing	Aspirin Beta blockers (bronchospasm) Cholinergic medications Cholinergic mushroom Irritant gases: chlorine, smoke, occupational hypersensitivity	Bronchospasm asthma Cardiac asthma Foreign body Cystic fibrosis Pneumonia Anaphylaxis Carcinoid

*T = tachycardia; B = bradycardia; R = reflex bradycardia initially.
†Includes barbiturates and benzodiazepines.
Abbreviations: CNS = central nervous system; CVA = cerebrovascular accident; GI = gastrointestinal; ICP = intracranial pressure; IV = intravenous; MAOI = monoamine oxidase inhibitor; PAT = paroxysmal atrial tachycardia; PCP = phencyclidine.

TABLE 7. **Toxic Effects of Central Nervous System Depressants***

General Manifestations	CNS Depressants
Bradycardia	Alcohols and glycols (S-H)
Bradypnea†	Anticonvulsants (S-H)
Shallow respirations	Antidysrhythmics (S-H)
Hypotension	Antihypertensives (S-H)
Hypothermia	Barbiturates (S-H)
Flaccid coma	Benzodiazepines (S-H)‡
Miosis	Butyrophenones (Syly)
Hypoactive bowel sounds	Beta-adrenergic blockers (Syly)
	Calcium channel blockers (Syly)
Frozen addict syndrome§	Digitalis (Syly)
	Opioids (O)‖¶
	Lithium (mixed)
	Muscle relaxants
	Phenothiazines (Syly)
	Nonbarbiturate, benzodiazepine sedative hypnotics (S-H)‖ (chloral hydrate, glutethimide, methaqualone, methyprylone, ethchlorvynol, bromide)
	Tricyclic antidepressants late (Syly)

*CNS depressants are cholinergics (C), opioids (O) and sedative hypnotics (S-H), and sympatholytic agents (Syly). The hallmarks of CNS depressant activity are lethargy, sedation, stupor, and coma.

†Barbiturates may produce an initial tachycardia.

‡Benzodiazepines rarely produce coma that interferes with cardiorespiratory functions.

§The "frozen addict" syndrome is due to a neurotoxin resulting from improper synthesis of an analogue of meperidine. Its manifestations are similar to those of the permanent type of parkinsonism.

‖Convulsions are produced by codeine, propoxyphene (Darvon), meperidine (Demerol), glutethimide, phenothiazines, methaqualone, and tricyclic or cyclic antidepressants.

¶Pulmonary edema is common with opioids and sedative hypnotics.

TABLE 8. **Toxic Effects of Central Nervous System Stimulants***

General Manifestations	CNS Stimulants
Tachycardia	Amphetamines (Sy)
Tachypnea and dysrhythmias	Anticholinergics (Ach)†
Hypertension	Cocaine (Sy)
Convulsions	Camphor (mixed)
Spastic coma‡	Ergot alkaloids (Sy)
Toxic psychosis	Isoniazid (mixed)
Mydriasis (reactive)	Lithium (mixed)
Agitation and restlessness	Lysergic acid diethylamine (LSD) (H)
Moist skin	Hallucinogens (H)
Tremors	Mescaline and synthetic analogues
	Metals (arsenic, lead, mercury)
	Methylphenidate (Ritalin) (Sy)
	MAOIs (Sy)
	Pemoline (Cylert) (Sy)
	Phencyclidine (H)§
	Salicylates (mixed)
	Strychnine (mixed)
	Sympathomimetics (Sy) (phenylpropanolamine, theophylline, caffeine, thyroid)
	Withdrawal from ethanol, beta-adrenergic blockers, clonidine, opioids, sedative hypnotics (W)

*CNS stimulants are anticholinergics (Ach), hallucinogens (H), sympathomimetics (Sy), and withdrawal (W). The hallmarks of CNS stimulant activity are convulsions and hyperactivity.

†Anticholinergics produce dry skin and mucosa and decreased bowel sounds.

‡Flaccid coma eventually develops after seizures.

§Phencyclidine may produce miosis.

tation of myoglobin), cardiotoxicity, and lack of proven clinical effectiveness. Alkalization with or without diuresis with sodium bicarbonate ($NaHCO_3$) at 1 to 2 mEq per kg in 15 mL of D5W (5% dextrose in water) per kg may be used in the therapy of weak acid intoxications, such as with salicylates (severe salicylate poisoning can require hemodialysis, which avoids complications of fluid overload), long-acting barbiturates (LABs) (e.g., phenobarbital), 2,4-dichlorophenoxyacetic acid, chlorpropamide, methotrexate, and methanol. Additional boluses of 0.5 mEq per kg can be administered to maintain alkalization, but blood pH values higher than 7.55 should be avoided. Many clinicians use the alkalization without the diuresis because of the danger of fluid overload. Hemodynamic status, fluids, blood gases and electrolytes, and glucose must be closely monitored during these procedures. See sodium bicarbonate ($NaHCO_3$) in Table 12. Saline diuresis, but not forced diuresis, is used in lithium intoxications.

Dialysis

Dialysis is an extrarenal means of removing certain substances from the body and can substitute for the kidney when renal failure occurs. Dialysis is not the first measure instituted; however, it may be lifesaving later in the course of a severe intoxication. It is needed in only a minority of intoxicated patients.

Peritoneal dialysis utilizes the peritoneum as the membrane for dialysis. It is only one twentieth as effective as hemodialysis. It is easier to use and less hazardous to the patient but also less effective in

TABLE 9. **Toxic Effects of Hallucinogens***

General Manifestations	Hallucinogens
Tachycardia and dysrhythmias	Amphetamines
	Anticholinergics
Tachypnea	Carbon monoxide
Hypertension	Cardiac glycosides
Hallucinations, usually visual	Cocaine
	Ethanol
Disorientation	Hydrocarbon inhalation (abuse)
Panic reaction	Hydrocarbon inhalation (occupational)
Toxic psychosis	Lysergic acid diethylamide
Moist skin	Marijuana
Mydriasis (reactive)	Mescaline (peyote)
Hyperthermia	Mescaline-amphetamine hybrids†
Flashbacks	Metals (chronic mercury, arsenic)
	Mushrooms (psilocybin)
	Phencyclidine
	Plants (morning glory seeds, nutmeg)

*There is considerable overlap in this category; however, the major hallmark manifestation is hallucinations.

†The mescaline-amphetamine hybrids are methylene dioxymethamphetamine (MDMA, Ecstasy, Adam) and methylene dioxyamphetamine (MDA, Eve), which have been associated with deaths.

TABLE 10. **Effects of Toxins on Autonomic Nervous System**

General Manifestations	Agents
Anticholinergic	
Tachycardia, dysrhythmias rare	Antihistamines
Tachypnea	Antispasmodic GI preparations
Hypertension (mild)	Antiparkinsonian preparations
Hyperthermia	Atropine
Hallucinations	Cyclobenzaprine (Flexeril)
Mydriasis (unreactive)	Mydriatic ophthalmologic agents
Flushed skin	Over-the-counter sleep agents
Dry skin and mouth	Plants (*Datura* species), mushrooms
Hypoactive bowel sounds	Phenothiazines (early)
Urinary retention	Scopolamine
Lilliputian hallucinations	Tricyclic or cyclic antidepressants (early)
Cholinergic	
Bradycardia (muscarinic)	Bethanechol
Tachycardia (nicotinic)	Carbamate insecticides (carbaryl)
Miosis (muscarinic)	Edrophonium
Diarrhea (muscarinic)	Organophosphate insecticides (malathion, parathion)
Hypertension (variable)	Parasympathetic agents (physostigmine, pyridostigmine)
Hyperactive bowel sounds	Toxic mushrooms (*Amanita muscaria, Clitocybe* species)
Excess urination (muscarinic)	
Excess salivation (muscarinic)	
Lacrimation (muscarinic)	
Bronchospasm (muscarinic)	
Muscle fasciculations (nicotinic)	
Paralysis (nicotinic)	

removing the toxin; thus, it is seldom used except for small infants.

Hemodialysis is the most effective means of dialysis but requires experience with sophisticated equipment. Blood is circulated past a semipermeable membrane by an extracorporeal method. Substances are removed by diffusion down a concentration gradient. Anticoagulation with heparin is necessary.

Hemodialysis is contraindicated when (1) the substance is not dialyzable, (2) effective antidotes are available, (3) hemodynamic instability (e.g., shock) is present, and (4) coagulopathy is present because heparinization is required.

The patient-related criteria for dialysis are (1) anticipated prolonged coma and the likelihood of complications, (2) renal compromise (toxin excreted or metabolized by kidneys and dialyzable chelating agents in heavy metal poisoning), (3) laboratory confirmation of lethal blood concentration, (4) lethal-dose poisoning with an agent with delayed toxicity or known to be metabolized into a more toxic metabolite (e.g., ethylene glycol, methanol), and (5) hepatic impairment when the agent is metabolized by the liver and clinical deterioration occurs despite optimal supportive medical management.

Dialyzable substances diffuse easily across the dialysis membrane and have the following characteristics: (1) a small molecular weight (less than 500 and preferably less than 350); (2) a Vd of less than 1 liter per kg; (3) low PB, less than 50%; (4) high water solubility (low lipid solubility); and (5) high plasma concentration and a toxicity that correlates reasonably with the plasma concentration (Tables 13 and 14).

Hemodialysis also has a role in correcting disturbances that are not amenable to appropriate medical management. These are easily remembered by the "vowel" mnemonic:

A = refractory acid-base disturbances
E = refractory electrolyte disturbances
I = intoxication with dialyzable substances (e.g., ethanol,* ethylene glycol,* isopropyl alcohol,* methanol,* lithium,* salicylates,* and theophylline); dialysis is rarely indicated with aminoglycosides, carbamazepine, phenobarbital, and phenytoin
O = overhydration
U = uremia (renal failure)

Complications of dialysis include hemorrhage, thrombosis, air embolism, hypotension, infections, electrolyte imbalance, thrombocytopenia, and removal of therapeutic medications.

Hemoperfusion

Hemoperfusion is the parenteral form of oral AC therapy. Heparinization is necessary. The patient's blood is routed extracorporeally through an outflow arterial catheter and then through a filter-adsorbing cartridge (charcoal or resin) and returned through a venous catheter. High flow rates (e.g., 300 mL per minute) through the filter are used to maximize the efficient use of the filter. Cartridges must be changed every 4 hours. Blood glucose, electrolytes, calcium, albumin, complete blood count (CBC), platelets, and serum and urine osmolarity must be carefully monitored. This procedure has extended extracorporeal removal to a large range of substances that were formerly either poorly dialyzable or nondialyzable. It is not limited by molecular weight, water solubility, or protein binding. However, hemoperfusion is limited by a Vd greater than 400 liters, plasma concentration, and rate of flow through the filter. AC cartridges are primarily used for hemoperfusion in the United States. Analysis of studies using hemodialysis and hemoperfusion indicates that use of these techniques does not reduce morbidity or mortality substantially except in certain cases (e.g., with theophylline). Hemoperfusion may be recommended in combination with hemodialysis (e.g., for paraquat, electrolyte disturbances).

The contraindications are similar to those for hemodialysis.

The patient-related criteria for use of hemoperfusion are (1) anticipated prolonged coma and the likelihood of complications, (2) laboratory confirmation of lethal blood concentrations, (3) lethal-dose poisoning with an agent with delayed toxicity or known to be

*Toxins for which hemodialysis is preferred to hemoperfusion.

TABLE 11. **Common Poisons and Their Recommended Antidotes**

Toxin	Antidote
Acetaminophen (in many analgesics)	*N*-acetylcysteine
Anticholinergics (antihistamines, plants, GI medications)	Physostigmine (use with caution)
Anticoagulants (in rodenticides)	Vitamin K_1
Antimony (ant paste)	Dimercaprol (BAL), penicillamine
Arsenic (ant traps)	Dimercaprol (BAL), penicillamine
Benzodiazepines	Flumazenil (Romazicon)
Beta blockers	Glucagon
Bismuth (GI medication)	Dimercaprol (BAL)
Botulism	Botulism antitoxin
Calcium channel blockers	Atropine
Carbamate insecticide	Calcium gluconate
Carbon monoxide	100% oxygen, hyperbaric oxygen
Chloroquine (Aralen) (antimalarial)	Diazepam (Valium)
Cyanide (fruit stone seeds, nitroprusside for hypertension, plastic fires, metal polishes)	Lilly cyanide kit; contains amyl nitrite, sodium nitrite, sodium thiosulfate Investigative vitamin B_{12a}
Digoxin, digitoxin in plants	Fragment antibody (Digibind)
Ethylene glycol (antifreeze)	Ethanol
Fluoride (rodenticides)	Calcium gluconate
Gold (antirheumatoid)	Dimercaprol (BAL)
Gyromitra mushrooms	Pyridoxine
Hydralazine (antihypertensive)	Pyridoxine
Hydrofluoric acid (for etching glass)	Local calcium gluconate jelly Soak in magnesium sulfate
Iron (dietary supplements)	Deferoxamine (Desferal)
Isoniazid (antituberculous)	Pyridoxine
Lead (old paints and plaster, dust)	Calcium disodium edetate (EDTA) Dimercaprol (BAL), DMSA
Mercury (fungicides, thermometers)	Dimercaprol (BAL), penicillamine, DMSA
Methanol (antifreeze, "dry gas")	Ethanol
Nitrites, dyes (causing methemoglobinemia)	Methylene blue
Opioids	Naloxone (Narcan)
Organophosphate insecticides	Atropine, pralidoxime
Phencyclidine (abused, "angel dust")	Ammonium chloride *not* recommended
Phenobarbital	Sodium bicarbonate
Phenothiazine (causing dystonic reaction)	Diphenhydramine (Benadryl)
Phenylurea rodenticide (Vacor)	Nicotinamide
Salicylate	Sodium bicarbonate
Snake bite venom	Antivenom
Spider bite venom, *Latrodectus* (black widow)	Antivenom
Tricyclic and cyclic antidepressants	Sodium bicarbonate
Withdrawal	
Opioids	Methadone, clonidine
Barbiturates	Phenobarbital
Benzodiazepines	Diazepam
Ethanol	Benzodiazepines
Other sedative hypnotics	Phenobarbital or diazepam

Abbreviations: BAL = British antilewisite; DMSA = dimercaptosuccinic acid (succimer); EDTA = ethylenediaminetetra-acetic acid.

metabolized into a more toxic metabolite, and (4) hepatic impairment when an agent is metabolized by the liver and there is clinical deterioration despite optimal supportive medical management.

Limited data are available to determine which toxicities are best treated with hemoperfusion. However, hemoperfusion has proved useful in glutethimide intoxication, barbiturate overdose even with SA barbiturates (SABs), carbamazepine, phenytoin, theophylline intoxication, and chlorophenothane (DDT). See Tables 13 and 14.

Complications include hemorrhage, thrombocytopenia, hypotension, infection, leukopenia, depressed phagocytic activity of granulocytes, decreased immunoglobulin levels, hypoglycemia, hypothermia, hypocalcemia, pulmonary edema, and air and charcoal embolism.

Plasmapheresis

Plasmapheresis consists of removal of a volume of blood. All the extracted components are returned to the blood except the plasma, which is replaced with a colloidal protein solution. Clinical data related to guidelines and efficacy in toxicology are limited. Centrifugal and membrane separators of cellular elements are used. Plasmapheresis can be as effective as hemodialysis or hemoperfusion for toxins with high protein binding and may be useful for removal of toxins not filtered by hemodialysis and hemoperfusion. It has been used in certain diseases such as myeloma, idiopathic thrombocytopenia, systemic lupus erythematosus, rheumatoid arthritis, and myasthenia gravis.

Use of plasmapheresis has been reported anecdot-

Text continued on page 1200

TABLE 12. **Initial Doses of Antidotes for Common Poisonings**

Antidote	Use	Dose	Route	Adverse Reactions (AR) and Comments
***N*-acetylcysteine** (NAC, Mucomyst). Stock level to treat 70-kg adult for 24 h: seven vials, 20%, 30 mL.	Acetaminophen, carbon tetrachloride (experimental).	140 mg/kg loading, followed by 70 mg/kg q 4 h for 17 doses.	PO	Nausea, vomiting. Dilute to 5% with sweet juice or flat cola.
Atropine. Stock level to treat 70-kg adult for 24 h: 1 gm (1 mg/mL in 1 or 10 mL).	Organophosphate and carbamate pesticides.	*Child:* 0.02–0.05 mg/kg repeated q 5–10 min to maximum of 2 mg as necessary until cessation of secretions. *Adult:* 1–2 mg q 5–10 min as necessary. Dilute in 1–2 mL of 0.89% saline for endotracheal instillation. *IV infusion dose:* Place 8 mg of atropine in 100 mL of D5W or saline. Concentration = 0.08 mg/mL. Dose range = 0.02–0.08 mg/kg/h or 0.25–1 mL/kg/h. Severe poisoning may require supplemental IV atropine intermittently in doses of 1–5 mg until drying of secretions occurs.	IV or ET	Tachycardia, dry mouth, blurred vision, and urinary retention. Ensure adequate ventilation before administration.
Calcium chloride (10%). Stock level to treat 70-kg adult for 24 h: 5–10 vials, 1 gm (1.35 mEq/mL).	Hypocalcemia, fluoride, calcium channel blockers.	0.1–0.2 mL/kg (10–20 mg/kg) slow push q 10 min up to maximum of 10 mL (1 gm). Because calcium response lasts 15 min, some patients may require continuous infusion of 0.2 mL/kg/h up to maximum of 10 mL/h during monitoring for dysrhythmias and hypotension.	IV	Administer slowly with BP and ECG monitoring and have magnesium available to reverse calcium effects. **AR:** Tissue irritation, hypotension, dysrhythmias resulting from rapid injection. Contraindication: Digitalis glycoside intoxication.
Calcium gluconate (10%). Stock level to treat 70-kg adult for 24 h: 5–10 vials, 1 gm (0.45 mEq/mL).	Hypocalcemia, fluoride, calcium channel blockers, hydrofluoric acid, black widow envenomation.	0.3–0.4 mL/kg (30–40 mg/kg) slow push; repeat as needed up to maximum dose of 10–20 mL (1–2 gm).	IV	Same as for calcium chloride.
Calcium gluconate gel. Stock level: 3.5 gm.	Hydrofluoric acid.	2.5 gm of USP powder added to 100 mL of water-soluble lubricating jelly (e.g., K-Y Jelly, Lubifax) (or 3.5 gm into 150 mL). Some use 6 gm of calcium carbonate in 100 gm of lubricant. Place injured hand in surgical glove filled with gel; or apply q 4 h. If pain persists, calcium gluconate injection may be needed (following).	Dermal	Powder is available from Spectrum Pharmaceutical Company in California: 1-800-772-8786. Commercial preparation of calcium gluconate gel is available from Pharmascience in Montreal, Quebec: 514-340-1114.
Infiltration of calcium gluconate.	Hydrofluoric acid.	Dose: Infiltrate each square cm of affected dermis or subcutaneous tissue with about 0.5 mL of 10% calcium gluconate using a 30-gauge needle. Repeat as needed to control pain.	Infiltrate	
Cyanide antidote kit. Stock level to treat 70-kg adult for 24 h: two Lilly Cyanide Antidote kits.	Cyanide; hydrogen sulfide (nitrites are given only; do not use sodium thiosulfate for hydrogen sulfide). Individual portions of the kit can be used in certain circumstances (consult PCC).	Amyl nitrite: 1 crushable ampule for 30 s of every minute. Use new ampule q 3 min. May omit step if venous access is established.	Inhalation	If methemoglobinemia occurs, do not use methylene blue to correct this because it releases cyanide.

Table continued on following page

TABLE 12. **Initial Doses of Antidotes for Common Poisonings** *Continued*

Antidote	Use	Dose	Route	Adverse Reactions (AR) and Comments
Cyanide antidote kit. Stock level to treat 70-kg adult for 24 h: two Lilly Cyanide Antidote kits.	Cyanide; hydrogen sulfide (nitrites are given only; do not use sodium thiosulfate for hydrogen sulfide). Individual portions of the kit can be used in certain circumstances (consult PCC).	Sodium nitrite: *Child:* 0.33 mL/kg 3% solution if hemoglobin level is not known, otherwise follow tables with product. *Adult:* up to 300 mg (10 mL). Dilute nitrite in 100 mL of 0.9% saline, administer slowly at 5 mL/min. Slow infusion if fall in BP.	IV	If methemoglobinemia occurs, do not use methylene blue to correct this because it releases cyanide.
	Do not use sodium thiosulfate for hydrogen sulfide. Individual portions of the kit can be used in certain circumstances (consult PCC).	Sodium thiosulfate: *Child:* 1.6 mL/kg 25% solution; may be repeated q 30–60 min to a maximum of 12.5 gm or 50 mL in *adult.* Administer over 20 min.	IV	**AR:** Nausea, dizziness, headache; tachycardia, muscle rigidity, and bronchospasm (rapid administration).
Dantrolene sodium (Dantrium). Stock level to treat 70-kg adult for 24 h: 700 mg in 35 vials (20 mg per vial).	Malignant hyperthermia.	2–3 mg/kg IV rapidly. Repeat loading dose q 10 min, if necessary up to a maximal total dose of 10 mg/kg. When temperature and heart rate decrease, slow the infusion to 1–2 mg/kg q 6 h for 24–48 h until all evidence of malignant hyperthermia syndrome has subsided. Follow with oral doses of 1–2 mg/kg qid for 24 h as necessary.	IV or PO	Available as 20-mg lyophilized dantrolene powder for reconstitution, which contains 3 gm of mannitol and sodium hydroxide in 70-mL vials. Mix with 60 mL of sterile distilled water without a bacteriostatic agent and protect from light. Use within 6 h after reconstituted. **AR:** Hepatotoxicity occurs with cumulative dose of 10 mg/kg; thrombophlebitis (best given in central line).
Deferoxamine (DFO, Desferal). Stock level to treat 70-kg adult for 24 h: 12 vials (50 mg per ampule).	Iron (100 mg of DFO binds 8.5–9.3 mg of iron).	IV infusion of 15 mg/kg/h (3 mL/kg/h: 500 mg in 100 mL D5W), maximum of 6 gm/d. Rates of >45 mg/kg/h if conc >1000 μg/dL.	IV preferred; avoid therapy >24 h	Hypotension (minimized by avoiding rapid infusion rates). DFO challenge test (50 mg/kg) is unreliable if negative.
Diazepam (Valium). Stock level to treat 70-kg adult for 24 h: 200 mg.	Any intoxication that provokes seizures when specific therapy is not available, for example, amphetamines, PCP, barbiturate and alcohol withdrawal, chloroquine poisoning.	*Adult:* 5–10 mg (maximum of 20 mg) at a rate of 5 mg/min until seizure is controlled. May be repeated two or three times. *Child:* 0.1–0.3 mg/kg up to 10 mg slowly over 2 min.	IV	**AR:** Confusion, somnolence, coma, hypotension. Intramuscular absorption is erratic. Establish airway and administer 100% oxygen and glucose.
Digoxin-specific Fab antibodies (Digibind). Stock level to treat 70-kg adult for 24 h: 20 vials.	Digoxin, digitoxin, oleander tea with any of the following: (1) imminent cardiac arrest or shock, (2) hyperkalemia of >5.0 mEq/L, (3) serum digoxin of >10 ng/mL (adult) or >5 ng/mL (child) at 8–12 h after ingestion in adults, (4) digitalis delirium, (5) ingestion of more than 10 mg in adult or 4 mg in child, (6) bradycardia or second- or third-degree heart block unresponsive to atropine, (7) life-threatening digitoxin or oleander poisoning.	1. *Amount (total mg) ingested known* multiplied by bioavailability (0.8) = body burden. The body burden divided by 0.6 (0.6 mg of digoxin is bound by one vial of 40 mg of Fab) = number of vials needed. 2. *If amount is unknown but the steady-state serum concentration is known in ng/mL:* *Digoxin:* ng/mL × (Vd = 5.6 L/kg) × wt (kg) = μg body burden. Body burden divided by 1000 = mg body burden/0.6 = number of vials needed. *Digitoxin:* ng/mL × (Vd = 0.56 L/kg) × wt (kg) = body burden. Body burden divided by 1000 = mg body burden/0.6 = number of vials needed. 3. *If the amount is not known,* agent is administered in life-threatening situations as 10 vials (400 mg) IV in saline over 30 min in adults. If cardiac arrest is imminent, administer 20 vials (adult) as a bolus.	IV	Administer by infusion over 30 min through a 0.22-μm filter. If cardiac arrest is imminent, may administer by bolus injection. Consult PCC for more details. **AR:** Allergic reactions (rare), return of condition being treated with digitalis glycoside.

Dimercaprol (BAL in oil). Stock level to treat 70-kg adult for 24 h: 1200 mg (four ampules, 100 mg/mL 10% in oil in 3-mL ampule).	Chelating agent for arsenic, mercury, lead, antimony, bismuth, chromium, copper, gold, nickel, tungsten, and zinc.	3–5 mg/kg q 4 h, usually for 5–10 d.	Deep IM	**AR:** Local injection site pain and sterile abscess, nausea, vomiting, fever, salivation, hypertension, and nephrotoxicity (alkalize urine).
Diphenhydramine (Benadryl). Antiparkinsonian action. Stock level to treat 70-kg adult for 24 h: five vials (10 mg/mL, 10 mL each).	Used to treat extrapyramidal symptoms and dystonia induced by phenothiazines, PCP, and related drugs.	*Child:* 1–2 mg/kg IV slowly over 5 min up to maximum of 50 mg, followed by 5 mg/kg per 24 h PO divided q 6 h in children up to 300 mg per 24 h. *Adult:* 50 mg IV followed by 50 mg PO qid for 5–7 d. Note: Symptoms abate within 2–5 min after IV administration.	IV and PO	Fatal dose, 20–40 mg/kg. **AR:** Dry mouth, drowsiness.
Ethanol (ethyl alcohol). Stock level to treat 70-kg adult for 24 h: three bottles 10% (1 L each).	Methanol, ethylene glycol.	10 mL/kg loading dose concurrently with 1.4 mL/kg (average) infusion of 10% ethanol. (Consult PCC for more details.)	IV	**AR:** Nausea, vomiting, sedation. Use 0.22-μm filter if preparing from bulk 100% ethanol.
Flumazenil (Romazicon). Stock level to treat 70-kg adult for 24 h: 10 vials (0.1 mg/mL, 10 mL).	Benzodiazepines.	Administer 0.2 mg (2 mL) over 30 s. (Pediatric dose not established, 0.01 mg/kg.) Wait 3 min for a response. If desired consciousness is not achieved administer 0.3 mg (3 mL) over 30 s. Wait 3 min for response. If desired consciousness is not achieved administer 0.5 mg (5 mL) over 30 s at 60-s intervals up to a maximal cumulative dose of 3 mg (30 mL) (1 mg in children). Because effects last only 1–5 h, if there is a response monitor carefully over next 6 h for resedation. If multiple repeated doses, consider a continuous infusion of 0.2–1 mg/h.	IV	It is not recommended to improve ventilation. Its role in CNS depression needs to be clarified. It should not be used routinely in comatose patients. It is *contraindicated* in cyclic antidepressant intoxications, stimulant overdose, long-term benzodiazepine use (may precipitate life-threatening withdrawal), if benzodiazepines are used to control seizures, in head trauma. **AR:** Nausea, vomiting, facial flushing, agitation, headache, dizziness, seizures, and death.
Folic acid (Folvite). Stock level to treat 70-kg adult for 24 h: two 100-mg vials.	Methanol or ethylene glycol (investigational).	1 mg/kg up to 50 mg q 4 h for 6 doses.	IV	Uncommon.
Glucagon. Stock level to treat 70-kg adult for 24 h: 100 mg (10 vials, 10 units).	Beta blockers, calcium channel blockers, hypoglycemic agents.	*Adult:* 5–10 mg, then infuse 1–5 mg/h. *Child:* 0.05–0.1 mg/kg, then infuse 0.07 mg/kg/h. Large doses up to 100 mg per 24 h have been used.	IV	**AR:** Hyperglycemia, nausea, vomiting. Dissolve in D5W, not in 0.9% saline. Do not use diluent in package because of possible phenol toxicity.
Magnesium sulfate. Stock level to treat 70-kg adult for 24 h: approximately 25 gm (50 mL of 50% or 200 mL of 12.5%).	Torsades de pointes.	*Adult:* 2 gm (20 mL of 20%) over 20 min. If no response in 10 min, repeat and follow by continuous infusion 1 gm/h. *Child:* 25–50 mg/kg initially, maintenance with 30–60 mg/kg per 24 h (0.25–0.50 mEq/kg per 24 h) up to 1000 mg per 24 h. (Dose not studied in controlled fashion.)	IV	Use with caution if there is renal impairment.
Methylene blue. Stock level to treat 70-kg adult for 24 h: five ampules (10 mg per 10 mL).	Methemoglobinemia.	0.1–0.2 mL/kg of 1% solution, slow infusion, may be repeated q 30–60 min.	IV	**AR:** Nausea, vomiting, headache, dizziness.

Table continued on following page

TABLE 12. **Initial Doses of Antidotes for Common Poisonings** *Continued*

Antidote	Use	Dose	Route	Adverse Reactions (AR) and Comments
Nalmefene (Revex). Stock level: not established.	Narcotic antagonist.	The dose for opioid overdose as bolus in adults is 0.5–1 mg q 2 min up to a total of 2 mg IV. May also be given IM or SC. In patients with renal failure, administer over 1 min. In postoperative opioid depression reversal IV 0.1–0.5 μg/kg every 2 min as needed and may repeat up to a total dose of 1 μg/kg.	IV, IM, SC	Role in comatose patients and opioid overdose is not clear. It is 16 times more potent than naloxone; duration of action is up to 8 h (half-life 10.8 h compared with naloxone, 1 h). Clinical trials in more than 1750 patients have not shown significant adverse reactions.
Naloxone (Narcan). Stock level to treat 70-kg adult for 24 h: 3 vials (1 mg/mL, 10 mL).	Comatose patient; ineffective ventilation or adult respiratory rate <12 rpm; opioids.	In suspected overdose administer IV 0.1 mg/kg in a child younger than 5 y up to 2 mg. In older children and adults administer 2 mg q 2 min up to a total of 10–20 mg. Can also be administered into the ET tube. If no response by 10 mg, a pure opioid intoxication is unlikely. If opioid abuse is suspected, restraints should be in place before administration, initial dose 0.1 mg to avoid withdrawal and violent behavior. The initial dose is then doubled every minute progressively to a total of 10 mg. A continuous infusion has been advocated because many opioids outlast the short half-life.	IV, ET	Larger doses of naloxone may be required for more poorly antagonized synthetic opioid drugs: buprenorphine, codeine, dextromethorphan, fentanyl, pentazocine, propoxyphene, diphenoxylate, nalbuphine, new potent designer drugs, or long-acting opioids such as methadone. **Complications:** Although naloxone is safe and effective, there are rare reports of complications (in less than 1% of cases) of pulmonary edema, seizures, hypertension, cardiac arrest, and sudden death. The infusions are titrated to avoid respiratory depression and opioid withdrawal manifestations. Tapering of infusions can be attempted after 12 h and when the patient's condition has been stabilized.
Physostigmine (Antilirium). Stock level to treat 70-kg adult for 24 h: 10 ampules (2 mL each).	Anticholinergic agents (not routinely used, indicated only with life-threatening complications).	*Child:* 0.02 mg/kg slow push to maximum of 2 mg q 30–60 min. *Adult:* 1–2 mg q 5 min to maximum of 6 mg.	IV	**AR:** Bradycardia, asystole, seizures, bronchospasm, vomiting, headaches. Do not use for cyclic antidepressants.
Pralidoxime (2-PAM, Protopam). Stock level to treat 70-kg adult for 24 h: 12 vials (1 gm per 20 mL).	Organophosphates.	*Child ≤ 12 y:* 25–50 mg/kg maximal (4 mg/kg/min); *older than 12 y:* 1–2 gm per dose in 250 mL of 0.89% saline over 5–10 min. Maximal 200 mg/min. Repeat q 6–12 h for 24–48 h. Maximal adult dose 6 gm/d. Alternative: Main infusion 1 gm in 100 mL of 0.9% saline at 5–20 mg/kg/h (0.5–12 mL/kg/h) up to maximal 500 mg/h or 50 mL/h. Titrate to desired response. End point is absence of fasciculations and return of muscle strength.	IV	**AR:** Nausea, dizziness, headache; tachycardia, muscle rigidity, bronchospasm (rapid administration).

Pyridoxine (vitamin B_6). Stock level to treat 70-kg adult for 24 h: four ampules (50 mg in 5-mL or 250 mg in 25-mL vial).	Seizures caused by isoniazid or *Gyromitra* mushrooms; ethylene glycol (investigational).	Isoniazid (INH): *Unknown amount ingested:* 5 gm (70 mg/kg) in 50 mL of D5W over 5 min with diazepam 0.3 mg/kg IV at rate of 1 mg/min in child or 10 mg per dose at rate up to 5 mg/min in adults. Use different site (synergism). May repeat q 5–20 min until seizure controlled. Up to 375 mg/kg has been given (52 gm). *Known amount ingested:* 1 gm for each gram of INH ingested over 5 min with diazepam (dose above). *Gyromitra* mushrooms: 25 mg/kg for child or 2–5 gm for adult over 15–30 min to maximum of 20 gm. Ethylene glycol: 100 mg daily.	IV	After seizure is controlled, administer remainder of pyridoxine at 1 gm per 1 gm of INH or total 5 gm as infusion over 60 min. **AR:** Uncommon; do not administer in same bottle as sodium bicarbonate. For *Gyromitra* mushrooms, some use 25 mg/kg PO early when mushroom is suspected.
Sodium bicarbonate ($NaHCO_3$). Stock level to treat 70-kg adult for 24 h: 10 ampules or syringes (500 mEq).	Tricyclic antidepressant (TCA) cardiotoxicity (wide QRS >0.10 s, ventricular tachycardia, severe conduction disturbances); metabolic acidosis; phenothiazine cardiotoxicity.	1–2 mEq/kg undiluted as a bolus. If no effect on cardiotoxicity, repeat twice a few minutes apart. An infusion of $NaHCO_3$ may follow to keep blood pH at 7.5–7.55 but not higher.	IV	Monitor serum sodium and potassium and blood pH because fatal alkalemia and hypernatremia have been reported. Continuous infusion of bicarbonate by itself is of limited usefulness in setting of TCA intoxication because of delayed onset. Prophylactic $NaHCO_3$ has not been encouraged.
	Salicylate: To keep blood pH 7.5–7.55 (not >7.55) and urine pH 7.5–8.0. Alkalinization is recommended if salicylate concentration >40 mg/dL in acute poisoning and at lower levels if symptomatic in chronic intoxication. 2 mEq/kg raises blood pH 0.1 unit.	*Adult* with clear physical signs and laboratory findings of acute moderate or severe salicylism: bolus 1–2 mEq/kg followed by infusion of 100–150 mEq $NaHCO_3$ added to 1 L of 5% dextrose at rate of 200–300 mL/h. *Child:* Bolus same as adult followed by 1–2 mEq/kg in infusion of 20 mL/kg/h 5% dextrose in 0.45% saline. Add potassium when patient voids. Rate and amount of the initial infusion, if patient is volume depleted: 1 h to achieve urine output of 2 mL/kg/h and urine pH of 7–8. In mild cases without acidosis and with urine pH of >6, administer 5% dextrose in 0.9% saline with 50 mEq/L or 1 mEq/kg $NaHCO_3$ as maintenance to replace ongoing renal losses. If acidemia and pH <7.2, add 2 mEq/kg as loading dose followed by 2 mEq/kg q 3–4 h to keep pH at 7.5–7.55. If acidemia, recommend isotonic $NaHCO_3$, three ampules to 1 L of D5W at 10–15 mL/kg/h or sufficient to produce normal urine flow and a urine pH of 7.5 or higher.	IV	Monitor both urine pH and blood pH. Do not use urine pH alone to assess the need for alkalinization because of the paradoxical aciduria that may occur. Adjust the urine pH to 7.5–8 by ($NaHCO_3$) infusion. After urine output established add potassium, 40 mEq/L.
	Long-acting barbiturates: phenobarbital, mephobarbital (Mebaral), metharbital (Gemonil), primidone (Mysoline). Note: Alkalinization is not effective for the shorter and intermediate-acting barbiturates.	2 mEq/kg during the first hour or 100 mEq in 1 L of D5W with 40 mEq/L potassium at rate of 100 mL/h in adults. Adequate potassium is necessary to accomplish alkalinization.	IV	Additional $NaHCO_3$ and potassium chloride may be needed. Adjust the urine pH to 7.5–8 by ($NaHCO_3$) infusion.

Abbreviations: BP = blood pressure; D5W = 5% dextrose in water; ET = by endotracheal route; PCC = poison control center; PCP = phencyclidine; rpm = respirations per minute; USP = U.S. Pharmacopeia.

TABLE 13. **Considerations for Hemodialysis or Hemoperfusion**

Serious Ingestions

Immediately notify the nephrologist. Compounds that are ingested in potentially lethal doses in which rapid removal may improve the prognosis include

- Amatoxins from *Amanita phalloides* mushroom: any amount with symptoms
- Arsenic trioxide: 120 mg in adults
- Ethylene glycol: 1.4 mL/kg 100% solution or equivalent
- Methanol: 6 mL/kg 100% solution or equivalent
- Paraquat: 1.5 gm in adults
- Diquat: 1.5 gm in adults
- Mercuric chloride: 1.0 gm in adults

Dialyzable Substances

Alcohol*	Isoniazid
Ammonia	Lithium*
Amphetamines	Meprobamate
Anilines	Paraldehyde
Antibiotics	Potassium*
Barbiturates (long-acting)*	Procainamide
Boric acid	Quinidine
Bromides*	Quinine*
Calcium	Salicylates*
Chloral hydrate*	Strychnine
Fluorides	Thiocyanates
Iodides	

Nondialyzable Substances

Anticholinergics	Glutethimide
Antidepressants (cyclic and MAOIs)	Hallucinogens
	Methyprylon (Noludar)†
Barbiturates (short-acting)	Methaqualone†
Benzodiazepines	Opioids including heroin
Digitalis and related drugs	Phenothiazine
Ethchlorvynol	Phenytoin

*Most useful.
†Controversial.

ally in the following intoxications: propranolol (30% removed); levothyroxine (30% removed); salicylate (10% removed); and digoxin, phenobarbital, prednisolone, and tobramycin (less than 10% removed). Complications include infection, allergic reactions including anaphylaxis, hemorrhagic disorders, thrombocytopenia, embolus and thrombus, hyper- and hypovolemia, dysrhythmias, syncope, tetany, paresthesia, pneumothorax, adult respiratory distress syndrome, and seizures.

Supportive Care, Observation, and Therapy of Complications

The Comatose Patient or Patient with Altered Mental Status

If airway protective reflexes are absent, endotracheal intubation is indicated. If respirations are ineffective, ventilation with 100% oxygen is instituted. If a cyanotic patient fails to respond to oxygen, the presence of methemoglobinemia should be suspected. A reagent strip test for blood glucose should be performed to detect hypoglycemia and the specimen sent to the laboratory for confirmation.

Glucose. Glucose is administered if the glucose reagent strip visually reads less than 150 mg per dL. Venous rather than capillary blood should be used for the reagent strip if the patient is in shock or is hypotensive.

Hypoglycemia accompanies many poisonings, including those with ethanol (especially in children), clonidine (Catapres), insulin, organophosphates, salicylates, sulfonylureas, and the fruit or seed of a Jamaican plant called akee. If hypoglycemia is present or suspected, glucose is administered immediately as an intravenous bolus in the following doses: neonate, 10% glucose (5 mL per kg); child, 25% glucose at 0.25 gram per kg (2 mL per kg); and adult, 50% glucose at 0.5 gram per kg (1 mL per kg).

Large amounts of glucose given rapidly to nondiabetic patients may cause transient reactive hypoglycemia and hyperkalemia and may accentuate damage in ischemic cerebrovascular and cardiac tissue. If focal neurologic signs are present, it may be prudent to withhold glucose, because hypoglycemia rarely causes focal signs (less than 10%).

Thiamine. This agent is administered to avoid precipitating the thiamine deficiency encephalopathy (Wernicke-Korsakoff syndrome) in alcohol abusers and in malnourished patients. The overall incidence of thiamine deficiency in ethanol abusers is 12%. Thiamine at 100 mg intravenously (IV) should be administered around the time of the glucose administration but not necessarily before the glucose, because it is more important to correct the hypoglycemia. The clinician should be prepared to manage anaphylaxis associated with thiamine, but it is extremely rare.

Naloxone. This reverses CNS and respiratory depression, miosis, bradycardia, and decreased GI peristalsis caused by opioids acting through mu, kappa, and delta receptors. It also affects endogenous opioid peptides (endorphins and enkephalins), which accounts for the variable responses reported in intoxications with ethanol, BZPs, clonidine, captopril (Capoten), and valproic acid and in spinal cord injuries. There is a high sensitivity for predicting a response if pinpoint pupils and circumstantial evidence of opioid abuse (e.g., track marks) are present.

In suspected overdose in a child younger than 5 years, naloxone is administered IV in a dose of 0.1 mg per kg up to 2 mg; in older children and adults administer 2 mg every 2 minutes for 5 doses up to a total of 10 mg. Naloxone can also be administered into an endotracheal tube. If there is no response after 10 mg has been given, pure opioid intoxication is unlikely. If opioid abuse is suspected, restraints should be in place before the administration of naloxone, and it is recommended that the initial dose be 0.1 to 0.2 mg to avoid withdrawal and violent behavior. The initial dose is then doubled every minute progressively to a total of 10 mg. Naloxone may unmask concomitant sympathomimetic intoxication as well as withdrawal.

Larger doses of naloxone may be required for more poorly antagonized synthetic opioid drugs: buprenorphine (Buprenex), codeine, dextromethorphan, fen-

TABLE 14. **Plasma Drug Concentrations Above Which Removal by Extracorporeal Measures May Be Indicated***

Drug	Plasma Concentration	Protein Binding (%)	Vd (L/kg)	Method of Choice
Amanitin	Not available	25	1.0	HP
Ethanol	500–700 mg/dL	0	0.3	HD
Ethchlorvynol	150 μg/mL	35–50	3–4	HP
Ethylene glycol	25–50 μg/mL	0	0.6	HD
Glutethimide	100 μg/mL	50	2.7	HP
Isopropyl alcohol	400 mg/dL	0	0.7	HD
Lithium	4 mEq/L	0	0.7	HD
Meprobamate	100 μg/mL	0	NA	HP
Methanol	50 mg/dL	0	0.7	HD
Methaqualone	40 μg/dL	20–60	6.0	HP
Other barbiturates	50 μg/dL	50	0–1	HP
Paraquat	0.1 mg/dL	Poor	2.8	HP>HD
Phenobarbital	100 μg/dL	50	0.9	HP>HD
Salicylates	80–100 mg/dL	90	0.2	HD>HP
Theophylline		0	0.5	
Chronic	40–60 μg/mL			HP
Acute	80–100 μg/mL			HP
Trichloroethanol	250 μg/mL	70	0.6	HP

*In mixed or chronic drug overdoses, extracorporeal measures may be considered at lower drug concentrations.

Abbreviations: HP = hemoperfusion; HD = hemodialysis; HP>HD = hemoperfusion preferred over hemodialysis.

Modified from Winchester JF: Active methods for detoxification. *In* Haddad LM, Winchester JF (eds): Clinical Management of Poisoning and Drug Overdose, 2nd ed. Philadelphia, WB Saunders Co, 1990, pp 148–167; Balsam L, Cortitsidis GN, Fienfeld DA: Role of hemodialysis and hemoperfusion in the treatment of intoxications. Contemp Manage Crit Care 61–71, 1990.

tanyl, pentazocine (Talwin), propoxyphene (Darvon), diphenoxylate, nalbuphine (Nubain), new potent "designer" drugs, or long-acting opioids such as methadone.

Indications for a continuous infusion include a second dose for recurrent respiratory depression, exposure to poorly antagonized opioids, a large overdose, and decreased opioid metabolism (e.g., impaired liver function). A continuous infusion has been advocated because many opioids outlast the short half-life ($t_{1/2}$) of naloxone (30 to 60 minutes). The naloxone infusion hourly rate is equal to the effective dose required to produce a response (improvement in ventilation and arousal). An additional dose may be required in 15 to 30 minutes as a bolus. The infusions are titrated to avoid respiratory depression and manifestations of opioid withdrawal. Tapering of infusions can be attempted after 12 hours and when the patient's condition has been stabilized.

Complications: Although naloxone is safe and effective, there are rare reports (in less than 1% of cases) of complications of pulmonary edema, seizures, hypertension, cardiac arrest, and sudden death.

Role Not Clarified

Nalmefene (Revex). This long-acting parenteral opioid antagonist, approved by the FDA, is undergoing investigation but its role for comatose patients and in opioid overdose is not clear. It is 16 times more potent than naloxone, and its duration of action is up to 8 hours ($t_{1/2}$ of 10.8 hours, compared with 1 hour for naloxone).

Flumazenil (Romazicon). This agent is a pure competitive BZP antagonist. It has been demonstrated to be safe and effective for BZP-induced sedation. It is not recommended to improve ventilation. Its role in CNS depression needs to be clarified. It should not be used routinely for comatose patients and is not an essential ingredient of the coma therapeutic regimen. It is contraindicated in cyclic antidepressant intoxications, in stimulant overdose, in long-term BZP use (may precipitate life-threatening withdrawal), if BZPs are used to control seizures, and in head trauma. There have been reports of seizures, dysrhythmias, and death.

Convulsions

Convulsions may be the direct effect of the toxin or secondary to hypoxia or other metabolic or electrolyte disturbances.

Specific therapy should be administered, for example, 100% oxygen for CO, calcium for ethylene glycol–produced hypocalcemia, intravenous glucose for intoxications that induce hypoglycemia, and pyridoxine and diazepam for isoniazid seizures and *Gyromitra* mushroom toxicity. Seizures in patients receiving lithium, salicylates, or theophylline may indicate toxic concentrations in the brain that require hemodialysis or hemoperfusion.

As anticonvulsants, diazepam and lorazepam are the agents of choice, but recurrent or persistent seizures require the use of phenobarbital and possibly neuromuscular blockers (as adjuncts), pentobarbital coma, or general anesthesia. Rapid intravenous injection of propylene glycol, the vehicle in BZP and phenytoin intravenous preparations, may cause dysrhythmias, hypotension, apnea, and shock. Therefore, the clinician should inject slowly (Table 15), administer with cardiac and blood pressure monitoring, and be prepared with ventilatory support to treat apnea. The patient should be monitored throughout the infusion and until 60 minutes after its completion. The propylene glycol vehicle may add to the toxicity in ethylene glycol intoxications. PEG, the vehicle for lorazepam, can be nephrotoxic when used long term. See Table 15 for anticonvulsant doses in children. Table 16 gives the treatment of status epilepticus.

BZPs enhance the activity of γ-aminobutyric acid (GABA), the major inhibitory neurotransmitter. Respiratory depression and hypotension occur in about 10% of patients.

Diazepam enters the brain rapidly and acts within seconds, but its duration of action is only 20 to 30 minutes. BZPs are administered directly or as close to the intravenous puncture site as possible to avoid adherence to tubing. They should be administered slowly. See Tables 15 and 16.

Lorazepam (Ativan) is a BZP but has a slower onset of action (2 to 3 minutes compared with seconds) and a longer duration of action (2 to 12 hours compared with 20 to 30 minutes) than diazepam. See Tables 15 and 16.

Midazolam (Versed) depresses all levels of the CNS through increased action of GABA. The $t_{1/2}$ is 2 to 4 hours, and the duration of sedation is 30 minutes to 2 hours, although its effects may last for 10 hours or more after infusion. The dosage is 0.05 to 0.1 mg per kg IV, with a maximum of 2.5 mg per dose over 2 minutes. Respiratory arrest may occur if it is given rapidly or in excessive doses. Although not approved by the FDA, it has been used safely and effectively in status epilepticus refractory to standard anticonvulsants.

Phenytoin stabilizes neuronal membranes and reduces sodium influx and calcium passage through the membranes. Phenytoin is effective as a single agent in termination of 56 to 80% of seizures, but with toxic and metabolic disturbances this rate falls to 40%. Phenytoin does not enhance the activity of GABA and therefore is not effective against cocaine, isoniazid, *Gyromitra* mushroom, and theophylline intoxications that interfere with GABA. Normal saline 0.89% (not glucose, which causes crystallization) is used to dilute the agent to a concentration of 10 mg per mL. A 0.22-μm filter should be placed on the intravenous line. Phenytoin acts within 20 minutes. Determine a phenytoin level 30 to 60 minutes after administration.

Phenobarbital interferes with the transmission of impulses from the thalamus to the cortex by enhancing the effect of GABA. A loading dose of 20 mg per kg gives a serum level of 20 μg per mL. The disadvantage of phenobarbital is its slow absorption by the brain parenchyma; 10 to 20 minutes is required for its anticonvulsive effects. It also has a long $t_{1/2}$ of 50 to 100 hours and alters the mental status for prolonged periods. It is the drug of choice for barbiturate withdrawal. The serum phenobarbital concentration is determined 30 to 60 minutes after administration.

Neuromuscular blockers or general anesthesia: If anticonvulsants fail to control seizures within 1 hour after their onset, the patient may require neuromuscular blockade and assisted ventilation. Refractory convulsions may be managed by general anesthesia with halothane. These agents are not anticonvulsants and require monitoring by electroencephalogram (EEG) for nonmotor brain seizure activity.

Pentobarbital anesthesia requires intubation, ven-

TABLE 15. **Common Anticonvulsant Therapy**

Agent	Dose	Maximal Rate of Delivery	Duration of Action
Children			
Diazepam IV	Initial 0.3 mg/kg Repeat 10–15 min Maximum 5 mg <5 y, 10 mg >5 y	1 mg/min	20–30 min
Phenytoin IV	15–20 mg/kg Maximum 30 mg/kg or 25 mg/min	1 mg/kg/min	6 h
Phenobarbital IV	10–20 mg/kg Maximum 40 mg/kg or 30 mg/min	1 mg/kg/min	6–8 h
Lorazepam IV	Initial 0.05–0.1 mg/kg Repeat 0.05 mg/kg	1 mg/min	2–12 h
Adults			
Diazepam IV	Initial 5–10 mg Repeat 10–15 min Maximum 30 mg	5 mg/min	20–30 min
Phenytoin IV	Initial 20 mg/kg Maximum 30 mg/kg	50 mg/min*	6 h
Phenobarbital IV	Initial 20 mg/kg Maximum 1200 mg	100 mg/min	6–8 h
Lorazepam IV	Initial 2–10 mg Repeat 10–15 min Maximum 10 mg	2 mg/min	2–12 h

*For adults with cardiopulmonary disease, administer less than 25 mg/min.

TABLE 16. **Management of Status Epilepticus**

Time	Procedure
0–5 min, immediate measures	1. Assess cardiorespiratory function; implement appropriate life support. 2. Take history, and perform neurologic and physical examination. 3. Continuously monitor vital signs; notify personnel for potential endotracheal intubation. 4. Obtain blood specimens for anticonvulsant drug levels, glucose, BUN, creatinine, calcium, magnesium, electrolytes, complete blood count, metabolic screen, drug screen, ABGs. Obtain EEG if possible.
6–9 min, initial treatment	5. Start IV infusion. If hypoglycemia confirmed or blood glucose determination unavailable, administer to adult 50 mL of 50% (25 gm) glucose, 100 mg of thiamine, 1–2 gm of magnesium to alcoholic or malnourished patients (child: 2 mL/kg 25% glucose).
10–45 min	6. For adult, infuse diazepam, 0.15–0.25 mg/kg, up to 30 mg total, not faster than 5 mg/min (child: 0.1–1.0 mg/kg up to 5 mg), or infuse lorazepam, 0.1 mg/kg, up to 10 mg total, not faster than 2 mg/min (child: 0.05–0.5 mg/kg, range 1–4 mg). 7. For adult, begin infusion of phenytoin, 18–20 mg/kg, not faster than 50 mg/min (child: 18–20 mg/kg, not faster than 1 mg/kg/min or 25 mg/min). This may take 20–40 min total; carefully monitor ECG, respiration, and blood pressure. If patient is receiving phenytoin, give 9 mg/kg. 8. If seizures persist, give additional phenytoin, 5 mg/kg, not faster than 50 mg/min (child: 1 mg/kg/min), and, if needed, another 5 mg/kg until a maximum of 30 mg/kg has been given.
46–60 min, refractory	9. If seizures persist, intubate and ventilate; for adult, administer phenobarbital, 20 mg/kg, not faster than 100 mg/min IV (child: 20 mg/kg, not faster than 1 mg/kg/min).
>1 h	10. If seizures persist, administer pentobarbital anesthesia, 5 mg/kg at 25 mg/min, followed by 0.5–3 kg/h; or general anesthesia with isoflurane should be implemented (anesthesiology assistance required); or propofol (Diprivan) anesthesia (anesthesiology assistance required); or midazolam: for adult, 5–10 mg bolus, not faster than 4 mg/min, followed by 0.05–0.4 mg/kg/h. Neuromuscular blockers, if needed; they are adjuncts, not anticonvulsants.

Abbreviations: ABGs = arterial blood gases; BUN = blood urea nitrogen; ECG = electrocardiogram; EEG = electroencephalogram.

Data from Watson C: Status epilepticus. Clinical features, pathophysiology, and treatment. West J Med *156*:558–559, 1991; Jagonda A, Riggio S: Refractory status epilepticus in adults. Ann Emerg Med *22*:1337–1348, 1993; and Cascarino GB: Generalized convulsive status epilepticus. Mayo Clin Proc *71*:787–792, 1996.

tilatory support, hemodynamic monitoring, preferably with a Swan-Ganz catheter, and continuous EEG monitoring. The loading dose is 5 mg per kg at an infusion rate of 25 mg per kg per minute, followed by maintenance at 2.5 mg per kg per hour to achieve an EEG that shows a suppression-burst pattern. Recurrent seizures are treated with a 50-mg bolus followed by an increase in the maintenance infusion to 0.5 mg per kg per hour. Tapering is recommended after 12 to 24 hours of EEG control at a rate of 0.5 to 1 mg per kg per hour every 4 to 6 hours.

Status epilepticus refers to a seizure episode that lasts for more than 30 minutes or a series of seizures during which the victim does not regain consciousness between seizures. After 90 minutes of seizure activity, CNS neuron damage occurs, electrolyte abnormalities develop, lactic acidosis develops within 30 minutes (it normalizes within 1 hour after the seizures cease), and convulsions become more difficult to control.

Substances that cause refractory seizures include alcohol, amphetamines, amoxapine (Asendin), cocaine, isoniazid, lead (chronic lead encephalopathy), and theophylline.

Complications of prolonged seizures include hypoxia, hypoglycemia, hyperthermia, hypotension, dysrhythmias, rhabdomyolysis and myoglobinemia, pulmonary and cerebral edema, and disseminated intravascular coagulation. In addition, leukemoid reactions and cerebrospinal fluid (CSF) pleocytosis develop.

The treatment of status epilepticus is outlined in Table 16.

Pulmonary Edema

Pulmonary edema complicating poisoning may be cardiac or noncardiac. See Table 6 for causes of pulmonary edema.

In underlying cardiac disorders, left atrial pressure and pulmonary capillary hydrostatic pressure are increased. This is accompanied by congestive heart failure. Fluid overload during forced diuresis may be a factor, particularly if the intoxicants have an antidiuretic effect (e.g., opioids, barbiturates, salicylates). Some toxic agents produce increased pulmonary capillary permeability, and other agents may cause a massive sympathetic discharge resulting in neurogenic pulmonary edema (e.g., opioids, salicylates). Management consists of fluid administration monitored by a Swan-Ganz catheter, administration of diuretics, use of vasopressors with afterload reduction, and use of inotropic agents and oxygen. If renal failure is present, hemodialysis may be necessary.

The noncardiac type of pulmonary edema occurs with inhaled toxins, such as ammonia, chlorine, and oxides of nitrogen, or with drugs, such as salicylates, opioids, paraquat, and intravenous ethchlorvynol (Placidyl). This type does not respond to cardiac support measures and requires oxygen with intensive respiratory management, using mechanical ventilation with positive end-expiratory pressure (PEEP) if necessary.

Hypotension and Circulatory Shock

Hypotension and circulatory shock may be caused by heart failure resulting from myocardial depression, hypovolemia (from fluid loss or venous pooling), decrease in peripheral vasculature resistance (adrenergic blockage), or loss of vasomotor tone occurring with CNS depression. See Table 6 for causes of hypotension.

Management consists of correction of hypoxia, volume expansion, correction of acidosis, rewarming in hypothermia, correction of electrolyte disturbances, and treatment of dysrhythmias producing hypotension and vasopressors, if necessary.

Vasopressors may be considered earlier if there is danger of fluid overload. Dopamine infused at 2 to 20 μg per kg per minute is the vasopressor usually chosen. However, for agents producing alpha-receptor blockage that are antidopaminogenic (e.g., PTZs, tricyclic antidepressants), norepinephrine, an alpha agonist, is preferable and is infused at 4 to 8 μg per minute in adults (0.1 to 1.0 μg per kg per minute in children) titrated every 5 to 10 minutes to the desired effect. Epinephrine infusion at 1 μg per kg per minute titrated to the desired response may also be used. Vasopressors may be used in combination. Norepinephrine and epinephrine are the agents of choice in severe hypotension.

Treatment is required for cardiac dysrhythmias that contribute to hypotension and poor perfusion (usually with rates lower than 40 per minute or above 180 per minute in adults). A wide QRS interval is treated immediately with an $NaHCO_3$ bolus. Table 17 shows specific agents for cardiotoxic intoxications.

Hypothermic hypotension does not respond to fluids but does respond to warming. In hypothermia with a body temperature of 32°C (90°F), a systolic blood pressure of 70 to 90 mm Hg would be expected.

Cerebral Edema

Cerebral edema or increased intracranial pressure in intoxicated patients is produced by hypoxia, hypercapnia, hypotension, hypoglycemia, and drug-impaired capillary integrity. Computed tomography (CT) may aid in diagnosis. Cerebral edema is managed by attempting to control cerebral blood volume to maintain mean arterial pressure (MAP) between 60 and 90 mm Hg and cerebral perfusion pressure between 50 and 70 mm Hg. The cerebral perfusion pressure is calculated as the difference between the MAP and the intracranial pressure. Inappropriate secretion of antidiuretic hormone may play a role in some poisonings, including those involving acetylsalicylic acid, barbiturates, carbamazepine (Tegretol), chlorpropamide (Diabinese), indomethacin (Indocin), opioids (especially morphine), sympathomimetics, tolbutamide (Orinase), and tricyclic antidepressants.

Management consists of correction of the ABGs, metabolic abnormalities, and blood pressure, as well as monitoring of intake and output, urine specific gravity, the patient's daily weight, serum electrolytes, blood urea nitrogen (BUN), creatinine, hemoglobin, and hematocrit. In addition, a chest radiograph and cranial CT scan should be obtained. Assessment by a neurosurgeon is advised; intracranial pressure monitors are helpful but may be associated with complications.

If the sodium value is low enough to produce major CNS symptoms, the serum sodium level should be raised 5 to 10 mEq per liter to correct symptoms. Furosemide (Lasix) is administered in a dose of 0.25 to 0.5 mg per kg, and concentrated sodium chloride, 6 mEq per kg, is given to raise the serum sodium value by 10 mEq per liter.

The increased intracranial pressure may be reduced by giving 20% mannitol, 0.5 to 1.0 gram per kg (100 grams in 500 mL of D5W, infused over a 30-minute period, acts in minutes and peaks in 90 minutes).

Hyperventilation to a carbon dioxide tension (PCO_2) of 25 mm Hg (not below 25) reduces intracranial pressure within 2 to 30 minutes. Hypocapnia produces pH-mediated cerebrovascular vasoconstriction that decreases the cerebral blood flow 5% for each millimeter fall in PCO_2. However, respiratory support with PEEP raises the intracranial pressure.

The head should be elevated 30 degrees if the vital signs are stable.

Fluid administration to correct dehydration and for daily maintenance should be minimized.

Most current studies have demonstrated no improvement in functional outcome in head injury with high-dose corticosteroids, but they reduce edema around a tumor or abscess.

Pentobarbital, in a loading dose of 5 to 30 mg per kg IV, is given to stabilize the membranes, to decrease neuronal metabolism, and to suppress bursts as seen on the EEG.

Table 17. **Specific Therapy for Cardiotoxic Ingestions**

Toxic Ingestion	Specific Therapy	Vasopressor
Beta-adrenergic antagonist	Glucagon	Epinephrine
	Amrinone (Inocor) Isoproterenol	Dobutamine
Calcium channel blocker	Calcium Glucagon Sodium bicarbonate Amrinone	Dopamine Dobutamine Isoproterenol
Alpha-adrenergic antagonist	Norepinephrine or phenothiazine	Phenylephrine
Cyclic antidepressants	Sodium bicarbonate	Norepinephrine Phenylephrine
Cholinergic agents	Atropine	Dopamine
Opioids	Naloxone	Dopamine
Magnesium	Calcium	Dopamine

Hypertension

Hypertension in a young person is more significant than that in a chronically hypertensive individual. Hypertension associated with poisonings is initially transient and does not require therapy. However, an emergency hypertensive crisis, although rare, can develop during alcohol withdrawal, cocaine and other sympathomimetic drug overdose, opioid withdrawal, MAOI drug and food interaction and overdose, and sudden discontinuation of antihypertensive therapy.

Acute emergency hypertensive crisis is defined as a diastolic blood pressure greater than 120 to 130 mm Hg or, more important, associated with target organ damage. Manifestations of target organ damage are classified as cardiac (pulmonary edema, myocardial ischemia or infarction), CNS (mental status changes, coma, convulsions or cerebrovascular accident), renal (hematuria, azotemia), and retinopathy (papilledema, hemorrhages).

Acute emergency hypertensive crisis is managed with nitroprusside, 10 μg per kg per minute for no longer than 10 minutes and then 0.3 to 2 μg per kg per minute (maximal dose 2 μg per kg per minute). Therapy at higher rates or for more than 48 to 72 hours or renal insufficiency may cause accumulation of thiocyanate, a toxic metabolite, and the thiocyanate level should be determined at 48 hours of therapy. Thiocyanate poisoning (paresthesia, tinnitus, blurred vision, delirium) is treated with 25% sodium thiosulfate, 1.65 mL per kg, without sodium nitrite and without waiting for laboratory confirmation. Diazoxide or longer acting antihypertensives are usually not recommended because they have a prolonged duration of action. See Table 18.

If focal neurologic signs are present, treatment for mild or moderate hypertension is omitted and CT is performed.

Dysrhythmias

Cardiac dysrhythmias can occur with poisoning. A wide QT interval occurs with PTZs, and a wide QRS complex occurs with tricyclic antidepressants, quinine, or quinidine overdose. Digitalis, cocaine, cyanide, propranolol, theophylline, and amphetamines are among the more frequent toxic causes of dysrhythmias. Normalization of metabolic disturbances and adequate oxygenation correct many of the dysrhythmias; antidysrhythmic drugs or a cardiac pacemaker or cardioversion may be required in other cases.

Life-threatening hemodynamically unstable ventricular dysrhythmias should receive direct current (DC) conversion. Synchronized DC conversion should be used with caution in digitalis intoxication because of the tendency to produce ventricular fibrillation. This is an indication for Fab. If DC conversion is used in digitalis intoxications, start with the lowest electrical dose.

For less urgent ventricular tachycardia, intravenous lidocaine at 1 to 3 mg per kg with electrocardiogram (ECG) and blood pressure monitoring may be used.

Tricyclic antidepressant overdose with evidence of cardiac toxicity such as wide QRS tachycardia should be treated with a bolus of $NaHCO_3$ at 2 mEq per kg IV.

Primary therapy for torsades de pointes consists of magnesium sulfate, 2 grams slowly IV as a 20% solution over 1 minute, followed by an infusion of 1 gram per hour. In children the dose is 25 to 50 mg per kg. Overdrive pacing may also be used. If hemodynamic compromise is present, DC conversion is used. Class I and class III antidysrhythmic agents should be avoided. See Table 6 for etiologic factors and Table 12 for dosages.

Unstable bradycardia and second- and third-degree heart block should be managed in an emergency with a transvenous or external pacemaker. Less urgent cases in which the patient is unstable, with bradycardia (syncope, hypotension), are treated with atropine at 0.01 to 0.03 mg per kg IV (minimum, 0.1 mg) or isoproterenol at 1 to 10 μg per minute IV. Hypothermia with a body temperature of 32 to 35°C (90 to 95°F) is associated with bradycardia, with a heart rate of 40 to 50 beats per minute, which becomes normal on rewarming.

Unexplained cardiac arrest in a young person warrants examination for drugs hidden in the bowel, vagina, or rectum (as in "body packing" or "body stuffing").

Specific antidotal therapy and vasopressors for cardiac toxicity are listed in Table 17.

Renal Failure

Renal failure may be due to tubular necrosis as a result of hypotension or hypoxia or a direct effect of the poison (e.g., salicylate, paraquat, acetaminophen, carbon tetrachloride) or heavy metals on the tubular cells. With hemoglobinuria or myoglobinuria, hemoglobin or myoglobin may precipitate in the renal tubules and produce renal failure.

The mechanisms of renal damage by toxin include

- Acute tubular necrosis, which is due to prolonged ischemia, nephrotoxic agents, heavy metals, aminoglycosides (which act on proximal tubules), and radiographic contrast media (in patients older than 65 years, those with diabetes mellitus)
- Drug-induced acute interstitial nephritis (e.g., penicillins, sulfonamides, nonsteroidal anti-inflammatory drugs [NSAIDs])
- Inter-renal deposition of pigment (myoglobinuria often associated with rhabdomyolysis, hemoglobinuria)

TABLE 18. **Antihypertensive Drugs for Emergency Use**

Drug	Adult Dose	Pediatric Dose
Nitroprusside	0.3–2 mg/kg/min; 10 μg/kg/min can be given for 10 min initially	Same
Phentolamine	2.5–5 mg IV slowly	0.02–0.1 mg/kg IV slowly
Labetalol	20 mg IV q 10 min	0.5 mg/kg IV followed by 0.25 mg/kg q 2 h
Diazoxide	1–3 mg/kg IV, maximum of 150 mg IV q 5–15 min until desired effect; repeat q 4–24 h	Same

- Any significant hypotension or ischemia caused by a toxin

Rhabdomyolysis

Rhabdomyolysis (muscle necrosis) occurs with prolonged immobilization on a hard surface, violent muscle activity, prolonged convulsions, myositis, and some metabolic myopathies. Destruction of the muscle membrane causes lysis or leakage of the muscle cytoplasmic constituents including myoglobin. Rhabdomyolysis has more than 150 causes but occurs most frequently with intoxications by amphetamines, ethanol, heroin, cocaine, and phencyclidine.

Myoglobinemia and myoglobinuria may occur with or without rhabdomyolysis. The creatine kinase level is often higher than 10,000 units. Rhabdomyolysis may result in myoglobinuria, in which myoglobin can precipitate in the renal tubules and cause renal failure, compartment syndrome, disseminated intravascular coagulation, and metabolic abnormalities.

Management of myoglobinuria consists of fluid diuresis to produce a urine output of 3 to 5 mL per kg per hour or 200 to 350 mL per hour and administration of furosemide at 2 to 5 mg per kg up to 200 mg in adults and mannitol, 0.5 gram per kg of a 20% solution (25 grams in adults), over 30 minutes, if necessary. Alkalization of the urine to pH greater than 7.0 by adding $NaHCO_3$ to intravenous fluids is controversial but should be considered if acidosis is present or if there are high levels of potassium. Any associated electrolyte abnormalities, metabolic acidosis, and hyperthermia should be corrected, with institution of monitoring as appropriate.

Acute Hepatic Failure

Acute fulminant hepatic failure is a clinical syndrome resulting from massive necrosis of liver cells leading to encephalopathy and severe impairment of hepatic function. The encephalopathy is usually present and prior liver disease is usually absent. The condition is potentially reversible. Acute hepatic encephalopathy is a universal feature of acute hepatic failure (AHF). Onset is abrupt, usually within 5 to 7 days of massive hepatic failure. Cerebral edema occurs in 75 to 80% of patients whose condition progresses to coma and is the leading cause of death. The most frequent cause is infectious. Other frequent causes include hepatotoxic drugs. The mechanisms of toxin-induced hepatotoxicity are as follows:

- Direct hepatocellular damage by phallotoxins binding to hepatocyte membranes (e.g., *A. phalloides*)
- Metabolic conversion of acetaminophen to a hepatotoxic intermediate metabolite (*N*-acetyl-*p*-benzoquinonimine [NAPQI])
- A vascular disturbance such as hepatic vein thrombosis (pyrrolizidine alkaloids)

The clinical and morphologic presentations are

Acute hepatitis: methyldopa, isoniazid, phenytoin, NSAIDs, lovastatin

Cholestasis: androgens, oral contraceptives, erythromycin estolate, metronidazole (Flagyl), chlorpropamide, chlorpromazine, increased alkaline phosphatase and bilirubin

Hepatic necrosis: acetaminophen, carbon tetrachloride, *A. phalloides,* yellow phosphorus

Chronic hepatitis: methyldopa, arsenic, isoniazid, halothane

The laboratory and clinical evidence does not become apparent until at least 24 to 36 hours after exposure to the toxin. If the hepatic damage is severe, the bilirubin and prothrombin time continue to worsen after 2 to 3 days. Metabolic acidosis and hypoglycemia are signs of poor prognosis.

Vasodilators of the microcirculation of the liver (e.g., NAC) may affect nitric oxide–induced control of vascular tone and increase oxygen delivery to the liver. Many patients appear to benefit from administration of NAC as an antidote for acetaminophen (APAP) toxicity. In addition, NAC prolongs survival, allowing orthotopic liver transplantation (OLT) in patients with APAP toxicity and in patients with AHF of other toxic and nontoxic causes. Hepatotoxicity is aggravated in chronic alcoholics and patients chronically receiving enzyme inducer drugs such as anticonvulsants.

Criteria for OLT in fulminant liver failure are listed in Table 19. Mortality without treatment is greater than 80% and with OLT is 60 to 80%. This indicates 20% unnecessary OLT procedures. The mortality with lesser grade encephalopathy is only 20%.

Temperature Disturbances

Although the most frequent cause of temperature elevation in toxicologic emergencies is infection (usu-

TABLE 19. **Criteria for Predicting Death and the Need for Liver Transplantation**

Cause	Criteria
Acetaminophen poisoning	pH <7.3 regardless of grade of encephalopathy* or prothrombin time >100 s Serum creatinine >3.4 mg/dL (300 μmol/L) or >2 mg/dL In patients with grade 3 or 4 encephalopathy Bilirubin >20 mg/dL
All other causes	Prothrombin time >100 s (regardless of grade of encephalopathy) or any three of the following (regardless of grade of encephalopathy): • Age younger than 10 y or older than 40 y • Liver failure caused by non-A, non-B hepatitis or halothane-induced hepatitis, or idiosyncratic drug reaction • Duration of jaundice >7 d before onset of encephalopathy or >2 d after onset of encephalopathy • Prothrombin time >50 s • Bilirubin >17.5 mg/dL (300 μmol/L)

*Encephalopathy classification: grade 1 = confused or altered mood; grade 2 = inappropriate behavior or drowsiness (mild obtundation); grade 3 = stuporous but arrestable, markedly confused behavior; grade 4 = coma with or without decerebrate posturing unresponsive to painful stimuli.

Modified from O'Grady JG, Alexander GJM, Hayllar KM, Williams R: Early indicators of prognosis in fulminant hepatic failure. Gastroenterology *97*:439–445, 1989; and Caraceni P, Van Thiel DH: Acute liver failure. Lancet *345*(8943):163–169, 1995. © by The Lancet Ltd, 1995.

ally secondary to aspiration pneumonia), elevations are often not associated with the prostaglandin mechanisms of fever. See Table 6 for causes of temperature elevation.

Hyperthermia in toxicologic emergencies is due to excess muscle activity, hypermetabolic state, interferences with oxidative phosphorylation, and impaired dissipation of heat. It occurs in anticholinergic, sympathomimetic overdoses (i.e., with cocaine) and ethanol withdrawal. Toxicologic temperature elevations require external cooling measures, control of excess muscular activity such as convulsions, and, in malignant hyperthermia, dantrolene and bromocriptine. Antipyretics are not useful in these cases.

Hyperthermia syndromes involve life-threatening elevations of temperature. The syndromes are characterized by altered mental state, rigidity, metabolic acidosis, and temperature elevation, except in the serotonin syndrome.

The neuroleptic malignant syndrome is an idiosyncratic reaction occurring in patients receiving neuroleptic medications (PTZs and butyrophenones).

Malignant hyperthermia (MH) is associated with drug interactions—for example, when synthetic opioids (e.g., meperidine) or tricyclic antidepressants are administered to patients receiving MAOIs.

The serotonin syndrome may occur with or without hyperthermia. It occurs in patients receiving MAOIs who take serotonergic drugs (meperidine, clomipramine) or serotonin inhibitors (fluoxetine [Prozac], sertraline [Zoloft], paroxetine [Paxil]) without a drug-free interval of at least 5 weeks.

Management of hyperthermia consists of the following measures:

1. The offending agent is immediately discontinued. Hyperventilation with 100% humidified cooled oxygen at high gas flow rates, at least 10 liters per minute, is instituted.
2. A BZP is required to allow the patient to tolerate the cooling measures, such as an ice bath. It reduces motor activity and muscle tone and protects the patient from seizures (e.g., with cocaine, amphetamines).
3. Acid-base and electrolyte disturbances are corrected. Hyperkalemia is common and, if life-threatening, should be treated with hyperventilation, calcium bicarbonate, and intravenous glucose and insulin. If it is refractory, hemodialysis may be necessary.
4. Simultaneously, active cooling of the patient (e.g., with intravenous cold saline, not lactated Ringer's); lavage of the stomach, bladder, and rectum with cold saline; and use of a hypothermic blanket are begun. The core body temperature should be monitored.
5. Dysrhythmias usually respond to treatment of acidosis and hyperkalemia. Antidysrhythmic agents may be used if needed, with the exception of calcium channel blockers (which may cause hyperkalemia and cardiovascular collapse).
6. ABGs, creatine kinase, electrolytes and calcium, clotting, core temperature, serum and urine myoglobin, and urine output should be determined and monitored. Monitoring with a central line may be optimal.
7. Dantrolene sodium, a phenytoin derivative, inhibits calcium release from the sarcoplasmic reticulum, resulting in decreased muscle contraction.

Dantrolene, which acts peripherally, used with dopamine agonists, bromocriptine mesylate, or amantadine hydrochloride (Symmetrel), which acts centrally, has been reported to be successful in combination with cooling and good supportive measures in MH. Dantrolene does not reverse the rigidity or psychomotor disturbances resulting from the central dopamine blockade and is therefore often used in combination with bromocriptine.

The dose of dantrolene is 2 to 3 mg per kg given IV as a bolus and then 1 mg per kg per minute, with incremental increases (average dose 2 to 5 mg per kg). The loading dose is repeated every 10 minutes (maximum total dose 10 mg per kg) or until the signs of MH (e.g., tachycardia, rigidity, increased end-tidal carbon dioxide, and temperature elevation) are controlled. Hepatotoxicity occurs at doses higher than 10 mg per kg. To prevent recurrence, a dose of 1 mg per kg is administered every 6 hours for 24 to 48 hours after the episode. After that, oral dantrolene is used at 1 mg per kg every 6 hours for 24 hours as necessary. Thrombophlebitis is a potential complication after dantrolene administration. The drug is best administered into a central vein.

8. Bromocriptine mesylate at 2.5 to 10 mg PO or through a nasogastric tube three times a day or amantadine at 100 mg twice a day has been used; there are no scientific data concerning the efficacy of these agents, but the use of either seems theoretically reasonable. They are to be used with dantrolene.

Hypothermia means a temperature below 95°F (35°C). It may occur when an overdose (e.g., of a CNS depressant) interferes with physiologic responses (vasoconstriction, muscle activity) when the victim is exposed to a cool environment. Hypothermia is frequently associated with hypoglycemia. See Table 6 for potential causes.

The management depends on body temperature and hemodynamic stability. Glucose is administered if the patient is hypoglycemic. In severe hypothermia, there may be bradycardia with a heart rate of 40 to 50 beats per minute, and hypotension (70 to 90 mm Hg systolic) should not be vigorously treated or fluid overload may occur. Management consists of rewarming by the following methods:

1. Body temperatures of 32 to 35°C (89.6 to 95°F) with stable hemodynamics are managed by increasing the body's heat production with gradual external rewarming at 1°C per hour, for example, by wrapping in insulated material such as blankets, offering warm liquids if the patient is alert, and providing a warm environment.
2. Body temperatures of 30 to 32°C (86 to 89.6°F)

with stable hemodynamics require transfer of heat to the patient, for example, with heated blankets, warmed intravenous solutions (D5W 0.9% saline warmed to 37 to 43°C), and warmed humidified oxygen. Cardiac monitoring should be carried out.

3. Body temperatures of 30 to 32°C (86 to 89.6°F) with unstable hemodynamics necessitate the initiation of active core rewarming in addition to the preceding measures, for example, with heated humidified oxygen (42 to 45°C), a warming bath (40 to 41°C), and heated GI irrigation (gastric lavage and colonic enemas). Vital signs must be monitored.

4. Body temperatures below 30°C (86°F) require rapid rewarming by invasive procedures because of the danger of ventricular fibrillation; for example, peritoneal lavage with heated dialysate (40 to 42°C), extracorporeal blood rewarming, or thoracotomy and mediastinal lavage with heated fluids can be used. Vital signs require close monitoring.

The Agitated, Violent, and Psychotic Victim

Violence is aggressive assault or combativeness. Agitation is uncontrollable restlessness or excessive excitability. Psychosis is a mental derangement that may cause violence or aggression. Affected patients may harm themselves and others. See Table 4 for a classification of the severity of the effects of stimulants.

The causes of violence may be psychiatric, situational frustration, and organic diseases. Most patients labeled as violent are schizophrenic, especially of the paranoid type (30 to 40%). Organic violent behavior usually occurs in patients older than 40 years without a previous psychiatric history. The patients are disoriented, lethargic, or stuporous and have visual hallucinations or illusions and abnormal vital signs. No patient with physical restraints should be placed on a gurney. Physical restraints should not be used for psychiatric patients.

Drugs and chemicals may produce violence or precipitate violent psychosis in a patient with an underlying psychiatric disorder. Agents with which this occurs most frequently include amphetamines, anticholinergics (scopolamine, jimsonweed), cocaine, ethanol (intoxication, intolerance, and withdrawal), hallucinogens, phencyclidine, sedative hypnotics (intoxication or withdrawal), and occupational chemicals including sulfides and mercury.

The differential diagnosis requires exclusion of hypoxia, hypoglycemia, electrolyte disturbances, and metabolic and endocrine disorders. In one review, hypoglycemia accounted for 9% for violent patients. The diaphoretic violent patient usually has an organic cause of the disorder (e.g., hypoglycemia, sepsis, withdrawal, heatstroke, myocardial infarction, or pulmonary edema).

If physical restraints are needed, the reason must be recorded (e.g., to facilitate evaluation or because there is a psychiatric or personality disorder or a need to administer medication to prevent harm to the patient and/or others). Physical restraints should be monitored frequently (at least every 15 minutes, and the monitoring should be documented) to prevent neurovascular sequelae and to avoid rhabdomyolysis. Figure 1 shows a seclusion and restraint record.

Pharmacologic restraints include haloperidol and other agents and rapid tranquilization. Haloperidol (Haldol) produces competitive blockade of the postsynaptic dopamine receptors, depresses the cortex and hypothalamus, and has strong alpha-adrenergic and anticholinergic blocking activity. Do not use the long-acting decanoate salt of haloperidol.

The dose of haloperidol for young adults varies from 0.5 to 5 mg PO three times a day or 2 to 5 mg intramuscularly (IM) every 4 to 8 hours, as needed. The doses may be increased rapidly. For prompt control use 5 to 10 mg, repeated every 30 to 60 minutes for 8 doses. The maximum oral daily dose is 100 mg; the maximum intramuscular dose 0.1 mg per kg per day. If parenteral administration is used initially, it should be changed to the oral route as soon as possible. Doses higher than 10 mg do not increase effectiveness. The initial dose for the elderly patient should be decreased to 0.5 to 2.0 mg.

The side effects of haloperidol are primarily dystonic reactions, although the neuroleptic malignant syndrome has been described after a single dose. Avoid haloperidol in the presence of pregnancy, lactation, lithium (encephalopathic interaction), phencyclidine intoxication, withdrawal syndromes, and intoxications with drugs with anticholinergic properties. Haloperidol and PTZs both have undesirable anticholinergic and alpha-blocking effects.

Alternatives are lorazepam, thiothixene (Navane), fluphenazine (Prolixin), and droperidol (which causes hypotension). Chlorpromazine is not advised because of its alpha-adrenergic blocking effect, which causes orthostatic hypotension.

When rapid tranquilization is used, the patient should be advised that the medication will have a calming effect. A combination of antipsychotic medication with lorazepam is more effective than antipsychotic medication alone. Core psychotic symptoms do not respond to a few doses but require weeks of therapy. See Table 20.

Most patients respond to a combination of haloperidol at 5 mg IM or thiothixene at 10 mg and lorazepam at 5 mg IM in the same syringe. The medication is administered hourly. Most patients respond to 1 to 3 doses. The use of antipsychotic medications IV in the emergency department has not been well studied. The dosage should be reduced to half for patients older than 65 years.

Investigational Procedures Used in Toxicologic Emergencies

Extracorporeal membrane oxygenation has been considered for management of shock in tricyclic antidepressant and quinidine poisoning.

Intra-aortic balloon counterpulsation has been considered for management of poisoning caused by beta-adrenergic blockers, calcium channel blockers, and medications that cause a temporary decrease in coronary perfusion.

Name of Patient ______________________ Chart # ______________________

Date ______________ Seclusion Time in ______________ Time out ______________

Physician order obtained Dr. ______________________ Date ______________________

Limbs circle 1 2 3 4 Time in ______________ Time out ______________ Date ______________

The following measures to alter the patient's behavior have failed

[ ] Patient has been removed from stimuli

[ ] Patient has been encouraged to express feeling in usual manner

[ ] Staff has been assigned to listen to patient

[ ] Patient has been offered noncompetitive tasks to complete

[ ] Patient has been medicated

[ ] Other Specify ______________________

Reason for seclusion and restraint explained to patient.

____

Behavior necessitating restraint ______________________

____

Vital signs on admission to seclusion P __________ R __________ Temp __________ BP __________ Time __________

Name of physician (write clearly) ______________________

Nurse ______________________

Date	Time	Seclusion Room	VS q 15 min	Bath Room	Fluids (cc)	Food	Limb RA LA RL LL Waist	Circulation	Range of motion	Staff sign.

Figure 1. Seclusion and restraint record.

Surfactant has been considered for potential use in hydrocarbon aspiration and inhalation injuries and in near-drowning. In a study of aspirated hydrocarbons in animals it was found to be detrimental.

Transplantation of lungs has been tried unsuccessfully for paraquat poisoning.

Nondepolarizing neuromuscular blocking agents have produced prolonged paralysis when used in combination in a patient receiving corticosteroids.

Laboratory and Radiographic Studies

Initial studies should include an ECG for dysrhythmias or conduction delays (resulting from cardiotoxic medications); a chest radiograph for aspiration pneumonia (if there is a history of loss of consciousness, unarousable state, vomiting) and noncardiac pulmonary edema; and electrolyte and glucose concentrations in the blood. The anion gap (AG) should be calculated, and acid-base and ABG profiles (if the patient has respiratory distress or altered mental status) and serum osmolality assay should be obtained. See Table 21 for appropriate testing on the basis of clinical toxicologic presentation. All laboratory specimens should be carefully labeled, timed, and dated. For potential legal cases a "chain of custody" must be established. Assessment of the laboratory studies may give a clue to the etiologic agent.

Electrolyte, Acid-Base, and Osmolality Disturbances

Electrolyte and acid-base disturbances are evaluated and corrected. Metabolic acidosis (low pH with a low $Pa\text{CO}_2$ and low HCO_3^-) with an increased AG is seen with many agents in overdose.

Metabolic Acidosis and the Anion Gap. The AG is an estimate of the anions other than chloride and HCO_3^- necessary to counterbalance the positive charge of sodium. The AG gives a clue to the underlying disorder, compensation, and complications.

The AG is calculated from the standard serum electrolytes by subtracting the total carbon dioxide (which reflects the actual measured HCO_3^-) and chloride from the sodium: $Na^+ - (Cl^- + HCO_3^-) =$ AG. Potassium is usually not used in the calculation because it may be hemolyzed and is an intracellular cation. The lack of an AG disturbance does not exclude a toxic basis for the disorder.

The normal gap was found to be 8 to 12 mEq per liter by flame photometry. However, a lower normal AG of 7 ± 4 mEq per liter has been determined by newer techniques (e.g., use of ion-selective electrodes or coulometric titration). Some studies have found the AG to be relatively insensitive for determining the presence of toxins.

It is important to recognize the AG toxins salicylates, methanol, and ethylene glycol because they have specific antidotes and hemodialysis is effective in management.

A list of the potential causes of increased AG, decreased AG, or no AG is shown in Table 22. The most common cause of a decreased AG is laboratory error. Lactic acidosis produces the largest AG and can result from any poisoning that causes hypoxia, hypoglycemia, or convulsions.

TABLE 20. **Rapid Tranquilization of the Violent Patient**

Type	Tranquilization*
Schizophrenia, mania, or other psychosis	Lorazepam 2–4 mg IM combined with haloperidol 5 mg IM or thiothixene 10 mg IM OR Thiothixene 10 mg IM or 20 mg concentrate OR Haloperidol 5 mg IM or 10 mg concentrate OR Loxapine 10 mg IM or 25 mg concentrate PO
Personality disorder	Lorazepam 1–2 mg PO q 1–2 h or 2–4 mg (0.5 mg/kg) IM q 1–2 h
Alcohol withdrawal	
Agitation, tremors, abnormal VS	Chlordiazepoxide 25–50 mg PO q 4–6 h
Older than 65 y, liver disease	Lorazepam 2 mg PO q 2 h
Extreme agitation	Lorazepam 2–4 mg IM q h RT if not controlled
Cocaine or amphetamine	Mild to moderate agitation, thiothixene 10 mg PO q 8 h Severe agitation, thiothixene 10 mg IM or 20 mg concentrate or haloperidol 5 mg IM or 10 mg concentrate
Phencyclidine	
Mild hyperactivity, tension, anxiety, excitement	Diazepam 10–30 mg PO OR Lorazepam 2–4 mg IM (0.05 mg/kg)
Severe agitation, excitement, hallucinations, bizarre behavior	Haloperidol 5–10 mg IM q 30–60 min

*All doses given q 30–60 min, half the dose for those older than 65 y.
Abbreviations: RT = rapid tranquilization; VS = vital signs.
Modified from Dubin WR, Weiss KJ: Handbook of Psychiatric Emergencies. Springhouse, PA, Springhouse Corp, 1991, p 31.

TABLE 21. **Patient Condition/Systemic Toxin and Appropriate Tests**

Condition/ Toxin	Tests
Comatose	Toxicologic tests (acetaminophen, sedative hypnotic, ethanol, opioids, benzodiazepines) Glucose, ammonia, CT, CSF analysis
Respiratory toxin	Spirometry, ABGs, chest radiography, monitor O_2 saturation
Cardiac toxin	ECG 12-lead and monitoring, echocardiogram, serial cardiac enzymes, hemodynamic monitoring
Hepatic toxin	Enzymes (AST, ALT, GGT), ammonia, albumin, bilirubin, glucose, PT, APTT, amylase
Nephrotoxin	BUN, creatinine, electrolytes (Na^+, K^+, Mg^{2+}, Ca^{2+}, PO_4^{3-}), serum and urine osmolarity, 24-h urine for heavy metals, CK, serum and urine myoglobin, urinalysis, and urinary sodium
Bleeding	Platelets, PT, APTT, bleeding time, fibrin split products, fibrinogen type and match blood

Abbreviations: ALT = alanine aminotransferase; AST = aspartate aminotransferase; CSF = cerebrospinal fluid; CT = computed tomography; GGT = γ-glutamyltransferase; PT = prothrombin time; APTT = activated partial thromboplastin time; ABGs = arterial blood gases.

Other blood chemistry derangements that suggest certain intoxications are shown in Table 23.

Serum Osmolal Gaps. The serum *osmolality* is a measure of the number of molecules of solute per kilogram of solvent, or mOsm per kg of water. The *osmolarity* is solute per liter of solution, or mOsm per liter of water at a specified temperature. Osmolarity is usually a calculated value and osmolality is usually a measured value. They are considered interchangeable when 1 liter equals 1 kilogram. The normal serum osmolality is 280 to 290 mOsm per kg. Serum for the freezing point osmolarity measurement and serum electrolyte specimens for calculation should be drawn simultaneously.

The serum osmolal gap is defined as the difference between the measured osmolality determined by the freezing point method and the calculated osmolarity determined as follows: the serum sodium value multiplied by 2 plus the BUN divided by 3 (0.1 molecular weight [MW] of BUN), plus the blood glucose value divided by 20 (0.1 MW of glucose). This gap estimate is usually within 10 mOsm of the simultaneously measured serum osmolality. Ethanol, if present, may be included in the equation to eliminate its

TABLE 22. **Potential Causes of Metabolic Acidosis**

No Gap Hyperchloremic	Increased Gap Normochloremic	Decreased Gap
Acidifying agents	Methanol	Laboratory error†
Adrenal insufficiency	Uremia*	Intoxication (bromine, lithium)
Anhydrase inhibitors	Diabetic ketoacidosis*	Protein abnormal
Fistula	Paraldehyde,* phenformin	Sodium low
Osteotomies	Isoniazid	
Obstructive uropathies	Iron	
Renal tubular acidosis	Lactic acidosis†	
Diarrhea, uncomplicated*	Ethanol,* ethylene glycol*	
Dilutional hyperchloremia	Salicylates, starvation, solvents	
Sulfamylon		

*Indicates hyperosmolar situation. Studies have found that the anion gap may be relatively insensitive for determining the presence of toxins.
†Lactic acidosis caused by carbon monoxide, cyanide, hydrogen sulfide, hypoxia, ibuprofen, iron, isoniazid, ischemia, phenformin, salicylates, seizures, or theophylline.

TABLE 23. **Blood Chemistry Derangements in Toxicology**

Derangement	Toxin or Disease
Acetonemia without acidosis	Acetone or isopropyl alcohol
Hypomagnesemia	Ethanol, digitalis
Hypocalcemia	Ethylene glycol, oxalate, fluoride
Hyperkalemia	Beta blockers, acute digitalis, renal failure
Hypokalemia	Diuretics, salicylism, sympathomimetics, theophylline, corticosteroids, chronic digitalis
Hyperglycemia	Diazoxide, glucagon, iron, isoniazid, organophosphate insecticides, phenylurea insecticides, phenytoin, salicylates, sympathomimetic agents, thyroid, vasopressors
Hypoglycemia	Beta blockers, ethanol, insulin, isoniazid, oral hypoglycemic agents, salicylates
Elevated CK	Amphetamines, ethanol, cocaine, phencyclidine
Elevated creatinine and normal BUN	Isopropyl alcohol, diabetic ketoacidosis

influence on the osmolality; the ethanol concentration divided by 4.6 (0.1 of ethanol MW) is added to the equation. See Table 24.

Calculated mOsm =

$$2Na^{+} + \frac{\text{BUN (mg/dL)}}{3} + \frac{\text{blood glucose (mg/dL)}}{20} + \frac{\text{ethanol (mg/dL)}}{4.6}$$

The osmolal gap is valid for a hemodynamically intact individual; it is not valid in shock and the postmortem state. Metabolic disorders such as hyperglycemia, uremia, and dehydration increase the osmolarity but usually do not cause gaps greater than 10 mOsm per kg.

A gap greater than 10 mOsm per kg suggests that unidentified osmolal-acting substances are present: acetone, ethanol, ethylene glycol, ethchlorvynol, glycerin, isopropyl alcohol, isoniazid, ethanol, mannitol, methanol, $NaHCO_3$ (1 mEq per kg raises osmolality by 2 mOsm per liter), and trichloroethane. Alcohols and glycols should be sought when the degree of obtundation exceeds that expected from the blood ethanol concentration (BEC) or when other clinical conditions exist, such as visual loss (methanol), metabolic acidosis (methanol and ethylene glycol), and renal failure (ethylene glycol).

A falsely elevated osmolal gap may be produced by other low-molecular-weight un-ionized substances (acetone, dextran, dimethyl sulfoxide, diuretics, ethyl ether, mannitol, sorbitol, trichloroethane), diabetic ketoacidosis, hyperlipidemia, and unmeasured electrolytes (e.g., magnesium).

False-negative results can occur when a normal osmolal gap is reported in the presence of alcohol or glycol poisoning if the parent compound is already metabolized—as, for example, when the osmolal gap is measured after a significant time has elapsed since ingestion. In alcohol and glycol intoxications, an early osmolar gap is due to the relatively nontoxic parent drug, and delayed metabolic acidosis and an increased AG are due to the more toxic metabolites.

The serum concentration (mg per dL) = mOsm gap × MW of substance divided by 10.

See Table 24.

Radiographic Studies

Chest and neck radiographs are obtained for pathologic conditions such as aspiration pneumonia and pulmonary edema, for localization of foreign bodies, and to determine the location of the endotracheal tube.

Abdominal radiographs are obtained to detect radiopaque substances. A mnemonic for radiopaque substances seen on abdominal radiographs is CHIPES: C, chlorides and chloral hydrate; H, heavy metals (arsenic, barium, iron, lead, mercury, zinc); I, iodide; P, Play Doh, Pepto-Bismol, or phenothiazine (which does not always show up on an abdominal radiograph if already dissolved); E, enteric-coated tablets; S, sodium, potassium, and other elements in tablet form (bismuth, calcium, potassium) and solvents containing chlorides (e.g., carbon tetrachloride).

Toxicologic Studies

In the average toxicologic laboratory, false-negative results occur at a rate of 10 to 30% and false-positive results at a rate of 0 to 10%. Table 25 lists test interactions that should be considered.

The predictive value of a positive result is about 90%. A negative result of a toxicology screen does not

TABLE 24. **Alcohols and Glycols**

Alcohol or Glycol	1 mg/dL in Blood Raises Osmolality (mOsm/L) by	Molecular Weight	Conversion Factor*
Ethanol	0.228	40	4.6
Methanol	0.327	32	3.2
Ethylene glycol	0.190	62	6.2
Isopropanol	0.176	60	6.0
Acetone	0.182	58	5.8
Propylene glycol	Not available	72	7.2

*Example: methanol osmolality. Subtract the calculated osmolarity from the measured serum osmolality (freezing point method) = osmolar gap × 3.2 (0.1 molecular weight) = estimated serum methanol concentration.

TABLE 25. **Factors Interfering with Common Toxicologic Testing**

Drug or Toxin	Method*	Factors Causing False-Positives or Interferences
Acetaminophen	SC	Salicylate, methylsalicylate (can increase level 10% in μg/mL), phenol, salicylamide, bilirubin, renal failure (each 1 mg/dL increase in creatinine = 30 μg/mL acetaminophen)
	GC	Phenacetin
	HPLC	Cephalosporins, sulfonamides
	IA	Phenacetin
Amphetamines (*d*-amphetamines)	GC	Other volatile stimulant amines, meperidine metabolites, antihistamine metabolites
	IA	Phenylpropanolamine, ephedrine, fenfluramine, isometheptene, isoxsuprine, phentermine, phenmetrazine, doxepin,† labetalol, *l*-amphetamine in Vicks inhalers, ranitidine, ritodrine, benzathine penicillin‡ (FPIA)
	TLC	See amines just listed
Barbiturates	IA	NSAIDs produce false-negatives
Benzodiazepines	IA	Oxazepam, temazepam, alprazolam; NSAIDs produce false-negatives
Chloride	SC	Bromide (0.8 mEq of Cl = 1 mEq of Br)
Cocaine	IA	"Coca teas" (benzoylecgonine)
	TLC	Urochromes and endogenous acids
Creatinine	SC	Ketoacidosis may increase creatinine up to 2–3 mg/dL in end-point assays, cephalosporins, creatinine with rhabdomyolysis
Digoxin	IA	Endogenous digoxin-like natriuretic substances in newborn (1 ng/mL), renal failure (1 ng/mL), cross-reacting metabolites in renal failure (2 ng/mL), pregnancy, liver disease, oleander and other plant glycosides, digoxin-binding antibody (Fab)
Ethanol	SC	Other alcohols, ketones (by oxidation methods); isopropanol (by enzyme methods); *Candida albicans* and *Proteus*, ethanol production
Ethylene glycol	SC	Other glycols, propylene glycol in IV phenytoin, diazepam and others, triglycerides
	GC	Propylene glycol: falsely lowers value by interfering with internal standard
Iron	SC	Deferoxamine falsely lowers TIBC 15%; lavender-topped Vacutainer tube has EDTA, binds and lowers iron
Isopropanol	GC	Isopropanol in skin disinfectants may produce elevations in blood concentration up to 40 mg/dL but usually trivial
Lithium	Any method	Green-topped Vacutainer (heparin) tube with lithium may elevate lithium 6–8 mEq/L
Marijuana	IA	Passive inhalation of marijuana smoke can produce a urine level of marijuana metabolites of 20 μg/mL
11-Nor-9-carboxyltetra-hydrocannabinol	TLC	Melanin, steroids, methadone, antihistamines
Methemoglobinemia	SC	Sulfhemoglobinemia (10% cross-positive by co-oximeter), methylene blue (2 mg/kg transient false positive 15% methemoglobin level), hyperlipidemia (triglyceride 6000 mg/dL = methemoglobin 28.6%)
Opioids (morphine or codeine)	IA	Cross-reactive with hydrocodone, hydromorphine, oxycodone, 6-monoacetylmorphine, two poppy seed bagels for 16 h, one lemon poppy seed muffin, Vicks Formula 44
	TLC	Hydrocodone, dextromethorphan
Osmolarity	Any	Lavender-topped Vacutainer tubes (EDTA) 15 mOsm/L, gray-topped Vacutainer tubes (fluoride-oxalate) 150 mOsm/L, blue-topped Vacutainer tubes (citrate) 10 mOsm/L Falsely normal if vapor pressure methods used
Phencyclidine, dextromethorphan	IA	Phencyclidine analogues, phenothiazines, diphenhydramine, antihistamines, methadone, meperidine
Salicylates	SC	Phenothiazines, acetaminophen, ketosis, salicylamide, diflunisal, accumulated salicylate metabolites in renal failure (10% increased) Decreased or altered salicylate by bilirubin; phenylketones
	GC	Methylsalicylate, eucalyptol, theophylline
	HPLC	Antibiotics, theophylline
Theophylline	SC	Diazepam, caffeine, accumulated theophylline metabolites in renal failure
	HPLC	Acetazolamide, cephalosporins, endogenous xanthines and accumulated theophylline metabolites in renal failure
	IA	Caffeine, accumulated theophylline metabolites in renal failure

*All assays within a methodologic group are not equivalent. Performance depends on the specific brand or formulation.

†Doxepin gives unconfirmed amphetamine by Abbot Adx test. The test is negative if not confirmed by thin-layer chromatography (data from Merigen KS, Browning R, Kellerman A: Doxepin causing false-positive urine test for amphetamine. Ann Emerg Med *22:*1370, 1993).

‡Benzathine salt of phenoxypenicillin with Syva EMIT I polyclonal assay (data from Berthier M, Bonneau D, Mura P, et al: Benzathine as a cause for a false-positive test result for amphetamines. J Pediatr *127:*669–670, 1995).

Abbreviations: EDTA = ethylenediaminetetraacetic acid; FPIA = fluorescent polarization immunoassay; GC = gas chromatography (interferences more common with older methods); HPLC = high-performance liquid chromatography; IA = immunoassay; NSAIDs = nonsteroidal anti-inflammatory drugs; SC = spectrochemical; TIBC = total iron-binding capacity; TLC = thin-layer chromatography.

Adapted from Olsen KR: Poisoning & Drug Overdose, 2nd ed. Norwalk, CT, Appleton & Lange, 1994, pp 37–38.

exclude poisoning. The negative predictive value of toxicologic screening is about 70%. For example, the following BZPs may not be detected by routine screening tests for BZP: alprazolam (Xanax), clonazepam (Klonopin), temazepam (Restoril), and triazolam (Halcion).

The "toxic" urine screen is a qualitative urine test for several common drugs, usually substances of abuse (cocaine and metabolites, opioids, amphetamines, BZPs, barbiturates, phencyclidine). Results are usually available within 2 to 6 hours. Because these tests may vary in different hospitals and communities, the physician should determine exactly which substances are included in the toxic urine screen of the laboratory used.

It is always advisable to determine the plasma acetaminophen level in any intentional overdose situation, as there are no clinical manifestations to guide the decision about treatment except the plasma acetaminophen level more than 4 hours after ingestion. For best results, the treatment should be started within 8 hours.

Ethylene glycol, red blood cell cholinesterase, and serum cyanide assays are not readily available.

For certain ingestions quantitative blood levels should be obtained at specific times after ingestion to avoid spurious low values in the distribution phase that result from incomplete absorption. Table 26 lists the times after ingestion when the quantitative tests should be obtained (the elimination phase). It is always wise to obtain serial quantitative tests to follow the trend because the peak may be delayed.

The detection time is the number of days after intake of a substance during which a person would be expected to excrete detectable levels of the substance or metabolite in urine. In general, urine detection is possible for 1 to 3 days after cocaine exposure, 2 to 4 days after heroin (the presence of monoacetylmorphine is diagnostic of heroin use but is detectable for only 12 hours after use), and 2 to 4 days after phencyclidine; if use is chronic, double the time.

Nontoxic Ingestions (Table 27)

Criteria for nontoxic ingestion are as follows:

- There is absolute identification of the product.
- There is absolute assurance that a single product was ingested.
- There is assurance that there is no signal word from the Consumer Product Safety Commission on the container's label.
- The amount ingested is known to a good approximation.
- It is possible to call back at frequent intervals to determine whether symptoms have developed.
- The exposed person is free of symptoms.
- If the exposed person is younger than 1 year or older than 6 years, a satisfactory explanation of the circumstances is necessary to exclude chemical maltreatment by the caretaker in the former case and to exclude a "cry for help" indicating an intolerable home situation in the latter case.

COMMON POISONS

Acetaminophen (*N*-acetyl-*p*-aminophenol [APAP], Tylenol, called paracetaminol in the United King-

TABLE 26. **Substances with Which Quantitative Blood Values May Be Necessary***

Substance	Specimen	Time After Ingestion to Obtain Specimen	Toxic Concentration
Acetaminophen (see "Acetaminophen" above)	Serum	>4 h	>150 μg/mL at 4 h
Carboxyhemoglobin	Blood	Stat	Extrapolate
Carbamazepine	Serum	Stat	>12 μg/mL
Digoxin	Serum	6–8 h	>2 ng/mL adult, >4 ng/mL child
Ethanol	Serum	0.5–1 h	>80 mg/dL (800 μg/mL)
Ethylene glycol	Serum	0.5–1 h	>20 mg/dL (200 μg/mL)
Iron			
Liquid	Serum	2 h	>350 μg/dL (3.5 μg/mL)
Tablet	Serum	4 h	>350 μg/dL (3.5 μg/mL)
Isopropanol	Serum	0.5–1 h	>50 mg/dL (500 μg/mL)
Lithium	Serum	8–12 h	>1.5 mEq/L
Methanol	Serum	0.5–1 h	>20 mg/dL (200 μg/mL)
Methemoglobin	Blood	Stat	>30%
Paraquat	Plasma	8 h	>1 μg/mL within 24 h
Phenobarbital	Serum	Stat	>40 μg/mL
Phenytoin	Serum	1–2 h	>20 μg/mL
Primidone	Serum	Stat	>12 μg/mL
Salicylate	Serum	After 6 h	>30 mg/dL (300 μg/mL)
Theophylline			
Liquid	Serum	1 h	>20 μg/mL
Regular tablet	Serum	1–3 h	>20 μg/mL
Slow release	Serum	3–10 h	>20 μg/mL

*Note that serial levels are needed to follow the trend in all cases. Because of delayed peak times, a single blood or plasma level is not sufficient to exclude intoxication.

TABLE 27. **Substances Usually Nontoxic When Ingested (Unless Ingested in Very Large Quantity)**

Abrasives	Lipstick
Acne preparations	Lubricants
Adhesives	Lysol disinfectant spray (70% ethanol), not the bowl cleaner
A and D ointment	Magic Marker
Air fresheners	Makeup (eye, liquid facial)
Ajax cleanser	Mascara (domestic)
Aluminum foil	Massengill disposable douches
Antacids	Matches (book type, three books)
Antibiotic ointments	Mineral oil (unless aspirated)
Antiperspirants	Miracle-Gro plant food
Ashes (wood, fireplace)	Newspaper
Automobile wax	Nutrasweet
Baby products, cosmetics	PAAS Easter egg dyes (after 1980)
Baby wipes	Paints (indoor latex acrylic)
Ballpoint pen inks	Paste, library type
Bath oil (castor oil and perfume)	Pencil lead (graphite)
Bathtub floating toys	Perfumes*
Battery (conventional, if bitten)	Preparation H suppository or ointment
Bleach, less than 5%	Saccharin
Body conditioners	Sachets (essential oils)
Bubble bath soaps (detergents)	Shampoo (liquid)
Calamine lotion	Shaving creams and lotions
Clotrimazole (Lotrimin) cream	Shoe polish
Dehumidifying packets (silica or charcoal)	Silica gel
Deodorants (spray and refrigerator)	Silly Putty
Deodorants (underarm)	Soaps and soap products
Detergents (phosphate type, anionic)	Soil
Dishwashing liquid soap (not automatic electric dishwasher)—Mr. Clean, Dawn, Joy, Tide, Wisk	Spackles
Disposable diapers—if not aspirated	Starch
Easter egg dyes	Sunscreen and suntan preparations
Erasers	Sweetening agents (saccharin, aspartame)
Etch A Sketch	Teething rings (fluid may have unsterile water and bacteria)
Eye makeup: pencil, shadow, mascara	Thermometers (mercury, alcohol)
Fabric softener	Toilet water*
Felt-tipped markers and pens	Toothpaste (even with fluoride)
Fertilizer (nitrogen, phosphoric acid, and potash; no insecticide or herbicides)	Vaseline
Fingernail polish	Vitamins (even with fluoride)
Finger paint	Warfarin (single dose, <0.5%)
Lanolin	Watercolor paint
Latex paint	Windex glass cleaner with ammonia
Laxatives	

*May contain high amounts of ethanol.

dom). *Toxic mechanism:* At therapeutic doses of APAP, less than 5% is metabolized by cytochrome P-450IIE1 to a toxic reactive oxidizing metabolite, *N*-acetyl-*p*-benzoquinonimine. In overdose, sufficient glutathione is not available to reduce the excess NAPQI into a nontoxic conjugate, and it forms covalent bonds with hepatic intracellular proteins to produce centrilobular necrosis and, by a similar mechanism, renal damage. *Toxic dose:* The therapeutic dose is 10 to 15 mg per kg per dose with a maximum of 5 doses per 24 hours and a maximal total daily dose of 2.5 grams. The acute single toxic dose is greater than 140 mg per kg, possibly greater than 200 mg per kg in children. Factors affecting the cytochrome P-450 enzymes (enzyme inducers such as anticonvulsants [barbiturates, phenytoin], isoniazid, alcoholism) and factors that decrease glutathione stores (e.g., alcoholism, malnutrition, human immunodeficiency virus [HIV] infection) contribute to the toxicity of APAP. Chronic alcoholics who ingest APAP at 3 to 4 grams per day for a few days can have depleted glutathione stores and require NAC therapy at blood APAP levels 50% below hepatotoxic levels on the nomogram (Figure 2). *Kinetics:* Onset of action occurs in 0.5 to 1 hour, the peak plasma concentration occurs in 20 to 90 minutes but usually 2 to 4 hours after an overdose, and the duration is 4 to 6 hours. The Vd is 0.9 liter per kg. PB is low, less than 50% (albumin); $t_{1/2}$ is 1 to 3 hours. The route of elimination is hepatic metabolism to an inactive nontoxic glucuronide conjugate and inactive nontoxic sulfate metabolite by two saturable pathways, and less than 5% is metabolized to the reactive metabolite NAPQI. In children younger than 6 years, metabolic elimination occurs to a greater degree by conjugation with the sulfate pathway, which may be hepatoprotective. *Manifestations:* The four phases of the intoxication's clinical course may overlap, and the absence of a phase does not exclude toxicity. Phase I occurs within 0.5 to 24 hours after ingestion and may consist of a few hours of malaise, diaphoresis, nausea, and vomiting, or there may be no symptoms. CNS depression or coma

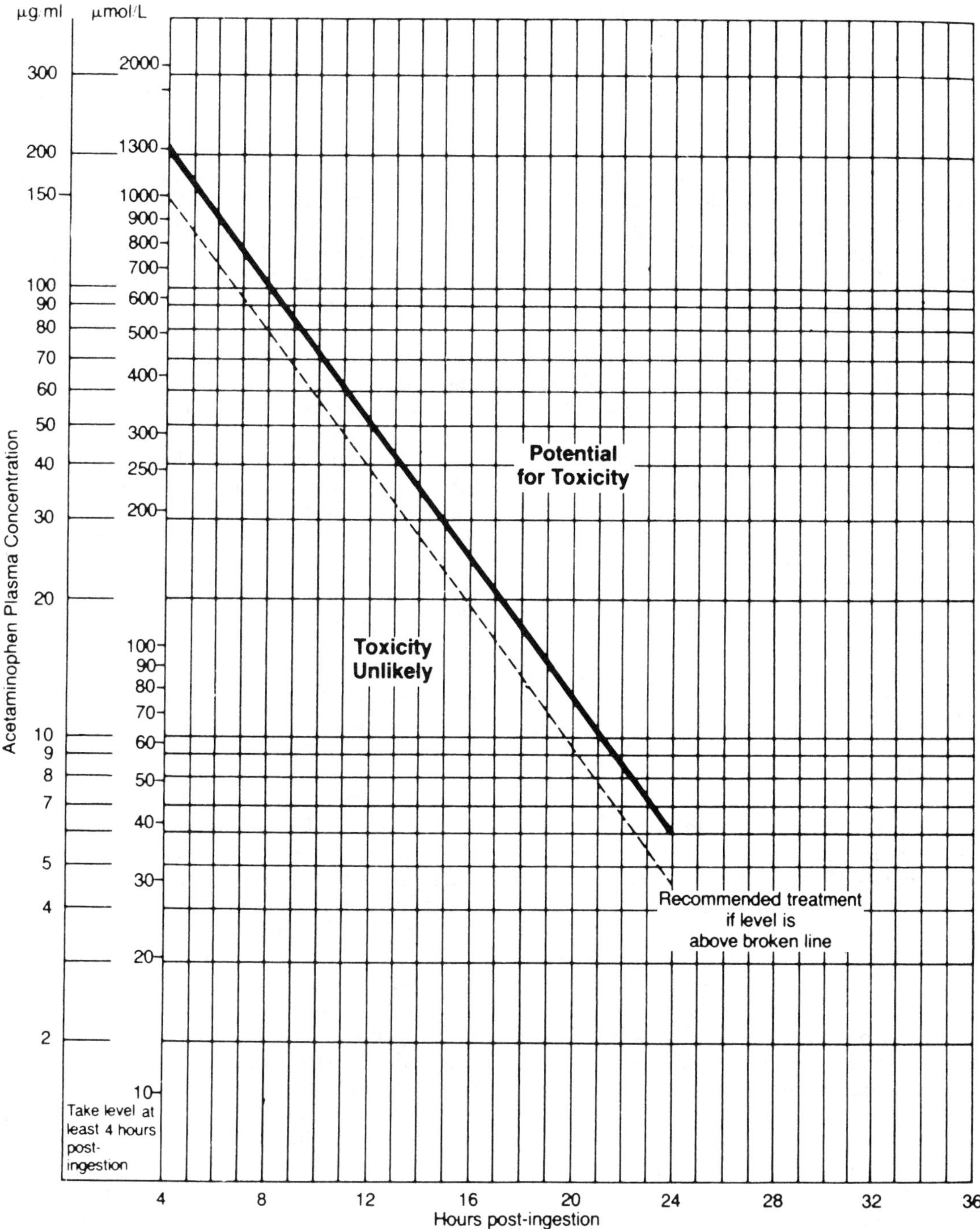

Figure 2. Nomogram for acetaminophen intoxication. Start *N*-acetylcysteine therapy if levels and time coordinates are above the lower line on the nomogram. Continue and complete therapy even if subsequent values fall below the toxic zone. The nomogram is useful only in acute, single ingestions. Levels in serum drawn before 4 hours may not represent peak levels. (From Rumack BH, Matthew H: Acetaminophen poisoning and toxicity. Reproduced by permission of Pediatrics, Vol 55, Page 871, Figure 2, Copyright 1975.)

is not a feature. Phase II occurs 24 to 48 hours after ingestion and is a period of diminished symptoms. The liver enzymes aspartate aminotransferase (AST) (earliest) and alanine aminotransferase (ALT) may increase as early as 4 hours or as late as 36 hours after ingestion. Phase III occurs in 48 to 96 hours, with peak liver function abnormalities at 72 to 96 hours. The degree of elevation of the hepatic enzyme values does not correlate with outcome. Recovery starts in about 4 days unless hepatic failure develops. Less than 1% of patients develop fulminant hepatotoxicity. Phase IV occurs in 4 to 14 days, with hepatic enzyme abnormalities reaching resolution. If extensive liver damage has occurred, sepsis and disseminated intravascular coagulation may ensue. Death can occur at 7 to 14 days. Transient renal failure may develop at 5 to 7 days with or without evidence of hepatic damage. Rare cases of myocarditis and pancreatitis have been reported. *Management:* (1) GI decontamination: Emesis may be useful within 30 minutes. However, it may interfere with the retention of AC and NAC. Gastric lavage is not necessary if AC is administered early. Studies have indicated that AC is useful within 4 hours after ingestion. MDAC has not been well studied. AC does adsorb NAC if they are given together, but this is not clinically important. However, if AC must be given along with NAC, the administration of AC must be separated from that of NAC by 1 to 2 hours to avoid vomiting. Use of a saline sulfate cathartic in adults is recommended because it can enhance the activity of the sulfate metabolic pathway, which may be hepatoprotective. (2) NAC (Table 28; also see Table 12): NAC, a derivative of the amino acid cysteine, acts as a sulfhydryl donor for glutathione synthesis and may enhance the nontoxic sulfation pathway, resulting in conjugation of NAPQI. Oral NAC should be administered within the first 8 hours after a toxic amount of APAP has been ingested. NAC may be started while the results of the blood tests for the acetaminophen plasma concentration (APC) are awaited, but there is no advantage to giving it before 8 hours. If the APC at more than 4 hours after ingestion is above the lower line on the modified Rumack-Matthew nomogram (see Figure 2), continue the full 17-dose maintenance course. Repeated blood specimens should be obtained 4 hours after the initial level if it is greater than 20 μg per mL because of unexpected delays in the peak caused by food and coingestants. An intravenous preparation (see Table 28) has been used in Europe and Canada for about 20 years but is not approved in the United States (studies are in progress). There have been a few anaphylactoid reactions and deaths with the intravenous route. *Variations in therapy:* (a) In patients with chronic alcoholism it is recommended that NAC be administered at 50% below the lower toxic line on the nomogram. (b) If emesis occurs within 1 hour after NAC administration, the dose should be repeated. To help prevent emesis, use the proper dilution from 20 to 5% NAC, and serve in a palatable vehicle in a covered container with a straw. If this is unsuccessful, administer through a nasogastric tube or a fluoroscopically placed nasoduodenal tube by a slow drip over 30 to 60 minutes. Antiemetics may be used if necessary: metoclopramide (Reglan) at 10 mg per dose IV a half-hour before NAC (child: 0.1 mg per kg with a maximum of 0.5 mg per kg per day) or, as a last resort, ondansetron (Zofran) at 32 mg (0.15 mg per kg) by infusion over 15 minutes, repeated for 3 doses if necessary. The side effects of ondansetron are anaphylaxis and increases in liver enzyme values. (c) Some investigators recommend variable durations of NAC therapy, stopping the therapy if the APC becomes nondetectable in serial determinations and the liver enzymes (ALT and AST) remain normal after 36 hours. (d) Time of administration: There is a loss of efficacy if NAC is initiated more than 8 to 10 hours after ingestion, but the loss is not complete and NAC may be initiated 36 or more hours after ingestion. Late treatment (after 24 hours) has been shown to decrease the morbidity and mortality in fulminant liver failure caused by acetaminophen and other etiologic agents. (e) An extended-release caplet (ER is embossed on the caplet) contains 325 mg of immediate-release and 325 mg of delayed-release formulations. A single serum APAP determination 4 hours after ingestion can underestimate the dose because the extended-release formulation can yield secondary delayed peaks. In overdoses of extended-release formulation, it is recommended that additional APAP levels at 4-hour intervals after the initial level be obtained. If any peak is in the toxic zone, initiate therapy. (3) Pregnancy: It is recommended that pregnant patients with toxic plasma concentrations of APAP receive NAC therapy to prevent hepatotoxicity in both fetus and mother. The available data suggest no teratogenicity caused by NAC or APAP. (4) Chronic intoxication: Indications for NAC therapy are a history of ingestion of 3 to 4 grams for several days, elevated liver enzyme (AST and ALT) values, and chronic alcoholism or use of chronic enzyme inducers. (5) Specific support care may be needed to treat liver failure, pancreatitis, transient renal failure, and myocarditis. (6) Liver transplantation has a definite but limited role in acute APAP overdose. According to a retrospective analysis, a continuing rise in the prothrombin time (4-day peak: 180 seconds), pH less than 7.3 (2 days after overdose), serum creatinine greater than 3.3 mg per dL, severe hepatic encephalopathy, and a disturbed coagulation factor VII/V ratio of more than 30% suggest a poor prognosis and may be indicators for hepatology consultation for consideration of OLT. (7) Extracorporeal measures are not expected to be of benefit. *Laboratory investigations:* The therapeutic reference range is 10 to 20 μg per mL. For toxic levels see the nomogram in Figure 2. Appropriate reliable methods for analysis are radioimmunoassay, high-performance liquid chromatography (HPLC), and gas chromatography.

TABLE 28. **Protocol for *N*-acetylcysteine Administration**

Route	Loading Dose	Maintenance Dose	Course Duration (h)	FDA Approval
Oral	140 mg/kg	70 mg/kg q 4 h	72	Yes
Intravenous—England, Canada	150 mg/kg over 15 min	50 mg/kg over 4 h followed by 100 mg/kg over 16 h	20	No
Intravenous—investigational in United States	140 mg/kg	70 mg/kg q 4 h	48	No

Spectroscopic assays often give falsely elevated values. Cross-reactions: Bilirubin, salicylate, salicylamide, diflunisal, phenols, and methyldopa increase the APAP level. Each 1 mg per dL increase in creatinine increases the APAP plasma level 30 μg per mL. Monitoring: If a toxic APAP level is present, monitor the liver profile (including AST, ALT, bilirubin, prothrombin time), serum amylase, blood glucose, CBC, platelet count, phosphate, electrolytes, bicarbonate, ECG, and urinalysis. *Disposition:* All cases of intentional ingestion require a serum APAP level obtained 4 hours or more after ingestion. Patients who ingest more than 140 mg per kg should receive therapy within 8 hours after ingestion or until the results of the APC determination 4 hours after ingestion are known.

Amphetamines (illicit methamphetamine ["ice"], diet pills, various trade names). *Analogues:* 3,4-methylenedioxymethamphetamine (MDMA; known as Ecstasy, XTC, Adam) and 3,4-methylenedioxyamphetamine (MDEA; known as Eve). Other similar stimulants are phenylpropanolamine and cocaine. *Toxic mechanism:* Amphetamines have a direct CNS stimulant effect and a sympathetic nervous system effect by releasing catecholamines from alpha- and beta-adrenergic nerve terminals but inhibiting their reuptake. Phenylpropanolamine stimulates only the beta-adrenergic receptors. *Toxic dose:* Child, 1 mg per kg dextroamphetamine; adult, 5 mg per kg. A dose of 12 mg per kg has been reported to be lethal. *Kinetics:* Amphetamine is a weak base with a pK_a of 8 to 10. Onset of action is in 30 to 60 minutes. Peak effects occur at 2 to 4 hours. The $t_{1/2}$ is pH-dependent; it is 8 to 10 hours with acidic urine (pH less than 6.0) and 16 to 31 hours with alkaline urine (pH greater than 7.5). The Vd is 2 to 3 liters per kg. Elimination is 60% hepatic to a hydroxylated metabolite that may be responsible for psychotic effects. Excretion by the kidney is 30 to 40% at alkaline urine pH and 50 to 70% at acidic urine pH. *Manifestations:* Effects are seen within 30 to 60 minutes after ingestion. Restlessness, irritation and agitation, tremors and hyper-reflexia, and auditory and visual hallucinations occur. Dilated but reactive pupils, cardiac dysrhythmias (supraventricular and ventricular), tachycardia, and hyperpyrexia may precede seizures, convulsions, hypertension, paranoia, violence, intracranial hemorrhage, rhabdomyolysis, myoglobinuria, psychosis, and self-destructive behavior. Paranoid psychosis and cerebral vasculitis occur with chronic abuse. *Management* (similar to that for cocaine): (1) Provide supportive care: blood pressure and cardiac thermal monitoring and seizure precautions. Diazepam is also administered (see Table 12). (2) GI decontamination: Administer AC and MDAC. (3) Treat anxiety, agitation, and convulsions with diazepam. If diazepam fails to control seizures, use neuromuscular blockers and monitor the EEG for nonmotor seizures. Avoid neuroleptics (PTZs and butyrophenone), which can lower the seizure threshold. (4) Cardiovascular disturbances: Hypertension and tachycardia are usually transient and can be managed by titration of diazepam. Nitroprusside may be used for hypertensive crisis; use a maximal infusion rate of 10 μg per kg per minute for 10 minutes, followed by 0.3 to 2 μg per kg per minute. Myocardial ischemia is managed by oxygen, vascular access, BZPs, and nitroglycerin. Aspirin and thrombolysis are not routinely recommended because of the danger of intracranial hemorrhage. Delayed hypotension can be treated with fluids and vasopressors if needed. Life-threatening tachydysrhythmias may respond to an alpha blocker (e.g., phentolamine at 5 mg IV for adults and 0.1 mg per kg IV for children) and a short-acting beta blocker (esmolol at 500 μg per kg IV over 1 minute for adults and 300 to 500 μg per kg IV over 1 minute for children). Ventricular dysrhythmias may respond to lidocaine or, in a severely hemodynamically compromised patient, immediate synchronized electrical cardioversion. (5) Treat rhabdomyolysis and myoglobinuria with fluids, alkaline diuresis, and diuretics. (6) Treat hyperthermia with external cooling and cool 100% humidified oxygen. (7) If focal neurologic symptoms are present, consider a diagnosis of a cerebrovascular accident and perform CT of the head. (8) Treat paranoid ideation and threatening behavior with rapid tranquilization. (See the earlier discussion of violent patients.) (9) The patient is observed for suicidal depression, which may follow intoxication and may require suicide precautions. (10) Extracorporeal measures are of no benefit. *Laboratory investigations:* Monitoring: ECG and cardiac monitoring is instituted, and monitoring is also indicated for ABGs and oxygen saturation, electrolytes, blood glucose, BUN, creatinine, creatine kinase and cardiac fraction (if chest pain), and liver profile; evaluate for rhabdomyolysis, and check urine for myoglobin, cocaine and metabolites, and other substances of abuse. The peak plasma concentration is 10 to 50 ng per mL 1 to 2 hours after ingestion of 10 to 25 mg. The toxic plasma concentration is 200 ng per mL. Cross-reactions occur with amphetamine derivatives (e.g., methylenedioxyamphetamine derivative [MDA], Ecstasy), brompheniramine, chlorpromazine, ephedrine, phenylpropanolamine, phentermine, phenmetrazine, ranitidine, and Vicks Inhaler (*l*-desoxyephedrine) and may give false-positive results. *Disposition:* Symptomatic patients should be observed in a monitored unit until the symptoms resolve and then observed for a short time after resolution for relapse.

Anticholinergic Agents. Drugs with anticholinergic properties include antihistamines (H_1 blockers); neuroleptics (PTZs); tricyclic antidepressants; antiparkinsonism drugs (trihexyphenidyl [Artane], benztropine [Cogentin]); over-the-counter sleep, cold, and hay fever medicines (methapyrilene); ophthalmic products (atropine); products of common plants including jimsonweed *(Datura stramonium),* deadly nightshade *(Atropa belladonna),* and henbane *(Hyoscyamus niger)* and antispasmodic agents for the bowel (atropine derivatives). *Toxic mechanism:* By competitive inhibition, anticholinergic agents block the action of acetylcholine on postsynaptic cholinergic receptor sites. The mechanism involves primarily the peripheral and CNS muscarinic receptors. *Toxic dose:* Toxic amounts of atropine are 0.05 mg per kg in a child and greater than 2 mg in adults. The minimal estimated lethal dose of atropine is greater than 10 mg in adults and greater than 2 mg in 2-year-old children. Other synthetic anticholinergic agents are less toxic, with the fatal dose varying from 10 to 100 mg. *Kinetics:* The onset of action with intravenous administration occurs in 2 to 4 minutes; peak effects on salivation after an intravenous or intramuscular dose occur in 30 to 60 minutes. The onset after ingestion is in 30 to 60 minutes, peak action occurs in 1 to 3 hours, and the duration is 4 to 6 hours, but symptoms are prolonged with overdose or sustained-release preparations. *Manifestations:* Anticholinergic signs: hyperpyrexia ("hot as a hare"), mydriasis ("blind as a bat"), flushing of skin ("red as a beet"), dry mucosa and skin ("dry as a bone"), "Lilliputian-type" hallucinations and delirium ("mad as a hatter"), coma, dysphagia, tachycardia, moderate hypertension, and rarely convulsions and urine retention. *Management:* (1) If respiratory failure occurs, use intubation and assisted ventilation. (2) For GI decontamination, emesis should be avoided in a diphenhydramine overdose because of rapid onset of action and the possibility of seizures. Use AC if bowel sounds are present; MDAC is not recommended. (3) Control seizures with BZPs (diazepam or lorazepam). (4) Use of physostigmine (see Table 12) is not routine and is reserved for reversal of life-threatening anticholinergic effects refractory to conventional treatments. This drug should be administered with adequate monitoring and resuscitative equipment available; it should be avoided if a tricyclic antidepressant is present. (5) Relieve urine retention by catheterization to avoid reabsorption. (6) If cardiac dysrhythmias are present, treat supraventricular tachycardia only if the patient is unstable. Control ventricular dysrhythmias with lidocaine or cardioversion. (7) Control hyperpyrexia by external cooling. (8) Hemodialysis and hemoperfusion are not effective. *Laboratory investigations:* These include ABGs (in respiratory depression), electrolytes, glucose, and ECG monitoring. Anticholinergic drugs and plants having anticholinergic effects are not routinely included in screens for substances of abuse. *Disposition:* Symptomatic patients should be observed in a monitored unit until the symptoms resolve and then observed for a short time after resolution for relapse.

Antihistamines (H_1-receptor antagonists). Antihistamines include the H_1-blocker "sedating anticholinergic" type. A single adult dose includes (1) ethanolamines: diphenhydramine (Benadryl), 25 to 50 mg, child 1 mg per kg; dimenhydrinate (Dramamine), 50 mg; and clemastine (Tavist), 1.34 to 2.68 mg; (2) ethylenediamines: tripelennamine (Pyribenzamine), 25 to 50 mg, child 1 mg per kg; (3) alkylamines: chlorpheniramine (Chlor-Trimeton), 4 to 8 mg, child 0.9 mg per kg; brompheniramine (Dimetane), 4 to 8 mg, child 0.125 mg per kg; (4) piperazines: cyclizine (Marezine), 50 mg; hydroxyzine (Atarax), 50 to 100 mg, child 0.6 mg per kg; meclizine (Antivert), 50 to 100 mg; and (5) promethazine (Phenergan), 12.5 to 25 mg, child 0.1 mg per kg.

THE H_1-BLOCKER SEDATING ANTIHISTAMINES. Many of these agents are used in combination with other medication, such as acetaminophen, aspirin, codeine, dextromethorphan, ephedrine, phenylephrine, phenylpropanolamine, and pseudoephedrine. *Toxic mechanism:* H_1 sedating-type antihistamines produce blockade of cholinergic muscarinic receptors (anticholinergic action) and depress or stimulate the CNS; in large overdoses, some have a cardiac membrane–depressant effect (e.g., diphenhydramine) and cause alpha-adrenergic receptor blockade (e.g., promethazine). *Toxic dose:* For diphenhydramine, the estimated toxic oral amount in a child is 15 mg per kg and the potential lethal amount is 25 mg per kg. In an adult the potential lethal amount is 2.8 grams. Ingestion of five times the single dose of an antihistamine is toxic. *Kinetics:* Onset is in 15 to 30 minutes to 1 hour, peak effects occur in 1 to 4 hours; PB is 75 to 80%; Vd is 3.3 to 6.8 liters per kg; and $t_{1/2}$ is 3 to 10 hours. Elimination is 98% hepatic by *N*-demethylation. Interactions with erythromycin, ketoconazole (Nizoral), and derivatives produce excessive blood levels and ventricular dysrhythmias. *Manifestations:* Exaggerated anticholinergic effects, jaundice (cyproheptadine), coma, seizures, dystonia (diphenhydramine), rhabdomyolysis (doxylamine), and in large doses cardiotoxic effects (diphenhydramine) may be seen. *Management and disposition* (see "Anticholinergic Agents"): $NaHCO_3$ at 1 to 2 mEq per kg IV may be useful for myocardial depression and QRS prolongation.

THE NONSEDATING SINGLE-DAILY-DOSE ANTIHISTAMINES. Single adult doses include terfenadine (Seldane), 10 mg; astemizole (Hismanal), 10 mg, child 0.6 mg per kg; loratadine (Claritin), 10 mg; and fexofenadine (Allegra), 60 mg. *Toxic mechanism:* These agents produce peripheral H_1 blockade and do not possess anticholinergic and sedating actions. They can produce prolonged QT intervals and torsades de pointes if blood levels are elevated because of impaired hepatic function, or interactions with enzyme-inhibiting drugs (cimetidine, ketoconazole and derivatives, or macrolide antibiotics). Loratadine and fexofenadine have not been reported to have these drug interactions. *Toxic dose:* An adult with an overdose of 3360 mg of terfenadine developed ventricular tachycardia and fibrillation that responded to lidocaine and defibrillation; a 1500-mg overdose produced hypotension. Cases of delayed serious dysrhythmias (torsades de pointes) have been reported with more than 200 mg of astemizole. *Kinetics:* Onset occurs in 1 hour, peak effects occur in 4 to 6 hours, and duration is greater than 24 hours. These drugs are more than 90% protein bound. Plasma $t_{1/2}$ is 3.5 hours. Metabolism is in the GI tract and liver. Only 1% is excreted unchanged, 60% in feces and 40% in urine. The chemical structure of these medications prevents entry into the CNS. *Manifestations:* Overdose produces headache, nausea, confusion, and serious dysrhythmias (e.g., torsades de pointes). *Management:* (1) Obtain an ECG and establish cardiac monitoring. Treat dysrhythmias with standard agents. Torsades de pointes is best treated with magnesium sulfate at 4 grams or 40 mL of a 10% solution given IV over 10 to 20 minutes (see Table 12) and countershock if the patient fails to respond. (2) GI decontamination with AC is advised. *Disposition:* All children who ingest nonsedating antihistamines or adults who ingest more than the therapeutic maximal dose require close cardiac monitoring for torsades de pointes for at least 24 hours. Patients receiving concurrent macrolide antibiotics or ketoconazole should not continue to take these while receiving terfenadine or astemizole. Medical evaluation is required for chronic use of this combination.

Barbiturates. Barbiturates are used as sedatives, anesthetic agents, and anticonvulsants. *Toxic mechanism:* Barbiturates are GABA agonists (they increase chloride flow and inhibit depolarization). They enhance the CNS depressant effect and depress the cardiovascular system. *Toxic dose:* (1) The short-acting barbiturates (SABs) (including the intermediate-acting agents) and their hypnotic doses are amobarbital (Amytal), 100 to 200 mg; aprobarbital (Alurate), 50 to 100 mg; butabarbital (Butisol), 50 to 100 mg; butalbital (Sandoptal), 100 to 200 mg; pentobarbital (Nembutal), 100 to 200 mg; and secobarbital (Seconal), 100 to 200 mg. They cause toxicity at lower doses than longer-acting barbiturates (LABs) and have a minimal toxic dose of 6 mg per kg; the fatal adult dose is 3 to 6 grams. (2) The LABs include mephobarbital (Mebaral), 50 to 100 mg, and phenobarbital (Luminal), 100 to 200 mg. These agents have a minimal toxic dose greater than 10 mg per kg; the fatal adult dose is 6 to 10 grams. A general rule is that an amount 5 times the hypnotic dose is toxic and 10 times the hypnotic dose is potentially fatal. Methohexital and thiopental are ultra-short-acting (USA) parenteral preparations and are not discussed. *Kinetics:* Barbiturates are enzyme inducers. (1) SABs are highly lipid soluble, penetrate the brain readily, and have shorter elimination times. Onset is in 10 to 30 minutes, the peak occurs in 1 to 2 hours, the duration is 3 to 8 hours. The Vd is 0.8 to 1.5 liters per kg. The pK_a is about 8. Mean $t_{1/2}$ varies from 8 to 48 hours. (2) LABs have longer elimination times and may be used as anticonvulsants. Onset is in 20 to 60 minutes, the peak occurs in 1 to 6 hours or, in an overdose, 10 hours, and the duration is greater than 8 to 12 hours. The Vd is 0.8 liter per kg. The pK_a of phenobarbital is 7.2, and alkalization of urine promotes its excretion. The $t_{1/2}$ is 11 to 120 hours. *Manifestations:* In mild intoxication, the initial symptoms resemble those of alcohol intoxication and include ataxia, slurred speech, and depressed cognition. Severe intoxication causes slow respirations, coma, and loss of reflexes (except pupillary light reflex). Hypotension (venodilatation), hypothermia, and hypoglycemia occur, and death is by respiratory arrest. Bullous skin lesions ("barb burns") over pressure points may be present. Barbiturates can precipitate an attack of acute intermittent porphyria. *Management:* (1) Establish and maintain the vital functions. Intense supportive care including intubation and assisted ventilation should dominate the management. All stuporous and comatose patients should have glucose, thiamine, and naloxone given IV and be admitted to the ICU. (2) GI decontamination: Avoid emesis, especially in SAB ingestions. AC with a single-dose cathartic, followed by MDAC (0.5 gram per kg) every 2 to 4 hours, has been shown to reduce the serum $t_{1/2}$ of phenobarbital by 50%, but its effect on the clinical course is undetermined. (3) Fluid management: Administer fluids to correct dehydration and hypotension. Vasopressors may be necessary to correct severe hypotension and hemodynamic monitoring may be needed. Observe carefully for signs of fluid overload. (4) Alkalization (ion trapping) is used for phenobarbital (pK_a 7.2) but not for SABs. $NaHCO_3$, 1 to 2 mEq per kg IV in 500 mL of 5% dextrose for adults or 10 to 15 mL per kg for children during the first hour, followed by sufficient bicarbonate to keep the urine pH at 7.5 to 8.0, enhances excretion of phenobarbital and shortens the $t_{1/2}$ by 50% (see Table 12). Diuresis is not advocated because of the danger of cerebral or pulmonary edema. (5) Hemodialysis shortens the $t_{1/2}$ to 8 to 14 hours and charcoal hemoperfusion shortens the $t_{1/2}$ to 6 to 8 hours. Both may be effective for both LABs and SABs. If the patient does not respond to supportive measures or if the phenobarbital plasma concentration is greater than 150 µg per mL, both procedures may be tried to shorten the $t_{1/2}$. (6) Treat any bullae as local second-degree skin burns. (7) Treat hypothermia. *Laboratory investigations:* Most barbiturates are detected by routine drug screens and can be measured in most hospital laboratories. Monitor barbiturate levels, ABGs, and a toxicology screen including acetaminophen and ethanol, glucose, electrolytes, BUN, creatinine, creatine kinase, and urine pH. Minimal toxic plasma levels are greater than 10 µg per mL for SABs and greater than 40 µg per mL for LABs. Fatal levels are 30 µg per mL for SABs and greater than 80 to 150 µg per mL for LABs. SABs and LABs can be detected in urine 24 to 72 hours after ingestion and LABs up to 7 days. *Disposition:* All comatose patients should be admitted to the ICU. Awake and oriented patients with an overdose of an SAB should be observed for at least 6 asymptomatic hours, and those with an overdose of an LAB for at least 12 asymptomatic hours. In an intentional overdose, psychiatric clearance is needed before discharge. Chronic use can lead to tolerance, physical dependence, and withdrawal and requires follow-up.

Benzodiazepines. BZPs are used as anxiolytics, sedatives, and relaxants. *Toxic mechanism:* GABA agonists produce CNS depression and increase chloride flow, inhibiting depolarization. *Toxic dose:* In the elderly the therapeutic dose should be reduced by 50%. BZPs have an additive effect with other CNS depressants. (1) For long-acting (LA) BZPs ($t_{1/2}$ greater than 24 hours), the maximal therapeutic doses are chlordiazepoxide (Librium), 50 mg; clorazepate (Tranxene), 30 mg; clonazepam, 20 mg; diazepam (Valium), 10 mg or 0.2 mg per kg for children; flurazepam (Dalmane), 30 mg; and prazepam (Centrax), 20 mg. (2) Short-acting (SA) BZPs ($t_{1/2}$ 10 to 24 hours) include alprazolam, 0.5 mg, and lorazepam, 4 mg or 0.05 mg per kg for children, which act similarly to the LABZPs. (3) The BZPs that are ultra short acting (USA) ($t_{1/2}$ less than 10 hours) are more toxic and include temazepam, 30 mg; triazolam, 0.5 mg; midazolam, 0.2 mg per kg; and oxazepam (Serax), 30 mg. (4) In overdoses: LABZPs: Ingestions of 10 to 20 times the therapeutic dose (greater than 1500 mg of diazepam or 2000 mg of chlordiazepoxide) have resulted in mild coma without respiratory depression. Fatalities are rare, and most patients recover within 24 to 36 hours after overdose with LABZPs and SABZPs. Asymptomatic patients who have taken nonintentional overdoses of less than five times the therapeutic dose may be observed. USABZPs have produced respiratory arrest and coma within 1 hour after ingestion of 5 mg of triazolam and death with ingestion of as little as 10 mg. Midazolam and diazepam administered by rapid intravenous injection have produced respiratory arrest. *Kinetics:* Onset of CNS depression is usually in 30 to 120 minutes, and the peak usually occurs within 1 to 3 hours with the oral route. The Vd is 0.26 to 6 liters per kg (for LABZPs, 1.1 liter per kg). PB is 70 to 99%. *Manifestations:* Ataxia, slurred speech, and CNS depression may be seen. Deep coma leading to respiratory depression suggests the presence of SABZPs or should prompt a search for other causes. *Management:* (1) GI decontamination: Emesis should be avoided. Gastric lavage (within 1 hour) and AC are advised if the ingestion was recent. (2) Supportive treatment should be provided but intubation and assisted ventilation are rarely required. (3) Flumazenil (see Table 12) is a specific BZP receptor antagonist that blocks chloride flow and is an inhibitor of neurotransmitters. It reverses sedative effects of BZPs, zolpidem (Ambien), and endogenous BZPs associated with hepatic encephalopathy. It is not recommended to reverse BZP-induced hypoventilation. It should be used with caution in overdoses if there is possible BZP dependence (because it can precipitate life-threatening withdrawal), if a cyclic antidepressant is suspected, or if the patient has a known seizure disorder. *Laboratory investigations:* Most BZPs can be detected in urinary drug screens. Quantitative blood levels are not useful. The BZPs usually not detected in urinary screens include alprazolam, clonazepam, flunitrazepam,* lorazepam, lormetazepam,* midazolam, oxazepam, temazepam, and triazolam. BZPs may not be detected if the dose is less than 10 mg, elimination is rapid, or there are different or no metabolites. Cross-reactions occur with NSAIDs (tolmetin, naproxen, etodolac, and fenoprofen). *Disposition:* Comatose patients should be admitted to the ICU. If the overdose was intentional, psychiatric clearance is needed before discharge. Chronic use can lead to tolerance, physical dependence, and withdrawal.

*Not available in the United States.

Beta-Adrenergic Blockers (beta blockers). Beta blockers are used in the treatment of hypertension and a number of systemic and ophthalmic disorders. Lipid-soluble drugs have CNS effects, active metabolites, a longer duration of action, and interactions with other drugs (e.g., propranolol). Cardioselectivity is lost in overdoses. Intrinsic partial agonist agents (e.g., pindolol) may initially produce tachycardia and hypertension. A cardiac membrane–depressive effect (quinidine-like) occurs with overdose but not therapeutic doses (e.g., metoprolol, sotalol). The alpha-blocking effect is weak (e.g., labetalol). Properties of beta blockers include the factors listed in Table 29. *Toxic mechanism:* Beta blockers compete with the catecholamines for receptor sites and block receptor action in the bronchi and the vascular smooth muscle and myocardium. *Toxic dose:* Ingestions of more than twice the maximal recommended daily therapeutic dose are considered toxic (see Table 29). Ingestion of propranolol at 1 mg per kg by a child may produce hypoglycemia. Fatalities have been reported in adults who have ingested 7.5 grams of metoprolol. The most toxic agent is sotalol, and the least toxic, atenolol. *Kinetics:* Regular release usually causes symptoms within 2 hours. Propranolol's onset of action is in 20 to 30 minutes; the peak is at 1 to 4 hours but may be delayed with coingestants and sustained-release preparations. The duration is 4 to 6 hours but in overdoses may be 24 to 48 hours and longer with the sustained-release type. With sustained-release preparations the onset may be delayed 6 hours and the peak 12 to 16 hours; the duration may be 24 to 48 hours. The regular preparation with the longest $t_{1/2}$ is nadolol (12 to 24 hours) and with the shortest is esmolol (5 to 10 minutes). PB is variable, ranging from 5 to 93%. The Vd is 1 to 5.6 liters per kg. Atenolol, nadolol, and sotalol have enterohepatic recirculation. *Manifestations:* See toxic properties and Table 29. Lipid-soluble agents produce coma and seizures. Bradycardia and hypotension are the major symptoms and may lead to cardiogenic shock. Intrinsic partial agonists may initially cause tachycardia and hypertension. Bronchospasm may occur in patients with reactive airway disease with any beta blocker because the selectivity is lost in overdoses. ECG changes include atrioventricular (AV) conduction delay and frank asystole. Membrane-depressant effects produce prolonged QRS and QT intervals, which may result in torsades de pointes. Sotalol produces a prolonged QT. Hypoglycemia (blocking of catecholamine counter-regulatory mechanisms) and hyperkalemia may occur, especially in children. *Management:* (1) Establish and maintain vital functions. Establish vascular access, obtain a baseline ECG, and institute continuous cardiac and blood pressure monitoring. Have a pacemaker available. Hypotension is treated with fluids initially, although it usually does not respond. Frequently, glucagon and cardiac pacing are needed. Cardiology

TABLE 29. **Pharmacologic and Toxic Properties of Beta Blockers***

Name	Dose	Lipid Solubility	Intrinsic Sympathomimetic Activity (Partial Agonist)	Membrane-Stabilizing Effect	Cardiac Selectivity (Beta-Selective)	Alpha Blocker
Acebutolol (Sectral)	Maximal daily dose 800 mg, therapeutic plasma level 200–2000 ng/mL	Moderate	+	+	+	+
Alprenolol†	Maximal daily dose 800 mg, therapeutic plasma level 50–200 ng/mL	Moderate	2+	+	–	–
Atenolol (Tenormin)	Maximal daily dose 100 mg, therapeutic plasma level 200–500 ng/mL	Low	–	–	2+	–
Betaxolol (Kerlone)	Maximal daily dose 20 mg, therapeutic plasma level NA	Low	+	–	+	–
Carteolol (Cartrol)	Maximal daily dose 10 mg, therapeutic plasma level NA	No	+	–	–	–
Esmolol (Brevibloc) (class II antidysrhythmic, by intravenous route only)		Low	–	–	+	–
Labetalol (Trandate)	Maximal daily dose 800 mg, therapeutic plasma level 50–500 ng/mL	Low	+	±	–	+
Levobunolol (eye drops 0.25% and 0.5%)	Maximal daily dose 20 mg, therapeutic plasma level NA	No	–	–	–	–
Metoprolol (Lopressor)	Maximal daily dose 450 mg, therapeutic plasma level 50–100 ng/mL	Moderate	–	–	2+	–
Nadolol (Corgard)	Maximal daily dose 320 mg, therapeutic plasma level 20–400 ng/mL	Low	–	–	–	–
Oxprenolol†	Maximal daily dose 480 mg, therapeutic plasma level 80–100 ng/mL	Moderate	2+	+	–	–
Pindolol (Visken)	Maximal daily dose 60 mg, therapeutic plasma level 50–150 ng/mL	Moderate	3+	±	–	–
Propranolol (Inderal) (class II antidysrhythmic)	Maximal daily dose 360 mg, therapeutic plasma level 50–100 ng/mL	High	–	2+	–	–
Sotalol (Betapace) (class III antidysrhythmic)	Maximal daily dose 480 mg, therapeutic plasma level 500–4000 ng/mL	Low	–	–	–	–
Timolol (Blocadren)	Maximal daily dose 60 mg, therapeutic plasma level 5–10 ng/mL	Low	–	±	–	–

*– indicates no effect; + indicates mild effect; 2+ indicates moderate effect; 3+ indicates severe effect; ± indicates no effect or mild effect; NA indicates not available.

†Not available in the United States.

consultation should be sought. (2) GI decontamination is done initially with AC and a single-dose cathartic. MDAC is recommended for symptomatic patients with ingestions of beta blockers with enterohepatic recirculation or sustained release (no data). Gastric lavage is done at less than 1 hour after ingestion. If gastric lavage is done, use of prelavage atropine (0.02 mg per kg for a child and 0.5 mg for an adult) and cardiac monitoring is recommended. Whole-bowel irrigation should be considered in large overdoses with sustained-release preparations (although no studies have been done). (3) Cardiovascular disturbances: A cardiology consultation should be obtained. Class IA (procainamide, quinidine) and class III (bretylium) antidysrhythmic agents are not recommended. Bradycardia in asymptomatic, hemodynamically stable patients requires no therapy. It is not predictive of the future course. If the patient is unstable (has hypotension or high-degree AV block), use atropine at 0.02 mg per kg up to 2 mg in adults, glucagon, and a pacemaker. In ventricular tachycardia, use overdrive pacing. A wide QRS interval may respond to $NaHCO_3$ (see Table 12). Torsades de pointes (associated with sotalol) may respond to magnesium sulfate (see Table 12) and overdrive pacing. Prophylactic magnesium for a prolonged QT interval has been suggested, but there are no supporting data. Do not use epinephrine, because an unopposed alpha effect may occur. Hypotension and myocardial depression are managed by correction of dysrhythmias, use of the Trendelenburg position, and administration of fluids, glucagon, and/or amrinone (Inocor). Hemodynamic monitoring may be needed to manage fluid therapy. Glucagon (see Table 12) is the initial drug of choice. It works through adenylate cyclase and bypasses catecholamine receptors, so it is not affected by beta blockers. It increases cardiac contractility and heart rate. It is given as an intravenous bolus of 5 to 10 mg* over 1 minute, followed by continuous infusion at 1 to 5 mg per hour (in children, 0.15 mg per kg followed by 0.05 to 0.1 mg per kg per hour). In large doses and in infusion therapy use D5W, sterile water, or saline as the diluent to reconstitute glucagon in place of the 0.2% phenol diluent provided with some drugs. Effects are seen within minutes. Glucagon can be used with other agents such as amrinone. Amrinone inhibits the enzyme phosphodiesterase, which metabolizes cyclic adenosine monophosphate (AMP). A bolus of 0.15 to 2 mg per kg (0.15 to 0.4 mL per kg) is administered IV followed by infusion of 5 to 10 μg per kg per minute. (4) Treat hypoglycemia with intravenous glucose and emergency hyperkalemia with calcium (avoid if digoxin is present), bicarbonate, and glucose. (5) Control convulsions with diazepam or phenobarbital. (6) If bronchospasm is present, give $beta_2$ nebulized bronchodilators and aminophylline. (7) Extraordinary measures include intra-aortic balloon pump support. (8) Extracorporeal measures: Hemodialysis for poisonings with atenolol, acebutalol, nadolol, and sotalol (low Vd, low PB) may be helpful, particularly with evidence of renal failure. It is not effective for intoxication with propranolol, metoprolol, and timolol. (9) Investigational: Prenalterol has successfully reversed both bradycardia and hypotension (it is not available in the United States). *Laboratory investigations:* Measurement of blood levels is not readily available or useful. (For propranolol the toxic level is greater than 2 ng per mL.) Monitoring: ECG and cardiac monitoring is recommended, as well as monitoring of blood glucose and electrolytes, BUN and serum creatinine, and ABGs if respiratory symptoms are present. *Disposition:* Asymptomatic patients with a history of overdose require a baseline ECG and continuous cardiac monitoring for at least 6 hours with regular-release preparations and for 24 hours with sustained-release preparations. Symptomatic patients should be observed with cardiac monitoring for 24 hours. If seizures, abnormal rhythm, or vital signs indicate, the patient should be admitted to the ICU.

Calcium Channel Blockers. These agents are used in the treatment of effort angina, supraventricular tachycardia, and hypertension. *Toxic mechanism:* Calcium channel blockers reduce the influx of calcium through the slow channels in membranes of the myocardium, the AV nodes, and vascular smooth muscles, resulting in peripheral, systemic, and coronary vasodilatation, impaired cardiac conduction, and depression of cardiac contractility. All calcium channel blockers have vasodilatory action, but only bepridil, diltiazem, and verapamil depress myocardial contractility and cause AV block. *Toxic dose:* Any ingested amount greater than the maximum daily dose has the potential of being severely toxic. The maximum oral daily doses are amlodipine (Norvasc), 10 mg; bepridil (Vascor), 400 mg; diltiazem (Cardizem), 360 mg (toxic dose greater than 2 grams), 6 mg per kg in children; felodipine (Plendil), 10 mg; isradipine (DynaCirc), 20 mg; nicardipine (Cardene), 120 mg; nifedipine (Procardia), 120 mg, 0.9 mg per kg per day in children; nimodipine (Nimotop), 360 mg; nitrendipine (Baypress),* 80 mg; and verapamil (Calan), 480 mg, 4 to 8 mg per kg in children. *Kinetics:* Onset of action of regular-release preparations varies: verapamil, 60 to 120 minutes; nifedipine, 20 minutes; diltiazem, 15 minutes after ingestion. The peak effect for verapamil is at 2 to 4 hours, for nifedipine 60 to 90 minutes, and for diltiazem 30 to 60 minutes; however, the peak action may be delayed for 6 to 8 hours. The duration is up to 36 hours. With sustained-release preparations the onset is usually at 4 hours but may be delayed; the peak effect is at 12 to 24 hours; and concretions and prolonged toxicity can develop. The $t_{1/2}$ for hepatic elimination varies from 3 to 7 hours. The Vd varies from 3 to 7 liters per kg. *Manifestations:* Hypotension, bradycardia, and conduction disturbances occur 30 minutes to 5 hours after ingestion. A prolonged PR interval is an early and constant finding and may occur at therapeutic doses. Torsades de pointes has been reported. All degrees of blocks may occur and may be delayed 12 to 16 hours. Lactic acidosis may be present. Calcium channel blockers do not affect intraventricular conduction, so the QRS interval is usually not affected. Hypocalcemia is rarely present. Hyperglycemia may be present because of calcium-dependent insulin release. Mental status changes, headaches, seizures, hemiparesis, and CNS depression may occur. Calcium channel blockers may precipitate respiratory failure in Duchenne's muscular dystrophy. *Management:* (1) Establish and maintain vital functions. Obtain a baseline ECG, and institute continuous cardiac and blood pressure monitoring. A pacemaker should be available. Cardiology consultation should be sought. (2) GI decontamination: AC is recommended, and MDAC may be useful (no data are available). If a large sustained-release preparation is involved, MDAC for 48 to 72 hours and whole-bowel irrigation may be useful, but the effectiveness has not been investigated. (3) If the patient is symptomatic, immediate cardiology consultation should be obtained because a pacemaker and hemodynamic monitoring may be needed. (4) If a heart block occurs, atropine is rarely effective and isoproterenol may produce vasodilatation. Consider the use of a pacemaker early.

*Exceeds dosage recommended by the manufacturer.

*Not available in the United States.

(5) Treat hypotension and bradycardia with positioning, fluids, calcium gluconate or calcium chloride, glucagon, amrinone, and ventricular pacing. Calcium gluconate or calcium chloride (see Table 12): Avoid calcium salts if digoxin is present. Calcium usually reverses depressed myocardial contractility but may not reverse nodal depression or peripheral vasodilatation. Calcium chloride is used as a 10% solution at 0.1 to 0.2 mL per kg up to 10 mL in an adult, or calcium gluconate as a 10% solution at 0.3 to 0.4 mL per kg, up to 20 mL in an adult, administered IV over 5 to 10 minutes. Monitor for dysrhythmias, hypotension, and serum calcium. The aim is to increase the calcium value 4 mg per dL to a maximum of 13 mg per dL. The calcium response lasts 15 minutes and may require repeated doses or a continuous calcium gluconate infusion (0.2 mL per kg per hour, up to a maximum of 10 mL per hour). If calcium fails, try glucagon (see Table 12) for its positive inotropic or chronotropic effect or both. Amrinone, an inotropic agent, may reverse calcium channel blockers. The effective dose is 0.15 to 2 mg per kg (0.15 to 0.4 mL per kg) by intravenous bolus followed by infusion of 5 to 10 μg per kg per minute. (6) Hypotension: Fluids, norepinephrine, and epinephrine may be required for hypotension. Amrinone and glucagon have been tried alone and in combination. Dobutamine and dopamine are often ineffective. (7) Extracorporeal measures (e.g., hemodialysis and charcoal hemoperfusion) are not considered useful. (8) Patients receiving digitalis and calcium channel blockers run the risk of digitalis toxicity because calcium channel blockers increase digitalis levels. (9) Extraordinary measures such as the intra-aortic balloon pump and cardiopulmonary bypass have been used successfully. (10) Hyperglycemia does not require insulin therapy. *Laboratory investigations:* Specific drug levels are not easily available and are not useful. Monitor blood glucose, electrolytes, calcium, ABGs, pulse oximetry, creatinine, BUN, hemodynamics, ECG, and cardiac function. *Disposition:* With intoxications involving regular-release preparations monitoring is indicated for at least 6 hours, and with those involving sustained-release preparations, for 24 hours after alleged ingestion. For intentional overdose, psychiatric clearance is needed. Symptomatic patients should be admitted to the ICU.

Carbon Monoxide. CO is an odorless, colorless gas produced by incomplete combustion; it is an in vivo metabolic breakdown product of methylene chloride used in paint removers. *Toxic mechanism:* The affinity of CO for hemoglobin is 240 times greater than that of oxygen; it shifts the oxygen dissociation curve to the left, which impairs hemoglobin release of oxygen to tissues, and inhibits the cytochrome oxidase system. *Toxic dose and manifestations:* See Table 30. CO exposure and manifestations: Exposure to 0.5% for a few minutes is lethal. Contrary to popular belief, the skin rarely shows a cherry-red color in the living patient. Sequelae correlate with the level of consciousness at presentation. ECG abnormalities may be noted. Creatine kinase is often elevated; rhabdomyolysis and myoglobinuria may occur. The carboxyhemoglobin (COHb) level expresses as a percentage the extent to which CO has bound with the total hemoglobin. This may be misleading in the anemic patient. The patient's presentation is more reliable than the COHb level. In Table 30, the manifestations listed for each level are in addition to those already listed at the preceding level. Note that 0.01% = 100 parts per million (ppm). A level greater than 40% is usually associated with obvious intoxication. The COHb may not correlate reliably with the severity of the intoxication, and attempts to link symptoms to specific levels of COHb are frequently inaccurate. *Kinetics:* The natural metabolism of the body produces small amounts of COHb, less than 2% for nonsmokers and 5 to 9% for smokers. CO is rapidly absorbed through the lungs. The rate of absorption is directly related to alveolar ventilation. Elimination occurs through the lungs. The $t_{1/2}$ of COHb in room air (21% oxygen) is 5 to 6 hours; in 100% oxygen, 90

TABLE 30. **Carbon Monoxide Exposure and Possible Manifestations**

CO in Atmosphere (%)	Duration of Exposure (h)	COHb Saturation (%)	Manifestations
<0.0035 (35 ppm)	Indefinite	3.5	None
0.005–0.01 (50–100 ppm)	Indefinite	5	Slight headache, decreased exercise tolerance
Up to 0.01 (100 ppm)	Indefinite	10	Slight headache, dyspnea on vigorous exertion; driving skills may be impaired
0.01–0.02 (100–200 ppm)	Indefinite	10–20	Dyspnea on moderate exertion; throbbing, temporal headache
0.02–0.03 (200–300 ppm)	5–6	20–30	Severe headache, syncope, dizziness, visual changes, weakness, nausea, vomiting, altered judgment
0.04–0.06 (400–600 ppm)	4–5	30–40	Vertigo, ataxia, blurred vision, confusion, loss of consciousness
0.07–0.10 (700–1000 ppm)	3–4	40–50	Confusion, tachycardia, tachypnea, coma, convulsions
0.11–0.15 (1100–1500 ppm)	1.5–3	50–60	Cheyne-Stokes respiration, coma, convulsions, shock, apnea
0.16–0.30 (1600–3000 ppm)	1.0–1.5	60–70	Coma, convulsions, respiratory and heart failure, death
>0.40 (>4000 ppm)	Few minutes		Death

Abbreviation: COHb = carboxyhemoglobin.

minutes; and in hyperbaric oxygen at 3 atmospheres of oxygen, 20 to 30 minutes. *Management:* (1) Adequately protect the rescuer. Remove the patient from the contaminated area. Establish vital functions. (2) The mainstay of treatment is administration of 100% oxygen via a non-rebreathing mask with an oxygen reservoir or endotracheal tube. Give 100% oxygen to all patients until the COHb level is 2% or less. Assisted ventilation may be necessary. (3) Monitor ABGs and COHb. Determine the present COHb level and extrapolate to the COHb level at the time of exposure using the $t_{1/2}$ of COHb in different percentages of ambient oxygen (see kinetics just discussed). Note: A near-normal COHb level does not exclude significant CO poisoning, especially if measured several hours after the termination of exposure or if oxygen has been administered before obtaining the sample. (4) The exposed pregnant woman should be kept in 100% oxygen for several hours after the COHb level is almost zero because COHb concentrates in the fetus and oxygen is needed longer to ensure elimination of CO from the fetal circulation. Monitor the fetus. CO and hypoxia are teratogenic. (5) Metabolic acidosis should be treated with sodium bicarbonate only if the pH is below 7.2 after correction of hypoxia and adequate ventilation. Acidosis shifts the oxygen dissociation curve to the right and facilitates oxygen delivery to the tissues. (6) Use of the hyperbaric oxygen (HBO) chamber: The decision must be made on the basis of availability of a hyperbaric chamber, the ability to handle other acute emergencies that may coexist, extrapolated COHb level, and the severity of the poisoning. The standard of care for persons exposed to CO has yet to be determined, but most authorities recommend HBO therapy with any of the following guidelines: (a) if HBO therapy is not readily available, a COHb greater than 40%, or if HBO therapy is readily available, COHb greater than 25%; (b) if the patient is unconscious or has a history of loss of consciousness or seizures; (c) if cardiovascular dysfunction (clinical ischemic chest pain or ECG evidence of ischemia) is present; (d) if there is metabolic acidosis; (e) if symptoms persist despite 100% oxygen therapy; (f) if there is an initial COHb level greater than 15% in a child, in a patient with cardiovascular disease, or in a pregnant woman; or (g) if there are signs of maternal or fetal distress regardless of COHb level. Management of CO toxicity in infants and fetuses is a special problem because fetal hemoglobin has greater affinity for CO than does adult hemoglobin. A neurologic-cognitive examination has been used to help determine which patients with low CO levels should receive more aggressive therapy. Testing should include the following: general orientation memory testing (address, phone number, date of birth, present date) and cognitive testing (serial 7s, digit span, forward and backward spelling of three-letter and four-letter words). Patients with delayed neurologic sequelae or recurrent symptoms for up to 3 weeks may benefit from HBO treatment. (7) Treat seizures and cerebral edema. *Laboratory investigations:* ABGs may show metabolic acidosis and normal oxygen tension. If there is significant poisoning, monitor the ABGs, electrolytes, blood glucose, serum creatine kinase and cardiac enzymes, renal function, and liver function. Obtain a urinalysis and test for myoglobinuria. Obtain a chest radiograph if there has been smoke inhalation or use of an HBO chamber is being considered. ECG monitoring is needed especially if the patient is older than 40 years, has a cardiac history, or has moderate to severe symptoms. Determine the blood ethanol level and conduct toxicology studies on the basis of symptoms and circumstances. Monitor COHb during and at the end of therapy. The pulse oximeter has two wavelengths and overestimates oxyhemoglobin saturation in CO poisoning. The true oxygen saturation is determined by blood gas analysis measuring the oxygen bound to hemoglobin. The co-oximeter measures four wavelengths and separates out COHb and the other hemoglobin-binding agents from oxyhemoglobin. Fetal hemoglobin has a greater affinity for CO than does adult hemoglobin, and the COHb may be falsely elevated as much as 4% in young infants. *Disposition:* Patients with no or mild symptoms (after exposures of less than 5 minutes) who become asymptomatic after a few hours of oxygen therapy and have a CO level below 10%, normal findings on physical examination and on neurologic-cognitive examination, and normal ABG parameters may be discharged but instructed to return if there are any signs of neurologic dysfunction. Patients with CO poisoning requiring treatment need follow-up neuropsychiatric examinations.

Caustics and Corrosives. The U.S. Consumer Products Safety Commission labeling recommendations on containers for acids and alkalis indicate the potential for producing serious damage: caution (weak irritant), warning (strong irritant), danger (corrosive). Some common acids with corrosive potential are acetic acid (>50%), calcium oxide, formic acid, glycolic acid (>10%), hydrochloric acid (>10%), mercuric chloride, nitric acid (>5%), oxalic acid (>10%), phosphoric acid (>60%), sulfuric acid (battery acid) (>10%), zinc chloride (>10%), and zinc sulfate (>50%). Some common alkalis with corrosive potential include ammonia (>5%), calcium carbide, calcium hydroxide (dry), potassium hydroxide (lye) (>1%), and sodium hydroxide (lye) (>1%). *Toxic mechanism:* Acids produce mucosal coagulation necrosis and an eschar and may be systemically absorbed, but with the exception of hydrofluoric acid they do not penetrate deeply. Injury to the gastric mucosa is more likely, although specific sites of injury for acids and alkalis are not clearly defined. Alkalis produce liquefaction necrosis and saponification and penetrate deeply. The esophageal mucosa is more likely to be damaged. Oropharyngeal and esophageal damage by solids is more frequent than by liquids. Liquids produce superficial, circumferential burns and gastric damage. *Toxic dose:* The toxicity is determined by concentration, contact time, and pH. Significant injury is more likely at pH values less than 2 or greater than 12, stricture at pH 14, prolonged contact time, and large volumes. *Manifestations:* The absence of oral burns does not exclude the possibility of esophageal or gastric damage. General clinical findings include stridor; dysphagia; drooling; oropharyngeal, retrosternal, and epigastric pain; and ocular and oral burns. Alkali burns are yellow, soapy, frothy lesions. Acid burns are gray-white in color and later form an eschar. Abdominal tenderness and guarding may be present if there is perforation. *Management:* Bring the container; the substance must be identified and the pH of the substance, vomitus, tears, and saliva tested. *Ingestion, ocular, and dermal management:* (1) Prehospital and initial hospital management: If ingestion occurs, all GI decontamination procedures are contraindicated except for immediate rinsing, removal of the substance from the mouth, and then dilution with small amounts (sips) of milk or water. Check for ocular and dermal involvement. Contraindications to oral dilution are dysphagia, respiratory distress, obtundation, and shock. If ocular involvement occurs, immediately irrigate with tepid water for at least 30 minutes, perform fluorescein staining of the eye, and consult an ophthalmologist. If dermal involvement occurs, immediately remove contaminated clothes and irrigate the skin with tepid water for at least 15 minutes. Consult with a burn specialist. (2) For acid ingestion, some authorities advocate placement of a small flexible nasogastric tube and aspiration within 30 minutes after ingestion. (3) The patient should receive only intravenous fluids after dilution until endoscopy consultation is obtained. (4) Endoscopy is valuable for predicting damage and the risk of stricture. The indications are controversial: some authorities recommend its use in all caustic ingestions regardless of symptoms, whereas others are selective, using clinical features such as vomiting, stridor, and drooling and oral or facial lesions as criteria. Endoscopy is indicated for all symptomatic patients or those with intentional ingestions. Endoscopy may be done immediately if the patient is symptomatic but is usually done 12 to 48 hours after ingestion. After 72 hours there is increased risk of perforation. (5) Corticosteroids may be ineffective and are considered mainly for second-degree circumferential burns. If a corticosteroid is used, start hydrocortisone sodium succinate given IV at 10 to 20 mg per kg per day within 48 hours and change to oral prednisolone at 2 mg per kg per day. Continue prednisolone for 3 weeks, and then taper the dose. (6) Provide tetanus prophylaxis. Antibiotics are not useful prophylactically. (7) An esophagogram is not useful in the first few days and may interfere with endoscopic evaluation; later, it may be used to assess the severity of damage. (8) Investigative therapy includes agents to inhibit collagen formation and the use of intraluminal stents. (9) Esophageal and gastric outlet dilatation may be needed if there is evidence of stricture. Bougienage of the esophagus has, however, been associated with brain abscess. Interposition of a colon segment may be necessary if dilatation fails to provide a passage of adequate size. *Inhalation management* requires immediate removal of the patient from the environment, administration of humid supplemental oxygen, and observation for airway obstruction and noncardiac pulmonary edema. Obtain radiographic and ABG evaluation when appropriate. Intubation and respiratory support may be required. Certain caustics produce systemic disturbances; formaldehyde causes metabolic acidosis; hydrofluoric acid, hypocalcemia and renal damage; oxalic acid, hypocalcemia; phenol, hepatic and renal damage; and pitric acid, renal injury. *Laboratory investigations:* If acid has been ingested, determine the acid-base balance and electrolytes. If there are pulmonary symptoms, use chest radiography, ABGs, and pulse oximetry. *Disposition:* Infants and small children should be medically evaluated and observed. Admit all symptomatic patients. Admit to the ICU if there are severe symptoms or danger of airway compromise. After endoscopy, if there is no damage, the patient may be discharged when oral feedings are tolerated. Intentional exposures require psychiatric evaluation before discharge.

Cocaine (benzoylmethylecgonine). Cocaine is derived from the leaves of *Erythroxylon coca* and *Truxillo coca.* A body packer is a person who conceals many small packages of cocaine contraband in the GI tract or other areas for illicit transport. A body stuffer spontaneously ingests substances for the purpose of hiding evidence. *Toxic mechanism:* Cocaine directly stimulates CNS presynaptic sympathetic neurons to release catecholamines and acetylcholine, blocks presynaptic reuptake of the catecholamines, blocks the sodium channels along neuronal membranes, and increases platelet aggregation. Long-term use depletes the CNS of dopamine. *Toxic dose:* The maximal mucosal local anesthetic therapeutic dose is 200 mg or 2 mL of 10% solution. Psychoactive effects occur at 50 to 95 mg; cardiac and CNS effects occur at 1 mg per kg. The potential fatal dose is 1200 mg intranasally, but death has occurred with 20 mg parenterally. *Kinetics:* See Table 31. Cocaine is well absorbed by all routes including nasal insufflation and oral, dermal, and inhalation routes. It is metabolized by plasma and liver cholinesterase to the inactive metabolites ecgonine methyl ester and benzoylecgonine. Plasma pseudocholinesterase is congenitally deficient in 3% of the population and decreased in fetuses, in young infants, in elderly persons, in pregnancy, and in liver disease. Persons with this enzyme deficit are at increased risk for life-threatening cocaine toxicity. The PB is 8.7%; the Vd, 1.2 to 1.9 liters per kg; 10% is excreted unchanged. Cocaine and ethanol undergo liver synthesis to form cocaethylene, a metabolite with a $t_{1/2}$ three times longer than that of cocaine. This metabolite may account for some of cocaine's cardiotoxicity and appears to be more lethal than cocaine or ethanol alone. *Manifestations:* (1) CNS: euphoria, hyperactivity, agitation, convulsions, intracranial hemorrhage; (2) eye-ear-nose-throat: mydriasis, septal perforation; (3) cardiovascular: cardiac dysrhythmias, hypertension and hypotension (in severe overdose), chest pain (occurs frequently but only 5.8% of affected patients have

TABLE 31. **Different Routes and Kinetics of Cocaine**

Type	Route	$t_{1/2}$ (min)	Onset	Peak (min)	Duration (min)
Cocaine leaf	Oral, chew	NA	20–30 min	45–90	240–360
Hydrochloride	Insufflation	78	1–3 min	5–10	60–90
	Ingested	54	20–30 min	50–90	Sustained
	Intravenous	36	30–120 s	5–11	60–90
Freebase, crack	Smoked	—	5–10 s	5–11	Up to 20
Coca paste	Smoked	—	Unknown		

true myocardial ischemia and infarction); (4) hyperthermia (vasoconstriction, increased metabolism); (5) GI: ischemic bowel perforation if the drug was ingested; (6) rhabdomyolysis, myoglobinuria, and renal failure; (7) premature labor and abruptio placentae; (8) in prolonged toxicity, suspect body cavity packing; (9) mortality resulting from cerebrovascular accidents, coronary artery spasm and myocardial injury, and lethal dysrhythmias. *Management:* (1) Supportive care: Blood pressure, cardiac, and thermal monitoring and seizure precautions are instituted. Diazepam is the agent of choice for treatment of cocaine toxicity with agitation, seizures, dysrhythmias; the dose is 10 to 30 mg IV at 2.5 mg per minute for adults and 0.2 to 0.5 mg per kg at 1 mg per minute up to 10 mg for a child. (2) GI decontamination: If cocaine was ingested, administer AC. MDAC may absorb cocaine leakage in body stuffers or body packers. Whole-bowel irrigation with PEG solution has been used in body packers and stuffers if the contraband is in a firm container. If packages are not visible on an abdominal radiograph, a contrast study and/or ultrasonography can help to confirm successful passage. PEG may desorb the cocaine from AC. Cocaine in the nasal passage can be removed with an applicator dipped in a non–water-soluble product (lubricating jelly). (3) In body packers and stuffers, secure venous access and have drugs readily available to treat life-threatening manifestations until contraband is passed in the stool. Surgical removal may be indicated if a packet does not pass the pylorus, in a symptomatic body packer, or in intestinal obstruction. (4) Cardiovascular disturbances: Hypertension and tachycardia are usually transient and can be managed by careful titration of diazepam. Nitroprusside may be used for management of hypertensive crisis. Myocardial ischemia is managed by oxygen, vascular access to administer intravenous medications, BZPs, and nitroglycerin. Use of aspirin and thrombolytic agents is not routinely recommended because of danger of intracranial hemorrhage. Dysrhythmias are usually supraventricular tachycardias and do not require specific management. Adenosine is ineffective. Life-threatening tachydysrhythmias may respond to phentolamine, in a dose of 5 mg given as an intravenous bolus in adults, or 0.1 mg per kg in children, at 5- to 10-minute intervals. Phentolamine also relieves coronary artery spasm and myocardial ischemia. Electrical synchronized cardioversion should be considered for hemodynamically unstable dysrhythmias. Lidocaine is not recommended initially but may be used after 3 hours for ventricular tachycardia. Wide complex QRS ventricular tachycardia may be treated with $NaHCO_3$ at 2 mEq per kg as a bolus. Beta-adrenergic blockers are not recommended. (5) Treat anxiety, agitation, and convulsions with diazepam. If diazepam fails to control seizures, use neuromuscular blockers and monitor the EEG for nonmotor seizures. (6) Hyperthermia: Administer external cooling and cool humidified 100% oxygen. Neuromuscular paralysis to control seizures reduces temperature. Dantrolene and antipyretics are not recommended. (7) Treat rhabdomyolysis and myoglobinuria with fluids, alkaline diuresis, and diuretics. (8) If the patient is pregnant, monitor the fetus and observe for threatened spontaneous abortion. (9) Treat paranoid ideation and threatening behavior with rapid tranquilization. (See the earlier section on violent patients, page 1208.) Observe the patient for suicidal depression that may follow intoxication and may require suicide precautions. (10) If focal neurologic manifestations are present, consider a diagnosis of cerebrovascular accident and perform CT. (11) Extracorporeal measures are of no benefit. *Laboratory investigations:* Monitoring: ECG and cardiac monitoring is instituted, as well as monitoring of ABGs and oxygen saturation, electrolytes, blood glucose, BUN, creatinine, creatine kinase and cardiac function if chest pain is present, liver profile, rhabdomyolysis and urine for myoglobin, and urine for cocaine and metabolites and other substances of abuse. Abdominal radiography or ultrasonography is performed for assessment in body packers. A urine sample collected more than 12 hours after cocaine intake contains little or no cocaine. If cocaine is present, it has been used within the past 12 hours. Cocaine's metabolite benzoylecgonine may be detected within 4 hours after a single nasal insufflation and up to 48 to 114 hours after use. Intravenous drug users should have HIV and hepatitis virus testing. Cross-reactions with herbal teas, lidocaine, and droperidol may give false-positive results with some laboratory methods. *Disposition:* Patients with mild intoxication or a brief seizure that does not require treatment who become asymptomatic may be discharged after 6 hours with appropriate psychosocial follow-up. If there are cardiac or cerebral ischemia manifestations, monitor in the ICU. Body packers and stuffers require ICU care until passage of the contraband.

Cyanide. Some sources of cyanide: (1) Hydrogen cyanide (HCN) is a by-product of burning plastic and wools and is produced in residential fires and salts in ore extraction. (2) Nitriles, such as acetonitrile (present in artificial nail removers), are metabolized in the body to produce cyanide. (3) Cyanogenic glycosides in the seeds of fruit stones (as amygdalin in apricots, peaches, apples) in the presence of intestinal β-glucosidase form cyanide (the seeds are harmful only if the capsule is broken). (4) Sodium nitroprusside, the antihypertensive vasodilator, contains five cyanide groups. *Toxic mechanism:* Cyanide blocks the cellular electron transport mechanism and cellular respiration by inhibiting the mitochondrial ferricytochrome oxidase system and other enzymes. This results in cellular hypoxia and lactic acidosis. *Toxic dose:* The ingestion of 1 mg per kg or 50 mg of HCN can produce death within 15 minutes. The lethal dose of potassium cyanide is 200 mg. Five to 10 mL of 84% acetonitrile is lethal. The permissible exposure limit for volatile HCN is 10 ppm, and 300 ppm is fatal in minutes. *Kinetics:* Cyanide is rapidly absorbed by all routes. In the stomach it forms hydrocyanic acid. The PB is 60%; the Vd, 1.5 liters per kg. Cyanide is detoxified by metabolism in the liver via the mitochondrial endogenous thiosulfate-rhodanese pathway, which catalyzes the transfer of sulfur to cyanide to form irreversibly the less toxic thiocyanate, which is excreted in the urine. The $t_{1/2}$ for cyanide elimination from the blood is 1.2 hours. Cyanide is also detoxified by reacting with hydroxocobalamin (vitamin B_{12a}) to form cyanocobalamin (vitamin B_{12}). Elimination is through the lungs. *Manifestations:* HCN has the distinctive odor of bitter almonds (odor of silver polish). The clinical findings are flushing, hypertension, headache, hyperpnea, seizures, stupor, cardiac dysrhythmias, and pulmonary edema. Cyanosis is absent or appears late. Various ECG abnormalities may be present. *Management:* (1) Protect rescuers and attendants. Immediately administer 100% oxygen and continue during and after the administration of the antidote. If cyanide is inhaled, remove the patient from the contaminated atmosphere. Attendants should not administer mouth-to-mouth resuscitation. (2) Cyanide antidote kit (see Table 12): The clinician must decide whether to use any or all components of the kit. The mechanism of action of the antidote kit is to form methemoglobin (MetHb), which has a greater affinity for cyanide than the cytochrome oxidase system and forms cyanomethemoglobin. The cyanide is transferred from MetHb by sodium thiosulfate, which provides a sulfur atom that is converted by the rhodanese-catalyzed enzyme reaction (thiosulfate sulfurtransferase) to convert cyanide into the relatively nontoxic sodium thiocyanate, which is excreted by the kidney. Procedure for using the antidote kit: Step 1, use of amyl nitrite inhalant Perles, is only a temporizing measure (forms only 2 to 5% MetHb) and can be omitted if venous access is established. Administer 100% oxygen and the inhalant for 30 seconds of every minute. Use a new Perle every 3 minutes. Step 2, administration of sodium nitrite ampule, is not necessary in poisonings associated with residential fires, smoke inhalation, nitroprusside, or acetonitrile. Sodium nitrite is administered IV to produce MetHb of 20 to 30% at 35 to 70 minutes after administration. For adults, 10 mL of a 3% solution of sodium nitrite (child, 0.33 mL per kg of 3% solution) is diluted to 100 mL with 0.9% saline and administered slowly IV at 5 mL per minute. If hypotension develops, slow the infusion. Step 3, administration of sodium thiosulfate, is useful alone in smoke inhalation, nitroprusside toxicity, and acetonitrile toxicity and should not be used at all in hydrogen sulfide poisoning. For adults, administer 12.5 grams of sodium thiosulfate or 50 mL of 25% solution (for children, 1.65 mL per kg of 25% solution) IV over 10 to 20 minutes. If cyanide-related symptoms recur, repeat antidotes in 30 minutes as half of the initial dose. The dosage regimen for children on the package insert must be carefully followed. One hour after antidotes are administered, the MetHb level should be obtained and should not exceed 20%. Methylene blue should not be used to reverse excessive MetHb. (3) GI decontamination after oral ingestion by gastric lavage and AC is recommended but is not very effective (1 gram binds only 35 mg of cyanide). (4) Treat seizures with intravenous diazepam. Correct acidosis with $NaHCO_3$ if it does not resolve rapidly with therapy. (5) Treat metabolic acidosis with $NaHCO_3$. (6) There is no role for the HBO chamber, hemodialysis, or hemoperfusion. (7) Other antidotes: In France, hydroxocobalamin (vitamin B_{12a}) is used (it exchanges its hydroxyl with free cyanide to form cyanocobalamin). It has proved effective when given immediately after exposure in large doses of 4 grams (50 mg per kg) or 50 times the amount of cyanide in the exposure with 8 grams of sodium thiosulfate (it has FDA orphan drug approval). *Laboratory investigations:* Obtain and monitor ABGs, oxygen saturation, blood lactate (which takes 0.5 hour), blood cyanide (which takes hours), hemoglobin, blood glucose, and electrolytes. Lactic acidemia, decreases in the arterial-venous oxygen difference, and bright red color of the venous blood are manifestations of toxicity. If smoke inhalation is the possible source of exposure, obtain COHb and MetHb concentrations. The cyanide level in whole blood for a smoker is less than 0.5 μg per mL; with exposures with flushing and tachycardia, 0.5 to 1.0 μg per mL; with obtundation, 1.0 to 2.5 μg per mL; and with coma and death, greater than 2.5 μg per mL. *Disposition:* Asymptomatic patients should be observed for a minimum of 6 hours. Patients who ingest nitrile compounds must be observed for 24 hours. Patients requiring antidote administration should be admitted to the ICU.

Digitalis. Cardiac glycosides are found in cardiac medication, common plants, and the skin of *Bufo* species of toad. More than 1 to 3 mg may be found in a few leaves of oleander or foxglove. *Toxic mechanism:* Cardiac glycosides inhibit the enzyme Na^+, K^+-ATPase, leading to intracellular potassium loss, increased intracellular sodium-producing phase 4 depolarization, increased automaticity, and ectopy. Increased intracellular calcium and potentiation of contractility occur. Pacemaker cells are inhibited and the refractory period is prolonged, leading to AV blocks. Vagal tone is increased. *Toxic dose:* The digoxin total digitalizing dose is 0.75 to 1.25 mg or 10 to 15 μg per kg in patients older than 10 years and 40 to 50 μg per kg in those younger than 2 years; 30 to 40 μg per kg at 2 to 10 years of age produces a therapeutic serum concentration of 0.6 to 2.0 ng per mL. The acute single toxic dose is more than 0.07 mg per kg or more than 2 to 3 mg in adults; however, 2 mg in a child or 4 mg in an adult usually produces mild toxicity. Serious and potentially fatal overdoses are greater than 4 mg in a child and greater than 10 mg in an adult. Digoxin clinical toxicity is usually associated with serum digoxin levels of 3.5 ng per mL or more in adults. Patients at greatest risk of overdose include those with cardiac disease, electrolyte abnormalities (low potassium, low magesium, low thyroxine, high calcium), or renal impairment and those receiving amiodarone, quinidine, erythromycin, tetracycline, calcium channel blockers, and beta blockers. *Kinetics:* Digoxin is a metabolite of digitoxin. With oral ingestion, onset occurs within 1 to 2 hours, peak levels occur at 2 to 3 hours, and peak effects occur at 3 to 4 hours; the duration is 3 to 4 days. In overdose, the typical onset is at 30 minutes with peak effects in 3 to 12 hours. With intoxications due to intravenous use, onset is in 5 to 30 minutes, the peak level occurs immediately, and the peak effect occurs at 1.5 to 3 hours. Elimination is 60 to 80% renal. The Vd is 5 to 6 liters per kg. The cardiac-to-plasma ratio is 30:1. The elimination $t_{1/2}$ is 30 to 50 hours. After an acute ingestion overdose, the serum concentration does not reflect the tissue concentration for at least 6 hours or more, and steady state is reached 12 to 16 hours after the last dose. *Manifestations:* These may be delayed 9 to 18 hours. (1) GI effects: Nausea and vomiting are always present in acute ingestion and may occur in chronic ingestion. (2) Cardiovascular effects: The "digitalis effect" on the ECG consists of scooped ST segments and PR prolongation. In overdose, any dysrhythmia or block is possible, but none is characteristic. Bradycardia occurs in acute overdose in patients with healthy hearts or tachycardia with existing heart disease, or in chronic overdose. Ventricular tachycardia is seen only in severe poisoning. (3) CNS effects are headaches, visual disturbances, and colored-halo vision. (4) Potassium disturbances: Hyperkalemia is a predictor of serum digoxin concentrations greater than 10 ng per mL and is associated with a 50% mortality rate without treatment. In one review, if serum potassium was less than 5.0 mEq per liter, the survival rate was 100%; if 5 to 5.5 mEq per liter, 50% of the patients survived; and if greater than 5.5 mEq per liter, all died. Hypokalemia is commonly seen with chronic intoxication. Patients with normal digitalis levels may have toxicity in the presence of hypokalemia. (5) Chronic intoxications are more likely to produce scotoma, color perception disturbances, yellow vision, halos, delirium, hallucinations or psychosis, tachycardia, and hypokalemia. *Management:* Obtain a cardiology consultation and have a pacemaker readily available. (1) GI decontamination: Use caution with vagal stimulation, and avoid emesis and gastric lavage. Administer AC; if a nasogastric tube is required for AC therapy, consider pretreatment with atropine (0.02 mg per kg for a child and 0.5 mg for an adult). MDAC may interrupt enterohepatic recirculation of digitoxin and adsorb active metabolites. (2) Digoxin-specific antibody fragment (Fab, Digibind), 40 mg, binds with 0.6 mg of digoxin and is then excreted through the kidneys. It decreases digoxin 50-fold. (See Table 12.) Indications include life-threatening hemodynamically unstable dysrhythmias (ventricular dysrhythmias or rapid deterioration of clinical findings); ingestions greater than 4 mg in a child and 10 mg in an adult; serum potassium greater than 5.0 mEq per liter produced by cardiac glycoside toxicity; serum digoxin toxicity (more than 10 ng per mL in adults or more than 5 ng per mL in children) 6 to 8 hours after acute ingestion; and unstable severe bradycardia or second- or third-degree blocks unresponsive to atropine. This agent is also useful in digitalis delirium with thrombocytopenia and in treatment of life-threatening digitoxin and oleander poisoning. Empirical digoxin-specific Fab fragment therapy may be administered as a bolus through a 22-μm filter if there is a critical emergency. If the clinical situation is less urgent, administer over 30 minutes. The empirical dose is 10 vials for adults and 5 vials or children.

Calculation of dose: The amount (total mg) of digoxin known to have been ingested multiplied by 80% bioavailability (0.8) = body burden. If the agent was given as liquid capsules or IV, do not multiply by 0.8. The body burden divided by 0.6 (0.6 mg of digoxin is bound by 1 vial of 40 mg of Fab) = number of vials needed. If the amount is unknown but the steady-state serum concentration is known, for digoxin:

$$\text{Digoxin (ng/mL)} \times \text{Vd (5.6 L/kg)} \times \text{weight (kg)} = \text{body burden } (\mu g)$$

$$\text{Body burden}/1000 = \text{body burden in mg}$$

$$\text{Body burden}/0.6 = \text{number of vials needed}$$

For digitoxin:

$$\text{Digitoxin (ng/mL)} \times \text{Vd (0.56 L/kg)} \times \text{weight (kg)} = \text{body burden}$$

$$\text{Body burden}/1000 = \text{body burden in mg}$$

$$\text{Body burden}/0.6 = \text{number of vials needed}$$

(3) Antidysrhythmic agents and a pacemaker should be used only if Fab therapy fails. The onset of action is within 30 minutes. Complications of Fab therapy are mainly related to withdrawal of digoxin and worsening heart failure and include hypokalemia, decreased glucose (if low glycogen stores), and aller-

gic reactions (rare). Digitalis administered after Fab therapy is bound and may be inactivated for 5 to 7 days. (4) For ventricular tachydysrhythmias, correct electrolyte disturbances and administer lidocaine or phenytoin. For torsades de pointes, administer 20 mL of 20% magnesium sulfate given IV slowly over 20 minutes, or 25 to 50 mg per kg in a child, and titrate to control the dysrhythmia. Discontinue magnesium if hypotension, heart block, or a decrease in deep tendon reflexes occurs. Magnesium should be used with caution if renal impairment is present. Ventricular pacing should be reserved for patients who fail to respond to Fab. (5) Do not use antidysrhythmics of classes IA, IC, II, and IV or agents that increase conduction time (e.g., procainamide, bretylium, diltiazem, beta blockers). Class IB drugs can be used. (6) Cardioversion should be used with caution; start at a setting of 5 to 10 joules and pretreat with lidocaine, if possible, because it may precipitate ventricular fibrillation or asystole. (7) Treat unstable bradycardia and second- and third-degree AV block with atropine. If the patient is unresponsive, use Fab. A pacemaker should be available if the patient fails to respond. Avoid isoproterenol, which causes dysrhythmias. (8) Electrolyte disturbances: Potassium disturbances are due to a shift, not a change, in total body potassium. Treat hyperkalemia (potassium level greater than 5.0 mEq per liter) with Fab only. Never use calcium, and do not use insulin or glucose. Do not use $NaHCO_3$ concomitantly with Fab because it may produce severe life-threatening hypokalemia. Sodium polystyrene sulfonate (Kayexalate) should not be used. Treat hypokalemia with caution because this condition may be cardioprotective. (9) Extracorporeal procedures are ineffective. Hemodialysis is used for severe or refractory hyperkalemia. *Laboratory investigations:* Monitor baseline ECG and continuous cardiac function and blood glucose, electrolytes, calcium, magnesium, BUN, and creatinine levels. Measure initial digoxin levels more than 6 hours after ingestion because earlier values do not reflect the tissue distribution. Obtain free (unbound) serum digoxin concentrations after Fab therapy because the free (unbound) digoxin decreases and reflects the true level. Cross-reactions: An endogenous digoxin-like substance cross-reacts in most common immunoassays (not with HPLC), and values as high as 4.1 ng per mL have been reported in newborns, in patients with chronic renal failure or abnormal immunoglobulins, and in the third trimester of pregnancy. *Disposition:* Consult with a poison control center and cardiologist experienced with the use of digoxin-specific Fab fragments. All patients with significant dysrhythmias, symptoms, an elevated serum digoxin concentration, or elevated serum potassium level should be admitted to the ICU. Fab fragments and pacemaker therapy should be readily available. Asymptomatic patients with nontoxic levels should have studies repeated in 12 hours.

Ethanol (grain alcohol). See Table 32. *Toxic mechanism:* Ethanol has a CNS hypnotic and anesthetic effect produced by a variety of mechanisms, including membrane fluidity and effect on the GABA system. It promotes cutaneous vasodilatation (contributes to hypothermia), stimulates secretion of gastric juice (potentially causing gastritis), inhibits secretion of the antidiuretic hormone, inhibits gluconeogenesis (potentially causing hypoglycemia), and influences

TABLE 32. **Summary of Alcohol and Glycol Features***

Feature	Alcohol			Ethylene Glycol
	Methanol	*Isopropanol*	*Ethanol*	
Principal uses	Gas line Antifreeze Sterno Windshield wiper deicer	Solvent Jewelry cleaner Rubbing alcohol	Beverage Solvent	Antifreeze Deicer
Odor	None	None	Yes	None
Specific gravity	0.719	0.785	0.789	1.12
Fatal dose	1 mL/kg, 100% mortality	3 mL/kg, 100% mortality	5 mL/kg, 100% mortality	1.4 mL/kg
Hepatic enzyme	Alcohol dehydrogenase	Alcohol dehydrogenase	Alcohol and acetaldehyde dehydrogenases	Alcohol dehydrogenase
Toxic metabolite(s)	Formate, formaldehyde	Acetone	Acetaldehyde	Glyoxylic acid, oxalate
Drunkenness	±	2+	2+	1+
Metabolic change		Hyperglycemia	Hypoglycemia	Hypocalcemia
Metabolic acidosis	4+	0	1+	2+
Anion gap	4+	±	2+	4+
Ketosis	Ketobutyric acid	Acetone	Hydroxybutyric acid	None
GI tract	Pancreatitis	Hemorrhagic gastritis	Gastritis	
Visual	Blindness, pink optic disk			
Crystalluria	0	0	0	+
Pulmonary edema				+
Renal failure				+
Molecular weight	32	60	46	62
Osmolality†	0.337	0.176	0.228	0.190

*0 indicates no effect; + indicates mild effect; ± indicates no effect or mild effect; 2+ indicates moderate effect; 4+ indicates severe effect.

†1 mL/dL of substances raises the freezing point osmolarity of serum. The validity of the correlation of osmolality with blood concentrations has been questioned. Inebriation index: methanol < ethanol < ethylene glycol < isopropanol.

fat metabolism (potentially causing lipidemia). *Toxic dose:* 1 mL per kg of absolute or 100% ethanol or 200-proof ethanol (proof defines alcohol concentration in beverages) results in a blood ethanol concentration (BEC) of 100 mg per dL. The potentially fatal dose is 3 grams per kg for children or 6 grams per kg for adults. Children frequently have hypoglycemia at a BEC greater than 50 mg per dL. *Kinetics:* Onset of action occurs 30 to 60 minutes after ingestion, peak action is at 90 minutes on an empty stomach, and the Vd is 0.6 liter per kg. The major route of elimination (more than 90%) is by hepatic oxidative metabolism. The first step involves the enzyme alcohol dehydrogenase (ADH), which converts ethanol to acetaldehyde. The kinetics in this step are zero order at a constant rate (regardless of the level) of 12 to 20 mg per dL per hour (12 to 15 mg per dL per hour in nonalcoholic drinkers, 15 mg per dL per hour in social drinkers, 30 to 50 mg per dL per hour in alcoholics, and 28 mg per dL per hour in children). At a low BEC (less than 30 mg per dL), the metabolism is by first-order kinetics. In the second step of metabolism the acetaldehyde is metabolized by acetaldehyde dehydrogenase to acetic acid. In subsequent steps, acetic acid is metabolized via the Krebs citric acid cycle to carbon dioxide and water. The enzyme steps are dependent on nicotinamide adenine dinucleotide, which interferes with gluconeogenesis. Only 2 to 10% of ethanol is excreted unchanged by the kidneys. BEC and amount ingested can be estimated by the following equations (SG indicates specific gravity):

$$\text{BEC (mg/dL)} = \frac{\text{amount ingested (mL)} \times \text{\% ethanol in product} \times \text{SG (0.79)}}{\text{Vd (0.6 L/kg)} \times \text{body weight (kg)}}$$

$$\text{Dose (amount ingested)} = \frac{\text{BEC (mg/dL)} \times \text{Vd (0.6)} \times \text{body weight (kg)}}{\text{\% ethanol} \times \text{SG (0.79)}}$$

Manifestations: See Table 33. (1) Acute: BECs over 30 mg per dL produce euphoria; over 50 mg per dL, incoordination and intoxication; over 100 mg per dL, ataxia; over 300 mg per dL, stupor; and over 500 mg per dL, coma. Levels of 500 to 700 mg per dL may be fatal. Children frequently have hypoglycemia at a BEC above 50 mg per dL. (2) Chronic alcoholic patients tolerate a higher BEC, and correlation with manifestation is not valid. A rapid interview for alcoholism uses the CAGE questions: C, Have you felt the need to cut down? A, Have others annoyed you by criticizing your drinking? G, Have you felt guilty about your drinking? E, Have you ever had a morning eye-opening drink to steady your nerves or get rid of a hangover? Two affirmative answers indicate probable alcoholism. *Management:* Inquire about trauma and disulfiram (Antabuse) use. (1) Protect from aspiration and hypoxia. Establish and maintain vital functions. The patient may require intubation and assisted ventilation. (2) GI decontamination plays no role. (3) If the patient is comatose, administer IV 50% glucose at 1 mL per kg in adults and 25% glucose at 2 mL per kg in children. Thiamine, 100 mg IV, is administered if the patient has a history of chronic alcoholism, malnutrition, or suspected eating disorders and to prevent Wernicke-Korsakoff syndrome. Naloxone has produced a partial inconsistent response and is not recommended for known alcoholic CNS depressants. (4) General supportive care: Administer fluids to correct hydration and hypotension; correct electrolyte abnormalities and acid-base imbalance. Vasopressors and plasma expanders may be necessary to correct severe hypotension. Hypomagnesemia is frequently present in chronic alcoholics. In hypomagnesemia administer a loading dose of 2 grams of a 10% magnesium sulfate solution given IV over 5 minutes in the ICU with blood pressure and cardiac monitoring and have 10% calcium chloride on hand in case of overdose. Follow with constant infusion of 6 grams of 10% magnesium sulfate over 3 to 4 hours. Be cautious with magnesium administration if renal failure is present. (5) Hypothermic patients should be warmed. See general treatment of poisoning. (6) Hemodialysis may be used in severe cases when conventional therapy is ineffective (rarely needed). (7) Treat repeated or prolonged seizures with diazepam. Brief "rum fits" do not require long-

TABLE 33. **Clinical Signs in the Intolerant Ethanol Drinker**

Ethanol (mg/dL)	Blood (μg/mL)	Concentration* (mmol/L)	Manifestations† in Nonalcoholics
>25	>250	>5.4	Euphoria
>47	>470	>10.2	Mild incoordination, sensory and motor impairment
>50	>500	>10.8	Increased risk of motor vehicle accidents
>100	>1000	>21.7	Ataxia (legal toxic level in many localities)
>150	>1500	>32.5	Moderate incoordination, slow reaction time
>200	>2000	>43.4	Drowsiness and confusion
>300	>3000	>65.1	Severe incoordination, stupor, blurred vision
>500	>5000	>108.5	Flaccid coma, respiratory failure, hypotension; may be fatal

*Ethanol concentrations are sometimes reported as percents. Note that mg% is not equivalent to mg/dL because ethanol weighs less than water (specific gravity 0.79). A 1% ethanol concentration is 790 mg/dL and 0.1% is 79 mg/dL.

†There is a great variation in individual behavior at particular blood ethanol levels. Behavior is dependent on tolerance and other factors.

term anticonvulsant therapy. Repeated seizures or focal neurologic findings may warrant skull radiography, lumbar puncture, and CT of the head, depending on the clinical findings. (8) Treat withdrawal with hydration and large doses of chlordiazepoxide (50 to 100 mg) or diazepam (2 to 10 mg) IV; these may be repeated in 2 to 4 hours. Large doses of BZPs may be required for delirium tremors. Withdrawal can occur in the presence of an elevated BEC and can be fatal if untreated. *Laboratory investigations:* The BEC should be specifically requested and followed. (Gas chromatography or a Breathalyzer test gives rapid reliable results if there is no belching or vomiting; enzymatic methods do not differentiate between the alcohols.) Monitor ABGs, electrolytes, and glucose; determine anion and osmolar gaps (measure by freezing point depression, not vapor pressure); and check for ketosis. See discussion of general management. The AG increases 1 mg per kg for each 4.5 mg per dL BEC. Obtain a chest radiograph to determine whether aspiration pneumonia is present. Perform renal and liver function tests and obtain bilirubin levels. *Disposition:* Clinical severity (e.g., whether intubation or assisted ventilation is needed or aspiration pneumonia is present) should determine the level of hospital care needed. Young children with significant accidental exposure to alcohol (calculated to reach a BEC of 50 mg per dL) should have BEC measured and blood glucose levels monitored for hypoglycemia frequently for 4 hours after ingestion. Patients with acute ethanol intoxication seldom require admission unless a complication is present. However, intoxicated patients should not be discharged until they are fully functional (can walk, talk, and think independently), have had suicide potential evaluated, have a proper environment to which they can be discharged, and have a sober escort. Extended liability means that a physician can be held liable for subsequent injuries or death of an intoxicated patient who has been allowed to sign out against medical advice. No patient can sign out with an altered mental status.

Ethylene Glycol. Ethylene glycol is found in solvents, windshield deicer, antifreeze (95%), and air-conditioning units and has contaminated imported wines. Ethylene glycol is a sweet-tasting, colorless, water-soluble liquid with a sweet aromatic aroma. *Toxic mechanism:* Ethylene glycol is oxidized by ADH to glycolaldehyde and then is metabolized to glycolic acid and glyoxylic acid. Glyoxylic acid is metabolized to oxalic acid. Ethylene glycol metabolites are metabolized via pyridoxine-dependent pathways to glycine, benzoic acid, and hippuric acid and by thiamine- and magnesium-dependent pathways to α-hydroxyketoadipic acid. The metabolites of ethylene glycol produce a profound metabolic acidosis, increased AG, hypocalcemia, deposition of oxalate crystals in tissues, and renal damage. *Toxic dose:* The ingestion of 0.1 mL of 100% ethylene glycol per kg can result in a toxic serum ethylene glycol concentration (SEGC) of 20 mg per dL, a level that requires ethanol therapy, the antidote. Ingestion of 3.0 mL of 100% solution by a 10-kg child or 30 mL of 100% ethylene glycol by an adult produces an SEGC of 50 mg per dL (8.1 mmol per liter), a concentration that requires hemodialysis. The fatal amount is 1.4 mL of 100% solution per kg. *Kinetics:* Absorption by dermal, inhalation, and ingestion routes. Ethylene glycol is rapidly absorbed from the GI tract. Onset is in 30 minutes to 12 hours, and the peak level usually occurs at 2 hours. Without ethanol the $t_{1/2}$ is 3 to 8 hours; with ethanol, 17 hours; and with hemodialysis, 2.5 hours. The Vd is 0.65 to 0.8 liter per kg. For metabolism, see the toxic mechanism discussion. Renal clearance is 3.2 mL per kg per minute. About 20 to 50% is excreted unchanged in the urine. The following equations can be used for calculating SEGC and the amount ingested (SG indicates specific gravity):

Calculation of SEGC:

$$0.12 \text{ mL/kg of } 100\% = \text{SEGC } 10 \text{ mg/dL}$$

SEGC (mg/dL) =

$$\frac{\text{amount ingested (mL)} \times \%\text{ EG} \times \text{SG (1.12)}}{\text{Vd (0.65 L/kg)} \times \text{weight (kg)}}$$

Amount ingested (mL) =

$$\frac{\text{SEGC (mg/dL)} \times 0.65 \text{ L/kg} \times \text{weight (kg)}}{\%\text{ EG} \times \text{SG (1.12)}}$$

Manifestations: Phase I: The onset is 30 minutes to 12 hours after ingestion or longer with concomitant ethanol ingestion. The patient acts inebriated at an SEGC of 50 to 100 mg per dL. Hypocalcemia, tetany, and calcium oxalate and hippuric acid crystals in the urine may be observed within 4 to 8 hours but are not always present. Early, before metabolism of ethylene glycol, an osmolal gap may be present. Later, the metabolites of ethylene glycol produce changes starting 4 to 12 hours after ingestion, including an AG, metabolic acidosis, coma, convulsions, cardiac disturbances, and pulmonary and cerebral edema. Oral mucosa and urine fluoresce under Wood's light if "antifreeze" ethylene glycol has been ingested. Phase II: After 12 to 36 hours, cardiopulmonary deterioration occurs with pulmonary edema and congestive heart failure. Phase III: This occurs in 36 to 72 hours; oliguric renal failure resulting from oxalate crystal deposition and from tubular necrosis predominates, and pulmonary edema occurs. Phase IV: Neurologic sequelae occur 6 to 10 days after ingestion. They include facial diplegia, hearing loss, bilateral visual disturbances, elevated CSF pressure with or without elevated protein and pleocytosis, vomiting, hyper-reflexia, dysphagia, and ataxia. *Management:* (1) Establish and maintain the vital functions. Protect the airway and use assisted ventilation, if necessary. (2) GI decontamination has a limited role, with only gastric lavage within 30 to 60 minutes after ingestion. AC is not effective. (3) Obtain baseline serum electrolytes and calcium, glucose, ABGs, ethanol, SEGC (difficult to obtain, often takes more than 48 hours), and methanol concentrations. In the first few hours determine the measured serum osmolality and compare it with the calculated osmolarity (see "Serum Osmolal Gaps"). (4) If seizures occur, exclude hypocalcemia and treat with intravenous diazepam. If hypocalcemic seizures occur, treat with 10 to 20 mL of 10% calcium gluconate (0.2 to 0.3 mL per kg for children) slowly IV and repeat as needed. (See Table 12.) (5) Correct metabolic acidosis with $NaHCO_3$ given IV. (6) Ethanol therapy (see Table 12): The enzyme ADH has 10 times greater affinity for ethanol than ethylene glycol. Therefore, ethanol blocks the metabolism of ethylene glycol at BECs of 100 to 150 mg per dL. Initiate therapy if there is a history of ingestion of 100% ethylene glycol at 0.1 mL per kg, if the SEGC is more than 20 mg per dL, if there is an osmolar gap not accounted for by other alcohols or factors (e.g., hyperlipidemia) (see "Serum Osmolal Gaps"), if there is metabolic acidosis with an increased AG, or if there are oxalate crystals in the urine or positive results on fluorescence testing of urine for antifreeze, and while awaiting hemodialysis. Ethanol should be administered IV (the oral route is less reliable) to produce a BEC of 100 to 150 mg per dL. The loading dose is derived from the formula 1 mL of 100% ethanol per kg = a BEC of 100 mg per dL (which protects against metabolism of ethylene glycol). Therefore, 10 mL of 10% ethanol is administered IV concomitantly with a maintenance dose of 10% ethanol of 2.0 mL per kg per hour (alcoholic), 0.83 mL per kg per hour (nondrinker), or 1.4 mL per kg per hour (social drinker). Increase the infusion rate of 10% ethanol to 2 to 3.5 mL per kg per hour when the patient is receiving hemodialysis. (7) Hemodialysis: Obtain a nephrology consultation. Early hemodialysis is indicated if the ingestion was potentially fatal, if the SEGC is more than 50 mg per dL (some recommend hemodialysis at levels of more than 25 mg per dL), if severe acidosis or electrolyte abnormalities occur despite conventional therapy, or if congestive heart failure or renal failure is present. Hemodialysis reduces the ethylene glycol $t_{1/2}$ from 17 hours with ethanol therapy to 3 hours. Continue therapy (ethanol and hemodialysis) until the SEGC is less than 10 mg per dL or undetectable, the glycolate level is undetectable, the acidosis has cleared, there are no mental disturbances, the creatinine level is normal, and the urine output is adequate. This may require 2 to 5 days. (8) Adjunctive therapy: Thiamine (100 mg per day [children 50 mg] slowly over 5 minutes IV or IM and repeated every 6 hours) and pyridoxine (50 mg IV or IM every 6 hours) have been recommended until intoxication is resolved but have not been extensively studied. Folate may be given at 50 mg IV (in children, 1 mg per kg)* every 4 hours for 6 doses. (9) Therapy with 4-methylpyrazole given PO at 15 mg per kg, followed by 5 mg per kg in 12 hours and then 10 mg per kg every 12 hours until levels of the toxin are not detectable blocks ADH without causing inebriation.

*Exceeds dosage recommended by the manufacturer.

Laboratory investigations: Monitor blood glucose, electrolytes, urinalysis (look for oxalate ["envelope"] and monohydrate ["hemp seed"] crystals and for urine fluorescence), and ABGs. Obtain ethylene glycol and ethanol levels and determine plasma osmolarity (use freezing point depression method), calcium, BUN, and creatinine. An SEGC of 20 mg per dL is toxic (ethylene glycol levels are difficult to obtain). If possible, obtain a glycolate level. Fluorescence testing: The oral mucosa and urine (do not put in a glass tube) fluoresce under Wood's light if antifreeze ethylene glycol is present. Cross-reactions: Propylene glycol, a vehicle in many liquids and intravenous medications (phenytoin, diazepam), other glycols, and triglycerides may produce spurious ethylene glycol levels. *Disposition:* All patients who ingest significant amounts of ethylene glycol should be referred to the emergency department. If the SEGC cannot be obtained, follow-up for 12 hours, monitoring the osmolal gap, acid-base parameters, and electrolytes, is recommended to rule out development of metabolic acidosis with an AG.

Hydrocarbons. The lower the viscosity and surface tension or the greater the volatility, the greater the risk of aspiration. Volatile substance abuse has resulted in the "sudden sniffing death syndrome," most likely caused by dysrhythmias. *Toxicologic classification and toxic mechanism:* All systemically absorbed hydrocarbons can lower the myocardial threshold for development of dysrhythmias produced by endogenous and exogenous catecholamines. (1) Petroleum distillates are aliphatic hydrocarbons. Toxic dose: Aspiration of a few drops produces chemical pneumonitis, but these substances are poorly absorbed from the GI tract and produce no systemic toxicity by this route. Examples are gasoline, kerosene charcoal lighter fluid, mineral spirits (Stoddard's solvent), and petroleum naphtha. (2) Aromatic hydrocarbons are six-carbon ringed structures that produce CNS depression and in chronic abuse may have multiple organ effects. Examples are benzene (which in chronic intoxications produces leukemia), toluene, styrene, and xylene. The ingested seriously toxic dose is 20 to 50 mL in an adult. (3) Halogenated hydrocarbons are aliphatic hydrocarbons with one or more halogen substitutions (Cl, Br, Fl, or I). They are highly volatile and abused as inhalants. They are well absorbed from the GI tract, produce CNS depression, and have metabolites that can damage the liver and kidneys. Examples are methylene chloride (which may be converted to CO in the body), dichloroethylene (which also causes a disulfiram reaction ["degreaser's flush"] when associated with consumption of ethanol), and 1,1,1-trichloroethane (Glamorene Spot Remover, Scotchgard, typewriter correction fluid) (acute lethal oral dose 0.5 to 5 mL per kg). (4) Dangerous additives to the hydrocarbons include those in the mnemonic CHAMP: C, camphor (demothing agent); H, halogenated hydrocarbons; A, aromatic hydrocarbons; M, metals (heavy); and P, pesticides. Exposure to these agents may warrant gastric emptying with a small-bore nasogastric lavage tube. (5) Heavy hydrocarbons have high viscosity, low volatility, and minimal GI absorption, so gastric decontamination is not necessary. Examples are asphalt (tar), machine oil, motor oil (lubricating oil, engine oil), home heating oil, and petroleum jelly (mineral oil). (7) Mineral seal oil (e.g., signal oil), found in furniture polishes, is a low-viscosity, low-volatility oil with minimal absorption that never warrants gastric decontamination. It can produce severe pneumonia if aspirated. *Management of hydrocarbon ingestion:* (1) Asymptomatic patients who ingested small amounts of petroleum distillates may be observed at home by reliable caretakers for development of signs of aspiration (cough, wheezing, tachypnea, and dyspnea) with telephone contact for 4 to 6 hours. (2) Inhalation of any hydrocarbon vapors in a closed space can produce intoxication. Remove the victim from the environment, and administer oxygen and respiratory support. (3) GI decontamination is not advised in ingestions of hydrocarbons that usually do not cause systemic toxicity (petroleum distillates, heavy hydrocarbons, mineral seal oil). For hydrocarbons that cause systemic toxicity in small amounts (aromatic hydrocarbons, halogenated hydrocarbons), pass a small-bore nasogastric tube (these substances are liquids) and aspirate if appropriate time has not elapsed (absorption with aromatic and halogenated hydrocarbons is complete in 1 to 2 hours) and spontaneous vomiting has not occurred. Patients with altered mental status should have the airway protected because of concern over uncontrolled vomiting. Although some toxicologists advocate ipecac-induced emesis under medical supervision instead of small-bore nasogastric gastric lavage, we do not. AC is suggested, but there are no reliable data concerning its effectiveness, and it may produce vomiting. AC may, however, be useful for adsorbing toxic additives or coingestants. (4) The symptomatic patient who is coughing, gagging, choking, or wheezing on arrival has probably already aspirated. Offer supportive respiratory care, maintain the airway, provide assisted ventilation, offer supplemental oxygen with monitoring of pulse oximetry, measure ABGs, obtain a chest radiograph and ECG, and admit to the ICU. A chest radiograph for aspiration may be positive as early as 30 minutes, and almost all are positive within 6 hours. If bronchospasm occurs, administer a nebulized beta-adrenergic agonist and intravenous aminophylline if necessary. Avoid epinephrine because of the susceptibility to dysrhythmias. If cyanosis is present that does not respond to oxygen and the Pa_{O_2} is normal, suspect methemoglobinemia that may require therapy with methylene blue (see Table 12). Corticosteroids and prophylactic antimicrobial agents have not been shown to be beneficial. (Fever or leukocytosis may be produced by the chemical pneumonitis itself.) It is not necessary to surgically treat pneumatoceles that develop because they usually resolve. Most infiltrations resolve spontaneously in 1 week except for lipoid pneumonia, which may last up to 6 weeks. Dysrhythmias may require alpha- and beta-adrenergic antagonists or cardioversion. (5) There is no role for enhanced elimination procedures. (6) Methylene chloride is metabolized in several hours to CO. See the section on treatment of CO poisoning. Give 100% oxygen, and monitor serial COHb levels, ECG, and pulse oximetry. (7) Halogenated hydrocarbons are hepatorenal toxins; therefore, monitor hepatorenal function. *N*-acetylcysteine therapy may be useful if there is evidence of hepatic damage. (8) Investigational: Surfactant has been used for hydrocarbon aspiration in an animal study of aspirated hydrocarbons and was found to be detrimental. Extracorporeal membrane oxygenation has been used successfully in a few patients with life-threatening respiratory failure. *Laboratory investigations:* Monitor ECG continuously; ABGs; liver, pulmonary, and renal function; serum electrolytes; and serial chest radiographs. *Disposition:* Asymptomatic patients with small ingestions of petroleum distillates can be managed at home. Symptomatic patients with abnormal results on chest radiograph, oxygen saturation, or ABGs should be admitted. If the patient becomes asymptomatic, oxygenation is normal, and repeated radiographs are normal, the patient can be discharged.

Iron. There are more than 100 over-the-counter iron preparations for supplementation and treatment of iron deficiency anemia. *Toxic mechanism:* Toxicity depends on the amount of elemental (free) iron available in various salts (gluconate 12%, sulfate 20%, fumarate 33%, lactate 19%, and chloride 21%, of elemental iron), not on the amount of the preparation. Locally, iron is corrosive and may cause fluid loss, hypovolemic shock, and perforation. Excessive free iron in the blood is directly toxic to the vasculature and leads to the release of vasoactive substances, which produce vasodilatation. In overdose, iron deposits injure mitochondria in the liver, the kidneys, and the myocardium. The exact mechanism of cellular damage is not clear. *Toxic dose:* The therapeutic dose of elemental iron is 6 mg per kg per day. Elemental iron at 20 to 40 mg per kg per dose may produce mild self-limited GI symptoms, a dose of 40 to 60 mg per kg produces moderate toxicity, more than 60 mg per kg produces severe toxicity and is potentially lethal, and more than 180 mg per kg is usually fatal without treatment. Children's chewable vitamins with iron have from 12 to 18 mg of elemental iron per tablet or per 0.6 mL of liquid drops. These preparations rarely produce toxicity unless extremely large quantities are ingested. The following equation can be used to calculate the amount of elemental iron ingested:

$$\text{Elemental iron (mg/kg)} = \frac{\text{number of tablets ingested} \times \text{\% elemental iron}}{\text{body weight (kg)}}$$

Kinetics: Absorption occurs chiefly in the upper small intestine, usually with iron in the ferrous (+2) state absorbed into the mucosal cells, where it is oxidized to the ferric (+3) state and bound to ferritin. Iron is slowly released from ferritin into the plasma to become bound to transferrin and transported to specific tissues for production of hemoglobin (70%), myoglobin (5%), and cytochrome. About 25% of iron is stored in the liver and spleen. In overdoses, larger amounts of iron are absorbed because of direct mucosal corrosion. There is no mechanism for additional elimination of iron (normal elimination is 1 to 2 mg per day) except through bile, sweat, and blood loss. *Manifestations:* Serious toxicity is unlikely if the patient remains asymptomatic for 6 hours, has a normal white blood cell count and glucose, and has a negative abdominal radiograph. Iron intoxication usually follows a multiphasic course. A phase may be omitted entirely. Phase I: GI mucosal injury occurs 30 minutes to 12 hours after ingestion. Vomiting starts 30 minutes to 1 hour after ingestion and is persistent. Hematemesis and bloody diarrhea, abdominal cramps, fever, hyperglycemia, and leukocytosis occur. Enteric-coated tablets may pass through the stomach without causing symptoms. Acidosis and shock can occur within 6 to 12 hours. Phase II is a latent period of apparent improvement over 8 to 12 hours after ingestion. Phase III is the systemic toxicity phase (12 to 48 hours after ingestion) with cardiovascular collapse and severe metabolic acidosis. Phase IV (2 to 4 days after ingestion) is characterized by hepatic injury associated with jaundice, elevated liver enzymes, prolonged prothrombin time, and kidney injury with proteinuria and hematuria. Pulmonary edema, disseminated intravascular coagulation, and *Yersinia enterocolitica* sepsis can occur. In phase V (4 to 8 weeks after ingestion), sequelae of the pyloric outlet or intestinal stricture may cause obstruction or anemia secondary to blood loss. *Management:* (1) GI decontamination: Induce emesis immediately in ingestions of elemental iron greater than 40 mg per kg if the patient has not already vomited. Gastric lavage with 0.9% saline is less effective than emesis because of the large size of the tablets but may be useful if chewed tablets and liquid preparations are involved. AC is ineffective. Obtain an abdominal radiograph after emesis or lavage to determine the success of gastric emptying procedures. Children's chewable vitamins and liquid iron are not radiopaque. If radiopaque iron is still present, consider whole-bowel irrigation with PEG solution (see the section on evaluation and general management). (2) In extreme cases, removal by endoscopy or surgery may be necessary because coalesced iron tablets can produce hemorrhagic infarction in the bowel and perforation peritonitis. (3) Deferoxamine (DFO) (see Table 12): About 100 mg of DFO binds only 8.5 to 9.35 mg of free iron in the serum in transit. The DFO infusion rate (the intravenous route is preferred) should not exceed 15 mg per kg per hour or 6 grams daily, but higher rates (up to 45 mg per kg per hour) and larger daily amounts have been administered and tolerated in extreme cases of iron poisoning (greater than 1000 μg per dL). The deferoxamine-iron complex is hemodialyzable if renal failure develops. Indications for chelation therapy are any of the following: serious clinical intoxication (severe vomiting and diarrhea [often bloody], severe abdominal pain, metabolic acidosis, hypotension, or shock); symptoms that persist or progress to more serious toxicity; estimate of elemental iron ingestion that is quite high and presence of symptoms; and serum iron (SI) greater than 500 μg per dL. Chelation should be performed as early as possible, within 12 to 18 hours, to be effective. Start the infusion slowly and gradually increase to avoid hypotension. Successful chelation results in a urine color change from a positive vin rosé color to a normal color. Adult respiratory distress syndrome has developed in patients receiving high doses of DFO for several days; therefore, avoid prolonged infusions over 24 hours. The end points of treatment are absence of symptoms and clearing of the urine that was originally a positive vin rosé color. In a diagnostic chelation test, DFO, 50 mg per kg in children or 1 gram in adults IM, produces a vin rosé color (ferroxime-iron complex) of the urine within 3 hours. This is not a reliable test for elevated SI levels; however, obtain a baseline urine sample for comparison with subsequent specimens. (4) Supportive therapy: Intravenous bicarbonate may be needed to correct the metabolic acidosis. Hypotension and shock treatment may require fluid volume expansion, vasopressors, and blood transfusions. Attempt to keep the urine output at more than 2 mL per kg per hour. Coagulation abnormalities and overt bleeding require blood products and vitamin K. (5) Treatment in pregnant patients is similar to that in any others with iron poisoning. (6) Extracorporeal measures: Hemodialysis and hemoperfusion are not effective. Exchange transfusion has been used in single cases of massive poisoning in children. *Laboratory investigations:* Iron poisoning produces AG metabolic acidosis. Monitor the CBC, blood glucose, SI, stools and vomitus for occult blood, electrolytes, acid-base balance, urinalysis results and urine output, liver function tests, BUN, and creatinine. If GI bleeding occurs, obtain the blood type and match blood. SI measured at the proper time correlates with the clinical findings. The lavender-top Vacutainer tube contains ethylenediaminetetraacetic acid (EDTA), which falsely lowers the SI. Obtain the SI before administering DFO. SI levels at 2 to 6 hours of less than 350 μg per dL predict an asymptomatic course; levels of 350 to 500 μg per dL are usually associated with mild GI symptoms; levels above 500 μg per dL predict a 20% risk of shock and serious iron intoxication with phase III manifestations. A follow-up SI after 6 hours may not be elevated even in severe poisoning; however, an SI at 8 to 12 hours is useful for excluding delayed absorption from a bezoar or sustained-release preparation. The total iron-binding capacity is not a necessary study. Abdominal radiographs can visualize adult iron tablet preparations before they dissolve. A negative radiograph does not exclude iron poisoning. Iron sepsis: Patients who develop high fevers and signs of sepsis after iron overdose should have blood and stool cultures checked for *Y. enterocolitica*. *Disposition:* Observe the patient who is asymptomatic or has minimal symptoms for persistence and progression of symptoms or development of signs of toxicity (GI bleeding, acidosis, shock, altered mental state). A patient with mild self-limited GI symptoms who becomes asymptomatic or has no signs of toxicity for 6 hours is unlikely to have a serious intoxication and can be discharged after psychiatric clearance, if needed. Patients with moderate or severe toxicity should be in the ICU.

Isoniazid (isonicotinic acid hydrazide, INH, Nydrazid). INH is a hydrazide derivative of vitamin B_3 (nicotinamide) used as an antituberculosis drug. *Toxic mechanism:* INH produces pyridoxine deficiency by doubling the excretion of pyridoxine (vitamin B_6) and by inhibiting the interaction of pyridoxal 5-phosphate (the active form of pyridoxine) with L-glutamic acid decarboxylase to form GABA, the major CNS neurotransmitter inhibitor, resulting in seizures and coma. INH blocks the conversion of lactate to pyruvate, resulting in profound lactic acidosis. *Toxic dose:* The therapeutic dose is 5 to 10 mg per kg (maximum of 300 mg) daily. A single acute dose of 15 mg per kg lowers the seizure threshold, 35 to 40 mg per kg produces spontaneous convulsions, more than 80 mg produces severe toxicity, and 200 mg per kg is an obligatory convulsant. Malnourished persons, those with a previous seizure disorder or alcoholism, and slow acetylators are more susceptible to INH toxicity. In chronic intoxication, 10 mg per kg per day produces hepatitis in 10 to 20% of patients, but doses of 3 to 5 mg per kg per day affect less than 2%. *Kinetics:* Rapid absorption from intestine occurs in 30 to 60 minutes, onset is in 30 to 120 minutes, with a peak level of 5 to 8 μg per mL within 1 to 2 hours. The Vd is 0.6 liter per kg; PB is minimal. Elimination is by liver acetylation to a hepatotoxic metabolite, acetylisoniazid, which is then hydrolyzed to isonicotinic acid. Slow acetylators show a $t_{1/2}$ of 140 to 300 minutes (mean 5 hours) and eliminate 10 to 15% unchanged in the urine. Most (45 to 75%) whites and 50% of African blacks are slow acetylators and with chronic use (without pyridoxine supplements) may develop peripheral neuropathy. Fast acetylators show a $t_{1/2}$ of 35 to 110 minutes (mean 80 minutes) and excrete 25 to 30% of the drug unchanged in the urine. About 90% of Asians and patients with diabetes mellitus are fast acetylators and may develop hepatitis with chronic use. In overdose and hepatic disease, the serum $t_{1/2}$ may increase. INH inhibits the metabolism of phenytoin, diazepam, phenobarbital, carbamazepine, and prednisone. These drugs also interfere with the metabolism of INH. Ethanol may decrease the INH $t_{1/2}$ but may increase its toxicity. *Manifestations:* Within 30 to 60 minutes, nausea, vomiting, slurred speech, dizziness, visual disturbances, and ataxia are present. Within 30 to 120 minutes, the major clinical triad of severe overdose develops: (1) refractory convulsions (90% of overdose patients have one or more seizures), (2) coma, and (3) resistant severe AG lactic acidosis (secondary to convulsions), and metabolic blocks, often with pH of 6.8. Acidosis occurs after seizures. *Management:* (1) Control seizures: Administer pyridoxine, 1 gram for each gram of isoniazid ingested (see Table 12). If the dose ingested is unknown, give at least 5 grams (70 mg per kg) of pyridoxine IV. Pyridoxine is administered in 50 mL of D5W or 0.9% saline over 5 minutes IV. Do not administer in the same bottle as for $NaHCO_3$. Repeat intravenous pyridoxine every 5 to 20 minutes until seizures are controlled. Total doses of pyridoxine up to 52 grams have been safely administered. However, patients given 132 and 183 grams of pyridoxine have developed a persistent crippling sensory neuropathy. Some authorities recommend prophylactic pyridoxine if there is a history of ingestion of 80 mg of INH per kg. Administer diazepam concomitantly with pyridoxine but at a different site. They work synergistically. Administer diazepam IV at 0.3 mg per kg slowly at rate of 1 mg per minute in children or 10 mg per dose slowly at rate of 5 mg per minute in adults. After the seizures are controlled, administer the remainder of the pyridoxine (1 gram per gram of INH), or total dose of 5 grams, as an infusion drip over 60 minutes. Do not use phenobarbital (it increases INH metabolism to toxic metabolites) or phenytoin (it interferes with INH metabolism and is not effective). (2) In asymptomatic patients or patients without seizures, pyridoxine should be considered prophylactically in gram-for-gram doses with large overdoses (80 mg per kg per dose or more) of INH (there are no supporting studies, however). (3) In comatose patients, pyridoxine administration may result in rapid regaining of consciousness. (4) Correction of the acidosis and control of the seizures may occur spontaneously with pyridoxine administration. Administer $NaHCO_3$ if acidosis persists. (5) GI decontamination: After the patient is stabilized, or if the patient is asymptomatic, gastric lavage may be performed after recent (less than 1 hour) ingestion with protection of the airway, if necessary. AC may be administered. (6) Hemodialysis is rarely needed because of antidotal therapy and the short $t_{1/2}$ but may be used as an adjunct for uncontrollable acidosis and seizures. Hemoperfusion has not been adequately evaluated. Diuresis is ineffective. *Laboratory investigations:* INH produces AG metabolic acidosis. Therapeutic levels are 5 to 8 μg per mL, and acute toxic levels are more than 20 μg per mL. Monitor the blood glucose (hyperglycemia is common), electrolytes (hyperkalemia is frequent), bicarbonate, ABGs, liver function tests (elevations occur with chronic exposure), BUN, and creatinine. *Disposition:* Asymptomatic or mildly symptomatic patients who become asymptomatic may be observed in the emergency department for 4 to 6 hours. Larger amounts of INH may warrant pyridoxine and longer periods of observation. Patients with intentional ingestions require psychiatric evaluation before discharge. Patients with convulsions or coma should be admitted to the ICU.

Isopropanol (IP or rubbing alcohol, solvents, lacquer thinner). Coma has occurred in children sponged for fever with isopropanol. See Table 32. *Toxic mechanism:* Isopropanol is a gastric irritant. It is metabolized to acetone, a CNS and myocardial depressant. It inhibits gluconeogenesis. Normal propyl alcohol is related to isopropanol but is more toxic. *Toxic dose:* The toxic dose is 0.5 to 1 mg of 70% isopropanol per kg (1 mL of 70% isopropanol per kg produces a blood isopropyl alcohol concentration [BIPC] of 70 mg per dL). The CNS depressant effect is twice that of ethanol. *Kinetics:* Onset is within 30 to 60 minutes and the peak effect occurs at 1 hour after ingestion. Elimination is renal. Isopropyl alcohol is metabolized to acetone. The Vd is 0.6 liter per kg. The BIPC and amount ingested can be estimated by using equations in ethanol kinetics and an SG of 0.785 for isopropanol:

$$\text{BIPC (mg/dL)} = \frac{\text{amount ingested (mL)} \times \text{\% isopropyl alcohol in product} \times \text{SG (0.79)}}{\text{Vd (0.6 L/kg)} \times \text{body weight (kg)}}$$

$$\text{Dose (amount ingested)} = \frac{\text{BIPC (mg/dL)} \times \text{Vd (0.6 L/kg)} \times \text{body weight (kg)}}{\text{\% ethanol} \times \text{SG (0.79)}}$$

Manifestations: Ethanol-like inebriation with an acetone odor of the breath, gastritis occasionally with hematemesis, acetonuria, and acetonemia without systemic acidosis are seen. CNS depressant effects include lethargy at 50 to 100 mg per dL and coma at 150 to 200 mg per dL; ingestion of more than 240 mg per dL is potentially fatal in adults. Hypoglycemia and seizures may occur. *Management:* (1) Protect the airway with intubation and administer assisted ventilation if necessary. If the patient is hypoglycemic, administer glucose. Supportive treatment is similar to that for ethanol. (2) GI decontamination has no role. (3) Hemodialysis in life-threatening overdose is rarely needed. Consult a nephrologist if the BIPC is greater than 250 mg per dL. *Laboratory investigation:* Monitor isopropyl alcohol levels, acetone, glucose, and ABGs. The osmolal gap increases 1 mOsm per 5.9 mg per dL of isopropyl alcohol and 1 mOsm per 5.5 mg per dL of acetone. Absence of excess acetone in the blood (normal, 0.3 to 2 mg per dL) within 30 to 60 minutes or excess acetone in the urine within 3 hours excludes the possibility of significant isopropanol exposure. *Disposition:* Symptomatic patients with concentrations greater than 100 mg per dL require at least 24 hours of close observation for resolution and should be admitted. If the patient is hypoglycemic, hypotensive, or comatose, admit to the ICU.

Lead. Lead is an environmental toxin. Acute lead intoxication is rare and is usually caused by inhalation of lead, resulting in severe intoxication and often death. It may be produced by burning lead batteries or using a heat gun to remove lead paint. It also results from exposure to high concentrations of organic lead (e.g., tetraethyl lead). Chronic lead poisoning occurs most often in children 6 months to 6 years of age who are exposed in their environment and in adults in certain occupations. See Table 34. In the United States, the percentage of children 1 to 5 years of age with a venous blood lead level (VBPb) greater than 10 μg per dL decreased from 88.2% in a survey of 1976 to 1980 to 8.9% in survey of 1988 to 1991 as a result of measures to reduce lead in the environment, particularly by reducing leaded gasoline. However, an estimated 1.7 million children between 1 and 5 years old have blood lead levels greater than 10 μg per dL, and more than 1 million workers in over 100 different occupations are exposed to lead. *Toxic dose in chronic lead poisoning:* An intake of more than 5 μg per kg per day in children or more than 150 μg per day in adults can give toxic screen levels of lead. In 1991, the Centers for Disease Control and Prevention (CDC) recommended routine screening for children. The CDC recommended a VBPb or a capillary blood lead determination for all children. In children a VBPb greater than 10 μg per dL was determined by the CDC to be a threshold of concern (it was 25 μg per dL in 1985). The average VBPb in the United States is 4 μg per dL. In occupational exposure (see Table 34) a VBPb greater than 40 μg per dL is indicative of increased lead absorption in adults. *Toxic mechanism:* Lead affects the sulfhydryl enzyme systems of the proteins, the immature CNS, the enzymes of heme synthesis, vitamin D conversion, the kidneys, the bones, and growth. Lead alters the tertiary structure of cell proteins, denaturing them and causing death. Risk factors are mouthing behavior of infants and children and excessive oral behavior (pica), living in the inner city, a poorly maintained home, and poor nutrition (e.g., low calcium and iron). Use of the CDC questionnaire is recommended at every pediatric visit. See Table 35. If any answers to the CDC questionnaire are positive, obtain a blood screening test for lead. However, studies have suggested that to be more accurate in identifying lead exposure the questionnaire would have to be modified for each community because it has had poor sensitivity (40%) and specificity (60%). *Sources of lead* (Table 36): (1) The primary source of lead is deteriorating lead-based paint, which forms leaded dust. Lead concentrations in indoor paint were not reduced to safer levels (0.06%) until 1978. Lead can

TABLE 34. **Occupations Associated with Lead Exposure**

Lead production or smelting	Instructor or janitor at firing range
Production of illicit whiskey	Demolition of ships and bridges
Brass, copper, and lead foundries	Battery manufacturing
Radiator repair	Machining or grinding lead alloys
Scrap handling	Welding of old painted metals
Sanding of old paint	Thermal paint stripping of old buildings
Lead soldering	Ceramic glaze and pottery mixing
Cable stripping	

Modified from Rempel D: The lead-exposed worker. JAMA *262*:532–534, 1989. Copyright 1989, American Medical Association.

TABLE 35. **CDC Questionnaire: Priority Groups for Lead Screening**

1. Children 6–72 mo old (was 12–36 mo) who live in or are frequent visitors to older deteriorated housing built before 1960
2. Children 6–72 mo old who live in housing built before 1960 with recent, ongoing, or planned renovation or remodeling
3. Children 6–72 mo old who are siblings, housemates, or playmates of children with known lead poisoning
4. Children 6–72 mo old whose parents or other household members participate in a lead-related industry or hobby
5. Children 6–72 mo old who live near active lead smelters, battery recycling plants, or other industries likely to result in atmospheric lead release

also be produced by improper interior or exterior home renovation (scraping or demolition). (2) The use of leaded gasoline (limited in 1973) resulted in residues from leaded motor vehicle emissions. Lead persists in the soil near major highways and deteriorating homes and buildings. Vegetables grown in contaminated soil may contain lead. (3) Oil refineries and lead-processing smelters are other sources. (4) Food cans produced in Mexico contain lead solder (95% do not in the United States). (5) Lead pipes (until 1950) and pipes with lead solder (until 1986) deliver lead-containing drinking water (calcium deposits, however, may offer some protection). Water at the consumer's tap should have a lead level less than 15 ppb (parts per billion). See Table 37. (6) Occupational exposure (see Table 34): Occupational Safety and Health Administration (OSHA) standards require employers to provide showering and clothes-changing facilities for persons working with lead; however, businesses with less than 25 employees are exempt from regulation. The OSHA lead standard of 1978 set a limit of 60 μg per dL for occupational exposure to lead. At a blood lead level of 60 μg per dL, a worker should be removed from lead exposure and not allowed back until the level is below 40 μg per dL. Many authorities think that this level should be lower. The lead residue on workers' clothes may represent a hazard to their families. Others occupationally exposed to lead include plumbers, pipefitters, lead miners, auto repairers, shipbuilders, printers, steel welders and cutters, construction workers, and those in rubber product manufacturing. (7) Other sources are leaded pots to make molds and "kusmusha" tea. (8) Hobbies (see Table 38) associated with lead exposure include making stained glass windows, lead fish sinkers, or curtain weights, which may pose additional hazard if ingested and retained by children; imported pottery with ceramic glaze can leach large amounts of lead into acids (e.g., citrus fruit juices). (9) Some "traditional" folk remedies or cosmetics contain lead: "Azarcon por empacho" ("Maria Louisa," 90 to 95% lead trioxide), a bright orange powder (used in Hispanic culture, especially Mexican, for digestive problems and diarrhea); "Greta" (4 to 90% lead), a yellow powder for "empacho" ("empacho" refers to a variety of GI symptoms; used in Hispanic cultures, especially Mexican); "Payloo-ah,"

TABLE 36. **Product Lead Content by Dry Weight**

Product	Lead (%)	Product	Lead (%)
Plastic additives	2.0	Construction material	0.1
Priming inks	2.0	Fertilizers	0.1
Plumbing fixtures	2.0	Toys and recreational games	0.1
Solder	0.6	Curtain weights	0.1
Pesticides	0.1	Fishing weights	0.1
Stained glass came	0.1	Glazes, enamels, frits	0.06
Wine bottle foils	0.1	Paint	0.06

TABLE 37. **Agency Regulations and Recommendations for Lead Content**

Agency	Specimen	Acceptable Level	Comments
CDC	Blood, child	10 μg/dL	Investigate community
OSHA	Blood, adult	60 μg/dL	Medical removal from work
OSHA	Air	50 μg/m³	PEL
	Air	0.75 mg/m³	Tetraethyl or tetramethyl
ACGIH	Air	150 μg/m³	TWA
EPA	Air	1.5 μg/m³	3-mo average
EPA	Water	15 μg/liter (ppb)	5 ppb circulating
EPA	Food	100 μg/d	Advisory
FDA	Wine	300 ppm	Plan to reduce to 200 ppm
EPA	Soil and dust	50 ppm	
CPSC	Paint	600 ppm (0.06%)	By dry weight

Abbreviations: ACGIH = American Conference of Governmental Industrial Hygienists; CDC = Centers for Disease Control and Prevention; CPSC = Consumer Products Safety Commission; EPA = Environmental Protection Agency; FDA = Food and Drug Administration; OSHA = Occupational Safety and Health Administration; PEL = permissible exposure limit (highest level over 8-h workday); ppb = parts per billion; ppm = parts per million; TWA = time-weighted average (air concentration for 8-h workday and 40-h workweek).

TABLE 38. **Hobbies Associated with Lead Exposure**

Casting of ammunition
Collecting antique pewter
Collecting or painting lead toys (e.g., soldiers and figures)
Ceramics or glazed pottery
Refinishing furniture
Making fishing weights
Home renovation
Jewelry making (lead solder)
Glassblowing (lead glass)
Bronze casting
Printmaking and other fine arts (when lead white, flake white, chrome yellow pigments are involved)
Liquor distillation
Hunting and target shooting
Painting
Car and boat repair
Burning lead-painted wood
Making stained lead glass
Copper enameling

an orange-red powder for rash and fever (used in Southeast Asian cultures, especially northern Laos Hmong immigrants); "Alkohl" (Al-kohl, kohl, suma, 5 to 92% lead), a black powder (used in Middle Eastern, African, and Asian cultures as a cosmetic and umbilical stump astringent); "Farouk," an orange granular powder with lead (Saudi Arabian); "Bint Al Zahab," used to treat colic (Saudi Arabian); "Surma" (23 to 26% lead), a black powder used in India as a cosmetic and to improve eyesight; "Bali goli," a round black bean that is dissolved in "grippe water" (used by Asian and Indian cultures to aid digestion). (10) Substance abuse: The synthesis of amphetamines includes lead acetate, which may not be removed before use. Lead poisoning as a result of sniffing organic lead gasoline has been reported. *Kinetics:* Absorption of lead is 10 to 15% of the ingested dose in adults; in children up to 40% is absorbed, especially when iron deficiency anemia is present. Inhalation absorption is rapid and complete. The Vd in blood (0.9% of total body burden) is 95% in red blood cells; the $t_{1/2}$ is 35 to 40 days; $t_{1/2}$ in soft tissue, 45 days; and $t_{1/2}$ in bone (99% of the lead), 28 years. Lead is eliminated via the stool (80 to 90%); kidneys (10%; 80 μg per day); and hair, nails, sweat, and saliva. Organic lead is metabolized in the liver to inorganic lead; 9% is excreted in the urine per day. Lead passes through the placenta to the fetus and is present in breast milk. *Manifestations:* See Table 39. Adverse health effects include (1) Hematologic: Lead inhibits δ-aminolevulinic acid dehydratase early in the synthesis of heme (which has been associated with CNS symptoms) and ferrochelatase (which transfers iron to ferritin for iron incorporation into protoporphyrin to produce heme); anemia is a late finding. Decreased heme synthesis starts at more than 40 μg per dL. Basophilic stippling occurs in 20% of persons with severe lead poisoning. (2) Neurologic: segmental demyelination and peripheral neuropathy, usually of motor type (wrist and ankle drop), occur in workers. A VBPb greater than 70 μg per dL (usually greater than 100 μg per dL) produces encephalopathy in children (a symptom mnemonic is PAINT: P, persistent forceful vomiting and papilledema; A, ataxia; I, intermittent stupor and lucidity; N, neurologic coma and refractory convulsions; T, tired and lethargic). Decreased cognitive abilities have been associated with a VBPb higher than 10 μg per dL; behavior problems and decreased attention span and learning abilities have been reported. IQ scores may begin to decrease at 15 μg per dL. In adults, peripheral neuropathies and "lead gum lines" at the dental border of the gingiva occur. Encephalopathy is rare in adults. (3) Renal nephropathy with damaged capillaries and glomeruli is seen at VBPb greater than 80 μg per dL, but renal damage and hypertension have been observed with low VBPb levels. Lead reduces excretion of uric acid, and high-level exposure is associated with hyperuricemia and "saturnine gout," Fanconi's syndrome (aminoaciduria and renal tubular acidosis), and tubular fibrosis. A linear association between hypertension and 30 μg per dL has been reported. (4) Reproductive effects include spontaneous abortion, transient delay in development (catch-up age 5 to 6 years), a decreased sperm count, and abnormal sperm morphology. Lead is transmitted across the placenta in 75 to 100% of cases and is teratogenic. (5) Metabolic: Decreased cytochrome P-

TABLE 39. **Summary of Lead-Induced Health Effects in Adults and Children**

Blood Lead Level (μg/dL)	Age Group	Health Effect
>100	Adult	Encephalopathic signs and symptoms
>80	Adult	Anemia
	Child	Encephalopathy
		Chronic nephropathy (e.g., aminoaciduria)
>70	Adult	Clinically evident peripheral neuropathy
	Child	Colic and other GI symptoms
>60	Adult	Female reproductive effects
		CNS disturbances and symptoms (i.e., sleep disturbances, mood changes, memory and concentration problems, headaches)
>50	Adult	Decreased hemoglobin production
		Decreased performance on neurobehavioral tests
		Altered testicular function
		GI symptoms (i.e., abdominal pain, constipation, diarrhea, nausea, anorexia)
	Child	Peripheral neuropathy
>40	Adult	Decreased peripheral nerve conduction
		Hypertension, age 40–59 y
		Chronic neuropathy
>25	Adult	Elevated erythrocyte protoporphyrin in males
15–25	Adult	Elevated erythrocyte protoporphyrin in females
	Child	Decreased intelligence and growth
>10	Fetus/child	Preterm delivery
		Impaired learning
		Reduced birth weight
		Impaired mental ability

From Implementation of the Lead Contamination Control Act of 1988. MMWR Morb Mortal Wkly Rep *41*:288–290, 1992.

450 (which alters metabolism of drugs and endogenously produced substances), decreased activation of cortisol, and decreased growth caused by interference with vitamin conversion (25-hydroxyvitamin D to 1,25-dihydroxyvitamin D) have been seen at VBPb of 20 to 30 μg per dL. (6) Other abnormalities of thyroid, cardiac, and hepatic function occur in adults. Abdominal colic is seen in children with a level greater than 50 μg per dL. *Management:* The basis of treatment is removal of the source. Cases of poisoning in children should be reported to the local health department, and cases of occupational poisoning to OSHA. Control the exposure by identifying and abating the source, improving housekeeping by wet mopping and using a high-phosphate detergent solution, allowing cold water to run for 2 minutes before using it for drinking, and planting shrubbery in contaminated soil to keep children away. (1) GI decontamination: Lead does not bind to AC. Do not delay chelation therapy for complete GI decontamination in severe cases. Whole-bowel irrigation has been used before treatment. Some authorities recommend abdominal radiography followed by GI decontamination, if necessary, before switching to oral therapy. (2) Supportive care includes measures to deal with refractory seizures (continue antidotal therapy, diazepam, and possibly neuromuscular blockers), hepatic and renal failure, and intravascular hemolysis. Treat seizures with diazepam, followed by neuromuscular blockers if needed. (3) Chelation therapy is used for children with levels above 45 μg per dL and adults with levels above 80 μg per dL or at lower levels with a positive lead mobilization test. See Table 40. Dimercaprol (BAL, British antilewisite) is a peanut oil–based dithiol (two sulfhydryl molecules) that combines with one atom of lead to form a heterocyclic stable ring complex. It is usually reserved for cases in which VBPb is above 70 μg per dL. It chelates red blood cell–bound lead and enhances its elimination through the urine and bile. It crosses the blood-brain barrier. About 50% of patients have adverse reactions including an unpleasant metallic taste in the mouth, pain at the injection site, sterile abscesses, and fever. Edetate calcium disodium (ethylene diaminetetra-acetic acid, $CaNa_2EDTA$, Calcium Disodium Versenate) is a water-soluble chelator given IM (with 0.5% procaine) or IV. The calcium in the compound is displaced by divalent and trivalent heavy metals, which form a soluble complex that is stable at physiologic pH (but not at acid pH) and enhances clearance in the urine. It is usually administered IV, especially in severe cases. It must not be administered until adequate urine flow is established. It may redistribute lead to the brain; therefore, BAL is started at VBPb levels exceeding 55 μg per dL in children and 100 μg per dL in adults. Phlebitis occurs at concentrations above 0.5 mg per mL. Alkalization of the urine may be helpful (see Table 12). $CaNa_2EDTA$ should not be confused with sodium EDTA (disodium edetate), which is used to treat hypercalcemia; inadvertent use may produce severe hypocalcemia. Succimer (dimercaptosuccinic acid [DMSA], Chemet), a derivative of BAL, is an oral agent approved by the FDA in 1991 for chelation in children with a VBPb above 45 μg per dL. The recommended dose is 10 mg per kg given every 8 hours for 5 days and then every 12 hours for 14 days (see Table 12). DMSA is under investigation to determine its role in children with VBPb less than 45 μg per dL. Although not approved for adults, it has been used in adults at the same dosage. Monitor the CBC, liver transaminases, and urinalysis for toxicity. D-Penicillamine is given at 20 to 40 mg per kg per day, not to exceed 1 gram per day. It is an oral chelator used to enhance the urinary elimination of lead; it is not FDA approved and has a 10% adverse reaction rate. Succimer is preferred. D-Penicillamine is used in adults with minimal symptoms but high VBPb levels. A VBPb above 70 μg per dL or clinical symptoms suggesting encephalopathy in children indicate a potential life-threatening emergency. Management should be accomplished in a medical center with a pediatric ICU by a multidisciplinary team including a critical care specialist, toxicologist, neurologist, and neurosurgeon, with careful monitoring of neurologic parameters, fluid status,

TABLE 40. **Pharmacologic Chelation Therapy for Lead Poisoning**

Drug	Route	Dose	Duration	Precautions	Monitor
Dimercaprol (BAL in oil)	IM	3–5 mg/kg q 4–6 h	3–5 d	G6PD deficiency Concurrent iron therapy	AST and ALT
$CaNa_2EDTA$ (Calcium Disodium Versenate)	IM or IV	50 mg/kg/d	5 d	Inadequate fluid intake Renal impairment	Urinalysis BUN Creatinine
D-Penicillamine (Cuprimine)	PO	10 mg/kg/d; increase to 30 mg/kg over 2 wk	6–20 wk	Penicillin allergy Concurrent iron therapy Lead exposure Renal impairment	Urinalysis BUN Creatinine CBC
2,3-Dimercaptosuccinic acid (DMSA; succimer)	PO	10 mg/kg per dose tid for 5 d 10 mg/kg per dose bid for 14 d	19 d	AST and ALT elevations Concurrent iron therapy G6PD deficiency Lead exposure	AST and ALT

Abbreviations: BAL = British antilewisite; G6PD = glucose-6-phosphate dehydrogenase; AST = aspartate aminotransferase; ALT = alanine aminotransferase; BUN = blood urea nitrogen; CBC = complete blood count; EDTA = ethylenediaminetetra-acetic acid.

and intracranial pressure if necessary. These patients need close monitoring for hemodynamic instability. Adequate hydration should be maintained to ensure renal excretion of lead. Monitor fluids, renal and hepatic function, and electrolytes. While measures to ensure adequate urine flow are implemented, therapy should be initiated with intramuscular dimercaprol (BAL) only (25 mg per kg per day divided into 6 doses). Four hours later, a combination of a second dose of BAL given IM with $CaNa_2EDTA$ (50 mg per kg per day) given IV as a single dose infused over several hours or as a continuous infusion is administered. The double therapy is continued until VBPb is less than 40 μg per dL. Therapy is continued for 72 hours and followed by one of two alternatives: either parenteral therapy with the two drugs ($CaNa_2EDTA$ and BAL) for 5 days or continued therapy with $CaNa_2EDTA$ alone if there is a good response and VBPb is below 40 μg per dL. If a report on VBPb has not been obtained, continue therapy with both BAL and EDTA for 5 days. In patients with lead encephalopathy, parenteral chelation should be continued with both drugs until the patient is clinically stable before changing therapy. Mannitol and dexamethasone can reduce the cerebral edema, but removal of the lead is essential, and the role of these agents in lead encephalopathy is not clear. Avoid surgical decompression to reduce cerebral edema. If BAL and $CaNa_2EDTA$ are used together, a minimum of 2 days with no treatment should elapse before considering another 5-day course of therapy. Repeat the 5-day course with $CaNa_2EDTA$ alone if the blood lead level remains above 40 μg per dL or in combination with BAL if it is above 70 μg per dL. If a third course is required, unless there are compelling reasons, wait at least 5 to 7 days before administration. Continue chelation therapy at all costs. After chelation therapy, a period of equilibration of 10 to 14 days should be allowed, and repeated determinations of VBPb concentrations should be obtained. If the patient is stable enough for oral intake, oral succimer at 30 mg per kg per day in three divided doses for 5 days followed by 20 mg per kg per day in two divided doses for 14 days has been suggested, but data are limited. Continue therapy until VBPb is less than 20 μg per dL in children or 40 μg per dL in adults. Chelators combined with lead are hemodialyzable in the event of renal failure. *Laboratory investigations:* (1) A classification of blood lead concentrations in children is given in Table 41. (2) The lead mobilization test is used to determine the chelatable pool of lead. It consists of the administration of 25 mg per kg in children or 1 gram in adults as a single dose deeply IM with 0.5% procaine diluted 1:1 or as an infusion. Empty the bladder and collect the urine for 24 hours (3 days if there is renal impairment). A modified 8-hour collection may be obtained. If the ratio of micrograms of lead excreted in the urine to the milligrams of $CaNa_2EDTA$ administered is greater than 0.6, it represents an increased lead body burden, and therapeutic chelation is indicated. However, many authorities consider this test of little importance in making the decision about chelation. The use of x-ray fluorescence of bone as an alternative to determine the lead burden is being tested. (3) Evaluate the CBC, serum ferritin, VBPb, erythrocyte protoporphyrin (greater than 35 μg per dL indicates lead poisoning as well as iron deficiency and other causes), electrolytes, serum calcium and phosphorus, urine, BUN, and creatinine. Abdominal and long bone radiographs are not routine but may be useful in certain circumstances for identifying radiopaque material in bowel and lead lines in proximal tibia (these occur after prolonged exposure in association with VBPb above 50 μg per dL). Serial VBPb measurements are obtained on days 3 and 5 during treatment, 7 days after chelation therapy, then every 1 to 2 weeks for 8 weeks, and then every month for 6 months. Stop the intravenous infusion at least 1 hour before obtaining blood for lead determination. (4) Neuropsychologic tests are difficult to conduct in young children but should be considered at the end of treatment, especially to determine auditory dysfunction. *Disposition:* All patients with levels above 70 μg per dL or who are symptomatic should be admitted to the hospital. If a child is hospitalized, all lead hazards must be removed before allowing the child to return home. The source must be eliminated by environmental and occupational investigations.

TABLE 41. **Classification of Blood Lead Concentrations in Children**

Blood Lead Level (μg/dL)	Classification	Recommended Interventions
<9	I	None
10–14	IIa	Community intervention Repeat blood lead determination in 3 mo
15–19	IIb	Individual case management Environmental counseling Nutritional counseling Repeat blood lead determination in 3 mo
20–44	III	Medical referral Environmental inspection and/or abatement Nutritional counseling Repeat blood lead determination in 3 mo
45–69	IV	Environmental inspection and/or abatement Nutritional counseling Pharmacologic therapy: oral succimer or parenteral $CaNa_2EDTA$ Repeat q 2 wk for 6–8 wk, monthly for 4–6 mo
>70	V	Hospitalization in intensive care unit Environmental inspection and/or abatement Pharmacologic therapy: dimercaprol given IM alone initially, then dimercaprol given IM and $CaNa_2EDTA$ together; repeat every week

The local health department should be involved in the management of children with lead poisoning, and OSHA in occupational lead poisoning. Consultation with the poison control center and/or an experienced toxicologist is necessary when chelation therapy is used. Follow-up VBPb concentrations should be obtained within 1 to 2 weeks, then every 2 weeks for 8 weeks, and then monthly for 6 months if the patient required chelation therapy. All patients with VBPb values above 10 μg per dL should undergo follow-up evaluation at least every 3 months until 2VBPb is 10 μg per dL or 3VBPb is less than 15 μg per dL.

Lithium (Li, Eskalith, Lithane). Lithium is an A-1 alkali metal whose primary use is in the treatment of bipolar psychiatric disorders. Most intoxications are chronic overdoses. One gram of lithium carbonate contains 189 mg of lithium; a regular tablet, 300 mg or 8.12 mEq; and a sustained-release preparation, 450 mg or 12.18 mEq. *Toxic mechanism:* The brain is the primary target organ of toxicity, but the mechanism is unclear. Lithium may interfere with physiologic functions by acting as a substitute for cellular cations (sodium and potassium), depressing neural excitation and synaptic transmission. *Toxic dose:* A lithium dose of 1 mEq per kg (40 mg per kg) results in a serum lithium concentration of about 1.2 mEq per liter. The therapeutic serum lithium concentration in acute mania is 0.6 to 1.2 mEq per liter and for maintenance 0.5 to 0.8 mEq per liter. Serum lithium levels are usually obtained 12 hours after the last dose. The toxic dose is determined by clinical manifestations and serum levels after the distribution phase. Acute ingestion of twenty 300-mg tablets (300 mg increases the serum lithium concentration by 0.2 to 0.4 mEq per liter) in adults may produce serious intoxication. Chronic intoxication is produced by any state that increases lithium reabsorption. Risk factors that predispose to chronic lithium toxicity are febrile illness, impaired renal function, hyponatremia, advanced age, lithium-induced diabetes insipidus, dehydration, vomiting and diarrheal illness, concomitant drugs (thiazide and spironolactone diuretics, NSAIDs, salicylates, angiotensin-converting enzyme inhibitors [captopril], and selective serotonin reuptake inhibitors [SSRIs] [e.g., fluoxetine and antipsychotic drugs]). *Kinetics:* GI absorption is rapid and peaks in 2 to 4 hours after regular-release preparations, and complete absorption occurs by 6 to 8 hours. Absorption may be delayed 6 to 12 hours after ingestion of sustained-release preparations. The onset of toxicity may occur at 1 to 4 hours after acute overdose but is usually delayed because lithium enters the brain slowly. The Vd is 0.5 to 0.9 liter per kg. Lithium is not protein bound. The $t_{1/2}$ after a single dose is 9 to 13 hours; at steady state it may be 30 to 58 hours. The renal handling of lithium is similar to that of sodium, by glomerular filtration and reabsorption (80%) in the proximal renal tubules. Adequate sodium must be present to prevent lithium reabsorption. More than 90% of lithium is excreted by the kidney unchanged, 30 to 60% within 6 to 12 hours. Alkalization of the urine increases clearance. *Manifestations:* It is important to distinguish among side effects and acute, acute in a patient on chronic therapy, and chronic intoxications. Chronic is the most common and dangerous type of intoxication. (1) Side effects of lithium include fine tremor, GI upset, hypothyroidism, polyuria and frank diabetes insipidus, dermatologic manifestations, and cardiac conduction deficits. Lithium is teratogenic. (2) Toxic effects: Patients with acute poisoning may be asymptomatic with an early high serum lithium concentration of 9 mEq per liter and deteriorate as the serum level falls 50% and lithium is distributed to the brain and the other tissues. The onset of nausea and vomiting may occur within 1 to 4 hours, but the systemic manifestations are usually delayed several more hours. It may take as long as 3 to 5 days for serious symptoms to develop. Acute toxicity is manifested by neurologic findings including weakness, fasciculations, altered mental state, myoclonus, hyper-reflexia, rigidity, coma, and convulsions with limbs in hyperextension. Cardiovascular effects are nonspecific and occur at therapeutic doses: flat T or inverted T waves, AV block, and prolonged QT interval. Lithium is not a primary cardiotoxin. Cardiogenic shock is secondary to CNS toxicity. Chronic intoxication is associated with manifestations at lower serum lithium concentrations. There is some correlation with manifestations especially at higher serum lithium concentrations. See Table 42. Permanent neurologic sequelae can result from lithium intoxication. *Management:* (1) Establish and maintain vital functions. Institute seizure precautions and treat seizures, hypotension, and dysrhythmias. Restore normothermia. (2) Evaluation: Examine for ri-

TABLE 42. **Classification of Severity of Chronic Lithium Intoxication**

Classification	Manifestations	Blood Concentration (mEq/L)*
Subacute or pretoxic	Apathy, fine tremor, vomiting and diarrhea, weakness	<1.2
Mild intoxication	Lethargy, drowsiness; hypertonia, hyper-reflexia; muscle rigidity, dysarthria; ataxia, apathy, nystagmus	1.2–2.5
Moderate intoxication	Impaired consciousness; severe fasciculations; coarse tremor, severe ataxia; myoclonus, paresthesias; diabetes insipidus; electrocardiographic changes; renal tubular acidosis; paralysis, blurred vision	2.5–3.5
Severe intoxication	Muscle twitching, coma; severe myoclonic jerking; cardiac dysrhythmias; seizures, spasticity, shock	>3.5

*Plasma lithium concentrations (not an absolute correlation).

Modified from El-Mallakh RS: Treatment of acute lithium toxicity. Vet Hum Toxicol *26*:31–35, 1984.

gidity and signs of hyper-reflexia, and monitor hydration status, renal function (BUN, creatinine), and electrolytes, especially sodium. Inquire about use of diuretics and other drugs that increase the serum lithium concentrations, and discontinue them. If the patient is receiving chronic therapy, discontinue the lithium. Obtain serial serum lithium concentrations every 4 hours until the concentration peaks and there is a downward trend toward an almost therapeutic range, especially with sustained-release preparations. Monitor vital signs including temperature and ECG, and conduct serial neurologic examinations including mental status and urine output. Obtain a nephrology consultation if there is a chronic and elevated serum lithium level (above 2.5 mEq per liter), a large ingestion, or altered mental state. (3) Fluid and electrolyte therapy: An intravenous line should be established, and hydration and electrolyte balance restored. Determine the serum sodium level before administration of 0.89% saline fluid in chronic overdoses, because hypernatremia may be present as a result of diabetes insipidus. Although current evidence indicates that an initial 0.89% saline infusion (at 200 mL per hour) enhances excretion of lithium, once hydration, output, and normonatremia are established, administer 0.45% saline and slow the infusion (to 100 mL per hour). (4) GI decontamination: Gastric lavage is useful only after recent acute ingestion and is not necessary after chronic intoxication. AC is ineffective. With slow-release preparations, whole-bowel irrigation may be useful, but this has not been proved. Sodium polystyrene sulfonate, an ion exchange resin, in a dose of 15 to 50 grams PO every 4 to 6 hours, may be useful in preventing absorption and in enhancing the removal in acute massive overdoses, but it is difficult to administer. The data are based on a few uncontrolled studies. (5) Hemodialysis is the most efficient method of removing lithium from the vascular compartment. It is the treatment of choice for severe intoxications with an altered mental state and seizures and in anuric patients. Long "runs" are used until the serum lithium level is below 1 mEq per liter, because of extensive re-equilibration. Monitor the serum lithium level every 4 hours after dialysis for rebound. Repeated and prolonged hemodialysis may be necessary. Expect a lag in neurologic recovery. *Laboratory investigations:* Monitor CBC (lithium causes significant leukocytosis), renal dysfunction, thyroid dysfunction (chronic intoxication), ECG, and electrolytes. Determine the serum lithium concentrations every 4 hours until there is a downward trend to near the therapeutic range. The levels do not always correlate with the manifestations but are more predictive in severe intoxications. A value above 3.0 mEq per liter with chronic intoxication and altered mental state indicates severe toxicity. Patients with a value above 9 mEq per liter after an acute overdose may be asymptomatic. Cross-reactions: The green-top Vacutainer specimen tube containing heparin spuriously elevates the serum lithium value 6 to 8 mEq per liter. *Disposition:* An acute asymptomatic lithium overdose cannot be medically cleared on the basis of a single lithium level. Patients should be admitted if they have any neurologic manifestations (altered mental status, hyper-reflexia, stiffness, or tremor). Patients should be admitted to the ICU if they are dehydrated, have renal impairment, or have a high or rising lithium level.

Methanol (wood alcohol). The concentration of methanol in Sterno fuel is 4% (it also contains ethanol), in windshield washer fluid 30%, and in gas line antifreeze 100%. *Toxic mechanism:* Methanol is metabolized by hepatic ADH to formaldehyde and formate. Formate produces tissue hypoxia, metabolic lactic acidosis, and retinal damage. Formate is converted by folate-dependent enzymes to carbon dioxide. *Toxic dose:* The minimum toxic amount is approximately 100 mg per kg. One tablespoonful (15 mL) of 40% methanol was lethal for a 2-year-old child and can cause blindness in an adult. The lethal oral dose is 30 to 240 mL of 100% methanol (20 to 150 grams). The toxic blood methanol concentration (BMC) is above 20 mg per dL, the very serious toxicity and potentially fatal level, greater than 50 mg per dL. The BMC and amount ingested can be estimated using the following equations and an SG for methanol of 0.719:

$$\text{BMC (mg/dL)} = \frac{\text{amount ingested (mL)} \times \text{\% methanol in product} \times \text{SG (0.719)}}{\text{Vd (0.6 L/kg)} \times \text{body weight (kg)}}$$

$$\text{Dose (amount ingested)} = \frac{\text{BMC (mg per dL)} \times \text{Vd (0.6 L/kg)} \times \text{body weight (kg)}}{\text{\% ethanol} \times \text{SG (0.719)}}$$

Kinetics: Onset of effect can be within 1 hour but is typically delayed 12 to 18 hours by metabolism to toxic metabolites. It may be delayed longer if ethanol is ingested concomitantly. Onset may be up to 72 hours in infants. The peak blood methanol concentration occurs at 1 hour. The Vd is 0.6 liter per kg (total body water); $t_{1/2}$ is 8 hours (with ethanol blocking it is 30 to 35 hours, and with hemodialysis, 2.5 hours). For metabolism see the section on toxic mechanism. Elimination is renal. *Manifestations:* Slow metabolism may delay onset for 12 to 18 hours in adults or longer if ethanol is ingested concomitantly. Methanol may produce inebriation, a formaldehyde odor on the breath, hyperemia of the optic disk, violent abdominal colic, "snow" vision, blindness, and shock. Later, worsening acidosis, hypoglycemia, and multiple organ failure develop; death results from complications of intractable acidosis and cerebral edema. Methanol produces an osmolal gap (early), and its metabolite formate produces AG metabolic acidosis (later). Absence of an osmolar gap or AG does not always rule out methanol intoxication. *Management:* (1) Protect the airway by intubation to prevent aspiration, and administer assisted ventilation as needed. Administer 100% oxygen if needed. Consult with a nephrologist early regarding the need for hemodialysis. (2) GI decontamination procedures have no role. (3) Treat metabolic acidosis vigorously with $NaHCO_3$ at 2 to 3 mEq per kg IV. Large amounts may be needed. (4) Ethanol therapy and hemodialysis (see Table 12): Classically, ethanol therapy was started if the blood methanol concentration was above 20 mg per dL, and hemodialysis was added if the concentration was above 50 mg per dL, but values less than 25 mg per dL are currently used as an indication for hemodialysis. Ethanol therapy: ADH has 100 times greater affinity for ethanol than methanol. Therefore, ethanol blocks the metabolism of methanol at a blood methanol concentration of 100 to 150 mg per dL. Initiate therapy to block metabolism if there is a history of ingestion of 0.4 mL of 100% methanol per kg, if the blood methanol level is above 20 mg per dL or the patient has an osmolar gap that is not accounted for, or if the patient is symptomatic or acidotic with an increased AG and/or hyperemia of the optic disk. (See Table 12.) Hemodialysis increases the clearance of both methanol and formate 10-fold over renal clearance. Continue to monitor methanol levels and/or formate levels for rebound every 4 hours after the procedure. Toxicologists and nephrologists have recommended early hemodialysis at blood methanol levels greater than 25 mg per dL because it significantly shortens the course of the intoxication and provides better outcomes. Other indications for early hemodialysis are significant metabolic acidosis, electrolyte abnormalities despite conventional therapy, and the presence of visual or mental symptoms. A serum formate level greater than 20 mg per dL has also been used as a criterion for hemodialysis. If hemodialysis is used, increase the infusion rate of 10% ethanol to 2.0 to 3.5 mL per kg per hour. Obtain the BEC and glucose every 2 hours. Continue therapy with both ethanol and hemodialysis until a blood methanol level is undetectable, there is no acidosis, and there are no mental or visual disturbances. This may require 2 to 5 days. (5) Treat hypoglycemia with intravenous glucose. (6) A bolus of folinic acid and folic acid has been used successfully in animal investigations to enhance formate metabolism to carbon dioxide and water. Administer leucovorin (Wellcovorin) at 1 mg per kg up to 50 mg IV every 4 hours for several days. (7) 4-Methylpyrazole inhibits ADH and is being investigated for use in methanol and ethylene glycol poisoning (see dosage under ethylene glycol management). It has been approved for use in the United States. (8) Obtain ophthalmologic consultation initially and at follow-up. *Laboratory investigations:* Methanol is detected on drug screens if specified. Monitor methanol and ethanol levels every 4 hours, electrolytes, glucose, BUN, creatinine, amylase, and ABGs. Formate levels correlate more closely than blood methanol levels with severity of intoxication and should be obtained if possible. If methanol levels are not available, the osmolal gap × 3.2 can be used to estimate the blood methanol levels in mg per dL. *Disposition:* All patients who ingest significant amounts of methanol should be referred to the emergency department for evaluation and determination of blood methanol concentration. Ophthalmologic follow-up of all intoxications should be arranged.

Monoamine Oxidase Inhibitors. MAOIs include MAO-A inhibitors, the hydrazine phenelzine sulfate (Nardil; dose 60 to 90 mg per day), isocarboxazid (Marplan; 10 to 30 mg per day), and the nonhydrazine tranylcypromine (Parnate; 20 to 40 mg per day). The MAO-B inhibitor selegiline (deprenyl, Eldepryl; 10 mg per day), an antiparkinsonism agent, does not have toxicity similar to that of MAO-A and is not discussed. MAOIs are used to treat severe depression. *Toxic mechanism:* MAO enzymes are responsible for the oxidative deamination of both endogenous and exogenous catecholamines. MAO-A in the intestinal wall also metabolizes tyramine in food. MAOIs permanently inhibit MAO enzymes until a new enzyme is synthesized at 14 days or later. The toxicity results from the accumulation, potentiation, and prolongation of the catecholamine action followed by profound hypotension and cardiovascular collapse. *Toxic dose:* Toxicity begins at 2 to 3 mg per kg, and fatalities occur at 4 to 6 mg per kg. Death has occurred after a single dose of tranylcypromine of 170 mg in an adult. *Kinetics:* Structurally, MAOIs are related to amphetamines and catecholamines. The hydrazine peak level occurs at 1 to 2 hours; elimination is by hepatic acetylation metabolism and excretion of inactive metabolites in the urine. The nonhydrazine peak level is at 1 to 4 hours, and elimination is by hepatic metabolism to active amphetamine-like metabolites. The onset of symptoms in overdoses is delayed 6 to 24 hours after ingestion, peak activity occurs at 8 to 12 hours, and the duration is 72 hours or longer. Peak MAOI effect occurs in 5 to 10 days, and effects last as long as 5 weeks. *Manifestations:* (1) Acute ingestion overdose: Phase I consists of an adrenergic crisis in which onset of effects is delayed for 6 to 24 hours and the peak may not be reached until 24 hours. Manifestations start as hyperthermia, tachycardia, tachypnea, dysarthria, transient hypertension, hyper-reflexia, and CNS stimulation. Phase II consists of neuromuscular excitation and sympathetic hyperactivity with increased temperature (above 104°F [40°C]), agitation, hyperactivity, confusion, fasciculations, twitching, tremor, masseter spasm, muscle rigidity, acidosis, and electrolyte abnormalities. Seizures and dystonic reactions may occur. The pupils are mydriatic and sometimes nonreactive, with a "Ping-Pong gaze." Phase III, CNS depression and cardiovascular collapse, occurs in severe overdose as the catecholamines are depleted. Symptoms usually resolve within 5 days but may last 2 weeks. Phase IV consists of secondary complications; rhabdomyolysis, cardiac dysrhythmias, multiple organ failure, and coagulopathies. (2) Biogenic interactions usually occur while therapeutic doses of MAOIs are given or shortly after they are discontinued, before the new MAO enzyme is synthesized. The onset occurs within 30 to 60 minutes after exposure. The following substances have been implicated: indirect-acting sympathomimetics (e.g., amphetamines); serotonergic drugs, opioids (e.g., meperidine, dextromethorphan), tricyclic antidepressants, and SSRIs (fluoxetine, sertraline, paroxetine); and tyramine-containing foods (wine, beer, avocados, cheese, caviar, chocolate, chicken liver) and L-tryptophan. SSRIs should not be started for at least 5 weeks after MAOIs have been discontinued. In mild cases, usually caused by foods, headache and hypertension develop and last for several hours. In severe cases, malignant hypertension and malignant hyperthermia syndromes consisting of hypertension or hyperthermia, altered mental state, skeletal muscle rigidity, shivering (often beginning in the masseter muscle), and seizures may occur. The serotonin syndrome, which may be due to inhibition of serotonin metabolism, has clinical manifestations similar to those in malignant hyperthermia and may occur with or without hyperthermia or hypertension. (3) Clinical findings in chronic toxicity include tremors, hyperhidrosis, agitation, hallucinations, confusion, and seizures and can be confused with withdrawal syndromes. *Management:* (1) MAOI overdose: GI decontamination with ipecac-induced emesis should not be used because it may aggravate the food-MAOI interaction hypertension. Use gastric lavage and AC or AC alone. If the patient is admitted to the hospital and is well enough to eat, order a nontyramine diet. Extreme agitation and seizures can be controlled with BZPs and barbiturates. Phenytoin is ineffective. Nondepolarizing neuromuscular blockers (not depolarizing succinylcholine) may be needed in severe cases of hyperthermia and rigidity. If there is severe hypertension (catecholamine-mediated), use phentolamine, a parenteral alpha blocking agent, at 3 to 5 mg IV, or labetalol, a combination of an alpha blocking agent and beta blocker, as a 20-mg intravenous bolus. If malignant hypertension with rigidity is present, use short-acting nitroprusside and BZP. Hypertension is often followed by severe hypotension, which should be managed with fluid and vasopressors. Caution: Vasopressor therapy should be administered at lower doses than usual because of an exaggerated pharmacologic response. Norepinephrine is preferred to dopamine, which requires release of intracellular amines. Cardiac dysrhythmias are treated with standard therapy but are often refractory, and cardioversion and pacemakers may be needed. For malignant hyperthermia, administer dantrolene (see Table 12), a nonspecific peripheral skeletal relaxing agent that inhibits the release of calcium from the sarcoplasm. Dantrolene is reconstituted with 60 mL of sterile water without bacteriostatic agents; do not use glass equipment, protect from light, and use within 6 hours. The loading dose of dantrolene is 2 to 3 mg per kg given IV as a bolus, which is repeated until the signs of malignant hyperthermia (tachycardia, rigidity, increased end-tidal carbon dioxide, and increased temperature) are controlled. The maximum total dose is 10 mg per kg to avoid hepatotoxicity. When malignant hyperthermia subsides, give 1 mg dantrolene per kg IV every 6 hours for 24 to 48 hours; then give 1 mg per kg PO every 6 hours for 24 hours to prevent recurrence. There is a danger of thrombophlebitis after peripheral dantrolene administration, and it should be given through a central line if possible. In addition, provide external cooling and correct metabolic acidosis and electrolyte disturbances. BZP can be used for sedation. Dantrolene does not reverse central dopamine blockade; therefore, give bromocriptine mesylate at 2.5 to 10 mg PO or through a nasogastric tube three times a day. Treat rhabdomyolysis and myoglobinuria with fluid diuresis, furosemide, and alkalization. Hemodialysis and hemoperfusion are of no proven value. (2) Biogenic amine interactions are managed symptomatically as for overdose. For the serotonin syndrome, cyproheptadine, a serotonin blocker, may be given at 4 mg PO every hour for 3 doses, or methysergide (Sansert) at 2 mg PO every 6 hours for 3 doses may be used, but their efficacy is not proved. *Laboratory investigations:* Monitor ECG, cardiac parameters, creatine kinase, ABGs, pulse oximetry, electrolytes, blood glucose, and acid-base balance. *Disposition:* All patients who ingest more than 2 mg per kg should be admitted to the hospital for 24 hours of observation and monitoring in the ICU because the life-threatening manifestations may be delayed. Patients with drug or dietary interactions that are mild may not require admission if symptoms subside within 4 to 6 hours and they remain asymptomatic. Patients with symptoms that persist or require active intervention should be admitted to the ICU.

Opioids (narcotic opiates). Opioids are used for analgesia, as antitussives, and as antidiarrheal agents and are illicit agents (heroin, opium) used in substance abuse. Tolerance, physical dependence, and withdrawal may develop. *Toxic mechanism:* At least four main opioid receptors have been identified. Mu is considered the most important for central analgesia and depression. Kappa and delta are predominant in spinal analgesia. The sigma receptors may mediate dysphoria. Death is due to dose-dependent CNS respiratory depression or is secondary to apnea, pulmonary aspiration, or noncardiac pulmonary edema. The mechanism of noncardiac pulmonary edema is unknown. *Toxic dose:* This depends on the specific drug, route of administration, and degree of tolerance. For therapeutic and toxic doses, see Table 43. In children, respiratory depression has been produced by 10 mg of morphine or methadone, 75 mg of meperidine, and 12.5 mg of diphenoxylate. Infants younger than 3 months are more susceptible to respiratory depression. Reduce the dose by 50%. *Kinetics:* Oral onset of the analgesic effect of morphine is at 10 to 15 minutes; the effect peaks in 1 hour, and the duration is 4 to 6 hours, but with sustained-release preparations (e.g., MS Contin), the duration is 8 to 12 hours. Opioids are 90% metabolized in the liver by hepatic conjugation and 90% excreted in the urine

TABLE 43. **Doses, Onset, and Duration of Action of Common Opioids**

Drug	Oral Dose: Adult	Oral Dose: Child	Onset of Action (min)	Duration of Action (h)	Adult Fatal Dose
Camphored tincture of opium (0.4 mg/mL), paregoric	25 mL	0.25–0.50 mL/kg	15–30	4–5	NA
Codeine	30–180 mg (>1 mg/kg is toxic in a child, above 200 mg in adult; >5 mg/kg fatal in a child)	0.5–1 mg/kg	15–30	4–6	800 mg
Dextromethorphan	15 mg 10 mg/kg is toxic	0.25 mg/kg	15–30	3–6	NA
Diacetylmorphine (heroin)	60 mg Street heroin is less than 10% pure	NA	15–30	3–4	100 mg
Diphenoxylate (Lomotil)	5–10 mg 7.5 mg is toxic in a child, 300 mg is toxic in adult	NA	120–240	14	300 mg
Fentanyl (Sublimaze, Duragesic transdermal)	0.1–0.2 mg	0.001–0.002 mg/kg	7–8	0.5–2	1.0 mg
Hydrocodone (Hycodan, Vicodin)	5–30 mg	0.15 mg/kg	30	3–4	100 mg
Hydromorphone (Dilaudid)	4 mg	0.1 mg/kg	15–30	3–4	100 mg
Meperidine (Demerol)	100 mg	1–1.5 mg/kg	10–45	3–4	350 mg
Methadone (Dolophine)	10 mg	0.1 mg/kg	30–60	4–12	120 mg
Morphine	10–60 mg Oral dose is six times parenteral dose; MS Contin (sustained-release)	0.1–0.2 mg/kg	<20	4–6	200 mg
Oxycodone (Percodan)	5 mg	NA	15–30	4–5	NA
Pentazocine (Talwin)	50–100 mg	NA	15–30	3–4	NA
Propoxyphene (Darvon)	65–100 mg 100 mg hydrochloride = 65 mg of napsylate, toxic at 10 mg/kg	NA	30–60	2–4	700 mg

Abbreviation: NA = not available.

as inactive compounds. The Vd is 1 to 4 liters per kg; PB is 35 to 75%. The typical plasma $t_{1/2}$ of opiates is 2 to 5 hours, but that of methadone is 24 to 36 hours. Morphine metabolites include morphine-3-glucuronide (M3G) (inactive) and morphine-6-glucuronide (M6G) (active) and normorphine (active). Meperidine is rapidly hydrolyzed by tissue esterases into the active metabolite normeperidine, which has twice the convulsant activity of meperidine. Heroin (diacetylmorphine) is deacetylated within minutes to the metabolite 6-monacetylmorphine (6MAM), the presence of which is diagnostic of heroin use, and morphine. Propoxyphene (Darvon) has a rapid onset, and death has occurred within 15 to 30 minutes after a massive overdose. Propoxyphene is metabolized to norpropoxyphene, an active metabolite with convulsive, cardiac dysrhythmic, and heart block effects. Symptoms of diphenoxylate (Lomotil) intoxication appear within 1 to 4 hours. It is metabolized into the active metabolite difenoxin, which is five times more active as a recurrent respiratory depressant. Death has been reported in children after a single tablet. *Manifestations:* (1) Initial or mild intoxication produces miosis, dull facial expression, drowsiness, partial ptosis, and "nodding" (head drops to chest and then bobs up). Larger amounts produce the classic triad of miotic pupils (exceptions follow), respiratory depression, and depressed level of consciousness (flaccid coma). The blood pressure, pulse, and bowel sounds are decreased. (2) Dilated pupils do not exclude opioid intoxication. Some exceptions to miosis include dextromethorphan (which paralyzes the iris), fentanyl, meperidine, and diphenoxylate (rarely). Physiologic disturbances including acidosis, hypoglycemia, hypoxia, and postictal state or a coingestant may also produce mydriasis. (3) Usually the muscles are flaccid, but increased muscle tone may be produced by meperidine and fentanyl (chest rigidity). (4) Seizures are rare but can occur with codeine, meperidine, propoxyphene, and dextromethorphan. Hallucinations and agitation have been reported. (5) Pruritus and urticaria caused by histamine release of some opioids or by sulfites may be present. (6) Noncardiac pulmonary edema often occurs after resuscitation and naloxone administration, especially with intravenous abuse. (7) Cardiac effects include vasodilatation and hypotension. A heart murmur in a person who is addicted to an intravenous drug suggests endocarditis. Propoxyphene can produce delayed cardiac dysrhythmias. (8) Fentanyl is 100 times more potent than morphine and can cause chest wall muscle rigidity. Some of its derivatives are 2000 times more potent than morphine. *Management:* (1) Provide supportive care, particularly an endotracheal tube and assisted ventilation. Temporary ventilation may be provided by bag-valve-mask with 100% oxygen. Begin cardiac monitoring; establish intravenous access; and obtain specimens for ABGs, glucose, electrolyte,

BUN, creatinine, CBC, coagulation profile, and liver function determinations, a toxicology screen, and urinalysis. (2) GI decontamination: Do not induce emesis. Administer AC if bowel sounds are present. Cathartics may be used because of opioid-induced decreased GI mobility and constipation. (3) Naloxone (Narcan) (see Table 12): If addiction is suspected, restrain the patient first; then administer 0.1 mg of naloxone and double the dose every 2 minutes until the patient responds or 10 to 20 mg has been given. If addiction is not suspected, give 2 mg every 2 to 3 minutes to total of 10 to 20 mg. It is essential to determine whether there is a complete response to naloxone (mydriasis, improvement in ventilation), because administration of this drug is a diagnostic therapeutic test. A continuous naloxone infusion may be appropriate using the "response dose" every hour. Repeated doses of naloxone may be necessary because the effects of many opioids can last much longer than that of naloxone (30 to 60 minutes). Methadone intoxication may require a naloxone infusion for 24 to 48 hours. Half of the response dose may have to be repeated in 15 to 20 minutes after starting the infusion. Acute iatrogenic withdrawal on administration of naloxone to a dependent patient should not be treated with morphine or other opioids. Naloxone's effects are limited to 30 to 60 minutes (shorter than those of most opioids), and withdrawal effects subside in a short time. (4) Nalmefene (Revex), an FDA-approved long-acting (4 to 8 hours) pure opioid antagonist, is being investigated, but its role in acute intoxication is unclear. It may have a role in place of naloxone infusion but could produce prolonged withdrawal. (5) Noncardiac pulmonary edema does not respond to naloxone, and the patient requires intubation, assisted ventilation, PEEP, and hemodynamic monitoring. Fluids should be given cautiously in opioid overdose because they stimulate antidiuretic hormone. (6) If the patient is comatose, give 50% glucose (3 to 4% of comatose opioid-overdose patients have hypoglycemia) and thiamine before naloxone. If the patient has seizures unresponsive to naloxone, administer diazepam and examine for other metabolic (hypoglycemia, electrolyte disturbances) and structural disorders. (7) Hypotension is rare and should prompt a search for another cause. (8) If the patient is agitated, exclude hypoxia and hypoglycemia before considering opioid withdrawal. (9) Complications to consider include urine retention, constipation, rhabdomyolysis, myoglobinuria, hypoglycemia, and withdrawal. *Laboratory investigations:* For overdoses, monitor ABGs, blood glucose, and electrolytes; obtain chest radiographs and an ECG. For drug abusers, consider testing for hepatitis B, syphilis, and HIV antibody (HIV testing usually requires consent). Blood opioid concentrations are not useful. They confirm the diagnosis (morphine therapeutic 65 to 80 ng per mL, toxic greater than 200 ng per mL) but are not useful for making a therapeutic decision. Cross-reactions can occur with Vicks Formula 44, poppy seeds on bagels, and other opioids (codeine and heroin are metabolized to morphine). Naloxone in a dose of 4 mg IV was not associated with a positive enzyme multiple immunoassay technique (EMIT) urine screen at 60 minutes, 6 hours, or 48 hours. *Disposition:* If a patient responds to intravenous naloxone, careful observation for relapse and the development of pulmonary edema is required, with cardiac and respiratory monitoring for 6 to 12 hours. Patients requiring repeated doses of naloxone or an infusion or who develop pulmonary edema require ICU admission and cannot be discharged from the ICU until they are symptom-free for 12 hours. With intravenous administration, complications are expected to be present within 20 minutes after injection, and discharge after 4 symptom-free hours has been recommended. Adults with oral overdose have a delayed onset of toxicity and require observation for 6 hours. Children with oral opioid overdose should be admitted to the hospital for 24 hours of observation because of delayed toxicity. Restrain the patient who attempts to sign out against medical advice after treatment with naloxone, at least until psychiatric evaluation.

Organophosphates and Carbamates. Sources of cholinergic intoxication are insecticides, medications (carbamates), and some mushrooms. Examples of organophosphate (OP) insecticides are malathion (Cythion; low toxicity, median lethal dose [LD_{50}] 2800 mg per kg), chlorpyrifos (Dursban; moderate toxicity, LD_{50} 250 mg per kg), and parathion (high toxicity, LD_{50} 2 mg per kg); carbamate insecticides are carbaryl (Sevin; low toxicity, LD_{50} 500 mg per kg), propoxur (Baygon; moderate toxicity, LD_{50} 95 mg per kg), and aldicarb (Temik; high toxicity, LD_{50} 0.9 mg per kg). Carbamate medicinals include neostigmine and physostigmine (Antilirium). Cholinergic compounds also include the dreaded "G" nerve war weapons Tubun (GA), Sarin (GB), Soman (GB), and VX. *Toxic mechanism:* (1) OPs phosphorylate the active site on red blood cell acetylcholinesterase and pseudocholinesterase in the serum (3% of the general population has a deficiency) and other organs, causing irreversible inhibition. There are two types of OP action: direct action by the parent compound (e.g., tetraethyl pyrophosphate) and indirect action by the toxic metabolite (e.g., paraoxon or malaoxon). (2) Carbamates (esters of carbonic acid) cause reversible carbamylation of the active site of the enzymes. When a critical amount of cholinesterase is inhibited by more than 50% from baseline, acetylcholine accumulates, causing transient stimulation of conduction and, soon after, paralysis of conduction, through cholinergic synapses and sympathetic terminals (muscarinic effect), the somatic nerves, the autonomic ganglia (nicotinic effect), and CNS synapses. (3) Major differences of the carbamates from OPs: Carbamate toxicity is less severe and the duration is shorter; carbamates rarely produce overt CNS effects (poor CNS penetration); with carbamates the acetylcholinesterase returns to normal rapidly, so blood values are not useful even in confirming the diagnosis; with carbamates, pralidoxime, the enzyme regenerator, may not be necessary in the management of mild intoxication (e.g., carbaryl), but atropine is required. *Toxic dose:* Parathion's minimal lethal dose is 2 mg in children and 10 to 20 mg in adults. The lethal dose of malathion is greater than 1375 mg per kg (it is 1000 times less toxic than parathion) and that of chlorpyrifos is 25 grams, and they are unlikely to cause death. *Kinetics:* Absorption is by all routes. The onset of acute ingestion toxicity occurs as early as 3 hours, usually before 12 hours, and always before 24 hours. Lipid-soluble agents absorbed by the dermal route (e.g., fenthion) may have a delayed onset to more than 24 hours after exposure. Inhalation toxicity occurs immediately after exposure. Massive ingestion can produce intoxication within minutes. The effects of the thions (e.g., parathion, malathion) are delayed because they undergo hepatic microsomal oxidative metabolism to their toxic metabolites, oxons (e.g., paraoxon, malaoxon). The $t_{1/2}$ of malathion is 2.89 hours and of parathion is 2.1 days. The metabolites are eliminated in the urine, and the presence of *p*-nitrophenol in the urine is a clue up to 48 hours after exposure. *Manifestations:* Many OPs produce a garlic odor on the breath, from the gastric contents, or from the container. Diaphoresis, excessive salivation, miosis, and muscle twitching are helpful clues. (1) Early, a cholinergic (muscarinic) crisis develops and consists of parasympathetic nervous system activity. DUMBELS is a mnemonic for the manifestations of defecation, cramps, and increased bowel mobility; urinary incontinence; miosis (mydriasis may occur in 20%); bronchospasm and bronchorrhea; excess secretion; lacrimation; and seizures. Bradycardia, pulmonary edema, and hypotension may be present. (2) Later, sympathetic and nicotinic effects occur consisting of muscle weakness and fasciculations (eyelid twitching is often present), adrenal stimulation and hyperglycemia, tachycardia, cramps in muscles, and hypertension (mnemonic MATCH). Finally, paralysis of the skeletal muscles ensues. (3) CNS effects are headache, blurred vision, anxiety, ataxia, delirium and toxic psychosis, convulsions, coma, and respiratory depression. Cranial nerve palsies have been noted. Delayed hallucinations may occur. (4) Delayed respiratory paralysis and neurologic and neurobehavioral disorders have been described after exposure to certain OPs or with dermal exposure. The "intermediate" syndrome consists of paralysis of proximal and respiratory muscles developing 24 to 96 hours after the successful treatment of OP poisoning. A delayed distal polyneuropathy has been described with certain OPs (e.g., tri-*o*-cresyl phosphate [TOCP], bromoleptophos, methomidophous). (5) Complications include aspiration, pulmonary edema, and adult respiratory distress syndrome. *Management:* (1) Safeguard health care personnel with protective clothing (masks, gloves, gowns, goggles, and respiratory equipment or hazardous material suits as necessary). General decontamination consists of isolation, bagging, and disposal of contaminated clothing and other articles. Establish and maintain vital functions. Institute cardiac and oxygen saturation monitoring. Intubation and assisted ventilation may be needed. Suction secretions until atropinization drying is achieved. (2) Specific decontamination: Dermal: Prompt removal of clothing and cleansing of all affected areas of skin, hair, and eyes are indicated. Ocular: Irrigation with copious amounts of tepid water or 0.9% saline is performed for at least 15 minutes. GI: If ingestion is recent, use gastric lavage with airway protection, if necessary, and administer AC. (3) Antidotes: Atropine sulfate (see Table 12) is both a diagnostic and a therapeutic agent. Atropine counteracts the muscarinic effects but is only partially effective for the CNS effects (seizures and coma). Use preservative-free atropine (no benzyl alcohol). If the patient is symptomatic (bradycardia or bronchorrhea may be present), administer a test dose of 0.02 mg per kg for a child or 1 mg for an adult IV. If there are no signs of atropinization (tachycardia, drying of secretions, and mydriasis), immediately administer atropine at 0.05 mg per kg for a child or 2 mg for an adult every 5 to 10 minutes as needed to dry the secretions and clear the lungs. Beneficial effects are seen within 1 to 4 minutes, and the maximal effect occurs in 8 minutes. The average dose in the first 24 hours is 40 mg, but 1000 mg or more has been required in severe cases. Glycopyrrolate (Robinul) may be used if atropine is not available. Maintain the maximal dose for 12 to 24 hours; then taper it and observe for relapse. Poisoning, especially with lipophilic agents (e.g., fenthion, chlorfenthion), may require weeks of atropine therapy. The alternative is a continuous infusion of 8 mg of atropine in 100 mL of 0.9% saline at rate of 0.02 to 0.08 mg per kg per hour (0.25 to 1.0 mL per kg per hour) with additional 1- to 5-mg boluses as needed to dry the secretions. Pralidoxime chloride (2-PAM) has antinicotinic, antimuscarinic, and possibly CNS effects. Concomitant use of this agent may require a reduction in the dose of atropine (see Table 12). It acts to reactivate the phosphorylated cholinesterases by binding the phosphate moiety on the esteric site and displacing it. It should be given early before "aging" of the phosphate bond produces tighter binding. However, reports indicate that 2-PAM is beneficial even several days after the poisoning. Improvement is seen within 10 to 40 minutes. The initial dose of 2-PAM is 1 to 2 grams in 250 mL of 0.89% saline over 5 to 10 minutes, for a maximum of 200 mg per minute (in adults), or 25 to 50 mg per kg (in children younger than 12 years), for a maximum of 4 mg per kg per minute. Repeat every 6 to 12 hours for several days. An alternative is a continuous infusion of 1 gram in 100 mL of 0.89% saline at 5 to 20 mg per kg per hour (0.5 to 12 mL per kg per hour) up to 500 mg per hour, with titration to the desired response. The maximum adult daily dose is 12 grams. Cardiac monitoring and blood pressure monitoring are advised during and for several hours after the infusion. The end point is absence of fasciculations and return of muscle strength. (4) Contraindicated drugs: Do not use morphine, aminophylline, barbiturates, opioids, phenothiazine, reserpine-like drugs, parasympathomimetics, or succinylcholine. (5)

Non-cardiac pulmonary edema may require respiratory support. (6) Seizures may respond to atropine and 2-PAM, but the effect is not consistent and anticonvulsants may be required. (7) Cardiac dysrhythmias may require electrical cardioversion or antidysrhythmic therapy if the patient is hemodynamically unstable. (8) Extracorporeal procedures are of no proven value. *Laboratory investigations:* Monitor chest radiograph, blood glucose (nonketotic hyperglycemia occurs frequently), ABGs, pulse oximetry, ECG, blood coagulation status, liver function, hyperamylasemia (pancreatitis has been reported), and the urine for the metabolite alkyl phosphate *p*-nitrophenol. Draw blood for red blood cell cholinesterase determination before giving pralidoxime. In mild poisoning, this value is 20 to 50% of normal; in moderate poisoning, 10 to 20% of normal; and in severe poisoning, 10% of normal (more than 90% depressed). A postexposure rise of 10 to 15% in the cholinesterase level determined by at least 10 to 14 days after exposure confirms the diagnosis. *Disposition:* Asymptomatic patients with a normal examination after 6 to 8 hours of observation may be discharged. If intentional poisoning occurred, psychiatric clearance is required for discharge. Symptomatic patients should be admitted to the ICU. Observation of patients with milder carbamate poisoning, even those requiring atropine, for 6 to 8 hours without symptoms may be sufficient to rule out significant toxicity. If work place exposure occurred, notify OSHA.

Phencylidine (PCP, "angel dust," "peace pill," "hog"). PCP is an arylcyclohexylamine related to ketamine and chemically related to the PTZs. It is a "dissociative" anesthetic that has been banned in the United States since 1979 and is now an illicit substance, with at least 38 analogues. It is inexpensively manufactured by "kitchen" chemists and is mislabeled as other hallucinogens. Improperly synthesized PCP may release cyanide when heated or smoked and can cause explosions. *Toxic mechanism:* PCP action is complex and not completely understood. It inhibits neurotransmitters and causes loss of pain sensation without depressing the CNS respiratory status. It stimulates alpha-adrenergic receptors and may act as a "false" neurotransmitter. The effects are sympathomimetic, cholinergic, and cerebellar stimulation. *Toxic dose:* The usual dose in "joints" is 100 to 400 mg weight; joints or leaf mixture, 0.24 to 7.9%, 1 mg per 150 leaves; tablets, 5 mg (usual street dose). CNS effects at 1 to 6 mg produce hallucinations and euphoria; 6 to 10 mg produces toxic psychosis and sympathetic stimulation, 10 to 25 mg produces severe toxicity, and more than 100 mg has resulted in fatality. *Kinetics:* PCP is a lipophilic weak base with a pK_a of 8.5 to 9.5. It is rapidly absorbed when smoked and snorted, poorly absorbed from the acid stomach, and rapidly absorbed from the alkaline media of the small intestine. It is secreted enterogastrically and is reabsorbed in the small intestine. The onset of action when it is smoked is at 2 to 5 minutes, with a peak in 15 to 30 minutes. The onset is at 30 to 60 minutes when it is taken PO and immediate when it is taken IV. Most adverse reactions in overdose begin within 1 to 2 hours. Its duration of action at low doses is 4 to 6 hours, and normality returns in 24 hours; in large overdoses, fluctuating coma may last 6 to 10 days. The $t_{1/2}$ is 1 hour (in overdose, 11 to 89 hours). The Vd is 6.2 liters per kg, and the PB is 70%. It is eliminated by gastric secretion, liver metabolism, and 10% urinary excretion of conjugates and free PCP. Renal excretion may be increased 50% with urinary acidification. PCP concentrates in brain and adipose tissue. *Manifestations:* The classic picture is one of bursts of horizontal, vertical, and rotary nystagmus, which is a clue (occurs in 50% of cases); miosis; hypertension; and fluctuating altered mental state. There is a wide spectrum of clinical presentations. (1) Mild intoxication: A dose of 1 to 6 mg produces drunken and bizarre behavior, agitation, rotary nystagmus, and black stare. Violent behavior and sensory anesthesia make these patients insensitive to pain, self-destructive, and dangerous. Most are communicative within 1 to 2 hours, are alert and oriented in 6 to 8 hours, and recover completely in 24 to 48 hours. (2) Moderate intoxication: A dose of 6 to 10 mg produces excess salivation, hypertension, hyperthermia, muscle rigidity, myoclonus, and catatonia. Recovery of consciousness occurs in 24 to 48 hours and complete recovery in 1 week. (3) Severe intoxication: A dose of 10 to 25 mg results in opisthotonos, decerebrate rigidity, convulsions, prolonged fluctuating coma, and respiratory failure. This category involves a high rate of medical complications. Recovery of consciousness occurs in 24 to 48 hours, with complete normality in 1 month. (4) Medical complications include apnea, aspiration pneumonia, cardiac arrest, hypertensive encephalopathy, hyperthermia, intracerebral hemorrhage, psychosis, rhabdomyolysis and myoglobinuria, and seizures. Loss of memory and flashbacks last for months. PCP-induced depression and suicide have been reported. (5) Fatalities occur with ingestions of greater than 100 mg and with serum levels higher than 100 to 250 ng per mL. *Management:* Observe the patient for violent, self-destructive, bizarre behavior and paranoid schizophrenia. Patients should be placed in a low sensory environment, and dangerous objects removed from the area. (1) GI decontamination is not effective because PCP is rapidly absorbed from the intestines. Avoid overtreating mild intoxication. Administer AC initially and MDAC every 4 hours, because PCP is secreted into the stomach even if it is smoked or snorted. Continuous gastric suction is not routine but may be useful (with protection of the airway) in severe toxicity (stupor or coma), because the drug is secreted into the gastric juice. (2) Protect patients from harming themselves or others. Physical restraints may be necessary, but use them sparingly and for the shortest time possible because they increase the risk of rhabdomyolysis. Avoid metal restraints such as handcuffs. For behavioral disorders and toxic psychosis, diazepam is the agent of choice. Pharmacologic intervention includes diazepam in a dose of 10 to 30 mg PO or 2 to 5 mg IV initially;

titrate upward to 10 mg, but up to 30 mg may be required. See the section on management of the violent patient (page 1208). The "talk-down" technique is usually ineffective and dangerous. Avoid PTZs and butyrophenones in the acute phase because they lower the convulsive threshold; however, they may be needed later for psychosis. Haloperidol (Haldol) administration has been reported to produce catatonia. (3) Seizures and muscle spasms are controlled with diazepam in a dose of 2.5 mg, up to 10 mg. (4) Hyperthermia (temperature above 38.5°C [101.3°F]) is treated with external cooling measures. (5) Hypertension is usually transient and does not require treatment. In an emergency hypertensive crisis (blood pressure above 200/115 mm Hg) use nitroprusside, 0.3 to 2 μg per kg per minute. The maximal infusion rate is 10 μg per kg per minute for only 10 minutes. (6) Acid ion-trapping diuresis is not recommended because of the danger of myoglobin precipitation in the renal tubules. (7) Rhabdomyolysis and myoglobinuria are treated by correcting volume depletion and ensuring a urine output of at least 2 mL per kg per hour. Alkalization is controversial because of PCP reabsorption. (8) Hemodialysis is beneficial if renal failure occurs; otherwise, the extracorporeal procedures are not beneficial. *Laboratory investigations:* Marked elevation of the creatine kinase level may be a clue to PCP intoxication. Values of greater than 20,000 units have been reported. Monitor result of urinalysis and test urine for myoglobin with *o*-toluidine blood reagent strip. A 3+ or 4+ test result and less than 10 red blood cells per high-power field on microscopic examination suggest myoglobinuria. Measure for PCP in the gastric juice, where it is concentrated 10 to 50 times higher than in blood or urine. Monitor blood for creatine kinase, uric acid (an early clue to rhabdomyolysis), BUN, creatinine, electrolytes (hyperkalemia), and glucose (20% of intoxications involve hypoglycemia); also monitor urine output, liver function tests, ECG, and ABGs if there are any respiratory manifestations. PCP blood concentrations are not helpful. A level of 10 ng per mL produces excitation, 30 to 100 ng per mL coma, and greater than 100 ng per mL, seizures and fatalities. PCP may be detected in the urine of the average user for 10 to 14 days or up to 3 weeks after the last dose. With chronic use it can be detected for more than 1 month. The analogue of PCP may not test positive for PCP in the urine. Cross-reactions: Bleach and dextromethorphan may cause false-positive urine test results on immunoassay; doxylamine, a false-positive result on gas chromatography. *Disposition:* All patients with coma, delirium, catatonia, violent behavior, aspiration pneumonia, sustained hypertension (blood pressure above 200/115 mm Hg), and significant rhabdomyolysis should be admitted to the ICU until they are asymptomatic for at least 24 hours. If patients with mild intoxication are mentally and neurologically stable and become asymptomatic (except for nystagmus) for 4 hours, they may be discharged in the company of a responsible adult. All patients must be assessed for risk of suicide before discharge. Drug counseling and psychiatric follow-up should be arranged. Patients should be warned that episodes of disorientation and depression may continue intermittently for 4 weeks or more.

Phenothiazines and Nonphenothiazines: Neuroleptics. *Toxic mechanism:* Neuroleptics have complex mechanisms of toxicity including (1) block of the postsynaptic dopamine receptors, (2) block of peripheral and central alpha-adrenergic receptors, (3) block of cholinergic muscarinic receptors, (4) a quinidine-like antidysrhythmic and myocardial depressant effect in large overdose, (5) a lowered convulsive threshold, and (6) an effect on hypothalamic temperature regulation. See Table 44. *Toxic dose:* Extrapyramidal reactions, anticholinergic effects, and orthostatic hypotension may occur at therapeutic doses. See Table 44 for therapeutic doses. The toxic amount is not established, but the maximum daily therapeutic dose may result in significant side effects, and twice this amount is potentially fatal. Chlorpromazine (Thorazine), the prototype, may produce serious hypotension and CNS depression at doses above 200 mg (17 mg per kg) in children and 3 to 5 grams in adults. Fatalities have been reported after ingestion of 2.5 grams of loxapine and mesoridazine and 1.5 grams of thioridazine. *Kinetics:* These agents are lipophilic and have unpredictable GI absorption. Peak levels occur 2 to 6 hours after ingestion and have enterohepatic recirculation. The mean serum $t_{1/2}$ in phase I is 1 to 2 hours and the biphasic $t_{1/2}$ is 20 to 40 hours. The PB is 92 to 98%. Chlorpromazine has oral onset at 30 to 60 minutes, peak effect at 2 to 4 hours, and a duration of 4 to 6 hours. With sustained-release preparations, the onset is at 30 to 60 minutes and the duration is 6 to 12 hours. The PB is 95%; the Vd, 10 to 40 liters per kg. Elimination is by hepatic metabolism, which results in multiple metabolites (some are active). Metabolites may be detected in urine months after chronic therapy. Only 1 to 3% is excreted unchanged in the urine. *Manifestations:* (1) PTZ overdose effects: Anticholinergic symptoms may be present early but are not life-threatening. Miosis is usually present (80%) if the PTZ has strong alpha-adrenergic blocking effect (e.g., chlorpromazine), but if there is strong anticholinergic activity, mydriasis may occur. Agitation and delirium rapidly progress to coma. Major problems are cardiac toxicity and hypotension. The cardiotoxic effects are seen more commonly with thioridazine and its metabolite mesoridazine. These agents have produced the largest number of fatalities in PTZ overdoses. Cardiac conduction disturbances include prolonged PR, QRS, and QT_C intervals; U and T wave abnormalities; and ventricular dysrhythmias including torsades de pointes. Seizures occur mainly in patients with convulsive disorders or with loxapine overdose. Sudden death in children and adults has been reported. (2) Idiosyncratic dystonic reactions are most common with the piperidine group. The reaction is not dose-dependent and consists of opisthotonos, torticollis, orolingual dyskinesia, and oculogyric crisis (painful upward

TABLE 44. **Neuroleptic Daily Doses and Properties: Comparison of Effects***

Compound/Dose	Effects: *Antipsychotic*	*Anticholinergic*	*Extrapyramidal*	*Hypotensive and Cardiotoxic*	*Sedative*
Phenothiazine					
Aliphatic†	1+	3+	2+	**2+**	3+
Chlorpromazine (Thorazine), 20–50 mg adult dose, range 20–2000 mg per 24 h					
Promethazine (Phenergan), 25–50 mg adult dose, range 25–200 mg per 24 h					
Piperazine‡	3+	1+	3+	1+	1+
Fluphenazine (Prolixin), 2.5–10 mg adult dose, range 2.5–20 mg per 24 h					
Perphenazine (Trilafon), 4–16 mg adult dose, range 10–30 mg per 24 h					
Prochlorperazine (Compazine), 5–10 mg adult dose, range 15–40 mg per 24 h					
Trifluoperazine (Stelazine), 2–5 mg adult dose, range 1–40 mg per 24 h					
Piperidine†	1+	2+	1+	3+	3+
Mesoridazine (Serentil), 25–100 mg adult dose, range 150–400 mg per 24 h					
Thioridazine (Mellaril), 25–100 mg adult dose, range 150–300 mg per 24 h					
Nonphenothiazine					
Butyrophenone‡	3+	1+	3+	1+	1+
Haloperidol (Haldol), 0.5–5.0 mg adult dose, range 1–100 mg per 24 h					
Dibenzoxazepine‡	3+	1+	3+	1+	2+
Loxapine (Loxitane), 10–50 mg adult dose, range 60–100 mg per 24 h					
Dihydroindolone‡	3+	1+	3+	1+	1+
Molindone (Moban), 5–25 mg adult dose, range 50–225 mg per 24 h					
Thioxanthenes‡	3+	1+	3+	3+	1+
Thiothixene (Navane), 2–15 mg adult dose, range 5–80 mg per 24 h					
Chlorprothixene (Taractan), 5–60 mg adult dose, range 75–200 mg per 24 h					

*1+ indicates very low activity; 2+, moderate activity; 3+, very high activity. Bold indicates major effect. Equivalent doses: 100 mg of chlorpromazine or thioridazine = 50 mg of mesoridazine = 15 mg of loxapine or prochlorperazine = 10 mg of molindone or perphenazine = 5 mg of thiothixene = 2 mg of fluphenazine or haloperidol.

†Low antipsychotic potency.

‡High antipsychotic potency.

gaze). It occurs more frequently in children and women. (3) Neuroleptic malignant syndrome occurs in patients receiving chronic therapy and is characterized by hyperthermia, muscle rigidity, autonomic dysfunction, and altered mental state. One case has been reported with acute overdose. (4) The loxapine syndrome consists of seizures, rhabdomyolysis, and renal failure. *Management:* (1) Establish and maintain the vital functions. All patients with overdose require venous access, 12-lead ECG (to measure intervals), cardiac and respiratory monitoring, and seizure precautions. Monitor core temperature to detect a poikilothermic effect. The comatose patient may require intubation and assisted ventilation, 100% oxygen, intravenous glucose, naloxone, and 100 mg of thiamine. (2) GI decontamination: Emesis is not recommended. Gastric lavage may be useful but is not necessary if AC or a cathartic is administered promptly. MDAC has not been proved beneficial. A radiograph of the abdomen may be useful, if the PTZ is radiopaque. Haloperidol and trifluoperazine are most likely to be radiopaque. Whole-bowel irrigation may be useful when a large number of pills is visualized on a radiograph or sustained-release preparations are involved, but this modality has not been investigated for management of PTZ toxicity. (3) Treat convulsions with diazepam or lorazepam. A loxapine overdose may result in status epilepticus. If nondepolarizing neuromuscular blockade is required, use pancuronium (Pavulon) or vecuronium (Norcuron) (not succinylcholine [Anectine], which may cause malignant hyperthermia), and monitor the EEG during paralysis. (4) Dysrhythmias: Monitor with serial ECG. Treat unstable rhythms with electrical cardioversion. AVOID class IA anti-dysrhythmic drugs (procainamide, quinidine, and disopyramide). Hypokalemia predisposes to dysrhythmias and should be corrected aggressively. Supraventricular tachycardia with hemodynamic instability is treated with electrical cardioversion. The role of adenosine has not been defined. Avoid calcium channel blockers and beta blockers. QRS interval prolongation is treated with $NaHCO_3$ at 1 to 2 mEq per kg by intravenous bolus given over a few minutes. Torsades de pointes is treated with 2 grams of a 20% magnesium sulfate solution given IV over 2 to 3 minutes; if there is no response in 10 minutes, this is repeated and followed by a continuous infusion of 5 to 10 mg per minute, or an infusion of 50 mg per minute is given for 2 hours, followed by an infusion of 30 mg per minute given over 90 minutes twice a day for several days, as needed. The dose in children is 25 to 50 mg per kg initially with a maintenance dose of 30 to 60 mg per kg per 24 hours (0.25 to 0.50 mEq per kg per 24 hours), up to 1000 mg per 24 hours. Monitor serum magnesium: Ventricular tachydysrhythmias: If the patient is stable, lidocaine is the agent of choice. If the patient is unstable, electrical cardioversion is used. Heart blocks with hemodynamic instability should be managed with temporary cardiac pacing. (5) Hypotension is treated with the Trendelenburg position, 0.89% saline, and, in refractory cases or if there is danger of fluid overload, administration of vasopressors. The vasopressor of choice is the alpha-adrenergic agonist norepinephrine, 0.1 to 0.2 μg per gram per minute and titrated to response. Epinephrine and dopamine should not be used because beta-receptor stimulation in the presence of alpha-receptor blockade may provoke dysrhythmias, and PTZs are antidopaminergic. (6) Treat hypothermia or hyperthermia with external warming or cooling measures. Do not use antipyretic drugs. (7) Management of the neuroleptic malignant syndrome includes discontinuing the offending agent, aggressively reducing the temperature with passive and active cooling measures, correcting electrolyte and metabolic imbalances, and administering dantrolene sodium (see Table 12 and the section on malignant hyperthermia syndrome management). The loading dose is 2 to 3 mg per kg given IV as a bolus, and the loading dose is repeated until the signs of the syndrome (tachycardia, rigidity, and temperature elevation) are controlled. The maximum total dose is 10 mg per kg. (8) Idiosyncratic dystonic reaction can be treated with diphenhydramine at 1 to 2 mg per kg per dose given IV over 5 minutes up to a maximum of 50 mg IV; a response is noted within 2 to 5 minutes. Follow with oral doses for 5 to 7 days to prevent recurrence. (9) Extracorporeal measures (hemodialysis, hemoperfusion) are not effective in enhancing removal of these agents. *Laboratory investigations:* Monitor ABGs, renal and hepatic function, electrolytes, blood glucose, and creatine kinase and myoglobinemia in neuroleptic malignant syndrome. Most of these agents are detected by routine screens. A positive ferric chloride test of the urine occurs if there is a sufficient blood level; however, it is not specific (salicylates and phenolic compounds also give a positive result). Quantitative serum levels are not useful in management. Cross-reactions with EMIT tests occur with cyclic antidepressants. PTZs give false-negative pregnancy urine test results using human chorionic gonadotropin as the indicator and false-positive test results for urinary porphyrins, the indirect Coombs test, urobilinogen, and amylase. *Disposition:* Asymptomatic patients should be observed for at least 6 hours after gastric decontamination. Symptomatic patients with cardiotoxicity, hypotension, or convulsions should be admitted to the ICU and monitored for 48 hours.

Salicylates (acetylsalicylic acid, aspirin, salicylic acid). *Toxic mechanism:* The primary toxic mechanisms include (1) direct stimulation of the medullary chemoreceptor trigger zone and respiratory center; (2) uncoupling of oxidative phosphorylation; (3) inhibition of the Krebs cycle enzymes; (4) inhibition of vitamin K–dependent and –independent clotting factors; (5) alteration of platelet function; and (6) inhibition of prostaglandin synthesis. *Toxic dose:* Acute mild intoxication occurs at a dose of 150 to 200 mg per kg (tinnitus, dizziness), moderate intoxication at 200 to 300 mg per kg, and severe intoxication at 300 to 500 mg per kg (CNS manifestations). An acute salicylate plasma concentration (SPC) higher than 30 mg per dL (usually over 40 mg per dL) may be associated with clinical toxicity. Chronic intoxication occurs at ingestions of more than 100 mg per kg per day for more than 2 days because of cumulative kinetics. Methyl salicylate (oil of wintergreen) is the most toxic form of salicylate; 1 mL of 98% methyl salicylate contains 1.4 grams of salicylate. Fatalities have occurred with ingestion of 1 teaspoonful in a child and 1 ounce in adults. It is found in topical ointments and liniments (18 to 30%). *Kinetics:* Acetylsalicylic acid is a weak acid, with a pK_a of 3.5; salicylic acid has a pK_a of 3.0. Salicylic acid is absorbed from the stomach and small bowel and dermally. Onset of action is within 30 minutes. Methyl salicylate and effervescent tablets are absorbed more rapidly. An SPC is detectable within 15 minutes after ingestion and the peak occurs in 30 to 120 minutes but may be delayed 6 to 12 hours in large overdoses, in overdoses with enteric-coated and sustained-release preparations, and if concretions develop. The therapeutic duration of action is 3 to 4 hours but is markedly prolonged in an overdose. The $t_{1/2}$ of salicylic acid is 3 hours after a 300-mg dose, 6 hours after a 1-gram overdose, and over 10 hours after a 10-gram overdose. The Vd is 0.13 liter per kg for salicylic acid but increases as the SPC increases. PB is up to 90% for salicylic acid at pH 7.4 at a therapeutic SPC, 75% at an SPC above 40 mg per dL, 50% at an SPC of 70 mg per dL, and 30% at an SPC of 120 mg per dL. Elimination includes Michaelis-Menten hepatic metabolism by three saturable pathways: (1) glycine conjugation to salicyluric acid (75%), (2) saturable glucuronyltransferase to salicyl phenol glucuronide (10%), and (3) salicyl aryl glucuronide (4%). Nonsaturable pathways involve hydrolysis to gentisic acid (<1%), and 10% is excreted unchanged. Acidosis increases the severity by increasing the nonionized salicylate that can move into the brain cells. In kidneys the un-ionized salicylic acid undergoes glomerular filtration and the ionized portion undergoes secretion in proximal tubules and passive reabsorption in the distal tubules. Renal excretion of salicylate is enhanced by alkaline urine. *Manifestations:* Ingestion of concentrated topical salicylic acid preparations (e.g., Compound W) can cause caustic mucosal injury to the GI tract. The possibility of occult salicylate overdose should be considered in any patient with an unexplained acid-base disturbance. Acute overdose: (1) Minimal symptoms—tinnitus, dizziness, and difficulty hearing—may occur at a high therapeutic SPC of 20 to 30 mg per dL. Nausea and vomiting may occur immediately as a result of local gastric irritation. (2) Phase I consists of mild manifestations (1 to 12 hours after ingestion at a 6-hour SPC of 45 to 70 mg per dL). Nausea and vomiting followed by hyperventilation are usually present within 3 to 8 hours after acute overdose. Hyperventilation with an increase in both rate (tachypnea) and depth (hyperpnea) is present but may be subtle. It results in a mild respiratory alkalosis (serum pH greater than 7.4 and urine pH greater than 6.0). Some patients may have lethargy, vertigo, headache, and confusion. Diaphoresis is prominent. (3) Phase II involves moderate manifestations (12 to 24 hours after ingestion at a 6-hour SPC of 70 to 100 mg per dL). Serious metabolic disturbances including a marked respiratory alkalosis, followed by AG metabolic acidosis, and dehydration occur. The pH may be normal, elevated, or depressed, with a urine pH less than 6.0. Other metabolic disturbances may include hypoglycemia or hyperglycemia, hypokalemia, decreased ionized calcium, and increased BUN, creatinine, and lactate. Mental disturbances (confusion, disorientation, hallucinations) may occur. Hypotension and convulsions have been reported. (4) Phase III involves severe intoxication (more than 24 hours at a 6-hour SPC of 100 to 130 mg per dL). In addition to the preceding clinical findings, coma and seizures develop and indicate severe intoxication. Pulmonary edema may occur. Metabolic disturbances include metabolic acidemia (pH less than 7.4) and aciduria (pH less than 6.0). In adults, alkalosis may persist until terminal respiratory failure occurs. (5) In children younger than 4 years, a metabolic or mixed metabolic acidosis and respiratory alkalosis develop within 4 to 6 hours, because these children have less respiratory reserve and accumulate lactate and other organic acids. Hypoglycemia is more common in children. (6) Fatalities occur at a 6-hour SPC greater than 130 to 150 mg per dL and result from CNS depression, cardiovascular collapse, electrolyte imbalance, and cerebral edema. Chronic salicylism is more serious than acute intoxication, and the 6-hour SPC does not correlate with the manifestations. It usually occurs with therapeutic errors in young children or the elderly with underlying illness, and the diagnosis is delayed because it is not recognized. Noncardiac pulmonary edema is a frequent complication in the elderly. The mortality rate is about 25%. Chronic salicylate poisoning in children may mimic Reye's syndrome. It is associated with exaggerated CNS findings (hallucinations, delirium, dementia, memory loss, papilledema, bizarre behavior, agitation, encephalopathy, seizures, and coma). Hemorrhagic manifestations, renal failure, and pulmonary and cerebral edema may occur. The metabolic picture is that of hypoglycemia and mixed acid-base derangements. A chronic SPC higher than 60 mg per dL with metabolic acidosis and an altered mental state is extremely serious. *Management:* Treatment is started on the basis of clinical and metabolic findings, not on the basis of salicylate levels. Continuous monitoring of the urine pH is essential for successful alkalization treatment. Always obtain an acetaminophen plasma level. (1) Establish and maintain vital functions. If the mental state is altered, administer glucose, naloxone, and thiamine in standard doses. Depending on the severity, the initial studies include an immediate and a 6-hour postingestion SPC, ECG and cardiac monitoring, pulse oximetry, urine assays (analysis, pH, specific gravity, and ferric chloride test), chest radiography, ABGs, blood glucose, electrolytes and AG calculation, calcium (ionized), magnesium, renal and liver profiles, and prothrombin time. Test gastric contents and stool for occult blood. Bismuth and magnesium salicylate preparations may be radiopaque on radiographs. A nephrologist should be consulted for moderate, severe, or chronic intoxication. (2) GI decontamination: Gastric lavage and AC are useful (each gram of AC binds 550 mg of salicylic acid) if a toxic dose was ingested up to 12 hours before because of factors with salicylism that delay absorption, such as food, enteric-coated tablets, pylorospasm, concretions, and coingestants. "It's never too late to aspirate salicylate." MDAC effectively reduces the $t_{1/2}$ and should be administered every 4 hours. Concretions may occur with massive (usually greater than 300 mg per kg) ingestions, and if blood levels fail to decline, prompt contrast radiography of the stomach may reveal concretions that must be removed by repeated lavage, whole-bowel irrigation, endoscopy, or gastrostomy. (3) Fluids and electrolytes (Table 45): Shock: Establish perfusion and vascular volume with 5% dextrose in 0.89% saline; then proceed with correction of dehydration and alkalization. Fluids and bicarbonate: In acute moderate or severe salicylism (see Table 45), adults should receive a bolus of 1 to 2 mEq per kg of $NaHCO_3$ followed by an infusion of 100 to 150 mEq of $NaHCO_3$ added to 500 to 1000 mL of 5% dextrose and administered over 60 minutes. Children should receive a bolus of 1 to 2 mEq of $NaHCO_3$ per kg followed by an infusion of 1 to 2 mEq per kg added to 20 mL per kg of 5% dextrose administered over 60 minutes. Add potassium to the intravenous infusion after the patient voids. Attempt to achieve a target urine output of more than 2 mL per kg per hour and a target urine pH of more than 7. The initial infusion is followed by subsequent infusions (two to three times normal maintenance) of 200 to 300 mL per hour in adults or 10 mL per kg per hour in children. If the patient is acidotic and the serum pH is less than 7.15, an

TABLE 45. **Fluid and Electrolyte Treatment of Salicylate Poisoning**

Type of Salicylism	Metabolic Disturbance	Blood pH	Urine pH	Hydrating Solution	Amount of $NaHCO_3$ (mEq/L)	Amount of Potassium (mEq/L)
Mild	Respiratory alkalosis	>7.4	>6.0	5% dextrose 0.45% saline	50 (adult) 1 mEq/kg (child)	20
Moderate						
Chronic	Respiratory alkalosis	>7.4	<6.0	D5W	100 (adult)	40
Child younger than 4 y	Metabolic acidosis	<7.4			1–2 mEq/kg (child)	
Severe						
Chronic	Metabolic acidosis	<7.4	<6.0	D5W	150 (adult)	60
Child younger than 4 y	Respiratory alkalosis				2 mEq/kg (child)	
CNS depressant coingestant	Respiratory acidosis	<7.4	<6.0	D5W	100–150*	60

*Hypoventilation must be corrected.
Abbreviation: D5W = 5% dextrose in water.
Modified from Linden CH, Rumack BH: The legitimate analgesics, aspirin and acetaminophen. *In* Hansen W Jr (ed): Toxic Emergencies. New York, Churchill Livingstone, 1984, p 118.

additional 1 to 2 mEq per kg $NaHCO_3$ is given over 1 to 2 hours, and persistent acidosis may require $NaHCO_3$ at 1 to 2 mEq per kg every 2 hours. Adjust the infusion rate, the amount of bicarbonate, and the electrolytes to correct serum abnormalities and to maintain the targeted urine output and urinary pH. Most authorities believe that the diuresis is not as important as the alkalization or MDAC. Carefully monitor for fluid overload in those at risk of pulmonary and cerebral edema (e.g., the elderly) and because of inappropriate secretion of antidiuretic hormone. In patients with mild intoxication who are not acidotic and whose urine pH is greater than 6, administer 5% dextrose in 0.45% saline, with $NaHCO_3$ at 50 mEq per liter or 1 mEq per kg as maintenance to replace ongoing renal losses. (4) Alkalization: $NaHCO_3$ is administered to produce a serum pH of 7.4 to 7.5 and urine pH above 7. Carbonic anhydrase inhibitors (e.g., acetazolamide [Diamox]) should not be used. If the patient is acidotic, additional bicarbonate may be required. About 2 mEq per kg raises the blood pH by 0.1. In children, alkalization may be a difficult problem because of the organic acid production and hypokalemia. Hypokalemic and fluid-depleted patients cannot undergo adequate alkalization. Alkalization is usually discontinued in asymptomatic patients with an SPC below 30 to 40 mg per dL but is continued in symptomatic patients regardless of the SPC. A decreased serum bicarbonate with a normal or high blood pH indicates respiratory alkalosis predominating over metabolic acidosis, and the bicarbonate should be administered cautiously. An alkalemia (pH of 7.40 to 7.50) is not a contraindication to bicarbonate therapy because these patients have a significant base deficit in spite of the elevated blood pH. (5) Potassium is added (20 to 40 mEq per liter) to the infusion after the patient voids. In severe, late, and chronic salicylism, potassium at 60 mEq per liter may be needed. When the serum potassium level is below 4.0 mEq per liter, add 10 mEq per liter over the first hour. If the patient has hypokalemia (less than 3 mEq per liter), flat T waves, and U waves, administer 0.25 to 0.5 mEq per kg up to 10 mEq per hour. Administer potassium with ECG monitoring. Recheck the serum potassium value after each rapidly administered dose. A paradoxical urine acidosis (alkaline serum pH and acidic urine pH) indicates that potassium is probably needed. (6) Convulsions are treated with diazepam or lorazepam, but rule out hypoglycemia, low ionized calcium, cerebral edema, or hemorrhage with CT. If tetany develops, discontinue the $NaHCO_3$ therapy and administer 10% calcium gluconate at 0.1 to 0.2 mL per kg. (7) Pulmonary edema management consists of fluid restriction, high forced inspiratory oxygen (FIO_2), mechanical ventilation, and PEEP. (8) Cerebral edema management consists of fluid restriction, elevation of the head, hyperventilation, osmotic diuresis, and dexamethasone. (9) Administer vitamin K_1 parenterally to correct an increased prothrombin time of more than 20 seconds and coagulation abnormalities. If there is active bleeding, administer fresh plasma and platelets as needed. (10) Hyperpyrexia is managed by external cooling measures, not antipyretics. (11) Hemodialysis is the method of choice for removing salicylates because it corrects the acid-base, electrolyte, and fluid disturbances as well. Indications for hemodialysis include acute poisoning with an SPC greater than 100 to 130 mg per dL without improvement after 6 hours of appropriate therapy; chronic poisoning with cardiopulmonary disease and an SPC as low as 40 mg per dL with refractory acidosis, severe CNS manifestations (coma and seizures), and progressive deterioration, especially in the elderly; impairment of vital organs of elimination; clinical deterioration in spite of good supportive care, repeated doses of AC, and alkalization; and severe refractory acid-base or electrolyte disturbances despite appropriate corrective measures. *Laboratory investigations:* In all intentional salicylate overdoses, the acetaminophen plasma level should be determined after 4 hours. (1) Continuously monitor ECG, urine output, urine pH, and specific gravity. Every 2 to 4 hours in severe intoxication, monitor SPC, glucose (in salicylism, CNS hypoglycemia may be present despite a normal serum glucose level), electrolytes, ionized calcium, magnesium and phosphorus, AG, ABGs, and pulse oximetry. Daily, monitor BUN, creatinine, liver function tests, and prothrombin time. (2) In the *ferric chloride test,* 1 mL of boiled urine containing 2 or 3 drops of 10% ferric chloride turns purple if salicylates are present. This is a nonspecific test and is positive for ketones (if the sample is not boiled), PTZs, and phenolic compounds in urine. (3) SPC: The therapeutic value is less than 10 mg per dL for analgesia and 15 to 30 mg per dL for an anti-inflammatory effect. Mild toxicity occurs at values above 30 mg per dL (tinnitus, dizziness), severe toxicity above 80 mg per dL (CNS changes). Cross-reaction: Diflunisal (Dolobid) results in a falsely high SPC. The Done nomogram (Figure 3) has been used as a predictor of expected severity after an acute single ingestion. The nomogram is not useful for chronic intoxications; for enteric-coated aspirin; or for methyl salicylate, phenyl salicylate, or homomethyl salicylate intoxications. The blood sample for use with the Done nomogram should be obtained 6 hours or more after ingestion. *Disposition:* There are limitations of SPCs, and patients are managed on the basis of clinical and laboratory findings. Patients who are asymptomatic should be monitored for a minimum of 6 hours and longer if an ingestion of enteric-coated tablets, a massive overdose, or suspicion of concretions is involved. Those who remain asymptomatic with an SPC below

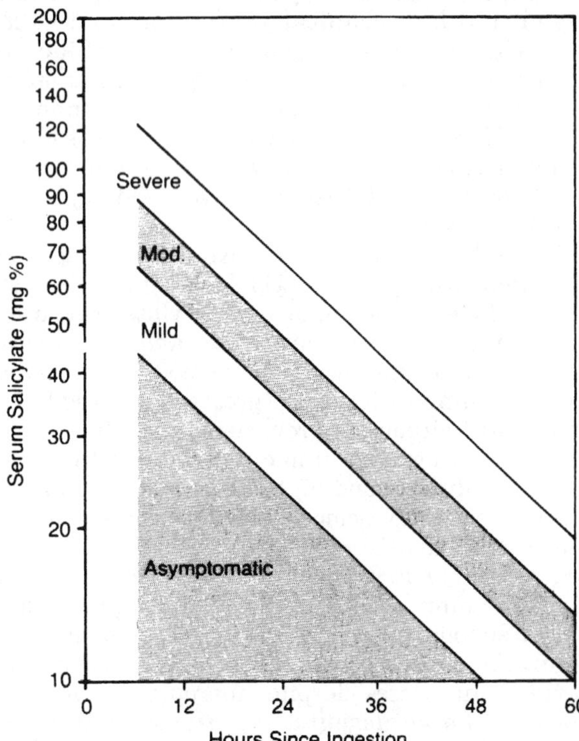

Figure 3. The Done nomogram for salicylate intoxication. For limitations of use, see *Laboratory Investigations.* (Redrawn from Done A: Salicylate intoxication: Significance of measurements of salicylate in blood in cases of acute ingestion. Reproduced by permission of Pediatrics, Vol 26, Page 800, Figure 3, Copyright 1960.)

35 mg per dL may be discharged after psychiatric evaluation, if indicated. Patients with chronic salicylate intoxication, acidosis, and an altered mental state should be admitted to the ICU. Patients with acute ingestion, an SPC below 60 mg per dL, and mild symptoms may be able to receive adequate treatment in the emergency department. Patients with moderate or severe intoxications should be admitted to the ICU.

Theophylline. Theophylline is a methylxanthine alkaloid similar to caffeine and theobromine. Aminophylline is 80% theophylline. It is used in the acute treatment of asthma, pulmonary edema, chronic obstructive pulmonary disease, and neonatal apnea. *Toxic mechanism:* The proposed mechanisms of action include phosphodiesterase inhibition, adenosine receptor antagonism, inhibition of prostaglandins, and increases in serum catecholamines. Theophylline stimulates the CNS, respiratory, and emetic centers and reduces the seizure threshold; has positive cardiac inotropic and chronotropic effects; acts as a diuretic; relaxes smooth muscle and causes peripheral vasodilatation but cerebral vasoconstriction; increases gastric secretions and GI mobility; and increases lipolysis, glycogenolysis, and gluconeogenesis. *Toxic dose:* A single dose of 1 mg per kg produces a theophylline plasma concentration (TPC) of approximately 2 μg per mL. The therapeutic range is usually 10 to 20 μg per mL. An acute, single dose above 10 mg per kg yields mild toxicity; above 20 mg per kg, moderate toxicity; and above 50 mg per kg, serious, potentially fatal toxicity. Fatalities occur at lower doses in chronic toxicity, especially with risk factors (see discussion of kinetics). The following equation can be used to estimate TPC:

$$\text{TPC} = \frac{\text{dose (mg ingested)}}{\text{weight (kg)} \times \text{Vd (0.45 L/kg)}}$$

Kinetics: The pK_a is 9.5. Absorption from stomach and upper small intestine is complete and rapid, with onset in 30 to 60 minutes. Peak TPC levels occur within 1 to 2 hours after ingestion of liquid preparations, 2 to 4 hours after regular tablets, and 7 to 24 hours after slow-release formulations. The Vd is 0.3 to 0.7 liter per kg. The PB is 40 to 60% in adults, mainly to albumin, and with low albumin, free active theophylline is increased. Elimination is 90% by hepatic metabolism to the active metabolite 2-methylxanthine. The $t_{1/2}$ is 3.5 hours in a child and 4 to 6 hours in an adult. It is shorter in smokers and those taking enzyme inducer drugs. Elimination: Only 8 to 10% is excreted unchanged in the urine. Risk factors that produce a longer $t_{1/2}$ include age younger than 6 months or older than 60 years, enzyme inhibitor drugs (e.g., calcium channel blockers, oral contraceptives), H_2 blockers (e.g., cimetidine), ciprofloxacin (Cipro), erythromycin and macrolide antibiotics, isoniazid, hyperthermia (persistent temperature above 102°F [38.5°C]), viral illness, liver impairment, heart failure, chronic obstructive pulmonary disease, and influenza vaccine. *Manifestations:* Acute toxicity generally correlates with blood levels; chronic toxicity does not. See Table 46. (1) Acute single-agent regular-release overdose (see Table 46): Vomiting and occasionally hematemesis occur at a low TPC. CNS stimulation results in restlessness, muscle tremors, and protracted tonic-clonic seizures, but coma is rare. Convulsions are a sign of severe toxicity and are usually preceded by GI symptoms (except with sustained-release and chronic intoxications). Cardiovascular disturbances include cardiac dysrhythmias (supraventricular tachycardia) and transient hypertension with mild overdoses but hypotension and ventricular dysrhythmias with severe intoxications. Rhabdomyolysis and renal failure are occasionally seen. Children tolerate higher serum levels, and cardiac dysrhythmias and seizures occur at a TPC greater than 100 μg per mL. Metabolic disturbances, including hyperglycemia, pronounced hypokalemia, hypocalcemia, hypomagnesemia, hypophosphatemia, increased serum amylase, and elevation of uric acid, may occur. (2) Chronic intoxication occurs when multiple doses of theophylline are taken over 24 hours or when an interacting drug or illness interferes with theophylline metabolism. It is more serious and difficult to treat than acute intoxication. Cardiac dysrhythmias and convulsions may occur at a TPC of 40 to 60 μg per mL, and there is less correlation with TPC. The seizures occur without warning and are protracted, are repetitive, and may progress to status epilepticus. Vomiting and typical metabolic disturbances do not occur. (3) Differences in slow-release preparations: Few or no GI symptoms occur; peak concentrations and convulsions may be delayed up to 12 to 24 hours after ingestion, and convulsions occur without warning. *Management:* (1) Establish and maintain vital functions. If coma, convulsions, and vomiting occur, the patient should be intubated immediately. Obtain the TPC, and repeat TPC determination every 2 to 4 hours to establish peak absorption; the presence of a theophylline bezoar should be suspected if the TPC fails to decline. A nephrologist should be consulted about charcoal hemoperfusion. (2) GI decontamination in acute overdose: Induce emesis. Gastric lavage can be done less than 1 hour after ingestion but may not be necessary if AC is available. AC is the agent of choice for decontamination and is administered in a dose of 1 gram per kg to all patients, followed with MDAC at 0.5 gram per kg every 2 to 4 hours until the TPC is less than 20 μg per mL. MDAC is effective in acute, chronic, and intravenous overdoses. AC shortens the $t_{1/2}$ by about 50%. AC may be indicated up to 24 hours after ingestion. Whole-bowel irrigation with a polyethylene-electrolyte solution given PO or via nasogastric tube has been recommended for massive overdose, possible concretions, and slow-release preparations, but its value is unproved. Whole-bowel irrigation may cause theophylline to be desorbed from AC. If intractable vomiting occurs, administer an antiemetic, metoclopramide (Reglan; 0.1 mg per kg in adults), droperidol (Inapsine; 2.5 to 10 mg IV), or ondansetron (Zofran; 8 to 32 mg IV). Ondansetron, however, inhibits metabolism of theophylline. (3) Control convulsions with lorazepam or diazepam and phenobarbital. Phenytoin is ineffective. The convulsions in chronic intoxication are often refractory and may require, in addition to anticonvulsants, neuromuscular paralyzing agents, sedation, assisted ventilation, and EEG monitoring. (4) Hypotension is treated with fluids and vasopressors, if necessary. Norepinephrine at 0.05 μg per kg per minute is preferred over dopamine as the vasopressor. (5) Dysrhythmias: Supraventricular tachycardia with hemodynamic instability requires cardioversion. Low-dose beta blockers may be used but not for patients with reactive airway disease or hypotension. Adenosine is ineffective. For ventricular dysrhythmias, correct electrolyte disturbances. Lidocaine is the agent of choice but has the potential to cause seizures at toxic concentrations. Cardioversion may be needed. (6) Hematemesis is managed with sucralfate (Carafate) at 1 gram four times daily and/or aluminum hydroxide–magnesium hydroxide (Maalox Therapeutic Concentrate) at 30 mL every 2 hours and blood replacement, if necessary. Histamine H_2 blockers that are enzyme inhibitors are not used. (7) Correct fluid and metabolic disturbances. Hyperglycemia does not require insulin therapy. Hypokalemia should be corrected cautiously, as it may reflect largely an intracellular shift and not total body loss. Usually, adding 40 mEq of potassium to a liter of fluid suffices. Monitor the serum potassium value closely. (8) Charcoal hemoperfusion is the management of choice for serious intoxications. Hemoperfusion can increase the clearance two- to threefold over hemodialysis, but hemodialysis can be used if hemoperfusion is not available. Criteria for use of hemoperfusion are life-threatening events such as convulsions or dysrhythmias; intractable vomiting refractory to antiemetics; acute intoxications with TPC greater than 80 to 100 μg per mL, greater than 70 μg per mL 4 hours after an overdose

TABLE 46. **Theophylline Blood Concentrations and Acute Toxicity**

Plasma Concentration (μg/mL)	Toxicity Degree	Manifestations
8–10	None	Bronchodilatation
10–20	Mild	Therapeutic range: nausea, vomiting, nervousness, respiratory alkalosis, tachycardia
15–25		Mild manifestations of toxicity in 35% of cases
20–40	Moderate	GI complaints and CNS stimulation Transient hypertension, tachypnea, tachycardia Some manifestations of toxicity in 80% of cases
>60	Severe	Convulsions, dysrhythmias Hypokalemia, hyperglycemia
>100		Ventricular dysrhythmias, protracted convulsions, hypotension, acid-base abnormalities

with a slow-release formulation, or greater than 40 to 60 μg per mL in chronic intoxication; and acute or chronic overdoses with TPC above 40 μg per mL, especially if the patient has risk factors that lengthen the $t_{1/2}$ (see the discussion of kinetics). *Laboratory investigations:* Monitor vital signs, pulse oximetry, ABGs, hemoglobin, hematocrit (for GI hemorrhage), ECG and cardiac parameters, renal and hepatic function, electrolytes, blood glucose, acid-base balance, and serum albumin. Test gastric contents and stools for occult blood. The TPC should be determined after ingestion of liquid preparations within 1 to 2 hours, regular-release formulations within 2 to 4 hours, and slow-release formulations at 4 hours. Check the serum albumin level (a decrease in albumin level may cause manifestations of toxicity despite a normal TPC). A single TPC determination may be misleading; therefore, repeat the TPC measurement every 2 to 4 hours to determine the trend until a declining pattern is reached and then monitor every 4 to 6 hours until the TPC is below 20 μg per mL. *Disposition:* Patients with mild symptoms and a TPC lower than 20 μg per mL may be treated in the emergency department and discharged when asymptomatic for a few hours. Anyone with an acute ingestion with a TPC above 35 μg per mL should be admitted to a monitored bed with seizure precautions and suicide precautions if needed. If there are neurologic or cardiotoxic effects or the TPC is above 50 μg per mL, admit the patient to the ICU. An overdose of a slow-release preparation, regardless of symptoms or initial TPC, requires admission, monitoring, AC, and MDAC. In patients receiving chronic therapy, toxicity may occur at a lower TPC, and these patients should not be discharged until they are asymptomatic for several hours.

Tricyclic and Cyclic Antidepressants. Traditionally, tricyclic antidepressants have been an important cause of pharmaceutical overdose fatalities (more than 100 in 1992). The mortality has been reduced from 15% in the 1970s to less than 1% in the 1990s through a better understanding of their pathophysiology and improvements in management. See Table 47. *Toxic mechanism:* The major mechanisms of toxicity of the tricyclic antidepressants are central and peripheral anticholinergic effects, peripheral alpha-adrenergic blockade, quinidine-like cardiac membrane–stabilizing action blocking the fast

TABLE 47. **Cyclic Antidepressants: Daily Doses and Major Properties***

Generic Name	Adult Daily Dose (mg)	Therapeutic Range (ng/mL)	Half-life (h)	Toxicity		
				Antichol	*CNS*	*Cardiac*
Tricyclic antidepressants: Major toxicity is cardiac						
Tertiary amines demethylated into secondary active amine metabolites						
Amitriptyline (Elavil)	75–300	120–250	31–46	3+	3+	3+
Imipramine (Tofranil)	75–300	125–250	9–24	3+	3+	2+
Doxepin (Sinequan)	75–300	30–150	8–24	3+	3+	2+
Trimipramine (Surmontil)	75–200	10–240	16–18	3+	3+	2+
Secondary amines metabolized into inactive metabolites						
Nortriptyline (Pamelor)†	75–150	50–150	18–93	2+	3+	3+
Desipramine (Norpramin)	75–200	75–160	14–62	1+	3+	3+
Protriptyline (Vivactil)	20–60	70–250	54–198	2+	3+	3+
Newer cyclic antidepressants						
Tetracyclic agent produces a high incidence of cardiovascular disturbances and seizures						
Maprotiline (Ludiomil)	75–300	—	30–60	1+	2+	3+
Triazolopyridine, a noncyclic agent, produces less serious cardiac and CNS toxicity						
Trazodone (Desyrel)	50–600	700	4–7	1+	1+	1+
Monocyclic aminoketone produces seizures in doses >600 mg						
Bupropion (Wellbutrin)	200–400	—	8–24	1+	3+	1+
Dibenzazepine						
Clomipramine (Anafranil)	100–250	200–500	21–32	2+	2+	2+
Dibenzoxazepine produces syndrome of convulsions, rhabdomyolysis, and renal failure						
Amoxapine (Asendin)	150–300	200–500	6–10	1+	3+	2+

*Other drugs with similar structures are cyclobenzaprine (Flexeril), a muscle relaxant (similar to amitriptyline) and carbamazepine (Tegretol), an anticonvulsant (similar to imipramine); however, they cause less cardiac toxicity. 1+ indicates mild effect; 2+ indicates moderate effect; 3+ indicates severe effect.

†Not available in the United States.

Abbreviations: Antichol = anticholinergic effect; CNS = central nervous system effect (primarily seizures); Cardiac = cardiac effect.

inward sodium channels, and inhibition of synaptic neurotransmitter reuptake in the CNS presynaptic neurons. The tetracyclic, monocyclic aminoketone dibenzoxazepine possesses convulsive activity and less cardiac toxicity in overdoses. Triazolopyridine has less serious cardiac and CNS toxicity. *Toxic dose:* The therapeutic dose of imipramine is 1.5 to 5 mg per kg; a dose of less than 3 to 5 mg per kg may be mildly toxic; 10 to 20 mg per kg may be life-threatening, although doses of less than 20 mg per kg have produced few fatalities; more than 30 mg per kg is associated with 30% mortality; and at doses higher than 70 mg per kg, survival is rare. Doses of 375 mg in a child and as little as 500 to 750 mg in an adult have been fatal. In adults, 5 times the maximal daily dose is toxic and 10 times the maximal daily dose is potentially fatal. Major overdose symptoms are associated with plasma concentrations above 1 μg per mL (1000 ng per mL). Relative dosage equivalents are amitriptyline 100 mg = amoxapine 125 mg = desipramine 75 mg = doxepin 100 mg = imipramine 75 mg = maprotiline 75 mg = nortriptyline 50 mg = trazodone 200 mg. See Table 47. *Kinetics:* Cyclic antidepressants are lipophilic. They are rapidly absorbed from the alkaline small intestine, but absorption may be prolonged and delayed in massive overdose owing to anticholinergic action. Onset varies from less than 1 hour (30 to 40 minutes) rarely to 12 hours. The peak serum levels are reached in 2 to 8 hours, and the peak effect is in 6 hours but may be delayed 12 hours because of erratic absorption. The clinical effects correlate poorly with plasma levels. Cyclic antidepressants are highly protein bound to plasma glycoproteins (98% at pH 7.5 and 90% at pH 7.0); the Vd is 10 to 50 liters per kg. The $t_{1/2}$ varies from 10 hours for imipramine to 81 hours for amitriptyline and 100 hours for nortriptyline. The active metabolites have considerable $t_{1/2}$ values. Elimination is by hepatic metabolism. The tertiary amines are metabolized to active demethylated secondary amine metabolites. The active secondary amine metabolites undergo 15% enterohepatic recirculation and are metabolized over a period of days to nonactive metabolites. The intestinal bacterial flora may reconstitute the active metabolites. Only 3% of an ingested dose is excreted in the urine unchanged. *Manifestations:* On arrival, previously alert, oriented patients may suddenly become comatose, have a seizure, develop hemodynamically unstable dysrhythmias within minutes, and die. Most patients with severe toxicity develop symptoms within 1 to 2 hours but onset may be delayed 6 hours after an overdose. (1) Small overdoses produce early anticholinergic effects, agitation, and transient hypertension, which are not life-threatening. (2) Large overdoses produce depression of CNS and myocardium, convulsions, and hypotension. Death usually occurs within the first 2 to 6 hours after ingestion. (3) ECG screening tools for use in tricyclic antidepressant toxicity include QRS greater than 0.10 second (seizures are likely) and QRS greater than 0.16 second (50% of patients developed ventricular dysrhythmias—life-threatening in 20% of the cases—and seizures); a terminal 40 milliseconds of the QRS axis greater than 120 degrees in the right frontal plane; and an R wave greater than 3 mm as measured by the right arm lead. The quinidine cardiac membrane–stabilizing effect produces depression of myocardium, conduction disturbances, and ECG changes. The peripheral alpha-adrenergic blockade produces hypotension. *Management:* (1) Establish and maintain vital functions. Even if the patient is asymptomatic, establish intravenous access, monitor vital signs and neurologic status, obtain a baseline 12-lead ECG, and continue cardiac monitoring for at least 6 hours from admission or 8 to 12 hours after ingestion. Measure the QRS interval every 15 minutes. (2) GI decontamination: Do not induce emesis, and omit gastric lavage if AC is available. If the mental state is altered, protect the airway. AC with cathartic at 1 gram per kg is recommended immediately and repeated once (0.5 mg per kg) in 4 hours without a cathartic. A clinical benefit of MDAC has not been demonstrated. (3) Control seizures. Alkalization does not control seizures; use diazepam or lorazepam. Status epilepticus (as may occur with amoxapine) may require high-dose barbiturates or neuromuscular blockers with intravenous diazepam. If this is not successful, paralysis is induced by short nondepolarizing neuromuscular blockers such as vecuronium, with intubation and assisted ventilation. A bolus of $NaHCO_3$ is recommended as an adjunct to correct the acidosis produced by the seizures. (4) Cardiovascular management consists of administration of $NaHCO_3$ (see Table 12). A dose of 1 to 2 mEq per kg is given undiluted as a bolus and repeated twice a few minutes apart, if needed, for sodium loading and alkalization, which increases PB. The sodium loading overcomes the sodium channel blockage and is more important than the alkalization, which increases the PB from 90 to 98%. Indications include a QRS complex greater than 0.12 second, ventricular tachycardia, severe conduction disturbances, metabolic acidosis, coma, and seizures. An infusion of $NaHCO_3$ may follow to keep the blood pH at 7.5 to 7.55. The continuous infusion by itself is of limited usefulness for controlling dysrhythmias because of its delayed onset of action. Bolus therapy is given as needed. Hyperventilation alone has been advocated, but the pH elevation is not so instantaneous and there is compensatory renal excretion of bicarbonate; therefore, it is not recommended. The combination of hyperventilation and $NaHCO_3$ has produced fatal alkalemia and is not recommended. Monitor the serum potassium (the sudden increase in blood pH can aggravate or precipitate hypokalemia), serum sodium, ionized calcium (hypocalcemia may occur with alkalization), and blood pH. (5) Specific cardiovascular complications should be treated as follows: For management of hypotension, norepinephrine, a predominantly alpha-adrenergic drug, is preferred to dopamine. Hypertension that occurs early rarely requires treatment. Sinus tachycardia usually does not require treatment. Supraventricular tachycardia with hemodynamic instability requires synchronized electrical cardioversion, starting at 0.25 to 1.0 watt-second per kg, after sedation. Ventricular tachycardia that persists after alkalization requires intravenous lidocaine or countershock if the patient is hemodynamically unstable. Ventricular fibrillation should be treated with defibrillation. Torsades de pointes is treated with 20% magnesium sulfate solution given IV, 2 grams over 2 to 3 minutes, followed by a continuous infusion of 1.5 mL of 10% solution or 5 to 10 mg per minute (see Table 12). For bradydysrhythmias, atropine is contraindicated because of the anticholinergic activity. Isoproterenol at 0.1 μg per kg per minute with caution may produce hypotension. If the patient is hemodynamically unstable, use a pacemaker. (6) Extraordinary measures such as intra-aortic balloon pump and cardiopulmonary bypass have been successful. (7) Investigational: Use of Fab fragments specific for tricyclic antidepressants has been successful in animals. Prophylactic $NaHCO_3$ to prevent dysrhythmias is being investigated. (8) Contraindicated: Physostigmine has produced asystole. Flumazenil has produced seizures. *Laboratory investigations:* Monitoring: If altered mental status or ECG abnormalities are present, obtain ABGs, institute ECG monitoring, perform chest radiography, and determine blood glucose, serum electrolytes, calcium, magnesium, BUN and creatinine, liver profile, creatine kinase, and urine output; in severe cases, hemodynamic monitoring is indicated. Levels of tricyclic and cyclic antidepressants below 300 ng per mL are therapeutic, levels above 500 ng per mL indicate toxicity, and levels above 1000 ng per mL indicate serious poisoning and are associated with QRS widening. *Disposition:* Admission to the ICU for 12 to 24 hours is essential for any patient with an antidepressant overdose who meets any of the following criteria: ECG abnormalities (except sinus tachycardia), altered mental state, seizures, respiratory depression, or hypotension. Caution: In 25% of fatal cases the patients were alert and awake at presentation. Low-risk patients are those who do not have the preceding symptoms at 6 hours after ingestion, those who present with minor transient manifestations such as sinus tachycardia and subsequently become and remain asymptomatic for a 6-hour period, and asymptomatic patients who remain asymptomatic for 6 hours. These patients may be discharged if the ECG remains normal and they have normal bowel sounds, have AC therapy repeated once, and undergo psychiatric counseling. Children younger than 6 years with nonintentional (accidental) exposures should be referred to the emergency department for monitoring, observation, and AC therapy.

Section 18

Appendices and Index

REFERENCE INTERVALS FOR THE INTERPRETATION OF LABORATORY TESTS

method of
WILLIAM Z. BORER, M.D.
Thomas Jefferson University Hospital
Philadelphia, Pennsylvania

Most of the tests performed in a clinical laboratory are quantitative in nature. That is, the amount of a substance present in blood or serum is measured and reported in terms of concentration, activity (e.g., enzyme activity) or counts (e.g., blood cell counts). The laboratory must provide reference intervals to assist the clinician in the interpretation of laboratory results. These reference intervals comprise the physiologic quantities of a substance (concentrations, activities, or counts) to be expected in healthy persons. Deviation above or below the reference range may be associated with a disease process, and the severity of the disease process may be associated with the magnitude of the deviation. Unfortunately, a sharp demarcation rarely exists to distinguish between physiologic and pathologic values, and the time of transition between the two is often gradual as the disease process progresses.

The terms "normal" and "abnormal" have been used to describe the laboratory values that fall inside and outside the reference range, respectively. Use of these terms is inappropriate, because no good definition of normality exists in the clinical sense and because the term "normal" may be confused with the statistical term "Gaussian." Reference ranges are established from statistical studies in groups of healthy volunteers. These study subjects must be free of disease, but they may have lifestyles or habits that result in variations in certain laboratory values.

TABLE 1. **Base SI Units**

Property	Base Unit	Symbol
Length	meter	m
Mass	kilogram	kg
Amount of substance	mole	mol
Time	second	s
Thermodynamic temperature	kelvin	K
Electric current	ampere	A
Luminous intensity	candela	cd
Catalytic amount	katal	kat

TABLE 2. **Derived SI Units and Non-SI Units Retained for Use with SI Units**

Property	Unit	Symbol
Area	square meter	m^2
Volume	cubic meter liter	m^3 L
Mass concentration	kilogram/cubic meter gram/liter	kg/m^3 g/L
Substance concentration	mole/cubic meter mole/liter	mol/m^3 mol/L
Temperature	degree Celsius	C = K − 273.15

Examples of these variables include diet, body mass, exercise, and geographic location. Age and gender may also affect reference values.

When the data from a large cohort of healthy subjects fit a Gaussian distribution, the usual statistical approach is to define the reference limits as two standard deviations above and below the mean. By definition, the reference range excludes the 2.5% of the population with the lowest values and the 2.5% with the highest values. Non-Gaussian distributions are handled by different statistical methods, but the result is similar in that the reference range is defined by the central 95% of the population. In other words, the probability is 1 in 20 that a healthy person will have a laboratory result that falls outside the reference range. If 12 laboratory tests are performed, the probability increases to about 50% that at least one

TABLE 3. **Standard Prefixes**

Prefix	Multiplication Factor	Symbol
yocto	10^{-24}	y
zepto	10^{-21}	z
atto	10^{-18}	a
femto	10^{-15}	f
pico	10^{-12}	p
nano	10^{-9}	n
micro	10^{-6}	u
milli	10^{-3}	m
centi	10^{-2}	c
deci	10^{-1}	d
deca	10^{1}	da
hecto	10^{2}	h
kilo	10^{3}	k
mega	10^{6}	M
giga	10^{9}	G
tera	10^{12}	T

of the results will be outside the reference range. This means that all healthy persons are likely to have a few laboratory results that are unexpected. The clinician must then integrate these data with other clinical information such as the history and physical examination to arrive at an appropriate clinical decision.

The reference intervals for many tests (especially enzyme and immunochemical measurements) vary with the method used. Accordingly, each laboratory must establish reference intervals that are appropriate for the methods used.

SI UNITS

During the 1980s a concerted effort was made to introduce SI units (le Système International d'Unités). The rationale for conversion to SI units is sound. Laboratory data are scientifically more informative when the units are based on molar concentration rather than on mass concentration. For example, the conversion of glucose to lactate and pyruvate or the binding of a drug to albumin is more easily understood in units of molar concentration. Another example is illustrated as follows:

Conventional Units

1.0 gram of hemoglobin:

- Combines with 1.37 mL of oxygen
- Contains 3.4 mg of iron
- Forms 34.9 mg of bilirubin

SI Units

4.0 mmol of hemoglobin:

- Combines with 4.0 mmol of oxygen
- Contains 4.0 mmol of iron
- Forms 4.0 mmol of bilirubin

The use of SI units would also enhance the standardization of nomenclature to facilitate global communication of medical and scientific information. The units, symbols, and prefixes employed in the International System are shown in Tables 1, 2, and 3.

Unfortunately, problems have arisen with the implementation of SI units in the United States. Their introduction in 1987 prompted many medical journals to report laboratory values in both SI and conventional units in anticipation of complete conversion to SI units in the early 1990s. The lack of a coordinated effort toward this goal has forced a retrenchment on the issue. Physicians continue to think and practice using laboratory results expressed in conventional units, and few if any American hospitals or clinical laboratories exclusively use SI units. Complete conversion to SI units is not likely to occur in the foreseeable future, yet most medical journals will probably continue to publish both sets of units. For this reason the values in the tables of reference ranges in this appendix are given in both conventional units and SI units.

TABLES OF REFERENCE INTERVALS

Some of the values included in the tables that follow have been established by the Clinical Laboratories at Thomas Jefferson University Hospital, Philadelphia, Pennsylvania, and have not been published elsewhere. Other values have been compiled from the sources cited in the references. These tables are provided for information and educational purposes only. Laboratory values must always be interpreted in the context of clinical data derived from other sources including the medical history and physical examination. Users must exercise individual judgment when employing the information provided in this appendix.

Reference Intervals for Hematology

Test	Conventional Units	SI Units
Acid hemolysis (Ham test)	No hemolysis	No hemolysis
Alkaline phosphatase, leukocyte	Total score 14–100	Total score 14–100
Cell counts		
Erythrocytes		
Males	4.6–6.2 million/mm^3	4.6–6.2 × 10^{12}/L
Females	4.2–5.4 million/mm^3	4.2–5.4 × 10^{12}/L
Children (varies with age)	4.5–5.1 million/mm^3	4.5–5.1 × 10^{12}/L
Leukocytes, total	4500–11,000/mm^3	4.5–11.0 × 10^9/L
Leukocytes, differential counts*		
Myelocytes	0%	0/L
Band neutrophils	3–5%	150–400 × 10^6/L
Segmented neutrophils	54–62%	3000–5800 × 10^6/L
Lymphocytes	25–33%	1500–3000 × 10^6/L
Monocytes	3–7%	300–500 × 10^6/L
Eosinophils	1–3%	50–250 × 10^6/L
Basophils	0–1%	15–50 × 10^6/L
Platelets	150,000–400,000/mm^3	150–400 × 10^9/L
Reticulocytes	25,000–75,000/mm^3 (0.5–1.5% of erythrocytes)	25–75 × 10^9/L

Reference Intervals for Hematology *Continued*

Test	Conventional Units	SI Units
Coagulation tests		
Bleeding time (template)	2.75–8.0 min	2.75–8.0 min
Coagulation time (glass tube)	5–15 min	5–15 min
D-Dimer	<0.5 μg/mL	<0.5 mg/L
Factor VIII and other coagulation factors	50–150% of normal	0.5–1.5 of normal
Fibrin split products (Thrombo-Welco test)	<10 μg/mL	<10 mg/L
Fibrinogen	200–400 mg/dL	2.0–4.0 g/L
Partial thromboplastin time, activated (aPTT)	20–35 s	20–35 s
Prothrombin time (PT)	12.0–14.0 s	12.0–14.0 s
Coombs' test		
Direct	Negative	Negative
Indirect	Negative	Negative
Corpuscular values of erythrocytes		
Mean corpuscular hemoglobin (MCH)	26–34 pg/cell	26–34 pg/cell
Mean corpuscular volume (MCV)	80–96 μm^3	80–96 fL
Mean corpuscular hemoglobin concentration (MCHC)	32–36 g/dL	320–360 g/L
Haptoglobin	20–165 mg/dL	0.20–1.65 g/L
Hematocrit		
Males	40–54 mL/dL	0.40–0.54
Females	37–47 mL/dL	0.37–0.47
Newborns	49–54 mL/dL	0.49–0.54
Children (varies with age)	35–49 mL/dL	0.35–0.49
Hemoglobin		
Males	13.0–18.0 g/dL	8.1–11.2 mmol/L
Females	12.0–16.0 g/dL	7.4–9.9 mmol/L
Newborns	16.5–19.5 g/dL	10.2–12.1 mmol/L
Children (varies with age)	11.2–16.5 g/dL	7.0–10.2 mmol/L
Hemoglobin, fetal	<1.0% of total	<0.01 of total
Hemoglobin A_{1C}	3–5% of total	0.03–0.05 of total
Hemoglobin A_2	1.5–3.0% of total	0.015–0.03 of total
Hemoglobin, plasma	0.0–5.0 mg/dL	0.0–3.2 μmol/L
Methemoglobin	30–130 mg/dL	19–80 μmol/L
Sedimentation rate (ESR)		
Wintrobe: Males	0–5 mm/h	0–5 mm/h
Females	0–15 mm/h	0–15 mm/h
Westergren: Males	0–15 mm/h	0–15 mm/h
Females	0–20 mm/h	0–20 mm/h

*Conventional units are percentages; SI units are absolute cell counts.

Reference Intervals* for Clinical Chemistry (Blood, Serum, and Plasma)

Analyte	Conventional Units	SI Units
Acetoacetate plus acetone		
Qualitative	Negative	Negative
Quantitative	0.3–2.0 mg/dL	30–200 μmol/L
Acid phosphatase, serum (thymolphthalein monophosphate substrate)	0.1–0.6 U/L	0.1–0.6 U/L
ACTH (see Corticotropin)		
Alanine aminotransferase (ALT) serum (SGPT)	1–45 U/L	1–45 U/L
Albumin, serum	3.3–5.2 g/dL	33–52 g/L
Aldolase, serum	0.0–7.0 U/L	0.0–7.0 U/L
Aldosterone, plasma		
Standing	5–30 ng/dL	140–830 pmol/L
Recumbent	3–10 ng/dL	80–275 pmol/L
Alkaline, phosphatase (ALP), serum		
Adult	35–150 U/L	35–150 U/L
Adolescent	100–500 U/L	100–500 U/L
Child	100–350 U/L	100–350 U/L
Ammonia nitrogen, plasma	10–50 μmol/L	10–50 μmol/L
Amylase, serum	25–125 U/L	25–125 U/L
Anion gap, serum, calculated	8–16 mEq/L	8–16 mmol/L
Ascorbic acid, blood	0.4–1.5 mg/dL	23–85 μmol/L
Aspartate aminotransferase (AST) serum (SGOT)	1–36 U/L	1–36 U/L
Base excess, arterial blood, calculated	0 ± 2 mEq/L	0 ± 2 mmol/L
Bicarbonate		
Venous plasma	23–29 mEq/L	23–29 mmol/L
Arterial blood	21–27 mEq/L	21–27 mmol/L

Table continued on following page

Reference Intervals* for Clinical Chemistry (Blood, Serum, and Plasma) *Continued*

Analyte	Conventional Units	SI Units
Bile acids, serum	0.3–3.0 mg/dL	0.8–7.6 μmol/L
Bilirubin, serum		
Conjugated	0.1–0.4 mg/dL	1.7–6.8 μmol/L
Total	0.3–1.1 mg/dL	5.1–19.0 μmol/L
Calcium, serum	8.4–10.6 mg/dL	2.10–2.65 mmol/L
Calcium, ionized, serum	4.25–5.25 mg/dL	1.05–1.30 mmol/L
Carbon dioxide, total, serum or plasma	24–31 mEq/L	24–31 mmol/L
Carbon dioxide tension (P_{CO_2}), blood	35–45 mm Hg	35–45 mm Hg
β-Carotene, serum	60–260 μg/dL	1.1–8.6 μmol/L
Ceruloplasmin, serum	23–44 mg/dL	230–440 mg/L
Chloride, serum or plasma	96–106 mEq/L	96–106 mmol/L
Cholesterol, serum or EDTA plasma		
Desirable range	<200 mg/dL	<5.20 mmol/L
LDL cholesterol	60–180 mg/dL	1.55–4.65 mmol/L
HDL cholesterol	30–80 mg/dL	0.80–2.05 mmol/L
Copper	70–140 μg/dL	11–22 μmol/L
Corticotropin (ACTH), plasma, 8 AM	10–80 pg/mL	2–18 pmol/L
Cortisol, plasma		
8:00 AM	6–23 μg/dL	170–630 nmol/L
4:00 PM	3–15 μg/dL	80–410 nmol/L
10:00 PM	<50% of 8:00 AM value	<50% of 8:00 AM value
Creatine, serum		
Males	0.2–0.5 mg/dL	15–40 μmol/L
Females	0.3–0.9 mg/dL	25–70 μmol/L
Creatine kinase (CK), serum		
Males	55–170 U/L	55–170 U/L
Females	30–135 U/L	30–135 U/L
Creatine kinase MB isoenzyme, serum	<5% of total CK activity <5% ng/mL by immunoassay	<5% of total CK activity <5% ng/mL by immunoassay
Creatinine, serum	0.6–1.2 mg/dL	50–110 μmol/L
Estradiol-17β, adult		
Males	10–65 pg/mL	35–240 pmol/L
Females		
Follicular	30–100 pg/mL	110–370 pmol/L
Ovulatory	200–400 pg/mL	730–1470 pmol/L
Luteal	50–140 pg/mL	180–510 pmol/L
Ferritin, serum	20–200 ng/mL	20–200 μg/L
Fibrinogen, plasma	200–400 mg/dL	2.0–4.0 g/L
Folate, serum	3–18 ng/mL	6.8–41 nmol/L
Erythrocytes	145–540 ng/mL	330–1220 nmol/L
Follicle-stimulating hormone (FSH), plasma		
Males	4–25 mU/mL	4–25 U/L
Females, premenopausal	4–30 mU/mL	4–30 U/L
Females, postmenopausal	40–250 mU/mL	40–250 U/L
Gamma-glutamyltransferase (GGT), serum	5–40 U/L	5–40 U/L
Gastrin, fasting, serum	0–100 pg/mL	0–100 mg/L
Glucose, fasting, plasma or serum	70–115 mg/dL	3.9–6.4 nmol/L
Growth hormone (hGH), plasma, adult, fasting	0–6 ng/mL	0–6 μg/L
Haptoglobin, serum	20–165 mg/dL	0.20–1.65 g/L
Immunoglobulins, serum (see table of Reference Intervals for Tests of Immunologic Function)		
Iron, serum	75–175 μg/dL	13–31 μmol/L
Iron binding capacity, serum		
Total	250–410 μg/dL	45–73 μmol/L
Saturation	20–55%	0.20–0.55
Lactate		
Venous whole blood	5.0–20.0 mg/dL	0.6–2.2 mmol/L
Arterial whole blood	5.0–15.0 mg/dL	0.6–1.7 mmol/L
Lactate dehydrogenase (LD), serum	110–220 U/L	110–220 U/L
Lipase, serum	10–140 U/L	10–140 U/L

Reference Intervals* for Clinical Chemistry (Blood, Serum, and Plasma) *Continued*

Analyte	Conventional Units	SI Units
Lutropin (LH), serum		
Males	1–9 U/L	1–9 U/L
Females		
Follicular phase	2–10 U/L	2–10 U/L
Midcycle peak	15–65 U/L	15–65 U/L
Luteal phase	1–12 U/L	1–12 U/L
Postmenopausal	12–65 U/L	12–65 U/L
Magnesium, serum	1.3–2.1 mg/dL	0.65–1.05 mmol/L
Osmolality	275–295 mOsm/kg water	275–295 mOsm/kg water
Oxygen, blood, arterial, room air		
Partial pressure ($Pa{O_2}$)	80–100 mm Hg	80–100 mm Hg
Saturation ($Sa{O_2}$)	95–98%	95–98%
pH, arterial blood	7.35–7.45	7.35–7.45
Phosphate, inorganic, serum		
Adult	3.0–4.5 mg/dL	1.0–1.5 mmol/L
Child	4.0–7.0 mg/dL	1.3–2.3 mmol/L
Potassium		
Serum	3.5–5.0 mEq/L	3.5–5.0 mmol/L
Plasma	3.5–4.5 mEq/L	3.5–4.5 mmol/L
Progesterone, serum, adult		
Males	0.0–0.4 ng/mL	0.0–1.3 mmol/L
Females		
Follicular phase	0.1–1.5 ng/mL	0.3–4.8 mmol/L
Luteal phase	2.5–28.0 ng/mL	8.0–89.0 mmol/L
Prolactin, serum		
Males	1.0–15.0 ng/mL	1.0–15.0 μg/L
Females	1.0–20.0 ng/mL	1.0–20.0 μg/L
Protein, serum, electrophoresis		
Total	6.0–8.0 g/dL	60–80 g/L
Albumin	3.5–5.5 g/dL	35–55 g/L
Globulins		
$Alpha_1$	0.2–0.4 g/dL	2.0–4.0 g/L
$Alpha_2$	0.5–0.9 g/dL	5.0–9.0 g/L
Beta	0.6–1.1 g/dL	6.0–11.0 g/L
Gamma	0.7–1.7 g/dL	7.0–17.0 g/L
Pyruvate, blood	0.3–0.9 mg/dL	0.03–0.10 mmol/L
Rheumatoid factor	0.0–30.0 IU/mL	0.0–30.0 kIU/L
Sodium, serum or plasma	135–145 mEq/L	135–145 mmol/L
Testosterone, plasma		
Males, adult	300–1200 ng/dL	10.4–41.6 nmol/L
Females, adult	20–75 ng/dL	0.7–2.6 nmol/L
Pregnant females	40–200 ng/dL	1.4–6.9 nmol/L
Thyroglobulin	3–42 ng/mL	3–42 μg/L
Thyrotropin (hTSH), serum	0.4–4.8 μIU/mL	0.4–4.8 mIU/L
Thyrotropin-releasing hormone (TRH)	5–60 pg/mL	5–60 ng/L
Thyroxine (FT_4), free, serum	0.9–2.1 ng/dL	12–27 pmol/L
Thyroxine (T_4), serum	4.5–12.0 μg/dL	58–154 nmol/L
Thyroxine-binding globulin (TBG)	15.0–34.0 μg/mL	15.0–34.0 mg/L
Transferrin	250–430 mg/dL	2.5–4.3 g/L
Triglycerides, serum, after 12-hour fast	40–150 mg/dL	0.4–1.5 g/L
Triiodothyronine (T_3), serum	70–190 ng/dL	1.1–2.9 nmol/L
Triiodothyronine uptake, resin (T_3RU)	25–38%	0.25–0.38
Urate		
Males	2.5–8.0 mg/dL	150–480 μmol/L
Females	2.2–7.0 mg/dL	130–420 μmol/L
Urea, serum or plasma	24–49 mg/dL	4.0–8.2 nmol/L
Urea nitrogen, serum or plasma	11–23 mg/dL	8.0–16.4 nmol/L
Viscosity, serum	1.4–1.8 × water	1.4–1.8 × water
Vitamin A, serum	20–80 μg/dL	0.70–2.80 μmol/L
Vitamin B_{12}, serum	180–900 pg/mL	133–664 pmol/L

*Reference values may vary depending upon the method and sample source used.

Reference Intervals for Therapeutic Drug Monitoring (Serum)

Analyte	Therapeutic Range	Toxic Concentrations	Proprietary Name(s)
Analgesics			
Acetaminophen	10–20 μg/mL	>250 μg/mL	Tylenol Datril
Salicylate	100–250 μg/mL	>300 μg/mL	Aspirin Bufferin
Antibiotics			
Amikacin	25–30 μg/mL	Peak >35 μg/mL Trough >10 μg/mL	Amikin
Gentamicin	5–10 μg/mL	Peak >10 μg/mL Trough >2 μg/mL	Garamycin
Tobramycin	5–10 μg/mL	Peak >10 μg/mL Trough >2 μg/mL	Nebcin
Vancomycin	5–35 μg/mL	Peak >40 μg/mL Trough >10 μg/mL	Vancocin
Anticonvulsants			
Carbamazepine	5–12 μ/mL	>15 μg/mL	Tegretol
Ethosuximide	40–100 μg/mL	>150 μg/mL	Zarontin
Phenobarbital	15–40 μg/mL	40–100 ng/mL (varies widely)	Luminal
Phenytoin	10–20 μg/mL	>20 μg/mL	Dilantin
Primidone	5–12 μg/mL	>15 μg/mL	Mysoline
Valproic acid	50–100 μg/mL	>100 μg/mL	Depakene
Antineoplastics and Immunosuppressives			
Cyclosporine	50–400 ng/mL	>400 ng/mL	Sandimmune
Methotrexate, high-dose, 48-hour	Variable	>1 μmol/L, 48 h after dose	
Tacrolimus (FK-506), whole blood	3–10 μg/L	>15 μg/L	Prograf
Bronchodilators and Respiratory Stimulants			
Caffeine	3–15 ng/mL	>30 ng/mL	
Theophylline (aminophylline)	10–20 μg/mL	>20 μg/mL	Elixophyllin Quibron
Cardiovascular Drugs			
Amiodarone (obtain specimen more than 8 hours after last dose)	1.0–2.0 μg/mL	>2.0 μg/mL	Cordarone
Digitoxin (obtain specimen 12–24 hours after last dose)	15–25 ng/mL	>35 ng/mL	Crystodigin
Digoxin (obtain specimen more than 6 hours after last dose)	0.8–2.0 ng/mL	>2.4 ng/mL	Lanoxin
Disopyramide	2–5 μg/mL	>7 μg/mL	Norpace
Flecainide	0.2–1.0 ng/mL	>1 ng/mL	Tambocor
Lidocaine	1.5–5.0 μg/mL	>6 μg/mL	Xylocaine
Mexiletine	0.7–2.0 ng/mL	>2 ng/mL	Mexitil
Procainamide	4–10 μg/mL	>12 μg/mL	Pronestyl
Procainamide plus NAPA	8–30 μg/mL	>30 μg/mL	
Propranolol	50–100 ng/mL	Variable	Inderal
Quinidine	2–5 μg/mL	>6 μg/mL	Cardioquin Quinaglute
Tocainide	4–10 ng/mL	>10 ng/mL	Tonocard
Psychopharmacologic Drugs			
Amitriptyline	120–150 ng/mL	>500 ng/mL	Elavil Triavil
Bupropion	25–100 ng/mL	Not applicable	Wellbutrin
Desipramine	150–300 ng/mL	>500 ng/mL	Norpramin
Imipramine	125–250 ng/mL	>400 ng/mL	Tofranil
Lithium (obtain specimen 12 hours after last dose)	0.6–1.5 mEq/L	>1.5 mEq/L	Lithobid
Nortriptyline	50–150 ng/mL	>500 ng/mL	Aventyl Pamelor

Reference Intervals* for Clinical Chemistry (Urine)

Analyte	Conventional Units	SI Units
Acetone and acetoacetate, qualitative	Negative	Negative
Albumin		
Qualitative	Negative	Negative
Quantitative	10–100 mg/24 hr	0.15–1.5 μmol/day
Aldosterone	3–20 μg/24 hr	8.3–55 nmol/day
δ-Aminolevulinic acid (δ-ALA)	1.3–7.0 mg/24 hr	10–53 μmol/day
Amylase	<17 U/hr	<17 U/hr
Amylase/creatinine clearance ratio	0.01–0.04	0.01–0.04
Bilirubin, qualitative	Negative	Negative
Calcium (regular diet)	<250 mg/24 hr	<6.3 nmol/day
Catecholamines		
Epinephrine	<10 μg/24 hr	<55 nmol/day
Norepinephrine	<100 μg/24 hr	<590 nmol/day
Total free catecholamines	4–126 μg/24 hr	24–745 nmol/day
Total metanephrines	0.1–1.6 mg/24 hr	0.5–8.1 μmol/day
Chloride (varies with intake)	110–250 mEq/24 hr	110–250 mmol/day
Copper	0–50 μg/24 hr	0.0–0.80 μmol/day
Cortisol, free	10–100 μg/24 hr	27.6–276 nmol/day
Creatine		
Males	0–40 mg/24 hr	0.0–0.30 mmol/day
Females	0–80 mg/24 hr	0.0–0.60 mmol/day
Creatinine	15–25 mg/kg/24 hr	0.13–0.22 mmol/kg/day
Creatinine clearance (endogenous)		
Males	110–150 mL/min/1.73 m^2	110–150 mL/min/1.73 m^2
Females	105–132 mL/min/1.73 m^2	105–132 mL/min/1.73 m^2
Cystine or cysteine	Negative	Negative
Dehydroepiandrosterone		
Males	0.2–2.0 mg/24 hr	0.7–6.9 μmol/day
Females	0.2–1.8 mg/24 hr	0.7–6.2 μmol/day
Estrogens, total		
Males	4–25 μg/24 hr	14–90 nmol/day
Females	5–100 μg/24 hr	18–360 nmol/day
Glucose (as reducing substance)	<250 mg/24 hr	<250 mg/day
Hemoglobin and myoglobin, qualitative	Negative	Negative
Homogentisic acid, qualitative	Negative	Negative
17-Ketogenic steroids		
Males	5–23 mg/24 hr	17–80 μmol/day
Females	3–15 mg/24 hr	10–52 μmol/day
17-Hydroxycorticosteroids		
Males	3–9 mg/24 hr	8.3–25 μmol/day
Females	2–8 mg/24 hr	5.5–22 μmol/day
5-Hydroxyindoleacetic acid		
Qualitative	Negative	Negative
Quantitative	2–6 mg/24 hr	10–31 μmol/day
17-Ketosteroids		
Males	8–22 mg/24 hr	28–76 μmol/day
Females	6–15 mg/24 hr	21–52 μmol/day
Magnesium	6–10 mEq/24 hr	3–5 mmol/day
Metanephrines	0.05–1.2 ng/mg creatinine	0.03–0.70 mmol/mmol creatinine
Osmolality	38–1400 mOsm/kg water	38–1400 mOsm/kg water
pH	4.6–8.0	4.6–8.0
Phenylpyruvic acid, qualitative	Negative	Negative
Phosphate	0.4–1.3 g/24 hr	13–42 mmol/day
Porphobilinogen		
Qualitative	Negative	Negative
Quantitative	<2 mg/24 hr	<9 μmol/day
Porphyrins		
Coproporphyrin	50–250 μg/24 hr	77–380 nmol/day
Uroporphyrin	10–30 μg/24 hr	12–36 nmol/day
Potassium	25–125 mEq/24 hr	25–125 mmol/day
Pregnanediol		
Males	0.0–1.9 mg/24 hr	0.0–6.0 μmol/day
Females		
Proliferative phase	0.0–2.6 mg/24 hr	0.0–8.0 μmol/day
Luteal phase	2.6–10.6 mg/24 hr	8–33 μmol/day
Postmenopausal	0.2–1.0 mg/24 hr	0.6–3.1 μmol/day
Pregnanetriol	0.0–2.5 mg/24 hr	0.0–7.4 μmol/day
Protein, total		
Qualitative	Negative	Negative
Quantitative	10–150 mg/24 hr	10–150 mg/day
Protein/creatinine ratio	<0.2	<0.2

Table continued on following page

Reference Intervals* for Clinical Chemistry (Urine) *Continued*

Analyte	Conventional Units	SI Units
Sodium (regular diet)	60–260 mEq/24 hr	60–260 mmol/day
Specific gravity		
Random specimen	1.003–1.030	1.003–1.030
24-hour collection	1.015–1.025	1.015–1.025
Urate (regular diet)	250–750 mg/24 hr	1.5–4.4 mmol/day
Urobilinogen	0.5–4.0 mg/24 hr	0.6–6.8 μmol/day
Vanillylmandelic acid (VMA)	1.0–8.0 mg/24 hr	5–40 μmol/day

*Values may vary depending on the method used.

Reference Intervals for Toxic Substances

Analyte	Conventional Units	SI Units
Arsenic, urine	<130 μg/24 hr	<1.7 μmol/d
Bromides, serum, inorganic	<100 mg/dL	<10 mmol/L
Toxic symptoms	140–1000 mg/dL	14–100 mmol/L
Carboxyhemoglobin, blood:	saturation	
Urban environment	<5%	<0.05
Smokers	<12%	<0.12
Symptoms		
Headache	>15%	>0.15
Nausea and vomiting	>25%	>0.25
Potentially lethal	>50%	>0.50
Ethanol, blood	<0.05 mg/dL <0.005%	<1.0 mmol/L
Intoxication	>100 mg/dL >0.1%	>22 mmol/L
Marked intoxication	300–400 mg/dL 0.3–0.4%	65–87 mmol/L
Alcoholic stupor	400–500 mg/dL 0.4–0.5%	87–109 mmol/L
Coma	>500 mg/dL >0.5%	>109 mmol/L
Lead, blood		
Adults	<25 μg/dL	<1.2 μmol/L
Children	<15 μg/dL	<0.7 μmol/L
Lead, urine	<80 μg/24 hr	<0.4 μmol/day
Mercury, urine	<30 μg/24 hr	<150 nmol/day

Reference Intervals for Tests Performed on Cerebrospinal Fluid

Test	Conventional Units	SI Units
Cells	<5/mm^3; all mononuclear	<5 × 10^6/L, all mononuclear
Protein electrophoresis	Albumin predominant	Albumin predominant
Glucose	50–75 mg/dL (20 mg/dL less than in serum)	2.8–4.2 mmol/L (1.1 mmol less than in serum)
IgG	<8% of total protein	<0.08 of total protein
Children under 14	<14% of total protein	<0.14 of total protein
Adults		
IgG index		
$\left(\dfrac{\text{CSF/serum IgG ratio}}{\text{CSF/serum albumin ratio}}\right)^*$	0.3–0.6	0.3–0.6
Oligoclonal banding on electrophoresis	Absent	Absent
Pressure, opening	70–180 mm H_2O	70–180 mm H_2O
Protein, total	15–45 mg/dL	150–450 mg/L

**Abbreviation:* CSF = cerebrospinal fluid.

Reference Intervals for Tests of Gastrointestinal Function

Test	Conventional Units
Bentiromide	6-hour urinary arylamine excretion greater than 57% excludes pancreatic insufficiency
β-Carotene, serum	60–250 ng/dL
Fecal fat estimation	
Qualitative	No fat globules seen by high-power microscope
Quantitative	<6 gm/24 h (>95% coefficient of fat absorption)
Gastric acid output	
Basal	
Males	0.0–10.5 mmol/hr
Females	0.0–5.6 mmol/hr
Maximum (after histamine or pentagastrin)	
Males	9.0–48.0 mmol/hr
Females	6.0–31.0 mmol/hr
Ratio: basal/maximum	
Males	0.0–0.31
Females	0.0–0.29
Secretin test, pancreatic fluid	
Volume	>1.8 mL/kg/hr
Bicarbonate	>80 mEq/L
D-Xylose absorption test, urine	>20% of ingested dose excreted in 5 hours

Reference Intervals for Tests of Immunologic Function

Test	Conventional Units	SI Units
Complement, serum		
C3	85–175 mg/dL	0.85–1.75 g/L
C4	15–45 mg/dL	150–450 mg/L
Total hemolytic (CH_{50})	150–250 U/mL	150–250 U/mL
Immunoglobulins, serum, adult		
IgG	640–1350 mg/dL	6.4–13.5 g/L
IgA	70–310 mg/dL	0.70–3.1 g/L
IgM	90–350 mg/dL	0.90–3.5 g/L
IgD	0.0–6.0 mg/dL	0.0–60 mg/L
IgE	0.0–430 ng/dL	0.0–430 μg/L

Lymphocyte subsets, whole blood, heparinized

Antigen(s) Expressed	*Cell Type*	*Percentage*	*Absolute Cell Count*
CD3	Total T cells	56–77%	860–1880
CD19	Total B cells	7–17%	140–370
CD3 and CD4	Helper-inducer cells	32–54%	550–1190
CD3 and CD8	Suppressor-cytotoxic cells	24–37%	430–1060
CD3 and DR	Activated T cells	5–14%	70–310
CD2	E rosette T cells	73–87%	1040–2160
CD16 and CD56	Natural killer (NK) cells	8–22%	130–500

Helper/suppressor ratio: 0.8–1.8

Reference Values for Semen Analysis

Test	Conventional Units	SI Units
Volume	2–5 mL	2–5 mL
Liquefaction	Complete in 15 min	Complete in 15 min
pH	7.2–8.0	7.2–8.0
Leukocytes	Occasional or absent	Occasional or absent
Spermatozoa		
Count	$60–150 \times 10^6$ mL	$60–150 \times 10^6$ mL
Motility	>80% motile	>0.80 motile
Morphology	80–90% normal forms	>0.80–0.90 normal forms
Fructose	>150 mg/dL	>8.33 mmol/L

SELECTED REFERENCES

Drug Evaluations Annual. Chicago, American Medical Association, 1994.

Bick R L, (Ed): Hematology — Clinical and Laboratory Practice. St Louis, Mosby–Year Book, 1993.

Borer WZ: Selection and use of laboratory tests. *In* Tietz NW, Conn RB, Pruden EL (eds): Applied Laboratory Medicine. Philadelphia, WB Saunders Co, 1992, pp 1–5.

Campion EW: A retreat from SI units. N Engl J Med *327*:49, 1992.

Friedman RB, Young DS: Effects of Disease on Clinical Laboratory Tests, 3rd ed. Washington, DC, AACC Press, 1997.

Henry JB: Clinical Diagnosis and Management by Laboratory Methods, 19th ed. Philadelphia, WB Saunders Co, 1996.

Hicks JM, Young DS: DORA 97–99: Directory of Rare Analyses. Washington, DC, AACC Press, 1997.

Jacob DS, Demott WR, Grady HJ, et al (eds): Laboratory Test Handbook, 4th ed. Baltimore, Williams & Wilkins, 1996.

Kaplan LA, Pesce AJ: Clinical Chemistry — Theory, Analysis, and Correlation, 3rd ed. St Louis, Mosby–Year Book, 1996.

Kjeldsberg CR, Knight JA: Body Fluids: Laboratory Examination of Amniotic, Cerebrospinal, Seminal, Serous and Synovial Fluids, 3rd ed. Chicago, ASCP Press, 1993.

Laposata M: SI Unit Conversion Guide. Boston, NEJM Books, 1992.

Scully RE, McNeely WF, Mark EJ, McNeely BU: Normal reference laboratory values. N Engl J Med *327*:718–724, 1992.

Speicher CE: The Right Test: A Physician's Guide to Laboratory Medicine, 2nd ed. Philadelphia, WB Saunders Co, 1993.

Tietz NW (ed): Clinical Guide to Laboratory Tests, 3rd ed. Philadelphia, WB Saunders Co, 1995.

Wallach J: Interpretation of Diagnostic Tests: A Synopsis of Laboratory Medicine, 6th ed. Boston, Little, Brown, 1996.

Young DS: Implementation of SI units for clinical laboratory data. Ann Intern Med *106*:114–129, 1987.

Young DS: Determination and validation of reference intervals. Arch Pathol Lab Med *116*:704–709, 1992.

Young DS: Effects of Drugs on Clinical Laboratory Tests, 4th ed. Washington, DC, AACC Press, 1995.

Young DS: Effects of Preanalytical Variables on Clinical Laboratory Tests, 2nd ed. Washington, DC, AACC Press, 1997.

NEW DRUGS FOR 1997

method of
PAULA PIETRUCHA-DILANCHIAN, PHARM.D.
Memorial Hospital–Pasadena
Pasadena, Texas

Drug								
Generic Name	*Trade Name (Manufacturer)*	**Dosage Form**	**Strength**	**Average Dosage Range**	**FDA Rating***	**Approved Use**	**Approval Date**	**Classification**
Anagrelide	Agrylin (Roberts Pharmaceuticals)	Capsule	0.5 mg, 1 mg	0.5 mg qid–1 mg bid	1-P	Platelet reducer for treatment of essential thrombocytopenia	Mar 97	Platelet-reducing agent
Ardeparin	Normiflo (Wyeth Laboratories)	Injectable	5000 U, 10,000 U	50 anti-Xa U/kg SC every 12 h	1-S	Prevention of deep venous thrombosis that may lead to pulmonary embolism following knee replacement surgery	May 97	Low-molecular-weight heparin
Becaplermin	Regranex (Ortho-McNeil)	Gel	0.01%	Based on ulcer and tube size; see specific tables in package insert for dosing	Biological	Treatment of lower extremity diabetic neuropathic ulcers that extend into the subcutaneous tissue or beyond and have adequate blood supply	Dec 97	Biological
Bromfenac	Duract (Wyeth)	Capsule	25 mg	25 mg PO every 6–8 h as needed for short-term (less than 10 days) management of pain; total daily dose not to exceed 150 mg	1-S	Short-term management of pain	Jul 97	Nonsteroidal anti-inflammatory drug
Cefdinir	Omnicef (Parke-Davis)	Capsule Powder	300 mg 125 mg/5 mL	300 mg PO bid or 600 mg once daily; children with otitis media: 7 mg/kg bid or 14 mg/kg once daily	1-S	Treatment of community-acquired pneumonia, acute exacerbations of chronic bronchitis, acute bacterial otitis media, acute maxillary sinusitis, pharyngitis/tonsillitis, and uncomplicated skin and skin structure infections	Dec 97	Cephalosporin, third-generation
Cerivastatin	Baycol (Bayer Corporation)	Tablet	0.2 mg, 0.3 mg	0.3 mg PO once daily in evening	1-S	Adjunct to diet for the reduction of elevated total and LDL-cholesterol levels in patients with primary hypercholesterolemia and mixed dyslipidemia (Fredrickson types IIa and IIb)	Jun 97	HMG-CoA reductase inhibitor

Table continued on following page

Drug								
Generic Name	*Trade Name (Manufacturer)*	**Dosage Form**	**Strength**	**Average Dosage Range**	**FDA Rating***	**Approved Use**	**Approval Date**	**Classification**
Clopidogrel	Plavix (Sanofi)	Tablet	75 mg	75 mg PO once daily	1-P	Reduction of atherosclerotic events in patients with atherosclerosis	Nov 97	Antiplatelet
Dacliximab	Zenapax (Roche)	Injection	25 mg/5 mL	1 mg/kg IV over 15 min every 2 wk for five doses	Biological	Prophylaxis of acute organ rejection in patients receiving renal transplants	Dec 97	Biological
Delavirdine	Rescriptor (Pharmacia & Upjohn)	Tablet	100 mg	400 mg PO three times daily	1-P	Treatment of HIV-1 infection in combination with appropriate antiretroviral agents when therapy is warranted	Apr 97	Antiviral
Dolasetron	Anzemet (Hoechst Marion Roussel)	Injectable Tablet	20 mg/mL 50 mg, 100 mg	Injectable: chemotherapy-induced nausea/vomiting: 1.8 mg/kg; postoperative nausea: 12.5 mg in adults, 0.35 mg/kg in children Tablet: chemotherapy: 100 mg for adults and 1.8 mg/kg for pediatric patients; prevention of postoperative nausea: 100 mg 2 h before surgery (adults), 1.2 mg/kg 2 h before surgery (children)	1-S	Prevention of chemotherapy-induced and postoperative nausea and vomiting	Sep 97	Antiemetic
Emedastine	Emandine (Alcon)	Ophthalmic solution	0.05%	1 drop in affected eye(s) up to four times a day	1-S	Allergic conjunctivitis	Dec 97	Antihistamine
Eprosartan	Teveten (SmithKline Beecham)	Not available	Not available	Under FDA review	1-S	Mild to moderate hypertension	Dec 97	Angiotensin II receptor antagonist
Fenoldopam	Corlopam (Neurex)	Injectable	10 mg/mL	0.03–0.1 μg/kg/min initially up to 1.6 μg/kg/min infusion	1-S	In-hospital, short-term use in the management of severe hypertension when rapid, reversible reduction of blood pressure is indicated	Sep 97	Antihypertensive
Fomepizole	Antizol (Orphan Medical)	Injection	1 gm/mL	Loading dose of 15 mg/kg, then 10 mg/kg every 12 h for 4 doses, then 15 mg/kg every 12 h thereafter until ethylene glycol levels are below 20 mg/dL	1-S	Ethanol alternative for the early or late treatment of ethylene glycol intoxication	Dec 97	Alcohol dehydrogenase inhibitor

Grepafloxacin	Raxar (Glaxo Wellcome)	Tablet	200 mg	400–600 mg once daily	1-S	Chronic bronchitis, community-acquired pneumonia, uncomplicated gonorrhea, nongonococcal urethritis/cervicitis	Nov 97	Fluoroquinolone
Imiquimod	Aldara (3M Pharmaceuticals)	Cream	5.000%	Apply topically three times a week	1-S	Treatment of external genital and perianal warts/condylomata acuminata in adults	Feb 97	Immune response modifier
Interferon alfacon-1	Infergen (Amgen)	Injection	9 μg, 15 μg	9 μg SC three times a week for 24 wk	Biological	Chronic hepatitis C virus infection in adults with compensated liver disease	Oct 97	Biological
Irbesartan	Avapro (Bristol-Myers Squibb/Sanofi)	Tablet	75 mg, 150 mg, 300 mg	150–300 mg PO daily	1-S	Treatment of hypertension	Sep 97	Angiotensin II receptor antagonist
Letrozole	Femara (Novartis Pharmaceuticals)	Tablet	2.5 mg	2.5 mg PO once daily	1-S	Treatment of advanced breast cancer in postmenopausal women	Jul 97	Antiestrogen
Nelfinavir	Viracept (Agouron)	Tablet, powder for suspension	250 mg	Adults: 750 mg PO three times a day; pediatric: 20–30 mg/kg three times a day	1-P	Treatment of HIV infection when therapy is warranted	Mar 97	Antiviral
Oprelvekin	Neumega (American Home Products)	Injection	5 mg/mL	50 μg/kg SC once daily for 3 wk	Biological	Reduction of thrombocytopenia and need for platelet transfusion in cancer patients receiving chemotherapy	Nov 97	Biological
Pramipexole	Mirapex (Pharmacia & Upjohn)	Tablet	0.125 mg, 0.25 mg, 1 mg, 1.5 mg	1.5–4.5 mg daily in three divided doses	1-S	Treatment of signs and symptoms of idiopathic Parkinson's disease	Jul 97	Anti-parkinsonian
Quetiapine	Seroquel (Zeneca)	Tablet	25 mg, 100 mg, 200 mg	50–400 mg PO divided into two or three doses daily	1-S	Treatment of manifestations of psychotic disorders	Sep 97	Atypical antipsychotic
Raloxifene	Evista (Lilly)	Tablet	60 mg	60 mg PO once daily	1-P	Prevention of osteoporosis in postmenopausal women	Dec 97	Estrogen receptor modulator
Repaglinide	Prandin (Novo Nordisk)	Tablet	0.5 mg, 1 mg, 2 mg	0.5–2 mg PO before each meal	1-P	Treatment of Type 2 diabetes	Dec 97	Oral hypoglycemic agent
Rituximab	Rituxan (Genentech)	Injection	10 mg/mL	375 mg/m^2 IV once weekly for four doses	Biological	Treatment of patients with relapsed or refractory low-grade or follicular, CD20$^+$ B-cell non-Hodgkin's lymphoma	Nov 97	Biological
Ropinirole	Requip (SmithKline Beecham)	Tablet	0.25 mg, 0.5 mg, 1 mg, 2 mg, 5 mg	1–8 mg PO three times daily	1-S	Treatment of signs and symptoms of idiopathic Parkinson's disease	Sep 97	Anti-parkinsonian
Sibutramine	Meridia (Knoll)	Capsule	5 mg, 10 mg, 15 mg	10–15 mg once daily	1-S	Management of obesity	Nov 97	Appetite suppressant

Table continued on following page

Drug								
Generic Name	*Trade Name (Manufacturer)*	**Dosage Form**	**Strength**	**Average Dosage Range**	**FDA Rating***	**Approved Use**	**Approval Date**	**Classification**
Tamsulosin	Flomax (Boehringer Ingelheim)	Capsule	0.4 mg	0.4–0.8 mg PO daily	1-S	For treatment of signs and symptoms of benign prostatic hyperplasia	Apr 97	$Alpha_1$-adrenoceptor antagonist
Tazarotene	Tazorac (Allergan)	Gel	0.05%, 0.1%	Apply once daily in evening	1-S	Resistant plaque psoriasis and acne	Nov 97	Retinoid
Tiagabine	Gabitril (Abbott Labs)	Tablet	4 mg, 12 mg, 16 mg, 20 mg	32–56 mg PO daily in 2–4 divided doses	1-S	As adjunctive therapy for partial seizures in adults and children ≥12 years of age	Sep 97	Anticonvulsant
Tiludronate	Skelid (Sanofi Winthrop Pharmaceuticals)	Tablet	240 mg	400 mg PO once daily	1-S	Treatment of Paget's disease of the bone	Mar 97	Bisphosphonate
Toremifene	Fareston (Schering)	Tablet	60 mg	60 mg PO daily	1-S	Treatment of metastatic breast cancer in postmenopausal women with estrogen receptor-positive/receptor-unknown tumors	May 97	Antiestrogen
Troglitazone	Rezulin (Parke-Davis)	Tablet	200 mg, 400 mg	200–600 mg PO once daily	1-P	Type 2 diabetes in patients whose hyperglycemia is inadequately controlled despite insulin therapy	Jan 97	Antidiabetic agent
Trovafloxacin	Trovan (Pfizer)	Tablet Injection	100 mg, 200 mg 5 mg/mL	100–300 mg once daily	1-S	Community-acquired pneumonia, other upper respiratory infections; chlamydial infections; gonorrhea; gynecologic, pelvic, and urinary infections; skin and skin structure infections	Dec 97	Fluoroquinolone
Zolmitriptan	Zomig (Zeneca)	Tablet	2.5 mg, 5 mg	2.5 mg PO every 2 hr, not to exceed 10 mg/24 h	1-S	Treatment of migraine headaches	Nov 97	Antimigraine agent

Abbreviations: HIV = human immunodeficiency virus; HMG-CoA = 3-hydroxy-3-methylglutaryl coenzyme A; LDL = low-density lipoprotein.
*1 = new molecular entity; P = priority review drug; S = standard drug review.

NOMOGRAM FOR THE DETERMINATION OF BODY SURFACE AREA OF CHILDREN AND ADULTS

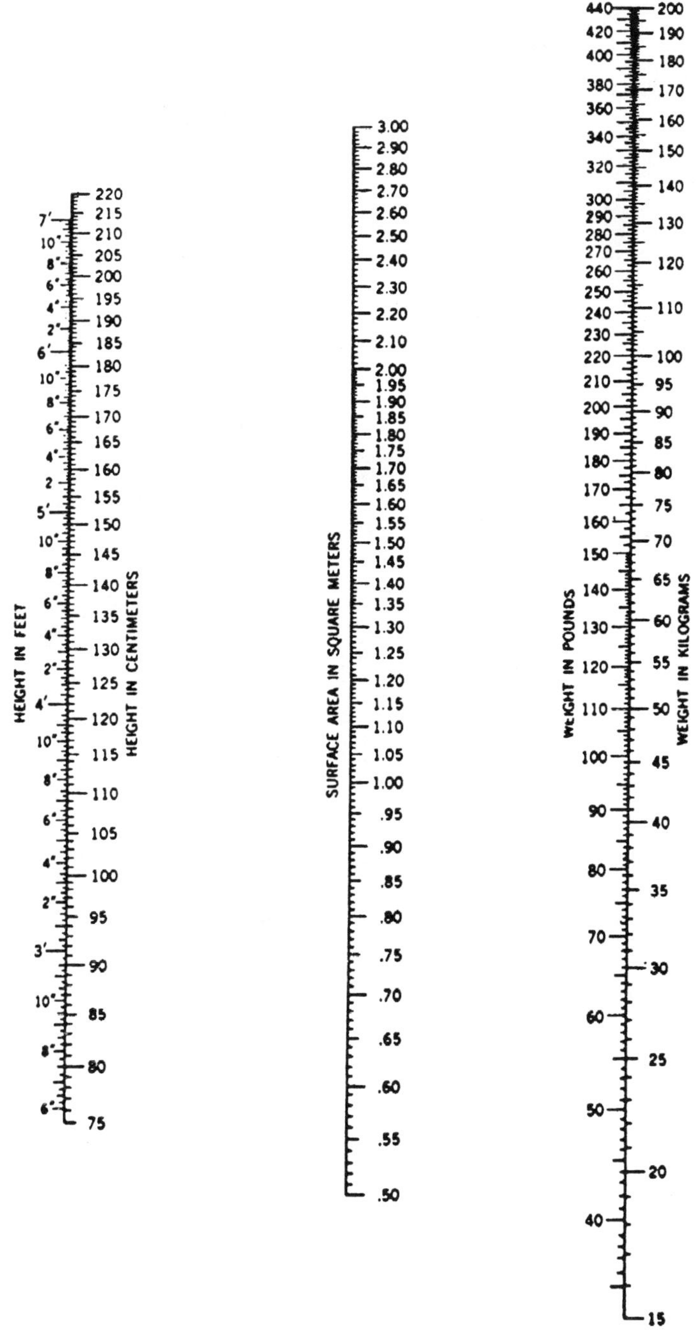

From Boothby WM, Sandiford RB: Boston Med Surg J *185*:337, 1921.

Index

Note: Page numbers in *italics* refer to illustrations; page numbers followed by t refer to tables; page numbers followed by n indicate notes.

ISBN 0-7216-7224-8